Sleisenger and Fordtran's
Gastrointestinal and Liver Disease

10th Edition   Volume 2

PATHOPHYSIOLOGY • DIAGNOSIS • MANAGEMENT

Mark Feldman, MD

William O. Tschumy Jr., MD, Chair of Internal Medicine
Director, Internal Medicine Residency Program
Texas Health Presbyterian Hospital Dallas
Clinical Professor of Internal Medicine
University of Texas Southwestern Medical School
Dallas, Texas

Lawrence S. Friedman, MD

Professor of Medicine
Harvard Medical School
Professor of Medicine
Tufts University School of Medicine
Boston, Massachusetts
The Anton R. Fried, MD, Chair
Department of Medicine
Newton-Wellesley Hospital
Newton, Massachusetts
Assistant Chief of Medicine
Massachusetts General Hospital
Boston, Massachusetts

Lawrence J. Brandt, MD

Professor of Medicine and Surgery
Albert Einstein College of Medicine
Emeritus Chief
Division of Gastroenterology
Montefiore Medical Center
Bronx, New York

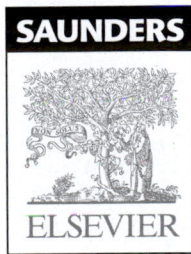

SAUNDERS

ELSEVIER

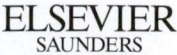

ELSEVIER
SAUNDERS

1600 John F. Kennedy Blvd.
Ste 1800
Philadelphia, PA 19103-2899

SLEISENGER AND FORDTRAN'S GASTROINTESTINAL
AND LIVER DISEASE, 10TH EDITION

ISBN: 978-1-4557-4692-7
Volume 1 Part Number: 9996097102
Volume 2 Part Number: 9996097161

Notices

Knowledge and best practice in this field are constantly changing. As new research and experience broaden our understanding, changes in research methods, professional practices, or medical treatment may become necessary.

Practitioners and researchers must always rely on their own experience and knowledge in evaluating and using any information, methods, compounds, or experiments described herein. In using such information or methods they should be mindful of their own safety and the safety of others, including parties for whom they have a professional responsibility.

With respect to any drug or pharmaceutical products identified, readers are advised to check the most current information provided (i) on procedures featured or (ii) by the manufacturer of each product to be administered, to verify the recommended dose or formula, the method and duration of administration, and contraindications. It is the responsibility of practitioners, relying on their own experience and knowledge of their patients, to make diagnoses, to determine dosages and the best treatment for each individual patient, and to take all appropriate safety precautions.

To the fullest extent of the law, neither the Publisher nor the authors, contributors, or editors assume any liability for any injury and/or damage to persons or property as a matter of products liability, negligence or otherwise, or from any use or operation of any methods, products, instructions, or ideas contained in the material herein.

Copyright © 2010, 2006, 2002, 1998, 1993, 1989, 1983, 1978, 1973 by Elsevier.

Chapter 82: Hepatitis E by Rakesh Aggarwal and Krzysztof Krawczynski is in public domain.

Library of Congress Cataloging-in-Publication Data

Sleisenger and Fordtran's gastrointestinal and liver disease (Feldman)
  Sleisenger and Fordtran's gastrointestinal and liver disease : pathophysiology/diagnosis/management / [edited by] Mark Feldman, Lawrence S. Friedman, Lawrence J. Brandt.—Tenth edition.
    p. ; cm.
  Gastrointestinal and liver disease
  Includes bibliographical references and index.
  ISBN 978-1-4557-4692-7 (2 volume set, hardcover : alk. paper)—ISBN 9996097102 (v. 1 : alk. paper)—ISBN 9996097161 (v. 2 : alk. paper)
  I. Feldman, Mark, 1947- editor. II. Friedman, Lawrence S. (Lawrence Samuel), 1953- editor. III. Brandt, Lawrence J., editor. IV. Title. V. Title: Gastrointestinal and liver disease.
  [DNLM: 1. Gastrointestinal Diseases. 2. Liver Diseases. WI 140]
  RC801
  616.3'3—dc23
                                                                    2014016501

Senior Content Strategist: Suzanne Toppy
Senior Content Development Specialist: Dee Simpson
Publishing Services Manager: Anne Altepeter
Senior Project Manager: Cindy Thoms
Senior Book Designer: Lou Forgione

Printed in United States of America

Last digit is the print number: 9 8 7 6 5 4 3 2 1

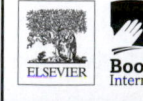
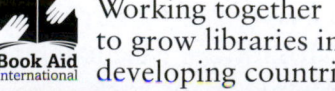

To our wives—Barbara Feldman, Mary Jo Cappuccilli, and Lois Brandt; from whom we stole the time necessary to edit this textbook. With gratitude and love.

CONTRIBUTORS

Abier Abdelnaby, MD
Associate Professor of Surgery
University of Texas Southwestern
  Medical Center
Dallas, Texas
Diseases of the Anorectum

Julian A. Abrams, MD
Assistant Professor of Medicine,
  Department of Medicine
Columbia University College of
  Physicians and Surgeons
New York, New York
*Adenocarcinoma of the Stomach and
Other Gastric Tumors*

Nada A. Abumrad, PhD
Department of Medicine
Center for Human Nutrition
Washington University
St. Louis, Missouri
*Digestion and Absorption of Dietary Fat,
Carbohydrate, and Protein*

Nezam H. Afdhal, MD
Professor of Medicine
Harvard Medical School
Division of Gastroenterology
Liver Center
Beth Israel Deaconess Medical Center
Boston, Massachusetts
Gallstone Disease

Rakesh Aggarwal, MD, DM
Professor, Gastroenterology
Sanjay Gandhi Postgraduate Institute of
  Medical Sciences
Lucknow, India
Hepatitis E

Karin L. Andersson, MD
Hepatologist
Gastrointestinal Unit
Massachusetts General Hospital
Instructor in Medicine
Harvard Medical School
Boston, Massachusetts
*Acalculous Biliary Pain, Acute Acalculous
Cholecystitis, Cholesterolosis, Adenomyomatosis,
and Gallbladder Polyps*

Jane M. Andrews, MBBS, PhD
Clinical Associate Professor
Head IBD Service and Education
Department of Gastroenterology and
  Hepatology
Royal Adelaide Hospital and University
  of Adelaide
Adelaide, Australia
*Small Intestinal Motor and Sensory Function
and Dysfunction*

Farshid Araghizadeh, MD
Professor of Surgery
Department of Surgery
Chief, Section of Colon and Rectal
  Surgery
University of Texas Southwestern
  Medical Center
Dallas, Texas
Ileostomy, Colostomy, and Pouches

Olga C. Aroniadis, MD
Senior Fellow, Gastroenterology
Albert Einstein College of Medicine
Montefiore Medical Center
Bronx, New York
Vascular Disorders of the Gastrointestinal Tract

Fernando Azpiroz, Prof, MD, PhD
Professor of Medicine
Universitat Autonoma de Barcelona
Chief, Gastroenterology Department
Univerisyt Hopsital Vall d'Hebron
Centro de Investigacion Biomedica en
  Red de Enfermedades Hepaticas y
  Digestivas (Ciberehd)
Barcelona, Spain
Intestinal Gas

Bruce R. Bacon, MD
James F. King MD Endowed Chair in
  Gastroenterology, Professor of
  Internal Medicine
Division of Gastroenterology and
  Hepatology
Saint Louis University School of
  Medicine,
St. Louis, Missouri
Hemochromatosis

William F. Balistreri, MD
Director, Pediatric Liver Care Center
Gastroenterology, Hepatology, and
  Nutrition
Children's Hospital Medical Center
Cincinnati, Ohio
Other Inherited Metabolic Disorders of the Liver

Todd H. Baron, MD
Professor of Medicine
Director of Advanced Therapeutic
  Endoscopy
Division of Gastroenterology and
  Hepatology
University of North Carolina
School of Medicine
Chapel Hill, North Carolina
*Endoscopic Treatment of Pancreatic Disease
Endoscopic and Radiologic Treatment of
Biliary Disease*

Bradley A. Barth, MD
Associate Professor, Pediatrics
University of Texas Southwestern
  Medical Center
Dallas, Texas
*Anatomy, Histology, and Developmental Anomalies
of the Pancreas*

Lee M. Bass, MD
Assistant Professor of Pediatrics
Gastroenterology, Hepatology and
  Nutrition
Ann and Robert H. Lurie Children's
  Hospital of Chicago
Northwestern University Feinberg
  School of Medicine
Chicago, Illinois
*Anatomy, Histology, Embryology, and
Developmental Anomalies of the Small and
Large Intestine*

John T. Bassett, MD
Deputy Chief Gastroenterology
Internal Medicine
Walter Reed National Military Medical
  Center
Bethesda, Maryland
Hepatitis A

Anne E. Becker, MD, PhD
Maude and Lillian Presley Professor of
  Global Health and Social Medicine
Department of Global Health and Social
  Medicine
Harvard Medical School
Associate Professor of Psychiatry,
  Department of Psychiatry
Massachusetts General Hospital
Boston, Massachusetts
Feeding and Eating Disorders

Alex S. Befeler, MD
Professor of Internal Medicine
Medical Director Liver Transplantation
Division of Gastroenterology and
  Hepatology
Saint Louis University
St. Louis, Missouri
Hepatic Tumors and Cysts

Taft P. Bhuket, MD
Assistant Clinical Professor of
  Medicine, Division of
  Gastoenterology
University of California, San Francisco
San Francisco, California
Chief of Gastroenterology
Director of Endoscopy
Chief of Staff
Alameda Health System
Oakland, California
Diverticular Disease of the Colon

L. Ashley Blackshaw, PhD
Professor of Enteric Neuroscience
Blizard Institute
Queen Mary University of London
London, United Kingdom
*Small Intestinal Motor and Sensory Function
and Dysfunction*

Boris Blechacz, MD, PhD
Assistant Professor of Medicine,
  Gastroenterology, Hepatology, and
  Nutrition
MD Anderson Cancer Center
Houston, Texas
*Tumors of the Bile Ducts, Gallbladder,
and Ampulla*
Tumors of the Small Intestine

Diego V. Bohórquez, PhD
Postdoctoral Fellow
Department of Medicine
Duke University Medical Center
Durham, North Carolina
Gastrointestinal Hormones and Neurotransmitters

Lawrence J. Brandt, MD
Professor of Medicine and Surgery
Albert Einstein College of Medicine
Emeritus Chief
Division of Gastroenterology
Montefiore Medical Center
Bronx, New York
Vascular Disorders of the Gastrointestinal Tract
Intestinal Ischemia
Probiotics and Fecal Microbiota Transplant

George A. Bray, MD
Boyd Professor
Clinical Research
Pennington Biomedical Research Center
Louisiana State University
Baton Rouge, Louisiana
Obesity

Robert S. Bresalier, MD
Professor of Medicine
Lydia and Birdie J. Resoft Distinguished
  Professor in Gastrointestinal
  Oncology
Gastroenterology, Hepatology, and
  Nutrition
The University of Texas MD Anderson
  Cancer Center,
Houston, Texas
Tumors of the Small Intestine
Colorectal Cancer

Stuart M. Brierley, PhD
NHMRC R.D. Wright Biomedical
  Fellow; Discipline of Physiology,
  Faculty of Health Sciences
Discipline of Medicine, Faculty of
  Health Sciences
The University of Adelaide
Department of Gastroenterology and
  Hepatology
Royal Adelaide Hospital
Adelaide, Australia
*Small Intestinal Motor and Sensory Function
and Dysfunction*

Robert S. Britton, PhD
Adjunct Associate Research Professor
Department of Internal Medicine,
  Division of Gastroenterology and
  Hepatology
Saint Louis University School of
  Medicine
St. Louis, Missouri
Hemochromatosis

Simon J.H. Brookes, PhD
Professor of Human Physiology
Flinders Medical Science and
  Technology, School of Medicine
Flinders University
Adelaide, Australia
*Colonic Motor and Sensory Function
and Dysfunction*

Alan L. Buchman, MD, MSPH
Professor of Medicine and Surgery
Medical Director of Intestinal
  Rehabilitation/Transplant Center
Division of Gastroenterology
Northwestern University Feinberg
  School of Medicine
Chicago, Illinois
Short Bowel Syndrome

Robert L. Carithers, Jr., MD
Professor of Medicine
University of Washington
Director, Liver Care Line
University of Washington Medical
  Center
Seattle, Washington
Alcoholic Liver Disease

Andres F. Carrion, MD
Division of Hepatology
University of Miami Miller School of
  Medicine
Miami, Florida
Liver Transplantation

Scott Celinski, MD
Division of Surgical Oncology
Baylor University Medical Center
Dallas, Texas
Abdominal Abscesses and Gastrointestinal Fistulas

Francis K.L. Chan, MD, DSc
Professor of Medicine
Institute of Digestive Disease
Chinese University of Hong Kong
Hong Kong, China
Peptic Ulcer Disease

Shivakumar Chitturi, MD
Staff Specialist
Gastroenterology and Hepatology Unit
Canberra Hospital
Garran, Australia
*Hepatic Drug Metabolism and Liver Disease
Caused by Drugs*

Daniel C. Chung, MD
Associate Professor of Medicine
Harvard Medical School
Director, GI Cancer Genetics Program
GI Unit and Cancer Center
Massachusetts General Hospital
Boston, Massachusetts
Cellular Growth and Neoplasia

Raymond T. Chung, MD
Director of Hepatology, Vice Chief,
  Gastroenterology
Massachusetts General Hospital
Boston, Massachusetts
*Bacterial, Parasitic, and Fungal Infections of the
Liver, Including Liver Abscesses*

Robert H. Collins, Jr., MD
Director, Hematologic Malignancies/
    Blood and Marrow Transplantation
    Program
Professor of Internal Medicine
University of Texas Southwestern
    Medical Center
Dallas, Texas
Gastrointestinal Lymphomas

Marcello Costa, MD
Matthew Flinders Distinguished
    Professor and Professor of
    Neurophysiology
Physiology
Flinders University
Adelaide, Australia
*Colonic Motor and Sensory Function
and Dysfunction*

Diane W. Cox, PhD
Professor of Medical Genetics
University of Alberta
Faculty of Medicine
Edmonton, Alberta, Canada
Wilson Disease

Sheila E. Crowe, MD
Professor of Medicine
Division of Gastroenterology
Department of Medicine
University of California, San Diego
San Diego, California
Helicobacter pylori Infection

Albert J. Czaja, MD
Professor Emeritus of Medicine
Gastroenterology and Hepatology
Mayo Clinic College of Medicine
Rochester, Minnesota
Autoimmune Hepatitis

Brian G. Czito, MD
Associate Professor
Radiation Oncology
Duke University Medical Center
Durham, North Carolina
Radiation Injury

Paul A. Dawson, PhD
Professor
Division of Pediatric Gastroenterology,
    Hepatology, and Nutrition
Emory University School of Medicine
Atlanta, Georgia
Bile Secretion and the Enterohepatic Circulation

Gregory de Prisco, MD
Director of Emergency Radiology
Baylor University Medical Center
Dallas, Texas
Abdominal Abscesses and Gastrointestinal Fistulas

Kenneth R. DeVault, MD
Professor and Chair of Medicine
Mayo Clinic
Jacksonville, Florida
Symptoms of Esophageal Disease

Adrian M. Di Bisceglie, MD
Badeeh A. and Catherine V. Bander
    Chair in Internal Medicine
Chairman and Professor of Internal
    Medicine
Chief of Hepatology
Saint Louis University
St. Louis, Missouri
Hepatic Tumors and Cysts

Philip G. Dinning, PhD
Associate Professor
Senior Medical Scientist
Flinders University
Departments of Gastroenterology
    and Surgery
Flinders Medical Center
Adelaide, Australia
*Colonic Motor and Sensory Function
and Dysfunction*

Iris Dotan, MD
Sackler Faculty of Medicine
Tel Aviv University
Head, IBD Center
Gastroenterology and Liver Diseases
Tel Aviv Sourasky Medical Center
Tel Aviv, Israel
Mucosal Immunology and Inflammation

J. Marcus Downs, MD
Program Director
Colon and Rectal Surgery
Parkland and Presbyterian Hospitals
Dallas, Texas
Diseases of the Anorectum

Douglas A. Drossman, MD
Professor Emeritus of Medicine and
    Psychiatry
Center for Functional GI and Motility
    Disorders
University of North Carolina
President
Center for Education and Practice of
    Biopsychosocial Care
Chapel Hill, North Carolina
Biopsychosocial Issues in Gastroenterology

Kerry B. Dunbar, MD, PhD
Assistant Professor of Medicine
Department of Medicine—Division of
    Gastroenterology and Hepatology
University of Texas Southwestern
    Medical School
Staff Physician
Department of Medicine—
    Gastroenterology Section
VA North Texas Healthcare System—
    Dallas VA Medical Center
Dallas, Texas
*Diverticula of the Pharynx, Esophagus, Stomach,
and Small Intestine*
Abdominal Hernias and Gastric Volvulus

John E. Eaton, MD
Instructor of Medicine
Department of Internal Medicine
Division of Gastroenterology and
    Hepatology
Mayo Clinic
Rochester, Minnesota
Primary Biliary Cirrhosis

Ellen C. Ebert, MD
Professor of Medicine
University of Medicine and Dentistry of
    New Jersey
New Brunswick, New Jersey
*Gastrointestinal and Hepatic Manifestations of
Systemic Diseases*

David E. Elliott, MD, PhD
Department of Internal Medicine
Carver College of Medicine
University of Iowa
Department of Internal Medicine
Veterans Administrattion Health Care
    System
Iowa City, Iowa
Intestinal Worms

B. Joseph Elmunzer, MD
Division of Gastroenterology
University of Michigan Medical School
Ann Arbor, Michigan
Biliary Tract Motor Function and Dysfunction

Grace H. Elta, MD
Division of Gastroenterology
University of Michigan Medical School
Ann Arbor, Michigan
Biliary Tract Motor Function and Dysfunction

Silvia Degli Esposti, MD
Associate Professor of Medicine
Director of Fellowship Pathway in
    Women's Gastrointestinal Diseases
Warren Alpert Medical School of
    Brown University
Director
Center for Women's Gastrointestinal
    Medicine
Women's Medicine Collaborative
Miriam Hospital
Providence, Rhode Island
*Gastrointestinal and Hepatic Disorders in the
Pregnant Patient*

Michael B. Fallon, MD
Professor of Medicine
Gastroenterology, Hepatology and
    Nutrition
The University of Texas Health Science
    Center at Houston
Houston, Texas
*Hepatic Encephalopathy, Hepatorenal Syndrome,
Hepatopulmonary Syndrome, and Other Systemic
Complications of Liver Disease*

Geoffrey C. Farrell, MD
Professor of Hepatic Medicine
Australian National University
Senior Staff Hepatologist
The Canberra Hospital
Woden, Australia
*Hepatic Drug Metabolism and Liver Disease
Caused by Drugs*

Jordan J. Feld, MD
Assistant Professor of Medicine
Toronto Western Hospital Liver Centre
Scientist
Sandra Rotman Centre for Global
    Health
University of Toronto
Toronto, Ontario, Canada
Hepatitis Caused by Other Viruses

Marc D. Feldman, MD
Clinical Professor
Department of Psychiatry
Adjunct Professor
Department of Psychology
University of Alabama
Tuscaloosa, Alabama
Factitious Gastrointestinal Disease

Mark Feldman, MD
William O. Tschumy, Jr., MD, Chair of
    Internal Medicine
Director, Internal Medicine Residency
    Program
Texas Health Presbyterian Hospital
    Dallas
Clinical Professor of Internal Medicine
University of Texas Southwestern
    Medical School
Dallas, Texas
Gastrointestinal Stromal Tumors (GISTs)
Gastritis

Lincoln Eduardo Ferreira, MD, PhD
Director of Digestive Endoscopy Unit
Gastrointestinal and Hepatology
Hospital Universitario of UFJF
Hosptial Monte Sinai
Juiz de For A
Minas Gerais, Brazil
Endoscopic Treatment of Pancreatic Disease

Paul Feuerstadt, MD
Clinical Instructor
Yale University School of Medicine
Yale-New Haven Hospital
New Haven, Connecticut
Intestinal Ischemia

Laurel Fisher, MD
Associate Professor
Division of Gastroenterology
Department of Internal Medicine
University of Michigan Medical School
Ann Arbor, Michigan
Intestinal Ulcerations

Alexander C. Ford, MD
Associate Professor and Honorary
    Consultant Gastroenterologist
Leeds Gastroenterology Institute
St. James's University Hospital
Leeds, West Yorkshire, United
    Kingdom
Irritable Bowel Syndrome

John S. Fordtran, MD
Internal Medicine
Division of Gastroenterology
Baylor University Medical Center
Dallas, Texas
Factitious Gastrointestinal Disease

Chris E. Forsmark, MD
Professor of Medicine
University of Florida College of
    Medicine
Gainesville, Florida
Chronic Pancreatitis

Amy E. Foxx-Orenstein, DO
Professor of Medicine
Mayo Clinic
Scottsdale, Arizona
Ileus and Pseudo-obstruction

Frank K. Friedenberg, MD
Professor of Medicine
Gastroenterology
Temple University School of Medicine
Philadelphia, Pennsylvania
Gastroesophageal Reflux Disease

Lawrence S. Friedman, MD
Professor of Medicine
Harvard Medical School
Professor of Medicine
Tufts University School of Medicine
Boston, Massachusetts
The Anton R. Fried, MD, Chair
Department of Medicine
Newton-Wellesley Hospital
Newton, Massachusetts
Assistant Chief of Medicine
Massachusetts General Hospital
Boston, Massachusetts
Chronic Abdominal Pain
*Acalculous Biliary Pain, Acute Acalculous
Cholecystitis, Cholesterolosis, Adenomyomatosis,
and Gallbladder Polyps*

Manish K. Gala, MD
Research Fellow in Medicine
Harvard Medical School
Clinical and Research Fellow
Gastrointestinal Unit
Massachusetts General Hospital
Boston, Massachusetts
Cellular Growth and Neoplasia

Robert E. Glasgow, MD
Associate Professor
Section Chief
Gastrointestinal and General Surgery
Vice Chairman
Clinical Operations and Quality
Department of Surgery
University of Utah
Salt Lake City, Utah
Treatment of Gallstone Disease

Gregory J. Gores, MD
Executive Dean for Research
Professor of Medicine
Division of Gastroenterology and
    Hepatology
Mayo Clinic
Rochester, Minnesota
*Tumors of the Bile Ducts, Gallbladder,
and Ampulla*

Norton J. Greenberger, MD
Clinical Professor of Medicine
Harvard Medical School
Senior Physician
Brigham and Women's Hospital
Boston, Massachusetts
Foreword

David A. Greenwald, MD
Professor of Clinical Medicine
Albert Einstein College of Medicine
Associate Division Director
Gastroenterology Fellowship Program
    Director
Division of Gastroenterology and Liver
    Diseases
Albert Einstein College of Medicine/
    Montefiore Medical Center
Bronx, New York
Protein-Losing Gastroenteropathy

Evan B. Grossman, MD
Assistant Professor of Medicine
Division of Gastroenterology and
    Hepatology
SUNY Downstate Medical Center
Brooklyn, New York
Nutritional Management

Yael Haberman, MD, PhD
Fellow
Pediatric Gastroenterology, Hepatology,
    and Nutrition
Cincinnati Children's Hospital Medical
    Center
Cincinnati, Ohio
Eosinophilic Disorders of the Gastrointestinal Tract

Charles F. Haines, MD
Division of Infectious Diseases
Department of Medicine
The Johns Hopkins University School of
    Medicine
Baltimore, Maryland
Infectious Enteritis and Proctocolitis

Heinz F. Hammer, MD
Associate Professor
Gastroenterology and Hepatology
Medical University
Chief of Internal Medicine
Privatklinik Kastanienhof
Graz, Austria
Maldigestion and Malabsorption

Shawn M. Hancock, DO
Clinical Instructor
Advanced Endoscopy Fellow
Gastroenterology and Hepatology
University of Wisconsin School of
    Medicine and Public Health
Madison, Wisconsin
Foreign Bodies, Bezoars, and Caustic Ingestions

Stephen A. Harrison, MD
Chief of Hepatology
Medicine, Division of Gastroenterology
Brooke Army Medical Center
Fort Sam Houston, Texas
Nonalcoholic Fatty Liver Disease

David J. Hass, MD
Assistant Clinical Professor of Medicine
Division of Digestive Diseases
Yale University School of Medicine
New Haven, Connecticut
Complementary and Alternative Medicine

Colin Hill, PhD, DSc
Professor of Microbial Food Safety
Alimentary Pharmabiotic Centre
School of Microbiology
University College Cork
Cork, Ireland
Enteric Microbiota

Christoph Högenauer, MD
Associate Professor of Medicine
Department of Internal Medicine
Medical University of Graz
Graz, Austria
Maldigestion and Malabsorption

Sohail Z. Husain, MD
Associate Professor of Pediatrics
University of Pittsburgh and the
    Children's Hospital of Pittsuburgh
    of UPMC
Pittsburgh, Pennsylvania
*Anatomy, Histology, and Developmental Anomalies
of the Pancreas*

Christopher D. Huston, MD
Associate Professor
Departments of Medicine,
    Microbiology, and Molecular
    Genetics
University of Vermont College of
    Medicine
Attending Physician
Medicine and Infectious Diseases
Fletcher Allen Health Care
Burlington, Vermont
Intestinal Protozoa

Steven H. Itzkowitz, MD
Professor of Medicine and Oncological
    Sciences
Division of Gastroenterology
Department of Medicine
Icahn School of Medicine at Mount Sinai
New York City, New York
Colonic Polyps and Polyposis Syndromes

Dennis M. Jensen, MD
Professor of Medicine
Medicine—Gastroenterology
David Geffen School of Medicine
University of California, Los Angeles
Staff Physician
Medicine—Gastroenterology
VA Greater Los Angeles Healthcare
    System
Key Investigator
Director, Human Studies Core and GI
    Hemostasis Research Unit
CURE Digestive Diseases Research
    Center
Los Angeles, California
Gastrointestinal Bleeding

Robert T. Jensen, MD
Chief, Cell Biology Section
Digestive Diseases Branch, NIDDK
National Institutes of Health
Bethesda, Maryland
Neuroendocrine Tumors

D. Rohan Jeyarajah, MD, PA
Director, Surgical Oncology
Director, HPB Fellowship Program
Methodist Dallas Medical Center
Dallas, Texas
*Diverticula of the Pharynx, Esophagus, Stomach,
and Small Intestine*
Abdominal Hernias and Gastric Volvulus

Peter J. Kahrilas, MD
Gilbert H. Marquartd Professor in
    Medicine
Northwestern University
Feinberg School of Medicine
Chicago, Illinois
*Esophageal Neuromuscular Function and
Motility Disorders*

Patrick S. Kamath, MD
Professor of Medicine
Gastroenterology and Hepatology
Consultant
Gastroenterology and Hepatology
Mayo Clinic
Rochester, Minnesota
Overview of Cirrhosis
Portal Hypertension and Variceal Bleeding

David A. Katzka, MD
Professor of and Consultant in
    Medicine
Mayo Clinic
Rochester, Minnesota
*Esophageal Disorders Caused by Medications,
Trauma, and Infection*

Debra K. Katzman, MD
Professor of Pediatrics
Senior Associate Scientist
Research Institute
Division of Adolescent Medicine
Department of Pediatrics
The Hospital for Sick Children
University of Toronto
Toronto, Ontario, Canada
Feeding and Eating Disorders

Jonathan D. Kaunitz, MD
Professor
Medicine and Surgery
University of California, Los Angeles
School of Medicine
Staff Physician
Medicine
West Los Angeles Veterans Affairs
   Medical Center
Los Angeles, California
Gastric Secretion

Sarah A. Kearney, MD
Division of Adolescent Medicine
Department of Pediatrics
The Hospital for Sick Children
University of Toronto
Toronto, Ontario, Canada
Feeding and Eating Disorders

Ciarán P. Kelly, MD
Professor of Medicine
Gastroenterology
Harvard Medical School
Fellowship Program Director
Gastroenterology
Beth Israel Deaconess Medical Center
Boston, Massachusetts
Celiac Disease
*Antibiotic-Associated Diarrhea and Clostridium
difficile Infection*

Colleen R. Kelly, MD
Clinical Assistant Professor of Medicine
Women's Medicine Collaborative
Alpert Medical School of Brown
   University
Providence, Rhode Island
Food Poisoning

Arthur Y. Kim, MD
Division of Infectious Diseases
Massachusetts General Hospital
Assistant Professor of Medicine
Harvard Medical School
Boston, Massachusetts
*Bacterial, Parasitic, and Fungal Infections of the
Liver, Including Liver Abscesses*

Kenneth L. Koch, MD
Professor of Medicine
Department of Medicine
Chief, Section on Gastroenterology
Wake Forest University School of
   Medicine
Winston-Salem, North Carolina
*Gastric Neuromuscular Function and
Neuromuscular Disorders*

Kris V. Kowdley, MD
Clinical Professor of Medicine
Gastroenterology
University of Washington
Director of Research
Director, The Liver Center of Excellence
Digestive Disease Institute
Virginia Mason Medical Center
Seattle, Washington
*Primary Sclerosing Cholangitis and Recurrent
Pyogenic Cholangitis*

Krzysztof Krawczynski, MD, PhD
Distinguished Consultant and Team
   Leader
Division of Viral Hepatitis
Centers for Disease Control and
   Prevention
Atlanta, Georgia
Hepatitis E

J. Thomas Lamont, MD
Physician
Division of Gastroenterology
Beth Israel Deaconess Medical Center
Professor
Harvard Medical School,
Boston, Massachusetts
*Antibiotic-Associated Diarrhea and Clostridium
difficile Infection*

Carmen Landaverde, MD
Transplant Hepatologist
Hepatology Division
Baylor University Medical Center
Dallas, Texas
Hepatitis D

Anne M. Larson, MD
Director
Swedish Liver Center
Swedish Health Systems
Seattle, Washington
*Gastrointestinal and Hepatic Complications of Solid
Organ and Hematopoietic Cell Transplant*

James Y.W. Lau, MD
Professor of Surgery
Surgery
The Chinese University Hong Kong
Director
Endoscopy Centre
Prince of Wales Hospital
Hong Kong, China
Peptic Ulcer Disease

Jessica LeBlanc, MD
Dermatology Resident
Dermatology
Indiana University
Indianapolis, Indiana
*Oral Diseases and Oral-Cutaneous Manifestations
of Gastrointestinal and Liver Disease*

Edward L. Lee, MD
Professor and Chair
Department of Pathology
Howard University College of Medicine
Howard University Hospital
Washington, DC
Gastritis

Anthony J. Lembo, MD
Associate Professor of Medicine
Harvard Medical School
Division of Gastroenterology
Beth Israel Deaconess Medical Center
Boston, Massachusetts
Constipation

Mike A. Leonis, MD, PhD
Associate Professor
Pediatrics
University of Cincinnati College of
   Medicine
Attending Physician
Cincinnati Children's Hospital Medical
   Center
Cincinnati, Ohio
Other Inherited Metabolic Disorders of the Liver

James H. Lewis, MD
Professor of Medicine, Director of
   Hepatology
Division of Gastroenterology
Georgetown University Medical Center
Washington, DC
*Liver Disease Caused by Anesthetics, Chemicals,
Toxins, and Herbal Preparations*

Hsiao C. Li, MD
Assistant Professor
Internal Medicine
University of Texas Southwestern
   Medical Center
Dallas, Texas
Gastrointestinal Lymphomas

Gary R. Lichtenstein, MD

Professor of Medicine
Division of Gastroenterology
Raymond and Ruth Perelman School of
    Medicine of the University of
    Pennsylvania
Director, Center for Inflammatory
    Bowel Disease
Department of Medicine
Hospital of the University of
    Pennsylvania
Philadelphia, Pennsylvania
Ulcerative Colitis

Rodger A. Liddle, MD

Professor of Medicine
Department of Medicine
Duke University Medical Center
Chief, Gastroenterology
Medicine
Veterans Affairs Medical Center
Durham, North Carolina
Gastrointestinal Hormones and Neurotransmitters

Steven D. Lidofsky, MD, PhD

Professor of Medicine
University of Vermont
College of Medicine
Director of Hepatology
Fletcher Allen Health Care
Burlington, Vermont
Jaundice

Keith D. Lindor, MD

Executive Vice Provost and Dean
College of Health Solutions
Arizona State University
Professor of Medicine
Gastroenterology and Hepatology
Mayo Clinic Hospital
Phoenix, Arizona
Primary Biliary Cirrhosis

Mark E. Lowe, MD, PhD

Professor and Vice-Chairman
Pediatrics
University of Pittsburgh Medical School
    and Children's Hospital of Pittsburgh
    of UPMC
Pittsburgh, Pennsylvania
*Hereditary, Familial, and Genetic Disorders of the
Pancreas and Pancreatic Disorders in Childhood*

Ryan Madanick, MD

Assistant Professor of Medicine
Division of Gastroenterology and
    Hepatology
University of North Carolina
School of Medicine
Chapel Hill, North Carolina
*Anatomy, Histology, Embryology, and
Developmental Anomalies of the Esophagus*

Matthias Maiwald, MD, PhD

Consultant in Microbiology
Department of Pathology and
    Laboratory Medicine
KK Women's and Children's Hospital
Adjunct Associate Professor
Department of Microbiology
National University of Singapore
Adjunct Associate Professor
Duke-NUS Graduate Medical School
Singapore
Whipple's Disease

Carolina Malagelada, MD, PhD

Attending Gastroenterologist
Digestive Diseases Department
Hospital Universitari Vall d'Hebron
Autonomous University of Barcelona
Barcelona, Spain
Nausea and Vomiting

Juan-R. Malagelada, MD

Associate Professor of Medicine
Autonomous University of Barcelona
Consultant
Digestive Diseases Department
Hospital Universitari Vall d'Hebron
Barcelona, Spain
Nausea and Vomiting

Akiva Marcus, MD, PhD

Division of Gastroenterology and Liver
    Disease
Albert Einstein College of Medicine
Montefiore Medical Center
Bronx, New York
*Digestion and Absorption of Dietary Fat,
Carbohydrate, and Protein*

Lawrence A. Mark, MD, PhD

Assistant Professor
Dermatology
Indiana University School of Medicine
Indianapolis, Indiana
*Oral Diseases and Oral-Cutaneous Manifestations
of Gastrointestinal and Liver Disease*

Paul Martin, MD

Chief, Division of Heaptology
University of Miami
Miami, Florida
Liver Transplantation

Joel B. Mason, MD

Professor of Medicine and Nutrition
Divisions of Gastroenterology and
    Clinical Nutrition
Tufts Medical Center
Director
Vitamins and Carcinogenesis
    Laboratory
USDA Human Nutrition Research
    Center at Tufts University
Boston, Massachusetts
*Nutritional Principles and Assessment of the
Gastroenterology Patient*

Jeffrey B. Matthews, MD

Dallas B. Phemister Professor and
    Chairman
Surgery
The University of Chicago
Chicago, Illinois
*Surgical Peritonitis and Other Diseases of the
Peritoneum, Mesentery, Omentum, and Diaphragm*

†Lloyd Mayer, MD

Mucosal Immunology and Inflammation

Craig J. McClain, MD

Professor of Medicine
University of Louisville
Director, Gastroenterology
Robley Rex VA Medical Center
Louisville, Kentucky
Alcoholic Liver Disease

George B. McDonald, MD

Professor of Medicine
Division of Gastroenterology
University of Washington
Member
Clinical Research Division
Fred Hutchinson Cancer Research
    Center
Seattle, Washington
*Gastrointestinal and Hepatic Complications of Solid
Organ and Hematopoietic Cell Transplant*

Frederick H. Millham, MD

Associate Clinical Professor of Surgery
Harvard Medical School
Boston, Massachusetts
Chair of Surgery
South Shore Hospital
Weymouth, Massachusetts
Visiting Surgeon
Massachusetts General Hospital
Boston, Massachusetts
Acute Abdominal Pain

Ginat W. Mirowski, DMD, MD
Adjunct Associate Professor
Department of Oral Pathology Medicine
  Radiology
Indiana University School of Dentistry
Indianapolis, Indiana
*Oral Diseases and Oral-Cutaneous Manifestations
of Gastrointestinal and Liver Disease*

Joseph Misdraji, MD
Associate Professor of Pathology
Department of Pathology
Massachusetts General Hospital
Boston, Massachusetts
*Embryology, Anatomy, Histology, and
Developmental Anomalies of the Liver*

Jason S. Mizell, MD
Assistant Professor
Department of Surgery
University of Arkansas for Medical
  Sciences
Little Rock, Arkansas
Intestinal Obstruction

Douglas R. Morgan, MD
Associate Professor of Medicine
Division of Gastroenterology,
  Hepatology, and Nutrition
Department of Medicine
Vanderbilt Institute for Global Health
Vanderbilt University
Nashville, Tennessee
Helicobacter pylori Infection

John Magaña Morton, MD
Associate Professor
Surgery
Stanford University Medical Center
Stanford, California
Surgical and Endoscopic Treatment of Obesity

Sean J. Mulvihill, MD
Professor
Department of Surgery
Associate Vice President for Clinical
  Affairs
Health Sciences Center
CEO
University of Utah Medical Group
University of Utah
Salt Lake City, Utah
Treatment of Gallstone Disease

Fatiha Nassir, PhD
Division of Gastroenterology and
  Hepatology
University of Missouri
School of Medicine
Columbia, Missouri
*Digestion and Absorption of Dietary Fat,
Carbohydrate, and Protein*

Moises Ilan Nevah, MD
Assistant Professor of Medicine
Gastroenterology, Hepatology, and
  Nutrition
University of Texas Health Science
  Center at Houston
Houston, Texas
*Hepatic Encephalopathy, Hepatorenal Syndrome,
Hepatopulmonary Syndrome, and Other Systemic
Complications of Liver Disease*

Jeffrey A. Norton, MD
Professor of Surgery
Department of Surgery
Stanford University School of Medicine
Stanford, California
Neuroendocrine Tumors

Kjell Oberg, MD, PhD
Professor
Department of Endocrine Oncology
University Hospital
Uppsala, Sweden
Adjunct Professor
Department of Surgery
Vanderbilt University
Nashville, Tennessee
Neuroendocrine Tumors

John O'Grady, MD
Professor
Institute of Liver Studies
King's College Hospital
London, United Kingdom
Acute Liver Failure

Roy C. Orlando, MD
Mary Kay and Eugene Bozymski and
  Linda and William Heizer
  Distinguished Professor of
  Gastroenterology
Medicine
University of North Carolina at
  Chapel Hill
Chapel Hill, North Carolina
*Anatomy, Histology, Embryology, and
Developmental Anomalies
of the Esophagus*

Mark T. Osterman, MD
Assistant Professor of Medicine
Hospital of the University of
  Pennsylvania
Presbyterian Medical Center of
  Philadelphia
Philadelphia, Pennsylvania
Ulcerative Colitis

Manisha Palta, MD
Assistant Professor
Radiation Oncology
Duke University
Durham, North Carolina
Radiation Injury

Stephen J. Pandol, MD
Professor of Medicine
University of California, Los Angeles
Director, Pancreatic Research
Cedars-Sinai Medical Center
Los Angeles, California
Pancreatic Secretion

John E. Pandolfino, MD
Hans Popper Professor of Medicine
Northwestern University
Feinberg School of Medicine
Chief
Division of Gastroenterology and
  Hepatology
Northwestern Medicine
Chicago, Illinois
*Esophageal Neuromuscular Function and
Motility Disorders*

Neal C. Patel, MD
Assistant Professor of Medicine
Division of Gastroenterology
Mayo Clinic
Scottsdale, Arizona
Esophageal Tumors

V.S. Periyakoil, MD
Director, Palliative Care Education and
  Training
Clinical Associate Professor
Medicine
Stanford University School of Medicine
Stanford, California
*Palliative Care for Patients with Gastrointestinal
and Hepatic Disease*

Robert Perrillo, MD
Senior Hepatologist
Hepatology Division
Baylor University Medical Center
Dallas, Texas
Hepatitis B
Hepatitis D

Patrick R. Pfau, MD
Professor, Chief of Clinical
  Gastroenterology
Section of Gastroenterology and
  Hepatology
University of Wisconsin School of
  Medicine and Public Health
Madison, Wisconsin
Foreign Bodies, Bezoars, and Caustic Ingestions

Jonathan Potack, MD
Assistant Professor of Medicine
Division of Gastroenterology
Department of Medicine
Icahn School of Medicine at Mount
  Sinai
New York, New York
Colonic Polyps and Polyposis Syndromes

Daniel S. Pratt, MD
Clinical Director, Liver Transplantation
Gastrointestinal Unit
Massachusetts General Hospital
Assistant Professor of Medicine
Harvard Medical School
Boston, Massachusetts
Liver Chemistry and Function Tests

Michael Quante, MD
Internal Medicine II
Technische Universität München
Munich, Germany
Adenocarcinoma of the Stomach and Other Gastric Tumors

Eamonn M.M. Quigley, MD
Professor of Medicine
Weill Cornell Medical College
David M. Underwood Chair of
    Medicine in Digestive Disorders
Houston, Texas
Small Intestinal Bacterial Overgrowth

B.S. Ramakrishna, MBBS, MD, DM, PhD
Director
Institute of Gastroenterology
SRM Institutes for Medical Science
Chennai, Tamil Nadu, India
Tropical Diarrhea and Malabsorption

Francisco C. Ramirez, MD
Professor of Medicine
Division of Gastroenterology
Mayo Clinic
Scottsdale, Arizona
Esophageal Tumors

Mrinalini C. Rao, PhD
Professor
Physiology and Biophysics, and
    Department of Medicine, Division of
    Gastroenterology and Hepatology
University of Illinois at Chicago
Chicago, Illinois
Intestinal Electrolyte Absorption and Secretion

Satish S.C. Rao, MD, PhD
Professor of Medicine
Chief, Gastroenterology/Hepatology
Director, Digestive Health Center
Medical College of Georgia
Georgia Regents University
Augusta, Georgia
Fecal Incontinence

John F. Reinus, MD
Professor of Clinical Medicine
Department of Medicine
Albert Einstein College of Medicine
Chief of Clinical Hepatology
Division of Gastroenterology and Liver
    Diseases
Montefiore Medical Center
Bronx, New York
Gastrointestinal and Hepatic Disorders in the Pregnant Patient

David A. Relman, MD
Thomas C. and Joan M. Merigan
    Professor
Departments of Medicine, and
    Microbiology and Immunology
Stanford University
Stanford, California
Chief of Infectious Diseases
Veterans Affairs Palo Alto Health Care
    System
Palo Alto, California
Whipple's Disease

Joel E. Richter, MD
Professor and Director
Division of Digestive Diseases and
    Nutrition
Director
Joy McCann Culverhouse Center for
    Swallowing Disorders
University of South Florida
Tampa, Florida
Gastroesophageal Reflux Disease

Eve A. Roberts, MD
Adjunct Professor
Paediatrics, Medicine, and
    Pharmacology
University of Toronto
Adjunct Scientist
Genetics and Genome Biology
Hospital for Sick Children Research
    Institute
Associate
Division of Gastroenterology,
    Hepatology, and Nutrition
The Hospital for Sick Children
Toronto, Ontario, Canada
Wilson Disease

Andrew S. Ross, MD
Section Chief
Gastroenterology
Virginia Mason Medical Center
Director, Therapeutic Endoscopy Center
    of Excellence
Digestive Disease Institute
Virginia Mason Medical Center
Seattle, Washington
Primary Sclerosing Cholangitis and Recurrent Pyogenic Cholangitis

Marc E. Rothenberg, MD, PhD
Director, Division of Allergy and
    Immunology
Department of Pediatrics
Cincinnati Children's Hospital Medical
    Center
Director, Division of Allergy and
    Immunology
Department of Pediatrics
University of Cincinnati
Cincinnati, Ohio
Eosinophilic Disorders of the Gastrointestinal Tract

Jayanta Roy-Chowdhury, MBBS
Professor
Departments of Medicine and Genetics
Albert Einstein College of Medicine
New York, New York
Liver Physiology and Energy Metabolism

Namita Roy-Chowdhury, PhD
Professor
Departments of Medicine and Genetics
Albert Einstein College of Medicine
Bronx, New York
Liver Physiology and Energy Metabolism

Bruce A. Runyon, MD
Director of Hepatology
University of California Medical Center,
    Santa Monica
Santa Monica, California
Clinical Professor of Medicine
Division of Digestive Diseases
David Geffen School of Medicine at
    UCLA
Los Angeles, California
Ascites and Spontaneous Bacterial Peritonitis

Michael A. Russo, MD
Assistant Professor of Pediatrics
Division of Pediatric Gastroenterology,
    Hepatology, and Nutrition
University of Texas Southwestern
    Medical School
Dallas, Texas
Attending Physician
Children's Medical Center of Dallas at
    Legacy
Plano, Texas
Anatomy, Histology, and Developmental Anomalies of the Stomach and Duodenum

Hamid M. Said, PhD
Professor and Vice-Chair
Medicine
University of California, Irvine
Irvine, California
Intestinal Digestion and Absorption of Micronutrients

Hugh A. Sampson, MD
Professor of Pediatrics
Pediatrics
Icahn School of Medicine at Mount
  Sinai
New York, New York
Food Allergies

Bruce E. Sands, MD
Dr. Burril B. Crohn Professor of
  Medicine
Department of Medicine
Icahn School of Medicine at Mount
  Sinai
Chief of the Dr. Henry D. Janowitz
  Division of Gastroenterology
Mount Sinai Medical Center
New York, New York
Crohn's Disease

Jayashree Sarathy, PhD
Visiting Research Assistant Professor
Physiology and Biophysics
University of Illinois at Chicago
Chicago, Illinois
Assistant Professor
Biological Sciences
Benedictine University
Lisle, Illinois
Intestinal Electrolyte Absorption and Secretion

George A. Sarosi, Jr., MD
Associate Professor
Robert H. Hux, MD Professor
Surgery
University of Florida College of
  Medicine
Staff Surgeon
Surgical Service
NF/SG VAMC
Gainesville, Florida
Appendicitis

Thomas J. Savides, MD
Professor of Clinical Medicine
Division of Gastroenterology
University of California, San Diego
La Jolla, California
Gastrointestinal Bleeding

Mark A. Schattner, MD
Associate Clinical Member
Medicine
Memorial Sloan-Kettering Cancer
  Center
Associate Professor of Clinical Medicine
Medicine
Joan and Sanford I. Weill Medical
  College of Cornell University
New York, New York
Nutritional Management

James M. Scheiman, MD
Professor
Division of Gastroenterology
Department of Internal Medicine
University of Michigan Medical School
Ann Arbor, Michigan
Intestinal Ulcerations

Lawrence R. Schiller, MD
Attending Physician
Digestive Health Associates of Texas
Baylor University Medical Center
Dallas, Texas
Diarrhea

Mitchell L. Schubert, MD
Professor of Medicine and Physiology
Virginia Commonwealth University
  Health System
Chief, Section of Gastroenterology
McGuire Veterans Affairs Medical
  Center
Richmond, Virginia
Gastric Secretion

Cynthia L. Sears, MD
Professor of Medicine
Johns Hopkins University School of
  Medicine
Baltimore, Maryland
Infectious Enteritis and Proctocolitis

Joseph H. Sellin, MD
Professor of Medicine
Division of Gastroenterology
Baylor College of Medicine
Chief of Gastroenterolgy
Ben Taub General Hospital
Houston, Texas
Diarrhea
Intestinal Electrolyte Absorption and Secretion

M. Gaith Semrin, MD, MBBS
Assistant Professor
Pediatric Gastroenterology and
  Nutrition
University of Texas Southwestern
  Medical Center
Children's Medical Center—Dallas
Dallas, Texas
*Anatomy, Histology, and Developmental Anomalies
of the Stomach and Duodenum*

Vijay H. Shah, MD
Professor of Medicine and Physiology
Chair
Division of Gastroenterology and
  Hepatology
Mayo Clinic
Rochester, Minnesota
Overview of Cirrhosis
Portal Hypertension and Variceal Bleeding

Fergus Shanahan, MD
Professor and Chair
Medicine
University College Cork
National University of Ireland
Cork, Ireland
Enteric Microbiota

G. Thomas Shires, MD
John P. Thompson Chair
Surgical Services
Texas Health Presbyterian Hospital
  Dallas
Dallas, Texas
*Pancreatic Cancer, Cystic Pancreatic Neoplasms,
and Other Nonendocrine Pancreatic Tumors*

Corey A. Siegel, MD
Assistant Professor of Medicine and the
  Dartmouth Institute for Health Policy
  and Clinical Practice
Hanover, New Hampshire
Director
Dartmouth-Hitchcock Inflammatory
  Bowel Disease Center
Geisel School of Medicine
Lebanon, New Hampshire
Crohn's Disease

Maria H. Sjogren, MD
Senior Hepatologist
Gastroenterology
Walter Reed National Military Medical
  Center
Bethesda, Maryland
Hepatitis A

Rhonda F. Souza, MD
Professor of Medicine
Division of Gastroenterology
VA North Texas Healthcare System
University of Texas Southwestern
  Medical Center
Dallas, Texas
Barrett's Esophagus

Cedric W. Spak, MD
Physician
Infectious Diseases
Baylor University Medical Center
Dallas, Texas
Abdominal Abscesses and Gastrointestinal Fistulas

Stuart Jon Spechler, MD
Chief, Division of Gastroenterology
VA North Texas Healthcare System
Professor of Medicine, Berta M. and
  Cecil O. Patterson Chair in
  Gastroenterology
University of Texas Southwestern
  Medical Center
Dallas, Texas
Barrett's Esophagus

William M. Steinberg, MD
Clinical Professor of Medicine
George Washington University
Washington, DC
Acute Pancreatitis

Andrew H. Stockland, MD
Physician
Division of Vascular and Interventional
  Radiology
Mayo Clinic
Rochester, Minnesota
*Endoscopic and Radiologic Treatment of
Biliary Disease*

Neil H. Stollman, MD
Associate Clinical Professor
Department of Medicine, Division of
  Gastroenterology
University of California, San Francisco
San Francisco, California
Chairman
Department of Medicine
Alta Bates Summit Medical Center
Oakland, California
Diverticular Disease of the Colon

Frederick J. Suchy, MD
Chief Research Officer Director, The
  Children's Hospital Research Institute
Pediatrics
Children's Hospital Colorado
Professor of Pediatrics and Associate
  Dean for Child Health Research
Pediatrics
University of Colorado School of
  Medicine
Aurora, Colorado
*Anatomy, Histology, Embryology, Developmental
Anomalies, and Pediatric Disorders of the
Biliary Tract*

Christina M. Surawicz, MD
Professor of Medicine
Medicine, Division of Gastroenterology
University of Washington
Seattle, Washington
Probiotics and Fecal Microbiota Transplant

Jan Tack, MD, PhD
Professor of Medicine, Head of
  Department
TARGID (Translational Research Center
  for Gastrointestinal Disorders)
University of Leuven
Head of Clinic
Gastroenterology
University Hospitals Leuven
Leuven, Belgium
Dyspepsia

Nicholas J. Talley, MD, PhD
Pro Vice-Chancellor and Professor
Faculty of Health
University of Newcastle,
Newcastle, New South Wales, Australia
Irritable Bowel Syndrome

Scott Tenner, MD
Clinical Professor of Medicine
Division of Gastroenterology
State University of New York
Brooklyn, New York
Acute Pancreatitis

Narci C. Teoh, MBBS, PhD
Professor
Gastroenterology and Hepatology
  Academic Unit of Internal Medicine,
  ANU Medical School
The Australian National University
Canberra, Capital Territory, Australia
*Hepatic Drug Metabolism and Liver Disease
Caused by Drugs*

Christopher C. Thompson, MD
Director of Therapeutic Endoscopy
Division of Gastroenterology,
  Hepatology, and Endoscopy
Brigham and Women's Hospital
Associate Professor of Medicine
Harvard Medical School
Boston, Massachusetts
Surgical and Endoscopic Treatment of Obesity

Dawn M. Torres, MD
Chief, Hepatology
Gastroentrology Service, Department of
  Medicine
Walter Reed National Military Medical
  Center
Bethesda, Maryland
Nonalcoholic Fatty Liver Disease

Timothy M. Trebble, MD
Consultant Gastroenterologist
Departments of Gastroenterology and
  Nutrition
Portsmouth Hospitals Trust
Portsmouth, United Kingdom
*Intestinal Digestion and Absorption of
Micronutrients*

Richard H. Turnage, MD
Professor and Chair
Department of Surgery
University of Arkansas for Medical
  Sciences
Little Rock, Arkansas
Intestinal Obstruction

Dominique Charles Valla, MD
Coordinator, DHU Unity
Service d'Hepatologie
Hôpital Beaujon
Clichy, France
Professor
Hepatology
Université Paris Diderot
Paris, France
Vascular Diseases of the Liver

John J. Vargo II, MD
Associate Professor of Medicine
Cleveland Clinic Lerner College of
  Medicine
Gastroenterology and Hepatology
Vice Chairman, Digestive Disease
  Institute
Cleveland Clinic
Cleveland, Ohio
*Preparation for and Complications of
Gastrointestinal Endoscopy*

Axel von Herbay, MD
Professor of Pathology
Doctor of Medicine
Professor of Pathology
Faculty of Medicine
University of Heidelberg
Heidelberg, Germany
Whipple's Disease

Arnold Wald, MD
Professor of Medicine
Division of Gastroenterology and
  Hepatology
University of Wisconsin School of
  Medicine and Public Health
Madison, Wisconsin
Other Diseases of the Colon and Rectum

David Q.-H. Wang, MD, PhD
Associate Professor of Medicine,
  Biochemistry and Molecular Biology
Division of Gastroenterology and
  Hepatology, Department of Internal
  Medicine
Saint Louis University School of
  Medicine
St. Louis, Missouri
Gallstone Disease

Heiner Wedemeyer, MD
Professor
Gastroenterology, Hepatology and
  Endocrinology
Hannover Medical School
Hannover, Germany
Hepatitis C

Jennifer T. Wells, MD
Hepatology Division
Baylor University Medical Center
Dallas, Texas
Hepatitis B

Barry K. Wershil, MD
Professor
Pediatrics
Northwestern University Feinberg
    School of Medicine
Chief, Division of Gastroenterology,
    Hepatology, and Nutrition
Pediatrics
Ann and Robert H. Lurie Children's
    Hospital of Chicago
Chicago, Illinois
*Anatomy, Histology, Embryology, and
Developmental Anomalies of the Small and
Large Intestine*

David C. Whitcomb, MD, PhD
Professor, and Chief, Division of
    Gastroentrology, Hepatology, and
    Nutrition
Medicine, Cell Biology and Molecular
    Physiology, and Human Genetics
University of Pittsburgh and UPMC
Pittsburgh, Pennsylvania
*Hereditary, Familial, and Genetic Disorders of the
Pancreas and Pancreatic Disorders in Childhood*

C. Mel Wilcox, MD, MSPH
Professor of Medicine
Division of Gastroenterology and
    Hepatology
University of Alabama at Birmingham
Birmingham, Alabama
*Gastrointestinal Consequences of Infection with
Human Immunodeficiency Virus*

Lalan S. Wilfong, MD
Department of Internal Medicine
Division of Hematology/Oncology
Texas Health Presbyterian Hospital
    Dallas
Dallas, Texas
*Pancreatic Cancer, Cystic Pancreatic Neoplasms,
and Other Nonendocrine Pancreatic Tumors*

Christopher G. Willett, MD
Professor and Chairman
Radiation Oncology
Duke University
Durham, North Carolina
Radiation Injury

Stephan G. Wyers, MD
Assistant Professor of Surgery
University of Chicago Pritzker School
    of Medicine
General Surgery
University of Chicago Medical Center
Chicago, Illinois
*Surgical Peritonitis and Other Diseases of the
Peritoneum, Mesentery, Omentum, and Diaphragm*

Joseph C. Yarze, MD
Clinical Associate Professor of Medicine
Albany Medical College
Albany, New York
Consultant
Gastroenterology Associates of
    Northern New York
Medical Co-Director
Gastrointestinal Center
Glens Falls Hospital
Glens Falls, New York
Chronic Abdominal Pain

FOREWORD

The tenth edition of *Sleisenger and Fordtran's Gastrointestinal and Liver Disease: Pathophysiology/Diagnosis/Management* continues as the benchmark textbook of gastroenterology and hepatology. It is authoritative, comprehensive, and, although encyclopedic in its coverage, very readable. The editors have done an excellent job ensuring that the organization of chapters is uniform. Thus, chapters have sections on epidemiology, etiology, pathology, pathophysiology, clinical features, diagnosis, differential diagnosis, treatment, and prognosis. This uniform format allows readers to search easily for information under different subheadings to find answers to their questions. As noted in the Preface, the content of the book has changed dramatically in the 42 years since the first edition was published in 1973. Whereas the first edition had 115 chapters and the tenth edition has 132, the additional 17 chapters belie the masterly job the contributors and editors have done in preserving references not only to classic articles but also to the important new advances that have occurred between publications of successive editions. This newer material also includes references that have been updated to include articles published into 2014. As also noted in the Preface, some of the new chapters include up-to-date discussions of enteric microbiota, probiotics and fecal transplantation, and factitious gastrointestinal diseases. An outstanding feature of the textbook is the clarity and detail of the tables and the high quality of the photomicrographs.

The tenth edition of "Sleisenger and Fordtran" will continue to be a premier textbook, as was the case with its predecessors, and will be especially useful to medical residents, gastroenterology fellows, and gastroenterologists. Finally, I can personally attest to the remarkable advances that have been made, as I was author of the chapter on eosinophilic gastroenteritis in the second edition of the textbook, and reading the same chapter in the tenth edition underscores the important advances that have been made in our understanding of the molecular basis as well as the pathophysiology of this and related disorders.

Norton J. Greenberger, MD
Boston, Massachusetts

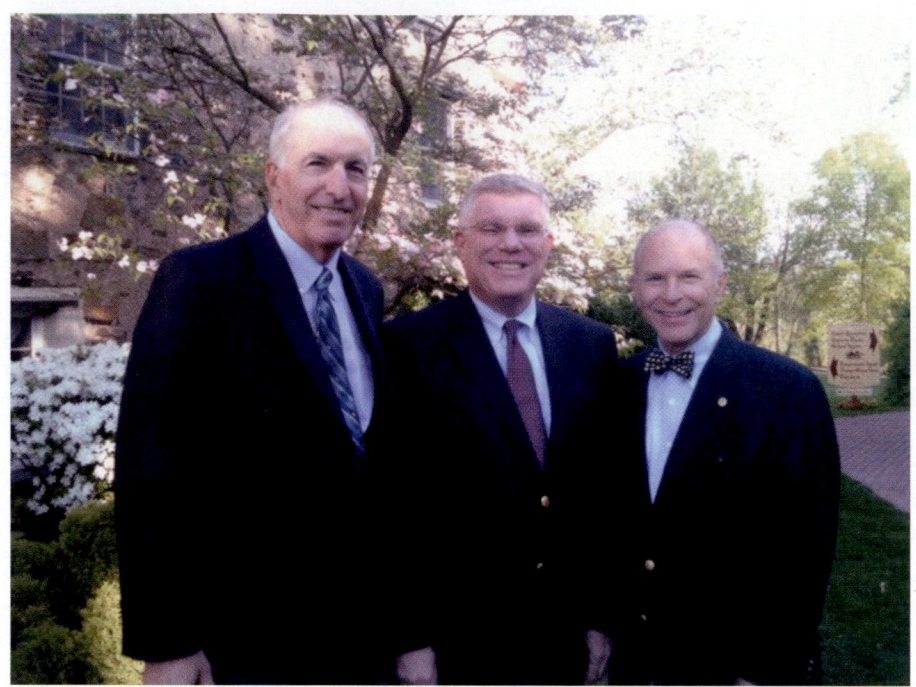

From left: Mark Feldman, MD; Lawrence S. Friedman, MD; Lawrence J. Brandt, MD.

PREFACE

The tenth edition of *Sleisenger and Fordtran's Gastrointestinal and Liver Disease: Pathophysiology/Diagnosis/Management* is among a select group of textbooks that have been valuable to readers over a long time span. Work by its founding editors, Marvin Sleisenger and John S. Fordtran, began more than four decades ago and culminated in the publication of the first edition, *Gastrointestinal Disease*, in 1973. Much has happened in the field of gastroenterology since then, and each edition of the text has methodically incorporated these exciting advances into its pages. Advances have included clearer understanding of the basic mechanisms of health and disease at a cellular, subcellular, genetic, and molecular level; a much clearer comprehension of the pathophysiology of GI and liver diseases; the introduction of numerous diagnostic tests and procedures (many of which displaced now outmoded tests and procedures); combining diagnostic with therapeutic endoscopy; developing many novel pharmaceutical agents and drug classes for conditions that previously had no such treatments; applying laparoscopic surgery in many common GI disorders; and so much more.

Over its 42-year lifespan, the textbook has had six editors: Marvin H. Sleisenger and John S. Fordtran (founding editors), as well as Mark Feldman, Bruce F. Scharschmidt, Lawrence S. Friedman, and Lawrence J. Brandt. These editors have had the good fortune to engage hundreds of superb author-contributors from around the globe who generously shared their knowledge and expertise with readers of the book. The editors also have had the luxury of stalwart support from a highly competent and professional publishing company, Elsevier, throughout the life of the book.

When the first edition of *Gastrointestinal Disease* was published in 1973, it was quite different from this, the tenth edition. The first edition was printed in a single volume of less than 1600 pages, with well over 200 of these pages devoted to a single entity—peptic ulcer disease. There were 115 chapters in the first edition, compared with 132 chapters in the tenth edition. Besides its two founding editors, the first edition had 55 contributors, compared with 217 contributors in the tenth edition. The first edition was written almost entirely by authors based in the United States, whereas authors from 15 countries have contributed to the pages of the tenth edition. The vast majority of chapters in the first edition were written by a single author, whereas most chapters now have two authors. And perhaps most important, there was no coverage of liver diseases in the first edition, or even in the four subsequent editions, until the sixth edition—renamed *Gastrointestinal and Liver Disease: Pathophysiology/Diagnosis/Management*—was published in 1998. In 2007, the British Medical Association awarded the eighth edition of the book its First Prize in the field of gastroenterology.

The first edition was available to readers in print format only, and color was used sparingly. As time went on, the book became available in CD-ROM and then online via a secure website. Enhanced use of color allowed improved depictions of endoscopic images and histopathology. Today the contents of the tenth edition are available on handheld devices such as smartphones, iPads, and Kindles. The online version of the tenth edition also incorporates dozens of video clips that illustrate diagnostic and therapeutic approaches in the field, with narrative descriptions of the procedures. The authors are greatly appreciative of Gregory G. Ginsberg, Christopher J. Gostout, Michael L. Kochman, Ian D. Norton, and the team at Elsevier for allowing our readers access to these valuable educational videos.

Fortunately, with the help of our distinguished contributors, the content of the textbook remains unparalleled. Comparing the contents of the first with the tenth editions, one can appreciate the striking advances in the field. Many conditions that now constitute the core of gastroenterology practice were not even known to exist in 1973. Furthermore, comparing the hepatology section in the sixth edition (1998) with that in the current edition is a striking tribute to the discoveries that have improved the diagnosis and therapy of liver disease, particularly with respect to the panorama of drugs to treat chronic viral hepatitis.

The tenth edition includes three notable chapters not included in earlier editions. An entire chapter, authored by Fergus Shanahan, has been devoted to Enteric Microbiota and another, authored by Christina Surawicz and Lawrence J. Brandt, to Probiotics and Fecal Microbiota Transplantations. These additions reflect our increasing knowledge about the bowel flora and our emerging understanding of the role of intestinal microbiota in the pathogenesis and treatment of a variety of GI (and other) diseases, most notably *Clostridium difficile* colitis. The editors are also delighted to welcome back John S. Fordtran who, along with Marc D. Feldman, has written a scholarly chapter on Factitious Gastrointestinal Disease, a group of disorders that can be most challenging for clinicians to diagnose and treat. Additional changes since the ninth edition are expansions of the chapter on Surgical Treatment of Obesity to include endoscopic treatment, and the chapter on Complications of Gastrointestinal Endoscopy to include preparation for endoscopy; combination of the chapters on Peptic Ulcer Disease and Treatment of Peptic Ulcer Disease into a single chapter; a new chapter on Overview of Cirrhosis; separation of the chapter on Hepatitis B and D into two chapters; and separation of the chapters on Digestion and Absorption of Nutrients and Vitamins into one on Digestion and Absorption of Macronutrients and one on Digestion and Absorption of Micronutrients. We are delighted to welcome many new authors, as well as returning authors, to the tenth edition.

Finally, the editors gratefully acknowledge the capable and spirited roles of Kate Dimock, Suzanne Toppy, Deidre (Dee) Simpson, and Cindy Thoms at Elsevier for facilitating the publication of the tenth edition. Without their support and vision, the editors would have fallen short of the high standards that were set by the founding editors and to which we remain committed.

Mark Feldman, MD
Lawrence S. Friedman, MD
Lawrence J. Brandt, MD

CONTENTS

SECTION V
Esophagus

SECTION VI
Stomach and Duodenum

SECTION X
Small and Large Intestine

SECTION XI
Additional Treatments for Patients with Gastrointestinal and Liver Disease

VIDEO CONTENTS

ABBREVIATION LIST

AASLD	American Association for the Study of Liver Diseases	HEV	Hepatitis E virus
ACG	American College of Gastroenterology	Hgb	Hemoglobin
ACTH	Corticotropin	HIV	Human immunodeficiency virus
AFP	Alpha fetoprotein	HLA	Human leukocyte antigen
AIDS	Acquired immunodeficiency syndrome	HPV	Human papillomavirus
ALT	Alanine aminotransferase	HSV	Herpes simplex virus
APACHE	Acute Physiology and Chronic Health Examination	Hp	*Helicobacter pylori*
ASGE	American Society for Gastrointestinal Endoscopy	IBD	Inflammatory bowel disease
		IBS	Irritable bowel syndrome
		ICU	Intensive care unit
AST	Aspartate aminotransferase	INR	International normalized ratio
ATP	Adenosine triphosphate	IV	Intravenous
BICAP	Bipolar electrocoagulation	LDH	Lactate dehydrogenase
BMI	Body mass index	MELD	Model for End-Stage Liver Disease
CCK	Cholecystokinin	MEN	Multiple endocrine neoplasia
CEA	Carcinoembryonic antigen	MRA	Magnetic resonance angiography/angiogram
CF	Cystic fibrosis	MRCP	Magnetic resonance cholangiopancreatography
CO_2	Carbon dioxide	MRI	Magnetic resonance imaging
COX	Cyclooxygenase	NG	Nasogastric
CT	Computed tomography	NPO	Nil per os (nothing by mouth)
CTA	Computed tomography angiography/angiogram	NSAIDs	Nonsteroidal antiinflammatory drugs
DIC	Disseminated intravascular coagulation	O_2	Oxygen
DNA	Deoxyribonucleic acid	PBC	Primary biliary cirrhosis
EBV	Epstein-Barr virus	PCR	Polymerase chain reaction
EGD	Esophagogastroduodenoscopy	PET	Positron emission tomography
EGF	Epidermal growth factor	PPI	Proton pump inhibitor
ERCP	Endoscopic retrograde cholangiopancreatography	PSC	Primary sclerosing cholangitis
		PSS	Progressive systemic sclerosis
EUS	Endoscopic ultrasonography	PUD	Peptic ulcer disease
FDA	U.S. Food and Drug Administration	RA	Rheumatoid arthritis
FNA	Fine-needle aspiration	RNA	Ribonucleic acid
GERD	Gastroesophageal reflux disease	SBP	Spontaneous bacterial peritonitis
GGTP	Gamma glutamyl transpeptidase	SIBO	Small intestinal bacterial overgrowth
GI	Gastrointestinal	SLE	Systemic lupus erythematosus
GIST	GI stromal tumor	SOD	Sphincter of Oddi dysfunction
H&E	Hematoxylin & eosin	TB	Tuberculosis
HCG	Human chorionic gonadotropin	TG	Triglyceride(s)
H2RA	Histamine-2 receptor antagonist	TNF	Tumor necrosis factor
HAART	Highly active antiretroviral therapy	TNM	Tumor Node Metastasis (staging)
HAV	Hepatitis A virus	TPN	Total parenteral nutrition
HBV	Hepatitis B virus	UC	Ulcerative colitis
HCV	Hepatitis C virus	US	Ultrasonography
HDV	Hepatitis D virus	USA	United States of America
HELLP	*Hemolysis, elevated liver enzymes, low platelet count*	WBC	White blood cell
		WHO	World Health Organization
		ZES	Zollinger-Ellison syndrome

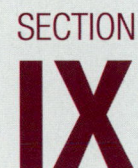

SECTION

IX

Liver

Embryology, Anatomy, Histology, and Developmental Anomalies of the Liver

JOSEPH MISDRAJI

Knowledge of embryology, anatomy, and histology of the liver is basic to understanding pathologic processes. Some developmental anomalies of the biliary tract and liver are discussed in Chapter 62.

EMBRYOLOGY

The liver develops at 3 to 4 weeks' gestation as an outgrowing diverticulum of proliferating endodermal cells from the ventral wall of the foregut in response to signals from the adjacent developing heart (Fig. 71-1).[1,2] In the fourth week, 2 buds can be recognized in the hepatic diverticulum: the cranial bud becomes the liver and the hilar biliary tract, whereas the caudal bud develops into a superior bud that forms the gallbladder and cystic duct and an inferior bud that forms the ventral pancreas.[3,4]

Initially, the liver bud is separated from the mesenchyme of the septum transversum by basement membrane.[1] Shortly, however, the basement membrane surrounding the liver bud is lost, E-cadherin expression is down-regulated in hepatic cells, and cells delaminate from the bud and invade the septum transversum as cords of hepatoblasts—bipotential cells that differentiate into hepatocytes and cholangiocytes.[2,5,6] As they invade the septum transversum mesenchyme, the hepatoblasts intermingle with endothelial cells; this interaction is necessary to support hepatic morphogenesis.[1]

Hepatocytic differentiation involves the development of abundant rough endoplasmic reticulum and the Golgi apparatus needed for synthesis of secreted proteins such as albumin, the best characterized marker of nascent hepatocytes. Hepatic differentiation is highly dependent on signals from the cardiogenic mesoderm and septum transversum mesenchyme, which produce fibroblast growth factor (FGF) and bone morphogenetic protein (BMP), respectively.[2,5] These factors may be important in development. For example, in the absence of FGF signaling from the cardiac mesoderm, the ventral endoderm develops into pancreas,[1] but too high a concentration of FGF

results in differentiation toward lung.[7] The control of hepatocytic differentiation is complex and involves several transcription factors at various stages of development. For example, GATA4 and forkhead box A (FoxA) are involved in developmental "competence" because they have the ability to interact with compacted chromatin and act as "pioneer" factors that can mark domains of chromatin as competent to be expressed in response to later developmental cues.[6,7] These cells can now respond to extracellular signals, such as FGFs secreted by cardiogenic mesoderm, that induce hepatic fate.[7] The transcription factor Prox1 may be involved in down-regulation of E-cadherin, because mutant hepatoblasts maintain high levels of E-cadherin and fail to degrade the matrix surrounding the liver bud.[6] The terminal differentiation of hepatocytes requires the overlapping interaction of a group of transcription factors including hepatocyte nuclear factor 1β (HNF1β), HNF1α, FoxA2, HNF4α1, HNF6, and liver receptor homolog-1 (LRH-1).[6,7] These cross-regulating factors form a dynamic transcriptional network by binding to each other's promoters as well as to the promoters of other hepatic transcription factors, creating synergistic interdependence as hepatocyte maturation proceeds.[7] The contribution of Wnt signaling and β-catenin is complex and stage dependent. During early development, canonical Wnt/β-catenin signaling represses hematopoietically expressed homeobox (Hhex), another early transcription factor in hepatic development; therefore, early in the process, Wnt must be suppressed in the anterior endoderm to facilitate commitment of the endoderm to a hepatic fate. After specification, Wnt signaling promotes hepatogenesis.[6,8]

The extrahepatic biliary system develops originally as a solid structure that becomes recanalized at the end of the fifth week.[3] It may develop ab initio, however, as a hollow structure, refuting the concept that biliary atresia results from a failure of the bile duct to recanalize.[9] Extrahepatic biliary tract development may require the expression of sex-determining region Y-box 17 (SOX17), which is regulated by the homolog of hairy/enhancer-of-split (Hes-1); absence of Hes-1 results in the differentiating of bile duct cells to a pancreatic phenotype.[6]

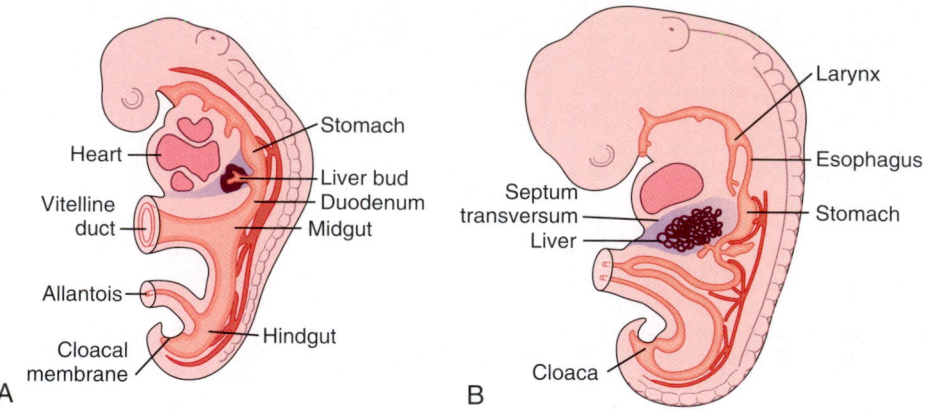

FIGURE 71-1. Embryology of the liver. *A,* At the 3-mm embryo stage, the liver bud forms in response to signals from the developing heart. *B,* At the 5-mm stage, the hepatoblasts penetrate the septum transversum.

Another transcription factor that may be involved in extrahepatic biliary development is Hhex; in Hhex-null embryos, the bile duct is replaced by tissue that resembles duodenum.[6] Either the extrahepatic and intrahepatic biliary systems merge at the hepatic hilum, or they maintain luminal continuity from the start.[9]

Intrahepatic biliary development begins at 6 weeks when a subset of hepatoblasts close to the portal mesenchyme strongly express biliary-specific antigens (see Chapter 62).[10] These biliary precursor cells form a continuous single layered ring around the portal mesenchyme, called the *ductal plate*. This plate becomes partly bilayered in the next step with the cells closest to the portal mesenchyme maintaining a biliary phenotype, and those closest to the parenchyma resembling hepatoblasts, a process known as *transient asymmetry*.[11,12] A period of remodeling follows in which focal dilatations appear between the 2 cell layers and eventually form lumens. The parts of the ductal plate not involved in the formation of ducts regress by apoptosis, and, around the time of birth, the remaining ducts are incorporated into the portal mesenchyme.[10] Incorporation and elongation of ducts begins in the hilum and extends to the periphery of the liver.[11,12] At birth, the most peripheral small portal tracts require an additional 4 weeks before the ductal plates develop into bile ducts.[9] Similarly, bile canaliculi develop their fully mature appearance during the perinatal and early postnatal period, even though the major bile transporters are expressed at the mid-gestational age.[9]

The switch in phenotype of hepatoblasts to cholangiocytes requires the coordinated activity of various signaling systems and transcription factors. The earliest sign of biliary differentiation is expression of Sox9, a transcription factor that regulates the timing of biliary duct development.[6] The Wnt/β-catenin signaling system may also play a temporal role in the commitment of hepatoblasts to biliary epithelial cells.[8] HNF-6 and HNF1β are other transcription factors that regulate biliary differentiation; mice deficient in these factors show cystic dysgenesis of the biliary tract as well as abnormalities in the hepatic arterial branches,[11] suggesting that biliary tract development is tightly linked to hepatic arteriogenesis. The developing ducts produces vascular endothelial growth factor (VEGF), which cooperates with angiopoietin-1 produced by hepatoblasts to promote arterial vasculogenesis and recruit mural pericytes to the developing arteries.[11] The maintenance of duct structure during the elongation phase requires that mitoses be aligned uniformly along the axis of the duct, a process called *planar cell polarity* that is controlled by noncanonical Wnt signaling and that is defective in fibropolycystic liver disease.[11]

Two signaling systems have emerged as critical to biliary differentiation and restriction of biliary differentiation to a periportal location. Transforming growth factor (TGF)-β generated by portal mesenchyme stimulates hepatoblasts to switch to a biliary phenotype, and TGF-β is greater near the portal vein and less in the parenchyma.[11,12] The Notch pathway is also involved in bile duct development; Jagged1 expressed in portal vein mesenchyme interacts with Notch2 on hepatoblasts to induce biliary differentiation at the expense of hepatocyte differentiation.[11-13] Notch signaling is also instrumental in biliary tubulogenesis. In its absence, formation of the ducts beyond the monolayer ductal plate is impaired.[6] Mutations in the gene that codes for Jagged1 are associated with Alagille syndrome (see Chapter 62).

Investigations into the origin of mesenchymal cells in the liver have determined that mesothelial cells and submesothelial cells migrate inward from the liver surface and give rise to stellate cells, portal fibroblasts, and perivascular mesenchymal cells.[14,15] Mesenchymal cells from the septum transversum may also contribute to the formation of hepatic stellate cells.[15] Kupffer cells presumably originate from the yolk sac because their presence in fetal liver precedes bone marrow development.[2]

Hepatic Stem Cells and Maturational Lineages

The existence of hepatic stem cells has been debated, with the assumption that hepatic stem cells are hepatoblasts. More recently, hepatic stem cells have been recognized as cells that give rise to hepatoblasts.[16] In this model, hepatic stem cells are self-renewing cells that express epithelial cell adhesion molecule (EpCAM), neural cell adhesion molecule (NCAM), and cytokeratin 19 and weakly express albumin but not AFP.[16,17] They are found in the ductal plates in fetal livers and in the canals of Hering in adult livers.[16,17]

When human hepatic stem cells are grown in culture, they produce cords of cells interspersed with clear channels, presumed to be hepatoblasts with canaliculi. These cells more strongly express albumin, express EpCAM, AFP, and intracellular adhesion molecule (ICAM)-1, have reduced cytokeratin 19 expression, and lose NCAM.[16] Hepatoblasts are diploid bipotent cells that give rise to hepatocyte and cholangiocyte lineages and are the transit amplifying cells of the liver.[17] They are present throughout the parenchyma of fetal and neonatal livers, and in small groups at the ends of canals of Hering in adult livers.[16] They are reduced in number with advancing age.[17]

Committed progenitor cells are diploid, unipotent, immature cells that give rise to only one adult cell type. They are either intermediate hepatocytes that express albumin and hepatic enzymes or small cholangiocytes that line canals of Hering, intrahepatic bile ducts, and bile ductules.[17] Finally, diploid adult cells can undergo 6 or 7 rounds of division before reaching subcultivation capacity.[17]

Vascular Development

During early development, there are 3 major venous systems in the embryo—2 extraembryonic and 1 intraembryonic. The extraembryonic venous systems are the omphalomesenteric (vitelline) and umbilical (placental) veins, and the intraembryonic system includes the cardinal veins that drain the venous blood of the embryo to the heart.[18] All of these systems converge into the sinus venosus, a quadrangular cavity that is incorporated into the heart. The developing liver eventually incorporates the vitelline and umbilical veins.[18]

The vitelline veins run from the yolk sac to the heart, and as the liver invades them, the midsection of the veins becomes capillarized.[19] The 2 vitelline veins become connected by various anastomoses, and portions of their inferior segments regress and other portions form a single portal vein; remnants of the right and left vitelline circulations persist as the right and left intrahepatic portal circulations in the adult liver.[18,19] Whereas the definitive right portal vein derives from the right vitelline vein, the definitive left portal vein derives from the portal sinus, explaining why the left portal vein begins with a horizontal segment.[18] The superior segment of the left vitelline vein regresses and the superior segment of the right vitelline vein becomes the common hepatic vein, which is incorporated into the inferior vena cava.[19]

The umbilical veins run from the placenta to the heart and during fetal life are the predominant afferent vessels that supply the liver.[18] During the 6- to 7-mm stage of human development, part of the left umbilical vein becomes the ductus venosus, a large branchless channel that shunts placenta-derived arterial blood from the umbilical vein to the inferior vena cava, thereby bypassing the liver[18]; the remainder of the left umbilical vein and the right umbilical vein disappear. After birth, the obliterated prehepatic segment of the left umbilical vein becomes the round ligament of the liver (ligamentum teres hepatis) in the free edge of the falciform ligament, and the ductus venosus collapses and becomes the ligamentum venosum.[18]

The arterial supply of the liver begins as an offshoot from the celiac trunk at around the eighth week of gestation. By the 10th week, the first arterial radicles are visible in the central portion of the liver, and by the fifteenth week, they reach the periphery of the liver.[18] As discussed earlier, the development of the arterial supply is closely coordinated with that of the bile duct. The processes of vasculogenesis and vascular remodeling are dependent on stage-specific expression of the VEGF and angiopoietin-1 by ductal plate cells and hepatoblasts, respectively, and by their receptors in developing endothelial and perivascular smooth muscle cells.[20]

Sinusoidal development occurs between the fifth and twelfth weeks of gestation. Before that, the capillaries between hepatocyte plates lack fenestrae or other characteristics of sinusoids.[18] During development, the sinusoids acquire fenestrae, lose expression of the typical endothelial markers CD34 and CD31, and become invested by a perisinusoidal matrix rich in tenascin and poor in laminins.[18] These alterations may be necessary to adapt the liver to its hematopoietic function during fetal life.[18] The mechanisms that control the growth and maturation of sinusoidal endothelial cells are not well defined, although a role for Wnt signaling has been suggested.[6]

ANATOMY

Parietal peritoneum covers the liver except for the bare area, where the liver comes in direct contact with the diaphragm and is suspended by fibrous tissue and the hepatic veins.[21] The peritoneal reflections that surround the bare area comprise the superior and inferior coronary ligaments and the right and left triangular ligaments, which attach the liver to the diaphragm; these avascular attachments are not true ligaments but are in continuity with Glisson's capsule.[22]

Traditionally, 4 lobes are distinguished in the liver based on its external appearance: right, left, caudate, and quadrate. On the anterior surface, the falciform ligament divides the liver into the right and left anatomic lobes. On the inferior surface, the quadrate lobe is defined by the gallbladder fossa, porta hepatis, and ligamentum teres hepatis. The caudate lobe is delineated by the inferior vena cava groove, porta hepatis, and ligamentum venosum fissure.[23] Although these lobes are convenient and well known, they are not true functional lobes.[22]

The true right and left lobes of the liver are of roughly equal size and are divided not by the falciform ligament, but by a plane passing through the bed of the gallbladder and the notch of the inferior vena cava. This plane, which has no external indications, is called the *Cantlie line*.[21,23] Based on arterial blood supply, portal venous blood supply, biliary drainage, and hepatic venous drainage, the liver is divided into right and left functional lobes, each of which is divided into 2 segments, and these are further subdivided into 2 subsegments.[21] Several systems of subdivision have been proposed, but the most widely used systems are those of Couinaud, which follows the distribution of the portal and hepatic veins,[24] and Healey and Schroy, which is based on the distribution of bile ducts.[25] In these systems, the subsegments are assigned numbers from 1 to 8, with the caudate lobe being subsegment 1 and the others following in a clockwise pattern (Fig. 71-2).[23]

The liver receives approximately 70% of its blood supply and 40% of its oxygen from the portal vein and 30% of its blood supply and 60% of its oxygen from the hepatic artery.[26] The portal vein is formed from the confluence of the superior mesenteric vein and the splenic vein. At the hilum, the portal vein divides into right and left branches, on which the right and left lobes of the liver are based.[22,27] Although Couinaud's scheme holds that the right and left portal veins branch supply 8 venous territories, the number of second-order branches of the right and left portal veins varies greatly.[28] The hepatic artery commonly arises from the celiac trunk, although occasionally it arises from the superior mesenteric artery.[27] A common variant is a left hepatic artery that branches from the left gastric artery and a right hepatic artery branch that arises from the superior mesenteric artery.[27] Within the hilum, the hepatic artery lies anterior to the portal vein and to the left of the bile duct. In the liver, the arteries, portal veins, and bile ducts are surrounded by a fibrous sheath, the Glissonian sheath, whereas the hepatic veins lack this structure.[21] Three major hepatic veins drain into the inferior vena cava, although in 60% to 85% of persons, the left and middle veins unite to enter the inferior vena cava as a single vein.[21,22,27]

The extrahepatic biliary tract is composed of the common hepatic duct, cystic duct, gallbladder, and right and left hepatic ducts. The right and left hepatic ducts drain the right and left lobes of the liver, respectively. The fusion of the right and left hepatic ducts gives rise to the common hepatic duct. The caudate lobe usually drains to the origin of the left hepatic duct or to the right hepatic duct. The cystic duct usually drains into the lateral aspect of the common hepatic duct below its origin to form the bile duct.[29]

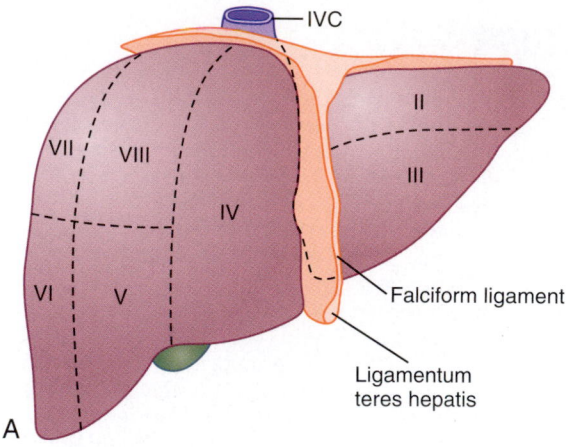

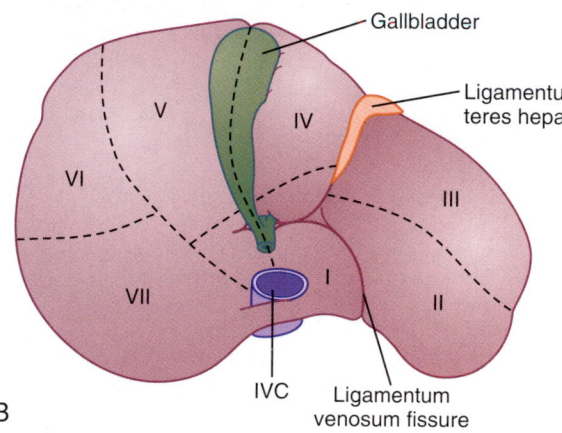

FIGURE 71-2. Segmental anatomy of the liver based on the Couinaud terminology. Eight segments are identified. *A,* Anterior view. *B,* Inferior view. IVC, inferior vena cava.

Nerves

Sympathetic or adrenergic nerve fibers form a rich plexus around blood vessels and, to a lesser extent, bile ducts.[30] Fibers from the plexus supply the lobules where they run along sinusoidal walls, predominantly in the periportal region.[30] Parasympathetic (cholinergic) nerve fibers innervate extrahepatic and intrahepatic branches of the hepatic artery, portal vein, and hepatic vein, but only a few fibers reach hepatocytes.[30,31] Intrinsic nerves regulate hepatic blood flow, sinusoidal microcirculation, biliary physiology, and metabolism. Since the advent of liver transplantation, however, the importance of the hepatic nervous system has been questioned, given the adequate functioning of the denervated allograft.[31,32]

Lymphatics

Superficial lymphatics from the convex surface of the liver run through the right or left triangular ligament and the falciform ligament. They cross the diaphragm to enter precardiac, superior phrenic, and juxtaesophageal lymph nodes or travel alongside the right or left inferior phrenic artery to the celiac nodes.[33] Superficial lymphatics from the visceral surface of the liver mostly run to the hepatic lymph nodes. From the caudate lobe, lymph vessels drain into precaval nodes. Deep lymphatic vessels leave the liver at the porta hepatis to drain into the foraminal node at the epiploic foramen and the superior

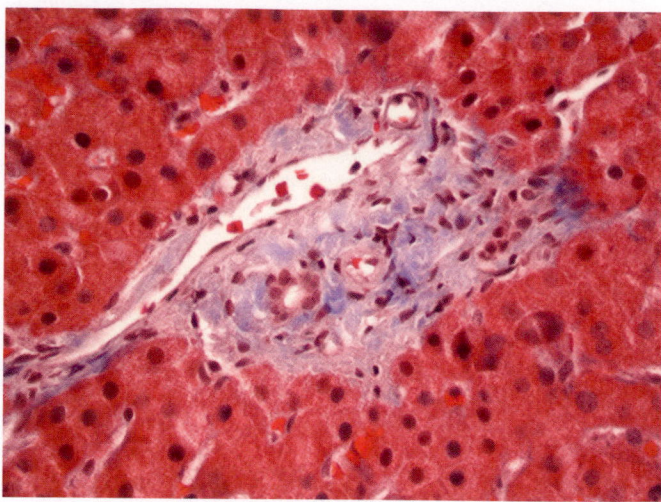

FIGURE 71-3. Histology of the liver showing a normal portal tract with a portal vein *(upper left)* and paired arteriole and bile duct *(center)*; the bile duct is to the left of the arteriole in this portal tract. (Masson trichrome, ×200.)

pancreatic nodes. Lymphatic vessels that leave the liver with the hepatic veins continue in the wall of the inferior vena cava.[33]

HISTOLOGY

The majority of the liver is composed of hepatocytes arranged in plates or "muralium" one or two cells thick, separated by sinusoids (see also Chapter 72). Hepatocytes appear as polygonal cells with round nuclei of varying sizes with frequent binucleate cells. Portal tracts within the parenchyma contain a branch of the hepatic arteriole, portal vein, and bile duct running together as a triad and accompanied by nerve fibers and lymphatic vessels (Fig. 71-3). Terminal hepatic arterioles and terminal portal venules originate from portal tracts and supply blood to the sinusoids. The sinusoids lead mixed portal and arterial blood from the portal tract to the terminal hepatic venules (also known as *central veins*). These terminal hepatic venules drain into sublobular veins, then into hepatic veins, and eventually to the vena cava.

The terminal portal venules do not possess a muscle layer and so have no inlet sphincters at their junction with sinusoids; however, the nuclei of large endothelial cells at that junction bulge into the lumen and, by means of contraction, these cells control the flow of blood into the sinusoids.[32] A similar outlet sphincter-like activity occurs at the site where the sinusoid connects with the terminal hepatic vein.[32] In contrast to terminal portal venules, terminal hepatic arterioles are invested by smooth muscle and are capable of forming presinusoidal sphincters.[32]

Sinusoidal endothelial cells are the primary barrier between blood and hepatocytes (see Chapter 72 and Fig. 72-1). They are a unique type of endothelial cell in that they have fenestrations, have a limited capacity for endocytosis, and lack a basal lamina.[26] The size of the fenestrae in the lobular periphery differs from that in the center of the lobule.[34] Contraction of actin filaments within endothelial cells controls the pore size, which in turn is controlled by calcium and calmodulin.[34] Kupffer cells are macrophages that also line sinusoids and have the capacity to phagocytose large particles.[34] They are more numerous, larger, and more phagocytically active in the periportal than perivenular region.[26] Their major role is to clear blood of senescent red blood cells and toxic endogenous and exogenous substances.[34] Apart from phagocytosis, Kupffer cells handle low-density lipoproteins and produce lymphokine mediators that direct hepatocyte protein synthesis, inflammatory mediators, and hepatocyte-protective prostaglandins.[32]

Hepatic stellate cells were formerly known as "Ito cells," or fat-storing cells; they are perisinusoidal cells that are sites of fat metabolism and vitamin A storage.[32] They encircle the sinusoidal wall and may regulate the width of the lumen. When hepatic stellate cells are activated, they transform into myofibroblasts that express desmin and smooth muscle actin.[26]

A perisinusoidal space, the space of Disse, remains between the sinusoidal lining and the vascular pole of hepatocytes and communicates with the sinusoidal space through multiple fenestrations.[32] This space contains plasma and collagen types I, III, IV, and V, which act as the scaffolding of the organ.[32] The space of Mall is a space between the periportal hepatocytes and portal connective tissue. Lymphatic fluid accumulates in the space of Disse and then passes into the space of Mall before draining into lymphatic vessels.[26,35] Lymphatic vessels form a network in the portal spaces in association with branches of the hepatic artery.[32]

One aspect of the hepatocyte borders the sinusoid and another borders the bile canaliculus. The canaliculi direct bile to the terminal canals of Hering, which are lined partly by hepatocytes and partly by cholangiocytes.[36] The canals of Hering do not stop at the limiting plate of the portal tract but extend into the periportal region of the lobule. The canals of Hering pass into bile ductules, which are lined entirely by cholangiocytes.[36] The ductules in turn connect to the smallest interlobular bile ducts. Interlobular bile ducts connect to septal bile ducts, which connect to hepatic bile ducts. Histologically, the smaller ducts are lined by cuboidal cells, whereas the larger ducts are lined by columnar epithelial cells.

Organization of the Liver Parenchyma

The classic lobule of the liver was described in 1833 by Kiernan as a hexagon with a central vein at its center and portal tracts at 3 corners. Because many glands have a duct as the center of their functional unit, Mall envisioned the basic unit of the liver to be the portal unit, defined at its center by a portal tract and at its periphery by central veins.[32] The liver acinus was defined in 1954 by Rappaport as the parenchyma around terminal afferent portal and arterial vessels that supply this group of hepatocytes with blood. At the periphery of the acinus lies the terminal hepatic venule (the "central vein"), which drains several acini.[32] In this model, the following 3 zones exist: (1) the periportal zone, or zone 1, which is supplied by blood with high oxygen content; (2) the intermediate zone (zone 2); and (3) the perivenular zone (zone 3), which receives blood that is relatively low in oxygen content.[32] The acinus represents a functional and a structural unit that facilitates the description of lesions such as bridging necrosis and fibrosis (Fig. 71-4) (see Chapters 74 and 80).[26]

In 1982, Matsumoto and Kawakami presented a view of liver architecture based on its angioarchitecture.[37] In this concept, the portal and hepatic venous systems are divided into a conducting portion, which delivers and drains blood from the parenchyma, and a parenchymal portion, which is the basis for the primary lobule. The parenchymal portion of the portal and hepatic venous systems consists of minute side branches that originate as orderly rows along the terminal branches of the conducting portion. The portal venous branches divide several times more often than the hepatic venous branches, thereby creating a larger number of portal venous channels for each hepatic venous channel. The final

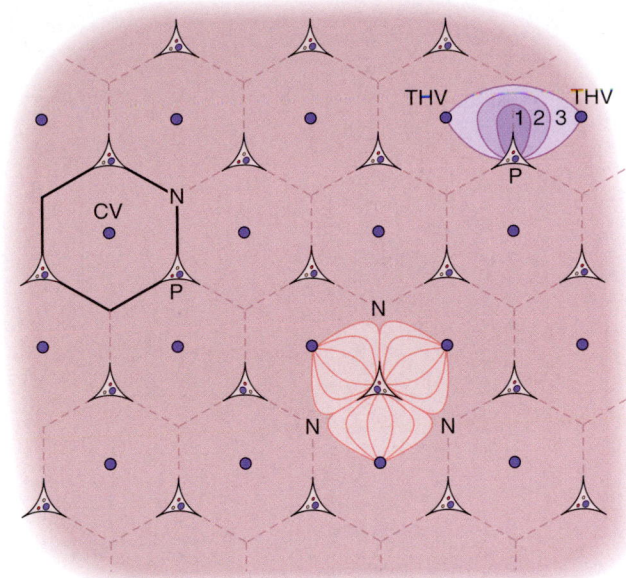

FIGURE 71-4. Schematic drawing of the liver architecture. At the left is the classic hepatic lobule, with the central vein as its center and portal tracts at 3 corners. Toward the middle is the portal unit, with the portal tract at its center, and central veins and nodal points at its periphery. At the right is the liver acinus, the center of which is the terminal afferent vessel (in the portal tract) and the periphery of which is drained by the terminal hepatic venule, or central vein. Zones 1, 2, and 3 extending from the portal tract to the terminal hepatic venule are shown. CV, central vein; N, nodal point; P, portal tract; THV, terminal hepatic venule.

ramifications of the portal venous system are known as *septal branches*. The "central vein," meanwhile, is actually 6 to 8 draining venules that individually face a corresponding inflow unit. The conical cluster of hepatocytes fed by a septal branch and drained by a hepatic vein branch forms a "primary lobule." Several primary lobules together form a classic lobule.

Matsumoto and Kawakami also noted that the sinusoids that arise from the septal branches have a transverse course near the portal tract before turning radially to the central vein, and this bed of transverse sinusoids forms a sickle-shaped "inflow front" for perfusion of the lobule that differs from the linear supply proposed by the acinus model (Fig. 71-5).[37] The convex aspect of the sickle abuts a portal tract, its arms extend along septal branches, and the concave aspect faces the central vein. This arrangement defines two zones: the peripheral part of the classic lobule composed of adjoining sickle-shaped areas and the centrilobular portion bound by these sickle-shaped areas. Immunohistochemical studies of hepatic enzymes highlight the presence of a continuous periportal network around portal tracts and terminal afferent vessels and a distinct concentric perivenous area around the central vein, supporting the idea that the liver architecture resembles the classic lobule more than the acinus.[38] The functional heterogeneity in the lobule has been referred to as "metabolic zonation," a concept that may explain how seemingly opposing metabolic functions coexist in the liver.[39] Gluconeogenesis, for example, occurs largely in the periportal region, whereas glycolysis is mostly centrilobular. This metabolic zonation is maintained by the Wnt/β-catenin pathway: the activation of β-catenin signaling induces expression of genes associated with centrilobular hepatocytes and repression of the periportal genetic program.[39]

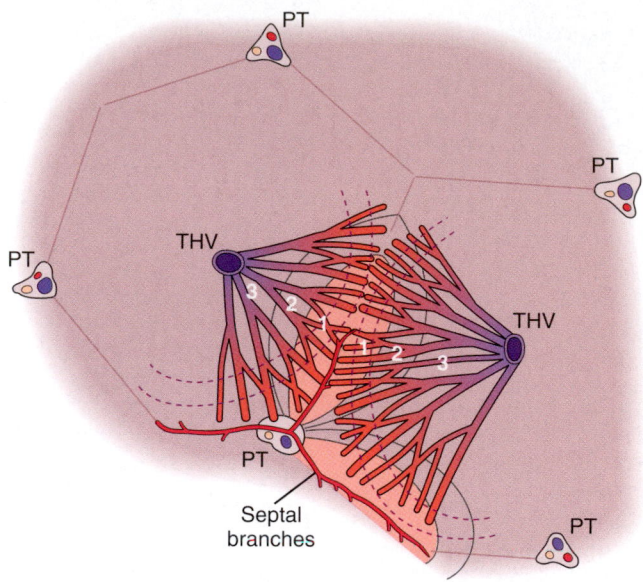

FIGURE 71-5. Drawing that compares liver blood flow in the 3 zones of the acinus model with Matsumoto and Kawakami's concept of liver architecture. According to this model, sinusoids that abut the portal tracts and terminal afferent vessels (septal branches) form a hemodynamically equipotential sickle-shaped perfusion front *(dotted lines)*. This model conforms to the concept of the classic lobule rather than to the acinus. Zones 1, 2, and 3 of the hepatic acinus are labeled. PT, portal tract; THV, terminal hepatic venule.

DEVELOPMENTAL ANOMALIES
(See Chapter 62)

Riedel's Lobe

Riedel's lobe denotes a prominent right liver lobe that extends below the level of the umbilicus. Riedel's lobe is an anatomic variation that occurs more often in women than in men. It may be mistaken for an abdominal mass. Liver biochemical test levels are normal, and the diagnosis is established by US.[40]

Abernethy Malformation

The Abernethy malformation is a congenital extrahepatic portocaval shunt. Two types of shunts are known to occur. In a type 1 shunt, portal blood is diverted completely into the inferior vena cava, with absence of the portal vein. This type of shunt occurs more often in girls than in boys; is associated with other congenital abnormalities such as cardiac defects,

biliary atresia, and polysplenia; may manifest with hypergalactosemia, hyperbilirubinemia, hyperammonemia, or variceal bleeding; and may be complicated by the formation of hepatic tumors such as focal nodular hyperplasia.[41] Type 1 Abernethy malformation can be further divided into subtype 1a, in which the superior mesenteric vein and the splenic vein do not join and thus there is no anatomic portal vein, and subtype 1b, in which the superior mesenteric vein and splenic vein do join to form a portal vein, which then drains into a systemic vein.[41,42] In type 2 Abernethy malformation, the portal vein is intact, but a side-to-side anastomosis with the inferior vena cava leads to shunting; technically, therefore, type 2 is not a true absence of the portal vein. A type 2 shunt occurs in both girls and boys and is not associated with other malformations.[42,43]

KEY REFERENCES

Full references for this chapter can be found on www.expertconsult.com.

1. Duncan SA. Mechanisms controlling early development of the liver. Mech Dev 2003; 120:19-33.
6. Si-Tayeb K, Lemaigre FP, Duncan SA. Organogenesis and development of the liver. Dev Cell 2010; 18:175-89.
16. Zhang L, Theise N, Chua M, et al. The stem cell niche of human livers: Symmetry between development and regeneration. Hepatology 2008; 48:1598-607.
17. Turner R, Lozoya O, Wang Y, et al. Human hepatic stem cell and maturational liver lineage biology. Hepatology 2011; 53:1035-45.
21. Skandalakis JE, Skandalakis LJ, Skandalakis PN, et al. Hepatic surgical anatomy. Surg Clin North Am 2004; 84:413-35.
23. Rutkauskas S, Gedrimas V, Pundzius J, et al. Clinical and anatomical basis for the classification of the structural parts of liver. Medicina (Kaunas, Lithuania) 2006; 42:98-106.
24. Couinaud C. Le foie. Etudes anatomiques et chirurgicales. Paris: Masson & Cie; 1957.
26. Malarkey DE, Johnson K, Ryan L, et al. New insights into functional aspects of liver morphology. Toxicol Pathol 2005; 33:27-34.
27. Deshpande RR, Heaton ND, Rela M. Surgical anatomy of segmental liver transplantation. Br J Surg 2002; 89:1078-88.
32. Sasse D, Spornitz UM, Maly IP. Liver architecture. Enzyme 1992; 46:8-32.
34. David H, Reinke P. The concept of the "perisinusoidal functional unit" of the liver—Importance to pathological processes. Exp Pathol 1987; 32:193-224.
37. Matsumoto T, Kawakami M. The unit-concept of hepatic parenchyma—A re-examination based on angioarchitectural studies. Acta Pathol Jpn 1982; 32(Suppl 2):285-314.

NAMITA ROY-CHOWDHURY AND JAYANTA ROY-CHOWDHURY

CHAPTER OUTLINE

LIVER CELL TYPES AND ORGANIZATION

Liver cells can be classified into 3 groups: parenchymal cells include hepatocytes and bile duct epithelia, sinusoidal cells are composed of hepatic sinusoidal endothelial and Kupffer cells (hepatic macrophages), and perisinusoidal cells consist of hepatic stellate cells and pit cells. Hepatocytes comprise 60% of the adult liver cell population, representing approximately 78% of the tissue volume (see Chapter 71).[1]

Parenchymal Cells

Hepatocytes

Hepatocytes are large polyhedral cells approximately 20 to 30 μm in diameter.[2] Consistent with their high synthetic and metabolic activity, hepatocytes are enriched in organelles, and ≈30% are binucleate. Hepatocytes are polarized epithelial cells. Their plasma membranes have 3 distinct domains: (1) the sinusoidal surface (≈37% of the cell surface) that comes in direct contact with plasma through the fenestrae of the specialized hepatic sinusoidal endothelial cells, (2) the canalicular surface (≈13% of the cell surface) that encloses the bile canaliculus, and (3) contiguous surfaces. By analogy with glandular epithelia, the sinusoidal, canalicular, and contiguous plasma membrane domains are also termed *basolateral*, *apical*, and *lateral surfaces*, respectively.[3] The sinusoidal and canalicular surfaces contain microvilli, which greatly extend the surface area of these domains. The space between the endothelia and the sinusoidal villi is termed the *space of Disse*. There is a bidirectional exchange of liquids and solutes between the plasma and hepatocytes at the sinusoidal surface. In many cases, the molecular transfer is augmented by proteins that promote facilitated diffusion or energy-consuming active transport. The canalicular domains of two adjacent hepatocytes are sealed at the periphery by tight junctions (desmosomes), thereby delimiting the bile canaliculus, which is the beginning of the biliary drainage system (see Chapter 62). In contrast to the bidirectional flow at the sinusoidal surface, flow from hepatocytes into the bile canaliculi is predominantly unidirectional.

Plasma Membranes

The plasma membranes consist of lipid bilayers composed of glycerophospholipids, cholesterol, and sphingolipids that provide a barrier to water and most polar substances.[3,4] The inner and outer leaflets of the plasma membrane differ in lipid, protein, and carbohydrate composition, reflecting their functional differences. Protein molecules within the leaflets mediate transport of specific molecules and serve as a link with cytoskeletal structures and the extracellular matrix. Hepatocyte plasma membranes consist of 36% lipid, 54% protein, and 10% carbohydrate by dry weight. Outer leaflets of hepatocyte plasma membranes are enriched in carbohydrates.

Lipid rafts are microdomains (≈50 nm in diameter) of the outer leaflets of the plasma membrane that are highly enriched in cholesterol and sphingolipids.[5] These are coupled to cholesterol-rich microdomains in the inner leaflet by an unknown mechanism. Raft lipids and associated proteins diffuse together laterally on the membrane surface. Some surface receptors become associated with the rafts on ligand binding, or they can lead to "clustering" of smaller rafts into larger ones. Lipid rafts are important in signal transduction, apoptosis, cell adhesion and migration, cytoskeletal organization, and protein sorting during both exocytosis and endocytosis (see later). Certain viruses enter cells via the lipid rafts.

Membrane proteins perform receptor, enzyme, and transport functions.[6] Integral membrane proteins traverse the lipid bilayer once or multiple times or are buried in the lipid. Additional "extrinsic" protein molecules are associated with plasma membrane. Membrane proteins can rotate or diffuse laterally but usually do not flip-flop from one leaflet to another.

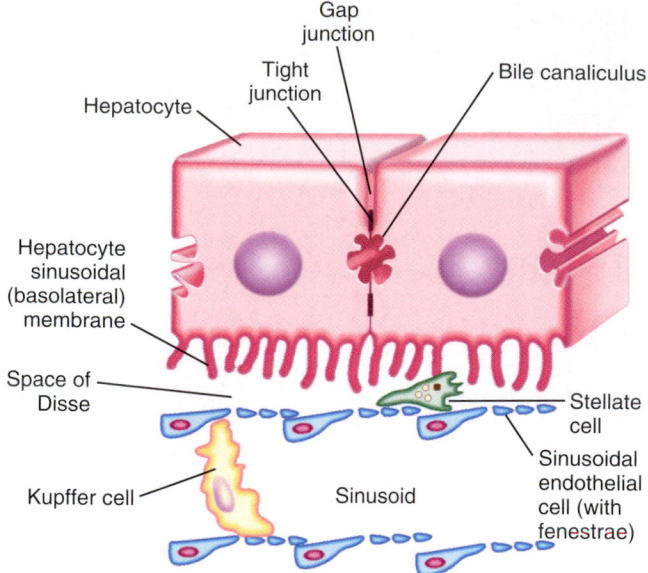

FIGURE 72-1. The spatial relationship among the different cell types of the liver. Sinusoidal plasma comes in direct contact with hepatocytes in the space of Disse. The endothelial cells are fenestrated and lack a basement membrane. Kupffer cells are located in the lumen of the sinusoid, where they are in direct contact with the sinusoidal endothelial cells and portal blood. Stellate cells are situated between the endothelial cells and hepatocytes, and come in direct contact with both cell types. The hepatocytes are joined with each other by tight junctions and the communicating gap junctions. The canalicular domain of the plasma membrane of two adjacent hepatocytes encloses the bile canaliculus.

Concentration of specific membrane proteins is maintained by a balance between their synthesis and degradation by shedding of membrane vesicles, proteolytic digestion within the membrane, or internalization into the cell. Receptor proteins internalized into the cell may be degraded or recycled to the cell surface.

Cell Junctions. Hepatocytes are organized into sheets (seen as chords in 2-dimensional sections) by occluding ("tight"), communicating ("gap"), and anchoring junctions (Fig. 72-1). Tight junctions or desmosomes form gasket-like seals around the bile canaliculi, thereby permitting a concentration difference of solutes between the cytoplasm and bile canaliculus. Desmosomes are specialized membrane structures that anchor intermediate filaments to the plasma membrane and link cells together. Gap junctions are subdomains of contiguous membranes of hepatocytes that comprise about 3% of the total surface membrane. They consist of hexagonal particles with hollow cores, termed *connexons*, made up of 6 connexin molecules.[7] Connexons of one cell are joined to those of an adjacent cell to form a radially symmetrical cylinder that can open or close the central channel. Gap junctions are involved in nutrient exchange, synchronization of cellular activities, and conduction of electrical impulses.

Cytoskeleton

The hepatocyte cytoskeleton supports the organization of subcellular organelles, cell polarity, intracellular movement of vesicles, and molecular transport.[8,9] It comprises microfilaments, microtubules, and intermediate filaments, as well as the cytoskeleton-associated proteins.[10] Intermediate filaments are polymers of fibrous polypeptides (cytokeratins and lamins)

that provide structural support to the cells. In addition, vimentin is expressed by hepatocytes in tissue culture, and neurofilaments appear in injured hepatocytes and form Mallory bodies (also termed *Mallory-Denk bodies* or *Mallory's hyaline*). Hepatocytes express two cytokeratins, CK8 and CK18. Bile duct epithelial cells express these proteins and CK19. Plectin is a giant protein that cross-links intermediate filaments to each other and to the plasma membrane, microtubules, and actin filaments.

Microtubules are hollow tubular structures (with an outer diameter of 24 nm) that consist of polymerized dimers of α- and β-tubulin; they are involved in intracellular transport and cellular organization.[11,12] Microtubules serve as tracks to the movement of cytoplasmic vesicles, mediated by ATPase-powered motor proteins, kinesin, dynein, and dynamin. Depolymerization of the microtubules by colchicine inhibits plasma protein secretion without affecting protein synthesis. Microtubules participate in cellular organization by interacting with the Golgi apparatus, intermediate filaments, and F-actin.[13] They also maintain the integrity of the surface membrane during canalicular contraction.[14]

Microfilaments are composed of double-helical F-actin strands, which are polymers of G-actin. A large number of actin-associated proteins control the polymerization, depolymerization, and splicing of F-actin. Together with myosins, actins maintain the integrity of the cell matrix, facilitate bile canalicular contraction, and control tight junction permeability. Microfilaments are also important in receptor-mediated endocytosis and various transport processes. Collapse of the cellular structure of hepatocytes during apoptosis and formation of apoptotic bodies may be related to remodeling of the actin cytoskeleton of hepatocytes.[15]

Nucleus

Nuclei of hepatocytes are relatively large and have prominent nucleoli. The 2 concentric nuclear membranes are stabilized by networks of intermediate filaments, 1 inside the inner membrane and 1 outside the outer membrane.[16] The outer nuclear membrane is in direct continuity with the endoplasmic reticulum (ER) membranes. The perinuclear space between the 2 nuclear membranes surrounds the nucleus and is continuous with the ER lumen. The nuclear membrane contains pores through which molecules are selectively transported to and from the cytoplasm. The ribonuclear protein (RNP) network and the perinucleolar chromatin radiate from the nucleolus.

The nuclear chromatin contains the chromosomes and associated proteins. The chromosomes comprise a series of genes, interspersed with intragenic DNA. The DNA is transcribed into RNA, which undergoes multiple processing steps, giving rise to messenger RNA (mRNA) molecules that are translocated across the nuclear pores into the cytoplasm, where they become associated with ribosomes. Nuclear DNA also encodes additional RNA types that have accessory roles in protein synthesis and other functions. Ribosomal RNAs (rRNAs) are encoded by DNA within the nucleolus. Transfer RNA (tRNA) binds to amino acids and provides a necessary link between the nucleic acid code and sequential amino acid incorporation in the growing protein chain during translation. Other RNAs are involved in the processing of mRNA, rRNA, and tRNA molecules. Just before cell division, both the DNA and protein components of chromatin are duplicated. The two copies of each duplicated chromosome are separated and distributed precisely so that the 2 daughter cells each receive a complete set of genes.

Transport between the Nucleus and Cytoplasm. Pores of the nuclear envelope are associated with a large number of proteins organized in an octagonal symmetry.[17] The nuclear pore complex (NPC) is a large macromolecular assembly that protrudes into both the cytoplasm and the nucleoplasm. Bidirectional nucleocytoplasmic transport occurs through the central aqueous channel in NPCs.[18] Histones, DNA and RNA polymerases, transcription factors, and RNA-processing proteins are selectively transported into the nucleus from the cytoplasm, where they are synthesized, whereas tRNAs and mRNAs are synthesized in the nucleus and exported to the cytoplasm through the NPCs.

Often, the export and import processes are interrelated. For example, ribosomal proteins are imported into the nucleus from the cytoplasm and, after assembly with ribosomal RNA, are exported to the cytoplasm as a ribosomal subunit. Proteins containing nuclear localization motifs that consist of specific cationic amino acid sequences are recognized by pore complex receptors termed *importins* or *karyopherins*, and are rapidly transported into the nucleus via an energy-consuming process powered by specific ATPase and GTPase enzymes. In other cases, large molecules diffuse slowly through the nuclear pores and are retained in the nucleus by binding to specific intranuclear sites. Molecules that are smaller than 5 kd diffuse freely across the nuclear pores.

Endoplasmic Reticulum

The ER is the largest intracellular membrane compartment, consisting of membranous tubules or flattened sacs (cysternae) that enclose a continuous lumen or space and extend throughout the cytoplasm.[19] The domain of ER in which active protein synthesis occurs has attached ribosomes and is termed the *rough ER*. The other domain, termed *smooth ER*, is devoid of ribosomes and is the site of lipid biosynthesis, detoxification, and calcium regulation. The nuclear envelope is a specialized domain of the ER.[20]

Golgi Complex

The Golgi complex consists of a stack of flat sac-like membranes (cysternae) that are dilated at the margins.[21] Many proteins synthesized in the rough ER are transported to the Golgi apparatus in protein-filled transition vesicles. The aspect of the Golgi complex facing the ER is the *cis face*; the opposite side is termed the *trans face*. Glycoproteins are thought to be transported between the Golgi sacs via shuttle vesicles. The highly mannosylated glycosyl moiety of proteins that are *N*-glycosylated in the ER are processed in the Golgi sacs into mature forms. Some other proteins are *O*-glycosylated in the Golgi complex. These proteins are then sorted for transport to appropriate cellular organelles (see later discussion of exocytosis and endocytosis).[22]

Lysosomes

Lysosomes consist of a system of membrane-bound sacs and tubules that contain hydrolytic enzymes that are active at pH 4.5 to 5.[23,24] The ATPase-powered proton pump maintains the acid pH by importing hydrogen ions into the lysosomal lumen.[23] Lysosomal enzymes are glycoproteins with *N*-linked oligosaccharides. Following synthesis in the ER, the carbohydrate moieties are modified in the Golgi apparatus, where their mannose residues are phosphorylated. Recognition of these mannose 6-phosphate (M6P) groups by the M6P receptor in *trans*-Golgi stacks[25] results in their segregation and translocation into late endosomes, which transform into lysosomes.[26,27] By degrading damaged organelles, lipids, and long-lived proteins, lysosomes play a critical role in maintaining

cellular homeostasis and providing an energy source during cellular stress (see later).

Mitochondria

Mitochondria constitute about 20% of the cytoplasmic volume of hepatocytes and are responsible for cellular respiration.[28-30] Mitochondria are dynamic organelles that undergo changes in number, size, shape, and distribution during their life cycle and in response to intra- and extracellular cues. Division of a preexisting mitochondrion is followed by cycles of fission and fusion that lead to individual mitochondria or organization into a mitochondrial network.[31] When solitary mitochondria are injured and depolarized, they are selectively surrounded by isolation membranes, eventually leading to the formation of autophagosomes that fuse to lysosomes, and the cargoes are degraded by hydrolytic enzymes.[32] By selectively degrading damaged mitochondria, autophagy maintains the integrity of the mitochondrial population, which is essential for the well being of cells (see later).

Mitochondria contain the enzymes of the tricarboxylic acid cycle, fatty acid oxidation, and oxidative phosphorylation.[33] They conserve the energy generated by oxidation of substrates as high-energy phosphate bonds of ATP. In addition, parts of the urea cycle, gluconeogenesis, fatty acid synthesis, regulation of intracellular calcium concentration, and heme synthesis take place in the mitochondria. Mitochondria play a key role in regulating nonselective autophagy[34] and apoptosis (see later).[35]

The outer smooth surface membrane of the mitochondrion is functionally different from the inner membrane, which is highly folded to form cristae. Mitochondria are positioned at major sites of ATP utilization by translocation along microtubules. In addition to soluble enzymes, the mitochondrial matrix includes large intramitochondrial granules that store calcium and other ions and smaller granules that contain mitochondrial ribosomes. Mitochondrial DNA, embedded within the matrix, encodes a number of mitochondrial proteins; the remaining mitochondrial proteins are encoded by nuclear genes.

Glycolysis and fatty acid oxidation in the mitochondria generate chemical intermediates that feed into the citric acid cycle of energy-yielding reactions (see later).[36,37] The citric acid cycle breaks down acetyl coenzyme A (acetyl-CoA) into 3 molecules of nicotinamide adenine dinucleotide (NADH), 1 molecule of flavin adenine dinucleotide ($FADH_2$), and 2 molecules of carbon dioxide. Electrons derived from NADH and $FADH_2$ drive an electron transport pathway in the inner mitochondrial membrane, leading to ATP production. Passage of electrons across the inner mitochondrial membrane to the space between the inner and outer membrane generates a proton gradient that drives ATP synthesis.[38]

Peroxisomes

Peroxisomes are spherical-appearing structures that enclose a matrix that contains a lattice or crystalline core.[39] Peroxisomes are abundant in hepatocytes and are thought to be essential for life. Several oxidative catabolic reactions, as well as anabolic reactions, take place in peroxisomes, which provide important links between the metabolism of carbohydrates, lipids, proteins, fats, and nucleic acids.

Exocytosis and Endocytosis

Exocytosis and endocytosis are pathways involved in exporting, importing, and intracellular trafficking of molecules. Addition of new proteins and lipids to the plasma membrane by exocytosis and removal of membrane components into cytoplasmic compartments by endocytosis keep the cell surface in a state of dynamic polarization. During exocytosis, secreted proteins, synthesized in the ER, pass sequentially through the *cis-*, *medial-*, and *trans-*Golgi stacks and the *trans-*Golgi network and finally appear at the cell surface.[40,41] This vectorial transport through the Golgi stacks occurs via vesicles that are coated by proteins termed *coatamers* or COP (COPI and COPII), which are distinct from clathrin (see later).[42,43] Guanosine triphosphate-guanosine diphosphate (GTP-GDP) exchange factors and GTP-activating proteins that are specific for each type of vesicle stimulate membrane binding and catalytic activation of small GTPases.

Once bound to the membrane, GTPases induce recruitment of COP proteins. In the ER, the first coat protein to be recruited is COPII, and vesicular/tubular clusters are formed. These clusters are thought to coalesce to form a complex tubular network termed the *ER/Golgi intermediate compartment*. Acquisition of COPI proteins by the membranes of this tubular network results in the formation of vesicles that carry out bidirectional protein transport to and from the Golgi stacks. Some vesicles that emerge from the exit side of the Golgi apparatus, termed the *trans-Golgi network* (TGN), can transport multiple protein molecules simultaneously and release them together into the extracellular medium. Other types of vesicles that carry membrane proteins and enzymes destined for specific intracellular organelles also pass through this secretory pathway. These vesicles are sorted at the TGN, and vesicles carrying specific cargo are delivered to appropriate target organelles.[44]

Endocytosis is the import of extracellular macromolecules by processes that include pinocytosis, phagocytosis, receptor-mediated endocytosis (RME), and caveolar internalization.[45] *Pinocytosis* refers to nonselective bulk-phase uptake of extracellular fluid via engulfment by plasma membrane invaginations. *Phagocytosis* is the ingestion of particles as well as regions of the cell surface. In contrast to these nonspecific modes of uptake, RME is a mechanism of uptake of specific molecules (ligands). After the ligands bind to their specific cell surface receptors, the ligand-receptor complexes concentrate in "pits" that are coated on the cytoplasmic surface by 3-pronged structures (triskelions) composed of 3 heavy chains and 3 light chains of clathrin. The assembled coats consist of a geometric array of 12 pentagons and a variable number of hexagons, depending on the size of the coat. The coated pits pinch off into the underlying cytoplasm as coated vesicles.[46] In the next step, the vesicles lose their clathrin coat and are termed *endosomes*. Endosomal vesicles travel along microtubules and can take 3 distinct pathways. Some endosomes return to the cell surface, and the contained ligand-receptor complexes are secreted out of the cells by a process termed *diacytosis*. Transferrin is a prototype ligand for diacytosis. Some other ligands, such as immunoglobulin (Ig)A oligomers, may traverse the cells to be secreted into bile along with the receptor. This process is termed *transcytosis*.[47]

The best studied type of RME is the classical endocytotic pathway, in which the interior of the endosome is acidified by the action of a proton pump, thereby leading to ligand-receptor uncoupling.[48] By uncertain mechanisms, the dissociated ligands and receptors are sorted into different vesicles. The ligand-containing vesicles proceed to lysosomes, where the ligand is degraded by lysosomal hydrolases. A majority of the ligand-free receptors translocate to the cell surface and replenish the receptor pool. Some receptors, such as the insulin receptor, are rapidly degraded in lysosomes. In addition to the recruitment of clathrin, initiation of the formation of endocytotic vesicles requires adaptor proteins, particularly AP-2, which localizes between the lipid bilayer and clathrin.

Non-scaffold proteins, such as the GTPases and dynamin, are also important in the conversion of a coated pit to a coated vesicle. This function of dynamin requires association with the protein amphiphysin. In addition to physiologic ligands, many viruses use receptor-mediated endocytosis to enter cells.

Internalization via caveolae is another pathway by which macromolecules can enter cells. Binding of caveolin to the cytoplasmic aspect of cholesterol-rich lipid rafts on the plasma membrane generates 50- to 60-nm flask-shaped invaginations of the plasma membrane. These invaginations bud off into the cytoplasm to form vesicles, termed *caveolae* or *plasmalemmal vesicles*. Caveolae perform various functions, including signal transduction, calcium regulation, non–clathrin-dependent internalization, and transcytosis. Glucosyl phosphatidylinositol (GPI)-anchored proteins, the β-adrenergic receptor, and tyrosine kinase are concentrated in caveolae.[49]

Bile Duct Epithelial Cells

Bile duct epithelial cells, or cholangiocytes, comprise large and small subpopulations of cells, the volumes of which correlate roughly with the diameter of the intrahepatic bile ducts (see Chapter 62). The large cholangiocytes have a relatively more developed ER and a lower nucleus-to-cytoplasmic ratio than do the small cholangiocytes.[50] The paucity of expression of cytochrome P450 (CYP)–dependent mono-oxygenase activity imparts a survival advantage to the small cholangiocytes against injury by chemicals. For example, CYP2E1-mediated formation of toxic intermediates of carbon tetrachloride leads to the loss of large cholangiocyte function after administration of the pro-toxin, whereas the small cholangiocytes are resistant to the toxic injury.

Bile ducts are not mere passive conduits for biliary drainage but play an active role in the secretion and absorption of biliary components and regulation of the extracellular matrix composition. Cholangiocytes are highly polarized. A sodium-dependent bile salt transporter (ABAT), located at the apical (luminal) surface of cholangiocytes, mediates the uptake of conjugated bile acids by cholangiocytes, whereas an alternatively spliced truncated form of the protein (ASBT), located at the basolateral surface, mediates the efflux of the bile acids in a sodium-independent manner. The sodium-dependent glucose transporter (SGLT1), located at the apical domain, and GLUT1, a facilitative glucose transporter on the basolateral domain, are responsible for glucose reabsorption from bile. Aquaporin-1 at the apical and basolateral surfaces constitute water channels that may mediate hormone-regulated transport of water into bile by cholangiocytes. The purinergic receptor (P_{2u}) stimulates chloride ion efflux. Activation of apical P_{2u} by ATP, which is secreted into the bile by hepatocytes, mobilizes Ca^{2+} stores, thereby stimulating Cl^- efflux from cholangiocytes. The large, but not the small, cholangiocytes express secretin and somatostatin receptors, the chloride/bicarbonate exchanger, and the cystic fibrosis transmembrane regulator, which may enable this population of cholangiocytes to modulate water and electrolyte secretion in response to secretin and somatostatin (see also Chapter 64).[51]

Sinusoidal Cells

Hepatic Sinusoidal Endothelial Cells

Hepatic sinusoidal endothelial cells (HSECs) account for 20% of total liver cells. These cells are distinguished by the fenestrae (pores) in their flat, thin extensions that form sieve plates. Unlike capillary endothelial cells, HSECs do not form intracellular junctions and simply overlap each other (see Fig. 72-1B). The presence of fenestrae and the absence of a basement membrane permit plasma to enter the space of Disse and come in direct contact with the sinusoidal surface of hepatocytes.[52] Diameters of the fenestrae are actively controlled by the actin-containing components of the cytoskeleton in response to changes in the chemical milieu.[53] Therefore, the specialized endothelial lining of hepatic sinusoids serves as a selective barrier between the blood and the hepatocytes. HSECs can secrete prostaglandins and a wide variety of proteins, including interleukin (IL)-1, IL-6, interferon, TNF-α, and endothelin.

Kupffer Cells

Kupffer cells are specialized tissue macrophages that account for 80% to 90% of the total population of fixed macrophages in the body. These cells are derived from bone marrow stem cells or monocytes and are highly active in removing particulate matter and toxic or foreign substances that appear in the portal blood from the intestine.[54] Kupffer cells are located in the sinusoidal lumen and are in direct contact with endothelial cells (see Fig. 72-1). They possess bristle-coated micropinocytic vesicles, fuzzy-coated vacuoles, and worm-like structures that are special features of cells that are active in pinocytosis and phagocytosis. An abundance of lysosomes reflects their prominent role in degrading substances taken up from the bloodstream. Kupffer cells secrete a variety of vasoactive toxic mediators, which may be involved in host defense mechanisms and in pathophysiologic processes in some liver diseases, and increase in number and activity in chemical, infectious, or immunologic injury to the liver.[55]

Perisinusoidal Cells

Hepatic Stellate Cells

Hepatic stellate cells (HSCs) are also known as *Ito cells*, *vitamin A–storing cells*, *fat-storing cells*, or *lipocytes*. These cells are a part of the stellate cell system, which includes similar cells in the pancreas, lung, kidney, and intestine. Hepatic stellate cells are located between the endothelial lining and hepatocytes (see Fig. 72-1). These mesenchymal cells represent 5% to 8% of all liver cells and are important sources of paracrine, autocrine, juxtacrine, and chemoattractant factors that maintain homeostasis in the microenvironment of the hepatic sinusoid. Microfilament and microtubule-enriched flat cytoplasmic extensions of quiescent stellate cells store vitamin A–enriched lipid droplets and spread out parallel to the endothelial lining, contacting several cells.[56] HSCs express receptors for retinol-binding protein (RBP), which mediates the endocytosis of RBP-retinol complexes.[57]

After chronic liver injury, the slender star-shaped HSCs become activated to elongated myofibroblasts. They lose retinoids and up-regulate the synthesis of extracellular matrix components, such as collagen, proteoglycan, and adhesive glycoproteins. Stellate cell activation is the central event in hepatic fibrosis (see Chapter 74).[58] Activation of HSCs is initiated by paracrine stimulation by neighboring HSECs, Kupffer cells, and hepatocytes, as well as platelets and leukocytes. Endothelial cells participate in activation by producing cellular fibronectin and by converting the latent form of transforming growth factor (TGF)-β to its active, profibrogenic form. Binding of TGF-β to its receptor on HSCs plays a critical role in stellate cell activation. Binding of bacterial lipopolysaccharides (LPS) arriving to the liver from the intestine to Toll-like receptor 4 (TLR4) enhances the effect of TGF-β on HSCs by two different mechanisms.[59] First, increased chemokine expression by stellate cells results in chemotaxis of Kupffer cells, which secrete TGF-β. Second, LPS binding to TLR4

activates nuclear factor kappa B (NF-κB) via the adapter protein MyD88 (myeloid differentiation response protein), thereby down-regulating the TGF-β pseudoreceptor Bambi (bone morphogenic protein and the activin membrane-bound inhibitor) and sensitizing the HSCs to TGF-β signaling. The 3-dimensional structure of the extracellular matrix modulates the shape, proliferation, and function of HSCs, probably by signal transduction via binding to cell surface integrins, followed by changes in cytoskeleton assembly.

Activation of HSCs leads to several discrete changes in cell behavior, such as proliferation, contractility, overexpression of extracellular matrix proteins (e.g., collagens I, III, IV, V, and VI, laminin, tenascin, undulin, hyaluronic acid, proteoglycans), matrix degradation by release of metalloproteinases, and release of leukocyte chemoattractants and cytokines. The overall number of HSCs increases during fibrosis because of a change in the balance between proliferation and apoptosis, which is influenced by soluble growth factors and the matrix.

Pit Cells

Pit cells, the natural killer (NK) cells of the liver, are located mainly within the sinusoidal lumen, close to Kupffer cells. They have the appearance of large lymphocytes and are adherent to the sinusoidal wall, often anchored with villous extensions (pseudopods).[60] In the human liver, pit cells have pronounced polarity, abundant cytoplasm containing dense granules, a conspicuous cytocenter, and a locomotory shape characterized by hyaloplasmic pseudopods and a uropod (a tail-like structure that forms on the trailing end of a moving cell). The cytoplasmic granules appear as pits by microscopy, hence the name *pit cells*. Pit cells are short-lived and are replenished from extrahepatic sources.

In common with circulating NK cells, the pit cells express OX-8 antigen, and some express asialoganglioside ganglio-tetrasylceramide (asialo-GMr1). Pit cells do not express the pan–T-cell marker, OX-19, which is expressed by circulating NK cells. Although the source of pit cells remains debated, they are antigenically related to NK cells of other viscera. Pit cells have tumor cell–killing activity in the liver and are also thought to remove virus-infected liver cells. Their per-cell cytolytic activity is greater than that of circulating NK cells. Pit cells may also have a role in controlling the growth and differentiation of liver cells and possibly in liver graft rejection.[61]

INTEGRATION OF THE FUNCTIONS OF THE DIFFERENT CELL TYPES

Functional integration of the various groups of liver cells occurs through direct cell-to-cell communication (e.g., via gap junctions), paracrine secretion that affects neighboring cells, cell signaling, interaction with the extracellular matrix, and generalized response to endocrine and metabolic fluxes.[62] Hepatocytes and HSECs lack a continuous basement membrane, and the spatial relationship of the cells is maintained through interaction with the extracellular matrix. Anchoring to the extracellular matrix is important for the survival of hepatocytes, provides traction for movement, and permits liver cells to receive signals from matrix components and matrix-bound growth factors. Hepatic extracellular matrix components are produced during development along the migration path of the hepatocytes and exhibit unique patterns of distribution and organization. HSCs, hepatocytes, and, to some extent, HSECs are major producers of the extracellular matrix in the liver. Excess deposition of connective tissue causes changes in hemodynamic properties and eventually impairs liver function.[58]

Cell-Matrix Interactions

Cell-matrix interactions in the liver are important in maintaining hepatocyte morphology and proliferation. For example, when plated on a flat layer of collagen, hepatocytes synthesize DNA at a level that is 4-fold higher than when they are grown on gels composed of basement membrane proteins. The type of matrix determines the level of expression of albumin and other hepatocyte-specific gene products in cultured hepatocytes.[62,63] Cell-cell and cell-matrix interactions determine the level of synthesis and deposition of hepatic extracellular matrix proteins by the various types of liver cells. Such interactions also modulate the production of specific enzymes and their inhibitors that mediate remodeling of the extracellular matrix.

Integrin and non-integrin receptors mediate the interaction of liver cells with extracellular matrix. Integrins bind to extracellular matrix proteins at specialized cell attachment sites that often contain the arginine-glycine-aspartate motif, thereby resulting in attachment of the extracellular matrix to the intracellular cytoskeleton network. This attachment results in changes in cell shape, spreading, and migration. Integrins also influence cell proliferation, differentiation, survival, apoptosis, and gene expression via signal transduction.[64,65]

Components of the Extracellular Matrix

Components of the extracellular matrix include collagens, noncollagenous glycoproteins, and proteoglycans. The liver contains 5 types of collagen (I, III, IV, V, and VI) and 7 classes of noncollagenous glycoproteins (fibronectin, laminin, entactin/nidogen, tenascin, thrombospondin, SPARC [secreted protein, acidic, and rich in cysteine], and undulin). Hepatic extracellular matrix also includes a large number of proteoglycans and glycosaminoglycans, such as membrane-associated syndecan, thrombomodulin, and betaglycan, and extracellular matrix–associated versican, biglycan, decorin, fibromodulin, and perlecan.[62,66]

REGENERATION AND APOPTOSIS OF LIVER CELLS

Regeneration

Normal adult hepatocytes divide infrequently, with fewer than 1 in 10,000 hepatocytes undergoing mitosis at any given time—yet the liver possesses a unique capacity to replace tissue mass after liver injury or loss of liver mass. The capacity of the liver to regulate its own growth is evident after liver transplantation, when the size of the transplanted organ increases or decreases as appropriate to the size of the recipient.[67]

Following resection of two thirds of the liver in rats, the residual liver cells proliferate and restore the liver mass within days to weeks. Although generally termed "regeneration," this process is, in fact, restorative hyperplasia because the total liver mass, rather than the lobulated anatomic configuration, is reconstituted. In the rat, DNA synthesis peaks at 24 hours after partial hepatectomy, when approximately 35% of hepatocytes are in cell cycle. Cell division occurs 6 to 8 hours after DNA synthesis. The time frame of DNA synthesis varies from species to species; in mice, maximum DNA synthesis occurs 36 to 40 hours after hepatic resection. Because 80% to 95% of

hepatocytes undergo mitosis, liver mass is restored after 1 or 2 cell divisions. All classes of hepatocytes, including diploid, tetraploid, and octaploid cells, participate in this quasi-synchronized proliferation, either by mitosis of mononucleated cells or by cytokinesis of binucleated or tetranucleated hepatocytes, after DNA synthesis in all nuclei. Interestingly, adult hepatocytes, rather than liver progenitor cells, contribute to liver regeneration after partial hepatectomy. Only when the proliferation of adult hepatocytes is inhibited because of toxic or physical injuries do progenitor cells, often termed *oval cells*, proliferate. The oval cells are thought to give rise to both hepatocytes and bile duct epithelial cells.[68]

After liver injury, early signals for hepatocyte replication come from nonparenchymal cells (see Fig. 72-2B).[69,70] LPS and intestine-derived cytokines stimulate Kupffer cells and HSECs to produce TNF-α and IL-6 via signaling through TNF receptor and TLRs. Growth factors, such as hepatic growth factor (HGF), are released from stores in the hepatic matrix and are secreted by HSCs, whereas EGF is secreted into portal blood by epithelial cells of the proximal small intestine and salivary glands.[70] Hormones, such as tri-iodothyronine (T_3), insulin, and nonrepinephrine, are important cooperative factors in liver regeneration.[71] The role of mitogen-activated protein kinases (MAPK), such as c-Jun N-terminal kinase (JNK), is of interest both for regulation of regeneration and apoptosis. Following stress or mitogenic signaling, there is activation of a cascade of kinases (MAPK kinase kinase (MKKK) → MAPK kinase (MKK) → MAPK). MKK4 and MKK7 phosphorylate JNK, which is promitotic, whereas MKK3 and MKK6 activate p38, which inhibits entry into the cell cycle. Down-regulation of MKK4 results in reciprocal up-regulation of MKK7, which is a strong activator of JNK; this increases the ability of transplanted hepatocytes to proliferate in vivo and makes them partly resistant to Fas-mediated apoptosis (see later).[72] MPKK4 has been identified as a master regulator of cell cycle entry and progression during liver regeneration.[72]

Replication of nonparenchymal cells lags behind that of hepatocytes by 24 to 72 hours. Initially, the newly proliferated hepatocytes form clusters, first in zone 1 and later in other zones of the liver (see Chapter 71). Regenerating endothelial cells invade these clusters and restore the single-cell-thick liver plates.

Early as well as late changes occur in the expression of extracellular matrix components and the enzymes that modulate them. The mitotic phase is mostly completed in 3 days, and the liver mass is restituted in about 7 days. Liver cells return to their quiescent state when the liver mass is restored to within 10% of the original size. A balance between mitosis and apoptosis fine-tunes the restoration of hepatic mass. The strictly self-limited nature of hepatocyte replication suggests that strong regulatory pressures favor replicative repression. The ability of the liver to regulate its size is dependent on hormonal or metabolic signals generated outside the liver, as well as internal signals generated within the liver.[68] Signals for cessation of growth of the regenerating liver are understood less well than those that govern replication.

Gene Expression During Regeneration

The regenerative process is a cascade of events that move cells from their resting G_0 phase through the G_1 phase, S (DNA synthesis) phase, G_2 phase, and then to M (mitotic cell division) phase (Fig. 72-2A) (see Chapter 1). Expression of a large number of genes is induced or down-regulated after partial hepatectomy at transcriptional or post-transcriptional levels.[69,71] The sequence of activation of various genes during liver regeneration has been elucidated by studies using partial hepatectomy and gene knockout mice that lack specific

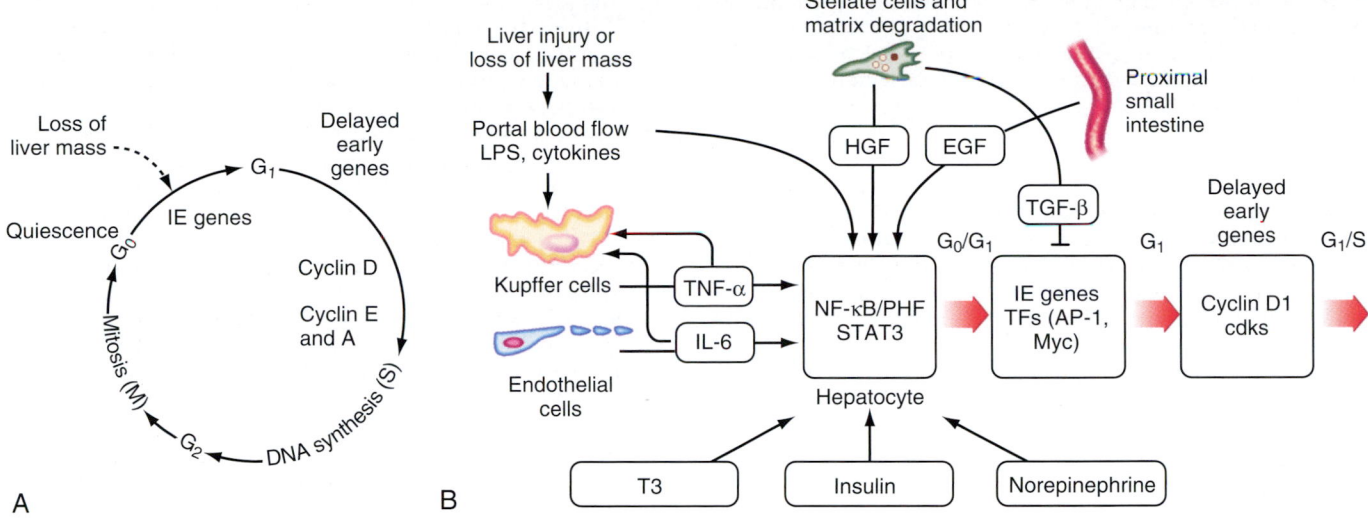

FIGURE 72-2. *A,* The cell cycle of hepatocytes in response to liver injury or loss of liver mass. Quiescent hepatocytes (G_0) rapidly enter G_1 after loss of liver mass (e.g., partial hepatectomy), along with expression of immediate early (IE) genes. This phase is followed sequentially by the expression of delayed early genes and cyclins. DNA synthesis (S phase) reaches a peak in 24 hours in rats and 36 to 40 hours in mice. Shortly thereafter, the cell enters G_2 and undergoes mitosis (M). *B,* The sequence of signals that leads to liver regeneration following liver damage or partial hepatectomy. Intestine-derived lipopolysaccharides (LPS) and cytokines in the portal venous blood activate Kupffer cells and endothelial cells, which release TNF-α and interleukin (IL)-6. These signals lead to activation of nuclear factor (NF)-κB, also known as post hepatectomy factor (PHF), and STAT3 (signal transducer and activator of transcription-3), without the need for new protein synthesis. Hepatic growth factor (HGF) is released by hepatic stellate cells and may also be derived from storage sites following matrix degradation. EGF secreted by proximal small intestinal and salivary gland epithelial cells, as well as insulin, triiodothyronine (T3), and norepinephrine, serves as cooperative factors for transition of hepatocytes through G_1 to the S phase. IE genes and transcription factors (TFs), including AP-1 and Myc, are expressed as the hepatocyte enters the initial phase of G_1. Delayed early genes and cyclins are expressed later in G_1. Transforming growth factor (TGF)-β, which inhibits hepatocyte DNA synthesis, is blocked during the proliferative phase. Removal of the block at the end of the cell cycle may be one of the factors that permit the hepatocyte to return to the quiescent state. AP-1, activator protein-1; cdks, cyclin-dependent kinases. *(Data from Taub R. Liver regeneration: From myth to mechanism. Nat Rev Mol Cell Biol 2004; 5:836-47.)*

cytokines. These genes include cell cycle genes, metabolic genes, genes coding for extracellular matrix proteins, growth factors, cytokines, and transcription factors. Chronologically, these genes can be grouped into immediate early genes, delayed early genes, and cell cycle–associated genes. Expression of these genes is modulated by signal transduction pathways that receive and transduce stimuli for cell replication and tissue remodeling. Expression of genes involved with acute-phase and defense responses increase rapidly in the early phases. Gene expression needed for cell proliferation and DNA replication become up-regulated in middle phase, whereas a number of genes involved in cell adhesion are up-regulated as regeneration progresses toward completion. Interestingly, those involved in amino acid and lipid metabolism are down-regulated during liver regeneration.[73]

Immediate Early Genes

Immediate early genes are activated almost immediately after partial hepatectomy, without the need for protein synthesis. Many of these immediate early genes are involved in metabolic processes not directly linked to DNA synthesis. In addition to the proto-oncogenes, c-*fos*, c-*jun*, c-*myc*, and c-*ets*, the immediate early genes include those that code for transcription factors, such as NF-κB, STAT3 (signal transducer and activator of transcription), activator protein-1 (AP-1), C/EBPβ (CCAAT enhancer binding protein β), insulin-like growth factor–binding protein-1, phosphatases, cyclic adenosine monophosphate (cAMP)-responsive promoter element modulator (CREM), X-box–binding protein 1 (XBP-1), and

metabolic enzymes such as phosphoenolpyruvate carboxykinase (PEPCK) and glucose-6-phosphatase.

In the quiescent liver, NF-κB remains in the cytosol and is inactivated by binding to its inhibitor (IκB). Binding of TNF to its cell surface receptor initiates a signaling cascade that culminates in phosphorylation of IκB, causing the release of NF-κB and its translocation to the nucleus and resulting in transcriptional activation of more than a dozen genes likely to be involved in the immediate early response. The gene for IL-6 is one of the target genes of NF-κB. IL-6 is a strong inducer of STAT3 activation and is thought to play an important role in hepatic regeneration. C/EBPα expression is down-regulated during liver regeneration, whereas C/EBPβ expression is induced. C/EBPα may repress hepatocyte replication by inhibiting the proteolytic degradation of the cell cycle inhibitor p21 and by reducing E2F complexes containing the retinoblastoma protein p107. On the other hand, C/EBPβ activates the expression of mitogen-activated protein kinase phosphatase (MKP-1), Egr-1 transcription factor, and the cell cycle proteins cyclin B and E. CREM and XBP-1 participate in the regulation of liver regeneration through their effect on cAMP-responsive genes.

Delayed Early Genes

Delayed early genes are transcribed after the immediate early gene response but before the cell cycle genes reach maximum levels of expression. Expression of these genes occurs during the $G_0 \rightarrow G_1$ phase transition and is dependent on protein synthesis. This group of genes includes those that encode

HRS/SRp40 (a splicing factor and modulator of alternative splicing of RNA transcripts) and the anti-apoptotic gene, bcl-x. In contrast, the pro-apoptotic genes BAK, BAD, and BAX are initially down-regulated after partial hepatectomy and are induced at a later time.

Cell Cycle Genes

Cyclins and cyclin-dependent kinases (cdks) are expressed during cell cycle progression from the G_1 through S to M phase. During the G_1 phase, cdks catalyze the phosphorylation of retinoblastoma gene protein (pRb), causing its dissociation from the E2F family of proteins. This dissociation eliminates the repression of gene expression by pRb. In regenerating mouse liver cyclin D1, mRNA is expressed before DNA synthesis, whereas the expression of cyclin E mRNA coincides with DNA synthesis. Cyclin D1 forms a complex with cdk4, which causes phosphorylation of pRb, resulting in E2F activation. Cyclin D1 may also sequester the cell cycle inhibitor p27.

Integration of Cytokine and Growth Factors in Regeneration

The early, reversible phase of liver regeneration, during which hepatocytes can enter the cell cycle by moving from the quiescent G_0 state to early G_1 phase, is termed *priming*.[69] This phase is initiated by the effect of cytokines, the best studied of which include TNF-α and IL-6. Generation of reactive oxygen species as a consequence of the acute metabolic changes and release of LPS that occur in response to the loss of hepatic functional mass may have a role in triggering the initial cytokine response. During priming, NF-κB and STAT3 are activated, and AP-1 and C/EBP are expressed. Together, these factors lead to the immediate early gene expression response after partial hepatectomy (see earlier). The priming events sensitize hepatocytes to growth factors. In the absence of growth factors, the cells cannot move past a certain "restriction point" in G_1.

The second phase of liver regeneration, termed *progression*, requires HGF and TGF-α as well as cyclins D1 and E. During the progression phase, the cells move past the restriction point in G_1 to S and beyond.

When the peak level of cyclin D1 expression is reached, cells progress autonomously through the cell cycle, without further need for growth factors. Expression of HGF, TGF-α, and probably EGF increase after partial hepatectomy. These factors are the direct mitogens for liver regeneration. EGF binds to both the EGF receptor and the TGF-α receptor, and c-met is the receptor for HGF. Growth hormone, thyroid hormones, and parathormone are permissive for liver regeneration, whereas insulin and norepinephrine are considered adjuvant factors.[69]

Major sources of HGF in the liver are Kupffer cells and HSCs. HGF is produced as a single 87- to 90-kd pro-protein by nonparenchymal cells and is cleaved into approximately 64-kd and 32-kd peptides that form heterodimers.[68,69] HGF mRNA levels are increased 12 to 24 hours after partial hepatectomy in rats. Elevated levels of HGF have been observed in the serum of patients with fulminant hepatic failure, thus suggesting an important role for HGF in regeneration of human liver. C-met, the HGF receptor, is a heterodimer consisting of a 145-kd β chain and a 45-kd α chain, linked by disulfide bonds. The two polypeptide chains of c-met are also derived from proteolytic cleavage of a single precursor protein. The β chain contains the transmembrane region and the intracellular tyrosine kinase domain. HGF binding to the extracellular domain of c-met activates tyrosine kinase, thereby initiating a signal transduction pathway.

Apoptosis

Programmed cell death, or *apoptosis*, is an integral part of hepatic regeneration. Apoptosis is involved in a fine-tuning and remodeling process that results in reconstruction of the hepatic architecture and removal of damaged, senescent, or supernumerary cells, without altering the cellular microenvironment. Loss of function of pro-apoptotic proteins, overexpression of anti-apoptotic proteins, or loss of apoptotic signaling in cells can lead to the survival of DNA-damaged cells, leading in turn to several forms of cancer.[74]

Apoptotic signals can originate within the cells through mechanisms that sense DNA damage and inappropriate proliferative signals. In other cases, the apoptotic signals come from other cells in at least 3 ways.[75] First, cells recognized as foreign or as pathogens may receive apoptotic signals from immune mediator cells. Second, the nurturing signals of neighboring cells or extracellular matrix may be lost, thus resulting in apoptosis of anchor-dependent cells. Third, some cells undergo apoptosis in response to certain growth factors such as TGF-β1.

In contrast to necrosis, apoptosis is an active process that culminates in cell death. During the latent phase of apoptosis, the cell undergoes molecular and biochemical change but remains morphologically intact. In the execution phase, a series of dramatic structural changes take place that culminate in the fragmentation and condensation of the cell into membrane-enclosed apoptotic bodies. Initially, a variety of stimuli, including DNA damage, growth factor withdrawal, toxins, or radiation, trigger the apoptotic pathway. The signal is transduced by a series of defined protein-protein interactions Finally, cell death is executed by the activation of specific proteases called *caspases* that cleave multiple substrates, leading to DNA fragmentation, chromatin condensation, cell shrinkage, and membrane blebbing. The apoptotic cell may be phagocytosed or simply lose contact with neighboring cells. Apoptosis does not cause an acute inflammatory reaction. All these morphologic features of apoptosis contrast with those of necrosis, in which the cell swells and releases proinflammatory material into the neighboring space.[74]

The two major apoptotic pathways include activation of cell surface death receptors[75] and mitochondrial permeability transition.[76] At least 6 different cell surface molecules can function as death receptors. One of the best characterized death receptors is Fas (also known as *Apo1* or *CD95*). Fas belongs to the family of TNF receptors. Binding of Fas to Fas ligand leads to an interaction between the cytoplasmic domain of the Fas receptor and the death domain of the adaptor protein, FADD (Fas-associated protein with death domain), which in turn recruits and activates procaspase-8. Once activated, caspase-8 activates downstream caspases such as caspase-3. The second major pathway involves mitochondria and is triggered by various toxic insults. Either Bax or Bak opens channels and thereby releases the electron transport protein cytochrome c and other proteins from the intermembranous space into the cytoplasm. Cytochrome c binds the scaffolding protein Apaf-1. The C-terminal portion of Apaf1 is a negative regulator of apoptosis. The N-terminal region contains a caspase recruitment domain and an ATPase domain. Binding of cytochrome c and deoxyadenosine triphosphate (dATP) removes the negative regulatory influence of the C-terminus of Apaf-1, thereby permitting binding and autoactivation of caspase-9. Activated caspase-9, in turn, activates caspases-3 and -7, thus initiating cell death. In addition, permeabilization of the mitochondrial outer membrane results in the loss of function of the electron transport chain, which is essential for most mitochondrial functions, including ATP generation.

Genes involved in apoptosis are actively expressed in the regenerating liver. These genes include the inducing genes c-*fos*, c-*jun*, c-*myc*, *TP53*, *Bax*, *Bad*, *Bak*, and *TGF-β*; the apoptosis inhibitory genes, *Bcl-2*, *Bcl-X$_L$*, *TRPM-2/clusterin*; and the *Rb* gene. Some of these genes are also involved in cell proliferation through regulation of the cell cycle.

AUTOPHAGY

Autophagy (from the Greek, meaning "self-eating") is an essential prosurvival catabolic process within the lysosome that maintains cellular homeostasis and quality control by selectively degrading damaged ER, peroxisomes, mitochondria, and ribosomes and promoting basal turnover of long-lived proteins.[77] Autophagy provides cytoprotection during cellular stress, such as nutrient deprivation, growth factor withdrawal, oxidative stress, infection, hypoxia, and cancer. Free fatty acids (FFAs) and amino acids produced by lipolytic and proteolytic digestion provide energy sources and material for synthesis of new proteins during cellular stress, thereby buying time for cells to recover.[78] In infectious diseases, autophagy helps clear intracellular pathogens (xenophagy) and plays a role in antigen presentation and regulation of inflammatory responses.[79] The autophagic machinery is also used as an alternative pathway of secretion, whereby specific proteins (e.g., IL-1A) can be secreted, bypassing the conventional pathway through the Golgi apparatus.[79] On the other hand, the autophagic machinery can be co-opted by viruses for their replication.[80] Autophagy and its disorders are widely implicated in cancer and metabolic, neurodegenerative, cardiovascular, and pulmonary diseases, as well as in energy metabolism and physiologic responses to exercise and aging.[81] Three principal routes of autophagic degradation are distinguished based on the mode of cargo delivery to lysosomes: macroautophagy, microautophagy, and chaperone-mediated autophagy (CMA).

Macroautophagy consists of enclosure of components of cell organelles and proteins inside a double-layer membrane structure termed *autophagosome* (AP) that is trafficked to lysosomes, with which it fuses, resulting in digestion of its cargo by lysosomal enzymes.[77] Steps of this process include initial nucleation of pre-autosomal membranes (phagophores), which elongate with contribution of membranes from the ER, mitochondria, and plasma membrane, eventually enclosing the cargo within the AP vesicle. The AP is translocated to lysosomes along microtubules, powered by dynein motors. The AP "matures" by fusion with late endosomes and then fuses with lysosomes, where the contents are degraded. Macroautophagy is controlled by products of a number of autophagy genes (*Atg*) that were first identified in yeasts. Initial nucleation of phagophores is controlled by two macromolecular complexes, mTor (mammalian target of rapamycin)-Atg13-ULK1 (mTORC1) and a Beclin-1 interacting complex consisting of Beclin-1, Bcl-2 (an autophagy inhibitor), Vps34 (a class III phosphatidylinositol 3-kinase [PI3]), and Atg14L (autophagy activator). In the presence of growth factors and nutritional signals (e.g., amino acids leucine, glutamine, tyrosine, phenylalanine, proline, methionine, tryptophan, histidine) that stimulate the class I PI3-AKT pathway, mTORC1 negatively regulates a complex consisting of UNC-51–like kinase 1 (ULK1), ATG13, ATG101, and FIP200. Conversely, nutrient depletion or energy exhaustion inhibits mTORC1, permitting ULK1 activation, which is crucial in initiating phagophore nucleation. Stimulation of the Beclin-1 interacting complex generates phosphatidylinositol-3-phosphate, which promotes phagophore membrane formation. Elongation of phagophore membranes requires two interacting

ubiquitin-like conjugation systems: the ATG5-ATG12 system and the microtubule-associated protein light chain 3 (LC3-ATG8) system. LC3-I, the cytosolic form of LC3 becomes conjugated with phosphatidylethanolamine, forming the AP membrane-associated form, LC3-II. Visualization of the discrete LC3-II puncta by immunofluorescence analysis indicates autophagosome formation.

The AP vesicles are then translocated to lysosomes along microtubules, powered by dynein motor proteins. Autophagosomes mature by fusing with late endosomes before fusing with lysosomes. The fusion step involves proteins such as ESCRT, SNAREs, Rab7, and the class C Vps proteins Rubicon (RUN domain Beclin-1 interacting cysteine-rich containing) and localizes to the late endosome and lysosome, negatively regulating the maturation of AP and late endosomes. Failure of the fusion step may result in the accumulation of AP vesicles in the cell. Expression of a number of positive and negative regulators of autophagy is modulated post-transcriptionally by several non-coding microRNAs (miRNAs).[82] Because autophagy provides survival benefit to many cancer cells, understanding the role of different miRNAs in specific malignant neoplasms is relevant to designing chemotherapy of cancer (see Chapter 1).

In microautophagy, the cargo is internalized into the lysosomes by invagination of the lysosomal membrane. In contrast to macroautophagy, through which the AP is formed within the cytosol, in microautophagy the vesicles form the lysosomal membrane that sequesters areas of the surrounding cytosol as it invaginates toward the lumen.[83] Much less is known about the mechanistic basis of microautophagy than other forms of autophagy. Notably, selective degradation of specific proteins has been observed in both macroautophagy and microautophagy, which cannot be explained by simple sequestration of cytosol or organellar fragments either in the AP or in lysosomal invaginations. The determinants of selectivity in different autophagic pathways include peptide motifs,[84] covalent modifications (e.g., ubiquitination), derivatization (e.g., acetylation, phosphorylation), recognition by specific receptors (e.g., p62, NBR1), and biding to molecular chaperones and co-chaperones that can deliver specific proteins for degradation through each of the 3 autophagic pathways.[85]

CMA consists of several steps[85]: (1) binding of cytosolic hsc70 (heat shock cognate protein 70 kd), aided by co-chaperones, to the KFERQ-like targeting motif in substrate proteins; (2) delivery of the substrate–chaperone complex to LAMP-2A (lysosome-associated membrane protein type 2A); (3) unfolding of the substrate protein; (4) organization of LAMP-2A molecules into a multimeric translocation complex on the lysosomal membrane; (5) translocation of the substrate protein across the lysosomal membrane, assisted by the lysosome-resident form of hsc70; and (6) degradation of the substrate by the lysosomal proteases. The concentration of LAMP-2A on lysosomal membranes is rate limiting for substrate binding, whereas assembly of the LAMP-2A into a translocation complex is rate limiting for translocation into the lysosome. Following internalization of the substrate, the translocation complex disassembles into monomers. Both the assembly and disassembly require chaperone proteins.

During periods of stress or nutrient deprivation, autophagy maintains cellular biosynthetic capacity and ATP levels by generating amino acids for de novo protein synthesis and supplying energy by providing substrates for the tricarboxylic acid cycle (see later). Lipid droplets within hepatocytes are sequestered inside AP before fusion with lysosomes (lipophagy), where lipid hydrolysis generates FFA for energy homeostasis of the cell.[86] Similar release of FFAs by lipophagy within HSCs leads to fibrogenesis.[87]

Autophagy can protect as well as kill a cell, depending on the death signal. For example, embryonic mouse fibroblasts with loss of macroautophagy due to deletion of *atg5* are sensitized to caspase-dependent apoptosis from the death receptor ligands Fas and TNF-α, but are resistant to death from menadione and ultraviolet light because of the activation of CMA.[88]

PROTEIN SYNTHESIS AND DEGRADATION IN THE LIVER

Hepatic Gene Expression

Compared with most organs, the liver expresses a large number of genes. Over 90% of plasma proteins and about 15% of the total protein mass of the body are produced in the liver.[89] As in all mammalian cells, gene expression is initiated by transcription of the gene into an RNA transcript, mediated by RNA polymerase II. The nascent RNA is modified by capping of the 5'-terminus with 7-methylguanosine, excision of the noncoding intervening sequences (introns), splicing together of the coding sequences (exons), and, in most cases, addition of polyadenylate at the 3'-end. The processed mRNA is actively transported out of the nucleus. In the cytoplasm, association of the mRNA with the 40s ribosomal subunit and methionine RNA requires several initiation factors, a cap-binding protein, and ATP hydrolysis.

Once this initiation complex is formed, the 60s ribosomal subunit is recruited and polypeptide chain elongation proceeds as specific tRNAs recognize corresponding codons and sequentially attach appropriate amino acids. Chain elongation requires elongation factors and energy provided by GTP hydrolysis. Cessation of translation at the stop codons requires recognition by a termination factor. In most cases, the nascent protein is processed by cleavage of an amino terminal signal peptide. Many proteins undergo further proteolytic cleavage, cotranslational glycosylation, and modification of the carbohydrate moieties in the Golgi apparatus, before being secreted or transported to other intracellular organelles (see earlier).

Gene expression is regulated at multiple levels. Gene transcription is regulated by the state of the chromatin, which determines the accessibility of specific genes to the transcription machinery, and binding of specific transcription factors that promote or repress gene transcription. Post-transcriptional regulation can involve differential splicing, modulation of mRNA stability and efficiency of translation, protein folding, association with self or other proteins, and phosphorylation or other forms of protein modification. Modulation of protein degradation is another important mechanism that regulates net protein content.

Some genes expressed in hepatocytes, loosely termed "housekeeping genes," are expressed in many other organs as well. In addition, the expression of many other genes occurs preferentially or uniquely in the liver. Expression of these liver-specific genes permits the liver to perform essential functions of the body, including secretion of plasma proteins, gluconeogenesis, glycogen storage, glucose metabolism, cholesterol homeostasis, bile salt production, and detoxification of endogenous metabolites and exogenous substances. A series of *cis*-acting elements in specific genes mediate their hepatocyte-preferred expression.[90] These *cis*-acting DNA elements bind different families of HNFs. Although none of these factors is entirely liver-specific, high levels of liver-preferred gene expression occur only in the presence of combinatorial interaction of these transcription factors. Maintenance of hepatocyte-enriched expression of specific transcription factors involves cross-regulation by other unrelated liver-enriched transcription factors. Some of the transcription factors involved in hepatocyte specificity are also important in hepatic tissue specification during embryogenesis. Many of the transcription factors are normally located in the cytoplasm. Binding of hormones or cytokines to their respective cell surface receptors causes conformational changes in the cytoplasmic domain of these receptors, often through phosphorylation. Such conformational changes lead to a series of events that eventually lead to the translocation of specific transcription factors to the nucleus and their binding to the respective *cis*-acting elements in the regulatory regions of genes. Therefore, extracellular signals are transduced to a series of intracellular events, culminating in the induction or repression of gene expression.

Regulation of gene transcription is the most important, but not the only, mechanism of modulation of gene expression. Stability of the RNA, translational regulation, and post-translational modifications can all affect the steady-state concentration, intracellular or extracellular location, and activity of a given gene product. The major plasma proteins synthesized and secreted by the liver are shown in Table 72-1.

Nuclear Receptors

Modulation of metabolic pathways and detoxicating mechanisms according to the needs of the body often requires coordinated up-regulation or repression of the expression of a set of genes. In many cases, such coordination is mediated by nuclear receptors, such as retinoid X receptor (RXR), liver X-receptor (LXR), farnesoid X-receptor (FXR), constitutive androstane receptor (CAR), peroxisome proliferator activator receptor (PPAR), and thyroid hormone receptor (TR).[91] For example, expression of proteins that mediate bilirubin uptake by hepatocytes, intracellular storage of bilirubin, glucuronidation of bilirubin, and bile canalicular excretion of bilirubin glucuronides may all be regulated by CAR. Nuclear receptors mediate induction or repression of genes by small nonprotein molecules. For example, phenobarbital binds to CAR in the cytoplasm, leading to the translocation of CAR to the nucleus and thereby resulting in simultaneous induction of multiple genes that have CAR-binding elements in their *cis*-regulatory regions. Similarly, bile acids bind to FXR, fibrates bind to PPAR, and thyroid hormones bind to TR. In most cases, nuclear receptors function by forming heterodimers with RXR, although some nuclear receptors can function as homodimers.

Protein Folding

Proteins that are destined for export to intracellular membranes or secretion into the plasma are translocated into the ER, where folding takes place prior to secretion through the Golgi apparatus.[92] The ER contains a number of molecular chaperones and folding catalysts that promote efficient folding. All chaperones enable and promote protein folding and assembly, but their specific functions differ. Many chaperones work in tandem with one other. Some molecular chaperones bind to nascent chains as they emerge from the ribosome and protect aggregation-prone hydrophobic regions. Other chaperones are involved in later stages of folding, particularly for complex proteins that include oligomeric species and multimolecular assemblies.

In addition to promoting proper folding, chaperones play an important role in the "quality control" of proteins, through a complex series of glycosylation and deglycosylation processes and prevention of misfolded proteins from being secreted from the cell.[93] The unfolded or misfolded proteins are targeted for degradation through the ubiquitin-proteasome

TABLE 72-1 Some Serum Proteins Produced by the Liver

Protein	Molecular Weight (Daltons)	Function	Association with Liver Disease	Levels During an cute-Phase Response
α_1-Acid glycoprotein (orosomucoid)	40,000	Inhibits proliferating response of peripheral lymphocytes to mitogens	—	Increased
Albumin	66,500	Binding protein, osmotic regulator	Decreased in chronic liver disease	Decreased
AFP	66,300	Binding protein	Increased in hepatocellular carcinoma	Decreased
α_1-Antichymotrypsin	68,000	Inhibits chymotrypsin-like serine proteinase	—	Increased
α_1-Antitrypsin (α_1-AT)	54,000	Inhibits elastin	Missense mutations are associated with liver disease	Increased
Ceruloplasmin	132,000	Ferroxidase	Decreased in Wilson disease	Increased
Complement C3	185,000	Complement pathway	—	Increased
Complement C4	200,000	Complement pathway	—	Increased
C-reactive protein	118,000	Binds pathogens and damaged cells to initiate their elimination	—	Increased
Ferritin	450,000	Intracellular iron storage	Increased in hemochromatosis	Increased
Fibrinogen	340,000	Precursor to fibrin in hemostasis, wound healing	Decreased in chronic liver disease	Increased
Haptoglobin	≈100,000	Binds hemoglobin released by hemolysis	—	Increased
Serum amyloid A	9000	Unknown	—	Increased
Transferrin	79,500	Iron-binding protein	—	Decreased

Data from Katz N, Jungermam K. Metabolic heterogeneity of the liver. In: Tavoloni N, Berk PD, editors. Hepatic transport and bile secretion: Physiology and pathophysiology. New York: Raven Press; 1993. p 55; and Putnam FW. Progress in plasma proteins. In: The plasma proteins: Structure, function, and genetic control. Orlando, Fla.: Academic Press; 1984. p 45.

pathway.[94] Up to half of all polypeptide chains fail to satisfy the quality control mechanism in the ER, and for some proteins, such as the cystic fibrosis transmembrane conductance regulator (CFTR), the success rate is even lower. The proportion of molecules that misfold is increased greatly in mutant proteins with amino acid substitutions. Some molecular chaperones are able to rescue misfolded proteins to enable them to have a second chance to fold correctly. Under some circumstances, chaperones can solubilize proteins that have aggregated because of misfolding. In some cases, energy for such active intervention may be derived from ATP hydrolysis. Many molecular chaperones, such as the heat shock protein (HSP), are up-regulated in stressful situations, when protein misfolding is more prone to occur.

In addition to molecular chaperones, several classes of folding catalysts accelerate steps in the folding process. For example, peptidylprolyl isomerases increase the rate of cis/trans isomerization of peptide bonds involving proline residues, and protein disulfide isomerases enhance formation and reorganization of disulfide bonds within proteins.

Protein Catabolism

Like protein synthesis, proteolysis is a major process that contributes to the body protein turnover. The autophagic-lysosomal pathway (see earlier) and the ubiquitin/proteasome

pathway are the two major mechanisms of protein degradation. The ubiquitin/proteasome pathway is the principal mechanism for turnover of normally short-lived proteins in mammalian cells.[95] ER chaperones, such as Hsp70, and chaperone-like proteins survey the conformations of nascent polypeptides in the ER. The chaperone proteins and lectins that bind to N-glycans of glycoproteins facilitate protein folding. Perturbations in protein folding trigger a signaling cascade, termed the *unfolded protein response* (UPR), which produces cellular stress. A substantial fraction of normal proteins may be misfolded or incompletely processed. Misfolding is greatly enhanced for some proteins harboring missense mutation but can also be caused by protein modifications, such as oxidative damage. Misfolded proteins expose hydrophobic domains that are normally buried inside the folded molecule, and intermolecular binding of these hydrophobic patches cause protein aggregation. If the misfolding is not corrected despite the binding of chaperones and lectins, the proteins are ejected from the ER to the cytoplasm. In the case of some proteins, hydrophobic interaction leads to chaperone-mediated formation of aggregates that are transported to the microtubule organization center near the nucleus, forming aggregosomes that enter autophagosomes for eventual lysosomal degradation by a process termed *chaperone-mediated selective autophagy* (CASA).[96] P62, an aggregate-forming protein, is recruited to the polyubiquitinated aggregates. If the aggregates are not efficiently cleared by autophagy, they accumulate in cells and cause proteinopathy. Known examples in hepatocytes include intracellular hyaline bodies in hepatocellular carcinoma and Mallory-Denk bodies in alcoholic hepatitis.[97]

Misfolded proteins that remain soluble or do not form large aggregates are ubiquitinated during or soon after entering the cytoplasm and degraded by the 26S proteasome by a process termed *ER-associated degradation* (ERAD).[98] Ubiquitin is a small protein that can link covalently to itself or to other proteins, either as monomers or as chains of polyubiquitin. Ubiquitin is added to a target protein by ubiquitin-activating, ubiquitin-conjugating, and ubiquitin-ligating enzymes. The first function attributed to ubiquitin was the covalent binding to misfolded proteins, thereby directing proteasome-dependent proteolysis. Ubiquitin and ubiquitin-related proteins are also known to direct specific proteins through the endocytotic pathway by modifying cargo proteins, as well as by regulating components of the cytoplasmic protein trafficking machinery. By regulating the turnover of mitotic cyclins, ubiquitination plays an important role in cell cycle regulation.[99,100] A subset of endocytosed proteins must be conjugated to ubiquitin as a trigger for internalization from the plasma membrane.[101,102]

HEPATIC NUTRIENT METABOLISM

The liver is at the hub of numerous metabolic pathways. The liver provides energy continuously to the entire body through its ability to store and modulate the availability of systemic nutrients.[103] In turn, the metabolic function of the liver is regulated by hormones secreted by the pancreas, adrenals, thyroid, and adipose tissue, as well as neuronal inputs. A liver–adipose tissue–brain-pancreas axis,[104] as well as a gut-brain-liver axis,[105] orchestrates the management of the energy supply to body tissues. In addition to serving as a store for excess energy as lipids, the adipose tissue, particularly visceral fatty tissue that drains into the portal circulation, plays an active role in hepatic energy metabolism by releasing FFAs into plasma and releasing a series of adipokines that either increase or decrease insulin sensitivity in the liver and other tissues.[104] During nutrient absorption (fed state), the liver regulates nutrient flux as the absorbed nutrients are metabolized, modified for storage in the liver and fatty tissue, or made available to other organs as an energy source. During fasting, the energy supply is maintained from the stored fuel and by synthesis. Starvation induces breakdown of TG in adipose tissues into FFAs and glycerol. FFAs reduce insulin sensitivity, thereby affecting glucose metabolism in muscles and the liver. FFAs bind and activate PPARs in liver and other tissues, thereby affecting gene expression.[106] In the hepatocyte, most of the acetyl-CoA produced by oxidation of FFA is used to synthesize ketone bodies (e.g., acetoacetate, β-hydroxybutyrate) that are released into circulation and used as an energy source by many peripheral tissues. The glycerol released by TG hydrolysis is used by the liver for the synthesis of glucose, which is the only source of energy for neurons and red blood cells (RBCs), or of TG. The TG is packaged into very-low-density lipoproteins (VLDL) and returns to the adipose tissue (see later).[107]

The role of a gut-brain-liver axis in glucose homeostasis has also been established.[105] In rats, lipids arriving in the intestine give rise to long-chain fatty CoA by the action of acyl-CoA synthase, which sends an afferent signal to the nucleus of the solitary tract in the hindbrain through the vagus nerve. This signal leads to *N*-methyl-ᴅ-aspartate ion channel–dependent glutamatergic neurotransmission through the efferent vagal fibers that supply the liver, thereby resulting in a reduction in glucose production by the liver that precedes the actual post-absorptive glucose influx from the intestine. Therefore, the rapid gut-brain-liver communication helps prevent excessive fluctuation of the blood glucose level. Unfortunately, this mechanism becomes inoperative with continued intake of excessive calories for several days.[108]

Carbohydrate

Glucose is the primary energy source for the brain, erythrocytes, muscle, and renal cortex. Maintaining adequate circulating levels of glucose is essential for the central nervous system, which normally uses glucose as its major metabolic fuel. After a person fasts for 24 to 48 hours, the brain can use ketones as a metabolic fuel, thereby reducing its glucose requirement by 50% to 70%.[108] The liver is the principal organ that maintains total carbohydrate stores by synthesizing glycogen and generating glucose from precursors.[109] Glucose is synthesized from nonoxidative metabolic products of glucose (pyruvate and lactate) that are generated predominantly by RBCs and from amino acid precursors that are derived predominantly from muscle during prolonged starvation or exercise.

Regulation of Glucose Uptake and Efflux from the Hepatocyte

Glucose is a critical molecule in the metabolic pathway because it can be converted to amino acids, fatty acids, or glycogen, the major storage form of glucose. Glucose enters hepatocytes via the glucose transporter-2, which facilitates the diffusion of glucose across the sinusoidal membrane.[110] Glucose transporter-2 differs from other members of the glucose transporter family in that it is independent of metabolic conditions or insulin levels. Because of the low-affinity, high-capacity characteristics of glucose transporter-2, intrahepatic glucose concentration is determined by the plasma glucose level, which, in turn, is regulated by glucokinase activity (see later).[111] Glucose transporter-1, which is present in the brain, RBCs, and hepatocytes, particularly in zone 3, is a low-capacity, high-affinity glucose transporter that permits glucose uptake by hepatocytes when the circulating glucose concentration is low. Increased expression of glucose transporter-1 during fasting enhances glucose uptake by hepatocytes. Hepatocellular glucose homeostasis is maintained by interlinking pathways that are regulated by multiple signals that prevent competing pathways from operating at the same time.[112] Figure 72-3 illustrates these pathways and the modulating influences that control the metabolic flux of glucose and other sugars, such as fructose.

Formation of Glucose-6-Phosphate

Rapid conversion of glucose to glucose-6-phosphate (glucose-6-P) modulates the glucose concentration within the hepatocyte, thereby regulating influx or efflux of glucose from the hepatocyte.[109] Glucose-6-P is a nodal branch point compound that can enter 3 independent metabolic pathways: (1) synthesis of glycogen, which can be mobilized rapidly during fasting; (2) anaerobic glycolysis via the Embden-Meyerhof pathway, which generates pyruvate or lactate as a substrate for the tricarboxylic acid (Krebs) cycle in mitochondria; or (3) the pentose-phosphate shunt, which generates reducing equivalents necessary for anaerobic glycolysis and fatty acid synthesis. The pentose-phosphate shunt is regulated by the activity of mitochondrial glucose-6-P dehydrogenase.[110] Conversion of glucose to glucose-6-P is catalyzed by hexokinase, which accepts several different hexose substrates, and glucokinase (GK, also termed *hexokinase type 4* or *D*), which is expressed

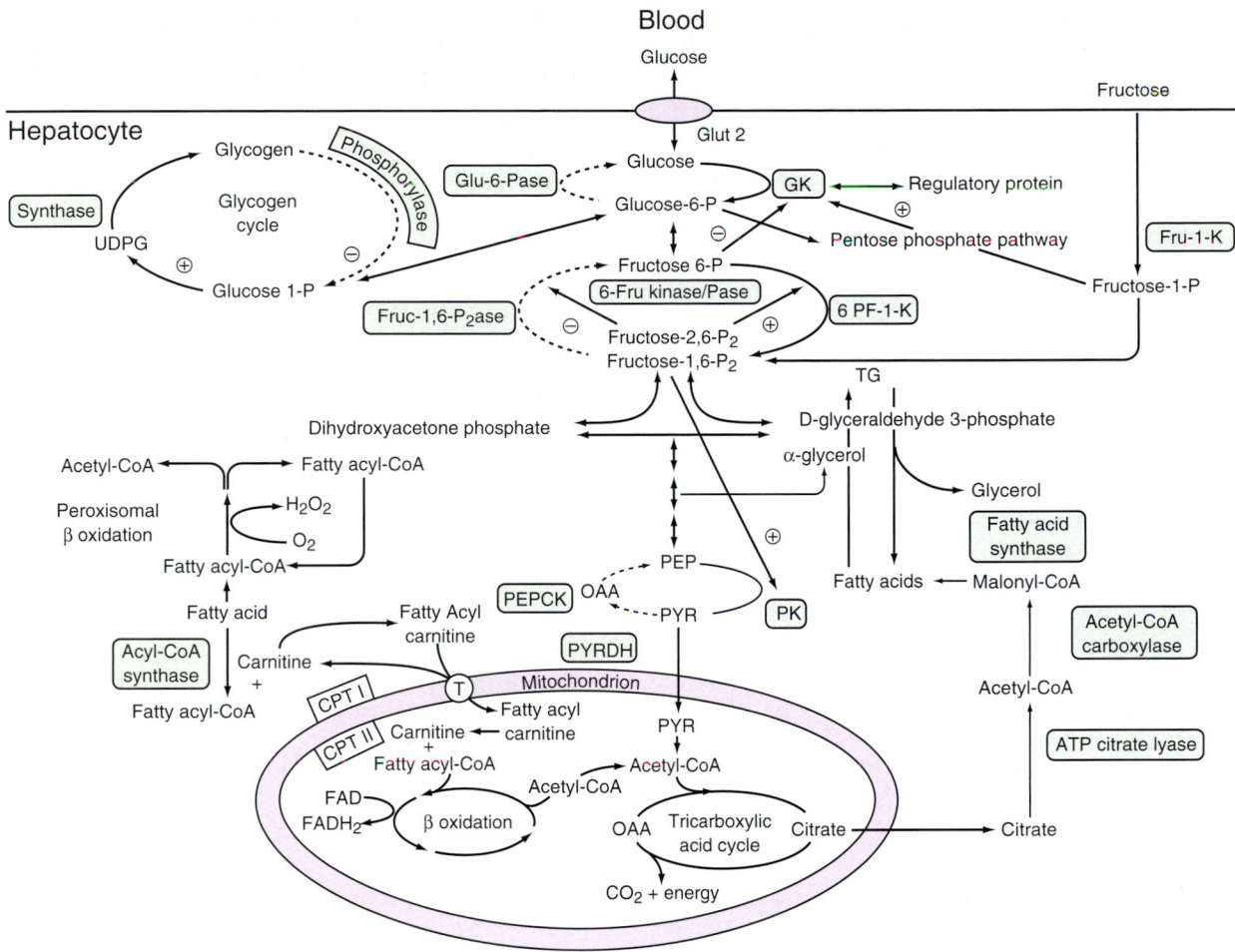

FIGURE 72-3. Hepatic carbohydrate and lipid metabolism. Gluconeogenic pathways are identified by *dashed lines*. 6-Fru Kinase/Pase, 6-phosphofructo-2-kinase/fructose-2,6-biphosphatase; 6 PF-1-K, 6-phosphofructo-1-kinase; CoA, coenzyme A; CPT, carnitine palmitoyltransferase; FAD, flavine adenine dinucleotide; FADH2, reduced flavine adenine dinucleotide; Fru-1-K, hepatic fructokinase; Fruc-1,6-P2ase, fructose-1,6-biphosphatase; Fructose-1-P, fructose-1-phosphate; Fructose-1,6-P2, fructose-1,6-diphosphate; Frucose-2,6-P2, fructose-2,6-diphosphate; Fructose 6-P, fructose-6-phosphate; GK, glucokinase; Glucose-6-P, glucose-6-phosphate; Glu-6-Pase, glucose-6-phosphatase; Glut 2, glucose transporter 2; OAA, oxaloacetate; PEP, phosphoenol pyruvate; PEPCK, phosphoenol pyruvate carboxykinase; PK, pyruvate kinase; PYR, pyruvate; PYRDH, pyruvate dehydrogenase; T, carnitine:acylcarnitine transferase; UDPG, uridine diphosphate glucose. *(Data from Piklis SJ, Granner DK. Molecular physiology of the regulation of hepatic gluconeogenesis and glycolysis. Annu Rev Physiol 1992; 54:885-909.)*

predominantly in the liver and pancreas and is specific for glucose.[113]

A low-affinity, high-capacity system, GK is not inhibited by the reaction product, glucose-6-P. Therefore, the level of GK activity regulates hepatocellular glucose concentration, which determines the net uptake of glucose by hepatocytes from hepatic sinusoidal plasma. GK is activated by insulin and inhibited by glucagon.[108] Mutations in the GK gene are associated with rare cases of maturity-onset diabetes of young adults (MODY).[113] Fructose-1-phosphate modulates GK activity by regulating the inhibitory activity of a GK regulatory protein.[114] The regulation of GK by fructose is thought to prevent futile cycling between glucose and glucose-6-P that consumes ATP. Starvation decreases GK activity, thereby promoting glucose efflux from the hepatocyte.

Conversion of Glucose-6-Phosphate to Glucose

Conversion of glucose-6-P to glucose is catalyzed by glucose-6-phosphatase (glu-6-Pase), a multisubunit enzyme with its active site located within the ER lumen.[115] Therefore, glucose-6-P has to traverse the ER membrane to be dephosphorylated. Inherited deficiency of glu-6-Pase causes glycogen storage disease type Ia (see Chapter 77).[115] Glucose-6-P transport is mediated by a microsomal transport protein, which, when defective, causes type Ib glycogen storage disease. As expected, glu-6-Pase activity is increased by starvation, resulting in an increase in hepatocellular glucose concentration and consequent efflux of glucose into the sinusoidal space by the bidirectional glucose transporter-2.

Glucose-6-P can enter the pentose monophosphate shunt that generates the reduced form of nicotinamide dinucleotide phosphate (NADPH). The other possible metabolic fate of glucose-6-P is conversion to fructose 6-P, which can enter the fructose 6-P-fructose 1,6-diphosphate (fructose-1,6-P2) pathway. Fructose-1,6-P2 modulates the activity of pyruvate kinase (PK), which can affect substrate cycling in the subsequent pyruvate (PYR)-phosphoenol pyruvate (PEP) pathway. These opposing enzyme reactions regulate the formation of gluconeogenesis precursors and glycolysis.

The relative production of fructose 6-P and fructose-1,6-P$_2$ is regulated by the opposing action of 6-phosphofructo-1-phosphokinase (6-PK-1-K) and fructose-1,6-bisphosphatase (fruc-1,6$_2$Pase).[109] Within this cycle is a unique enzyme: 6-phosphofructo-2-kinase/fructose-2,6-biphosphatase (6-fru kinase/Pase). This enzyme, which combines the properties of both a 6-PF-2K and its corresponding phosphorylase enzyme activity, produces the regulatory product fructose-2,6-P$_2$. Fructose-2,6-P$_2$ is a potent activator of 6-PF-1-K and inhibitor of fruc-1,6$_2$Pase; moreover, it favors the formation of the fructose-1,6-P$_2$ product. The enzyme is regulated by both hormonal and nutrient regulations and serves as another modulator of glucose metabolism. During starvation, when fructose-2,6-P$_2$ levels are low, gluconeogenesis is enhanced. On the other hand, high levels of 6-fru kinase/Pase found during refeeding and insulin administration promote glycolysis and fatty acid synthesis. The phosphorylation status of the 6-fru kinase/Pase is regulated by the cAMP-dependent kinase site and phosphatase 2A activity.

From fructose-1,6-P$_2$, a sequence of 4 biochemical reactions leads to the formation of PEP with generation of 8 molecules of ATP.[103] PEP can then be metabolized into PYR as part of the third regulatory cycle in glucose metabolism. Pyruvate kinase, which transforms PEP to PYR, generates two ATP molecules. PYR is another nodal branch point, from which it can undergo further metabolism in mitochondria to form acetyl-CoA. Thereafter, it can undergo aerobic metabolism by the tricarboxylic acid cycle. In this pathway, PYR may be metabolized ultimately to water and CO_2, with the production of 15 molecules of ATP per molecule of PYR. Other products of the tricarboxylic acid cycle are also precursors for fatty acid (citrate) or amino acids by means of oxaloacetate formation. Fructose-1,6-P$_2$ is also an inducer of PK.[116] In the reverse reaction, PYR is metabolized to oxaloacetate, which is a precursor to the amino acid L-aspartate. Oxaloacetate is converted by the energy-dependent activity of phosphoenolpyruvate carboxykinase (PEPCK), an important regulator of gluconeogenesis. PEPCK expression is inhibited by insulin at the transcriptional level[108,116] and is up-regulated during fasting and in diabetes mellitus.

Hepatic Metabolism of Galactose and Fructose

Lactose, a major disaccharide present in human and cow milk, is split into glucose and galactose. Galactose can be converted to glucose-6-P, after which it can be used for glycogen synthesis; or it can be oxidized further to form PYR or acetyl-CoA for additional energy generation or fatty acid synthesis.[103] Galactose is initially phosphorylated by galactokinase to form galactose-1-phosphate (galactose-1-P). In the presence of uridine diphosphoglucose (UDPG), further metabolism by uridyltransferase forms glucose-1-phosphate (glucose-1-P) and UDP-galactose. UDP-galactose can be epimerized by UDP-glucose-4-epimerase to form UDP-glucose, which is a precursor to glucose-1-P. Glucose-1-P can be converted to glucose-6-P. Therefore, like glucose, galactose can participate in the glycolytic pathway.

Fructose, an abundant sugar in the diet, is absorbed by the intestinal epithelium by a sodium-independent carrier distinct from the intestinal glucose transporter (see Chapter 102). It is converted to fructose-1-phosphate (fructose-1-P) by hepatic fructokinase (Fru-1-K), using either ATP or GTP as a cofactor. Fructose-1-P activates GK activity by removing the inhibitory regulatory protein. Fructose-1-P does not enter the glucogenic pathway but is further metabolized by fructose-1-phosphate aldolase to form two trioses: dihydroxylacetone phosphate and glyceraldehyde-3-phosphate. Dihydroxylacetone phosphate may be isomerized to glyceraldehyde phosphate and enter the glycolytic pathway or may be reduced to glyceraldehyde-3-phosphate and provide the glycerol backbone for triacylglycerol and phospholipids. Glyceraldehyde-3-phosphate may be combined with dihydroxylacetone phosphate by aldolase B ultimately to form fructose-1,6-P$_2$. Depending on the metabolic requirements of the liver, fructose-1,6-P$_2$ can be used for gluconeogenesis and glycogen synthesis or may be subjected to glycolysis, ultimately resulting in the formation of lactate. Because fructose enters the carbohydrate cycle at the second regulatory step, fructose is a better substrate for lipogenesis in the liver than is glucose. Aldolase B deficiency results in hereditary fructose intolerance as a result of excess fructose-1-P build-up. Treatment consists of avoidance of sucrose and fructose in the diet.

Glycogen Formation

Glycogen stored in the liver is the main source of rapidly available glucose for the glucose-dependent tissues, such as RBCs, retina, renal medulla, and brain.[117] Hepatic glycogen stores contain up to a 2-day supply of glucose before gluconeogenesis occurs, mainly from lactate, a 3-carbon end-product of anaerobic glucose metabolism.[103,118] Hepatic gluconeogenesis produces up to 240 mg of glucose a day, which is approximately twice the metabolic need of the RBCs, retina, and brain. The 3-carbon precursors generated by anaerobic metabolism from muscle, intestine, liver, or RBCs may account for up to 50% of the glycogen pool formed during nonabsorptive states. Alanine, another major glucose precursor, is generated by the catabolism of muscle proteins, which is a major cause of muscle wasting during prolonged fasting. Glycogen stored in muscle is used locally and cannot be exported out of the cell because muscles lack glu-6-Pase. The relative contribution of each of the precursors to glycogen synthesis depends on the nutritional status, amount, and route of glucose administration (oral vs. IV) and on hormonal regulation.

Rapid switching between glycogen synthesis and breakdown is mediated by a cascade of enzymes that are regulated by local nutrients and hormones.[103] Glycogen phosphorylase, which is activated by phosphorylation, catalyzes the breakdown of glycogen subunits, and glycogen synthase, which is activated by dephosphorylation, catalyzes the addition of UDP-glucose to the expanding glycogen chain. In addition, glucose and glucose-6-P are allosteric activators of the synthase enzyme, whereas glucose binding inactivates the phosphorylase.

Glycogen exists as two distinct populations consisting of proglycogen, with a molecular weight of approximately 4×10^5, and macroglycogen, with a molecular weight of 1×10^7, the concentrations of which depend on the relative activities of enzymes favoring proglycogen formation (phosphorylase and debranching enzymes) and those favoring glycogenin formation (branching enzymes). The ability of glycogenin to initiate the formation of glycogen is important in hepatic carbohydrate metabolism. The existence of these two distinct pools of glycogen permits subtle control of glucose levels, and their relative contributions could have a physiologic role in disease states such as diabetes mellitus.

Regulation of Glycolytic-Gluconeogenic Pathways

The glycolytic-gluconeogenic pathways are regulated by hormonal signals and the relative availability of nutrients. Insulin up-regulates the expression of genes that encode the glycolytic enzymes and represses the expression of metabolic enzymes responsible for gluconeogenesis. Glucagon, catecholamines, corticosteroids, and growth hormone increase cellular cAMP levels, thereby augmenting the gluconeogenic pathway. In many cases, post-transcriptional mRNA stabilization or degradation, post-translational phosphorylation or end-product inhibition, or allosteric modulation contributes to the relative abundance or activity of specific enzymes.[109,116] Glucose and fructose modulate the enzyme activities by direct inhibition or by allosteric modulation of the enzymes. In the fed state, high activity of GK, 6-PF-1-K, and PK induced by insulin favors formation of PYR, with low activity of PEPCK and other gluconeogenic enzymes. During fasting, the fall in plasma insulin levels removes the inhibition of the gluconeogenic enzymes PEPCK and fruc-1,6-P$_2$ase. Simultaneously, an increase in glucagon and β-adrenergic agonists raises intracellular cAMP levels, leading to inhibition of 6-PK-2 kinase activity and stimulation of fruc-2,6-Pase, thereby reducing fructose-2,6-P$_2$ concentration and activation of fruc-1,6$_2$Pase, with a net increase in gluconeogenesis. After a prolonged fast, gluconeogenesis is further stimulated by an increase in the supply of substrate and alterations in the concentration of various enzymes.

Carbohydrate Metabolism in Cirrhosis

Patients with cirrhosis have an increased frequency of hyperglycemia and relative hyperinsulinemia.[119] The hyperglycemia may be explained by decreased glucose uptake by muscle and reduced glycogen storage in liver and muscle. These changes lead to insulin resistance, which causes an increase in plasma insulin levels. Other causes of relative insulin resistance include increased serum FFA levels that can inhibit glucose uptake by muscle, altered second messenger activity after insulin binds to its receptor, and increased serum concentrations of cytokines that result from elevated serum levels of LPS. Increased levels of glucagon and catecholamines may be contributing factors. The net result is impaired nonoxidative use of glucose with decreased storage of glycogen and impaired uptake of glucose by muscle, thereby causing a relative insulin-resistant state similar to that found in patients with diabetes mellitus and obesity.

Lipid

Fatty acids are an important energy source for the liver and serve as an efficient fuel store within and outside the liver, because oxidation of fatty acids yields the highest ATP production of any metabolic fuel.[103] In addition, most organs are capable of using fatty acids as a fuel.[120] The liver plays a central role in regulating the body's total fatty acid needs. Excess glucose can be converted to fatty acid for future use and stored at distal sites such as adipose tissue and delivered by lipoproteins (see later). TGs are stored in the cytoplasm of hepatocytes, where they are enclosed in a monolayer of phospholipids to form lipid droplets, which are important in the energy balance of the cell and the whole organism. Under conditions of excess lipid accumulation in the hepatocyte—for example, in overnutrition—the risk of acquiring insulin resistance increases. Lipid droplet formation may require a family of PPARα-induced ER proteins, termed *fat-inducing transcripts 1 and 2* (FIT-1 and FIT-2).[121] Beta oxidation of fatty acids in mitochondria and peroxisomes has different physiologic consequences.[122] Furthermore, fatty acids are structural components of cell membranes and are important in cellular function and cell anchoring. The regulation of fatty acid synthesis and transport of fatty acids to other organs in association with lipoproteins constitutes another critical role of the liver in managing the metabolic needs of the entire body.

Fatty Acid Synthesis

Fatty acid synthesis occurs in the cytosol and is regulated closely by the availability of acetyl-CoA, which forms the basic subunit of the developing fatty acid carbon chain.[103]

Acetyl-CoA is synthesized predominately in mitochondria and is derived mainly from carbohydrate metabolism, with a small fraction coming from amino acids. Acetyl-CoA is condensed with oxaloacetate to form citrate, which is exported from the mitochondria and is then cleaved by the cytosolic ATP citrate lyase to produce oxaloacetate and acetyl-CoA. Conversion of acetyl-CoA to malonyl-CoA by the action of acetyl-CoA carboxylase is the first step in fatty acid synthesis. Acetyl-CoA carboxylase is the key enzyme in regulating fatty acid synthesis because it provides the necessary building blocks for elongation of the fatty acid carbon chain.[123]

Malonyl-CoA is used by a set of enzymatic activities contained within a single peptide chain that comprises the remarkable fatty acid synthase system.[103] Malonyl-CoA binds to acyl carrier protein (ACP). Catalytic activity is contained within two distinct domains that catalyze sequential condensation, reduction, dehydrogenation, and reduction, which constitute the fatty acid synthetic cycle. Two NADPH molecules are required for each 2-carbon unit that is added to the growing fatty acid chain. After completion of the first cycle, the 4-carbon butyl group is transferred from ACP to a peripheral thiol, thereby allowing it to accept the next malonyl-CoA group to restart the entire cycle. The cycle continues for an additional 6 or 7 rounds until a carbon-16 (palmitate) or carbon-18 (stearate) fatty acid is synthesized. Fatty acid-CoA is then released and used for other metabolic pathways.

Further elongation of the fatty acid chain can occur either in the mitochondrion or within the microsomal membrane.[103] In the mitochondrion, the first step is mediated by enoyl-CoA reductase. Microsomal elongation uses malonyl-CoA to increase the size of fatty acyl-CoA in a process that involves 4 separate enzymatic reactions. The elongation ability of microsomes is tissue dependent and serves the needs of specific organs. The fatty acid chain elongates until an appropriate length has been achieved, and the fatty acid is then esterified with glycerol to form TG. These newly formed TG can be transported by lipoproteins to distal sites for storage and use. In situations of excess carbohydrates, PYR can be converted to acetyl-CoA by the mitochondrial pyruvate dehydrogenase complex to serve as fatty acid precursors, although lipogenesis from carbohydrates consumes about 25% of the energy contained in the carbohydrates.

Beta Oxidation of Fatty Acids

Fatty acid beta oxidation is an important source of energy for many organs, including the liver. Beta oxidation occurs in mitochondria and peroxisomes, and the process requires transport of substrates across the membranes delimiting these organelles.

Mitochondrial Beta Oxidation

Fatty acids are translocated across the mitochondrial membranes by first undergoing fatty acyl-CoA formation by the activity of distinct fatty acyl-CoA synthetases that are specific for short-, medium-, or long-chain fatty acids in the mitochondrial outer membrane.[103,124] In the inner mitochondrial membrane, conjugation of fatty acyl-CoA with carnitine is catalyzed by carnitine palmitoyltransferase I, with formation of fatty acyl carnitine, which is translocated into the mitochondrion, in exchange for free carnitine, by an integral inner membrane protein, fatty acyl carnitine:carnitine translocase.[125] Inside the mitochondrion, a reverse reaction mediated by carnitine palmitoyltransferase II releases fatty acyl-CoA, which is now a substrate for beta oxidation. The first step that is unique to beta oxidation is formation of *trans*-enol fatty acid, which is generated by acyl-CoA dehydrogenase. Acyl-CoA dehydrogenase transfers two electrons to flavin adenine dinucleotide

(FAD), which then transfers them to the electron transport chain in the mitochondrion. 3-Keto fatty acyl-Co then undergoes a series of sequential reactions to acetyl-CoA and fatty acyl-CoA, which undergo another round of beta oxidation. Acetyl-CoA can enter the tricarboxylic acid cycle, thereby generating 12 ATP, or it can enter the 3-hydroxyl-3-methylglutaryl (HMG)-CoA cycle to form ketone bodies. Only mitochondria in the liver are capable of forming ketone bodies. Regulation of mitochondrial beta oxidation lies with fatty acylcarnitine formation, which is catalyzed by carnitine palmitoyltransferase I.[125] Malonyl-CoA, the basic subunit of fatty acid synthesis, is a potent inhibitor of carnitine palmitoyltransferase I, and therefore prevents beta oxidation and fatty acid synthesis from occurring concurrently.

Peroxisomal Beta Oxidation

Peroxisomes have lesser capacity than mitochondria for beta oxidation of fatty acid. The relative contribution of peroxisomes to beta oxidation depends on the fatty acid chain length and administration of peroxisome proliferators. In contrast to fatty acid oxidation in the mitochondrion, initial fatty acyl-CoA formation within the peroxisome does not require fatty acyl carnitine formation for entry into peroxisomes. During the next metabolic step, in which *trans*-enoyl fatty acyl-CoA is formed, another difference is that electrons produced are transferred to FAD to form $FADH_2$, which is then transferred directly to oxygen to form hydrogen peroxide. Hydrogen peroxide is detoxified by catalase to form water and oxygen. (In the mitochondrion, electrons are delivered to the mitochondrial electron transport system that ultimately generates water and ATP.) The significance of this difference is that both lack of ATP production and generation of hydrogen peroxide in the peroxisomes, in the presence of transitional metals, can yield toxic hydroxyl radicals and can promote lipid peroxidation and oxidant injury.

NADH generated in subsequent reactions has to be removed from the peroxisomes, whereas in mitochondria, NADH can enter the electron transport cycle and generate additional ATP molecules. Peroxisomal enzymes can metabolize only long-chain fatty acids with a minimal chain length of 10 carbons and a maximal length of 24 carbons. As in mitochondria, beta oxidation in peroxisomes proceeds similarly by 2-carbon acetyl-CoA cleavage until octanoyl-CoA is formed. Octanoyl-CoA is then combined with carnitine to form fatty acyl carnitine, which can be transported by the mitochondrial inner membrane transporter and undergo completion of beta oxidation. Acyl-CoA formed in peroxisomes by beta oxidation of fatty acids can diffuse out of the peroxisomes after formation of acetyl carnitine.[125]

The regulation of peroxisomal metabolism of fatty acids appears to be solely at the level of substrate availability, which may be regulated by a family of soluble fatty acid binding proteins present in the cytosol of all cells. The peroxisomal pathway provides a supply of acetyl-CoA that does not require citrate formation and that can be used in fatty acid synthesis. Because the initial electron transfer is not coupled to the mitochondrial electron transport system, peroxisomal fatty acid oxidation is less efficient than mitochondrial beta oxidation and may provide a means of eliminating fatty acids with energy loss. Peroxisomes proliferate on administration of a large number of hypolipidemic agents, such as clofibrate, with a resulting 5- to 10-fold increase in the relative contribution of peroxisomal fatty acid beta oxidation. Because peroxisomal beta oxidation produces less ATP than does beta oxidation in mitochondria, a relative increase in peroxisomal fatty acid beta oxidation can lead to a reduction in lipid mass and to weight loss. The hydrogen peroxide generated by this pathway

can be used by catalase for the oxidation of substrates such as ethanol.

Increased TG synthesis, reduced synthesis of lipid transport proteins (see later), and a decreased level of beta oxidation can result in the accumulation of fat within hepatocytes (steatosis), as in alcoholic steatosis, which occurs when a large percentage of the total caloric intake is derived from ethanol. Alteration in the redox potential with excess NADH produced by ethanol metabolism results in an increased NADH/NAD ratio, which favors the formation of α-glycerol phosphate, which in turn promotes TG formation. In addition, a decrease in NAD content in mitochondria may reduce fatty acid beta oxidation, thereby contributing to fatty acid accumulation.[126]

Lipoproteins

Apolipoproteins (apo), which are synthesized by the liver, in combination with TG, phospholipids, cholesterol, and cholesteryl esters, constitute circulating lipoproteins, which mediate the transport of lipids from the liver into the plasma and from the plasma into the liver and other tissues. The liver also expresses cell surface receptors for circulating lipoproteins and modulates plasma levels of these important macromolecules.[127]

Types

Lipoproteins were originally classified according to their relative density, which is inversely related to their particle size. In increasing order of density, they are: chylomicrons, very-low-density lipoproteins (VLDL), intermediate-density lipoproteins (IDL), low-density lipoproteins (LDL), and high-density lipoproteins (HDL). Density differences in these particles reflect the type and amount of specific lipids and the proportion of protein present within these lipoprotein fractions.[127] Specific apolipoproteins bind lipids to form lipoproteins, which are modified by enzymes in plasma or endothelial cells and act as ligands for specific lipoprotein receptors that mediate their uptake by target tissues.

The lipid components are in constant dynamic flux because of delivery of lipids and cholesterol to cells, transfer to other lipoproteins (mediated by lipid transfer proteins), and catalysis by lipolytic enzymes. TG are the major lipids contained in chylomicrons that are generated in the intestinal epithelial cells and VLDL produced in the liver. They are the energy source for peripheral tissues and components of cellular membrane structures. Cholesterol is the major lipid in LDL and HDL. Cholesterol, unlike TG, is not used as a fuel source but as a structural component of membranes and as a precursor for steroid hormones. Trafficking of cholesterol is usually in the form of cholesteryl ester, which is generated in the plasma by the activity of lecithin-cholesterol acyltransferase (LCAT) (see later).

Tangier's disease, a rare autosomal recessive disorder characterized by the accumulation of cholesteryl esters in reticuloendothelial cells, including the tonsils, thymus, and lymph nodes, as well as liver, spleen, and gallbladder, in combination with the near absence of serum HDL cholesterol, is now recognized to be caused by mutations in the gene encoding ATP-binding cassette transporter A1 (*ABCA1*), a member of the ABC supergene family.[128] Affected patients classically present with enlarged, orange-colored tonsils and have a 4- to 6-fold increased risk of atherosclerotic heart disease. The location of the transporter at the plasma membrane suggests that it mediates the active transport ("flipping") of cholesteryl ester from the inner to the outer leaflet of the plasma membrane, from which it can be transferred to apolipoproteins and secreted (see Chapter 36).[128]

Apolipoproteins

The major apolipoproteins associated with TG transport are apoB-100, which is synthesized in the liver, and apoB-48, which is synthesized in the intestine.[129] Both proteins are translated from the same mRNA. In human intestinal epithelium, the apoB mRNA undergoes post-transcriptional RNA editing, which generates a stop codon by cytidine deamination that results in the translation of a form of apoB that is approximately 48% of the size of the full-length apoB-100 generated in the liver. The carboxy-terminal domain that is absent in apoB-48 is essential for binding to the LDL receptor. Unlike the apoB-100-containing VLDL, chylomicron remnants, which contain apoB-48, are rapidly cleared from plasma and do not give rise to LDL.[129]

ApoC is synthesized predominately in the liver, with minor expression in the intestine and other organs, and is composed of 3 different gene products that may inhibit the uptake of chylomicron remnants by the liver. ApoC-1 is a minor component of VLDL, HDL, and IDL and is of unknown function. ApoC-II is present in VLDL, IDL, HDL, and chylomicrons and is an essential activator of lipoprotein lipase (LPL) (see later). Inherited deficiency of apoC-II causes hypertriglyceridemia. ApoC-III is present in IDL, HDL, and chylomicrons and may be an inhibitor of LPL activity.[130]

ApoE is synthesized in the liver and is found on all lipoproteins. ApoE is important for removal of lipoprotein remnants in the serum, can bind to the LDL receptor and other membrane proteins, and is important in targeting lipoproteins to specific receptors on peripheral cells. Three major alleles of the apoE gene exist (ε2, ε3, and ε4), with the ε3 allele being the most abundant and the ε2/ε3 genotype being the most frequent. Each allele possesses a different ability to bind to the LDL receptor. Absence of apoE leads to reduced clearance of chylomicron and VLDL remnants, resulting in elevated plasma levels and a consequent increase in the risk of atherosclerosis.[131] ApoE is also important in lipid transport in the central nervous system, especially after neuronal injury. Inheritance of a single apoε4 allele is associated with the onset of Alzheimer's disease 6 to 8 years earlier than that associated with the ε3/ε3 genotype.[132]

ApoA-I and -II are synthesized in the liver and intestine. ApoA-I is the major component of HDL lipoproteins. In a lipid-poor state, apoA-I accepts cholesterol from the cell membrane. ApoA-I is a key activator of LCAT, which enhances cholesterol esterification in the plasma, and the absence of a specific conserved region in apoA-I causes loss of its LCAT activating property. ApoA-II is another component of HDL. ApoA-IV is a minor constituent synthesized in the intestine.[133]

Lipolytic Enzymes and Lipid Transport Proteins

LPL is synthesized in fat and muscle cells and is located in the luminal surface of the capillary bed of adipose, lung, and muscle tissues.[134] LPL catalyzes lipolysis of TG present in VLDL, chylomicrons, or HDL. LPL is stimulated by fasting, fatty acids, hormones, and catecholamines. Patients who are homozygous for LPL deficiency present with severe hypertriglyceridemia in childhood and pancreatitis.

Hepatic TG lipase (HTGL) is another member of the lipase family. It is synthesized in the liver and binds to the luminal surface of hepatic endothelial cells. It is involved in lipolysis of VLDL or IDL and thus plays a major role in LDL formation. HDL may be another substrate for HTGL activity. Inherited deficiency of LPL leads to accumulation of large particles containing both apoB-100 and apoB-48, with almost complete absence of smaller apoB-containing lipoprotein. In animal studies, inhibition of HTGL results in accumulation of VLDL and IDL, with the enrichment of HDL in TG.

In plasma, lipid exchange between particles is facilitated by the activity of LCAT and cholesteryl ester transfer protein (CETP).[134] LCAT is synthesized in the liver, and apoA-I is a cofactor for LCAT activity. CETP is synthesized predominantly in the liver and circulates in association with HDL. CETP mediates the exchange of cholesteryl esters from HDL and TG from chylomicrons or VLDL. The activity of LCAT, in combination with the lipid transfer proteins, CETP and phospholipid transfer protein (PLTP), is essential for the transfer of cholesterol from nonhepatic tissue to the liver.[134]

Intestinal and Hepatic Lipid Transport

The liver functions as the hub for receiving fatty acids and cholesterol from the diet and peripheral tissues, packages them into lipoprotein complexes, and releases the complexes into the circulation (Fig. 72-4). Following absorption by intestinal epithelial cells, fatty acids are formed into TG, and cholesterol is esterified. The lipids are packaged into nascent chylomicrons composed predominantly of TG (85% to 92%), phospholipids (6% to 12%), cholesteryl ester (1% to 3%), fat-soluble vitamins, and the following apolipoproteins (1% to 3%): apoB-48, apoA-I, apoA-II, and apoA-IV.[135] Nascent chylomicrons enter the interstitial space and are carried into the systemic venous circulation via the thoracic duct. In the interstitial space, chylomicrons acquire apoC-II, which activates LPL, thereby promoting TG release. TG release may be reduced by acquisition of apoC-III, which may inhibit LPL activity. The addition of apoE is critical for targeting the chylomicron remnant, which can then be taken up by hepatocytes through the chylomicron remnant receptor.

Release of TG by LPL and extraction by peripheral tissues increases the relative cholesteryl ester concentration in chylomicron remnants, which are taken up by hepatocytes via a hepatocyte membrane transporter that recognizes a binding domain on apoE. The endocytosed chylomicron remnants are targeted to lysosomes, where they are degraded. Inherited mutations of the binding domain of apoE reduce chylomicron remnant clearance. When chylomicron excretion is delayed, as occurs with mutations of the binding domain of apoE or reduced LPL activity or apoC-II levels, chylomicron remnants that accumulate in the serum may be taken up by endothelial cells or macrophages, which transform into foamy cells, which are precursors of fatty streaks and atheromas. Increased VLDL secretion resulting from excess fatty acid absorption can also compete with the chylomicron remnant uptake system.

Fatty acids released from adipocytes by the action of intracellular hormone-sensitive lipase are bound to serum albumin and transported to other tissues including the liver, where they are used for synthesis of phospholipids and TG.[136] The liver synthesizes cholesterol from low-molecular-weight precursors. Hepatic cholesterol synthesis is regulated by the rate-limiting enzyme HMG-CoA reductase. Lipids are exported from the liver as VLDL particles, which are the major carriers of plasma TG during nonabsorptive states.[103] Lipids may be stored temporarily in the liver as lipid droplets and cholesteryl esters, excreted directly into bile, or metabolized into bile acids. During nutrient deprivation, FFA released by lipolysis of adipose tissues are taken up by hepatocytes, resulting in an increased number of lipid droplets within hepatocytes. The lipid droplets become enclosed into autophagosomes, probably through recruitment of LC3, which initiates the formation of the limiting membrane through ATG7-dependent conjugation (see earlier). This process, termed *lipophagy*, leads to lysosomal hydrolysis of fat, releasing FFA as well as reducing the hepatic lipid load.[86] Decreased autophagy in the liver with

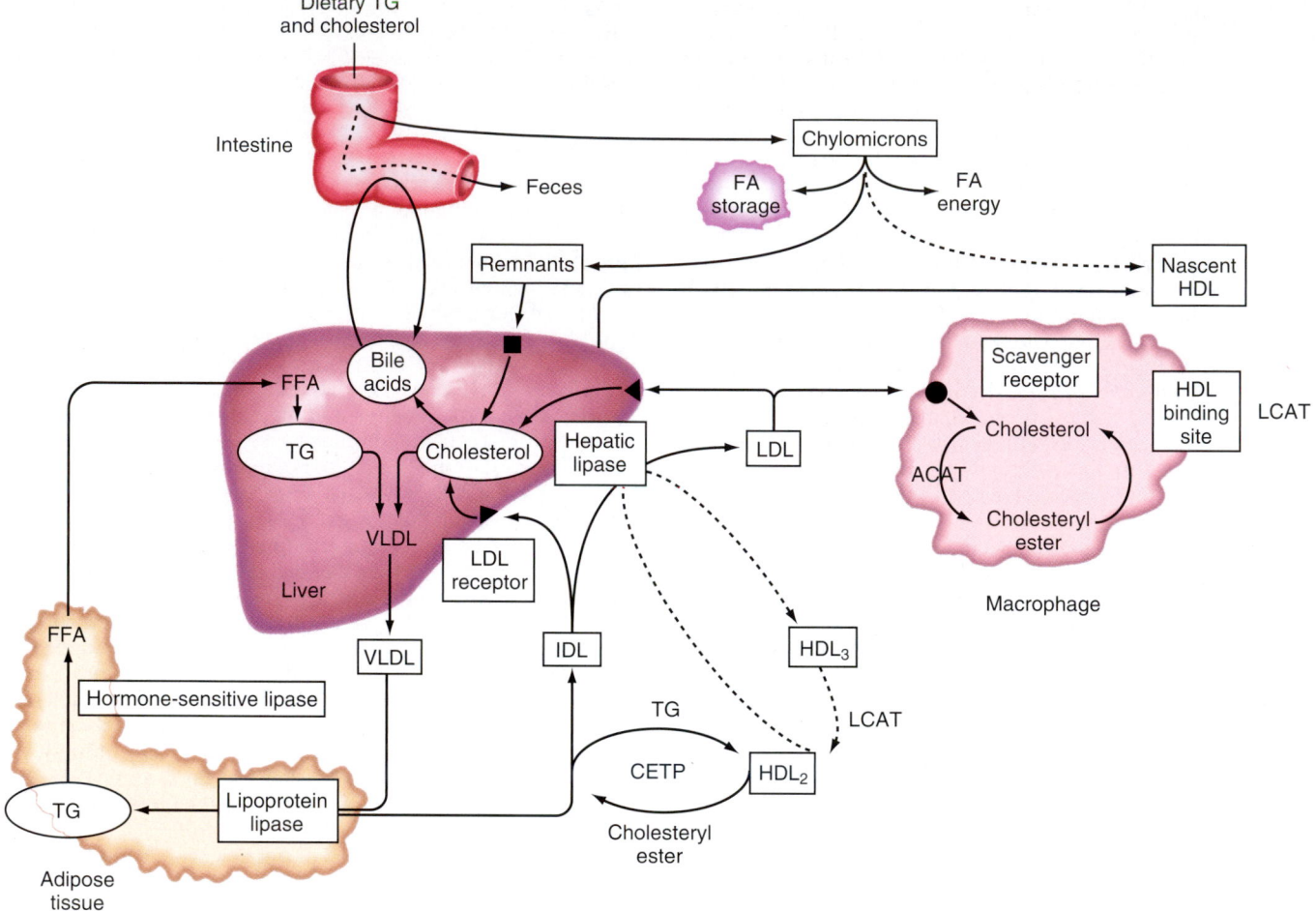

FIGURE 72-4. Lipoprotein metabolism. ACAT, acylcholesterol acyltransferase; CETP, cholesteryl ester transfer protein; FA, fatty acid; FFA, free fatty acid; HDL, high-density lipoproteins; IDL, intermediate-density lipoproteins; LCAT, lecithin-cholesterol acyltransferase; LDL, low-density lipoproteins; VLDL, very-low-density lipoproteins. *(Modified from Shepherd J. Lipoprotein metabolism. An overview. Drugs 1994; 47[Suppl 2]:1-10.)*

aging may contribute to hepatic lipid accumulation,[81] which could account in part for the rising incidence of the metabolic syndrome (see Chapter 87).[137]

The liver is the major site of sterol excretion from the body and is the site of bile acid synthesis. The coordinated input, synthesis, and excretion of sterols require complex regulation of multiple enzymatic pathways. Bile acids returning to the liver via the enterohepatic circulation modulate these enzyme activities. Bile acids recycle 20 to 30 times per day via the enterohepatic circulation and use specific transmembrane transporters at apical and basolateral domains of hepatocyte plasma membrane, as well as intracellular binding proteins.[138] In the terminal ileum, a great majority of the bile acid molecules are reabsorbed via a sodium-dependent bile acid transporter. Bile acids are also important in micellization of fats for intestinal absorption and as coactivators of bile acid–dependent lipase activity. FXR, a member of the sterol nuclear receptor family, binds to and is activated by bile salts. Heterodimers of activated FXR and RXR modulate the coordinated regulation of multiple genes that encode key bile salt transporters, such as the sodium-dependent taurocholate pump (NTCP) at the sinusoidal domain of hepatocytes, bile salt export pump (BSEP) at the canalicular domain, intestinal bile acid transporter (IBAT) in the terminal ileum, and cholesterol-7α-hydroxylase in hepatocytes (see Chapter 64).[139]

Transport of ApoB-Containing Lipoproteins

In the fasting state, VLDL, which is synthesized in the liver, replaces chylomicrons as the major transporter of TG and cholesterol. In addition to the full-length apoB-100, VLDL contains TG (taken up from plasma or synthesized in the liver), cholesteryl esters (exogenous or endogenous), and phospholipids.[140] During fasting, fatty acids in VLDL are derived predominantly from the activity of hormone-sensitive lipase in adipocytes, whereas after a meal, dietary fatty acids are the major source. Fatty acids may be taken up by hepatocytes by passive diffusion or via fatty acid transport proteins in the sinusoidal domain of the cell membrane. In hepatocyte cytosol, fatty acids are stored bound to the abundant 12-kd fatty acid binding protein (FABP) family, which may direct fatty acids to specific subcellular targets, such as the smooth ER for VLDL synthesis or peroxisomes for beta oxidation. FABPs are transcriptionally regulated by peroxisome proliferating agents (e.g., fibrates), suggesting that their role is physiologic in global lipid metabolism.

ApoB-100 is the predominant transport carrier in VLDL; apoC-I, C-II, C-III, and apoE arise from other lipoproteins within the serum. ApoB-100 synthesis and VLDL secretion are regulated by the availability of cotransported lipids and sterols in the smooth ER. ApoB-100 synthesis may change dramatically without alteration in apoB-100 mRNA levels.[141] Following synthesis in the smooth ER, apoB-100 interacts with newly synthesized TG and cholesteryl esters that enter the ER via specific membrane transporters. The apoB-lipid complex is translocated into the lumen, transported through the Golgi apparatus, and secreted into the sinusoidal space as VLDL. When the lipid components are not available, apoB-100 undergoes degradation in the ER. During periods of low plasma TG levels, the liver secretes smaller IDL-like particles or even LDL-type particles.

In the plasma, the activity of LPL and HTGL removes TG from VLDL, generating progressively smaller and denser IDL and LDL particles. Conversion of IDL to LDL requires the activity of apoE. LDL particles become enriched in cholesteryl esters, both by removal of TG and acquisition of cholesteryl esters from other lipoproteins, predominantly HDL, with release of apoC to HDL. LDL is subsequently removed from the circulation by LDL receptors in the liver and peripheral tissues. Subpopulations of VLDL that begin as large VLDL undergo lipolysis and are converted to IDL, which is taken up via the LDL receptor.

Transport of ApoA-Containing High-Density Lipoproteins

HDL, another major class of lipoproteins secreted by the liver, appears to have a protective role against atherosclerosis. HDL is a heterogeneous population of lipoproteins that can be separated by sophisticated analytic centrifugation techniques. Nascent HDL is formed in the liver and intestine by lipolysis of VLDL and chylomicrons, respectively, with modification by peripheral tissue. The major protein constituents of HDL are apoA-I and apoA-II, with minor amounts of apoA-IV, apoC, apoE, and others.[142] In humans, apoA-I is synthesized in the liver and intestine. Nascent apoA-containing lipoprotein complexes that appear as discoid particles can be transformed into HDL particles in the serum by the action of LCAT and the lipid transfer proteins CETP and PLTP.

The HDL$_3$ subclass is particularly important because these cholesterol-poor particles are able to deliver cholesterol extracted from peripheral membranes and provide a substrate for plasma LCAT activity. Cholesteryl esters formed by LCAT are extremely hydrophobic and move into the core of the lipoprotein complex, thereby providing space on the surface of the lipoprotein for extraction of additional cholesterol from cell membranes. This complex enlarges with increasing amounts of cholesteryl esters, which are able to accommodate apoC-II and C-III, thereby resulting in HDL$_2$ formation. CETP removes esterified cholesterol from HDL in exchange for TG, which are eventually hydrolyzed by HTGL, thereby regenerating small HDL. Acquisition of apoC-II also promotes LPL activity, thus increasing lipolysis.[134]

The movement of apolipoproteins between HDL and chylomicrons allows the recycling of lipids and proteins between these two pools. Cholesterol and phospholipids are also transferred to the chylomicrons as TG are released by LPL activity to local tissues. As the remnant is further processed, apoC-II and apoC-III, phospholipids, and cholesterol are transferred back to HDL. TG that are transferred from VLDL and chylomicrons to HDL are more accessible to lipolysis by endothelial-based lipases because of their smaller size. With the removal of TG, these particles revert to HDL$_3$ and apoC-II, after which apoC-II and apoE recycle to chylomicrons and VLDL.

Lipoprotein Receptors

The major lipoprotein receptors for LDL, chylomicron remnants, HDL, and the scavenger receptor are members of the larger LDL receptor supergene family.[143] These receptors share 4 major structural features: (1) cysteine-rich complement-type repeats, (2) EGF precursor-like repeats, (3) a transmembrane domain, and (4) a cytoplasmic domain.[144]

Low-Density Lipoprotein Receptor

The LDL receptor exists as an oligomeric surface glycoprotein that plays a pivotal role in LDL clearance and cholesterol homeostasis. It binds ligands at the cell surface, after which the ligand-receptor complex is internalized via the classic endocytotic pathway. The ligand dissociates from the receptor in acidic endosomal vesicles. Subsequently, the ligand is delivered to lysosomes for degradation and the receptor returns to the surface. The LDL receptor is present on all cell types; however, the liver contains approximately 70% of the total body pool of LDL receptors. The LDL receptor recognizes apoE and apoB-100, but not apoB-48. ApoE-containing chylomicron remnants, VLDL, LDL, IDL, and HDL can all be taken up via the LDL receptor. Almost two thirds of LDL is cleared by this receptor. Homozygous deficiency of the functional LDL receptor occurs in approximately 1 in 1 million persons and is associated with accelerated atherosclerosis manifesting in childhood (familial hypercholesterolemia).[143]

Very-Low-Density Lipoprotein Receptor

The VLDL receptor has a high-sequence homology with the LDL receptor but is expressed predominantly in extrahepatic tissues such as heart, muscle, and fat. Unlike the LDL receptor, the VLDL receptor does not bind to apoB and may serve specifically to take up TG-rich apoE-containing lipoproteins, such as VLDL or IDL.[143,144]

Chylomicron Remnant Receptor

The chylomicron remnant receptor accepts apoE as a ligand. Chylomicron remnants are removed from the circulation exclusively by the liver, probably because these large complexes can penetrate the unique sinusoidal vascular space. The multifunctional α_2-macroglobulin/LDL receptor-related protein (LRP) is the chylomicron remnant receptor.[145] LRP is present in liver, brain, and muscle. In cultured cells, LRP is able to mediate the endocytosis of apoE-containing chylomicron remnants. Mice that lack LRP in the liver do not have hepatic chylomicron remnant uptake, confirming that LRP is the major chylomicron remnant receptor. Unlike the LDL receptor, LRP is able to bind a number of unrelated ligands, such as lipoprotein, proteinase-inhibitor complex, and protein-lipid complex.

Low-Density Lipoprotein Scavenger Receptor

Ligands for the scavenger receptor A (SR-A) include lipopolysaccharides, polyanionic lipids, and LDL in which some of the free lysine residues have been chemically modified.[146] These receptors exist in two forms as trimeric integral membrane glycoproteins in endothelial cells, macrophages, and Kupffer cells. Oxidized LDL is internalized via the scavenger receptors but is metabolized poorly in macrophages, leading to the accumulation of cholesteryl esters within the cell. Monocytes, which migrate into lipid-enriched atherosclerotic lesions, can also be induced to express SR-A.

High-Density Lipoprotein Receptor

A high-affinity HDL binding protein has been identified in the plasma membrane of hepatocytes, macrophages, adrenal cells, and adipocytes.[146] These receptors appear to recognize specifically apoA present in HDL particles. The HDL receptor does not mediate endocytosis but allows only selective delivery of lipids to and from the HDL lipoproteins. By mediating the transfer of cholesterol from the plasma membrane to the HDL lipoprotein, the HDL receptor facilitates reverse cholesterol transport. The HDL receptor is a class B scavenger receptor referred to as *SR-B1*.[142] This receptor is most abundant in the liver, ovary, and adrenal glands—organs previously shown to be the principal sites of cholesterol uptake from HDL in vivo. HDL is a major source of cholesterol secreted in bile. Overexpression of SR-B1 in mouse liver increases biliary cholesterol secretion and reduces plasma HDL.[147] Conversely, deficiency of this receptor results in decreased biliary cholesterol secretion.[148]

Derangement of Lipid Metabolism in Liver Disease

The most common lipid abnormality in patients with chronic liver disease is hypertriglyceridemia (plasma levels of 250 to 500 mg/dL), which is found in patients with alcoholic or viral liver disease and tends to resolve when the liver disease improves. Excess ethanol ingestion causes predominantly hypertriglyceridemia, due to increased fatty acid synthesis, and decreased beta oxidation of fatty acids, resulting from increased NADH production by alcohol metabolism. Moderate alcohol ingestion is associated with increased HDL$_3$ levels, which may reduce the risk of atherosclerosis. LDL, HDL, and total serum cholesterol levels decrease progressively, with cirrhosis advancing from Child-Pugh class A to class C (see Chapters 73, 74, and 92). The serum cholesterol level may be a useful prognostic marker in patients with noncholestatic liver diseases.[149]

Cholestatic disorders manifest with a distinct pattern of dyslipoproteinemia because of the retention of cholesterol, phospholipids, and bile salts that are normally secreted in bile.[150] A prolonged increase in total serum cholesterol and lipid levels, as seen in PBC, can be associated with formation of xanthomata (see Chapter 91). Within the LDL fraction of the serum of cholestatic patients, 3 distinct lipoproteins can be identified, namely, β$_2$-lipoprotein (TG rich), also known as *lipoprotein Y (LP-Y), lipoprotein X (LP-X),* and *normal LDL.* LP-Y appears to be a remnant of a TG-rich lipoprotein that is distinct from IDL. Cholestatic patients with elevated TG levels often have clear (not lipemic) serum because most of the TG are contained in LP-Y and LDL. LP-X is a complex composed of equimolar amounts of excess phospholipid and cholesterol in combination with albumin and certain members of the apoC family. The phospholipid flippase activity of multidrug resistance protein-3 (MDR3), also termed *ATP-binding cassette protein B4* (see Chapter 64), is essential for LP-X formation. Mice lacking mdr2 (the murine homolog of MDR3) are unable to form LP-X during cholestasis caused by complete bile duct obstruction.[151]

In patients with chronic parenchymal liver disease, plasma cholesteryl ester levels are often reduced, a finding that suggests that LCAT activity is diminished because of impaired hepatic synthesis. Alternatively, decreased LCAT activity may result from reduced apoC-II levels or release of cholesteryl ester hydrolase from damaged hepatocytes, with conversion of cholesteryl esters to cholesterol. Chronic dyslipoproteinemia in these patients can also lead to alterations in cellular membrane lipids, resulting in formation of abnormal RBCs, such as echinocytes, and altered membrane function with potential pathophysiologic consequences.

KEY REFERENCES

Full references for this chapter can be found on www.expertconsult.com.

3. Zegers MMP, Hoekstra D. Mechanisms and functional features of polarized membrane traffic in epithelial and hepatic cells. Biochem J 1998; 336:257-69.
7. Vinken M, Henkens T, De Rop E, et al. Biology and pathobiology of gap junctional channels in hepatocytes. Hepatology 2008; 47:1077-88.
18. Nakielny S, Dreyfuss G. Transport of proteins and RNAs in and out of the nucleus. Cell 1999; 99:677-90.
35. Newmeyer DD, Ferguson-Miller S. Mitochondria: Releasing power for life and unleashing the machineries of death. Cell 2003; 112:481-90.
45. Conner SD, Schmid SL. Regulated portals of entry into the cell. Nature 2003; 422:37-44.
53. Xie G, Wang X, Wang L, et al. Role of differentiation of liver sinusoidal endothelial cells in progression and regression of hepatic fibrosis in rats. Gastroenterology 2012; 142:918-27.
58. Hernandez-Gea V, Friedman SL. Pathogenesis of liver fibrosis. Annu Rev Pathol 2011; 6:425-56.
62. Bedossa P, Paradis V. Liver extracellular matrix in health and disease. J Pathol 2003; 200:504-15.
69. Taub R. Liver regeneration: From myth to mechanism. Nat Rev Mol Cell Biol 2004; 5:836-47.
75. Yin XM, Ding WX. Death receptor activation-induced hepatocyte apoptosis and liver injury. Curr Mol Med 2003; 3:491-508.
77. Choi AM, Ryter SW, Levine B. Autophagy in human health and disease. N Engl J Med 2013; 368:651-62.
91. Karpen SJ. Nuclear receptor regulation of hepatic function. J Hepatol 2002; 36:832-50.
104. Anghel SI, Wahli W. Fat poetry: A kingdom for PPAR gamma. Cell Res 2007; 17:486-511.
111. Nordlie RC, Foster JD, Lange AJ. Regulation of glucose production by the liver. Annu Rev Nutr 1999; 19:379-406.
127. Tiwari S, Siddiqi SA. Intracellular trafficking and secretion of VLDL. Arterioscler Thromb Vasc Biol 2012; 32:1079-86.

When appropriately ordered and interpreted, serum biochemical tests, the so-called "liver function tests" or "liver chemistries," can be useful in the evaluation and management of patients with liver disorders. The term *liver biochemical tests* is preferable to *liver function tests* because the most commonly used tests—the aminotransferases and alkaline phosphatase—do not measure a known function of the liver. These tests have the potential to identify liver disease, distinguish among types of liver disorders, gauge the severity and progression of liver dysfunction, and monitor response to therapy. Understanding the shortcomings of these tests, however, is important. No test can accurately assess the liver's total functional capacity; biochemical tests measure only a few of the thousands of biochemical functions performed by the liver. Furthermore, considered individually, these tests lack sensitivity and specificity for liver injury; a battery of tests must be used to evaluate the liver. The standard battery of tests that is most helpful in assessing liver disease includes total and direct bilirubin, albumin, prothrombin time, and the serum enzymes: ALT, AST, alkaline phosphatase (ALP), and occasionally GGTP and 5′ nucleotidase (5′NT). Interpretation of these results in concert with careful history taking and a physical examination may suggest a specific type of liver injury, thereby allowing a directed evaluation, risk assessment for surgical procedures, and estimation of prognosis. Other more specialized tests include quantitative tests of liver function and a growing number of options to assess the degree of hepatic fibrosis.

BILIRUBIN (See Chapter 21)

Metabolism

Bilirubin is a breakdown product of heme (ferroprotoporphyrin IX). About 4 mg/kg body weight of bilirubin is produced each day, nearly 80% from the breakdown of hemoglobin in senescent red blood cells and prematurely destroyed erythroid cells in the bone marrow and the remainder from the turnover of hemoproteins such as myoglobin and cytochromes distributed throughout the body.[1] The initial steps of bilirubin metabolism occur in reticuloendothelial cells, predominantly in the spleen. Heme is converted to biliverdin by the microsomal enzyme heme oxygenase. Biliverdin is then converted to bilirubin by the cytosolic enzyme biliverdin reductase.

Bilirubin formed in the reticuloendothelium is lipid soluble and virtually insoluble in water. In order to be transported in blood, unconjugated bilirubin must be solubilized. The process is initiated by reversible, noncovalent binding to albumin, which has both high-affinity and lower-affinity binding sites for unconjugated bilirubin. The unconjugated bilirubin-albumin complex passes readily through the fenestrations in the endothelium lining the hepatic sinusoids into the space of Disse, where the bilirubin dissociates from albumin and is taken up by hepatocytes via a protein-mediated, facilitated process, possibly mediated by a liver-specific organic anion transport protein.

After entering the hepatocyte, unconjugated bilirubin is bound in the cytosol to a number of proteins, including proteins in the glutathione S-transferase superfamily.[2] These proteins serve to reduce efflux of bilirubin back into the serum and present the bilirubin for conjugation. The enzyme uridine-5′-diphosphate (UDP) glucuronyl transferase found in the endoplasmic reticulum solubilizes bilirubin by conjugating it to glucuronic acid to produce bilirubin monoglucuronide and diglucuronide.[3] The now hydrophilic bilirubin diffuses to the canalicular membrane for excretion into the bile canaliculi. Conjugated bilirubin is transported across the canalicular membrane by the multidrug resistance-associated protein 2 (MRP2) via an ATP-dependent process.[4] This is the only energy-dependent step in bilirubin metabolism and explains why even patients with fulminant hepatic failure have a predominantly conjugated hyperbilirubinemia. Once in the bile, conjugated bilirubin passes undisturbed until it reaches the distal ileum and colon, where bacteria containing β-glucuronidases hydrolyze conjugated bilirubin to unconjugated bilirubin, which is further reduced by bacteria to colorless urobilinogen.[5] The urobilinogen is either excreted unchanged, oxidized and excreted as urobilin (which has an orange color), or absorbed passively by the intestine into the portal system. The majority of the absorbed urobilinogen is re-excreted by the liver. A small percentage filters across the renal glomerulus and is excreted in urine. Unconjugated bilirubin is never found in urine because in the serum it is bound to albumin and not filtered by the glomerulus. The presence of bilirubin in urine indicates conjugated hyperbilirubinemia and hepatobiliary disease.

Measurement

The terms *direct* and *indirect bilirubin*, which correspond roughly to conjugated and unconjugated bilirubin, respectively, derive from the original van den Bergh reaction.[6] Serum bilirubin is still measured in clinical laboratories by some modification of this method.[7] In this assay, bilirubin is exposed to diazotized sulfanilic acid. The conjugated fraction of bilirubin reacts promptly, or "directly," with the diazo reagent without the need for an accelerant and thereby allows measurement of the conjugated bilirubin fraction by photometric analysis within 30 to 60 seconds. The total bilirubin is measured 30 to 60 minutes after the addition of an accelerant such as alcohol or caffeine. The unconjugated, or indirect, fraction is then determined by subtracting the direct component from the total bilirubin.

Newer and more accurate methods of measuring bilirubin, such as high-performance liquid chromatography, have been developed but are not generally available because they are more difficult to perform and do not add additional information beyond that provided by the diazo method in most clinical situations. These newer methods allow the identification of delta bilirubin—conjugated bilirubin tightly linked to albumin through covalent binding. Delta bilirubin is found in cases of prolonged and severe elevation of serum conjugated bilirubin levels, and because of the strength of the covalent binding, delta bilirubin has the half-life of albumin, 14 to 21 days, which far exceeds the usual serum half-life of bilirubin of 4 hours. The identification of delta bilirubin explains why the decline in serum bilirubin in some patients with prolonged jaundice seems to lag behind clinical recovery and why some patients with conjugated hyperbilirubinemia do not have bilirubinuria.

Using the diazo method, normal values of total serum bilirubin are between 1.0 and 1.5 mg/dL, with 95% of a normal population falling between 0.2 and 0.9 mg/dL.[8] Normal values for the indirect component are between 0.8 and 1.2 mg/dL. The diazo method, however, tends to overestimate the amount of conjugated bilirubin, particularly within the normal range. As a result, "normal" ranges for conjugated bilirubin have crept upward over time. In general, if the direct acting fraction is less than 15% of the total, the bilirubin can be considered to be entirely indirect. The most frequently reported upper limit of normal for conjugated bilirubin is 0.3 mg/dL. The presence of even a mild increase in conjugated bilirubin in the serum should raise the possibility of liver injury. The measurement and fractionation of serum bilirubin in patients with jaundice does not allow differentiation between parenchymal (hepatocellular) and obstructive (cholestatic) jaundice.

The magnitude and duration of hyperbilirubinemia have not been critically assessed as prognostic markers. In general, the higher the serum bilirubin level in patients with viral hepatitis, the greater the hepatocellular damage and the longer the course of disease. Patients may die, however, of acute liver failure with only a modest elevation of serum bilirubin. Total serum bilirubin correlates with poor outcomes in alcoholic hepatitis and is a critical component of the MELD score, which is used to estimate survival of patients with end-stage liver disease (see later and Chapter 97).

Approach to the Patient with an Elevated Level

Hyperbilirubinemia may be the result of overproduction of bilirubin through excessive breakdown of hemoglobin; impaired hepatocellular uptake, conjugation, or excretion of bilirubin; or regurgitation of unconjugated and conjugated bilirubin from damaged hepatocytes or bile ducts. The presence of conjunctival icterus suggests a total serum bilirubin level of at least 3.0 mg/dL but does not allow differentiation between conjugated and unconjugated hyperbilirubinemia. Tea- or cola-colored urine may indicate the presence of bilirubinuria and thus conjugated hyperbilirubinemia.

The evaluation of the patient with an isolated elevation of the serum bilirubin level is quite different from that of the patient with an elevated bilirubin associated with elevated liver enzyme levels; the latter suggests either a hepatocellular or cholestatic process, as discussed later. The first step in the evaluation of a patient with an isolated elevation of the serum bilirubin level is to fractionate the bilirubin to determine if it is conjugated or unconjugated (Fig. 73-1). If less than 15% of the total is conjugated, one can be assured that virtually all the serum bilirubin is unconjugated. Overproduction of bilirubin as a result of excessive breakdown of hemoglobin can occur

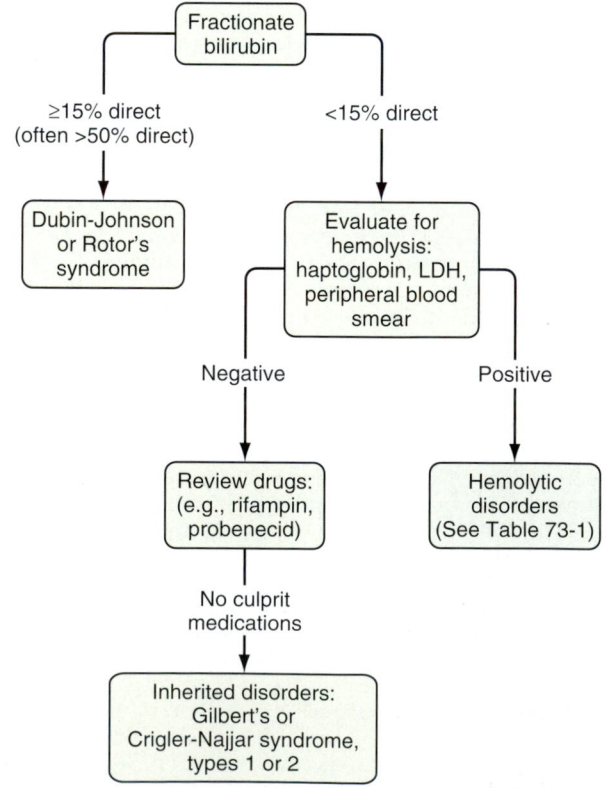

FIGURE 73-1. Evaluation of an isolated elevation of the serum bilirubin level.

TABLE 73-1 Causes and Mechanisms of Isolated Hyperbilirubinemia in Adults

Cause	Mechanism
Indirect Hyperbilirubinemia	
Hemolytic Disorders	Overproduction of bilirubin
Inherited	
Red cell enzyme defects (e.g., glucose-6-phosphate dehydrogenase deficiency)	
Sickle cell disease	
Spherocytosis and elliptocytosis	
Acquired	
Drugs and toxins	
Hypersplenism	
Immune mediated	
Paroxysmal nocturnal hemoglobinuria	
Traumatic: macro- or microvascular injury	
Ineffective Erythropoiesis	Overproduction of bilirubin
Cobalamin deficiency	
Folate deficiency	
Profound iron deficiency	
Thalassemia	
Drugs: Rifampin, Probenecid	Impaired hepatocellular uptake of bilirubin
Inherited Conditions	Impaired conjugation of bilirubin
Crigler-Najjar syndrome types I and II	
Gilbert's syndrome	
Other	
Hematoma and massive blood transfusion	Overproduction of bilirubin
Direct Hyperbilirubinemia	
Inherited Conditions	
Dubin-Johnson syndrome	Impaired excretion of conjugated bilirubin
Rotor's syndrome	

with any of a number of inherited or acquired disorders (Table 73-1). The patient's medication history should be reviewed for drugs that can cause impaired hepatocellular uptake of bilirubin. If no cause is identified, a genetic enzyme deficiency that results in impaired conjugation of bilirubin, the most common of which is Gilbert's syndrome, is likely.

As discussed in Chapter 21, Gilbert's syndrome is common, with a reported frequency of 6% to 12% (see Table 21-2). A mutation in the TATAA element in the 5′ promoter region of the UDP glucuronyl transferase gene results in a reduction in enzyme activity to approximately one third of normal. The mildly elevated indirect serum hyperbilirubinemia seen in Gilbert's syndrome is of no clinical consequence. This benign clinical course contrasts with those of much rarer conditions, Crigler-Najjar syndrome types I and II (see Table 21-2). The mutations in these conditions result in significantly reduced UDP glucuronyl transferase activity: less than 10% in Crigler-Najjar type II and complete absence of enzyme activity in Crigler-Najjar type I, leading to much greater elevations of

unconjugated serum bilirubin to levels that carry an increased risk of kernicterus.

When isolated hyperbilirubinemia is associated with a conjugated fraction of over 15%, and typically over 50%, the diagnosis is either the uncommon Dubin-Johnson syndrome or the even rarer Rotor's syndrome (see Fig. 73-1, Table 21-2, and Table 64-5). The defect in Dubin-Johnson syndrome is in the gene that encodes MRP2. A 2012 study has suggested that the defect in Rotor's syndrome is due to coexisting deficiencies of the organic anion transporting polypeptides OATP1B1 and OATP1B3 (see Chapter 64).[9] In both syndromes, excretion of conjugated bilirubin across the bile canalicular membrane is reduced, resulting in an increase in the conjugated serum bilirubin level. Neither syndrome is associated with adverse clinical outcomes. Additional genetic disorders of bile acid transport that may be associated with hyperbilirubinemia are discussed in Chapters 64 and 77.

AMINOTRANSFERASES

The serum aminotransferases (also called *transaminases*), the most sensitive markers of acute hepatocellular injury, have been used to identify liver disease since the 1950s.[10] ALT (formerly serum glutamic pyruvic transaminase, or SGPT) and AST (formerly serum glutamic oxaloacetic transaminase, or SGOT) catalyze the transfer of the α-amino groups of alanine and L-aspartic acid, respectively, to the α-keto group of ketoglutaric acid. AST, found in cytosol and mitochondria, is widely distributed throughout the body; it is found, in order of decreasing concentration, in liver, cardiac muscle, skeletal muscle, kidney, brain, pancreas, lung, leukocytes, and erythrocytes. ALT, a cytosolic enzyme also found in many organs, is present in greatest concentration by far in the liver and is, therefore, a more specific indicator than AST of liver injury. Increases in serum values of the aminotransferases reflect either damage to tissues rich in these enzymes or changes in cell membrane permeability that allow ALT and AST to leak into serum; hepatocyte necrosis is not required for the release of aminotransferases, and the degree of elevation of the aminotransferases does not correlate with the extent of liver injury.[11]

Aminotransferases have no function in serum and act like other serum proteins. They are distributed in plasma and interstitial fluid and have half-lives measured in days. The activity of ALT and AST at any moment reflects the relative rate at which they enter and leave the circulation. They are probably cleared by cells of the reticuloendothelial system, with AST cleared more rapidly than ALT.

Normal values for aminotransferases in serum vary widely among laboratories, but values gaining general acceptance are equal to or below 30 U/L for men and 19 U/L for women. The inter-laboratory variation in the normal range is the result of technical issues; no reference standards exist to establish the upper limits of normal for serum ALT and AST levels. Therefore, each reference laboratory is responsible for identifying a locally defined reference population or for using a normal range first established in the 1950s.[10] The normal range is defined as the mean of the reference population plus 2 standard deviations; approximately 95% of a uniformly distributed population will fall within this "normal" range. Some investigators have recommended revisions of normal values for the aminotransferases with adjustments for sex and BMI, but others have raised concern about the potential costs and unclear benefits of implementing such a change.[12-16] A longitudinal analysis observed that serum levels of ALT decrease with age, independent of sex, alcohol use, BMI, diabetes mellitus, serum TG levels, and other factors known to affect ALT levels, thereby prompting the investigators to suggest that clinicians consider a patient's age, especially in older adults, when interpreting serum ALT levels.[17] A serum aminotransferase level below the lower limit of normal is of no clinical importance; it has been reported in patients with chronic kidney disease on hemodialysis and is believed to be caused in part by vitamin B_6 deficiency.

Approach to the Patient with an Elevated Level

Serum aminotransferase levels are typically elevated in all forms of liver injury; levels up to 300 U/L are nonspecific. In certain circumstances the degree and pattern of elevation of the aminotransferases, evaluated in the context of a patient's characteristics, symptoms, and physical examination findings, can suggest particular diagnoses and direct the subsequent evaluation (Box 73-1). The differential diagnosis of marked

---

BOX 73-1 Causes of Elevated Serum Aminotransferase Levels*

Chronic, Mild Elevations, ALT > AST (<150 U/L or 5 × normal)
Hepatic Causes
α_1-Antitrypsin deficiency
Autoimmune hepatitis
Chronic viral hepatitis (B, C, and D)
Hemochromatosis
Medications and toxins
Steatosis and steatohepatitis
Wilson disease

Nonhepatic Causes
Celiac disease
Hyperthyroidism

Severe, Acute Elevations, ALT > AST (>1000 U/L or >20-25 × normal)
Hepatic Causes
Acute bile duct obstruction
Acute Budd-Chiari syndrome
Acute viral hepatitis
Autoimmune hepatitis
Drugs and toxins
Hepatic artery ligation
Ischemic hepatitis
Wilson disease

Severe, Acute Elevations, AST > ALT (>1000 U/L or >20-25 × normal)
Hepatic Cause
Medications or toxins in a patient with underlying alcoholic liver injury

Nonhepatic Cause
Acute rhabdomyolysis

Chronic, Mild Elevations, AST > ALT (<150 U/L, <5 × normal)
Hepatic Causes
Alcohol-related liver injury (AST/ALT > 2:1, AST nearly always <300 U/L)
Cirrhosis

Nonhepatic Causes
Hypothyroidism
Macro-AST
Myopathy
Strenuous exercise

*Virtually any liver disease can cause moderate aminotransferase elevations (5-15 × normal).

---

elevations of aminotransferase levels (>1000 U/L) includes viral hepatitis (A to E), toxin or drug-induced liver injury, ischemic hepatitis, and less commonly, autoimmune hepatitis, acute Budd-Chiari syndrome, fulminant Wilson disease, and acute obstruction of the biliary tract.

The ratio of AST to ALT in serum is helpful in a few specific circumstances—perhaps most importantly in the recognition of alcoholic liver disease. If the AST level is less than 300 U/L, a ratio of AST to ALT of more than 2 suggests alcoholic liver disease, and a ratio of more than 3 is highly suggestive of alcoholic liver disease.[18] The ratio results from a deficiency of pyridoxal 5'-phosphate in patients with alcoholic liver disease; ALT synthesis in the liver requires pyridoxal phosphate more than does AST synthesis.[19] When a patient with chronic alcoholic liver disease sustains a superimposed liver injury, particularly acetaminophen hepatotoxicity, the aminotransferase levels can be strikingly elevated, yet the AST/ALT ratio is maintained.

An increased ratio of AST to ALT may also be seen in muscle disorders. The degree of elevation is typically less than 300 U/L, but in rare cases, such as rhabdomyolysis, levels typically observed in patients with acute hepatocellular disease can be reached. In cases of acute muscle injury, the AST/ALT ratio may initially be greater than 3:1, but the ratio quickly declines toward 1:1 because of the shorter serum half-life of AST.[20] The ratio typically is close to 1:1 in patients with chronic muscle diseases.

Although the AST/ALT ratio is typically less than 1 in patients with chronic viral hepatitis and nonalcoholic fatty liver disease (NAFLD), a number of investigators have observed that, as cirrhosis develops, the ratio rises and may become greater than 1. Studies have shown that an AST/ALT ratio of greater than 1 as an indicator of cirrhosis in patients with chronic hepatitis C has a high specificity (94% to 100%) but a relatively low sensitivity (44% to 75%).[21] The increase in AST/ALT ratio with the development of cirrhosis is believed to result from impaired functional hepatic blood flow, with a consequent decrease in hepatic sinusoidal uptake of AST.[22]

The majority of patients evaluated for elevated serum aminotransferase levels are asymptomatic and have mild elevations (≤5-fold) identified during routine screening. The first step in the evaluation of mildly elevated serum aminotransferase levels is to repeat the test to confirm persistence of the elevated value. If the aminotransferase level remains elevated, the recommended evaluation is illustrated in Figure 73-2. The next step is to take a careful history focused on identifying all of the patient's medications, including over-the-counter (OTC) medications, complementary and alternative medications (CAM), and substances of abuse. Correlating the use of medications temporally with the laboratory abnormalities will sometimes reveal a specific culprit. Almost any medication, including OTC medications, CAM, and substances of abuse, has the potential to elevate serum aminotransferase levels. Relatively common offending agents include NSAIDs, antibiotics, hydroxymethylglutaryl-coenzyme A reductase inhibitors, antiepileptics, and antituberculous medications (see Chapter 88). The association between use of a medication and liver enzyme elevations is readily established by stopping the medication and observing return of the enzyme levels to normal. Rechallenge with the suspect medication followed by a rise in serum aminotransferase levels is confirmatory but often not undertaken. Muscle disease should also be excluded by obtaining serum creatine kinase and aldolase levels.

The next step in the evaluation is to assess the patient for the more common and treatable causes of liver disease, including chronic hepatitis B and C, hemochromatosis, autoimmune hepatitis, Wilson disease, and NAFLD. Although autoimmune hepatitis is commonly considered a disease of young to

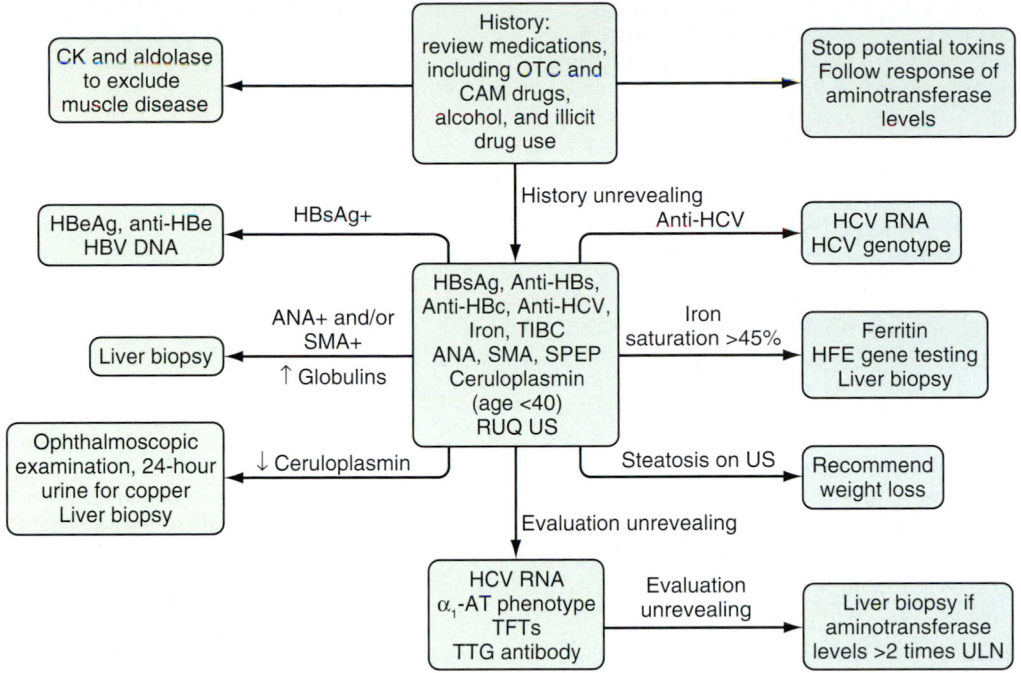

FIGURE 73-2. Evaluation of asymptomatic elevation of serum aminotransferase levels. a₁-AT, a₁-antitrypsin; ANA, antinuclear antibodies; Anti-HBc, antibody to hepatitis B core antigen; Anti-HBe, antibody to hepatitis B e antigen; Anti-HBs, antibody to hepatitis B surface antigen; Anti-HCV, antibody to HCV; CAM, complementary and alternative medicines; CK, creatine kinase; HBeAg, hepatitis B e antigen; HBsAg, hepatitis B surface antigen; HFE, hemochromatosis; OTC, over-the-counter; RUQ, right upper quadrant; SMA, smooth muscle antibodies; SPEP, serum protein electrophoresis; TIBC, total iron binding capacity, TFTs, thyroid function tests; TTG, tissue transglutaminase; ULN, upper limit of normal.

middle-aged women, it also is seen in men and has been reported in all ethnic groups (see Chapter 90). The clinical onset of Wilson disease is usually between 5 and 25 years of age; the diagnosis should be considered initially in all patients age 40 or younger and those older than age 40 with aminotransferase elevations that remain unexplained after other causes are excluded (see Chapter 76). NAFLD is the most common cause of elevated serum aminotransferase levels in the United States (see Chapter 87), but there is no specific laboratory test for NAFLD.

If testing for the more common causes fails to provide a diagnosis, the less common causes of liver disease, such as α₁-antitrypsin deficiency, and extrahepatic causes of persistently elevated liver enzyme levels, such as thyroid disease and celiac disease, should be sought. A meta-analysis of 11 studies has shown that undetected celiac disease is a potential cause of otherwise unexplained elevated serum aminotransferase levels in 3% to 4% of cases.[23] If testing for these disorders is negative, the decision to perform a liver biopsy is determined by the degree of aminotransferase elevation, with the recognition that the results of the biopsy are unlikely to alter management.

ALKALINE PHOSPHATASE

The term *alkaline phosphatase* applies generally to a group of isoenzymes distributed widely throughout the body.[24] The isoenzymes of greatest clinical importance in adults are in the liver and bone because these organs are the major sources of serum ALP. Other isoenzymes originate from the placenta, small intestine, and kidneys. In the liver, ALP is found on the canalicular membrane of hepatocytes; its precise function is undefined. ALP has a serum half-life of approximately 7 days,

and although the sites of degradation are unknown, clearance of ALP from serum is independent of either patency of the biliary tract or functional capacity of the liver. Hepatobiliary disease leads to increased serum ALP levels through induced synthesis of the enzyme and leakage into the serum, a process mediated by bile acids.[25]

A number of individual physiologic variations in serum ALP levels have been identified. Patients with blood groups O and B have elevations in serum ALP levels caused by release of intestinal ALP after a fatty meal.[26] This observation is the basis for the recommendation by some authorities that the serum ALP level be checked in the fasting state. An increased serum ALP level of intestinal origin is seen in benign familial elevation of the serum ALP. Serum ALP values vary with age. Male and female adolescents have serum ALP levels twice the level seen in adults; the level correlates with bone growth, and the increase in serum is in bone ALP. Although the level of serum ALP increases after 30 years of age in both men and women, the increase is more pronounced in women than in men; a healthy 65-year-old woman has a serum ALP level 50% higher than that of a healthy 30-year-old woman.[27] The reason for this difference is not known. In a person with isolated elevation of the serum ALP level, the serum GGTP or 5′NT are used to distinguish a liver origin from bone origin of the ALP elevation (see later). A low serum ALP level may occur in patients with Wilson disease, especially those presenting with fulminant hepatitis and hemolysis, possibly because of reduced activity of the enzyme owing to displacement of the cofactor zinc by copper (see Chapter 76).

GGTP

GGTP is found in the cell membranes of a wide distribution of tissues including liver (both hepatocytes and

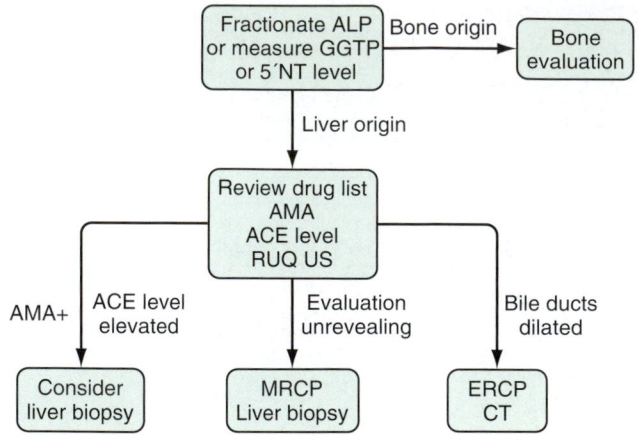

FIGURE 73-3. Evaluation of an isolated elevation of the serum alkaline phosphatase level. ACE, angiotensin-converting enzyme; ALP, alkaline phosphatase; AMA, antimitochondrial antibodies; 5′NT, 5′ nucleotidase; RUQ, right upper quadrant.

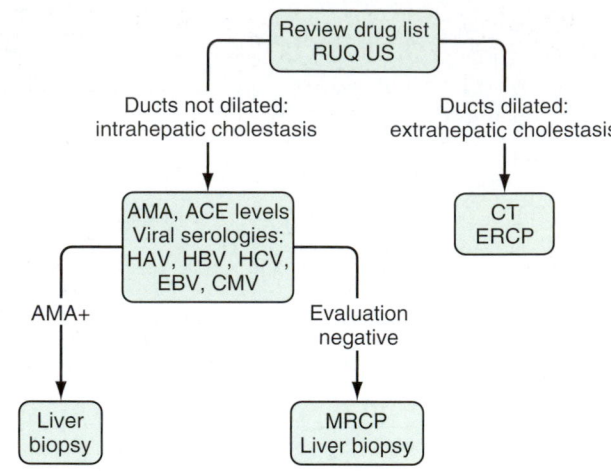

FIGURE 73-4. Evaluation of cholestatic liver enzyme elevations. ACE, angiotensin-converting enzyme; AMA, antimitochondrial antibodies; CMV, cytomegalovirus; RUQ, right upper quadrant.

cholangiocytes), kidney, pancreas, spleen, heart, brain, and seminal vesicles. It is present in the serum of healthy persons. Serum levels are not different between men and women and do not rise in pregnancy. Although an elevated serum GGTP level has high sensitivity for hepatobiliary disease, its lack of specificity limits its clinical utility. The primary use of serum GGTP levels is to identify the source of an isolated elevation in the serum ALP level; GGTP is not elevated in bone disease (Fig. 73-3).[28] GGTP is elevated in patients taking phenytoin, barbiturates, and some drugs used in HAART, including nonnucleoside reverse transcriptase inhibitors and the protease inhibitor abacavir.[29,30]

Serum GGTP levels are also elevated in patients who drink alcohol, and some experts have advocated use of the GGTP level for identifying unreported alcohol use (see Chapter 86). The sensitivity of an elevated serum GGTP level for alcohol use ranges from 52% to 94%, but a low specificity limits its usefulness for this purpose.[31] One study has suggested an association between high serum GGTP levels and the risk of hepatocellular carcinoma.[32] The GGTP level had a negative predictive value of 97.9%—higher than that for ALP, total bilirubin, ALT, and AST—for detecting bile duct stones in patients undergoing laparoscopic cholecystectomy.[33] An isolated GGTP level was associated with an elevated mortality risk in 560,000 insurance applicants and with metabolic syndrome, diabetes mellitus, and cardiovascular disease.[34]

5′-Nucleotidase

5′NT is associated with the canalicular and sinusoidal plasma membranes; its function is undefined. 5′NT is also found in the intestine, brain, heart, blood vessels, and endocrine pancreas. Serum levels of 5′NT are unaffected by sex or race, but age affects the level; values are lowest in children and increase gradually, reaching a plateau at approximately 50 years of age. As with GGTP, the primary role of the serum 5′NT level is to identify the organ source of an isolated serum ALP elevation (see Fig. 73-3). The 5′NT level is not increased in bone disease and is primarily increased in hepatobiliary disease.

Approach to the Patient with an Elevated Level

The first step in the evaluation of a patient with an isolated and asymptomatic elevation of the serum ALP is to identify the tissue source (see Fig. 73-3). The most precise way of doing this is via fractionation through electrophoresis; each isoenzyme of ALP has different electrophoretic mobilities.[35] Tests used in the past that involved heat and urea denaturation of ALP are neither sensitive nor specific. An acceptable alternative method is to check either the serum GGTP or 5′NT level; elevation of either verifies that the elevated ALP is the result of hepatobiliary disease. A normal 5′NT level, however, does not rule out the possibility of hepatobiliary disease, because the 5′NT and ALP do not necessarily increase in parallel in early or mild hepatic injury, thus making GGTP the preferred test.

The primary value of an elevated serum level of ALP of liver origin is to allow the recognition of a cholestatic disorder (i.e., a disorder associated with impaired bile flow, often with jaundice). In general, a serum ALP elevation out of proportion to the level of the aminotransferases suggests a cholestatic disorder (see Chapter 21). A 4-fold elevation of the serum ALP is seen in approximately 75% of patients with chronic cholestasis, both intrahepatic or extrahepatic, whereas lesser elevations are nonspecific and can occur in a wide range of conditions. Figures 73-3 and 73-4 illustrate the recommended evaluation of cholestatic liver enzymes—either an isolated ALP elevation (see Fig. 73-3) or a disproportionate elevation of the ALP compared with the aminotransferases (Fig. 73-4).

Central to the evaluation of an elevated ALP level is imaging of the biliary tract. Absence of dilated intrahepatic bile ducts focuses the search on intrahepatic causes of cholestasis (Box 73-2), whereas dilated ducts should lead to an evaluation of extrahepatic causes of cholestasis (Box 73-3). As with elevated aminotransferase levels, the evaluation of intrahepatic causes of cholestatic liver enzymes begins with a carefully taken history of medication use, including OTC medications, CAM, and drugs of abuse, and temporal correlation of their use with elevation of the liver enzyme levels. Withdrawal of the offending agent and resolution of the liver enzymes is sufficient to confirm the diagnosis, and a liver biopsy is generally not required. The rate of improvement can be slow, and if bile duct destruction has developed ("vanishing bile duct syndrome"), the changes may be irreversible.

PBC is a classic autoimmune disease. The immunologic injury is characterized by T cell–mediated destruction of the intrahepatic bile ducts. Although predominantly a disease of middle-aged women, with a median age at diagnosis of

---

BOX 73-2 Intrahepatic Causes of Cholestatic Liver Enzyme Elevations in Adults

Drugs*
Bland cholestasis
    Anabolic steroids
    Estrogens
Cholestatic hepatitis
    Angiotensin-converting enzyme inhibitors: captopril,
        enalapril
    Antimicrobials: amoxicillin-clavulanic acid, ketoconazole
    Azathioprine
    Chlorpromazine
    NSAIDs: sulindac, piroxicam
Granulomatous hepatitis
    Allopurinol
    Antibiotics: sulfonamides
    Antiepileptics: carbamazepine, phenytoin
    Cardiovascular agents: hydralazine, procainamide,
        quinidine
    Phenylbutazone
Vanishing bile duct syndrome
    Amoxicillin-clavulanic acid
    Chlorpromazine
    Dicloxacillin
    Flucloxacillin
    Macrolides

PBC

PSC

Granulomatous Liver Disease
Infections
    Brucellosis
    Fungal: histoplasmosis, coccidioidomycosis
    Leprosy
    Q fever
    Schistosomiasis
    TB, *Mycobacterium avium* complex, bacillus
        Calmette-Guérin
Sarcoidosis
Idiopathic granulomatous hepatitis

Other
    Crohn's disease
    Heavy metal exposure: beryllium, copper
    Hodgkin's disease

Viral Hepatitis
HAV and HEV
HBV and HCV, including fibrosing cholestatic hepatitis
EBV
Cytomegalovirus

Idiopathic Adulthood Ductopenia

Genetic Conditions
Progressive familial intrahepatic cholestasis
    Type 1 (formerly Byler's disease)
    Type 2
    Type 3
Benign recurrent intrahepatic cholestasis
    Type 1
    Type 2
CF

Malignancy
Hepatocellular carcinoma
Metastatic disease
Paraneoplastic syndrome
    Non-Hodgkin's lymphoma
    Prostate cancer
    Renal cell cancer

Infiltrative Liver Disease
Amyloidosis
Lymphoma

Intrahepatic Cholestasis of Pregnancy

TPN

Graft-versus-Host Disease

Sepsis

*Categorized by histologic pattern. Drug lists are not meant to be comprehensive.

---

approximately 50 years, 5% to 10% of affected patients are men. The reported age range is 22 to 93 years. Antimitochondrial antibodies (AMA) are found in serum in 95% of patients and are diagnostic; a liver biopsy that demonstrates characteristic histologic findings is confirmatory (see Chapter 91).

PSC is a disease of altered immunity marked by inflammation and fibrosis of the intra- or extrahepatic bile ducts, or both. The disorder is strongly associated with IBD and is found most commonly in younger men. The diagnosis is confirmed by cholangiography, either MRCP or ERCP (see Chapter 68).

Granulomatous liver disease can be caused by a number of disorders (see Box 73-2). Infectious etiologies must be excluded because treatment for many of the other causes of granulomatous liver disease is immunosuppressive therapy. Sarcoidosis is the most common etiology. The diagnosis is based on an elevated angiotensin-converting enzyme (ACE) level and typical extrahepatic manifestations. Hepatic involvement, however, is uncommonly the impetus for initiating therapy for sarcoidosis (see Chapter 36).

Viral hepatitis, particularly cases caused by EBV and cytomegalovirus (CMV), can manifest with a prominent cholestatic liver enzyme pattern (see Chapter 83). A number of familial conditions produce intrahepatic cholestasis (see Table

64-5). Progressive forms of these disorders manifest in childhood, whereas the benign forms—benign recurrent intrahepatic cholestasis types 1 and 2—can manifest for the first time in adulthood. Other intrahepatic causes of cholestatic liver enzymes are listed in Box 73-2.

If imaging shows intrahepatic ductal dilatation, the evaluation focuses on the extrahepatic biliary tract to identify an intrinsic or extrinsic cause of biliary obstruction (see Box 73-3). The evaluation often includes an ERCP for tissue acquisition and placement of a biliary stent if obstruction is present (see Chapter 70). CT provides assessment for an extrinsic process, and tissue acquisition can be performed with CT or EUS guidance.

TESTS OF HEPATIC SYNTHETIC FUNCTION

Albumin

Quantitatively, the most important plasma protein, albumin, accounts for 75% of the plasma colloid oncotic pressure and is synthesized exclusively by hepatocytes. The average adult produces approximately 15 g/day and has 300 to 500 g of albumin distributed in body fluids. The liver has the ability to double the rate of synthesis in the setting of rapid albumin loss or a dilutional decrease in the serum albumin concentration.[36] The half-life of albumin is 14 to 21 days; the site of degradation is not known. Albumin synthesis is regulated by changes in nutritional status, osmotic pressure, systemic inflammation, and hormone levels.[37] Therefore, the differential diagnosis of serum hypoalbuminemia, in addition to hepatocellular dysfunction, includes malnutrition, excessive loss from protein-losing enteropathy or nephrotic syndrome, chronic systemic inflammatory conditions, and hormonal imbalances.

The long half-life of albumin in serum accounts for its unreliability as a marker of hepatic synthetic function in acute liver injury. Serum albumin levels less than 3 g/dL in a patient with newly diagnosed hepatitis should raise suspicion of a chronic process. Serum albumin is an excellent marker of hepatic synthetic function in patients with chronic liver disease and cirrhosis, with the exception of patients with cirrhosis and ascites, who may have normal or increased albumin production but an increased volume of distribution that results in a low serum albumin level. Albumin has no utility as a screening test in patients for whom there is low suspicion of liver disease; a study in which the serum albumin level was measured in 449 consecutive patients yielded 56 abnormal results, of which only 2 (0.4%) were of clinical importance.[38]

Prothrombin Time

Clotting is the end result of a complex series of enzymatic reactions involving clotting factors, all of which are produced in the liver except factor VIII, which is produced by vascular endothelial cells. The prothrombin time is a measure of the rate at which prothrombin is converted to thrombin, reflecting the extrinsic pathway of coagulation. Factors involved in the synthesis of prothrombin include II, V, VII, and X. The INR is used to express the degree of anticoagulation on warfarin therapy. The INR standardizes prothrombin time measurement according to the characteristics of the thromboplastin reagent used in a particular laboratory; the initial measurement is expressed as an international sensitivity index (ISI), which is then used in calculating the INR. Because the ISI is validated only for patients taking a vitamin K antagonist, concern has been raised about the validity of using the ISI (and INR) in patients with chronic liver disease.[39] Two studies have demonstrated, in fact, that the ISI, as currently determined, is not accurate for calculating the INR in patients with cirrhosis, and the investigators have proposed that specific ISI and INR determinations using control patients with liver disease be used to eliminate inter-laboratory variability in calculating the INR in patients with cirrhosis.[40,41]

A prolonged prothrombin time can be caused by a number of conditions besides reduced hepatic synthetic function: congenital deficiency of clotting factors, vitamin K deficiency (vitamin K is required for normal functioning of factors II, VII, IX, and X), and DIC. DIC can be identified by measuring a factor VIII level in serum; the level is decreased in DIC and normal or increased in liver disease. Vitamin K deficiency is identified by demonstrating that IV administration of vitamin K (e.g., 10 mg) leads to improvement in the prothrombin time; a 30% or more improvement in the prothrombin time is consistent with hypovitaminosis K. Oral vitamin K may not be absorbed by the intestine in patients with jaundice (see Chapter 94).

Measurement of the prothrombin time in patients with liver disease is most useful in cases of acute liver disease. Unlike the serum albumin, the prothrombin time allows an assessment of current hepatic synthetic function; factor VII has the shortest serum half-life (6 hours) of all the clotting factors. The prothrombin time has prognostic value in patients with acute acetaminophen- and nonacetaminophen-related liver failure (see Chapter 95), as well as alcoholic hepatitis (see Chapter 86). The INR, along with total serum bilirubin and creatinine levels, are components of the MELD score, which is used to allocate donor organs for liver transplantation (see Chapter 97). The MELD score accurately predicts survival in patients with decompensated cirrhosis (see later).

The prothrombin time is not an accurate measure of bleeding risk in patients with cirrhosis, because it assesses only the activity of procoagulant clotting factors, not anticoagulants such as protein C and antithrombin, the production of which is also reduced in cirrhosis. The partial thromboplastin time (PTT) assesses the intrinsic pathway of the coagulation cascade. The PTT can be prolonged in patients with advanced cirrhosis, but prolongation of the PTT is less sensitive than the PT for detecting coagulopathy.

TESTS TO DETECT HEPATIC FIBROSIS

Although liver biopsy is the standard for the assessment of hepatic fibrosis, noninvasive measures of hepatic fibrosis have been developed and show promise (see Chapter 74).[42] These measures include single serum biochemical markers that potentially reflect the activity level of hepatic fibrogenesis (hyaluronan is the best to date) and multiparameter tests aimed at detecting and staging the degree of hepatic fibrosis (>20 such tests are described in the literature).

Hyaluronan is a glucosaminoglycan produced in mesenchymal cells and widely distributed in the extracellular space. Typically degraded by hepatic sinusoidal cells, serum levels of hyaluronan are elevated in patients with cirrhosis as a result of sinusoidal capillarization (see Chapter 92). A fasting hyaluronan level greater than 100 mg/L had a sensitivity of 83% and specificity of 78% for the detection of cirrhosis in patients with a variety of chronic liver diseases.[43] Hyaluronan has been shown to be useful for identifying advanced fibrosis in patients with chronic hepatitis C, chronic hepatitis B, alcoholic liver disease, and nonalcoholic steatohepatitis.[44] Preoperative serum hyaluronan levels also have been shown to correlate with the development of hepatic dysfunction after hepatectomy.[45]

FibroTest (marketed as FibroSure in the United States) is the best evaluated of the multiparameter blood tests. The test incorporates haptoglobin, bilirubin, GGTP, apolipoprotein A-1, and α_2-macroglobulin and has been found to have high positive and negative predictive values for diagnosing advanced fibrosis in patients with chronic hepatitis C (see Chapter 80). One study showed that use of a more sensitive index cut-off had a sensitivity of 90%, specificity of 36%, positive predictive value of 88%, and negative predictive value of 40% for the diagnosis of bridging fibrosis in patients with chronic hepatitis C.[46] The test has similar performance characteristics in patients with chronic hepatitis B and alcoholic liver disease and has been shown to predict advanced fibrosis in patients taking methotrexate for psoriasis.[47] The newer FIBROSpect II assay incorporates hyaluronate, tissue inhibitor of metalloproteinase 1, and α_2-macroglobulin. In a group of patients with chronic hepatitis C, FIBROSpect II had a sensitivity of 72% and a specificity of 74% for identifying advanced fibrosis.[48]

Transient elastography, marketed as FibroScan, as well as acoustic force radiation impulse elastography, uses US waves to measure hepatic stiffness noninvasively (see Chapter 74). Central to the development of this technique were the principles that fibrosis leads to increased stiffness of hepatic tissue and that a shear wave will propagate faster through stiff material than through elastic material.[49] The US transducer emits a low-frequency (50 Hz) shear wave, and the amount of time required for the wave to go through a set "window" of tissue is measured.[50] The window of tissue is 1 cm by 4 cm—100 times the area of an average liver biopsy. A meta-analysis showed that transient elastography performed best at differentiating cirrhosis from absence of cirrhosis but was less accurate for the estimation of lesser degrees of fibrosis.[51] Transient elastography has been shown to be accurate for identifying advanced fibrosis in patients with chronic hepatitis C, PBC, hemochromatosis, NAFLD, and recurrent chronic hepatitis after liver transplantation[52-55] and was approved by the FDA in 2013 for use in patients with liver disease.

Magnetic resonance elastography (MRE) is another noninvasive technique that has been approved by the FDA. The shear elasticity of the liver is measured after low-frequency (65 Hz) waves are transmitted into the right lobe of the liver. In one study,[56] MRE was found to be superior to transient elastography for staging liver fibrosis in patients with a variety of chronic liver diseases.

QUANTITATIVE LIVER FUNCTION TESTS

Quantitative function tests have been developed in the hope of evaluating the excretory or detoxification capacity of the liver more specifically than the serum bilirubin level. Unfortunately, although these tests lead to improved sensitivity, their lack of specificity and often cumbersome methodology have limited their widespread acceptance, except in research settings.

Indocyanine Green Clearance

Indocyanine green (ICG) is a nontoxic dye that is cleared exclusively by the liver; 97% of an administered dose (0.64 to 6.4 mol/kg given as an IV bolus) is excreted unchanged into bile. ICG can be measured directly by spectrophotometry. Noninvasive methods (dichromatic earlobe densitometry and fingertip optical sensors) generate data that appear to correlate well with levels determined by blood sampling. Possible uses of ICG include the assessment of hepatic dysfunction, measurement of hepatic blood flow, and prediction of clinical outcomes in patients with liver disease. Unfortunately, measurement of ICG has proved to be insensitive for detecting hepatic dysfunction and is inaccurate for measuring blood flow in patients with cirrhosis because of decreased ICG extraction by the diseased liver. Although ICG measurement has shown some promise for predicting outcomes in certain clinical situations such as burn patients, it has not been employed widely outside of research protocols.[57]

Galactose Elimination Capacity

The galactose elimination capacity (GEC) has been studied as a measure of functional hepatic mass. Galactose is given as a single IV bolus (0.5 g/kg), and blood samples are collected. Patients with cirrhosis and chronic hepatitis have reduced galactose clearance from serum as compared with healthy controls. In a study of 781 patients with newly diagnosed cirrhosis and a decreased GEC, the GEC was a strong predictor of short- and long-term all-cause and cirrhosis-related mortality.[58]

Caffeine Clearance

Caffeine clearance tests quantify functional hepatic capacity by assessing the activity of cytochrome P450 1A2, N-acetyltransferase, and xanthine oxidase. Caffeine is given orally (200 to 366 mg), and levels are measured in blood, urine, saliva, breath, or scalp hair. The alternative methods correlate well with the plasma clearance method. Tobacco use increases caffeine clearance, and drug interactions can affect results. Increasing age correlates with decreased caffeine clearance. Overnight salivary caffeine clearance has been shown to correlate with ICG measurements and galactose clearance as well as with results of the aminopyrine breath test (see later).[59]

Lidocaine Metabolite Formation

Lidocaine is metabolized to its major metabolite monoethylglycinexylidide (MEGX) by the hepatic cytochrome P450 system.[60] Serum samples are taken 15, 30, and 60 minutes after IV administration of lidocaine (1 mg/kg). Neither MEGX formation nor galactose elimination was found to be superior to the Child-Turcotte-Pugh (CTP) (see Chapter 92) or MELD (see Chapter 97) score in predicting prognosis in patients with cirrhosis secondary to viral hepatitis (see later).[61] Other studies have suggested that a decline in MEGX concentration correlates well with histologic worsening in patients with chronic liver disease.[62]

Aminopyrine Breath Test

The ^{15}C and ^{14}C aminopyrine breath tests (ABTs) measure hepatic mixed-function oxidase mass. The radioactive methyl groups of aminopyrine undergo demethylation and eventual conversion to labeled CO_2, which is then exhaled and can be measured. After an overnight fast, a known dose of ^{15}C aminopyrine (1 to 2 µCi) is administered orally, and breath samples are taken every 30 minutes for 4 hours; some investigators check a single sample at either 1 or 2 hours. Healthy subjects excrete 6.6% ± 1.3% of the administered dose in the breath in 2 hours; patients with hepatocellular injury excrete considerably less. The degree of decrease in excretion of aminopyrine overlaps considerably in patients with all types of severe liver disease, including cirrhosis, chronic hepatitis, alcoholic liver disease, and hepatocellular carcinoma.[63] Although data have been conflicting regarding the ability of this test to predict survival in patients with chronic liver disease, a study in 2012 of 50 patients showed that the ABT accurately predicted the risk of disease progression in patients with HCV-related chronic hepatitis.[64]

BILE ACIDS

Bile acids are synthesized from cholesterol in hepatocytes, conjugated to glycine or taurine, and secreted into bile (see Chapter 64). After passage into the small intestine, most bile acids are actively reabsorbed. The liver efficiently extracts bile acids from the portal blood. In healthy persons, all bile acids in serum emanate from the reabsorption of bile acids in the small intestine. Maintenance of normal serum bile acid concentrations depends on hepatic blood flow, hepatic uptake, secretion of bile acids, and intestinal transit. Serum bile acids are sensitive but nonspecific indicators of hepatic dysfunction and allow some quantification of functional hepatic reserve. Serum bile acid levels correlate moderately well with the results of ABTs in patients with chronic hepatitis.[65] Unfortunately, the correlation between serum bile acid levels and the histologic severity of chronic hepatitis and alcoholic liver disease is poor.[66] Serum bile acid levels are elevated in patients with cholestatic liver diseases but normal in patients with Gilbert's syndrome and Dubin-Johnson syndrome and can be used to make the distinction. Although decreased serum bile acid levels are highly specific indicators of liver dysfunction, they are not as sensitive as initially hoped.

SPECIFIC APPLICATIONS OF LIVER BIOCHEMICAL TESTING

Liver biochemical tests have been used to monitor for and assess the severity of drug-induced liver injury, assess operative risk, identify candidates for liver transplantation, and direct donor organ allocation.

Drug-Induced Liver Injury

Most drugs that are hepatotoxic cause idiosyncratic liver injury, defined as injury that is unpredictable, occurs at therapeutic drug levels, and is infrequent (see Chapter 88). The estimated frequency of idiosyncratic drug-induced liver injury for any particular medication ranges from 1 in 1000 to 1 in 100,000. These reactions are marked by a variable latency period ranging from 5 to 90 days, or even longer.[67] Other drugs produce dose-dependent toxicity. These injuries are predictable, have a high incidence, and generally have a well-understood mechanism. Acetaminophen is the classic example of a drug that causes dose-dependent liver injury. The dose of acetaminophen exceeds 15 g, almost 4 times the recommended daily dose, in 80% of cases. Acetaminophen doses within the therapeutic range (<4 g/day) can be sufficient to cause liver injury in susceptible persons, such as those who use ethanol chronically. The King's College criteria identify patients with

a poor prognosis from acetaminophen-induced liver injury: those with an arterial pH below 7.3 or those with an INR above 6.5, serum creatinine level above 3.4 g/dL, and stage 3 to 4 hepatic encephalopathy (see Chapters 88 and 95).[68]

Most occurrences of drug-induced liver injury are mild and respond promptly to drug withdrawal with complete resolution. Isolated elevation of the serum aminotransferase levels, even to values greater than 3 times the upper limit of normal, is associated with a positive outcome. When aminotransferase elevations are associated with clinical jaundice (so-called Hy's Law, after the late Dr. Hyman Zimmerman), the risk of mortality is increased to as high as 10% (see Chapter 88).[69]

Surgical Candidacy and Organ Allocation

Patients with acute and chronic liver disease are potentially at increased risk of morbidity and mortality if they undergo surgery. The risk depends on the etiology of the liver disease, severity of the liver disease, and planned operation. Although routine preoperative liver biochemical testing is not recommended in otherwise healthy people, the identification of unexpected elevated liver enzyme levels should prompt a postponement of surgery until the cause of the abnormalities has been identified. A retrospective analysis found that patients with acute viral hepatitis who undergo laparotomy had an operative mortality rate of approximately 9.5%.[70] Elective surgery should be postponed in patients with acute hepatitis. The surgical risk in patients with chronic hepatitis correlates with the severity of histologic inflammation in the liver. Those with only portal inflammation and interface hepatitis have low operative risk, whereas those with panlobular hepatitis have an increased risk. The etiology of chronic hepatitis does not influence outcome.

Examination of histology is also critical in assessing the surgical risk in patients with alcoholic liver disease. Hepatic steatosis alone is associated with a low operative risk, whereas alcoholic hepatitis is associated with a mortality rate as high as 55% in patients undergoing portosystemic shunt surgery, for example. A period of abstinence of 3 to 6 months before elective surgery is recommended in these patients. Few data exist for surgical risk in patients with NAFLD, but the mortality rate appears to correlate with the severity of steatosis in patients undergoing liver resection. Steatohepatitis may carry a higher risk than that for steatosis.

An estimated 10% of patients with advanced liver disease undergo surgery in the last two years of their lives. Cirrhosis is associated with increased operative risk, particularly with certain types of surgery, including cardiothoracic surgery, hepatic resection, and other abdominal operations. The data evaluating the surgical risk in these patients were derived retrospectively but point consistently toward the usefulness of the CTP scoring system for predicting perioperative mortality. Two studies performed more than 10 years apart examined mortality after abdominal surgery in cirrhotic patients and reported nearly identical rates of mortality for patients with Child-Pugh class A, B, and C cirrhosis: 10%, 30% to 31%, and 76% to 82%, respectively,[71,72] although lower mortality rates have been reported with greater use of laparoscopic surgery at an expert center.[73] In general, surgery may be undertaken in patients with Child-Pugh class A cirrhosis, whereas the medical condition of patients with Child-Pugh class B cirrhosis should be optimized prior to planned surgery. The mortality rate in patients with Child-Pugh class C cirrhosis is prohibitive, and surgery should be avoided.

The MELD score was created originally to predict survival in patients with cirrhosis and portal hypertension undergoing placement of a transjugular intrahepatic portosystemic shunt

(TIPS).[74] The score has subsequently been validated as an accurate predictor of survival in patients with advanced liver disease. The MELD score incorporates 3 objective variables into a mathematical formula: $9.57 \times \log_e(\text{creatinine}) + 3.78 \times \log_e(\text{total bilirubin}) + 11.2 \times \log_e(\text{INR}) + 6.43$. The working range is 6 to 40, and the score has been shown to correlate with mortality in patients undergoing surgery other than liver transplantation, including hepatic resection, other abdominal procedures, and cardiac surgery.[75-77] MELD is used most often for prioritizing the allocation of donor organs for liver transplantation.[78] Since implementation of the MELD score for prioritizing organ allocation, the number of deaths among patients on the wait list has decreased, suggesting that use of the MELD score is achieving its primary goal—allocation of organs to the sickest patients first (see Chapter 97).

KEY REFERENCES

Full references for this chapter can be found on www.expertconsult.com.

13. Prati D, Taioli E, Zanella A, et al. Updated definitions of healthy ranges for serum alanine aminotranferase levels. Ann Intern Med 2002; 137:1-10.

14. Kim HC, Nam CM, Jee SH, et al. Normal serum aminotransferase concentration and risk of mortality from liver diseases: Prospective cohort study. BMJ 2004; 328:983.

16. Kunde SS, Lazenby AJ, Clements RH, et al. Spectrum of NAFLD and diagnostic implications of the proposed new normal range for serum ALT in obese women. Hepatology 2005; 42:650-6.

20. Nathwani RA, Pais S, Reynolds TB, et al. Serum alanine aminotransferase in skeletal muscle diseases. Hepatology 2005; 41:380-2.

24. Kaplan M. Alkaline phosphatase. Gastroenterology 1972; 62:452-68.

40. Bellest L, Eschwege V, Poupon R, et al. A modified international normalized ratio as an effective way of prothrombin time standardization in hepatology. Hepatology 2007; 46:528-34.

41. Tripodi A, Chantarangkul V, Prirnignani M, et al. The international normalized ratio calibrated for cirrhosis normalizes prothrombin time results for model for end-stage liver disease calculation. Hepatology 2007; 46:520-7.

42. Martínez SM, Crespo G, Navasa M, et al. Noninvasive assessment of liver fibrosis. Hepatology 2011; 53:325-35.

44. Kaneda H, Hashimoto E, Yatsuji S, et al. Hyaluronic acid levels can predict severe fibrosis and platelet counts can predict cirrhosis in patients with nonalcoholic fatty liver disease. J Gastroenterol Hepatol 2006; 21:1459-65.

46. Poynard T, McHutchison J, Manns M, et al. Biochemical surrogate markers of liver fibrosis and activity in a randomized trial of peginterferon alpha-2b and ribavirin. Hepatology 2003; 38:481-92.

51. Friedrich-Rust M, Martens S, Sarrazin C, et al. Performance of transient elastography for the staging of liver fibrosis: A meta-analysis. Gastroenterology 2008; 134:960-74.

61. Addario L, Scaglione G, Tritto G, et al. Prognostic value of quantitative liver function tests in viral cirrhosis: A prospective study. Eur J Gastroenterol Hepatol 2006; 18:713-20.

67. Lee WM. Drug-induced hepatotoxicity. N Engl J Med 2003; 349:474-85.

72. Mansour A, Watson W, Shayani V, et al. Abdominal operation in patients with cirrhosis: Still a major surgical challenge. Surgery 1997; 122:730-6.

74. Kamath PS, Kim WR. The model for end-stage liver disease (MELD). Hepatology 2007; 45:797-805.

78. Wiesner R, Edwards E, Freeman R, et al. Model for end-stage liver disease (MELD) and allocation of donor livers. Gastroenterology 2003; 124:91-6.

PATRICK S. KAMATH AND VIJAY H. SHAH

Cirrhosis, a final pathway for a wide variety of chronic liver diseases (Box 74-1), is a pathologic entity defined as diffuse hepatic fibrosis with the replacement of the normal liver architecture by nodules. The rate of progression of chronic liver disease to cirrhosis may be quite variable, from weeks in patients with complete biliary obstruction to decades in patients with chronic hepatitis C. Cirrhosis is 1 of the leading causes of mortality in the United States and particularly afflicts persons in the most productive years of their lives. The protean complications of cirrhosis (Box 74-2) are discussed in other chapters.

PATHOGENESIS

The liver cell type most implicated in the pathogenesis of liver fibrosis is the hepatic stellate cell. In normal liver, the hepatic stellate cell is viewed as a pericyte that lies albuminal to the sinusoidal endothelial cell in the space of Disse[1] (see Chapter 71). On activation, a hepatic stellate cell transforms into a myofibroblast (Fig. 74-1).[2] Activation is characterized by increases in the expression of smooth muscle actin, motility, and contractility. Most importantly for the development of liver fibrosis, the stellate cell begins to generate various forms of matrix, which lead to liver fibrosis.[2] Fibronectin is the earliest form of matrix produced by stellate cells, which ultimately produce other forms of matrix, including collagen 1.[3] Matrix deposition in turn leads to further hepatic stellate cell activation and changes in the hepatic angioarchitecture.[3] The canonical pathways that are most implicated in activation of the hepatic stellate cell include kinase activation pathways mediated through platelet-derived growth factor (PDGF), transforming growth factor (TGF)-β, and integrin signaling pathways.

In addition to the hepatic stellate cell, other cells, including the portal fibroblast,[4] may ultimately culminate in the myofibroblast phenotype that deposits collagen matrix. The portal fibroblast resides closer than hepatic stellate cells to the portal tract and is implicated in the liver fibrosis that develops in response to portal-based, cholestatic injury, as in PBC and PSC.[4] It is hypothesized that epithelial cell injury in the periportal region leads to transformation of portal fibroblasts into myofibroblasts.

Cell types other than myofibroblasts are also important in the fibrosis process. For example, epithelial cell injury is the initiating step in most forms of liver injury that leads to fibrosis. Injury to epithelial cells, either through apoptosis, inflammation, or sterile necrosis, culminates in the recruitment and activation of hepatic stellate cells.[5] The macrophage is also important in fibrosis owing to release of inflammatory cytokines, which in turn lead to transactivation of hepatic stellate cells into myofibroblasts. Studies have also indicated an important role for the sinusoidal endothelial cell in fibrosis development. Sinusoidal endothelial cells act through autocrine and paracrine signaling pathways to participate in angiogenesis. Angiogenesis may lead to fibrosis through paracrine release of hepatic stellate cell activating molecules from angiogenic sinusoidal endothelial cells. Therefore, multiple cell types in the liver participate in fibrogenesis, although the hepatic stellate cell is most directly implicated in this process because of its abundant capacity to produce matrix.

DIAGNOSIS

Although cirrhosis is strictly speaking a histologic diagnosis (Fig. 74-2), a combination of clinical, laboratory, and imaging features can help confirm a diagnosis of cirrhosis. Several physical findings suggestive of cirrhosis result in part from alterations in the metabolism of estrogen by the cirrhotic liver. An intense red coloration of the thenar and hypothenar eminences suggests palmar erythema. Terry's nails are characterized by proximal nail bed pallor, which can also involve the entire nail plate, with predominant involvement of the thumb and index finger. Clubbing of the fingernails may result from the presence of arteriovenous shunts in the lung as a result of portal hypertension. Gynecomastia is the enlargement of the male breast with palpable tissue. Spider telangiectasias (or angiomata) are dilated arterioles characterized by a prominent central arteriole with radiating vessels. Compression of the central arteriole with a pinhead results in blanching followed by reformation of the "spider" after release of pressure on the arteriole. In general, more than 2 to 3 spider telangiectasias are considered abnormal. Dilated abdominal veins (caput medusae) with flow away from the umbilicus, toward the inferior vena cava in the infraumbilical area and toward the superior vena cava in the supraumbilical area, suggest intrahepatic portal hypertension. On the other hand, dilatation of veins in the flank with blood draining toward the superior vena cava suggests inferior vena caval obstruction. Parotid enlargement is also a feature of cirrhosis, especially alcoholic cirrhosis.

BOX 74-1 Causes of Cirrhosis

Viral
HBV
HCV
HDV

Autoimmune
Autoimmune hepatitis
PBC
PSC

Toxic
Alcohol
Arsenic

Metabolic
α_1-Antitrypsin deficiency
Galactosemia
Glycogen storage disease
Hemochromatosis
Nonalcoholic fatty liver disease and steatohepatitis
Wilson disease

Biliary
Atresia
Stone
Tumor

Vascular
Budd-Chiari syndrome
Cardiac fibrosis

Genetic
CF
Lysosomal acid lipase deficiency

Iatrogenic
Biliary injury
Drugs: high-dose vitamin A, methotrexate

BOX 74-2 Principal Complications of Cirrhosis

Portal Hypertension
Ascites
Variceal bleeding

Malignancy
Cholangiocarcinoma
Hepatocellular carcinoma

Bacterial Infections
Bacteremia
Clostridium difficile infection
Cellulitis
Pneumonia
SBP
Urinary tract infection

Cardiopulmonary Disorders
Cardiomyopathy
Hepatic hydrothorax
Hepatopulmonary syndrome
Portopulmonary hypertension

GI Disorders
GI bleeding
    Nonvariceal
    Variceal
Protein-losing enteropathy
Venous thrombosis

Renal Disorders
Hepatorenal syndrome
Other causes of acute kidney injury

Metabolic Disorders
Adrenal insufficiency
Hypogonadism
Malnutrition
Osteoporosis

Neuropsychiatric Disorders
Depression
Hepatic encephalopathy

Hematologic Disorders
Anemia
Hypercoagulability
Hypersplenism
Impaired coagulation

Unclear Etiology
Erectile dysfunction
Fatigue
Muscle cramps

Patients with a history of chronic liver disease with gastroesophageal varices, ascites, or hepatic encephalopathy are likely to have cirrhosis, and liver biopsy is not essential in such cases for confirming cirrhosis. In patients with a diagnosis of chronic liver disease without these complications, physical findings of an enlarged left hepatic lobe with splenomegaly, along with the cutaneous stigmata of liver disease described earlier, suggest cirrhosis, especially in the setting of thrombocytopenia and impaired hepatic synthetic function (e.g., hypoalbuminemia, prolongation of the prothrombin time). If physical and laboratory findings are not suggestive of cirrhosis, imaging studies can help make a diagnosis of cirrhosis. A small nodular liver with splenomegaly and intra-abdominal collaterals and the presence of ascites on abdominal US (or other cross-sectional imaging study) suggests cirrhosis (Fig. 74-3). A number of commercially available tools combine hematologic parameters, liver biochemical tests, and serologic markers to determine the degree of hepatic fibrosis.[6] In general, these tools are useful in discriminating early from late stages of fibrosis, but not between individual stages of fibrosis (see Chapters 73 and 80).

Where available, transient elastography (or fibroelastography), acoustic radiation force impulse (ARFI) elastography (another form of ultrasound elastography),[6] or magnetic resonance elastography (MRE) can help confirm a diagnosis of cirrhosis. On transient elastography, a liver stiffness measurement (measured in kilopascals) of greater than 14 kPa suggests cirrhosis, with values greater than 21 kPa associated with portal hypertension and its complications.[7] ARFI imaging values greater than 2.6 m/sec also suggest cirrhosis; moreover, ARFI imaging is more easily performed than transient elastography.[6] On MRE, liver stiffness values greater than 5.9 kPa suggest cirrhosis, and a liver biopsy is typically not required to confirm the diagnosis. Increasing spleen stiffness on ultrasound elastography or MRE is associated with the onset of portal hypertension.[8]

Liver biopsy has long been the gold standard for diagnosing cirrhosis but may be associated with costs and procedure-related risks, albeit infrequently (see Chapter 21). The major concerns regarding the use of a liver biopsy to diagnose cirrhosis includes sampling error and interobserver disagreement in the estimation of the extent of fibrosis. The ideal combination of clinical findings and routine laboratory tests to determine whether a patient has cirrhosis without the need

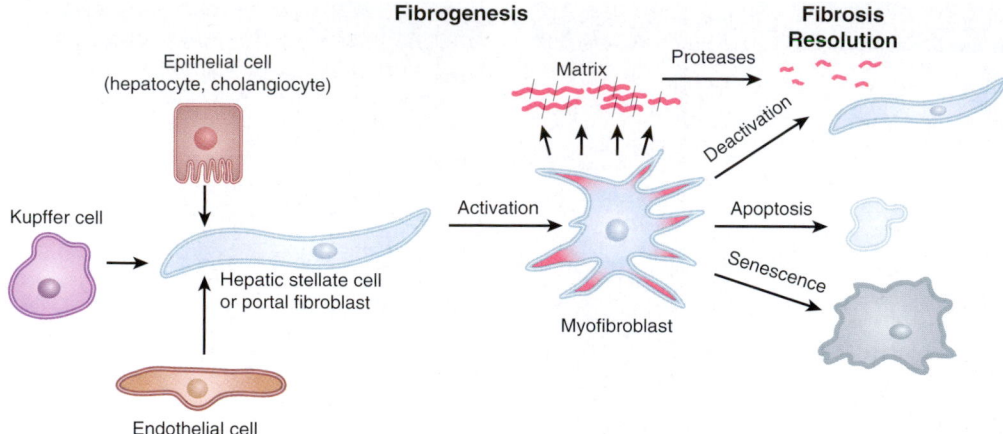

FIGURE 74-1. Schematic overview of the pathogenesis of fibrosis and reversal of fibrosis in cirrhosis. Epithelial cell injury in combination with cytokine release by Kupffer cells and paracrine molecule release by sinusoidal endothelial cells leads to activation of hepatic stellate cells (or portal fibroblasts) into myofibroblasts. Reversal of fibrosis results from myofibroblast deactivation, apoptosis, or senescence. Matrix proteases can also achieve fibrosis resolution (see text for details).

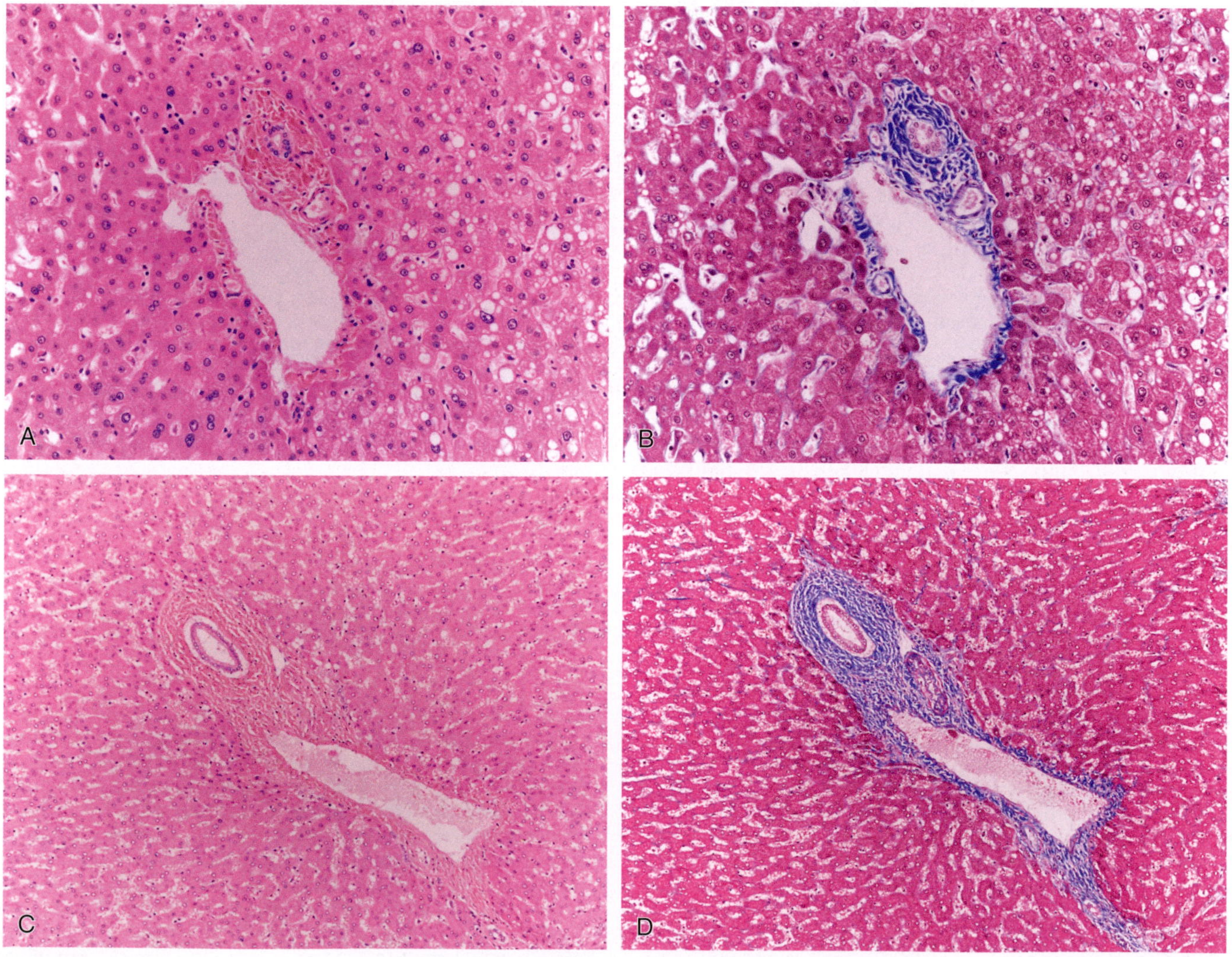

FIGURE 74-2. Histologic stages of hepatic fibrosis. *A,* A normal portal tract containing a portal vein branch, hepatic artery branch, and interlobular bile duct. The acinar parenchyma shows mild steatosis but no fibrosis. This is stage 0 fibrosis. (H&E.) *B,* A Masson's tri-chrome stain highlights in blue a normal (minimal) amount of collagen in a portal tract in stage 0. *C,* In stage 1 (of 4), there is a significant increase in collagen (fibrosis) in the portal tract. (H&E.) *D,* The fibrosis in stage 1 is highlighted in blue by a Masson's trichrome stain. The fibrosis expands the portal tract but does not involve the surrounding periportal acinar parenchyma.

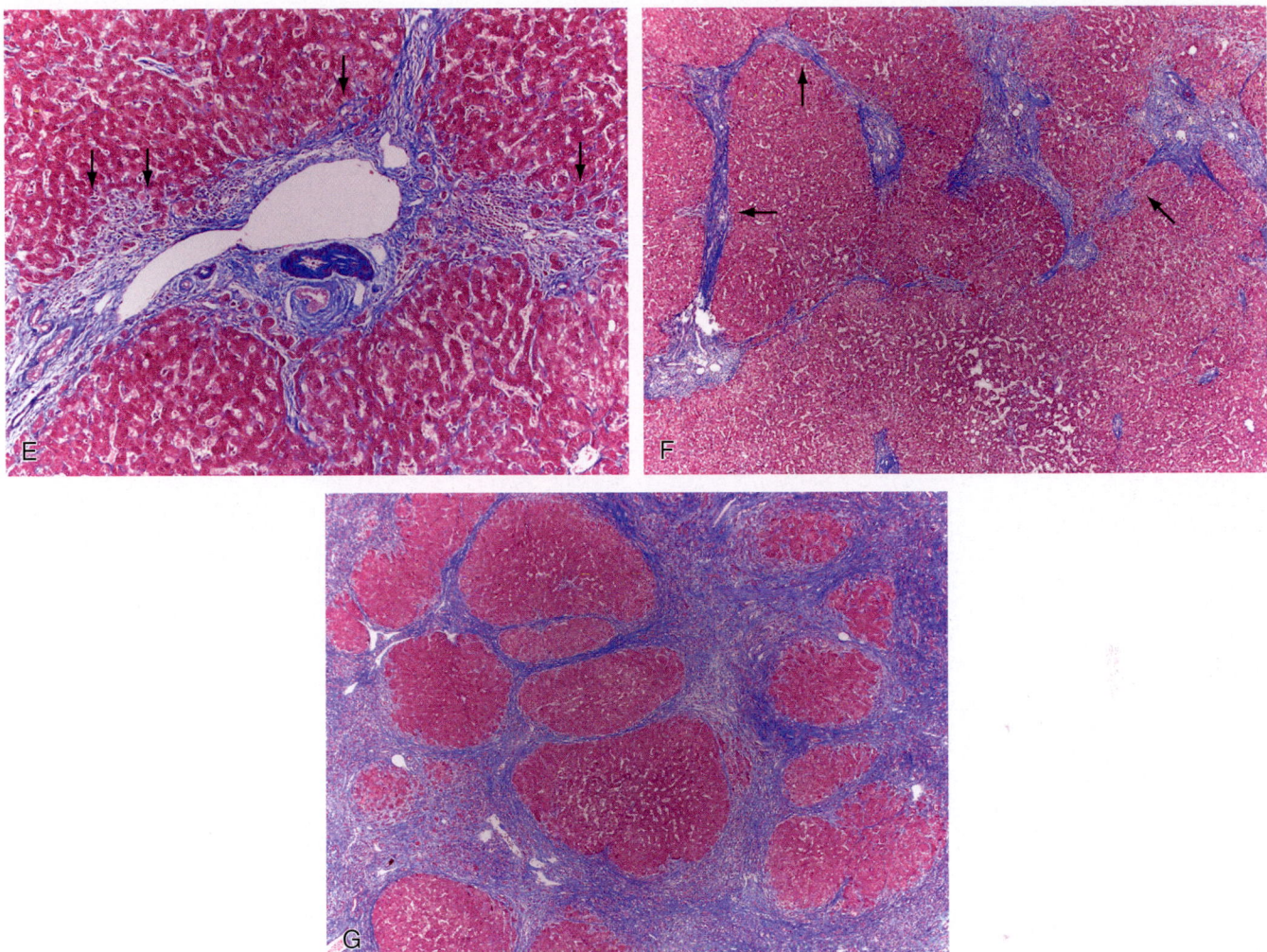

FIGURE 74-2, cont'd *E,* Periportal fibrosis characterizes stage 2. Expansion of the portal tract by fibrosis in blue is seen. The collagen is not confined to the portal tract but also extends to involve the surrounding periportal acinar parenchyma *(arrows).* (Masson's trichrome stain.) *F,* In stage 3, bridging fibrosis is seen. Multiple portal tracts demonstrate increased fibrosis in blue and connect with one another, forming fibrous bridges *(arrows).* (Masson's trichrome stain.) *G,* In cirrhosis (stage 4), the normal liver architecture is completely distorted and replaced by regenerative nodules that are separated by fibrous septa in blue. (Masson's trichrome stain.) *(Images courtesy Taofic Mounajjed, MD, Rochester, Minn.)*

for a liver biopsy has been addressed in a systematic fashion.[9] The most commonly used scoring systems are outlined in Table 74-1. A serum AST/platelet ratio index (APRI) of greater than 2 suggests cirrhosis, as does a Bonacini cirrhosis discriminant score of 7 or greater. A Bonacini score of less than 3, or a Lok index of less than 0.2, argues against a diagnosis of cirrhosis. Ascites and a platelet count of less than $160,000/mm^3$ render the diagnosis of cirrhosis more likely, whereas the absence of hepatomegaly or a firm liver, or a platelet count of $160 \times 10^3/mm^3$ or greater, makes cirrhosis unlikely.

NATURAL HISTORY

Cirrhosis may be classified broadly as *compensated* or *decompensated.* The development of complications of variceal hemorrhage, ascites, encephalopathy, jaundice, or hepatocellular carcinoma characterizes decompensated cirrhosis. In compensated cirrhosis, these complications are absent. Four clinical stages of cirrhosis have been proposed, with stages 1 and 2 representing compensated cirrhosis, and stages 3 and 4 representing decompensated cirrhosis. Stage 1 cirrhosis is characterized by absence of both ascites and varices; stage 2 cirrhosis is characterized by the presence of varices without bleeding and the absence of ascites; stage 3 cirrhosis is characterized by ascites with or without esophageal varices; and stage 4 cirrhosis is characterized by variceal bleeding with or without ascites. In the future, it is possible that staging of cirrhosis will consider not only clinical and histologic parameters, but also hemodynamic and biological data.[10]

Most deaths in patients with cirrhosis occur as a result of hepatic decompensation; however, in the compensated stages, the most common cause of death is cardiovascular disease, followed by stroke, malignancy, and renal disease.[11] Complications of portal hypertension, hepatocellular carcinoma (HCC),

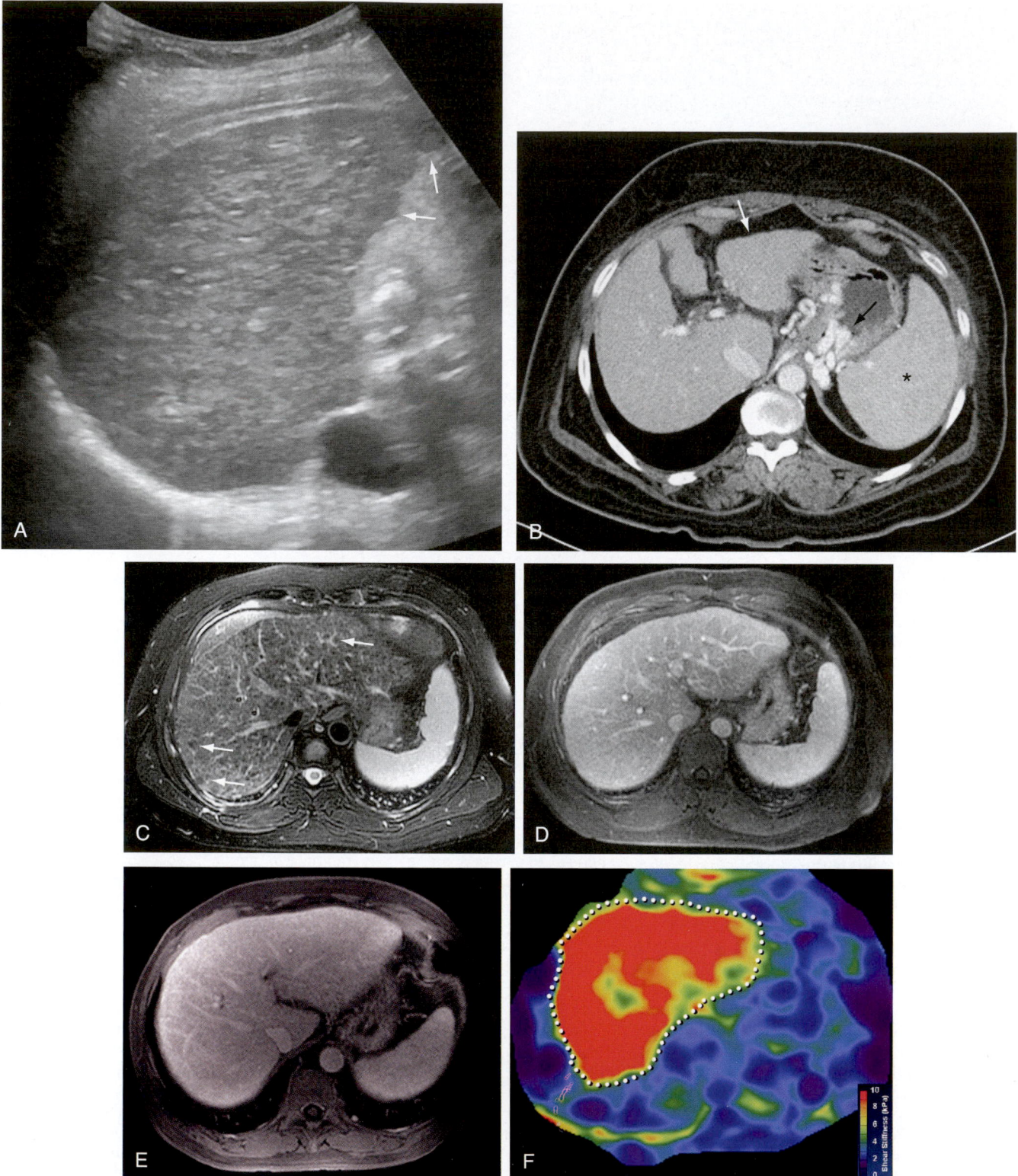

FIGURE 74-3. Imaging in cirrhosis. *A,* A transverse US image of the right lobe of liver demonstrates the characteristic heterogeneous liver parenchyma with surface nodularity *(arrowheads). B,* Axial contrast-enhanced CT image shows a nodular left lobe of the liver *(white arrow).* Note the gastric and esophageal varices *(black arrow)* and splenomegaly *(asterisk). C,* T2-weighted and *D,* contrast-enhanced T1-weighted MRIs show hypointense siderotic nodules *(white arrows)* and an enlarged left lobe and splenomegaly. *E,* A contrast-enhanced MRI shows a heterogeneous liver with an enlarged left lobe. *F,* A stiffness map from magnetic resonance elastography shows increased stiffness of the liver *(dotted outline),* with a mean stiffness value of 9.2 kilopascals. The normal liver stiffness value is less than 2.93 kilopascals. *(F, From Yin M, Talwalker JA, Glaser KJ, et al. Assessment of hepatic fibrosis with magnetic resonance elastography. Clin Gastroenterol Hepatol 2007; 5:1207-13.e2. Other images courtesy Sudhakar Venkatesh, MD, Rochester, Minn.)*

TABLE 74-1 Commonly Used Scores for Predicting Cirrhosis

AST/platelet ratio index (APRI)*

(AST/upper limit of normal AST) × (100/platelet count [×10^3/mm^3])

Bonacini cirrhosis discriminant score (CDS)†

Platelet score + ALT/AST ratio score + INR score

Score	Platelets (×10^3/mm^3)	ALT/AST ratio	INR
0	>340	>1.7	<1.1
1	280-340	1.2-1.7	1.1-1.4
2	220-279	0.6-1.19	>1.4
3	160-219	<0.6	-
4	100-159	-	-
5	40-99	-	-
6	<40	-	-

Lok index‡

exp (log odds) / [1 + exp(log odds)]

log odds = − 5.56 − (0.0089 × platelet count [×10^3/mm^3]) + (1.26 × AST/ALT ratio) + (5.27 × INR)

*Higher values of the APRI increase the likelihood of cirrhosis, and lower values decrease the likelihood of cirrhosis.

†The modified Bonacini CDS has a range of possible values from 0 to 11; higher scores identify patients with a higher likelihood of cirrhosis, and lower scores identify patients with a lower likelihood of cirrhosis.

‡The Lok index is an odds ratio normalized to possible values between 0 and 1; a higher fraction (i.e., probability) increases the likelihood of cirrhosis, whereas a lower fraction reduces the likelihood of cirrhosis. (See also http://www.haltctrial.org/cirrhosis.html.)

Adapted from Udell JA, Wang CS, Tinmouth J, et al. Does this patient with liver disease have cirrhosis? JAMA 2012; 307:832-42, with permission.

and sepsis[12] are the usual causes of mortality in patients with decompensated cirrhosis.

PROGNOSIS

Liver-related mortality is the eighth leading disease cause of death in the United States. Among persons 45 to 64 years of age, cirrhosis is the third leading cause of death. As compared with the general population, persons with compensated cirrhosis have a 5-fold increased risk of death, whereas patients with decompensated cirrhosis have a 10-fold increased risk. The median survival in patients with compensated cirrhosis is 9 to 12 years, compared with 2 years in those with decompensated cirrhosis.

In a nationwide Danish population study, the overall survival probability in patients with cirrhosis was 66% at 1 year, 38% at 5 years, and 22% at 10 years.[13] The majority of deaths were related to cirrhosis. Most deaths among patients with compensated cirrhosis occurred as a result of transition to a decompensated state. In the Danish study,[13] the median survival in patients without complications was 48 months, with a 1-year survival rate of 83% in those with compensated cirrhosis, 80% in those with variceal bleeding, 71% in those with ascites, 51% in those with ascites and variceal bleeding, and 36% in those with hepatic encephalopathy.

Prognosis depends not only on the clinical stage of the disease but also on the presence of comorbidities. Generic scores to determine mortality risk include the Child-Turcotte-Pugh score (Child-Pugh class) and the MELD score and its modifications (see Chapters 73 and 97), as well as von Willebrand factor levels[14] (see Chapter 94). Levels of von Willebrand factor antigen above 315% are associated with a higher risk of decompensation. Measuring the hepatic vein pressure gradient (HVPG) (see Chapter 92) is a useful tool to assess prognosis but is invasive and expensive, making repeated measurements impractical.

Infection and renal failure are commonly associated with mortality in patients with cirrhosis (see Chapters 93 and 94). Patients with an infection have a 4-fold increase in mortality compared with cirrhotic patients without an infection.[15] Patients with renal failure have a 7- to 8-fold increased risk of death compared with patients without renal failure.[16]

Because the majority of deaths in patients with cirrhosis are due to progression to a decompensated state, it is important to determine the risk of progression to decompensated cirrhosis. The 10-year probability of decompensation from a compensated state is 58%. The annual rate of decompensation varies with the etiology of liver disease; it is 4% for patients with HCV-related cirrhosis, 6% to 10% in those with alcoholic cirrhosis (and even higher if they continue to drink actively), and 10% in those with HBV-related cirrhosis.[17] The risk of decompensation is also associated with the serum albumin level, MELD score, and HVPG. An HVPG less than 10 mm Hg has a 90% negative predictive value for the development of clinical decompensation over 4 years.[18] An increase in MELD score and a decrease in the serum albumin level are also associated with decompensation.

TREATMENT

Management of compensated cirrhosis includes surveillance for HCC with US of the liver every 6 months (see Chapter 96), screening for esophageal varices by upper GI endoscopy (see Chapters 20 and 92), cessation of alcohol use, weight loss, and other lifestyle changes, although the cost-effectiveness of screening for HCC has been questioned.[19] Immunization against HAV, HBV, pneumococcal pneumonia, and influenza is recommended. Live-attenuated vaccines are not contraindicated in patients with cirrhosis. Delaying the progression of compensated cirrhosis to a decompensated state may be achieved by treating the underlying cause of cirrhosis (e.g., chronic hepatitis B and C),[20] abstinence from alcohol, and weight loss. The use of low molecular weight heparin has been reported to delay decompensation even in patients without portal vein thrombosis.[21]

In general, acetaminophen may be used in persons with cirrhosis in doses of up to 2 g daily (see Chapter 88). Aspirin and other NSAIDs should be avoided in patients with decompensated cirrhosis, including those with ascites. Aminoglycosides are contraindicated, but other antibiotics are acceptable, as are statins for treatment of hyperlipidemia. In patients with diabetes mellitus, oral hypoglycemic agents may be used if the cirrhosis is compensated, but in patients with decompensated cirrhosis, insulin is preferred. Patients with cirrhosis have protein-calorie malnutrition, and frequent high-calorie small meals, as well as bedtime snacks, are recommended. Fat-soluble vitamins and zinc levels require monitoring, with replacement if required.

Problems that occur in patients with cirrhosis for which there are no clear management solutions include fatigue, muscle cramps, and sexual dysfunction. Fatigue is a major factor in reducing a patient's quality of life and may be a manifestation of covert encephalopathy. Fatigue is more common in patients with obesity, depression, and sleep apnea. A search for reversible causes of fatigue, including anemia and thyroid disease, should be conducted. Muscle cramps also impair the patient's quality of life and are independent of age, disease severity, and diuretic use. Unfortunately, no effective therapy is available to alleviate muscle cramps. Erectile dysfunction is a common problem, but agents like phosphodiesterase inhibitors typically used for the treatment of erectile dysfunction may be ineffective in patients with cirrhosis. Finally, depression occurs in 30% to 40% of patients with cirrhosis, especially in those patients with hepatitis C, and is associated with obesity, diabetes mellitus, and sleep disorders. Selective serotonin reuptake inhibitors and mirtazapine are safe and effective agents for the treatment of depression in patients with cirrhosis.

In the future, treatment of cirrhosis will involve reversal of hepatic fibrosis and prevention of hepatic decompensation using a combination of drugs aimed at reducing portal pressure and hepatic inflammation.[22]

Reversal of Fibrosis

Evidence to indicate that fibrosis is reversible has come from clinical observations in humans and experimental studies in animal models of liver fibrosis. Human evidence that fibrosis is reversible is based on the observation that fibrosis improves in response to control of the underlying disease process. For example, patients with liver fibrosis secondary to chronic biliary obstruction in whom the obstruction is relieved show improvement in hepatic histology. The same occurs in patients who have undergone successful therapy for chronic viral hepatitis.

In animal models, genetic disruption of fibrogenic signaling pathways prevents or reverses liver fibrosis (or both).[23] A number of compounds have also been shown to reverse or prevent liver fibrosis in animal models,[23] but fibrosis is easier to prevent or reverse in animal models than in humans.

Specific factors and pathways that have been studied as mediators of fibrosis reversal include angiotensin, nuclear receptors, receptor tyrosine kinases, integrins, and matrix degrading proteases.[24] These pathways broadly aim to reverse the myofibroblast state of hepatic stellate cells by inducing senescence, deactivation, or apoptosis (see Fig. 74-1)[24] and have been studied in preclinical models; however, evidence of their clinical utility in humans is as yet lacking.

A number of limitations have precluded successful antifibrosis therapy in humans. One limitation is the lack of effective tools to precisely assess fibrosis noninvasively.[24] Despite advances in US elastography and MRE, most clinical trials still require liver biopsy, which is invasive and unappealing to patients. Resolution of fibrosis may take years to achieve, further complicating trial design. Additionally, development of fibrosis is a multifactorial process, and it is challenging to target the correct cell selectively with a specific pharmacologic intervention. Finally, although earlier stages of fibrosis may be amenable to resolution, advanced stages of fibrosis may not be reversible, owing to fixed angioarchitectural changes.

KEY REFERENCES

Full references for this chapter can be found on www.expertconsult.com.

1. Iwakiri Y, Grisham M, Shah V. Vascular biology and pathobiology of the liver: Report of a single-topic symposium. Hepatology 2008; 47:1754-63.
2. Lee UE, Friedman SL. Mechanisms of hepatic fibrogenesis. Best Pract Res Clin Gastroenterol 2011; 25:195-206.
3. Yaqoob U, Cao S, Shergill U, et al. Neuropilin-1 stimulates tumor growth by increasing fibronectin fibril assembly in the tumor microenvironment. Cancer Res 2012; 72:4047-59.
8. Colecchia A, Montrone L, Scaioli E, et al. Measurement of spleen stiffness to evaluate portal hypertension and the presence of esophageal varices in patients with HCV-related cirrhosis. Gastroenterology 2012; 143:646-54.
9. Udell JA, Wang CS, Tinmouth J, et al. Does this patient with liver disease have cirrhosis? JAMA 2012; 307:832-42.
10. Garcia-Tsao G, Friedman S, Iredale J, et al. Now there are many (stages) where before there was one: In search of a pathophysiological classification of cirrhosis. Hepatology 2010; 51:1445-9.
11. Asrani SK, Kamath PS. Natural history of cirrhosis. Curr Gastroenterol Rep 2013; 15:308.
12. Bajaj JS, O'Leary JG, Reddy KR, et al. Second infections independently increase mortality in hospitalized patients with cirrhosis: The North American consortium for the study of end-stage liver disease (NACSELD) experience. Hepatology 2012; 56:2328-35.
13. Jepsen P, Vilstrup H, Andersen PK, et al. Comorbidity and survival of Danish cirrhosis patients: A nationwide population-based cohort study. Hepatology 2008; 48:214-20.
15. Arvaniti V, D'Amico G, Fede G, et al. Infections in patients with cirrhosis increase mortality four-fold and should be used in determining prognosis. Gastroenterology 2010; 139:1246-56, 1256 e1-5.
17. Jepsen P, Ott P, Andersen PK, et al. Clinical course of alcoholic liver cirrhosis: A Danish population-based cohort study. Hepatology 2010; 51:1675-82.
18. Ripoll C, Groszmann R, Garcia-Tsao G, et al. Hepatic venous pressure gradient predicts clinical decompensation in patients with compensated cirrhosis. Gastroenterology 2007; 133:481-8.
19. Jepsen P, Ott P, Andersen PK, et al. Risk for hepatocellular carcinoma in patients with alcoholic cirrhosis: A Danish nationwide cohort study. Ann Intern Med 2012; 156:841-7, W295.
22. Tsochatzis EA, Bosch J, Burroughs AK. New therapeutic paradigm for patients with cirrhosis. Hepatology 2012; 56:1983-92.
24. Schuppan D, Pinzani M. Anti-fibrotic therapy: Lost in translation? J Hepatol 2012; 56(Suppl 1):S66-74.

Hemochromatosis

BRUCE R. BACON AND ROBERT S. BRITTON

Trousseau was the first to describe a case of hemochromatosis in the French pathology literature in 1865.[1] Almost 25 years later, in 1889, von Recklinghausen, thinking that the disease was a blood disorder that caused increased skin pigmentation, introduced the term *hemochromatosis*.[1] In 1935, Sheldon published a description of all 311 cases of the disease that had been reported in the world's literature to that point, including several from his own records. He recognized that hemochromatosis was an inborn error of iron metabolism and that all the pathologic manifestations of the disease were caused by increased iron deposition in the affected organs.[1] In 1976, Simon and coworkers[2] demonstrated that the gene for hereditary hemochromatosis (HH) was linked to the HLA region on the short arm of chromosome 6. The benefit of early diagnosis on survival was shown in a classic paper by Niederau and colleagues,[3] who demonstrated that if HH was identified and treated before the development of cirrhosis or diabetes mellitus, survival of affected patients was equivalent to that of an age- and gender-matched population.

In 1996, the *HFE* gene was identified on chromosome 6, thereby permitting genetic testing for the two major mutations (C282Y, H63D) that are responsible for *HFE*-related HH.[4] Several prospective population studies have shown that the frequency of the C282Y homozygous state is approximately 1 in 250 in white populations of northern European descent.[5] It is now recognized that C282Y homozygosity has incomplete clinical penetrance, with a strong male predominance for symptomatic disease.[6] HH is characterized by increased intestinal iron absorption that results from low expression of the iron-regulatory protein hepcidin.[5-7] In addition to the discovery of *HFE* and hepcidin, several additional genes and proteins involved in the regulation of iron homeostasis have been identified, contributing to a better understanding of cellular iron uptake and release. Also, numerous clinical and pathophysiologic studies have been performed and have led to improved diagnosis, better family screening, and new insights into normal and abnormal iron homeostasis. *HFE*-related HH is a common autosomal recessive disorder of iron metabolism; if it is diagnosed early and treated appropriately, every patient with the disorder can have a normal lifespan. Publications from the AASLD and the European Association for the Study of the Liver (EASL) provide expert guidelines for the evaluation and management of HH.[8,9]

CAUSES OF IRON OVERLOAD

HH comprises several inherited disorders of iron homeostasis characterized by increased intestinal iron absorption that results in tissue iron deposition (Box 75-1). The older terms "primary hemochromatosis" and "idiopathic hemochromatosis" are no longer used. The liver is always the principal recipient of most of the absorbed iron and is always involved in symptomatic HH. The most common form of HH by far is *HFE*-related HH.[5-7,10-12] It is an autosomal recessive disorder usually identified in adults of northern European ancestry. Most patients who present with HH are homozygous for the C282Y mutation of *HFE*, although some persons (about 10%) who are compound heterozygotes (C282Y/H63D) also have iron overload.

Other inherited forms of iron overload, classified as non-*HFE*-related HH, are juvenile hemochromatosis and iron overload resulting from mutations in the genes for hepcidin (*HAMP*), transferrin receptor 2 (*TFR2*), or ferroportin (*SLC40A1*).[13] Juvenile HH is characterized by rapid iron accumulation. Mutations in two different genes have been shown to cause forms of juvenile HH. The more common mutation occurs in the *HJV* gene on chromosome 1q; this gene encodes a protein called *hemojuvelin*. Mutations in *HAMP* also produce a form of juvenile HH; hepcidin is a hepatic peptide that acts to down-regulate iron absorption (see later). Mutations of the gene *TFR2* produce an autosomal recessive form of HH that is clinically similar to *HFE*-related HH. How these *TFR2* mutations result in iron overload is not yet known; they possibly cause abnormal iron sensing by hepatocytes, the predominant site of TFR2 expression. A rare autosomal dominant form of HH results from two categories of mutations in the gene for the iron transporter ferroportin.[14] "Loss-of-function" mutations decrease the cell surface localization of ferroportin, thereby reducing its ability to export iron. The result is iron deposition primarily in macrophages, and this disorder is sometimes termed *ferroportin disease*. The second category

Hereditary Hemochromatosis
HFE-Related Hereditary Hemochromatosis (Type 1)
C282Y homozygosity
C282Y/H63D compound heterozygosity
Other HFE mutations

Non–HFE-Related Hereditary Hemochromatosis
Hemojuvelin (HJV) mutations (type 2A)
Hepcidin (HAMP) mutations (type 2B)
Transferrin receptor 2 (TFR2) mutations (type 3)
Ferroportin (SLC40A1) mutations (type 4)
  Loss-of-function mutations
  Gain-of-function mutations
African iron overload

Secondary Iron Overload
Iron-Loading Anemias
Aplastic anemia
Chronic hemolytic anemia
Pyridoxine-responsive anemia
Pyruvate kinase deficiency
Sideroblastic anemia
Thalassemia major

Parenteral Iron Overload
Iron-dextran injections
Long-term hemodialysis
Red blood cell transfusions

Chronic Liver Disease
Alcoholic liver disease
Hepatitis B
Hepatitis C
Nonalcoholic steatohepatitis
Porphyria cutanea tarda
Portacaval shunt

Insulin Resistance Syndrome with Iron Overload

Dietary Iron Overload

Miscellaneous
Aceruloplasminemia
Congenital alloimmune hepatitis (neonatal hemochromatosis)
Congenital atransferrinemia

includes "gain-of-function" ferroportin mutations that abolish hepcidin-induced ferroportin internalization and degradation; the distribution of excess iron is similar to that in HFE-related HH, primarily within parenchymal cells.

African iron overload occurs primarily in sub-Saharan Africa and is now considered to be the result of a non–HFE-related genetic trait that can be exacerbated by dietary iron loading.[15] Some persons who manifest African iron overload consume an iron-rich fermented maize beverage, but iron overload also can occur in people who do not drink this beverage. In most cases, iron-loaded Kupffer cells are prominent in African iron overload; by contrast, Kupffer cells are relatively spared in HFE-related HH. A similar form of iron overload has been suggested to occur in African Americans,[16] and further investigations are needed to determine the genetic basis, prevalence, and clinical consequences of this condition.

Persons who absorb excessive amounts of iron as a result of an underlying cause other than any of the previously mentioned inherited defects have *secondary iron overload*[12] (see Box 75-1). Causes of secondary iron overload include disorders of ineffective erythropoiesis, liver disease (in some cases), increased oral intake of iron, or the rare condition congenital atransferrinemia. Both HH and secondary iron overload

should be distinguished from *parenteral iron overload*, which is always iatrogenic and which leads to iron deposition that is found initially in the reticuloendothelial system. In patients with ineffective erythropoiesis who require red blood cell transfusions, parenchymal and reticuloendothelial iron overload coexist because these people have a stimulus for increased iron absorption and receive iron in the form of red blood cell transfusions. Congenital alloimmune hepatitis is responsible for most cases of neonatal hemochromatosis.[17] In these cases, immune-mediated liver injury in the fetus is associated with the development of iron overload. Treatment with IV immunoglobulin during pregnancy markedly slows or prevents the development of this condition.

PATHOPHYSIOLOGY

The pathophysiologic mechanisms of HH fall into the following 4 main categories: (1) increased intestinal absorption of dietary iron, (2) decreased expression of the iron-regulatory hormone hepcidin, (3) altered function of HFE protein, and (4) iron-induced tissue injury and fibrogenesis.

Intestinal Iron Absorption

An increase in intestinal iron absorption is a pathogenic characteristic of *HFE*-related HH.[5-7,11] Understanding the pathogenesis of HH, therefore, requires a review of the determinants of duodenal iron absorption. Because there are no important physiologic mechanisms to regulate iron loss, iron homeostasis depends on a tight linkage between body iron requirements and intestinal iron absorption. Nearly all absorption of dietary iron occurs in the duodenum, where iron may be taken up as either ionic iron or heme.[18] The absorption of both forms of iron is increased in patients with *HFE*-related HH.

Absorption of ionic iron across the enterocyte occurs in two stages: uptake across the apical membrane and transfer across the basolateral membrane (Fig. 75-1A). Before uptake, ionic iron must be reduced from the ferric to the ferrous state; this step is accomplished by ferric reductases that are expressed on the luminal surface of duodenal enterocytes. The ferrous iron crosses the apical membrane via divalent metal transporter 1 (DMT-1). Iron taken up by the enterocyte may be stored as ferritin (and excreted in the feces when the senescent enterocyte is sloughed) or transferred across the basolateral membrane to the plasma. This latter process occurs via the transporter ferroportin. The basolateral transfer of iron requires oxidation of iron to the ferric state by the ferroxidase hephaestin. Uptake of heme occurs by a transporter whose identity remains uncertain. Once internalized, the heme is degraded and the liberated iron is handled by the enterocyte in the same manner as absorbed ionic iron. Patients with *HFE*-related HH demonstrate increased basolateral transfer of iron from the enterocytes to the plasma. This increased transfer may be the driving force behind the increased intestinal iron absorption that is characteristic of HH. Some studies of patients with *HFE*-related HH have demonstrated higher duodenal expression of ferroportin and DMT-1. The major regulator of intestinal iron absorption is the peptide hormone hepcidin.

Hepcidin

Hepcidin is an iron-regulatory hormone that plays a central role in iron homeostasis by coordinating iron absorption, mobilization, and storage to meet the iron requirements of erythropoiesis and other iron-dependent processes[18-21] (see Fig. 75-1B). Hepcidin is expressed predominantly in

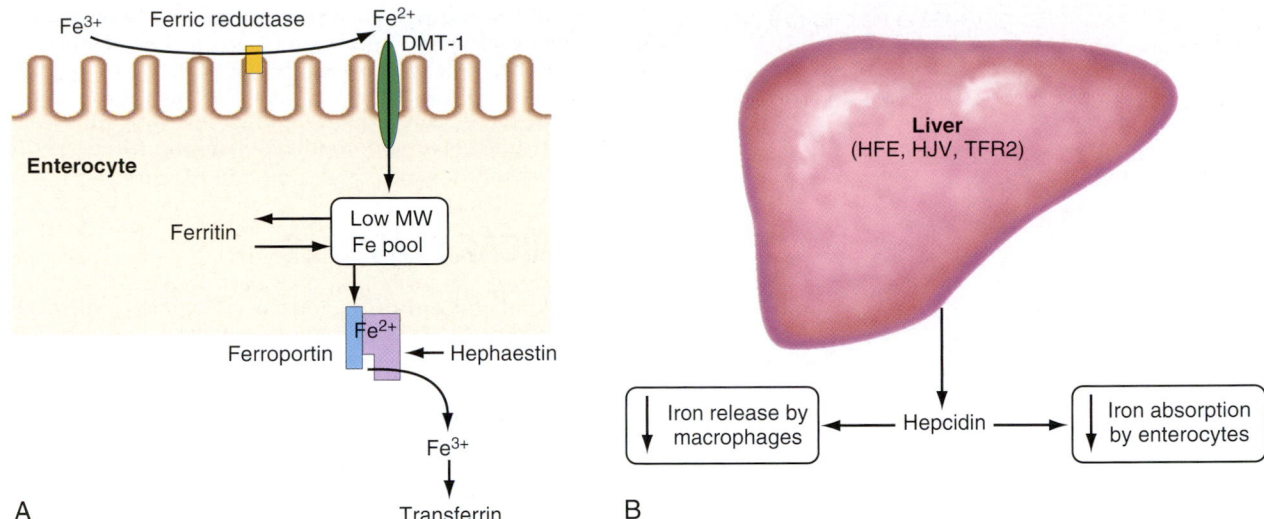

FIGURE 75-1. Iron absorption pathway in duodenal enterocytes and the role of hepcidin. *A,* Duodenal enterocytes are the major site of iron absorption. Before uptake, dietary ionic iron requires reduction from the ferric (Fe^{3+}) to the ferrous (Fe^{2+}) state. This is accomplished by ferric reductases that are expressed on the luminal surfaces of enterocytes. Ferrous iron is taken up by the apical divalent metal transporter 1, (DMT-1). Iron may be stored within the cell as ferritin, and then lost with the sloughed senescent enterocyte, or transferred across the basolateral membrane to the plasma. This latter process occurs via the transporter ferroportin and requires oxidation of iron back to the ferric state by the ferroxidase hephaestin. *B,* Hepcidin is produced by the liver and secreted into the blood. HFE protein, hemojuvelin (HJV), and transferrin receptor 2 (TFR2) may participate in the hepatic iron-sensing mechanism that regulates hepcidin expression. Hepcidin reduces iron release by macrophages (and thereby increases macrophage iron stores) and also reduces iron absorption by duodenal enterocytes to reduce the amount of dietary iron in the circulation. In *HFE*-related hereditary hemochromatosis, loss of functional HFE protein leads to aberrant hepatocellular sensing of plasma iron, inappropriately low levels of hepcidin, diminished macrophage iron stores, and greater duodenal iron absorption. MW, molecular weight.

hepatocytes and is secreted into the circulation. It binds to ferroportin, which is highly expressed on macrophages and the basolateral surface of enterocytes, thereby causing ferroportin to be internalized and degraded, thus inhibiting iron export. Hepcidin expression is regulated by total body iron, erythropoiesis, hypoxia, and inflammation. Excess iron and inflammation induce hepcidin expression, which, in turn, results in decreased intestinal iron absorption and diminished iron release from macrophages. By contrast, hepcidin expression is decreased by iron deficiency, erythropoiesis, and hypoxia, with resulting increases in iron absorption from the intestine and release of iron from macrophages.

In all types of HH, iron overload results from impairment in the hepcidin regulatory pathway. In humans and mice, mutations or knockout of the genes for HFE, hemojuvelin, hepcidin, or TFR2 decrease hepcidin expression, with a resulting increase in intestinal iron absorption via upregulation of ferroportin levels.[18-23] Studies have revealed that iron-induced regulation of hepcidin expression involves a bone morphogenetic protein 6 (BMP6)-dependent signaling pathway.[18,20,21] BMP6 binds to specific receptors on hepatocytes, thereby triggering SMAD protein-dependent activation of hepcidin expression. Selective inhibition of BMP signaling abrogates iron-induced upregulation of hepcidin. Hemojuvelin is a BMP co-receptor and facilitates the binding of BMP6 to its receptor; knockout of the hemojuvelin gene markedly decreases BMP6 signaling and hepcidin expression, and causes iron overload.

The inflammatory cytokine interleukin-6 up-regulates hepcidin via signal transducer and activator of transcription-3 (STAT3) signaling, causing iron retention in macrophages and decreased intestinal iron absorption. The resulting hypoferremia plays a major causal role in the anemia of chronic disease.[18-21] Reactive oxygen species inhibit hepcidin expression via a CCAAT/enhancer binding protein α

(C/EBPα)-mediated mechanism, which may contribute to the hepatic iron loading associated with alcoholic liver disease and chronic hepatitis C.[24] The development of minihepcidins—small peptides that mimic the action of hepcidin—opens the possibility of a new therapeutic approach for iron overload disorders caused by a low hepcidin state.[25]

HFE Protein

Studies of HFE protein structure and function were a direct consequence of the cloning of the *HFE* gene. The *HFE* gene encodes a 343–amino acid protein consisting of a 22–amino acid signal peptide, large extracellular domain, single transmembrane domain, and short cytoplasmic tail (Fig. 75-2).[4] The extracellular domain of HFE protein consists of 3 loops (α_1, α_2, and α_3), with intramolecular disulfide bonds within the second and third loops. The structure of the HFE protein is similar to that of other major histocompatibility complex (MHC) class I proteins, but evidence indicates that HFE protein does not participate in antigen presentation. Like MHC class I molecules, however, HFE protein is physically associated with β_2-microglobulin (see Fig. 75-2). The major mutation responsible for HH results in the substitution of tyrosine for cysteine at amino acid 282 in the α_3 loop (C282Y) and abolishes the disulfide bond in this domain.[4] Loss of this disulfide bond interferes with the interaction of HFE protein with β_2-microglobulin, and the C282Y mutant protein demonstrates decreased presentation at the cell surface, increased retention in the endoplasmic reticulum, and accelerated degradation. A second mutation associated with HH results in the change of a histidine to an aspartate at position 63 in the α_1 chain (H63D), but this mutation has less biological impact than the C282Y mutation. Like persons with HH, *Hfe*-knockout mice manifest higher hepatic iron levels, elevated transferrin saturation (TS), increased

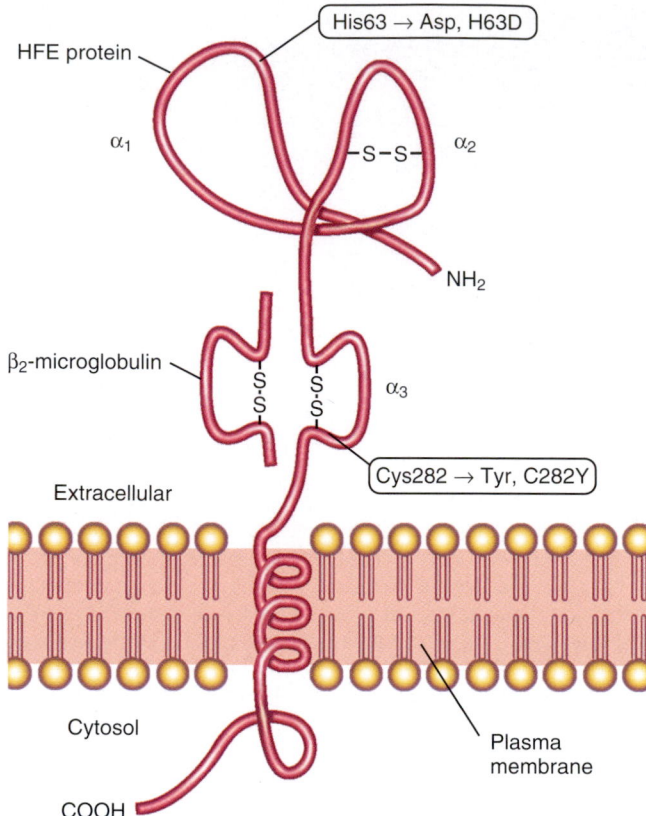

FIGURE 75-2. Schematic model of HFE protein in association with β_2-microglobulin at the cell surface. The 3 extracellular domains of HFE protein are designated α_1, α_2, and α_3. β_2-Microglobulin is physically associated with the α_3 domain. HFE protein also contains a transmembrane domain and a short intracellular domain. Positions of the 2 common HFE mutations, C282Y and H63D, are shown.

intestinal iron absorption, and relative sparing of iron loading in reticuloendothelial cells.

Despite intensive investigation, the molecular mechanisms by which HFE influences iron-dependent regulation of hepcidin remain unclear.[26] HFE can bind to the classic transferrin receptor TFR1,[18] and this interaction could be involved in iron sensing and hepcidin regulation. In addition, both HFE and TFR2 may interact with hemojuvelin, thereby suggesting another way that these proteins might play a role in iron-dependent BMP6 signaling to hepcidin.

Iron-Induced Tissue Injury and Fibrosis

Another major pathophysiologic mechanism in HH relates to the liver damage that results from iron overload. In patients with advanced HH, hepatic fibrosis and cirrhosis are the principal pathologic findings. A number of studies of experimental hepatic iron overload have identified iron-dependent lipid peroxidation and associated impairment of membrane-dependent functions of mitochondria, microsomes, and lysosomes.[27] A relationship between iron-induced lipid peroxidation and fibrosis has been shown in several studies.[28,29] One hypothesis is that iron-induced lipid peroxidation occurs in hepatocytes and causes hepatocellular injury or death. Kupffer cells may become activated by products released from injured iron-loaded hepatocytes and produce profibrogenic cytokines, which can, in turn, stimulate hepatic stellate cells

to synthesize larger amounts of collagen, thereby leading to pathologic fibrosis.[28,29]

Studies of iron-induced tissue damage in organs other than the liver, such as the heart, pancreas, and endocrine glands, have been limited. Studies in myocardial cells have shown functional abnormalities resulting from iron-induced peroxidation.[30]

CLINICAL FEATURES

Many patients with *HFE*-related HH come to medical attention without any symptoms or physical findings. They are identified as homozygous relatives of probands during family screening studies or by the results of serum iron studies in routine screening blood chemistry panels (Table 75-1).[31,32] Nevertheless, the clinician should know the typical clinical manifestations in patients who do present with symptomatic disease. Most patients with symptomatic *HFE*-related HH are 40 to 50 years of age at the time of detection. Although C282Y homozygosity is distributed equally between men and women, the clinical penetrance is much lower in women, as a result of iron loss from normal menses and childbirth, as well as possible gender-related disease modifier genes (Table 75-2).[33-38]

When patients present with symptoms, the most common are weakness and lethargy, arthralgias, abdominal pain, and loss of libido or potency in men.[3,39] Patients with *HFE*-related HH may have nonspecific right upper quadrant abdominal pain that is most likely caused by hepatic capsular distention. Hepatomegaly is found on physical examination in a majority of patients; splenomegaly and other complications of chronic liver disease, including ascites, edema, and jaundice, may be present. Diabetes mellitus has decreased in frequency with earlier diagnosis of hemochromatosis and is typically not seen in the absence of cirrhosis (see later). Detection of the often subtle bronzed or slate-gray skin pigmentation of *HFE*-related HH requires astuteness on the part of the clinician (see later). Organ damage and symptoms are usually related to the extent of iron loading. When patients are identified prospectively by either family or population screening, the frequency of patients who are asymptomatic increases dramatically.[33-38]

All patients with *HFE*-related HH who have an elevated serum ferritin value should also have increased hepatic iron stores, but the extent of hepatic iron loading is often not high enough to cause liver damage. In the late 1960s, cirrhosis was found in more than 50% of the patients identified with HH[3]; in studies from the 1970s through the 1990s, cirrhosis was found in only 5% to 10% of patients.[31,32] Subsequent population screening studies have reported an even lower frequency of cirrhosis in C282Y homozygotes.[34,37,38] Serum aminotransferase elevations are usually mild. With regular phlebotomy and depletion of excess iron stores, elevated liver enzyme values typically revert to normal. When *HFE*-related HH is diagnosed and treated before the development of hepatic fibrosis or cirrhosis, long-term hepatic abnormalities do not develop. When *HFE*-related HH is detected after cirrhosis has developed, however, hepatocellular carcinoma can occur even after successful phlebotomy,[40] thereby emphasizing the importance of early diagnosis and treatment.

Other clinical manifestations that can occur relate to the level of iron loading in nonhepatic organs. In older series, diabetes mellitus was a common complication of pancreatic iron loading,[3] but in subsequent series in which the diagnosis of *HFE*-related HH was made earlier in its course, diabetes mellitus has rarely been present.[31,32] Other endocrinologic abnormalities are loss of libido and impotence in men, owing to both primary testicular failure and gonadotropin insufficiency resulting from the effects of iron on pituitary function,[41]

TABLE 75-1 Clinical Features of Hereditary Hemochromatosis in 3 Studies from Different Time Periods

	1959-1983[3]	Before 1990[31]	1990-1995[32]
Variable			
Case selection method	Symptomatic index cases, family screening	Family screening by HLA typing	Screening chemistry panels, family screening
Number of patients	163	37	40
Men	145	19	26
Women	18	18	14
Mean age (yrs)	46	Men: 49	Men: 46
		Women: 53	Women: 47
Age range (yrs)	18-77	11-79	23-73
Symptoms (%)			
Weakness or lethargy	83	19	25
Abdominal pain	58	3	3
Arthralgias	43	40	13
Loss of libido, impotence (% of men)	38	32	12
None	9	46	73
Findings (%)			
Hepatomegaly	83	3	13
Skin pigmentation	75	9	5
Diabetes mellitus	55	11	5
Elevated liver enzymes	62	27	33
Cirrhosis	69	3	13*

*Five of 40 patients had cirrhosis; 1 had concomitant chronic hepatitis C, and 1 had alcoholic liver disease.

TABLE 75-2 Clinical Penetrance of C282Y Homozygosity in Women and Men

Finding	Women (%)	Men (%)
Iron-overload–related disease*[38]	1	28
Liver fibrosis[33,36-38]	0-5	11-18
Cirrhosis[33,34,36-38]	0-2	1-12
Abnormal metacarpophalangeal joints[33,36,38]	2-12	4-26

*Defined as iron overload accompanied by at least 1 of the following conditions: hepatocellular carcinoma, liver fibrosis or cirrhosis, characteristic arthropathy, raised serum aminotransferase levels, or diagnosis due to symptoms of hereditary hemochromatosis.

and occasionally hypothyroidism; adrenal function is typically normal. Other endocrinologic effects can occur as a result of complications of cirrhosis (see Chapter 94).

Cardiac manifestations occur rarely because patients are now diagnosed earlier in the course of *HFE*-related HH than in the past. Cardiomyopathy, atrial and ventricular dysrhythmias, and heart failure can occur.[42] Characteristic of the arthropathy of *HFE*-related HH are changes in the second and third metacarpophalangeal joints. Joint space narrowing, chondrocalcinosis, subchondral cyst formation, osteopenia, and swelling of the joints may be seen.[39] Unfortunately, the arthritic symptoms of *HFE*-related HH typically do not improve with phlebotomy. The skin pigmentation of *HFE*-related HH, which can be subtle, is characterized by either a bronze discoloration due to predominant melanin pigmentation or a gray pigmentation resulting from iron deposition in the basal layers of the epidermis.[39] The frequency of certain infections, including those caused by *Vibrio vulnificus*, *Listeria*

monocytogenes, *Yersinia enterocolitica*, and *Yersinia pseudotuberculosis*, is more common in iron-loaded patients, although still rare.

DIAGNOSIS

The requirements for diagnosis of HH have changed since the availability of HFE mutation analysis. As in the past, the disorder should be considered in any patient with typical symptoms or abnormal screening iron test results. If the physical examination or family history raises suspicions, then the appropriate serum iron tests along with HFE mutation analysis should be obtained. With the advent of genetic testing, the need for liver biopsy has diminished. In symptomatic patients, as discussed earlier, the most common symptoms are fatigue, malaise, right upper quadrant abdominal pain, and arthralgias. Less commonly, symptoms of chronic liver disease, diabetes mellitus, and heart failure are identified. Because many of these symptoms are nonspecific or are related to other common diseases, HH is often overlooked by clinicians.

In the early 1990s, patients with HH commonly presented after the discovery of abnormal results of screening blood chemistry tests obtained as part of routine health maintenance or for another reason.[32] Many commercial laboratories added iron and total iron-binding capacity (TIBC), with TS calculated as iron ÷ TIBC × 100%, to their panel of screening serum chemistry tests, and in many patients, a TS was obtained inadvertently even though the test had not been specifically ordered. In 1 series, 62% of patients newly identified between 1990 and 1995 came to medical attention in this way.[32] Another 14% of cases were identified through screening of family members of a known proband. Therefore, up to 75% of patients came to medical attention by way of screening laboratory tests. The majority of these patients were asymptomatic and had no physical findings of HH, and the frequency of end-stage complications of *HFE*-related HH, such as cirrhosis and diabetes mellitus, was much lower than that reported in earlier series of patients who presented with symptoms of the disease.[32] In 1998, the Health Care Finance Administration (now the Centers for Medicare and Medicaid Services) stopped providing reimbursement for screening tests of any kind, and since then, fewer American patients with HH have been identified through routine screening.

When the possibility of *HFE*-related HH has been considered, the diagnosis is relatively straightforward. Measurements of serum iron and TIBC (or transferrin), with calculation of TS, and serum ferritin should be obtained (Table 75-3). Studies have shown that it is not necessary for blood samples to be drawn in the fasting state. A TS value greater than 45% is an early phenotypic manifestation of *HFE*-related HH. As a result, TS may be a more sensitive and specific test for *HFE*-related HH than serum ferritin, which can be normal in young persons with *HFE*-related HH or elevated in unaffected persons for a variety of reasons, including various types of necroinflammatory liver disease (e.g., chronic viral hepatitis, alcoholic liver disease, nonalcoholic steatohepatitis), certain malignancies, and other inflammatory conditions. An elevated serum ferritin level with a normal TS value in a person who has an inflammatory disorder generally suggests that the person does not have *HFE*-related HH. On the other hand, an elevated TS value with a normal ferritin value in a young person does not exclude *HFE*-related HH. A large North American population screening study demonstrated that 1 in 227 white persons was homozygous for the C282Y mutation, but only 57% and 88% of the female and male homozygotes, respectively, had an elevated ferritin value.[35] This finding indicates that a higher proportion of C282Y homozygotes do not

express iron overload than had previously been thought. The proportion of the non-expressing cohort that will subsequently show evidence of iron loading is uncertain. In a longitudinal follow-up study of patients identified by genetic screening, progressive iron loading, as indicated by rising serum ferritin levels, developed in 40% of C282Y homozygotes.[43]

As soon as serum iron parameters have been determined to be abnormal, *HFE* mutation analysis should be performed. If the patient is a C282Y homozygote or a compound heterozygote (C282Y/H63D) and has a serum ferritin level lower than 1000 ng/mL and normal liver enzyme values, a liver biopsy is not needed.[8,44-46] If, however, the serum ferritin value is higher than 1000 ng/mL or liver enzymes are elevated, liver biopsy is indicated. If liver biopsy is determined to be appropriate, sufficient tissue for histopathologic evaluation and biochemical measurement of the hepatic iron concentration (HIC) should be obtained. With the advent of genetic testing, liver biopsy is performed solely to assess the damage (if any) to the liver. A proposed algorithm for evaluating people for possible *HFE*-related HH is shown in Figure 75-3.

When a liver biopsy specimen is obtained, Perls' Prussian blue stain is used for the determination and localization of storage iron. Iron stores in *HFE*-related HH are typically found in periportal hepatocytes, with little or no iron found in Kupffer cells (Fig. 75-4).[47] In patients with a higher HIC, iron distribution becomes panlobular, and storage iron can be seen in Kupffer cells and bile duct cells. Grade 1 or 2 Perls' Prussian blue staining can be seen in specimens from normal livers or specimens from patients with very early HH confirmed by *HFE* mutation analysis. Grade 3 stainable iron occasionally can be seen in specimens from patients with alcoholic cirrhosis or end-stage liver disease, in which iron staining correlates poorly with HIC. In the absence of other disorders, grade 3 to 4 stainable iron in an *HFE* pattern is consistent with *HFE*-related HH.

In addition to histochemical staining, biochemical iron measurement in the liver is important (see Table 75-3). Typically, patients with *HFE*-related HH who present with symptoms have a HIC greater than 10,000 μg/g (dry weight) (normal < 1500 μg/g); HIC values may be more than 30,000 μg/g. Fibrosis and cirrhosis are usually not seen until the HIC exceeds 20,000 μg/g.[48] In patients with both *HFE*-related HH and other forms of chronic liver disease, such as alcoholic liver disease or chronic viral hepatitis, increased fibrosis or cirrhosis can occur at a much lower HIC and at a younger age.[49,50] In asymptomatic or younger patients with early *HFE*-related HH, HIC is increased to a lesser degree and often is much less than 10,000 μg/g.

A common diagnostic dilemma occurs when it is not clear whether a patient has liver disease with abnormal iron parameters or *HFE*-related HH with elevations in serum liver enzyme levels. In this setting, HFE mutation analysis is extremely useful. If the patient is a C282Y homozygote or a compound heterozygote (C282Y/H63D), the iron loading is most likely caused predominantly by the genetic abnormality. On the other hand, if the patient has underlying non-HH liver disease, is a C282Y heterozygote, is an H63D heterozygote or H63D homozygote, or has neither HFE mutation, the iron loading is likely to be caused by the underlying liver disease, perhaps with a minor contribution from the *HFE* genotype. In the past, the hepatic iron index (HIC in μmol/g ÷ the patient's age in years) was used to distinguish HH (>1.9) from secondary iron overload (≤1.9).[48] With HFE mutation analysis, the value of the hepatic iron index has diminished.

CT, MRI, and magnetic susceptibility testing have all been proposed as techniques to quantify the HIC without the need for a liver biopsy (Fig. 75-5). Magnetic susceptibility testing is available in only a few centers in the United States and Europe

TABLE 75-3 Representative Iron Measurements in Serum and Liver and HFE Mutation Analysis Findings in Patients with Phenotypic *HFE*-Related Hereditary Hemochromatosis

Test	Normal Value/ Result	Value/Result in *HFE*-Related Hemochromatosis
Serum		
Iron		
(μg/dL)	60-180	180-300
(μmol/L)	11-32	32-54
Transferrin saturation (%)	20-45	45-100
Ferritin		
Men (ng/mL; μg/L)	20-200	300-3000
Women (ng/mL; μg/L)	15-150	250-3000
Liver		
Iron staining	0, 1+	3+, 4+
Iron concentration		
(μg/g dry weight)	300-1500	3000-30,000
(μmol/g dry weight)	5-27	53-536
Hepatic iron index ([μmol/g dry weight] ÷ age in years)	<1.1	>1.9
HFE Mutation Analysis		
	wt/wt C282Y/wt H63D/wt	C282Y/C282Y C282Y/H63D

wt, wild-type.

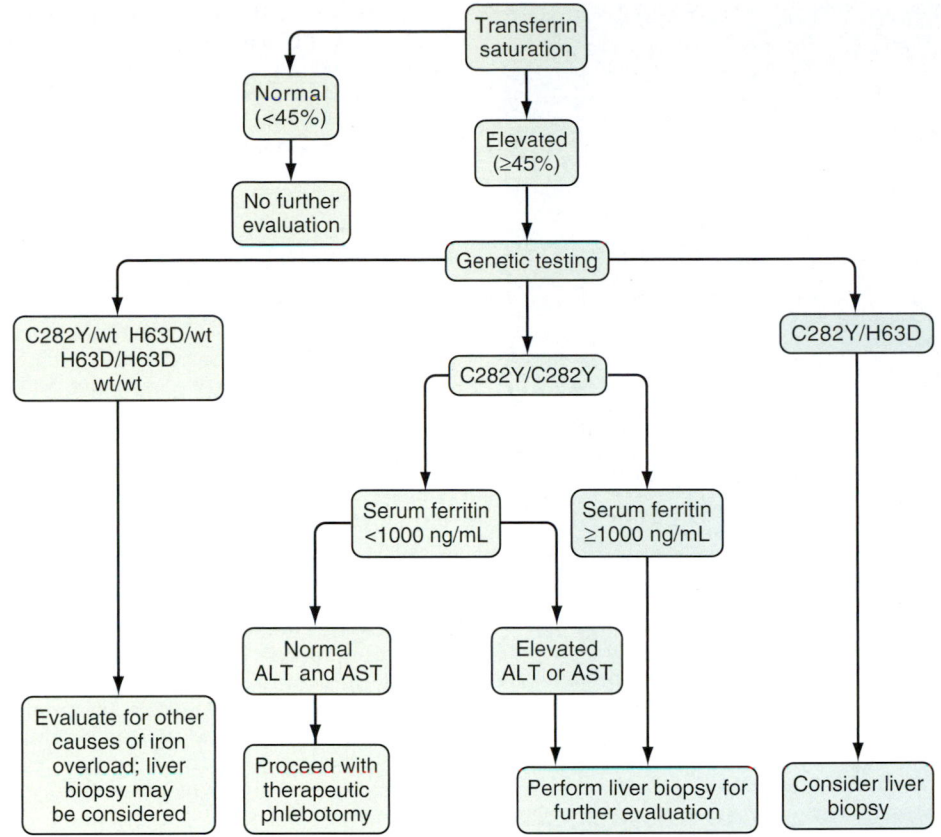

FIGURE 75-3. Algorithm for the evaluation of possible *HFE*-related hereditary hemochromatosis in a person with a negative family history. wt, wild-type.

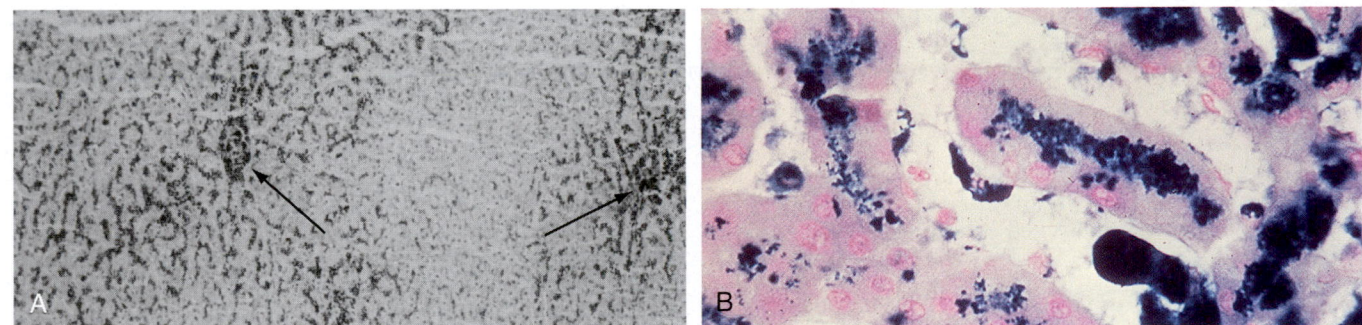

FIGURE 75-4. Histopathology of *HFE*-related hereditary hemochromatosis. *A*, This liver biopsy specimen was obtained from a 47-year-old C282Y homozygous woman who presented with a transferrin saturation of 63% and a serum ferritin level of 1190 ng/mL. The hepatic iron concentration was 9840 µg/g with a hepatic iron index of 3.7. At low power, iron deposition is seen to be much greater in the periportal zone (acinar zone 1) *(arrows)* than in the centrilobular zone (acinar zone 3). (Perls' Prussian blue; ×100.) *B*, At a higher magnification of a specimen from another patient with *HFE*-related hereditary hemochromatosis, iron deposition is seen to be primarily in hepatocytes arranged in cords, with less iron accumulation in reticuloendothelial (Kupffer) cells that line the intervening sinusoids. In patients with higher hepatic iron concentrations, iron deposition becomes panlobular, and storage iron can be seen in the Kupffer cells and bile duct cells. (Perls' Prussian blue.) *(A, Courtesy Elizabeth M. Brunt, MD, St. Louis; B, courtesy Edward Lee, MD, Washington, D.C.)*

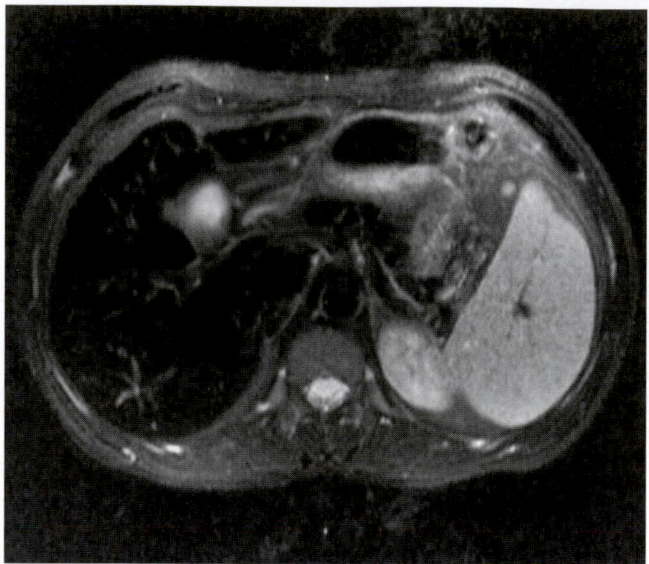

FIGURE 75-5. MRI of a patient with hemochromatosis. This T2-weighted image shows low signal intensity in the liver due to the magnetic susceptibility effects of iron, compared with normal signal intensity in the spleen. In secondary iron overload the spleen would also have low signal intensity due to increased iron deposition in reticuloendothelial cells.

BOX 75-2 Treatment of *HFE*-Related Hereditary Hemochromatosis

Perform phlebotomy of 500 mL (1 unit) of whole blood weekly unless the hematocrit value drops below 37%.
Check the transferrin saturation and ferritin levels at 2- to 3-month intervals to monitor response (optional).
When the iron stores are depleted (ferritin between 50 and 100 ng/mL and transferrin saturation <50%), proceed to maintenance phlebotomy of 1 unit of whole blood every 2 to 3 months. Aim to keep the transferrin saturation below 50%; if successful, the ferritin level should remain between 50 and 100 ng/mL.

---

as a research tool. In early studies, CT and MRI were generally not reliable for detecting mild iron overload, but newer MRI techniques have shown improved sensitivity.[51,52]

TREATMENT AND PROGNOSIS

The treatment of *HFE*-related HH is relatively straightforward; most patients can be treated with routine therapeutic phlebotomy (Box 75-2). Ideally, diagnosis and initiation of treatment should begin before the development of hepatic fibrosis or cirrhosis; if they are, patients will have a normal lifespan. Each unit of whole blood (500 mL) contains approximately 200 to 250 mg of iron, depending on the hemoglobin concentration; therefore, C282Y homozygotes who have 10 to 20 g of excess storage iron require extended phlebotomy regimens (40 to 80 units of blood removed). Most patients can tolerate weekly phlebotomy of 1 unit of whole blood, and occasional younger patients can tolerate the removal of 2 or 3 units per week. Treatment with a PPI reduces intestinal absorption of non-heme iron and may decrease the phlebotomy requirement.

Some older patients and occasional patients with a coexisting underlying hematologic disorder resulting in anemia can tolerate phlebotomy of only 0.5 unit per week or every other week. The iron-chelating drug deferoxamine is used in patients with *HFE*-related HH and cardiac manifestations or in patients who cannot tolerate phlebotomy. Deferoxamine, 20 to 50 mg/kg/day, is administered 5 days per week as a continuous subcutaneous infusion (over a 12-hour period each day) via a portable pump. Deferasirox (Exjade), a once-daily oral iron chelator, appears to be effective in the treatment of HH based on the results of a phase 1/2 trial.[53] Negative aspects of therapy with deferasirox include potentially serious side effects (hepatic failure, GI bleeding, renal injury) and expense, especially when compared with phlebotomy.

The FDA has approved another oral iron chelator, deferiprone (Ferriprox), to treat patients with thalassemia who have iron overload due to blood transfusions and an inadequate response to prior chelation therapy. Deferiprone is associated with agranulocytosis in about 1.7% of treated patients and has not undergone clinical trials in patients with HH. Therefore, phlebotomy remains the therapy of choice for HH, and in patients who cannot tolerate phlebotomy, iron chelation with deferoxamine may be utilized.

Although not absolutely necessary, obtaining a TS value and serum ferritin level every 2 to 3 months is useful for predicting the eventual return of iron stores to normal. Typically, the serum ferritin level falls progressively as hepatic iron stores decrease, whereas TS usually remains elevated until just before iron stores return to normal. In uncomplicated cases, the ferritin level drops by about 30 ng/mL with each unit of blood removed.

When the iron stores have reached a level in the low-normal range, the serum ferritin level should be between 50 and 100 ng/mL and the TS less than 50%. At this point, maintenance phlebotomies every 2 to 3 months are required in most patients. The rate of reaccumulation of iron varies among individuals, and patients may require regular maintenance phlebotomy at more or less frequent intervals. Occasional patients do not reaccumulate iron, for reasons that are unknown.

The prognosis for patients with *HFE*-related HH is improved significantly by therapeutic phlebotomy.[3,54,55] Life expectancy is reduced in patients who present with cirrhosis or diabetes mellitus, and the risk of death from hepatocellular carcinoma is increased in patients with *HFE*-related HH. Hepatocellular cancer is usually seen only in patients who already have cirrhosis. Established cirrhosis typically does not reverse with phlebotomy, but many patients will have a decrease in hepatic fibrosis with aggressive treatment.[36] Unfortunately, neither arthritis nor hypogonadism improves; however, management of diabetes mellitus may become easier after iron removal.

The value of screening for hepatocellular carcinoma in cirrhotic patients with HH is controversial because the cost-effectiveness of the screening approaches has not been validated. Most authorities suggest US or CT and a serum AFP measurement every 6 months in cirrhotic patients with *HFE*-related HH. With improved methods of detection and treatment of small, early hepatocellular carcinomas (e.g., radiofrequency ablation, chemoembolization, resection, and liver transplantation), screening seems to be reasonable (see Chapter 96).

When diagnosis and treatment are delayed and complications of end-stage liver disease develop, liver transplantation (LT) may be undertaken (see also Chapter 97). In the era before HFE genotyping was available, studies addressing the outcome of iron-loaded patients after LT reported that the survival rate was substantially lower than that for other patients. Significant hepatic iron loading is now known to occur in 35% to 78% of patients with end-stage liver disease, regardless of the cause of cirrhosis.[56] Only about 10% of patients with iron overload and end-stage liver disease are C282Y homozygotes.[57] Two studies have analyzed post-LT outcome in patients with confirmed *HFE*-related HH and found 5-year survival rates of 34% and 55%, which were lower than the overall post-LT survival rate of 72% to 75%.[58,59] The most common causes of death were infections, cardiovascular complications, and recurrence of hepatocellular carcinoma. The 5-year survival rate for patients with non-HH iron overload was higher (63%) than that for patients with *HFE*-related HH (34%) but still somewhat reduced compared with the survival rate of all patients undergoing LT.[58] If iron overload of any cause is diagnosed early, it should be treated to reduce the chance of death following LT.

Unfortunately, *HFE*-related HH or secondary iron overload resulting from liver disease is often not diagnosed before LT. One factor that may contribute to the increased post-LT mortality in patients with undiagnosed or untreated *HFE*-related HH is the extent of iron deposition in extrahepatic sites, such as the heart. A high index of suspicion for iron overload in patients with end-stage liver disease should lead to improved diagnosis and prompt institution of phlebotomy or iron-chelation therapy before LT. These changes in management should reduce the frequency of postoperative complications and improve long-term post-LT survival.

FAMILY SCREENING

When a proband with *HFE*-related HH has been identified and therapy has been initiated, the clinician still has a responsibility to the patient's family.[60] Assessment of both *HFE* genotype and phenotype (serum ferritin and TS) is recommended for all first-degree relatives of a proband. Relatives identified as C282Y homozygotes or compound heterozygotes (C282Y/H63D) who have elevated serum ferritin levels should undergo therapeutic phlebotomy. Liver biopsy should be utilized to detect potential fibrosis or cirrhosis in C282Y homozygotes or compound heterozygotes with ferritin levels greater than 1000 ng/mL or if another concomitant liver disease is suspected. Relatives who are C282Y heterozygotes are not at risk for progressive iron overload. For children of a proband, *HFE* genotyping of the other parent is recommended, although the possibility of genetic discrimination and stigmatization of this person must be acknowledged and considered. If the other parent does not carry the C282Y or H63D mutation (i.e., *HFE* genotype of wild type/wild type), then the children are not at risk for iron loading and need not undergo *HFE* genotyping.

For children or other relatives who are C282Y homozygotes or compound heterozygotes with normal serum ferritin levels, it is appropriate to measure serum ferritin levels yearly and initiate phlebotomy therapy when ferritin values become elevated.

KEY REFERENCES

Full references for this chapter can be found on www.expertconsult.com.

4. Feder J, Gnirke A, Thomas W, et al. A novel MHC class 1-like gene is mutated in patients with hereditary haemochromatosis. Nat Genet 1996; 13:399-408.
5. Adams P, Barton J. Haemochromatosis. Lancet 2007; 370:1855-60.
6. Olynyk J, Trinder D, Ramm G, et al. Hereditary hemochromatosis in the post-HFE era. Hepatology 2008; 48:991-1001.
8. Bacon BR, Adams PC, Kowdley KV, et al. Diagnosis and management of hemochromatosis: 2011 practice guideline by the American Association for the Study of Liver Diseases. Hepatology 2011; 54:328-43.
9. EASL clinical practice guidelines for HFE hemochromatosis. J Hepatol 2010; 53:3-22.
11. Pietrangelo A. Hereditary hemochromatosis: Pathogenesis, diagnosis, and treatment. Gastroenterology 2010; 139:393-408.
13. Pietrangelo A. Non-HFE hemochromatosis. Hepatology 2004; 39:21-9.
15. Gordeuk V. African iron overload. Semin Hematol 2002; 39:263-9.
18. Andrews N. Forging a field: The golden age of iron biology. Blood 2008; 112:219-30.
20. Babitt JL, Lin HY. The molecular pathogenesis of hereditary hemochromatosis. Semin Liver Dis 2011; 31:280-92.
21. Ganz T, Nemeth E. Hepcidin and iron homeostasis. Biochim Biophys Acta 2012; 1823:1434-43.
29. Philippe M, Ruddell R, Ramm G. Role of iron in hepatic fibrosis: One piece in the puzzle. World J Gastroenterol 2007; 13:4746-54.
34. Beutler E, Felitti V, Koziol J, et al. Penetrance of 845G→A (C282Y) HFE hereditary haemochromatosis mutation in the USA. Lancet 2002; 359:211-8.
35. Adams P, Reboussin D, Barton J, et al. Hemochromatosis and iron-overload screening in a racially diverse population. N Engl J Med 2005; 352:1769-78.
38. Allen K, Gurrin L, Constantine C, et al. Iron-overload-related disease in HFE hereditary hemochromatosis. N Engl J Med 2008; 358:221-30.

Copper, a component of several essential enzymes, is toxic to cells when present in excess. Dietary intake of copper generally exceeds the trace amount required physiologically, and mechanisms to control influx and efflux from cells must maintain an appropriate balance. Two human disorders of copper transport are known: *Menkes disease*, an X-linked defect in transport of copper from the intestine that leads to generalized copper deficiency, and *Wilson disease*, an autosomal recessive disorder of copper overload. Wilson disease was first described in 1912, by Kinnear Wilson, as a familial disease characterized by progressive, lethal neurologic dysfunction with liver cirrhosis and a corneal abnormality, the Kayser-Fleischer ("KF") ring.[1] Wilson also observed that some younger siblings of typical patients died of liver disease without experiencing neurologic abnormalities. In this disease, inadequate hepatic copper excretion leads to copper accumulation in the liver, brain, kidney, and cornea. The estimated prevalence in most populations is on the order of 1 in 30,000.

COPPER METABOLISM

Dietary copper is absorbed in the upper intestine. Loosely bound to albumin and to histidine, copper is distributed to a variety of tissues. Portal blood flow directs most copper to the liver. Trace amounts of copper are required for essential enzymes that affect connective tissue and elastin cross-linking (lysyl oxidase), free radical scavenging (superoxide dismutase), electron transfer (cytochrome oxidase), pigment production (tyrosinase), and neurotransmission (dopamine β-monooxygenase). Molecular copper is never free within a cell. Copper in hepatocytes and other cells is bound to metallochaperones, low molecular weight proteins that specifically deliver copper to a target molecule. Metallothioneins and glutathione also bind intracellular copper.

In the liver, copper is incorporated into apoceruloplasmin to produce ceruloplasmin (also called holoceruloplasmin). More than 90% of the copper in plasma is an integral part of ceruloplasmin, an α_2-glycoprotein that contains 6 molecules of copper and has a molecular weight of 132 kd. The normal serum concentration of ceruloplasmin in adults, as measured by immunochemical or enzymatic techniques, is 200 to 400 mg/L, rising from a very low level at birth to 300 to 500 mg/L in the first years of life. Because it is an acute-phase reactant, ceruloplasmin is elevated by inflammation (including inflammatory hepatic disease), pregnancy, and the use of exogenous estrogen. The majority of ingested copper is excreted via the bile; a very small fraction is excreted in urine. When intestinal or liver cells are overloaded with copper, metallothioneins, a class of low molecular weight cysteine-rich proteins, are induced and sequester copper in a nontoxic form. The normal pathways of copper transport in the body and in the hepatocyte are shown in Figures 76-1 and 76-2.

MOLECULAR PATHOGENESIS

An understanding of the pathogenesis of Wilson disease increased dramatically with the cloning of the gene associated with Menkes disease and the one associated with Wilson disease. The abnormal gene in Menkes disease (*ATP7A*), which was cloned by using a chromosomal breakpoint in an affected female patient, was found to be related to bacterial copper-resistance genes. Cloning of the gene mutated in Wilson disease (*ATP7B*) was accomplished by a combination of linkage analysis, physical mapping of the relevant region of chromosome 13q14, and recognition of its extensive homology with the Menkes disease gene.[2,3] The coding region of the gene is 4.1 kilobases in length, with messenger RNA (mRNA) of about 8 kilobases; the gene is distributed over 80 kilobases. The product, ATP7B (known as the *Wilson ATPase*), is a membrane-bound P_1-type ATPase that consists of 1443 amino acid residues and has a molecular mass of 160 kd. The structure[2,4] has 6 copper-binding units, a phosphorylation domain, an ATP-binding region, and 8 transmembrane domains (Fig. 76-3). All functionally important regions of the gene are conserved between bacteria and yeast. Mutations in the *ATP7B* gene result in retention of copper in the liver. The Long-Evans

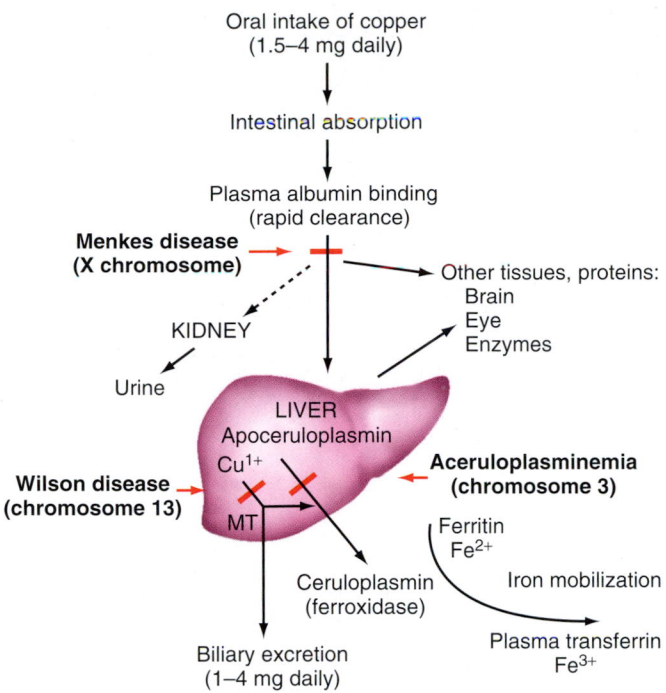

FIGURE 76-1. Simplified overview of the pathways for copper ion transport and the steps affected in genetic disorders of copper metabolism. MT, metallothioneins. *(Modified from Cox DW. Genes of the copper pathway. Am J Hum Genet 1995; 56:828-34.)*

cinnamon (LEC) rat and the toxic milk (tx) mouse have mutations in their homologous *ATP7B* genes and are thus suitable models for the study of Wilson disease mechanisms and therapy.[5,6]

Although *ATP7A* is expressed in many tissues, the gene that is abnormal in Wilson disease is expressed predominantly in the liver and kidney, with minor expression in brain, lungs, and placenta.[2] The Wilson ATPase has at least 2 intracellular functions: participating in the synthesis of enzymatically active ceruloplasmin and expediting biliary excretion of copper. It is localized in the trans-Golgi network and trafficks to cytoplasmic vesicles in the presence of increased copper. When intracellular copper concentrations are elevated, the Wilson ATPase is found near the apical (bile canalicular) membrane in hepatocytes, consistent with its proposed function of facilitating excretion of copper via bile.[7] Evidently, the Wilson ATPase also serves a sensing function for ambient hepatocellular copper concentration.

Additional proteins are involved in the intracellular disposition of copper. Loosely bound to intracellular metallochaperones (also called *copper chaperones*), copper is transported to specific proteins, such as superoxide dismutase in the cytoplasm and various copper-containing proteins in mitochondria. The metallochaperone antioxidant 1 copper chaperone (ATOX1) transports copper to the Wilson ATPase. The interactome for the Wilson ATPase includes COMMD1, glutaredoxin, dynactin p62, PLZF (promyelocytic leukemia zinc finger) protein, clusterin (apolipoprotein j), and possibly the Niemann-Pick protein C1, in addition to ATOX1. The gene *COMMD1* (initially called *MURR1*) was identified through the study of inherited hepatic copper toxicosis in Bedlington terriers.

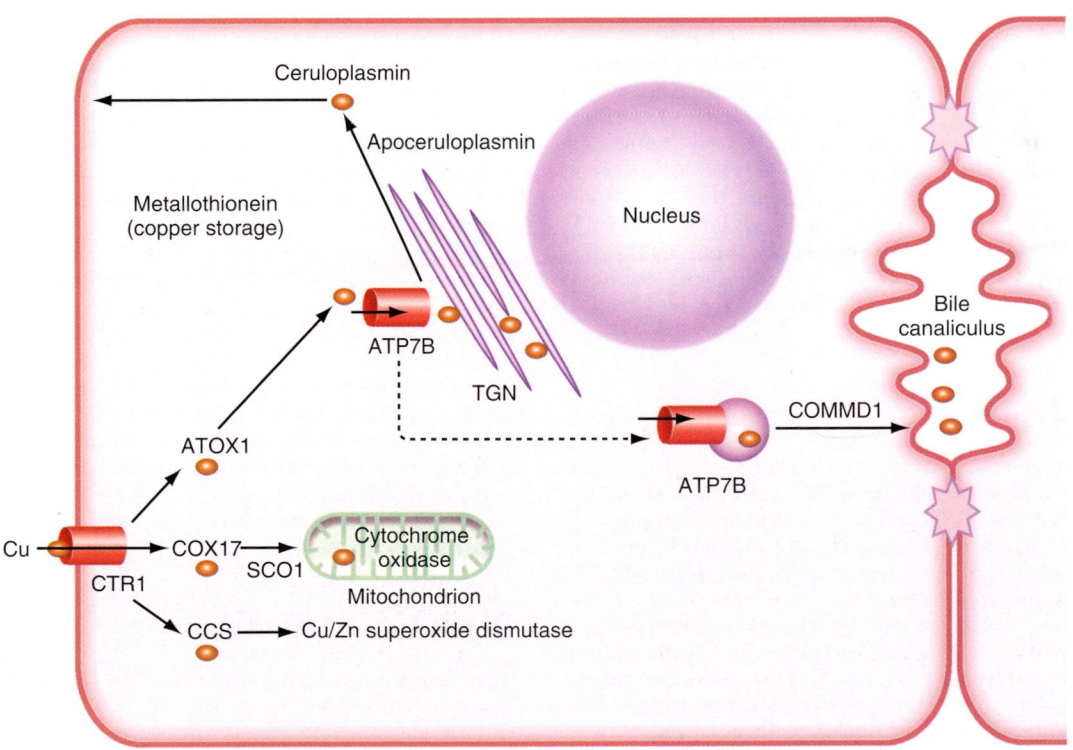

FIGURE 76-2. Model of a hepatocyte showing the major proteins in the copper transport pathway. Low molecular weight copper (Cu) chaperones (ATOX1 [antioxidant 1 copper chaperone], COX17 [cytochrome c oxidase 17], and CCS [copper chaperone for superoxide dismutase]) deliver copper to specific target proteins (ATP7B, cytochrome oxidase, and superoxide dismutase, respectively). SCO1 (synthesis of cytochrome c oxidase 1) transports copper across the mitochondrial membrane. ATP7B (shown as a channel) trafficks from the trans-Golgi network (TGN) to cytoplasmic vesicles that deliver copper to the bile canaliculus. COMMD1 may be involved in the excretion of copper into bile.

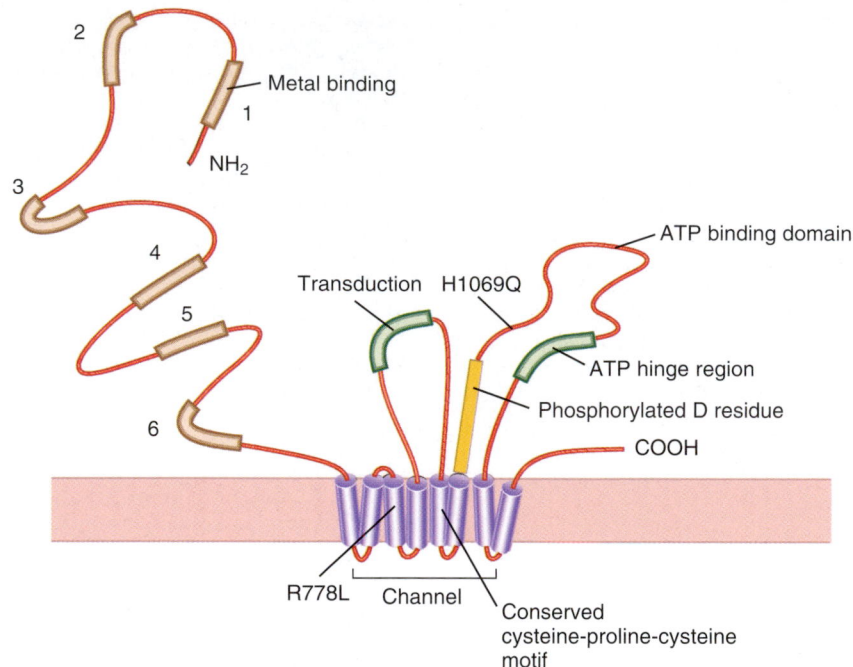

FIGURE 76-3. A model of the Wilson ATPase, the product of *ATP7B*. The domains conserved in both the Menkes ATPase and the Wilson ATPase include the metal-binding domain, copper-binding units 1 to 6, which are shown as tan cylinders, and the transduction domain and ATP hinge region, which are shown as green cylinders. Numerous mutations occur in functionally important regions. The positions of common missense mutations, H1069Q and R778L, are shown. *(Model modified from Bull PC, Cox DW. Wilson disease and Menkes disease: New handles on heavy-metal transport. Trends Genet 1994; 10:246-52.)*

Affected dogs show clinical variability that ranges from death or hepatic disease at 2 to 3 years of age to less severe chronic disease to a high hepatic copper level. The proposed defective canine gene was identified by positional cloning; the gene has a deletion of one exon in some,[8] but not all, affected dogs. Although the gene responsible for the excess copper remains to be identified, the disease in Bedlington terriers has highlighted other genes that may be involved in response to excess copper. While its function with respect to disposition of copper remains unclear, COMMD1 appears to facilitate elimination of excess copper. COMMD1 interacts not only with the Wilson ATPase, but also with the X-linked inhibitor of apoptosis (XIAP), which can also bind copper.[9]

PATHOLOGY

In the earliest stages before cirrhosis develops, histologic findings in the liver include steatosis, focal necrosis, glycogenated nuclei in hepatocytes, and sometimes apoptotic bodies. As parenchymal damage progresses, possibly through repeated episodes of lobular necrosis, periportal fibrosis develops. Cirrhosis is usually macronodular.

Early in the course of Wilson disease, hepatocellular copper is bound mainly to metallothionein and is distributed diffusely in the cytoplasm of hepatocytes; therefore, histochemical stains for copper are negative. As the disease progresses, the copper content exceeds the storage capacity of metallothionein, and copper is deposited in lysosomes. Lysosomal aggregates of copper can be detected by special staining techniques for copper or copper-binding protein (e.g., rubeanic acid or orcein, respectively). In the cirrhotic liver, some areas may have no stainable copper at all. If the clinical presentation mimics autoimmune hepatitis (see later), a liver biopsy specimen may reveal classic histologic features such as

interface hepatitis. Inflammation may be severe. Mallory-Denk bodies may be found. In patients who present with Wilsonian fulminant hepatic failure (see later), histologic findings confirm preexisting liver disease, often cirrhosis, and parenchymal copper is located mainly in Kupffer cells rather than hepatocytes.

Changes in hepatocellular mitochondria, identified with electron microscopy, are an important feature in Wilson disease.[10] The mitochondria vary in size, and the numbers of dense bodies in mitochondria may be increased. The most striking change is dilatation of the tips of the mitochondrial cristae as a result of separation of the inner and outer membranes of the cristae, with widening of the intercristal space until the appearance is irregularly cystic. The crista resembles a tennis racquet if only the tip is dilated. This finding, although not entirely specific for Wilson disease, can be helpful diagnostically, even in young and minimally affected patients. Involvement of hepatocytes may be not uniform, and abnormalities may be found in some hepatocytes in some lobules and not in others. The mitochondrial changes are probably a consequence of oxidative damage from excessive copper in hepatocytes.[11]

CLINICAL FEATURES

The clinical presentation of Wilson disease is variable. Wilson disease can present clinically at any age. Hepatic Wilson disease has been identified in 1- to 2-year-old patients and in patients older than age 60. Nevertheless, most patients present between 3 and 55 years of age. The clinical presentation may be as chronic or fulminant liver disease, a progressive neurologic disorder without clinically prominent hepatic dysfunction, isolated acute hemolysis, or psychiatric illness. The clinical variability often makes confirmation of the diagnosis difficult.[12,13]

Hepatic Presentation

The hepatic presentation of Wilson disease is more common in younger patients than in older patients. Wilson disease should be considered as a possible diagnosis in any child, symptomatic or not, with hepatomegaly, persistently elevated serum aminotransferase levels, or evidence of fatty liver. Symptoms may be vague and nonspecific, such as fatigue, anorexia, or abdominal pain. Occasional patients present with a self-limited clinical illness that resembles acute hepatitis, with malaise, anorexia, nausea, jaundice, elevated serum aminotransferase levels, and abnormal coagulation test results. Some patients have a history of self-limited jaundice, likely caused by unexplained hemolysis. Patients may present with severe, established chronic liver disease with hepatosplenomegaly, ascites, congestive splenomegaly, a low serum albumin level, and persistently abnormal coagulation test results. Rare patients have isolated splenomegaly without hepatomegaly. Many of these findings relate to portal hypertension as a consequence of Wilson disease rather than to the metabolic disorder itself.

Wilson disease may present in children and young adults with clinical liver disease indistinguishable from autoimmune hepatitis.[14] As in autoimmune hepatitis, the onset may be acute. Fatigue, malaise, arthropathy, and rashes may occur; laboratory findings include elevated aminotransferase levels, a greatly increased serum immunoglobulin (Ig)G concentration, and detectable nonspecific autoantibodies, such as antinuclear antibodies and smooth muscle (anti-actin) antibodies. Wilson disease must be specifically ruled out because the treatment of the 2 diseases is entirely different. With appropriate treatment, the long-term outlook for patients with Wilson disease that manifests as autoimmune hepatitis appears to be favorable, even if cirrhosis is present.

Wilson disease may present as fulminant hepatic failure, with severe coagulopathy and encephalopathy. Acute intravascular hemolysis is usually present, and renal failure may develop. Because underlying liver disease has not been suspected, acute liver failure due to viral hepatitis is usually the working diagnosis. In contrast to acute liver failure, Wilsonian fulminant hepatic failure is typically characterized by disproportionately low aminotransferase levels (usually much less than 1500 U/L) at the onset of clinically apparent disease. The serum alkaline phosphatase level is in the normal range or even low for the patient's age, and the serum bilirubin level is often disproportionately elevated as a result of hemolysis. In adults who present with Wilsonian fulminant hepatic failure, a calculation based on simple biochemical tests (in "American" units) can be helpful in making the diagnosis, specifically the combination of a ratio of the alkaline phosphatase to the total bilirubin level of less than 4 and a ratio of AST to ALT level of greater than 2.2.[15] The serum ceruloplasmin level is not diagnostically informative in this situation (see later). Slit-lamp examination may reveal Kayser-Fleischer rings. Urinary copper excretion is greatly elevated. These patients require urgent liver transplantation because they do not respond well to chelation treatment; albumin dialysis and related techniques may serve as temporary procedures until liver transplantation can be performed (see later).[16] This presentation of Wilson disease is not rare, and affected patients account for approximately 3% of persons transplanted for acute liver failure (see Chapters 95 and 97).

Recurrent bouts of hemolysis may predispose to the development of gallstones. Cirrhosis, if present, may be a further predisposing factor. Children with unexplained cholelithiasis, particularly bilirubinate stones, should be tested for Wilson disease. Compared with other chronic liver diseases, Wilson disease is infrequently complicated by hepatocellular carcinoma; however, patients may have an increased propensity to abdominal malignancies,[17] and hepatocellular carcinoma has been reported in a child with Wilson disease.

In patients who have predominantly hepatic disease, evidence of subtle neurologic involvement can often be found. Mood disturbance (mainly depression, but sometimes impulsive or neurotic behavior), deterioration in school performance or handwriting, and clumsiness may be identified by careful direct questioning. A soft whispery voice (hypophonia) is another early feature of neurologic involvement.

Neurologic Presentation

The neurologic presentation of Wilson disease tends to occur in the second and third decades or later but has been reported in children as young as 6 to 10 years of age. Most patients with a neurologic presentation have hepatic involvement, albeit often asymptomatic. Neurologic involvement follows 2 main patterns: movement disorder or rigid dystonia. Movement disorders tend to occur earlier and include tremors, poor coordination, and loss of fine motor control. Spastic dystonic disorders generally develop later, with mask-like facies, rigidity, gait disturbance, and pseudobulbar involvement such as dysarthria, drooling, and swallowing difficulty. Rarely, patients present with peripheral neuropathy or dysautonomia. Seizures are uncommon, and intellect is not impaired. Imaging of the brain is important for assessing neurologic Wilson disease, and results may be abnormal in the absence of overt neurologic symptoms. MRI is the most sensitive modality.[18]

Psychiatric Presentation

As many as 20% of patients may present with purely psychiatric symptoms. These symptoms are highly variable, although depression is common. Phobias and compulsive behaviors have been reported; aggressive or antisocial behavior may also be found.

Ocular Signs

The classic Kayser-Fleischer ring is caused by copper deposition in Descemet's membrane of the cornea. Copper is actually distributed throughout the cornea, but fluid-streaming favors accumulation near the limbus, especially at the superior and inferior poles, and eventually circumferentially around the iris. Kayser-Fleischer rings are visible on direct inspection only when iris pigmentation is light and copper deposition is heavy. A careful slit-lamp examination is mandatory. Copper deposition in the lens (sunflower cataract), which does not interfere with vision, may be seen on slit-lamp examination and, like Kayser-Fleischer rings, disappears with chelation therapy. Kayser-Fleischer rings may be absent in 40% to 60% of patients with exclusively hepatic involvement and in presymptomatic patients. Most patients with a neurologic or psychiatric presentation of Wilson disease have Kayser-Fleischer rings; only 5% do not. Kayser-Fleischer rings are not specific for Wilson disease; they may be found occasionally in patients with other types of chronic liver disease, usually with a prominent cholestatic component, such as PBC, PSC, or familial cholestatic syndromes. In rare persons with incidental Kayser-Fleischer rings, Wilson disease should be excluded.

Involvement of Other Systems

Wilson disease can be accompanied by various extrahepatic disorders apart from neurologic disease. Episodes of hemolytic anemia can result from the sudden release of copper into the blood. Renal disease, mainly Fanconi syndrome, may be prominent. Findings include microscopic hematuria, aminoaciduria, phosphaturia, and defective acidification of the urine. Nephrolithiasis has also been reported. Arthritis, mainly affecting the large joints, may occur as a result of synovial copper accumulation. Other musculoskeletal problems include osteoporosis and osteochondritis dissecans. A so-called osseomuscular presentation has been reported mainly in India. Vitamin D–resistant rickets may develop as a result of the renal damage. Copper deposition in skeletal muscle can cause rhabdomyolysis. Copper deposition in the heart can lead to cardiomyopathy or cardiac arrhythmias. Sudden death in Wilson disease has been attributed to cardiac involvement but is rare. Endocrine disorders can occur. Hypoparathyroidism has been attributed to copper deposition. Amenorrhea and testicular problems appear to result from Wilson disease itself, not from cirrhosis. Infertility or repeated spontaneous abortion may signal Wilson disease. Pancreatitis, possibly resulting from copper deposition in the pancreas, may also occur.

DIAGNOSIS

The patient with the classic combination of chronic liver disease, tremor or dystonia, and Kayser-Fleischer rings is readily diagnosed on clinical grounds, but such patients are uncommon. A diagnostic scoring system has been proposed[19] but has been evaluated only in children. Suggestive clinical symptoms are often the main prerequisite for diagnosing Wilson disease, and laboratory investigations may provide confirmation. Kayser-Fleischer rings should be sought through a careful slit-lamp examination, repeated if necessary. Lack of Kayser-Fleischer rings does not exclude the diagnosis of Wilson disease. Serum aminotransferase levels are usually mildly to moderately elevated. Serum levels of AST may be much higher than those of ALT, possibly reflecting damage to hepatocyte mitochondria.

Tests

A summary of biochemical features in Wilson disease in comparison with normal persons is shown in Table 76-1. The classic feature of a very low ceruloplasmin concentration has proved less typical than previously thought, partly because hepatic inflammation may be sufficient to elevate serum ceruloplasmin levels. Also, the normal range for serum ceruloplasmin is increased in very young children. The method of measuring ceruloplasmin is likely the most important reason

for finding normal ceruloplasmin levels in patients with Wilson disease. Immunologic methods, which are used in most laboratories, measure both apoceruloplasmin and holoceruloplasmin and typically overestimate the true amount of functional ceruloplasmin in plasma. The oxidase assay, although technically less convenient for laboratories that perform automated testing, provides a more reliable measure of ceruloplasmin for diagnosis because the assay measures enzymatically active, copper-containing ceruloplasmin. This method permits an accurate estimate of non–ceruloplasmin-bound copper[20] and can also indicate possible early copper deficiency in treated patients.[21]

Serum ceruloplasmin measurement by itself is not a sufficient diagnostic test for Wilson disease. A low serum level of ceruloplasmin is not unique to Wilson disease; synthesis of ceruloplasmin may be reduced in other types of chronic liver disease, intestinal malabsorption, nephrotic syndrome, and malnutrition. Furthermore, a subnormal ceruloplasmin concentration is found in at least 10% of heterozygotes for Wilson disease. Almost complete absence of ceruloplasmin is found in hereditary aceruloplasminemia, a rare autosomal recessive condition that is associated with neurologic, retinal, and pancreatic degeneration caused by iron accumulation in the brain, retina, and pancreas.[22] Anemia and an elevated plasma ferritin level are observed. Aceruloplasminemia has confirmed the important function of ceruloplasmin as a ferroxidase that oxidizes iron for transport from ferritin to transferrin. Targeted disruption of the ceruloplasmin gene in a mouse model has confirmed the critical role of ceruloplasmin in transporting iron out of cells.[23] Rarely, patients with Wilson disease who undergo rigorous chelation therapy over decades may resemble those with hereditary aceruloplasminemia if ceruloplasmin oxidase activity is reduced to undetectable levels.[24] The concurrence of Wilson disease and mutation-confirmed hereditary hemochromatosis has been reported.[25,26]

In patients with Wilson disease, the serum copper concentration is low, in parallel with the low serum ceruloplasmin level. The non–ceruloplasmin-bound copper concentration, which can be estimated by subtracting the amount of copper associated with ceruloplasmin from the total serum copper, is elevated. The amount of ceruloplasmin-bound copper (in µg/dL) is estimated by multiplying the serum ceruloplasmin (in mg/dL) by 3.15 (the amount of copper, in µg, per mg of ceruloplasmin). In normal persons the non–ceruloplasmin-bound copper concentration is less than 15 µg/dL. For results reported under the conventions of the Système Internationale, the conversion factor is the same, but reference values are converted to µg/L (by multiplying by 10); total serum copper reported in µmol/L must be converted to µg/L by multiplying that value by 63.5, the molecular weight of copper. In Wilson disease, the concentration of non–ceruloplasmin-bound copper is more than 20 µg/dL (200 µg/L), and even 10 times higher in patients with fulminant hepatic failure with intravascular hemolysis. The usefulness of this calculation, which is highly dependent on the accuracy of the copper and ceruloplasmin measurements, has not been validated as a diagnostic criterion. Methods are being developed to measure non–ceruloplasmin-bound copper concentration directly, and their diagnostic value is being assessed.[27,28] What is measured is not actually "free" copper, because copper in the plasma compartment is always loosely bound to albumin and various amino acids, and the notion of "exchangeable copper" has been suggested.

Serum uric acid and phosphate concentrations may be low in patients with untreated Wilson disease, reflecting renal tubular dysfunction. Urinalysis may show microscopic hematuria; if possible, aminoaciduria, phosphaturia, and proteinuria should be quantified.

TABLE 76-1 Biochemical Parameters in Normal Adults and in Patients with Wilson Disease

	Normal Adults	Wilson Disease*
Serum ceruloplasmin (mg/L)	200-350	0-200
Serum copper (µg/L) (µmol/L)	700-1520 11-24	190-640 3-10
Basal 24-hr urinary copper (µg/day) (µmol/day)	<40 ≤0.6	40-10,000 >0.6
Liver copper (µg/g dry weight)	20-50	>250 (possibly >70)

*For all the assays, results in homozygotes and heterozygotes may overlap.

Studies of basal urinary copper excretion, preferably with 3 separate 24-hour collections, have proved useful for diagnosis. Urinary copper excretion reflects the non–ceruloplasmin-bound copper concentration in plasma. The collection must be complete, and the volume and total creatinine excretion should be measured; precautions against contamination with copper in the collection process are essential. The basal 24-hour urinary copper excretion is elevated at least 2 to 3 times normal in the vast majority of patients; however, the conventional diagnostic criterion of greater than 100 µg/day (>1.6 µmol/day), although typical, is not sufficiently sensitive. A patient with a basal 24-hour urinary copper excretion of greater than 40 µg/day (>0.6 µmol/day) requires further investigation for Wilson disease.[29] Heterozygotes usually have a normal basal 24-hour urinary copper excretion, although the value may be borderline abnormal in some cases. Although a normal person may excrete as much as 20 times the baseline level of copper after administration of D-penicillamine, a patient with symptomatic Wilson disease will excrete considerably more. In the standard provocative test with administration of D-penicillamine, urinary copper excretion of 25 µmol (1600 µg) or more per 24 hours is diagnostic of Wilson disease; however, the test lacks sensitivity for diagnosing Wilson disease and for identifying presymptomatic affected siblings.[30]

Hepatic tissue copper concentration, which usually is measured by neutron activation analysis or atomic absorption spectrometry, may provide important diagnostic information. A hepatic copper content greater than 250 µg per g dry weight of liver is considered diagnostic of Wilson disease. On the basis of a large series of genetically diagnosed patients, a value of greater than 70 µg per g dry weight has been proposed as a better diagnostic threshold, although some specificity is lost.[31] Hepatic parenchymal concentrations of less than 40 µg per g dry weight in a large enough sample are regarded as strong evidence against a diagnosis of Wilson disease. Liver biopsy samples must be collected without extraneous copper contamination, but in general, ordinary disposable liver biopsy needles can be used. Importantly, the sample submitted must be adequate, at least 1 cm in length. In the early stages of Wilson disease, when copper is distributed diffusely in the liver cell cytoplasm, this measurement may clearly indicate hepatic copper overload. In later stages of hepatic Wilson disease, the measurement of hepatic copper is less reliable because copper is distributed unequally in the liver (see earlier). Moreover, liver biopsy may not be safe in such patients because of coagulopathy or ascites; transjugular biopsy may be performed, or hepatic copper measurement may be omitted. Some heterozygotes have minor elevations of liver tissue copper. An elevated hepatic copper concentration is not specific for Wilson disease; patients with chronic cholestasis or Indian childhood cirrhosis may have elevated hepatic copper levels.

Approach

In view of the numerous available diagnostic tests, a methodical approach is required. The classic patient with Wilson disease, whether displaying hepatic or neurologic findings, may be considered to be someone between 6 and 40 years of age with a serum ceruloplasmin level less than 5 mg/dL (<50 mg/L) and definite Kayser-Fleischer rings. Many patients are not classic. Age is no longer a meaningful diagnostic criterion. In the presence of chronic liver disease (indicated by hepatomegaly or biochemical abnormalities) or typical neurologic symptoms, the combination of a low serum ceruloplasmin level (<140 mg/L)[32] and elevated basal 24-hour urinary copper excretion (>40 µg/day) is highly suggestive of Wilson disease. The measurement of 24-hour urinary copper

excretion after administration of D-penicillamine may be definitive. Typical ocular findings complete the clinical diagnosis but are not essential. A percutaneous liver biopsy is useful for assessing the severity of liver damage and measuring parenchymal copper concentration, which is regarded by some to be the sine qua non for the diagnosis of Wilson disease. This procedure, however, may have to be delayed in patients with severe liver dysfunction. Other clinical entities in the differential diagnosis must be appropriately excluded. Ultimately, molecular genetic analysis is the only convincing and reliable diagnostic procedure.

Mutation Analysis

More than 500 reported mutations in the *ATP7B* gene have been detected in many different populations since the original mutations were described. These mutations are recorded in the Wilson Disease Mutation Database (http://www.wilsondisease.med.ualberta.ca/database.asp),[33] which includes references and population sources. The usual approach to detection of a mutation is high-throughput sequencing of either selected or all exons of the gene, supplemented by sequencing of the promoter region, close examination of exon/intron boundaries, and exclusion of large deletions by multiplex ligation-dependent probe amplification (MPLA) technology. Although identification of a mutation is technically straightforward, care must be taken that the change detected causes disease and is not a rare normal variant, particularly for single amino acid missense mutations. Because of the similarity between yeast and mammalian copper transport systems, yeast and cell assay systems have been developed for the functional assessment of variants.[34-36] Alternatively, structural changes in the Wilson ATPase protein due to a gene alteration can be assessed in silico. Of the various algorithms available for this purpose, the SIFT (sorting intolerant from tolerant) score (which predicts whether an amino acid substitution affects function) works best for *ATP7B* and its gene product.[37] Most patients with Wilson disease are compound heterozygotes, with a different mutation of *ATP7B* on each allele. The identification of one mutation may be adequate to confirm the diagnosis, if characteristic clinical symptoms and biochemical features are present and if the one mutation detected is clearly established as a disease-causing mutation. Complete genetic characterization is preferred. With current analytical techniques, two mutations can be found in more than 95% of affected patients.

The majority of mutations in *ATP7B* identified to date are missense mutations. Small deletions, insertions, nonsense, and splice-site mutations occur throughout the gene. Large gene deletions, which are found in about 20% of patients with Menkes disease, occur rarely, and the mutation spectrum for *ATP7A* in Menkes disease is different from that for *ATP7B*.[38] Various ethnic groups have different specific mutations. The histidine1069glutamine (H1069Q) mutation is present, at least in the heterozygous state, in 35% to 75% of Europeans with Wilson disease.[39] Exon 8 of the gene is particularly rich in mutations in European populations. The mutation arginine-778leucine (R778L) is common in Chinese populations. Mutation detection is more challenging in Japanese and Mediterranean populations, in which no mutation is present in high frequency. In populations with ethnic homogeneity or in which a limited spectrum of mutations is established, testing strategies can identify the mutations in most patients. A prominent example is Sardinia, where the disease frequency is 1 in 7000 live births,[40] and a mutation in the 5′-untranslated region (5′-UTR) predominates. In populations with a limited number of mutations, use of a customized "Wilson disease chip"[41] may be cost-effective.

Genetic diagnosis is important for identifying simple heterozygotes. Someone who is clinically normal, has only mild signs of the disease, or has a late age of onset could be a heterozygote carrying only one mutated allele. Heterozygotes have not been known to develop clinical disease or require treatment. Data suggest, however, that it is equally likely that such a person has an atypical presentation of Wilson disease.

Efforts to identify clear patterns of correlation between genotype and phenotype have been largely disappointing in Wilson disease, given its complex pathophysiology. Nevertheless, important genotype-phenotype correlations exist. *ATP7B* mutations resulting in absent or totally nonfunctional Wilson ATPase are associated with severe, usually hepatic, disease.[42,43] Gene deletions, duplications, nonsense mutations, and splice-site mutations are predicted to prevent the formation of the gene product almost completely and thus to produce a severe defect. Such truncating mutations are associated with absent holoceruloplasmin production and early onset of clinical disease[44] or with Wilsonian fulminant hepatic failure.[45] The common H1069Q mutation tends to be associated with neurologic disease and later onset[46]; however, this mutation has been reported in homozygotes as young as 9 years of age with hepatic disease. The positions of this and R778L (see earlier) are shown in Figure 76-3. Many mutations occur in exons 5-10 and exons 13-20,[42,47] which encode copper-binding unit 6, transmembrane segments, and the ATP loop.

With the opportunity of confirming a diagnosis of Wilson disease by direct identification of mutations, the spectrum of manifestations of Wilson disease has been found to be even wider than previously recognized. No individual biochemical test is reliable for the identification of patients. In some cases, even all combinations of tests prove inadequate for a diagnosis. The use of molecular tests in patients with any clinical symptoms of the disease may soon become routine and is already feasible as the primary diagnostic intervention in populations in which the repertoire of *ATP7B* mutations is relatively limited (e.g., Iceland, Sardinia, Gran Canaria in the Canary Islands, the Aegean island of Kalymnos). Such populations may also be suitable for local newborn screening programs. Mutation analysis should also be carried out to distinguish asymptomatic patients from heterozygotes.

Presymptomatic Diagnosis of First-Degree Relatives

If mutations have been identified in a patient, mutational analysis is easily carried out in first-degree relatives by direct testing for the mutations found in the patient. If mutations have not been identified, accurate diagnosis can be achieved using markers flanking the gene. The most useful genetic markers are stretches of dinucleotides or trinucleotides that show extensive variability in the normal population, so that parents within any one family will carry different alleles of these markers. This variability allows the tracking of the disease gene as it segregates within families, as shown in Figure 76-4. It is important that informative markers flank the gene, because an erroneous diagnosis could result if markers on only one side of the gene are informative and a recombinant event has occurred close to the gene. The combination of markers, or haplotype, reliably indicates the genetic status within the family. According to marker studies or genetic diagnosis, an occasional person considered as a result of biochemical testing to have a high probability of being a presymptomatic patient has been shown to be a heterozygote. Therefore, confirmation of the genotype is highly recommended before treatment is initiated. Conversely, if the clinical diagnosis of a heterozygote is uncertain, genetic diagnosis can be highly informative.

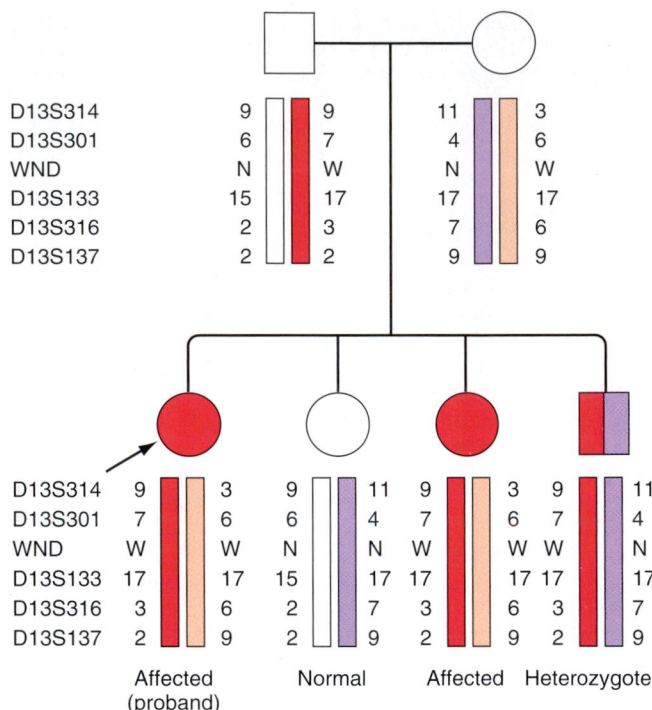

FIGURE 76-4. Diagnostic use of polymorphic DNA microsatellite markers for siblings of a confirmed patient with Wilson disease. DNA markers are listed on the left in centromeric to telomeric order. Three markers are usually sufficient for an unambiguous result: D13S314, D13S301, and D13S316. Numbers represent alleles of each marker listed. The proband (arrow) and presymptomatic sibling confirmed as affected are shown as filled circles.

In the absence of genetic analysis, screening should include physical examination, liver biochemical tests, serum copper and ceruloplasmin measurements, a basal 24-hour urinary copper determination, and a careful slit-lamp examination. Children 6 years of age or younger who appear to be unaffected should be rechecked at yearly intervals over the next 5 to 10 years. Genetic screening with the use of flanking markers, or by direct mutation analysis, however, is the most reliable way to identify an affected first-degree relative when the patient's DNA is available for mutation analysis. For deceased patients, tissue from autopsy or biopsy material can be used.

Accumulating data indicate that the incidence of Wilson disease in children of patients with Wilson disease is higher than predicted. Therefore, screening of all first-degree relatives, not just siblings, is recommended.

TREATMENT

Three treatments for Wilson disease are generally recognized: D-penicillamine, trientine, and zinc (Table 76-2).[48] Chelation with tetrathiomolybdate remains experimental. With effective lifelong chelation treatment, most patients live normal, healthy lives. Starting treatment early is critical, and the outcome is best for patients in whom the disease is diagnosed and treatment begun when the patient is presymptomatic. Whether routine institution of chelation or zinc therapy in infancy (<2 years old) is advantageous or deleterious remains unknown. Likewise, the potential role of gene transfer therapy remains

TABLE 76-2 Recommendations for the Treatment of Wilson Disease

Drug	Dose*	Tests for Monitoring Efficacy	Tests for Monitoring Side Effects
D-penicillamine (+ pyridoxine 25 mg daily)	Initial: 1-1.5 g/day (adults) or 20 mg/kg/day (children) divided into 2 or 3 doses Maintenance: 0.75-1 g/day as needed to maintain cupruresis	24-hour urinary copper: 200-500 µg (3-8 µmol)/day as target; estimated non–ceruloplasmin-bound copper <200 µg/L Estimated non–ceruloplasmin-bound copper <100 µg/L	Complete blood count; urinalysis; skin examination
Trientine[†]	Initial: 1-1.2 g/day divided into 2 or 3 doses[‡] Maintenance: Same	Same as for D-penicillamine Same as for D-penicillamine	Complete blood count; iron studies
Zinc	Initial: 50 mg elemental zinc 3 times daily (adults)[§] Maintenance: titrate the dose based on efficacy monitoring data[¶]	24-hour urinary copper: <75 µg (1.2 µmol)/day as target Estimated non–ceruloplasmin-bound copper <100 µ/L	Serum zinc level Serum AST and ALT levels

*All medications should be taken before or after mealtime if possible, but the timing of the dose may have to be adjusted to enhance consistent adherence to treatment.
[†]Requires refrigeration.
[‡]The dose of trientine in children is not established (≈20 mg/kg/day).
[§]The dose of zinc in children is not established. Typical dosing is 25 mg of elemental zinc 3 times daily until adult stature (≈50 kg body weight) is achieved, when the adult dose of 50 mg of elemental zinc 3 times daily is used. The dose is not well defined for children younger than 5 years. The dose in children can also be titrated to achieve optimal 24-hr urinary copper excretion.
[¶]The 24-hour urinary copper excretion reflects total body copper load and thus can be used to monitor zinc treatment even though zinc does not cause cupruresis; some groups prefer to use the estimated non–ceruloplasmin-bound copper determination as a guide.

uncertain.[49] Dietary treatment alone is ineffective, but most patients should eliminate copper-rich foods from the diet. These foods include organ meats, shellfish, nuts, chocolate, and mushrooms. Vegetarians require specific dietary counseling. If the concentration of copper in the patient's drinking water is believed to be high, the water should be analyzed and a copper-removing device installed in the plumbing system.

D-penicillamine, introduced in 1956 by J.M. Walshe, is effective in most patients with Wilson disease. Penicillamine, which is the sulfhydryl-containing amino acid cysteine substituted with 2 methyl groups, greatly increases urinary excretion of copper; only the D-penicillamine form is used clinically. Studies in the LEC rat model indicate that D-penicillamine inhibits the accumulation of copper in hepatocellular lysosomes and solubilizes copper for mobilization from these particles, but not from cytoplasmic metallothioneins.[50] In addition to its chelating action, D-penicillamine inhibits collagen cross-linking and has some immunosuppressive properties. The neurologic status of patients with mainly neurologic symptoms may worsen initially after treatment with D-penicillamine is started[51]; most, but not all, recover with continued use of D-penicillamine. Substituting trientine or zinc reduces this risk. A febrile reaction with rash and proteinuria develops in some patients within 7 to 10 days of beginning treatment. Although D-penicillamine can be restarted slowly, along with glucocorticoids, changing to an alternative chelator is preferred.

D-penicillamine, although highly effective, can cause serious side effects. Adverse reactions involving the skin include various types of rashes, pemphigus, and elastosis perforans serpiginosa. Hypothyroidism has been reported. Other side effects vary from minor (loss of taste, GI upset, arthralgias) to severe (proteinuria, leukopenia, thrombocytopenia). Aplastic anemia occurs rarely and does not always reverse when D-penicillamine is stopped. Nephrotic syndrome, Goodpasture syndrome, a myasthenia syndrome, and a systemic disease that resembles SLE have all been reported. These severe side effects require immediate discontinuation of D-penicillamine and use of a different chelator. Whether lifelong treatment with D-penicillamine is free of adverse consequences is not yet clear. Patients who have taken D-penicillamine for 30 to 40 years may have chronic skin changes with loss of elastic tissue. Whether the antifibrotic effect weakens other connective tissues is not known. Theoretically, chronic depletion of other trace metals may occur. In view of these side effects, D-penicillamine should be used in the lowest effective dose.

Trientine, or triethylene tetramine dihydrochloride (2,2,2-tetramine), the official short name of which is "trien," is the usual second-line treatment for patients who are intolerant of D-penicillamine. Trientine differs chemically from D-penicillamine in lacking sulfhydryl groups. Copper is chelated by forming a stable complex with the 4 constituent nitrogens in a planar ring. Trientine increases urinary copper excretion and may interfere with intestinal absorption of copper. Trientine is a less potent chelator than D-penicillamine, but the difference is not clinically important. Trientine produces little significant toxicity in patients with Wilson disease—apart from causing occasional gastritis and inducing iron deficiency, apparently by chelating dietary iron. Bone marrow suppression is rare. Adverse effects of D-penicillamine resolve and do not recur during treatment with trientine.[52] Neurologic worsening after treatment with trientine is begun has rarely been reported. Trientine is highly effective, even in patients with advanced liver fibrosis or as initial treatment in children.[53]

Oral zinc, used in Europe since the 1970s,[54] has been investigated extensively as a treatment modality in North America. Its mechanism of action is entirely different from that of the chelators. In pharmacologic doses, zinc interferes with the absorption of copper from the GI tract and increases the excretion of copper in the stool. The postulated mechanism of action is through the induction of metallothionein in enterocytes. The metallothionein has a greater affinity for copper than for zinc and preferentially binds copper from the intestinal contents. Once bound, the copper is not absorbed but is lost in the feces as enterocytes are shed during normal turnover. Additionally, zinc may interfere with lipid peroxidation and enhance the availability of glutathione.

Problems with zinc therapy include gastritis, which is a common side effect, and uncertainty about dosing. Using a zinc salt other than zinc sulfate may minimize gastritis; any zinc salt is equally acceptable for the treatment of Wilson disease. Food interferes with the effectiveness of zinc, and some investigators recommend that no food be eaten for one hour before or after a dose of zinc is taken. This dosing regimen tends to increase the severity of gastritis and may be sufficiently inconvenient to compromise compliance, as in adolescents. An alternative approach is to be less rigorous about avoiding zinc at mealtimes and to titrate the dose according to the urinary copper excretion or serum–ceruloplasmin-bound copper concentration. Treatment with zinc appears to have few other side effects.[55] Rare patients experience a deterioration in hepatic Wilson disease when started on zinc. Additionally, zinc may have immunosuppressant effects and reduce leukocyte chemotaxis. Studies in rats suggest a possible interference with bone formation. Long-term studies indicate that zinc is more effective in neurologic Wilson disease than in hepatic Wilson disease.[51,56] Despite interest in use of zinc as primary therapy for hepatic Wilson disease, its best role is as maintenance therapy.

For patients who present with decompensated chronic liver disease, combining zinc with a conventional chelator (preferably trientine) has become a popular treatment strategy even in the absence of extensive validation. The 2 types of treatments must be temporally dispersed through the day, with at least 4 to 5 hours between administration of the 2 drugs, or else they may neutralize each other. This intensive short-term induction regimen is best suited to patients with severe hepatic or neurologic disease[57] and remains semi-investigational. Some patients with severe hepatic Wilson disease fail on this regimen and require urgent liver transplantation, arrangements for which should be in place.

Ammonium tetrathiomolybdate, an experimental drug, may be especially suitable for treatment of severe neurologic Wilson disease because, unlike D-penicillamine, it is not associated with early neurologic deterioration.[58] Tetrathiomolybdate interferes with the absorption of copper from the intestine and binds to plasma copper with high affinity. Unlike D-penicillamine, tetrathiomolybdate has been found in LEC rats to remove copper from metallothionein at low doses; at higher doses, an insoluble copper complex is deposited in the liver.[59] Although tetrathiomolybdate is regarded as nontoxic, bone marrow suppression and hepatotoxicity are noteworthy adverse effects. Little is known about where the mobilized copper and molybdate may be deposited. The optimal dose and length of treatment, as well as long-term adverse effects, require further study. Such a potent copper-binding drug could produce copper deficiency.

Antioxidants may be a useful adjunct for preventing tissue damage. Studies in copper-loaded animals and in patients with Wilson disease indicate that copper enhances free radical production in tissues and may thereby cause liver damage. Oxidative damage may be reflected in DNA strand breaks in the brains of LEC rats.[60] Oxidative effects of excess copper may contribute to the development and progression of liver damage.[61] The antioxidant α-tocopherol may be beneficial adjunctive treatment for patients with severe hepatic decompensation.

For pregnant patients with Wilson disease, treatment must be continued throughout pregnancy. Postpartum hepatic decompensation may occur if treatment is stopped completely during pregnancy. Although many pregnancies during treatment with D-penicillamine have been successful, the drug is officially classified as a teratogen. Occasional reports of severe collagen defects in the offspring of a patient treated with D-penicillamine may be caused in part by copper deficiency as a result of prolonged aggressive treatment, as well as the teratogenic effects of D-penicillamine.[62] Treatment with zinc may be less likely to produce adverse effects on developing collagen in the fetus. The safety of trientine during pregnancy is unknown, apart from favorable anecdotal reports. Judicious reduction of the dose of D-penicillamine or trientine by approximately 25% of the pre-pregnancy dose is advisable, especially if delivery by cesarean section is anticipated.

PROGNOSIS

Patients with clinically evident Wilson disease are generally regarded as having a good prognosis if the disease is diagnosed promptly and treated consistently. An asymptomatic first-degree relative who is diagnosed on biochemical or genetic grounds and treated before any sign of clinical impairment generally has the best long-term outlook. Patients with early hepatic disease have a generally favorable prognosis as long as treatment is consistent and well tolerated. Severe neurologic disease may not entirely resolve on treatment.

The role of liver transplantation in Wilson disease is limited (see Chapters 95 and 97). Fulminant hepatic failure in a patient with Wilson disease necessitates liver transplantation. Some patients with severe liver disease that is unresponsive to drug therapy may also proceed to liver transplantation. The outcome is favorable, with one year survival rates of 80% to 90% and excellent survival beyond one year.[63] Severe neurologic disease may improve after liver transplantation, but experience is conflicting,[12] and liver transplantation cannot be recommended for neurologic Wilson disease. Patients with neurologic or psychiatric manifestations of Wilson disease appear to have poor outcomes after liver transplantation and adhere poorly to medical regimens.[64] Therefore, liver transplantation should be reserved for patients who present with severe, decompensated liver disease that is unresponsive to therapy or with fulminant hepatic failure. Live-donor liver transplantation, even when the graft is from a family member who is a heterozygote, yields adequately functioning grafts.[65,66] If the donor is the brother or sister of the patient, mutational analysis of his or her *ATP7B* gene should be performed to exclude presymptomatic Wilson disease.

Patients who stop taking chelating treatment have a poor prognosis. New neurologic abnormalities, such as dysarthria, may develop. Rapidly progressive hepatic decompensation has been observed and occurs on average within 3 years, and as early as 8 months, after treatment is stopped. The liver damage is usually refractory to reinstitution of chelation therapy. Such patients require liver transplantation.

The quality of life of patients with Wilson disease may be compromised by drug toxicity. Anecdotal observations suggest that damage to collagen may accrue over decades in patients who are maintained indefinitely on D-penicillamine, but the risk has not been assessed adequately. Deficiencies in trace metals may develop with the use of any chelator, but whether these deficiencies are clinically important is not yet clear. Abnormal iron metabolism, leading to hepatic iron overload and anemia, can be predicted if serum ceruloplasmin oxidase activity is zero. Patients should be encouraged to maintain a healthy lifestyle, including avoidance of alcohol and obesity.

KEY REFERENCES

Full references for this chapter can be found on www.expertconsult.com.

2. Bull PC, Thomas GR, Rommens JM, et al. The Wilson disease gene is a putative copper transporting P-type

ATPase similar to the Menkes gene. Nat Genet 1993; 5:327-37.

12. Roberts EA, Schilsky ML. Diagnosis and treatment of Wilson disease: An update. Hepatology 2008; 47:2089-111.

15. Korman JD, Volenberg I, Balko J, et al. Screening for Wilson disease in acute liver failure: A comparison of currently available diagnostic tests. Hepatology 2008; 48:1167-74.

31. Ferenci P, Steindl-Munda P, Vogel W, et al. Diagnostic value of quantitative hepatic copper determination in patients with Wilson's disease. Clin Gastroenterol Hepatol 2005; 3:811-18.

33. Kenney SM, Cox DW. Sequence variation database for the Wilson disease copper transporter, ATP7B. Hum Mutat 2007; 28:1171-7.

36. Hsi G, Cullen LM, Macintyre G, et al. Sequence variation in the ATP-binding domain of the Wilson disease transporter, ATP7B, affects copper transport in a yeast model system. Hum Mutat 2008; 29:491-501.

42. Thomas GR, Forbes JR, Roberts EA, et al. The Wilson disease gene: Spectrum of mutations and their consequences. Nat Genet 1995; 9:210-7.

43. Wilson DC, Phillips MJ, Cox DW, Roberts EA. Severe hepatic Wilson's disease in preschool-aged children. J Pediatr 2000; 137:719-22.

44. Merle U, Weiss KH, Eisenbach C, et al. Truncating mutations in the Wilson disease gene ATP7B are associated with very low serum ceruloplasmin oxidase activity and an early onset of Wilson disease. BMC Gastroenterol 2010; 10:8.

48. Wiggelinkhuizen M, Tilanus ME, Bollen CW, et al. Systematic review: Clinical efficacy of chelator agents and zinc in the initial treatment of Wilson disease. Aliment Pharmacol Ther 2009; 29:947-58.

51. Weiss KH, Gotthardt DN, Klemm D, et al. Zinc monotherapy is not as effective as chelating agents in treatment of Wilson disease. Gastroenterology 2011; 140:1189-98.

63. Emre S, Atillasoy EO, Ozdemir S, et al. Orthotopic liver transplantation for Wilson's disease: A single-center experience. Transplantation 2001; 72:1232-6.

Other Inherited Metabolic Disorders of the Liver

MIKE A. LEONIS AND WILLIAM F. BALISTRERI

Metabolic liver diseases may manifest as acute, life-threatening illnesses in the neonatal period or as chronic liver disease in adolescence or adulthood, with progression to liver failure, cirrhosis, or hepatocellular carcinoma. In a 2013 report of the Scientific Registry of Transplant Recipients, 13% of all liver transplants in the United States were performed because of complications resulting from metabolic liver disease.[1,2] When the pediatric population alone was analyzed, approximately 20% of the liver transplants performed in children over the 2-year period from 2009 to 2011 were for complications of metabolic liver disease.[1,2] Nontransplant treatment options have become available that may, in certain cases, obviate the need for liver transplantation.[3,4]

CLINICAL FEATURES OF METABOLIC LIVER DISEASE

The diverse presenting features of metabolic liver disease are listed in Box 77-1. Certain metabolic liver diseases in young patients may mimic other illnesses, such as acute infections and intoxications. By contrast, the older patient with metabolic liver disease may present with symptoms of chronic liver disease. Because metabolic diseases can resemble multiple other disorders, a high index of suspicion is required. Evaluation of any infant presenting with cholestasis should include a consideration of metabolic liver disease. Any patient with progressive neuromuscular disease, developmental delay, or regression of developmental milestones also requires evaluation. Metabolic liver disease should be an immediate consideration in patients of all ages with elevated serum aminotransferase levels, hepatomegaly, acidosis, hypoglycemia, ascites, bleeding diathesis, hyperammonemia, coma, recurrent vomiting, or poor weight gain.

A detailed history can often raise the possibility of metabolic liver disease. A family history of consanguinity, multiple miscarriages, or early infant deaths may suggest a metabolic derangement. Close relatives with undiagnosed liver disease, progressive neurologic or muscle disease, or undiagnosed developmental delays should also raise suspicion. Introduction of certain foods may correlate with the onset of symptoms, as in patients with urea cycle defects, galactosemia, or fructosemia. A history of specific dietary aversions may be revealing.

Recommended initial screening tests are listed in Box 77-2. Because patients with metabolic liver disease often present with acute and recurrent symptoms, diagnostic studies should

Symptoms

Coma
Developmental delay
Growth failure
Hyperammonemic symptoms
Hypoglycemic symptoms
Neurologic or motor skill deterioration
Recurrent vomiting
Seizures

Signs

Ascites
Abdominal distention
Cardiac dysfunction
Cataracts

Dysmorphic features
Hepatomegaly
Hypotonia
Jaundice
Short stature
Splenomegaly
Unusual odors

Other Findings

Acidosis
Acute liver failure
Cholestasis
Coagulopathy
Ketosis
Rickets

Serum

Albumin
Alkaline phosphatase
Amino acids
Aminotransferases
Ammonia
Anion gap calculation
Bile acids
Coagulation profile
Electrolytes
Ferritin
Fractionated bilirubin

GGTP
Glucose
Lactate[†]
Peripheral blood smear
Pyruvate[†]
Uric acid[†]

Urine

Bile acids
Organic acids
Orotic acid
Reducing substances

*Specimens of serum and urine obtained during acute episodes should be saved for later studies.
[†]Obtain if the patient is acidotic or has neurologic symptoms.

be obtained when the patient is experiencing symptoms, because the characteristic laboratory abnormalities for many of these illnesses may normalize between acute episodes. In enigmatic cases, serum and urine samples should be obtained during the acute illness and saved (frozen) for definitive studies, if available. A liver biopsy can be valuable. In addition to biopsy specimens for standard histology, a frozen specimen should be saved for biochemical assessment and a sample prepared for later electron microscopic study to look at the subcellular organelles, which may exhibit characteristic changes in some metabolic disorders. The increasing availability of molecular diagnostic testing allows genotypic evaluation for some diseases to complement phenotypic diagnosis.

α_1-ANTITRYPSIN DEFICIENCY

Deficiency of α_1-antitrypsin (α_1-AT) is transmitted in an autosomal recessive fashion and leads to an increased risk of lung and liver disease. This deficiency is one of the most common genetic diseases in the world and the second most common metabolic disease affecting the liver (after hereditary hemochromatosis [see Chapter 75]).[5]

Pathophysiology

The prototypical member of the serpin family of protease inhibitors (Pis), α_1-AT binds with and promotes the degradation of serine proteases in the serum and tissues. The most important serine protease is neutrophil elastase, which is inhibited by α_1-AT through formation of a tight 1:1 α_1-AT-to-elastase complex. Two mechanisms likely contribute to the premature development of pulmonary emphysema in affected patients: (1) loss of serum α_1-AT activity, as occurs in the most common form of α_1-AT deficiency, leading to uninhibited neutrophil elastase activity and (2) buildup in the lung of α_1-AT Z polymers that are proinflammatory to neutrophils.[6,7]

Allelic α_1-AT mutant variants produce Pi gene products that can be distinguished from the normal product by electrophoretic methods; the normal allelic representation is designated PiM. The PiZ variant produces a mutant α_1-AT Z protein that contains a single amino acid replacement of glutamine with a lysine residue as a result of a mutation at position 342 of the α_1-AT *(SERPINA1)* gene. Homozygosity at the PiZ allele is the most common and classic pathologic form of α_1-AT deficiency and is capable of leading to liver and lung disease. In addition, more than 100 naturally occurring variants of α_1-AT have been described. Although most of these variants are either of no clinical significance or are extremely rare, additional variants—PiS(iiyama), PiM(duarte), and PiM(malton)—have been reported to be associated with liver injury and even cirrhosis, especially in persons who are heterozygous for the PiM(duarte) PiZ allele.[6,8-11]

α_1-AT is produced almost exclusively in the rough endoplasmic reticulum (ER) of hepatocytes and is targeted to the secretory pathway via the Golgi apparatus. Structural misfolding and polymerization of the mutant α_1-AT Z protein causes its aberrant retention in the hepatocyte ER, failure of progression through the secretory pathway, and diminished intracellular degradation. In persons with the phenotype PiZZ, serum α_1-AT activity levels are reduced to less than 15% of normal; this loss of function accounts for the development of pulmonary disease. The rate of intracellular degradation may itself be genetically determined and may influence the expression of disease; α_1-AT Z appears to be degraded more slowly in the ER of PiZZ patients who are susceptible to liver disease than in PiZZ patients who are not susceptible to liver disease.[12]

Studies of transgenic mice that express the human α_1-AT Z gene suggest a gain-of-function mechanism in which retention in the ER and accumulation in hepatocytes of mutant α_1-AT Z is responsible for hepatotoxicity.[13] Multiple intracellular signaling pathways, including caspase activation, ER stress responses, and the autophagic response, are activated by the retention of malformed proteins in the ER.[14] Autophagy is an intracellular degradative pathway that targets proteins and organelles for destruction during development as well as at times of stress or nutrient deprivation. Other genetic and environmental modifiers of the ER "quality control" process for handling mutant α_1-AT Z protein are undoubtedly involved and account for the wide variation in clinical phenotype observed in the hepatic presentation of PiZZ patients.[15]

Clinical Features

Although the prevalence of the classic α_1-AT deficiency allele, PiZ, is highest in populations derived from northern European ancestry, many racial subgroups are affected worldwide, and millions of persons have combinations of deficiency alleles (i.e., PiSS, PiSZ, or PiZZ).[6,16] In the United States, the overall prevalence of deficiency allele combinations is approximately 1 in 490 (i.e., 1 in 1058 for PiSS, 1 in 1124 for PiSZ, and 1 in 4775 for PiZZ).[17] Mounting evidence suggests that heterozygous α_1-AT deficiency states can contribute to the development of cirrhosis and chronic liver failure in adults through mechanisms similar to those encountered with the

PiZZ phenotype.[8-10,18] In addition, the heterozygous α_1-AT deficiency state may contribute to worsening of chronic liver disease caused by HCV infection or nonalcoholic fatty liver disease in adults, as well as cholestatic liver diseases in children.[15,18-21]

In the most unbiased epidemiologic study of α_1-AT deficiency to date, reported by Sveger,[22] 200,000 Swedish infants were screened for α_1-AT deficiency, 184 were found to have abnormal allelic forms of α_1-AT (127 PiZZ, 2 PiZnull, 54 PiSZ, and 1 PiSnull), and 6 (5 PiZZ and 1 PiSZ) died in early childhood, but only 2 of cirrhosis. About 10% of newborns with α_1-AT deficiency (PiZZ) present with cholestasis, and as many as 50% continue to have elevated serum aminotransferase levels at age 3 months; most are clinically asymptomatic.[22,23] Liver disease does not develop in patients with null α_1-AT phenotypes, whereas early-onset emphysema develops in all of them.[24] Therefore, the prognosis for patients with liver disease manifesting in infancy as a result of α_1-AT deficiency (PiZZ) is highly variable. Even children in whom cirrhosis develops can have a highly variable progression to end-stage liver disease (ESLD), which infrequently leads to liver transplantation.[25] Moreover, siblings with PiZZ have a variable degree of liver involvement; in a study reported by Hinds and colleagues, 5 of 7 children with PiZZ requiring liver transplantation had siblings with PiZZ who lacked persistent liver involvement.[26] Therefore, environmental or additional genetic factors must be involved in determining the severity of liver disease in α_1-AT deficiency.[27,28] One such genetic modifier is the ER mannosidase I gene, an allelic variant of which was associated with an earlier age of onset of ESLD.[29]

Of 150 patients with α_1-AT deficiency from Sveger's original study[22] who subsequently underwent evaluation at age 16 and 18 years, none had clinical signs of liver disease. Elevated serum aminotransferase or GGTP levels were found in fewer than 20% of patients with a PiZZ phenotype and in fewer than 15% of those with a PiSZ phenotype.[23] By the third decade of life, analysis of this same cohort of affected persons showed that 6% of PiZZ and 9% of PiSZ patients had a marginal increase in serum ALT levels.[30] An analysis of 647 patients with a PiZZ phenotype found that 49% had slight increases in aminotransferases when a stricter cutoff for normal levels was used, suggesting small amounts of ongoing liver injury.[31]

Although liver disease is often mild during infancy and childhood, patients with α_1-AT deficiency have an increased risk for developing cirrhosis during adulthood; 42% of all PiZZ patients have histologic evidence of cirrhosis at autopsy.[32,33] A study of 57 PiZZ adults with lung disease revealed that 63% had findings of chronic liver disease by conventional laboratory tests of liver function and liver US.[34] Moreover, homozygous α_1-AT deficiency raises the risk of hepatocellular carcinoma, especially in men older than 50 years.[33] The diagnosis of α_1-AT deficiency should be considered in any patient presenting with noninfectious chronic hepatitis, hepatosplenomegaly, cirrhosis, portal hypertension, or hepatocellular carcinoma.

Histopathology

Histopathologic features of α_1-AT deficiency change as the patient ages. In infancy, liver biopsy specimens may show bile duct paucity, bile duct proliferation, intracellular cholestasis with or without giant cell transformation, mild inflammatory changes, or steatosis, with few of the characteristic periodic acid–Schiff (PAS)-positive, diastase-resistant globules.[28] These inclusions, which result from polymerized α_1-AT Z protein, are most prominent in periportal hepatocytes and may also be seen in Kupffer cells. Immunohistochemistry with monoclonal

antibody to α_1-AT Z can also be performed to verify the diagnosis. As the patient ages, these changes may resolve completely or progress to chronic hepatitis or cirrhosis.

Diagnosis

α_1-AT is considered a hepatic acute-phase reactant, and its release may be stimulated by stress, injury, pregnancy, or neoplasia. Because these factors can influence α_1-AT production, even in patients with the PiZZ phenotype, the diagnosis of α_1-AT deficiency should be based on phenotype analysis and not solely on the serum α_1-AT level.[35] A liver biopsy specimen, although not universally recommended, should confirm the diagnosis. Commercial tests are available to detect the most common mutant alleles by PCR analysis of genomic DNA. In addition, a resequencing molecular array chip is available for rapid sequencing of the entire *SERPINA1* gene to allow identification of rare mutant alleles.[36]

Screening guidelines to diagnose α_1-AT deficiency in asymptomatic persons have been proposed.[37] Adults with chronic lung disease and siblings of affected patients with lung or liver disease should be targeted for screening, and appropriate education and genetic counseling should be offered to patients with α_1-AT deficiency identified by screening.[28]

Treatment

The initial treatment of α_1-AT deficiency is symptomatic care. The importance of providing fat-soluble vitamins when indicated, adequate nutrition, and counseling to avoid smoking and second-hand smoke cannot be overemphasized. Animal models of α_1-AT deficiency suggest that NSAIDs may be uniquely toxic to the PiZZ liver by increasing the burden of accumulated mutant protein in the liver; this observation, however, has not been validated in human studies.[11] The role of neonatal screening for α_1-AT deficiency is still not settled, although early diagnosis leads to a beneficial effect on smoking practices. If effective therapy for liver disease caused by α_1-AT deficiency becomes available, neonatal screening may become more useful for preventing the need for liver transplantation.

Although progression to ESLD is uncommon, α_1-AT deficiency is the most common metabolic liver disease for which liver transplantation is performed. Besides replacing the injured organ, transplantation corrects the metabolic defect, thereby preventing further progression of systemic disease. Between 1995 and 2004, 161 children and 406 adults underwent liver transplantation for ESLD associated with α_1-AT deficiency in the United States; of these, 4.4% of the children and fewer than 1% of the adults were African Americans. Five-year patient survival rates following liver transplantation for the pediatric and adult patients with α_1-AT deficiency were 83% and 90%, respectively.[38] Liver transplantation using grafts from donors with unrecognized α_1-AT deficiency appears to have an outcome comparable to that for transplantation using grafts without α_1-AT deficiency.[39] Although data are lacking on the risk of hepatocellular carcinoma in patients with liver disease due to α_1-AT deficiency, a prudent approach is to follow the AASLD guidelines for surveillance: liver US every 6 months in patients with cirrhosis, significant fibrosis, or persistently high aminotransferase elevations.[40]

Replacement therapy with purified α_1-AT is the only treatment option approved by the FDA for lung disease associated with α_1-AT deficiency. Patients who receive replacement therapy have a slower rate of decline in lung tissue and function than untreated patients.[41] This therapy does not benefit α_1-AT deficiency–associated liver disease.

Small molecule chemical chaperones such as phenylbutyric acid (PBA) markedly increase secretion of α_1-AT Z in experimental in vitro and in vivo models of α_1-AT deficiency[42]; however, PBA was not of statistical benefit in a small human trial.[43] Another pharmacologic approach in the early stages of investigation involves the use of autophagy-enhancer agents, such as rapamycin or carbamazepine, to increase autophagy in the liver and thereby increase the degradation of α_1-AT mutant Z protein polymers.[11,44,45]

α_1-AT deficiency is one of many diseases for which reconstitution of the normal genotype through gene therapy has been successful in mouse models; however, these results have not been extended to human studies. Approaches to inhibiting transcription or translation of the mutant α_1-AT Z protein using small interfering (si)RNAs or ribozymes have been successful in animal models, and human trials have begun.[11]

GLYCOGEN STORAGE DISEASES

More than 10 distinct inborn disorders of glycogen metabolism have been described, but only 3 are associated with serious liver disease: glycogen storage disease (GSD) types I, III, and IV.[46,47] Other GSDs may cause hepatomegaly or liver histologic changes but generally do not cause clinically important liver disease. The overall incidence of GSD types I, III, and IV is estimated to range from 1 in 50,000 to 1 in 100,000 population.

Glycogen metabolism occurs in many tissues, but the areas of clinical importance are the muscle, liver, and polymorphonuclear neutrophils. The body uses glycogen to store glucose and as a ready reserve when systemic glucose is required (see Chapter 72). Glycogen is composed of long-chain glucose molecules arranged in a linear 1,4 linkage. From 8% to 10% of the glucose molecules are attached in a 1,6 linkage to form branching chains, which permit efficient storage of glucose while minimizing the impact on intracellular osmolality. The substrates for glycogen synthesis, glucose-6-phosphate (Glu-6-P) and glucose-1-phosphate (Glu-1-P), are derived from several pathways, including fructose and galactose metabolic cycles, as well as gluconeogenesis and glycogenolysis (Fig. 77-1).

Through the action of uridine diphosphate glucose (UDPG) pyrophosphorylase and glycogen synthase, Glu-1-P is metabolized to UDPG and glycogen sequentially. The 1,4 linkages can be converted to 1,6 linkages by the actions of branching enzymes. Amylo-1,6-glucosidase is a debranching enzyme that can release 8% to 10% of the glucose stored in glycogen. The remaining glucose is released as Glu-1-P through the action of phosphorylase *a* and is converted to Glu-6-P by phosphoglucomutase. Phosphorylase exists in an active (*a*) and an inactive (*b*) form; protein kinase is responsible for the conversion of phosphorylase *b* to *a*. Protein kinase is stimulated by epinephrine, glucagon, and fasting, and thereby increases glycogenolysis. High levels of glucose influence the conversion of phosphorylase *a* back to phosphorylase *b*, thereby decreasing glycogenolysis. Glycogen synthase also exists in active (*a*) and inactive (*b*) forms. Phosphorylase *a* inhibits the conversion to glycogen synthase *a*, thereby reducing glycogen synthesis. High levels of glycogen favor the formation of glycogen synthase *b*.[47]

Type I

GSD type I, the most common inborn error of glycogen metabolism, results from deficiency of a 2-component enzyme system involved in the transport of Glu-6-P from the cytosol into the ER by Glu-6-P translocase (encoded by

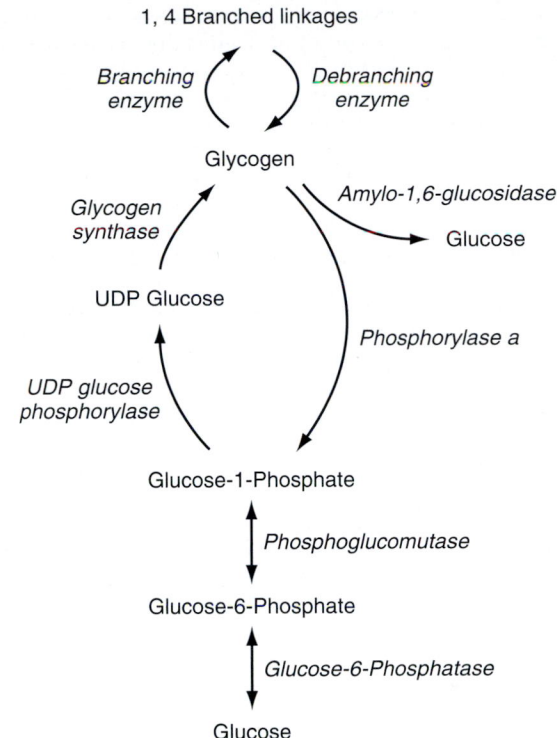

FIGURE 77-1. Pathway of glycogen synthesis and glycogenolysis. Enzymes are shown in *italics*. UDP, uridine diphosphate.

the ubiquitously expressed *SLC37A4* gene) and subsequent cleavage of Glu-6-P by glucose-6-phosphatase (Glu-6-Pase, encoded by the *G6PC1* gene), located on the luminal side of the ER. Clinical and molecular genetic observations have disclosed 2 subtypes of GSD type I, Ia and Ib, that account for virtually all cases.[48] The clinical phenotype with respect to liver disease is similar in the 2 forms; however, patients with GSD type Ib often have intermittent severe neutropenia and neutrophil dysfunction, making them prone to recurrent episodes of severe bacterial infections and Crohn's-like intestinal disease.[49,50] Loss-of-function of an isoform of Glu-6-Pase encoded by the *G6PC3* gene, although also ubiquitously expressed, leads to severe congenital neutropenia type 4, an autosomal recessive condition.[51]

Disruption of the function of Glu-6-Pase (type Ia) or Glu-6-P translocase (type Ib) inhibits the utilization of glucose by gluconeogenesis, glycogenolysis, and the metabolism of fructose or galactose.[52] This inability to release stored glucose leads to hypoglycemia within 90 to 180 minutes of the last orally ingested glucose. Lactate and fatty acid metabolism and glycolytic pathways are then used as sources of energy.

Clinical Features

Most patients with GSD type I present in infancy with symptoms of metabolic derangement, such as lethargy, seizures, or coma as a result of profound hypoglycemia or metabolic acidosis, a protruding abdomen caused by hepatomegaly, muscular hypotonia, and delayed psychomotor development.[53]

Physical signs invariably include hepatomegaly, usually with a normal-sized spleen. Patients in whom the disease is poorly controlled for a long time exhibit short stature and growth failure and may be prone to adiposity. Delayed bone age and reduced postpubertal bone mineral density are common.[54] Xanthomas can appear after puberty and localize to the elbows, knees, buttocks, or nasal septum, the last leading to epistaxis. Patients with GSD type I are susceptible to a wide spectrum of brain damage that may result in epilepsy, hearing loss, and abnormal neuroradiologic findings, most likely as a result of recurrent episodes of hypoglycemia.[55]

Other metabolic derangements can be seen. Lactic acid levels can reach 4 to 8 times normal; the accompanying metabolic acidosis may manifest as muscle weakness, hyperventilation, malaise, headache, or recurrent fever. Serum ATP and phosphorus levels are low, secondary to an increase in purine synthesis and the inability to release phosphorus from Glu-6-P. Hyperuricemia is common and may lead to gout, arthritis, or progressive nephropathy. Nephromegaly secondary to increased glycogen deposition is common, and with advancing age, progressive renal disease, hypertension, and renal failure requiring dialysis and transplantation may develop.[53] Because of hypoglycemia, patients have chronically high serum levels of glucagon with depressed levels of insulin. Hypertriglyceridemia and hypercholesterolemia are present in both GSD Ia and GSD Ib (but more prominently in GSD Ia) and may account for the greater frequency of xanthoma formation.[56] Hypercalcemia during acute metabolic decompensation has been observed.[57]

Patients with GSD type Ib often also have severe intermittent neutropenia and neutrophil dysfunction as well as high platelet counts. Crohn's-like IBD often occurs in patients with GSD type Ib at the time of severe neutropenia, and patients are prone to severe bacterial infections, with abscess formation throughout the body.[49] No correlation has been found between the severity of bacterial infections or degree of neutropenia and the molecular defect in Glu-6-P transport activity in humans with GSD type Ib, suggesting that other as yet unknown factors, such as modifying genes, define the ultimate disease phenotype.[58] A child with GSD type Ib who developed ESLD with complications from cirrhosis and who subsequently underwent liver transplantation has been reported.[59]

Hepatic Involvement

Hepatomegaly in GSD type I results from increased glycogen storage in the liver, as well as a large degree of fatty infiltration; the latter likely develops because of a wide array of perturbations in lipid metabolism, including increased free fatty acid flux into the liver.[56] Patients demonstrate mild elevations in serum aminotransferase levels but generally do not develop cirrhosis or liver failure.

Hepatocellular adenomas develop in 22% to 75% of patients, as early as 3 years of age but most commonly in the second decade of life, and tend to increase in both size and number as the patient ages (see Chapter 96).[60] Adenomas in GSD type I differ from sporadic adenomas in that hepatic nuclear factor 1α inactivation is not observed in the former.[61] In rare instances, adenomas can transform to hepatocellular carcinoma; unfortunately, serum AFP and carcinoembryonic antigen levels and features of the lesions on hepatic imaging are not predictive of malignant transformation.[60,62,63] Whether poor metabolic control increases the risk of hepatocellular adenoma formation in patients with GSD type Ia is controversial.[64,65] In some patients, hepatocellular adenomas have been demonstrated to regress and disappear after adequate nutritional therapy, but in general, the course is unpredictable, especially in nonadherent patients.[60,62] Because of the unreliability of imaging and serum marker levels in predicting malignant transformation in this patient population, whether resection of an adenoma or liver transplantation is preferable is uncertain.[66]

Diagnosis

Hepatic glycogen content is elevated in patients with GSD type I, and the most accurate diagnostic measure is direct analysis of enzyme activity performed on fresh, rather than frozen, liver tissue. Analysis of fresh liver tissue is important to avoid disrupting microsomal Glu-6-Pase activity.[67] Fasting serum glucose and lactate levels, a positive glucagon response test result, and the response to fructose or galactose administration (patients with GSD type I do not show the expected rise in serum glucose concentration after administration of glucagon or either sugar) often provide supportive evidence but may not yield a definitive diagnosis. DNA analysis–based approaches that integrate biochemical features and the presence or absence of persistent neutropenia in patients with GSD type Ib have been proposed and may provide a diagnostic alternative to liver biopsy.[68]

Treatment

Patients with undiagnosed or undertreated GSD type I are at increased risk of death, usually from hypoglycemic comas, seizures, metabolic acidosis, or, in those with GSD type Ib, sepsis from neutropenia.[53] Rarely, hepatocellular carcinoma is a cause of death. Management centers on preventing the acute metabolic derangements and potential long-term complications and enabling the patient to attain normal psychological development and a good quality of life.[67,69]

Consensus guidelines for the management of GSD type I have been proposed.[67,69] Biomedical targets for good metabolic control include a preprandial blood glucose level higher than 63 to 77 mg/dL (3.5 to 4.3 mmol/L), urine lactate-to-creatinine ratio higher than 0.06, high-normal serum uric acid level, venous blood base excess higher than 5 mmol/L, bicarbonate level higher than 20 mmol/L, serum triglyceride level lower than 6 mmol/L, and BMI between 0 and 2 standard deviations of normal. In addition, for GSD type Ib, demonstrating a normal fecal α₁-AT level is desirable (see Chapter 30).[67,70] Because optimal glycemic control is not always possible and the risk of severe hypoglycemia is high if delivery of glucose is interrupted inadvertently, serum lactate levels should be kept at the high end of normal, because lactate is an alternative fuel for the brain.

Nutritional supplementation has become the mainstay of therapy for GSD type I. Frequent, high-carbohydrate, daytime feedings, such as uncooked cornstarch, or continuous nighttime drip feedings, or both, allow the steady release of glucose and lead to improved metabolic control and normalized growth and development.[56,70] The serum glucose level should be maintained above 70 mg/dL (3.9 mmol/L). Uncooked cornstarch in a dose of 2 g/kg every 6 hours (6 to 8 mg of glucose/kg/min) has been suggested; however, alternative regimens have been implemented successfully.

For infants, when the diagnosis of GSD type I is confirmed, a formula that does not contain fructose or galactose should be prescribed. Frequent daytime feedings and continuous nocturnal administration are required, with a rate of delivery needed to maintain euglycemia of approximately 8 mg/kg/min. Morning feedings should be given soon after discontinuation of the nighttime drip to avoid hypoglycemia. As solids are introduced, high-carbohydrate foods should be emphasized. These patients require special attention during acute illnesses that may affect oral intake or metabolism, because they can become hypoglycemic quickly.

Prophylaxis with antibiotics (e.g., trimethoprim/sulfamethoxazole) is recommended for patients with GSD type Ib and severe neutropenia or recurrent bacterial infections.[69] Granulocyte colony stimulating factor (GCSF) has been used with success in patients with GSD type Ib to improve hematologic parameters and neutrophil function and reduce the morbidity associated with severe bacterial infections.[71] Splenomegaly may worsen with GCSF therapy, and bone marrow aspiration before and during GCSF therapy may be prudent, given rare instances of acute myelogenous leukemia (AML) in patients with GSD type Ib.[69] Both GCSF and IBD raise the risk of osteopenia, and bone density should be monitored.

Adenoviral-mediated gene replacement therapy of recombinant Glu-6-Pase in both murine and canine models of GSD type Ia deficiency, which has all of the major features of GSD type Ia in humans, has led to encouraging results and may be an option in humans in the future.[72,73] Hepatocyte transplantation, with the use of standard post-transplantation immunosuppression, has been performed successfully in an 18-year-old male adolescent with GSD type Ib, with euglycemia maintained up to 2 years.[74] Liver transplantation has corrected the metabolic error in patients with GSD type I and permitted catch-up growth, even in patients in the third decade of life.[75,76] Neutrophil counts and function, however, are only variably improved after liver transplantation in patients with GSD type Ib.[75]

Type III

GSD type III results from deficiency of glycogen-debranching enzyme (GDE) and leads to the accumulation of limit dextrin units, which restrict subsequent glucose release by phosphorylase. Because deficiency of GDE does not interfere with metabolism of Glu-6-P, patients with GSD type III still have effective mechanisms for gluconeogenesis. Therefore, the clinical course is milder than in patients with GSD type I, and patients are able to fast for longer periods; most survive into adulthood. In infancy, however, GSD type III may be indistinguishable from GSD type I.

GDE is encoded by a single gene and possesses 2 independent catalytic activities, an amylo-1,6-glucosidase and oligo-1,4→1,4 glucan transferase. Both of these activities are deficient in the 2 main clinical subtypes of GSD type III, types IIIa and IIIb. Differential expression of 4 major GDE mRNA isoforms in liver and muscle tissue distinguishes the 2 types: type IIIa affects liver and muscle and accounts for 80% of patients, and type IIIb affects the liver only and accounts for 15% of patients. Although subtype-specific mutations in the GDE gene have increasingly been identified, the molecular basis for this differential tissue-specific expression of GDE is unknown, and no clear genotype-phenotype correlations have been identified.[77,78] Rare isolated loss of 1 of the 2 GDE activities has been observed (i.e., glucosidase activity in type IIIc and transferase activity in type IIId).[77]

Clinical Features

Persons with GSD type III typically exhibit hypoglycemia, hepatomegaly, and growth failure. Liver enlargement results from increased glycogen deposition, not fatty infiltration. The liver may show fibrotic septa that rarely lead to frank cirrhosis and liver failure. Serum lactate and uric acid levels are normal, and aminotransferase levels are increased only moderately until advanced liver disease occurs. Hyperlipidemia may be present but is not as pronounced as in GSD type I. Patients have normal responses to fructose and galactose loading.

Patients with GSD type III may also display progressive (skeletal, cardiac, and bulbar) muscle weakness, which worsens with activity, and muscle wasting.[77,79] Nephromegaly is not seen, but ventricular hypertrophy or cardiac arrhythmias may occur; frequent cardiac evaluation and monitoring are recommended.[77] The diagnosis can be made by direct enzyme analysis of muscle or liver tissue or peripheral leukocytes. Mutation analysis of the GDE gene is complicated but increasingly utilized, with a sequencing strategy that focuses on common mutation locations and ethnic variability.[77] Hepatocellular adenomas develop in approximately 25% of patients, and isolated reports of cirrhosis leading to hepatocellular carcinoma have been reported.[62,77,80] A naturally occurring canine model of GSD type IIIa with liver and muscle features similar to those in humans has been characterized.[81]

Treatment

A high-protein, low-carbohydrate diet has been suggested to normalize metabolic activity, ensure normal growth, normalize muscle function, and minimize hepatomegaly. This diet provides adequate substrates for gluconeogenesis while reducing the need for glycogen storage. Patients with refractory hypoglycemia or persistent hepatomegaly may require a nighttime continuous infusion or cornstarch therapy, as used for GSD type I. Liver transplantation has been successful but is usually not necessary for patients with GSD type III, even in those with evidence of cirrhosis, as long as liver synthetic function remains well preserved.[77]

Type IV

Deficiency of the branching enzyme is seen in GSD type IV, a rare syndrome also known as *amylopectinosis*. Glycogen and amylopectin accumulate in hepatocytes, leading to hepatomegaly, abdominal distention, and failure to thrive, most commonly during infancy. Signs of liver disease, when present, predominate later in the course of the disease. Several variable forms of GSD type IV have been observed—a severe congenital form that manifests as fetal hydrops, neonatal hypotonia, or fetal death[82]; a childhood subtype that manifests as cardiomyopathy and abnormal neuromuscular development; and other milder, nonprogressive presentations of hepatic disease that do not lead to cirrhosis and are not associated with skeletal muscle or neurologic involvement.[83] Genotype-phenotype analyses of the branching enzyme gene have revealed a high degree of molecular heterogeneity without clear clinical associations.[83,84]

Hypoglycemia is relatively uncommon, and responses to fructose and galactose challenges are normal. Serum lactate and pyruvate levels are normal, and aminotransferase levels are only moderately elevated until more severe liver involvement becomes apparent. Progressive macronodular cirrhosis is present with an abundance of PAS-positive deposits (amylopectin) in hepatocytes (Fig. 77-2). Cirrhosis may progress to liver failure, and, rarely, adenomas and hepatocellular carcinoma may develop.[85] The diagnosis of GSD type IV can be made by direct enzyme analysis of liver tissue or fibroblasts.

Most patients die within the first 3 years of life if the disease is untreated. Diets high in protein and low in carbohydrate have been associated with improved growth but have had little effect on liver involvement. Liver transplantation has been used successfully and results in correction of the metabolic error and normal growth for most patients; however, persistence of amylopectin deposits in the heart (with progressive cardiomyopathy leading to death) and leukocytes has been described for a small subset of patients.[86]

CONGENITAL DISORDERS OF GLYCOSYLATION

Congenital disorders of glycosylation (CDGs) comprise a group of inherited defects in the enzymes that synthesize the glycan moiety of glycoproteins or the macromolecules that affect intracellular trafficking and functioning of

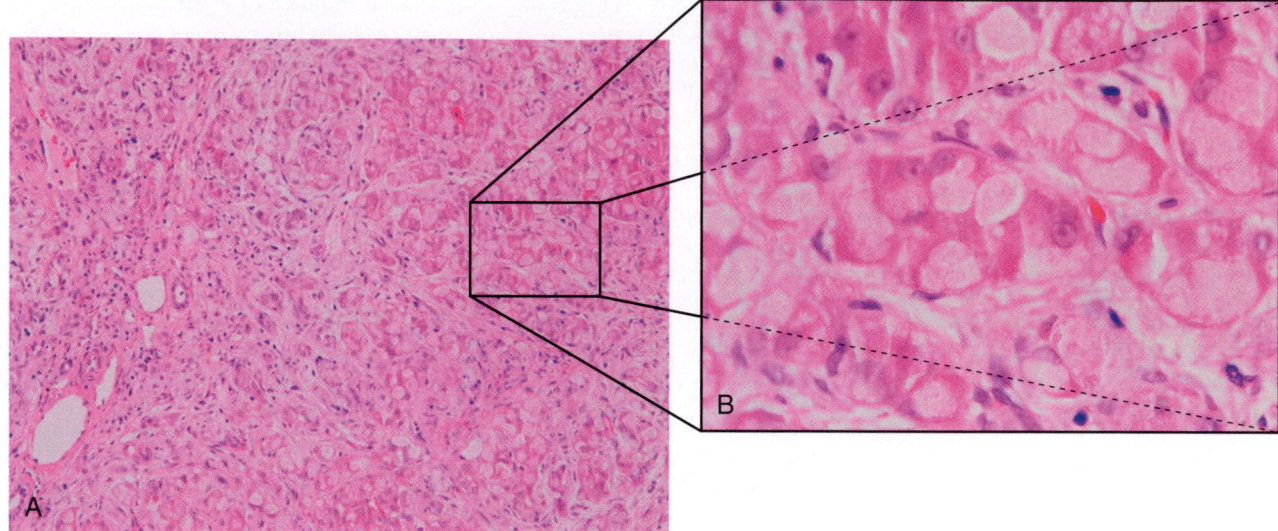

FIGURE 77-2. Histopathology of a liver biopsy specimen from a patient with glycogen storage disease type IV. *A,* At low power, the loss of the normal trabecular hepatic architecture is seen. (H&E, ×20.) *B,* A higher power photomicrograph shows the accumulation of "ground-glass" cytoplasmic inclusions within the hepatocytes; this finding is a consequence of abnormal intracellular processing of amylopectin-like material. (H&E, ×100.)

glycoproteins.[87,88] The CDGs can be divided into 4 groups: (1) disorders of protein *N*-glycosylation, (2) disorders of protein *O*-glycosylation, (3) disorders of lipid glycosylation, and (4) disorders of other glycosylation pathways and of multiple glycosylation pathways.[89] More than 60 CDGs involving both asparagine (*N*)- and serine/threonine (*O*)-linked protein glycosylation have been reported.[88] The clinical spectrum is broad, impacting every organ system. Many of these disorders lead to dysfunction of the liver, intestine, or both.[87-89]

Protein glycosylation is complex and involves multiple enzymatic steps and subcellular compartments.[88] Secretory glycoproteins with altered carbohydrate moieties in patients with CDGs include coagulation factors, albumin and other binding proteins, growth hormone, apolipoproteins, insulin, and thyroxine-binding globulin.[90] Because protein glycosylation occurs in all cells, it is not surprising that patients with a CDG exhibit multisystem abnormalities, often dominated by central nervous system manifestations.

In general, potential glycosylation disorders can be assessed with biochemical biomarkers; however, markers do not identify the genetic defect. Serum transferrin is the best marker for detecting most disorders affecting the *N*-glycosylation pathway.[88]

Hepatic dysfunction is usually mild in patients with CDG and usually does not lead to symptoms. Mild hepatic steatosis and fibrosis typically are seen on light microscopy; on electron microscopy, lysosomal vacuoles, termed *myelosomes*, with concentric electron-dense membranes and variable electron-lucent and electron-dense material, are noted. Patients uncommonly can progress to liver failure, with micronodular cirrhosis noted at autopsy.

A simplified nomenclature system[89,91,92] employs a non-italicized gene name followed by CDG; for example, CDG-Ia is PMM2-CDG (see later).[88] Two main groups of protein *N*-glycosylation disorders, I and II, have been delineated on the basis of characteristic isoelectric focusing patterns of serum transferrin, a marker protein for this group of disorders.[87] Group I disorders involve aberrant processing of lipid-linked oligosaccharides before transfer to protein targeted for glycosylation and include the 3 most common and best characterized types of CDG (types Ia, Ib, and Ic). Clinical features

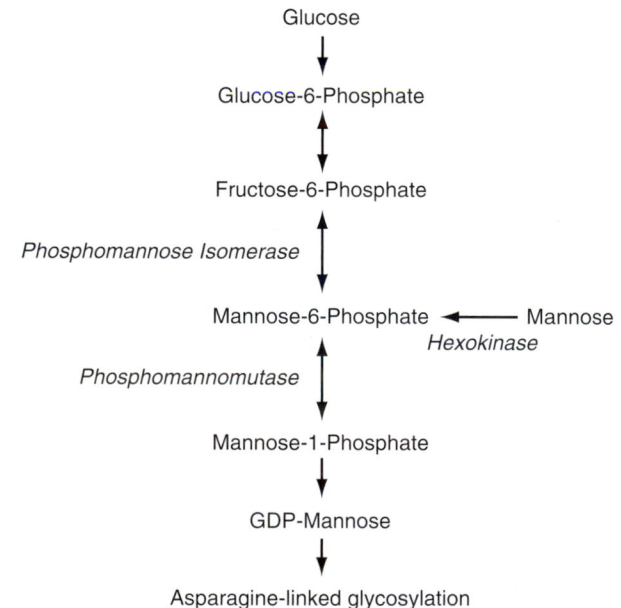

Glucose
↓
Glucose-6-Phosphate
↕
Fructose-6-Phosphate
Phosphomannose Isomerase ↕
Mannose-6-Phosphate ← Mannose
Hexokinase
Phosphomannomutase ↕
Mannose-1-Phosphate
↓
GDP-Mannose
↓
Asparagine-linked glycosylation

FIGURE 77-3. Pathway of mannose metabolism. Enzymes are shown in *italics*. GDP, guanosine diphosphate.

in common among these 3 disorders are protein-losing enteropathy, coagulopathy (both procoagulant and anticoagulant states), feeding difficulties, and hepatomegaly.[87,88,93,94] In patients with genetic diseases affecting protein *N*-glycosylation in the ER, liver symptoms in distinct subtypes of autosomal recessive disease have been reported to overlap those of polycystic liver disease (see Chapter 96).[95]

CDG type Ia (PMM2-CDG) is caused by defects in phosphomannomutase (PMM), an enzyme that converts mannose-6-phosphate to mannose-1-phosphate (Fig. 77-3). Multiple distinct mutations have been found in the *PMM2* gene; most patients are compound heterozygotes for mutations that likely preserve some residual PMM enzymatic activity, thereby suggesting that complete loss of PMM activity is incompatible with life. Targeted disruption of the *Pmm2* gene in the mouse leads to early embryonic lethality.[96,97] Patients with PMM2-CDG typically have severe neurologic abnormalities, dysmorphisms (inverted nipples, abnormal fat distribution, and esotropia), and congenital hepatic fibrosis and steatosis.[98]

Patients with CDG type Ib (MPI-CDG) have a defect in phosphomannose isomerase (PMI), which converts fructose-6-phosphate to mannose-6-phosphate (see Fig. 77-3). In addition to intractable diarrhea, protein-losing enteropathy, and congenital hepatic fibrosis, recurrent episodes of hyperinsulinemic hypoglycemia and cyclic vomiting have been reported.[99] Neurologic symptoms are usually absent, and dysmorphic features are less common than in CDG type Ia. Many patients with CDG type Ib have been treated effectively with dietary mannose, making CDG type Ib the only specifically treatable form of CDG, although liver fibrosis can develop despite improvement in clinical symptoms.[88,100,101]

Transient hepatomegaly, without congenital hepatic fibrosis, has been noted in patients with CDG type Ic (ALG6-CDG); otherwise, the clinical features of CDG type Ic are similar to but milder than those of CDG type Ia.[88,89,91,92] Patients with CDG type Ih (ALG8-CDG) may also manifest protein-losing enteropathy with chronic diarrhea, hepatic fibrosis, and variable degrees of hepatic dysfunction.[102] Children with untyped cases of CDG have been found to have isolated cryptogenic chronic liver disease, mild coagulopathy, and mild portal fibrosis and focal steatosis on liver biopsy specimens.[103]

Group II CDGs involve defects that affect the processing of *N*-linked glycoproteins.[88,89,91,92] Most types result from defects in enzymes involved in the trimming of protein-bound oligosaccharides and the subsequent addition of terminal sugars. Patients have marked dysmorphic features and severe developmental delay. Two infants with hepatosplenomegaly, progressive jaundice, severe epilepsy, recurrent infections, and heart failure have been shown to have mutations in a subunit of the conserved oligomeric Golgi complex that result in disruption of glycosylated protein intracellular trafficking.[104] Another CDG type II disorder with liver involvement has been reported in an infant with recurrent infections, chronic diarrhea, progressive cirrhosis, and normal hepatic excretory and synthetic function.[104]

Any patient with unexplained congenital hepatic fibrosis, protein-losing enteropathy, or a procoagulant tendency should be evaluated for CDG. Initial screening is with a serum transferrin level with isoelectric focusing, followed by confirmatory enzymatic analysis in fibroblasts, leukocytes, or liver tissue.[88,89,97] If the diagnosis of CDG type Ib is confirmed, oral mannose therapy should be initiated.

PORPHYRIAS

The porphyrias are a diverse group of metabolic diseases that result from deficiencies in enzymes involved in the heme synthetic pathway.

Pathophysiology

The metabolic pathways of heme synthesis are essentially the same in the 2 tissues in which heme synthesis primarily occurs, the liver (15% to 20%) and the bone marrow (75% to 80%), although synthetic control may be different in the 2 tissues. The rate-limiting step in hepatic heme synthesis begins with the conversion of glycine and succinyl coenzyme A (CoA) to 5-aminolevulinic acid (ALA) by the action of ALA synthase (Fig. 77-4). ALA synthase activity is decreased by the end-product of the pathway, heme, and is increased by substances that induce hepatic cytochrome P450 enzymes. Six additional

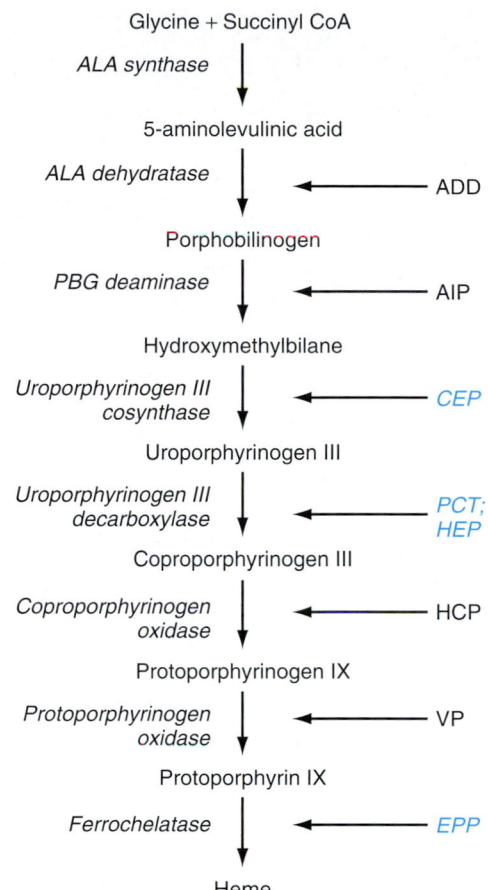

FIGURE 77-4. Pathway of heme synthesis. The location of the enzymatic deficiency in the various forms of porphyria is noted. On the left, the enzymes are shown in *italics*. On the right, abbreviations for the cutaneous porphyrias are shown in *italics and blue*, and those for the acute porphyrias are shown in roman typeface. ADD, 5-aminolevulinic acid (ALA) dehydratase deficiency; AIP, acute intermittent porphyria; CEP, congenital erythropoietic porphyria; EPP, erythropoietic protoporphyria; HCP, hereditary coproporphyria; HEP, hepatoerythropoietic porphyria; PBG, porphobilinogen; PCT, porphyria cutanea tarda; VP, variegate porphyria.

enzymatic steps convert ALA to protoporphyrin IX (see Fig. 77-4). In the final step of the pathway, protoporphyrin IX is coupled to ferrous iron by ferrochelatase to create heme. Enzyme deficiencies arising from any of the 8 steps of the heme synthetic pathway lead to clinically apparent porphyria.[105]

The porphyrias are commonly classified according to clinical features into 2 main groups, acute porphyrias, which are characterized by dramatic and potentially life-threatening neurologic symptoms, and cutaneous porphyrias, which typically cause few or no neurologic symptoms but instead give rise to a variety of severe skin lesions (Table 77-1). In 5 of the porphyrias, the liver is the major site of expression; in 2 others, both the liver and bone marrow are involved; and in 1, only the bone marrow is involved.

Acute Porphyrias

The symptoms and signs of the acute neurovisceral attacks that occur in the 4 acute porphyrias vary considerably. Abdominal pain is present in more than 90% of patients, followed in frequency by tachycardia and dark urine in about

TABLE 77-1 The Porphyrias

Acute Porphyrias	Enzymatic Defect	Mode of Inheritance	Clinical Findings	Site of Expression	Substances Detected in Urine and Stool
Acute intermittent porphyria	PBG deaminase	Autosomal dominant	Neurologic	Liver	Urine: ALA < PBG
ALA dehydratase deficiency	ALA dehydratase	Autosomal recessive	Neurologic	Liver	Urine: ALA
Hereditary coproporphyria	Coproporphyrinogen oxidase	Autosomal dominant	Neurologic, cutaneous	Liver	Urine: ALA > PBG, coproporphyrin Stool: coproporphyrin
Variegate porphyria	Protoporphyrinogen oxidase	Autosomal dominant	Neurologic, cutaneous	Liver	Urine: ALA > PBG, coproporphyrin Stool: coproporphyrin, protoporphyrinogen
Cutaneous Porphyrias					
Congenital erythropoietic porphyria	Uroporphyrinogen III cosynthase	Autosomal recessive	Cutaneous	Bone marrow	Urine and stool: coproporphyrin I
Erythropoietic protoporphyria	Ferrochelatase	Various	Cutaneous, rarely neurologic	Liver, bone marrow	Urine: none Stool: protoporphyrin, coproporphyrin
Hepatoerythropoietic porphyria	Uroporphyrinogen III decarboxylase	Autosomal recessive	Cutaneous	Liver, bone marrow	Urine: uroporphyrin, 7-carboxylate porphyrin Stool: isocoproporphyrin
Porphyria cutanea tarda	Uroporphyrinogen III decarboxylase	Autosomal dominant or acquired	Cutaneous	Liver	Urine: uroporphyrin, 7-carboxylate porphyrin Stool: isocoproporphyrin

ALA, 5-aminolevulinic acid; PBG, porphobilinogen.

80% of patients. Neuropsychiatric features include hysteria, depression, psychosis, confusion, hallucinations, seizures, and coma, although little evidence suggests that chronic psychiatric illness occurs. Other features are constipation, extremity pain, paresthesias, nausea, vomiting, urinary retention, hypertension, peripheral sensory deficits (often in a "bathing trunk" distribution), and weakness leading to ascending paralysis or quadriplegia. These neurologic attacks appear to be related to the overproduction of ALA and porphobilinogen (PBG), which leads to higher serum and tissue levels of these neurotoxic products.

Acute episodes are about 5 times as common in women as in men and may be precipitated by many factors, most commonly drugs, alcohol ingestion, and smoking.[106,107] Steroids, sex hormones, and medications that stimulate hepatic cytochrome P450 enzymes, perhaps by increasing the requirements for heme production, are often identified as precipitants.[108] Other inciting factors are fasting, infections, and pregnancy; some women report greater problems during the luteal phase of their menstrual cycles. The disease is clinically latent in 65% to 80% of patients.

ALA dehydratase deficiency is a rare syndrome with autosomal recessive transmission in which the enzyme activity is less than 3%. The enzyme activity is 50% of normal in carriers, who are asymptomatic. Affected patients have severe, recurrent neurologic attacks that may be life threatening. They excrete large amounts of ALA in their urine. Liver transplantation was reported to result in complete resolution of symptoms in one patient with ALA dehydratase deficiency.[109]

The 3 remaining acute porphyrias—acute intermittent porphyria (AIP), hereditary coproporphyria (HCP), and variegate porphyria (VP)—result from partial deficiency of the enzymes PBG deaminase, coproporphyrinogen oxidase, and protopor-

phyrinogen oxidase, respectively. All 3 disorders are inherited in an autosomal dominant fashion with variable expression. AIP is the most common of the 3 conditions, occurring in 5 to 10 per 100,000 people, and manifests primarily as derangements in the autonomic nervous system or as a psychiatric disorder.[106,110] VP is more common in South Africa than elsewhere. Although HCP and VP give rise to neurologic symptoms similar to those of AIP, cutaneous lesions also occur in HCP and predominate in VP.[111]

Cutaneous Porphyrias

The cutaneous porphyrias differ from the acute porphyrias in that affected patients exhibit few or no neurologic symptoms. In these illnesses, excess porphyrins or porphyrinogens are deposited in the upper dermal capillary walls, where these photoreactive compounds cause tissue damage that manifests as cutaneous vesicles and bullae in areas exposed to light or excessive mechanical manipulation. Scarring, infection, pigment changes, and hypertrichosis can follow and even lead to severe mutilation.

Porphyria cutanea tarda (PCT), the most common of the porphyrias, typically involves an 80% reduction in activity of the enzyme uroporphyrinogen decarboxylase. Patients usually present after 20 years of age. Two types of PCT are recognized. Type I PCT affects 80% of patients and is a sporadic (acquired) form in which the enzyme deficiency is restricted to the liver. Type II, which affects the other 20% of patients, is familial and inherited in an autosomal dominant fashion with incomplete penetrance; the enzyme deficiency occurs in all tissues.[105] Symptoms develop in fewer than 10% of patients with type II PCT. Type I PCT is associated strongly with high alcohol intake, estrogen therapy, and systemic illnesses, including SLE, diabetes mellitus, chronic kidney disease, and AIDS. For unclear reasons, concomitant HCV infection is strongly associated with expression of PCT (see Chapter 80).[112,113] The frequency of mutations of the *HFE* gene, which causes hereditary hemochromatosis, is increased in patients with types I and II PCT, and these mutations are thus susceptibility factors for clinical expression of the PCT phenotype (see Chapter 75).[112,114] Iron overload enhances oxidation of uroporphyrinogen to uroporphomethene, an inhibitor of uroporphyrinogen-decarboxylase activity, thereby explaining the association of increased oxidative stress and the unmasking of the PCT phenotype.[105,115] This association is consistent with pathologic findings in liver biopsy specimens from patients with PCT, of whom 80% have siderosis, 15% have cirrhosis, and most have evidence of iron overload. A patient in whom hepatocellular carcinoma developed has been reported to have unsuspected underlying PCT and hereditary hemochromatosis with bridging fibrosis.[116] Patients usually do not show signs of overt clinical liver disease, apart from elevated serum aminotransferase levels.

Hepatoerythropoietic porphyria (HEP) is a rare form of porphyria with a pathogenesis similar to that of PCT. HEP results from homozygous uroporphyrinogen decarboxylase deficiency, yielding less than 10% of normal enzyme activity. The cutaneous lesions, which resemble those of PCT, are typically severe and mutilating. The disease usually manifests in the first year of life. As the patient ages, the dermatologic manifestations may subside, but liver disease, characterized by a nonspecific hepatitis, worsens. Mutation analysis of the uroporphyrinogen decarboxylase gene has revealed no clear genotype-phenotype correlations.[117]

Congenital erythropoietic porphyria (CEP) is a rare form of porphyria with autosomal recessive transmission that is caused by deficiency of uroporphyrinogen III cosynthase, which mainly affects erythropoietic tissue. Patients typically present in the first year of life with blisters and disfiguring skin lesions in exposed areas and may present with pink urine and photosensitivity. As patients age, erythrodontia, a pathognomonic red or brownish discoloration of the teeth, is commonly seen. CEP can be distinguished clinically from HEP by the presence in some cases of a Coombs-negative hemolytic anemia, which can be quite severe. Splenomegaly is common. Gain-of-function mutations in the ALA synthase 2 *(ALAS2)* gene in patients with CEP suggest that *ALAS2* is a modifier gene for CEP disease by increasing the flux of ALA production.[118]

Erythropoietic protoporphyria (EPP) is caused by partial deficiency of the enzyme ferrochelatase (FECH), the final step in the heme synthetic pathway. EPP is the second most common type of porphyria and has been thought to be inherited in an autosomal dominant manner with variable penetrance. Patients with EPP and asymptomatic carriers exhibit FECH enzyme activities of 30% to 40% and 50%, respectively, even though both groups inherit a defective FECH allele. Autosomal recessive forms of EPP, in which two copies of a defective FECH allele are inherited, are recognized.[119,120]

Although the bone marrow is the predominant source of excess protoporphyrin, with a variable contribution from the liver and other tissues, the skin is the primary site of deposition of this phototoxic compound in patients with EPP. Therefore, the principal clinical manifestation is exquisite photosensitivity, which may present during infancy and can lead to a wide spectrum of symptoms (e.g., itching, burning, pain) and to scars and lichenification of the skin. Vesicles are rare. Patients with EPP may have a mild hypochromic, microcytic anemia.

Clinical liver disease, which develops in 5% to 10% of patients with EPP, results from progressive hepatic accumulation of protoporphyrin.[121] Liver disease typically occurs after age 30 but has been described in children. The liver appears black and nodular, with hepatocellular necrosis, portal inflammation, cholestasis, and extensive deposits of dark brown pigment in hepatocytes, Kupffer cells, and biliary structures; birefringence of pigment deposits is seen on polarization microscopy.[122] Of 57 patients with EPP followed for more than 20 years in one study,[123] 50% had normal serum aminotransferase levels and liver histologic findings. Of the remaining patients, cirrhosis occurred in 7 and liver failure developed in 2. Liver disease is not believed to be secondary to alcohol consumption, viral infections, or external toxins, although these insults can worsen liver function.[124] Genetic heterogeneity in the FECH gene has been noted in multiple studies.[105]

Hepatic Involvement

Hepatic involvement in porphyria is variable; in general, patients with acute porphyria may have elevated serum aminotransferase and bile acid levels, with further increases during acute episodes. Liver biopsy specimens may show steatosis and iron deposition. Although these changes are minor, patients with acute porphyria are at increased risk for the development of hepatocellular carcinoma.[125] PCT and HEP are more commonly associated with hepatic complications, including liver enlargement with fatty infiltration, inflammation, and granulomatous changes. Siderosis and fibrosis may lead to cirrhosis and liver failure. The risk of hepatocellular carcinoma is increased only slightly in patients with these disorders.[116] The patterns of liver injury in CEP are similar to those in PCT and HEP.[126]

Diagnosis

The approach to the diagnosis of the porphyrias is summarized in Table 77-1. Clinical features alone are usually not specific enough to confirm a diagnosis or distinguish among the various forms of porphyrias. The diagnosis of porphyria should be considered in patients with recurrent bouts of severe abdominal pain, dark urine, constipation, and neuropsychiatric disturbances or in patients with typical dermatologic findings. To differentiate among the different porphyrias, urine and stool samples should be obtained for porphyrin studies and a urine specimen collected for quantitative ALA and PBG determinations.

In AIP, excretion of PGB and ALA (PGB more than ALA) in dark urine is common during porphyric attacks, but the levels may be normal during asymptomatic periods and in prepubertal patients. Patients with HCP and VP excrete high levels of ALA and PBG in the urine; in contrast to those with AIP, these patients excrete more ALA than PGB. A "spot" urine test to detect urinary PGB is recommended to diagnose the acute porphyrias, except for the rare patient with ALA dehydratase deficiency.[127] Fecal coproporphyrins are increased in both HCP and VP, whereas only in VP is the amount of fecal protoporphyrin also increased.

Mutation analysis is available for each porphyria, and direct assays of heme synthesizing enzymes are being developed.[105,128] A large number of gene mutations have been identified for several acute porphyrias, including AIP, VP, and HCP. Given the high degree of genetic heterogeneity, the lack of clear genotype-phenotype correlations, and the failure to find mutations in 5% to 10% of families with available techniques, however, genetic testing is not recommended as a general screening tool.[105] If a mutation that causes porphyria has been identified in a particular subject, however, screening of asymptomatic family members has a sensitivity and specificity of nearly 100% for that family and may be helpful, together with appropriate genetic counseling. Enzyme activity measurement is less helpful than genetic testing because the variable tissue expression of many of the heme synthesizing enzymes.

Treatment

The overall survival of patients with acute porphyria is good. Consensus guidelines for the treatment of acute porphyria attacks are available.[127] Treatment is based on avoidance of drugs and other precipitating factors. Generous fluid and glucose administration is recommended during acute attacks and can elicit the "glucose effect" that diminishes ALA synthase activity. IV administration of hematin, a congener of heme, has been shown to decrease the drive for heme synthesis and its excessive by-products and, in serious attacks, is more effective than glucose administration alone.[129] Hematin can also have a dramatic effect on neurologic symptoms, especially if given early in an attack, with clinical improvement often occurring within 1 to 2 days.[127] Women in whom symptoms are affected by the phases of their menstrual cycle can show improvement while taking oral contraceptives. Dietary supplementation with vitamin C and E may minimize the oxidative damage in plasma and neutrophils in women with VP.[130] Liver transplantation has been attempted for several of the porphyrias, with mixed results, perhaps in part because of reaccumulation of toxic metabolites in the graft due to continued excess bone marrow production.[105,127,131-133] Because of the increased frequency of hepatocellular carcinoma, patients with AIP should undergo standard surveillance for this tumor (see Chapter 96).[127]

Because of the wavelengths of light absorbed by the porphyrins, patients affected by porphyria are at risk from exposure to sunlight as well as household and fluorescent lights. Patients must use special sunscreen lotions that block rays in the 400- to 410-nm range. Skin trauma should be minimized as much as possible; early treatment of skin infections can decrease scarring. Special screens may be especially useful for protection against indoor lighting. Some patients have incurred severe or lethal internal burns during surgery, including liver transplantation; therefore, appropriate precautions must be taken.[134]

Treatment of PCT initially consists of removal of any offending agent. Historically, treatment has included phlebotomy to decrease iron overload and hepatic siderosis. This approach may provide relief of cutaneous symptoms in 4 to 6 months. Chloroquine complexes with uroporphyrin and facilitates its excretion, but the drug is potentially hepatotoxic.[105,134] In a head-to-head comparison of phlebotomy and chloroquine therapy for PCT, no significant differences were observed between treatments except for better compliance with the use of chloroquine.[135] The efficacy of chloroquine has been variable in patients with PCT who are homozygous for mutations in the *HFE* gene; for these patients, phlebotomy should be first-line therapy.[136,137] A pilot study of the iron chelator deferasirox in patients with cutaneous findings from PCT showed improvement of skin lesions, urinary porphyrin, and serum ferritin levels.[138] Treatment strategies for HEP are similar to, but have not been as successful as, those for PCT.

Blood transfusions and administration of hematin, charcoal, and cholestyramine all have led to clinical improvement in patients with EPP, but long-term resolution has not been demonstrated.[105] Oral β-carotene may improve sunlight intolerance.[105] One report of a 63-year-old man with severe cholestatic liver disease caused by EPP showed complete biochemical and histologic resolution of cholestasis with the use of blood transfusions, hematin, cholestyramine, and ursodeoxycholic acid. Subsequently, the patient underwent bone marrow

transplantation, with apparently complete resolution of EPP.[139] Liver transplantation has been accomplished in patients with EPP and ESLD, with mixed results; the erythropoietic defect persists.[140-142] A retrospective review of all 20 patients with EPP who have undergone liver transplantation in the United States revealed unique perioperative complications, including light-induced tissue damage in 4 patients and neuropathy in 6, as well as recurrent EPP-associated liver disease in 65% of patients who survived more than 2 months. Overall patient and graft survival rates were statistically similar to those for all other patients transplanted in the United States during the same period.[140] A European study of 34 liver transplant recipients for EPP-associated liver disease had similar results.[142] Therefore, liver transplantation must be considered symptomatic therapy, except in patients with fulminant hepatic failure, given the high risk of recurrent disease in the graft and the added risk of intraoperative photodynamic injury to internal organs.[140,143] Bone marrow transplantation after liver transplantation has been performed successfully in a child with EPP-induced ESLD.[144]

Splenectomy, which lengthens the lifespan of circulating red blood cells and decreases the erythropoietic drive, has been effective in many patients with CEP. Frequent blood transfusions or hematin infusions inhibit the stimulus for heme production, thereby diminishing or eliminating the cutaneous manifestations of the disease.[145] Bone marrow transplantation has proved curative in severely affected patients.[145,146]

TYROSINEMIA

Four known human diseases are caused by enzymatic deficiencies in the catabolic pathway for the amino acid tyrosine: alkaptonuria and hereditary tyrosinemia (HT) types I, II, and III. Although all of the enzymes involved in this pathway are found in the liver, only HT-1 leads to progressive liver dysfunction.[147] Formerly known as hepatorenal tyrosinemia, HT-1 also affects other organ systems, in particular the kidneys and peripheral nerves. A disease with autosomal recessive transmission, HT-1 has a worldwide incidence of about 1 in 100,000. The incidence is much greater in northern Europe (1 per 8000) and in the Saguenay-Lac-St. Jean region of Quebec, Canada (1 per 1846), where a founder effect has been documented.[148] Advances in our understanding of the pathophysiology of the disease process and new treatment options, such as an inhibitor of an early step in the degradation pathway, have improved the clinical course for affected persons dramatically.

Pathophysiology

The pathway for tyrosine metabolism is shown in Figure 77-5. The enzymatic defect in patients with tyrosinemia has been identified in fumarylacetoacetate hydrolase (FAH), the final step in the tyrosine degradation process. More than 30 mutations in FAH have been found in patients with HT-1, but no clear correlation between FAH genotype and HT-1 phenotype has been found.[147] FAH deficiency leads to accumulation of the upstream metabolites fumarylacetoacetate (FAA) and maleylacetoacetate (MAA), which are then converted to the toxic intermediates succinylacetoacetate (SAA) and succinylacetone (SA). FAA has been shown to deplete blood and liver of glutathione, the consequence of which may be augmentation of the mutagenic potential of FAA. SA inhibits renal glucose and amino acid transport and the degradation of ALA to PBG, probably via direct modification of amino acids in enzyme active sites. SA also inhibits DNA ligase activity in fibroblasts isolated from patients with HT-1.[149] Over time, the

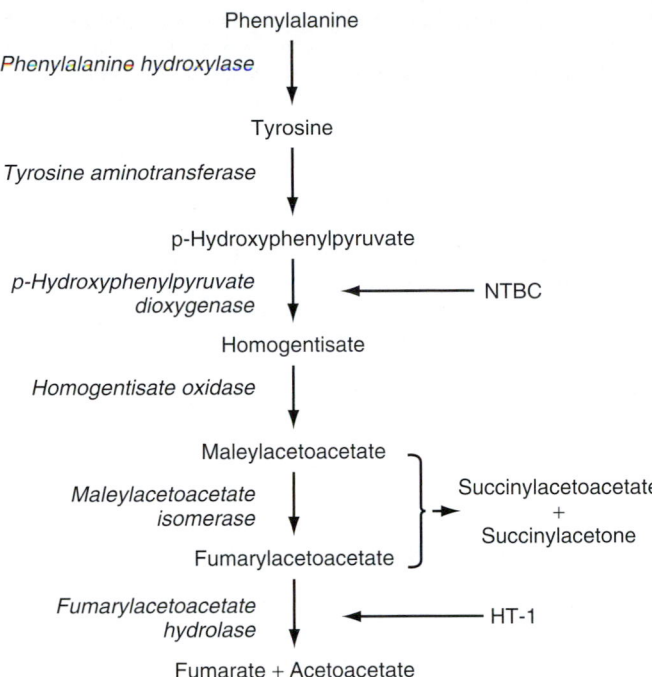

Phenylalanine

Phenylalanine hydroxylase

Tyrosine

Tyrosine aminotransferase

p-Hydroxyphenylpyruvate

p-Hydroxyphenylpyruvate dioxygenase ← NTBC

Homogentisate

Homogentisate oxidase

Maleylacetoacetate

Maleylacetoacetate isomerase → Succinylacetoacetate + Succinylacetone

Fumarylacetoacetate

Fumarylacetoacetate hydrolase ← HT-1

Fumarate + Acetoacetate

FIGURE 77-5. Pathway of tyrosine metabolism. The location of the enzymatic defect in hereditary tyrosinemia type 1 (HT-1) and the site of action of 2-(2-nitro-4-trifluoro-methylbenzoyl)-1,3-cyclohexanedione (NTBC) are shown. Enzymes are shown in *italics*.

combined effects of high levels of FAA and SA on the integrity of DNA and cellular repair mechanisms may account for increased chromosomal breakage in fibroblasts isolated from patients with HT-1, as well as an increased risk of hepatocellular carcinoma.[150]

Clinical and Pathologic Features

Patients with HT-1 present either acutely with liver failure or with chronic liver disease, with or without hepatocellular carcinoma. In the acute form of HT-1, patients manifest liver disease in the first 6 months of life; symptoms include those associated with severe hepatic synthetic dysfunction, such as hypoglycemia, ascites, jaundice, and bleeding diathesis, as well as anorexia, vomiting, and irritability. Laboratory studies show elevations of serum aminotransferase, GGTP, and bilirubin levels and decreased levels of coagulation factors. Serum tyrosine, methionine, and AFP levels are elevated. Analysis of the urine may reveal phosphaturia, glucosuria, hyperaminoaciduria, renal acidosis, and increased excretion of SA, SAA, ALA, and phenolic acids. The acute form of HT-1 is potentially fatal within the first 2 years of life. In a multicenter study, van Spronsen and associates showed that 77% of patients with tyrosinemia presented before the age of 6 months.[151] The 1- and 2-year survival rates were 38% and 29%, respectively, if patients presented between birth and 2 months of age, and 74% and 74%, respectively, if they presented between 2 and 6 months. Survival for both time intervals rose to 96% if the first symptoms appeared after age 6 months. The cause of death was usually recurrent bleeding and liver failure; however, hepatocellular carcinoma and neurologic crisis accounted for some deaths.

Patients with the chronic form of HT-1 classically have symptoms that are similar to, but milder than, those of the acute presentation; serum aminotransferase levels as well as plasma tyrosine and methionine levels may be within the normal range. These patients usually present after 1 year of age with hepatomegaly, rickets, nephromegaly, hypertension, and growth retardation. They also are likely to have neurologic problems and to develop hepatocellular carcinoma.

The pathologic changes in the liver differ in the acute and chronic forms of the disease. In the acute form, the liver may appear enlarged with a pale nodular pattern or may be shrunken, firm, and brown. Micronodular cirrhosis, fibrotic septa, bile duct proliferation and plugging, steatosis, pseudoacinar and nodular formations, and giant cell transformation may be found on histologic examination. Varying amounts of FAH enzyme activity have been found in liver tissue from patients with HT-1 as a result of spontaneous reversion of FAH gene mutations. Patients with the chronic form of the disease have a higher level of reversion and a lower frequency of liver dysplasia.[147,151] In an analysis of mutations in the FAH gene in members of 13 unrelated families with HT-1, no mutation type predominated, and no correlation between genotype and phenotype was observed.[152] In the chronic form of tyrosinemia, the liver appears enlarged, coarse, and nodular. In histologic specimens, micronodular and macronodular cirrhosis may be present, as may steatosis, fibrotic septa, and a mild lymphoplasmacytic infiltrate. Cholestasis is less pronounced than in the acute form of HT-1. Large- or small-cell dysplasia may be present, reflecting premalignant changes. Because of the nodular changes, identification of progression to hepatocellular carcinoma can be difficult. The serum AFP value is elevated before hepatocellular carcinoma develops, and measurement of AFP is not helpful in the diagnosis. Imaging is required to screen for hepatocellular carcinoma.

Renal involvement is nearly universal in patients with tyrosinemia. Findings include a decreased glomerular filtration rate, proximal renal tubular dysfunction, nephromegaly, phosphaturia (which is responsible for the development of rickets), glucosuria, and aminoaciduria. The toxic metabolites SA and SAA are thought to have a direct effect on kidney function. Some patients progress to renal failure and require renal transplantation.[153] One third of patients develop cardiomyopathy, most commonly interventricular septal hypertrophy, which is reversible with either medical or surgical management of the disease.[154]

The neurologic manifestations may be the most concerning feature in older patients with tyrosinemia; affected patients may experience porphyria-like symptoms.[155] In a study of 20 children with HT-1 and 104 neurologic crises, the most common symptoms were pain (96%), hypertonia (76%), vomiting and ileus (69%), weakness (29%), and diarrhea (12%).[155] A neurologic crisis has been considered to be a frequent cause of death, but the onset of a neurologic crisis may not be associated with worsening liver disease.

Diagnosis

The diagnosis of tyrosinemia should be suspected in any child with neonatal liver disease or a bleeding diathesis or in any child older than 1 year with undiagnosed liver disease, rickets, or a hepatic mass. The diagnosis is suggested by increased serum tyrosine, methionine, phenylalanine, and AFP levels. Elevated serum and urine SA and urine ALA levels are regarded as pathognomonic for tyrosinemia. The diagnosis can be confirmed with an assay for FAH in lymphocytes, erythrocytes, skin fibroblasts, or liver tissue.[147,156] Molecular genetic approaches and targeted mutation analysis are becoming more widely available.

Prenatal diagnosis can be performed by determining SA levels in amniotic fluid or by measuring FAH activity in chorionic villus biopsy specimens. If the specific gene mutation in a family is known, early genetic diagnosis can be made from chorionic villus biopsy specimens as well.[157,158] Improved newborn screening methodologies have been developed that measure SA in addition to amino acid levels in dried blood specimens. Newborn screening programs for hepatorenal tyrosinemia have used an isotope dilution liquid chromatography tandem mass spectrometry assay of pooled dried blood samples.[159]

Treatment

In the past, the treatment of tyrosinemia was based on dietary restriction of tyrosine and phenylalanine intake, which was shown to reverse renal damage and improve metabolic bone disease despite progression of liver disease. An adequate intake of these amino acids, however, is needed to ensure normal growth and development. Liver transplantation has become a mainstay of therapy for patients with tyrosinemia. The transplant corrects the phenotype and normalizes FAH activity and liver function. Additionally, the biochemical profiles normalize and kidney disease abates, with improvement in glomerular filtration rate, tubular acidosis, and hypercalcemia in most patients.[160,161] Abnormal renal size and architecture persist after liver transplantation, and many patients continue to excrete SA despite normal serum values.[160,161]

In 1992, Lindstedt and associates published data on the treatment of tyrosinemia with the herbicide 2-(2-nitro-4-trifluoro-methylbenzoyl)-1,3-cyclohexanedione (NTBC).[162] Later, Holme and Lindstedt published the results of a large, long-term study of 220 patients with HT-1 who were treated with this agent for up to 7 years.[163] NTBC, known as nitisinone (Orfadin), is a potent inhibitor of 4-hydroxyphenylpyruvate dioxygenase, one of the initial steps in tyrosine metabolism (see Fig. 77-5). Blocking the degradation of tyrosine to its downstream toxic metabolites (FAA, SA, and SAA) was postulated to lead to improved hepatic function. Treated patients exhibited improved liver synthetic function, as reflected by a shortening of the prothrombin time, as well as decreased serum aminotransferase levels and a reduction in liver parenchymal heterogeneity and nodules on imaging. In addition, serum AFP and ALA levels decreased and renal tubular dysfunction reversed.[164] Therefore, elevated AFP levels in a patient receiving NTBC therapy should raise concern about the patient's nonadherence to therapy or the development of hepatocellular cancer.[165]

Long-term results have demonstrated continued improvement in all parameters noted in the earlier report, as well as a lower risk for the development of hepatocellular carcinoma in patients who started therapy and were free of the tumor before age 2.[163] No patient withdrew from the study because of adverse side effects of the drug. Transient thrombocytopenia and neutropenia as well as ocular symptoms suggestive of corneal irritation have been noted rarely. Cognitive impairment resulting in learning problems may be a complication of long-term use of NTBC in this patient population, possibly from the effects of chronic hypertyrosinemia.[166]

In a study from Quebec, only 4 of 35 patients treated with NTBC underwent liver transplantation.[167] One patient underwent a transplant because of concern about the heterogeneous texture of the liver (suggestive of cirrhosis) shown by US coupled with a persistent moderate elevation in the serum AFP level. At resection, this child was found to have a small nodule with hepatocellular dysplasia. The 31 remaining patients were monitored while receiving NTBC therapy for up to 3 years, and none experienced neurologic crises or deterioration of liver disease.

In the United States, the need for liver transplantation for children with HT-1 has decreased and age at transplantation has increased since 2000, reflecting early diagnosis and treatment with NTBC.[168] Use of NTBC requires careful clinical and biochemical monitoring. A rapid liquid chromatography coupled with negative electrospray ionization tandem mass spectrometry method has been developed and validated for the quantification of NTBC in heparinized human plasma.[169] This method is suitable for following patients treated with NTBC; therapeutic concentrations range from 20 to 120 μM.[169]

Therapy with NTBC has significantly improved the clinical course of patients with HT-1 who are treated at an early age.[170-173] For those in whom therapy is initiated at a later age, NTBC offers a palliative benefit, although the risk of hepatocellular carcinoma is still high. Greater experience with NTBC is required to assess the relative costs, long-term outcome, and possible adverse effects of long-term therapy.[166] Early diagnosis, achieved by inclusion of HT-1 in neonatal screening programs, may allow prompt initiation of effective therapy with NTBC and avoidance of liver transplantation.

UREA CYCLE DEFECTS

The urea cycle consists of 5 enzymes that, through several steps, process ammonia derived from amino acid metabolism to urea. Genetic defects in each of these enzymes have been reported, and their overall incidence has been estimated to be 1 in 20,000 to 1 in 30,000.[174] Although the syndromes related to the urea cycle defects (UCDs) are not associated with serious liver injury, the basic genetic defect is located within the liver, and the manifestations can mimic those of other metabolic liver diseases.

Pathophysiology

The steps of the urea cycle are illustrated in Figure 77-6. Carbamyl phosphate synthetase (CPS) I forms carbamyl phosphate from ammonium and bicarbonate. This step requires the cofactor N-acetyl glutamate, which is synthesized from N-acetyl CoA and glutamic acid by N-acetyl glutamate synthetase. Ornithine transcarbamylase (OTC) combines carbamyl phosphate with ornithine to form citrulline. A second nitrogen enters the cycle as aspartate, which combines with citrulline by the action of argininosuccinate synthetase (AS) to form argininosuccinate. Argininosuccinate is converted to arginine and fumarate by argininosuccinase, or argininosuccinate lyase (AL). Arginase then catalyzes the breakdown of arginine to urea and ornithine in the final step of the pathway. Several amino acid transporters, such as citrin, an aspartate/glutamate carrier protein that supplies aspartate to the urea cycle, are involved in shuttling metabolites into the urea cycle.[175]

CPS II, through the pyrimidine synthetic pathway, leads to the formation of orotic acid. Excess carbamyl phosphate can be used by this pathway if a block occurs distal to OTC in the metabolic pathway. Excess nitrogen in the form of amino acids can be shunted to alternative pathways of waste-nitrogen excretion by the medicinal use of sodium benzoate and sodium phenylacetate, leading to the generation of hippurate and phenylacetylglutamine, respectively.

Enzymatic defects have been identified in all 5 steps of the urea cycle. Deficiency of 4 of the enzymes is transmitted through autosomal recessive inheritance, whereas OTC deficiency is transmitted as an X-linked trait. More than 340 different mutations in the OTC gene give rise to OTC deficiency, the most common UCD.[176] Numerous defects in the other enzymes or amino acid transporters of the cycle (e.g., N-acetylglutamate synthetase or citrin) have been characterized as well.[177-179] Moreover, numerous mRNA

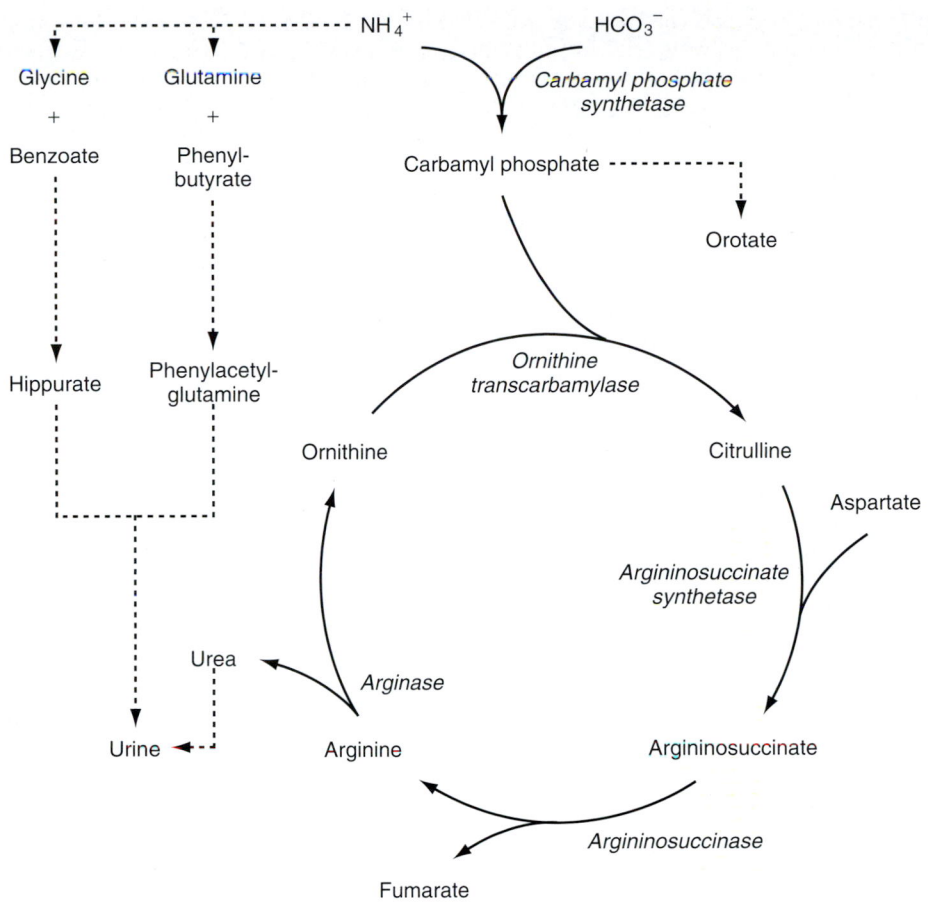

FIGURE 77-6. The urea cycle. Alternative pathways that are used therapeutically for waste nitrogen disposal are also illustrated (dotted lines). Enzymes are shown in *italics*.

instability mutations have been found in patients with CPS I deficiency.[180]

A UCD has two main biochemical consequences: Arginine becomes an essential amino acid (except in arginase deficiency [see later]), and nitrogen accumulates in a variety of molecules, some of which can have deleterious toxic effects.

Clinical Features

The spectra of clinical presentations in patients with any of the UCDs are virtually identical; in the neonatal period, these disorders usually manifest as acute life-threatening events. Contrary to the commonly held belief that UCDs are primarily disorders of the newborn period, two reports of the clinical presentation and outcome data of 260 and 183 patients with UCDs revealed that two thirds of patients present later than 30 days of age, even when female OTC carriers are excluded from the analysis.[181,182] Late-onset adult presentations, in some cases associated with an illness or dietary changes, have also been described.[183,184] Affected infants appear normal for the first 24 to 72 hours until they are exposed to their first feeding, which provides the initial protein load that fosters ammonia production. Symptoms include irritability, poor feeding, vomiting, lethargy, hypotonia, seizures, coma, and hyperventilation, all secondary to hyperammonemia.[181,185] Initially, neonates are often mistakenly thought to have sepsis, despite the absence of perinatal risk factors, and diagnostic laboratory testing is delayed.[186] Plasma ammonia levels should be obtained whenever an evaluation for sepsis is initiated in a neonate; levels may exceed 2000 μmol/L (3400 mg/dL), with normal levels of 50 μmol/L (85 mg/dL) or less.

For all age groups, overall survival decreases as the peak plasma ammonia level rises for a given episode of hyperammonemia, with survival rates of 98% and 47% for peak ammonia levels of less than 200 μmol/L and greater than 1000 μmol/L, respectively.[187] Newborns have a survival rate of 73% after their presenting episode of hyperammonemia, whereas patients older than 30 days of age have a survival rate of 98%. Male patients with OTC deficiency have a survival rate of 91% following an episode of hyperammonemia, a rate significantly less than those (93% to 98%) of all other forms of UCDs. Blood gas analysis shows respiratory alkalosis secondary to the hyperventilation caused by the effects of ammonia on the central nervous system. Blood urea nitrogen levels are typically low but can be elevated during times of dehydration or hypoperfusion. Serum levels of liver enzymes are usually normal or minimally elevated. Severe hepatomegaly can occur in early-onset forms of AL deficiency.[174]

OTC deficiency is the most common UCD (55%), followed by argininosuccinic aciduria (AL deficiency, 16%) and citrullinemia (AS deficiency, 14%).[182] Male patients with OTC deficiency have been diagnosed as late as 40 years of age with varied phenotypic presentations. As many as 10% of female carriers of OTC deficiency can have symptoms, which may be severe and fatal, although most female carriers have no symptoms or report only nausea after high-protein meals.[188] Late-onset CPS deficiency has also been described,[189] and the adult form of AS deficiency is relatively common in Japan.[178]

TABLE 77-2 Laboratory Values in Urea Cycle Defects

Enzyme Deficiency	Ammonia (Plasma)	Citrulline (Serum)	Argininosuccinate (Urine or Serum)	Orotic Acid (Urine)	Arginine/Ornithine (Serum)
Carbamyl phosphate synthetase	↑-↑↑↑	↓	↓	↓	↓
Ornithine transcarbamylase	↑-↑↑↑	↓	↓	↑↑	↓
Argininosuccinate synthetase	↑-↑↑↑	↑↑↑	↓	Normal-↑	↓
Argininosuccinase	↑-↑↑↑	↑↑↑	↑↑↑	Normal-↑	↓
Arginase	↑	↑↑	↑↑	Normal-↑	↑↑

Symptoms and signs of late-onset UCDs, especially OTC and CPS deficiencies, include episodic irritability, lethargy, or vomiting; self-induced avoidance of protein such as milk, eggs, and meats; and short stature or growth delays. Neurologic symptoms, which can also be episodic, include ataxia, developmental delays, behavioral abnormalities, combativeness, biting, confusion, hallucinations, headaches, dizziness, visual impairment, diplopia, anorexia, and seizures.[181] Acute hyperammonemic episodes can resemble Reye's syndrome (see Chapter 88). Such episodes can be precipitated by high-protein meals, viral or bacterial infections, medications, trauma, or surgery. Infants may present after being weaned from breast milk to infant formulas, which have a higher protein content. Patients with OTC and CPS deficiencies have been reported to present in the postpartum period with acute decompensation and death.[190,191]

Citrin deficiency is caused by mutations in the *SLC25A13* gene and is associated with both adult-onset type 2 citrullinemia and neonatal intrahepatic cholestasis resulting from citrin deficiency (NICCD), a syndrome that primarily affects newborns in East Asia.[178,192-195] A case of citrin deficiency in an infant of European descent who presented with poor weight gain and a bleeding diathesis, and without cholestasis, has been reported, expanding the clinical spectrum of presentations of citrin deficiency.[196] NICCD is associated with hyperaminoacidemia (elevated citrulline, methionine, and tyrosine levels) and cholestasis.[178,197] Hypergalactosemia and elevated acylcarnitine levels also may be observed.[198] Hepatic steatosis may be seen in the liver histologically.[199] In most patients with NICCD, all biochemical abnormalities resolve spontaneously or with minimal dietary restrictions (e.g., the use of lactose-free formulas); however, several affected infants have required liver transplantation before 1 year of age.[192] Therefore, jaundiced infants with multiple abnormal newborn metabolic screen results (e.g., elevation of blood phenylalanine, methionine, or galactose levels) must be observed closely because of the risk for development of ESLD caused by NICCD; a chubby face outside the realm of normal may be a diagnostic clue.[200] The diagnosis can be made by sequence analysis of the *SLC25A13* gene or by failure to detect citrin protein in peripheral lymphocytes.[193-195,201]

Diagnosis

A high index of suspicion is required for prompt diagnosis of UCDs. Symptoms can mimic those of other acute neonatal problems, such as infections, seizures, and pulmonary or cardiac disease. Later presentations can mimic other behavioral, psychiatric, or developmental disorders. The first clue may be an elevated serum ammonia level with normal serum aminotransferase levels and without metabolic acidosis. Therefore, if a UCD is considered, the following laboratory measurements should be obtained: serum ammonia, arterial blood gases, urine organic acids, serum amino acids, and urinary orotic acid; Table 77-2 reviews the expected results.

Urinary organic acid profiles are typically normal in UCDs. The plasma amino acid profiles are distinctive, with abnormal levels of arginine, ornithine, and citrulline. Citrulline levels are barely detectable in OTC or CPS deficiencies but markedly raised in AS and AL deficiencies. AL deficiency can be distinguished from AS deficiency by the finding of argininosuccinic acid in the plasma and urine. OTC deficiency is differentiated from CPS deficiency by excessive urinary excretion of orotic acid. Direct enzyme analysis can be performed and can be useful in patients who have a partial deficiency or who present in adulthood. Early neonatal diagnosis leads to improved survival, so prenatal enzyme and genetic linkage analysis can be carried out in family members of known carriers to aid in early diagnosis.[202] An *N*-carbamoyl-glutamic acid test has been advocated for all patients presenting with a suspected UCD while further testing is carried out; patients with *N*-acetylglutamate synthase deficiency, one of the less common UCDs, have a significant drop in plasma ammonia levels within 8 hours of receiving an oral dose of *N*-carbamoyl glutamic acid, a structural analog of *N*-acetyl glutamic acid.[203,204] An allopurinol loading test, which leads to excretion of orotic acid in amounts that are 10- to 20-fold greater than normal in heterozygote female carriers of OTC deficiency, is nonspecific, and the results must be interpreted with caution; some patients with mitochondrial disease or defects in pyrimidine metabolism may have a positive result.[205] Liver biopsy specimens typically show hepatocyte pallor due to glycogen accumulation and minimal fatty infiltration; fibrosis or cirrhosis are uncommon findings but have been reported.[206,207]

Treatment

All external protein intake should be discontinued in infants presenting acutely with UCDs. Serum ammonia levels should be restored to normal. The use of oral lactulose to lower the nitrogen load has not been studied in this patient population. Given the extremely high ammonia levels often encountered, continuous arteriovenous hemodialysis or hemofiltration is frequently required, but exchange transfusions and peritoneal dialysis are ineffective. Alternative pathways for waste nitrogen disposal should be employed, specifically IV administration of sodium benzoate and sodium phenylacetate; however, sodium benzoate should be used with caution in patients with cirrhosis, because a paradoxical rise in blood ammonia levels has been observed.[208] Oral phenylbutyrate can be substituted for phenylacetate to improve palatability.

Arginine, carnitine, and long-chain fatty acids are usually present in low levels in these patients and should be supplemented.[185,209] Low-dose arginine (100 mg/kg/day) together with an ammonia scavenger is effective in repleting arginine stores, maintaining low ammonia levels, and minimizing liver enzyme elevations compared with high-dose arginine (500 mg/kg/day), although consensus guidelines recommend an intermediate dose of arginine (250 mg/kg/day).[185,210] Once the patient stabilizes, low levels of dietary protein, 0.5 to 1 g/kg, may be introduced, with progressive increases as tolerated to provide sufficient protein for growth and tissue repair while minimizing urea production. Long-term therapy and protein restriction are then tailored to the patient; those with a severe disorder may need essential amino acids to supplement their protein intake.[185,209]

The outcome for patients who present with hyperammonemic coma and a delayed diagnosis is poor.[187] The level of ammonia at the time of the first hyperammonemic episode is a rough guide to the eventual neurodevelopmental outcome.[211] The sooner the hyperammonemia is treated and the correct diagnosis is made, the better the long-term survival, although for patients who survive the neonatal period, the median survival without liver transplantation is less than 4 years and is associated with severe developmental delay and neurologic morbidity.[186] With optimal dietary and medical management, patients may still have repeated hyperammonemic crises, often during intercurrent viral infections. Symptomatic female OTC heterozygotes also benefit from therapy, which leads to fewer hyperammonemic episodes and a reduced risk of further cognitive decline.[212]

Patients with a UCD and deterioration or lack of improvement despite therapy have undergone either orthotopic or auxiliary liver transplantation successfully (see Chapter 97), with normalization of enzyme activity and ammonia levels, restored ability to tolerate a normal diet, and 5-year survival rates of 90%.[213,214] Liver transplantation, if considered, should be done before neurologic damage is permanent, because the patient's neurologic status does not improve after transplantation. Developmental outcomes appear to be improved in those transplanted in the first year of life compared with historical controls who have not undergone transplantation.[215] The metabolic condition of the patients normalizes completely, and neurologic status does not worsen after transplantation.[189] Hepatocyte transplantation has been successful in improving metabolic function in patients with a UCD and has been applied successfully as a bridge to auxiliary liver transplantation.[216] For patients without severe neurologic compromise before liver transplantation, this therapeutic approach may be worthwhile. The annual cost of care for patients with a UCD is likely to be reduced dramatically after liver transplantation.

The importance of identifying the deleterious mutation in a patient with a UCD will likely become increasingly important not only as a means of allowing carrier testing and prenatal diagnosis, but also as an aid to treatment decisions. For example, patients with a mutation that results in the most severe OTC deficiency (e.g., abolished enzyme activity) may benefit preferentially from immediate liver transplantation to prevent severe mental retardation or death, whereas those with a mutation that leads to milder disease may be better managed medically with dietary restrictions and ammonia scavengers to facilitate growth before possible liver transplantation.

Arginase Deficiency

At least 2 forms of arginase activity occur in humans. Arginase I (AI) predominates in the liver and red blood cells, and arginase II (AII) is found predominantly in kidney and prostate. Arginase deficiency involving AI is the least common of the UCDs. Hyperammonemia is unusual in affected persons, but

hyperammonemic coma and death have been reported.[217] Clinical features are distinct from those of the other UCDs. The disease is characterized by indolent deterioration of the cerebral cortex and pyramidal tracts, leading to progressive dementia and psychomotor retardation, spastic diplegia progressing to quadriplegia, seizures, and growth failure. The syndrome is often confused with cerebral palsy.[218,219] One report describes a 20-year-old patient with arginase deficiency who, in addition to the typical neurologic findings, had liver cirrhosis and associated hepatocellular carcinoma.[219]

Laboratory studies may reveal elevated blood arginine values, mild hyperammonemia, and a mild increase in urine orotic acid excretion. Varying amounts of urea are still produced in these patients secondary to the compensatory elevated expression of AII in the kidneys that ameliorates the clinical disorder. The diagnosis is confirmed by enzymatic analysis, which can be performed prenatally on cord blood samples. Treatment consists of protein restriction and, when needed, sodium phenylbutyrate.[218]

BILE ACID SYNTHESIS AND TRANSPORT DEFECTS

The pathways for bile acid synthesis and the mechanism of bile acid transport within the hepatobiliary system are complex, involving several enzymes and transport processes located in multiple subcellular fractions of the hepatocyte (see Chapter 64). With advances in molecular biology, genetics, and mass spectrometry, several different inborn errors in bile acid synthesis and transport have been identified as causes of clinical disease.[220,221] The classification of these disorders has been clarified, particularly in the clinically heterogeneous subset of cases that comprise progressive familial intrahepatic cholestasis (PFIC) syndromes. For some of the disorders, this progress has led to improved diagnosis and life-saving therapy.

PFIC refers to a heterogeneous group of autosomal-recessive disorders that disrupt bile formation and present with cholestasis of hepatocellular origin. Historically, the diagnosis of PFIC has been imprecise; broad criteria included the presence of chronic, unremitting intrahepatic cholestasis, exclusion of identifiable metabolic or anatomic disorders, and characteristic clinical, biochemical, and histologic features.[220] Other symptoms and signs are severe pruritus, hepatomegaly, wheezing and cough, short stature, delayed sexual development, fat-soluble vitamin deficiency, and cholelithiasis. Affected persons exhibit severe and progressive intrahepatic cholestasis, usually manifesting within the first few months of life and often proceeding to cirrhosis and ESLD by the second decade of life.

Specific types of PFIC due to defective bile acid synthesis or transport have been identified, and each is associated with mutations in enzymes or hepatocellular transport-system genes involved in bile formation. With the discovery of these specific defects and the development of sophisticated biochemical and molecular methodology and gene mutation analysis, precise characterization is now possible using techniques such as mass spectrometry, the JaundiceChip, and DNA sequencing by capillary electrophoresis.[36,222] These complementary tests allow rapid, sensitive, and cost-effective bile acid profiling and mutation screening to aid clinical diagnosis in patients with intrahepatic cholestasis. Patients believed previously to have idiopathic neonatal hepatitis or an undiagnosed familial hepatitis syndrome may now be diagnosed accurately. An estimated 3% to 5% of patients with idiopathic cholestasis may have defects in bile acid synthesis and

TABLE 77-3 Inborn Errors of Bile Acid Synthesis and Transport*

Defects in Bile Acid Synthesis

Alterations of the enzymes involved in modification of the steroid ring	3β-hydroxy-Δ5-C$_{27}$-steroid oxidoreductase deficiency *(HSD3B7)*
	Δ^4-3-oxosteroid 5β-reductase deficiency *(AKR1D1)*
	Oxysterol 7α-hydroxylase deficiency *(CYP7B1)*
	Cholesterol 7α-hydroxylase deficiency *(CYP7A1)*
	12α-hydroxylase deficiency *(CYP8B1)*
Alterations of the enzymes involved in modification of the side chain	CTX-sterol 27-hydroxylase deficiency *(CYP27A1)*
	2-methylacyl-CoA racemase deficiency *(AMACAR)*
	Bile acid–CoA: *N*-acyl amino acid transferase deficiency *(BAAT)*
	Bile acid–CoA ligase deficiency *(BACL; SLC27A5)*
	Sterol 25-hydroxylase deficiency *(CH25H)*
Organelle or cell injury	Peroxisomal biogenesis disorders
	Zellweger's syndrome
	Rhizomelic chondrodysplasia punctata
	Neonatal adrenoleukodystrophy
	Infantile Refsum's disease
	Disorders with loss of a single peroxisomal function
	Generalized hepatic synthetic dysfunction
	Fulminant hepatic failure (multiple causes)
	Neonatal iron storage disease
	Tyrosinemia

Defects in Bile Acid or Phospholipid Transport

	PFIC type I: FIC1 deficiency *(ATP8B1,* or *FIC1)*
	Byler's disease
	Benign recurrent intrahepatic cholestasis
	Greenland familial cholestasis
	PFIC type II: BSEP deficiency *(ABCB11)*
	PFIC type III: MDR3 deficiency *(ABCB4)*

*Corresponding genes are shown in *italics.*
BSEP, bile salt export pump; MDR, multidrug resistance protein; PFIC, progressive familial intrahepatic cholestasis.
Adapted from reference 221.

transport.[221] Table 77-3 lists the known errors of primary and secondary bile acid synthesis and transport.

Bile Acid Synthesis Defects

Defects in bile acid synthesis due to mutations in genes that encode the enzymes responsible for primary bile acid formation may have profound effects on hepatic and GI function and integrity. The 8 known defects in bile acid synthesis that have been described result in highly variable phenotypic expression: (1) familial, progressive infantile, or late-onset cholestasis ("PFIC-like"); (2) fat-soluble vitamin malabsorption; and (3) variable degrees of neurologic involvement (see Table 77-3).[221,223,224] Typical biochemical abnormalities detected in patients with bile acid synthetic defects include elevated serum aminotransferase and conjugated bilirubin levels with normal GGTP levels; serum cholesterol concentrations are also usually normal. Bile acid synthesis defects have been identified in 2% of approximately 11,000 screened cases of idiopathic cholestatic liver disease in infants and children.[221]

These disorders respond well to replacement and displacement therapy.[220,221] Such therapy is based on the principle that inborn errors of bile acid biosynthesis lead to underproduction of normal trophic and choleretic primary bile acids and overproduction of hepatotoxic primitive bile acid metabolites.[221,225] Bile acids found in patients with inborn errors also act as cholestatic agents by inhibiting canalicular ATP-dependent bile acid transport, the rate-limiting step in the overall process of bile acid transport across the canalicular membrane.[226] Patients with some of the bile acid synthetic defects have been treated effectively with the primary bile acid (cholic acid) and ursodeoxycholic acid supplementation.[221,227]

Replacement therapy using cholic acid bypasses the enzymatic block and provides negative feedback to earlier steps in the synthetic pathways, and ursodeoxycholic acid displaces toxic bile acid metabolites and serves as a hepatobiliary cytoprotectant.[227]

Diagnosis

Marked alterations in urinary, serum, and biliary bile acid composition and concentration may be found in infants and children with severe liver disease of any etiology. Therefore, determining whether these changes are primary or secondary to the liver dysfunction may be difficult, and a detailed biochemical evaluation is necessary. Initially, defects in bile acid synthesis were discovered with the use of liquid secondary ionization mass spectrometry; specifically, fast atom bombardment ionization mass spectrometry allows direct analysis of bile acids from a drop of urine.[221] More advanced mass spectrometry approaches, including electrospray ionization tandem mass spectrometry, as well as gene sequencing techniques, have subsequently been applied. The mass spectra generated permit accurate identification of the absence of primary bile acids and presence of atypical bile acids specific to each primary defect.[221,228]

Disorders of Enzymes Involved in Modification of the Steroid Ring

The most common inborn error of bile acid biosynthesis is 3β-hydroxy-Δ^5-C$_{27}$-steroid dehydrogenase/isomerase (3β-HSD) deficiency. This disorder is caused by deficient activity of the second step in the bile acid synthetic pathway, the conversion of 7α-hydroxycholesterol into 7α-hydroxy-4-cholesten-3-one.[221] This reaction is catalyzed by a microsomal 3β-hydroxy-Δ^5-C_{27}-steroid oxidoreductase; deficiency of this enzyme results in the accumulation of 7α-hydroxycholesterol within the hepatocyte. The normal primary bile acids (cholic acid) are not formed; instead, C_{24}-bile acids that retain the 3β-hydroxy-Δ^5-structure are synthesized. Affected patients may present with pruritus, jaundice, hepatomegaly, steatorrhea, and fat-soluble vitamin deficiencies.[221,223,225] A report of 3β-HSD deficiency in adults not only highlights the clinical utility of homozygosity mapping in diagnosing autosomal recessive metabolic disorders, but also illustrates the wide variation in expressivity that occurs in 3β-HSD deficiency[229] and underscores the need to consider a bile acid synthetic defect as a possible cause of liver disease in patients of all ages.

Δ^4-3-Oxosteroid 5β-reductase (AKR1D1) deficiency was first described in monochorionic twins born with marked and progressive cholestasis.[230] This cytosolic enzyme is responsible for the conversion of 7α-hydroxy- and 7α,12α-dihydroxy-4-cholesten-3-one into the corresponding 3-oxo-5β(H) analogs. Deficiency of Δ^4-3-oxosteroid 5β-reductase usually leads to neonatal cholestasis, which rapidly progresses to synthetic dysfunction and liver failure.[230,231] Cholesterol 7a-hydroxylase (CYP7A1) deficiency is associated with hypertriglyceridemia and gallstone disease in adults; it does not present as cholestatic disease.[221]

Disorders of Enzymes Involved in Side-Chain Modification

Aberrant bile acid side chain hydroxylation and oxidation may be manifested as neurologic disease and/or fat-soluble vitamin malabsorption; in general, liver disease is mild in affected patients (see Table 77-3).[221,232]

Cerebrotendinous xanthomatosis (CTX), sterol-27-hydroxylase deficiency, is a rare autosomal recessive neurologic disease. CTX is characterized by bilateral juvenile cataracts and chronic diarrhea, followed by progressive neurologic dysfunction, hypercholesterolemia, atherosclerosis, and accumulation of cholesterol and cholestanol in tissues (brain, tendons).[233,234] CTX is caused by a mutation in the sterol 27-hydroxylase gene (CYP27A1)[235] and has been treated with chenodeoxycholic acid (CDCA) (see Chapters 64 and 65).[236] In 1 series, 5 children with CTX showed dramatic improvement in biochemical and electroencephalographic abnormalities and resolution of diarrhea during CDCA therapy. In addition, no further delay in motor development was noted; 3 patients showed an improved intelligence quotient.[237] In another series of patients treated with CDCA, those patients who started treatment after 25 years of age had worse outcomes, more limited ambulation, and more cognitive impairment; some continued to deteriorate despite CDCA treatment.[236] Therefore, prompt diagnosis and initiation of CDCA treatment is important in preventing neurologic damage and deterioration. After significant neurologic pathology is established, the effect of treatment is limited and deterioration may continue.[236]

2-Methylacyl Co-A racemase (AMACR) deficiency has been identified in an infant presenting with mildly elevated liver enzyme levels and low serum 25-hydroxy-vitamin D and vitamin E concentrations.[238]

Finally, bile acid synthesis culminates in conjugation with glycine and taurine, and genetic defects in conjugation and amidation have been identified using mass spectrometry analysis of urine, bile, and serum samples and sequence analysis of the genes encoding bile acid–CoA:amino acid N-acyltransferase (BAAT) and bile acid–CoA ligase (gene symbol SLC27A5).[232] Affected persons exhibit fat-soluble vitamin deficiency and growth failure, indicating the importance of bile acid conjugation in lipid absorption. In some patients, liver disease with features of a cholangiopathy has been present.[232]

Peroxisomal Disorders

Peroxisomes are responsible for beta oxidation in the final steps of bile acid synthesis to yield the primary bile acids, cholic acid and chenodeoxycholic acid. Defects in peroxisomal assembly and function have a significant impact on bile acid synthesis, because peroxisomes contain multiple enzymes required for the oxidation and conjugation of bile acids.[221,239] The peroxisomopathies encompass a diverse group of genetic disorders caused by impairment in one or more peroxisomal functions. These disorders are subdivided into 3 main groups: (1) peroxisome biogenesis disorders (PBDs) that cause multiple abnormalities, (2) single peroxisomal protein (enzyme) deficiencies that result in limited dysfunction, and (3) single peroxisomal substrate transport deficiencies.[240] PBDs comprise a group of disorders that share similar clinical and biochemical features; this group includes Zellweger's syndrome, neonatal adrenoleukodystrophy (NALD), infantile Refsum's disease (IRD), and rhizomelic chondrodysplasia punctata (RCDP), which is characterized by severe rhizomelic shortening of the limbs, severe skeletal abnormalities, cataracts, and facial abnormalities.[239]

PBDs are caused by defects in any of at least 14 different PEX genes, which encode proteins involved in peroxisome assembly and proliferation.[241] The single peroxisomal enzyme deficiency group consists of D-bifunctional protein and phytanoyl-CoA hydroxylase (adult Refsum's disease) deficiencies, among others.[240] The single peroxisomal substrate transport deficiency group consists of only one disease, X-linked adrenoleukodystrophy (X-ALD).[240]

These neurometabolic diseases are highly variable in age of onset and severity. The spectrum includes death in infancy, rapid functional decline, slow decline over a long term, and an apparently stable course.[242] Leukoencephalopathy may be detected on cerebral MRI.[242,243]

Liver histologic changes are frequent in patients with peroxisomal disorders.[244] Hepatotoxic metabolites, specifically the bile acid synthesis intermediates di- and trihydroxycholestanoic acids (DHCA and THCA), are responsible for the liver injury.[244] These compounds interfere with critical physiologic processes, including mitochondrial oxidative phosphorylation.

Zellweger's (cerebrohepatorenal) syndrome is a primary disorder of peroxisome biogenesis.[240,245] The multiple features include distinctive dysmorphic features (hypertelorism, large anterior fontanelle, deformed earlobes), neonatal hypotonia, impaired hearing, retinopathy, cataracts, seizures, and skeletal changes. Hepatomegaly is common, and the progressive liver disease that develops in patients with Zellweger's syndrome is similar to that identified in other errors of bile acid synthesis.[246] Peroxisome biogenesis involves more than 13 PEX genes and requires the targeting and importation of cytosolic proteins into the peroxisomal membrane and matrix. Importation of proteins fated for the peroxisomal matrix requires guidance from 1 of 2 peroxisome-targeting signals, PTS1 and PTS2. Patients with Zellweger spectrum disorders display defects in the importation of proteins that use PTS1 and PTS2, whereas patients with RCDP have a defect in the importation of proteins that use PTS2.[239]

The most common disorder of peroxisomes, ALD, is included in the second group of peroxisomopathies. This disorder results from a defect in the peroxisomal adrenoleukodystrophy protein (ALDP), which is a member of the ATP-binding cassette (ABC) superfamily of membrane transporters (see Chapter 64).[247] NALD, a distinct genetic disorder of autosomal recessive inheritance, must be distinguished from Zellweger's syndrome and X-ALD; all 3 conditions lead to storage of very-long-chain fatty acids.[248] Clinical features in NALD, present at birth, include hypotonia, severe psychomotor delay, and failure to thrive.

All of these disorders are associated with multiple clinical abnormalities and a wide range of biochemical abnormalities. They are diagnosed through a combination of biochemical and histologic assessment, such as a search for very-long-chain fatty acids and ultrastructural abnormalities in tissue biopsy specimens.[249] DNA testing for PBDs may be used for carrier testing of relatives, early prenatal diagnosis or preimplantation genetic diagnosis, and counseling in families with a risk of recurrence for one of these disorders.[241]

Bile Acid Transport Defects

The study of intrahepatic cholestasis syndromes has enhanced our understanding of hepatic excretory function and bile acid metabolism. The spectrum of diseases associated with mutations in genes involved in bile acid transport physiology is large and growing. The precise terminology used to describe these disorders continues to evolve as well (see Table 77-3). Specific disorders of bile acid transport defects include familial intrahepatic cholestasis 1 (FIC1) disease, bile salt export pump (BSEP) disease, and multidrug resistance protein 3 (MDR3) disease.[220,250,251] Diagnosis is based on clinical manifestations, cholangiography, and liver histology, including immunostaining for BSEP and MDR3 deficiencies. Specific tests must also be conducted to exclude other causes of cholestasis. Serum GGTP activity is normal in patients with FIC1 disease and BSEP deficiency but elevated in patients with MRD3 deficiency. Diagnosis has been aided by the development of a resequencing chip that efficiently identifies the most common disease-causing mutations.[36,222]

FIC1 disease (also called *PFIC type I*) encompasses a continuum comprising intermediate phenotypes of at least 2 disease states: Byler's disease, which generally presents in infancy and leads to progressive cholestasis often associated with severe pruritus, and benign recurrent intrahepatic cholestasis (BRIC) type I, which gives rise to recurrent episodes of intrahepatic cholestasis beginning in childhood or adulthood that can last days to months and resolve spontaneously without causing detectable lasting liver damage.[220,250] The occurrence of extrahepatic features in patients with FIC1 disease, including chronic diarrhea, deafness, and pancreatic insufficiency, suggests a biological cell function for FIC1.

In patients with FIC1 disease, serum GGTP and cholesterol levels are normal or mildly elevated, and levels of bile acids are elevated in the serum and low in the bile. Serum aminotransferase and bilirubin levels are mildly elevated as well. Impaired bile acid transport in the intestine may account for the striking malabsorption and diarrhea in some patients. These intestinal clinical features do not resolve after liver transplantation. Histology of liver tissue from patients with FIC1 disease typically shows bland canalicular cholestasis, with varying degrees of hepatocellular ballooning and giant cell transformation; portal fibrosis and eventually cirrhosis may be seen later in the course of the disease. (The liver histology of patients with BRIC-1 is normal between episodes.) On electron microscopic evaluation of liver tissue from patients with FIC1 disease, characteristic coarse, granular bile deposits are seen in the canaliculus ("Byler's bile").[169,220,251,252]

FIC1 disease is caused by mutations in the *ATP8B1* gene (initially named the *FIC1* gene) that encodes the FIC1 protein,

a P-type adenosine triphosphatase (ATPase) involved in ATP-dependent aminophospholipid transport.[253,254] FIC1 protein is expressed on the hepatocyte canalicular membrane and in many other organs, including the intestine and pancreas. FIC1 is responsible for maintaining the enrichment of phosphatidylserine and phosphatidylethanolamine on the inner leaflet of the plasma membrane. This transporter thereby plays a role in maintaining canalicular membrane integrity, including microvilli formation. Abnormal protein function is postulated to indirectly disrupt the biliary secretion of bile acids, which explains the reduced biliary bile acid concentrations found in patients with FIC1 disease.[251] Impaired ATP8B1 function also leads to down-regulation of the farnesoid X receptor (FXR), a nuclear receptor involved in the regulation of bile acid metabolism, with subsequent down-regulation of BSEP protein in the liver and up-regulation of bile acid synthesis and of the apical sodium bile salt transporter (ASBT) in the intestine (see Chapter 64).[251] Severe mutations in *ATP8B1* lead to progressive early-onset FIC1 disease, whereas mutations that are predicted to affect protein structure minimally are seen more commonly in patients with BRIC type 1.[253] Patients with Greenland familial cholestasis also have distinct defects in the FIC1 gene, as do other kindreds of Dominican and Saudi descent.[253]

BSEP disease (also called *PFIC type II*) is caused by a wide spectrum of mutations in the *ABCB11* gene, which encodes an ABC protein that serves as the canalicular BSEP,[255] the major transport protein governing the secretion of bile acids from hepatocytes into bile. BSEP, which is expressed exclusively in hepatocytes, is localized to the canalicular membrane and is thus responsible for the bile salt-dependent bile flow, governing the transport of monovalent bile acids (see Chapter 64).

Patients with the progressive form of BSEP disease present with high serum bile acid levels, but low or low-normal serum GGTP levels, and usually have intense pruritus, jaundice, poor weight gain, and hepatosplenomegaly.[250,256-258] In addition, a genetically distinct form of BRIC (type II) is associated with mutations in *ABCB11*. Patients with BRIC-II commonly have cholelithiasis and lack extrahepatic manifestations.[259] In addition, genetic polymorphisms are linked to intrahepatic cholestasis of pregnancy (see Chapter 39) and drug-induced liver injury (see Chapter 88).[255,260]

Early in the course of BSEP disease, nonspecific giant cell hepatitis is found on histologic examination of the liver, and on electron microscopy amorphous bile deposits are seen in the canaliculi. For unclear reasons, patients with clinically severe, nonremitting intrahepatic cholestasis ascribed to *ABCB11* mutations associated with absence or severe deficiency of BSEP expression have an increased risk of developing malignancies of the hepatobiliary system, such as hepatoblastoma, hepatocellular carcinoma, and cholangiocarcinoma.[261-264] Three children who underwent orthotopic liver transplantation for severe BSEP deficiency had post-transplantation episodes of cholestatic dysfunction that mimicked the original disease. Remission of all episodes was achieved by intensifying their immunosuppressive regimens. The phenotypical recurrence of the disease correlated with the presence of high titers of circulating antibodies against BSEP that inhibited transport by BSEP in vitro. When administered to rats, these antibodies targeted the bile canaliculi and impaired bile acid secretion.[263-266]

MDR3 disease (also called *PFIC type III*) is caused by mutations in the *ABCB4* gene that encodes the MDR3 glycoprotein, an ABC phosphatidylcholine translocase expressed on the canalicular membrane of hepatocytes.[267] This phospholipid translocator is involved in biliary phospholipid (phosphatidylcholine) excretion. MDR3 deficiency is thought to lead to cholestasis via decreased excretion of cytoprotective biliary phospholipids, leaving an increased pool of cytotoxic, detergent biliary bile acids that are not inactivated by phospholipids and giving rise to subsequent bile duct damage and proliferation and release of GGTP into the serum.

Patients with MDR3 disease present with several disease phenotypes as well, ranging from neonatal cholestasis to the later presentation of cirrhosis, intrahepatic and gallbladder lithiasis, intrahepatic cholestasis of pregnancy, adult-onset ductopenic cholestatic liver disease, drug-induced cholestasis, and some cases of transient neonatal cholestasis, adult idiopathic cirrhosis, and cholangiocarcinoma.[268-270] Patients with MDR3 deficiency present with high serum levels of GGTP and bile acids as well as bile ductular proliferation on routine microscopy. Some female patients with intrahepatic cholestasis of pregnancy have been shown to be heterozygous carriers of a mutation in *ABCB4*; other nongenetic factors are likely required for full expression of the disease.[268,271]

Other chronic intrahepatic cholestatic diseases include North American Indian childhood cirrhosis (NAICC), cholestasis-lymphedema syndrome (Aagenaes syndrome),[272] neonatal icthyosis and sclerosing cholangitis syndrome, and arthrogryposis-renal dysfunction-cholestasis (ARC) syndrome. Each is characterized by the presence of disease-causing loci that are genetically distinct from those that cause FIC1, BSEP, or MDR3 disease. For example, a single-point mutation in the cirhin gene encodes a nucleolar protein of unknown function in patients with NAICC.[273] In addition, mutations in the claudin-1 and *VPS33B* (vacuolar protein sorting 33B) genes have been identified in patients with neonatal icthyosis and sclerosing cholangitis and in ARC syndromes, respectively; both of these genes encode proteins that are important in membrane fusion events.[274,275]

Treatment

Medical management of patients with disorders of bile acid transport is directed towards the prevention of growth failure, reduction of pruritus, and monitoring for complications of chronic liver disease.[220] Supportive treatment requires supplementation of fat-soluble vitamins (A, D, E, and K) and administration of medium-chain TGs, which are absorbed independently of bile acids. Therapy with ursodeoxycholic acid may be effective in reducing pruritus and improving liver biochemical test levels in up to 50% of patients with PFIC, regardless of serum GGTP levels.[276] Amelioration of pruritus with cholestyramine, opioid antagonists, rifampin, and phototherapy has been variably effective with a short duration of benefit at best. Surgical approaches such as ileal exclusion and partial external biliary diversion have provided satisfactory symptomatic relief to some patients by decreasing the bile acid pool and pruritus, especially in patients with PFIC types I and II.[277-279] Long-term improvement in pruritus and growth has been reported in 6 pediatric patients treated with biliary diversion. If all else fails, liver transplantation leads to good overall outcomes, with normalization of bile acid synthesis and growth, even in patients who receive a live-donor organ from a potentially heterozygous parent.[280]

CF

Liver disease can be the presenting symptom of CF in the newborn, and CF-associated liver disease (CFALD) has been associated with meconium ileus. Other risk factors for CFALD include male sex, pancreatic insufficiency, and a CF transmembrane regulator (CFTR) genotype associated with severe disease (see Chapter 57).[281-284]

Clinical and Pathologic Features

CFALD may become more common as the mean age of survival for patients with CF rises; however, liver involvement is not universal and seems to peak during adolescence. Although CF has been identified in fewer than 2% of patients with neonatal cholestasis, the diagnosis should be considered in any infant who presents with neonatal cholestasis. Up to 30% of patients may have clinical or symptomatic liver disease after the neonatal period.[281,282,285]

Hepatobiliary diseases noted in patients with CF can be grouped into 3 categories (Table 77-4). The pathognomonic lesion of CF, focal biliary cirrhosis (FBC), presumably results from defective function of the CFTR protein, which is expressed in bile duct epithelial cells. Obstruction of small bile ducts leads to chronic inflammatory changes, bile duct proliferation, and portal fibrosis. At autopsy, FBC has been identified in 25% to 30% of patients older than 1 year of age.[286] Progression to multilobular biliary cirrhosis occurs in 5% to 10% of patients with CF and leads to symptoms associated with portal hypertension, such as splenomegaly and variceal bleeding.[281,282,285] Hepatic steatosis also develops in roughly half of patients but does not appear to correlate with outcome. Biliary abnormalities range from microgallbladder, which is largely asymptomatic and is found in up to 20% of patients, to cholelithiasis and cholangiocarcinoma.[282] The presence of liver disease does not necessarily correlate with the severity of pulmonary disease.

Pathophysiology

The pathogenesis of CFALD is complex. The development of CFALD is related to the CFTR defect in cholangiocytes.[284]

TABLE 77-4 Hepatobiliarys Disease in Patients with CF

Specific to CF	Hepatic
	    Focal biliary cirrhosis with inspissation
	    Multilobular biliary cirrhosis with
	      inspissation
	Biliary
	    Microgallbladder
	    Mucocele
	    Mucous hyperplasia of the gallbladder

Secondary to extrahepatic disease	Hepatic lesions associated with
	    cardiopulmonary disease
	    Centrilobular necrosis
	    Cirrhosis
	Pancreatic lesions
	    Fibrosis (leading to bile duct
	      compression/stricture)

Increased in frequency in patients with CF	Hepatic
	    Drug hepatotoxicity
	    Fatty liver
	    Neonatal cholestasis
	    Viral hepatitis
	Biliary
	    Biliary sludge
	    Cholangiocarcinoma
	    Cholelithiasis
	    Sclerosing cholangitis

Modified from Balistreri WF. Liver disease in infancy and childhood. In: Schiff ER, Sorrell MF, Maddrey WC, editors. Schiff's diseases of the liver. 9th ed. Philadelphia: Lippincott-Raven; 1999. p 1379.

CFTR is expressed exclusively in cholangiocytes, not in hepatocytes; therefore, altered CFTR protein function on the apical membrane of cholangiocytes, in combination with altered biliary transport, leads to retention of toxic bile acids. CFTR dysfunction has been shown to lead to fibrotic liver disease in a murine model.[287] Although all patients with CF express defective CFTR in cholangiocytes, not all develop CFALD. There is no association between specific CFTR mutations and CFALD.[288] The variable occurrence and clinical course of liver disease in patients with CF suggest that other genetic or environmental factors are involved in disease expression.[289-292] For example, the α_1-AT Z allele has been shown to be a risk factor for liver disease and portal hypertension in patients with CF.[292] Also, elevated concentrations of endogenous ursodeoxycholic acid (UDCA) have been documented in patients with CF without liver disease, thereby raising the possibility that UDCA may protect against liver injury in these patients.[293] The hepatic expression of certain genes correlates with the severity of fibrosis in patients with CFALD.[290] Differential expression of a number of genes is associated with hepatic fibrogenesis, including down-regulation of collagens, matrix metalloproteinases, and chemokines, thereby providing evidence of a transcriptional basis for the pathogenesis of CFALD.

Diagnosis

The diagnosis of liver disease in patients with CF can be difficult because the presenting signs are subtle. Hepatomegaly, which is present in approximately 30% of patients, has been shown to correlate with the presence of cirrhosis and is often the first indication of liver disease. Liver biochemical test levels may remain relatively normal despite histologic evidence of cirrhosis. Biopsy of the liver can be helpful; liver fibrosis predicts the development of clinically significant liver disease.[294] Because of the focal distribution of histologic abnormalities, however, sampling error may occur. US can detect biliary abnormalities as well as heterogeneous or nodular liver parenchyma; however, a normal study does not exclude significant hepatic fibrosis.[295,296] Measurement of liver stiffness by transient elastography or acoustic radiation force impulse imaging has been utilized to stage liver fibrosis in patients with CF.[297-299]

Treatment

Few trials have assessed the effectiveness of UDCA therapy, and evidence to justify its routine use in CF is insufficient.[300,301] In some patients with CF, however, treatment with UDCA improves liver biochemical test levels, but the evidence that the drug halts progression to cirrhosis is inconclusive.[302]

Because patients with CF rarely have true hepatocellular dysfunction, the role of liver transplantation in this patient population remains controversial, particularly given the scarcity of donor livers. The optimal timing of liver transplantation, if this option is considered, is also unclear, and guidelines are needed. Some studies have shown stable or improved lung function, better nutritional status, and increased quality of life in patients with CFALD after liver transplantation, whereas other studies have found no improvement in long-term survival after liver transplantation.[285,291,303-309] Long-term outcomes following liver transplantation are acceptable but are inferior to the outcomes of transplantation for other diseases. One study suggested that liver transplantation was neither beneficial nor detrimental to pulmonary function in patients with CF.[310] Liver transplantation should likely be reserved for CF patients with evidence of hepatic decompensation or advanced complications of ESLD.[284] A portosystemic shunt can be an effective treatment in patients with variceal bleeding; long-term outcomes are comparable to those for patients who undergo liver transplantation.[311]

MITOCHONDRIAL LIVER DISEASES

A large number of liver diseases have been attributed to defects in mitochondrial function. In addition to defects in mitochondrial enzymes involved in the urea cycle or energy metabolism, several mitochondrial hepatopathies involve respiratory chain/oxidative phosphorylation/electron transport defects or alterations in mitochondrial DNA (mtDNA) levels. The mitochondrial genome is especially vulnerable to oxidative injury not only because of its spatial relationship to the respiratory chain, but also because of its lack of protective histones and of an adequate excision and recombination repair system. mtDNA is inherited almost entirely from the maternal ovum; therefore, many primary mitochondrial deficiencies are inherited in a dominant fashion. Many nuclear genes, however, such as DNA polymerase-γ (POLG), thymidine kinase 2 (TK2), deoxyguanosine kinase (DGUOK), SCO1, BCS1L, and MPV17, encode proteins critical to maintaining proper amounts of mtDNA and to allowing normal mitochondrial respiratory function. Most mitochondrial diseases with primary involvement of the liver are caused by nuclear rather than mitochondrial gene mutations.[312]

Mitochondrial respiratory chain disorders can affect 1 in 20,000 children, with liver involvement occurring in 10% to 20% of patients.[312,313] Striking heterogeneity of clinical features, ranging from single-organ involvement to multisystem disease, can lead to a delayed or missed diagnosis and can confound therapeutic decision making, for example, with respect to the advisability of liver transplantation. This heterogeneity of clinical presentations is likely due to the observations that (1) mitochondrial quantity and function are uniquely influenced by both nuclear and mtDNA, and (2) cells in various tissues can contain different mixtures of normal and abnormal mitochondrial genomes (heteroplasmy).[312]

The diagnosis of a mitochondrial respiratory chain defect should be considered in a patient with liver disease who has unexplained neuromuscular symptoms, including a seizure disorder; involvement of seemingly unrelated organ systems; a rapidly progressive course; or a chronic course that proves to be a diagnostic dilemma.[312] In about 80% of patients, symptoms appear before age 2. The plasma lactate level and the ratio of lactate to pyruvate are often elevated, especially when the presentation is insidious.[312] Given the complex array of tests that are useful for establishing a diagnosis of a mitochondrial hepatopathy, a tiered approach to the diagnostic workup has been proposed. The results of early screening tests, such as an acylcarnitine profile or urine organic acid levels, may provide clues to abnormalities in energy metabolism and may subsequently guide confirmatory testing to establish a molecular diagnosis.[312] In selected cases, next-generation or targeted exomic sequencing of a patient's mitochondrial genes and a subset of nuclear genes may lead to a definitive diagnosis.[314,315]

Infantile liver failure has been reported in numerous mitochondrial disorders, including cytochrome c oxidase deficiency, caused by mutations in the SCO1 or BCS1L genes; succinyl-CoA enzyme deficiency, caused by mutations in the SUCLG1 genes; mutations in the TRMU gene encoding the mitochondrial-specific tRNA-modifying enzyme; and mutations in the TSFM gene encoding the mitochondrial translation elongation factor EFTs.[312,316-318] Key features of these disorders typically include a lactic acidemia and an elevated ratio of plasma lactate to pyruvate levels. Infants with Alpers-Huttenlocher syndrome (progressive neuronal degeneration in childhood with liver disease ascribed to mitochondrial dysfunction) experience vomiting, hypotonia, seizures, and liver failure, often beginning by 6 months of age. Frequently, the liver disease is unsuspected clinically and becomes evident late in the course of the disease. Alpers-Huttenlocher syndrome has been shown to be caused by mutations in *POLG* and in the *FARS2* gene encoding a mitochondrial phenylalanyl transfer RNA synthetase.[319,320] Alternatively, in mtDNA depletion syndrome (caused by mutations in the *POLG*, *DGUOK*, or *MPV17* genes), hypoglycemia, acidosis, and liver failure develop early in infancy, and neurologic abnormalities are less prominent.[312,321]

Navaho neurohepatopathy has been shown to be caused by mtDNA depletion and a defect in the *MPV17* gene product, which is involved in mtDNA maintenance and regulation of oxidative phosphorylation.[312,322,323] Other multisystemic mitochondrial diseases with liver involvement are Pearson's marrow-pancreas syndrome (caused by large deletions of mtDNA segments) and chronic diarrhea and intestinal pseudo-obstruction with liver involvement.[312,322]

Liver biopsy specimens in mitochondrial disorders typically show macrovesicular and microvesicular steatosis, with increased density and occasional swelling of mitochondria on electron microscopy. Immunohistochemical techniques are used more frequently (e.g., to diagnose cytochrome c oxidase deficiency). Cholestasis may be present, and conditions associated with chronic liver disease can show micronodular cirrhosis. Lactic acidemia may be constant, intermittent, or absent in mitochondrial disorders.[324] Direct measurement of the enzymatic activity of the respiratory chain electron transport protein complexes can be performed on frozen tissue from the organ that expresses the clinical disease, although skin fibroblasts and lymphocytes may also be used. Few academic centers around the world can perform the assays for mitochondrial respiration (polarographic studies) or mtDNA analysis.

No known effective therapy has been developed for mitochondrial respiratory chain disorders that alters the course of disease. Strategies proposed to delay the progression of these disorders include the use of antioxidants such as vitamin E or ascorbic acid; electron acceptors and cofactors, such as coenzyme Q10, thiamine, or riboflavin; and supplements proposed to work by other mechanisms, such as carnitine, creatine, or succinate. A Cochrane systemic review, however, failed to show any clear evidence to support their general use in mitochondrial disorders, but specific diseases, such as coenzyme Q deficiency, may respond to treatment.[322,325] Liver transplantation is generally contraindicated in these patients, given the dire outcome and high frequency of severe extrahepatic organ involvement.[322]

KEY REFERENCES

Full references for this chapter can be found on www.expertconsult.com.

5. Silverman GA, Pak SC, Perlmutter DH. Disorders of protein misfolding: Alpha-1-antitrypsin deficiency as prototype. J Pediatr 2013; 163:320-6.
36. Liu C, Aronow B, Jegga A, et al. Novel resequencing chip customized to diagnose mutations in patients with inherited syndromes of intrahepatic cholestasis. Gastroenterology 2007; 132:119-26.
48. Matern D, Seydewitz H, Bali D, et al. Glycogen storage disease type I: Diagnosis and phenotype/genotype correlation. Eur J Pediatr 2002; 161:S10-19.
88. Freeze HH. Understanding human glycosylation disorders: Biochemistry leads the charge. J Biol Chem 2013; 288:6936-45.
89. Jaeken J. Congenital disorders of glycosylation. Handb Clin Neurol 2013; 113:1737-43.
110. Siegesmund M, van Tuyll van Serooskerken AM, Poblete-Gutierrez P, et al. The acute hepatic porphyrias: Current status and future challenges. Best Pract Res Clin Gastroenterol 2010; 24:593-605.
147. Sinderman KL, Trahms C, Scott CR. Tyrosinemia type 1. In: Pagon RA, Adam MP, Bird TD, et al, editors. GeneReviews(™). Seattle: University of Washington; 2006. pp 1993-2013. (Updated 2011, Aug 25.).
163. Holme E, Lindstedt S. Tyrosinaemia type I and NTBC (2-(2-nitro-4-trifluoromethylbenzoyl)-1,3-cyclohexanedione). J Inherit Metab Dis 1998; 21:507-17.
185. Haberle J, Boddaert N, Burlina A, et al. Suggested guidelines for the diagnosis and management of urea cycle disorders. Orphanet J Rare Dis 2012; 7:32.
227. Gonzales E, Gerhardt MF, Fabre M, et al. Oral cholic acid for hereditary defects of primary bile acid synthesis: A safe and effective long-term therapy. Gastroenterology 2009; 137:1310-20.
235. Bjorkhem I. Cerebrotendinous xanthomatosis. Curr Opin Lipidol 2013; 24:283-7.
264. Jara P, Hierro L, Martinez-Fernandez P, et al. Recurrence of bile salt export pump deficiency after liver transplantation. N Engl J Med 2009; 361:1359-67.
282. Colombo C, Russo M, Zazzeron L, et al. Liver disease in cystic fibrosis. J Pediatr Gastroenterol Nutr 2006; 43:S49-55.
310. Miller MR, Sokol RJ, Narkewicz MR, et al. Pulmonary function in individuals who underwent liver transplantation: From the US Cystic Fibrosis Foundation registry. Liver Transpl 2012; 18:585-93.
322. Lee WS, Sokol RJ. Mitochondrial hepatopathies: Advances in genetics, therapeutic approaches and outcomes. J Pediatr 2013; 163:942-8.

MARIA H. SJOGREN AND JOHN T. BASSETT

Hepatitis A is the most common form of acute viral hepatitis worldwide.[1] It is a self-limited infection caused by a cytopathic single-stranded RNA virus without an envelope transmitted primarily by the fecal-oral route by contaminated food or water and sometimes resulting in epidemic outbreaks.[1,2] HAV was first characterized in 1973 when scientists detected the virus in stools of human volunteers who were infected with HAV.[3] The ensuing development of sensitive and specific serologic assays for the diagnosis of HAV infection and the isolation of HAV in cell culture[4] permitted understanding of the epidemiology of HAV infection and, ultimately, control of the disease.

VIROLOGY

In 1982, HAV was classified as an enterovirus belonging to the Picornaviridae family. Subsequent determination of the sequence of HAV nucleotides and amino acids led to the creation of a new genus, *Hepatovirus*.[5] HAV has an icosahedral shape, measures 27 to 28 nm in diameter, and is able to survive in acidic environments but is inactivated when heated to 85°C for 1 minute. HAV is capable of surviving in sea water (4% survival rate), dried feces at room temperature for 4 weeks (17% survival), and live oysters for 5 days (12% survival).[6] HAV has only 1 known serotype and no antigenic cross-reactivity with the hepatitis B, C, D, or E virus, or the GBV-C agent (see Chapters 79 to 83). The HAV genome consists of a positive-sense RNA that is 7.48 kb long, single-stranded, and linear (Fig. 78-1).

The onset of HAV replication in cell culture systems takes from weeks to months. Primate cells, including African green monkey kidney cells, primary human fibroblasts, human diploid cells, and fetal rhesus kidney cells, are favored for cultivation of HAV in vitro. Two conditions control the outcome of HAV replication in cell culture.[7] The first is the genetic makeup of the virus; HAV strains mutate in distinct regions of the viral genome as they become adapted to cell culture. The second is the metabolic activity of the host cell at the time of infection. Cells in culture, although infected simultaneously, initiate HAV replication in an asynchronous manner. This asynchronicity may be caused by differences in the metabolic activity of individual cells, but definitive evidence of cell-cycle dependence of HAV replication is lacking.[8]

An initial step in the life cycle of a virus is its attachment to a cell surface receptor. The location and function of these receptors determine tissue tropism. Little is known about the mechanism of entry of HAV into cells. Some work has suggested that HAV could infect cells by a surrogate-receptor binding mechanism (involving a nonspecified serum protein). HAV infectivity in tissue culture has been shown to require calcium and to be inhibited by the treatment of the cells with trypsin, phospholipases, and β-galactosidase.[9] A surface glycoprotein, HAVcr-1, on African green monkey kidney cells has been identified as a receptor for HAV. Blocking of HAVcr-1 with specific monoclonal antibodies prevents infection of otherwise susceptible cells. Experimental data suggest that HAVcr-1 not only serves as an attachment receptor but also may facilitate uncoating of HAV and its entry into hepatocytes.[10]

Once HAV enters a cell, the viral RNA is uncoated, cell host ribosomes bind to viral RNA, and polysomes are formed. HAV is translated into a large polyprotein of 2227 amino acids. This polyprotein is organized into 3 regions: P1, P2, and P3. The P1 region encodes structural proteins VP1, VP2, VP3, and a putative VP4. The P2 and P3 regions encode nonstructural proteins associated with viral replication (see Fig. 78-1).

The HAV RNA polymerase copies the plus RNA strand. The RNA transcript in turn is used for translation into proteins, which are used for assembly into mature virions. Down-regulation of HAV RNA synthesis appears to occur as defective HAV particles appear.[11] In addition, a group of specific RNA-binding proteins has been observed during persistent infection.[12] The origin and nature of these proteins is unknown, but they exert activity on the RNA template and are believed to play a regulatory role in the replication of HAV.[13]

Human HAV strains can be grouped into 4 different genotypes (I, II, III, and VII), whereas simian strains of HAV belong to genotypes IV, V, and VI.[14] Despite the nucleotide sequence heterogeneity, the antigenic structure of human HAV is highly conserved among strains. The HAV VP1/2A and 2C genes are thought to be responsible for viral virulence, as demonstrated

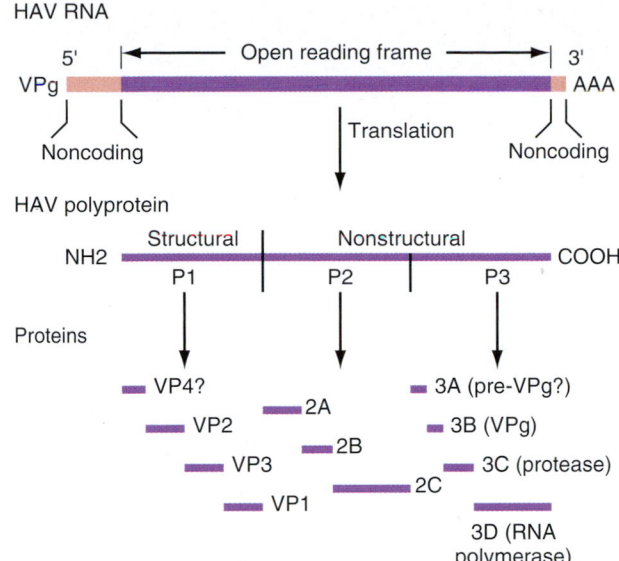

HAV RNA

HAV polyprotein

Proteins

FIGURE 78-1. Genomic organization of HAV. VP, viral protein; VPg, 5′ terminal protein. *(From Levine JE, Bull FG, Millward-Sadler GH, et al. Acute viral hepatitis. In: Millward-Sadler GH, Wright R, Arther MJP, editors. Wright's liver and biliary disease. 3rd ed. London: WB Saunders; 1992. p 679.)*

by experiments in which the genotypes and phenotypes of viruses were compared after animals were infected with 1 of 14 chimeric virus genomes derived from 2 infectious cDNA clones that encoded a virulent HAV isolate and an attenuated HAV isolate (HM175 strain), respectively.[15]

Among the many strains of HAV, the HM175 and CR326 human HAV strains were used for production of commercially available vaccines. In 1978, strain HM175 was isolated from human feces from Australian patients in a small outbreak of hepatitis A. CR326 was isolated from Costa Rican patients infected with HAV. The nucleotide and amino acid sequences showed 95% identity between the 2 strains. Vaccines prepared from these strains are thought to provide protection against all relevant human strains of HAV.

Variations in the HAV genome are thought to play a role in the development of fulminant hepatic failure (FHF) during acute HAV infection. The 5′ untranslated region of the HAV genome was sequenced in serum samples from 84 patients with HAV infection, including 12 with FHF.[16] The investigators observed fewer nucleotide substitutions in the HAV genome from patients with FHF than in those from patients without FHF ($P < 0.001$). The differences were most prominent between nucleotides 200 and 500, suggesting that nucleotide variations in the central portion of the 5′ untranslated region influence the clinical severity of HAV infection.

EPIDEMIOLOGY

Acute hepatitis A is a reportable infectious disease in all 50 states, as well as the District of Columbia, and in U.S. territories. Incidence has declined by over 90% since 1995. In 2010, 1670 cases of acute HAV infection were reported, corresponding to a rate of infection of 0.5 per 100,000, compared with 4 per 100,000 in 2001. Considering the underreporting of cases and the occurrence of asymptomatic infections, the true number of HAV infections in 2010 was calculated to be 17,000, down from 93,000 in 2001.[17] The decrease in rates of HAV infection is due in part to expanded use of the HAV vaccine

(see later). In 2006, the Centers for Disease Control and Prevention (CDC) recommended routine vaccination of children in all 50 states. Although the impact of HAV vaccination has been profound, vaccination coverage rates for HAV remain below rates for other routine childhood vaccines.[18] Historically, the highest rate of reported disease has been among children aged 5 to 14 years. Because of the rapid rate of decline of disease in children, however, rates are now similar among age groups, with adults aged 20 to 44 having the highest rate of disease in 2006.[19] A 2010 publication of 1158 cases of HAV infection reported from 2005 to 2007 identified the principal risk factor as international travel in 45.8%, contact with someone infected with HAV in 14.8%, contact with an employee or child in a daycare center in 7.6%, exposure during a food or waterborne outbreak in 7.2%, a history of illicit drug use in 4.3%, and, in men, a history of having sexual relations with other men in 3.9% of cases.[17]

HAV infection generally follows 1 of 3 epidemiologic patterns.[20] In countries where sanitary conditions are poor, most children are infected at an early age. Although earlier seroepidemiologic studies routinely showed that 100% of preschool children in these countries had detectable antibody to HAV (anti-HAV) in serum, presumably reflecting previous subclinical infection, subsequent studies have shown that the average age of infection has risen rapidly to 5 years and older, when symptomatic infection is more likely. For example, 82% of 1393 Bolivian school children were shown to have detectable anti-HAV, but when they were stratified into 2 groups according to family income, a significant difference was found between the groups: 95% of children from low-income families, but only 56% of children from high-income families, had detectable anti-HAV.[21]

The second epidemiologic pattern is seen in industrialized countries, where the prevalence of HAV infection is low among children and young adults. In the United States, prior to universal HAV vaccination, the prevalence of anti-HAV was about 10% in children but 37% in adults.[22] Data from the third National Health and Nutrition Examination Survey III (NHANES III) indicate that 31% of the overall U.S. population had serologic evidence of prior HAV infection before implementation of HAV vaccination—specifically, 9% of children aged 6 to 11, 19% of young adults aged 20 to 29, 33% of middle-aged adults aged 40 to 49, and 75% of those older than 70.[23]

The third epidemiologic pattern is observed in closed or semiclosed communities, such as some isolated communities in the South Pacific, where HAV is capable (through epidemics) of infecting the entire population, which then becomes immune. Thereafter, newborns remain susceptible until the virus is reintroduced into the community.

The primary route of transmission of HAV is the fecal-oral route, by either person-to-person contact or ingestion of contaminated food or water. Although rare, transmission of HAV by a parenteral route has been documented after transfusion of blood[24,25] or blood products.[26] Cyclical outbreaks among people who inject drugs (PWID) and users of noninjection illicit drugs and among men who have sex with men (up to 10% may become infected in outbreak years) have been reported.[27] Table 78-1 provides information about the detection of HAV and its infectivity in human body fluids.[28-35] From 11% to 22% of patients with acute hepatitis A require hospitalization, with an average length of stay of 4.6 days, costing on average $7926 per patient in 2004. In 1 outbreak involving 43 persons, the total cost was approximately $800,000. On average, 27 workdays are lost per adult case of hepatitis A. In adolescents and adults, the combined direct and indirect costs associated with HAV infection in the United States totaled roughly $93 million in 2006, compared with $488.8 million in 1997.[27,36,37] The decline in costs is a direct result of the dramatic

TABLE 78-1 Detection of HAV and Infectivity of Human Secretions or Excretions

Secretion/Excretion	Comment	References
Stool	The main source of infection. HAV is detectable during the incubation period and for several weeks after the onset of disease. After the onset of symptoms, HAV is detectable in 45% and 11% of fecal specimens collected during the first and second weeks of illness, respectively, whereas HAV RNA (by PCR assay) is detectable for 4 to 5 months.	28, 29
Blood	Viremia is present during the incubation period. Blood collected 3 and 11 days before the onset of symptoms has caused post-transfusion infection in recipients. Chronic viremia does not occur.	30, 31
Bile	HAV has been detected in the bile of chimpanzees infected with HAV.	32
Urine	HAV is detected in low titer during the viremic phase. A urine sample was reported to be infectious after oral inoculation. Urine contaminated with blood was also infectious.	33, 34
Nasopharyngeal	Unknown in humans. HAV has been identified in the oropharynx of experimentally infected chimpanzees.	35
Semen, vaginal fluid	Uncertain. HAV may be detectable during the viremic phase.	—

reduction in the number of infections seen since the introduction of the HAV vaccine and changes in vaccination policies in the United States.

PATHOGENESIS

After HAV is ingested and survives gastric acid, it traverses the small intestinal mucosa, reaches the liver via the portal vein, and is taken up by hepatocytes. In hepatocytes, virus particles replicate, assemble, and are secreted into the biliary canaliculus, from which they pass into the bile duct and back to the small intestine, with eventual excretion in the feces. The enterohepatic cycles of the virus life cycle continue until neutralizing antibodies and other immune mechanisms interrupt the cycle.[38,39]

The pathogenesis of HAV-associated hepatocyte injury is not completely defined. The lack of injury to cells in cell culture systems suggests that HAV is not cytopathic. Immunologically mediated cell damage is more likely. The emergence of anti-HAV could result in hepatic necrosis during immunologically mediated elimination of HAV.

CLINICAL FEATURES

Infection with HAV does not result in chronic infection, only in an acute self-limited episode of hepatitis. Rarely, acute hepatitis A can have a prolonged or a relapsing course, and occasionally profound cholestasis can occur.[40] The incubation period is commonly 2 to 4 weeks, rarely up to 6 weeks. The mortality rate is low in previously healthy persons. Morbidity can be substantial in adults and older children.

The most common clinical feature of cases of hepatitis A reported to the CDC in 2010 was jaundice in 68.1% of patients. The rates of hospitalization and death were 42.5% and 1%, respectively, possibly reflecting a reporting bias in favor of more severe cases. Adults and older adults are more likely to have profound hepatocellular dysfunction, require hospitalization, and have higher mortality rates.[41] The increased morbidity and mortality in older adults may be due to the reduced regenerative capacity of the liver with advanced age, increased

comorbidity, and a decline in immune function, including decreased antibody affinity to antigens.[42] By contrast, the rate of hospitalization in a younger population of active-duty U.S. Armed Forces members with acute HAV infection from 1991 to 2011 was 1.3 per 100,000 person-years. Because of a 1996 Department of Defense directive to provide HAV vaccine to all active-duty and reserve members, with the goal of immunization of the entire force by end of 1998, the rate of hospitalization fell from 2000 to 2011 to 0.2 to 0.7 per 100,000 patient-years.[43]

Patients with HAV infection usually present with 1 of the following 5 clinical patterns: (1) asymptomatic without jaundice; (2) symptomatic with jaundice and self-limited after approximately 8 weeks; (3) cholestatic, with jaundice lasting 10 weeks or more[40]; (4) relapsing, with 2 or more bouts of acute HAV infection occurring over a 6- to 10-week period; and (5) FHF. Children younger than 2 years are usually asymptomatic; jaundice develops in only 20% of them, whereas symptoms develop in most children (80%) 5 years or older. HAV infection with prolonged cholestasis is a rare variant but occasionally leads to invasive diagnostic procedures (inappropriately) because the diagnosis of acute hepatitis may not be readily accepted in patients who have jaundice for several months, even in the presence of detectable anti-HAV of the immunoglobulin (Ig)M class (see later).[40] A relapsing course is observed in some 10% to 15% of patients with acute hepatitis A within a 6-month period after acute illness has resolved; however, this variant (or any other) does not result in the development of chronic HAV infection.[44] Shedding of HAV in stool has been documented during the relapse phase.[45] Neither the cholestatic variant nor relapsing hepatitis A is associated with an increase in mortality.

In a retrospective observational multicenter study of 47 patients with acute HAV infection, during the prodrome phase (from 3 to 30 days after infection), the most common symptoms were fever (87%), malaise (74%), and jaundice (62%).[2] Additional prodromal symptoms include fatigue, weakness, anorexia, nausea, vomiting, and abdominal pain. Less common symptoms are fever, headache, arthralgias, myalgias, and diarrhea.[46] Dark urine precedes other symptoms in approximately 90% of infected persons; this symptom occurs within 1 to 2 weeks of the onset of prodromal symptoms. Symptoms of hepatitis may last from a few days to 2 weeks and usually decrease with the onset of clinical jaundice. Right upper quadrant tenderness and mild liver enlargement are found on physical examination in 85% of patients; splenomegaly and cervical lymphadenopathy are each present in 15%.

Complete clinical recovery is achieved in 60% of affected persons within 2 months and in almost everyone by 6 months. The overall prognosis of acute hepatitis A in otherwise healthy adults is excellent. Potentially fatal complications (e.g., FHF) develop in a small minority of patients.[47]

Acute hepatitis A, unlike hepatitis E, is not associated with a higher mortality rate in pregnant women. However, in a retrospective review of 13 cases of acute HAV infection during the second and third trimesters of pregnancy, gestational complications, including premature contractions, premature rupture of membranes, placental separation, and vaginal bleeding, developed in 9 patients (69%). In 8 of these patients, complications led to preterm labor at a median of 34 gestational weeks (range, 31 to 37 weeks).[48]

Acute HAV infection must be differentiated by appropriate serologic testing from other causes of acute viral hepatitis, autoimmune hepatitis, and other causes of acute nonviral hepatitis. In some cases the diagnosis may be difficult to make because the patient may harbor another viral infection, such as chronic hepatitis B or chronic hepatitis C, with superimposed acute HAV infection.

Fulminant Hepatitis A

FHF due to HAV is rarely seen in children, adolescents, or young adults. The case-fatality rate in 2008 was calculated by the CDC to be 0.02 per 100,000 population, with the highest mortality rates in persons older than 75 (0.12 deaths per 100,000 population). Mortality rates were similar among blacks and other non-whites, who had rates slightly higher than those of whites. From 2004 to 2008, the mortality rate of acute hepatitis A was consistently higher among male patients than female patients.[49] In addition to age, risk factors for FHF and mortality include underlying liver disease and chronic viral hepatitis.[50] Clinical predictors of FHF-associated mortality in a 2012 study were a serum creatinine level greater than 2 mg/dL, total bilirubin greater than 9.6 mg/dL, and albumin less than 2.5 g/L. Of these predictors, a serum creatinine level greater than 2 mg/dL had the best sensitivity and specificity for predicting FHF and mortality.[2] Acute liver failure caused by HAV becomes manifest in the first week of illness in about 55% of affected patients and during the first 4 weeks in 90%; the onset of FHF rarely occurs after 4 weeks of illness.[47] Late hepatic failure has been reported to occur in 1 patient 79 days after the onset of symptoms of HAV infection, with long-term survival achieved after live-donor liver transplantation (see Chapter 97).[51]

The contribution of HAV infection to acute liver failure has been reported to be greater in populations classified as hyperendemic for HAV. In a report from India, where 276 patients with FHF were seen between 1994 and 1997, 10.6% of the cases among adults were caused by HAV. HAV had been responsible for only 3.5% of cases among 206 patients with FHF seen in the same community from 1978 to 1981.[52] Although 2 reports since the late 1990s have described a decline in the number of cases of acute viral hepatitis among patients with FHF in the United States,[53,54] this decline is attributable principally to the control of HBV infection.

Extrahepatic Manifestations

Extrahepatic manifestations are less frequent in acute HAV infection than in acute HBV infection and consist most commonly of an evanescent rash (14%) and arthralgias (11%) and uncommonly of leukocytoclastic vasculitis, glomerulonephritis, and arthritis, in which immune-complex disease is believed to play a pathogenic role. Cutaneous vasculitis is typically seen on the legs and buttocks; skin biopsies reveal the presence of IgM anti-HAV and complement in blood vessel walls. The arthritis also appears to have a predilection for the lower extremities. Both vasculitis and arthritis have been associated with cryoglobulinemia, although cryoglobulinemia in general is more frequently associated with HCV infection. Cryoglobulins in acute hepatitis A have been shown to contain IgM anti-HAV. Other rare extrahepatic manifestations that may be immune-complex related include toxic epidermal necrolysis, fatal myocarditis, renal failure in the absence of liver failure, optic neuritis, transverse myelitis, polyneuritis, and cholecystitis. Hematologic complications include thrombocytopenia, aplastic anemia, and red-cell aplasia. Patients with more protracted illness appear to have a higher frequency of extrahepatic manifestations.

Autoimmune Hepatitis after Acute Hepatitis A

Several viruses have been reported to trigger the onset of autoimmune hepatitis (AIH) (see Chapter 90). In rare cases, acute hepatitis A has been followed by the development of type 1 AIH. AIH also may result in the detection of IgM anti-HAV for a prolonged period of time. Genetic predisposition is thought to play a role.[55-57]

DIAGNOSIS

Acute hepatitis A is clinically indistinguishable from other forms of viral hepatitis. The diagnosis of infection is based on detection of specific antibodies against HAV (anti-HAV) in serum (Fig. 78-2). A diagnosis of acute hepatitis A requires demonstration of IgM anti-HAV in serum. The test result is positive from the onset of symptoms[58] and usually remains positive for about 4 months.[59] Some patients may have low

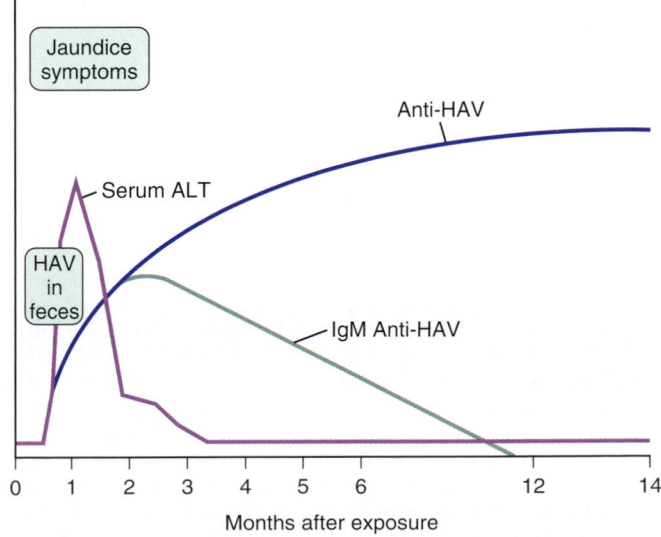

FIGURE 78-2. Typical course of a case of acute hepatitis A. Anti-HAV, antibody to HAV; IgM, immunoglobulin M. *(From Hoofnagle JH, DiBisceglie AM. Serologic diagnosis of acute and chronic viral hepatitis. Semin Liver Dis 1991; 11:73-83.)*

levels of detectable IgM anti-HAV for more than a year after the initial infection.[59] IgG anti-HAV is also detectable at the onset of the disease, remains present usually for life, and after clinical recovery is interpreted as a marker of previous HAV infection (as demonstrated by a positive result on a commercial assay for total anti-HAV and negative result for IgM anti-HAV).

Testing for HAV RNA is limited to research laboratories. HAV RNA has been detected in serum, stool, and liver tissue. Viral RNA can be amplified by PCR methodology.[60] With a PCR assay, HAV RNA has been documented in human sera for up to 21 days after the onset of illness.[26] The use of HCV RNA testing has been described in a report of 76 French patients with acute HAV infection seen between January 1987 and April 2000[61]; 19 had FHF, 10 of whom required liver transplantation and 1 of whom died while awaiting liver transplantation. The HAV RNA status was determined in 39 of the 50 patients in whom sera and clinical data were available, including the 19 with FHF. HAV RNA was detected in 36 of these 50 patients (72%). The presence of low-titer HAV RNA in patients with severe acute hepatitis may signal an ominous prognosis and the need for early referral for liver transplantation. As in other studies, HAV genotype did not seem to play a role in the severity of clinical manifestations.[62]

PREVENTION AND TREATMENT

Recommendations concerning immunoprophylaxis against HAV were published by the CDC in December 1999 for persons in groups at increased risk for hepatitis A or its adverse consequences. In 2006, these recommendations were updated by the Advisory Committee on Immunization Practices (ACIP), which specifically recommended routine vaccination of children in the United States.[27] The overall strategy is to protect persons from disease and to lower the U.S. incidence of HAV infection. The available monovalent vaccines were initially licensed for use in children older than age 2 but are now licensed for use after age 12 months.[27,63] The decline in incidence rates not surprisingly has been greater in children than in adults, effectively removing children as a high-risk population and potentially removing the primary reservoir for the virus in the United States.[19,27] Box 78-1 lists the populations now considered to be at highest risk of HAV infection. In June 2012, the WHO recommended deferring large-scale vaccination programs in highly endemic countries where almost all persons are asymptomatically infected with HAV in childhood, thereby effectively preventing clinical hepatitis A in adolescents and adults. In countries with intermediate HAV endemicity (or in those with high endemicity and rapidly improving socioeconomic status), a relatively large proportion of the adult population is susceptible to HAV infection, and

large-scale hepatitis A vaccination is likely to be cost-effective and is recommended. In countries with low or very low endemicity, the WHO has recommended targeted vaccination to provide individual health benefits. Groups for which vaccination should be offered include travelers to areas of intermediate or high endemicity, persons who require lifelong blood product transfusions, men who have sex with men, persons with chronic liver disease, workers in contact with non-human primates, and persons who inject drugs.[64]

No specific medications are available to treat acute hepatitis A; symptomatic treatment is the rule. Historically, attention to sanitation and administration of serum immune globulin (IG) have been the mainstays of preventing HAV infection. The availability of excellent HAV vaccines has rendered use of IG for preexposure prophylaxis unnecessary. Furthermore, in June 2007, the HAV vaccine was approved for use in postexposure prophylaxis of immunocompetent persons, 12 months to 40 years of age, without chronic liver disease.[65] This new indication for the HAV vaccine was based on results of a study that compared the efficacy of the HAV vaccine with that of IG for postexposure prophylaxis against HAV infection. Clinical hepatitis A developed in 4.4% of subjects in the vaccine group compared with 3.3% of those in the IG group.[66] Analysis revealed no statistical difference between the 2 groups (95% confidence interval, 0.70 to 2.67) but likely excluded persons with asymptomatic infection. In the vaccine group, 162 persons with IgM HAV in serum were excluded, compared with 50 persons in the IG group, because of either lack of symptoms or absence of an elevated serum ALT level of at least 2 times the upper limit of normal. The possibility exists that a number of persons with asymptomatic hepatitis A still posed an infectious risk to others. Although both HAV vaccine and IG appear to be effective when administered within 2 weeks of exposure to HAV, advantages of the HAV vaccine include long-term protection (when a second dose is subsequently administered), a good safety record, and wide availability.[67]

Taking into account data from Canada and the United Kingdom, where the HAV vaccine has been used for postexposure prophylaxis since the early 2000s, the ACIP concluded that the HAV vaccine is safe and comparable to IG in protecting recipients against clinical hepatitis A. The ACIP guidelines allow persons who have recently been exposed to HAV, and who have not been vaccinated previously, to be given a single dose of single-antigen HAV vaccine or IG (0.02 mL/kg) as soon as possible within 2 weeks of exposure. The standard vaccine schedule is detailed in Table 78-2.[65] Although IG is considered safe, the perception is widespread that it poses a risk because it is a blood-derived product. IG can cause fever and myalgias, just as the vaccine can, but pain at the injection site is usually more pronounced with IG than with the vaccine. Postexposure prophylaxis with IG can be administered at the same time as initiation of active immunization with the vaccine.[67]

The HAV vaccine was first licensed in the United States in 1995; 2 inactivated HAV vaccines are commercially available. Extensive use of the vaccines in clinical trials and postmarketing surveillance support the safety and efficacy of these products. HAVRIX is manufactured by GlaxoSmithKline Biologicals, Rixensart, Belgium, and VAQTA is manufactured by Merck & Co Inc., West Point, Pennsylvania. Both vaccines are derived from HAV grown in cell culture. The final products are purified and formalin-inactivated; they contain alum as an adjuvant. The basic difference between the 2 commercially available vaccines is the HAV strain used for preparation. HAVRIX was prepared with the HM175 strain, whereas VAQTA was prepared with the CR326 strain.[68,69] The difference is of little practical importance because both vaccines are safe and immunogenic. The doses and schedule of immunization

---

BOX 78-1 Groups at High Risk of HAV Infection

Healthy persons who:
  Travel to endemic areas
  Work in occupations for which the likelihood of exposure is high
  Have infected family members
  Adopt infants or children from an endemic areas
Men who have sex with men
Persons who have tested positive for HIV
Persons with chronic liver disease
Persons with a clotting factor disorder
People who inject drugs or users of noninjection illicit drugs

TABLE 78-2 Recommended Regimens for Hepatitis A Vaccination*

Vaccine	Schedule	Age (yr)	Dose	Volume (mL)	Dosing Schedule
HAVRIX	Standard	1-18	720 ELU	0.5	0, 6-12 months
	Standard	>18	1440 ELU	1	0, 6-12 months
	Accelerated	≥1	Single age-appropriate dose	Age appropriate	≥2 weeks prior to travel[†]
	Postexposure prophylaxis	≥1	Single age-appropriate dose	Age appropriate	<2 weeks after exposure[†]
VAQTA	Standard	1-18	25 U	0.5	0, 6-18 months
	Standard	>18	50 U	1	0, 6-18 months
	Accelerated	≥1	Single age-appropriate dose	Age appropriate	≥2 weeks prior to travel[†]
	Postexposure prophylaxis[‡]	≥1	Single age-appropriate dose	Age appropriate	<2 weeks after exposure[†]
TWINRIX	Standard	≥18	720 ELU HAV, 20 mg HBV	1	0, 1, 6 months
	Accelerated	≥18	720 ELU HAV, 20 mg HBV	1	0, 7, 21-30 days[†]

*Vaccines are injected intramuscularly into the deltoid muscle.
[†]Timing of the booster dose (necessary for long-term protection): VAQTA, 6 mo; HAVRIX, 6-12 mo; TWINRIX, 12 mo.
[‡]Not FDA approved.
ELU, enzyme-linked immunoassay (ELISA) units; U, units.

are shown in Table 78-2. After vaccination with HAVRIX, anti-HAV is estimated to remain detectable in serum for approximately 20 years; immunity may last longer.[70] Among adults, the most common local side effects have been soreness at the injection site (56%), headache (14%), and malaise (7%). In children, the most common side effects have been soreness at the injection site (15%), feeding problems (8%), headache (4%), and induration at the injection site (4%).[27]

In the United States, through November 2012, the Vaccine Adverse Event Reporting System received 20,057 reports of unexplained adverse events after immunization with the HAV vaccine alone or in combination with other vaccines. Of the 20,057 reports, 1230 were considered serious and included Guillain-Barré syndrome, immune thrombocytopenic purpura, elevated serum aminotransferase levels, and seizures in children.[27] No reported serious event, however, could be attributed definitively to the HAV vaccine, and the reported rates did not exceed the expected background rates. For example, the general population incidence of Guillain-Barré syndrome ranges from 0.5 to 2.4 cases per 100,000 person-years, and among adult HAV vaccine recipients, the incidence of Guillain-Barré was 0.2 cases per 100,000 person-years.[27]

A combined formulation of hepatitis A and B vaccines (TWINRIX, GlaxoSmithKline Biologicals, Rixensart, Belgium) is available and has an excellent record of efficacy and safety.[71] Although some long-term studies have shown persistence of anti-HAV in children and adolescents, seroconversion rates for TWINRIX are apparently lower in children aged 1 to 6 than those for standard monovalent vaccines.[72] Currently, therefore, TWINRIX is approved only for persons 18 years of age and older.

As a result of the reduction in endemic cases of hepatitis A in the United States, the largest proportion of patients who now become infected with HAV are nonimmune adults traveling to endemic areas. Even if medical advice is sought before travel, the time is usually insufficient for completing the standard immunization schedule. HAVRIX and VAQTA are approved by the FDA for use in an accelerated vaccination schedule before planned travel. If given at least 2 weeks before travel, a single dose of either monovalent vaccine results in protective anti-HAV titers.[65] In 2008, the FDA also approved an accelerated vaccination schedule for TWINRIX that can be completed within 30 days, with a booster at 12 months, after studies showed equivalent protection when TWINRIX was compared with standard and alternative schedules of the individual monovalent vaccines. After 1 year, HAV seroconversion

rates were 100%, and HBV seroconversion rates were 96.4% to 100% with TWINRIX.[73,74] The TWINRIX accelerated schedule is being considered for use in new inmates at U.S. correctional facilities, where high-risk activities place the inmates at risk for both HAV and HBV infections.[75] Dosing schedules are shown in Table 78-2.

Another population that may have increased risk of contracting HAV infection appears to be close contacts of newly arriving international adoptees. In 2009, the CDC provided updated recommendations for use of the HAV vaccine in this population after receiving case reports of new HAV infections among persons in close contact with new international adoptees, including a case of fulminant hepatitis A in a nontraveling household contact of an asymptomatic adoptee from Ethiopia. From 1998 to 2008, some 18,000 children were adopted from foreign countries by families in the United States; 99.8% of those children were from counties considered to be of high or intermediate endemicity for HAV. Given these data, the CDC now recommends vaccination of all previously unvaccinated persons who anticipate close personal contact with an international adoptee from a country of high or intermediate endemicity during the first 60 days following arrival of the adoptee in the United States.[76]

Immunization against Hepatitis A Virus in Patients with Chronic Illnesses

Persons with chronic liver disease are at increased risk of HAV-related morbidity and mortality if they acquire HAV infection. Therefore, preexposure prophylaxis with the HAV vaccine has been recommended for patients with chronic liver disease who are susceptible to HAV.[77] This recommendation should be extended to patients awaiting liver transplantation as well as those who have already undergone liver transplantation, although the immunogenicity of the HAV vaccine is reduced in such persons.[78]

An episode of acute hepatitis in a patient with underlying chronic liver disease poses the risk of considerable morbidity and mortality. Although current guidelines recommend immunization against HAV for all patients with chronic liver disease,[27] the results of several cost-effectiveness analyses have been conflicting. A report published in 2000 found that saving the life of one patient with HCV infection through HAV vaccination would cost $23 million Canadian dollars,[79] although some of the assumptions in this report have been challenged.[80] Two other studies of patients with chronic hepatitis C showed a decided benefit to immunization against HAV.[81,82] The methods used in these studies were dissimilar, and some analyses may have been insensitive to the incidence of HAV or may have underestimated the economic and societal costs of a case of FHF. Universal immunization against HAV during childhood, before the possible occurrence of chronic liver disease, offers the greatest promise of preventing HAV infection.[83]

Patients infected with HIV should be vaccinated against HAV. The response to vaccination, however, may be reduced because of a blunted immune system. Earlier studies suggested HAV seroconversion rates above 97% in HIV-infected children on antiretroviral therapy[84]; however, another study found that a CD4+ count of less than 25/mm³, and an HIV viral load of more than 400 copies/mL, predicted a reduced seroconversion rate.[85] Although the discrepancies among studies can be explained in part by different sensitivities of assays for anti-HAV, it appears that the more immunosuppressed a person is, the less likely the person is to respond to vaccination. In this population, consideration should be given to checking post-vaccination IgG anti-HAV titers to assess immunity. Small studies have shown limited additional benefit to a third dose of HAV vaccine in persons who fail to respond to the standard vaccine schedule.[85]

KEY REFERENCES

Full references for this chapter can be found on www.expertconsult.com.

2. MacKinney-Novelo I, Barahona-Garrido J, Castillo-Albarran F, et al. Clinical course and management of acute hepatitis A infection in adults. Ann Hepatol 2012; 11:652-7.
23. Bell BP, Kruszon-Moran D, Shapiro CN, et al. Hepatitis A virus infection in the United States: Serologic results from the Third National Health and Nutrition Examination Survey. Vaccine 2005; 23:5798-806.
27. Centers for Disease Control and Prevention (CDC). Prevention of hepatitis A through active or passive immunization. MMWR Recomm Rep 2006; 55:1-23.
38. Jeong SH, Lee HS. Hepatitis A: Clinical manifestations and management. Intervirology 2010; 53:15-9.
41. Carrion AF, Martin P. Viral hepatitis in the elderly. Am J Gastroenterol 2012; 107:691-7.
43. Armed Forces Health Surveillance Center (AFHSC). Hospitalizations for hepatitis A, B, and C, active component, U.S. Armed Forces, 1991-2011. MSMR 2012; 19:18-21.
49. National Center for Health Statistics, Health Data Interactive. www.cdc.gov/nchs/hdi.htm. Accessed on 30 December 2012.
50. Vogt TM, Wise ME, Bell BP, et al. Declining hepatitis A mortality in the United States during the era of hepatitis A vaccination. J Infect Dis 2008; 197:1282-8.
63. American Academy of Pediatrics Committee on Infectious Disease. Hepatitis A vaccine recommendations. Pediatrics 2007; 120:189-99.
64. WHO position paper on hepatitis A vaccines—June 2012. Wkly Epidemiol Rec 2012; 87:261-76.
66. Victor JC, Monto AS, Surdina TY, et al. Hepatitis A vaccine versus immune globulin for postexposure prophylaxis. N Engl J Med 2007; 357:1685-94.
71. Centers for Disease Control and Prevention (CDC). FDA approval for a combined hepatitis A and B vaccine. MMWR Morb Mortal Wkly Rep 2001; 50:806-7.
76. Centers for Disease Control and Prevention (CDC). Advisory Committee on Immunization Practices. Updated recommendations from the Advisory Committee on Immunization Practices (ACIP) for use of hepatitis A vaccine in close contacts of newly arriving international adoptees. MMWR Morb Mortal Wkly Rep 2009; 58:1006-7.

JENNIFER T. WELLS AND ROBERT PERRILLO

An estimated 400 million persons in the world today are chronically infected with HBV. The majority of these individuals will not experience complications, but 15% to 40% will have serious sequelae such as cirrhosis or hepatocellular carcinoma (HCC), and many will die prematurely.[1,2] In the United States, the rate of acute liver failure attributable to hepatitis B has been declining, as has the number of cases listed for transplantation for chronic liver failure.[3,4] This decline is most likely due to broader vaccination and use of antiviral therapy. Unfortunately, these favorable trends are counterbalanced by a continuing increase in new cases of chronic hepatitis B and HCC.[4,5]

Effective vaccines against HBV have been available since the early 1980s, but perinatal and early life exposures continue to be major sources of infection in much of the developing world because of limited resources that preclude a policy of universal vaccination for newborns. From a global perspective, widespread implementation of early-life vaccination programs in high- and intermediate-risk countries will ultimately have the greatest impact on liver disease–related mortality in future generations. Promiscuous heterosexual contact and injection drug use account for most new cases of hepatitis B in adults in low-prevalence areas such as the United States and Western Europe. Even in these areas, however, a further reduction in the incidence of acute infections will remain a challenge in the future because people who inject drugs and promiscuous heterosexuals greatly underutilize vaccination.

EPIDEMIOLOGY

Geographic Distribution and Sources of Infection

The prevalence of HBV infection varies markedly around the world. In highly endemic regions, such as Southeast Asia (excluding Japan), China, and much of Africa, 8% or more of the population are chronic HBV carriers, and the lifetime risk of infection ranges from 60% to 80%.[6] In these high-risk areas, perinatal transmission and horizontal spread among children are the major means of transmission. Approximately 60% of the world's population reside where HBV is highly endemic.[7] Regions of intermediate risk include parts of southern and Eastern Europe, the Middle East, Japan, the Indian subcontinent, much of the former Soviet Union, and northern Africa. In these areas, the lifetime risk of infection is between 20% and 60%. Horizontal transmission occurs among a broad age range, but neonatal exposure is also presumed to be common. Areas of low prevalence include North America, Western Europe, certain parts of South America, and Australia, where the lifetime risk of HBV infection is less than 20% and transmission is primarily horizontal between young adults. Sexual transmission is the main mode of transmission in Europe and North America, but injecting drug use continues to be a major contributor to new cases as well.[8]

Perinatal transmission accounts for the majority of new infections in the world and is believed to account for as many as half of all hepatitis B surface antigen (HBsAg)-positive carriers. Sixty percent to 90% of hepatitis B e antigen (HBeAg)–positive mothers transmit the infection to their offspring, whereas mothers who are positive for antibody to HBeAg (anti-HBe) transmit the disease less frequently (5% to 15%) (see later). Fortunately, the incidence of new infections and childhood HCC has diminished greatly in countries such as Taiwan where universal vaccination has been in place for decades.[9]

Infectivity

HBV is transmitted efficiently by percutaneous and mucous membrane exposure to infectious body fluids. The virus is 50 to 100 times as infectious as HIV and 10 times as infectious as HCV. HBeAg seropositivity indicates a higher risk not only of transmission from mother to child, but also after needlestick exposure and in the setting of household contact. HBV DNA has been detected by sensitive techniques such as PCR methodology in most body fluids, except for stool that has not been contaminated with blood. Although HBV replicates primarily in hepatocytes, the presence of replicative intermediates and virally encoded proteins in other sites, such as the adrenal gland, testis, colon, nerve ganglia, and skin, suggests that a vast extrahepatic reservoir for infectious virus exists.[10] Small amounts of HBV DNA have been demonstrated in peripheral mononuclear cells and liver tissue years after apparent resolution of chronic infection.[11,12] Extrahepatic localization of low levels of replicating virus explains the relatively high rate of HBV transmission from organ donors positive for antibody to hepatitis B core antigen (anti-HBc) (see later).[13]

Prevalence

Estimates of chronic HBV infection report a prevalence of 2.2 million persons in the United States.[14] This number is approximately 1 million higher than formerly believed. The older figure of 1.25 million persons was an underestimate because of changing immigration patterns since the 1980s and an underrepresentation of certain minority groups in the National Health and Nutrition Examination Survey (NHANES) study. Nearly 15 million Asians live in the United States, and even a conservative estimate of the prevalence of HBV infection such as 5% would raise the overall number of HBV carriers in the United States by more than 750,000. Of all immigrants to the United States between 1974 and 1998, an estimated 60% were born in regions of intermediate or high HBV prevalence. This finding explains why more than 90% of chronic HBV infections in the United States are imported[14] (Fig. 79-1).

In contrast to the growth of new cases of chronic hepatitis B, a decline in acute cases of hepatitis B since the 1990s has been the result of universal vaccination of newborns, adult vaccination programs for high-risk persons, changes in sexual lifestyle, refinements in blood screening procedures, and the availability of virus-inactivated blood components.[15] Health care workers have experienced a striking decline in HBV infection owing to high rates of vaccination.[16]

In the United States and much of the developed world, however, the highest incidence of acute cases continues to be in sexually active young adults.[17] Since 1995, approximately 40% of cases of acute hepatitis B reported to the CDC were caused by intimate contact among heterosexuals. Fifteen percent to 20% were due to injecting drug use, and 12% occurred in men who have sex with men. No identifiable source of exposure was demonstrated in approximately 15% of cases.[18] Cases of hepatitis B continue to result from hemodialysis, acupuncture, artificial insemination, and, rarely, blood transfusion, but these cases account for a small

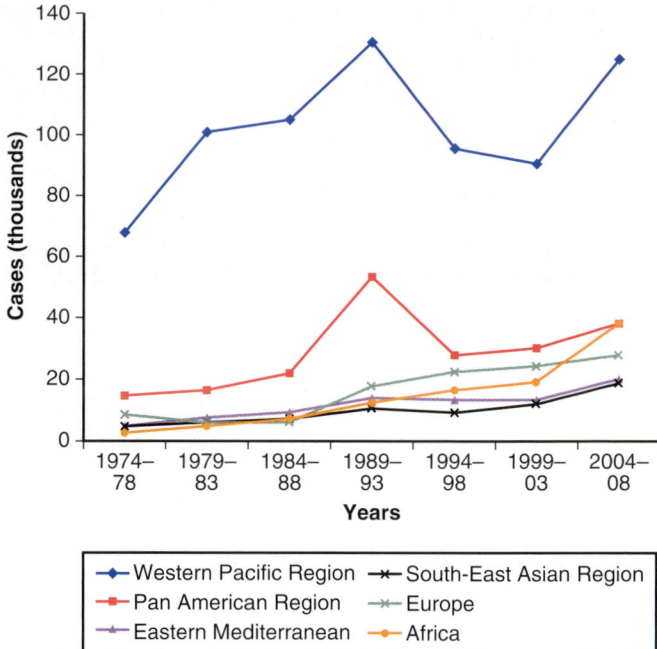

FIGURE 79-1. Estimated number of cases of chronic HBV infection imported into the USA by WHO region of origin, from 1974 to 2008. *(Modified from Mitchell T, Armstrong GL, Hu DJ, et al. The increasing burden of imported chronic hepatitis B—United States, 1974-2008. PLoS One 2011; 6:e27717 with permission of author.)*

contribution to the overall number of newly established acute infections.

Data from the CDC indicate that more than 95% of pregnant women in the United States are tested for HBsAg, and infant vaccine coverage levels are up to 93%. Despite these encouraging figures, however, the CDC also estimates that approximately 1000 new cases of hepatitis B in newborns each year are due to a missed birth dose or failure to complete the vaccine schedule.[19]

Several distinct trends in prevalence are noted when the results of the CDC-sponsored NHANES survey between 1988 and 1994 are compared with those obtained from 1999 to 2006. Although the prevalence of past and present infection was not different in the 2 groups as a whole, a significant decrease in the prevalence of infection was found in persons 6 to 19 and 20 to 49 years of age for the more recent time interval. Additionally, although the prevalence among foreign-born children continued to be higher than that among children born in the United States, it decreased by approximately 85%, most likely because of universal vaccination programs in the native countries of foreign-born children.[20] Little difference in prevalence was found in foreign-born and native adults 50 years of age and older.

CLINICAL OUTCOMES

Acute Hepatitis B

The age at which a person becomes infected with HBV is a principal determinant of the clinical outcome. Perinatal exposure leads to the chronic HBV carrier state in as many as 95% of persons because of immunologic tolerance to the virus (see later). By contrast, children exposed during the first 5 years of life have a 30% chance of developing chronic HBV. Only 2%

to 5% of adults with an intact immune system become chronically infected.[21]

Two thirds of patients with acute hepatitis B have an asymptomatic or subclinical illness that goes unrecognized. In the other one third, acute hepatitis, ranging from mild to moderate in severity, develops, with acute liver failure occurring in 1%. Although uncommon, hepatitis B accounts for 7% of all cases of acute liver failure and approximately 400 deaths annually in the United States.[3,22] Rapid viral elimination may result in clearance of HBsAg from serum by the time of initial presentation. In these cases, the accurate diagnosis of acute hepatitis B may require testing with immunoglobulin (Ig) M anti-HBc (see later).

The rate of spontaneous survival in acute liver failure caused by HBV is only approximately 20%. Liver transplantation has resulted in survival rates of 50% to 60%. Recurrent disease in the allograft is uncommon because of administration of hepatitis B immune globulin (HBIG) and orally administered antiviral agents (see later and Chapter 97).

Chronic Hepatitis B

Progressive liver disease (including cirrhosis and HCC) can be expected to develop in one quarter to one third of people who acquire infection in the first few years of life. An estimated 15% to 25% of predominately middle-aged or older male patients with acquisition of infection early in life ultimately die of liver-related causes. Outcomes are related to host (age, male gender, genetic background, immune status) and viral (serum HBV DNA level, HBV genotype, mutation patterns) factors. HCC is 4 times as likely to develop in males as in females.

The presence of active viral replication and long-standing necroinflammatory liver disease caused by HBV strongly influences the rate of progression to cirrhosis. The major determinant of survival is the severity of the liver disease when the patient first comes to medical attention.[23] Cirrhosis is associated with decreased survival and an increased frequency of HCC. Prior to the advent of antiviral therapy, 5- and 20-year survival rates of 55% and 25%, respectively, were reported in patients with HBV-related cirrhosis, compared with 97% and 63%, respectively, for those with mild (noncirrhotic) disease.[24] In one study, an 84% 5-year survival rate was reported for patients with compensated HBV-related cirrhosis, compared with 14% for patients with cirrhosis complicated by ascites, jaundice, encephalopathy, or a history of variceal bleeding (see Chapters 74 and 92).[25] Multivariate analyses in several large cohort studies have identified age, ascites, hyperbilirubinemia, and renal dysfunction as correlating independently with survival in patients with HBV-related cirrhosis. Therefore, early hepatic decompensation is an indication for antiviral therapy as well as assessment for liver transplantation (see later).

Clearance of HBsAg from serum in patients with HBV-related cirrhosis has been associated with an excellent prognosis, including improvement in liver histology and function, a decreased chance of viral reactivation, and improved long-term survival.[23] HBsAg clearance, however, is not an absolute safeguard against the future development of HCC in persons who have preexisting cirrhosis.[26]

VIROLOGY

HBV is a small DNA virus that belongs to the Hepadnaviridae family. Other members of this virus family are human HBV-like agents that infect the woodchuck, ground and tree squirrels, woolly monkey, crane, heron, Ross goose, and duck. HBV is a small (3.2-kilobase [kb]) virus with a DNA genome that has a relaxed, circular, partially double-stranded configuration (Fig. 79-2). The genome is composed of 4 open reading frames (ORFs) and has a compact design in which several genes overlap and use the same DNA to encode different viral proteins. The 4 viral genes components include the core, surface, X, and polymerase genes. The core gene encodes the core nucleocapsid protein, which is important in viral packaging and production of HBeAg. The surface gene encodes the pre-S1, pre-S2, and S proteins (comprising the large [L], middle [M], and small [S] surface proteins). The X gene encodes the X protein, which has transactivating properties and may be important in hepatic carcinogenesis. The polymerase gene has a large ORF (≈800 amino acids) and overlaps the entire length of the surface ORF. It encodes a large protein with functions that are critical for packaging and DNA replication (including priming, RNA- and DNA-dependent DNA polymerase, and RNase H activities).

Viral Replication

Although HBV is a DNA virus, replication occurs through an RNA intermediate and requires an active viral reverse transcriptase/polymerase enzyme (Fig. 79-3). The mutation rate is higher for HBV than for other DNA viruses (an estimated 10^{13} to 10^{15} point mutations per day).[27] Complete HBV genomic sequencing has identified a large number of mutations within the HBV genome, many of which are silent or do not alter the amino acid sequence of encoded proteins. Because of genomic overlap, however, some of the silent mutations in 1 ORF (e.g., the polymerase gene) may result in an amino acid substitution in an overlapping ORF (surface gene), although with uncertain clinical implications.

HBV replication begins with encapsidation of the pregenomic RNA through complex interactions between host and viral proteins. HBV DNA polymerase reverse transcribes the pregenomic RNA into a negative-strand HBV DNA, which in turn serves as the template for positive-strand synthesis to form a partially double-stranded genome. Concurrent with HBV DNA synthesis, the nucleocapsid undergoes maturation and, through an incompletely understood mechanism, interacts with the S protein to initiate viral assembly in the endoplasmic reticulum. S protein is synthesized in the endoplasmic reticulum, where monomer aggregates that exclude host membrane proteins subsequently bud into the lumen as subviral particles. When formed, HBsAg undergoes glycosylation in the endoplasmic reticulum and the Golgi apparatus. Noninfectious subviral particles (spherical and filamentous forms of HBsAg) are secreted in great abundance when compared with mature virions. These subviral HBsAg particles exceed virions in number by a variable factor of 10^2 to 10^5 and can accumulate up to concentrations of several hundred micrograms per milliliter of serum.[28]

Genotypes

A genetic classification based on comparisons of complete genomes has demonstrated 10 genotypes (designated A through J) and numerous subtypes of HBV (Box 79-1).[29] These classifications are defined as a divergence in the entire HBV genomic sequence of 8% or more. Genotype A is the predominant genotype in northern Europe and the United States. Genotypes B and C are confined to populations in eastern Asia and the Far East, but changes in immigration patterns have resulted in an influx of Asian HBV carriers with these genotypes into the United States.[30] Genotype D is found worldwide but is especially prevalent in the Mediterranean area, Middle East, and south Asia. Genotype E is indigenous to western

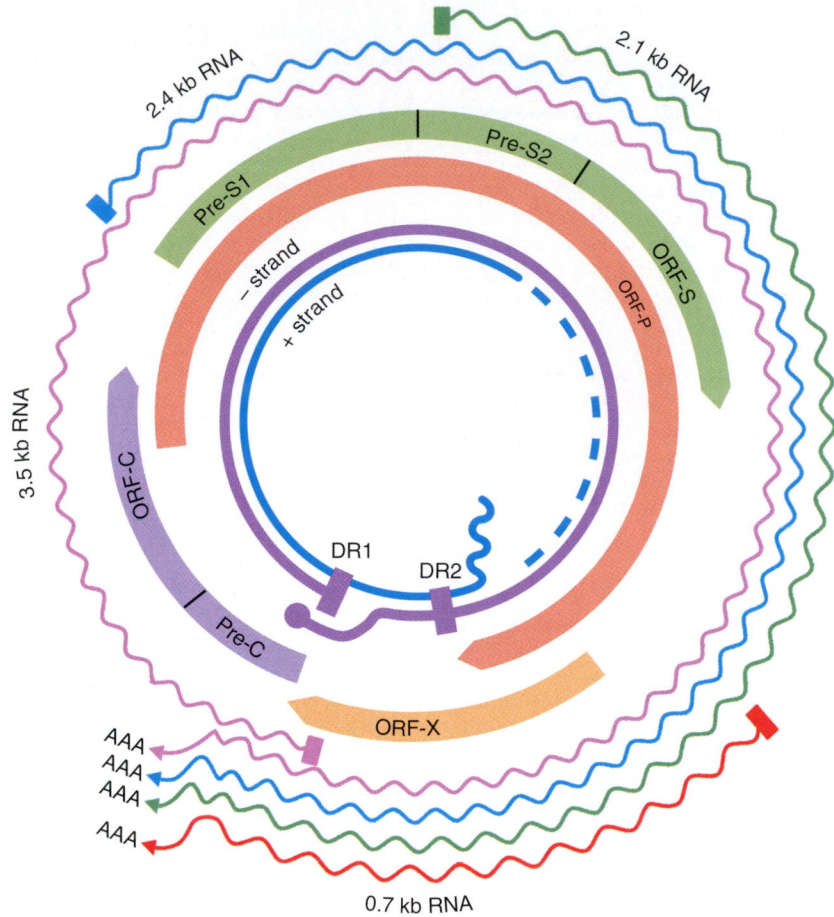

FIGURE 79-2. The molecular structure and organization of HBV. Note the overlapping open reading frames (ORFs) of the viral genome and its major transcripts *(wavy lines)*. The genome is partially double stranded with 4 overlapping ORFs, or genes. The S gene encodes the viral surface envelope protein (hepatitis B surface antigen, HBsAg) and is composed of the pre-S1, pre-S2, and S regions. The core gene (C) consists of the precore (Pre-C) and core regions, which give rise to the hepatitis B e antigen (HBeAg) and core protein, respectively. The polymerase (P) gene overlaps the entire S gene, and mutations in this region may, in theory, give rise to changes in the HBsAg protein that affect neutralization by antibody to HBsAg. The fourth gene (X) codes for an incompletely understood protein, HBX. Two 11-base-pair direct repeats (DR1 and DR2) are required for strand-specific HBV DNA synthesis during viral replication.

sub-Saharan areas, and genotype F prevails in Central America. Cases of genotype G have been reported in the United States and France. Genotype H has been described in Mexico. Genotypes I and J are the most recently discovered and have been observed in Vietnam and the Ryukyu Islands in Japan, respectively.[29]

Clinical associations appear to exist with the various genotypes (see Box 79-1). The strongest clinical associations appear to be that (1) HBeAg seroconversion occurs earlier in patients with HBV genotype B than in those with genotype C, and (2) the response to therapy with interferon (IFN) is better with genotypes A and B than with C and D (see later).[31] The viral genotype also has implications for the frequency of precore and core mutations (see later) and may have an effect on the frequency of HCC. There is no compelling evidence that genotypes affect the HBV DNA response to nucleoside analogs (see later).

The clinical associations with the various genotypes have not led to specific recommendations on routine testing because genotype classification does not generally lead to a difference in management. One exception to this rule, however, occurs when a patient is being considered for IFN therapy. In patients who are suitable candidates based on age and other factors

(see later), genotype testing may have clinical value because genotypes A and B are associated with higher rates of a sustained virologic response and HBsAg clearance.[32]

Mutations

The vast majority of mutations in the HBV genome that are identified by comparing nucleotide sequences with those of wild-type HBV are silent or do not alter the amino acid sequence in a particular ORF. Some mutations have potentially important disease associations, however, and are described below.

Hepatitis B Surface Antigen Gene

HBsAg gene mutants result from a primary mutation in the HBsAg gene or a mutation in the overlapping DNA polymerase gene during nucleoside antiviral therapy (see later). Once the mutation appears, mutated virions can become selected immunologically as the dominant form of the virus.

Mutations in the HBsAg gene between amino acid positions 124 to 147 are potentially important because this region of the HBsAg gene includes the major "a" epitope that binds

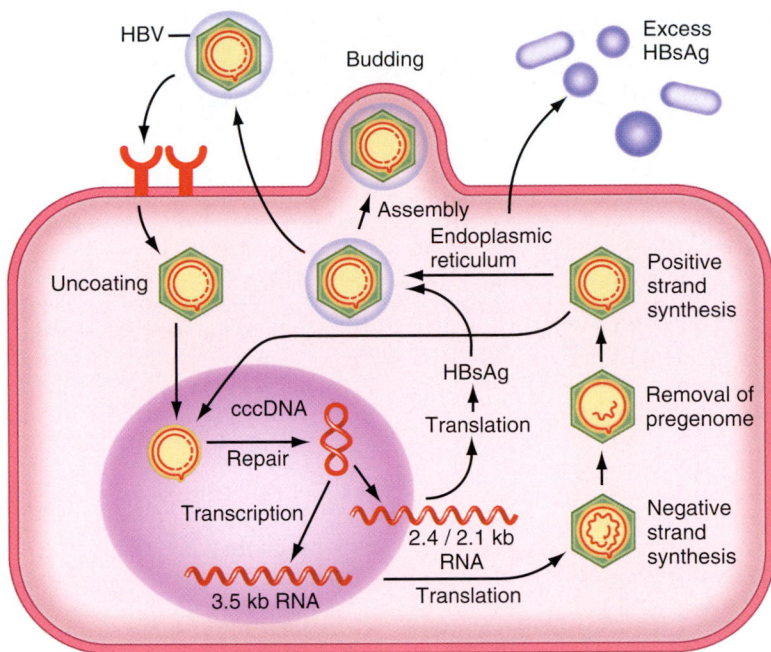

FIGURE 79-3. Life cycle of HBV. The receptor for viral entry has not been identified, but studies have suggested that sodium taurocholate cotransporting polypeptide is likely to be the receptor for binding the pre-S1 HBsAg protein.* Once inside the hepatocyte, the virus undergoes uncoating, and the HBV genome enters the nucleus, followed by repair of the single-stranded DNA strand and formation of the covalently closed circular (ccc) DNA template. Viral transcripts are formed for the hepatitis B surface antigen (HBsAg), DNA polymerase, X protein, and RNA pregenome; the pregenome and polymerase are incorporated into the maturing nucleocapsid and removed after translation. The surface protein enveloping process occurs in the endoplasmic reticulum. Some of the nonenveloped nucleocapsid recirculates back to the nucleus, and the cycle begins again. Excess tubular and spherical forms of HBsAg are secreted in great abundance and outnumber complete virions in serum by a factor of 10^3 or more.

*Yan H, Zhong G, Xu G, et al. Sodium taurocholate cotransporting polypeptide is a functional receptor for human hepatitis B and D virus. Elife 2012; 1:e00049.

to neutralizing antibody to HBsAg (anti-HBs). The mutation can lead to failure to detect HBsAg by commercial assays, which depend on binding to anti-HBs, and to failure of neutralization by HBIG or of vaccination.

Infection with HBsAg gene-mutant HBV is accompanied by detection of anti-HBc. Serum HBV DNA levels can be as varied as they are in HBsAg carriers (see later). These mutants need to be distinguished from cases of "occult" hepatitis B, which has been linked to cryptogenic cirrhosis and an increased risk of HCC.[33,34] In occult HBV infection, HBsAg-negative persons have detectable HBV DNA in serum.[33] Some of these persons may lack evidence of other serologic markers of infection (e.g., anti-HBc). Occult HBV infection is considered to be due to active suppression of viral replication by the host immune system; as a result, when HBV DNA is detectable in serum, it is present in low levels (<200 IU/mL).

Large-scale vaccination programs in regions endemic for HBV have revealed a 2% to 3% frequency of vaccine-escape HBsAg mutants. It remains controversial whether or not these mutants will be further selected in the future, thereby leading to widespread vaccine failure, but most available evidence does not support this scenario. The importance of HBsAg gene mutants for HBIG failure is less controversial. Such escape mutants are detected in as many as 50% of HBIG-treated patients in whom recurrent HBV infection develops after liver transplantation, and the frequency of their occurrence appears to correlate with the length of time over which HBIG is repeatedly administered.[35]

Precore, Basal Core Promoter, and Core Genes

Mutations in the precore and basal core promoter regions of the HBV genome can influence the production of HBeAg. A precore mutation results in a stop codon at nucleotide 1896 that abolishes the synthesis of HBeAg,[36] whereas mutations in the basal core promoter at nucleotides 1762 and 1764 decrease HBeAg synthesis by approximately 70% while maintaining pregenomic RNA levels.[37] Both types of mutations have been observed in cases of severe hepatitis, which has been attributed to the loss of the immune-tolerizing effects of HBeAg antigen (see later). The presence of core promoter mutations has been linked to an increased risk of HCC, and a higher prevalence has been found in patients infected with HBV genotype C.[29] Precore and basal core promoter mutants have been described in the same patients and are particularly common in Asian and European patients with chronic hepatitis B.[38] A large serosurvey of HBV carriers residing in the United States has found that precore and core promoter mutations are common (frequencies of 27% and 44%, respectively). Both mutant forms of HBV were observed to occur far more commonly in HBeAg-negative patients (precore mutation in 38% of HBeAg-negative vs. 9% of HBeAg-positive patients; core promoter mutation in 51% vs. 36%).[39] In addition to these mutations, upstream mutations in the core gene can influence immunologic responses to HBV. Core gene mutations have been shown to block recognition of HBV by cytotoxic T lymphocytes (CTLs), a key mode of viral clearance. Therefore, the mutations contribute to HBV immune escape and possibly influence the response to IFN.[40] Core gene mutations within the immunodominant epitopes of the HBV nucleocapsid also can affect CD4+ T-cell reactivity.[41]

In patients with perinatally acquired chronic hepatitis B, a prolonged immune tolerant phase with minimal to absent hepatic necroinflammatory activity is typically seen for the first 20 to 30 years of HBV infection. Sequencing studies have shown stable core gene sequences during this phase. Precore mutations are also uncommon during this phase. Core gene mutations become more common as patients pass from the immune active phase and undergo HBeAg seroconversion, at which time a growing number of mutations are observed in the region of the core gene that includes many B- and T-cell epitopes. Both precore stop codon mutants and core gene mutants have been associated with a poor response to IFN therapy.

HBV DNA Polymerase

The polymerase gene encodes a DNA polymerase enzyme needed for encapsidation of viral RNA into core particles, conversion of the pregenomic viral RNA into a negative strand of viral DNA (reverse transcription), and conversion of this first HBV DNA strand into a second DNA strand of positive polarity. In general, the HBV reverse transcriptase function of the polymerase gene is highly conserved because major mutations that impair the efficiency of viral replication lead to selection pressure against such variants. As indicated earlier, HBV has low replication fidelity, however, meaning that it has a propensity to mispair nucleotide bases when it reverse transcribes viral RNA to DNA. HBV DNA polymerase also lacks any proofreading activity, so it cannot repair its mistakes. Therefore, when a nucleotide base is misplaced, it remains in the growing viral DNA strand as a base mutation, and the new HBV DNA genome has a different sequence from the original (wild-type) genome. The overall error rate of HBV DNA polymerase is estimated to be 1 per 10,000 nucleotides copied, which translates to the potential for 10 million base-pair errors per day in an infected person. All possible single-base mutations can be produced in a 24-hour period, although many such mutations will yield nonviable viruses.[42]

Single or double nucleotide substitutions alter the amino acid sequence in the reverse transcriptase domain of the HBV DNA polymerase enzyme, thereby decreasing binding of drugs to its active site on the enzyme. Mutations in the HBV polymerase gene can lead to clinically apparent resistance to nucleoside analog therapy whenever there is both decreased susceptibility to the antiviral drug and sufficient replication fitness to allow continued propagation in the expanding viral population (or "quasispecies").

High levels of viral replication and high mutability of the virus allow the preexistence of single and even double polymerase mutants as a minor component of the viral quasispecies even before antiviral therapy is begun. Because of the limitations in sensitivity of currently available molecular assays (e.g., the line probe assay), these mutants are not detectable until they constitute at least 5% to 10% of the entire viral population. Ultradeep pyrosequencing is a research technique with the ability to detect HBV mutants that constitute less than 1% of the total population.[43]

Persistent infection with drug-resistant HBV has been associated with progression of disease and blunting of hepatic histologic improvement with antiviral therapy.[44] Severe flares of hepatitis have also been reported after the emergence of drug-resistant mutants,[45] and acquisition of these mutants may lead to rapidly progressive liver disease after liver transplantation.[46] Horizontal transmission of these mutants also has been described.

PATHOGENESIS

HBV is generally not a cytopathic virus, and the severity of HBV-associated liver disease is considered to be related to the intensity of the host immunologic response to the virus. Whereas both cellular and humoral immune responses are needed for effective clearance and long-term protection against reinfection, the cellular immune response appears to be the arm principally involved in the pathogenesis of disease. The immunologic response to HBV encompasses both an innate, or nonspecific, response (e.g., natural killer cells and IFNs) and an adaptive immune response, including antibodies to viral antigens, HLA class II–restricted CD4+ T cells, and HLA class I–restricted CD8+ cytotoxic T cells (CTLs).[47] Induction of the antigen-specific T-cell response is thought to occur in lymphoid organs, where the host T cells encounter viral peptide antigens (or epitopes) that are presented by antigen-presenting cells such as dendritic cells, B cells, and macrophages. This process results in the maturation and expansion of T cells that are specific for these viral epitopes and is followed by their migration to the liver, where they perform their effector function.

During acute HBV infection, most HBV DNA molecules are cleared rapidly from the liver via noncytopathic mechanisms mediated by cytokines that are released initially by cells of the innate immune system[48] and later by liver-infiltrating HBV-specific CD8+ cells. Cell-mediated immune responses are efficient in self-limited infection because the responses are vigorous, multispecific, and oriented toward type 1 helper T-cell functions. Persons with chronic HBV infection, by contrast, exhibit infrequent, narrowly focused, and weak HBV-specific T-cell responses.[49] In chronic hepatitis B, the majority of mononuclear cells in liver infiltrates of patients with chronic hepatitis B at any given time are non–antigen specific.[50]

CD8+ CTLs are thought to contribute to the disease process in the liver and result in apoptosis of infected hepatocytes. To be recognized by the CD8+ CTLs, targeted hepatocytes must present viral epitopes as short peptides that have been endogenously processed and fit within the peptide-binding groove of the class I major histocompatibility complex (MHC) molecules.[51] The binding of the CTL T-cell receptor to the peptide-MHC complex on the hepatocyte surface can then result in the direct killing of the infected cell and release of potent antiviral cytokines by the activated CTL. Recognition by MHC class II–restricted CD4[+] helper T cells requires the appropriate presentation of viral peptides in the context of class II MHC molecules. The CD4[+] cells produce antiviral cytokines and provide help in neutralizing antibody production. Antibody neutralization limits intrahepatic spread of virus during primary infection and serves an important role in preventing reinfection.

NATURAL HISTORY

Four phases of HBV infection have been described: immune tolerance, immune clearance, the inactive carrier state, and reactivation (Fig. 79-4). These consecutive phases are much more likely to be apparent in patients with acquisition of chronic hepatitis B early in life.

The *immune tolerance* phase is often the earliest phase to be recognized when there is a history of infection at birth or the first few years of life. It is characterized by HBeAg positivity, high levels of HBV DNA ($\geq 10^7$ IU/mL), low or normal levels of serum aminotransferases, and minimal or no necroinflammation or fibrosis in the liver. During this phase, the rates of HBeAg loss are low. Experiments in transgenic mice suggest that HBeAg induces a state of immunologic tolerance to HBV in neonates.[52] Perinatal transmission of HBeAg is considered to be one of several potential mechanisms behind the immune-tolerance phase.[53]

The *immune active* phase often begins after several decades of HBV infection and is characterized by elevated serum aminotransferase levels, lower HBV DNA levels than in the immune tolerance phase, and histologic evidence of chronic hepatitis. The trigger mechanisms for this apparent immunologic activation against HBV are poorly understood, but CD8[+] CTL-mediated lysis of infected hepatocytes has been shown to occur. The duration of the immune active phase varies and frequently is many years. Continued efforts by the host immune system against the virus may result in HBeAg seroconversion (loss of HBeAg with the development of anti-HBe in serum). The mean annual rate of spontaneous HBeAg seroconversion generally ranges from 8% to 15% in older children or adults with elevated serum ALT levels; however, the rate is considerably lower among Asian children and immunocompromised persons.[23]

HBeAg seroconversion does not always indicate quiescent disease, however. As many as 30% of persons who undergo HBeAg seroconversion enter into a subsequent phase of active disease that is caused by the selection of HBeAg-negative

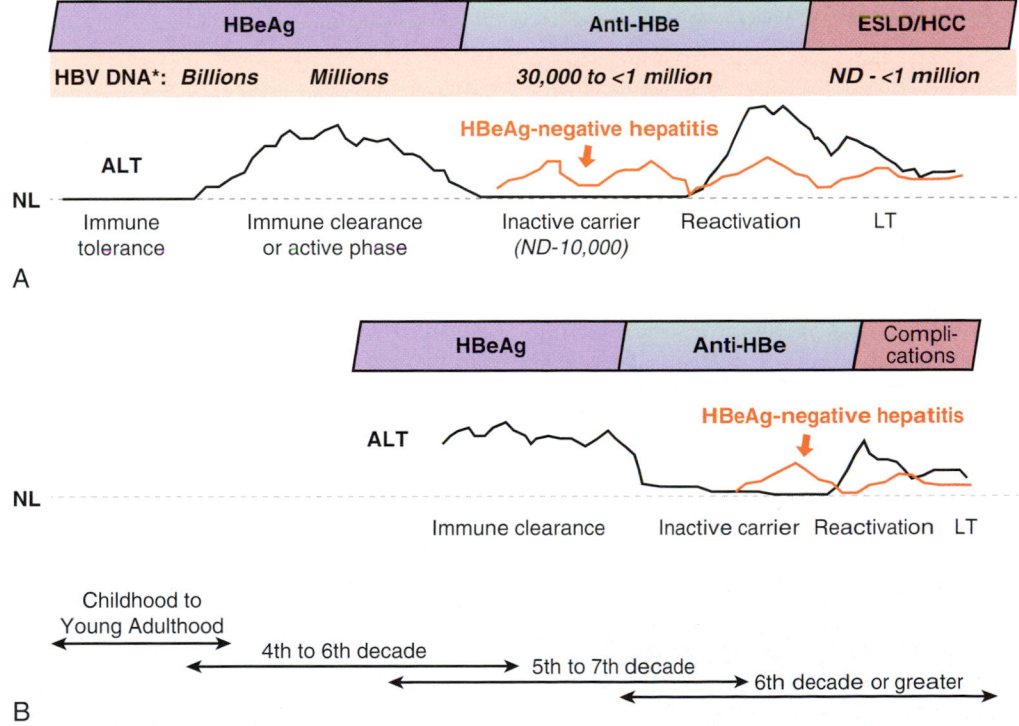

FIGURE 79-4. Natural history of chronic HBV infection in patients with early-life (A) and adult (B) acquisition of the infection. *A*, In patients who are infected early in life, the first phase is that of immune tolerance. After decades of normal (NL) serum ALT and high HBV DNA levels, this immune-tolerant phase evolves to a hepatitis B e antigen (HBeAg)-positive immune active phase of variable duration. Ultimately, patients enter a spontaneous or therapeutically-induced inactive carrier state, which can last indefinitely. At the time of HBeAg seroconversion, however, immunologic pressure may select for a viral mutant (precore, core promoter, or both), which is incapable of producing HBeAg antigen. Viral and serum ALT levels typically fluctuate during this stage (HBeAg-negative hepatitis). If the patient is not treated, late disease complications often occur. *B*, Persons who acquire the infection in adulthood do not enter into an immune-tolerant phase. Otherwise, the serologic and laboratory features are the same as those for persons who acquire HBV infection early in life. Because of the compressed time scale of events, however, HBeAg-negative chronic hepatitis B and late-stage complications are observed less frequently. The relative time dimensions of each phase are shown; note that there may be significant overlap. *Levels of serum HBV DNA in copies/mL. ESLD, end-stage liver disease; HCC, hepatocellular carcinoma; LT, liver transplantation; ND, nondetectable.

mutants (precore mutation, core promoter mutantion, or a combination of both).[54] At least 50% of these persons demonstrate multiple fluctuations in HBV DNA and aminotransferase levels each year, and recognition of active disease and exclusion of the inactive HBsAg carrier state (see later) may require serial assessments of both serum HBV DNA and aminotransferase levels.

The majority of patients who undergo HBeAg seroconversion, however, enter into a third phase (*inactive HBV carrier stage*) that is characterized by normalization of serum ALT and low (<2000 IU/mL) or nondetectable serum HBV DNA levels (see Fig. 79-4). Over time, hepatic necroinflammation and fibrosis subside.[55] The inactive HBsAg carrier phase may last a lifetime, but some patients ultimately develop *reactivation*, which may occur spontaneously because of a loss of immunologic control over viral replication or may be due to immunosuppressive drug therapy (see later). Reactivation is defined by the reappearance of high levels of HBV DNA in serum, with or without HBeAg seroreversion, and often a noticeable rise in serum ALT levels.

If the immune active phase of hepatitis B remains untreated, cirrhosis can be anticipated to develop in at least 20% of cases. Various factors have been determined to increase the risk of cirrhosis, and, of these, older age, male gender, the stage of fibrosis at presentation, and ongoing HBV replication are perhaps the most important clinically. Combined infection with HDV (see Chapter 81), HCV (see Chapter 80), or HIV, as well as concomitant alcohol abuse, has also been linked to a higher rate of development of cirrhosis and HCC.

When cirrhosis develops, 2 major complications may occur: hepatic decompensation and HCC. The estimated annual frequency of developing hepatic decompensation in HBV-associated cirrhosis is 5% to 8%, whereas that of HCC is 2% to 4%.[56] Factors associated with an increased risk of HCC include male gender, age 45 years or greater, having a first-degree relative with HCC, the presence of cirrhosis, HBeAg positivity, reversion from anti-HBe to HBeAg positivity, and increased HBV DNA levels regardless of the HBeAg state.[57] Some studies suggest that core promoter mutations (which are generally associated with higher levels of viral replication) and genotype C are additive risk factors for a high rate of eventual transformation to HCC.[58] HCC can still develop in HBsAg-positive persons with none of the identified risk factors, but less frequently. In addition, HCC can occur in cirrhotic patients who have undergone HBsAg seroconversion, and all patients with cirrhosis need continued surveillance (Box 79-2 [see Chapter 96]).[59]

BOX 79-2 Populations of Persons with HBV Infection for which Surveillance for Hepatocellular Carcinoma (HCC) is Recommended or Uncertain

Recommended
Asian male HBV carriers over age 40
Asian female HBV carriers over age 50
HBV carriers with a family history of HCC
HBV carriers born in Africa and over age 20
HBV carriers with cirrhosis
Patients with high serum levels of HBV DNA and ongoing liver injury

Uncertain
African Americans
HBV carriers in immune-tolerant phase (see text and Fig. 79-4)
HBV carriers with concomitant HDV infection, HCV infection, or nonalcoholic steatohepatitis
HBV carriers younger than age 40 (males) or 50 (females)

Serum ALT as a Surrogate Marker for Disease Activity

The serum ALT level has been used conventionally as a measure of disease activity in patients with chronic hepatitis B. A serum ALT level within the normal laboratory reference range, however, has been shown to be an imperfect surrogate marker for lack of disease activity. Clinical laboratories base their range of normal values on donors without known liver disease, but this population may include obese persons, alcohol consumers, and diabetics, each of whom tends to expand the supposedly upper limit of normal. In fact, all-cause and liver-related mortality is increased when the serum ALT level exceeds 20 U/L in women and 30 U/L in men, and these values should be accepted as the upper limits of the normal range (see Chapter 73).[60] Studies in Asia and the United States have shown that as many as 20% to 30% of Asian HBV carriers with persistently normal serum ALT levels and serum HBV DNA levels over 2000 IU/mL (roughly equivalent to 10,000 copies/mL) have grade 2 or greater inflammation and stage 2 or greater fibrosis (on scales of 0 to 4) on a liver biopsy specimen.[61] HBeAg-negative Asian HBV carriers with high-normal serum ALT levels by standard reference ranges tend to be older, have a greater frequency of serum HBV DNA levels in excess of 2000 IU/mL, and have a higher frequency of basal core promoter HBV mutations—all features that can be associated with adverse long-term outcomes.[62] Therefore, liver biopsy or a noninvasive determination of hepatic fibrosis can be a useful tool to ensure that the severity of underlying liver disease is not underestimated in such persons (see Chapter 73).

HBV DNA Level and Long-Term Complications

Population-based Asian cohort studies have established that the serum HBV DNA level is the single best predictor of future progression to cirrhosis and HCC in HBV-infected persons.[63,64] In the prospective REVEAL-HBV natural history cohort study, more than 3600 untreated HBsAg carriers from Taiwan were followed for more than 11 years. Of these, 60% were male, 40% were older than age 50, 85% were HBeAg negative, and 95% had normal serum ALT levels using standard reference ranges. The calculated relative risks for cirrhosis and HCC were shown to correlate with the level of HBV DNA on entry into the study when compared with a reference population of HBsAg carriers with undetectable serum HBV DNA by PCR assay.[64] Even serum HBV DNA levels as low as 10,000 copies/mL (equivalent to 2000 IU/mL) were associated with a higher relative risk of cirrhosis and HCC. The relative risk was highest (hazard ratio of 10) in persons with a serum HBV DNA level that was greater than 100,000 copies/mL and intermediate (hazard ratio of 3.8) in persons in whom the serum HBV DNA level decreased spontaneously from greater than 100,000 copies/mL at the time of enrollment to less than 10,000 copies/mL at the last point of follow-up. These data can be interpreted to mean that both the duration and level of viremia are important risk factors for the development of HCC. The data also suggest that suppression of serum HBV DNA levels, whether spontaneously or as a result of antiviral therapy, lowers the risk of HCC.

Some authorities recommend that Asian men 50 years of age or older with serum HBV DNA levels 100,000 copies/mL or greater receive long-term therapy with a nucleoside (or nucleotide) analog to prevent HCC, even if serum ALT values are normal.[65] Additional support for this recommendation can be found in a landmark study in which more than 600 Asian patients with advanced fibrosis and a serum HBV DNA level greater than 100,000 copies/mL were randomized in a ratio of 2:1 to active treatment with the nucleoside analog lamivudine or placebo.[66] Disease progression and HCC occurred significantly more frequently in the group of patients randomized to placebo.

CLINICAL AND PATHOLOGIC FEATURES

Acute Hepatitis B

The incubation period of acute hepatitis B varies from a few weeks to 6 months (average, 60 to 90 days), depending on the amount of replicating virus in the inoculum. The disease may be more severe in patients coinfected with other hepatitis viruses and in those with established underlying liver disease.[67] Acute infections are heralded by malaise, nausea, vomiting, and a serum sickness-like prodrome of fever, arthralgias or arthritis, and rash, which is most commonly maculopapular or urticarial, in 10% to 20% of patients. This prodrome results from circulating HBsAg–anti-HBs complexes that activate complement and are deposited in the synovium and walls of cutaneous blood vessels. These features generally abate before the manifestations of liver disease and peak serum aminotransferase elevations are observed. Jaundice develops in only about 30% of patients.

Clinical symptoms and jaundice generally disappear after 1 to 3 months. In general, elevated serum ALT levels and serum HBsAg titers decline and disappear together, and in approximately 80% of cases, HBsAg disappears by 12 weeks after the onset of illness. Persistence of HBsAg after 6 months implies development of a carrier state, with only a small likelihood of recovery during the next 6 to 12 months.

Serum aminotransferase levels of 1000 to 2000 U/L are typical during acute hepatitis B, with the ALT higher than the AST level. In patients with icteric hepatitis, the rise in serum bilirubin levels often lags behind the rise in ALT levels. The peak ALT level does not correlate with prognosis, and the prothrombin time (INR) is the best indicator of prognosis. If acute liver failure develops, patients usually present within 4 weeks of the onset of symptoms and have associated multiorgan dysfunction, coagulopathy, encephalopathy, and high mortality rates if they are not treated by prompt antiviral therapy and liver transplantation. Patients older than 40 years appear to be more susceptible than younger persons to "late-onset" liver failure, which occurs several months after the onset of acute symptoms and is associated with encephalopathy and renal dysfunction. The pathogenic mechanisms of this severe form of HBV-related hepatitis are poorly understood but are presumed to involve massive immune-mediated lysis of infected hepatocytes and possibly impaired regeneration of new hepatocytes (see Chapter 95).

Chronic Hepatitis B

A history of acute or symptomatic hepatitis is often lacking in patients with chronic HBV infection. When symptoms are present, fatigue tends to predominate over other constitutional symptoms, such as poor appetite and malaise. Patients may remain asymptomatic even during periods of reactivated hepatitis. In other instances, particularly when superimposed on cirrhosis, reactivation of HBV infection may be associated with frank jaundice and signs of liver failure.

Physical examination may be normal, or hepatosplenomegaly may be found. In decompensated cirrhosis, spider telangiectasias, jaundice, ascites, and peripheral edema are common. During exacerbations of disease, serum ALT levels may be as high as 1000 U/L or more, and the clinical and laboratory picture is indistinguishable from that of acute hepatitis B, including the presence in serum of IgM anti-HBc in some cases. Progression to cirrhosis should be suspected whenever hypersplenism, hypoalbuminemia (in the absence of nephropathy), or prolongation of the prothrombin time is found. The serum AST level is typically higher than the serum ALT level in patients with advanced cirrhosis.

Extrahepatic Manifestations

Although uncommon, extrahepatic syndromes can occur with acute or, more commonly, chronic hepatitis B and are important to recognize because they may occur without clinically apparent liver disease and can be mistaken for independent disease processes in other organ systems. The pathogenesis is not completely understood but likely involves an aberrant immunologic response to extrahepatic viral proteins.[68] Many of the extrahepatic manifestations are observed in association with circulating immune complexes that activate serum complement. Serum complement levels are generally low, and antiviral therapy may be beneficial in reducing the amount of immunologically activating viral antigens.

Arthritis-Dermatitis

The dermatitis-arthritis prodromal manifestations of acute hepatitis B must be distinguished from inflammatory forms of arthritis, because glucocorticoid therapy, if mistakenly given to these patients, can lead to enhanced HBV replication, and abrupt withdrawal of these agents may be associated with a flare in disease activity.

Polyarteritis Nodosa

As many as 30% of patients with polyarteritis nodosa are infected with HBV, but the disorder develops in less than 1% of patients with chronic HBV infection. This association has been reported predominantly in North America and Europe and not observed in Asia, where HBV is acquired perinatally. Typical features include arthralgias, fever, rash, abdominal pain, renal disease, hypertension, mononeuritis multiplex, and central nervous system abnormalities. Plasmapheresis may be useful, and therapeutic responses have also been observed with antiviral agents, given alone or in combination with plasmapheresis.

Glomerulonephritis

Several types of glomerular lesions have been described in patients with chronic HBV infection; membranous glomerulonephritis and membranoproliferative glomerulonephritis are the most common.[69] Renal biopsy specimens have demonstrated immune-complex deposition and cytoplasmic inclusions in the glomerular basement membrane. Nephrotic syndrome is the most common presentation of HBV-associated glomerulonephritis. The diagnosis requires the presence of immune-complex glomerulonephritis in a renal biopsy specimen and the demonstration of glomerular deposits of 1 or more HBV antigens, such as HBsAg, HBcAg, or HBeAg, by immunohistochemistry. The renal disease typically resolves in months to several years in children. Resolution may occur after HBeAg seroconversion. The natural history of HBV-related glomerulonephritis in adults has not been well defined, but several reports suggest that glomerular disease is often slowly and relentlessly progressive.[70] Successful treatment has been accomplished with IFN-α and has been linked to long-term control of HBV replication.[71] Therapy with nucleos(t)ide analogs has also resulted in improved renal function and diminished proteinuria.[72]

Cryoglobulinemia

Type II cryoglobulins consist of a polyclonal IgG and monoclonal IgM, whereas type III cryoglobulins contain polyclonal IgG and rheumatoid factor. Type II and type III cryoglobulinemia have been associated with hepatitis B, but the association is uncommon. Cryoglobulinemia may be associated with systemic vasculitis (purpura, arthralgias, peripheral neuropathy, and glomerulonephritis) but is often paucisymptomatic or asymptomatic. Nucleos(t)ide analog therapy has been used successfully to treat symptomatic cryoglobulinemia.[73]

Histopathologic Features

Chronic HBV infection is characterized by mononuclear cell infiltration in the portal tracts. Periportal inflammation often leads to the disruption of the limiting plate of hepatocytes (interface hepatitis), and inflammatory cells often can be seen at the interface between collagenous extensions from the portal tracts and liver parenchyma (referred to as *active septa*). During reactivated hepatitis B, lobular inflammation is more intense and reminiscent of that seen in acute viral hepatitis. Steatosis is not a feature of chronic hepatitis B, as it is of chronic hepatitis C.

The only histologic feature noted on routine light microscopy that is specific for chronic hepatitis B is the presence of ground-glass hepatocytes (Fig. 79-5). This morphologic finding results from accumulation of HBsAg particles (20 to 30 nm in diameter) in the dilated endoplasmic reticulum. Because of high levels of cysteine in HBsAg, ground-glass cells have a high affinity for certain dyes, such as orcein, Victoria blue, and aldehyde fuchsin. Ground-glass hepatocytes may also be seen in HBV carriers, in whom they may be detected in up to 5% of cells. When present in abundance, ground-glass hepatocytes often indicate active viral replication.[74] Immunofluorescence and electron microscopic studies have shown HBcAg inside the hepatocyte nuclei of affected cells. During periods of intense hepatitis activity, cytoplasmic core antigen staining is generally observed. After successful treatment of HBV infection with a nucleos(t)ide analog, the cytoplasmic core antigen staining often disappears, but nuclear core antigen staining

due to persistence of the HBV cccDNA trancriptional template may remain.

Acute Flares

Chronic hepatitis B is often punctuated by sudden flares of disease activity that are characterized by a precipitous increase in serum aminotransferase levels. Although a uniform biochemical definition of a flare is lacking, it has frequently been described as an increase in serum ALT levels to at least 2 to 3 times the baseline value and at least 100 IU/mL. Flares are an important part of the natural history of hepatitis B because they can lead to histologic progression when they occur repeatedly and are moderate or severe. Acute flares in chronic hepatitis B occur in association with a number of circumstances and clinical situations (Table 79-1). Most flares are preceded by an increase in viral replication, which stimulates an enhanced cellular immune response that targets virus-infected hepatocytes. The mechanisms behind the increase in viral replication are unknown in many instances and are presumed to be due to weakening of immune control over viral replication or replication-fit viral mutants such as core promoter mutants or drug-resistant mutant HBV (see earlier). Irrespective of the cause of the increased viral replication, however, the biochemical abnormalities usually occur coincident to or immediately after an increase in serum HBV DNA levels.

Spontaneous Flares

Spontaneous flares have been observed in patients with HBeAg-positive chronic hepatitis B, in whom they occur in 5% to 10% of patients annually, and in those with HBeAg-negative chronic hepatitis B, in whom fluctuations of both serum HBV DNA and ALT levels are common. It is not clear if severe physical or emotional stress can weaken the immune system and lead to a secondary increase in viral replication.

In persons who acquire HBV infection early in life, flares become more common during adulthood, presumably because of a breakdown in immune tolerance to HBV.[75] In this situation, the flares are almost certainly host derived rather than virally mediated, and although poorly understood, they are

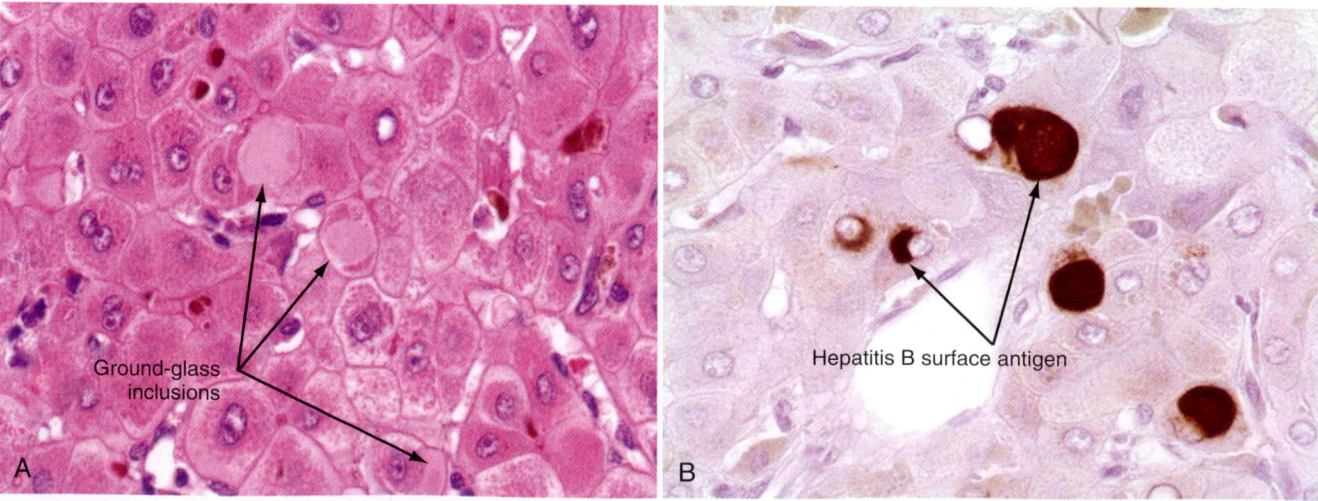

FIGURE 79-5. Histopathology of HBV infection. *A,* Photomicrograph showing ground-glass inclusions in hepatocytes. These inclusions represent large amounts of hepatitis B surface antigen (HBsAg) in the endoplasmic reticulum. (H&E, ×630.) *B,* Immunohistochemical stain for HBsAg. Note that the brownish inclusions correspond to the ground-glass inclusions seen in *A.* (×630.) *(Courtesy Dr. Gist Farr, New Orleans, La.)*

TABLE 79-1 Causes of Hepatitis Flares in Patients with Chronic Hepatitis B

Cause of Flare	Comment
Spontaneous	Factors that precipitate viral replication are unclear
Immunosuppressive therapy	Flares are often observed during withdrawal of the agent; preemptive antiviral therapy is required
Antiviral therapy for HBV	
Interferon	Flares are often observed during the second to third month of therapy in 30% of patients; may herald virologic response
Nucleoside analog	
During treatment	Flares are no more common than with placebo
Drug-resistant HBV	Severe consequences can occur in patients with advanced liver disease
On withdrawal	Flares are caused by the rapid re-emergence of wild-type HBV; severe consequences can occur in patients with advanced liver disease
HIV treatment	Flares can occur as a result of the direct toxicity of HAART or with immune reconstitution; HBV increases the risk of antiretroviral drug hepatotoxicity
Genotypic variation	
Precore and core promoter mutants	Fluctuations in serum ALT levels are common with precore mutants
Superinfection with other hepatitis viruses	May be associated with suppression of HBV replication

most likely the result of a change in the regulation of viral antigen-specific T cells.[53]

Immunosuppressive Therapy–Induced Flares

Reactivation of hepatitis B with flares of serum aminotransferase levels is a well-recognized complication of cytotoxic or immunosuppressive therapy, including conventional cancer chemotherapy and potent biologic response modifiers that are used to treat rheumatic, GI, and skin disorders.[76] Although many drugs have been reported to induce HBV reactivation, they tend to fall into one of several classes of agents (Table 79-2). Suppression of the normal immunologic responses to HBV during therapy leads to enhanced viral replication and is thought to result in widespread infection of hepatocytes. On discontinuation of immunosuppressive medications, as occurs with cancer chemotherapy, immune competence is restored and infected hepatocytes are rapidly destroyed. In general, the more potent the immunosuppression, the higher the level of viral replication and, thus, the greater the potential for serious clinical consequences. Postmortem studies of liver tissue from patients with severe liver injury have documented sparse staining of viral antigens, suggesting that the patients were in an active state of immune clearance.[77]

The literature provides ample evidence for HBV reactivation leading to severe hepatitis, death from acute liver failure, and delay or inability to continue treatment for the underlying disease. When reactivation occurs in the setting of cancer chemotherapy or systemic treatment for a severe autoimmune disorder, the patient may not be eligible for salvage liver transplantation. A growing body of evidence shows benefit to screening all patients in need of immunosuppressive drug therapy for HBsAg and anti-HBc and prophylactically treating HBsAg-positive patients with antiviral therapy.[78] Whenever indicated, antiviral therapy should be started at least 1 week before the immunosuppressive drug therapy is initiated. Clinical outcomes are much better when prophylaxis is provided as compared with on-demand antiviral therapy after reactivation has become clinically apparent.[78] In a prospective, randomized controlled study of lamivudine treatment of HBsAg-positive lymphoma patients undergoing chemotherapy, reactivated HBV infection developed in 53% of the "watchful-waiting" group but 0% of the prophylactically

treated group.[79] Nucleos(t)ide analog therapy should be given for 6 to 12 months after completion of therapy. Lamivudine can be used successfully when immunosuppressive therapy of finite duration is given.[78] When immunosuppressive therapy is given indefinitely for conditions other than cancer or when the patient has a baseline serum HBV DNA level of 2000 IU/mL or more, a nucleos(t)ide analog with high antiviral potency and a high genetic barrier to resistance (e.g., entecavir, tenofovir) is recommended.

The vast majority of patients reported to have immunosuppressive therapy–induced HBV reactivation have been positive for HBsAg in serum before treatment, but some studies have described the reappearance of HBsAg in patients who were initially positive only for anti-HBs, anti-HBc, or both. This event is called *reverse HBsAg seroconversion* and is particularly apt to happen with bone marrow or hematopoietic stem cell transplantation or the use of rituximab, a B-cell depleting drug (see Chapter 35).[80] Therefore, antiviral therapy is generally recommended for anti-HBc-positive patients in these clinical situations. A management dilemma exists when an HBsAg-negative/anti-HBc-positive patient is treated with immunosuppressive drug therapy in other circumstances, because adequate studies are lacking in these situations. Whether these patients are best managed by prophylactic antiviral treatment or serial HBV DNA monitoring with early treatment if there is an increase in the serum HBV DNA level of at least 1 $\log_{10}$ IU/mL is controversial.

There have been numerous reports of HBV reactivation after the use of TNF-α inhibitor therapy. TNF-α inhibits HBV replication in vitro, and all drugs that block this proinflammatory cytokine have been associated with HBV reactivation.[81] In one large retrospective series from Spain, HBV reactivation occurred in 39% of HBsAg-positive patients and 5% of anti-HBc-positive patients given TNF-α inhibitors.[81] Reactivation occurs considerably more frequently with infliximab than with adalimumab or etanercept, possibly owing to the high peak levels associated with infliximab, as well as its ability to induce complete elimination of TNF-α.[82] The importance given to these drugs as a potential cause of reactivation cannot be overemphasized, because they are usually administered for prolonged periods, millions of patients are being treated with these agents in the United States alone, and they are used for a diverse number of medical conditions, including

TABLE 79-2 Drugs Known to Be Associated with Hepatitis B Reactivation*

Category	Agent	Drug Class	Common Indications
Antineoplastic			
	Busulfan	Alkylating agent	Solid tumors, leukemia
	Chlorambucil	Alkylating agent	Leukemia, lymphoma
	Cisplatin	Platinum complex	Solid tumors
	Cyclophosphamide	Alkylating agent	Solid tumors, leukemia
	Docetaxel	Taxoid	Breast cancer
	Doxorubicin	Anthracycline	Leukemia, lymphoma
	Imatinib	TK inhibitor	Leukemia
	Melphalan	Alkylating agent	Leukemia, lymphoma
	Methotrexate	Antimetabolite	Leukemia, lymphoma
	Temozolmide	Alkylating agent	Brain cancer
	Thalidomide	Immunomodulatory	Solid tumors
	Vinblastine	Vinca alkaloid	Solid tumors, lymphoma
	Vincristine	Vinca alkaloid	Solid tumors, lymphoma
Endocrinologic			
	Cortisone	Glucocorticoid	Hormone replacement
	Betamethasone		Immune suppression
	Dexamethasone		Immune suppression
	Hydrocortisone		Hormone replacement
	Methylprednisolone		Immune suppression
	Prednisolone		Immune suppression
	Prednisone		Immune suppression
	Triamcinolone		Immune suppression
Immunomodulatory			
	Adalimumab	TNF-α inhibitor	Rheumatic disease, plaque psoriasis
	Azathioprine	Thiopurine	Autoimmune disease, transplantation
	Certolizumab	TNF-α inhibitor	Crohn's disease, RA
	Etanercept	TNF-α inhibitor	Rheumatic disease, plaque psoriasis
	Infliximab	TNF-α inhibitor	Crohn's disease, UC, RA, AS, psoriatic arthritis
	Natalizumab	Anti–alpha 4 integrin	Multiple sclerosis
	Rituximab	B-cell depleting agent	ITP, lymphoma, leukemia, transplantation
Anti-rejection			
	Cyclosporine	Calcineurin inhibitor	Transplantation
	Everolimus	mTor inhibitor	
	Mycophenolate mofetil	Antimetabolite	
	Sirolimus	mTor inhibitor	
	Tacrolimus	Calcineurin inhibitor	

*Partial list of agents.
AS, ankylosing spondylitis; ITP, immunologic thrombocytopenic purpura; mTor, mammalian target of rapamycin; TK, tyrosine kinase.

RA, ankylosing spondylitis, IBD, psoriasis, and several other autoimmune disorders.

Reactivated hepatitis B also occurs in patients who are given immunosuppressive medications to prevent organ transplant rejection. All HBsAg-positive and anti-HBc-positive transplant recipients should be considered to be at risk for HBV reactivation, with bone marrow and hematopoietic stem cell recipients having the highest level of risk (see Chapter 35). Post-transplantation treatment of organ rejection and graft-versus-host disease further contributes to this risk. In the setting of liver transplantation, indefinite nucleos(t)ide analog therapy is generally administered when grafts from anti-HBc-positive donors are given to previously nonexposed or anti-HBc-positive recipients.[83] A few cases have been reported in which the use of anti-HBc-positive livers given to lamivudine-treated recipients resulted in de novo hepatitis due to lamivudine-resistant HBV mutants.[84] Some experts routinely recommend the use of higher genetic barrier nucleos(t)ide analogs in the setting of anti-HBc-positive liver donation.

Antiviral Therapy–Induced Flares

Antiviral treatment of chronic hepatitis B can be associated with ALT increases and flares of hepatitis in several circumstances. Flares may occur during IFN or nucleos(t)ide analog therapy, after withdrawal of nucleos(t)ide analogs or glucocorticoid therapy, and in association with lamivudine-, adefovir-, entecavir-, or telbivudine-resistant mutants.

During Interferon Therapy. IFN-induced flares of chronic hepatitis B occur in approximately one third of treated patients and result from the immunostimulatory properties of the drug. Flares occur with conventional and pegylated formulations of IFN (see later and Chapter 80) and have been reported to occur more frequently in patients infected with HBV genotype A than with other genotypes. This finding may explain the higher rate of sustained virologic response and HBsAg clearance in IFN-treated patients with genotype A infection. Serum ALT flares have been shown to be a predictor of sustained virologic response and may be especially important in achieving a sustained virologic remission in patients with a high level of viremia.[85] Flares tend to be particularly common in patients who have decompensated liver disease, with rates as high as 50% reported in one series.[86] Flares that occur in patients with advanced liver fibrosis have frequently been associated with clinical deterioration, and, as a result, IFN is generally considered to be contraindicated in patients with cirrhosis.

During Nucleos(t)ide Analog Therapy. The registration studies for all nucleos(t)ide analogs have detected ALT flares during treatment in approximately 10% of patients, and these flares were no more common or severe than those occurring in nontreated patients. Whether a reduction in viral burden results in a transient restoration of immune competence is controversial, but the interaction does not appear to be clinically important. Aminotransferase increases are generally brief, even with continuation of therapy.

After Withdrawal of Nucleos(t)ide Analog. Serum ALT flares occur in approximately 20% of patients after withdrawal of nucleos(t)ide analog therapy. These flares are thought to be caused by rapid resurgence of wild-type HBV, and although generally well tolerated, they too may be associated with serious clinical exacerbations in patients with advanced liver disease. Reinstitution of the original therapy is usually associated with a decline in HBV DNA levels.

During Antiretroviral Therapy. Serum ALT flares occur in patients coinfected with HIV and HBV who receive HAART.[87] The cause of these flares can be multifactorial. One of the most common causes is immunologic reconstitution due to the effectiveness of antiretroviral therapy.[88] Patients with low CD4 counts before HAART therapy and high HBV DNA levels are often at greatest risk for this syndrome, and acute liver failure may occasionally result.[89]

Lamivudine resistance is less important as a cause of flares in HBV/HIV coinfected patients, because most patients in developed nations are now taking tenofovir or combination therapy with tenofovir and emtrictabine instead (see later). HBV infection increases the risk of hepatotoxicity from antiretroviral therapy, usually within 6 months after the initiation of treatment, and hepatotoxicity should be suspected if aminotransferase elevations occur despite an appropriate decline in HBV DNA levels. Affected HIV-infected patients may also be particularly susceptible to ALT flares because of a higher risk of infection with other hepatitis viruses.

Flares Associated with Genotypic Variation

Chronic infection with precore mutant HBV is often associated with periodic flares of liver cell necrosis interspersed with periods of normal serum ALT and low serum HBV DNA levels.[54] These flares have been attributed to rises in the concentration of precore mutants in the liver and changes in the ratio of concentrations of precore to wild-type HBV.

Mutations at the basal core promoter region of the HBV genome are associated with increased histologic evidence of liver inflammation and viral replication.[90] Multiple exacerbations of hepatitis resulting from reactivated HBV infection have been described in patients with basal core promoter mutations, either alone or in association with precore mutations.

Flares Caused by Infection with Other Viruses

Patients with chronic HBV infection may exhibit severe flares in serum aminotransferase levels and even frank liver failure when superinfected with another hepatotropic virus, such as HAV, HCV, or HDV. Increased mortality has been reported when HDV superinfection is superimposed on chronic hepatitis B, and chronic HDV infection is often associated with multiple fluctuations in serum aminotransferase levels (see Chapter 81).

Acute hepatitis C superimposed on chronic hepatitis B has been reported to be as clinically severe as HDV superinfection and has been associated with high rates of liver failure (34%) and death (10%).[91] In a study involving 240 Chinese HBV carriers, those who became superinfected with HEV had a significantly higher rate of complications, including liver failure and death (33% vs. 2%), when compared to those who became superinfected with HAV.[92] Because a vaccine for HEV is not commercially available, these data underscore the importance of clinical vigilance for acute hepatitis E in the right setting and consideration for early treatment with IFN if there is serologic confirmation of infection in an established HBV carrier (see Chapter 82).

DIAGNOSIS

HBsAg appears in serum 2 to 10 weeks after exposure to HBV and before the onset of symptoms or elevation of serum aminotransferase levels. In self-limited acute hepatitis, HBsAg usually becomes undetectable after 4 to 6 months. Persistence of HBsAg for more than 6 months implies evolution to chronic HBV infection.

The disappearance of HBsAg is followed several weeks later by the appearance of anti-HBs. In most patients, anti-HBs persists for life and provides long-term immunity. In some patients, anti-HBs may not become detectable after disappearance of HBsAg, but these patients do not appear to be susceptible to recurrent HBV infection.[93] Anti-HBs may not be detectable during a window period of several weeks to months after the disappearance of HBsAg. During this period, the diagnosis of acute HBV infection is made by the detection of IgM anti-HBc in serum.

Coexistence of HBsAg and anti-HBs in serum has been reported in approximately 10% to 20% of HBV carriers. The mechanisms of this finding are not clear but most likely relate to antibody formed against minor variants of the HBsAg protein. The presence of these heterotypic antibodies is not associated with specific risk factors or changes in clinical course and may occur in patients with or without active liver disease and viral replication.

Anti-HBc is detectable in acute and chronic HBV infection. During acute infection, anti-HBc is predominantly of the IgM class and is usually detectable for 4 to 6 months after an acute episode of hepatitis and rarely for up to 2 years. IgM anti-HBc may become detectable during exacerbations of chronic hepatitis B and is often used as a surrogate for active viral replication. Anti-HBc of the IgG class is found in persons who recover from acute hepatitis B and also is the form found in those who progress to chronic infection.

In low endemic areas of the world such as the United States, isolated anti-HBc in serum has been detected in 1% to 4% of the general population. Less than 5% of these patients can be anticipated to have HBV DNA detectable in serum and therefore occult viremia.[94] By contrast, isolated anti-HBc may be found in more than 50% of patients in highly endemic regions of the world, and 10% to 30% of patients with this finding may have HBV DNA detectable in serum.[95,96] Isolated reactivity for anti-HBc may occur in a number of other clinical situations also (Table 79-3). Perhaps the most clinically important to recognize is a false-positive test result, which is usually very weakly reactive and may not be reproducible. Failure to appreciate this possibility in patients who have no apparent risk of exposure to HBV may result in needless consultation, inappropriate exclusion from vaccination, and, unfortunately,

TABLE 79-3 Possible Interpretations of an Isolated Positive Test Result for Antibody to Hepatitis B Core Antigen

Interpretation	Comments
Remote infection	Most common cause; particularly common in endemic areas of the world where acquisition of infection early in life is frequent. Patients may have HBV DNA detectable in serum
False-positive result	Weakly positive. May be nonreproducible in a different clinical laboratory
Window period of acute hepatitis B	Seen relatively infrequently due to increased sensitivity of current anti-HBs assays
Occult infection	HBV DNA detectable in serum and liver tissue

Anti-HBs, antibody to hepatitis B surface antigen.

rejection of the person from blood or organ donation. Such individuals often have a primary rather than anamnestic response to HBV vaccination.

HBeAg is a viral protein that is found in serum early during acute HBV infection. HBeAg reactivity usually disappears at the time of or soon after the peak in serum aminotransferase levels, and persistence of HBeAg 3 or more months after the onset of illness indicates a high likelihood of transition to chronic HBV infection. The finding of HBeAg in the serum of an HBsAg-positive carrier indicates a high level of viral replication and greater infectivity for intimate contacts. With a commercially available PCR assay, nearly 90% of patients with HBeAg-positive chronic hepatitis B have been found to have serum HBV DNA levels persistently above 10^5 copies/mL, with a mean value of 8.37 $\log_{10}$ (>10^8 copies/mL).[97] Serum HBV DNA values can be as high as $10^{12\text{-}13}$ during the immune tolerance phase. By contrast, anti–HBe-positive patients have much lower serum HBV DNA levels (10^5 to 10^8 copies/mL), with the highest values being found in those with persistently or intermittently elevated serum ALT levels.

HBV DNA can be measured in serum with qualitative or quantitative assays. Most clinical laboratories in the United States use a quantitative PCR method that is capable of detecting less than 400 copies/mL. The Cobas TaqMan (Roche Molecular Diagnostics, Pleasanton, Calif.) is commonly used and can reliably determine HBV DNA levels over a linear range from 25 IU/mL (≈100 copies/mL) to 10^8 IU/mL. A number of non–PCR-based assays are available, but they are less useful clinically.

The quantification of serum HBV DNA is commonly used to evaluate a patient's candidacy for antiviral therapy and to monitor response during treatment. Patients with a high serum HBV DNA level (>10^9 copies/mL) at baseline respond less commonly to therapy with IFN than do those with lower levels.[98] By contrast, baseline serum HBV DNA levels have not been shown to correlate with response to nucleos(t)ide analog therapy because of the more potent inhibition of viral replication by these agents. Monitoring of HBV DNA levels at key intervals such as 12 and 24 weeks of therapy allows one to predict the likelihood of HBeAg clearance with both pegylated IFN and nucleos(t)ide analog therapy.[99,100] In the past, reappearance of HBV DNA in serum during treatment predominantly suggested that drug resistance had occurred.[101] Such is not the case, however, with high-genetic-barrier nucleos(t)ide

analog therapy during which the reemergence of HBV DNA often indicates poor adherence to therapy.[102]

Qualitative PCR has been reported to be an even more sensitive method than quantitative PCR for detecting HBV DNA. Use of qualitative PCR has altered traditional concepts about the clearance of HBV DNA from serum in acute and chronic HBV infection. For example, small amounts of HBV DNA can be detected in serum and peripheral mononuclear cells years after recovery from acute or chronic hepatitis B.[103] Qualitative PCR for HBV DNA has a relatively limited role in clinical decision making, however, and suffers from poor standardization of assay techniques.

Assays for quantification of HBsAg have become commercially available and are licensed in Europe and Asia (Architect Assay, Abbott Diagnostics, Chicago, Ill.; Elecys II assay, Roche Molecular Diagnostics). These assays are available for research purposes in the United States and are likely to become commercially available. Clinical trials in both HBeAg-positive and HBeAg-negative patients have demonstrated a rapid decline in HBsAg concentration during IFN therapy and a much slower decline during the first few years of nucleos(t)ide analog therapy. In HBeAg-negative hepatitis B, a decrease in HBsAg concentration of 0.5 log at week 12 or 1 log at week 24 of IFN therapy has been found to provide better prediction of a sustained virologic response than does the decline in serum HBV DNA levels.[104] High negative predictive values at week 12 (>90%) have led to proposal of a stopping rule that would avoid needless extension of IFN therapy and lead to initiation of a different treatment regimen. The data are less clear for patients with HBeAg-positive chronic hepatitis B. Although the HBsAg kinetic data provide promising insights, there is no consensus on how serial measurement of HBsAg should be used. The rate of decline of HBsAg concentration has been found to vary according to HBV genotype, and the proposed stopping rule is unlikely to be applicable to all genotypes.[105]

TREATMENT

Seven drugs are approved for the treatment of chronic hepatitis B. Five of these agents are nucleos(t)ide analogs that suppress HBV replication through an inhibitory effect on the viral DNA polymerase. Nucleos(t)ide analogs have excellent oral bioavailability and a good safety record and are far more potent inhibitors of viral replication than IFN-α. They have proved to be particularly useful in the management of patients with decompensated cirrhosis, because even small doses of IFN can lead to worsening liver failure and severe infections. IFN therapy is used much less frequently because of its adverse effects, but continued interest in this agent stems from the fact that it is both immunostimulatory as well as antiviral. Moreover, IFN induces a more rapid decline in HBsAg concentration and a higher rate of HBsAg clearance.

Goals

The primary treatment goals for patients with chronic hepatitis B are to forestall progression of liver disease, prevent late complications (cirrhosis, liver failure, and HCC), and increase survival. All of these objectives are achievable with long-term suppression of viral replication with either IFN-α or nucleos(t)ide analogs. Unfortunately, less than 10% of patients with potentially treatable chronic hepatitis B are estimated to be given antiviral therapy. Missed opportunities for HBV screening and poor appreciation of the indications for treatment are the major impediments.[106,107]

Cultural Barriers

More than two thirds of immigrant populations with chronic hepatitis B were born in areas of the world where hepatitis B is highly endemic. Many of these persons do not seek health care, and the possibility of hepatitis B is often not explored when they do.

Significant cultural barriers to the effective management of these patients exist. Appreciation of these barriers is critical because the potential impact on future health and financial resources needed to care for late complications of hepatitis B are immense. One of the greatest barriers to acceptance of antiviral therapy is the limited proficiency in English language skills that leads to isolation and may negatively influence government support to an individual or community. Asian immigrants, for example, often own small businesses or have jobs in which insurance is not provided, thus preventing them from having access to care. If they are able to obtain medical care, the health care provider often is not able to communicate with first-generation immigrants in their native tongues, further leading to distrust, confusion, and embarrassment. Cultural, religious, and stigmatizing beliefs may impede care. These barriers may be overcome, however, with sensitivity on the part of the care provider. Whenever possible, the provider should arrange for a translator or seek the assistance of someone who speaks the patient's native language.[108]

Choice of Agent

In deciding on the appropriate type of therapy for a patient with chronic hepatitis B, the physician should consider the serum ALT level, serum HBV DNA level, and liver histology, if available, as well as the expense of treatment, potential for adverse events, age of the patient, and presence of other comorbid conditions (Table 79-4). Moreover, before starting antiviral therapy, the patient should be committed to having serial blood samples and assessments.

The latest generation of nucleos(t)ide analogs such as tenofovir and entecavir have a high genetic barrier to resistance and, therefore, can be used as monotherapy. Accordingly, these agents are generally preferred as first-line treatment when available (Table 79-5). In emerging nations, lamivudine and adefovir are often used as first-line therapy owing to financial constraints and limited availability of the newer oral agents.

IFN and nucleos(t)ide analogs each have advantages and disadvantages that should be considered when making a treatment decision (see Table 79-4). One major advantage of IFN is that treatment is limited to 1 year or less, and virologic responses tend to be quite durable, especially in patients with HBeAg-positive hepatitis B. The shorter time required for treatment may be an important factor for some patients.

Definitions of Response

Phase 3 drug registration trials for nucleos(t)ide analogs utilized predefined biochemical, virologic, and histologic end points to evaluate the response to treatment. Biochemical response required normalization of serum ALT levels, virologic response required a sustained disappearance of HBV DNA from serum for at least 6 months after treatment, and histologic response required a 2-point or greater improvement in the necroflammatory score without worsening fibrosis. HBeAg seroconversion to anti-HBe, rather than HBeAg disappearance alone, was used as an additional virologic end point to minimize the chance of virologic relapse.

Some of the large clinical trials of IFN used a virologic end point of HBeAg loss rather than HBeAg seroconversion, and the persistent detection of low levels of serum HBV DNA (<2000 IU/mL) was allowed in the definition of a sustained virologic response, because nondetectable HBV DNA occurs less frequently with IFN-based therapy than with nucleos(t)ide therapy. These less stringent requirements did not preclude a durable response to IFN in approximately 80% of HBeAg-positive patients when evaluated years later.[109] This durability has been hypothesized to be due to a continued immunoregulatory effect of IFN after treatment discontinuation. A sustained decline of serum HBV DNA levels to less than 2000 IU/mL was also included as a primary end point in many of the IFN trials in patients with HBeAg-negative hepatitis B. Long-term follow-up of these patients has indicated a higher rate of relapse when compared with HBeAg-positive patients, but sustained responses have been reported in 30% of the HBeAg-negative patients.

Irrespective of the type of antiviral therapy used, the best assurance that late relapses will not occur is provided by the

TABLE 79-4 Positive and Negative Factors to Consider in the Decision to Treat Hepatitis B with Peginterferon or a Nucleoside or Nucleotide Analog

Agent	Positive Factors	Negative Factors
Peginterferon	Finite duration of treatment Durable off-treatment response More rapid disappearance of HBsAg Immunostimulatory as well as intrinsically antiviral Better tolerability compared with its use in hepatitis C	Inconvenience of subcutaneous injection Frequent side effects Clearance of HBsAg in a small minority of patients depending on genotype Potential risk of ALT flares in patients with advanced liver fibrosis Relative contraindication in patients > age 60 or those with comorbid illnesses
Nucleoside or nucleotide analog	Negligible side effects Convenience; ready acceptance by patients Potent inhibition of virus replication Reduced drug resistance with the third-generation nucleoside analogs	Slight risk of nephropathy with nucleotide analogs (adefovir, tenofovir) Drug expense can be considerable during long-term use Long or indefinite treatment needed for both HBeAg-positive and HBeAg-negative patients Access issues in developing nations

HBsAg, hepatitis B surface antigen.

TABLE 79-5 Choice of Nucleoside or Nucleotide Analog for HBV Infection

Clinical Situation	First-Line Therapy	Second-Line Therapy	Comment
Treatment naïve	Entecavir or tenofovir	Telbivudine	Discontinue telbivudine if HBV DNA is still detected in serum at week 24
Prior lamivudine or telbivudine exposure	Switch to tenofovir	Entecavir	Entecavir resistance is facilitated by resistance to either lamivudine or telbivudine
Proved lamivudine resistance	Switch to tenofovir	Add adefovir*	Addition of adefovir late in the course may not control viral replication
Proved adefovir resistance	Switch to entecavir	Tenofovir	Slight reduction in drug susceptibility to tenofovir
Primary drug failure with both lamivudine and adefovir†	Switch to tenofovir or entecavir	Telbivudine	Suspect poor adherence if lamivudine had been used; see telbivudine precaution above
Proved entecavir resistance	Switch to tenofovir	Add adefovir*	—
Proved telbivudine resistance	Switch to tenofovir	Add adefovir*	—
Persistent low-level viremia during treatment with high-genetic-barrier drug	Continue tenofovir or entecavir or switch to the other	None	Nonadherence is possible; resistance testing may be needed
Treatment naïve, decrease in GFR (60-90 mL/min)	Entecavir	Telbivudine	Discontinue telbivudine if HBV DNA is still detected at week 24

*Whenever a high-genetic-barrier drug option is not available.
†See text for definition of primary drug failure.
GFR, glomerular filtration rate.

disappearance of HBsAg, with or without seroconversion to anti-HBs; this occurrence comes closest to a clinical cure of hepatitis B. Unfortunately, this more stringent end point occurs uncommonly with IFN and is even more rarely achieved with nucleos(t)ide analog therapy despite the greater antiviral potency of the latter.

Nucleoside and Nucleotide Analogs

The vast majority of previously untreated ("treatment-naïve") patients are treated with 1 or more nucleos(t)ide analogs rather than IFN. Between 70% and 85% of HBeAg-positive patients will become HBV DNA negative during the first year of treatment.[110] The rate is as high as 85% to 95% after 2 years of therapy when drugs associated with a high genetic barrier to resistance are used. A small group of patients may still have HBV DNA detectable in serum after several years of therapy with high-genetic-barrier nucleos(t)ide analogs even though the clinical and biochemical response persists. The reason for the persistence of serum HBV DNA in these patients is not well understood, but the HBV DNA level is almost always below 2000 IU/mL, and drug-resistant mutants have not been demonstrated in this situation; most experts recommend continuing treatment with the same drug with a high genetic barrier to resistance.

The lack of side effects and excellent resistance profiles of the orally available antiviral agents are especially important properties because HBeAg seroconversion occurs slowly and often requires treatment for years or for an indefinite duration. Despite a rapid decline in serum HBV DNA levels on nucleos(t)ide analog therapy, only 20% to 25% of treated patients achieve HBeAg seroconversion after 1 year of treatment. The rate rises to 40% after 5 years of continuous treatment provided that the patient remains adherent and viral resistance does not occur.[111] Long-term or maintenance therapy is particularly likely to be necessary in patients with HBeAg-negative hepatitis B because relatively high rates of relapse have been demonstrated after drug withdrawal despite years of treatment during which HBV DNA has remained nondetectable.

From 15% to 20% of patients with HBeAg-positive hepatitis B have a virologic relapse, including reappearance of HBeAg as well as HBV DNA, within 1 year of treatment discontinuation. Continuation of nucleos(t)ide analog therapy for several months beyond the period when HBeAg seroconversion is first detected diminishes the chance of relapse.[112] Treatment for a minimum of 6 months after HBeAg seroconversion has been recommended by all the international liver societies. Even when this practice has been followed, however, some studies have reported relapse rates as high as 30% to 50% in Asian patients with HBeAg-positive chronic hepatitis B.[113] The reasons for differences in relapse rates in various studies are not clear, but interstudy differences in HBV genotype and patient-related factors, such as the duration of infection, may be potential explanations.

Lamivudine

Owing to a high rate of resistance, lamivudine is no longer recommended as first-line therapy except in persons who require only short-term therapy, such as patients undergoing cancer chemotherapy. Prolonged lamivudine resistance has been associated with a blunted histologic response and more frequent hepatitis flares. The drug is still used widely as first-line therapy in developing countries. Before starting antiviral therapy in patients born in endemic areas for hepatitis B, care should be taken to inquire if antiviral therapy had ever been taken previously. In such patients, it may be best not to use entecavir because of the high likelihood that the patient had been exposed to lamivudine, prior exposure to which may predispose the patient to entecavir resistance (see later).

Adefovir Dipivoxil

Adefovir was licensed by the FDA a few years after lamivudine became available and was used frequently because it was effective against both wild-type and lamivudine-resistant HBV. Because of its limited potency, however, primary treatment failure (<1 log decline in the serum HBV DNA level at week 12) was observed in 30% of patients. Resistance to this drug due to 1 or 2 nucleotide substitutions in HBV DNA was documented in nearly 30% of patients by the end of 5 years of continuous therapy.[114]

Although adefovir use in the United States has largely been supplanted by tenofovir (see later), adefovir is still used widely outside of this country as primary therapy or whenever lamivudine resistance has emerged. In such cases, it is often used in combination with lamivudine in patients with advanced disease, because lamivudine is capable of suppressing adefovir-resistant mutants. Adefovir has the disadvantage of potential nephrotoxicity and should not be used in patients with preexisting compromised renal function.

Entecavir

Entecavir is a nucleoside analog that is more potent than lamivudine or adefovir and has a much higher genetic barrier to resistance, requiring an additional DNA polymerase mutation superimposed on the backbone of preexisting lamivudine-resistant mutations. This situation is rare in treatment-naïve patients, thus explaining the fact that resistance has been found in only 2% of treatment-naïve patients during 5 years of continuous treatment. In phase 3 clinical trials, an entecavir dose of 0.5 mg was used in treatment-naïve HBeAg-positive and HBeAg-negative patients, whereas 1 mg was used in patients who were resistant to lamivudine. The latter strategy is not recommended any longer because of a shortened time to acquisition of entecavir resistance in lamivudine-resistant patients[115]; tenofovir should be used instead (see later). The benefits of long-term use of entecavir include progressive regression of fibrosis, reversal of the features of cirrhosis, and a decreased incidence of HCC.[116,117]

Telbivudine

Telbivudine is a nucleoside analog that has been shown to be more potent than lamivudine in both HBeAg-positive and HBeAg-negative patients. Unfortunately, after 2 years of treatment, genotypic resistance was found in 25% of HBeAg-positive patients and 11% of HBeAg-negative patients, respectively. The highest rates of virologic response, and, conversely, the lowest rates of resistance, were found in patients who achieved nondetectable HBV DNA levels at 24 weeks of treatment. This drug shares cross resistance with lamivudine and should never be used as replacement therapy in lamivudine-resistant patients.

Telbivudine has fallen out of favor as a first-line treatment for HBV infection in the United States because of an unacceptably high rate of resistance when used as monotherapy. Resistance can be avoided in most instances, however, by careful attention to patient selection. The package insert states that this drug is only indicated in HBeAg-positive patients with a baseline serum HBV DNA level less than 10^9 copies/mL and a baseline serum ALT level greater than 2-fold elevated, and patients who are HBeAg-negative should have a serum HBV DNA level less than 10^7 copies/mL. Moreover, the drug should be discontinued if HBV DNA is still detected at week 24 of treatment. These recommendations on patient selection and early discontinuation of treatment are based on observations from the pivotal registration trial in which meeting these thresholds was predictive of low resistance and high virologic response. For example, if HBV DNA is not detectable at week 24 of treatment, telbivudine can be continued because drug resistance is much less common (3% to 4%) after 2 years of treatment.

Data collected on more than 500 HBeAg-positive and HBeAg-negative patients with chronic hepatitis B have revealed an increase in glomerular filtration rate (GFR) of 14.9 mL/min from baseline to 4 years of treatment. Improvement in renal function was observed in the first year of treatment and was sustained during subsequent years. Most of the improvement was confined to patients with minimal renal impairment (GFR of 60 to 90 mL/min) at baseline, and the renal functional improvement was not related to the degree of viral suppression.[118] Therefore, the drug may be a safer alternative to adefovir or tenofovir in patients with preexisting renal impairment or those who are predisposed to this risk (e.g., obese patients with diabetes mellitus and hypertension).

Tenofovir Disoproxil Fumarate

Tenofovir is similar chemically to adefovir, but it has significantly more antiviral potency. Although head-to-head comparisons are not available, tenofovir may have slightly greater antiviral potency than entecavir. It is associated with a few safety issues, however, that are not found with entecavir. Tenofovir therapy has rarely been associated with decreased bone density in HIV-infected patients. As with adefovir, renal tubular damage and Fanconi syndrome have been observed in rare instances, and the elderly or persons with preexisting mild renal disease may be at particular risk.

Remarkably, resistance to tenofovir has not occurred after 5 years of treatment in either HBeAg-positive or HBeAg-negative patients. In a study that included more than 300 patients, 240 weeks of tenofovir-based therapy was associated with significant histologic regression, including reversal of cirrhosis in 74% of patients with pretreatment cirrhosis.[111] High serum HBV DNA levels (>10^9 copies/mL), previously considered a treatment challenge when resistance-prone antiviral agents are used, are suppressed to undetectable levels in more than 90% of patients during long-term treatment.[111,119] Because of its high genetic barrier to resistance and strong antiviral potency, tenofovir is used frequently as first-line therapy, particularly in cases of heavy prior exposure to lamivudine, known lamivudine resistance, or suboptimal response to adefovir.

Emtricitabine

Structurally similar to lamivudine, emtricitabine also inhibits HBV DNA polymerase and HIV reverse transcriptase. It is not FDA approved for use in hepatitis B, either alone or in a combined tablet with tenofovir that is commonly used for HIV infection. Because of its structural similarity to lamivudine, it shares the same resistance profile.

HBV DNA Monitoring

Patients who undergo treatment with a nucleos(t)ide analog should be followed with serial ALT and HBV DNA assessments at 4-month intervals during the first year of treatment.[100] Once the HBV DNA level is nondetectable or less than 2000 IU/mL, follow-up intervals can be extended to every 6 months provided that the patient is taking a drug with a high genetic barrier to resistance and has demonstrated adherence to therapy.

As mentioned earlier, not all patients have nondetectable HBV DNA within the first several years of treatment even with drugs that have a high genetic barrier to resistance. In such cases, continuing the antiviral agent is reasonable, with the expectation of an eventual response or maintenance of virologic remission. In cases in which low-level viremia persists during maintenance treatment with a low-genetic-barrier drug such as lamivudine, adefovir, or telbivudine, switching to tenofovir is most appropriate. Entecavir is an equally suitable alternative if the patient fails to clear HBV DNA on adefovir (see Table 79-5).

Drug Failure

Primary drug failure at 12 weeks of treatment or a 1-log or greater increase in HBV DNA level (virologic breakthrough) is rarely seen with entecavir and tenofovir and usually indicates that the patient is not taking the drug appropriately. Based on a database of prescription utilization, at least 10% to 15% of patients fail to take their medication appropriately and miss 1 or more doses each month.[120] Patients who experience early treatment failure or virologic breakthrough at any time should be questioned carefully in a culturally sensitive manner about drug adherence, and treatment goals should be reinforced.

Virologic breakthrough can also be due to drug resistance with low-genetic-barrier nucleos(t)ide analogs. *Genotypic resistance* is the term that describes the finding of a nucleotide substitution in the HBV DNA polymerase gene that has been associated with clinical evidence of drug resistance. Mutations that have commonly been associated with antiviral drug resistance can be detected by a commercially available reverse hybridization assay (InnoLipa, Innogenetics, Belgium). This method can only detect HBV mutants that have been proved to be associated with drug resistance. Furthermore, to be detectable, the drug-resistant mutant HBV has to constitute at least 10% of the viral population. Ultradeep pyrosequencing is a research method for detecting minor HBV variants that constitute less than 1% of the total HBV quasispecies.[121] As a result of its greatly enhanced sensitivity, this method may ultimately provide clues as to why some adherent patients fail to become negative for serum HBV DNA after several years of treatment.

If a patient is unknowingly continued on the same therapy after genotypic resistance is detected, virologic rebound (defined as an increase in serum HBV DNA levels to >100,000 copies, or 20,000 IU/mL) will follow, and subsequently the serum ALT level will become elevated. Rescue therapy can modify this sequence of events if the patient is switched to a second agent that lacks cross resistance to the original drug (see Table 79-5). Preferably, the second agent should be a high-genetic-barrier drug. In clinical practice, tenofovir monotherapy has been used successfully in cases of lamivudine, adefovir, or entecavir resistance.[122] Entecavir could be used for adefovir resistance. When neither tenofovir nor entecavir is available, another alternative would be to add a second low-genetic-barrier nucleos(t)ide analog that is effective against the original drug-resistant mutant. The disadvantage of this approach is that combined therapy is more cumbersome and expensive than switching to a high-genetic-barrier drug.

Interferon

Both standard and pegylated forms of IFN-α are available. They have similar immunologic effects, but pegylated IFN has greater antiviral potency and is better tolerated.[123] Pegylated IFN is used more frequently worldwide. The FDA-approved duration of therapy is 48 weeks at a dose of 180 μg for both HBeAg-positive and HBeAg-negative chronic hepatitis B.

Predictors of response are the same for both types of IFN. Patients with baseline ALT values of at least 2 to 3 times the upper limit of normal, an HBV DNA level less than 10^9 IU/mL, and genotype A or B respond more frequently than patients without these features. Because ALT flares may occur during therapy, IFN is contraindicated in patients with even mildly decompensated cirrhosis and must be used with caution in patients with clinically stable cirrhosis.

Loss of HBsAg occurs in approximately 5% of HBeAg-positive patients within the first 6 months after completion of treatment.[31] This rate compares with rates of disappearance of HBsAg in 5% of patients treated for 96 weeks with entecavir and 3% of those on tenofovir for 48 weeks.[124,125] Although these differences may seem minimal, sustained responses to IFN are often associated with incremental HBsAg loss during long-term follow up, a finding that has not been demonstrated for nucleos(t)ide analogs.[109,126] A 3-year follow-up study of patients who lost HBeAg and had sustained virologic response after a year of pegylated IFN-α demonstrated that initial responders with HBV genotypes A or B had the highest rates of durable virologic response (96% and 86%, respectively) and the highest rate of HBsAg clearance (58% and 14%, respectively).[109] By contrast, the same end points were achieved, respectively, in only 76% and 6% of initial responders with genotype D. Unlike nucleos(t)ide analogs, IFN use is not associated with drug resistance.

The more rapid decline in HBsAg concentration during IFN treatment of both HBeAg-positive and HBeAg-negative hepatitis B (see earlier) is thought to reflect immune-mediated elimination of HBV cccDNA (the genomic template for viral transcription). These differences in viral kinetics emphasize that the mechanisms of action of the 2 major classes of antiviral agents differ and provides a rationale for the use of combined IFN and nucleoside analog therapy.

Combination Interferon and Nucleos(t)ide Analog Therapy

From a conceptual standpoint, treatment with the combination of IFN and a nucleos(t)ide analog may prove to be more effective than either drug alone and may permit a shorter course of nucleos(t)ide analog therapy, thereby reducing the risk of viral resistance to low-genetic-barrier drugs. Three large multicenter studies evaluated responses to a combination of pegylated IFN and lamivudine compared with IFN alone. Although suppression of HBV DNA was greater in the combined-therapy arms, the response was not sustained after discontinuation of treatment.[31,127,128] Trials of pegylated IFN combined with entecavir or tenofovir are in progress, as are studies in which sequential therapy, starting with a nucleos(t)ide analog, is given.[129] It is hoped that IFN combined with a high-genetic-barrier nucleos(t)ide analog given for a longer interval than previously reported may be a more effective approach than prior treatment regimens.

Guidelines

Consensus guidelines for the treatment of hepatitis B have been published by the AASLD, Asian-Pacific Association for the Study of the Liver, and European Association for the Study of the Liver.[102,130,131] The recommendations made in the 3 sets of published guidelines have many similarities. In general, they recommend treatment of persons who have both biochemical evidence of liver injury and serum HBV DNA levels in excess of 20,000 IU/mL in HBeAg-positive patients and greater than 2000 IU/mL in HBeAg-negative patients.[132] Nucleos(t)ide analog therapy is recommended specifically as first-line treatment in patients with decompensated cirrhosis. Emphasis also is given to the treatment of patients with serum ALT levels that are at least double the upper limit of normal, although some experts disagree with setting arbitrary serum ALT and HBV DNA thresholds.[132] The guidelines indicate that treatment decisions ideally should be made in the context of moderately severe disease (stage 2 or greater fibrosis). Liver biopsy is no longer mandated in the AASLD guidelines but is encouraged whenever doubt about the extent of disease exists. Noninvasive assessment of fibrosis, such as US (e.g., transient) elastography and MR elastography, can be helpful in situations in which a liver biopsy is either not possible or contraindicated (see Chapters 73, 74, and 80).[133]

The guidelines recommend continuing treatment for 6 to 12 months after HBeAg seroconversion to minimize the chance of virologic relapse. Defining the duration of treatment remains an even greater challenge in patients with HBeAg-negative hepatitis because of the absence of secure virologic end points. It is worth noting that although the published treatment guidelines are helpful in assessing the need for treatment, their reliance on grade A evidence (randomized controlled clinical trials) has led to the absence of definitive recommendations in special patient populations for which the data have been less stringently acquired.

Special Populations

Pregnant Women

HBV infection may still develop in 5% to 10% of appropriately immunized newborns of HBV-infected mothers and may occur when vaccination is delayed or incomplete (see later). Preliminary studies have shown that infected spermatozoa or maternal oocytes are associated with HBsAg-expressing embryos.[134] Threatened preterm labor, premature rupture of maternal membranes, and detection of HBV in the placenta have also been linked to intrapartum transmission.[135]

There are only 2 reasons to treat HBsAg-positive pregnant women: to forestall disease progression in the mother or to prevent breakthrough infection in newborns of highly viremic mothers. Epidemiologic studies have shown that HBeAg-positive mothers with a serum HBV DNA level greater than 10^6 or 10^8 copies/mL present a significantly higher risk of maternal transmission to the neonate even when properly immunized at birth.[136,137] Several studies, most of which were neither prospective nor randomized and controlled in design, have shown that treatment of such highly viremic mothers in the third trimester reduces the rate of neonatal breakthrough infection.[137] Many experts have recommended administering antiviral therapy during the last trimester and even continuing it for a brief period after delivery to avoid postpregnancy flares of disease caused by recovery of immunologic function.[138]

None of the current antiviral agents is licensed for use in pregnancy. Telbivudine and tenofovir are considered category B drugs by the FDA (defined as a lack of animal embryologic toxicity without studies in humans). Lamivudine is a category B drug in HIV-infected pregnant women but a category C drug in HBV-infected women (defined as embryotoxic or teratogenic in animals, without study in humans). A large amount of safety data exists for lamivudine in HIV-infected mothers, and there is increasing data on tenofovir (category B) in the U.S. Antiretroviral Pregnancy Registry.[139] Of the more than 10,000 reported pregnancies in which the mother received an oral nucleos(t)ide analog, 95% had HIV infection, and less than 1% had HBV monoinfection. Nevertheless, the overall

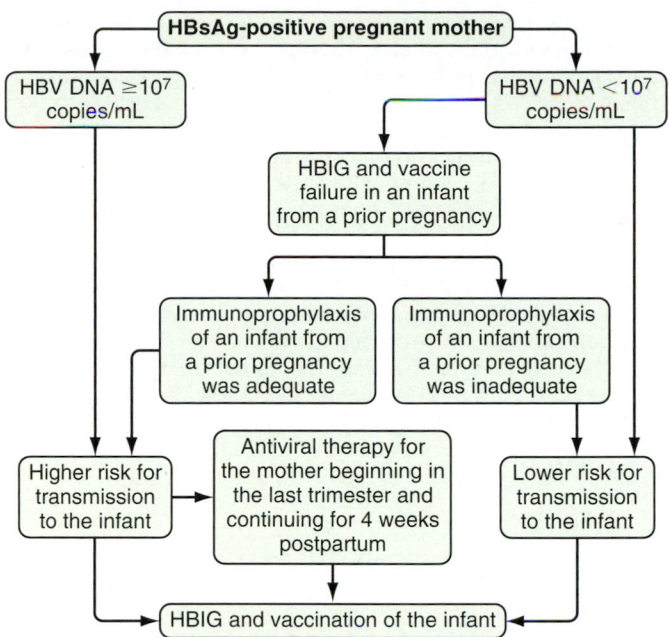

FIGURE 79-6. Algorithm for the treatment of hepatitis B surface antigen (HBsAg)-positive mothers during pregnancy. The goal of treatment in highly viremic mothers is to lower the serum HBV DNA level by several $\log_{10}$ IU/mL by the time of delivery to minimize the chance of newborn infection. The choice of antiviral agent is less important if treatment of the mother is not needed long term. In the event that the treatment needs to be continued after delivery, the patient should be started on a high–genetic-barrier drug initially or switched to one immediately after delivery. See text for further details about drug selection. HBIG, hepatitis B immune globulin.

frequency of birth defects in the infants of these women has not been shown to be significantly different from that reported in the general U.S. population.

Women who are of child-bearing age should be warned not to become pregnant while undergoing treatment with a nucleos(t)ide analog. If pregnancy occurs during treatment, however, the risk of drug withdrawal and subsequent ALT flares must be balanced against the slight uncertainty of harmful effects to the fetus. Figure 79-6 shows a proposed algorithm for the treatment of HBsAg-pregnant mothers with a high level of viremia. Because lamivudine has an excellent safety record and the most extensive use during pregnancy, its use can been recommended for highly viremic mothers. The risk of developing drug-resistant HBV can be anticipated to be small because of the need for short-term treatment. Telbivudine has also been used successfully during pregnancy to prevent neonatal infection from highly viremic HBeAg-positive mothers and has an FDA status B classification.[137] Tenofovir is another reasonable choice not only because of its category B status, but also because it is more potent than lamivudine or telbivudine. IFN is contraindicated during pregnancy because of its antiproliferative effects. Breast-feeding is not contraindicated in infants of HBsAg-positive women. Mothers who remain on a nucleos(t)ide analog after delivery, however, are advised not to breast-feed because of a small amount of maternal transfer of drug to the newborn.[140]

Severe Acute Hepatitis

Because of the high rate (>95%) of complete immunologic recovery from acute hepatitis B, definitive recommendations about drug treatment cannot be made. Some experts recommend nucleos(t)ide analog therapy when HBeAg remains detectable in serum for more than 10 to 12 weeks because of the high likelihood of evolution to chronic HBV infection without treatment. It has been suggested that persons with acute viral hepatitis complicated by an increase in the INR above 1.5 and deep jaundice persisting for more than 4 weeks should receive antiviral therapy.[141] Antiviral treatment of patients with hepatitis B–induced acute liver failure is recommended in the practice guidelines of the AASLD because of the safety of nucleos(t)ide analog therapy and the need for liver transplantation in many of these patients.[130]

The duration of antiviral therapy is not established for severe or life-threatening acute hepatitis. It has been recommended that therapy continue for 3 months after HBsAg seroconversion or at least 12 months after HBeAg seroconversion if HBsAg loss does not occur.[102]

Cirrhosis

Nucleos(t)ide analog therapy has been shown to be safe in patients with cirrhosis and has made a major difference in the care of patients with advanced liver disease. Antiviral therapy with a high-genetic-barrier drug is preferred in all cases of HBV-related cirrhosis. Marked improvement in hepatic function and regression of fibrosis, including reversal of the histologic features of cirrhosis, has been shown after prolonged viral suppression with entecavir and tenofovir.[111] Nucleos(t)ide analog therapy has been associated with a remarkable decline in the need for liver transplantation in patients with HBV-associated chronic liver failure.[142] HCC may still occur in cirrhotic patients who have lost HBsAg, and regular US surveillance should be continued in these persons (see Chapter 96).[143] The mechanisms behind such late development of HCC have not been defined, but continued hepatocyte regeneration is likely to have a promotional effect on tumorigenesis, and cumulative chromosomal damage from integrated viral sequences may also play a role.[144]

HBV-HIV Coinfection

With improved control of HIV disease with HAART, liver disease has emerged as one of the leading causes of death in patients with HIV infection (see Chapter 34).[145] Antiviral therapy for moderate to severe hepatitis B should be considered for all HIV-HBV coinfected patients, irrespective of the CD4 count. Guidelines enacted by the Department of Health and Human Services suggest that early antiretroviral therapy for all patients who are to undergo treatment for hepatitis B is not required.[146] Entecavir treatment is associated with a decline in HIV RNA levels and is not recommended for use in patients who are not receiving concomitant HIV treatment.[147] In patients with a CD4 count less than $350/mm^3$, the use of agents with activity against both HIV and HBV, such as lamivudine and tenofovir, is recommended. Combination therapy with either emtricitabine and tenofovir or lamivudine and tenofovir should ideally be used to avoid or delay the development of HIV resistance to tenofovir.

HBV-HCV Coinfection

When compared with monoinfected patients, HBV-HCV–coinfected patients tend to have more severe liver injury and a higher probability of cirrhosis.[148] Limited data are available, however, to define the best approach to treatment in this group of patients. The typical patient is positive for HCV RNA but negative for HBV DNA in serum. Close monitoring has been recommended before and after treatment is initiated, because some patients exhibit alternating viremia, and in some instances resurgence of HBV replication has been documented after successful treatment of hepatitis C.[149] The optimal therapy for patients who are positive in serum for both HBV DNA and HCV RNA is also unclear. In such instances, the authors have had success in treating both infections simultaneously with a combination of a nucleos(t)ide analog, pegylated IFN-α, and ribavirin. What effect direct-acting antiviral agents for hepatitis C will have on the treatment of combined HBV and HCV infection remains to be explored (see Chapter 80).

Urgent Treatment

Hepatitis B seldom needs to be treated immediately. There are clinical situations, however, for which prompt or even urgent therapy is required to forestall disease progression, decrease morbidity, or clinically stabilize the patient. Antiviral therapy for hepatitis B should be started as soon as possible whenever a patient with active disease has advanced liver fibrosis or potentially life-threatening disease (Table 79-6). The strongest

TABLE 79-6 Indications for Prompt or Urgent Treatment of Hepatitis B

	Indications	Preferred Agent	Principal Supportive Data
Cirrhosis*			
Decompensated	Clinical stabilization; minimizing risk for recurrence post transplant	Entecavir (0.5 mg) or tenofovir (300 mg)[†]	Open label; multiple large case series
Borderline compensated	Forestalling disease progression; avoidance of transplantation	As above	Undefined
Well compensated	As above	As above	Randomized controlled trials
Acute Liver Failure			
HBV reactivation	Minimizing further liver injury; reducing risk of recurrence after liver transplantation, if needed	Entecavir (0.5 mg) or tenofovir (300 mg)[†]	Open label with comparison with historical controls
Severe acute hepatitis	Minimizing further liver injury and enhancing full recovery	Consider lamivudine or telbivudine[‡]	Small case series

*It has been the author's (RP) practice to use maintenance antiviral therapy for all HBsAg-positive patients with cirrhosis to prevent reactivation of hepatitis B.
[†]Daily dose should be adjusted according to the patient's renal function, as indicated in the manufacturer's recommendations.
[‡]Either agent can be used if the anticipated duration of therapy is 6 months or less.

evidence of benefit for antiviral treatment is for advanced fibrosis, cirrhosis, and decompensated chronic hepatitis B. The data are less certain for reactivation of chronic hepatitis B and even less so for acute severe hepatitis, because available studies have been small and mostly retrospective in nature. The benefit of antiviral treatment for severe acute hepatitis B associated with liver failure remains particularly problematic because disparate rates of efficacy have been reported and HBV DNA may be present in low levels or even nondetectable when the patient is first seen. Based on the expectation that antiviral therapy may be beneficial and will not be harmful, however, a controlled clinical trial is no longer ethically justified.

PREVENTION

Immunoprophylaxis against HBV is of 2 types: passive immunization using HBIG and active immunization using inactive HBsAg. Active immunization gives long-term immunity, whereas passive immunization confers only immediate and short-lived protection.

Hepatitis B Immune Globulin

HBIG is prepared from plasma that is known to contain high titers of anti-HBs. Numerous clinical trials have established the efficacy of HBIG in preventing HBV infection in high-risk persons, such as hemodialysis patients, sexual partners of patients with hepatitis B, and newborn infants of HBsAg-positive mothers within 12 hours of birth along with simultaneous vaccination. HBIG licensed in the United States has an anti-HBs titer of 1:100,000. In Europe, several preparations of HBIG with different concentrations and pharmacokinetic properties are available. HBIG is safe, although rare anaphylactic reactions can occur. Myalgias, rash, and arthralgias have also been reported and are believed to result from formation of antigen-antibody complexes.

Hepatitis B Vaccine

Currently marketed HBV vaccines make use of recombinant DNA technology by introducing the gene for HBsAg (S gene) into the genome of yeast. The 2 vaccines available in the United States are Recombivax HB (Merck, licensed in 1986) and Engerix-B (GlaxoSmithKline, licensed by SmithKline Beecham in 1989). No serious side effects of the HBV vaccine have been reported. Aluminum hydroxide is used as an adjuvant in both vaccines. Because thimerosal, a preservative used in the vaccines, contains mercury, thimerosal-free vaccines have become available, especially for use in infants. The HBV vaccine is administered intramuscularly in the deltoid muscle of adults and the anterolateral thigh of infants and neonates. Because the vaccines contain HBsAg only, anti-HBs is the sole antibody produced. Consequently, vaccinees who test positive for anti-HBc after vaccination should be considered to have either resolved infection or active infection depending on the results of reflex testing for HBsAg.

The vaccines typically achieve an anti-HBs titer greater than 100 mIU/mL. Antibody titers greater than 100 mIU/mL confer 100% protection against HBV infection, and a lower antibody titer (up to 10 mIU/mL) is seroprotective in most instances. Peak antibody titers and persistence of antibody levels vary among different persons. The titers drop steadily over the first 2 years after vaccination, sometimes to levels less than 10 mIU/mL. Two studies in different populations have demonstrated that anti-HBs titers decrease to nonprotective levels in at least 25% to 50% of recipients over a period of 5 to 10 years.[150]

Although protective anti-HBs response rates after HBV vaccination occur in approximately 90% of patients, a number of factors can impede an adequate antibody response. Smoking; obesity; injection into the buttock; chronic liver disease; presence of HLA-DR3, DR7, and DQ2 alleles; absence of the HLA-A2 allele; and extremes of age may be associated with reduced immunogenicity. Such "hyporesponders" may benefit from a higher dose of vaccine. Response rates are also lower in immunocompromised patients, such as transplant recipients, patients receiving chemotherapy, and those with end-stage liver disease. Only 50% to 60% of patients on hemodialysis respond adequately to vaccination. Therefore, patients with chronic kidney disease should be vaccinated early in the course of their disease, before renal disease progresses, to ensure optimal response to vaccination. Five percent to 8% of HBV vaccine recipients do not achieve detectable anti-HBs levels ("nonresponders").

Because HBV vaccination results in strong immunologic memory capable of preventing infection even in patients with low or undetectable antibody titers, recommendations do not call for a booster vaccine dose in immunocompetent adults and children. Booster doses are, however, recommended for patients undergoing hemodialysis, in whom anti-HBs titers should be tested annually and a booster dose given if the titer is lower than 10 mIU/mL.[151] Data from a study in Taiwan demonstrated a surprisingly high rate of HBsAg positivity in adolescents who were vaccinated at birth, especially those born to HBeAg-positive mothers who did not receive HBIG or had less than 4 doses of vaccine. The suggestion was made that a booster dose may be needed at age 15 or older in such highly exposed individuals.[152] Confirmation of this finding would have important implications.

Vaccination Schedule

The typical vaccination schedule is 0, 1, and 6 months. The first 2 doses have no effect on the final anti-HBs titer. The third dose acts as a booster to achieve a high anti-HBs titer. In immunocompromised patients and those undergoing hemodialysis, 4 vaccine doses are recommended, with the fourth dose given to ensure the highest possible anti-HBs titer. If vaccination is interrupted, the second dose should be administered as soon as possible after the first.[153] If the third dose is not given on schedule, it should be given at least 2 months after the second dose.

In the United States and elsewhere, the HBV vaccine is administered to all children and infants as a part of the universal immunization program. Unfortunately, although more than 160 countries have proposed and approved universal vaccination, not all have the financial resources to sponsor a national health program that incorporates affordable or free vaccination.[154]

Combination HBV vaccines with diphtheria-pertussis-tetanus (DPT) and *Haemophilus influenzae* type B (Hib) (DTPw-HB/Hib) are in use for immunization of infants. The other component antigens do not reduce the immunogenicity against HBV.[155] Adolescents who have not been vaccinated in infancy or childhood should also be vaccinated.

Postexposure and Perinatal Prophylaxis

Table 79-7 lists recommendations for prophylaxis after exposure to a known HBsAg-positive source. Postexposure vaccination should be considered for any percutaneous, ocular, or mucous membrane exposure. The type of immunoprophylaxis is determined by the HBsAg status of the source and the

TABLE 79-7 Recommended Postexposure Prophylaxis for HBV According to the Vaccination Status of the Exposed Person

Vaccination Status of Exposed Person	Recommended Prophylaxis
Unvaccinated	HBIG (0.06 mL/kg) and initiate the hepatitis B vaccine series
Previously vaccinated: Known responder*	None
Known nonresponder	HBIG × 2 doses (1 month apart) *OR* HBIG × 1 dose and initiate revaccination
Antibody response unknown	Test for anti-HBs If adequate*: No treatment If inadequate†: HBIG × 1 dose and give vaccine booster dose

*Anti-HBs titer ≥ 10 mIU/mL.
†Anti-HBs titer < 10 mIU/mL.
Anti-HBs, antibody to hepatitis B surface antigen; HBIG, hepatitis B immune globulin; HBsAg, hepatitis B surface antigen.

vaccination-response status of the exposed person. If a patient is a known responder to previous vaccination, then nothing need be done.

Bivalent Vaccine

A combined HAV and HBV vaccine has been licensed commercially (TWINRIX, GlaxoSmithKline, Research Triangle Park, N.C.) and has been shown to be highly immunogenic and protective against both infections. This vaccine offers ease of administration for persons at increased risk of both HAV and HBV infection (e.g., world travelers, men who have sex with men) and in patients with underlying chronic liver disease.[156]

Recommendations

In 2008, the CDC extended its original recommendations for routine HBsAg screening to include persons born in countries in which the prevalence of hepatitis B exceeds 2%.[153] In 2011, the CDC added a recommendation for HBV vaccination in persons 19 to 59 years of age with diabetes mellitus type 1 or 2. Health care professionals may vaccinate diabetics 60 years of age or older after assessing their risk of exposure.[157]

The CDC has revised its recommendations for health care providers and students chronically infected with hepatitis B.[158] In general, the CDC suggests that such persons can maintain their current form of practice. They do not recommend notification of patients of the caregivers' HBV status, nor do they broadly recommend antiviral therapy. Another basic recommendation is that all health care providers and students receive the HBV vaccine followed by testing for anti-HBs to verify immunity. If anti-HBs is not detectable, reflex testing with anti-HBc and HBsAg is the suggested next step and will allow identification of those persons with active HBV infection.

In the past, the CDC did not recommend prevaccination screening for health care providers and students who perform exposure-prone tasks (i.e., surgical procedures in which access is difficult and a needlestick injury may occur). In the 2012 guidelines, the CDC recommended that persons who perform exposure-prone procedures and those at high risk for HBV infection (e.g., those born in endemic regions of the world)

undergo prevaccination testing for hepatitis B.[158] This recommendation is not considered necessary for providers and students who do not perform exposure-prone procedures. It is further recommended that for surgeons who are found to be HBV carriers, including oral surgeons, obstetricians/gynecologists, surgical residents, and others who perform exposure-prone procedures, their procedures should be reviewed by a duly constituted expert review panel with balanced perspective that will oversee the procedures and practice of the individual. A serum HBV level of 1000 IU/mL (equivalent to 5000 copies/mL) is a suggested appropriate threshold for review by the expert panel. Regular activities can be maintained if a lower or undetectable HBV DNA level is documented by regular testing at least every 6 months. Spontaneous fluctuations above the threshold may require that the health care provider or student abstain from performing exposure-prone procedures until retested and, if positive at this level again, "reasonable" steps are taken; the term *reasonable* is meant to include antiviral therapy.

The 2012 CDC guidelines strongly emphasize the need for strict confidentiality but admit that confidentiality may not be possible. It may be difficult to implement all of these guidelines at institutions that lack the necessary infrastructure or for health care providers who perform exposure-prone procedures and choose not to receive antiviral therapy.

KEY REFERENCES

Full references for this chapter can be found on www.expertconsult.com.

1. Kowdley KV, Wang CC, Welch S, et al. Prevalence of chronic hepatitis B among foreign-born persons living in the United States by country of origin. Hepatology 2012; 56:422-33.
29. Lin CL, Kao JH. The clinical implications of hepatitis B virus genotype. Recent advances. J Gastroenterol Hepatol 2011; 26(Suppl 1):123-30.
59. Bruix J, Sherman M. Management of hepatocellular carcinoma: An update. Hepatology 2011; 53:1020-2.
76. Manzano-Alonso ML, Castellano-Tortajada G. Reactivation of hepatitis B virus infection after cytotoxic chemotherapy or immunosuppressive therapy. World J Gastroenterol 2011; 17:1531-7.
81. Perez-Alvarez R, Diaz-Lagares C, Garcia-Hernandez F, et al. Hepatitis B virus (HBV) reactivation in patients receiving tumor necrosis factor (TNF)-targeted therapy: Analysis of 257 cases. Medicine (Baltimore) 2011; 90:359-71.
98. Buster EH, Hansen BE, Lau GK, et al. Factors that predict response of patients with hepatitis B e antigen-positive chronic hepatitis B to peginterferon-alfa. Gastroenterology 2009; 137:2002-9.
102. European Association for the Study of the Liver. EASL clinical practice guidelines: Management of chronic hepatitis B virus infection. J Hepatol 2012; 57:167-85.
105. Chan HL, Thompson A, Martinot-Peignoux M, et al. Hepatitis B surface antigen quantification: Why and how to use it in 2011—A core group report. J Hepatol 2011; 55:1121-31.
106. Hu KQ, Pan CQ, Goodwin D. Barriers to screening for hepatitis B virus infection in Asian Americans. Dig Dis Sci 2011; 56:3163-71.
111. Marcellin P, Gane E, Buti M, et al. Regression of cirrhosis during treatment with tenofovir disoproxil fumarate for chronic hepatitis B: A 5-year open-label follow-up study. Lancet 2013; 381:468-75.

118. Wang Y, Thongsawat S, Gane EJ, et al. Efficacy and safety of continuous 4-year telbivudine treatment in patients with chronic hepatitis B. J Viral Hepat 2013; 20:e37-46.

120. Chotiyaputta W, Peterson C, Ditah FA, et al. Persistence and adherence to nucleos(t)ide analogue treatment for chronic hepatitis B. J Hepatol 2011; 54:12-8.

137. Pan CQ, Duan ZP, Bhamidimarri KR, et al. An algorithm for risk assessment and intervention of mother to child transmission of hepatitis B virus. Clin Gastroenterol Hepatol 2012; 10:452-9.

157. Centers for Disease Control and Prevention. Use of hepatitis B vaccination for adults with diabetes mellitus: Recommendations of the Advisory Committee on Immunization Practices (ACIP). MMWR Morb Mortal Wkly Rep 2011; 60:1709-11.

158. Centers for Disease Control and Prevention (CDC). Updated CDC recommendations for the management of hepatitis B virus-infected health-care providers and students. MMWR Recomm Rep 2012; 61:1-12.

CHAPTER OUTLINE

More than 200 million people worldwide have been infected with HCV.[1,2] In the United States, conservative estimates suggest that more than 5 million people live with HCV.[3] Unfortunately, HCV successfully evades the host immune response in 50% to 90% of acutely infected persons, thus leading to chronic infection in the majority of cases. The natural history of hepatitis C varies greatly; reasons for this heterogeneity remain incompletely understood but are related to viral, host, and environmental factors. Chronic HCV infection can lead to cirrhosis and hepatocellular carcinoma (HCC). The incidence of these complications has risen dramatically in the 2000s but is expected to decline by 2030. In fact, whereas HCV-related mortality increased dramatically after 1995, the rate has reached a plateau since 2002.[4,5] Complications of HCV-related cirrhosis are the leading indication for liver transplantation in the United States and Europe.

Chronic hepatitis C is the only chronic viral infection that can be cured by antiviral therapy. Importantly, successful antiviral treatment can prevent short- and long-term complications of HCV infection in many patients.[6] Up to 80% of patients infected with HCV genotype 1 who tolerate treatment with pegylated interferon-α (IFN-α), ribavirin, and a first-generation HCV protease inhibitor achieve a sustained virologic response (SVR), defined as absence of HCV RNA in serum 3 to 6 months after discontinuation of treatment; an SVR is almost always associated with durable eradication of

the virus.[7,8] From 60% to 90% of genotype 2- and 3-infected patients achieve an SVR with pegylated IFN-α and ribavirin. Substantial progress in understanding the mechanisms of virus entry into the hepatocyte, replication, and the host immune response has led to the development of new therapeutic agents that target the steps in the viral lifecycle. Several new direct-acting antiviral agents (DAAs) are in advanced clinical development and are leading to the availability of IFN-free antiviral regimens for all HCV genotypes, with cure rates well above 90%.

VIROLOGY

Structure

The HCV virion has been visualized by electron microscopy and is an enveloped virus 50 nm in diameter.[9] The 2 envelope proteins, E1 and E2, heterodimerize and assemble into tetramers, which create a smooth outer layer. This layer has a "fishbone" configuration with icosahedral symmetry. The envelope proteins are anchored to a host cell–derived lipid bilayer envelope membrane that surrounds the nucleocapsid. The nucleocapsid is believed to be composed of multiple copies of the core protein and forms an internal icosahedral viral coat that encapsulates the genomic RNA.[10] HCV circulates in various forms in the serum of an infected host, including (1) virions that are bound to very-low-density and low-density lipoproteins and appear to represent the infectious fraction, (2) virions bound to immunoglobulins, and (3) free virions.

---

*Dr. Jacqueline G. O'Leary and Dr. Gary L. Davis contributed to this chapter in previous editions of this book.

Genomic Organization

HCV is a single-stranded positive-sense RNA virus that belongs to the Flaviviridae family and has been classified as the sole member of the genus *Hepacivirus*.[11] The genome of HCV contains approximately 9600 nucleotides with an open reading frame (ORF) that encodes 1 large viral polypeptide precursor of about 3000 amino acids. The HCV ORF is flanked upstream by a 5′ untranslated region (UTR) that functions as an internal ribosome entry site (IRES) to direct cap-independent translation (i.e., without the addition of an extra ribonucleotide to the 5′ end of the viral messenger RNA) and downstream by a 3′ UTR that is critical for initiation of new RNA strand synthesis.[12] The 5′ and portions of the 3′ UTR are the most conserved parts of the HCV genome.

Viral Replication and Life Cycle

Although peripheral blood mononuclear cells, B cells, T cells, and dendritic cells have been reported to support HCV replication, hepatocytes are the major site of viral replication.[13,14]

Significant progress has been made since 2000 in the understanding of how HCV binds and enters the hepatocyte (Fig. 80-1).[15] HCV entry involves the attachment of envelope proteins E1 and E2 to cell surface molecules. The expression and function of CD81, a member of the tetraspan superfamily, are essential for HCV entry into hepatocytes.[16] In addition, human scavenger receptor class B type 1 (SR-B1), a selective importer of cholesteryl esters from high-density lipoproteins (HDL) into cells, has been shown to interact with E2 and is essential for HCV entry.[17] Whereas CD81 and SR-B1 are required early in the process of viral entry, claudin-1 (CLDN1), a tight junction component that is highly expressed on hepatocytes, and occludin are required later in the cell entry process.[18,19] Heparin sulfated proteoglycans and low-density lipoproteins (LDL) have also been shown to be involved in HCV cell entry.[20,21] Additional cellular factors and receptors suggested to be required for viral entry include EGF[22] and Niemann-Pick C1-Like 1 (NPC1L1), a cholesterol uptake receptor. NPC1L1 is an HCV entry factor that can be modified by therapeutic intervention—for example, with the FDA-approved NPC1L1 antagonist ezetimibe, which blocks HCV uptake in vitro via a

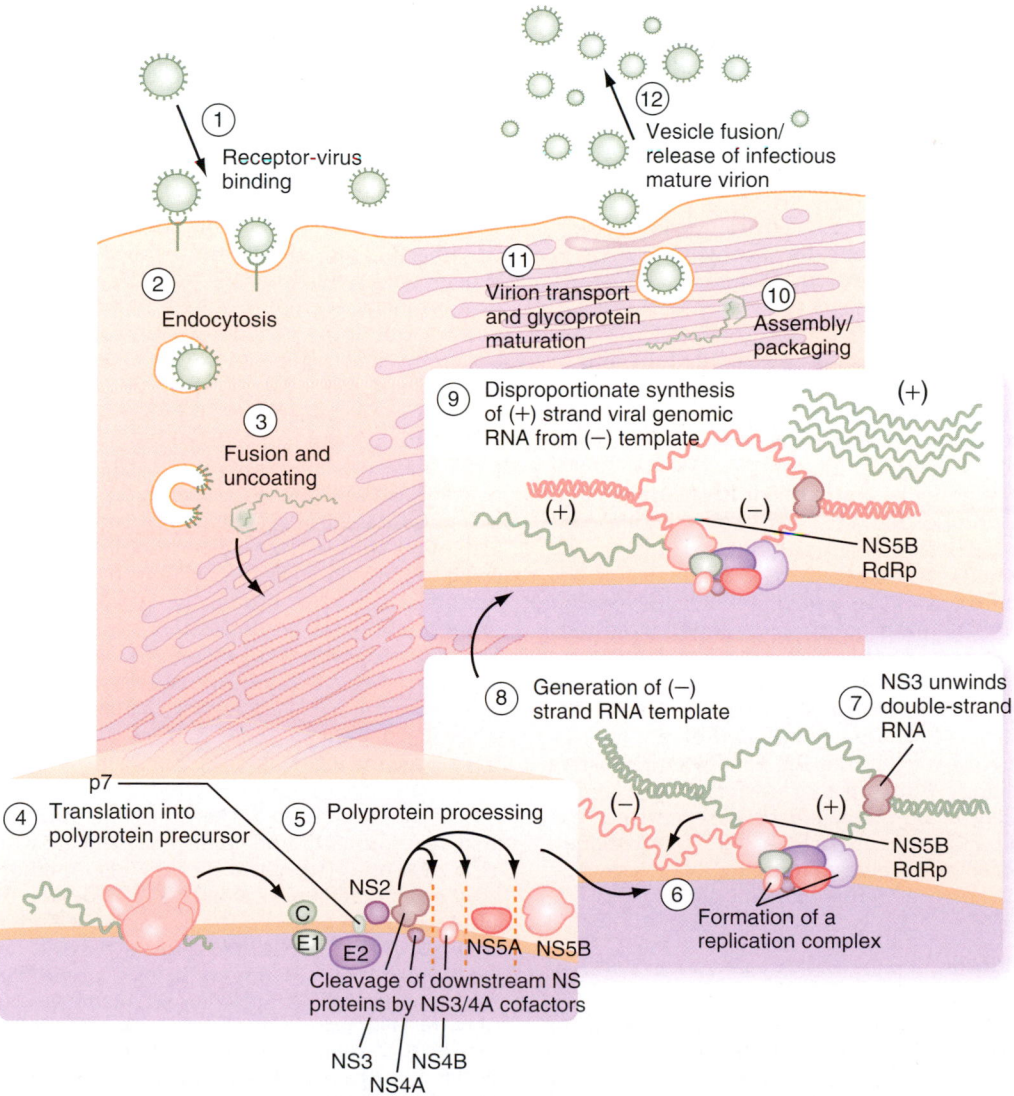

FIGURE 80-1. Putative life cycle of HCV. (See text for details and Fig. 80-2 for functions of the HCV proteins.) NS, nonstructural; RdRp, RNA-dependent RNA polymerase. *(Reproduced with permission from Pawlotsky JM, Chevaliez S, McHutchison JG. The hepatitis C virus life cycle as a target for new antiviral therapies. Gastroenterology 2007; 132:1979-98.)*

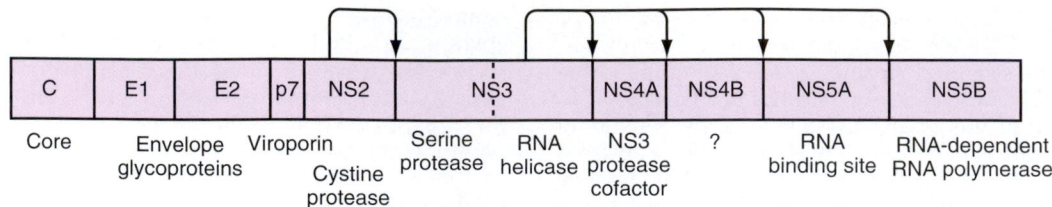

FIGURE 80-2. Schematic representation of the HCV polyprotein. The structural proteins C (core), E1, and E2 (envelope proteins) are cleaved from the polyprotein by the host signal peptidase. p7, a viroporin protein, is cleaved by the endoplasmic reticulum signal peptidase and forms an ion channel that is essential for assembly and release of infectious virions. The NS2 cysteine protease auto-catalytically cleaves itself from the polyprotein. The NS3 protease cleaves the remainder of the nonstructural proteins: NS3 (serine protease and RNA helicase), NS4A (NS3 protease cofactor), NS4B, NS5A (RNA binding site), and NS5B (RNA-dependent RNA polymerase).

virion cholesterol-dependent step prior to virion-cell membrane fusion.[18,23]

Once HCV attaches to the cell, endocytosis of the bound virion is presumed to occur, as with other flaviviruses. A pH drop in the vesicle causes conformational changes in the glycoproteins that lead to fusion of the viral and cellular membranes[24] and release of viral RNA into the cytoplasm. In the cytosol, the 5' UTR contains several highly conserved and structured domains that function as an IRES, which directs the RNA to its docking site on the endoplasmic reticulum and mediates cap-independent internal initiation of HCV polyprotein translation by recruiting both cellular proteins, including eukaryotic initiation factors (eIF) 2 and 3, and viral proteins.[25]

The large polyprotein generated by translation of the HCV genome is co- and post-translationally processed proteolytically into at least 11 viral proteins, including both structural (nucleocapsid [C], or p21; envelope 1 [E1], or gp31; and envelope 2 [E2], or gp70) and nonstructural (NS2, NS3, NS4A, NS4B, NS5A, and NS5B) proteins (Fig. 80-2). The functions of these specific proteins are described later in the chapter.

After polyprotein processing, NS4B expression causes the membrane alterations that are seen on electron microscopy as a membranous web.[26] The replication complex associates viral proteins, cellular components, and nascent RNA strands and is essential for HCV replication. HCV replication is catalyzed by the NS5B RNA-dependent RNA polymerase (RdRp). The positive-strand genomic RNA serves as a template for the synthesis of a negative-strand intermediate. Negative-strand RNA serves as a template for production of numerous strands of RNA of positive polarity that are used for polyprotein translation and synthesis of new intermediates of replication and that are packaged into new virus particles.[27]

Finally, viral particle formation is initiated by the interaction of the core protein with genomic RNA in the endoplasmic reticulum.[28] By analogy with pestiviruses, HCV packaging and release are likely to be inefficient because much of the virus remains in the cell. Following release, viral particles may infect adjacent hepatocytes or enter the circulation, where they are available for infection of another cell or host.

Virus Protein Function

The large polyprotein generated by translation of the HCV genome is cleaved by cellular and viral proteases to form structural and nonstructural proteins. The structural proteins are separated from the nonstructural proteins by the short membrane peptide p7, which is believed to be a viroporin, a protein that plays a role in viral particle maturation and release.[29] At least 1, and possibly 3, alternative reading frame proteins (ARFP, or F for "frameshift") exists.[30] The exact

number of alternative reading frames, the number of proteins that result, and the functions of the proteins are not known.[30] One such protein is 17 kd in size; it can be expressed in vitro, and antibodies to it have been found in infected patients.

The crystal structures of most of the ORF proteins have been elucidated and have been helpful in understanding protein interactions and functions. Although these proteins are most important for viral replication, some also interact with host proteins and may facilitate persistence of the virus by impairing the immune response.

The core protein is first cleaved from the large polypeptide and then further processed by a host signal peptidase.[27] In infectious HCV virions, core protein forms the viral nucleocapsid and binds RNA; it has many other functions as well. Core protein has been found attached to lipid rafts and the endoplasmic reticulum, and it translocates into the nucleus. When core protein attaches to lipid rafts, it recruits nonstructural proteins, thereby resulting in the assembly of infectious virions. Core protein can also interact with the host immune system by inactivating the RNA silencing activity of Dicer, a cellular endoribonuclease that produces small interfering RNA to bind and target HCV RNA for destruction by the cell.[31] Core protein can also bind to Janus kinase-1 (JAK1) and JAK2 and alter the activation of signal transducer activator of transcription (STAT) proteins, leading to impairment of IFN production.[32] Extracellularly, core protein inhibits T-cell activation and proliferation, possibly by down-regulating co-stimulatory molecules on dendritic cells.[33] Specific polymorphisms in core protein have also been associated with intracellular lipid accumulation[34]; this may be the result of facilitation of phosphorylation of insulin receptor substrate-1 (IRS-1), thereby leading to insulin resistance.[35] Mutations in core protein have also been associated with an increased risk of HCC in patients; core protein alone can cause HCC in transgenic mice.[36]

E1 and E2 proteins are cleaved from the polypeptide by host signal peptidase.[37] The 2 proteins form highly glycosylated heterodimers and then tetramers that are essential for viral assembly (see earlier). They also mediate cell entry by binding to surface receptors.[38] Subsequently, they are responsible for fusion between the host cell membrane and the viral envelope. Because E1 and E2 are expressed on the surface of the virion, they are targets of host antibodies. The first 27 amino acids of E2 form hypervariable region 1 (HVR1); alterations in HVR1 are believed to be an attempt by the virus at antibody-mediated immune evasion.

P7 is cleaved by the endoplasmic reticulum signal peptidase and forms an ion channel. This viroporin protein is essential for efficient assembly and release of infectious virions but not for cell entry. Because p7 is needed later in the viral life cycle, cleavage of the polypeptide is delayed.[39]

NS2 complexes with NS3 and zinc to form a cysteine protease, with 2 composite active sites, that autocatalytically cleaves NS2 from NS3.[40] No other function of NS2 has been discovered to date. NS3 has several functions in addition to complexing with NS2 for autocatalytic cleavage of the NS2-NS3 site.[40] Its function as a serine protease is markedly enhanced by its association with NS4A. The enzyme results in cleavage of the polyprotein at the NS3-NS4A, NS4A-NS4B, NS4B-NS5A, and NS5A-NS5B sites.[41,42] The NS3 protease also cleaves and thereby destroys the function of Cardif and TRIF (Toll/interleukin receptor domain-containing adapter-inducing IFN-β), which are intermediates in 2 separate pathways of host-cell IFN secretion in response to viral infection.[43-45] This property may have a significant effect in impairing the host response to HCV infection. Finally, a portion of the NS3 protein functions as a helicase that unwinds viral RNA as well as host DNA. The helicase function is dependent on ATP, may require dimerization of NS3, and progresses in discrete steps like an inchworm.[46] NS4A complexes with NS3 and functions to stabilize the protease and helicase activities and anchor the complex to the endoplasmic reticulum membrane.[41,47] It also regulates hyperphosphorylation of NS5A.[48] The only known function of NS4B is to induce the formation of the membranous web on which HCV transcription occurs.[49] NS5A binds zinc and forms homodimers that are bound to the endoplasmic reticulum membrane.[47] NS5A is essential for viral replication and is believed to provide an RNA-binding site within the replication complex.[50] In addition, NS5A inhibits apoptosis in infected cells,[51,52] and some mutations confer improved sensitivity to IFN therapy.[53] NS5B is the viral RNA-dependent RNA polymerase.[41] The crystal structure elucidates the tunnel of the enzyme that directs single-stranded RNA into the active site.[54] It can synthesize both negative-strand HCV RNA templates and positive-strand HCV RNA genomes.

Genotypes and Quasispecies

HCV has an inherently high mutational rate that results in considerable heterogeneity throughout the genome. This high mutational rate is in part a consequence of the RNA-dependent RNA polymerase of HCV, which lacks 3'- to 5'-exonuclease proofreading ability that ordinarily would remove mismatched nucleotides incorporated during replication. An average of 1 error occurs for every 10^4 to 10^5 nucleotides copied. This phenomenon is favored by a high viral turnover rate; 10^{10} to 10^{12} virions are produced per day.[55] The estimated half-life of HCV in serum is only about 45 minutes.[56] A substantial proportion of newly synthesized viral genomes have alterations. Because of the functional differences in HCV proteins, genetic variation in some parts of the genome confers advantages by evading or inhibiting the host immune system, whereas other mutations may be lethal to the virus if they lead to defective replication machinery. Therefore, genetic variation is distributed irregularly along the genome. Each new genetic variant is produced in a single cell and may or may not spread through the liver and into the serum. The result is not only genetic diversity in the serum, but also compartmentalization of variant virions in different parts of the liver and perhaps in extrahepatic sites.

Because of the vast genetic variation, a classification scheme was devised whereby viral sequences are given a genotype and subtype. The first division used to describe the genetic heterogeneity of HCV is the viral *genotype*, which refers to genetically distinct groups of HCV isolates that have arisen during the evolution of the virus. Nucleotide sequencing has shown variation of up to 34% between genotypes.[57] The most conserved region (5' UTR) has a maximum

nucleotide sequence divergence of 9% between genotypes, whereas the highly variable regions that encode the envelope proteins (E1 and E2) exhibit a nucleotide sequence divergence of 35% to 44% between genotypes. The sequences cluster into 6 major genotypes (designated by numbers), with sequence similarities of 60% to 70%, and more than 70 *subtypes* (designated by a lower-case letter) within these major genotypes, with sequence similarities of 77% to 80%.[57] In this scheme, the first variant, which was cloned by Choo and colleagues, is designated type 1a.[58] The HCV genotype is an intrinsic characteristic of the infecting HCV strain and does not change over time; therefore, the genotype only needs to be determined once in an infected person. Mixed-genotype infections may be seen and reflect either coinfection with more than 1 HCV virus or methodological problems in genotype testing. In addition, intergenotypic HCV recombinants have been described[59]; these are thought to arise because of recombination between different genotypes in patients with repeated exposure. The recombination events have been reported to occur in or between NS2 and NS3.[60]

Global geographic differences exist in the distribution of HCV genotypes, as well as in the mode of acquisition. In the United States, genotype 1a is the most prevalent, accounting for approximately 57% of HCV infections, followed by genotype 1b in 17%, genotype 2 in 14%, genotype 3 in 7%, and genotype 4, 5, or 6 in less than 5%.[61] Racial differences are seen in the prevalence of genotypes; approximately 90% of African Americans are infected with HCV genotype 1, whereas only 70% of whites and 71% of Hispanics are infected with genotype 1.[62] In Europe, the most prevalent genotype is 1b (47%), followed by 1a (17%), 3 (16%), and 2 (13%).[2] Genotype 4 is found mainly in Egypt, the Middle East, and Central Africa.[63] In Egypt, approximately 15% of the population is infected with HCV, and more than 90% have HCV genotype 4. Because of the high prevalence in Egypt, genotype 4 represents 20% of the world's HCV-infected population. Genotype 5, although originally isolated in South Africa, is also seen in specific regions of France, Belgium, and Spain.[64] Genotype 6 is found predominantly in Asia. The distribution of genotypes is ever changing with immigration and alterations in the primary modes of viral transmission. Therefore, the frequencies of viral genotypes change over time.

An important clinical correlation with HCV genotype is response to treatment (see later). HCV genotype does not, however, appear to influence the severity of liver disease, as defined by the stage of fibrosis, or the likelihood of progression of acute to chronic HCV infection.

The second component of genetic heterogeneity is *quasispecies* generation.[57] Quasispecies are closely related, yet heterogeneous, sequences of HCV RNA within a single infected person that result from mutations that occur during viral replication. The rate of nucleotide changes varies significantly among the different regions of the viral genome. The highest proportion of mutations is found in the E1 and E2 regions, particularly in HVR1. Even though this region represents only a minor part of the E2 region, it accounts for approximately 50% of the nucleotide changes and 60% of the amino acid substitutions within the envelope region.

The development of quasispecies may be 1 mechanism by which the virus escapes the host's immune response and establishes persistent infection.[65] During acute infection or during treatment, the lack of quasispecies is associated with viral clearance, and the development of numerous quasispecies is associated with viral persistence.[66] In acute disease, patients in whom genetic variation in the HVR1 region develops after antibody seroconversion progress to chronic disease, whereas those in whom such genetic variation does not develop are more likely to achieve viral clearance.[65] Genetic variation before seroconversion does not correlate with outcome, indicating that quasispecies formation results from antibody-mediated immune pressure. Interestingly, no intrinsically IFN-resistant variants of HCV have been defined, indicating that both viral and host factors play important roles in determining whether the virus persists or is cleared. An increased number of quasispecies has also been associated with more rapid progression to cirrhosis and the development of HCC.[67]

EPIDEMIOLOGY

Incidence and Prevalence

The worldwide seroprevalence of HCV infection, based on detection of antibody to HCV (anti-HCV), is estimated to be 3%, with more than 170 million people infected chronically. The overall worldwide prevalence increased from 1990 to 2010.[1] Marked geographic variation exists, with infection rates ranging from 1.3% to 1.6% in the United States to 15% in Egypt. In 2002, between 3.2 and 5 million persons were infected with HCV in the United States,[68] but the incidence of HCV has declined continually since 1994.[5] The highest prevalence in different age groups shifted from 35 to 44 years (2.5%) to 55 to 64 years in 2005 (2.7%).[1] It has therefore been recommended that all persons born between 1945 and 1965 be tested for anti-HCV.[69] The prevalence is higher in males (2.1%) than in females (1.1%), and in African Americans (3%) than in whites (1.5%). Other risk factors for HCV infection are injection drug use,[70] blood transfusion before 1992, more than 50 lifetime sexual partners, and family income below the poverty level. The prevalence of HCV infection in the United States may be underestimated because the National Health and Nutrition Examination Survey (NHANES) data did not evaluate persons who are homeless, incarcerated, or in the military. Trends in the epidemiology of HCV infection suggest an increase in prevalence in young drug-using persons.[71]

Worldwide, 3 different epidemiologic patterns of HCV infection have emerged. They are (1) previous exposure through health care with a peak prevalence in older persons; (2) exposure through IV drug use, the major risk factor since data first became available in about 1960, with a peak prevalence among middle-aged persons; and (3) ongoing high levels of infection in areas where high rates of infection occur in all age groups.

Given the factors that influence viral diversity (see earlier), estimating the site of origin and age of HCV by phylogenetic analysis is difficult. The best estimate is that HCV originated in western and sub-Saharan Africa.[72] Subsequent global spread probably occurred coincident with trade and human migration. Evolution of the virus led to a geographic distribution of genotypes, so that genotypes 1, 2, and 3 are most common in North America and Europe, genotype 4 is most common in the Middle East, and genotype 6 is most common in Southeast Asia. In Japan, HCV transmission transitioned from constant to exponential growth in the 1920s, and the prevalence of HCV infection is highest in older persons.[73] In Japan, and later in southern and Eastern Europe, health care–related procedures—particularly reuse of contaminated syringes—played a major role in viral spread. In the United States, Australia, and other developed countries, peak prevalence is in persons 40 to 49 years of age, and analysis of risk factors suggests that most HCV transmission occurred between the mid-1980s and the mid-1990s, through IV drug use. In Egypt, the spread of HCV increased exponentially from the 1930s to the 1980s because of mass vaccination campaigns with reuse of medical equipment.[63] In Egypt and other developing countries, high rates of

infection are observed in all age groups, suggesting that an ongoing risk of HCV acquisition exists.

In the United States, the incidence of acute hepatitis C is falling. The peak incidence was estimated to be 180,000 cases per year in the mid-1980s, but the rate declined to less than 20,000 cases.[74] Many factors have contributed to the falling incidence of acute hepatitis C. In the 1980s, when blood was purchased from donors, 2% to 10% of blood units were infected with HCV, leading to a high rate of transfusion-acquired HCV infection.[75] The institution of volunteer blood donation, creation of recombinant clotting factors, and implementation of HCV blood testing (between 1990 and 1992) dramatically decreased transfusion-acquired HCV infection.

An important mechanism of transmission worldwide has been the lack of sterilization of medical instruments such as syringes. Although the incidence of HCV transmission by medical instruments has also decreased markedly, the risk has not been eliminated, even in the United States. New HCV infections in the United States and other developed countries occur primarily as a result of injection drug use.

Transmission

Modes of transmission of HCV can be divided into percutaneous (blood transfusion and needlestick inoculation) and nonpercutaneous (sexual contact and perinatal exposure). Patients are often unwilling to disclose percutaneous risk factors, and therefore "nonpercutaneous" transmission may represent occult percutaneous exposure.

Percutaneous Transmission

Blood transfusion (before the introduction of screening) and injection drug use are the most clearly documented risk factors for HCV infection. Following the introduction of anti-HCV screening of blood donors between 1990 and 1992, the number of transfusion-related cases of HCV infection declined sharply to the point that less than 1 case occurs per 2,000,000 units transfused. In many countries, blood products are assayed directly for HCV RNA by "mini-pool" testing. Implementing HCV RNA testing has basically eliminated transmission of HCV by blood transfusions.[76]

Injection drug use has always been the major route of HCV acquisition in the United States and accounts for an increasingly large portion of cases, at least two thirds of new cases of HCV infection.[70] The frequency of HCV infection in persons who inject drugs (PWID) ranges from 57% to 90%.[70] Although risk factors for HBV and HIV infection overlap with those for HCV infection, the prevalence of HCV infection in this population is the highest among the 3 viruses. The majority of PWID become anti-HCV positive within 6 months of initiating injection drug use with shared paraphernalia.

Chronic hemodialysis is also associated with increased rates of HCV infection. The frequency of anti-HCV in patients on hemodialysis ranges from less than 10% in the United States to 55% to 85% in Jordan, Saudi Arabia, and Iran.[77] Serologic assays for anti-HCV may underestimate the frequency of HCV infection in this relatively immunocompromised population, and virologic assays may be necessary for accurate diagnosis.[78]

Transmission may occur from infected patients to health care workers. Anti-HCV seroconversion rates are approximately 0.3% to 4% in longitudinal studies of health care workers after percutaneous inoculation from anti-HCV–positive sources, although the risk is dependent on the type of needle (hollow vs. solid, infusion vs. withdrawal), volume of inoculum, depth of injury, time the body fluid has spent ex vivo, level of viremia (viral load), and HIV status of the inoculating body fluid.[79-81] Although less common, transmission of HCV also may occur from health care workers to patients.[82] Because acute HCV infection is often subclinical, nosocomial transmission may occur with greater frequency than has been recognized previously. Strict adherence to universal precautions to protect health care workers and patients is critically important. At this time, no treatment is effective for postexposure prophylaxis, and no data support such treatment even if it were available.

Nonpercutaneous Transmission

Nonpercutaneous modes of HCV transmission include sexual practices and childbirth. Available evidence indicates that transmission by nonpercutaneous routes occurs but is inefficient. From 10% to 20% of patients with HCV infection report that their only risk factor is sexual exposure to a partner with HCV infection. Most seroepidemiologic studies, however, have demonstrated anti-HCV in only a small proportion of sexual contacts of infected persons. In a large prospective study of monogamous seronegative partners of HCV-infected patients who denied anal intercourse and intercourse during menstruation, no instances of HCV transmission of a virus with the same gene sequence occurred over a 10-year period of time.[83] Similarly, a study in which 500 anti-HCV–positive persons and their long-term heterosexual partners were followed identified only 3 couples (0.6%) with concordant viral strains.[84] The calculated maximum HCV transmission rate was 1 per 190,000 sexual contacts. Therefore, many of the cases presumed to be the result of sexual transmission are likely the result of other, perhaps unreported or unrecognized, exposures. If the index sexual partner is infected with HIV or the partners engage in high-risk sexual practices (e.g., anal intercourse), however, the transmissibility of HCV is likely increased.[85]

The incidence of acute hepatitis C has been reported to have increased in HIV-infected men having sex with men in the 2000s in different regions of the world, including the United States, Australia, and Europe.[86] Permucosal risk factors including specific sexual practices and mucosally administered drugs have been suggested to be responsible for the increase in incidence.

Compared with the high efficiency of perinatal transmission of HBV infection (see Chapter 79), the risk of perinatal transmission of HCV infection is low, averaging 5.1% to 6.7% for HCV-monoinfected patients and 2 to 3 times higher for HCV-HIV coinfected patients.[87,88] Mothers with a high serum level of HCV RNA (high viral load) are more likely to transmit HCV to their infants, a finding that may explain why infants born to mothers with HCV-HIV coinfection are at higher risk of HCV infection. Interestingly, the use of HAART in HCV-HIV coinfected mothers may decrease the risk of perinatal transmission of both HIV and HCV.[88] Data regarding the risk associated with vaginal delivery as opposed to cesarean delivery are uncontrolled, but evidence for a higher risk of HCV transmission with vaginal delivery is unconvincing. This issue remains controversial, and some authorities recommend elective cesarean section before membrane rupture.[87]

Although little data exist, the risk of HCV transmission from breastfeeding is negligible to small. The CDC and international societies have concluded that breastfeeding by HCV-infected mothers is generally safe.[2,89] Because anti-HCV can be acquired passively by the infant, testing for HCV RNA is required if the diagnosis of HCV infection is suspected. Infants of infected mothers should not undergo serologic testing for anti-HCV before 18 months of age, because maternal antibodies may persist in the infant's serum and lead to diagnostic confusion.

Sporadic HCV Infection

The source of transmission is unknown in up to one third of cases of HCV infection. Such sporadic HCV infection probably results from an undisclosed or unrecognized percutaneous route of infection. This presumption is supported by the observation that intranasal cocaine use is not considered a major risk factor for HCV transmission (although it was considered a risk factor in the past).[90] HCV infection can be acquired from non-commercial tattooing and body piercing when equipment is reused, shared, or improperly sterilized. Commercial tattooing is now well controlled and likely conveys little risk of HCV infection. Iatrogenic transmission of HCV is well documented in a variety of circumstances, most notably via contaminated multi-use vials and inadequately sterilized multi-use instruments and syringes, as seen with schistosomal treatment campaigns in Egypt.[91]

PATHOGENESIS

Determinants of persistence of HCV include (1) the evasion of immune responses through several viral mechanisms, (2) inadequate induction of the innate immune response, (3) insufficient induction or maintenance of an adaptive immune response, (4) the production of viral quasispecies, and (5) the induction of immunologic tolerance.[92] Chronic hepatitis develops in 50% to 90% of persons with acute HCV infection. In the minority of patients in whom acute HCV resolves, an early and multispecific T-cell response occurs.[93] This response can be detected up to 20 years after resolution of infection[94] and may contribute to protection in case of subsequent exposures to HCV. Although the immune response is essential in preventing viral persistence, in those without viral clearance, the immune response mediates hepatic cell destruction and fibrosis.

Viral Mechanisms

In chronically infected patients, the pathogenesis of liver damage is largely immune mediated. In a small subset of immunocompromised HCV-infected patients among both HIV-infected patients and organ transplant recipients, however, a syndrome termed *fibrosing cholestatic hepatitis* develops (see Chapter 97).[95,96] Such cases are thought to result from direct viral hepatotoxicity of infected cells, because viral levels are typically greater than 30 million copies/mL and hepatocytes contain enormous concentrations of virus and viral proteins.[97] Survival in such patients is poor.

The majority of patients with HCV infection have a variable immune response that, although inadequate to eradicate acute infection, appears to regulate the vigor of persistent infection and avoid the development of fibrosing cholestatic hepatitis. The immune response to HCV is incompletely understood because animal models are not readily available,[98] and most studies in humans rely on observations in peripheral blood rather than the hepatic immune environment.

Immune-Mediated Mechanisms

HCV infection elicits an immune response in the host that involves both an initial innate response and a subsequent adaptive response. The innate response is the first line of defense against the virus and includes several arms such as natural killer (NK) cell activation and cellular antiviral mechanisms triggered by pathogen-associated molecular patterns (PAMPs) recognized by the cell.[99] These processes can lead to apoptosis of infected cells within the first few hours of infection. NK cells, as the effector cells of the innate immune system, also produce TNF-β and IFN-α, cytokines that are critical for dendritic cell maturation and subsequent induction of adaptive immunity. NK cells can also attack virus-infected cells directly, as do other immune cells by different effector molecules.[100] Subsequently, however, the virus initiates a number of mechanisms that undermine the ability of the host to control the infection.

Virus-related disruption of the innate, and later adaptive, immune response occurs at several levels. NK cell function is slowed possibly because NK cell–mediated cytotoxicity and production of cytokines are interrupted when the HCV E2 protein binds its cellular receptor CD81.[101] Expression of TNF-related apoptosis-inducing ligand (TRAIL) on NK cells correlates with disease activity in both acute[102] and chronic[103] hepatitis C, thereby suggesting that NK cells have a direct role in the immunopathogenesis of hepatitis C. PAMPs activate several cellular processes including the JAK-STAT pathway and Toll-like receptor-3 (TLR-3), activation of both of which ultimately results in production of cellular IFNs and IFN-regulated factors that convey antiviral properties to the cell. NS3/4 protease degrades TRIF, an essential intermediate in this pathway, and cleaves IFN promoter stimulator-1 (IPS-1), an intermediate in the signaling cascade, to activate IFN when retinoic inducible gene-1 (RIG-1) binds viral intermediates.[104] In addition, HCV core protein promotes STAT-1 degradation, inhibits STAT-1 phosphorylation, promotes suppressor of cytokine signaling (SOCS) induction (an inhibitor of JAK-STAT signaling), and impairs IFN-stimulated gene factor-3 (ISGF3), a heterotrimer of STAT-1, STAT-2, and IFN-β promoter stimulator (IRF-9) from binding to the promoter regions of IFN-stimulated response elements (ISRE), thereby inhibiting transcription of IFN response genes. Even when IFN response genes are activated, NS5A and E2 both can disrupt protein kinase R (PKR) function to suppress translation, thereby allowing viral replication to continue.[104] In addition, NS5A inhibits 2′-5′-oligoadenylate synthetase (OAS), which is expressed in response to HCV infection and leads to HCV RNA degradation. Taken together, HCV is able to disrupt the innate immune response at several levels, and these strategies appear to be pivotal in establishing the chronicity of infection.

The ability of HCV to impair the innate immune response prevents development of a vigorous adaptive immune response to the infection. NK cells do not adequately activate dendritic cells, and as a result, the priming of CD8+ and CD4+ T cells in HCV-infected patients is inadequate.[105] Even if an adequate T-cell response is created, HCV-infected patients have a large number of regulatory T cells in their portal tracts[106]; intrahepatic immune regulation by these cells has not been demonstrated but is presumed.

HCV-specific T cells are enriched at the site of viral replication, with an increased number in the liver when compared with the peripheral blood.[107] CD8+ lymphocytes predominate, suggesting that cytotoxic T lymphocytes are the main perpetrators of hepatocellular injury. The T-cell immune response in the liver may result in direct lysis of infected cells and inhibition of viral replication by secreted antiviral cytokines.[92]

Whereas the cellular immune response plays a pivotal role in the pathogenesis of HCV infection, the importance of the humoral immune response is less clear. Antibodies to viral proteins are produced and do not appear to correlate with the stage of infection or immune reactivity. Furthermore, administration of high-titer HCV-enriched or HCV-specific immunoglobulin has little effect on viral levels or persistence in humans.

In summary, viral products play an integral role in the immune regulation that leads to chronic infection instead of viral clearance. Both the virus and the immune response probably play a role in the development of hepatocellular injury.

CLINICAL FEATURES

Acute Hepatitis C

HCV accounts for an estimated 20% of cases of acute hepatitis. Acute hepatitis C is rarely seen in clinical practice, because nearly all cases are asymptomatic. Within 7 to 21 days after viral transmission, HCV RNA becomes detectable in serum.[108] Longer incubation periods can occur, especially in cases in which only a small amount of virus has been transmitted. These data suggest that the duration of the incubation period may vary between different transmission routes. HCV RNA levels rise rapidly in serum after infection, followed by a delayed increase in serum ALT levels 4 to 12 weeks after infection, indicating hepatic injury. Serum ALT levels frequently reach values more than 10 times the upper limit of normal, with concomitant rises in the serum bilirubin level[109] (Fig. 80-3). Some patients also develop clinical symptoms 2 to 12 weeks after viral transmission, but the majority of patients remain asymptomatic during the acute phase, and most infected persons do not become aware of their disease. Therefore, it is not easy to investigate the early phase of HCV infection. Several studies have investigated patients recruited during the acute symptomatic phase of HCV infection, and 80% of the patients have presented with diverse symptoms.[110] Even in symptomatic patients, however, most of the clinical symptoms are nonspecific. Commonly reported symptoms include fatigue, nausea, abdominal pain, loss of appetite, mild fever, itching, and myalgia. Jaundice, which is the most specific liver-related symptom, develops in 50% to 84% of patients with clinically overt acute HCV infection. Fulminant acute hepatitis C has been reported in only single cases, in contrast to infections with other hepatotropic viruses (see Chapter 95). The presentation may be more apparent and the clinical course more severe when acute HCV infection occurs in patients who drink large amounts of alcohol or have coinfection with HBV or HIV.

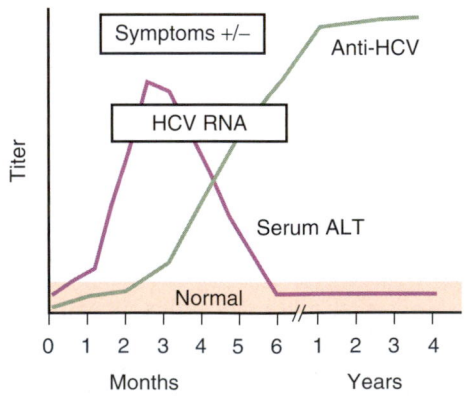

FIGURE 80-3. Typical course of acute HCV infection followed by recovery. Symptoms may or may not be present during acute infection. Anti-HCV, antibody to HCV. *(Modified from the Centers for Disease Control and Prevention, www.cdc.gov/hepatitis/Resources/Professionals/Training/Serology/training.htm#one.)*

The rate of viral persistence after acute infection ranges from 45% to more than 90%. Age and gender clearly influence the risk of chronicity, with younger and female patients having the lowest rates of chronicity. Other factors that may play a role include the source of infection and size of inoculum (chronicity may be less common in PWID than in those who acquire HCV infection by blood transfusion), immune status of the host (chronicity rates are higher in persons with immunodeficiency states such as agammaglobulinemia and HIV infection), and the patient's race (rates of viral persistence are higher in African Americans than in whites and Hispanic Americans in the United States).[111] Finally, the rate of spontaneous clearance is higher in symptomatic patients in whom jaundice develops during acute infection than in those who remain asymptomatic.[112]

Single nucleotide polymorphisms (SNPs) close to the interleukin 28B (IL28B) gene have been found to be associated with the outcome of acute hepatitis C. The IL28B gene is located on chromosome 19 and encodes IFN-λ-3. Ge and colleagues reported a significant role for a specific SNP in the IL28B gene region (rs12979860 CC) in the response to pegylated IFN-α–based therapy for chronic hepatitis C in 2009.[113] Shortly thereafter, Thomas and colleagues identified a major contribution for the same SNP in spontaneous clearance of acute HCV infection.[114] Subsequently, these findings were confirmed by other investigators in different cohorts.[112,115] An association between clearance of acute HCV infection and the IL28B genotype may differ, however, between symptomatic and asymptomatic patients, because the CC IL28B polymorphism was associated with spontaneous recovery only in nonicteric patients in a cohort of East German women exposed to HCV in a single-source outbreak in the late 1970s.[112]

Chronic Hepatitis C

Serum ALT levels are usually elevated in patients with chronic HCV infection. Because levels commonly fluctuate, however, as many as half of patients may have a normal ALT level at any given time.[116] The ALT level may remain normal for prolonged periods of time in about 20% of cases, although transient elevations occur even in these cases.[116] Persistently normal ALT levels are more common in women, and such cases typically are associated with lower serum HCV RNA levels and less inflammation and fibrosis on liver biopsy specimens.

Most patients with chronic hepatitis C are asymptomatic before the onset of advanced hepatic fibrosis. Patients who have been diagnosed with chronic infection, however, often complain of fatigue or depression, and they consistently score lower than HCV-negative persons in all aspects of health-related quality of life (HRQOL).[117] Whether the decrease in HRQOL is related to viral factors, social factors (e.g., IV drug use), social stigmatization, or worry related to the diagnosis itself is unclear. Nevertheless, HRQOL scores improve if the patient achieves a sustained response to antiviral therapy. Less common symptoms may include arthralgias, paresthesias, myalgias, sicca syndrome, nausea, anorexia, and difficulty with concentration. The severity of these symptoms may be, but is not necessarily, related to the severity of the underlying liver disease.

Extrahepatic Manifestations

Patients with HCV infection may present with extrahepatic conditions, or these manifestations may occur in patients known to have chronic hepatitis C. Classification of the

---

BOX 80-1 **Extrahepatic Manifestations of HCV Infection**

Proved
Autoimmune thyroiditis
B-cell non-Hodgkin's lymphoma
Lichen planus
Mixed cryoglobulinemia
Monoclonal gammopathies
Porphyria cutanea tarda

Possible
Chronic polyarthritis
Diabetes mellitus
Idiopathic pulmonary fibrosis
Non-cryoglobulinemic nephropathies
Sicca syndrome
Thyroid cancer
Renal cell carcinoma
Vitiligo

---

extrahepatic manifestations of HCV is shown in Box 80-1 and is based on the strength of available data to prove a correlation. Types 2 and 3 cryoglobulinemia, characterized by polyclonal immunoglobulin (Ig)G plus monoclonal IgM and polyclonal IgG plus polyclonal IgM, respectively, can both be caused by HCV infection. Among HCV-infected patients, 19% to 50% have cryoglobulins in serum, but clinical manifestations of cryoglobulinemia are reported in only 5% to 10% of these patients and are more common in patients with cirrhosis. Symptoms and signs include fatigue, arthralgias, arthritis, purpura, Raynaud's phenomenon, vasculitis, peripheral neuropathy, and nephropathy. The diagnosis is clear when a rheumatoid factor is detected, cryoglobulins are present, and complement levels are low in serum; however, the reliability of cryoglobulin measurements is dependent on proper handling and processing of the sample.[118]

Glomerular disease generally manifests as cryoglobulinemic nephropathy, membranoproliferative glomerulonephritis (MPGN), and membranous nephropathy. Cryoglobulinemic nephropathy manifests as hematuria, proteinuria, edema, and renal insufficiency of varying degrees, and on renal biopsy specimens it has features of MPGN. At diagnosis, 20% of patients with type 2 cryoglobulinemia have renal involvement, and renal involvement develops in another 35% to 60% over time. In about 15% of patients, cryoglobulinemic nephropathy progresses to end-stage kidney disease requiring dialysis.

Therapy should be considered in patients with symptomatic cryoglobulinemia. Cryoglobulinemia resolves in patients who achieve an SVR with pegylated IFN and ribavirin therapy (see later). Unfortunately, patients with significant renal involvement are at a disadvantage with respect to antiviral therapy, because administration of ribavirin is generally contraindicated if the creatinine clearance is less than 50 mL/min. In these patients, treatment with rituximab should be considered.[119] The effectiveness and safety of rituximab either alone or in combination with pegylated IFN-α and ribavirin in hepatitis C has been shown in prospective clinical trials.[119] Prednisone, cyclophosphamide, other chemotherapeutic agents, and plasmapheresis have been used with variable success; however, these approaches do not treat the underlying HCV infection. If cryoglobulinemia and renal disease improve with such treatment, then subsequent treatment of the HCV infection with pegylated IFN-α and ribavirin should be reconsidered.

Patients with vasculitis due to HCV infection may benefit from low-dose interleukin-2 therapy. This cytokine may promote the survival of immunosuppressive regulatory T cells.[120]

HCV infection is associated with the development of B cell non-Hodgkin's lymphoma and monoclonal gammopathy of uncertain significance.[121] The relative risk of lymphoma is small (1.28) in the United States.[122] The most prevalent forms of lymphoma found in patients infected with HCV are follicular lymphoma, chronic lymphocytic lymphoma, lymphoplasmacytic lymphoma, and marginal zone lymphoma.[121] Type 2 cryoglobulinemia evolves into lymphoma over time in 8% to 10% of patients. Despite the known association of HCV infection with lymphoma, HCV RNA does not integrate into the host genome and cannot be considered a typical oncogenic virus. Rather, HCV shows lymphotropism and may facilitate the development and selection of abnormal B-cell clones by chronic stimulation of the immune system. In addition, genetic rearrangements in B cells, specifically the $Bcl2/J_H$ rearrangement and the t(14;18) translocation, have been found in HCV-infected patients in some,[123] but not all,[124] studies.

Other extrahepatic manifestations of HCV infection include porphyria cutanea tarda, lichen planus, and sicca syndrome. In addition, insulin resistance and diabetes mellitus have been thought to be associated with HCV infection, although the association has been questioned. The SVR to antiviral therapy for HCV infection is reduced in insulin-resistant patients; however, if HCV can be eradicated, insulin resistance often improves, an observation that further supports the relationship between HCV infection and insulin resistance.[125] Although associations between HCV infection and both thyroid cancer and idiopathic pulmonary fibrosis have been described, data about the effect of HCV eradication on disease progression are lacking (see Box 80-1). A myriad of other conditions have been observed in association with HCV infection, but a true link has not been firmly established for these disorders.

Although not associated with disease, seropositivity for autoantibodies (e.g., antinuclear antibodies with a titer greater than 1:40 in 9%, smooth muscle antibodies with a titer greater than 1:40 in 20%, anti-liver-kidney microsomal antibodies in 6%) is found in many HCV-infected persons.[126] The diagnosis of an autoimmune condition in a patient with HCV infection, however, can never be based on serology alone.

The spectrum of extrahepatic manifestations may adversely impact the overall survival of HCV-infected persons. The prospective Taiwanese population-based Risk Evaluation of Viral Load Elevation and Associated Liver Disease/Cancer (R.E.V.E.A.L.-HCV) study in which almost 24,000 adults 30 to 65 years of age were followed demonstrated that HCV-infected persons had not only increased liver-related mortality, but also higher mortality from extrahepatic diseases compared with anti-HCV–negative persons.[127]

DIAGNOSIS

Several immunologic and molecular assays are used to detect and monitor HCV infection. The presence of anti-HCV in high titer in serum (generally an enzyme immunoassay [EIA] ratio > 9) indicates exposure to the virus but does not differentiate among acute, chronic, and resolved infection. Anti-HCV usually persists for many years in patients after spontaneous resolution of infection or an SVR following antiviral therapy. Anti-HCV titers may decline over time, however, and can become undetectable 5 to 20 years after HCV clearance.[128,129] Serologic assays are used initially for diagnosis, whereas virologic assays are required for confirming infection, monitoring response to treatment, and evaluating immunocompromised patients.

Indirect Assays

EIAs detect antibodies against different HCV antigens. The time course of the development of symptoms, detection of anti-HCV, and appearance of HCV RNA after acute infection is shown in Figure 80-3. Three generations of EIAs have been developed. The third-generation EIAs detect antibodies against HCV core, NS3, NS4, and NS5 antigens as early as 7 to 8 weeks after infection, with sensitivity and specificity rates of 99%.[130] Despite ongoing viral replication, serologic test results can be negative in patients who are on hemodialysis or are immunocompromised. Because the performance characteristics of third-generation EIAs are so good, confirmation with a recombinant immunoblot assay (RIBA) is no longer required. Instead, patients who are anti-HCV positive should undergo HCV RNA testing to determine if they have active viremia or have cleared the infection.

Direct Assays

Quantitative, highly sensitive, "real-time" HCV RNA tests represent the state of the art for determining HCV viremia in anti-HCV–positive persons.[131] The lower limit of detection of most assays varies from 10 to 15 international units (IU)/mL.[132] These assays have a linear dynamic range of 1 to 7 $\log_{10}$ IU/mL and are the preferred testing method in practice. Transcription-mediated amplification (TMA) is also extremely sensitive, but available assays are not quantitative in the lower dynamic range of the test. The advantages of these very sensitive tests include positivity within 1 to 3 weeks after acute infection and detection of low-level residual infection during antiviral therapy.

A disadvantage of all quantitative tests is the lack of comparability among different assays. Although conversion to a standard IU/mL concentration attempted to resolve such discrepancies, results are still variable. Conversion factors vary from 0.9 copies/mL to 5.2 copies/mL per IU/mL reported. For this reason, the same laboratory and assay should be used during antiviral treatment, when comparisons of levels at different points in time are critical to decision making about treatment. Moreover, it is important for treatment decisions when response-guided algorithms are applied (see later) that the laboratory report detectable but not quantifiable test results. Very low levels of viremia that cannot be quantified are associated with lower SVR rates with pegylated IFN, ribavirin, and an HCV protease inhibitor than undetectable HCV RNA,[133] and this important information must be available to allow determination of the optimal treatment duration for each patient.

A cheaper and faster alternative to nucleic acid testing for HCV RNA to confirm HCV viremia is the HCV core antigen assay. Fully automated immunoassays have been developed that detect the HCV core antigen, and the assays have been proved to be robust across HCV genotypes and in different patient populations,[134,135] but with major limitations in sensitivity. Therefore, the assay cannot be used to monitor response to antiviral therapy and make decisions regarding response-guided therapy. If viremia needs just to be confirmed, however, HCV core antigen testing is a reasonable alternative to HCV RNA testing.

HCV Genotype

Identifying the genotype of HCV can be accomplished by several methods. The most accurate method is PCR methodology and direct sequencing of the NS5B or E1 region; however, this approach is not practical in clinical practice. HCV genotyping can be done by evaluating type-specific antibodies and has a 90% concordance in immunocompetent patients when results are compared with sequence analysis of the HCV genome. Testing can also be accomplished with reverse hybridization to genotype-specific probes, restriction fragment length polymorphism analysis, or PCR amplification of the 5' noncoding region of the HCV genome. These tests have 92% to 96% concordance with the correct genotype; genotype 1 is identified with the highest accuracy. Because of mutations in the regions studied, errors in subtype identification occur in 10% to 25% of cases regardless of the technique used. A line-probe assay (Inno-LIPA) using genotype-specific probes for reverse transcription of the 5' portion of the HCV genome is the most popular commercial assay for HCV genotyping.

Selection of Serologic and Virologic Tests

For patients at low risk for HCV infection, a negative result of an EIA for anti-HCV is sufficient to exclude HCV infection. A positive anti-HCV result is sufficient to confirm the diagnosis if the serum ALT level is elevated. If the serum ALT level is not elevated, HCV RNA should be measured. In high-risk patients, such as those with an elevated ALT level who have a known risk factor for HCV, have experienced recent exposure, or are either immunocompromised or on dialysis, a positive anti-HCV result is sufficient to confirm HCV infection; if the anti-HCV result is negative, then HCV RNA testing should be done.[89]

LIVER BIOPSY AND NONINVASIVE ASSESSMENT OF FIBROSIS

The risk of progressive hepatic injury from HCV infection varies considerably, with some patients showing little or no progression after decades of infection and others progressing rapidly to cirrhosis.[136] Therefore, an assessment of the degree of liver injury is usually advisable. This assessment is usually done by percutaneous liver biopsy (Box 80-2), but indirect and noninvasive methods to assess liver fibrosis are used frequently instead of liver biopsy. In some centers, liver biopsies are performed primarily to exclude other causes of liver disease.

Several scoring systems have been used to quantify hepatic injury into discrete grades of inflammation and stages of fibrosis (Fig. 80-4). The first system used was the Histology Activity Index (HAI) described by Knodell and colleagues. The components of this system include periportal inflammation and necrosis (graded as 0 to 10), lobular inflammation and necrosis (0 to 4), portal inflammation (0 to 4), and fibrosis (0 to 4). This scoring system combines inflammation and fibrosis into 1 score. Scheuer created a simplified scoring system that separates grade from stage: Portal inflammation and interface hepatitis (0 to 4), lobular activity (0 to 4), and fibrosis stage (0 to 4). The Ishak system is a modification of Knodell's system but separates histologic grade from stage. Ishak's fibrosis

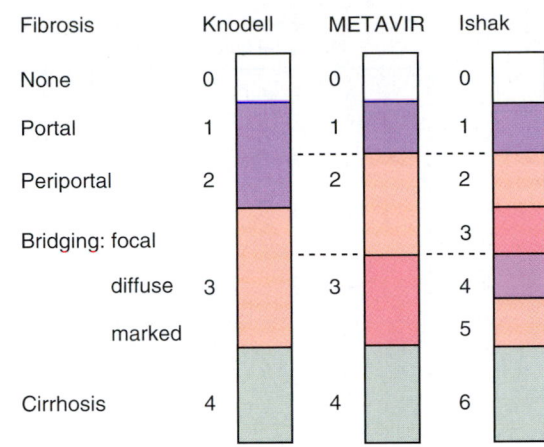

FIGURE 80-4. Comparison of the Knodell, METAVIR, and Ishak hepatic fibrosis staging systems. The METAVIR staging system is similar to the Scheuer system. Portal, periportal, bridging, and cirrhosis describe the degree (stage) of fibrosis (see also Fig. 80-5).

scores range from 0 to 6 (1 or 2, portal fibrotic expansion; 3 or 4, bridging fibrosis; 5 or 6, cirrhosis) (see Fig. 80-4). The higher number of gradations of fibrosis has made the Ishak system popular for scoring progression of fibrosis in clinical trials. The METAVIR scoring system is the most popular in practice; it is simpler than all the aforementioned systems (Fig. 80-5). Inflammation is graded from 0 to 4 (none, mild, moderate, and severe), and fibrosis is staged from 0 to 4 (1, portal fibrotic expansion; 2, portal fibrosis with septa formation; 3, bridging fibrosis; 4, cirrhosis) (see Fig. 80-4).

Although examination of liver biopsy specimens is still considered the standard for establishing the grade of inflammation and stage of fibrosis, limitations of liver biopsy include (1) associated morbidity (pain occurs in as many as 30% in some series, and hemorrhage or bile leak occurs in 0.3% of patients) and mortality (0.03%); (2) cost; (3) poor patient acceptance; (4) intraobserver and interobserver variability in the interpretation of findings (with current scoring systems, intraobserver and interobserver concordance for staging fibrosis among hepatopathologists is ≈ 90% and 85%, respectively); (5) inaccuracy in interpretation of findings, particularly for the diagnosis of cirrhosis (with a false-negative rate of 15%); and (6) sampling error (a 33% difference in 1 stage of fibrosis and 2.4% difference in 2 stages of fibrosis is seen in simultaneously obtained biopsy specimens from the right and left hepatic lobes).[137,138] Interobserver and intraobserver variability is increased when inexperienced pathologists use a complicated scoring system to evaluate liver tissue. Sampling error is especially common when small biopsy specimens are obtained. A biopsy should be done with at least a 16-gauge needle, be 15 to 20 mm or more in length, and contain at least 6 portal triads, although 11 or greater is considered optimal.[139,140]

Because of the limitations of liver biopsy, several noninvasive tests to estimate fibrosis have been developed (Table 80-1). FibroSure (or FibroTest) is a noninvasive measure of fibrosis that creates a composite score, adjusted for gender and age, derived from the serum levels of α_2-macroglobulin, haptoglobin, apolipoprotein A-1, GGTP, and total bilirubin.[138] The test accurately categorizes patients with stage 0 and 1 fibrosis and those with cirrhosis; however, it is less useful in patients with intermediate scores. The AST-to-platelet ratio index (APRI) is used primarily to diagnose or exclude cirrhosis.[141] In an initial evaluation, 81% of cirrhotic patients were accurately

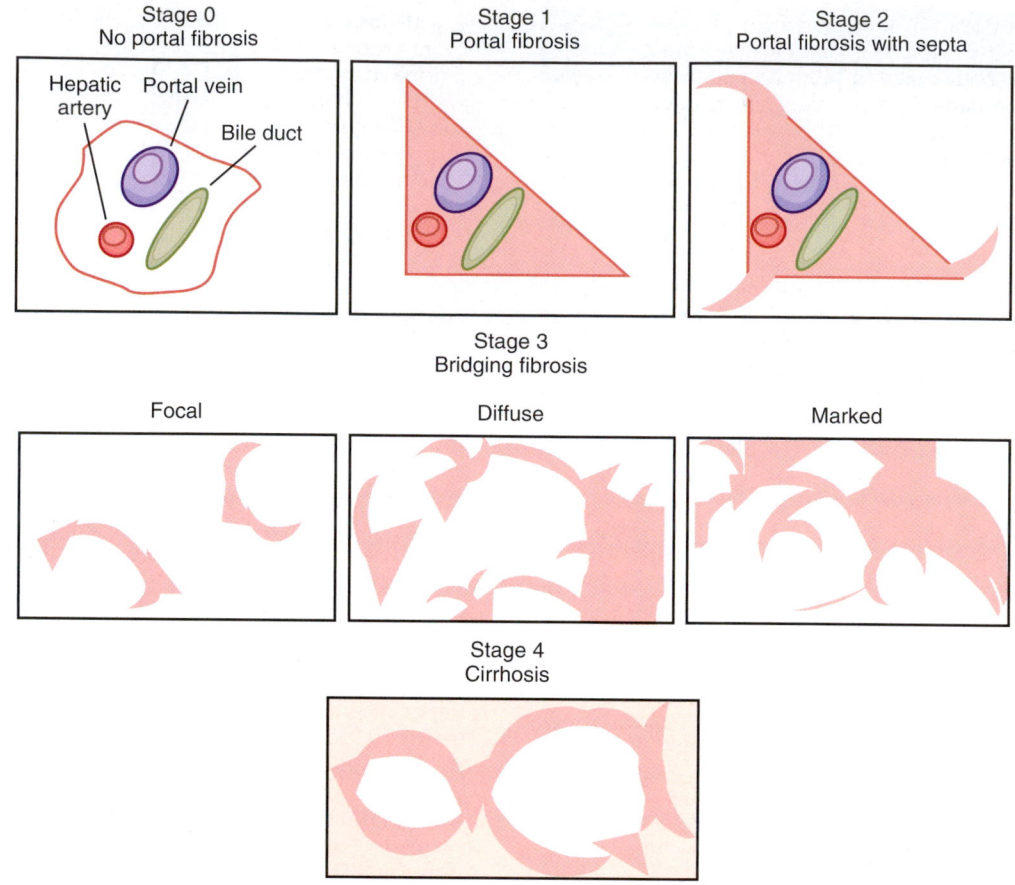

FIGURE 80-5. Visual depictions of fibrosis staging (METAVIR system) in patients with chronic hepatitis C (see Fig. 80-4). A diagnosis of cirrhosis requires the presence of nodule formation.

TABLE 80-1 Accuracy of Noninvasive Tests for Predicting Hepatic Fibrosis in Patients with Hepatitis C

Test	Number of Patients Studied	Fibrosis Staging System	Histologic Fibrosis (F) Stages Compared	Sensitivity (%)*	Specificity (%)*	PPV for Fibrosis-Cirrhosis (%)	Test Accuracy (%)†
APRI	270	Ishak	F0-2 vs. F3-6	41	95	88	70
			F0-4 vs. F5-6	89	75	57	77
FibroSure	339	METAVIR	F0-1 vs. F2-4	100	22	50	57
			F0-2 vs. F3-4	70	95	91	84
Transient elastography (Fibroscan)	327	METAVIR	F0-1 vs. F2-4	56	91	88	68
			F0-3 vs. F4	86	96	78	94

*Sensitivity and specificity for distinguishing higher stages of fibrosis from lower stages of fibrosis.
†Accuracy = (sensitivity)(prevalence) + (specificity)(1 − prevalence).
APRI, AST-to-platelets ratio index; PPV, positive predictive value.
From Wai CT, Greinson JT, Fontana RJ, et al. A simple noninvasive index can predict both significant fibrosis and cirrhosis in patients with chronic hepatitis C. Hepatology 2003; 38:518-26; Imbert-Bismut F, Ratziu V, Pieroni L, et al. Biochemical markers of liver fibrosis in patients with hepatitis C virus infection: A prospective study. Lancet 2001; 357:1069-75; and Ziol M, Handra-Luca A, Kettaneh A, et al. Noninvasive assessment of liver fibrosis by measurement of stiffness in patients with chronic hepatitis C. Hepatology 2005; 41:48-54.

categorized with a score of 0.5 or less; however, the index does not discriminate among lower levels of fibrosis. Different techniques and instruments (e.g., transient elastography, acoustic radiation force impulse imaging, magnetic resonance elastography) are now available to determine liver stiffness. The most frequently used system is transient elastography (Fibroscan) to assess liver elasticity, which correlates inversely with the amount of hepatic fibrosis. In a meta-analysis, the area under the receiver operating curve (an estimate of accuracy) of Fibroscan for predicting cirrhosis was 0.94.[142] Combining transient elastography with serum markers increases the accuracy of predicting fibrosis and cirrhosis and may avoid liver biopsy in many patients.[143,144] Although noninvasive testing has improved dramatically, all available tests have limitations. Most importantly, the degree of hepatic inflammation is not assessed by these tests, and inflammation may significantly alter test results. Moreover, although cirrhosis is accurately predicted by several noninvasive tests, the finer discrimination of the fibrosis score is not as reliable as examination of liver biopsy specimens.

Regardless of the degree of serum aminotransferase elevations, a determination of the stage of liver fibrosis, either by liver biopsy or noninvasive methods, is recommended in patients undergoing initial assessment of chronic hepatitis C. Liver biopsy is not required when cirrhosis is already suggested by clinical findings (e.g., ascites, splenomegaly, spider telangiectasias, low platelet count, prolonged prothrombin time) or imaging (e.g., nodularity of the liver, evidence of portal hypertension). It is also not indicated following successful antiviral therapy, although histology generally improves significantly over time following eradication of HCV (see later). Surveillance for HCC and varices is recommended for all patients with cirrhosis (see Chapters 92 and 96).

NATURAL HISTORY

Once chronic HCV infection is established, spontaneous HCV clearance rarely occurs. Chronic hepatitis C can cause continuous liver damage, resulting in liver cirrhosis and subsequently HCC (Fig. 80-6). The individual course of liver disease is highly variable. Patients may report symptoms such as right abdominal discomfort, nausea, fatigue, myalgia, arthralgias, or weight loss. All of these clinical features are uncharacteristic, however, and are not associated with the severity of liver injury. Most liver-related symptoms are restricted to patients with advanced cirrhosis.

The most feared complication of chronic HCV infection is liver-related mortality due to decompensated liver cirrhosis or development of HCC. Studies published since the 1990s have shown remarkably different frequency rates of cirrhosis. Whereas very low rates of cirrhosis were reported in some cohorts like young women infected in the late 1970s,[115] cirrhosis has been described in up to 69% of patients in hospital-based settings.[146] In a meta-analysis, Thein and colleagues calculated that in a large number of studies that have been published, cirrhosis developed on average in 16% of patients within 20 years after the onset of HCV infection.[147] Cirrhosis

was attributable to HCV infection in 27% of cases, with a wide range among studies (14% to 62%) that can be explained by regional differences and the presence of cofactors.[111,148]

A key challenge in clinical practice is to identify persons with a low risk for disease progression who may not require immediate antiviral therapy. Several factors reported to influence the liver-related outcomes of chronic hepatitis C remain controversial (Table 80-2; see next section). Still, some of these factors may help estimate the risk of cirrhosis and identify groups of patients who require antiviral treatment.

Factors Associated with Progression

Age is one of the most important risk factor for fibrosis progression in chronic HCV infection (see Table 80-2). A longer duration of infection has also been associated with a higher stage of liver fibrosis, but HCV infection acquired during childhood seems to follow a milder course.[149] Overall, the development of HCV-related cirrhosis seems to be a dynamic process that accelerates exponentially with increasing age. The mechanisms by which progression of fibrosis accelerates with aging are not well defined. Changes in the regenerative capacity of the liver, alterations in the immune system, and telomere shortening may play roles. A higher risk for fibrosis progression in patients older than 40 years has been described

TABLE 80-2 Factors Associated with Progression of Hepatic Fibrosis in Patients with Chronic HCV Infection

Established	Possible	Not Associated
Age > 40 years	Increased hepatic iron concentration	Viral genotype
Alcohol consumption	Male gender	Viral load
HBV coinfection	Serum ALT level	
HIV coinfection		
Immunosuppressed state		
Insulin resistance		
Marijuana use		
Obesity		
Schistosomiasis		
Severe hepatic necroinflammation		
Smoking		
White race		

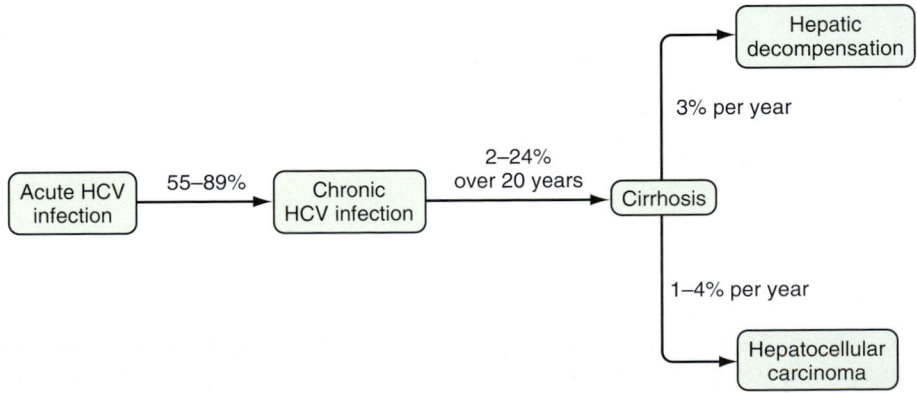

FIGURE 80-6. Natural history of HCV infection. Hepatic decompensation includes ascites, hepatic encephalopathy, variceal hemorrhage, hepatorenal syndrome, or hepatic synthetic dysfunction.

in patients with various causes of liver disease.[150] Some studies, but not others, have suggested that older age in general, and more specifically older age at the time of infection, is a risk factor for progression of fibrosis.[151-153] Overall, cirrhosis has been predicted to develop in most patients with hepatitis C by about 65 years of age, irrespective of the age at infection.[154]

Some studies have suggested that the mode of viral transmission may influence the degree of liver damage; however, the role of the route of transmission in fibrosis progression remains controversial. By contrast, female gender seems to be protective, and fibrosis progression is much faster in HCV-infected men, thereby suggesting that hormonal factors may be important in the regulation of liver fibrosis.[155] Genetic factors also play a role in the development of cirrhosis. Histologic activity and the incidence of cirrhosis are lower in African Americans than in Caucasians.[156] Several specific genes have been suggested to be involved in fibrosis progression; these include certain variants of the HLA class I and II antigens.[157] A cirrhosis risk score based on polymorphisms in 7 genes has been proposed for patients with hepatitis C[158]; this score was able to predict fibrosis progression in patients with initially mild chronic hepatitis C.[159]

Elevated serum aminotransferase levels are used widely as a surrogate for ongoing intrahepatic inflammation, and elevated serum ALT levels during chronic hepatitis C are associated with an increased risk of liver fibrosis progression.[160] Lower progression rates of fibrosis are reported in patients with normal serum ALT levels, but normal levels do not exclude the possibility of fibrosis progression.[116]

Viral factors have also been associated with disease progression in hepatitis C. Differences in the natural history of hepatitis C have been reported for different HCV genotypes. Several studies have described accelerated disease progression in patients infected with HCV genotype 3,[161] which is consistent with higher reported mortality rates in patients infected with HCV genotype 3.[162] Flares of hepatitis seem to occur more frequently in HCV genotype 2 infection and may result in a more severe course of liver disease.[163] By contrast, viral load is not related to the degree of liver damage or fibrosis.[164]

Hepatic steatosis is a histologic hallmark of chronic hepatitis C. Several studies have shown that steatosis is linked to the stage of liver fibrosis in patients with chronic HCV infection.[161] Some studies suggest that HCV infection itself can trigger hepatic steatosis as well as nonalcoholic steatohepatitis, and HCV infection may cause insulin resistance. There is also evidence for a direct association between HCV infection and hepatic steatosis. The strongest association exists between HCV genotype 3 infection and steatosis, and a direct molecular effect has been shown in a mouse model in which HCV genotype 3 is expressed.[165]

Mild to moderately increased hepatic iron stores are associated with more advanced liver fibrosis. A consistent relationship between C282Y or H63D heterozygosity (see Chapter 75) and increased progression of fibrosis in patients with HCV infection has not been established, however. A reduction in hepatic iron concentrations does not reduce the risk of progression of fibrosis or improve the response to antiviral treatment.[166]

Excessive alcohol consumption is clearly an independent major cause of cirrhosis, and chronic alcohol intake of more than 50 g/day is associated with a remarkable increase in the risk of cirrhosis in HCV-infected patients. On the other hand, coffee consumption has been reported to have a beneficial effect on overall mortality from HCV infection in population-based studies, and drinking coffee has been associated with a more favorable course of liver disease in general.[167] Freedman

and colleagues have also shown that greater coffee consumption correlates with a lower stage of liver fibrosis, as well as less steatosis and insulin resistance and lower serum ALT levels; the best outcomes occur in persons who drink 3 or more cups per day.[167] Drinking more than 3 cups of coffee per day also increases the likelihood of SVR to antiviral treatment with pegylated IFN and ribavirin.[168]

Hepatocellular Carcinoma

The incidence of HCC has been rising rapidly in the industrial countries since the 1980s (see Chapter 96). In the United States, the incidence of HCC is 3 times higher than in 1975,[169] and the global HCV epidemic has contributed to the rising incidence of HCC worldwide. Overall, chronic hepatitis C is responsible for approximately 25% of cases of HCC worldwide, with particularly high prevalence rates in East Asia.[73] Because the development of HCC in HCV-infected patients is an indolent and age-dependent process, the peak incidence of HCV-related HCC has not been reached yet in Europe and the United States, where the majority of infections occurred in the 1970s and 1980s. In some European countries such as Italy, however, the peak rate of HCC-related mortality may have been reached.[170] In contrast to chronic hepatitis B, HCC due to HCV usually does not develop in noncirrhotic livers, although HCC may be detected in some patients in whom cirrhosis has not yet developed. Lok and colleagues reported an HCC incidence rate of 0.8% per year in noncirrhotic patients with chronic hepatitis C who had advanced liver fibrosis[171]; however, the risk is much higher in patients with cirrhosis, with a rate of 1.4% to 4.9% per year.[171-173] The overall 5-year risk of HCC has been reported to be as high as 7% to 30% in patients with HCV-related cirrhosis.[174,175] The appearance of HCC frequently is the first clinical complication of HCV-related cirrhosis and occurs before hepatic decompensation becomes evident.

Risk factors for the development of HCC in patients with chronic HCV infection are similar to those associated with the development of cirrhosis. For example, older age is related to a higher frequency of HCC, and male gender and substantial alcohol consumption are well-established risk factors. Moreover, type 2 diabetes mellitus has been identified as an important independent risk factor.[176,177] Coinfection with HBV increases the risk of HCC. Importantly, there are synergistic interactions among the various risk factors that enhance the overall risk for HCC. There is little doubt that genetic factors also contribute to development of HCC. Kumar and colleagues performed a genome-wide association study in 721 persons with HCV-related HCC and showed that a SNP (rs2596542) at the gene encoding MICA (major histocompatibility class I polypeptide-related sequence A) was strongly associated with the development of HCC in HCV-infected persons.[178]

TREATMENT

IFN-α monotherapy was approved for the treatment of chronic hepatitis C, then known as *non-A, non-B hepatitis*, before HCV was even identified. Substantial advances have been made since then with the introduction of prolonged treatment periods, longer-acting pegylated formulations of IFN, and the oral guanosine analog ribavirin. In 2011, the first DAAs, telaprevir and boceprevir, were approved for the treatment of chronic HCV genotype 1 infection, and in 2013, simeprevir, another protease inhibitor, and sofosbuvir, a nucleotide polymerase inhibitor, were approved. Elucidation of the mechanisms of HCV replication has led to the development of additional classes of DAAs, including NS5A inhibitors and nucleoside, as well non-nucleoside inhibitors of the HCV polymerase.[25] At least 30 different DAAs active against HCV are in clinical development. Ultimately, the availability of IFN-free regimens will lead to a complete shift in the treatment paradigm of hepatitis C. As treatment evolves, the choice of agents will be increasingly highly individualized based on the availability of DAAs, HCV genotype, and stage of liver disease.

Goals

The primary goal of therapy for HCV infection is eradication of the virus. A consequence of achieving this goal is prevention of liver-related deaths associated with the development of decompensated cirrhosis and HCC. SVR—the absence of detectable virus in blood 12 to 24 weeks after completion of therapy—is an excellent surrogate marker for the resolution of HCV infection. Late relapses are rare. Long-term follow-up studies confirm sustained responses in more than 98% of cases if the patient is HCV RNA negative in serum 24 weeks after completion of antiviral therapy.[7,8] SVR is also associated with a reduction in hepatic inflammation and regression of fibrosis (Fig. 80-7).[179] Moreover, an improvement in HRQOL has been documented in successfully treated patients.[180]

Antiviral treatment prevents the development of clinical endpoints. A significant reduction of liver-related death and hepatic decompensation can be observed even in patients who already have advanced liver fibrosis.[181-183] A benefit in the reduction in the incidence of HCC has also been documented for patients who respond during antiviral therapy but experience a virologic relapse after treatment.[184] An SVR is also associated with improved overall survival in patients who had advanced fibrosis or liver cirrhosis at the time of therapy.[6] By contrast, low-dose IFN-α maintenance treatment for 3 to 4 years in patients who did not achieve viral clearance with standard IFN-based or pegylated IFN-based treatment regimens does not prevent disease progression or reduce the incidence of hepatic decompensation or HCC.[185]

Virologic Response

Although SVR is considered the endpoint of therapy, other indicators of response are often monitored during therapy because they may help guide and refine treatment. A rapid virologic response (RVR), defined as undetectable HCV RNA in serum after the first 4 weeks of antiviral therapy, identifies those patients who are most sensitive to treatment and is associated with an 80% to 90% SVR rate in HCV genotype 1–infected patients who complete 48 weeks of therapy or in HCV genotype 2– or 3–infected patients who complete 24 weeks of therapy.[2] An extended rapid virologic response (eRVR) is defined as negative HCV RNA in serum from week 4 to week 12 of therapy and has been used in treatment trials with the protease inhibitor telaprevir (see later). An early virologic response (EVR), defined as a greater than 2-log drop in viral load at 12 weeks of therapy, is needed to continue therapy beyond 12 weeks, because the absence of an EVR predicts failure of treatment in more than 98% of cases. An EVR can be subdivided further into a complete EVR (cEVR), defined as undetectable HCV RNA in serum at 12 weeks of therapy, and a partial EVR (pEVR), defined as a greater than 2-log decrease in the level of HCV RNA in serum despite residual detectable HCV RNA after 12 weeks of therapy. An end-of-treatment response (ETR) is defined as undetectable HCV RNA in serum at the end of treatment; a small and variable proportion of patients with an ETR will relapse when treatment is stopped. The absence of an ETR is considered nonresponse to treatment with pegylated IFN and ribavirin.

Different additional definitions of on-treatment virologic responses have been proposed. Revised, more descriptive, standardized nomenclature to define treatment response in therapies against hepatitis C has also been suggested.[186] These definitions are based on the time of response assessment (e.g., week 2, week 4) and the degree of virologic response (e.g., HCV RNA undetectable, detectable but not quantifiable, positive).

Drugs

Interferons

IFN-based regimens have been the cornerstone of antiviral therapy for HCV infection since the late 1980s. IFNs are naturally occurring glycoproteins that exert a wide array of antiviral, antiproliferative, and immunomodulatory effects. Pegylated IFNs consist of IFN bound to a molecule of polyethylene glycol (PEG) of varying length. The large size of the molecule increases the half-life of the IFN, thereby allowing once-weekly dosage. Two pegylated IFNs are licensed for use in the United States and elsewhere. The first is 40-kd peginterferon alfa-2a, used in a fixed dose of 180 μg per week. The second is 12-kd peginterferon alfa-2b, prescribed according to the patient's body weight in a dose of 1.5 μg/kg per week. Pegylated IFNs have replaced standard IFN, used in the past, and have resulted in a significant increase in the SVR.[187]

Ribavirin

Ribavirin is an oral guanosine analog with activity against DNA and RNA viruses. When ribavirin is used in combination with IFN, the ETR improves and the relapse rate decreases. Several mechanisms to explain the synergistic effect of ribavirin when administered in combination with IFN have been proposed, including (1) alterations of the cytokine milieu

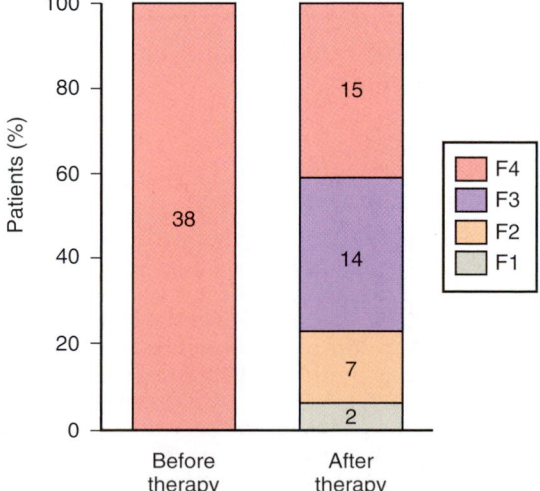

FIGURE 80-7. Reversal of cirrhosis in 38 patients with chronic hepatitis C who achieved a sustained virologic response to antiviral therapy. F1 to F4 indicate stages of fibrosis, with F4 being cirrhosis. *(Redrawn from D'Ambrosio R, Aghemo A, Rumi MG, et al. A morphometric and immunohistochemical study to assess the benefit of a sustained virological response in hepatitis C virus patients with cirrhosis. Hepatology 2012; 56:532-43.)*

leading to a change from a type 2 T-helper cell (Th2) to a Th1 immune response; (2) depletion of intracellular guanosine triphosphate through inhibition of the host enzyme inosine monophosphate dehydrogenase (IMPDH); (3) inhibition of the action of the HCV RNA-dependent RNA polymerase; (4) induction of lethal mutagenesis during HCV RNA replication, and (5) increasing responsiveness to type I IFNs.[188] Ribavirin generally is well tolerated, although it results in a dose-dependent hemolytic anemia. The dose administered is based on the patient's weight, and the patient's Hgb level must be monitored during treatment. Furthermore, in patients with a history of cardiopulmonary disease who cannot tolerate a sudden fall in the Hgb level, ribavirin must be used with caution, if at all. In addition, ribavirin is teratogenic; patients taking ribavirin and their partners are required to avoid pregnancy during therapy and for 6 months after cessation of the drug. Ribavirin has a long cumulative half-life in serum and is excreted by the kidneys; as a result, it can lead to severe side effects, particularly hemolysis, in patients with kidney disease. The dose of ribavirin must be adjusted for renal function, and the drug should be administered with extreme caution to patients with a creatinine clearance less than 50 mL/min. Ribavirin is not removed by hemodialysis.

Direct-Acting Antiviral Agents

Novel DAAs against hepatitis C include compounds that target the HCV protease, the HCV NS5A protein, and the HCV polymerase. These drugs inhibit HCV replication by interfering with the respective step in the HCV life cycle.

HCV protease inhibitors ("…previrs") generally have high antiviral potency but differ in respect to the development of resistance. Most of the compounds show better response rates in HCV genotype 1b than in genotype 1a infection.[189] Boceprevir and telaprevir are 2 protease inhibitors that were approved by the FDA in 2011. Simeprevir became available in 2014. Simeprevir and the protease inhibitor faldaprevir have important advantages compared with boceprevir and telaprevir in terms of side effect profile and dosing schedule. Most of the other HCV protease inhibitors in clinical development are not being developed in the context of IFN-containing regimens but as part of novel IFN-free regimens (see later).[190]

NS5A inhibitors ("…asvirs") are characterized by very high antiviral potency at picomolar doses. The cross-genotype efficacy of these agents varies. Limited data on the efficacy of these drugs are available in patients with non-genotype 1 HCV. Ledipasvir was the first NS5A inhibitor approved by the FDA in 2014 (see later).

HCV polymerase inhibitors ("…buvirs") are categorized as nucleoside or nucleotide analog and non-nucleoside polymerase inhibitors. Non-nucleoside polymerase inhibitors are the weakest class of compounds against HCV because of a low barrier to resistance. Most drugs in this class are active mainly against HCV genotype 1b and to a lesser extent against HCV genotype 1a. They are being developed to be used only in combination with other DAAs, mainly with protease inhibitors and NS5A inhibitors. Different domains in the polymerase protein can be targeted by non-nucleoside polymerase inhibitors, and theoretically, use of a combination of different non-nucleoside polymerase inhibitors is possible. Importantly, there is also no cross-resistance between drugs targeting different polymerase domains.[191]

Nucleoside analogs are active across all HCV genotypes and have a high barrier to resistance. Nucleoside analog resistant variants may emerge but have very low fitness and do not expand rapidly. They cause a chain termination and thereby block HCV replication. A triphosphorylated agent is usually required for activity. The first compound tested in a large number of patients was mericitabine.[192,193] Unfortunately, the compound has only a modest antiviral activity, and relapses after treatment and breakthroughs during treatment have been observed frequently in phase 2 trials when mericitabine has been used in combination with protease inhibitors. The first approved nucleotide NS5B polymerase inhibitor was sofosbuvir (see later).[194]

Acute Hepatitis C

Although postexposure prophylaxis against HCV is not effective, early treatment of acute HCV infection is effective.[195] Various cohort studies have demonstrated high (>85%) response rates if acute hepatitis C is treated with IFN alone early after acquisition.[195] Because a substantial proportion of patients may clear the infection spontaneously without any antiviral intervention, different strategies have been proposed to avoid unnecessary treatment with IFN.[110,195] The patient's *IL28B* genotype can provide an indication as to whether a patient is more or less likely to recover spontaneously[196,197]; however, the positive predictive value of *IL28B* testing is below 90%, and treatment decisions cannot be based solely on the patient's *IL28B* genotype. A prospective randomized trial compared immediate treatment of acute hepatitis C with pegylated IFN alone and a delayed approach of starting combination therapy with pegylated IFN-α and ribavirin after 12 weeks in those patients who did not become HCV RNA negative spontaneously.[198] Delayed therapy resulted in a lower SVR rate on an intention-to-treat analysis but gave similar response rates on an "adherence-to-therapy" analysis. Therefore, delayed therapy is effective, but early treatment has advantages because fewer patients are lost to follow-up. A reasonable approach for managing acute hepatitis C is to monitor the serum HCV RNA for 4 to 8 weeks before early monotherapy with pegylated IFN is considered. Treatment may be delayed in particular in patients who carry the favorable *IL28B* CC genotype. Delayed therapy is then still effective. Whether ribavirin is needed in this situation is still a matter of debate. Treatment of acute hepatitis C in the context of HIV coinfection is similar to that for patients with HCV monoinfection, even though in this situation, most experts prefer early immediate therapy to delayed treatment.[199] The role of novel DAAs in the treatment of acute hepatitis C needs to be defined.

Chronic Hepatitis C

Pegylated Interferon and Ribavirin

Until 2011, the standard of care for the treatment of HCV infection was the combination of a pegylated IFN administered subcutaneously once per week and ribavirin taken orally in divided doses daily. The dose of IFN is the same for all HCV genotypes. The daily dose of ribavirin is based on the patient's weight for genotypes 1 and 4 (13.3 mg/kg/day in 2 divided doses). Different recommendations exist regarding the optimal dose of ribavirin for patients infected with HCV genotype 2 or 3 infection: either a fixed dose at 800 mg per day (in 2 divided doses)[89] or a body-weight adjusted dose.[2] Different doses of ribavirin have also been used in IFN-free DAA combination regimens. Pegylated IFN-α and ribavirin treatment is administered for 48 weeks in patients with HCV genotype 1 or 4 infection and 24 weeks in those with HCV genotype 2 or 3 infection. In HCV genotype 1–infected patients, treatment should be stopped if an EVR is not achieved. The SVR for HCV genotype 1–infected patients is 42% to 52%.[2,89,200,201]

Some patients may not require the standard duration of treatment to achieve an SVR. Patients with HCV genotypes 2 or 3 infection may achieve an SVR in some cases with just 12 to 16 weeks of treatment.[7] If a truncated course of treatment is anticipated, the patient should be given a ribavirin dose based on weight rather than a fixed dose of 800 mg/day and should only be treated with a shortened course if an RVR is achieved. Similarly, patients with HCV genotype 1 infection may be treated for only 24 weeks if they have a low baseline HCV viral load (<400,000 IU/mL) and if they achieve an RVR. A longer-than-standard course of therapy appears to be helpful in HCV genotype 1–infected patients who have a slow response to antiviral therapy. In patients with a pEVR, extending the duration of therapy from 48 to 72 weeks improves the SVR rate from 30% to 45.5% (with use of weight-based ribavirin).[2,89]

The best predictor of response to pegylated IFN and ribavirin is the rate of the initial fall in serum HCV RNA levels during treatment. The highest SVRs occur in patients with an RVR, followed respectively by those with a cEVR, those with a pEVR, and those without an EVR. Pretreatment factors associated with a greater chance of an SVR include infection with non–genotype 1 HCV, a low baseline serum HCV RNA level, absence of bridging fibrosis or cirrhosis on a liver biopsy specimen, age younger than 40 years, absence of obesity, lack of hepatic steatosis or insulin resistance, absence of HIV infection, and white race (Fig. 80-8).

As noted earlier, a SNP close to the *IL28B* gene is associated with response to pegylated IFN–based antiviral therapy.[113,202] The frequency of the favorable rs12979860 CC genotype varies in different regions worldwide. Although the CC genotype is highly prevalent in Asian populations, the TT genotype is more common in persons of African origin, explaining in part the lower response rates to antiviral therapy in African American populations.[203]

Of the known pretreatment variables that affect response to therapy, the most powerful predictor is the HCV genotype. HCV genotype 2 is the most responsive to therapy. Response rates for HCV genotype 3 infection are similar to those for HCV genotype 2, but HCV genotype 3–infected patients with a high viral load have been shown to have lower response rates. HCV genotype 4 infection is associated with an SVR similar to that for genotype 1.

Pegylated Interferon, Ribavirin, and a First-Generation Protease Inhibitor

Five pivotal phase 3 studies on therapy of chronic hepatitis C with pegylated IFN-α, ribavirin, and either boceprevir or telaprevir led to the approval of the 2 protease inhibitors in 2011.[204-208] So-called triple therapy is based on a response-guided treatment approach, which means that the treatment duration is based on the virologic response at week 4 of protease inhibitor therapy. If the HCV RNA is undetectable at that time point, the overall duration of treatment can be shortened in treatment-naïve (i.e., previously untreated) patients without cirrhosis to 24 weeks (telaprevir) or 28 weeks (boceprevir). Patients with cirrhosis should always be treated for 48 weeks. A 4-week "lead-in" course of pegylated IFN and ribavirin is used before boceprevir therapy is added, whereas triple therapy is initiated from the start if telaprevir is used. Telaprevir is given for 12 weeks only, whereas boceprevir can be added for the entire course of antiviral therapy, with few exceptions.

Triple therapy led to an increase in response rates of 25% to 30% in treatment-naïve patients and of 3- to 4-fold in patients who had previously failed to respond to pegylated IFN and ribavirin. Most guidelines considered relapsers after pegylated IFN and ribavirin with some degree of liver fibrosis or with cirrhosis to be ideal candidates for triple therapy; 70% to 85% will achieve an SVR.[89] Cure rates were still disappointing (<15%), however, in previous nonresponders (null responders) with cirrhosis and other factors associated with a poor response. Since 2011, various baseline and on-treatment parameters were found to be associated with an SVR with triple therapy and were used to individualize therapy (Table 80-3). For example, a patient with a previous null response, HCV genotype 1a infection, and cirrhosis had a low chance of achieving an SVR on triple therapy.[187] The pegylated IFN/ribavirin "lead-in" phase was used to identify patients with a minimal response who were unlikely to respond to continuation of the regimen.

Patients treated in phase 3 trials have in general been carefully selected, and subjects with comorbidities have generally been excluded. Moreover, hepatitis C registration studies included only a small proportion of patients with cirrhosis, who are in most urgent need of therapy but who also may

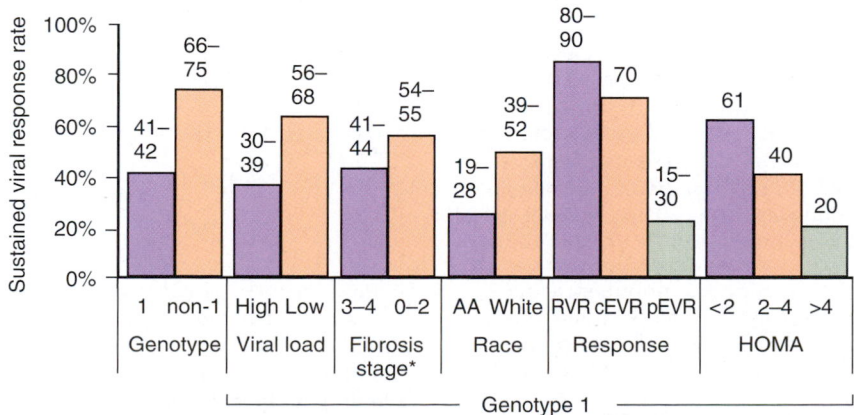

FIGURE 80-8. Sustained virologic response to pegylated interferon and weight-based ribavirin in relation to patient and virus characteristics. AA, African American; cEVR, complete early virologic response; high viral load, ≥ 400,000 IU/mL; HOMA, homeostatic model assessment, a measure of insulin resistance (higher value indicates greater insulin resistance); IU, international units; low viral load, < 400,000 IU/mL; pEVR, partial early virologic response; RVR, rapid virologic response. *METAVIR system.

TABLE 80-3 Factors Associated with Response to Triple Therapy with Pegylated Interferon-α, Ribavirin, and a Protease Inhibitor

Pretreatment		
Host		**Comments**
	IL28B genotype	Lower response rates in patients with the T allele of the rs12979860 SNP; less important with triple therapy than with dual therapy with pegylated IFN-α and ribavirin
	Stage of liver disease	Lower response rates in patients with advanced fibrosis/cirrhosis
	Serum LDL level	Higher SVR in patients with high serum LDL levels (telaprevir only)
	Genetic background	Lower response rates in non-white populations; higher response rates in Asian patients
Viral		
	HCV genotype 1 subtype	Lower response rates in HCV genotype 1a-infected patients than in genotype 1b-infected patients. Subtype is especially important in patients with other poor response factors
	Baseline viral load	Slightly lower SVR rates in patients with high baseline HCV RNA levels (>2 × 10^6 IU/mL)
On Treatment		
	Virologic response during pegylated IFN/ribavirin "lead-in" phase	Response after 4 weeks is associated with SVR in both treatment-naïve and treatment-experienced patients; may identify patients who will not need protease inhibitor-containing treatment
	Virologic response during triple therapy	Response-guided therapy based on the response after 4 weeks of protease inhibitor treatment; stopping rules are based on weeks 4, 8, and 12 responses during protease inhibitor therapy
	Anemia, decline in Hgb level	Higher response rates in patients in whom anemia or a Hgb decline > 3 mg/dL develops

IL28B, interleukin-28B; IU, international units; LDL, low-density lipoprotein; SNP, single nucleotide polymorphism; SVR, sustained virologic response.

suffer most from therapy-associated side effects. Experiences from real-world settings have demonstrated that triple therapy was highly effective in patients with advanced liver disease, but the frequency of serious adverse events was much higher in patients with cirrhosis treated outside of controlled clinical trials than in those treated in clinical trials. In France, more than 600 patients were included in an early-access program, and treatment-related serious adverse events occurred in 40% to 50% of patients treated with boceprevir or telaprevir.[209] Approximately one quarter of patients discontinued therapy during the first 16 weeks of therapy. A few fatal cases were also reported, mainly due to serious infectious complications. Anemia was a frequent side effect that occurred during both boceprevir and telaprevir therapy. Grade 3 or 4 anemia was observed in about 10% of patients despite the frequent use of erythropoietin (56% to 66%), and blood transfusions were necessary in up to 15% of cases. These findings are consistent with other reports demonstrating that the antiviral efficacy of triple therapy is effective, but that side effects are more frequent than in the phase 3 studies. In particular, management of anemia is time consuming and costly.[210] A platelet count below 110,000/mm^3 was associated with treatment failure or hospitalization.

Pegylated Interferon, Ribavirin, and Other Direct-Acting Antiviral Agents

Several DAAs have been tested in phase 2 and phase 3 trials in combination with pegylated IFN and ribavirin (Table 80-4). The main advantages over the first-generation HCV protease inhibitors are better tolerability and use in IFN-sparing or IFN-free regimens. A higher proportion (>80%) of patients treated with the protease inhibitors simeprevir[211] and

TABLE 80-4 Relative Properties of Classes of Direct-Acting Antiviral Agents in Clinical Development

Drug Class	Properties		
	Potency	Pan-genotypic efficacy	Barrier to resistance
Protease inhibitors (second generation)	++ - +++	+ - ++	+ - ++
Non-nucleos(t)ide polymerase inhibitors	+ - ++	±	±
Nucleos(t)ide polymerase inhibitors	+ - +++	+++	++ - +++
NS5A inhibitors	+++	+ - ++	+ - ++

+, lowest; +++, highest.

faldaprevir[212,213] achieve an extended RVR (negative HCV RNA at weeks 4 and 12), and therefore qualify for shortened therapy, than with first-generation protease inhibitors. Simeprevir was approved by the FDA in 2013 but is less effective in patients infected with HCV genotype 1a that contains a Q80K NS3 polymorphism. A fixed (i.e., not response-guided) 12 weeks of a combination of pegylated IFN and ribavirin plus sofosbuvir led to response rates of 90% in patients infected with HCV genotypes 1, 4, 5, and 6,[214] thereby allowing reduced exposure to IFN. Sofosbuvir was also approved in 2013. Combinations of IFN and other DAAs such as daclatasvir have also shown an increase in virologic response rates for HCV genotype 2 and 3.

Interferon-Free Therapies

In contrast to most other chronic viral infections, cure of HCV infection is possible. HCV has an entirely cytosolic life cycle; therefore, suppression of viral replication in the absence of resistance can cure HCV-infected cells. Combinations of novel DAAs that target different steps in the HCV life cycle (see Fig. 80-1) have led to cure of HCV infection in vitro[215] and in small animal models.[216] The first proof-of-concept study showing an SVR in 4 patients with chronic hepatitis C with an IFN-free DAA combination therapy was published in 2012.[217] The compounds investigated in that study were the HCV NS5A inhibitor daclatasvir and the HCV NS3 protease inhibitor asunaprevir. Nevertheless, this combination failed to induce an SVR in 7 of 9 patients infected with HCV genotype 1a, demonstrating that the efficacy of all-oral combination regimens may differ among HCV genotypes. By contrast, therapy with daclatasvir and asunaprevir was highly successful in a study performed in Japan that only enrolled patients infected with HCV genotype 1b, with 10 of 10 patients achieving an SVR.[218] Several other trials have confirmed cure of patients with chronic hepatitis C with various IFN-free treatment regimens.[214,219-221]

The HCV polymerase inhibitor sofosbuvir has been used in combination with ribavirin in patients with HCV genotype 2 or 3 infection,[214,219,222] and the majority of patients with HCV genotype 2 or 3 infection have been cured with just 3 months of therapy. It has also become evident that HCV genotype 2 responds much better to IFN-free sofosbuvir-based therapy than HCV genotype 3 and that patients with cirrhosis have 20% to 30% lower SVRs. This finding is concerning because IFN-free therapies are urgently awaited for patients with decompensated cirrhosis who cannot be treated with IFN. Surprisingly, and for unexplained reasons, women have responded better than men to sofosbuvir-based IFN-free therapy. In one trial,[214] standard pegylated IFN-α plus ribavirin therapy, as a control arm, was as effective as sofosbuvir and ribavirin (67% SVR each). This finding may be important in resource-limited settings, because the newer therapies are more expensive than IFN-based therapy. Prolongation of sofosbuvir-ribavirin therapy from 12 weeks to up to 24 weeks increased SVR rates in various subgroups (e.g., patients with HCV genotype 3 infection and cirrhosis), and the FDA approved a 24-week course for treatment of HCV genotype 3 infection. Importantly, no sofosbuvir-resistant variants have been selected during therapy. All treatment failures were due to relapses after the end of therapy, and not a single patient showed primary treatment failure.

Other IFN-free regimens are being studied, including the combination of sofosbuvir and simeprevir in genotype 1 HCV infection. It is likely that HCV genotype 1 will become the most easy-to-cure genotype, and that most HCV genotype 2 will also be cured with the newer therapies. Treatment of HCV genotype 3 infection may remain a challenge because few alternative compounds are yet in development.

Ledipasvir, an NS5A inhibitor with potent activity against genotype 1 HCV, has been formulated in a fixed-dose combination with sofosbuvir and is highly effective in treatment-naive and treatment-experienced patients, even in those with cirrhosis.[122a,122b]

The combination was approved by the FDA in 2014 for HCV genotype-1 infection in a fixed dose of ledipasvir 90 mg and sofosbuvir 400 mg once daily for 12 weeks in treatment-naive patients and treatment-experienced patients without cirrhosis and for 24 weeks in treatment-experienced patients

with cirrhosis. In treatment-naive patients without cirrhosis, the duration of treatment can be shortened to 8 weeks if the HCV RNA level is less than 6 million IU/mL. SVR rates are well above 90%.

Daclatasvir in combination with sofosbuvir has proved effective in genotypes 1-, 2-, and 3-infected patients.[122c] Also promising in genotype 1-infected patients has been the combination of paritaprevir (a protease inhibitor), boosted by ritonavir, plus ombitasvir (an NS5A inhibitor) and dasabuvir (an NS5B non-nucleoside inhibitor).[122d] This regimen is effective in both treatment-naive patients and prior null responders with or without cirrhosis. As noted earlier, the combination of daclatasvir and asunaprevir is highly effective in genotype 1b-infected patients and also in genotypes 4-, 5-, and 6-infected patients but less effective in genotype 1a-infected patients.[122e] Other drugs and drug combinations are under study (Table 80-5).

Indications and Contraindications

Antiviral therapy should be considered in all patients with chronic hepatitis C. In most cases, the decision as to whether or not to proceed with treatment is based on the patient's desire and need for therapy. The degree of need is a subjective risk-benefit or cost-benefit decision that is made after considering the stage of disease, presence or absence of favorable factors for a response to treatment, and comorbid conditions that might preclude any potential benefit of eradication of the virus. As treatments have become more effective, these decisions have become easier, and more patients have been considered to be appropriate candidates. Physicians who are not comfortable with administering and monitoring the therapy should refer patients to a gastroenterologist or hepatologist experienced in treating patients with hepatitis C, but the new all-oral regimens are relatively easy to prescribe and monitor.[89]

The best time to treat a patient with chronic hepatitis C is before the development of cirrhosis, because response rates are better and the risk of later complications of cirrhosis can be eliminated if treatment is successful. Treatment of patients with decompensated cirrhosis can still be successful but should only be undertaken by an experienced clinician. Managing patients with decompensated cirrhosis who are treated for HCV infection is labor intensive and requires reductions in dose because of cytopenias in 50% to 75% of cases, as well as administration of growth factors in some cases; however, the treatment is generally poorly tolerated and an all-oral regimen is preferable.

Relative and absolute contraindications to IFN and ribavirin therapy are listed in Box 80-3. In general, more patients with relative contraindications to treatment have been treated successfully as practitioners have gained experience and familiarity with the treatment. Many relative contraindications to therapy may resolve over time or as a result of a specific intervention. A few absolute contraindications remain. Because ribavirin is a teratogen, unwillingness of the patient and his or her partner to practice adequate contraception and avoid pregnancy during treatment or for 6 months after the discontinuation of therapy is an absolute contraindication to starting or continuing treatment. Any severe or uncontrolled psychiatric condition is considered an absolute contraindication to therapy. If a patient's psychiatric disorder is treated appropriately and is stable, however, the patient may become a candidate for HCV therapy. Severe cardiac or pulmonary disease is an absolute contraindication to HCV therapy because of the risk of worsening tissue hypoxia if severe hemolytic anemia occurs because of ribavirin. Moreover, in most patients with severe comorbid disease, successful

TABLE 80-5 Direct-Acting Antiviral Agents for HCV Infection*

Agent	Genotype(s)	Dose†	Comment
Protease Inhibitors			
Boceprevir	1	800 mg three times daily	Used in combination with pegylated interferon and ribavirin; no longer recommended
Telaprevir	1	1125 mg twice daily	Used in combination with pegylated interferon and ribavirin; no longer recommended
Simeprevir	1 and 4	150 mg once daily	Used in combination with pegylated interferon and ribavirin or with sofosbuvir
Paritaprevir	1 and 4	150 mg once daily	Used in combination with ombitasvir and dasabuvir; ritonavir boosted
Asunaprevir	1 and 4	200 mg twice daily	Used in combination with daclatasvir or with daclatasvir and BMS-791325
Grazoprevir	1, 2, 4-6	100 mg once daily	Used in combination with elbasvir
Non-nucleos(t)ide Polymerase Inhibitors			
Dasabuvir	1 and 4	250 mg twice daily	Used in combination with paritaprevir and ombitasvir
BMS-791325	1	75 mg twice daily	Used in combination with daclatasvir and asunaprevir
Nucleos(t)ide Polymerase Inhibitor			
Sofosbuvir	1-6	400 mg once daily	Used in combination with pegylated interferon and ribavirin (all genotypes) or with ribavirin alone (genotypes 2 and 3) or with simeprevir (genotypes 1 and 4) or with daclatasvir (all genotypes) or with ledipasvir (genotypes 1, 3, and 4) or with GS-5861 (under study)
NS5A Inhibitors			
Daclatasvir	1-6	60 mg once daily	Used in combination with sofosbuvir (genotypes 1-6) or with pegylated interferon and ribavirin (genotype 4) or with asunaprevir (with or without BMS-791325; under study)
Ledipasvir	1, 3, and 4	90 mg once daily	Used in combination with sofosbuvir
Ombitasvir	1 and 4	25 mg once daily	Used in combination with paritaprevir and dasabuvir
Elbasvir	1-6	50 mg once daily	Used in combination with grazoprevir
GS-5816	1-6	100 mg once daily	Used in combination with sofosbuvir

*Some agents have not been approved by the FDA as of 2015; additional drugs are under study.
†The preferred regimen and duration of treatment may vary depending on HCV genotype, presence or absence of cirrhosis, or nonresponse to prior therapy for HCV infection.

BOX 80-3 Contraindications to Therapy with Pegylated Interferon and Ribavirin

Absolute
Acute pancreatitis
Autoimmune hepatitis
Comorbid conditions that markedly limit life expectancy
History of hypersensitivity to one of the drugs
Organ transplant (except liver)
Pregnancy or unwillingness to use birth control during and for 6 months after treatment
Severe cardiac disease
Severe pulmonary disease
Uncontrolled psychiatric condition
Uncontrolled seizure disorder

Relative
Active alcohol or drug abuse
Active infection
Baseline Hgb level < 10 g/dL (for ribavirin)
Baseline neutrophil count < 1500/mm³
Baseline platelet count < 90,000/mm³
Creatinine clearance < 50 mL/min (use ribavirin with extreme caution)
Decompensated cirrhosis
Hemoglobinopathy
Ophthalmologic disorders
Other autoimmune conditions
Uncontrolled hyperthyroidism or hypothyroidism

---

antiviral therapy would offer no survival benefit. Patients with an underlying autoimmune condition are at risk of experiencing an exacerbation of the condition on pegylated IFN. Although previously considered an absolute contraindication, an autoimmune disorder should probably be considered a strong relative contraindication, and the risk of an exacerbation of the underlying autoimmune disease must be weighed against the potential benefit of clearing the HCV infection.[2,89]

Monitoring and Safety

Before antiviral therapy is started, baseline liver biochemical test levels, a complete blood count (CBC), and a thyroid-stimulating hormone (TSH) level should be obtained. A pregnancy test is required in women before ribavirin is initiated. The HCV genotype and serum HCV RNA level are necessary to determine the dose of ribavirin and duration of therapy (see earlier).

Most hematologic side effects, particularly hemolytic anemia, occur within the first month of therapy that includes IFN and ribavirin, and initially a CBC should be performed weekly. Approximately 10% of patients will have a fall in Hgb levels to less than 10 g/dL, with a mean decrease of approximately 3 g/dL. After the first month, a serum ALT level and a CBC should be obtained monthly, and a TSH level should be obtained every 3 months when IFN is used. Drug doses should be reduced according to the severity of side effects.

A serum HCV RNA level should be obtained at baseline in all patients. Assessment of the decline in HCV RNA level during treatment predicts the likelihood of an SVR, can be used to determine the duration of therapy (see earlier), and is essential for determining treatment duration in HCV genotype 1–infected patients treated with IFN-based therapy. Therefore, quantitative HCV RNA levels should be drawn at baseline and at weeks 4 and 12. If HCV RNA is still detectable in serum at week 12, a level should also be drawn at week 24. If an SVR is achieved, HCV RNA testing should be performed annually for at least 2 years. In nonresponders or relapsers in whom no additional treatment is considered, follow-up testing should be similar to that in patients who receive no treatment, with at least yearly check-ups and laboratory testing and a repeat liver biopsy every 4 to 5 years to assess disease progression, particularly if retreatment is considered.

A reduction in the dose of pegylated IFN is required in 26% to 36% of patients and of ribavirin in 19% to 38%, depending on the initial dose and anticipated duration of therapy. Neutropenia, anemia, and thrombocytopenia are the most frequent reasons for reductions in dose. To ensure maximal response rates, dose reductions should be avoided, and the patient's adherence to therapy should be encouraged.

The most frequent side effects of IFN include flu-like symptoms (in > 90% of patients) and alopecia (in 10% to 30%). Flu-like side effects are common but usually do not necessitate dose adjustments. Other adverse events include depression and hypothyroidism or hyperthyroidism. Because adherence to therapy is an important factor in optimizing efficacy, the various drug-related toxicities—in particular, psychiatric symptoms and thyroid dysfunction—should be managed medically as soon as they are detected.

With ribavirin, anemia, cough, pharyngitis, insomnia, dyspnea, pruritus, rash, nausea, and anorexia are the most common side effects. The most serious side effects are anemia and teratogenic effects. Hemolytic anemia is reversible and usually resolves within the first month after therapy is stopped. If anemia is severe or slow to recover, the patient's iron stores should be assessed by laboratory testing.

Administration of hematopoietic growth factors (e.g., erythropoietin, filgrastim) may enable a patient to continue full-dose pegylated IFN and ribavirin. Use of growth factors may improve the patient's subjective well-being but has not been shown to have an effect on response to antiviral treatment.[2,89]

Telaprevir can cause a troubling rash (that requires discontinuation of the drug in up to 12% of patients), pruritus, GI distress, anal pain, and anemia. The major side effects of boceprevir are anemia, nausea, vomiting, and dysgeusia. Both protease inhibitors have a low genetic barrier to resistance but are inhibitors of cytochrome P450 3A and the drug transporter P-glycoprotein and thus interact with many other drugs. Simeprevir may cause a photosensitivity reaction and an elevation in serum bilirubin levels. Side effects of sofosbuvir appear to be mild. In general, side effects with the newer all-oral regimens that do not include ribavirin appear to be mild and well-tolerated.

HCV-HIV Coinfection

Patients with HCV-HIV coinfection are likely to progress more rapidly to cirrhosis than do HCV-monoinfected patients, and therefore treatment of HCV infection should always be considered in this group.[223] Patients are at even higher risk of progression of fibrosis if they are female, older than 33 years of age, have an increase in the CD4$^+$ count of less than 100/mm^3 with HAART, continue to have a detectable HIV viral load during antiretroviral therapy, or have untreated HCV infection.

The clinical benefit of successful antiviral therapy of hepatitis C has also been demonstrated in HIV coinfected persons.[224]

SVR rates to pegylated IFN and ribavirin therapy, however, were lower in HCV-HIV coinfected patients in clinical trials than in HCV-monoinfected historical controls.[225] Response rates to triple therapy with either telaprevir[226] or boceprevir[227] were not very different from results in monoinfected patients, and therefore, triple therapy has been recommended in HIV-HCV coinfected patients with HCV genotype 1 infection. Newer IFN-free regimens are likely to be preferable. Ideally, therapy for HCV infection should be started before antiretroviral therapy for HIV is initiated. When HCV therapy cannot be started first, zidovudine, stavudine, and didanosine should not be used in combination with ribavirin because of the additive risk of mitochondrial toxicity. Drug-drug interaction of antiretroviral therapies with HCV protease inhibitors also need to be considered. Otherwise, contraindications to antiviral therapy for HCV infection in HCV-HIV–coinfected patients do not differ from those for monoinfected patients.

Treatment of coinfected patients will evolve with the availability of newer IFN-free regimens. All regimens in clinical development are also tested in coinfected persons.

Liver Transplant Recipients

Complications of chronic hepatitis C are the most common indication for liver transplantation (see Chapter 97). Patients who have detectable HCV RNA in serum at the time of liver transplantation almost universally experience HCV reinfection of the allograft. Reducing HCV RNA to undetectable levels before transplantation may prevent reinfection in some cases,[228,229] but therapy with IFN-α–based regimens is complicated in patients with advanced cirrhosis and can be associated with significant morbidity and even mortality. Patients with a MELD score higher than 18 or patients with ascites should not be treated with IFN-α.[2]

The natural history of hepatitis C after liver transplantation is characterized by a more rapid progression of liver fibrosis. At least 25% of patients will develop cirrhosis within 5 to 10 years after transplantation.[230] Once cirrhosis is established, transplanted patients show an accelerated natural history, with decompensation rates of as high as 40% after 12 months. Some data suggest that the outcome of hepatitis C after liver transplantation has worsened in the 2000s.[231] Across different countries and transplantation programs, the 5-year post-transplantation survival rate for patients with hepatitis C is significantly lower than those of patients who underwent liver transplantation for other chronic liver diseases. Factors associated with graft loss in HCV-infected patients include an older donor age, steatosis of the donor organ, specific immunosuppressive regimens, female sex, high necroinflammatory activity in the allograft 1 year after transplantation, and high HCV viral loads.[230,231] Additional factors thought to influence the long-term outcome of graft HCV infection include herpesvirus infections,[232] the degree of HLA matching, and the matching of the *IL28B* genotypes of the donor and recipient.[233-235] Cellular immune responses by both T cells and NK cells are thought to play a major role in the pathogenesis of chronic hepatitis C after transplantation. HCV-specific T-cell responses have been linked with improved histologic and clinical outcomes and are also associated with spontaneous HCV clearance after liver transplantation.[236]

Immunosuppressive therapies have been suggested to influence the outcome of graft HCV infection. The 2 approved calcineurin inhibitors, cyclosporine and tacrolimus, have been studied extensively in liver transplant recipients with HCV infection.[237] Some earlier studies suggested that immunosuppression with cyclosporine might be associated with a better histologic outcome of graft hepatitis C; however, the vast majority of subsequent studies did not identify major differences between cyclosporine and tacrolimus in the outcome of HCV infection after liver transplantation.[237] Conversely, a retrospective study of more than 8000 HCV-positive liver-transplanted persons showed that death, graft failure, liver failure owing to recurrent disease, and acute cellular rejection were slightly more frequent in the cyclosporine-treated group than in the tacrolimus-treated group.[238] Nevertheless, to avoid HCV reinfection, it may be helpful to employ a cyclosporine-based immunosuppressive regimen in the early phase after transplantation, because cyclosporine has a clear additive antiviral effect in vitro.[239] Moreover, some studies have suggested that immunosuppression with cyclosporine enhances SVR rates in liver transplant patients treated with pegylated IFN-α and ribavirin.[240] Finally, cyclosporine may have advantages concerning drug-drug interactions as novel HCV protease inhibitors are explored; for example, cyclosporine blood levels are less affected than tacrolimus levels when coadministered with telaprevir.[241]

The use of glucocorticoids after transplantation of HCV-infected patients has also been a matter of debate. Glucocorticoids increase HCV replication in vitro by up-regulation of distinct HCV entry factors.[242] Clearly, repeated administration of high doses of glucocorticoids to treat rejection is associated with more rapid fibrosis progression and poor long-term outcome of graft HCV infection and should be avoided.[243] Several studies have confirmed a strong correlation between glucocorticoid bolus therapy of acute rejection episodes and severe recurrence of hepatitis C.[230] Low-dose glucocorticoids, however, may not necessarily have to be avoided in patients with HCV infection after liver transplantation.

The impact of other immunosuppressive agents including mycophenolate mofetil, azathioprine, and IL-2 inhibitors on HCV recurrence remains controversial. Study results have been conflicting, and large, high-quality prospective studies with long-term follow-up are lacking. Therefore, no recommendation can be given regarding preferential use or avoidance of any of these compounds.

Antiviral treatment after transplantation with pegylated IFN-α–based regimens is possible and can lead to cure of HCV infection. Importantly, HCV clearance after transplantation is associated with an improved long-term outcome.[244] Therapies are associated with serious side effects, however, and tolerability of treatment is low. SVR rates for pegylated IFN plus ribavirin are between 30% and 50% depending on the viral genotype, donor and recipient *IL28B* genotypes, and stage of liver disease.[245] Treatment is better tolerated more than 1 year post transplantation than immediately after transplantation, but reductions in drug doses are required in most patients. Few patients tolerate full doses of ribavirin because of the renal dysfunction associated with calcineurin inhibitors.

Triple therapy with pegylated IFN, ribavirin, and a protease inhibitor also increases SVR rates after liver transplantation, but therapy has been even more challenging because of the increased frequency of serious adverse events, in particular anemia and infections, and drug-drug interactions between immunosuppressive agents and the protease inhibitor.[246-248] IFN-free therapies should lead to a complete paradigm shift in the treatment of post-transplant hepatitis C. Serious complications of hepatitis C, such as fibrosing cholestatic hepatitis (see Chapter 97), may be managed in the future by potent antiviral combination therapies.[249]

KEY REFERENCES

Full references for this chapter can be found on www.expertconsult.com.

1. Hanafiah KM, Groeger J, Flaxman AD, et al. Global epidemiology of hepatitis C virus infection: New estimates of age-specific antibody to HCV seroprevalence. Hepatology 2013; 57:1333-42.
2. European Association for the Study of the Liver. EASL Clinical Practice Guidelines: Management of hepatitis C virus infection. J Hepatol 2011; 55:245-64.
5. Razavi H, ElKhoury AC, Elbasha E, et al. Chronic hepatitis C virus (HCV) disease burden and cost in the United States. Hepatology 2013; 57:2164-70.
6. van der Meer AJ, Veldt BJ, Feld JJ, et al. Association between sustained virological response and all-cause mortality among patients with chronic hepatitis C and advanced hepatic fibrosis. JAMA 2012; 308:2584-93.
25. Scheel TK, Rice CM. Understanding the hepatitis C virus life cycle paves the way for highly effective therapies. Nat Med 2013; 19:837-49.
89. Ghany MG, Nelson DR, Strader DB, et al. An update on treatment of genotype 1 chronic hepatitis C virus infection: 2011 Practice Guideline by the American Association for the Study of Liver Diseases. Hepatology 2011; 54:1433-44.
198. Deterding K, Gruner N, Buggisch P, et al. Delayed versus immediate treatment for patients with acute hepatitis C: A randomised controlled non-inferiority trial. Lancet Infect Dis 2013; 13:497-506.
201. McHutchison JG, Lawitz EJ, Shiffman ML, et al. Peginterferon alfa-2b or alfa-2a with ribavirin for treatment of hepatitis C infection. N Engl J Med 2009; 361:580-93.
204. Poordad F, McCone J Jr, Bacon BR, et al. Boceprevir for untreated chronic HCV genotype 1 infection. N Engl J Med 2011; 364:1195-206.
206. Jacobson IM, McHutchison JG, Dusheiko G, et al. Telaprevir for previously untreated chronic hepatitis C virus infection. N Engl J Med 2011; 364:2405-16.
211. Fried MW, Buti M, Dore GJ, et al. Once-daily simeprevir (TMC435) with pegylated interferon and ribavirin in treatment-naive genotype 1 hepatitis C: The randomized PILLAR study. Hepatology 2013; 58:1918-29.
214. Lawitz E, Gane EJ. Sofosbuvir for previously untreated chronic hepatitis C infection. N Engl J Med 2013; 369:678-9.
219. Jacobson IM, Gordon SC, Kowdley KV, et al. Sofosbuvir for hepatitis C genotype 2 or 3 in patients without treatment options. N Engl J Med 2013; 368:1867-77.
220. Poordad F, Lawitz E, Kowdley KV, et al. Exploratory study of oral combination antiviral therapy for hepatitis C. N Engl J Med 2013; 368:45-53.
225. Naggie S, Sulkowski MS. Management of patients coinfected with HCV and HIV: A close look at the role for direct-acting antivirals. Gastroenterology 2012; 142:1324-34.

CARMEN LANDAVERDE AND ROBERT PERRILLO

Hepatitis D (delta) virus (HDV) was discovered by Rizzetto and associates in 1977, as a unique nuclear antigen in the hepatocytes of patients infected with HBV.[1] The antigen was identified subsequently as a novel pathogen and was linked to severe chronic hepatitis B and fulminant HBV infection. The HDV particle, termed the *delta agent*, was found to consist of a small RNA genome encapsidated by HBV envelope proteins.[2] It has been called a defective virus because it is dependent on the presence of the hepatitis B surface antigen (HBsAg) for replication in an infected individual.

EPIDEMIOLOGY

HDV is distributed globally with wide variations in prevalence. At least 5% of HBV carriers worldwide are estimated to be infected with HDV, thus making the global burden of HDV infection between 15 and 20 million cases.[3] The highest prevalence is seen in northern parts of South America, the Mediterranean basin, Central Africa, and the Middle East (Fig. 81-1). HDV is highly endemic in developing nations, such as Central Africa, parts of the Middle East, and the Amazon basin, where HBV remains poorly controlled.[4] Intermediate prevalence is seen in much of Eastern Europe, Turkey, and Central and South America.[5] In the past, the prevalence of HDV infection was considered low in Northern Europe and North America, where HDV infection was confined primarily to people who inject drugs (PWID); additional special-risk groups included persons infected with HIV, on hemodialysis, with hemophilia, and with other high-risk behaviors, such as promiscuous sexual activity. A prevalence of HDV infection of 14.5% has been reported in European patients coinfected with HIV and HBV, thereby confirming that the prevalence of HDV in special-risk groups can be substantial.

Increased rates of immigration from Eastern Europe, Africa, and Asia are thought to account for a resurgence of HDV infection in Northern Europe, which traditionally has been considered to be a low-prevalence area.[6] The prevalence of HDV began to diminish in Europe at the end of the 1980s[5];

the rate of infection among HBsAg-positive blood donors in the United States at that time was reported to be 3.8%.[7] Many epidemiologists believed that the epidemic of HDV, which started in Europe in the 1970s, was coming to an end. This conclusion was supported by data from an epidemiologic study in Italy that showed the prevalence of HDV infection in HBV carriers to be 8.3% in 2000, compared with 25% in the early 1970s.[8-10] In the 2000s, however, no further decline in the prevalence of HDV infection has been noted. Data from a multicenter study in 2006 to 2007 indicated that the overall prevalence of HDV infection in Italy remained unchanged from a rate of 8.1% in 1997. The same study found a prevalence of 14.3% in incident cases of chronic HBV infection, pointing to a resurgence of HDV infection.[11]

HDV continues to be a health burden in Europe, despite a decline in incidence in various European countries, due in large part to an increase in the rate of immigration of persons from endemic areas.[12,13] Epidemiologic data indicate that a shift has occurred in the groups most affected by HDV: from young persons who acquired the infection through high-risk behavior or through a blood transfusion to 2 major groups—older, domestic patients with advanced liver disease who survived acute infection in the 1970s or 1980s and immigrants from endemic areas who may have contracted infection through traditional high-risk behaviors, including unsterile vaccination techniques (Fig. 81-2).[5,13-15] HDV infection continues to be an important problem among PWID in various regions of Europe.[4,8,16] Likewise, there is a high burden of HDV among PWID in the United States, as shown in a study from Baltimore in 2006, which revealed a 50% prevalence of concomitant HDV infection in chronically HBV-infected PWID.[17] Information on the epidemiology of HBV in North America is limited and suggests that the prevalence of HDV infection among chronic HBV carriers is highly variable, ranging from less than 1% to 30%.[18-21] The results from the National Health and Nutrition Examination Survey (NHANES) in 2003-2004 demonstrated a 3.6% prevalence of HDV infection among HBsAg-positive persons, and a study from the Northern California Network in 2010 revealed a 6.3% rate of HDV infection in HBsAg carriers.[22]

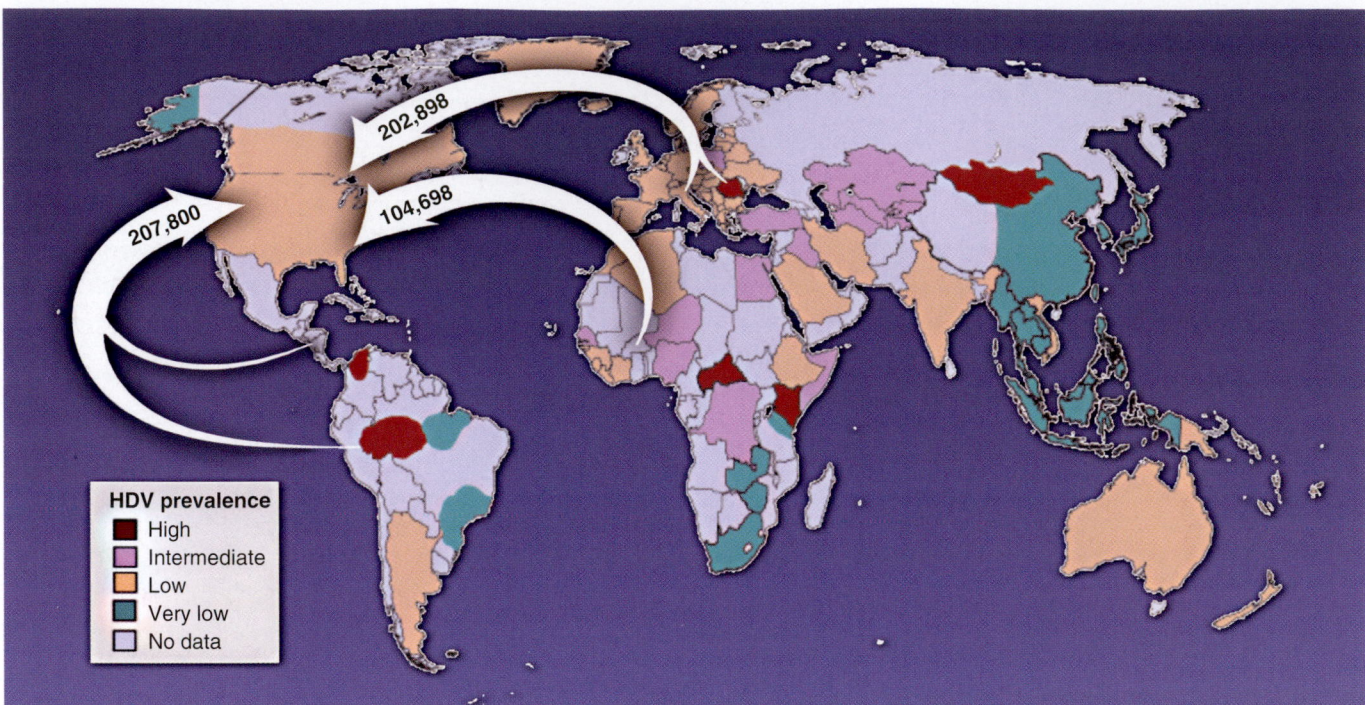

FIGURE 81-1. Worldwide prevalence of HDV infection and immigration patterns to the United States from endemic regions of the world (1974-2008). The numbers within the *arrows* indicate the total number of hepatitis B surface antigen-positive immigrants who are estimated to have come to the United States from various regions during this period. Changing immigration patterns are likely to account for a greater prevalence of HDV infection in the United States than previously considered.

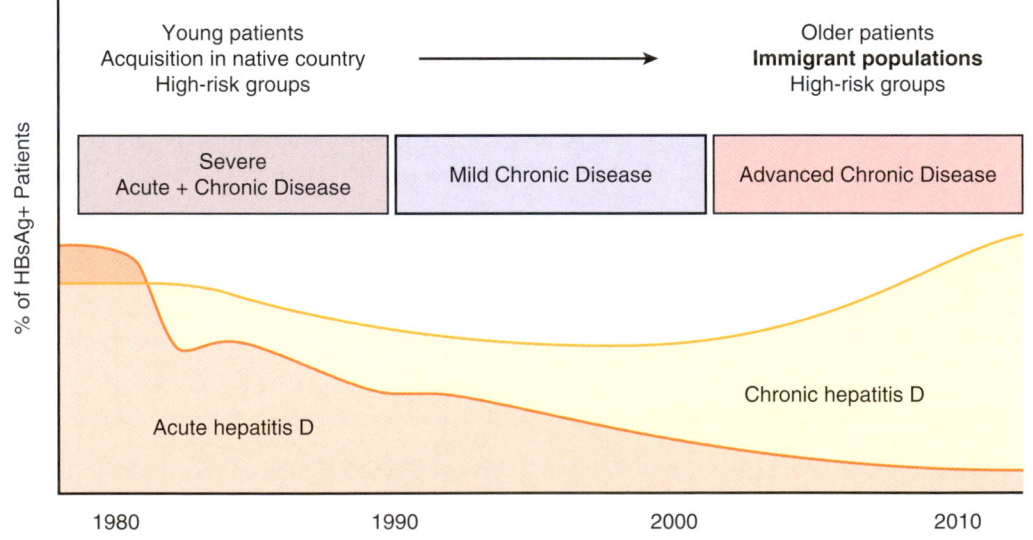

FIGURE 81-2. Timeline of the changing epidemiology of HDV infection since the late 1970s. HDV had a dramatic acute appearance in the early to mid-1980s, and many of the patients were young, from countries with a high prevalence of HDV infection, or identified as being in high-risk groups (e.g., people who inject drugs). Since that time, many of the patients with severe liver injury have died because of the infection, and many of those with initially mild hepatitis have developed advanced liver disease and its complications. With changing immigration patterns in Europe and the United States (see Fig. 81-1), more cases of chronic HDV infection are being seen in persons who have relocated from high-prevalence areas. HBsAg, hepatitis B surface antigen.

VIROLOGY

HDV is a unique agent that bears no similarity to other transmissible agents that infect animals. The complete virion is 36 nm in size, making it slightly smaller than the complete HBV virion. In fact, the HDV genome, a 1.7-kb circular single-stranded RNA of negative polarity, shares several features, such as intramolecular base pairing and autocatalytic RNA segments, with plant viroids.[23,24] The unique genome is the smallest of any animal virus.

Unlike plant viroids, HDV RNA encodes a protein, hepatitis delta antigen (HDAg). HDV RNA has 6 open reading frames, or genes. One encodes the HDAg, but the others do not seem to be actively transcribed. The virion is a spherical particle that consists of the HDV genome complexed with 2 structural proteins, short and long HDAg, to form a ribonucleoprotein that is encapsidated by the HBV envelope protein, composed of host lipids and the 3 envelope proteins (large, medium, and small HBsAg) (see Chapter 79).[25] The protein envelope protects the HDV RNA-HDAg complex and facilitates HDV infectivity. The pre-S1 moiety of the large HBsAg contains the receptor-binding domain, which through a process of myristoylation allows HDV entry into susceptible hepatocytes.[26,27] It appears that the antigenic loop of all 3 envelope proteins is also necessary for viral entry.[28] The protein envelope is not required for replication of HDV and is the only helper function provided by HBV. Once HDV with its HBV envelope protein enters the host hepatocyte, the HDV RNA-HDAg complex migrates to the nucleus. Viral replication then proceeds in the nucleus according to a double-rolling model, aided by host DNA-dependent RNA polymerases.[29-32]

During translation, 2 forms of HDAg (encoded by the same regions of RNA) are produced, a short form (HDAg-S) and a long form (HDAg-L). HDAg-L has 19 to 20 more amino acids than HDAg-S. The additional amino acids in HDAg-L are incorporated by a process of RNA editing, another unique aspect of the HDV genome.[33] Interestingly, HDAg-S and HDAg-L have opposite effects on viral replication: HDAg-S acts as a facilitator and HDAg-L as an inhibitor.[34] HDAg-L plays a pivotal role in virion assembly, however, and post-translational modification of HDAg-L by prenylation of the cysteine residue at the C-terminus is essential to its ability to bind to HBsAg.[35] The extent of RNA editing determines the amount of HDAg-L formed and consequently influences the rate of replication. The viral life cycle is also influenced by post-translational modifications of HDAg-S, because phosphorylation, methylation, and sumoylation of HDAg-S at different sites affect the rate of viral replication.[36-38] Ultimately, the intracellular ratio of HDAg-S to HDAg-L and post-translational modifications of HDAg determine the rate of replication, assembly, and transport from infected hepatocytes.

Because it has a unique genome, HDV is classified in a separate genus of the Deltaviridae family. No other virus has been identified in this genus. The current consensus is that HDV is a satellite virus. Satellite viruses are subviral particles that carry a distinct nucleic acid, usually RNA, that requires a helper virus for transmission and multiplication. In addition, the nucleic acid of satellite viruses is distinct from the nucleic acid of helper viruses. No other animal virus has been identified as a satellite virus.

Eight genotypes of HDV have been identified.[39] Genotype 1 is the most prevalent overall and the most common in Europe, Mediterranean countries, the Middle East, North Africa, and North America.[4,40,41] Genotype 2 is reported mostly in East and Northern Asia and is associated with milder liver disease than that seen with genotype 1.[42,43] Genotype 3 has been isolated from epidemics in the northern part of South America.[44] Genotype 4 has been found in Taiwan and Japan.[42,45] Genotypes 5 to 8 are found mainly in West and Central Africa.[4] Different genotypes of HDV may interact variably with different HBV genotypes. Whether the interaction between HDV and HBV genotypes increases the severity of HDV infection is unclear, although infection with HDV genotype 3 and HBV genotype F has been reported to cause severe hepatitis.[46]

PATHOGENESIS

The pathogenesis of HDV-induced liver disease remains poorly understood. Because HBV is not known to be directly cytotoxic, the severity of combined infection with HBV and HDV may be attributed either to a direct cytotoxic effect of HDV or an enhanced immune response against the 2 viruses. Direct cytotoxicity of HDV has been questioned on the basis of studies in transgenic mice. Mice expressing either HDAg-L or HDAg-S show no evidence of hepatocyte injury. The lack of a direct cytotoxic effect also is supported by the observation that liver transplant recipients who express HDAg in their allografts do not manifest evidence of cellular damage.[47] Instead, several lines of evidence indicate the pathogenic mechanism of HDV-induced liver damage is most likely related to the immunologic response to HDV. First, patients with inactive HDV disease demonstrated HDV-specific proliferative CD4 responses to HDAg.[48] Second, a higher frequency of CD4⁺ T cells that contain a cytolytic protein, perforin, has been noted in HDV-infected persons as compared with monoinfected persons with hepatitis B or C and correlates with disease activity.[49] Third, HDV interferes with alpha interferon signaling by blocking tyrosine kinase 2 activation, suggesting that the virus has the ability to block innate immune responses, thereby leading to viral persistence.[50] Also, the occurrence of prominent necroinflammatory changes in the liver and presence of several circulating autoantibodies, such as antibodies to liver-kidney microsome (anti-LKM), thymocytes, and nuclear lamin C, also suggest a role for immune-mediated liver injury. One fact is certain: the ability of HDV to cause hepatic necrosis is determined by coexpression of HBV, as occurs after liver transplantation when HDV becomes pathogenic only if HBV infection also recurs.[47]

DIAGNOSIS

The most useful markers of HDV infection include HDAg, antibody to HDAg (anti-HDV), HDV RNA, and immunohistochemical staining of HDAg in liver tissue. Detection of HDV RNA by reverse transcriptase PCR (RT-PCR) amplification is the most sensitive diagnostic technique (Table 81-1).

HDV RNA

HDV RNA can be detected with qualitative and quantitative HDV RNA PCR assays. The introduction of the real-time PCR technique in 2004 has led to improved in-house and commercial assays for HDV RNA, with detection limits as low as 10 copies/mL.[51] The sensitivity and reliability of the available assays vary, however, because of the use of different primers and the variability in the RNA region being amplified. There is no standardized assay for HDV RNA measurement. In the United States, a real-time PCR assay that can be used for quantification of HDV RNA has become available through the CDC.

HDV RNA is the earliest marker to appear during the course of HDV infection and may be found in the absence of other markers.[52] The diagnosis of active HDV infection is established by the presence of immunoglobulin (Ig)M anti-HDV and confirmed with serum HDV RNA by a PCR assay. Higher levels of HDV RNA in serum may be associated with more severe disease. The level of HDV RNA in serum can be a reliable marker for monitoring the efficacy of treatment and documenting viral eradication, provided that the same assay is used throughout (see later). HDV RNA also can be detected in hepatocytes by hybridization techniques, which are generally less sensitive than PCR assays. The real-time RNA assay can quantify HDV RNA in both serum and liver, and a correlation has been found between HDV RNA levels in serum and liver. The technique and the observations made require validation.[53]

TABLE 81-1 Diagnostic Markers for HDV Infection, Their Importance, and Potential Weaknesses

Diagnostic Markers and Their Importance	Potential Weaknesses
IgG anti-HDV	
Positive in all persons exposed to HDV; persists long term, even after viral clearance May indicate active or past infection; not a neutralizing antibody	May not be elevated in immunocompromised persons
IgM anti-HDV	
Positive in acute infection; negative in past infection May be used as a surrogate marker for HDV replication Decrease in titers and subsequent clearance in chronic HDV infection is a predictor of spontaneous or therapy-induced remission	Often persists in chronic infection, particularly with active liver disease Neither 100% sensitive nor specific for HDV replication
HDAg	
Can be demonstrated in hepatocytes by immunohistochemical staining	The reliability of immunochemistry decreases as the disease becomes chronic The presence of high titers of neutralizing antibodies (anti-HDV) interferes with detection of HDAg Less sensitive than molecular assays
HDV RNA (qualitative)	
Marker of HDV replication Positive in all patients with chronic HDV infection Negative in spontaneous or treatment-induced viral clearance	Variability in the HDV genome and assay primers influences the sensitivity of HDV RNA detection No WHO standardized assay
HDV RNA (quantitative)	
Used to measure the level of HDV RNA in serum Useful method for predicting and monitoring treatment response	HDV RNA may be present at a lower titer than the limit of detection (as low as 10 copies/mL) Levels do not reflect the grade or stage of liver disease May be useful for monitoring patients during therapy with interferon, but there is no WHO standardized assay Results may differ significantly among laboratories
HBsAg (quantitative)	
May be useful for predicting or monitoring treatment response during therapy with interferon, because a falling titer heralds HBsAg loss and hence HDV RNA clearance	Confined to research laboratories in the United States but commercially licensed in Asia and Europe

HBsAg, hepatitis B surface antigen; HDAg, hepatitis D antigen; IgG, immunoglobulin G; IgM, immunoglobulin M.

Hepatitis D Antigen

The HDV genomic product, HDAg, is another marker of HDV infection. HDAg can be demonstrated in hepatocytes by immunohistochemical staining, but the reliability of this method decreases as the HDV infection becomes chronic. Measurement of HDAg in serum is also problematic because of the presence of high titers of neutralizing antibodies, which can interfere with detection of HDAg.

Antibody to HDV

The most readily available marker of HDV infection has been anti-HDV. Two antibody tests are commercially available, and both can be detected in actively infected patients: IgM anti-HDV and total anti-HDV, which is composed of both IgM and IgG anti-HDV. IgM anti-HDV appears in serum at the time of acute infection, and IgG anti-HDV develops later in the course. IgM anti-HDV often persists as the disease progresses to chronicity and is detectable in high titers in patients with chronic HDV infection. It is frequently regarded as a marker of serious liver damage.[54] As the infection evolves from the acute to the chronic phase, the type of IgM antibody also changes from a

> **BOX 81-1** Persons Who Should Be Clinically Suspected of Having HDV Infection*
>
> HBsAg-positive immigrants from regions that are moderately to highly endemic for HDV
> HBsAg carriers with a history of injection drug use
> Persons with chronic hepatitis B and rapid evolution to cirrhosis or hepatocellular carcinoma
> HBsAg carriers who are persistently HBV DNA negative but have active liver disease
> Persons with an unexplained acute flare of chronic hepatitis B that is not due to acute hepatitis A or C or reactivation of hepatitis B
>
> *Initial screening with anti-HDV is recommended.
> Anti-HDV, antibody to HDV; HBsAg, hepatitis B surface antigen.

monomeric (S) form to a multimeric (19S) form. IgG anti-HDV persists for a long time in immunocompetent persons and may indicate either chronic or previous HDV infection. Some patients with IgG anti-HDV may not have active infection and therefore test negative for HDV RNA (Box 81-1).[55]

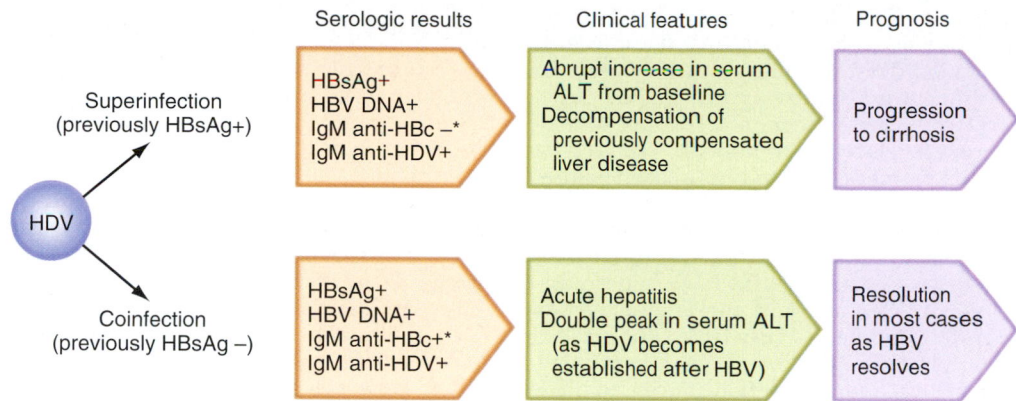

* Distinguishing feature between superinfection and coinfection.

FIGURE 81-3. Serologic results, clinical features, and prognosis of HDV superinfection and coinfection with HDV and HBV. anti-HBc, antibody to hepatitis B core antigen; anti-HDV, antibody to hepatitis D virus; HBsAg, hepatitis B surface antigen; IgM, immunoglobulin M.

NATURAL HISTORY

Because of the obligate relationship of HDV to HBV infection, the natural history of HDV infection depends on the clinical course of HBV. Two distinct types of HDV infections are possible: *coprimary infection* (or coinfection), in which infection of HBV and HDV occurs simultaneously, and *superinfection*, in which HDV infection is superimposed on established chronic HBV infection. These 2 different disease states can usually be distinguished by serologic and genomic testing for both viruses (Fig. 81-3).

Early epidemiologic studies suggested that HDV infection aggravates the severity of HBV infection in coinfected persons, but subsequent reports have disputed this claim.[56] In a European multicenter study on prognostic factors in 366 patients with chronic hepatitis B and compensated cirrhosis, HDV infection did not influence the prognosis.[57] In a long-term follow-up study of 302 patients with chronic hepatitis B (76 with HDV infection), HDV infection was not an independent predictor of mortality.[58] Therefore, HDV infection appears to have a varying influence on the course of hepatitis B and is not necessarily associated with severe hepatitis. The severity of HDV infection may vary with the frequency of HDV in a population, level of HBV viremia, and interactions between specific HBV and HDV genotypes.

Coprimary infection is seen most often in PWID. Because HBV infection resolves in a majority of patients, HDV also resolves in most patients, and the risk of chronicity after coprimary infection is less than 5%. Some data suggest, however, that coinfection with HDV enhances the risk of fulminant hepatitis B.[59]

Superinfection of HDV in an HBV carrier can lead to severe hepatitis and acute decompensation of preexisting liver disease. Affected patients often express a high level of HDV viremia because high serum levels of HBsAg readily protect the replicating HDV genome. Superinfection may also coincide with a decline in serum HBV DNA levels because HDV replication inhibits HBV replication.[60] HDV proteins inhibit HBV replication by two mechanisms: repression of enhancers contained within the HBV genome and transactivation of the alpha interferon–inducible MxA gene.[61] In a study involving 185 patients with HDV superinfection, HDV RNA was detectable in 63 of 64 patients with acute HDV infection, but HBV DNA was detectable in only 40%.[60] Rarely, HDV

superinfection may lead to disappearance of HBsAg and appearance of antibody to HBsAg (anti-HBs).[60] In contrast to coprimary infection, chronic HDV infection develops frequently after HDV superinfection. HDV superinfection evolves to chronic HDV infection in 70% of patients and is characterized by persistent HDV viremia and detectable HDV RNA in serum. Although the clinical course of chronic HDV infection varies, persistent replication of HDV and HBV often leads to progressive hepatitis and cirrhosis within a few years. More rapid clinical progression leading to end-stage liver disease within 2 years may be seen in some PWID; hepatocellular carcinoma (HCC) also may develop.[62,63] Patients with compensated cirrhosis from HDV have a 3-fold increase in HCC risk compared with patients with cirrhosis from HBV monoinfection.[64] This increased risk was further demonstrated in a 28-year follow-up Italian study, in which HCC developed in 15% of 46 patients with HDV infection.[65]

In patients with a triple infection with HBV, HDV, and HCV, HDV infection often tends to be dominant because it can inhibit viral replication of both HBV and HCV.[66] One study reported that HCV RNA and markers of HBV replication were persistently absent in serum in 80% of patients with markers of active HDV infection (HDV RNA, HDAg, or IgM anti-HDV).[67] A longitudinal study conducted in Italy that evaluated the virologic patterns in patients with triple infection, however, demonstrated wide fluctuations in viremia for both HBV and HCV virus, and in some patients the HDV RNA positivity also fluctuated.[68] Furthermore, in a study from Spain that evaluated HDV and HBV viremia longitudinally, persistence of HDV RNA in the absence of HBV DNA was seen in only 20% of cases. Fluctuating activity of both or of one of the two viruses was noted in more than 50% of the patients.[69] These data indicate that HDV infection is a far more dynamic disease than had previously been appreciated.

CLINICAL FEATURES

HDV and HBV coprimary infection typically manifests as self-limited acute hepatitis (see Chapter 79). Some patients may demonstrate a double peak in serum aminotransferase levels because of a delay in HDV replication after HBV replication. Markers detectable in serum at the time of acute hepatitis include IgM antibody to hepatitis B core antigen (anti-HBc), IgM anti-HDV, HDV RNA, HBV DNA, and HBsAg. Acute hepatitis usually resolves in a few weeks, with a gradual return of liver biochemical test levels to normal. As the infection resolves, HDV RNA and HBV DNA titers steadily decrease, and anti-HBs appears after the disappearance of HBsAg. Occasionally, IgM anti-HDV may persist after anti-HBs appears and serum aminotransferase levels return to normal.

HDV superinfection manifests clinically as acute hepatitis in an otherwise stable chronic HBV carrier. Clinically, HDV superinfection can mimic a spontaneous flare of chronic HBV infection. These two diagnostic possibilities can usually be differentiated easily because patients with HDV superinfection have detectable HDV RNA and IgM anti-HDV in serum as well as a corresponding decline in serum HBV DNA instead of an increase that is typical of a hepatitis B flare. Determining whether an HDV infection is a superinfection or acute coinfection depends on whether the HBV infection is chronic or acute; the distinguishing serologic feature of acute hepatitis B is the presence of IgM anti-HBc in serum.

TREATMENT

Despite developments in the treatment of HBV monoinfection (see Chapter 79), results of therapy for HDV-HBV infection have been disappointing. HDV is the least common cause of chronic viral hepatitis worldwide, but it is the most severe form and ironically the one for which new and effective treatments have been slowest to develop. The only therapeutic option available is interferon-α (IFN-α), the efficacy of which is related to the dose and duration of treatment. Nucleoside and nucleotide analogs, currently the mainstays of treatment for HBV infection, are not effective in HDV infection. The lack of efficacy of nucleos(t)ide analogs may be explained in part by the observation that nucleos(t)ide analogs have unpredictable and slow effects on HBsAg concentration[70,71] and seldom lead to disappearance of HBsAg, the only HBV protein that is required by HDV.

Interferon

The rate of sustained HDV clearance after a 1- or 2-year course with high doses of conventional IFN-α (9 million units 3 times a week) varies but overall is low (≈20%).[72,73] Patients with disease of short duration or without cirrhosis are most likely to respond.

Recommendations from an Italian workshop include the use of pegylated IFN-α for 48 to 72 weeks.[74] The sustained virologic response (SVR) rates with pegylated IFN-α alone for at least 48 weeks have been reported to be between 17% and 47%, with relapse rates of 2% to 14%.[75-80] A negative HDV RNA at 6 months from the end of treatment has been found to be a reliable predictor of SVR (OR = 20; 95% CI, 2-195; P = 0.01).[80] However, a long-term follow-up study of IFN-treated patients who were negative for HDV RNA in serum 6 months after the end of treatment reported a 56% virologic relapse rate (9 of 16 patients).[80a] Because the ultimate goal of treatment is the eradication of both HBV and HDV, some authorities have advocated that therapy be continued as long as possible in responders and preferably until the loss of HBsAg occurs.[72] Sustained disappearance of HDV RNA and HBsAg, accompanied by regression of liver fibrosis, has been reported after continuous therapy with IFN-α, 5 million units daily, for 12 years.[81] Monitoring HBsAg concentration may allow prediction of how long therapy will need to be continued to ensure disappearance of HBsAg (Fig. 81-4).[82]

Combination Antiviral Therapy

Lamivudine therapy for 48 weeks used in conjunction with IFN-α does not improve response rates compared with interferon alone.[83] The Hep-Net International Delta Hepatitis Intervention Trial (HIDIT) is a large multicenter study that evaluated the efficacy of 48 weeks of treatment with peginterferon alfa-2a, 180 μg once weekly, in combination with the nucleotide analog adefovir dipivoxil compared with either

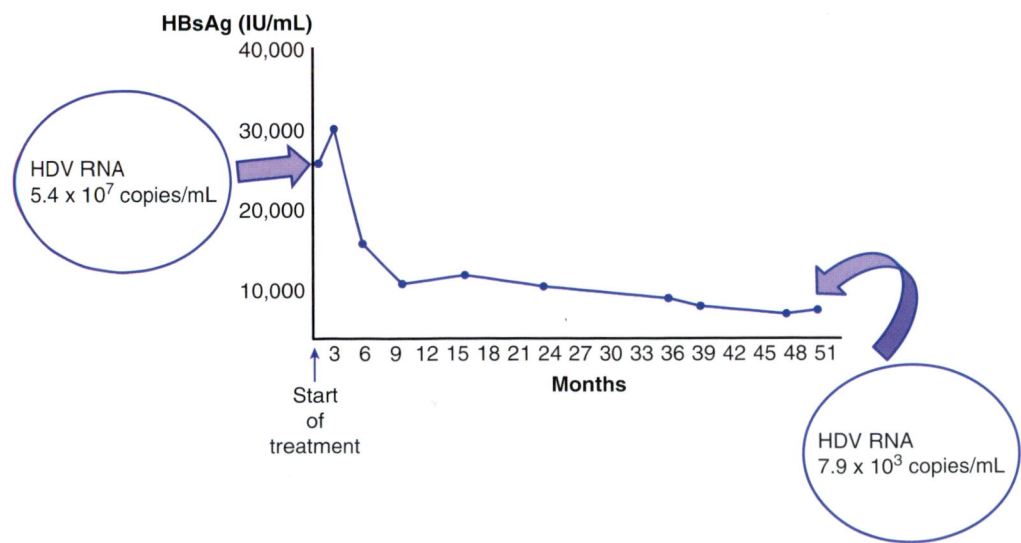

FIGURE 81-4. Time course of hepatitis B surface antigen (HBsAg) concentration during prolonged therapy with peginterferon alfa-2a in a 28-year-old woman with HDV infection. HBsAg concentration was measured by the Elecys II assay (Roche Diagnostics, Penberg, Germany) and HDV RNA by the CDC (Atlanta, Georgia). Note that there is a slow decline in HBsAg concentration and a nearly 4-log decrease in HDV RNA levels. Because of the high rate of relapse with 1 to 2 years of peginterferon alfa-2a therapy, some investigators feel that only eradication of HBsAg will ensure a cure of the HDV infection.

drug alone.[78] The proportion of patients who had sustained HDV RNA clearance at week 72 with peginterferon alfa-2a alone and with combination therapy was similar (26% vs. 31%), whereas none of those treated with adefovir alone achieved HDV RNA clearance[78]; however, combination therapy led to a more marked decrease in HBsAg levels (0.89 $\log_{10}$ IU per mL vs. 0.2 $\log_{10}$ for IFN alone and no change with adefovir alone). Furthermore, HBsAg clearance occurred in 2 patients in the combination treatment arm compared with none in the other 2 groups by week 72.[78] The HIDIT-2 multicenter study compared the efficacy of pegfinterferon alfa-2a plus tenofovir with peginterferon and placebo for 96 weeks to determine whether a longer duration of therapy with a more potent nucleotide analog results in improved efficacy. Unfortunately, sustained virologic response rates (29% and 21%, respectively) were neither statistically different between the two treatment arms nor greater than those reported in the earlier HIDIT trial.[83a]

Novel Drugs

Several therapies are under investigation that target key steps in the HDV life cycle. A class of drugs called *prenylation inhibitors* are the closest to clinical application. Prenylation of the HDAg is critical to virion assembly. Prenylation inhibitors have been developed as anticancer therapies, and several have been shown to have antiviral effects on HDV replication in both in vitro and in vivo study models.[84,85] Importantly, production of HDV genotype 3, which is associated with particularly severe clinical disease, has been shown to be as sensitive to prenylation inhibition in vitro as is the more broadly distributed HDV genotype 1.[81] A phase 2 study of one of these agents (lonafarnib) as a treatment for chronic HDV infection is ongoing at the National Institutes of Health (www.clinicaltrials.gov). If the use of prenylation inhibitors is found to suppress HDV RNA in clinical trials and not associated with serious safety concerns, further trials in combination with IFN therapy are likely to occur.

PREVENTION

Because the ability of HDV to infect a host depends on the preexistence of HBsAg, vaccination against HBV confers protection against HDV. Groups of persons who exhibit a high rate of HDV infection, such as PWID, should be targeted for vaccination. An HDV vaccine would be an important step forward in regions of the world endemic for HBV. Experiments in a woodchuck hepatitis model have demonstrated that HDV infection can be prevented when woodchuck hepatitis virus (WHV) and HDV are inoculated simultaneously in uninfected animals but not in those that are already chronic carriers of the WHV.[86]

KEY REFERENCES

Full references for this chapter can be found on www.expertconsult.com.

5. Rizzetto M, Ciancio A. Epidemiology of hepatitis D. Semin Liver Dis 2012; 32:211-19.
6. Hughes SA, Wedemeyer H, Harrison PM. Hepatitis delta virus. Lancet 2011; 378:73-85.
12. Wedemeyer H, Heidrich B, Manns MP. Hepatitis D virus infection—Not a vanishing disease in Europe! Hepatology 2007; 45:1331-2; author reply 1332-3.
15. Buti M, Homs M, Rodriguez-Frias F, et al. Clinical outcome of acute and chronic hepatitis delta over time: A long-term follow-up study. J Viral Hepat 2011; 18:434-42.
17. Kucirka LM, Farzadegan H, Feld JJ, et al. Prevalence, correlates, and viral dynamics of hepatitis delta among injection drug users. J Infect Dis 2010; 202:845-52.
25. Taylor JM. Hepatitis delta virus. Virology 2006; 344:71-6.
39. Le Gal F, Gault E, Ripault MP, et al. Eighth major clade for hepatitis delta virus. Emerg Infect Dis 2006; 12:1447-50.
50. Pugnale P, Pazienza V, Guilloux K, et al. Hepatitis delta virus inhibits alpha interferon signaling. Hepatology 2009; 49:398-406.
51. Olivero A, Smedile A. Hepatitis delta virus diagnosis. Semin Liver Dis 2012; 32:220-7.
69. Schaper M, Rodriguez-Frias F, Jardi R, et al. Quantitative longitudinal evaluations of hepatitis delta virus RNA and hepatitis B virus DNA shows a dynamic, complex replicative profile in chronic hepatitis B and D. J Hepatol 2010; 52:658-64.
73. Yurdaydin C. Treatment of chronic delta hepatitis. Semin Liver Dis 2012; 32:237-44.
78. Wedemeyer H, Yurdaydin C, Dalekos GN, et al. Peginterferon plus adefovir versus either drug alone for hepatitis delta. N Engl J Med 2011; 364:322-31.
81. Lau DT, Kleiner DE, Park Y, et al. Resolution of chronic delta hepatitis after 12 years of interferon alfa therapy. Gastroenterology 1999; 117:1229-33.
82. Manesis EK, Schina M, Le Gal F, et al. Quantitative analysis of hepatitis D virus RNA and hepatitis B surface antigen serum levels in chronic delta hepatitis improves treatment monitoring. Antivir Ther 2007; 12:381-8.
85. Bordier BB, Ohkanda J, Liu P, et al. In vivo antiviral efficacy of prenylation inhibitors against hepatitis delta virus. J Clin Invest 2003; 112:407-14.

RAKESH AGGARWAL AND KRZYSZTOF KRAWCZYNSKI

Hepatitis E is a form of viral hepatitis caused by HEV. The disease, often acute, self-limited, and associated with icterus, was first recognized in the 1980s, when sera collected during a large epidemic in Delhi, India, in 1955,[1] and during another epidemic in Kashmir, India, in 1978,[2] were found to lack serologic markers of HAV and HBV.[3] In retrospect, it appears that several hepatitis outbreaks that occurred around the world in the 18th and 19th centuries had epidemiologic features resembling those of hepatitis E epidemics.[4] HEV was identified in 1983 by immune electron microscopy,[5] and its genome was cloned and sequenced in early 1990s.[6] HEV infection was initially believed to be limited to humans residing in developing countries; however, the subsequent discovery of HEV-like genomic sequences ("swine HEV") in pig sera[7] and occasional locally acquired human cases caused by HEV genetically related to swine HEV in developed countries[8] indicate a broader host range and geographical distribution than previously thought.

VIROLOGY

HEV, currently placed in the genus Hepevirus in the family Hepeviridae,[9] is a 32- to 34-nm diameter, nonenveloped, icosahedral virion. It has an approximately 7.2-kilobase-long, single- and positive-stranded, polyadenylated RNA genome with 3 open reading frames (ORFs)[10] that encode viral nonstructural proteins, the viral capsid protein, and a protein of unknown function (Fig. 82-1). The capsid protein exhibits a protruding domain that is involved in the binding of HEV to susceptible cells and contains neutralization epitopes.[11] The virus grows poorly in vitro, and the mechanisms of its entry into, replication in, and release from host cells remain uncertain.

Phylogenetic analysis of human HEV isolates reveals 4 geographically distinct genotypes (genotypes 1 to 4; Table 82-1), with divergence in nucleotide sequences exceeding 20% among them.[12] Genotype 1 includes isolates from Asia and Africa, and genotype 2 includes 1 strain from Mexico and some isolates from western Africa; both of these genotypes are restricted to humans and have been associated with waterborne disease outbreaks.

Genotypes 3 and 4 circulate in several animal species, particularly in pigs; HEV genotype 3 causes human disease in Europe, United States, and South America, and HEV genotype 4 causes human disease in China, Taiwan, Japan, and Vietnam. In geographical regions where human cases with HEV genotype 3 or 4 infection are reported, swine isolates of HEV belong to the same genotype. In addition, swine and human HEV strains in these regions often show greater genetic similarity with each other than with swine and human HEV isolates from other parts of the world, suggesting zoonotic transmission to humans.[13] Swine HEV identified in India, a highly endemic area, however, is genetically different from the HEV in patients from the same geographic region.[14] Natural infection of pigs with swine HEV occurs by the fecal-oral route, usually at 2 to 4 months of age, and is associated with transient viremia and no clinical manifestations, although liver biopsy specimens may show mild hepatitis.[7] A similar infection has been detected among deer and wild boars.

HEV-like genomic sequences have also been identified in other mammals, including the rat, mongoose, rabbit, and ferret[13]; however, the potential of these isolates to cause human disease remains unclear. Cows, sheep, and goats show detectable antibodies to HEV (anti-HEV),[13] but isolation of HEV genomic material from these species has not been reported. HEV-like genomic sequences have been recovered from chickens and turkeys[15]; the infectious agents appear to be noninfectious to mammals and are classified as a separate genus ("avian HEV") in the family Hepeviridae.[9] Identification of HEV-like viruses in bats, ferrets, and fish suggests that additional reclassification of HEV-like viruses may be necessary.[16] Despite their considerable genomic heterogeneity, all HEV genotypes show extensive serologic cross-reactivity and belong to a single serotype.

EPIDEMIOLOGY

Two distinct epidemiologic patterns of infection and human disease caused by HEV are observed: (1) genotype 1 or 2 HEV disease in areas of high endemicity and (2) genotype 3 or 4 disease in areas of lower endemicity.

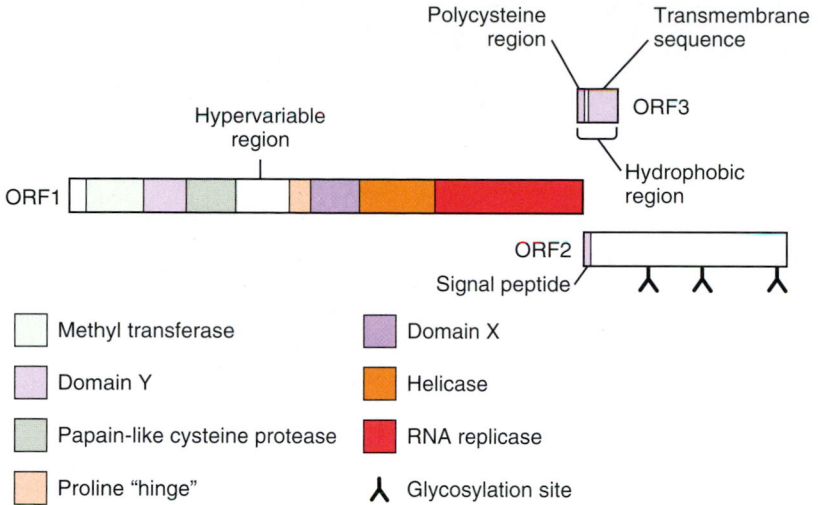

FIGURE 82-1. The genome of HEV. The 3 open reading frames—ORF1, ORF2, ORF3—are shown.

TABLE 82-1 HEV Genotypes and Their Geographic Distribution

Genotype	Human Cases	Animal Cases
1	South, Southeast and Central Asia, Africa	—
2	Mexico, Western Africa	—
3	USA, South America, Europe (France, Spain, UK, the Netherlands), Japan	USA, China, Japan, Southeast Asia, Australia, New Zealand, South America
4	China, Taiwan, Japan, Vietnam	India, China, Taiwan, Japan

BOX 82-1 Features of HEV Genotypes 1 and 2

Acute infection with no evidence of chronicity
Large outbreaks involving up to several thousand persons in developing countries
Frequent sporadic cases
Disease is more common among young adults
Fecal-oral transmission, usually through contaminated water
Highest attack rates are among young adults aged 15 to 40 years, with relative sparing of children
Infrequent person-to-person transmission
No evidence of parenteral or sexual transmission
Greater likelihood of severe disease (liver failure) with high mortality rates (15% to 25%) in pregnant women, especially in the third trimester
Mother-to-newborn (transplacental) transmission is known to occur

Genotypes 1 and 2

In developing countries of Asia (Indian subcontinent, southeast and central Asia), the Middle East, Africa, parts of South America, and Mexico, HEV is highly endemic.[17,18] In these areas, human HEV infection occurs in the form of disease outbreaks[1,2,18-20] and frequent cases of sporadic disease (Fig. 82-2). The outbreaks can be quite large, causing several hundred to several thousand cases, with overall population incidence rates ranging from 1% to 15%, and higher in adults (3% to 30%) than in children (0.2% to 10%) and in men than in women. Characteristically, the rates of disease and mortality are high in pregnant women. The epidemics vary from single-peaked, short-lived outbreaks to prolonged, multipeaked epidemics lasting more than 1 year. In these areas, hepatitis E accounts for up to 50% to 70% of cases of sporadic acute hepatitis; these cases are demographically and clinically similar to those observed during disease outbreaks.

The predominant route of transmission of HEV infection in these areas is fecal-oral. Most reported outbreaks have been related to consumption of fecally contaminated drinking water (Box 82-1), as supported by the results of epidemiologic investigations and demonstration of HEV RNA in waste water, sewage, and drinking water. The outbreaks frequently follow heavy rains and floods, but some are related to decreased flow in rivers during hot summers, with a consequent increase in the risk of water contamination. Genotypes 1 and 2 HEV, the prevalent genotypes in human cases of hepatitis E in these regions, appear not to cause either natural or experimental infection in animals; therefore, the likely source of contamination of water sources is human feces, either from persons with clinical disease or with subclinical HEV infection. The duration of fecal excretion of the virus by clinical cases is usually short. Although data on subclinical HEV genotype 1 infection in humans in endemic regions are scant, viral excretion has been demonstrated during subclinical HEV infection in an experimental macaque model.[21]

Person-to-person transmission of HEV appears uncommon during both epidemic and sporadic settings,[22,23] with secondary attack rates among household contacts of only 0.7% to 2.2%, with some exceptions.[24] Vertical transmission from pregnant mothers to newborn babies is well documented.[25] One study showed evidence of transmission of HEV by blood transfusion,[26] but further data are needed to determine the frequency of transmission by this mode.

Seroprevalence rates in highly endemic areas are generally higher than those in developed countries. In India, the seroprevalence rate increases during young adulthood to about 40%

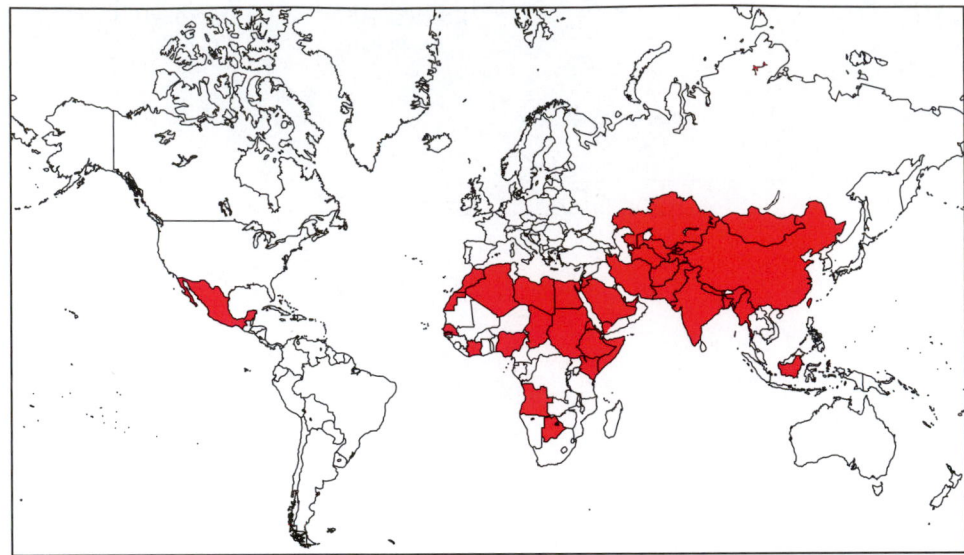

FIGURE 82-2. Geographic distribution of areas where HEV genotype 1 and 2 infection is highly endemic *(red areas)*.

in adults.[27] These rates are lower, however, than those expected from the high frequency of clinical disease and outbreaks and from the nearby universal detection of antibody to HAV by adolescence in the same area. These observations suggest the possibility of a reduction in HEV antibody titers or their disappearance with time. By contrast, in Egypt, anti-HEV is commonly found in children, and the seroprevalence rate of anti-HEV reaches 70% or more in young adults,[28] although epidemics of disease are not known; these findings are poorly understood, although infection with an attenuated or animal strain of HEV or differences in environmental conditions have been proposed as possible explanations.

Genotypes 3 and 4

In Europe, North America, developed countries in Asia (Japan, Taiwan), Australia, and New Zealand, hepatitis E has been reported in the form of case reports and case series and accounts for less than 1% of cases of acute viral hepatitis. A considerable proportion of these infrequent cases are related to travel to HEV-endemic regions, but some cases are caused by autochthonous (locally-acquired) HEV infection.[29] The autochthonous cases in low-endemicity areas have mostly been related to HEV genotype 3, except for a few cases in Japan and Taiwan that were caused by HEV genotype 4.

In a series from the United Kingdom,[29] patients with HEV infection most often presented with features of liver disease such as jaundice, but some patients had an anicteric illness with nonspecific symptoms or asymptomatic serum aminotransferase elevations. The number of cases appeared to peak in the spring and summer, and disease appeared to be more common in residents of coastal and estuarine areas. Case series with similar characteristics have been described from southwest France and the Netherlands.[30,31]

The source and route of infection in autochthonous hepatitis E in areas of low endemicity remain unclear. The available evidence suggests that most such cases are related to zoonotic transmission from pigs (or other animals) by the oral route. Such transmission could occur through consumption of undercooked animal meat, close contact with infected animals, or contamination of water supplies from animal feces. Definite animal-to-human transmission of HEV has been shown to occur in Japan, where hepatitis E developed in members of 2 families after ingestion of uncooked deer meat; the viral

genomic sequences obtained from these cases were similar to those retrieved from leftover meat.[32] Genomic sequences from human cases of hepatitis E in various areas of low endemicity had close molecular similarity to swine isolates of HEV in the same area. HEV genomic sequences have been isolated from pig livers and pig liver sausages in Japan, the United States, and France and have been closely related to those from human cases of hepatitis E in these countries.[33,34] Consumption of raw or undercooked shellfish from HEV-contaminated waters has also been implicated.

Anti-HEV seroprevalence rates in areas where HEV genotype 3 autochthonous hepatitis is diagnosed have varied widely among studies, even within the same country, in part because of differences in the assays used. Reported seroprevalence rates among healthy people of 21% in the United States[35] and 16% in the United Kingdom[29] appear quite high compared with the relatively infrequent occurrence of clinical disease. Subclinical HEV infection with HEV genotype 3 is known to occur[36] and could account in part for this observation; other possibilities include serologic cross-reactivity with other agents, exposure to animal reservoirs of HEV-like viruses, or false-positive serologic results.

Table 82-2 highlights differences in the epidemiologic and clinical features of HEV genotypes 1 and 3 infections.

In China, outbreaks of hepatitis E were common in the past; however, in the 2000s, no outbreaks have been reported and sporadic cases have been caused mainly by HEV genotype 4. These findings appear to represent an epidemiologic transition from a high-endemicity pattern to a low-endemicity pattern.

PATHOGENESIS

Current understanding of virologic, serologic, and pathologic events during acute HEV infection (Fig. 82-3) is based on data from experimentally infected primates, 2 human volunteers, and a few patients. The sequence of events between the ingestion of HEV and its reaching the liver remains unclear. The incubation period ranges from 2 to 10 days. In volunteers, HEV was detected in feces approximately 1 week before the onset of illness. In clinical cases, viremia and fecal shedding of the virus have lasted until about 2 and 4 weeks, respectively, after the onset of illness. In experimentally infected

TABLE 82-2 Comparison of Epidemiologic and Clinical Features Associated with HEV Genotypes 1 and 3

Characteristic	Genotype 1	Genotype 3
Epidemiologic patterns of human disease	Large epidemics, small outbreaks, and frequent sporadic cases	A small proportion of cases with sporadic acute hepatitis
Persons affected	Young, otherwise healthy persons; males > females	Mostly elderly, often with other comorbid conditions; males > females
Animal-to-human transmission	Not reported	Demonstrated; a likely mode of transmission through consumption of undercooked meat or close contact with animals
Water-borne transmission	Well known to occur; most common route	Unknown
Animal reservoir	No	Yes (pigs, wild boars, deer)
Severity	Variable severity, including fulminant hepatic failure; severe disease is particularly more common in pregnant women	Severity and poor outcome are related to comorbid conditions
Chronic infection	Not known to occur after acute infection	Immunosuppressed persons; transplant recipients receiving immunosuppressive drugs

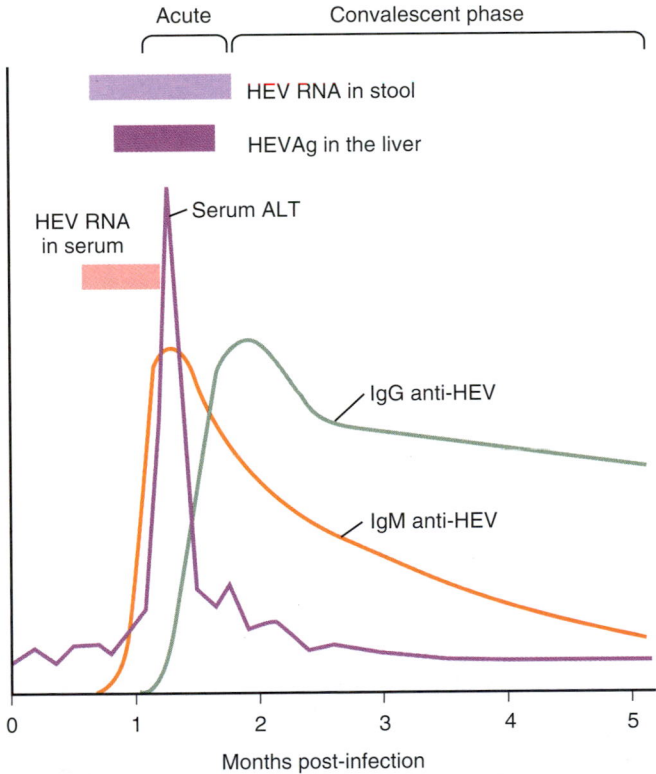

FIGURE 82-3. Typical course of HEV infection (based on studies in human subjects and in experimentally infected primates). anti-HEV, antibody to HEV; Ag, antigen; IgG, immunoglobulin G; IgM, immunoglobulin M.

primates, HEV RNA appears in serum, bile, and feces a few days before the elevation of serum ALT levels. HEV antigen (HEVAg) expression in hepatocytes is seen within 7 days after infection, can involve more than 50% of cells, and declines sharply as serum ALT levels increase.[37] Elevation of serum ALT and appearance of histopathologic changes in the liver generally correspond with the appearance of anti-HEV in serum.

Available evidence suggests that HEV is noncytopathic. This conclusion, along with temporal concordance of the HEV-specific immune response with the onset of liver pathology, suggests that liver injury in hepatitis E is immune mediated, as is the case in hepatitis B and C. Data on cellular immune events during HEV infection are relatively limited. Patients with acute hepatitis E show CD4+ and CD8+ T-cell responses to HEV proteins,[38-41] although the quality and strength of these responses have varied among studies, which used different techniques. In some studies, the responses have been weaker in patients with fulminant hepatitis than in those with nonfulminant disease.[42] Also, the HEV-specific T-cell responses appeared to decline with time. In addition, changes in natural killer cells, natural killer T cells, and regulatory T cells have been reported.[43] Gene expression data from experimentally HEV-infected chimpanzees suggest that the infection may induce an innate immune response and that adaptive immunity seems to be less important for clearance of the virus.[44] Occurrence of chronic HEV infection in immunosuppressed persons suggests a role for T-cell responses in viral clearance.

Histopathologic changes in acute hepatitis E are similar to those of other forms of acute hepatitis and include ballooned hepatocytes, acidophilic bodies, focal parenchymal necrosis, and inflammatory infiltrates in the lobules and expanded portal tracts. Some patients have prominent cholestasis, characterized by canalicular bile stasis and gland-like transformation of parenchymal cells, with less marked hepatocytic changes.[45] Infiltration of liver with CD8+ T cells has been shown.[46] Severe disease is associated with submassive or massive necrosis and collapse of liver parenchyma. Chronic HEV genotype 3 viremia is associated with evidence of prolonged liver inflammation and injury and can progress to chronic hepatitis and cirrhosis over time.[47]

The reason for severe liver damage during pregnancy, especially during the third trimester, remains unknown, although immune and hormonal factors have been suspected to play a role. These factors have included a bias in helper T cell type 1/type 2 (Th1/Th2) cytokine balance in favor of Th2 cytokines,[48] suppression of nuclear factor kappa B p65 in both peripheral blood mononuclear cells and liver tissue from such patients,[49] a higher viral load,[50] a higher ratio of interleukin (IL)-12 to IL-10,[50] and a reduced expression of progesterone receptors and progesterone-induced blocking factor.[50]

The pathogenesis and course of disease may differ among HEV genotypes. HEV genotype 1 or 2 infection during pregnancy is associated with a greater frequency of severe disease. Chronic infection has been observed only with HEV genotype 3.

CLINICAL FEATURES

Acute Hepatitis E

The most common recognizable form of HEV genotype 1 and 2 infection is acute icteric hepatitis, with clinical features (Box 82-2) resembling acute hepatitis A or B (see Chapters 78 and 79).[51] The illness begins insidiously with a prodromal phase with varying combinations of flu-like symptoms, fever, chills, abdominal pain, anorexia, aversion to smoking, vomiting, clay-colored stools, dark urine, diarrhea, arthralgias, and a transient macular skin rash. These prodromal symptoms are replaced in 1 to 7 days with jaundice, dark urine, light stool color, and itching, which last up to a few weeks. Physical examination reveals jaundice, a mildly enlarged, soft, and slightly tender liver, and at times splenomegaly. Laboratory test abnormalities include bilirubinuria, conjugated hyperbilirubinemia, and marked elevations in serum levels of ALT, AST, and GGTP. Serum ALT elevations may precede symptoms, and the magnitude of the elevation does not correlate with the severity of liver injury. Mild leukopenia and relative lymphocytosis may occur. US may show a mildly enlarged liver, increase in hepatic parenchymal echogenicity, gallbladder wall edema, prominence of portal venules, and a slightly enlarged spleen; its main purpose is exclusion of biliary obstruction as the cause of jaundice.

Acute hepatitis E is usually self-limited. A few patients have a prolonged course with marked cholestasis (cholestatic hepatitis), including persistent jaundice lasting 2 to 6 months, prominent itching, and marked elevation of the serum alkaline phosphatase level, ultimately with spontaneous resolution. Case-fatality rates in highly endemic areas have ranged from 0.5% to 4% in hospital-based data and 0.07% to 0.6% in population surveys during outbreaks.[18]

Some HEV-infected persons have only nonspecific symptoms resembling those of an acute viral febrile illness with serum aminotransferase elevations but without jaundice (anicteric hepatitis), and some remain entirely asymptomatic; these forms appear to be more common in children. Anicteric and asymptomatic infections may occur more frequently than icteric disease, because a large proportion of HEV-seropositive persons in endemic areas do not recall ever having had jaundice. In a small proportion of patients, the disease is severe and associated with subacute or fulminant hepatic failure.

Pregnant women, particularly those in the second or third trimester, are affected more frequently during hepatitis E outbreaks than are others in the population and have a worse outcome, with mortality rates of 5% to 25%. In an epidemic in Kashmir, India, clinical hepatitis E developed in 17.3% of pregnant women (8.8%, 19.4%, and 18.6% of those in trimesters 1, 2, and 3, respectively), compared with 2.1% of nonpregnant women and 2.8% of men of similar age.[52] Fulminant hepatic failure developed in approximately 22% of the affected pregnant women, with an increased frequency of abortions, stillbirths, and neonatal deaths.

In geographic areas where HEV genotype 3 infection is observed, the manifestations are generally similar, except that the patients are generally older and more likely to have history of alcohol use and other coexisting illnesses.[8,30,31] Both in Europe and the United States, retrospective serologic testing has identified cases of hepatitis E among patients who had originally been diagnosed as having drug-induced hepatitis.[53] Intriguing reports of a wide variety of neurologic manifestations among persons with HEV genotype 3 infection have been described[54]; such manifestations are even less frequent in areas where HEV genotype 1 predominates.

Chronic Hepatitis E

Chronic infection with HEV, with persistent viremia and fecal excretion lasting for several months to years, can occur[55]; all the cases have been reported from areas of low endemicity and have been associated with HEV genotype 3 infection. Such persistent infection is limited to immunosuppressed patients, including organ-transplant recipients, those receiving cancer chemotherapy, and HIV-infected persons. These patients may have clinical symptoms of liver disease, often high serum ALT and AST levels, and evidence of continuing inflammation in liver tissue. Over time, progressive liver damage and fibrosis may lead to development of cirrhosis,[47] although data are inadequate to determine the frequency of this complication.

The predominant route of acquisition of infection in such cases appears to be similar to those for autochthonous cases in areas of low endemicity. Transmission via the grafted organ and blood transfusion has been considered but appears unlikely.

DIAGNOSIS

The diagnosis of human HEV infection is based either on detection of HEV RNA in stool and serum specimens using a reverse transcription-PCR assay or on demonstration of a virus-specific host immune response (see Fig. 82-3).[56] Detection of HEV RNA relies solely on in-house tests, because no commercial assay is available yet. Enzyme immunoassays (EIAs) for the detection of immunoglobulin (Ig)M and IgG antibodies to HEV have been developed using recombinant HEV proteins expressed in *Escherichia coli* or insect cells, synthetic peptides corresponding to immunogenic epitopes of HEV, and protein expressed from a synthetic gene encoding multiple linear antigenic epitopes from the ORF2 and ORF3 regions.[57-59]

The presence in serum of IgM anti-HEV strongly suggests acute infection, whereas detection of IgG anti-HEV indicates the convalescent phase or past infection. IgM anti-HEV appears in the early phase of clinical illness, lasts 4 to 5 months, and can be detected in 80% to 100% of cases during outbreaks of hepatitis E. IgG anti-HEV appears a few days after IgM

BOX 82-2 Clinical Features of Acute Hepatitis E

Incubation period of 2 to 10 weeks
Varying clinical manifestations:
    Anicteric hepatitis
    Icteric hepatitis
    Severe hepatitis leading to fulminant hepatic failure
    Inapparent, asymptomatic infection
Clinical illness similar to that with other types of acute viral hepatitis (except among pregnant women)
Milder illness in children
Low mortality rate (0.07% to 0.6%) (except in pregnant women; see Table 82-2)

anti-HEV and remains detectable for at least one to several years; the exact duration of its persistence is not known.

Although several commercial kits for the detection of IgM and IgG anti-HEV are available in various countries, none is currently licensed for clinical use in the United States. Use of different target antigens from different HEV strains produced using different expression systems makes the results of various tests noncomparable; in one study, the sensitivities of 6 IgM anti-HEV assays varied from 72% to 98%, and the specificities varied from 78% to 96%.[60] Efforts are in progress to identify a test that can be validated against a panel of well-characterized sera from around the world.

TREATMENT AND PREVENTION

Acute hepatitis E is usually self-limited, and only supportive care is needed. Patients with acute or acute-on-chronic liver failure need admission to an ICU, measures to control cerebral edema, and consideration for liver transplantation (see Chapter 95). In pregnant women, a benefit to the termination of pregnancy has not been proved; postpartum hemorrhage resulting from deranged coagulation requires treatment with fresh-frozen plasma.

In chronic HEV infection, withdrawal or reduction in dose of immunosuppressive drugs leads to disappearance of HEV viremia in about one third of patients. In small case series of patients with chronic hepatitis E, treatment with either ribavirin or pegylated interferon α-2a or 2b for 3 to 12 months has shown moderate success in achieving virologic response (no detectable HEV RNA in serum 3 to 6 months after treatment is stopped)[61,62]; results of controlled trials are not available.

Prevention of hepatitis E in endemic areas depends primarily on the supply of clean drinking water and strict attention to sewage disposal. In an epidemic setting, measures to improve the quality of water—as simple as boiling water—have led to a rapid decline in the number of new cases. Use of immune globulin manufactured in endemic areas for pre- or postexposure prophylaxis has not been associated with a significant reduction in disease incidence. In areas of low endemicity, zoonotic transmission can be avoided through emphasis on thorough cooking of pork and avoidance of undercooked meats; these measures may be particularly important for immunosuppressed persons.

Experimental studies in HEV-susceptible primates using various candidate vaccines containing different recombinant HEV capsid proteins have shown evidence of protection against hepatitis and viremia, although viral excretion was not prevented.[63] Two of these vaccines have undergone human trials. An experimental HEV DNA vaccine has also shown promising results in cynomolgus macaques.[64]

The first vaccine to undergo efficacy trials in humans contained a recombinant truncated HEV capsid protein produced in insect cells as virus-like particles (VLPs) and aluminum hydroxide as an adjuvant. In a phase 2, double-blind, randomized placebo-controlled safety and efficacy trial, nearly 2000 young adults (>99% male) in Nepal[65] were randomly assigned to receive 3 doses of either this vaccine or a matched placebo (at 0, 1, and 6 months) and were actively followed for 2 years. The vaccine showed 95.5% protective efficacy against clinical acute hepatitis E after 3 doses. All vaccinated subjects had a high IgG anti-HEV level at 1 month after the third vaccine dose, but the proportion declined to 56% by the end of follow-up.

The second vaccine consists of a 239–amino acid–long truncated ORF2 protein, which has been expressed in E. coli

and forms 23-nm VLPs. In a large population-based trial in southern China with more than 110,000 volunteers, administration of 3 doses showed a protective efficacy against clinical acute hepatitis E of 100% during a 13-month follow-up period.[66] This vaccine has recently been approved for marketing in China.

HEV vaccines are likely to be useful for travelers to regions where hepatitis E is highly endemic and for pregnant women and persons with chronic liver disease who reside in such regions. Further data on the efficacy and safety of these vaccines among high-risk groups (pregnant women, patients with chronic liver disease, and immunosuppressed persons), efficacy in the postexposure setting and against HEV genotype 3 disease, duration of protective efficacy, and effect on subclinical HEV infection and fecal shedding of the virus are needed before their widespread use can be recommended.

KEY REFERENCES

Full references for this chapter can be found on www.expertconsult.com.

1. Vishwanathan R. Infectious hepatitis in Delhi (1955-56): A critical study: Epidemiology. Indian J Med Res 1957; 45:1-29.
2. Khuroo M. Study of an epidemic of non-A, non-B hepatitis: Possibility of another human hepatitis virus distinct from post-transfusion non-A, non-B type. Am J Med 1980; 68:818-23.
7. Meng XJ, Purcell R, Halbur P, et al. A novel virus in swine is closely related to the human hepatitis E virus. Proc Natl Acad Sci U S A 1997; 94:9860-5.
8. Dalton HR, Bendall R, Ijaz S, et al. Hepatitis E: An emerging infection in developed countries. Lancet Infect Dis 2008; 8:698-709.
12. Lu L, Li C, Hagedorn CH. Phylogenetic analysis of global hepatitis E virus sequences: Genetic diversity, subtypes and zoonosis. Rev Med Virol 2006; 16:5-36.
13. Meng XJ. From barnyard to food table: The omnipresence of hepatitis E virus and risk for zoonotic infection and food safety. Virus Res 2011; 161:23-30.
18. Aggarwal R, Naik S. Epidemiology of hepatitis E: Current status. J Gastroenterol Hepatol 2009; 24:1484-93.
29. Dalton H, Stableforth W, Thurairajah P, et al. Autochthonous hepatitis E in Southwest England: Natural history, complications and seasonal variation, and hepatitis E virus IgG seroprevalence in blood donors, the elderly and patients with chronic liver disease. Eur J Gastroenterol Hepatol 2008; 20:784-90.
52. Khuroo M, Teli M, Skidmore S, et al. Incidence and severity of viral hepatitis in pregnancy. Am J Med 1981; 70:252-5.
55. Kamar N, Garrouste C, Haagsma EB, et al. Factors associated with chronic hepatitis in patients with hepatitis E virus infection who have received solid organ transplants. Gastroenterology 2011; 140:1481-9.
56. Aggarwal R. Diagnosis of hepatitis E. Nat Rev Gastroenterol Hepatol 2013; 10:24-33.
65. Shrestha M, Scott R, Joshi D, et al. Safety and efficacy of a recombinant hepatitis E vaccine. N Engl J Med 2007; 356:895-903.
66. Zhu FC, Zhang J, Zhang XF, et al. Efficacy and safety of a recombinant hepatitis E vaccine in healthy adults: A large-scale, randomised, double-blind placebo-controlled, phase 3 trial. Lancet 2010; 376:895-902.

CHAPTER OUTLINE

A number of viruses may be hepatotropic in that viremia is occasionally associated with elevations in serum aminotransferase levels and viral replication may occur in hepatocytes, but little, if any, liver disease ensues. Such viruses include hepatitis G virus (HGV) and the GB agents, TT virus (TTV), Sanban virus, Yonban virus, SEN virus, and TTV-like minivirus. Other novel agents such as the NV-F virus-like agent, which may exacerbate the severity of chronic hepatitis C, have been reported, but little is known about them.

Other viral diseases may sometimes involve the liver as part of a systemic infection. The agents of such infections include HIV (see Chapter 34), EBV, cytomegalovirus (CMV), HSV, varicella-zoster virus (VZV), the virus that causes severe acute respiratory syndrome (SARS), parvovirus B19, and human herpesvirus 6 (HHV-6). Infection with any of these viruses may rarely lead to severe, sometimes fatal, liver disease.

HEPATITIS G AND GB AGENT INFECTION

During the long search for the cause of transfusion-associated non-A, non-B hepatitis (see Chapter 80), the GB agent (GBV) and HGV were discovered and later shown to be 2 isolates of the same virus. A 35-year-old surgeon with the initials GB developed an acute icteric hepatitis. When his serum was serially inoculated into healthy marmosets, they too developed hepatitis. Analysis of the marmosets infected with derivations of the GB serum led to the identification of 2 distinct viruses, labeled *GBV-type A (GBV-A)* and *GBV-type B (GBV-B)*.[1] A third virus closely related to the GB agents was subsequently identified by the same investigators from a human sample and was classified as *GBV-C*.[2] At approximately the same time, another group independently identified a virus from the serum of a patient with cryptogenic non-A-to-E hepatitis, which they named *HGV*.[3] Subsequent studies revealed 96% homology between the genomes of HGV and GBV-C, indicating that they were actually 2 strains of the same virus.[4] Because large epidemiologic studies have not demonstrated any association between infection with GBV-C/HGV and acute or chronic hepatitis, the use of the term "hepatitis G virus" has been questioned. In fact, even the index patient ("GB") was subsequently shown to be infected with HCV as the cause of his liver disease. For clarity, GBV-C/HGV will be referred to as *GBV-C*.

Virology

GBV-C is a positive-strand RNA virus with a genome of 9400 nucleotides encoding approximately 2900 amino acids and is classified as a member of the Flaviviridae family. There has been a proposal to establish a new genus, *Pegivirus* (pe for persistent, G for G or GB), to include GBV-A, GBV-C, and the bat virus GBV-D, within the Flaviviridae family.[5,6] GBV-B would be included with HCV in the *Hepacivirus* genus. GBV-C shares 44% and 28% nucleotide homology with GBV-A and GBV-B, respectively, and has 5 known genotypes with distinct global geographic distributions.[4] Although similar in many respects to HCV, GBV-C shares only 27% nucleotide homology with HCV, and the 2 viruses are clearly distinct.

The GBV-C genome is organized like that of HCV. One long open reading frame encodes a single large polyprotein with structural proteins encoded at the 5' aminoterminus and nonstructural proteins encoded at the 3' carboxyterminus. A nontranslated region at the 5' end serves as an internal ribosomal entry site (IRES), allowing translation of the uncapped messenger RNA.[7]

The structural proteins differ between HCV and GBV-C. Two glycoproteins—E1 and E2—predicted to compose the GBV-C viral envelope are cleaved from the polyprotein, likely by a host cell signal peptidase. Whereas HCV E1 and E2 have 5 and 11 N-linked glycosylation sites, GBV-C E1 and E2 have only 1 and 3 such sites, respectively.[8] Perhaps of greater importance, amino acid polymorphisms do not cluster in the

*Acknowledgment: E. Jenny Heathcote, MD, contributed to this chapter in previous editions of the textbook.

hypervariable region of GBC-C E2, as they do in HCV E2. The hypervariable region of HCV E2 is thought to account in part for the ability of HCV to evade immune attack and cause persistent infection. This difference in E2 polymorphisms may account for the 60% to 75% rate of chronic HCV infection, compared with only 25% in GBV-C infection.

The GBV-C genome does not encode a core protein, but biophysical and electron microscopic studies suggest that the virus does have a nucleocapsid structure, presumably with a core protein.[9] Some GBV-C-infected patients have antibodies that react with a synthetic peptide that corresponds to the region immediately proximal to the E1 coding region, suggesting that GBV-C may have a truncated core protein at the amino terminus of the genome.

In contrast to the structural differences, the GBV-C non-structural proteins—designated NS1, NS2, and so on—are similar to those of HCV, including a zinc-dependent thiol protease that cleaves NS2 from NS3, a serine protease at the amino terminus of NS3 that probably cleaves all downstream proteolytic sites, and an RNA helicase (as in all positive-strand RNA viruses) that is also found in NS3 downstream from the protease region. NS4A likely serves as a cofactor for the NS3 protease. The NS5A protein is believed to interact with double-strand RNA protein kinase, and NS5B serves as the RNA-dependent RNA polymerase.[10]

Another important difference between GBV-C and HCV may be tissue tropism. Negative-strand RNA (indicating the presence of active viral replication) has been demonstrated in liver tissue during HCV infection, implying hepatotropism, but has not been clearly demonstrated during GBV-C infection. Negative-strand RNA, however, has been demonstrated in peripheral blood mononuclear cells (PBMCs), bone marrow, and spleens of patients with GBV-C infection, suggesting that GBV-C is a lymphotropic virus.[11] The demonstration of replication of a GBV-C clone in CD4+ T cells confirms that GBV-C is able to replicate in lymphocytes and may help explain the interaction between GBV-C and HIV infection (see later).

GBV-C can be grown in cell culture and has been proposed as a model for studying HCV. Persistent GBV-C infection has been achieved in marmosets, which provide a small animal model of HCV infection in which antiviral agents can be studied.[12] GBV-B has been proposed as a better model for HCV infection than GBV-C because GBV-B causes acute and rarely chronic hepatitis in tamarins and marmosets.[13] Therefore, although the GB viruses do not cause overt human liver disease, they may be useful tools to study HCV infection.

Epidemiology

GBV-C is found worldwide. At least 5 genotypes have been identified, each with a specific geographic distribution: genotype 1 predominates in West Africa, genotype 2 in Europe and the United States, genotype 3 in parts of Asia, genotype 4 in Southeast Asia, and genotype 5 in South Africa.[14]

The development of GBV-C E2 antibodies correlates with loss of GBV-C viremia and suggests past exposure and clearance of GBV-C infection.[15] Evidence of current and past GBV-C infection is found frequently in persons with parenteral risk factors and also is common among volunteer blood donors. Between 14% and 38% of persons with frequent exposures to blood are viremic with GBV-C, whereas 50% to 70% of such persons are seropositive for E2 antibodies.[16] Up to 16% of healthy blood donors are positive for E2 antibodies, with much lower rates of active viremia.[17] Past or current GBV-C viremia is found as often in blood donors with a normal serum ALT level as in donors rejected because of an elevated serum ALT level.[18] Consequently, GBV-C transmission is not

prevented by exclusion of donors with a normal ALT value. GBV-C also has been shown to be transmitted sexually and vertically much more frequently than HCV, and the risk may vary with the GBV-C genotype.[19] No evidence exists for hepatitis or other clinical sequelae in infected babies.[20] Because both GBV-C and HCV are transmitted parenterally, GBV-C–HCV coinfection is common. GBV-C viremia is present in about 20% of HCV-infected persons, and 80% of the remaining subjects are seropositive for antibodies to E2.[10] These findings suggest that the rate of natural clearance of GBV-C is higher (≈75%) than that for HCV (≈25%).

Clinical Features

Although GBV-C is detected in many patients with non-A-to-E acute and chronic hepatitis and may persist for years, it does not appear to cause liver (or any other) disease, even in immunocompromised persons.[18,21-23] In fact, patients with HCV-HIV coinfection with GBV-C viremia have been reported to have reduced hepatic fibrosis and inflammation compared with GBV-C–negative cohorts, possibly through inhibition of T-cell activation by the virus.[24] Nor does GBV-C appear to negatively affect the response to treatment of chronic HCV or hepatitis B virus (HBV) infection,[23] with 1 study reporting higher rates of sustained virologic response in HCV-infected patients coinfected with GBV-C treated with peginterferon-based therapy.[25] GBV-C infection does not affect the outcome of liver transplantation, even though liver transplant recipients have high rates of GBV-C viremia, probably because of their high transfusion requirements.[26]

The duration of GBV-C infection may depend on the immune status and age of the host. As with HBV infection, childhood acquisition of GBV-C appears to lead to chronic infection, whereas sexual transmission in immunocompetent adults typically leads to rapid clearance of viremia.[27] Chronic GBV-C infection also is more likely to develop in HIV-infected persons than in non–HIV-infected persons.[28] In contrast to HCV infection, the development of antibodies to GBV-C E2 seems to protect against reinfection.[29] No associations between GBV-C and hepatocellular carcinoma,[30] non-Hodgkin's lymphoma,[31] aplastic anemia, or lichen planus[32] have been documented.

Diagnosis

Because GBV-C rarely causes disease in humans, diagnostic tests are not widely available and generally are reserved for research purposes. GBV-C RNA can be detected by using PCR methodology with commercially available primers. A test for GBV-C antibody, to document past infection, is also available.

GB Virus Type C and HIV

Once GBV-C was shown not to cause liver disease, interest in this virus diminished. In 1998, however, 2 independent groups of investigators observed that among a small number of HIV-infected persons, lower HIV viral loads as well as slower progression to AIDS and death correlated with the presence of GBV-C viremia (Fig. 83-1).[29,33] Subsequently, larger studies have confirmed this finding in varied populations and have suggested that HIV–GBV-C–coinfected persons have a better prognosis than HIV-monoinfected persons.[33-37] In addition, coinfected persons respond better to antiretroviral therapy, with a more rapid increase in CD4 counts and suppression of HIV viral load.[37,38] Children infected with GBV-C at birth also have a reduced risk of contracting HIV via vertical transmission, independent of the mother's GBV-C status.[39,40] Notably,

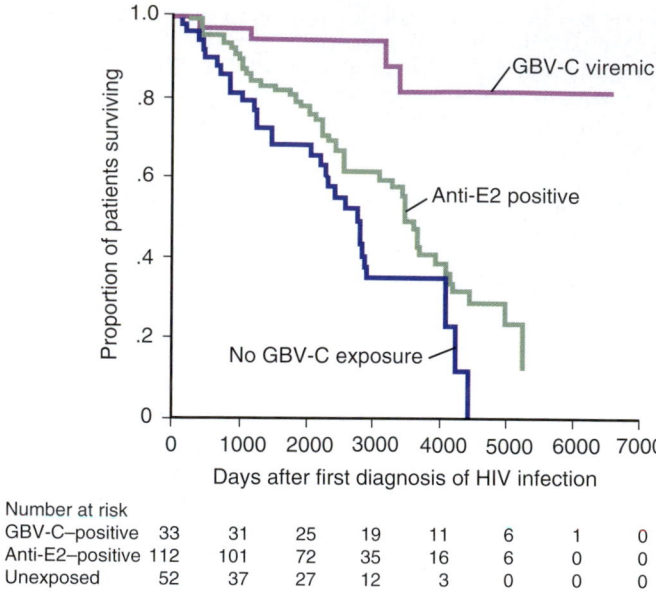

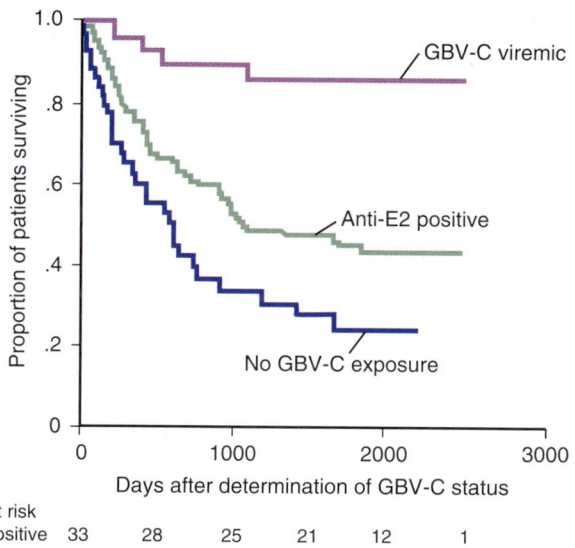

Number at risk

GBV-C–positive	33	31	25	19	11	6	1	0
Anti-E2–positive	112	101	72	35	16	6	0	0
Unexposed	52	37	27	12	3	0	0	0

Number at risk

GBV-C–positive	33	28	25	21	12	1
Anti-E2–positive	112	65	44	38	24	0
Unexposed	52	21	11	9	4	0

FIGURE 83-1. Survival according to GBV-C status in patients with HIV infection. Survival from the time of diagnosis of HIV infection (A) and survival from the time the blood sample was drawn to determine the GBV-C status (B) are shown in relation to the GBV-C status. For both measures, the patients who were sero-positive for GBV-C RNA had significantly better survival. Anti-E2, antibody to E2 glycoprotein. (From Tillmann HL, Heiken H, Knapik-Botor A, et al. Infection with GB virus C and reduced mortality among HIV-infected patients. N Engl J Med 2001; 345:715-24.)

a study of blood transfusion recipients showed that HIV-infected persons who contracted GBV-C infection had improved survival, thereby suggesting a possible role for GBV-C infection as a therapeutic intervention.[41] Some studies, however, have not confirmed a protective effect of GBV-C infection in HIV-infected persons.[42-46] The discrepant results

may relate to differences in the HIV-inhibitory effect of different GBV-C genotypes and the duration of GBV-C infection[47]: the longer the duration of GBV-C infection, the greater the benefit on HIV progression.[36] The viral interaction may work in both directions. In a longitudinal study of coinfected persons, GBV-C viral titers increased during effective HAART and fell with interruptions in HAART, suggesting that HIV may also inhibit GBV-C.[48] Although GBV-C does not affect the outcome of HCV monoinfection, a study of the effect of GBV-C infection on the progression of liver disease in HIV-HCV coinfected persons found that patients with current or past GBV-C infection had a lower risk of cirrhosis and hepatic complications but no difference in survival compared with patients without GBV-C infection.[49]

Why HIV–GBV-C coinfected persons have an improved response to HAART is unknown. HIV replication is diminished in PBMCs that are infected with both HIV and GBV-C, and a higher inoculum of HIV is required to infect cells already infected with GBV-C. The NS5A protein of GBV-C has been shown to down-regulate the expression of the HIV co-receptor CXCR4, and the E2 protein of GBV-C interferes with early steps in the HIV life cycle, including viral entry and replication.[50-53] An understanding of the interaction may lead to identification of novel therapeutic targets for HIV, and some investigators have even proposed active GBV-C infection as an anti-HIV strategy.[54,55] In addition to virologic inhibition, immune mechanisms, including GBV-C-induced stimulation of HIV-inhibitory cytokines, endogenous interferon production, and reduced T-cell activation, have been proposed.[56-59]

Treatment

Because GBV-C infection is not associated with clinical liver disease, no treatments have targeted GBV-C specifically. In HIV–HCV–GBV-C coinfected persons, peginterferon and ribavirin treatment led to sustained GBV-C clearance in 31% of patients, with no observable subsequent effect on the course of HCV or HIV infection.[60] In patients coinfected with GBV-C and HCV who were treated with interferon and ribavirin, GBV-C RNA disappeared from serum during therapy but reappeared in all patients following discontinuation of therapy.[61] Importantly, no effect of GBV-C infection was observed on the response to treatment of HCV infection.[62]

TT VIRUS INFECTION

TTV was first identified in 1977, by the use of representational difference analysis in a patient (with the initials TT) in Japan who had acute post-transfusion non-A-to-G hepatitis.[63] TTV is also referred to as the transfusion-transmitted and Torque-Teno virus.

Virology

TTV is a non-enveloped, single-stranded, negative-polarity, circular DNA virus. It is closely related to a family of animal viruses known as Circoviridae, which have not been associated with human disease. TTV is the first human single-stranded circular DNA virus to be identified and does not fit precisely into any known virus family. Other TTV-like viruses were subsequently discovered and together make up the human Anellovirus family.

The TTV genome is 3965 nucleotides long and contains at least 3 overlapping open reading frames. Three messenger

RNAs (mRNAs) are expressed by TTV; each mRNA is translated from 2 start codons, leading to the production of 6 viral proteins. One protein product of the largest mRNA (3.0 kb) functions as the capsid protein and also serves as a replicase enzyme. The product of the second open reading frame interferes with host nuclear factor kappa B signaling, but its role in viral replication is unknown.[64] TTV displays remarkable genomic sequence diversity, even among isolates found in an individual patient.[65] At least 23 genotypes have been identified, with greater than 30% sequence divergence among isolates. Some genotypes differ in sequence by greater than 50%, and genotype prevalence rates vary geographically.[66]

TTV is believed to be hepatotropic on the basis of the observation that viral levels are higher in the liver than in the serum of infected patients. TTV has also been identified within hepatocytes, and shown to replicate, by in situ hybridization and PCR; however, no or only minor morphologic changes have been seen in cells with positive hybridization signals.[67] TTV has also been shown to replicate in stimulated PBMCs and bone marrow cells.[68]

Epidemiology

TTV is found worldwide and is common. Initial studies documented infection in 1% to 40% of healthy blood donors.[69] As more inclusive primers have been used to detect differing genotypes, the reported prevalence among blood donors has increased dramatically, approaching 100% in some studies.[70] The prevalence of TTV infection increases with age but appears to reach a plateau by early childhood.[71] TTV is also found in a variety of nonhuman primate species.

TTV is transmitted effectively by all parenteral routes; high prevalence rates have been documented in hemophiliacs, people who inject drugs, patients on hemodialysis, and organ transplant recipients.[72] TTV has also been shown to be transmitted enterically, and high TTV DNA titers are present in the feces of viremic patients. Fecal-oral spread may account for the high prevalence in low-risk, healthy blood donor populations.[70]

Clinical Features

Although TTV was associated with acute hepatitis in the patient in whom it was first identified, other studies have not supported a causal association between TTV and liver disease.[73,74] In the original study,[63] viremia was detected 6 weeks after exposure and 2 weeks before a rise in serum ALT levels. The viral DNA was cleared from serum, as documented by PCR testing, and serum ALT levels subsequently returned to normal. Viremia may persist for years in both immunocompetent and immunosuppressed persons. Most infected persons have no biochemical or histologic evidence of liver disease.[73,75] Like GBV-C, TTV does not appear to alter the natural history or response to treatment of either chronic HCV or HBV infection.[76,77] A report that TTV infection may increase the risk of hepatocellular carcinoma in patients with chronic HCV infection remains to be confirmed.[78]

Treatment

Formal studies of treatment of TTV infection have not been performed. A small study of HCV-TTV-coinfected patients showed that TTV infection had no effect on sustained virologic response of HCV to therapy with peginterferon and ribavirin. Although TTV viremia cleared after therapy in 6 of 10 patients, 4 of the 6 relapsed within 6 months.[79]

SANBAN, YONBAN, AND SEN VIRUS AND TTV-LIKE MINIVIRUS INFECTIONS

Since the discovery of TTV in 1997,[63] several similar viruses with a small DNA genome have been isolated in Japan and named *Sanban, Yonban,* and *TTV-like minivirus (TLMV)*. These viruses have been divided into 29 genotypes, with sequence divergence of greater than 30%.[80] Like TTV, they are readily transmitted parenterally and can also be passed by the fecal-oral route. None has been clearly associated with human liver disease to date.

In 1999, a novel virus was identified in an HIV-positive person (with the initials SEN) who had post-transfusion hepatitis of unknown etiology. This virus was found with the use of degenerative primers from the prototype TTV. The SEN virus is a small, nonenveloped, single-stranded DNA virus, but unlike that of TTV, the SEN genome is linear. Nucleotide sequencing has shown 50% homology with the prototype TTV, but only 30% of amino acids are homologous. Sequencing of multiple isolates has demonstrated sequence divergence of 15% to 50%.[81]

Like TTV, SEN virus is transmitted both parenterally and by the fecal-oral route.[82] Vertical transmission occurs but in most cases does not lead to chronic infection. Natural clearance of both perinatally and parenterally acquired SEN virus does not appear to protect against reinfection.[83] The prevalence varies markedly and is highest among patients with parenteral risk factors, particularly those coinfected with HCV.[84] The prevalence among healthy blood donors is approximately 2% in the United States and 10% in Japan.[85]

The clinical significance of SEN infection remains controversial. One study of patients with post-transfusion non-A-to-E hepatitis suggested that SEN was the cause in a majority (11 of 12) of cases. SEN viremia persisted for more than 1 year in 45% of those infected; however, clinical hepatitis did not develop in a majority (86%) of transfused patients who acquired SEN infection. None of the patients with hepatitis had a fulminant course, nor did chronic liver disease or cirrhosis develop during follow-up.[86] Other reports and case series have identified SEN or TTV viremia in patients with both fulminant and chronic hepatitis or hepatocellular carcinoma, but causation has been difficult to establish.[87] Most studies have shown neither an association between SEN or any of the other viruses in this group and human disease, nor an effect of these viruses on the course or response to treatment for chronic viral hepatitis.[82,88]

SYSTEMIC VIRAL INFECTIONS THAT MAY INVOLVE THE LIVER

EBV

EBV infection is common and covers a wide spectrum of clinical presentations. Most infants and children are either asymptomatic or have mild, nonspecific complaints, whereas adolescents and adults typically present with the triad of pharyngitis, fever, and lymphadenopathy.[89] Although usually subclinical, liver involvement is nearly universal in patients with EBV mononucleosis and ranges from serum aminotransferase elevations to rare cases of fulminant and even fatal hepatitis.[90]

Up to 90% of patients with acute mononucleosis have serum aminotransferase and lactate dehydrogenase elevations 2 to 3 times the upper limit of normal. The enzyme levels typically rise over a 1- to 2-week period, and peak levels are usually less than 5-fold the upper limit of normal, much lower than those normally seen in patients with acute hepatitis A, B, D, or E.[91] Elevated levels of alkaline phosphatase are common, and mild hyperbilirubinemia is observed in as many as 45% of cases.[91,92] In most patients, liver biochemical test levels normalize within 1 month, often before complete resolution of clinical symptoms.[93] As with infectious mononucleosis, EBV hepatitis tends to be more severe in adults older than age 30 than in younger adults and children.[94] Elderly patients occasionally present with jaundice, fever, and right upper quadrant pain that may be confused with extrahepatic biliary obstruction.[95] Although jaundice may be caused by viral-induced cholestasis, autoimmune hemolytic anemia should be excluded in hyperbilirubinemic patients. Cholestatic jaundice with pruritus may be observed in young women with EBV infection who continue taking oral contraceptive pills.

Fatal, fulminant EBV hepatitis has been described in both immunocompetent and immunocompromised persons and appears to be associated with a greater than usual EBV viral burden, particularly in T cells as opposed to B cells.[96] A small minority of patients develops a chronic active form of EBV infection at the time of initial infection, which resembles infectious mononucleosis, with involvement of liver, lungs, and other organs, and which does not resolve and may be life-threatening. High levels of EBV DNA are found in the blood, with associated fever, hepatitis, and lymphadenopathy.[97] Treatment with immunosuppressive agents may induce remission, but only stem cell transplantation has been reported to be curative.[97] In addition to chronic active EBV, a hemophagocytic syndrome characterized by fever, hepatosplenomegaly, hepatic synthetic dysfunction, cytopenias, and marked hyperferritinemia (>10,000 µg/L) may develop in patients with EBV infection. The syndrome, also known as *hemophagocytic lymphohistiocytosis (HLH)*, is caused by natural killer T-cell dysregulation, leading to lymphocyte proliferation and activation with uncontrolled hemophagocytosis and cytokine production. The syndrome is associated with primary or reactivated EBV infection and is also seen in the context of hematologic malignancies and collagen vascular diseases.[98] Successful treatment has been reported with immunosuppressive therapy with glucocorticoids or cyclosporine, or both, chemotherapy, and peripheral stem cell transplantation. Although rare, the syndrome is usually severe and may be fatal.[99]

EBV hepatitis is a relatively infrequent cause of acute hepatitis in adults, accounting for just 0.85% of 1995 cases of hepatitis reported at a tertiary center. Notably, only a minority (12%) had clinical features of infectious mononucleosis, but all had lymphocytosis and 88% had splenomegaly. Mild thrombocytopenia may also be seen.[100] The Monospot test is sensitive for the detection of heterophile antibodies but is not a specific test for EBV infection. Levels of EBV-specific immunoglobulin (Ig)M antibodies peak early in serum and may persist for many months, at which point IgG antibodies appear. Findings on abdominal US are usually nonspecific and may include hepatosplenomegaly, lymphadenopathy, and possibly gallbladder wall thickening, which has been reported to portend more severe liver disease.[101] Liver biopsy is rarely necessary for diagnosis and, if done, shows portal and sinusoidal mononuclear cell infiltration with no disruption of hepatic architecture; multinucleated giant cells are not a feature. In more severe cases, focal hepatic necrosis may be evident. In situ hybridization or PCR testing of biopsy samples may be used to confirm the diagnosis, but immunohistochemistry for EBV proteins is rarely positive.[102]

No specific treatment for EBV hepatitis exists. Acyclovir inhibits EBV replication and reduces viral shedding from the nasopharynx but has no effect on clinical symptoms or outcome.[103] Improvement in acute and chronic EBV hepatitis has been reported with ganciclovir treatment, but this approach has not been well studied.[104] Liver transplantation has been performed for fulminant EBV hepatitis. EBV rarely causes hepatitis after liver transplantation but has been associated with post-transplantation lymphoproliferative disease (see Chapter 35). EBV DNA is commonly found in the blood after liver transplantation, but viral titers are not associated with symptoms or complications.[105] Similarly, although EBV DNA can be isolated from the liver in the setting of post-transplant graft hepatitis, it is not associated with graft survival or other outcomes (see Chapter 97).[106] By contrast, high levels of HHV-6 DNA have been associated with graft hepatitis with impaired graft survival.[106] In a patient with chronic EBV hepatitis after kidney transplantation, treatment with rituximab has been reported to lead to improvement in serum liver enzyme levels and hepatic pathology.[107]

Cytomegalovirus

CMV is the largest member of the Herpesviridae family and, like other herpesviruses, persists lifelong in a latent, nonreplicative state after resolution of primary infection. Consequently, clinical disease caused by CMV may occur as a primary infection or, more commonly, as reactivation of latent infection,[108] particularly in immunocompromised persons.

In immunocompetent children and adults, primary CMV infection is usually subclinical but may cause a mononucleosis-like illness. Liver involvement is common and is characterized by mild to moderate serum aminotransferase (88%) and alkaline phosphatase (64%) elevations with or without hepatosplenomegaly.[109] Although the clinical course is mild in most patients, rare instances of granulomatous cholestatic CMV hepatitis, with or without jaundice, and even massive, fatal hepatic necrosis have been described.[110] In addition to the congenital CMV syndrome (jaundice, hepatosplenomegaly, thrombocytopenic purpura, and severe neurologic impairment), CMV is a common cause of neonatal hepatitis.[111] A number of case reports also suggest a possible association between CMV infection and acute portal vein thrombosis; however, the mechanism is unclear.[112]

Disseminated, life-threatening CMV infection with multiorgan involvement may develop in patients with impaired cell-mediated immunity (see Chapters 34 and 35). Hepatobiliary involvement by CMV is common in patients with AIDS and may manifest as hepatitis, pancreatitis, or acalculous gangrenous cholecystitis.[113] CMV also may cause AIDS-associated cholangiopathy, which manifests with chronic cholestasis and mimics PSC clinically and radiographically.[114] Patients may have papillary stenosis alone or in combination with intra- or extrahepatic (or both) biliary stricturing and dilatation (Fig. 83-2 [see also Fig. 34-8]). Antiviral therapy has no effect on this syndrome, but papillotomy, with or without placement of a biliary stent, may lead to symptomatic improvement.[113] Organ transplant recipients are also at risk for aggressive CMV hepatitis, including fibrosing cholestatic hepatitis (see Chapter 97), but for unclear reasons cholangiopathy does not develop in these patients.[115] CMV hepatitis can be difficult to distinguish from graft rejection in liver transplant recipients.[116]

The diagnosis of CMV infection is based on results of serologic studies, liver biopsy, or both. In acute primary CMV infection, IgM antibodies to CMV are present. For patients with reactivation of latent CMV, "shell vial" assays, which use monoclonal antibodies to detect CMV antigens, or direct CMV antigenemia testing are necessary. Because CMV viremia precedes organ involvement, testing for CMV antigenemia or

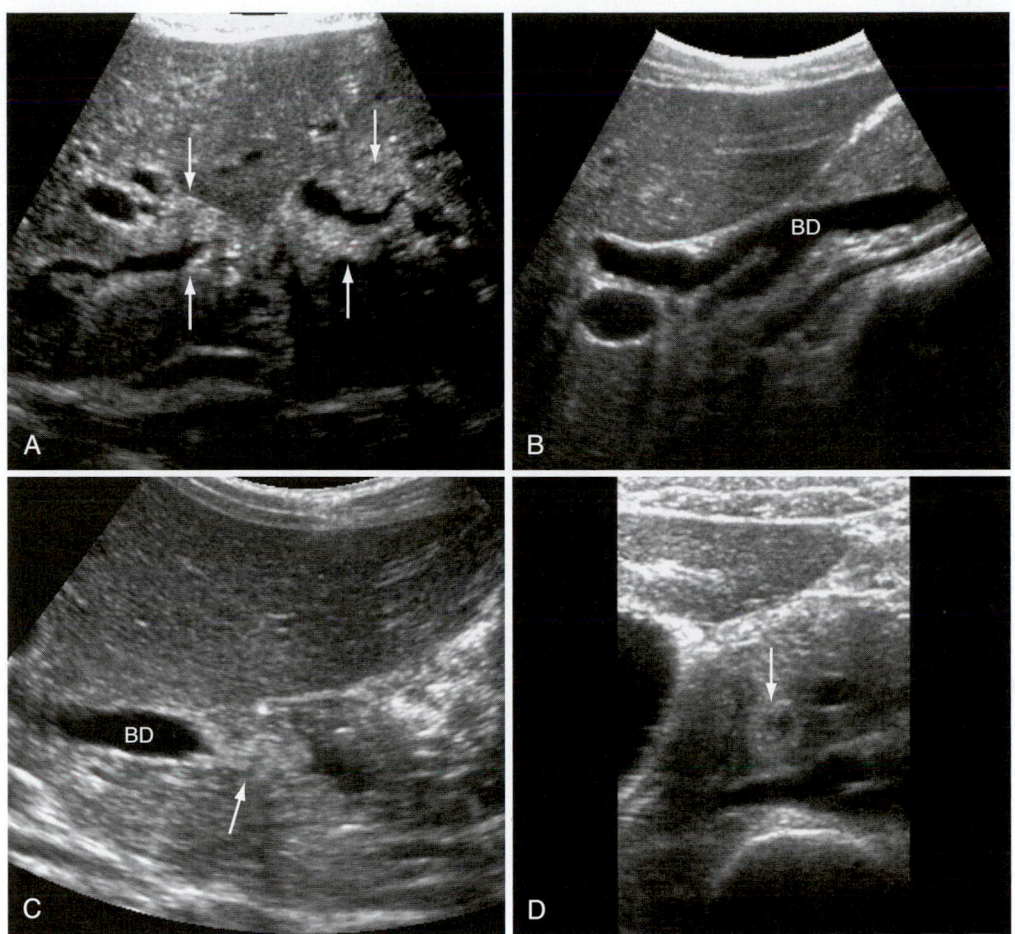

FIGURE 83-2. US findings in AIDS cholangiopathy and cytomegalovirus infection. *A,* A thick rind of echogenic tissue *(arrows)* surrounds the central portal triads and causes irregular narrowing of the intrahepatic bile ducts. *B,* The bile duct (BD) is dilated, and its wall is minimally irregular. *C,* The dilated BD tapers abruptly at an echogenic, inflamed ampulla *(arrow)*, indicative of papillary stenosis. *D,* The ampulla *(arrow)* is enlarged and echogenic, as viewed transversely in the caudal aspect of the pancreatic head.

CMV PCR testing of blood is a useful screening tool in immunocompromised patients.[117] Multinucleated giant cells with mononuclear portal and parenchymal inflammatory infiltrates and cholestasis are commonly seen on liver biopsy specimens. Large nuclear inclusions, sometimes referred to as "owl's eye" inclusions, may be seen in hepatocytes or biliary epithelial cells (Fig. 83-3).

With mild CMV disease in an immunocompetent adult, treatment is unnecessary. In immunocompromised patients, antiviral therapy is indicated. Ganciclovir, a guanosine nucleoside analog with a much longer intracellular half-life than that of acyclovir, has proved to be most effective. The major toxicity is bone marrow suppression, particularly granulocytopenia. Because viremia correlates with disease outcome, ganciclovir should be continued until CMV antigenemia is undetectable.[118] For patients resistant to or intolerant of ganciclovir, alternative agents include foscarnet and cidofovir.

HSV

HSV typically causes mucocutaneous vesicular oral or genital lesions; visceral involvement may occur in certain clinical settings. HSV hepatitis is seen in neonates, pregnant women, and immunocompromised persons and can be aggressive and life-threatening.[119] Cases of severe HSV hepatitis in immunocompetent persons have been reported as well.[120] Severe hepatitis

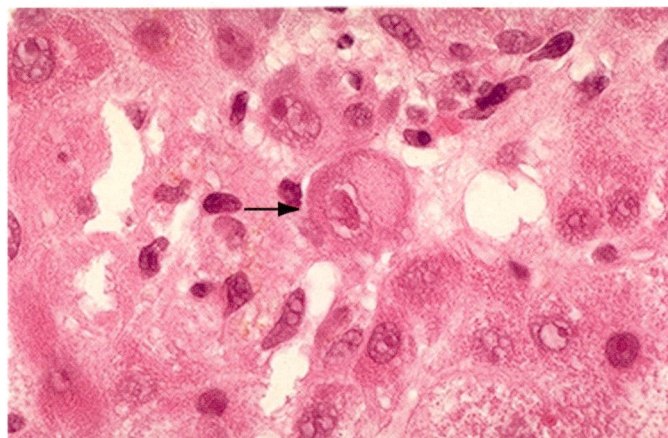

FIGURE 83-3. Histopathology of cytomegalovirus hepatitis. In the center *(arrow)* is a large hepatocyte with a large nucleus that contains an "owl's eye" inclusion. (H&E.) *(Courtesy Maha Guindi, MD, Toronto, Canada.)*

with multiorgan involvement and, often, adrenal insufficiency may develop in neonates exposed to infected maternal genital secretions at the time of delivery.[121] Risk factors for severe disease and the need for liver transplantation include the lack of skin lesions, positive HSV by PCR testing, thrombocytopenia, and liver synthetic dysfunction.[122] In pregnant women, HSV hepatitis usually has a fulminant course. The disease is most common in late gestation, typically (in 65% of patients) in the third trimester. Mucocutaneous lesions are present in only 50% of cases, and a high index of clinical suspicion is important to ensure timely diagnosis.[123] Maternal and perinatal mortality rates approach 40%, and in the largest series, 25% of patients were diagnosed only at autopsy. Early diagnosis and initiation of antiviral therapy are critical.[124]

Mild, asymptomatic liver enzyme elevations may be seen in 14% of immunocompetent patients with acute genital HSV infection. By contrast, immunocompromised patients may present with fulminant hepatitis.[125] Hepatitis is more common with acute infection than with reactivation and presents with fever, leukopenia, and markedly elevated serum aminotransferase levels. Coagulopathy, including DIC, and jaundice may be seen. Of reported cases, only 50% had a rash at presentation, and 58% were diagnosed at autopsy.[126] Risk factors for progression to death or liver transplantation include male gender, age over 40 years, ALT over 5000 U/L, platelet count less than 75,000/mm^3, and lack of antiviral therapy.[126]

Liver biopsy is essential for diagnosis, particularly in pregnancy. The transjugular route may be required because liver failure may develop rapidly, precluding percutaneous biopsy. Focal or extensive hemorrhagic or coagulative necrosis, with few inflammatory infiltrates, is seen. Intranuclear (Cowdry A type) inclusions may be identified in hepatocytes at the margins of the necrosis. In addition, some periportal multinucleated hepatocytes show a ground-glass appearance suggestive of viral inclusions (Fig. 83-4).[127] Electron microscopy, immunohistochemical staining, and PCR techniques can be used to confirm the diagnosis.[128] Serum PCR testing has been reported to allow rapid diagnosis with early institution of therapy.[129]

HSV hepatitis constitutes an emergency, and empirical therapy should be instituted pending diagnostic confirmation. High-dose IV acyclovir (at least 10 mg/kg every 8 hours) is

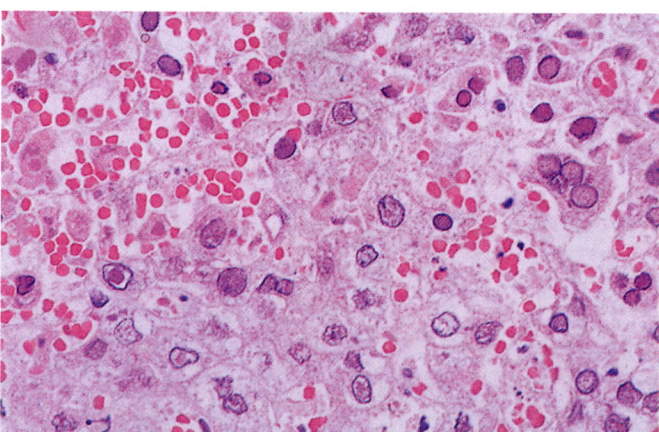

FIGURE 83-4. Histopathology of HSV hepatitis. At the edge of a necrotic zone, some hepatocytes are multinucleated, and many nuclei contain eosinophilic viral (Cowdry type A) inclusions. (H&E.) *(From Lucas SB. Other viral and infectious diseases and HIV-related liver disease. In: Burt AD, Portmann BC, Ferrell LD, editors. Pathology of the liver. 5th ed. London: Churchill Livingstone; 2007. p 446.)*

effective and appears to be safe in pregnancy.[130] Prolonged therapy may be required because severe relapse has been reported.[120] Although successful liver transplantation has been reported, transplant outcomes for HSV hepatitis have been disappointing, with just a 38% 1-year survival rate in the European transplant registry.[131]

Varicella-Zoster Virus

Like HSV infection, VZV infection occasionally can be complicated by hepatitis. Serum liver enzyme levels may be elevated in up to 3.4% of children with chickenpox; however, clinically significant hepatitis has been reported only rarely.[132] Although VZV reactivation in adults usually is limited to the skin, dissemination with liver, lung, and pancreatic involvement may occur.[133] Rarely, visceral involvement has been reported to develop before cutaneous manifestations in bone marrow or solid organ transplant recipients. If visceral involvement is suspected, treatment with high-dose IV acyclovir should be instituted.

Other Viruses

A number of other viruses have been reported to involve the liver, ranging from mild hepatitis to fulminant liver failure. During the 2003 outbreak of severe acute respiratory syndrome (SARS), elevated serum aminotransferase levels were commonly observed during the acute illness. Subsequently, cases of SARS hepatitis were reported in 3 patients in whom the coronavirus that causes SARS was demonstrated in the liver by reverse transcriptase–PCR techniques; no viral particles were seen on electron microscopy. All 3 cases fulfilled the WHO criteria for SARS. Examination of liver tissue revealed marked apoptosis, ballooning of hepatocytes, and moderate lobular lymphocytic infiltration.[134]

Parvovirus B19 is a common childhood exanthem that may also precipitate aplastic anemia. Liver enzyme elevations have been described, and rare cases of hepatitis with synthetic dysfunction or even fulminant liver failure have been reported in both immunocompetent and immunocompromised persons.[135-137] The frequency of parvovirus B19 exposure has been reported to be increased in patients with HBV and HCV infection, and some studies have reported an association with worse hepatic outcomes[138]; however, this has not been a universal finding.[139] Diagnosis is made using serologic tests for IgM and IgG parvovirus B19 antibodies or detection of viral DNA in blood or liver tissue by PCR methodology.

HHV-6 has also been associated with hepatitis and fulminant liver failure, most commonly in the setting of reactivation after liver transplantation, including presentation as syncytial giant cell hepatitis.[140-142] Nonspecific liver biochemical abnormalities are common in many viral illnesses, including influenza, Middle East respiratory syndrome, and Ebola virus infection, and rare instances of frank hepatitis may occur.[143]

KEY REFERENCES

Full references for this chapter can be found on www.expertconsult.com.

18. Alter HJ, Nakatsuji Y, Melpolder J, et al. The incidence of transfusion-associated hepatitis G virus infection and its relation to liver disease. N Engl J Med 1997; 336:747-54.

35. Tillmann HL, Heiken H, Knapik-Botor A, et al. Infection with GB virus C and reduced mortality among HIV-infected patients. N Engl J Med 2001; 345:715-24.

36. Williams CF, Klinzman D, Yamashita TE, et al. Persistent GB virus C infection and survival in HIV-infected men. N Engl J Med 2004; 350:981-90.

41. Vahidnia F, Petersen M, Stapleton JT, et al. Acquisition of GB virus type C and lower mortality in patients with advanced HIV disease. Clin Infect Dis 2012; 55:1012-9.

49. Berzsenyi MD, Bowden DS, Kelly HA, et al. Reduction in hepatitis C-related liver disease associated with GB virus C in human immunodeficiency virus coinfection. Gastroenterology 2007; 133:1821-30.

75. Charlton M, Adjei P, Poterucha J, et al. TT-virus infection in North American blood donors, patients with fulminant hepatic failure, and cryptogenic cirrhosis. Hepatology 1998; 28:839-42.

82. Akiba J, Umemura T, Alter H, et al. SEN virus: Epidemiology and characteristics of a transfusion-transmitted virus. Transfusion 2005; 45:1084-8.

98. Park HS, Kim DY, Lee JH, et al. Clinical features of adult patients with secondary hemophagocytic lymphohistiocytosis from causes other than lymphoma: An analysis of treatment outcome and prognostic factors. Ann Hematol 2012; 91:897-904.

99. Rouphael NG, Talati NJ, Vaughan C, et al. Infections associated with haemophagocytic syndrome. Lancet Infect Dis 2007; 7:814-22.

100. Vine LJ, Shepherd K, Hunter JG, et al. Characteristics of Epstein-Barr virus hepatitis among patients with jaundice or acute hepatitis. Aliment Pharmacol Ther 2012; 36:16-21

108. Goodgame RW. Gastrointestinal cytomegalovirus disease. Ann Intern Med 1993; 119:924-35.

126. Norvell J, Blei A, Jovanovic B, et al. Herpes simplex virus hepatitis: An analysis of the published literature and institutional cases. Liver Transpl 2007; 13:1428-34.

132. Feldman S, Crout J, Andrew M. Incidence and natural history of chemically defined varicella-zoster virus hepatitis in children and adolescents. Scand J Infect Dis 1997; 29:33-6.

138. Toan NL, Song le H, Kremsner PG, et al. Co-infection of human parvovirus B19 in Vietnamese patients with hepatitis B virus infection. J Hepatol 2006; 45:361-9.

141. Potenza L, Luppi M, Barozzi P, et al. HHV-6A in syncytial giant-cell hepatitis. N Engl J Med 2008; 359:593-602.

Bacterial, Parasitic, and Fungal Infections of the Liver, Including Liver Abscesses

ARTHUR Y. KIM AND RAYMOND T. CHUNG

The liver serves as the initial site of filtration of absorbed intestinal luminal contents and is particularly susceptible to contact with microbial antigens of all varieties. In addition to infection by viruses (see Chapters 78 to 83), the liver can be affected by (1) spread of bacterial or parasitic infection from outside the liver; (2) primary infection by spirochetal, protozoal, helminthic, or fungal organisms; or (3) systemic effects of bacterial or granulomatous infections.

BACTERIAL INFECTIONS INVOLVING OR AFFECTING THE LIVER

Gram-Positive and Gram-Negative Bacteria

A number of extrahepatic infections can lead to derangements in hepatic function, ranging from mild abnormalities of liver biochemical test results to frank jaundice and, rarely, hepatic failure.

Toxic Shock Syndrome: Staphylococcus aureus or Group A Streptococci

Toxic shock syndrome is a multisystem disease caused by toxic shock syndrome toxins, which are superantigens that cause T-cell activation and massive cytokine release. Originally described in association with serious infections caused by *Staphylococcus aureus*, this syndrome is now more frequently a complication of group A streptococcal infections, particularly necrotizing fasciitis.[1] Risk factors for *S. aureus* toxic shock syndrome include tampon use and surgical wound infection. Typical findings include a scarlatiniform rash, mucosal hyperemia, hypotension, vomiting, and diarrhea.[2] Hepatic involvement is almost always present and can range from elevations of serum aminotransferase levels to jaundice and extensive necrosis. Histologic findings in the liver include microabscesses and granulomas. The diagnosis is confirmed by culture of toxigenic *Streptococcus pyogenes* or *S. aureus* from the wound, blood, or other body sites. For wound infections or necrotizing fasciitis, surgical intervention is critical. Clindamycin, in conjunction with another active agent, is recommended to interfere with bacterial toxin production. Antibiotics effective against *S. aureus* include nafcillin for methicillin-sensitive isolates and vancomycin or linezolid for methicillin-resistant isolates, whereas penicillin remains active against *S. pyogenes*. IV immunoglobulin may have a benefit in the setting of toxic shock associated with *S. pyogenes*.[3]

Clostridium perfringens

Clostridial myonecrosis involving *Clostridium perfringens* usually is a mixed anaerobic infection that results in the rapid development of local wound pain, abdominal pain, and diarrhea. The skin lesions become discolored and even bullous, and gas gangrene spreads rapidly, leading to a high mortality rate. Jaundice may develop in up to 20% of patients with gas gangrene and is predominantly a consequence of massive intravascular hemolysis caused by an exotoxin elaborated by the bacterium.[4] Evidence of liver involvement may include abscess formation and gas in the portal vein. Hepatic involvement does not appear to affect mortality. The presence of clostridial bacteria portends a poor prognosis in persons with cirrhosis.[5] Surgical débridement with wide excision is essential; penicillin and clindamycin are effective antibiotics.

Actinomyces

Actinomycosis is caused most commonly by *Actinomyces israelii*, a Gram-positive anaerobic bacterium. Although cervicofacial infection is the most frequent manifestation of actinomycotic infection, GI involvement occurs in 13% to 60% of patients.[6,7] Hepatic involvement is present in 15% of cases of abdominal actinomycosis and is believed to result from metastatic spread from other abdominal sites. Common presenting manifestations of actinomycotic liver abscess include fever, abdominal pain, and anorexia with weight loss.[8,9] The course is more indolent than that seen with the usual causes of pyogenic hepatic abscess (see later) and thus may be mistaken for a tumor.[8] Fistula formation and invasion of other surrounding tissues such as the pleural space can occur. Anemia, leukocytosis, an elevated erythrocyte sedimentation rate, and an elevated serum alkaline phosphatase level are nearly universal. Radiographic findings are nonspecific; multiple abscesses may be seen in both lobes of the liver.

The diagnosis is based on aspiration of an abscess cavity and either visualization of characteristic sulfur granules or positive results on an anaerobic culture. Most abscesses resolve with a prolonged course of IV penicillin or oral tetracycline. Large abscesses can be drained percutaneously or resected surgically.[10]

Listeria

Hepatic invasion in adult human *Listeria monocytogenes* infection is uncommon. One report described 34 cases of listeriosis involving the liver, ranging from solitary to multiple abscesses and acute and granulomatous hepatitis.[11] Hepatic histologic features include multiple abscesses and granulomas. Predisposing conditions include immunosuppression, diabetes mellitus, and underlying liver disease, including cirrhosis, hemochromatosis, and chronic hepatitis. The diagnosis of disseminated listerial infection is based on a positive culture result from blood or isolation from an aspirate in the case of a liver abscess. Cholecystitis with *L. monocytogenes* has also been described.[12] Treatment is with ampicillin or penicillin, often with gentamicin for synergy.[13]

Shigella and Salmonella

Several case reports have described cholestatic hepatitis attributable to enteric infection with *Shigella*.[14,15] Histologic findings in the liver have included portal and periportal infiltration with polymorphonuclear leukocytes (neutrophils), hepatocyte necrosis, and cholestasis.

Typhoid fever, caused by *Salmonella typhi*, is a systemic infection that frequently involves the liver. Elevation of serum aminotransferase levels is common, whereas the serum bilirubin level may rise in a minority of cases.[16] Some patients may present with an acute hepatitis-like picture, characterized by fever and tender hepatomegaly.[17] Cholecystitis and liver abscess may complicate hepatic involvement with *S. typhi* infection.[18]

Hepatic damage by *S. typhi* appears to be mediated by bacterial endotoxin, although organisms can be visualized within the liver tissue. Endotoxin may produce focal necrosis, a periportal mononuclear infiltrate, and Kupffer cell hyperplasia in the liver. These changes resemble those seen in Gram-negative sepsis. Characteristic typhoid nodules scattered throughout the liver are the result of profound hypertrophy

and proliferation of Kupffer cells. The clinical course can be severe, with a mortality rate approaching 20%, particularly with delayed treatment or in patients with other complications of *Salmonella* infection. Severe typhoid fever with jaundice and encephalopathy may be differentiated from acute liver failure by the presence of an elevated serum alkaline phosphatase level, mild hypoprothrombinemia, thrombocytopenia, hepatomegaly, and an AST level greater than the ALT level.[19] Ciprofloxacin and ceftriaxone are first-line agents for the treatment of typhoid fever.

S. paratyphi A and B (*Salmonella enterica* serotypes paratyphi A and B) are the predominant causes of paratyphoid fever. As in typhoid fever, abnormalities in liver biochemical test results, particularly elevated serum aminotransferase levels, with or without hepatomegaly, are common.[20] Liver abscess is a rare complication.[21] Treatment is with a third-generation cephalosporin or a fluoroquinolone.

Yersinia

Infection with *Yersinia enterocolitica* manifests as ileocolitis in children and as terminal ileitis or mesenteric adenitis in adults. Arthritis, cellulitis, erythema nodosum, and septicemia may complicate *Yersinia* infection. Most patients with complicated disease have an underlying comorbid condition, such as diabetes mellitus, cirrhosis, or hemochromatosis. Excess tissue iron, in particular, may be a predisposing factor because growth of the *Yersinia* bacterium is enhanced by iron.

The subacute septicemic form of the disease resembles typhoid fever or malaria. Multiple abscesses are distributed diffusely in the liver and spleen. In some cases, the occurrence of *Y. enterocolitica* liver abscesses may lead to the detection of underlying hemochromatosis.[22,23] The mortality rate is approximately 50%. Fluoroquinolones are the preferred antibiotics.

Gonococci

In approximately 50% of patients with disseminated gonococcal infection, serum alkaline phosphatase levels are elevated, and in 30% to 40% of patients, AST levels are elevated.[24] Jaundice is uncommon.

The most common hepatic complication of gonococcal infection is the Fitz-Hugh–Curtis syndrome, a perihepatitis that is believed to result from direct spread of the infection from the pelvis (see later).[24] Clinically, patients describe a sudden, sharp pain in the right upper quadrant (RUQ). The pain may be confused with that of acute cholecystitis or pleurisy. Most patients have a history of pelvic inflammatory disease. The syndrome is distinguished from gonococcal bacteremia by a characteristic friction rub over the liver and negative blood culture results. The diagnosis is made by vaginal culture for gonococci. The overall prognosis of gonococcal infection appears to be unaffected by the presence of perihepatitis.[25] Although resistance to various antibiotics is of increasing concern, ceftriaxone remains the antibiotic of choice. Presumed coinfection with *Chlamydia trachomatis* should be treated empirically (see later).

Legionella

Legionella pneumophila, a fastidious Gram-negative bacterium, is the cause of legionnaires disease. Although pneumonia is the predominant clinical manifestation, abnormal liver biochemical test results are frequent, with elevations in serum aminotransferase levels in 50%, alkaline phosphatase levels in 45%, and bilirubin levels in 20% of cases (but usually without jaundice). Involvement of the liver does not influence clinical outcome. Liver histologic changes include microvesicular steatosis and focal necrosis; organisms can be seen occasionally. The diagnosis is confirmed by detection of a direct fluorescence antibody in the serum or sputum or of antigen in the urine.[26] The antibiotic of choice is azithromycin or a fluoroquinolone.

Burkholderia pseudomallei (Melioidosis)

Burkholderia pseudomallei is a soil-borne and water-borne Gram-negative bacterium that is found predominantly in Southeast Asia. The clinical spectrum of melioidosis ranges from asymptomatic infection to fulminant septicemia with involvement of the lungs, GI tract, and liver. Histologic changes in the liver include inflammatory infiltrates, multiple microabscesses, and focal necrosis. Organisms can be visualized with a Giemsa stain of a liver biopsy specimen. With chronic disease, granulomas may be seen. Some liver abscesses may demonstrate a "honeycombing" appearance on CT.[27] Abscesses may need to be drained or débrided, and ceftazidime or meropenem is the initial drug of choice, followed by a prolonged course of trimethoprim/sulfamethoxazole, with or without doxycycline.[28]

Brucella

Brucellosis may be acquired from infected pigs, cattle, goats, and sheep (*Brucella suis*, *Brucella abortus*, *Brucella melitensis*, and *Brucella ovis*, respectively) and typically manifests as an acute febrile illness. Hepatic abnormalities are seen in a majority of infected persons, and jaundice may be present in severe cases. Typically, multiple noncaseating hepatic granulomas are found in liver biopsy specimens; less often, focal mononuclear infiltration of the portal tracts or lobules is seen.[29] Rarely, brucellosis also may produce hepatosplenic abscesses.[30,31] The diagnosis can be made by isolation of the organism from a cultured specimen of liver tissue and is confirmed by serologic testing in combination with a history of exposure to animals. Surgical drainage may be required for management of *Brucella* abscesses. The combination of streptomycin and doxycycline is the most effective antimicrobial therapy.

Coxiella burnetii (Q Fever)

Infection by *Coxiella burnetii*, typically acquired by inhalation of animal dusts, causes the clinical syndrome of Q fever, which is characterized by relapsing fevers, headache, myalgias, malaise, pneumonitis, and culture-negative endocarditis. Liver involvement is common.[32] The predominant abnormality is an elevated serum alkaline phosphatase level, with minimal elevations of AST or bilirubin levels. The histologic hallmark in the liver is the presence of characteristic fibrin ring granulomas. The diagnosis is confirmed by serologic testing for complement-fixing antibodies.[33] Treatment with doxycycline is usually effective.

Bartonella (Oroya Fever)

Endemic to Colombia, Ecuador, and Peru, *Bartonella bacilliformis* is a Gram-negative coccobacillus that causes an acute febrile illness accompanied by jaundice, hemolysis, hepatosplenomegaly, and lymphadenopathy. Centrilobular necrosis of the liver and splenic infarction may occur. As many as 40% of patients die of sepsis or hemolysis. Prompt treatment with chloramphenicol in combination with penicillin, clindamycin, or trimethoprim/sulfamethoxazole prevents fatal complications.[34]

Bacillary Angiomatosis and AIDS

Bacillary angiomatosis is an infectious disorder that primarily affects persons with AIDS or other immunodeficiency states. The causative agents have been identified as the Gram-negative bacilli *Bartonella henselae* and, in some cases, *Bartonella quintana*.[35] Infection is frequently associated with exposure to cats.

Bacillary angiomatosis is characterized most commonly by multiple blood-red papular skin lesions, but disseminated infection with or without skin involvement has also been described.[36] The causative bacilli can infect liver, lymph nodes, pleura, bronchi, bones, brain, bone marrow, and spleen. Additional manifestations include persistent fever, bacteremia, and sepsis. Hepatic infection should be suspected when serum aminotransferase levels are elevated in the absence of other explanations.

Hepatic infection in persons with bacillary angiomatosis may manifest as peliosis hepatis, or blood-filled cysts (see Chapter 85). Histologically, peliosis in patients with AIDS is characterized by an inflammatory myxoid stroma containing clumps of bacilli and dilated capillaries surrounding the blood-filled peliotic cysts. Increasingly, the diagnosis of *Bartonella* infection is by PCR-based methods.[37] Bacillary angiomatosis responds uniformly to therapy with erythromycin. For visceral infection, prolonged treatment with erythromycin or doxycycline should be administered.[35]

Bacterial Sepsis and Jaundice

Jaundice may complicate systemic sepsis caused by Gram-negative or Gram-positive organisms. Exotoxins and endotoxin liberated in overwhelming infection can directly or indirectly, through cytokines such as TNF-α, inhibit the transport of bile acids and other organic anions across the hepatic sinusoidal and bile canalicular membranes, thereby leading to intrahepatic cholestasis (see Chapter 21).[38] Serum bilirubin levels can reach 15 mg/dL or higher. The magnitude of the jaundice does not correlate with mortality. Results of cultures of liver biopsy specimens usually are negative.

Chlamydia

Fitz-Hugh–Curtis Syndrome

Although perihepatitis was first associated with gonococcal salpingo-oophoritis (see earlier), it is now most frequently associated with *Chlamydia trachomatis* infection. The presentation is similar to perihepatitis caused by gonococcal infection, with RUQ pain accompanying a urogenital infection such as pelvic inflammatory disease. The diagnosis can be made by direct visualization at laparoscopy or laparotomy and supported by pathologic demonstration of endometritis, salpingitis, and microbiologic detection of *C. trachomatis* in the genital tract. Liver biochemical test results are generally normal. The treatment of choice should follow guidelines for treatment of *C. trachomatis* or pelvic inflammatory disease.[39]

Rickettsiae

Rocky Mountain Spotted Fever

Mortality from Rocky Mountain spotted fever, a systemic tick-borne rickettsial illness, has decreased considerably as a result of prompt recognition of the classic maculopapular rash in association with fever and an exposure history. A small subset of patients, however, present with multiorgan manifestations and have a high mortality rate.[40] A characteristic severe vasculitis develops in these patients and is believed to be the result of a microbe-induced coagulopathy. Hepatic involvement is frequent in multiorgan disease. In one postmortem study, rickettsiae were identified in the portal tracts of 8 of 9 fatal cases. Portal tract inflammation, portal vasculitis, and sinusoidal erythrophagocytosis were consistent findings, but hepatic necrosis was negligible. The predominant clinical manifestation was jaundice; elevations of serum aminotransferase and alkaline phosphatase levels varied. Jaundice probably results from a combination of inflammatory bile ductular obstruction and hemolysis and is associated with increased mortality.[32,41]

Ehrlichiae

Ehrlichiae are rickettsiae that parasitize leukocytes. In the United States, human monocytic ehrlichiosis is caused principally by *Ehrlichia chaffeensis* and, less often, by *Ehrlichia canis*. Human granulocytic anaplasmosis (formerly known as human granulocytic ehrlichiosis) is caused by *Anaplasma phagocytophilum*.[32,42] In contrast to Rocky Mountain spotted fever, a rash is often absent. Hepatic involvement is seen in more than 80% of cases, usually in the form of mild, transient serum aminotransferase elevations. More marked aminotransferase elevations may occur occasionally, in association with cholestasis, hepatosplenomegaly, and liver failure. Liver injury is attributable to proliferation of organisms within hepatocytes and provocation of an immune response. Focal necrosis, fibrin ring granulomas, and cholestatic hepatitis can be observed. A mixed portal tract infiltrate and lymphoid sinusoidal infiltrate are usually seen. The disease generally resolves with appropriate antibiotic therapy with doxycycline.[43]

Spirochetes

Leptospirosis

Leptospirosis is one of the most common zoonoses in the world, and the causative organism has a wide range of domestic and wild animal reservoirs. Humans acquire the spirochete by contact with infected urine or contaminated soil or water. In humans, disease can occur as anicteric leptospirosis or as Weil's syndrome.

Anicteric leptospirosis accounts for more than 90% of cases and is characterized by a biphasic illness. The first phase begins, often abruptly, with viral illness-like symptoms associated with fever, leptospiremia, and conjunctival suffusion, which serves as an important diagnostic clue. Following a brief period of improvement, the second phase in 95% of cases is characterized by myalgias, nausea, vomiting, abdominal tenderness, and, in some cases, aseptic meningitis.[44] During this phase, a few patients have elevated serum aminotransferase and bilirubin levels with hepatomegaly.

Weil's syndrome is a severe icteric form of leptospirosis and constitutes 5% to 10% of all cases. The first phase of this illness is often marked by jaundice, which may last for weeks. During the second phase, fever may be high, and hepatic and renal manifestations predominate. Jaundice may be marked, with serum bilirubin levels approaching 30 mg/dL (predominantly conjugated). Serum aminotransferase levels usually do not exceed 5 times the upper limit of normal.[45] Acute tubular necrosis often develops and can lead to renal failure, which may be fatal. Hemorrhagic complications are frequent and are the result of capillary injury caused by immune complexes.[44] Spirochetes are seen in renal tubules in a majority of autopsy specimens but rarely are found in the liver. Hepatic histologic findings generally are nonspecific and do not include necrosis. Altered mitochondria and disrupted membranes in hepato-

cytes on electron microscopy suggest the possibility of a toxin-mediated injury.

The diagnosis of leptospirosis is made on clinical grounds in conjunction with a positive result of a blood or urine culture specimen in the first and second phase, respectively. Serologic testing confirms the diagnosis when culture results are unrevealing. Doxycycline is effective if given within the first several days of illness. Most patients recover without residual organ impairment.

Syphilis

Secondary Syphilis

Liver involvement is characteristic of secondary syphilis.[46] The frequency of hepatitis in secondary syphilis ranges from 1% to 50%.[46,47] Symptoms and signs are usually nonspecific, including anorexia, weight loss, fever, malaise, and sore throat. A characteristic pruritic maculopapular rash involves the palms and soles. Jaundice, hepatomegaly, and tenderness in the RUQ are less common. Almost all patients exhibit generalized lymphadenopathy. Biochemical testing generally reveals low-grade elevations of serum aminotransferase and bilirubin levels, with a disproportionate elevation of the serum alkaline phosphatase level; isolated elevation of the alkaline phosphatase is common.[48] Proteinuria may be present.

Histologic examination of the liver in syphilitic hepatitis generally discloses focal necrosis in the periportal and centrilobular regions. The inflammatory infiltrate typically includes neutrophils, plasma cells, lymphocytes, eosinophils, and mast cells.[46,47] Kupffer cell hyperplasia may be seen, but bile ductule injury is rare. Granulomas may be seen. Spirochetes may be demonstrated by silver staining in as many as 50% of patients. Resolution of these findings without sequelae follows treatment with penicillin.

Tertiary (Late) Syphilis

Tertiary syphilis is now rare. Although hepatic lesions are common in late syphilis, most patients are asymptomatic. Some patients describe anorexia, weight loss, fatigue, fever, or abdominal pain. The characteristic hepatic lesion in tertiary syphilis is the gumma, which can be single or multiple. It is necrotic centrally, with surrounding granulation tissue consisting of a lymphoplasmacytic infiltrate and endarteritis; exuberant deposition of scar tissue may occur, giving the liver a lobulated appearance (hepar lobatum). If hepatic involvement is unrecognized, hepatocellular dysfunction and portal hypertension with jaundice, ascites, and gastroesophageal varices can ensue. Hepatic gummas may resolve after therapy with penicillin.[49]

Lyme Disease

Lyme disease is a multisystem disease caused by the tick-borne spirochete *Borrelia burgdorferi*. Predominant manifestations are dermatologic, cardiac, neurologic, and musculoskeletal. Hepatic involvement has been described. Among 314 patients, abnormal liver biochemical test results with generally increased serum aminotransferase and lactate dehydrogenase levels were seen in 19%.[50] Clinical findings include anorexia, nausea and vomiting, weight loss, RUQ pain, and hepatomegaly, usually within days to weeks of the onset of illness and often accompanied by the sentinel rash, erythema migrans.[51]

In early stages of the illness, the spirochetes are believed to disseminate hematogenously from the skin to other organs, including the liver.[32] Histologic examination of the liver in

Lyme hepatitis reveals hepatocyte ballooning, marked mitotic activity, microvesicular fat, Kupffer cell hyperplasia, a mixed sinusoidal infiltrate, and intraparenchymal and sinusoidal spirochetes.[52]

The diagnosis of Lyme disease is confirmed with serologic studies in patients with a typical clinical history. Hepatic involvement tends to be more frequent in disseminated disease but does not appear to affect overall outcome, which is excellent in primary disease after institution of treatment with oral doxycycline, amoxicillin, clarithromycin, or azithromycin.[53] Ceftriaxone is the drug of choice for late disease.[43,52]

TB and Other Mycobacteria

Granulomas are found in liver biopsy specimens in approximately 25% of persons with pulmonary TB and 80% of those with extrapulmonary TB. Tuberculous granulomas can be distinguished from sarcoid granulomas by central caseation, acid-fast bacilli, and the presence of fewer granulomas, with a tendency to coalesce.[54] Multiple granulomas in the liver also may be seen following vaccination with Bacille Calmette-Guérin, especially in persons with an impaired immune response. Patients with multiple granulomas caused by TB rarely have clinically significant liver disease. Occasionally, tender hepatomegaly is found. Jaundice with elevated serum alkaline phosphatase levels may occur in miliary infection. The treatment of tuberculous granulomatous disease of the liver is the same as that for active pulmonary TB—namely, 4-drug therapy.[55] Hepatic involvement in *Mycobacterium avium* complex infection is discussed in Chapter 34.

PARASITES (Tables 84-1 and 84-2)

Protozoa (see also Chapter 113)

Malaria

An estimated 300 to 500 million persons in more than 100 countries are infected with malaria each year. The liver is affected during 2 stages of the malarial life cycle: first in the pre-erythrocytic phase, and then in the erythrocytic phase, which coincides with clinical illness.

The *Plasmodium* Life Cycle

The life cycle of the prototypical malarial parasite is illustrated in Figure 84-1. Malarial sporozoites injected by an infected mosquito circulate to the liver and enter hepatocytes. Maturation to schizonts ensues. When the schizont ruptures, merozoites are released into the bloodstream, where they enter erythrocytes. The major species of *Plasmodium* responsible for malaria differ with respect to the number of merozoites released and the maturation times. Infection by *Plasmodium falciparum* and *Plasmodium malariae* is not associated with a residual liver stage after the release of merozoites, whereas infection by *Plasmodium vivax* and *Plasmodium ovale* is associated with a persistent exoerythrocytic stage, the hypnozoite, which persists in the liver and, when activated, can divide and mature into schizont forms. *Plasmodium knowlesi* has been identified as a fifth species capable of infecting humans and occasionally results in severe manifestations including jaundice, hepatic dysfunction, and acute kidney injury.[56]

The extent of hepatic injury varies with the malarial species (most severe with *P. falciparum*) and the severity of infection. Unconjugated hyperbilirubinemia most commonly is seen as a result of hemolysis, but hepatocellular dysfunction is also possible, leading to conjugated hyperbilirubinemia. Moderate

TABLE 84-1 Classification of Parasitic Diseases of the Liver and Biliary Tract by Pathologic Process

Pathologic Process	Diseases
Liver Disease	
Granulomatous hepatitis	Capillariasis
	Fascioliasis
	Schistosomiasis
	Strongyloidiasis
	Toxocariasis
Portal fibrosis	Schistosomiasis
Hepatic abscess or necrosis	Amebiasis
	Toxoplasmosis
Cystic liver disease	Echinococcosis
Peliosis hepatis	Bacillary angiomatosis
Reticuloendothelial Disease	
Kupffer cell infection or hyperplasia	Babesiosis
	Malaria
	Toxoplasmosis
	Visceral leishmaniasis
Biliary Tract Disease	
Cholangitis	Clonorchiasis/opisthorchiasis
	Fascioliasis
Biliary hyperplasia	Ascariasis
	Clonorchiasis
	Cryptosporidiosis
	Fascioliasis
Cholangiocarcinoma	Clonorchiasis/opisthorchiasis

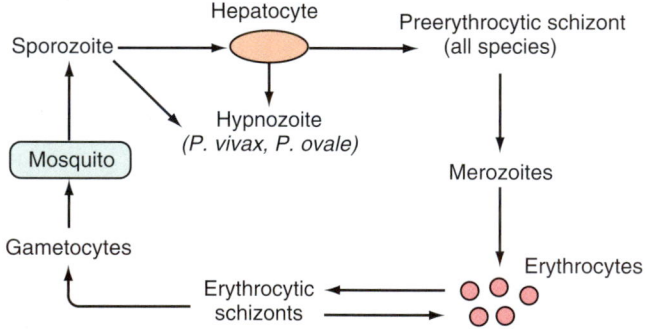

FIGURE 84-1. The life cycle of *Plasmodium* species.

elevations of serum aminotransferase and 5′-nucleotidase levels may be observed.[57] Synthetic dysfunction (e.g., prolongation of the prothrombin time, hypoalbuminemia) may be seen as well. In severe falciparum malaria, hypoglycemia and lactic acidosis are late and life-threatening complications.[58] Reversible reductions in portal venous blood flow have been described during the acute phase of falciparum malaria, presumably as a consequence of micro-occlusion of portal venous branches by parasitized erythrocytes.[59]

Histopathologic Features

In acute falciparum malaria in a previously unexposed person, hepatic macrophages hypertrophy, and large quantities of malarial pigment (the result of hemoglobin degradation by the parasite) accumulate in Kupffer cells, which phagocytose parasitized and unparasitized erythrocytes.[60] Histopathologic features include Kupffer cell hyperplasia with pigment

TABLE 84-2 Parasitic Diseases of the Liver and Biliary Tract

Disease (Cause)	Endemic Areas	Predisposing Factors	Pathophysiology	Manifestations	Diagnosis	Treatment*
Protozoans						
Amebiasis (*Entamoeba histolytica*) (see also Chapter 113)	Worldwide, especially Africa, Asia, Mexico, South America	Poor sanitation, sexual exposure	Hematogenous spread and tissue invasion, abscess formation (see Fig. 84-10)	Fever, RUQ pain, peritonitis, elevated right hemidiaphragm, rupture	Cysts in stool, serology (e.g., ELISA, CIE, IHA), hepatic imaging	Metronidazole 750 mg (oral or IV) 3 times daily × 7-10 days or tinidazole 2 g × 3 days, followed by iodoquinol 650 mg 3 times daily × 20 days or diloxanide furoate 500 mg 3 times daily × 10 days or aminosidine (paromomycin) 25-35 mg/kg/day in 3 divided doses × 7-10 days
Malaria (*Plasmodium falciparum, P. malariae, P. vivax, P. ovale, P. knowlesi*)	Africa, Asia, South America	Blood transfusion, IV drug use	Sporozoite clearance by hepatocytes; exoerythrocytic replication in the liver	Tender hepatomegaly, splenomegaly, rarely hepatic failure (*P. falciparum*)	Identification of the parasite on a blood smear	*P. falciparum*: chloroquine (chloroquine-sensitive), mefloquine, or quinine and either doxycycline or clindamycin; or pyrimethamine-sulfadoxine (Fansidar); or atovaquone/proguanil (chloroquine-resistant); or an artesiminin *P. malariae*: chloroquine *P. vivax, P. ovale, P. knowlesi*: chloroquine and primaquine (chloroquine-sensitive) or mefloquine and primaquine (chloroquine-resistant)†
Babesiosis (*Babesia* spp.)	United States	Exposure to deer tick	Hemolysis with multiorgan involvement	Fever, anemia, hepatosplenomegaly, abnormal liver test results, hemoglobinuria	Identification of the parasite on a blood smear, PCR	Azithromycin 500 mg on day 1, then 250 mg daily and atovaquone 750 mg bid × 7-10 days or clindamycin 300-600 mg IV every 6 hr or 600 mg orally every 8 hr and quinine 650 mg every 8 hr × 7-10 days
Visceral leishmaniasis (*Leishmania donovani*)	Eurasia, Central America, South America	Immunosuppression (AIDS, organ transplantation)	Infection of RE cells	Fever, weight loss, hepatosplenomegaly, secondary bacterial infection, skin hyperpigmentation (kala-azar)	Amastigotes seen in the spleen, liver, or bone marrow	Pentavalent antimonial (stibogluconate sodium and meglumine antimoniate) 20 mg/kg/day × 28 days; or liposomal amphotericin B (IV) 3 mg/kg/day on days 1-5, 14, and 21; or aminosidine (paromomycin) 16-20 mg/kg/day × 21 days; or pentamidine isethionate, 2-4 mg/kg/day for up to 15 days; or miltefosine 2.5 mg/kg/day × 28 days
Toxoplasmosis (*Toxoplasma gondii*)	Worldwide	Congenital infection, immunosuppression (AIDS, organ transplantation)	Replication in the liver leading to inflammation, necrosis	Fever, lymphadenopathy, occasionally hepatosplenomegaly, atypical lymphocytosis	Serology (IF, ELISA), isolation of the organism in the tissue	Pyrimethamine 100 mg loading dose followed by 25-50 mg/day; plus sulfadiazine 2-4 g/day in 4 divided doses; or clindamycin 300 mg 4 times daily, plus folinic acid 10-25 mg daily for 2-4 wk
Nematodes						
Toxocariasis (*Toxocara canis, T. cati*)	Worldwide	Exposure to dogs or cats, especially for children < 5 yr	Migration of larvae to the liver (visceral larva migrans)	Granuloma formation with eosinophilia	Larvae in tissue, serology (ELISA)	Albendazole 10 mg/kg/day × 5 days or mebendazole 100-200 mg twice daily × 5 days
Hepatic capillariasis (*Capillaria hepatica*)	Worldwide	Exposure to rodents	Migration of larvae to the liver; inflammatory reaction to eggs	Acute, subacute hepatitis, tender hepatomegaly, occasionally splenomegaly, eosinophilia	Adult worms or eggs in a liver biopsy specimen (see Fig. 84-2)	Supportive; possibly dithiazine iodide, sodium stibogluconate, albendazole, or thiabendazole

Continued

TABLE 84-2 Parasitic Diseases of the Liver and Biliary Tract—cont'd

Disease (Cause)	Endemic Areas	Predisposing Factors	Pathophysiology	Manifestations	Diagnosis	Treatment*
Ascariasis (*Ascaris lumbricoides*)	Tropical climates	Ingestion of raw vegetables	Migration of larvae to the liver; invasion of the bile ducts by adult worms	Abdominal pain, fever, jaundice, biliary obstruction, granulomas	Ova or adult in stool or contrast study	Albendazole 400 mg × 1 dose; or mebendazole 100 mg twice daily × 3 days; or pyrantel pamoate 11 mg/kg up to 1 g; or ivermectin 200 µg/kg × 1 dose
Strongyloidiasis (*Strongyloides stercoralis*)	Asia, Africa, South America, Southern Europe, USA	Immunosuppression (AIDS, chemotherapy, organ transplantation) predisposes to hyperinfection	Larval penetration from the intestine to the liver	Hepatomegaly, occasionally jaundice, larvae in the portal tract or lobule	Larvae in the stool or duodenal aspirate	Ivermectin 200 µg/kg/day × 2 days; or albendazole 400 mg/day × 3 days
Trichinosis (*Trichinella spiralis*)	Temperate climates	Ingestion of undercooked pork	Hematogenous dissemination to the liver	Occasionally jaundice, biliary obstruction, larvae in hepatic sinusoids	History, eosinophilia, fever, muscle biopsy	Glucocorticoids for allergic symptoms; albendazole 400 mg twice daily × 10-15 days; or mebendazole 200 mg/day × 10-15 days
Trematodes						
Schistosomiasis (*Schistosoma mansoni, S. japonicum*)	Asia, Africa, South America, Caribbean	Travelers exposed to bodies of fresh water	Fibrogenic host immune response to eggs in the portal vein	*Acute:* eosinophilic infiltrate *Chronic:* hepatosplenomegaly, presinusoidal portal hypertension, granulomas	Ova in the stool, rectal or liver biopsy	Praziquantel 40-60 mg/kg in 2-3 divided doses × 1 day; or oxamniquine for *S. mansoni* (not readily available) Acute toxemic schistosomiasis: praziquantel 40-60 mg/kg in 2-3 divided doses × 1 day + glucocorticoids
Fascioliasis (*Fasciola hepatica*)	Worldwide	Cattle or sheep raising; ingestion of contaminated watercress	Migration of larvae through the liver; penetration of the bile ducts or surgery	*Acute:* fever, abdominal pain, jaundice, hemobilia *Chronic:* hepatomegaly	Ova in the stool, flukes in the bile ducts at ERC	Triclabendazole 10 mg/kg × 1 dose
Clonorchiasis and opisthorchiasis (*Clonorchis sinensis, Opisthorchis viverrini, O. felineus*)	Southeast Asia, China, Japan, Korea, Eastern Europe	Ingestion of raw fresh-water fish	Migration through the ampulla; egg deposition in the bile ducts	Biliary hyperplasia, obstruction, sclerosing cholangitis, stone formation, cholangiocarcinoma	Ova in the stool, flukes in the bile ducts at ERC or surgery	Praziquantel 75 mg/kg in 3 divided doses × 1 day
Cestodes						
Echinococcosis (*Echinococcus granulosus, E. multilocularis*)	Worldwide	Cattle and sheep raising (*E. granulosus*)	Migration of larvae to the liver; encystment (hydatid cyst)	Tender hepatomegaly, fever, eosinophilia, cyst rupture, biliary obstruction	Serology (ELISA, IHA), hepatic imaging	Surgical resection or percutaneous drainage. Perioperative albendazole 400 mg twice daily continuing × 8 wk

*All drugs are given orally unless otherwise specified.
†For dosing guidelines for malaria, please refer to http://www.cdc.gov/malaria/pdf/treatmenttable.pdf.
CIE, counterimmunoelectrophoresis; ELISA, enzyme-linked immunosorbent assay; ERC, endoscopic retrograde cholangiography; IF, immunofluorescence; IHA, indirect hemagglutination assay; RE, reticuloendothelial; RUQ, right upper quadrant.

deposition and a mononuclear infiltrate. Hepatocyte swelling and centrizonal necrosis may be seen. All abnormalities are reversible with treatment.

Clinical Features

Only the erythrocytic stage of malaria is associated with clinical illness. Symptoms and signs of acute infection typically develop 30 to 60 days following exposure and include fever, which often is hectic, malaise, anorexia, nausea, vomiting, diarrhea, and myalgias. Jaundice caused by hemolysis is common in adults, especially in heavy infection with *P. falciparum*. In general, hepatic failure is seen only in association with concomitant viral hepatitis or with severe *P. falciparum* infection.[61,62] One series identified evidence of hepatic encephalopathy in 15 of 86 patients with falciparum malaria and jaundice; 4 cases were fatal.[61] Tender hepatomegaly with splenomegaly is common. Cytopenias are common in acute infection. The differential diagnosis includes viral hepatitis, gastroenteritis, amebic liver abscess, yellow fever, typhoid, TB, and brucellosis.

Diagnosis

The diagnosis of acute malaria rests on the clinical history, physical examination, and identification of parasites on peripheral thin and thick blood smears. Because the number of parasites in the blood may be small, repeated smear examinations should be performed by an experienced examiner when the index of suspicion is high. *P. knowlesi* may resemble *P. malariae* in morphology, and PCR-based tests may help distinguish these two species.[56] Rapid antigen detection assays are available but have yet to be implemented widely.[63]

Treatment

The treatment of acute malaria depends on the species of parasite and, for falciparum infection, the pattern of chloroquine resistance. Chloroquine generally is effective in areas endemic for chloroquine-sensitive species. Resistant falciparum infections can be treated with mefloquine alone; quinine and either doxycycline or clindamycin; pyrimethamine-sulfadoxine (Fansidar); a combination of atovaquone and proguanil; or artemisinin derivatives, including artemisinin, artemether, and artesunate.[64] For *P. vivax* and *P. ovale* infections, the addition of primaquine (in persons without glucose-6-phosphate dehydrogenase deficiency) to chloroquine or mefloquine is indicated to eliminate the exoerythrocytic hypnozoites in the liver.[65]

Hyperreactive Malarial Splenomegaly (Tropical Splenomegaly Syndrome)

In endemic areas, repeated exposure to malaria may lead to an aberrant immunologic response characterized by overproduction of B lymphocytes, circulating malarial antibody, and increased levels of circulating immune complexes, resulting in dense hepatic sinusoidal lymphocytosis and stimulation of the reticuloendothelial cell system. The clinical picture includes massive splenomegaly, markedly elevated antimalarial antibody levels, and high serum immunoglobulin (Ig)M levels. Severe debilitating anemia caused by hypersplenism, especially in women of childbearing age, can result.[66] Variceal bleeding is uncommon but may result from portal hypertension consequent to markedly increased splenic and portal venous blood flow. Treatment consists of lifelong antimalarial therapy and blood transfusions.

Babesiosis

Babesiosis, caused by *Babesia* species, is a malaria-like illness transmitted by the deer tick *Ixodes scapularis*.[67] The disease is endemic to coastal areas of the Northeast and areas of the Midwest in the United States. Clinical features include fever, anemia, mild hepatosplenomegaly, abnormalities on liver biochemical tests, hemoglobinuria, and hemophagocytosis on bone marrow biopsy specimen. The disease is especially severe in asplenic and immunocompromised patients. In rare cases, marked pancytopenia occurs. Hepatic involvement reflects the severity of the systemic illness but generally is not severe. Uncomplicated cases are treated with a combination of the following active agents: (1) oral azithromycin, 500-mg single dose followed by 250 mg once daily, plus atovaquone, 750 mg twice daily, for 7 to 10 days; or (2) oral clindamycin, 600 mg 3 times daily, in combination with quinine, 650 mg 3 times daily, for 7 to 10 days. In severe cases, clindamycin may be given IV, and partial or complete exchange transfusion should be considered.[43]

Leishmaniasis

Visceral leishmaniasis is caused by *Leishmania donovani* and is endemic in Mediterranean countries, central Asia, the former Soviet Union, the Middle East, China, India, Pakistan, Bangladesh, Africa, Central America, and South America.[68] This entity should be considered in immigrants, returning travelers, and military personnel from these areas. Amastigotes are ingested by the sand fly (*Lutzomyia* in the New World, *Phlebotomus* in the Old World) and become flagellated promastigotes. Following injection into the human host, the promastigotes are phagocytosed by macrophages in the reticuloendothelial system, where they multiply.

Histopathologic Features

In visceral leishmaniasis, organisms usually can be found in mononuclear phagocytes of the liver, spleen, bone marrow, and lymph nodes. Proliferation of Kupffer cells is often seen, and amastigotes (Leishman-Donovan bodies) can be detected within these cells.[69] Occasionally, parasite-bearing cells aggregate within noncaseating granulomas.[70] Hepatocyte necrosis can range in degree from mild to severe. Healing is accompanied by fibrous deposition, and occasionally the liver takes on a cirrhotic appearance. Nevertheless, complications of chronic liver disease are rare.

Clinical Features

Visceral infection caused by *L. donovani* begins with a papular or ulcerative skin lesion at the site of the sand fly bite. Following an incubation period of 2 to 6 months (sometimes years), intermittent fevers, weight loss, diarrhea (of bacillary, amebic, or leishmanial origin), and progressive painful hepatosplenomegaly develop, often accompanied by pancytopenia and a polyclonal hypergammaglobulinemia. Secondary bacterial infections resulting from suppression of reticuloendothelial cell function are important causes of mortality and include pneumonia, pneumococcal infection, and TB.

Physical findings include hepatomegaly, massive splenomegaly, jaundice or ascites in severe disease, generalized lymphadenopathy, and muscle wasting.[71] Cutaneous gray hyperpigmentation, which prompted the name *kala-azar* (black fever), is characteristically seen in patients in India. Oral and nasopharyngeal nodules resulting from granuloma formation also may be seen.

Diagnosis

The diagnosis is based on the history, physical examination, and microscopic demonstration of amastigotes by a Wright or Giemsa stain of affected tissue samples. The highest yield (90%) comes from aspiration of the spleen. Liver biopsy is less risky and associated with a yield nearly as great as that of splenic aspiration. The yield of bone marrow aspirates is 80% and may be higher with a longer time of observation[72] and higher than that of lymph node aspirates. Culture requires specialized media and may take several weeks. Serologic testing (enzyme-linked immunosorbent assay [ELISA], immunofluorescence, direct agglutination) can be used to support a presumptive diagnosis of visceral leishmaniasis but is insensitive, particularly in immunocompromised hosts.[73] The leishmanin skin test (Montenegro test) is not helpful in acute visceral disease. PCR-based testing of blood or other tissue may also be useful for diagnosis as well as monitoring.[74]

Treatment

Pentavalent antimonial compounds are the drugs of choice for all forms of leishmaniasis. Parenteral sodium stibogluconate and meglumine antimoniate are available through the CDC for treatment of infections in the United States. Treatment with antimonials should be administered for at least 4 weeks. Alternative parenteral agents include liposomal amphotericin B and aminosidine (paromomycin).[75] Patients with AIDS and leishmaniasis often fail to respond to or relapse following treatment with conventional regimens.[73] Miltefosine, a phosphocholine analog administered orally, has shown promise in visceral leishmaniasis, with a reported cure rate of 82% to 97%.[76,77]

Toxoplasmosis

Toxoplasmosis, caused by *Toxoplasma gondii*, is found worldwide. In the United States, serologic surveys suggest that exposure to *T. gondii* has decreased from 14% to 9% among persons ages 12 to 49.[78] The infection may be transmitted congenitally or occur as an opportunistic infection that causes cerebral mass lesions in patients with AIDS. Oocysts of *T. gondii* in soil, water, or contaminated meat are ingested and mature in the intestinal tract of humans to become sporozoites, which penetrate the intestinal mucosa, become tachyzoites, and circulate systemically, invading a wide array of cell types.[79] Hepatic involvement has been observed in severe, disseminated infection.

Clinical Features

Although most primary infections are asymptomatic, acquired toxoplasmosis can manifest as a mononucleosis-like illness with fever, chills, headache, and regional lymphadenopathy.[80] Hepatomegaly, splenomegaly, and minimal elevations of serum aminotransferase levels are uncommon findings.[81,82] Infections of immunocompromised hosts can result in pneumonia, myocarditis, encephalitis, and, rarely, hepatitis.[79,83] Toxoplasmosis can produce atypical lymphocytosis, an otherwise unusual feature of parasitic disease.

Diagnosis

The diagnosis is best made by detecting specific IgM or IgG antibody using highly specific indirect immunofluorescence or an enzyme immunoassay.[84] Specialized histologic staining techniques and tissue culture systems can provide adjunctive diagnostic support. PCR analysis of serum and liver also can be helpful in ambiguous cases.[85]

Treatment

Antibiotic therapy should be administered to all persons with severe symptomatic infection and to immunocompromised or pregnant patients with acute uncomplicated infection. Treatment consists of a combination of pyrimethamine and sulfadiazine, plus folinic acid to minimize hematologic toxicity, for 2 to 4 weeks.[79]

Helminths (see also Chapter 114)

Nematodes (Roundworms)

Nematodes are nonsegmented roundworms that have a thick cuticle covering the body. Toxocariasis and capillariasis manifest with major hepatobiliary features, whereas ascariasis, strongyloidiasis, and trichinosis affect the liver less frequently or less severely.

Toxocariasis

Toxocara canis and *Toxocara cati* infect dogs and cats, respectively. Infection occurs worldwide, especially in children, and is acquired when embryonated eggs in soil or contaminated food are ingested. The eggs hatch in the small intestine and release larvae that penetrate the intestinal wall, enter the portal venous circulation, and reach the liver and systemic circulation. Blocked by narrowing vascular channels, the immature worms bore through vessel walls and migrate through the tissues, where they cause hemorrhagic, necrotic, and secondary inflammatory responses. When larvae become trapped in tissue, they provoke granuloma formation with a predominance of eosinophils. Tissue larvae may remain in inflammatory capsules or granulomas for months to years. The liver, brain, and eye are affected most frequently.[86]

Clinical Features. Most infected persons are asymptomatic. Two clinical syndromes are recognized: (1) visceral larva migrans and (2) "occult" infections associated with nonspecific symptoms, including abdominal pain, anorexia, fever, and wheezing.[86]

Visceral larva migrans is seen most commonly in children with a history of pica. Findings include fever, hepatomegaly, urticaria, leukocytosis with persistent eosinophilia, hypergammaglobulinemia, and elevated blood group isohemagglutinins.[86] Toxocariasis has been implicated in the development of chronic cholestatic hepatitis[87] as well as pyogenic liver abscess.[88] Pulmonary manifestations include asthma and pneumonitis. Neurologic involvement can result in focal or generalized seizures, encephalopathy, and abnormal behavior.[86] Ocular larva migrans often is associated with granulomatous lesions, vitritis, uveitis, visual loss, and strabismus.[89]

Diagnosis. The possibility of toxocariasis should be considered in persons with a history of pica, exposure to dogs or cats, and persistent eosinophilia.[90] Stool studies are not useful for toxocariasis, because these organisms do not produce eggs in humans, nor do they remain in the GI tract. A definitive diagnosis is made by identification of the larvae in affected tissues, although blind biopsies are not routinely recommended.[91] The finding of an eosinophilic granuloma may be specific for visceral larva migrans.[92] A liver biopsy may be necessary to differentiate visceral larva migrans from hepatic capillariasis (see later). A strongly positive result on an ELISA using larval antigens provides support for the diagnosis.

Treatment. Treatment is primarily supportive because visceral larva migrans is generally self-limited. If required, antihelminthic therapy with albendazole, 10 mg/kg/day in 2 divided doses for 5 days, or mebendazole, 100 to 200 mg twice daily for 5 days, may be used. Severe pulmonary, cardiac, ophthalmologic, or neurologic manifestations may warrant use of systemic glucocorticoids.[91]

Hepatic Capillariasis

Human infection with *Capillaria hepatica* is rare. Infection with *C. hepatica* is acquired by ingesting soil, food, or water contaminated with embryonated eggs. Larvae released in the cecum penetrate the intestinal mucosa, enter the portal venous circulation, and lodge in the liver. Four weeks after infection, adult worms disintegrate, releasing eggs into the hepatic parenchyma and producing an intense inflammatory reaction with macrophages, eosinophils, and giant cells. Resolution is accompanied by marked peri-egg fibrosis.

Clinical Features. Hepatic capillariasis typically manifests as acute or subacute hepatitis. Findings include fever, nausea, vomiting, diarrhea or constipation, anorexia, myalgias, arthralgias, tender hepatomegaly, and occasionally splenomegaly. Laboratory investigation may reveal leukocytosis with eosinophilia; mild elevations of serum AST, alkaline phosphatase, and bilirubin levels; anemia; and an increased erythrocyte sedimentation rate. A chest x-ray may show pneumonitis.[93]

Diagnosis. The diagnosis is established by detection of adult worms or eggs in the liver (Fig. 84-2). Histologic findings in the liver include necrosis, fibrosis, and granulomas.[94] A finding of *C. hepatica* eggs in stools is not indicative of acute infection and probably reflects passage of undercooked liver from an infected animal.

Treatment. Treatment of hepatic capillariasis has, in general, been unsuccessful. Anecdotal benefit has been reported in end-stage cases with therapy with dithiazanine iodide, sodium stibogluconate, albendazole, or thiabendazole.[94]

Ascariasis

Ascaris lumbricoides infects at least 1 billion persons, particularly in areas of lower socioeconomic standing.[95] Humans are infected by ingesting embryonated eggs, usually adherent to raw vegetables. The eggs hatch in the small intestine, and the larvae penetrate the mucosa, enter the portal circulation, and reach the liver, pulmonary artery, and lungs; they grow in the alveolar spaces, are regurgitated and swallowed, and become mature adults in the intestine 2 to 3 months after ingestion. Then the cycle repeats itself.

Clinical Features. Symptoms generally occur in persons with a large worm burden; most infected persons are asymptomatic. Cough, fever, dyspnea, wheezing, substernal chest discomfort, and hepatomegaly may occur in the first 2 weeks. Chronic infection more frequently is characterized by episodic epigastric or periumbilical pain. If the worm burden is particularly heavy, small bowel complications such as obstruction, intussusception, volvulus, perforation, or appendicitis may occur.[96] Fragments of disintegrating worms within the biliary tract can serve as nidi for the development of biliary calculi.[97] Preexisting disease of the biliary tract or pancreatic duct can predispose the patient to migration of the worm into the bile ducts, with development of obstructive jaundice, cholangitis, or intrahepatic abscesses.[95,98]

Diagnosis. A history of regurgitating a worm or passing a large worm (15 to 40 cm long) in the stool suggests ascariasis. In the absence of such a history, the diagnosis is made by identification of characteristic eggs in stool specimens. Larvae may also be identified in sputum and gastric washings and in liver and lung biopsy specimens. In patients with biliary or pancreatic symptoms, US, MRCP, or ERCP is performed. ERCP also allows extraction of the worm.[99] A chest x-ray may show an infiltrate, and eosinophilia may be present.

Treatment. One of the following regimens may be used: (1) a single dose of albendazole, 400 mg; (2) mebendazole, 100 mg twice daily for 3 days; (3) pyrantel pamoate, 11 mg/kg to a maximum of 1 g; or (4) a single dose of ivermectin, 200 µg/kg.[100] Intestinal or biliary obstruction may require endoscopic or surgical intervention.

Strongyloidiasis

Strongyloides stercoralis is prevalent in the tropics and subtropics, southern and eastern Europe, and the United States. Infection is usually asymptomatic. Humans are infected by the filariform larvae, which penetrate intact skin, are carried to the lungs, migrate through the alveoli, and are swallowed to reach the intestine, where maturation ensues. Autoinfection can occur if the rhabditiform larvae transform into infective filariform larvae in the intestine; reinfection occurs by penetration of the bowel wall or perianal skin. Symptomatic infection results from a heavy infectious burden or infection in an immunocompromised patient. In the latter case, a hyperinfection syndrome may result from dissemination of filariform larvae into tissues that usually are not infected.[101]

Clinical Features. Acute infection can lead to a pruritic eruption, followed by fever, cough, wheezing, abdominal pain, diarrhea, and eosinophilia. In immunocompromised patients, the hyperinfection syndrome may be characterized by invasion of any organ, including the liver, lung, and brain. Hyperinfection should be considered particularly in the setting of sepsis caused by multiple organisms found in intestinal flora, a consequence of burrowing of larvae through the intestinal mucosa.[102] When the liver is affected, features include jaundice and cholestatic liver biochemical test abnormalities. A liver biopsy specimen may show periportal inflammation, eosinophilic granulomatous hepatitis, or both. Larvae may be observed in intrahepatic bile canaliculi, lymphatic vessels, and small branches of the portal vein.[101]

Diagnosis. Serologic tests include counterimmunoelectrophoresis and ELISA and can be used for post-treatment evaluation.[103] The diagnosis of active infection is firm when larvae are identified in the stool or intestinal biopsy specimens. An

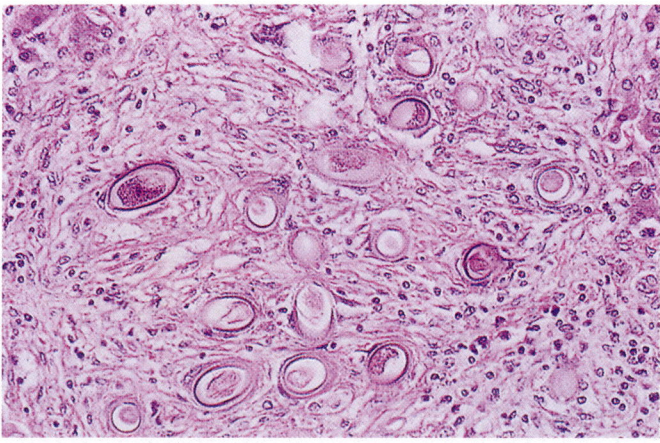

FIGURE 84-2. Histopathology of hepatic capillariasis. Intrahepatic granulomas may be seen surrounding numerous eggs. (H&E.) *(From Burt AD, Portmann BC, Ferrell LD, editors. MacSween's pathology of the liver. 6th ed. London: Churchill Livingstone; 2012. p 436.)*

obstructive hepatobiliary picture in a person with known strongyloidiasis should alert the clinician to the possibility of dissemination.

Treatment. For treatment of acute infection, the drug of choice is ivermectin, 200 mg/kg/day for 2 days. Clearance rates are high. An alternative agent is albendazole, 400 mg/day for 3 days for adults and children older than 2 years of age, but retreatment may be necessary, and this drug is less effective for disseminated disease. The hyperinfection syndrome requires longer courses of treatment than those used for the primary acute infection.[104]

Trichinosis

Humans may be infected with *Trichinella spiralis* by eating raw or undercooked pork bearing larvae, which are released in the small intestine, penetrate the mucosa, and disseminate through the systemic circulation. Larvae can be found in the myocardium, cerebrospinal fluid, brain, and, less commonly, liver and gallbladder. The larvae then reenter the circulation and reach striated muscle, where they become encapsulated.

Clinical Features. Clinical manifestations occur when the worm burden is high and include diarrhea, fever, myalgias, periorbital edema, and leukocytosis with marked eosinophilia. Rarely, larvae can be seen invading hepatic sinusoids on examination of a liver biopsy specimen. Jaundice may result from biliary obstruction. Hepatic complications may be associated with fatal cases.[105]

Diagnosis. The diagnosis is suggested by a characteristic history in a patient with fever and eosinophilia. Serologic assays for antibody to *Trichinella* may not be helpful in the acute phase of infection but can be useful after 2 weeks.[106] Muscle biopsy may help to confirm the diagnosis. DNA-based tests are investigational.

Treatment. Treatment consists of glucocorticoids to relieve allergic symptoms, followed by antihelminthic treatment with albendazole, 400 mg twice daily for 10 to 15 days, or mebendazole, 200 mg/day for 10 to 15 days.[106]

Trematodes (Flukes)

Schistosomiasis (Bilharziasis)

About 230 million persons worldwide are infected with trematodes of the genus *Schistosoma*. *Schistosoma mansoni* is found in the Western Hemisphere, Africa, and the Middle East; *S. haematobium* is found in Africa and the Middle East; *S. japonicum* and *S. mekongi* are found in the Far East; and *S. intercalatum* is found in parts of central Africa. The last 2 species are much less common than the other 3 and cause liver disease and colonic disease, respectively.[107,107a]

The Schistosomal Life Cycle. The infectious cycle is initiated by penetration of the skin by free cercariae in fresh water (Fig. 84-3). The cercariae reach the pulmonary vessels within 24 hours, pass through the lungs, and reach the liver, where they lodge, develop into adults, and mate. Adult worms then migrate to their ultimate destinations in the inferior mesenteric venules (*S. mansoni*), superior mesenteric venules (*S. japonicum*), or veins around the bladder (*S. haematobium*). These locations correlate with the clinical complications associated with each species. Each female fluke can lay 300 to 3000 eggs daily. The eggs are deposited in the terminal venules and eventually migrate into the lumen of the involved organ, after which they are expelled in the stool or urine. Eggs remaining in the organ provoke a robust granulomatous response. Excreted eggs hatch immediately in fresh water and liberate early intermediate miracidia that infect their snail hosts. The miracidia transform into cercariae within the snails and then

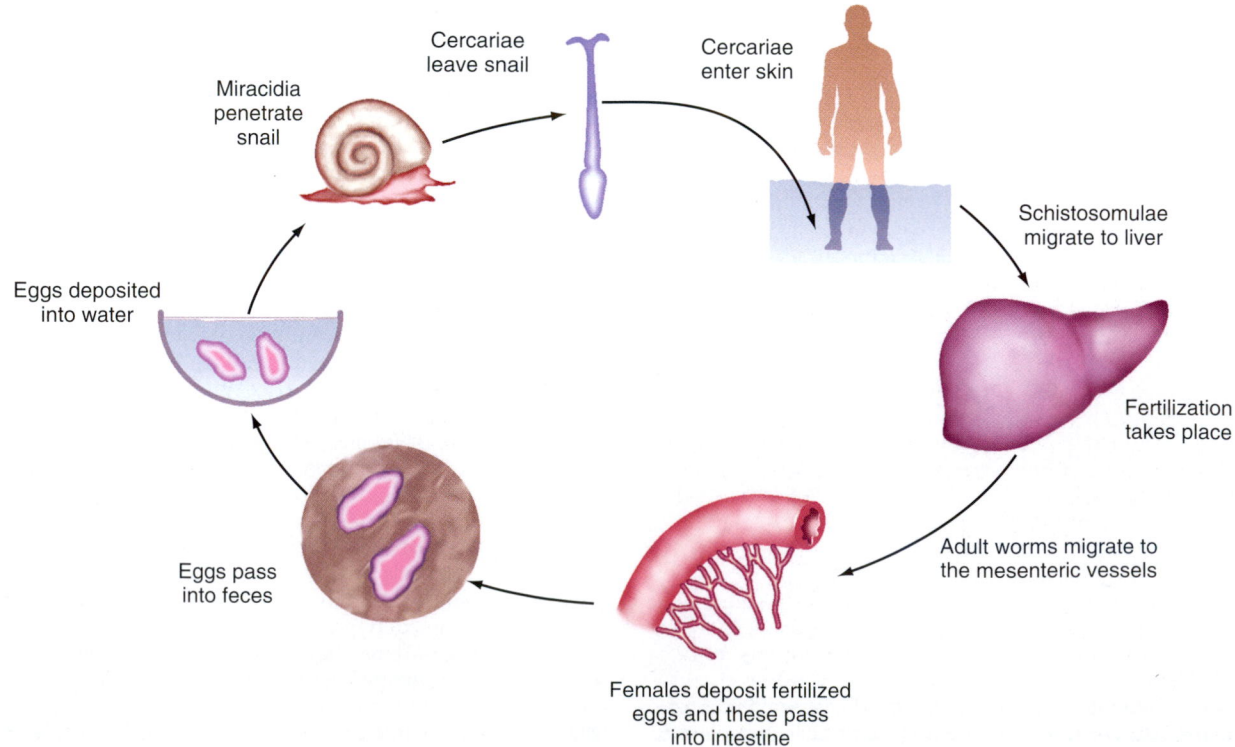

FIGURE 84-3. The life cycle of *Schistosoma* species. *(From Gitlin N, Strauss R. Atlas of clinical hepatology. Philadelphia: WB Saunders; 1995. p 72.)*

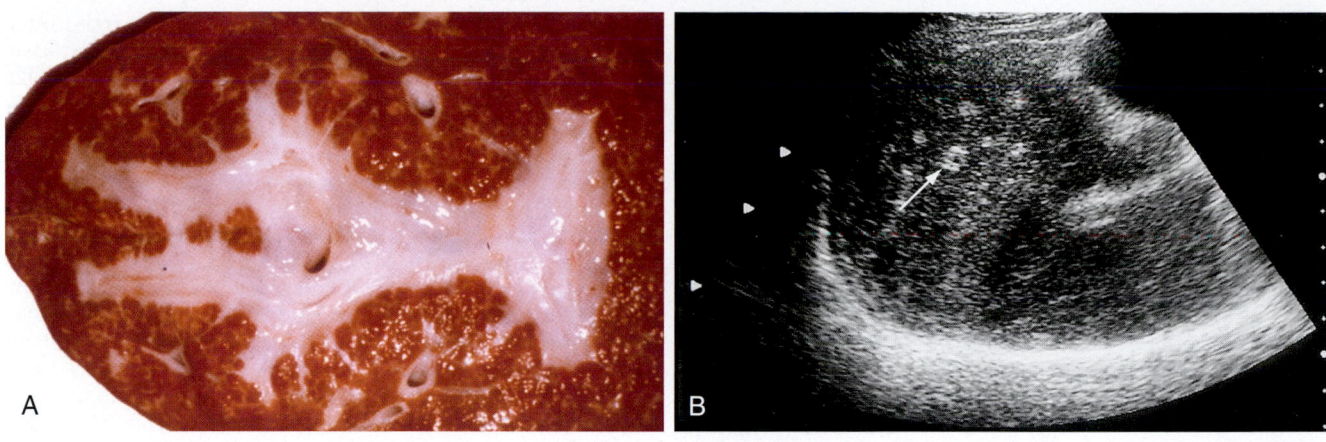

FIGURE 84-4. Pipestem fibrosis. *A*, Liver resection specimen demonstrating characteristic pipestem fibrosis due to long-term infection with *Schistosoma mansoni*. *B*, US image of the liver from a patient with schistosomiasis demonstrating the pipestem fibrosis, seen as echodense circles surrounding vessels *(arrow)*. (A, *Courtesy Dr. Fiona Graeme-Cook, Boston, Mass.;* B, *courtesy Dr. Mark Feldman, Dallas, Tex.)*

are released into the water, from which they may again infect humans.[107]

Clinical Features. Acute toxemic schistosomiasis (Katayama syndrome or Katayama fever), presumably a consequence of the host immunologic response to mature worms and eggs, occurs approximately 4 to 6 weeks after exposure. Manifestations include headache, fever, chills, cough, diarrhea, myalgias, arthralgias, tender hepatomegaly, and eosinophilia.

Untreated acute schistosomiasis invariably progresses to chronic disease. Mesenteric infection leads to hepatic complications, including periportal fibrosis, presinusoidal occlusion, and, ultimately, portal hypertension, as a result of the inflammatory reaction to eggs deposited in the liver. The development of periportal fibrosis appears to be related to production of TNF-α.[108] The lungs and central nervous system may be affected when eggs or adult worms pass through the liver into the systemic circulation, especially in *S. japonicum* infection; pulmonary hypertension and cor pulmonale may result.[109] With severe schistosomal infection, portal hypertension becomes progressive, leading to gastroesophageal varices, splenomegaly, and rarely ascites.

Chronic schistosomal infection may be complicated by increased susceptibility to *Salmonella* infections.[110] Hepatitis B or hepatitis C viral coinfection also is common in persons living in endemic areas and may accelerate the progression of liver disease and development of hepatocellular carcinoma.[111] In African intestinal schistosomiasis, pseudopolyps of the colon may develop, leading in some cases to protein-losing colopathy and formation of an inflammatory mass in the descending colon.

Laboratory findings in chronic schistosomiasis include anemia from recurrent luminal GI bleeding or hypersplenism, leukocytosis with eosinophilia, an elevated erythrocyte sedimentation rate, and increased serum IgE levels. Results of liver biochemical tests generally are normal until the disease is at an advanced stage.

Diagnosis. The possibility of acute schistosomiasis should be considered in a patient with a history of exposure, abdominal pain, diarrhea, and fever. Multiple stool examinations for ova may be required to confirm the diagnosis because results frequently are negative in the early phase of disease. Serologic testing using counterimmunoelectrophoresis or ELISA cannot distinguish between past infection and active disease but may be useful in a returned traveler. Sigmoidoscopy or colonoscopy may reveal rectosigmoid or transverse colon

involvement and may be useful in chronic disease, when few eggs pass in the feces. US and liver biopsy are useful for demonstrating periportal ("pipestem" or "clay pipestem") fibrosis (Fig. 84-4), but not for diagnosing acute infection because of their insensitivity for detecting schistosomal eggs.[112] CT may show low-attenuation rings around main portal vein branches with marked enhancement with contrast.[113]

Treatment. Praziquantel, 40 mg/kg for *S. mansoni* or *S. haematobium* and 60 mg/kg for *S. japonicum* or *S. mekongi* given in 1 day in 2 to 3 divided doses 4 hours apart, is the therapeutic agent of choice. Oxamniquine is an effective alternative agent for *S. mansoni* infection in patients who cannot tolerate praziquantel, but it is no longer readily available. Treatment of acute toxemic schistosomiasis often requires prednisone to suppress immune-mediated helminthicidal or drug reactions, in conjunction with praziquantel at the dose appropriate for the particular species for 3 to 6 days.[107] Retreatment after 2 to 3 months is often necessary after Katayama fever.[114]

Band ligation or injection sclerotherapy of varices is effective in controlling variceal bleeding (see Chapter 92). Management of advanced chronic schistosomal liver disease may require placement of a distal splenorenal shunt or esophagogastric devascularization with splenectomy. Fortunately, since the advent of praziquantel, complicated schistosomal liver disease has become uncommon.

Fascioliasis

Fascioliasis is endemic in parts of Europe and Latin America, North Africa, Asia, the Western Pacific, and some parts of the United States. Fascioliasis is caused by the sheep liver fluke *Fasciola hepatica*. Eggs passed in the feces of infected mammals into fresh water give rise to miracidia that penetrate snails and eventually emerge as mobile cercariae, which attach to aquatic plants such as watercress. Hosts become infected when they consume plants containing encysted metacercariae, which then bore into the intestinal wall, enter the abdominal cavity, penetrate the hepatic capsule, and eventually settle in the bile ducts, where they attain maturity. Mature flukes release eggs that are passed in the host's feces to complete the life cycle.[115]

Clinical Features. Three phases (or syndromes) are recognized: acute or invasive, chronic latent, and chronic obstructive.[116] The acute phase corresponds to the migration of young flukes through the liver and is marked by fever, pain in the RUQ, and eosinophilia. Urticaria with dermatographia and nonspecific GI symptoms are common. Physical examination often reveals fever and a tender, enlarged liver. Splenomegaly is seen in as many as 25% of cases, but jaundice is rare and liver biochemical test abnormalities are mild.[117] Eosinophilia can be profound, with eosinophils sometimes exceeding 80% of the differential leukocyte count.[118]

The latent phase corresponds to the settling of the flukes into the bile ducts and can last for months to years. Affected patients may experience vague GI symptoms. Eosinophilia persists, and fever can occur.[117]

The chronic obstructive phase is a consequence of intrahepatic and extrahepatic bile ductal inflammation and hyperplasia evoked by adult flukes. Recurrent biliary pain, cholangitis, cholelithiasis, and biliary obstruction may result. Blood loss from epithelial injury occurs, but overt hemobilia is rare. Liver biochemical testing commonly demonstrates a pattern suggestive of biliary obstruction.[119] Long-term infection may lead to biliary cirrhosis and secondary sclerosing cholangitis, but no convincing association with biliary tract or hepatic malignancy has been demonstrated.[120]

Diagnosis. The diagnosis should be considered in a patient with prolonged fever, abdominal pain, diarrhea, tender hepatomegaly, and eosinophilia. Because eggs are not passed during the acute phase, diagnosis depends on the detection of antibody by counterimmunoelectrophoresis or ELISA. In the latent and chronic phases, a definitive diagnosis is based on the detection of eggs in stool, duodenal aspirate specimens, or bile.[121] On occasion, US or ERCP demonstrate flukes in the gallbladder and bile duct.[122] If one member of a family is diagnosed with fascioliasis, all household members should be evaluated.

Hepatic histologic findings include necrosis and granulomas with eosinophilic infiltrates and Charcot-Leyden crystals. Eosinophilic abscesses, epithelial hyperplasia of the bile ducts, and periportal fibrosis may be seen.[123]

Treatment. The drug of choice is triclabendazole, 10 mg/kg given once orally. Praziquantel, mebendazole, and albendazole are not effective for fascioliasis. Other medications that are potentially efficacious are bithionol and nitazoxanide.[115]

Clonorchiasis and Opisthorchiasis

Clonorchis sinensis, *Opisthorchis viverrini*, and *Opisthorchis felineus* are trematodes of the family Opisthorchiidae. Infection by *C. sinensis* and *O. viverrini* is widespread in East and Southeast Asia and is linked to lower socioeconomic status. *O. felineus* infects humans and domestic animals in Eastern Europe. All 3 have similar life cycles and result in similar clinical manifestations. Eggs are passed in the feces into fresh water, consumed by snails, and hatch as free-swimming cercariae, which seek and penetrate fish or crayfish and encyst in skin or muscle as metacercariae. The mammalian host is infected when it consumes raw or undercooked fish. The metacercariae excyst in the small intestine and migrate into the ampulla of Vater and bile ducts, where they mature into adult flukes. Infection can be maintained for 2 decades or longer.[121]

Clinical Features. In general, acute infection is clinically silent. Occasional symptoms include fever, abdominal pain, and diarrhea. Chronic manifestations correlate with the fluke burden and are dominated by hepatobiliary features: fever, pain in the RUQ, tender hepatomegaly, and eosinophilia. If the worm burden in the bile ducts is heavy, chronic or intermittent biliary obstruction can ensue, with frequent cholelithiasis, cholecystitis, jaundice, and, ultimately, recurrent pyogenic cholangitis (see Chapter 68). Liver biochemical test results, especially serum alkaline phosphatase and bilirubin levels, are elevated. Long-standing infection leads to exuberant

inflammation, resulting in periportal fibrosis, marked biliary epithelial hyperplasia and dysplasia, and, ultimately, a substantially increased risk of cholangiocarcinoma.[121,124] Cholangiocarcinoma resulting from clonorchiasis or opisthorchiasis tends to be multicentric and arises in the secondary biliary radicles of the hilum of the liver. Cholangiocarcinoma should be suspected in infected persons with weight loss, jaundice, epigastric pain, or an abdominal mass (see Chapter 69).

Diagnosis. The diagnosis of clonorchiasis or opisthorchiasis is made by detection of characteristic fluke eggs in the stool, except late in the disease when biliary obstruction has supervened. In these cases, the diagnosis is made by identifying flukes in the bile ducts or gallbladder at surgery or in bile obtained by postoperative drainage or percutaneous aspiration (Fig. 84-5). Endoscopic or intraoperative cholangiography reveals slender, uniform filling defects within intrahepatic ducts that are alternately dilated and strictured, mimicking sclerosing cholangitis. Serologic methods of diagnosis cannot distinguish between past or current infection.[115]

Treatment. All patients with clonorchiasis or opisthorchiasis should receive praziquantel, which is uniformly effective in a dose of 75 mg/kg in 3 divided doses over 1 day. Side effects are uncommon and include headache, dizziness, and nausea. After treatment, dead flukes may be seen in the stool or biliary drainage. When the burden of infecting organisms is high, the dead flukes and surrounding debris or stones may cause biliary obstruction, necessitating endoscopic or surgical drainage.[115]

Cestodes (Tapeworms)

Echinococcosis

Infections with *Echinococcus granulosus* can be found worldwide in areas where dogs are used to help raise livestock. *Echinococcus multilocularis* is distributed in northern North America and Eurasia, whereas *Echinococcus vogeli* is found in scattered areas of Central and Latin America.

The Echinococcal Life Cycle. Infection occurs when humans eat vegetables contaminated by dog feces that contain embryonated eggs. The eggs hatch in the small intestine and liberate oncospheres that penetrate the mucosa and migrate via vessels or lymphatics to distant sites. The liver is the most common destination (70%), followed by the lungs (20%), kidney, spleen, brain, and bone. In these organs, a hydatid

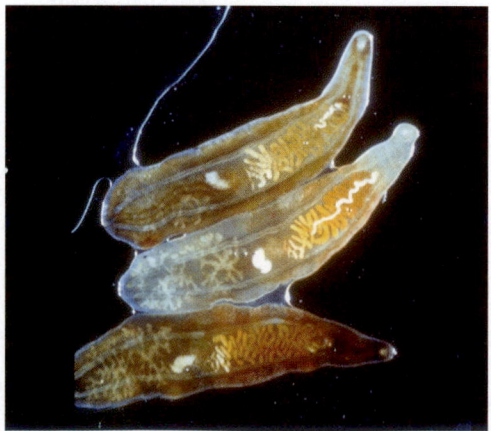

FIGURE 84-5. *Clonorchis sinensis.* (Courtesy Dr. Fiona Graeme-Cook, Boston, Mass.)

cyst develops by vesiculation and produces thousands of protoscolices. The cyst wall contains 3 layers: an outer adventitial layer, which is host-derived and can calcify, and intermediate acellular and inner germinal layers, which are worm-derived. A protoscolex is produced asexually within small secondary cysts that develop from the inner layer. Rupture of the hydatid cyst releases the viable protoscolices, which set up daughter cysts in secondary sites. The adult *Echinococcus* tapeworm consists of a scolex, which contains a rostellum with 20 to 50 hooklets and 4 suckers, a neck, and an immature, mature, and gravid proglottid. Dogs acquire the infection by consuming organs of sheep, cattle, or other livestock bearing the hydatid cyst.

Clinical Features. Most patients with a hydatid cyst in the liver have no symptoms. As the cysts of *E. granulosus* grow within the liver (Fig. 84-6), they begin to cause low-grade fever, pain, tender hepatomegaly (usually affecting the right hepatic lobe), and eosinophilia. If the cysts grow large enough, they may rupture spontaneously or after trauma into the lungs, thereby leading to dyspnea and hemoptysis. More extensive rupture into the peritoneum or lungs may lead to a life-threatening anaphylactic reaction to the cyst contents. Rupture into the biliary tract can cause cholangitis and obstruction; marked eosinophilia may be present. Superinfection of the hepatic cysts can lead to pyogenic liver abscesses in up to 20% of patients with hepatic disease. Rare complications of hydatid cysts or cyst rupture include pancreatitis, portal hypertension, Budd-Chiari syndrome, and rupture into the pericardial sac.

E. multilocularis is highly invasive; infection leads to formation of solid masses in the liver that are easily confused with cirrhosis or carcinoma. *Alveolar hydatid disease* is the term applied to hepatic nodules that appear on microscopy as alveoli-like microvesicles.[125] Daughter cysts bud from the germinal membrane in an uncontrolled manner, with "invasion" of the surrounding liver parenchyma by the scolices. Infection of bile ducts and vessels and necrosis of parenchyma may result in cholangitis, liver abscess, sepsis, portal hypertension, hepatic vein occlusion, and biliary cirrhosis. Unfortunately, infection generally is not diagnosed until the lesions are inoperable because of extensive invasion or distant metastatic disease, and mortality rates are high, approaching 90%.[125]

Infection with *E. vogeli* has clinical features intermediate between those of infections caused by the other 2 species and is characterized by multiple fluid-filled cysts containing daughter cysts and protoscolices. Although not as aggressive as *E. multilocularis* infection, *E. vogeli* infection can spread to contiguous sites.

Diagnosis. A history of exposure in a patient with hepatomegaly and an abdominal mass is highly suggestive of hepatic echinococcosis, but the most important diagnostic tools are imaging and serology. Ring-like calcifications in up to one fourth of hepatic cysts are visible on plain abdominal films in patients infected with *E. granulosus*. The sensitivity and specificity of both US and CT in confirming the diagnosis are high (Fig. 84-7).[126] Both modalities can demonstrate intracystic septations and daughter cyst formation in about half of the cysts. Contrast-enhanced CT may display avascular cysts with ring enhancement. Percutaneous aspiration of the cyst had traditionally been discouraged because of concern about anaphylactic reactions. Encouraging reports, however, suggest that under carefully controlled conditions, with use of thin needles and concomitant antihelminthic therapy, percutaneous aspiration for diagnosis and therapy may be safe.[127,128] The detection of protoscolices or acid-fast hooklets in the cyst fluid confirms the diagnosis.[129] An ELISA is the best serologic assay for diagnosis, with a sensitivity of 84% to 90%.[130] Assays for detecting circulating antigen are likely to provide additional diagnostic benefit in the future. The Casoni skin test, used in the past, is nonspecific and no longer recommended.

E. multilocularis infection can be diagnosed with a combination of ELISA and CT, which often shows scattered areas of calcified necrotic tissue. In *E. vogeli* infection, CT demonstrates polycystic lesions in the liver or peritoneal space.

Treatment. In the past, accessible cysts in younger persons were always treated surgically, and surgery is still considered the preferred treatment in many cases. The goal has been removal of the cestode without disruption of cyst contents. Care must be taken to isolate the cyst and to inject cidal agents

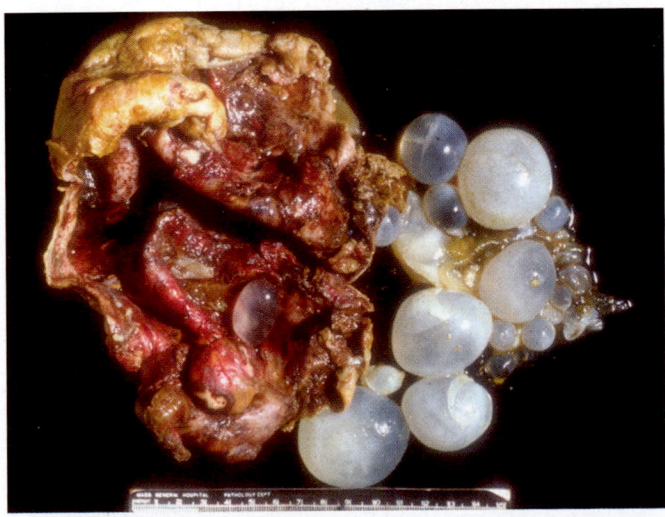

FIGURE 84-6. Liver resection specimen of a hydatid cyst caused by *Echinococcus granulosus*. Multiple daughter cysts are seen. (*Courtesy Dr. Fiona Graeme-Cook, Boston, Mass.*)

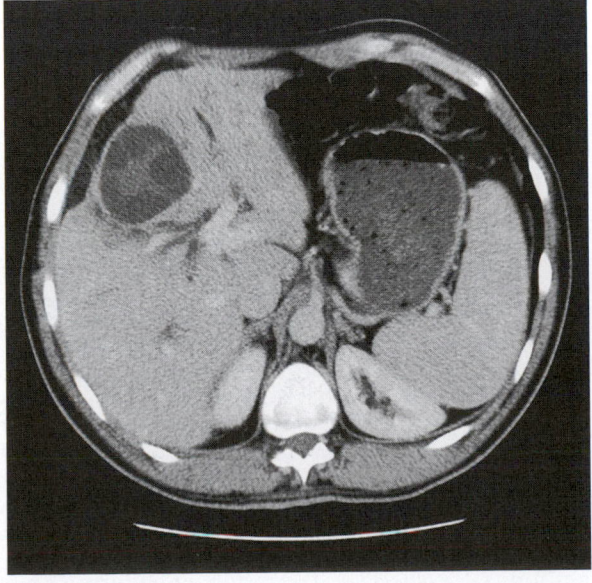

FIGURE 84-7. CT showing the typical appearance of a hydatid cyst in the liver. (*Courtesy Dr. Mukesh Harisinghani, Boston, Mass.*)

before the cyst is aspirated. Successful approaches have included cystectomy, endocystectomy, omentoplasty, and marsupialization. A laparoscopic approach is feasible in some cases. In complicated cases, hepatic lobectomy or hemihepatectomy may be necessary. Calcified cysts need not be removed.

Promising data indicate that careful percutaneous drainage is a safe and effective alternative to surgery for the treatment of complicated cysts.[131] In addition to surgery or drainage, administration of an antihelminthic, such as albendazole, 10 mg/kg/day for 8 weeks, is recommended.[132] Puncture, *a*spiration, *i*njection (of a scolicidal agent), and *re*-aspiration (PAIR) can be performed safely with long-term control of echinococcal cysts.[128] Injection of hydatid liver cysts with albendazole has also been described.[127] Therefore, nonsurgical approaches are now available for management of hydatid cysts. The decision between surgical and nonsurgical techniques depends on the extent and type of lesions.[133] Cysts that cannot be treated surgically or percutaneously should be treated with albendazole, preferably, or mebendazole. Large doses and prolonged treatment are required (e.g., albendazole 10 mg/kg daily in 2 divided doses for 28 days, repeated 3 or 4 times, with 2-week breaks between courses).

Surgical resection is curative in up to one third of cases of *E. multilocularis* infection. In most cases the disease is advanced when the diagnosis is made. In such cases, palliative drainage procedures or long-term treatment with albendazole or other benzimidazole carbamates may prolong survival.[125,134] Surgery appears to be the most effective approach to the management of *E. vogeli* infection.

FUNGI

Candidiasis

Candida species may cause invasive systemic infection with hepatic involvement in severely immunocompromised persons (see Chapters 34 and 35). The liver can become infected by *C. albicans* and related species in the setting of disseminated multiorgan disease. Most disseminated infections occur in leukemic patients undergoing high-dose chemotherapy and become clinically evident during the period of recovery from severe neutropenia. In several series, hepatic candidiasis was present in 51% to 91% of predominantly leukemic patients with disseminated candidiasis.[135,136] Disease is often overwhelming, with a high mortality rate.[136]

Other, less frequent, presentations in the compromised host include isolated or focal hepatic or hepatosplenic candidiasis.[137] Focal candidiasis is believed to result from colonization of the GI tract by *Candida*, which disseminates locally following the onset of neutropenia and mucosal injury caused by high-dose chemotherapy.[137] Resulting fungemia of the portal vein seeds the liver and leads to formation of hepatic microabscesses and macroabscesses.

In either focal or disseminated candidiasis involving the liver, clinical features include fever, abdominal pain and distention, nausea, vomiting, diarrhea, and tender hepatomegaly. The serum alkaline phosphatase level is almost invariably elevated, with varying elevations in serum aminotransferase and bilirubin levels. CT and MRI of the abdomen are sensitive tests to detect hepatic or splenic abscesses, which often are multicentric (Fig. 84-8).[138,139] In cases diagnosed antemortem, liver biopsy or laparoscopy reveals macroscopic nodules, necrosis with microabscesses, and characteristic yeast or hyphal forms of *Candida*.[140] The results of cultures of biopsy material are negative in most cases. PCR methodology has been used to diagnose hepatic candidiasis.[141]

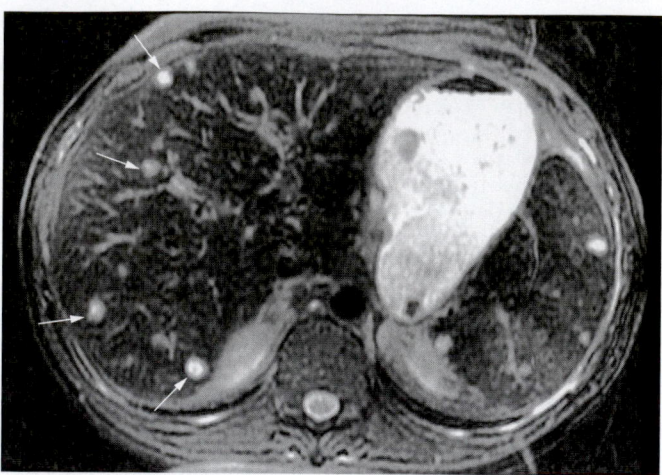

FIGURE 84-8. T2-weighted MRI showing the characteristic small high-intensity foci *(arrows)* of hepatosplenic candidiasis. *(Courtesy Dr. Mukesh Harisinghani, Boston, Mass.)*

Response rates to therapy with IV amphotericin B are better (almost 60%) for focal hepatic candidiasis than for disseminated disease. The success of treatment is currently far from optimal, however. Alternatives to amphotericin B are fluconazole, liposomal amphotericin, and IV echinocandins such as caspofungin, micafungin, or anidulafungin.[142] Adjunctive glucocorticoids may speed recovery from the inflammatory response that accompanies disseminated candidiasis as neutrophils return.[143] The widespread use of prophylactic fluconazole in high-risk patients has resulted in lower rates of fatal visceral fungal infection while promoting a shift toward infections caused by other fungi resistant to this agent.[144]

Histoplasmosis

Infection with *Histoplasma capsulatum* is acquired through the respiratory tract and in most cases is confined to the lungs. Severely immunocompromised persons (e.g., those with AIDS), however, are predisposed to disseminated histoplasmosis (see Chapter 34). The liver can be invaded in both acute and chronic progressive disseminated histoplasmosis. Fever, oropharyngeal ulcers, hepatomegaly, and splenomegaly may be present in patients with chronic disease.[145] In children with acute hepatic disease, which appears to be an extension of primary pulmonary infection, marked hepatosplenomegaly is universal and is associated with high fever and lymphadenopathy. In one series of 111 cases of disseminated histoplasmosis, serum ALT levels were elevated in 39%, AST levels were elevated in 27%, and alkaline phosphatase levels were greater than 200 U/L in 55%.[146] Hepatosplenomegaly is present in approximately 30% of adults with acute disease (often the AIDS-defining illness).

Yeast forms can be identified in liver biopsy specimens with standard H&E staining. The silver methenamine method is superior for detecting yeast forms in areas of caseating necrosis or in granulomas. The organism is difficult to culture and almost never grows from biopsy specimens. Serologic testing for complement-fixing antibodies is therefore helpful in confirming the diagnosis. In immunocompromised persons who may not be capable of mounting an antibody response, detection of *H. capsulatum* antigens in urine and serum can be useful.[147] Treatment options include therapy with amphotericin B, fluconazole, or itraconazole.

LIVER ABSCESS

Pyogenic

In the past, most cases of pyogenic liver abscess were a consequence of appendicitis complicated by pylephlebitis (portal vein inflammation) in a young patient. This presentation is uncommon today as a result of earlier diagnosis and effective antibiotic therapy. Most cases now are cryptogenic or occur in older men with underlying biliary tract disease.[148] Predisposing conditions include malignancy, immunosuppression, diabetes mellitus, and previous biliary surgery or interventional endoscopy.

Pathogenesis

Infections of the biliary tract (e.g., cholangitis, cholecystitis) are the most common identifiable source of liver abscess. Infection may spread to the liver from the bile duct, along a penetrating vessel, or from an adjacent septic focus (including pylephlebitis). Pyogenic liver abscess may arise as a late complication of endoscopic sphincterotomy for bile duct stones or within 3 to 6 weeks of a surgical biliary-intestinal anastomosis.[149] Pyogenic liver abscesses may complicate recurrent pyogenic cholangitis, which is found predominantly in East and Southeast Asia and is characterized by recurring episodes of cholangitis, intrahepatic stone formation, and, in many cases, biliary parasitic infections (see earlier and Chapter 68). Less commonly, liver abscess is a complication of bacteremia arising from underlying abdominal disease, such as diverticulitis, appendicitis, perforated or penetrating peptic ulcer, GI malignancy, IBD, or peritonitis, or rarely from bacterial endocarditis or penetration of a foreign body through the wall of the colon. The risk of liver abscess may be increased in patients with underlying diabetes mellitus or cirrhosis.[150,151] Occasionally, a pyogenic liver abscess may be the presentation of a hepatocellular or gallbladder carcinoma or a complication of chemoembolization or percutaneous ablation of a hepatic neoplasm.[152]

In approximately 40% of cases of pyogenic liver abscess, no obvious source of infection can be identified. Oral flora have been proposed to be a potential source in such cases, particularly in patients (often alcoholics) with severe periodontal disease.

Microbiology

Most pyogenic liver abscesses are polymicrobial. The bacterial organisms that have been cultured from liver abscesses are listed in Box 84-1. The most frequently isolated organisms are *Escherichia coli* and *Klebsiella, Proteus, Pseudomonas,* and *Streptococcus* species, particularly the *Streptococcus milleri* group. Certain virulent strains of *Klebsiella pneumoniae* can cause liver abscess in the absence of underlying hepatobiliary disease, often with metastatic infection.[153] With improved cultivation methods and earlier diagnosis, the number of cases caused by anaerobic organisms has increased. The most commonly identified anaerobic species are *Bacteroides fragilis* and *Fusobacterium necrophorum*; anaerobic streptococci have also been identified. Pyogenic abscess associated with recurrent pyogenic cholangitis may be caused by *Salmonella typhi*. *Clostridium* and *Actinomyces* species are uncommon causes of liver abscess, and rare cases are caused by *Yersinia enterocolitica, Pasteurella multocida, Haemophilus parainfluenzae,* and *Listeria* species. Septic melioidosis also has been described. Liver abscesses caused by *Staphylococcus aureus* infection are most common in children and patients with septicemia or other conditions associated with impaired host resistance, including

---

BOX 84-1 Organisms That May Be Isolated from the Abscess and the Blood in Patients with a Pyogenic Liver Abscess

Gram-Negative Aerobic Bacteria
Escherichia coli
Klebsiella pneumoniae
Enterobacter spp.
Pseudomonas spp.
Citrobacter spp.
Morganella spp.
Proteus spp.
Salmonella spp.
*Serratia marcescens**
Yersinia spp.*
*Burkholderia pseudomallei**
*Capnocytophaga canimorsus**
*Pasteurella multocida**
*Achromobacter xylosoxidans**

Gram-Positive Aerobic Bacteria
Enterococcus spp.
Streptococcus pyogenes

Staphylococcus aureus
Streptococcus milleri group
*Listeria monocytogenes**
*Bacillus cereus**

Anaerobic Bacteria
Bacteroides spp.
Fusobacterium spp.
Streptococcus spp.
Peptostreptococcus spp.
Peptococcus spp.
Prevotella spp.*
Clostridium spp.*
Actinomyces spp.*

Others
Candida spp.
Mycobacterium tuberculosis

*Rare.

---

chronic granulomatous disease.[154] Fungal abscesses of the liver may occur in immunocompromised hosts, particularly those with a hematologic malignancy (see earlier).

Clinical Features

In the preantibiotic era, patients with a pyogenic liver abscess typically presented with acutely spiking fevers, pain in the RUQ, and, in many cases, shock. After the introduction of antibiotics, the presentation of pyogenic liver abscess became less acute. Today's presentation often is insidious, particularly in older adult patients, and is characterized by malaise, low-grade fever, anorexia, weight loss, and dull abdominal pain that may increase with movement. Symptoms may be present for 1 month or more before a diagnosis is made. Multiple abscesses are typical when biliary disease is the source and are associated with a more acute systemic presentation, often with sepsis and shock, than is the case with solitary abscesses. When an abscess is situated near the dome of the liver, pain may be referred to the right shoulder, or a cough resulting from diaphragmatic irritation or atelectasis may be present.

Physical examination usually discloses fever, hepatomegaly, and liver tenderness, which is accentuated by movement or percussion. Splenomegaly is unusual, except with a chronic abscess. Ascites is rare, and in the absence of cholangitis, jaundice is present only late in the course of the illness. Portal hypertension may follow recovery if the portal vein has been thrombosed. Laboratory findings include anemia, leukocytosis, an elevated erythrocyte sedimentation rate, and abnormal liver biochemical test results, especially an elevated serum alkaline phosphatase level.

Diagnosis

Blood culture specimens will identify the causative organism in at least 50% of cases.[155] Direct cultures of aspirated fluid are useful for identification of the organism and determination of antibiotic susceptibility and should be sent for both aerobic and anaerobic culture.[156] Chest x-rays may show elevation of the right hemidiaphragm and atelectasis. US and CT are the initial imaging modalities of choice. Abscesses as small as

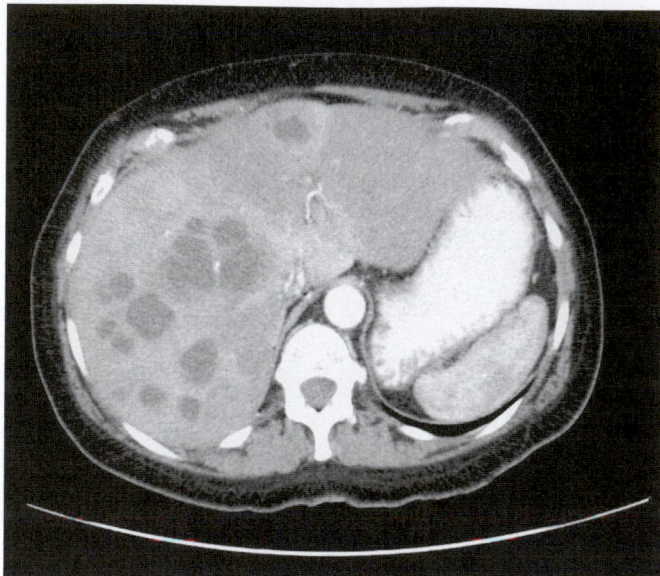

FIGURE 84-9. CT showing multiple pyogenic abscesses in the liver. *(Courtesy Dr. Mukesh Harisinghani, Boston, Mass.)*

1 cm in diameter can be detected. US is inexpensive and accurate and can guide needle aspiration of the abscess. Culture specimens of aspirated material yield positive results in 90% of cases (although the yield probably is lower if the patient has been receiving antibiotics). CT is also accurate, with a sensitivity approaching 100%, but is more expensive than US. Hepatic abscesses are usually hypodense on a CT and may display a rim of contrast enhancement in less than 20% of cases (Fig. 84-9). CT permits precise localization of an abscess, assessment of its relationship to adjacent structures, and detection of gas in the abscess, which is associated with increased mortality.

An abscess must be distinguished from other mass lesions in the liver, including cystic lesions, benign and malignant neoplasms, soft tissue tumors (neurofibroma, leiomyoma, and malignant fibrous histiocytoma), focal nodular hyperplasia, and hemangiomas (see Chapter 96), as well as inflammatory pseudotumors. MRI is more sensitive than CT for detecting small abscesses, which have low signal intensity on T1-weighted images and high signal intensity on T2-weighted images and enhance with gadolinium. ERCP is indicated in patients with imaging evidence of biliary stones or prominent cholestasis.[157] Rarely, arteriography may be of value in distinguishing an abscess from a tumor.

Inflammatory pseudotumor of the liver (also called *plasma cell granuloma*) is a rare, benign lesion characterized by proliferating fibrous tissue infiltrated by inflammatory cells. The cause is unknown. Affected persons (typically young men) often have a history of recent infection, but a causative infectious agent is rarely isolated from the lesion. Additional associated disorders include chronic inflammatory and autoimmune disorders, particularly ascending cholangitis and PSC, as well as diabetes mellitus, Sjögren's syndrome, gout, UC, Crohn's disease, HIV infection, EBV infection, and acute myeloblastic leukemia. Patients typically present with intermittent fever, abdominal discomfort, vomiting, diarrhea, weight loss, and malaise and have hepatomegaly, RUQ tenderness, and jaundice on physical examination. Portal hypertension may develop. Laboratory findings also are similar to those associated with liver abscess, including polyclonal hyperglobulinemia in 50% of cases, and imaging studies generally are

interpreted as showing a tumor or an abscess. Treatment generally has been by surgical resection of the lesion, although some patients may recover spontaneously or after treatment with antibiotics or glucocorticoids, once the diagnosis is made on the basis of needle biopsy findings.[158,159]

Prevention and Treatment

Pyogenic liver abscesses are best prevented by prompt treatment of acute biliary and abdominal infections and by adequate drainage of infected intra-abdominal collections under appropriate antibiotic coverage. Treatment of a hepatic abscess requires antibiotic therapy directed at the causative organism(s) and, in most cases, drainage of the abscess, usually percutaneously with imaging guidance. An indwelling drainage catheter may be placed in the abscess until the cavity has resolved, particularly for lesions greater than 5 cm in size, although intermittent needle aspiration may be as effective as continuous catheter drainage for smaller lesions.[160,161] With multiple abscesses, only the largest abscess may need to be aspirated; smaller lesions often resolve with antibiotic treatment alone, but rarely, each lesion may need drainage. For a small abscess, antibiotic therapy without drainage may suffice. Biliary decompression is essential when a hepatic abscess is associated with biliary tract obstruction or communication and may be accomplished through the endoscopic or transhepatic route (see Chapter 70). Surgical drainage of a hepatic abscess may be necessary in patients with incomplete percutaneous drainage, unresolved jaundice, renal impairment, a multiloculated abscess, or a ruptured abscess.[162] A laparoscopic approach may be feasible in select cases.

Initial antibiotic coverage, pending culture results, should be broad in spectrum, such as a third-generation cephalosporin, or fluoroquinolone plus metronidazole, to cover anaerobic organisms. If amebiasis is suspected, metronidazole should be started before aspiration is performed (see later). Alternative regimens include combinations of a beta-lactam and beta-lactamase inhibitor active against enteric organisms, including anaerobes. After culture results and sensitivity profiles have been obtained, IV antibiotic therapy directed at the specific organism(s) should be administered until a clinical response to therapy is demonstrated, followed by an oral regimen for up to 6 weeks.[163] For streptococcal infections, the use of high-dose oral antibiotics for 6 months may be preferable.

The mortality rate for patients with hepatic abscesses treated with antibiotics and percutaneous drainage has improved since the 1980s.[162,164] A worse prognosis is associated with a delay in diagnosis, multiple abscesses, multiple organisms cultured from blood, a fungal cause, shock, jaundice, hypoalbuminemia, a pleural effusion, an underlying biliary malignancy, multiorgan dysfunction, sepsis, or other associated medical diseases.[162,165-169] Complications of pyogenic liver abscess include empyema, pleural or pericardial effusion, portal or splenic vein thrombosis, rupture into the pericardium, thoracic and abdominal fistula formation, and sepsis. Metastatic septic endophthalmitis occurs in as many as 10% of diabetic patients with a liver abscess caused by *Klebsiella pneumoniae*.[170]

Amebic

Amebiasis occurs in 10% of the world's population and is most common in tropical and subtropical regions (see also Chapter 113).[171,172] Endemic areas include Africa, Southeast Asia, Mexico, Venezuela, and Colombia. In the United States, it is a disease of young, often Hispanic adults. Amebic liver abscess is the most common extraintestinal manifestation of amebiasis. Compared with affected persons who reside in an endemic area, persons in whom an amebic liver abscess develops after travel to an endemic area are older and more likely to be male, have marked hepatomegaly, and have a large abscess or multiple abscesses. The occurrence of an amebic liver abscess in a person who has not traveled to or resided in an endemic area should raise the suspicion of underlying immunosuppression, particularly AIDS.[173,174] Other persons at increased risk include inpatients in residential institutions and men who have sex with men. Host factors that contribute to the severity of disease include younger age, pregnancy, malnutrition, alcoholism, glucocorticoid use, and malignancy.

Pathogenesis

During its life cycle, *Entamoeba histolytica* exists as trophozoite or cyst forms (Fig. 84-10). After infection, amebic cysts pass through the GI tract and become trophozoites in the colon, where they invade the mucosa and produce typical "flask-shaped" ulcers. The organism is carried by the portal vein circulation to the liver, where an abscess may develop. Occasionally, organisms travel beyond the liver and can establish abscesses in the lung or brain. Rupture of an amebic liver abscess into the pleural, pericardial, and peritoneal spaces can also occur.

Clinical Features

Amebic liver abscess is 10 times as common in men as in women and is rare in children.[171] An amebic liver abscess is more likely than a pyogenic liver abscess to be associated with an acute presentation. Symptoms are present on average for 2 weeks by the time a diagnosis is made. A latency period between intestinal and subsequent liver infection of up to many years is possible, and less than 10% of patients report an antecedent history of bloody diarrhea with amebic dysentery.

Pain is typically localized to the RUQ but may be localized to the right chest, epigastrium, or right shoulder. Fever is nearly universal but may be intermittent. Malaise, myalgias, and arthralgias are common. Jaundice is uncommon and signifies a poor prognosis. Pulmonary symptoms and signs may be present, but a pericardial rub and peritonitis are rare. Occasionally a friction rub is heard over the liver. Laboratory features resemble those found in pyogenic abscess. Coinfection with bacterial pathogens is uncommon. Rare complications of amebic abscesses can include intraperitoneal, intrathoracic, and pericardial rupture and multiorgan failure.

Diagnosis

The diagnosis of amebic liver abscess is based on clinical suspicion, hepatic imaging, and serologic testing. The organism is isolated from the stool in only 50% of patients. Hepatic imaging studies cannot distinguish a pyogenic from an amebic liver abscess (Fig. 84-11). An amebic abscess is commonly localized to the right hepatic lobe, close to the diaphragm, and is usually single (Table 84-3).[175] Available serologic tests include an ELISA and indirect hemagglutination, cellulose acetate precipitin, counterimmunoelectrophoresis, immunofluorescent antibody, and rapid latex agglutination tests. Serologic test results must be interpreted in the clinical context because serum antibody levels may remain elevated for years after recovery or cure. The sensitivity of these tests is approximately 95%, and the specificity is more than 95%. False-negative results may occur within the first 10 days of infection.[172] PCR-based tests to detect amebic DNA and an ELISA to detect amebic antigens in serum are available in the research setting.[176,177]

Aspiration of an amebic abscess should be performed if the diagnosis remains uncertain. The presence of a reddish-brown pasty aspirate ("anchovy paste" or "chocolate sauce") is typical; trophozoites rarely are identified. Aspiration also may be considered when no response to antibiotic therapy has occurred after 5 to 7 days or when an abscess in the left lobe of the liver is close to the pericardium.[178,179]

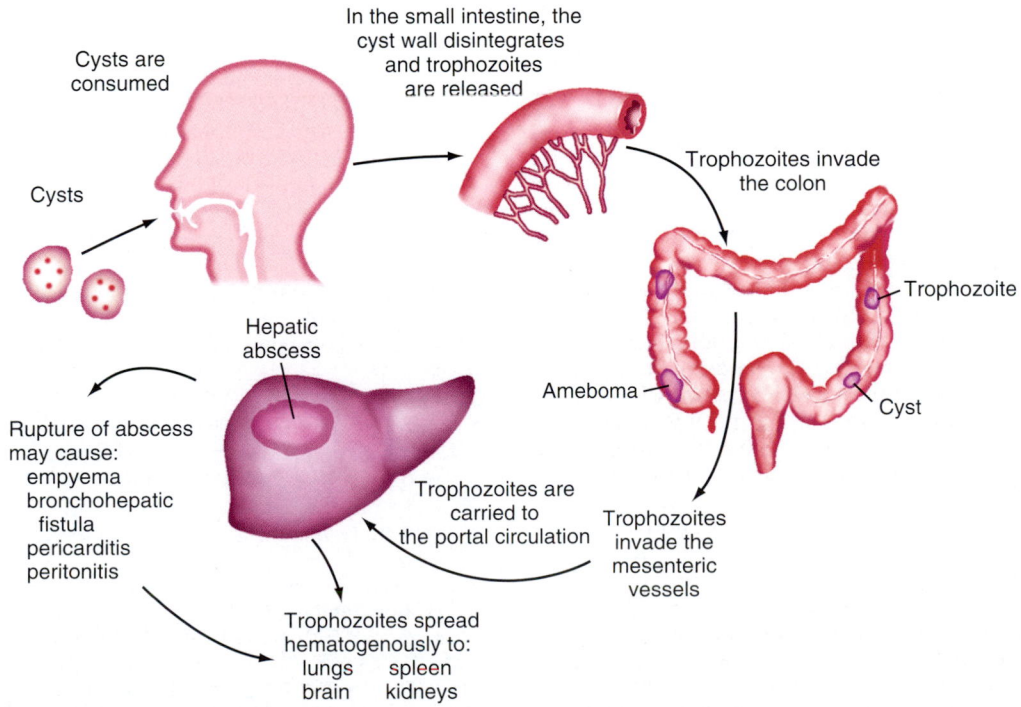

FIGURE 84-10. The life cycle of *Entamoeba histolytica* in amebiasis. *(From Gitlin N, Strauss R. Atlas of clinical hepatology. Philadelphia: WB Saunders; 1995. p 64.)*

TABLE 84-3 Comparisons of Pyogenic and Amebic Liver Abscess

Parameter	Pyogenic Liver Abscess	Amebic Liver Abscess
Number	Often multiple	Usually single
Location	Either lobe of liver	Usually right hepatic lobe, near the diaphragm
Presentation	Subacute	Acute
Jaundice	Mild	Moderate
Diagnosis	US or CT ± aspiration	US or CT and serology
Treatment	Drainage (if technically feasible) + IV antibiotics (see text)	Metronidazole, 750 mg 3 times daily for 7-10 days orally or IV; or tinidazole, 2 g orally for 3 days, followed by iodoquinol, 650 mg orally 3 times daily for 20 days; diloxanide furoate, 500 mg orally 3 times daily for 10 days; or aminosidine (paromomycin) 25-35 mg/kg/day orally in 3 divided doses for 7-10 days

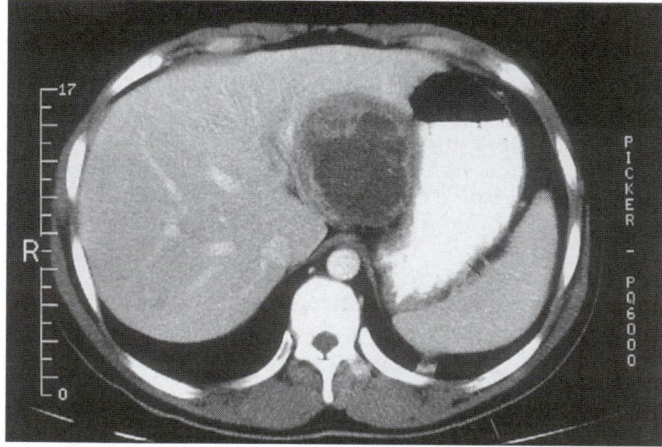

FIGURE 84-11. CT showing a large amebic abscess in the left lobe of the liver. *(Courtesy Dr. Mark Feldman, Dallas, Tex.)*

Treatment

Standard therapy consists of metronidazole, 750 mg 3 times daily by mouth or, if necessary, IV for 7 to 10 days. Tinidazole or chloroquine may be substituted for metronidazole. The response to treatment usually occurs within 96 hours. Following a course of metronidazole, most authorities recommend the addition of an oral luminal amebicide—such as iodoquinol, 650 mg 3 times daily for 20 days; diloxanide furoate, 500 mg 3 times daily for 10 days; or aminosidine (paromomycin), 25 to 35 mg/kg daily in 3 divided doses for 7 to 10 days—to eradicate residual amebae in the gut.[180] The development of a vaccine against *E. histolytica* has been hampered in part because natural infection does not result in long-term immunity.

KEY REFERENCES

Full references for this chapter can be found on www.expertconsult.com.

11. Scholing M, Schneeberger PM, van den Dries P, Drenth JP. Clinical features of liver involvement in adult patients with listeriosis. Review of the literature. Infection 2007; 35:212-18.

29. Akritidis N, Tzivras M, Delladetsima I, et al. The liver in brucellosis. Clin Gastroenterol Hepatol 2007; 5:1109-12.

65. Galappaththy GN, Tharyan P, Kirubakaran R. Primaquine for preventing relapse in people with *Plasmodium vivax* malaria treated with chloroquine. Cochrane Database Syst Rev 2013; CD004389.

77. Bhattacharya SK, Sinha PK, Sundar S, et al. Phase 4 trial of miltefosine for the treatment of Indian visceral leishmaniasis. J Infect Dis 2007; 196:591-8.

100. Keiser J, Utzinger J. Efficacy of current drugs against soil-transmitted helminth infections: Systematic review and meta-analysis. JAMA 2008; 299:1937-48.

101. Greaves D, Coggle S, Pollard C, et al. Strongyloides stercoralis infection. BMJ 2013; 347:f4610.

107. Alm EW, Zimbler D, Callahan E, Plomaritis E. Patterns and persistence of antibiotic resistance in faecal indicator bacteria from freshwater recreational beaches. J Appl Microbiol 2014; 117:273-85.

121. Marcos LA, Terashima A, Gotuzzo E. Update on hepatobiliary flukes: Fascioliasis, opisthorchiasis and clonorchiasis. Curr Opin Infect Dis 2008; 21:523-30.

131. Khuroo MS, Wani NA, Javid G, et al. Percutaneous drainage compared with surgery for hepatic hydatid cysts. N Engl J Med 1997; 337:881-7.

134. Craig P. Echinococcus multilocularis. Curr Opin Infect Dis 2003; 16:437-44.

144. Kontoyiannis DP, Luna MA, Samuels BI, Bodey GP. Hepatosplenic candidiasis. A manifestation of chronic disseminated candidiasis. Infect Dis Clin North Am 2000; 14:721-39.

170. Fang CT, Lai SY, Yi WC, et al. *Klebsiella pneumoniae* genotype K1: An emerging pathogen that causes septic ocular or central nervous system complications from pyogenic liver abscess. Clin Infect Dis 2007; 45:284-93.

173. Karp CL, Auwaerter PG. Coinfection with HIV and tropical infectious diseases. I. Protozoal pathogens. Clin Infect Dis 2007; 45:1208-13.

175. Lodhi S, Sarwari AR, Muzammil M, et al. Features distinguishing amoebic from pyogenic liver abscess: A review of 577 adult cases. Trop Med Int Health 2004; 9:718-23.

180. Salles JM, Salles MJ, Moraes LA, Silva MC. Invasive amebiasis: An update on diagnosis and management. Expert Rev Anti Infect Ther 2007; 5:893-901.

Vascular Diseases of the Liver*

DOMINIQUE CHARLES VALLA

Vascular disorders of the liver are characterized by a primary alteration in blood or lymphatic vessels, which excludes the vascular changes secondary to parenchymal or biliary diseases. Primary alterations consist of obstruction, fistula, aneurysm, or absence (due to agenesis or disappearance) affecting the large or small vessels (or both). This chapter reviews a heterogeneous group of disorders of the hepatic vasculature as well as liver involvement in cardiovascular disease. Vasculitis involving the liver is discussed in Chapter 36.

BUDD-CHIARI SYNDROME

Budd-Chiari syndrome (BCS) is defined as the obstruction of hepatic veins or terminal inferior vena cava (IVC).[1-3] The term *obliterative hepatocavopathy* has been coined to designate obstruction of the IVC or of the hepatic vein ostia in the IVC and has been suggested to be distinct from BCS[4]; however, this distinction has not been widely accepted. Primary BCS arises from a venous anomaly, whereas secondary BCS arises from an initial lesion outside the veins.

Epidemiology

BCS is a rare disease. In Sweden, prevalence rates in 1990 to 2001 were estimated to be 1.4 per million population.[5] There is a slight female predominance. The median age at diagnosis was 37 in one case series.[6] The incidence of BCS in Asia may

be higher. BCS accounted for 17% of hospital admissions for liver-related disease in Kathmandu, Nepal, from 1990 to 1992.[7]

Risk factors for BCS consistently identified in Western patients are shown in Table 85-1.[3] In a study from 2009, one risk factor was found in 84% of patients and two or more risk factors in 48%. A local risk factor (e.g., venous anomaly) was found in only 5% of patients.[6]

Etiology

The causes of BCS are listed in Box 85-1. Myeloproliferative disorders have accounted for 41% of patients with primary BCS,[8] a much higher proportion than in patients with nonsplanchnic venous thrombosis (see Chapter 36).[9] In patients with BCS and a myeloproliferative disorder, portal hypertension may lead to normalization of the blood cell counts. A primary deficiency in protein C, protein S, or antithrombin is difficult to establish as a cause of BCS, because these coagulation inhibitors are decreased nonspecifically by liver disease.[3] Several genetic polymorphisms in coagulation or fibrinolysis factors have been associated with an increased risk of BCS, but their clinical relevance is still uncertain.[10] In Asia, a myeloproliferative disorder, paroxysmal nocturnal hemoglobinuria, and oral contraceptive use are rarely implicated in BCS.[11-14] In Nepal, an unexplained association between obstruction of the terminal IVC and extreme poverty has been shown[7]; the overwhelming representation of this cause may lead to lack of recognition of other causes.

Secondary BCS is related to several mechanisms: (1) invasion by a malignant tumor or alveolar echinococcosis, (2) compression by cysts or focal nodular hyperplasia, usually without clinically significant liver disease, (3) compression

---

*William E. Stevens, MD, and Abhitabh Patil, MD, contributed to this chapter in previous editions of the textbook.

TABLE 85-1 Frequencies of Acquired and Inherited Risk Factors for Budd-Chiari Syndrome and Acute Portal Vein Thrombosis in European Cohort Studies

Risk Factor*	Budd-Chiari Syndrome (n=163)[6] % with Risk Factor	Acute Portal Vein Thrombosis (n=102)[28] % with Risk Factor
Myeloproliferative neoplasms	39	21
JAK2 mutation V617F	29	16
Antiphospholipid syndrome	25	8
Paroxysmal nocturnal hemoglobinuria	19	0
Factor V Leiden mutation	12	3
Factor II (prothrombin) mutation G20210A	3	14
Protein C deficiency	4	1
Protein S deficiency	3	5
Antithrombin deficiency	3	2
Hyperhomocysteinemia	22	11
Recent pregnancy	6	1
Recent oral contraceptive use	33	44
Systemic disease†	23	4
>1 risk factor	46	52
Local factor‡	6	21

*Not all patients were assessed for each risk factor.
†Including connective tissue disease, IBD, Behçet disease, and HIV infection.
‡Acute pancreatitis, intra-abdominal focus of infection, or abdominal trauma.
JAK2, Janus kinase 2.

and inflammation due to polycystic liver disease or liver abscesses, and (4) blunt abdominal or thoracic trauma.[3]

Pathogenesis

A territory corresponding to at least 2 major hepatic veins needs be obstructed before clinical manifestations of BCS develop.[15] The pattern and speed of the occlusive process varies among the major veins and from patient to patient.[4,15] Following initial thrombosis, a vein may transform into a fibrous cord or undergo wall thickening, a process that affects a variable length of the vein and causes varying degrees of narrowing. Short-length stenosis may simulate a membrane. Often, the occlusion predominates at the ostia of a major hepatic vein into the IVC and the adjacent portion of the IVC.[4] A collateral circulation develops, draining into the neighboring patent intra- and extrahepatic veins. When the IVC is obstructed, collaterals form from the lumbar and azygos veins. Such collaterals, coursing subcutaneously, provide a ready clue to the diagnosis. Restoration of hepatic venous drainage through large collaterals may alleviate all symptoms and signs and carries a good prognosis.[15]

Increased hepatic venous and sinusoidal pressures translate into sinusoidal distension and congestion, predominantly in the centrilobular area, and cause ascites formation. Outflow tract obstruction reduces the low-pressure portal venous inflow. Due to stasis and an underlying prothrombotic condition, intra- and extrahepatic portal vein thrombosis is common.[16] A decrease in hepatic blood flow causes ischemic coagulative necrosis and apoptosis, predominantly in the central parts of the lobules, leading to liver dysfunction or liver failure.[16] Subsequently, the loss of hepatocytes results in so-called parenchymal extinction, with replacement of liver cells with connective tissue.[16] Regions of the liver with a preserved blood supply undergo hypertrophy, as is commonly the case for segment I (Spiegel lobe), for which the venous drainage is preserved because its drainage is independent of the major hepatic veins. Areas deprived of portal venous inflow but with enhanced arterial inflow undergo regenerative changes, which can be microscopic (regenerative foci or nodular regenerative hyperplasia) or macroscopic (regenerative macronodules or focal nodular hyperplasia).[16] Fibrosis typically bridges together central areas, eventually leading to venocentric cirrhosis. Associated portal venous obstruction also induces portoportal or portovenous fibrosis. Asynchronous involvement of the diverse venous and portal structures explains the considerable variation of one area of the liver from another.[16]

Clinical Features

The spectrum of clinical presentation ranges from a completely asymptomatic disease to fulminant hepatic failure to chronic liver disease.[6,17] Major features include ascites, abdominal pain, and fever. All complications of chronic liver disease may occur, including GI bleeding, bacterial infections, hepatorenal syndrome, and encephalopathy.[6,17] Serum aminotransferase, creatinine, bilirubin, and albumin levels, as well as the

Hypercoagulable States
Antiphospholipid syndrome
Antithrombin deficiency
Factor V Leiden mutation
Methylenetetrahydrofolate reductase TT677 polymorphism
Myeloproliferative neoplasm
Oral contraceptives
Paroxysmal nocturnal hemoglobinuria
Postpartum thrombocytopenic purpura
Pregnancy
Protein C deficiency
Protein S deficiency
Prothrombin gene mutation G20210A
Sickle cell disease

Infections
Aspergillosis
Filariasis
Hydatid cysts (*Echinococcus granulosus* or *E. multilocularis*)
Liver abscess (amebic or pyogenic)
Pelvic cellulitis
Schistosomiasis
Syphilis
TB

Malignancies
Adrenal carcinoma
Hepatocellular carcinoma
Leiomyosarcoma
Leukemia
Lung cancer
Myxoma
Renal carcinoma
Rhabdomyosarcoma

Miscellaneous
Behçet's disease
Celiac disease
Dacarbazine therapy
IBD
Laparoscopic cholecystectomy
Membranous obstruction of the vena cava
Polycystic liver disease
Sarcoidosis
Trauma to abdomen or thorax

prothrombin time, are variably altered.[6,17] A moderate increase in serum alkaline phosphatase levels is common. Blood cell counts are influenced by the underlying cause of BCS. In patients with a myeloproliferative disorder, blood cell counts are usually normal or decreased due to marked hypersplenism.[6,18] The contrast between normal blood cell counts and severe portal hypertension suggests that a myeloproliferative disorder is present.

Diagnosis and Natural History

Abdominal imaging with Doppler US, CT, or MRI show variable findings in the hepatic veins and IVC (Fig. 85-1), including (1) lack of visibility, (2) dilatation upstream due to a complete or partial obstruction of the terminal portion, (3) diffuse narrowing and irregularity, and (4) transformation into a cord-like remnant. Collateral veins draining peripheral segments of a venous territory into another vein, either hepatic or extrahepatic, are usual. The size, course, and location of these collaterals are diverse.[15] Additional findings are common (see Fig. 85-1): (1) a combination of liver sectorial atrophy and hypertrophy, including segment I enlargement; (2) ascites, portosystemic collaterals, and enlargement of the spleen; (3) patchy enhancement in the arterial and portal phases, which disappears at the late phase, a pattern indicating decreased portal perfusion due to stasis; (4) a marked nodular enhancement in the arterial phase with disappearance in the portal and late phases, without washout, corresponding to regenerative macronodules, some of which have a central scar (Fig. 85-2).[16] On the other hand, some regenerative nodules may show washout.[19]

Because of the variable presentation, the diagnosis of BCS should be suspected in any patient with acute or chronic liver disease, particularly when a cause of BCS is present. The diagnosis is based on direct or indirect evidence of hepatic vein or IVC obstruction.[1-3] The differential diagnosis includes sinusoidal obstruction syndrome (see later), constrictive pericarditis (see later), and cirrhosis (see Chapter 74). As a rule, the accuracy of Doppler US in showing hepatic venous outflow tract obstruction is excellent and depends mostly on the operator's experience and clinical suspicion. MRI and multidetector CT are excellent alternatives. MRI is particularly useful for the characterization of hepatic nodules (see Fig. 85-2). Liver biopsy is not required for diagnosis, except in a BCS variant in which large hepatic veins and the IVC are patent and small veins are thrombosed and in patients with a presentation that mimics cirrhosis when the hepatic veins are not visible on imaging. Direct (transhepatic) or retrograde (transjugular) hepatic

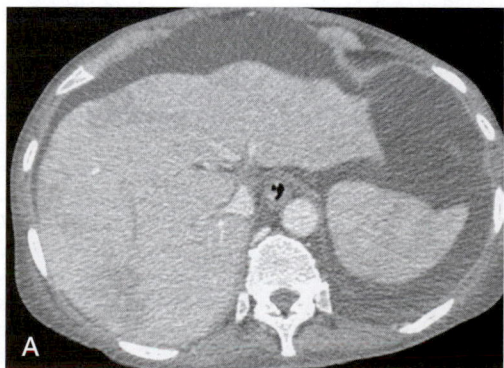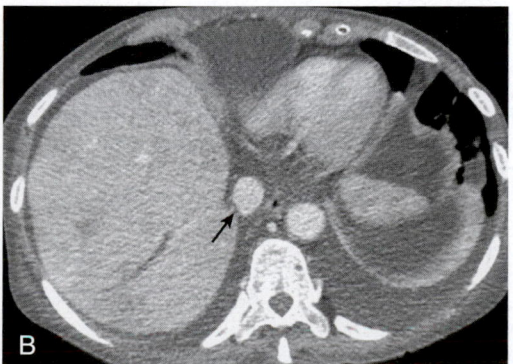

FIGURE 85-1. CT in a patient with Budd-Chiari syndrome. The venous phase of vascular enhancement is shown. The liver is dysmorphic (better seen in *A*) and enhances in an inhomogeneous fashion. Ascites is present. The hepatic veins are visible as slender, unenhanced structures converging toward an enhanced patent inferior vena cava (most prominent in *B*) *(arrow)*.

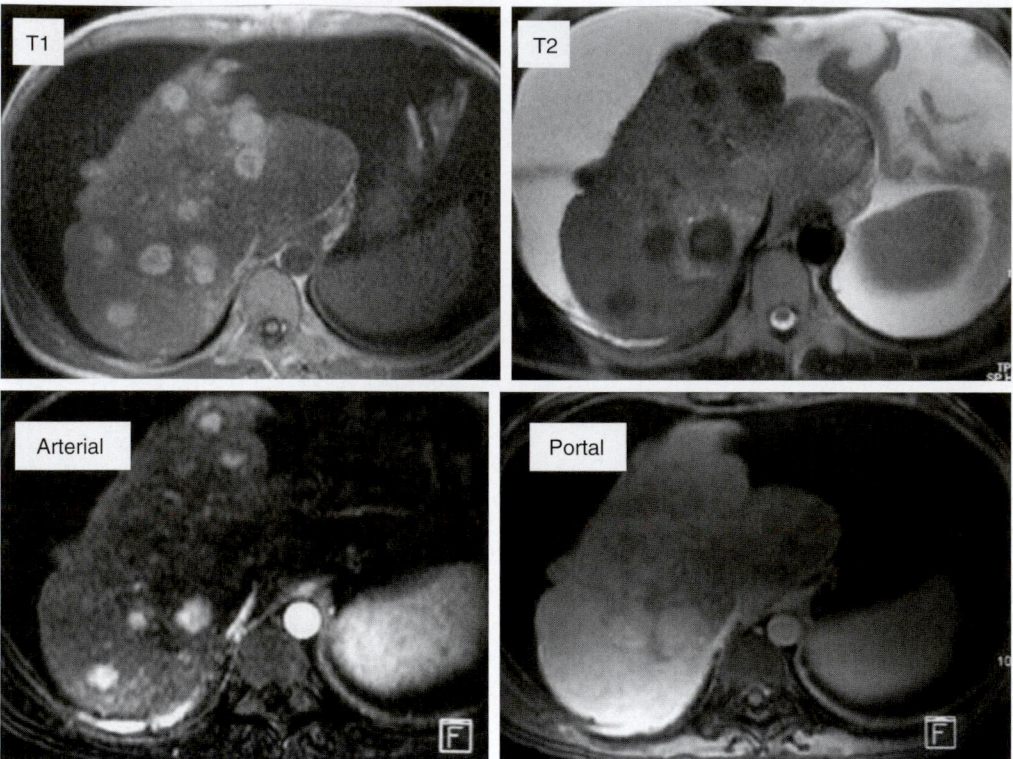

FIGURE 85-2. MRI in a patient with Budd-Chiari syndrome. Numerous regenerative macronodules less than 2 cm in diameter are hyperintense in the T1-weighted sequence and hypointense in the T2-weighted sequence. Marked enhancement of the nodules is seen in the arterial phase, with isointensity in the portal venous phase.

venography is almost never needed for making the diagnosis, but when combined with venous pressure measurements, venography allows percutaneous therapy (see later). Differentiating benign regenerative macronodules from hepatocellular carcinoma often requires US-guided liver biopsy.[19]

The underlying cause of BCS should be identified to determine prognosis and implement appropriate therapy (see Box 85-1). A recommended evaluation for the underlying cause[1,3] should include a general examination for a systemic disease, imaging for secondary BCS, a complete blood cell count, assessment for the *JAK2* V617F mutation, flow cytometry of blood cells for paroxysmal nocturnal hemoglobinuria, factor V Leiden and prothrombin G20210A gene mutations, and a lupus anticoagulant and anti–β_2-glycoprotein I antibodies for antiphospholipid syndrome. Determination of antithrombin, protein C, and protein S levels is warranted only if the prothrombin level is normal. Bone marrow biopsy should be considered when *JAK2* testing for V617F is negative. Identification of one causative factor should not stop the search for other factors.[3]

The natural history of BCS is not well known in the late phase. Early studies suggested that 90% of the patients would die from liver disease within 3 years of diagnosis. Subsequent data have indicated that patients with asymptomatic disease have an excellent medium- and long-term outcome. Patients with IVC obstruction are at high risk of developing hepatocellular carcinoma (see Chapter 96).[19]

Treatment

According to a widely accepted treatment algorithm,[1-3] all patients with primary BCS should receive anticoagulation and specific therapy for the underlying disease. The implementation of routine anticoagulation has been accompanied by a marked improvement in outcome.[20] Guidelines for anticoagulation in cases of venous thromboembolism should be followed.[21] Patients with manifestations of portal hypertension (ascites, variceal bleeding, encephalopathy) should receive medical or endoscopic therapy as appropriate, according to standard recommendations for patients with cirrhosis (see Chapters 92 and 94). It is still a matter of debate as to whether asymptomatic patients with a short stenosis of a major hepatic vein or IVC should undergo percutaneous angioplasty. In symptomatic patients, venous lesions amenable to percutaneous angioplasty should be investigated and treated accordingly. When symptoms and signs are not well controlled, or angioplasty is not feasible, a transjugular intrahepatic portosystemic shunt (TIPS) should be placed, generally through a transcaval approach (see Chapter 92). When the patient does not improve with TIPS, or TIPS proves unfeasible or fails, a surgical portacaval shunt or liver transplantation should be considered (see Chapters 92 and 97). Because medical, interventional, and surgical management may prove difficult, patients with BCS should be referred to specialized centers with expertise.[1,3]

Long-term results achieved with this algorithm have been reported.[22] At a median follow-up of 4 years, 20% of the patients had died and 80% were alive; a fourth had survived on medical therapy, about 5% were alive after percutaneous angioplasty and stenting, about 40% were alive after TIPS, and about 10% were alive after liver transplantation. Anticoagulation therapy, given to 85% of patients, was associated with a bleeding rate of 17%. Portal hypertension was the main cause of bleeding, followed by intracranial hemorrhage. The rate of bleeding-related deaths was 2%, similar to that in patients anticoagulated for venous thromboembolism in general. It is unclear whether the above treatment algorithm applies to Asian patients, who have different causes of BCS and a predominance of IVC obstruction. In a report from China, percutaneous recanalization was associated with excellent rates of technical success (95%) and 10-year survival (73%).[23]

Prognostic factors include the Child-Turcotte-Pugh or MELD scores (see Chapters 92 and 97).[22,24] These scores are of little utility, however, for guiding management in an individual patient.[24] Major concerns for patients surviving long term are hepatocellular carcinoma and complications of the underlying disease.[1,3,19]

EXTRAHEPATIC PORTAL VEIN OBSTRUCTION

Extrahepatic portal vein obstruction (EHPVO) may or may not extend into the intrahepatic portal veins.[1,25] Secondary EHPVO may be caused by malignant invasion, compression, or encasement of the portal vein. Primary EHPVO is comprised of acute portal vein thrombosis (PVT) and portal cavernoma. Acute PVT is characterized by the presence of a thrombus, shown on imaging as solid material in the lumen of the portal vein, in the absence of a cavernoma; whether the recent onset of symptoms should be added to these criteria has been debated. The subsequent transformation of an acutely thrombosed portal vein into a portal cavernoma has frequently been referred to as chronic PVT. Portal cavernoma is characterized by the disappearance of the normal portal vein and its replacement by a network of portoportal collaterals. Whether a portal cavernoma is always preceded by thrombosis remains unclear. When a portal cavernoma is found in a child, a congenital malformation should also be considered. Therefore, EHPVO is the preferred general designation for all conditions leading to obstruction of the portal vein. The term of *chronic PVT* is better reserved for those cases in which the initial stage of acute PVT has been well documented; *portal cavernoma* is otherwise the more appropriate descriptive term.[1,25]

An autopsy study in Sweden found the prevalence of EHPVO to be as high as 1.0%.[26] In another Swedish study based on hospital discharge diagnoses, however, the prevalence was much lower (3.7 per 100,000 population).[27] The difference between these 2 estimates suggests that EHPVO commonly develops at a late stage of many diseases. Chronic liver disease and abdominal malignancy are each found in about one third of patients.[26,27]

Acute Portal Vein Thrombosis in the Absence of Cirrhosis

Etiology

According to a prospective study in 2010, one risk factor for venous thrombosis is found in 67% of patients with acute PVT, and two such factors are found in 18%.[28] A local factor (e.g., vascular anomaly or injury) was identified in only 25% of patients. Furthermore, one third of the patients with a local factor also had a systemic risk factor for thrombosis.[28] Therefore, as for primary BCS, acute PVT is usually associated with multiple systemic risk factors, while local factors generally are unrecognized. Risk factors for PVT are shown in Table 85-1, and the potential causes are listed in Box 85-2. Unlike BCS, PVT has been associated with similar factors in Western and Asian studies.[3,12,14,18,27-30] Myeloproliferative disorders account for 25% to 35% of cases.[8] By contrast with primary BCS, oral contraceptives, paroxysmal nocturnal hemoglobinuria, and factor V Leiden mutation have not been clearly associated with PVT, whereas the prothrombin G20210A gene mutation appears to be particularly frequent.[29]

BOX 85-2 Causes of Portal Vein Thrombosis

Hypercoagulable States
Antiphospholipid syndrome
Antithrombin deficiency
Factor V Leiden mutation
Methylenetetrahydrofolate reductase TT677 polymorphism
Myeloproliferative neoplasm
Nephrotic syndrome
Oral contraceptives
Paroxysmal nocturnal hemoglobinuria
Pregnancy
Prothrombin gene mutation G20210A
Protein C deficiency
Protein S deficiency
Sickle cell disease

Infections
Appendicitis
Cholangitis
Cholecystitis
Diverticulitis
Liver abscess (amebic or pyogenic)
Schistosomiasis
Umbilical vein infection

Inflammatory Diseases
Behçet's disease
IBD
Pancreatitis

Complications of Therapeutic Interventions
Alcohol injection
Colectomy
Endoscopic sclerotherapy
Fundoplication
Gastric banding
Hepatic chemoembolization
Hepatobiliary surgery
Islet cell injection
Liver transplantation
Peritoneal dialysis
Radiofrequency ablation of hepatic tumor(s)
Splenectomy
TIPS procedure
Umbilical vein catheterization

Impaired Portal Vein Flow
Budd-Chiari syndrome
Cirrhosis
Cholangiocarcinoma
Hepatocellular carcinoma
Nodular regenerative hyperplasia
Pancreatic carcinoma
Sinusoidal obstruction syndrome

Miscellaneous
Bladder cancer
Choledochal cyst
Living at high altitude

TIPS, transjugular intrahepatic portosystemic shunt.

Pathogenesis

Local factors associated with PVT can be classified into 3 main categories: (1) inflammatory foci, particularly acute pancreatitis,[31] as well as bacterial cholangitis, appendicitis, and diverticulitis; (2) injury to the portal, splenic, or mesenteric veins (e.g., splenectomy, blunt abdominal trauma); and (3) stasis of blood in the portal venous bed due to cirrhotic or non-cirrhotic intrahepatic block.[32] The trigger for the development of PVT usually remains unknown. The thrombotic occlusion is extremely variable in degree (partial or complete) and extent (involving only the portal vein or one of its two branches or the splenic or superior mesenteric vein [or both]). Independent of the local factor, acute PVT is often associated with a marked systemic inflammatory response syndrome. Superinfection with bacteria, however, is uncommon. By contrast, an infected thrombus ab initio is characteristic of septic pylephlebitis. Commonly encountered species include *Bacteroides* spp., *Escherichia coli*, or *Streptococcus* spp.[32,33]

As long as the thrombus does not reach the mesenteric venous arches, the intestine appears to be protected from ischemia.[34] Intestinal ischemia and necrosis, when they develop, may well be related to intense arterial vasoconstriction in response to extensive mesenteric venous thrombosis.[32,34] There is no evidence of ischemic injury to the liver unless the hepatic artery is also obstructed or circulatory shock occurs, in which case a liver infarct develops. Hepatic blood flow is maintained because of increased arterial blood flow and rapid opening of portoportal collaterals that permit blood flow around the obstructed segment of the portal vein.[32] These collaterals can be demonstrated within hours or days of the onset of PVT.

Clinical Features

At the stage of uncomplicated acute PVT, severe abdominal pain is a major feature and is often accompanied by a steady fever. By contrast, physical examination is unremarkable at this stage. A spiking fever with chills suggests septic pylephlebitis. Blood counts may show nonspecific changes, mostly reflecting the systemic inflammatory response syndrome (which may be marked) or the underlying blood disease. Liver biochemical test results usually show no alterations or minor transient changes.

Diagnosis and Natural History

Abdominal imaging usually shows the thrombus as solid material filling the lumen of the portal vein and extending variably into portal vein branches or to the splenic and superior mesenteric veins (Fig. 85-3).[3] Doppler US shows the absence of flow in the portal vein and is preferred to US alone

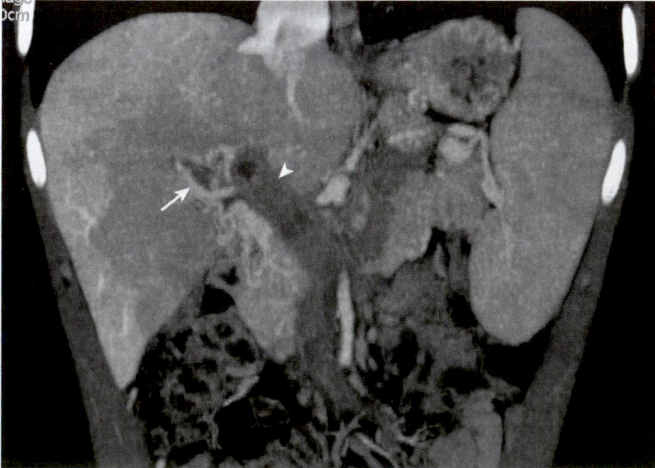

FIGURE 85-3. CT in a patient with acute portal vein thrombosis. The portal venous phase is shown and demonstrates vascular enhancement. The portal and mesenteric veins are enlarged and lack enhancement *(arrowhead)*. Dilated veins are seen in the porta hepatis, particularly in the gallbladder wall *(arrow)*.

because the thrombus is not always hyperechoic at the early stage. Contrast-enhanced CT is most accurate for showing the filling defect in the portal vein lumen. When the thrombus is less than 30 days old, unenhanced images appear as hyperattenuated material. When the thrombus is limited to a branch of the portal vein, there is increased enhancement at the arterial phase in the liver corresponding to the thrombosed branch.[32] Patchy enhancement in the arterial phase ("mosaic pattern") may predominate in the peripheral areas of the liver and persist during the portal venous phase, with homogenous enhancement in the late phase. This pattern reflects portal blood stasis.[32] The collateral vessels that enhance in the portal phase can be demonstrated within a couple of days of the onset, particularly in the gallbladder wall.[32] MRI provides information similar to that of CT on the luminal filling defect and perfusion changes but may not be available on an emergency basis. A diffusely thickened intestinal wall is usually found in uncomplicated PVT, likely corresponding to congestion induced by intestinal outflow tract obstruction. The intestinal mucosa enhances homogeneously. A small amount of ascitic fluid may be detected on imaging in the absence of intestinal ischemia.[28]

The natural history of acute PVT is not known. When noninvasive imaging was not available in the past for the assessment of acute abdominal pain, most cases of acute PVT escaped attention. EHPVO was recognized at the time of a late complication related to portal hypertension.[35] The limited data available show that spontaneous recanalization of the portal vein is unlikely to occur in patients with symptomatic acute PVT.[3,32,36] Whether acute PVT may develop in the absence of symptoms, and whether asymptomatic PVT may regress, remain unanswered questions.

Intestinal ischemia usually occurs in patients whose pain lasts for several days. The occurrence of ascites or rectal bleeding usually heralds intestinal ischemia. Signs of multiorgan dysfunction, acidosis, or lactic acidemia are major indicators of severe intestinal involvement requiring surgical exploration.[3,32] On abdominal imaging, homogeneous or heterogeneous hypoattenuated or hyperattenuated intestinal wall thickening and intestinal dilatation, abnormal or absent wall enhancement, and mesenteric stranding, as well as ascites, pneumatosis cystoides, and portal venous gas, suggest intestinal ischemia or necrosis.[37] Decreased wall enhancement and dilatation of the lumen have been proposed as criteria for differentiating transmural infarction from nontransmural ischemia.[38] The spontaneous development of ischemic intestinal necrosis appears to be invariably fatal; however, some patients with nontransmural intestinal ischemia may recover spontaneously and are recognized subsequently when presenting with an intestinal stricture.[39] Venous intestinal infarction is a major cause of short bowel syndrome (see Chapters 106 and 118).

Demonstrating solid material in the portal vein lumen is sufficient for establishing a diagnosis of acute PVT, once a malignant cause of portal vein obstruction has been ruled out. Evidence for malignant obstruction includes demonstration of a tumor in the vicinity of the portal vein, enhancement of endoluminal material in the arterial phase, or neoplastic cells on biopsy specimens of the endoluminal material. The enhancement of the gallbladder wall combined with pain and a systemic inflammatory response syndrome may suggest an erroneous diagnosis of acute cholecystitis (see Fig. 85-3).

Treatment

Early initiation of anticoagulation is associated with complete and partial recanalization of the portal vein in about 40% and 15% of patients with acute PVT, respectively.[28,36] Extension of thrombosis in the portal venous system is prevented, as are intestinal ischemia and necrosis.[28,36] Complications of anticoagulation therapy appear to be uncommon.[28,35] Even at a later stage of intestinal ischemia, anticoagulation may increase survival.[40,41]

Recanalization of the portal vein is unlikely to occur beyond 6 months of the initiation of anticoagulation, if it has not already been achieved.[28] Splenic or mesenteric veins may continue to recanalize after at least 1 year of anticoagulation.[28] Data are still insufficient, however, for recommending prolongation of anticoagulation beyond 6 to 12 months. The extension of the thrombus, and the type of underlying prothrombotic condition, must be taken into account when a decision is made to prolong anticoagulation.[1,3] Thrombolytic therapy, usually given after anticoagulation has failed, has achieved recanalization rates similar to those for anticoagulation. Rates of adverse events and mortality, however, are particularly high.[36] Therefore, the benefit-to-risk ratio of thrombolytic therapy is generally not considered acceptable in patients with acute PVT.[1,3] Indications for surgery for intestinal ischemia are discussed in Chapter 118.

In patients with uncomplicated acute PVT, long-term overall survival is relatively good, whether or not recanalization has occurred.[3,32] The prognosis depends primarily on the underlying disease.[32,42] The presence of ascites (detected on imaging) and splenic vein involvement have been identified as independent predictors of non-recanalization; no patient with both features has experienced recanalization.[28] In patients with acute intestinal ischemia due to mesenteric venous thrombosis, the overall in-hospital mortality rate has averaged 44%, highlighting the severity of this condition.[43] Intestinal infarction due to venous thrombosis is responsible for short bowel syndrome and a high rate of delayed mortality. Early initiation of anticoagulation therapy is likely critical to preventing this dreaded complication.[28]

Portal Cavernoma

Causes of portal cavernoma and of acute PVT in adults are similar except for a lower proportion of local factors recognized at the stage of portal cavernoma.[35] In adults, therefore, a workup for an underlying cause similar to that for primary BCS is recommended.[1,3] Caution should be taken in interpreting decreased levels of coagulation inhibitors and low levels of anticardiolipin antibodies, because they are common and nonspecific findings in patients with a portal cavernoma.[3,32] In children, prothrombotic conditions are less frequently encountered,[44-47] whereas underlying vascular malformations are common, suggesting that a congenital defect is often a contributing factor, as are prior umbilical cannulation and infection.[46,47]

A cavernoma does not protect a patient from nor relieve portal hypertension. Portoportal collaterals arise from preexisting veins in the porta hepatis and pancreas. These collaterals can be considerably developed or limited. Collaterals that emanate from the bile duct veins can produce deformity of the bile ducts, a condition named portal hypertensive biliopathy or portal cholangiopathy.[48] These biliary changes may rarely be accompanied by evidence of cholestasis. In the absence of preexisting liver disease, liver structure and function remain normal because the cavernoma restores, at least partially, the abolished portal venous inflow to the liver, while hepatic arterial inflow increases.[32] Liver biopsy specimens usually show no abnormalities.[32] In patients with normal liver biochemical test results and normal or near-normal liver biopsy findings, however, a portal cavernoma is associated with atrophy of the peripheral segments of the liver (left liver lobe, segments VI and VII) and hypertrophy of the central segments (segments

I and IV) (see Chapter 71), suggesting impaired perfusion of the former.[49] Sinusoidal dilatation of unclear pathogenesis,[50] as well as regenerative hepatocellular changes or minimal portal fibrosis,[51] can be seen on liver biopsy specimens. Plasma levels of coagulation factors and inhibitors are decreased,[52] and these alterations are increased by portosystemic shunting but ameliorated by portal reperfusion.[53] Minimal hepatic encephalopathy is common.[54] Overall, however, the impact of a portal cavernoma on liver function appears to be limited.

Most patients have no symptoms or signs until they present with GI bleeding related to portal hypertension.[42] Otherwise, the diagnosis is usually made fortuitously by finding an enlarged spleen, esophageal varices, or thrombocytopenia. The most conspicuous laboratory findings are related to hypersplenism. Liver biochemical test levels are usually normal or near normal, although plasma levels of coagulation factors and inhibitors can be moderately decreased.[42] Biliary manifestations include pain and cholecystitis related to biliary stones.[55] Mild to moderate increases in the serum GGTP and alkaline phosphatase levels are common even in the absence of portal cholangiopathy. Conversely, patients with cholangiopathy often have normal liver biochemical test results. US and CT or MRI, with and without contrast enhancement, show the replacement of the portal vein by a network of convoluted channels (Fig. 85-4).[49,56] Liver findings may include atrophy of the periphery and hypertrophy of the central part of the liver and hypervascular nodules in the arterial phase, without washout during the later phases; these findings correspond to benign regenerative nodules.[49,56]

Data on the natural history of portal cavernomas are limited. GI bleeding related to portal hypertension is the most frequent complication, followed by recurrent venous thrombosis, mostly in the portal venous territory.[42] A past history of bleeding and moderate to large esophageal varices are independent risk factors for GI bleeding, and an underlying prothrombotic condition is an independent risk factor for recurrent thrombosis.[42] Biliary complications affect about 25% of patients, mostly those with biliary dilatation[55]; however, chronic cholestasis is unusual.

The diagnosis has been made easy by modern imaging modalities.[1,3] There are some pitfalls, however, mainly related to an atypical aspect of the cavernoma; some patients have a

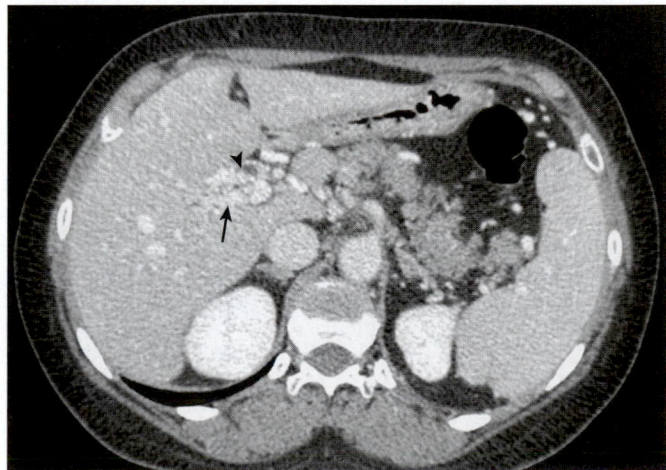

FIGURE 85-4. CT in a patient with a portal cavernoma. The portal venous phase with vascular enhancement is shown. The portal vein bifurcation is not visible and is replaced by serpiginous structures that enhance during the portal venous phase and represent the cavernoma *(arrow)*. Structures that enhance in the wall of the bile duct correspond to biliary veins *(arrowhead)*.

large portal collateral vein that runs straight in the small omentum and that can be mistaken as a normal portal vein. In rare patients, the appearance is that of a solid mass that causes biliary obstruction. The differential feature is the enhancement of the "pseudotumor" in the portal phase of the study.[57]

The therapeutic challenge is to balance the increased risks of bleeding and thrombosis. Based on limited data, anticoagulation therapy is not associated with an increased risk or severity of GI bleeding, as compared with the absence of anticoagulation therapy.[42] There is circumstantial evidence that anticoagulation therapy effectively prevents recurrent thrombosis.[1,3] Therefore, patients without esophageal varices and with a strong risk factor for thrombosis may benefit from anticoagulation therapy. In other patients, the decision regarding long-term anticoagulation should be made on an individual basis, taking into account the prothrombotic potential of the underlying condition and the likelihood of adherence to therapy.[1,3] Recurrent bleeding related to portal hypertension can be prevented with a nonselective β-adrenergic blocking agent or endoscopic variceal ligation.[58] The feasibility of a surgical portocaval shunt or TIPS is limited, and their long-term patency rates are unknown.[1,3] Portal hypertension can be managed as in patients with cirrhosis (see Chapter 92). When feasible, a meso-Rex shunt has provided excellent results in children, in whom it is the preferred option,[53] but experience in adults is lacking (see Chapter 92).

Mortality in patients with a portal cavernoma is related mostly to the underlying condition, not to the complications of portal hypertension.[3,32] Involvement of the superior mesenteric vein is an independent predictor of a poor long-term outcome.[30,59]

PORTAL VEIN THROMBOSIS IN PATIENTS WITH CIRRHOSIS

PVT is found in 5% to 25% of patients with cirrhosis.[60,61] The risk of PVT is independently related to multiple factors: a high MELD or Child-Turcotte-Pugh score, a decreased blood flow velocity in the portal vein, and inherited prothrombotic factors (e.g., prothrombin gene G20210A mutation).[60-62] In contrast to noncirrhotic PVT, the thrombus is usually nonocclusive.[60] Portal cavernoma is uncommon.

The manifestations of PVT must be differentiated from the circumstances that led to its recognition. Many patients have no acute symptoms when PVT is found on routine US. On the other hand, extension to the superior mesenteric vein may induce intestinal ischemia.[62]

PVT in patients with cirrhosis has been associated with a small liver and complications of liver disease.[62,63] A causal role for PVT in these complications, however, is questionable,[63] and the impact of PVT on pre–liver transplant survival, independent of the severity of liver disease, is minimal or absent.[60,64] On the other hand, PVT makes liver transplantation more difficult[60] and is associated with decreased posttransplant survival.[64]

Differentiating PVT unassociated with hepatocellular carcinoma from PVT due to malignant invasion is challenging. Features that suggest malignant invasion are a markedly increased diameter of the vein, a contiguous tumor in the liver, endoluminal enhancement in the arterial phase of imaging or arterial signals recorded on Doppler US, and malignant cells detected on biopsy specimens of the endoluminal material.[3]

Two treatment options are available: anticoagulation and TIPS.[60,61,65,66] Controlled clinical trials are lacking, however, and the actual benefit of these 2 approaches is unclear. With respect to anticoagulation, complete recanalization can be expected in about 40% of patients, and the risk of severe bleeding is not significant. The type of anticoagulant (low molecular weight heparin or an oral vitamin K antagonist) and duration of treatment to achieve an optimal result remain to be studied.[65,66] There is evidence for improved recanalization rates with early initiation of therapy.[66] Laboratory targets and the optimal approach to monitoring also remain unclear. TIPS seems to be feasible when intrahepatic portal venous branches are visible on imaging and is followed by recanalization in over 50% of patients in the absence of anticoagulation therapy.[60,61]

A randomized controlled trial in patients with Child-Pugh class B to C cirrhosis showed that enoxaparin given for 48 weeks was well tolerated, completely prevented the development of PVT, and prevented decompensation and death.[67] These findings lend support to the notion that thrombosis of intrahepatic portal and hepatic venous branches is a determinant of both extrahepatic PVT and decompensation in patients with cirrhosis.[63,68] Confirmation of these findings by other groups is needed before prophylactic anticoagulation in patients with cirrhosis can be recommended.

IDIOPATHIC NONCIRRHOTIC PORTAL HYPERTENSION

Idiopathic noncirrhotic portal hypertension (INCPH) is a syndrome characterized by portal hypertension, patent hepatic veins and extrahepatic portal vein, absence of an identifiable cause of intrahepatic noncirrhotic portal hypertension, and absence of cirrhosis and of a cause of cirrhosis.[69] Well-characterized causes of intrahepatic portal hypertension include schistosomiasis and congenital hepatic fibrosis (see Chapters 62 and 84) and sinusoidal obstruction syndrome (veno-occlusive disease) (see later). INCPH overlaps with various entities characterized either by portal hypertension and unusual histopathologic findings (e.g., noncirrhotic portal fibrosis, idiopathic portal hypertension, hepatoportal sclerosis) or purely histopathologic features (e.g., obliterative portal venopathy, nodular regenerative hyperplasia, perisinusoidal fibrosis).

Conditions associated with INCPH can be classified into 4 categories[69,70]: (1) prolonged exposure to certain drugs and toxins, including purine analogs (e.g., didanosine, azathioprine, 6-thioguanine) and oxaliplatin; (2) immune disorders including connective tissue diseases, common variable immunodeficiency, and HIV infection; (3) prothrombotic conditions including myeloproliferative disorders, antiphospholipid syndrome, and protein S deficiency; and (4) genetic anomalies including Turner syndrome, telomerase disease, and Adams-Oliver syndrome. Familial aggregation also suggests that INCPH may result from a developmental anomaly that could have a genetic basis,[69,70] but over half the cases remain unexplained.[70,71]

Liver biopsy specimens may show a variety of lesions.[70] A primary alteration may be obstruction of the intrahepatic portal venules, with sinusoidal dilatation, regenerative hepatocellular changes, and perisinusoidal or portal fibrosis as consequences. Alternatively, the primary damage may be to the hepatic sinusoids. It is likely that neither small samples obtained at needle biopsy of the liver nor examination of explanted livers with advanced disease provide sufficient clues to the cause of INCPH.[70] Obliterative portal venopathy is characterized by a complete loss of portal veins in most portal tracts (Fig. 85-5), a marked thickening of the venous wall, replacement of portal venules by numerous small

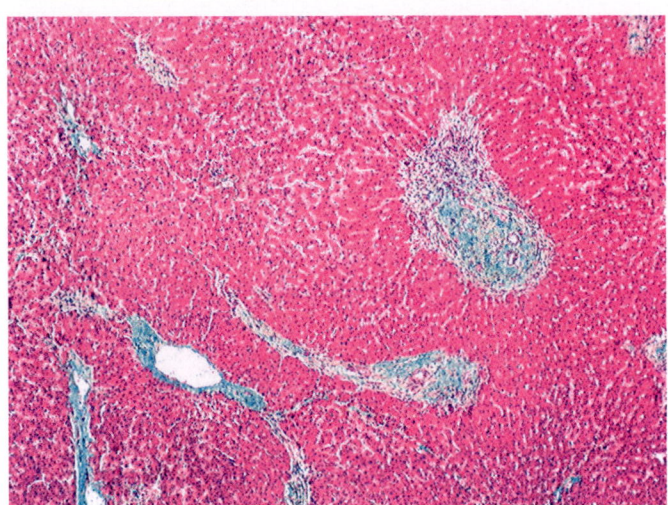

FIGURE 85-5. Histopathology of obliterative portal venopathy. Sclerotic portal tracts devoid of patent venules, irregularly distributed in a noncirrhotic parenchyma, are seen. (Masson trichrome stain, ×40.)

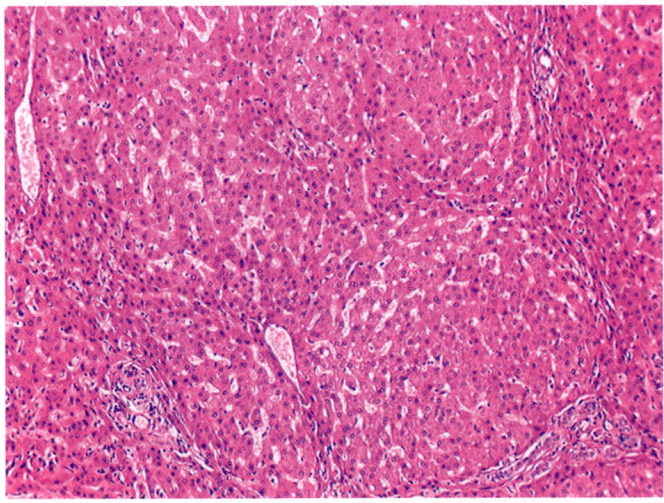

FIGURE 85-6. Histopathology of nodular regenerative hyperplasia. Small regenerative nodules within the acini are surrounded by atrophic hepatocytes in a nonfibrous parenchyma. (H&E, ×100.)

vascular structures, regarded as equivalent to a microscopic cavernoma, and dilated, thin-walled microscopic vessels in an ectopic location in the vicinity of portal tracts.[70,71] Typically, there is little or no lobular or portal inflammation. Slender bridging septa are common and are prominent in the related entity of incomplete septal fibrosis.[69] Frank nodular regenerative hyperplasia is characterized by a widespread distribution of regenerative nodules and atrophic plates of hepatocytes at their periphery (Fig. 85-6). Scattered, less well-defined areas of regenerative changes of hepatocytes are common.[70] It remains to be established that nodular regenerative hyperplasia is always associated with obliterative changes in the portal veins.[71] Calcifications are often seen in extrahepatic portal vein, suggesting a primary disease of the portal venous wall.[72] The incidence of extrahepatic PVT is high.

The lesions described constitute a block to intrahepatic portal flow that causes portal hypertension. The hepatic venous pressure gradient (see Chapter 92) is typically normal but may be increased because the site of the block is not always exclusively presinusoidal.[71] As for BCS and EHPVO, an enlarged hepatic artery and regenerative macronodules (focal nodular regenerative hyperplasia-like nodules) are common.[72]

The clinical presentation is similar to that of EHPVO, with pure portal hypertension but without ascites or liver failure. Nevertheless, some patients have come to liver transplantation because of advanced liver disease, often with a misdiagnosis of cirrhosis.[69,70] Enlargement of the spleen is often conspicuous. On the other hand, obliterative portal venopathy can be found in patients in whom features of portal hypertension are inconspicuous or lacking.

Laboratory tests usually show a mild to moderate increase in serum aminotransferase, GGTP, and alkaline phosphatase levels. Abnormalities of the serum bilirubin, albumin, and coagulation factor levels are common, but marked changes are unusual.[69-71] Blood counts characteristically show features of marked hypersplenism.

On abdominal imaging, intrahepatic portal venous abnormalities (reduced caliber, occlusive thrombosis, and lack of visibility), focal nodular hyperplasia-like nodules, and perfusion disorders are common. Atrophy of segment IV of the liver is much less common than in patients with cirrhosis. EHVPO may be found at presentation.

In the absence of EHPVO, the diagnosis requires exclusion of cirrhosis. The principal distinctions are the absence of a cause for cirrhosis and preserved liver function despite severe portal hypertension. Liver biopsy is required. An expert pathologist and abundant liver tissue for examination are crucial.[70] When EHVPO is also present, portal hypertension should not be attributed solely to the infrahepatic block.

Portal hypertension can be managed as in patients with cirrhosis (see Chapter 92). Treatment of associated conditions is probably of benefit. The rationale for using anticoagulation therapy includes the frequent association with prothrombotic conditions, a high risk of superimposed extrahepatic PVT, anecdotal reports of marked improvement in liver function with therapy, and the extrapolation of data on the prevention of PVT with anticoagulation in patients with cirrhosis.[67] The benefit-to-risk ratio of this approach is unknown, and caution is needed when considering anticoagulation therapy.[69] Liver transplantation is an option for patients with advanced liver disease.[69]

Limited data are available on the outcome and prognosis. Portal hypertension does not appear to be an important cause of mortality.[69] De novo PVT occurs in 20% to 40% of patients within 5 years of follow-up; a prothrombotic condition is a risk factor for PVT.[70] The actual impact of PVT on outcome is unknown. Short- and medium-term outcomes appear to be good and much better than those in patients with cirrhosis. In the long term, however, advanced liver disease may complicate the course of 10% of patients.[70,71] Baseline prognostic factors are still unknown. The risk of developing hepatocellular carcinoma is unclear.[69]

SINUSOIDAL OBSTRUCTION SYNDROME (HEPATIC VENO-OCCLUSIVE DISEASE)

Sinusoidal obstruction syndrome (SOS) is characterized by destruction of sinusoidal endothelial cells predominantly in the central part of the hepatic lobule, with focal obstruction of sinusoidal lumens and resulting congestion.[3,73] In many, but not all, cases, nonthrombotic occlusion of the central hepatic veins is also present (hence the original designation of veno-occlusive disease [VOD]). In practice, the diagnostic criteria are clinical, rather than histologic, and have therefore produced some confusion (see later).

Etiology

SOS is due almost exclusively to agents that are toxic to both bone marrow progenitor cells and sinusoidal endothelial cells.[3,73] These agents include irradiation of the liver area, chemotherapy, immunosuppressive agents, and plant alkaloids related to pyrrolizidine (see Chapters 35 and 89). The most common settings for SOS are conditioning for hematopoietic cell transplantation (HCT), chemoradiation for abdominal organ malignancy, immunosuppression with purine derivatives, and chemotherapy with oxaliplatin for metastatic colorectal cancer to the liver.[74] Epidemics related to the consumption of flour contaminated with alkaloid-containing plants, as well as sporadic cases related to herbal teas or contaminated herbal remedies, still occur (see Chapter 89).[3,73] Causative agents are transformed in the liver and detoxified by glutathione. Sinusoidal endothelial cells appear to be more sensitive than hepatocytes to the toxic effects of the transformed drugs, possibly related to lower stores of glutathione in sinusoidal endothelial cells.[3,73] Changes similar to SOS have been described in liver transplant recipients in the absence of exposure to azathioprine. Several arguments suggest that endothelialitis related to graft rejection is the cause of this particular entity (see Chapter 97).[75]

In the context of HCT, risk factors for the development of SOS are underlying liver disease (particularly iron overload and viral hepatitis), administration of female sex hormones to prevent uterine bleeding, use of high-intensity regimens (particularly those containing busulfan or cyclophosphamide), and use of gemtuzumab ozogamicin. The frequency of SOS is 20% on average.[3,73]

Pathology

Sinusoidal dilatation and a loss of hepatocytes in the centrilobular area are the 2 major histopathologic features (Fig. 85-7). Their severity varies greatly from patient to patient.[3,73] Occasionally, sinusoidal congestion is so marked as to mimic peliosis hepatitis (see later). Endothelial damage in the central veins manifests as a rounding of the cells, followed by subendothelial edema and hemorrhage, producing the characteristic eccentric narrowing of the lumen. Central vein damage is more marked in areas where sinusoidal dilatation is more severe. Fibrosis of veins and sinusoids produces various degrees of occlusion. Characteristically the periportal area, portal tracts, and portal vessels remain intact. Studies in the monocrotaline rat model of SOS have indicated that the earliest lesion occurs in sinusoidal endothelial cells and that repopulation with bone marrow–derived endothelial progenitor cells is instrumental in repairing sinusoidal lesions.[3,73] The acute development of sinusoidal obstruction induces abrupt ischemia, as well as portal hypertension related to a postsinusoidal block.[3,73]

Clinical Features and Diagnosis

Clinical and laboratory manifestations of SOS closely mimic those of BCS, with a range from asymptomatic, to acute with conspicuous ischemic necrosis of the liver, to subacute or chronic with ascites. Liver dysfunction of varying severity is common. On imaging, the liver is enlarged with a mosaic pattern suggestive of altered perfusion similar to that seen in BCS. Gross changes in the flow pattern in the portal and hepatic veins, as well as hepatic arteries, are nonspecific.[3,73] In

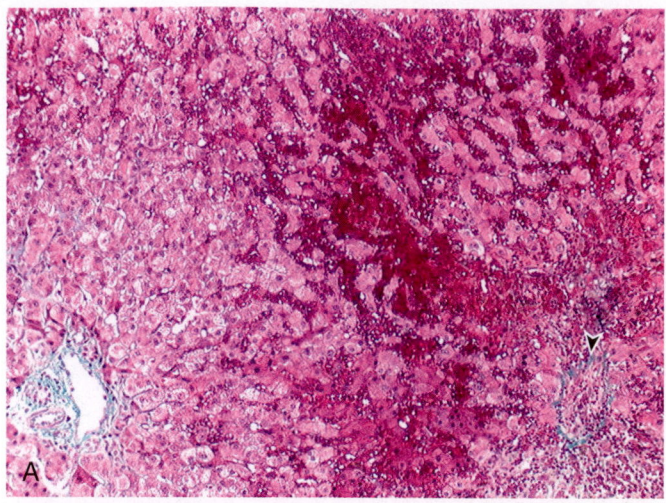
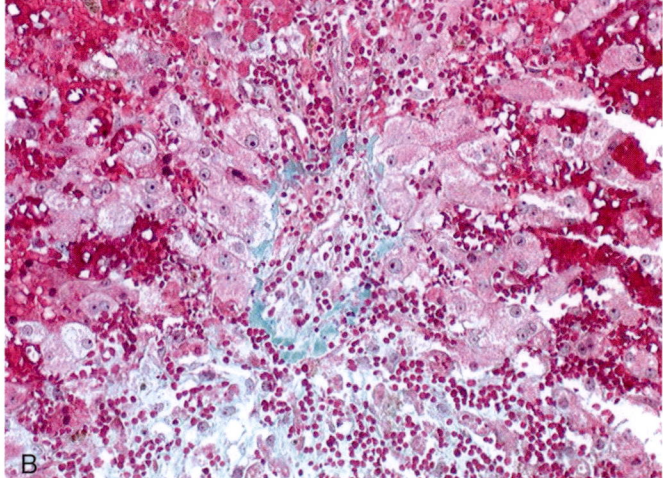

FIGURE 85-7. Histopathology of acute sinusoidal obstruction syndrome. *A,* Massive centrilobular and mid-lobule congestion with obliteration of a terminal hepatic vein *(arrowhead)* is seen. (Masson trichrome stain, ×100.) *B,* A higher-power image shows obliteration of the terminal hepatic vein by subendothelial edema and fine collagen tissue. (×250.)

the setting of HCT, symptoms and signs usually develop within the first 2 months after conditioning, but not more than 100 days after conditioning. Liver biopsy specimens after 100 days may still show features of SOS, albeit in association with another condition (e.g., graft-versus-host disease, viral hepatitis).[3,73] As a rule, the diagnosis of SOS can only be established with liver biopsy, after patency of large hepatic veins and the IVC is shown on imaging. The differential diagnosis of the histopathologic finding includes right-sided heart failure (see later), BCS due to pure small hepatic vein thrombosis, and pure sinusoidal dilatation or peliosis hepatis. In the context of HCT, liver biopsy is difficult to obtain, and clinical diagnostic criteria have been proposed, generally incorporating weight gain or ascites, increased serum bilirubin levels, and the absence of other causes of liver dysfunction, particularly sepsis and graft-versus-host disease.[3,76] The hepatic venous pressure gradient is increased.[3,73] The clinical features are nonspecific, however, and may relate to preexisting liver disease, such as transfusion-related viral hepatitis and iron overload, drug toxicity, hematologic disease, alcoholic liver disease, or metabolic syndrome.

Treatment

Treatment options for SOS have been evaluated mainly in the context of HCT. Prevention relies on decreasing the intensity of conditioning regimens.[3,73] None of the drugs proposed for primary prophylaxis has shown a clear benefit in survival rates. There is limited evidence that defibrotide, a novel oligodeoxyribonucleotide with anti-ischemic, antithrombotic, and thrombolytic activity, decreases the incidence of SOS.[77] None of the options proposed for established SOS has been supported by convincing data, although defibrotide is widely used in the HCT setting because of its favorable safety profile.[3,73] Bevacizumab has been reported to protect against oxaliplatin-related SOS.[74,78]

The occurrence of SOS has a negative impact on overall outcome. Serum bilirubin or aminotransferase elevations are major determinants of immediate prognosis.[76] In HCT recipients, features of SOS have been associated with early mortality rates ranging from 0% to 67%, but the contribution of SOS to mortality is difficult to delineate in these frail patients with multiorgan failure.[3,73] In patients receiving oxaliplatin for metastatic colorectal cancer, the occurrence of SOS increases the incidence of complications after hepatic resections.[78] A favorable benefit-to-risk ratio still exists for preoperative chemotherapy to reduce the size of hepatic metastases but not as adjuvant therapy for resectable metastasis.[78] Long-term sequelae of SOS include pericentral fibrosis, nodular regenerative hyperplasia, and focal nodular hyperplasia.[3,73,79] The latter 2 appear to be nonspecific consequences of the uneven alterations in intrahepatic perfusion and arterialization.

CONGENITAL PORTOSYSTEMIC SHUNTS

Congenital portosystemic shunts (CPSS) are characterized by a large communication between the portal venous system and the systemic venous circulation in the absence of parenchymal or biliary disease.[3,80,81] This entity has also been referred to as the *Abernethy malformation*, of which 2 types have been described: type 1 is characterized by the absence of a detectable portal vein (an end-to-side shunt), and type 2 is characterized by a still demonstrable portal vein (side-to-side shunt) (see Chapter 71). The type 2 CPSS are further divided according to the intrahepatic or extrahepatic location of the shunt.[80] The associations that suggest that type 1 CPSS are congenital malformations are the female predominance and the frequent occurrence with situs inversus, polysplenia, and congenital heart defects. The etiology of type 2 CPSS is unclear. The prevalence of CPSS has been estimated to be 1 in 30,000.[80] A systematic review was able to find only about 320 reported.[81]

Closure of CPSS is usually followed by reperfusion of the liver with a structure resembling a normal portal vein, thereby suggesting that the term "portal vein agenesis" is inappropriate for characterizing this entity.[80] The clinical expression is related to portosystemic shunting and deprivation of portal blood inflow to the liver. Portosystemic shunting explains why some patients present with hepatic encephalopathy, primary pulmonary arterial hypertension, or hypoxemia due to hepatopulmonary syndrome (see Chapter 94). Portal blood deprivation explains the liver hyperarterialization and regenerative changes, including nodular regenerative hyperplasia and regenerative macronodules, that have been reported as adenomas or focal nodular hyperplasia. There are anecdotal reports of hepatocellular carcinoma, although causality is difficult to ascertain.[80,81]

Among reported cases of CPSS, one third have had anomalies related to hyperammonemia or neurologic anomalies. The spectrum of neurologic involvement has ranged from changes in brain imaging and subtle abnormalities on neuropsychological testing to learning disabilities and overt encephalopathy. Such a mode of presentation can occur late in life.[80,81] Liver tumors have accounted for one fourth of the reported cases. Their characteristics can be typical of benign regenerative macronodules or focal nodular hyperplasia. Completely benign nodules can have a heterogeneous appearance and not remain stable in size or features. Portopulmonary and hepatopulmonary syndrome occur in a lower proportion of cases.[80,81] Liver dysfunction and ascites are extremely uncommon.

The diagnosis of CPSS is based on their demonstration by abdominal imaging (US, contrast-enhanced CT, or MRI).[3,80] In patients presenting with unexplained brain dysfunction, the demonstration of hyperammonemia or signal intensity of the lesion on MRI is most useful in suggesting portosystemic shunting. The diagnosis of CPSS should be considered in neonates who screen positive for galactosemia. In patients with multiple regenerative macronodules, CPSS should be routinely considered, as should hereditary hemorrhagic telangiectasia (see later).

Specific treatment for CPSS should be considered in patients with portosystemic encephalopathy, hepatopulmonary syndrome, or portopulmonary hypertension. Shunt closure can be performed with percutaneous interventional radiology techniques or surgically.[80] Even when the portal vein lumen cannot be identified prior to the procedure, portal reperfusion to the liver can be achieved following closure of the shunt.[80] When the preprocedural portal venous pressure is high and the portal vein is not demonstrated, progressive banding of the shunt may be an option. The possibility of closing a shunt should limit the need for liver transplantation. In a patient with regenerative macronodules, surgical resection or liver transplantation should not be considered unless hepatocellular carcinoma or marked dysplasia has been demonstrated unequivocally. Moreover, compensatory hypertrophy of the remnant liver following resection may be considerably slower than in the absence of a portosystemic shunt.

Outcomes are excellent following closure of CPSS for encephalopathy, portopulmonary hypertension, or hepatopulmonary syndrome, as well as for large liver nodules, which decrease in size.[80] A handful of cases of hepatocellular carcinoma have been reported in association with CPSS, and monitoring with repeated abdominal imaging is probably warranted.[3,80,81]

ISCHEMIC HEPATITIS

Because *hepatitis* refers to inflammation of the liver, the term *ischemic hepatitis* is a misnomer, because inflammation is typically not present. A more physiologic term would be *hypoxic hepatitis*, because the primary cause of this syndrome is tissue hypoxia, which may be the result of hypoperfusion from cardiac failure, systemic hypoxemia from respiratory failure, or increased oxygen requirements from sepsis.[82] The name *ischemic hepatitis* is used, however, because of clinical similarities to other forms of acute hepatitis and the characteristic pathologic feature of acute centrilobular necrosis. Ischemic hepatitis is probably the most commonly encountered form of vascular liver disease.

Etiology

Of all cases of extreme serum AST elevations (to > 3000 U/L), ischemic hepatitis accounts for about half.[83] The most common cause of ischemic hepatitis is cardiovascular disease, which accounts for more than 70% of cases, followed in frequency by respiratory failure and sepsis, each of which accounts for less than 15% of cases.[82] Hypotension is documented as a precipitating factor in more than 50% of patients with ischemic hepatitis but does not need to be evident for ischemic hepatitis to occur. Hypotension often is clinically apparent as a result of acute myocardial infarction, severe heart failure, or sepsis but may be less obvious following a transient arrhythmia or silent coronary ischemic event. The presence of heart failure significantly increases the likelihood that a drop in cardiac output from any cause will result in ischemic hepatitis. More than 80% of cases of ischemic hepatitis occur in the setting of heart failure.[84] Acute trauma, hemorrhage, burns, and heat stroke can also cause ischemic hepatitis, but the likelihood is substantially less in the absence of underlying heart disease.

Clinical Features and Diagnosis

Ischemic hepatitis often is first considered when extreme serum aminotransferase elevations are detected in a patient hospitalized for problems not primarily associated with the liver. Findings on physical examination are usually dominated by the underlying precipitating medical condition. The patient's mental status is often altered because of diminished cerebral perfusion. Laboratory studies show extreme elevations of the aminotransferase levels (>3000 U/L). The serum LDH level is profoundly elevated, often more so than the ALT, and an ALT/LDH ratio of less than 1.5 is more typical of ischemic hepatitis than of viral hepatitis.[85] The prothrombin time may be prolonged by 2 or 3 seconds, and the serum bilirubin level is often mildly increased, with peak levels seen after the aminotransferase levels peak. Serum creatinine and blood urea nitrogen levels are often elevated because of acute tubular necrosis. Characteristically, serum aminotransferase levels peak 1 to 3 days after the hemodynamic insult and return to normal within 7 to 10 days.

The differential diagnosis of this type of severe acute injury includes acute hepatitis caused by viral infections, autoimmunity, toxins, and medications (see Chapter 73). Liver biopsy specimens, although usually unnecessary, reveal bland, centrilobular necrosis with preservation of the hepatic architecture (Fig. 85-8). Occasionally a definitive diagnosis of ischemic hepatitis can be difficult to make, but the typical prompt rise in serum aminotransferase and LDH levels followed by a rapid fall within a few days is more characteristic of ischemic hepatitis than of other causes of severe acute liver injury (Fig. 85-9).[86]

Treatment

Most cases of ischemic hepatitis are transient and self-limited. In the most severely affected patients, ischemic hepatitis is just one manifestation of multiorgan failure and signals a poor prognosis. Fulminant hepatic failure resulting from ischemic hepatitis is uncommon but is more likely to occur when chronic heart failure or cirrhosis is also present. The overall prognosis depends primarily on the severity of the underlying predisposing condition, not the severity of the liver disease. No specific therapy exists for ischemic hepatitis, and treatment is directed at improving cardiac output and systemic oxygenation.

CONGESTIVE HEPATOPATHY

The effects of heart failure on the liver predictably include decreased hepatic blood flow, increased hepatic vein pressure,

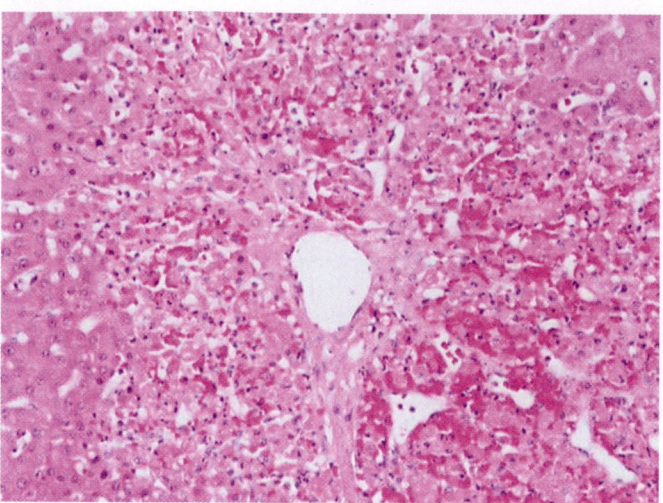

FIGURE 85-8. Histopathology of ischemic hepatitis. This low-power photomicrograph demonstrates centrilobular necrosis, loss of hepatocytes, and sinusoidal congestion with red blood cells, but only a scant inflammatory infiltrate. Perivenular fibrosis is evident. (H&E.) *(Courtesy Dr. Pamela Jensen, Dallas, Tex.)*

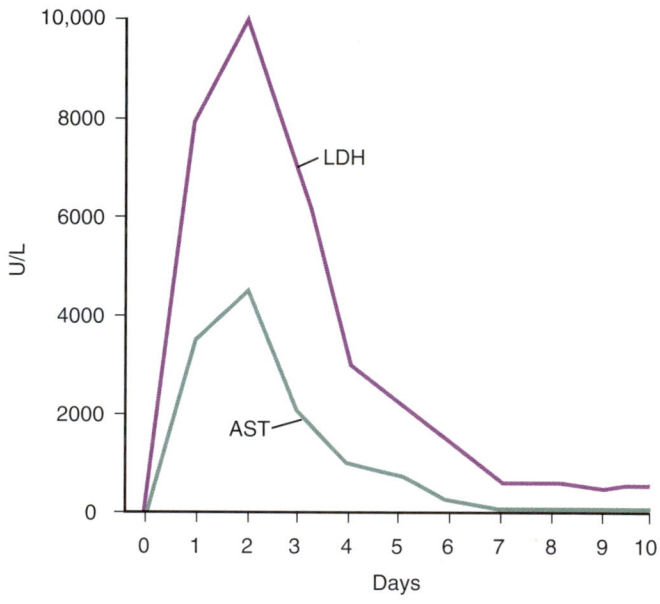

FIGURE 85-9. A frequently observed course of serum AST and LDH levels in ischemic hepatitis. *(Adapted from Gitlin NG, Serio KM. Ischemic hepatitis: Widening horizons. Am J Gastroenterol 1992; 7:831-6.)*

and decreased arterial oxygen saturation.[87] Right-sided heart failure results in transmission of increased central venous pressure from the heart directly to the hepatic sinusoids. The result is centrilobular congestion and sinusoidal edema that further decrease oxygen delivery. The injurious effects of superimposed ischemic hepatitis are common in these patients. The acute and chronic damage results in progressive centrilobular fibrosis. Sinusoidal hypertension and congestion can lead to the development of ascites, with a characteristically high serum-ascites albumin gradient and a high protein concentration (see Chapter 93).

Clinically, the symptoms and signs of heart failure are the predominant features. Dull right upper quadrant pain in association with hepatomegaly is common. The liver may be pulsatile if tricuspid regurgitation is present, and hepatojugular reflux is often apparent on compression over the liver. Spider telangiectasias and varices are usually not present, and variceal bleeding caused by congestive hepatopathy alone does not occur. Mild elevation of the serum bilirubin level (to < 3 mg/dL) is common, and jaundice is seen in fewer than 10% of patients, occurring in those with severe or acute heart failure.[88] The prothrombin time is prolonged in more than 75% of cases and usually is resistant to therapy with vitamin K. Other liver biochemical test levels are often normal or only mildly elevated. Liver test results improve slowly or normalize with effective therapy of the underlying heart failure. US is useful in excluding other hepatobiliary diseases. Typical CT findings in congestive hepatopathy include hepatomegaly, ascites, dilatation of the IVC and hepatic veins, and inhomogeneous hepatic enhancement during the portal phase of contrast administration.

The histologic features of congestive hepatopathy include atrophy of hepatocytes, sinusoidal distention, and centrilobular fibrosis (Fig. 85-10). Centrilobular necrosis, consistent with ischemic hepatitis, is frequent in liver biopsy specimens that show congestive hepatopathy and usually correlates with recent hypotension.[89] Bridging fibrosis typically extends between central veins (rather than between portal tracts) to produce a pattern of "reverse lobulation" characteristic of cardiac cirrhosis. The distribution of fibrosis throughout the liver is highly variable and correlates with focal sinusoidal thrombosis, with obliteration of central and portal veins that leads in turn to localized ischemia, parenchymal extinction, and fibrosis.[90]

The presence of congestive hepatopathy does not affect the prognosis in patients with heart failure; the mortality rate is determined primarily by the severity of the underlying cardiac disease. Occasionally, paracentesis may be needed to alleviate tense ascites, but therapy is generally directed at improving cardiac disease.

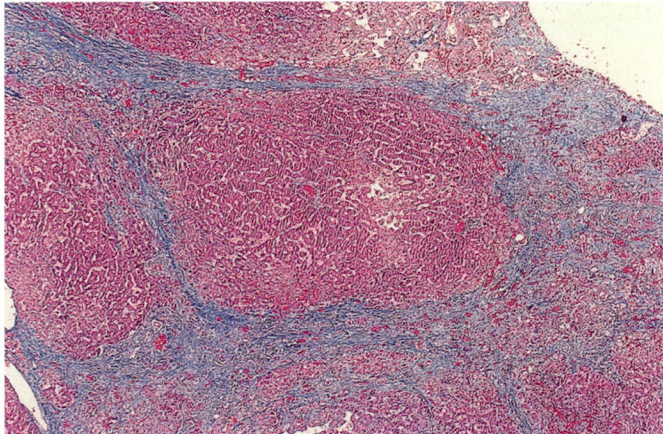

FIGURE 85-10. Histopathology of cardiac cirrhosis. This low-power view shows a portal tract in the center of a regenerative nodule and fibrotic bands bridging central veins. The size of the scar and the presence of the nodule attest to the long-term course of the fibrotic process. Even at low power, the bland nature of the cirrhosis is apparent. No inflammatory cells are evident. The sinusoids are dilated and congested. (Masson trichrome stain.) *(Courtesy Dr. Edward Lee, Washington, D.C.)*

ISCHEMIC CHOLANGIOPATHY

Ischemic cholangiopathy (IC) is the designation for the biliary changes that result from impaired arterial blood flow.[91] The term *ischemic cholangitis* is also used, although inflammation is not a primary mechanism. Circumstances in which arterial blood supply to the bile ducts is compromised are mostly iatrogenic and include liver transplantation, surgery on the liver and bile ducts, arterial chemotherapy, and embolization.[91] The disease may develop in survivors of intensive care for septic shock or trauma.[92] Systemic causes of arterial disease account for a small proportion of cases; polyarteritis nodosa and primary or secondary antiphospholipid syndrome are the most typical examples.[93] Although IC is relatively common in the setting of liver transplantation, overall it is a rare condition.

Bile ducts receive blood almost exclusively from arteries, many of which are branches of the common hepatic artery; others (e.g., diaphragmatic branches) penetrate the liver through the capsule, away from porta hepatis. Extensive anastomoses between these arteries open whenever one arterial branch is obstructed, explaining why ligation or embolization of an isolated large artery is generally harmless. The peribiliary arteriolar plexus also acts as a collateral pathway. Ischemia to the bile duct occurs when the collaterals are prevented from providing compensation,[94] as may happen early after liver transplantation (due to dissection of the liver) or when the small arterial vessels of the peribiliary plexus are obstructed, as by arteritis, toxic injury from infusion of floxuridine (FUDR), or embolization with small-sized particles. In hereditary hemorrhagic telangiectasia, diversion of blood from the peribiliary plexus is thought to cause biliary ischemia (see later). Nonocclusive ischemia to the bile ducts is thought to occur in patients in whom cholangiopathy develops following a stay in the intensive care unit for shock.[91]

The initial stage of IC consists of ischemic necrosis of the biliary mucosa, which leads to biliary cast formation. Subsequently, full-thickness ischemia of the bile duct wall occurs and may result in necrosis with extravasation of bile and formation of collections (bilomas) in the liver parenchyma or porta hepatis. Later, ischemic areas undergo fibrous transformation, resulting in biliary strictures.[91]

Acutely, IC is heralded by pain, systemic inflammatory reaction syndrome, and cholestatic jaundice. This initial phase, which develops a few days to a few weeks after the ischemic insult, may be unrecognized. Presentation at a later stage is generally with cholestatic features or bacterial cholangitis.[91] Bile duct imaging with MRI or direct cholangiography initially shows finely irregular, dilated bile ducts with filling defects corresponding to the casts. Later, bilomas may develop and may or may not be superinfected. At a late stage, multiple strictures of extra- and intrahepatic ducts mimic those of PSC (see Chapter 68). Strictures are often particularly marked at the termination of right and left bile ducts and proximal portion of the common bile duct.[91]

Diagnosis relies heavily on a setting in which the arterial blood supply to the bile ducts is likely to be impaired and the demonstration of bile duct changes compatible with IC.[91] MR cholangiography is the test of choice for demonstrating biliary casts, bilomas, and biliary strictures. The main differential diagnosis during the initial phase of IC includes biliary stones and abscesses and in the late phase primary or secondary sclerosing cholangitis. The diagnosis can be difficult to make when the ischemic insult to the bile ducts escapes attention, as may occur during a stay in an ICU.[92] After liver transplantation, monitoring of arterial blood flow with Doppler US is the cornerstone of early diagnosis of hepatic arterial impairment (see Chapter 97).

In the transplant setting, prevention and early correction of impaired arterial blood flow is of utmost importance (see Chapter 97). Early recognition of hepatic arterial impairment allows early correction, either by percutaneous radiologic intervention or surgery. In other settings, the treatment in supportive. Liver transplantation is the only definitive therapy. In the absence of liver transplantation, the outcome of diffuse IC is extremely poor.[91] Causes of death are liver failure and sepsis. The outcome of localized ischemic stenosis may be better, except when the main bile duct is involved.

IDIOPATHIC SINUSOIDAL DILATATION AND PELIOSIS HEPATIS

Idiopathic sinusoidal dilatation is characterized by widening of hepatic sinusoidal lumens in the absence of a postsinusoidal block or infiltration of the sinusoids by abnormal cells or substances (Fig. 85-11A).[50,95,96] Peliosis hepatis is similar to idiopathic sinusoidal dilatation and is characterized by a "lake-forming," hemorrhagic dilatation of the sinusoids (see Fig. 85-11B).[97] Peliosis hepatis shares etiologic and clinical features with idiopathic sinusoidal dilation but is less common and more severe.

Conditions reported to be associated with idiopathic sinusoidal dilatation can be separated into the following 4 categories[50,95,96]: (1) portal venous inflow impairment, including EHVPO, obliterative portal venopathy, CPSS, and sarcoidosis; (2) neoplasia, including hepatic metastases, renal cell carcinoma, and Hodgkin's disease; (3) non-neoplastic conditions associated with systemic inflammatory reaction syndrome, including Castleman's disease, Crohn's disease, RA, Takayasu arteritis, SLE, sarcoidosis, infections with intracellular microbes, acute bacterial pyelonephritis, and *Bartonella henselae* infection; and (4) exposure to certain drugs and toxins, including thiopurines and oxaliplatin. Oral contraceptives have been associated with sinusoidal dilatation, although often in combination with other causative conditions.[95] Overall, the incidence of idiopathic sinusoidal dilatation is low but likely underestimated.

The lumens of the sinusoids are widened and may appear empty or filled with erythrocytes. The endothelial cells have a normal appearance in most cases. The hepatocellular plates bordering the dilated sinusoids are commonly atrophic. Other regions of the liver may demonstrate regenerative hepatocytes or frank nodularity and perisinusoidal fibrosis.[50,95,96] The mechanism underlying sinusoidal dilatation is unknown. A role for interleukin-6 has been suggested but remains unproved.

Clinical manifestations are usually lacking. Whether abdominal pain can be a manifestation of the condition or simply a trigger for the investigation that discloses it is uncertain. Liver biochemical test levels are generally mildly abnormal. Other laboratory features reflect associated conditions.[50,95,96] A particular imaging feature seen on CT or MRI is vague heterogeneity of the liver, particularly in the peripheral subcapsular areas. On the arterial and portal phases, the enhancement follows a mosaic or vaguely nodular pattern. Late-phase images show a homogeneous parenchyma.[98] Imaging findings may be unremarkable.

The mosaic pattern of enhancement following IV injection of a contrast agent appears to be specific for sinusoidal dilatation once other causes of an altered perfusion pattern have been excluded. Histologically, peliosis hepatis can be distinguished from sinusoidal dilatation by the following

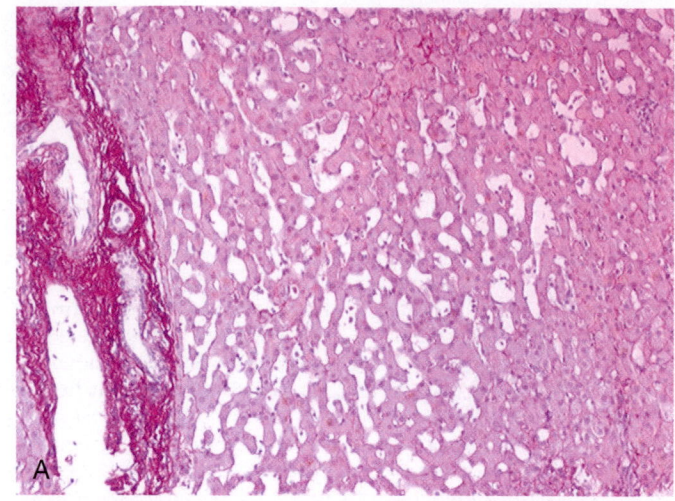
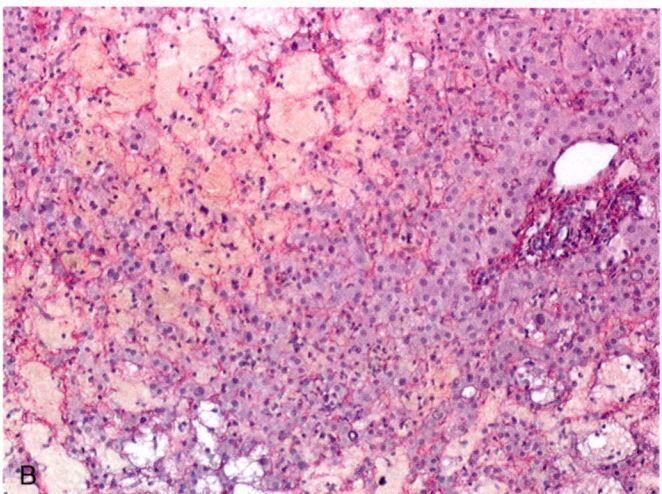

FIGURE 85-11. Histopathology of sinusoidal dilatation and peliosis hepatis. *A,* Pure noncongestive sinusoidal dilatation with continuous hepatocytes plates and sinusoid walls. *B,* Peliosis hepatitis with lobular blood cysts surrounded by interrupted hepatocytes plates and sinusoid walls. (Picrosirius-hemalun stain, ×100.)

contrasting features: round lake-like blood collections, random locations of the dilated area in the hepatic lobule, and destruction of the sinusoidal lining with erythrocytes found in the space of Disse. SOS is distinguished by the associated lesions of the central veins and the clinical context, although the distinction from peliosis hepatis may be impossible.

There is no specific treatment for either disorder. For sinusoidal dilatation, the outcome of the hepatic disease is excellent, and prognosis is related to any associated condition. For peliosis hepatitis, severe complications have occasionally been reported, including portal hypertension, liver failure, liver rupture, and death.

HEPATIC ARTERY ANEURYSM AND ATHEROSCLEROSIS

A hepatic artery aneurysm (HAA) is characterized by a localized blood-filled balloon-like bulge in the wall of an artery. HAAs are uncommon, but they are the second leading category of visceral artery aneurysms (after splenic artery aneurysms) and account for more than 20% of cases. A true aneurysm is one that involves all 3 layers of the wall of an artery (intima, media, and adventitia). A majority of true HAAs are isolated, saccular, extrahepatic lesions involving the full arterial wall. In the past, HAAs were mainly mycotic (infectious) in etiology, but today they typically result from atherosclerosis, mediointimal degeneration, trauma, and, less commonly, infection. Other rare causes of true HAAs are vasculitides (e.g., polyarteritis nodosa, SLE, Takayasu arteritis, Kawasaki disease) and connective tissue disorders (e.g., Marfan syndrome, Ehlers-Danlos syndrome, hereditary hemorrhagic telangiectasia [see later]).[99] Approximately half of HAAs are pseudoaneurysms, or false aneurysms, characterized by blood leaking out of the vessel but confined by the surrounding tissue. Pseudoaneurysms usually result from trauma as a result of a liver biopsy, transhepatic biliary drainage, cholecystectomy, hepatectomy, or liver transplantation.[100]

Symptoms of HAA include epigastric or right subchondral pain, but most affected persons are asymptomatic until the aneurysm ruptures. Rarely, a pulsatile right upper quadrant mass or thrill may be detected. Patients may present with rupture into the biliary tract, with hemobilia, epigastric pain, and jaundice; rupture into the portal vein, with portal hypertension and variceal bleeding; or rupture into the peritoneal cavity, with abdominal pain and shock. The mortality rate from rupture of a HAA is more than 30%. Nonatherosclerotic aneurysms and multiple HAAs carry an increased risk of rupture and should be treated. Although the risk of rupture of an aneurysm is independent of its size, atherosclerotic aneurysms greater than 2 cm in diameter should also be treated.[99]

Doppler US studies and CT readily demonstrate HAAs, but angiography is especially useful for defining these lesions, accessing the collateral circulation, and planning treatment. Hepatic artery pseudoaneurysms are treated effectively by angiographic embolization.[100] True extrahepatic aneurysms may be treated with embolization, provided that the presence of collateral circulation, distance from the gastroduodenal artery, absence of cirrhosis, and patency of the portal vein can be confirmed, but surgical resection of the aneurysm may be preferable to minimize the risk of hepatic infarction.[101]

Despite its frequency in the general population, atherosclerosis is rarely a cause of liver disease. Intimal thickening and atherosclerosis in hepatic arteries are less common and occur later in life than is typical for coronary arteries.[102] Hepatic infarction resulting from atherosclerosis alone is rare. The dual blood supply to the liver undoubtedly confers protection from ischemia. Nevertheless, atherosclerosis is the primary cause of approximately one third of HAAs (see earlier).[101] In addition, because the bile duct derives all of its blood supply from the hepatic artery, atherosclerosis can result in IC with biliary strictures and obstruction (see earlier).[103] The presence of atherosclerosis occasionally prevents the use of a donor liver for transplantation. Atherosclerosis makes arterial anastomoses technically more difficult to secure and may predispose the liver to ischemic injury during transport and reperfusion.

HEREDITARY HEMORRHAGIC TELANGIECTASIA

Hereditary hemorrhagic telangiectasia (HHT), or Osler-Weber-Rendu disease, is a genetic disorder with autosomal dominant inheritance, characterized by widespread cutaneous, mucosal, and visceral telangiectasias (see Chapters 20 and 37).[104] HHT is reported to affect 1 to 2 per 10,000 population.

Most patients have mutations in one of the two known disease-related genes that encode endoglin (HHT1) and activin A receptor type II-like 1 (HHT2), both of which are involved in the transforming growth factor (TGF)-β pathway. Mutations in the *Smad4* gene can cause a rare syndrome that combines juvenile polyposis and HHT; additional genes have been found on chromosomes 5 and 7.[104] Hepatic vascular malformations (HVMs) are found in 44% to 74% of patients with HHT and are more frequent in those with the HHT2 genotype than with the HHT1 genotype.[3] The penetrance increases with age, and the mean age of patients with HVMs is 52 years. Women are more commonly affected than men.[105,106]

The abnormal blood vessels in HHT result in a direct artery-to-vein connection.[104] Vascular malformations affect the liver diffusely although haphazardly. They encompass a spectrum from microscopic telangiectasias to large arteriovenous shunts.[105,106] Vascular malformations increase in size in about 20% of patients by approximately 4 years.[105] Three types of shunting may occur and coexist[3,105,106]: (1) hepatic artery-to-hepatic vein shunting can induce a decrease in systemic vascular resistance and high cardiac output, eventually evolving to heart failure; (2) hepatic artery-to-portal vein shunting can produce portal hypertension; and (3) portal vein-to-hepatic vein shunting, the rarest form, may lead to hepatic encephalopathy. Shunting of blood may produce IC (see earlier) and mesenteric ischemia.[105,106] There is a marked increase in hepatic arterial blood flow and accordingly in the size of hepatic arteries.[105,106] By causing uneven parenchymal perfusion, shunting of blood and portal venous inflow deprivation are likely responsible for nodular regenerative hyperplasia, regenerative macronodules, and focal nodular hyperplasia that develop in areas with preserved inflow of hyperarterialized blood.[105,106]

High-output heart failure and complications of portal hypertension are the most common manifestations of HVMs. GI bleeding in patients with portal hypertension is more frequently related to intestinal telangiectasias than to ruptured gastroesophageal varices (see Chapter 37).[105] A systolic bruit may be heard in the hepatic area. An acute presentation with severe cholangitis related to IC is uncommon. An exceptional picture of acute or fulminant liver failure is related to acute ischemic necrosis of large bile ducts (also referred to as "acute disintegration" of the liver).[3] Increased serum alkaline phosphatase and GGTP levels, with a normal serum bilirubin level, are common. These abnormalities are not necessarily associated with large bile duct damage.[105,106]

In patients with HVMs, abdominal imaging usually shows a heterogeneous, enlarged, dysmorphic liver and patchy enhancement during the arterial phase.[105,106] Enhancement of the hepatic veins in the arterial phase indicates severe hepatic artery–to–hepatic vein shunting. The hepatic artery is markedly enlarged. Regenerative macronodules and focal nodular hyperplasia may have a typical massive and homogeneous enhancement during the arterial phase while reaching an attenuation similar to that of the surrounding parenchyma during the later phases. Purely benign nodules may occasionally be extremely heterogeneous and even show washout in the late phase.[105,106] Recognizing HHT in patients with hepatic anomalies relies on comprehensive history taking and a thorough physical examination for telangiectasias. HHT should be considered in patients with multiple focal nodular hyperplasias. Genetic testing is needed to diagnose sporadic cases. Recognizing HVMs in patients with known or suspected HHT is based mostly on indirect evidence of arteriovenous shunting on imaging, with early enhancement of the hepatic veins during the arterial phase and an enlarged hepatic artery. US is the recommended initial examination.[3,105] Liver biopsy, which is hazardous in such patients, is rarely needed once a diagnosis of HHT with liver involvement has been made.[3] The probability that hepatic nodules are benign regenerative nodules or focal nodular hyperplasia is highest in this setting, whereas biliary disease is likely to be IC in HHT-related HVMs.

Asymptomatic patients with HVMs do not require treatment. Management of patients with high-output cardiac failure requires aggressive therapy.[3] In patients with complications of portal hypertension, the guidelines for patients with cirrhosis may be applied (see Chapter 92).[3] In patients failing to respond to the first-line intensive symptomatic therapy, second-line therapeutic options include bevacizumab therapy,[107] staged embolization, and liver transplantation.[3] Of these options, only the last one is definitive, and each of these options carries a significant risk of potentially fatal complications. Over 90% of patients with HVMs are asymptomatic. Still, rates of complications and death are 3.6 and 1.1 per 100 person-years, respectively.[105] There is a correlation between a Doppler US–based grading of hepatic involvement and clinical outcome.[105] Cardiac failure and portal hypertension have occurred at a rate of 1.4 and 1.2 per 100 person-years, respectively.[105] Cardiac failure and portal hypertension are each responsible for half of the fatalities related to HVMs.[105] About two thirds of patients show a complete response to intensive first-line therapy for complicated HVMs and therefore do not need embolization or liver transplantation.[105] Survival rates close to 90% have been reported after liver transplantation; liver transplantation for heart failure achieves better results than for portal hypertension.[108]

KEY REFERENCES

Full references for this chapter can be found on www.expertconsult.com.

8. Smalberg JH, Arends LR, Valla DC, et al. Myeloproliferative neoplasms in Budd-Chiari syndrome and portal vein thrombosis: A meta-analysis. Blood 2012; 120:4921-8.

19. Moucari R, Rautou PE, Cazals-Hatem D, et al. Hepatocellular carcinoma in Budd-Chiari syndrome: Characteristics and risk factors. Gut 2008; 57:828-35.

22. Seijo S, Plessier A, Hoekstra J, et al. Good long-term outcome of Budd-Chiari syndrome with a step-wise management. Hepatology 2013; 57:1962-8.

28. Plessier A, Darwish-Murad S, Hernandez-Guerra M, et al. Acute portal vein thrombosis unrelated to cirrhosis: A prospective multicenter follow-up study. Hepatology 2010; 51:210-8.

42. Condat B, Pessione F, Hillaire S, et al. Current outcome of portal vein thrombosis in adults: Risk and benefit of anticoagulant therapy. Gastroenterology 2001; 120:490-7.

50. Kakar S, Kamath PS, Burgart LJ. Sinusoidal dilatation and congestion in liver biopsy: Is it always due to venous outflow impairment? Arch Pathol Lab Med 2004; 128:901-4.

53. Lautz TB, Keys LA, Melvin JC, et al. Advantages of the meso-Rex bypass compared with portosystemic shunts in the management of extrahepatic portal vein obstruction in children. J Am Coll Surg 2013; 216:83-9.

55. Llop E, de Juan C, Seijo S, et al. Portal cholangiopathy: Radiological classification and natural history. Gut 2011; 60:853-60.

61. Sochatzis EA, Senzolo M, Germani G, et al. Systematic review: Portal vein thrombosis in cirrhosis. Aliment Pharmacol Ther 2010; 31:366-74.

67. Villa E, Camma C, Marietta M, et al. Enoxaparin prevents portal vein thrombosis and liver decompensation in patients with advanced cirrhosis. Gastroenterology 2012; 143:1253-60 e1-4.

70. Cazals-Hatem D, Hillaire S, Rudler M, et al. Obliterative portal venopathy: Portal hypertension is not always present at diagnosis. J Hepatol 2011; 54:455-61.

74. Rubbia-Brandt L, Lauwers GY, Wang H, et al. Sinusoidal obstruction syndrome and nodular regenerative hyperplasia are frequent oxaliplatin-associated liver lesions and partially prevented by bevacizumab in patients with hepatic colorectal metastasis. Histopathology 2010; 56:430-9.

80. Bernard O, Franchi-Abella S, Branchereau S, et al. Congenital portosystemic shunts in children: Recognition, evaluation, and management. Semin Liver Dis 2012; 32:273-87.

91. Deltenre P, Valla DC. Ischemic cholangiopathy. Semin Liver Dis 2008; 28:235-46.

105. Buscarini E, Leandro G, Conte D, et al. Natural history and outcome of hepatic vascular malformations in a large cohort of patients with hereditary hemorrhagic telangiectasia. Dig Dis Sci 2011; 56:2166-78.

Alcoholic liver disease remains a challenging enigma for basic scientists and clinicians. Despite extensive research since the 1950s, many important facets of this disease have yet to be resolved. Paramount among these important questions are the following: (1) Why does cirrhosis develop in only a small fraction of heavy alcohol abusers? (2) What is the pathogenesis of severe alcoholic liver disease? (3) What are the most effective treatments for patients with severe alcoholic liver disease?

EPIDEMIOLOGY

Excessive consumption of alcohol is the third leading preventable cause of death in the United States.[1] The total costs of alcohol abuse amount to $223.5 billion annually, most of which are related to lost productivity and motor vehicle collisions.[2] Alcohol use also is the third leading risk factor for global disease burden (Fig. 86-1); for persons 15 to 49 years of age, it is the leading risk factor for mortality and disease burden in the world.[3]

Alcohol abuse is the most common etiology of cirrhosis in the developed world. It is the underlying cause of 44% of liver disease deaths in the United States, resulting in 13,000 deaths annually and exceeding those for hepatitis C, the second most common fatal liver disease in this country.[4-6] In Europe and the United States combined, alcoholic liver disease and its complications account for 50,000 deaths each year.[7]

Numerous studies have shown that alcoholic liver disease develops in women after a shorter duration of drinking and with a lower daily alcohol intake than in men.[8,9] Population-based surveys have documented that men usually must drink 40 to 80 g of alcohol daily and women must drink 20 to 40 g daily for 10 to 12 years to achieve a significant risk of liver disease.[8-10] Table 86-1 illustrates the alcohol content of various beverages sold in the United States, their typical serving sizes, and the daily alcohol intake, for at least 10 years, that puts both men and women at risk for the development of alcoholic liver disease.[11]

SPECTRUM OF DISEASE

Chronic alcohol abuse can result in a spectrum of liver injury that ranges from mild fatty infiltration to cirrhosis and hepatocellular carcinoma (Fig. 86-2).[12-15] Fat accumulation in liver cells, the earliest and most predictable response to alcohol ingestion, is seen in 90% of heavy drinkers.[15] Although fatty liver generally is a benign condition that reverses quickly with abstinence, cirrhosis can develop within 5 years in 10% of patients who continue to drink heavily.[16] More important than steatosis is the development of necroinflammation and fibrosis (alcoholic hepatitis, or steatohepatitis) that occurs in approximately 10% to 35% of heavy drinkers. Alcoholic hepatitis is an important clinical entity for the following reasons: (1) patients with severe disease have extremely high short-term mortality rates, (2) they also can develop portal hypertension in the absence of cirrhosis, and (3) this entity is a well-documented precursor of cirrhosis, with a long-term risk 9 times higher than that for patients with fatty liver alone.[16,17] With continued alcohol abuse, a fine mesh-like pattern of fibrosis (micronodular cirrhosis) develops in 8% to 20% of heavy drinkers. Over time, this lesion can evolve to include

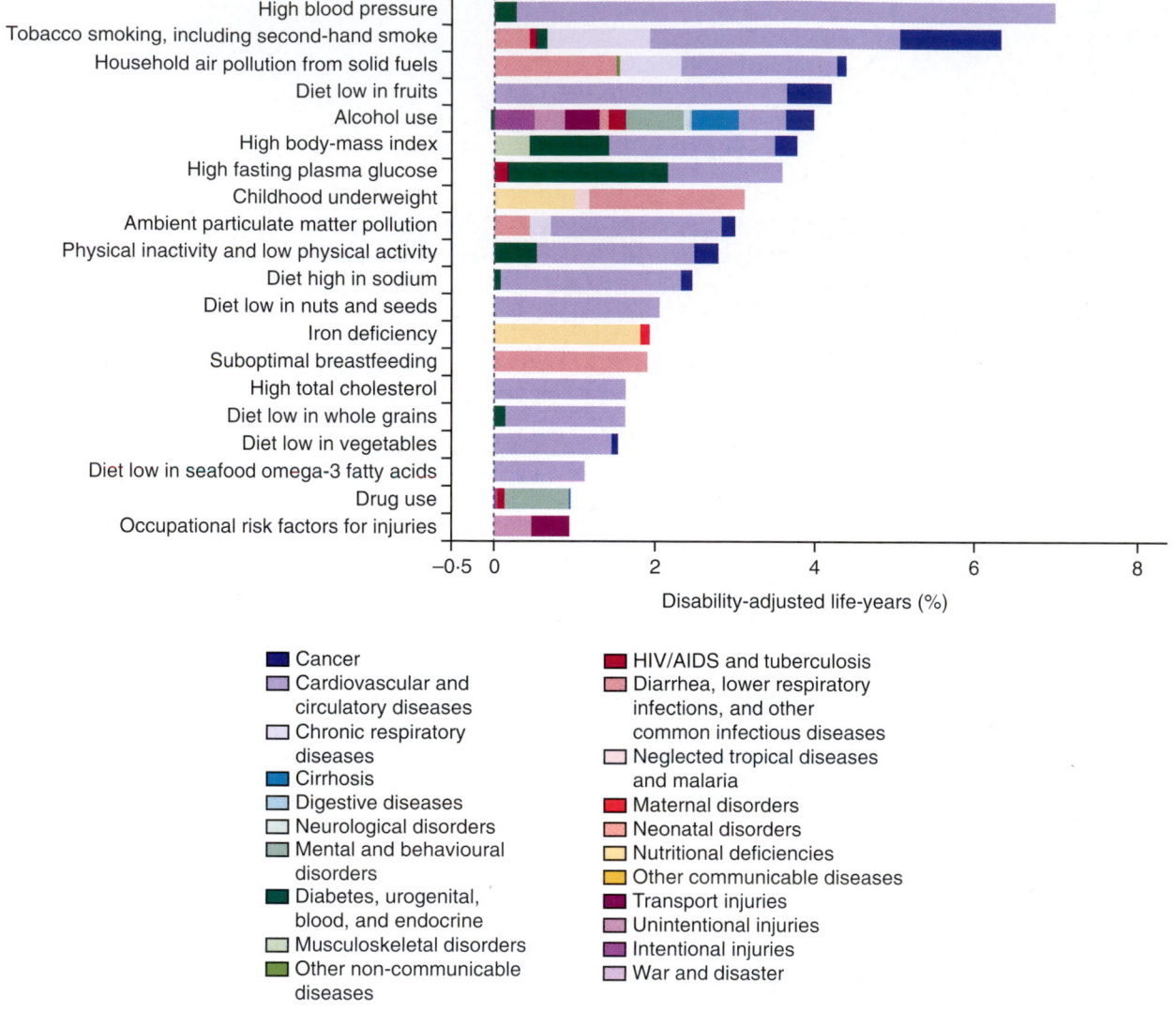

FIGURE 86-1. Burden of disease in 2010 attributable to risk factors, expressed as a percentage of global disability-adjusted life years. Alcohol use is fifth on the list. *(Adapted from Lim SS, Vos T, Flaxman AD, et al. A comparative risk assessment of burden of disease and injury attributable to 67 risk factors and risk factor clusters in 21 regions, 1990-2010: A systematic analysis for the Global Burden of Disease 2010. Lancet 2010; 380:2224-60.)*

TABLE 86-1 Alcohol Content of Various Beverages					
				Daily Intake Needed to Exceed Threshold for Alcoholic Liver Disease*	
Beverage	**Approximate Alcohol Content**	**Serving Size**	**Amount of Alcohol**	**Men**	**Women**
Beer	5%	12 oz	14.02 g	3-6 cans	1.5-3 cans
Wine	12%	5 oz	14.02 g	3-6 glasses	1.5-3 glasses
Hard liquor	40%	1.5 oz	14.02 g	3-6 drinks	1.5-3 drinks

*Alcohol intake of 40-80 g/day for men and 20-40 g/day for women for 10 years.

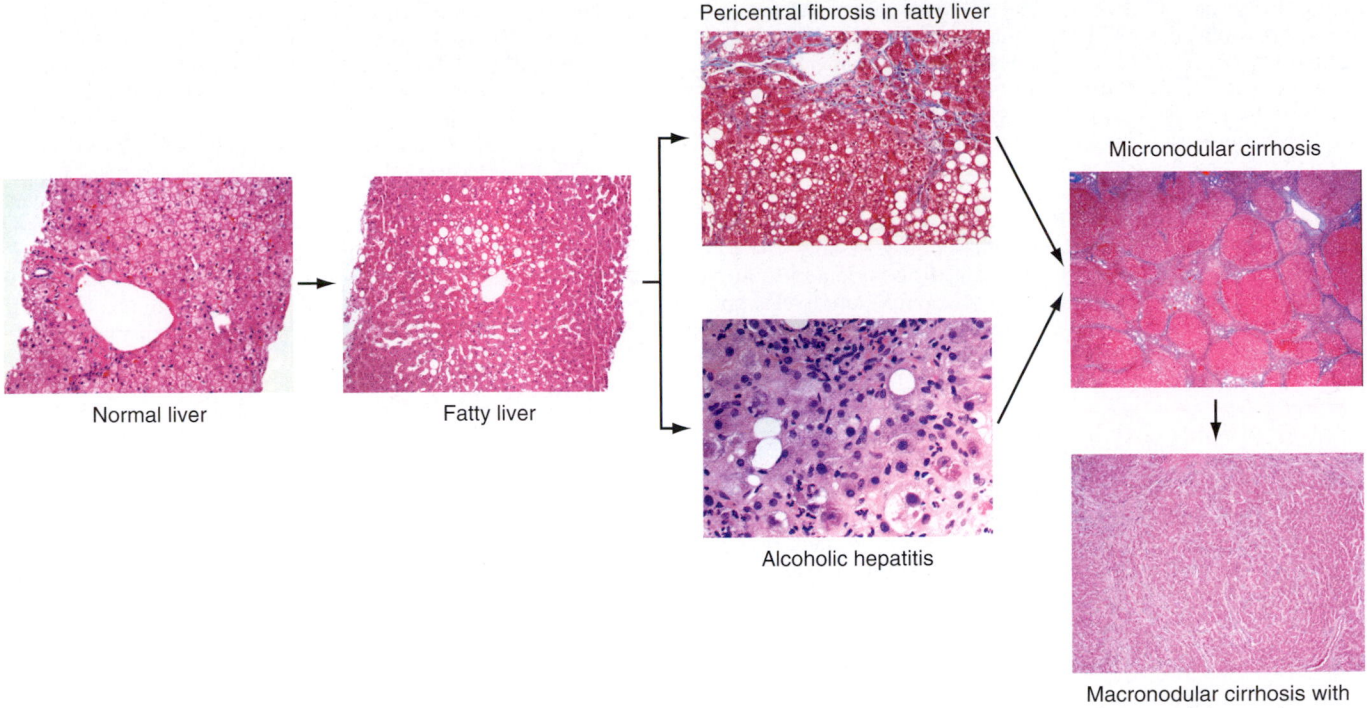

Pericentral fibrosis in fatty liver

Micronodular cirrhosis

Normal liver

Fatty liver

Alcoholic hepatitis

Macronodular cirrhosis with hepatocellular carcinoma

FIGURE 86-2. Histopathologic spectrum of alcoholic liver disease.

broad bands of fibrosis that separate large nodules of liver tissue (macronodular cirrhosis)[14]; hepatocellular carcinoma typically develops in this setting.[18]

PATHOGENESIS

Ethanol Metabolism and Toxic Metabolites

The liver is the main organ responsible for ethanol metabolism; other organs such as the stomach contribute to much lesser degrees. Ethanol is metabolized by 3 major systems in the liver: alcohol dehydrogenase (ADH), cytochrome P450 2E1 (CYP2E1), and, of least importance, catalase.[19] ADH is the primary enzyme system responsible for metabolism of ethanol at low concentrations, whereas CYP2E1 contributes at higher concentrations of ethanol (>10 mM) and is induced by exposure to ethanol. Both ADH and CYP2E1 convert ethanol to acetaldehyde, which is then converted by aldehyde dehydrogenase (ALDH) to acetate. Acetaldehyde is a highly reactive and potentially toxic compound that is responsible for many of the systemic toxic effects of alcohol, such as nausea, headaches, and flushing.

Acetaldehyde also is postulated to play an etiologic role in alcoholic liver disease. Acetaldehyde can form adducts with reactive residues on proteins or small molecules (e.g., cysteines). These chemical modifications can alter or interfere with normal biological processes and can be directly toxic to the cell. Modified molecules may also stimulate the host's immune response and cause autoimmune-like manifestations. Antibodies against such oxidatively modified proteins have been reported in both human and animal models of alcoholic liver disease.[20] An example is the hybrid adduct of malondialdehyde and acetaldehyde (MAA), unique to alcohol exposure, which induces an immune reaction in human alcoholics and in animal models.[20] Acetaldehyde also has been shown to impair mitochondrial glutathione transport and to sensitize

hepatocytes to TNF-mediated killing.[21] Lastly, acetaldehyde disrupts intestinal barrier function, leading to endotoxemia and proinflammatory cytokine production.

In addition to forming cytotoxic metabolites such as acetaldehyde, ethanol metabolism can alter the cellular oxidation-reduction (redox) state, thereby modulating liver injury. Specifically, the oxidation of ethanol uses nicotinamide adenine dinucleotide (NAD$^+$) as an electron acceptor and thereby causes a shift in the ratio of reduced NAD (NADH) to NAD$^+$ to a more reduced state.[19] This change in the redox state can impair normal carbohydrate and lipid metabolism; multiple effects ensue, including a decrease in the supply of ATP to the cell and an increase in hepatic steatosis.

Other Metabolic Mechanisms

Oxidative Stress

Oxidative stress is an imbalance between pro-oxidants and antioxidants. Reactive oxygen species (ROS) and reactive nitrogen species (RNS) are products of normal metabolism and can be beneficial to the host (e.g., by contributing to bacterial killing).[22] Overproduction of ROS and RNS or inadequate antioxidant defenses (e.g., low levels of vitamins, selenium, mitochondrial glutathione), or both, can lead to liver injury. Oxidative stress in alcoholic liver disease is usually documented by detection of one of several indirect markers: (1) protein oxidation (e.g., protein thiol or carbonyl products), (2) lipid oxidation (e.g., isoprostanes, malondialdehyde), (3) DNA oxidation (e.g., oxodeoxyguanosine), or (4) depletion or induction of antioxidant defenses (e.g., vitamin E, glutathione, thioredoxin).[23]

The stimulus for oxidative stress in the liver comes from multiple sources. In hepatocytes, CYP2E1 activity increases after alcohol consumption—in part because of stabilization of messenger RNA (mRNA). The CYP2E1 system leaks electrons to initiate oxidative stress.[22] CYP2E1 is localized in the hepatic lobule in areas of alcohol-induced liver injury. Moreover, overexpression of CYP2E1 in mice and in HepG2 cells (a human hepatoma cell line) in vitro leads to enhanced alcohol hepatotoxicity.[24,25] Nonparenchymal cells and infiltrating inflammatory cells (e.g., polymorphonuclear neutrophils) are another major source of pro-oxidants that are used for normal cellular processes, such as killing invading organisms. Major enzyme systems for pro-oxidant production in Kupffer cells include NAD phosphate (NADPH) oxidase and inducible nitric oxide synthase (iNOS). Mice deficient in NADPH oxidase or mice treated with the drug diphenyleneiodonium sulfate, which blocks NADPH oxidase, are resistant to ethanol-induced liver injury.[26] Infiltrating neutrophils use enzyme systems such as myeloperoxidase to generate hypochlorus acid ($HOCl^-$, a halide species that causes oxidative stress) and RNS.

Oxidative stress can mediate liver injury through at least 2 major pathways: direct cell injury and cell signaling. Direct cell injury is indicated by markers such as lipid peroxidation and DNA damage. An even greater role is played by signaling pathways; for example, activation of transcription factors such as nuclear factor kappa B (NF-κB) plays a critical role in the production of cytokines such as TNF.

Mitochondrial Dysfunction

Mitochondria are the major consumers of molecular oxygen and major generators of ROS in the liver. Mitochondrial dysfunction is well documented in alcoholic liver disease and contributes to oxidative stress.[27]

Mitochondrial abnormalities in alcoholic liver disease include megamitochondria observed on light and electron microscopy and functional mitochondrial abnormalities as documented by an abnormal ^{13}C ketoacid breath test result (ketoacids are metabolized by mitochondria). Short-term administration of alcohol causes increased hepatic superoxide generation in liver mitochondria, with an increased flow of electrons along the respiratory electron transport chain. The increased $NADH/NAD^+$ ratio caused by ethanol intake favors superoxide generation.[22] Because hepatic mitochondria lack catalase, glutathione plays a critical role in protecting mitochondria against oxidative stress. Mitochondria do not make glutathione but instead import it from the cytosol. In alcoholic liver disease, the transport of glutathione into mitochondria is impaired, and selective mitochondrial glutathione depletion is observed. Glutathione depletion also sensitizes the liver to the toxic effects of TNF, and TNF also impairs mitochondrial function.

Normal mitochondrial function requires continuous exchange of substrate between the cytosol and the mitochondrial matrix, and this process is catalyzed by specific exchangers within the inner mitochondrial membrane. On the other hand, exchange of most water-soluble metabolites between the cytosol and the intermembrane space occurs through the voltage-dependent anion channel (VDAC) in the mitochondrial outer membrane. Alcohol-mediated closure of the VDAC limits free diffusion of metabolites into the intermembrane space and causes mitochondrial dysfunction.[28] This is likely a cause of global alterations in mitochondrial function related to alcohol abuse and alcoholic liver disease.

Hypoxia

The centrilobular area of the hepatic lobule (the functional unit of the liver [see Chapter 71]) has the lowest oxygen tension and greatest susceptibility to hypoxia. Chronic alcohol intake increases oxygen uptake by the liver and increases the lobular oxygen gradient. A chronic intragastric feeding model in rats has been used to define the mechanisms that underlie hepatic hypoxia and the association of these mechanisms with cycling of urinary alcohol levels (UALs).[29] At high UALs, hepatic hypoxia is observed, along with reduced ATP levels; the $NADH/NAD^+$ ratio is shifted to the reduced state; and, hypoxia-inducible factor (HIF) genes are up-regulated. When UALs fall, reperfusion injury occurs, with free radical formation and peak liver enzyme release from hepatocytes. Hepatocyte-specific HIF-1α has been shown to be up-regulated in alcohol-fed mice and to play a role in hepatic lipid accumulation.[30] While HIF and HIF-regulated proteins appear to be up-regulated in the liver during alcohol feeding, intestinal HIF is markedly down-regulated. The down-regulation of intestinal HIF appears to play a role in the increase in intestinal permeability, with subsequent endotoxemia and liver injury. Indeed, one mechanism of the beneficial action of the probiotic agent *Lactobacillus* GG in experimental alcoholic liver disease appears to be the maintenance of intestinal HIF.[31]

Impaired Proteasome Function

The 26S ubiquitin-proteasome pathway is the primary proteolytic pathway of eukaryotic cells (see Chapter 72). This pathway controls the levels of numerous proteins involved in gene regulation, cell division, and surface receptor expression, as well as the stress response and inflammation. The proteasome system is considered a cellular defense mechanism because it also removes irregular and damaged proteins generated by mutations, translational errors, or oxidative stress.[32] Animal studies have demonstrated that chronic ethanol feeding results in a significant decrease in proteolytic activity of the proteasome; this decreased activity can lead to abnormal protein accumulation, including accumulation of oxidized proteins.[33] The decrease in proteasome function correlates significantly with the level of hepatic oxidative stress. Hepatocytes from alcoholics contain large amounts of ubiquitin in the form of cellular inclusions, or Mallory-Denk (or simply Mallory) bodies, which accumulate because they are not degraded efficiently by the proteasome.[34] As hepatocytes die as a result of proteasome inhibition, they inappropriately release cytokines such as interleukin (IL)-8 and IL-18. IL-8 recruits neutrophils and probably plays a role in neutrophil infiltration in alcoholic hepatitis, whereas IL-18 sustains inflammation in the liver.[35]

Abnormal Metabolism of Methionine, S-Adenosylmethionine, and Folate

In mammals, the liver plays a central role in methionine metabolism; nearly half of the daily intake of methionine is metabolized in the liver (Fig. 86-3). The first step in methionine metabolism is the formation of S-adenosylmethionine (SAMe) in a reaction catalyzed by methionine adenosyltransferase (MAT). Activity of this enzyme is depressed in alcoholic liver disease.[36-38] SAMe is the principal biological methyl donor through the transmethylation pathway, the precursor of aminopropyl groups used in polyamine biosynthesis, and a precursor of glutathione through its conversion to cysteine along the transsulfuration pathway.

Deficiency of SAMe in patients with alcoholic liver disease was first noted in the early 1980s, when it was observed that alcoholic subjects had delayed clearance of an oral bolus of methionine (presumably because of blocked conversion of methionine to SAMe).[37,38] Functional MAT activity was subsequently shown to be subnormal in liver biopsy specimens from alcoholic subjects. Exogenous administration of SAMe corrects the deficiency and attenuates the severity of many experimental forms of liver injury.

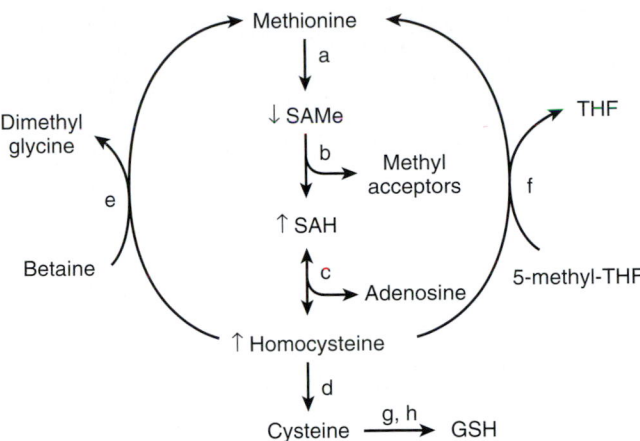

FIGURE 86-3. Hepatic methionine metabolism. Chronic alcohol consumption causes *S*-adenosylmethionine (SAMe) deficiency and an increase in *S*-adenosylhomocysteine (SAH) and homocysteine levels. a, methionine adenosyltransferase; b, enzymes involved in transmethylation reactions, including phosphatidylethanolamine *N*-methyltransferase; c, SAH hydrolase; d, cystathionine B-synthase; e, betaine-homocysteine methyltransferase; f, methionine synthetase; g, glutamate-cysteine synthetase; h, glutathione (GSH) synthetase; THF, tetrahydrofolate; ↑↓, effects of alcohol.

In models of alcohol-induced hepatotoxicity, SAMe has been shown to maintain mitochondrial glutathione levels. Depletion of mitochondrial glutathione is thought to be one pathogenic factor in the development of alcoholic liver disease, and SAMe, but not other glutathione prodrugs, prevents mitochondrial glutathione depletion in experimental alcoholic liver disease (possibly by protecting mitochondrial glutathione transport systems).[39] The antioxidant response element (ARE) is an essential component of upstream regulatory sequences present on many genes that provide hepatoprotection, including most phase II detoxification enzymes (see Chapter 88). NF-E2-related factor 2 (Nrf2) is a critical transcription factor that binds to the ARE and plays a key role in cellular responses to stress via the Keap1-Nrf2-ARE pathway. In experimental cholestatic liver disease, Nrf2 binding decreases, and this occurrence is partially prevented with SAMe therapy. Therefore, SAMe therapy may help maintain glutathione levels as well as induce other antioxidant pathways by maintaining appropriate Nrf2 binding.[40,41] SAMe also decreases lipopolysaccharide (LPS)-stimulated TNF release and increases IL-10 release in a monocyte cell line.[36] Similarly, in rats fed a diet to induce SAMe deficiency, serum TNF levels increase and sensitivity to endotoxin-induced hepatotoxicity, which can be blocked by injection of SAMe, increases markedly. These data support the concept that SAMe may have direct hepatoprotective functions and may modify LPS-stimulated cytokine production.

Although serum SAMe levels are decreased in patients with alcoholic liver disease, levels of the downstream products *S*-adenosylhomocysteine (SAH) and homocysteine are elevated.[37,38,42] Elevated SAH levels have been shown to sensitize hepatocytes to TNF-mediated destruction, and SAH may be a critical physiologic sensitizer of TNF-mediated killing in liver injury.[42] Homocysteine and SAH can be removed by giving betaine, which facilitates regeneration of methionine from homocysteine. Folic acid also can play a critical role in the regeneration of homocysteine to methionine by means of 5-methyltetrahydrofolate (5-MTHF).[43] Folic acid deficiency enhances the development of alcohol-induced liver injury in micropigs, and alcohol feeding interferes with normal folic acid metabolism in multiple different pathways—from impaired intestinal uptake to increased renal excretion.[43] Collectively, the data support a role for altered methionine-transmethylation-transsulfuration metabolism in alcoholic liver disease and link these pathways to TNF hepatotoxicity.[38]

Immune and Inflammatory Mechanisms

Gut-Liver Axis and Dysregulated Cytokine Production

It is now generally accepted that the intestinal flora and gut-derived toxins play a critical role in the development of alcoholic liver disease and its complications (Fig. 86-4).[44] Indeed, germ-free rodents or rodents treated with antibiotics to "sterilize the gut" are resistant to nutritional and toxin-induced liver injury. Early studies showed that cirrhosis developed in rats fed a choline-deficient diet and that the cirrhosis could be prevented by oral neomycin.[45] When endotoxin was added to the water supply, however, neomycin no longer prevented the development of liver injury and fibrosis.[45] Subsequently, antibiotics, prebiotics, and probiotics have all been used to prevent experimental alcohol-induced liver injury.[46] Numerous clinical studies have also demonstrated that plasma endotoxin levels are significantly elevated in patients with various stages of alcoholic liver disease—fatty liver, hepatitis, and cirrhosis—when compared with healthy control subjects. Ethanol-induced endotoxemia observed in experimental rodent models of alcoholic liver disease also provides support for the essential role of LPS in the development of liver injury.

Alcohol-induced intestinal barrier dysfunction and endotoxemia are multifactorial events, with altered microflora and impaired intestinal integrity among the causal factors (see Fig. 86-4). Alcohol promotes the overgrowth of Gram-negative bacteria in the intestines of patients with chronic alcohol abuse. Studies on intestinal flora from alcoholics in an inpatient treatment program demonstrated altered microflora composition, with decreased numbers of *Bifidobacterium* spp. and *Lactobacillus* spp.[47] Two animal studies have documented altered intestinal flora with chronic alcohol feeding. Intestinal bacterial overgrowth of both aerobic and anaerobic bacteria after 3 weeks of intragastric alcohol feeding has been demonstrated in an animal model of alcoholic liver disease.[48] Hepatic steatosis and steatohepatitis occurred simultaneously with translocation of live bacteria into the systemic circulation. Importantly, prebiotic therapy attenuated liver injury. In a second study, mice were fed alcohol for 8 weeks.[49] Major changes in intestinal flora occurred relatively late in the disease process, whereas changes in intestinal barrier function and endotoxemia occurred much earlier. Fecal pH increased in association with alterations in intestinal flora, and probiotic therapy for the final 2 weeks effectively treated liver disease (decrease in serum liver enzyme levels, reduction in endotoxemia, and correction of intestinal trefoil factor and tight junction proteins). In both studies, alcohol intake decreased levels of critical intestinal antimicrobial peptides.

Alcohol and its metabolite acetaldehyde induce intestinal permeability to various macromolecules including LPS in both human subjects and animal models of alcoholic liver disease.[38] Translocation of LPS across the intestinal epithelial barrier has been attributed to disruption of intestinal barrier integrity. Indeed, decreased tight junction (ZO-1) protein levels were observed in sigmoid colonic biopsy specimens of human alcoholics when compared with healthy controls. This finding was attributed to an increase in microRNA (miRNA)-212 expression observed in alcoholic subjects compared with controls.[50] Alcohol-induced oxidative stress and generation of nitric

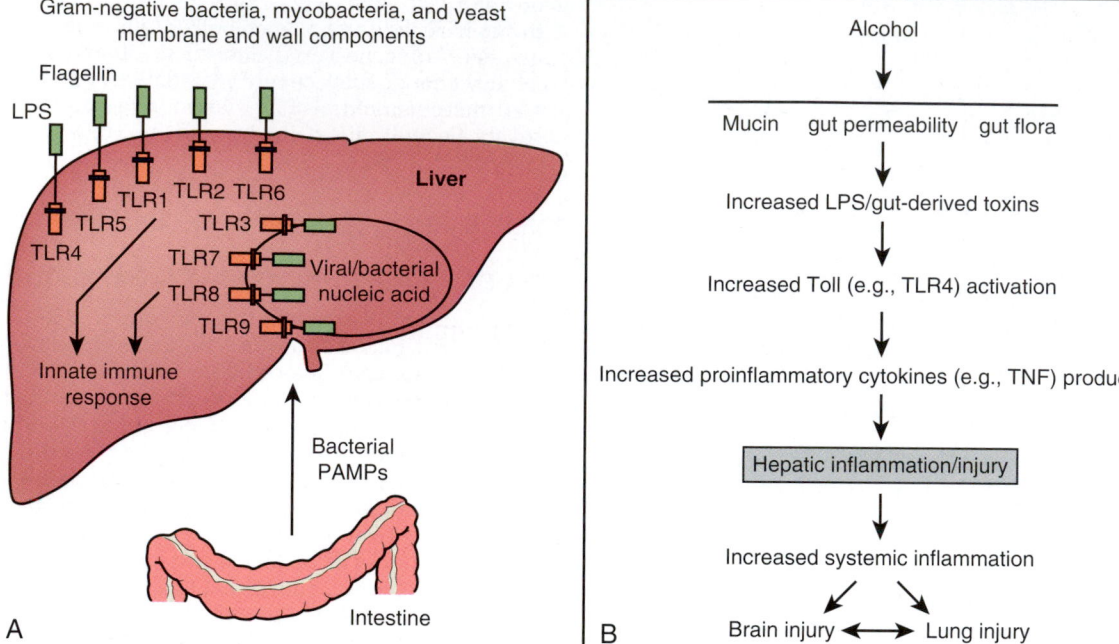

FIGURE 86-4. The gut-liver axis. *A,* Under certain circumstances, gut-derived pathogen-associated molecular patterns (PAMPs), including lipopolysaccharide (LPS), lipopeptides, flagellin, unmethylated DNA and double-stranded RNA, other components of Gram-negative bacteria, and other microbiota, translocate from the intestine into the portal vein and to the liver. In the liver, they are recognized by specific recognition receptors, the Toll-like receptors (TLRs). This results in initiation of an innate immune response, production of inflammatory mediators, and subsequent liver injury. *B,* Alcohol alters gut-barrier function, thereby promoting bacteria and LPS translocation, TLR activation, cytokine production (e.g., TNF), liver injury, and potentially other organ injury, including brain inflammation, which may stimulate further alcohol consumption.

oxide in the intestines of experimental animals, leading to loss of tight junction integrity, intestinal leakiness, endotoxemia, hepatic inflammation, and liver injury, have also been reported.[51] Multiple laboratories have also reported increased intestinal permeability in experimental animal models of alcoholic liver disease due to redistribution and decreased expression of intestinal tight junction proteins.[38] Increased intestinal production of proinflammatory cytokines, such as TNF-α and IL-6, can also contribute to alcoholic endotoxemia by altering tight junction morphology and distribution, thereby creating a self-perpetuating vicious cycle that can amplify bacterial translocation.[52]

Increased plasma and hepatic concentrations of proinflammatory cytokines (e.g., TNF-α) are consistently observed in rodent models of alcoholic liver disease and are stimulated in large part by gut-derived toxins (see Fig. 86-4). Toll-like receptor 4 (TLR-4) activation by endotoxin results in recruitment of the adaptor molecules MyD88 and Toll/IL-1 receptor (TIR) domain–containing adapter inducing interferon-β (TRIF), which each activate separate downstream signaling cascades. Data suggest that the MyD88-independent pathway (TRIF) is more important in the development of experimental alcoholic liver disease, whereas nonalcoholic steatohepatitis appears to signal through the MyD88-dependent pathway.[53]

Dysregulated cytokine metabolism in human alcoholic liver disease has been recognized since the 1980s, with the initial observation that peripheral blood monocytes from patients with alcoholic hepatitis have significantly increased basal and LPS-stimulated TNF production.[54,55] Serum concentrations of TNF-inducible cytokines and chemokines, such as IL-6, IL-8, IL-18, monocyte chemoattractant protein 1 (MCP-1), and others, are elevated in patients with alcoholic hepatitis or cirrhosis, and the levels often correlate with markers of the

acute-phase response, reduced liver function, and poor clinical outcomes.[54]

This enhanced cytokine response to a physiologic stimulus such as LPS is termed *priming.* Increased serum or urinary levels of neopterin and other markers indicate that monocytes and Kupffer cells are primed in alcoholic liver disease. This priming for LPS-stimulated TNF production has been reproduced in vitro by culturing monocyte cell lines with relevant concentrations of alcohol. This response appears to be mediated, at least in part, by induction of CYP2E1 and oxidative stress.[56] Not only are levels of proinflammatory cytotoxic cytokines increased in alcoholic liver disease, but also monocyte and Kupffer cell production of protective anti-inflammatory cytokines, such as IL-10, is decreased.[57]

Several strategies have been devised to decrease cytokine production or activity in an attempt to block or attenuate liver injury. Examples include antibiotics to modulate intestinal flora and LPS, gadolinium chloride to destroy Kupffer cells, and antioxidants such as glutathione prodrugs to inhibit cytokine production. Each of these strategies has been successful in attenuating alcohol-induced liver injury in rats.[54] Administration of prebiotics such as oat bran or probiotics has also been shown to decrease endotoxemia in experimentally induced alcoholic liver injury. Moreover, anti-TNF antibody has been used to prevent liver injury in alcohol-fed rats,[58] and alcoholic liver injury does not develop in mice that lack the TNF type I receptor.[59]

Hepatocytes normally are resistant to TNF killing. Hepatocytes from rats fed alcohol or hepatocytes incubated in alcohol are sensitized to TNF killing, however.[24,60] Some potentially relevant mechanisms for this sensitization include mitochondrial depletion of glutathione, accumulation of SAH, and proteasome inhibition. Therefore, in alcoholic liver disease, monocytes and Kupffer cells are primed to increase production of TNF, and hepatocytes are sensitized to TNF killing. These processes are closely intertwined with previously described mechanisms such as oxidative stress, mitochondrial dysfunction, abnormal metabolism of methionine, and dysfunction of proteasomes.

Immune Responses to Altered Hepatocellular Proteins

Alcoholic hepatitis may persist histologically for many months after exposure to ethanol has ceased, suggesting an ongoing immune or autoimmune response. Autoimmune reactions are now well documented in patients with alcoholic liver disease, with autoantibodies directed against phospholipids, alcohol dehydrogenase, heat shock protein, and other potential antigens. Patients with alcoholic liver disease are at increased risk for the development of immune responses directed at neoantigens generated from the interactions of metabolites of alcohol (e.g., acetaldehyde or hydroxyethyl radicals) with liver proteins. Some studies have also linked genetic susceptibility and autoimmunity in alcoholic liver disease.[61]

Gender and Genetic Factors

Because the development of liver injury varies among people who drink the same amount of alcohol, great interest exists in possible gender-associated and genetic predisposition to alcoholic liver disease. Female gender is a well-accepted risk factor for the development and rapid progression of alcoholic liver disease.[8,9] Studies in rats or mice chronically fed alcohol also have demonstrated that females are more susceptible than males to liver injury. Risk factors for the development of liver disease in females appear to include sex hormone levels, endotoxemia, lipid peroxidation, chemokines, and NF-κB activation. These risk factors are critical for determining "safe" levels of alcohol consumption in women. Indeed, many authorities consider any amount of alcohol above 20 g a day to be a risk factor for the development of liver disease in women.

Genetic polymorphisms in alcohol-metabolizing systems such as CYP2E1 and ADH have been postulated to play a role in the development of alcoholic liver disease. None of these polymorphisms, however, adequately explains the diverse pathologic responses seen among patients with alcoholic liver disease. Polymorphisms in the promoter regions of cytokines TNF and IL-10 have also been reported to predispose affected persons to the development of alcoholic liver disease and are under active study.[62] A sequence variation (rs738409) within the gene coding for patatin-like phospholipase encoding 3 (PNPLA3) has been found to modulate steatosis, necroinflammation, and fibrosis in NAFLD, and this same variant has been shown to be a robust genetic risk factor for progressive alcoholic liver disease.[62]

Epigenetic mechanisms that regulate gene expression primarily involve alterations to the chromatin structure via DNA and histone modifications, without changes to the underlying DNA sequence. Alcohol administration to experimental animals has been demonstrated to result in epigenetic alterations in the liver, including posttranslational histone modifications and DNA methylation.[63-65] Histone acetylation is a key component in the regulation of gene expression and is associated with enhanced transcriptional activity, whereas deacetylation is typically associated with transcriptional repression. Steady-state levels of acetylation of the core histones result from the balance between the opposing activities of histone acetyltransferases (HATs) and histone deacetylases (HDACs). Binge alcohol exposure has been shown to significantly alter mRNA expression of liver class I, II, and IV HDACs.[66] These data strongly support a major pathogenic role for binge alcohol-induced alterations in HDACs that regulate the expression of genes that are relevant for hepatic steatosis. Another type of epigenetic effect is miRNA, small noncoding RNA molecules that regulate gene expression posttranscriptionally. Several miRNAs have been linked to both alcoholic liver disease and hepatocellular carcinoma as either biomarkers or molecular mediators. For example, miRNA 155 has been shown to modulate LPS-induced TNF-α production in Kupffer cells and TNF production in macrophages from patients with alcoholic liver disease.[67]

Emerging Mechanisms

At least 3 factors deserve recognition as emerging mechanisms of liver injury. The first factor is the endoplasmic reticulum (ER) stress response, which is induced by the accumulation of unfolded or misfolded proteins. To deal with the ER stress response, cells activate a series of signaling pathways termed the *unfolded protein response* (UPR), which can be either protective (usually in the short term) or detrimental (usually in the long term). One of the effects of a prolonged UPR can be increased production of TGs and cholesterol, leading to fatty liver. Some potential inducers of the ER stress in alcoholic liver disease include elevated homocysteine levels, acetaldehyde adducts, and oxidative stress.[68]

A second factor is the endogenous cannabinoids, which are ubiquitous lipid-signaling molecules that mediate their effects by specific cannabinoid receptors, CB1 and CB2. Studies have demonstrated that inhibition of CB1 receptors can cause weight loss and attenuate fatty liver and hyperlipidemia in animal models of obesity and steatohepatitis. Moreover, CB1 blockade reduces hepatic fibrosis in a variety of animal models of cirrhosis.[69]

Malnutrition has reemerged as a third factor of interest. Alterations in micronutrients, such as vitamins A, D, and zinc, as well as macronutrients, such as dietary fat, are increasingly recognized to play a role in the development and progression of alcoholic liver disease.[67] Decreased serum zinc levels, inadequate dietary zinc intake, and altered zinc metabolism are well documented in alcoholic liver disease.[70] Zinc plays a critical role in a host of metabolic pathways, including the function of zinc-finger proteins. Oxidative stress can cause zinc to be released from zinc-finger proteins and lead to loss of functional activity. Therefore, nutrient modulation may be a way of protecting against or treating alcoholic liver disease.

Fibrosis

The development of hepatic fibrosis, leading to cirrhosis, indicates major progression of alcoholic liver disease and represents a maladaptive wound healing response (see Chapter 74). The development of fibrosis is a dynamic state, with constant remodeling of scar tissue; fibrosis may regress with discontinuation of exposure to alcohol. The activated stellate cell (myofibroblast) is the major source of collagen production in the liver; it normally exists in a quiescent state and serves as a major storehouse for vitamin A. With activation, the stellate cell assumes a myofibroblast-like contractile phenotype and produces collagen. The cytokine TGF-β is a major stimulus for stellate cell activation and collagen production. Selected other cytokines implicated in the activation of stellate cells include platelet-derived growth factor and connective tissue growth factor (see Chapter 92). Whereas the hepatic stellate cell is considered the major origin of myofibroblasts, other resident cells (portal fibroblasts), bone-marrow derived mesenchymal cells, and cells undergoing epithelial-to-mesenchymal transition (EMT) have been postulated as sources of myofibroblasts as well.[71] Importantly, TLR-4 signaling in hepatic stellate cells plays a major role in stellate cell activation, myofibroblast chemokine secretion, interactions between myofibroblasts and Kupffer cells, and sensitization of myofibroblasts to TGF-β signaling.[72]

Oxidative stress also plays a major role in stellate cell activation, and a variety of antioxidants can block both stellate cell activation and collagen production in vitro. Serum levels of 4-hydroxynonenal, a specific product of lipid peroxidation, are elevated in patients with alcoholic liver disease and up-regulate both procollagen type I and tissue inhibitor of metalloproteinase-1 (TIMP-1) gene expression. Matrix metalloproteinase-1 plays a major role in degrading type I collagen. TIMP-1 levels also are elevated in alcoholic liver disease. The result appears to be an increase in stellate cell activation and collagen production on the one hand and a decrease in matrix degradation on the other hand.[73-75]

The main extracellular matrix protein associated with fibrosis is collagen type I, but other extracellular matrix proteins also accumulate, including fibrin and fibrinogen. The liver is the major organ that regulates the fibrin coagulation system. Fibrin metabolism is regulated via 2 pathways, coagulation and fibrinolysis (see Chapter 94).[19] Inhibition of fibrinolysis by plasminogen activator inhibitor-1 (PAI-1) can cause fibrin extracellular matrix to accumulate, even in the absence of enhanced fibrin deposition by the thrombin cascade. Hepatic injury in models of liver disease often involves dysregulation of the coagulation cascade and fibrinolysis, resulting in the formation of fibrin clots in the hepatic sinusoids.[19] Fibrin clots block blood flow within the hepatic parenchyma, thereby causing microregional hypoxia and subsequent hepatocellular death.[19] In summary, important cross-talk between cell types (e.g., stellate and Kupffer cells) and major metabolic pathways (e.g., wound healing, clotting, innate immunity) play a critical role in both the early and late stages of fibrosis.

DIAGNOSIS OF ALCOHOL ABUSE

Alcohol abuse should be suspected in a patient with a history of heavy alcohol intake, organ system damage, or a history of an excessive frequency of falls, lacerations, or fractures. Only 10% of patients with drinking problems are identified by primary care providers.[76] Owing to delays in diagnosis and treatment, many patients have cirrhosis by the time they are referred to a gastroenterologist.[77] Underdiagnosis is common in teenagers and older patients and is of particular concern in women of childbearing age.[78,79] The first step to insure more timely diagnosis of alcohol abuse is the uniform application of screening tools in various practice settings. Three such tools are now in common use: the 10-item AUDIT (*A*lcohol *U*se *D*isorders *I*dentification *T*est); the 3-item AUDIT-C consumption questions; and the 4-item CAGE (need to *c*ut down, *a*nnoyed by criticism, *g*uilty after drinking, need for an *e*ye-opener in the morning) questionnaire.[80,81] An alternative approach is the use of a single question: "How many times in the past year have you had x or more drinks a day?" ($x = 5$ for men, 4 for women) to identify persons with risk drinking.[80] Specific tools have also been developed for use in pregnant women.[79] Regardless of which instrument is chosen, it is important that physicians incorporate systematic screening into their practices.[82] An excellent guide to various screening strategies is available at http://pubs.niaaa.nih.gov/publications/Practitioner/CliniciansGuide2005.pdf.

Ongoing interest has centered on developing laboratory tests that can reliably identify patients with problem drinking. Although not as sensitive as screening questions, such tests are particularly useful in patients suspected of drinking who deny alcohol use. Blood or breath alcohol measurements are the most sensitive and specific indicators of recent alcohol use, particularly among binge drinkers.[83] The major limitation of these tests is the short half-life of ethanol in blood, urine, and breath. As a result, efforts have focused on developing biomarkers of alcohol abuse that are detectable over longer periods of time. The most specific of these biomarkers is carbohydrate-deficient transferrin (CDT).[84] Even higher sensitivity and specificity for alcohol abuse has been reported by combining CDT with mean corpuscular erythrocyte volume (MCV) and serum GGTP levels.[85] Measurement of 2 alcohol metabolites, phosphatidylethanol and ethyl glucuronide, also shows promise in detecting recent alcohol use.[86] Urinary ethyl glucuronide appears to be a particularly useful test for monitoring patients before and after liver transplantation.[87] An innovative approach under investigation is the development of transdermal sensors to monitor alcohol use continuously.[88]

DIAGNOSIS OF ALCOHOLIC LIVER DISEASE

History

Most patients with fatty liver are asymptomatic. Although patients with alcoholic hepatitis and cirrhosis may be asymptomatic, many present with a variety of complaints including anorexia, nausea and vomiting, weakness, jaundice, weight loss, abdominal pain, fever, and diarrhea.

Physical Examination

The most detailed clinical information on alcoholic liver disease in the United States comes from studies of hospitalized patients who were assigned the diagnosis on the basis of classic histologic features.[89,90] The most common physical finding in patients with fatty liver and alcoholic hepatitis is hepatomegaly, which is detectable in more than 75% of patients, regardless of disease severity. Patients with alcoholic hepatitis and cirrhosis may also have hepatic tenderness, an audible bruit over the liver, spider telangiectasias, splenomegaly, and peripheral edema. Jaundice and ascites, which are found in approximately 60% of patients, are more frequent in patients with severe disease (Table 86-2). Various degrees of hepatic encephalopathy can be seen, usually in the most severely ill patients. Some patients with alcoholic hepatitis have a fever, with temperatures as high as 104°F, that can persist for weeks (likely mediated by proinflammatory cytokines such as IL-1 and TNF).

In patients with well-compensated cirrhosis, the physical examination can be normal; however, most patients have obvious hepatomegaly and splenomegaly. As the disease progresses, the liver decreases in size and has a hard and nodular consistency. Patients with decompensated cirrhosis typically have muscle wasting, ascites, spider telangiectasias, palmar erythema, and Dupuytren's contractures. Enlarged parotid and lacrimal glands are often seen, and severely ill patients may have Muercke's lines or white nails. Patients with hepatopulmonary syndrome often have digital clubbing (see Chapters 74 and 92).

Laboratory Features

Only one third of hospitalized patients with fatty liver have laboratory abnormalities, which usually consist of mild increases in serum AST and ALT levels. As illustrated in

TABLE 86-2 Symptoms and Signs in Hospitalized Patients with Alcoholic Liver Disease

	Mild Disease (n = 89)	Moderate Disease* (n = 58)	Severe Disease† (n = 37)	Overall
Hepatomegaly	84.3	94.7	79.4	86.7
Jaundice	17.4	100	100	60.1
Ascites	30.3	79.3	86.5	57.1
Hepatic encephalopathy	27.3	55.2	70.3	44.6
Splenomegaly	18.0	30.9	39.4	26.0
Fever	18.0	31.0	21.6	22.8

*Moderate disease was defined by a serum bilirubin level > 5 mg/dL.
†Severe disease was defined by a bilirubin level > 5 mg/dL and a prolonged prothrombin time > 4 seconds.
Data from Mendenhall CL. Alcoholic hepatitis. Clin Gastroenterol 1981; 10:417-41.

TABLE 86-3 Laboratory Values in Hospitalized Patients with Alcoholic Liver Disease

Laboratory Test	Mean Value		
	Mild Disease (n = 89)	Moderate Disease* (n = 58)	Severe Disease† (n = 37)
Hematocrit value (%)	38	36	33
Mean corpuscular volume (fL)	100	102	105
WBC count (per mm³)	8000	11,000	12,000
Serum AST level (U/L)	84	124	99
Serum ALT level (U/L)	56	56	57
Serum alkaline phosphatase level (U/L)	166	276	225
Serum bilirubin level (mg/dL)	1.6	13.5	8.7
Prolongation of prothrombin time (seconds)	0.9	2.4	6.4
Serum albumin level	3.7	2.7	2.4

*Moderate disease was defined by a serum bilirubin level > 5 mg/dL.
†Severe disease was defined by a bilirubin level > 5 mg/dL and a prolonged prothrombin time > 4 seconds.
Data from Mendenhall CL. Alcoholic hepatitis. Clin Gastroenterol 1981; 10:417-41.

Table 86-3, surprisingly modest elevations of serum aminotransferase levels are seen in patients with alcoholic hepatitis and cirrhosis, even when the disease is severe.[89,90] Serum AST levels are almost always less than 300 to 500 U/L and typically are associated with trivial elevation of serum ALT levels, resulting in an AST/ALT ratio greater than 2. A ratio greater than 2 is characteristic of alcoholic liver disease, in part because of deficiency of pyridoxal 5′ phosphate (a cofactor of aminotransferases) in alcoholic patients (see Chapters 21 and 73). Serum alkaline phosphatase levels can range from normal to values greater than 1000 U/L. Serum bilirubin levels range from normal to 20 to 40 mg/dL, and serum albumin levels may be normal or depressed to a value as low as 1.0 to 1.5 g/dL. Most patients with alcoholic liver disease are anemic and have some degree of thrombocytopenia. By contrast, the WBC count is usually normal or elevated, occasionally to levels consistent with a leukemoid state. Severely ill patients usually have marked prolongation of the prothrombin time—often expressed as the INR (see Chapter 94)—and often have elevated serum creatinine values.

Histopathology

The clinical diagnosis of alcoholic liver disease is quite sensitive and specific; therefore, liver biopsy is usually not needed to establish the diagnosis. A liver biopsy is useful, however, in selecting patients for clinical trials, determining the severity of hepatic injury, and clarifying the diagnosis in atypical cases (see Fig. 86-2). Centrilobular and perivenular fatty infiltration is seen in most persons who drink more than 60 g of alcohol daily. Classic histologic features of alcoholic hepatitis include ballooning degeneration of hepatocytes, alcoholic hyaline (Mallory-Denk bodies) within damaged hepatocytes, and a surrounding infiltrate composed of polymorphonuclear leukocytes.[12,13,15] Most patients have moderate to severe fatty infiltration. Varying degrees of fibrosis may be present, and many patients exhibit an unusual perisinusoidal distribution of fibrosis, at times with partial or complete obliteration of the terminal hepatic venules (sclerosing hyaline necrosis).[15,17] Cirrhosis can be identified by the presence of nodules of hepatic tissue that are completely surrounded by fibrous tissue.

Alcoholic cirrhosis typically is micronodular or mixed micro- and macronodular (see Chapter 74). In patients with coexisting alcoholic hepatitis, alcoholic hyaline is almost universal, and sclerosing hyaline necrosis and moderate to severe fatty infiltration are common. In patients with alcoholic cirrhosis who abstain from alcohol for long periods, a frequent finding is a gradual transformation to macronodular cirrhosis, which is indistinguishable from cirrhosis caused by other forms of liver disease.[14,15,17]

Conditions That May Resemble Alcoholic Liver Disease

Although the clinical diagnosis of alcoholic liver disease usually is quite straightforward, the similarity of the clinical and histologic features with those of other disorders sometimes causes diagnostic confusion. The most commonly encountered conditions that have clinical or histologic features in common with alcoholic liver disease are nonalcoholic fatty liver disease (NAFLD), hereditary hemochromatosis, and Budd-Chiari syndrome.

Nonalcoholic Fatty Liver Disease

NAFLD is the most difficult condition to distinguish from alcoholic liver disease. There is considerable overlap between the histologic features of NAFLD and alcoholic liver disease.[15] As a consequence, the distinction between the 2 conditions requires careful clinicopathologic correlation. Patients with alcoholic liver disease typically manifest clinical features of more advanced liver disease. Patients with NAFLD are more likely to have features of the metabolic syndrome, including peripheral insulin resistance, obesity, hypertension, and dyslipidemia, although these features are not invariably present.[91,92] They also should have a weekly alcohol intake of less than 21 drinks for men and 14 for women.[93] When a patient's alcohol intake is questionable, differentiating the 2 conditions can be difficult, if not impossible. The use of structured questionnaires to assess alcohol intake is recommended in this situation (see Chapter 87).[93]

Hereditary Hemochromatosis

On occasion, distinguishing patients with alcoholic liver disease and secondary iron overload from those with liver disease caused by hereditary hemochromatosis can be difficult. Patients with end-stage liver disease from alcoholic cirrhosis can have elevated serum iron and ferritin levels and increased hepatic iron levels suggestive of hereditary hemochromatosis.[94] To complicate matters further, 15% to 40% of patients with hereditary hemochromatosis consume more than 80 g of alcohol daily.[95]

The overlapping clinical features of hereditary hemochromatosis and alcoholic liver disease include hepatomegaly, testicular atrophy, cardiomyopathy, and glucose intolerance. Testing for mutations in the gene for hereditary hemochromatosis and measuring the hepatic iron index are the best methods for differentiating the two conditions. Few patients with alcoholic cirrhosis and iron overload are homozygous for the C282Y or heterozygous for the C282Y and H63D *HFE* genes, and few have a hepatic iron index value greater than 1.9 (see Chapter 75).[94,96]

Budd-Chiari Syndrome

Occasional patients with severe alcoholic liver disease can be misdiagnosed as having acute Budd-Chiari syndrome (hepatic vein thrombosis) on the basis of rapid clinical deterioration,

marked hepatomegaly, caudate lobe hypertrophy, and failure to visualize the hepatic veins by Doppler US.[97] Careful evaluation of these patients usually reveals clinical and biochemical features typical of severe alcoholic hepatitis. Patent hepatic veins usually can be demonstrated by venography. Liver biopsy also is useful in distinguishing the characteristic histologic features of alcoholic liver disease from those of Budd-Chiari syndrome. Failure to recognize alcoholic hepatitis as the underlying cause of the liver disease before initiating anticoagulation or performing portacaval shunt surgery or a transjugular intrahepatic shunt procedure can result in high mortality rates (see Chapter 85).[97]

COFACTORS THAT MAY INFLUENCE PROGRESSION OF ALCOHOLIC LIVER DISEASE

A number of factors have been reported to have an adverse effect on the progression of liver disease in chronic alcoholics. The most important of these are chronic HCV infection, obesity, and smoking.

Chronic Hepatitis C

Between one fourth and one third of patients with alcoholic liver disease also have hepatitis C.[98] Liver disease is more severe, advanced disease develops at a younger age, and survival is shorter in patients with both alcoholic liver disease and HCV infection than in those with either disease alone.[6,80,82,98] The relative risk of cirrhosis is 10- to 30-fold higher among heavy drinkers with chronic hepatitis C (Fig. 86-5).[99,100] In

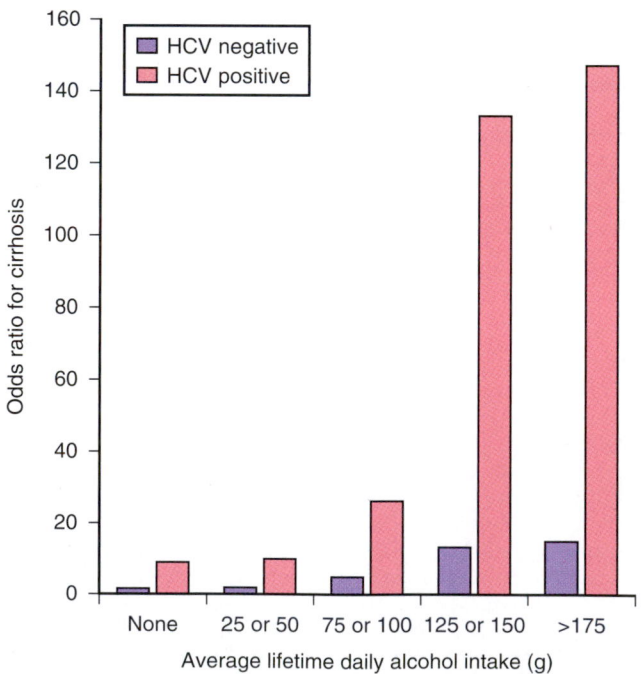

FIGURE 86-5. Odds ratios for developing cirrhosis in patients who chronically drink varying amounts of alcohol, based on the presence or absence of HCV infection. *(Data from Corrao G, Lepore AR, Torchio P, et al. The effect of drinking coffee and smoking cigarettes on the risk of cirrhosis associated with alcohol consumption. A case-control study. Provincial Group for the Study of Chronic Liver Disease. Eur J Epidemiol 1994; 10:657-64.)*

addition, alcohol and HCV act synergistically in the development of hepatocellular carcinoma (see Chapters 80 and 96).[100-102]

Obesity and Smoking

Obesity is also an independent risk factor for disease progression in alcoholic hepatitis and alcoholic cirrhosis.[80,82,103,104] Patients with alcoholic cirrhosis who are overweight also appear to be at increased risk of developing hepatocellular carcinoma.[101] Cigarette smoking also has been shown to accelerate the progression of fibrosis and risk of hepatocellular carcinoma.[80,99,105]

PROGNOSIS

The prognosis for individual patients with alcoholic liver disease depends on the degree of pathologic injury, patient's nutritional status, complications of advanced liver disease, presence of other comorbid conditions such as obesity and HCV infection, and patient's ability to discontinue destructive patterns of drinking. Patients with fatty liver have the best outcome, those with alcoholic hepatitis or cirrhosis have an intermediate outcome, and those with cirrhosis combined with alcoholic hepatitis have the worst outcome (Fig. 86-6).[106] Estimating the prognosis of patients with alcoholic liver disease is particularly important for determining the need for specific drug therapy in patients with severe alcoholic hepatitis and liver transplantation in those with alcoholic cirrhosis (see later).

Alcoholic Hepatitis

Patients with alcoholic hepatitis account for almost 1% of hospital admissions in the United States. Almost 7% during their initial hospitalization, and 40% with severe disease, die within 6 months of clinical presentation.[1,107] Clinical features associated with severe disease include hepatic encephalopathy, marked prolongation of the prothrombin time, elevation of the serum bilirubin level above 25 mg/dL, and development of renal insufficiency.

A number of models have been shown to predict short-term prognosis in these often critically ill patients.[108] Maddrey and colleagues discovered a simple formula they called the *discriminant function* (DF), which proved useful in identifying patients with poor short-term survival rates.[109] A modification of the original DF (mDF) calculated as [4.6 × prothrombin time − control value (seconds)] + serum bilirubin (mg/dL)] has proved useful in identifying patients with a poor prognosis who should be considered for specific drug therapy.[110] Three prospective studies have demonstrated that patients with mDF values of 32 or greater have a poor prognosis, with 1-month mortality rates of 35% to 50%.[110-112] As a result, the mDF has been incorporated into the selection criteria for most therapeutic trials involving patients with alcoholic hepatitis. The prognosis of patients with mDF values of 32 or greater can be further stratified by the presence of encephalopathy and development of acute kidney injury (Fig. 86-7).[110,113] Two other prognostic models, the MELD score (see Chapter 97) and the Glasgow alcoholic hepatitis score, have been shown to predict survival in patients with severe alcoholic hepatitis.[114,115] Although none is perfect, each of these models appears to be effective in selecting patients for medical therapy.[80,82,108]

The short-term survival of patients with mDF values less than 32 have ranged from 83% to 100% in various studies.[108] To determine the prognosis of all patients with alcoholic hepatitis more accurately, a new scoring system has been proposed that separates patients into 3 groups with predicted 3-month survival rates of 25%, 70%, and 100% on the basis of patient's *a*ge, serum *b*ilirubin, *I*NR, and serum *c*reatinine level (ABIC score).[116]

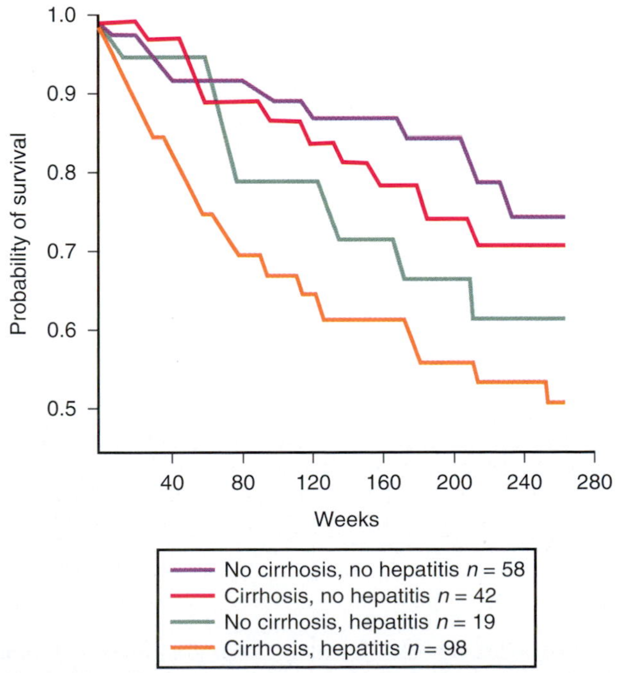

FIGURE 86-6. Survival of patients with alcoholic liver disease stratified by histologic severity of disease. *(From Orrego H, Black JE, Blendis LM, Medline A. Prognosis of alcoholic cirrhosis in the presence or absence of alcoholic hepatitis. Gastroenterology 1987; 92:208-14, with permission.)*

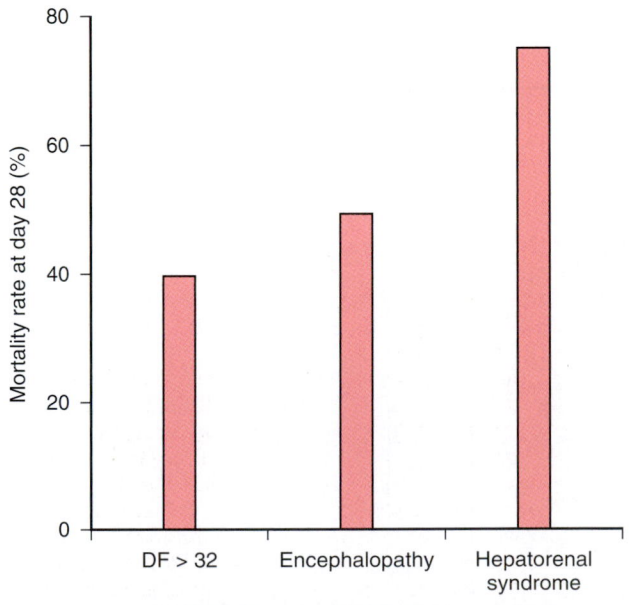

FIGURE 86-7. Mortality rate at day 28 in patients with severe alcoholic hepatitis who had a discriminant function (DF) score greater than 32, spontaneous hepatic encephalopathy, or hepatorenal syndrome. See text for calculation of DF. *(Data from references 110 and 113.)*

Alcoholic Cirrhosis

The 5-year mortality rate of patients with alcoholic cirrhosis ranges from 60% to 85%.[117] Within 15 years, 90% of patients can be expected to die if they do not undergo liver transplantation.[118] Prognosis among individual patients is dependent on the development of various complications. One-year mortality is 15% to 20% in patients with no complications, 20% following variceal bleeding, 30% after the development of ascites, 50% in those with variceal bleeding and ascites, and 65% following the development of hepatic encephalopathy.[117] The clinical tool used most widely to determine prognosis in patients with alcoholic cirrhosis is the Child-Turcotte-Pugh (CTP) score (Child-Pugh class). Although it has limitations, the CTP score been adopted widely for risk-stratifying patients with cirrhosis because of its simplicity and ease of use (see Chapters 92 and 97). Five-year survival rates for patients with alcoholic cirrhosis vary dramatically based on the CTP score at the time of clinical presentation (Fig. 86-8).[119,120]

Other models that have been used to predict prognosis in patients with alcoholic cirrhosis are the Beclere model and the MELD score. The Beclere model includes the serum bilirubin level, serum albumin level, patient's age, and presence or absence of hepatic encephalopathy.[119] The MELD model, which is useful for predicting short-term survival in groups of patients with various liver diseases, is the system used for allocation of donor livers in the United States (see Chapter 97).

Acute-on-Chronic Liver Failure

Patients with stable, compensated cirrhosis can gradually develop complications or suddenly develop jaundice and coagulopathy with rapid development of ascites or encephalopathy (or both), a syndrome referred to as *acute-on-chronic liver failure*.[117,121,122] The 3 most common precipitating factors are superimposed alcoholic hepatitis due to an increase in alcohol intake, viral infections, and drug toxicity.

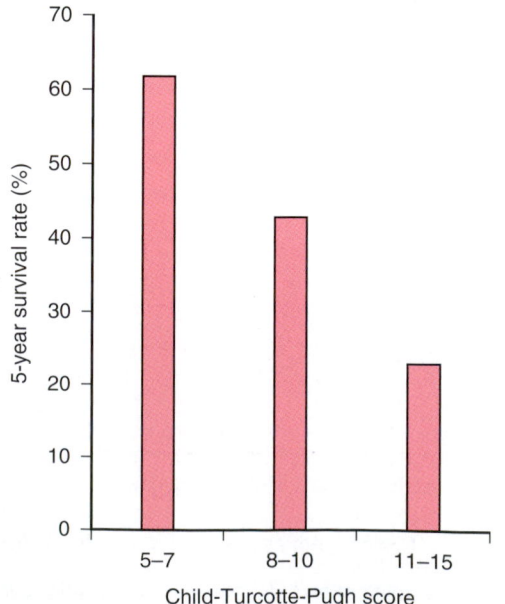

FIGURE 86-8. Five-year survival rates in patients with alcoholic cirrhosis according to their Child-Turcotte-Pugh scores. *(Data from references 119 and 120.)*

Acute Viral Illness

Patients with alcoholic cirrhosis are vulnerable to sudden decompensation from infection with hepatotropic viruses including hepatitis A, B, and E and nonhepatotropic viruses such as influenza A (see Chapters 78, 79, 82, and 83).[121] The potential for sudden deterioration from these infections underscores the importance of routine immunizations.[123]

Hepatotoxic Drugs

Sudden and unexplained clinical deterioration in patients with alcoholic cirrhosis can also result from ingestion of hepatotoxic medications and herbal remedies. The morbidity and mortality associated with these conditions are considerable. Because of induction of CYP2E1, drinkers are uniquely susceptible to acetaminophen hepatotoxicity. Chronic alcoholics who take excessive amounts of this drug over a period of days to weeks for relief of a headache, toothache, or other minor pain can undergo sudden deterioration of their clinical condition.[124] The clinical features in these patients are indistinguishable from those of alcoholic liver disease, with one obvious exception: serum AST values are frequently more than 1000 U/L, much higher than expected in patients with alcoholic liver disease. Because liver injury has occurred by the time of hospitalization, acetaminophen levels are not helpful for diagnosis or management. Recognition of the cause of the unusually elevated serum aminotransferase levels comes from careful questioning of the patient and family about acetaminophen ingestion in the days to weeks before hospitalization. Sudden clinical deterioration in a patient with alcoholic cirrhosis can also result from an idiosyncratic hepatotoxic reaction to a number of other drugs and herbal medications (see Chapters 88 and 89).[125,126]

Hospitalized Patients with Decompensated Cirrhosis or Acute-on-Chronic Liver Failure

Patients hospitalized with decompensated cirrhosis or acute-on-chronic liver failure are inordinately predisposed to infection and the subsequent development of hepatic encephalopathy, sepsis, acute kidney injury, and multiorgan failure.[127,128] The 90-day mortality rate of patients who require ICU management for 3 or more failing organ systems due to these complications exceeds 90%.[129] The prognosis of patients hospitalized in an ICU is more accurately reflected by the Sequential Organ Failure Assessment (SOFA) score than by the CTP and other liver-related scores.[80,129,130]

Hepatocellular Carcinoma

The true frequency of hepatocellular carcinoma in patients with alcoholic cirrhosis is unclear.[131] Although alcoholic liver disease has been long considered to be the leading cause of hepatocellular carcinoma in the United States and Europe, many of the affected patients were infected with HCV. Studies in the 2000s suggest that the incidence of hepatocellular carcinoma is 2 to 3 times higher in patients with alcoholic liver disease and no evidence of HCV infection than in the normal population.[18] The risk of hepatocellular carcinoma shows a strong correlation with alcohol intake and is roughly doubled in those with concurrent HCV infection (Fig. 86-9).[102] The risk of hepatocellular carcinoma is higher in men than women and increases with age.[101] Given the ongoing risk of hepatocellular carcinoma, lifetime surveillance with US every 6 months is recommended for all patients with alcoholic cirrhosis (see Chapter 96).[131]

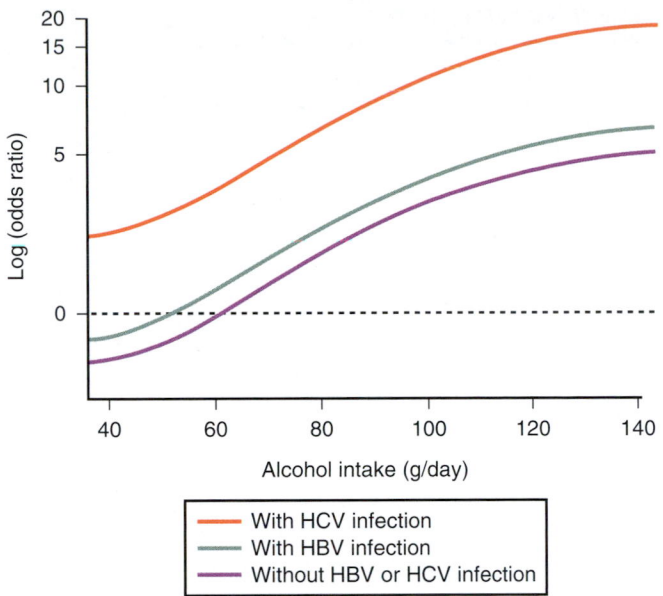

FIGURE 86-9. Odds ratio for hepatocellular carcinoma according to alcohol intake (g/day) and presence or absence of HCV or HBV infection. *(From El-Serag HB. Epidemiology of viral hepatitis and hepatocellular carcinoma. Gastroenterology 2012; 142:1264-73, with permission.)*

TREATMENT

Abstinence and Lifestyle Modification

Abstinence from continued excessive drinking is the most important predictor of survival in patients with alcoholic cirrhosis.[80,82,118,120,132] The 3-year survival rate is 70% to 80% among patients who abstain or dramatically reduce their excessive drinking, compared with only 20% to 30% in those who continue to drink heavily (Fig. 86-10).[132] Reducing, but not completely stopping, alcohol consumption also has been shown to improve survival.[118] The question is how best to achieve these goals effectively.

The first steps are to identify excessive drinking, determine the severity of the drinking problem, and assess the patient's motivation for change. Patients may experience risk drinking, alcohol abuse, or dependence (Fig. 86-11).[2] Patients with risk drinking without dependence respond well in primary care settings to brief interventions that result in reduced consumption and a reduction in alcohol-related harm and mortality.[80,133] Brief interventions have also been effective in reducing alcohol intake in pregnant women with a subsequent reduction in fetal mortality.[79] Most patients seen in acute care settings by a gastroenterologist have alcohol abuse or dependence. Although a brief intervention may be very effective in an individual patient, the majority of patients need referral to a qualified alcohol and substance abuse counselor for assessment and specialty treatment if they are to have the best opportunity to achieve long-term remission. From 20% to 30% of patients remain abstinent for one year after a single course of treatment, and another 10% reduce their intake to the point that they no longer experience adverse consequences from their drinking.[2]

Three oral medications (disulfiram, acomposate, naltrexone) and an extended-release injectable form of naltrexone have been approved by the FDA to treat alcohol dependence. Pharmacotherapy with these agents is modestly effective; however, all have side effects and are underutilized.[2,80,82]

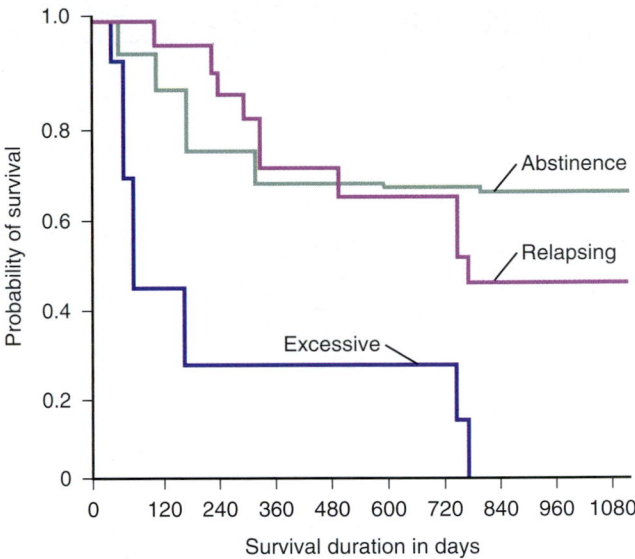

FIGURE 86-10. Survival curves in patients with severe alcoholic cirrhosis during the 3 years following hospital discharge according to alcohol consumption during this period: abstinence, patients who were abstinent; relapsing, patients with one or more periods of abstinence alternating with one or more periods of excessive consumption; excessive, patients with excessive consumption of alcohol at the first follow-up point. Survival differed significantly between patients who were abstinent and those who were drinking excessively (P < 0.001). *(Modified with permission of Veldt BJ, Laine F, Guillygomarc'h A, et al. Indication of liver transplantation in severe alcoholic liver cirrhosis: Qualitative evaluation and optimal timing. J Hepatol 2002; 36:93-8.)*

Baclofen, a gamma aminobutyric acid (GABA) B-receptor agonist, shows promise as the first safe and effective agent to improve abstinence and decrease the likelihood of relapse in patients with alcoholic cirrhosis.[80,134] Given the limited efficacy of the currently available medications to prevent relapse, a number of new approaches are under active investigation.[135] Involvement in mutual support groups, such as Alcoholic Anonymous (AA), can reduce the risk of relapse, primarily by building social support for sobriety.[2] An excellent guide to various treatment strategies is available at http://pubs.niaaa.nih.gov/publications/Practitioner/CliniciansGuide2005.pdf.

The goal of intervention should be sustained abstinence, which improves the histologic features of alcoholic liver injury, reduces portal pressure, and slows progression to cirrhosis.[80,82] In two thirds of patients, significant clinical improvement can be seen within 3 months.[82] Within 2 years many patients achieve complete clinical and biochemical recovery, regain lost muscle mass, and can safely stop diuretics and other liver-related medicines.[136] Although reducing alcohol intake to "safe" levels does reduce mortality and morbidity, only 10% of persons are able to maintain safe levels of drinking over an extended period of time.[2] Three fourths of patients have a relapse within 1 year. Longitudinal care by the treatment program is important. Clinicians can also help by providing regular visits in a nonjudgmental manner and ongoing counseling and support of the longer-term treatment goals.[2]

It is also important to address obesity and smoking, 2 comorbidities associated with progression of alcoholic liver disease (see earlier). The majority of alcoholics smoke cigarettes, a risk factor for more severe alcoholic liver disease. In addition, smoking and alcohol act synergistically to increase

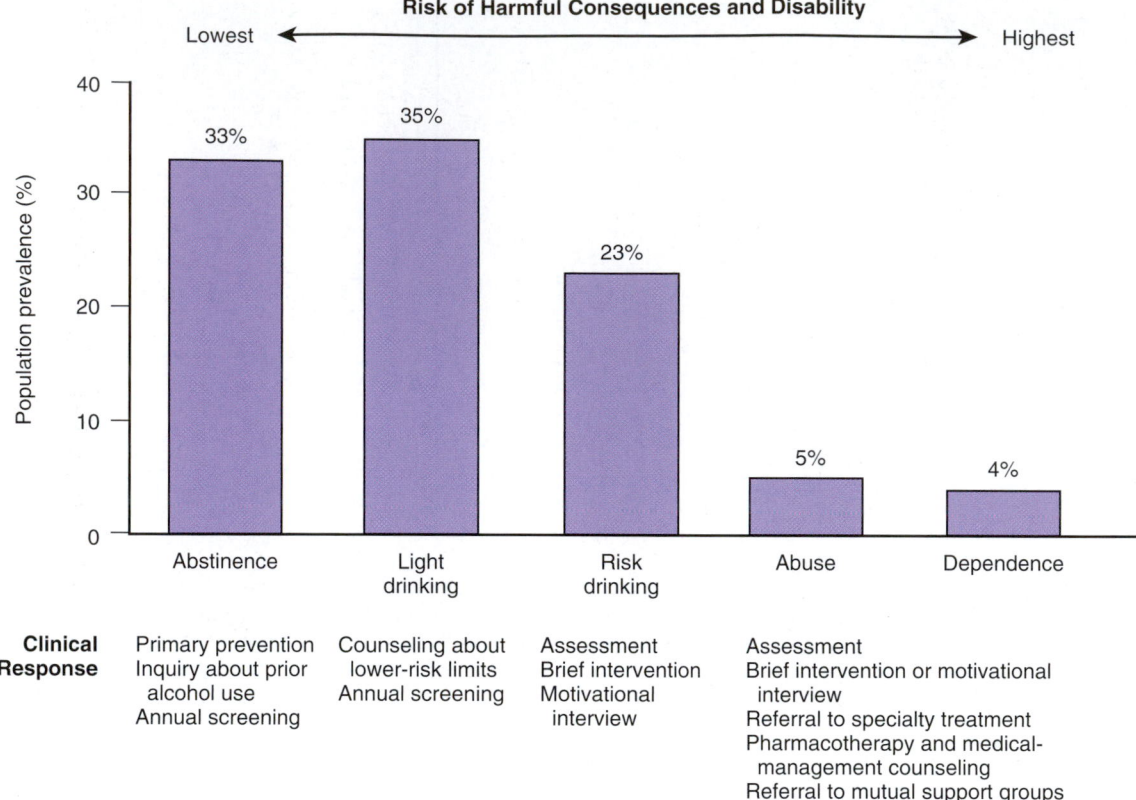

FIGURE 86-11. Continuum of risk for harmful consequences and disability associated with alcohol use and possible clinical responses. Risk drinking is defined as an average of 15 or more standard drinks weekly or 5 or more on one occasion for men and 8 or more drinks weekly or 4 or more on one occasion for women and persons older than age 65. Persons in remission from an alcohol-use disorder remain at risk for recurrent drinking and adverse consequences. *(From Friedmann PD. Clinical practice. Alcohol use in adults. N Engl J Med 2013; 368:365-73, with permission.)*

the risk of cardiovascular disease and hepatocellular carcinoma.[80,105] Smoking cessation is particularly important in patients being considered for liver transplantation. Smoking after the transplant increases the risk of cardiovascular complications and cardiovascular and sepsis-related deaths.[105] In addition, cigarette smoking increases the risk of de novo extrahepatic malignancies, such as laryngeal, pharyngeal, and lung cancer, which are leading causes of late deaths after liver transplantation (see Chapter 97).[105]

Nutritional Support

Malnutrition is a widespread clinical problem among patients with alcoholic liver disease. Every patient with moderate to severe alcoholic hepatitis or cirrhosis shows some signs of malnutrition. The presence of malnutrition is associated with higher rates of liver-related complications and mortality. Malnutrition has also been associated with longer ICU stays, longer durations of hospitalization, and higher mortality rates after liver transplantation.[137] Provision of adequate nutritional support is the most frequently overlooked aspect of the management of patients with alcoholic liver disease.

Accurate assessment of the nutritional status of patients with liver disease can be quite difficult. Many of the tests typically used for this purpose are influenced by either the liver disease or alcohol consumption. Visceral proteins such as albumin and prealbumin are produced in the liver and correlate better with the severity of liver disease than with nutritional status. Anthropometric measurements such as BMI and the creatinine-height index are unreliable in patients with

altered renal function and fluid retention.[136,137] The subjective global assessment (SGA) of protein energy malnutrition, a simple bedside tool, often reveals obvious malnutrition, particularly in patients with muscle wasting and ascites.[136-138] Measurement of handgrip strength and middle arm muscle mass also can be helpful in assessing the nutritional status of these patients.[137,138]

Adequate nutritional support is critical to the management of patients with severe alcoholic hepatitis. In 2 large Veterans Administration studies, the 6-month mortality rate correlated in a dose-response fashion with voluntary dietary intake (Fig. 86-12).[136] Despite this knowledge and expert care by nutritionists and hepatologists, two thirds of the patients failed to consume the recommended caloric intake of 2500 kcal/day.[136] It is typical for patients with severe alcoholic hepatitis to spend extended periods of time in the hospital with inadequate nutritional intake. These patients often have little or no appetite for prolonged periods and are deprived of adequate nutrition by their caregivers because of dietary restrictions of salt, water, and protein, as well as intermittent interruption of all nutritional support for various procedures. Patients with severe alcoholic hepatitis often experience a hypermetabolic state with a higher-than-normal resting energy expenditure. Because of the vital need for adequate nutrition in these often critically ill patients, we do not hesitate to place an NG feeding tube if the patient cannot voluntarily ingest at least 2500 kcal/day, even when esophageal varices are present.[136,139] Glucocorticoid therapy can increase voluntary dietary intake, but providing adequate calories through enteral feeding provides the same 1-month survival benefit with significantly lower

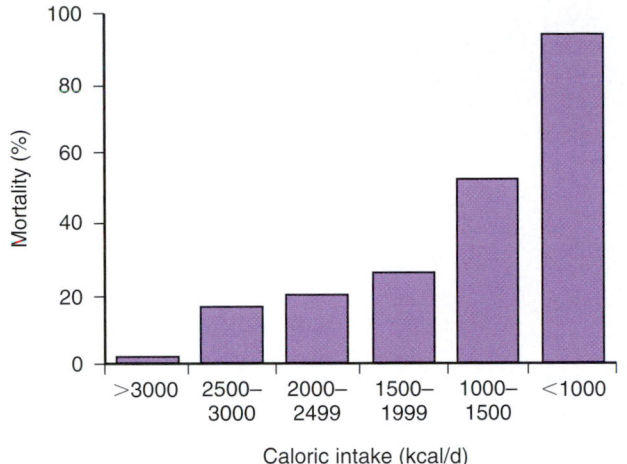

FIGURE 86-12. Relationship between voluntary caloric intake and mortality in patients with severe alcoholic hepatitis. *(From McClain CJ, et al. Alcoholic liver disease and malnutrition. Alcohol Clin Exp Res 2011; 35:815-20, with permission.)*

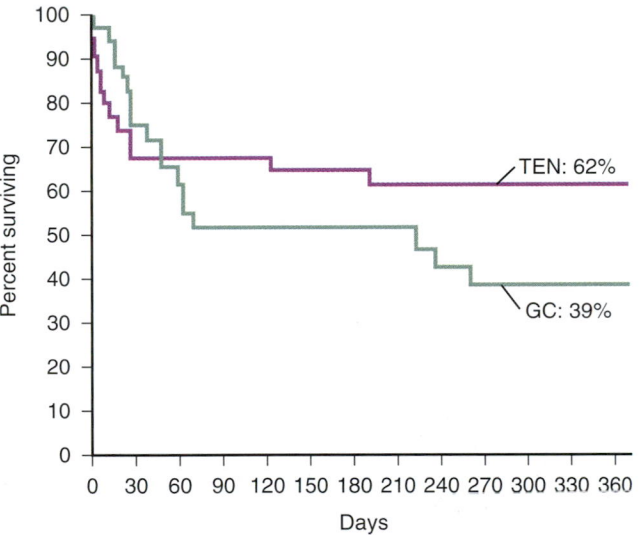

FIGURE 86-13. Probability of survival for one year after randomization of 72 patients with severe alcoholic hepatitis to total enteral nutrition (TEN) or to glucocorticoid therapy (GC). Survival in one year was statistically great for TEN (P = 0.028). *(From Cabre E, Rodriguez-Iglesias P, Caballeria J, et al. Short- and long-term outcome of severe alcohol-induced hepatitis treated with steroids or enteral nutrition: A multicenter randomized trial. Hepatology 2000; 32:36-42, with permission.)*

mortality at 1 year (Fig. 86-13).[89,140] Furthermore, in patients who are provided adequate enteral nutrition, *N*-acetylcysteine offers no improvement in 1- and 6-month survival rates.[141]

Patients with stable cirrhosis have nutritional deficiencies almost as severe as those found in patients with alcoholic hepatitis.[136] The frequency of malnutrition increases with the severity of disease. For example, the risk of profound malnutrition increases from 45% in patients with Child-Pugh class A cirrhosis to 95% in those with Child-Pugh class C cirrhosis.[136,137] Patients with cirrhosis who require hospitalization have a substantially higher prevalence of malnutrition compared with general medical inpatients and have significantly longer hospital stays and a 2-fold higher risk of in-hospital mortality.[142] Even in patients with stable, compensated cirrhosis, malnutrition is associated with higher 1-year mortality (20% vs. 0%) and complication rates (65% vs. 13%).[137,138]

Hepatic glycogen stores are depleted in patients with cirrhosis. As a result, these patients exhibit an early starvation mode after only 12 hours of fasting compared with 48 hours in normal persons. Therefore, even short periods of inadequate nutrition can result in peripheral muscle proteolysis, which contributes to protein malnutrition. Patients with decompensated cirrhosis also can be hypermetabolic. Not surprisingly, the protein intake recommended for patients with cirrhosis is higher than that for healthy adults.[138,139] The positive impact of judicious nutritional supplements in patients with cirrhosis is illustrated by a randomized trial that showed that a nighttime snack of 700 kcal each evening resulted in an accrual of 2 kg of lean tissue over 12 months.[143]

The increased nutritional requirements and the vulnerability to early starvation in cirrhotic patients underscore the importance of limiting the duration of protein restriction in patients with encephalopathy to a maximum of 24 to 48 hours. Prolonged protein restriction has no beneficial effect on encephalopathy and can be nutritionally catastrophic (see Chapter 94).[136,138,144] If, despite appropriate medical therapy, standard enteral formulas lead to encephalopathy, a branched-chain amino acid–enriched formula can be given as a supplement to meet nitrogen needs.[136,139] Patients with alcoholic liver disease can also have a plethora of vitamin and mineral deficiencies.[136,137] In addition to the commonly recognized deficiencies in folate and B vitamins, deficiencies in fat-soluble vitamins (A, D, and E) and minerals (magnesium, selenium, and zinc) are common causes of symptoms and physical findings in these patients.[137] Zinc deficiency, for example, may be an important component of the skin lesions, night blindness, mental irritability, confusion and hepatic encephalopathy, anorexia, altered taste and smell, hypogonadism, and altered wound healing so commonly seen in patients with alcoholic liver disease.[145] Assessment and judicious correction of each of these deficiencies is an important aspect of the care of these patients.

The nutritional status of patients at the time of liver transplantation is also important. Morbid obesity and severe malnutrition are each predictors of poor outcomes.[146] Among persons transplanted in the United States since 1990, extremes of BMI (<18.5 and > 40) were more common in patients with alcoholic liver disease than in patients transplanted for other conditions. Severely malnourished patients had longer lengths of stay, a higher retransplantation rate, and diminished survival.[146] The observation that diminished cross-sectional area of the psoas muscle as measured by CT shows a strong correlation with poor survival following liver transplantation confirms the importance of malnutrition in these patients and may offer a means of more systematic and objective detection of this condition in future transplant candidates.[147]

Therapy for Alcoholic Hepatitis

Glucocorticoids

Glucocorticoid therapy was first demonstrated to provide a short-term survival benefit for patients with severe alcoholic hepatitis in a small U.S. prospective randomized multicenter trial in 1989.[110] Each of the patients enrolled had a clinical diagnosis of alcoholic hepatitis and either an mDF greater than 32, spontaneous hepatic encephalopathy, or both. Patients were excluded if they had active GI bleeding requiring blood transfusions, active infection requiring antibiotic treatment, preexisting chronic renal disease with a serum creatinine level greater than 2 mg/dL (175 µmol/L), or obvious contraindications to glucocorticoid therapy. Treatment consisted of 28

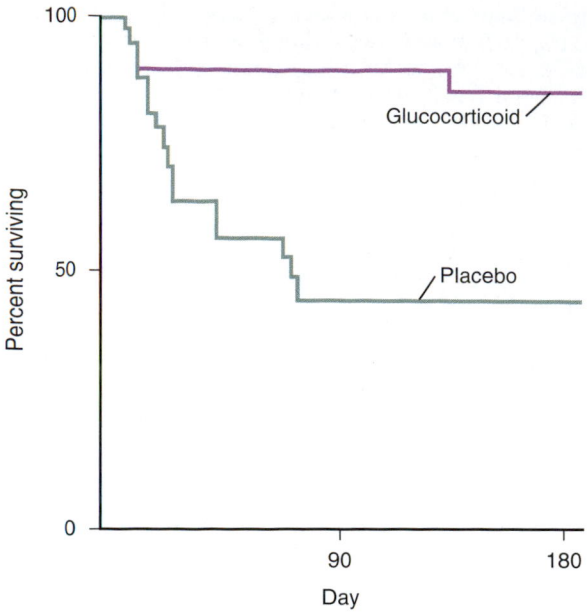

FIGURE 86-14. Survival in 61 patients with alcoholic hepatitis randomly assigned to receive glucocorticoid therapy or placebo. Survival rates at 6 months were 84% in the glucocorticoid treatment group and 45% in the placebo group (P = 0.002). *(From Raymond MJ, Poynard T, Rueff B, et al. A randomized trial of prednisone in patients with severe alcoholic hepatitis. N Engl J Med 1992; 326:507, with permission.)*

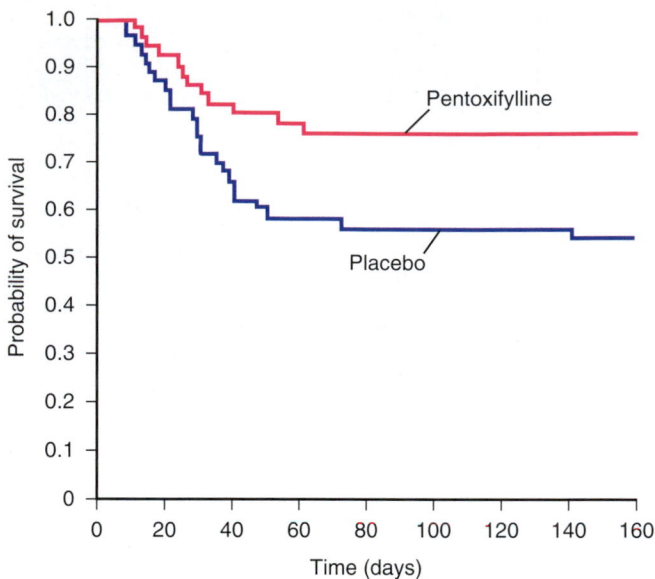

FIGURE 86-15. Probability of survival in 101 patients with alcoholic hepatitis treated with pentoxifylline *(red line)* or placebo *(blue line)* (P = 0.037). *(From Akriviadis E, Botla R, Briggs W, et al. Pentoxifylline improves short-term survival in severe acute alcoholic hepatitis: A double blind, placebo-controlled trial. Gastroenterology 2000; 119:1637-48, with permission.)*

days of methylprednisolone 32 mg daily followed by a 2-week taper. The 28-day mortality among patients who received prednisolone was only 6%, compared with 35% among the placebo-treated control subjects. Among patients with encephalopathy at study entry, the 28-day mortality rate was 7% compared with 47%.[110] These findings were confirmed and expanded shortly thereafter by a second trial from France, which required the presence of either an mDF greater than 32 or encephalopathy as well as histologic confirmation of alcoholic hepatitis (Fig. 86-14).[111]

Since the publication of these two studies,[110,111] 3 important observations have been made regarding glucocorticoid therapy in patients with severe alcoholic hepatitis: (1) the 2-month survival of glucocorticoid-treated patients has remained remarkably constant in subsequent clinical trials, (2) many patients do not respond to glucocorticoid therapy, and (3) glucocorticoids can be used safely in patients with active infection at the time of hospitalization, if there is a rapid clinical response to treatment.

The 2-month mortality rate of patients randomly assigned to glucocorticoid therapy in most relevant clinical trials has been approximately 20%.[148] This reproducible response is helpful to those designing clinical trials that compare newer treatments with glucocorticoid therapy. It also is a useful benchmark for persons who read reports of these newer forms of therapy. Studies that have reported a markedly diminished glucocorticoid response typically have included much sicker patients than those enrolled in the original trials.

A blunted response to glucocorticoid therapy is seen in more than 25% of patients with severe alcoholic hepatitis.[149] These patients have a grim prognosis, with fewer than 25% surviving 6 months. The 6 variables that help predict this outcome include the patient's age, presence of renal insufficiency, baseline values for serum albumin, prothrombin time, and serum bilirubin, and the change in bilirubin level after 7 days of treatment (the Lille model).[150] The underlying reasons

for treatment failure are probably multifactorial. Some patients have an intrinsic resistance to glucocorticoid therapy.[151] Two agents, basiliximab and theophylline, which enhance sensitivity to glucocorticoid in vitro, offer theoretical promise for overcoming this intrinsic resistance to glucocorticoids.[151,152] Although less well characterized, two other factors critical to an optimal response to glucocorticoid therapy are good renal function and adequate nutritional intake. Patients enrolled in the original studies, which showed the best outcomes with glucocorticoid therapy, had minimal renal disease.[110,111] A dramatic reduction in survival among glucocorticoid-treated patients has been reported in studies that included patients with renal impairment.[112,149,150] For example, patients who participated in the development of the Lille model had baseline serum creatinine levels as high as 6.7 mg/dL.[149,150] The importance of dietary intake was illustrated in a small pilot study of glucocorticoids plus enteral nutrition, in which the response was so dramatic that glucocorticoids could be safely tapered within 2 weeks in many of the patients.[153]

Infection has long been considered a contraindication to glucocorticoid therapy in patients with severe alcoholic hepatitis. If taken at face value, 25% of patients would be eliminated from consideration of treatment[154]; however, a prospective study has shown that if an infection can be effectively treated, glucocorticoids can be used safely.[154]

Pentoxifylline

Pentoxifylline is a safe and effective alternative to glucocorticoid therapy in patients with severe alcoholic hepatitis. In the original placebo-controlled trial demonstrating the efficacy of this agent, only 12 patients (24.5%) who received pentoxifylline died, compared with 24 (46%) who received placebo (Fig. 86-15). Pentoxifylline therapy was associated with a significant decrease in the frequency of hepatorenal syndrome as a cause of death and was well tolerated, with no major side effects.[155] A subsequent small study has confirmed these findings.[156] In this trial, the 30-day mortality rate in the patients who received pentoxifylline was half of that in the control subjects who received placebo (20% vs. 40%). Furthermore, renal failure was the cause of death in only 10% of the pentoxifylline recipients, compared with 70% among the control subjects.[156]

Two other studies have explored other options for pentoxifylline. In the first study,[157] the possibility of switching patients to pentoxifylline if they failed to respond to glucocorticoid therapy was examined. A total of 29 patients who did not show a significant change in the serum bilirubin level after 7 days of glucocorticoid therapy were switched to pentoxifylline. The outcome of these patients was compared with that of 58 nonresponders who continued glucocorticoids. The 2-month mortality rate of the pentoxifylline-treated patients (36%) did not differ from that of the control subjects who continued glucocorticoids (32%).[157]

The final and most intriguing trial was a direct comparison of pentoxifylline and glucocorticoid therapy. In this trial,[158] 68 patients with a clinical diagnosis of alcoholic hepatitis and an mDF greater than 32 were randomly allocated to receive treatment with prednisolone or pentoxifylline. The 60-day mortality rate in the glucocorticoid recipients was 35% compared with 15% in those who received pentoxifylline. Hepatorenal syndrome developed in 6 patients in the glucocorticoid group compared with none in the pentoxifylline group. If confirmed, these data could transform standard management of patients with severe alcoholic hepatitis.

Combination Therapy

Combination therapy including glucocorticoids and another agent has been explored in 2 trials. In the first, glucocorticoid therapy was compared with treatment with glucocorticoids plus a 5-day course of IV N-acetylcysteine. Although a high proportion of patients in the glucocorticoid group (24%) died within the first 30 days compared with 8% in the combination therapy group, and hepatorenal syndrome developed in twice as many in the former group, no difference in survival at 90 or 180 days was found.[159]

The second, and perhaps most disappointing, trial compared the combination of glucocorticoids plus pentoxifylline with glucocorticoid monotherapy.[160] The 30-day mortality rate in the patients in the combination group was 28% compared with 26% in the patients who received only glucocorticoids. The 6-month mortality rate was also comparable in the 2 groups of patients. Hepatorenal syndrome was the cause of death in only 1 of 10 patients (10%) in the combination therapy group compared with 4 of 9 (44%) in the glucocorticoid group. Although patients with renal failure were excluded, this group of patients was quite ill, with a mean mDf score of 75, compared with mDF scores in the low to mid-40s in the original trials of glucocorticoids.[110,111] Furthermore, a significant treatment effect could easily have been missed because of the small size of the study,

Drugs of Unlikely Benefit and Promising New Agents Under Investigation

A number of other therapeutic agents have been studied in patients with alcoholic hepatitis, including androgenic steroids, propylthiouracil, antioxidants, and anti-TNF agents. None has been shown to improve survival.[1,4,80-82,108] The National Institutes of Health has funded 4 grants to evaluate novel mechanisms and new therapies for alcoholic hepatitis. Two programs are using IL-1 inhibitors, based in part on very high IL-1 levels in the serum of alcoholic hepatitis patients and the fact that IL-1 receptor blockade attenuates experimental alcoholic hepatitis. One study combines IL-1 inhibitor therapy

with pentoxifylline and zinc. Another center plans to study a caspase inhibitor, which is thought to block apoptotic cell death in severe alcoholic hepatitis. For more moderate alcoholic hepatitis, a probiotic approach is being used, as well as an oral agent that inhibits intestinal absorption of endotoxin.

Recommendations

Glucocorticoid therapy can result in dramatic improvement in survival in carefully selected patients with severe alcoholic hepatitis.[110,111] Three factors limit their usefulness: (1) a number of patients are not candidates for therapy because of obvious contraindications, (2) a substantial number of patients fail to respond, and (3) glucocorticoids have limited efficacy in patients with chronic kidney disease or acute kidney injury and do not appear to prevent the development of hepatorenal syndrome. Therefore, in patients who have contraindications to glucocorticoid therapy or any degree of renal disease, pentoxifylline appears to be safer and more effective. Figure 86-16 illustrates the factors that should be taken into account when glucocorticoid and pentoxifylline therapy are considered in patients with severe alcoholic hepatitis. Although combination therapies are attractive in theory, we do not feel that the existing data support their use.

Therapy for Alcoholic Cirrhosis

Abstinence is the only treatment that clearly improves survival in patients with alcoholic cirrhosis. A variety of

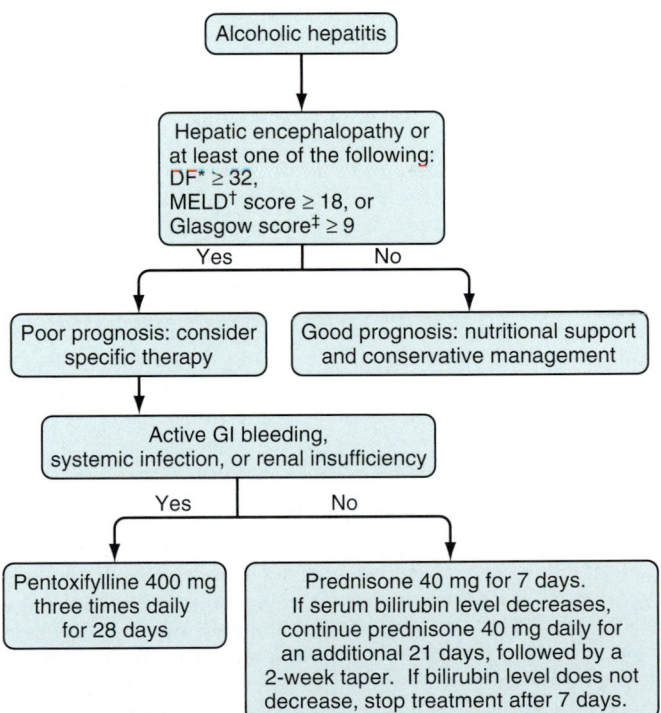

FIGURE 86-16. Algorithm for the management of patients with alcoholic hepatitis. *The DF is calculated as follows: 4.6 (prothrombin time of patient − prothrombin time of control) + serum bilirubin level (in mg/dL). †The MELD score is based on the serum bilirubin level, INR, and serum creatinine level (see Chapter 92). ‡The Glasgow alcoholic hepatitis score is based on the patient's age, WBC count, blood urea nitrogen level, ratio of prothrombin time to a control value, and serum bilirubin level. DF, discriminant function. On-line calculators for these various models are available at http://www.lillemodel.com.

treatments for which there is a specific rationale have been investigated over the years. Examples include silymarin, SAMe, betaine, colchicine, androgenic steroids, lecithin, vitamin E, and pentoxifylline. None has been shown to improve survival (see Chapter 74).[4,80]

Liver Transplantation

Alcoholic cirrhosis is the second most common indication for liver transplantation in the United States and Europe.[161] The outcome following liver transplantation is quite favorable (see Chapter 97).[162] Three factors that reduce survival after transplantation are concurrent HCV infection, smoking, and a return to destructive patterns of drinking.[105,162-164] Although almost half of the transplant recipients drink some alcohol after the operation, few return to destructive patterns of alcohol use.[165] A multidisciplinary approach both before and after transplantation, including addiction specialists, psychiatrists, and transplant professionals, appears to offer the best opportunity for patients with alcoholic liver disease to achieve a long-term high quality of life after transplantation.[166,167]

Many patients with apparently advanced alcoholic cirrhosis can recover to the degree that liver transplantation is not required if they can abstain from drinking (see Fig. 86-10).[132] Because the benefits of abstinence can be so dramatic, requiring a period of abstinence before proceeding with transplantation is reasonable; however, if patients do not show evidence of significant recovery within 3 months, they are unlikely to survive without transplantation.[161] Referral to a transplant center at that time for further evaluation of their alcoholism and candidacy for transplantation gives patients the best opportunity to be placed on the transplant waiting list after the traditional 6-month waiting period required by most transplant centers and insurance companies.

Patients with a CTP score greater than 11 despite at least 6 months of abstinence have improved survival with liver transplantation (Fig. 86-17).[119] Evidence of a survival benefit following transplantation is less clear for patients with milder degrees of alcoholic cirrhosis, unless they have hepatocellular carcinoma. Patients with CTP scores of 5 to 7 do not benefit from liver transplantation.[119] Patients with CTP scores of 8 to 10 who were randomized to receive immediate transplantation, compared with those who were randomized to be observed expectantly, showed a lower 2-year survival rate (73% vs. 80%), primarily because of a high risk of postoperative malignancy.[168]

Patients with severe alcoholic hepatitis have not been considered to be appropriate candidates for liver transplantation because of recent drinking, the fear that they will return to drinking after the operation, and the assumption that many will recover with abstinence or appropriate medical therapy.[1,4,82] These assumptions have been challenged by a study in which carefully selected patients with severe alcoholic hepatitis who failed to respond to glucocorticoid therapy were shown to have a dramatic improvement in survival with early liver transplantation compared with matched controls (Fig. 86-18).[169]

Optimal Management

Reducing the substantial morbidity and mortality associated with alcohol abuse will only occur if the global medical community makes a major commitment to early diagnosis of alcohol misuse. Systematic application of alcohol questionnaires at all points of entry into medical care will be required to achieve this goal. Government programs that

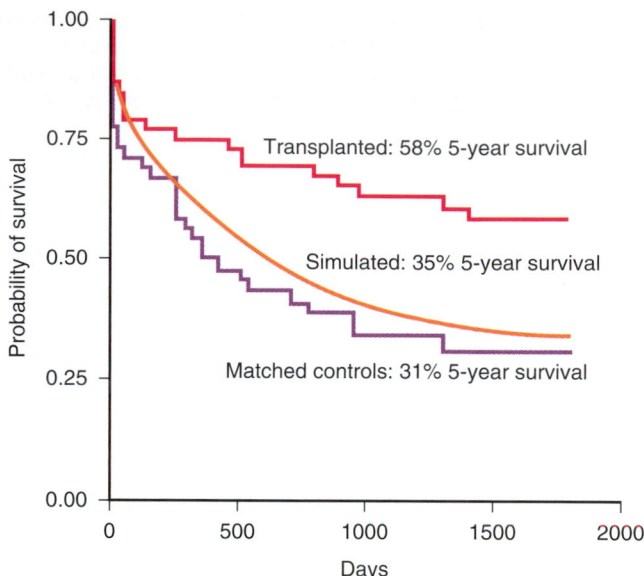

FIGURE 86-17. Improved probability of survival over 5 years in patients with alcoholic cirrhosis and Child-Turcotte-Pugh scores of 11 to 15 following 6 months of abstinence from alcohol and liver transplantation *(top line)*, compared with matched control subjects (P = 0.008) and simulated control subjects (i.e., predicted from a model) (P = 0.001). *(Modified from Poynard T, Naveau S, Doffoel M, et al. Evaluation of efficacy of liver transplantation in alcoholic cirrhosis using matched and simulated controls: 5-year survival. Multi-centre group. J Hepatol 1999; 30:1130-7.)*

provide frequent monitoring and swift, certain, and modest sanctions for violations also show promise in reducing arrests for driving under the influence of alcohol and domestic violence.[170]

For patients with stable cirrhosis, maintaining abstinence is the most important aspect of management, because no drugs have been shown to improve survival. Nutritional support with evening snacks can be beneficial. All patients should receive recommended vaccinations. In addition, they should undergo regular surveillance for hepatocellular carcinoma and screening for esophageal varices as appropriate (see Chapters 92 and 96). In addition, weight control and cessation of smoking are important.

For hospitalized patients with alcoholic hepatitis or cirrhosis, electrolyte disturbances and vitamin deficiencies should be corrected and withdrawal symptoms treated when present. During the first few days of admission, the patient should be offered a nutritious diet if the patient's mental status is adequate. Patients with severe alcoholic hepatitis should receive enteral feedings to ensure adequate caloric and protein intake. In patients with severe alcoholic hepatitis who do not have a systemic infection or GI bleeding, a short course of glucocorticoid therapy should be considered. An alternative strategy is the use of pentoxifylline, especially in patients with marginal renal function or hepatorenal syndrome. Given the extremely poor prognosis of patients hospitalized with multiple organ failure, palliative care teams should be involved within the first few days after admission to provide appropriate support for both patients and families. Liver transplantation is effective in providing prolonged survival with excellent quality of life in carefully selected patients with alcoholic cirrhosis and potentially in patients with severe alcoholic hepatitis who fail to respond to medical therapy.

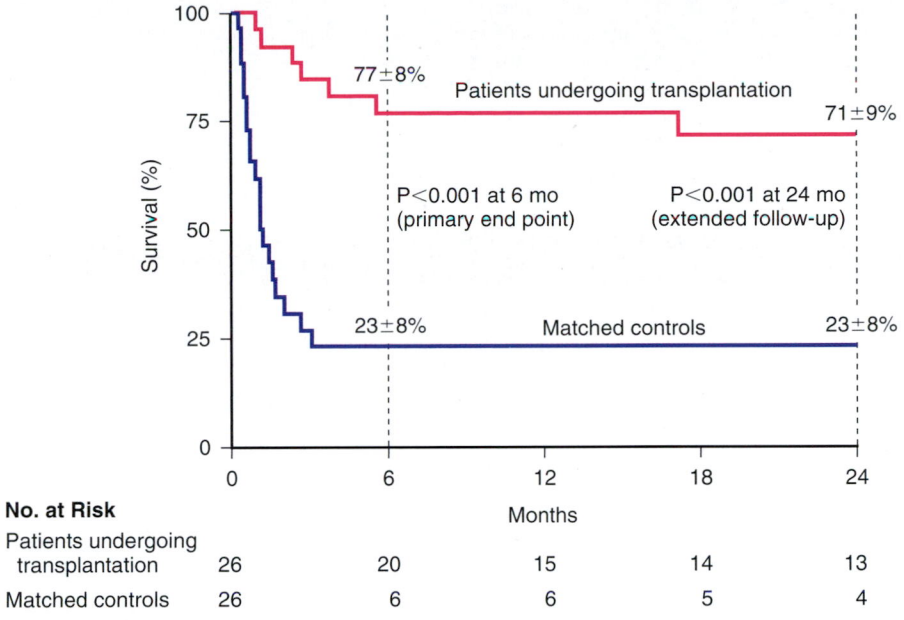

FIGURE 86-18. Kaplan-Meier estimates of survival in patients with severe alcoholic hepatitis who failed glucocorticoid therapy and underwent early liver transplantation compared with matched controls who did not undergo liver transplantation. *(From Mathurin P, Moreno C, Samuel D, et al. Early liver transplantation for severe alcoholic hepatitis. N Engl J Med 2011; 365:1790-800, with permission.)*

KEY REFERENCES

Full references for this chapter can be found on www.expertconsult.com.

2. Friedmann PD. Clinical practice. Alcohol use in adults. N Engl J Med 2013; 368:365-73.
19. Beier JI, Arteel GE, McClain CJ. Advances in alcoholic liver disease. Curr Gastroenterol Rep 2011; 13:56-64.
44. Purohit V, Bode JC, Bode C, et al. Alcohol, intestinal bacterial growth, intestinal permeability to endotoxin, and medical consequences: Summary of a symposium. Alcohol 2008; 42:349-61.
53. Szabo G, Bala S. Alcoholic liver disease and the gut-liver axis. World J Gastroenterol 2010; 16:1321-9.
62. Stickel F, Hampe J. Genetic determinants of alcoholic liver disease. Gut 2012; 61:150-9.
66. Kirpich I, Ghare S, Zhang J, et al. Binge alcohol-induced microvesicular liver steatosis and injury are associated with down-regulation of hepatic HDAC 1, 7, 9, 10, 11 and up-regulation of HDAC 3. Alcohol Clin Exp Res 2012; 36:1578-86.
80. European Association for the Study of the Liver. EASL clinical practical guidelines: Management of alcoholic liver disease. J Hepatol 2012; 57:399-420.

82. O'Shea RS, Dasarathy S, McCullough AJ, et al. Alcoholic liver disease. Hepatology 2010; 51:307-28.
108. Singal AK, Shah VH. Alcoholic hepatitis: Prognostic models and treatment. Gastroenterol Clin North Am 2011; 40:611-39.
117. Jepsen P, Ott P, Andersen PK, et al. Clinical course of alcoholic liver cirrhosis: A Danish population-based cohort study. Hepatology 2010; 51:1675-82.
132. Veldt B, Laine F, Guillygomarc'h A, et al. Indication of liver transplantation in severe alcoholic liver cirrhosis: Quantitative evaluation and optimal timing. J Hepatol 2002; 36:93-8.
143. Plank LD, Gane EJ, Peng S, et al. Nocturnal nutritional supplementation improves total body protein status of patients with liver cirrhosis: A randomized 12-month trial. Hepatology 2008; 48:557-66.
150. Louvet A, Naveau S, Abdelnour M, et al. The Lille model: A new tool for therapeutic strategy in patients with severe alcoholic hepatitis treated with steroids. Hepatology 2007; 45:1348-54.
168. Vanlemmens C, Di Martino V, Milan C, et al. Immediate listing for liver transplantation versus standard care for Child-Pugh stage B alcoholic cirrhosis: A randomized trial. Ann Intern Med 2009; 150:153-61.
169. Mathurin P, Moreno C, Samuel D, et al. Early liver transplantation for severe alcoholic hepatitis. N Engl J Med 2011; 365:1790-800.

The global obesity epidemic has dramatically increased the prevalence of nonalcoholic fatty liver disease (NAFLD), such that it is the most common cause of chronic liver disease in Western nations. Although NAFLD is associated with cardiovascular disease, obstructive sleep apnea, vitamin D deficiency, type 2 diabetes mellitus, and other manifestations of the metabolic syndrome, the most clinically relevant subset of patients with NAFLD in terms of liver-specific outcomes are those with nonalcoholic steatohepatitis (NASH). Ludwig and colleagues coined the term *NASH* in 1980 to describe a cohort of middle-aged patients with elevated serum liver enzyme levels who had evidence of alcoholic hepatitis on liver biopsy specimens in the absence of alcohol consumption.[1] Subsequent study led to the popular "2-hit" hypothesis by which sequential progression from isolated fatty liver (IFL) to NASH involved an initial lesion of hepatic steatosis followed by a second "hit" of oxidative stress resulting in liver injury.[2] It is now recognized that patients who have steatohepatitis on liver biopsy specimens are at risk of progression to cirrhosis, and our understanding of the pathogenesis of NAFLD has evolved from the 2-hit hypothesis and has suggested new therapeutic approaches.

NONALCOHOLIC FATTY LIVER AND STEATOHEPATITIS

Epidemiology

Because the majority of patients with NAFLD are asymptomatic, the prevalence of NAFLD in the United States and globally is not completely defined, although several studies have suggested a wide range of prevalence rates of 2.8% to 46%.[3] The prevalence of NAFLD is rising in concert with rising rates of obesity and diabetes mellitus, with an estimated 33.8% of the population meeting criteria for obesity and 10.6% for type 2 diabetes mellitus.[4] Prevalence estimates vary widely depending on the information available in a given population and the diagnostic criteria that are used to establish the diagnosis (i.e., liver biochemical test levels, imaging results, liver biopsy findings).

The first estimates of the prevalence of NASH came from autopsy studies, in which steatohepatitis was found in 18.5% of markedly obese and 2.7% of lean persons.[5] Advanced fibrosis was seen in 13.8% of the markedly obese subjects compared with 6.6% of the lean ones. High rates of NAFLD and NASH among obese persons were subsequently confirmed in a study of patients undergoing bariatric surgery, in which the prevalence rates of NAFLD and NASH were as high as 91% and 37%, respectively.[6]

The Dallas Heart Study used MR spectroscopy in more than 2200 adults to identify a 31% prevalence of NAFLD in a cohort of asymptomatic persons.[7,8] Subsequent population-based cohort studies from China, Japan, and Korea have reported a prevalence of NAFLD ranging from 10% to 24% using US.[9-11] The largest study to date using US followed by hepatic histology was in a cohort of asymptomatic middle-aged patients from San Antonio, Texas, and revealed a 46% prevalence of NAFLD and a 12.2% prevalence of NASH.[12] Most cases of NAFLD are discovered in middle age during the fourth to sixth decades of life, although NAFLD has also been described with increasing frequency in children and adolescents, among whom the frequency of overweight and obesity has been reported to be 30%.[13] A comparison of data in 12,715 patients 12 to 19 years of age, obtained from the National Health and Examination Surveys (NHANES) from 1988 to 1994 and 2007 to 2010, demonstrated an increase in the prevalence of pediatric NAFLD from 3.9% to 10.7%.[14]

Most relevant studies have reported NAFLD to be more common in men than women and have described a later peak in prevalence in women,[15] suggesting a relationship to sex hormones and menopause.[16] NAFLD, and specifically NASH, is often associated with diabetes mellitus, which is associated with a 60% to 76% frequency of NAFLD and a 22% frequency of NASH.[12,17] NAFLD is considered to be the hepatic manifestation of the metabolic syndrome as defined by the presence of 3 or more of the following: abdominal obesity, hypertriglyceridemia, low high-density lipoprotein (HDL) levels, hypertension, and an elevated fasting plasma glucose (see also Chapter 7).[18]

An understanding of the role of ethnicity is evolving. Early evidence from the Dallas Heart Study, among others, suggested that ethnicity was important, with Hispanics showing the highest prevalence of NAFLD (45%) compared with Caucasians (33%) and African Americans (24%). Similar findings have been reported by others,[12] with a prevalence of 58.3% in Hispanics, 44% in Caucasians, and 35% in African Americans. The reason for these trends appears to be multifactorial. A study by the NASH Clinical Research Network (CRN) found Hispanics with NASH to be younger, less active, and more likely to consume a diet higher in carbohydrates compared with Caucasians.[19] Another study compared disease severity between Hispanic and Caucasian age-, sex-, and total body fat–matched patients with NASH and found disease severity to be similar, with a trend toward greater hepatic fibrosis in diabetic Hispanic patients.[20]

Lifestyle is an important factor, and increased consumption of high-fructose corn syrup and sugar-containing sodas, coupled with a sedentary lifestyle, has been associated with higher rates of NAFLD and specifically NASH.[12] Genetic influences on the development of NAFLD may prove to be equally important. Single nucleotide polymorphisms (SNPs) from specific genes have been found to be associated with an increased risk of NAFLD. The first of these SNPs to be identified was in the patatin-like phospholipase domain–containing protein-3 (PLPLA3) gene located on chromosome 22q13 and known to encode adiponutrin, a 481–amino acid protein that mediates triacylglycerol synthesis.[21] The allelic variant rs738409 results in a change from isoleucine to methionine at position 148 (I148M) and was shown to be associated with increased hepatic steatosis as well as inflammation.[22] Interestingly, this variant was more common in Hispanics, followed by Caucasians and African Americans. A subsequent study confirmed the association of the I148M SNP with hepatic steatosis, NASH, and even fibrosis, and a 2011 meta-analysis demonstrated an odds ratio (OR) of 3.26 (95% CI, 2.14-4.95) for NASH and 3.25 (95% CI, 2.86-3.70) for hepatic fibrosis for persons with the I148M SNP.[23]

Other genetic mutations have been found to be associated with NAFLD, including 2 SNPs (rs2854117 and rs2854116) that affect the insulin response element in the gene encoding apolipoprotein C3 (APOC3). APOC3 is known to regulate plasma TG concentrations, and these 2 SNPs were found to be associated with NAFLD in a study of Asian Indian men of normal weight,[24] although subsequent studies in other ethnic groups failed to confirm this association.[25-27] Numerous other genetic polymorphisms have been studied, including those encoding microsomal TG transfer protein (MTP), superoxide dismutase 2 (SOD 2), TNF-α, and transforming growth factor (TGF)-β and have shown at least some association with hepatic steatosis and steatohepatitis.[28]

Definitions and Associations

Macrovesicular fat accumulation in more than 5% of hepatocytes is the defining feature of NAFLD. The majority of patients with NAFLD have IFL, which is defined as hepatic steatosis in the absence of significant necroinflammation or fibrosis (Fig. 87-1). Hepatocyte ballooning degeneration and lobular inflammation of a mixed inflammatory cell infiltrate are required to meet criteria for NASH, and Mallory-Denk (or Mallory) bodies, iron deposition, ductular reaction, megamitochondria, periodic acid–Schiff diastase-resistant Kupffer cells, and vacuolated nuclei in periportal hepatocytes may also be seen (Fig. 87-2).[29] Fibrosis, if present, is predominantly perisinusoidal and pericellular ("chicken-wire" fibrosis) in acinar zone 3, although it may extend to portal and periportal regions with disease progression (Box 87-1). Alcoholic steatosis and steatohepatitis (alcoholic hepatitis) is histologically indistinguishable from IFL and NASH (see Chapter 86), although expert pathologists recognize more fibro-occlusive venous lesions and bile stasis in alcoholic steatohepatitis.[30] Pediatric NAFLD is a somewhat distinct histologic entity marked by portal-based chronic inflammation and fibrosis, with less frequent findings of hepatocyte ballooning degeneration and Mallory-Denk bodies.[31]

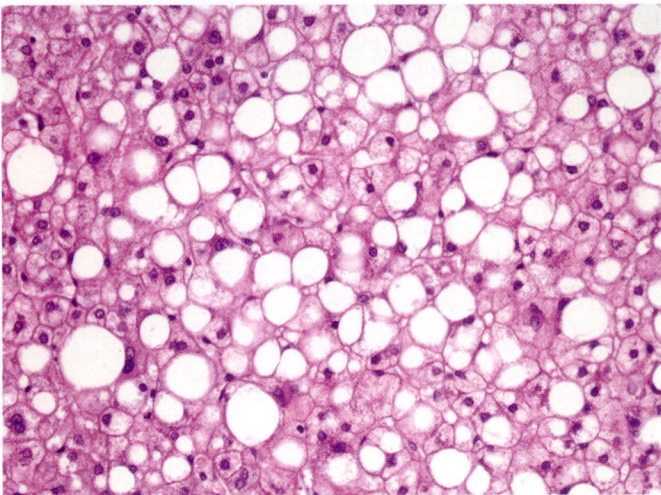

FIGURE 87-1. Histopathology of fatty liver. The characteristic feature is diffuse macrovesicular steatosis without significant necroinflammation or fibrosis. Glycogenated nuclei are common. (H&E.) *(Courtesy Dr. Gregory Y. Lauwers, Boston, Mass.)*

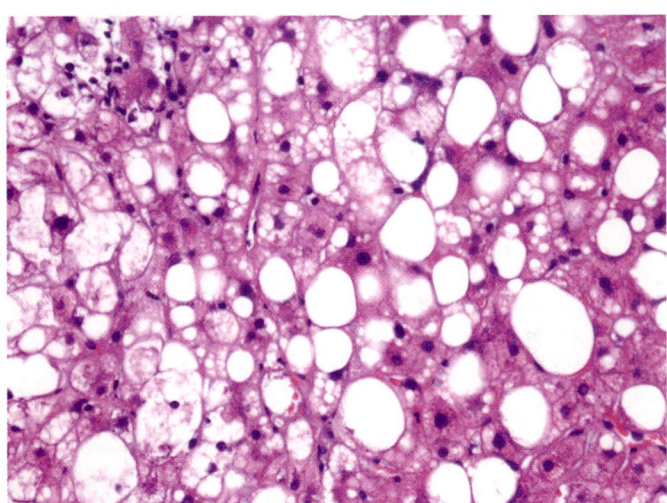

FIGURE 87-2. Histopathology of nonalcoholic steatohepatitis. Diffuse or perivenular macrovesicular steatosis is present. Lobular inflammation consists of neutrophils, lymphocytes, and other mononuclear cells. Hepatocyte ballooning and necrosis of varied degrees are hallmark features. Glycogenated nuclei are present. Mallory-Denk bodies, which may be small, sparse, and inconspicuous, are seen. (H&E.) *(Courtesy Dr. Gregory Y. Lauwers, Boston, Mass.)*

To reach consensus on the pathologic classification of NASH, the Pathology Committee of the National Institutes of Health NASH CRN proposed a scoring system incorporating 14 histologic features in 2005.[32] The NAFLD activity score (NAS) combines the unweighted sum of scores for steatosis, lobular inflammation, and hepatocellular ballooning on a scale of 0 to 8 (Table 87-1). A score of 0 to 2 is most suggestive of "not-NASH," and a score of 5 or greater suggests that NASH is present. Although the NAS is primarily a research tool, and NASH is not defined by an absolute score, NAS provides a framework to accurately detect changes in disease activity with therapy.

BOX 87-1 Histopathologic Features of Nonalcoholic Fatty Liver Disease

Present in All or Most Cases
Macrovesicular steatosis
  Diffuse or centrilobular steatosis; degree may correlate
    with BMI
Parenchymal inflammation
  Polymorphonuclear neutrophils, lymphocytes, other
    mononuclear cells
Hepatocyte necrosis
Ballooning hepatocyte degeneration

Observed with Varied Frequencies
Perivenular, perisinusoidal, or periportal fibrosis (37%-84%),
  moderate to severe in 15%-50%; most prevalent in zone 3
  (perivenular)
Cirrhosis (7%-16% on index biopsy specimen)
Mallory-Denk bodies
Glycogenated nuclei
Lipogranulomas
Stainable hepatic iron

TABLE 87-1 NAFLD Activity Score on a Liver Biopsy Specimen

Steatosis	
5%	1
5%-33%	2
33%-66%	3
Ballooning	
None	0
Few	1
Many	2
Lobular Inflammation	
Mild	1
Moderate	2
Severe	3
Total Score	
0-2	Likely not NASH
3-4	Intermediate
5-8	Likely NASH

NAFLD, nonalcoholic fatty liver disease; NASH, nonalcoholic steatohepatitis.

BOX 87-2 Causes of Fatty Liver Disease

Acquired Metabolic Disorders
Diabetes mellitus
Dyslipidemia
Kwashiorkor and marasmus
Obesity
Rapid weight loss
Starvation

Cytotoxic and Cytostatic Drugs
L-Asparaginase
Azacitidine
Bleomycin
Cisplatin
5-Fluorouracil
Methotrexate
Tetracyclines (inhibit mitochondrial beta oxidation)

Other Drugs and Toxins
Amiodarone
Camphor
Chloroform
Cocaine
Ethanol
Ethyl bromide
Estrogens
Glucocorticoids
Griseofulvin
HAART (zidovudine, stavudine, didanosine)
Lycopodium serratum (Jin bu huan, an herbal supplement)
Nifedipine
Nitrofurantoin
NSAIDs (piroxicam, ibuprofen, indomethacin, sulindac)
Tamoxifen
Valproic acid

Metals
Antimony
Barium salts
Chromates
Mercury
Phosphorus
Rare earth metals of low atomic number
Thallium compounds
Uranium compounds

Inborn Errors of Metabolism
Abetalipoproteinemia
Familial hepatosteatosis
Galactosemia
Glycogen storage disease
Hereditary fructose intolerance
Homocystinuria
Systemic carnitine deficiency
Tyrosinemia
Weber-Christian syndrome
Wilson disease

Surgical Procedures
Biliopancreatic diversion
Extensive small bowel resection
Jejunoileal bypass

Miscellaneous Conditions
Industrial exposure to petrochemicals
IBD
Jejunal diverticulosis with bacterial overgrowth
Partial lipodystrophy
TPN

Other conditions may promote hepatic steatosis (Box 87-2). TPN, rapid weight loss, or starvation can lead to hepatic steatosis. Similarly, surgeries that lead to rapid and extreme intestinal malabsorption and weight loss, such as extensive small bowel resection, biliopancreatic diversion, or jejunoileal bypass (see Chapter 8), have been associated with hepatic steatosis. Medications including amiodarone, valproic acid, methotrexate, tamoxifen, glucocorticoids, certain antiretrovirals, and tetracyclines have also been implicated, as have systemic conditions such as Wilson disease, abetalipoproteinemia, and lipodystrophy.

Pathogenesis

The 2-hit hypothesis proposed by Day and colleagues in 1988 (see earlier) has provided a framework for our current understanding of the increasingly complicated steps that lead to hepatic steatosis, steatohepatitis, and fibrosis. Given the variety of conditions that have been associated with NAFLD, a single pathogenic mechanism cannot account for all cases. The 2-hit hypothesis states that dysregulation of fatty acid metabolism leads to steatosis, which is associated with several cellular adaptations and altered signaling pathways that render hepatocytes vulnerable to a second hit. The second insult may be 1 or more environmental or genetic perturbations that cause hepatocyte necrosis and inflammation. In a minority of cases, incompletely defined factors activate a fibrogenic cascade that leads eventually to cirrhosis.

Hepatic Steatosis

Hepatic steatosis is the hallmark histologic feature of NAFLD and is the net result of excessive accumulation of free fatty acid (FFA). Normally, FFA is supplied to the liver through intestinal absorption (in the form of chylomicron remnants) or from lipolysis of adipose tissue, where FFA is stored as TGs. In the liver, FFA is oxidized by mitochondria, esterified into TGs, synthesized into phospholipids and cholesteryl esters, and secreted from the liver as very-low-density lipoprotein (VLDL). Fatty acid metabolism is under tight regulatory control by catecholamines, glucagon, growth hormone, and insulin. Hepatic TG accumulation occurs when fatty acid metabolism shifts to favor net lipogenesis, rather than lipolysis. This shift occurs when the amount of FFA supplied to the liver from the intestine or adipose tissue exceeds the amount needed for mitochondrial oxidation, phospholipid synthesis, and synthesis of cholesteryl esters. TGs also accumulate in the liver when synthesis of lipoprotein decreases or export of lipids from the liver is impeded (see also Chapter 72).

Insulin resistance from excessive accumulation of FFA is thought to be a primary factor in the development of steatosis in most patients with NAFLD. Laboratory and clinical evidence supports the association of peripheral insulin resistance and hyperinsulinemia with NAFLD, even in lean patients without obvious glucose intolerance.[33,34] This complicated process involves an accumulation of toxic lipid metabolites, including diacylglycerol, ceramides, and fatty acyl-CoA, in muscle cells, which, in turn, leads to insulin signaling defects and impaired skeletal muscle glucose metabolism. Elevated glucose levels subsequently activate carbohydrate response element-binding protein, while elevated insulin levels promote de novo lipogenesis via activation of sterol regulatory element–binding protein 1 (SREBP-1).[35]

The excess and dysfunctional visceral adipose tissue seen in NAFLD further promotes insulin hypersecretion secondary to insulin resistance. The increased secretion of specific proinflammatory cytokines, such as TNF-α, interleukin (IL)-6, resistin, visfatin, and plasminogen activator inhibitor-1, has been described, along with decreased secretion of the anti-inflammatory cytokine adiponectin. Serum adiponectin levels are reduced in obesity, insulin resistance, diabetes mellitus, and the metabolic syndrome and have been shown to be correlated negatively with the severity of NASH.[36] The degree of adipose tissue insulin resistance, as defined by the nonesterified fatty acid concentration multiplied by the fasting serum insulin level (rather than the absolute amount of visceral adiposity), is more important in determining the severity of NAFLD than are serum adiponectin levels.[37]

Leptin is another peptide that is secreted by adipocytes and thought to potentiate insulin resistance, thereby leading to hepatic steatosis (see Chapter 4). Leptin is a satiety hormone that controls food intake and energy regulation via insulin signaling and regulation of glucose metabolism in peripheral tissues and may play an important role in regulating the partitioning of fat between mitochondrial beta oxidation and TG synthesis in the liver.[38] Severe steatosis and steatohepatitis develop in leptin-deficient (ob/ob) mice. Obesity in humans

is associated with relative leptin resistance and high leptin levels, which may contribute to the genesis of steatosis by a negative impact on insulin signaling or may be a consequence of the chronic hyperinsulinemia associated with obesity. Several studies have examined the relationship between serum leptin levels and NAFLD, with conflicting results.[39,40]

Research into the pathogenesis of NAFLD has addressed the role of nuclear hormone receptors, particularly as they affect bile acid metabolism and intestinal absorption of dietary lipids and lipid-soluble vitamins, as well as glucose and lipid homeostasis (see Chapter 64). Bile acids absorbed from the distal ileum bind to these nuclear hormone receptors. The most studied nuclear hormone receptor is the farnesoid X receptor (FXR), which has been identified as the master regulator of bile acid synthesis. Activation of FXR has been shown to decrease de novo lipogenesis, impair VLDL synthesis and assembly, and increase beta oxidation of FFA.[41] Other nuclear hormone receptors such as G protein–coupled receptor (TGR-5), liver X receptor (LXR), and liver receptor homolog-1 (LRH-1) may prove to be equally important regulators of glucose and lipid homeostasis, although they have been less well studied.[42]

Genetic influences are also thought to be important in the development of hepatic steatosis. As discussed earlier, SNPs for the genes that influence lipid metabolism, including those that encode PNPLA3 (adiponutrin), APOC3, and MTP, have been associated with NAFLD. Genome-wide association studies have suggested that SNPs in 2 additional genes, lipid phosphate phosphatase-related protein type 4 (*LPPR-4*) and solute carrier family 38 member 8 (*SLC38A8*), are associated with NAFLD in adolescents.[43] Genetic variants that promote insulin resistance or impaired glucose metabolism may also be uncovered, although few relevant studies have been performed to date.

Steatohepatitis

Although insulin resistance and hyperinsulinemia are pivotal to the development of steatosis, consensus is lacking on the subsequent insults that lead to steatohepatitis and fibrosis in some patients. Isolated steatosis may be considered an adaptive mechanism designed to mitigate the effects of long-chain saturated fatty acids within the liver. If the protective processes are overwhelmed or faulty, lipotoxicity can develop, potentially activating numerous signaling pathways in the liver and resulting in hepatocyte apoptosis and stellate cell activation. The precise signaling pathways are still being uncovered, but several key pathways have been defined.

Increased levels of FFA can be directly toxic to hepatocytes through a number of mechanisms. An increased FFA concentration leads to lysosomal destabilization and stimulation of TNF-α, as well as sustained up-regulation of peroxisomal proliferator–activated receptor (PPAR)-α.[44] These events promote fatty acid oxidation and disposal and may increase oxidative stress through the production of dicarboxylic acid derivatives. Chronic oxidative stress is believed to be central to the pathogenesis of alcohol-related liver damage and has been shown to be important in NAFLD. Activation of microsomal enzymes, including cytochrome P450 2E1, in patients with NAFLD[45] and mitochondrial production of reactive oxygen species in a murine model of NAFLD[46] suggest that chronic oxidative stress and lipid peroxidation may also be central to the pathogenesis of NAFLD.

FFA can also be directly toxic to cellular membranes, lead to the formation of toxic fatty acid ethyl ethers, and cause overall disruption of mitochondrial function, thereby overwhelming the overlapping protective mechanisms designed to combat FFA hepatotoxicity. These protective mechanisms include a variety of interrelated pathways, the purpose of which is to limit damage from hepatic insults.

Hepatic progenitor cells (HPCs) are typically quiescent cells that are thought to be part of the repair processes available to respond to liver injury. HPCs provide a secondary source of hepatocytes via a hedgehog ligand–mediated epithelial-to-mesenchymal transformation (EMT).[47] EMT makes hepatocytes less vulnerable to apoptosis, although their activation also indirectly activates hepatic stellate cells to promote hepatic fibrosis via a ductular reaction that is seen in small bile ductules filled with stromal and inflammatory cells.[48]

The hedgehog signaling pathway activation leads to the conversion of quiescent hepatic stellate cells into myofibroblasts, which in turn produce chemoattractants for natural killer T (NKT) cells.[49] NKT cells secrete profibrotic cytokines that further activate myofibroblasts. The stage of fibrosis has been correlated directly with the degree of hedgehog pathway activation in patients with NASH, and mouse model studies have demonstrated promisingly that hedgehog pathway inhibition can reverse liver fibrosis.[50]

Autophagy is another housekeeping process within hepatocytes that involves autodigestion of unwanted proteins and organelles (see Chapter 72). Aging causes diminished autophagy, and in NAFLD autophagy appears to be down-regulated in settings of obesity and insulin resistance as well as exposure to SFAs in vitro.[51] The net result is decreased removal of damaged mitochondria, enhanced oxidative stress, increased endoplasmic reticulum stress, activation of Jun N-terminal kinase (JNK)/c-Jun signaling, and worsening of insulin resistance. Autophagy may also influence hepatic stellate cells and protect against apoptosis.[52]

While the pathways above promote endoplasmic reticulum stress, excessive SFAs independently affect the endoplasmic reticulum by triggering an adaptive process called the *unfolded protein response*. Typically this response leads to the induction of autophagy, but in the setting of prolonged exposure to SFAs, stress sensor proteins such as activated transcription factor-6 (ATF6), inositol-requiring enzymes-1 (IRE1), and PKR-like endoplasmic reticulum kinase are induced and activate apoptotic pathways via JNK.[53,54] The net result is increased endoplasmic reticulum stress, which in turn may activate the hedgehog pathway, resulting in increased hepatic fibrinogenesis.[55]

Endotoxin and endotoxin-mediated cytokine release are suspected in the pathogenesis of alcoholic steatohepatitis, in which increased serum levels of bacterial endotoxin and lipopolysaccharide (LPS) stimulate hepatic production of TNF-α,

IL-6, and IL-8 and activate an inflammatory response that leads to hepatic necrosis[56] (see Chapter 86). The role of intestinal microflora in the development of NAFLD is becoming clearer. Bacterial endotoxin may contribute to the development of NAFLD in some circumstances. Additional data suggest that the intestinal microbiota in patients with NASH is distinct.[57] SIBO in the setting of a surgical jejunoileal bypass or duodenal switch procedure (performed in the past to treat obesity) has been associated with the development of NASH, the risk of which was reduced with antibiotics or even reversed with revision of the surgical procedure (see Chapters 3, 8, and 105).[58-60]

In addition to bariatric surgery, obesity and fructose consumption have been linked to intestine-derived endotoxin in humans.[61,62] Yang and colleagues have demonstrated that ob/ob mice with steatosis are highly vulnerable to endotoxin-induced hepatocyte damage, and NASH rapidly develops in these animals after exposure to low doses of bacterial LPS.[63] Vitamin D deficiency similarly promotes endotoxin exposure and has been associated with NAFLD.[64] The net result of increased endotoxin, particularly from Gram-negative bacteria, is activation of Kupffer cells via Toll-like receptor 4, which in turn up-regulates several inflammatory pathways including JNK and nuclear factor kappa B (NF-κB) and releases proinflammatory cytokines such as TNF-α and IL-1β.

The exact interplay of all the proposed pathogenic factors remains to be elucidated. An understanding of the pathogenesis of NAFLD as of 2015 is summarized in Figure 87-3.

Clinical Features and Diagnosis

The clinical and laboratory features of NAFLD are summarized in Table 87-2. NAFLD usually is discovered incidentally because of elevated liver biochemical test levels or the finding of hepatic steatosis on imaging. Most patients with NAFLD are asymptomatic, but some may describe vague right upper quadrant pain, fatigue, and malaise. Hepatomegaly is commonly seen but often is difficult to appreciate on physical examination because of obesity. Stigmata of chronic liver disease, such as splenomegaly, spider telangiectasias, and ascites, are limited to those patients with cirrhosis. To establish a diagnosis of NAFLD, alcoholic liver disease must be excluded, and the diagnosis of NAFLD should be entertained only in the absence of significant alcohol use (consumption of < 20 to 40 g of alcohol per day in most clinical studies).

A mild to moderate (1.5- to 4-fold) elevation of the serum AST or ALT level, or both, is common, although levels seldom exceed 10 times the upper limit of normal. The serum ALT

TABLE 87-2 Symptoms, Signs, and Laboratory Features of Nonalcoholic Fatty Liver Disease

Symptoms	Signs	Laboratory Features
Common		
None (48%-100% of patients)	Hepatomegaly	2- to 4-fold elevation of serum ALT and AST levels AST/ALT ratio < 1 in most patients Serum alkaline phosphatase level slightly elevated in one third of patients Normal serum bilirubin, serum albumin, and prothrombin time Elevated serum ferritin level
Uncommon		
Vague right upper quadrant pain Fatigue Malaise	Splenomegaly Spider telangiectasias Palmar erythema Ascites	Low-titer (<1:320) antinuclear antibodies

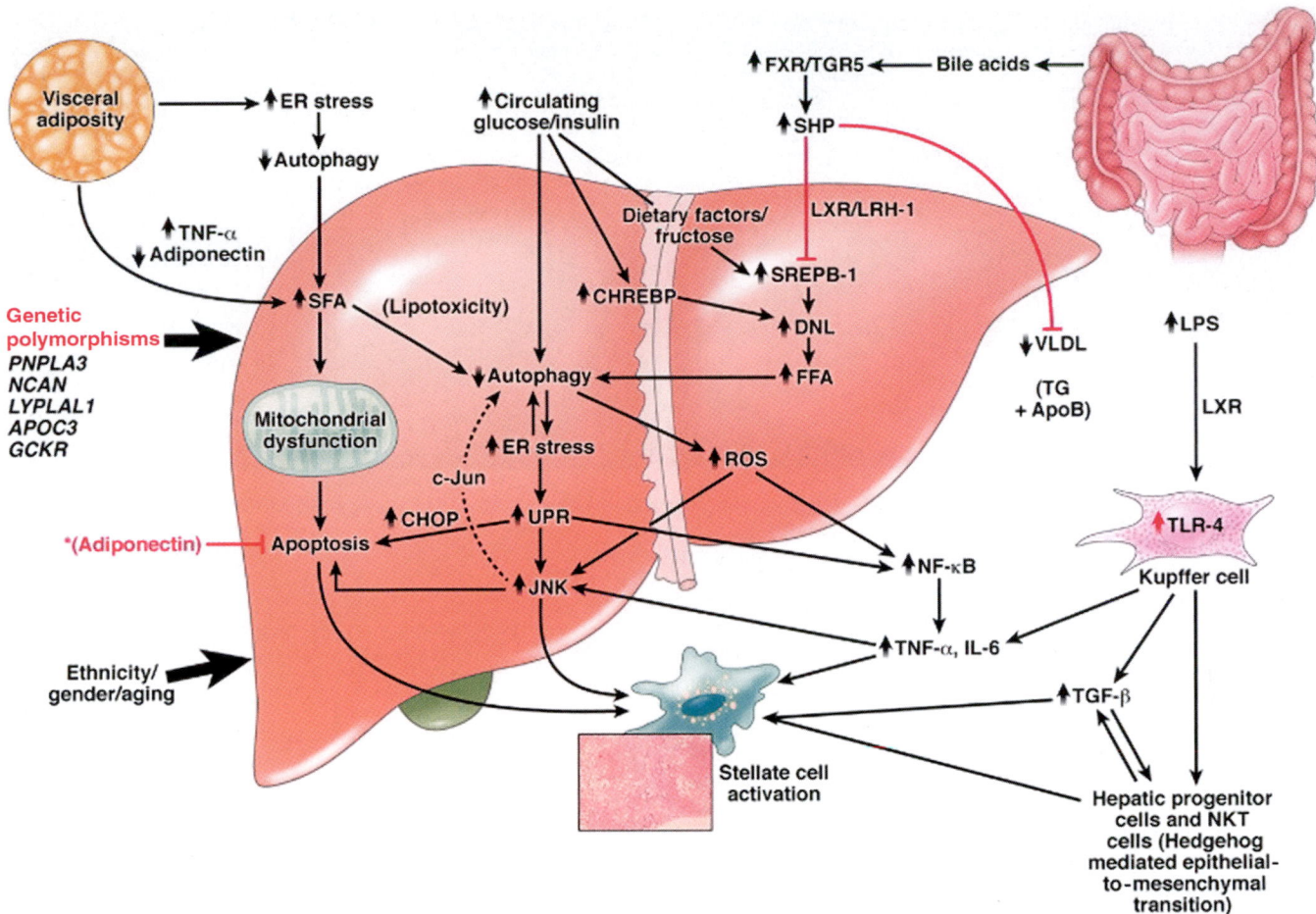

FIGURE 87-3. Proposed pathogenesis of nonalcoholic steatohepatitis integrating obesity and insulin resistance with bile acid metabolism, lipotoxicity, autophagy, endoplasmic reticulum stress, apoptosis, and hepatic progenitor cell transformation and stellate cell activation resulting in hepatic steatosis, necroinflammation, and fibrosis (see text for details). ApoB, apolipoprotein B; *APOC3*, apoprotein C3; Bax, Bcl-2-associated X protein; CHOP, CCAAT/enhancer-binding protein homologous protein; CHREBP, carbohydrate-responsive element binding protein; DNL, de novo lipogenesis; FXR, farsenoid X receptor; *GCKR*, glucokinase (hexokinase 4) regulator; IL-6, interleukin-6; JNK, Jun N-terminal kinase; LPS, lipopolysaccharide; LRH-1, liver receptor homolog 1; LXR, liver X receptor; *LYPLAL1*, lysophospholipase-like1; *NCAN*, gene encoding neurocan; NF-κB, nuclear factor kappa B; NKT, natural killer T; *PNPLA3*, patatin-like phospholipase domain containing 3; ROS, reactive oxygen species; SFA, saturated fatty acid; SREPB-1, sterol regulatory element-binding protein 1; TGF-β, transforming growth factor beta; TLR-4, Toll-like receptor-4; UPR, unfolded protein response; VLDL, very low-density lipoprotein. *(From Torres DM, Williams CD, Harrison SA. Features, diagnosis and treatment of nonalcoholic fatty liver disease. Clin Gastronterol Hepatol 2012; 10:837-58.)*

level is usually greater than the AST level, in contrast to the pattern of alcoholic hepatitis, in which the AST level is at least 2-fold higher than the ALT level (see Chapters 73 and 86). A large retrospective study of patients with NAFLD demonstrated a mean serum ALT level of 83 and AST of 63 U/mL, respectively.[65] Serum alkaline phosphatase and GGTP levels may be elevated, but the serum bilirubin level, prothrombin time, and serum albumin level are typically normal, except in patients with cirrhosis.

Up to one fourth of patients with NAFLD may have antinuclear antibodies (ANA) in low titers (<1:320); laboratory tests for other chronic liver disease are negative.[66] NAFLD can exist in concert with HCV, although HCV infection by itself can promote hepatic steatosis (see Chapter 80). Serum and hepatic iron levels may be elevated in patients with NAFLD. In particular, the serum ferritin level may be elevated in 20% to 50% of patients with NAFLD and may be a marker of more advanced disease. A serum ferritin level more than 1.5 times the upper limit of normal has been independently associated

with a higher NAS in a study of 628 adult patients with NAFLD,[67] although the frequency of genetic hemochromatosis is not increased in patients with NAFLD, who demonstrate predominantly Kupffer cell (secondary) iron overload on liver biopsy specimens.[68] Clinical and laboratory findings do not correlate with the histologic severity of NAFLD, and the entire histologic spectrum of NAFLD, including cirrhosis, can be seen in patients with normal or near-normal serum aminotransferase levels.[69]

Imaging studies often are obtained during the evaluation of unexplained liver biochemical abnormalities or suspected NAFLD (see Chapter 73). Hepatic US may reveal a "bright" liver of increased echogenicity, consistent with hepatic steatosis (Fig. 87-4). Fatty liver also can be documented by abdominal CT (a fatty liver is lower in density than the spleen) and by MRI, with which fat appears bright on T1-weighted imaging. Areas of relative sparing of fat may be seen on imaging studies. A study that assessed the sensitivities of MRI, abdominal CT, and US for distinguishing advanced NASH

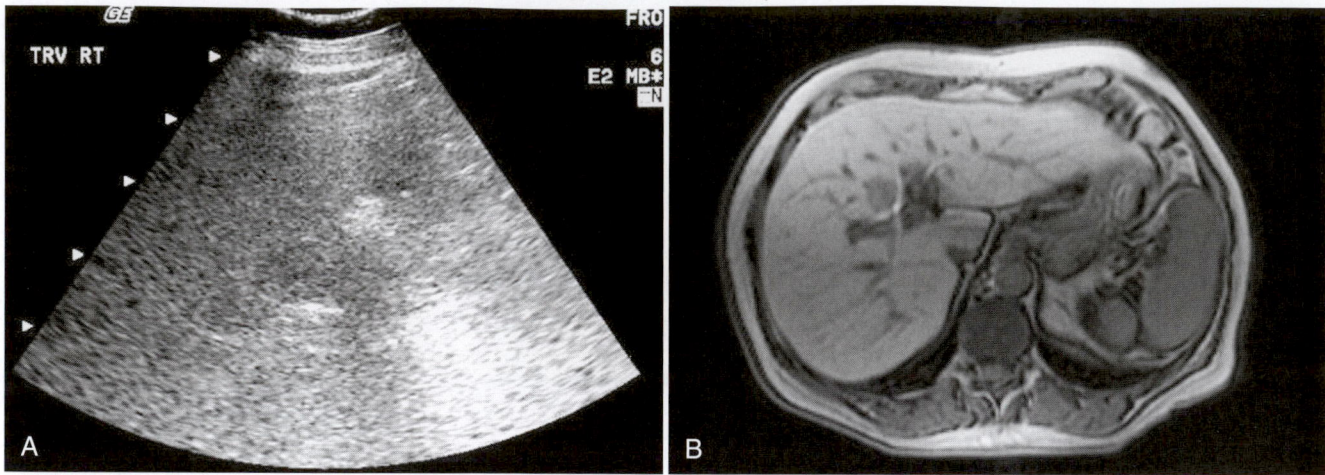

FIGURE 87-4. Imaging studies of fatty liver. *A,* US demonstrating increased echogenicity. *B,* T1-weighted MRI demonstrating a "bright" liver. *(Courtesy Dr. Mukesh Harisinghani, Boston, Mass.)*

from simple steatosis showed that US and CT had sensitivity rates of 100% and 93%, respectively, for detecting hepatic fat involving greater than 33% of the liver, with positive predictive values of 62% and 76%, respectively.[70] No imaging modality, however, was able to distinguish simple steatosis from more advanced forms of NAFLD. Traditional cross-sectional imaging studies may support the diagnosis of NAFLD but cannot predict the severity of disease and cannot replace liver biopsy for establishing the diagnosis with certainty.

Role of Liver Biopsy

Although the diagnosis of NAFLD is relatively easy to make when hepatic steatosis is seen on cross-sectional imaging and other chronic liver diseases have been excluded, a liver biopsy is still required to identify patients with NASH. In practice, most patients with NAFLD do not undergo a liver biopsy. Liver biopsy is an invasive procedure associated with rare but severe complications, including hemorrhage and even death, and undertaking liver biopsies in 20% to 30% of the general population is not feasible (see Chapter 21). The ability to distinguish NASH from IFL is critical because patients with NASH are at risk of progression to cirrhosis. The ideal approach would be to select patients for whom liver biopsy might influence management through more aggressive treatment, participation in clinical trials, or screening for hepatocellular carcinoma in the setting of cirrhosis (Fig. 87-5). Advanced imaging techniques as well as laboratory tests and scoring systems have been studied as a means of identifying high-risk patients who should undergo liver biopsy or as potential noninvasive markers of steatohepatitis or fibrosis.

Imaging to Detect Fibrosis

Newer imaging techniques have been successful in identifying hepatic fibrosis (see also Chapters 73, 74, and 80). The most studied and widely available has been transient elastography (Fibroscan; Echosens, Paris, France), which uses a low-amplitude shear wave that propagates through the liver parenchyma. The speed at which the wave moves is correlated with liver stiffness, measured in kilopascals. Advantages of this noninvasive technique include relative simplicity, ease of use, and patient acceptance. Optimal cutoff values to predict fibrosis stage have varied among studies, and limitations include decreased accuracy in the setting of obesity, narrow

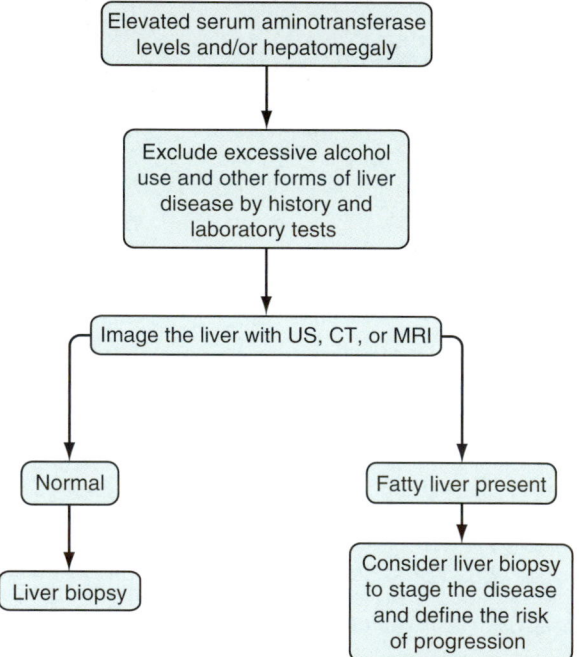

FIGURE 87-5. Algorithm for the diagnostic approach to the patient with suspected nonalcoholic fatty liver disease (NAFLD). The diagnosis of NAFLD is based on clinical and histologic criteria. Most patients are evaluated because of elevated serum aminotransferase levels and/or hepatomegaly. The diagnosis of NAFLD should be considered when excessive alcohol use is absent and laboratory test results exclude other causes of liver disease. Imaging studies may demonstrate fatty liver. Liver biopsy is the standard means of diagnosis and the only test that can reliably differentiate simple steatosis from NASH, although noninvasive methods for assessing fibrosis are emerging.

intercostal spaces, extrahepatic cholestasis, hepatic venous congestion, and acute inflammation.[71,72] An "XL" probe has been developed to increase diagnostic accuracy in obese persons, and one study reported successful measurements in 57% of the cases in which the standard M probe had failed.[73]

Another US-based method that has proved useful in assessing fibrosis in NAFLD is acoustic radiation force impulse

(ARFI) elastography. This technology measures the velocity of a short-duration, high-intensity acoustic pushing pulse in the liver. Pilot trials have suggested accuracy similar to that of US elastography, with an area under the receiver operating curve (AUROC) of 0.973 in a trial of 54 Japanese NAFLD patients.[74]

MR elastography (MRE) combines MRI with elastography and has been accurate in staging NAFLD fibrosis in early studies. MRE appears to be better than transient elastography in differentiating mild from moderate to severe fibrosis, with a sensitivity of 86% and a specificity of 85% in a study of 35 normal volunteers and 50 patients with chronic liver disease.[75] Another study of patients with NAFLD demonstrated a good correlation between MRE stiffness measurements and hepatic histology.[76] Disadvantages to MRE include high cost and limited availability.

Biomarkers and Scoring Systems

Progress has been made in developing simple, noninvasive, and quantitative tests to estimate the presence and degree of steatohepatitis or hepatic fibrosis. The most studied single marker for identifying NASH is cytokeratin-18 (CK-18), a marker of apoptosis. A study by Wieckowski and colleagues demonstrated sensitivity and specificity rates of 91% and 93%, respectively, with an AUROC of 0.93, using a cutoff value of 380 U/L.[77] Subsequent studies, including a meta-analysis of 9 studies, demonstrated lower sensitivity and specificity rates of 78% and 87%, respectively, with an AUROC of 0.82.[78] The test is not commercially available and does not appear to have enough sensitivity and specificity to be used alone as a predictive marker of NASH.

Other biomarkers that have been studied include the apoptosis markers CK-18 fragments and soluble Fas. When used in combination in a study of 95 patients with NAFLD, these markers demonstrated a sensitivity of 88% and a specificity of 89%, with an AUROC of 0.93, for distinguishing NASH from absence of NASH.[79] Another pilot study compared CK-18 alone with a newer assay (M65 enzyme-linked immunoassay [ELISA]) that measured both cleaved and uncleaved CK-18 and demonstrated a sensitivity of 100% and specificity of 80% for the combination.[80] These results were supported by a subsequent of study of 147 biopsy-proved patients with NAFLD and 37 controls.[81] The M65 ELISA is also not commercially available and requires validation prior to widespread application. The terminal peptide of procollagen III (PIIINP) has been investigated as a single biomarker of hepatic fibrosis in a study of 172 patients with NAFLD and was able to distinguish among IFL, NASH, and advanced fibrosis, with an AUROC of 0.83 to 0.85.[82]

Clinical scoring systems have also been investigated for the ability to predict either NASH or advanced fibrosis. (Box 87-3) These scoring systems employ clinical or laboratory variables ranging from readily available tests, such as serum liver enzyme levels and the platelet count, to surrogate markers of necroinflammation or fibrosis, such as apolipoprotein A-1 or tissue inhibitor of metalloproteinase 1 (TIMP-1) levels.

The major clinical scoring systems studied in NAFLD include FibroSURE (FibroTest), Fibrometer, NAFLD fibrosis score, Fib-4, AST-to-platelet ratio index (APRI), BARD, European Liver Fibrosis Score (ELF), NASHTest, and AST/ALT ratio. Comparison of the accuracy of these tests in terms of positive and negative predictive values generally has demonstrated that the more complex and expensive tests (e.g., TIMP-1, FibroSURE, ELF) are equivalent to the more easily obtained clinical and laboratory tests (e.g., APRI, AST/ALT ratio) that can be calculated during an office visit. These tests are best at predicting either absent or advanced fibrosis

---

BOX 87-3 Risk Factors for Advanced* Nonalcoholic Fatty Liver Disease

Clinical
Older age (>50 years)
Obesity
Diabetes mellitus/insulin resistance
Ethnicity (e.g., Hispanics)
Hypertension

Laboratory
AST/ALT ratio > 1
Serum ALT level > twice the upper limit of normal

Histologic
Necroinflammatory activity (hepatocyte ballooning degeneration, necrosis)
Stainable iron
Fibrosis

*Nonalcoholic steatohepatitis and advanced fibrosis.

(cirrhosis) and are less helpful for estimating intermediate stages of fibrosis. For example, the FibroSURE test was highly sensitive for detecting bridging fibrosis and cirrhosis in a study of 167 patients with NAFLD, with a cutoff value of 0.70 demonstrating a 73% positive predictive value and a specificity of 98% for advanced fibrosis.[83] A cutoff value of 0.30 had a negative predictive value of 90% for advanced fibrosis. Unfortunately, 33% of patients had a FibroSURE score between 0.30 and 0.70, in which range the test was inaccurate for assessing the stage of fibrosis. Therefore, patients with a score in this range would need a liver biopsy for accurate staging.

The NAFLD fibrosis score is a commonly used clinical scoring algorithm that incorporates age, BMI, hyperglycemia, AST/ALT ratio, platelet count, and serum albumin level.[84] A low cutoff value for this score has been shown to have a high negative predictive value of 88% to 93%, and a high cutoff value has shown a good positive predictive value of 82% to 90%. One in 4 scores is indeterminate, and a liver biopsy is therefore required for accurate staging. A study investigating the utility of US or the NAFLD fibrosis score in the NHANES 1988 to 1994 cohort suggested that the NAFLD fibrosis score may predict increased mortality as well as advanced hepatic fibrosis[85]; death was due predominantly to cardiovascular causes.

Natural History

The natural history of NAFLD is determined in large part by the histopathology at baseline, which distinguishes IFL from NASH and quantifies the amount of fibrosis. The prognosis in patients with steatosis in the absence of hepatocyte necrosis and fibrosis clearly is favorable, with little potential for histologic or clinical progression.[86,87] Patients with IFL are thought to have mortality rates similar to that of the general population, whereas an established diagnosis of NASH portends a reduced life expectancy from cardiovascular, malignancy, or liver-related causes.[88,89] The finding of NASH with fibrosis suggests a worse prognosis compared with NASH without fibrosis, and additional factors that predict progression of fibrosis include the presence of diabetes mellitus, severe insulin resistance, cigarette smoking, weight gain greater than 5 kg, and rising serum ALT and AST levels.[90,91] Rates of fibrosis progression are quite variable, and no clinical or laboratory data appear to predict the disease course reliably. The best estimates to date predict an approximately 11% rate of progression to cirrhosis over a 15-year period (Fig. 87-6).[92]

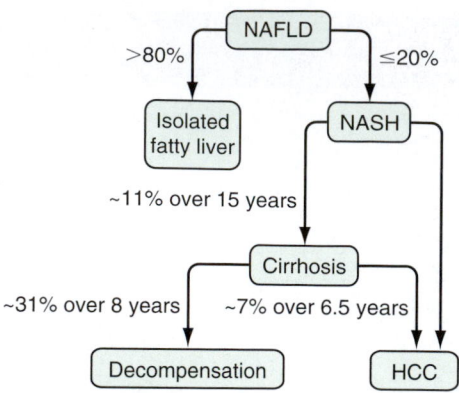

FIGURE 87-6. Natural history of nonalcoholic fatty liver disease (NAFLD), including isolated fatty liver and nonalcoholic steatohepatitis (NASH). Isolated fatty liver rarely if ever progresses to cirrhosis and is not associated with an increased risk of death compared with the general population. NASH is associated with an increased risk of death due to cardiovascular disease, malignancy, and cirrhosis and its complications. Progression of fibrosis in NASH is associated with diabetes mellitus, severe insulin resistance, higher BMI, weight gain > 5 kg, cigarette smoking, and rising serum aminotransferase levels. HCC, hepatocellular carcinoma. *(Adapted from Torres DM, Williams CD, Harrison SA. Features, diagnosis and treatment of nonalcoholic fatty liver disease. Clin Gastroenterol Hepatol 2012; 10:837-58.)*

NAFLD and alcoholic hepatitis are similar histologically but differ substantially in clinical outcomes (see Chapter 86). The 5-year survival rate of patients with alcoholic hepatitis is only 50% to 75% because of the large proportion of patients (>50%) in whom cirrhosis and its complications develop. The long-term survival of patients with NASH has been reported to be significantly better than the long-term survival of patients with alcoholic hepatitis.[93]

In patients in whom NAFLD-associated cirrhosis develops, the outcome may be similar to that for other causes of cirrhosis. NAFLD is the likely cause of many cases of cryptogenic cirrhosis[94] and may be associated with the development of hepatocellular carcinoma.[95] One study showed that the 5- to 10-year outcome of NAFLD-associated cirrhosis was similar to that for HCV-associated cirrhosis, although hepatocellular carcinoma was less common in the patients with NAFLD than in those with HCV infection.[96] The importance of hepatocellular carcinoma as a complication of NASH is rising due to the increasing prevalence of NASH; data suggest that hepatocellular carcinoma will develop in approximately 7% of patients with NASH cirrhosis over 6.5 years of follow-up.[97,98] Age, obesity, diabetes mellitus, and iron deposition all appear to be risk factors for development of hepatocellular carcinoma in patients with NASH.[99] Reports of hepatocellular carcinoma developing in patients with noncirrhotic NASH pose a difficult diagnostic dilemma because it is not feasible to screen such a large population with imaging every 6 months. One French study has suggested that coexisting metabolic syndrome and NASH in the presence of little or no hepatic fibrosis may provide a substrate for the development of hepatocellular carcinoma.[100]

Associated Disorders

In addition to the metabolic syndrome, diabetes mellitus, and vitamin D deficiency, cardiovascular disease, obstructive sleep apnea, colonic adenomas, hypothyroidism, polycystic ovary syndrome, pancreatic steatosis, and elevated serum uric acid levels have been reported to be associated with NAFLD. Cardiovascular disease has been shown to be the primary cause of death in this population. NAFLD appears to be an independent risk factor for cardiovascular disease (OR, 2.05; 95% CI, 1.81-2.31).[101]

Obstructive sleep apnea is common is the general population, with an estimated prevalence of 1% to 4% and higher rates (25% to 35%) reported in obese populations. Chronic intermittent hypoxia has been associated with a high NAS and increased hepatic fibrosis in a cohort of morbidly obese patients undergoing bariatric surgery.[102] Obese patients with obstructive sleep apnea have been reported to have a greater than 90% prevalence of NAFLD, and 50% of patients with NAFLD have symptoms suggestive of obstructive sleep apnea.[103]

Vitamin D deficiency is found in populations with NAFLD independent of age, gender, serum TG levels, or glucose levels[104] and may even correlate with disease severity.[105] There are no prospective studies to suggest that vitamin D replacement may improve NAFLD or NASH, but it is common in clinical practice to check vitamin D levels in patients with NAFLD and prescribe vitamin D if levels are low.

A population-based study in Korea[106] and a prospective study in China[107] have demonstrated a higher prevalence of colonic adenomas, as well as advanced neoplasia such as cancer, high-grade dysplasia, or villous histology in patients with NAFLD. NASH histology was more strongly correlated with adenoma detection in Asian studies but not in the largest U.S. study,[108] which demonstrated an increase in adenomatous polyps in all patients with NAFLD.[108]

Treatment

The optimal therapy for NAFLD has not been established. Clinical trials to date have been marked by small numbers of patients as well as varying inclusion criteria and end points. Although improvements in metabolic parameters, liver enzyme levels, or steatosis on imaging are readily determined in clinical trials, histologic improvement in steatosis, inflammation, and fibrosis is the ultimate goal of treatment. A 2-point improvement in the NAS, with 1 of the points coming from a reduction in hepatocyte ballooning degeneration, may indicate a successful intervention.[109] Improvement in fibrosis (which is not part of the NAS) is also desirable, although it is difficult to conduct trials of adequate length to allow improvement in fibrosis. Multiyear trials are rarely seen; most trials have been 6 to 12 months in duration. Standard treatment of NAFLD has consisted of weight loss, removal of potentially offending drugs and toxins, and control of associated metabolic disorders, including diabetes mellitus and hyperlipidemia (Table 87-3).

Lifestyle Modification

Lifestyle modification is often divided into calorie reduction, with a goal of weight loss, macronutrient modification, and physical activity, including aerobic and resistance activity. Most studies of calorie restriction include an exercise component, making it difficult to assess whether diet or exercise is more beneficial.

Intensive nutritional counseling may lead to sustained weight loss and significant histologic improvement in some patients.[110] In a small but well-designed prospective study of 31 patients with NASH who were randomized to lifestyle modification (diet, exercise, and behavior modification) or a control group consisting of a basic education class about diet and exercise,[111] those randomized to lifestyle modification had a 9.3% reduction in body weight compared with 0.2% in the

TABLE 87-3 Treatment Options for Patients with Nonalcoholic Fatty Liver Disease (NAFLD) and Nonalcoholic Steatohepatitis (NASH)

Option	Effect	Comments
Diet		
Moderate calorie restriction; aim to reduce daily calories by 500-750 kcal and achieve weight loss of 7%-10%	Improves most histopathologic features of NASH	Data are lacking for fibrosis improvement; only ≈ 40% of patients were able to achieve this goal in clinical trials
Eliminate or significantly reduce saturated fatty acids and high-fructose corn syrup from diet	Fructose increases lipogenesis via activation of pyruvate dehydrogenase and transcriptional activation of sterol regulatory element-binding protein 1	Prospective trials demonstrating biochemical and histologic benefit of fructose reduction are lacking, although fructose consumption is a risk factor for NAFLD
Consider omega-3 fatty acid supplementation	May decrease hepatic steatosis; improves TG levels	The optimal dose is unclear, but some benefit may be seen with ≈ 1 g daily; treatment for 1 year or longer is associated with reduced risk of cardiovascular death, sudden cardiac death, all-cause mortality, and nonfatal cardiac events
Consider regular coffee consumption, 2-3 cups daily	Decreases risk of hepatic fibrosis	Optimal amount is unclear, but data suggest at least 2 cups daily
Exercise		
Moderate exercise 4-5 times weekly for 30-45 minutes each time	Improves insulin resistance, liver enzyme levels, and steatosis by imaging	No studies have assessed the effect on NASH histopathology; weight loss is not expected without associated dietary modification
Resistance training 3 times weekly; total exercise time ≈ 45 minutes	Improves insulin resistance and steatosis imaging modestly	Likely best combined with aerobic exercise and diet
Pharmacotherapy		
Vitamin E 800-1000 IU daily	Improves NASH when used for 2 years; no improvement in fibrosis	Validation studies in diabetics and various ethnic groups are needed to confirm a benefit; may increase risk of prostate cancer
Pioglitazone 30-45 mg daily	Improves NASH when used for 6 months to 2 years; may improve fibrosis	Expect a 4-kg weight gain; possible increased risk of heart failure, and osteoporosis; not approved by FDA for NASH treatment; limit use to patients with stage 2 fibrosis or greater who have failed to improve with dietary measures and exercise
Pentoxifylline 400 mg three times daily	Improves NASH and fibrosis	Small pilot trial data only
Statins	Limited data on histopathology	Safe in patients with NAFLD; reduces risk of cardiovascular disease
Bariatric Surgery		
RYGB, LAGB, sleeve gastrectomy	Improves or resolves NASH in 60%-80% of cases; likely improves fibrosis	Lack of randomized controlled trials; use with caution in cirrhotic patients

LAGB, laparoscopic adjustable gastric banding; RYGB, Roux-en-Y gastric bypass.
Adapted from Torres DM, Williams CD, Harrison SA. Features, diagnosis and treatment of nonalcoholic fatty liver disease. Clin Gastroenterol Hepatol 2012; 10:837-58.

control group; repeat liver biopsies at 1 year demonstrated a significant improvement in the NAS in the lifestyle modification group compared with the control group.

Preliminary evidence has suggested that low-carbohydrate, calorie-restricted approaches improve insulin sensitivity and decrease hepatic TG content more than high-carbohydrate caloric restriction, despite comparable weight loss.[112] Another study, however, compared different lifestyle modification approaches (low-fat diet, low-carbohydrate diet, exercise, and control arms) and found that all of these approaches led to some hepatic histologic improvement, which correlated with weight loss.[113]

Limiting saturated fatty acids and high-fructose corn syrup may also be beneficial because diets high in saturated fatty acids and fructose have been associated with NASH.[114] A large retrospective study has correlated daily fructose consumption with hepatic fibrosis stage,[115] although no prospective trials have demonstrated histologic improvement with fructose restriction.

There are no prospective data to support omega-3 fatty acid supplementation in NASH patients; however, circumstantial and secondary evidence suggests a benefit. A meta-analysis of 9 studies with a total of 355 patients demonstrated that omega-3 supplementation improves hepatic steatosis, although no histologic data were available.[116] Reduction in hepatic steatosis occurred in the absence of weight loss with an average daily dose of 1 g of omega-3 fatty acid. Omega-3 supplementation was shown to reduce all-cause mortality as well as the risk of a cardiovascular event or death in a large meta-analysis of 11 randomized controlled trials involving 39,044 patients.[117] In the absence of an ideal therapy, omega-3 supplementation may be a reasonable part of a lifestyle modification regimen for the average patient with NAFLD.

In large retrospective studies, caffeinated coffee intake has been found to have a protective effect against hepatic fibrosis in alcoholic liver disease[118] as well as chronic hepatitis C.[119] Preliminary study suggests that this finding is true for NAFLD as well.[120] This benefit has been seen with 1 to 2 cups of caffeinated coffee daily and did not appear to carry over to other caffeinated beverages, decaffeinated coffee, or espresso in a study of patients undergoing bariatric surgery.[121]

As a general rule, alcohol use should be discouraged, and evidence strongly indicates that heavy alcohol use, as defined by more than 3 drinks per day, increases the likelihood of hepatic injury. The effects of "light" or "moderate" alcohol intake are controversial, with conflicting results in several cross-sectional and retrospective studies. Current expert opinion recommends against "even light alcohol consumption" in the absence of prospective data.[122]

Physical activity is another lifestyle intervention that can be recommended alone or in concert with nutritional counseling. Patients with NAFLD and specifically NASH are more sedentary and have less cardiovascular fitness than the general population. A pilot trial of 19 obese patients with NAFLD showed that after 4 weeks of aerobic training 3 times per week, visceral adipose tissue volume, intrahepatic TG content, and plasma FFA concentrations all improved in the absence of weight reduction.[123] This result was corroborated in another small trial of 18 obese patients[124] as well as a meta-analysis that suggested exercise alone improves hepatic steatosis.[125] Resistance training may also be of benefit, and in 18-week pilot trial, resistance exercise 45 to 60 minutes 3 times per week modestly improved intrahepatic TG content as well as insulin resistance independent of weight loss.[126]

Although lifestyle modification appears beneficial in patients with NAFLD, no single particular lifestyle intervention can be recommended, and no single approach is likely to be suitable for all patients.[127] Adequate weight loss of 5% to 10% is difficult to achieve, and even more difficult to sustain over time. A reduction in the intake of high-fructose corn syrup and an increase in the intake of omega-3 fatty acids and caffeinated coffee are intriguing adjuvants to a multidisciplinary approach that includes caloric reduction and increased physical activity. Tri-society practice guidelines of the American Gastroenterological Association, AASLD, and ACG recommend weight loss of at least 3% to 5%, either with a hypocaloric diet or in conjunction with increased physical activity, and note that weight loss of up to 10% may be required to improve hepatic necroinflammation in patients with NAFLD.[128]

Weight Loss Surgery

Bariatric surgery leads to massive weight loss and improves insulin sensitivity, normalizes some of the metabolic abnormalities involved in the pathogenesis of NAFLD, decreases the hepatic expression of mediators of liver inflammation and fibrosis, and improves hepatic histology in patients with NAFLD.[129-131] The majority of trials demonstrating a benefit to bariatric surgery were of adequate size but uncontrolled, leading to inconclusive findings in a 2001 Cochrane review on bariatric surgery for NASH[132] and the tri-society guidelines,[128] which noted that it is premature to consider bariatric surgery specifically to treat NASH. Overly rapid weight loss seen with the older bariatric surgical procedures can exacerbate steatohepatitis in morbidly obese patients; therefore, the rate

of weight loss and serial liver biochemical test results should be monitored carefully in patients on a weight reduction regimen. Given the expense and invasive nature of bariatric surgery, this intervention should be reserved for patients with noncirrhotic NASH and comorbid medical conditions.

Pharmacotherapy

A myriad of pharmacologic approaches have been investigated in the treatment of NAFLD. None is yet of proved value.

Weight Loss Medications

A limited number of medical therapies are available for weight loss, and even fewer have been studied in patients with NAFLD. The most studied such agent to date is orlistat, a reversible inhibitor of pancreatic and gastric lipase. Orlistat promotes modest weight loss through intestinal fat maldigestion and is available by prescription (Xenical, Roche) as well as in a lower dose over the counter (Alli, GlaxoSmithKline). Pilot trials were promising, but subsequent larger randomized controlled trials demonstrated similar degrees of weight loss in the group assigned orlistat and that assigned placebo.[133,134] A weight loss of 9% was shown to be the threshold required to produce histologic improvement in steatosis and necroinflammation in both treatment arms. Case reports of cholelithiasis, cholestasis, and rarely hepatic injury prompted the FDA to issue a post-marketing warning for orlistat in 2009. This warning, combined with an only modest weight loss effect and side effects of oily stools and potential malabsorption of other medications, has limited the usefulness of this drug.

Other weight loss agents have either not been studied in NAFLD (phentermine) or have been removed from clinical trials secondary to adverse effects (rimonibant, sibutramine). Newer agents just coming on the market such as lorcaserin and phentermine/topamax in combination remain to be investigated.

Antioxidants

Medications that reduce the generation of reactive oxygen species in the liver and reduce oxidative stress are another potential avenue for therapy. The most studied antioxidants are vitamin E, vitamin C, and betaine.

Vitamin E, an inexpensive yet potent antioxidant, has been examined as an agent for the treatment of NAFLD in pediatric and adult patients, with varying results. In all studies, vitamin E was well tolerated, and most studies showed modest improvements in serum aminotransferase levels and the US appearance of the liver,[135] but infrequently histologic findings.[136,137] Although a pilot trial showed a benefit to vitamin E and C together for hepatic fibrosis, a larger randomized controlled trial did not show improvement in hepatic fibrosis despite significant improvement in steatosis, inflammation, and ballooning degeneration (when compared with placebo). In a large pediatric trial, vitamin E was no better than placebo (or metformin) in improving serum liver enzyme levels or hepatic histology, with the exception of ballooning degeneration.[138] In light of the potentially negative effects of vitamin E on cardiovascular health,[139] all-cause mortality,[140] and prostate cancer rates,[141] caution should be exercised in treating NAFLD with vitamin E until better studies are available. The tri-society practice guidelines[128] recommend vitamin E 800 IU/day as a first-line therapy in nondiabetic adults with biopsy-proved NASH but caution against use of vitamin E in diabetic patients or patients with NAFLD without a liver biopsy.

Betaine, a metabolite of choline that raises *S*-adenosyl methionine levels and decreases cellular oxidative damage, has shown promise in mouse models.[142] A pilot study investigating betaine as a therapeutic agent for NASH demonstrated an improvement in only hepatic steatosis.[143]

Diabetes Medications

The association between hyperinsulinemic insulin resistance and NAFLD provides a logical target for treatment. Metformin, thiazolidinediones (TZDs), and incretin mimetics are all diabetes medications that have been investigated in the treatment of NASH. Metformin, a biguanide that reduces hyperinsulinemia and improves hepatic insulin sensitivity, reduces hepatomegaly and hepatic steatosis in ob/ob mice,[144] but results in both adult and human NAFLD have been less impressive.[145,146] The use of metformin is currently not recommended as a therapy for NAFLD or NASH.

TZDs are potent PPAR-γ agonists. PPAR-γ is a nuclear receptor that is expressed in adipose tissue, muscle, and liver. In adipocytes, PPAR-γ promotes cell differentiation and decreases lipolysis and FFA release. TZDs improve insulin resistance by increasing glucose disposal in muscle and decreasing hepatic glucose output. Treatment with troglitazone, a first-generation TZD, was associated with biochemical and histologic improvements in patients with NASH, but troglitazone subsequently was withdrawn from the market because of rare but serious hepatotoxicity (see Chapter 88). Rosiglitazone and in particular pioglitazone are TZDs with low rates of hepatotoxicity and have been investigated in several large well-designed randomized controlled trials in which treatment was well tolerated and associated with improvement in insulin resistance, normalization of liver biochemical test levels, and histologic improvement in most patients.[141,147-149] Several drawbacks to TZD therapy may limit their widespread use in NASH, however. Continued treatment appears to be necessary, because subsequent studies demonstrated recurrence of NASH off therapy.[150] Long-term therapy with either agent is problematic because of an associated average weight gain of 3 to 4 kg. Rosiglitazone has been linked to increased rates of myocardial infarction, for which an FDA black box warning was placed. Retrospective study has linked both agents to increased fracture rates and decreased bone mineral density.[151] Because of these issues, TZDs cannot be recommended for all patients with NASH, although use of pioglitazone in diabetic patients with histologically advanced NASH seems reasonable. The tri-society guidelines agree that pioglitazone can be used to treat biopsy-proved NASH but emphasize that the long-term safety and efficacy have not been established in this population.[128]

Incretin mimetics have been less well studied in patients with NASH but have shown preliminary promise. Exenatide and liraglutide are glucagon-like protein-1 receptor agonists that improve insulin sensitivity and serum glucose levels and promote modest weight loss. Exenatide in particular has shown promise in animal models[152] and human pilot trials.[153,154] Nausea has been a limiting factor in the pilot trials, although a once-weekly formulation of exenatide may mitigate this side effect.

Cytoprotective Agents

Cytoprotective agents are thought to prevent apoptosis and down-regulate the inflammatory cascade. Ursodeoxycholic acid (UDCA) (see Chapter 91) is a cytoprotective agent that has been investigated with mixed results in randomized controlled trials. The largest placebo-controlled trial demonstrated equal improvement in patients receiving UDCA and placebo.[155] In a subsequent trial, UDCA plus vitamin E improved hepatic steatosis and serum aminotransferase levels.[156] Two other trials also demonstrated modest improvement in serum liver enzyme levels, but histology was not studied in one of the trials[157] and only lobular inflammation improved in the other.[158] These two studies[157,158] used high-dose UDCA, which has been associated with increased mortality in patients with PSC. The tri-society practice guidelines do not recommend routine use of UDCA.[128]

Pentoxifylline (PTX) is another cytoprotective agent studied in NASH that has been shown to inhibit proinflammatory cytokines, including TNF-α, leading to reduced production of reactive oxygen species.[159] Two pilot trials as well as the largest randomized controlled trial for NASH to date[160] have shown varying degrees of histologic improvement as well as improved serum liver enzyme levels and reduced insulin resistance. The controlled trial involved 55 patients with NASH and demonstrated a 1.6-point improvement in the NAS in PTX-treated patients compared with a 0.1-point improvement in the patients receiving placebo. A second smaller randomized controlled trial of 30 patients showed improvement in steatosis and ballooning degeneration with PTX, although the improvement was not statistically better than that for the placebo group.[161]

Lipid-Lowering Agents

Because patients with NASH often have coexisting hyperlipidemia, the use of lipid-lowering agents has been studied as a potential dual-target therapy to address both conditions. The most commonly prescribed agents for hyperlipidemia are statins, which inhibit 3-hydroxy-3-methylglutaryl-coenzyme A (HMG-CoA) reductase, a primary enzyme in cholesterol biosynthesis (see Chapter 64). Statins have shown modest benefit in pilot trials.[162-165] Larger trials without the surrogate end points of serum liver enzyme levels and improved hepatic steatosis have also suggested a benefit.[166,167] For now, statins can be recommended to treat concomitant hyperlipidemia in patients with NASH, but further study is needed before statins can be recommended as primary therapy for NASH. Ezetimibe is another lipid-lowering agent that has shown benefit in improving hepatic histology in animal models[168] as well as one pilot trial in 24 patients with NAFLD.[169]

Other Therapies

Phlebotomy has been investigated because high serum iron and ferritin levels have been identified in some patients with NAFLD in the absence of genetic hemochromatosis, and serum iron indices have been associated with the severity of NAFLD.[67] Increased serum iron indices are thought to be a by-product of hepatic inflammation, rather than a contributor to the pathogenesis of NAFLD, but a few small studies have suggested that iron depletion may have a therapeutic role in NAFLD by decreasing plasma insulin, glucose, and serum aminotransferase levels.[170,171] The primary limitation of these studies is the lack of histologic inclusion criteria and end points. Further investigation is necessary before phlebotomy can be recommended.

Angiotensin-receptor blockers (ARBs) are used routinely for the treatment of hypertension, heart failure, and chronic kidney disease, conditions that may be found in patients with NAFLD. In animal models, ARBs have been shown to inhibit hepatic stellate cell activity, leading to a reduction in hepatic fibrosis in obese mice.[172] One human pilot trial suggested a similar benefit, but a larger randomized controlled trial of losartan in addition to rosiglitazone failed to produce any additional histologic benefit beyond that seen with rosiglitazone alone.[173]

Other novel therapeutic approaches may be derived from advances in our understanding of the pathogenesis of NASH. Alterations in intestinal flora and SIBO are thought to contribute to NASH and may be novel targets for therapy. Similarly, modulation of autophagy via such agents as carbamazepine, or of bile acid metabolism with obeticholic acid, an FXR agonist,[174] requires further study. Caspase inhibitors are being investigated as well; preliminary results of a phase 2 study of 1 such agent has suggested a benefit in hepatic histology as well as serum liver enzyme levels.[175]

Liver Transplantation

NASH cirrhosis is currently the third most common indication for liver transplantation after cirrhosis caused by HCV and alcoholic liver disease (see Chapter 97). It is expected to become the number 1 indication for liver transplantation by the 2020s.[176] Comorbid conditions limit eligibility for transplantation, and although 30-day mortality following liver transplantation is higher for patients with NASH cirrhosis, 1- to 3-year mortality rates are similar to those for other indications for liver transplantation.[177,178] An increased rate of cardiovascular events in patients with NASH cirrhosis undergoing liver transplantation has been reported, particularly in the perioperative period, as compared with patients who are transplanted for alcoholic cirrhosis (OR, 4.12; 95 CI, 1.91-8.90).[179] The majority of patients have recurrent steatosis 5 years after transplantation, although cirrhosis has been reported to develop in only 5%.[180]

Hepatic steatosis in donor grafts is common, with one third to one half of potential cadaveric donor livers having steatosis.[181] Transplanted steatotic livers have been associated with primary graft nonfunction and poorer overall outcomes.[182] Grafts with less than 30% steatosis are acceptable for use, and those with more than 60% fat are generally considered unacceptable. Those with an intermediate degree of steatosis (30% to 60%) are evaluated on a case-by-case and center-dependent basis. Liver biopsy with expert consultation by a pathologist prior to harvesting the organ can be useful for determining donor acceptability.

FOCAL FATTY LIVER

In contrast to NAFLD, which is a diffuse parenchymal process, focal fatty liver is a localized or patchy process that simulates a space-occupying lesion in the liver on imaging studies. This condition has been recognized increasingly in adults and children as a result of the improved sensitivity of abdominal imaging. Focal fatty liver has characteristic patterns on CT: usually a nonspherical shape, absence of mass effect, and CT attenuation values consistent with those of soft tissue.[183] The density of focal fatty liver is close to that of water, unlike that of liver metastases, which have a density that is closer to that of hepatocytes. US and MRI can help confirm a diagnosis of focal fatty liver (Fig. 87-7). A presumptive diagnosis of focal fatty liver should not be made when a mass effect, areas of mixed hypo- and hyperechogenicity, an irregular shape, or a history of malignancy is present. In such cases, US-guided fine-needle biopsy is recommended. No evidence exists to suggest that the pathogenesis of focal fatty liver is similar to that of NAFLD. In fact, the pathogenesis of focal fatty liver is uncertain and may involve altered venous blood flow to the liver, tissue hypoxia, or intestinal malabsorption of lipoprotein. In the absence of accompanying liver disease, the lesion often regresses. No specific treatment is necessary.

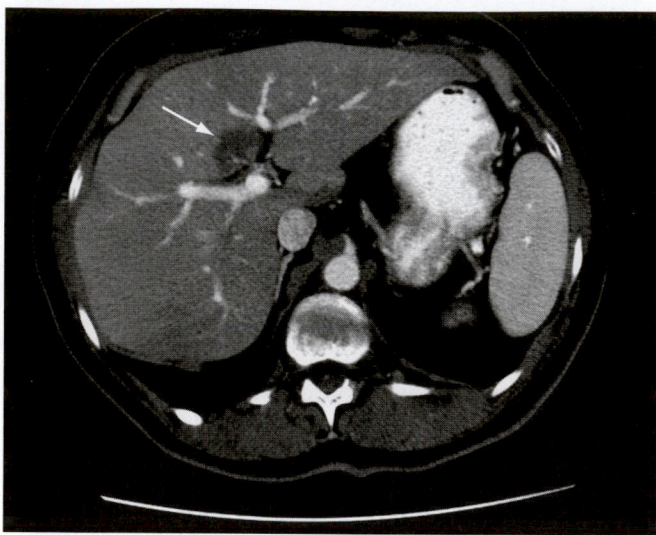

FIGURE 87-7. CT demonstrating fatty liver *(arrow)*. The characteristic features are the nonspherical shape, absence of a mass effect (i.e., compression of the surrounding tissue), and CT attenuation values consistent with those of soft tissue. US studies and MRI also may confirm the diagnosis of focal fatty liver. *(Courtesy Dr. Mukesh Harisinghani, Boston, Mass.)*

KEY REFERENCES

Full references for this chapter can be found on www.expertconsult.com.

2. Day CP, James OFW. Steatohepatitis: A tale of two "hits"? Gastroenterology 1998; 114:842-5.
7. Browning JD, Szczepaniak LS, Dobbins R, et al. Prevalence of hepatic steatosis in an urban population in the United States: Impact of ethnicity. Hepatology 2004; 40:1387-95.
12. Williams CD, Stengel J, Asike MI, et al. Prevalence of nonalcoholic fatty liver disease and nonalcoholic steatohepatitis among a largely middle-aged population utilizing ultrasound and liver biopsy: A prospective study. Gastroenterology 2011; 140:124-31.
15. Torres DM, Williams CD, Harrison SA. Features, diagnosis, and treatment of nonalcoholic fatty liver disease. Clin Gastro Hepatol 2012; 10:837-58.
24. Petersen KF, Dufour S, Hariri A, et al. Apolipoprotein C3 gene variants in nonalcoholic fatty liver disease. N Engl J Med 2010; 362:1082-9.
29. Brunt EM, Janney CG, Di Bisceglie AM, et al. Nonalcoholic steatohepatitis: A proposal for grading and staging the histologic lesions. Am J Gastroenterol 1999; 94:2467-74.
32. Kleiner D, Brunt EM, Van Natta M, et al. Design and validation of a histological scoring system for nonalcoholic fatty liver disease. Hepatology 2005; 41:1313-21.
51. Amir M, Czaja MJ. Autophagy in nonalcoholic steatohepatitis. Expert Rev Gastroenterol Hepatol 2011; 5:159-66.
61. Abu-Shanab A, Quigley EM. The role of the gut microbiota in nonalcoholic fatty liver disease. Nat Rev Gastroenterol Hepatol 2010; 7:691-701.
84. Angulo P, Hui JM, Marchesini G, et al. The NAFLD fibrosis score: A noninvasive system that identifies liver fibrosis in patients with NAFLD. Hepatology 2007; 45:846-54.
89. Soderberg C, Stal P, Askling J, et al. Decreased survival of subjects with elevated liver function tests during a 28-year follow-up period. Hepatology 2010; 51:595-602.

127. Zivkovic A, German J, Sanyal A. Comparative review of diets for the metabolic syndrome: Implications for nonalcoholic fatty liver disease. Am J Clin Nutr 2007; 86:285-300.

128. Chalasani N, Younossi Z, Lavine JE, et al. The diagnosis and management of non-alcoholic fatty liver disease: Practice guidelines by the American Gastroenterological Association, American Association for the Study of Liver Disease, and the American College of Gastroenterology. Gastroenterology 2012; 142:1592-609.

137. Sanyal AJ, Chalasani N, Kowdley KV, et al. Pioglitazone, vitamin E or placebo for nonalcoholic steatohepatitis. N Engl J Med 2010; 362:1675-85.

176. Charlton MR, Burns JM, Pederson RA, et al. Frequency and outcomes of liver transplantation for nonalcoholic steatohepatitis in the United States. Gastroenterology 2011; 141:1249-53.

CHAPTER

88

Hepatic Drug Metabolism and Liver Disease Caused by Drugs

SHIVAKUMAR CHITTURI, NARCI C. TEOH, AND GEOFFREY C. FARRELL

CHAPTER OUTLINE

HEPATIC DRUG METABOLISM

Role of the Liver in Drug Elimination

By virtue of the portal circulation, the liver is highly exposed to drugs and other toxins absorbed from the intestine. Most drugs tend to be lipophilic compounds that are readily taken up by the liver but cannot be easily excreted unchanged in bile or urine. The liver is well equipped to handle these agents by an adaptable (inducible) series of metabolic pathways. These pathways include those that alter the parent molecule (*phase 1*), synthesize conjugates of the drug or its metabolite with a more water-soluble moiety (e.g., sugar, amino acid, sulfate molecule [*phase 2*]), and excrete in an energy-dependent manner the parent molecule, its metabolites, or conjugates into bile (*phase 3*). For any given compound, 1, 2, or all 3 steps may be necessary for drug elimination. Expression and subcellular location of the proteins (enzymes, membrane transporters) that mediate these steps are controlled by a set of nuclear receptors that function as transcriptional regulators and co-regulators, thereby accounting for coordinated regulation of the 3 phases of hepatic drug elimination.

Pathways of Drug Metabolism

Phase 1 pathways of drug metabolism include oxidation, reduction, and hydrolytic reactions.[1,2] The products can be readily conjugated or excreted without further modification.

Cytochrome P450

Most type 1 reactions are catalyzed by microsomal drug oxidases, the key component of which is a hemoprotein of the cytochrome P450 (CYP) gene superfamily. The apparent promiscuity of drug oxidases toward drugs, environmental toxins, steroid hormones, lipids, and bile acids results from the existence of multiple closely related CYP proteins. More than 20 CYP enzymes are present in the human liver.[2]

The reaction cycle involves binding of molecular oxygen to the iron in the heme prosthetic group, with subsequent reduction of oxygen by acceptance of an electron from nicotinamide adenine dinucleotide phosphate (NADPH) cytochrome P450 reductase, a flavoprotein reductase. The resulting "activated oxygen" is incorporated into the drug or another lipophilic compound. Reduction of oxygen and insertion into a drug substrate ("mixed-function oxidation") generates chemically reactive intermediates, including free radicals, electrophilic "oxy-intermediates" (e.g., unstable epoxides, quinone imines), and reduced (and therefore reactive) oxygen species (ROS). The quintessential example is the CYP2E1-catalyzed metabolite of acetaminophen, N-acetyl-p-benzoquinone imine (NAPQI), an oxidizing and arylating metabolite responsible for acetaminophen hepatotoxicity. Other quinone compounds are potential reactive metabolites of troglitazone, quinine, and methyldopa. Likewise, hepatic metabolism of some plant toxins can generate potentially hepatotoxic epoxide metabolites of diterpenoids (see Chapter 89).[3] ROS contribute significantly to tissue injury, particularly by involvement in generating oxidative stress and triggering tissue stress responses and cell death pathways, as discussed later.

The hepatic content of CYP proteins is higher in acinar zone 3 than in zone 1. Localization of CYP2E1 is usually confined to a narrow rim of hepatocytes 1 to 2 cells thick around the terminal hepatic venule. This explains in part the zonality of hepatic lesions produced by drugs and toxins such as acetaminophen and carbon tetrachloride, which are converted to reactive metabolites.

Genetic and Environmental Determinants of Cytochrome P450 Enzymes

Pharmacogenetics and Polymorphisms of Cytochrome P450 Expression. The hepatic expression of each CYP enzyme is genetically determined. This finding largely explains the 4-fold or greater differences in rates of drug metabolism among healthy subjects. Some CYPs, particularly minor forms, are also subject to polymorphic inheritance, so occasional persons completely lack the encoded protein.[2] One example is CYP2D6, which metabolizes debrisoquine and perhexiline. Poor metabolizers lack CYP2D6 and accumulate perhexiline with usual doses; lack of CYP2D6 is the critical determinant in serious adverse effects of perhexiline, including chronic hepatitis and cirrhosis.[4] Other examples include CYPs 2C9 and 2C19, which affect the metabolism of S-warfarin, omeprazole, tolbutamide, and phenytoin and of S-mephenytoin, respectively[2]; 3% of white populations and 15% of Asians are poor metabolizers of S-mephenytoin.

Developmental Regulation and Constitutive Expression. Expression of several CYPs is developmentally regulated. During adult life, expression of some CYPs declines slightly (by up to 10%) with advancing age, but this change is minor compared with the effects of genetic variation, environmental influences, and liver disease. Gender differences in the expression of CYPs 3A4 and 2E1 may explain the slightly enhanced metabolism of certain drugs (erythromycin, chlordiazepoxide, midazolam) in women, but whether this difference contributes to the increased risk of hepatic drug reactions in women remains unclear.

Nutrition and Disease-Related Changes. A person's nutritional status influences the expression of certain CYPs, both in health and with liver disease.[1,2,5,6] Expression of CYP2E1 is increased by obesity, high fat intake, and fasting.[2,6] Diseases that alter expression of hepatic CYPs include diabetes mellitus (increased CYP2E1), hypothyroidism (decreased CYP1A), and hypopituitarism (decreased CYP3A4).[2] Cirrhosis is associated with decreased levels of total cytochrome P450 and also with reduced hepatic perfusion; the result is a decrease in the clearance of drugs like propranolol that are metabolized rapidly by the liver.[2] The effects of cirrhosis vary, however, among individual CYP families (Table 88-1) and with the type of liver disease (e.g., CYP3A4 levels are preserved with cholestatic but lowered with hepatocellular liver disease).

Adaptive Response and Enzyme Induction. Exposure to lipophilic substances results in an adaptive response that usually

TABLE 88-1 Cytochrome P450 (CYP) Isoenzymes Involved in Phase I Drug Metabolism in Humans

CYP Isoenzyme	Substrates	Effect of Liver Disease on CYP Activity
CYP1A2	Caffeine, theophylline, clonazepam	↓↓↓
CYP2A6	Halothane, methoxyflurane	↓↓
CYP2C9	Diclofenac, losartan, warfarin	↓
CYP2C19	Citalopram, diazepam, omeprazole	↓↓↓
CYP2D6	Codeine, haloperidol, metoprolol	↔
CYP2E1	Enflurane, halothane, acetaminophen	↓
CYP3A4	Amiodarone, carbamazepine, cyclosporine, terfenadine	↓↓↓

involves transient liver cell injury (discussed later) as well as synthesis of new enzyme protein, a process termed *enzyme induction*. The molecular basis for genetic regulation of constitutive and inducible expression of the major human hepatic cytochrome P450, CYP3A4, has been determined.[7] Agents such as rifampin interact with the pregnane X-receptor (PXR), a member of the orphan nuclear receptor family of transcriptional regulators.[7] Activated PXR and the analogous constitutive androstane receptor (CAR) in turn bind to cognate nucleotide sequences upstream to the CYP3A4 structural gene within a "xenobiotic-regulatory enhancer module" (XREM). This interaction regulates the CYP3A4 promoter downstream and ultimately the transcription of CYP3A4 protein. Similar control mechanisms apply to several other CYP pathways,[7,8] particularly those involved with bile acid synthesis.[7]

Common examples of microsomal enzymes induced by environmental agents include the effect of smoking cigarettes and cannabis on CYP1A2[8] and of alcohol on CYP2E1 and possibly CYP3A4.[9] Several drugs are potent inducers of CYP enzymes. Isoniazid induces CYP2E1, whereas phenobarbital and phenytoin increase expression of multiple CYPs.[2] Rifampin is a potent inducer of CYP3A4, as is hypericum,[10] the active ingredient of St. John's wort, a commonly used herbal medicine, thereby causing interactions between conventional medicines and a complementary and alternative medicine (CAM) preparation.

The implications for drug-induced liver disease are 2-fold. First, enzyme induction often involves more than the CYP system, possibly because of PXR and CAR activation, including changes in bile acid metabolism and liver growth. This observation could account for increases in serum alkaline phosphatase and γ-glutamyl transpeptidase (GGTP) levels, which reflect "hepatic adaptation" to chronic drug ingestion. Second, the influence of one drug on expression and activity of drug metabolizing enzymes and drug elimination (phase 3) pathways can alter metabolism or disposition of other agents. Such drug-drug interactions are important pharmacologically and may be relevant to mechanisms of drug-induced liver injury (DILI).

Inhibition of Drug Metabolism. Some chemicals inhibit drug metabolism. In persons taking more than one medication, for example, competition for phase 2 pathways such as glucuronidation and sulfation facilitates the presentation of unconjugated drug to the CYP system. This mechanism appears to explain in part why agents like zidovudine and phenytoin lower the dose threshold for acetaminophen-induced hepatotoxicity.

Other Pathways of Drug Oxidation

In addition to CYP enzymes, mitochondrial electron transport systems can generate tissue-damaging reactive intermediates during drug metabolism. Examples include nitroradicals from nitrofuran derivatives (nitrofurantoin, cocaine). Subsequent electron transfer by flavoprotein reductases into molecular oxygen generates superoxide and other ROS. Some anticancer drugs (e.g., doxorubicin, imidazole antimicrobials) can participate in other oxidation-reduction (redox) cycling reactions that generate ROS.

Phase 2 (Conjugation) Reactions

Phase 2 reactions involve formation of ester links to the parent compound or a drug metabolite to form highly water-soluble conjugates that can be excreted readily in bile or urine. The responsible enzymes include glucuronyl transferases, sulfotransferases, glutathione S-transferases, and acetyl and amino acid N-transferases. Conjugation reactions are also regulated by CAR and other nuclear transcription factors and can be retarded by depletion of their rate-limiting cofactors, such as glucuronic acid and inorganic sulfate. The relatively low capacity of these enzyme systems restricts the efficacy of drug elimination when substrate concentrations exceed enzyme saturation. In general, drug conjugates are nontoxic, and phase 2 reactions are considered to be detoxification reactions, with exceptions. For example, some glutathione conjugates can undergo cysteine S-conjugate beta-lyase-mediated activation to highly reactive intermediates. In general, conjugation reactions are little affected by liver disease, with the possible exception of some reduction of enzyme activity and resulting drug clearance in patients with decompensated cirrhosis; this effect is relevant to selection of major analgesics (morphine rather than meperidine) and hypnotics (oxazepam rather than diazepam). Little is known about the regulation of such enzymes or their potential significance for DILI.

Phase 3 Pathways

Phase 3 involves secretion of drugs, drug metabolites, or their conjugates into bile. Several transporters participate in these pathways that involve adenosine triphosphate (ATP)-binding cassette (ABC) proteins and are powered by energy from ATP hydrolysis (see Chapter 64). ABC transport proteins are widely distributed in nature and include the cystic fibrosis transmembrane conductance regulator (CFTR) (see Chapters 57 and 77) and the canalicular and intestinal copper transporters (see Chapter 76).

Multidrug resistance protein 1 (MDR1, gene symbol *ABCB1*) is highly expressed on the apical (canalicular) plasma membrane of hepatocytes, where it transports cationic drugs, particularly anticancer agents, into bile. Another family of ABC transporters, the multidrug resistance–associated proteins (MRPs), is also expressed in the liver. At least 2 members of this family excrete drug (and other) conjugates from hepatocytes: MRP3 (gene symbol *ABCC3*) on the basolateral surface

facilitates passage of drug conjugate into the sinusoidal circulation, and MRP2 (gene symbol *ABCC2*), expressed on the canalicular membrane, pumps endogenous compounds (e.g., bilirubin diglucuronide, leukotriene-glutathionyl conjugates, glutathione) and drug conjugates into bile. The bile salt export pump (BSEP) and MDR3 (gene symbol *ABCB4* in humans and *Mdr2* in mice) are other canalicular transporters concerned, respectively, with bile acid and phospholipid secretion into bile. Polymorphisms involving these genes are associated with human cholestatic liver diseases. BSEP interacts with several drugs (see Chapter 64).[11]

Regulation of the membrane expression and activity of these drug elimination pathways is complex. Altered expression or impaired activity (by competition between agents, changes in membrane lipid composition, or damage from reactive metabolites or covalent binding) could lead to drug accumulation, impairment of bile flow, or cholestatic liver injury. These effects have been demonstrated for estrogens,[12,13] troglitazone,[14] terbinafine,[15] and flucloxacillin[16] and may have wider mechanistic importance for drug-induced cholestasis and other forms of liver injury.[11]

Effect of Liver Disease on Drug Metabolism

In considering the safety of prescribing medications in patients with liver disease, health care providers need to understand the hepatic extraction ratio of the drug (its rate of uptake and metabolism), drug disposition (hepatic, renal, other), pathways of hepatic drug metabolism (if any), and potential interactions between drug effects (pharmacodynamics) and complications of the liver disease. In light of the complexity of hepatic drug handling, it is fortunate that most drugs are safe to use in most patients with liver disease. The contexts that give rise to concern are liver disease associated with reduced hepatic blood flow (cirrhosis and portal hypertension), in which case hepatic clearance of drugs with high clearance will be reduced, and poor metabolic (synthetic) function of the liver. In addition to patients awaiting liver transplantation, those with alcoholic hepatitis and cirrhosis, severe autoimmune hepatitis (AIH), and hepatitis C with hepatic decompensation are at risk. In such patients, oral doses of high-clearance compounds must be reduced substantially because there may be 2- to 10-fold increases in systemic bioavailability resulting from the reduced "first-pass" hepatic clearance. The best example is propranolol, usually prescribed in such patients to lower portal venous pressure and reduce the risk of variceal bleeding (see Chapter 92). Instead of doses used for cardiovascular indications (160 to 320 mg daily), the usual starting dose in a patient with cirrhosis should be 10 to 20 mg daily. Other high-clearance compounds affected by severe liver disease include meperidine, tricyclic antidepressants, and salbutamol.

The pathways of hepatic drug metabolism and elimination most affected by liver disease are those involving CYPs (see Table 88-1). As mentioned earlier, cholestatic forms of liver disease have little effect on CYP3A4 and therefore minimally affect hepatic metabolism of commonly used drugs like glucocorticoids, angiotensin-converting enzyme (ACE) inhibitors, cyclosporine, and protease inhibitors. Drugs that rely on hepatic elimination through biliary excretion are not affected much by liver disease, with the exception of cancer chemotherapeutic agents; patients with jaundice are at increased risk of liver injury from such agents. By contrast, liver disease has much less effect on conjugation pathways (phase 2 drug metabolism), a property that can be exploited in the choice of sedatives or major analgesics (see later).

Drugs known to precipitate liver complications should be avoided; for example, patients with cirrhosis have impaired creatinine clearance and are at risk of developing renal failure with gentamicin. Another challenge is the appropriate choice of a sedative, as in a patient with alcoholic cirrhosis during alcohol withdrawal. Diazepam is a poor choice in this setting because it is metabolized extensively by CYPs; its clearance is delayed and hepatic encephalopathy may be precipitated by its use. Alternatively, oxazepam, a benzodiazepine that is metabolized by conjugation alone, is a safer choice. Other unwanted drug effects that may occur in patients with liver disease but are not usually related to hepatic drug metabolism include exaggerated effects on clotting factor synthesis (although warfarin metabolism is not usually affected by liver disease), sodium and water retention by nonsteroidal anti-inflammatory drugs (NSAIDs, which also confer a high risk of GI bleeding), metabolic acidosis or profound hypoglycemia by metformin and other oral hypoglycemic agents, and hypotension after administration of an ACE inhibitor or major tranquilizer. Acetaminophen appears to be the safest analgesic agent to use in cirrhosis (see later). In general, however, most commonly used agents (antimicrobials, antiviral agents for hepatitis B virus [HBV], hepatitis C virus [HCV], including direct antiviral agents, antiepileptics, antidepressants, antihypertensives, statins, and oral contraceptives) are safe to use in patients with liver disease.

LIVER DISEASE CAUSED BY DRUGS

Definitions and Importance

Drugs are a relatively common cause of liver injury, which usually is defined by abnormalities of liver biochemical test levels, particularly an increase in the serum alanine aminotransferase (ALT), alkaline phosphatase, or bilirubin level, to more than twice the upper limit of normal (ULN). DILI can be difficult to define in clinical practice, because the biochemical tests used to detect liver injury may also be elevated as part of a hepatic adaptive response. Indeed, evidence indicates that some forms of hepatic adaptation to drugs follow an earlier transient process of self-limiting liver injury, followed in turn by operation of innate immunity.[17] Further, the severity of DILI varies from minor nonspecific changes in hepatic structure and function to acute liver failure, cirrhosis, and liver cancer.

The term *drug-induced liver disease* should be confined to cases in which the nature of liver injury has been characterized histologically. With the exception of acetaminophen, anticancer drugs, and some botanical or industrial hepatotoxins, most cases of DILI represent *adverse drug reactions* or *hepatic drug reactions*. These effects are noxious and unintentional and occur at recommended doses. The latent period is longer (typically 1 week to 3 or 6 months) than that for direct hepatotoxins (hours to a few days), and extrahepatic features of drug hypersensitivity may be present.

Although DILI is a relatively uncommon cause of jaundice or acute hepatitis in the community, it is an important cause of more severe acute liver disease, particularly among older adults. The overall mortality rate among patients hospitalized for DILI is approximately 10%[18] but varies greatly for individual drugs.[19,20] Reported frequencies of individual hepatic drug reactions are underestimated because of the inadequacy of spontaneous reporting.[19,20] With reliable prospective and epidemiologic techniques, the frequency (or risk) of most types of DILI is between 1 per 10,000 and 1 per 100,000 persons exposed.[21] Because these responses to drug exposure are clearly rare and unpredictable, they are often termed *idiosyncratic drug reactions*. Their rarity blunts diagnostic acumen because most clinicians will see few if any cases and therefore do not have an appropriate level of clinical suspicion. This

concern applies especially to complementary and alternative medicines (CAM) (see Chapter 89). Failure to withdraw the causative agent after the onset of symptoms of drug hepatitis or inadvertent reexposure to such a drug is a common and avoidable factor in acute liver failure attributable to DILI.[1,22-24] Another challenge is that DILI includes an array of clinical syndromes and pathologic findings that mimic known hepatobiliary diseases. Furthermore, although individual agents (and some drug classes) typically produce a characteristic "signature syndrome," they can also be associated with other and sometimes multiple clinicopathologic syndromes.

DILI is one of the most common reasons for withdrawal of an approved drug. The subject therefore has medico-economic, legal, and regulatory ramifications. Because most types of idiosyncratic hepatic drug reactions are infrequent, serious hepatotoxicity is not usually detected until post-marketing surveillance is conducted. Historically, drugs with a reputation for potential hepatotoxicity have usually been replaced by more acceptable alternatives. Examples include troglitazone, the prototypical thiazolidinedione, and bromfenac, an NSAID, both of which were withdrawn owing to fatal hepatotoxicity.[1,22,24,25]

The burgeoning number of available conventional medications and CAM preparations now includes many hundreds that can be cited as rare causes of DILI. This poses several challenges to clinicians,[1,5,22-25] including concern about what constitutes an adequate level of patient information at the time a drug is prescribed and the reliability of evidence linking an individual agent to a particular type of liver injury.[1,26-28] Another development is the appreciation that in the context of complex medical situations, drug toxicity can interact with other causes of liver injury (see earlier). Noteworthy examples of such situations are bone marrow transplantation, cancer chemotherapy, highly active antiretroviral therapy (HAART) for human immunodeficiency virus (HIV) infection/acquired immunodeficiency syndrome (AIDS), use of antituberculosis drugs in patients with chronic viral hepatitis, rifampin hepatitis in patients with PBC, and nonalcoholic fatty liver disease (NAFLD)—particularly nonalcoholic steatohepatitis (NASH)—precipitated by tamoxifen.

Epidemiology

Frequency, or *risk,* the number of adverse reactions for a given number of persons exposed, is the best term for expressing how common a drug reaction is. Time-dependent terms such as *incidence* and *prevalence* are not appropriate because the frequency is not linearly related to the duration of exposure. For most reactions, the onset occurs within a relatively short exposure time, or latent period, although some forms of chronic liver disease occur months or years later. The frequency of DILI is derived from post-marketing surveillance reports submitted to the manufacturers or adverse drug reaction monitoring bodies. In the United States, following approval by the U.S. Food and Drug Administration (FDA), drug companies are required to report serious adverse events (any incident resulting in death, a threat to life, hospitalization, or permanent disability [Code of Federal Regulations]). Surveillance becomes a more passive process, however, when a drug is approved for marketing, and physicians and pharmacists are encouraged to file voluntary written reports through the MedWatch program. Nevertheless, MedWatch receives reports for fewer than 10% of adverse drug reactions,[19] and in France fewer than 6% of hepatic adverse drug reactions are reported.[20] The situation may be somewhat better in Sweden, but the annual incidence of adverse drug reactions of 2.2 per 100,000 in the population over the age of 15 is still much lower than the predicted incidence of 14 per 100,000.[20]

The electronic tool for drug-induced serious hepatotoxicity (eDISH) is a graphic instrument that can help identify participants in clinical trials who may be at risk of severe liver disease. Both at-a-glance laboratory data (especially serum aminotransferase and bilirubin levels) for all participants and time-course data for individual patients can be obtained for further scrutiny (see http://www.fda.gov/downloads/Drugs/ScienceResearch/ResearchAreas/ucmD76777.pdf).

Case Definition: Which Agent?

At least 300 agents have been implicated in DILI.[5] The evidence for most drugs, however, is confined to individual or small numbers of case reports, especially in letters to scientific journals or regulatory authorities or in small observational series. Therefore, for most agents, the evidence that they could cause liver injury is circumstantial and incomplete. Reports often lack pathologic definition, full exclusion of other disorders (for older reports), and logistic imputation of causality, especially with respect to temporal associations (see later).[1,5,25] Overall, probably fewer than 50 agents have been reliably implicated as causes of DILI (i.e., implicated in at least 20 cases). In general, agents used most commonly in clinical practice and in the community, including antimicrobials, antineoplastic agents, and NSAIDs, are those that have been implicated in causing DILI. The challenge of identifying the culprit drug among multiple candidates is discussed later.[1,18,21,22,26]

Frequencies of Hepatic Drug Reactions

Because of incomplete reporting, frequencies of hepatic drug reactions are often underestimated. These estimated frequencies are also crude indicators of risk because of the inherent inaccuracies of case definitions (see later)[1,5,25] and because case recognition and reporting depend on the skill and motivation of observers. The increased interest of prescribers when initial cases of DILI have been described, together with inappropriate prescribing (e.g., prolonged use of bromfenac, which was approved only for 7 days of use, and overprescribing of flucloxacillin and amoxicillin–clavulanic acid in some countries) can give rise to apparent "mini-epidemics." More appropriate epidemiologic methods applied to hepatotoxicity have included prescription event monitoring, record linkage, and case-control studies. Prescription event monitoring and record linkage have been used to estimate the frequency of liver injury with some antimicrobials (erythromycins, sulfonamides, tetracyclines, flucloxacillin, amoxicillin-clavulanate) and NSAIDs.[26]

Epidemiologic studies confirm the rarity of DILI with currently used agents. For NSAIDs, the risk of liver injury is between 1 and 10 per 100,000 persons exposed.[1,18,21,22] Amoxicillin–clavulanic acid has been associated with cholestatic hepatitis in 1 to 2 per 100,000 exposed persons,[1,18,21,22,24] and low-dose tetracyclines have caused hepatotoxicity in less than 1 case per million persons exposed.[1,18,21,22] The frequency of liver injury may be higher for agents that exert a metabolic type of hepatotoxicity. For example, isoniazid causes liver injury in up to 2% of persons exposed; the risk depends on the patient's age and gender, concomitant exposure to other agents, and presence of HBV and possibly HCV infections.[27] For some drugs in which other host factors play an etiopathogenic role, case-control studies have been used to define attributable risk. Examples include the association of aspirin with Reye's syndrome and of oral contraceptives with liver tumors and hepatic vein thrombosis.

In the 1970s, the late Hyman Zimmerman hypothesized a relationship between the frequency and severity of serum ALT elevations that indicate liver injury and the risk of severe

hepatotoxicity.[22] According to "Hy's rule," elevations of serum ALT levels to 3-fold or more above the ULN with an associated increase in the serum bilirubin concentration ($\geq 2 \times$ ULN), without an elevation of serum alkaline phosphatase ($<2 \times$ ULN), indicate a potential for the drug to cause acute liver failure at a rate of about 10% of the number of cases of jaundice. Therefore, if 2 cases of jaundice associated with DILI are observed in a phase 3 clinical trial experience of 2500 patients, approximately 1 case of acute liver failure would be expected for every 12,500 subjects who were prescribed the drug during the marketing phase.

Importance of Drugs as a Cause of Liver Disease

Hepatotoxicity accounts for less than 5% of cases of jaundice or acute hepatitis in the community and for even fewer cases of chronic liver disease.[1,22] However, drugs are an important cause of more severe types of liver disease and for liver disease in older people. They account for 10% of cases of severe hepatitis admitted to the hospital in France[22] and for 43% of cases of hepatitis among patients 50 years of age or older.[23] Drugs account for more than half of the cases of acute liver failure referred to special units in the United States[23] and between 20% and 75% of cases of acute liver failure in other industrialized countries.[21,23] The pattern of agents incriminated varies among countries; for example, herbal medicines are a relatively more common cause in Asian countries than in other countries (Chapter 89); herbal medicines account for over a quarter of DILI cases in South Korea.[29]

In most cases of DILI, drugs are the sole cause of hepatic damage. In other cases, drugs increase the relative risk for types of liver disease that may occur in the absence of drug exposure. Examples include salicylates in Reye's syndrome, oral contraceptive steroids in hepatic venous thrombosis, methotrexate in hepatic fibrosis associated with alcoholic liver disease and NAFLD, and tamoxifen in NAFLD/NASH. Predisposition of patients with preexisting liver disease to DILI is minimal (see earlier), but some interesting potential interactions between chronic HCV infection and several groups of drugs and between chronic HBV infection and antituberculosis chemotherapy are now reasonably established. On the other hand, liver failure may be more likely to develop if the patient with a hepatic drug reaction (e.g., to amoxicillin–clavulanic acid) usually associated with a good outcome has underlying chronic liver disease.

Risk Factors

For dose-dependent hepatotoxins like acetaminophen and methotrexate and for some idiosyncratic reactions that are partly dependent on dose (e.g., bromfenac, tetracyclines, dantrolene, tacrine, oxypenicillins), the factors that influence the risk of DILI include drug dose (doses of ≥ 50 mg are more likely to be associated with DILI),[30] blood level of the drug, and duration of intake. For idiosyncratic reactions, however, host determinants are central to liver injury. The most critical determinant is likely to be genetic predisposition, but other "constitutional" and environmental factors can influence the risk of liver injury, as summarized in Table 88-2. The most important factors are age,[21] gender, exposure to other substances, a history or family history of previous drug reactions, other risk factors for liver disease, and concomitant medical disorders.

Genetic Factors

As with other types of drug reaction, genetic determinants predispose to DILI[28] (e.g., penicillin allergy). The contention

TABLE 88-2 Factors Influencing the Risk of Liver Diseases Caused by Drugs

Factor	Examples of Drugs Affected	Influence
Genetic factors	Halothane, phenytoin, sulfonamides Amoxicillin-clavulanic acid, flucloxacillin, abacavir Valproic acid	Multiple cases in families Strong HLA association Familial cases; association with mitochondrial enzyme deficiencies
Age	Isoniazid, nitrofurantoin, halothane, troglitazone Valproic acid, salicylates	Age > 60 years: increased frequency, increased severity More common in children
Gender	Halothane, minocycline, nitrofurantoin Amoxicillin-clavulanic acid, azathioprine	More common in women, especially in cases with chronic hepatitis More common in men
Dose	Acetaminophen, aspirin, some herbal medicines Tetracycline, tacrine, oxypenicillins Methotrexate, vitamin A	Blood levels are directly related to the risk of hepatotoxicity Idiosyncratic reactions, with partial relationship to dose Total dose, dosing frequency, and duration of exposure are related to the risk of hepatic fibrosis
Other drugs	Acetaminophen Valproic acid Anticancer drugs	Isoniazid, zidovudine, and phenytoin lower the dose threshold and increase the severity of hepatotoxicity Other antiepileptic drugs increase the risk of hepatotoxicity Interactive vascular toxicity
History of other drug reactions	Isoflurane, halothane, enflurane Erythromycins Diclofenac, ibuprofen, tiaprofenic acid Sulfonamides, COX-2 inhibitors	Instances of cross-sensitivity have been reported among members of each drug class but are rare
Excessive alcohol use	Acetaminophen Isoniazid, methotrexate	Lowered dose threshold, poorer outcome Increased risk of liver injury, hepatic fibrosis
Nutritional status: Obesity Fasting	Halothane, troglitazone, tamoxifen, methotrexate Acetaminophen	Increased risk of liver injury, hepatic fibrosis Increased risk of hepatotoxicity
Preexisting liver disease	Hycanthone, pemoline Antituberculosis drugs, ibuprofen	Increased risk of liver injury Increased risk of liver injury with chronic hepatitis B and C
Other diseases/conditions: Diabetes mellitus HIV/AIDS Renal failure Organ transplantation	Methotrexate Sulfonamides Tetracycline, methotrexate Azathioprine, thioguanine, busulfan	Increased risk of hepatic fibrosis Increased risk of hypersensitivity Increased risk of liver injury, hepatic fibrosis Increased risk of vascular toxicity

that atopic patients may be at increased risk of some types of drug hepatitis is unproven, however. Genetic factors determine the activity of drug-activating and antioxidant pathways, encode pathways of canalicular bile secretion, and modulate the immune response, tissue stress responses, and cell death pathways. Documented examples of drugs associated with a familial predisposition to adverse hepatic drug reactions are few and include valproic acid and phenytoin.[1,24,28] Inherited mitochondrial diseases are a risk factor for valproic acid–induced hepatotoxicity.[31] Some forms of

DILI, particularly drug-induced hepatitis and granulomatous reactions, can be associated with the drug reaction with eosinophilia and systemic symptoms (DRESS) syndrome (see later) (Table 88-3).

Initial studies showed only no or weak associations between specific human leukocyte antigen (HLA) haplotypes and some types of DILI. More recently, large genome-wide association studies (GWAS) have revealed stronger associations between specific HLA haplotypes and hepatotoxicity associated with several drugs, including flucloxacillin,

TABLE 88-3 Genetic Variants Associated with Drug-Induced Liver Injury (DILI)

Drug	Category	Allele(s)*	Odds Ratio (CI) for DILI
Flucloxacillin	Antibiotic	HLA-B*5701	81 (23-285)
Ticlopidine	Antiplatelet agent	HLA-A*3303	36.5 (7.3-184)
Lumiracoxib	NSAID	HLA-DQA1*0102; DRB5*0101; DQB1*0602; **DRB1*1501**	6.3 (4.1-9.6)
Diclofenac	NSAID	*ABCC2* (MRP2) C24T	6 (2.4-17)
Ximelagatran	Thrombin inhibitor	HLA-DRB1*0701	4.4
Sex hormones	Various	*ABCB11* (BSEP) V444A	1.7-4
Amoxicillin-clavulanic acid	Antibiotic	HLA-DRB5*0101; DQB1*0602; **DRB1*1501**	2.3 (1.0-5.26)

*Alleles in bold are the most important in the pathogenesis of DILI for the particular drug.
ABC, ATP-binding cassette; BSEP, bile salt export pump; CI, confidence intervals; MRP2, multidrug resistance-associated protein 2.

amoxicillin–clavulanic acid (see later), lapatinib, ximelagatran, and lumiracoxib (see Table 88-2).[28,32-34]

Age

Most hepatic drug reactions are more common in adults than in children. Exceptions include valproic acid hepatotoxicity, which is most common in children younger than 3 years of age and rare in adults, and Reye's syndrome, in which salicylates play a key role. As discussed later, both are examples of mitochondrial toxicity.[31] In adults, the risk of isoniazid-associated hepatotoxicity is greater in persons older than age 40. Similar observations have been made for nitrofurantoin, halothane, etretinate, diclofenac, and troglitazone.[1,5,18,21] The increased frequency of adverse drug reactions in older adults is largely the result of increased exposure, polypharmacy, and altered drug disposition.[1,5,18,21] In addition, clinical severity of hepatotoxicity increases strikingly with age, as exemplified by fatal reactions to isoniazid and halothane.

Gender

Women are particularly predisposed to drug-induced hepatitis, a difference that cannot be attributed simply to increased exposure. Examples include toxicity caused by halothane, nitrofurantoin, sulfonamides, flucloxacillin, minocycline, and troglitazone.[1,22] Drug-induced chronic hepatitis caused by nitrofurantoin, diclofenac, or minocycline has an even more pronounced female preponderance.[22] Conversely, equal sex frequency or even male preponderance is common for some cholestatic drug reactions (e.g., amoxicillin–clavulanic acid). Azathioprine-induced liver disease is more likely to develop in male renal transplant recipients than in female recipients.[35]

Concomitant Exposure to Other Agents

Patients who are taking multiple drugs are more likely to experience an adverse reaction than those who are taking one agent.[1,5,25] The mechanisms include enhanced CYP-mediated metabolism of the second drug to a toxic intermediate (see Toxic Mechanisms of Liver Injury). Examples discussed later include toxicity caused by acetaminophen, isoniazid, valproic acid, other anticonvulsants, and anticancer drugs. Alternatively, drugs may alter the disposition of other agents by

reducing bile flow or competing with canalicular pathways for biliary excretion (phase 3 drug elimination). This mechanism may account for apparent interactions between oral contraceptive steroids and other drugs to produce cholestasis. Drugs or their metabolites may also interact in mechanisms of cellular toxicity and cell death that involve mitochondrial injury, intracellular signaling pathways, activation of transcription factors, and regulation of hepatic genes involved in controlling the response to stress and injury that triggers pro-inflammatory and cell death processes.[6,36]

Previous Drug Reactions

A history of an adverse drug reaction generally increases the risk of reactions to the same drug and also to some other agents (see later). Nevertheless, instances of cross-sensitivity to related agents in cases of DILI are surprisingly uncommon. Examples of cross-sensitivity between drugs (or drug classes) include the haloalkane anesthetics (see Chapter 89), erythromycins, phenothiazines and tricyclic antidepressants, isoniazid and pyrazinamide, and some NSAIDs. A crucial point is that a previous reaction to the same drug is a major risk factor for an increase in the severity of DILI.[22] A 2011 Spanish study examined the risk of DILI in a person who has previously experienced DILI (with a different drug).[37] Recurrent DILI was infrequent (1.2%), with most cases related to the use of structurally similar drugs or drugs with similar targets. Some exhibited features consistent with AIH, raising the possibility that immune-mediated processes may be mechanistically involved or that the correct diagnosis was actually AIH.

Alcohol

Chronic excessive alcohol ingestion decreases the dose threshold for, and enhances the severity of, acetaminophen-induced hepatotoxicity and increases the risk and severity of isoniazid hepatitis, niacin (nicotinic acid, nicotinamide) hepatotoxicity, and methotrexate-induced hepatic fibrosis.

Nutritional Status

Obesity is strongly associated with the risk of halothane hepatitis and is an independent risk factor for NASH and hepatic fibrosis in persons taking methotrexate or tamoxifen. Fasting also predisposes to acetaminophen hepatotoxicity,[38] and a role for under-nutrition has been proposed in isoniazid hepatotoxicity.[39]

Preexisting Liver Disease

In general, liver diseases like alcoholic cirrhosis and cholestatic disorders do not predispose to adverse hepatic reactions (see earlier). Exceptions include toxicity to some anticancer drugs, niacin, pemoline, and hycanthone. Preexisting liver disease is a critical determinant of methotrexate-induced hepatic fibrosis. Patients with chronic HBV infection[27] and possibly those with chronic HCV infection or HIV/AIDS appear to be at heightened risk of liver injury during antituberculosis or HAART therapy,[40] after exposure to ibuprofen and possibly other NSAIDs, after myeloablative therapy in preparation for bone marrow transplantation (resulting in sinusoidal obstruction syndrome [see later]),[41] and possibly after taking antiandrogens like flutamide and cyproterone acetate.[42] A particularly strong association is reported between HCV infection and the risk of liver injury during HAART; the risk may be increased 2- to 10-fold.[43-45]

Other Diseases

Rheumatoid arthritis appears to increase the risk of salicylate hepatotoxicity, and a curious unexplained observation is that sulfasalazine hepatitis is more common in patients with rheumatoid arthritis than in those with IBD.[5,24,25,46,47] Diabetes mellitus, obesity, and chronic kidney disease predispose to methotrexate-induced hepatic fibrosis, whereas HIV/AIDS confers a heightened risk of sulfonamide hypersensitivity.[46-48] A retrospective cohort study found that the age- and sex-standardized incidence of drug-induced acute liver failure in patients with diabetes mellitus was 0.08 to 0.15 per 1000 person-years, irrespective of the therapeutic agent used (the number using troglitazone was small); the incidence was highest (≈0.3 per 1000) during the first 6 months of exposure.[47] Renal transplantation is a risk factor for azathioprine-associated vascular injury, whereas kidney disease predisposes to tetracycline-induced fatty liver.[22] Finally, sinusoidal obstruction syndrome induced by anticancer drugs is more common after bone marrow transplantation[41] and in persons with HCV infection.[1,5,22,24,25,43]

Pathophysiology

Toxic Mechanisms of Liver Injury

Direct Hepatotoxins and Reactive Metabolites

Highly hepatotoxic chemicals injure key subcellular structures, particularly mitochondria and the plasma membrane. The injury arrests energy generation, dissipates ionic gradients, and disrupts the physical integrity of the cell. This type of overwhelming cellular injury does not apply to currently relevant hepatotoxins, most of which require metabolic activation to mediate damage to liver cells. The resulting reactive metabolites can interact with critical cellular target molecules, particularly those with nucleophilic substituents such as thiol-rich proteins and nucleic acids. Together with ROS, they act as oxidizing species within the hepatocyte to establish oxidative stress, a state of imbalance between pro-oxidants and antioxidants. ROS are also key signaling molecules that mediate biological responses to stress, as discussed later. Alternatively, reactive metabolites bind irreversibly to macromolecules, particularly proteins and lipids. Such covalent binding may produce injury by inactivating key enzymes or by forming protein-drug adducts that could be targets for immunodestructive processes that cause liver injury. Notwithstanding these comments, there is increasing evidence that "direct hepatotoxins" like acetaminophen activate innate immune mechanisms in the liver in response to stress with release of damage (or danger)-activated molecular patterns (DAMPs); the latter (as well as bacterial products like endotoxin, a pathogen-associated molecular pattern [PAMP]) trigger Toll-like receptors to activate pro-inflammatory and cell death pathways (see Chapter 72).[49]

Oxidative Stress and the Glutathione System

The liver is exposed to oxidative stress by the propensity of hepatocytes to reduce oxygen, particularly in mitochondria and also in microsomal electron transport systems (e.g., CYP2E1), and by NADPH oxidase–catalyzed formation of ROS and nitroradicals in Kupffer cells, endothelial cells, and stimulated polymorphonuclear leukocytes (neutrophils) and macrophages. To combat oxidative stress, the liver is well endowed with antioxidant mechanisms, including micronutrients (e.g., vitamin E, vitamin C), thiol-rich proteins (e.g., metallothionein, ubiquinone), metal-sequestering proteins (e.g., ferritin), and enzymes that metabolize reactive metabolites (e.g., epoxide hydrolases), ROS (e.g., catalase, superoxide dismutase), and lipid peroxides (e.g., glutathione peroxidases). Glutathione (L-γ-glutamyl-L-cysteinyl-glycine) is the most important antioxidant in the mammalian liver.[36]

Hepatocytes are the exclusive site of glutathione synthesis. Hepatic levels of glutathione are high (5 to 10 mmol/L) and can be increased by enhancing the supply of cysteine for glutathione synthesis; this mechanism is the cornerstone of thiol antidote therapy for acetaminophen poisoning. Hepatocyte glutathione synthesis increases in response to pro-oxidants, as occurs when CYP2E1 is overexpressed as a result of signaling via the redox-sensitive transcription factor Nrf.[6,36,50,51] Glutathione synthesis, via expression of the rate-limiting enzyme glutamate cysteine ligase (CGL), is also a response to mitochondrial injury by agents such as acetaminophen. Glutathione in its reduced form (GSH) is a critical cofactor for several antioxidant pathways, including thiol-disulfide exchange reactions and glutathione peroxidase. Glutathione peroxidase has a higher affinity for hydrogen peroxide than does catalase, and it disposes of lipid peroxides, free radicals, and electrophilic drug metabolites. GSH is also a cofactor for conjugation reactions catalyzed by the glutathione S-transferases involved with phase 3 transport of drug metabolites into bile. Other reactions proceed nonenzymatically. In turn, the products include glutathione-protein mixed disulfides and oxidized glutathione. The latter can be converted back to glutathione by proton donation catalyzed by glutathione reductase.

Normally, most glutathione within the hepatocyte is in the reduced state, indicating the importance of this pathway for maintenance of the redox capacity of the cell. The reduced form of NADPH is an essential cofactor for glutathione reductase; NADPH formation requires ATP, thereby illustrating a critical link between mitochondrial integrity and the energy-generating capacity of the liver and its ability to withstand oxidative stress. Glutathione is also compartmentalized within the hepatocyte, with the highest concentrations found in the cytosol. Adequate levels of glutathione are essential in mitochondria, where ROS are constantly being formed as a minor by-product of oxidative respiration and in response to some drugs or metabolites that interfere with the mitochondrial respiratory chain. Mitochondrial glutathione is maintained by active uptake from the cytosol, a transport system that is altered by chronic ethanol exposure and in some forms of lipotoxicity (e.g., with cholesterol) and is therefore another potential target of drug toxicity.[36]

Biochemical Mechanisms of Cellular Injury

Mechanisms once thought to be central to hepatotoxicity, such as covalent binding to cellular enzymes and peroxidation of membrane lipids, are no longer regarded as exclusive pathways of cellular damage. Rather, oxidation of proteins, phospholipid fatty acyl side chains (lipid peroxidation), and nucleosides appears to be a component of the biochemical stress that characterizes toxic liver injury. In one experiment, healthy volunteers were administered a variety of low-molecular-weight heparins known to cause transient serum ALT elevations.[17] In addition to aminotransferase increases in over 90% of cases, markers of subcellular (cytosol, mitochondrial) injury and apoptosis (M30, a fragmentation product of cytokeratins 8 and 18), as well as microRNA (miRNA)-122, DNA, and high-mobility group protein B1 (HMGB1), increased; the last is a DAMP released in necrosis. The authors concluded that heparins as a class caused self-limited and mild necrosis with secondary activation of an innate immune response. Secondary reactions, including post-translational modification of proteins via adenosine diphosphate (ADP) ribosylation or protease activation, cleavage of DNA by activation of endogenous endonucleases, and disruption of lipid membranes by activated phospholipases may also play a role in DILI.[6] Some of these catabolic reactions could be initiated by a rise in the cytosolic ionic calcium concentration $[Ca^{2+}]_i$ as a result of increased Ca^{2+} entry or release from internal stores in the endoplasmic reticulum and mitochondria.[6,36] The potential role of endoplasmic reticulum stress in DILI is less well defined.[52,53]

The concept that hepatotoxic chemicals cause hepatocyte cell death by a biochemical final common pathway (e.g., activation of catalytic enzymes by a rise in $[Ca^{2+}]_i$) has proved inadequate to explain the diverse processes that can result in lethal hepatocellular injury. Rather, a variety of processes can damage key organelles, thereby causing intracellular stress that activates signaling pathways and transcription factors. Mitochondrial injury, particularly that signaled via activation of the c-Jun N-terminal kinase (JNK), appears to be critically involved with acetaminophen and most likely several other hepatotoxins.[49,54-56] In turn, the balance between these factors can trigger the onset of cell death or facilitate protection of the cell, as discussed later.

Types of Cell Death

Apoptosis. Apoptosis is an energy-dependent, genetically programmed form of cell death that typically results in controlled deletion of individual cells. In addition to its major roles in developmental biology, tissue regulation, and carcinogenesis, apoptosis is important in toxic, viral, and immune-mediated liver injury.[57-60] The ultrastructural features of apoptosis are cell and nuclear shrinkage, condensation and margination of nuclear chromatin, plasma membrane blebbing, and ultimately fragmentation of the cell into membrane-bound bodies that contain intact mitochondria and other organelles. Engulfment of these apoptotic bodies by surrounding epithelial and mesenchymal cells conserves cell fragments that contain nucleic acid and intact mitochondria. These fragments are then digested by lysosomes and recycled without release of bioactive substances. As a consequence, apoptosis in it purest form (usually found only in vitro) does not incite an inflammatory tissue reaction. The cellular processes that occur in apoptosis are often mediated by caspases, a family of proteolytic enzymes that contain a cysteine at their active site and cleave polypeptides at aspartate residues; non–caspase-mediated programmed cell death has also been described in experimental hepatotoxicity.

Apoptosis rarely if ever is the sole form of cell death in common forms of liver injury like ischemia-reperfusion injury, cholestasis, and toxic liver injury, all of which are typically associated with at least some necrosis and a hepatic inflammatory response. Whether or not activation of pro-death signals causes cell death depends on several factors, including pro-survival signals, the rapidity of the process, the availability of glutathione and ATP, and the role of other cell types.[6,57-60]

The operation of hepatocellular apoptosis can be determined by detection of the caspase-3-cleaved fragmentation product (M30) of cytokeratin 8 and 18, which is specific to hepatocytes. Hepatocytes undergo apoptosis when pro-apoptotic intracellular signaling pathways are activated, either because of toxic biochemical processes within the cell (intrinsic pathway) or because cell surface receptors are activated to transduce cell death signals (external pathway). Pro-apoptotic receptors are members of the tumor necrosis factor (TNF)-α receptor superfamily, which possess a so-called death domain. These receptors include Fas, for which the cognate ligand is Fas-ligand (Fas-L), TNF-R1 receptor (cognate ligand is TNF), and *TNF-related apoptosis-inducing ligand* (TRAIL) receptors (cognate ligand is TRAIL). In addition to model hepatotoxins like quinone, menadione, and hydrogen peroxide, some drugs (e.g., acetaminophen, plant diterpenoids) have been shown to be converted into pro-oxidant reactive metabolites, thereby initiating the following sequence: CYP-mediated metabolism to form reactive metabolites → glutathione depletion → mitochondrial injury with release of cytochrome *c* and operation of the mitochondrial membrane permeability transition (MPT) → caspase activation → apoptosis.

Mitochondria play a pivotal role in pathways that provoke or oppose apoptosis.[55,57,58,60] In the external pathway, activation of the death domain of pro-apoptotic receptors recruits adapter molecules, Fas-associated death domain (FADD) and TNF receptor–associated death domain (TRADD), which bind and activate procaspase 8 to form the death-inducing signaling complex (DISC). In turn, caspase 8 cleaves Bid, a pro-apoptotic member of the B cell lymphoma/leukemia (Bcl-2) family, to tBid. Then, tBid causes translocation of Bax to the mitochondria, where it aggregates with Bak to promote permeability of the mitochondria.[57] Release of cytochrome c and other pro-death molecules, including Smac (which binds caspase inhibitor proteins, such as inhibitor of apoptosis proteins [IAPs]) and apoptosis-inducing factor (AIF, also known as *Apaf*)[58] allows formation of the "apoptosome," which activates caspase 9 and eventually caspase 3 to execute cell death (Fig. 88-1). Intracellular stresses in various sites release other mitochondrial permeabilizing proteins (e.g., Bmf from the cytoskeleton and Bim from the endoplasmic reticulum), whereas members of the Bcl-2 family, Bcl-2 and Bcl-X_L antagonize apoptosis and serve as survival factors by regulating the integrity of mitochondria; the protective mechanism is not yet fully understood but involves in part myeloid cell leukemia sequence 1 (Mcl-1). Stress-activated protein kinases, particularly JNK, are also be pro-apoptotic[59] by targeting Mcl-1 degradation and phosphorylating and inactivating the mitochondrial protective protein Bcl-X_L.

Execution of cell death by apoptosis usually occurs via activation of caspase 3, but more than 1 caspase-independent pathway of programmed cell death has been described.[60] Stresses to the endoplasmic reticulum can bypass mitochondrial events by activation of caspase 12, which in turn activates caspase 9 independently of the apoptosome. The final steps of programmed cell death are energy dependent. Therefore, depletion of ATP abrogates the controlled attempt at "cell suicide," resulting instead in necrosis (see later) or an overlapping pattern that has been designated as "apoptotic necrosis" or "necrapoptosis."[61,62] Furthermore, when apoptosis is

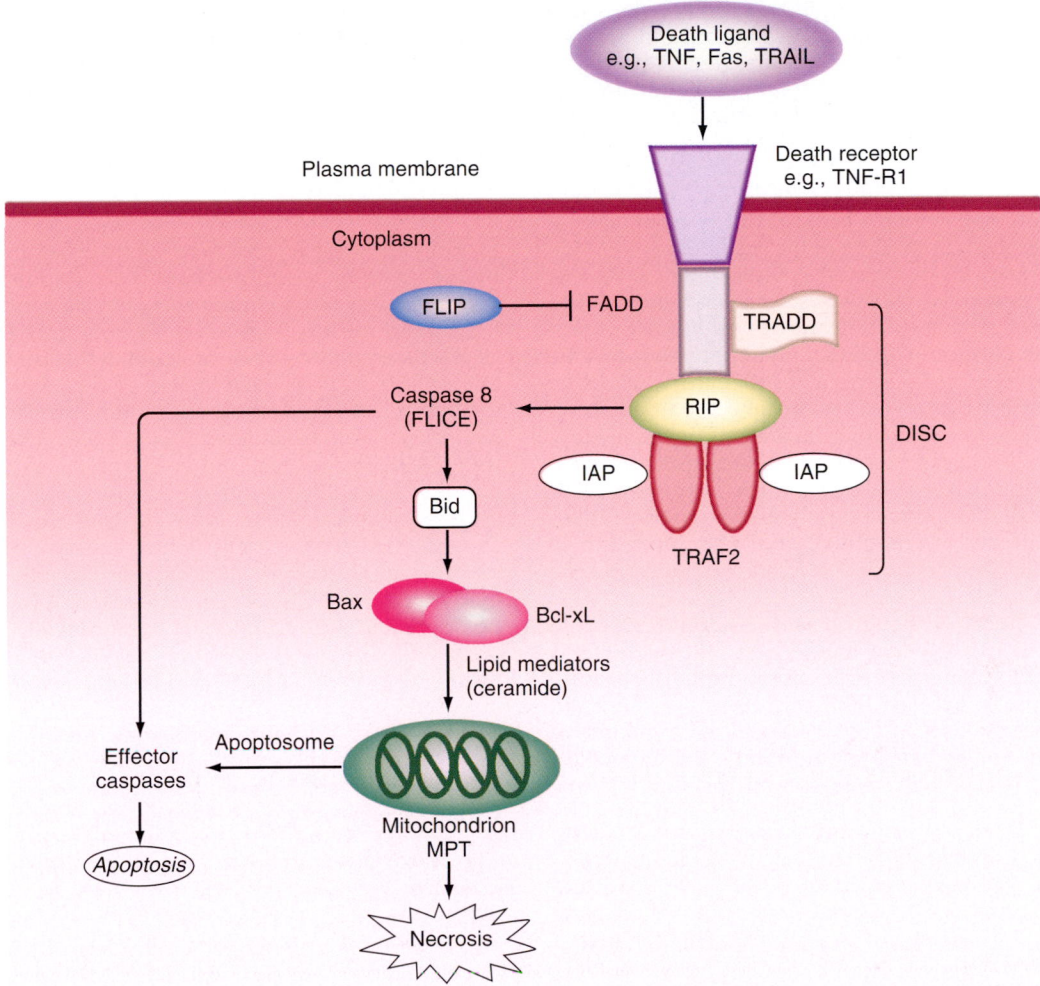

FIGURE 88-1. Apoptosis and necrosis pathways in mammalian cells. See text for details. Bcl, B-cell lymphoma/leukemia family (Bax, Bid, and Bcl-xL are members); DISC, death-inducing signaling complex; FADD, Fas-associated death domain; FLIP, FLICE-inhibitory proteins; IAP, inhibitor of apoptosis proteins; MPT, mitochondrial permeability transition; RIP, receptor-interacting protein; TNF, tumor necrosis factor; TNF-R1, TNF receptor-1; TRADD, TNF receptor–associated death domain; TRAF2, TNF receptor–associated factor-2; TRAIL, TNF-related apoptosis ligand.

massive, the capacity for rapid phagocytosis can be exceeded, and "secondary" necrosis can occur.[62]

Intracellular processes and activation of pro-apoptotic death receptors are not mutually exclusive pathways of cell death in toxic liver injury. In fact, drug toxicity could predispose the injured hepatocyte to apoptosis mediated by TNF-R or Fas-operated pathways by several mechanisms, including blockade of nuclear factor kappa B (NF-κB), which usually is a hepatoprotective transcription factor in hepatocytes, and inhibition of purine and protein synthesis. Furthermore, activation of Kupffer cells (e.g., by endotoxin) and recruitment of activated inflammatory cells can increase production of TNF.

Caspase inhibition is an important protective mechanism against cell death. Such anti-apoptotic pathways include chemical blockade of the cysteine thiol group by nitric oxide (NO) or ROS and cellular depletion of glutathione.[6] Protein inhibitors include IAP family members, heat shock proteins (HSPs), and FLICE (caspase-8)-inhibitory proteins (FLIP).[57-59] FLIP inhibit caspase-8 activation as a decoy for FADD binding. Bcl-2 and Bcl-X$_L$ inhibit mitochondrial permeability, whereas phosphatidylinositol 3-kinase/Akt phosphorylates caspase 9 and activates NF-κB.

Necrosis. In contrast to apoptosis, necrosis has been conceptualized as a relatively uncontrolled process that can result from extensive damage to the plasma membrane with disturbance of ion transport, dissolution of membrane potential, cell swelling, and eventually rupture of the cell. Drug-induced injury to the mitochondrion can impair energy generation, whereas MPT can release stored Ca^{2+} into the cytosol and perturb other ionic gradients. Mitochondrial enzymes appear to be a particular target of NAPQI, the reactive metabolite of acetaminophen (see earlier), as has been demonstrated both in rodent models and in human acetaminophen hepatotoxicity, in which mitochondrial injury with fragmentation of nuclear DNA by the released endonucleases has been documented.[63] The initial mitochondrial injury can also activate various signaling pathways (JNK, glycogen synthase kinase [GSK]-3β), thereby leading to further mitochondrial dysfunction.[55] Reye's syndrome–like disorders (e.g., toxicity caused by valproic acid, some nucleoside analogs [fialuridine, didanosine, zidovudine, zalcitabine], possibly "ecstasy") may also result from mitochondrial injury. Mitochondrial injury can result in cell death by either apoptosis or necrosis[61,62]; the type of cell death pathway may depend primarily on the energy state of the cell, as well as the rapidity and severity of the injury process. In the presence of ATP, cell death can proceed by apoptosis, but when mitochondria are de-energized, the mechanism of cell death is necrosis. This apparent dichotomy between cell death processes is probably artificial, and apoptosis and necrosis more likely represent the morphologic and mechanistic ends of a spectrum of overlapping cell death processes.[36,62]

One important way in which necrosis differs from apoptosis is that uncontrolled dissolution of the cell liberates DAMPs (e.g., HMGB1) and macromolecular breakdown products, including lipid peroxides, aldehydes, and eicosanoids. The latter products act as chemoattractants for circulating leukocytes, which then partake in the inflammatory response in the hepatic parenchyma. Even before cell death occurs, oxidative stress produced during drug toxicity can up-regulate adhesion molecules and chemokines that are expressed or secreted by endothelial cells. These processes contribute to recruitment of the hepatic inflammatory response, which is prominent in some types of DILI. Lymphocytes, polymorphonuclear leukocytes (neutrophils and eosinophils), and macrophages also may be attracted to the liver as part of a cell-mediated immune reaction.[64]

Role of Oxidative Stress. Although severe oxidative stress in hepatocytes, particularly when focused on mitochondria, is likely to induce necrosis, lesser (or more gradual) exposure can trigger apoptosis because ROS and oxidative stress can activate Fas signaling, JNK and other kinases, p53, and microtubular assembly and impair protein folding, thereby resulting in an unfolded protein response by the endoplasmic reticulum.[64]

Oxidative stress also may amplify cell death processes by uncoupling of the mitochondrial respiratory chain, release of cytochrome c, or massive oxidation and export of glutathione (intact glutathione is required for Fas signaling). Conversely, oxidative stress may protect against apoptosis in some circumstances through inhibition of caspase or activation of NF-κB. As a result of these opposing effects, predicting the consequences of hepatic oxidative stress in terms of liver injury is not easy.

Role of Hepatic Non-parenchymal Cells and the Innate Immune Response

In addition to migratory cells, activation of non-parenchymal liver cell types is likely to play an important role in drug and toxin-induced liver injury. Kupffer cells function as resident macrophages and antigen-presenting cells, whereas dendritic cells and NK T cells are also resident in the liver and play a role in antigen processing and innate immunity. Some of the toxic effects of activated Kupffer cells, as well as of recruited leukocytes, may be mediated by release of cytokines like TNF, interleukin (IL)-1β, and Fas-L, which under some circumstances can induce cell death in hepatocytes by apoptosis or necrosis.[62] In addition, activated Kupffer cells release ROS, nitroradicals, leukotrienes, and proteases. It has been suggested, however, that the sterile inflammatory response is not completely unhelpful and could aid in clearing cell debris and paving the way for tissue repair.[65]

Endothelial cells of the hepatic sinusoids or terminal hepatic veins are vulnerable to injury by some hepatotoxins because of their low glutathione content. Such hepatotoxins include the pyrrolizidine alkaloids, which are an important cause of the sinusoidal obstruction syndrome (hepatic veno-occlusive disease) (see Chapter 85).[66] Other types of drug-induced vascular injury may be caused primarily by involvement of the sinusoidal endothelial cells.

Hepatic stellate cells are the principal liver cell type involved in matrix deposition in hepatic fibrosis. Stellate cells are activated in methotrexate-induced hepatic fibrosis. The possibility that vitamin A, ROS, or drug metabolites can transform stellate cells into collagen-synthesizing myofibroblasts is of considerable interest.

Immunologic Mechanisms

In addition to the activation of innate inflammatory processes in the liver by toxic mechanisms, adaptive immunologic mechanisms could account for certain aspects of idiosyncratic DILI. Immune attack involves liganding of death receptors, as discussed earlier, or porin-mediated introduction of granzyme.[36,67] The most convincing evidence for drug allergy includes (1) delayed onset after initial exposure and accelerated onset after rechallenge, (2) hepatic inflammatory infiltrates with neutrophils and eosinophils, and (3) fever, rash, lymphadenopathy, peripheral eosinophilia, and involvement of other organs. In some types of drug hepatitis, the liver is clearly implicated as part of a systemic hypersensitivity reaction, as described later for the DRESS syndrome (formerly the reactive metabolite syndrome). Why the liver is the predominant site of injury in some persons, whereas other organs are involved in other persons is unclear; genetic factors relevant to tissue-specific gene expression could be involved.

One possible immunopathogenic mechanism for DILI is the *altered antigen concept,* in which an initial interaction between drug metabolites and cellular proteins results in the formation of neoantigens (haptens) or drug-protein adducts. An example is the formation of trifluoroacetylated (TFA) adducts after exposure to halothane or other haloalkane anesthetics (see Chapter 89). For these adducts to initiate tissue-damaging immune responses (1) processing should be presented in an immunogenic form (e.g., by Kupffer cells, in association with major histocompatibility complex [MHC] molecules); (2) appropriately responsive CD4+ T cells must be present to provide help to induce an immune response; and (3) the drug-derived antigen, together with a class II MHC molecule, must be expressed on the target cells in order to attract CD8+ (cytotoxic) T cells. That bile duct epithelial cells are more likely to express class II MHC antigens may explain why they are possible targets in drug-induced cholestatic hepatitis.

Although antibodies directed against TFA-protein adducts circulate in the majority of patients following recovery from halothane-induced liver injury,[68] the specificity and pathogenicity of these antibodies remain in doubt. Another way in which circulating drug-induced antibodies could result in immune-mediated lysis of hepatocytes is through molecular mimicry of host enzymes.[69] Experimental evidence suggests that for diclofenac antibody-dependent cell-mediated immunity could operate as a mechanism for DILI.[70]

A second type of immunopathogenic mechanism is dysregulation of the immune system, termed *drug-induced autoimmunity.*[71] This mechanism can lead to the formation of drug-induced autoantibodies (e.g., anti–liver-kidney microsome [LKM] antibodies) directed against microsomal enzymes. For tienilic acid, CYP2C9 is the target of anti-LKM, whereas after halothane hepatitis, anti-LKM are directed against CYP2E1. Non–tissue specific autoantibodies, such as antinuclear and smooth muscle antibodies, may be detected in patients with nitrofurantoin, methyldopa, or minocycline hepatitis. Like spontaneous autoimmunity, drug-induced autoimmunity may involve genetic predisposition through anomalies of immune tolerance.

Clinicopathologic Features

Classification

Hepatic drug reactions mimic all known liver diseases, but classification is often difficult because of overlap among categories. Although a classic ("signature") syndrome is associated with many individual agents, a given drug may be associated with more than one clinicopathologic syndrome. Furthermore, the clinical and laboratory features of liver disease and the hepatic histologic findings may be discordant. Therefore, although recognition of specific patterns or syndromes is vital to the diagnosis of DILI, the chronologic relationship between administration of the drug and liver injury is more important.

Drugs are often divided into dose-dependent, or predictable, hepatotoxins and dose-independent, or unpredictable (idiosyncratic), hepatotoxins. Dose-dependent hepatotoxins generally require metabolic activation to toxic metabolites or interfere with subcellular organelles and biochemical processes at key sites, such as mitochondria or canalicular bile secretion.[12] Liver injury produced by dose-dependent hepatotoxins usually occurs after a short latent period (hours), is characterized by zonal necrosis or microvesicular steatosis, and can be reproduced in other species. By contrast, idiosyncratic hepatotoxins cause a wide range of histologic changes and do not reliably cause injury in other species; in addition, the latent period before the onset of injury is variable in duration. The distinction between dose-dependent and idiosyncratic hepatotoxins is blurred with agents like dantrolene, tacrine, perhexiline, flucloxacillin, cyclophosphamide, nucleoside analogs, bromfenac, anticancer drugs, and cyclosporine. Liver injury caused by each of these drugs is partly dose dependent, but reactions occur in only a small proportion of exposed persons.

Two general types of mechanisms may account for idiosyncratic hepatotoxicity: metabolic idiosyncrasy and immunoallergy. *Metabolic idiosyncrasy* refers to the susceptibility of rare persons to hepatotoxicity from a drug that in conventional doses is usually safe. Such susceptibility may result from genetic or acquired differences in drug metabolism or canalicular secretion, mitochondrial defects, or cell death receptor signaling. *Immunoallergy* indicates involvement of the immune system in mediating the response to a drug. These two mechanisms may be interrelated (see Metabolic Idiosyncrasy). Other pathogenic mechanisms may include indirect mediation of liver injury, as in vascular and possibly hyperthermic changes produced by cocaine, ecstasy, intraarterial fluxoridine, and possibly anesthetics (see Chapter 89).

The most practical classification of drug hepatotoxicity is based on clinical and laboratory features and liver histology, as summarized in Table 88-4. This classification provides a framework for discussing drug-induced hepatic disease in comparison with other hepatobiliary disorders but is imperfect because the clinical and pathologic features are not always congruent. Moreover, much overlap between categories exists, particularly in the spectrum from severe necrosis (which may result from dose-dependent or idiosyncratic hepatotoxicity) to focal necrosis with lobular inflammation (hepatitis) to cholestasis. Many drugs produce a spectrum of syndromes from hepatitis to cholestasis, and some authorities include a further category of mixed cholestatic-hepatocellular reactions. Granulomatous hepatitis is associated with liver biochemical test abnormalities that are usually indistinguishable from those typical of hepatitis, cholestasis, or mixed reactions.

Drugs can alter liver biochemical test results without causing significant liver injury. Such adaptive responses include hyperbilirubinemia associated with rifampin, cyclosporine, and indinavir and raised serum GGTP and alkaline phosphatase levels associated with phenytoin and warfarin.[1,22] The latter effect is probably attributable to microsomal enzyme induction. For other agents, transient ALT or aspartate aminotransferase (AST) elevations are probably related to hepatocellular necrosis (discussed earlier for heparins), but with some agents, such as isoniazid, the distinction between adaptation and minor injury is blurred; adaptation in such cases may be a response to oxidative injury. Conversely, liver tumors or hepatic fibrosis may develop insidiously without significant abnormalities of liver biochemical tests—the former in association with sex steroids or vinyl chloride monomer and the latter with methotrexate, arsenic, or hypervitaminosis A.

The duration of the disorder is another consideration in classifying DILI. In general, chronic liver disease is much less commonly attributable to drugs and toxins than are acute reactions,[24] but not to consider drugs as a possible etiology of chronic liver disease can lead to a missed diagnosis, with serious clinical consequences.[24,25] In contrast to most other types of hepatic pathobiology, drugs and toxins constitute the most important cause of vascular disorders of the liver. Drugs also have been associated with chronic cholestasis, chronic hepatitis, steatohepatitis, hepatic fibrosis, cirrhosis, and benign and malignant liver tumors.

Histopathologic Features

Although no pathognomonic hallmarks of DILI have been identified, certain histologic patterns are suggestive.[72] These patterns include zonal necrosis or microvesicular steatosis (which accompanies mitochondrial injury) and mixed histologic features of hepatocellular necrosis and cholestasis. Necrotic lesions that are disproportionately severe compared with the clinical picture also indicate a possible drug cause, whereas destructive bile duct lesions, prominent neutrophils, and eosinophils (at least 25% of inflammatory cells) are suggestive of drug-induced cholestatic hepatitis. Hepatic granuloma formation is another common type of hepatic drug reaction. In cases of steatohepatitis, hepatic fibrosis, or liver tumors, no specific clues to a drug cause have been recognized, although sex steroids increase the vascularity of hepatic tumors and are frequently associated with sinusoidal dilatation or peliosis hepatis. Drug-induced steatohepatitis caused by amiodarone and perhexilene tends to be associated with severe lesions that more closely resemble alcoholic hepatitis than NASH.[73] Other drugs (e.g., tamoxifen, methotrexate) cause lesions that are indistinguishable from NASH associated with diabetes mellitus and the metabolic syndrome.[22,24]

Although detection of "signature" lesions support a diagnosis of DILI, most patients with DILI are not subjected to liver biopsy unless the reaction is severe or unexpected or improvement fails to occur after cessation of the drug. One particular situation in which liver histology is often sought is consideration of a diagnosis of AIH, although in this circumstance, liver histology may not be as helpful as desired. In a 2011 study, 4 expert hepatopathologists reviewed 35 cases of AIH and 28 cases of DILI. The interobserver agreement was only 46% for histology alone and increased to 60% to 71% if both clinical and pathologic features were considered. Although the ability to distinguish DILI from AIH improved considerably if a combination of histologic features was used, these observations highlight the potential limitations of histologic appraisal in this setting.[74]

Clinical Features

The history and physical examination can provide important clues to the diagnosis of hepatic drug reactions. Most

TABLE 88-4 Clinicopathologic Classification of Drug-Induced Liver Disease

Category	Description	Implicated Drugs: Examples
Hepatic adaptation	No symptoms; raised serum GGTP and AP levels (occasionally raised ALT) Hyperbilirubinemia	Phenytoin, warfarin, heparins Rifampin, HIV protease inhibitors
Dose-dependent hepatotoxicity	Symptoms of hepatitis; zonal, bridging, and massive necrosis; serum ALT level > 5-fold increased, often > 2000 U/L	Acetaminophen, nicotinic acid, amodiaquine, hycanthone
Other cytopathic toxicity, acute steatosis	Microvesicular steatosis, diffuse or zonal; partially dose dependent, severe liver injury, features of mitochondrial toxicity (lactic acidosis)	Valproic acid, didanosine, HAART agents, fialuridine, L-asparaginase, some herbal medicines
Acute hepatitis	Symptoms of hepatitis; focal, bridging, and massive necrosis; serum ALT level > 5-fold increased; extrahepatic features of drug allergy in some cases	Isoniazid, dantrolene, nitrofurantoin, halothane, sulfonamides, phenytoin, disulfiram, acebutolol, etretinate, ketoconazole, terbinafine, troglitazone
Chronic hepatitis	Duration > 3 months; interface hepatitis, bridging necrosis, fibrosis, cirrhosis; clinical and laboratory features of chronic liver disease; autoantibodies with some types of reaction	Nitrofurantoin, etretinate, diclofenac, minocycline, nefazodone (see Table 88-6)
Granulomatous hepatitis	Hepatic granulomas with varying hepatitis and cholestasis; raised serum ALT, AP, GGTP levels	Allopurinol, carbamazepine, hydralazine, quinidine, quinine (see Table 88-5)
Cholestasis without hepatitis	Cholestasis, no inflammation; serum AP levels > twice normal	Oral contraceptives, androgens
Cholestatic hepatitis	Cholestasis with inflammation; symptoms of hepatitis; raised serum ALT and AP levels	Chlorpromazine, tricyclic antidepressants, erythromycins, amoxicillin–clavulanic acid, cyproterone acetate
Cholestasis with bile duct injury	Bile duct lesions and cholestatic hepatitis; clinical features of cholangitis	Chlorpromazine, flucloxacillin, dextropropoxyphene
Chronic cholestasis:	Duration > 3 months	
Vanishing bile duct syndrome (VBDS)	Paucity of small bile ducts; resembles PBC but AMA negative	Chlorpromazine, flucloxacillin, trimethoprim/sulfamethoxazole
Sclerosing cholangitis	Strictures of large bile ducts	Intra-arterial floxuridine, intralesional scolicidals
Steatohepatitis	Steatosis, focal necrosis, Mallory's hyaline, pericellular fibrosis, cirrhosis; chronic liver disease, portal hypertension	Perhexiline, amiodarone, tamoxifen
Fibrosis and cirrhosis	Fibrosis, nodular regeneration (Other features [e.g., interface hepatitis, steatohepatitis, paucity of bile ducts, cholestasis] depend on etiology.)	Methotrexate, cyproterone acetate; also see VBDS, chronic hepatitis, steatohepatitis
Vascular disorders	Sinusoidal obstruction syndrome, nodular regenerative hyperplasia, others	Many (see Table 88-10)
Tumors	Hepatocellular carcinoma, adenoma, angiosarcoma, others	Many (see Chapter 96)

AMA, antimitochondrial antibodies; AP, alkaline phosphatase.

important is the temporal pattern of disease evolution in relation to exposure to drugs or toxins. Identification of specific risk factors for hepatotoxicity (e.g., chronic excessive alcohol intake in a person taking acetaminophen) and the presence of systemic features of drug hypersensitivity may indicate the correct diagnosis. Systemic features include fever, rash, mucositis, eosinophilia, lymphadenopathy, a mononucleosis-like syndrome, bone marrow suppression, vasculitis, renal failure, pneumonitis, and pancreatitis. These features may be part of a characteristic syndrome thought to have a genetic basis and likely mediated by formation of drug metabolites that act as haptens to initiate an immunodestructive tissue reaction, termed the *DRESS syndrome*. Reactivation of viral infections, notably human herpesvirus 6 or 7 (HHV-6, HHV-7) and Epstein-Barr virus infections, has also been implicated in the pathogenesis.[75,76] Further, the detection of HHV-6 has been proposed as a diagnostic marker for the DRESS syndrome.

DRESS (Drug Reaction with Eosinophilia and Systemic Symptoms) Syndrome

Drugs implicated as a cause of DRESS syndrome include sulfonamides, aminopenicillins, fluoroquinolones, clozapine, anticonvulsants (phenytoin, lamotrigine, phenobarbital, carbamazepine, valproic acid), minocycline, protease inhibitors (nevirapine, abacavir), pentoxyphilline, some NSAIDs, and Chinese herbal medicines.[75] Risk factors for DRESS syndrome include a family history of an affected first-degree relative (increases the risk to 1 in 4) and a personal history of drug allergy, including to aspirin. Use of other drugs, such as glucocorticoids or valproic acid, at the time the new agent is started increases the risk 4- to 10-fold. The presence of a disorder associated with immune dysregulation (e.g., systemic lupus erythematosus) increases the risk 10-fold, whereas HIV/AIDS increases the risk 100-fold.

The illness characteristically begins between 1 and 12 weeks (typically 2 to 4 weeks) after the drug is started; "sentinel symptoms" include fever, pharyngitis, malaise, periorbital edema, headache or otalgia, rhinorrhea, and mouth ulcers. A severe drug rash is an essential feature. Erythematous reactions are usual and may evolve to toxic epidermal necrolysis or erythema multiforme, often with mucositis (Stevens-Johnson syndrome). Early abnormalities on blood testing include neutrophilia and elevated levels of acute-phase reactants; atypical lymphocytosis and eosinophilia may be noted later. Hepatic reactions are found in about 13% of cases. Findings include cholestasis, acute hepatitis, and granulomas. Other features include lymphadenopathy (16%), nephritis (6%), pneumonitis (6%), and more severe hematologic abnormalities (5%). In a literature review of cases reported as DRESS syndrome or drug hypersensitivity reactions from 1997 to 2009, 172 reactions involving 44 drugs were documented.[75] Although skin involvement was present in all cases, features associated with "probable" or "definite" cases of DRESS syndrome were eosinophilia, liver involvement (abnormal liver biochemical test results in 59%, hepatomegaly in 12%), fever, and lymphadenopathy.[75]

Latent Period to Onset

For idiosyncratic reactions, a latent period occurs between starting the drug and the onset of clinical and laboratory abnormalities. This period is commonly 2 to 8 weeks for immunoallergic types of drug hepatitis (e.g., DRESS syndrome) and often 6 to 20 weeks or longer for agents like isoniazid, dantrolene, and troglitazone. Occasionally, liver injury may become evident after discontinuation of the causative agent; for oxypenicillins and amoxicillin–clavulanic acid, the onset of hepatotoxicity may occur as long as 2 weeks after the end of therapy. In other cases, hepatotoxicity is rare after the first exposure to a drug but more frequent and more severe after subsequent courses. Examples include halothane, nitrofurantoin, and dacarbazine. A history of a previous reaction to the drug in question (inadvertent rechallenge) may, therefore, be the key to the diagnosis of DILI.

Dechallenge and Rechallenge

Another aspect of the temporal relationship between ingestion of a drug and hepatotoxicity is the response to discontinuation of the drug, or *dechallenge*. Dechallenge should be accompanied by discernible and progressive improvement within days or weeks of stopping the incriminated agent. Exceptions occur with ketoconazole, troglitazone, etretinate, and amiodarone; with these agents, reactions may be severe, and clinical recovery may be delayed for months. Although some types of drug-induced cholestasis also can be prolonged, failure of jaundice to resolve in a suspected drug reaction most often is indicative of an alternative diagnosis. Rarely, deliberate rechallenge may be used to confirm the diagnosis of DILI or prove involvement of one particular agent when the patient has been exposed to several drugs; however, this approach is potentially hazardous. In a series of 88 cases where DILI developed following drug challenge, severe hepatocellular injury with jaundice occurred in 14, and 2 died.[77] Therefore, rechallenge should be undertaken only with a fully informed and consenting (in writing) patient and preferably with the approval of an institutional ethics committee.

Diagnosis

In the absence of specific diagnostic tests, diagnosis of DILI requires clinical suspicion, a thorough drug history, careful consideration of the temporal relationships between drug ingestion and liver disease, and exclusion of other disorders. The objective weighing of evidence for and against an individual agent—*causality assessment*—is a probabilistic form of diagnosis.[78,79] Several clinical scales that incorporate and weigh various features of hepatic adverse drug reactions have been described.[25,80,81] A liver biopsy may be indicated in some cases to exclude other diseases and to provide further clues to a drug etiology. Rechallenge is currently the standard test for DILI but is hardly ever used in practice. Future strategies include the use of in vitro tests to provide confirmatory evidence for particular drugs.[68-70,73,78,80] There is increasing interest in toxicogenomic methods for the diagnosis of DILI. These methods encompass studies of transcriptomics, metabonomics, and proteomics (measuring circulating messenger RNA [mRNA] or miRNA, metabolites, and cellular proteins, respectively).[82,83] In some studies, toxicogenomic changes preceded elevations in serum aminotransferase levels, thereby raising the hope that these changes could serve as biomarkers of early DILI.[84]

Physician Awareness

Physician awareness is critical for the diagnosis of DILI. The sources of potential hepatotoxins include prescribed medications, over-the-counter drugs (e.g., ibuprofen), CAM preparations (see Chapters 89 and 131), recreational drugs (e.g., cocaine, ecstasy) or self-poisoning, and environmental contaminants in food and water supplies, the home, the workplace, and the community. Unfortunately, patients and physicians do not always heed early nonspecific symptoms associated with reactions to hepatotoxic drugs. For example, preventable deaths from liver failure still occur decades after the recognition that isoniazid can cause drug hepatitis (see later).[85] Although continuing education and availability of information about potentially hepatotoxic drugs are important issues, physicians have a professional and legal obligation to inform patients about possible adverse drug reactions. Experience suggests that drug reactions may not be mentioned as a diagnosis in physicians' discharge notes in over half the cases.

Drug toxicity should be considered a possibility in cases of obscure or poorly explained liver disease, particularly in cases with mixed or atypical patterns of cholestasis and hepatitis; cholestasis in which common causes have been excluded, especially in older adults; and histologic features suggestive of a drug etiology. In such cases, the drug history must be addressed as a special investigation, with attention paid to additional sources of information (household members, primary care providers), household drugs, non-prescribed medications, and environmental toxins (see Chapter 89). LiverTox is a web-based searchable database of information relating to liver injury resulting from the use of prescription and nonprescription drugs (see http://www.livertox.nih.gov/).

Exclusion of Other Disorders

Other diseases must be excluded before hepatobiliary disease can be ascribed to a drug. For acute and chronic hepatocellular reactions, viral and autoimmune causes of hepatitis and vascular and metabolic disorders must be considered. Some cases of acute hepatitis E have been mislabeled as cases of DILI.[86] Some types of drug-induced chronic hepatitis are associated with autoantibodies and superficially resemble AIH. An approach to the correct diagnosis is described later (see Nitrofurantoin). Drug-induced cholestasis should be considered only when biliary obstruction has has been excluded by imaging. In older patients, and particularly when drug exposure does not include agents known to cause cholestasis, cholangiography (e.g., magnetic resonance imaging [MRCP], endoscopic retrograde cholangiography [ERCP]) is obligatory, as is liver biopsy.

Extrahepatic Features

The constellation of rash, eosinophilia, and other organ involvement is relatively specific for an adverse drug reaction as a cause of liver disease (DRESS, see earlier). Because these findings are present in only a minority of cases, their absence is not helpful. In particular, drugs that cause idiosyncratic liver injury by nonimmunologic mechanisms are not usually associated with extrahepatic features. Specific diagnostic tests for individual drug-induced liver diseases have been described[68] but are not generally accepted or available. In the case of dose-dependent hepatotoxins, blood levels may be helpful (see later).

Chronologic Relationships

For most drugs, the chronologic relationship among drug ingestion, onset, and resolution of liver injury remains the most important consideration in diagnosis. The criteria for temporal eligibility include the relationship of drug ingestion to onset, course of the reaction after discontinuation of the drug, and response to readministration of the drug.[1,22-25] Inadvertent rechallenge may have occurred already. The rechallenge is regarded as positive if the serum ALT or alkaline phosphatase level increases at least 2-fold.[18,22,25] Deliberate rechallenge (discussed earlier) may be considered to ascertain whether a drug that is important for an individual patient (e.g., amiodarone for refractory ventricular tachycardia) is responsible for hepatotoxicity.

Which Drug?

New and nonproprietary compounds should arouse particular suspicion. For patients who are taking multiple drugs, the agent started most recently before the onset of liver injury is most likely to be responsible. If that agent is unlikely to be the culprit and another well-known hepatotoxin is being taken, the latter is the more likely culprit. When possible, the most likely hepatotoxin or all therapeutic agents should be discontinued. If the patient improves, the drugs that are unlikely to be responsible can be carefully reintroduced.

Indications for Liver Biopsy

Liver biopsy may be helpful in difficult cases, especially when temporal relationship between the ingestion of a known hepatotoxic agent and the onset of liver injury is unclear. In practice, for example, the onset of jaundice within 2 to 6 weeks of starting an agent such as amoxicillin–clavulanic acid or of acute hepatitis in the presence of other features of DRESS syndrome in a person taking nevirapine as part of HAART would be contexts where the suspicion of a drug etiology is so strong that liver biopsy is unnecessary. Conversely, substantially abnormal liver biochemical test levels (e.g., a serum ALT level elevated more than 5-fold) in a person who has one or more autoantibodies suggestive of AIH and has been taking a statin or other cardiovascular drug for 3 to 6 months may constitute a clinical challenge that often can be resolved only by liver biopsy. The medical community may benefit when new instances or patterns of DILI are adequately defined; this benefit may persuade the clinician (but not always the informed patient) to proceed with a liver biopsy in equivocal cases.

Considerations in Patients with Viral Hepatitis

Patients with chronic hepatitis B or C may be at higher risk of liver injury from antituberculosis chemotherapy, ibuprofen and possibly other NSAIDs, anticancer drugs, and HAART compared with persons without viral hepatitis.[43] A more common clinical problem is the finding of a serum ALT level greater than 300 U/L at a routine office visit in a patient with previous levels less than 150 U/L. In patients with hepatitis C, the rise in serum ALT is more likely due to DILI than to a spontaneous change in the activity of the hepatitis C, particularly when the ALT level is greater than 1000 U/L. The most commonly implicated agents are acetaminophen taken in moderate doses under conditions of increased risk (e.g., fasting, alcohol excess, use of other medication) and CAM preparations (see Chapter 89). Clinical suspicion is essential for recognizing DILI so that appropriate advice can be given. Determination of serum acetaminophen levels may be useful in difficult cases, but levels (particularly undetectable levels) can be difficult to interpret in the context of regular ingestion, as opposed to a single episode of self-poisoning (see later).

Prevention and Management

With the exception of acetaminophen hepatotoxicity, little effective treatment for DILI is available, other than liver transplantation for liver failure. Special emphasis must be placed on prevention and early detection of liver injury as well as on prompt withdrawal of the offending agent. Safe use of over-the-counter agents such as acetaminophen, NSAIDs, and CAM preparations is important. Clear and open communication between the physician and patient and appropriate recommendations about dose limitations could prevent most instances of liver injury from these agents.

Most drugs associated with DILI are idiosyncratic hepatotoxins for which liver injury rarely occurs. Avoiding overuse of these drugs can minimize the overall frequency of adverse hepatic reactions; antibiotics such as amoxicillin–clavulanic acid and flucloxacillin are pertinent examples. Similarly, polypharmacy should be avoided when possible. Post-marketing surveillance of new drugs is critical, and all physicians should participate in reporting adverse effects to monitoring agencies.

For dose-dependent hepatotoxins, prevention depends on adherence to dosage guidelines or use of blood levels. This approach has virtually abolished some forms of DILI, such as tetracycline-induced fatty liver, aspirin hepatitis, and methotrexate-induced hepatic fibrosis. In cases with specific risk factors, strategies to prevent toxicity are essential (e.g., avoid use of valproic acid with other drugs in the very young; do not prescribe methotrexate to persons who consume alcohol in excess). Moderate doses of acetaminophen are contraindicated in heavy drinkers and after fasting,[38] and administration of halothane should not be repeated within 28 days or in persons suspected of previous sensitivity to a haloalkane anesthetic (see Chapter 89).

Early detection is also critical. Patients should be warned to report any untoward symptoms, particularly unexplained nausea, malaise, right upper quadrant abdominal pain, lethargy, or fever. These nonspecific features may represent the prodrome of drug-induced hepatitis. They are an indication for liver biochemical testing and, if the results suggest liver injury, for cessation of treatment.

A more difficult issue is whether regular (protocol) screening with liver biochemical tests should be performed when a drug is prescribed. Although authors and drug manufacturers often recommend such screening, the efficiency and cost-effectiveness of this approach are unknown. The onset of liver injury is often rapid, rendering once-a-month or every-second-week screening futile. Furthermore, 7.5% of persons who receive placebo in clinical trials have persistently raised serum ALT levels. If liver biochemical test levels are monitored, the level of abnormality at which a drug should be discontinued is uncertain, as illustrated by isoniazid, which causes some liver biochemical test abnormality in 30% of exposed subjects. Generally, the recommendation is that isoniazid be stopped if serum ALT levels exceed 250 U/L or more than 5 times the ULN, but elevation of the serum bilirubin or albumin concentration, prolongation of the prothrombin time, or any pertinent symptoms provides a clearer indication to stop the drug. Conversely, a rise in the serum GGTP level or a minor elevation in the serum alkaline phosphatase level usually indicates hepatic adaptation rather than liver injury. We do not routinely recommend protocol screening except for methotrexate, but this approach could be useful for agents such as valproic acid, isoniazid, pyrazinamide, ketoconazole, dantrolene, thiazolidinediones, and synthetic retinoids, either because the onset of liver injury may be delayed and gradual in some cases or because such screening can emphasize the hepatotoxic potential of these drugs to patients and physicians. Ultrasound elastography (see Chapters 73 and 74) and possibly liver biopsy has a role in the assessment of hepatic fibrosis in patients who take methotrexate (see later).

Active management of DILI includes removal of the drug and administration of antidotes. In practice, treatment usually is confined to discontinuation of the hepatotoxic drug. Failure to discontinue a drug that is the cause of liver injury is the single most important factor leading to poor outcomes like acute liver failure and chronic liver disease.[24,25] For ingested toxins (e.g., metals, acetaminophen), removal of the unabsorbed drug by aspirating stomach contents may be appropriate. Methods to remove absorbed toxins (charcoal hemodialysis, forced diuresis) are ineffective. Thiol replacement therapy, usually with N-acetylcysteine (NAC), is indicated as an antidote for acetaminophen poisoning (see later).

Beyond discontinuation of the offending agent, the management of DILI is symptomatic and supportive. In cases of acute liver failure, NAC can be used, but hepatic transplantation should be considered earlier rather than at an advanced stage (see Chapter 97).[23] Ursodeoxycholic acid has shown some promise in managing drug-induced cholestasis, but

glucocorticoids are ineffective. Glucocorticoids have little role in the cases of drug-induced hepatitis and are ineffective in chlorpromazine-, methyldopa-, and isoniazid-induced hepatitis and in drug-induced fulminant hepatic failure. Case reports attest to the occasional effectiveness of glucocorticoids in protracted cases of hepatitis caused by etretinate, allopurinol, diclofenac, or ketoconazole.[1] Glucocorticoids should be reserved for atypical and refractory cases, particularly those associated with vasculitis.

DOSE-DEPENDENT HEPATOTOXICITY

Few dose-dependent hepatotoxins are clinically relevant today. Examples include acetaminophen, some herbal medicines, plant and fungal toxins, amodiaquine, hycanthone, vitamin A, methotrexate, cyclophosphamide, anticancer drugs, carbon tetrachloride, phosphorus, and metals (especially iron, copper, and mercury).

Acetaminophen

General Nature, Frequency, and Predisposing Factors

Acetaminophen (paracetamol) is safe in recommended therapeutic doses of 1 to 4 g daily, but hepatotoxicity produced by self-poisoning with acetaminophen has been recognized since the 1960s. Despite the effectiveness of thiol-based antidotes, acetaminophen remains the most common cause of DILI in most countries and an important cause of acute liver failure.[23,87] Parasuicide (suicide attempt) and suicide are the usual reasons for overdose. Although controversial,[88] hepatologists and pediatricians see cases of acetaminophen poisoning that have arisen through what Zimmerman and Maddrey termed *therapeutic misadventure*.[89] This occurrence is especially common in persons who habitually drink alcohol to excess and has also been recognized after daily ingestion of moderate therapeutic doses (10 to 20 g over 3 days) of acetaminophen in adults and children who are fasting or malnourished[38] or who are taking drugs that interact with the metabolism of acetaminophen.[89]

Single doses of acetaminophen that exceed 7 to 10 g (140 mg/kg body weight in children) may cause liver injury, but this outcome is not inevitable. Severe liver injury (serum ALT level > 1000 U/L) or fatal cases usually involve doses of at least 15 to 25 g, but because of inter-individual variability, survival is possible even after ingestion of a massive single dose of acetaminophen (>50 g).[90] Among persons with an untreated acetaminophen overdose, severe liver injury occurred in only 20%, and among those with severe liver injury, the mortality rate was 20%.[90] Conversely, among heavy drinkers, daily acetaminophen doses of 2 to 6 g have been associated with fatal hepatotoxicity.[88-91]

Risk factors for acetaminophen-induced hepatotoxicity are summarized in Table 88-5. Children are relatively resistant to acetaminophen-induced hepatotoxicity,[92] possibly because of their tendency to ingest smaller doses, greater likelihood of vomiting, or biological resistance. However, liver injury has been reported with intravenous acetaminophen use in children (usually due to dosing errors).[93] Therapeutic misadventure after multiple doses, especially during fasting and when weight-based recommendations have been exceeded, has a high mortality rate.[94] By contrast, the presence of underlying liver disease does not predispose to acetaminophen hepatotoxicity.

Self-poisoning with acetaminophen is most common in young women, but fatalities are most frequent in men, possibly because of alcoholism and late presentation.[87,91,95] The time of presentation is critical because thiol therapy given within

TABLE 88-5 Risk Factors for Acetaminophen-Induced Hepatotoxicity

Factor	Relevance
Age	Children may be more resistant than adults
Dose	Minimal hepatotoxic dose: 7.5 g (≈100 mg/kg) in adults, 150 mg/kg in children
	Severe toxicity possible with a dose > 15 g
Blood level of acetaminophen	Influenced by dose, time after ingestion, gastric emptying
	Best indicator of risk of hepatotoxicity (see text and Fig. 88-2)
Chronic excessive alcohol ingestion	Toxic dose threshold is lowered; worsens prognosis (also related to late presentation); nephrotoxicity common
Fasting	Toxic dose threshold is lowered— therapeutic misadventure (see text)
Concomitant medication	Toxic dose threshold is lowered— therapeutic misadventure; worsens prognosis (e.g., isoniazid, phenytoin, zidovudine)
Time of presentation	Late presentation or delayed treatment (>16 hours) predicts a worse outcome

12 hours of acetaminophen poisoning virtually abolishes significant liver injury (see later). Therapeutic misadventure is also associated with a worse outcome.[88] Concomitant use of agents such as phenobarbital, phenytoin, isoniazid, and zidovudine increases the risk of hepatotoxicity. These drugs promote the oxidative metabolism of acetaminophen to NAPQI by inducing CYP2E1 (for isoniazid) or CYP3A4 (for phenytoin) or by competing with glucuronidation pathways (for zidovudine). Alcohol and fasting have dual effects by enhancing expression of CYP2E1 and by depleting hepatic glutathione. Fasting also may impair acetaminophen conjugation by depleting cofactors for the glucuronidation and sulfation pathways.[38]

Acetaminophen hepatotoxicity produces zone 3 hepatic necrosis, with extension into submassive (bridging) or panacinar (massive) necrosis in severe cases. Inflammation is minimal, and recovery is associated with complete resolution without fibrosis. The zonal pattern of acetaminophen-induced necrosis is related to the mechanism of hepatotoxicity, particularly the role of CYP2E1, which is expressed in zone 3, and to lower levels of glutathione in zone 3 hepatocytes than in hepatocytes in the other zones.

Clinical Course, Outcomes, and Prognostic Indicators

In the first 2 days after acetaminophen self-poisoning, features of liver injury are not present. Nausea, vomiting, and drowsiness are often due to concomitant ingestion of alcohol and other drugs. After 48 to 72 hours, serum ALT levels may be elevated, and symptoms such as anorexia, nausea and

vomiting, fatigue, and malaise may occur. Hepatic pain may be pronounced. Repeated vomiting, jaundice, hypoglycemia, and other features of acute liver failure, particularly coagulopathy and hepatic encephalopathy, characterize severe cases. The liver may shrink as a result of severe necrosis. Serum levels of ALT are often between 2000 and 10,000 U/L. These high levels can help clinch the diagnosis in complex settings, as may occur with alcoholic patients and those with viral hepatitis.[89]

Indicators of a poor outcome[87,88,91,95] include grade IV hepatic coma, acidosis, severe and sustained impairment of coagulation factor synthesis, renal failure, and a pattern of falling serum ALT levels in conjunction with a worsening prothrombin time (see Chapter 95). Renal failure reflects acute tubular necrosis or hepatorenal syndrome. Myocardial injury also has been attributable to acetaminophen toxicity.[90] Death occurs between 4 and 18 days after the overdose and generally results from cerebral edema and sepsis complicating hepatic and multiorgan failure. A majority of patients recover completely. Cases of apparent chronic hepatotoxicity rarely have been attributed to continued ingestion of acetaminophen (2 to 6 g/day), usually in a susceptible host such as a heavy drinker or a person with preexisting unrecognized liver disease.[1,22] Rare cases of acetaminophen hypersensitivity, typically involving skin or lung, have been reported in association with liver injury.[96]

Treatment

In patients who present within 4 hours of ingesting an excessive amount of acetaminophen, the stomach should be emptied with a wide-bore gastric tube. Osmotic cathartics or binding agents have little if any role in management. The focus of management is on identifying patients who should receive thiol-based antidote therapy and, in those with established severe liver injury, assessing the patient's candidacy for liver transplantation.

Blood levels of acetaminophen should be measured at the time of presentation. Because of delayed gastric emptying, however, blood levels within 4 hours of ingestion may underestimate the extent of exposure. After 4 hours, acetaminophen blood levels give a reliable indicator of the risk of liver injury in patients with an acute overdose (not in those with a therapeutic misadventure). The risk of liver injury is then estimated by reference to the Prescott nomogram (Fig. 88-2).[90] Indications for antidote therapy include a reliable history of major poisoning (>10 g) or blood acetaminophen levels in the moderate- or high-risk bands on the monogram, or both.[90,95] At-risk patients should be hospitalized for monitoring.

Hepatic necrosis occurs only when glutathione concentrations fall below a critical level, thereby allowing NAPQI to produce liver injury. Administration of cysteine donors stimulates hepatic synthesis of glutathione. Many cysteine precursors or thiol donors could be used, but NAC has become the agent of choice. Oral administration is preferred in the United States,[87,90] with a loading dose of 140 mg/kg followed by administration of 70 mg/kg every 4 hours for 72 hours. This regimen is highly effective despite the theoretical disadvantage that delayed gastric emptying and vomiting may reduce intestinal absorption of NAC. In Europe and Australia, NAC is administered by slow bolus intravenous injection followed by infusion (150 mg/kg over 15 minutes in 200 mL of 5% dextrose, with a second dose of 50 mg/kg 4 hours later if blood acetaminophen levels indicate a high risk of hepatotoxicity, and a total dose over 24 hours of 300 mg/kg).[90] The intravenous regimen is also now available in the United States and approved for patients who cannot tolerate oral NAC.[97] The intravenous route may be associated with a higher rate of

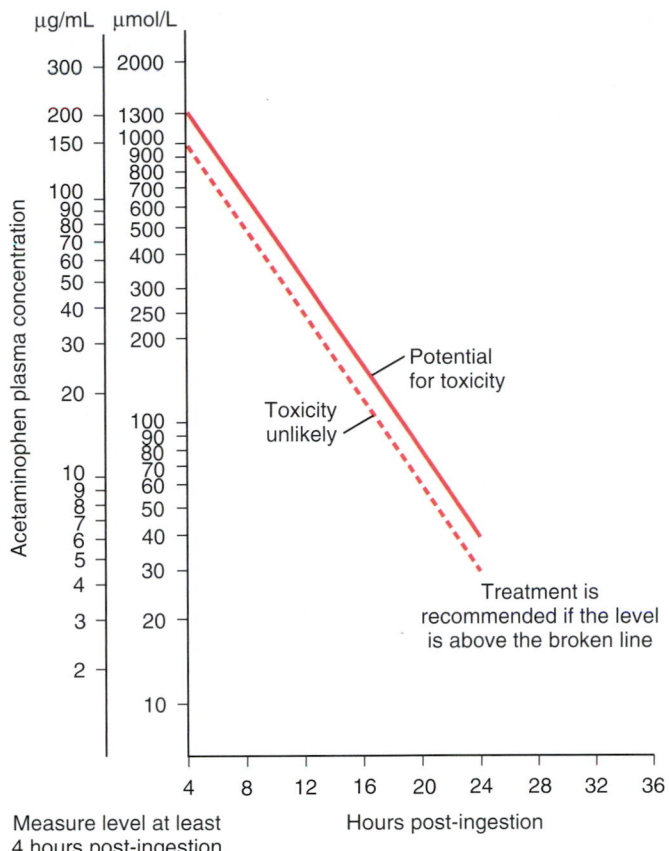

Measure level at least
4 hours post-ingestion

FIGURE 88-2. Acetaminophen toxicity nomogram. The risk of hepatotoxicity correlates with the plasma acetaminophen level and the time after ingestion. *(From Smilkstein MJ, Knapp GL, Kulig KW, et al. Efficacy of oral N-acetylcysteine in the treatment of acetaminophen overdose. Analysis of the National Multicenter Study [1976-1985]. N Engl J Med 1988; 319:1557-62.)*

prospects for successful psychological rehabilitation (see Chapter 97).[95] There are issues relating to poor adherence and self-harm post transplantation that cannot be predicted accurately by pretransplant assessment.[99] In several series, about 60% of listed patients have been transplanted, and survival rates have exceeded 70%.[95]

Prevention

Safe use of acetaminophen involves adherence to the recommended maximum dose for healthy adults and children and education about the risk factors that lower the toxic dose threshold. Acetaminophen doses of more than 2 g/day are contraindicated in heavy drinkers, in those taking other medications (particularly phenytoin, zidovudine, and isoniazid), and during fasting. Prolonged use of acetaminophen requires caution in patients with severe cardiorespiratory disease or advanced cirrhosis. Use of acetaminophen for self-poisoning continues despite attempts at public education about the risks involved. The chances of harm from a suicidal gesture may be reduced by the sale of acetaminophen in smaller package sizes and in blister packs, which hamper ready access to the tablets or capsules.[100,101]

Other Causes

Some hepatotoxins are not as clearly dose dependent as acetaminophen but cause cytopathic or cytotoxic changes like extensive hydropic change, diffuse or zonal microvesicular steatosis, and zonal necrosis.[1,22] Injury likely represents *metabolic idiosyncrasy,* in which the drug or one of its metabolites accumulates and interferes with protein synthesis or intermediary metabolism, or both. The mitochondrion often appears to be the main subcellular target, and other metabolically active tissues can be involved. Pancreatitis and renal tubular injury may accompany severe liver injury caused by valproic acid, tetracycline, and HAART, and metabolic acidosis with a shock-like state is common. This presentation was first recognized with intravenous high-dose tetracycline (>2 g/day for more than 4 days) in pregnant women, men taking estrogens, or patients in renal failure.[22] With appropriate dose limitations, this reaction is entirely preventable.

Niacin (Nicotinic Acid)

Hepatotoxicity associated with niacin, or nicotinic acid, has been noted since the 1960s. When used to treat hypercholesterolemia, niacin has been an important cause of liver injury.[102] It is a dose-dependent hepatotoxin; liver injury usually occurs at doses that exceed 2 g/day, but in rare instances, low-dose (500 mg/day) sustained-release niacin has been implicated in fulminant hepatic failure. Patients on sulfonylurea drugs and those with preexisting liver disease, particularly alcoholic hepatitis, are at increased risk. No association with age, diet, or insulin-managed diabetes mellitus has been recognized. The symptoms of liver injury begin as early as 1 week to as long as 4 years after the drug is started. The clinicopathologic spectrum encompasses mild and transient increases in serum ALT levels, jaundice, acute hepatitis, and cholestasis. Liver injury resolves completely when the drug is stopped. Liver biopsy shows hepatic necrosis and centrilobular cholestasis. Well-documented cases of fulminant hepatitis, some necessitating liver transplantation, also have been attributed to niacin. Substituting one niacin preparation for another without a dose adjustment should be avoided; switching from immediate- to sustained-release preparations requires a 50% to 70% reduction in the dose of niacin. Doses of sustained-release niacin should not exceed 2 g/day.[103]

hypersensitivity reactions because of the higher systemic blood levels achieved.[1] Adverse reactions to NAC are common but usually mild[98]; however, they can be occasionally severe, with rash, angioedema, and shock. Therefore, NAC must be administered under close supervision and only for appropriate indications. In patients known to be sensitized to NAC, methionine is probably just as effective but is not available in a commercial preparation; it must be made up fresh and often causes vomiting.[90]

Cases of acetaminophen-induced severe liver injury are virtually abolished if NAC is administered within 16 hours of acetaminophen ingestion.[87,90,95] After 16 hours, thiol donation is unlikely to affect the development of liver injury because oxidation of acetaminophen to NAPQI with consequent oxidation of thiol groups is complete and mitochondrial injury and activation of cell death pathways are likely to be established. Nevertheless, NAC has also been reported to decrease the mortality associated with acetaminophen-induced hepatotoxicity when administered 16 to 36 hours after self-poisoning,[87,90,95] possibly because NAC stabilizes vascular reactivity in patients with liver failure. Therefore, administration of NAC is recommended for patients with a late presentation after acetaminophen overdose.

Liver transplantation is a therapeutic option for select patients in whom liver failure develops after acetaminophen poisoning.[99] The selection of cases is based on the prognostic indicators discussed earlier and is strongly influenced by the

Valproic Acid (Sodium Valproate)

Valproic acid–associated hepatic injury occurs almost exclusively in children, particularly those younger than 3 years of age. Also at risk are persons with a family history of a mitochondrial enzyme deficiency (particularly involving the urea cycle or long-chain fatty acid metabolism) (see Chapter 77), Friedreich's ataxia, or Reye's syndrome or with a sibling affected by valproic acid hepatotoxicity. Another risk factor is multiple drug therapy. Cases in adults have been described rarely. Genetic analysis of 17 patients with valproic acid hepatotoxicity revealed mutations within the mitochondrial polymerase γ gene (POLG) in nearly half (8 of 17) of the subjects, and these mutations carried a greater than 20-fold increased risk of valproic acid–associated liver injury compared with population-matched controls.[104] The overall risk of liver injury among persons taking valproic acid varies from 1 per 500 persons exposed among high-risk groups (children younger than 3, polypharmacy, genetic defects of mitochondrial enzymes) to less than 1 in 37,000 among low-risk groups.[105]

No relationship exists between valproic acid toxicity and dose, but blood levels of valproic acid tend to be high in half of affected persons. The metabolite 4-en-valproic acid, produced by CYP-catalyzed metabolism of valproic acid, is a dose-dependent hepatotoxin in animals and in vitro. The concept has emerged that valproic acid is an occult dose-dependent toxin in which accumulation of a hepatotoxic metabolite (favored by co-exposure to CYP-inducing antiepileptic agents) produces mitochondrial injury in a susceptible host (e.g., young children, especially those with partial deficiencies of mitochondrial enzymes).[106] Valproic acid also inhibits synthesis of carnitine, a cofactor in mitochondrial fatty acid beta oxidation (and also for valproic acid).

Symptoms begin within 4 to 12 weeks, are often nonspecific, and include lethargy, malaise, poor feeding, somnolence, worsening seizures, muscle weakness, and facial swelling. In typical cases, features of hepatotoxicity follow, including anorexia, nausea, vomiting, right upper quadrant abdominal discomfort, and weight loss.[105,106] When jaundice ensues, hypoglycemia, ascites, coagulopathy, and encephalopathy indicate liver failure with imminent coma and death. In some cases, a neurologic syndrome characterized by ataxia, mental confusion, and coma predominates, with little evidence of hepatic involvement. In other cases, fever and tender hepatomegaly suggestive of Reye's syndrome may be present (see later); such cases tend to have a better prognosis. Additional extrahepatic features may include alopecia, hypofibrinogenemia, thrombocytopenia, and pancreatitis. The terminal phase is often indicated by renal failure, hypoglycemia, metabolic acidosis, and severe bacterial infection.

Laboratory features include modest elevations of serum bilirubin and aminotransferase levels; the AST level is usually higher than the ALT level. A profound decrease in clotting factor levels, hypoalbuminemia, and raised serum ammonia levels are common. A small liver with increased echogenicity suggestive of steatosis or extensive necrosis is seen on hepatic imaging. Histologic examination shows submassive or massive hepatic necrosis in two thirds of cases with either zonal or generalized microvesicular steatosis.[106] Ultrastructural studies indicate conspicuous mitochondrial abnormalities.

Treatment is supportive. Small nonrandomized studies have shown that intravenous L-carnitine supplementation can reduce hyperammonemia and improve survival in severe cases.[107] Liver transplantation has been performed successfully, but poor outcomes have been recorded, particularly in children, implying that case selection must be individualized.[108] Prevention depends on adherence to prescribing guidelines, including avoiding valproic acid in combination with other drugs in the first 3 years of life and in children who may have mitochondrial enzyme abnormalities. Pretreatment screening for POLG mutations is recommended for high-risk groups.[109] Liver biochemical test abnormalities develop in at least 40% of patients on valproic acid and are therefore an unreliable predictor of severe hepatotoxicity. Warning patients and parents about the need to report any adverse symptoms during the first 6 months of valproic acid therapy is most important.

Antiretroviral Agents

Abnormal liver biochemical test levels and clinical evidence of liver disease are common in patients with HIV/AIDS. Potential causes include HBV or HCV infection, other hepatobiliary infections, lymphoma and other tumors, and possibly effects of HIV infection itself. The frequency of hepatic injury with HAART (which often includes 3 or 4 agents) is at least 10%.[40,44,110,111] The agents used can be broadly categorized as nucleoside (or nucleotide) and non-nucleoside reverse transcriptase inhibitors, protease inhibitors, fusion inhibitors, integrase inhibitors, and CCR5 blockers. Because HIV coinfection with HBV or HCV increases the risk of hepatotoxicity, all patients should be screened for viral hepatitis before starting HAART.[112]

Nucleoside (or Nucleotide) Reverse Transcriptase Inhibitors

Nucleoside or (nucleotide) reverse transcriptase inhibitors are also weak inhibitors of mitochondrial DNA polymerase gamma in vitro; the order of their potency is as follows: zalcitabine > didanosine > stavudine > lamivudine > zidovudine > abacavir.[113] The mechanisms of hepatotoxicity may also involve oxidative stress, resulting in further deletion of mitochondrial DNA and the consequences of impaired oxidative phosphorylation, fatty acyl beta oxidation, and insulin resistance. Abacavir can cause liver injury as part of a systemic hypersensitivity reaction, which occurs within the first 6 weeks and is linked to a particular HLA haplotype (HLA-B*5701). Excluding patients carrying this polymorphism has practically abolished the risk of hypersensitivity reactions to abacavir (0% vs. 2.7% in controls).[114]

In clinical studies, zidovudine, didanosine, and stavudine are the agents implicated most often in liver injury.[111,113,115] Risk factors for mitochondrial drug toxicity among persons with HIV infection include obesity, female gender, pregnancy, and co-prescription of didanosine and stavudine.[111,113,115] Hallmarks of mitochondrial hepatotoxicity include extensive microvesicular or macrovesicular steatosis (or both), lactic acidosis, and liver biochemical test abnormalities with progression to acute liver failure. Asymptomatic hyperlactatemia is common (especially with stavudine) among persons treated with HAART, but life-threatening lactic acidosis with hepatic steatosis is rare, with an estimated risk of 1.3 per 1000 person-years of antiretroviral use. The onset is a median of 6 months (range, 3 to 17 months) after treatment is started. The often nonspecific symptoms include nausea, vomiting, diarrhea, dyspnea, lethargy, and abdominal pain. Extrahepatic manifestations, such as myopathy or peripheral neuropathy, and in severe cases pancreatitis and renal failure, may follow the onset of the lactic acidosis and liver injury. Discontinuation of the drug is mandatory but does not prevent fatalities. Nevertheless, the overall mortality rate is low. One suggested approach to prevention is to monitor therapy by coupling serum ALT and

AST testing with serial measurements of the HIV load and CD4 count. Any new aminotransferase elevation should be followed immediately by measurement of serum lactate, muscle, and pancreatic enzyme levels.[115]

Over 60 cases of noncirrhotic portal hypertension have been associated with nucleoside reverse transcriptase inhibitors.[116,117] Most cases involved didanosine alone or in combination with stavudine.[118] Features of portal hypertension, namely variceal bleeding, ascites, and splenomegaly, are usually present, but hepatic encephalopathy and liver failure are uncommon. The majority (>75%) of those affected have been men who had already achieved virologic suppression and had been exposed to these agents for a period of 13 to 111 months. Nodular regenerative hyperplasia and portal vein thrombosis are the main histologic lesions. Postulated mechanisms include sinusoidal endothelial cell injury and thrombophilia. Discontinuation of didanosine does not lead to reversal of portal hypertension.

Non-nucleoside Reverse Transcriptase Inhibitors

Non-nucleoside reverse transcriptase inhibitors occasionally cause hepatitis as part of a hypersensitivity reaction within the first 6 weeks of use.[111,119,120] Reactions are usually accompanied by peripheral and tissue eosinophilia, rash, and lymphadenopathy. Resolution occurs within 4 weeks of discontinuing the drug.[119] Nevirapine has also been implicated in several instances of severe hepatotoxicity when used for postexposure prophylaxis.[121,122] Nevirapine hepatotoxicity has been associated with a specific HLA haplotype and increases in CD4 counts; specific CD4 thresholds have been established (>400 cells/mm^3 and >250 cells/mm^3 for men and women, respectively). The FDA received 12 reports of such hepatotoxic reactions between 1997 and 2000; 1 patient had acute liver failure requiring liver transplantation, 7 had clinical features of hepatitis, and 4 others had elevated serum aminotransferase levels without symptoms. The recommended 2-week dose escalation regimen was not adhered to in some of the cases.[123] Sequential toxicity with nevirapine followed by efavirenz has been reported in an HIV-HCV coinfected person.[124]

Protease Inhibitors

Elevation of serum liver enzyme levels occurs commonly with protease inhibitors, but clinical hepatitis is infrequent. The agents most often implicated in liver injury are ritonavir and indinavir. The latter also may be associated with unconjugated hyperbilirubinemia in 7% of treated persons, a finding that is of no clinical consequence (see Chapter 21).[25] Severe acute hepatitis may occur rarely. The association with peripheral or tissue (in liver biopsy specimens) eosinophilia in some cases suggests an immunoallergic basis for liver injury.[125] Acute hepatitis also has been reported in 2.9% to 30% of persons who take ritonavir. Liver injury is associated with high (>400 mg/day) ritonavir doses but not with regimens that include low-dose ritonavir. The course of the illness is generally mild, and the liver injury responds favorably to drug withdrawal. Rarely, acute liver failure may develop; in these cases, liver histologic examination has shown severe microvesicular steatosis, cholestasis, and extensive fibrosis.

Several studies have addressed the potential influence of underlying chronic viral hepatitis on the toxicity of protease inhibitors. Although hepatotoxicity appeared to be more common in the setting of chronic viral hepatitis, liver injury was rapidly reversible in most cases; this observation suggests that the overall effect of protease inhibitors in co-infected persons is not detrimental.[126] Many protease induce or inhibit CYP3A4, thereby causing important drug-drug interactions.[127] Immune reconstitution after successful HAART can lead to reactivation of chronic hepatitis B infection.

Aspirin

Aspirin has occasionally been associated with major increases in serum ALT levels suggestive of drug hepatitis, but hepatotoxicity occurs only when blood salicylate concentrations exceed 25 mg/100 mL.[128] Individual susceptibility factors include hypoalbuminemia, active juvenile rheumatoid arthritis, and systemic lupus erythematosus. Most cases of aspirin-induced hepatotoxicity have been identified by biochemical testing, rather than clinical features. If present, symptoms usually begin within the first few days or weeks of high-dose aspirin therapy. Acute liver failure and fatalities have been rare. Resolution occurs rapidly after drug withdrawal, and salicylates can be reintroduced at a lower dose. All salicylates appear to carry hepatotoxic potential, so there is no advantage to replacing aspirin with another salicylate. Liver biopsy specimens reveal a nonspecific focal hepatitis with hepatocellular degeneration and hydropic changes. Steatosis is not usually present, and the absence of steatosis distinguishes aspirin hepatotoxicity from Reye's syndrome.

Reye's syndrome has been linked with the use of aspirin in febrile children. Although Reye's syndrome is not simply a form of DILI, aspirin plays an important role in its multifactorial pathogenesis. Reye's syndrome usually occurs between 3 and 4 days after an apparently minor viral infection. It is characterized by acute encephalopathy and hepatic injury, the latter documented by a 3-fold or greater rise in serum aminotransferase or ammonia levels and by characteristic histologic findings. Because of effective public health campaigns against the use of aspirin in young febrile children, the incidence of Reye's syndrome has declined markedly, but cases still occur.[129] Misdiagnosis in the past of cases that subsequently were diagnosed as inborn errors of metabolism that mimic Reye's syndrome may account in part for the apparent decline in the incidence of Reye's syndrome.

Patients with juvenile rheumatoid arthritis (Still's disease) or systemic lupus erythematosus appear to be at particular risk of Reye's syndrome. Clinical and laboratory features of chronic liver disease do not develop in affected persons, and features of drug allergy are not present. Management requires suspecting the correct diagnosis and reducing the dose (or discontinuation) of aspirin. Recovery is usually rapid. Aspirin can be used again in lower doses, but other NSAIDs have displaced the use of high-dose aspirin for most conditions.

Other Drugs

L-Asparaginase is an antileukemic drug that often causes hepatotoxicity that is usually reversible but can result in liver failure associated with diffuse microvesicular steatosis.[130]

Amodiaquine, a 4-aminoquinolone antimalarial agent, has been associated with fatal hepatotoxicity (≈1 : 15,000 exposed) and agranulocytosis.[131,132] Toxicity may be related to the total dose of the drug. It is no longer used for prophylaxis but is widely used in Africa in combination with artesunate. Amodiaquine should be reserved for cases of chloroquine-resistant falciparum malaria, and dose recommendations should be strictly observed.

Hycanthone, an antischistosomal agent, caused dose-dependent hepatotoxicity when used in the past. Risk factors for hepatotoxicity included concomitant administration of phenothiazines or estrogens, preexisting liver injury, and bacterial infection.[133]

DRUG-INDUCED ACUTE HEPATITIS

The term *acute hepatitis* is used to describe lesions characterized by the presence of hepatic inflammation with conspicuous hepatocyte cell death or degeneration. More severe lesions include zonal and bridging necrosis or massive (panlobular) hepatic necrosis; these lesions may be associated with acute (fulminant or subfulminant) hepatic failure.[1,22] Acute hepatitis accounts for nearly 50% of reported adverse drug reactions involving the liver,[18-21] and potential causative agents are numerous.[1,22,24,133,134]

Two broad types of drug hepatitis are those cases with clinical and laboratory features consistent with drug allergy (immunoallergic reactions) and those without such features; the latter type could be the result of metabolic idiosyncrasy. Partial dose dependence, a relationship between hepatitis and metabolism of the drug, and histologic or ultrastructural features consistent with chemical toxicity are often found. The clinical and laboratory features that suggest one or the other type of drug hepatitis are summarized in Table 88-6. Nitrofurantoin is discussed as an example of immunoallergy, and isoniazid is used to illustrate metabolic idiosyncrasy. Other relatively frequent examples of drug hepatitis are described briefly, including those associated with granulomatous reactions and chronic hepatitis.

Immunoallergic Reactions

Nitrofurantoin

Nitrofurantoin is a urinary antiseptic agent that has long been associated with hepatic injury.[135] This reaction occurs at a frequency of 0.3 to 3 cases per 100,000 exposed persons.[136,137] The risk increases with age, particularly after the age of 64. Two thirds of acute cases occur in women, and the female-to-male ratio is 8:1 for chronic hepatitis.[136,137] The range of liver diseases associated with nitrofurantoin includes acute hepatitis, occasionally with features of cholestasis, hepatic granulomas, chronic hepatitis with autoimmune phenomena, acute liver failure, and cirrhosis.[136,137] Causality has been proved by rechallenge, and no relationship to dose has been observed; cases have been described after ingestion of milk from a nitrofurantoin-treated cow.[138]

The relative frequencies of hepatocellular and cholestatic or mixed reactions and of acute and chronic hepatitis caused by nitrofurantoin have been the subject of debate. The nature of the adverse reactions covers a spectrum of biochemical and histologic features that have no apparent relevance to the patient's clinical outcome. Chronicity depends mostly on the duration of drug ingestion, which has been less than 6 weeks in acute cases but more than 6 months in 90% of chronic cases.[136,137] Patients with chronic hepatitis often have

TABLE 88-6 Drug-Induced Acute Hepatitis: Immunoallergic Reaction versus Metabolic Idiosyncrasy

Characteristic	Immunoallergic Reaction	Metabolic Idiosyncrasy
Frequency	<1 case per 10,000 persons exposed	1-50 cases per 10,000 persons exposed
Gender predilection	Women, often ≥ 2:1	Variable, slightly more common in women
Latent period to onset of hepatitis	Fairly constant, 2-10 weeks	More variable, 2-24 weeks, occasionally > 1 year
Relationship to the dose	None	Usually none, but drugs with daily doses > 50 mg/day are overrepresented in cases of DILI
Interactions with other agents	None	Alcohol; occasionally other drugs (e.g., isoniazid with rifampin)
Course after stopping the drug	Prompt improvement (rare exceptions [e.g., minocycline])	Variable; occasionally slow improvement or deterioration (e.g., troglitazone)
Positive rechallenge	Always; often fever within 3 days	Usual (in two thirds of cases), abnormal liver biochemical test levels in 2-21 days
Fever	Usual; often initial symptom, part of prodrome	Infrequent, less prominent
Extrahepatic features (rash, lymphadenopathy)	Common	Rare

Eosinophilia
   Blood
   Tissue
	
	33%-67% of cases
	Usual, pronounced
		
		<10% of cases
		Common but mild

Autoantibodies	Often present	Rarely present
Examples	Nitrofurantoin, phenytoin, methyldopa, sulfonamides, etretinate, minocycline	Isoniazid, pyrazinamide, ketoconazole, dantrolene, troglitazone

DILI, drug-induced liver injury.

continued taking nitrofurantoin despite symptoms attributable to an adverse drug effect or have been exposed to another course of the drug after previous toxicity. The mortality rate for chronic nitrofurantoin hepatitis is 20%, compared with 5% to 10% for acute hepatitis.[136]

The latent period between initial exposure to the drug and the onset of liver disease ranges from a few days to 6 weeks. Early symptoms may be nonspecific (e.g., fever, myalgia, arthralgia, fatigue, malaise, anorexia, weight loss) and are followed by more specific features of hepatitis like nausea and vomiting, hepatic pain or discomfort, dark urine, jaundice, and, occasionally, pruritus. Rash occurs in 20% of affected persons, and lymphadenopathy may be present. Pneumonitis, which may be complicated by pulmonary fibrosis, can develop concurrently with hepatitis in 20% of cases and is suggested by cough and dyspnea. Rarely, liver failure develops, with ascites, coagulopathy, and encephalopathy. In patients with chronic hepatitis, clinical findings (e.g., hepatosplenomegaly, muscle wasting, ascites) may suggest chronic liver disease.

Liver biochemical testing may show pronounced elevation of serum ALT levels, but more often the pattern is mixed, with increases in the serum alkaline phosphatase level as well. In other cases, the results suggest cholestasis. Serum bilirubin levels tend to be increased in proportion to the severity of the reaction. In contrast to most types of acute drug hepatitis, serum albumin concentrations often are low. Hypergammaglobulinemia is more likely in patients with chronic hepatitis than in those with acute hepatitis.[136] Eosinophilia occurs in 33% of cases. Autoantibodies (antinuclear antibodies and smooth muscle antibodies) are present in some patients with acute hepatitis and in 80% of those with chronic hepatitis. The presence of autoantibodies can make differentiation of nitrofurantoin-induced fulminant hepatitis from AIH challenging.[139] In contrast to AIH, the frequency of HLA-B8 and HLA-DRw3 in nitrofurantoin-induced fulminant hepatitis is not increased.[136,137] A 2010 study from the Mayo Clinic documented striking imaging changes in nearly three quarters of patients with nitrofurantoin-induced fulminant hepatitis; these changes included confluent fibrosis, fibrotic bands, and lobar or diffuse liver atrophy.[140]

Treatment consists of supportive measures. Glucocorticoids have no role, even in patients with chronic hepatitis with autoimmune features. Recovery is rapid after nitrofurantoin is discontinued. Monitoring liver biochemical tests in users of nitrofurantoin is unlikely to be useful or cost effective.

Other Drugs

Methyldopa was one of the first drugs reported to cause immunoallergic drug hepatitis. Cases are now rare because better antihypertensive agents are available and methyldopa is not used except in pregnancy.[141] Hepatic reactions vary from abnormal liver biochemical test levels in asymptomatic persons, severe acute hepatitis, granuloma formation, and cholestasis to chronic hepatitis with bridging necrosis and cirrhosis. The female predilection, clinical and laboratory changes, course, and extrahepatic features of drug allergy are similar to those for nitrofurantoin.

Phenytoin causes severe acute drug hepatitis in less than 1 per 10,000 persons exposed.[142] Incidence rates are equal in men and women, and cases can occur in childhood. African Americans may be affected more often than Europeans. Rash, fever, eosinophilia, lymphadenopathy, a pseudomononucleosis syndrome, and other allergic features are common. The clinical features are suggestive of immunoallergy as part of the DRESS syndrome. An individual or familial enzymatic defect that leads to reduced disposal of phenytoin arene oxide has been detected among patients with phenytoin reactions.[142]

This finding implicates a possible metabolic factor in the pathogenesis of phenytoin toxicity.

A mortality rate of up to 40% has been reported in patients with phenytoin-induced hepatitis, but the rate has been much lower (13%) in more recent studies. Some deaths are due to liver failure, whereas others are the result of severe systemic hypersensitivity, bone marrow suppression, exfoliative dermatitis, or vasculitis involving the skin and kidney. Rare hepatic reactions include cholestatic hepatitis and bile duct injury. The most common association with phenytoin therapy is a hepatic adaptive response with microsomal enzyme induction; at least two thirds of patients have raised serum GGTP levels, and one third exhibit raised serum alkaline phosphatase levels. On histopathologic examination, ground-glass cytoplasm, which represents hypertrophied smooth endoplasmic reticulum, is usually present in hepatocytes.

Barbiturates, including phenobarbital, are rarely associated with acute hepatitis. Described cases have been similar to phenytoin reactions; fever and rash are usual, and the rate of mortality due to liver failure is high. Among newer antiepileptic drugs, lamotrigine,[143] felbamate,[144] and topiramate[145] have been associated with acute liver failure.

Sulfonamides are a cause of drug hepatitis that is relatively common with combination drugs such as trimethoprim/sulfamethoxazole (co-trimoxazole).[146] Trimethoprim alone has been associated with some cases of cholestatic hepatitis; the estimated risk is 1.4 cases per 100,000 exposed persons.[146] Reactions to trimethoprim/sulfamethoxazole resemble those associated with trimethoprim more closely than they resemble sulfonamide reactions; cholestasis or cholestatic hepatitis is more common than hepatitis. Patients with HIV/AIDS are predisposed to sulfonamide hypersensitivity. Some other drugs have a sulfa moiety that differs from that of sulfonamides and that may increase the risk of inadvertent cross-sensitivity reactions; for example, celecoxib, a cyclooxygenase (COX)-2 inhibitor, has been observed to cause severe hepatitis in 2 women with a history of sulfonamide sensitivity. Likewise, sulfonylureas (e.g., gliclazide) have rarely been associated with drug hepatitis with features of immunoallergy.[147]

The latent period between exposure to the drug and the onset of sulfonamide hepatitis is 5 to 14 days, and clinical features often include fever, rash, mucositis (Stevens-Johnson syndrome), lymphadenopathy, and vasculitis (i.e., features of DRESS syndrome). Reactions may be severe, and deaths have occurred. The serum ALT level is usually increased to a greater degree than the serum alkaline phosphatase level, but mixed or cholestatic reactions occur. A few cases of hepatic granuloma formation and of chronic hepatitis also have been associated with sulfonamides.

Sulfasalazine has been associated with cases of often severe acute hepatitis.[148] A study of 10 cases of liver injury in patients with inflammatory arthritis suggested that this complication may be more frequent than appreciated (0.4%).[149] Although the sulfonamide moiety has been held responsible, this assumption has been challenged by a report of recurrent hepatitis after exposure to mesalamine (mesalazine).[150] This finding implicates the salicylate moiety, and like salicylate (discussed earlier), sulfasalazine hepatotoxicity is more common in patients with rheumatoid arthritis than in those with IBD. Other presentations include chronic hepatitis with autoimmune features following 21 months of therapy and granulomatous hepatitis.[151,152]

Minocycline and other tetracyclines used in conventional low doses are a rare but important cause of drug hepatitis,[153] including cases that have resulted in acute liver failure requiring liver transplantation.[154] Minocycline is one of the few agents in current use that can lead to drug-induced AIH, as discussed later.

Disulfiram (Antabuse) has rarely been associated with acute hepatitis, occasionally leading to liver failure.[155] Disulfiram hepatitis usually is easy to distinguish from alcoholic hepatitis by the 10-fold or greater elevation of serum ALT activity.

β-Adrenergic blocking agents have rarely been incriminated in hepatotoxicity. Acebutolol, carvedilol, labetalol, and metoprolol have each been associated with cases of acute hepatitis, some of which were severe; some cases were proved by rechallenge. Data are insufficient to determine whether or not immunoallergy is likely.

The calcium channel blockers nifedipine, verapamil,[156] diltiazem,[157] and amlodipine[158] have good safety records, but rare cases of acute hepatitis with a short incubation period (5 days to 6 weeks) and other features of immunoallergy have been reported.

Of the angiotensin II receptor blocking agents, irbesartan has been linked to 2 reports of cholestasis.[159,160] In both patients, jaundice developed within 1 month of the start of therapy. Liver biochemical testing showed predominant cholestasis, and histologic examination confirmed marked cholestasis in both and an inflammatory infiltrate and eosinophils in one case. Clinical resolution occurred when the medication was stopped, but liver biochemical abnormalities persisted for more than 1 year in one case. Biliary ductopenia is a rare complication. Other angiotensin II receptor blockers implicated in cases of acute hepatitis or cholestatic hepatitis include losartan, valsartan, and candesartan.[161-163]

ACE inhibitor–induced liver disease is a rare but important complication of this widely prescribed class of drugs. The incidence has been estimated to be 9 per 100,000 patients treated. Reactions to captopril (the oldest and possibly most hepatotoxic representative) and enalapril usually manifest as cholestatic hepatitis, but hepatocellular or mixed hepatocellular reactions can occur.[164,165] Features of hypersensitivity (DRESS syndrome) such as fever, rash, and eosinophilia have been observed in patients with captopril hepatotoxicity.[164] Histologic examination reveals marked centrilobular cholestasis with eosinophilic portal infiltrates.[164] Liver biochemical abnormalities usually resolve after withdrawal of the drug, but resolution may take up to 6 months in some cases. Fulminant hepatic failure has been attributed to lisinopril, whereas fosinopril has been associated with bland cholestasis.[166] Ramipril has been implicated in 3 cases of cholestatic liver injury, 1 of which progressed to biliary cirrhosis.[167] Biliary ductopenia has been observed with enalapril.[168]

Hydroxymethylglutaryl–coenzyme A (HMG-CoA) reductase inhibitors (commonly known as "statins") are not strongly associated with important hepatic injury, although literature reports and data contributed to drug safety surveillance authorities appear to be discordant. With lower low-density lipoprotein (LDL) cholesterol targets being recommended, higher statin doses are being used. A dose-related rise in serum aminotransferase levels develops in 1% to 3% of statin users.[169] A minor (<2-fold) rise in the serum ALT and AST levels (without symptoms) is the most common manifestation of liver injury with the statins. These elevations usually reverse rapidly with statin withdrawal and also if therapy is *not* interrupted. Lovastatin,[170] pravastatin,[171] atorvastatin,[172] simvastatin,[173] and rosuvastatin[174] have been implicated in a few reports of acute hepatitis or cholestatic hepatitis.[175,176] Older data estimated the risk of statin-related DILI at less than 1 per million person-years, but Swedish registry data in 2012 suggested a much higher frequency (1.2 per 100,000).[176]

In the Swedish registry,[176] atorvastatin was most often implicated as a cause of statin hepatoxicity (41% of cases), but the overall frequency of DILI was highest for fluvastatin (17 per 100,000 person-years compared with 0.5 to 2.9 per 100,000 person-years for the other statins). Most hepatic reactions occurred within 3 to 4 months. One third of the patients had jaundice, and 2 deaths occurred from acute liver failure. Positive rechallenge was documented in 3 cases. Rechallenge with the same statin is not recommended, but an alternative statin was used successfully in 5 cases (suggesting a lack of class effect). With respect to the pattern of liver injury, cholestatic/mixed reactions were associated more often with atorvastatin (57%) than simvastatin (25%). Use of some statins in combination with gemfibrozil is associated with an increased rate of myositis but apparently not with an increased rate of DILI. A few small case series have noted an association between statin therapy and AIH, but the level of evidence for causality is unconvincing. These drugs are used for about 15% of the population, so it would be expected that a proportion of patients in whom AIH develops will be taking them. Instances of resolution of AIH following discontinuation of statins are not conspicuous in existing case reports and small series.

Prescribing guidelines for statins invariably warn about the risk of liver injury when these agents are prescribed to persons with preexisting liver abnormalities. Nevertheless, evidence that fatty liver (or NASH), hepatitis C, or other common liver disorders predispose to DILI is lacking (see earlier). Moreover, a controlled trial of high-dose pravastatin in patients with preexisting liver disease demonstrated the safety of statins in this setting.[177] Similar conclusions were reached in the Dallas Heart Study, in which statin users were no more likely to exhibit serum ALT elevations than nonusers.[178] Likewise, statin hepatotoxicity has been unrelated to the serum ALT level at baseline in other retrospective studies[179,180] and has even been shown to reduce overall progression of hepatic fibrosis.[180] Finally, patients with raised ALT levels not receiving statins were more likely to develop cardiovascular events (30%) than those treated with these agents (10%; 68% relative risk reduction).[181] Monitoring serum aminotransferase levels had previously been recommended, but this requirement has been reversed by the FDA based on the recommendations of expert panels that concluded that patients with NAFLD are not at increased risk of statin hepatotoxicity and that routine monitoring of serum aminotransferase levels is not warranted.[182]

Unlike vitamin A (see Chapter 89), synthetic retinoids like etretinate are not predictable hepatotoxins, but the latter has been associated with abnormal liver biochemical test results in 10% to 25% of treated patients.[183] Levels normalized with dose reduction, thereby suggesting partial dose dependency. Several cases of acute hepatitis have been attributed to etretinate, some confirmed by rechallenge.[183] Most patients were women older than age 50; 2 cases were associated with chronicity, and 1 patient responded to glucocorticoids. Etretinate has been superseded by acitretin, another synthetic retinoid that has also been associated with a few instances of acute hepatitis, including cases associated with bile duct injury, progressive hepatic fibrosis, and (rarely) fulminant hepatic failure (after acitretin overdose).[184-186]

Gastric acid suppression drugs have an excellent safety record, although rare adverse hepatic reactions have been reported. The histamine H_2 receptor antagonists oxmetidine and ebrotidine were withdrawn because of hepatotoxicity. Cimetidine, ranitidine, and famotidine have been associated with cases of acute hepatitis, mostly mild and often with cholestatic features. Some cases have been proved by rechallenge. Features of immunoallergy were present in some of the cimetidine reactions. Cases of hepatotoxicity have been attributed to the PPIs omeprazole, lansoprazole, and pantoprazole; these reports have been isolated, and causality was not established unequivocally in some of the cases.[187]

Zafirlukast, a leukotriene receptor antagonist effective against asthma, has been reported to cause severe liver injury, with several instances of acute liver failure.[188] Montelukast has been implicated in a few cases of acute hepatitis or cholestatic hepatitis.[189]

Ticlopidine, an antiplatelet agent, has been associated with more than 30 reports of hepatotoxicity. Liver histology has shown bland cholestasis in most cases and occasionally microvesicular steatosis; cholestatic hepatitis with bile duct injury also has been reported. Japanese subjects carrying a specific HLA haplotype (A*3303) and certain cytochrome polymorphisms (CYP2B6*1H or *1J) are at an increased risk of ticlopidine hepatotoxicity (see Table 88-3).[190] Clopidogrel has become preferred to ticlopidine, but clopidogrel also can cause hepatocellular or mixed hepatocellular-cholestatic liver injury.[191,192]

Metabolic Idiosyncrasy

Isoniazid

Isoniazid-induced liver injury has been characterized since the 1970s, but deaths still occur.[193-196] Hepatitis develops in about 21 per 1000 persons exposed to isoniazid; 5% to 10% of cases are fatal. The risk and severity of isoniazid hepatitis increase with age; the risk is 0.3% in the third decade of life and increases to 2% or higher after age 50.[193,194] Overall frequency rates are the same in men and women, but 70% of fatal cases are in women; black and Hispanic women may be at particular risk.[193,194] The risk of toxicity is not related to the dose or blood level of isoniazid. The role of genetic factors has been controversial. Associations have been described with specific genes that code for enzymes involved in aspects of drug metabolism or detoxification (CYP2E1, N-acetyltransferase, glutathione-S-transferase), but data are conflicting.[197-199] Chronic excessive alcohol intake increases the frequency and severity of isoniazid hepatotoxicity,[193,194] as may rifampin and pyrazinamide.[200] Concomitant use of pyrazinamide or acetaminophen has been associated with several cases that were fatal or led to liver transplantation.[201] Some studies have found that the risk of liver injury from isoniazid and other antituberculosis drugs is increased among persons with chronic HBV infection, but reports are conflicting.[201] Malnutrition may play a role in isoniazid hepatotoxicity in some countries. Likewise, in patients with HCV or HIV infection (or both), the risk of significant serum ALT elevations during antituberculosis treatment is increased severalfold; successful antiviral treatment of HCV infection has allowed the safe reintroduction of antituberculosis drugs.

Serum ALT levels increase in 10% to 36% of persons taking isoniazid in the first 10 weeks. The elevations typically are minor and resolve spontaneously. In persons in whom hepatitis develops, the latent period from exposure to disease ranges from 1 week to more than 6 months (median, 8 weeks), and, in severe cases, 12 weeks.[193,194] Reexposure to isoniazid may be associated with an accelerated onset, although the experience in India is that gradual reintroduction of isoniazid and rifampin can be achieved in most cases after the hepatitis has resolved. Prodromal symptoms occur in one third of patients and include malaise, fatigue, and early symptoms of hepatitis (e.g., anorexia, nausea, vomiting). Jaundice appears several days later and is the only feature in about 10% of cases. Fever, rash, arthralgias, and eosinophilia are uncommon.

Liver biochemical testing indicates hepatocellular injury; serum AST levels exceed serum ALT levels in half of patients. Serum bilirubin levels usually are elevated; values that are increased more than 10-fold indicate a poor prognosis. In one study,[193] one third of patients had a prolonged prothrombin time, and 60% of these cases were fatal. Liver biopsy samples generally show hepatocellular injury, which is focal in approximately 50% of cases, often with marked hydropic change in residual hepatocytes. In the remaining cases, hepatocellular necrosis is zonal, submassive, or massive, with inflammation confined to the portal tracts. Cholestasis and lobular regeneration suggestive of early cirrhosis are rare features.

Cases with a fatal outcome have been associated with a longer duration of treatment or continued ingestion of isoniazid after the onset of symptoms.[193,194] Most deaths from isoniazid hepatitis are preventable if patients report symptoms early in the course and isoniazid is discontinued. In the United States, isoniazid hepatotoxicity is second only to acetaminophen as an indication for liver transplantation for DILI.[201] Children are less susceptible than adults, but serious hepatotoxicity can occur in children; over a 10-year period (1987 to 1997), 8 children were transplanted for isoniazid hepatotoxicity in the United States (0.2% of pediatric liver transplants).[202]

Recovery is rapid if isoniazid is discontinued before severe liver injury is established. Management of liver failure is supportive; liver transplantation is indicated in the most severe cases. Prevention is the most appropriate way to avoid isoniazid hepatotoxicity, and determining whether the risks of isoniazid therapy outweigh those of latent tuberculosis is critical. Other regimens are gaining favor for treating latent tuberculosis infection. A 4-month course of rifampin has been associated with improved compliance and a lower rate of hepatotoxicity than a standard course of isoniazid.[203] The optimal approach to monitoring a patient for isoniazid toxicity is uncertain; every-other-week or monthly monitoring of serum ALT levels will not always prevent the rapid onset of severe hepatotoxicity. Effective prevention depends on awareness of early symptoms, no matter how nonspecific.

Other Antituberculosis and Antifungal Drugs

Other Antituberculosis Drugs

Most cases where rifampin has been implicated in liver injury have occurred in patients who are also taking isoniazid, but a few cases have occurred with rifampin monotherapy in persons with underlying liver disease.[204]

Pyrazinamide (and a related agent, ethionamide) has long been known to be a dose-dependent hepatotoxin. The drug is now used in lower doses (1.5 to 2 g/day) because of the emergence of resistant strains of mycobacteria. Hepatotoxicity in patients who are taking combinations that include isoniazid and pyrazinamide may be particularly severe.[195] Monitoring of serum ALT levels during therapy is recommended. Cross-sensitivity among isoniazid, pyrazinamide, and ethionamide may occur. Treatment of latent tuberculosis with the combination of pyrazinamide and rifampin, levofloxacin, or ethambutol has been associated with an increased risk of hepatic injury.[205,206]

Antifungal Drugs

Ketoconazole is associated with raised serum aminotransferase levels in 5% to 17% of treated patients.[207,208] Symptomatic hepatitis occurs in 7 to 20 of 100,000 exposed persons. Women (with a female-to-male ratio of 2:1) and persons older than 40 years of age are particularly susceptible to liver injury.[207-209] Concurrent use of drugs (e.g., lovastatin) that share similar metabolic pathways of elimination (CYP3A4) with ketoconazole can lead to hepatotoxicity.[210] Reactions are usually mild but can be severe, with rare cases of acute liver failure.[211] Persons who have received multiple course of ketoconazole can present with acute hepatitis and even anaphylaxis within 1 to 3 days when reexposed to this agent.[212]

The mortality rate is 3% to 7%.[207,208] The onset of toxicity is within 6 to 12 weeks and rarely after the drug is stopped. Toxicity is unrelated to the dose of the drug. Continued ingestion of ketoconazole after the onset of symptoms leads to an adverse outcome. Jaundice occurs in 50% of patients in whom acute hepatitis develops, and up to one third may present with nonspecific symptoms like nausea, anorexia, and vomiting. Fever, rash, eosinophilia, and other immunoallergic characteristics are rare. The pattern of liver biochemical test levels is primarily hepatocellular or mixed, and cholestatic hepatitis or bland cholestasis may occur.[207] Jaundice usually resolves within 12 weeks, but resolution may take months.[207,208] Cirrhosis is a rare complication following acute hepatic injury.[213]

Terbinafine is used to treat onychomycosis. Several cases of cholestatic hepatitis attributed to terbinafine have been reported.[214] The frequency of hepatotoxicity is 2 to 3 cases per 100,000 persons exposed.[214] The onset is usually within 4 to 6 weeks. Liver biopsy specimens show hepatocyte degeneration and canalicular cholestasis with variable portal tract inflammation. Recovery is usual with discontinuation of the drug, although prolonged cholestasis with ductopenia have been reported. Ursodeoxycholic acid has been used to hasten recovery when cholestasis is protracted.[215] Other presentations include sinusoidal obstruction syndrome in a liver transplant recipient[216] and 16 reports to the FDA of fulminant liver failure possibly linked to terbinafine[217]; the frequency of the latter outcome has been estimated to be 1 per million persons exposed.[218]

Fluconazole and itraconazole appear to be less hepatotoxic than ketoconazole and terbinafine[219]; elevations of liver biochemical test levels occur in fewer than 5% of patients. Rare cases of severe hepatic necrosis have been ascribed to fluconazole, but other causes were not excluded. Instances of acute liver failure associated with itraconazole have been reported.[220-222] Among more than 69,000 patients who received an oral antifungal agent, ketoconazole and itraconazole were most often associated with liver injury; the relative risks were 228 and 17.7, respectively, in comparison with nonusers.[223]

Serum aminotransferase levels are elevated in 20% of voriconazole recipients. Overt clinical hepatitis has been noted in patients receiving voriconazole in a liver intensive care unit and has led to discontinuation of the drug.[224]

Antidiabetic Drugs

Thiazolidinediones

Troglitazone was the first peroxisome proliferator–activated receptor-γ (PPARγ) agonist used in type 2 diabetes mellitus. Elevated serum aminotransferase levels were noted in 0.5% to 1.9% of recipients in early trials, which failed to reveal serious hepatotoxicity.[225] Reports of acute liver failure emerged in the post-marketing phase, in which troglitazone was associated with more than 75 instances of fatal hepatotoxicity or liver failure requiring hepatic transplantation.[226] Most cases occurred in older women and obese persons, the common phenotype of people with type 2 diabetes mellitus. Evidence that preexisting liver disease or other drugs predispose to troglitazone hepatotoxicity is lacking, although a progressive course in one patient was attributed to concurrent use of simvastatin and troglitazone.[227] Mitochondrial injury is favored as the mechanism of hepatic injury, but other mechanisms (e.g., reactive metabolites, inhibition of BSEP) have been proposed.[228]

The onset of troglitazone hepatotoxicity was often as late as 9 to 12 months after treatment was started[229,230]; rare cases had a much earlier onset (8 days).[231] Presenting features included nausea, fatigue, jaundice, vomiting, and symptoms of liver failure. Progression to acute liver failure was often

rapid, and in some cases, deterioration continued despite discontinuation of troglitazone.[232] Histologic examination of liver biopsy specimens, explanted livers, or autopsy material showed submassive or massive hepatic necrosis, with post-collapse scarring, bile duct proliferation, and some eosinophils.[233] Severe cholestasis also was reported,[234] as is sometimes observed with other causes of fulminant hepatic failure (e.g., valproic acid) and does not necessarily imply a pathogenic mechanism different from that in cases not associated with cholestasis. Troglitazone was withdrawn in 1999.

Serious liver injury is rare with the second-generation thiazolidinediones rosiglitazone and pioglitazone. In clinical trials, a raised serum ALT level (to >3 × ULN) was reported in 0.25% of patients treated with rosiglitazone and 0.26% treated with pioglitazone.[226] Six reports of hepatotoxicity associated with rosiglitazone have been published.[235] This agent has now been withdrawn owing to cardiotoxicity.

Pioglitazone has been implicated in acute hepatocellular injury.[235] Cholestatic hepatitis with bile duct injury was observed in 2 cases.[236] Most patients have recovered after discontinuing pioglitazone. Acute liver failure is a rare complication,[237] but a series of cases compiled by the FDA noted a high case-fatality rate (80%).[238] Causality has been questioned by the manufacturers,[239,240] who cited the known background incidence of liver complications in patients with diabetes mellitus and other confounding factors. By contrast, a French pharmacovigilance study concluded that the risk of hepatic reactions with these drugs was similar to that reported with other oral hypoglycemic drugs.[241] Before commencing treatment, the FDA recommends that liver biochemical test levels be measured; the pretreatment serum ALT level should be less than 2.5 times the ULN. Monitoring the serum ALT level every 2 months during the first year of therapy and periodically thereafter is advised. If ALT levels remain persistently elevated (>3 × ULN), the thiazolidinedione should be discontinued. Symptoms suggestive of hepatitis should be assessed immediately. Persons in whom jaundice developed with troglitazone should not take other thiazolidinediones.[242]

Other Oral Hypoglycemic Drugs

Hepatocellular liver injury was common with older sulfonylureas like carbutamide, metahexamide, and chlorpropamide.[243] Contemporary drugs (tolbutamide, tolazamide, glimepiride, and glibenclamide) may rarely cause cholestasis or cholestatic hepatitis.[244,245] Hypersensitivity phenomena (fever, skin rash, eosinophilia [DRESS syndrome]) were present in some cases, as would be expected in view of the structural relationship between sulfonylureas and sulfonamides. Most cases resolved after withdrawal of the drug, but chronic cholestasis progressing to vanishing bile duct syndrome (VBDS) has been described with tolbutamide and tolazamide. Fatal liver failure has been reported in 2 cases, 1 of whom had underlying cirrhosis. Gliclazide[32,246] and glibenclamide also have been associated with hepatocellular liver injury and, with the latter drug, hepatic granulomas.[245] Metformin, acarbose, repaglinide, and human insulin have rarely been associated with liver injury.

Drugs Used for Psychiatric and Neurologic Disorders

Several neuroleptic agents have been associated with drug hepatitis. Some reactions appear to be immunoallergic, whereas others conform to the pattern of apparent metabolic idiosyncrasy, depending on the structure of the drug. Such reactions have been reported for commonly used antidepressants, such as fluoxetine,[247,248] paroxetine,[249] venlafaxine,[250] trazodone,[251] tolcapone,[252] and nefazodone.

Antidepressants

Monoamine Oxidase Inhibitors. Iproniazid was one of the first drugs associated with acute hepatitis. Reactions occurred in 1% of recipients and were often severe, with instances of fatal fulminant liver failure. The hydrazine substituent (which iproniazid shares in part with isoniazid, ethionamide, pyrazinamide, and niacin) was determined to be hepatotoxic moiety.[253] Phenelzine and isocarboxazid have also been associated with occasional instances of hepatocellular injury, but monoamine oxidase inhibitors are now prescribed infrequently.

Tricyclic Antidepressants. Tricyclic antidepressants bear a structural resemblance to the phenothiazines and are occasional causes of cholestatic or, less commonly, hepatocellular injury. Recovery following cessation of the drug is usual, but prolonged cholestasis has been observed with amitriptyline[254] and imipramine.[255]

Selective Serotonin Reuptake Inhibitors (SSRIs) and Other Modern Antidepressants. SSRIs have a better overall safety profile than tricyclic antidepressants. Liver enzyme elevations have been observed in asymptomatic persons taking fluoxetine and paroxetine.[247] A few reports of acute and chronic hepatitis have been attributed to the use of SSRIs.[247,248] Acute hepatitis has been documented with mirtazapine, a noradrenergic and specific serotonergic antidepressant.[256] Nefazodone (now withdrawn) has been associated with cases of subacute liver failure.[257] Centrilobular, massive, or submassive hepatic necrosis was observed on liver histology. Trazodone has been implicated in causing acute and chronic hepatocellular injury.[251,258] The onset can be delayed as long as 18 months or can occur within 5 days of the start of the drug.[259] Occasional reports described severe hepatotoxicity with combinations of antidepressants or with antidepressants used in combination with other neuroleptic agents.[260,261] Drug regulatory authorities have been alerted about hepatic adverse events (including acute liver failure) with atomoxetine, a norepinephrine reuptake inhibitor. Only a few of the reported cases have been linked conclusively with the drug; all showed a pattern of acute hepatocellular injury.[262,263]

Other Neurologic Drugs

Tolcapone, a catechol-O-methyltransferase (COMT) inhibitor used in Parkinson's disease, has been associated with at least 4 cases of acute liver failure.[264] All were women older than 70 years of age who presented with jaundice and high serum ALT levels. Centrilobular necrosis was observed on liver histologic examination at autopsy in one case. Post-marketing surveillance has identified 3 additional patients with acute hepatocellular injury caused by tolcapone. The general consensus, however, is that tolcapone is safe if patients are monitored appropriately. FDA guidelines recommend serum ALT testing every 2 to 4 weeks for the first 6 months. Thereafter, the frequency of testing is left to the discretion of the treating doctor. Patients in whom signs of hepatic impairment or a rise in the serum ALT level (at least 1 to 2 × ULN) develop should be monitored closely; persistent serum ALT elevations (>2 × ULN) are an indication to discontinue the drug. Another COMT inhibitor, entacapone, has only rarely been associated with significant liver injury.[265]

Alpidem,[266] zolpidem,[267] and bentazepam[268] are sedative hypnotics that have been implicated in hepatotoxicity. In 3 reported cases of bentazepam hepatotoxicity, the clinicopathologic pattern resembled chronic hepatitis, but without autoantibodies or other immunologic features.[268]

Tacrine is a reversible choline esterase inhibitor used in Alzheimer's disease. Serum ALT elevations (>3 × ULN) are seen in 25% of patients, more often in women than in men;

levels are elevated more than 20-fold in 2% of patients.[269] The liver enzyme changes resolve with discontinuation of tacrine. A dose effect has not been observed. Symptoms are rare; only nausea and vomiting correlate with major serum ALT elevations. In liver biopsy specimens from 3 patients, steatosis and mild lobular hepatitis were observed. In one study,[269] minor degrees of hepatocellular injury were noted in up to 50% of cases, but tolerance eventually developed. There are isolated reports of jaundice, indicating a rare potential for more severe hepatotoxicity. Although the mechanism of liver injury is unclear, metabolic idiosyncrasy seems likely. No genetic factors have as yet been identified.[270] Mitochondrial injury has been implicated in an animal model of tacrine hepatotoxicity.

Dantrolene, a skeletal muscle relaxant used to treat spasticity, causes hepatitis in about 1% of exposed persons, with a case-fatality rate of approximately 28%.[271] Most affected patients have been older than 30 years of age. One third of patients are asymptomatic, and the remainder present with jaundice and symptoms of hepatitis. Hepatocellular necrosis, often submassive or massive, has been noted on liver biopsy specimens.[271] When therapy with dantrolene is initiated, liver biochemical tests should be monitored every 2 weeks. Liver enzyme elevations are an indication to stop dantrolene.

Other neurotropic drugs and muscle relaxants implicated as idiosyncratic hepatotoxins include tizanidine (a centrally acting muscle relaxant), alverine (a smooth muscle relaxant),[272] and riluzole.[273] Patients with cirrhosis who take tizanidine are at risk of hypotension; levels of this CYP1A2-metabolized drug are increased as a consequence of diminished cytochrome activity (see Table 88-1).[274] Riluzole is approved for treating amyotrophic lateral sclerosis. Increased serum ALT levels were reported in 1.3% to 10% of trial participants. Two cases of acute hepatitis with microvesicular steatosis have since been reported, with onset 4 and 8 weeks, respectively, after commencement.[273,275] Rarely, hepatocellular injury may be delayed for as long as 6 months. Liver biochemical test elevations resolved rapidly after riluzole was discontinued.

NSAIDs

NSAIDs rarely cause DILI, with or without immunoallergic features and with varying degrees of hepatocellular injury and cholestasis. Bromfenac was withdrawn because of severe hepatotoxicity.[276] Although only a 7-day course was recommended, most of those affected had used bromfenac for over 90 days.

Although COX-2 inhibitors are less likely to cause upper GI toxicity than conventional NSAIDs, they are not necessarily safer than the latter group of drugs with respect to the risk of liver injury.[277] A small number of cases of acute hepatitis (some severe) have been reported in association with nimesulide and celecoxib. Lumiracoxib was associated with severe hepatotoxicity[277,278] and was withdrawn from use. Overall, celecoxib has a low potential for liver injury. In a review of 14 controlled trials, the frequency of hepatic dysfunction (0.8%) was not significantly different from that in placebo-treated patients (0.9%).[279] Increased serum aminotransferase levels often occurred in persons taking diclofenac concurrently. When serious hepatocellular injury was attributed to celecoxib, female gender was a predisposing factor.[280] The onset of symptoms was between 4 days and 4 weeks after the drug was started. Liver biochemical abnormalities were consistent with a pattern of hepatocellular or mixed liver injury. Eosinophilia and skin rash suggestive of DRESS syndrome occurred in some patients. Most patients recovered within 1 to 4 months of discontinuation of the drug. Acute

TABLE 88-7 Drug-Induced Granulomatous Hepatitis: Major Causative Agents, Frequency, Risk Factors, Clinicopathologic Features, and Outcomes

Causative Agent*	Frequency	Risk Factors	Clinicopathologic Features	Outcomes
Carbamazepine	16:100,000 treatment-years	Age > 40 years, no gender predilection	Two thirds of cases show granulomatous hepatitis; the remainder show acute hepatitis, cholangitis; no features of drug allergy	No reported fatality, rapid recovery
Phenylbutazone	1:5000 exposed	No age or gender predilection	Severe acute hepatitis, cholestasis and bile duct injury are also reported; features of drug allergy are common; occasionally vasculitis	Mortality rate 25%, particularly in cases with hepatocellular necrosis
Allopurinol	Rare (<40 cases)	Older men, black race, renal failure, use of thiazides	Acute hepatitis, cholestatic hepatitis, bile duct injury are also frequent; rash (exfoliative dermatitis), nephritis, vasculitis are usual	Mortality rate 15%, especially with vasculitis
Hydralazine	Rare	Older patients, possibly slow acetylators	Other types of reaction are also common: acute hepatitis, cholestatic hepatitis, cholangitis; features of drug allergy are uncommon; vasculitis is not described	Reactions severe, but no mortality reported
Quinine	Rare	No recognized risk factors	Acute hepatitis occurs in two thirds of cases; rash, interstitial pneumonitis, positive Coombs test, thrombocytopenia	Good prognosis

*Other drugs that have been reliably reported to cause granulomatous hepatitis include quinidine, phenytoin (usually with vasculitis), sulfonamides (usually with vasculitis), nitrofurantoin, aspirin, papaverine, procainamide, sulfasalazine, mesalamine, and glyburide. Single case reports have implicated many other agents, as referred to briefly in the text.

liver failure is a rare complication.[281] Celecoxib should not be administered to persons with documented sulfonamide allergy because of published reports of cross-reactivity and toxicity.

Nimesulide, an NSAID with COX-2 selectivity, has been linked to several cases of acute hepatitis and fatal hepatic failure,[282] especially in women, although the risk of liver injury is small.[283] The onset of symptoms is between 1 to 15 weeks (occasionally up to 8 months after the drug is started). Hypersensitivity features with peripheral eosinophilia may occur. Liver histology shows centrilobular or bridging necrosis and occasionally bland cholestasis. Resolution usually has occurred within 2 to 17 months of stopping nimesulide.

DRUG-INDUCED GRANULOMATOUS HEPATITIS

Granulomatous reactions are a common type of DILI,[152,245,284-286] and drugs account for 2% to 29% of cases of granulomatous hepatitis (see Chapter 36). The number of drugs and foreign compounds associated with hepatic granulomas exceeds 40 (Table 88-7). Not all of these agents is associated with systemic inflammation or with persuasive evidence of causality. Many (e.g., halothane, methyldopa, nitrofurantoin, troglitazone, amiodarone, amoxicillin–clavulanic acid) are more commonly associated with other patterns of liver injury. Some of these associations may be fortuitous.

The clinical picture is heralded by fever and systemic symptoms (e.g., malaise, headache, myalgias) from 10 days to 4 months after the start of treatment. Hepatomegaly and hepatic tenderness are common; splenomegaly is present in 25% of patients. Extrahepatic features of drug hypersensitivity are common, as is eosinophilia (30%). The pattern of liver biochemical test levels is typically mixed because of the infiltrative nature of hepatic granulomas and the frequent presence of some hepatocellular necrosis or cholestasis. For several drugs that cause granulomatous hepatitis, continued exposure leads to more severe types of liver disease such as cholestatic hepatitis, with or without bile duct injury and hepatic necrosis (Table 88-7). Small-vessel vasculitis is another potential complication and may involve the kidneys, bone marrow, skin, and lungs; the mortality rate is high.

DRUG-INDUCED CHRONIC HEPATITIS

Chronic hepatitis is defined as hepatitis that continues for more than 6 months. For drug reactions, however, the definition often has been made inappropriately on hepatic histologic features alone. The histologic features include interface hepatitis, bridging necrosis, and fibrosis. Because these features may be present as early as 6 weeks after the onset of severe reactions, they do not confirm chronicity. The diagnosis of chronic hepatitis is more convincing when clinical or biochemical evidence of hepatitis has been present for more than 3 months and when clinical and laboratory features of chronic liver disease or histologic evidence of established hepatic fibrosis are present. Drugs are an uncommon cause of chronic hepatitis (Table 88-8), because the most commonly implicated agents (e.g., oxyphenisatin,[1] methyldopa) are now rarely used, and the proportion of cases caused by viral hepatitis has increased.

TABLE 88-8 Drug-Induced Chronic Hepatitis: Causative Agents, Risk Factors, Clinicopathologic Features, and Outcomes

Causative Agent*	Risk Factors	Clinicopathologic Features	Outcomes
Nitrofurantoin	Age > 40 years; 90% of cases in women; continued ingestion after onset	Clinical features of chronic hepatitis, liver failure; some cases with features of cholestasis; 20% with pneumonitis; hyperglobulinemia usual, ANA, SMA	Mortality rate 10%
Methyldopa	Age > 50 years; 80% of cases in women; repeated courses, continued ingestion in sensitized patient	Jaundice, diarrhea, liver failure; hyperglobulinemia, ANA, SMA positive; protracted course	High mortality rate
Diclofenac	Age > 65 years; most cases in women	Clinical features of chronic hepatitis, liver failure; hyperglobulinemia, ANA, SMA	Response to glucocorticoids in a few cases
Minocycline	Young women; prolonged use of drug	Often part of drug-induced systemic lupus erythematosus syndrome (arthritis, rash, rarely nephritis); hyperglobulinemia, ANA	Cases may be severe, with a fatal outcome or need for liver transplantation; glucocorticoid treatment may be indicated
Isoniazid	Age > 50 years; continued drug ingestion after onset; duration of therapy	Severe and fatal cases with cirrhosis; no immune phenomena	High mortality rate or need for liver transplantation
Dantrolene	Age > 30 years; dose, duration of therapy	Jaundice, liver failure; no immune phenomena	High mortality rate
Etretinate	Age > 50 years; two thirds in women	Jaundice, weight loss, liver failure; deterioration after stopping drug	Response to glucocorticoids in 2 reported cases
Acetaminophen	Regular intake at moderate doses (2-6 g/day); alcohol, fasting, other drugs	No features of chronic liver disease, no autoimmune phenomena; these are cases of chronic toxicity	Rapid normalization of liver biochemical test levels after the drug is stopped

*Several other agents, including sulfonamides, aspirin, halothane, cimetidine, methotrexate, trazodone, fluoxetine, fenofibrate, and germander, have been mentioned as associated with chronic hepatitis, but evidence of causation is not robust. In the past, causes included oxyphenisatin and tienilic acid, which are no longer available.
ANA, antinuclear antibodies; SMA, smooth muscle antibodies.

Chronic hepatitis is more common in women (≈4-fold) than men. Older patients appear to be at greater risk (as in the case of nitrofurantoin), and the reaction is virtually unknown in children. Drugs associated with chronic hepatitis more commonly cause acute hepatitis, and the latent period to recognition tends to be longer in cases of chronic hepatitis; therefore, the duration of drug ingestion may be a risk factor for chronic hepatitis. In a 2009 study, the mean duration of use in patients in whom chronic hepatitis or liver-related morbidity and mortality occurred after an episode of DILI was significantly greater than the duration in those in whom an adverse outcome did not occur (153 vs. 53 days).[287]

Two syndromes of drug-induced chronic hepatitis may occur. In the first, cases appear to be identical to acute hepatitis but more severe, more prolonged, or later in onset, perhaps as a result of failure of recognition. These cases may appropriately be termed *chronic toxicity*. Clinical and laboratory features of chronic liver disease are rare, and hallmarks of autoimmunity are absent. Management consists of withdrawal of the drug and treatment of liver failure (see Table 88-8).

The second syndrome more closely resembles AIH, based on the presence of spider telangiectasias, a firm liver edge, splenomegaly, and potential for liver failure. Ascites, bruising, variceal hemorrhage, and hepatic encephalopathy are common. In addition to raised serum ALT and bilirubin levels, hypoalbuminemia and hyperglobulinemia are usual.

The prothrombin time is prolonged in severe cases. Autoantibodies, particularly antinuclear and smooth muscle antibodies, are frequent. In contrast to idiopathic AIH, other hallmarks of autoimmunity like a history of other autoimmune diseases and genetic predisposition indicated by HLA-B8 and HLA-DRw3 alleles are not found. Immunosuppressive treatment is not indicated; the clinical condition improves spontaneously after withdrawal of the causative drug. In individual cases, glucocorticoids occasionally appear to hasten recovery, but immunosuppressive therapy can usually be discontinued, in contrast to the majority (65%) of patients with AIH, in whom discontinuation is followed eventually by relapse.[140]

Diclofenac

Diclofenac is one of the world's most prescribed NSAIDs and appears to be at least as safe as comparable agents. In clinical trials, elevations of serum aminotransferase levels (>3 × ULN and >10 × ULN) were noted in 3.1% and 0.5%, respectively, but liver disease–related hospitalizations were infrequent (0.023%).[288] Other studies have estimated the risk of significant hepatotoxicity to be 1 to 5 per 100,000 persons exposed, or 0.4 per 1 million defined daily doses; the latter rate is minimally greater than that for phenylbutazone (0.2 per 1 million) and piroxicam (0.3 per 1 million) but less than that for benoxaprofen (12.6 per 1 million) and bromfenac (now withdrawn). More than 200 cases of diclofenac hepatitis have been reported,[289] including several proved by inadvertent rechallenge. Only 4 cases have been fatalities, and 5 cases can reasonably be regarded as chronic hepatitis. Genetic susceptibility to diclofenac hepatotoxicity has been documented.[290,291] In these cases, polymorphisms have been observed in genes that affect metabolic pathways that lead to formation of reactive metabolites of the drug and affect biliary excretion. Immune responses to drug metabolite–protein adducts have been identified.[290,291]

The risk of hepatitis is increased in women and with aging. A prodromal illness characterized by anorexia, nausea, vomiting, and malaise heralds the onset of liver injury, which usually occurs within 3 months (range, 1 to 11 months) of the start of treatment. Fever and rash occur in 25% of patients.[289] Liver biochemical test results reflect acute hepatitis with or without cholestasis. Reactions tend to be severe, with jaundice occurring in 50% of cases. Liver biopsy specimens reveal acute lobular hepatitis, and in severe cases, bridging or confluent necrosis, interface hepatitis, and fibrous expansion of the portal tracts have been noted. The prognosis is usually good; resolution occurs after discontinuation of the drug. Cases of drug-induced chronic hepatitis have been described in which the clinical and laboratory features (ascites, hypoalbuminemia, hyperglobulinemia, jaundice) suggested AIH, although the frequency of autoantibodies is unclear. These cases usually improve spontaneously after discontinuation of the drug, but glucocorticoids have been used successfully in a few protracted cases.[292] Cross-sensitivity with other NSAIDs seems to be rare but has been reported with ibuprofen and tiaprofenic acid.[292] The rarity of severe diclofenac-induced hepatotoxicity makes liver biochemical monitoring unrealistic. Patients need to be advised to report adverse effects, and clinicians must be aware that diclofenac can cause both acute and chronic hepatitis.

Minocycline

Minocycline has been associated with rare cases of drug-induced systemic lupus erythematosus syndrome (rash, polyarthritis, hyperglobulinemia, and antinuclear antibodies), chronic hepatitis with autoimmune features, and both syndromes in the same patient.[293,294] The onset often occurs after treatment with minocycline for more than 6 months, and young women appear to be particularly affected. In the United States, minocycline is the most common drug associated with idiosyncratic drug hepatotoxicity in children.[295] The reactions are severe; some patients have died or required liver transplantation. Progression to cirrhosis has been reported.[296] The course may be prolonged after the drug is discontinued; several patients have been treated with glucocorticoids.[294]

DRUG-INDUCED ACUTE CHOLESTASIS

Importance, Types of Reactions, and Diagnosis

Cholestatic drug reactions include acute cholestasis with or without hepatitis, cholestatic hepatitis with cholangitis, and chronic cholestasis, either with a VBDS resembling PBC (see Chapter 91) or with biliary strictures reminiscent of sclerosing cholangitis (see Chapter 68).[297,298] Clinical and biochemical features of drug-induced cholestasis resemble those of several other hepatobiliary disorders, and clinicians must take a thorough drug history from all patients with cholestasis. Prompt discontinuation of a causative agent prevents an adverse outcome and avoids unnecessary invasive investigations or surgery.

The clinical syndrome of cholestasis is characterized by pruritus, dark urine, pale stools, and, in more serious cases, jaundice. Liver biochemical test results show a predominant elevation of serum alkaline phosphatase level (with a lesser increase in serum ALT level), elevation of GGTP and 5'-nucleotidase levels, and conjugated hyperbilirubinemia. The serum ALT level may be elevated up to 8-fold as a result of either the toxic effects of acute bile retention on hepatocellular integrity or concomitant "hepatitis." In such cases, the ratio of the relative increases in serum ALT and alkaline phosphatase levels (based on multiples of the upper limits of normal) is typically less than 2:1.[297] Cases of mixed cholestasis and hepatitis are highly suggestive of a drug reaction.

Hepatobiliary imaging is critical to exclude biliary obstruction and a hepatic or pancreatic mass lesion. In the absence of such findings, drug-induced cholestasis is more likely, and a liver biopsy is often advisable. Certain histologic features suggest a hepatic drug reaction, whereas others (e.g., edema of the portal tracts) suggest biliary obstruction. When the temporal relationship to drug ingestion indicates a high probability of a drug reaction, particularly when the agent is known to be potentially hepatotoxic, the incriminated drug should be discontinued and the patient observed for improvement.

Management should focus on symptom relief, with particular attention to pruritus (see Chapter 91).[297-299] Pruritus is often ameliorated with cholestyramine. In intractable cases, ursodeoxycholic acid has shown promise.[299,300] Rifampin, phototherapy, plasmapheresis, and morphine receptor antagonists (e.g., naloxone, naltrexone, nalmefene) have been used as third-line therapies.[299] Glucocorticoids have no role. Phenobarbital and antihistamines are usually ineffective or cause oversedation.

Cholestasis without Hepatitis

Cholestatic reactions are characterized by the retention of bile in canaliculi, Kupffer cells, and hepatocytes, with minimal inflammation or hepatocellular necrosis. Synonyms are pure, canalicular, or bland cholestasis. Cholestasis without hepatitis reflects a primary disturbance in bile flow. Sex steroids are the typical causative agents. Some drugs generally associated with cholestatic hepatitis (e.g., amoxicillin–clavulanic acid, sulfonamides, griseofulvin, ketoconazole, tamoxifen, warfarin, ibuprofen)[297,298] occasionally produce bland cholestasis. Cyclosporine is associated with liver biochemical test abnormalities; the features resemble those of cholestasis, but hyperbilirubinemia usually is predominant.[1] The reaction is mild and reverses rapidly with dose reduction. Tacrolimus can also cause cholestasis,[301] whereas sirolimus has been implicated in cases of mild acute hepatitis.[302]

Steroids

Oral Contraceptive Steroids

The frequency of cholestasis with oral contraceptive steroids (OCS) is 2.5 per 10,000 women exposed. OCS-associated cholestasis is partly dose dependent and less likely with low-dose than high-dose estrogen preparations.[303] Genetic factors contribute to the high frequency of this complication among women in Chile and Scandinavia.[298] Persons with a history of cholestasis of pregnancy are also at risk (50%) (see Chapter 39). The estrogenic component is most likely responsible and is mediated through impaired functioning of BSEP or canalicular transport of water (or both).[304] Polymorphisms within genes relating to canalicular transport (e.g., ABCB4, ABCB11) also underlie some cases of oral contraceptive–induced cholestasis (also see Chapter 64).[305,306] Symptoms develop 2 to 3 months, rarely as late as 9 months, after OCS are started. A mild transient prodrome of nausea and malaise may occur and is followed by pruritus and jaundice. The serum alkaline phosphatase level is moderately elevated, and serum aminotransferase levels are increased transiently, occasionally to levels exceeding 10 times the ULN. The serum GGTP level is often normal. Recovery is usually prompt, within days to weeks after cessation of the drug. Chronic cholestasis is rare.[298] Acute hepatitis is also an uncommon complication.[307]

Hormone replacement therapy (HRT) is safe in patients with liver disease. Jaundiced patients, however, may experience an increase in serum bilirubin levels, and liver biochemical tests should be monitored in HRT users with liver disease.[298]

Anabolic Steroids

At high doses, anabolic steroids often produce reversible bland cholestasis, usually within 1 to 6 months after the start of treatment. Recovery usually follows drug withdrawal, but protracted cholestasis with biliary ductopenia can occur. Rarely, anabolic steroid use can cause an acute hepatocellular pattern of injury.[308]

Both OCS and the 17-alkylated anabolic steroids are associated with cholestasis, vascular lesions, and hepatic neoplasms. The strength of these associations with individual lesions varies. Benign hepatic neoplasms, except hemangiomas,[309] are clearly associated with use of OCS, whereas their association with hepatocellular carcinoma is controversial.[310] By contrast, hepatocellular carcinoma is well documented in anabolic steroid users (see Chapter 96). Likewise, hepatic and portal vein thrombosis is an established adverse effect of OCS but not of anabolic steroids, whereas peliosis hepatis is seen more often with the latter than with OCS (see Chapter 85).

Cholestasis with Hepatitis

Cholestasis with hepatitis is a common type of hepatic drug reaction and is characterized by conspicuous cholestasis and hepatocellular necrosis. Histologic lesions in the liver include lobular and portal tract inflammation, often with neutrophils and eosinophils as well as mononuclear cells. This type of reaction overlaps with drug-induced acute hepatitis (occasionally resulting in acute liver failure), cholestasis without hepatitis, and cholestasis with bile duct injury. Causative agents include chlorpromazine; antidepressants and other psychotropic agents; erythromycins, other macrolides, and related ketolide antibiotics (telithromycin,[311] clindamycin,[312] sulfonamides, oxypenicillins,[313] ketoconazole [see earlier])[219]; sulfonylureas; sulindac[314]; ibuprofen; phenylbutazone; piroxicam[315]; captopril[316]; flutamide[317]; enalapril[168]; pravastatin[171]; atorvastatin[172]; ticlopidine[318]; ciprofloxacin and other fluoroquinolones[319]; and metformin.[320]

Chlorpromazine

Chlorpromazine hepatitis, the prototypical drug-induced cholestatic hepatitis,[321] has been recognized since the 1950s, and cases still occur. The full spectrum of hepatic reactions includes asymptomatic liver biochemical test abnormalities in 20% to 50% of recipients and rare cases of fulminant hepatic necrosis. The frequency of cholestatic hepatitis varies from 0.2% to 2.0%, depending on the type of study; the lower value probably is representative of the risk in the general population. No relationship to dose or to underlying liver disease has been recognized. Female predominance is evident. Reactions do not appear to be more common with increasing age but are rare in children.

The onset of cholestatic hepatitis is generally 1 to 6 weeks after the start of chlorpromazine and occasionally 5 to 14 days after its discontinuation. Accelerated onset occurs with rechallenge. A prodromal illness of fever and nonspecific symptoms is usual and is followed by GI symptoms and jaundice. Pruritus is common and occurs later with chlorpromazine hepatitis than with drug-induced cholestasis without hepatitis. In a small proportion of affected patients, right upper quadrant abdominal pain is severe. Rash is infrequent. Serum bilirubin, ALT, and alkaline phosphatase levels are increased. Eosinophilia is present in 10% to 40% of patients. Most patients recover completely: one third within 4 weeks, another third between 4 and 8 weeks, and the remainder after 8 weeks.[300,321] In about 7% of cases, full recovery has not occurred by 6 months (see later).

Amoxicillin–Clavulanic Acid

Over 150 cases of cholestatic hepatitis have been attributed to amoxicillin–clavulanic acid. The overall frequency is 1.7 cases per 10,000 prescriptions.[36] Male gender, increasing age (older than 55 years), and prolonged duration of use are risk factors.[322] The clavulanic acid component has been implicated because similar lesions have been noted with ticarcillin–clavulanic acid,[323] whereas amoxicillin rarely causes liver disease.[324]

The onset of symptoms is within 6 weeks (mean, 18 days) but can be delayed up to 6 weeks after stopping the drug. Features of hypersensitivity such as fever, rash, and eosinophilia are seen in 30% to 60% of patients. Liver histology shows cholestasis with mild portal inflammation. Bile duct injury (usually mild) and perivenular cholestasis with lipofuscin deposits are often present. Other histologic features include hepatic granulomas, biliary ductopenia, and cirrhosis.[325] Most patients recover in 4 to 16 weeks; fatal outcomes are rare. A strong association with the HLA-DRB1*1501-DRB5*0101-DQB1*062 haplotype and, more recently, with single nucleotide polymorphisms within the HLA class I region[326] supports the view that immunologic idiosyncrasy mediated through HLA class I and II antigens may be involved in the pathogenesis. The presence of the HLA class II haplotype, however, has no influence on the clinical characteristics, severity, and outcome of the disease. On the other hand, patients with the HLA-DRB1*07 family of alleles are less likely to develop liver injury (odds ratio, 0.18 to 2.6) compared with nonaffected treated persons or untreated control subjects.[327] The risk of liver injury is also increased over 2-fold in persons carrying certain glutathione *S*-transferase genotypes (the double-null genotype, T1 and M1), indicating that defects in detoxification may contribute to hepatotoxicity.[328]

Fluoroquinolones

Almost all currently used fluoroquinolones have been implicated in causing liver injury, with the highest frequencies attributed to levofloxacin and moxifloxacin.[329] Trovafloxacin was withdrawn because of hepatotoxicity. As a group, the fluoroquinolones have been associated with acute hepatocellular, cholestatic, and mixed reactions.[330] The onset can be rapid (median, 8 days; range, 1 to 39 days) but occasionally can be delayed up to 30 days after completion of the course of antibiotic. Hypersensitivity features may be present. Resolution usually follows discontinuation of the drug, but instances of acute liver failure, chronic cholestasis, and VBDS have been recorded.[319]

Cholestatic Hepatitis with Bile Duct Injury

Bile duct (cholangiolytic) injury is observed with several drugs that cause cholestatic hepatitis, such as chlorpromazine[300] and flucloxacillin.[313] The severity of bile duct injury may be a determinant of the VBDS (see later).[323,331] Clinical features may resemble those of bacterial cholangitis, with upper abdominal pain, fever, rigors, tender hepatomegaly, jaundice, and cholestasis. Liver biochemical test levels are typical of cholestasis. Compounds associated with this syndrome include carbamazepine,[332] dextropropoxyphene[333] and methylenediamine, an industrial toxin responsible for Epping jaundice, an outbreak of jaundice associated with the ingestion of bread made from contaminated flour (see Chapter 89).[334]

Dextropropoxyphene

Dextropropoxyphene is an opioid analgesic used alone or in compound analgesics. It has caused cholestasis with bile duct injury in at least 25 reported cases,[333] some proved by inadvertent rechallenge. A female predominance has been recognized. The onset of symptoms is usually within 2 weeks. The illness is often heralded by abdominal pain that may be severe and simulates other causes of cholangitis. Jaundice is usual. ERCP shows normal bile ducts. Liver biopsy specimens demonstrate cholestasis with expansion of the portal tracts by inflammation and mild fibrosis; portal tract edema also may be present. Other features include irregularity and necrosis of the biliary epithelium, together with an infiltrate of neutrophils and eosinophils on the outer surface of bile ducts. Bile ductule proliferation is universal. Recovery is the rule, with liver biochemical test levels normalizing within 1 to 3 months.[333]

DRUG-INDUCED CHRONIC CHOLESTASIS

DILI is considered to be chronic when typical liver biochemical changes last longer than 3 months[298]; earlier definitions required the presence of jaundice for more than 6 months or anicteric cholestasis (raised alkaline phosphatase and GGTP levels) for more than 12 months after the implicated agent was stopped.[297] Drug-induced chronic cholestasis is uncommon but has been ascribed to more than 45 compounds.[297-299,321,335-337] Chronicity complicates some 7% of cases of chlorpromazine hepatitis (see earlier)[300] and is a feature in 10% to 30% of cases of flucloxacillin hepatitis.[298] Chronicity has been reported in less than 5% of cases of erythromycin hepatitis[336] and in only isolated instances for other agents (e.g., tetracycline,[337] amoxicillin–clavulanic acid,[338] ibuprofen,[339] trimethoprim/sulfamethoxazole,[340] ciprofloxacin [see earlier]).[341]

Chronic cholestasis always is preceded by an episode of acute cholestatic hepatitis. The episode of acute cholestatic hepatitis tends to be severe and occasionally is associated with Stevens-Johnson syndrome.[339] The severity of bile duct lesions at the time of the initial hepatic reaction is a critical determinant of a chronic course.[331] Other possible mechanisms include continuing toxic or immunologic destruction of the biliary epithelium.[335] The hepatic histologic lesion is characterized by a paucity of smaller (septal, interlobular) bile ducts and ductules, often with residual cholestasis, and portal tract inflammation directed against injured bile ducts. This process may lead to an irreversible loss of biliary patency and VBDS.[342]

Clinical features are those of chronic cholestasis. Pruritus is the dominant symptom and is often severe. Continuing jaundice, dark urine, and pale stools are possible but not invariable findings and may resolve despite persistence of liver biochemical abnormalities. In severe cases, intestinal malabsorption, weight loss, and bruising caused by vitamin K deficiency may occur; xanthelasma, tuberous xanthomata, and other complications of severe hypercholesterolemia have also been noted. Firm hepatomegaly may be found on physical examination, but splenomegaly is unusual unless portal hypertension develops. Antimitochondrial antibodies are not usually present. Most cases resolve, but there are rare reports of severe biliary ductopenia and biliary cirrhosis.[297,298]

Flucloxacillin

Flucloxacillin is an important cause of drug-induced hepatitis in Europe, Scandinavia, and Australia.[313,343] Flucloxacillin-induced hepatotoxicity is usually severe, and several deaths have resulted from the systemic features and associated cholestatic hepatitis. The course is prolonged, and a high proportion of cases result in chronic cholestasis and VBDS.[343] GWAS of 51 patients with flucloxacillin hepatotoxicity and 282 controls showed a strong association (odds ratio, 80.6) between HLA-B*5701 and the risk of liver injury.[344] Other oxypenicillins (cloxacillin and dicloxacillin) are less often associated with cholestasis.[313,345] Acute hepatocellular injury has been reported with oxacillin.[346]

Fibrotic Bile Duct Strictures

Fibrotic strictures of the larger bile ducts can cause chronic cholestasis. Theses strictures have been observed with intralesional formalin therapy of hepatic hydatid cysts and intraarterial infusion of floxuridine for metastatic colorectal carcinoma. After several months of floxuridine infusion, the frequency of toxic hepatitis or bile duct injury, or both, has been as high as 25% to 55%, but the frequency has declined considerably (to ≈5%) with modern treatment schedules.[347] Acalculous cholecystitis also may occur. ERCP and MRCP show strictures, typically in the bile duct and the left and right hepatic ducts. Unlike PSC, the bile duct and the smaller intrahepatic bile ducts are spared. Ischemia has been the suspected pathogenesis, and toxicity to biliary epithelial cells is another possibility. Recovery may occur after floxuridine is discontinued. Some patients require dilation or stenting of biliary strictures.

DRUG-INDUCED STEATOHEPATITIS AND HEPATIC FIBROSIS

Steatohepatitis is a form of chronic liver disease in which fatty change is associated with focal liver cell injury, Mallory's hyaline, focal inflammation of mixed cellularity, including neutrophils, and progressive hepatic fibrosis in a pericentral (zone 3) and pericellular distribution.[348] Alcohol is a common etiologic factor. NASH is associated with insulin resistance, diabetes mellitus, obesity, and several drugs (e.g., perhexiline maleate, amiodarone).[349] In addition to causing steatohepatitis or chronic injury to liver cells or bile ducts, some exogenous compounds promote hepatic fibrogenesis directly, most likely through effects on hepatic nonparenchymal cells, especially stellate cells. Compounds that stimulate hepatic fibrosis include arsenic, vitamin A, and methotrexate.

Amiodarone

Amiodarone is an iodinated benzofuran antiarrhythmic drug that has several adverse effects involving the lungs, thyroid, and other organs. Hepatotoxicity is among the most serious complication and encompasses a spectrum of abnormalities from abnormal liver biochemical tests in 15% to 80% of patients to clinically significant liver disease, including rare cases of acute liver failure in 0.6%. Acute hepatitis has been reported with intravenous amiodarone; the toxic ingredient is likely to be the vehicle (polysorbate 80), because oral amiodarone has been successfully reinstituted in these cases.[350-355] It has been contended that ischemic hepatitis rather than drug toxicity is the actual diagnosis in these cases.[356] In longer-term users, steatohepatitis can develop; cirrhosis develops in 15% to 50% of patients with hepatotoxicity.[351,352]

A notable feature of amiodarone-induced liver disease is that progression of disease may occur despite discontinuation of amiodarone.[352,355] Amiodarone is highly concentrated in the liver, and after a few weeks of treatment, the drug accounts for as much as 1% of the wet weight of the liver. The iodine content absorbs radiation, so that the liver appears opaque on CT[355]; although odd, this appearance is not clinically significant.

Hepatic storage of amiodarone also produces phospholipidosis, a storage disorder characterized by enlarged lysosomes stuffed with whorled membranous material (myeloid bodies). In animals fed amiodarone, development of phospholipidosis is time and dose dependent.[353] Phospholipidosis may result from the direct inhibition of phospholipase or from the formation of nondegradable drug-phospholipid complexes and appears to have no relationship to the development of NASH and hepatocyte injury. Other occasional hepatic abnormalities include granuloma formation and acute liver failure, apparently due to severe acute hepatitis or a Reye's syndrome–like illness.[357] Amiodarone, by virtue of its physicochemical properties, is concentrated in mitochondria and may interrupt mitochondrial electron transport.[358] In rats and mice, treatment with amiodarone produces microvesicular steatosis, augments mitochondrial production of ROS, and causes lipid peroxidation.[359]

Chronic liver disease is detected only 1 year or more (median, 21 months) after amiodarone is started. The duration of treatment and possibly the total dose,[357,360] but not the incremental dose, are related to the development of chronic liver disease. Cases of cirrhosis with low-dose amiodarone have been documented.[361] The frequency of other toxic effects of amiodarone (most of which are thought to be dose dependent) is increased in patients with liver disease.[360]

Patient complaints include fatigue, nausea and vomiting, malaise, weight loss, and abdominal swelling due to ascites. Hepatomegaly, jaundice, bruising, and other features of chronic liver disease may be present. Liver biochemical test abnormalities include increased aminotransferase levels (up to 5 × ULN) and minor increases in serum alkaline phosphatase levels. The ratio of serum AST to ALT levels is close to unity and thus differs from the ratio seen in patients with alcoholic hepatitis. In severe cases, hyperbilirubinemia, hypoalbuminemia, and prolongation of the prothrombin time are evident. Diagnosing the cause of liver biochemical test elevations and hepatomegaly is often difficult in patients taking amiodarone, and a liver biopsy may be indicated. The histologic changes in the liver include phospholipidosis, steatosis, focal necrosis with Mallory's hyaline, infiltration with neutrophils, and pericellular fibrosis.[352] Cirrhosis is often present.

Prevention and management of amiodarone-induced liver disease are problematic because liver biochemical test abnormalities are common in patients who take amiodarone, particularly in those with heart failure. Further, the frequency of amiodarone hepatotoxicity does not appear to differ between patients with and without baseline serum ALT elevations, and amiodarone should not be withheld in patients with an elevated serum ALT level.[362] In asymptomatic or less severe cases, abnormalities resolve in 2 weeks to 4 months after amiodarone is discontinued. In cases of severe liver disease, the mortality rate is high.[352,360] Cessation of amiodarone therapy does not always result in clinical improvement, presumably because of prolonged hepatic storage of amiodarone, and in one study, outcome was worse (usually from fatal arrhythmias) in patients who discontinued amiodarone than in those who did not.[352] Although serial liver biochemical testing is recommended,[360] whether such testing is adequate to prevent serious amiodarone hepatotoxicity and reduce overall mortality is unknown.

Tamoxifen and Other Causes of Drug-Induced Steatohepatitis

For agents reported to be associated with steatohepatitis since the 1990s, causality has been difficult to prove,[363] particularly because NASH is frequent among patients with the metabolic syndrome (see Chapter 87). Calcium channel blockers have rarely been associated with steatohepatitis,[364] and methyldopa has been reported to be associated with cirrhosis in obese middle-aged women[365]; however, these associations may have been fortuitous. Other drugs, including estrogens[366] and glucocorticoids,[367] may precipitate NASH in predisposed persons because of their effects on the risk factors for NASH, including insulin resistance, type 2 diabetes mellitus, obesity, and hypertriglyceridemia. On the other hand, the association between NASH and tamoxifen is much stronger.

Tamoxifen is an estrogen receptor ligand used widely in treating breast cancer. Several forms of liver injury have been attributed to tamoxifen[368]: cholestasis, hepatocellular carcinoma,[369] peliosis hepatis,[370] acute hepatitis, massive hepatic necrosis,[368] steatosis, and steatohepatitis, occasionally with cirrhosis.[371-373] In one series of 66 women with breast cancer who had received tamoxifen for 3 to 5 years, 24 showed imaging evidence of hepatic steatosis.[372] The median time to development of steatosis is around 2 years.[374] Seven other patients have been found to have steatohepatitis after taking tamoxifen for 7 to 33 months.[371]

The metabolic profile of women with imaging evidence of hepatic steatosis (or histologic proof of steatohepatitis) during tamoxifen therapy appears similar to that of most patients with NASH; half have been obese, and the increase in body mass index has correlated with hepatic steatosis. Tamoxifen can induce hypertriglyceridemia, another risk factor for NASH. Reduction in the severity of hepatic steatosis has been documented with bezafibrate, a PPARα agonist.[375] Therefore, tamoxifen may play a synergistic role with other metabolic factors in causing steatohepatitis. This hypothesis is supported by results of an Italian tamoxifen chemoprevention trial in which fatty liver or steatohepatitis was noted mainly in overweight or obese women with the metabolic syndrome.[376]

Physicians need to be aware of the high frequency (≈30%) of hepatic steatosis or steatohepatitis, as determined by hepatic imaging or liver biopsy, in women who receive tamoxifen. Tamoxifen recipients should be monitored for this adverse effect by physical examination (to detect hepatomegaly) and liver biochemical testing; some authors also advocate annual hepatic imaging (by US or CT).[377] Liver biopsy may be indicated to establish the severity of the disorder, particularly if liver biochemical test abnormalities do not resolve after tamoxifen is discontinued or, in some cases, to exclude metastatic breast cancer. Many patients improve after tamoxifen is discontinued, but whether treatment should always be withdrawn permanently is not clear, particularly because the effect of tamoxifen on survival from breast cancer is impressive. Optimizing body weight is desirable because there is a 3-fold future risk of developing abnormal glucose tolerance.[378] An alternative option to bezafibrate is to use exemstane (or another aromatase inhibitor), which can lower serum triglyceride levels, instead of tamoxifen.

Toremifene, an analog of tamoxifen, is associated with a lower frequency (<10%) of steatosis or steatohepatitis than occurs with tamoxifen.[377] Raloxifene, a selective estrogen receptor modulator, has been implicated in one report of steatohepatitis and another of acute hepatocellular injury accompanied by eosinophilia,[379] but causality could not be established conclusively in this case because preexisting liver disease (NASH) could not be excluded. Perhexiline maleate and coralgil (4,4'-diethylaminoethoxyhexestrol) are definite causes of steatohepatitis and have been withdrawn from the market.[363]

Cyproterone Acetate

Cyproterone acetate (CPA) is a steroidal antiandrogen used for prostate cancer, acne, hirsuitism, and paraphilias and as a component of some oral contraceptives. Serious DILI occurs in 2% to 5% of patients treated with antiandrogens for metastatic prostate cancer, and although the nonsteroidal agents flutamide and bicalutamide are most often implicated, reactions to CPA are often particularly severe. Mean latency is just under 6 months, and reported reactions to CPA include jaundice (nature unspecified), hepatitis, cholestatic hepatitis, and mixed reactions.[380,381] Although 90% of CPA-related instances of DILI resolve slowly (over 6 months), cases of cirrhosis and hepatocellular carcinoma have been reported. Serial liver biochemical test monitoring has been recommended,[382] but there is no evidence to support the efficacy of this approach in preventing severe reactions. Patients treated with CPA and other antiandrogens should be warned to report new symptoms that could indicate liver injury.

Methotrexate

Methotrexate is a dose-dependent toxin. In high doses, methotrexate can result in bone marrow suppression, mucocutaneous reactions, pneumonitis, and hepatotoxicity. In the 1950s, previous methotrexate treatment of acute childhood leukemia was complicated by severe hepatic fibrosis and cirrhosis and a few cases of hepatocellular carcinoma. In the 1960s, the use of methotrexate for psoriasis was associated with hepatic fibrosis and cirrhosis in up to 25% of cases. Since then, a clearer picture of methotrexate as a dose-dependent promoter of hepatic fibrosis has emerged, particularly in persons who drink alcohol excessively or have preexisting liver disease. Guidelines have been instituted for scheduled pretreatment and interval liver biopsies to monitor the safety of methotrexate therapy.

Methotrexate is now usually used as a low-dose weekly regimen in managing rheumatoid arthritis, psoriasis, and other immunologic conditions, including IBD. The problem of methotrexate hepatotoxicity has largely been overcome by avoiding daily dosing and reducing the weekly dose to 5 to 15 mg.[383-385]

Risk Factors

Risk factors for methotrexate-induced hepatic fibrosis are listed in Table 88-9; dose, alcohol intake, and preexisting liver disease are the most important.[384,385] Total dose, incremental dose, dose interval, and duration of methotrexate therapy each influence the risk of hepatic fibrosis. After the cumulative ingestion of 3 g of methotrexate, the chance of histologic progression is 20%, but only 3% of patients have advanced hepatic fibrosis.[386] Obesity and diabetes mellitus are important risk factors for hepatic fibrosis, because they predispose to NASH

and are associated with induction of CYP2E1. The strong association between NASH and methotrexate in causing liver injury during long-term, low-dose methotrexate treatment has been highlighted,[387] as has the possibility that methotrexate itself can cause a pattern of injury resembling steatohepatitis. Increasing age, impaired renal function, and concomitant use of certain drugs decrease elimination of methotrexate or facilitate tissue uptake by displacing methotrexate from plasma protein-binding sites. Pharmacogenetic factors may also contribute. SNPs within genes involving folate metabolism and methotrexate transport into or out of red blood cells have also been linked to hepatotoxicity.[388]

Psoriasis and rheumatoid arthritis are associated with hepatic abnormalities that range from abnormal liver biochemical test levels (25% to 50% of cases) and minor histologic changes (50% to 70%) to fibrosis (11%) and cirrhosis (1%). In patients with psoriasis, alcoholism often is a complicating factor, and in a meta-analysis,[385] alcohol consumption was the most important determinant of advanced hepatic fibrosis in patients treated with methotrexate; the risk of progressive hepatic fibrosis was 73% in persons who drank more than 15 g of alcohol daily, compared with 26% in those who did not.

Whether low-dose (5 to 15 mg) methotrexate given as a single weekly dose can cause hepatic fibrosis has been debated.[383-385] The available data are limited by a lack of controlled studies in which liver histologic findings were evaluated; the lack of pretreatment evaluation of liver histology is a particularly serious deficiency in view of the high frequency of liver biochemical abnormalities among patients with rheumatoid arthritis and psoriasis. The conclusion has been reached that contemporary regimens can promote hepatic fibrosis, at least at the ultrastructural level, but cases of clinically significant liver disease are now virtually unknown. Repeat liver biopsies in some series have shown a reduction in fibrosis despite continuation of methotrexate in lower doses,[386] so although methotrexate remains a potential cause of liver disease, advanced hepatic fibrosis is in large part preventable.

Clinicopathologic Features

Liver biochemical test abnormalities are common among patients who take methotrexate, but advanced hepatic fibrosis occasionally can develop in the absence of such abnormalities. Likewise, nausea, fatigue, and abdominal pain are common adverse effects, but patients with hepatic fibrosis are typically asymptomatic unless complications of liver failure or portal hypertension develop. A firm liver edge, hepatomegaly, splenomegaly, and ascites may be noted. Liver biochemical test levels are either normal or show nonspecific changes, including minor elevations of serum ALT and GGTP levels. In more advanced cases, hypoalbuminemia and thrombocytopenia are present, but jaundice and coagulation disturbances are rare.

Liver histologic findings are graded according to the system of Roenigk, which has been useful in analyzing the published literature (also see Chapter 24).[385] In this system, grades I and II indicate a variable amount of steatosis, nuclear pleomorphism, and necroinflammatory activity, but no fibrosis. Higher grades reflect increasing degrees of fibrosis as follows: grade IIIa, few septa; grade IIIb, bridging fibrosis; and grade IV, cirrhosis. The pattern of hepatic fibrosis includes pericellular fibrosis, a feature of both alcoholic steatohepatitis and NASH; the possibility that methotrexate itself causes steatohepatitis or accentuates fibrogenesis among persons with underlying "primary NASH" has been suggested.[387] Cases of hepatic fibrosis with a relative paucity (or complete absence) of portal and lobular inflammation have been reported.

TABLE 88-9 Risk Factors for Methotrexate-Induced Hepatic Fibrosis

Risk Factor	Importance	Implications for Prevention
Age	Increased risk > 60 years, possibly related to reduced renal clearance and/or a biological effect on fibrogenesis	Care in use of methotrexate in older adults
Dose	Incremental dose Dose frequency Duration of therapy Cumulative (total) dose	5-15 mg/wk is safe Weekly bolus (pulse) safer than daily schedules Consider a liver biopsy every 2 years Consider a liver biopsy after each 2 g of methotrexate
Alcohol consumption	Increased risk with daily levels > 15 g (1-2 drinks)	Avoid methotrexate use if intake is not curbed Consider a pretreatment liver biopsy in a patient with a relevant history
Obesity	Increased risk	Consider a pretreatment and interval liver biopsies
Diabetes mellitus	Increased risk in obese persons (type 2 diabetes mellitus)	Consider a pretreatment and interval liver biopsies
Preexisting liver disease	Greatly increased risk, particularly related to alcohol, obesity, and diabetes mellitus (NASH)	Pretreatment liver biopsy is mandatory Avoid methotrexate, or schedule interval biopsies according to the severity of hepatic fibrosis, total dose, and duration of methotrexate therapy Monitor liver biochemical tests during therapy.
Systemic disease	Risk is possibly greater with psoriasis than rheumatoid arthritis (may depend on preexisting liver disease, alcohol intake)	None
Impaired renal function	Increased risk because of reduced clearance	Reduce dose; greater caution with use of methotrexate
Other drugs	NSAIDs, vitamin A, and arsenic may increase the risk Folate supplementation decreases risk	Greater caution with use; monitor liver biochemical tests Concurrent folate therapy is recommended
Genetic factors	Increased risk of liver injury is associated with SNPs related to genes involved in methotrexate transport into and out of red blood cells and in folate metabolism	Future strategies could involve pretreatment genetic screening

NASH, nonalcoholic steatohepatitis; SNPs, single nucleotide polymorphisms.

Outcome and Prevention

Serious clinical sequelae (portal hypertension, liver failure, hepatocellular carcinoma) resulting from methotrexate-induced liver disease are now rarely seen. In a study of 32 patients with IBD receiving methotrexate (mean dose, 2.6 g; follow-up period, 131 weeks), minor liver histologic changes were common, but advanced hepatic fibrosis was rare. Cases that have come to liver transplantation have generally been associated with suboptimal supervision of methotrexate therapy.[389] Cases of severe hepatic fibrosis (Roenigk grades IIIb and IV) are often associated with lack of progression and even improvement after dose reduction or cessation of methotrexate.[386] In less severe cases, a balanced judgment must be made about the appropriateness of continuing or discontinuing methotrexate. An interval liver biopsy after an additional 2 years or 2 g of methotrexate may be judicious in a patient who is found to have minor hepatic fibrosis earlier. Recommendations for preventing methotrexate-induced hepatic fibrosis have been made.[384,390] If possible, methotrexate should be avoided when the risk of liver injury is high. Persons treated with methotrexate should abstain from alcohol, and those who

drink more than 100 g of ethanol per week should not be given methotrexate.[384,385,390] A pretreatment liver biopsy is indicated only if the liver biochemistry is abnormal or if the history (e.g., alcoholism) and clinical features (e.g., hepatomegaly, risk factors for NASH) indicate possible underlying liver disease.[73] The risk of methotrexate hepatotoxicity when used for indications besides rheumatoid arthritis and psoriasis has been reassuringly low; a meta-analysis in 2012 showed that the risk of liver injury (defined by serum aminotransferase levels > 2 × ULN) for patients with IBD receiving methotrexate was 0.9 per 100 person-months, with low rates of discontinuation due to toxicity.[391]

To monitor progress during treatment, liver biochemical testing is recommended but is problematic because of the lack of specificity and sensitivity of the tests. An international panel of rheumatologists has proposed guidelines for patients receiving methotrexate.[392] These guidelines include gradual dose escalation of methotrexate, co-prescription of folic acid, and checking serum ALT and AST levels as well as blood counts and a serum creatinine level every 1 to 1.5 months until a stable dose of methotrexate is reached and every 1 to 3 months thereafter. If the ALT or AST level rises to 3 times

TABLE 88-10 Types of Drug-Induced Hepatic Vascular Disorders*

Disorder	Clinicopathologic Features	Outcomes	Implicated Etiologic Agents
Sinusoidal obstruction syndrome (veno-occlusive disease)	Abdominal pain, tender hepatomegaly, ascites, liver failure; occasionally chronic liver disease, other signs of portal hypertension	High mortality rate; some cases may evolve into nodular regenerative hyperplasia	Especially in bone marrow transplantation: 6-thioguanine, busulfan; dactinomycin, azathioprine, mitomycin; pyrrolizidine alkaloids
Nodular regenerative hyperplasia	Portal hypertension, encephalopathy—especially after variceal bleeding; diagnosed by histology	Relatively good prognosis	Anticancer drugs: busulfan, dactinomycin; azathioprine, didanosine
Noncirrhotic portal hypertension	Splenomegaly, hypersplenism, varices; ascites if associated hepatocellular disease	Prognosis depends on cause and associated liver injury	Vitamin A, methotrexate, azathioprine, arsenic, vinyl chloride, anticancer drugs, didanosine
Peliosis hepatis	May be an incidental finding; hepatomegaly, hepatic rupture, liver failure; diagnosed from appearances at surgery, vascular imaging	Prognosis depends on cause and complications	Anabolic steroids, azathioprine, 6-thioguanine
Sinusoidal dilatation	Hepatomegaly, abdominal pain	May regress after stopping oral contraceptives	Oral contraceptive steroids

*Also see Chapter 85.

ULN, methotrexate should be stopped, but the drug can be reintroduced at a lower dose if the liver biochemical tests normalize. A persistently elevated serum ALT or AST level greater than 3 times ULN, decreasing serum albumin level, or hepatomegaly warrants investigation by liver biopsy.

Liver biopsy is recommended after a cumulative dose of 4 g of methotrexate or duration of therapy of 2 years.[385] Other authors have suggested a slightly higher threshold (5 g) for liver biopsy.[393] Whether a liver biopsy is necessary in patients with normal liver biochemical test levels and without major risk factors for hepatic fibrosis remains unclear.[386] Some authors have suggested a lower threshold for liver biopsy (cumulative dose of 1.5 g and after every 1 g of methotrexate thereafter) for patients with no risk factors for hepatotoxicity.[394] Although histologic assessment of liver fibrosis remains the gold standard, noninvasive methods of monitoring using serum biomarkers (e.g., procollagen peptide-3 levels) and imaging techniques (e.g., ultrasound [transient] elastography) are being evaluated.[395]

DRUG-INDUCED VASCULAR TOXICITY

Drugs and chemical toxins are the most common causes of hepatic vascular injury,[396] which include several unusual types of liver disease, including sinusoidal obstruction syndrome (formerly veno-occlusive disease, a form of hepatic venous outflow obstruction), peliosis hepatis (dilatation and destruction of hepatic sinusoids), noncirrhotic portal hypertension, and nodular regenerative hyperplasia. The mechanism of injury is primarily dose-dependent toxicity to sinusoidal and other vascular endothelial cells, particularly when drugs are used in combination or concurrently with radiotherapy. Activation of inflammatory cells may also be important. Individual drugs (e.g., azathioprine) have been associated with more than one vascular syndrome, and the various disorders overlap and may evolve from one type to another. Vascular toxicity may give rise to a continuum of disorders, each resulting from injury to different components of the hepatic vasculature. The essential features of hepatic vascular disorders are summarized in Table 88-10 (also see Chapter 85). Hepatic imaging and measurement of portal pressure play a role in the diagnosis of these conditions; some, particularly nodular regenerative hyperplasia, are difficult to confirm in needle biopsy specimens.

Azathioprine

Hepatic complications of azathioprine, although rare (<0.1%), may be severe, diverse, and often late in onset. Many cases occur in complex medical situations, particularly organ transplantation, in which activation of the immune system, viral infections, and other agents may increase the risk of hepatotoxicity. The central role of azathioprine has been confirmed in some cases by positive rechallenge or resolution after the drug was stopped.[397,398] Disturbances associated with azathioprine include bland cholestasis, cholestatic hepatitis with bile duct injury,[398,399] zonal necrosis, and vascular toxicity.[397] Vascular toxicity may give rise to the diverse syndromes of sinusoidal obstruction syndrome, peliosis hepatis, nodular regenerative hyperplasia, and noncirrhotic portal hypertension.[397,399,400] Hepatocellular carcinoma with focal glycogenosis also has been reported with long-term use.

Cholestatic hepatitis is the most common presentation. Other cases have been associated with zone 3 necrosis and congestion, suggesting acute vascular injury, and azathioprine shares the vascular toxicity of other thiopurines. All of the hepatic vascular syndromes have been associated with azathioprine, particularly after organ transplantation. Nodular regenerative hyperplasia and sinusoidal obstruction syndrome have also been reported in patients receiving azathioprine for IBD and other medical conditions.[396]

There is no relationship of toxicity with dose or duration of therapy, but men are almost exclusively involved in cases of hepatic vascular injury following renal transplantation. Cholestatic reactions present within 2 weeks to 22 months, but vascular toxicity is recognized later, typically 3 months to 3 years (occasionally >9 years) after transplantation.[400] Cases of later onset are the result of delayed recognition and tend to present with complications of portal hypertension (e.g., ascites, liver failure). Recovery can occur in such cases,[398] but the overall mortality rate is high.

Successful substitution with 6-mercaptopurine has been achieved in cases of azathioprine hepatotoxicity.[401] In contrast to azathioprine, 6-mercaptopurine causes dose-dependent hepatocellular necrosis that has been fatal in a few cases. Other rare presentations include cholestasis[5] and hepatoportal sclerosis with portal hypertension.[402]

LIVER TUMORS

Several associations between pharmacologic and environmental agents and benign and malignant liver tumors have been described, but causality has been difficult to prove because of the rarity of these associations. For some sex steroid–related tumors, as well as for vinyl chloride–induced angiosarcoma, the relative risk attributable to the causative agent has been determined. The major tumors of interest include cavernous hemangioma, focal nodular hyperplasia, hepatic adenoma, hepatocellular carcinoma, angiosarcoma, hepatoblastoma, cholangiocarcinoma, mixed carcinosarcoma, and epithelioid hemangioendothelioma (see Chapter 96).

KEY REFERENCES

Full references for this chapter can be found on www.expertconsult.com.

33. Russmann S, Jetter A, Kullak-Ublick GA. Pharmacogenetics of drug-induced liver injury. Hepatology 2010; 52:748-61.
52. Dara L, Ji C, Kaplowitz N. The contribution of endoplasmic reticulum stress to liver diseases. Hepatology 2011; 53:1752-63.
65. Jaeschke H, Williams CD, Ramachandran A, Bajt ML. Acetaminophen hepatotoxicity and repair: The role of sterile inflammation and innate immunity. Liver Int 2012; 32:8-20.
75. Cacoub P, Musette P, Descamps V, et al. The DRESS syndrome: A literature review. Am J Med 2011; 124:588-97.
86. Davern TJ, Chalasani N, Fontana RJ, et al. Acute hepatitis E infection accounts for some cases of suspected drug-induced liver injury. Gastroenterology 2011; 141:1665-72.
97. Bebarta VS, Kao L, Froberg B, et al. A multicenter comparison of the safety of oral versus intravenous acetylcysteine for treatment of acetaminophen overdose. Clin Toxicol (Phila) 2010; 48:424-30.
104. Stewart JD, Horvath R, Baruffini E, et al. Polymerase gamma gene *POLG* determines the risk of sodium valproate–induced liver toxicity. Hepatology 2010; 52:1791-6.
112. Nunez M. Clinical syndromes and consequences of antiretroviral-related hepatotoxicity. Hepatology 2010; 52:1143-55.
116. Chang HM, Tsai HC, Lee SS, et al. Noncirrhotic portal hypertension associated with didanosine: A case report and literature review. Jpn J Infect Dis 2012; 65:61-5.
277. Chitturi S, Farrell GC. Lessons from lumiracoxib: Are cyclooxygenase-2 inhibitors less hepatotoxic than non-selective non-steroidal anti-inflammatory drugs? J Gastroenterol Hepatol 2012; 27:993-4.
326. Lucena MI, Molokhia M, Shen Y, et al. Susceptibility to amoxicillin-clavulanate-induced liver injury is influenced by multiple HLA class I and II alleles. Gastroenterology 2011; 141:338-47.
329. Paterson JM, Mamdani MM, Manno M, et al. Fluoroquinolone therapy and idiosyncratic acute liver injury: A population-based study. CMAJ 2012; 184:1565-70.
344. Daly AK, Donaldson PT, Bhatnagar P, et al. HLA-B*5701 genotype is a major determinant of drug-induced liver injury due to flucloxacillin. Nat Genet 2009; 41:816-19.
374. Saphner T, Triest-Robertson S, Li H, Holzman P. The association of nonalcoholic steatohepatitis and tamoxifen in patients with breast cancer. Cancer 2009; 115:3189-95.
388. Barker J, Horn EJ, Lebwohl M, et al. Assessment and management of methotrexate hepatotoxicity in psoriasis patients: Report from a consensus conference to evaluate current practice and identify key questions toward optimizing methotrexate use in the clinic. J Eur Acad Dermatol Venereol 2011; 25:758-64.

Liver Disease Caused by Anesthetics, Chemicals, Toxins, and Herbal Preparations

JAMES H. LEWIS

CHAPTER OUTLINE

The use of complementary and alternative medicine (CAM) preparations continues to increase, and reports of liver injury from potentially hepatotoxic herbal agents, dietary supplements, and weight loss products continue to appear (see Chapter 131).[1-4] Although halothane hepatitis is now largely of historical interest in Western nations,[5] it remains in use elsewhere, with ongoing reports of acute liver injury.[6,7] In contrast to the largely unpredictable hepatotoxicity seen with more modern anesthetics and most other medicinal agents (see Chapter 88), liver damage caused by occupationally and environmentally encountered chemical compounds and other toxins often is more predictable, dose related, and predominantly cytotoxic.[5,8,9] Industrial exposure to hepatotoxic chemicals is a far less frequent occupational hazard today than in the past in industrialized nations, but reports of toxicity from chemical agents, as well as metals, pesticides, adulterated cooking oils, and botanical toxins, have not disappeared, especially from developing countries,[10] nor has the risk of hepatic carcinogenesis been eliminated.[11] Mushroom poisoning appears to be on the rise, with silibilin emerging as a potential antidote.[12] Still, a substantial percentage of emergency liver transplants for acute liver failure are due to mycelism, herbal preparations, and various chemical compounds (see Chapters 95 and 97).[13,14]

ANESTHETIC AGENTS

The volatile inhalational anesthetics in current use are derivatives of some of the most potent chemical hepatotoxins developed for medicinal purposes. Chloroform, the original haloalkane anesthetic, has long been abandoned but remains an important experimental hepatotoxin, as does carbon tetrachloride (another chlorinated aliphatic hydrocarbon), which found use as an early vermifuge and is still employed as a household reagent in some parts of the world. Halothane (fluothane), introduced in 1956 as a safer, nonexplosive alternative to ether, is a haloalkane compound that produced a well-described but rare syndrome of acute hepatotoxicity, usually after repeat exposure.[15,16] The anesthetics that followed—methoxyflurane, enflurane, isoflurane—all have been implicated as a cause of similar injury, albeit less commonly for enflurane and isoflurane than for halothane; even fewer instances have been reported for the newest agents, sevoflurane and desflurane,[17,18] because of their proportionally lower degree of metabolism.[19] Halothane is no longer produced in the United States but continues to be used in other countries and is a case study in the elucidation of immunologic-mediated liver injury.[20]

Halothane

The retrospective National Halothane Study, cited in the past as the basis for exonerating halothane as a cause of hepatotoxicity,[21] is now considered flawed.[5] Nearly 1000 cases of halothane hepatotoxicity were reported worldwide during the 1960s and 1970s.[16,22] A fairly uniform clinical picture of postoperative fever, eosinophilia, jaundice, and hepatic necrosis occurred a few days to weeks after administration of anesthesia, usually after repeat exposure to halothane, and the case-fatality rate was high (Box 89-1). Rare cases of halothane-induced liver injury were reported after workplace exposure among anesthesiologists, surgeons, nurses, and laboratory staff and after halothane sniffing for "recreational" use; in affected persons, antibodies to trifluoroacetylated (TFA) proteins were demonstrated, indicating previous exposure.[23]

Two types of postoperative liver injury have been associated with halothane. A minor form (type 1) is seen in 10% to 30% of patients in whom mild, asymptomatic, self-limited elevations in serum ALT levels develop between the first and 10th postoperative days; the risk of hepatotoxicity is higher after 2 or more exposures to halothane than with subsequent use of alternative agents such as enflurane, isoflurane, and desflurane. Evidence of immune activation is lacking in these patients,[24] in whom the ALT elevations generally reverse rapidly.

The major form of halothane-induced hepatotoxicity (type 2) is a rare, dose-independent, severe hepatic drug reaction with elements of immunoallergy and metabolic idiosyncrasy (see Box 89-1). After an initial exposure to halothane, the frequency of this form of toxicity is only about 1 per 10,000,[25] but the rate increases to approximately 1 per 1000 after 2 or more exposures, especially when the anesthetic agent is readministered within a few weeks.[5] Typically, zone 3 (centrilobular) hepatic necrosis is seen histologically.[26] The case-fatality rate ranged from 14% to 71% in the pre–liver transplantation era[5] and remains high in developing countries where halothane is still used.[6,7]

Risk Factors

Host-related risk factors for halothane hepatitis are listed in Box 89-1. The reaction is rare in childhood[18]; patients younger than 10 years of age represent only about 3% of the total, and cases in persons younger than 30 years account for less than 10%.[18,22] In a 2008 Iranian series, 60% of patients were older than 40, with none being younger than 18.[6] The liver injury tends to be more severe in persons older than 40. Two thirds of cases have been in women, and repeat exposure to halothane (especially within a few weeks or months) is documented in as many as 90% of cases.[5] The time between exposures can be as long as 28 years,[27] although after repeat exposure, hepatitis is earlier in onset and more severe. Obesity is another risk factor, possibly because of storage of halothane in body fat. The induction of cytochrome P450 (CYP) enzymes (especially CYP2E1) that metabolize halothane to its toxic intermediate has been produced experimentally with phenobarbital, alcohol, and isoniazid; valproate inhibits and phenytoin has no specific effect on halothane hepatotoxicity.[5] Inhibition of CYP2E1 by administration of a single dose of disulfiram has been suggested as a means of preventing halothane hepatitis by inhibiting the production of the metabolite responsible for neoantigen formation.[28]

Familial predisposition to halothane-induced liver injury has been reported.[29] Serum antibodies to volatile anesthetics have been found in pediatric anesthesiologists,[23] who, like patients with halothane hepatitis, had higher levels of serum autoantibodies to CYP2E1 and to endoplasmic reticulum protein 58 (ERp58) than those found in general anesthesiologists and control subjects who had never been exposed to inhalational anesthetics. The autoantibodies, however, are not thought to have a role in pathogenesis.[5]

Pathology

In a study of 77 cases of halothane hepatitis reviewed by the Armed Forces Institute of Pathology,[26] various degrees of liver injury were seen, depending on the severity of the reaction. Massive or submassive necrosis involving zone 3 was present in all autopsy specimens, whereas biopsy material revealed a broader range of injury—from spotty necrosis in about one third of cases to sharply demarcated zone 3 necrosis in two

---

BOX 89-1 Epidemiologic, Clinical, and Histopathologic Features of Halothane Hepatitis

Epidemiologic Features
Estimated incidence
  After first exposure: 0.3 to 1.5 per 10,000
  After multiple exposures: 10 to 15 per 10,000
Female-to-male ratio 2-3 : 1
Latent period to first symptom
  After first exposure: 6 days (11 days to jaundice)
  After multiple exposures: 3 days (6 days to jaundice)

Risk Factors
Older age (>40 years)
Female gender
Two or more exposures (documented in 60%-90% of cases)
Obesity
Familial predisposition
Induction of CYP2E1 by phenobarbital, alcohol, or isoniazid

Clinical Features
Jaundice is the presenting symptom in 25% (range of serum bilirubin: 3-50 mg/dL)
Fever (75%; precedes jaundice in 75%); chills (30%)
Rash (10%)
Myalgias (20%)
Ascites, renal failure, and/or GI hemorrhage (20%-30%)
Eosinophilia (20%-60%)
Serum ALT and AST levels: 25-250× ULN
Serum alkaline phosphatase level: 1-3× ULN

Histopathologic Features
Zone 3 massive hepatic necrosis (30%); submassive necrosis (70%; autopsy series)
Inflammation usually less marked than in viral hepatitis
Eosinophilic infiltrate (20%)
Granulomatous hepatitis (occasional)

Course and Outcome
Mortality rate (pretransplantation era): 10%-80%
Symptoms can resolve within 5-14 days
Full recovery can take 12 weeks or longer
Chronic hepatitis is not well documented

Adverse Prognostic Findings
Age > 40 years
Obesity
Short duration to onset of jaundice
Serum bilirubin level > 20 mg/dL
Coagulopathy

CYP2E1, cytochrome P450 2E1.
ULN, upper limit of normal.
From references 5, 6, 17, and 18.

thirds. The inflammatory response is less severe than in acute viral hepatitis.

Pathogenesis

Approximately one third of halothane is metabolized via oxidative pathways via CYP2E1 and 2A6, and less than 1% is metabolized via reduction.[7] Hepatic injury occurs by 1 or more of 3 potential mechanisms: hypersensitivity, production of hepatotoxic metabolites, and hypoxia, in decreasing order of importance.[5] Evidence for the role of hypersensitivity is found in the increased susceptibility and shortened latency after repeat exposure, hallmark symptoms and signs of drug allergy (fever, rash, eosinophilia, and granuloma formation), and detection of neoantigens and antibodies. Halothane oxidation yields TFA, which is generated by the reaction between lysine and halothane metabolites and which acts on hepatocyte proteins to produce neoantigens that are responsible for the major form of injury.[7] By contrast, reductive pathways produce free radicals that can act as reactive metabolites that may have a role in causing minor injury.[30] Zimmerman suggested that halothane injury most likely results from immunologic enhancement of zone 3 necrosis produced by the reductive metabolites.[5] Accordingly, the hepatotoxic potential of halothane depends on the susceptibility of the patient and on factors that promote production of hepatotoxic or immunogenic metabolites.[5] A murine model of halothane hepatotoxicity has been developed and demonstrates female susceptibility based on an increase in levels of gamma interferon, possibly mediated through female hormones, and an increase in natural killer cell activity.[31,32]

Course and Outcome

Mortality rates for halothane hepatitis were high in early series; since then, successful treatment has been achieved with liver transplantation when necessary.[33] When spontaneous recovery occurs, symptoms usually resolve within 5 to 14 days, and recovery is complete within several weeks.[5] Immunosuppressive agents have only rarely been reported to improve the outcome.[18] It is doubtful that halothane causes chronic hepatitis.[5] Adverse prognostic factors include age older than 40 years, obesity, severe coagulopathy, serum bilirubin level greater than 20 mg/dL, and a shorter interval to onset of jaundice.[5,6,22,25]

The best treatment is prevention, specifically avoidance of reexposure, especially when a previous reaction has occurred. A history of a prior reaction to halothane contraindicates repeat use of halothane.[6,33] Attempts to demonstrate a protective role for zinc, disulfiram, and other compounds against halothane hepatitis have been reported in animal models,[28,34] but none has yet to be of proved value in humans.

Other Anesthetic Agents

The likelihood that individual haloalkane anesthetics will cause liver injury appears to be related to the extent to which they are metabolized by hepatic CYP enzymes: 20% to 30% for halothane, greater than 30% for methoxyflurane, 2% for enflurane, less than 1% for sevoflurane, and 0.2% or less for isoflurane and desflurane.[19] Accordingly, the estimated frequency of hepatitis from the newer agents is much less than that for halothane (Table 89-1).

Methoxyflurane caused hepatotoxicity and a high frequency of nephrotoxicity that led to its withdrawal.[35] Enflurane caused a clinical syndrome similar to that for halothane, with the onset of fever within 3 days and jaundice in 3 to 19 days after anesthesia[36,37]; the estimated incidence of enflurane-induced liver injury was about 1 in 800,000 exposed patients.[17]

Despite its low rate of metabolism,[19] several instances of isoflurane-associated liver injury have been reported.[38-42] In one case, cross-sensitivity was suspected 22 years after initial exposure to enflurane.[39] TFA liver proteins have been detected in patients with suspected isoflurane liver toxicity.[40]

The newest haloalkane anesthetics, desflurane and sevoflurane, appear to be nearly free of adverse hepatic effects. Desflurane undergoes minimal biotransformation and is not associated with the development of TFA antibodies in exposed rats.[19] Only isolated reports of liver injury in patients receiving desflurane anesthesia have been published.[43] The biotransformation of sevoflurane also is minimal, and only rare reports have implicated this agent in postoperative hepatic dysfunction.[44,45] Ether, nitrous oxide, and cyclopropane apparently are devoid of significant hepatotoxic potential because of their lack of halogen moieties,[5] and ketamine has only rarely been reported to cause hepatic injury.[46,47] Propofol is considered largely free of hepatotoxic effects, even in patients with cirrhosis.[47]

Jaundice in the Postoperative Period

From 25% to 75% of patients undergoing surgery experience postoperative hepatic dysfunction, ranging from mild elevations in liver biochemical test levels to hepatic failure, with postoperative jaundice reported in nearly 50% of patients with underlying cirrhosis (see Chapter 21).[48] Patients undergoing upper abdominal surgical procedures are at highest risk of postoperative liver dysfunction (see Chapter 73), as well as pancreatitis, cholecystitis, and bile duct injury, because of impaired blood flow to the liver.[48] Box 89-2 lists many causes of postoperative jaundice and hepatic dysfunction, broadly divided into hepatocellular injury, cholestasis, and indirect hyperbilirubinemia. Drugs that may cause hepatotoxicity in this setting include antibiotics (e.g., erythromycin, amoxicillin–clavulanic acid, trimethoprim/sulfamethoxazole,

TABLE 89-1 Hepatotoxic Anesthetics Other Than Halothane

Anesthetic	Percent Metabolized	Incidence of Hepatotoxicity	Cross-Reactivity with Other Haloalkanes	Other Clinical Features
Methoxyflurane	>30	Low	Yes	Nephrotoxicity
Enflurane	2	1 in 800,000	Yes	Similar to halothane
Isoflurane	0.2	Rare	Yes	Similar to halothane
Desflurane	<0.2	Few reports	Yes	Cardiac toxicity, malignant hyperthermia
Sevoflurane	Minimal	Rare	Uncertain	None reported

TABLE 89-2 Comparative Features of Causes of Acute Postoperative Liver Injury

Feature	Haloalkane Anesthetic Toxicity	Ischemic Hepatitis	Postoperative Cholestasis
Incidence	Rare	Not uncommon	Common
Latency	2-15 days	Within 24 hours	A few days
Fever, rash, eosinophilia	Present	Absent	Absent
Serum ALT/AST (× ULN)	25-200×	Can exceed 200× (AST≫ALT)	Minimal or normal
Jaundice	Common	Rare	Common (direct hyperbilirubinemia)
Histology	Zone 3 necrosis	Coagulative necrosis, sinusoidal congestion	Bile plugs, cholestasis
Mortality	High	Varies with diagnosis	Not from liver disease
Recovery time	Up to 12 weeks	10-12 days with supportive care	Variable, may be prolonged
Risk factors			
Age	Adults, age > 40 years	Any	Any
Gender	F > M 2:1	F = M	F = M
Body weight	Obese	Any	Any
Hypotension	May or may not be present	Documented in 50%	Absent

F, female; M, male; ULN, upper limit of normal.

BOX 89-2 Causes of Postoperative Hepatic Dysfunction

Hepatocellular Injury (predominant serum ALT elevation, with or without hyperbilirubinemia)
Acute transfusion-associated viral hepatitis
Hepatic allograft rejection
Hepatic artery thrombosis
Inhalational anesthetics—halothane, others
Ischemic hepatitis (shock liver)
Other drugs—antihypertensives (e.g., labetalol), heparin
Unrecognized chronic liver disease—NASH, hepatitis C, other disorders
Cholestatic Jaundice (elevated serum alkaline phosphatase ± ALT; direct hyperbilirubinemia)
Acalculous cholecystitis
Benign postoperative cholestasis
Bile duct injury—following cholecystectomy or liver transplantation
Bile duct obstruction—gallstones, pancreatitis
Cardiac bypass of prolonged duration
Cholangitis
Drugs—amoxicillin-clavulanic acid, chlorpromazine, erythromycin, telithromycin, trimethoprim/sulfamethoxazole, warfarin, others
Hemobilia
Microlithiasis (biliary sludge)
Prolonged TPN
Sepsis
Indirect Hyperbilirubinemia (serum alkaline phosphatase and ALT often normal)
Gilbert's syndrome
Hemolytic anemia (G6PD deficiency, other causes)
Multiple transfusions
Resorbing hematoma

G6PD, glucose-6-phosphate dehydrogenase; NASH, nonalcoholic steatohepatitis.
From references 1, 5, and 48.

fluoroquinolones) as well as the halogenated anesthetics discussed earlier. Table 89-2 contrasts the features of halogenated anesthetic-induced hepatitis, ischemic hepatitis (shock liver) (see Chapter 85), and cholestatic injury in the early postoperative period.

CHEMICALS

Commercial and Industrial Agents

Among the tens of thousands of chemical compounds in commercial and industrial use, several hundred are listed as causing liver injury by the National Institute for Occupational Safety and Health (NIOSH), as published in their *Pocket Guide to Chemical Hazards*.[49] The National Library of Medicine maintains a database of chemical toxins in its Toxicology and Environmental Health Information Program (TEHIP),[50] as do other sources.[51] Toxic exposure to chemical agents occurs most often from inhalation or absorption by the skin and less often from absorption by the GI tract after oral ingestion or through a parenteral route. Because most chemical toxins are lipid soluble, when absorbed they can easily cross biological membranes to reach their target organ(s), including the liver.[8-10] Hepatotoxic chemical exposure (as with carbon tetrachloride and phosphorus) usually results in an acute cytotoxic injury that typically consists of 3 distinct phases, similar to those observed after an acetaminophen overdose or ingestion of toxic mushrooms (Table 89-3).[5,8] Less commonly, acute cholestatic injury may occur.[52] Many chemicals (e.g., vinyl chloride) also are carcinogenic, and hepatic malignancies have been part of the clinicopathologic spectrum of chemical injury (Box 89-3).[1] Although liver injury is the dominant toxicity for some agents, hepatic damage may be only one facet of more generalized toxicity for other agents.[8]

TABLE 89-3 Phases of Illness after Ingestion of Various Hepatotoxins

Phase	Toxin			
	Acetaminophen	**Phosphorus**	**Amanita phalloides**	**Carbon Tetrachloride**
Phase I (1-24 Hours)				
Onset of toxicity	Immediate	Immediate	Delayed 6-20 hr	Immediate
Anorexia, nausea, vomiting, diarrhea	+	++++	++++	+
Shock	−	+	±	−
Neurologic symptoms	−	+	±	−
Phase II (24-72 Hours)				
Asymptomatic latent period	+	±	+	+
Phase III (>72 Hours)				
Jaundice	+	+	+	+
Hepatic failure	+	+	+	+
Renal failure	+	+	+	+
Maximum serum AST and ALT (× ULN)	1000	<10-100	500	500
Zonal necrosis	3	1	3	3
Steatosis	−	++++	+	+
Case-fatality rate	5%-15%	25%-50%	20%-25%	20%-25%

ULN, upper limit of normal.

Adapted from Zimmerman HJ. Hepatotoxicity. The adverse effects of drugs and other chemicals on the liver. 2nd ed. Philadelphia: Lippincott Williams & Wilkins; 1999.

BOX 89-3 Clinicopathologic Spectrum of Chemical Hepatotoxins

Acute Injury
Necrosis
Carbon tetrachloride and other haloalkanes
Cocaine, "ecstasy," phencyclidine
Haloaromatics, nitroaromatics, nitroaliphatics
Hydrochlorofluorocarbons
Phosphorus, iron, copper salts, inorganic arsenic

Microvesicular Steatosis
Boric acid
Chlordecone
Cocaine
Dimethylformamide
Hydrazine
Hypoglycin
Thallium
Toluene, xylene

Cholestasis
Alpha-naphthylisocyanate
Aniline—rapeseed oil
Dinitrophenol
Methylene dianiline
Paraquat

Subacute Injury
Necrosis
Trinitrotoluene

Sinusoidal Obstruction Syndrome
Pyrrolizidine alkaloids, arsenic, thorium dioxide

Toxic Cirrhosis
Hexachlorobenzene, polychlorinated biphenyls
Tetrachlorethane

Peliosis Hepatis
Dioxin

Chronic Injury
Cirrhosis
Chloroaliphatics, trinitrotoluene, arsenic, pyrrolizidine alkaloids

Hepatoportal Sclerosis
Arsenic, vinyl chloride

Neoplasia
Hepatocellular Carcinoma
Arsenic, aflatoxins, thorium dioxide

Angiosarcoma
Vinyl chloride, thorium dioxide, arsenic

Hemangioendothelioma
Arsenic

From references 1, 5, 8, 9, 15, and 52.

Carbon Tetrachloride and Other Chlorinated Aliphatic Hydrocarbons

Carbon tetrachloride (CCl_4) is a classic example of a zone 3 hepatotoxin that causes necrosis leading to hepatic failure (see Table 89-3). Injury is mediated by its metabolism to a toxic trichloromethyl radical catalyzed by CYP2E1.[13,53] Alcohol potentiates the injury through induction of this cytochrome.[5]

Most cases have been the result of industrial or domestic accidents, such as inhalation of CCl_4-containing dry cleaning fluids that are used as household reagents or ingestion of these compounds by alcoholics who mistake them for potable beverages.[5,54] At the cellular level, direct damage to cellular membranes results in leakage of intracellular enzymes and electrolytes, leading in turn to calcium shifts and lipid peroxidation.[15] Hepatic steatosis develops as a result of triglyceride

TABLE 89-4 Relative Hepatotoxicity of Haloalkane Compounds

Compound	Relative Toxicity
Carbon tetrachloride	++++
Tetrachlorethane	++++
Chloroform	++
Trichloroethylene	+ to ++
1,1,2-Trichloroethane	+ to ++
Tetrachloroethylene	+
1,1,1-Trichloroethane	+
Dibromomethane	±
Dichloromethane	±
Methylchloride	–

Scale from ++++, maximal injury, to –, trivial or no injury.
From references 5 and 8.

accumulation caused by haloalkylation-dependent inhibition of lipoprotein micelle transport out of the hepatocyte.[53] CCl$_4$ is more toxic than other haloalkanes and haloalkenes because toxicity correlates inversely with the level of bond dissociation energy, number of halogen atoms, and chain length (Table 89-4).[5,53] In older series, complete clinical and histologic recovery from CCl$_4$-induced liver damage was the rule with modest exposures, but supervening acute tubular necrosis and GI hemorrhage were associated with a case-fatality rate of 10% to 25%.[5,8] Activation of endonucleases, causing chromosomal damage and mutations, may result in carcinogenesis.[53] CCl$_4$ continues to play an important role in studies of hepatoprotection.[55]

Chloroform (trichloromethane) remains an important experimental hepatotoxin, although its use as an anesthetic has long been abandoned (see earlier).[5,8,10] Hepatic injury, including chronic hepatitis, has been reported with 1,1,1-trichloroethane,[56] which has been used as an inhaled treatment for trigeminal neuralgia, and instances of jaundice and hepatic necrosis are described in as many as 10% of workers exposed to the compound during its manufacture.[10]

Hydrochlorofluorocarbons (HCFCs) have been associated with liver injury in several industrial workers exposed to dichlorotrifluoroethane (HCFC-123) and 1-chlorotetrafluoroethane (HCFC-124), both of which are metabolized to reactive trifluoroacetyl halide intermediates similar to those implicated in halothane toxicity.[57] Zone 3 necrosis is present on liver biopsy specimens, and autoantibodies against CYP2E1 or P58 protein disulfide isomerase isoform are detected in the serum of many affected persons. As with halothane, liver toxicity may be potentiated by ethanol.[58]

Vinyl Chloride and Other Chlorinated Ethylenes

In the past, exposure to vinyl chloride monomer (VCM), or monochloroethylene, occurred in polymerization plants where vinyl chloride was heated to form polyvinyl chloride (PVC) in the manufacture of plastics; the toxic gas containing VCM was inhaled in this process.[5,11] Vinyl chloride is ubiquitous in the environment and has been estimated by the

Environmental Protection Agency to exist in at least 10% of toxic waste sites.[9] Although PVC appears to be nontoxic, long-term exposure to VCM has led to chronic liver injury, including nodular subcapsular fibrosis, sinusoidal dilatation, peliosis hepatis, and periportal fibrosis associated with portal hypertension.[5,8] Nonalcoholic fatty liver disease, including lipogranulomas, has been described in 80% of nonobese chemical workers with high exposure levels to VCM; some of these workers continued to have nonalcoholic steatohepatitis up to 6 years later.[59]

Vinyl chloride is carcinogenic[60] and is classified as a group I carcinogen by the International Agency for Research on Cancer.[11] Angiosarcoma develops after a mean latency of 25 years after exposure; the risk is related to the duration and extent of contact.[61] Alcohol appears to enhance the hepatocarcinogenicity of vinyl chloride, in rodents and possibly in humans, by inducing CYP2E1, which converts vinyl chloride to a toxic or carcinogenic metabolite (e.g., 2-chloroethylene oxide).[5] A history of vinyl chloride exposure was found in 15% to 25% of all cases of hepatic angiosarcoma reported in the late 1970s,[8] and strict hygienic measures instituted in 1974 resulted in a marked decrease in the frequency of angiosarcoma; however, persons with the highest exposure still have a 4-fold increased risk of developing periportal hepatic fibrosis, which may be a precursor to angiosarcoma.[62] Persons previously exposed to vinyl chloride should undergo regular clinical examinations for early detection of liver tumors, and those with known chronic liver disease or high levels of exposure should undergo regular hepatic imaging. Persons who work in PVC plants should undergo regular monitoring of liver biochemical test levels, and those with persistent abnormalities should be removed from workplace exposure.[62] High serum levels of hyaluronic acid were correlated with the development of angiosarcoma in 26 of 82 workers occupationally exposed to PVC in Kentucky.[63]

Nonhalogenated Organic Compounds

Benzene has been associated with minor hepatic injury in animals. Toluene led to steatosis and necrosis in a "glue sniffer,"[64] has been associated with acute fatty liver of pregnancy, and has caused elevations in serum GGTP levels after industrial exposure. Xylene can cause mild hepatic steatosis, and styrene (vinyl benzene) has led to elevated serum aminotransferase levels after prolonged exposure.[8] Elevated levels of serum cytokeratin 18 and proinflammatory cytokines have been found in workers with suspected toxicant-associated steatohepatitis exposed to acrylonitrile, styrene, and other elastomers or polymers and might serve as another potential biomarker of occupational liver injury.[65]

Trinitrotoluene and Other Nitroaromatic Compounds

Trinitrotoluene (TNT), or nitroglycerin, was first observed to be hepatotoxic during World War I, when severe acute and subacute hepatic necrosis developed in munitions workers in England, Germany, and the United States; the case-fatality rate was more than 25%.[5,8] The frequency of hepatotoxicity during World War II was lower, with approximately 1 in 500 workers affected, but the estimated frequencies of methemoglobinemia and aplastic anemia were 50 times higher.[8] Subacute hepatic necrosis followed 2 to 4 months of regular exposure to TNT. Percutaneous absorption was the major source of exposure. In some patients, rapidly progressive liver failure and death occurred within days to months, with massive hepatic necrosis at autopsy. In others, the subacute injury progressed over several months to micronodular cirrhosis and portal hypertension. The relatively low incidence of injury suggests that formation of a toxic metabolite was involved.[5] Nitrobenzene and dinitrobenzene also were observed to be hepatotoxic during World War I. As with TNT, excessive exposure led to methemoglobinemia.[8]

Nitroaliphatic Compounds

Nitromethane, nitroethane, and nitropropane cause variable degrees of hepatic injury. 2-Nitropropane (2-NP) has caused fatal massive hepatic necrosis after occupational exposure as a solvent, fuel additive, varnish remover, and rocket propellant. Toxic hepatitis associated with the chronic inhalation of propane and butane also has been reported.[66]

Polychlorinated Biphenyls and Other Halogenated Aromatic Compounds

Polychlorinated biphenyls (PCBs) are synthetic chlorinated aromatic hydrocarbons created from mixtures of trichloro-, tetrachloro-, pentachloro-, and hexachloro-derivatives of biphenyls, naphthalenes, and triphenyls that have been used in the manufacture of electrical transformers, condensers, capacitors, insulating materials for electrical cables, and industrial fluids. More than 100 different congeners have been synthesized.[11] Acute and chronic hepatotoxicity from PCB exposure seen during World War II resembled that caused by TNT.[8,9] Inhalation of toxic fumes released by the melting of PCBs and chloronaphthalene mixtures during soldering of electrical materials was the most common means of exposure.[5] The severity of liver injury correlated with the number of chlorine molecules.[8] Liver damage appeared as early as 7 weeks after ongoing exposure and was accompanied by anorexia, nausea, and edema of the face and hands. Acne-like skin lesions (chloracne) usually preceded hepatic injury. Once jaundice appeared, death occurred within 2 weeks in fulminant cases, which were characterized by massive necrosis (so-called acute yellow atrophy), or after 1 to 3 months in subacute cases. Cirrhosis developed in some persons who survived the acute injury.[5] Availability of PCBs declined significantly from a peak in the 1970s owing to a ban on production because of their health and environmental hazards,[67] although many are still in use.[11]

Polybrominated biphenyls (PBBs) appear to be even more toxic than PCBs. Consumption of milk and meat from livestock given feed mistakenly contaminated by a PBB led to hepatomegaly and minor elevations in liver enzyme levels in exposed persons.[8]

Miscellaneous Chemical Compounds

Dimethylformamide is a solvent used in the synthetic resin and leather industries that causes dose-related massive hepatic necrosis in animals[68] and is capable of producing focal hepatic necrosis and microvesicular steatosis in humans.[8] Most persons exposed for more than 1 year have symptomatic disease that slowly resolves when they are removed from the workplace.[8] Disulfiram-like symptoms can occur.[69] Alcohol use, HBV infection, and a high body mass index are risk factors.[70] Dimethylacetamide hepatotoxicity is well described in animals, with only rare reports after human exposure.[11,71]

Hydrazine and its derivatives used in jet and rocket fuel cells are also experimental hepatotoxins and carcinogens and have been reported to cause hepatic steatosis in animals[5] and reversible injury in humans after inhalation.[72] Bromoalkanes and iodoalkanes, used in insecticides and aircraft fuels, have rarely caused hepatic injury.[8] Ethylene dibromide (dibromoethane) has led to zone 3 hepatic necrosis after ingestion in attempted suicide and to fatal hepatotoxicity associated with

nephrotoxicity and cardiotoxicity following occupational exposure or inadvertent poisoning.[73]

Pesticides

Although exposure to insecticides, herbicides, and other pesticides is common, acute liver injury resulting from these compounds, many of which are chlorinated hydrocarbons, is rare.[5,8] Evidence that dichlorodiphenyl-trichloroethane (DDT) and other organochlorines (aldrin, amitrole, chlordane, dieldrin, lindane, mirex) lead to liver damage or carcinogenicity is limited,[5] but a study in 2012 has suggested a possible relationship with hepatocellular carcinoma.[74] Agent Orange (2.4-dichlorophenoxyacetic acid), the defoliant widely used in Vietnam, has been reported to cause acute hepatitis after chronic exposure, although contaminating dioxins have been suggested to be responsible for the toxic effects.[75,76] Moreover, chronic liver injury among Vietnam veterans is more likely to have been related to viral infections or alcohol than to Agent Orange,[76] and hepatocarcinogenesis is more likely to have been related to chronic hepatitis B.[77]

Ingestion of or dermal exposure to dichloride dimethyldipyridilium (paraquat) has been implicated in several instances of hepatotoxicity as a result of attempted suicide and homicide.[78] Patients may present with severe vomiting and profuse diarrhea leading to hypokalemia and often have evidence of oral, pharyngeal, and esophageal caustic injury after ingestion. Death results from a combination of renal, respiratory, cardiac, and hepatic failure; mortality rates are as high as 70%, and death often occurs within the first 48 hours. Histopathologic changes include zone 3 necrosis followed by injury to small- and medium-sized interlobular bile ducts.[79] Treatment with charcoal hemoperfusion in conjunction with cyclophosphamide, dexamethasone, furosemide, and vitamins B and C—the so-called Caribbean scheme—has been attempted, but persons who ingest more than 45 mL are likely to die with or without this treatment.[78] In animals, N-acetylcysteine and silymarin may be protective.[80]

Chlordecone (Kepone) has been shown to impair biliary excretion and lipid transport and storage,[81] but neurologic toxicity appears to dominate the clinical injury. Occupational exposure has led to hepatic steatosis and elevated serum aminotransferase levels. Trivial hepatic enzyme abnormalities have been seen in persons heavily exposed to chloretone.[8] Hexachlorobenzene in contaminated grain has been associated with an epidemic of porphyria cutanea tarda and liver injury.[8]

Inorganic arsenic has long been used as a homicidal or suicidal agent, and toxic exposure in the past also followed ingestion of Fowler's solution (arsenic trioxide), used as a treatment for psoriasis and asthma.[5,8] Organic arsenic is present in seafood, whereas inorganic forms are found mainly in contaminated ground and well water[11] and homemade alcohol.[5] Doses greater than 3 g can cause death in 1 to 3 days, but hepatic injury generally is overshadowed by GI, neurologic, and vascular effects, leading ultimately to central nervous system (CNS) depression and vascular collapse.[5] A lesion resembling hepatic sinusoidal obstruction syndrome (veno-occlusive disease) can develop,[8] and noncirrhotic portal hypertension developed in more than 90% of 248 patients who consumed contaminated drinking water for up to 15 years.[82]

Occupational exposure to inorganic arsenic is still observed among vineyard workers, farmers, and gold miners,[83] although its use as an insecticide has been curtailed since the 1940s. Lumber treated with chromated copper arsenate as a preservative may be an additional source of exposure.[84] The clinical syndrome associated with arsenicosis includes skin lesions (blackfoot disease), anemia, diabetes mellitus, hearing loss, neurobehavioral disorders, and cardiovascular diseases, in addition to benign and malignant liver disease.[85] Chronic hepatic injury, including cirrhosis and noncirrhotic portal hypertension, may be a precursor to hepatic neoplasms, such as angiosarcomas, hemangioendotheliomas, and hepatocellular carcinomas, after exposure of more than 10 years.[11,86] Increased serum levels of EGF receptor have been found in patients with liver cancer who overexpress this biomarker following exposure to arsenic.[87] Treatment with thiol chelators has had variable success in cases of prolonged exposure, and coadministration of antioxidants, such as vitamins C and E, may be of added benefit.[88]

METALS

Iron

Most of the 5000 cases of accidental iron poisoning in the United States each year occur in young children who mistake iron supplements for candy.[5] Ferrous sulfate tablets contain 20% elemental iron by weight, and the severity of injury correlates with the dose ingested.[8] Ingestion of less than 20 mg/kg of elemental iron is unlikely to produce serious toxicity, whereas doses of more than 200 mg/kg can be fatal.[5] Severe injury has been seen only with serum iron concentrations above 700 mg/dL measured within the first 12 hours after ingestion.[89] Iron, per se, is not hepatotoxic, but ferric and ferrous ions can act through free radicals and lipid peroxidation to cause membrane disruption and necrosis.[90] Clinically evident liver injury is uncommon, but zone 1 necrosis occurs in the most severe cases.[5] Clinical illness is characterized by sequential phases of GI injury, subsidence of symptoms, and overt hepatotoxicity accompanied by renal failure.[91] Deferiprone, an oral iron chelator, was implicated in causing worsening hepatic fibrosis in a long-term study of patients with thalassemia[92]; however, these findings were not confirmed by subsequent histopathologic analysis,[93] and injury from this agent appears unlikely. Hyperbaric oxygen treatment of acute iron intoxication has been effective in an animal model[94] and may offer a potential therapy in cases of human poisonings.

Phosphorus

Poisoning by white phosphorus has been rare since its use in firecrackers and matches was outlawed in the mid-20th century.[8] Cases reported since then usually have been the result of ingestion of rat or roach poison.[5] Shortly after ingestion, vomiting, GI bleeding, convulsions, shock, and death occur within 24 hours. Phosphorescence of the vomitus and stools and a typical garlic-like odor on the breath are characteristic, when present. The predominant hepatic lesion is steatosis and necrosis, most prominent in the periportal region. Serum aminotransferase levels generally are no higher than 10 times the upper limit of normal.[5]

Copper

Acute poisoning by copper leads to a syndrome resembling iron toxicity. Ingestion of toxic amounts (1 to 10 mg) usually is seen with suicidal intent, especially on the Indian subcontinent.[8,90] Vomiting, diarrhea, and abdominal pain accompanied by a metallic taste are seen during the first few hours after ingestion. GI tract erosions, renal tubular necrosis, and rhabdomyolysis often accompany zone 3 hepatic necrosis by the second or third day. Jaundice results from both hepatic injury and acute hemolysis caused by high blood copper levels.[8] The mortality rate is 15%, with early deaths resulting from shock and circulatory collapse and late deaths resulting from hepatic and renal failure.[5]

Thorium Dioxide

Thorotrast is a colloidal suspension of radioactive thorium dioxide that was used as an IV contrast medium for radiographic procedures in the first half of the 20th century, with more than 50,000 persons having been exposed.[5] Thorotrast was subsequently found to cause hepatic angiosarcomas and cholangiocarcinomas after latency periods of 20 to 40 years. The long latency is thought to be due in part to the uneven distribution of radionuclides and the limited range of the alpha particles being emitted.[95] Histologically, thorium dioxide is found in Kupffer cells and macrophages as dark brown refractile granules, the identity of which can be confirmed by spectrographic analysis.[53] As with arsenic, reports of hepatic sinusoidal obstruction syndrome and a Budd-Chiari–like syndrome also have appeared.[1] Given the extraordinarily long half-life (hundreds of years) of the compound, exposed persons remain at risk for the development of leukemia, in addition to hepatocellular cancer,[96] and require life-long monitoring because hepatic malignancies have occurred in approximately 20% of those exposed.[97]

Others

Although cadmium produces hepatic necrosis and cirrhosis in laboratory animals,[98] evidence is lacking that exposure to cadmium causes important human injury.[5] Several metals are associated with apoptosis, which might explain their potential for hepatotoxicity.[99] Beryllium has led to midzonal liver necrosis as a result of phagocytosis of insoluble beryllium phosphate by Kupffer cells.[5] Chronic industrial exposure (usually by inhalation of high concentrations of oxide or phosphorus mixtures) is associated with the formation of hepatic (and pulmonary) granulomas.[8] Therapy with chelating agents and antioxidants has been used in animal models of beryllium toxicity.[100] Lead hepatotoxicity may be seen as part of the larger symptom complex of abdominal pain, constipation, and encephalopathy that occurs with chronic ingestion or environmental exposure.[101]

ADULTERATED COOKING OILS AND CONTAMINATED FOODS

A number of contaminated foodstuffs and cooking oils have been associated with epidemics of hepatotoxicity. They are now largely of historical interest only.

The Spanish toxic oil syndrome occurred in 1981 after exposure of up to 100,000 Spaniards to rapeseed cooking oil that was contaminated by anilines and acetanilides. Nearly 20,000 persons became ill, many with hepatic injury and jaundice, and approximately 2500 died.[102] Among 332 patients followed for up to 8 years, hepatic injury developed in 43%, usually at the onset of a multisystem disease. A mixed cholestatic-hepatocellular injury pattern was seen, with jaundice or hepatomegaly in fewer than 20%. After an 8-year follow-up, liver disease persisted in only 4 patients.[102]

Epping jaundice refers to an epidemic of toxic liver injury that occurred in Epping, England, in 1965.[8,52,103] The outbreak involved 84 persons who had eaten bread contaminated with methylenedianiline that had spilled onto the floor of a van carrying flour. The clinical syndrome consisted of abdominal pain, fever, and chills, followed by cholestatic jaundice resembling that seen with biliary obstruction; eosinophilia was seen in about half the cases. Liver biopsy specimens revealed Kupffer cell hyperplasia with portal inflammation but little or no necrosis.[8] Most persons recovered in 4 to 6 weeks, with jaundice lasting up to 4 months in a few. The mechanism of injury was thought to be a chemically induced cholangitis, possibly as a result of a hypersensitivity reaction. Cholangiocarcinoma developed later in 1 patient.[103]

Yusho oil disease in western Japan, and a related epidemic referred to as *yu-cheng* in Taiwan, involved nearly 2000 persons who had eaten rice prepared in oil contaminated by PCBs, dioxins, and polychlorinated dibenzofurans in 1968.[104] The disease was characterized by chloracne, skin hyperpigmentation, eyelid edema, and neuropathy, with jaundice reported in approximately 10% of patients. Exposed persons still harbored high levels of these agents nearly 3 decades after the outbreak.[104]

Hexachlorobenzene contamination of wheat in the 1950s led to an epidemic of toxic porphyria cutanea tarda and severe liver disease involving more than 3000 Turkish Kurds, with a mortality rate that exceeded 10%. This fungicide had been added to seed grain that was used for food during a famine.[8,52]

DRUGS OF ABUSE

Cocaine

Cocaine is a dose-dependent hepatotoxin.[8] Acute cocaine intoxication affects the liver in 60% of patients, and many affected persons have markedly elevated serum ALT levels (>1000 U/L). Associated features include rhabdomyolysis, hypotension, hyperpyrexia, DIC, and renal failure.[5,8] Hepatic injury probably is the result of toxic metabolites (e.g., norcocaine nitroxide) formed by CYP2E1 and CYP2A,[105] and enhanced hepatotoxicity is seen in persons who regularly consume alcohol.[8] In animals, pretreatment with *N*-acetylcysteine decreases the risk of cocaine hepatotoxicity,[106] although the usefulness of *N*-acetylcysteine for treating human cocaine-induced hepatic injury has not been determined.

Others

"Ecstasy" (3,4-methylenedioxymethamphetamine) is a euphorigenic and psychedelic amphetamine derivative that can lead to hepatic necrosis as part of a heat stroke–like syndrome resulting from exhaustive dancing in hot nightclubs ("raves").[107] The injury can be fatal and has necessitated liver transplantation in some instances.[108,109] The role of CYP enzymes in the toxicity of this and other so-called designer drugs may relate to specific genetic polymorphisms of CYP2D6 or other cytochromes.[110]

Phencyclidine ("angel dust") is another stimulant that can lead to hepatic injury as part of a syndrome of malignant hyperthermia that produces zone 3 hepatic necrosis, congestion, and collapse, with high serum AST and ALT levels reminiscent of ischemic hepatitis.[111]

BOTANICAL AND ENVIRONMENTAL HEPATOTOXINS

Examples of hepatotoxic mushrooms, fruits, and other foodstuffs, including grains and nuts contaminated by fungal mycotoxins or other potentially injurious compounds, are listed in Table 89-5.

Mushrooms

Poisonous varieties of mushrooms number approximately 100 among the more than 5000 species, but only about 32 have been associated with fatalities. More than 8000 mushroom poisonings were reported in the United States in 2004.[112] Greater than 90% of cases of fatal poisoning are caused by *Amanita phylloides* (death cap) or *Amanita verna* (destroying angel), found in the Pacific Northwest and eastern United States.[113] A fatal outcome can follow ingestion of a single 50-g (2-oz) mushroom; the toxin is one of the most potent and lethal in nature.[114] Alpha-amatoxin is thermostable, can resist drying for years, and is not inactivated by cooking. Rapidly absorbed through the GI tract, the amatoxin reaches hepatocytes through the enterohepatic circulation and inhibits production of messenger RNA and protein synthesis, leading in turn to cell necrosis. A second toxin, phalloidin, is responsible for the severe gastroenteritis that precedes hepatic and CNS injury.[115] Phalloidin disrupts cell membranes by interfering with polymerization of actin. A latent period of 6 to 20 hours after ingestion of a mushroom precedes the first symptoms of intense abdominal pain, vomiting, and diarrhea. Hepatocellular jaundice and renal failure occur over the next 24 to 48 hours and are followed by confusion, delirium, convulsions, and eventually coma by 72 hours.[5,115] The characteristic hepatic lesion is steatosis and zone 3 hepatic necrosis, with nucleolar inclusions seen on electron microscopy.[8]

In a case series of 8 patients,[116] the mean serum AST level was 5488 U/L (range, 1486 to 12,340), ALT 7618 (range, 3065 to 15,210), and bilirubin 10.5 mg/dL (range, 1.8 to 52), with peak levels on days 4 and 5. Acute kidney injury requiring dialysis developed in 1 patient, and 3 exhibited encephalopathy. Mortality rates traditionally have been high, especially when the serum ALT level exceeds 1000 U/L, and emergency liver transplantation often is required[116]; however, some

TABLE 89-5 Botanical and Environmental Hepatotoxins

Agent	Toxic Component	Type of Injury	Comment
Ackee fruit	Hypoglycin	Microvesicular steatosis	Jamaican vomiting sickness
Aspergillus flavus	Aflatoxin B1	Acute hepatitis, portal hypertension	Hepatocarcinogenic
Aspergillus tamari	Cyclopiazonic acid	Acute hepatitis	—
Cycasin	Methylazoxymethanol	Acute hepatitis	—
Toxic mushrooms	Alpha-amatoxin, phalloidin	Fulminant hepatic failure	Resembles APAP injury

APAP, *N*-acetyl-*p*-aminophenol (acetaminophen).

patients survive with conservative management, which includes NG lavage with activated charcoal, IV penicillin G, N-acetylcysteine (using a standard oral or IV protocol (see Chapter 88), along with milk thistle (*Silybum marianum*) (see Chapter 131).[115] The use of these therapeutic modalities is not always effective, and in a large review of 2108 cases over a 20-year period in the United States and Europe,[117] penicillin G, either alone or in combination with other therapy, demonstrated limited benefit. No role for glucocorticoids has been found, but plasmapheresis or hemoperfusion has been beneficial in some instances.[118] In a 2012 study, the addition of IV silibinin (isolated from milk thistle) in a loading dose of 5 mg/kg, followed by 20 mg/kg continuous infusion for 24 hours, given with standard supportive measures, proved effective in reducing mortality to less than 10% in nearly 1500 cases.[12] These results prompted the authors to recommend silibinin as the antidote of choice.

Other Foodstuffs

The unripe fruit of the ackee tree *(Blighia sapida)*, native to Jamaica, contains a hepatotoxin, hypoglycin A, that produces a clinical syndrome of GI distress and microvesicular steatosis known as *Jamaican vomiting sickness*, which resembles Reye's syndrome (see Chapter 88).[8,52,119] Cholestatic jaundice has been described after chronic ingestion.[120]

Cycasin is a potent hepatotoxin and hepatocarcinogen found in the fruit of the cycad tree (*Cycas circinalis, Cycas revoluta*). A small epidemic of acute hepatic injury attributable to the ingestion of cycad nuts was reported from Japan. The purported toxin is methylazoxymethanol, which normally is eliminated or rendered inactive in preparing the nuts before ingestion.[8]

Aflatoxins are a family of mycotoxins found in *Aspergillus flavus* and related fungi that are ubiquitous in tropical and subtropical regions. They contaminate peanuts, cashews, soybeans, and grains stored under warm, moist conditions and are well-known hepatotoxins and hepatocarcinogens.[5,8] Aflatoxin B1, a potent inhibitor of RNA synthesis, is the most hepatotoxic member of the family. Reactive metabolites are formed by CYP enzymes, and malnutrition is a possible potentiating factor (perhaps because of the depletion of glutathione). When consumed in large quantities, aflatoxin B1 is responsible for a clinical syndrome characterized by fever, malaise, anorexia, and vomiting, followed by jaundice. Portal hypertension with splenomegaly and ascites may develop over the next few weeks. In large epidemics, mortality rates have approached 25% and correlate with the dose ingested.[8] Zone 3 hepatic necrosis without inflammation is the characteristic lesion. Other histologic findings include cholestasis, microvesicular steatosis, and bile duct proliferation.[8]

The risk of hepatocellular carcinoma (HCC) correlates with the amount of aflatoxin consumed, especially in sub-Saharan Africa and eastern China, where wheat often exceeds rice as a staple in the diet (see Chapter 96).[8] Alcohol and possibly exposure to DDT (see earlier) may play an enhancing role in hepatocarcinogenesis.[121] An even more important cofactor may be HBV.[122] The frequency of a mutation in the *TP53* tumor suppressor gene correlates with the development of HCC in these regions, but this mutation is rare in HCC from Western countries (see Chapter 96).[122]

VITAMINS AND HERBAL PREPARATIONS

The use of vitamins, dietary supplements, nutraceuticals, and herbal remedies is an important aspect of CAM and continues to increase (see Chapter 131).[123] In the United States, alternative medicines were used by 38% of adults and nearly 12% of children in 2007,[124] with nearly 20% of the population having taken CAM at the same time as conventional prescriptions.[125] The use of herbal products is popular among patients with chronic liver disease,[126,127] despite the absence of formal controlled clinical trials to assess safety and efficacy in this setting.[128] In a population-based survey of 1040 patients with a wide array of chronic liver diseases (including 18% with cirrhosis), current use of CAM was listed by 27.3%.[126] The most commonly used products were vitamins and other dietary supplements in 18% and herbal remedies in 16.8%. CAM had been prescribed by a physician in 24% to 32% of respondents.[126]

Many so-called health foods, dietary and weight-loss supplements, and herbal products are potent hepatotoxins that have led to acute liver failure and the need for emergency liver transplantation.[13,14,129,130] Preparations containing anabolic androgenic steroids may cause severe cholestatic liver injury,[129-132] and other safety concerns involving such dietary supplements persist, despite the enactment of the Dietary Supplement Health and Education Act in 1994.[128,133,134]

Vitamin A

Among vitamin supplements, vitamin A remains the most important hepatotoxin. Vitamin A (retinol) is a dose- and duration-dependent hepatotoxin capable of causing injury ranging from asymptomatic elevations in serum aminotransferase levels with minor hepatic histologic changes to perisinusoidal fibrosis leading to noncirrhotic portal hypertension and, in some cases, cirrhosis.[135] Approximately one third of the U.S. population is estimated to take vitamin supplements containing vitamin A, with as many as 3% of products providing a daily dose of at least 25,000 IU. Hypervitaminosis A usually is the result of self-ingestion, rather than intentional overdose, and all age groups are represented.[136] The average daily dose of vitamin A in reported cases of liver disease has been nearly 100,000 IU over an average duration of 7.2 years, for a mean cumulative dose of 229 million IU, but liver injury has been described with daily doses of 10,000 to 45,000 IU,[137] and cirrhosis has occurred after a daily intake of 25,000 IU for at least 6 years.[135,137] On the other hand, long-term use of low-dose vitamin A supplements (250 to 5000 retinol equivalents per day) does not appear to be toxic.[138]

Because of the long half-life of vitamin A in the liver (50 days to 1 year),[137,139] the fibrotic process may continue because of the slow release of hepatic vitamin A stores despite discontinuation of oral intake of the vitamin.[140] Genetic factors may play a role, and apparent familial hypervitaminosis A has occurred in 4 siblings who ingested large doses as treatment for congenital ichthyosis.[141] Vitamin A toxicity has been reported in native Alaskans who ingest large amounts of fresh polar bear liver,[135] which is plentiful in arctic predators but does not cause them hepatic injury.[142] Water-soluble, emulsified, and solid formulations of vitamin A are up to 10 times as toxic as oil-based preparations because of higher peak plasma levels, higher hepatic concentrations, and less fecal loss with the water-miscible formulations.[143]

Hepatotoxicity from vitamin A has been attributed to activation of hepatic stellate cells, the body's principal storage site of the vitamin. Resulting hyperplasia and hypertrophy produce sinusoidal obstruction and increased collagen synthesis, leading in turn to portal hypertension.[144] Rare cases of peliosis hepatis also have been attributed to hypervitaminosis A. Ethanol interferes with the conversion of beta carotene, a precursor of vitamin A, to retinol, and the combination of ethanol and beta carotene has resulted in hepatotoxicity in various experimental models.[145]

Liver biopsy specimens show increased storage of vitamin A, seen as characteristic greenish autofluorescence after irradiation with ultraviolet light.[135] The excess vitamin A is stored initially in stellate cells that lie in the space of Disse and become hyperplastic and hypertrophic. The enlarged clear stellate cells compress the hepatic sinusoids, giving rise to a "Swiss cheese" or honeycombed appearance.[135] Hepatocellular injury usually is minor, with microvesicular steatosis and focal degeneration and without significant necrosis or inflammation. Hepatic fibrosis in a perisinusoidal distribution can arise from activated stellate cells that transform into myofibroblasts. In a widely cited series,[135] cirrhosis was present in 59%, chronic hepatitis in 34%, microvesicular steatosis in 21%, perisinusoidal fibrosis in 14%, and peliosis in 3% of cases.

In affected patients, hepatomegaly is common, and in severe cases, splenomegaly, ascites, and esophageal variceal bleeding may be features.[5,129] Hypervitaminosis A also can involve the skin and CNS.[5] Liver biochemical test abnormalities, present in two thirds of cases, are nonspecific, with only modest elevations in serum aminotransferase and alkaline phosphatase levels.

The diagnosis of vitamin A toxicity rests on a dietary and medication history and clinical suspicion. Plasma vitamin A levels may be normal, and the diagnosis is supported by the demonstration of increased hepatic stores of vitamin A and characteristic histologic findings.[146] The diagnosis may be delayed for several years if hepatotoxicity is not recognized or is misdiagnosed.[135,137]

Symptoms resolve and liver enzymes normalize gradually after discontinuation of vitamin A ingestion in less severe cases, but deterioration may continue in cases of severe intoxication, particularly when cirrhosis is already present.[137] Features of liver failure and cirrhosis at the time of diagnosis indicate a poor prognosis, and liver transplantation may be required.[5] Alcohol can potentiate hepatotoxicity and should be avoided. Vitamin A supplements generally should be avoided in other types of liver disease because of possible accentuation of hepatic injury and fibrosis.[145] Severe liver injury rarely has been reported with the use of acitretin, a vitamin A metabolite.[147]

Herbal Remedies and Nutritional Supplements

The increasing use of CAM is well described in patients with liver disease (see Chapter 131).[126,127,148] Silymarin (*Silybum marianum*, milk thistle) is the most commonly used herbal preparation among these patients,[148] and although it appears to be quite safe,[149] if not effective,[150] an increasing number of reports of hepatotoxicity from several classes of herbal and weight-reduction agents have paralleled the rise in use of CAM therapies.[1,129,151] Indeed, the prevalence of hepatotoxicity from herbal and dietary supplements in drug-induced liver injury registries is appreciable, ranging from 2% to 10% in westernized nations[2] and as high as 73% in Asian centers.[3,152-154] Warnings have been issued for several agents, and in a few instances, the FDA and other health authorities have requested their removal from the marketplace (e.g., kava kava, ephedra [ma huang], Lipokinetix, and Hydroxycut in the United States[155] and germander in France[2] [see later]). Any patient with liver disease should be questioned about the ingestion of herbal remedies; Estes and colleagues,[130] for example, documented the use of several commonly promoted herbal agents (including Lipokinetix, skullcap, ma huang, chaparral, and kava kava) in 50% of 20 patients with acute liver failure over a 2-year period.

Table 89-6 lists herbal remedies associated with hepatotoxicity; however, the case reports and other sources on which the list is based have come under increasing scrutiny and criticism by Teschke and colleagues.[151,156-158] Although some cases have had well-documented hepatic injury, others have been more poorly confirmed and have not considered other relevant factors.[2] For example, several herbal formulations are known to have been contaminated by hepatotoxic substances, an occurrence that is probably more common than currently appreciated.[159,160] According to a tabulation of 60 herbal hepatotoxins compiled by Teschke and colleagues,[151] when stringent, liver-specific causality assessment methodologies are applied to the cases under review, many cases cannot be substantiated, and the published findings have been called into question.[156,157,161] Similarly, the accuracy of spontaneous herbal toxicity reports submitted to pharmacovigilance databases has been questioned.[162,163] Indeed, the FDA Center for Food Safety and Applied Nutrition's Adverse Event Reporting System (CAERS) database of dietary botanical supplements purported to have caused hepatic and other organ toxicity contains a relatively small number of reports, thereby leading the authors to conclude that validation of cases may be incomplete.[163] Given that the production and review standards for herbal products and dietary supplements are not as strict as for pharmaceutical products,[128] it should not be surprising that a

---

TABLE 89-6 Hepatotoxic Herbal Remedies, Dietary Supplements, and Weight Loss Products

Remedy	Popular Uses	Source	Hepatotoxic Component	Type of Liver Injury
Ayurvedic herbal medicine	Multiple	Multiple	Uncertain (may contain heavy metal contaminants)	Hepatitis
Barakol	Anxiolytic	*Cassia siamea*	Uncertain	Reversible hepatitis or cholestasis
Black cohosh	Menopausal symptoms	*Cimicifuga racemosa*	Uncertain	Hepatitis (causality uncertain)
"Bush tea"	Fever	*Senecio, Heliotropium, Crotalaria* spp.	Pyrrolizidine alkaloids	SOS
Cascara	Laxative	*Cascara sagrada*	Anthracene glycoside	Cholestatic hepatitis

Continued

TABLE 89-6 Hepatotoxic Herbal Remedies, Dietary Supplements, and Weight Loss Products—cont'd

Remedy	Popular Uses	Source	Hepatotoxic Component	Type of Liver Injury
Chaparral leaf (greasewood, creosote bush)	"Liver tonic," burn salve, weight loss	*Larrea tridenta*	Nordihydroguaiaretic acid	Acute and chronic hepatitis, FHF
Chaso/onshido	Weight loss	—	*N*-nitro-fenfluramine	Acute hepatitis, FHF
Chinese medicines (traditional) Jin bu huan	Sleep aid, analgesic	*Lycopodium serratum*	?Levo-tetrahydropalmitine	Acute or chronic hepatitis or cholestasis, steatosis
Ma huang	Weight loss	*Ephedra* spp.	Ephedrine	Severe hepatitis, FHF
Shou-wu-pian	Anti-aging, neuroprotection, laxative	*Polygonum multiflorum* Thunb (fleeceflower root)	?Anthraquinone	Acute hepatitis or cholestasis
Syo-saiko-to	Multiple	*Scutellaria* root	Diterpenoids	Hepatocellular necrosis, cholestasis, steatosis, granulomas
Comfrey	Herbal tea	*Symphytum* spp.	Pyrrolizidine alkaloid	Acute SOS, cirrhosis
Germander	Weight loss, fever	*Teucrium chamaedry, T. capitatum, T. polium*	Diterpenoids, epoxides	Acute and chronic hepatitis, FHF, ?autoimmune injury
Greater celandine	Gallstones, IBS	*Chelidonium majus*	Isoquinoline alkaloids	Cholestatic hepatitis, fibrosis
Green tea leaf extract	Multiple	*Camellia sinensis*	?Catechins	Hepatitis (causality questioned)
Herbalife	Nutritional supplement, weight loss	—	Various; ?ephedra	Severe hepatitis, FHF
Hydroxycut	Weight loss	*Camellia sinensis*, among other constituents	Uncertain	Acute hepatitis, ?FHF
Impila	Multiple	*Callilepsis laureola*	Potassium atractylate	Hepatic necrosis
Kava kava	Anxiolytic	*Piper methysticum*	Kava lactone, pipermethystine	Acute hepatitis, cholestasis, ?FHF
Kombucha	Weight loss	Lichen alkaloid	Usnic acid	Acute hepatitis
Limbrel (Flavocoxid)	Osteoarthritis	Plant bioflavonoids	Baicalin, ?epicatechin	Acute mixed hepatocellular-cholestatic injury
Lipokinetix	Weight loss	Lichen alkaloid	Usnic acid	Acute hepatitis, jaundice, FHF
Mistletoe	Asthma, infertility	*Viscus album*	Uncertain	Hepatitis (in combination with skullcap)
Oil of cloves	Dental pain	Various foods, oils	Eugenol	Zonal necrosis
Pennyroyal (squawmint oil)	Abortifacient	*Hedeoma pulegoides, Mentha pulegium*	Pulegone, monoterpenes	Severe hepatocellular necrosis
Prostata	Prostatism	Multiple	Uncertain	Chronic cholestasis
Sassafras	Herbal tea	*Sassafras albidum*	Safrole	HCC (in animals)
Senna	Laxative	*Cassia angustifolia*	Sennoside alkaloids; anthrone	Acute hepatitis
Skullcap	Anxiolytic	*Scutellaria*	Diterpenoids	Hepatitis
Valerian	Sedative	*Valeriana officinalis*	Uncertain	Elevated liver enzymes

FHF, fulminant hepatic failure; HCC, hepatocellular carcinoma; SOS, sinusoidal obstruction syndrome.
Citations for individual agents can be found in references 1, 2, 4, 5, 8, 129, 151, 164, 166, 174, 177, 194, 211, and 213.

number of groups have called for increased regulation regarding the manufacture, quality control, safety, and efficacy of these products in the United States and abroad.[2,133,164-166] With these caveats in mind, the clinicopathologic features of hepatotoxicity caused by the compounds discussed later are derived from the best available evidence.[1,2,4,151,155,164,166]

Pyrrolizidine Alkaloids

Pyrrolizidine alkaloids are found in approximately 3% of all flowering plant species throughout the world, and ingestion of such plants, often as medicinal teas or in other formulations, can produce acute and chronic liver disease, including sinusoidal obstruction syndrome (SOS), in humans and livestock.[167] SOS was first reported in the 1950s as a disease of Jamaican children, manifesting with acute abdominal distention, marked hepatomegaly, and ascites—a triad that resembles Budd-Chiari syndrome (see Chapter 85).[8] The disease was linked to consumption of "bush tea," made largely from plants of *Senecio*, *Heliotropium*, and *Crotalaria* species taken as a folk remedy for acute childhood illnesses and was characterized histologically by centrilobular hepatic congestion with occlusion of the hepatic venules, leading to congestive cirrhosis. Comfrey (*Symphytum officinale*) remains commercially available even though it is a dose-dependent hepatotoxin.[167] In Afghanistan, ingestion of pyrrolizidine alkaloid–contaminated grains and bread led to a large epidemic of SOS, affecting 8000 persons and innumerable sheep.[8]

Hepatotoxic pyrrolizidine alkaloids are cyclic diesters, and some forms (e.g., fulvine, monocrotaline) cause both liver and lung injury. The mechanism of injury is postulated to be impairment of nucleic acid synthesis by reactive metabolites of pyrrolizidine alkaloids generated by hepatic microsomes, leading in turn to progressive loss of sinusoid cells and sinusoidal hemorrhage, as well as injury to the endothelium of the terminal hepatic venule, with deposition of fibrin.[167]

SOS causes acute, subacute, and chronic injury. The acute form is characterized by zone 3 necrosis and sinusoidal dilatation, leading to a Budd-Chiari–like syndrome with abdominal pain and the rapid onset of ascites within 3 to 6 weeks of ingestion. In Jamaica, the course was rapidly fatal in 15% to 20% of affected persons. Approximately half of the patients with the acute form recovered spontaneously; transition to a more chronic form of injury occurred in the remainder.[5,8] In the subacute and chronic forms, central fibrosis and bridging between central veins led to a form of cirrhosis similar to that seen with chronic passive hepatic congestion (so-called cardiac cirrhosis). At one time, this form of injury accounted for one third of the cases of cirrhosis seen in Jamaica, with death often resulting from complications of portal hypertension in as few as 1 to 3 years.[8] Certain pyrrolizidine alkaloids, such as comfrey extracts, are hepatocarcinogenic and, like aflatoxins, induce mutations of the *TP53* gene.[167]

Germander

The blossoms of plants from the Labiatae family (*Teucrium chamaedrys*) were used for years in herbal teas and in the mid-1980s as capsules for weight reduction in France, until several dozen cases of liver injury, including fatal hepatic failure,[168,169] forced its withdrawal from the French marketplace in 1992. Most patients were middle-aged women who had ingested germander for 3 to 18 weeks, with consequent development of acute hepatocellular injury, often with jaundice. The injury usually resolved within 1.5 to 6 months after the germander was discontinued, with prompt recurrence after rechallenge in many persons. The cause of germander hepatotoxicity is an interplay between toxic metabolites and immunoallergic

mechanisms. Germander is composed of several compounds, including glycosides, flavonoids, and furan-containing diterpenoids, all of which are converted by the CYP system (especially CYP3A) to reactive metabolites. Covalent binding to cellular proteins, depletion of hepatic glutathione, apoptosis, and cytoskeleton membrane injury (bleb formation) cause cell disruption in animal models. Epoxide hydrolase on plasma membranes is a target of germander antibodies, which have been found in the sera of patients who have consumed germander teas over long periods of time.[170] Reports of liver injury also have appeared with other species of *Teucrium*, including *Teucrium capitatum*[171] and *Teucrium polium*.[172]

Chaparral

The dried leaf of the desert shrub chaparral (*Larrea tridentata*), also known as greasewood or creosote bush, is ground into a tea or used in capsules or tablets for various ailments. Multiple reports of hepatitis have appeared; most cases have occurred within 1 to 12 months of use and resolved within a few weeks to months of discontinuation.[173] Among the 13 cases reported to the FDA,[173] acute hepatocellular or cholestatic injury was observed, with 2 cases of fulminant hepatitis requiring liver transplantation and 4 cases of progression to cirrhosis. Renal toxicity and rash can accompany liver injury. The active ingredient, nordihydroguaiaretic acid, an inhibitor of cyclooxygenase and lipoxygenase pathways, is the likely cause of hepatic injury, although the mechanism also may involve phytoestrogen-induced effects on the liver.[130] A case of recurrence on rechallenge suggests a possible role for immunoallergy.[174]

Pennyroyal

The leaves of pennyroyal (the common name for 2 related plant species, *Hedeoma pulegoides* and *Mentha pulegium*) are used to make oils (squawmint oil), tablets, and home-brewed mint teas. The plant contains pulegone and smaller amounts of other monoterpene ketones. Oxidative metabolites of pulegone (e.g., menthofuran) bind to cellular proteins and deplete hepatic glutathione, thereby leading to liver injury.[175] Cases of hepatocellular injury, including fatal necrosis, were associated with GI and CNS toxicity within a few hours of ingestion. In animals, inhibition of pulegone metabolism by the CYP system with disulfiram and cimetidine has limited pennyroyal hepatotoxicity.[176] The use of *N*-acetylcysteine may protect against pennyroyal toxicity in human cases.[175]

Chinese Herbal Medications

Most traditional Chinese medicines are composed of several different herbal compounds and usually are dominated by one main ingredient referred to as the "king herb."[2] The traditional preparations discussed are among the best characterized with respect to hepatotoxicity.

Jin bu huan (*Lycopodium serratum*) is a traditional herbal remedy that has been used as a sedative and analgesic for more than 1000 years.[174] Numerous cases of hepatic injury have appeared,[177,178] with a mean latency of 20 weeks (range, 7 to 52 weeks) after the start of jin bu huan in recommended doses. Associated symptoms and signs included fever, fatigue, nausea, pruritus, abdominal pain, hepatomegaly, and jaundice. Liver biopsy specimens from a small number of patients showed a range of histopathologic changes, including lobular hepatitis with prominent eosinophils, mild hepatitis with microvesicular steatosis, and fibrotic expansion of the portal tracts. The injury resolved within a mean of 8 weeks (range, 2 to 30 weeks) but could recur on rechallenge.[177] The only predisposing factor was female gender. Serum ALT levels were increased 20- to 50-fold, with minor increases in the alkaline phosphatase level, except in one patient with cholestasis. Hyperbilirubinemia was prominent in the more severe cases. A case of chronic hepatitis has been described. The mechanism of injury may involve levotetrahydropalmatine, a neuroactive metabolite with structural similarity to pyrrolizidine alkaloids. The FDA has banned the importation of jin bu huan anodyne tablets into the United States.[174]

Syo-saiko-to (xiao-chai-hu-tang, dai-saiko-to) contains *Scutellaria* root (skullcap), which is a postulated hepatotoxin.[179] The spectrum of liver injury has included hepatocellular necrosis, microvesicular steatosis, cholestasis, granuloma formation, and a flare of autoimmune hepatitis.[177,180] Reversible acute hepatitis or cholestasis has followed the consumption of shou-wu-pian, a product derived from *Polygonum multiflorum*.[181]

Ma huang, derived from plants of *Ephedra* species, has been reported to cause acute, sometimes severe, hepatitis, including acute liver failure.[2,130,182,183] The active constituent, ephedrine, also has been linked to severe adverse cardiovascular and CNS effects, including fatalities, when used as a stimulant and weight loss aid.[184] The FDA has issued a ruling that ephedra-containing products present an unreasonable risk and should be avoided.[185]

Weight Loss Products

Chaso and onshido are Chinese herbal dietary weight loss supplements that were reported to cause severe liver injury, with a mean serum ALT level of 1978 U/L (range, 283 to 4074 U/L), in 12 patients.[186] Fulminant hepatic failure developed in 2 persons; 1 died, and the other survived after receiving a liver transplant. The suspected hepatotoxic ingredient was N-nitroso-fenfluramine, a derivative of the appetite suppressant fenfluramine, which was withdrawn from the U.S. market in 1997.[187]

Another dietary supplement used for weight loss, LipoKinetix (composed of norephedrine, sodium usniate [usnic acid], diiodothyronine, yohimbine, and caffeine) has been associated with acute hepatitis, including fulminant hepatic failure requiring liver transplantation.[130,188] In a case series of 7 previously healthy patients (4 women, 3 men; mean age, 27 years), acute hepatitis developed after a latent period of less than 4 weeks in 5 patients and 8 to 12 weeks in the other 2. Mean serum ALT levels were 4501 U/L (range, 438 to 14,150 U/L), and mean serum bilirubin levels were 6.5 mg/dL (range, 2.2 to 14.6 mg/dL). No evidence of immunoallergy was evident. All of the patients recovered spontaneously, with normalization of serum ALT and bilirubin levels within 4 months.[188] Fulminant hepatic failure necessitating emergency liver transplantation was reported in a previously healthy 28-year-old nonobese woman who had taken an over-the-counter preparation of usnic acid for weight loss,[189] suggesting that this agent may be the hepatotoxic component of LipoKinetix. Usnic acid also is a component of Kombucha tea, which has been associated with hepatic injury.[174] Usnic acid is a potent inhibitor of CYP2C19 and CYP2C9 and may interact with other medications or supplements to produce hepatotoxic drug-drug interactions.[190]

Herbalife is another nutritional supplement reported to cause severe liver injury, including the need for liver transplantation.[191,192] A mixed hepatic infiltrate with eosinophils and lymphocytes was seen on liver biopsy specimens, along with other changes, including necrosis, cholestasis, and sinusoidal obstruction. A positive rechallenge reaction was observed in a number of patients after their liver biochemical abnormalities had normalized.[191]

Hydroxycut is a weight loss supplement that was recalled from the U.S. market in 2009, after an FDA review of reports found that this slimming aid was associated with nearly 2 dozen spontaneous reports of possible hepatotoxicity.[193,194] Two patients required liver transplantation, and 1 died. One of its active ingredients, green tea leaf extract (*Camellia sinensis*), despite being used widely for millennia,[195] has been implicated in liver injury.[196] A safety review of green tea by the U.S. Pharmacopeia[197] found that a relationship with liver injury was possible, although the study used the Naranjo causality scale, which is not specific for assessing hepatotoxicity, and the association has been called into question.[156,198] Although the FDA did not identify a specific hepatotoxic component, Hydroxycut was reformulated with caffeine as the principal ingredient and has been reintroduced into the marketplace without subsequent reports of liver injury.

Kava Kava

Kava kava is a natural sedative and antianxiety agent derived from the root of the pepper plant (*Piper methysticum*). This herbal product has been the subject of an FDA consumer alert[174] after it was banned in the European Union and Canada[199] because of severe hepatotoxicity, including fatal liver failure.[130,200] A review of 78 cases of hepatic injury reported to the FDA included 11 cases of liver failure requiring liver transplantation and 4 deaths.[201] Other investigators, however, have questioned the validity of the causality assessment used by regulators, and only rare instances of hepatotoxicity have been found when a more accurate liver-specific causality scale is used.[158,202] Although kavalactone has been shown to inhibit CYP enzymes, deplete hepatic glutathione, and possibly inhibit cyclooxygenase,[201] the hepatotoxic component may be the major kava alkaloid pipermethystine. Contamination of the raw material by molds has been cited as an alternative explanation for hepatotoxicity,[160,203] but no evidence for aflatoxicosis has been found.[204] Induction of apoptosis and mitochondrial toxicity are the suspected hepatotoxic mechanisms.[205]

Black Cohosh

Black cohosh (*Actaea racemosa* and *Cimicifuga racemosa*), used for menopausal symptoms, has been implicated in reports of possible hepatic injury,[206] although causality has been questioned.[207] A meta-analysis in 2011 that included 5 studies involving more than 1100 women found no evidence for an adverse effect of the isopropanolic extract of black cohosh on the liver.[208]

Other Herbals

Greater celandine extract (*Chelidonium majus*) is regarded as hepatotoxic; its toxic component appears to be isoquinolone alkaloids.[209] *Polygonum multiflorum* Thunb is suspected as a cause of more than 2 dozen instances of severe hepatocellular injury at one Korean hospital.[210] Flavocoxid, a blend of plant-derived bioflavonoids, is a medical food prescribed for osteoarthritis. It is an uncommon cause of hepatotoxicity among cases contained within the U.S. Drug-Induced Liver Injury Network registry.[211] Four middle-aged women developed acute hepatocellular injury within 1 to 3 months of the start of usage. All were reported to recover after the product was discontinued.

Indian Ayurvedic herbal products have been in use for centuries to treat a variety of ailments.[2] Although some of the preparations purchased via the internet have been contaminated with potentially hepatotoxic heavy metals, such as lead, mercury, iron, and arsenic,[159] instances of documented liver injury from unadulterated formulations are rare.[212]

The hepatotoxic potential of green tea extracts that contain catechins (composed of polyphenolic flavonoids) was examined by investigators from the U.S. Drug-Induced Liver Injury Network.[213] The investigators found that nearly 40% of 73 herbal and dietary supplements that did not list catechins as an ingredient actually contained one or more of these compounds. This finding highlights the difficulties in determining the composition of various herbal and dietary supplements. Moreover, the investigators found no statistical differences in hepatic injury patterns, disease severity, or results of causality assessment when hepatotoxic herbal and dietary supplements containing catechins were compared with those not containing catechins. These results call into question whether green tea extracts or catechins are truly hepatotoxic by themselves.[213]

Hepatoprotection by Herbal Compounds

In contrast to the cases of hepatotoxicity seen with the herbal products, dietary supplements, and weight loss aids discussed in this chapter, an entire field of study has been devoted to the hepatoprotective properties of nutraceuticals and other phytomedicines against liver injury induced by various chemicals, drugs, and other hepatotoxins, including acetaminophen and carbon tetrachloride.[214-218]

KEY REFERENCES

Full references for this chapter can be found on www.expertconsult.com.

1. Lewis JH, Kleiner DE. Hepatic injury due to drugs, herbal compounds, chemicals and toxins. In: Burt AD, Portmann BC, Ferrell LD, editors. MacSween's pathology of the liver. 6th ed. Philadelphia: Churchill Livingstone Elsevier; 2012. pp 645-760.
2. Bunchorntavakul C, Reddy KR. Review article: Herbal and dietary supplement hepatotoxicity. Aliment Pharmacol Ther 2013; 37:3-17.
4. Stickel F, Kesselbohm K, Weimann R, et al. Review of liver injury associated with dietary supplements. Liver Int 2011; 31:595-605.
5. Zimmerman HJ. Hepatotoxicity. The adverse effects of drugs and other chemicals on the liver. 2nd ed. Philadelphia: Lippincott Williams & Wilkins; 1999.
8. Zimmerman HJ, Lewis JH. Chemical- and toxin-induced hepatotoxicity. Gastroenterol Clin North Am 1995; 24:1027-45.
9. Tolman K, Sirrine R. Occupational hepatotoxicity. Clin Liver Dis 1998; 2:563-89.
14. Reuben A, Koch DG, Lee WM, Acute Liver Failure Study Group. Drug-induced acute liver failure: Results of a U.S. multicenter, prospective study. Hepatology 2010; 52:2065-76.
48. Faust TW, Reddy KR. Postoperative jaundice. Clin Liver Dis 2004; 8:151-66.
53. Mandibusan MK, Odin M, Eatmond DA. Postulated carbon tetrachloride mode of action: A review. J Environ Sci Health C Environ Carcinog Ecotoxicol Rev 2007; 25:185-209.
90. Britton R. Metal-induced hepatotoxicity. Semin Liver Dis 1996; 16:3-12.
115. Rengstorff DS, Osorio RW, Bonacini M. Recovery from severe hepatitis caused by mushroom poisoning without liver transplantation. Clin Gastroenterol Hepatol 2003; 1:392-6.
120. Mohi-ud-din R, Lewis JH. Drug- and chemical-induced cholestasis. Clin Liver Dis 2004; 8:95-132.
126. Ferrucci LM, Bell BP, Dhotre KB, et al. Complementary and alternative medicine use in chronic liver disease patients. J Clin Gastroenterol 2010; 44:e40-45.
128. Frankos VH, Street DA, O'Neill RK. FDA regulation of dietary supplements and requirements regarding adverse event reporting. Clin Pharmacol Ther 2010; 87:239-44.
151. Teschke R, Wolff A, Frenzel C, et al. Herbal hepatotoxicity: A tabular compilation of reported cases. Liver Int 2012; 32:1543-56.

CHAPTER

90
Autoimmune Hepatitis

ALBERT J. CZAJA

Autoimmune hepatitis (AIH) is a disease of unknown cause characterized by the presence of interface hepatitis (Fig. 90-1) and lymphoplasmacytic infiltration (Fig. 90-2) on histologic examination, hypergammaglobulinemia, and autoantibodies.[1] Diagnosis requires the exclusion of other chronic liver diseases that have similar features, including Wilson disease, chronic viral hepatitis, drug-induced liver disease, nonalcoholic fatty liver disease, and the immune cholangiopathies of PBC and PSC.[2] Centrilobular (Rappaport zone 3) necrosis (Fig. 90-3) may indicate an early pattern of injury before the development of interface hepatitis[3,4] or a spontaneous exacerbation of chronic disease.[5]

EPIDEMIOLOGY

AIH has a global distribution,[6-9] and it affects all ages[10-13] and both genders.[14-16] In Sweden, 76% of patients are women,[17] and in the United States, women outnumber men by 3.5 : 1.[14] Men may have an earlier age of onset (peak incidence in late teens) than women (peak incidence after menopause).[17] The prevalence of AIH among white Scandinavians is 0.85 to 1.9 cases per 100,000 persons per year, and its point prevalence is 10.7 to 16.9 cases per 100,000 persons per year.[17,18] In the United States, AIH affects 100,000 to 200,000 persons, and it accounts for 2% to 3% of the pediatric and 4% to 6% of the adult liver transplantations performed in Europe and the United States.[1]

The occurrence of AIH varies among ethnic groups, and it has been associated with genetic predispositions that can differ between races and between age groups within races.[19] The prevalence of AIH is greatest among North American and northern European white persons (or derivative populations), who have a high frequency of HLA-DRB1*03 and HLA-DRB1*04.[20] All populations are susceptible to AIH, which has

been well described in Africans, Canadian Aboriginals, Chinese, Egyptians, Europeans, Iranians, Japanese, Mexicans, Saudi Arabians, South Americans, South Asians, and Turks.[21-27] The prevalence of AIH is as high as 43 per 100,000 persons in Alaskan natives[28] and as low as 5.6 per 100,000 persons in Brunei Darussalam.[29]

PATHOPHYSIOLOGY

AIH is a consequence of genetic predisposition, antigenic exposures, and various factors that affect autoantigen display, immunocyte activation, and effector cell proliferation (Fig. 90-4).[30-33] Proposed triggering factors include infectious agents, drugs, and toxins. The lag time between exposure to the antigenic trigger and the onset of the disease can be long, and the triggering agent is not needed to perpetuate the disorder. The CD4+ helper T cell is the principal effector cell, and its activation is the initial step in the pathogenic pathway.

Molecular mimicry of a foreign antigen by a self-antigen is the most common explanation for the loss of self-tolerance, but this mechanism has not been established in autoimmune disease.[30-33] Genetic factors influence autoantigen presentation and CD4+ helper T-cell recognition. The antigen-binding groove of the class II molecule of the major histocompatibility complex (MHC) is encoded by alleles that determine the groove's configuration and ability to activate immunocytes. The susceptibility alleles of AIH in white North Americans and northern Europeans reside on the DRB1 gene and are DRB1*0301 and DRB1*0401 (see Fig. 90-4).[20,34,35]

Different ethnic groups have different susceptibility alleles, but these alleles may still encode the antigen binding groove similarly ("shared motif") and support the presentation of the same or similar antigens.[20,34,35] The critical shared motif in white North American and northern European patients with

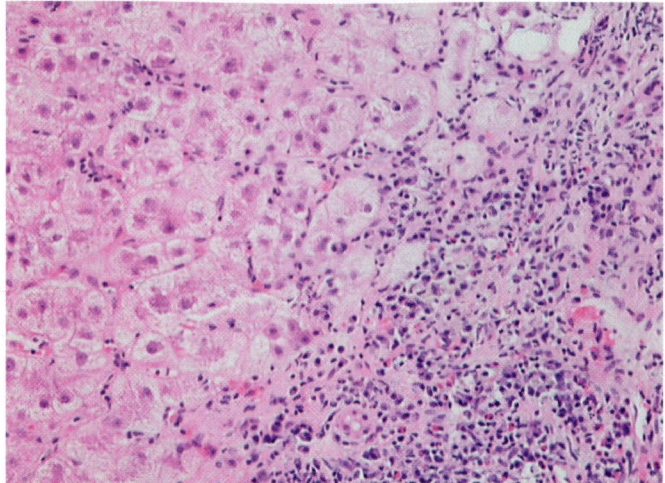

FIGURE 90-1. Histopathology of interface hepatitis. The limiting plate of the portal tract is disrupted by a lymphoplasmacytic infiltrate. This histologic pattern is the hallmark of autoimmune hepatitis, but it is not disease specific. (H&E, ×200.)

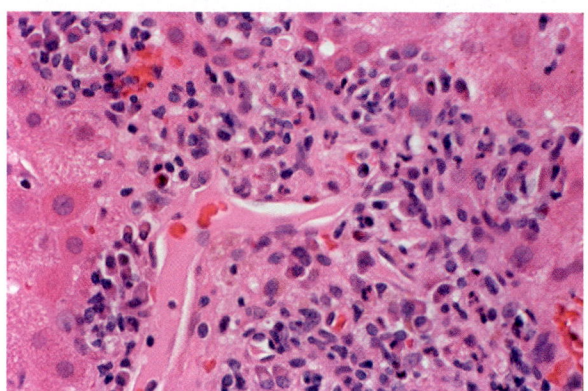

FIGURE 90-2. Histopathology of lymphoplasmacytic infiltration. Plasma cells denoted by perinuclear halos are present in the portal tract and extend into the liver parenchyma with the interface hepatitis. (H&E, ×200.)

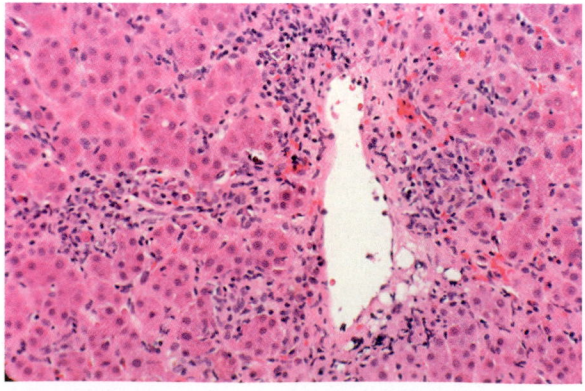

FIGURE 90-3. Histopathology of centrilobular zone 3 necrosis with hepatocyte rosettes. Mononuclear inflammatory cells surround the terminal hepatic venule and are diffusely distributed in the hepatic parenchyma. The hepatic architecture is disorganized, and hepatocyte rosettes are in the perivenular area. (H&E, ×200.)

AIH is a 6–amino acid sequence represented by the code LLEQKR.[20,34,35] This sequence is located between positions 67 and 72 of the DRβ polypeptide chain of the class II MHC molecule, and lysine (K) in position 71 is the critical determinant of susceptibility. DRB1*0301 and DRB1*0401 encode identical amino acid sequences in the DRβ67-72 region and affect susceptibility similarly.

DRB1*0404 and DRB1*0405 are the susceptibility alleles in Mexican, Japanese, mainland Chinese, and Argentinean adults and encode a sequence similar to that in white North American and northern European patients, except for arginine (R) instead of lysine (K) at the DRβ71 position.[34,35] Arginine is a positively charged amino acid that is structurally similar to lysine, and its substitution for lysine should not greatly alter the antigen-binding properties of the class II MHC molecule. Antigenic peptides are selected for display by the nature of the amino acids that interact with residues within the antigen-binding groove (see Fig. 90-4).[35] The critical 6–amino acid motif in AIH restricts the range of peptides that can be accommodated. Multiple self-antigens or foreign antigens may satisfy the minimal structural requirements and serve as immunogenic peptides.

DRB1*1301 is associated with AIH in Argentina,[36] Brazil,[22,37] Venezuela,[38] and Peru,[39] and this allele encodes ILEDER at positions DRβ67-72. Glutamic acid (E), aspartic acid (D), and glutamic acid (E) are at positions DRβ69, DRβ70, and DRβ71, respectively, in the class II MHC molecule, and the presence of these critically located but negatively charged amino acid residues negates the universality of the "shared motif" hypothesis. Susceptibility to AIH in different regions and ethnic groups may relate to indigenous factors or agents favored by certain genetic phenotypes that are outside those found in white North American and northern European patients.[34,35] In South America, DRB1*1301 is associated with protracted HAV infection,[40] and persons with this allele may be "selected" from their environment to have prolonged exposure to viral and hepatic antigens that favor the development of AIH. An understanding of the individual susceptibility allele in different geographic regions may be useful in tracking the cause of the disease.

Genetic promoters inside and outside the MHC can affect disease occurrence and clinical phenotype, either in synergy with the principal susceptibility factors or in lieu of them (see Fig. 90-4).[32,34,35] Polymorphisms of the TNF-α gene (*TNFA*2*),[41] the cytotoxic T lymphocyte antigen 4 gene (*CTLA4*),[42] and *Fas* gene promoter at position −670 (*TNFRSF6*)[43] have been associated with increased immune reactivity, disease severity, and early progression to cirrhosis in white North American and northern European patients. Constellations of autoimmune promoters, as yet undefined, may individualize the disease by affecting its occurrence, clinical phenotype, and outcome. These genetic promoters of AIH are not disease specific, and they are not uniformly important in all ethnic groups.[44-48]

Liver cell destruction is accomplished by either cell-mediated cytotoxicity, antibody-dependent cell-mediated cytotoxicity, or a combination of both mechanisms (see Fig. 90-4).[30-32] Cell-mediated cytotoxicity depends on the clonal expansion of CD8+ cytotoxic T cells that accomplish liver cell injury through the release of lymphokines. This mechanism is regulated by type 1 cytokines, and the −308 polymorphism of *TNFA*2* may facilitate this pathway.[41] Antibody-dependent cell-mediated cytotoxicity is regulated by type 2 cytokines, and the natural killer cell accomplishes liver cell destruction by binding its Fc receptor with an antigen-antibody complex on the hepatocyte surface.[30-32] The predominant mechanism depends on the phenotypic differentiation of the CD4+ helper T cell, which in turn reflects the cytokine milieu. The cytokine milieu may reflect polymorphisms of the cytokine genes that

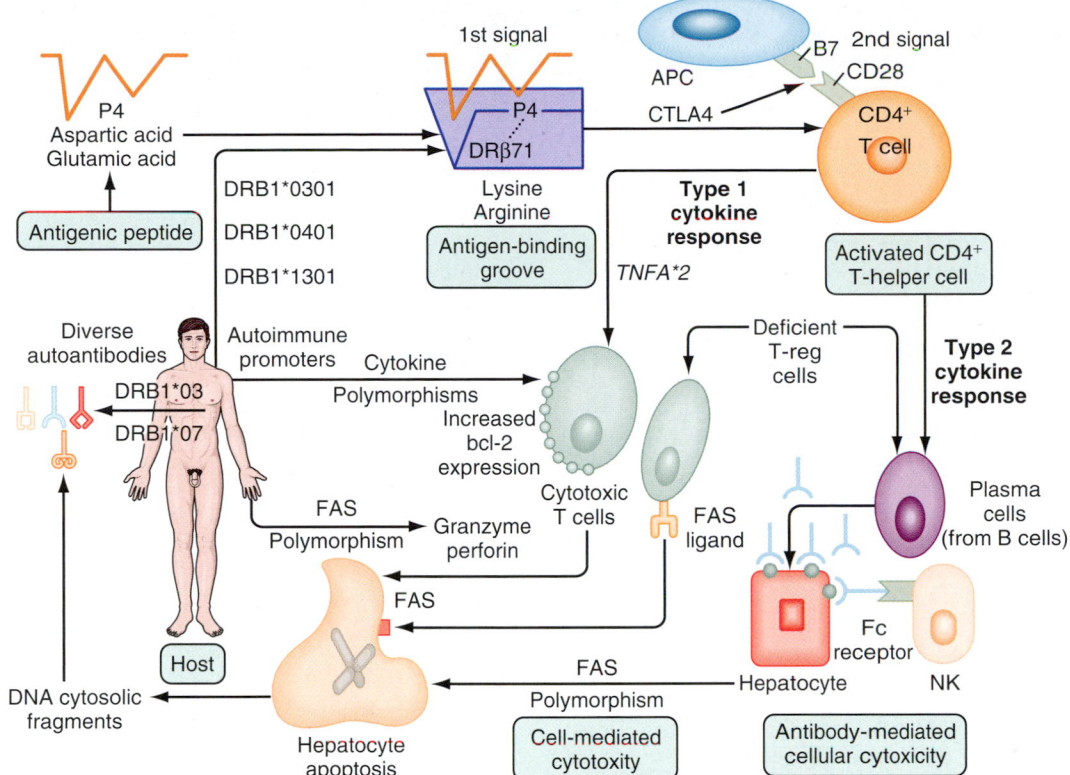

FIGURE 90-4. Interactive mechanisms that contribute to the development of autoimmune hepatitis in white North American and northern European adults. The initial stimulus for immune activity is an antigenic peptide *(upper left corner)* that has a negatively charged aspartic acid or glutamic acid at a position within its structure (P4) that can form a salt bridge with a positively charged lysine or arginine residue at position 71 within the DR beta polypeptide chain (DRβ71) of the antigen binding groove of the class II DR molecule of the major histocompatibility complex *(top center)*. The DR molecule-antigen complex of the antigen-presenting cell (APC) then interacts with the antigen receptor of a CD4+ T-helper cell (interaction not shown), and the first co-stimulatory signal is completed (1st signal). The CD28 molecule on the surface of the CD4+ T-helper cell ligates with the B7 ligand on the surface of the APC, and the second co-stimulatory signal (2nd signal) is completed *(upper right corner)*. The activated CD4+ T-helper cell can then differentiate and proliferate along type 1 and type 2 cytokine pathways *(middle right)*. Deficiencies in the function or amount of cytotoxic T lymphocyte antigen 4 (CTLA4) can enhance the strength of the 2nd signal. Differentiation along the type 1 cytokine pathway can be promoted by polymorphisms of the tumor necrosis factor gene *(TNFA*2)* and tumor necrosis factor receptor superfamily gene *(FAS)*, resulting in cell-mediated cytotoxicity by sensitized liver-infiltrating cytotoxic T cells and increased hepatocyte apoptosis *(middle bottom)*. The apoptosis of hepatocytes can, in turn, release DNA cytosolic fragments that contribute to the production of diverse collateral autoantibodies *(middle left)*. Autoantibody expression is, in part, host dependent and influenced by the susceptibility alleles DRB1*03 and DRB1*07. Host genetic predispositions are also important in encoding the antigen-binding groove of the class II DR molecule through the actions of DRB1*0301, DRB1*0401, and DRB1*1301 alleles and in generating autoimmune promoters (cytokine and FAS polymorphisms) that enhance cell-mediated cytotoxicity and hepatocyte apoptosis. The enhanced expression of the anti-apoptotic protein (bcl-2) on the surface of cytotoxic T cells can protect them from programmed cell death and perpetuate their autoreactivity *(middle)*. The cytokine pathways can be enhanced by deficiencies in the actions of T-regulatory cells (T-reg cells), which have suppressive effects that can be reversed by glucocorticoid treatment. Differentiation of B cells into plasma cells, via the type 2 cytokine response of activated CD4+ T-helper cells, can result in immunoglobulin production that, in turn, generates an antibody-mediated cellular toxicity. Natural killer (NK) cells with Fc receptors are directed against complexes of immunoglobulin with normal hepatocyte membrane constituents. *(Adapted from Czaja AJ. Autoimmune hepatitis—Part A: Pathogenesis. Expert Rev Gastroenterol Hepatol 2007; 1:113-128.)*

favor excessive production of some modulators, such as TNF-α, or deficient production of others.

Defects in the counter-regulatory cytokine milieu may also reflect reduced numbers of intrahepatic natural killer T (NKT) cells[49,50] and the failure of T-regulatory (T-reg) cells (CD4+CD25+ cells) to modulate CD8+ T-cell proliferation and cytokine production.[32,51] The recruitment and intrahepatic trafficking of cytotoxic T lymphocytes may be enhanced by the up-regulation of chemokines such as CXCL16, and perivascular hepatic stellate cells may transform into myofibroblasts in response to inflammatory activity, thereby stimulating fibrogenesis.[32] The matrix proteins accumulate in the liver tissue and retard the counteractive degradative actions of

matrix metalloproteinases as stellate cells continue to be activated in an autocrine fashion by transforming growth factor (TGF)-β.[52]

Perturbations in the counter-regulatory mechanisms that influence cell-mediated cytotoxicity, antibody-dependent cell-mediated cytotoxicity, inflammatory cell response, and apoptosis of effector and target cell populations are the bases for the occurrence and severity of AIH. They constitute pathways that can be targeted by evolving pharmacologic, molecular, and cellular interventions.[53-60] Uncertainty about the role of T-reg cells in the pathogenesis of AIH exemplifies the clarifications that are still required to improve the design of these future therapies.[61] Apoptosis is the principal mechanism of hepatocyte death, and the histologic manifestations are a consequence of receptor-mediated overactive apoptosis (mainly through Fas-Fas ligand interactions).

CLINICAL FEATURES

Symptoms and Physical Findings

The clinical features of AIH typically reflect the inflammatory activity of the liver disease, the acuteness of the presentation, or the complications of cirrhosis.[2,62] Cholestatic features may be present, but they do not dominate the clinical picture. Pruritus, hyperpigmentation, and weight loss virtually exclude the diagnosis. Similarly, manifestations of liver decompensation, such as ascites, hepatic encephalopathy, and variceal bleeding, are uncommon findings at initial presentation in Western countries.

Ready fatigability is the most common symptom (seen in 86% of adult patients). Hepatomegaly is the most common physical finding (78%), and jaundice is found in 69% of patients with severe disease. Splenomegaly can be present in patients with and without cirrhosis (56% and 32%, respectively), as can spider telangiectasias. As many as 25% to 34% of patients are asymptomatic at initial consultation,[63,64] and 25% of adults have a normal physical examination.[2] The discordance between the severity of inflammatory activity and the presence of symptoms is most common in children, whose clinical status frequently does not accurately reflect the severity of the underlying liver disease. The clinical phenotype of autoimmune hepatitis at presentation has been changing as the disease is being recognized at earlier stages and with nonclassic manifestations.

Concurrent extrahepatic immune-mediated diseases are recognized in 14% to 44% of patients, and the variable frequencies probably relate to the age group at risk.[2,6,10,11,65,66] Patients aged 60 years or older have concurrent thyroid disorders or rheumatic conditions more commonly than adults aged 30 years or younger (42% vs. 13%).[11] By contrast, adults aged 30 or younger have UC or autoimmune hemolysis more frequently than patients aged 60 or older (13% vs. 0%).[11]

Autoimmune thyroiditis, Graves' disease, and RA are the most common concurrent conditions, but celiac disease is present in 2% to 4% of patients and important to recognize and treat.[67,68] In some instances, the rheumatic (RA, SLE), GI (celiac disease, IBD), and endocrinologic (Graves' disease, autoimmune thyroiditis) disorders obscure the presence of the AIH, and it is essential to look beyond these manifestations for the treatable liver disease.[2,10,11,66,69,70] Patients with multiple endocrine organ failure, mucocutaneous candidiasis, and ectodermal dystrophy have autoimmune polyendocrinopathy-candidiasis–ectodermal dystrophy (APECED), and 10% to 15% have AIH.[71]

Laboratory Findings

Serum AST, ALT, and gamma globulin levels reflect the severity of disease and immediate prognosis. Sustained severe elevations indicate a poor outcome unless therapy is started. Untreated patients with serum AST levels 10-fold or more than the upper limit of normal (ULN) or serum AST levels 5-fold or more than the ULN in conjunction with serum gamma globulin levels 2-fold or more than the ULN have a mortality rate as high as 40% within 6 months.[1] Less severe laboratory abnormalities are associated with a better immediate prognosis.[62,64] Mild AIH may still progress, and the laboratory indices reflective of mild inflammatory activity are unable to predict disease behavior in individual patients. The 10-year

survival of untreated patients with mild AIH is 67%,[72] and 26% to 70% of asymptomatic patients become symptomatic.[63,64] Hyperbilirubinemia is present in 83% of patients, but the serum bilirubin level is 3-fold or more than the ULN in only 46%. Similarly, the serum alkaline phosphatase level is commonly increased (81%), but elevations are more than 2-fold the ULN in only 33% and more than 4-fold the ULN in only 10%.[73] The hypergammaglobulinemia of AIH is polyclonal, and the immunoglobulin (Ig)G fraction predominates.[74] The diagnosis of AIH is suspect without hypergammaglobulinemia.[75] Cryoglobulinemia may be present, but symptomatic cryoglobulinemia is rare.

Serology

The serologic tests essential for diagnosis are assays for antinuclear antibodies (ANA), smooth muscle antibodies (SMA), and antibodies to liver-kidney microsome type 1 (anti-LKM1) (Table 90-1).[1,2,76-80] SMA and ANA have neither disease nor organ specificity, and their performance parameters as diagnostic markers of AIH are best if they are detected together. The presence of both SMA and ANA by indirect immunofluorescence has a sensitivity of 43%, specificity of 99%, and diagnostic accuracy of 74%.[81] Antibodies to LKM1 are usually present in the absence of SMA and ANA. They have a specificity of 99% and diagnostic accuracy of 57% by indirect immunofluorescence, but they are present in only 1% to 4% of North American adults with AIH.[81] The production of anti-LKM1 has been associated with HLA DQB1*0201, which is in tight linkage disequilibrium with HLA DRB1*07, and variation in the occurrence of these antibodies in different populations may reflect the regional prevalence of these genetic factors.[82,83]

SMA, ANA, and anti-LKM1 are detected by indirect immunofluorescence assays using rodent tissues or Hep-2 cell lines or by enzyme immunoassays using microtiter plates with adsorbed recombinant or highly purified antigens.[84] The indirect immunofluorescence assays are labor- and time-intensive, subject to intra-observer variation, and not antigen specific. They have been the cornerstone for diagnosing AIH, and the performance parameters of these assays have been well described.[81,84] Enzyme immunoassays are replacing indirect immunofluorescence in clinical laboratories, but their performance parameters are less well defined.[81,84] They are quite antigen specific, but the recombinant antigens used in these assays are not necessarily the same antigens detected by indirect immunofluorescence. Consequently, results of one assay cannot be equated with the results of the other assay.[84]

Serologic tests of additional diagnostic value are atypical perinuclear antineutrophil cytoplasmic antibodies (atypical pANCA)[77] and IgA antibodies to tissue transglutaminase or endomysium.[77,78] Atypical pANCA are common in type 1 AIH, PSC, and UC.[77,78] They are directed against antigens within the nucleus, rather than the cytoplasm, of granulocytes, and the reactivities localize to the proteins within the lamina of the nucleus.[85] Atypical pANCA have been useful in evaluating patients who lack the conventional autoantibodies.[77,78] IgA A antibodies to tissue transglutaminase or endomysium are valuable in excluding celiac disease, which can occur with AIH or be associated with liver disease that resembles AIH.[67,78,86]

Serologic tests that have prognostic as well as diagnostic implications are antibodies to soluble liver antigen (anti-SLA), actin (anti-actin), and asialoglycoprotein receptor (anti-ASGPR) (see Table 90-1).[87,88] Antibodies to SLA are directed against a transfer ribonucleoprotein (tRNP$^{(ser)sec}$) involved in the transport of selenocysteine,[89] and this antigenic target has been named SEPSECS (Sep [O-phosphoserine] tRNA:Sec

TABLE 90-1 Serologic Markers of Autoimmune Hepatitis

Autoantibodies	Antigenic Target	Clinical Implications
ANA	Multiple nuclear antigens	Type 1 AIH Variably expressed with SMA
SMA	Actin (F and G) Non-actin components (14%)	Type 1 AIH Variably expressed with ANA
Anti-LKM1	CYP2D6 (main epitope, 193-212 amino acid sequence)	Type 2 AIH Usually exclusive of ANA, SMA Mainly in children Associated with HLA DRB1*07
Anti-SLA	Transfer ribonucleoprotein (tRNP$^{(ser)sec}$); renamed Sep [O-phosphoserine] tRNA:Sec [selenocysteine] tRNA synthase (SEPSECS)	Diagnostic specificity of 99% for AIH Associated with HLA DRB1*0301 and anti-Ro/SSA Of prognostic value (severe disease, relapse, treatment dependence)
Atypical pANCA	Nuclear lamina proteins	Present in 50%-92% of type 1 AIH Absent in type 2 AIH Associated with PSC and UC
Anti-actin	Actin (F and G)	Present in 86% of AIH with SMA Of possible prognostic value (assay dependent) Double reactivities to actin and α-actinin are associated with severe disease
Anti-asialoglycoprotein receptor	Asialoglycoprotein receptor (recombinant H1 subunit in investigational EIA)	Associated with histologic activity and relapse after drug withdrawal Disappears with effective treatment
Anti-liver cytosol type 1	Formiminotransferase cyclodeaminase	Frequently concurrent with anti-LKM1 (32%) Mainly in young patients (≤20 years of age) Associated with concurrent immune diseases, severe liver inflammation, and rapid progression to cirrhosis Rare in North American patients

Anti-LKM1, antibodies to liver kidney microsome type 1; anti-SLA, antibodies to soluble liver antigen; AIH, autoimmune hepatitis; ANA, antinuclear antibodies; CYP2D6, cytochrome P450 2D6; EIA, enzyme immunoassay; pANCA, perinuclear antineutrophil cytoplasmic antibodies; Ro/SSA, ribonucleoprotein/Sjögren's syndrome A protein; SMA, smooth muscle antibodies.

[selenocysteine] tRNA synthase).[90] Antibodies to SLA are closely associated with HLA DRB1*03, and patients with anti-SLA have severe disease and relapse after drug withdrawal.[91,92] Antibodies to ribonucleoprotein/Sjögren's syndrome A antigen (anti-Ro/SSA) occur in 98% of patients with anti-SLA, and the pathologic implications of this tight association are unclear.[93,94] Antibodies to SLA are present in 15% of patients with AIH in the United States.[95]

Antibodies to actin have mainly a diagnostic function and have high specificity for AIH (see Table 90-1).[96] Whereas 99% of patients with anti-actin also have SMA, 14% of patients with AIH and SMA lack anti-actin.[97] Consequently, the diagnosis of AIH may not be supported by testing only for anti-actin. The preferred assay for anti-actin has not been determined, and diagnostic results and prognostic implications are assay dependent.[80,97] An investigational assay assessing "double reactivities" against actin and α-actinin, a component of the actin molecule, may identify patients with a severe form of AIH and poor outcome.[98,99]

Antibodies to ASGPR are closely associated with histologic activity and also identify 88% of persons who relapse after drug withdrawal (possibly because of residual hepatic inflammation) (see Table 90-1).[78,100] These antibodies may prove useful in defining a treatment end point by supplementing liver tissue examination. Antibodies to ASGPR occur as commonly in AIH as SMA and ANA, and their behavior can be monitored in most patients.[87,100] The ASGPR receptor is composed of 2 subunits (H1 and H2), and an enzyme immunoassay based on recombinant H1, which contains most of the antigenic sites found on the natural receptor, may prove useful in diagnosing the disease and monitoring the treatment response.[79,101]

Antibodies to liver cytosol type 1 (anti-LC1) target formiminotransferase cyclodeaminase,[102] and the recombinant human antigen has been used in murine models of experimental AIH (see Table 90-1).[103,104] Thirty-two percent of patients with anti-LKM1 also express anti-LC1, and anti-LC1 have been associated with early age of disease onset, concurrent immune diseases, severe liver inflammation, and rapid progression to cirrhosis. Antibodies to LC1 are rarely found in North American patients with AIH.[87]

New autoantibodies continue to be characterized in the hope of improving diagnostic specificity and prognostic value.[78,79,87] Antibodies to chromatin, double-stranded DNA, histones, lactoferrin, and *Saccharomyces cerevisiae* have all been evaluated in this effort with varying success, and none has been incorporated into the standard diagnostic repertoire.[77]

Histology

Interface hepatitis is the hallmark of AIH, but it is a nondiscriminating feature (see Fig. 90-1).[105] Virus-related, drug-induced, hereditary, and metabolic causes of the liver injury must still be excluded.[2] Lymphocytic or lymphoplasmacytic inflammation, hepatocyte rosetting, emperiopolesis (penetration of one cell into and through a larger cell), and hepatocyte swelling are other common findings.[105,106] Panacinar hepatitis can be seen during an acute onset or relapse after treatment withdrawal.[105,107] Bridging necrosis and multi-acinar necrosis are indicative of severe inflammatory activity.[105]

Plasma cells are abundant at the interface and throughout the acinus, but only 66% of patients with AIH have plasma cells in groups or sheets in the portal tract (see Fig. 90-2).[108] The presence of plasma cells in conjunction with moderate to severe interface hepatitis has a specificity of 81% and positive predictability of 68% for AIH.[108] Lymphoid aggregates surround and infiltrate bile ducts in 7% to 9% of specimens, and they probably represent an exuberant inflammatory response that does not preclude the diagnosis.[109-111]

Centrilobular necrosis is found in 29% of patients with AIH, and it occurs with similar frequency in patients with and without cirrhosis (see Fig. 90-3).[5] The classic histologic features of interface hepatitis, lymphoplasmacytic infiltration, and hepatocyte rosettes[106,112] may be present with centrilobular necrosis in patients with an acute presentation.[5] Sequential tissue examinations in patients with an acute presentation and centrilobular necrosis have demonstrated transition to the typical pattern of interface hepatitis during the course of the disease.[3]

In patients with acute severe (fulminant) AIH, massive hepatic necrosis is common, and it is typically associated with centrilobular hemorrhagic necrosis or classic interface hepatitis.[113] A lymphoplasmacytic infiltration around the central vein with hepatocyte drop-out or necrosis is present in 93% of these patients ("centrilobular perivenulitis"), and lymphoid aggregates (in 50%) and plasma cell infiltration (in 90%) constitute the histologic diagnosis of acute severe (fulminant) AIH.[113]

DIAGNOSIS

An international panel codified the diagnostic criteria of AIH in 1992, and an expanded panel updated them in 1999.[114] The propensity for an acute, rarely fulminant, presentation has been recognized,[115] and the requirement for 6 months of disease activity to establish chronicity has been waived.[114] Cholestatic histologic changes, including bile duct injury and ductopenia, are incompatible findings, but minor biliary changes do not preclude the diagnosis.[110,111]

Clinical Criteria

The definite diagnosis of AIH requires exclusion of other similar diseases, laboratory findings that indicate substantial immune reactivity, and histologic features of interface hepatitis (Fig. 90-5).[114] A probable diagnosis is justified when

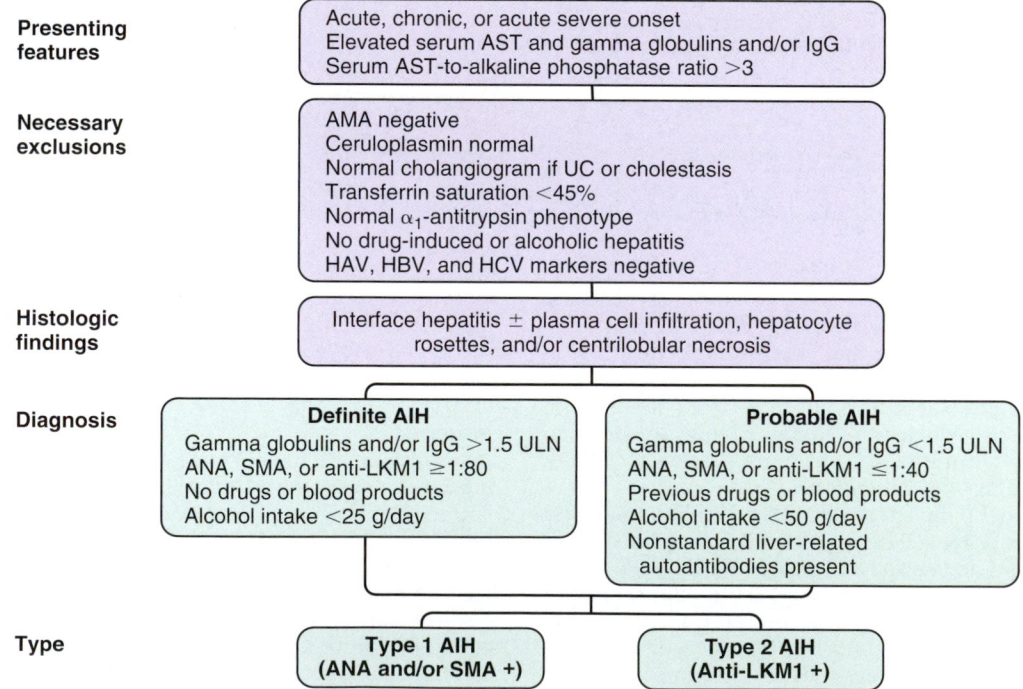

FIGURE 90-5. Diagnostic algorithm for autoimmune hepatitis (AIH). The diagnosis requires predominant elevation of the serum AST level and exclusion of other hepatic diseases (especially PBC, PSC, Wilson disease, hemochromatosis, α1-antitrypsin deficiency, drug-induced or alcoholic hepatitis, and viral hepatitis). Antimitochondrial antibodies (AMA) should be absent; cholangiography should be negative in patients with concurrent UC or cholestasis; and the serologic markers of HAV, HBV, and HCV should be negative. Interface hepatitis should be present on histologic examination, and laboratory manifestations of immune reactivity should be evident by abnormal elevation of the serum gamma globulin and/or immunoglobulin (Ig)G level and the presence of antinuclear antibodies (ANA), smooth muscle antibodies (SMA), or antibodies to liver-kidney microsome type 1 (anti-LKM1). The degree of immune reactivity and the presence of confounding etiologic factors, such as alcohol and drug or blood product exposure, distinguish definite from probable AIH. Classification as type 1 AIH or type 2 AIH is based on the type of autoantibodies that predominate in the disease. ULN, upper limit of normal.

findings are compatible with AIH but insufficient for a definite diagnosis (see Fig. 90-5).[114] Patients who lack conventional autoantibodies but who have antibodies to ASGPR, SLA, actin, or liver cytosol type 1 are classified as having probable disease.[114]

Scoring Criteria

The original scoring system proposed by the International Autoimmune Hepatitis Group (IAIHG) accommodates the diverse manifestations of AIH and renders an aggregate score that reflects the net strength of the diagnosis before and after glucocorticoid treatment (Table 90-2).[114] By weighing each

component of the syndrome, atypical features can be identified and biases associated with isolated inconsistencies can be avoided. The original scoring system ensures the comparability of study populations in clinical trials, provides a comprehensive template for systematically assessing all features of the disease, and accommodates the diagnosis of AIH in patients with few or atypical manifestations (see later). The original scoring system is not a discriminative diagnostic index, and it should not be used to distinguish AIH from other liver diseases. The scoring system was developed as a research tool, and the value of its clinical application is to ensure a uniform evaluation of each patient and to support clinical judgment.

A simplified scoring system has been developed to ease clinical application and is based on 4 clinical components that include the presence and level of autoantibody expression by indirect immunofluorescence, serum IgG concentration, histologic features, and viral markers (Table 90-3).[74] The original scoring system has greater sensitivity for the diagnosis than the simplified system (100% vs. 95%), but the simplified system has greater specificity (90% vs. 73%) and predictability (92% vs. 82%).[116] Whereas the original scoring system is useful for evaluating patients in whom every component must be assessed because of few or atypical findings, the simplified scoring system is useful for excluding AIH in patients with mixed immune and non-immune features.

The scoring systems have not been validated by prospective clinical trials, and the diagnosis by a score never overrides clinical judgment. Furthermore, the designations of "definite" and "probable" AIH are arbitrary, and patients with probable

TABLE 90-2 Revised Original Scoring System for the Diagnosis of Autoimmune Hepatitis

Category	Variable	Score
Gender	Female	+2
AP/AST	>3	−2
	<1.5	+2
Gamma globulin or IgG level	>2.0 times ULN	+3
	1.5-2.0 times ULN	+2
	1.0-1.5 times ULN	+1
	<1.0 times ULN	0
ANA, SMA, or anti-LKM1 titer	>1:80	+3
	1:80	+2
	1:40	+1
	<1:40	0
AMA	Positive	−4
Viral markers	Positive	−3
	Negative	+3
Drug history	Yes	−4
	No	+1
Alcohol consumption	<25 g/day	+2
	>60 g/day	−2
HLA	DR3 or DR4	+1
Concurrent immune disease	Thyroiditis, UC, synovitis, others	+2
Other liver-defined autoantibodies	Anti-SLA, anti-actin, anti-LC1, atypical pANCA	+2
Histologic features	Interface hepatitis	+3
	Plasmacytic infiltrate	+1
	Rosettes	+1
	None of above	−5
	Biliary changes	−3
	Other features	−3
Treatment response	Complete	+2
	Relapse	+3

Pretreatment Score		
Definite diagnosis		>15
Probable diagnosis		10-15

Post-treatment Score		
Definite diagnosis		>17
Probable diagnosis		12-17

AMA, antimitochondrial antibodies; ANA, antinuclear antibodies; anti-LC1, antibodies to liver cytosol type 1; anti-LKM1, antibodies to liver-kidney microsome type 1; anti-SLA, antibodies to soluble liver antigen; AP/AST (or AP/ALT), ratio of serum alkaline phosphatase level to serum AST (or serum ALT) level; IgG, immunoglobulin G; pANCA, perinuclear antineutrophil cytoplasmic antibodies; SMA, smooth muscle antibodies; ULN, upper limit of normal.
Adapted from Alvarez F, Berg PA, Bianchi FB, et al. International Autoimmune Hepatitis Group report: Review of criteria for diagnosis of autoimmune hepatitis. J Hepatol 1999; 31:929-38. Used with permission from Elsevier BV.

TABLE 90-3 Simplified Scoring System for the Diagnosis of Autoimmune Hepatitis

Category	Variable	Score
Autoantibodies*		
ANA or SMA	1:40	+1
Anti-LKM1	≥1:80	+2
	≥1:40	+2
Anti-SLA	Positive	+2
Immunoglobulin Level		
Immunoglobulin G	>1 × ULN	+1
	>1.1 × ULN	+2
Histologic Findings		
Morphologic features	Compatible with autoimmune hepatitis	+1
	Typical of autoimmune hepatitis	+2
Viral Disease		
Absence of viral hepatitis	No viral markers	+2
Pretreatment Aggregate Score		
Definite diagnosis		≥7
Probable diagnosis		6

*Autoantibody titers as determined by indirect immunofluorescence.
ANA, antinuclear antibodies; anti-LKM1, antibodies to liver-kidney microsome type 1; anti-SLA, antibodies to soluble liver antigen; SMA, smooth muscle antibodies; ULN, upper limit of normal.
Adapted from Hennes EM, Zeniya M, Czaja AJ, et al. Simplified diagnostic criteria for autoimmune hepatitis. Hepatology 2008; 48:169-76. Used with permission of John Wiley & Sons.

AIH typically have valid disease but with less pronounced inflammatory changes.[75]

CLASSIFICATION AND VARIANTS

Two types of AIH have distinctive serologic profiles.[117] Neither has been ascribed a unique cause, specific treatment strategy, or special type of behavior. The terms are useful as clinical descriptors and as research designations to ensure homogeneous study populations. In addition, AIH may present in nonclassic ways and may occur as part of an overlap syndrome with other disorders.

Type 1 Autoimmune Hepatitis

Type 1 AIH is characterized by SMA, ANA, or both (see Fig. 90-5).[1,2,62] Antibodies to actin have greater specificity, but less sensitivity, than SMA for the diagnosis of AIH.[78] Atypical pANCA are found in as many as 90% of patients with type 1 AIH (often in high titer) and typically are absent in type 2 AIH.[78]

Type 1 AIH can occur at any age and in either gender.[2,10,11] The disease has been described in infants and probably is underdiagnosed in the elderly. The female-to-male ratio is 3.5 : 1, and concurrent extrahepatic immunologic diseases are common (14% to 44%).[2] Autoimmune thyroiditis (in 12% of cases), Graves' disease (in 6% of cases), UC (in 6% of cases), RA, pernicious anemia, systemic sclerosis, Coombs-positive hemolytic anemia, celiac disease, autoimmune thrombocytopenic purpura, symptomatic cryoglobulinemia, leukocytoclastic vasculitis, nephritis, erythema nodosum, SLE, or fibrosing alveolitis may be occur with AIH as single or multiple diseases at presentation or later. Cholangiography is warranted to exclude PSC in all patients who have concurrent UC or prominent features of cholestasis (see Chapter 68).[2,118]

Type 1 AIH is associated with an abrupt onset of symptoms in 40% of cases and may manifest in an acute severe (fulminant) fashion.[4,115] Clinical features of chronic disease are lacking in 8% of patients, in whom the presentation is indistinguishable from that of acute viral or toxic hepatitis. The target autoantigen of type 1 AIH is unknown. HLA DRB1*0301 and HLA DRB1*0401 are independent risk factors for the disease in white North Americans and northern Europeans.[20,34,35] Over 80% of white patients in Great Britain and the United States possess either HLA DRB1*0301, DRB1*0401, or both, compared with 42% of the unaffected white population. In South America, especially in children, DRB1*1301 is the principal susceptibility allele.[36,37]

Type 2 Autoimmune Hepatitis

Type 2 AIH is characterized by the expression of anti-LKM1 (see Fig. 90-5).[2,62,119] Most affected persons are children (aged 2 to 14 years), but in Europe, especially in Germany and France, 20% of patients are adults.[119] In the United States, type 2 AIH is rare, and only 4% of patients older than 18 years have anti-LKM1.[120] The regional differences in prevalence may relate to ethnic differences in the genetic predisposition to the disease.[121]

Type 2 patients are younger than type 1 patients and may have different clinical and laboratory features.[62,119] Concurrent autoimmune diseases are common and include autoimmune thyroiditis, vitiligo, and type 1 diabetes mellitus. As with type 1 AIH, an acute or fulminant presentation is possible and important to recognize and treat early.[115] Susceptibility to type 2 AIH has been associated with DQB1*0201, DRB1*07,

and DRB1*03.[82] DQB1*0201 is in strong linkage disequilibrium with DRB1*07, and DRB1*03 and has been proposed as the principal genetic determinant of the disease.[82] The expression of anti-LKM1 has been associated with DRB1*07, and various aspects of type 2 AIH may have different genetic determinants.[122]

The target antigen of type 2 AIH is cytochrome P450 2D6 (CYP2D6).[123] CYP2D6 has 5 epitopes that are recognized by anti-LKM1.[124] The amino acid sequence spanning positions 193 to 212 of the CYP2D6 molecule is the target of anti-LKM1 in 93% of patients. Homologies exist between CYP2D6 and the genomes of the hepatitis C virus, cytomegalovirus, and herpes simplex type 1 virus.[124] These molecular mimicries may result in cross-reacting antibodies and support the hypothesis that repeated viral infections may break self-tolerance and cause AIH.[31]

Nonclassic Presentations

AIH can be discovered in asymptomatic persons[63,64] and patients with acute severe (fulminant) presentations.[115] Manifestations may also vary in different ethnic groups.[6-9] Diagnostic criteria must be flexible to accommodate these diverse nonclassic presentations to ensure prompt recognition and proper therapy.

Asymptomatic Patients

AIH can be asymptomatic in 34% to 45% of patients.[63,64] Histologic findings of moderate to severe interface hepatitis (91% vs. 95%) and fibrosis (41% vs. 44%) are similar in asymptomatic and symptomatic patients, respectively, and 26% to 70% of asymptomatic patients become symptomatic.[63,64] Asymptomatic patients can improve spontaneously, but spontaneous improvement is unpredictable, usually incomplete, and slow to evolve.[72] Progression to cirrhosis and liver failure are possible during the observation interval,[72] and the 10-year survival of untreated asymptomatic patients with mild AIH is less than that of treated patients with severe symptomatic AIH (67% vs. 98%).[72] The inflammatory activity of AIH can fluctuate spontaneously, and by definition AIH is aggressive and warrants treatment regardless of symptom status or mild disease severity. Treatment-related side effects occur in 12%, and this possibility can deter the institution of conventional glucocorticoid treatment in asymptomatic patients.[72] Budesonide (3 mg 3 times daily) in combination with azathioprine (1 to 2 mg/kg daily) may be better tolerated in uncomplicated, noncirrhotic patients with mild disease than are the prednisone-based regimens.[125,126]

Acute Severe (Fulminant) Presentation

AIH can have an acute severe or fulminant presentation that can be mistaken for acute viral or toxic hepatitis.[115] The acute presentation may reflect a spontaneous flare of preexisting chronic disease, an abruptly emergent disease of new onset, chronic disease with a superimposed infection or toxic injury ("acute-on-chronic disease"), or an acute disease that follows previous viral infection or treatment with immune-modifying drugs.[115] The percentage of cases of an acute severe (fulminant) presentation of AIH is 6% in North American adults with acute liver failure.[113]

The acute severe (fulminant) presentation is characterized by the presence of severe liver inflammation manifested by marked serum aminotransferase elevations and histologic changes that frequently include massive hepatic necrosis, lymphoid follicles, plasma cell infiltration, and centrilobular necrosis (central perivenulitis).[113,127] Difficulties in diagnosis relate mainly to the frequency with which typical laboratory and histologic findings are absent. The serum IgG level is normal in 25% to 39% of patients with acute severe (fulminant) AIH, and ANA are absent or weakly positive (titers ≤ 1:40) in 29% to 39%.[128,129] The international diagnostic scoring systems can support the clinical diagnosis in difficult cases.[115,116,130]

CT or MRI of the liver may indicate ascites, splenomegaly, and surface nodularity characteristic of advanced fibrosis and preexisting chronic liver disease,[131] and a heterogeneous reduction in hepatic attenuation on unenhanced CT scan may indicate acute severe (fulminant) AIH.[132,133] Heterogeneous hypoattenuated areas within the liver are present in 65% of patients with acute liver failure associated with AIH and only 5% of patients with late-admission virus-induced acute liver failure.[133]

Glucocorticoid therapy is effective in 36% to 100% of patients,[134] and the range of success probably reflects the promptness of diagnosis and treatment.[135] Failure to improve within 2 weeks of glucocorticoid therapy or worsening of the clinical or laboratory manifestations of liver inflammation and cholestasis at any time justifies a liver transplantation evaluation (see later).[136,137] Liver transplantation is effective in patients with an acute severe (fulminant) presentations, and the 5-year patient and graft survival rates are 56% and 51%, respectively.[138]

Non-Caucasian Patients

The descriptions of AIH have evolved mainly from experiences in white patients from Australia, northern Europe, and North America, and persons of other ethnicity or geographic location may have genetic, etiologic, cultural, and socioeconomic factors that alter their phenotype at presentation.[19,139] In the United States, African American, Hispanic, and Asian American patients have a high frequency of cirrhosis at diagnosis (>50%), and their responses to glucocorticoid treatment may also differ from that of white patients.[140,141] Outside the United States, non-Caucasian patients may have chronic indolent and unsuspected disease (Canadian Aboriginal populations),[25] distinctions in phenotype, severity, and outcome by age group (South American and Japanese populations),[22,27,142] frequent acute-on-chronic disease (South Asian populations),[143,144] and glucocorticoid-resistant cholestatic manifestations (Canadian-Aboriginal, Turkish, and Middle Eastern populations).[8,21,25]

African American patients with AIH have cirrhosis at presentation more commonly than white American patients (57% to 85% vs. 38%),[139,140] and they typically are younger at the onset of disease.[140] Liver failure is more common at presentation (38% vs. 9%); the need for liver transplantation is greater (51% vs. 23%); and the overall mortality rate of AIH is higher (24% vs. 6%).[139] African American men commonly have a poor treatment outcome,[139] and the 5-year graft survival of African Americans after transplantation is also lower than that for white Americans (60% vs. 68%).[145] Similarly, Asian American patients with AIH frequently have cirrhosis at presentation and an even higher mortality rate from their disease than blacks.[141,146] By contrast, Hispanic American patients with AIH, who have similar frequencies of cirrhosis at presentation[141] and the same socioeconomic issues as African Americans,[147] have a survival rate that is superior to that of African Americans and similar to or better than that of non-Hispanic whites with AIH.[147,148] The experiences among these ethnic groups in the United States probably reflect genetic differences in the behavior of the disease and in the pharmacogenomics of the drug therapy. They may also indicate differences in education,

medical awareness, cultural attitudes, and insurance coverage that impact health care access.[149-151]

Autoantibody-Negative Autoimmune Hepatitis

Thirteen percent of adults with chronic hepatitis of undetermined cause satisfy international criteria for the diagnosis of AIH but lack ANA, SMA, and anti-LKM1.[130,152-155] These patients commonly are designated as having cryptogenic chronic hepatitis and may be excluded from therapies of potential benefit. Autoantibody-negative patients are similar in age, gender, frequency of concurrent immunologic diseases, histologic features, and laboratory findings to patients with classic AIH.[130,152,155] Furthermore, they have similar frequencies of HLA-B8, DRB1*03, and A1-B8-DRB1*03, and they respond as well to glucocorticoid treatment as do their autoantibody-positive counterparts.[152-154] These persons may have an autoantibody outside the conventional testing battery, autoantibodies that have been suppressed or delayed in expression, or a signature autoantibody that is as yet undiscovered.[130,156]

Liver diseases such as Wilson disease, celiac-related liver disease, and drug-induced liver disease may closely resemble autoantibody-negative AIH and must be excluded by appropriate clinical history, laboratory tests, and histologic assessment.[130,155] Serologic evaluation for atypical pANCA and anti-SLA can reclassify 15% to 20% of autoantibody-negative patients as classic AIH.[95,130,155] IgA antibodies to tissue transglutaminase or endomysium support the diagnosis of celiac-related liver disease,[130,155] whereas the late appearance of conventional autoantibodies in patients seronegative at presentation strengthens the possibility of AIH.[156]

The comprehensive diagnostic scoring system of the IAIHG can be useful in supporting the possibility of AIH before and after glucocorticoid therapy in autoantibody-negative patients.[114,116,130,155] All autoantibody-negative patients who are candidates for AIH because of the confident exclusion of alternative diagnoses should undergo a monitored 3-month treatment trial of glucocorticoids. Improvement has occurred in 67% to 87% of treated cases consistent with the diagnosis of AIH.[130]

Drug-Induced Autoimmune-Like Hepatitis

Nine percent of patients diagnosed with AIH have a drug-induced liver injury (see Chapter 88).[157] Minocycline, nitrofurantoin, methyldopa, dihydralazine, halothane, tienilic acid, and oxiphenistatin have been well documented to induce a liver disease that is indistinguishable from classic AIH.[158] Multiple other medications, supplements, and toxins have also been implicated in the occurrence of drug-induced autoimmune-like hepatitis,[158] and immune-modulating drugs, such as recombinant interferon-α, antibodies to CTLA4, and pulsed methylprednisolone, may facilitate the emergence of "latent" AIH.[158]

Minocycline and nitrofurantoin are the principal drugs in current practice that can induce an acute idiosyncratic liver injury that resembles AIH, and they account for 90% of cases.[157,159] Most patients with drug-induced autoimmune-like hepatitis are women (80% to 90%); jaundice develops in 69%; 18% are 65 or older; an acute onset is typical (median onset from drug exposure, 42 days; range, 20 to 117 days); and features of hypersensitivity (fever, rash, and eosinophilia) are present in 15% to 20%.[158] Histologic features include interface hepatitis with portal and periportal lymphocytes, plasma cells, and eosinophils. Findings that especially favor drug-induced injury are portal neutrophils and intercellular cholestasis, whereas portal and intra-acinar plasma cells, hepatocyte rosettes, and emperiopolesis (active penetration of one cell into another cell) favor AIH.[106] Hepatic fibrosis may be present, but cirrhosis is rare in drug-induced autoimmune-like hepatitis.[157,158]

Causality assessment by codified diagnostic scales and structured expert opinion has been flawed, and the diagnosis of drug-induced autoimmune-like hepatitis is best made by clinical judgment.[158-161] Keys to the diagnosis are the temporal sequence between the drug exposure and onset of disease and the disease behavior after drug withdrawal. Drug-induced autoimmune-like hepatitis typically resolves after discontinuation of the drug, and it does not recur.[157,158] Classic AIH is self-perpetuating and does not resolve after discontinuation of the drug.

Drug-induced autoimmune-like hepatitis is commonly treated with glucocorticoids in addition to drug withdrawal because of the uncertainty of the diagnosis and the severity of the presentation.[157,158] Resolution is characteristic, and recurrence (denoting AIH) or nonrecurrence (denoting drug-induced autoimmune-like hepatitis) after glucocorticoid withdrawal can support the final diagnosis.[158] Patients with AIH commonly relapse after glucocorticoid withdrawal (50% to 87%),[158,162] and recurrent disease, while indicative of AIH, does not exclude the possibility that drug exposure converted a preexisting latency for AIH into a fully expressed classic phenotype.[158,163]

Overlap Syndromes

Patients with AIH who have cholestatic features currently lack an official designation and established treatment strategy.[118,130,164-166] Their principal phenotype is AIH, but they have secondary features of a cholestatic liver disease. These patients have findings that suggest PBC, PSC, or a cholestatic syndrome indistinguishable from AMA-negative PBC or small-duct PSC (Table 90-4).[118,166-168] The frequency of the overlap syndromes ranges from 7% to 18% depending on the presumed nature of the cholestatic component,[118,164] and the frequency of a complete glucocorticoid response lessens with increasing degree of cholestasis.[164,165]

Rigid boundaries across which the manifestations of classic disease cannot occur are impossible to establish, especially because the manifestations that are common in one disease are not specific for that disease.[118] Accordingly, the validity of the overlap syndromes as distinct pathologic entities remains unclear. This uncertainty has justified the position statement by the IAIHG that patients with atypical manifestations be classified by their predominant diagnosis and not by their overlapping features.[166] The clinical manifestations and outcomes of these syndromes vary by the predominant disease, and patients with predominantly AIH with features of PBC or PSC must be distinguished from patients with predominantly PBC or PSC with features of AIH.[118] The rarity of an overlap syndrome between PBC and PSC supports the hypothesis that the overlap syndromes are mainly classic diseases with atypical features rather than concurrent diseases.

Overlap with PBC

Patients with AIH who have AMA and histologic features of bile duct injury have an overlap syndrome with PBC (see Table 90-4).[118,164-166,169] Antibodies against the PBC-specific mitochondrial antigens may be present[170]; histologic features of cholangitis, including destructive cholangitis ("florid duct lesion"), may be seen[169]; and copper staining of hepatic tissue indicative of cholestasis may be observed.[73] The frequency of this overlap syndrome ranges from 2% in patients initially diagnosed as having AIH to 19% in patients initially diagnosed as having PBC (see Chapter 91).[118,164,171] This discrepancy in part relates to the common use of a diagnostic scoring system for AIH in patients with PBC, whereas the diagnosis of PBC in patients with AIH relies on other indices.[118] Importantly, diagnostic scoring systems for AIH were not developed to define overlap syndromes, and their use in this clinical context is discouraged.[118,166]

TABLE 90-4 Overlap Syndromes of Autoimmune Hepatitis

	Autoimmune Hepatitis with Overlapping Features of:		
	PBC	**PSC**	**Cholestasis**
Clinical and laboratory features	AMA + Serum AP frequently > 2-fold ULN	AMA − Serum AP frequently > 2-fold ULN IBD common Abnormal cholangiogram (except in small-duct disease)	AMA − Serum AP frequently > 2-fold ULN No UC Normal cholangiogram
Histology	Destructive cholangitis Ductopenia Cholestasis	Ductopenia Cholangiolar proliferation Swollen fibrotic portal tracts	Lymphoplasmacytic portal and acinar infiltrates Lymphocytic destructive cholangitis Swollen hepatocytes
Treatment	Prednisone (10 mg daily) in combination with azathioprine (50 mg daily) if AP ≤ 2 × ULN Prednisone (10 mg daily) in combination with azathioprine (50 mg daily) and low-dose UDCA (13-15 mg/kg daily) if AP > 2 × ULN and/or florid duct lesions	Prednisone (10 mg daily) in combination with azathioprine (50 mg daily) and low-dose UDCA (13-15 mg/kg daily)	Prednisone (10 mg daily) in combination with azathioprine (50 mg daily) and/or low-dose UDCA (13-15 mg/kg daily) depending on AP level and histologic features

AMA, antimitochondrial antibodies; AP, alkaline phosphatase level; UDCA, ursodeoxycholic acid; ULN, upper limit of normal.

The "Paris criteria," promulgated in 1998 as a guideline for the diagnosis of this overlap syndrome,[169] have been largely incorporated into the recommendations of the European Association for the Study of the Liver (EASL).[166,172] The Paris criteria require the presence of at least 2 of 3 recognized hallmarks of each disease. The 3 hallmarks of AIH are a serum ALT level 5 times the ULN or greater, IgG level twice the ULN or greater or positive test for SMA, and histologic features of moderate to severe interface hepatitis. The 3 hallmarks of PBC are serum alkaline phosphatase level twice the ULN or greater or GGTP 5 times the ULN or greater, positive test for AMA, and histologic evidence of florid duct lesions.[169] The sensitivity and specificity of the Paris criteria for the overlap syndrome of AIH and PBC were 92% and 97%, respectively, using clinical judgment as the gold standard.[173] The inclusion of patients who fail to satisfy the Paris criteria but who respond to glucocorticoids has been proposed as a supplemental diagnostic criterion.[171] The diagnostic guidelines promulgated by the EASL require the presence of interface hepatitis in all persons designated as having an AIH-PBC overlap syndrome.[166,172]

The clinical course of the overlap syndrome with PBC and its response to treatment depend mainly on the predominant components of the disease. Patients who have high serum AST levels, serum alkaline phosphatase levels less than 2-fold the ULN, moderate to severe interface hepatitis on histologic examination, and high diagnostic scores for AIH ("AIH-predominant disease") commonly respond to glucocorticoid therapy. By contrast, patients who have serum alkaline phosphatase levels twice the ULN or greater, serum GGTP 5 times the ULN or greater, and florid bile duct lesions on histologic examination ("PBC-predominant disease") commonly respond to low-dose ursodeoxycholic acid (≤15 mg/kg daily) in combination with glucocorticoids (prednisone, prednisolone, or budesonide).[118,164,174] This combination regimen has induced laboratory resolution (67% vs. 27%) and prevented progressive hepatic fibrosis (100% vs. 50%) more commonly than in patients treated with low-dose ursodeoxycholic acid or prednisone alone.[174] The 5-year liver transplant-free survival rate has been 100%, and the 10-year survival rate has been 92%.[173] The combination regimen of low-dose ursodeoxycholic acid and glucocorticoids has been endorsed by the EASL with the understanding that the recommendation is not evidence based.[166,172]

AMA can be detected in 18% of patients with AIH in the absence of cholestatic features and can appear, disappear, or persist during the course of the disease without evolution to PBC or the need for alternative therapy.[175,176] Histologic changes of bile duct injury are required in addition to AMA and other classic features of AIH to designate an overlap form of AIH.

Overlap with PSC

Histologic changes of lymphocytic, pleomorphic, or fibrous cholangitis; cholestatic laboratory findings; concurrent IBD; or failure to respond to glucocorticoids constitute indications for cholangiography in patients who have AIH.[118,164,165] The absence of characteristic cholangiographic changes does not preclude the diagnosis of PSC, because small-duct disease may be present (see Table 90-4) (see Chapter 68).[177,178] MR cholangiography has demonstrated unsuspected PSC in 8% of adults with AIH, and the possibility of PSC must be evaluated in all persons with AIH and disease refractory to glucocorticoid therapy.[179] Hepatic fibrosis may produce biliary changes that resemble intrahepatic PSC by MR cholangiography, and the occurrence of small-duct PSC in patients with otherwise classic AIH is low.[180]

The frequency of PSC in patients with AIH and cholestatic features is 6% to 11%,[118,177,181] and the frequency of AIH in patients with PSC who are assessed for AIH by the comprehensive scoring system of the IAIHG is 8% to 17%.[118,182,183] Children with AIH may also have unsuspected bile duct changes. Autoimmune sclerosing cholangitis is a disorder described in children who have the clinical phenotype of AIH but abnormal findings on cholangiographic studies.[184] IBD is frequently absent, and unlike adults with AIH and PSC, these children frequently respond to conventional glucocorticoid therapy.[184]

Treatment is empirical and includes prednisone alone or a lower dose of prednisone in combination with azathioprine.[118,185] Ursodeoxycholic acid (≤15 mg/kg daily) has also been used in conjunction with glucocorticoids depending on whether hepatitic or cholestatic features predominate.[118,164,165,183] Other immunosuppressive agents used have included cyclosporine, tacrolimus, and mycophenolate mofetil, but there has been no evidence of a consistent benefit from these drugs.[186]

Patients may respond to conventional glucocorticoid therapy if the features of AIH predominate, the stage of PSC is early, and PSC is limited to a histologic pattern of mild bile duct injury.[118,185] High-dose ursodeoxycholic acid (28 to 30 mg/kg daily) should be avoided because liver toxicity and hepatic failure may occur, possibly because of expansion of the bile acid pool with lithocholic acid.[187,188] The combination regimen of low-dose ursodeoxycholic acid and glucocorticoids has been recommended by the EASL,[166,172] based mainly on a small single-center experience.[183] The guidelines developed by the AASLD recommend the use of glucocorticoids and other immunosuppressive agents,[166,186] but the drug preferences are not specified and the use of ursodeoxycholic acid is not promulgated. Each society indicates that their recommendations are not evidence based. All therapies are empirical and directed against the predominant disease. Treatment regimens require close monitoring and individualized adjustments.

Patients with AIH and PSC show improved laboratory and histologic features to normal or near-normal less frequently (22% vs. 64%), deteriorate during therapy more often (33% vs. 10%), and die of liver failure or require liver transplantation more commonly (33% vs. 8%) than patients with classic AIH after comparable treatment with conventional glucocorticoid regimens.[118,167,183,189] Fibrosis usually progresses, and cirrhosis develops in 75% within 12 years.[190] Patients with the overlap syndrome of AIH and PSC may have a better outcome than patients with classic PSC.[166]

Overlap with Cholestatic Features

Eight percent of patients with AIH have histologic features of bile duct injury and laboratory changes of cholestasis in the absence of AMA and cholangiographic changes of PSC (see Table 90-4 and Chapter 91).[109,164] This variant form is probably a heterogeneous category that encompasses patients with atypical, early, or transitional features of classic disease. Patients with AMA-negative PBC and small-duct PSC are probably the principal members of this category.[118,166] Persons with the cholestatic variant are inconsistently responsive to glucocorticoids alone, low-dose ursodeoxycholic acid alone, or glucocorticoids in combination with low-dose ursodeoxycholic acid.[109,118,164] Limited experience suggests that these treatments can improve the clinical and laboratory abnormalities but not the histologic changes. As in all the overlap syndromes, treatment is empirical and not evidence based. Management with glucocorticoids alone, low-dose ursodeoxycholic acid alone, or glucocorticoids in combination with low-dose ursodeoxycholic acid can be considered depending on the degree of cholestasis.[118,165] Treatment strategies typically

TABLE 90-5 Indications for Glucocorticoid Treatment in Autoimmune Hepatitis*

	Urgent Indications	Nonurgent Indications
Clinical	Incapacitating symptoms Clinical progression Acute presentation (de novo and spontaneous exacerbation of preexisting disease) Acute severe presentation with liver failure	Mild or no symptoms No clinical progression
Laboratory	AST ≥ 10-fold ULN AST ≥ 5-fold ULN and gamma globulins ≥ 2-fold ULN	AST < 10-fold ULN with or without elevated gamma globulins or IgG
Histologic	Moderate to severe interface hepatitis Bridging necrosis Multilobular necrosis Centrilobular necrosis	Mild interface hepatitis

*All patients with autoimmune hepatitis are candidates for glucocorticoid therapy regardless of symptom status or disease severity, and the decision to treat an individual patient should be based on clinical judgment. Sepsis and active GI bleeding are contraindications to treatment.
IgG, immunoglobulin G; ULN, upper limit of normal.

mirror those used in the overlap syndromes with PBC and PSC.[166]

Histologic findings of bile duct injury, including destructive cholangitis, may be seen in classic AIH in the absence of other cholestatic features.[110,111] These changes are commonly isolated and transient, and they probably represent collateral damage associated with severe inflammatory activity. They do not constitute an overlap syndrome, nor do they change the diagnosis or affect the treatment strategy.

TREATMENT

Indications

All patients with AIH are candidates for treatment (Table 90-5).[1,72,80,126] The urgency rather than the need for treatment may be the only variable in making the decision to treat. Fragile patient populations, especially the elderly and pregnant women, require individualized treatment regimens that are well monitored,[9,126,191] and asymptomatic patients with mild disease may be observed initially to document disease behavior before starting drug therapy.[1,7,9,72,126,191]

The urgency for treatment is based on the severity of the clinical, laboratory, and histologic manifestations of liver inflammation.[62] Patients with an acute severe (fulminant) presentation,[115] those with serum AST or ALT elevations 10-fold or more than the ULN or serum AST or ALT levels 5-fold or more than the ULN with serum gamma globulin levels 2-fold or more than the ULN, and those with histologic features of bridging necrosis or multi-acinar collapse warrant immediate therapy. The 6-month mortality rate of untreated patients with these findings is as high as 40%.[192] Patients with less severe AIH have less immediate risk of clinical deterioration, progression to cirrhosis, or liver failure, and the need for treatment is less urgent.[72]

Drug Regimens

Prednisone (30 mg daily tapered over a 4-week induction period to 10 mg daily) in combination with azathioprine (50 mg daily) is the preferred treatment strategy (Table 90-6).[1]

TABLE 90-6 Preferred First-Line Treatment Regimens in Autoimmune Hepatitis

Combination Therapy		Single-Drug Therapy
Prednisone (or Prednisolone)	Azathioprine	Prednisone (or Prednisolone)
Induction Phase		
30 mg daily × 1 wk 20 mg daily × 1 wk 15 mg daily × 2 wk	50 mg daily 50 mg daily 50 mg daily	60 mg daily × 1 wk 40 mg daily × 1 wk 30 mg daily × 2 wk
Maintenance Phase		
10 mg daily until end point	50 mg daily until end point	20 mg daily until end point
Ideal Candidates		
All noncytopenic, nonpregnant patients Patients with preexisting obesity, diabetes mellitus, osteopenia, hypertension, or emotional instability		Patients with: Cytopenia Absent TPMT activity Pregnancy Azathioprine intolerance Active malignancy Acute severe (fulminant) onset

TMPT, thiopurine methyltransferase.

Therapy with prednisone alone (60 mg daily tapered over a 4-week induction period to 20 mg daily) is as effective as the combination regimen, but it is associated with a higher frequency of glucocorticoid-related side effects than the combination regimen (44% vs. 10%).[1,193-195] Treatment with prednisone alone is warranted mainly in pregnant patients and in those with severe cytopenia, absent thiopurine methyltransferase activity, or azathioprine intolerance.[193,194]

Prednisolone is preferred in Europe because it does not require intrahepatic conversion to the active metabolite and achieves a faster peak plasma concentration (1.3 ± 0.7 hours vs. 2.6 ± 1.3 hours) and greater systemic bioavailability ($99 \pm 8\%$ vs. $84 \pm 13\%$) than prednisone.[194,196] These attributes have not been associated with differences in outcome,[194] but they have justified the preference for prednisolone in the treatment of acute severe (fulminant) AIH.[115] Azathioprine adds little to the acute regimen because its therapeutic effect emerges slowly.[194,195]

Budesonide is a next-generation glucocorticoid with 90% or better hepatic first-pass clearance and metabolites devoid of glucocorticoid activity.[126,194,197] Budesonide (3 mg 3 times daily) in combination with azathioprine (1 to 2 mg/kg daily) normalized serum AST and ALT levels more commonly (47% vs. 18%) and with fewer side effects (28% vs. 53%) than the combination regimen with prednisone (40 mg daily, tapered to 10 mg daily) when administered as first-line therapy for 6 months in a large randomized clinical trial.[125]

The frequency of histologic resolution and the durability of the response to budesonide are unknown.[125,194] Furthermore, budesonide has not been useful as a rescue therapy for prednisone-refractory AIH; its low systemic availability may complicate the management of concurrent nonhepatic immune-mediated diseases; and typical glucocorticoid-induced side effects have developed in patients with cirrhosis.[194] Nevertheless, budesonide in combination with azathioprine is emerging as an alternative first-line treatment, and it may be most appropriate in noncirrhotic, treatment-naïve patients with uncomplicated AIH or in patients with obesity, diabetes mellitus, hypertension, and osteoporosis that might be worsened by therapy with prednisone.[126,194,197]

Drug Actions

Prednisone is a prodrug that is converted in the liver to prednisolone by 11β-hydroxysteroid dehydrogenase type 1 (11β-HSD1).[194,198] Prednisolone is the active metabolite responsible for the therapeutic and toxic effects of the medication, and its actions are modulated in part by the degree of protein-binding within the circulation.[193,194] Protracted hypoalbuminemia or hyperbilirubinemia can increase the concentrations of unbound prednisolone in the blood and enhance its actions and toxicities.[193] Advanced liver disease can decrease the conversion of prednisone to prednisolone, but this reduction has not been sufficient to impact treatment outcomes in patients with cirrhosis.[194] Impaired hepatic conversion of prednisone to prednisolone is a consideration when treating patients with acute severe (fulminant) AIH.[115]

Glucocorticoids limit T-cell activation mainly by inhibiting cytokine production and the expression of adhesion molecules.[194,199] Glucocorticoids are lipophilic and can diffuse into the cytosol of cells to bind the glucocorticoid receptor. The complex of drug and receptor then translocates to the nucleus where it suppresses cytokine gene expression and reduces the activity of nuclear factor (NF)-κB (nuclear factor kappa-light chain enhancer of activated B cells).[194,196] Production of the intracytoplasmic inhibitor of NF-κB (IBκ) is increased by prednisolone, and nuclear coactivator proteins necessary for the transcription of cytokines are depleted. Type 1 and type 2 cytokine pathways are affected, and both cellular and humoral immune responses are blunted.[194]

Prednisolone also impairs the production of adhesion molecules necessary for the attraction of inflammatory cells to sites of tissue damage, and it induces the apoptosis of lymphocytes.[194,200] These anti-inflammatory actions limit the recruitment of immune cells to the liver and reduce the extent of liver damage.[194] Prednisolone can also prevent hepatic

fibrosis by limiting the production of TGF-β, the transformation of hepatic stellate cells into myofibroblasts, and the interference of metalloproteinase inhibitors on the degradation of fibrillar collagen.[52] Repeated administration of glucocorticoids is required to achieve results in AIH because of a short biological half-life (mean half-life, 3.2 ± 1 hours).[194]

Azathioprine is a purine antagonist that mainly blocks the proliferation of lymphocytes.[195,201,202] It is converted to 6-mercaptopurine (6-MP) in blood by a nonenzymatic, glutathione-based pathway. The intermediate metabolite, 6-MP, is then converted in the liver to either 6-thioguanine nucleotides by hypoxanthine guanine phosphoribosyl transferase, 6-thiouric acid by xanthine oxidase, or 6-methylmercaptopurine by thiopurine methyltransferase (TPMT).[195] The 6-thioguanines are the active metabolites that interfere with purine nucleotide synthesis within the cell cycle, and they thereby impair proliferation of rapidly dividing T and B lymphocytes.[195] The 6-thioguanine nucleotides also inhibit the expression of genes affecting inflammatory activity, promote the apoptosis of activated lymphocytes, and decrease the number of natural killer cells within the liver.[195,202-204]

The integrity of the xanthine oxidase and TPMT pathways influences the amount of the 6-MP that is converted to the 6-thioguanine nucleotides or the inactive metabolites, 6-MP and 6-methylmercaptopurine.[195,201,202] These pathways in turn influence the therapeutic (antiproliferative and anti-inflammatory) and toxic (myelosuppressive) actions of the medication. Drugs that inhibit xanthine oxidase activity (e.g., allopurinol) or a deficiency in TPMT activity can increase the therapeutic efficacy and the toxicity of the 6-thioguanine nucleotides.

The plasma concentrations of the azathioprine metabolites peak 3.8 hours after an oral dose of the parent drug, and 6-MP is eliminated from the plasma within 8 hours (plasma half-life, 1.9 ± 0.6 hours).[195] The full immunosuppressive action of azathioprine can take 3 months or longer to achieve because the nuclear incorporations and cell line transformations required for a pharmacologic effect evolve slowly. Azathioprine is used mainly in combination with prednisone as a glucocorticoid-sparing agent. It can be used as a sole drug in AIH to maintain the improvements achieved by the glucocorticoids (see later).[195]

Budesonide is metabolized in the liver mainly through the mediation of the cytochrome CYP3A4, and its two main metabolites, 6 β-hydroxy budesonide and 16 α-hydroxy prednisolone, lack glucocorticoid activity.[194] Budesonide has anti-inflammatory and immunosuppressive properties similar to those of conventional glucocorticoids. The anti-inflammatory effects are accomplished by inhibiting the release of the chemokines (CXCL1, CXCL8) and interleukin (IL)-6 from neutrophils and by modulating the expression of the chemokine receptor, CXCR2. The immune suppressive effects are accomplished by reducing the production of cytokines, including TNF-α and interferon γ, and by inhibiting the activation and proliferation of T lymphocytes. The plasma half-life of budesonide in adults is 2.8 ± 1.1 hours, and the systemic availability after oral administration is $10.7\% \pm 4.3\%$. Equivalencies in the anti-inflammatory and antiproliferative actions of budesonide, prednisone, and prednisolone cannot be assumed when treating AIH.[194]

Drug-Related Side Effects

Cosmetic changes, such as facial rounding, dorsal hump formation, obesity, acne, striae, alopecia, and facial hirsutism, occur in 80% of patients after 2 years of treatment with prednisone or prednisolone, regardless of the treatment regimen used (combination or monotherapy).[193,194] Severe side effects include osteopenia with vertebral compression, diabetes mellitus, cataracts, emotional instability, opportunistic infections, pancreatitis, and hypertension. Severe complications are uncommon and develop only after protracted therapy (>18 months) and on the regimen with the higher dose of prednisone (20 mg daily). Azathioprine with prednisone is preferred to a higher dose of prednisone alone because the combination produces fewer glucocorticoid-related side effects during comparable periods of treatment (10% vs. 44%).[1] Treatment must be discontinued prematurely in 13% of patients, mainly because of intolerable obesity, cosmetic changes, brittle diabetes mellitus, or osteoporosis with vertebral compression.[193]

Treatment with azathioprine can be complicated by cholestatic liver disease, nausea, emesis, rash, pancreatitis, arthralgias, opportunistic infections, and cytopenia.[193,195] Five percent of patients treated with azathioprine develop early adverse reactions (nausea, vomiting, arthralgias, fever, skin rash, or pancreatitis) that warrant its discontinuation. The overall frequency of azathioprine-related side effects in patients treated with 50 mg daily is 10%, and the side effects typically improve after the dose is reduced or the therapy is discontinued.[193] Cytopenia is the most common consequence of treatment; bone marrow failure is rare. Cytopenia occurs in 46% of patients, and severe hematologic abnormalities occur in 6%.[193,195,205] These toxicities are not predictable by either genotyping or phenotyping for TPMT activity, and the most common association with cytopenia in these patients is cirrhosis and presumed hypersplenism associated with portal hypertension.[205-207]

Teratogenicity is a theoretical complication of therapy with azathioprine (see Chapter 115).[193,195] Azathioprine has been administered successfully in pregnant women with AIH, pregnant mothers with IBD, and women who have conceived while taking azathioprine after liver transplantation. Furthermore, multiple large clinical studies have indicated that therapy with azathioprine is safe in pregnant women with IBD. Nevertheless, azathioprine has been associated with congenital malformations in pregnant mice, and these defects have included cleft palate, skeletal anomalies, hydrops fetalis, reduced thymic size, anemia, and hematopoietic depression. Furthermore, the placenta is only a partial barrier to the metabolites of azathioprine, and low levels of 6-thioguanine are detectable in the newborns of mothers treated for Crohn's disease. Azathioprine is designated a category D drug for pregnancy (see Chapter 39), and its use can be avoided during pregnancy in women with AIH. Azathioprine is not an essential medication in the treatment of AIH and can be discontinued during pregnancy, in which case the liver disease can be managed successfully by adjustments in the dose of prednisone. The activity of AIH frequently improves during pregnancy, and less medication is required. The disease exacerbates after delivery in 12% to 86% of cases, and standard full-dose therapy should be resumed.

Oncogenicity is another possible complication of therapy with azathioprine (see Chapter 115).[193,195,208] The incidence of extrahepatic neoplasms is 1 per 194 patient-years; the probability of tumor occurrence is 3% after 10 years; and the risk of malignancy is 1.4-fold greater than normal. The low but increased risk of malignancy does not contraindicate azathioprine therapy in AIH but emphasizes the importance of maintaining strict indications for treatment.

Blood TPMT activity is significantly lower in patients with AIH and intolerance to azathioprine than in patients with uncomplicated courses of treatment.[206] Similar findings have been described in patients with IBD and rheumatic conditions (see Chapter 115). These observations have suggested that routine screening of the blood TPMT level may identify persons with AIH at risk for azathioprine-related complica-

tions. The blood TPMT activity level, however, has not been predictive of toxicity in individual patients. Genotypic and phenotypic screening for blood TPMT activity has not reduced the frequency of azathioprine-induced side effects in patients with AIH compared with unscreened patients,[205-207] nor has the occurrence of azathioprine-related side effects been associated with below-normal levels of TPMT activity.[205] Near-zero enzyme activity occurs rarely in otherwise normal persons (0.3% to 0.5%), and the value of screening to detect this unusually low enzyme deficiency remains uncertain, especially because some patients with low levels do not exhibit azathioprine toxicity.[205] Testing for blood TPMT activity seems most appropriate in patients with preexisting or progressive cytopenias and in those subjected to doses of azathioprine higher than the conventional schedule of 50 mg daily.[1,193] Avoidance of azathioprine in patients with preexisting or progressive cytopenias (leukocyte count < 2.5×10^9/L or platelet count < 50×10^9/L) and close monitoring (at 3-month intervals) of the blood leukocyte and platelet counts in all patients taking the drug may be the best preventive strategy.[1]

The high hepatic first-pass clearance of budesonide, which protects against the development of glucocorticoid-related side effects, is diminished in cirrhosis, and budesonide-treated patients with cirrhosis can develop the same complications associated with conventional glucocorticoid therapy.[194] Furthermore, it can be difficult to switch patients already treated with prednisone to budesonide without incurring severe glucocorticoid-withdrawal symptoms or exacerbating concurrent nonhepatic immune-mediated diseases.[194]

PROGNOSIS AND OUTCOMES

Prognostic Indices

Problematic patients can be identified by their clinical phenotype at presentation and by their response to conventional glucocorticoid therapy.[126] A score of 12 or more points at presentation by the MELD score (see Chapter 97) identifies 97% of persons who will fail conventional glucocorticoid therapy, die of liver failure, or require liver transplantation, and the specificity of this score for treatment failure is 68%.[209] Young adults with AIH (18 to 40 years of age) have a frequency of treatment failure that exceeds 20%, and they commonly (56%) have HLA DRB1*0301.[10] By contrast, patients older than 40 respond well to conventional glucocorticoid therapy (frequency of treatment failure, 7%), and they commonly (41%) have HLA DRB1*0401.[10] The presence of anti-SLA at presentation identifies persons with AIH who invariably relapse after glucocorticoid withdrawal, and antibodies to SLA are strongly (86%) associated with HLA DRB1*0301.[91] These antibodies may be surrogate markers for a genetic propensity for severe disease and long-term treatment dependence.[91,92]

The early response to glucocorticoid therapy can also identify problematic patients with AIH.[126] Patients with AIH and multilobular collapse on histologic assessment in whom at least one laboratory feature of liver inflammation or function, especially pretreatment hyperbilirubinemia, fails to improve within 2 weeks of starting glucocorticoid therapy invariably develop liver failure within 6 months.[136] Similarly, patients with acute icteric presentations in whom the U.K. End-Stage Liver Disease (UKELD) score fails to improve by at least 2 points within 7 days of initiating glucocorticoid therapy have poor outcomes (frequency of death, liver transplantation, or need for alternative therapy of 85%).[137] Patients in whom laboratory tests and liver histology fail to improve to normal or nearnormal within 12 months of standard treatment have higher frequencies of progression to cirrhosis (54% vs. 18%)

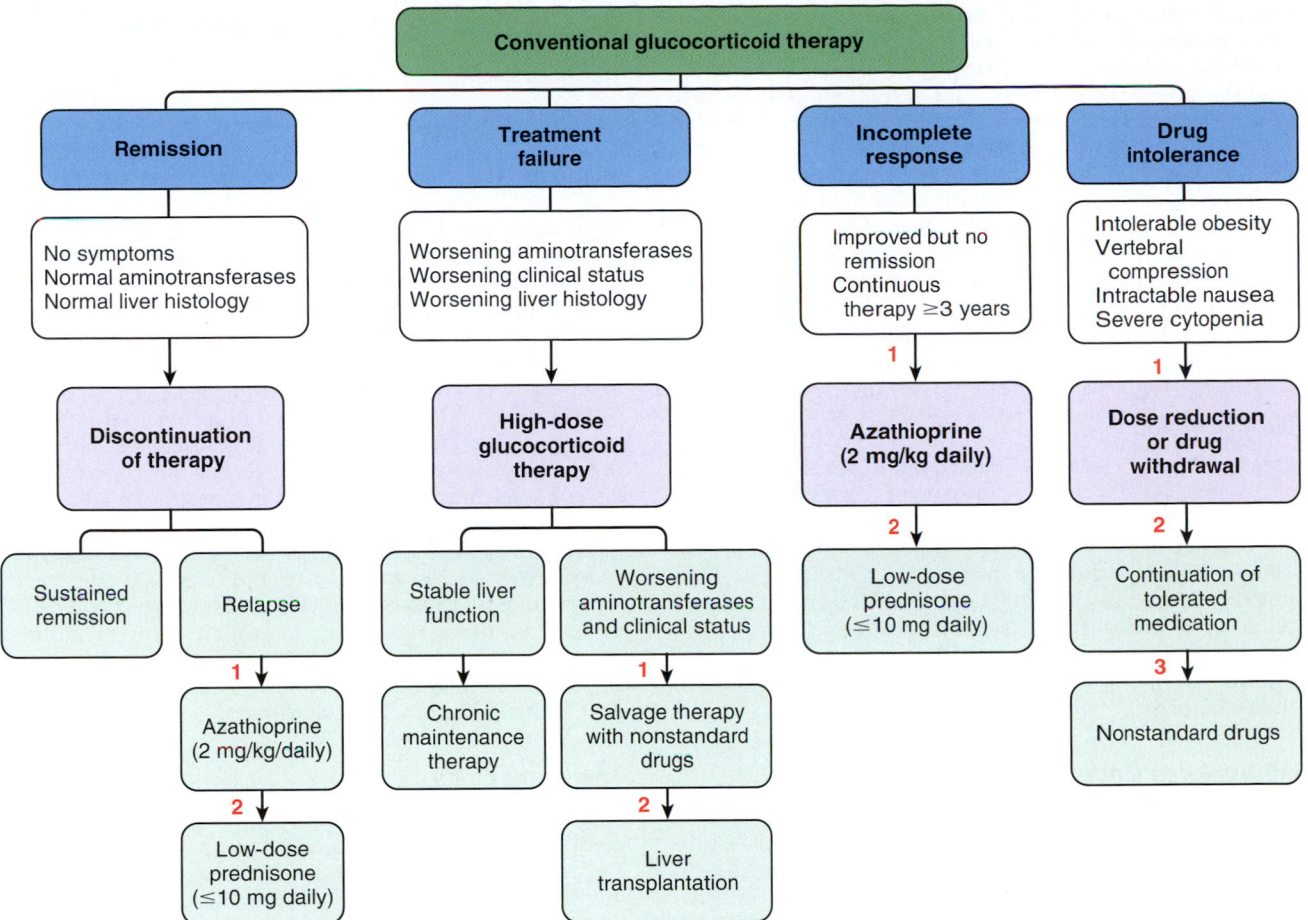

FIGURE 90-6. Algorithm for the treatment of autoimmune hepatitis. Patients who satisfy indications for glucocorticoid therapy are given prednisone in combination with azathioprine or a higher dose of prednisone alone (conventional glucocorticoid therapy) (see Table 90-6). Treatment is continued until the criteria for a treatment end point are met. Possible end points are remission, treatment failure, incomplete response, and drug intolerance (*dark blue panels*). Therapy can then be discontinued, increased in dose, or reduced in dose according to the response (*light blue panels*). Responses to the dose adjustments determine the need for other actions, numbered sequentially in order of preference (*light green panels*).

and need for liver transplantation (15% vs. 2%) than patients who respond more rapidly.[210] The clinical phenotype at presentation and the disease dynamics during therapy should prompt close surveillance and early institution of dose-adjusted or alternative therapies.[126,211]

Outcomes of Treatment

Remission

Remission connotes absence of symptoms, resolution of all laboratory indices of liver inflammation, and improvement in histology to normal or inactive cirrhosis (Fig. 90-6).[1,80,126,212] Evaluation of liver tissue before drug withdrawal is essential to establish remission because histologic activity may be present in 55% of patients who satisfy other requirements for remission.[1,126] Histologic improvement lags behind clinical and laboratory resolution by 3 to 8 months, and treatment should be extended for at least this period to compensate for the lag.

Prednisone alone or in combination with azathioprine induces clinical, laboratory, and histologic remission in 65% of patients within 3 years.[1,62,126,211,213] Laboratory improvement commonly occurs within 3 to 12 months,[214,215] remission is usually achieved within 22 months,[62,126,162] and immediate

survival is enhanced.[214,216-218] The 10-year life expectancies for treated patients with and without cirrhosis are 89% and 90%, respectively, in tertiary referral centers.[214,216] The overall 10-year survival rate in these centers is 93% and is comparable to that of an age- and sex-matched cohort from the population at large (94%).[214,216] In nontransplant centers, the survival rates from liver-related death or liver transplantation are 91% and 70% after 10 and 20 years, respectively, and the standardized mortality ratio for all-cause death is 1.63.[215] Twenty-one percent of patients sustain their remission for a median of 76 months after drug withdrawal, and this result justifies the effort to stop therapy in all patients who satisfy remission criteria.[162]

Relapse

Patients who enter remission commonly experience an exacerbation after drug withdrawal (see Fig. 90-6).[62,162,213] Relapse is defined as the reappearance of histologic disease after discontinuation of drug therapy. An increase in the serum AST level to more than 3-fold the ULN after discontinuation of medication is invariably associated with interface hepatitis on histologic examination. This biochemical change is sufficient to diagnose relapse without requiring liver tissue examination.[126]

Relapse occurs in 50% of patients within 6 months of discontinuing therapy, and most patients (70% to 86%) experience an exacerbation within 3 years.[162,212,219] Reinstitution of the original treatment induces another remission, but relapse commonly recurs after termination of therapy. Repeated relapse and retreatment is associated with cumulative morbidity and mortality. Cirrhosis develops more commonly (38% vs. 4%; P = 0.004)[220]; death from hepatic failure or the need for liver transplantation occurs more often (20% vs. 0%; P = 0.008)[220]; and drug-induced side effects are more frequent (70% vs. 30%; P = 0.01) in persons who relapse than in those who sustain remission after drug withdrawal.[193] The frequencies of each complication increase with each subsequent relapse and re-treatment.

Treatment Failure

Treatment failure connotes deterioration during therapy despite compliance with the treatment regimen (see Fig. 90-6).[62,209,211,213] It is characterized by worsening of the serum AST or bilirubin level by at least 67% of previous values, progressive histologic activity, or the onset of ascites or encephalopathy. Histologic assessment is required for evaluation, and the accuracy of the original diagnosis must be reconfirmed or an alternative diagnosis considered. Nine percent of patients deteriorate during glucocorticoid therapy and experience treatment failure.[62,209,211,213]

Incomplete Response

An incomplete response connotes improvement that is insufficient to satisfy remission criteria (see Fig. 90-6).[62,211,213] Failure to achieve full clinical, laboratory, and histologic resolution after 3 years of conventional glucocorticoid treatment indicates that remission is unlikely. Thirteen percent of patients with AIH experience an incomplete response.[62,213]

Drug Toxicity

Drug toxicity justifies premature withdrawal of medication or a reduction in dose (see Fig. 90-6).[62,126,211,213] Thirteen percent of patients with AIH experience treatment-ending drug-induced complications, commonly manifested as intolerable cosmetic changes (striae, obesity, cushingoid appearance), osteopenia, or diabetes mellitus.[193]

Other Complications

Cirrhosis develops in 7% to 40% of treated patients, depending on the frequencies of relapse, treatment failure, and incomplete response.[216,221] Esophageal varices develop in 13% of patients with cirrhosis, and upper GI bleeding of any cause occurs in 6% within 5 years of treatment.[222] The frequency of hepatocellular carcinoma in patients with cirrhosis is 1% to 9%, and the annual rate of occurrence is 1.1% to 1.9% (see later).[208] The standardized incidence ratio for hepatocellular carcinoma in AIH is 23.3 (95% CI, 7.5-54.3) in Sweden,[223] and the standardized mortality ratio for hepatobiliary cancer is 42.3 (95% CI, 20.3-77.9) in New Zealand.[224] The principal risk factor for hepatocellular cancer is longstanding cirrhosis, and patients at risk are characterized mainly by cirrhosis for 10 or more years, manifestations of portal hypertension, persistent liver inflammation, and immunosuppressive therapy for 3 or more years.[208,225] Extrahepatic malignancies of diverse cell types occur in 5% of patients with AIH,[208] and the standardized incidence ratio is 2.7 (95% CI, 1.8-3.9) in New Zealand.[224] Non-melanoma skin cancers are most common.[226]

Management of Suboptimal Responses

Relapse

Long-term maintenance therapy with azathioprine (2 mg/kg daily) is the preferred management strategy after the first relapse of AIH.[1,80,126,211] Conventional therapy with prednisone and azathioprine is restarted and continued until clinical and laboratory resolution is achieved (see Fig. 90-6). The dose of azathioprine is then increased to 2 mg/kg daily as the dose of prednisone is reduced. Azathioprine is continued indefinitely as a chronic maintenance regimen, and 80% of patients are able to suppress disease activity over a 10-year period of observation. An alternative strategy after the first relapse is to suppress liver inflammation by using daily low-dose prednisone (see Fig. 90-6). Eighty-seven percent of patients can be managed long term on prednisone at doses of 10 mg or less per day (median dose, 7.5 mg/day). The dose is titrated to the lowest level needed to prevent symptoms and to maintain serum AST levels below 3-fold the ULN.

Treatment after relapse does not need to be indefinite. The probability of achieving a treatment-free state after previous relapse and retreatment is 28%.[162] Patients who have had inactive disease for at least 1 year after relapse can be withdrawn cautiously from maintenance therapy in a well-monitored, gradual fashion, and the medication can be reapplied at full dose if the laboratory indices worsen.

Treatment Failure

Treatment failure is managed by administering high doses of prednisone alone (60 mg daily) or prednisone (30 mg daily) in conjunction with azathioprine (150 mg daily) for at least 1 month (Fig. 90-7).[1,62,126,211,213,227] The doses of medication are then reduced by 10 mg of prednisone and 50 mg of azathioprine for each month of clinical and laboratory improvement until conventional maintenance doses of medication are achieved (prednisone, 20 mg daily, or prednisone, 10 mg daily, with azathioprine, 50 mg daily).[126,211] Each schedule induces clinical and biochemical improvement in 70% of patients within 2 years. Histologic resolution occurs in only 20%, and long-term therapy is frequently necessary. These patients are at risk of liver failure and serious drug toxicity. Liver transplantation must be considered at the first sign of hepatic failure (most commonly, the development of ascites).

Alternative management strategies for treatment failure have included the administration of calcineurin inhibitors (cyclosporine or tacrolimus) and mycophenolate mofetil (see Fig. 90-7).[126,195,197,211,213] In each instance, experience has been limited, and the drugs have been used for off-label indications. Experience with cyclosporine as a salvage therapy (2 to 5 mg/kg daily, with trough levels between 100 and 300 ng/mL) indicates that a positive response of any degree can be achieved in 93% of problematic patients, whereas a negative response, defined as no response, noncompliance, or drug intolerance, occurs in 7%.[126,195,197,211] Experience with tacrolimus as a salvage therapy (0.5 mg daily in patients with cirrhosis and 1 mg daily in patients without cirrhosis to as high as 3 mg twice daily; median serum levels, 3 ng/mL; range, 1.7 to 10.7 ng/mL) indicates that a positive response of any degree can be achieved in 98% of problematic patients, whereas a negative response, defined as no response or treatment-ending drug intolerance, occurs in 2%.[126,195,197,211]

Problems with the calcineurin inhibitors in AIH include the theoretical risk of enhancing the autoreactive response by diminishing the negative selection of activated lymphocytes, risk of serious drug-induced complications, especially neurotoxicity, failure of these drugs to prevent or treat AIH that

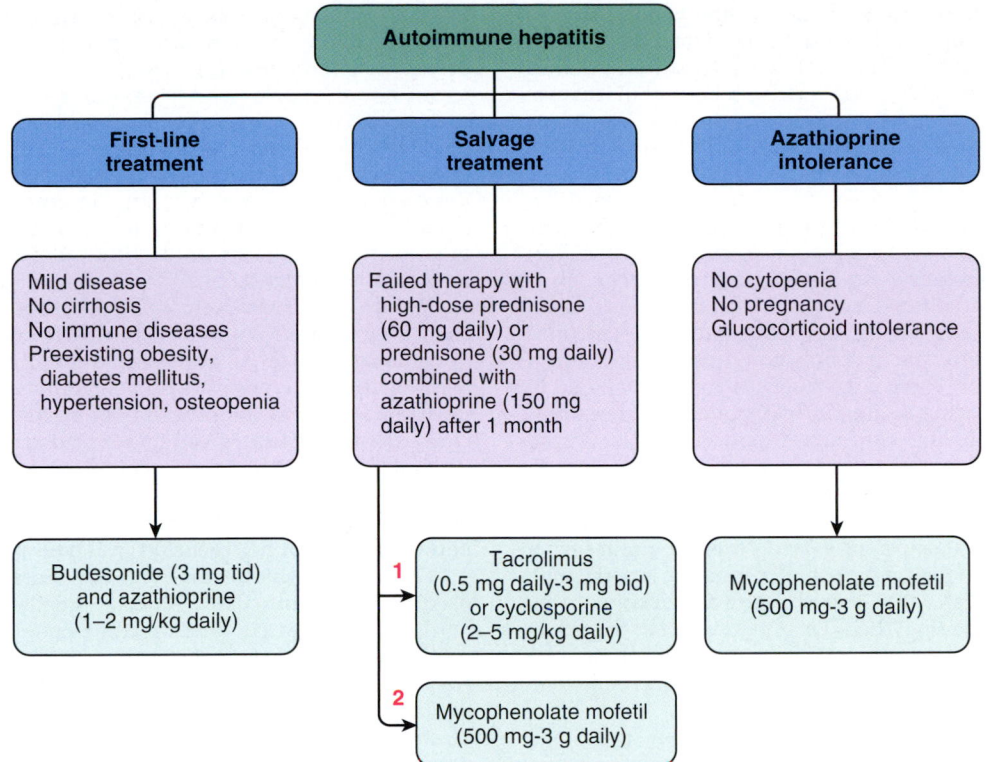

FIGURE 90-7. Nonstandard treatments for suboptimal responses of autoimmune hepatitis to conventional glucocorticoid regimens. The selection of a nonstandard medication depends on the therapeutic objective, which may be to start therapy in treatment-naïve patients (first-line treatment), rescue patients with glucocorticoid-refractory disease (salvage treatment), or manage patients with azathioprine intolerance *(dark blue panels)*. Clinical circumstances direct each treatment strategy *(light blue panels)*. Budesonide in combination with azathioprine can be considered as a first-line therapy in selected patients *(light green panel)*. Treatment-naïve persons with mild, asymptomatic, uncomplicated, and early-stage disease are candidates for this therapy, as are persons whose preexisting obesity, diabetes mellitus, hypertension, or osteopenia could be worsened by therapy with prednisone (or prednisolone). High-dose prednisone alone or in combination with azathioprine for at least 1 month is the preferred treatment for patients whose disease worsens during conventional glucocorticoid therapy. Continued worsening or failure to improve laboratory indices on continuous high-dose treatment justifies consideration of salvage therapy sequentially with a calcineurin inhibitor (preferred) or mycophenolate mofetil *(light green panels)*. Azathioprine intolerance in patients who require a glucocorticoid-sparing agent and who do not have cytopenia and are not pregnant can be considered for therapy with mycophenolate mofetil *(light green panel)*. The nonstandard therapies are unlicensed for use in autoimmune hepatitis, and their institution for these off-label indications requires careful consideration, patient selection, and monitoring.

recurs or develops de novo after liver transplantation (see later), and lack of anti-inflammatory properties that might be useful in managing complex immune-mediated diseases such as AIH.[126,195]

Mycophenolate mofetil is a next-generation purine antagonist, and it has been used in small single-center experiences as first-line and salvage therapy for AIH (usual starting dose, 1 g daily increased to 1.5 to 2 g daily; dose range, 500 mg to 3 g daily) in combination with a glucocorticoid (see Fig. 90-7).[56,126,195,197,211,227,228] In a compilation of experiences, a positive response of any degree was achieved in 47% of treated patients, whereas a negative response, defined as no response or drug intolerance, occurred in 53%.[126,195,197,211] Complete glucocorticoid withdrawal was possible in 40% of patients, and the frequency of treatment-ending side effects, including cytopenia, was 15%. Patients treated for azathioprine intolerance improved more commonly than patients treated for refractory AIH (58% vs. 12%), and mycophenolate mofetil seems to be more effective in rescuing patients from azathioprine toxicity than from their liver disease.[126,195] Mycophenolate mofetil in combination with prednisolone has normalized serum AST, ALT, and gamma globulin levels in 88% of treatment-naïve patients treated for up to 92 months; glucocorticoids were withdrawn in 58% usually within 8 months; and serious side effects occurred in only 3%.[228] Mycophenolate mofetil can be effective as first-line therapy for AIH when combined with prednisolone, but a preference for this regimen over conventional treatment has not been established.

Mycophenolate mofetil is expensive, associated with side effects (including cytopenia in 3% to 34% of treated patients), and deleterious during pregnancy.[56,126,195,197,211] Mycophenolate mofetil can disturb the migration of the fetal cranial neural crest and result in facial, cranial, and cardiac malformations in the human fetus. The use of this drug for off-label indications in AIH must be highly individualized and carefully monitored.

Incomplete Response

Protracted conventional therapy that has failed to induce full clinical, laboratory, and histologic resolution within 3 years is associated with a diminishing benefit-to-risk ratio, and it justifies an alternative treatment strategy that is drug sparing (see

Fig. 90-6).[126,210] The administration of azathioprine (2 mg/kg daily) as the sole drug or a low-dose prednisone regimen is a reasonable approach.[126,191] The goal of treatment is to reduce and stabilize disease activity on a drug schedule that is well tolerated.

Drug Toxicity

Most side effects associated with prednisone and azathioprine therapy are reversible with reduction in the dose or discontinuation of the offending drug, and consequences such as cataracts, diabetes mellitus, hypertension, and obesity have effective therapies (see Fig. 90-6).[193] The most serious consequences of treatment are vertebral compression and severe myelosuppression.[193] These consequences are best avoided by instituting bone-sparing regimens in all patients at the start of therapy and monitoring complete blood counts at regular intervals.[1] Preemptive efforts to maintain bone density in the vulnerable elderly population is especially important, and treatment with bisphosphonates, calcium and vitamin D supplements, and a regular weight-bearing exercise program can improve tolerance to the treatment.[1,193] Complete blood counts must be performed at 3- to 6-month intervals throughout the duration of azathioprine therapy, and the dose should be reduced or the drug discontinued if cytopenia develops.[1,126,193] Pretreatment testing for TPMT activity will identify the 0.3% to 0.5% of patients with absent activity.

Treatment can usually be continued with the single tolerated drug (prednisone or azathioprine) in an adjusted dose (see Fig. 90-6).[62,193,213] The calcineurin inhibitors and mycophenolate mofetil have been used as glucocorticoid-sparing agents; mycophenolate mofetil has been administered to noncytopenic patients with azathioprine intolerance; and budesonide in combination with azathioprine is a consideration in fragile treatment-naïve patients at risk of glucocorticoid complications.[126,195] Drug selection, adjunctive treatments, surveillance programs, and alternative interventions should be considered prior to any commitment to therapy, and they must be tailored to the patient's anticipated needs.

TUMOR SURVEILLANCE

Hepatocellular carcinoma and extrahepatic malignancies are possible consequences of long-standing cirrhosis and immunosuppressive therapy.[208] The annual rate of occurrence of hepatocellular carcinoma in patients with AIH and cirrhosis is 1.1% to 1.9%, and this rate is insufficient to justify a formal tumor surveillance strategy.[208,229,230] Patients with AIH who are at risk of hepatocellular carcinoma have had cirrhosis for 10 or more years, manifestations of portal hypertension, persistent liver inflammation, and immunosuppressive therapy for 3 or more years.[225] Hepatic US every 6 months in such patients is a reasonable consideration.[208] Extrahepatic malignancies of diverse cell types occur in 5% of patients with AIH, and this risk may relate to the nature and duration of immunosuppressive therapy (see earlier).[208] Routine health screening measures should be applied.

LIVER TRANSPLANTATION

Liver transplantation is effective in the treatment of AIH with features of liver failure (see Chapter 97).[1,62,213] Five-year survival rates for patients and grafts range from 83% to 92%, and the actuarial 10-year survival rate after transplantation is 75%.[1] AIH recurs in 8% to 12% of transplanted patients at 1 year and 36% to 68% at 5 years.[231,232] AIH develops de novo in

1% to 7% of patients who are observed for 0.1 to 9 years after transplantation for non-autoimmune liver disease, and it occurs most commonly in children.[231,232] The appearance of autoantibodies may herald the emergence of de novo AIH, and antibodies to glutathione S-transferase T1 have been reported to herald its occurrence.[231,232] Acute rejection, glucocorticoid-resistant rejection, and chronic rejection occur more commonly in patients undergoing transplantation for AIH than for other conditions, and patients with AIH may be more difficult than others to withdraw from glucocorticoids after liver transplantation.[231,232]

Recurrent AIH is frequently mild, but it can progress to cirrhosis and graft failure.[231] Glucocorticoid therapy alone or in combination with azathioprine should be instituted. Anti-rejection drugs have neither prevented nor consistently treated recurrent AIH, and they should not be the basis of therapy.[231] Other treatment strategies have included the substitution of mycophenolate mofetil for azathioprine, a change in the calcineurin inhibitor, and the use of rapamycin for refractory disease.[231] Retransplantation has been necessary in some patients, and AIH has recurred in the new graft.[231]

De novo AIH is treated with the same regimens that are used for recurrent AIH.[231] Glucocorticoids must be increased in dose or restarted, and azathioprine or mycophenolate mofetil can be added to the regimen while maintaining conventional immunosuppressive therapy. The calcineurin inhibitors can be switched, and rapamycin has been used successfully in one patient. Laboratory indices improve in all patients by at least 50% after 1 month, the need for retransplantation is 8%, and the 4-year survival rate is 95%.

KEY REFERENCES

Full references for this chapter can be found on www.expertconsult.com.

1. Manns MP, Czaja AJ, Gorham JD, et al. Diagnosis and management of autoimmune hepatitis. Hepatology 2010; 51:2193-213.
19. Czaja AJ. Genetic factors affecting the occurrence, clinical phenotype, and outcome of autoimmune hepatitis. Clin Gastroenterol Hepatol 2008; 6:379-88.
56. Czaja AJ. Nonstandard drugs and feasible new interventions for autoimmune hepatitis: Part I. Inflamm Allergy Drug Targets 2012; 11:337-50.
57. Czaja AJ. Nonstandard drugs and feasible new interventions for autoimmune hepatitis: Part II. Inflamm Allergy Drug Targets 2012; 11:351-63.
60. Lapierre P, Beland K, Yang R, et al. Adoptive transfer of ex vivo expanded regulatory T cells in an autoimmune hepatitis murine model restores peripheral tolerance. Hepatology 2013; 57:217-27.
61. Peiseler M, Sebode M, Franke B, et al. FOXP3+ regulatory T cells in autoimmune hepatitis are fully functional and not reduced in frequency. J Hepatol 2012; 57:125-32.
80. Czaja AJ, Manns MP. Advances in the diagnosis, pathogenesis, and management of autoimmune hepatitis. Gastroenterology 2010; 139:58-72.
113. Stravitz RT, Lefkowitch JH, Fontana RJ, et al. Autoimmune acute liver failure: Proposed clinical and histological criteria. Hepatology 2011; 53:517-26.
125. Manns MP, Woynarowski M, Kreisel W, et al. Budesonide induces remission more effectively than prednisone in a controlled trial of patients with autoimmune hepatitis. Gastroenterology 2010; 139:1198-206.
126. Czaja AJ. Advances in the current treatment of autoimmune hepatitis. Dig Dis Sci 2012; 57:1996-2010.

158. Czaja AJ. Drug-induced autoimmune-like hepatitis. Dig Dis Sci 2011; 56:958-76.

166. Boberg KM, Chapman RW, Hirschfield GM, et al. Overlap syndromes: The International Autoimmune Hepatitis Group (IAIHG) position statement on a controversial issue. J Hepatol 2011; 54:374-85.

194. Czaja AJ. Drug choices in autoimmune hepatitis: Part A—Steroids. Expert Rev Gastroenterol Hepatol 2012; 6:603-15.

195. Czaja AJ. Drug choices in autoimmune hepatitis: Part B—Nonsteroids. Expert Rev Gastroenterol Hepatol 2012; 6:617-35.

211. Selvarajah V, Montano-Loza AJ, Czaja AJ. Systematic review: Managing suboptimal treatment responses in autoimmune hepatitis with conventional and nonstandard drugs. Aliment Pharmacol Ther 2012; 36:691-707.

JOHN E. EATON AND KEITH D. LINDOR*

CHAPTER OUTLINE

PBC is an autoimmune liver disease that generally affects middle-aged women and is the most common chronic cholestatic liver disease in adults in the United States. PBC is characterized by progressive intrahepatic duct destruction, which leads to cholestasis, complications and symptoms related to cholestasis, cirrhosis, and portal hypertension. Despite the designation of PBC, most patients do not have "cirrhosis" on liver biopsy specimens at the time of diagnosis. Evidence for an immunologic cause of PBC includes the presence of activated T cells in areas of bile duct destruction, presence of highly specific autoantibodies that react with antigens localized on biliary epithelial cells, and association of PBC with other disorders thought to be autoimmune in nature. The presence of antimitochondrial antibodies (AMA) in serum is highly characteristic of the disease.

EPIDEMIOLOGY

PBC occurs worldwide and predominantly in women, with a female-to-male ratio of 9:1. The diagnosis of PBC usually is made between the ages of 30 and 60 years, with a range of 21 to 93 years. The disease has been documented in even younger patients—2 teenagers 15 and 16 years of age, respectively.[1] Until the early 1970s, PBC was considered a rare condition that manifested with persistent jaundice and almost inevitably progressed to end-stage liver disease. A better understanding

of its pathogenesis, along with subsequent clinical and epidemiologic studies, has modified current concepts regarding this condition. PBC seems to be more common than was formerly believed because of increasing awareness of the disease and because asymptomatic patients are identified through the widespread use of screening tests such as determination of serum cholesterol and liver biochemical test levels in otherwise healthy persons.

The reported prevalence of PBC varies among countries, with a range of 19 cases per 1 million population in Israel to 402 cases per 1 million population in Olmsted County, Minnesota.[2] The view that PBC is more prevalent in North America and Europe has been challenged by data from China that suggest the prevalence of PBC is similar in China to that in other geographic areas.[3] Whether the difference in prevalence is real or a result of different methodologies used to detect the disease is unknown. Inconsistency in case definition and case finding methods, as well as imprecision in defining the study area, populations evaluated, and dates of diagnosis, particularly in earlier reports, makes comparisons among studies difficult. Estimates of the annual incidence of PBC range from 0.7 to 49 per 1 million population. Both the prevalence and incidence of PBC have been suggested to increase over time[2]; however, a nationwide population-based study conducted in Iceland between 2 periods (1991-2000 vs. 2001-2010) revealed a stable incidence and prevalence of PBC, confirming data from Olmsted County, Minnesota.[4,5]

In the United States,[5] the age-adjusted reported incidence of PBC per 1 million person-years is 45 for women and 7 for men (27 overall). The reported prevalence per 1 million population is 654 for women and 121 for men (402 overall). Similar values have been reported in Canada.[6]

---

*Paul Angulo, MD, contributed to this chapter in prior editions of the textbook. The authors also thank Jayant A. Talwalkar, MD, for his contribution to this chapter.

PATHOGENESIS

Although the etiology of PBC remains unknown, it is likely an immune mediate process that occurs as a result of complex interactions between the environment and genetically susceptible persons. Several features of PBC suggest an autoimmune pathogenesis. The evidence includes the intense humoral and cellular response to an intracytoplasmic antigen, presence of highly specific AMAs, involvement of T lymphocytes in the destruction of bile ducts, and numerous defects in immunologic regulation. Like other autoimmune diseases, PBC has a clear female predominance. PBC is associated with an increased incidence of autoimmune disease of other types in both patients with PBC and their first-degree relatives.[7,8] PBC seems to be triggered by an immune-mediated response to 1 or more allo- or autoantigens, which leads to progressive destruction of bile ducts, chronic cholestasis, and eventual biliary cirrhosis. Indeed, lymphocyte recruitment and homing to the liver through a variety of chemokines appears to be an important step in the pathogenesis of PBC.[9] Immunohistochemical phenotyping of inflammatory cells surrounding the bile ducts shows a combination of CD4[+] and CD8[+] T lymphocytes, accompanied by B lymphocytes and natural killer cells. Bile duct destruction is induced directly by the cytotoxicity of CD4[+] and CD8[+] T cells in contact with biliary epithelium. B lymphocytes are relatively uncommon in the inflammatory reaction but sometimes can be seen in clusters. Intracellular adhesion molecules (e.g., intracellular adhesion molecule-1 [ICAM-1]) are strongly expressed on many epithelial cells, particularly in areas of lymphocyte damage; these molecules may facilitate the interaction between destructive lymphocytes and their targets and have been found in cholangiocytes of patients with PBC.[10] In the early biliary lesions of PBC, eosinophilic infiltration and granulomas often are seen. PBC is principally a disease of the small intrahepatic bile ducts, with loss of biliary epithelial cells that line these ducts and resulting cholestatic damage. PBC is not restricted to the liver; abnormalities of salivary and lacrimal glands with an associated cellular phenotypic change similar to that seen in the biliary epithelial cells also occur. As of 2012, 4 inducible and 5 genetically modified mouse PBC models were described.[11]

Autoantibodies

AMA were described for the first time in patients with PBC in the 1960s and continue to be regarded as the most sensitive and specific immunologic hallmark of the disease. AMA are directed to the E2 component of the pyruvate dehydrogenase complex (PDC-E2), the E2 unit of the branched-chain 2-oxo-acid dehydrogenase complex (BCOADC-E2), and the E2 subunit of the 2-oxo-glutarate dehydrogenase complex (OGDC-E2). Other AMA recognize the E1a subunit of PDC (PDC E1a) and the dihydrolipoamide dehydrogenase–binding protein (E3BP) of PDC. These molecules all are located on the inner mitochondrial membranes. At least 1 of these components usually reacts with AMA in a patient with PBC. The most frequent antigen against which AMA are directed is PDC-E2; PDC-E2–reacting antibodies are present in 90% to 95% of PBC sera.[12]

AMA do not appear to be cytotoxic: (1) They persist after liver transplantation without evidence of disease recurrence; (2) disease severity is unrelated to antibody titer; (3) they are not always present in PBC; and (4) they develop in animal models after the injection of recombinant PDC-E2 protein, but without resulting bile duct destruction or inflammation. Furthermore, the different types and numbers of mitochondrial antigens recognized by Western immunoblot analysis at the time of the patient's presentation are independent of the stage of the liver disease and not associated with specific clinical, biochemical, histologic, and immunologic features or with the Mayo risk score (see later).[13] Although AMA are predominantly of the IgG1 and IgG3 classes, most patients who have PBC exhibit polyclonal elevation of serum IgM levels; the IgM is not directed at mitochondrial or nuclear antigens. This phenomenon is suggestive of polyclonal activation of the B cell compartment with an associated failure of isotype switching, representing aberrant B-cell activation.[14]

Antinuclear antibodies (ANA) are present in nearly half of patients with PBC and in up to 85% of patients with AMA-negative PBC (see later). The most relevant immunofluorescent reactivities of ANA in patients with PBC are anti-multiple nuclear dots antibodies ([anti-MND], with the molecular target being a 100-kd soluble protein called Sp100), anticentromere antibodies, and antinuclear envelope antibodies. The immunofluorescence pattern of the antinuclear envelope antibodies is characterized as rim-like and membranous; its molecular targets are structural components of the nuclear pore complex, such as gp210 and nucleoprotein p62, and of the nuclear membrane, such as lamin B receptors. Antibodies against the nuclear pore protein gp210 (anti-gp210) are found in 25% of patients with AMA-positive PBC and in up to 50% of those with AMA-negative PBC. ANA with the MND and rim-like and membranous patterns, which are relatively rare or absent in normal and pathologic controls, are strongly associated with PBC and can be considered to be surrogate markers of PBC in AMA-negative patients.[15-17] The specificity of anti-gp210 for PBC when detected by immunoblotting is greater than 99%. Antibodies to p62 (anti-p62) are found in approximately 25% of patients and are also highly specific for PBC. Anti-p62 antibodies seem to be mutually exclusive with anti-gp210 antibodies. Furthermore, anti-gp210 and possibly anti-p62 also offer prognostic information in that they seem to be associated with aggressive disease and a poor prognosis.[15,18,19]

Genetic Factors

The occurrence of PBC in relatives of affected persons and of abnormalities of cell-mediated immunity in first-degree relatives of patients with PBC suggests a genetic association. This association is supported further by the finding that PBC exhibits a higher concordance rate in monozygotic than dizygotic twin pairs, suggesting a genetic component to disease susceptibility and expression of the susceptibility through genes that regulate the immune response.[20]

Genome-wide association studies have identified over 20 potential PBC risk loci. Such loci appear to be involved in key immunoregulatory factors and roles, such as T-cell differentiation, Toll-like receptors, TNF signaling, interleukin-12, and other cytokine signaling pathways.[3,21-23] Many loci in PBC are associated with other autoimmune diseases such as celiac disease and multiple sclerosis, which suggests a role for common pathways across these diseases.[24] HLA class II class genes DQB1, DPB1, DRB1, and DRA have been linked with PBC.[21] HLA-DRB1*08 has been associated with PBC susceptibility in European and Asian cohorts, whereas HLA-DRB1*11 appears to be protective.[25,26]

Apoptosis

It has been suggested that dysregulation in apoptosis can lead to loss of tolerance and the development of autoimmune diseases by 3 possible mechanisms. First, impaired or enhanced clearance of apoptotic cells can lead to an enhanced inflammatory response or an accumulation of autoimmunogenic fragments. Second, genetic defects in apoptosis can result in autoimmunity by interfering with tolerogenic deletion of lymphocytes. Third, apoptosis is a common event that can occasionally lead to abnormal autoantigen presentation, which can result in autoimmunity.[27]

An important role of apoptosis in the pathogenesis of PBC is emerging.[28-30] During apoptosis, cholangiocytes (unlike other epithelial cells) translocate intact, immunologically active, PDC-E2 to apoptotic bodies called *apoptopes*.[28] PDC-E2 can then react with circulating immune complexes that are processed by antigen-presenting cells, which present the epitope(s) to T cells, thereby leading to specific T- and B-cell activation and targeting of the biliary epithelial cells.[30] In addition, when these biliary apoptopes are cultured with macrophages from patients with PBC in the presence of AMA, an inflammatory reaction ensues that may result in apoptosis of surrounding cells.[29] These observations may explain in part the selectivity of PBC for small- and medium-sized bile ducts. Furthermore, these findings could explain in part the mechanism of ursodeoxycholic acid (UDCA), an agent that has been shown to suppress apoptosis, and its ability to delay progression of PBC (see later).[31]

Molecular Mimicry

Molecular mimicry between host autoantigens and unrelated exogenous proteins is 1 of the hypotheses to explain how autoantibodies to self-proteins arise, break tolerance, and lead to autoimmune disease. Molecular mimicry of an extrinsic protein produced by an infectious agent has long been suggested as a possible initiating event in PBC. Microorganisms produce a multitude of foreign antigens that collectively constitute the major determinants recognized by the immune system. These antigens potentially include a variety of carbohydrates, lipids, and proteins that can be recognized by specific receptors on inflammatory cells. In PBC, PDC-E2 appears to be an ideal candidate for foreign antigens to mimic. PDC-E2, particularly its inner lipoyl domain, is highly conserved among bacteria, yeasts, and mammals. Autoimmune phenomena in PBC could result from peptides that mimic T-cell epitopes of microbial proteins and that are derived from, and presented by, abnormally expressed HLA class II molecules. Infectious agents incriminated in the immune response in PBC include various bacteria, including *Escherichia coli*, and viruses.[32] Interestingly, patients with PBC are more likely to have had a urinary tract infection within the 5 years preceding the diagnosis of PBC compared with matched controls.[33] A population-based study detected a seasonal variation in the time of diagnosis of PBC with a peak in June.[34] This finding led the authors to suggest that a seasonally variant agent, such as an infectious organism, is involved in the pathogenesis of PBC.[34]

Xenobiotics and Other Implicated Agents

Xenobiotics are foreign compounds that may alter self-proteins by inducing a change in the molecular structure of the native protein sufficient to induce an immune response. The immune response may then result in the recognition of both the modified and the native proteins. PBC sera have been shown to react strongly against PDC-E2 modified with synthetic chemicals such as 2-octynoic acid and 2-nonynoic acid, which are found in a variety of products and have been shown to induce PBC-like liver lesions when given to animals.[35-37] In addition, AMA-positive PBC serum appears to react with xenobiotic modified PDC-E2 structures including 6,8-bis (acetylthio) octanoic acid.[38,39]

Several epidemiologic studies have found an association between tobacco smoking and PBC.[40] A French study of 223 patients with PBC demonstrated an independent association between smoking and advanced fibrosis (Metavir stage F3-F4 [see Chapter 80]). In addition, each pack-year of smoking was associated with a 5% increase in the likelihood of advanced fibrosis.[41] Consequently, patients with PBC who smoke should be counseled about this added risk.

CLINICAL FEATURES

Asymptomatic Disease

Widespread use of screening laboratory tests has led to diagnosis of PBC at an asymptomatic stage in up to 60% of patients with this disorder. Such patients are found incidentally to have an elevated serum alkaline phosphatase level and AMA during routine health evaluations or during investigation of an unrelated complaint, such as a clinical manifestation of an autoimmune disease known to be associated with PBC. Some asymptomatic persons with AMA and normal results of liver biochemical tests are found to have features on liver biopsy specimens that are diagnostic of or consistent with PBC; symptoms, signs, and laboratory evidence of chronic cholestasis eventually develop in these persons. Most patients found to have AMA on screening, however, do not ultimately prove to have PBC.[12]

Symptomatic Disease

The typical patient with symptomatic disease (Table 91-1) is a middle-aged woman with a complaint of fatigue or pruritus. Other symptoms include right upper quadrant abdominal pain, anorexia, and jaundice. Fatigue, although relatively nonspecific, is considered to be the most disabling symptom by many patients. Despite the high prevalence of fatigue in PBC, patients may underreport this symptom to their physicians. An increased level of fatigue is often found in those with more advanced liver disease and with other comorbidities, and the etiology of fatigue is often multifactorial.[42] Fatigue often persists throughout the disease course, and higher fatigue levels have been associated with an increased risk of death and need for liver transplantation.[43,44] Patients with noncirrhotic

TABLE 91-1 Symptoms and Signs of PBC at Presentation

Symptom or Sign	Frequency (%)
Fatigue	21-85
Pruritus	19-55
Hyperpigmentation	25
Hepatomegaly	25
Splenomegaly	15
Xanthelasma	10
Jaundice	3-10
Right upper quadrant pain	8
None	25-61

PBC exhibit altered sleep patterns compared with healthy controls. Their sleep onset is often delayed, and this pattern is associated with both diminished quality of sleep and quality of life.[45]

Pruritus may occur at any point, early or late, in the course of the disease or intermittently throughout the course. Pruritus is generally intermittent during the day, most troublesome in the evening and at night, and often resolves as the disease progresses. In some patients, however, severe, intractable pruritus can develop in earlier stages of the disease and may require liver transplantation for effective management. Pruritus in cholestatic liver disease may be mediated in part by lysophosphatidic acid and the enzyme autotoxin, which leads to the production of lysophosphatidic acid from lysophosphatidylcholine. Serum levels of lysophosphatidic acid and activity of autotaxin have been shown to correlate with the severity of pruritus.[46] In a population-based study of 770 patients with PBC from England, the cumulative risk of developing pruritus was 19%, 45%, and 57% at 1, 5, and 10 years, respectively.[47]

Most patients with PBC do not have jaundice at the time of diagnosis. Jaundice occurs later in the course of the disease and usually is persistent and associated with a worse prognosis. Symptoms also may relate to fat-soluble vitamin deficiency, bone pain with or without spontaneous fractures, or an associated autoimmune disease (Table 91-2). Symptoms and signs of advanced liver disease, such as ascites, bleeding from gastroesophageal varices, and encephalopathy, typically occur late in the course of PBC.

On physical examination, the most common signs are skin hyperpigmentation (caused by deposition of melanin), hepatosplenomegaly, xanthelasma, and, in more advanced disease, jaundice. Symptoms appear to be less frequent in men than in women, and autoimmune manifestations, especially Sjögren's syndrome, also are less frequent in men. Otherwise, PBC is identical clinically in men and in women.

Associated Diseases

Many of the diseases found frequently in patients with PBC (see Table 91-2) are thought to be related to disturbances in immune mechanisms. These associated disorders include Sjögren's syndrome (characterized by dry eyes [keratoconjunctivitis sicca] and dry mouth), scleroderma and its variants, RA, some cutaneous disorders, renal tubular acidosis, and thyroiditis (see Chapter 36).

The frequency of malignancy is increased in patients with PBC. An increased risk of breast cancer in women with PBC was found in earlier studies but was not confirmed by a subsequent meta-analysis. The risk of hepatocellular carcinoma is an important malignancy associated with PBC, and the risk is nearly 19-fold higher than that in the general population (see Chapter 96).[48]

DIAGNOSIS

The diagnosis of PBC is established when 2 out of 3 of the following criteria are met: chronic cholestatic liver biochemical test elevation (typically with alkaline phosphatase ≥ 1.5 times the upper limit of normal), elevated serum AMA (titer ≥ 1:40), or a liver biopsy consistent with PBC. A liver biopsy is typically not required (see later).[12]

Biochemical Features

Liver biochemical test results show a cholestatic picture. Almost all patients have increased serum levels of alkaline phosphatase and GGTP. Serum aminotransferase (AST, ALT) levels are mildly elevated (usually <3 times the upper limit of normal); marked elevations (>5 times normal) are distinctly unusual and may suggest an autoimmune hepatitis-PBC overlap syndrome (see Chapter 90) or coexisting viral hepatitis. Serum bilirubin levels usually are normal in early stages of PBC and increase slowly over the course of the disease; levels ultimately may exceed 20 mg/dL. A high serum bilirubin level, low serum albumin, and prolonged prothrombin time indicate a poor prognosis and advanced disease. Serum immunoglobulin levels, especially IgM, are increased, as are serum levels of bile acids.[12]

Serologic Tests

Indirect immunofluorescence, immunoblotting, and an enzyme-linked immunosorbent assay (ELISA) can detect AMA. Indirect immunofluorescence is by far the most commonly used serologic test and detects AMA in 90% to 95% of patients with PBC; however, indirect immunofluorescence testing requires interpretation by a skilled observer, and the result may be interpreted erroneously as negative for AMA in some patients with PBC. Immunoblotting and ELISA have sensitivity and specificity rates higher than 95% for the detection of AMA in PBC and can detect AMA in patients with PBC who are AMA negative by direct immunofluorescence testing. Other autoantibodies found in patients with PBC include rheumatoid factor (70%), smooth muscle antibodies (66%), ANA (50%), and antithyroid (antimicrosomal, antithyroglobulin) antibodies (41%).

Histopathologic Features

One of the earliest histologic changes associated with PBC may be a loss of the canals of Hering, which can be demonstrated by biliary cytokeratin 19 staining.[49] Damage to the epithelial cells of the small bile ducts can also be appreciated early in the disease course (Figs. 91-1 and 91-2A and B). The most important and only diagnostic clue in many cases is ductopenia, defined as the absence of interlobular bile ducts

TABLE 91-2 Diseases Associated with PBC	
Disease	**Frequency (%)**
Keratoconjunctivitis sicca (Sjögren's syndrome)	72-100
Renal tubular acidosis	50-60
Arthritis/arthropathy	4-42
Gallstones	33
Autoimmune thyroiditis	15-20
PSS and its variants*	15-19
Cutaneous disorders—lichen planus, discoid lupus, pemphigoid	11
Celiac disease	1-7
Hepatocellular carcinoma	1-3

*Includes CREST (calcinosis, Raynaud's phenomenon, esophageal dysmotility, sclerodactyly, telangiectasia).

in greater than 50% of portal tracts. The florid duct lesion, in which the epithelium of the interlobular and segmental bile ducts degenerates segmentally, with formation of poorly defined, noncaseating epithelioid granulomas, is nearly diagnostic of PBC but is found in a relatively small number of cases, mainly in early stages.

The 2 most popular histologic staging systems are those proposed by Ludwig and colleagues and Scheuer, which classify the disease in 4 stages. Both systems describe progressive pathologic changes beginning initially in the portal areas surrounding the bile ducts and culminating in cirrhosis. Ludwig stage 1 disease is characterized by inflammatory destruction of the intrahepatic septal and interlobular bile ducts that range up to 100 μm in diameter. These lesions often are focal and described as *florid duct lesions*, characterized by marked inflammation and necrosis around a bile duct. The portal tracts usually are expanded by lymphocytes, with only sparse neutrophils or eosinophils seen. In stage 2 disease (see Fig. 91-2*A*), the inflammation extends from the portal tract into the hepatic parenchyma; this lesion is called *interface hepatitis* or (formerly) *piecemeal necrosis*. Destruction of bile ducts, with proliferation of bile ductules, can be seen. Stage 3 disease is characterized by scarring and fibrosis. Lymphocytic involvement of the portal and periportal areas, as well as the hepatic parenchyma, can be seen, but the hallmark of this stage is the presence of fibrosis without regenerative (or regenerating) nodules. Stage 4 disease is characterized by cirrhosis with fibrous septa and regenerative nodules (see Fig. 91-2*B*).[50]

Most patients with PBC demonstrate histologic progression of the liver disease; a few patients have a prolonged course of histologic stability, and only rare patients have sustained regression. A time course Markov model has been used to describe the rate of histologic progression over time (Table 91-3).

In a patient with AMA, the combination of a serum alkaline phosphatase level greater than 1.5 times the upper limit of normal plus a serum AST level less than 5 times the upper limit of normal is highly predictive for a diagnosis of PBC.[12] Therefore, a liver biopsy is not necessary in the majority of patients and should be reserved if AMA-negative PBC or an alternative diagnosis, such as small-duct PSC (see Chapter 68) or overlap with autoimmune hepatitis (see Chapter 90), is being considered.[50]

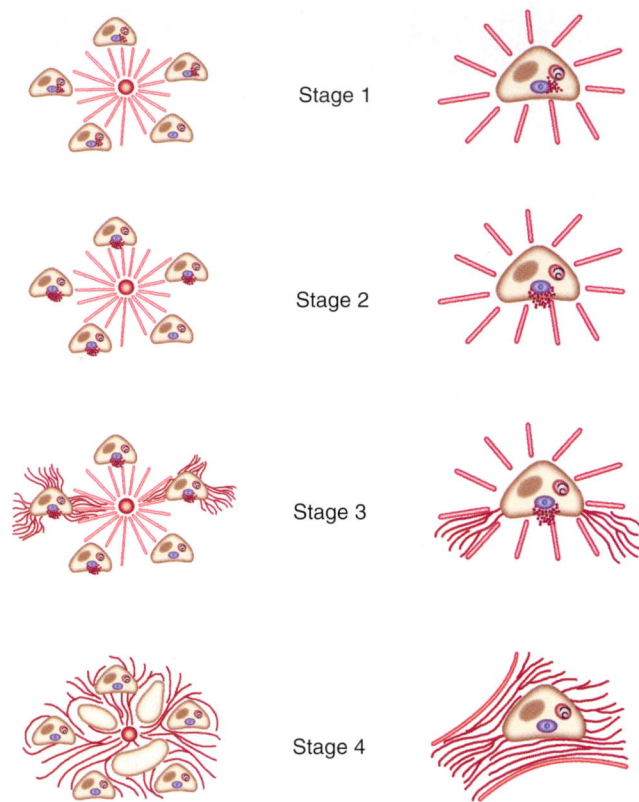

FIGURE 91-1. Schematic representation of the staging system of PBC (Ludwig's classification). The *left side* of the schematic shows 5 portal tracts surrounding a central vein at each stage. The *right side* shows a larger single portal tract at each stage (the bile ductule is *blue*). In stage 1, the inflammation is confined to the portal tract, focused on the bile duct. In stage 2, the inflammation extends into the hepatic parenchyma (interface hepatitis or piecemeal necrosis). In stage 3, fibrosis is present; in stage 4, cirrhosis is present.

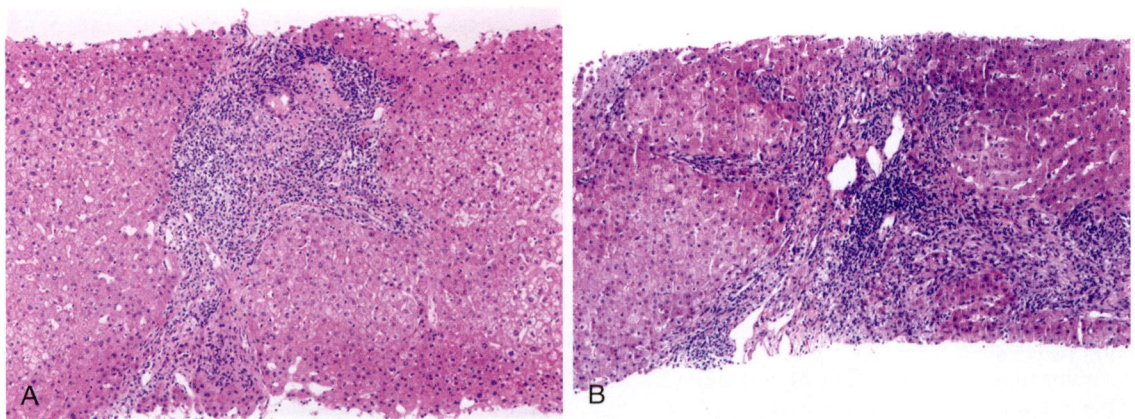

FIGURE 91-2. Histopathology of PBC. *A,* Photomicrograph of stage 2 PBC. Mononuclear inflammatory cells expand the portal tracts, with some disruption of the limiting plates (interface hepatitis). The bile ducts are surrounded by inflammatory cells, and no fibrosis is evident. (H&E, ×100.) *B,* Photomicrograph of stage 4 PBC. Cirrhosis, with areas of fibrosis surrounding the hepatic parenchyma, is present. A dense mononuclear inflammatory infiltrate is still seen in the portal tract, with interface hepatitis. (H&E, ×100.)

TABLE 91-3 Time Course of Histologic Progression to a Higher Stage in Patients with PBC

Histologic Progression*	Initial Histologic Stage		
	1	2	3
1 year	41	43	35
2 years	62	62	50

*Percent of patients in whom the histologic stage increases at 1 year and 2 years.

BOX 91-1 Independent Predictors of Survival in Patients with PBC in Various Clinical Studies

Clinical
Age
Ascites
Edema
Hepatomegaly
Variceal bleeding

Laboratory
Serum albumin level
Serum alkaline phosphatase level
Serum bilirubin level
Prothrombin time

Liver Histology
Cholestasis
Cirrhosis
Fibrosis
Mallory's hyaline

Imaging Studies

Cross-sectional imaging with US, CT, or MRI is useful for excluding biliary obstruction and plays a key role in the diagnostic evaluation of patients presenting with cholestatic liver biochemical test elevations (see Chapter 21) and surveillance for hepatocellular carcinoma among patients with cirrhosis (see Chapter 96). In addition to increased liver echogenicity and signs of portal hypertension, several imaging findings appear to be common in patients with PBC. Nearly two thirds of patients with PBC have a periportal "halo" sign (T1-and T2-weighted hypointensity centered around portal venous branches) and intraabdominal lymphadenopathy on MRI.[51] Stable periportal adenopathy is important to recognize to avoid undue concern about underlying malignancy; however, large, bulky adenopathy should raise the question of associated malignancy. Elastography is utilized increasingly for the noninvasive assessment of hepatic fibrosis (see Chapters 73 and 74). US-based transient elastography is a device that utilizes an ultrasonic transducer mounted on the axis of a vibrator that transmits an elastic shear wave through organ tissue. The velocity of the wave propagation is measured and translated into a measure of tissue stiffness (in units of kilopascals). Results of transient elastography correlate well with the stage of hepatic fibrosis, and its performance in PBC is similar to that in other chronic liver disorders. In addition, liver stiffness has been shown to be an independent prognostic factor in PBC.[52,53] MR elastography has also been used for noninvasive assessment of fibrosis but requires validation in large cohorts of PBC patients.

NATURAL HISTORY

The natural history of PBC has been described in patients with symptoms attributable to PBC, as well as in asymptomatic patients who have normal or abnormal liver biochemical test levels. Prognostic models useful in predicting survival in an individual patient have been developed.

Asymptomatic Disease

A series published in 1996[54] reported on 29 patients with AMA (in a titer of 1:40 or greater), normal liver biochemical test levels, and no symptoms of liver disease. Liver histology was compatible with or diagnostic of PBC in 24 patients (83%) and normal in only 2 patients. The entire cohort of patients was followed for a median of 17.8 years (range, 11 to 24 years). Liver biochemical test values became persistently abnormal in 24 patients (83%), and persistent symptoms attributable to PBC, including fatigue, pruritus, and right upper abdominal discomfort, developed in 22 (76%). Five patients died, none

because of liver disease, after a median period of 11.7 years (range, 6.4 to 16.8 years) from the first positive AMA result. The median time from the first positive AMA result to persistent liver biochemical abnormalities was 5.6 years (range, 0.9 to 19 years). Four of 10 patients who underwent a second liver biopsy during a median follow-up of 11.4 years (range, 1.3 to 14.3 years) showed progression of disease stage, but cirrhosis or portal hypertension did not develop in any of the patients during the follow-up period.[54] This study showed clearly that asymptomatic patients who have AMA and normal liver biochemical test levels can have early PBC; with time, clinically obvious PBC may develop. These patients may represent a subgroup of patients with PBC whose natural history is different from that in the general PBC patient population.

Several reports have described the natural history of asymptomatic patients who have AMA, abnormal liver biochemical test levels consistent with cholestasis, and liver histologic features diagnostic of or compatible with PBC. Asymptomatic patients have less advanced disease than that typically seen in symptomatic patients.[55] A median survival of approximately 10 years has been reported for this group of patients. Patients who remain asymptomatic for several years may have a significantly longer survival than that of symptomatic patients, but their life expectancy is still less than that of an age- and gender-matched population. Symptoms of PBC will develop in approximately 40% of the initially asymptomatic patients within 5 to 7 years of follow-up, and most asymptomatic patients ultimately will become symptomatic if the follow-up period is long enough (95% after 20 years).[55] When symptoms develop, life expectancy falls significantly and is the same as that for other symptomatic patients. The mortality rate for liver-related causes is significantly higher in initially symptomatic patients than in initially asymptomatic patients; however, an excess rate of non–liver-related mortality in initially asymptomatic patients has been reported to decrease the median survival in these patients to that in initially symptomatic patients.[55]

Symptomatic Disease

When compared with asymptomatic patients, patients with PBC who have symptoms of chronic cholestasis show a more rapid progression to end-stage liver disease and have a worse prognosis. Several independent predictors of a poor prognosis have been identified in this group of patients (Box 91-1).

The manifestations of portal hypertension and its complications in patients with PBC are similar to those in other forms of cirrhosis (see Chapters 74, 92, 93, and 94). Most patients with PBC and portal hypertension have cirrhosis; however, portal hypertension can be found in some patients with PBC and moderate to severe hepatic inflammation without cirrhosis on a liver biopsy specimen. Development of gastroesophageal varices is an ominous sign that is observed in approximately one third of patients with PBC during extended follow-up. Approximately 40% of these patients will experience 1 or more episodes of variceal bleeding within 3 years of developing varices and, as a group, have a decreased survival rate. It is important to note that varices can occur, albeit rarely, in patients with early-stage (1-2) PBC. The frequency of varices in patients with stages 1 and 2 PBC at a large referral center was 6%.[56] Although a variety of predictors have been suggested (male gender, elevated serum bilirubin, prolonged prothrombin time, and low serum albumin), the optimal approach to identifying persons with early-stage PBC at an increased risk of varices remains unclear.[56]

Predicting Survival

When untreated, PBC may follow a course that extends over a 15- to 20-year period. In patients with a serum bilirubin level greater than 10 mg/dL, however, the average life expectancy is reduced to 2 years. In order to predict survival in patients with PBC, prognostic models, some of which rely on Cox's proportional hazards analysis, have been developed. Among these models, the Mayo risk score (http://www.mayoclinic.org/gi-rst/mayomodel2.html), based on the patient's age, serum bilirubin level, serum albumin level, prothrombin time, edema score, and need for diuretics, has been cross-validated and is widely used for predicting survival and guiding referral of patients for liver transplantation.[12] Although all the prognostic models are of help in clinical decision making, they should not replace clinical judgment in determining the optimal timing of liver transplantation in an individual patient.

AMA-NEGATIVE PBC

AMA-negative PBC is the designation for those patients who clinically, biochemically, and histologically appear to have the classic features of PBC but are found not to have AMA in serum by indirect immunofluorescence or immunoblotting techniques. Of patients who have PBC by all other criteria, 5% are confirmed to be AMA negative.[12]

Most patients with AMA-negative PBC have ANA (perinuclear/rim-like or MND pattern) or smooth muscle antibodies (or both). Although these patients may be distinguished by the lack of AMA in serum, the specific AMA antigen PDC-E2 is expressed on the apical region of their biliary epithelium, as occurs in AMA-positive patients—an observation suggesting that the pathogenesis of both conditions may be identical. In fact, AMA-negative and AMA-positive patients have similar clinical, laboratory, and histologic features. When regulatory T cells and the subgroup of T cells suggested to have a role in the genesis of autoimmune disease were examined in patients with PBC, no difference was found between those who had and those who did not have AMA.[57]

When a patient with AMA-negative PBC is evaluated, other diseases that may manifest in a similar manner should be excluded. The absence of AMA makes liver biopsy mandatory to look for features of PBC and rule out other liver diseases. Also, imaging by MRCP is essential to identify other cholangiopathies such as PSC. Liver biopsy and MRCP, along with selected laboratory tests, will allow the exclusion of conditions that should be considered in the differential diagnosis, such as celiac disease, hepatitis C, sarcoidosis, small-duct PSC, and IgG4-associated autoimmune cholangitis (see Chapter 68).

Patients with AMA-negative PBC tend to follow a clinical course and demonstrate a therapeutic response to UDCA similar to those in AMA-positive patients.[57] Patients with AMA-negative PBC should be treated with UDCA in a dose of 13 to 15 mg/kg/day (see later).

TREATMENT

A large number of published controlled and uncontrolled trials have evaluated various drugs in PBC. These drugs can be classified according to their mechanisms of action as bile acids, immunosuppressive, anti-inflammatory, cupruretic, or antifibrotic. In addition to treating the underlying disease, a key component of caring for PBC patients is recognition, prevention, and treatment of disease-related complications.

Ursodeoxycholic Acid

UDCA, the 7-β epimer of chenodeoxycholic acid, occurs naturally in small quantities in human bile (<4% of total bile acids). It was first introduced for the dissolution of radiolucent gallstones in the 1970s and is the only medication approved by the FDA for treatment of PBC. Several mechanisms for the protective actions of UDCA have been proposed, including enhancement of hepatic secretion; inhibition of the absorption of toxic, hydrophobic, endogenous bile salts; stabilization of hepatocyte membranes against toxic bile salts; inhibition of apoptosis and fibrosis; replacement of endogenous bile acids, some of which may be hepatotoxic, with the nonhepatotoxic UDCA; and reduction in the expression of major histocompatibility complex (MHC) class II antigens.[58] During UDCA therapy, a variable increase in the concentration of total bile acids in serum is observed. The proportion of UDCA in serum and bile increases to approximately 50% of total bile acids, and the proportion of endogenous bile acids, such as cholic, chenodeoxycholic, deoxycholic, and lithocholic acids, declines consequently (see Chapter 64).[58] The degree of enrichment of the bile acid pool with UDCA is similar in all histologic stages of PBC and correlates with improvement in liver biochemical test levels and the Mayo risk score.

Because of its safety and high rate of patient adherence to treatment with the drug, UDCA has received the most attention of any drug used to treat PBC. Treatment with UDCA leads to rapid and long-lasting improvements in liver biochemistries and a decrease in the histologic severity of interface hepatitis, inflammation, cholestasis, bile duct paucity, and bile duct proliferation.[59-61] UDCA significantly decreases the risk of development of gastroesophageal varices and ascites and delays progression to cirrhosis.[62,63] The predicted probability that cirrhosis will develop after 5 years of therapy with UDCA for patients with stage 1, 2, or 3 disease at diagnosis is 4%, 12%, and 59%, respectively; at 10 years of therapy with UDCA, the probability of cirrhosis is 17%, 27%, and 76%, respectively.[63] These figures suggest a beneficial effect of UDCA on delaying progression to cirrhosis, as compared with disease progression in the absence of treatment. Moreover, UDCA reduces proliferation of colonic epithelial cells, and its long-term use in patients with PBC significantly reduces the probability that colorectal adenomas will recur following removal.[64]

When an effective dose of UDCA (13 to 15 mg/kg/day) has been used and an appropriate number of patients received treatment for a sufficient period of time in randomized controlled trials, UDCA has been shown clearly to improve survival free of liver transplantation (Fig. 91-3).[65] A meta-analysis that included only randomized controlled trials in

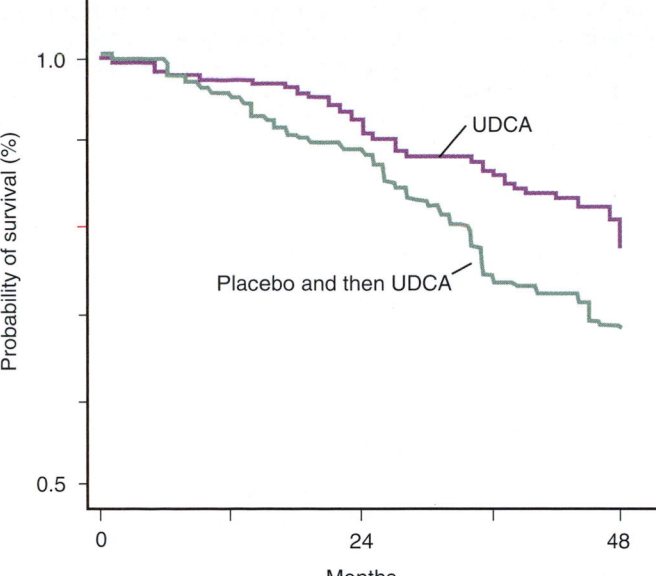

FIGURE 91-3. Survival in 548 patients with PBC. The probability of survival was significantly greater in patients who received treatment with ursodeoxycholic acid (UDCA) for 4 years than in those who first received placebo for two years and then received UDCA (P < 0.001; relative risk, 1.92; 95% CI, 1.30-2.82). *(Adapted from Poupon R, Lindor KD, Cauch-Dudek K, et al. Combined analysis of French, American and Canadian randomized controlled trials of ursodeoxycholic acid therapy in primary biliary cirrhosis. Gastroenterology 1997; 113:884-90.)*

which the doses of UDCA administered and the duration of follow-up were adequate concluded that the frequency of liver transplantation was reduced significantly, with a marginally significant reduction in the rate of death or liver transplantation, but that the rate of death alone was not reduced in the group of patients who received UDCA.[66] In addition, in the sensitivity analyses that included studies that administered placebo as control, long-term studies (>48 months), and large-sized studies (>100 patients), long-term treatment with UDCA reduced the frequencies of liver transplantation and of death or liver transplantation significantly.[66]

Several reports have provided further data on the long-term effects of UDCA in PBC. A study of 192 patients with PBC treated with UDCA for a mean of 6.7 years found that patients with PBC who have a biochemical response by the Barcelona criteria (decrease in serum alkaline phosphatase level of at least 40% from baseline or to normal) after 1 year of treatment had a survival rate better than that predicted by the Mayo risk score and similar to that of a historical control population.[67] Another prospective cohort study of 136 patients found that those patients who had a biochemical response to UDCA (Paris criteria, see later) and who were not fatigued had a 9-year survival rate identical to that of controls.[44] In the same study, non-treatment with UDCA was associated with an increased risk of death.[44] A report that evaluated the effect of UDCA on hepatocellular carcinoma found that, compared with the general population, the increased risk in UDCA-treated patients with PBC was 3-fold, in contrast to an 8-fold increased risk in patients with PBC not treated with UDCA.[68] A few studies have failed to demonstrate a survival benefit in UDCA-treated patients with PBC, but several flaws in study design, most notably small numbers of patients enrolled and

use of suboptimal doses of UDCA, preclude meaningful conclusions.

The most cost-effective dose of UDCA in patients with PBC is 13 to 15 mg/kg/day, which can be given in 1 or 2 divided doses taken with meals. In patients also taking cholestyramine, UDCA should be taken at least 2 hours before or after cholestyramine to ensure intestinal absorption.

There remains a subset of patients who do not respond to UDCA. A lower response rate is observed in men and in patients diagnosed at an earlier age (50% response rate if diagnosed before age 30 compared with a 90% response rate if diagnosed after age 70).[69] A variety of criteria to assess responsiveness to UDCA have been proposed based on changes in serum liver biochemical test levels, principally improvement in alkaline phosphatase. The Paris criteria have been recognized as the best validated and easiest to use criteria after 6 months of UDCA.[70] The original Paris criteria were a decrease in the serum alkaline phosphatase level to less than 3 times the upper limit of normal and in the serum AST level to less than 2 times the upper limit of normal plus a normal bilirubin level. When the Paris and other criteria are applied at 3, 6, and 12 months after initiating UDCA, they remain predictive of long-term outcomes (liver-related death, liver transplantation, and complications related to cirrhosis); assessment of the biochemical response at the sixth month may be more accurate than assessment at month 12.[71] When modified Paris criteria— normal serum total bilirubin level and both an alkaline phosphatase and AST level less than 1.5 times the upper limit of normal after 1 year of UDCA—were applied to patients with early-stage PBC, no evidence of disease progression was observed after a mean follow-up of 7 years.[72] Clearly, the biochemical response to UDCA is predictive of long-term clinical outcomes, and nonresponders to UDCA represent a group of patients with an unmet therapeutic need.

Other Drugs

Prednisolone and Prednisone

Prednisolone and prednisone may improve serum alkaline phosphatase and aminotransferase levels and liver histologic features in patients with PBC, at least in the short term. Unfortunately, the development of side effects with glucocorticoids, particularly a reduction in bone mass, precludes their use in the treatment of PBC.[73]

Budesonide

Budesonide is a glucocorticoid, structurally related to 16α-hydroxyprednisolone, with extensive first-pass hepatic metabolism and minimal systemic availability. In a randomized multicenter trial, 79 patients with noncirrhotic (stage 1 to 3) PBC were enrolled, and 41 were randomized to treatment with oral budesonide (6 mg daily) in combination with UDCA (15 mg/kg/day), whereas 36 received UDCA alone.[74] At 3 years of treatment, the combination of budesonide and UDCA led to greater histologic improvement than UDCA alone. Side effects of glucocorticoids led to discontinuation of treatment in only 1 patient, and 7 other patients reported mild glucocorticoid-related side effects. In an earlier open-label study, 22 patients with PBC who had experienced a suboptimal response to UDCA for a number of years were treated with oral budesonide (3 mg 3 times daily) for 1 year.[75] The addition of budesonide to treatment with UDCA was associated with improvement in serum liver enzyme levels, without affecting other important prognostic markers such as the bilirubin level and Mayo risk score. In that study, the addition of budesonide was associated with a significant worsening of osteoporosis and cosmetic effects, particularly in those patients with more advanced (stage 3 to 4) PBC.[75] Collectively, the data suggest that budesonide may be of potential benefit for patients with early-stage PBC but is associated with important systemic glucocorticoid-related adverse events in patients with more advanced-stage disease. Therefore, before budesonide can be recommended for the treatment of PBC, appropriately designed controlled trials of long-term duration are necessary.

Methotrexate

Patients with PBC who demonstrated biochemical and histologic improvement with methotrexate therapy have been described in observational studies. In a placebo-controlled trial of methotrexate for PBC, methotrexate in a dose of 7.5 mg a week for up to 6 years was not only of no benefit, but also was associated with more unfavorable outcomes than was observed with placebo. A large randomized trial evaluating UDCA (15 mg/kg/day) plus methotrexate (15 mg/m^2 of body surface area weekly, maximal dose of 20 mg/week) compared with UDCA plus placebo has been reported.[76] In that study, 265 patients with PBC and a serum bilirubin level below 3 mg/dL were assigned to 1 of the 2 treatment groups; the mean period of study was 7.5 years. The hazard ratio for death with or without liver transplantation was no better in the methotrexate-UDCA combination group than in the UDCA-placebo group. Therefore, methotrexate should not be recommended routinely as monotherapy or as an adjuvant to UDCA.

Farnesoid X Receptor Agonists

The farnesoid X receptor (FXR) is a nuclear receptor expressed in the liver, kidneys, adrenal glands, and intestine and plays a key role in bile acid metabolism, liver regeneration, and inflammation. Obeticholic acid (INT-747) is a novel, first-in-class FXR agonist that is 100 times as potent as the natural FXR ligand, chenodeoxycholic acid. Preclinical data have suggested that obeticholic acid has antifibrotic and choleretic properties.[77] An international double-blind, placebo-controlled parallel study examined the effects of obeticholic acid among patients with PBC who were on concurrent UDCA and had serum alkaline phosphatase levels at least 1.5 times the upper limit of normal.[78] In that study, 161 patients were randomized to placebo or 3 different doses of obeticholic acid (10 mg, 25 mg, or 50 mg) in addition to UDCA. After 12 weeks, serum liver biochemical test levels were significantly improved in the groups that received the study drug compared with placebo, and the serum alkaline phosphatase level in the treatment groups decreased by 21% to 25%. Pruritus was the most common adverse effect, but the frequency of pruritus in the group that received the lowest dose of the study drug was similar to that for the group receiving placebo (50%).[78] Additional clinical trials will clarify the role of FXR agonists in the management of PBC.

Other Medications and Combination Therapy

Other medications such as D-penicillamine, azathioprine, chlorambucil, cyclosporine, malotilate, tetracycline, tacrolimus, thalidomide, and silymarin have been evaluated for the treatment of PBC, but no convincing evidence of efficacy has been reported for any of these agents and some were associated with serious adverse events. None of these medications can be recommended for the treatment of PBC. Ten trials of varying methodological quality have examined the use of colchicine in PBC; these trials have been systematically reviewed,

and no effect on mortality, liver transplantation, histologic progression, or liver biochemical test levels was observed.[79]

Small pilot open-label studies of short duration have been reported for rituximab, fenofibrate, bezafibrate, mycophenolate mofetil, rifampin, lamivudine plus zidovudine (Combivir), and sulindac. Although some improvement in liver biochemical test levels was observed with these medications, none of these agents can be recommended outside of clinical trials.

The use of combination therapy with drugs that have different properties has been evaluated in open-label and controlled trials. Combinations studied have included UDCA and methotrexate, UDCA and colchicine, cyclosporine and prednisone, chlorambucil and prednisolone, UDCA and prednisone or prednisolone, UDCA and sulindac, and UDCA, prednisone, and azathioprine. Although some improvement in liver biochemical test levels in the short term has been reported with some of these combinations, the small numbers of patients enrolled, short follow-up periods, and risk of drug-related side effects do not allow recommendation of any of these combinations for the treatment of PBC without further supporting evidence. Furthermore, none of these combinations seems to be more effective than UDCA alone. A small study examined the effects of UDCA, budesonide, and mycophenolate mofetil in 15 patients with noncirrhotic PBC who had a suboptimal biochemical response to UDCA after at least 1 year of monotherapy. All the patients received concurrent calcium, vitamin D, and a bisphosphonate. After 3 years, there was significant biochemical and histologic improvement without any reported side effects or change in bone density.[80] These encouraging results require confirmation in larger controlled trials.

MANAGEMENT OF COMPLICATIONS OF CHRONIC CHOLESTASIS

Bone Disease

Bone disease with a predisposition to spontaneous fracturing is a common complication of chronic cholestatic liver disease. In North America, most patients with bone disease from cholestasis have osteoporosis rather than osteomalacia. Osteoporosis is defined as defective bone formation, whereas osteomalacia is defective bone mineralization resulting from vitamin D deficiency. Women with PBC lose bone mass at a rate approximately twice that seen in age-matched controls, and this accelerated bone loss is the result of decreased formation rather than increased resorption of bone. Osteoporosis in PBC involves perturbations of bone remodeling, and the cause is multifactorial and poorly understood. It likely involves a multitude of factors including insulin-like growth factor-1 deficiency, hypogonadism, cholestasis, genetic susceptibility such as vitamin D receptor gene polymorphisms, decreased vitamin D levels, and use of concurrent medications, such as immunosuppressive therapy in the post-transplant setting.[81]

Dual-energy x-ray absorptiometry and dual-photon absorptiometry are noninvasive techniques that quantify bone mass accurately. From 14% to 52% of patients with PBC have osteoporosis, as defined by a T-score below −2.5 in either the lumbar spine or the femoral neck, and approximately 10% have severe bone disease, as defined by a Z-score below −2 (the *T-score* is the number of standard deviations below the mean peak value in young gender-matched normal subjects, whereas the *Z-score* is the number of standard deviations below mean normal values corrected for age and gender).[81] The risk of osteoporosis (T-score below −2.5) is 8 times higher in patients with PBC than in a gender-matched population, whereas the risk of severe bone disease (Z-score below –2) is 4 times higher in patients with PBC than in a healthy age- and gender-matched population.[82] Testing for osteoporosis is indicated at the time of diagnosis of PBC, among those who have experienced a fragility fracture or are receiving a prolonged course (>3 months) of glucocorticoids, and before liver transplantation.[81] Repeat testing every 2 to 3 years in at-risk persons has been recommended.[12]

In patients with PBC, as in the general population, older age, postmenopausal status, and lower BMI are independent risk factors for the development of osteoporosis. In patients with PBC, however, the severity of osteoporosis increases as liver disease advances; bone mass in patients with stage 1 or 2 PBC is similar to that in a normal age- and gender-matched population, but bone mass is significantly lower in patients with stage 3 or 4 disease.[82] Higher serum bilirubin levels, possibly as an indication of more advanced PBC, correlate significantly with a higher rate of bone loss.[82] The reported cumulative frequency of all fractures and vertebral fractures in patients with PBC is 21% and 11%, respectively.[83] Risk assessment tools such as the WHO Fracture Risk Assessment Tool (http://www.shef.ac.uk/FRAX/) are used frequently by general practitioners to assess the 10-year probability of major osteoporotic hip fractures among individual patients based on their risk factors, including the presence of chronic liver disease. The clinical utility of FRAX in subjects with PBC remains undefined and requires additional study.

Treatment of the bone disease includes adequate exercise and supplemental calcium (1200 to 1500 mg daily orally) and vitamin D (600 to 800 IU daily orally, or if deficiency is present, 25,000 to 50,000 IU orally once or twice a week). The bisphosphonate alendronate improves bone mass significantly in patients with PBC when compared with placebo.[81] Parenteral bisphosphonates (zoledronic acid, pamidronate, and ibandronate) have been found to be safe and effective in patients with PBC in a small retrospective study and should be considered for patients with a contraindication (e.g., gastroesophageal varices) to oral bisphosphonate therapy.[84]

Treatment with estrogens significantly prevents loss of bone mass in postmenopausal patients with PBC and was not associated with worsening cholestasis in a series of 46 patients with PBC who received estrogen treatment for a mean period of almost 5 years.[81] Because of the carcinogenic properties of estrogens and the risk of thromboembolism, they are not considered first-line agents. Raloxifene, a selective estrogen receptor modulator, is as an alternative to estrogen replacement therapy for postmenopausal osteoporosis. Other therapeutic options for osteoporosis that have not been widely studied in PBC include denosumab, strontium ranelate, and teriparatide.

Fat-Soluble Vitamin Deficiency

Most patients with PBC and fat-soluble vitamin deficiency have advanced liver disease with jaundice. Fat-soluble vitamin deficiency is almost always caused by malabsorption resulting from decreased amounts of bile salts in the intestinal lumen. Vitamin A and D levels and the prothrombin time should be checked annually in patients with PBC with a serum bilirubin level greater than 2 mg/dL.[12]

Vitamin D deficiency should be excluded in patients with PBC by measurement of the serum level of 25-hydroxyvitamin D, a major metabolite of vitamin D. When vitamin D deficiency is encountered, vitamin D in a dose of 25,000 to 50,000 IU, given orally once or twice a week, is usually sufficient to achieve a normal serum vitamin D level. Because 25-hydroxylation of vitamin D is normal in patients with PBC, vitamin D (rather than the more expensive 25-hydroxyvitamin D or 1,25-hydroxyvitamin D) can be prescribed.

Vitamin A deficiency, which can cause reduced night vision, may occur in patients with PBC. When blood levels of vitamin A are low and the patient is symptomatic, replacement therapy with oral vitamin A, 100,000 IU daily for 3 days, and then 50,000 IU daily for 14 days, should be instituted. If patients are deficient but asymptomatic, a dose of 25,000 to 50,000 IU 2 or 3 times a week is sufficient. The adequacy of replacement therapy is assessed by repeating serum vitamin A assays and evaluating the patient for darkness adaptation, if indicated.

Vitamin K deficiency occurs with severe cholestasis and is manifested by a prolonged prothrombin time. A trial of oral vitamin K, 5 to 10 mg daily, should be given to determine if the prothrombin time improves. If it does, the patient should be maintained on a water-soluble vitamin K, 5 mg per day.

Deficiency of vitamin E has been reported in a few patients with PBC. Typically, vitamin E deficiency causes a neurologic abnormality that primarily affects the posterior columns and is characterized by areflexia, loss of proprioception, and ataxia. In patients with chronic cholestasis and low serum levels of vitamin E, oral replacement therapy with high-dose vitamin E (100 mg daily) may halt progression of neuropathy.

Hyperlipidemia

Lipid abnormalities are found in up to 85% of patients with PBC (see Chapter 72). High-density lipoprotein (HDL) levels usually are elevated most prominently in the early stages of PBC. As the disease progresses, HDL levels decrease and low-density lipoprotein (LDL) levels increase; despite this, the risk of myocardial infarction and stroke does not appear to be increased.[12] Xanthelasmas (deposits of cholesterol in the skin) may develop in some patients with hyperlipidemia and can be troublesome.

Among patients with PBC who would benefit from lipid-lowering therapy, the use of statins appears to be safe and has not been associated with deterioration of liver function.[85] Therapy with UDCA has been shown to lower LDL levels in patients with PBC and has been useful in some patients with xanthelasmas. Surgical removal of xanthelasmas is seldom successful, and such attempts should be avoided.

Pruritus

The cause of pruritus in patients with PBC remains incompletely understood (see earlier). Various agents may provide symptomatic relief (Table 91-4). The bile acid-binding resin cholestyramine was the first medication described to alleviate this symptom. Therapy with cholestyramine is successful in a majority of patients who can tolerate the unpleasant side effects of bad taste, bloating, and occasional constipation. The recommended total dose is 3 to 12 g/day orally, and the drug is most effective when one half of the dose is given 30 minutes before and one half is given 30 minutes after breakfast, to permit maximal bile acid binding as the gallbladder empties. All drugs that can potentially bind to cholestyramine should be taken several hours before or after the cholestyramine. Colesevelam has a higher bile acid binding capacity and fewer side effects than cholestyramine; however, a small randomized controlled trial demonstrated that despite a significant reduction in serum bile acid levels, colesevelam was not more effective than placebo at improving pruritus.[86]

Not all patients with pruritus are helped by cholestyramine. The antibiotic rifampin also is effective in relieving the pruritus of PBC. A majority of patients respond to rifampin, and benefit occurs within one week of the start of therapy. The

TABLE 91-4 Medical Therapy of Cholestasis-Associated Pruritus

Drug	Oral Regimen	Efficacy	Adverse Effects
Cholestyramine	3-4 g 30 min before meals and 2 hours apart from UDCA	Beneficial in most patients	Fat malabsorption, decreased intestinal absorption of other medications, constipation
Rifampin	150-300 mg twice daily	Beneficial in some, but not all, controlled trials to date	Inducer of hepatic enzymes involved in drug metabolism, potential hepatotoxicity, red-orange discoloration of urine and secretions
UDCA	13-15 mg/kg/day	Beneficial in intrahepatic cholestasis of pregnancy	No major toxicity reported
Naltrexone	50 mg daily	Beneficial in small controlled trials	Opiate withdrawal symptoms, rare hepatotoxicity
Antihistamines: Diphenhydramine Hydroxyzine	25-50 mg 4 times a day 25 mg 3 times a day	Rarely provide significant relief apart from sedation	Drowsiness

UDCA, ursodeoxycholic acid.

starting dose is 150 mg twice daily orally; occasionally, higher doses are needed. Rifampin induces drug-metabolizing enzymes, so caution is needed when concurrent drugs are administered. Rifampin has been associated with reversible liver injury in up to 15% of patients.

Occasionally, treatment with UDCA alleviates pruritus, although on occasion pruritus may worsen with initiation of UDCA. In warm countries, exposure to ultraviolet light without sun block can alleviate pruritus, and not surprisingly, the pruritus of PBC subsides during the summer months. The hypothesis has been proposed that pruritus may be related to the release of endogenous opioids. The opiate receptor antagonist naloxone has shown a clear benefit in a double-blind trial.[87] Oral opiate receptor antagonists such as nalmefene and naltrexone have led to amelioration of pruritus in patients with PBC, although further trials are needed to evaluate their safety. The serotonin reuptake inhibitor sertraline, 75 to 100 mg orally, has been associated with relief of pruritus as assessed by a visual analog scale and healing of excoriations.[88] Because of their sedative effects, antihistamines such as diphenhydramine and hydroxyzine are helpful for treating the insomnia associated with pruritus, which is always more troublesome at night. The pruritus of PBC is almost always cured by liver transplantation, which is a viable option for patients with severe intractable pruritus (see later).

Steatorrhea

Steatorrhea can occur in patients with advanced PBC. Several causes have been described. The most important cause is decreased bile acid delivery with insufficient micellar concentration of bile acids in the small intestine. Occasionally, exocrine pancreatic insufficiency can be found as part of a widespread glandular dysfunction seen in some patients with PBC. Coexisting celiac disease has been reported in a small number of patients with PBC, and SIBO may be the cause of steatorrhea in some patients with PBC and scleroderma. Because each of these causes has specific and different treatments, determining the exact cause of steatorrhea is important. Patients with decreased intestinal bile acid concentrations usually benefit from substitution of medium-chain TGs for long-chain TGs in their diets and a decrease in total fat intake (see Chapter 104). Patients with exocrine pancreatic insufficiency will benefit from pancreatic replacement therapy (see Chapter 59); patients with celiac disease require gluten withdrawal from the diet (see Chapter 107); and patients with SIBO should receive intermittent broad-spectrum oral antibiotic therapy (see Chapter 105).

LIVER TRANSPLANTATION

The best therapeutic alternative for patients with end-stage PBC is liver transplantation. The major manifestations of chronic liver disease that should prompt an evaluation for liver transplantation in patients with other causes of chronic liver disease apply to patients with PBC. These indications include complications related to portal hypertension. In patients with PBC, the development of complications associated with chronic cholestasis, such as a poor quality of life secondary to disabling fatigue, intractable pruritus, and severe muscle wasting, as well as persistent increases in the serum bilirubin level in the absence of hepatic malignancy, should prompt clinicians to consider referral for liver transplantation, even in patients without cirrhosis.

Data from the United Network for Organ Sharing show a clear trend toward decreased rates of liver transplantation for PBC.[89] From 1995 to 2006, the absolute number of liver transplants in the United States increased an average of 249 cases per year, but the absolute number of transplants performed for PBC decreased by an average of 5.4 cases per year.[89] This trend has also been observed in Europe.[90] Because UDCA is now prescribed nearly universally to patients with PBC, the decline in the number of liver transplants for PBC is likely related to a reduction in disease progression from UDCA.

Liver transplantation clearly improves survival, as well as quality of life, for patients with PBC. One-year survival rates after liver transplantation are higher than 90%, with 5-year survival rates of 80% or higher in most transplant centers. Outcomes following live-donor liver transplantation appear to be comparable with 5-year survival rates following deceased-donor liver transplantation, with low rates of PBC recurrence (see later).[91] The advent of prognostic models has helped identify factors that predict survival. The Mayo risk score (http://www.mayoclinic.org/gi-rst/mayomodel2.html [see earlier]) is superior to the Child-Turcotte-Pugh score in predicting survival. The MELD score (http://www.mayoclinic.org/meld/mayomodel6.html) is also a reliable measure of mortality risk in patients with end-stage liver disease, including PBC, and is used as a disease severity index to determine organ allocation priorities (see Chapter 97).[92]

PBC may recur after liver transplantation. The frequency of recurrent PBC varies among centers and ranges from 0% to 35%. PBC typically recurs 3 to 6 years after liver transplantation, and the risk of recurrent PBC increases with time. Liver biochemical test levels in recurrent PBC may be normal or mildly elevated. AMA may persist after liver transplantation, and AMA levels do not correlate with recurrent PBC. Therefore, the diagnosis of recurrent PBC relies heavily on the histologic features. Tacrolimus-based immunosuppression has been the most consistently identified risk factor for disease recurrence. Recurrent PBC following liver transplantation does not seem to decrease survival significantly, although in some studies a small proportion of patients had graft failure. UDCA may play a role in treatment of recurrent PBC, and its use has been associated with improvement in liver biochemical test levels.[93]

KEY REFERENCES

Full references for this chapter can be found on www.expertconsult.com.

4. Baldursdottir TR, Bergmann OM, Jonasson JG, et al. The epidemiology and natural history of primary biliary cirrhosis: A nationwide population-based study. Eur J Gastroenterol Hepatol 2012; 24:824-30.
11. Concepcion AR, Medina JF. Approaches to the pathogenesis of primary biliary cirrhosis through animal models. Clin Res Hepatol Gastroenterol 2012; 36:21-8.
22. Mells GF, Floyd JA, Morley KI, et al. Genome-wide association study identifies 12 new susceptibility loci for primary biliary cirrhosis. Nat Genet 2011; 43:329-32.
29. Lleo A, Bowlus CL, Yang GX, et al. Biliary apotopes and anti-mitochondrial antibodies activate innate immune responses in primary biliary cirrhosis. Hepatology 2010; 52:987-98.
34. McNally RJ, James PW, Ducker S, James OF. Seasonal variation in the patient diagnosis of primary biliary cirrhosis: Further evidence for an environmental component to etiology. Hepatology 2011; 54:2099-103.
41. Corpechot C, Gaouar F, Chretien Y, et al. Smoking as an independent risk factor of liver fibrosis in primary biliary cirrhosis. J Hepatol 2012; 56:218-24.
44. Jones DE, Al-Rifai A, Frith J, et al. The independent effects of fatigue and UDCA therapy on mortality in primary biliary cirrhosis: Results of a 9-year follow-up. J Hepatol 2010; 53:911-7.
48. Liang Y, Yang Z, Zhong R. Primary biliary cirrhosis and cancer risk: A systematic review and meta-analysis. Hepatology 2012; 56:1409-17.
50. Selmi C, Bowlus CL, Gershwin ME, Coppel RL. Primary biliary cirrhosis. Lancet 2011; 377:1600-9.
52. Corpechot C, Carrat F, Poujol-Robert A, et al. Noninvasive elastography-based assessment of liver fibrosis progression and prognosis in primary biliary cirrhosis. Hepatology 2012; 56:198-208.
69. Carbone M, Mells G, Pells G, et al. Sex and age are determinants of the clinical phenotype of primary biliary cirrhosis and response to ursodeoxycholic acid. Gastroenterology 2013; 144:560-9.
71. Zhang LN, Shi TY, Shi XH, et al. Early biochemical response to ursodeoxycholic acid and long-term prognosis of primary biliary cirrhosis: Results of a 14-year cohort study. Hepatology 2013; 58:264-72.
72. Corpechot C, Chazouilleres O, Poupon R. Early primary biliary cirrhosis: Biochemical response to treatment and prediction of long-term outcome. J Hepatol 2011; 55:1361-7.
77. Lindor KD. Farnesoid X receptor agonists for primary biliary cirrhosis. Curr Opin Gastroenterol 2011; 27:285-8.
91. Kaneko J, Sugawara Y, Tamura S, et al. Long-term outcome of living donor liver transplantation for primary biliary cirrhosis. Transpl Int 2012; 25:7-12.

Portal Hypertension and Variceal Bleeding

VIJAY H. SHAH AND PATRICK S. KAMATH

Variceal hemorrhage, hepatic encephalopathy, and ascites—the major complications of cirrhosis of the liver (see Chapters 74, 93, and 94)—result from portal hypertension, defined as an increase in hepatic sinusoidal pressure to 6 mm Hg or greater. Portosystemic collaterals decompress the hypertensive hepatic sinusoids and give rise to varices at the gastroesophageal junction and elsewhere.

NORMAL PORTAL CIRCULATION

The portal venous system carries capillary blood from the esophagus, stomach, small and large intestine, pancreas, gallbladder, and spleen to the liver. The portal vein is formed by the confluence of the splenic vein and the superior mesenteric vein behind the neck of the pancreas.[1] The inferior mesenteric vein usually drains into the splenic vein. The left gastric vein, also called the left coronary vein, usually drains into the portal vein at the confluence of the splenic vein and superior mesenteric vein (Fig. 92-1). The portal vein is approximately 7.5 cm in length and runs dorsal to the hepatic artery and bile duct into the hilum of the liver. The uppermost 5 cm of the portal vein does not receive any tributaries.[2] In the hilum of the liver, the portal vein divides into the left and right portal vein branches, which supply the left and right sides of the liver,

respectively. The umbilical vein drains into the left portal vein, and the cystic vein from the gallbladder drains into the right portal vein. The portal venules drain into hepatic sinusoids that, in turn, are drained by the hepatic veins into the inferior vena cava. The left and middle hepatic veins usually join and drain into the inferior vena cava separately but adjacent to the confluence of the right hepatic vein with the inferior vena cava. The caudate lobe drains separately into the inferior vena cava (see Chapter 71).

The circulatory system of the normal liver is a high-compliance, low-resistance system that is able to accommodate a large blood volume, as occurs after a meal, without substantially increasing portal pressure. The liver receives a dual blood supply from the portal vein and the hepatic artery that constitutes nearly 30% of total cardiac output. Portal venous blood derived from the mesenteric venous circulation constitutes approximately 75% of total hepatic blood flow, whereas the remainder of blood to the liver is derived from the hepatic artery, which provides highly oxygenated blood directly from the celiac trunk of the aorta. Portal vein–derived and hepatic artery–derived blood flow converge in high-compliance, specialized vascular channels termed *hepatic sinusoids*. A dynamic and compensatory interplay occurs between hepatic blood flow derived from the portal vein and that from the hepatic artery. When portal venous blood flow to the liver is diminished, as occurs in portal vein thrombosis, arterial inflow increases in an attempt to maintain total hepatic blood flow at a constant level. Similarly, after hepatic artery occlusion, portal venous inflow increases in a compensatory manner. This autoregulatory mechanism, aimed at maintaining total hepatic blood flow at a constant level, is termed the *hepatic arterial buffer response.*

The sinusoids are highly permeable and thus facilitate the transport of macromolecules to the parenchymal hepatocytes that reside on the extraluminal side of the endothelial cells. The hepatic sinusoids are highly permeable because they lack a proper basement membrane and because the endothelial cells that line the sinusoids contain fenestrae. Other unique aspects of the hepatic sinusoids are the space of Disse, a virtual space located extraluminal to the endothelial cell and adjacent to the hepatocyte, and its cellular constituents, the hepatic stellate cell (HSC) and the Kupffer cell (Fig. 92-2; see also Chapters 71 and 74). These 2 cell types probably play an

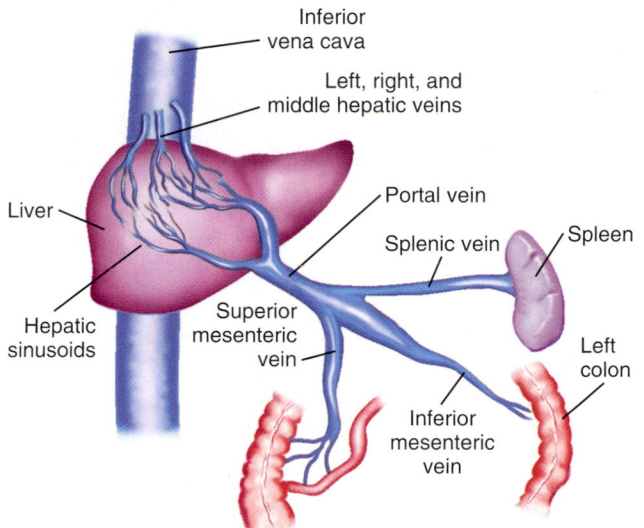

FIGURE 92-1. Anatomy of the portal circulation. Blood vessels that constitute the portal circulation and hepatic outflow tracts are depicted.

important role, in concert with the endothelial cell, in regulating sinusoidal hemodynamics and homeostasis and may contribute to the sinusoidal derangements that occur in portal hypertension. Under basal conditions, HSCs maintain a quiescent phenotype and accumulate vitamin A. On activation, however, as occurs in cirrhosis and portal hypertension, these cells are postulated to develop contractile abilities that permit them to function as sinusoidal pericytes. Kupffer cells contribute to vascular homeostasis by generating cytokines with potent cellular and vasoregulatory actions, including TNF. Endothelial cells and smooth muscle cells in nonsinusoidal hepatic vessels such as the portal venule and the terminal hepatic venule are important in hepatic vasoregulation, particularly in the normal liver, where HSCs are quiescent, not activated, and presumably less contractile.

Many studies have established the important role of nitric oxide (NO), derived from endothelial NO synthase (eNOS), in hepatic vasodilatation. Shear stress, caused by the frictional force of blood within the sinusoids, is one of the most potent physiologic stimuli of eNOS-derived NO production in hepatic sinusoids. By contrast, endothelin-1 (ET-1), also released by endothelial cells, promotes hepatic vasoconstriction by binding to ET-A receptors located on HSCs. ET-1 also appears to be generated within HSCs themselves and promotes HSC contraction through an autocrine loop. Of interest, ET-1 may alternatively bind to ET-B receptors on endothelial cells. This signaling pathway paradoxically promotes vasodilatation by activating eNOS. Other vascular mediators implicated in hepatic vasoregulation include carbon monoxide generated by the heme oxygenase system, the sympathetic adrenergic agonist norepinephrine, the renin-dependent vasoconstrictor angiotensin, prostaglandins, thromboxane, leukotrienes, and hydrogen sulfide. Of these mediators, angiotensin is of particular interest because it is a potent constrictor of HSCs and is released in increased amounts in cirrhosis owing to systemic sympathetic hyperactivity.

HEMODYNAMIC PRINCIPLES OF PORTAL HYPERTENSION

In cirrhosis, as well as in most noncirrhotic causes of portal hypertension, portal hypertension results from changes in

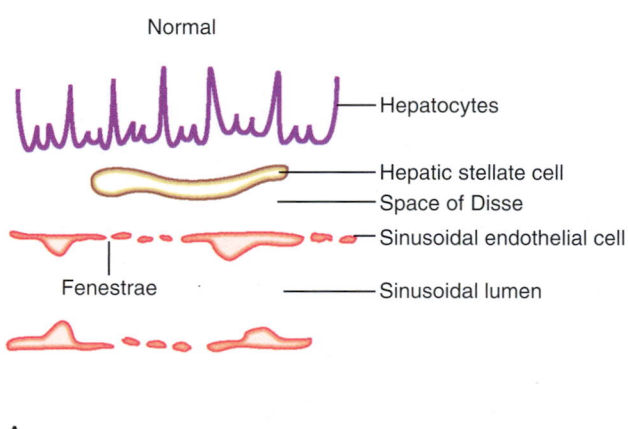

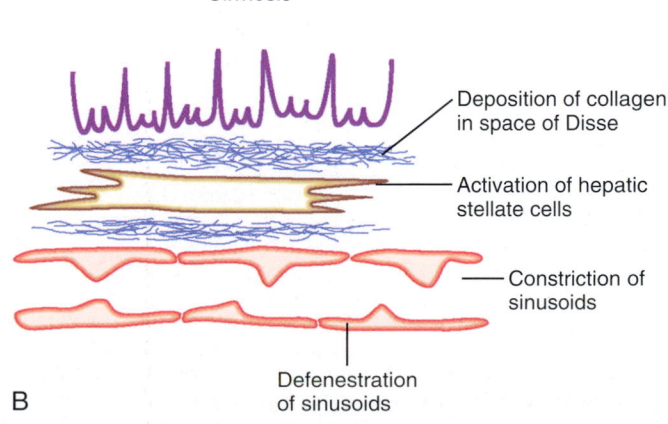

FIGURE 92-2. Anatomy of the hepatic microvasculature. *A,* Normal sinusoidal microanatomy is depicted. The sinusoidal lumen is lined by fenestrated sinusoidal endothelial cells that allow the transport of macromolecules to the abluminal space of Disse. Quiescent hepatic stellate cells reside within this space, adjacent to hepatocytes and endothelial cells. *B,* In cirrhosis, a number of changes occur in the hepatic microcirculation, including loss of fenestrae in endothelial cells (defenestration), constriction of sinusoids, and activation of hepatic stellate cells with ensuing deposition of collagen and increased contractility.

portal resistance in combination with changes in portal inflow. The influence of flow and resistance on pressure can be represented by the formula for Ohm's law:

$$\Delta P = F \times R$$

in which the pressure gradient in the portal circulation (*ΔP*) is a function of portal flow (*F*) and resistance to flow (*R*). Increases in portal resistance or portal flow can contribute to increased pressure. Portal hypertension almost always results from increases in both portal resistance and portal flow (Fig. 92-3). One exception is an arteriovenous fistula (AVF), which in the initial stages causes portal hypertension largely through an increase in portal flow in the absence of an increase in resistance. The mechanism of the increase in portal resistance depends on the site and cause of portal hypertension; in the

Western world, the most common cause is liver cirrhosis (see later). Because of the increase in hepatic resistance and the decrease in hepatic compliance, small changes in flow that do not increase pressure in the normal liver can have a prominent stimulatory effect on portal pressure in the cirrhotic liver. The increase in portal venous inflow is part of a generalized systemic derangement termed the *hyperdynamic circulatory state*. Collateral vessels that dilate and new vascular sprouts that form connect the high-pressure portal venous system with lower-pressure systemic veins. Unfortunately, this process of angiogenesis and collateralization is insufficient for normalizing portal pressure and actually causes complications of portal hypertension, such as esophageal varices.[3]

The changes in portal flow and resistance also can be viewed as originating from mechanical and vascular factors. Mechanical factors include the fibrosis and nodularity of the

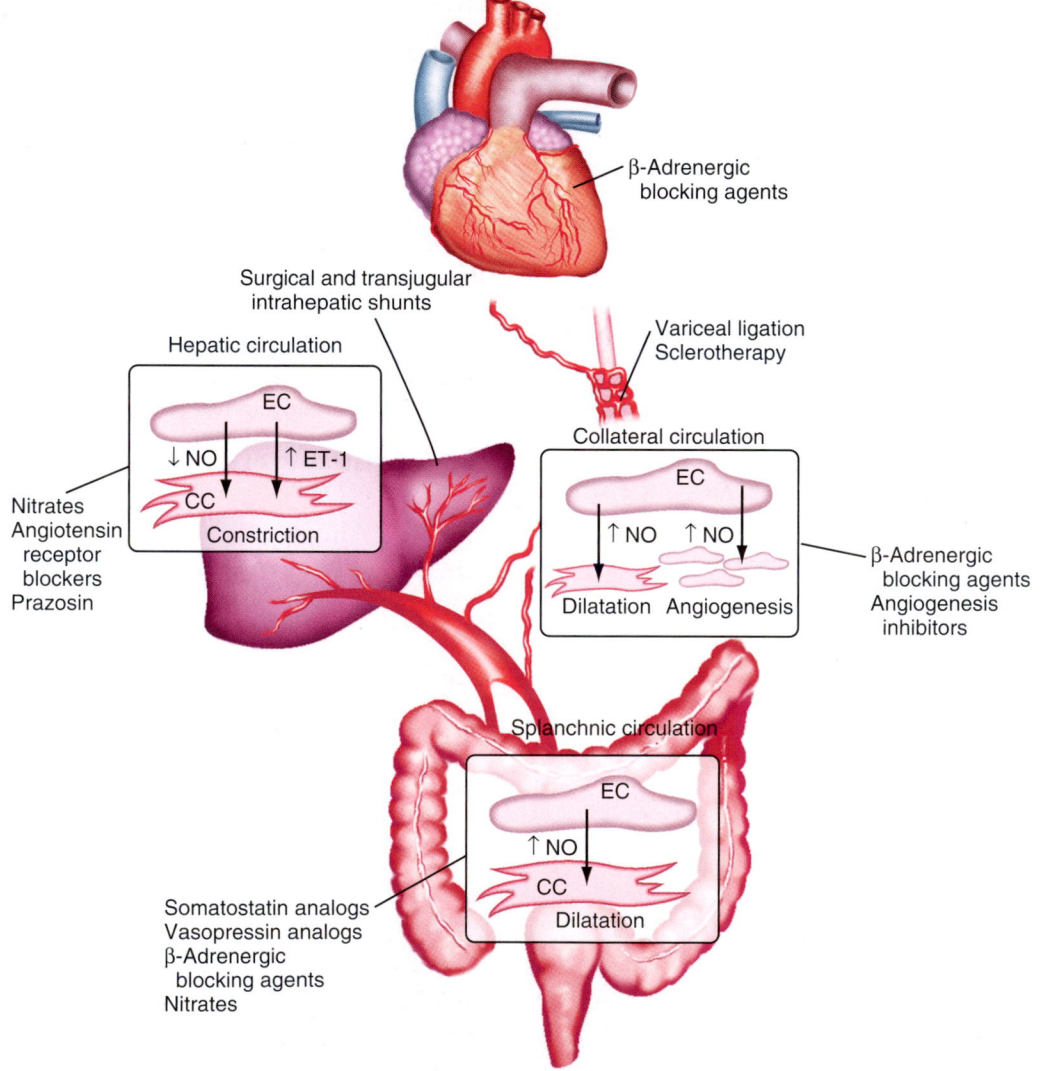

FIGURE 92-3. Vascular disturbances in portal hypertension and sites of action of portal pressure-reducing therapies. Portal hypertension typically results from increased resistance, usually from within the liver, in combination with increased portal venous flow. The increase in hepatic resistance results from mechanical factors in combination with dynamic vasoconstriction mediated by decreased nitric oxide (NO) production and increased endothelin-1 (ET-1) production. The increase in portal venous flow occurs as a result of vasodilatation in the splanchnic circulation that is mediated by increased NO production. A collateral circulation, including esophageal varices, develops between the hypertensive portal vasculature and systemic venous system; however, these collaterals are inadequate to decompress the hypertensive portal circulation fully. Collateral vessel development is mediated by dilatation of existing collateral vessels, as well as the development of new blood vessels and sprouts (angiogenesis). Therapies aimed at the different sites of hemodynamic disturbances are shown. CC, contractile cell (e.g., hepatic stellate cell, vascular smooth muscle cell); EC, endothelial cell.

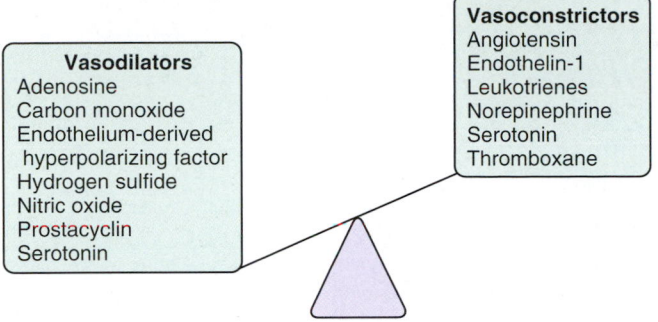

Vasodilators	**Vasoconstrictors**
Adenosine	Angiotensin
Carbon monoxide	Endothelin-1
Endothelium-derived	Leukotrienes
hyperpolarizing factor	Norepinephrine
Hydrogen sulfide	Serotonin
Nitric oxide	Thromboxane
Prostacyclin	
Serotonin	

FIGURE 92-4. Representative vasodilator and vasoconstrictor molecules implicated in portal hypertension. Increased levels of vasodilators and decreased levels of vasoconstrictors lead to splanchnic vasodilatation (not shown). Conversely, decreased levels of vasodilators and increased levels of vasoconstrictors are implicated in intrahepatic vasoconstriction in portal hypertension (shown).

cirrhotic liver, with distortion of the vascular architecture and the remodeling that is recognized to occur in the systemic and splanchnic vasculature in response to the chronic increases in flow and shear stress that characterize the hyperdynamic circulatory state. Vascular factors include intrahepatic vasoconstriction, which contributes to increased intrahepatic resistance, and the splanchnic and systemic vasodilatation that accompanies the hyperdynamic circulatory state. The vascular factors that contribute to portal hypertension are particularly important because they are reversible and dynamic and therefore compelling targets for experimental therapies (Fig. 92-4). Conversely, effective therapies for the fixed, mechanical component of portal hypertension caused by scar, regenerative nodules, and vascular remodeling are currently lacking. Indeed, most available therapies for portal hypertension focus on correction of hemodynamic alterations in the portal circulation.[4,5] Other agents reduce the increased intrahepatic resistance (see later).

Increased Intrahepatic Resistance

In cirrhosis, increased portal resistance occurs in great part as a result of mechanical factors that reduce vessel diameter. In addition to regenerative nodules and fibrotic bands, these mechanical factors include capillarization of the sinusoids and swelling of cells, including hepatocytes and Kupffer cells. As discussed earlier, however, reduced hepatic vessel diameter resulting in increased portal resistance, even when caused by cirrhosis, is not a purely mechanical phenomenon.[6] Hemodynamic changes in the hepatic circulation also contribute to increased intrahepatic resistance.[7,8] These changes are characterized by hepatic vasoconstriction and impaired responses to vasodilatory stimuli. The increase in intrahepatic resistance is determined largely by changes in vessel radius, with small reductions in vessel radius causing prominent increases in resistance. Blood viscosity and vessel length also can influence resistance, albeit to a much smaller extent. The factors that regulate resistance can be viewed in the context of Poiseuille's law:

$$R = 8\eta L / \pi r^4$$

in which R is resistance, ηL is the product of blood viscosity and vessel length, and r is vessel radius.

Although vasoactive changes were estimated initially to account for 10% to 30% of the increase in portal resistance in cirrhosis, subsequent studies have suggested that these figures actually may underestimate the contribution of hepatic vasoconstriction to the increased resistance observed in the cirrhotic liver. In noncirrhotic causes of portal hypertension, the increase in resistance may occur at sites upstream (prehepatic) or downstream (posthepatic) of the liver, as in portal vein thrombosis and hepatic vein thrombosis, respectively (Fig. 92-5). Furthermore, the site of increased intrahepatic resistance can be further delineated as the sinusoids (sinusoidal), upstream from the sinusoids within the portal venules (presinusoidal), or downstream from the sinusoids in the hepatic venules (postsinusoidal), as in alcoholic cirrhosis, schistosomiasis, and sinusoidal obstruction syndrome, respectively. Pressure is increased only in the portal circulation behind the site of increased resistance, and in isolated portal vein thrombosis, hepatic function frequently remains largely preserved despite prominent portal hypertension.

Most evidence suggests that a decrease in the production of the vasodilator NO and an increase in the production of the vasoconstrictor ET-1 jointly contribute to the increase in hepatic vascular resistance. In experimental models of cirrhosis, the bioavailability of hepatic NO is diminished because of a reduction in the production of NO by endothelial cells.[7,9,10] A similar paradigm is observed in the human cirrhotic liver.[11] Most relevant studies indicate that the reduction in NO production occurs not through a reduction in hepatic eNOS levels[9,10] but through defects in the steps necessary to activate existing eNOS. For example, increases in the production of the eNOS-inhibiting protein caveolin-1 have been observed in experimental models of cirrhosis[10] and in human cirrhosis. Another pathway that contributes to deficient generation of NO by eNOS is a reduction in the level of AKT (protein kinase B) phosphorylation of eNOS and up-regulation of the eNOS inhibiting protein GRK (G protein–coupled receptor kinase) in the cirrhotic liver.[12] Irrespective of the mechanism of deficiency, the lack of availability of NO is thought to allow HSCs, which are activated and highly contractile in liver cirrhosis, to constrict the sinusoids that they envelop, thereby increasing portal pressure. The role of the HSCs in this process remains controversial, however, because evidence is mixed regarding whether the site of the increase in intrahepatic resistance in cirrhosis is the sinusoids, where stellate cells reside, or the pre- or postsinusoidal venules (or both), which are devoid of stellate cells and in which endothelial cells signal smooth muscle cells. Furthermore, increasing evidence points toward diverse origins of these myofibroblastic cells within the cirrhotic sinusoids, with portal myofibroblasts as well as HSCs postulated to play important roles.[13] Therapies that target myofibroblast migration, including targeted kinase inhibitors such as sorafenib, are a compelling approach by limiting the density of these contractile cells within the hepatic sinusoids (see Chapter 96).[14,15] The contribution of HSCs to hepatic angiogenesis may also be an important target for treating fibrosis and portal hypertension.[16]

In clinical practice, NO can be delivered by NO donor agents such as mononitrates. NO donor agents exert their beneficial effects in part by relaxing the actively contractile stellate cells.[17,18] The systemic actions of these agents, however, tend to cause side effects and exacerbate the hyperdynamic circulatory state. In studies using a liver-specific NO donor compound, increased intrahepatic vascular resistance could be corrected by the generation of additional NO and consequent relaxation of HSCs, but, unfortunately, human studies have not been promising.[19,20] In cirrhosis, in fact, deficient endothelial cell NO generation may be accompanied by

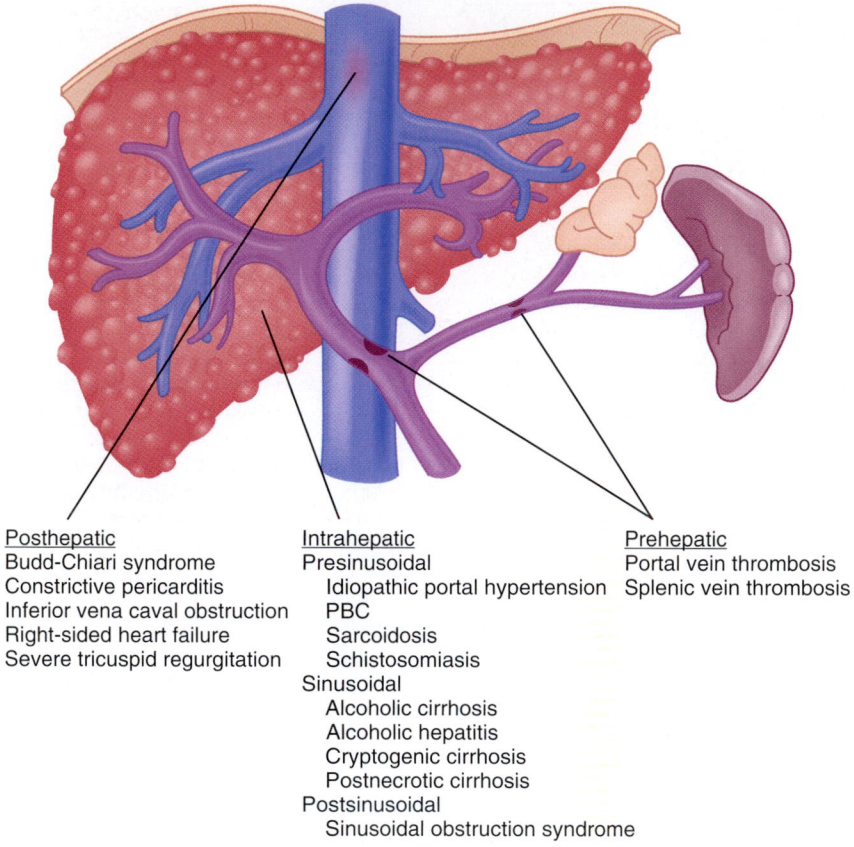

Posthepatic
Budd-Chiari syndrome
Constrictive pericarditis
Inferior vena caval obstruction
Right-sided heart failure
Severe tricuspid regurgitation

Intrahepatic
Presinusoidal
 Idiopathic portal hypertension
 PBC
 Sarcoidosis
 Schistosomiasis
Sinusoidal
 Alcoholic cirrhosis
 Alcoholic hepatitis
 Cryptogenic cirrhosis
 Postnecrotic cirrhosis
Postsinusoidal
 Sinusoidal obstruction syndrome

Prehepatic
Portal vein thrombosis
Splenic vein thrombosis

FIGURE 92-5. Classification of portal hypertension. The different sites of increased resistance to portal flow (posthepatic, intrahepatic, and prehepatic) and associated diseases are shown. Many diseases cause a mixed pattern. Portal hypertension rarely can occur exclusively as a result of increased portal blood flow, as occurs with an arteriovenous shunt (not shown).

impaired stellate cell relaxation in response to NO,[21] perhaps because of diminished response of the NO second messenger cyclic guanosine monophosphate (cGMP) in activated cells.[17] In this situation, a prominent beneficial effect of NO donors is less predictable. Human and experimental studies suggest that statins may activate eNOS in liver and thereby reduce portal hypertension.[22]

Excessive ET-1 also contributes to increased intrahepatic vasoconstriction in portal hypertension through vasoconstrictive effects in the liver, presumably by enhancing HSC contractility.[23,24] In experimental models, ET-1 protein and receptor expression are increased, most notably in HSCs and endothelial cells.[23,25,26] In humans with portal hypertension, plasma and liver ET-1 levels also are increased.[27] The reason for activation of the ET-1 system in portal hypertension is not known, but this effect may be secondary to transforming growth factor (TGF)-β, a key fibrogenic growth factor.[26] The variable effects of ET antagonists in experimental models of portal hypertension, as well as the possible hepatotoxicity of these compounds, have limited enthusiasm for studies of these agents in humans.[28] Somatostatin, which reduces portal pressure by constricting the splanchnic circulation, may also act by inhibiting ET-1–dependent HSC contraction.[29]

Other vasoactive mediators, including cysteinyl leukotrienes, thromboxane, angiotensin, and hydrogen sulfide, have also been implicated in the development of increased intrahepatic resistance in cirrhosis.[30,31] Attempts to reduce portal pressure using pharmacologic agents that inhibit angiotensin activation of HSC contraction have met with mixed results.[32]

Promising approaches for human evaluation include statins and targeted kinase inhibitors such as sorafenib.[20,22]

Hyperdynamic Circulation

In addition to the increases in portal resistance discussed earlier, a major factor in the development and perpetuation of portal hypertension is an increase in portal venous flow, or the hyperdynamic circulation. The term *portal venous inflow* indicates the total blood that drains into the portal circulation, not the blood flow in the portal vein itself, which may actually be diminished in portal hypertension because of portosystemic collateral shunts. The hyperdynamic circulation is characterized by peripheral and splanchnic vasodilatation, reduced mean arterial pressure, and increased cardiac output. Vasodilatation, particularly in the splanchnic bed, permits an increase in inflow of systemic blood into the portal circulation.[33]

Splanchnic vasodilatation is caused in large part by relaxation of splanchnic arterioles and ensuing splanchnic hyperemia. Studies of experimental portal hypertension have demonstrated that splanchnic vascular endothelial cells are primarily responsible for mediating splanchnic vasodilatation and enhanced portal venous inflow through excess generation of NO.[34-42] This excess generation of NO and ensuing vasodilatation, hyperdynamic circulation, and hyperemia in the splanchnic and systemic circulation contrasts with the hepatic circulation, in which NO deficiency contributes to increased intrahepatic resistance.

Some of the increase in NO production probably occurs from shear stress–dependent and shear stress–independent increases in the expression of eNOS, which can be corrected in part by β-adrenergic blocking agents (beta blockers).[40,43-48] Activation of existing eNOS by cytokines or mechanical factors also seems to contribute to excess systemic and splanchnic NO generation through pathways that include eNOS phosphorylation and protein interactions.[45-49] The physiologic stimuli that mediate this process are not well understood but may include ET-1, which is increased in the serum of patients with portal hypertension, and the cytokine TNF-α because inhibitors of TNF-α improve portal pressure and the splanchnic circulatory disturbances in both human and experimental portal hypertension; however, TNF-α inhibitors are not safe for use in patients with advanced liver disease with high MELD scores (see later and Chapter 97).[50] TNF-α may be derived from intestinal endotoxin, and intestinal decontamination appears to correct the hyperdynamic circulation in humans, thereby suggesting a link with intestinal inflammation.[51] Studies have linked intestinal microbes and lipopolysaccharide (LPS) with portal hypertensive hemodynamics.[52] Vascular endothelial growth factor (VEGF) has also been implicated in this process by excessively activating eNOS.[53] In humans with portal hypertension, therapeutic inhibition of NOS has met with mixed clinical results.[54,55]

Other mediators that may contribute to systemic and splanchnic vasodilatation include anandamide, an endogenous vasodilatory cannabinoid,[56-58] heme oxygenase,[18,59-61] cyclooxygenase,[62] and agonists of the innate immune system such as LPS.[52] Compelling evidence also supports a primary defect in smooth muscle cells in portal hypertension, perhaps because of defects in potassium channels.[63-67] In fact, many pharmacologic therapies for portal hypertension target the splanchnic arteriolar smooth muscle cells, rather than endothelial cells, to reduce splanchnic vasodilatation. For example, octreotide, a synthetic analog of somatostatin, causes marked but transient reductions in portal pressure by contracting splanchnic smooth muscle cells, thereby limiting portal venous inflow, especially after meals. Nonselective beta blockers and vasopressin also reduce portal pressure by constricting splanchnic arterioles and thereby reducing portal venous inflow. Because intrahepatic resistance persists, therapies targeted against the increase in portal venous inflow usually do not normalize portal pressure entirely but often blunt the prominent increases in portal venous inflow that occur in response to a meal. Combination therapy with an agent that reduces increased intrahepatic resistance, such as a nitrate, and an agent that reduces portal venous inflow, such as a beta blocker, are more effective in reducing portal pressure than is either agent alone. Carvedilol as a single agent has combined effects of beta blockade and relaxation of intrahepatic sinusoidal vessels.[68]

Collateral Circulation and Varices

The portal vein–systemic collateral circulation develops and expands in response to elevation of the portal pressure.[69] Blood flow in the low volumes that normally perfuse these collaterals and flow toward the portal circulation is reversed in portal hypertension because the increased portal pressure exceeds systemic venous pressure. Therefore, flow is reversed in these collateral vessels, and blood flows out of the portal circulation toward the systemic venous circulation. The sites of collateral formation are the distal esophagus and proximal stomach, where gastroesophageal varices are the major collaterals formed between the portal venous system and systemic venous system; the umbilicus, where the vestigial umbilical vein communicates with the left portal vein and

gives rise to prominent collaterals around the umbilicus (caput medusae); the retroperitoneum, where collaterals, especially in women, communicate between the ovarian vessels and iliac veins; and the rectum, where the inferior mesenteric vein connects with the pudendal vein and rectal varices develop.

Four distinct zones of venous drainage at the gastroesophageal junction are particularly relevant to the formation of esophageal varices.[70] The gastric zone, which extends for 2 to 3 cm below the gastroesophageal junction, comprises veins that are longitudinal and located in the submucosa and lamina propria. They come together at the upper end of the cardia of the stomach and drain into short gastric and left gastric veins. The palisade zone extends 2 to 3 cm proximal to the gastric zone into the lower esophagus. Veins in this zone run longitudinally and in parallel in 4 groups corresponding to the esophageal mucosal folds. These veins anastomose with veins in the lamina propria. The perforating veins in the palisade zone do not communicate with extrinsic (periesophageal) veins in the distal esophagus. The palisade zone is the dominant watershed area between the portal and systemic circulations. More proximal to the palisade zone in the esophagus is the perforating zone, where there is a network of veins. These veins are less likely to be longitudinal and are termed *perforating veins* because they connect the veins in the esophageal submucosa and the external veins. The truncal zone, the longest zone, is approximately 10 cm in length, located proximal to the perforating zone in the esophagus, and usually characterized by 4 longitudinal veins in the lamina propria.

Veins in the palisade zone in the esophagus are most prone to bleeding because no perforating veins at this level connect the veins in the submucosa with the periesophageal veins. Varices in the truncal zone are unlikely to bleed, because the perforating vessels communicate with the periesophageal veins, allowing the varices in the truncal zone to decompress. The periesophageal veins drain into the azygos system, and as a result, an increase in azygos blood flow is a hallmark of portal hypertension. The venous drainage of the lower end of the esophagus is through the coronary vein, which also drains the cardia of the stomach, into the portal vein.

The fundus of the stomach drains through short gastric veins into the splenic vein. In the presence of portal hypertension, varices may therefore form in the fundus of the stomach. Splenic vein thrombosis usually results in isolated gastric fundal varices. Because of the proximity of the splenic vein to the renal vein, spontaneous splenorenal shunts may develop and are more common in patients with gastric varices than in those with esophageal varices.[71,72]

The predominant collateral flow pattern in intrahepatic portal hypertension is through the right and left coronary veins, with only a small portion of flow through the short gastric veins. Therefore, most patients with an intrahepatic cause of portal hypertension have esophageal varices or gastric varices in continuity with esophageal varices. Unfortunately, portal hypertension caused by cirrhosis generally persists and progresses despite the development of even an extensive collateral circulation. Progression of portal hypertension results from (1) the prominent obstructive resistance in the liver, (2) resistance within the collaterals themselves, and (3) continued increase in portal vein inflow. The collateral circulatory bed develops through a combination of angiogenesis, the development of new blood vessels, and dilatation and increased flow through preexisting collaterals.[3,73] VEGF, a key NO stimulatory growth factor, may contribute to both the angiogenic and collateral vessel responses.[60,74] Inhibition of VEGF or NO may attenuate the collateral vessel propagation by inhibiting angiogenic responses in experimental models of portal hypertension and collateralization.[73-78] Beta blockers and octreotide may act in part by constricting collateral vessels.[79-82] Attempts to inhibit VEGF and angiogenesis have focused on targeted kinase inhibitors.[53]

The development of gastroesophageal varices requires a portal pressure gradient of at least 10 mm Hg. Furthermore, a portal pressure gradient of at least 12 mm Hg is thought to be required for varices to bleed; other local factors that increase variceal wall tension are also needed[83] because not all patients with a portal pressure gradient of greater than 12 mm Hg bleed. Factors that influence variceal wall tension can be viewed in the context of Laplace's law:

$$T = Pr/w$$

where T is variceal wall tension, P is the transmural pressure gradient between the variceal lumen and esophageal lumen, r is the variceal radius, and w is the variceal wall thickness. When the variceal wall thins and the varix increases in diameter and pressure, the tolerated wall tension is exceeded and the varix ruptures. These physiologic observations are manifested clinically by the observation that patients with larger varices (r) in sites of limited soft tissue support (w), with elevated portal pressure (P), tend to be at greatest risk for variceal rupture from variceal wall tension (T) that becomes excessive. One notable site in which soft tissue support is limited is at the gastroesophageal junction. The lack of tissue support and high vessel density may contribute to the greater frequency of bleeding from varices at the gastroesophageal junction. Laplace's law also has implications for the relevance of pharmacologic therapies aimed at reducing portal pressure. A reduction in portal pressure reduces the variceal transmural pressure gradient, thereby reducing the risk that variceal wall tension will become excessive and that varices will rupture. Clinically, a reduction in the hepatic venous pressure gradient to less than 12 mm Hg almost eliminates the risk of variceal hemorrhage. The changes in portal pressure and local variceal factors, however, are dynamic and influenced by a number of physiologic (an increase in intra-abdominal pressure, meal-induced increases in portal pressure), diurnal (circadian changes in portal pressure), and pathophysiologic (acute alcohol use) factors; moreover, portal pressure and esophageal variceal pressure may vary at different times.

MEASUREMENT OF PORTAL PRESSURE

Portal pressure may be measured indirectly or directly. The most commonly used method of measuring portal pressure is determination of the hepatic vein pressure gradient (HVPG), which is an indirect method. Measurement of splenic pulp pressure and direct measurement of the portal vein pressure are infrequently used approaches because they are invasive and cumbersome. Variceal pressure also can be measured but is not routinely performed in clinical practice. Measurement of liver stiffness using ultrasound (e.g., transient) fibroelastography or magnetic resonance elastography (MRE) may indicate the presence of portal hypertension but cannot yet be used to measure portal pressure (see Chapters 73 and 74).

Hepatic Vein Pressure Gradient

The HVPG is the difference between the wedged hepatic venous pressure (WHVP) and free hepatic vein pressure (FHVP). The HVPG has been used to assess portal hypertension since its first description in 1951,[84] and has been validated as the best predictor for the development of complications of portal hypertension.

Measurement of the HVPG requires passage of a catheter into the hepatic vein under radiologic guidance until the catheter can be passed no further, that is, until the catheter has been "wedged" in the hepatic vein. The catheter can be passed into the hepatic vein through the femoral vein or using a transjugular venous approach. The purpose of wedging the catheter is to form a column of fluid that is continuous between the hepatic sinusoids and the catheter. Therefore, the measured pressure of fluid within the catheter reflects hepatic sinusoidal pressure. One of the drawbacks of using a catheter that is wedged in the hepatic vein is that the WHVP measured in a more fibrotic area of liver may be higher than the pressure measured in a less fibrotic area because of regional variation in the degree of fibrosis. Using a balloon-occluding catheter in the right hepatic vein to create a stagnant column of fluid in continuity with the hepatic sinusoids eliminates this variation in measurement of WHVP because the balloon catheter measures the WHVP averaged over a wide segment of the liver.[85] The pressure in the hepatic vein following deflation of the balloon is the FHVP.

HVPG measurement is not effective for detecting presinusoidal causes of portal hypertension. For example, in portal hypertension secondary to portal vein thrombosis, the HVPG is normal. Moreover, the HVPG may underestimate sinusoidal pressure in PBC and other presinusoidal causes of portal hypertension.[86] Therefore, the HVPG is accurate for detecting only sinusoidal and postsinusoidal causes of portal hypertension.

The HVPG represents the gradient between the pressure in the portal vein and the intra-abdominal inferior vena caval pressure (FHVP). By contrast, using the right atrial pressure as a reference for intra-abdominal pressure gives rise to an erroneous estimation of hepatic sinusoidal pressure.[87]

An elevation in intra-abdominal pressure increases both WHVP and FHVP equally, so that the HVPG is unchanged. The advantage of the HVPG is that variations in the "zero" reference point have no impact on the HVPG.[88] The HVPG is measured at least 3 times to demonstrate that the values are reproducible. Total occlusion of the hepatic vein by the inflated balloon to confirm that the balloon is in a wedged position is demonstrated by injecting contrast into the hepatic vein. A sinusoidal pattern should be seen, with no collateral circulation to other hepatic veins. The contrast washes out promptly with deflation of the balloon. Correct positioning of the balloon is also demonstrated by a sharp increase in the recorded pressure on inflation of the balloon. The pressure then becomes steady until the balloon is deflated, when the pressure drops sharply. In experienced hands, measurement of the HVPG is highly reproducible, accurate, and safe.

Measurement of the HVPG has been proposed for the following indications: (1) to monitor portal pressure in patients taking drugs used to prevent variceal bleeding, (2) as a prognostic marker,[89] (3) as an end point in trials using pharmacologic agents for the treatment of portal hypertension,[90] (4) to assess the risk of hepatic resection in patients with cirrhosis, and (5) to delineate the cause of portal hypertension (i.e., presinusoidal, sinusoidal, or postsinusoidal [Table 92-1]), usually in combination with venography, right-sided heart pressure measurements, and transjugular liver biopsy. Although the indication for HVPG measurement with the most potential for widespread use is monitoring the efficacy of therapies to reduce portal pressure, HVPG monitoring is not done routinely in clinical practice because no controlled trials have yet demonstrated its usefulness.[91]

Splenic Pulp Pressure

Determination of splenic pulp pressure is an indirect method of measuring portal pressure and involves puncture of the splenic pulp with a needle catheter. Splenic pulp pressure is elevated in presinusoidal portal hypertension, when the

TABLE 92-1 Use of Hepatic Vein Pressure Gradient in the Differential Diagnosis of Portal Hypertension

Type of Portal Hypertension	WHVP	FHVP	HVPG
Prehepatic	Normal	Normal	Normal
Presinusoidal	Normal	Normal	Normal
Sinusoidal	Increased	Normal	Increased
Postsinusoidal	Increased	Normal	Increased
Posthepatic Heart failure Budd-Chiari syndrome	Increased —	Increased Hepatic vein cannot be cannulated	Normal —

FHVP, free hepatic vein pressure; HVPG, hepatic vein pressure gradient; WHVP, wedged hepatic venous pressure.

HVPG is normal. Because of the potential risk of complications, especially bleeding, associated with splenic puncture, however, the procedure is rarely used.

Portal Vein Pressure

Direct measurement of the pressure in the portal vein is also a rarely used method that can be carried out through a percutaneous transhepatic route, transvenous approach, or, rarely, intraoperatively (although anesthesia can affect portal pressure). The transhepatic route requires portal vein puncture performed under US guidance. A catheter is then threaded over a guidewire into the main portal vein. With increasing use of the transjugular intrahepatic portosystemic shunt (TIPS) (see later), radiologists have gained expertise in puncturing the portal vein and measuring portal vein pressure by a transjugular route. Direct portal pressure measurements are carried out when HVPG cannot be measured, as in patients with occluded hepatic veins caused by the Budd-Chiari syndrome in whom a surgical portosystemic shunt is being contemplated[92] or in patients with intrahepatic, presinusoidal causes of portal hypertension, such as idiopathic portal hypertension, in which the HVPG may be normal.

Endoscopic Variceal Pressure

Varices rupture and bleed when the expanding force of intravariceal pressure exceeds variceal wall tension. Measurement of the difference between intravariceal pressure and pressure within the esophageal lumen (the transmural pressure gradient across the varices) is potentially a more important indicator of bleeding risk than measurement of HVPG,[93,94] especially in patients with portal vein thrombosis and other causes of portal hypertension associated with a normal HVPG.

Variceal pressure can be measured by various ways: insertion of a needle connected to a pressure transducer, use of a miniature pneumatic pressure sensitivity gauge at the tip of the endoscope, or manometry using an endoscopic balloon. Patients with previous variceal bleeding have been demonstrated to have higher variceal pressures than those in patients without previous bleeding.[95] A variceal pressure greater than 18 mm Hg during a bleeding episode is associated with failure to control bleeding and predicts early rebleeding.[96] Moreover, patients on pharmacologic therapy who show a decrease in variceal pressure of greater than 20% from baseline have a low probability of bleeding, as compared with patients who do not

demonstrate a greater than 20% decrease in variceal pressure, in whom the risk of variceal bleeding is 46%.[95] In general, techniques for measuring variceal pressure are still investigational and have not been found suitable for routine clinical use.

DETECTION OF VARICES

Upper GI Endoscopy

Upper GI endoscopy is the most commonly used method to detect varices. The consensus is that all patients with cirrhosis of the liver should be screened for esophageal varices by endoscopy. In patients in whom no varices are detected on initial endoscopy, endoscopy to screen for varices should be repeated in 2 to 3 years. If small varices are detected on the initial endoscopy, endoscopy should be repeated in 1 to 2 years.[97,98] None of the various noninvasive methods of determining which patients benefit most from endoscopic screening is accurate enough to recommend for routine use in clinical practice.[99] The role of noninvasive markers in predicting the risk of large esophageal varices requires study in large multicenter trials. Preliminary data suggest that wireless video capsule endoscopy (see Chapter 20)[100] and CT imaging are alternative screening modalities in patients who are not candidates for upper endoscopy. Moreover, CT screening may be more cost-effective than endoscopy.[101]

Endoscopic grading of esophageal varices is subjective. Various criteria have been used to try to standardize the reporting of esophageal varices. The best known of these criteria are those compiled by the Japanese Research Society for Portal Hypertension. The descriptors include red color signs, color of the varix, form (size) of the varix, and location of the varix.[102] Red color signs include red "wale" markings, which are longitudinal whip-like marks on the varix; cherry-red spots, which usually are 2 to 3 mm or less in diameter; hematocystic spots, which are blood-filled blisters 4 mm or greater in diameter; and diffuse redness. The color of the varix can be white or blue. The form of the varix at endoscopy is described most commonly. Esophageal varices may be small and straight (grade I), tortuous and occupying less than one third of the esophageal lumen (grade II), or large and occupying more than one third of the esophageal lumen (grade III). Varices can be in the lower third, middle third, or upper third of the esophagus. Of all of the aforementioned descriptors, the size of the varices in the lower third of the esophagus is the most important. The size of the varices in the lower third of the esophagus is determined during withdrawal of the endoscope (Fig. 92-6). Small varices are less than 5 mm in diameter, whereas large varices are greater than 5 mm in diameter.[102,103] As a point of reference, any varix larger in diameter than an open pinch biopsy forceps is likely to be greater than 5 mm in diameter. Patients with large esophageal varices, Child-Pugh class C cirrhosis (see later), and red color signs on varices have the highest risk of variceal bleeding within 1 year.[104] The increase in bleeding risk attributable to the presence of red color signs, however, is not independent of the risk associated with large variceal size. Therefore, prophylactic treatment to prevent variceal bleeding is recommended in all patients with large esophageal varices irrespective of the presence or absence of red color signs (see later).

US

US examination of the liver with Doppler study of the vessels has been used widely to assess patients with portal hypertension. Features suggestive of portal hypertension on US include

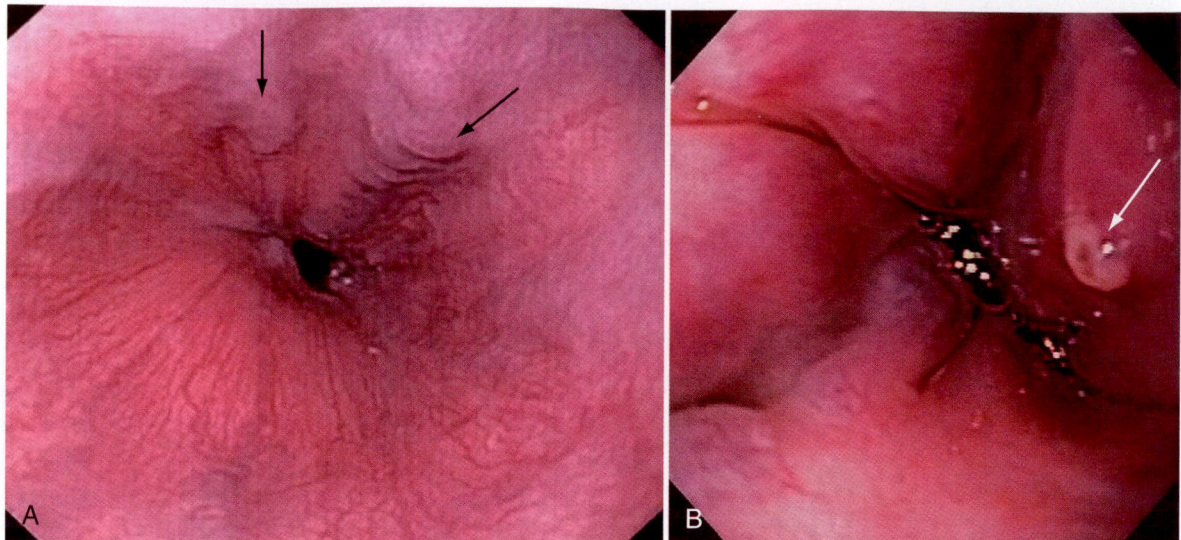

FIGURE 92-6. Endoscopic appearances of esophageal varices. *A,* Upper GI endoscopy demonstrates dilated and straight veins (small esophageal varices) in the distal esophagus *(arrows). B,* Upper GI endoscopy demonstrates large esophageal varices, greater than 5 mm in diameter, with a fibrin plug *(arrow)* indicating the site of a recent bleed.

splenomegaly, portosystemic collateral vessels, and reversal of the direction of flow in the portal vein (hepatofugal flow). Some studies have demonstrated that a portal vein diameter greater than 13 mm and the absence of respiratory variations in the splenic and mesenteric veins are sensitive but nonspecific markers of portal hypertension.[105,106] These criteria are not used routinely in clinical practice in most centers. US examination can detect thrombosis of the portal vein, which appears as nonvisualization or cavernous transformation (a cavernoma) of the portal vein; the latter finding indicates an extensive collateral network in place of the portal vein.[107] Splenic vein thrombosis also can be demonstrated. Although Doppler US is clinically useful in the initial evaluation of portal hypertension, the technique is not widely used to provide quantitative assessments of the degree of portal hypertension. US elastography of the liver and spleen may be useful in detecting portal hypertension but is not sufficiently sensitive to recommend as a modality to monitor decreases in portal pressure in patients on pharmacotherapy (see Chapter 73).[108] In one study, however, liver stiffness was the single best noninvasive variable for identifying patients most likely to have large esophageal varices, especially when combined with a low platelet count and increased spleen size.[109] A combination of liver and spleen stiffness measured by acoustic radiation force impulse (ARFI) elastography may also identify patients at risk for esophageal varices.[110]

CT

CT is useful for demonstrating many features of portal hypertension, including abnormal configuration of the liver, ascites, splenomegaly, and collateral vessels (Figs. 92-7 and 92-8). Detection of varices may be an emerging indication for CT. The detection of fundal varices by multidetector CT (MDCT) is at least as accurate as EUS (see later). CT is especially helpful in distinguishing submucosal from perigastric fundal varices[111] and is considered a less invasive alternative to conventional angiographic portography in assessing portosystemic collaterals. Nevertheless, CT is not yet a recommended screening method for detecting large esophageal varices but may ultimately be confirmed as a cost-effective method of screening for varices and preferable to endoscopy by patients.[101]

MRI

Gadolinium-enhanced MRI is a potentially useful method of detecting esophageal varices.[112] In addition, MRI can be used to measure portal and azygos blood flow, which is increased in patients with portal hypertension.[113] MRI provides excellent detail of the vascular structures of the liver and can detect portal venous thrombosis and spleen stiffness in patients with portal hypertension. Unlike US elastography, MR elastography can accurately assess the stiffness of fatty livers.[114] The role of MRI in the assessment of portal hypertension requires further study.

EUS

EUS examination (endosonography) using radial or linear array echo-endoscopes or EUS mini-probes passed through the working channel of a diagnostic endoscope has been applied to the evaluation of patients with varices. EUS has been used to study several aspects of esophageal varices, including the cross-sectional area of varices to identify patients at increased risk of bleeding[83]; size of and flow in the left gastric vein, azygos vein, and paraesophageal collaterals; changes after endoscopic therapy; and recurrence of esophageal varices following variceal ligation (see later).[115] Endosonography can be combined with endoscopic measurement of transmural variceal pressure to allow estimation of variceal wall tension, which is a predictor of variceal bleeding (see earlier).[116-118] Endosonography may be used to target varices for sclerotherapy or glue injection.[119]

CAUSES OF PORTAL HYPERTENSION

The usual classification of causes of portal hypertension is based on the site of increased resistance to portal blood flow—namely, prehepatic, intrahepatic, and posthepatic—and is outlined in Figure 92-5. Intrahepatic sites of increased resistance can be presinusoidal, sinusoidal, or postsinusoidal. Many causes of portal hypertension are associated with an increase in resistance at more than one site. For example, alcoholic cirrhosis may be associated with increased resistance at the

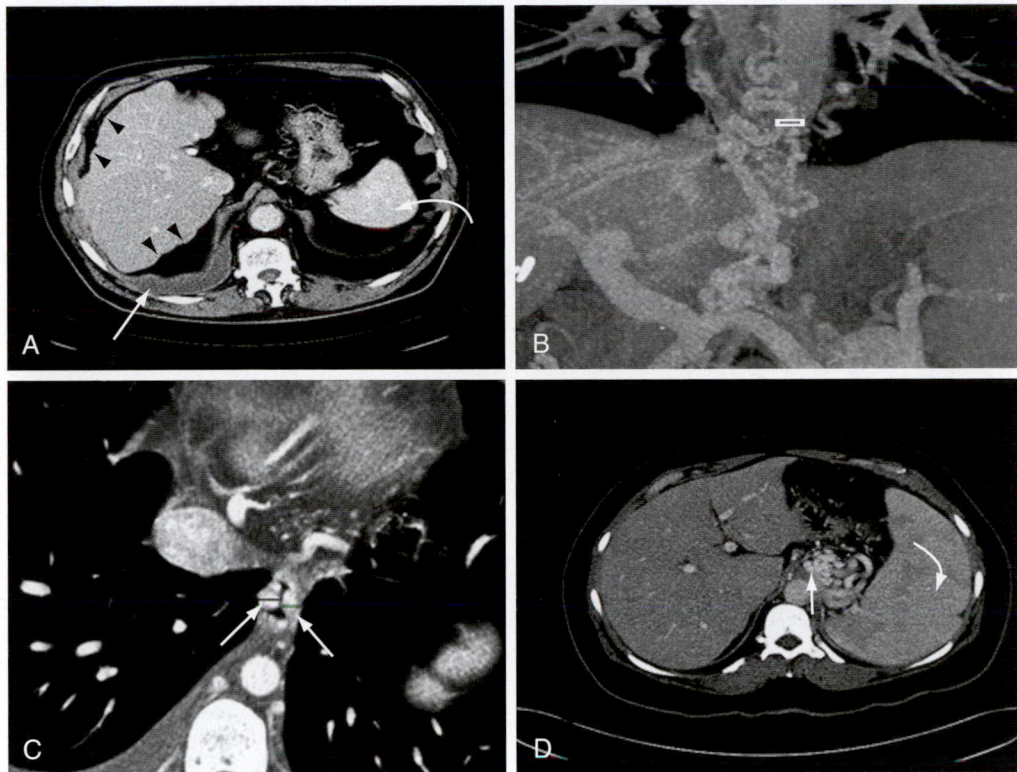

FIGURE 92-7. Abdominal CT in patients with portal hypertension. *A,* Image showing an irregular contour of the liver typical of cirrhosis *(arrowheads).* A small right pleural effusion is evident *(straight arrow).* The liver is hypointense relative to the spleen *(curved arrow),* typical of fatty infiltration of the liver in alcoholic cirrhosis. *B,* Coronal section of a CT showing contrast-enhanced esophageal varices *(cursor). C,* Image showing 2 large esophageal varices *(arrows)* 5 mm and 6 mm in diameter. Varices are almost opposed to each other. *D,* Image showing a tuft of gastroesophageal collaterals *(straight arrow).* The enlarged spleen is also seen *(curved arrow).*

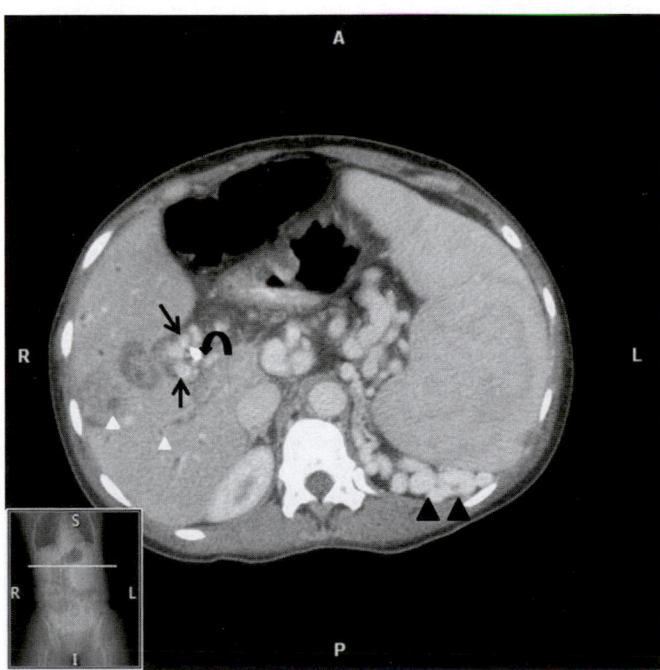

FIGURE 92-8. CT showing choledochal varices *(arrows)* surrounding a stent in the bile duct *(curved arrow).* Dilated bile ducts *(white arrowheads)* and perisplenic varices *(black arrowheads)* are also seen.

BOX 92-1 Causes of Portal Hypertension

Common
Cirrhosis
Schistosomiasis
Extrahepatic portal vein thrombosis
Idiopathic portal hypertension
Cardiac fibrosis

Less Common
Nodular regenerative hyperplasia
Partial nodular transformation of the liver
Fibropolycystic liver disease
Sarcoidosis
Malignancy
Splanchnic arteriovenous fistula
Hereditary hemorrhagic telangiectasia

presinusoidal, sinusoidal, and postsinusoidal levels. Therefore, classification based on the site of resistance may not be possible for all diseases that cause portal hypertension. A more useful classification is clinically based and considers common and less common causes of portal hypertension (Box 92-1).

Common Causes

Cirrhosis

Complications related to portal hypertension are the usual clinical manifestations of cirrhosis of the liver (see Chapter 74).

Although all causes of cirrhosis are associated with portal hypertension, some features are disease specific. In alcoholic liver disease, elevation of the portal pressure is accurately reflected by the HVPG; moreover, portal hypertension may occur in the absence of cirrhosis but is more marked when cirrhosis is present. Perivenular lesions implicated in the pathogenesis of noncirrhotic alcoholic liver injury account for the presinusoidal component of portal hypertension in these patients (see Chapter 86).[120] Autoimmune hepatitis also may be associated with portal hypertension in the absence of cirrhosis[121]; however, the risk of variceal bleeding is low in patients with autoimmune hepatitis (see Chapter 90). In patients with hemochromatosis, portal hypertension may be seen even before cirrhosis; the severity of portal hypertension increases with increasing fibrosis. Patients with hemochromatosis may bleed from varices despite an HVPG less than 12 mm Hg, indicating a presinusoidal component of portal hypertension. Phlebotomy therapy in patients with hemochromatosis may result in a decrease in portal hypertension (see Chapter 75).[122] In patients with PBC as well, portal hypertension may occur before cirrhosis has developed. The risk of variceal bleeding increases with an increase in the histologic stage of the disease.[123] In earlier stages of PBC, portal hypertension is predominantly presinusoidal, but as the disease progresses, a sinusoidal component develops. Therefore, the HVPG may underestimate portal pressure in patients with PBC.[86] Treatment of PBC with ursodeoxycholic acid may result in a decrease in portal pressure (see Chapter 91). Portal hypertension occurs in patients with PSC (see Chapter 68) and in those with biliary strictures (see Chapter 70). A long duration of biliary obstruction usually is required, although portal hypertension has been known to develop in a few months in patients with chronic bile duct obstruction caused by chronic alcoholic pancreatitis (see Chapter 59).[124] Portal hypertension in patients with biliary obstruction regresses following relief of the biliary obstruction. Signs of portal hypertension are present in 25% of patients at the time of diagnosis of NAFLD with advanced fibrosis or cirrhosis; however, portal hypertension may occur even in the absence of fibrosis if steatosis is extensive (see Chapter 87).[125]

Schistosomiasis

Schistosomiasis may be the most common cause of portal hypertension worldwide (see Chapter 84). Bleeding from esophageal varices is a major cause of death in patients with hepatosplenic schistosomiasis. Portal hypertension results from presinusoidal obstruction caused by deposition of eggs of *Schistosoma mansoni* and *Schistosoma japonicum* in the presinusoidal portal venules. The host reaction results in granulomatous inflammation, which causes presinusoidal and periportal fibrosis.[126] The fibrosis that results is sometimes called "clay pipestem" or simply "pipestem" fibrosis and is usually associated with sustained heavy infection. The periportal collagen deposition leads to progressive obstruction of portal blood flow, portal hypertension, and variceal bleeding, along with splenomegaly and hypersplenism. Lobular architecture usually is preserved. Coinfection with hepatitis B or C virus in patients with hepatic schistosomiasis can result in more rapid progression of fibrosis, hepatic failure, and an increased risk of hepatocellular carcinoma.[127]

In the initial stages of schistosomiasis, the HVPG is normal owing to the presinusoidal nature of the obstruction. Some patients with schistosomiasis and portal hypertension may also have portal vein thrombosis. Patients with schistosomiasis often undergo portosystemic shunt surgery to treat variceal bleeding, with excellent long-term outcomes.

Extrahepatic Portal Vein Thrombosis

Extrahepatic portal vein thrombosis is a prehepatic, presinusoidal cause of portal hypertension and a common cause of portal hypertension in children (see Chapter 85). The most common causes of portal vein thrombosis include hematologic disorders such as polycythemia vera or other myeloproliferative neoplasms. Other causes include a prothrombotic state, such as antithrombin, protein C, or protein S deficiency; antiphospholipid syndrome (or antiphospholipid antibody syndrome); paroxysmal nocturnal hemoglobinuria; oral contraceptive use; a neoplasm, usually intra-abdominal; an inflammatory disease, such as pancreatitis, IBD, or diverticulitis; abdominal trauma; and postoperative states, especially post splenectomy. Portal vein thrombosis may develop in up to 25% of patients with cirrhosis.[128] The association with hepatocellular carcinoma may not be as strong as previously thought. Isolated splenic vein thrombosis caused by a pancreatic neoplasm or pancreatitis usually is not associated with a thrombophilia. Umbilical vein sepsis may be an etiologic factor in children with portal vein thrombosis, but even in these cases, an associated prothrombotic state may be an additional predisposing factor.

Acute and subacute portal vein thrombosis usually does not manifest with variceal bleeding.[1] Chronic portal vein thrombosis is suggested by nonvisualization of the portal or splenic vein and an extensive collateral circulation on imaging studies. Patients may present with nonspecific symptoms or with variceal bleeding and hypersplenism. Bleeding is usually from gastroesophageal varices but may be from duodenal varices and, rarely, other ectopic sites. Gallbladder varices have also been described in patients with portal vein thrombosis.[129]

The treatment of chronic portal vein thrombosis is symptomatic, with the aim of controlling variceal bleeding or preventing recurrent variceal bleeding. Patients in whom esophageal varices are not large, and a thrombophilia is detected, are best managed with anticoagulation because in these patients the benefits of anticoagulation outweigh the risks.[130] Local or systemic thrombolytic therapy is seldom required and is generally reserved for patients in whom an acute portal vein thrombus extends into the superior mesenteric vein, with danger of impending intestinal ischemia. Endoscopic therapy is used to control acute variceal bleeding and to prevent recurrent bleeding. Use of pharmacologic agents such as beta blockers to prevent variceal bleeding is probably also effective in patients with portal vein thrombosis, but this approach has not been well studied. Patients with portal vein thrombosis have lower mortality and morbidity rates from variceal bleeding than those reported in patients with cirrhosis and variceal bleeding, owing to the lack of coagulopathy and synthetic liver dysfunction. Surgical portosystemic shunt procedures are carried out in patients in whom bleeding cannot be controlled by conservative measures. If a suitable vein is not available for anastomosis, a large collateral vein may be anastomosed to a systemic vein.[131] The mesenterico–left portal venous bypass discussed later is especially effective because it preserves portal blood flow and avoids hepatic encephalopathy while decompressing the portal venous system.[132] Placement of a TIPS is possible in many patients with chronic portal vein thrombosis and cirrhosis, with excellent long-term patency.[133]

Idiopathic Portal Hypertension

Idiopathic portal hypertension is uncommon in Western countries but is common in parts of Asia such as India and Japan. This disorder is diagnosed when portal pressure is elevated in the absence of significant histologic changes in the liver or extrahepatic portal vein obstruction.[134] A liver biopsy specimen from affected patients may be entirely normal,[135] although increased concentrations of ET-1 have been noted in the periportal hepatocytes, portal venules, and hepatic sinusoids of patients with idiopathic portal hypertension.[136] Various terms used (rather loosely) to describe idiopathic portal hypertension include *hepatoportal sclerosis*, *noncirrhotic portal fibrosis*, and *Banti's syndrome*.[137,138] Some authors include nodular regenerative hyperplasia and incomplete septal fibrosis under the broad term *idiopathic portal hypertension*.[139] Use of the term is probably best restricted to portal hypertension in patients in whom no hepatic lesion is found on light microscopy and the portal venous system is patent. The term *hepatoportal sclerosis* is used when there is obliterative portal venopathy with subendothelial thickening of the intrahepatic portal veins; thrombosis and recanalization of these veins may follow. Fibrosis of the portal tracts is prominent later in the course.

The cause of idiopathic portal hypertension is unclear in a majority of patients, although chronic arsenic intoxication, exposure to vinyl chloride, and hypervitaminosis A have been implicated (see Chapter 89). These etiologic factors are present in only a minority of patients. The dominant clinical features of the condition are variceal bleeding and hypersplenism related to a markedly enlarged spleen. Liver biochemical test levels are usually normal, although the serum alkaline phosphatase level may be mildly elevated. Ascites is uncommon. The HVPG in this disorder is usually normal because the site of increased resistance is presinusoidal.[140] Surgical portosystemic shunts are well tolerated in these patients, although hepatic encephalopathy may occur on long-term follow-up.[135] Liver transplantation is rarely required in these patients, but patients with idiopathic portal hypertension may have reduced survival.[141] Hypersplenism in idiopathic portal hypertension is seldom severe enough to require a splenectomy.

Cardiac Fibrosis

Cardiac fibrosis (or cardiac cirrhosis) has been recognized in patients with long-standing passive congestion of the liver due to heart failure and increasingly in patients with complex congenital heart disease who have had corrective surgery in childhood and live beyond the second decade of life (see Chapter 85). Cirrhosis occurs especially in patients who have undergone a Fontan procedure, which allows systemic venous blood flow to enter the pulmonary artery and bypass the right ventricle. Long-term sequelae of the Fontan procedure include complications of portal hypertension and hepatocellular carcinoma; variceal bleeding may occur.

Less Common Causes

Nodular Regenerative Hyperplasia

Nodular regenerative hyperplasia is a histopathologic diagnosis characterized by atrophy of zone 3 hepatocytes and hypertrophy of zone 1 hepatocytes, without significant fibrosis (see Chapters 36 and 96).[142] This disorder has been recognized increasingly as a cause of portal hypertension and may even occur after liver transplantation.[143] Similar histologic changes may be seen in well-established Budd-Chiari syndrome.[144] The nodular hyperplasia may not be apparent on histologic examination unless a reticulin stain is carried out to demonstrate the micronodules. The changes are believed to result from an imbalance between hyperperfused areas of the liver, with resulting regenerative nodules, and poorly perfused areas, with resulting atrophy. Nodular regenerative hyperplasia is

associated with a variety of conditions, predominantly hematologic and rheumatologic (see Chapter 36). Mild elevation of the serum aminotransferase levels is seen. Portal hypertension manifesting as variceal bleeding is the predominant clinical presentation. Ascites also may develop in these patients, suggesting that an increase in sinusoidal pressure occurs.[145] Hepatocellular carcinoma does not occur, but liver transplantation may be required in some patients.

Partial Nodular Transformation of the Liver

Partial nodular transformation of the liver is an uncommon lesion that is characterized by large nodules in the perihilar region.[146] These nodules may be visible on imaging studies of the liver. The rest of the liver may be normal or may show changes of nodular regenerative hyperplasia. Liver biochemical test levels usually are normal. Like nodular regenerative hyperplasia, partial nodular transformation of the liver is believed to be related to an imbalance in portal perfusion of the liver, but the abnormality is restricted to the hilar branches, whereas in nodular regenerative hyperplasia the abnormality is more diffuse. Variceal bleeding is the predominant presentation, although patients with large nodules may experience abdominal pain. Hepatocellular carcinoma may rarely develop in a regenerative nodule. Treatment with a surgical portosystemic shunt is associated with good long-term results.

Fibropolycystic Liver Disease

Fibropolycystic liver disease is a term that encompasses Caroli's disease; Caroli's syndrome (or complex), which consists of Caroli's disease and congenital hepatic fibrosis; congenital hepatic fibrosis alone; and polycystic liver disease (see Chapter 96). Congenital hepatic fibrosis usually occurs in association with Caroli's disease of the liver, polycystic disease of the kidney, and medullary sponge kidney (see Chapter 62). The major manifestation of congenital hepatic fibrosis is variceal bleeding.[147] A portosystemic shunt may be placed in affected patients to treat refractory variceal bleeding, with a low long-term risk of hepatic encephalopathy. Patients with polycystic liver disease, whether associated with polycystic kidney disease or not, rarely present with portal hypertension (see Chapter 96)[148]; portal hypertension, if present, may decrease after treatment of the cysts.[149]

Sarcoidosis

Portal hypertension is an uncommon manifestation of hepatic sarcoidosis (see Chapter 36).[150] The site of increased intrahepatic resistance in patients with sarcoidosis seems to be postsinusoidal, in view of the elevated HVPG. In early disease, however, the resistance is predominantly at a presinusoidal level. Treatment with glucocorticoids may decrease portal hypertension in some patients with hepatic sarcoidosis.

Malignancy

Portal hypertension has been associated with leukemias, lymphomas, and systemic mastocytosis (see Chapters 31 and 36).[151] Portal hypertension may also occur in patients with hepatocellular carcinoma independent of the presence of cirrhosis (see Chapter 96). The pathogenesis of portal hypertension in patients with hepatocellular carcinoma is thought to be multifactorial; contributing factors include portal vein thrombosis, pressure by the tumor on the portal vein, and, in some cases, a hepatic artery–portal vein fistula. Esophageal varices may be seen in patients with hepatic metastases, although variceal bleeding is unusual.[152]

Splanchnic Arteriovenous Fistula

A splanchnic AVF should be suspected when the onset of ascites and variceal bleeding is acute, especially in the presence of an abdominal bruit. When a splanchnic artery ruptures into a mesenteric vein, the portal pressure increases acutely, reaching levels of systemic arterial pressure.[153] The result is acute portal hypertension with development of ascites and variceal bleeding. A bruit may be heard in the left upper quadrant of the abdomen with a splenic AVF and in the right upper quadrant with a hepatic artery–portal vein fistula. With a long-standing fistula, secondary perisinusoidal hepatic fibrosis related to an increase in portal venous inflow may develop. In the early stages, embolization or ligation of the fistula will ameliorate the portal hypertension. In late stages, however, portal fibrosis may be advanced, and portal hypertension may not correct completely with embolization of the fistula.

Hereditary Hemorrhagic Telangiectasia

Hereditary hemorrhagic telangiectasia (HHT), or Osler-Weber-Rendu disease, is an unusual cause of portal hypertension (see also Chapters 20, 36, and 85). Diagnostic criteria include mucocutaneous telangiectasias, epistaxis, AVFs of the viscera (usually lung or liver), and a family history of the disorder. Manifestations of HHT depend on the site of fistula formation. A fistula between the hepatic artery and hepatic vein manifests predominantly as biliary disease, mainly biliary strictures and cholangitis, and high-output cardiac failure. A fistula between the hepatic artery and portal vein results in portal hypertension and biliary strictures, whereas a fistula between the portal vein and hepatic vein, which is rare, results in hepatic encephalopathy.[154] Nodular regenerative hyperplasia, which develops in some patients with HHT, may worsen portal hypertension.[155] Treatment with bevacizumab may ameliorate the vascular lesions.[156]

CLINICAL ASSESSMENT

Patients with esophageal or gastric variceal bleeding present with hematemesis or melena (or both). Chronic blood loss is a more common presentation of portal hypertensive gastropathy or GI vascular ectasia. The classic presentation of patients with variceal bleeding is with effortless and recurrent hematemesis; the vomitus is described as dark red in color (see Chapter 20).

Portal hypertension should be suspected in all patients with GI bleeding and peripheral stigmata of liver disease (see Chapter 74)—namely, jaundice, spider telangiectasias, palmar erythema, Dupuytren's contractures, parotid enlargement, testicular atrophy, loss of secondary sexual characteristics, ascites, and encephalopathy. Splenomegaly is an important clue to the presence of portal hypertension, and the presence of ascites makes the presence of esophageal varices even more likely. A bruit may be heard in the left or the right upper quadrant in a patient with a splanchnic AVF. A venous hum may be heard in the epigastrium in a patient with portal hypertension and represents collateral flow in the falciform ligament.

Laboratory studies frequently reveal evidence of hepatic synthetic dysfunction, including prolongation of the prothrombin time, hypoalbuminemia, and hyperbilirubinemia, as well as anemia. Thrombocytopenia and leukopenia, reflecting hypersplenism and, in alcoholics, bone marrow suppression,

may be noted. Patients with severe bleeding may present with hypovolemic shock and renal insufficiency. Abdominal imaging studies frequently reveal splenomegaly, collateral vessels, abnormal liver echotexture and contour, and ascites.

TREATMENT

The treatment of portal hypertension is aimed either at reducing portal blood flow with pharmacologic agents, such as beta blockers or vasopressin and its analogs, or at decreasing intrahepatic resistance with pharmacologic agents, such as nitrates, or by radiologic or surgical creation of a portosystemic shunt. Treatment also may be directed at the varices with use of endoscopic or radiologic techniques.

Pharmacologic Therapy

The pharmacologic agents used in the treatment of portal hypertension are divided into 2 groups: those that decrease splanchnic blood flow and those that decrease intrahepatic vascular resistance (Box 92-2). The agents that decrease splanchnic blood flow acutely are vasopressin and its analogs and somatostatin and its analogs. β-Adrenergic blocking agents also decrease portal blood flow but are used only to prevent variceal bleeding and rebleeding. Agents that target intrahepatic vascular resistance include α-adrenergic blocking agents, angiotensin receptor blocking agents, and nitrates, but only carvedilol and nitrates are now considered for clinical use. Diuretics, by decreasing plasma volume, may reduce portal pressure but are not recommended if the patient does not have ascites. Metoclopramide and other gastric prokinetic agents may decrease intravariceal pressure by contracting the lower esophageal sphincter but have not been evaluated in clinical trials.

Vasopressin and Its Analogs

Vasopressin is an endogenous peptide hormone that causes splanchnic vasoconstriction, reduces portal venous inflow, and reduces portal pressure. This drug is associated with serious systemic side effects, however. By causing constriction of systemic vessels, vasopressin may result in necrosis of the bowel. Additionally, vasopressin has direct negative inotropic and chronotropic effects on the myocardium that lead to reduced cardiac output and bradycardia, respectively. An increase in cardiac afterload can result in myocardial infarction, and antidiuresis, resulting from the action of vasopressin on the kidney, can result in hyponatremia.

Terlipressin, or triglycyl-lysine-vasopressin, is a semisynthetic analog of vasopressin that is cleaved by endothelial

---

BOX 92-2 Drugs Used in the Treatment of Portal Hypertension

Drugs That Decrease Portal Blood Flow
Nonselective β-adrenergic blocking agents
Somatostatin and its analogs
Vasopressin and terlipressin

Drugs That Decrease Intrahepatic Resistance
α_1-Adrenergic blocking agents (e.g., prazosin)
Angiotensin receptor blocking agents
Nitrates

peptidases to release lysine vasopressin. Compared with vasopressin, terlipressin results in lower circulatory levels of the vasopressin analog and a lower rate of systemic side effects. Vasopressin and terlipressin have been used in combination with nitrates to decrease the risk of systemic side effects. Terlipressin is preferred over vasopressin because of its superior safety profile. In addition, an increase in survival has been demonstrated in patients with variceal bleeding treated with terlipressin.

Somatostatin and Its Analogs

Somatostatin is a 14–amino acid peptide. Five somatostatin receptors—SRTR 1 to SRTR 5—are recognized, but the actual distribution of the receptors in humans is not clear. Following IV injection, somatostatin has a half-life in the circulation of 1 to 3 minutes; therefore, longer-acting analogs of somatostatin have been synthesized. The best known of these analogs are octreotide, lanreotide, and vapreotide.[157] Somatostatin decreases portal pressure and collateral blood flow by inhibiting release of glucagon.[158] The optimal dose and duration of use of somatostatin have not been adequately studied. Following a single 250-µg bolus injection of somatostatin, portal and azygos blood flow decrease, but the effect lasts only a few minutes.[159] Use of higher doses is associated with a more impressive decrease in HVPG. Somatostatin also decreases portal pressure by decreasing postprandial splanchnic blood flow.[160] Following a variceal bleed, blood in the GI tract acts like a meal, leading to an increase in portal flow and elevation in the portal pressure; this elevation in pressure is ameliorated by the use of somatostatin.

Following IV administration, octreotide has a half-life in the circulation of 80 to 120 minutes. Its effect on portal pressure is not prolonged, however. Moreover, continuous infusion of octreotide does not decrease portal pressure despite decreasing the postprandial increase in portal pressure.[67,161] Long-acting octreotide does not reliably reduce portal pressure, and side effects with higher doses preclude use of this agent for the treatment of portal hypertension.[162]

Some randomized controlled trials support the view that somatostatin or octreotide may be equivalent in efficacy to terlipressin or sclerotherapy (see later) for controlling acute variceal bleeding. Also, early administration of vapreotide may be associated with improved control of bleeding, but without a significant reduction in mortality rate.[163] In clinical practice, somatostatin or octreotide administration is combined with endoscopic management of variceal bleeding (see later).

β-Adrenergic Blocking Agents

Nonselective β-adrenergic blocking agents have been used extensively since the landmark study of Lebrec and colleagues demonstrated the efficacy of these agents in preventing variceal rebleeding.[164] Nonselective beta blockers such as propranolol or nadolol are preferred. Blockade of β_1-adrenergic receptors in the heart decreases cardiac output. Blockade of β_2-adrenergic receptors, which cause vasodilatation in the mesenteric circulation, allows unopposed action of α_1-adrenergic receptors and results in decreased portal flow. The combination of decreased cardiac output and decreased portal flow leads to a decrease in portal pressure. Nadolol has advantages over propranolol in that it is excreted predominantly by the kidney, has low lipid solubility, and is associated with a lower risk of central nervous system side effects such as depression. The effectiveness of beta blockers is assessed most accurately by monitoring the HVPG; this

approach is not widely used in clinical practice. The acute hemodynamic response (decrease in HVPG to < 12 mm Hg, or by 10%) 20 minutes after administration of IV propranolol may be used to predict the long-term reduction in bleeding risk.[165] The benefit of beta blockers is reduced when hepatic function worsens.[166] The usual method of monitoring the efficacy of beta blockers is to observe a decrease in the heart rate, which is a measure of β_1-adrenergic receptor blockade. Despite adequate β_1-adrenergic receptor blockade, however, some patients might benefit from a further increase in the dose of beta blocker to increase the degree of β_2-adrenergic blockade. Raising the dose, however, results in more side effects and the likelihood that treatment will need to be withdrawn.[167]

In patients with refractory ascites, beta blocker use may be associated with increased mortality. Therefore, the drug needs to be discontinued in patients with ascites who have worsening renal function (see Chapter 93).[168]

Combined α- and β-Adrenergic Blocking Agents

Carvedilol is a drug that has both nonselective β-blocker and weak α-receptor blockade activity. α-Receptor activity normally increases resistance within the intrahepatic circulation. Therefore, blockade of the α-receptor decreases intrahepatic vascular resistance, which results in a further reduction in portal pressure. Carvedilol may be associated with hypotension and renal sodium retention and should be used cautiously in patients with Child-Pugh class C cirrhosis. Carvedilol is also known to have antioxidant as well as antiproliferative actions and may be superior to endoscopic variceal ligation in the prevention of a first variceal bleed.[68] In a 2013 study, patients with cirrhosis were randomized to either carvedilol 12.5 mg once daily or endoscopic variceal ligation performed every 2 weeks; carvedilol was associated with a lower bleeding risk (10% vs. 23%), but neither overall nor bleeding-related mortality was reduced. Additionally, carvedilol has been demonstrated to be equivalent to a combination of nadolol and isosorbide mononitrate in reducing variceal rebleeding, with fewer side effects.[169] Carvedilol is started in a dose of 6.25 mg once daily, and the dose is increased stepwise to a maximum of 25 mg daily. Dose increases are usually limited by arterial hypotension.[170]

Nitrates

Short-acting (nitroglycerin) or long-acting (isosorbide mononitrate) nitrates result in vasodilatation. The vasodilatation results from a decrease in intracellular calcium in vascular smooth muscle cells. Nitrates cause venodilatation, rather than arterial dilatation, and decrease portal pressure predominantly by decreasing portal venous blood flow. The effect on intrahepatic resistance is less impressive than generally has been believed. Nitroglycerin has been used in combination with vasopressin to control acute variceal bleeding. The rate of infusion of nitroglycerin is 50 to 400 µg per minute, provided that the systolic blood pressure is greater than 90 mm Hg; however, the combination of vasopressin and nitroglycerin is seldom used nowadays. Nitrates are no longer recommended, either alone or in combination with a beta blocker, for primary prophylaxis to prevent first variceal bleeds. For secondary prophylaxis (to prevent variceal rebleeding), isosorbide mononitrate may be added to a beta blocker if the beta blocker alone has not resulted in an appropriate decrease in HVPG. In the United States, it is unusual for patients to tolerate nitrates for any length of time because of side effects, especially hypotension and headaches.

Drugs That Decrease Intrahepatic Vascular Resistance

The ideal agent for treatment of portal hypertension would be a drug that selectively decreases intrahepatic vascular resistance without worsening systemic vasodilatation. Besides carvedilol and nitrates, agents that may decrease intrahepatic resistance include α_1-adrenergic blockers such as prazosin, but long-term administration of prazosin causes worsening of the systemic hyperdynamic circulation associated with portal hypertension and consequent sodium retention and ascites.[171] The addition of propranolol to prazosin may ameliorate the adverse effects of prazosin on the systemic circulation. Losartan, an angiotensin II receptor type I antagonist, causes a reduction in portal pressure without significant effects on the systemic circulation.[172] In randomized controlled trials of losartan or another angiotensin II receptor antagonist, irbesartan, however, portal pressure was not reduced significantly. In fact, renal function has worsened in patients given losartan or irbesartan.[173,174] ET-receptor blockers and liver-selective NO donors are promising investigational agents for therapies that target intrahepatic vascular resistance.[17] Simvastatin may decrease intrahepatic resistance and maintain hepatic blood flow while decreasing portal pressure.[22]

Endoscopic Therapy

Endoscopic therapy is the only treatment modality that is widely accepted for the prevention of variceal bleeding, control of acute variceal bleeding, and prevention of variceal rebleeding. Endoscopic variceal therapy includes variceal sclerotherapy and band ligation.

Sclerotherapy

Endoscopic sclerotherapy has largely been supplanted by endoscopic band ligation, except when poor visualization precludes effective band ligation of bleeding varices. Available evidence does not support emergency sclerotherapy as first-line treatment of variceal bleeding (Box 92-3).[175] The technique involves injection of a sclerosant into (intravariceal) or adjacent to (paravariceal) a varix. Some paravariceal injection usually takes place during attempted intravariceal therapy. The sclerosants used include sodium tetradecyl sulfate, sodium morrhuate, ethanolamine oleate, and absolute alcohol; the choice of a sclerosant is based on availability, rather than on superior efficacy of one agent over another.

BOX 92-3 Complications of Endoscopic Variceal Therapy*

During Procedure
Aspiration pneumonia
Retrosternal chest pain

Following Procedure
Bleeding
Esophageal dysmotility
Esophageal stricture
Esophageal ulcers
Mediastinitis
Perforation

Systemic (Usually with Sclerotherapy)
Mesenteric venous thrombosis
Pulmonary embolism
Sepsis

*Sclerotherapy and band ligation.

Complications of endoscopic sclerotherapy may arise during or after the procedure. During injection, the patient may experience some degree of retrosternal discomfort, which may persist after the procedure. More serious complications include sclerosant-induced esophageal ulcer-related bleeding, strictures, and perforation. The risk of ulcers caused by sclerotherapy may be reduced by use of oral sucralfate or a PPI after sclerotherapy.

Variceal Ligation

Endoscopic variceal ligation is the preferred endoscopic modality for control of acute esophageal variceal bleeding and prevention of rebleeding; however, the utility of band ligation in the treatment of gastric varices is limited. Variceal ligation is simpler to perform than injection sclerotherapy. The procedure involves suctioning of the varix into a cap fitted on the tip of an endoscope and deploying a band around the varix. The band strangulates the varix, thereby causing thrombosis. Multi-band devices can be used to apply several bands without requiring withdrawal and reinsertion of the endoscope. Varices at the gastroesophageal junction are banded initially, and then more proximal varices are banded in a spiral manner at intervals of approximately 2 cm; the endoscope is then withdrawn. Varices in the mid- or proximal esophagus do not need to be banded. Endoscopic variceal ligation is associated with fewer complications than sclerotherapy and requires fewer sessions to achieve variceal obliteration. Moreover, esophageal variceal ligation during an acute bleed is not associated with a sustained elevation in HVPG, as occurs with sclerotherapy.[176]

Endoscopic variceal ligation can cause local complications, including esophageal ulcers (Fig. 92-9), strictures, and dysmotility, albeit less frequently than does sclerotherapy. Banding-induced ulcers can be large and potentially serious if gastric fundal varices are banded. A PPI is usually recommended after variceal ligation, even though data to support PPI use are limited.

Detachable Snares and Clips

Detachable snares have generally been used in the treatment of large polyps in the colon. There is only limited experience with detachable snares for treatment of gastric varices. The "tails" on the detachable snare can interfere with visualization at endoscopy. Furthermore, traction on the varix during detachment of the snare can result in a variceal tear. The snares are technically difficult to apply, thereby limiting their widespread use in treatment of gastric varices. Snares are not superior to endoscopic variceal ligation in the treatment of esophageal varices, and the difficulty in application of snares makes them an unattractive option. Clips have also been used to treat large varices, especially at ectopic sites, but experience is limited (see Chapter 20).

Balloon Tamponade and Stents

From 10% to 15% of patients with an acute variceal bleeding are refractory to pharmacologic and endoscopic treatment. Balloon tamponade is used as a temporizing measure until TIPS can be carried out. Varices are easily compressed because they are superficial and thin-walled and the flow of blood is via submucosal vessels. The Sengstaken-Blakemore tube is a triple-lumen tube: one tube is for aspirating gastric contents, the other allows inflation of a gastric balloon to 200 to 400 mL in volume, and the third inflates an esophageal balloon. The Minnesota tube is a modified Sengstaken-Blakemore tube, with the modifications being a larger gastric balloon (500 mL)

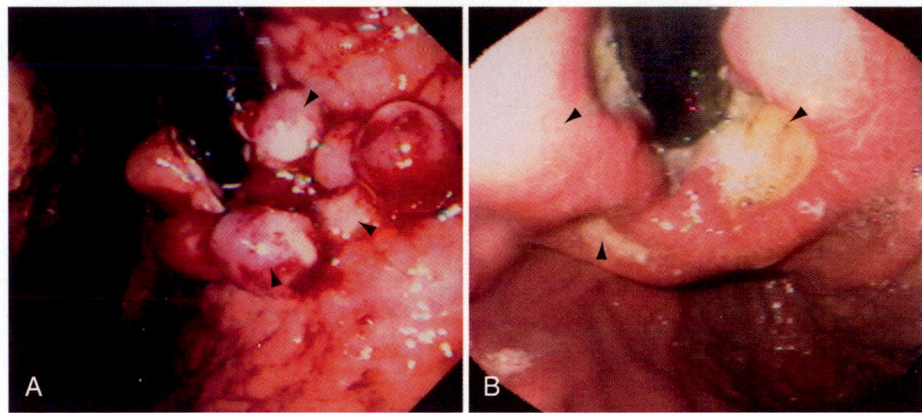

FIGURE 92-9. Endoscopic views of gastric varices and esophageal variceal ligation-related ulcers. *A,* The gastroesophageal junction is seen on a retroflexed view following ligation of multiple gastric varices *(arrowheads),* which resemble polyps. *B,* Upper endoscopy in the same patient 4 weeks later demonstrates ulcers at the sites of earlier variceal ligation *(arrowheads).*

and provision of an additional lumen for esophageal aspiration. The Linton-Nachlas tube has a single 600-mL gastric balloon with lumens for aspirating both the stomach and esophagus. Inflation of a gastric balloon alone is preferred with any of these tubes. Balloon tamponade can control bleeding for up to 24 hours in approximately 80% to 90% of patients. The risk of pulmonary aspiration is reduced by placement of an endotracheal tube. If bleeding cannot be controlled after placement of the tube, it is more important to reinflate and reposition the gastric balloon than to inflate the esophageal balloon.

Because of the risks associated with placement of tamponade balloons, self-expandable metallic covered stents have been used to tamponade esophageal varices. These stents may be left in place for up to 2 weeks and then removed. Preliminary results have been promising, and complications have been few[177]; however, experience with this device is limited. Whether self-expandable metallic stents are superior to balloon tamponade is the subject of ongoing trials.

Transjugular Intrahepatic Portosystemic Shunt

A *transjugular intrahepatic portosystemic shunt* (TIPS)—also referred to as a *transjugular intrahepatic portosystemic stent shunt* (TIPSS)—reduces elevated portal pressure by creating a communication between the hepatic vein and an intrahepatic branch of the portal vein. A percutaneous transjugular approach is used to insert the shunt. A TIPS functions as a side-to-side portacaval shunt and has been used to treat complications of portal hypertension, mainly variceal bleeding and refractory ascites, as well as Budd-Chiari syndrome, hepatic hydrothorax, and hepatorenal syndrome (see Chapters 85, 93, and 94). A TIPS can be placed by an interventional radiologist, with a mortality rate of less than 1% to 2%. TIPS placement usually is carried out with the patient under sedation. A platelet count greater than $60,000/mm^3$ and an INR less than 1.5 usually are recommended but are not essential in an emergency. Broad-spectrum antibiotic coverage is recommended when TIPS placement is carried out in a patient with PSC and as an emergency procedure.

For TIPS placement, the hepatic vein is cannulated through a transjugular approach, and using a Rosch needle, the portal vein is cannulated. A guidewire is then passed to connect the hepatic vein and a branch of the portal vein. Following dilation of the tract, a stent is placed and dilated as required

TABLE 92-2 Complications of Transjugular Intrahepatic Portosystemic Shunt Placement

Timing of Complication	Complication
Procedure-related (life-threatening)	Cardiopulmonary failure Carotid artery puncture injury Intraperitoneal hemorrhage Sepsis
Early post-procedure (1-30 days)	Cardiac arrhythmia Fever Hematoma at puncture site Hemolytic anemia Hepatic encephalopathy Pain at puncture site Progressive hepatic failure Pulmonary artery hypertension Shunt thrombosis Stent migration Reaction to contrast media
Late post-procedure (>30 days)	Hepatic encephalopathy Liver failure Portal vein thrombosis Progressive hepatic failure Shunt stenosis or thrombosis

Modified from Kamath PS, McKusick M. Transjugular portosystemic shunt (TIPS). Baillieres Clin Gastroenterol 1997; 11:327-49.

to reduce the portacaval pressure gradient (the pressure difference between the portal vein and the inferior vena cava at the confluence of the hepatic vein) to below 12 mm Hg (Fig. 92-10). A coated stent is typically used. This stent has an uncoated portion that anchors the stent to the portal vein and a polytetrafluoroethylene-coated portion that lines the tract in the liver parenchyma and the draining hepatic vein. The frequency of shunt stenosis is reduced when coated stents are used instead of uncoated stents.[178]

A TIPS can be placed successfully by an experienced operator in greater than 95% of cases.[179] Complications following the procedure are classified as procedure related, early (occurring within 30 days), or late (after 30 days) (Table 92-2). The

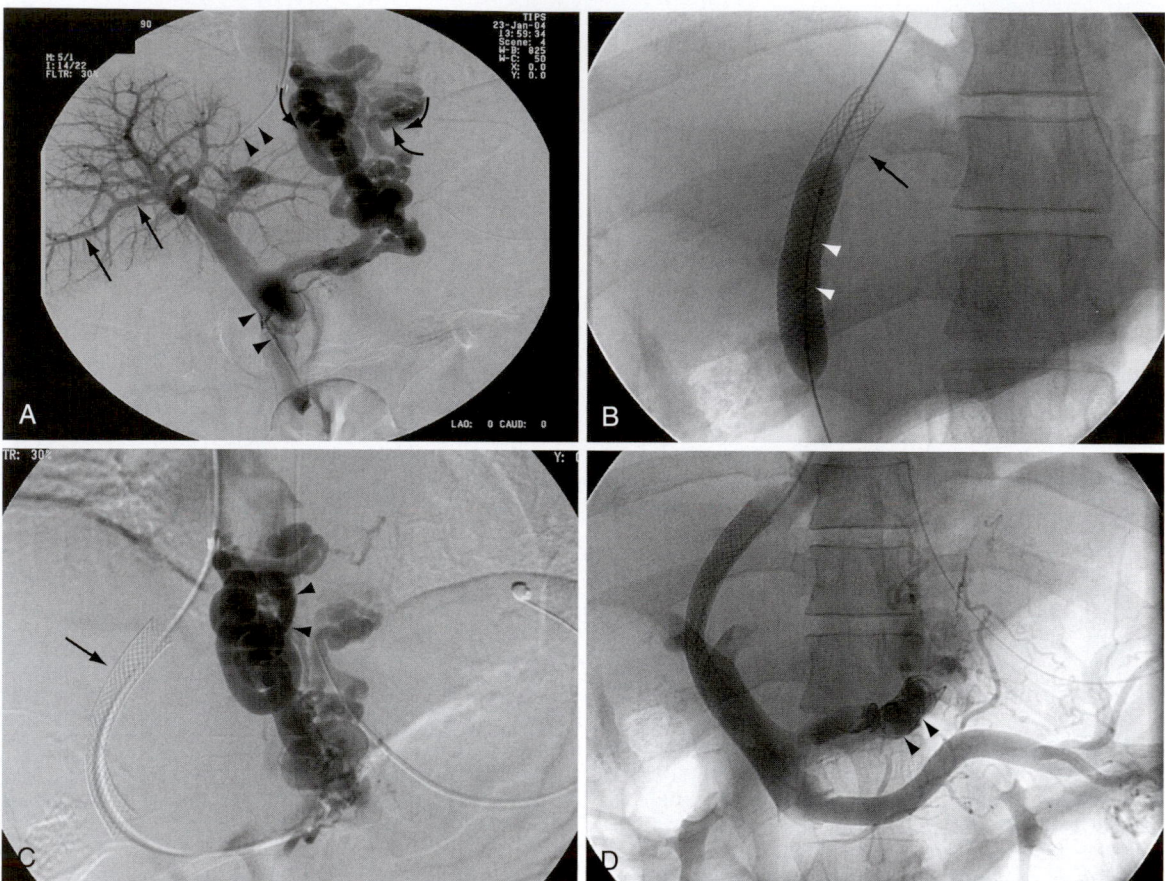

FIGURE 92-10. Creation of a transjugular intrahepatic portosystemic shunt (TIPS). *A,* Portogram with a catheter in the portal venous system *(arrowheads)*. The portal venous system is clearly outlined *(straight arrows)*. Gastroesophageal collaterals are also demonstrated *(curved arrows)*. *B,* A stent *(arrow)* has been placed to bridge the hepatic vein and the portal vein. A balloon *(arrowheads)* is being used to dilate the parenchymal tract within the liver. *C,* Following expansion of the stent *(arrow)*, injection into the portal vein demonstrates persistence of the gastroesophageal varices *(arrowheads)*. *D,* Following embolization of the varices with steel coils *(arrowheads)*, the intrahepatic portal vasculature is no longer demonstrated, indicating hepatofugal flow of portal blood through the shunt.

prevention and treatment of procedure-related, early, and late post-TIPS complications are outlined in Table 92-3.

TIPS for Portal Hypertension–Related Bleeding

The most common indication for placement of a TIPS is refractory variceal bleeding. TIPS has been used to control acute variceal bleeding and to prevent variceal rebleeding when pharmacologic and endoscopic therapies have failed, especially in patients with Child-Pugh class B or C cirrhosis, in whom bleeding is more likely to be refractory to therapy than in patients with Child-Pugh class A cirrhosis. The use of early TIPS (within 72 hours of control of variceal bleeding) in patients at high-risk of rebleeding (Child-Pugh class C, class B with active bleeding, or a MELD score > 18 and a transfusion requirement of > 4 units of red blood cells [RBCs]) is associated with a reduced rate of treatment failure and mortality, without an increased risk of hepatic encephalopathy, compared with continued pharmacologic and endoscopic therapy.[180] Prevention of variceal rebleeding and treatment of refractory ascites are the only indications for TIPS that have been subjected to controlled trials. When bleeding from varices cannot be controlled after 2 sessions of endoscopic therapy within a 24-hour period, TIPS placement is the usual salvage treatment. TIPS is also used to treat bleeding from isolated gastric fundal varices, for both control of bleeding and prevention of

rebleeding. A surgical portosystemic shunt may be preferred over a TIPS in patients with preserved synthetic liver function (Child-Pugh class A) in centers that have the surgical expertise (see later).

TIPS has been effective in the management of uncontrolled esophageal variceal bleeding in patients with decompensated cirrhosis of the liver.[181] Hemorrhage is controlled in more than 90% of patients, but the mortality rate in such patients is high—greater than 60% within 90 days. A similar outcome is observed in patients who undergo TIPS placement for refractory gastric variceal bleeding.[182]

In a meta-analysis of 12 randomized controlled trials that compared TIPS with endoscopic therapy, the rate of rebleeding was lower with TIPS, but the frequency of encephalopathy was higher, and no effect on survival was observed.[183] Therefore, TIPS cannot be recommended as a first choice for preventing variceal rebleeding; rather, it is reserved for patients who have failed endoscopic or pharmacologic therapy.

Follow-up Evaluation

The frequency of stenosis of a non-covered TIPS is high, ranging from 20% to 78% depending on the surveillance technique used and the definition of stenosis. This risk is reduced to about 15% with the use of a covered stent. Neither the

TABLE 92-3 Prevention and Treatment of Transjugular Intrahepatic Portosystemic Shunt-Related Complications

Complication	Prevention	Treatment
Inadvertent injury to carotid artery during jugular vein access	Perform with US guidance to facilitate venous access	Manual compression of the carotid puncture site to prevent hematoma
Hepatic capsular laceration during portal vein access	Avoid atrophic lobes and limit needle passes to 3-4 cm of excursion	Usually requires no treatment For severe hemorrhage, transfuse with blood products until stable; obtain an abdominal CT and surgical consultation
Extrahepatic puncture of portal venous system	Delineate the bifurcation of portal vein on preprocedure CT	Leave the catheter in place for a portogram; use as a guide for intrahepatic portal vein puncture Work quickly to establish a functioning shunt, then remove the errant catheter
Intrahepatic arterial or biliary puncture	Work centrally within the liver	Usually no treatment is required; remove the catheter and continue If a fistula develops, embolize the arterial feeder with steel coils
Sepsis after shunt placement	Give prophylactic antibiotics Adhere to strict sterile technique	Broad-spectrum antibiotics
Early shunt thrombosis	Avoid sharp angles when placing the stent Ends of the stent should not abut against the intima of the vein	Shunt venogram and clot lysis using a lytic agent delivered by the pulse-spray technique Extend the shunt to ensure stent coverage of the intrahepatic tract and to ensure an adequate length in hepatic and portal veins
Uncontrollable encephalopathy after shunt placement	Use a narrow shunt in high-risk patients	Reduce the diameter of the shunt with additional concentrically placed stents Embolize the shunt with steel coils
Shunt stenosis	Use a wider or covered stent Avoid bile duct injury	Dilation or atherectomy of the shunt Place an additional stent if necessary
Post-shunt liver failure	Avoid the procedure in patients with a MELD score ≥ 24	Consider early liver transplantation

Modified from Kamath PS, McKusick M. Transjugular portosystemic shunt (TIPS). Baillieres Clin Gastroenterol 1997; 11:327-49.

optimal interval nor the most cost-effective method of surveillance for TIPS stenosis has been determined. Doppler US evaluation generally is used to identify TIPS stenosis, but the negative predictive value of this approach is low and the positive predictive value is only acceptable. The best indicator that a TIPS has stenosed is recurrence of the problem that necessitated the TIPS. The only certain method of demonstrating shunt patency is by means of a TIPS venogram and measurement of the portacaval pressure gradient. An increase in the gradient to greater than 12 mm Hg warrants dilation of the stent or placement of an additional stent.

Selection of Patients

TIPS may worsen liver function by depriving the liver of portal venous blood, thereby increasing the risk of hepatic encephalopathy, with decreased survival in some patients. Therefore, the procedure should be used selectively. Emergency TIPS is clearly associated with a high mortality rate.[184,185] In patients in whom TIPS placement has been carried out to prevent variceal rebleeding, 30-day mortality rates may be as high as 44%. Factors associated with a poor prognosis include a serum ALT level greater than 100 U/L, serum bilirubin level greater than 3 mg/dL, and pre-TIPS hepatic

encephalopathy unrelated to bleeding.[185] Patients with a high Child-Turcotte-Pugh score (Table 92-4) also have reduced survival. The Child-Pugh classification has some limitations, however; for example, it does not discriminate survival well among patients within each Child-Pugh class. Furthermore, some parameters that make up the Child-Turcotte-Pugh score, such as ascites and encephalopathy, are assessed by subjective interpretation. The need for a more accurate method to assess survival in patients undergoing TIPS led to creation of the MELD score (see http://www.mayoclinic.org/gi-rst/mayomodel6.html and Chapter 97).[184] This mathematical model originally was composed of the serum creatinine level, INR, serum bilirubin level, and etiology of liver disease. Subsequently, the MELD formula was modified to include only the first 3 parameters (creatinine, INR, and bilirubin).[186] The MELD score has been widely validated for predicting survival in patients with cirrhosis, including patients who have undergone TIPS placement, and is more accurate for this purpose than the Child-Pugh classification.

Patients with a MELD score of 14 or less have an excellent survival rate after TIPS placement; therefore, TIPS may be carried out routinely in such patients when indicated (see earlier). Patients with a MELD score higher than 24 have reduced survival following TIPS placement, with a mortality

TABLE 92-4 Child-Turcotte-Pugh Scoring System and Child-Pugh Classification

Parameter	Numerical Score		
	1	2	3
Ascites	None	Slight	Moderate/severe
Encephalopathy	None	Slight/moderate	Moderate/severe
Bilirubin (mg/dL)	<2	2-3	>3
Albumin (g/dL)	>3.5	2.8-3.5	<2.8
Prothrombin time (seconds increased)	1-3	4-6	>6

Total Numerical Score	Child-Pugh Class
5-6	A
7-9	B
10-15	C

rate approaching 30% at 3 months. This high risk should be discussed with the patient before the procedure is undertaken. In the intermediate group with a MELD score ranging from 15 to 24, TIPS placement can be carried out depending on the patient's preference, physician's judgment, and likelihood of liver transplantation in the future. This approach has been validated independently.[187]

Balloon-Occluded Retrograde Transvenous Obliteration

Balloon-occluded retrograde transvenous obliteration (BRTO) of varices may be used to occlude gastric varices when a large splenorenal shunt is seen on abdominal cross-sectional imaging. The left renal vein is approached via the femoral vein, and the splenorenal shunt is then catheterized. Other approaches are via an existing TIPS or via a transjugular approach to the splenic vein. Following occlusion of the shunt with a balloon, the gastric varices are embolized with coils. Although ascites and splenomegaly can be aggravated following this procedure, these complications are easily managed.[188] The long-term durability of the occlusion is uncertain. BRTO has been used for both the prevention and control of gastric variceal bleeding.

Surgical Therapy

Surgical treatment of portal hypertension falls into 3 groups: non-shunt procedures, portosystemic shunt procedures, and liver transplantation. Surgical procedures (other than liver transplantation) are used as salvage therapy when standard management with pharmacologic and endoscopic therapy fails in patients with noncirrhotic causes of portal hypertension and in patients with Child-Pugh class A cirrhosis. Surgical treatment also may be considered early in the course of portal hypertension in patients who live at a great distance from centers that can manage variceal bleeding adequately or in whom cross-matching blood products (in case of bleeding) is difficult. How failure of standard therapy is defined depends on the specific circumstances of the patient's presentation, availability of surgical expertise, and outcome of conservative management. Liver transplantation should be considered in all patients with cirrhosis and variceal bleeding (see Chapter 97).

Non-shunt Procedures

Non-shunt procedures include esophageal transection and gastroesophageal devascularization. They are performed infrequently but may be required in selected cases.

Esophageal Transection

Esophageal transection, in which the esophagus is stapled and transected, is highly effective in controlling variceal bleeding and is associated with a lower risk of encephalopathy than that for portosystemic shunts. Esophageal transection was considered in the past when 2 sessions of endoscopic therapy had failed to control variceal bleeding within a 24-hour period.[85] Mortality rates are not improved over those observed with endoscopic sclerotherapy, however. With the advent of TIPS, esophageal staple transection is now seldom used.

Devascularization Procedures

Devascularization procedures typically have been used to prevent recurrent variceal bleeding in patients with extensive splenic and portal vein thrombosis when a suitable vein is not available for creation of a portosystemic shunt.[189] In the original operation described by Sugiura and Futagawa, both a thoracotomy and a laparotomy were carried out.[190] The operation is now carried out through an abdominal approach and combined with a splenectomy. The procedure consists of total devascularization of the greater curvature of the stomach combined with devascularization of the upper two thirds of the lesser curvature of the stomach and circumferential devascularization of the lower 7.5 cm of the esophagus. The rate of recurrent bleeding following this procedure is variable but may be as high as 40%, depending on the population being treated and duration of follow-up.

Portosystemic Shunts

With the increasing availability of TIPS, the use of surgical shunts for refractory variceal bleeding has declined markedly. In children, surgical shunts are carried out almost exclusively for refractory bleeding due to noncirrhotic portal hypertension, such as congenital hepatic fibrosis and portal vein thrombosis.[132] Surgical portosystemic shunts are categorized as selective shunts such as distal splenorenal shunts, partial shunts such as the side-to-side calibrated portacaval shunt, and total portosystemic shunts such as the side-to-side portacaval shunt or end-to-side portacaval shunt.

Selective Shunts

The most widely used selective shunt is the distal splenorenal shunt, originally described by Warren and colleagues.[191] With this shunt, only varices at the gastroesophageal junction and spleen are decompressed, and portal hypertension is maintained in the superior mesenteric vein and portal vein; therefore, variceal bleeding is controlled, but the risk of ascites persists. The shunt procedure involves a portal-azygos disconnection and subsequent anastomosis between the splenic vein and left renal vein in an end-to-side fashion (Fig. 92-11). The entire length of the pancreas must be mobilized, and the left adrenal vein must be ligated. The distal splenorenal shunt has been associated with control of variceal bleeding in approximately 90% of patients and a lower rate of hepatic encephalopathy than that reported for total shunts.[192]

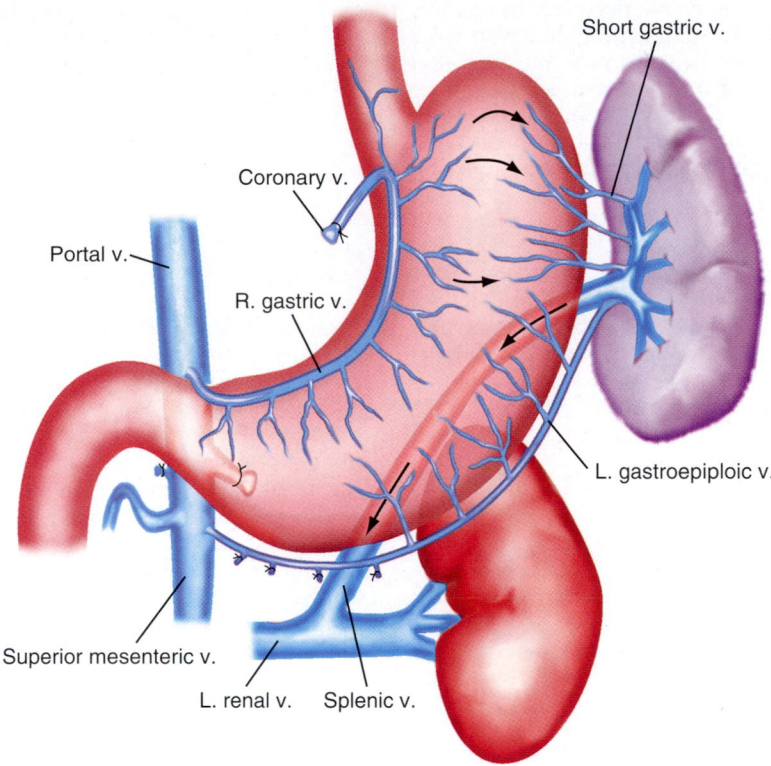

Short gastric v.

Coronary v.

Portal v.

R. gastric v.

L. gastroepiploic v.

Superior mesenteric v.

L. renal v.   Splenic v.

FIGURE 92-11. Distal splenorenal shunt. The anatomy following completion of a distal splenorenal shunt is depicted. For this procedure, the splenic vein (v.) is disconnected from the superior mesenteric vein and is separated from the pancreas; all its collaterals are ligated. The portal system is thus disconnected from the azygos system so that all flow from the gastroesophageal junction is through the short gastric veins into the splenic vein. The splenic vein is then anastomosed to the left renal vein in an end-to-side fashion.

Partial Portosystemic Shunts

A partial portosystemic shunt is carried out using a synthetic interposition graft between the portal vein and the inferior vena cava. When the shunt diameter is 8 mm, portal pressure is reduced below 12 mm Hg, and antegrade flow to the liver is maintained in most patients.[193] Rates of preventing variceal rebleeding and encephalopathy following this shunt are similar to those seen with a distal splenorenal shunt. As in patients who have had a distal splenorenal shunt, ascites may occur in approximately 20% of patients who have had a partial portosystemic shunt, because hepatic sinusoidal pressure is not reduced.[194,195]

Portacaval Shunts

End-to-side and side-to-side portacaval shunts have been described, but nowadays only the side-to-side portacaval shunt is in use.[196] Any portacaval shunt that is greater than 12 mm in diameter is likely to result in a total shunting of portal blood. A shunt with a diameter less than 12 mm is created with an interposition graft, or alternatively a direct vein-to-vein anastomosis may be constructed. Variceal bleeding, as well as ascites, is well controlled because the hepatic sinusoids are decompressed. Variceal rebleeding following a total shunt is seen in less than 10% of patients, but hepatic encephalopathy occurs in 30% to 40% of patients.[103] Liver transplantation in patients who have had a portacaval shunt is associated with increased operative morbidity and intraoperative transfusion requirements. The outcome of liver transplantation is not otherwise significantly different, however, from that for patients who have not had a portacaval shunt. Nevertheless, surgical portacaval shunts should be avoided in patients who are potential candidates for liver transplantation.

Mesenterico–Left Portal Venous Bypass

The mesenterico–left portal venous bypass, or Rex shunt, is carried out in patients with extrahepatic portal vein thrombosis if the intrahepatic portion of the portal vein is patent. With this procedure, portal blood flow is restored to the liver, thereby reducing the risk of hepatic encephalopathy or long-term learning disability in children. A jugular vein graft may be used to bridge the superior mesenteric vein to the intrahepatic portion of the left portal vein in the Rex recessus. (The Rex recessus is the location where the left portal vein divides to supply segments III and IV of the liver.) This surgery is the treatment of choice in children with extrahepatic portal vein thrombosis who have complications related to portal hypertension and in adults in whom portal vein thrombosis has developed late after liver transplantation.[132]

MANAGEMENT OF SPECIFIC LESIONS

Esophageal Varices

Natural History

Esophageal varices are present in approximately 40% of patients with cirrhosis and in as many as 60% of patients with cirrhosis and ascites.[103] In cirrhotic patients who do not have esophageal varices at initial endoscopy, new varices will develop at a rate of approximately 5% per year. In patients with small varices at initial endoscopy, progression to large varices occurs at a rate of about 10% per year and is related predominantly to the degree of liver dysfunction.[197] On the other hand, improvement in liver function in patients with alcoholic liver disease who abstain from alcohol is associated with a decreased risk, and sometimes even disappearance, of varices.[198]

Up to 25% of patients with newly diagnosed varices will experience variceal bleeding within 2 years.[197] The best clinical predictor of bleeding appears to be variceal size. The risk of bleeding in patients with varices less than 5 mm in diameter is 7% by 2 years, and the risk in patients with varices greater than 5 mm in diameter is 30% by 2 years.[197] Even more important, however, is the HVPG, because the risk of bleeding is virtually absent when the HVPG is below 12 mm Hg.[94] Nevertheless, measurement of HVPG is not routinely performed in clinical practice to assess bleeding risk.

Initial treatment is associated with cessation of bleeding in approximately 80% to 90% of patients.[197,199] Approximately half of patients with a variceal bleed stop bleeding spontaneously because hypovolemia leads to splanchnic vasoconstriction, which results in a decrease in portal pressure. Excessive transfusions may, in fact, increase the chance of rebleeding.[200] Active bleeding at endoscopy, a lower initial hematocrit value, higher serum aminotransferase levels, higher Child-Pugh class, bacterial infection, an HVPG above 20 mm Hg, and portal vein thrombosis are associated with failure to control bleeding at 5 days.[199,201-203] Of patients who have stopped bleeding, approximately one third will rebleed within the next 6 weeks. Of all rebleeding episodes, approximately 40% will take place within 5 days of the initial bleed.[204] Predictors of rebleeding include active bleeding at emergency endoscopy, bleeding from gastric varices, hypoalbuminemia, renal insufficiency, and an HVPG greater than 20 mm Hg.[197] The risk of death with acute variceal bleeding is 5% to 8% at 1 week and about 20% at 6 weeks.[197] Patients who rebleed early, have a MELD score over 18, require more than 4 units of packed RBC transfusions,[205] and in whom renal failure develops have the highest risk of death. Alcohol as the cause of cirrhosis, a higher serum bilirubin level, a lower serum albumin level, hepatic encephalopathy, and hepatocellular carcinoma are additional factors associated with an increased 6-week mortality rate.

Treatment of esophageal variceal bleeding is classified as either primary prophylaxis (i.e., prevention of variceal hemorrhage in patients who have never bled), control of acute variceal bleeding, or secondary prevention of rebleeding in patients who have survived an initial bleeding episode. Effective treatments to prevent the development of varices and ascites in patients with cirrhosis are not yet available, although beta blockers may slow enlargement of small varices into large varices.

Prevention of Bleeding

Pharmacologic Prevention

The utility of pre-primary prophylaxis—that is, the efficacy of beta blockers to prevent the formation of varices—has not been demonstrated.[85,206] Patients with Child-Pugh class C cirrhosis who have small varices may be considered for treatment with a beta blocker. All patients with large varices (diameter > 5 mm) should be considered for prophylactic therapy (primary prophylaxis) to prevent variceal bleeding. The presence of additional endoscopic signs such as red wales does not influence the decision regarding prophylactic therapy. The absolute risk reduction with beta blockers is approximately 10%, and the number needed to treat to prevent

1 variceal bleed is approximately 10 patients. The mortality rate is reduced from 28.4% in control patients to 23.9% in patients taking a beta blocker; the absolute risk reduction is 4.5%. The number of patients needed to be treated to prevent 1 death is approximately 22. In patients who do not bleed during therapy and who do not experience side effects, treatment should be continued indefinitely because withdrawal of a beta blocker can result in an increased risk of bleeding.[207,208] Patients who have an initial bleed while on a beta blocker have an increased risk of future bleeds and death even if variceal ligation is performed.[209]

The side effects of beta blocker treatment are probably overemphasized because only approximately 15% of patients need to discontinue the drug.[210] A baseline heart rate and blood pressure recording will help determine whether a patient is a candidate for pharmacologic treatment with a beta blocker. A resting heart rate of less than 55 to 60 beats per minute or a systolic blood pressure less than 90 mm Hg indicates that the patient is likely to be intolerant of beta blockers. In other patients, the HVPG ideally should be measured at baseline (Fig. 92-12). A long-acting preparation of propranolol or nadolol may be started; the usual starting dose of long-acting propranolol is 60 mg once daily and that of nadolol is 20 mg once daily. Because the risk of bleeding is greatest at night, the beta blocker should probably be administered in the evening.[113] The dose of propranolol or nadolol can be increased gradually every 3 to 5 days until the target heart rate of 25% below baseline or 55 to 60 beats per minute or the maximum tolerated dose is reached, provided that the systolic blood pressure remains above 90 mm Hg. The daily dose of long-acting propranolol or nadolol required to reach the target heart rate ranges from 40 to 160 mg. Patients with a decrease

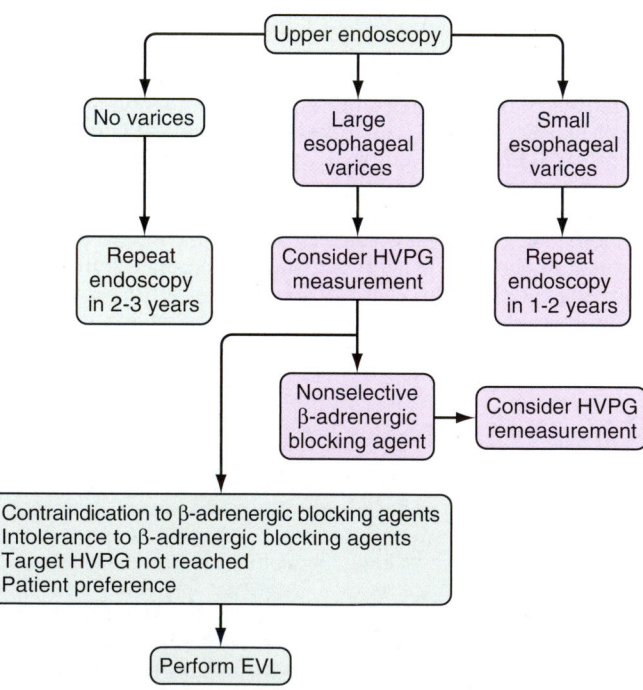

FIGURE 92-12. Algorithm for the primary prophylaxis of esophageal variceal hemorrhage in patients with cirrhosis. The hepatic vein pressure gradient (HVPG) may be measured in patients with large varices before a nonselective β-adrenergic blocking agent is started and remeasured one month after the maximum tolerated dose of the beta blocker is reached. The goal of treatment is to reduce the HVPG to < 12 mm Hg or by ≥ 20%. EVL, endoscopic variceal ligation.

in systolic blood pressure below 90 mm Hg are most likely to experience side effects. In patients with hypertension or coronary artery disease, carvedilol may be used in an initial dose of 6.25 mg daily; the dose is increased to a maximum of 25 mg daily. Side effects of and contraindications to carvedilol are similar to those for other nonselective beta blockers.

In patients on pharmacologic therapy, follow-up endoscopy is unnecessary unless GI bleeding occurs. In patients in whom the HVPG has decreased to less than 12 mm Hg, the risk of bleeding is virtually eliminated. Patients in whom the HVPG decreases by at least 20% have a risk of variceal bleeding of less than 10%. Unfortunately, only 30% to 40% of patients respond to a beta blocker; those with better liver function show the best response.[210] In patients who are intolerant of or who have contraindications to beta blockers, endoscopic prophylaxis should be pursued (see later). Unfortunately, patients who do not achieve a decrease in the HVPG to less than 12 mm Hg, or of greater than 20%, on a beta blocker may not respond well to endoscopic variceal ligation either.[211]

Endoscopic Prevention

The preferred method of endoscopic treatment is variceal band ligation. Prophylactic sclerotherapy for the prevention of variceal bleeding has been studied extensively but cannot be recommended.[212] Meta-analysis of the trials that compared endoscopic variceal ligation with a beta blocker demonstrated a lower bleeding risk with endoscopic variceal ligation, with no difference in mortality rates.[213] A subsequent study has suggested that nonbleeding-related mortality may actually be reduced by beta blockers.[214] Side effects with beta blockers are more frequent than with variceal ligation, but complications of variceal ligation can be potentially life threatening.

Nineteen randomized trials have compared endoscopic variceal ligation and nonselective beta blockers for the primary prevention of variceal bleeding in adults. Variceal band ligation is superior to beta blockers in reducing the risk of GI bleeding and variceal bleeding (RR, 0.69 and 0.67, respectively). This benefit is lost, however, when only high-quality trials are included in the analysis. Bleeding-related mortality is not different, suggesting that beta blockers may have benefits other than a reduction in bleeding risk.[215]

The risks and benefits of the options should be discussed with the patient and treatment individualized. Beta blockers are cheaper and more convenient to use and may potentially reduce the risk of bleeding from gastric varices and portal hypertensive gastropathy. Band ligation is the only option for patients with high-risk varices who have contraindications to beta blockers or who have not responded to or are intolerant of beta blockers. Combined use of a nonselective beta blocker and endoscopic variceal ligation as primary prophylaxis is not currently recommended.

Control of Acute Bleeding

Acute esophageal variceal bleeding constitutes a life-threatening emergency and requires management by a well-trained team of hepatologists, endoscopists, intensive care personnel, radiologists, and surgeons. Treatment is aimed at resuscitating the patient, controlling the bleeding, and preventing complications (see Chapter 20). Two large-bore IV access lines should be inserted immediately. RBCs should be transfused with the goal of maintaining the hematocrit value around 25%. A restrictive strategy of transfusing RBCs only when the Hgb level drops below 7 g/dL is associated with improved survival in patients with Child-Pugh class A and B cirrhosis, as compared with a strategy of transfusing when the Hgb level drops below 9 g/dL.[216] The optimal target INR and platelet count are not known.[217] Normal saline may be infused IV until packed RBCs are available for transfusion. In patients with active bleeding, the airway needs to be protected, and endotracheal intubation is advised. Antibiotics should be administered to all patients to prevent bacteremia and spontaneous bacterial peritonitis (see Chapter 93). Norfloxacin, 400 mg orally twice daily for 7 days, is the preferred choice.[218] When oral intake is not possible, IV ceftriaxone, 1 g every 24 hours for 7 days; ciprofloxacin, 400 mg every 12 hours; or levofloxacin, 500 mg every 24 hours is recommended. Infection is associated with a significantly increased risk of mortality and rebleeding.[219] The addition of treatment with recombinant factor VIIa to standard therapy has not been shown to improve control of bleeding.[220]

A combination of endoscopic therapy and pharmacologic therapy of variceal bleeding is superior to pharmacologic treatment alone. Pharmacologic agents should be started as early as possible; in some centers, they are started while the patient is being transferred by ambulance to the hospital. Somatostatin, octreotide, vapreotide, or terlipressin are the options for pharmacologic therapy. Vasoactive agents are associated with improved hemostasis and a shorter length of hospitalization. None of the agents studied seems to have a clear benefit over the others.[221] Therefore, the specific agent chosen depends on availability and physician preference. In the United States, octreotide has been the agent used most commonly. Terlipressin is the first choice in many other countries because it has been associated with improved survival.[222] Pharmacologic treatment should be continued for up to 5 days to prevent early rebleeding; however, a 2012 study has shown that a 24-hour course and a 72-hour course of terlipressin may be equally effective when used in conjunction with variceal ligation.[223]

Endoscopic therapy is carried out as soon as the patient is hemodynamically stabilized. At upper endoscopy, bleeding from esophageal varices is diagnosed if active bleeding from the varices is seen; signs of recent hemorrhage, such as a white fibrin plug or a red blood clot over a varix, are present; varices with risk signs for bleeding, such as a cherry-red spot, hematocystic spot, or red wale sign, are seen; or esophageal varices are seen in the absence of any other lesion that could give rise to GI bleeding. Endoscopic treatment is recommended at the time of initial endoscopy, and endoscopic variceal ligation is the preferred method.

At upper endoscopy, the actively bleeding varix is ligated (Fig. 92-13). Ligation initially should be at or immediately below the site of bleeding on the varix. Other large varices also should be banded during the same session. If active bleeding is not seen, ligation should be carried out beginning with varices at the gastroesophageal junction and proceeding proximally at intervals of 2 cm in a spiral fashion. If bleeding obscures the varices, then multiple bands are placed at the gastroesophageal junction circumferentially until bleeding can be controlled, but the long-term risks of esophageal stricture are increased in such cases. Bleeding can be controlled in up to 85% to 90% of patients with a combination of pharmacologic and endoscopic treatment.

Bleeding cannot be controlled in approximately 10% to 15% of patients, as defined by any of the following 3 criteria: (1) transfusion of 4 units of RBCs or more to maintain the hematocrit value above 25%, (2) inability to increase the systolic blood pressure by 20 mm Hg or to greater than 70 mm Hg, or (3) persistence of a heart rate greater than 100 beats per minute.[224] Rebleeding is defined as recurrence of bleeding after initial control for 24 hours during which the vital signs and Hgb level are stable. When 2 sessions of endoscopic treatment within a 24-hour period have failed to control variceal bleeding, salvage therapies such as TIPS should be carried out

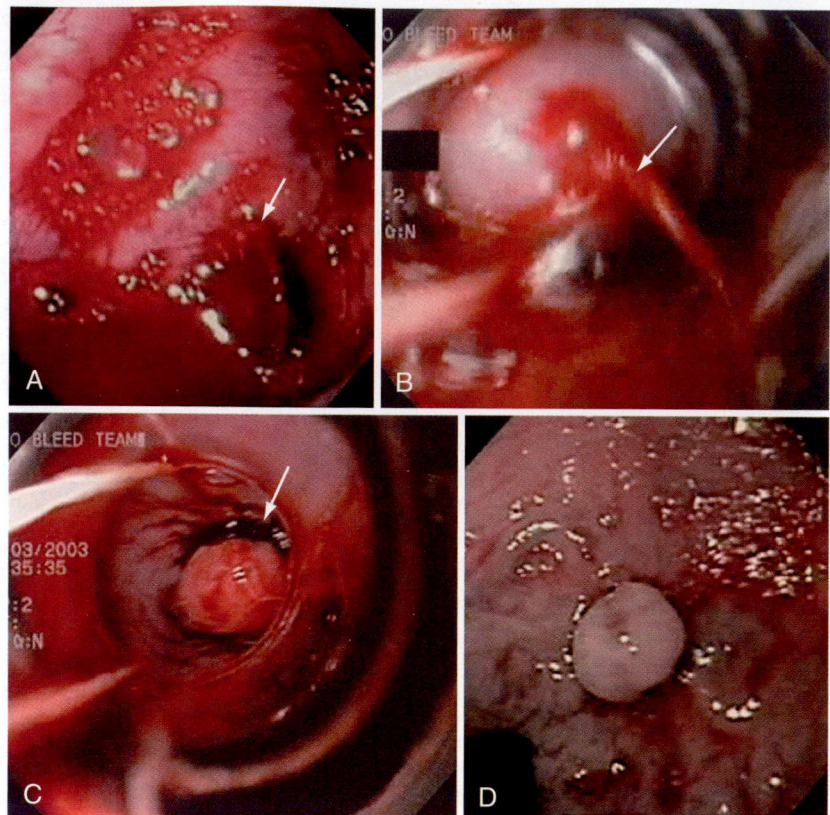

FIGURE 92-13. Band ligation for control of esophageal variceal bleeding. *A,* On upper endoscopy, an actively bleeding varix can be seen in the distal esophagus *(arrow). B,* With the variceal banding device in position, the varix is suctioned into the device at the site of active bleeding *(arrow). C,* After the band is in place *(arrow)* and the varix has been ligated, the bleeding has stopped. *D,* Visualization of the varix with the band in place, with complete control of bleeding. *(Images courtesy Dr. Louis M. Wong Kee Song, Rochester, Minn.)*

(Fig. 92-14), although the mortality rate in this group of patients is high. In the group of patients at high risk of treatment failure (Child-Pugh class C, Child-Pugh class B with active bleeding, or MELD score > 18 and requirement for transfusion of > 4 units of RBCs), TIPS carried out within 72 hours of the control of bleeding is associated with reduced rates of mortality and treatment failure.[180] Emergency surgical portosystemic shunts, although extremely effective in controlling variceal bleeding, have largely been abandoned because of high mortality rates. Balloon tamponade may be used to stabilize a patient until definitive treatment can be carried out.

Prevention of Rebleeding

All patients who have had a variceal bleed should receive prophylactic therapy (secondary prophylaxis) to reduce the risk of rebleeding, which otherwise occurs in up to 80% of patients at 2 years. Patients with cirrhosis should be evaluated for liver transplantation (see Chapter 97). Options for preventing variceal rebleeding are pharmacologic therapy, endoscopic therapy, and a portosystemic shunt (surgical or radiologic) or combinations of these therapies.

Combined therapy with endoscopic variceal ligation and a nonselective beta blocker is the preferred treatment, and long-acting propranolol or nadolol may be used. Ideally, the hemodynamic response to a beta blocker should be monitored with the goal of reducing the HVPG by greater than 20% or to less than 12 mm Hg. If these goals are not achieved, isosorbide mononitrate may be added. The extended-release form of isosorbide mononitrate is preferred, with an initial starting

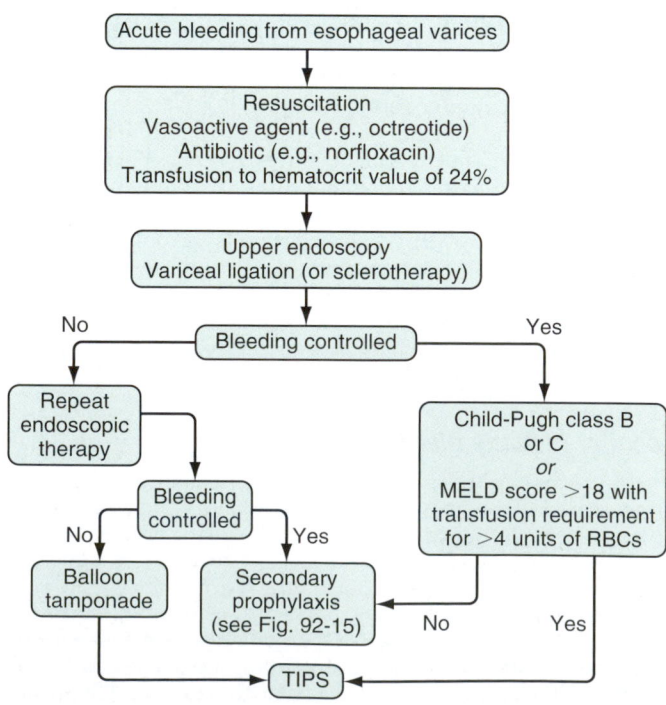

FIGURE 92-14. Algorithm for the management of bleeding esophageal varices. RBC, red blood cell; TIPS, transjugular intrahepatic portosystemic shunt.

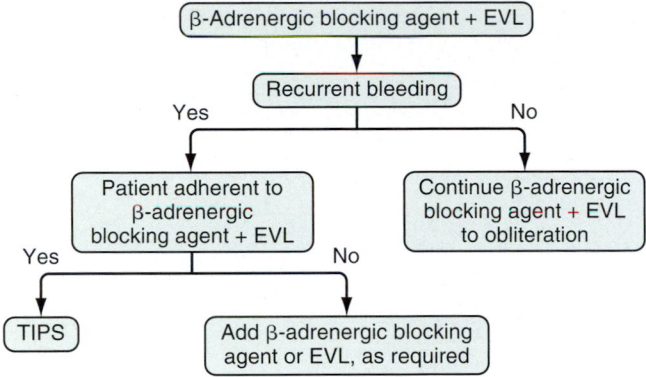

FIGURE 92-15. Algorithm for the prevention of recurrent variceal bleeding (secondary prophylaxis). EVL, endoscopic variceal ligation; TIPS, transjugular intrahepatic portosystemic shunt.

dose of 30 mg/day. Unfortunately, hypotension and headaches are common and require discontinuation of isosorbide mononitrate. The beneficial effect of long-term pharmacologic therapy may be restricted to patients with alcoholic cirrhosis who remain abstinent.[225]

Endoscopic variceal ligation alone may be performed to prevent variceal rebleeding in patients who have poor liver function and may not tolerate a beta blocker (Fig. 92-15). In practice, the first endoscopic session is carried out 7 to 14 days after the initial variceal ligation to control bleeding. Endoscopic therapy is then repeated at 3- to 4-week intervals; this approach has been suggested because bands might still be in place if endoscopy is repeated sooner. If the HVPG is monitored, a reduction in HVPG to less than 12 mm Hg or by greater than 20% should obviate the need for variceal ligation. For patients who bleed during pharmacologic treatment, variceal ligation should be carried out. Conversely, for patients who have undergone variceal ligation alone and experience recurrent bleeding, a beta blocker should be started, although in patients with a noncirrhotic cause of portal hypertension the addition of propranolol and isosorbide mononitrate to endoscopic variceal ligation does not reduce the risk of bleeding compared with variceal ligation alone.[226] On the other hand, in patients with cirrhosis on nadolol and isosorbide mononitrate, the addition of variceal ligation may not reduce the risk of rebleeding and mortality further[227]; these results have not been confirmed in the United States. Patients who have variceal rebleeding despite optimal pharmacologic and endoscopic treatment require a portosystemic shunt. Even in patients with Child-Pugh class A cirrhosis, a TIPS may be as effective as a distal splenorenal shunt, and the choice of therapy depends on local expertise.[228]

Gastric Varices

The most widely used classification of gastric varices is the Sarin classification.[229] According to this classification, type 1 gastroesophageal varices (GOV1) extend 2 to 5 cm below the gastroesophageal junction and are in continuity with esophageal varices; type 2 gastroesophageal varices (GOV2) are in the cardia and fundus of the stomach and in continuity with esophageal varices; varices that occur in the fundus of the stomach in the absence of esophageal varices are called isolated gastric varices type 1 (IGV1), whereas varices that occur in the gastric body, antrum, or pylorus are called isolated gastric varices type 2 (IGV2).

Approximately 25% of patients with portal hypertension have gastric varices, most commonly GOV1, which comprise

approximately 70% of all gastric varices. Intrahepatic causes of portal hypertension may be associated with both GOV1 and GOV2. Splenic vein thrombosis usually results in IGV1, but the most common cause of fundal gastric varices may be cirrhosis.

Natural History

Gastric varices typically occur in association with advanced portal hypertension. Bleeding is thought to be more common in patients with GOV2 and IGV1 than in those with other types of gastric varices; in other words, bleeding is more common from fundal varices than from varices at the gastro-esophageal junction. Whereas intraesophageal pressure is negative, intra-abdominal pressure is positive, and the transmural pressure gradient across gastric varices is smaller than that across esophageal varices. Gastric varices, however, tend to be larger in diameter than esophageal varices. Gastric varices are supported by gastric mucosa, whereas esophageal varices tend to be unsupported in the lower third of the esophagus. Therefore, gastric varices are likely to bleed only when they are large, as demonstrated in a study in which larger gastric varices (>20 mm in diameter) in patients with a MELD score above 17 were more likely than smaller ones to bleed.[230] Although gastric varices have been thought to bleed less frequently than esophageal varices, the bleeding rates probably are comparable if patients are matched for the severity of cirrhosis (Child-Turcotte-Pugh score).[229] In contrast with esophageal varices, bleeding from gastric varices has been described with an HVPG less than 12 mm Hg.[231,232] Gastric varices in continuity with esophageal varices may regress following treatment of the esophageal varices. When gastric varices persist despite obliteration of esophageal varices, the prognosis is poorer, probably because of the severity of liver disease.

Prevention of Bleeding

Unfortunately, there is a paucity of studies that have evaluated pharmacologic or endoscopic treatment for primary prophylaxis of gastric variceal hemorrhage, and recommendations are still based primarily on the guidelines for managing esophageal varices. Large gastric varices (>20 mm diameter), especially in patients with a MELD score above 17, are most likely to bleed. Because these gastric varices usually are associated with esophageal varices, pharmacologic treatment with a nonselective beta blocker may be initiated to prevent variceal hemorrhage. Cyanoacrylate glue injection may be more effective than beta blocker therapy in preventing gastric variceal bleeding[230] but is not currently recommended until confirmed by larger studies. TIPS is also not recommended for the primary prevention of gastric variceal bleeding. BRTO has been used in uncontrolled studies to prevent bleeding from gastric varices, with some success.

Control of Acute Bleeding

The approach to treating esophageal variceal hemorrhage also applies to acute gastric variceal hemorrhage and includes volume resuscitation, avoidance of overtransfusion, and antibiotic prophylaxis with norfloxacin, 400 mg twice daily for 7 days. Upper endoscopy is carried out after patients have been volume resuscitated and stabilized and often following endotracheal intubation to protect the airway. The endoscopic diagnosis of gastric variceal bleeding may be difficult because of pooling of blood in the fundus. A diagnosis of gastric variceal hemorrhage should be considered if bleeding is noted from a gastric varix (Fig. 92-16); blood is found to appear at the gastroesophageal junction or the gastric fundus; blood is found

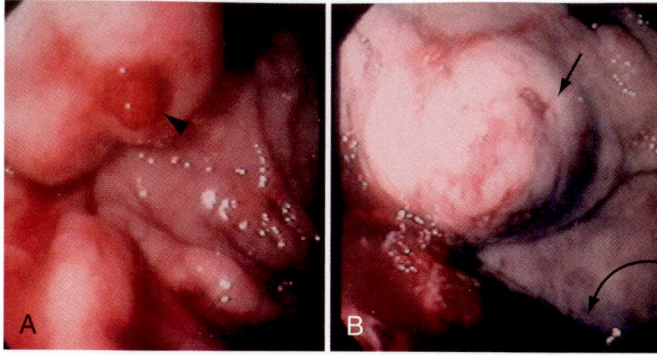

FIGURE 92-16. Gastric variceal bleeding. *A*, Active bleeding from a gastric varix *(arrowhead)* can be seen. *B*, Bleeding from the varix *(straight arrow)* is controlled following injection of sodium tetradecyl sulfate. Pooling of blood in the stomach is indicated by the *curved arrow*.

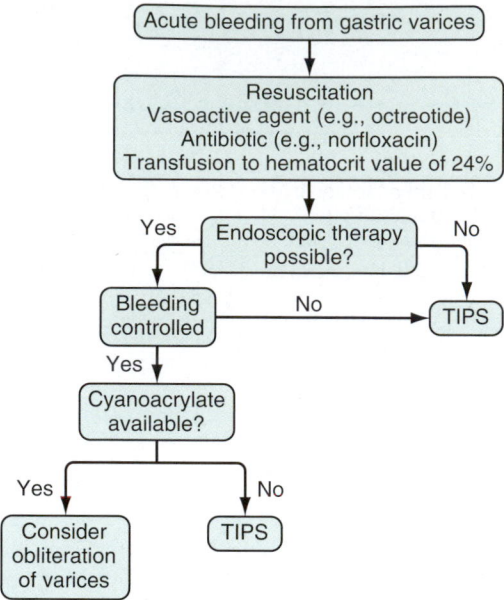

FIGURE 92-17. Algorithm for the management of bleeding gastric varices in patients with portal hypertension. TIPS, transjugular intrahepatic portosystemic shunt.

in the stomach and gastric varices with a "white nipple sign" (indicating a fibrin-platelet plug) are seen in the absence of other causes of bleeding; and gastric varices are noted in the absence of other lesions in the esophagus and stomach.[233]

Because controlled studies evaluating pharmacologic therapy for gastric variceal bleeding are lacking, the agents used are based on extension of the data relating to esophageal varices. Medical management with vasoactive agents should be started as early as possible, preferably at least 30 minutes before endoscopic therapy is carried out. The preferred endoscopic therapy for fundal gastric variceal bleeding is injection of polymers of cyanoacrylate, usually N-butyl-2-cyanoacrylate,[234,235] but these tissue adhesives are not currently available in the United States. Obliteration of the varices occurs when the injected cyanoacrylate adhesive hardens on contact with blood. The endoscope may be damaged by the glue, but the risk is minimized if silicone gel is used to cover the tip of the instrument, and suction is avoided for 15 to 20 seconds following injection.[236] The mucosa overlying the varix injected eventually sloughs, and the hardened polymer is extruded. Fortunately, the resulting ulcers occur late, and the risk of bleeding is lower than that associated with sclerotherapy-related ulcers. Cyanoacrylate injection has been found to be superior to both variceal band ligation and sclerotherapy using alcohol.[235] Complications of cyanoacrylate injection include bacteremia and variceal ulceration. Pulmonary and cerebral emboli have been reported on occasion, usually in patients with spontaneous large portosystemic or intrapulmonary shunts. Embolization probably occurs via spontaneous splenorenal shunts. Therefore, a combined approach using interventional radiology to occlude the shunt and endoscopic variceal glue injection is probably a safer strategy.[237]

For injection of GOV2 or IGV1, a retroflexed endoscopic approach is recommended. Sclerosants such as sodium tetradecyl sulfate, ethanolamine oleate, and sodium morrhuate are not particularly effective for control of gastric variceal bleeding.[238] When sclerotherapy is carried out for gastric varices, the volume of sclerosant required is larger than that used for esophageal varices, and fever and retrosternal pain are more common. It is much easier to obliterate GOV1 than GOV2 or IGV1. IGV1 are the most difficult gastric varices to obliterate and, when present, should prompt early consideration of definitive treatment such as portosystemic shunting if cyanoacrylate is not available.

Although some investigators recommend ligation of gastric varices up to 20 mm in diameter,[239] this recommendation is not supported by our experience. Band ligation of

varices greater than 10 mm in diameter is usually unsafe. Ligation is safest if the varices are in the cardia of the stomach. Because gastric fundal varices are covered by mucosa, drawing the entire varix into the ligation device is often not possible. Application of bands results in creation of a large ulcer on the varix, sometimes with disastrous results (see Fig. 92-9).

If endoscopic and pharmacologic therapies fail to control gastric variceal bleeding, then a Linton-Nachlas tube may be passed as a temporizing measure. Most patients in whom endoscopic and pharmacologic treatment fails to control gastric variceal bleeding will require a TIPS, which can control bleeding in greater than 90% of patients—a rate of efficacy equivalent to that for TIPS in controlling esophageal variceal bleeding (Fig. 92-17).[182,240]

Prevention of Rebleeding

Cyanoacrylate glue injection may be superior to nonselective beta blockers in preventing gastric variceal rebleeding.[241] In a small study, the 2-octyl-cyanoacrylate polymer (Dermabond) has been used to prevent gastric variceal rebleeding, with excellent results.[242] Patients require an average of 2 or 3 sessions for obturation of gastric varices with cyanoacrylate polymers. Detachable snares or BRTO may also be carried out to prevent gastric variceal bleeding

Limited data are available regarding use of surgical portosystemic shunts for the treatment of gastric varices in patients with cirrhosis. Two studies performed in patients with good liver function, most of whom had extrahepatic portal vein thrombosis, demonstrated excellent results, with a low long-term risk of bleeding and encephalopathy, after creation of a surgical shunt.[243,244] TIPS is also effective in preventing gastric variceal rebleeding. Because TIPS for this indication does not always result in a decrease in the size of gastric varices,[245] the target HVPG is uncertain in these patients.[232] Patients with an HVPG less than 12 mm Hg after TIPS are protected from esophageal variceal bleeding but have been known to bleed from gastric varices. Therefore, if the HVPG is reduced to a level below 12 mm Hg but gastric fundal varices are still prominent when contrast is injected into the portal vein (especially if the patient has bled from gastric fundal varices), the gastric varices may be embolized.

Ectopic Varices

Varices that occur at a site other than the gastroesophageal junction are termed *ectopic varices* and account for less than 5% of all varix-related bleeding episodes. Ectopic varices most commonly manifest with melena or hematemesis. They also may manifest with hemobilia, hematuria, hemoperitoneum, or retroperitoneal bleeding. The duodenum is a common site of ectopic varices, and varices typically are associated with portal vein obstruction, but in the West, the usual cause of duodenal varices is cirrhosis. The common occurrence of duodenal varices in patients with portal vein obstruction probably relates to the formation of collateral vessels around the thrombosed portal vein that connect pancreaticoduodenal veins to retroduodenal veins, which drain into the inferior vena cava.[246] In some of those patients with extrahepatic portal vein obstruction, varices form around the gallbladder and bile duct, giving rise to portal hypertensive cholangiopathy and biliary strictures (see Fig. 92-8).

The other common site of ectopic varices is peristomal in patients with IBD and PSC who have undergone a proctocolectomy with creation of an ileostomy.[247] Varices develop at the level of the mucocutaneous border of the stoma and are termed *stomal varices*. They are recognized by a bluish halo surrounding the stoma and by a dusky appearance and friable consistency of the stomal tissue; no obvious variceal lesions are seen. Bleeding from stomal varices is readily apparent on presentation.

Anorectal varices are reported in 10% to 40% of cirrhotic patients who undergo colonoscopy and must be distinguished from hemorrhoids (Fig. 92-18). Rectal varices are dilated superior and middle hemorrhoidal veins, whereas hemorrhoids are dilated vascular channels above the dentate line. Rectal varices collapse with digital pressure, but hemorrhoids do not.

Ectopic variceal bleeding should be considered in all patients with portal hypertension and overt GI bleeding (without an obvious bleeding source on endoscopy) or a drop in the Hgb level associated with abdominal pain and increasing abdominal girth. CT of the abdomen demonstrates layering of free fluid in the peritoneal cavity in patients who have intra-abdominal hemorrhage, typical of fresh blood mixed with ascitic fluid. The diagnosis of intra-abdominal hemorrhage secondary to ectopic variceal bleeding is confirmed by a paracentesis that yields bloody ascitic fluid with clots.

Management

In patients suspected of having ectopic variceal bleeding, vasoactive drugs may be administered initially to control the bleeding. If the bleeding ectopic varix is visualized at endoscopy, as typically is the case with duodenal or colonic varices, then endoscopic therapy can be carried out.[248] Endoscopic glue injection or band ligation is the preferred approach for bleeding duodenal varices. Colonic varices tend to be larger in diameter and may require application of hemostatic clips. Patients with bleeding stomal varices can be trained to compress the site locally if bleeding is obvious. Because bleeding from stomal varices is visible and detected early, the mortality rate for bleeding stomal varices is low.[249] Percutaneous sclerotherapy of the stomal varices may be carried out under US guidance.

At present, no recommendations support primary prophylaxis to prevent bleeding from ectopic varices. To prevent rebleeding from ectopic varices, pharmacologic treatment with a beta blocker is usually tried, although no studies are available to support this approach. If the portal vein is patent, then transhepatic embolization of stomal varices can be carried out (Fig. 92-19). Embolization of varices using a transhepatic approach can control bleeding in most patients with stomal varices. The rate of rebleeding is high, however, because portal hypertension persists. In patients in whom embolization fails to prevent rebleeding, TIPS placement may be considered.[250]

A surgical portosystemic shunt is recommended in patients with portal hypertension from extrahepatic portal vein thrombosis in which a vein suitable for a shunt is available. Placement of a nonselective portosystemic shunt, such as a portacaval shunt, mesocaval shunt, or proximal splenorenal shunt, should be carried out in a patient with stomal varices.

Patients with ectopic varices who present with intraperitoneal hemorrhage have a poor outcome because the diagnosis usually is not considered and is often made at laparotomy. Acute bleeding may be controlled by transhepatic obliteration or surgical ligation of the varices. In patients who are critically ill, a TIPS should be placed, followed by embolization of the bleeding varix.

Portal Hypertensive Gastropathy and Gastric Vascular Ectasia

Mucosal changes in the stomach in patients with portal hypertension include portal hypertensive gastropathy (PHG) and gastric vascular ectasia. In all likelihood, these lesions are distinct, as demonstrated by histologic features and differences in the response to a TIPS. An appearance analogous to PHG in the colon is termed *portal hypertensive colopathy* (see Chapter 37).

The diagnosis of PHG is based on the presence of a characteristic mosaic-like pattern of the gastric mucosa on endoscopic examination. This pattern is characterized by small polygonal areas with a depressed border. Superimposed on this mosaic-like pattern may be red point lesions that are usually greater than 2 mm in diameter. PHG is considered mild when only a mosaic-like pattern is present and severe when superimposed discrete red spots are also seen (Fig. 92-20).[251] The cause and pathogenesis of PHG are poorly understood. Development of PHG correlates with the duration of cirrhosis but not necessarily the degree of liver dysfunction. The frequency of PHG following endoscopic

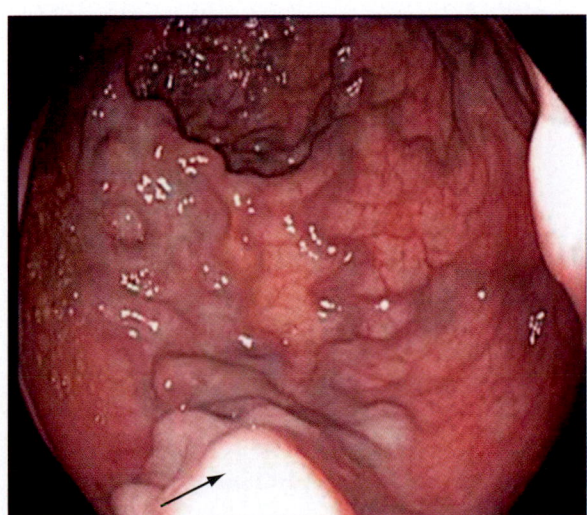

FIGURE 92-18. Endoscopic image of a colonic varix *(arrow)*.

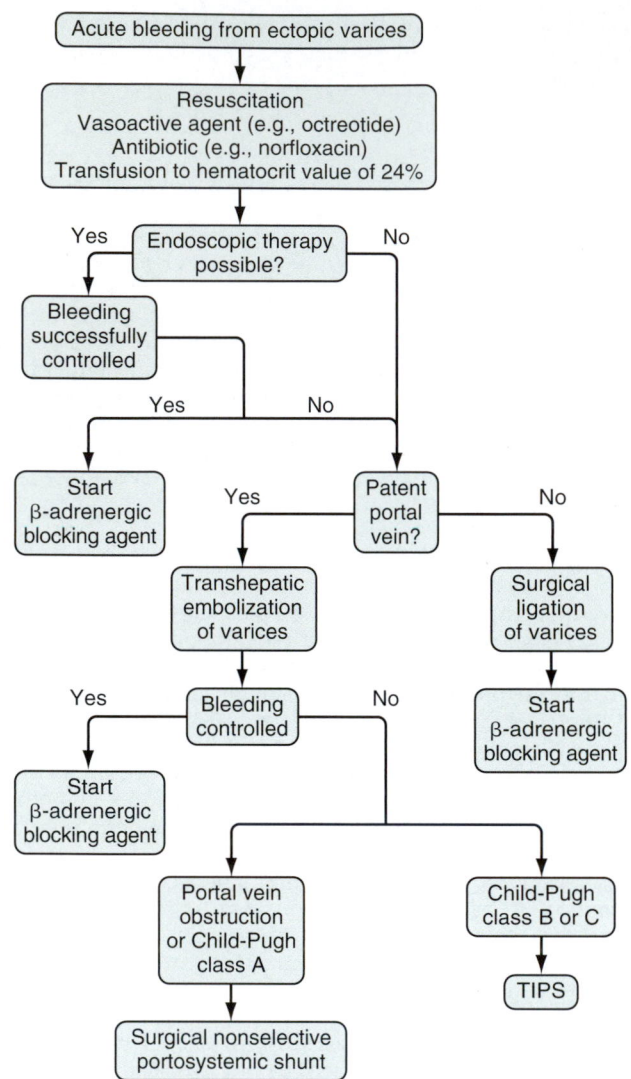

FIGURE 92-19. Algorithm for the management of bleeding from ectopic varices in patients with portal hypertension. TIPS, transjugular intrahepatic portosystemic shunt.

treatment of esophageal varices is increased, possibly a result of longer duration of portal hypertension in these patients.

In gastric vascular ectasia, aggregates of ectatic vessels can be seen on endoscopic examination as red spots without a mosaic background.[252] When the aggregates are confined to the antrum of the stomach, the term *gastric antral vascular ectasia* (GAVE) is used (see Chapters 20 and 37). If aggregates in the antrum are linear, the term *watermelon stomach* is used to describe the lesion (Fig. 92-21). When the red spots are distributed diffusely, in both the distal and the proximal stomach, the term *diffuse gastric vascular ectasia* is preferred.[253]

Distinguishing PHG from GAVE is sometimes difficult (Table 92-5). A background mosaic pattern and proximal distribution favor PHG. GAVE is less common, occurs in the absence of a background mosaic pattern, and typically is antral in location, although lesions may be present in the proximal stomach. Mucosal biopsies are recommended when the

TABLE 92-5 Comparison of Portal Hypertensive Gastropathy (PHG) and Gastric Antral Vascular Ectasia (GAVE)

Feature	PHG	GAVE
Distribution	Proximal stomach	Distal stomach
Mosaic pattern	Present	Absent
Red color signs	Present	Present
Findings on gastric mucosal biopsy		
Thrombi	−	+++
Spindle cell proliferation	+	++
Fibrohyalinosis	−	+++
Treatment	β-Adrenergic blocking agent ?APC TIPS	Endoscopic therapy ?Antrectomy ?Liver transplantation

APC, argon plasma coagulation; TIPS, transjugular intrahepatic portosystemic shunt.

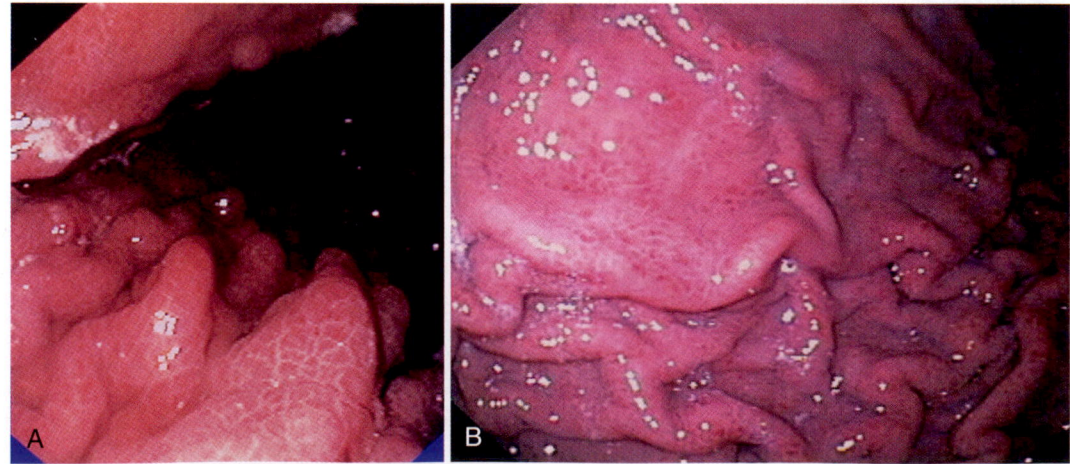

FIGURE 92-20. Endoscopic views of portal hypertensive gastropathy. *A*, Mild portal hypertensive gastropathy is characterized by a mosaic appearance without red color signs. *B*, Severe portal hypertensive gastropathy is characterized by superimposed red spots.

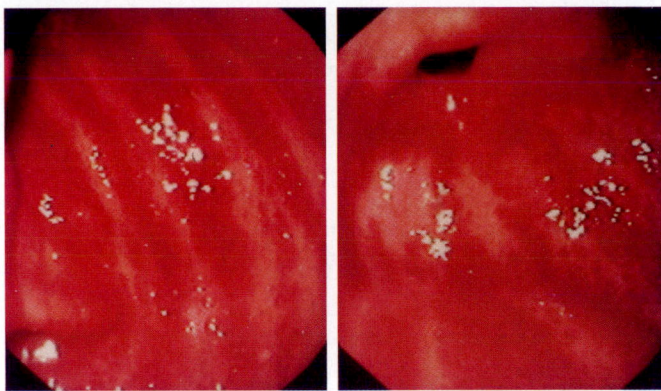

FIGURE 92-21. Endoscopic images of severe watermelon stomach (gastric antral vascular ectasia, GAVE).

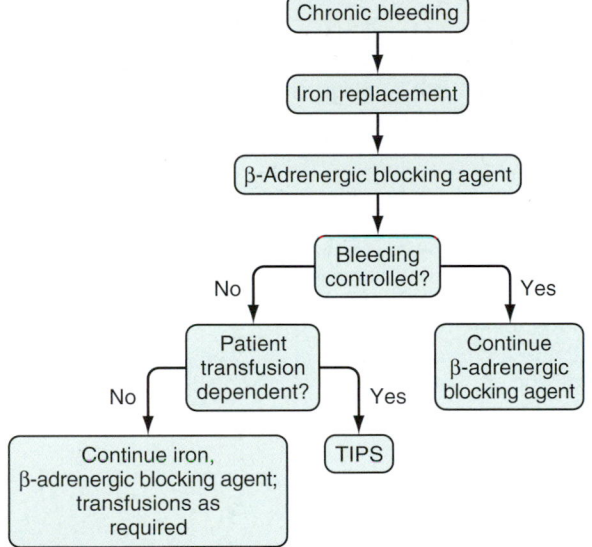

FIGURE 92-22. Algorithm for the management of chronic bleeding from portal hypertensive gastropathy. TIPS, transjugular intrahepatic portosystemic shunt.

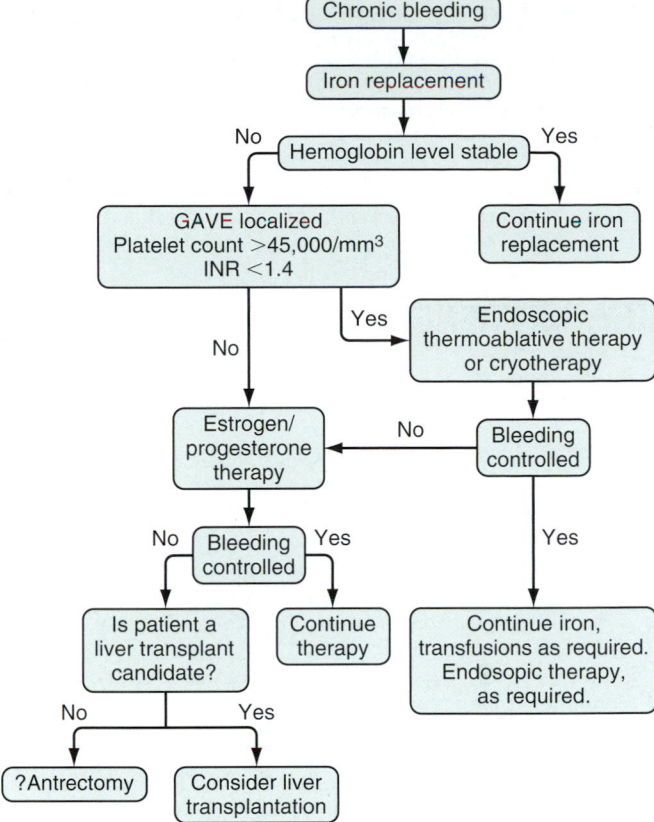

FIGURE 92-23. Algorithm for the management of chronic bleeding from gastric vascular antral ectasia (GAVE).

endoscopic diagnosis is uncertain. GAVE appears histologically as dilated mucosal capillaries with focal areas of fibrin thrombi or ectasia in combination with proliferation of spindle cells.[254] Similar ectatic lesions may be seen in the small bowel and may cause acute or chronic GI blood loss.

Management

PHG accounts for approximately one fourth of all cases of GI bleeding (acute and chronic) in patients with portal hypertension, but for less than 10% of all episodes of acute bleeding. The more common presentation is one of chronic, slow bleeding and anemia. Pharmacologic therapy to prevent bleeding (primary prophylaxis) in patients with severe portal hypertensive gastropathy is not currently recommended. Small studies have suggested that octreotide may be useful for controlling acute bleeding.[255] Beta blockers are recommended for preventing chronic blood loss in patients who have bled from severe PHG.[256,257] When patients are transfusion dependent despite beta blockade and iron supplementation, a TIPS may be inserted (Fig. 92-22). A TIPS decreases transfusion requirements and results in reversal of the mucosal lesions on endoscopic examination.[253]

Management of GAVE is more problematic. Initial treatment involves repletion of iron and RBC transfusions to treat symptomatic anemia. If lesions are localized, the platelet count is greater than approximately 45,000/mm[3], and the INR is less than 1.4, thermoablative therapy, as with argon plasma coagulation, may be helpful (Fig. 92-23). The usual settings for argon plasma coagulation are an energy level of 60 to 90 watts and a gas flow rate of 1 to 2 L per minute. If the coagulation parameters are suboptimal, thermal coagulation is associated with an increase in mucosal bleeding in many patients. It does not appear that use of the oral thrombopoietin receptor agonist eltrombopag, which increases the platelet count, is associated with a decrease in the risk of bleeding associated with procedures.[258] When the vascular ectasias are diffuse and extensive in the stomach, cryotherapy using liquid nitrogen or CO_2 may be used.[259] If endoscopic therapy fails, therapy with an oral estrogen-progesterone combination may be useful in reducing transfusion requirements.[260] The usual dose is estradiol, 35 µg, plus norethindrone, 1 mg, daily. Because the medication is taken daily, no risk of breakthrough vaginal bleeding exists. Rarely, painful gynecomastia may limit use of this combination in men. In the occasional patient with preserved hepatic synthetic function who continues to bleed despite thermoablative therapy and an estrogen-progesterone combination, a surgical antral resection may be carried out. TIPS does not reduce the bleeding risk in patients with GAVE and is associated with a substantial risk of hepatic encephalopathy[253]; therefore, TIPS placement is not recommended as therapy for GAVE. By contrast, GAVE is reversed with liver transplantation, even in the presence of portal hypertension, suggesting that GAVE is related to liver failure, rather than to portal hypertension.[55,261]

Other Nonvariceal Causes of Bleeding

Other causes of GI bleeding include peptic ulcers, Dieulafoy lesions, Mallory-Weiss tears, hemorrhoids, and portal hypertensive colopathy. The most common findings reported in patients with cirrhosis and lower GI bleeding are portal hypertensive colopathy and hemorrhoids, with diverticulosis a less common cause.[262] Patients with cirrhosis, especially alcoholic cirrhosis[263] are at increased risk of peptic ulcer bleeding,[264] but the risk of ulcer bleeding appears to decline with age.[265]

KEY REFERENCES

Full references for this chapter can be found on www.expertconsult.com.

15. Thabut D, Routray C, Lomberk G, et al. Complementary vascular and matrix regulatory pathways underlie the beneficial mechanism of action of sorafenib in liver fibrosis. Hepatology 2011; 54:573-85.
22. Abraldes JG, Albillos A, Banares R, et al. Simvastatin lowers portal pressure in patients with cirrhosis and portal hypertension: A randomized controlled trial. Gastroenterology 2009; 136:1651-8.
52. Zhu Q, Zou L, Jagavelu K, et al. Intestinal decontamination inhibits TLR4 dependent fibronectin-mediated cross-talk between stellate cells and endothelial cells in liver fibrosis in mice. J Hepatol 2012; 56:893-9.
68. Tripathi D, Ferguson JW, Kochar N, et al. Randomized controlled trial of carvedilol versus variceal band ligation for the prevention of the first variceal bleed. Hepatology 2009; 50:825-33.
109. Berzigotti A, Seijo S, Arena U, et al. Elastography, spleen size, and platelet count identify portal hypertension in patients with compensated cirrhosis. Gastroenterology 2013; 144:102-11.
110. Takuma Y, Nouso K, Morimoto Y, et al. Measurement of spleen stiffness by acoustic radiation force impulse imaging identifies cirrhotic patients with esophageal varices. Gastroenterology 2013; 144:92-101.
128. Maruyama H, Okugawa H, Takahashi M, et al. De novo portal vein thrombosis in virus-related cirrhosis: Predictive factors and long-term outcomes. Am J Gastroenterol 2013; 108:568-74.
139. Schouten JN, Garcia-Pagan JC, Valla DC, et al. Idiopathic noncirrhotic portal hypertension. Hepatology 2011; 54:1071-81.
155. Garcia-Tsao G. Liver involvement in hereditary hemorrhagic telangiectasia (HHT). J Hepatol 2007; 46:499-507.
167. Lui H, Stanley A, Forrest E, et al. Primary prophylaxis of variceal hemorrhage: A randomized controlled trial comparing band ligation, propranolol, and isosorbide mononitrate. Gastroenterology 2002; 123:735-44.
179. Fidelman N, Kwan SW, LaBerge JM, et al. The transjugular intrahepatic portosystemic shunt: An update. AJR Am J Roentgenol 2012; 199:746-55.
215. Buch P, Patel V, Ranpariya V, et al. Neuroprotective activity of *Cymbopogon martinii* against cerebral ischemia/reperfusion-induced oxidative stress in rats. J Ethnopharmacol 2012; 142:35-40.
216. Villanueva C, Colomo A, Bosch A, et al. Transfusion strategies for acute upper gastrointestinal bleeding. N Engl J Med 2013; 368:11-21.
218. Bernard B, Grange J, Khac E, et al. Antibiotic prophylaxis for the prevention of bacterial infections in cirrhotic patients with gastrointestinal bleeding: A meta-analysis. Hepatology 1999; 29:1655-61.
257. Panes J, Bordas J, Pique J, et al. Effects of propranolol on gastric mucosal perfusion in cirrhotic patients with portal hypertensive gastropathy. Hepatology 1993; 17:213-8.

Ascites is of Greek derivation ("askos") and refers to a bag or sack. The word is a noun and describes pathologic fluid accumulation within the peritoneal cavity. The adjective *ascitic* is used in conjunction with the word *fluid* to describe the liquid per se. Therefore, "ascitic fluid" is preferred to "ascites fluid."

PATHOGENESIS OF ASCITES

Cirrhotic Ascites

Ascites occurs in the setting of cirrhosis as a result of the sequence of events detailed in Figure 93-1. The most recent theory of ascitic fluid formation, the "peripheral arterial vasodilation hypothesis," proposes that both older hypotheses, the underfill and overflow theories, are correct, but that each is operative at a different stage.[1] The first abnormality that develops appears to be portal hypertension. Portal pressure increases above a critical threshold, and circulating nitric oxide levels increase. Nitric oxide leads to vasodilatation. As the state of vasodilatation worsens, plasma levels of vasoconstrictor sodium-retentive hormones increase, renal function deteriorates, and ascitic fluid forms—that is, hepatic decompensation occurs.

In the setting of volume overload in a patient with cirrhosis and ascites, the explanation for the neurohumoral excitation, which is characteristic of volume depletion, may relate to volume sensors. Animals have sophisticated systems for detecting and preserving vascular perfusion pressures and intravascular osmolality. An organism's ability to detect changes in intravascular volume (especially volume overload) is limited, however, and is linked to pressure receptors. This observation may explain, in part, the paradox of dramatic volume overload in the face of sympathetic nervous traffic and hormone levels that are indicative of intravascular volume depletion.

Noncirrhotic Ascites

The mechanism of fluid retention in patients with malignancy-related ascites depends on the location of the tumor. Peritoneal carcinomatosis appears to cause ascites through the production of proteinaceous fluid by tumor cells lining the peritoneum. Extracellular fluid enters the peritoneal cavity to reestablish oncotic balance. Fluid accumulates in patients with massive liver metastases because of portal hypertension caused by stenosis or occlusion of portal veins by tumor nodules or tumor emboli.[2] In patients with hepatocellular carcinoma, ascites arises because of the underlying cirrhosis-related portal hypertension, tumor-induced portal vein thrombosis, or both. Chylous ascites in patients with malignant lymphoma appears to be caused by lymph node obstruction by tumor and rupture of chyle-containing lymphatics.

Ascites can complicate high-output or low-output heart failure or nephrotic syndrome. As in cirrhosis, effective arterial blood volume appears to be decreased, and the vasopressin, renin-aldosterone, and sympathetic nervous systems are activated.[3] These changes lead to renal vasoconstriction and sodium and water retention. Fluid then "weeps" from the congested hepatic sinusoids as lymph, as in cirrhosis. TB, *Chlamydia* infection, and coccidioidomycosis probably cause ascites through the production of proteinaceous fluid, as in peritoneal carcinomatosis. SBP does not appear to cause fluid to accumulate; infection develops only in preexisting ascites.

In patients with pancreatic or biliary ascites, fluid accumulates by leakage of pancreatic juice or bile into the peritoneal cavity or forms secondary to a "chemical burn" of

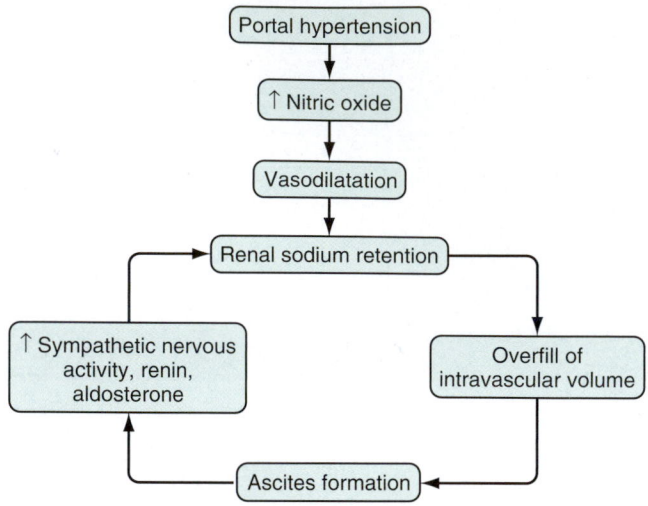

FIGURE 93-1. Pathogenesis of ascites in the setting of cirrhosis.

TABLE 93-1 Causes of Ascites	
Cause	**%**
Cirrhosis (with or without peritoneal infection)	85
Miscellaneous portal hypertension-related disorder (including 5% with two causes)	8
Cardiac disease	3
Peritoneal carcinomatosis	2
Miscellaneous nonportal hypertension–related disorders	2

Data from Runyon BA, Montano AA, Akriviadis EA, et al. The serum-ascites albumin gradient is superior to the exudate-transudate concept in the differential diagnosis of ascites. Ann Intern Med 1992; 117:215-20.

the peritoneum. After abdominal surgery, especially extensive retroperitoneal dissection, lymphatics may be transected and may leak lymph for varying amounts of time. The mechanism of development of ascites in this condition is similar to that for malignant chylous ascites, namely, lymphatic leak.

CLINICAL FEATURES

History

Most patients (≈85%) with ascites in the United States have cirrhosis. The 3 most common causes of cirrhosis are excess alcohol use, chronic hepatitis C, and nonalcoholic steatohepatitis (NASH) related in many cases to obesity. As the obesity epidemic evolves, NASH could become the most common cause of cirrhosis. Many patients have 2 of these conditions, and some have all 3.[4] In approximately 15% of patients with ascites, a nonhepatic cause of fluid retention is identified (Table 93-1).

Ascites frequently develops during a patient's first episode of decompensation of alcoholic liver disease. Ascites can develop early in alcoholic liver disease in the precirrhotic alcoholic hepatitis stage. At this stage, portal hypertension and the

resulting predisposition to sodium retention are reversible with abstinence from alcohol. Patients with precirrhotic alcoholic liver disease may lose their predisposition to fluid retention when they reduce or cease consumption of alcohol.

Evidence is accumulating that cirrhosis unrelated to alcohol use can also be reversible with effective therapy.[5] Whether a decompensated cirrhotic liver can revert to a normal liver, however, remains to be seen. Many patients with cirrhosis and ascites will ultimately require liver transplantation.

Patients with ascites should be questioned about risk factors for liver disease other than alcohol, such as injection drug use, blood transfusions prior to 1992, sex with a same-gender partner, acupuncture, tattoos, ear piercing, and country of origin. Commonly, the cause of ascites in a middle-aged or elderly woman is viral hepatitis–induced cirrhosis resulting from a remote, often forgotten blood transfusion. Another cause of "cryptogenic" cirrhosis and ascites is NASH from long-standing obesity.[6] Many patients who have been obese will spontaneously lose 50 or even 100 pounds after their liver disease decompensates. Unless the patient is questioned about lifetime maximum body weight and usual adult body weight, the possibility of NASH-related cirrhosis may not be considered. With careful history-taking and appropriate laboratory testing, the percentage of patients with cirrhosis who are now labeled cryptogenic is approaching zero (see Chapter 74).[6]

Patients with a long history of stable cirrhosis and the sudden development of ascites should be suspected of harboring a hepatocellular carcinoma that has precipitated the decompensation. Patients with ascites who have a history of cancer should be suspected of having malignancy-related ascites. Cancer in the past, however, does not guarantee a malignant cause of ascites. For example, patients with tobacco-related lung cancer and a history of alcohol abuse may have ascites due to cirrhosis. Breast, lung, colon, and pancreatic cancers are regularly complicated by ascites.[2] Abdominal pain is a helpful distinguishing feature. Malignancy-related ascites frequently is painful, whereas cirrhotic ascites usually is not, unless bacterial peritonitis or alcoholic hepatitis is superimposed.

A history of heart failure may raise the possibility of cardiac ascites. Alcoholic patients in whom ascites develops may have alcoholic cardiomyopathy or alcoholic liver disease, but usually not both.

Tuberculous peritonitis usually manifests as fever and abdominal pain. Many affected patients are immigrants from an endemic area. In the United States, more than half of the patients with tuberculous peritonitis have underlying alcoholic cirrhosis that may contribute to the formation of ascitic fluid.

Ascites may occur in patients with acute pancreatitis with necrosis or a ruptured pancreatic duct from chronic pancreatitis or trauma. Often, troublesome ascites also may develop in a small percentage of patients undergoing hemodialysis. Fitz-Hugh–Curtis syndrome caused by chlamydia or gonorrhea may cause inflammatory ascites in a sexually active woman. Patients in whom ascites and anasarca develop in the setting of diabetes mellitus should be suspected of having nephrotic ascites. Ascites in a patient with symptoms and signs of myxedema should prompt assessment of thyroid function. Serositis in a patient with a connective tissue disease may be complicated by ascites.[7]

Physical Examination

On the basis of the history and the appearance of the abdomen, the diagnosis of ascites is readily suspected and usually confirmed easily on physical examination. The presence of a full, bulging abdomen should lead to percussion of the flanks. If the degree of flank dullness is greater than usual (i.e., if the percussed air-fluid level is higher than that normally found on the lateral aspect of the abdomen with the patient supine), the examiner should check for "shifting." If flank dullness is absent, checking for shifting is unnecessary. Approximately 1500 mL of fluid must be present before dullness is detected.[8] If flank dullness is not present, the chance that the patient has ascites is less than 10%.[8] A fluid wave is not worth testing for.[8]

Gaseous distention of the bowel, a thick panniculus, and an ovarian mass can mimic ascites. Gaseous distention should be readily apparent on percussion. Ovarian masses usually cause tympanitic flanks with central dullness. The speed of increase in abdominal girth also can be helpful: ascites develops in days to weeks, whereas thickening of the omentum and panniculus takes months to years. An obese abdomen may be diffusely dull to percussion, and abdominal US may be required to determine if fluid is present. US can detect as little as 100 mL of fluid in the abdomen.

The presence of palmar erythema, large pulsatile spider telangiectasias, large abdominal wall collateral veins, or fetor hepaticus is suggestive of parenchymal liver disease and portal hypertension (see Chapter 74). The presence of large veins on the patient's back suggests inferior vena cava blockage. An immobile mass in the umbilicus, the Sister Mary Joseph nodule, is suggestive of peritoneal carcinomatosis.

The neck veins of patients with ascites should always be examined. Alcoholic cardiomyopathy with cardiac ascites can mimic cirrhosis with ascites; an elevated jugular venous pressure helps with this aspect of the differential diagnosis. Constrictive pericarditis is one of the few curable causes of ascites. Most patients with cardiac ascites have impressive jugular venous distention. Some have no visible jugular venous distention but such high central venous pressures that their bulging forehead veins rise to the top of their skulls. When present, peripheral edema in patients with liver disease is usually found in the lower extremities and occasionally may involve the abdominal wall. Patients with nephrotic syndrome or cardiac failure may have total body edema (anasarca).

DIAGNOSIS

Although the diagnosis of ascites may be suspected on the basis of the history and physical examination, final confirmation is based on successful abdominal paracentesis or detection of ascites on imaging. Determination of the cause of ascites is based on the results of the history, physical examination, and ascitic fluid analysis. In general, few other tests are required.

Abdominal Paracentesis

Indications

Abdominal paracentesis[9] with appropriate ascitic fluid analysis is probably the most rapid and cost-effective method of diagnosing the cause of ascites. Also, because of the possibility of ascitic fluid infection in a patient with cirrhosis admitted to the hospital, a surveillance paracentesis performed on admission may detect unexpected infection.[10] Not all patients with ascitic fluid infection are symptomatic; many have subtle symptoms, such as mild confusion noticed only by the family. An emergency department study has demonstrated that a physician's impression regarding the presence or absence of ascitic fluid infection is inaccurate.[11]

Detection of infection at an early asymptomatic stage may reduce mortality. Therefore, ascitic fluid should be sampled in all inpatients and outpatients with new-onset ascites and in all patients with ascites who are admitted to the hospital. Paracentesis should be repeated in patients (whether hospitalized or not) in whom symptoms, signs, or laboratory abnormalities suggestive of infection develop (e.g., abdominal pain or tenderness, fever, encephalopathy, hypotension, renal failure, acidosis, peripheral leukocytosis).

Contraindications

Few contraindications to paracentesis have been recognized. Coagulopathy is a potential contraindication; however, most patients with cirrhosis and ascites have coagulopathy, and if mild to moderate coagulopathy were viewed as a contraindication to paracentesis, few patients with cirrhosis would undergo this procedure.[12] Coagulopathy should preclude paracentesis only when clinically evident fibrinolysis or DIC is present.[12] These conditions occur in fewer than 1 per 1000 paracenteses. No data are available to support cutoff values for coagulation parameters beyond which paracentesis should be avoided. Overall coagulation is usually normal in the setting of cirrhosis, despite abnormal tests of coagulation, because there is a balanced deficiency of procoagulants and anticoagulants.[13] Even after multiple paracenteses, bloody ascites usually does not develop in patients with marked prolongation of the prothrombin time. Patients with cirrhosis and without clinically obvious coagulopathy simply do not bleed excessively from needlesticks unless a blood vessel is entered.[12]

Studies regarding complications of paracentesis in patients with ascites have documented no deaths or infections caused by paracentesis.[10,12] No episodes of hemoperitoneum or entry of the paracentesis needle into the bowel have been reported in these studies. Complications have included only abdominal wall hematomas in approximately 2% of paracenteses, even though 71% of the patients had an abnormal prothrombin time and 21% had a prothrombin time prolonged by more than 5 seconds.[12] Complication rates may be higher when paracentesis is performed by an inexperienced operator.

Transfusion of blood products (fresh frozen plasma or platelets) routinely before paracentesis in patients with cirrhosis and coagulopathy, presumably to prevent hemorrhagic complications, is not supported by data. Because a hematoma that necessitates blood transfusion develops in only approximately 1% of patients who undergo paracentesis without prophylactic transfusion of plasma or platelets, approximately 100 to 200 units of fresh frozen plasma or platelets would have to be given to prevent the transfusion of approximately 2 units of red blood cells (RBCs). In a prospective study of 1100 therapeutic paracenteses, no blood products were given prior to the procedure, nor were they needed after the procedure despite a platelet count as low as $19,000/mm^3$ [$0.19 \times 10^9/L$] and INR as high as 8.7.[14]

Patient Position and Choice of Needle and Entry Site

The volume of fluid in the abdomen and the thickness of the abdominal wall determine, in part, how the patient should be positioned in preparation for paracentesis. Patients with a large volume of ascites and thin abdominal wall can be "tapped" successfully in the supine position, with the head of the bed or examining table elevated slightly. Patients with less fluid can be placed in the lateral decubitus position and tapped in the midline or in the right or left lower quadrant while supine (see later). Patients with small amounts of fluid may be tapped successfully only in the face-down position or with US guidance.[15]

The choice of the site for inserting the needle has changed over the years because of the increasing prevalence of obesity and frequency of therapeutic paracentesis. Paracentesis in obese patients poses special challenges. In obese patients, the abdominal wall usually is substantially thicker in the midline than in the lower quadrants on US examination.[15] The abdominal wall may be even thicker than the length of a 3.5-inch paracentesis needle. Also, on physical examination, determining whether ascites is present or absent in the obese patient is frequently difficult. US examination is helpful in confirming the presence of fluid and in guiding the paracentesis needle. Preferably, the needle is inserted into the left lower quadrant, rather than the right lower quadrant, because the cecum may be distended with gas from lactulose therapy (see Chapter 94). Also, the right lower quadrant is more likely than the left to have a surgical scar (e.g., from an appendectomy). When therapeutic paracentesis is performed, more fluid can be obtained using a lower quadrant needle insertion site than a midline site.

The needle must be placed several centimeters from a surgical scar. The bowel may be adherent to the peritoneal surface of the abdomen near a scar, and a needle inserted there may enter the bowel.[10] A long midline scar precludes midline paracentesis. An appendectomy scar precludes a right lower quadrant site, in general.

I usually choose a site in the left lower quadrant 2 fingerbreadths (3 cm) cephalad and 2 fingerbreadths medial to the anterior superior iliac spine.[15] In a patient with multiple abdominal scars, US guidance may be required.

In a patient who is not overweight, I prefer to use a standard metal 1.5-inch, 22-gauge needle. Paracentesis in obese patients requires the use of a longer needle—for example, one that is 3.5 inches and 22 gauge. Steel needles are preferable to plastic-sheathed cannulas because plastic sheaths may shear off into the peritoneal cavity, with the potential to kink and obstruct the flow of fluid after the cannula is removed. Metal needles do not puncture the bowel unless the bowel is adherent to a scar or severe gaseous distention is present.

Technique

The optimal technique of diagnostic and therapeutic paracentesis has been reviewed in detail.[9]

Diagnostic Paracentesis

Drapes, gown, hat, and mask are optional, but sterile gloves should be used when paracentesis is performed. The skin is disinfected with an iodine solution. The skin and subcutaneous tissue should be infiltrated with a local anesthetic. The sterile package insert enclosing the gloves can be used as a sterile field on which to place syringes, needles, gauze, and other supplies. When sterile gloves are not used, ascitic fluid cultures frequently grow skin contaminants; a single viable organism will grow to detectable levels in blood culture bottles.

To prevent leakage of fluid after the needle is withdrawn, a special technique is required. The previously used term "Z tract" led to confusion about the precise technique. It does not involve manipulating the needle up and down, which could lead to tissue injury. The technique of needle insertion is accomplished by displacing (with one gloved hand) the skin approximately 2 cm downward and then slowly inserting the paracentesis needle mounted on the syringe held in the other hand. The hand holding the syringe stabilizes the syringe and retracts its plunger simultaneously. A steady hand and experience are needed. The skin is released only after the needle has penetrated the peritoneum and fluid flows. When the needle is ultimately removed, the skin resumes its original position and seals the needle pathway. (If the needle were inserted straight into the peritoneum from the skin surface, the fluid would leak out easily because the pathway would be straight.)

The needle should be advanced slowly through the abdominal wall in approximately 5-mm increments. Slow insertion allows the operator to see blood if a vessel is entered, so that the needle can be withdrawn immediately before further damage is done. Slow insertion also allows the bowel to move away from the needle, thereby avoiding bowel puncture. The syringe that is attached to the needle should be aspirated intermittently during insertion. If continuous suction is applied, bowel or omentum may be drawn to the end of the needle as soon as the needle enters the peritoneal cavity, thereby occluding flow and resulting in an apparently unsuccessful tap. Slow insertion also allows time for the elastic peritoneum to "tent" over the end of the needle and be pierced by it. The most common causes of an unsuccessful paracentesis are continuous aspiration during insertion of the needle and rapid insertion and withdrawal of the needle before the peritoneum is pierced. If the operator is certain that the needle tip is inserted far enough but no fluid is apparent, the syringe and needle can be twisted 90 degrees to pierce the peritoneum, thereby permitting flow of fluid.

Approximately 30 mL of fluid is obtained using one or more syringes. I prefer to use a 5- or 10-mL syringe for the initial portion of a diagnostic tap and then twist this syringe off the needle and replace it with a 20- or 30-mL syringe to obtain the remainder of the sample. The initial use of a small syringe allows the operator to have better control and to see fluid more easily as it enters the hub of the syringe. The syringe and attached needle are then pulled out of the abdomen, and the needle is removed and discarded. A sterile needle is then placed on the larger syringe, and an appropriate amount of fluid is inoculated into each of a pair of prepared blood culture bottles (see later). Usually, 5 to 10 mL is inoculated into 50-mL bottles, and 10 to 20 mL into 100-mL bottles. The next aliquot is placed into a "purple-top" ethylenediaminetetraacetic acid (EDTA) tube for a cell count, and the final aliquot is placed into a "red-top" tube for chemistries. Inoculating the culture bottles first with a sterile needle minimizes contamination. The fluid must be placed promptly into the anticoagulant-containing tube to avoid clotting; clotted fluid cannot be analyzed for cell count.

Therapeutic Paracentesis

Therapeutic paracentesis is similar to diagnostic paracentesis except that a larger-bore needle is used and additional equipment is required. In the patient who is not overweight, I prefer to use a standard metal 1.5-inch, 16- to 18-gauge needle. Obese patients may require a longer needle (e.g., 3.5 inches and 18 gauge). A set of 15-gauge 5-hole needles has been produced specifically for therapeutic abdominal paracentesis; these needles may replace the spinal needles generally used for paracentesis in obese patients. The 15-gauge needles have a removable sharp inner component and a blunt outer cannula; they range in length from 3.25 to 5.9 inches. A tiny scalpel nick is required to permit the large needle to enter the skin.

An old method of using a 60-mL syringe, stopcock, and collection bag is tedious; use of vacuum bottles (1 or 2 L) connected to the needle with noncollapsible tubing is much faster. Use of a pump is even faster than vacuum bottles. Unless the needle is allowed to drift subcutaneously, the needle (or blunt steel cannula) can be left in the abdomen during a therapeutic paracentesis without injury. Larger-bore needles or cannulas permit more rapid removal of fluid but leave larger defects if they enter vessels or the bowel inadvertently.

Once fluid is flowing, the needle should be stabilized to ensure steady flow. Not unusually, flow ceases intermittently.

With respiratory movement, the needle may gradually work its way out of the peritoneal cavity and into the soft tissue, and some serosanguineous fluid may appear in the needle hub or tubing. When this happens, the pump should be turned off or a clamp placed on the tubing connected to the vacuum bottle. The tubing should be removed from the needle and the needle twisted a few degrees. If flow does not resume, the needle should be twisted a bit more. If flow still does not resume, the needle should be inserted in 1- to 2-mm increments until brisk dripping of fluid from the needle hub is seen. The tubing can then be reattached and more fluid removed. Occasionally, fluid cannot be aspirated but drips from the needle hub. In this situation, fluid can be allowed to drip into a sterile container for collection, as in a lumbar puncture.

As the fluid is removed, the bowel and omentum draw closer to the needle and eventually block the flow of ascitic fluid. The patient must then be repositioned so that gravity causes the fluid to pool near the needle. It is useful to reposition the patient a few times during a total paracentesis to maximize the amount of fluid removed. Excessive manipulation of the needle should be avoided to minimize the risk of trauma to the bowel or blood vessels.

After samples of fluid are obtained for testing, a total of 2 to 4 L of fluid is removed to relieve the pressure of tense ascites in patients with new or diuretic-sensitive ascites. A sodium-restricted diet and diuretics are prescribed to reduce the fluid further. If a patient is known to be diuretic-resistant, a "total tap" is performed—that is, all of the fluid that is accessible is removed. If less is removed, the tap will need to be repeated soon (see later).

Ascitic Fluid Analysis

Gross Appearance

Non-neutrocytic (i.e., ascitic fluid polymorphonuclear neutrophil [PMN] count less than 250/mm³ [0.25 × 10⁹/L]) ascitic fluid is transparent and usually slightly yellow (Fig. 93-2). Ascitic fluid with a very low protein concentration may have no pigment and look like water. The opacity of many cloudy ascitic fluid specimens is caused by neutrophils. The presence of neutrophils leads to a shimmering effect when a glass tube containing the fluid is rocked back and forth in front of a light. Fluid with an absolute neutrophil count less than 1000/mm³ (1.0 × 10⁹/L) may be nearly clear. Fluid with a count greater than 5000/mm³ (5.0 × 10⁹/L) is quite cloudy, and fluid with a count greater than 50,000/mm³ (50.0 × 10⁹/L) resembles mayonnaise.

Ascitic fluid specimens frequently are blood-tinged or frankly bloody. An RBC count of 10,000/mm³ (10.0 × 10⁹/L) is the threshold for a pink appearance; lower concentrations result in clear or turbid fluid. Ascitic fluid with an RBC count greater than 20,000/mm³ (20.0 × 10⁹/L) is distinctly red. Many ascitic fluid specimens are bloody because of a traumatic tap; these specimens are blood-streaked and frequently clot unless the fluid is transferred immediately to the anticoagulant-containing tube for the cell count. By contrast, nontraumatic or remotely traumatic blood-tinged ascitic fluid is homogeneous and does not clot because it has already clotted and the clot has lysed. Some patients with portal hypertension have bloody hepatic lymph, resulting in bloody ascitic fluid—perhaps because of rupture of lymphatics that are under high pressure. Samples from patients with hepatocellular carcinoma are regularly bloody, but only about 10% of samples from patients with peritoneal carcinomatosis are red.[2] Although many physicians have the impression that TB results in bloody ascitic fluid, less than 5% of tuberculous samples are hemorrhagic in my experience.

Ascitic fluid frequently is lipid-laden. Lipid opacifies the fluid. The degree of opalescence of ascitic fluid ranges from slightly cloudy to completely opaque and chylous. Most opaque, milky fluid samples have a TG concentration greater than 200 mg/dL (2.26 mmol/L) and usually greater than 1000 mg/dL (11.30 mmol/L). Fluid that has the appearance of dilute skim milk has a TG concentration between 100 mg/dL (1.13 mmol/L) and 200 mg/dL (2.26 mmol/L). A substantial minority of cirrhotic ascitic fluid samples are neither transparent nor frankly milky. These opalescent samples have slightly elevated TG concentrations ranging from 50 mg/dL (0.56 mmol/L) to 200 mg/dL (2.26 mmol/L).[16] The opacity of these fluids does not have the shimmering characteristics of ascitic fluid with an elevated WBC count. The lipid usually layers out when a tube of ascitic fluid is placed in a refrigerator for 48 to 72 hours. In contrast to findings in older published reports, most patients with chylous or opalescent ascites have cirrhosis.[16,17]

Dark-brown fluid with a bilirubin concentration greater than that of serum usually indicates biliary perforation.[18] Deeply jaundiced patients have bile-stained ascitic fluid, but the bilirubin level and the degree of pigmentation are visually less than those of the corresponding serum. Pancreatic ascites may be pigmented because of the effect of pancreatic enzymes on RBCs. The RBCs may have to be centrifuged before the discolored supernatant is revealed. The degree of pigmentation ranges from tea-colored to jet black, as in pancreatic necrosis. Black ascitic fluid also may be found in patients with malignant melanoma.

Tests

The practice of ordering every available body fluid test on every ascitic fluid specimen is expensive and can be more confusing than helpful, especially when unexpectedly abnormal results are encountered. An algorithm for the analysis of ascitic fluid is shown in Figure 93-2. The basic concept is that screening tests are performed on the initial specimen; additional testing is performed only when necessary as indicated by the results of the screening tests. Further testing may require another paracentesis, but because most specimens consist of ascitic fluid resulting from uncomplicated cirrhosis, no further testing is needed in a majority of cases. Also, because laboratories frequently store the fluid for a few days, additional testing can often be ordered on the stored fluid.

On the basis of cost analysis, tests can be classified as routine, optional, unusual, and unhelpful (Table 93-2).[10] The cell count is the single most helpful ascitic fluid test. Only approximately 10 µL of fluid is required for a standard manual hemocytometer count. Therefore, if only 1 drop of fluid can be obtained, it should be sent for cell count. More fluid is almost always obtainable, however. The fluid should be submitted in an anticoagulant-containing tube (i.e., EDTA) to prevent clotting. Because the decision to begin empirical

TABLE 93-2 Ascitic Fluid Laboratory Tests

Routine	Optional	Unusual	Unhelpful
Cell count	Amylase	Bilirubin	Cholesterol
Albumin	Culture in blood	Cytology	Fibronectin
Total protein	culture bottles	TB smear,	Lactate
	Glucose	culture, and	pH
	Gram stain	PCR test	
	LDH	TG	

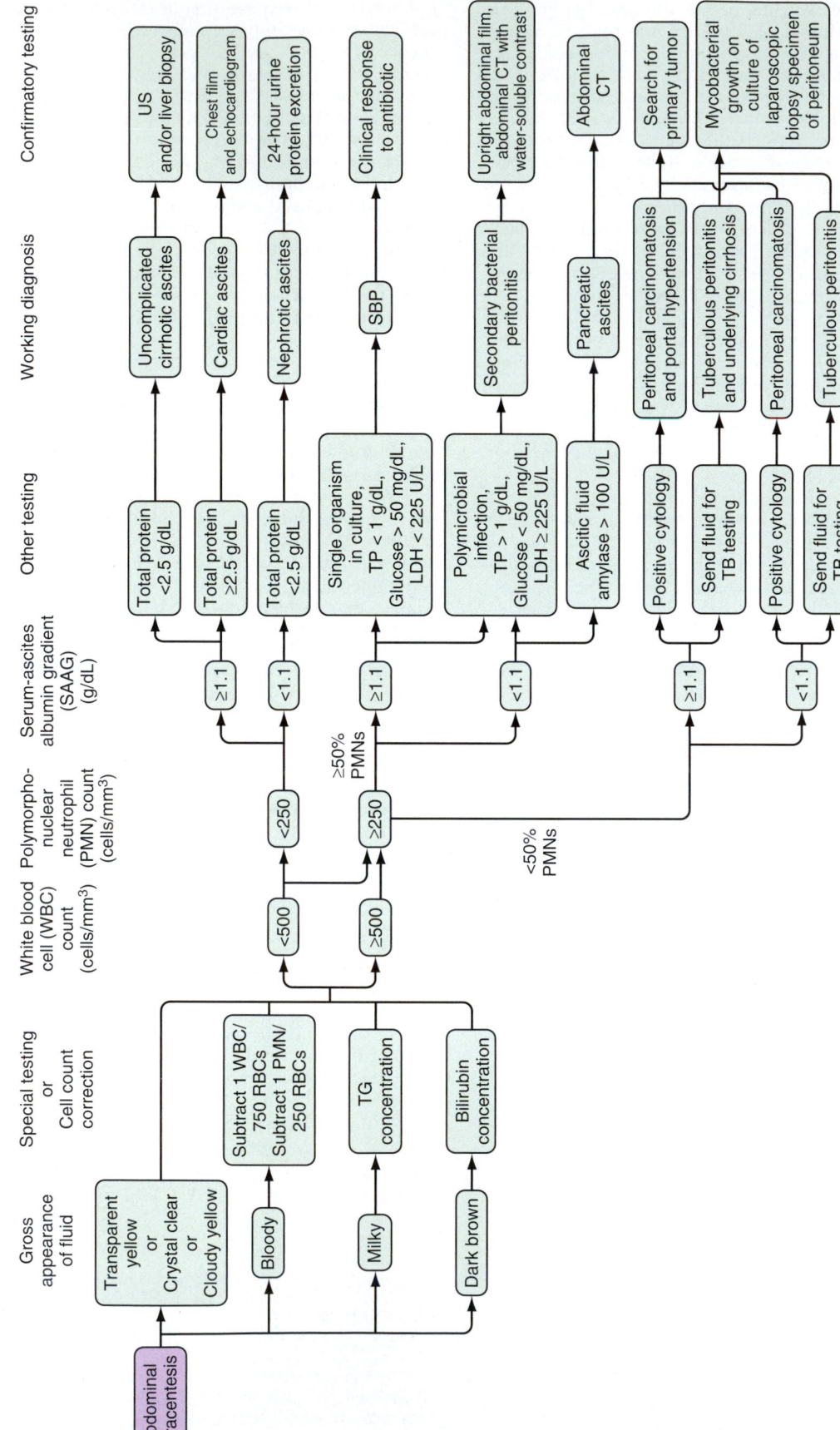

FIGURE 93-2. Algorithm for the approach to the differential diagnosis of ascites. PMN, polymorphonuclear neutrophil; RBC, red blood cell; TP, total protein.

protein concentrations are the most susceptible to spontaneous peritonitis.[29] During a 10-kg diuresis, however, the ascitic fluid total protein concentration doubles, and 67% of such patients with cirrhosis and ascites have a protein concentration greater than 2.5 g/dL (25 g/L) by the end of diuresis.[19] In almost one third of patients with malignancy-related ascites, the ascites is caused by massive liver metastases or hepatocellular carcinoma, and the ascitic fluid in these patients has a low protein concentration.[2] In cardiac ascites, the ascitic fluid protein concentration is usually greater than 2.5 g/dL (25 g/L).[30]

The SAAG classifies fluid by the presence or absence of portal hypertension and is much more physiologic and intuitive than the old exudate/transudate classification. The exudate/transudate method of classification of ascites places many patients with cirrhosis and ascites and all patients with cardiac ascites in the exudate category, and many patients with malignant ascites and essentially all patients with spontaneously infected ascites in the transudate category. Clearly, this method of classification is not useful.[24] The albumin gradient classifies cardiac ascites in the high-SAAG category, similar to ascites in cirrhosis. The high SAAG of cardiac ascites is presumably the result of high right-sided cardiac pressures. In patients with cardiac ascites, the SAAG may narrow with diuresis; such narrowing does not happen in patients with cirrhosis.

The combination of ascitic fluid total protein, glucose, and LDH is of value in distinguishing SBP from intestinal perforation with leakage of intestinal contents into ascites[31] (Fig. 93-3). Patients who have neutrocytic ascitic fluid, in whom the clinical picture suggests bacterial peritonitis (rather than peritoneal carcinomatosis or tuberculous peritonitis) and who meet 2 of the following 3 criteria, are likely to have surgical peritonitis and merit immediate radiologic evaluation to determine if intestinal perforation with leakage of intestinal contents into ascites has occurred: total protein greater than 1 g/dL (10 g/L), glucose less than 50 mg/dL (2.8 mmol/L), and LDH greater than the upper limit of normal for serum.[31]

Glucose

The glucose molecule is small enough to diffuse readily into body fluid cavities. Therefore, the concentration of glucose in ascitic fluid is similar to that in serum, unless glucose is being consumed by ascitic fluid WBCs or bacteria.[31] In early SBP, the ascitic fluid glucose concentration is similar to that of sterile fluid.[28] By contrast, in SBP detected late in its course (as well as in the setting of intestinal perforation into ascitic fluid), the ascitic fluid glucose concentration usually drops to 0 mg/dL (0 mmol/L) because of large numbers of stimulated neutrophils and bacteria.[31]

Lactate Dehydrogenase

The LDH molecule is too large to enter ascitic fluid readily from blood,[31] and the ascitic fluid concentration of LDH usually is less than half of the serum level in uncomplicated ascites in the setting of cirrhosis. In SBP, the ascitic fluid LDH level rises because of the release of LDH from neutrophils, and the ascitic fluid concentration is greater than that of serum. In

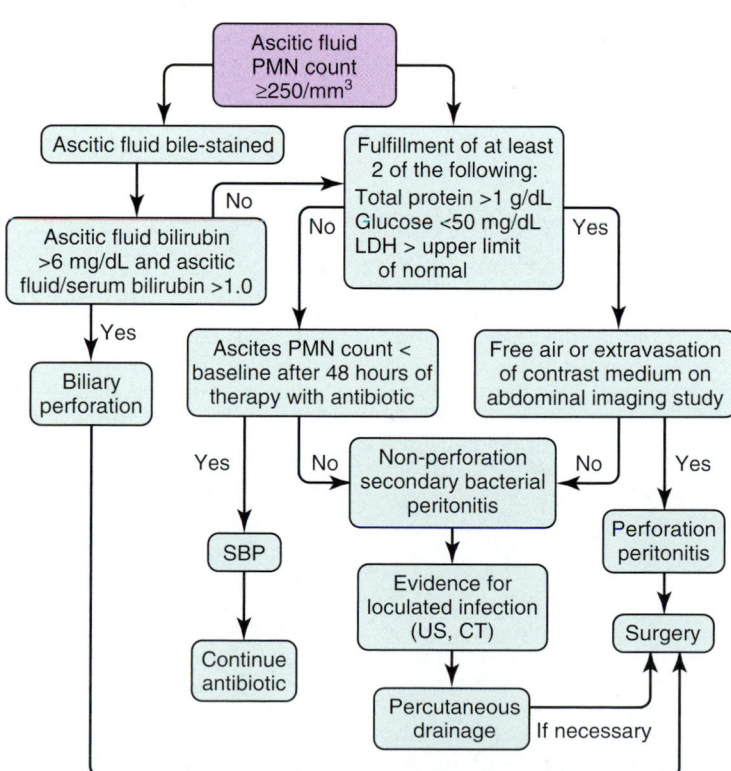

FIGURE 93-3. Algorithm for differentiating SBP from secondary bacterial peritonitis in patients with neutrocytic ascites (i.e., neutrophil count of ≥ 250 cells/mm³ [0.25 × 10⁹]) in the absence of hemorrhage into ascitic fluid, TB, peritoneal carcinomatosis, or pancreatitis. Antibiotic therapy should be started at the time peritonitis (ascitic fluid PMN count ≥ 250 cells/mm³) is detected. PMN, polymorphonuclear neutrophil. *(From Akriviadis EA, Runyon BA. The value of an algorithm in differentiating spontaneous from secondary bacterial peritonitis. Gastroenterology 1990; 98:127-33. Copyright 1990 by the American Gastroenterological Association, with permission.)*

secondary peritonitis, the LDH level is even higher than that seen in SBP and may be several-fold higher than the serum LDH level.[31]

Amylase

In uncomplicated ascites in the setting of cirrhosis, the ascitic fluid amylase concentration usually is half that of the serum value, approximately 50 U/L.[32] In patients with acute pancreatitis or intestinal perforation (with release of luminal amylase into the ascitic fluid), the fluid amylase concentration is elevated markedly, usually greater than 2000 U/L, and approximately 5-fold greater than simultaneous serum values.[31-33]

Gram Stain

Gram stains of body fluids demonstrate bacteria only when more than 10,000 bacteria/mL are present. The median concentration of bacteria in ascitic fluid in SBP is only 1 organism/mL, similar to the colony count in bacteremia.[26] Requesting an ascitic fluid Gram stain to detect bacteria in SBP is analogous to requesting a Gram stain of blood to detect bacteremia. Bacteria are detected on Gram stain only with overwhelming infection, as in advanced SBP or asplenic pneumococcal sepsis. Gram stain of ascitic fluid is most helpful in the diagnosis of free perforation of the intestine into ascitic fluid. In this setting, sheets of multiple different bacteria are found. Gram stain of the centrifuged sediment of 50 mL of ascites has a sensitivity of only 10% for visualizing bacteria in SBP.[26]

Smear and Culture for TB

A direct smear of ascitic fluid to detect mycobacteria is almost never positive because of the rarity of tuberculous peritonitis and the low concentration of mycobacteria in ascitic fluid in tuberculous peritonitis.[34] The older literature suggests that 1 L of fluid should be cultured. The largest centrifuge tube found in most laboratories, however, has a capacity of 50 mL. In general, only 1 50-mL aliquot of fluid is centrifuged, and the pellet is cultured. In contrast to a sensitivity of approximately 50% for ascitic fluid mycobacterial culture with optimal processing, laparoscopy with histology and culture of peritoneal biopsies has a sensitivity approaching 100% for detecting tuberculous peritonitis.[34] Tuberculous peritonitis can easily be confused with SBP, because both conditions are associated with abdominal pain and fever and half of the patients with tuberculous peritonitis have cirrhosis. A negative bacterial culture and predominance of mononuclear cells in the differential count, however, provide clues to the diagnosis of tuberculous peritonitis. DNA probes have become available to detect mycobacteria and probably will replace older methods of detection.[35] Nevertheless, cultures still will be required to determine susceptibility to antimicrobial agents.

Cytologic Examination

Cytologic studies can be expected to detect malignancy only when tumor cells line the peritoneal cavity and exfoliate into the ascitic fluid (i.e., in peritoneal carcinomatosis). In the past, massive liver metastases and hepatocellular carcinoma superimposed on cirrhosis were not recognized as causes of "malignant" ascites.[36] Cytologic studies should not be expected to detect tumor when the peritoneum is uninvolved, as in ascites resulting from portal hypertension in patients with hepatocellular carcinoma or massive liver metastases or from lymph node obstruction in patients with malignant lymphoma.[2] In one study in which the location and type of tumor that caused ascites were confirmed by a standard test, only approximately two thirds of patients with malignancy-related ascites were found to have peritoneal carcinomatosis, but nearly 100% of patients with peritoneal carcinomatosis were reported to have positive findings on cytologic examination of ascitic fluid; the remaining one third of patients with massive liver metastases, chylous ascites caused by lymphoma, or hepatocellular carcinoma had negative cytologic findings.[2] Therefore, the sensitivity of cytology is approximately 100% for detecting peritoneal carcinomatosis but much lower for detecting malignancy-related ascites caused by conditions other than peritoneal carcinomatosis. Cytologic studies should not be falsely positive if performed carefully; I have never encountered a false-positive result.

Because hepatocellular carcinoma rarely metastasizes to the peritoneum, a positive ascitic fluid cytology in a patient with hepatocellular carcinoma is unusual enough to be the subject of a case report.[37] Measurement of the serum AFP concentration (which is always higher in serum than in ascitic fluid) may be of value in detecting hepatocellular carcinoma; serum AFP is much more sensitive than ascitic fluid cytology for this purpose (see Chapter 96).[2] In malignancy-related ascites, the fluid may have an elevated PMN count, presumably because dying tumor cells attract neutrophils.[2] The elevated PMN count may cause confusion with SBP; however, a predominance of lymphocytes in malignancy-related ascites is usual. Flow cytometry and magnetic enrichment of ascitic fluid as an adjunct to cytology may further increase diagnostic accuracy.[38]

TG

A TG level should be measured in opalescent or frankly milky ascitic fluid (see Fig. 93-2). By definition, chylous ascites has a TG concentration greater than 200 mg/dL (2.26 mmol/L) and greater than the serum level; usually, the level is greater than 1000 mg/dL (11.30 mmol/L).[39] In sterile but slightly cloudy ascitic fluid specimens in the setting of cirrhosis, in the absence of an elevated cell count, the TG concentration is elevated: 64 ± 40 mg/dL (0.72 ± 0.45 mmol/L), compared with 18 ± 9 mg/dL (0.20 ± 0.10 mmol/L) in clear ascites in the setting of cirrhosis.[16]

Bilirubin

The bilirubin concentration should be measured in ascitic fluid that is dark brown. An ascitic fluid bilirubin level greater than 6 mg/dL (102 μmol/L) and greater than the serum level of bilirubin suggests biliary or proximal small intestinal perforation into ascitic fluid.[18,31]

Tests That Are Seldom Helpful

Tests that have been proposed to be helpful in the analysis of ascitic fluid but shown subsequently to be of no benefit include determination of pH, lactate, fibronectin, and cholesterol. The studies that attempted to validate the value of pH and lactate included small numbers of patients and used suboptimal culture techniques. In the 2 largest studies, which did not have some of the deficiencies of smaller, earlier studies, the ascitic fluid pH and lactate were found not to be helpful.[40,41] The pH was found to have no impact on decision making regarding the use of empirical antibiotic therapy.[40]

Fibronectin and cholesterol were proposed to be useful in detecting malignant ascites. The basic premise in studies of these markers was that ascitic fluid cytologic examination is insensitive. Unfortunately, the design of the studies was problematic, several subgroups of malignancy-related ascites (e.g., massive liver metastases, hepatocellular carcinoma with cirrhosis) were not considered, and appropriate control groups (e.g., patients with ascites caused by conditions other than cirrhosis or peritoneal carcinomatosis) were not included. Other studies have demonstrated that in patients with massive liver metastases, ascitic fluid fibronectin and cholesterol concentrations are not abnormally elevated.[42,43] Therefore, in patients with malignancy-related ascites and negative cytologic findings, these "humoral tests of malignancy" are usually negative. Additionally, patients with high-protein ascites in the absence of cirrhosis nearly always have ascitic fibronectin and cholesterol elevations despite the absence of malignancy.[2,42,43]

CEA in ascitic fluid was proposed as a helpful marker for detecting malignant ascites.[44] The study that attempted to validate this proposal, however, was flawed, and more studies, with various subgroups of patients, are required before testing for ascitic fluid CEA can be considered validated.

Measurement of adenosine deaminase has been proposed as a useful test for detecting peritoneal TB. In the United States, however, where greater than 50% of patients with tuberculous peritonitis have underlying cirrhosis, the adenosine deaminase level has been found to be too insensitive to be helpful.[34]

DIFFERENTIAL DIAGNOSIS OF ASCITES

Although cirrhosis is the cause of ascites in most patients with ascites evaluated by a primary care provider, a cause other than liver disease is found in approximately 15% of patients (see Table 93-1). Approximately 5% of patients have 2 causes of ascites (i.e., mixed ascites).[24] Usually, these patients have cirrhosis plus peritoneal carcinomatosis or tuberculous peritonitis (see Table 93-1). Because TB is potentially fatal but curable and frequently occurs in patients with cirrhosis and preexisting ascites, the physician must not assume that liver disease is the only cause of ascites in a febrile alcoholic patient if the ascitic fluid analysis is atypical. If the ascitic fluid lymphocyte count is unusually high, for example, tuberculous peritonitis may be present. Liver diseases other than cirrhosis (e.g., alcoholic hepatitis or fulminant hepatic failure) may cause ascites (see Table 93-1).

An algorithm for the differential diagnosis of ascites is shown in Figure 93-2. This proposed strategy is applicable to a majority of patients with ascites, including many with the causes listed in Table 93-1. Not every patient (including patients with rare causes of ascites) can be categorized readily with such an algorithm, however. Many patients with enigmatic ascites eventually are found to have 2 or even 3 causes of ascites (e.g., heart failure, cirrhosis caused by NASH, diabetic nephropathy). In these cases, the sum of predisposing factors leads to sodium and water retention, even though each factor alone may not be severe enough to cause fluid overload.

In most patients with ascites, cirrhosis is the cause. Cirrhotic ascites, especially when low in protein, is complicated frequently by SBP (see later).[29] Other forms of ascites are rarely complicated by spontaneous peritonitis.

The intestine can perforate, with spillage of contents in patients with ascites of any cause, cirrhosis or otherwise. The ascitic fluid analysis in intestinal perforation is dramatically different from that in SBP (see Fig. 93-3).[31,45] Distinguishing SBP from surgical peritonitis in a patient with cirrhosis is critical to the patient's survival; SBP is treated with antibiotics alone, whereas surgical peritonitis is treated with antibiotics and emergency surgical intervention (see Chapter 38).

Cancer accounts for fewer than 10% of cases of ascites (see Table 93-1). Not all cases of malignancy-related ascites are

---

BOX 93-2 Classification of Malignancy-Related Ascites

Hepatocellular carcinoma
Malignant Budd-Chiari syndrome (tumor emboli in hepatic veins)
Malignant lymph node obstruction
Massive liver metastases
Peritoneal carcinomatosis
Peritoneal carcinomatosis with massive liver metastases

---

caused by peritoneal carcinomatosis (see earlier); the characteristics of the ascitic fluid and the treatments differ depending on the pathophysiology of the ascites[2] (Box 93-2).

Heart failure accounts for less than 5% of cases of ascites. Cardiac ascites is characterized by a high albumin gradient, high ascitic fluid protein concentration, and normal blood hematocrit value.[30] The gradient may narrow with diuresis, in contrast to cirrhosis. Patients with cardiac ascites often have alcoholic cardiomyopathy, with cardiomegaly on a chest radiograph and 4-chamber enlargement of the heart on an echocardiogram. Clinically, heart failure may mimic cirrhosis, including the presence of small nonbleeding esophageal varices and hepatic encephalopathy.[46] Ascites in the setting of cirrhosis is characterized by a high albumin gradient, as in cardiac ascites, but a low protein concentration, and patients with cirrhosis and ascites have a lower mean blood hematocrit value of 32%.[30] Serum pro-brain-type natriuretic peptide also can be useful in distinguishing cardiac ascites from ascites due to cirrhosis. The median value is 6100 pg/mL in the former and only 166 pg/mL in the latter.[47]

In the United States, tuberculous peritonitis generally is a disease of Asian and Latin American immigrants to the West Coast, poor African Americans, and the elderly. Tuberculous peritonitis was a rare disease between 1955 and 1985, but it subsequently increased in prevalence because of the advent of AIDS.[48] Fifty percent of patients with tuberculous peritonitis have underlying cirrhosis (and thus mixed ascites). Although most patients with liver disease are not unusually predisposed to the hepatotoxicity of anti-TB drugs, they tolerate drug toxicity less well than do patients with a normal liver.[49] Underdiagnosis can lead to unnecessary deaths from untreated TB, whereas overdiagnosis and overtreatment of suspected but unproved tuberculous peritonitis may lead to unnecessary deaths from the hepatotoxicity of isoniazid and other anti-TB drugs. If the clinical circumstances (e.g., fever in an immigrant from an area endemic for TB) and results of the initial ascitic fluid analysis (high lymphocyte count) suggest TB, strong consideration should be given to an urgent laparoscopy with histologic examination and culture of peritoneal biopsy specimens. If at laparoscopy the peritoneum demonstrates the typical "millet-seed" and "violin-string" appearance, anti-TB therapy can be started immediately. Blind peritoneal biopsy may be performed in patients without cirrhosis; however, in patients with cirrhosis, the predictable presence of peritoneal collateral veins makes blind biopsy potentially hazardous, and laparoscopically guided biopsy is preferable. Suspected tuberculous peritonitis is one of the few remaining indications for diagnostic laparoscopy. Peritoneal coccidioidomycosis can mimic tuberculous peritonitis, including its appearance at laparoscopy, and can occur in patients without AIDS.[50] The high sensitivities of cytology for peritoneal carcinomatosis and US-guided biopsy for focal liver lesions have obviated the need for laparoscopy in detecting tumor, for all practical purposes.[2]

Pancreatic ascites, an uncommon condition, occurs in patients with clinically obvious severe acute pancreatitis or a history of chronic pancreatitis or pancreatic trauma (see Chapters 58 and 59).[32] Ordering an ascitic fluid amylase level on all ascitic fluid samples is unnecessary; the test is indicated only in patients in whom pancreatitis is suspected or the initial ascitic fluid is nondiagnostic (see Table 93-2). Patients with alcohol-related pancreatic ascites may also have underlying alcoholic cirrhosis. Pancreatic ascites frequently is neutrocytic and may also be complicated by bacterial infection. Patients with an ascitic fluid neutrophil count of 250/mm³ (0.25 × 10⁹/L) or greater merit empirical antibiotic coverage, at least until the cause of the elevated neutrophil count is explained.

Nephrogenous ascites is a poorly understood form of ascites that develops in patients undergoing hemodialysis.[51] On careful evaluation, most patients with ascites in the setting of hemodialysis are found to have another cause of ascites, usually cirrhosis from alcohol abuse or from hepatitis C. The presence of a second cause of fluid overload explains why these patients have ascites, whereas a majority of patients on dialysis do not. "Urine ascites," due to leakage of urine into the abdominal cavity, is most likely to result from a surgical complication and is characterized by a low protein concentration, low SAAG, and ascitic fluid-to-serum creatinine level ratio greater than 1.

Although the nephrotic syndrome used to be a common cause of ascites in children, it is rare in adults.[52] When it occurs in adults, a second cause of ascites usually is present, just as in nephrogenous ascites. The ascitic fluid is usually characterized by a low protein concentration and low SAAG and can be complicated by SBP.

Chlamydial (or rarely gonococcal) peritonitis should be suspected in sexually active young women with fever and neutrocytic, high-protein, low-gradient ascites and no evidence of liver disease. This infection responds rapidly to oral doxycycline and is one of the few curable causes of ascites.

In some patients, pathologic accumulation of fluid develops in the peritoneal cavity as a result of leakage from a ruptured viscus (e.g., "bile ascites" from a ruptured gallbladder).[18,31] The ascitic fluid analysis is critical to the preoperative diagnosis of this condition (see earlier and Fig. 93-3).

Chylous ascites develops when intra-abdominal lymphatics containing chyle rupture. Cirrhosis is the cause of chylous ascites in more than 90% of the patients whom I have encountered (see Table 93-1).[17,24] The high lymphatic flow and pressure are presumed to be the cause of lymphatic rupture in patients with cirrhosis. In addition, retroperitoneal surgery and radical pelvic surgery in patients with cancer can transect lymphatics and thereby lead to chylous ascites. In the past, this form of ascites was caused by a malignancy in nearly 90% of cases.[39]

Additional causes of ascites include ambulatory peritoneal dialysis, Budd-Chiari syndrome, myxedema, connective tissue disease, postoperative ascites, and rare entities. With the iatrogenic form of ascites associated with peritoneal dialysis, the patient is usually not under the care of a gastroenterologist. Although Budd-Chiari syndrome is regularly complicated by ascites, hepatic vein thrombosis is rare and accounts for less than 0.1% of cases of ascites (see Chapter 85). Ascites in patients with myxedema appears to be related to heart failure[53]; treatment of the hypothyroidism cures the fluid retention. Serositis with development of ascites may complicate systemic lupus erythematosus (see Chapter 36).[7]

Ascites after abdominal surgery (often after cholecystectomy in the setting of asymptomatic gallstones and abnormal liver biochemical test results) is a common mode of presentation of previously undiagnosed cirrhosis.[54] Resection of hepatocellular carcinoma in the setting of cirrhosis regularly leads to hepatic decompensation, which all too often starts a downward spiral ending in death.[55]

Aggressive hormone administration to induce ovulation can lead to ascites from ovarian hyperstimulation syndrome.[56]

Other rare causes of ascites include the POEMS syndrome (polyneuropathy, organomegaly, endocrinopathy, M component, and skin changes) and hemophagocytic syndrome.[57,58] The latter is a rare syndrome that usually occurs in patients with leukemia or lymphoma and can masquerade as decompensated cirrhosis.[58] Ascites that recurs or does not resolve after liver transplantation appears to be due to relative hepatic venous outflow obstruction or hepatitis C but frequently is enigmatic.[59,60]

COMPLICATIONS

Ascitic Fluid Infection, Including SBP

Ascitic fluid infection can be classified into 5 categories based on ascitic culture results, PMN count, and presence or absence of a surgical source of infection (Box 93-3). An abdominal paracentesis must be performed and ascitic fluid analyzed before a confident diagnosis of ascitic fluid infection can be made. A "clinical" diagnosis of infected ascitic fluid without a paracentesis is inadequate.

Classification

Of the 3 subtypes of spontaneous ascitic fluid infection, the prototype is SBP. The diagnosis of SBP is made when there is a positive ascitic fluid culture and an elevated ascitic fluid absolute PMN count (i.e., at least 250/mm³ [0.25 × 10⁹/L]) without evidence of an intra-abdominal surgically treatable source of infection.[10] When Correia and Conn coined the term *spontaneous bacterial peritonitis* in 1975, their goal was to distinguish this form of infection from surgical peritonitis.[61] Therefore, although many patients with SBP have a focus of infection (e.g., urinary tract infection or pneumonia), the diagnosis of SBP is still appropriate unless the focus requires surgical intervention (e.g., a ruptured viscus). I have not encountered a convincing case of polymicrobial SBP; all of the patients presumed to have SBP in whom ascitic fluid cultures initially grew more than 1 organism eventually were found to have surgical peritonitis or an erroneous culture result (e.g., a pathogen plus a contaminant or 2 colony morphologies of 1 species of bacteria).

The criteria for a diagnosis of *monomicrobial non-neutrocytic bacterascites* (MNB) include (1) a positive ascitic fluid culture for a single organism, (2) an ascitic fluid PMN count lower than 250/mm³ (0.25 × 10⁹/L), and (3) no evidence of an intra-abdominal surgically treatable source of infection.[62] In the older literature, MNB was either grouped with SBP or labeled "asymptomatic bacterascites." Because many patients with bacterascites have symptoms, the modifier asymptomatic seems inappropriate.

Culture-negative neutrocytic ascites (CNNA) is diagnosed when (1) the ascitic fluid culture grows no bacteria, (2) the ascitic fluid PMN count is 250/mm³ (0.25 × 10⁹/L) or greater, (3) no antibiotics have been given (not even a single dose), and

---

BOX 93-3 Classification of Ascitic Fluid Infection

SBP
Monomicrobial non-neutrocytic bacterascites
Culture-negative neutrocytic ascites
Secondary bacterial peritonitis
Polymicrobial bacterascites (needle perforation of the bowel)

(4) no other explanation for an elevated ascitic PMN count (e.g., hemorrhage into ascites, peritoneal carcinomatosis, TB, or pancreatitis) can be identified.[63] This variant of ascitic fluid infection is seldom diagnosed when sensitive culture methods are used.[26]

Secondary bacterial peritonitis is diagnosed when (1) the ascitic fluid culture is positive (usually for multiple organisms), (2) the PMN count is 250/mm^3 (0.25 × 10^9/L) or greater, and (3) an intra-abdominal surgically treatable primary source of infection (e.g., perforated intestine, perinephric abscess) has been identified.[31,45] The importance of distinguishing this variant from SBP is that secondary peritonitis usually requires emergency surgical intervention (see Chapter 38).

Polymicrobial bacterascites is diagnosed when (1) multiple organisms are seen on Gram stain or cultured from the ascitic fluid and (2) the PMN count is lower than 250/mm^3 (0.25 × 10^9/L).[64] This diagnosis should be suspected when the paracentesis is traumatic or unusually difficult because of ileus or when stool or air is aspirated into the paracentesis syringe. Polymicrobial bacterascites is essentially diagnostic of intestinal perforation by the paracentesis needle.

Clinical Setting

The spontaneous variants of ascitic fluid infection—SBP, CNNA, and MNB—occur almost exclusively in the setting of severe liver disease. The liver disease usually is chronic (cirrhosis), but may be acute (fulminant hepatic failure) or subacute (alcoholic hepatitis). Cirrhosis of all causes can be complicated by spontaneous ascitic fluid infection. Spontaneous infection of noncirrhotic ascites is rare.

Essentially all patients with SBP have an elevated serum bilirubin level and prolonged prothrombin time because of advanced cirrhosis.[10] Ascites appears to be a prerequisite for the development of SBP. The peritonitis is unlikely to precede the development of ascites. Usually, the infection develops when the volume of ascites is at its maximum.

Secondary bacterial peritonitis and polymicrobial bacterascites can develop with ascites of any type. The only prerequisite, in addition to the presence of ascites, is an intra-abdominal surgical source of infection.[31] Such an infection can result from penetration of a needle into the bowel during attempted paracentesis.[64]

Pathogenesis

Currently available evidence suggests that the spontaneous forms of ascitic fluid infection are the result of overgrowth of a specific organism in the intestine, translocation of that microbe from the intestine to mesenteric lymph nodes, and resulting spontaneous bacteremia and subsequent colonization of susceptible ascitic fluid[65,66] (Fig. 93-4). When bacteria enter the fluid in the abdomen, by whatever route, a battle ensues between the virulence factors of the organism and the immune defenses of the host.[67] The ascitic fluid protein concentration does not change with development of spontaneous infection.[28] Low-protein ascitic fluid (e.g., protein content < 1 g/dL [10 g/L]) is particularly susceptible to SBP.[29] The endogenous antimicrobial (opsonic) activity of human ascitic fluid correlates directly with the protein concentration of the fluid.[66] Patients with deficient ascitic fluid opsonic activity are predisposed to SBP.[68] Patients with detectable ascitic fluid opsonic activity appear to be protected from SBP unless they are exposed to a particularly virulent organism (e.g., *Salmonella*).[67,68]

Studies in both patients and animals with cirrhosis demonstrate that MNB is common.[62,69] Pieces of bacterial DNA are

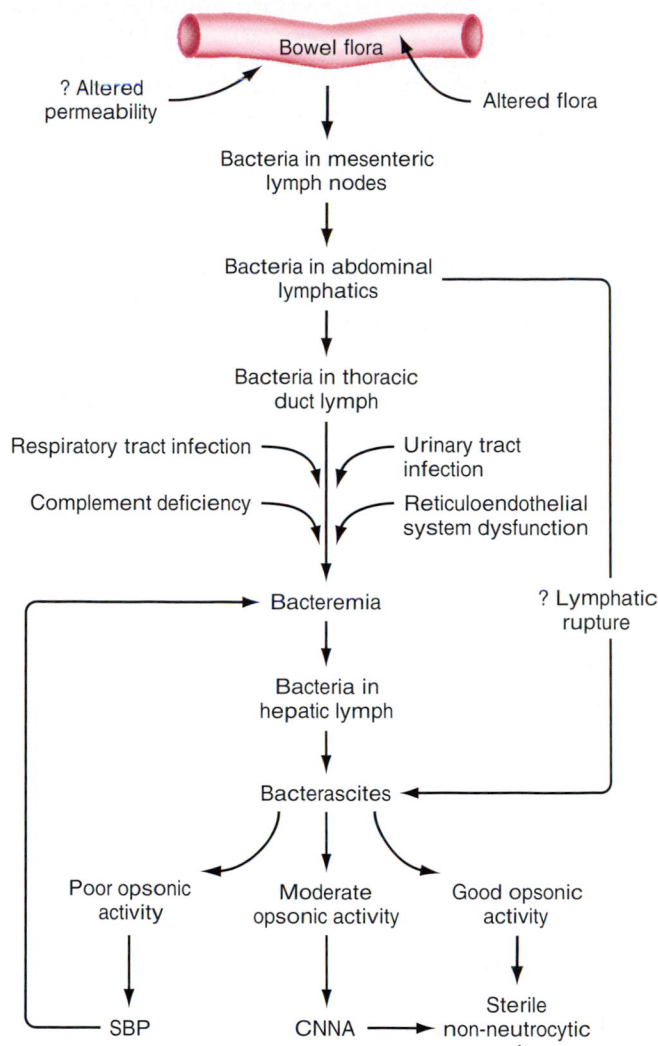

FIGURE 93-4. Proposed pathogenesis of spontaneous ascitic fluid infection. CNNA, culture-negative neutrocytic ascites.

commonly present in serum and ascitic fluid of patients with cirrhosis.[70] In both humans and rats, most episodes of bacterascites resolve without antibiotic treatment.[62,69] The fluid frequently becomes sterile without an increase in ascitic PMNs. Apparently, the host's defense mechanisms are able to eradicate the invading bacteria on most occasions. Uncontrolled infection probably develops only when the defenses are weak or the organism is virulent (see Fig. 93-4). Bacterascites probably is more common than SBP. Conceivably, ascitic fluid in the setting of cirrhosis is colonized regularly by bacteria, and almost just as regularly, the colonization resolves. The entry of PMNs into the fluid probably signals failure of the peritoneal macrophages to control the infection.[71] A majority of episodes of MNB appear to resolve in rats and humans with cirrhosis, whereas untreated SBP is frequently fatal. In summary, MNB probably represents an early stage of ascitic fluid infection, which can resolve or progress to CNNA or to SBP.

Most episodes of CNNA are diagnosed by insensitive culture methods for which the numbers of bacteria are insufficient to reach the threshold of detectability.[26] Inoculation of ascitic fluid into blood culture bottles can lead to detection of a single organism in the cultured aliquot of fluid, whereas the older method of culture by inoculation of agar plates and broth probably requires at least 100 organisms/mL (see earlier).[26] Even when optimal culture methods are used, however, a variable percentage of specimens of neutrocytic ascitic fluid grow no bacteria. A study of rapid sequential paracenteses (before the initiation of antibiotic treatment) in patients with CNNA demonstrated that, in most cases, the PMN count dropped spontaneously and the culture results remained negative in the second specimen.[72] When sensitive culture techniques are used, CNNA probably results from (1) previous antibiotic treatment (even 1 dose), (2) an inadequate volume of fluid inoculated, or (3) spontaneously resolving SBP in which the paracentesis is performed after all bacteria have been killed by host defenses but before the PMN count has normalized.

The pathogenesis of secondary bacterial peritonitis is more straightforward than that of SBP. When the intestine perforates, billions of bacteria flood into the ascitic fluid. In the absence of a frank perforation, bacteria may cross inflamed tissue planes and enter the fluid. The pathogenesis of polymicrobial bacterascites is also obvious.[64] A paracentesis needle enters the bowel, and the bowel contents are released into the ascites.

Symptoms and Signs

Although 87% of patients with SBP are symptomatic at the time the infection is diagnosed, the symptoms and signs of infection are often subtle, such as a slight change in mental status.[62] Without prompt paracentesis, the diagnosis and treatment of infected ascites may be delayed, often resulting in the death of the patient. The symptoms and signs manifested in all 5 variants of ascitic fluid infection are listed in Table 93-3.

Frequency

Since the 1980s, routine paracenteses at the time of hospitalization in patients with ascites have provided data regarding the frequency of ascitic fluid infection. In the 1980s, approximately 10% of patients with ascites were infected at the time of hospital admission; of the subgroup of patients with cirrhosis, about 27% were infected.[10] At present, because of measures to prevent SBP, the frequency has dropped significantly (see later). Of patients with culture-positive ascitic fluid, about two thirds have neutrocytic ascitic fluid (SBP), and one third have MNB.[62] The frequency of CNNA depends largely on the culture technique (see earlier). Polymicrobial bacterascites occurs in only 1 in 1000 paracenteses. Secondary bacterial peritonitis is found in only 0% to 2% of patients with ascites at the time of hospital admission.[10,31]

Bacteriology

Escherichia coli, streptococci (mostly pneumococci), and *Klebsiella* caused most episodes of SBP and MNB in the past in patients who were not receiving selective intestinal decontamination. Now more Gram-positive and resistant Gram-negative organisms are being isolated (Table 93-4).[73] Selective intestinal decontamination and recent exposure to antibiotics are causing a change in the bacteria isolated from patients in whom an ascitic fluid infection develops. We may encounter organisms for which we have no effective antibiotics.[74] The antibiotic susceptibility of bacteria that cause infections in patients with cirrhosis should be tested periodically in each hospital, and the preferred empirical antibiotic regimens should be adapted accordingly.[73]

CNNA is, by definition, culture-negative, and polymicrobial bacterascites is, by definition, polymicrobial. The most apparent difference between the spontaneous forms of ascitic fluid infection and the secondary forms (secondary peritonitis and polymicrobial bacterascites) is that the former always are monomicrobial and the latter usually are polymicrobial. Although older papers reported that anaerobic bacteria were present in approximately 6% of cases of SBP, the detection of anaerobes probably reflected unrecognized cases of secondary bacterial peritonitis. In more recent series, anaerobes have been found in approximately 1% of cases of SBP and MNB.[26,62]

Risk Factors

Patients with cirrhosis are unusually predisposed to bacterial infection because of multiple defects in immune defense. The concept that cirrhosis is a form of acquired immunodeficiency (in the generic sense) is relatively new. In a prospective study, a bacterial infection occurred in 34% of 405 patients with cirrhosis at the time of admission to the hospital or during the hospitalization.[75] Low ascitic fluid total protein concentrations, as well as the phagocytic (both motile and stationary)

TABLE 93-4 Pathogens in Ascitic Fluid Infection

	Frequency (%)*			
Organism	**SBP**	**Monomicrobial Non-Neutrocytic Bacterascites**	**Secondary Bacterial Peritonitis**	**SBP with SID**
Monomicrobial				
Escherichia coli	37	27	20	0
Klebsiella pneumoniae	17	11	7	7
Streptococcus pneumoniae	12	9	0	29
Streptococcus viridans	9	2	0	0
Staphylococcus aureus	0	7	13	0
Miscellaneous Gram-positive	14	30	0	50
Miscellaneous Gram-negative	10	14	7	7
Polymicrobial	1	0	53	7

*Data are reported as % of total patients in that group.
SID, selective intestinal decontamination.
Data from references 26, 31, 62, and Fernández J, Navasa M, Gómez J, et al. Bacterial infections in cirrhosis: Epidemiologic changes with invasive procedures and norfloxacin prophylaxis. Hepatology 2002; 35:140-8.

dysfunction associated with cirrhosis, are risk factors for bacterial infection.

Paracentesis itself has been proposed as a risk factor for ascitic fluid infection, but this theoretical risk has not been substantiated in prospective studies of paracentesis-related complications.[12] SBP is statistically more likely to be diagnosed on the first paracentesis than on subsequent taps.[12] Needle-induced ascitic fluid infections do not occur unless the bowel is penetrated by the paracentesis needle.[12,64] Fortunately, bowel penetration occurs in only 1 in 1000 taps. One would expect bacteria of the skin flora to be isolated more frequently if poor paracentesis technique were the cause of many cases of SBP; yet skin flora microorganisms are seldom isolated from ascitic fluid when sterile technique is used.[26] Iatrogenic peritonitis is most likely to occur when the paracentesis needle enters the bowel during a difficult paracentesis.

GI hemorrhage is an under-recognized risk factor for the development of spontaneous bacteremia and SBP (see Chapters 20 and 92). The cumulative probability of infection during a single hospitalization for bleeding is approximately 40%.[76] The risk appears to peak 48 hours after the onset of hemorrhage. The high risk of infection probably is mediated by a shock-induced increase in the translocation of bacteria from the intestine to extraintestinal sites. Urinary tract infections also constitute an under-recognized risk factor for SBP.[77]

Diagnosis

Timely diagnosis of ascitic fluid infection requires a high index of suspicion and a low threshold for performing a paracentesis. Clinical deterioration, especially fever or abdominal pain, in a patient with ascites should raise the suspicion of infection and prompt a paracentesis. If the ascitic fluid PMN count is elevated, the working diagnosis is ascitic fluid infection until proved otherwise. Although peritoneal carcinomatosis, pancreatitis, hemorrhage into ascites, and TB can lead to an elevated ascitic fluid PMN count, most cases of neutrocytic ascites are caused by bacterial infection. A predominance of PMNs in the WBC differential count lends further support to the diagnosis of infection. An elevated absolute ascitic fluid PMN count with a predominance of neutrophils in a clinical setting compatible with infection should prompt empirical antibiotic therapy (see later).

Although SBP is approximately 20 times as common as surgical peritonitis in a patient with ascites, secondary peritonitis should be considered in any patient with neutrocytic ascites (see Chapter 38).[45] Clinical symptoms and signs do not distinguish patients with secondary peritonitis from those with SBP (see Fig. 93-3).[31] Even with free perforation of the colon into ascitic fluid, a classic surgical abdomen does not develop. Peritoneal signs require contact of inflamed visceral and parietal peritoneal surfaces, and such contact does not occur when there is a large volume of fluid separating these surfaces. Intestinal perforation can be suspected and pursued if a specimen of ascites is neutrocytic and meets 2 of the following 3 criteria (see Fig. 93-3): (1) total protein greater than 1 g/dL (10 g/L), (2) glucose less than 50 mg/dL (2.8 mmol/L), and (3) LDH greater than the upper limit of normal for serum.[31] In the setting of a perforated viscus, cultures of ascitic fluid nearly always disclose multiple organisms, except in gallbladder rupture, which is usually monomicrobial.[18] Brown ascitic fluid with a bilirubin concentration that is greater than 6 mg/dL (102 µmol/L) and greater than the serum level is indicative of biliary or proximal small intestinal perforation into ascites.[18] An ascitic fluid amylase level that is greater than 5-fold that of the serum level also may be indicative of intestinal rupture (but not gallbladder rupture) with the release of luminal amylase.[31,32]

The initial ascitic fluid analysis is helpful in delineating which patients are likely to have a ruptured viscus (see Fig. 93-3). Within minutes of the detection of neutrocytic ascitic fluid, these patients should undergo abdominal CT to confirm and localize the site of rupture.[45] If perforation is documented, emergency surgical intervention is the next step. Timing is crucial; after septic shock occurs, death is nearly certain. Antibiotic therapy without surgical intervention in the treatment of a ruptured viscus is predictably unsuccessful.

In contrast to patients with peritonitis resulting from perforation of a viscus, patients with secondary peritonitis unrelated to perforation tend not to have a diagnostic initial ascitic fluid analysis.[31] The need to make the diagnosis of secondary peritonitis in patients without free perforation is less urgent, and there may be time to evaluate the response of the ascitic PMN count and fluid culture to treatment with antibiotics. It is best to repeat the paracentesis to assess the response to treatment after 48 hours of therapy; by 48 hours, the ascitic PMN count will be lower than the pretreatment value and the ascitic culture will be negative in essentially every patient with SBP who has been treated with an appropriate antibiotic.[31] Before 48 hours of treatment, the ascitic PMN count may rise to a value higher than baseline in either SBP or secondary peritonitis.[31] The culture remains positive in secondary peritonitis and becomes rapidly negative in SBP (see Fig. 93-3).[31] Whereas antibiotics alone cannot control secondary peritonitis, medical therapy cures SBP rapidly.[31]

Treatment

Patients with an ascitic fluid PMN count of 250/mm³ (0.25 × 10⁹/L) or greater and a clinical scenario compatible with ascitic fluid infection should receive empirical antibiotic treatment (Table 93-5).[10,78] Patients with hemorrhage into the ascitic fluid, peritoneal carcinomatosis, pancreatic ascites, or tuberculous peritonitis may have an elevated ascitic PMN count that is unrelated to SBP and usually do not require empirical antibiotic treatment. If they do receive antibiotics, the ascitic PMN count usually fluctuates randomly, in contrast to the dramatic reduction in PMN count typical of SBP. If the clinical picture is unclear initially, the physician should err on the side of antibiotic treatment (with a non-nephrotoxic antibiotic). If ascitic fluid cultures are negative, the antibiotic can be stopped after 48 hours. In patients with uninfected neutrocytic ascitic fluid (except those with hemorrhage), lymphocytes usually predominate in the ascitic fluid differential count, in contrast to those with SBP, in whom PMNs predominate. In patients with bloody ascitic fluid, a "corrected" PMN count should be calculated (as discussed earlier). Antibiotic therapy is not necessary for patients with bloody fluid unless the corrected ascitic fluid PMN count is 250/mm³ (0.25 × 10⁹/L) or greater.

The decision to begin empirical antibiotic treatment in patients with bacterascites must be individualized. Many episodes resolve without treatment[62]; however, the hospital mortality rate of 32% in patients when MNB is attributable, at least, in part, to infection.[62] Therefore, treatment appears to be warranted in many patients. By definition, the ascitic PMN count is lower than 250/mm³ (0.25 × 10⁹/L) in this variant of ascitic fluid infection, and the PMN count cannot be the only parameter on which to base the decision about empirical therapy. Most patients with MNB in whom the colonization does not resolve progress to SBP and have symptoms or signs of infection at the time of the paracentesis that documents bacterascites.[62] Therefore, patients with cirrhosis and ascites who have convincing symptoms or signs of infection should receive treatment regardless of the ascitic fluid PMN count. Empirical treatment can be discontinued after only 2 to 3

TABLE 93-5 Treatment of Ascitic Fluid Infection

Diagnosis	Treatment
SBP	5 days of IV antibiotic to which the organism is highly susceptible (e.g., cefotaxime 2 g every 8 hours empirically followed by more specific therapy after susceptibility results are available)
Monomicrobial non-neutrocytic bacterascites	5 days of IV antibiotic to which the organism is highly susceptible, if the patient is symptomatic or persistently culture-positive; not all patients with bacterascites require treatment
Culture-negative neutrocytic ascites	5 days of IV third-generation cephalosporin (e.g., cefotaxime 2 g every 8 hours)
Secondary bacterial peritonitis	Surgical intervention plus ≈ 2 weeks of IV cephalosporin (e.g., cefotaxime 2 g every 8 hours) plus an antianaerobic drug such as metronidazole*
Polymicrobial bacterascites	IV third-generation cephalosporin (e.g., cefotaxime 2 g every 8 hours) plus an antianaerobic drug such as metronidazole* Duration is determined by clinical response and serial ascitic fluid PMN counts and cultures

*Dose of IV metronidazole is 15 mg/kg × 1, then 7.5 mg/kg every 6 hours.
PMN, polymorphonuclear neutrophil.

days if the culture demonstrates no growth. Asymptomatic patients may not need treatment.[62] The paracentesis should be repeated for cell count and culture in patients without clinical evidence of infection, as soon as it is known that the initial culture result is positive. If the PMN count has risen to at least $250/mm^3$ ($0.25 \times 10^9/L$) or if symptoms or signs of infection have developed, antibiotics should be started. Culture results usually are negative in patients without a rise in the ascitic fluid PMN count on repeat paracentesis and without clinical evidence of infection, and these persons do not require antibiotics[62] because colonization has been eradicated by host immune defenses.

The physician will not know initially that the ascitic fluid culture is destined to be negative in a patient with CNNA; therefore, empirical antibiotic treatment should be started. When the preliminary culture demonstrates no growth, it is helpful to repeat the paracentesis after 48 hours of therapy to assess the response of the PMN count to antibiotics. A dramatic decline in PMN count (always below the baseline pretreatment value and frequently a reduction of more than 80%) confirms a response to treatment.[31] In such cases, a few more days of therapy is probably warranted. A stable ascitic fluid PMN count, especially with a predominance of lymphocytes and monocytes, suggests a nonbacterial (or mycobacterial) cause of ascitic fluid neutrocytosis, and the fluid should be sent for cytologic examination and mycobacterial culture. Because a negative culture result may be due to insensitive culture techniques, the prevalence of CNNA in a hospital that still uses older methods of culture (sending a tube or syringe of fluid to the laboratory) can be reduced by convincing the

microbiology laboratory to accept and process ascitic fluid submitted in blood culture bottles.[26]

Gram stain of the ascitic fluid is most helpful in detecting secondary peritonitis, in which multiple different bacterial forms are seen, but is of little value in guiding the choice of empirical antibiotic treatment for spontaneous ascitic infections (see earlier). I have found that use of the Gram stain did not help narrow the antibiotic coverage in even 1 patient of approximately 700 with SBP. Only approximately 10% of Gram stains demonstrate organisms in SBP.[26] If a Gram stain indicates secondary peritonitis, coverage for anaerobic flora, in addition to coverage for aerobic and facultative anaerobic flora, is required, as is an emergency search for the source of the infection (see Fig. 93-3 and Table 93-5).[31] Therefore, a positive Gram stain may lead to broader antibiotic coverage, rather than narrower coverage. Narrow coverage based on a misinterpretation of the significance of the results of the Gram stain may lead to uncontrolled infection and death before resistance of the isolated organism to the chosen antibiotic becomes apparent.

Until the results of susceptibility testing are available, relatively broad-spectrum antibiotic therapy is warranted in patients with suspected ascitic fluid infection. After sensitivities are known, the spectrum of coverage can usually be narrowed. The antibiotics that have been recommended for empirical treatment have changed over the years. In the late 1970s, the combination of ampicillin and gentamicin was promoted, but this recommendation was not based on susceptibility testing or efficacy data. One study has documented an adjusted odds ratio of 4.0 for aminoglycosides as a risk factor for renal dysfunction in patients with cirrhosis.[79] Evidence that newer aminoglycosides are less nephrotoxic than gentamicin is lacking.

Several antibiotics are now available for the treatment of ascitic fluid infection. Cefotaxime, a third-generation cephalosporin, has been shown in a controlled trial to be superior to ampicillin plus tobramycin for the treatment of SBP.[80] Fully 98% of causative organisms were susceptible to cefotaxime, which did not result in superinfection or nephrotoxicity.[80] Cefotaxime or a similar third-generation cephalosporin appears to be the treatment of choice for suspected SBP.[10] Anaerobic coverage is not needed.[26] Cefotaxime, 2 g IV every 8 hours, has been shown to result in excellent ascitic fluid levels (20-fold killing power after 1 dose).[81] In patients with a serum creatinine level greater than 3 mg/dL, the dosing interval may be extended to 12 hours.[81] Neither a loading dose nor an intraperitoneal dose appears to be necessary or appropriate. The clinician should, however, order the first dose "STAT," to avoid a delay in administration of the life-saving agent. More broad-spectrum antibiotics are warranted if local susceptibility testing demonstrates increasing resistance to third-generation cephalosporins.

Other Intravenous Antibiotics

Amoxicillin-clavulanic acid has been shown to be as effective as cefotaxime in a randomized trial but is not available in a parenteral formulation in the United States.[82] Other antibiotics have been recommended as well but have been less well studied than has cefotaxime. Some newer drugs have been used to treat SBP (without any data on antibiotic penetration into the ascitic fluid) on the basis of their spectrum of coverage and formulary constraints.

Intravenous Albumin

Renal impairment occurs in 33% of episodes of SBP.[83] SBP leads to increased intraperitoneal nitric oxide production, which in turn further increases systemic vasodilatation and promotes renal failure (see Chapter 94).[84] IV albumin (1.5 g/ kg of body weight at the time the infection is detected, and 1 g/kg on day 3) can increase intravascular volume and, in combination with cefotaxime, has been shown in a large randomized trial to reduce the risk of renal failure and improve survival compared with cefotaxime without albumin.[85] Albumin appears to be effective by decreasing systemic vasodilatation.[86] Because of the survival advantage, the use of IV albumin as an adjunct to antibiotic treatment has been recommended.[87]

Oral Antibiotics

Oral ofloxacin has been reported in a controlled trial to be as effective as parenteral cefotaxime in the treatment of SBP in patients who do not have vomiting, shock, bleeding, or renal failure.[88] The dose studied was 400 mg twice daily.[88] Another study has demonstrated the efficacy of IV ciprofloxacin, 200 mg every 12 hours for 2 days, followed by oral ciprofloxacin, 500 mg every 12 hours for 5 days.[89] Because of the possibility of fluoroquinolone resistance in patients receiving fluoroquinolones to prevent SBP (see later), however, the empirical use of a fluoroquinolone to treat suspected SBP should be avoided.[90] Fortunately, bacterial isolates from patients with SBP who were receiving fluoroquinolones for prophylaxis of this disorder remain susceptible to cefotaxime.[78]

Narrowing the Spectrum of Coverage

After the results of susceptibility testing are available, an antibiotic with a narrower spectrum of activity usually can be substituted for the broad-spectrum drug (e.g., pneumococci will usually be sensitive to penicillin, and many *E. coli* species will usually be sensitive to ampicillin).

Duration of Treatment

Infectious disease subspecialists generally recommend 10 to 14 days of antibiotic therapy for life-threatening infections; however, no data are available to support this duration of treatment in spontaneous ascitic fluid infections. The ascitic fluid culture becomes sterile after 1 dose of cefotaxime in 86% of patients.[31] After 48 hours of therapy, the ascitic fluid PMN count is always less than the pretreatment value in patients with a spontaneous ascitic fluid infection treated with appropriate antibiotics; frequently, an 80% reduction is observed at 48 hours.[31] A randomized controlled trial involving 100 patients has demonstrated that 5 days of treatment is as efficacious as 10 days in patients with SBP or CNNA.[91] I have been treating SBP and CNNA for 5 days since the late 1980s, with excellent results. The average duration of oral ofloxacin treatment was 8 days in the only published trial.[88]

Follow-up Paracentesis

On the basis of a large database of repeat paracenteses during and after the treatment of SBP,[31] a follow-up paracentesis does not appear to be needed if the setting (advanced cirrhosis with symptoms and signs of infection), bacterial isolate (monomicrobial with a characteristic organism), and response to treatment (dramatic reduction in symptoms and signs of infection) are typical.[31] Paracentesis should be repeated after 48 hours of treatment if the course is atypical.[31]

Treatment of Ascitic Fluid Infection Other Than SBP

Because of the predictable presence of anaerobes, patients with suspected secondary peritonitis require empirical antibiotic coverage that is broader in spectrum than that used for SBP. They also require an emergency evaluation to assess the need for surgical intervention (see earlier, Box 93-4, and Fig. 93-3). Cefotaxime plus metronidazole appears to provide excellent initial empirical therapy of suspected secondary peritonitis.[31]

Polymicrobial bacterascites (from needle perforation of the bowel) is tolerated relatively well. Peritonitis developed in only 1 in 10 patients with a needle perforation of the intestine with spillage of intestinal contents into ascitic fluid in the one relevant study.[64] The single episode of paracentesis-related peritonitis was not fatal. Patients with low-protein ascitic fluid appear to be at most risk for development of a PMN response and clinical peritonitis related to needle perforation of the intestine.[64] Most of the patients with a higher ascitic protein concentration (e.g., >1 g/dL [10 g/L]) did not receive antibiotics, yet did well. Many physicians, however, probably would feel uncomfortable in withholding antibiotic treatment if needle perforation is suspected. If a decision to treat is made, anaerobic coverage should be included (e.g., cefotaxime plus metronidazole [see Table 93-5]). Whether or not treatment is begun, a follow-up paracentesis is helpful (if it can be performed safely) to monitor the ascitic fluid PMN count and culture results. If a decision is made to defer antibiotic treatment initially and the number of organisms in the ascitic fluid does not decrease or the PMN count rises in the second specimen, antibiotic treatment should then be initiated (see Table 93-5).

Prognosis

In the past, 48% to 95% of patients with a spontaneous ascitic fluid infection died during the hospitalization in which the diagnosis was made, despite antibiotic treatment.[10,23] By 1991, mortality rates were low (<5% if antibiotics are administered in a timely fashion), probably because of earlier detection and treatment of infection, as well as the avoidance of nephrotoxic antibiotics.[91] The trial in which cefotaxime plus albumin was studied reported an inpatient mortality rate of 10%.[85] Even now, however, some patients are cured of their infection but die of liver failure or GI bleeding because of the severity of the underlying liver disease. In fact, spontaneous ascitic fluid infection is a marker of end-stage liver disease and has been proposed as an indication for liver transplantation in a patient who is otherwise a candidate.

To maximize survival, it is important that paracentesis is performed in all patients with ascites at the time of hospitalization, so that infection can be detected and treated promptly. The ascitic fluid cell count should be reviewed as soon as the results are available (≈60 minutes), and appropriate treatment should be instituted if indicated. The first dose of antibiotic should be given immediately. Because dipstick test results (see earlier) are available in 90 to 120 seconds, this tool may speed treatment of SBP and improve survival.[20,22]

Paracentesis should be repeated during the hospitalization if any manifestation of clinical deterioration develops, including abdominal pain, fever, change in mental status, renal failure, acidosis, peripheral leukocytosis, or GI bleeding. If the physician waits to perform a paracentesis until convincing symptoms and signs of peritoneal infection have developed, the infection is likely to be advanced by the time the diagnosis is made. No survivors of SBP have been reported when the diagnosis was made after the serum creatinine level had risen above 4 mg/dL (350 μmol/L).

Without surgical intervention, the mortality rate for secondary peritonitis in hospitalized patients with ascites approaches 100%. When secondary peritonitis is diagnosed early and treated with emergency laparotomy, the mortality rate is 50% to 67%.[31,45]

Prevention

The identification of risk factors for SBP (including an ascitic fluid protein concentration < 1.0 g/dL, variceal hemorrhage, and previous episode of SBP) has led to controlled trials of prophylactic antibiotics.[29,92-94] Norfloxacin, 400 mg/day orally, has been reported to reduce the risk of SBP in inpatients with low-protein ascites and those with previous SBP.[92,93] Norfloxacin, 400 mg orally twice daily for 7 days, helps prevent infection in patients with variceal hemorrhage[94] and is cost-effective in preventing recurrent SBP.[95] IV ceftriaxone 1 g daily for 7 days has been found to be even more effective than norfloxacin in the setting of GI bleeding; this regimen allows administration of antibiotics to patients who are vomiting blood.[96] Oral antibiotics select for resistant organisms in the intestinal flora in patients, and in animals these organisms can then cause spontaneous ascitic fluid infection.[90,97] Despite this concern, 2 randomized trials of primary prevention of ascitic fluid infection with prophylactic norfloxacin or ciprofloxacin have demonstrated a survival advantage for the antibiotic-treated patients (Table 93-6).[98-100]

Trimethoprim/sulfamethoxazole has also been shown to prevent SBP in an animal model and in patients; in animals survival was increased.[101,102] The recommended dose for patients is 1 double-strength tablet daily.[102]

Use of parenteral antibiotics to prevent endoscopic sclerotherapy–related or band ligation–related infections in nonbleeding patients does not appear to be warranted, as indicated by a controlled trial.[103] Active bleeding, not endoscopic treatment, appears to be the risk factor for ascitic fluid infection. On the other hand, bacterial infection is associated with failure to control variceal hemorrhage.[104] This observation provides additional incentive to try to prevent, detect, and treat infections aggressively in this setting to minimize mortality related not only to infection, but also to hemorrhage.

Cellulitis

Cellulitis of the lower extremities or abdominal wall is a common cause of soft tissue infection in obese patients with edema. One study has documented a 19% cumulative probability of cellulitis during hospitalization of patients with cirrhosis and ascites, compared with only a 4% likelihood of SBP.[105] Risk factors for cellulitis included obesity (which is increasing in frequency in patients with cirrhosis), homelessness, and greater degree of edema.[105] Another study has demonstrated a 22% risk of renal failure in patients with cellulitis and cirrhosis.[106] A high index of suspicion and low threshold for treatment with a first-generation cephalosporin or other antibiotic may help decrease morbidity and mortality from uncontrolled cellulitis.

Tense Ascites

Some patients with ascites do not seek medical attention until they can no longer breathe or eat comfortably because of the pressure of the intra-abdominal fluid on the diaphragm. Tense ascites requires urgent therapeutic paracentesis (see later). Contrary to folklore, tense ascites can be drained without untoward hemodynamic effects.[107] "Total paracentesis," even more than 22 L, has been demonstrated to be safe.[107] In the setting of tense ascites, therapeutic paracentesis improves venous return and hemodynamics; the myth of paracentesis-related hemodynamic catastrophes was based on anecdotal observations in small numbers of patients.

Pleural Effusions

Pleural effusions can occur in patients with cirrhosis and ascites. They usually are unilateral and right-sided but occasionally may be bilateral and larger on the right side than on the left. A unilateral left-sided effusion suggests TB. A large effusion in a patient with cirrhotic ascites is designated hepatic hydrothorax.[108] Most carefully studied patients with hepatic hydrothorax have been shown to have a small defect in the right hemidiaphragm. With large diaphragmatic defects, ascites may be undetectable on clinical examination despite a large pleural effusion.

The most common symptom associated with hepatic hydrothorax is shortness of breath. Infection of the fluid can occur, usually as a result of SBP and transmission of bacteria across the diaphragm.[109] The analysis of uncomplicated hepatic hydrothorax fluid is similar but not identical to that of ascitic fluid, because the pleural fluid is subject to hydrostatic pressures different from those that affect the portal bed. The total

TABLE 93-6 Prevention of SBP

Indication	Drug	Results
Prior SBP	Norfloxacin 400 mg orally once daily until death or liver transplantation	66% reduction in recurrence
Cirrhosis with GI hemorrhage	Norfloxacin 400 mg orally twice daily × 7 days, or	73% reduction in infection
	Ceftriaxone 1 g IV/day × 7 days	67% reduction in infection compared with norfloxacin
Cirrhosis with ascitic fluid total protein < 1.5 g/dL and either Child-Turcotte-Pugh score ≥ 9 and total bilirubin ≥ 3 mg/dL, or Creatinine ≥ 1.2 mg/dL, or Blood urea nitrogen ≥ 25 mg/dL, or Serum sodium ≤ 130 mEq/L	Norfloxacin 400 mg/day orally × 1 year	89% reduction in SBP 32% reduction in hepatorenal syndrome 52% increase in 3-month survival 25% increase in 1-year survival
Cirrhosis with ascitic fluid total protein < 1.5 g/dL	Ciprofloxacin 500 mg orally daily × 1 year	31% reduction in infection 30% improvement in survival

Data from references 92-94, 96, and 98.

protein concentration is higher (by ≈ 1.0 g/dL [10 g/L]) in the pleural fluid than in ascitic fluid.[108]

The treatment of hepatic hydrothorax was difficult until the transjugular intrahepatic portosystemic shunt (TIPS) became available (see later).[108] The effusions tend to occur in patients who are the least adherent to treatment regimens or in whom ascites is most refractory to therapy. Some authors have recommended chest tube insertion and sclerosing of the pleurae with tetracycline; however, chest tubes inserted to treat hepatic hydrothorax are usually difficult to remove,[110] Moreover, shortness of breath may recur when the tube is clamped, and fluid may leak around the insertion site of the tube. A peritoneovenous shunt (see later) can be considered when the patient with hepatic hydrothorax has large-volume ascites, but the shunt usually clots after a short time. Direct surgical repair of the diaphragmatic defect can be considered, but the patients typically are poor operative candidates. Video thoracoscopic suture of the hole in the diaphragm followed by pleurodesis has been reported to be successful.[111] Sodium restriction plus use of diuretics with intermittent thoracentesis is the safest and most effective first-line therapy of hepatic hydrothorax. TIPS placement has been reported to be successful and constitutes reasonable second-line treatment.[108] If the patient is a candidate for liver transplantation, proceeding with a transplant evaluation may be the best approach.

Abdominal Wall Hernias

Abdominal wall hernias are common in patients with ascites. They usually are umbilical or incisional and occasionally inguinal. Up to 20% of patients with cirrhosis and ascites have umbilical hernias at the time of hospitalization.[112] Some of these hernias incarcerate or perforate. Because of these potential complications, elective surgical treatment should be considered in a patient with a hernia and ascites. Insertion of mesh should be avoided because of the potential for the mesh to become infected. The ascitic fluid should be medically removed preoperatively because the hernia recurs in 73% of patients who have ascites at the time of hernia repair but in only 14% of those who have no ascitic fluid at the time of repair.[113] Nevertheless, hernia repair is not without hazard. Successful laparoscopic repair of a recurrent strangulated umbilical hernia has been described.[114] TIPS has also been reported to lead to good control of symptoms and may obviate the need for surgical repair.[115] Many transplant surgeons prefer to avoid repair of the hernia or postpone it until the time of liver transplantation. An elastic abdominal binder can be used as a temporizing measure to reduce pain and hernia enlargement.

Surgical repair of a hernia or TIPS should be performed urgently in patients with skin ulceration, crusting, or black discoloration and emergently for refractory incarceration or rupture. Rupture is the most feared complication of an umbilical hernia. If TIPS is used, it must be performed prior to bacteremia. Infection of the TIPS may be difficult to eradicate.

TREATMENT OF ASCITES

Appropriate treatment of ascites depends on the cause of fluid retention. Accurate determination of the etiology of ascites is crucial. The SAAG is helpful diagnostically and for therapeutic decision making. Patients with a low SAAG usually do not have portal hypertension and do not respond to salt restriction and diuretics (except for those with nephrotic syndrome). Conversely, patients with a high SAAG have portal hypertension and are usually responsive to these measures.[10]

Low-Albumin-Gradient Ascites

Peritoneal carcinomatosis is the most common cause of low-albumin-gradient ascites.[2] Peripheral edema in affected patients can be managed with diuretics. By contrast, patients without peripheral edema who receive diuretics lose only intravascular volume, without loss of ascitic fluid. The mainstay of treatment of nonovarian peritoneal carcinomatosis is outpatient therapeutic paracentesis. Patients with peritoneal carcinomatosis usually live only a few months. Patients with ovarian malignancy are an exception to this rule and may exhibit a good response to surgical debulking and chemotherapy.

Ascites caused by tuberculous peritonitis (without cirrhosis) is cured by anti-TB therapy. Diuretics do not speed weight loss unless the patient has underlying portal hypertension from cirrhosis. Pancreatic ascites may resolve spontaneously, require endoscopic placement of a stent in the pancreatic duct or operative intervention, or respond to treatment with somatostatin.[116] A postoperative lymphatic leak from a distal splenorenal shunt or radical lymphadenectomy also may resolve spontaneously but on occasion may require surgical intervention or placement of a peritoneovenous shunt. *Chlamydia* peritonitis is cured by doxycycline. Ascites caused by lupus serositis may respond to glucocorticoids.[7] Dialysis-related ascites may respond to aggressive dialysis.[51]

High-Albumin-Gradient Ascites

Cirrhosis is the most common cause of liver disease that leads to high-albumin-gradient ascites (see Table 93-1). Many patients with cirrhosis experience multiple insults to the liver, including excessive alcohol use, NASH, and chronic hepatitis C.[4] One of the most important steps in treating high-albumin-gradient ascites in a patient with alcoholic liver disease, with or without other causes of liver injury, is to convince the patient to stop drinking alcohol. In a period of months, abstinence from alcohol can result in healing of the reversible component of alcoholic liver disease, and the ascites may resolve or become more responsive to medical therapy.

Baclofen has been shown in a randomized controlled trial to reduce alcohol craving and alcohol consumption, specifically in patients with alcoholic liver disease.[117] It can be started at 5 mg orally 3 times daily and increased to 10 mg 3 times daily or even higher until craving is suppressed.

Similarly, patients with other forms of treatable liver disease (e.g., autoimmune hepatitis, chronic hepatitis B with reactivation, hemochromatosis, Wilson disease) should receive specific therapy for these diseases. Occasionally, cirrhosis due to causes other than alcohol or hepatitis B is reversible[5]; however, these diseases are usually less reversible than alcoholic liver disease, and by the time ascites is present, these patients may be better candidates for liver transplantation than for protracted medical therapy.

Hospitalization

Outpatient treatment of patients with small-volume ascites can be attempted initially. However, patients with large-volume ascites and those who are resistant to outpatient treatment frequently require hospitalization for definitive diagnosis and management.[10] Many of these patients also have GI hemorrhage, encephalopathy, infection, or hepatocellular carcinoma. An intensive period of inpatient education and treatment may be required to convince the patient that the prescribed diet and diuretics are actually effective and worth the effort to prevent future hospitalizations.

Precipitating Cause

Determining the immediate precipitant of ascites (e.g., dietary indiscretion or nonadherence to therapy with diuretics) may be of value. Ascites may be precipitated by IV saline given perioperatively or to treat variceal hemorrhage or by sodium bicarbonate tablets; in such cases the ascites may resolve without the need for long-term treatment.

Diet Education

Fluid loss and weight change are related directly to sodium balance in patients with portal hypertension–related ascites. In the presence of avid renal retention of sodium, dietary sodium restriction is essential. The patient and the food preparer should be educated by a dietitian about a sodium-restricted diet. Severely sodium-restricted diets (e.g., 500 mg [22 mmol] of sodium per day) are feasible (but not palatable) in an inpatient setting but unrealistic for outpatients. The dietary sodium restriction that I recommend for both inpatients and outpatients is 2000 mg (88 mmol) per day. Protein is not restricted unless the patient has hepatic encephalopathy refractory to 2 drugs on a vegetable protein diet (see Chapter 94).

Fluid Restriction

Indiscriminate restriction of fluid in the treatment of cirrhotic ascites is inappropriate and serves only to alienate patients, nurses, and dietitians. Sodium restriction, not fluid restriction, results in weight loss; fluid follows sodium passively. The chronic hyponatremia usually seen in patients with cirrhotic ascites is seldom morbid. Attempts to correct hyponatremia rapidly in this setting can lead to more complications than those related to the hyponatremia. Severe hyponatremia (e.g., serum sodium concentration < 120 mmol/L) does warrant fluid restriction in the patient with cirrhosis and ascites but fortunately occurs in only 1.2% of patients.[118] Unless the decline in sodium concentration is rapid, symptoms of hyponatremia usually do not develop in patients with cirrhosis until the serum sodium concentration is below 110 mmol/L.

Role of Bed Rest

Although bed rest has traditionally been prescribed, no controlled trials support this practice; bed rest was part of the treatment of heart failure in the past and was extrapolated to the treatment of cirrhotic ascites without data.[119] An upright posture may aggravate the plasma renin elevation found in most patients with cirrhosis and ascites and, theoretically, increase renal sodium retention. In all likelihood, however, strict bed rest is unnecessary and may lead to decubitus ulcer formation in emaciated patients.

Urine Sodium Excretion

Urinary sodium excretion is a helpful parameter to follow in patients with portal hypertension–related ascites. Because urine is the most important route of excretion of sodium in the absence of diarrhea or hyperthermia, and because dietary intake is the only source of nonparenteral sodium, dietary intake and urinary excretion of sodium should be roughly equivalent, if the patient's weight is stable. Nonurinary sodium losses are less than 10 mmol/day in these patients.[120] A suboptimal decline in body weight may be the result of inadequate natriuresis, failure to restrict sodium intake, or both. Monitoring 24-hour urinary sodium excretion and daily

weight will clarify the issue. Patients who are adherent to an 88 mmol/day sodium diet and who excrete more than 78 mmol/day of sodium in the urine should lose weight. If the weight is increasing despite urinary losses in excess of 78 mmol/day, one can assume that the patient is consuming more sodium than is prescribed in the diet.

Urine Sodium-to-Potassium Ratio

Although 24-hour urine specimens constitute the diagnostic standard, studies have demonstrated that random urine specimens tested for sodium-to-potassium ratios correlate well with 24-hour specimens.[121,122] When a random urine sodium-to-potassium ratio is greater than 1, the patient should lose fluid weight. Patients who do not lose weight despite a random urine sodium-to-potassium ratio greater than 1 probably are not adherent to the diet. Only the 10% to 15% of patients who have significant spontaneous natriuresis with urine sodium-to-potassium ratios greater than 1 can be considered for dietary sodium restriction as sole therapy of ascites (i.e., without diuretics).[10] When given a choice, however, most patients would prefer to take some diuretics with more liberal intake of sodium than to take no pills with severe restriction of sodium intake.

Avoidance of Urinary Bladder Catheters

Many physicians promptly insert a bladder catheter in hospitalized patients with cirrhosis to monitor urine output accurately. Unfortunately, many of these immunocompromised patients have urinary tract infections on hospital admission,[77] and urethral trauma from insertion of the catheter in the setting of cystitis can lead to bacteremia. Prolonged catheterization predictably leads to cystitis and possibly sepsis in these patients. A prospective study has confirmed the infectious consequences of these catheters.[123] I insert urinary catheters only briefly and only in the ICU setting; these portals of entry for bacteria should be removed as soon as possible.

Diuretics

Spironolactone is the mainstay of treatment for patients with cirrhosis and ascites but increases natriuresis slowly. Single-agent diuretic therapy with spironolactone requires several days to induce weight loss. Although spironolactone alone has been shown to be superior to furosemide alone in the treatment of ascites,[124] I prefer to start spironolactone and furosemide together on the first hospital day in initial doses of 100 mg and 40 mg, respectively, each taken once in the morning.[10] Amiloride, 10 mg/day, can be substituted for spironolactone; amiloride is less widely available and more expensive than spironolactone but more rapidly effective, and it does not cause gynecomastia. A newer potassium-sparing diuretic, eplerenone, has been used in the treatment of heart failure and does not cause gynecomastia, but studies of its use in cirrhosis are lacking.

The half-life of spironolactone is approximately 24 hours in normal control subjects but is markedly prolonged in patients with cirrhosis; almost 1 month is required to reach a steady state.[125] In view of its long half-life, dosing the drug multiple times per day is unnecessary. A loading dose may be appropriate but has not been studied. Single daily doses maximize adherence; 25-, 50-, and 100-mg spironolactone tablets are available generically. Furosemide also should be given once a day.[126]

If the combination of spironolactone, 100 mg/day (or amiloride, 10 mg/day) and furosemide, 40 mg/day orally, is ineffective in increasing urinary sodium or decreasing body weight, the doses of both drugs should be increased simultaneously as needed (e.g., spironolactone, 200 mg plus furosemide, 80 mg, then 300 mg plus 120 mg, and finally 400 mg plus 160 mg). In my experience, as well as in a randomized trial, starting both drugs at once speeds the onset of diuresis, whereas slowly increasing the daily dose of spironolactone to 400 mg or even higher before adding furosemide delays diuresis and results in hyperkalemia.[127]

The 100:40 ratio of the daily doses of spironolactone and furosemide usually maintains normokalemia. The ratio of doses can be adjusted to correct abnormal serum potassium levels. Occasionally, an alcoholic patient who has had no recent food intake will have hypokalemia at the time of admission (usually for alcoholic hepatitis) and for a variable interval thereafter. Such a patient should receive spironolactone alone until the serum potassium normalizes; furosemide can then be added. When combined with a sodium-restricted diet in a study of almost 4000 patients, the regimen of spironolactone and furosemide has been demonstrated to achieve successful diuresis in more than 90% of patients.[128]

IV diuretics cause acute decreases in the glomerular filtration rate in patients with cirrhosis and ascites and generally should be avoided.[129] Many patients are given IV furosemide when they are hospitalized because of failure of outpatient treatment of ascites in the setting of cirrhosis. The approach of switching from oral to IV administration is effective for heart failure, but in patients with cirrhosis, repeated doses of IV furosemide regularly lead to azotemia and then to an erroneous diagnosis of hepatorenal syndrome. The correct diagnosis is diuretic-induced azotemia, which resolves when the diuretics are withheld and fluid is administered IV. Some physicians give IV albumin with IV furosemide, but a randomized crossover study has shown no benefit to albumin in this setting.[130] Repeated IV dosing of furosemide appears to be too "harsh" for the patient with cirrhosis; oral diuretics are better tolerated.

If rapid weight loss is desired, therapeutic paracentesis should be performed (see later). No limit has been identified for acceptable daily weight loss in patients who have massive edema. As soon as the edema has resolved, a reasonable maximum weight loss is probably 0.5 kg/day.[131] Encephalopathy, a serum sodium concentration less than 120 mmol/L despite fluid restriction, and a serum creatinine level greater than 2.0 mg/dL (180 mmol/L) are indications to discontinue diuretics and reassess the patient. Abnormalities in potassium levels almost never prohibit diuretic use, because the ratio of the 2 diuretics can be readjusted. Patients with parenchymal renal disease (e.g., diabetic nephropathy) usually require relatively higher doses of furosemide and lower doses of spironolactone; otherwise, they develop hyperkalemia. Patients in whom complications develop despite a careful attempt at diuretic treatment usually require second-line therapy. Prostaglandin inhibitors (e.g., NSAIDs) should be avoided in patients with cirrhosis and ascites because they inhibit diuresis, may promote renal failure, and may cause GI bleeding.[132]

Reducing the quantity of fluid in the abdomen can improve the patient's comfort and prevent hepatic hydrothorax and hernias. Also, by concentrating the ascitic fluid, diuresis increases the opsonic activity of ascitic fluid 10-fold and theoretically may be of value in preventing spontaneous ascitic fluid infection.[133]

Blood Pressure

An issue that nurses regularly raise is whether diuretics should be withheld when a patient's blood pressure is low. No data exist to support this practice in the setting of cirrhosis.

Baseline blood pressure, mental status, and creatinine must be factored into the decision to continue, hold, or discontinue diuretics. The baseline blood pressure is usually low (e.g., 60 to 100 mm Hg systolic) in a patient with cirrhosis and ascites. Unless it has dropped rapidly or the patient has confusion or azotemia, diuretics should be given. Blood pressure correlates with survival in cirrhosis; if mean arterial pressure is 82 mm Hg or less, 2-year survival is only 20% compared with 70% for higher blood pressures.[134] A mean arterial pressure of 82 mm Hg correlates with a systolic blood pressure of approximately 100 mm Hg.

Beta blockers reduce survival in patients with refractory ascites, probably by reducing blood pressure.[135] Beta blockers should be stopped if blood pressure is less than 100 mm Hg systolic. Midodrine has been shown to increase blood pressure and increase survival in hypotensive patients with cirrhosis and ascites.[136] Midodrine can be started at 5 mg orally 3 times daily and titrated up to achieve an increase in blood pressure of approximately 10 mm Hg, a systolic blood pressure above 100 mm Hg, or both.

Goal of Inpatient Treatment

Hospitalized patients who are stable, with ascites as their major problem, can be discharged after they are demonstrated to be responding to the medical regimen and are normokalemic, are not azotemic, and have a normal or slightly to moderately reduced serum sodium level. In the past, patients with ascites frequently occupied hospital beds for prolonged durations because of uncertainty regarding the diagnosis and optimal treatment and because of iatrogenic complications. Complete resolution of ascites should not be a prerequisite for discharge from the hospital. Following discharge from the hospital, a patient should be seen in the outpatient setting within 7 to 14 days.

Role of Sodium Bicarbonate

Mild renal tubular acidosis develops in some patients with cirrhosis and ascites. Although oral sodium bicarbonate administration has been recommended in this setting, such treatment increases sodium intake dramatically and cannot be advocated in the absence of evidence to support its use.

Vaptans

The vaptans are a relatively new class of drugs that have been used in patients with cirrhosis to increase urinary water excretion.[137,138] Initially the focus of treatment with vaptans was an increase in serum sodium[137]; however, this is not a very important end point. Additionally, the largest randomized trial that included only patients with cirrhosis demonstrated that the vaptan was not clinically beneficial in long-term management of ascites in cirrhosis. Even more concerning was an increase in mortality in the vaptan-treated group.[138]

Outpatient Management

After discharge from the hospital, the patient's body weight, blood pressure at home (using a prescribed blood pressure cuff), orthostatic symptoms, and serum electrolyte, urea, and creatinine levels should be monitored. Random urine specimens for a sodium-to-potassium ratio can be collected to help guide treatment decisions. The subsequent frequency of follow-up evaluations is determined by the response to treatment and stability of the patient. I usually evaluate these patients every 1 to 4 weeks until they clearly are responding to treatment and are not experiencing problems. Intensive outpatient follow-up helps prevent subsequent hospitalizations.

Diuretic doses and dietary sodium intake are adjusted to achieve weight loss and negative sodium balance. Patients who are gaining fluid weight despite diuretic therapy should not be considered to have diuretic-resistant ascites (see later) until they are demonstrated to be adherent to the prescribed diet. Monitoring the urine sodium concentration provides insight into adherence. Patients who have a random urine sodium-to-potassium ratio greater than 1 should be losing weight if they are consuming less than 88 mmol of sodium per day. In my experience, most patients who initially are thought to be diuretic-resistant eventually are found to be nonadherent to the diet; they demonstrate weight gain and urinary sodium excretion as high as 500 mmol/day or more. Diet education is crucial to the successful management of such patients. Patients with truly diuretic-resistant ascites excrete nearly sodium-free urine despite maximal doses of diuretics. During long-term follow-up, abstinent alcoholic patients may become more sensitive to diuretics. In these cases, the dose of diuretics may be tapered and the drugs even discontinued.

Refractory Ascites

Refractory ascites is defined as ascites unresponsive to a sodium-restricted diet and high-dose diuretic treatment. Refractoriness may manifest as minimal or no weight loss despite diuretics or the development of complications of diuretics.[139] Studies have shown that ascites in the setting of cirrhosis is refractory to standard medical therapy in fewer than 10% of patients.[124,128]

Viable options for patients refractory to routine medical therapy include careful attention to medications, liver transplantation, serial therapeutic paracenteses, TIPS, and peritoneovenous shunts (Fig. 93-5).[10]

Careful Attention to Medications

Ascites can be made refractory by drugs that reduce blood pressure. These include beta blockers, acetylcholinesterase inhibitors, and angiotensin receptor blockers (see Fig. 93-5).[135] The risks versus benefits of each of these drugs must be considered carefully. If a patient's systolic blood pressure is below 100 mm Hg and azotemia is present, the beta blocker, acetylcholinesterase inhibitor, or angiotensin receptor blocker should be stopped. If ascites continues to be refractory to diuretics, midodrine can be added and carefully titrated upward to achieve the desired blood pressure and natriuresis. These simple steps can cause diuretic-resistant patients to become diuretic-sensitive.

Liver Transplantation

Liver transplantation should be considered among the treatment options for patients with cirrhosis and ascites—whether the fluid is diuretic-sensitive or diuretic-refractory (see Chapter 97). In many areas of the United States, patients with ascites are not offered transplantation until hepatorenal syndrome has developed (see Chapter 94). The 12-month survival rate for patients with ascites refractory to medical therapy is only 32%.[140] The survival rate following liver transplantation is much higher.

In patients who are candidates for liver transplantation, procedures that could make a future transplant difficult should be avoided. Surgery in the right upper quadrant causes adhesions that become vascularized and difficult to remove during transplant surgery.

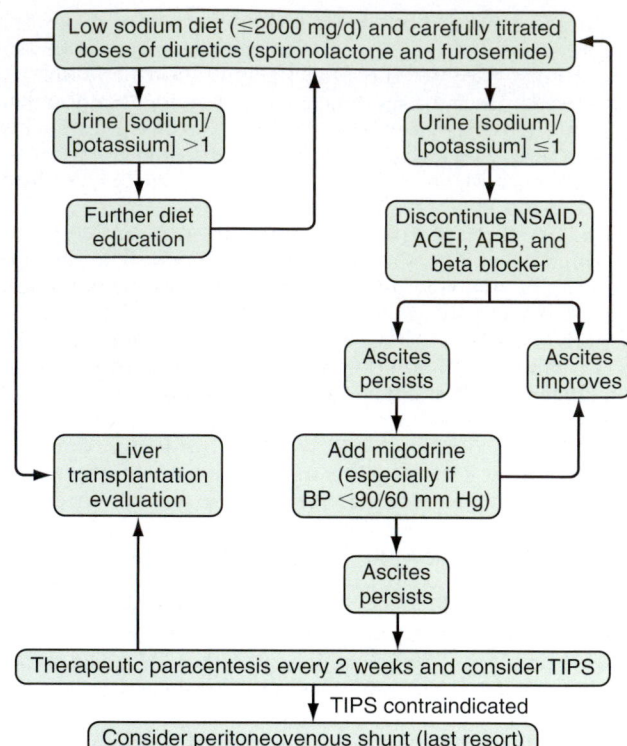

FIGURE 93-5. Algorithm for the treatment of patients with cirrhotic ascites. ACEI, angiotensin-converting enzyme inhibitor; ARB, angiotensin receptor blocker; TIPS, transjugular intrahepatic portosystemic shunt. *(Reproduced with permission from Such J, Runyon BA. Treatment of diuretic-resistant ascites in patients with cirrhosis. In: Basow DS, editor. UpToDate. Waltham, Mass.: UpToDate; 2013. Copyright © 2013 UpToDate, Inc. For more information, visit www.uptodate.com.)*

Serial Paracenteses

Therapeutic abdominal paracentesis is one of the oldest medical procedures. In the 1980s, after 2000 years of use, scientific data regarding large-volume paracentesis were reported, and patients were documented to tolerate large-volume paracentesis well, just as patients had in the 1940s and earlier.[141] In one large randomized controlled trial, therapeutic paracentesis plus IV infusion of colloid led to fewer minor (asymptomatic) changes in serum electrolyte and creatinine levels than those reported with diuretic therapy; however, no differences in morbidity or mortality rates could be demonstrated.[141] Therapeutic paracentesis now appears to be first-line therapy for patients in whom ascites is tense and second-line therapy for patients with cirrhosis whose ascites is refractory to diuretics (see Fig. 93-5).[10] The world record for volume of fluid removed at one time appears to be 41 L.[142]

Colloid Replacement

A controversial issue regarding therapeutic paracentesis is the role of colloid replacement. In one study, patients with tense ascites were randomized to receive IV albumin (10 g/L of fluid removed) or no albumin after therapeutic paracentesis.[143] More statistically significant (asymptomatic) changes in serum electrolyte, plasma renin, and serum creatinine levels developed in the patients who did not receive albumin than in those who received albumin, but no greater frequency of clinical morbidity or mortality was seen. Although another study has documented that the patients who have a postparacentesis rise in plasma renin levels have a decreased life expectancy compared with those who have stable renin levels, no study has demonstrated decreased survival rate in patients not given a plasma expander compared with patients given albumin after paracentesis.[144] The phrase "paracentesis-induced circulatory dysfunction" has been coined to describe the rise in plasma renin levels after paracentesis.[145]

The confusion regarding albumin infusion relates, in part, to the design of the relevant studies. In the studies from Barcelona, patients with "tense" ascites could be entered into the trial of albumin versus no albumin, and 31% of these patients were not even receiving diuretics.[142] It seems more appropriate to study the population in which repeated paracenteses are really needed, specifically the diuretic-resistant group, rather than all patients with tense ascites.[146] Another group of investigators has shown that patients with cirrhosis and diuretic-resistant ascites tolerate a 5-L paracentesis without a change in plasma renin levels.[147] My approach to patients with tense ascites is to take off enough fluid (4 to 5 L) to relieve intra-abdominal pressure and then to rely on diuretics to eliminate the remainder. To remove all of the fluid by paracentesis when most of it can be removed with diuretics seems inappropriate, partly because paracentesis removes opsonins, whereas diuresis concentrates opsonins.[133] Repeated therapeutic paracenteses should be reserved for the 10% of patients in whom diuretic treatment fails to relieve the ascites.

A meta-analysis has reported a survival advantage with albumin infusion after large-volume paracenteses.[148] Therefore, it seems reasonable to (1) avoid serial large-volume paracenteses in patients with diuretic-sensitive ascites, (2) withhold albumin after taps of 5 L or less, and (3) consider albumin infusion (6 to 8 g/L of fluid removed) after taps of larger volume in patients with diuretic-resistant ascites.[10,148]

A small randomized trial has shown that terlipressin may be equivalent to albumin after therapeutic paracentesis in preventing paracentesis-induced circulatory dysfunction; when this drug receives approval for use in the United States, and if further studies support its efficacy, terlipressin would be an alternative to albumin.[149]

Transjugular Intrahepatic Portosystemic Shunt (TIPS)

TIPS is a side-to-side portacaval shunt that is placed by an interventional radiologist (or hepatologist), usually with the use of local anesthesia. TIPS placement was first used for the treatment of refractory variceal bleeding, but it also has been advocated for diuretic-resistant ascites[150] (see Chapter 92). TIPS was received with great enthusiasm in the 1990s, similar to the enthusiasm for the peritoneovenous shunt in the 1970s. As with peritoneovenous shunting, TIPS was overused until serious complications and suboptimal efficacy were reported. Four large-scale randomized trials in patients with diuretic-resistant ascites have demonstrated consistently superior efficacy of TIPS over repeated paracenteses, but no survival advantage.[151-154] Several meta-analyses have confirmed the efficacy of TIPS but with a higher frequency of hepatic encephalopathy.[155-159] One meta-analysis has demonstrated a trend toward improved survival in patients undergoing TIPS placement.[156] Another meta-analysis, which analyzed individual patient data, did show improved transplant-free survival with TIPS.[159] Although TIPS dysfunction was common when an uncoated (or uncovered) stent was used, polytetrafluoroethylene-coated stents have been reported to improve patency and survival when compared with uncoated stents in a nonrandomized study and to improve patency, with no survival advantage, when compared with uncoated stents in a randomized trial.[160,161] Also, the 4 older TIPS trials

preceded development and implementation of the MELD score, which predicts 90-day mortality after TIPS placement (see Chapter 92). Trials using the coated stent and selecting patients according to their MELD scores may demonstrate a survival advantage for TIPS compared with repeated paracenteses.

TIPS also is useful in the treatment of hepatic hydrothorax and umbilical hernia.[116,126] A direct intrahepatic portosystemic shunt connects the portal vein directly to the inferior vena cava and has applicability in patients with Budd-Chiari syndrome (see Chapter 85).[162]

Peritoneovenous Shunt

In the mid-1970s, the peritoneovenous shunt was promoted as a new "physiologic" treatment for the management of ascites. Reports of shunt failure, fatal complications following shunt insertion, and randomized trials demonstrating no survival advantage have led to the relegation of this procedure to third-line therapy in patients with cirrhosis and ascites[10,128] (see Fig. 93-5). Patients who are not candidates for liver transplantation and who have a scarred abdomen that is not amenable to repeated paracenteses, who are not candidates for a TIPS, or in whom an attempt at TIPS placement has failed make up the small subset of candidates for a peritoneovenous shunt. A randomized trial has shown that even an uncoated TIPS stent has better "assisted patency" than a peritoneovenous shunt.[163]

Novel Treatments

Novel treatment options for patients with refractory ascites include weekly infusions of IV albumin, ascites reinfusion, ultrafiltration, terlipressin infusion (not available in the United States), partial splenic artery embolization, peritoneal-urinary drainage of the fluid using a surgically implanted pump, and percutaneous placement of a peritoneovenous shunt by an interventional radiologist.[164-171] More data are needed before these treatments can be recommended.

PROGNOSIS

Cirrhosis complicated by ascites is associated with significant morbidity and mortality, related, in part, to the severe underlying liver disease and, in part, to the ascites per se. In half of the patients in whom cirrhosis is detected before decompensation (i.e., development of ascites, jaundice, encephalopathy, or GI hemorrhage), ascites occurs within 10 years.[172] When ascites appears, the expected mortality rate is approximately 50% in just 2 years.[173] With liver transplantation, survival is improved dramatically.

KEY REFERENCES

Full references for this chapter can be found on www.expertconsult.com.

2. Runyon BA, Hoefs JC, Morgan TR. Ascitic fluid analysis in malignancy-related ascites. Hepatology 1988; 8:1104-9.
9. Runyon BA. Technique of diagnostic and therapeutic abdominal paracentesis. In: Basow DS, editor. UpToDate. Waltham, Mass.: UpToDate; 2012.
10. Runyon BA, AASLD Practice Guidelines Committee. Management of adult patients with ascites due to cirrhosis: An update. Hepatology 2009; 49:2087-107.
24. Runyon BA, Montano AA, Akriviadis EA, et al. The serum-ascites albumin gradient is superior to the

exudate-transudate concept in the differential diagnosis of ascites. Ann Intern Med 1992; 117:215-20.

26. Runyon BA, Canawati HN, Akriviadis EA. Optimization of ascitic fluid culture technique. Gastroenterology 1988; 95:1351-5.

45. Soriano G, Castellote J, Alvarez C, et al. Secondary bacterial peritonitis in cirrhosis: A retrospective study of clinical and analytical characteristics, diagnosis and management. J Hepatol 2010; 52:39-44.

65. Runyon BA, Squier SU, Borzio M. Translocation of gut bacteria in rats with cirrhosis to mesenteric lymph nodes partially explains the pathogenesis of spontaneous bacterial peritonitis. J Hepatol 1994; 21:792-6.

73. Fernandez J, Acevedo J, Castro M, et al. Prevalence and risk factors of infections by multiresistant bacteria in cirrhosis: A prospective study. Hepatology 2012; 55:1551-61.

91. Runyon BA, McHutchison JG, Antillon MR, et al. Short-course vs. long-course antibiotic treatment of spontaneous bacterial peritonitis: A randomized controlled trial of 100 patients. Gastroenterology 1991; 100:1737-42.

96. Fernandez J, Ruiz del Arbol L, Gomez C, et al. Norfloxacin vs. ceftriaxone in the prophylaxis of infections in patients with advanced cirrhosis and hemorrhage. Gastroenterology 2006; 131:1049-56.

117. Addolorato G, Leggio L, Ferrulli A, et al. Effectiveness and safety of baclofen for maintenance of alcohol abstinence in alcohol-dependent patients with liver cirrhosis: Randomised, double-blind controlled study. Lancet 2007; 370:1915-22.

127. Angeli P, Fasolato S, Mazza E, et al. Combined versus sequential diuretic treatment of moderate ascites in nonazotemic patients with cirrhosis. Gut 2010; 59:98-104.

135. Serste T, Melot C, Francoz C, et al. Deleterious effects of beta-blockers on survival in patients with cirrhosis and refractory ascites. Hepatology 2010; 52:1017-22.

137. Wong F, Blei AT, Blendis LM, Thuluvath PJ. A vasopressin receptor antagonist (VPA-985) improves serum sodium concentration in patients with hyponatremia: A multicenter, randomized, placebo-controlled trial. Hepatology 2003; 3:182-91.

159. Salerno F, Camma C, Enea M, et al. Transjugular intrahepatic portosystemic shunt for refractory ascites: A meta-analysis of individual patient data. Gastroenterology 2007; 133:825-34.

Hepatic Encephalopathy, Hepatorenal Syndrome, Hepatopulmonary Syndrome, and Other Systemic Complications of Liver Disease

MOISES ILAN NEVAH AND MICHAEL B. FALLON

Chronic liver disease and acute liver failure disrupt normal homeostasis and cause systemic manifestations that may dominate the clinical features of liver disease. Most of these extrahepatic syndromes are reversible with liver transplantation.

HEPATIC ENCEPHALOPATHY

The term *hepatic encephalopathy* (HE) encompasses a wide array of transient and subtle reversible neurologic and psychiatric manifestations usually found in patients with chronic liver disease and portal hypertension, but also seen in patients with acute liver failure. HE develops in 50% to 70% of patients with cirrhosis, and its occurrence is a poor prognostic indicator, with projected 1- and 3-year survival rates of 42% and 23%, respectively, without liver transplantation.[1] Symptoms may range from mild neurocognitive disturbances to overt coma.[2,3] HE is often triggered by an inciting event that results in a rise in the serum ammonia level. The precise underlying pathophysiologic mechanisms are not well understood, and

the mainstay of therapy is elimination of the precipitating event and excess ammonia.[4] Liver transplantation generally reverses HE.

Pathophysiology

A number of factors, occurring alone or in combination, have been implicated in the development of HE. These factors may differ in acute and chronic liver disease and include the production of neurotoxins, altered permeability of the blood-brain barrier, and abnormal neurotransmission (Fig. 94-1). The best-described neurotoxin involved in HE is ammonia, which is produced primarily in the colon, where bacteria metabolize proteins and other nitrogen-based products into ammonia. Enterocytes synthesize ammonia from glutamine.[4-6] Once produced, ammonia enters the portal circulation and, under normal conditions, is metabolized and cleared by hepatocytes. In cirrhosis and portal hypertension, reduced hepatocyte function and portosystemic shunting contribute to increased circulating ammonia levels. Arterial hyperammonemia is observed

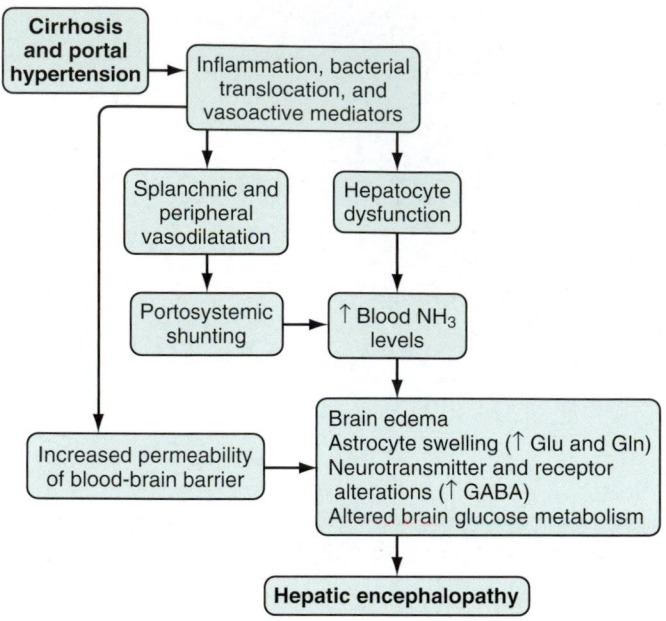

FIGURE 94-1. Proposed pathophysiology of hepatic encephalopathy. GABA, γ-aminobutyric acid; Gln, glutamine; Glu, glutamate; NH₃, ammonia.

in up to 90% of patients with HE, although serum levels are neither sensitive nor specific indicators of its presence. Increased permeability of the blood-brain barrier increases the uptake and extraction of ammonia by the cerebellum and basal ganglia.[7-9] Acute hyperammonemia appears to have a direct effect on brain edema, astrocyte swelling, and the transport of neurally active compounds such as myoinositol, thereby contributing to HE.[10-12]

Other alterations in HE affect neuronal membrane fluidity, central nervous system (CNS) neurotransmitter expression, and neurotransmitter receptor expression and activation.[13,14] The γ-aminobutyric acid (GABA)-benzodiazepine system has been the best studied. Although CNS benzodiazepine levels and GABA receptor concentrations are unchanged in animal models of HE, increased sensitivity of the astrocyte (peripheral-type) benzodiazepine receptor enhances activation of the GABA-benzodiazepine system.[15,16] This activation occurs in part through a feed-forward system in which production of neurosteroids (allopregnanolone and tetrahydrodeoxycorticosterone) by astrocytes further activates the GABA$_A$-benzodiazepine receptor system.[17,18] Other factors that influence CNS neurotransmission, including serotonin (5-hydroxytryptamine [5-HT]),[19-21] nitric oxide (NO), circulating opioid peptides, manganese, and increased oxygen free radical production, have also been postulated to contribute to HE.[4]

A 2010 study has demonstrated that distinct allelic mutations in the glutaminase gene increase the risk for overt HE, independent of hepatic synthetic function or the presence of minimal HE. This risk may be mediated by enhanced glutaminase transcriptional activity that results in increased levels of ammonia and glutamate.[22] Other work has found differences in colonic mucosal microbiota in cirrhotic patients with and without HE that could influence the production of substances that lead to the development of HE.[23] Finally, hyperammonemia, particularly in acute liver failure, also increases astrocyte glutamine production via glutamine synthetase. The rise in astrocyte glutamine and glutamate concentrations contributes to factors associated with CNS dysfunction.[5,24,25]

Clinical Features and Classification

HE may present as a spectrum of reversible neurocognitive symptoms and signs that range from mild changes in cognition to profound coma in patients with acute or chronic liver disease. HE is often precipitated by an inciting event (e.g., GI bleeding, electrolyte abnormalities, infections, medications, dehydration). The diagnosis of HE, therefore, requires careful consideration in the appropriate clinical situation. Occasionally, HE may be the initial presentation of chronic liver disease. Subtle findings in overt HE may include forgetfulness, alterations in handwriting, difficulty with driving, and reversal of the sleep-wake cycle.[26,27] As HE worsens, findings may include asterixis, agitation, disinhibited behavior, seizures, and coma. Other causes of altered mental status—particularly hypoglycemia, hyponatremia, medication ingestion, and structural intracranial abnormalities resulting from coagulopathy or trauma—should be considered and rapidly excluded in patients suspected of having HE.

There are 3 major types of HE: type A, associated with acute liver failure; type B, associated with portosystemic shunts in the absence of liver disease; and type C, associated with chronic and end-stage liver disease and portal hypertension.[3] Type C HE is the most common type and has historically been graded from 0 to 4 based on the West Haven criteria (Table 94-1).[28] A consensus report in 2011[29] proposed a new SONIC (Spectrum of Neurocognitive Impairment in Cirrhosis) nomenclature to reflect the wide spectrum of clinical findings and improve the clinical classification of HE for research studies.

Based on the SONIC classification, cirrhotic patients are divided into 3 categories: unimpaired, covert HE, and overt HE.[29] Unimpaired patients have no clinical, neurophysiologic, or neuropsychometric abnormalities. Patients with covert HE have minimal HE (clinically normal patients with abnormal cognition or neurophysiologic test results) or grade 1 HE by the West Haven criteria. Patients with overt HE have grade 2 HE or higher by the West Haven criteria (see Table 94-1). This classification eliminates the need to distinguish minimal HE from grade 1 HE, which has been difficult in clinical studies and takes advantage of the recognition that disorientation, specifically to time, is a distinct clinical feature that distinguishes grade 1 from grade 2 HE and distinguishes covert from overt HE.[2,30]

Diagnosis

No specific laboratory findings indicate the presence of HE definitively. Blood ammonia levels are commonly measured in patients with cirrhosis and portal hypertension but are not sensitive or specific for the presence of HE. Other factors such as GI bleeding, the ingestion of certain medications (e.g., diuretics, alcohol, narcotics, valproic acid),[15,31,32] the use of a tourniquet when blood is drawn, and delayed processing and cooling of a blood sample may raise the blood ammonia level irrespective of the presence of HE.[15] Measurement of arterial ammonia offers no advantage over venous ammonia levels in patients with chronic liver disease.[12,33-35] Blood ammonia levels may be a useful indicator of HE in the absence of cirrhosis and portal hypertension, as in patients with metabolic disorders that influence ammonia generation or metabolism, such as urea cycle disorders and disorders of proline metabolism (Box 94-1).[36,37]

The development of standardized neuropsychometric and neurocognitive tests has led to the recognition that routine evaluation is insensitive for the diagnosis of clinically relevant HE.[38-42] Simple tests such as the portosystemic encephalopathy syndrome test (PSET) and the Stroop test

TABLE 94-1 Clinical Stages of Hepatic Encephalopathy (HE): The West Haven Criteria and the Proposed Classification of the Spectrum of Neurocognitive Impairment in Cirrhosis (SONIC)

	West Haven Criteria		SONIC			
Grade	Intellectual Function	Neuromuscular Function	Classification	Mental Status	Special Tests	Asterixis
0	Normal	Normal	Unimpaired	Not impaired	Normal	Absent
Minimal	Normal examination findings; subtle changes in work or driving	Minor abnormalities of visual perception or on psychometric or number tests	Covert HE	Not impaired	Abnormal	Absent
1	Personality changes, attention deficits, irritability, depressed state	Tremor and incoordination				
2	Changes in sleep-wake cycle, lethargy, mood and behavioral changes, cognitive dysfunction	Asterixis, ataxic gait, speech abnormalities (slow and slurred)	Overt HE	Impaired	Abnormal	Present (absent in coma)
3	Altered level of consciousness (somnolence), confusion, disorientation, and amnesia	Muscular rigidity, nystagmus, clonus, Babinski sign, hyporeflexia				
4	Stupor and coma	Oculocephalic reflex, unresponsiveness to noxious stimuli				

From Ferenci P, Lockwood A, Mullen K, et al. Hepatic encephalopathy—Definition, nomenclature, diagnosis, and quantification: Final report of the working party at the 11th World Congresses of Gastroenterology, Vienna, 1998. Hepatology 2002; 35:716-21; and Bajaj JS, Cordoba J, Mullen KD, et al. The design of clinical trials in hepatic encephalopathy—An International Society for Hepatic Encephalopathy and Nitrogen Metabolism (ISHEN) consensus statement. Aliment Pharmacol Ther 2011; 33:739-47.

BOX 94-1 Differential Diagnosis of Hyperammonemia

Acute liver failure
Chronic kidney disease
Cigarette smoking
Cirrhosis
GI bleeding
Inborn errors of metabolism
  Proline metabolism disorders
  Urea cycle defects (e.g., carbamylphosphate synthetase I deficiency, ornithine transcarbamylase deficiency, argininosuccinate lyase deficiency, N-acetylglutamate synthetase deficiency)
Medications/toxins
  Alcohol
  Diuretics (e.g., acetazolamide)
  Narcotics
  Valproic acid
Muscle exertion and ischemia
Portosystemic shunts
Technique and conditions of blood sampling
  High body temperature
  High-protein diet
  Tourniquet use

evaluate the patient's attention, concentration, fine motor skills, and orientation and have been shown to be highly specific for the diagnosis of HE.[38,43,44] With the use of these tests, covert HE has been found to be common and to negatively influence a patient's quality of life and driving ability and to increase the risk of overt HE. Moreover, treatment of minimal HE improves quality of life, cognitive test results, and a patient's driving ability.[27,45,46]

A number of novel imaging and functional tests for the diagnosis of HE have also been studied. Magnetic resonance spectroscopy (MRS) and MR T1 mapping with partial inversion recovery (TAPIR) have been used to measure clinically relevant parameters quantitatively.[38,47] The critical flicker frequency test, a simple light-based test that assesses cerebral cortex function, has been shown to be a reliable marker of minimal HE. Whether these functional tests will become useful in clinical practice is still unknown.[39-41]

Treatment

Treatments for HE are directed primarily toward eliminating or correcting precipitating factors (e.g., bleeding, infection, hypokalemia, medications, dehydration), reducing blood ammonia levels, and avoiding the toxic effects of ammonia on the CNS. In the past, dietary protein restriction was considered an important component of the treatment of HE. Subsequent work has suggested that limiting protein-calorie intake is not beneficial in patients with HE.[48-50] Vegetable and dairy proteins may be preferable to animal proteins because of a more favorable calorie-to-nitrogen ratio. Although branched-chain amino acid supplementation may improve symptoms modestly, the benefits of such supplementation are not sufficient to justify its routine use.[4]

Nonabsorbable disaccharides have been the cornerstone of the treatment of HE. Oral lactulose or lactitol (the latter is not available in the United States) are metabolized by colonic bacteria to by-products that appear to have beneficial effects by causing catharsis and reducing intestinal pH, thereby inhibiting ammonia absorption.[51] These agents improve symptoms in patients with acute and chronic HE when compared with placebo but do not improve psychometric test performance or mortality. Side effects are common and include abdominal cramping, flatulence, diarrhea, and electrolyte imbalance. Lactulose may be administered per rectum (as an enema) to patients who are at increased risk of aspiration, although the efficacy of enema administration has not been evaluated.

Oral antibiotics have also been used to treat HE, with the aim of modifying the intestinal flora and lowering stool pH to enhance the excretion of ammonia. Antibiotics are generally used as second-line agents after lactulose or in patients who are intolerant of nonabsorbable disaccharides. Rifaximin given orally in a dose of 550 mg twice daily was approved in 2010 for the treatment of chronic HE and reduction in the risk of recurrence of overt HE in patients with advanced liver disease.[52,53] The tolerability and side-effect profile of rifaximin are superior to those of lactulose,[54-57] albeit at greater financial cost.[58] Other antibiotics, including neomycin, metronidazole, and vancomycin, have been studied in small trials and case series, but their effectiveness in patients with chronic HE is not established.

Several other agents that may modify intestinal flora and modulate the generation or intestinal absorption of ammonia have been evaluated as potential treatments for HE. Acarbose, an intestinal α-glucosidase inhibitor used to treat type 2 diabetes mellitus, inhibits the intestinal absorption of carbohydrates and glucose and results in their enhanced delivery to the colon. As a result, the ratio of saccharolytic to proteolytic bacterial flora is increased, and blood ammonia levels are decreased. A randomized controlled double-blind crossover trial has demonstrated that acarbose improves mild HE in patients with cirrhosis and adult-onset diabetes mellitus.[59] Similarly, probiotic regimens have been used to modify intestinal flora and diminish ammonia generation. Several studies have suggested that these agents may be beneficial in humans with mild HE.[60-66] A Cochrane Database review in 2011 was unable to conclude that probiotics improve clinically relevant outcomes.[67]

Strategies to enhance ammonia clearance may also be useful in the treatment of HE. Sodium benzoate, sodium phenylbutyrate, and sodium phenylacetate, all of which increase ammonia excretion in urine, are approved by the FDA for the treatment of hyperammonemia resulting from urea cycle enzyme defects and may improve HE in patients with cirrhosis (see Chapter 77). Administration of sodium benzoate, however, results in a high sodium load, and the efficacy of this agent is not clearly established.[4,68] The combination of IV sodium phenylacetate and sodium benzoate (Ammonul, Ucyclyd Pharma, Scottsdale, Ariz.) in patients with HE is being studied. Administration of zinc, which has been used because zinc deficiency is common in patients with cirrhosis[69-71] and because zinc increases the activity of ornithine transcarbamylase, an enzyme in the urea cycle, may also improve HE; however, clear efficacy has not been established. Extracorporeal albumin dialysis using the molecular adsorbent recirculating system (MARS) has resulted in a reduction in blood ammonia levels and improvement in severe HE in patients with acute-on-chronic liver failure (see Chapter 95).[72] Further studies are needed to clarify whether albumin dialysis has a role in treatment of HE. Finally, L-ornithine–L-aspartate (LOLA), a salt of the amino acids ornithine and aspartic acid that activates the urea cycle and enhances ammonia clearance, has been shown in several randomized controlled studies to improve HE compared with lactulose[73-75]; however, this agent is not available in the United States.

HEPATORENAL SYNDROME

The term *hepatorenal syndrome* (HRS) was first used in 1932 to describe acute kidney injury, mainly acute tubular necrosis (ATN) or interstitial nephritis, in a group of patients who had undergone biliary tract surgery.[76] As pathophysiologic mechanisms were better elucidated, HRS was found to be part of a cascade of events associated with intense dilatation of the splanchnic arterial vasculature in the setting of cirrhosis or acute liver injury and resulting in profound renal arterial vasoconstriction and progressive renal failure.[77] Histologically, the kidneys are normal in HRS. Function may be restored by correction of portal hypertension, liver transplantation, removal of the kidneys and transplantation of them into a noncirrhotic recipient, and, in some cases, medical therapy.[78-80]

Acute renal dysfunction occurs in 15% to 25% of hospitalized patients with cirrhosis.[81,82] HRS is found in 10% to 30% of such patients and appears to be an extension of the pathophysiology of prerenal azotemia and therefore potentially reversible.[81-83] The annual frequency of HRS in cirrhotic patients with ascites is roughly 8%[84] and, in some reports, as high as 40%.[85,86] HRS develops in approximately 30% of cirrhotic patients who are admitted with SBP or other infection (see Chapter 93), 25% who are hospitalized with severe alcoholic hepatitis, and 10% who require serial large-volume paracenteses.[87] The observation that morbidity and mortality remain high once the syndrome is established has led to a focus on the prevention, early diagnosis, and therapy of renal dysfunction in patients with cirrhosis.[84]

Pathophysiology

The pathophysiology of HRS is complex and incompletely characterized. Three important components contribute to the initiation and perpetuation of altered renal perfusion (Fig. 94-2): (1) arterial vasodilatation in the splanchnic and systemic circulation, (2) renal vasoconstriction, and (3) cardiac dysfunction.[88] These components influence renal function in concert and form the basis for current therapies and preventive strategies.

Splanchnic Arterial Vasodilatation

Splanchnic and systemic arterial vasodilatation is a hallmark of the progression of portal hypertension in patients with cirrhosis and leads to decreased effective circulating blood volume and ultimately to a decrease in blood pressure. This process is mediated by a number of endogenous substances, including nitric oxide (NO), carbon monoxide (CO), glucagon, prostacyclin, adrenomedullin, and endogenous opiates that are released or act locally in the vasculature in response to mechanical and inflammatory signals.[77,84,89,90] In the early stages of portal hypertension, increases in heart rate and cardiac output compensate for the decrease in effective circulatory volume and create a hyperdynamic circulation.[91] As liver disease and splanchnic vasodilatation progress, additional compensatory mechanisms are activated.

Renal Arterial Vasoconstriction

Splanchnic and systemic vasodilatation also lead to compensatory renal vasoconstriction and renal sodium and water retention, in turn leading to hyponatremia and ascites formation (see Chapter 93). These responses are mediated by stimulation of the sympathetic nervous system, activation of the renin-angiotensin-aldosterone system (RAAS), and

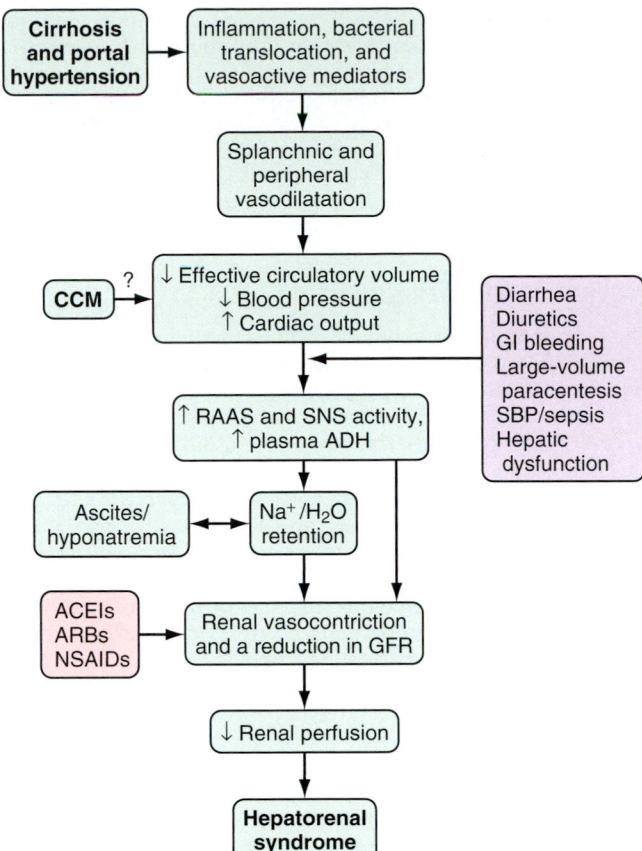

FIGURE 94-2. Proposed pathophysiology and triggers of hepatorenal syndrome. ACEIs, angiotensin-converting enzyme inhibitors; ADH, antidiuretic hormone; ARBs, angiotensin receptor blockers; CCM, cirrhotic cardiomyopathy; GFR, glomerular filtration rate; RAAS, renin-angiotensin-aldosterone system; SNS, sympathetic nervous system.

nonosmotic release and activity of arginine vasopressin (as a result of increased secretion and decreased clearance of arginine vasopressin and apparent increased expression of vasopressin-regulated water channels), as well as intrarenal events. Although the precise intrarenal mechanisms are speculative, altered production or action of endothelins, prostaglandins, kallikreins, and F2-isoprostanes may contribute to renal vasoconstriction.[85,92,93] Ultimately, the balance between vasoconstrictive responses in the kidney and systemic and splanchnic vasodilatation is lost, thereby leading to a prominent increase in renal vascular resistance, decrease in renal perfusion, and reduction in the glomerular filtration rate (GFR).[84,91] Finally, intense renal vasoconstriction may lead to tubular damage, and HRS can evolve from a functional syndrome to an organic disease.

Cardiac Dysfunction

Impaired cardiac function also may contribute to renal hypoperfusion in patients with HRS.[94] In one prospective study, HRS developed in cirrhotic patients with more severe arterial vasodilatation and lower cardiac output.[95] In another study of a cohort of patients who were treated for SBP, renal dysfunction (including HRS in some cases) developed in those with lower cardiac output and lower arterial pressure measurements associated with higher circulating levels of norepinephrine and renin plasma activity, despite effective treatment of

the infection.[96] These data demonstrate that cardiac output is impaired in patients with cirrhosis in whom HRS develops as compared with those in whom HRS does not develop and suggests that cardiac dysfunction may be an important additional factor in the pathogenesis of HRS. The relationship between cardiac dysfunction in patients with HRS and cirrhotic cardiomyopathy (see later) has not been studied.[97,98]

Clinical Features and Diagnosis

HRS is a functional disorder, and therefore, laboratory and imaging studies alone are not sufficient for making the diagnosis. A high index of clinical suspicion and exclusion of other potential causes of kidney injury are needed. The majority of patients with HRS are asymptomatic, although some may report decreased urine output. Acute kidney injury (AKI) decreases glomerular filtration rate (GFR) and increases the blood urea nitrogen (BUN) level and may result in HE as the initial clinical presentation of HRS.

The diagnostic criteria for HRS as defined by the International Ascites Club Consensus Workshop in 2007 include: (1) cirrhosis with ascites, (2) serum creatinine level higher than 1.5 mg/dL (133 μmol/L), (3) lack of improvement in the serum creatinine level to 1.5 mg/dL (133 μmol/L) or less after at least 2 days of diuretic withdrawal and volume expansion with albumin (1 g/kg of body weight/day, to a maximum of 100 g/day), (4) absence of shock, (5) lack of current or recent treatment with nephrotoxic drugs, and (6) absence of parenchymal kidney disease as indicated by proteinuria of more than 500 mg/day, microhematuria (>50 red blood cells/high-power field), or abnormal renal US findings (Box 94-2).[88]

Several aspects of the diagnosis of HRS deserve emphasis. First, in patients with no prior evidence or history of renal impairment, the diagnostic criteria for HRS include an increase in the serum creatinine level by 50% above baseline to a level higher than 1.5 mg/dL (133 μmol/L).[84] Although this definition is standardized, a subset of patients with cirrhosis and end-stage liver disease have a profound decrease in muscle mass and urea synthesis that may in turn result in reduced serum creatinine and BUN levels, thereby potentially delaying recognition of HRS.[87,99] Second, many medications, most notably diuretics, lactulose, angiotensin-converting enzyme inhibitors, angiotensin receptor blockers, and NSAIDs, may influence a patient's intravascular volume status and renal perfusion and should be identified expeditiously and discontinued in the setting of acute renal dysfunction. Third, even though SBP may not be accompanied by obvious symptoms and signs, HRS may develop in as many as 20% of affected patients.[100] Therefore, a low threshold for evaluating cirrhotic patients with ascites for the presence of SBP is required.

Because of the limited sensitivity of the serum creatinine level for the diagnosis of HRS, the Acute Dialysis Quality

---

BOX 94-2 Diagnostic Criteria for Hepatorenal Syndrome*

Cirrhosis with ascites
Serum creatinine level ≥ 1.5 mg/dL (133 μmol/L)
No or insufficient improvement in serum creatinine level (remains ≥ 1.5 mg/dL) 48 hr after diuretic withdrawal and adequate volume expansion with IV albumin
Absence of shock
No evidence of recent use of nephrotoxic agents
Absence of intrinsic renal disease

*As defined by the International Ascites Club Consensus Workshop in 2007 (Salerno F, Gerbes A, Ginès P, et al. Diagnosis, prevention and treatment of hepatorenal syndrome in cirrhosis. Gut 2007; 56:1310-8).

TABLE 94-2 Proposed Criteria for the Diagnosis of Kidney Dysfunction in Patients with Cirrhosis

Diagnosis	Criteria
Acute kidney injury	50% increase in the serum creatinine level from baseline in < 48 hours OR Rise of 0.3 mg/dL (26.4 μmol/L) in the serum creatinine level in < 48 hours
Chronic kidney disease	Glomerular filtration rate < 60 mL/min for > 3 months (using MDRD 6 formula)
Acute-on-chronic kidney disease	Glomerular filtration rate < 60 mL/min for > 3 months (using MDRD 6 formula) 50% increase in the serum creatinine level from baseline in < 48 hours or a rise of 0.3 mg/dL (26.4 μmol/L) in the serum creatinine level in < 48 hours

MDRD, Modification of Diet in Renal Disease.
From Nadim MK, Kellum JA, Davenport A, et al. Hepatorenal syndrome: The 8th international consensus conference of the Acute Dialysis Quality Initiative (ADQI) Group. Crit Care 2012; 16:R23.

Initiative (ADQI) Group has stratified AKI and renal dysfunction in cirrhotic patients into grades of increasing severity based on small changes in the GFR and serum creatinine level (Table 94-2).[101-103] The panel also proposed changing the nomenclature from *hepatorenal syndrome* to *hepatorenal disorders* to encompass all patients with end-stage liver disease/cirrhosis and concurrent kidney dysfunction.[101] Urinary biomarkers (e.g., interleukin [IL]-18, urinary neutrophil gelatinase-associated lipocalin [uNGAL]) may be able to distinguish acute tubular necrosis from other etiologies of renal failure in cirrhosis, but their role in clinical practice is not defined.[104-107]

Classification

HRS is classified into 2 types (types 1 and 2) on the basis of clinical characteristics and prognosis.[88] Type 1 HRS presents as a rapidly progressive form of renal dysfunction. Typically, the serum creatinine level doubles to a value higher than 2.5 mg/dL in a period of 2 weeks or less. Type 1 HRS is often triggered by an inciting event that causes a rapid decline in the hemodynamic parameters that maintain renal homeostasis in cirrhotic patients.[82] The most common triggers include severe bacterial infections,[108-110] GI bleeding, surgical procedures, and acute liver injury.[88,111,112] SBP is the main bacterial infection that predisposes cirrhotic patients to develop HRS.[84,109,113] Patients with high levels of inflammatory response markers, severe circulatory depression prior to the onset of infection, and adrenal insufficiency are most susceptible to the development of HRS.[114]

Type 2 HRS is more slowly progressive than type 1 HRS but still carries a median survival of only approximately 6 months. Type 2 HRS is observed in patients with severe ascites (diuretic resistant) and is characterized by serum creatinine levels lower than 2.5 mg/dL. The degree of arterial hypotension and circulatory dysfunction is less than that seen with type 1 HRS. Type 1 HRS may develop in patients with type 2 HRS following a triggering event.[84,85]

Many patients with cirrhosis and portal hypertension also have underlying chronic kidney disease, which complicates recognition of HRS even in the presence of underlying pathophysiologic mechanisms that favor the development of HRS.

Whether these patients should be considered to have a unique form of HRS (type 3) and whether they should be treated in a fashion similar to that for other patients with HRS have not been clearly defined.[85] Whether the more sensitive RIFLE (*R*isk, *I*njury, *F*ailure, *L*oss of kidney function, and *E*nd-stage kidney disease) classification of acute kidney injury will improve the diagnosis and therapy of kidney dysfunction in cirrhosis and alter outcomes in patients with HRS are areas of ongoing investigation (see Table 94-2).

Prevention and Treatment

The high mortality rate of HRS underscores the importance of prevention. Avoiding or addressing intravascular volume depletion (resulting from overdiuresis, diarrhea caused by lactulose, GI bleeding from gastroesophageal varices, or large-volume paracentesis without colloid administration), administration of nephrotoxic drugs (e.g., NSAIDs, certain antibiotics), and infection (SBP, bacteremia) is important. Specific guidelines for the primary and secondary prophylaxis of variceal bleeding, administration of colloid (albumin) to patients with a rising serum creatinine level after a large-volume paracentesis or with SBP, and prophylactic administration of antibiotics to patients at high risk of SBP or other infections and those hospitalized for GI bleeding have been published.[100,108,111,113] Routine invasive hemodynamic monitoring of cirrhotic patients with a rising serum creatinine level does not have a clear benefit and is not recommended.

The concept that specific treatment of HRS is possible and may improve survival has emerged since 2000. Current options include medical therapies, transjugular intrahepatic portosystemic shunt (TIPS) placement, and liver transplantation. Medical therapies for HRS are directed toward reversing the underlying splanchnic and systemic vasodilatation with vasoconstrictors, and increasing effective circulatory volume with the use of colloid. Such treatment is used as a temporizing measure until definitive treatment for liver disease (liver transplantation) or portal hypertension (TIPS) is undertaken or until an acute process (SBP, GI bleeding) has been reversed (Box 94-3).[115,116]

Medical Therapy

The use of vasoconstrictors with or without administration of colloid in patients with HRS was initially reported in the 1960s. Since then, several regimens, including terlipressin and albumin; midodrine, octreotide, and albumin; and norepinephrine and albumin, have been studied. Pooled analysis of published trials has confirmed that a goal-directed approach using vasoconstrictors improves kidney function in patients with HRS.[117,118]

Terlipressin is an IV-administered selective vasopressin 1 receptor agonist vasoconstrictor used in Europe and under review by the FDA for the treatment of type 1 HRS.[119,120] It has been evaluated in 4 randomized controlled trials and 2 meta-analyses.[81,121-133] In 2 multicenter studies of patients with type 1 HRS,[130,131] terlipressin in combination with albumin improved serum creatinine levels relative to albumin alone (30% to 43% vs. 8% to 13%), although survival was not significantly different in the 2 groups. In addition, in one study,[130] terlipressin was associated with a significantly increased rate of cardiovascular complications compared with albumin alone, highlighting the importance of close monitoring. The response to terlipressin in patients with type 1 HRS is greater in patients with less severe baseline renal dysfunction, thus supporting the early initiation of therapy. These studies indicate that administration of terlipressin in combination with albumin can improve renal function in patients with HRS.[134]

BOX 94-3 Management of Hepatorenal Syndrome (HRS)

Measures to prevent variceal bleeding (e.g., beta blockers, band ligation)
Pentoxifylline for severe alcoholic hepatitis
Prevention of HRS
  Avoid intravascular volume depletion (diuretics, lactulose, GI bleeding, large-volume paracentesis without adequate volume repletion)
  Judicious management of nephrotoxins (ACEIs, ARBs, NSAIDs, antibiotics)
  Prompt diagnosis and treatment of infections (SBP, sepsis)
  SBP prophylaxis
Treatment of HRS
  Stop all nephrotoxic agents (ACEIs, ARBs, NSAIDs, diuretics)
  Antibiotics for infections
  IV albumin—bolus of 1 g/kg/day on presentation (maximum dose, 100 g daily). Continue at dose of 20-60 g daily as needed to maintain central venous pressure between 10 and 15 cm H_2O
  Vasopressor therapy (in addition to albumin):
    Terlipressin*—start at 1 mg IV every 4 hr and increase up to 2 mg IV every 4 hr if baseline serum creatinine level does not improve by 25% at day 3 of therapy
    OR
    Midodrine and octreotide—begin midodrine at 2.5-5 mg orally 3 times daily and increase to a maximum dose of 15 mg 3 times daily. Titrate to an MAP increase of at least 15 mm Hg; begin octreotide at 100 μg subcutaneously 3 times daily and increase to a maximum dose of 200 μg subcutaneously 3 times daily, or begin octreotide at a 25-μg IV bolus and continue at a rate of 25 μg/hr
    OR
    Norepinephrine—0.1-0.7 μg/kg/min as an IV infusion. Increase by 0.05 μg/kg/min every 4 hr and titrate to an MAP increase of at least 10 mm Hg
  Duration of vasopressor treatment is generally a maximum of 2 weeks until reversal of hepatorenal syndrome or liver transplantation
Evaluation of patient for liver transplantation

*Not available in the USA.
ACEIs, angiotensin-converting enzyme inhibitors; ARBs, angiotensin receptor blockers; MAP, mean arterial pressure.
Data from References 81, 86, 100, 108, 111, 113, 115, 116, and 121-148.

Midodrine, an orally administered α_1-adrenergic agonist, and octreotide, a somatostatin analog that inhibits endogenous vasodilators,[135,136] have been used in combination with albumin for type 1 HRS in 3 small nonrandomized studies. In 2 studies, treatment with midodrine, titrated to cause a rise in mean arterial blood pressure, was associated with improved serum creatinine levels and improved survival compared with no treatment and was associated with few major side effects.[137-139] This regimen has the advantage of ease of administration and appears to have a favorable safety profile; however, its efficacy has not been established in randomized controlled trials.

Norepinephrine, a widely available IV-administered α_1-adrenergic agonist, in combination with albumin, has been proposed as an alternative to terlipressin on the basis of 2 small pilot studies.[140,141] In one study of 22 patients with type 1 or 2 HRS, norepinephrine appeared to be as effective and safe as terlipressin. Two small randomized clinical trials demonstrated equal efficacy and safety profiles for norepinephrine, the combination of midodrine and octreotide, and terlipressin for the treatment of HRS. Response rates ranged from 40% to 75%, and relapse rates were 20%.[142,143] Significant cardiovascular side effects, however, have been reported with the use of norepinephrine to treat HRS, and whether the efficacy and safety of norepinephrine are similar to those of terlipressin has not been fully defined.

Radiologic and Surgical Therapy

Transjugular Intrahepatic Portosystemic Shunt

TIPS is effective for the treatment of diuretic-resistant ascites, a precursor to type 2 HRS (see Chapter 93).[144] Four pilot studies have evaluated the use of TIPS in nontransplant candidates with type 1 or 2 HRS.[145-148] In these studies, serum creatinine levels declined, sodium excretion increased, and neurohumoral responses improved after TIPS, although survival was not affected. The major benefit was seen in patients with type 2 HRS. The use of midodrine, octreotide, and albumin followed by TIPS appeared to be effective in a small cohort of patients with type 1 HRS. An important limitation of the use of TIPS for HRS is the potential to worsen hepatic function in patients with decompensated cirrhosis.

Liver Transplantation

Liver transplantation is the only therapeutic modality that has the potential to reverse both liver dysfunction and HRS and should be considered in any patient found to have HRS (see Chapter 97).[77,78,84,149] Rates of postoperative complications and in-hospital mortality are higher in patients transplanted with HRS than in those transplanted without HRS,[89,149] and up to 35% of patients with HRS require long-term renal replacement therapy.[78] Still, the 3-year survival rate of patients transplanted with HRS is approximately 60% compared with 70% to 80% for patients transplanted without HRS. The duration, degree, and type (HRS or acute tubular necrosis) of renal dysfunction preoperatively may be independent predictors of survival,[101] and patients who require hemodialysis carry a mortality risk that is 1.77 times higher than that of patients who do not need dialysis.[149-151] In one study, patients with HRS who responded to treatment with a vasopressin analog prior to liver transplantation had outcomes similar to those of patients without HRS who underwent liver transplantation,[116] a finding that supports the use of such therapy as a bridge to liver transplantation. Larger trials are needed to confirm this observation.

Other Therapies

Extracorporeal albumin dialysis with MARS is an experimental therapeutic modality that enhances the removal of water-soluble and albumin-binding toxins from the circulation (see Chapter 95).[152] The results of one small randomized trial have supported the use of MARS to improve serum creatinine levels and survival rates in patients with HRS, although larger studies are needed to confirm these findings.[153,154] Several other vasoconstrictive medical therapies, including dopamine and octreotide in combination with albumin, have not improved the outcome of HRS, and in one study use of a nonselective endothelin receptor antagonist to inhibit intrarenal vasoconstriction in HRS proved deleterious.[155]

HEPATOPULMONARY SYNDROME AND PORTOPULMONARY HYPERTENSION

Cirrhosis and portal hypertension are accompanied by vascular alterations in multiple organs. In the pulmonary circulation, 2 distinct clinical entities, the hepatopulmonary syndrome (HPS) and portopulmonary hypertension (POPH), have been recognized. HPS occurs when pulmonary microvascular alterations impair gas exchange and is found in 5% to 30% of patients evaluated for liver transplantation.[156-159] POPH occurs when vasoconstriction and remodeling in resistance vessels increase pulmonary arterial pressures and is found in as many as 5% of patients with cirrhosis. The mechanisms whereby these 2 entities develop are incompletely characterized, although they occur in similar clinical settings and may share pathogenic pathways. The presence of HPS or POPH increases mortality in affected patients. No effective medical therapies are available for HPS, although liver transplantation reverses the syndrome in most patients. Medical therapies that improve pulmonary hemodynamics in patients with POPH have become available, but the specific role of liver transplantation in POPH is not clearly defined.[160-167]

Pathophysiology

Hepatopulmonary Syndrome

HPS is characterized by microvascular alterations and dilatation in the precapillary and capillary pulmonary arterial circulation. In human HPS, the production of vasodilatory substances within the pulmonary vasculature, most notably NO, is increased. Although increased circulating and pulmonary NO levels appear to be features of human HPS, improvement in oxygenation in response to acute inhibition of NO is variable,[168-171] and in advanced cases HPS may take more than 1 year to resolve after liver transplantation.[164] These findings suggest that other vasoactive mediators as well as vascular remodeling and angiogenesis in the pulmonary microvasculature may contribute to human disease. The finding that single nucleotide polymorphisms in angiogenic-related genes are more prevalent in patients with HPS than in those without HPS[172] supports a role for angiogenesis.

In experimental HPS induced by bile duct ligation in the rat, pulmonary NO overproduction has also been observed and is triggered by a series of pathophysiologic events. Increased biliary production and release of endothelin-1,[173] in conjunction with shear stress–induced pulmonary microvascular endothelin-B receptor overexpression, drives NO production by endothelin-1–mediated endothelial NO synthase (eNOS).[174,175] In addition, adherence of macrophages in the pulmonary vasculature results in the activation of a number of vasoactive pathways, including inducible NO synthase (iNOS)-derived NO production, heme oxygenase-1–derived carbon monoxide production, and vascular endothelial growth factor (VEGF)-mediated angiogenesis.[176-180] Endothelin receptor antagonists and inhibition of NOS, bacterial translocation, TNF-α, and heme oxygenase improve experimental HPS.[178-182]

Monocyte adhesion is driven by endothelin-B receptor activation, fracktalkine receptor overexpression, and TNF-α in the pulmonary microvasculature.[181,183] Accordingly, inhibition of endothelin-B activation, VEGF signaling, the fracktalkine pathway, and TNF-α signaling decreases macrophage accumulation and improves HPS (Fig. 94-3).[181,183-192]

Portopulmonary Hypertension

The mechanisms whereby POPH develops are poorly understood. Histologically, POPH shares the characteristic features of other forms of pulmonary arterial hypertension (PAH): medial proliferation and hypertrophy, plexiform arteriopathy, and in situ vascular thrombosis.[193-195] The precise role of portal hypertension in this process is not clear, however, and whether POPH shares pathophysiologic mechanisms with PAH is unknown. Studies have found that POPH, like PAH, is more

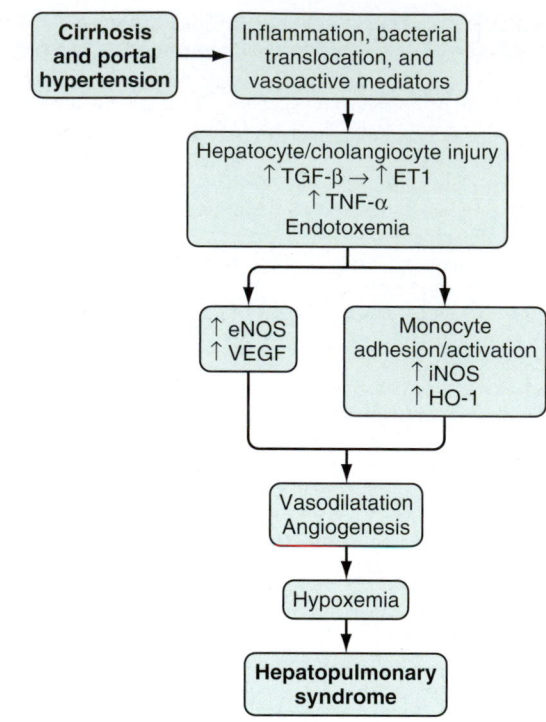

FIGURE 94-3. Proposed pathophysiology of hepatopulmonary syndrome. eNOS, endothelial nitric oxide synthase; ET1, endothelin-1; HO-1, heme oxygenase; iNOS, inducible nitric oxide synthase; TGF-β, transforming growth factor-β; VEGF, vascular endothelial growth factor.

common in women than men.[196] In addition, endothelin-1 and alteration in estrogen metabolism have been postulated to contribute to POPH.[197,198] By contrast, genetic polymorphisms in serotonin metabolism, which appear to increase vascular tone in a subset of patients with PAH, have not been found in patients with POPH.[199] Nevertheless, the observation that therapies used for PAH also appear to be effective for POPH supports the notion that downstream effector mechanisms are similar in the 2 disorders.

Clinical Features and Diagnosis

Hepatopulmonary Syndrome

HPS is defined as a widened age-corrected alveolar-arterial oxygen gradient (AaPO$_2$) on room air in the presence or absence of hypoxemia (normal AaPO$_2$ = 15 mm Hg, or 20 mm Hg in patients > 64 years) as a result of intrapulmonary vasodilation. A task force consensus statement has graded HPS on the basis of the degree of hypoxemia: mild (PaO$_2$ ≥ 80 mm Hg); moderate (PaO$_2$ > 60 to 80 mm Hg); severe (PaO$_2$ = 50 to 60 mm Hg), and very severe (PaO$_2$ < 50 mm Hg).[200] The frequency of HPS ranges from 5% to 35% in patients with cirrhosis who undergo evaluation for liver transplantation.[156,159,160,165] The presence of HPS significantly increases mortality in patients with cirrhosis. Moreover, survival of patients who undergo liver transplantation for HPS has been reported to be diminished compared with those without HPS, particularly when hypoxemia is severe.[201] More recent studies have found that survival of patients with HPS has improved after liver transplantation, even in those with severe disease.[202-204] This improvement may reflect advances in surgical techniques, the allocation of MELD exception points for advanced disease (see Chapter 97), and improved perioperative care.[164,205]

Patients with HPS present most commonly with respiratory complaints in the setting of chronic liver disease. Occasionally, HPS may be the initial manifestation of cirrhosis, and it also may be found in the setting of noncirrhotic and posthepatic portal hypertension, ischemic hepatitis, and chronic hepatitis in the absence of confirmed cirrhosis. A syndrome similar to HPS has been described in children with congenital abnormalities that divert hepatic blood from the pulmonary circulation.[206-208]

Classic clinical manifestations of HPS include platypnea (dyspnea worsened by an erect position and improved by a supine position) and orthodeoxia (exacerbation of hypoxia and hypoxemia in an upright position), both of which are relatively uncommon, and the insidious onset and slow progression of dyspnea, clubbing, and distal cyanosis.[156,160,209] Although clubbing and hypoxemia ($PaO_2 < 60$ mm Hg) in patients with liver disease in the absence of intrinsic cardiopulmonary disease are highly suggestive of HPS,[160] other clinical features are not reliable for detecting HPS. Many patients, particularly those with early HPS, are asymptomatic or have symptoms only on exertion. Cough has also been described as a presenting symptom of HPS.[210] In up to 70% of patients with HPS, marked hypoxemia occurs during sleep.[211] The severity of HPS appears to worsen over time, and marked nocturnal desaturation has been reported in patients with moderate wake-time hypoxemia.[211,212] In most studies, the presence or severity of HPS has not clearly correlated with the degree of hepatic dysfunction.[164,213]

The diagnosis of HPS requires a high degree of clinical suspicion, measurement of arterial blood gases, detection of intrapulmonary shunting, and exclusion of intrinsic cardiopulmonary disease as the cause of hypoxemia. The most sensitive test for the diagnosis of intrapulmonary shunting is contrast echocardiography,[214] which is performed by peripheral IV injection of agitated saline to produce microbubbles that are visualized during transthoracic echocardiography. Normally, microbubbles travel from the right ventricle to the lungs, where they are absorbed and do not reach the left ventricle. In patients with intracardiac shunting, microbubbles reach the left ventricle early (within 1 to 3 cardiac cycles after injection). In patients with intrapulmonary shunting, microbubbles reach the left ventricle in a delayed fashion (3 to 6 cardiac cycles after injection). Up to 60% of patients with cirrhosis have intrapulmonary vasodilatation on contrast echocardiography, but only a subset of patients have sufficient vasodilatation to cause abnormal arterial blood gas results and HPS.

In patients with pulmonary symptoms and hypoxemia who are found to have intrapulmonary shunting, intrinsic cardiopulmonary disease should be excluded. Chest radiography or CT and pulmonary function tests are generally performed in patients considered for liver transplantation. If potentially reversible cardiopulmonary disorders are detected, treatment is initiated, and the assessment of oxygenation is repeated. In the small subset of patients found to have severe hypoxemia ($PaO_2 < 60$ mm Hg) and both intrapulmonary shunting and significant cardiopulmonary disease, an abnormal technetium-labeled macroaggregated albumin scan that demonstrates a greater than 6% shunt fraction may confirm that HPS is contributing to the gas exchange abnormalities.[214-216]

Screening for HPS using pulse oximetry is a validated approach in patients being considered for liver transplantation. A value of less than 96% detects all patients with a PaO_2 below 70 mm Hg (sensitivity 100%, specificity 88%) (Fig. 94-4) and targets this subgroup of patients, who are likely to have moderate HPS, for further evaluation.[211,217] No practice guidelines for screening for HPS in liver transplantation candidates have been developed as of 2014.

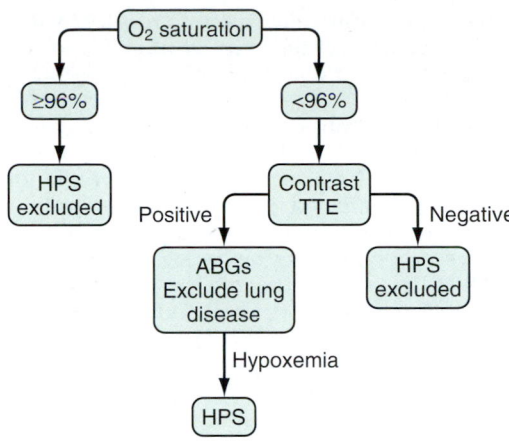

FIGURE 94-4. Approach to screening for hepatopulmonary syndrome (HPS) in potential candidates for liver transplantation. ABGs, arterial blood gases; TTE, transthoracic echocardiography.

Portopulmonary Hypertension

POPH is defined as the development of PAH in the setting of portal hypertension. The diagnostic criteria for POPH include the presence of PAH as defined by the WHO: mean arterial pulmonary pressure (mPAP) above 25 mm Hg at rest or 30 mm Hg with exercise; pulmonary capillary wedge pressure below 15 mm Hg; and pulmonary vascular resistance over 240 dynes • s • cm^{-5} occurring in the setting of pre-, intra-, and posthepatic portal hypertension (as evidenced by splenomegaly, thrombocytopenia, portosystemic shunts, or portal vein hemodynamic abnormalities).[157,218-220] POPH is generally graded according to the degree of elevation in mPAP, which correlates with the mortality risk associated with liver transplantation and influences decisions regarding therapy.[216] Mild POPH (mPAP = 25 to 35 mm Hg) is not associated with an increased operative risk for liver transplantation and may not require medical therapy. Moderate POPH (mPAP = 35 to 50 mm Hg) is associated with an increased operative risk for liver transplantation and is an indication for medical therapy. Severe POPH (mPAP > 50 mm Hg) is associated with a prohibitive operative mortality risk and is generally managed with medical therapy. POPH has been found in as many as 6% of cirrhotic patients who are evaluated for liver transplantation, and outcomes are worse for these patients than for cirrhotic patients without POPH.

The most common symptom associated with POPH is exertional dyspnea; other nonspecific symptoms such as orthopnea, fatigue, chest pressure, syncope, edema, and lightheadedness may also occur.[219] Characteristic physical examination features of PAH, including an elevated jugular venous pressure, loud second pulmonic heart sound, murmur of tricuspid regurgitation, and lower extremity edema, have been reported but are not sufficiently sensitive nor specific to be useful diagnostically. In cirrhotic patients, peripheral edema out of proportion to the degree of ascites should prompt consideration of right ventricular dysfunction secondary to pulmonary hypertension. In a number of studies, the majority of cirrhotic patients with significant POPH were asymptomatic.[162,221]

The diagnosis of POPH warrants a high degree of clinical suspicion, and all patients considered for liver transplantation as well as patients with suggestive symptoms or physical findings should be evaluated for POPH. Transthoracic echocardiography is the recommended screening test because it evaluates right-sided cardiac function and allows an estimation of right ventricular systolic pressure by evaluating the tricuspid regurgitant jet.[222] In addition, other causes of elevated right-sided cardiac pressures (e.g., secondary pulmonary hypertension, volume overload, a hyperdynamic circulation) should be considered and assessed. Methods for estimating right ventricular systolic pressure vary among centers, but in general, in the absence of significant pulmonary artery stenosis, an estimated right ventricular systolic pressure higher than 40 mm Hg or the presence of right ventricular abnormalities on echocardiography support further evaluation for POPH. The absence of both these findings essentially excludes POPH.[162] In all patients found to have echocardiographic features suggestive of POPH, pulmonary artery catheterization should be performed to establish the diagnosis and assess the severity of POPH. Findings on pulmonary artery catheterization are useful for distinguishing volume overload and a hyperdynamic circulation from POPH.

Treatment

Hepatopulmonary Syndrome

Treatment options for HPS are limited. No medical therapies have proved effective, although case reports and small case series have suggested that some treatments may improve oxygenation. Therefore, patients with well-preserved hepatic synthetic function who have hypoxemia are generally treated symptomatically until oxygenation worsens sufficiently to permit listing for liver transplantation based on an exception to the MELD score (see Chapter 97). Liver transplantation reverses HPS in most affected patients, although mortality after liver transplantation appears to be higher in patients with HPS than in those without HPS.[201,203,223,224]

Medical Therapy

A number of agents have been used empirically in patients with HPS or on the basis of data from experimental models.[168,216,225-227] Two small uncontrolled clinical studies and one randomized controlled trial have reported that garlic preparations improve oxygenation in patients with HPS.[225] Two small case series using pentoxifylline as a treatment for HPS have found conflicting results.[191,228] Oxygen supplementation is generally used in patients with HPS and resting or exercised-induced hypoxemia ($Pao_2 < 60$ mm Hg), although studies documenting a clinical benefit have not been performed.

Interventional Radiologic Therapy

Two radiologic techniques—TIPS[229] to lower portal pressure, and pulmonary angiography with embolization to occlude areas of intrapulmonary shunting[216]—have been described in case reports and small case series to improve HPS. These approaches are invasive and are not established to be effective. Therefore, the use of TIPS and angiography with embolization specifically to treat HPS is not generally recommended.[229,230] Pulmonary angiography has been considered in patients with severe hypoxemia to identify focal arteriovenous shunting that may be diminished with embolization. Little evidence to support such an approach is available, however, and arteriovenous shunting sufficient to cause hypoxemia and amenable to embolization may be detected instead by high-resolution CT.[216]

Liver Transplantation

Liver transplantation reverses HPS in as many as 80% of affected patients.[168] Hypoxemia may persist after transplantation, however, particularly when the hypoxemia is severe before transplantation, and may require more than 1 year to

resolve. Mortality also appears to be higher in patients with HPS who undergo liver transplantation than in patients transplanted without HPS, although this is not a consistent observation.[202-204] The increase in postoperative mortality is related in part to the severity of HPS, with 1 prospective study demonstrating that patients with profound hypoxemia ($Pao_2 < 50$ mm Hg) and marked intrapulmonary shunting (shunt fraction > 20%) had a significant increase in mortality.[164,165,201,223] In addition, unique complications such as transient worsening of hypoxemia following liver transplantation, the development of pulmonary hypertension, and embolic cerebrovascular events have been observed and may contribute to adverse postoperative outcomes. On the basis of the relationship between the severity of hypoxemia and poor outcomes in nontransplanted patients with HPS, MELD exception should be considered in patients with HPS and a resting Pao_2 less than 60 mm Hg, to increase their priority for transplantation.[203,223,224]

Portopulmonary Hypertension

Treatment of POPH has changed substantially since the early 2000s because of the availability of oral vasodilators to treat PAH. In general, liver transplantation is contraindicated in patients with moderate to severe POPH because of increased perioperative mortality resulting from poor right-sided cardiac function. The ability to lower pulmonary arterial pressures and decrease pulmonary vascular resistance with medications may decrease perioperative complications and allow liver transplantation to be performed in patients with POPH.

Medical Therapy

The therapy of POPH is largely empirical because there have been no randomized controlled trials evaluating therapy. In general, diuretics are used for volume overload, supplemental oxygen is provided if hypoxemia is present, and anticoagulation may be appropriate in the subset of patients with POPH who do not have hepatic decompensation, marked coagulopathy, or gastroesophageal varices. In one study, withdrawal of β-adrenergic blocker therapy improved right-sided cardiac function in patients with POPH, and some clinicians advocate treating varices with band ligation if feasible and withdrawing medical therapy for varices in patients with POPH.[231]

Case reports and series have shown benefit with prostacyclin analogs. Epoprostenol requires complicated IV administration, but newer agents (iloprost, treprostinil) are easier to administer.[167,221,232,233]

Oral endothelin receptor antagonists, including bosentan (a mixed endothelin-A and -B receptor antagonist)[234-236] and ambrisentan (an endothelin-A blocker),[237] have also been used in POPH. Bosentan may cause hepatotoxicity, which may be mediated by inhibitory effects on the canalicular bile salt export protein (see Chapter 64). Close monitoring of liver biochemical test levels and use of bosentan only in patients with well-compensated liver disease is advisable. Use of ambrisentan for POPH is increasing, although few data about its efficacy are available.[237]

Oral phsophodiesterase-5 inhibitors, including sildenafil, generally have been well tolerated in patients with POPH, although the magnitude of improvement in pulmonary arterial pressures has been modest. Long-acting phosphodiesterase-5 inhibitors (tadalafil and vardenafil) are under study.[238-242]

Liver Transplantation

Traditionally, moderate to severe POPH has been a contraindication to liver transplantation, particularly when the mPAP is higher than 40 to 50 mm Hg.[205] With the availability of oral agents to lower pulmonary pressures, consideration has been given to improving pulmonary hemodynamics with medical therapy followed by liver transplantation to attempt to reverse POPH.[243] Three case series have described such an approach.[232,244,245] Although results have varied among centers, POPH appears to have resolved in some patients after liver transplantation. A MELD exception can be considered in those patients with POPH who respond to medical therapy with an end mPAP below 35 mm Hg and PVR less than 400 dynes • s • cm⁻⁵.[243] Whether liver transplantation is an effective treatment for patients with POPH who respond to medical therapy and in which specific patient subgroups does POPH resolve completely remain to be clarified.

CIRRHOTIC CARDIOMYOPATHY

Systemic hemodynamic changes have been recognized in cirrhotic patients since the early 1900s. In the 1950s, a hyperdynamic circulation (decreased arterial blood pressure, decreased peripheral resistance, and increased cardiac output) was observed in patients with alcoholic liver disease and attributed to the effects of alcohol.[246] Subsequent studies documented vascular hyporesponsiveness to vasoconstrictors in patients with alcoholic liver disease, a finding also attributed to effects of alcohol on the heart and termed *alcoholic cardiomyopathy*.[247] More recently, specific vascular and cardiac abnormalities have been found in human and animal models of cirrhosis, independent of alcohol ingestion, and have led to the concept that cirrhosis itself triggers cardiac dysfunction, a disorder termed *cirrhotic cardiomyopathy* (CCM).[248]

Pathophysiology

Although diagnostic criteria for CCM have not been established, a consensus group during the 2005 Montreal World Congress of Gastroenterology proposed diagnostic and supportive criteria based on the 3 major pathophysiologic features observed: (1) structural and functional ventricular abnormalities; (2) an abnormal ventricular response in the presence of pharmacologic, physiologic, or surgical stress; and (3) cardiac electrophysiologic abnormalities (Fig. 94-5).[97,98,248-250]

The major structural and functional ventricular abnormalities found in histologic and echocardiographic studies are left ventricular hypertrophy and systolic and diastolic dysfunction.[98,251-254] The structural changes have been attributed to a hypertrophic response to the hyperdynamic circulation. Diastolic alterations are characterized by increased myocardial stiffness associated with myocardial hypertrophy, fibrosis, and subendothelial edema[255,256] and may precipitate and worsen ascites.[257-260] In addition, impaired systolic function and histologic injury to cardiomyocytes have been observed.[261] Whether the severity of hepatic synthetic dysfunction correlates with the degree of cardiac dysfunction is not clear.[262] The impaired ventricular response to stress and exercise observed in human and animal models of cirrhosis[98,248,251,253] has been attributed to impaired β-adrenergic signaling pathways that lead to subnormal chronotropic and contractile responses,[263-265] as well as to cardiomyocyte dysfunction resulting from overproduction of NO, carbon monoxide, and endocannabinoids.[266-271] Electrophysiologic abnormalities, most notably prolongation of the corrected QT interval (QTc), have also been observed in patients with CCM.[272,273] The degree of prolongation of the QTc appears to correlate with the severity of liver disease and may contribute to the dissociation between electrical and mechanical events in the heart and to cardiac dysfunction.[274] These abnormalities appear to improve after liver transplantation.

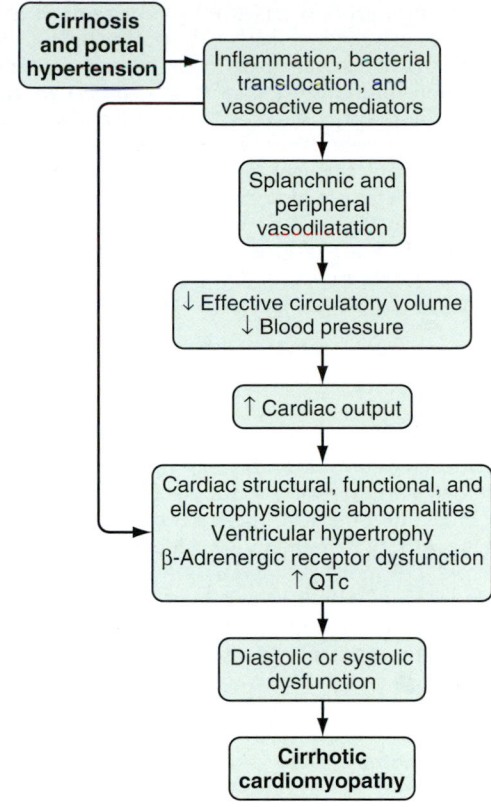

FIGURE 94-5. Proposed pathophysiology of cirrhotic cardiomyopathy. QTc, rate-corrected QT interval.

Clinical Features and Diagnosis

Because CCM typically becomes clinically detectable under circumstances of stress, the diagnosis is difficult to make and the process may not be recognized. Overt cardiac dysfunction may occur after common clinical interventions in cirrhosis. For example, a prospective multicenter analysis has shown that more than 10% of patients who undergo TIPS placement for refractory ascites exhibit signs of heart failure when compared with patients treated by repeated large-volume paracentesis.[275] Subsequent studies have revealed that both the severity of liver disease (as measured by the MELD score) and diastolic dysfunction 28 days after the procedure are independent predictors of death in patients with cirrhosis who are treated with a TIPS.[276-278] Similarly, in a case series of patients who underwent liver transplantation, 47% were found to have radiologic evidence of pulmonary edema within the first 24 hours after transplantation. Volume replacement was considered unlikely to be the sole culprit, suggesting that cardiac dysfunction may have played a role.[279,280] Diastolic dysfunction has shown a trend to worsen survival in cirrhotic patients, but multivariate analysis has revealed that age and degree of liver dysfunction are the main predictors of mortality.[260] Finally, in prospective studies, a lower cardiac output has been found in patients in whom HRS developed than in those in whom HRS did not, thereby supporting the role of cardiac dysfunction in HRS.[95,96]

No precise diagnostic criteria for CCM have been established because no baseline clinical, imaging, or biochemical findings have been found to definitively predict the development of overt cardiac dysfunction under stress.[281-285] The presence of QTc prolongation and echocardiographic evidence of diastolic dysfunction are readily detected but do not appear to correlate with the risk of development of cardiac dysfunction under stress. Serum levels of markers of cardiac dysfunction—brain natriuretic peptide, atrial natriuretic peptide, and troponin I—are elevated in patients with cirrhosis and appear to correlate with QTc prolongation, diastolic dysfunction, and the severity of liver disease. Evaluation of cardiac function under stress conditions with echocardiography or ventriculography has been reported, and cardiac function may be impaired but does not correlate clearly with subsequent clinical cardiac dysfunction. Further work is needed to define the role of serum markers and stress testing in the diagnosis of CCM.[284,285] In cirrhotic patients found to have evidence of heart failure, alternative causes of cardiac dysfunction, including coronary artery disease, valvular abnormalities, and other causes of cardiomyopathy, should be excluded.

Treatment

Therapy of volume overload in patients suspected of having CCM includes standard supportive measures and diuresis.[286] Use of preload and afterload reducing agents should be considered with caution because these agents may worsen hypotension in the setting of underlying systemic vasodilatation.[42,248] Inotropic and chronotropic agents do not appear to be of benefit.[97] In patients without overt heart failure but with electrocardiographic or echocardiographic features consistent with CCM, chronic use of aldosterone antagonists has been shown to improve echocardiographic features marginally,[286,287] and short-term administration of a noncardioselective β-adrenergic antagonist has been shown to improve QTc prolongation.[288] Whether these agents prevent or ameliorate cardiac dysfunction in response to stress is unknown.

The effects of liver transplantation on cardiac abnormalities in patients with cirrhosis have not been fully characterized. A small study has demonstrated that resting echocardiographic and stress radionuclide ventriculographic abnormalities found in patients with cirrhosis were improved or reversed after liver transplantation.[257,289] Further data are needed to determine whether CCM reverses after liver transplantation.

ENDOCRINE DYSFUNCTION

Cirrhosis has been linked to abnormalities in the endocrine system, including adrenal insufficiency, abnormal sex hormone metabolism, thyroid disease, and osteoporosis.

Adrenal Insufficiency

The recognition that adrenal insufficiency worsens outcomes in sepsis, a syndrome characterized by physiologic abnormalities seen in liver failure, has led to evaluation of adrenal dysfunction in patients with liver disease. Multiple studies have demonstrated the presence of relative adrenal insufficiency in critically ill patients with both compensated and decompensated cirrhosis, with reported frequencies of 10% to 92%.[78,290-296] The wide range in prevalence is a reflection of the absence of a standardized test to diagnose the entity in the cirrhotic population.[297] The presence of relative adrenal insufficiency has been associated with greater hemodynamic instability and increased mortality.[292,298] In 2 studies,[293,294] glucocorticoid therapy improved survival, but in 2 others[291,299] such therapy was associated with increased mortality secondary to GI bleeding and nosocomial and opportunistic infections. Two proposed pathophysiologic mechanisms for relative adrenal insufficiency include (1) impaired adrenal cortisol synthesis from cholesterol during stress, secondary to inadequate hepatic cholesterol production as a result of liver disease, and (2) increased circulating levels of endotoxins and proinflammatory cytokines.[300-302] No standardized diagnostic criteria have been developed to define relative adrenal insufficiency, and whether a subset of critically ill patients with liver disease may benefit from glucocorticoid treatment remains an area of active investigation.

Gonadal Dysfunction

Historical data have suggested a high frequency (70% to 80%) of central and peripheral hypogonadism in cirrhotic patients. Hypogonadism in this setting is associated with a decreased concentration of free or bioavailable testosterone in direct proportion to the degree of liver dysfunction.[303,304] Sex hormone–binding globulin (SHBG), which binds testosterone and 17β-estradiol in serum, has a lower affinity for estrogens than testosterone. In patients with cirrhosis, elevated concentrations of SHBG (with a resulting shift in the balance of hormones in favor of estrogens) and a decreased production of dehydroepiandrosterone sulfate (a precursor of androgenic hormones) may account for the "feminization syndrome" seen in male patients with cirrhosis.[304-306] Acute and chronic alcohol consumption is responsible for direct toxic effects on Leydig cells and for alterations of the hypothalamic-pituitary-gonadal axis. These alterations include a decrease in the serum concentration of luteinizing hormone and decreased responsiveness to gonadotropin-releasing hormone.[307,308] Spironolactone, which is frequently used to treat fluid overload, causes painful gynecomastia by displacing androgen from its receptor and binding protein and by increasing estradiol production and testosterone clearance.[309] Topical testosterone appears to improve muscle strength and survival in patients with chronic allograft failure after liver transplantation, but whether testosterone supplementation improves the symptoms and signs related to hypogonadism in pretransplantation cirrhotic patients is unknown.[310]

Thyroid Dysfunction

A number of thyroid abnormalities, including increased thyroid volume and decreased serum levels of free triiodothyronine, have been found in patients with cirrhosis. These alterations appear to correlate with the severity of liver disease, and the presence of thyroid disease may be a predictor of decreased survival.[311-314] In patients with hepatitis C or autoimmune liver disease, the incidence of hypothyroidism and autoimmune thyroid disease is increased.[315-317] The detection of HCV in thyroid cells raises the possibility of direct viral cytotoxicity.[318] Interferon-based treatment of viral hepatitis may cause thyroiditis and has been implicated in both hyper- and hypothyroidism in 10% to 15% of treated patients.[319] Whether routine screening for thyroid disease influences survival or quality of life is unknown.

Bone Disease

The frequency of osteoporosis among patients with all causes of chronic liver disease ranges from 12% to 55%.[320] Potential risk factors include cholestasis, a maternal history of hip fracture, progression of liver disease, alcohol consumption, lower BMI, oral glucocorticoid use for more than 3 months, and older patient age. Women with PBC have a 4-fold higher risk of developing osteoporosis and a 2-fold higher risk of bone fractures than age-matched controls (see Chapter 91).[321] Treatment with ursodeoxycholic acid does not influence bone density in patients with PBC,[322] but avoidance of glucocorticoids and improved nutrition appear to decrease the frequency of osteoporosis.[323] Bone mineral density is an appropriate screening tool for osteoporosis in patients with cirrhosis (especially PBC and PSC) and those who require more than 3 months of glucocorticoid therapy.[323-325] Treatment of osteoporosis in patients with chronic liver disease is based on studies of postmenopausal women and is an area of ongoing investigation. The use of calcium and vitamin D and of therapeutic bisphosphonates improves bone mineral density and appears not to have significant side effects.[325,326]

COAGULATION DISORDERS

Cirrhosis is commonly considered to be associated with a bleeding diathesis due to the frequent prolongation of the prothrombin time and thrombocytopenia. The interplay among abnormalities in both pro- and anticoagulant factors, however, may result not only in increased bleeding but also hypercoagulability.[327,328] The precise mechanisms for these clinical events are not fully characterized.[329]

Prolongation of the Prothrombin Time

The progressive loss of hepatocytes in cirrhosis leads to decreased synthesis of procoagulant factors, including vitamin K–dependent factors (II, VII, IX, X), factor V, and factor XI. The severity of clotting abnormalities, measured by the prothrombin time (PT), activated partial thromboplastin time (aPTT), and INR increases as liver disease progresses.[330] A prolonged PT alone is not generally considered to be a major risk factor for spontaneous bleeding in patients with cirrhosis but does increase the severity of bleeding when it occurs.[331] Common practice is to administer fresh frozen plasma (FFP), vitamin K, and occasionally recombinant factor VIIa to correct coagulopathy in patients with chronic liver disease, particularly in the setting of bleeding or prior to invasive procedures.[332] Clinical evidence that any of these measures reduces the severity of variceal bleeding, for example, is not strong.[333-335] Moreover, the volume of FFP (>6 units) required to achieve clinically significant reductions in the PT in cirrhosis has been associated with a significant increase in the risk of acute lung injury and volume overload.[336,337] Recombinant factor VIIa administration can normalize the PT, and one small uncontrolled study found that following its use, no patients required blood transfusions after liver biopsy.[338] Nevertheless, no placebo-controlled trial of recombinant factor VIIa in cirrhotic patients undergoing invasive procedures has been performed.

INR is also a key component of the MELD score used to predict survival and rank priority for liver transplantation in patients with liver disease (see Chapter 97).[339] One concern regarding the use of the INR in cirrhosis is the substantial inter-laboratory variability that occurs when using the standard international sensitivity index (ISI) to normalize varying sensitivities of thromboplastin reagents (see Chapter 73).[340] The difference in mean INR for a single patient sample assayed with different reagents may be as much as 25%. Adjusting the ISI calibration by using samples from patients with cirrhosis appears to eliminate this variation but is time-consuming and not widely used.[341] Therefore, INR has limitations both as a predictor of bleeding and as a factor in calculating the MELD score for prioritization of organ allocation.

Thrombocytopenia

Thrombocytopenia is a common feature in cirrhosis with portal hypertension and is generally associated with the presence of hypersplenism. Decreased hepatic thrombopoietin synthesis and direct bone marrow toxicity (e.g., from alcohol or HCV) may also lower the platelet count.[342] In addition to quantitative abnormalities, platelet thrombin generation appears to be impaired in cirrhosis, particularly at platelet counts below 50,000/mL, and may contribute to impaired clot formation.[343] On the other hand, cirrhotic patients have higher levels of von Willebrand factor (vWf) and lower levels of vWf-cleaving protease (VWFCP), which may promote platelet adhesion to the endothelium at the site of vascular injury.[344,345] Although platelet function, as assessed by measuring the bleeding time, is commonly impaired in patients with cirrhosis, neither prolongation of the bleeding time nor its correction with desmopressin administration influence the risk of bleeding.[346,347] As a general concept, thrombocytopenia itself does not appear to increase the risk of bleeding in patients with cirrhosis, and whether the administration of platelets influences bleeding risk in patients who undergo invasive procedures or decreases transfusion requirements in patients with variceal hemorrhage is uncertain. Nevertheless, common clinical practice is to administer platelet transfusions to achieve a platelet count of approximately 50,000/mm^3 prior to an invasive procedure and in the setting of active bleeding.[336,337]

Dysfibrinogenemia

Dysfibrinogenemia manifested either by hyper- or hypofibrinolysis is common in patients with cirrhosis. Hyperfibrinolysis reflected by elevated circulating levels of D-dimer and fibrinogen degradation products, and by prolongation of the clot lysis time, is seen in up to 46% of cirrhotic patients.[348,349] These abnormalities result from altered production of activators and inhibitors of fibrinolysis, activation of the coagulation cascade by endotoxemia, and decreased clearance of fibrinolytic proteins in the setting of hepatic synthetic dysfunction. One hypothesis is that hyperfibrinolysis becomes more severe as liver disease progresses and eventually results in overt DIC, further increasing the risk of bleeding. Chronic liver disease, however, has also been associated with hypofibrinolysis, including reduced levels of plasminogen and increased levels of plasminogen activator inhibitor.[350-352] Moreover, results of tests for individual pro- and antifibrinolytic factors are variable, and their measurement in patients with chronic liver disease has not been standardized or uniformly accepted. These findings highlight the complexity and uncertainty of assessing the clinical consequences of dysfibrinogenemia in patients with cirrhosis.[350] Antihyperfibrinolytic therapy with compounds such as ε-aminocaproic acid has been used to prevent blood loss in stable cirrhotic patients and during liver transplantation, but evidence to support the benefits of such an approach is limited.[353,354]

Endogenous Anticoagulants

In addition to decreasing production of procoagulant proteins, hepatic synthetic dysfunction in cirrhosis also impairs the production of endogenous anticoagulant proteins, including protein C, protein S, antithrombin, tissue plasminogen activator, and thrombomodulin.[355] These abnormalities may result in hypercoagulability and a risk of thrombosis. The risk of portal vein thrombosis, deep venous thrombosis, and pulmonary embolism has been reported to be increased in patients with chronic liver disease compared with non–liver disease controls.[356-358] A subset of these patients appear to have an underlying inherited or acquired cause of hypercoagulability, including factor V Leiden and prothrombin 20210A gene mutations, decreased protein C or S levels, and increased D-dimer levels that contribute to thrombosis.[359-362]

Anticoagulation has appeared to be safe and beneficial for patients with noncirrhotic portal vein thrombosis associated with gastroesophageal varices. Anticoagulation has also been reported to prevent portal vein thrombosis and hepatic decompensation in patients with cirrhosis. A small unblinded study showed that that patients with decompensated cirrhosis who received enoxaparin, 4000 IU/mL for 12 months, as prophylaxis against portal vein thrombosis had better clinical outcomes compared with patients who did not receive prophylaxis. This study highlights not only the impact of portal vein thrombosis on the natural history of cirrhosis, but also the paradox that treating the procoagulant state in patients with end-stage liver disease improves liver-related outcomes.[363] The role of anticoagulation therapy in the treatment and prevention of cirrhotic portal vein thrombosis and the question of whether hypercoagulability influences specific complications of cirrhosis remain unclear (see Chapter 85).[364,365]

Thromboelastography

Thromboelastography is a simple point-of-care test that assesses multiple components of hemostasis, including the cellular and plasmatic components of clot formation, strength, and stability. Studies using thromboelastography suggest that despite the thrombocytopenia and evidence of prolonged coagulation on standard laboratory-based assays, many patients with liver disease actually have a balanced homeostatic milieu in which coagulation may be normal or even enhanced.[366] Thromboelastography may also be useful as predictive test for establishing and determining the risk of rebleeding from esophageal varices.[367] The applicability and use of thromboelastography in daily clinical practice in patients with cirrhosis are yet to be established.

KEY REFERENCES

Full references for this chapter can be found on www.expertconsult.com.

22. Romero-Gómez M, Jover Ma, Del Campo JA, et al. Variations in the promoter region of the glutaminase gene and the development of hepatic encephalopathy in patients with cirrhosis: A cohort study. Ann Intern Med 2010; 153:281-8.
23. Bajaj JS, Hylemon PB, Ridlon JM, et al. Colonic mucosal microbiome differs from stool microbiome in cirrhosis and hepatic encephalopathy and is linked to cognition and inflammation. Am J Physiol Gastrointest Liver Physiol 2012; 303:G675-G685.
29. Bajaj JS, Cordoba J, Mullen KD, et al. Review article: The design of clinical trials in hepatic encephalopathy—An International Society for Hepatic Encephalopathy and Nitrogen Metabolism (ISHEN) consensus statement. Aliment Pharmacol Ther 2011; 33:739-47.
44. Bajaj JS, Thacker LR, Heuman DM, et al. The Stroop smartphone application is a short and valid method to screen for minimal hepatic encephalopathy. Hepatology 2013; 58:1122-32.
53. Bass NM, Mullen KD, Sanyal A, et al. Rifaximin treatment in hepatic encephalopathy. N Engl J Med 2010; 362:1071-81.
83. Martín–Llahí M, Guevara M, Torre A, et al. Prognostic importance of the cause of renal failure in patients with cirrhosis. Gastroenterology 2011; 140:488-96.
86. Salerno F, Gerbes A, Ginès P, et al. Diagnosis, prevention and treatment of hepatorenal syndrome in cirrhosis. Gut 2007; 56:1310-18.
97. Alqahtani S, Fouad T, Lee S. Cirrhotic cardiomyopathy. Semin Liver Dis 2008; 28:59-69.
101. Nadim MK, Genyk YS, Tokin C, et al. Impact of the etiology of acute kidney injury on outcomes following liver transplantation: Acute tubular necrosis versus hepatorenal syndrome. Liver Transpl 2012; 18:539-48.
103. Nadim MK, Kellum JA, Davenport A, et al. Hepatorenal syndrome: The 8th International Consensus Conference of the Acute Dialysis Quality Initiative (ADQI) Group. Crit Care 2012; 16:R23.
117. Velez JCQ, Nietert PJ. Therapeutic response to vasoconstrictors in hepatorenal syndrome parallels increase in mean arterial pressure: A pooled analysis of clinical trials. Am J Kidney Dis 2011; 58:928-38.
134. Gluud L, Christensen K, Christensen E, et al. Terlipressin for hepatorenal syndrome. Cochrane Database Syst Rev 2012; (9):CD005162.
164. Swanson K, Wiesner R, Krowka M. Natural history of hepatopulmonary syndrome: Impact of liver transplantation. Hepatology 2005; 41:1122-9.
216. Rodríguez-Roisin R, Krowka M. Hepatopulmonary syndrome—A liver-induced vascular disorder. N Engl J Med 2008; 358:2378-87.
366. Stravitz R. Potential applications of thromboelastography in patients with acute and chronic liver disease. Gastroenterol Hepatol 2012; 8:513-20.

Acute liver failure (ALF) is characterized by a sudden insult to the liver with catastrophic consequences, usually in the absence of preexisting liver disease. Coagulopathy and encephalopathy are the twin cardinal features that reflect the severity of liver injury, and both are required to make the clinical diagnosis of ALF, although significant coagulopathy in the absence of definite encephalopathy has been described as acute liver injury.[1] A number of subtypes reflect variability in clinical manifestations and prognosis.[2,3] The etiology may be drug-induced, viral, immunologic, ischemic, toxic, or unknown. The vast majority of patients have no evidence of preexisting liver disease, but 2 exceptions to this requirement have been made: (1) an acute presentation of Wilson disease in a young adult that presents in the setting of previously asymptomatic cirrhosis and (2) reactivation of HBV infection, either spontaneously or as a consequence of immunosuppression or chemotherapy.

ALF is a rare condition with an estimated 3000 cases per year in the United States. The risk is also low for each of the recognized causes. The risk in patients with hepatitis A or B is less than 1% and in those with an acetaminophen overdose, 0.2%. ALF is 1 of the most dramatic medical emergencies because it can lead to multiorgan failure within days or weeks, with almost no body system left unaffected. Cerebral edema has historically been 1 of the main determinants of outcome,[4] although data have demonstrated an unexplained but dramatic reduction in the frequency of cerebral edema. The acuity and severity of ALF requires a rapid multidisciplinary approach to management that has resulted in an overall survival rate of over 60%. Early recognition, improved intensive care protocols, and emergency liver transplantation (LT) have all contributed significantly to the improved outcomes, but so far, liver support devices have not proved beneficial.

DEFINITION

ALF is an umbrella term that has replaced prior descriptions, including fulminant hepatic failure, subfulminant hepatitis, and late-onset hepatic failure. The presence of clinical encephalopathy in the appropriate setting remains the essential requirement for the diagnosis of ALF. The definitions used have included a time limit between the onset of either symptoms or jaundice and the development of encephalopathy ranging from 8 weeks to 6 months. One categorization based on clinical patterns and outcome described 3 groups based on the time interval between the onset of jaundice and encephalopathy: hyperacute liver failure (7 days or less), ALF (8 to 28 days), and subacute liver failure (4 to 24 weeks).[2] Patients with hyperacute liver failure were more likely to develop cerebral edema and to recover without LT. At the other end of the spectrum, patients with subacute liver failure had less severe coagulopathy and a much lower propensity to cerebral edema but had poor outcomes. The utility of this categorization has been maintained despite the observed changes in the incidence of cerebral edema and improved outcomes independent of the use of LT. In the United States, the original definition of ALF (encephalopathy and coagulopathy within 8 weeks of the illness onset) is still widely used, especially in criteria for LT selection.[5]

In the 2000s, an entity entitled *acute-on-chronic liver failure* has gained widespread use but without consensus on the definition. A purist's definition is liver failure triggered by a type of insult that causes ALF but in a patient with preexisting liver disease. A broader definition attributes the deterioration to a range insults, including some associated with cirrhosis (e.g., variceal bleeding, sepsis).

TABLE 95-1 Etiology of Acute Liver Failure in Various Countries*

Cause	United Kingdom	United States	France	India	Japan	Spain
Acetaminophen	54	46	2	—	—	2
Drug reaction	7	12	15	5	—	17
Seronegative hepatitis	17	14	18	24	45	32
HAV or HBV	14	10	49	33	55	37
HEV	—	—	—	38	—	—
Other causes	8	18	16	—	—	12

*Percent of total cases in each country.

ETIOLOGY AND EPIDEMIOLOGY

The pattern of causation of ALF shows significant geographical variation, and in some areas the underlying etiologies have changed since the 1980s.[6,7] A consistent finding is a sizeable cohort of patients for whom no specific cause for ALF can be defined despite an exhaustive search (Table 95-1). This entity has been designated variably as seronegative hepatitis, non–A-E hepatitis, and hepatitis of indeterminate etiology. In some geographical areas, this group represent the single largest cohort of patients (up to 32% of cases). Middle-aged women and a subacute pattern of disease are overrepresented in this group. In the United States, a proportion of these cases were considered to be related to acetaminophen based on the detection of acetaminophen adducts, but this finding has not been reproduced elsewhere.[8] Unidentified toxins or autoimmune processes are other hypothetical underlying mechanisms.

The main identified viruses that cause ALF are hepatitis A, B, D, and E viruses. The risk of developing ALF following these infections has been estimated to be 0.1% to 4% of hospitalized cases.[9] The incidence of HAV- and HBV-related ALF has decreased, presumably as a consequence of vaccination programs and a range of effective antiviral drugs for HBV. The proportion of patients with hepatitis A or B among nonacetaminophen causes of ALF in the King's College Hospital series fell from 56% from 1973 to 1978 to only 17% from 2004 to 2008.[1] There is some evidence, however, of an increase in ALF in HBV carriers and reactivation of viral replication following chemotherapy or use of immunosuppression (see Chapter 79). Hepatitis E is common in parts of Asia and Africa and is being recognized increasingly in Western countries, where there is an observed association with porcine transmission (see Chapter 82). The risk of developing ALF after exposure to HCV appears to be very low, although well-documented cases have been reported.

Three patterns of ALF are associated with drugs: dose-related, idiosyncratic, and hypersensitivity reactions. The best example of a drug that causes dose-related toxicity is acetaminophen (or paracetamol, as it is widely known outside the United States), for which the amount ingested is among the determinants of risk for ALF. Idiosyncratic reactions are often referred to as *drug-induced liver injury* (DILI). In one prospective study of 300 cases of DILI, more than 100 different agents were implicated; 46% were antimicrobials and 15% were central nervous system agents. The mortality rate was 3% to 4% (see Chapter 88).[10] Halothane hepatitis, commonly encountered in the 1970s and 1980s and now mainly of historical interest, is an example of a hypersensitivity reaction; the risk

is negligible on first exposure but rises with subsequent administrations (see Chapter 89).

Drugs

Acetaminophen

Acetaminophen is a partially dose-dependent hepatotoxin with mortality highest at doses exceeding 48 g. Increased susceptibility to acetaminophen toxicity is recognized in people with liver enzyme induction as a consequence of antiepileptic therapy, regular alcohol consumption, and malnutrition. Acetaminophen is also a direct toxin to other organs, particularly the kidney and possibly heart and pancreas. N-acetylcysteine is the substrate for glutathione repletion and is an effective antidote to acetaminophen if administration is commenced within 16 hours of the ingestion of acetaminophen, when concentrations are above a time-dependent determinant of risk of liver injury. N-acetylcysteine is also beneficial in reducing the severity of liver injury with later administration (see Chapter 88).

Acetaminophen overdose is the most common cause of ALF in the United Kingdom and the United States.[6,11] In the United Kingdom, it is usually taken with suicidal or parasuicidal intent, and only 8% of cases in an early series were ascribed to therapeutic use.[12] In the United States, however, at least 48% of cases are considered to be secondary to unintentional overdosing.[13] Unintentional overdosing ("therapeutic misadventure") typically occurs over a period of days, whereas intentional overdoses can be a discrete episode or staggered over a period of time. In 1998, legislation was enacted in the United Kingdom to restrict over-the-counter access to acetaminophen, and this resulted in a nearly 50% reduction in cases of acute liver injury or failure in the King's College Hospital series.[1] In the United States, black box warnings on acetaminophen products and package labeling have been instituted.

Idiosyncratic Reactions

In the majority of cases, the diagnosis of DILI is made when there is a temporal relationship between exposure to the candidate drug and the development of ALF. About 10% of patients demonstrate features of hypersensitivity or drug reaction with eosinophilia and systemic symptoms (DRESS). In the King's College Hospital series of over 3300 patients with ALF, 190 were related to drugs other than acetaminophen; the most frequently encountered agents are listed in Table 95-2.[1] Halothane and the nonprescription drug methylenedioxy-N-methylamphetamine (MDMA, "ecstasy") were the 2 most

TABLE 95-2 Drugs or Drug Classes Associated with Acute Liver Failure at the King's College Hospital*		
	1973-1993 (*N* = 85)	1994-2008 (*N* = 105)
Halothane	53	2
Antituberculosis drugs	11	22
Anticonvulsants	4	12
Antibiotics	3	7
Antineoplastic agents	1	5
Antiretroviral drugs	0	4
MDMA (ecstasy)	0	17
NSAIDs	0	4
Combinations of drugs	2	6
Miscellaneous agents	11	26

*Number of cases for each drug is shown.
MDMA, methylenedioxy-N-methylamphetamine.
From Bernal W, Hyyrylainen A, Gera A, et al. Lessons from look-back in acute liver failure? A single centre experience of 3300 patients. J Hepatol 2013; 59:74-80.

common causes, with halothane encountered almost exclusively from 1973 to 1993 and MDMA seen only after 1994. Antituberculosis therapy, antibiotics, and anticonvulsants were the other main responsible drug categories, but the large size of the miscellaneous group reflects the wide range of potential causes of ALF. Among 141 U.S. LT recipients with drug-induced ALF, isoniazid (16%), propylthiouracil (9%), phenytoin (7%), and valproic acid (7%) were the most commonly identified causative medications.[14] The risk of developing ALF is low, ranging from 0.001% for NSAIDs to 1% for the combination of isoniazid and rifampin. Herbal remedies and dietary supplements can also cause ALF (see Chapters 89 and 131). Patients with drug-induced ALF are predominantly female (70%).

Viral Infections

HAV-related ALF has been seen predominantly in populations not routinely acquiring natural immunity through childhood infection. The risk of developing ALF correlates with the age of the patient at the time of infection. Data from the U.S. Acute Liver Failure Study Group, however, have indicated that the incidence of ALF is declining because of increased immunization against HAV.[15]

HBV causes ALF through a number of scenarios.[9] The classic presentation, which follows primary infection, results from an aggressive immune response against the virus but is becoming less common. Some cases have no serologic or virologic evidence of acute HBV at the time of presentation, other than immunoglobulin (Ig)M antibody to hepatitis B core antigen. A similar scenario can be encountered in patients with chronic hepatitis B infection at the point of seroconversion of hepatitis B e antigen (HBeAg) to antibody. An alternative mechanism of ALF is aggressive viral replication with high HBV DNA levels in serum, which can occur spontaneously or after initiation of immunosuppressive drugs (e.g., after hematopoietic stem cell or solid organ transplantation) or chemotherapy. This risk can be eliminated by the appropriate use of antiviral prophylaxis in patients at risk (see

Chapter 79). Hepatitis D virus is decreasing in incidence worldwide but previously was associated with the development of ALF as a result of both coinfection and superinfection with HBV (see Chapter 81).

Acute HEV infection is common in India and other tropical countries. It is a waterborne virus with an epidemiologic profile similar to that of HAV. HEV infection has developed a reputation for being dangerous in pregnant women, particularly during the third trimester. Although pregnant women are more likely to develop ALF, the outcome of ALF in persons with HEV infection is independent of sex, pregnancy status, and trimester of pregnancy (see Chapter 82).[16]

Unusual viral causes of ALF include HSV-1, 2, and 6, varicella-zoster virus, EBV, cytomegalovirus, and parvovirus B19. Of these viral causes, HSV is the most important to consider because early intervention with acyclovir can be effective; associated cutaneous lesions are seen in about 50% of cases (see Chapter 83).

Rare Causes

Pregnancy-Related Acute Liver Failure

ALF is an exceptionally rare complication of pregnancy, with an estimated incidence of 0.0008%.[17] The risk of developing ALF is highest in the first pregnancy and with a male fetus. Three discrete syndromes have been described: acute fatty liver of pregnancy, preeclampsia, and the HELLP syndrome, although in many cases the features overlap. Suggestive laboratory findings include high serum aminotransferase levels in patients with preeclampsia, high uric acid levels in those with acute fatty liver of pregnancy, and low platelet counts in those patients with the HELLP syndrome (see Chapter 39).

Vascular Causes

Hepatic vein thrombosis, or Budd-Chiari syndrome, can present as ALF. It is one of the few causes of ALF associated with an enlarged liver. The prognosis is poor in this setting, and the optimal management is LT. Ischemic hepatitis is now recognized as a relatively common cause of acute liver injury in a hospital setting but infrequently progresses to ALF (see Chapter 85).

Hyperthermia

Acute liver injury may occur in the setting of hyperthermia. The cause may be a drug reaction, and one of the more frequently encountered causative agents is the recreational drug ecstasy. Severe physical exertion in hot climates can also trigger ALF in association with evidence of damage to other organs, especially muscle, with evidence of rhabdomyolysis.

Autoimmune Hepatitis

ALF can be a presentation of classic autoimmune hepatitis, with strongly positive autoantibodies and elevated serum IgG levels. In this setting, autoimmune disease can be reasonably presumed to the true underlying etiology. Low titers of autoantibodies in association with less pronounced increases in IgG levels are often seen with the subacute pattern of ALF and are not reliably indicative of an autoimmune etiology (see Chapter 90).

Wilson Disease

An acute presentation of Wilson disease typically occurs in the second decade of life and accounts for up to 25% of cases. The diagnosis is usually suggested by unconjugated hyperbilirubinemia as a result of the associated hemolysis. Ascites is an early clinical feature, consistent with the presence of cirrhosis. Kayser-Fleischer rings are usually present. A similar clinical presentation is seen in previously treated patients who discontinue chelation therapy for a number of years. Ratios of serum alkaline phosphatase to total bilirubin below 4 and aspartate to ALT above 2.2 accurately distinguish Wilson disease from other causes of ALF (see Chapter 76).

Mushroom Poisoning

Poisoning with *Amanita phalloides* is seen most commonly in central Europe, South Africa, and the West Coast of the United States. Severe diarrhea and vomiting are characteristic early symptoms that develop within hours after ingestion of the mushrooms; liver failure develops 4 to 5 days later (see Chapter 89).

DIAGNOSIS

The diagnosis of ALF is clinical and based on the presence of encephalopathy in a patient with acute liver injury manifested by coagulopathy. The encephalopathy is usually overt and ranges from confusion to coma; however, psychometric testing may be needed in patients with subacute liver failure to detect subtle changes in mental state. Altered mental function secondary to hypoglycemia or uremia can occasionally be misinterpreted as encephalopathy.

Standard laboratory investigations include a complete blood count, coagulation tests, liver biochemical tests, serum electrolytes and tests of renal function, blood glucose, serum amylase, and arterial pH or serum lactate. These investigations allow an initial assessment of the severity of liver injury and direct management, whereas serial data aid the assessment of prognosis. To determine the etiology, an initial investigation should incorporate a screen for common viral agents and autoantibodies (Table 95-3).

Imaging of the liver with US and CT or MRI is routine practice but often yields little specific information. The typical early findings are a shrunken liver with no evidence of portal hypertension. Features of portal hypertension may be seen in subacute liver failure, and in this setting serial evaluation of liver volume can be helpful in assessing prognosis. Liver enlargement in the setting of ALF is unusual, except in Budd-Chiari syndrome, and should trigger consideration of malignant infiltration or alcoholic hepatitis as possible underlying diagnoses. Liver imaging can be informative in pregnancy-related ALF if it demonstrates fatty infiltration or the abnormal tissue perfusion patterns characteristic of acute fatty liver of pregnancy and preeclampsia, respectively.

The role of a liver biopsy in the diagnosis and management of ALF is limited. The characteristic findings of confluent necrosis and parenchymal collapse are nonspecific, and in subacute liver failure, sampling from a zone of regeneration may be unhelpful by revealing apparently healthy hepatic tissue that is not indicative of the likelihood of survival (Figs. 95-1 and 95-2). As a result, liver biopsy in patients with ALF is not performed routinely. The findings on biopsy may support specific diagnoses such as autoimmune hepatitis (characteristic inflammation), valproic acid toxicity (microvesicular steatosis), Wilson disease (cirrhosis, possible interface hepatitis, hepatocyte ballooning, steatosis), pregnancy-related syndromes (fatty infiltration characteristic of acute fatty liver of pregnancy or fibrin microthrombi and necrosis secondary to preeclampsia or eclampsia), and Budd-Chiari syndrome (venous congestion, sinusoidal dilatation). The strongest indication for a liver biopsy is to exclude malignant infiltration or

TABLE 95-3 Diagnostic Testing for the Etiology of Acute Liver Failure	
Etiology	**Diagnostic Test(s)**
Screen in All Cases	
HAV	IgM anti-HAV
HBV	HBsAg, IgM anti-HBc, HBV DNA
HEV	IgM anti-HEV
Acetaminophen	Drug levels in blood
Autoimmune hepatitis	Autoantibodies,* serum Ig levels
Test if Etiology Suspected	
Idiosyncratic drug reaction	Eosinophil count, liver histology
Acute fatty liver of pregnancy	US, serum uric acid level, liver histology
HELLP syndrome	Platelet count
Preeclampsia or eclampsia	Serum aminotransferase levels
Wilson disease	Urinary copper, serum ceruloplasmin level, serum alkaline phosphatase/bilirubin ratio, serum AST/ALT ratio, slit-lamp examination for Kayser-Fleischer rings
Budd-Chiari syndrome	Imaging of hepatic veins
Hepatic malignancy	Imaging of liver, liver histology
Ischemic hepatitis	Serum aminotransferase levels

*Antinuclear antibodies, smooth muscle antibodies; possibly antibodies to liver-kidney microsome type 1.
Anti-HBc, antibody to hepatitis B core antigen; HBsAg, hepatitis B surface antigen; Ig, immunoglobulin.

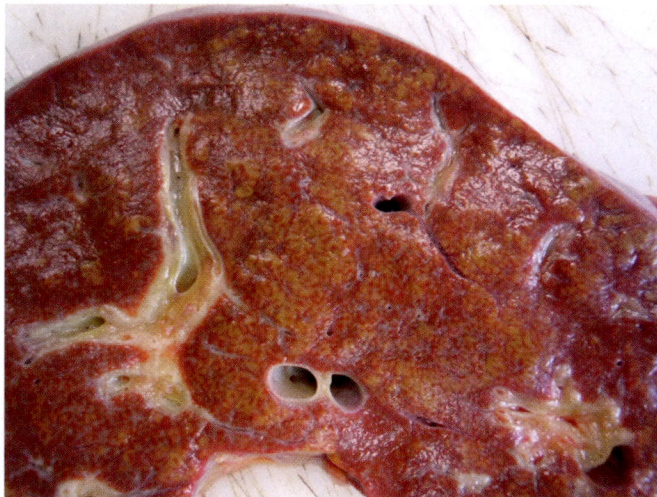

FIGURE 95-1. The cut surface of a liver removed at the time of liver transplantation in a patient with subacute liver failure. Areas of regeneration are lighter and yellowish in color compared with areas of necrosis. *(Image courtesy Dr. Yoh Zen, London, U.K.)*

alcoholic hepatitis in patients with hepatomegaly, especially if LT is under consideration (see later).

CLINICAL FEATURES

ALF can trigger catastrophic multiorgan failure. Jaundice is an expected finding but may not be prominent in patients presenting with hyperacute liver failure, especially acetaminophen-related liver injury. Other classic signs of liver failure notable by their absence are fetor hepaticus and tremor, the hallmark features of encephalopathy secondary to chronic liver disease; rarely, they are seen in patients with subacute liver failure. Ascites is characteristic of Wilson disease and Budd-Chiari syndrome and is seen in many patients with subacute liver failure, irrespective of the underlying etiology (see Fig. 95-2).

Encephalopathy

Encephalopathy is mandatory for a diagnosis of ALF. It is classically graded on a scale of 1 to 4. Patients with grades 1 or 2 encephalopathy exhibit degrees of drowsiness or disorientation, but they can be roused and will respond appropriately to verbal stimuli. Progression to grade 3 encephalopathy is often heralded by a period of extreme agitation before the patient becomes confused to the point of being able to respond only to simple commands. Grade 4 encephalopathy signifies

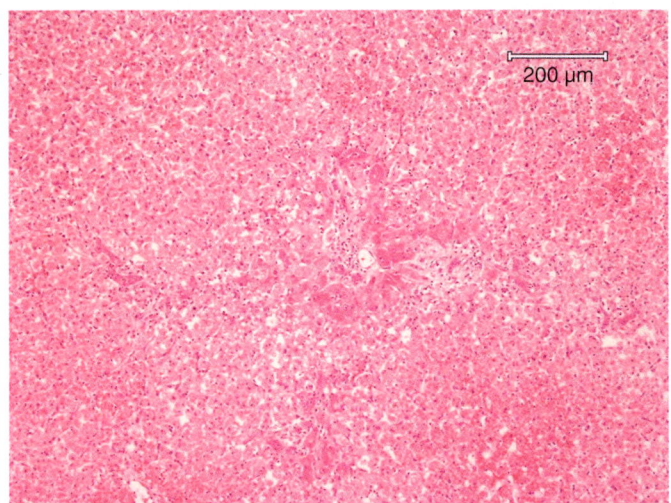

FIGURE 95-2. Histopathology of acetaminophen-related acute liver failure. The specimen is from a liver removed at transplantation. Confluent coagulative necrosis affects an entire lobule and spares a thin rim of periportal hepatocytes. A small portal tract is shown in the center of the figure. (H&E, ×100). *(Image courtesy Dr. Alberto Quaglia, London, U.K.)*

deep coma, with the patient responsive at best to painful stimuli. The briefest period between liver injury and the development of encephalopathy is 3 to 4 days, as demonstrated in patients with acetaminophen-induced ALF. With other etiologies, the point of onset and rate of progression of encephalopathy are variable and form the basis for the subclassification of ALF discussed earlier.

Intracranial Hypertension and Cerebral Edema

Cerebral edema has been a hallmark complication of ALF, major cause of death, and threat to successful LT. Early clinical studies suggested that cerebral edema developed in up to 80% of patients with grade 3 to 4 encephalopathy, but the risk was found not to be consistent across the spectrum of the disease, varying from 70% of patients with hyperacute liver failure to 55% of patients with ALF and only 15% of those with subacute liver failure.[2] Moreover, a large single-center review of acute liver injury and failure from King's College Hospital has confirmed a dramatic reduction in the frequency of intracranial hypertension, with a decline from 76% in 1984 to 1988 to only 20% in 2004 to 2008.[1]

The clinical features of cerebral edema include systemic hypertension, decerebrate posturing, hyperventilation, abnormal pupillary reflexes, and ultimately impairment of brainstem reflexes and functions. Papilledema is rarely observed. The outcome with medical management is usually either full recovery or death, although a few survivors with residual neurologic deficits have been described. Failure of neurologic recovery was observed during the early years of LT in ALF. CT of the brain shows characteristic changes but does not predict outcome, which is evaluated more accurately by direct intracerebral pressure monitoring (Fig. 95-3).

Hemodynamic Changes and Circulatory Failure

The hemodynamic changes in ALF are similar to those observed in systemic inflammatory response syndrome (SIRS) or septic shock.[18] The initial profile is of a hyperdynamic circulation, increased cardiac output, and reduced systemic peripheral vascular resistance. Progressive disease leads to circulatory failure either as a result of a falling cardiac output or an inability to maintain an adequate mean arterial pressure. This is a common cause of death in ALF as well as a barrier to successful LT. Cardiac arrhythmias occur and may be due to a definable precipitating event such as hypo- or hyperkalemia, acidosis, hypoxia, or cardiac irritation by a central venous catheter.

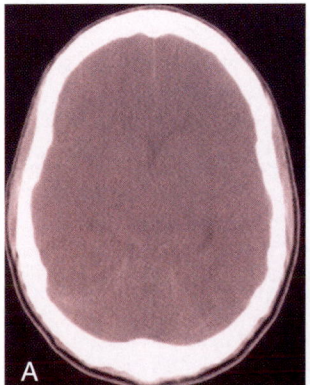
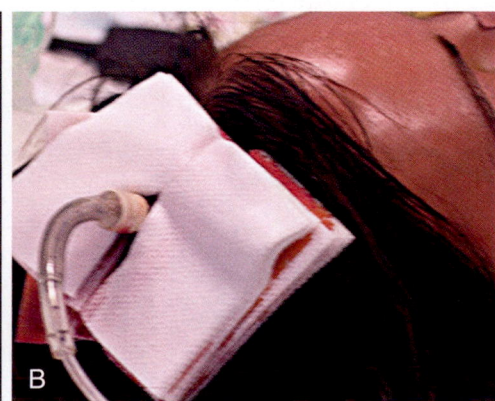
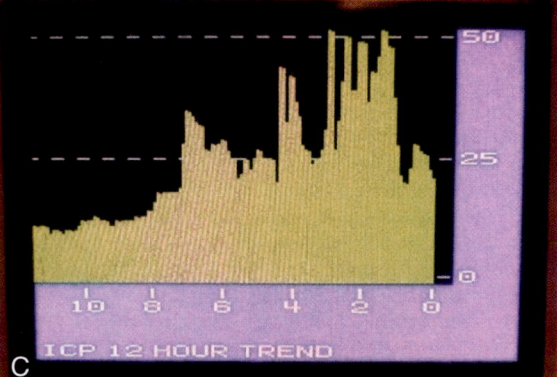

FIGURE 95-3. Neurologic testing in a patient with acute liver failure. *A,* CT of the brain showing severe swelling. *B,* Intracranial pressure (ICP) monitor in situ. *C,* Pressure tracing showing an elevated ICP (mm Hg). *(Image courtesy Dr. William Bernal, London, U.K.)*

Infection

Patients with ALF are notoriously prone to infection and have been found to have twice the risk when compared with similarly ill patients without liver disease. Infection is a common cause of death either independently or as a component of the circulatory and multisystem failure. Elements of immunosuppression, including defective neutrophil function, have been demonstrated across the spectrum of response to infection. Early clinical studies found that patients with grade 2 or higher encephalopathy had proved bacterial infection in up to 80% and fungal infection in 32% of cases.[19] The source of positive cultures included blood, urine, sputum, and vascular cannulae. The predominant bacteria were *Staphylococcus aureus*, *Streptococci*, and coliform bacteria, whereas *Candida* species accounted for most of the fungal infections. The fungal infections were particularly difficult to diagnose and were detected antemortem in only 50% of cases. Risk factors for both bacterial and fungal sepsis include coexisting renal failure, cholestasis, treatment with a barbiturate, and LT.

Renal Failure

Early studies of the natural history of ALF indicated that renal failure was present in 75% of patients following an acetaminophen overdose and 30% of patients with other etiologies.[3] Fundamental differences exist between acetaminophen-related and other causes of ALF. Renal failure after an acetaminophen overdose is a consequence of direct renal toxicity and develops early in the course of the illness and in parallel with liver injury. Early renal dysfunction may also be seen in Wilson disease, mushroom poisoning, and pregnancy-related syndromes. In most nonacetaminophen cases, renal failure tends to be a consequence of liver failure and develops later in the course of the disease, progressing from a stage of functional, or prerenal, failure (urinary sodium < 10 mmol/L, urine/plasma osmolarity ratio > 1.1) to acute tubular necrosis. Urea synthesis is impaired in ALF, and serum creatinine levels are preferred for monitoring renal function.

Hematologic Abnormalities

The liver is responsible for the synthesis of most of the coagulation factors (all except factor VIII, which is produced by endothelial cells), as well as some of the inhibitors of coagulation and fibrinolysis. After acute liver injury, circulating levels of fibrinogen, prothrombin, and factors V, VII, IX, and X fall, as rapidly becomes apparent because of the short half-life (measured in hours) of some of the factors. Functional parameters like the prothrombin time and the INR, as well as levels of an individual factor (e.g., factor V), are widely used as indicators of the severity of liver damage. In addition to decreased synthesis of coagulation factors by the liver, there is evidence of increased peripheral consumption. Overt DIC is occasionally observed, especially in the pregnancy-related syndromes.

Synthesis of anticoagulant proteins (e.g., proteins C and S), as well as antithrombin, is also decreased and often remains in physiologic balance with the levels of coagulation factors. This finding probably explains the clinical observation that patients with severe laboratory indicators of a coagulopathy may show little clinical evidence of bleeding.[20] In fact, the risk of bleeding is much more closely linked to the platelet count, and both quantitative and qualitative defects in platelet function are well described in ALF. Platelet counts below 100,000/mm^3 are seen in up to 70% of patients, whereas platelet aggregation is impaired. There is also evidence of increased platelet adhesiveness that may be due to increased levels of circulating von Willebrand factor.

A Coombs-negative hemolytic anemia is a characteristic of Wilson disease, and a Coombs-positive hemolytic anemia may be seen in ALF associated with autoimmune hepatitis. Aplastic anemia is associated with seronegative hepatitis in younger patients and may be related to parvovirus B19 infection. Erythrohemophagocytosis is an increasingly recognized occurrence in ALF and carries a poor prognosis.

APPROACH TO MANAGEMENT

Overall Strategy

Survival rates in ALF have improved dramatically, and over 60% of patients can be expected to survive the illness. The King's College Hospital experience from 1973 to 2008 has demonstrated that improvement in care and LT have independently contributed to an increase in overall survival from 16.7% to 62.2%, with rates of 86% for those undergoing LT and 48% for those managed medically.[1] Time is of the essence, and important benefit is derived from early recognition of ALF and early transfer to a specialist center, institution of monitoring, management of complications, and consideration of emergency LT in appropriate cases. A 12-point care plan is shown in Box 95-1.

BOX 95-1 12-Point Care Plan for Patients with Acute Liver Failure

1. Establish the diagnosis and assess the prognosis.
2. Consider liver transplantation; place the patient on the wait-list if the prognosis is poor.
3. Institute appropriate monitoring, especially hemodynamic and neurologic.
4. Monitor coagulation regularly. Prophylactic replacement of clotting factors is not advised unless an invasive procedure is planned. Treat bleeding with coagulation factors and platelets when appropriate.
5. Mechanically ventilate the patient when grade 3 encephalopathy develops.
6. Maintain a cerebral perfusion pressure > 55 mm Hg and intracranial pressure < 25 mm Hg. First-line therapy for cerebral edema is mannitol or hypertonic saline; second-line options include barbiturates, hypertonic saline, indomethacin, hyperventilation, and hypothermia.
7. Treat hemodynamic instability with fluid replacement and inotropic agents (norepinephrine, epinephrine) to maintain a mean arterial pressure > 90 mm Hg.
8. After mechanical ventilation for grade 3 encephalopathy, aim for a physiologic oxygen concentration and mild hypocapnia.
9. For renal dysfunction, institute early continuous renal replacement therapy; correct electrolyte abnormalities (e.g., hypokalemia, hypophosphatemia).
10. Perform daily culture surveillance; start broad-spectrum antibiotics if infection is suspected; begin a systemic antifungal agent in high-risk patients.
11. Monitor for hypoglycemia hourly; consider the possibility of functional adrenal insufficiency.
12. Protect the gastric mucosa with a PPI or H2RA; institute enteral feeding within 24 hours; otherwise start parenteral nutrition; consider the possibility of pancreatitis (especially in acetaminophen-related acute liver failure).

General Measures

In the nonspecialist setting, the priorities are adequate fluid resuscitation and protection of the airway in patients with advanced encephalopathy. Considerable evidence supports the importance of aggressive fluid resuscitation in patients with acetaminophen-related acute liver injury. Metabolic acidosis is an indicator of severe toxicity and is linked to a poor prognosis.[21,22] Survival prospects improve considerably, however, when the acidosis responds to early fluid resuscitation.[22] Patients with mushroom-related ALF probably benefit to a similar extent. The administration of parenteral vitamin K is common practice but is likely to have an impact in a minority of patients with protracted periods of jaundice prior to presentation.

N-acetylcysteine is well established in the management of an acetaminophen overdose and effective in preventing liver injury when administered within 15 hours of acetaminophen ingestion. *N*-acetylcysteine is indicated when the level of the drug in blood exceeds 1 of 2 curves: 1 for standard patients (the threshold is slightly lower in the United States than in the United Kingdom) and 1 for high-risk patients that includes those who have been taking an enzyme-inducing drug (e.g., antiepileptic therapy), consume alcohol regularly, or are malnourished. An extended role for *N*-acetylcysteine has been established in acetaminophen-induced acute liver injury in the United Kingdom,[23] but a double-blind, randomized controlled trial of *N*-acetylcysteine in 173 patients with nonacetaminophen causes of ALF conducted in the United States showed no difference in overall survival (70% vs. 66%)[24]; however, transplant-free survival was significantly better in patients with grade 1 to 2 encephalopathy at the time of randomization (see Chapter 88).

Fast-acting antiviral drugs effective against HBV (e.g., lamivudine, entecavir) are clearly indicated in patients with reactivated HBV infection and high levels of viremia and may also be beneficial in acute HBV infection, even though spontaneous rapid viral clearance from serum is expected (see Chapter 79).[25] Penicillin, and possibly silymarin, may be beneficial in patients with *Amanita phalloides* toxicity, particularly when administered soon after ingestion of the mushrooms (see Chapter 89).[26] D-penicillamine is not effective when encephalopathy develops in patients with Wilson disease but should be considered in patients with an acute presentation in the absence of encephalopathy (see Chapter 76). Similarly, in autoimmune hepatitis, glucocorticoid therapy rarely rescues the patient with established ALF and may complicate the process by predisposing to infection (see Chapter 90).[27]

PROGNOSIS

Understanding the prognosis in patients with ALF is pivotal to delivering an optimal management plan, specifically, the need to transfer a patient to a specialist center and determination of the likelihood of requiring LT. Three important determinants of outcome that are almost immediately apparent on presentation are the underlying etiology of ALF, age of the patient, and grade of encephalopathy. Another early indicator of a poor prognosis is a history of jaundice for more than 7 days before the onset of encephalopathy; most spontaneous survivors have the hyperacute category of ALF. The pattern and severity of organ failure as the disease progresses also gives insight into prognosis but at a stage of disease that may be too late to alter the outcome. Prognostication is also supported by a relatively small number of laboratory investigations. Various elements have been combined into prognostic models.

BOX 95-2 King's College Hospital Indicators of a Poor Prognosis in Acute Liver Failure

Acetaminophen Cases
Arterial pH < 7.25 more than 24 hours after drug ingestion*
All of the following:
    Prothrombin time > 100 sec or INR > 6.5
    Serum creatinine level > 3.4 mg/dL (300 µmol/L) or anuria
    Grade 3 to 4 encephalopathy

Nonacetaminophen Cases
Prothrombin time > 100 sec or INR > 6.7
Any 3 of the following:
    Unfavorable etiology (seronegative hepatitis or drug reaction)
    Age < 10 or > 40 years
    Acute or subacute category (duration of jaundice > 7 days)
    Serum bilirubin level > 17.5 mg/dL (300 µmol/L)
    Prothrombin time > 50 sec or INR > 3.5

*Subsequent modification: arterial pH < 7.25 or serum lactate > 3.0 mmol/L after adequate fluid resuscitation.

The King's College Hospital criteria published in 1989 were among the first prognostic models.[21] Different models were described for acetaminophen-induced and other etiologies of ALF (Box 95-2). The criteria have been subjected to 2 meta-analyses that reported an overall specificity of 82% for nonacetaminophen etiologies and 95% for acetaminophen-related ALF.[28,29] The analysis of nonacetaminophen etiologies involved 1105 patients in 18 studies and detected a higher specificity of 93% in patients with more advanced encephalopathy and 88% when the criteria were applied repeatedly in individual patients as the disease progressed.[28] The meta-analysis of 1960 acetaminophen-related cases in 14 studies indicated that the high level of specificity was weakened by a relatively low sensitivity of 58%,[29] due also in part to the non-dynamic application of the model, possibly because of the common practice of giving prophylactic fresh frozen plasma to these patients with a characteristically severe coagulopathy. The overall sensitivity for nonacetaminophen ALF was 85% prior to 1995, but fell to 58% after 2005, and was lowest in centers not offering LT.[28] Serum lactate levels, both at presentation and after initial resuscitation, predict survival in acetaminophen-related ALF but have been shown not to complement the criteria studied in the meta-analysis described earlier.[22,29]

The Clichy criteria are another set of parameters that have been effective determinants of outcome and continue to be used in France.[30] These criteria are based on factor V levels, with discriminatory values less than 20% in patients under 30 years of age and less than 30% in older patients. These criteria are applicable once grade 2 encephalopathy has developed.

The MELD score has been validated for use in prognostication in patients with chronic liver disease and has subsequently been applied in ALF (see Chapter 97).[31-33] The components of MELD (bilirubin, INR, serum creatinine) are well-recognized parameters of disease severity and have been incorporated into other prognostic models. A hybrid model developed in India combines classic indicators of prognosis (age > 50 years, jaundice-to-encephalopathy time > 7 days, prothrombin time > 35 seconds, and serum creatinine level > 1.5 mg/dL) with clinical complications associated with a poor outcome (advanced encephalopathy and cerebral edema).[34] A study from Germany has combined serum bilirubin, serum lactate, and etiology.[35] A more recently described prognostic model called the Acute Liver Failure Study Group

Index combines 3 classes of variables: clinical (coma grade), laboratory (INR, serum bilirubin, serum phosphorus), and a marker of apoptosis (M30).[36] This model was compared with both the King's College Hospital criteria and the MELD score and had a higher sensitivity of 86% but a relatively low specificity of 65%. The APACHE II score and Sequential Organ Failure Assessment (SOFA) index correlate well with outcome and may be better predictors in patients with acetaminophen-related ALF than the King's College criteria and MELD score.[37,38] A number of disease-specific prognostic models (for mushroom poisoning and for pregnancy) have also been described.[39-41]

The contribution of radiologic and histologic findings to the prognosis is relatively limited. Assessing the volume of viable hepatocytes may have prognostic value, with a critical mass of 25% to 40% suggested as being associated with a good prognosis. This approach is most reliable in hyperacute liver failure when the histologic changes are homogeneous and viable hepatocytes are likely to have evaded acute liver injury and thereby form the basis for clinical recovery. In the more slowly evolving syndromes, however, a map-like pattern emerges, with areas of regeneration interspersed with areas of collapse. Sampling from the area of regeneration might suggest that the liver is recovering, when in reality the prospects for survival are poor. Serial radiologic assessment of liver volume is valuable in patients with the subacute pattern of disease, particularly when the degree of encephalopathy and severity of coagulopathy may not be particularly marked.[42]

LIVER TRANSPLANTATION

LT is one of the main reasons why survival rates for ALF have increased from less than 20% in the 1970s to over 60% in the 2010s.[43-57] Data from the Scientific Registry of Transplant Recipients (SRTR) and the European Liver Transplant Registry (ELTR) have indicated that about 8% of overall organ utilization occurs in patients with ALF.[58,59] The King's College Hospital experience of 2095 patients admitted between 1973 and 2008 showed that 19% of patients with ALF and grade 2 or higher encephalopathy received liver transplants. Rates of LT for the most recent time period had increased to 53% for nonacetaminophen cases and 35% for acetaminophen cases.[1] The application of LT varies with the cause of ALF and in the United States is notably lower, at only 8%, for patients with acetaminophen-related ALF compared with about 40% for other etiologies.

Two fundamental approaches are used to select patients with ALF for LT. The first is to use indicators of a poor prognosis for wait-listing patients; however, use of these prognostic models creates clinical tensions that reflect the relative strengths and weakness of the models with respect to sensitivity and specificity. This approach relies on having a high level of confidence that an individual patient will benefit from LT in order to justify the use of a limited resource. Failure to list a patient for LT who subsequently dies because the model lacks sensitivity represents a missed opportunity for that patient. The second approach is to list all eligible patients and make the decision to transplant when a suitable donor organ becomes available. This approach favors the individual patient but risks unnecessary transplantation as well as diversion of scarce organs that could have been better used in different patient populations. The potential for "unnecessary transplantation" is significant and greatest for acetaminophen-related ALF, as illustrated by one U.S. study in which 59% of patients wait-listed for LT survived to leave the hospital after recovering function in their native livers.[13]

Donor organ allocation systems prioritize patients with ALF so that most patients receive transplants within 48 to 72 hours of wait-listing. In Europe, the average donor age is 41 years, and 89.6% of organs come from brain-dead donors.[59] About 70% of organs are ABO identical to the recipient and about 5% are incompatible.[59] Waiting times influence policy on the use of ABO-mismatched grafts, steatotic livers, livers from non–heart-beating deceased donors, and other suboptimal potential grafts (see Chapter 97). In Europe, auxiliary transplantation was at its peak from 1994 to 1998, when it accounted for 4% of LT activity; this figure has since fallen to 2%.[59] Auxiliary LT is intended to serve as a bridge to transplant-free survival, usually within 3 years of surgery. The outcomes are comparable to that for orthotopic transplants, and about 70% of patients recover enough function in the native liver to allow the graft to involute. Live-donor LT is well established in Asia, where deceased-donor donation is limited, but in Europe just under 1% of transplants have occurred after live donation.

The mortality rate on the wait-list is between 19% and 28% and is highest for acetaminophen-related ALF. In some of these patients, a suitable organ is never allocated, whereas in others a decision is made not to proceed to LT when the opportunity for transplantation arises because the patient has deteriorated to the point of being considered too sick to benefit from LT. The evidence supporting the latter decision is limited, but insight into this issue has emerged from 2 studies—an analysis using the United Network for Organ Sharing (UNOS) database of 1457 patients and an analysis of 310 patients listed at King's College Hospital.[60,61] These studies identified 5 clinical factors that correlate with outcome: BMI above 30, serum creatinine level above 2 mg/dL, recipient age older than 45 to 50 years, the need for inotropic support, and use of life support. These individual parameters are not clinically useful in identifying patients too ill to benefit from LT but performed better when grouped, and in the U.S. study, the survival rate was 81% when none was present but only 42% when 4 were present.[60]

The decision not to proceed with LT is therefore usually made on the basis of a number of clinical complications. Objective evidence of brainstem injury with established fixed and fully dilated pupils should preclude LT. In other patients with cerebral edema, however, no thresholds for cerebral perfusion or intracranial pressure have been validated to automatically exclude a patient from transplantation. With respect to infection, a pragmatic approach is not to contraindicate transplantation on the basis of a bacterial infection after 48 hours of appropriate antibiotic therapy. Confirmed systemic fungal infection, however, should contraindicate LT. A requirement for an inotropic agent is a surrogate marker of disease severity, and both the dose and the dynamics of dose escalation influence the decision to proceed with transplantation. Interpretation of these potential contraindications to transplantation varies with the age of the patient because younger patients are more resilient and more likely to recover following the procedure.

The overall 1-year patient survival rate following LT for ALF in Europe between 2004 and 2009 was 79%, and the graft survival rate was 73%.[59] The 1-year patient survival rate in the United States was similar (78.6%) with the use of deceased donors but numerically higher (87%) with the use of live donors.[58] After 1 year, the decline in survival is much less marked than in other patient cohorts undergoing LT, likely because patients with ALF are younger and have a much lower risk of recurrent disease that affects graft function. The etiology of the underlying disease did not correlate with outcome in the overall analysis of the ELTR data, but patients with acetaminophen-related ALF had a 24% greater risk of death.[59] Seronegative hepatitis or ALF of no definable cause was associated with a higher risk of primary graft nonfunction or early graft dysfunction. Survivors of LT for acetaminophen-related ALF received a graft about 2 days sooner than those who succumbed (day 4 vs. day 6 after drug ingestion).

TREATMENT OF COMPLICATIONS

Neurologic Complications

Encephalopathy is a consistent clinical feature of ALF, but in most patients few treatments are directed specifically to its management. The main exception is in patients with subacute liver failure who may benefit from the standard measures used in patients with chronic liver disease, including dietary protein restriction, lactulose, and nonabsorbable oral antibiotic therapy. Experimental approaches with branched-chain amino acids, the benzodiazepine antagonist flumazenil, and extracorporeal liver support devices (see later) have not resulted in a survival benefit and are not widely used. Therefore, the management of the encephalopathy is essentially that of the underlying liver disease. Protection of the patient's airway as encephalopathy progresses is important, and endotracheal intubation and mechanical ventilation are indicated once grade 3 encephalopathy develops. At this point, adequate analgesia and sedation are required, and propofol and fentanyl has been suggested as an appropriate combination.[20] In addition, propofol decreases the risk of seizure activity, which is frequently unrecognized in these patients.[62] At this point, additional measures to reduce the risk of cerebral edema are instituted, including minimization of tactile stimuli and movement, elevation of the head to 20% to 30%, and avoidance of rotation of the neck.

The main neurologic complication amenable to therapy is cerebral edema. Mannitol has been the mainstay of treatment of increased intracranial pressure, but hypertonic saline is now considered to be an alternative first-line therapy. These solutions act by increasing blood osmolality and reducing astrocyte swelling in the brain. The rapidity of the response to mannitol, however, suggests that it also functions by increasing cerebral blood. A rapidly delivered bolus of 0.25 to 0.5 mg/kg is recommended to obtain the maximal diuretic effect, which in anuric patients is achieved by manipulating the rate of fluid filtration. This process is repeated as determined by the pattern of clinical relapses until the serum osmolality exceeds 320 mOsm.[63] Hypertonic saline has the advantage over mannitol of increasing blood pressure. The induction of hypernatremia (serum sodium 145 to 155 mmol/L) has been shown to reduce intracranial pressure in a randomized controlled trial.[64]

Second-line therapeutic interventions have been described once the osmotic approach ceases to be effective in controlling intracranial pressure. Although there is little evidence that any of these interventions independently improves survival, these approaches can be effective bridges to LT. Hyperventilation can reduce surges in intracranial pressure, potentially at the cost of reducing cerebral blood flow, and it should probably only be used as an emergency measure in refractory cases.[63,65] Hypothermia (body temperature reduced to 32° to 33°C) reduces intracranial pressure and increases cerebral blood flow in ALF, but concerns include an increased risk of infection and aggravation of coagulopathy.[63,66] Other measures include phenobarbital (or sodium thiopental) and IV indomethacin.[67,68] Hepatectomy is occasionally considered as a final act of desperation because it predictably secures a period of improvement that lasts up to 18 to 24 hours. This strategy is usually undertaken to buy time when a potential donor organ has been identified for transplantation.[44]

In the advanced stages of these neurologic complications, the emphasis of management changes to the preservation of cerebral perfusion pressure, increased oxygen delivery to the brain, and manipulation of the neuronal microcirculation to promote cerebral oxygen extraction. The patient is now positioned with the trunk at 0 to 10 degrees to the horizontal. These adjustments are made to maintain a cerebral perfusion pressure greater than 50 mm Hg if possible.

Direct intracranial pressure monitoring is controversial and has not been subjected to clinical trials. The advantages of early detection of increases in intracranial pressure and the facility to optimize therapeutic intervention were considered to be significant when the frequency of cerebral edema was as high as 70% and the attendant mortality was also high. This perspective has changed with the dramatic reduction in the frequency of cerebral edema and its limited contribution to death. The risk of intracranial hemorrhage and the absence of evidence of improved survival were 2 of the arguments advanced against the routine use of direct intracranial pressure monitoring. A U.S. study found that the bleeding complication rate was reduced to 10% as compared with an earlier study but also that half of the bleeds were not associated with clinical sequelae.[69,70] Data from King's College Hospital indicate that about 30% of patients with ALF underwent direct intracranial pressure monitoring.[63] Further refinements since then have focused on patients who had some evidence of susceptibility to cerebral edema and who were being considered for LT. Monitoring should continue for 24 hours after LT or longer if early graft function is impaired. Alternatives to direct pressure monitoring, such as transcranial Doppler monitoring, are considered unsatisfactory.[63,71]

Infection

The consequence of the immunosuppression of ALF is a high frequency of bacterial and fungal infections that often lead to progressive multiorgan failure and death.[72] The classic clinical indicators of infection may be seen with SIRS, and detection of infection relies on intensive surveillance on a daily basis. Clinical trials of prophylactic antibiotics have demonstrated that systemic antibiotics reduce the frequency of culture-positive bacterial infection by half but at the cost of an increase in detection of highly resistant organisms in 10% of patients. Furthermore, the reduction in infection rates has not been accompanied by a significant improvement in major clinical outcomes, including rates of mortality and LT, or economic benefit (e.g., reduced duration of stay in ICU or in a hospital). Similarly, small bowel decontamination has not been effective in altering the pattern of infection.

The standard principles of prevention of infection apply to patients with ALF. The sites of infection and the causative organisms are similar to those for other critically ill patients, and the choice of antibiotics should reflect institutional antibiotic policy rather than the cause of the patient's illness. The use of prophylactic systemic antifungal therapy has not been subjected to formal assessment but should be considered in patients with recognized risk factors (e.g., renal failure, severe cholestasis, previous or concomitant barbiturate therapy, LT). The justification for this recommendation is the difficulty in detecting systemic fungal sepsis and the adverse implications for candidacy for LT if a diagnosis of systemic fungal infection is made. Again, the specifics of the antifungal regimen are generic to critically ill patients. Susceptibility to infection is another complication of ALF that persists after LT, and the treatment plan should be extended into this phase of management.

Hemodynamic Instability and Hypoxemia

Invasive hemodynamic monitoring is initiated routinely in patients with ALF, and current practice favors volumetric indices over pressure-derived variables.[63] When underfilling of the cardiovascular system is detected, appropriate combinations of colloid, crystalloid fluids, and blood products should be administered. Hypotension that occurs despite adequate intravascular volume is treated with vasopressor agents such as norepinephrine if the cardiac index exceeds 4.5 L/min/m² or epinephrine if the cardiac output needs to be boosted above this threshold. The initial stabilizing dose to achieve a mean arterial pressure above 60 mm Hg ranges from 0.2 to 2 mg/kg/min of norepinephrine and 0.2 to 1.8 mg/kg/min of epinephrine. Vasopressor agents may cause or aggravate hypoxia, and epoprostenol (prostacyclin) infused at a rate of 5 ng/kg/min has been shown to improve parameters of oxygen metabolism (delivery, consumption, and extraction ratio) when used in conjunction with both norepinephrine and epinephrine. Infusion of N-acetylcysteine, 10 mg/kg/min for 15 minutes followed by 0.2 mg/kg/min for 4 hours, causes less vasodilatation than epoprostenol, independently increases mean arterial pressure, and is as effective as epoprostenol in improving oxygen metabolism. The combination of epoprostenol and N-acetylcysteine is more beneficial to oxygen metabolism than either drug alone. Some patients who become resistant to inotropic agents have been shown to have a hypoadrenal profile that responds to hydrocortisone. A subnormal cosyntropin stimulation test or short tetracosactide test indicates the need for 200 to 300 mg of hydrocortisone daily for a period of about 1 week.[73]

The need for airway protection is the usual indication for intubation and initiation of controlled mechanical ventilation. Thereafter, hypoxemia and increasing oxygen requirements may develop secondary to atelectasis, infection, fluid overload, hemorrhage, or any combination of these factors. Early acute respiratory distress syndrome (ARDS) is seen particularly in acetaminophen-related ALF and is often associated with SIRS, pancreatitis, or cerebral edema. Pleural effusions are more typically encountered in subacute liver failure. It has been suggested that raised intra-abdominal pressure frequently compromises pulmonary function in ALF and should be monitored routinely.[63]

There are a number of potential conflicts between the optimal management of pulmonary complications and the control of intracranial hypertension and cerebral edema. Tracheal suction is a powerful tactile stimulus that may trigger a surge in intracranial pressure, but effective airway toilet is a priority in protecting the lungs from infection and should be managed by effective sedation. Positive end-expiratory pressure (PEEP) could delay venous drainage from the brain but in practice appears to be well tolerated in patients with cerebral edema.[63]

Renal Failure

An early fluid challenge is indicated in patients in whom oliguria or biochemical evidence of renal dysfunction develops. The prophylactic use of dopamine was common practice in the past but was not subjected to randomized controlled trials and has been challenged because of the profound vasodilatation typically seen early in ALF. Terlipressin is not indicated in patients with acetaminophen-related ALF, because the pattern of renal injury is acute tubular necrosis; in theory terlipressin might be effective for other indications, but no data are available to support this approach. Extracorporeal renal support has been required in 75% of cases of acetaminophen-induced ALF and 30% of cases due to other etiologies that have progressed to grade 3 to 4 encephalopathy.[4] The metabolic complexity of combined liver and renal failure suggests that early intervention with hemodialysis, preempting standard indications, is worth considering. Continuous filtration or dialysis systems are clearly preferred over intermittent hemodialysis because they are associated with less hemodynamic instability and run a lower risk of aggravating latent or established cerebral edema.[74,75] Established renal failure usually persists after LT, and recovery typically occurs sooner with nonacetaminophen etiologies of ALF.

The coagulopathy of ALF does not provide adequate clinical anticoagulation. Heparin or alternative anticoagulants are still required in patients on renal replacement therapy. The heparin doses required to prevent clotting and platelet depletion show considerable variation and should be monitored with functional assays such as the activated clotting time. Antithrombin supplementation in a dose of 3000 units prior to hemodialysis reduces heparin requirements. Epoprostenol infusions in doses of 2 to 5 ng/kg/min have proved superior to heparin anticoagulation in continuous systems with respect to the functional duration of the filters and the hemorrhagic complications that occur.

Coagulopathy

Prophylactic repletion of coagulation factors with fresh frozen plasma seems intuitive but is probably misguided. The potential advantages of a reduced bleeding risk have not been established by clinical studies. A controlled trial of fresh frozen plasma failed to demonstrate an improvement in survival and was thought to be detrimental in a minority of patients with a consumptive coagulopathy. Fresh frozen plasma administration interferes with the use of coagulation studies in the assessment of prognosis and monitoring of disease progression. Other potential disadvantages associated with aggressive repletion include fluid overload and hyperviscosity syndrome. Prophylactic fresh frozen plasma is used more commonly in anticipation of an invasive procedure (e.g., insertion of cannulae or intracranial pressure monitors) or LT. Fresh frozen plasma administration is clearly indicated in patients who are bleeding. It has been suggested that the details of management should be directed by patterns seen on thromboelastography (see Chapter 94).[20] Limited data are available on the utility of recombinant factor VIIa in ALF.[76] Thrombocytopenia is considered to be an important risk factor for hemorrhage, and maintenance of platelet counts above 50,000 to 70,000/mm³ has been recommended.

Metabolic Disorders

Hypoglycemia is common and can be mistaken for the onset of advanced encephalopathy. The symptoms and signs of hypoglycemia are often masked, and regular blood glucose monitoring is required, with administration of glucose as required. Metabolic acidosis is present in 30% of patients with ALF after an acetaminophen overdose and has been associated with a particularly high mortality of at least 90% if the arterial pH is below 7.30 on the second or subsequent days after the overdose.[21] Fluid resuscitation is first-line therapy, but persistence of the acidosis may be the indication to start filtration therapy. Metabolic acidosis is found in 5% of patients with other etiologies of ALF, occurs later in the disease process, and is also associated with a poor outcome. Increased serum lactate levels have been documented in patients with a metabolic acidosis and correlate inversely with mean arterial pressure, systemic vascular resistance, and oxygen extraction ratios. The hyperlactatemia may reflect tissue hypoxia resulting from impaired oxygen extraction due to microvascular shunting of blood away from actively respiring tissues. In most etiologies of ALF, alkalosis is the dominant acid-base abnormality and may be associated with hypokalemia. Hyponatremia may reflect sodium depletion in patients with vomiting and therefore responds to administration of IV saline, or it may be dilutional due to excessive antidiuretic hormone secretion or intracellular sodium shifts. Hypophosphatemia is encountered most frequently in acetaminophen-induced ALF when renal function is preserved. Replacement therapy is the appropriate management for hypokalemia, hypophosphatemia, and hypomagnesemia.

Nutritional Deficiencies

Although the standard patient with ALF is well nourished at the onset of the illness, the catabolic process can be profound. The catabolic rate increases further in patients with sepsis and those undergoing LT. Numerous theoretical problems, including ileus, aggravation of sepsis by IV feeding, and fluid restriction secondary to renal failure, limit nutritional options. In addition, the content of the nutritional supplementation may be influenced by the theoretical role of amino acid ratios in mediating encephalopathy, difficulty in lipid handling, and the desire to minimize protein in the GI tract. Enteral nutrition is desirable to help maintain the integrity of the small intestinal mucosa and should be titrated according to the volume of gastric aspirates and the development of diarrhea.

In practice, feeding is normally commenced within 24 hours of admission to an ICU, with a goal of 25 to 30 kcal/kg/day. The initial approach should be enteral via an NG tube. Pilot studies have shown that parenteral feeding is tolerated considerably better than would be expected from theoretical considerations. Lipid solutions (10%) are cleared from serum, and standard amino acid preparations do not appear to have a clinically relevant impact on encephalopathy. Continuous renal support systems give good flexibility with regard to the management of fluid loads, and assiduous attention to the maintenance of feeding lines keeps the septic complications within the expected frequency.

EXTRACORPOREAL LIVER SUPPORT

Attempts to improve survival in ALF using extracorporeal liver support devices extend back to the 1970s. A systematic review of published randomized trials using these devices up to September 2002 evaluated the outcome in a total of 353 patients and concluded that these systems had no effect on mortality.[77] Furthermore, no significant benefit in bridging patients to LT was identified. Since then, a small number of larger randomized controlled trials have been conducted, with mixed outcomes.

ALF was the conventional testing ground for these devices. It was an attractive patient group because of the rapid progression to either death or recovery. Nevertheless, trials of liver support devices are complicated by the fact that many patients are diverted to LT once a donor organ has been allocated and before the response to therapy with the device as a bridge to transplant-free survival can be evaluated. Therefore, an additional criterion for evaluating the devices evolved in later studies that assessed the ability of the devices to bridge patients to LT. Additional challenges in designing trials reflect the heterogeneity of ALF, particularly with respect to the capacity for hepatic regeneration.

The extracorporeal liver assist device (ELAD) system, based on C3a hepatocytes, was assessed in 24 patients with ALF, 17 of whom were considered to have potentially recoverable disease, and the survival rates were 78% and 75% for patients treated with and without ELAD, respectively.[78] An improved version of this device was subsequently developed, but it has not been evaluated specifically in ALF.

The bioartificial liver (BAL) based on porcine hepatocytes was assessed in a randomized controlled trial of 147 patients with ALF and 27 patients with primary graft nonfunction after LT. There was no overall difference in 30-day survival rates, which were 71% and 62% for BAL-treated and control patients, respectively.[79] There did appear, however, to be a significant benefit in terms of survival for a subgroup of patients with ALF with a defined etiology (acetaminophen, virus, other drug, or toxin). The 30-day survival rates in the patients who underwent LT were 89% in the BAL group and 80% in the control group, whereas in those not transplanted, 50% in the BAL group and 38% in the control group survived for 30 days. These differences were not statistically significant.[79] Despite some encouraging results in selected subgroups, this study was considered to be negative.

Liver support systems that do not use biological components include filtration techniques, albumin dialysis (e.g., molecular adsorbents recirculating system [MARS], single-pass albumin dialysis [SPAD]), charcoal or resin hemofiltration, and plasmapheresis. A large controlled study of charcoal hemoperfusion conducted in the 1980s failed to show an overall survival benefit.[4] In 75 patients with grade 3 encephalopathy randomized to either 5 or 10 hours of charcoal hemoperfusion, the respective survival rates were 51.3% and 47.2%. The 62 patients with grade 4 encephalopathy were randomized to 10 hours of therapy or to a control limb, and the respective survival rates were 39.3% and 31.0%. No further studies of charcoal hemoperfusion were undertaken, although charcoal columns were later included in some hybrid devices.

Despite being the most extensively used liver support device, data on MARS in ALF were initially limited. A small controlled study, for example, in patients with hyperacute liver failure demonstrated some hemodynamic benefit with therapy.[80] Subsequently, a large randomized controlled trial was carried out in France, where 110 patients were recruited over a 3-year period. The survival rate at 6 months was 85% in the MARS group compared with 76% in the control group.[81] In the patients with acetaminophen-related ALF, the survival differential was wider at 85% versus 69%, but this difference was not statistically significant. The majority of patients, however, were listed for LT with a median delay of only 16 hours, and 68% of the evaluated cohort received a liver transplant. Again, although the study was negative, the possibility of benefit from MARS could not be discounted based on trial design and the confounding effect of LT.

Randomized controlled trials of high-volume plasma exchange have been encouraging.[82,83] In one study,[83] 182 patients were randomized to standard medical therapy or, in addition, 3 days of high-volume plasma exchange. The survival rate was higher, at 59%, in the plasma-exchange group than in controls, who had a survival rate of 48%. The benefit was in transplant-free survival; plasma exchange did not improve survival after LT. This study needs to be interpreted with caution because it was conducted over an 11-year period, and the findings have yet to be reproduced.

KEY REFERENCES

Full references for this chapter can be found on www.expertconsult.com.

1. Bernal W, Hyyrylainen A, Gera A, et al. Lessons from look-back in acute liver failure? A single centre experience of 3300 patients. J Hepatol 2013; 59:74-80.

7. Sjogren M. Immunization and the decline of viral hepatitis as a cause of acute liver failure. Hepatology 2003; 38:554-6.

9. O'Grady JG. Acute liver failure. In: Bacon BR, O'Grady JG, Di Bisceglie AM, Lake JR, editors. Comprehensive clinical hepatology. 2nd ed. Philadelphia: Mosby Elsevier; 2005. pp 517-36.

11. Lee WM. Acute liver failure in the United States. Semin Liver Dis 2003; 23:217-26.

14. Russo MW, Galanko JA, Shrestha R, et al. Liver transplantation for acute liver failure from drug-induced liver injury in the United States. Liver Transpl 2004; 10:1018-23.

17. Ibdah JA, Bennett MJ, Rinaldo P, et al. A fetal fatty-acid oxidation disorder as a cause of liver disease in pregnant women. N Engl J Med 1999; 340:1723-31.

20. Stravitz RT, Kramer DJ. Management of acute liver failure. Nat Rev Gastroenterol Hepatol 2009; 6:542-53.

24. Lee WM, Hynan LS, Rossaro L, et al. Intravenous N-acetylcysteine improves transplant-free survival in early-stage non-acetaminophen acute liver failure. Gastroenterology 2009; 137:856-64.

25. Tillmann HL, Hadem J, Leifeld L, et al. Safety and efficacy of lamivudine in patients with severe acute or fulminant hepatitis B, a multicenter experience. J Viral Hepatol 2006; 13:256-63.

59. Germani G, Theocharidou E, Adam R, et al. Liver transplantation for acute liver failure in Europe: Outcomes over 20 years from the ELTR database. J Hepatol 2012; 57:288-96.

60. Barshes NR, Lee TC, Balkrishnan R, et al. Risk stratification of adult patients undergoing orthotopic liver transplantation for fulminant hepatic failure. Transplantation 2006; 81:195-201.

61. Bernal W, Cross TJ, Auzinger G, et al. Outcome after wait-listing for emergency liver transplantation in acute liver failure: A single centre experience. J Hepatol 2009; 50:306-13.

63. Auzinger G, Wendon J. Intensive care management of acute liver failure. Curr Opin Crit Care 2008; 14:179-88.

79. Demetriou AA, Brown RS Jr, Busuttil RW, et al. Prospective, randomized, multicenter controlled trial of a bioartificial liver in treating acute liver failure. Ann Surg 2002; 239:660-70.

96

Hepatic Tumors and Cysts*

ADRIAN M. DI BISCEGLIE AND ALEX S. BEFELER

CHAPTER OUTLINE

Hepatic mass lesions include tumors, tumor-like lesions, abscesses, cysts, hematomas, and confluent granulomas. Hepatic tumors may originate in the liver—from hepatocytes, bile duct epithelium, or mesenchymal tissue—or spread to the liver from primary tumors in remote or adjacent organs. In adults in most parts of the world, hepatic metastases are more common than primary malignant tumors of the liver, whereas in children, primary malignant tumors outnumber both metastases and benign tumors of the liver. Except for cavernous hemangiomas, benign hepatic tumors are rare in all geographic regions and in all age groups.

MALIGNANT TUMORS

Hepatocellular Carcinoma

Epidemiology

Hepatocellular carcinoma (HCC) is the most common primary malignant tumor of the liver. It is the fifth most common cancer in men and the eighth most common in women, and it ranks fourth in annual cancer mortality rates.[1,2] Information on incidence is derived from an increasing but still limited number of cancer registries, and it is possible to classify countries into broad risk categories only. Moreover, in low-income (developing) countries, especially in sub-Saharan Africa, HCC is underdiagnosed and underreported, in some cases by as much as 50%. Despite these sources of inaccuracy, HCC clearly has an unusual geographic distribution (Fig. 96-1). Moreover, the tumor is not necessarily uniformly common

throughout countries with a high incidence, such as China[3] and Mozambique.[4] The incidence of HCC has increased considerably in Japan since the 1980s, and lesser increases have been recorded in developed Western countries, including North America and Western Europe.[5] Interestingly, a study from Japan has shown that the rate of HCC began to decline in 2000, presumably because of the aging of the cohort of persons infected with HCV.[6] A similar downward trend has been noted in some European countries, including France and Italy.[7] By contrast, in the United States, HCC is the cancer that has been increasing in incidence most rapidly since 2000, at a time when other major cancers such as cancers of the lung, breast, prostate, and colon are decreasing.[8] Considerable racial and ethnic variation exits in the incidence of HCC in the United States. The incidence among Asians is highest, almost double that of white Hispanics and more than 4 times higher than that of whites.[9]

Migrants from countries with a low incidence to areas with a high incidence of HCC usually retain the low risk of their country of origin, even after several generations in the new environment. The consequences for migrants from countries with a high incidence to those with a low incidence differ, depending on the major risk factors for the tumor in their country of origin and whether chronic HBV infection, if this is the major risk factor, is acquired predominantly by the perinatal or horizontal route (see later and Chapter 79).[2,10,11]

Men are generally more susceptible than women to HCC. Male predominance is, however, more obvious in populations at high risk for the tumor (mean male-to-female ratio, 3.7 : 1.0) than in those at low or intermediate risk (2.4 : 1.0).[1,2] In industrialized countries, the number of men and number of women with HCC in the absence of cirrhosis are almost equal.

The incidence of HCC increases progressively with advancing age in all populations, although it tends to level off in the

---

*Professor Michael C. Kew contributed to this chapter in previous editions of the textbook.

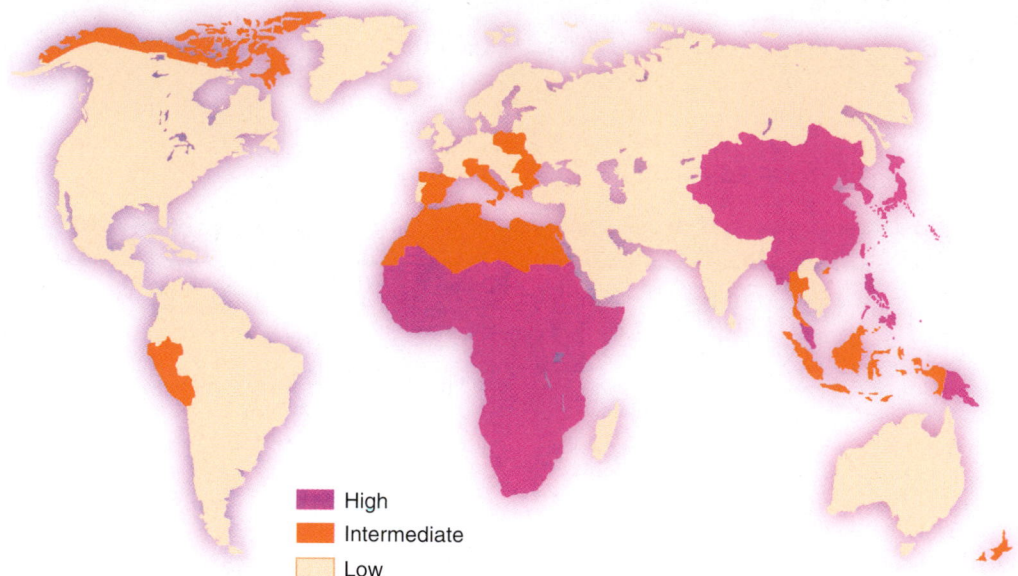

FIGURE 96-1. Incidence of hepatocellular carcinoma in different parts of the world. High, age-adjusted rate of more than 15 cases/100,000 population/year; intermediate, age-adjusted rate of 5 to 15 cases/100,000/year; low, age-adjusted rate of fewer than 5 cases/100,000/year.

oldest age groups.[1,2] In Chinese and particularly in black African populations, however, the mean age of patients with the tumor is appreciably younger than in other populations. This finding is in sharp contrast to the age distribution in Japan, where the incidence of HCC is highest in the cohort of men aged 70 to 79 years.[6] HCC is rare in children.[12,13]

Etiology and Pathogenesis

In contrast to many other malignancies, for which risk factors can only sometimes be identified, the immediate cause of HCC can usually be identified and is most commonly chronic viral hepatitis or cirrhosis. HCC is multifactorial in cause and complex in pathogenesis. Four major causative factors have been identified (Box 96-1). The differing blend of risk factors in various parts of the world may explain, in part, the diverse biological characteristics of HCC in various populations.[14]

Hepatitis B Virus

Some 387 million carriers of HBV exist in the world today, and HCC will develop in as many as 25% of them (see Chapter 79). HBV infection accounts for up to 80% of HCCs, which occur with high frequency in East Asian and African populations.[14,15] Persistent HBV infection antedates the development of HCC by several to many years, an interval commensurate with a cause-and-effect relationship between the virus and the tumor. Indeed, in at-risk populations, the HBV carrier state is largely established in early childhood by perinatal or horizontal infection.[16,17] Approximately 90% of children infected at this stage of life become chronic carriers of the virus, and these early-onset carriers face a lifetime relative risk for developing HCC of more than 100 compared with uninfected controls.[18]

An effective vaccine against HBV has been available since the early 1980s, and in countries where this vaccine has been included in the expanded program of immunization for a sufficient length of time, the HBV carrier rate among children has decreased by 10-fold or more. Studies in Taiwan, where universal immunization was started in 1984 and where the rate

of HBV carriage among children has decreased by more than 10-fold, have shown a 70% reduction in the mortality rate from HCC in children in the vaccinated age groups.[19] This finding gives promise for the ultimate eradication of HBV-induced HCC and provides further evidence of the causal role of the virus in the development of this tumor.

The precise mechanism by which HBV results in HCC is not known; however, the virus appears to be directly and indirectly carcinogenic.[20] HBV DNA is integrated into cellular DNA in approximately 90% of HBV-related HCCs.[21] The sites of chromosomal insertion appear to be random, and whether viral integration is essential for hepatocarcinogenesis is still

---

BOX 96-1 Risk Factors for Hepatocellular Carcinoma

Major Risk Factors
Chronic HBV infection
Chronic HCV infection
Cirrhosis
Dietary exposure to aflatoxin B_1

Other Liver Conditions
α_1-Antitrypsin deficiency
Hemochromatosis
Membranous obstruction of the inferior vena cava
Nonalcoholic fatty liver disease
Type 1 and type 2 glycogen storage disease
Type 1 hereditary tyrosinemia
Wilson disease

Inherited Conditions Not Associated with Liver Disease
Ataxia-telangiectasia
Hypercitrullinemia

Other Factors
Cigarette smoking
Diabetes mellitus
Oral contraceptive steroid use

uncertain. Possible direct carcinogenic effects include *cis*-activation of cellular genes as a result of viral integration, changes in the DNA sequences flanking the integrated viral DNA, transcriptional activation of remote cellular genes by HBV-encoded proteins (particularly the X protein), and effects resulting from viral mutations. The transcriptional activity of the HBV X protein may be mediated by interaction with specific transcription factors, activation of the mitogen-activated protein (MAP) kinase and Janus kinase/signal transducer and activator of transcription (JAK/STAT) pathways, an effect on apoptosis, and modulation of DNA repair. Studies have shown a clear link between the amount of HBV replication (measured as serum level of HBV DNA [viral load]) and subsequent risk of HCC. The long-term risk of HCC increases markedly in patients with serum HBV DNA levels higher than 10^4 copies/mL.[22] A randomized controlled trial of antiviral therapy has also shown a reduction in the incidence of HCC in association with reductions in serum levels of HBV DNA during therapy.[23]

Indirect carcinogenic effects are the result of the chronic necroinflammatory hepatic disease, in particular cirrhosis, induced by the virus. The increased hepatocyte turnover rate resulting from continuous or recurring cycles of cell necrosis and regeneration acts as a potent tumor promoter. In addition, the distorted architecture characteristic of cirrhosis contributes to the loss of control of hepatocyte growth, and hepatic inflammation generates mutagenic reactive oxygen species. Data from the REVEAL study in Taiwan have shown that genotype C of HBV and specific alleles of the basal core promoter and precore regions of the HBV genome are associated with a higher risk of HCC,[24] whereas in Alaska, genotype F has been more strongly associated with HCC.[25] The transgenic mouse model of Chisari and coworkers has provided indirect support for the role of prolonged hepatocyte injury in hepatocarcinogenesis.[26]

Hepatitis C Virus

Approximately 170 million people in the world today are chronically infected with HCV and are at greatly increased risk for the development of HCC. In Japan, Italy, and Spain, HCV is the single most common etiologic factor for HCC, and in other industrialized countries, HCV infection, often in combination with alcohol abuse, has emerged as a major cause of the tumor.[14,27] Patients with HCV-induced HCC generally are older than those with HBV-related tumors, and it is likely that the HCV infection is acquired mainly in adult life.

Almost all HCV-induced HCCs arise in cirrhotic livers, and most of the exceptions are in livers with chronic hepatitis and fibrosis. This observation strongly suggests that chronic hepatic parenchymal disease plays a key role in the genesis of HCV-related tumors. Because the HCV genome does not integrate into host DNA, the virus would have to exert a direct carcinogenic effect by some other means.

Long-term follow-up of a large group of patients with chronic hepatitis C and cirrhosis or bridging fibrosis found a cumulative 5-year incidence of HCC of just over 5%. The rate was higher among those with cirrhosis (7.0%) than those with bridging fibrosis at baseline (4.1%).[28] A multivariate analysis model showed that older age, black race, lower platelet count, presence of esophageal varices, and smoking were additional risk factors.

It has become apparent that successful treatment of chronic HCV infection, with a sustained virologic response (see Chapter 80), is associated with regression of hepatic fibrosis and a lower-than-expected rate of HCC.[29-31] Long-term maintenance therapy with peginterferon has not been successful in preventing HCC in patients with chronic hepatitis C.[32,33]

Cirrhosis

In all parts of the world, HCC frequently coexists with cirrhosis.[34] All causative forms of cirrhosis may be complicated by tumor formation. A long-term follow-up study of 2126 U.S. military veterans with cirrhosis found that HCC developed in 100 (4.7%) over an average period of 3.6 years.[34] The calculated rate was 1.3/100 patient-years. Risk factors for HCC included obesity, a low platelet count, and the presence of antibody to hepatitis B core antigen. A similar study from Italy found an incidence of HCC of 3.7/100 patient-years among cirrhotic persons with HCV infection and 2.0/100 patient-years among persons with HBV infection. Older age and male gender were confirmed as risk factors among patients with cirrhosis.[35] By contrast, a study from Denmark of more than 8000 patients with alcoholic cirrhosis found a 5-year cumulative risk of HCC of 1.0, suggesting that perhaps patients with this form of cirrhosis were at lower risk of HCC than, for example, those with HCV-related cirrhosis.[36]

Aflatoxin B_1

Dietary exposure to aflatoxin B_1, derived from the fungi *Aspergillus flavus* and *Aspergillus parasiticus*, is an important risk factor for HCC in parts of Africa and Asia. These molds are ubiquitous in nature and contaminate a number of staple foodstuffs in tropical and subtropical regions (see Chapter 89). Epidemiologic studies have shown a strong correlation between the dietary intake of aflatoxin B_1 and incidence of HCC.[37] Moreover, aflatoxin B_1 and HBV interact synergistically in the pathogenesis of HCC. Heavy dietary exposure to aflatoxin B_1 may contribute to hepatocarcinogenesis through an inactivating mutation of the third base of codon 249 of the *TP53* tumor suppressor gene.[38,39]

Other Liver Conditions

HCC develops in as many as 45% of patients with hemochromatosis (see Chapter 75).[40] Malignant transformation was thought previously to occur only in the presence of cirrhosis (and is certainly more likely to do so), but this complication also has been reported in patients without cirrhosis.[41] Excessive free iron in tissues may be carcinogenic, perhaps by generating mutagenic reactive oxygen species.[42] Further support for this theory comes from the observations that black Africans with dietary iron overload are at increased risk of HCC[43] and that rats fed a diet high in iron develop iron-free dysplastic foci and HCC in the absence of cirrhosis.[44] HCC develops occasionally in patients with Wilson disease, but only in the presence of cirrhosis (see Chapter 76).[45] Malignant transformation has been attributed to the cirrhosis but also may result from oxidant stress secondary to the accumulation of copper in the liver.[46] HCC also may develop in patients with other inherited metabolic disorders that are complicated by cirrhosis, such as α_1-antitrypsin deficiency and type 1 hereditary tyrosinemia, and in patients with certain inherited diseases in the absence of cirrhosis—for example, type 1 glycogen storage disease (see Chapter 77). HCC develops in approximately 40% of patients with membranous obstruction of the inferior vena cava, a rare congenital or acquired anomaly (see Chapter 85).

The roles of obesity, diabetes mellitus, and nonalcoholic fatty liver disease (NAFLD) have come to be recognized in the causation of HCC,[47-49] although the mechanisms whereby these overlapping conditions contribute to the development of HCC are unknown. Cirrhosis caused by nonalcoholic steatohepatitis appears to give rise to HCC less frequently than cirrhosis due to HCV but nevertheless appears to carry

TABLE 96-1 Symptoms and Signs of Hepatocellular Carcinoma

Symptom	Frequency (%)
Abdominal pain	59-95
Weight loss	34-71
Weakness	22-53
Abdominal swelling	28-43
Nonspecific GI symptoms	25-28
Jaundice	5-26
Sign	
Hepatomegaly	54-98
Ascites	35-61
Fever	11-54
Splenomegaly	27-42
Wasting	25-41
Jaundice	4-35
Hepatic bruit	6-25

significant risk.[50] Diabetes mellitus is also a risk factor for HCC, although it is not clear if the risk is independent of NAFLD or not.[51]

A statistically significant correlation between the use of oral contraceptive steroids and the occurrence of HCC has been demonstrated in countries in which the incidence of HCC is low and no overriding risk factor for development of the tumor is present.[52] Epidemiologic evidence of a link between cigarette smoking and the occurrence of HCC is conflicting, although most of the evidence suggests that smoking is a minor risk factor[53]; heavy smokers have an approximately 50% higher risk than nonsmokers. The incidence of HCC is increased in patients with HIV infection compared with controls in the general population, presumably because of the increased rate of chronic viral hepatitis in the HIV-positive population.[54]

Although the aforementioned risk factors have been identified, the precise mechanisms whereby they lead to HCC still need to be elucidated. Multiple cellular pathways are involved in causing unconstrained proliferation of hepatocytes and increased angiogenesis against a background of chronic liver disease. These pathways have become the targets for new molecular therapies against HCC (Box 96-2).[55]

Clinical Features

Although the typical clinical features of HCC are well recognized (including abdominal pain and weight loss in patients with cirrhosis), many patients are now diagnosed at an early stage when they have no specific symptoms or signs. This trend toward earlier diagnosis is probably the result of surveillance programs in patients with chronic liver disease (see later). In far-advanced disease, patients with HCC usually present with typical symptoms and signs, and diagnosis is easy. In addition, HCC often coexists with cirrhosis,[56] and the onset of HCC is marked by a sudden unexplained change in the patient's condition.

Patients with HCC often are unaware of its presence until the tumor has reached an advanced stage. The most common (and frequently first) symptom is right hypochondrial or epigastric pain. Other symptoms are listed in Table 96-1.

Physical findings vary with the stage of disease (see Table 96-1). Early in the course, evidence of cirrhosis alone may be present, or abnormal findings may be absent. When the tumor is advanced at the time of the patient's first medical visit, the liver is almost always enlarged, sometimes massively. Hepatic tenderness is common and may be profound, especially in the later stages. The surface of the enlarged liver is smooth, irregular, or frankly nodular. An arterial bruit may be heard over the tumor[57]; the bruit is heard in systole, rough in character, and not affected by changing the position of the patient.

BOX 96-3 Paraneoplastic Syndromes Associated with Hepatocellular Carcinoma

Carcinoid syndrome
Hypercalcemia
Hypertension
Hypertrophic osteoarthropathy
Hypoglycemia
Neuropathy
Osteoporosis
Polycythemia (erythrocytosis)
Polymyositis
Porphyria
Sexual changes—isosexual precocity, gynecomastia, feminization
Thyrotoxicosis
Thrombophlebitis migrans
Watery diarrhea syndrome

Although not pathognomonic, a bruit is a useful clue to the diagnosis of HCC. Less often, a friction rub may be heard over the tumor, but this sign is more characteristic of hepatic metastases or abscesses.

Ascites may be present when the patient is first seen or may appear with progression of the tumor. In most patients, ascites is the result of long-standing cirrhosis and portal hypertension (see Chapter 93), but in some cases it is caused by invasion of the peritoneum by the primary tumor or metastases or obstruction of the hepatic veins or superior vena cava.[58] The ascitic fluid may be blood stained. Splenomegaly, if present, reflects coexisting cirrhosis and portal hypertension.

Physical evidence of cirrhosis may also be noted. Severe pitting edema of the lower extremities extending up to the groins occurs when HCC has invaded the hepatic veins and propagates into and obstructs the inferior vena cava.[58] A Virchow-Trosier (supraclavicular) node, Sister Mary Joseph's (periumbilical) nodule, or enlarged axillary lymph node is rarely present.

Paraneoplastic Manifestations

Some of the deleterious effects of HCC are not caused by local effects of the tumor or metastases (Box 96-3). Each of the paraneoplastic syndromes in HCC is rare or uncommon. One of the more important is type B hypoglycemia, which occurs in less than 5% of patients, manifests as severe hypoglycemia early in the course of the disease,[58] and is believed to result from the defective processing by malignant hepatocytes of the precursor to insulin-like growth factor II (pre-IGF II).[59] By contrast, type A hypoglycemia is a milder form of glycopenia that occurs in the terminal stages of HCC (and other malignant tumors of the liver). It results from the inability of a liver extensively infiltrated by tumor, and often cirrhotic, to satisfy the demands for glucose by a large, often rapidly growing tumor and by the other tissues of the body.

Another important paraneoplastic syndrome is polycythemia (erythrocytosis), which occurs in less than 10% of patients with HCC.[60] This syndrome appears to be caused by the synthesis of erythropoietin or an erythropoietin-like substance by malignant hepatocytes.

Patients with HCC, especially the sclerosing variety, may present with hypercalcemia in the absence of osteolytic metastases. When hypercalcemia is severe, it may result in the typical complications of hypercalcemia, including drowsiness and lethargy. The probable cause is secretion of parathyroid hormone–related protein (PTHrP) by the tumor.[61]

Cutaneous paraneoplastic manifestations of HCC are rare except for pityriasis rotunda (circumscripta), which may be a useful marker of the tumor in black Africans. The rash consists of single or multiple, round or oval, hyperpigmented, scaly lesions on the trunk and thighs that range in diameter from 0.5 to 25 cm.[62]

Diagnosis

The gold standard for the diagnosis of HCC is pathology. For practical purposes (i.e., to apply treatment), HCC can only be diagnosed in the presence of an abnormality on imaging of the liver. Dysplastic nodules and even regenerative cirrhotic nodules can be seen on imaging studies and are potentially confused with HCC. Although enhancement patterns with dynamic imaging of dysplastic nodules and HCC are fairly specific (see later), some overlap occurs.[63,64] Nevertheless, there is a growing consensus that, based on guidelines from the major European and American hepatology societies and now backed by published experience, the diagnosis of HCC can be made in the appropriate clinical setting on the basis of specific imaging characteristics, with or without an elevated serum AFP level.[64-67]

Serum Tumor Markers

Serum tumor markers generally are not diagnostic for HCC by themselves but can be used in conjunction with imaging findings to diagnose HCC. Additionally, they may raise the suspicion of HCC and lead to more sensitive and serial imaging of the liver. Conventional liver biochemical tests do not distinguish HCC from other hepatic mass lesions or cirrhosis.

Many of the substances synthesized and secreted by HCC are not biologically active. Nevertheless, a few are produced by a sufficiently large proportion of tumors to warrant their use as serum markers for HCC. The most helpful of these markers is AFP.

Alpha Fetoprotein. AFP is an α_1-globulin normally present in high concentrations in fetal serum but in only minute amounts thereafter. Reappearance of high serum levels of AFP strongly suggests the presence of HCC (or hepatoblastoma [see later]),[68] especially in populations at risk for HCC.

Measurement of AFP can potentially be used for the diagnosis of HCC, surveillance, and prognostication. With regard to diagnosis, existing guidelines are based on biopsy or liver imaging and do not require use of AFP. Clearly, markedly elevated AFP levels (>10,000 ng/mL to > 1,000,000 ng/mL) can be considered diagnostic for HCC in an appropriate clinical context. Although there is no specific diagnostic cutoff, values above 400 ng/mL in association with a liver mass can be considered diagnostic in most cases.[69]

In the context of surveillance for HCC, the tumor must be detected at an early stage when potentially curative treatment can still be applied. Measurement of AFP has been used for early diagnosis but with sometimes disappointing results. For example, Marrero and colleagues studied a large group of patients with HCC and matched controls and found that the optimal cutoff value of serum AFP level that resulted in the greatest sensitivity was 10.9 ng/mL; still, the sensitivity of the test using this value was only 66%.[70] Therefore, routine use of AFP as part of a surveillance program for HCC has been largely abandoned.[33]

Serum AFP levels appear to have some prognostic utility, particularly with regard to liver transplantation, for which levels above 1000 ng/mL have been associated with poorer outcomes and higher rates of tumor recurrence. An AFP level higher than about 500 ng/mL predicts worse outcomes with liver transplantation compared with lower levels.[71] Attempts to correlate the degree of differentiation of HCC with production of AFP have produced conflicting results.

False-positive AFP results (for HCC) also may occur in patients with tumors of endodermal origin, nonseminomatous germ cell tumors, and pregnancy. A progressively rising serum AFP concentration is highly suggestive of HCC. Because both false-positive and false-negative results are obtained when AFP is used as a serum marker for HCC, the search for an ideal marker continues; however, alternative markers have not proved to be more useful than AFP.

Fucosylated Alpha Fetoprotein. AFP is heterogeneous in structure. Its microheterogeneity results from differences in the oligosaccharide side chain and accounts for the differential affinity of the glycoprotein for lectins. AFP secreted by malignant hepatocytes contains unusual and complex sugar chains that are not found in AFP produced by nontransformed hepatocytes. One variant, *Lens culinaris* agglutinin reactive fraction (AFP-L3), has been suggested to improve the specificity of AFP, particularly AFP serum levels from 10 to 200 ng/mL.[72,73] The recommended cutoff value for AFP-L3 to diagnose HCC is higher than 10%, although the specificity varies depending on the absolute level of AFP. Studies have not confirmed that AFP-L3 has greater sensitivity or specificity than AFP alone for the diagnosis of early HCC.[70,74] Therefore, AFP-L3 is not sufficiently validated to confirm the diagnosis of HCC without other supporting findings, such as suggestive imaging.

Des-γ-Carboxy Prothrombin. Serum concentrations of des-γ-carboxy prothrombin (DCP) (also known as prothrombin produced by vitamin K absence or antagonist II [PIVKA II]) are raised in most patients with HCC.[75] DCP is an abnormal prothrombin that is thought to result from a defect in the post-translational carboxylation of the prothrombin precursor in malignant cells.[76] DCP has been suggested to be a better marker than, or at least complementary to, AFP.[77-79] A large study in Western patients with HCV–related cirrhosis, however, did not confirm this finding.[74] Therefore, because appropriate diagnostic cutoff values are not well established, the precise role of DCP in the diagnosis of HCC still requires validation.

Other Markers. Multiple other potential serum markers for HCC are in the exploratory phase of evaluation, including glypican-3, Golgi protein 73, hepatocyte growth factor, insulin growth factor 1, transforming growth factor-β1, and proteomic profiling using surface-enhanced laser desorption/ionization time-of-flight (SELDI-TOF) mass spectrometry.[80-84] Serum levels of all of these novel markers have been shown to be elevated in patients with HCC compared with patients with chronic liver disease alone, but clear cutoff values and comparisons with other markers have not been established. Some of these markers may be complementary to conventional markers, although none of them has an established high-throughput method of measurement, as required for a clinical test. The roles of these markers in the diagnosis of HCC await further study.

Imaging

The diagnosis of HCC generally requires imaging evidence of a focal lesion in the liver, although large infiltrating lesions can also be diagnostic. Arterial hyperenhancement, particularly seen on dynamic contrast imaging of the liver, is observed because the blood supply of HCC comes from newly formed abnormal arteries (neoangiogenesis).[63,85,86] As a nodule transforms from low- to high-grade dysplasia and then to HCC, the primary blood supply shifts from portal to arterial; new abnormal arterial branches produce characteristic findings on dynamic contrast imaging of the liver.[67]

US. US detects most HCCs but may not distinguish this tumor from other solid lesions in the liver. Therefore, it is more effective as a tool for screening than for diagnosis. As with all imaging methods, the sensitivity increases with increasing size of the lesion. A systematic review of 8 studies using histologic reviews of liver explants has shown that US has fair sensitivity (pooled estimate, 48%; 95% confidence interval [CI], 34% to 62%) with good specificity (97%; 95% CI, 95% to 98%).[64] Advantages of US include safety, availability, and cost-effectiveness. Drawbacks include lack of standardization, examiner dependence, and limited sensitivity with certain body habituses, particularly obesity, and with fatty infiltration of the liver.

The US appearance of HCC is variable because it is influenced by the presence of fat, calcium, and necrosis. Smaller tumors (<5 cm) are most often hypoechoic and may demonstrate a thin peripheral fibrous capsule. Small HCCs can also be uniformly hyperechoic and therefore indistinguishable from focal fat and a hemangioma. With increased size there is generally increased complexity of the nodule.[87] Tumors located immediately under the right hemidiaphragm may be difficult to detect. US with Doppler technology is useful for assessing the patency of the inferior vena cava, portal vein and its larger branches, hepatic veins, and biliary tract.

Dynamic contrast-enhanced Doppler US with IV infusion of CO_2 microbubbles viewed with grayscale imaging and color Doppler US are refinements that, by characterizing hepatic arterial and portal venous flow in tumorous nodules, facilitate the diagnosis of malignant and benign hepatic nodules.[88] These techniques are generally not performed in the United States, owing to lack of approval by the FDA for noncardiac studies.

CT. Multiphase (also called dynamic) multidetector CT is the most popular imaging technique for the diagnosis of HCC.[64,87,88] In order to rely on CT or MRI for the diagnosis of HCC, certain technical specifications for imaging equipment, image acquisition, and dynamic contrast timing are necessary.[33,89] Dynamic contrast-enhanced CT can include noncontrast, arterial, portal venous, and delayed phases. The classic and most diagnostic pattern for HCC is a combination of enhancement in the arterial phase (with the uninvolved liver lacking enhancement), loss of central nodule enhancement compared with the enhancing uninvolved liver (washout), and capsular enhancement in the portal-venous and delayed phases (Fig. 96-2).[33,90] When the lesion is larger than 2 cm in diameter, this pattern has almost 100% specificity for HCC.[90-92] When the nodule is

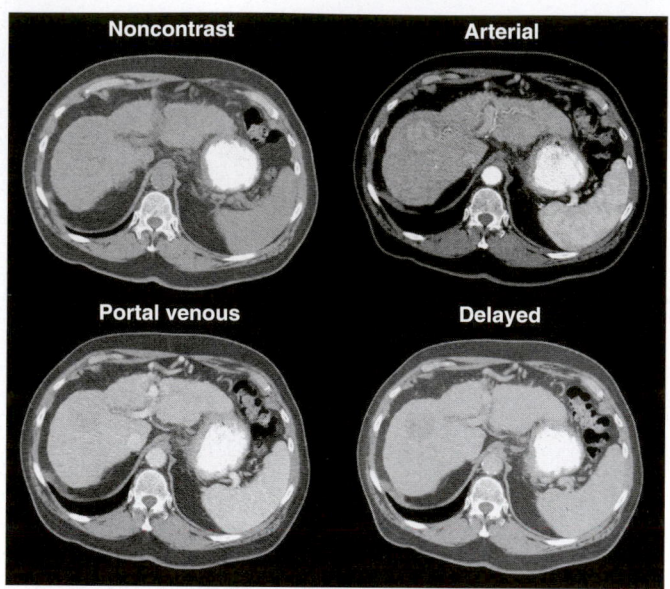

FIGURE 96-2. Dynamic CT of a patient with hepatocellular carcinoma showing no lesion in the noncontrast phase, an enhancing lesion in the right lobe of the liver in the arterial phase of contrast administration, and a faint lesion in the portal venous phase, seen better in the delayed phase.

1 to 2 cm, a diagnosis of HCC or high-grade dysplastic nodule can be made with a specificity greater than 95%.[33,93-95] CT often finds so-called hypervascular-only lesions, which enhance in the arterial phase and become isodense to the surrounding liver in the portal-venous and delayed phases. These lesions may be dysplastic nodules, arterial-portal shunts, atypical hemangiomas, HCC, intrahepatic cholangiocarcinoma, confluent fibrosis, or aberrant venous drainage. Only about 30% of nodules less than 2 cm in diameter are HCCs. Both HCCs and cholangiocarcinomas grow over time, whereas other nodules disappear or remain stable on follow-up studies. HCC may also have other patterns on CT, such as washout only on delayed imaging, a hypovascular nodule, or a fat-containing nodule.[67,96] Guidelines recommend biopsy of lesions larger than 1 cm and serial imaging for lesions smaller than 1 cm that do not have characteristic arterial enhancement and washout.[33] Overall, the pooled estimates of sensitivity and specificity of CT for detecting HCC are 67.5% (95% CI, 55% to 80%) and 92.5% (95% CI, 89% to 96%), respectively. Dynamic CT is also useful for detecting invasion into the portal or hepatic veins and identifying the location and number of tumors; these findings are critical for planning treatment (see later).

MRI. Dynamic MRI using gadolinium contrast agents provides another way of distinguishing HCC from normal liver tissue. The performance of MRI and the findings on multiphase contrast enhancement are similar to those described for CT (Fig. 96-3). Hyperintensity of a nodule on T2-weighted images is specific for HCC.[67,87] The pooled estimates of sensitivity and specificity of MRI for detecting HCC are 80.6% (95% CI, 70% to 91%) and 84.8% (95% CI, 77% to 93%), respectively.[64] MRI may be slightly superior overall to CT, although local expertise should dictate the choice of imaging technique. Close attention to technical specifications is essential.[89] Newer techniques that may improve the specificity of MRI for HCC, particularly in those with atypical vascular-enhancement patterns, include hyperintensity on diffusion-weighted images and lack of enhancement on late images utilizing hepatobiliary-specific contrast agents.

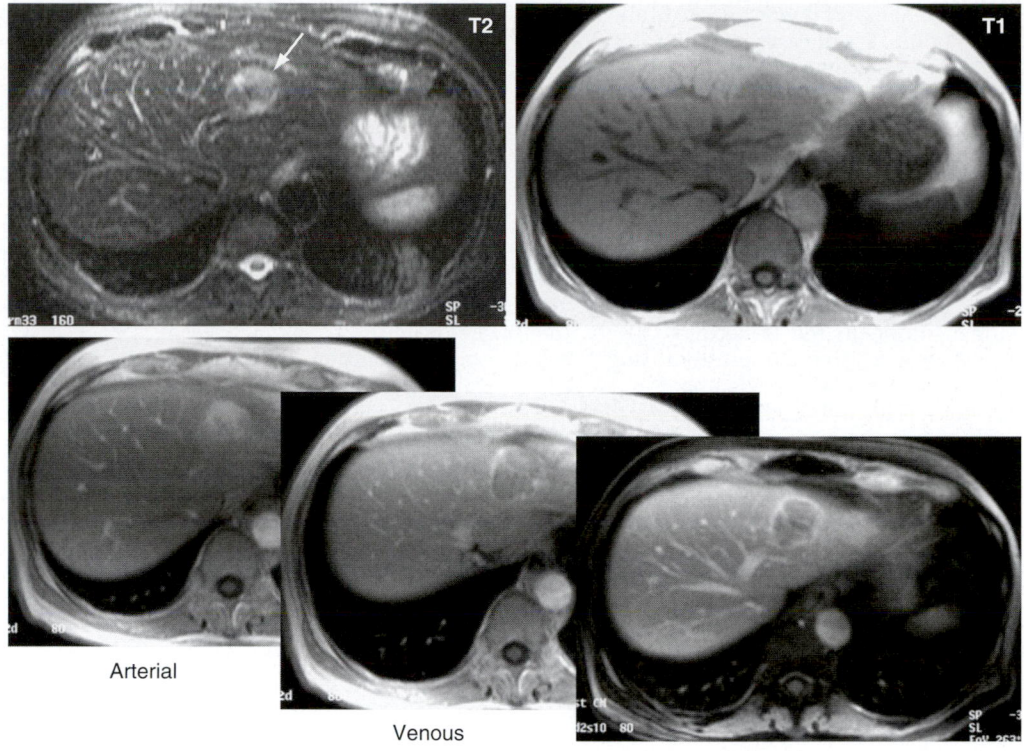

FIGURE 96-3. Multiphasic MRI of the liver showing hepatocellular carcinoma with characteristic features, including hyperintensity *(arrow)* on a T2-weighted image *(top left panel)* but not on a T1-weighted image *(top right panel)*, enhancement during the arterial phase of contrast administration *(bottom left panel)*, with central washout of contrast and capsular enhancement during the venous and delayed phases *(bottom middle and right panels)*.

PET. Whole-body fluorine-18-fluorodeoxyglucose (FDG) PET combined with CT (PET-CT) may have a role in the evaluation of some patients with HCC. The sensitivities of dynamic CT and MRI are superior to that of PET-CT. Several retrospective case series have shown that high avidity in the primary hepatic lesion predicts an increased risk of recurrence after potentially curative treatment. Once a diagnosis of HCC is made, staging involves imaging of the chest, usually with noncontrast CT, and imaging of other areas of the body based on clinical symptoms. Particularly if the tumor within the liver is beyond the Milan criteria, either bone scan or PET-CT can sometimes identify an unrecognized extrahepatic metastasis that would change the treatment plan. The use of PET-CT in HCC needs further study.

Hepatic Angiography. Since the advent of CT and MRI, the role of diagnostic hepatic angiography has been limited. Digital subtraction angiography is helpful for recognizing small hypervascular HCCs but may miss hypovascular tumors. Findings in HCC include arteries that are irregular in caliber and do not taper in the usual way, with smaller branches showing a bizarre pattern and delay in capillary emptying, which is seen as a blush. Angiography is essential for delineating the hepatic arterial anatomy in planning bland embolization, chemoembolization, and radioembolization of the tumor or infusion of cytotoxic drugs directly into the hepatic artery or its branches (see later).

Laparoscopy

Laparoscopy can be used to detect peritoneal and other extrahepatic spread, ascertain whether the nontumorous part of the liver is cirrhotic, and obtain biopsies under direct vision.

Pathology

Definitive diagnosis of HCC depends on demonstrating the typical histologic features. Suitable samples generally can be obtained by percutaneous biopsy or FNA. The yield and safety of the procedure can be increased by directing the needle under US or CT guidance. Laparoscopically directed biopsy is an alternative approach. Needle biopsy of the tumor carries a small but definite risk of spread along the needle track. Pathologic diagnosis of HCC is based on the recommendations of the International Consensus Panel. Immunostaining for glypican-3 (GPC3), heat shock protein HSP70, and glutamine synthetase or gene expression profiling (*GPC3*, *LYVE1* [encoding lymphatic vessel endothelial hyaluronan receptor-1], *BIRC5* [encoding baculoviral inhibitor of apoptosis repeat-containing-5, or survivin]) or both, is recommended to differentiate high-grade dysplastic nodules from early HCC.[97]

Gross Appearance

HCC may take 1 of 3 forms: nodular, massive, or diffusely infiltrating. The nodular variety of HCCs is most common and usually coexists with cirrhosis. It is characterized by numerous round or irregular nodules of various sizes scattered throughout the liver; some of the nodules are confluent. The massive type is characterized by a large circumscribed mass, often with small satellite nodules. This type of tumor is most prone to rupture and is more common in younger patients with a noncirrhotic liver. In the rare diffusely infiltrating variety, a large part of the liver is infiltrated homogeneously by indistinct minute tumor nodules, which may be difficult to distinguish from the regenerative nodules of cirrhosis that are almost invariably present. The portal vein and its branches are infiltrated by tumor in up to 70% of cases seen at autopsy; the hepatic veins and bile ducts are invaded less often.

Microscopic Appearance

HCC is classified histologically into well-differentiated, moderately differentiated, and undifferentiated (pleomorphic) forms.

Well-Differentiated Appearance. Despite the aggressive nature and poor prognosis of HCC, most tumors are well differentiated. Trabecular and acinar (pseudoglandular) varieties occur, sometimes in a single tumor. In the trabecular variety, the malignant hepatocytes grow in irregular anastomosing plates separated by often inconspicuous sinusoids lined by flat cells resembling Kupffer cells. The trabeculae resemble those of normal adult liver but often are thicker and may be composed of several layers of cells. Scanty collagen fibers may be seen adjacent to the sinusoid walls. The malignant hepatocytes are polygonal, with abundant, slightly granular cytoplasm that is less eosinophilic than that of normal hepatocytes. The nuclei are large and hyperchromatic with prominent nucleoli. Bile production is the hallmark of HCC, regardless of the pattern. Gland-like structures are present in the acinar variety. The structures are composed of layers of malignant hepatocytes surrounding the lumen of a bile canaliculus, which may contain inspissated bile. A tubular or pseudopapillary appearance may be produced by degeneration and loss of cells, or cystic spaces may form in otherwise solid trabeculae. The individual cells may be more elongated and cylindrical than in the trabecular variety.

Moderately Differentiated Appearance. Solid, scirrhous, and clear cell varieties of HCC are described. In the solid variety, the cells usually are small, although they vary considerably in shape. Pleomorphic multinucleated giant cells occasionally are present. The tumor grows in solid masses or cell nests. Evidence of bile secretion is rare, and connective tissue is inconspicuous. Central ischemic necrosis is common in larger tumors. In the scirrhous variety, the malignant hepatocytes grow in narrow bundles separated by abundant fibrous stroma. Duct-like structures are occasionally present. In most tumors, the cells resemble hepatocytes. In an occasional tumor, the malignant hepatocytes are predominantly or exclusively clear cells. More often, tumors contain areas of clear cells. The appearance of these cells results from a high glycogen or, in some cases, fat content.

Undifferentiated Appearance. The cells are pleomorphic and vary greatly in size and shape. The nuclei are also extremely variable. Large numbers of bizarre-looking giant cells are present and may be spindle shaped, resembling those of sarcomas. Globular hyaline structures may be seen in all types of HCC. These structures reflect the presence of AFP, α_1-antitrypsin, or other proteins. Mallory's hyaline occasionally is present.

Progenitor Cell HCC. A class of primary liver cancer appears to have its origins in progenitor cells, the stem cells of the liver, located in association with the canals of Hering (see Chapter 71). Progenitor cell activation is seen in association with chronic viral hepatitis and cirrhosis, presumably related to senescence of hepatocytes. These tumors may appear morphologically like typical HCC or mixed cholangiohepatocellular carcinoma. Tumor cells stain positively for cytokeratin 19, and the tumor appears to have a more aggressive course than typical HCC.[98]

Metastases

Extrahepatic metastases are present at autopsy in 40% to 57% of patients with HCCs.[99] The most common sites are the lungs (up to 50% in some reports) and regional lymph nodes ($\approx$20%). The adrenal glands are frequently involved.

Fibrolamellar Hepatocellular Carcinoma

The fibrolamellar variant of HCC typically occurs in young patients, has an approximately equal gender distribution, does not secrete AFP, is not caused by chronic hepatitis B or C, and almost always arises in a noncirrhotic liver.[100-102] The hepatocytes are characteristically plump, deeply eosinophilic, and encompassed by abundant fibrous stroma composed of thin, parallel fibrous bands that separate the cells into trabeculae or nodules. The cytoplasm is packed with swollen mitochondria and, in approximately half of the tumors, contains pale or hyaline bodies. Nuclei are prominent, and mitoses are rare. Fibrolamellar HCC has different immunohistochemical characteristics than usual HCC occurring either with or without cirrhosis; therefore, fibrolamellar HCC is much less likely to stain positively for GPC3, although expression of CK7 is more abundant.[103] Fibrolamellar HCC is more often amenable to surgical treatment and therefore generally carries a better prognosis than conventional HCC. It does not, however, respond to chemotherapy any better than other forms of HCC.

Staging

Accurate staging of HCC is necessary for prognostication and also to assist with selection of therapy. Determining the optimal staging system for HCC has been controversial, in part because it has to take into account both the severity of the underlying liver disease and the size and degree of spread of the tumor. As with all cancers, the TNM system can be used to stage HCC, but this system does not factor in the underlying liver disease. A study[104] comparing the usefulness of 7 staging systems, including the Okuda, TNM, Cancer of the Liver Italian Program (CLIP), Barcelona Clinic Liver Cancer (BCLC), Chinese University Prognostic Index (CUPI), Japanese Integrated Staging (JIS), and Group d'Etude et Traitement du Carcinome Hépatocellulaire (GETCH) systems in a cohort of patients from the United States, has found the BCLC staging system (Fig. 96-4) to have the best independent predictive power for survival. The BCLC system has been adopted by the AASLD for use in its practice guidelines on management of HCC.[33] This staging classification also includes a treatment schedule based on stage.[105]

Natural History and Prognosis

Symptomatic HCC carries a grave prognosis; in fact, the annual incidence and mortality rates for the tumor are almost identical. The main reasons for the poor outcome are the extent of tumor burden when the patient is first seen and the frequent presence of coexisting cirrhosis and hepatic dysfunction. The natural history of HCC in its florid form is one of rapid progression, with increasing hepatomegaly, abdominal pain, wasting, and deepening jaundice, and with death ensuing in 2 to 4 months. In industrialized countries, however, the tumor appears to run a more indolent course with longer survival times.[106] Rare cases of spontaneous tumor regression have been reported (see later).

Treatment

Important advances in the treatment of HCC have occurred since the 1980s and have resulted in improvement of the U.S. population-based 5-year survival rate to 18%[107]; these advances include randomized controlled trials that support the benefits of certain treatments such as chemoembolization and the

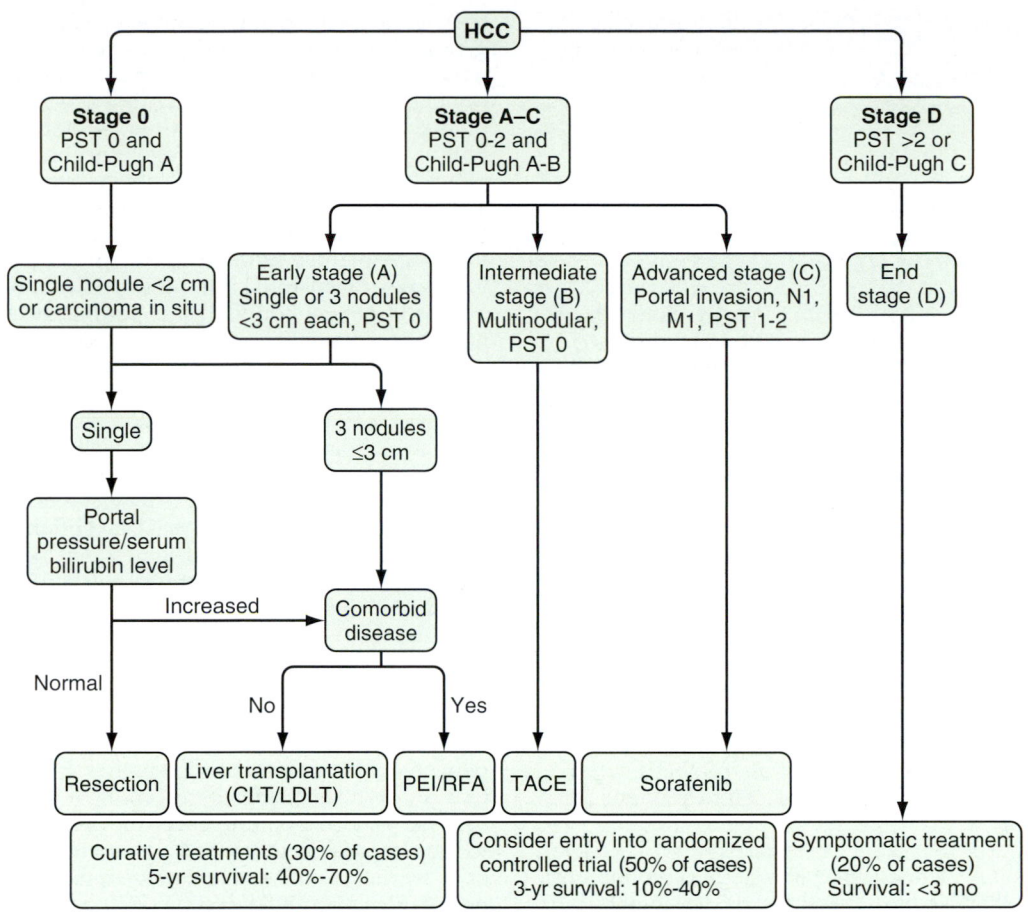

FIGURE 96-4. Barcelona Clinic Liver Cancer (BCLC) staging classification and treatment schedule. Staging is based on tumor size and spread, the patient's performance status (PST) on a scale of 0 (good) to > 2 (poor), and liver function as assessed by the Child-Pugh class (see Chapter 92). Patients with very early (stage 0) hepatocellular carcinoma (HCC) are optimal candidates for surgical resection. Patients with early (stage A) HCC are candidates for radical therapy (resection, cadaveric liver transplantation [CLT] or live-donor liver transplantation [LDLT]), or local ablation via percutaneous ethanol injection (PEI) or radiofrequency ablation (RFA). Patients with intermediate (stage B) HCC benefit from transarterial chemoembolization (TACE). Patients with advanced HCC, defined as the presence of macroscopic vascular invasion, extrahepatic spread, or cancer-related symptoms (PST 1 or 2) (stage C), benefit from sorafenib. Patients with end-stage disease (stage D) should receive symptomatic treatment. The treatment strategy will transition from one stage to another when treatment fails or is contraindicated. M, metastasis stage; N, nodal stage. *(Adapted from Llovet JM, Di Bisceglie AM, Bruix J, et al. Design and endpoints of clinical trials in hepatocellular carcinoma. J Natl Cancer Inst 2008; 100:698-711.)*

advent of the multikinase inhibitor sorafenib. Overwhelming evidence supports the superiority of liver transplantation over other therapies for patients with portal hypertension and cirrhosis (see Chapter 97). Because HCC is usually a combination of 2 diseases—the underlying liver disease (usually cirrhosis with varying degrees of decompensation) and the cancer itself—both factors must be taken into account when selecting treatment. When presented with a patient with HCC, the clinician should decide which is the best initial therapy: surgical resection or liver transplantation, if the patient is a candidate for either; ethanol or radiofrequency ablation (RFA), if possible, based on the size of the tumor; chemoembolization; and, if the tumor is too advanced, sorafenib or a clinical trial. Table 96-2 describes the treatment options for HCC. The BCLC staging classification and treatment schedule can help guide the clinician in choosing the most appropriate treatment (see Fig. 96-4).

Surgical Resection

Surgical therapy, whether by tumor resection or liver transplantation, offers the best chance of cure for HCC. For resection to be considered, the tumor should be confined to one lobe of the liver and favorably located, and ideally, the nontumorous liver tissue should not be cirrhotic. Expert surgical centers can achieve 5- and 10-year survival rates of 40% and 26%, respectively, with a mean tumor diameter of 8.8 cm in noncirrhotic patients.[108] Unfortunately, these patients represent less than 5% of Western cases.[109,110] Resection is also effective if the tumor is limited to the left lobe or a portion of the right lobe, thereby permitting a segmental resection if the patient has Child-Pugh class A cirrhosis, the serum bilirubin level is normal, and portal hypertension is not present (based on imaging, a normal platelet count, absence of varices on endoscopy, and a directly measured hepatic venous pressure gradient < 10 mm Hg).[109] Using these criteria, 5-year survival rates of 50% or better can be achieved. Patients with smaller and solitary tumors have better outcomes. In parts of the world where liver transplantation is not available, surgical resection is a viable option, particularly for Child-Pugh class A patients without portal hypertension and with a MELD score of 9 or less (see Chapters 21 and 97). All the tumor nodules need to be removed, with a negative margin of resection, and the patient needs to be left with enough functional

TABLE 96-2 Treatment Options for Hepatocellular Carcinoma

Modality	Comments
Surgical resection	Curative but limited to noncirrhotic patients and cirrhotic patients without portal hypertension May be technically difficult High recurrence rate
Liver transplantation	Successful in selected patients (Milan criteria; see text and Chapter 97) Requires lifelong immunosuppression Expensive and not available worldwide
Radiofrequency ablation or ethanol injection	Potentially curative for small tumors, including multiple tumors High recurrence rate
Transarterial chemoembolization (TACE)	Prolongs survival in unresectable tumors if hepatic function is preserved; not curative
Chemotherapy	No clear benefit; palliative only Drug toxicity is common
Targeted molecular therapies	Sorafenib is the first such agent shown to improve patient survival

liver volume (usually defined as $\geq$ 40%) to survive the postoperative period.[111-113] Overall, resection is feasible in only approximately 15% of patients. Resection performed at expert surgical centers carries an operative mortality rate of less than 5%, but at low-volume centers the mortality rate is almost 3 times greater.[114] Unfortunately, recurrence after resection occurs in more than 50% in the long term, and salvage liver transplantation is rarely possible.[115]

Liver Transplantation

Liver transplantation is performed in patients in whom the tumor is not resectable but is confined to the liver or in whom advanced cirrhosis and poor liver function preclude resection (see Chapter 97).[33] Liver transplantation is the ideal therapy for HCC because it provides the largest possible resection margin, removes the remaining liver, which is at high risk for de novo tumors, and replaces the dysfunctioning liver. Liver transplantation can fail in patients with extrahepatic tumor, which tends to grow rapidly under the influence of posttransplantation immunosuppression. Because the availability of donor livers is limited, the consensus is that the outcomes of liver transplantation for HCC should be similar to those for other indications for liver transplantation and superior to those for other treatments for HCC. Several large series have demonstrated that if one selects candidates based on the Milan criteria—a single lesion up to 5 cm in size or 2 to 3 lesions, each up to 3 cm, with no large-vessel vascular invasion or metastasis—the 5-year survival rate is 70% to 75%, and the tumor recurrence rate is 10% to 15%.[109,116-118] These criteria led to the HCC MELD exception pathway, which was adopted in the United States in 2002. As a result of the change, the frequency of HCC as an indication for liver transplantation rose from 4.6% to 26% of the total adult liver transplant population. Additionally, progression of the tumor beyond the Milan criteria before a patient undergoes transplantation has largely

been eliminated.[71,119] If the estimated time to transplantation is greater than 6 months, bridging therapy with RFA or transarterial chemoembolization can often be performed to prevent tumor growth beyond Milan criteria (see later). In other parts of the world, waiting times before transplantation remain critical, and when the waiting time increases to 1 year, as many as half of patients will not receive a transplant.[109] An analysis of 4-year survival rates for all patients transplanted in the United States has confirmed that overall outcomes for those transplanted with HCC are only minimally worse than for those transplanted for other indications.[71] Certain subgroups of patients do worse, including those with nodules 3 to 5 cm in diameter, a MELD score of 20 or greater, and a serum AFP level of 455 ng/mL or higher.

Some authorities have advocated expansion of the Milan criteria, provided that the tumor shrinks to within Milan criteria after application of locoregional therapy, based on similar prospective outcomes compared to those within the Milan criteria from small, single-center series, but these patients generally need a special exception from the regional review board in the United States.[120,121] Before these criteria can be widely adopted, a larger multicenter study is needed to confirm the outcomes and define which patients would benefit.

Local Ablation

Local ablative therapies are potentially curative treatments for patients with small tumors (usually < 3 to 5 cm in diameter) that are not amenable to resection or liver transplantation because of patient preference, the number and location of lesions, or significant hepatic dysfunction (Child-Pugh class B or C; see Fig. 96-4).[33] The first of these techniques available was percutaneous ethanol injection (PEI), a relatively effective and safe method that is still used and is most effective for lesions smaller than 2 cm and effective in those up to 3 cm in diameter.[122] PEI requires multiple sessions and, in patients with small tumors and preserved hepatic function, can lead to survival rates similar to those for surgical resection, although no randomized studies have been performed to demonstrate equivalent outcomes.[123] Complications are rare and include tumor seeding of the needle track. RFA has supplanted PEI because it is more effective, particularly with larger tumors (most effective in lesions up to 3 cm and effective in those up to 5 cm), requires fewer sessions, and has similar complication rates.[124] RFA can be performed percutaneously or by a laparoscopic or open surgical approach. Survival rates are similar to those for surgical resection, although recurrence rates are higher and complications are uncommon.[123,125] PEI is generally favored over RFA for lesions adjacent to a major vessel or large bile duct. PEI and RFA have been used to stabilize tumor growth in patients awaiting liver transplantation, but their use for this purpose is controversial and probably unnecessary, unless the waiting time for transplantation is more than 6 months or the tumor burden is near the limit of acceptability for transplantation.[109,126-128]

Chemoembolization

Transarterial chemoembolization (TACE) is a palliative treatment reserved for patients with relatively intact hepatic function (Child-Pugh class A or B with a total bilirubin level < 3 mg/dL), good performance status, and a tumor that is not amenable to local ablative treatments because of size, number, or location (see Fig. 96-4).[33] Six randomized trials and a meta-analysis have compared embolization or chemoembolization with supportive care and have shown overall improved survival with treatment.[129-135] TACE protocols vary greatly (e.g., in chemotherapeutic agents used, number of treatments, use of embolic agents) in clinical trials and clinical practice across the world. More recently, doxorubicin-eluting bead TACE has supplanted conventional TACE because of equal or better efficacy and a better side-effect profile.[136] Small studies using a combination of TACE and RFA or sorafenib have shown acceptable tolerability but no clear survival advantages compared with TACE alone. It is prudent to wait for large randomized clinical trials demonstrating a clear advantage to combination approaches before incorporating them into standard clinical practice. The effectiveness of TACE before liver transplantation has not been fully elucidated, but TACE can be considered if the waiting time for transplantation is more than 6 months or the tumor size is near the acceptable limit for transplantation.[137,138] Theoretically, TACE can be used to reduce the size of the tumor to make resection or transplantation possible (downstaging) or to allow a more conservative resection, although study results are mixed as to whether this approach is effective.[139,140]

Chemotherapy

A large number of anticancer drugs, including alkylating agents, antitumor antibiotics, antimetabolites, plant alkaloids, platinum derivatives, procarbazine, estrogen receptor modulators, and somatostatin, have been tried alone and in various combinations and by different routes of administration for the treatment of HCC, but response rates have invariably been less than 20% and no survival advantage has been demonstrated.[131,141] Several small-molecule, targeted anticancer agents have been developed and studied for the treatment of HCC. Sorafenib, an inhibitor of Raf kinase and the tyrosine kinase activity of vascular endothelial growth factor receptors (VEGFRs) and platelet-derived growth factor receptor (PDGFR), is the first of these new agents to show modest improvement in survival compared with supportive care.[142] The drug should be considered for patients with intact hepatic function (Child-Pugh class A or early class B) and portal vein thrombosis, extrahepatic tumor, or failure of other therapies (see Fig. 96-4). Other targeted agents, alone and in combination with each other and with traditional chemotherapy, are being studied. Patients with advanced hepatic dysfunction (Child-Pugh class C) or advanced tumor symptoms (Eastern Cooperative Oncology Group [ECOG] performance status > 2) have such a poor prognosis that only supportive care should be offered (see Fig. 96-4).[33]

New Alternative Techniques

Newer local ablative techniques including cryoablation, microwave ablation, and laser ablation are being studied in HCC, but these techniques have not been adequately compared with PEI and RFA; their use should be limited to clinical trials. Use of other local regional therapies including stereotactic radiotherapy and radioembolization with ^{90}Y microspheres should be limited to clinical trials or considered when chemoembolization is contraindicated, as in portal vein thrombosis, until these approaches are compared formally with chemoembolization.

Surveillance

Because symptomatic HCC seldom is amenable to surgical cure and responds poorly to conservative treatment, a pressing need exists to prevent the tumor or detect it at a presymptomatic stage when surgical intervention is still possible. An AASLD practice guideline published in 2005 and updated in 2011 provides recommendations for surveillance (Table 96-3).[65]

TABLE 96-3 Persons in Whom Surveillance for Hepatocellular Carcinoma (HCC) May Be Recommended

Patient Group	Annual Incidence of HCC
HBV carriers with cirrhosis	3%-8%
Patients with HCV-related cirrhosis	3%-5%
Patients with PBC and stage 4 fibrosis	3%-5%
Patients with hemochromatosis and cirrhosis	Unknown, probably > 1.5%
Patients with α_1-antitrypsin deficiency and cirrhosis	Unknown, probably > 1.5%
HBV carriers, Asian men > 40 yr	0.4%-0.6%
HBV carriers, Asian women > 50 yr	0.3%-0.6%
HBV carriers, family history of HCC	Unknown (higher than without family history)
HBV carriers, born in Africa	At least 0.5% (HCC occurs at a younger age)
Patients with hepatitis C and stage 3 fibrosis*	<1.5%
HBV carriers, < 40 yr (men) and < 50 yr (women)*	<0.2%
Patients with other causes of cirrhosis	Unknown

*The benefit of surveillance in this group is uncertain.
Adapted from Bruix J, Sherman M. Management of hepatocellular carcinoma: An update. Hepatology 2011; 53:1020-22.

Briefly, patients at high risk of developing HCC should be entered into a surveillance program in which surveillance for HCC is performed using US at 6-month intervals. AFP testing does not appear to increase the sensitivity of US surveillance but adds to the false-positive rate, so AFP testing should not be a part of the standard protocol. Other serum markers for HCC are unproved in the setting of screening, and their use should be limited to clinical studies. Although CT and MRI are effective imaging modalities for the diagnosis of HCC, they are not recommended for routine use in surveillance but may be considered if adequate US images cannot be obtained because of the patient's body habitus. Growing evidence suggests that surveillance for HCC in patients with cirrhosis improves outcome.[143]

Prevention

Although great progress has been achieved in the primary prevention of HBV-induced HCC with universal infant vaccination against HBV in many countries, the full impact of universal HBV vaccination on the occurrence of the tumor will not be realized for many years. A substantial reduction in the frequency of childhood HCC has been well demonstrated in Taiwan, where universal infant vaccination was adopted in the mid-1980s.[144] Similarly, in Alaska, introduction of universal infant vaccination against HBV in 1984 has eliminated HCC in Alaska Native children.[145] In the meantime, huge numbers of existing HBV carriers worldwide remain at risk for HCC, and little progress has been made in preventing malignant transformation in persons with chronic viral hepatitis. Additionally, a vaccine against HCV will not be available in the near future, and prevention of aflatoxin-induced tumors is far from becoming a reality, despite ongoing trials of chemopreventive agents.

Considerable interest has been expressed in the impact of antiviral therapy against HBV and HCV in reducing the incidence of HCC. One randomized controlled trial of long-term therapy of the nucleoside analog lamivudine compared with placebo in patients with chronic hepatitis B has shown a significant decrease in the frequency of clinical events in the treated group, including a decrease in the frequency of HCC (see Chapter 79).[23] Several large retrospective studies have shown a decrease in the frequency of HCC in patients treated successfully for chronic hepatitis C with interferon-based regimens (see Chapter 80).[29,30]

Intrahepatic Cholangiocarcinoma

Cholangiocarcinoma is a malignant neoplasm arising from the biliary duct epithelium. It often carries different names based on the particular portion of the biliary tract involved—small intrahepatic bile ducts (peripheral cholangiocarcinoma), hepatic duct bifurcation (perihilar cholangiocarcinoma, or Klatskin tumor), and extrahepatic bile ducts (bile duct carcinoma). The location of the tumor has a major impact on the presenting symptoms and treatment approach. Perihilar cholangiocarcinoma is classified with the intrahepatic group based on *International Classification of Diseases*, 9th revision (ICD-9), codes even though it is extrahepatic in origin and is the most common form.[146,147] This section will be limited to a discussion of true intrahepatic cholangiocarcinoma; extrahepatic cholangiocarcinoma including the perihilar type is discussed in Chapter 69.

Epidemiology

Intrahepatic cholangiocarcinoma represents approximately 10% to 20% of all primary liver cancers and up to 20% of cholangiocarcinomas. The geographic variation in prevalence rates is marked, ranging from 0.2 to 96/100,000 in men and from 0.1 to 38/100,000 in women, because of differences in the frequencies of known risk factors in various populations.[148] The highest incidence rates are found in parts of Asia, most notably certain regions of Thailand, Hong Kong, China, Japan, and Korea. Chronic infestation of the biliary tract with one of the liver flukes is thought to be the cause of these high rates (see Chapter 84).[149] The overall incidence rate in the United States is 0.85/100,000, with a 1.5-fold higher rate in men than women. The rate in whites is about equal to that in African Americans and about half that in Asians. Intrahepatic cholangiocarcinoma is rare before 40 years of age, and historically the worldwide approximate average age at presentation is 50 years. Epidemiologic data indicate that the age at presentation has shifted to more than 65 years. Additionally, the incidence and mortality rates are increasing worldwide.[146] Surveillance, Epidemiology, and End Results (SEER) registry data from the United States have shown a 165% increase between the late 1970s and the late 1990s.[148] This increase may be a result, in part, of the increased prevalence of cirrhosis, particularly HCV-associated cirrhosis.[150]

Etiology and Pathogenesis

Although the underlying predisposing factor for most cases of cholangiocarcinoma is unknown, a number of risk factors have been recognized. The strongest association is with *Opisthorchis viverrini*, a liver fluke endemic in parts of Southeast Asia and acquired by ingestion of raw or uncooked fish.[148,151,152] The association with *Clonorchis sinensis*, a related liver fluke, is weaker (see Chapter 84).[153] An association with the radiographic contrast agent thorium dioxide (Thorotrast), which was banned in the 1950s, has been well established.[154] PSC is linked to a diagnosis of cholangiocarcinoma at a young age, with a lifetime risk of 8% to 20% (see Chapter 68).[155-157] Congenital and acquired abnormalities of the biliary tract that may result in bile stasis, chronic inflammation, and infection (as in biliary atresia,[158] von Meyenburg complexes,[159] Caroli's disease,[160] choledochal cyst,[160] and intrahepatic cholelithiasis [hepatolithiasis]) have been associated with the development of cholangiocarcinoma (see Chapter 62). The previously discussed risk factors are most important for perihilar and extrahepatic bile duct cancer, although they probably play a role in intrahepatic cholangiocarcinoma also. Diabetes mellitus also seems to add to the risk for both types.[161] Cirrhosis, particularly caused by HCV and perhaps alcohol, also has been associated with cholangiocarcinoma.[150]

Malignant transformation of the bile duct cells generally occurs in an environment of inflammation or cholestasis (or both), usually as a result of one of the known risk factors. The proposal has been made that a combination of these environmental factors and genetic predisposition (e.g., defects in oncogenes or bile salt transporters) leads to an accumulation of genetic defects that results in carcinoma.[146,162] A polymorphism in the gene for the natural killer cell receptor G2D (NKG2D) has been associated with an increased risk of cholangiocarcinoma in patients with PSC.[163] At the molecular level, numerous changes have been described, including mutations of the *K-ras* gene, the gene for interleukin (IL)-6, and allelic loss or mutations of *TP53* and *p16*, as well as many others (see Chapter 69).

Clinical Features

Peripheral cholangiocarcinoma seldom produces symptoms until the tumor is advanced. The clinical features are then similar to those of HCC, including malaise, weight loss, abdominal pain, and jaundice, which may be more frequent and prominent than with HCC.[160,164]

Diagnosis

In patients with peripheral cholangiocarcinoma, often only the serum alkaline phosphatase level is elevated. CA 19-9 is the most frequently used serum tumor marker for cholangiocarcinoma but has significant limitations because CA 19-9 levels are also elevated in pancreatic, colorectal, gastric, and gynecologic cancers and in acute bacterial cholangitis (see Chapter 60).[165] CA 19-9 is always undetectable in the 7% of the population that is Lewis blood group negative. In patients with unexplained biliary obstruction without PSC, the sensitivity of CA 19-9 is 53%, and the negative predictive value is 72% to 92%, for a cutoff value of 100 U/mL. In patients with PSC, the sensitivity ranges from 38% to 89% and specificity from 50% to 98%. The addition of CEA probably does not improve the performance of CA 19-9 in the setting of PSC.

Initial imaging with US helps identify biliary obstruction. Dynamic contrast-enhanced CT or MRI further aids in localizing the lesion and determining the possibility of resection.[146,166] MRI with MRCP is a superior modality because of a higher sensitivity than CT for detecting lesions and localizing biliary obstruction. The tumor is hypointense on T1-weighted images and moderately intense on T2-weighted images. With dynamic contrast, the tumor generally has progressive enhancement in arterial, portal venous, and delayed phases, thereby helping to distinguish it from HCC, which usually has washout in the later 2 phases (see earlier). Endoscopic EUS with FNA of a lesion in patients without PSC has the advantage of improving sensitivity and specificity for the diagnosis of the primary lesion and nodal metastasis but the disadvantage of causing peritoneal seeding and, therefore, should be avoided if surgical resection is contemplated. Percutaneous biopsies also carry the risk of peritoneal seeding and are generally avoided if the tumor is potentially resectable.

Pathology

Peripheral cholangiocarcinoma usually is a large and solitary tumor, but it may be multinodular.[167] It is grayish-white, firm, and occasionally umbilicated and usually produces a focal hepatic mass; rarely, the tumor can grow alongside and infiltrate the bile ducts or occur as an intraductal papillary lesion.[166] The tumor is poorly vascularized and rarely bleeds internally or ruptures. Metastatic nodules may be distributed irregularly throughout the liver. The bile ducts peripheral to the tumor may be dilated, resulting in some cases in biliary cirrhosis. Metastases in regional lymph nodes occur in about 50% of cases.

Microscopically, cholangiocarcinoma exhibits acinar or tubular structures that resemble those of other adenocarcinomas.[167] Most tumors are well to moderately differentiated. Secretion of mucus may be demonstrable, but bile production is not seen. The tumor cells provoke a variable desmoplastic reaction, and in many tumors, the collagenized stroma may be the most prominent feature. Distinguishing the tumor from metastatic adenocarcinoma may be difficult, and some experts have advocated assuming that an adenocarcinoma in the liver is cholangiocarcinoma if no primary tumor can be found elsewhere.[168] Immunohistochemistry may be helpful, with cytokeratin (CK)7 usually staining strongly and CK20 staining negative or weakly. A panel of immunohistochemical stains is usually used to exclude common sites of metastatic adenocarcinoma, although metastasis from gallbladder, pancreas, and upper GI tract cancers needs to be excluded based on imaging and endoscopy, if indicated.[169]

Treatment and Prognosis

Early diagnosis of intrahepatic cholangiocarcinoma is unusual, and the annual mortality rate is almost identical to the annual incidence of the tumor.[160,164] Long-term survival after diagnosis in the United States based on the SEER database is dismal, with a 1-year survival rate of 28% and a 5-year survival rate less than 5%. The 5-year survival rate has not improved since the late 1980s.[148]

In a person with suspected or proved intrahepatic cholangiocarcinoma, staging is recommended to determine surgical resectability, which is the only opportunity for cure. The staging evaluation usually includes dynamic MRI of the abdomen and MRCP (or dynamic helical CT, if MRI is unavailable) and a chest x-ray or chest CT.[146] PET has been assessed in small series and does not clearly add to other modalities. EUS with FNA of suspicious lymph nodes may detect otherwise unrecognized metastasis in up to 20% of cases, but transduodenal or transgastric biopsy of the primary lesion should be avoided because of significant risk of needle track seeding.[166] Surgical resectability of intrahepatic cholangiocarcinoma

should be determined in conjunction with an experienced hepatobiliary surgeon and requires the ability to achieve clear surgical margins, which usually necessitates a major hepatectomy. Criteria for resection include absence of all the following: evidence of extrahepatic metastasis, main portal vein or hepatic artery invasion or encasement, bilateral segmental bile duct involvement, and contralateral hepatic lobar atrophy. Additionally, the patient must be medically fit to undergo surgery and have sufficient hepatic reserve. Without clear margins of resection, surgery provides benefits similar to those of endoscopic or biliary drainage. Patients well selected for surgical resection achieve a 1- to 2-year median survival and a 29% to 36% 5-year survival rate.

If resection is not possible and major biliary obstruction is present, biliary drainage, either endoscopic or percutaneous, should be performed, because drainage appears to improve symptoms and survival, although these outcomes generally apply to perihilar cholangiocarcinoma (see Chapter 70).[168] Placement of an expandable metal stent is generally preferred to plastic stents if the expected survival of the patient is more than 3 to 6 months.[146] The rates of response and survival following radiation therapy and chemotherapy are modest. A randomized trial showed a survival benefit of 3.6 months for locally advanced or metastatic biliary tract cancer with the combination of cisplatin and gemcitabine.[170] Photodynamic therapy in addition to biliary stent placement may provide benefit. Small case series suggest tumor responses and possibly improved survival for unresectable disease with conventional and drug-eluting bead TACE and transarterial radioembolization but have not been rigorously assessed. Liver transplantation alone or in combination with neoadjuvant and adjuvant chemotherapy results in unacceptably high recurrence rates and less than a 50% 5-year survival.

Hepatoblastoma

Epidemiology

In children, hepatoblastoma is the third most common malignant tumor and the most common malignant hepatic tumor. It occurs almost exclusively in the first 3 years of life; boys are affected twice as often as girls.[171,172]

Etiology and Pathogenesis

Hepatoblastoma may occur sporadically or in association with hereditary syndromes such as familial adenomatous polyposis (FAP) (see Chapter 126) and Beckwith-Wiedemann syndrome (characterized by macroglossia, macrosomia, midline abdominal wall defects, ear creases or pits, and neonatal hypoglycemia), suggesting a possible role for chromosomes 5 and 11 in the genesis of the tumor. Sporadic hepatoblastoma is not associated with any known environmental risk factor, and its pathogenesis is unclear. Most patients with hepatoblastoma have mutations of the FAP tumor suppressor gene, which down-regulates β-catenin, and a similar number have activating mutations of the β-catenin gene, raising the possibility that the Wnt signaling pathway plays a role in the development of the tumor.[173] Birth weight under 1500 g confers a relative risk for hepatoblastoma of approximately 20, although the mechanism is not known.[174]

Clinical Features

Most children with hepatoblastoma come to medical attention because of abdominal swelling.[175] Other reasons include failure to thrive, weight loss, poor appetite, abdominal pain, irritability, and intermittent vomiting and diarrhea. The tumorous liver almost always is enlarged and firm and may be tender. Its surface is smooth or nodular. Hepatoblastomas rarely rupture. Distant metastases are evident, usually in the lung, in 20% of patients at the initial visit.[176] The tumor occasionally causes isosexual precocity in boys as a result of the ectopic production of HCG.[177]

Diagnosis

AFP is present in high concentrations in the serum of 80% to 90% of patients with hepatoblastoma and is a useful clue to the diagnosis.[178] The few patients with a low serum AFP level appear to have a worse prognosis.[179] Anemia is common, as is thrombocytosis, which is attributed to raised serum thrombopoietin levels. Pulmonary metastases and, rarely, mottled calcification in the tumor may be seen on plain radiography. US is the most widely used initial imaging technique, although the findings are not specific. CT and MRI are used to define the extent of the tumor and plan definitive surgery. The tumor is seen as an avascular mass on hepatic arteriography.[180]

Pathology

Hepatoblastomas are the malignant derivatives of incompletely differentiated hepatocyte precursors. Their constituents are diverse, reflecting both the multipotentiality of their mesodermal origin and the progressive stages of embryonic and fetal development. Pathologists separate hepatoblastomas into subtypes based on their histopathologic appearance, each with a prognosis that can be risk stratified. The pure fetal type has an excellent prognosis, whereas the aggressive small-cell undifferentiated tumor has the worst prognosis and is usually assigned the most intensive therapeutic interventions.[174] The tumors usually are solitary, ranging in diameter from 5 to 25 cm, and always well circumscribed (about half are encapsulated). They vary in color, ranging from tan to grayish-white, and contain foci of hemorrhage, necrosis, and calcification. Vascular channels may be prominent on the capsular surface. Epithelial hepatoblastomas are solid, whereas tumors of the mixed variety often are separated into lobules by white bands of collagen tissue.

Two types of epithelial cells are present in the tumor.[181] Cells of the first type resemble fetal hepatocytes and are arranged in irregular plates, usually 2 cells thick, with bile canaliculi between individual cells and sinusoids between plates. Cells of the second type are embryonal and are less differentiated than the fetal type. Mixed hepatoblastomas contain mesenchymal tissue consisting of areas of a highly cellular primitive type of mesenchyme intimately admixed with epithelial elements. Cartilage and striated muscle may be present. Hepatoblastomas may show foci of squamous cells, with or without keratinization, and foreign body–type giant cells. Vascular invasion may be evident. Metastases most commonly involve lung, abdominal lymph nodes, and brain.

Treatment and Prognosis

Hepatoblastomas are rapidly progressive. If the lesion is solitary and sufficiently localized to be resectable, surgery often is curative, with 5-year survival rates as high as 75%.[175] The current practice is to pretreat the patient with cisplatin and doxorubicin, but platinum-based therapy is also widely used.[182] When the tumor is judged to be inoperable, neoadjuvant chemotherapy may reduce the size of the tumor sufficiently to permit resection. Encouraging results also have been obtained with liver transplantation in patients with bilobar multifocal tumors without extrahepatic extension.[183] If surgery is not possible or the tumor recurs after surgery, the prognosis

is generally poor. Liver transplantation plays an increasing role because of technical success with live-donor and split-liver transplantation.

Angiosarcoma

Epidemiology

Although rare, angiosarcoma is the most common malignant mesenchymal tumor of the liver.[184,185] It occurs almost exclusively in adults and is most prevalent in the sixth and seventh decades of life.[186,187] Men are affected 4 times as often as women.

Etiology and Pathogenesis

Despite its rarity, hepatic angiosarcoma is of special interest because specific risk factors have been identified, although no cause is discerned in most cases. In early reports, the tumor became evident approximately 20 years after exposure to thorium dioxide (see Chapter 89).[188] Angiosarcoma has also occurred in German vintners who used arsenic-containing insecticides and drank wine adulterated with arsenic.[189] A few patients with angiosarcoma had taken potassium arsenite (Fowler's solution) for many years to treat psoriasis.[190] Hepatic angiosarcoma in workers exposed to vinyl chloride monomer (VCM) was first reported in 1974.[186,191,192] The monomer is converted by enzymes of the endoplasmic reticulum to reactive metabolites that form DNA adducts and guanosine-to-adenine transitions in the K-ras and TP53 genes. Angiosarcomas have occurred after exposures of 11 to 37 years (or after shorter periods with a heavy initial exposure).[184] The mean age of patients at diagnosis is 48 years. In addition to angiosarcoma, persons exposed to VCM may be at increased risk of HCC and soft tissue sarcoma.

Clinical Features

The most common presenting symptom is upper abdominal pain. Other frequent complaints are abdominal swelling, rapidly progressing liver failure, malaise, weight loss, poor appetite, and nausea.[185,186] Vomiting occurs occasionally. The duration of symptoms generally ranges from 1 week to 6 months, but a few patients have had symptoms for as long as 2 years before seeking medical attention.

The liver almost always is enlarged and usually is tender. Its surface may be irregular, or a definite mass may be felt. An arterial bruit occasionally is heard over the enlarged liver. Splenomegaly may be present and is attributed to the hepatic fibrosis and consequent portal hypertension that may also complicate exposure to VCM. Ascites is frequent, and the fluid may be blood stained. The patient often has jaundice. Fever and dependent edema are less common. Approximately 15% of patients present with acute hemoperitoneum following tumor rupture. Rarely, pulmonary or skeletal metastases are present.

Diagnosis

A rising serum bilirubin level and other evidence of progressive hepatic dysfunction may be present, especially in the later stages of the tumor. In patients who were exposed to thorium dioxide, radiopaque deposits of the material may be evident in the liver and spleen.[188] One or more mass lesions may be demonstrated on US, CT, or MRI, but diffusely infiltrating tumor may not be visualized. Hepatic arteriography reveals a characteristic appearance.[193] The hepatic arteries are displaced by the tumor, which shows a blush and "puddling" during the middle of the arterial phase that persist for many seconds, except in the central area, which may be hypovascular.

Pathology

Angiosarcomas usually are multicentric.[194] Their hallmark is the presence of blood-filled cysts, although solid growth also is seen. The lesions are fairly well circumscribed but not encapsulated. Larger masses are spongy and bulge beneath Glisson's capsule.

The earliest microscopic change is the presence of hypertrophic sinusoidal lining cells with hyperchromatic nuclei in ill-defined loci throughout the liver. With progression of the lesion, sinusoidal dilatation and disruption of hepatic plates occur, and the malignant cells become supported by collagen tissue. Enlarging vascular spaces lined by malignant cells cause the tumor to become cavernous. The malignant endothelial cells usually are multilayered and may project into the cavity in intricate fronds and tufts supported by fibrous tissue. The fronds commonly are elongated with ill-defined borders. The cytoplasm is clear and faintly eosinophilic. Nuclei are hyperchromatic and vary greatly in size and shape; some cells are multinucleated. Evidence of phagocytosis may be seen. Foci of extramedullary hematopoiesis are common, and invasion of the portal and central veins occurs in most cases. Distant metastases are present in 50% of tumors.

Complications and Prognosis

Hepatic angiosarcomas grow rapidly, and the prognosis is poor; death ensues within 6 months. Patients may have thrombocytopenia resulting from entrapment of platelets within the tumor (Kasabach-Merritt syndrome), DIC with secondary fibrinolysis,[195] or microangiopathic hemolytic anemia as a result of fragmentation of erythrocytes within the tumor circulation.[196]

Treatment

Operative treatment is usually precluded by the advanced stage of the tumor. Even when surgery is undertaken, the patient commonly survives only 1 to 3 years, although long-term survival may be achieved in the few patients with a solitary tumor.[185] The results of irradiation and chemotherapy are poor.

Epithelioid Hemangioendothelioma

Epidemiology

Epithelioid hemangioendothelioma is a rare tumor with an estimated incidence of less than 0.1 per 100,000.[184] A series of 137 cases has been collected at a specialized referral center.[197] Two thirds of patients were female, and the tumor occurred at all ages in adulthood.

Clinical Features

Patients typically present with nonspecific symptoms such as abdominal pain and weight loss.

Diagnosis

Imaging studies show a characteristically highly vascular mass that may infiltrate throughout the liver. Case reports indicate that the tumor can be visualized on PET. Correct diagnosis requires histologic examination of tissue obtained by biopsy. Epithelioid hemangioendothelioma should be distinguished from infantile hemangioendothelioma, a not uncommon liver tumor of infancy that may be associated with abdominal distension, failure to thrive, heart failure, bronchiolitis, and even sudden infant death (see later). Type II infantile hemangioendothelioma tends to be more aggressive and may be indistinguishable from hepatic angiosarcoma in some cases.[198,199]

Pathology

Tumors are often multiple and may be diffuse throughout the liver. Histologically, they are characterized by the presence of dendritic and epithelioid cells that contain vacuoles, representing intracellular lumina. These cells stain positively for endothelial markers, such as factor VIII–related antigen, CD34, or CD31.

Complications and Prognosis

The tumor has low-grade malignant potential and must be distinguished from hemangiosarcoma, because it has a much better prognosis if treated appropriately and aggressively. Epithelioid hemangioendothelioma may metastasize, both within and beyond the liver.

Treatment

The primary treatment modality for epithelioid hemangioendothelioma is surgical, including resection or liver transplantation. Transplantation appears to be effective for this tumor, even in the presence of advanced or even metastatic disease. The tumor does not appear to be sensitive to radiation or chemotherapy.

Other Primary Malignant Tumors of the Liver

Undifferentiated (embryonal) sarcoma is a rare primary malignancy of the liver that occurs in both children and adults.[200,201] The tumor tends to be aggressive, but long-term survival can be achieved with radical surgery and chemotherapy.[202] Other rare neoplasms arising in the liver include liposarcoma,[203] primary lymphoma,[185,204] and rhabdomyosarcoma.[201]

Hepatic Metastases

Epidemiology and Etiology

The liver is the most frequent target for metastatic spread of tumors. Hepatic metastases occur in 40% to 50% of adult patients with extrahepatic primary malignancies.[205] Foremost among the reasons for the high frequency of hepatic metastases are the double blood supply of the liver and the presence of fenestrations in the sinusoidal endothelium that facilitate penetration of malignant cells into the hepatic parenchyma.[206] Hepatic metastases commonly originate from primary sites in the distribution of the portal venous system, including the pancreas, stomach, and colon. Outside this distribution, tumors of the lung and breast are the most common origins of hepatic metastases.

Clinical Features

Symptoms resulting from hepatic metastases often are absent or overshadowed by those of the primary tumor. Occasionally, the symptoms and signs attributable to metastases are the presenting manifestations of an asymptomatic primary tumor. In such cases, the likely symptoms are malaise, weight loss, and upper abdominal pain. Jaundice, when present, is seldom attributable to replacement of hepatic tissue by metastases. Depending on the extent of the metastatic disease, the liver may be enlarged, sometimes markedly. Its surface may be irregular, and umbilicated nodules may be felt by the examiner. A friction rub may be heard over hepatic metastases.

Diagnosis

CT is the most useful imaging technique.[207] Multiphase helical CT and CT during arterial portography are more sensitive than conventional CT. Dynamic contrast-enhanced Doppler US with IV infusion of CO_2 microbubbles also is useful for the diagnosis of hepatic metastases.[87] T1-weighted MRI may also be helpful, and iron oxide–enhanced MRI is even better. FDG PET-CT is helpful in identifying a liver mass as malignant and, more important, in locating extrahepatic disease that may influence treatment.

Pathology

Macroscopic Appearance

Hepatic metastases usually are multiple.[205] Their pathologic features vary, depending on the site of origin. Metastases are expansive, when they are discrete, or infiltrative. Individual metastases may reach a large size, and with multiple metastases, the liver may be greatly enlarged. Metastases commonly are gray-white and may show scattered hemorrhages or central necrosis. Individual metastases may be surrounded by a zone of venous stasis. Subcapsular lesions often are umbilicated. The dictum that cirrhotic livers are less likely than noncirrhotic livers to harbor metastatic deposits remains to be verified.

Microscopic Appearance

The microscopic features, including the degree of stromal growth, of most hepatic metastases duplicate those of the tumor of origin. Metastatic deposits usually are easily delineated from the surrounding liver tissue. Invasion of portal or hepatic veins may be seen, although less often than with HCC.[205] It may be difficult to distinguish metastatic adenocarcinoma from primary cholangiocarcinoma (see earlier).[168]

Treatment and Prognosis

The extent of replacement of liver tissue by metastases generally determines the patient's prognosis. The greater the tumor burden, the worse the outlook, with only approximately 50% of patients surviving 3 months after the onset of symptoms and less than 10% surviving more than 1 year.[208] Improved imaging modalities, advances in surgical techniques for resection, and new chemotherapeutic agents and regional therapies have made it possible to achieve long-term survival in individual patients. Long-term survival has been accomplished most often by resection of hepatic metastases in patients with colorectal cancer, a substantial number of whom have been cured or have obtained up to 20 years of disease-free survival.[208-210] Survival for 5 years can be achieved in up to 60% who undergo resection of a solitary colon cancer metastasis to the liver.[211] If the primary tumor has been removed completely and metastases are confined to the liver, resection of hepatic metastases should be considered. Liver transplantation, with or without chemotherapy, has been limited to a few patients with rare slow-growing malignancies such neuroendocrine tumors but is generally contraindicated. RFA is a valid therapy for colorectal metastases in patients who are unable to tolerate or refuse surgical resection. Other invasive methods of destroying metastases, such as ethanol injection, freezing with cryoprobes, and laser vaporization, warrant further study. Radiation therapy and intra-arterial infusion of cytotoxic drugs have limited roles.

BENIGN TUMORS

Hepatocellular Adenoma

Epidemiology

Hepatocellular adenomas (also termed hepatic adenomas and telangiectatic focal nodular hyperplasia or adenomas) are rare benign epithelial tumors of the liver that occur predominantly in women in the second to fifth decades of life. They are commonly associated with use of estrogen, including exogenous estrogens in oral contraceptive pills (OCPs), and can also be seen in the absence of exogenous estrogens and in men. The annual incidence of hepatic adenoma in OCP users is 30 to 40 per million compared with 1 to 1.3 per million in nonusers.[212] OCP use for more than 5 years, older age, and use of high-potency hormones all appear to increase the risk. Cessation of estrogens often leads to regression of an adenoma, adding support to their role in the pathogenesis. Hepatocellular adenomas have been associated with anabolic androgenic steroid use and FAP.

Hepatocellular adenomas are common in patients with glycogen storage disease type I, with a frequency of 22% to 75%, and type III, with a frequency of 25%. In this setting, there is a male predominance, and the diagnosis is usually made during childhood[213] (see Chapter 77).

The designation *liver adenomatosis* is usually applied to cases with multiple (arbitrarily > 10) hepatocellular adenomas and has been associated with germline and somatic mutations in hepatocyte nuclear factor-1α (HNF-1α) and with NAFLD in the adjacent liver parenchyma. It is not clear whether liver adenomatosis is a distinct entity, but it may be more difficult to manage clinically than a single or a few adenomas because of the high number of lesions.[214,215]

Etiology and Pathogenesis

Multiple genetic alterations have been identified in hepatocellular adenomas. Investigators in Bordeaux, France, proposed—and other groups have validated—a phenotypic-genotypic classification that divides hepatic adenomas into 4 groups[216,217] (Fig. 96-5). These groups have varying risks for transformation to HCC and implications for management. Bilallelic mutations of the TCF1 gene that encodes HNF-1α have been identified in 19% to 60% of patients with hepatic adenoma.[214,216,217] HNF-1α is implicated in hepatocyte differentiation and liver development.[214] Most of the mutations are somatic, although germline mutations associated with mature-onset diabetes of the young (MODY3), an autosomal dominant form of nonketotic diabetes mellitus presenting before age 25, are common in patients with liver adenomatosis (see earlier).[218] A second pathway, the Wnt pathway, which has also been implicated in 10% to 25% of HCCs, is activated in 12% to 14% of hepatocellular adenomas.[216,217,219] β-Catenin activation via this pathway appears to confer a higher risk of malignant transformation and is associated with glycogen storage disease and adenomas in male patients.[216,220] The third identified pathway for formation of hepatocellular adenomas includes acute inflammatory responses demonstrable by histologic examination of the tumor[216,220] and associated with obesity and alcohol (see Fig. 96-5). This group often has activation of the

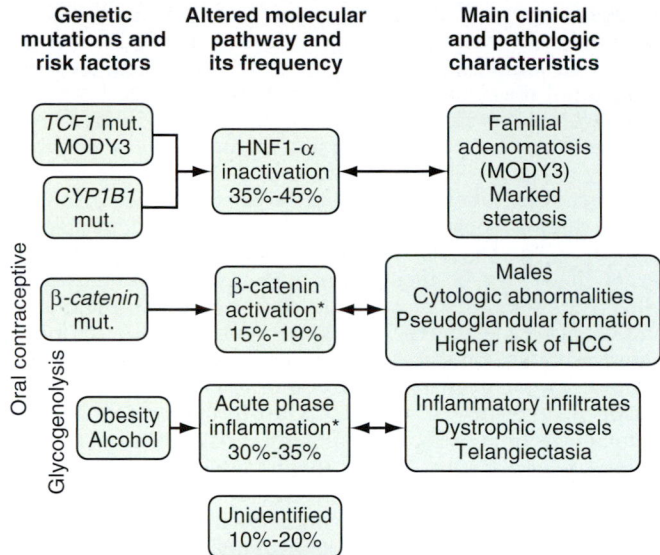

Genetic mutations and risk factors	Altered molecular pathway and its frequency	Main clinical and pathologic characteristics

FIGURE 96-5. Schematic representation of the different molecular pathways altered in hepatocellular adenoma. *Left,* Main risk factors and known genetic predispositions. *Center,* Altered molecular pathways and their frequencies. *Right,* Principal clinical and pathologic features of the types of adenomas. *Arrows* indicate the significant relationships. *Some tumors may be simultaneously β-catenin activated and inflammatory. CYP1B1, cytochrome P450 1B1; HCC, hepatocellular carcinoma; HNF-1α, hepatocyte nuclear factor 1α (gene symbol *TCF1*); MODY3, maturity-onset diabetes of the young type 3; mut, mutation. *(Adapted from Rebouissou S, Bioulac-Sage P, Zucman-Rossi J. Molecular pathogenesis of focal nodular hyperplasia and hepatocellular adenoma. J Hepatol 2008; 48:163-70.)*

IL-6 inflammatory signaling pathway, including STAT-3.[221] A small percentage of this group also exhibit β-catenin activation.

Clinical Features

Hepatocellular adenomas manifest in a number of ways. They may be found incidentally on abdominal imaging and produce no symptoms. Rarely, if large, they can be discovered during a routine physical examination. Approximately 25% of patients experience pain in the right hypochondrium or epigastrium. The pain usually is mild and ill defined but may be severe as a result of bleeding into or infarction of the tumor. If the liver is enlarged, the surface usually is smooth, and the liver may be slightly tender. The most alarming presentation is with severe abdominal pain and hypotension from acute hemoperitoneum following rupture of an adenoma. This complication is not uncommon, especially with tumors linked to OCP use, and carries an appreciable mortality rate.[222,223] Tumors that rupture generally are large (>5 cm) and solitary, although the most important determinant of rupture is a superficial location. Often, the affected woman is menstruating at the time; rupture also may occur during pregnancy.[224] The risk of malignant transformation is strongly associated with male gender, β-catenin activation, and a tumor diameter larger than 5 cm.

Diagnosis

Serum AFP concentrations are normal. The serum C-reactive protein (CRP) level and WBC count may be elevated with inflammatory adenomas. Historically, fine-needle biopsy has been useless because hepatocellular adenomas mimic normal hepatocytes microscopically. Core needle biopsy has also been of limited diagnostic value, although a definitive diagnosis can be made at expert centers with the use of immunohistochemical markers (see later).[225] Dynamic MRI with a hepatocyte-specific contrast agent such as gadobenate dimeglumin is the preferred imaging modality for diagnosis because it is most able to distinguish a hepatocellular adenoma from other benign or malignant masses in the liver; dynamic CT can also be helpful.[226,227] Because of the complexities associated with the differential diagnosis and the rarity of hepatocellular adenoma, imaging should be conducted at a center with expertise in diagnosing focal liver lesions. The tumor has a clearly defined margin and often has nearly parallel vessels entering it from the periphery ("spoke-wheel" appearance). Alternatively, the lesion may contain tortuous vessels coursing irregularly through it. On arterial-phase images, the tumor enhances irregularly, with areas of increased enhancement and focal avascularity as a result of hemorrhage or necrosis. On portal venous and delayed images, enhancement tends to decrease, and the lesion can be isointense or hypointense ("washout"). On late images using a hepatocyte-specific contrast agent, almost all hepatocellular adenomas are hypointense compared with focal nodular hyperplasias, which are the main consideration in the differential diagnosis and are hyper- or isointense (see later). HNF-1α–inactivated hepatocellular adenomas show diffuse signal dropout in the lesion on T1-weighted chemical shift sequences because of steatosis.[228] Inflammatory hepatocellular adenomas have marked hyperintensity on T2-weighted sequences, especially in the outer part of the lesions, as a result of sinusoidal dilatation and persistent enhancement in the delayed phases. The uninvolved liver in the inflammatory type often has evidence of steatosis.[228] β-Catenin–activated hepatocellular adenomas can have a poorly delineated scar. Surgical excision remains the gold standard for diagnosis (see later).

Pathology

Hepatocellular adenoma generally occurs as a solitary, relatively soft, light brown to yellow tumor. It is sharply circumscribed but does not have a true capsule, although a pseudocapsule is formed by compression of the surrounding liver tissue (Fig. 96-6A).[229] Hepatocellular adenomas arise in an otherwise normal liver, although hepatic steatosis is often seen in association with the inflammatory type. Most tumors are solitary, but multiple tumors can occur. Adenomas range in diameter from 1 to 30 cm. They are larger on average in women taking OCPs than in those not taking them; the lesions usually occupy a subcapsular position and project slightly from the surface of the liver. A pedunculated variety is occasionally seen. The cut surface of the tumor may show ill-defined lobulation but is never nodular or fibrotic. Foci of hemorrhage or necrosis are frequent, and bile staining may be evident.

Microscopically, hepatocellular adenoma may mimic normal liver tissue to an astonishing degree (see Fig. 96-6B).[229] The tumor is composed of sheets or cords of normal-looking or slightly atypical hepatocytes that show no features of malignancy. Few or no portal tracts or central veins are present, and bile ducts are conspicuously absent. Only an infrequent fibrous or vascular septum traverses the lesion. An essentially normal reticulin pattern is demonstrable throughout the adenoma. The HNF-1α–inactivated type often has intratumor steatosis and lacks inflammation. On immunohistochemistry, they do not stain with liver fatty acid–binding protein (L-FABP) compared with the surrounding liver and the other types.[216] The inflammatory type has scattered

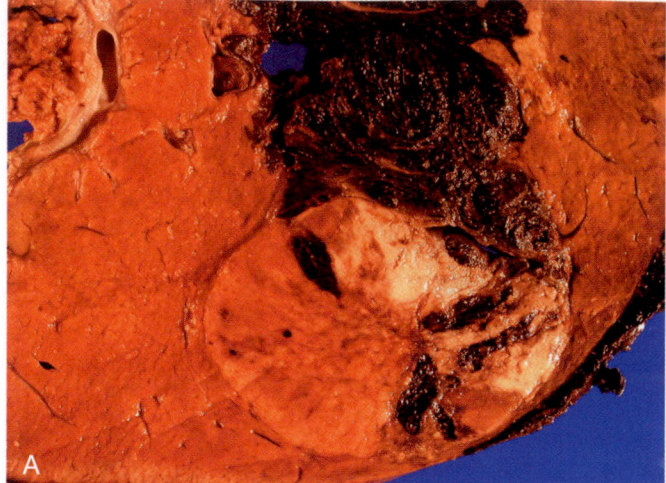

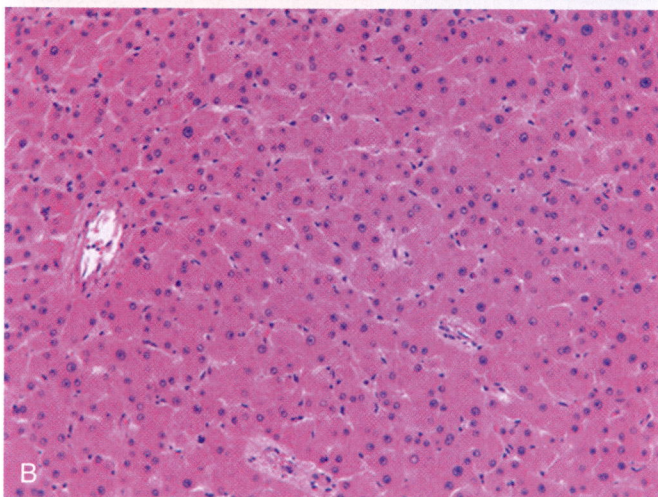

FIGURE 96-6. *A,* Surgical specimen of a large hepatocellular adenoma. The tumor is yellowish and slightly lobular, with a pseudocapsule and areas of necrosis and hemorrhage. *B,* Histopathology of a hepatocellular adenoma showing the resemblance to normal liver tissue, with cords of normal-looking, although generally slightly larger, hepatocytes, as well as Kupffer cells (but fewer in number than normal) lining the sinusoids. Bile ducts and central veins are not seen, but the presence of abnormal vascular structures is evident. (H&E.) *(A, Courtesy Elizabeth Brunt, MD, St. Louis, Mo.; B, courtesy Professor A.C. Paterson, Johannesburg, South Africa.)*

inflammatory infiltrates, thickened walled arteries with sinusoidal dilatation (peliosis), mild steatosis, and hemorrhage; in the past this type was called "telangiectatic focal nodular hyperplasia." The lesion stains with serum amyloid A (SAA) and with CRP.[216] The β-catenin–activated type has no steatosis, peliosis, or portal tract elements and forms pseudoglands with cytologic abnormalities. On immunohistochemistry, the hepatocyte nuclei stain for β-catenin, but this finding is often patchy, and diffuse staining with glutamine synthetase is preferred for diagnosis.[217] The unclassified type of hepatocellular adenomas do not stain for CRP, SAA, β-catenin, or glutamine synthetase and have normal L-FABP staining.[216,217]

Treatment and Prognosis

Historically, because of the danger that a hepatocellular adenoma may rupture and bleed, surgical treatment was always recommended.[229,230] Resection usually is feasible in an uncomplicated case. When rupture has occurred, emergency resection should be performed if possible. If resection cannot be accomplished, the hepatic artery should be ligated. Arterial embolization has also been used successfully to control hemorrhage from a ruptured adenoma, before surgery, or when surgery is not possible.[222] More recent series indicate that the risk of rupture is related to a size larger than 5 cm, although a few cases of hemorrhage have been reported in smaller lesions.[231] Therefore, resection is now recommended for lesions larger than 5 cm or those with evidence of hemorrhage or other symptoms. If the adenoma is not resected, pregnancy and exogenous estrogens should be avoided, although pregnancy without complications can be successful with careful monitoring for growth of the tumor, particularly for those smaller than 5 cm in diameter.[232] Transformation of a hepatocellular adenoma to HCC is a potential risk, with rates of 5% to 20% predominantly limited to adenomas larger than 5 cm in diameter and associated with β-catenin activation and male gender. Therefore, resection of an adenoma is recommended in persons with these risk factors. Advances in MRI and core needle biopsy typing of hepatocellular adenomas may improve the management of patients in the future.

The management of hepatic adenomatosis is problematic.[233] Often in these cases, the number of tumors is large, and they cannot be resected entirely. The size and gender risk factors for malignant transformation and rupture, however, seem to apply to patients with adenomatosis as well. The role of liver transplantation for adenomatosis is not clear.

Cavernous Hemangioma

Epidemiology

Cavernous hemangioma is the most common benign tumor of the liver and is found in as many as 7% of autopsies.[184] The lesion is thought to be a congenital malformation or hamartoma that increases in size, initially with growth of the liver and thereafter by ectasia. Cavernous hemangiomas affect persons of all ages, although they manifest most often in the third, fourth, and fifth decades of life. Women are predominantly affected (4:1 to 6:1) and often present at a younger age and with larger tumors in comparison with men. Cavernous hemangiomas may increase in size with pregnancy or the administration of estrogens and are more common in multiparous than in nulliparous women.

Clinical Features

The great majority of cavernous hemangiomas are small and asymptomatic and are discovered incidentally during imaging of the liver for another reason, at autopsy, or at laparotomy. Larger or multiple lesions produce symptoms.[234] Those larger than 4 cm in diameter are called giant cavernous hemangiomas, which may be as large as 27 cm. Upper abdominal pain is the most common complaint associated with giant cavernous hemangiomas and results from partial infarction of the lesion or pressure on adjacent tissues. Early satiety, nausea, and vomiting also may occur. Cavernous hemangiomas occasionally rupture. The only physical finding may be an enlarged liver. Occasionally, an arterial bruit is heard over the tumor. Arteriovenous shunting has been described with cavernous hemangiomas.

Thrombocytopenia resulting from sequestration and destruction of platelets in large hemangiomas (Kasabach-Merritt syndrome) is seen occasionally in infants but rarely in adults.[234,235] Malignant transformation has not been reported.

Diagnosis

Cavernous hemangiomas are often detected initially by US. The typical US appearance is an echogenic mass of uniform echodensity that lies in the posterior segment of the right lobe of the liver and is less than 3 cm in diameter.[184,236] Almost all cavernous hemangiomas can be diagnosed by contrast-enhanced CT or MRI with sequential scans.[237] The center of the lesion remains hypodense, whereas the peripheral zone, which varies in thickness and may have a corrugated inner margin, is enhanced. MRI has a high degree of specificity and a central role in the diagnosis of small hemangiomas (Fig. 96-7).[238,239] With small hemangiomas, the contrast material may assume a ring-shaped or C-shaped configuration, with an avascular center resulting from fibrous obliteration; this appearance is pathognomonic. Nuclear tagged red blood cell studies may be helpful in the diagnosis of cavernous hemangioma but are now largely of historical interest.

Because of the risk of severe bleeding, percutaneous needle biopsy should not be performed if a cavernous hemangioma is suspected. Moreover, a needle biopsy is of limited diagnostic value. Blunt abdominal trauma may sometimes result in rupture of a giant cavernous hemangioma.[240]

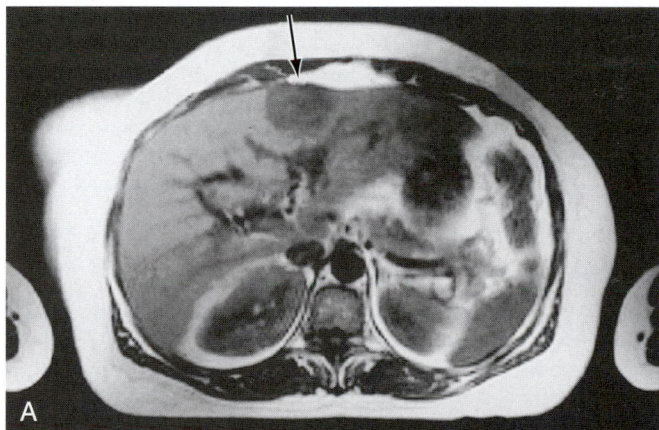

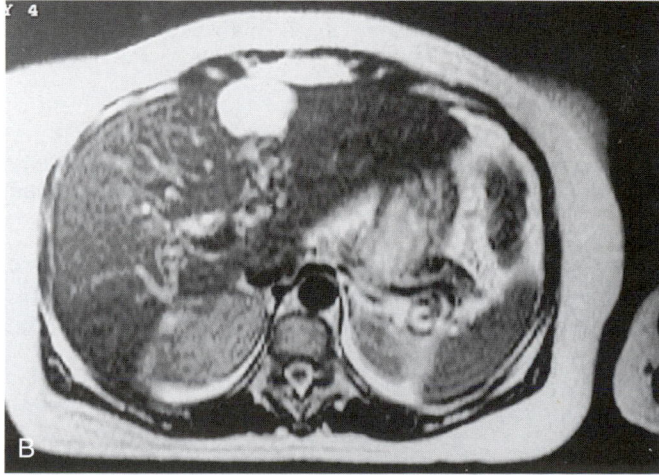

FIGURE 96-7. MRI of a small cavernous hemangioma in the liver *(arrow)*. *A*, T1-weighted image showing a rounded mass with a uniform increase in T1 signal intensity (low signal). *B*, Heavily T2-weighted image showing a mass with a uniform increase in signal intensity (bright signal relative to the water signal of cerebrospinal fluid). *(Courtesy Dr. P. Sneider, Johannesburg, South Africa.)*

Pathology

Cavernous hemangiomas usually are solitary lesions, although multiple tumors occur in 10% of patients.[100,229] Reddish-purple or bluish masses are seen under Glisson's capsule or deep in the substance of the liver. The larger lesions may be pedunculated. Cavernous hemangiomas are well circumscribed but seldom encapsulated. They may show central necrosis, and in some cases, the whole tumor is firm in consistency and grayish-white in appearance. Microscopically, hemangiomas are composed of multiple vascular channels of varying sizes lined by a single layer of flat epithelium and supported by fibrous septa.[184] The vascular spaces may contain thrombi. The demonstration of mast cells within hemangiomas suggests that mast cells may have a role in pathogenesis.[241] Sclerosing cavernous hemangiomas may sometimes be seen and probably represent natural involution of these lesions.

Occasionally, cavernous hemangiomas are associated with hemangiomas in other organs. They also may coexist with cysts in the liver or pancreas,[242] von Meyenburg complexes (see later and Chapter 62),[243] or focal nodular hyperplasia (see later).[244]

Treatment

The great majority of cavernous hemangiomas can safely be left untreated. Some controversy exists about allowing pregnancy or use of estrogen-containing medications in patients with a cavernous hemangioma, but most authorities consider these to be safe.[184,245] A cavernous hemangioma that is large but localized, and the cause of incapacitating symptoms, should be resected.[234] If resection is not feasible, reduction in the size of the tumor with relief of symptoms is rarely achieved with irradiation, arterial ligation, arteriographic embolization, or systemic glucocorticoids.[246,247] RFA has been used with some success. Liver transplantation is rarely needed.[248] If a cavernous hemangioma has ruptured, it may be necessary to embolize or clamp the hepatic artery to stop bleeding before proceeding with resection, although rupture is exceedingly rare.

Infantile Hemangioendothelioma

Epidemiology

Although rare, infantile hemangioendothelioma is the most common tumor of the liver in infants. Its importance stems from the high incidence of heart failure in infants with this tumor and the resulting high mortality rate. The tumor almost invariably manifests in the first 6 months of life and is twice as common in girls as in boys.[171,249] Hepatic hemangioendothelioma often coexists with hemangiomas in other organs, especially the skin (in ≈ 50% of patients).

Clinical Features

Small hemangioendotheliomas are usually asymptomatic. The presence of a large lesion is recognized clinically by the diagnostic triad of an enlarged liver, high-output heart failure, and multiple cutaneous hemangiomas.[249,250] The liver is larger than expected on the basis of the severity of the heart failure, and hepatomegaly persists after the heart failure has been treated successfully. When hemangioendotheliomas occur diffusely throughout the liver, as they usually do, their combined effect is to act as a large peripheral arteriovenous shunt. Shunts of this size are responsible for the heart failure. Approximately one third of patients have jaundice. Patients may be anemic, partly because of the dilutional effect of the increased circulating plasma volume that develops with large peripheral arteriovenous fistulas. A microangiopathic hemolytic anemia may contribute. In addition, thrombocytopenia may be present (Kasabach-Merritt syndrome). Malignant change is a rare complication.

Diagnosis

US may show one or more echogenic masses in the liver. Hepatic angiography is particularly helpful in diagnosis and shows stretching, but not displacement, of the intrahepatic arteries.[251] Abnormal vessels arise from the hepatic arteries and promptly opacify the liver, thereby giving rise to the characteristic blush of an arteriovenous shunt. The circulation time through the liver is short. Focal avascular areas may be evident when hemorrhage into or necrosis of the tumor has occurred. CT with enhancement and MRI are as specific as hepatic arteriography for the diagnosis of hemangioendotheliomas.[252] Percutaneous biopsy is contraindicated because of the danger of bleeding.

Pathology

Two types of infantile hemangioendothelioma are recognized. Type I lesions are often calcified and have a fibrous stromal separation (with bile ductules) between channels. Type II lesions have a more malignant and disorganized-appearing endothelial cell lining and no stromal bile ductules.[171,253] Infantile hemangioendotheliomas typically are multifocal and produce nodular deformity of the entire liver. The nodules range in size from a few millimeters to many centimeters and are well demarcated but not encapsulated. At laparotomy, the nodules can be seen to pulsate. They are reddish purple, although large tumors are gray to tan. They may show hemorrhages, fibrosis, or calcification.

Microscopically, infantile hemangioendothelioma is composed of layers of plump endothelial cells. A single layer characterizes the type I pattern, whereas several layers characterize the type II pattern. In some areas of the tumor, solid masses of mesoblastic primordial cells that differentiate early into vascular structures are observed. Fibrous septa may be prominent, and extramedullary hematopoiesis occurs frequently. Thrombosis may be followed by scarring and calcification.

Treatment and Prognosis

The course of infantile hemangioendothelioma is characterized by tumor growth during the early months of life, followed by gradual involution.[249] As noted earlier, type II infantile hemangioendothelioma may resemble hepatic angiosarcoma in both appearance and behavior in some cases.[198,199] Life-threatening aspects of the disorder are intractable heart failure and, to a lesser extent, consumptive coagulopathy or rupture of the tumor. Heart failure should be treated by conventional means initially, but if these measures fail, more aggressive treatment of the tumor, such as embolization, ligation of the hepatic artery, surgical resection, or liver transplantation, should be considered.[254,255] Use of glucocorticoids has been successful in many (but not all) patients,[256] whereas irradiation has seldom been beneficial. When the tumor is confined to one lobe, surgical resection is curative, even in the presence of cardiac failure.[249]

Other Tumors

Other rare benign tumors of the liver include angiomyolipoma,[257] bile duct adenoma,[258] biliary cystadenoma, and biliary adenofibroma.[259,260]

TUMOR-LIKE HEPATIC LESIONS

Focal Nodular Hyperplasia

Focal nodular hyperplasia is a circumscribed, usually solitary lesion composed of nodules of benign hyperplastic hepatocytes surrounding a central stellate scar.[261]

Epidemiology

Focal nodular hyperplasia is more common than hepatocellular adenoma. The lesion is seen more often in women than in men, although the gender difference is much less striking than that for hepatocellular adenoma. Focal nodular hyperplasia occurs at all ages, but most patients present in the third and fourth decades of life[250]; the age distribution is similar to that of hepatocellular adenomas, and the 2 lesions may coexist.

Pathogenesis

The cause of focal nodular hyperplasia is unknown. Abnormalities in arteries in small and medium-sized portal tracts have been described, suggesting a role for vascular malformation in the pathogenesis.[220,262] It has been described to occur with other vascular lesions, such as cavernous hemangioma, epithelioid hemangioendothelioma, and hereditary hemorrhagic telangiectasia.[263,264] A role for OCPs in the development of the lesion was suggested but has been disputed.[250] Nevertheless, some evidence suggests that focal nodular hyperplasia may be hormone dependent.[265,266] OCPs may accentuate the vascular abnormalities in focal nodular hyperplasia and cause the lesion to enlarge, become more symptomatic, and rarely rupture.

Clinical Features

Most of these lesions do not produce symptoms and are often discovered during upper abdominal imaging for other reasons or because an enlarged liver is felt on routine examination or found during abdominal surgery or at autopsy.[250,267,268] Patients may experience mild pain, particularly with bleeding into or necrosis of the lesion. Conditions and complications associated with focal nodular hyperplasia are listed in Box 96-4.

Diagnosis

Serum AFP levels are normal. The mass lesion seen on US and CT is not specific for focal nodular hyperplasia[269,270] unless the central scar and feeding artery are seen (Fig. 96-8). MRI may

---

BOX 96-4 Associations and Complications of Focal Nodular Hyperplasia

Associations
Cavernous hemangioma
Cavernous transformation of the portal vein
Congenital absence of the portal vein
Epithelioid hemangioendothelioma
Hereditary hemorrhagic telangiectasia
Liver transplantation (detection in graft)
Neonatal hepatic hemangioma
Spinal and pulmonary arteriovenous malformations

Complications
Budd-Chiari syndrome
Compression of the inferior vena cava

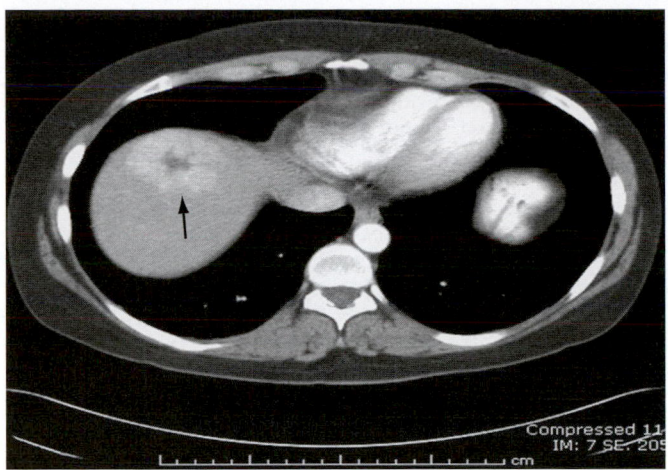

FIGURE 96-8. Contrast-enhanced CT of the liver during the arterial phase showing a typical focal nodular hyperplasia *(arrow)* with contrast enhancement of the mass lesion and the central stellate scar apparent by its lack of enhancement.

be useful for the diagnosis of focal nodular hyperplasia, and advances in the use of contrast agents for MRI have substantially improved the utility of this technique to diagnose focal nodular hyperplasia definitively. Liver-specific gadolinium-based MR contrast agents show focal nodular hyperplasia to be iso- to hyperintense relative to the liver parenchyma during the hepatobiliary phase of imaging, and rarely hypointense, with proved sensitivity greater than 90% for distinguishing focal nodular hyperplasia from hepatic adenomas. Gadoxetate disodium is thought to be the best choice of contrast agent for the diagnosis of focal nodular hyperplasia.[271]

Pathology

Focal nodular hyperplasia manifests as a firm, coarsely nodular, light brown or yellowish-gray mass of variable size, with a dense central stellate scar and radiating fibrous septa that divide the lesion into lobules.[272] The nodule may be small, resembling a cirrhotic nodule, or extremely large. The lesion of focal nodular hyperplasia usually occupies a subcapsular position and may be pedunculated. It generally is solitary. Larger lesions may show foci of hemorrhage or necrosis, although these features are seen less frequently than in hepatocellular adenomas. The fibrous septa sometimes are poorly developed, and the central scar may be absent. The lesion is sharply demarcated from the surrounding liver tissue, which is normal, but a true capsule is absent. Focal nodular hyperplasia is associated with hepatic hemangiomas in as many as 20% of cases.

Microscopically, focal nodular hyperplasia closely resembles a focal form of inactive cirrhosis. Individual hepatocytes are indistinguishable from those of normal liver but lack the usual cord arrangement in relation to sinusoids, central veins, and portal tracts. Kupffer cells are present. Characteristically, the fibrous septa contain numerous bile ductules and vessels. Other features include heavy infiltrations of lymphocytes and, to a lesser extent, plasma cells and histiocytes. Bile duct proliferation in portal tracts may also be evident. Branches of the hepatic artery and portal vein show various combinations of intimal and smooth muscle hyperplasia, subintimal fibrosis, thickening of the wall, occlusive luminal lesions, and thrombosis at times. Whether these vascular changes are primary or secondary is not known. Peliosis hepatis may be an associated lesion. The histologic features almost always make it possible to distinguish focal nodular hyperplasia from hepatocellular adenoma, although the distinction may be difficult to make, particularly in small biopsy specimens.

Treatment

Studies of the natural history of focal nodular hyperplasia indicate that most lesions remain stable or even regress or disappear after a long follow-up period.[273] Large symptomatic or complicated lesions should be resected, usually by segmental resection or enucleation. Recurrence after resection is rare. These lesions may also be treated with RFA. Otherwise, focal nodular hyperplasia should be left alone. If the lesion is not resected, discontinuation of OCPs is recommended and may result in regression of the lesion. Periodic US should be performed if a firm diagnosis of focal nodular hyperplasia has not been made, and a lesion that increases substantially in size should be resected. The available evidence argues against the notion that focal nodular hyperplasia is a premalignant condition.

Other Nodular Disorders

Nodular regenerative hyperplasia is characterized by nodularity of the liver without fibrosis[274] and may be associated with a number of diseases, such as RA and Felty's syndrome (see Chapter 36). Although generally diffuse, the nodularity occasionally is focal, in which case the lesion may be mistaken for a tumor. Patients with nodular regenerative hyperplasia typically present clinically with portal hypertension. Partial nodular transformation is characterized by nodules that are limited to the perihilar region of the liver. These patients also present with portal hypertension.

Macroregenerative nodules may occur in advanced cirrhosis or after massive hepatic necrosis. In the presence of cirrhosis, they are believed to be premalignant and may, in addition, be mistaken for hepatic tumors during hepatic imaging.[275]

Inflammatory pseudotumor is a rare entity, resulting from focal infection, that may be mistaken for a hepatic tumor (see Chapter 84).[276] It occurs particularly in young men, who present with intermittent fever, abdominal pain, jaundice, vomiting, and diarrhea. Leukocytosis, an elevated erythrocyte sedimentation rate, and polyclonal hyperglobulinemia are present in approximately 50% of patients. The lesion may be solitary or multiple and shows a mixture of chronic inflammatory cells, with plasma cells predominating. Focal fatty infiltration, or focal fatty sparing in the presence of diffuse fatty infiltration, may also be mistaken for a hepatic tumor (see Chapter 87).[277]

HEPATIC CYSTS

Hepatic cysts are abnormal fluid-filled spaces in the hepatic parenchyma and biliary tree. They are categorized into 3 main types: fibrocystic diseases of the liver, cystadenomas and cystadenocarcinomas, and hydatid cysts. Cystadenomas and cystadenocarcinomas are discussed in Chapter 69. Hydatid cysts are discussed in Chapter 84.

Fibrocystic diseases of the liver originate from abnormal persistence or defects in the progressive remodeling of the ductal plate during development, resulting in dilated fluid-filled spaces, including hepatic and choledochal cysts, portal fibrosis, and ductal plate malformations (see Chapter 62).[278,279] Fibrocystic disorders of the liver described here include simple hepatic cysts, polycystic liver disease (PCLD), fibrocystic disease associated with autosomal recessive polycystic kidney disease, von Meyenburg complexes, and Caroli's disease (type V choledochal cyst). (The other diseases are congenital hepatic fibrosis and type IV choledochal cysts; see Chapter 62.)

Simple Cysts

Simple hepatic cysts are thought to be congenital in origin and have a frequency of about 2.5% of the population.[280] They generally are smaller than 5 cm in diameter and can number up to 3 before being considered part of PCLD.[281] The cysts usually are asymptomatic and discovered incidentally during upper abdominal imaging. They occur more often in women than in men, and their prevalence increases with age. When symptomatic, they can produce complications similar to those of PCLD, including intracystic bleeding, infection, rupture, or compression of adjacent organs.

Typically, initial imaging with US, CT, or MRI provides an accurate diagnosis and distinguishes a simple cyst from a hydatid cyst and cystadenoma. Septations, papillary projections, or calcification should raise suspicion of an alternative diagnosis.[282] Asymptomatic solitary hepatic cysts should be left alone. If intervention is required because of symptoms, percutaneous aspiration and sclerosis with alcohol or doxycycline will almost always ablate the cyst, but recurrence is frequent.[281] An alternative approach is laparoscopic (or rarely, open surgical) fenestration, which is seldom followed by recurrence but has greater morbidity.

Polycystic Liver Disease

PCLD is a rare condition in which multiple cysts form in the hepatic parenchyma; usually it comes to clinical attention in adulthood (Fig. 96-9). PCLD usually presents in association with autosomal dominant polycystic kidney disease (ADPKD)[283,284] but can appear as isolated PCLD.[285,286]

The cysts range in diameter from a few millimeters to 10 cm or more. They contain clear, colorless, or straw-colored fluid and are lined by a single layer of cuboidal or columnar epithelium, resembling that of bile ducts.[283-287] Rarely, the cysts may be lined by squamous epithelium; these cysts may be complicated by the development of squamous cell carcinoma. In addition to the nature of the lining epithelium, evidence for a biliary origin of these cysts is suggested by the composition of the cystic fluid, which has a low glucose content and contains secretory immunoglobulin (Ig)A and GGTP. The cysts are thought to arise as a result of ductal plate malformation. This process gives rise to von Meyenburg complexes (see later), which become disconnected from the biliary tract during development and growth and dilate progressively to form cysts.

Epidemiology

PCLD is fairly common in patients with ADPKD. It occurs in approximately 24% of patients in the third decade of life to 80% in the sixth decade of life, but the kidney disease usually dominates the clinical course.[288] Cysts also may be present in the pancreas, spleen, and (less often) other organs. Symptomatic liver disease correlates with advancing age, severity of renal cysts, and renal dysfunction.[289] Women tend to have larger and more numerous cysts, and a correlation with the number of pregnancies has been found. The use of exogenous female sex hormones may accelerate the rate of growth and size of the cysts. PCLD may coexist with other fibrocystic liver diseases, such as congenital hepatic fibrosis (in which the patient is likely to present with portal hypertension), Caroli's disease, or von Meyenburg complexes.[283-287] PCLD is also associated with other conditions such as berry aneurysms, mitral valve prolapse, diverticular disease, and inguinal hernias.

Isolated PCLD not associated with ADPKD is rare, representing 7% of all PCLD in autopsy series.[290] It usually is asymptomatic.[291] Like ADPKD-associated PCLD, isolated PCLD is associated with pregnancy and appears to be more symptomatic in women than men.

Etiology and Pathogenesis

ADPKD is a common genetic disease with a frequency of 1:1000 in whites.[292] Two genes are responsible. The gene affected in ADPKD1 is *PKD-1*, which is located on chromosome 16q13-q23 and expresses a ubiquitous protein, polycystin-1.[293,294] The gene responsible for ADPKD2 is *PKD-2*, which is located on chromosome 4 and expresses polycystin-2. The 2 polycystins are transmembrane glycoproteins that complex and localize in the primary cilium, a microtubule-based structure found on renal and biliary tubule epithelium and thought to act as a flow sensor and regulator of Ca^{2+} influx.[295] Although the mutation is inherited as an autosomal dominant trait, a second somatic mutation is thought to be necessary to produce the monoclonally derived cysts.[296]

Isolated PCLD has been shown in North American and Finnish families to be linked to the gene *PRKCSH* (also known as protein kinase C substrate 80K-H) on chromosome 19p13.2-13.1 and to *SEC63* on chromosome 6q21, although other associated genes undoubtedly exist.[293,297,298] The gene products hepatocystin and SEC63p are thought to be involved in the folding and quality control of glycoproteins and protein translocation in the endoplasmic reticulum, respectively.[299] The genes appear to be autosomal dominant, and a second somatic mutation is thought to be needed to cause disease.

Clinical Features

The hepatic cysts in PCLD, whether or not they occur in association with renal cysts, rarely cause morbidity, and many

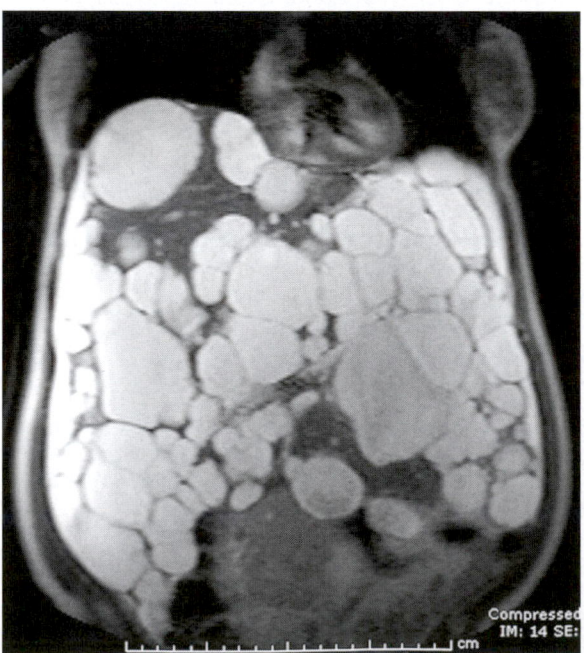

FIGURE 96-9. MRI of the abdomen in a patient with severe polycystic liver disease. This coronal T2-weighted image shows a massively enlarged liver with numerous bright fluid-filled cysts. *(Courtesy Dr. N. Cem Balci, St. Louis, Mo.)*

affected persons are asymptomatic.[283-287] The livers of these patients contain only a few cysts or cysts smaller than 2 cm in diameter. Symptoms occur in patients with more numerous and larger cysts (10% to 15% of patients, usually women), generally with markedly enlarged livers. Abdominal discomfort or pain, postprandial fullness, awareness of an upper abdominal mass, a protuberant abdomen, inability to bend over, and shortness of breath may be present. Severe pain may be experienced with rupture or infection of a cyst, bleeding into a cyst, or torsion of a pedunculated cyst. Jaundice is evident in approximately 5% of patients and is caused by compression of the major intrahepatic or extrahepatic bile ducts. Ascites, if present, is the result of portal hypertension, which generally is caused by associated congenital hepatic fibrosis but occasionally by compression of the hepatic veins by the cysts. Gastroesophageal variceal bleeding has rarely been reported.[300]

Diagnosis

Liver biochemical test results generally are normal, with intact hepatic function, although serum alkaline phosphatase and GGTP levels may be increased. The cysts contain high levels of the tumor marker CA 19-9, and serum levels of CA 19-9 may be elevated. A raised right hemidiaphragm may be evident on a plain x-ray of the chest in patients with severe PCLD. The diagnosis of PCLD is confirmed by US, CT, or MRI (see Fig. 96-9).

Treatment

On the rare occasions when cysts require treatment, fenestration (unroofing) should be performed.[283,301] Cyst fenestration originally was done at laparotomy but is now performed laparoscopically, thereby reducing morbidity.[302] A high recurrence rate is observed for cysts treated with fenestration, although symptomatic relief is usually durable. Cysts have also been treated by percutaneous injection of a sclerosing substance such as alcohol or doxycycline, but most patients have too many small cysts, so percutaneous injection should be reserved for those with a dominant cyst or excessive risk for surgery. Patients who fail to respond to cyst fenestration may be considered for partial hepatic resection if sufficient relatively uninvolved liver remains after surgery. The morbidity of this approach is substantial, and future liver transplantation may be more difficult after resection.[302] Liver transplantation (sometimes combined with renal transplantation) is associated with excellent outcomes and long-term survival but, because of the organ donor shortage, is generally reserved for patients with hepatic failure or severe symptoms that interfere with the patient's quality of life.[302] Several randomized clinical trials have demonstrated a modest reduction in cyst size and improvement in quality of life with treatment with a long-acting somatostatin analog, but the length of follow-up has been short.[144]

Autosomal Recessive Polycystic Kidney Disease

Fibrocystic liver disease may present in childhood as an autosomal recessive disorder that is usually rapidly fatal as a consequence of associated autosomal recessive polycystic kidney disease (ARPKD).[283,284] A proportion of patients maintain renal function into adulthood, however, and complications of the associated liver disease then predominate. The liver cysts are microscopic rather than macroscopic and present a clinical picture of congenital hepatic fibrosis. Complications of portal hypertension are the usual hepatic manifestations of the disease. The gene responsible for this disease, *PKHD1*, has been identified on chromosome 6p21-cen, and the ARPKD protein, fibrocystin, is predicted to be an integral receptor-like protein.[303] Many different mutations throughout the gene have been identified in patients with ARPKD.

von Meyenburg Complexes

von Meyenburg complexes (also known as biliary microhamartomas) are common and do not produce symptoms; they are small and usually multiple. Each complex is composed of cystically dilated intra- and interlobular bile ducts embedded in a fibrous stroma.[304,305] The cysts are lined by cuboidal or flat epithelium. They occur in almost all patients with congenital hepatic fibrosis and may coexist with Caroli's disease or ADPKD. von Meyenburg complexes are found in or adjacent to portal tracts and are believed to arise as a result of malformation of the ductal plate (see Chapter 62); they may be complicated by the development of peripheral cholangiocarcinoma.[306]

Caroli's Disease

Caroli's disease is a rare disorder characterized by congenital nonobstructive gross dilatation of the segmental intrahepatic bile ducts.[281] The disease has been included in the classification of choledochal cysts (as type V)[281,283] and may occur in association with medullary sponge kidney (in 60% to 80% of patients) or congenital hepatic fibrosis (see Chapter 62). Caroli's disease is believed to be caused by an intrauterine event that arrests ductal plate remodeling at the level of the larger intrahepatic bile ducts.[278] The resulting bile duct ectasia may be diffuse or localized. Both autosomal recessive and autosomal dominant modes of inheritance have been proposed. Caroli's disease affects men and women equally and usually becomes symptomatic in early adulthood; more than 80% of patients present with symptoms before 30 years of age.

Patients typically present with recurrent episodes of fever and abdominal pain caused by cholangitis. The liver often is enlarged. Ductal ectasia predisposes to bile stagnation, which in turn may lead to cholangitis, abscess formation, and septicemia.[307] Gallstones form in the ectatic ducts in one third of patients. The result of these complications may be cholangiocarcinoma, which develops in less than 10% of patients.

Caroli's disease usually is discovered when the liver is imaged during investigation of suspected cholangitis. Irregular dilatations of the larger intrahepatic bile ducts are seen.

Attacks of cholangitis require treatment with antibiotics. Endoscopic retrograde cannulation of the biliary system may be used to facilitate removal of sludge or stones from the accessible part of the biliary system, and the cysts may be drained by an endoscopic or percutaneous route. Liver resection for unilobar Caroli's disease and liver transplantation for diffuse Caroli's disease are associated with excellent long-term patient survival and a low rate of complications.[308]

APPROACH TO THE PATIENT WITH A HEPATIC MASS

The approach to the diagnosis of a mass in the liver will be influenced by the age and gender of the patient and the presence or absence of symptoms (Fig. 96-10). Making a definitive diagnosis of a mass in the liver solely on clinical grounds is seldom possible. Nevertheless, detailed history taking will provide important clues about the probable benign or malignant nature of the lesion.

The approach to a mass in the liver differs, depending on whether or not cirrhosis is present. In a noncirrhotic liver, masses may be found in the liver incidentally or because of symptoms; the main concern is cancer metastatic from elsewhere. Initial imaging studies such as US, CT, or MRI will indicate if the lesion is cystic. Cystic lesions should be investigated further and treated only if symptomatic or an echinococcal cyst or biliary cystadenoma is suspected, usually based on the complexity of the cyst wall, including calcification, septations, and daughter cysts (see Fig. 96-10A and Chapters 69 and 84).

Solid lesions in a noncirrhotic liver include a hemangioma, which can be confirmed by contrast-enhanced MRI. Hemangiomas generally show peripheral nodular enhancement in the arterial phase, with progressive centripetal filling in the portal venous and delayed phases. Focal nodular hyperplasia

shows intense homogenous enhancement on arterial phase, with a characteristic enhancing scar on delayed phase, by CT or MRI. By contrast, hepatocellular adenoma has less intense arterial enhancement and no central scar. Dynamic MRI with a hepatocyte-specific contrast agent and delayed imaging is helpful for distinguishing focal nodular hyperplasia from a hepatocellular adenoma because adenomas are hypointense on delayed phase images, whereas focal nodular hyperplasias are hyper- or isointense. If primary or metastatic malignancy is suspected because of the presence of underlying chronic liver disease, a prior or current malignancy, systemic symptoms or signs (e.g., weight loss), or an elevated serum tumor marker (AFP, CA 19-9), then a biopsy (with US or CT guidance) should be considered. Most metastases are less vascular

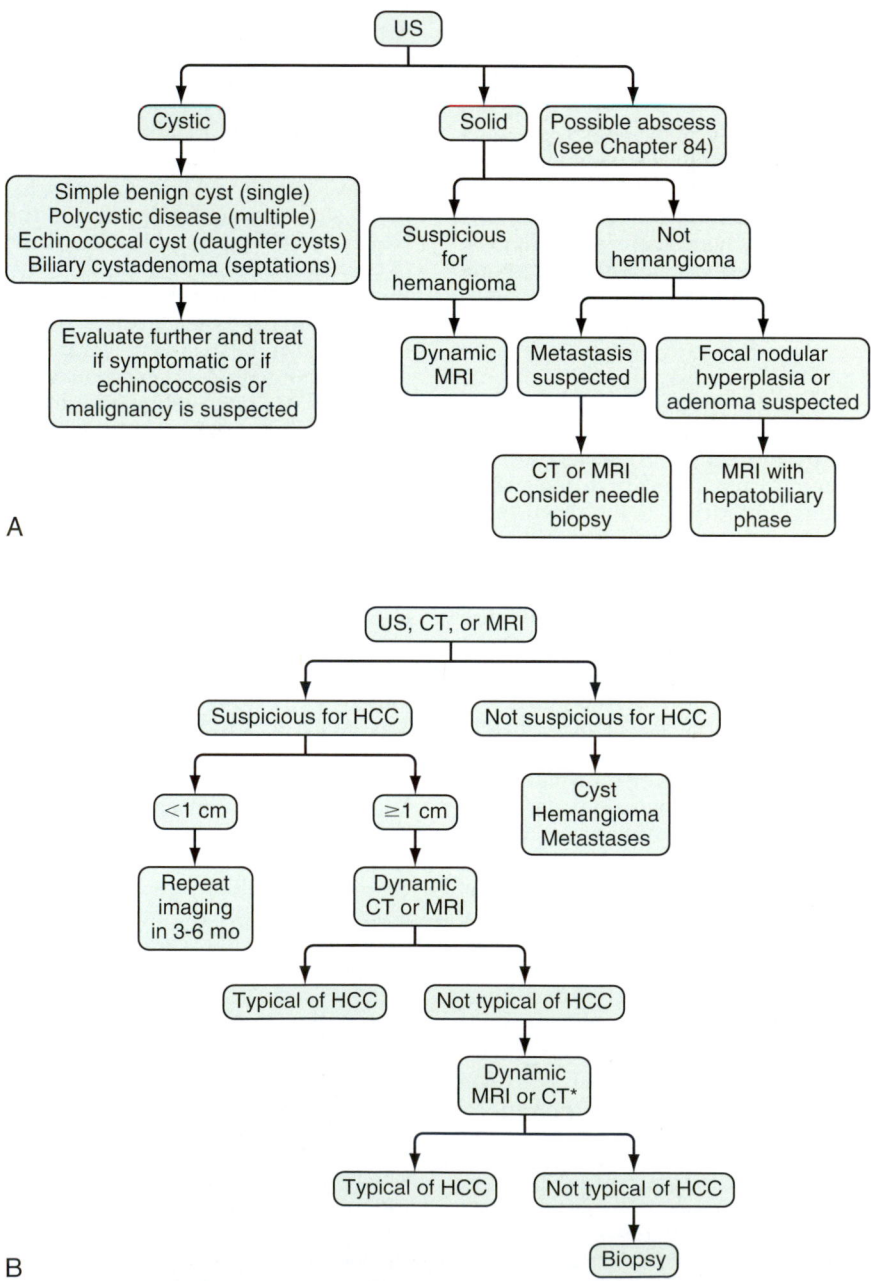

FIGURE 96-10. *A,* Algorithm for the approach to the management of a patient, not known to have cirrhosis, with a hepatic mass (often incidental, possibly symptomatic). *B,* Algorithm for the approach to the management of a patient with known or suspected cirrhosis and a hepatic mass (found on routine surveillance, because of symptoms, or because of an increasing AFP level). *Perform imaging modality not previously performed. HCC, hepatocellular carcinoma.

than HCC. A metastasis and peripheral cholangiocarcinoma often have peripheral rim enhancement on the arterial phase. If a biopsy is not performed or not diagnostic, then interval follow-up imaging studies are prudent unless the imaging findings are classic in appearance for focal nodular hyperplasia or hemangioma.

In a patient known to have cirrhosis, the presence of a nodule or mass should be presumed to be HCC until proved otherwise. AASLD practice guidelines provide criteria for the noninvasive diagnosis of HCC based on the vascularity of the tumor (see earlier). Contrast enhancement during the arterial phase of a multiphase CT or MRI study, with subsequent washout during the portal venous or delayed phase, is considered diagnostic of HCC if the lesion is larger than 1 cm in diameter. If the vascular enhancement pattern is atypical, a biopsy of the lesion should be considered. A high serum AFP level is strongly suggestive of HCC but may rarely occur with other GI malignancies, and its utility has been questioned. For a lesion smaller than 1 cm, interval imaging at 3 to 6 months is recommended. If determining whether a patient has underlying cirrhosis is impossible on clinical and imaging grounds, a biopsy of the nontumorous liver may be done. Although characteristic imaging features of HCC, hemangioma, and focal nodular hyperplasia have high diagnostic accuracy and can be relied on for treatment decisions, definitive diagnosis often depends on demonstrating the typical histologic features of the tumor.

KEY REFERENCES

Full references for this chapter can be found on www.expertconsult.com.

5. El-Serag H, Mason A. Rising incidence of hepatocellular carcinoma in the United States. N Engl J Med 1999; 340:745-50.

23. Liaw YF, Sung JJ, Chow WC, et al. Lamivudine for patients with chronic hepatitis B and advanced liver disease. N Engl J Med 2004; 351:1521-31.

33. Bruix J, Sherman M. Management of hepatocellular carcinoma: An update. Hepatology 2011; 53:1020-2.

47. Marrero JA, Fontana RJ, Fu S, et al. Alcohol, tobacco and obesity are synergistic risk factors for hepatocellular carcinoma. J Hepatol 2005; 42:218-24.

64. Colli A, Fraquelli M, Casazza G, et al. Accuracy of ultrasonography, spiral CT, magnetic resonance, and alpha-fetoprotein in diagnosing hepatocellular carcinoma: A systematic review. Am J Gastroenterol 2006; 101:513-23.

108. Bismuth H, Chiche L, Castaing D. Surgical treatment of hepatocellular carcinomas in noncirrhotic liver: Experience with 68 liver resections. World J Surg 1995; 19:35-41.

112. Ribero D, Curley SA, Imamura H, et al. Selection for resection of hepatocellular carcinoma and surgical strategy: Indications for resection, evaluation of liver function, portal vein embolization, and resection. Ann Surg Oncol 2008; 15:986-92.

123. Lencioni R, Cioni D, Crocetti L, et al. Early-stage hepatocellular carcinoma in patients with cirrhosis: Long-term results of percutaneous image-guided radiofrequency ablation. Radiology 2005; 234:961-7.

131. Llovet JM, Bruix J. Systematic review of randomized trials for unresectable hepatocellular carcinoma: Chemoembolization improves survival. Hepatology 2003; 37:429-42.

142. Llovet JM, Ricci S, Mazzaferro V, et al. Sorafenib in advanced hepatocellular carcinoma. N Engl J Med 2008; 359:378-90.

168. Khan SA, Thomas HC, Davidson BR, Taylor-Robinson SD. Cholangiocarcinoma. Lancet 2005; 366:1303-14.

216. Bioulac-Sage P, Laumonier H, Couchy G, et al. Hepatocellular adenoma management and phenotypic classification: The Bordeaux experience. Hepatology 2009; 50:481-9.

278. Desmet V. Congenital diseases of intrahepatic bile ducts: Variations on the theme "ductal plate malformation." Hepatology 1992; 16:1069-83.

287. Everson G. Hepatic cysts in autosomal dominant polycystic kidney disease. Am J Kidney Dis 1993; 22:520-5.

302. Drenth JP, Chrispijn M, Nagorney DM, et al. Medical and surgical treatment options for polycystic liver disease. Hepatology 2010; 52:2223-30.

CHAPTER OUTLINE

Although treatment of PBC with ursodeoxycholic acid and of chronic viral hepatitis with antiviral agents can favorably alter the outcome of some chronic liver diseases, once major complications of cirrhosis such as ascites or hepatic encephalopathy develop, treatment options are limited and typically do not extend life. Interventions such as variceal band ligation and transjugular intrahepatic shunt (TIPS) placement can effectively control life-threatening bleeding but do not abort progression of underlying cirrhosis (see Chapter 74). With some notable exceptions, as occur with abstinence from alcohol in decompensated alcoholic liver disease and antiviral therapy in advanced liver disease due to HBV infection, the course of clinically overt cirrhosis is almost invariably progressive. Even a previously well-compensated cirrhotic patient who experiences an index complication of liver disease can develop precipitous deterioration with "acute-on-chronic liver failure," leading to multiorgan involvement, frequently with sepsis and renal failure. The major indications for liver transplantation (LT) in adults are decompensated cirrhosis, unresectable primary hepatic malignancies, and acute liver failure.[1] Although the greatest challenge in LT remains the shortage of donor organs, recurrent disease, especially HCV infection, often diminishes the duration of survival of the recipient and the graft after an otherwise successful procedure. By contrast, oral antiviral agents in combination with hepatitis B immunoglobulin permit LT with a low likelihood of recurrent HBV infection.[2] Recurrence of nonviral liver disease is also recognized, albeit less severe than for HCV reinfection.[3] Effective immunosuppression has made graft rejection a less likely threat than disease recurrence.[4,5] The recognition that excessive immunosuppression is deleterious in HCV-infected recipients led to avoidance of overly vigorous use of glucocorticoids.[6] By contrast, more intensive immunosuppression may be necessary in liver transplant recipients with autoimmune liver disease.[7]

Deaths on the waiting list for LT reflect in large part the shortage of donor organs, the number of which is far outstripped by the number of potential recipients. Introduction of the MELD score for organ allocation in the United States achieved its stated aim of reducing the number of deaths on the waiting list.[8] The MELD score assigns organs to recipients on the basis of an objective measure of severity of liver disease (see later), with time on the waiting list no longer a determining factor. Although live-donor liver transplantation (LDLT) in adult recipients can potentially increase the available donor organ pool, potential risks to the donor have limited its application.[9] Other innovations such as splitting of a deceased-donor graft to share between 2 recipients and use of "extended-criteria" grafts, including those from older and non–heart-beating donors, have also expanded the organ supply, albeit modestly[10]; an increased frequency of biliary complications, however, is a consequence of the expanded donor criteria.[11] Efforts to expand the deceased-donor supply by public education programs have succeeded, although many potential organ donors remain unidentified. Although the shortage of donor organs will undoubtedly persist, and recurrence of the original disease remains a threat, the prospects for long-term survival are very good to excellent for most liver transplant recipients who otherwise would succumb to the underlying liver disease. The predicted 1-year survival rate for patients with decompensated cirrhosis is less than 10% without LT but approximately 85% to 90% at 1 year and 75% at 5 years after LT for most indications.[12]

Access to LT has transformed the management of advanced liver disease but has resulted in an expanding cohort of

---

*Dr. Hugo R. Rosen contributed to this chapter in previous editions of the textbook.

decompensated potential recipients requiring detailed medical attention.[13] The best outcomes following LT are obtained in recipients who have not already experienced multiple complications of liver disease[14]; therefore, referral is appropriate when a cirrhotic patient has had an index complication, such as the new onset of ascites. For at least some potential recipients, access to LDLT may avoid a lengthy waiting period with the risk of further and potentially life-threatening complications of liver disease.

In parallel with the evolution of LT, the care of transplant candidates with advanced disease has become an area of special expertise. The transplant hepatologist must combine the skills necessary to practice gastroenterology, multidisciplinary internal medicine, and intensive care. This skill set has been formally recognized by the development of a secondary subspecialty in transplant hepatology by the American Board of Internal Medicine.[15]

INDICATIONS

The major indications for LT in adults reflect the most frequent causes of cirrhosis (see Chapter 74), notably HCV infection, alcoholic liver disease, and to a lesser extent, HBV infection, PBC, PSC, autoimmune hepatitis, and hemochromatosis (Fig. 97-1) (see Chapters 68, 75, 79, 80, 90, and 91). An increasingly prominent indication is cirrhosis and hepatocellular carcinoma (HCC) due to nonalcoholic fatty liver disease (NAFLD), reflecting the high prevalence of obesity in the population. Many candidates for LT previously described as having "cryptogenic" cirrhosis are now considered to have NAFLD (see Chapter 87). An uncommon but important indication is acute liver failure (ALF), which has a high mortality rate in the absence of LT (see Chapter 95). The role of LT in primary hepatic malignancy has become better defined; a subset of patients with HCC have a high likelihood of cure with LT, and neoadjuvant and adjuvant therapies, including the oral chemotherapy agent sorafenib (a multitargeted tyrosine kinase inhibitor) are under active investigation (see Chapter 96).[16] Cholangiocarcinoma, the other major primary adult hepatic malignancy, had been regarded as a contraindication to LT because of its rapid and almost invariable recurrence, leading to dismal recipient survival rates; however, acceptable outcomes have been reported in a subset of patients with perihilar tumors who receive adjuvant external beam radiation and chemosensitization (see Chapter 69).[17] The major indication for pediatric LT is biliary atresia following a failed Kasai procedure (portoenterostomy) or delayed recognition of the diagnosis (see Chapter 62). Other major pediatric indications include α_1-antitrypsin deficiency and other metabolic disorders (see Chapter 77).

A diagnosis of cirrhosis per se is not an indication for LT, although a key issue in managing a cirrhotic patient is assessing whether LT will be needed in the future and when referral for a transplant evaluation is appropriate (Box 97-1). Other important aspects of care are anticipation of complications such as variceal bleeding (see Chapter 92) and surveillance for HCC (see Chapter 96).[13] LT should normally be recommended only when the limits of medical therapy for complications of cirrhosis have been reached. The risk of surgery must always be weighed against a realistic assessment of the potential recipient's prognosis in the absence of LT. For example, in a patient with decompensated cirrhosis caused by HBV infection, effective antiviral therapy may result in impressive clinical improvement, delaying or even obviating the need for LT (see Chapter 79). Similarly, abstinence from alcohol can result in resolution of signs of hepatic decompensation in a patient with alcoholic liver disease (see Chapter 86). Evaluation for LT should not be deferred, however, even when a potentially reversible component for hepatic decompensation is identified, because clinical improvement does not occur invariably and the course of chronic liver disease remains unpredictable. Although recognition of cirrhosis implies a risk of major complications and diminished life expectancy, a well-compensated cirrhotic patient can remain stable for a protracted period of time.[18] For example, in patients with well-compensated cirrhosis due to HCV infection, major complications of portal hypertension such as ascites and variceal hemorrhage occur in less than 30% of patients by 10 years (Fig. 97-2).[18] By contrast, once a complication supervenes, survival diminishes rapidly. For example, after the development of ascites refractory to diuretics, only 25% of patients survive beyond 1 year.[19] A prospective study of more than 200 Italian patients with HCV-related compensated cirrhosis followed for up to 17 years found that HCC was the most common complication of cirrhosis, occurring in 32% of patients, followed by ascites.[20] Zipprich and colleagues[21] observed that in patients with compensated cirrhosis, the median survival time was 2.6 times longer than that of patients with decompensated cirrhosis (78.7 months and 29.5 months, respectively). In addition, patients with decompensated cirrhosis had a 1-year mortality rate 3.7-fold higher than that of patients with compensated cirrhosis (20.2% and 5.4%, respectively).

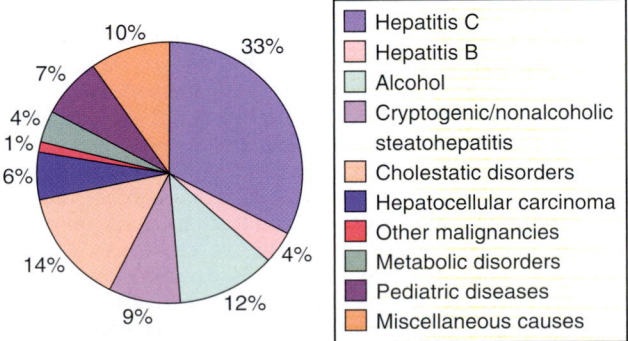

FIGURE 97-1. Proportion of liver transplants performed for specific indications, 1992 to 2007. *(From O'Leary JG, Lepe R, Davis GL. Indications for liver transplantation. Gastroenterology 2008; 134:1764-76, with permission.)*

Pie chart legend:
- Hepatitis C — 33%
- Hepatitis B — 4%
- Alcohol — 12%
- Cryptogenic/nonalcoholic steatohepatitis — 9%
- Cholestatic disorders — 14%
- Hepatocellular carcinoma — 6%
- Other malignancies — 1%
- Metabolic disorders — 4%
- Pediatric diseases — 7%
- Miscellaneous causes — 10%

BOX 97-1 Indications for Liver Transplantation

Acute liver failure
Complications of cirrhosis
    Ascites
    Chronic GI blood loss due to portal hypertensive gastropathy
    Encephalopathy
    Liver cancer
    Refractory variceal hemorrhage
    Synthetic dysfunction
Liver-based metabolic conditions with systemic manifestations
    α_1-Antitrypsin deficiency
    Familial amyloidosis
    Glycogen storage disease
    Primary oxaluria
    Tyrosinemia
    Urea cycle enzyme deficiencies
    Wilson disease
Systemic complications of chronic liver disease
    Hepatopulmonary syndrome
    Portopulmonary hypertension

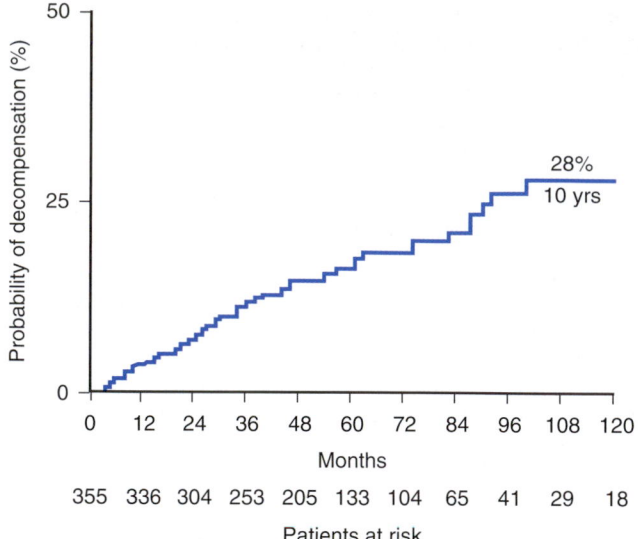

FIGURE 97-2. Probability of developing major complications (decompensation) in patients with well-compensated cirrhosis due to hepatitis C. *(From Fattovich G, Giustina G, Degos F, et al. Morbidity and mortality in compensated cirrhosis type C: A retrospective follow-up study of 384 patients. Gastroenterology 1999; 112:463-72, with permission.)*

The development of disease-specific predictive models based on the natural history of PBC (see Chapter 91) and PSC (see Chapter 68) can help clinical decision making for patients with these cholestatic disorders, which tend to progress in a fairly stereotypical fashion.[22] Before the introduction of the MELD score, analogous models had not been available for noncholestatic forms of cirrhosis, and the decision to refer a patient for LT was generally based on an estimate of disease severity using objective parameters such as the serum albumin level, as well as more subjective factors such as the presence of hepatic encephalopathy, as in the Child-Turcotte-Pugh score (see Chapter 92).

On clinical rather than biochemical grounds, important indications for LT remain severe disease reflective of hepatocellular failure, inferred by the presence of coagulopathy and jaundice; complications of portal hypertension such as refractory ascites and recurrent variceal bleeding; or the combination of portosystemic shunting and diminished hepatocellular function, as in hepatic encephalopathy (see Box 97-1). Deterioration in a patient's quality of life is not reflected adequately in predictive models, including the MELD score. Disabling symptoms such as pruritus, severe fatigue, incapacitating daytime sleepiness, and osteopenia in patients with cholestatic and other forms of cirrhosis, as well as recurrent bacterial cholangitis in those with PSC, are also important considerations. MELD "exceptions"—the addition of points to the "biological" MELD score—can be requested on a case-by-case basis from the local United Network for Organ Sharing (UNOS) Regional Review Board to facilitate LT. The awarding of extra points recognizes that although the MELD score has been a major advance in organ allocation, at least some patients may be disadvantaged by the use of purely objective parameters and exclusion of factors that were incorporated into older allocation schemes (e.g., intractable ascites, encephalopathy) or disabling symptoms that are disease specific. Ideally, LT should occur before a protracted period of disability reduces the likelihood that the recipient will return to full employment and normal social functioning.

LISTING CRITERIA AND POLICIES OF THE UNITED NETWORK FOR ORGAN SHARING

Organ allocation within the United States is administered by UNOS, which uses disease severity (not waiting time, as in the past) to assign a graft to a recipient. Prior to 2002, organ allocation was based on the Child-Turcotte-Pugh score (see Chapter 92). The MELD score (available at www.unos.org [http://optn.transplant.hrsa.gov/resources/MELDPELDCalculator.asp?index=98]) is a formula that incorporates the serum bilirubin level, creatinine level, and INR. It provides a numerical value (based on a log-transformed equation) that predicts the 3-month mortality rate without LT (e.g., 1.9% with a score < 9; 71.3% with a score of 40).[23] The MELD score also overcomes some of the inherent limitations of the Child-Turcotte-Pugh score, including limited discriminatory ability, subjective interpretation of parameters such as presence or absence of ascites on the basis of the physical examination, and the "ceiling effect" of the Child-Turcotte-Pugh score (i.e., no greater weight is given to a serum bilirubin level of 35 mg/dL than to a level of 3.5 mg/dL, even though a patient with the markedly higher bilirubin level clearly has more advanced liver disease). Inclusion of the serum creatinine level reflects its prognostic importance in patients with advanced liver disease. An analogous predictive model was developed and validated for children younger than 12 years of age with chronic liver disease (Pediatric End-stage Liver Disease [PELD] score). The main difference between the MELD and PELD scores is that the pediatric model does not incorporate serum creatinine but instead uses age, growth failure (≤ 2 standard deviations below the mean value for that age), and serum albumin level (also available at www.unos.org [http://optn.transplant.hrsa.gov/resources/MELDPELDCalculator.asp?index=99]).

ABSOLUTE AND RELATIVE CONTRAINDICATIONS

Contraindications to LT are continually evolving. Effective oral therapy now allows LT for HBV-related liver disease with a low likelihood of recurrence.[24] In stark contrast, retransplantation of debilitated recipients with a failing graft caused by recurrent HCV infection is usually futile and awaits more effective antiviral drug therapy to improve outcomes.[25] The introduction of antiretroviral therapy has permitted LT in HIV-infected recipients with decompensated liver disease, typically caused by either HCV or HBV infection.[26] Still, absolute and relative contraindications remain (Box 97-2). An absolute contraindication to LT implies that a successful outcome is so unlikely that transplantation should not be offered. A relative contraindication implies that the likelihood of a good outcome is suboptimal, although LT may still be considered in some patients. The role of LT in the management of HCC has become better defined with the recognition that a large tumor burden is associated with a high probability of metastatic spread postoperatively.[27] Tumor characteristics predictive of a poor outcome, most notably vascular invasion, may only be apparent once the explant is available, despite the sophistication of current imaging techniques. Although results of LT for cholangiocarcinoma have been poor because of a high rate of tumor recurrence, a subset of patients with perihilar tumors may benefit from multimodal therapy, including neoadjuvant chemotherapy along with concurrent external beam radiation, followed by LT in selected candidates in whom surgical exploration demonstrates stage I or II disease

BOX 97-2 Absolute Contraindications to Liver Transplantation

AIDS
Active alcoholism or substance abuse
Advanced cardiac or pulmonary disease
Anatomic abnormality that precludes liver transplantation
Cholangiocarcinoma
Extrahepatic malignancy
Fulminant hepatic failure with sustained ICP > 50 mm Hg or CPP < 40 mm Hg
Hemangiosarcoma
Persistent nonadherence
Uncontrolled sepsis

ICP, intracranial pressure; CPP, cerebral perfusion pressure (CPP = mean arterial pressure minus ICP).

(see Chapter 69).[28] Outcomes of LT remain poor for angiosarcoma, which is an absolute contraindication. By contrast, at least some patients with epithelioid hemangioendothelioma have been transplanted successfully despite an extensive tumor burden, with documented regression of extrahepatic metastases (see Chapter 96).

For an LT candidate with a prior extrahepatic malignancy, therapy of the malignancy needs to have been curative, with the resected specimen indicating a low likelihood of metastatic spread. A 2-year recurrence-free interval prior to LT is adequate for most nonhepatic malignancies, but a longer period following resection may be desirable for breast cancer, colon cancer, and malignant melanoma.[29] Myeloproliferative disorders frequently underlie Budd-Chiari syndrome (see Chapter 85), but fortunately evolution to acute leukemia is not accelerated following LT.[30]

Ongoing alcohol and recreational drug use remain absolute contraindications to LT. If continued abuse is a concern, random toxicology screening tests are appropriate. Although medicinal marijuana may be used legitimately for palliation, most transplant programs discourage its use because of concerns about the adherence of users to other therapies and possible pulmonary side effects, as well as evidence that use of marijuana may accelerate fibrosis in HCV-induced liver disease.[31] Cigarette smoking is prohibited in LT candidates because of its multiple adverse effects, including an association with hepatic artery thrombosis and malignancy postoperatively.[32] A history of prescription narcotic abuse is also a cause for concern because it may contribute to difficulties with pain management postoperatively. Non-narcotic alternatives should be encouraged for the management of chronic pain. NSAIDs are contraindicated in cirrhotic patients because of potential renal and GI toxicity. With increasing use of herbal compounds and other complementary and alternative medicines, a discussion of their unproved efficacy and unknown toxicities—with caution against their use after LT because of potential for drug interactions—is appropriate (see Chapters 89 and 131).[33]

The pre-LT evaluation frequently uncovers important comorbidities, typically cardiac and pulmonary. Patients with decompensated cirrhosis were previously considered to have a diminished risk of coronary artery disease (CAD) because of low afterload, reflecting peripheral vasodilatation, decreased hepatic synthesis of cholesterol, and increased circulating estrogen levels. Subsequent data have shown that cirrhotic patients have a prevalence of CAD at least equal to that of an age-matched control population.[34] Risk factors for CAD in cirrhotic patients include a high prevalence of diabetes mellitus. Additional risk factors for CAD in the post-LT period

include immunosuppressive drugs that contribute to systemic hypertension, hyperlipidemia, and obesity. Assessment of cardiac risk in cirrhotic patients may be inadequate because of poor physical stamina during routine stress testing. Administration of dobutamine mimics the physiologic effects of exercise and is used in stress echocardiography to exclude clinically significant CAD in LT candidates. Patients who reach 85% of their maximal predicted heart rate without an abnormality on stress echocardiography have a low likelihood of peri- and postoperative ischemic cardiac events.[35] Cardiac catheterization and coronary angiography should be performed if CAD cannot be confidently excluded by noninvasive testing. Discrete coronary artery stenoses can be managed by pre-LT angioplasty and stenting. Although coronary artery bypass grafting may be contraindicated because of a risk of perioperative morbidity and mortality in a patient with decompensated cirrhosis, successful bypass surgery may render a patient an acceptable candidate for LT. The pre-LT evaluation may overestimate cardiac performance, and impaired cardiac function may become apparent only after the protective effect of decreased systemic vascular resistance (typical of cirrhosis) is lost following LT, when afterload increases because of the hypertensive effects of the primary immunosuppressive agents or excessive volume repletion.[36] Specific etiologies of cirrhosis may be associated with extrahepatic manifestations that diminish long-term survival. For example, fatal cardiac arrhythmias may result in poorer survival in patients with hemochromatosis who undergo LT.[37]

Pulmonary evaluation in the LT candidate may reveal abnormal arterial oxygenation (see Chapter 94). Although severe chronic obstructive pulmonary disease or pulmonary fibrosis precludes LT, respiratory restriction as a result of ascites or diminished respiratory muscle strength caused by chronic illness is reversible and is not a contraindication to LT. Even patients who undergo LT for α_1-antitrypsin deficiency may show improvement in pulmonary function tests postoperatively.[38] Pulmonary artery hypertension (hemodynamically defined as mean pulmonary artery pressure [MPAP] $\geq$ 25 mm Hg and pulmonary vascular resistance $\geq$ 240 dynes $\bullet$ s $\bullet$ cm^{-5} by right heart catheterization) in a patient with established portal hypertension is known as *portopulmonary hypertension*. Importantly, moderate or severe portopulmonary hypertension (MPAP $\geq$ 35 mm Hg and MPAP $\geq$ 45 mm Hg, respectively) increases the mortality rate beyond that predicted by the MELD score and, if not improved by medical therapy, is a contraindication to LT.[39,40]

The hepatopulmonary syndrome (HPS) is characterized by the triad of chronic liver disease, pulmonary vascular dilatations (with right-to-left shunting), and hypoxemia.[41] The diagnosis is suggested by an arterial oxygen tension (Pao$_2$) less than 80 mm Hg on arterial blood gas obtained with the patient sitting upright, or an alveolar-arterial (A-a) oxygen gradient of 15 mm Hg or greater when breathing ambient air; in patients older than 65 years of age, a Pao$_2$ of 70 mm Hg or less and an A-a gradient of 20 mm Hg or greater are commonly used thresholds. LT candidates should be screened for HPS with pulse oximetry, using a threshold saturation of peripheral oxygen (Spo$_2$) value less than 96% at sea level (corresponding to a Pao$_2$ < 70 mm Hg). The sensitivity and specificity of pulse oximetry for diagnosing HPS are 100% and 88%, respectively; therefore, confirmatory evaluation should be performed in patients with a low Spo$_2$.[42] Definitive diagnosis is made by the demonstration of intrapulmonary vascular dilatations by contrast-enhanced echocardiography (which is the most sensitive technique), perfusion lung scanning with ^{99m}Tc-labeled macroaggregated albumin, or right heart catheterization with pulmonary arteriography. Detection of contrast in the left side of the heart within several beats after its appearance in the right atrium indicates intrapulmonary shunting. Predictors of potential reversibility of HPS after LT include younger age, a lesser degree of preoperative hypoxemia, and adequate correction of hypoxemia with inspiration of 100% oxygen (Pao$_2$ < 200 mm Hg).[43] In the majority of patients with HPS, hypoxemia resolves within several months after LT, although protracted ventilatory support may be required. Because of the potential for improvement with LT, extra MELD points may be allocated to a patient with HPS.

HPS must be distinguished from portopulmonary hypertension because the latter is associated with high perioperative mortality and frequently unchanged pulmonary hemodynamics despite LT. Specifically, a MPAP greater than 35 mm Hg, pulmonary vascular resistance greater than 300 dynes • s • cm^{-5}, and cardiac output less than 8 L/minute are indicative of a high perioperative risk because the patient will be unable to increase cardiac output appropriately in response to altered intra- and postoperative hemodynamics. Vasodilator therapy may reduce pulmonary arterial pressure and permit LT (see Chapter 94).[44]

Hepatic hydrothorax is transudative fluid in the pleural cavity, usually on the right side and often with relatively little ascites remaining in the abdominal cavity, as a result of portal hypertension (see Chapter 93). It can be difficult to manage, often requiring repeated thoracentesis or placement of a TIPS prior to LT.[45] Insertion of a permanent chest tube can lead to infection in the pleural cavity. Similarly, interventions such as pleurodesis or pleural decortication should be avoided.

Active uncontrolled extrahepatic infection is an absolute contraindication to LT. In decompensated cirrhosis, unexplained clinical deterioration, such as altered mental status or systemic hypotension in the absence of GI bleeding, must be presumed to reflect sepsis and is an indication to start antibiotics empirically. LT, however, may be the only option for patients with recurrent bacterial cholangitis complicating PSC (see Chapter 68). Repeated bouts of SBP need to be controlled by antibiotic therapy prior to LT (see Chapter 93). A particularly ominous finding is fungemia, which is typically impossible to eradicate in a debilitated cirrhotic patient and precludes LT. HIV infection is not a contraindication to LT per se; however, the HIV viral load must be undetectable at the time of transplantation, and the CD4$^+$ T-cell count should be greater than 100/μL in candidates who have never had an opportunistic infection and greater than 200/μL in those who have had an opportunistic infection.[46] Overall post-LT survival rates for HIV-infected patients are similar to those for non–HIV-infected transplant recipients but are worsened by HCV coinfection, inability of the patient to tolerate antiretroviral medications, and low CD4$^+$ T-cell counts.[47]

An important consideration in the LT candidate is the presence of vascular abnormalities that may increase the complexity of surgery. With increased surgical experience, such abnormalities, most notably portal vein thrombosis, are less likely to be an obstacle to LT. More extensive vascular thrombosis with involvement of the superior mesenteric vein may require extensive vascular reconstruction.[48] The presence of a prior portosystemic shunt, particularly a nonselective (side-to-side or end-to-side) portacaval shunt, increases the technical complexity of LT but is not a contraindication. TIPS, used to control manifestations of portal hypertension including variceal hemorrhage, intractable ascites, and hydrothorax without disrupting the vascular anatomy, is now the most frequently encountered shunt and does not usually present an operative challenge.

Age restrictions have been relaxed for LT candidates, although close attention must be paid to comorbid conditions in older patients. The presence of comorbidities not only increases perioperative mortality but may also diminish the likelihood that the recipient will be able to return to an active lifestyle, particularly because severe liver disease may cause more debility in older than in younger patients.[49] Because a subset of robust older recipients have good outcomes, candidates in their late 60s or even older who are otherwise in good health should not be precluded a priori from LT.

The differential diagnosis of renal insufficiency in patients with advanced liver disease includes hepatorenal syndrome, which is potentially reversible. Renal insufficiency has a detrimental effect on survival in cirrhotic patients and remains an important predictor of poor outcomes after LT (see Chapter 94).[50] Typically, renal dysfunction in patients with decompensated cirrhosis reflects a variety of insults, including sepsis, hypotension, and use of nephrotoxic medications. Assessment of the potential for renal function to improve following LT is critical. Inclusion of the serum creatinine level in the MELD score has resulted in an increased rate of combined liver-kidney transplants, with consequent depletion in the supply of kidneys for patients awaiting isolated deceased-donor kidney transplantation.[51] According to a consensus statement,[52] approval for combined liver-kidney transplantation should be granted to patients with any of the following criteria: (1) end-stage renal disease and symptomatic portal hypertension or a hepatic vein wedge pressure gradient of more than 10 mm Hg, (2) end-stage liver disease and chronic kidney disease with a glomerular filtration rate of 30 mL/min or less, (3) acute kidney injury including hepatorenal syndrome with a serum creatinine level greater than 2.0 mg/dL and dialysis for more than 8 weeks, and (4) end-stage liver disease and evidence of chronic kidney disease with renal biopsy findings demonstrating more than 30% glomerulosclerosis or 30% fibrosis.

An important reflection of impaired free-water handling in patients with decompensated cirrhosis is dilutional hyponatremia. Consequences of marked hyponatremia include altered mental status and an increased risk of calcineurin inhibitor–induced neurotoxicity after LT (see later). Incorporation of the serum sodium level in the MELD formula (MELDNa) may increase the prognostic accuracy of the MELD score, particularly in patients with relatively low MELD scores.[53,54]

Another consequence of decompensated cirrhosis is malnutrition. Loss of muscle mass increases the likelihood of perioperative morbidity, with the need for more protracted ventilatory support and poorer patient survival. Peripheral edema and ascites result in changes in body weight or anthropometric measurements, making them unreliable for assessing nutritional status in patients with advanced cirrhosis. More profound nutritional deficiencies may reflect the specific cause of cirrhosis, as in a malnourished alcoholic person with deficiency of multiple vitamins and electrolytes, or depletion of fat-soluble vitamins in cholestatic liver disease due to small intestinal malabsorption. Evaluation by a dietitian is an integral part of the pre-LT evaluation. Attempts to improve the nutritional status of LT candidates have included enteral and parenteral feeding, which may result in improvement of clinical outcomes, albeit modest.[55] An increasingly growing pool of obese LT candidates is raising concerns about the role of obesity in the pathogenesis of NAFLD and in postoperative mortality resulting from cardiovascular events, as well as postoperative complications such as wound infections.[56]

TRANSPLANTATION EVALUATION AND LISTING

Although details of the evaluation process vary by center, key elements include confirmation that LT is indicated for the

TABLE 97-1 Transplantation Evaluation Process

Step	Comment
Financial screening	Secure approval for the evaluation
Medical evaluation	As discussed in text
Hepatology evaluation	Confirm the diagnosis and optimize management
Laboratory testing	Assess hepatic synthetic function, serum electrolytes, renal function, viral serologies, markers of other causes of liver disease, tumor markers, ABO-Rh blood typing; 24-hour urine for creatinine clearance; urinalysis and urine drug screen
Cardiac evaluation	Electrocardiography and 2-dimensional echocardiography; stress testing and cardiology consult if risk factors are present and/or the patient is ≥ 40 yr
Hepatic imaging	US with Doppler to document portal vein patency, triple-phase CT or gadolinium MRI for tumor screening
General health assessment	Chest film, prostate-specific antigen level (men), Pap smear and mammogram (women), colonoscopy if the patient is ≥ 50 yr or has PSC
Transplantation surgery evaluation	Assess technical issues and discuss the risks of the procedure
Anesthesia evaluation	Required if operative risk is unusually high (i.e., the patient has portopulmonary hypertension, hypertrophic obstructive cardiomyopathy, previous anesthesia complications)
Psychiatry or psychology consultation	If there is a history of substance abuse, psychiatric illness, or adjustment difficulties
Social work evaluation	Address potential psychosocial issues and the possible effect of transplantation on the patient's personal and social supports
Financial and insurance counseling	Itemize the costs of transplantation and post-transplantation care; help develop a financial management plan
Nutritional evaluation	Assess the patient's nutritional status and provide patient education

Adapted from O'Leary JG, Lepe R, Davis GL. Indications for liver transplantation. Gastroenterology 2008; 134:1764-76, with permission.

management of the potential recipient's liver disease, exclusion of comorbidities severe enough to preclude transplantation, and identification of adequate emotional and social resources to undergo a major surgical procedure and continue on long-term immunosuppression afterward (Table 97-1). Approval is sought from the patient's insurance carrier before the extensive testing necessary for the LT evaluation is undertaken. The patient is typically seen during the pre-LT evaluation by a transplant surgeon, hepatologist, psychiatrist, dietitian, and social worker, with additional consultations as clinically indicated. As increasingly frailer and older candidates are evaluated, identifying potential causes of perioperative morbidity, such as carotid artery stenosis, is imperative. Detailed abdominal imaging is performed not only to screen for HCC, but also to uncover vascular abnormalities such as portal vein thrombosis that may make surgery technically challenging. Disease-specific issues need to be addressed, such as the likelihood of recidivism in an alcoholic patient or management of a large tumor burden in a patient with HCC. The appropriateness of LT is then discussed formally at a meeting of the patient selection committee. If the patient's candidacy is deemed to be appropriate, formal listing is undertaken with UNOS, followed by matching of recipients by blood type and weight with potential deceased donors. Once listed, a patient's priority for organ allocation is determined by the MELD score, either the "biological" score or with additional points awarded in specific circumstances such as HCC. The waiting time on the list is no longer a determining factor. With the seemingly intractable shortage of deceased-donor organs, the challenge has been to develop an equitable system of organ allocation and to ensure that hepatic allografts are not placed in recipients whose prognosis without LT remains good. Patients with a MELD score of less than 15 appear to have better survival without transplantation than with transplantation.[57] As shown in Figure 97-3, the MELD score has been found to correlate with the 3-month survival rate. Patients with a MELD score of less than 10 are ineligible for active listing with UNOS unless they receive extra points because of additional complications of liver disease, such as HCC or HPS (UNOS policies 3.6.4.4 and 3.5.5.1, available at www.unos.org).

Once the evaluation process is complete and the patient is accepted for LT, financial clearance is sought from the patient's private, state, or federal insurer. Unfortunately, criteria for coverage for LT vary among insurers; however, in the United States, if Medicare, the major federal payor, funds a particular indication, other insurance carriers generally follow suit.

DISEASE-SPECIFIC INDICATIONS

Alcoholic Liver Disease

Despite the high frequency of chronic HCV infection as an indication for LT (see later), alcoholic liver disease (ALD)

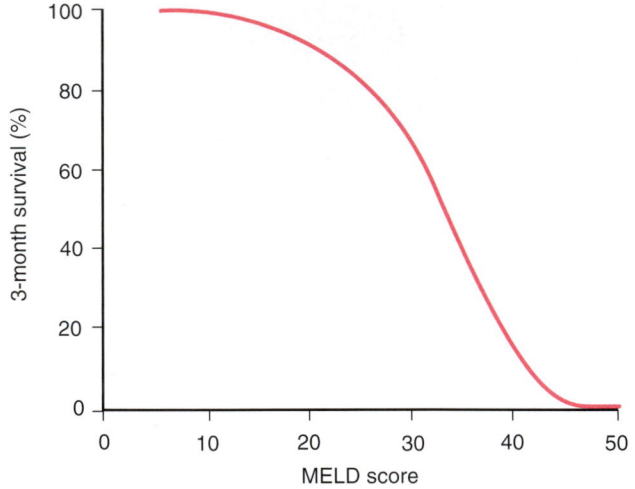

FIGURE 97-3. Relationship between the 3-month survival rate and the MELD score in patients with cirrhosis.

remains the most frequent cause of decompensated chronic liver disease (see Chapter 86).[58] Decompensated alcoholic cirrhosis is now firmly established as an appropriate indication for LT, despite some lingering controversy.[59] Concerns had included recidivism following LT, as well as potentially poor patient adherence. In addition, the large number of patients with ALD might outstrip the donor supply. These fears have not been confirmed, and even recipients with evidence of alcoholic hepatitis in the explant do not appear to have inferior post-LT survival rates, despite some earlier reports to the contrary.[60] Excellent graft and patient survival rates are the norm following LT for ALD.

Key factors in determining an alcoholic patient's candidacy for LT include recognition by the patient of the key role alcohol has played in the genesis of the liver disease, participation in some form of alcohol rehabilitation such as attendance at Alcoholics Anonymous, stable social support, and a defined period of abstinence prior to LT. Conventionally this period of abstinence has been 6 months, although rigorous studies have failed to confirm that this duration of abstinence confers a high likelihood of continued sobriety but have emphasized the importance of adverse factors such as social isolation or depression. Data have shown that up to 25% of patients with ALD listed for LT deemed to be abstinent continue to use alcohol; therefore, monitoring of adherence is prudent.[61] Despite these strategies, however, as many as 40% of alcoholic recipients resume alcohol use during long-term follow-up.[62] Surprisingly, graft loss or early death attributable to post-LT alcohol abuse has been uncommon. A higher rate of return to alcohol use is elicited by use of anonymous questionnaires or toxicology screening than by direct questioning of patients.

A particularly difficult dilemma arises in the alcoholic patient with severely decompensated liver disease and recent alcohol use in whom the likelihood of surviving without prompt LT is low. This dilemma persists because a significantly greater proportion of patients with severe alcoholic hepatitis (defined by a Maddrey's discriminant function score ≥ 32) that is nonresponsive to medical therapy with glucocorticoids (Lille score ≥ 0.45 after 7 days of medical therapy or continuous rise in the MELD score) have a higher rate of survival 6 months after LT compared with those who continue medical therapy (77% and 23%, respectively) (see Chapter 86).[60] In addition, post-LT outcomes are similar in patients with alcoholic hepatitis and those with alcoholic cirrhosis.[63]

Clearly enunciated criteria, including a contractual commitment by the patient to sobriety and active involvement in alcohol rehabilitation, ensure that selection is equitable. Patients who return to pathologic drinking after LT have more medical problems, including pneumonia, cellulitis, and pancreatitis, that can lead to graft loss and death.[64] In addition, alcoholic recipients are prone to develop de novo oropharyngeal and lung tumors, likely reflecting other aspects of an alcoholic lifestyle, most notably cigarette smoking.[65]

Hepatitis B

The availability of potent oral antiviral agents with low rates of resistance has resulted in a steady decline in LT for decompensated cirrhosis due to HBV infection.[66] In addition, HBV suppression prior to LT leads to a lower rate of recurrent HBV infection of the graft and improved survival after LT.[67] Effective prevention of graft reinfection in HBV-infected candidates has been a major triumph of LT. HBV recurrence was frequent and resulted in reduced patient and graft survival rates during the 1980s. Long-term high-dose hepatitis B immune globulin (HBIG) administration was the initial step in improving post-LT outcomes. Subsequently, HBIG administered in combination with the nucleoside analog lamivudine further decreased the rate of HBV recurrence. Lamivudine monotherapy for prevention of recurrent post-LT HBV infection was limited by frequent mutations in the HBV polymerase gene, with resulting resistance and graft reinfection (see Chapter 79).[68] Some groups have titrated HBIG doses according to trough serum levels of antibody to hepatitis B surface antigen (anti-HBs). Intramuscular administration of HBIG has been confirmed as an efficacious and less expensive alternative to IV HBIG regimens when used in combination with lamivudine. In addition, novel formulations of HBIG for subcutaneous administration are being evaluated.[69,70] Use of HBIG, however, is being curtailed and replaced by newer oral antiviral agents with a low risk of HBV resistance and a further decrease in post-LT HBV recurrence rates.[71] Emerging data support the efficacy of entecavir and tenofovir in preventing recurrence of hepatitis B after LT, and the use of these potent antiviral agents may obviate the need for HBIG.[72,73] A prospective study evaluating the efficacy of a combination of emtricitabine and tenofovir in preventing post-LT recurrence of HBV after discontinuation of HBIG endorses this approach.[74]

Hepatitis C

HCV is the most frequent indication for LT in North America and Western Europe. Recurrent HCV infection, however, leads to inferior graft and patient outcomes compared with LT for other major causes of cirrhosis. Analysis of serial liver biopsy specimens from liver transplant recipients with recurrent HCV infection demonstrates accelerated fibrosis and progression to cirrhosis.

Biopsy of the allograft helps identify recipients with recurrent HCV infection at increased risk of rapidly progressive disease. Less than 10% of patients with mild recurrent HCV infection at 1 year after LT progress to allograft cirrhosis within 5 years, whereas two thirds of those with at least moderately severe HCV infection at 1 year after LT develop cirrhosis.[75] Concern has been raised, however, that with longer follow-up, some patients with initially mild recurrent HCV infection will also progress. Berenguer and colleagues[76] evaluated serial protocol liver biopsy specimens to assess the histologic outcomes of 57 HCV genotype 1b–infected liver transplant recipients with an initially mild recurrence, defined as no or minimal hepatic fibrosis (fibrosis stage F0 or F1) during the first 3 years after LT (see Chapter 80).[76] They found

---

BOX 97-3 Factors Associated with Severe HCV Recurrence Following Liver Transplantation

Viral Factors
Absence of pretransplantation HBV coinfection
Cytomegalovirus coinfection
High serum HCV RNA levels before transplantation and within 2 weeks after transplantation
HCV genotype 1b

Immunosuppression
Multiple episodes of rejection (indicating a high cumulative prednisone dose)
Use of OKT3 to treat rejection

Other Factors
High TNF-α production in the graft
Impaired HCV-specific CD4+ T-cell responses
Ischemic-preservation injury
Nonwhite recipient

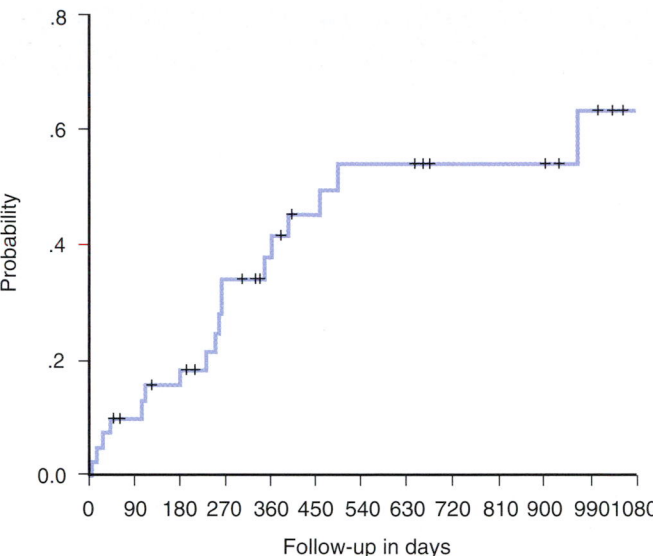

FIGURE 97-4. Probability of hepatic decompensation in 39 patients with cirrhosis resulting from recurrent hepatitis C following liver transplantation. *(From Berenguer M, Prieto M, Rayon JM, et al. Natural history of clinically compensated hepatitis C virus-related graft cirrhosis after liver transplantation. Hepatology 2000; 32:852-8, with permission.)*

that some degree of fibrosis at baseline appears to predict accelerated recurrent HCV infection.

A particularly ominous finding in liver transplant recipients with recurrent HCV infection is prominent biochemical and histologic cholestasis, a condition designated fibrosing cholestatic hepatitis (FCH), which is a precursor to allograft failure. The frequency of FCH is 5% to 10%, and HCV viremia during the first month after LT, HCV genotype 1 infection, and recipient interleukin (IL)-28B genotypes CT or TT are risk factors (see Chapter 80).[77,78] Histologically, FCH is characterized by extensive dense portal fibrosis with immature fibrous bands extending into sinusoidal spaces, ductal proliferation with hypercellularity, marked canalicular and cellular cholestasis, and moderate inflammation with mononuclear cells.[79] Histologic features, however, lack specificity for the diagnosis of FCH and may also be observed in recurrent HCV infection, acute cellular rejection, and chronic graft rejection. Treatment of FCH entails a reduction of immunosuppression and initiation of antiviral therapy.[5] In addition, conversion of tacrolimus- to cyclosporine-based immunosuppression has been suggested because the latter may have antiviral activity.[80]

Reported predictors of severe recurrent HCV infection have included a number of viral and nonviral factors (Box 97-3). Higher serum levels of HCV RNA before and immediately after LT, as well as the possibility of more rapid evolution of HCV quasispecies, have been implicated in aggressive recurrent HCV infection[76] (see Chapter 80). Older deceased-donor age is also an important risk factor. Episodes of acute cellular rejection, particularly if multiple, increase the severity of recurrent HCV infection. A major challenge is to distinguish recurrent HCV infection from graft rejection, because many of the histologic hallmarks of acute rejection, including bile duct injury, are also consistent with recurrent HCV infection. Examination of serial liver biopsy specimens may help clarify this issue and allow avoidance of inappropriate additional immunosuppression in the recipient with recurrent HCV infection rather than graft rejection.

Once recurrent HCV infection of the graft progresses to cirrhosis, hepatic decompensation is frequent. In contrast to recurrent HBV infection, effective prophylaxis against recurrent HCV infection has not been possible (Fig. 97-4).[5] Current treatment strategies generally fall into 3 categories: (1) pre-LT antiviral therapy, (2) preemptive therapy started in the early post-LT period before the development of clinically apparent acute HCV infection, and (3) post-LT therapy at the time of diagnosis of acute HCV infection or for established or severe chronic HCV infection.[5] The approach followed by most transplant centers has typically been to initiate antiviral therapy when evidence of clinically significant recurrent HCV infection is identified (as defined by either grade 3 or 4 [of 4] hepatic inflammation or a fibrosis stage of F2 or more). Increasingly, all-oral interferon- and ribavirin-free regimens with direct-acting antiviral agents (DAAs) are being used for the treatment of HCV infection (see Chapter 80).[81]

Recurrent HCV infection is a frequent cause of graft failure in liver transplant recipients, and the dilemma arises as to whether retransplantation is justified.[25] A subset of patients retransplanted for graft loss caused by recurrent HCV infection have reasonable survival rates in the absence of severe jaundice or renal failure at the time of retransplantation (see later).

DAAs are highly effective and now commonly used in clinical practice.[82-84] Emerging data support the efficacy of DAAs to treat recurrent HCV infection in liver transplant recipients.[85,86] Results of studies of combinations of DAAs in liver transplant recipients are eagerly awaited.

Acute Liver Failure

ALF is an uncommon but important indication for LT, owing to a low likelihood of spontaneous recovery. Excellent outcomes with prompt LT (unless major neurologic complications have occurred) are possible. ALF is defined by the onset of hepatic encephalopathy within 26 weeks of the initial recognition of acute liver disease (see Chapter 95). Despite an abrupt onset, antecedent chronic liver disease is absent, and hepatic recovery is possible. In the past, LT for ALF resulted in poorer patient survival rates than those for benchmark indications such as PBC. Subsequent experience, however, has shown that excellent patient survival rates are possible if ALF is identified early in its course and transplantation occurs before irreversible complications, especially neurologic, supervene.[87] The absence of papilledema on funduscopy and of typical findings on CT do not preclude the presence of cerebral edema

BOX 97-4 Criteria for Liver Transplantation in Acute Liver Failure

Criteria of King's College, London
Acetaminophen Cases
Arterial pH < 7.25 more than 24 hours after drug ingestion*
All of the following:
  Prothrombin time > 100 sec or INR > 6.5
  Serum creatinine level > 3.4 mg/dL (300 µmol/L) or anuria
  Grade 3 to 4 encephalopathy

Nonacetaminophen Cases
Prothrombin time > 100 sec or INR > 6.7
Any 3 of the following:
  Unfavorable etiology (seronegative hepatitis or drug reaction)
  Age < 10 or > 40 years
  Acute or subacute category (duration of jaundice > 7 days)
  Serum bilirubin level > 17.5 mg/dL (300 µmol/L)
  Prothrombin time > 50 sec or INR > 3.5

Criteria of Hôpital Paul-Brousse, Villejuif
Hepatic encephalopathy *and*
Factor V level < 20% in patients < age 30 yr *or*
Factor V level < 30% in patients ≥ age 30 yr

*Subsequent modification: arterial pH < 7.25 or serum lactate > 3.0 mmol/L after adequate fluid resuscitation.
From Keeffe EB. Liver transplantation: Current status and novel approaches to liver replacement. Gastroenterology 2001; 120:749-62, with permission.

TABLE 97-2 Comparison of Components of the Mayo Predictive Models for Survival in PBC and PSC

PBC	PSC
Serum bilirubin level	Serum bilirubin level
Serum albumin level	Serum albumin level
Patient's age	Patient's age
Prothrombin time	Serum AST level
Peripheral edema	History of variceal bleeding

Adapted from Murtaugh PA, Dickson ER, Van Dam GM, et al. Primary biliary cirrhosis: Prediction of short-term survival based on repeated patient visits. Hepatology 1994; 20:126-134; and Kim WR, Therneau TM, Wiesner RH, et al. A revised natural history model for primary sclerosing cholangitis. Mayo Clin Proc 2000; 75:688-694.

complicating worsening encephalopathy; therefore, direct intracranial pressure monitoring may be required to detect and manage this frequently lethal complication of ALF. Direct intracranial pressure monitoring can only be recommended, however, if local neurosurgical expertise and interest are available, because a high rate of complications has tempered enthusiasm for its use. Patients with ALF, regardless of etiology, should be promptly referred for urgent LT evaluation. Specific criteria to identify patients with ALF who are unlikely to recover spontaneously are shown in Box 97-4. The challenge in managing patients with ALF is to avoid unnecessary LT in those who will recover spontaneously, while not delaying it in patients in whom it is their only option for survival. The role of liver-assist devices in managing ALF, either as definitive therapy or as a "bridge to transplantation," remains an area of active investigation (see Chapter 95).

Cholestatic Liver Disease

PBC and PSC have been relatively common indications for LT, with a key role in the development of prognostic models, and PBC is a benchmark for patient and graft survival. The Mayo disease models to predict the course of cholestatic disorders (Table 97-2) have aided in determining the optimal timing of referral for LT (see Chapters 68 and 91). Patients with PBC and PSC should be referred for LT evaluation if their Mayo risk score predicts a 1-year survival rate of less than 95%. The models, however, do not take into account prominent and frequently disabling complications of cholestatic liver diseases, such as pruritus, osteopenia, or, in PSC, recurrent bouts of bacterial cholangitis and have now been superseded by the MELD score. Indications for LT in patients with cholestatic liver diseases are similar to those for patients with other chronic liver diseases. Additional MELD points may be granted to patients with PSC with either: (1) 2 or more episodes of culture-proved bacteremia within a 6-month period or (2) noniatrogenic septic complications of cholangitis, no identifiable correctable structural lesion, and absence of a biliary stent.[88] Despite the generally excellent results of LT for cholestatic disorders, PBC and PSC recur in approximately 25% of recipients at 10 years post LT.[89,90]

Biliary stricturing can be identified in a minority of recipients following LT for PSC.[3] Differentiation of recurrent disease from other causes of graft injury, such as chronic rejection or ischemia, may be difficult. Recurrent PSC results in nonanastomotic stricturing of the intrahepatic biliary tract. Although some improvement in symptoms can be obtained by balloon dilation and stent placement, long-term graft viability is reduced. Graft loss caused by recurrent PBC appears to be less frequent than that for PSC. Management of recurrent PBC entails excluding other causes of hepatic dysfunction. Primary immunosuppression with tacrolimus has been implicated in the recurrence of PBC by some but not all investigators. A controversial issue is whether colectomy reduces the risk of recurrent PSC in liver transplant recipients with PSC and IBD.[91]

Hepatic Malignancy

HCC is the most common primary hepatic malignancy in adults, typically occurring in the setting of cirrhosis. A notable exception is chronic HBV infection, in which HCC can arise in the absence of cirrhosis (see Chapter 96). HCC less than 2 cm in diameter discovered incidentally in an explant typically does not have an adverse effect on patient survival. The likelihood of tumor recurrence increases markedly, however, with greater tumor burden, vascular invasion, the presence of multiple lesions, and certain histologic features such as nuclear grade, microsatellitosis, and presence of giant or bizarre cells.[92] LT remains the definitive treatment of HCC; indeed, 24% of adult patients who received a liver allograft in the United States in 2009 had HCC (surpassed in frequency only by HCV infection, which accounted for 26% of adult LTs that year), reflecting the frequency of HCC in cirrhotic patients and the awarding of extra MELD points for HCC.[93]

Improvements in outcome of LT for HCC are attributable to better patient selection rather than adjuvant therapy.[94] The preoperative workup includes a bone scan and chest CT in addition to abdominal imaging. PET-based imaging is not accurate for staging early HCC. Portal vein occlusion in a patient with HCC is typically evidence of metastatic spread, which precludes LT. Generally accepted criteria for LT in patients with HCC include a tumor diameter of less than 5 cm if the tumor is solitary, or no more than 3 lesions, with the diameter of the largest lesion measuring no greater than 3 cm—the so-called Milan criteria, based on an initial experience from that city. Patients who meet the Milan criteria have a post-LT survival comparable to that for patients undergoing LT for decompensated cirrhosis in the absence of complicating HCC: 75% at 4 years.[95] Whether the Milan criteria are excessively restrictive, excluding potential recipients who might have done well with a low risk of tumor recurrence, remains controversial.[94] Expanded criteria have been proposed from the University of California, San Francisco (UCSF) to extend the limits of tumor size and number while preserving patient survival rates: specifically, a solitary tumor measuring 6.5 cm or less in diameter, or no more than 3 lesions, with the largest lesion measuring 4.5 cm or less and a total tumor diameter of 8 cm or less.[96,97] A meta-analysis, however, supports restriction of LT for HCC to patients who meet the Milan criteria rather than exceed them, although significant heterogeneity among included studies limits the strength of this conclusion.[98] With LDLT, recipients with HCC beyond Milan criteria had comparable survival to those meeting these criteria.[98] The comparable survival between patients undergoing LDLT for HCC under the Milan criteria and those undergoing LT under the expanded criteria reflects a reduction in waiting time for LT with a live donor. An international consensus statement, however, concluded that the Milan criteria remain the benchmark for selection of potential LT candidates with HCC.[99]

Adoption of the MELD score has resulted in proportionally more patients with HCC undergoing LT.[100] In addition, waiting times for patients with HCC to receive a deceased-donor organ have decreased significantly, and the number of patients removed from the waiting list because of progression of tumor has also decreased. In the most recent modification of the MELD score, patients with a solitary HCC measuring less than 2 cm do not receive additional MELD points, and patients with a solitary HCC measuring 2 to 5 cm or 3 nodules each measuring less than 3 cm receive 22 points. In addition, patients with HCC receive a 10% point increase for every 3 months on the waiting list.[101,102] Compared with prior allocation policies, fewer additional MELD points are now given for the diagnosis of HCC because of the relatively good short-term prognosis of patients with a small HCC.[100] Concern has been expressed that cirrhotic transplant recipients without HCC are now disadvantaged because of the preference given to patients with HCC. Importantly, when expanded criteria for LT (i.e., UCSF criteria) are used in patients with HCC, no additional MELD points are given to these patients.

Several adjuvant interventions have been reported in patients transplanted for HCC (see Chapter 96).[16] Recurrent tumor occurs frequently in the graft, so the rationale for adjuvant therapy is to eliminate hematogenous micrometastatic disease. Conventional systemic chemotherapy administered perioperatively as well as for varying durations before and after LT, and usually incorporating doxorubicin, is of uncertain benefit. One strategy to expand criteria for LT in HCC is to downstage the tumor with the use of neoadjuvant locoregional therapy so that the Milan criteria are met; whether this approach will ultimately improve patient survival remains to be determined.[97] For example, transarterial chemoembolization (TACE) is commonly employed to reduce tumor burden during the often protracted wait for LT. This intervention, however, can be hazardous in patients with decompensated cirrhosis, and its benefit in patients with favorable tumor characteristics remains to be confirmed. Radiofrequency ablation has also been used increasingly to manage HCC.

Confounding the management of the LT candidate with HCC is the frequent observation that the tumor burden in the explant is significantly underestimated by preoperative imaging studies. Nevertheless, a subset of patients with HCC can be cured by LT and would not have tolerated surgical resection of the tumor because of associated cirrhosis. The use of neoadjuvant treatments for HCC may reduce waiting list dropout rates. A Markov model has suggested that these interventions could be cost-effective when the time on the waiting list exceeds 6 months.[103,104]

One class of immunosuppressive agents, the mammalian target of rapamycin (mTOR) inhibitors (i.e., sirolimus and everolimus), has antineoplastic properties, and uncontrolled pilot studies have suggested lower tumor recurrence rates and improved survival in liver transplant recipients with HCC treated with sirolimus.[105,106] These results, however, have not been confirmed in randomized controlled trials, and therefore, current recommendations do not endorse the routine use of mTOR inhibitors to reduce the risk of HCC recurrence after LT.[99] Oral therapy for HCC with sorafenib in combination with sirolimus has been evaluated for treatment of recurrent HCC following LT, albeit only in small and uncontrolled preliminary studies. Conclusions about the efficacy of sorafenib in the treatment of post-LT recurrent HCC cannot be established at this time; however, there appear to be frequent side effects with sorafenib use in liver transplant recipients.[107,108]

Patients with the fibrolamellar variant of HCC, which is more common in younger adults without underlying cirrhosis, often present when the tumor burden is already large. Extensive resection can be tolerated because cirrhosis is absent, and LT may be performed in patients who have recurrent tumor after resection. Tumor recurrence after LT may be relatively indolent, and although not as infrequent as was once thought, survival rates are acceptable.[109]

Hepatoblastoma is a rare pediatric tumor that also occurs in the absence of underlying parenchymal liver disease. Initial management consists of surgical resection; adjuvant chemotherapy is indicated for metastatic disease, and LT is an option when the tumor cannot be resected (see Chapter 96).

Cholangiocarcinoma remains the only major primary hepatic tumor for which a definitive role for LT has been difficult to establish. Outcomes of LT for cholangiocarcinoma diagnosed preoperatively have been so poor that its presence had been regarded as a contraindication to LT, and even tumors discovered only incidentally in the explant have a high recurrence rate. A subset of patients with a perihilar tumor and absence of nodal involvement have an acceptable 5-year survival rate. The tumor burden, however, is frequently more extensive than suspected on imaging. The addition of en bloc pancreaticoduodenectomy to LT has not improved survival. Newer approaches to treatment include preoperative irradiation and chemotherapy, with careful intraoperative tumor staging followed by LT (see Chapter 69). A retrospective report evaluating the efficacy of neoadjuvant chemoradiation followed by LT for treatment of perihilar cholangiocarcinoma showed a 65% recurrence-free survival rate at 5 years, with the size of the tumor being an important determinant of recurrent disease (32% and 69% recurrence-free survival rates for patients with tumors measuring 3 cm or less and greater than 3 cm, respectively).[110]

Metabolic Disorders

Metabolic disorders amenable to LT (see Chapters 75 to 77) fall into 2 broad categories: diseases dominated clinically by obvious hepatocellular disease (e.g., Wilson disease, hemochromatosis) and those without clinical evidence of liver disease (e.g., primary hyperoxaluria, familial hypercholesterolemia). Metabolic disorders in general are more prominent in pediatric patients. Adult indications for LT include Wilson disease and hemochromatosis. Substantial improvement can occur following LT for Wilson disease in patients who present with neurologic involvement. A Wilsonian crisis with severe hemolysis is an indication for urgent LT because chelation therapy is ineffective. Compared with other forms of cirrhosis, hemochromatosis has been associated with poorer outcomes following LT because of cardiac and infectious complications. Ongoing studies are expected to clarify whether iron depletion in transplant candidates improves survival rates after LT.[111] Iron reaccumulation in the graft of transplanted hemochromatosis patients is a theoretical concern, but iron depletion is not typically required.[112] LT has also been performed as a curative procedure in combination with renal transplantation for primary hyperoxaluria, in which end-organ damage is confined to the kidney but the metabolic defect is hepatic. LT may be indicated in cases of multiple adenomas associated with glycogen storage disease and not only eliminates the risk of progression to HCC but also corrects the underlying metabolic disease (see Chapter 77).

Nonalcoholic Fatty Liver Disease

NAFLD is an increasingly frequent cause of cirrhosis and HCC (see Chapter 87). Morbid obesity (BMI > 40 kg/m^2) is commonly encountered in patients with NAFLD. Analysis of data from the UNOS registry has suggested that the risk of primary graft nonfunction is increased and short- and long-term survival is poorer in morbidly obese liver transplant recipients with various etiologies of end-stage liver disease.[113] When analyzed as an entire cohort and not stratified by BMI, however, patients with NAFLD have patient and graft survival rates that are comparable to those for other indications for LT.[114,115] Many of the key precipitants of NAFLD (obesity, hyperlipidemia, diabetes mellitus) are exacerbated by immunosuppression.[116] Recurrence of NAFLD after LT causes graft injury, although graft loss does not typically occur. De novo NAFLD after LT has also been described. In the absence of specific therapy for NAFLD, therapeutic efforts after LT should center on weight control, optimal diabetic management, and use of a lipid-lowering agent.

Vascular Disorders

Budd-Chiari syndrome, characterized by hepatic venous outflow obstruction, often mimics decompensated cirrhosis (see Chapter 85).[117] Good long-term results have been described in patients who undergo prompt TIPS or portosystemic shunt surgery, although LT is typically required if advanced fibrosis on a liver biopsy specimen is present. Despite the frequency of an underlying myeloproliferative disorder, accelerated progression to leukemia or bone marrow failure does not seem to occur after LT. Long-term anticoagulation is indicated in liver transplant recipients with Budd-Chiari syndrome.

Sinusoidal obstruction syndrome (SOS) is a similar disorder manifested by necrosis of zone 3 hepatocytes and fibrous obliteration of central venule lumens. Most commonly seen after hematopoietic cell transplantation (HCT), SOS may lead to hepatic failure and death in up to 25% of patients, despite an otherwise successful procedure. Although experience with LT for hepatic complications of HCT is limited,[118] LT appears to be the only intervention that consistently alters the course of advanced SOS. Similarly, LT has been shown to be effective in the management of severe post-HCT graft-versus-host disease with predominantly hepatic involvement (see Chapter 35). Patients with hypocoagulable (e.g., hemophilia A and B) as well as hypercoagulable (e.g., protein C and S deficiencies) hematologic disorders who undergo LT for other indications have been cured of these disorders owing to production of normal clotting factors by the graft and its vascular tissue.

Autoimmune Hepatitis

Failure of immunosuppression to arrest progression of autoimmune hepatitis with overt hepatic decompensation is an indication for LT (see Chapter 90).[119] In addition, the initial presentation of autoimmune hepatitis can be fulminant, requiring prompt LT, and a trial of glucocorticoid therapy may not be prudent because of the patient's decompensated state. The presence of HLA-DR3 is associated with a lower likelihood of a therapeutic response to immunosuppressive therapy in patients with autoimmune hepatitis compared with the presence of HLA-DR4. Excellent long-term survival is usual after LT for autoimmune hepatitis, although acute cellular rejection may occur more frequently than in recipients with other etiologies of cirrhosis. In addition, recurrent autoimmune hepatitis has been recognized increasingly and may require higher maintenance doses of immunosuppression. Recurrent disease mimics the features of disease in the native liver, with hypergammaglobulinemia and autoantibodies, and is generally glucocorticoid responsive. Graft survival is generally not diminished by recurrent autoimmune hepatitis.[3]

Others

A variety of other diagnoses are potential indications for LT (see Box 97-1). Adult polycystic disease with marked abdominal distention resulting from multiple hepatic cysts that are not amenable to resection has been treated successfully by LT (see Chapter 96). If chronic kidney disease is present, combined liver-kidney transplantation is indicated. Cerebral imaging is indicated to exclude intracranial aneurysms, which are a feature of this syndrome. Diseases with multiorgan involvement for which LT has been performed include Alagille syndrome, sarcoidosis, and amyloidosis (see Chapters 36 and 62). LT successfully arrests systemic manifestations of familial amyloid polyneuropathy. In addition, the explant, which is the source of the abnormal protein, is available for use in a "domino" fashion in an older recipient who will not live long enough for neurologic injury to develop.[120] Biliary cirrhosis associated with CF also has been managed successfully with LT, although patients remain at risk of infectious and other complications of this systemic disorder (see Chapters 57 and 77).

SURGICAL ASPECTS

Once a potential organ donor is identified, the local organ procurement organization coordinates harvesting and supplies pertinent donor medical information to centers with suitable potential recipients listed with UNOS. In contrast to other types of organ transplants, including kidney and hematopoietic cell, absence of HLA compatibility does not appear to affect liver graft survival. Donor-recipient matching is based primarily on ABO blood compatibility and recipient weight. In critically ill recipients, an ABO-incompatible organ may be implanted, with the recognition that graft survival may be diminished.[121] In addition to screening serologic studies and routine liver biochemical testing, particular attention is paid to the donor's medical history, including cardiovascular instability and need for vasopressor support before determination of brain death.

The typical deceased donor has had a catastrophic head injury or an intracerebral bleed, with brain death but without multisystem organ failure. Electrolyte imbalance and hepatic steatosis in the donor are predictors of graft nonfunction. A "donor risk index" has been derived to assess the likelihood of good graft function.[122] Key adverse factors include older donor age (especially > 60 years of age), use of a split or partial graft, and a non–heart-beating donor, from which the organs are harvested after the donor's cardiac output ceases, in contrast to the more typical deceased donation in which the organs are harvested prior to cardiovascular collapse. Use of non–heart-beating donors is associated with reduced rates of long-term graft survival and an increased risk of biliary complications and correlates with the duration of "warm ischemia" after cardiovascular collapse and before retrieval of the organ. With the critical shortage of deceased organ donors, expansion of the donor pool has included acceptance of donors 70 years of age and older. As noted earlier, however, use of older donors in recipients with HCV infection may lead to more severe recurrence of HCV infection, potentially limiting the use of older donors in at least some recipients.

The harvesting team makes a visual and, if necessary, histologic assessment of the donor organ. Particular attention is paid to anatomic variants in the hepatic artery that may complicate the graft arterial anastomosis in the recipient. Once donor circulation is interrupted, the organ is rapidly infused with cold preservation solution. Donor iliac arteries and veins are also retrieved in case vascular grafting is required. After its arrival at the recipient institution, further vascular dissection, with arterial reconstruction if necessary, is performed before implantation.

Splitting cadaveric donor livers either in situ during harvesting or ex vivo on return to the transplant center allows 2 recipients to receive portions of the organ if graft volume and quality are sufficient. An adult cadaveric liver is divided into 2 functioning grafts; the left lateral segment (segments 2 and 3) is used for a pediatric recipient, and segments 4 to 8 (the so-called right trisegment) are used for an adult recipient. Acceptable graft and patient survival rates can be obtained with split grafts, although high-risk unstable recipients may have poorer outcomes. Figure 97-5 shows the segmental anatomy of the liver, which is the basis of dissection for both split and living-donor LT.

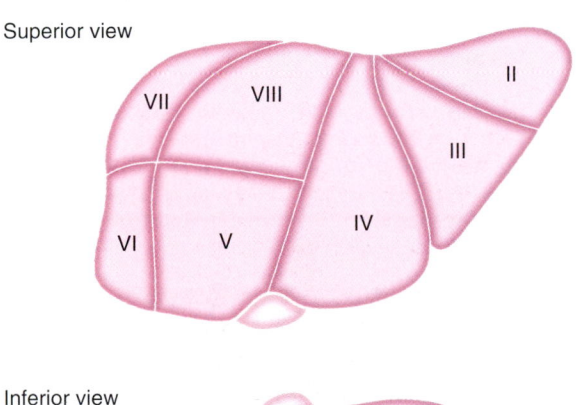

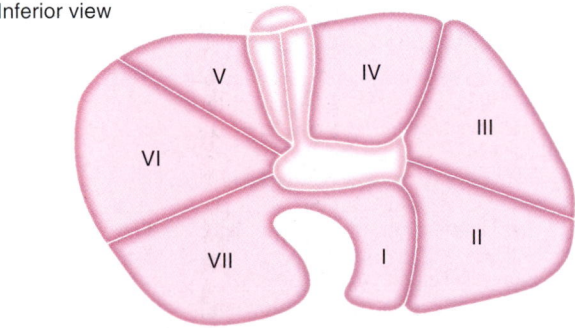

FIGURE 97-5. Segmental anatomy of the liver in the superior and inferior views. Segment VIII is visible only on the superior view, and segment I (caudate lobe) is visible only on the inferior view. *(From Keeffe EB. Liver transplantation: Current status and novel approaches to liver replacement. Gastroenterology 2001; 120:749-62, with permission.)*

Native Hepatectomy

Removal of the native liver is the most technically challenging part of deceased-donor LT. Previous abdominal surgery, especially a portosystemic shunt, and severe portal hypertension add to the complexity of hepatectomy, which is technically easier after placement of a TIPS compared with a surgical portosystemic shunt. Hilar dissection is performed to access the major hepatic vessels and devascularize the liver. Clamping of the portal vein during hepatectomy and liver implantation results in increased bleeding during dissection, mesenteric congestion, and production of lactate, whereas clamping of the inferior vena cava aggravates venous stasis and causes renal hypertension, with diminished venous return to the heart. To circumvent these problems, venovenous bypass is achieved by cannulation of the portal vein and inferior vena cava via the femoral vein and return of blood via the axillary vein to the right side of the heart. This technique is commonly performed in adults and older pediatric recipients. In some recipients, only a suprahepatic anastomosis to the vena cava is performed, the "piggyback" technique, in contrast to the more usual circumstance in which anastomosis to the vena cava is performed above and below the graft. The piggyback technique may be applicable if uninterrupted caval flow during LT is particularly beneficial, as in a recipient with cardiac instability, if a prior portosystemic shunt obviates the need for portal bypass or if the recipient is a pediatric patient in whom venovenous bypass may not be possible. The portal venous anastomosis is performed after portal bypass is terminated and is followed by the hepatic arterial anastomosis. Bile duct continuity is generally fashioned directly as a "duct-to-duct" anastomosis between the graft and recipient. Hepaticojejunostomy is the preferred anastomosis if there is intrinsic bile duct disease, such as PSC, or a major discrepancy in donor and recipient bile duct diameters. Microscopic surgical techniques facilitate the donor-recipient biliary and vascular anastomoses. Vascular anatomic anomalies increase the complexity of surgery further. In the past, a direct duct-to-duct anastomosis was typically stented by placement of a T-tube, with the added advantage of easy assessment of bile flow and its quality, as well as potential access for cholangiography postoperatively. The risk of a bile leak during subsequent removal of the T-tube, however, has led to its disuse.

The use of a live donor involves implantation of only a portion of the donor graft and is technically more challenging than using a whole cadaveric organ (see later). In contrast to orthotopic LT, in which the native liver is removed, auxiliary cadaveric LT is the placement of a graft without removal of the native liver. This technique has usually been performed in critically ill patients such as those with ALF who are too unstable to tolerate native hepatectomy.

Irrespective of the type of graft used, after the anastomoses are complete, the newly implanted graft is reperfused, with restoration of normal blood flow. The resulting release of vasoactive agents from pooled blood in the lower half of the body, however, can lead to lethal cardiovascular instability and tachyarrhythmias. Prompt bile production should occur if graft function is adequate. Hyperacute rejection is rare but devastating after LT and leads to rapid graft necrosis within hours and the need for urgent retransplantation.

Live-Donor Liver Transplantation

Extension of LDLT from pediatric recipients to adult recipients has remained controversial because of the magnitude of the risk to the donor in light of the large volume of donor liver required.[123] The potential donor is a healthy adult, typically a family member or close friend of the recipient, who volunteers to be evaluated. A series of checks and balances is necessary to ensure that the potential donor undergoes an adequate medical assessment and is not proceeding under duress. The potential recipient cannot be privy to details of the potential donor's evaluation. In most centers, a hepatologist not involved in the care of the recipient performs an assessment of the donor. Often an independent advocate is also appointed to safeguard the donor's interests. At each stage of the process, the potential donor is given the opportunity to withdraw from consideration.[124] Preoperative evaluation of the donor is best performed in 4 stages over a period of 1 to 3 months, with more invasive testing such as liver biopsy undertaken later in the evaluation (Box 97-5). After undergoing complete evaluation, only a relatively small proportion of potential donors are acceptable. One consequence of the evaluation of many potential donors has been the recognition that anatomic aberrations of the biliary and vascular system and unsuspected abnormalities on liver biopsy specimens are common in apparently healthy persons.

Right lobes (segments 5 to 8), extended right grafts (segments 4 to 8), or left hepatic grafts (segments 2 to 4) have been used successfully in adult-to-adult LDLT. Adult LDLT allows a reduction in waiting time and potentially mortality for recipients. An expected reduction in the risk of graft rejection because of receipt of a graft from a relative has not been confirmed, and a meta-analysis comparing recipients of deceased- and live-donor grafts has shown similar patient and graft survival and HCV recurrence rates.[125]

The overriding concern about LDLT is the consequences to the donor, including immediate perioperative morbidity and mortality, time lost from work, possible uninsurability in the future, and a lack of long-term follow-up data to ensure that hepatic resection and subsequent regeneration do not result in biliary or other abnormalities. The estimated mortality for live liver donors is different during the early postdonation period and long-term follow-up. For example, the risk of death for live liver donors within the first 90 days after donation has been estimated to be 1.7 per 1000, which is higher than the risk of death for healthy age-matched persons but not significantly different from the risk of death in live kidney donors. Cumulative long-term mortality estimates, however, are not different between live liver donors, live renal donors,

and healthy matched persons up to 11 years after donation.[126] Up to 38% of donors experience complications related to hepatic donation during the first 2 years that follow, including biliary leaks, bacterial infections, incisional hernias, pleural effusions, neurapraxia, surgical site infections, and intra-abdominal abscesses.[127]

IMMUNOSUPPRESSION

Immunosuppression is divided into induction (initial) and maintenance (long-term) phases. The goal of immunosuppression is to prevent graft rejection while avoiding morbidity due to its side effects.[128] Episodes of acute cellular and chronic ductopenic rejection require additional immunosuppression (see Chapter 35).[129]

The principal immunosuppressive agents, with route of administration, monitoring, and common adverse effects, are shown in Table 97-3, and drug-drug interactions in Box 97-6. The calcineurin inhibitors cyclosporine and tacrolimus form the basis for common induction and maintenance immunosuppressive regimens. Both agents, however, have substantial toxicity. Patients may be converted from a cyclosporine- to a tacrolimus-based regimen for glucocorticoid- or OKT3-refractory rejection (see later), late rejection (occurring > 6 months post LT), chronic ductopenic rejection, severe cholestasis, intestinal malabsorption of cyclosporine, or cyclosporine toxicity (hirsutism, gingivitis, severe hypertension). In chronic rejection, tacrolimus is less effective once the serum bilirubin levels rise above 10 mg/dL, underscoring the importance of early recognition. Although implicated in hepatic artery thrombosis as well as delayed wound healing and infections, sirolimus has been used as a calcineurin-sparing strategy in liver transplant recipients.[130] Basiliximab is a monoclonal antibody directed against the alpha subunit of the IL-2 receptor (CD25) and may be an alternative to glucocorticoids as an induction agent in LT.[131] Preliminary data support the efficacy of alemtuzumab (anti-CD52 monoclonal antibody) as a glucocorticoid-sparing induction agent; however, an increase in the frequency of infectious complications has been reported with its use.[132] Induction immunosuppression is tapered in the months following LT to avoid toxicity and lessen the risk of

---

BOX 97-5 Protocol for the Evaluation of Potential Living-Related Donors

Stage 1
Complete history and physical examination
Liver biochemical tests, blood chemistries, hematology, coagulation profile, urinalysis, AFP, CEA, and serologic tests for hepatitis A, B, and C, cytomegalovirus, EBV, and HIV
Abdominal US examination, chest film

Stage 2
Complete psychiatric and social evaluation
CT of the abdomen
Pulmonary function tests, echocardiography

Stage 3
Liver biopsy
Celiac and superior mesenteric angiography with portal phase*

Stage 4
MR cholangiography
Informed consent

*In stage 2, CT angiography is often done instead of standard angiography.
Adapted from Ghobrial RM, Amersi F, Busuttil RW. Surgical advances in liver transplantation. Living related and split donors. Clin Liver Dis 2000; 4:553-65, with permission.

BOX 97-6 Clinically Relevant Drug Interactions with Immunosuppressive Drugs

Drugs that increase blood levels of cyclosporine and tacrolimus:
  Antifungals: fluconazole, ketoconazole, itraconazole
  Antibiotics: clarithromycin, erythromycin
  Calcium channel blockers: diltiazem, verapamil
  Others: allopurinol, bromocriptine, metoclopramide
Drugs that decrease blood levels of cyclosporine and tacrolimus:
  Anticonvulsants: phenobarbital, phenytoin
  Antibiotics: nafcillin, rifampin
Drugs that increase nephrotoxicity of cyclosporine and tacrolimus:
  Gentamicin, ketoconazole, NSAIDs
Drugs that interact with mycophenolate mofetil:
  Acyclovir, ganciclovir (increase blood levels)
  Antacids (inhibit absorption)
  Cholestyramine (inhibits absorption)
Drugs that interact with azathioprine:
  Allopurinol, angiotensin-converting enzyme (ACE) inhibitors (increase hematologic toxicity)
  Warfarin (decreased anticoagulant effect)

TABLE 97-3 Immunosuppressive Agents Used in Liver Transplantation

Agent	Mode of Action	Monitoring	Toxic Effects
Cyclosporine	Calcineurin inhibitor: suppresses IL-2–dependent T-cell proliferation	Blood level	Renal, neurologic, hyperlipidemia, hypertension, hirsutism
Tacrolimus	Same as cyclosporine	Blood level	Renal, neurologic, diabetes mellitus
Prednisone	Cytokine inhibitor (IL-1, IL-2, IL-6, TNF, and IFN-γ)	None	Hypertension, diabetes mellitus, obesity, osteoporosis, infection, depression, psychosis
Azathioprine	Inhibition of T- and B-cell proliferation by interfering with purine synthesis	WBC count	Bone marrow suppression, hepatotoxicity
Mycophenolate mofetil	Selective inhibition of T- and B-cell proliferation by interfering with purine synthesis	WBC count	Diarrhea, bone marrow suppression
Sirolimus	Inhibition of late T-cell functions	Blood level	Neutropenia, thrombocytopenia, hyperlipidemia
OKT3 (Muromonab-CD3)	Blocking of T-cell CD3 receptor, preventing stimulation by antigen	CD3$^+$ count	Cytokine release syndrome, pulmonary edema, increased risk of infections
Basiliximab	Competitive inhibition of IL-2 receptor on activated lymphocytes	None	Hypersensitivity reactions

IFN, interferon; IL, interleukin.
Adapted from Everson GT, Karn I. Immediate post-operative care. In: Maddrey WC, Schiff ER, Sorrell MF, editors. Transplantation of the liver. 3rd ed. Philadelphia: Lippincott Williams & Wilkins; 2001. p 131.

recurrent disease, often by discontinuing maintenance glucocorticoids.[133]

POSTOPERATIVE COURSE

Initial Phase to Discharge from the Hospital

Because of the complexity of LT and the often markedly decompensated state of recipients, invasive monitoring with arterial and pulmonary venous lines is necessary in the first few postoperative days. If a T-tube is in place, dark copious bile provides evidence of satisfactory graft function. The patient's overall status, including neurologic recovery from anesthesia, urinary output, and cardiovascular stability, also reflects graft function. Routine antimicrobial prophylaxis includes bowel decontamination with oral nonabsorbable antibiotics, perioperative systemic broad-spectrum antibiotics, antifungal agents, and ganciclovir to prevent cytomegalovirus (CMV) infection. Markedly abnormal liver biochemical test levels are typical during the initial 48 to 72 postoperative hours and reflect a number of insults to the graft, including ischemia following harvesting and during preservation and subsequent reperfusion injury. The overall trend in serum aminotransferase levels should be downward, with a corresponding improvement in coagulopathy and a falling serum bilirubin level. Thrombocytopenia in the immediate postoperative period reflects a variety of processes, including residual splenomegaly, medications, and (importantly) reduced graft function.

Worrisome clinical features include scanty, pale bile if a T-tube has been used, metabolic acidosis, depressed mentation, and continued vasopressor support with worsening liver biochemical test levels. Hepatic artery thrombosis needs to be excluded promptly by Doppler US because it is an indication for urgent retransplantation. Hepatic artery thrombosis is more common in pediatric recipients because of the smaller size of the vessels. Antiplatelet therapy is administered to prevent hepatic artery thrombosis.[134] Primary nonfunction of the graft is also an indication for urgent retransplantation and is suggested by sluggish mentation, diminished urine output, cardiovascular instability, and coagulopathy. Donor characteristics associated with an increased likelihood of primary nonfunction include marked hepatic steatosis and profound hyponatremia. If graft function is adequate, however, vasopressor support can be tapered and extubation attempted, although the recipient who is markedly debilitated from advanced cirrhosis may require several days of ventilatory support. Poor graft function and renal insufficiency can also impede weaning.

During the first postoperative week, biochemical and coagulation test levels should steadily improve as ischemia and reperfusion injury resolve. Acute cellular rejection with graft dysfunction occurs at 1 week and beyond, with a rise in serum aminotransferase, alkaline phosphatase, and bilirubin levels. Because the biochemical features are nonspecific, liver biopsy is indicated to evaluate other diagnostic possibilities such as slowly resolving reperfusion injury, biliary tract obstruction, and cholestasis related to sepsis. Histologic findings characteristic of acute cellular rejection are bile duct injury, portal inflammation with eosinophils, and, with more severe injury, endotheliitis (Fig. 97-6). High doses of glucocorticoids (1000 mg of methylprednisolone or the equivalent) followed by a taper (200 to 20 mg/day) extending over several days constitute first-line therapy. A response is suggested by a return of liver biochemical test levels toward normal.

For the occasional patient with presumed acute cellular rejection who fails to respond to glucocorticoids, additional immunosuppression with the monoclonal antibody OKT3 (muromonab-CD3) may be necessary. Liver biopsy should be repeated before initiating more intensive therapy to confirm lack of a histologic response and to exclude other important causes of graft dysfunction, such as ischemia. The ability of

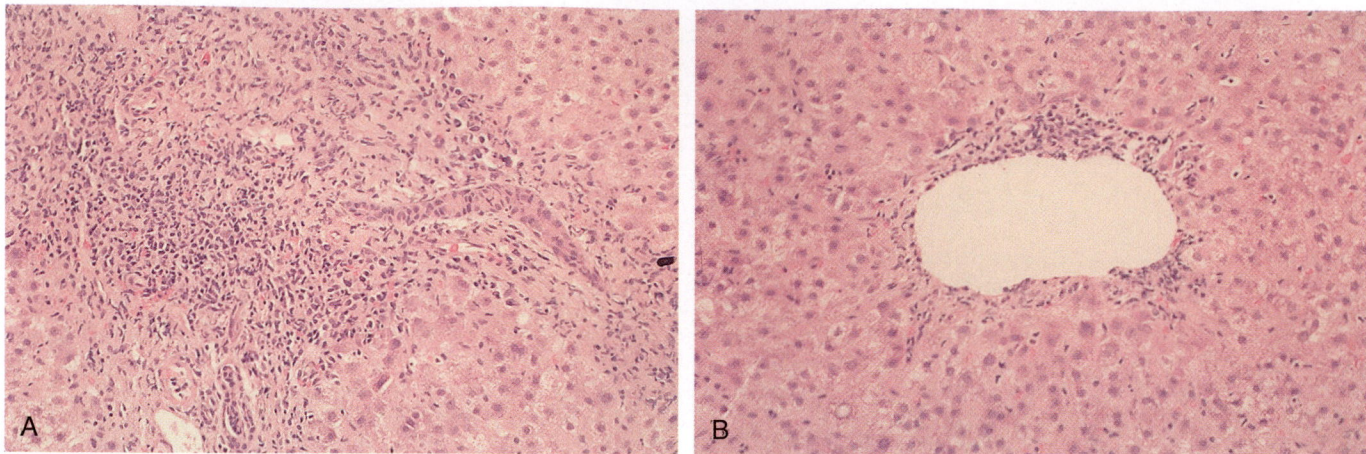

FIGURE 97-6. Histopathology of acute cellular rejection of a liver graft. *A,* The portal tract shows a lymphocytic and plasma cell infiltrate that spills over into the periportal hepatocytes and bile duct. *B,* The central vein shows attachment of lymphocytes to the endothelium (endotheliitis). *(From Cotran RS, Kumar V, Collins T, editors. Robbins' pathologic basis of disease. 6th ed. CD-ROM. Philadelphia: WB Saunders; 1999, with permission.)*

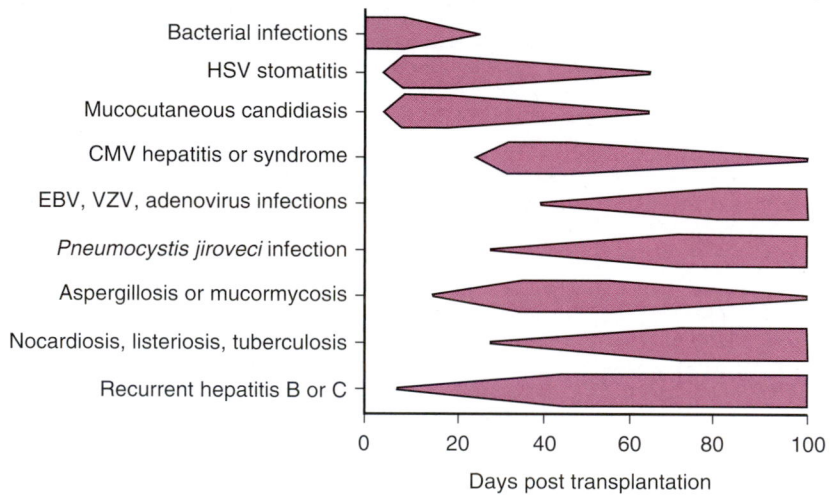

FIGURE 97-7. Time course of various infectious complications in liver transplant recipients. CMV, cytomegalovirus; VZV, varicella-zoster virus. *(Adapted from Everson GT, Kam I. Immediate post-operative care. In: Maddrey WC, Schiff ER, Sorrell MF, editors. Transplantation of the liver. 3rd ed. Philadelphia: Lippincott Williams & Wilkins; 2001. p 131.)*

recurrent HCV infection to mimic the histologic features of acute cellular rejection has led to reevaluation of the need to treat apparent acute cellular rejection aggressively under all circumstances. Routine (protocol) liver biopsies have also fallen out of favor because histologic evidence of acute cellular rejection can be noted in the absence of worsening graft function, with no apparent clinical significance.

In the first 3 to 4 weeks after LT, infections are typically bacterial and related to surgical complications such as intra-abdominal bleeding, bile leak, or wound infection. The timing of various infectious complications following LT is shown in Figure 97-7.

Other issues encountered during the first weeks following LT are listed in Box 97-7. Neurologic dysfunction can present as an acute confusional state or seizures, with a differential diagnosis that includes lingering effects of hepatic encephalopathy, electrolyte imbalance, poor graft function, sepsis, uremia, and side effects of medications. Of particular concern is the development of neurologic toxicity caused by the major

immunosuppressive agents. Management includes correcting electrolyte imbalances and reducing the dose of calcineurin inhibitors, which can be facilitated by the use of mycophenolate mofetil.[135] Overly rapid correction of hyponatremia perioperatively has been implicated in the genesis of central pontine myelinolysis, with evidence of osmotic demyelination on MRI. Diabetes mellitus can present for the first time postoperatively, and HCV infection increases the risk of diabetes mellitus in liver transplant recipients.[136] Post-LT renal impairment can reflect a number of factors, including slowly resolving pre-LT hepatorenal syndrome or renal failure due to other causes, intraoperative hypotension resulting in acute tubular necrosis, and (importantly) the nephrotoxic effects of cyclosporine and tacrolimus, which cause renal afferent arteriolar vasoconstriction with a reduction in glomerular filtration. Adjunctive therapy with mycophenolate mofetil allows a reduction in the doses of cyclosporine and tacrolimus while providing adequate immunosuppression. Short-term hemodialysis may be necessary until renal function improves.

BOX 97-7 Medical Complications in the Immediate Post-Transplantation Period

Infections
Bacterial
Viral
    Cytomegalovirus
    EBV
Fungal
    Aspergillosis, mucormycosis
    Candidiasis, torulopsosis
    Pneumocystis jiroveci pneumonia
Respiratory Complications
Acute respiratory distress syndrome
Hepatopulmonary syndrome
Pneumonia
Portopulmonary hypertension
Pulmonary edema
Acute Kidney Injury
Cardiovascular Diseases
Cardiomyopathy
Hemochromatosis
Idiopathic hypertrophic subaortic stenosis
Hypertension
Myocardial ischemia
Valvular heart disease
Neurologic Complications
Central nervous system hemorrhage
Central pontine myelinolysis
Ischemic events
Seizures
Coagulopathies
DIC
Thrombocytopenia
Diabetes Mellitus

From Everson GT, Karn I. Immediate post-operative care. In: Maddrey WC, Schiff ER, Sorrell MF, editors. Transplantation of the liver. 3rd ed. Philadelphia: Lippincott Williams & Wilkins; 2001, with permission.

Following Discharge from the Hospital

If the initial postoperative course has been smooth, planning for discharge is possible by the second week after LT. Recovery is often more protracted, particularly in debilitated recipients. Once discharged, patients are seen at frequent intervals during the first postoperative month. Liver biochemical test levels should normalize within a few weeks. Graft dysfunction is an indication for prompt liver biopsy to exclude acute cellular rejection. CMV becomes an important infectious consideration 3 or more weeks post LT.[137] Histologic features suggestive of CMV hepatitis include "owl's eye" inclusion bodies in the hepatocytes, as well as neutrophilic abscesses with focal necrosis of the parenchyma (see Chapter 83). Recipients who are CMV naïve are at increased risk of CMV infection, particularly if they receive a graft from a CMV-seropositive donor. These patients are candidates for more intensive antiviral prophylaxis. Oral ganciclovir or valganciclovir for a minimum of 3 months following LT is recommended for CMV prophylaxis.[138]

A distinction is made between asymptomatic CMV viremia, which may not require additional antiviral therapy, and CMV disease with systemic complaints such as fever, graft hepatitis, and diarrhea. CMV viremia is detected by PCR-based quantitative nucleic acid testing and by identification of CMV pp65 antigenemia.[138] Reactivation of CMV in a previously infected recipient tends to be less clinically severe than de novo infection. The diagnosis of tissue-invasive CMV disease requires confirmation by immunohistochemistry or in situ DNA hybridization techniques, because CMV viremia is not a reliable diagnostic finding in these cases.[138] High-dose IV ganciclovir is effective for treating CMV infection; however, viral resistance has been described. Oral valganciclovir is also a therapeutic option for milder CMV disease. IV ganciclovir is the preferred antiviral agent for patients with severe CMV infection or GI involvement (which may limit the bioavailability of oral antiviral agents). Treatment of CMV infection should be continued for at least 2 weeks and until complete resolution of symptoms with viral eradication is achieved.[138] Other therapies include CMV hyperimmune globulin and foscarnet. Not only is CMV infection an important cause of morbidity and mortality in liver transplant recipients, but it also has been implicated in other complications, notably chronic graft rejection and severe recurrent HCV infection.

Trimethoprim/sulfamethoxazole is prescribed to prevent *Pneumocystis jiroveci* infection. In patients intolerant of sulfa drugs, options include atovaquone, dapsone tablets, or inhaled pentamidine, although these agents are less effective than trimethoprim/sulfamethoxazole and have a narrower spectrum of protection against other opportunistic pathogens.[139] Prophylaxis needs to be continued for at least 1 year following LT.

Fungal infections pose a major threat to liver transplant recipients, particularly in the presence of marked debilitation, intensive immunosuppression for rejection, or retransplantation. Antifungal prophylaxis against invasive candidiasis for 7 to 14 days after LT, with either fluconazole or liposomal amphotericin B, is recommended for high-risk recipients.[140] Sites of infection are mucocutaneous (oral and esophageal), pulmonary, and intracerebral. Despite prolonged therapy with amphotericin, voriconazole, or itraconazole, a fatal outcome is usual with invasive fungal infection. A diagnosis of brain abscess due to *Aspergillus* implies a dismal prognosis. Superficial skin infections and simple colonization must be distinguished from invasive fungal infections, because topical antifungal agents such as nystatin or clotrimazole can eradicate the former. Similarly, bladder irrigation with amphotericin can cure candidal cystitis without the need for systemic antifungal therapy.

Although opportunistic infections are always a concern in liver transplant recipients, nonopportunistic infections also occur. Standard antibiotic therapy is appropriate for community-acquired respiratory infections, but a more extensive workup is indicated when symptoms are unusually severe or fail to resolve rapidly with treatment. Invasive diagnostic testing such as bronchoscopy or lumbar puncture with cultures may be necessary if clinically indicated. Enteric bacteremia may be an initial clue to hepatic artery thrombosis in an otherwise stable recipient. Reactivation of TB may present in an atypical fashion after LT.

Early recurrence of HCV infection may also become apparent during initial follow-up. As noted earlier, it is crucial to recognize that several histologic features of acute cellular rejection, such as bile duct inflammation and endotheliitis, may be mimicked by recurrent HCV infection (Table 97-4).

If a liver biopsy specimen shows features suggestive of biliary obstruction or if graft dysfunction is associated with clinical features of cholangitis such as fever and abdominal pain, a cholangiogram is necessary with MRCP because of its noninvasive nature and high degree of accuracy irrespective of the type of biliary anastomosis.[141] An anastomotic stricture in a choledochocholedochostomy is usually easily managed by endoscopic balloon dilation and temporary internal stenting (see Chapter 70). Surgical intervention is reserved for patients who do not respond to this approach, in which case conversion to a Roux-en-Y anastomosis is usual.

TABLE 97-4 Histologic Features of Recurrent HCV Infection versus Acute Cellular Rejection

Feature	Recurrent HCV Infection	Rejection
Time of onset after liver transplantation	Any time; onset usually within the first year	Usually within the first 2 months

Portal inflammation
  Lymphocytes
  Lymphoid aggregates
  Lymphoid follicles
  Eosinophils
	Most cases
	Bland, uniform
	Usually
	50% of cases
	Inconspicuous
		Always
		Activated
		Occasionally
		Rarely
		Almost always

Steatosis	Often	Never
Acidophilic bodies	Common	Uncommon
Bile ductule damage	About 50% of cases	Common
Atypical features	Cholestasis, ballooning degeneration without significant inflammation, marked ductular proliferation mimicking obstruction, granulomas	Prominent periportal and lobular necroinflammatory activity without subendothelial venular inflammation

From Rosen HR, Martin P. Liver transplantation. In: Schiff ER, Sorrell MF, Maddrey WC, editors. Schiff's diseases of the liver. 8th ed. Philadelphia: Lippincott-Raven; 1999. p. 1589.

A critical issue is distinguishing anastomotic from non-anastomotic biliary strictures caused by ischemia or other insult to the graft. The bile duct in the LT recipient is prone to ischemia because of its relatively tenuous arterial blood supply, and the development of a biliary stricture (unless it is obviously anastomotic) may reflect hepatic artery thrombosis. Ischemic stricturing is generally diffuse but can be predominantly hilar. Although temporizing measures such as balloon dilation may be attempted, such efforts are generally futile if hepatic artery thrombosis is present or stricturing is widespread and retransplantation will be required. Other causes of nonanastomotic stricturing include the use of an ABO-incompatible graft and protracted cold ischemia after harvesting. Biliary strictures can also be a feature of recurrent PSC.

LONG-TERM MANAGEMENT

General Preventive Measures

Long-term survival after LT is dependent on good general medical care of common disorders including hypertension, hyperlipidemia, and diabetes mellitus.[142] Once a recipient has stable graft and renal function, serial blood work including blood cell counts and serum liver biochemical tests, creatinine, and calcineurin inhibitor levels are obtained every few months and reviewed by the transplant center.

Systemic hypertension is a frequent complication of LT and is related to calcineurin inhibitor–induced renal vasoconstriction, as well as to the effects of other drugs such as glucocorticoids. Unfortunately, a reduction in immunosuppression is generally ineffective in ameliorating hypertension. Another contributing factor is mild renal insufficiency, which is frequent after LT. Initial antihypertensive therapy usually consists of a calcium channel blocker. Angiotensin-converting enzyme inhibitors and potassium-sparing diuretics are relatively contraindicated because of their propensity to accentuate hyperkalemia, which is frequent in liver transplant recipients, who often have renal tubular acidosis caused by the calcineurin inhibitor. Because cyclosporine and tacrolimus levels are increased by verapamil and diltiazem, nifedipine is the agent of choice. β-Adrenergic blocking agents are second-line antihypertensive agents; thiazide and loop diuretics are generally avoided because of concern about exacerbating renal insufficiency and electrolyte imbalance in the liver transplant recipient. Furosemide, however, is the diuretic of choice if fluid overload is present. In the minority of patients in whom hypertension is not controlled, a centrally acting agent such as clonidine may be introduced. For the occasional patient with intractable hypertension on cyclosporine-based immunosuppression, substitution of tacrolimus for cyclosporine may improve blood pressure control. Both cyclosporine and tacrolimus are nephrotoxic and accentuate impairment of renal function that may have existed perioperatively. Although acute nephrotoxicity may respond to interruption of or a reduction in the dose of these drugs, chronic renal impairment is usually irreversible. Drastic dose reductions of a calcineurin inhibitor may precipitate graft rejection and should be avoided. Cofactors implicated in advanced chronic kidney disease after LT include recurrent HCV infection with associated glomerulonephritis, diabetes mellitus, and systemic hypertension.[143] Renal transplantation may be considered in liver transplant recipients who become dialysis dependent after an otherwise successful LT.

Osteopenia is a frequent cause of morbidity in liver transplant recipients.[144] Although hepatic osteodystrophy is typically associated with cholestatic liver diseases, it is also common in patients with cirrhosis of other etiologies. Factors implicated in the pathogenesis of hepatic osteodystrophy include poor nutritional status, immobility, the calciuric effect of many diuretics, hypogonadism, and glucocorticoid use in patients with autoimmune hepatitis. In the initial several months after LT, osteopenia is accelerated further by high-dose glucocorticoid therapy as well as the other major immunosuppressive agents. Atraumatic fractures may occur in trabecular bone such as vertebrae or ribs. Bone mass increases after doses of immunosuppressive agents are reduced and mobility increases. Supplemental calcium and vitamin D are prescribed to patients with osteopenia, as is a bisphosphonate in patients with osteoporosis.

De novo malignancies are increased in frequency following LT.[145] Recipients need ongoing age-appropriate surveillance for common tumors such as breast, cervical, and colon cancer.[146] Screening for prostatic carcinoma by yearly digital rectal examination is recommended in male liver transplant recipients older than age 40. Screening with prostate-specific antigen (PSA) testing may also be considered on an individual basis; the incidence of prostate cancer in liver transplant recipients appears to be comparable to that in nontransplanted men. Screening for colorectal cancer by colonoscopy should also be performed every 3 to 5 years after age 50 in asymptomatic recipients; in patients with a history of PSC and UC, yearly colonoscopy with surveillance mucosal biopsies is recommended (see Chapters 68 and 116). Adherence to cervical cancer screening guidelines for the general population and screening female recipients older than age 40 for breast cancer by yearly mammography seem appropriate.[146] Other malignancies that are increased in frequency in organ transplant recipients include those of the skin, lung, liver, female genital tract, and GI tract. Alcoholic patients may be particularly prone to malignancies of the oropharynx (see Chapter 86).[147] Patients should be encouraged to use sunscreen regularly and have periodic examinations by a dermatologist.

Post-transplantation lymphoproliferative disorder (PTLD) varies from a low-grade indolent process to an aggressive neoplasm.[148] Uncontrolled proliferation of B cells after LT, typically in response to primary EBV infection, can be polyclonal or monoclonal. Pediatric recipients are at particular risk because of the absence of prior EBV infection. Intensive immunosuppression with OKT3 for severe rejection increases the risk of PTLD, which can present as a mononucleosis-like syndrome, lymphoproliferation, or malignant lymphoma. Clinical features suggestive of PTLD include lymphadenopathy, unexplained fever, and systemic symptoms such as weight loss. The majority of patients with PTLD present with extranodal masses, primarily involving the GI tract (stomach or intestine), lungs, skin, central nervous system, or hepatic allograft.[147] The WHO classifies PTLD into 4 main categories based on clinical, morphologic, immunophenotypic, and genetic features: benign polyclonal lymphoproliferation (early lesions), polymorphic PTLD, monomorphic PTLD, and classic Hodgkin's lymphoma–like PTLD. Management includes a reduction in immunosuppression and antiviral therapy directed against EBV, if present, with ganciclovir. Systemic chemotherapy, including the anti-CD20 monoclonal antibody rituximab, may be required in patients with malignant lymphoma.[147] The higher frequency of PTLD in pediatric recipients has led to surveillance by PCR methodology for EBV viremia and reduction in the level of immunosuppression in patients with a positive result before clinical features of PTLD occur. In addition, antiviral prophylaxis is prescribed for high-risk recipients, including those who are seronegative for EBV and received a graft from a seropositive donor. Chronic graft rejection is increased in frequency in survivors of PTLD because of reduction in the level of immunosuppression, which may be increased cautiously after PTLD is contained.

Hyperlipidemia is observed in up to half of liver transplant recipients, reflecting a number of factors including diabetes mellitus, obesity, renal dysfunction, and immunosuppressive agents, especially cyclosporine.[149] Pharmacologic therapy is indicated if hypercholesterolemia fails to improve with weight reduction and tight glycemic control. Pravastatin, a 3-hydroxy-3-methylglutaryl coenzyme-A-reductase inhibitor, is well tolerated and efficacious in liver transplant recipients.[150] Diabetes mellitus is common in liver transplant recipients and occurs in approximately one third of patients for the first time after transplantation. The pathogenesis is multifactorial; immunosuppressive therapy is a major factor because of the hyperglycemic effects of prednisone, cyclosporine, tacrolimus, azathioprine, and mycophenolate mofetil. HCV infection is also implicated. In most diabetic recipients, therapy with insulin is required. The high frequency of diabetes mellitus following LT has led to the development of glucocorticoid-sparing immunosuppressive regimens (see earlier).

A related problem is obesity, which is frequent even in liver transplant recipients who were profoundly malnourished preoperatively. Risk factors include glucocorticoid use, increased caloric intake, and decreased physical activity during recuperation from surgery. Immunosuppression with tacrolimus has been reported to result in less weight gain than occurs with cyclosporine; to a large extent, this difference may reflect the lower glucocorticoid doses used with tacrolimus. Management of obesity in this population includes a reduction in glucocorticoid doses and even complete withdrawal if possible. Use of mycophenolate mofetil may permit maintenance immunosuppression without glucocorticoids.

Excessive alcohol consumption (>20 g/day for women and > 30 g/day for men) is associated with poorer long-term survival after LT, regardless of the primary indication for transplantation.[151] Given the lack of data about the safety of more moderate alcohol consumption in liver transplant recipients, complete abstinence should be encouraged as a conservative approach.

Immunizations and Antibiotic Prophylaxis

Immunization against hepatitis A and B, influenza, pneumococcus, tetanus, and diphtheria is part of the standard pre-LT evaluation. A substantial proportion of patients may be unable to mount adequate antibody responses because of the immunosuppression associated with end-stage liver disease. Vaccines based on live or attenuated microorganisms (i.e., measles, mumps, rubella, oral polio, BCG, vaccinia, varicella-zoster) are contraindicated because of the risk of reactivation. Prophylactic antibiotics are recommended for any dental procedure, even basic cleaning.

Hepatic Retransplantation

Although improved immunosuppressive regimens have led to a lower rate of graft loss from chronic rejection, recurrence of the underlying liver disease has been recognized increasingly as a cause of graft failure, as illustrated most strikingly in HCV-infected recipients.[152] Understanding the full effect of recurrent disease, especially nonviral disease, on patient and graft survival will require studies with long-term follow-up. For example, although the rate of histologic recurrence of viral hepatitis is greatest in the first year following LT, recurrent PBC or PSC develops in less than 5% of patients by the first year, whereas more than 20% demonstrate histologic recurrence 10 years after LT.[153] As patients enter their second and third decades following LT, the number of patients who require retransplantation may deplete the donor pool further. This issue is compounded by the observation that patients who undergo retransplantation experience an approximate 20% overall reduction in the rate of survival but consume an increased amount of resources when compared with primary liver transplant recipients. On the basis of these considerations, a number of investigators have developed models to predict survival following retransplantation, especially for HCV infection.[154] For example, the liver transplant recipient with jaundice, graft failure caused by recurrent HCV infection, and renal failure has a markedly diminished likelihood of surviving retransplantation. In low-risk patients, retransplantation is associated with survival comparable to that for primary LT; however, determining whether retransplantation is justified in patients with high risk scores will require prospective studies and better treatments (e.g., for HCV).

Major challenges remain in LT, including the shortage of donor organs, threat of recurrent disease, and morbidity associated with lifelong therapeutic immunosuppression. Nevertheless, the availability of LT has transformed the lives of patients with advancing liver disease and their health care providers from an ultimately futile effort to manage the complications of cirrhosis into a life-prolonging and life-enhancing intervention.

KEY REFERENCES

Full references for this chapter can be found on www.expertconsult.com.

1. O'Leary JG, Lepe R, Davis GL. Indications for liver transplantation. Gastroenterology 2008; 134:1764-76.
13. Grewal P, Martin P. Pretransplant management of the cirrhotic patient. Clin Liver Dis 2007; 11:431-49.
39. Safdar Z, Bartolome S, Sussman N. Portopulmonary hypertension: An update. Liver Transpl 2012; 18:881-91.
47. Terrault NA, Roland ME, Schiano T, et al. Outcomes of liver transplant recipients with hepatitis C and human immunodeficiency virus coinfection. Liver Transpl 2012; 18:716-26.
54. Leise MD, Kim WR, Kremers WK, et al. A revised Model for End-Stage Liver Disease optimizes prediction of mortality among patients awaiting liver transplantation. Gastroenterology 2011; 140:1952-60.
60. Mathurin P, Moreno C, Samuel D, et al. Early liver transplantation for severe alcoholic hepatitis. N Engl J Med 2011; 365:1790-800.
72. Fung J, Cheung C, Chan SC, et al. Entecavir monotherapy is effective in suppressing hepatitis B virus after liver transplantation. Gastroenterology 2011; 141:1212-9.
98. Mazzaferro V, Bhoori S, Sposito C, et al. Milan criteria in liver transplantation for hepatocellular carcinoma: An evidence-based analysis of 15 years of experience. Liver Transpl 2011; 17(Suppl 2):S44-57.
99. Clavien PA, Lesurtel M, Bossuyt PM, et al. Recommendations for liver transplantation for hepatocellular carcinoma: An international consensus conference report. Lancet Oncol 2012; 13:e11-22.
100. Ioannou GN, Perkins JD, Carithers RL Jr. Liver transplantation for hepatocellular carcinoma: Impact of the MELD allocation system and predictors of survival. Gastroenterology 2008; 134:1342-51.
101. European Association for the Study of the Liver, European Organisation for Research and Treatment of Cancer. EASL-EORTC clinical practice guidelines: Management of hepatocellular carcinoma. J Hepatol 2012; 56:908-43.
110. Darwish Murad S, Kim WR, Harnois DM, et al. Efficacy of neoadjuvant chemoradiation, followed by liver transplantation, for perihilar cholangiocarcinoma at 12 US centers. Gastroenterology 2012; 143:88-98.
126. Muzaale AD, Dagher NN, Montgomery RA, et al. Estimates of early death, acute liver failure, and long-term mortality among live liver donors. Gastroenterology 2012; 142:273-80.
138. Kotton CN, Kumar D, Caliendo AM, et al. International consensus guidelines on the management of cytomegalovirus in solid organ transplantation. Transplantation 2010; 89:779-95.
147. Sampaio MS, Cho YW, Qazi Y, et al. Posttransplant malignancies in solid organ adult recipients: An analysis of the U.S. National Transplant Database. Transplantation 2012; 94:990-8.

Anatomy, Histology, Embryology, and Developmental Anomalies of the Small and Large Intestine

LEE M. BASS AND BARRY K. WERSHIL

ANATOMY

Macroscopic Features

Small Intestine

The small intestine is a specialized tubular structure within the abdominal cavity in continuity with the stomach proximally and the colon distally. The small bowel increases in length from about 250 cm in the term newborn to about 600 to 800 cm in the adult. The caliber of the small intestine gradually diminishes from proximal to distal, and there is a 4-fold reduction in surface area from the distal duodenum to the terminal ileum.

The duodenum is the most proximal portion of the small intestine. It begins with the duodenal bulb, travels in the retroperitoneal space around the head of the pancreas, and ends on its return to the peritoneal cavity at the ligament of Treitz. The biliary and pancreatic ducts join together 1 to 2 cm from the outer margin of the duodenal wall and drain into the second portion of the duodenum through the ampulla of Vater. In 5% to 10% of individuals, an accessory pancreatic duct, also known as the *duct of Santorini*, enters 1 to 2 cm proximal to the ampulla of Vater. The remainder of the small intestine is suspended within the peritoneal cavity by a thin broad-based mesentery that is attached to the posterior abdominal wall and allows relatively free but tethered movement of the small intestine within the abdominal cavity. The proximal 40% of the mobile small intestine is the jejunum, which occupies the left upper portion of the abdomen. The remaining 60% of small intestine is the ileum, and it is normally situated in the right side of the abdomen and upper part of the pelvis. There is no distinct anatomic demarcation between the jejunum and ileum, but the jejunum tends to be thicker, is more vascular, and has a greater diameter than the ileum.

The luminal surface of the small intestine has visible mucosal folds called the *plicae circularis* or *folds of Kerckring*. They are more numerous in the proximal jejunum, decrease in number distally, and are absent in the terminal ileum. Microscopic aggregates of lymphoid cells are scattered throughout the small intestine and make up the gastrointestinal-associated lymphoid tissue (GALT). Macroscopic lymphoid aggregates, or Peyer's patches, are more concentrated in the ileum and can be seen extending through to the serosa. Peyer's patches are more prominent in infancy and childhood and regress in size and number with advancing age.

The jejunum and ileum are freely mobile in the abdominal cavity and are attached to the posterior abdominal wall by the intestinal mesentery. The entire length of jejunum and ileum is suspended in this mesentery, except for the distal terminal ileum at the cecum, which is retroperitoneal. The mesentery is formed by a fan-shaped anterior reflection of the posterior peritoneum that extends from the left side of the body toward the right sacroiliac joint. The mesentery envelops a number of important structures, including the jejunum, ileum, jejunal and ileal branches of the superior mesenteric artery (SMA) and superior mesenteric vein (SMV), nerves, lacteals, lymph nodes, and a variable amount of fat.

The small bowel transitions to the colon at the ileocecal (IC) valve, which consists of 2 semilunar lips that protrude into the cecum. The IC valve functions like a flutter valve, allowing antegrade flow when a peristaltic wave is strong enough to overcome its resistance but preventing retrograde flow of colonic contents into the small intestine. The angulation between the ileum and cecum, supported by the superior and inferior ileocecal ligaments, is important to the function of the IC valve. The IC valve typically contracts when the cecum is overdistended to prevent ceco-ileal reflux. This explains why during colonoscopy, excessive distention of the cecum with air should be avoided, because this may lead to IC valve contraction, which can then hinder successful intubation of the ileum.

Colon and Rectum

The colon is a tubular structure about 30 to 40 cm in length at birth and measuring some 150 cm in the adult, or about one quarter the length of the small intestine. The colon begins at the IC valve and ends distally at the anal verge (Fig. 98-1). It consists of 4 segments: cecum and vermiform appendix, colon (ascending, transverse, and descending portions), rectum, and anal canal. The diameter of the colon is greatest in the cecum (7.5 cm) and narrowest in the sigmoid (2.5 cm) until it balloons in the rectum just proximal to the anal canal.

The colon is distinguished from the small intestine by several features. It is larger in caliber, mostly fixed in position, and has outer longitudinal muscle fibers that coalesce into 3 discrete bands called *taeniae*: the taenia liberis, taenia omentalis, and taenia mesocolica. Taeniae are located at 120-degree intervals around the colonic circumference and extend from the cecum to the proximal rectum. Outpouchings, or haustra, occur between the taeniae, giving the colon a sacculated and puckered appearance on its serosal surface. Semilunar folds characterize the mucosa between the haustra. Small sacs of peritoneum filled with adipose tissue, the appendices epiploicae, are found on the external surface of the colon. The

mesentery fully suspends the transverse colon and sigmoid colon, while the remainder of the colon has mesentery only on its free anterior surface. The appendix has a short mesentery called the *mesoappendix*.

The cecum is the most proximal portion of the colon. It is about 6 to 8 cm in length and breadth and lies in the right iliac fossa, projecting downward as a blind pouch below the entrance of the ileum. The large diameter of the cecum makes it susceptible to rupture with distal obstruction and permits tumors to grow quite large before producing symptoms of obstruction. The cecum is normally non-mobile because it is fixed in position by a small mesocecum; anomalous fixation exists in 10% to 20% of population, predominantly women, predisposing them to cecal volvulus.

The IC valve passes perpendicularly through the postero-medial wall of the cecum and consists of a superior and inferior fold arranged in an elliptical manner at the IC orifice. The appendiceal orifice is roughly 2.5 cm inferior to the IC valve, and the vermiform appendix is a blind outpouching extending from the cecum. Appendiceal anatomy is discussed further in Chapter 120.

The ascending colon is narrower than the cecum and extends about 12 to 20 cm from the level of the IC valve to the inferior surface of the posterior lobe of the liver, where it angulates left and forward, forming the hepatic flexure. The ascending colon is covered with peritoneum and thus is considered to reside in the retroperitoneum in about 75% of individuals.

At the hepatic flexure, the colon turns medially and anteriorly to emerge into the peritoneal cavity as the transverse colon, fully enveloped in mesentery. The transverse is the

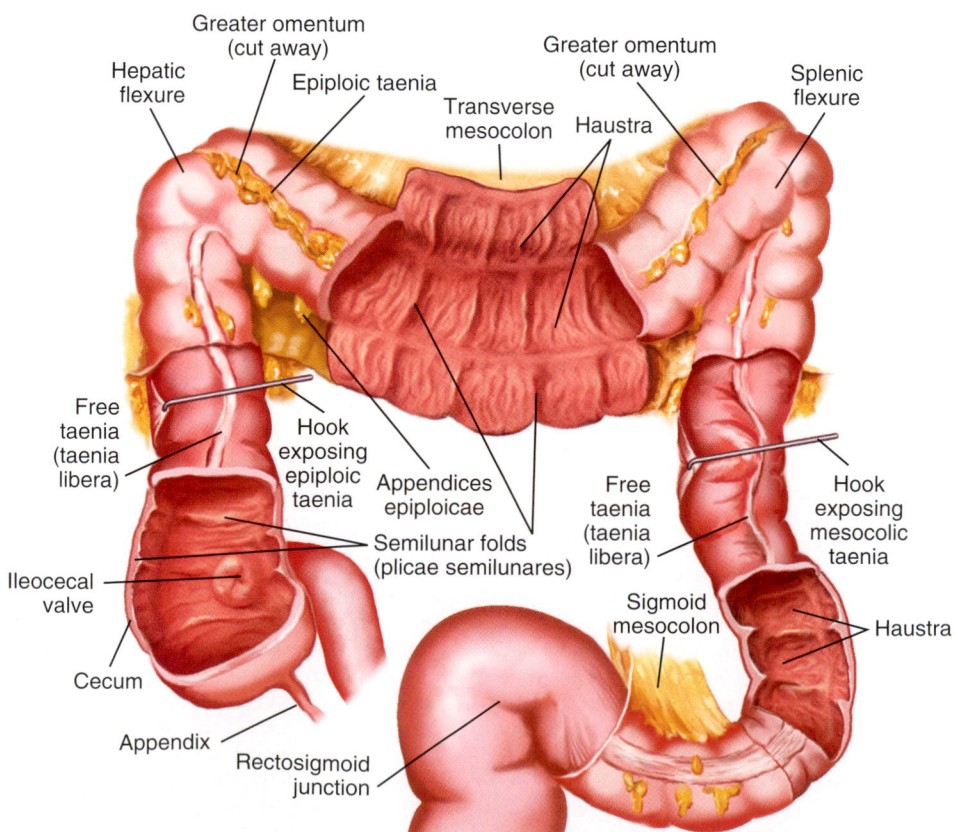

FIGURE 98-1. Macroscopic characteristics of the colon. Note the taeniae, haustra between the taeniae, the semilunar folds and the appendices epiploicae. (*Netter illustration from* www.netterimages.com. © *Elsevier Inc. All rights reserved.*)

longest (40 to 50 cm) and most mobile segment of the colon. It lies between the hepatic and splenic flexures and drapes itself across the anterior abdomen and anterior to the stomach. The phrenocolic ligament anchors the colon at the splenic flexure, but the transverse colon is so mobile that in the upright position it may actually dip down into the pelvis. Abdominal or pelvic surgery that results in adhesion formation can fix the position of the normally mobile transverse colon.

The descending colon is about 25 to 45 cm in length and travels posteriorly and then inferiorly in the retroperitoneal compartment to the pelvic brim. It emerges from the retroperitoneum into the peritoneal cavity as the sigmoid colon, an S-shaped redundant segment of variable length, tortuosity, and mobility. The mobility of the sigmoid colon renders it susceptible to volvulus, and because it is the narrowest part of the colon, tumors and strictures of this region typically cause obstructive symptoms early in the course of disease.

The rectum is 10 to 12 cm in length and begins at the peritoneal reflection, follows the curve of the sacrum passing down and posteriorly, and ends at the anal canal. The rectum narrows at its junction with the sigmoid, expanding proximal to the anus. The rectum lies entirely below the peritoneum in close relationship with the structure of the pelvis. The anorectal junction is 2 to 3 cm anterior to the tip of the coccyx. The rectum does not have sacculation, appendices epiploicae, or mesentery. The outer rectal wall is progressively thickened with prominent and anterior bands as it descends toward the anus. The luminal surface of the rectum has 3 transverse folds called the *valves of Houston*.

Anal Canal

The anal canal is 2 cm long in the infant and 4.5 to 5 cm long in the adult. It occupies the ischiorectal fossa, passing inferiorly and outward toward the anal opening. The anorectal junction is situated within the pelvic diaphragm and made up of the levator ani, coccygeus, and puborectalis muscles which encircle it; contraction of these muscles allows the anorectum to retain stool, and relaxation allows for defecation. The internal anal sphincter is made up of the circular smooth muscular layer of the intestine, which surrounds the upper three quarters of the canal. The external sphincter is made up of striated muscle; it surrounds the anal canal, and its fibers blend with those of the levator ani muscle to attach posteriorly to the coccyx and anteriorly to the perineal body. Distally, the anal verge represents the transition of anoderm to true skin. The mucosa of the distal 3 cm of the rectum and anal canal contains 6 to 12 redundant longitudinal folds called the *columns of Morgagni*, which terminate in the anal papillae. These columns are joined together by mucosal folds called the *anal valves*, which are situated at the dentate line. The *zona alba* is a white zone that demarcates the transition to typical squamous epithelium. The anatomy and function of these muscles are described in more detail in Chapter 129.

Vasculature

The proximal duodenum receives arterial blood from the right gastric artery, supraduodenal artery, right gastroepiploic artery, and superior and inferior pancreaticoduodenal arteries. Venous drainage is via the superior mesenteric vein (SMV) and the splenic and portal veins. The superior mesenteric artery (SMA) delivers oxygenated blood to the distal duodenum, jejunum and ileum, ascending colon, and proximal two thirds of the transverse colon. Branches of the inferior mesenteric artery supply the remainder of the colon. The arterial supply of the anal area is from the superior, middle, and inferior hemorrhoidal arteries, which are branches of the inferior

mesenteric, hypogastric, and internal pudendal arteries, respectively. Venous drainage of the anus is by both the systemic and portal systems. The internal hemorrhoidal plexus drains into the superior rectal veins and then into the inferior mesenteric vein, which, with the SMV, joins the splenic vein to form the portal vein. The distal anus drains by the external hemorrhoidal plexus through the middle rectal and pudendal veins into the internal iliac vein. (See Chapter 118 for discussion of the intestinal blood supply and its disorders.)

Lymphatic Drainage

Lymphatic drainage courses through the mesentery from villus lacteals and lymphatic follicles and converges at preaortic lymph nodes around the SMA and celiac artery. The lymphatic drainage of both the small intestine and colon follows their respective blood supplies to lymph nodes in the celiac, superior preaortic, and inferior preaortic regions. Lymphatic drainage proceeds to the cisterna chyli and then via the thoracic duct into the left subclavian vein. Proximal to the dentate line, lymphatic drainage is to the inferior mesenteric and periaortic nodes, whereas distal to the dentate line it flows to the inguinal lymph nodes. Therefore, inflammatory and malignant disease of the lower anal canal can manifest with inguinal lymphadenopathy.

Extrinsic Innervation

The autonomic nervous system—sympathetic, parasympathetic, and enteric—innervates the GI tract. The sympathetic and parasympathetic nerves constitute the extrinsic nerve supply and connect with the intrinsic nerve supply, which is composed of ganglion cells and nerve fibers within the intestinal wall. Innervation of the small intestine and colon is discussed in detail in Chapters 99 and 100, respectively.

Microscopic Features

General Considerations

The small and large intestine share certain histologic characteristics. The wall of the small intestine and colon is composed of 4 layers: mucosa (or mucous membrane), submucosa, muscularis (or muscularis propria), and adventitia (or serosa) (Fig. 98-2).

Mucosa

The mucosa consists of the glandular epithelium, lamina propria, and muscularis mucosae (Fig. 98-3A and B). The mucosa is thick and highly vascularized, although less so in distal portions. It has concentric folds (plicae circulares) that are also referred to as the *valves of Kerckring*. The surfaces of the mucosal folds are studded with villus projections, and these features combine to produce a 400- to 500-fold increase in mucosal surface area. An intestinal villus will typically project 0.5 to 1.5 mm into the lumen, and the height of the villus decreases from proximal to distal small intestine. Villi are wide and ridge shaped in the proximal duodenum, leaf shaped in the distal duodenum and proximal jejunum, and finger shaped in the remainder of intestine. The villi are covered with mature absorbing enterocytes interspersed with mucus-secreting goblet cells. Each villus contains an artery, vein, and central lacteal. A capillary bed forms along the epithelium, allowing for rapid clearance of absorbed nutrients, fluids, and electrolytes into the systemic circulation. To facilitate the absorptive process, capillary walls are fenestrated with diaphragmatic covers. The core of the villus also contains

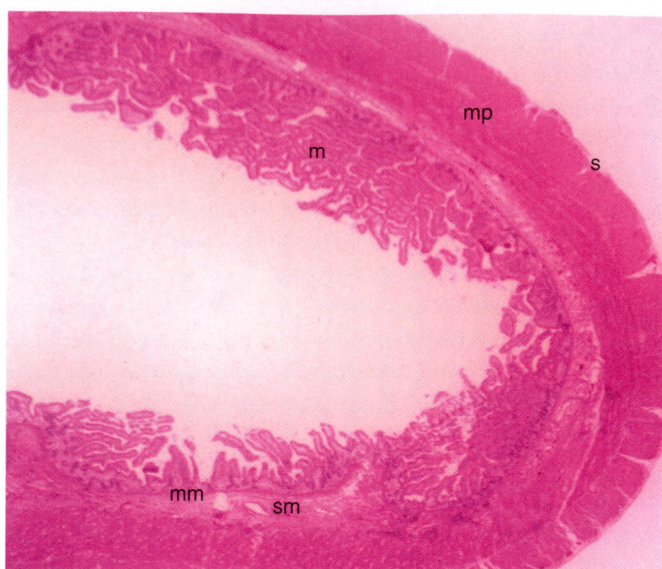

FIGURE 98-2. Photomicrograph of small intestine showing its general microscopic architecture. m, mucosa; mm, muscularis mucosae; mp, muscularis propria; s, serosa; sm, submucosa. (H&E, ×25.)

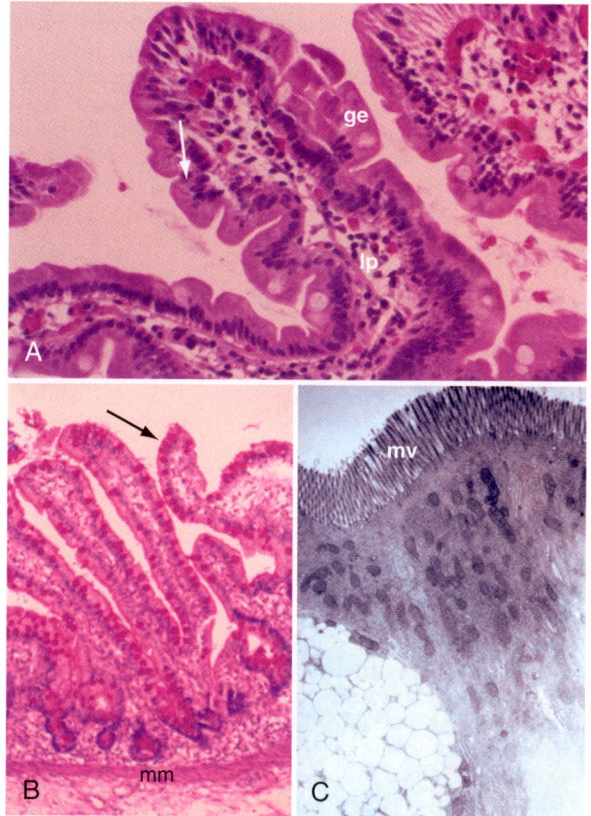

FIGURE 98-3. Histologic and electron microscopic photographs of small intestine. *A,* Components of the mucosa: ge, glandular epithelium; lp, lamina propria. Note the absorptive cells that appear as high columnar cells with eosinophilic cytoplasm *(arrow).* (H&E, ×250.) *B,* Goblet cells *(arrow)* and brush border are stained red. mm, muscularis mucosae. (Periodic acid–Schiff stain, ×150.) *C,* Microvilli *(mv)* are seen as delicate finger-like projections on electron microscopic examination, ×9000. *(C, Courtesy S. Teichberg, PhD.)*

nerve fibers, plasma cells, macrophages, eosinophils, and fibroblasts. The villi are surrounded by cylindrical structures called the *crypts of Lieberkühn,* which extend through the lamina propria to the muscularis mucosae. The crypts are lined with more immature epithelium that primarily functions as a secretory rather than an absorptive epithelium.

The epithelium of the small intestine is composed of various cell types: absorptive cells (columnar cells), secretory cells (goblet cells), undifferentiated cells, tuft cells, M cells, cup-like cells, and enteroendocrine cells. Crypts contain a similar cell population as the villi, with the addition of Paneth cells and stem cells.

The lamina propria is a layer of reticular connective tissue that provides the structural support for the mucosa, but it also contains many cellular elements important for absorption and immunity. The lamina propria is rich in arterioles, venules lacteals, nerve fibrils, and fibroblasts, lymphocytes, macrophages, neutrophils, eosinophils, and mast cells. The muscularis mucosae consists of a thin layer of smooth muscle only 3 to 10 cells thick at the boundary of the mucosa and submucosa.

Stem cells are pluripotential cells located at the base of the intestinal crypts. With intense mitotic activity, stem cells give rise to all types of mature intestinal epithelial cells and at the same time replenish themselves through self-renewal. Mucosal epithelial cells turn over every 5 to 7 days. Intestinal epithelial cells are mature by the time they reach the upper third of the villus. Paneth cells are the only cells that do not migrate. Undifferentiated cells have fewer intracellular organelles and microvilli than absorptive cells. The absorptive cells (see Fig. 98-3A) are high columnar cells with oval basal nuclei, eosinophilic cytoplasm, and a periodic acid–Schiff (PAS)-positive free surface, the brush border (see Fig. 98-3B). On electron microscopic examination, the brush border is seen to be composed of microvilli (see Fig. 98-3C), which are more numerous in the small intestinal than in the colonic epithelium. Enterocyte microvilli are estimated to increase the luminal surface area of the cell 14- to 40-fold.

Goblet cells are mucin-producing cells that are scattered among intestinal villi but are more common in the distal ileum and large intestine. Goblet cells are oval or round with flattened basal nuclei (Fig. 98-4A); their cytoplasm is basophilic, metachromatic (see Fig. 98-4B), and PAS positive (see Fig. 98-4C) and consists mostly of mucin-secreting granules. Mucin is secreted by 2 pathways: in a neutrally-mediated continuous manner, and by the active exocytosis of granules in response to extracellular stimuli.

Paneth cells are flask shaped with an eosinophilic granular cytoplasm and a broad base that is positioned against the basement membrane (Fig. 98-5). In the small intestine, Paneth cells are located exclusively in the crypts of Lieberkühn and secrete alpha-defensins, antimicrobial proteins, lysozyme, and phospholipase A, thought to be important in protection from infectious pathogens and function to maintain enteric homeostasis.[1]

Cup cells and tuft cells are 2 intestinal epithelial cell types with unidentified functions. Cup cells are present in villi and crypts largely limited to the ileum. Tuft cells are marked by a tuft of long microvilli projecting from the apical surface of the cell.

The mucosa also contains specialized cells called *enteroendocrine* or *neuroendocrine cells* (Fig. 98-6A) with specific endocrine functions. Intestinal endocrine cells are sparsely distributed and consist of 11 different cell types (Table 98-1). These are tall columnar cells present in both the crypts and villi and contain prominent secretory granules. The neuroendocrine cells have been divided histologically into argentaffin (i.e., their granules are able to reduce silver nitrate) or

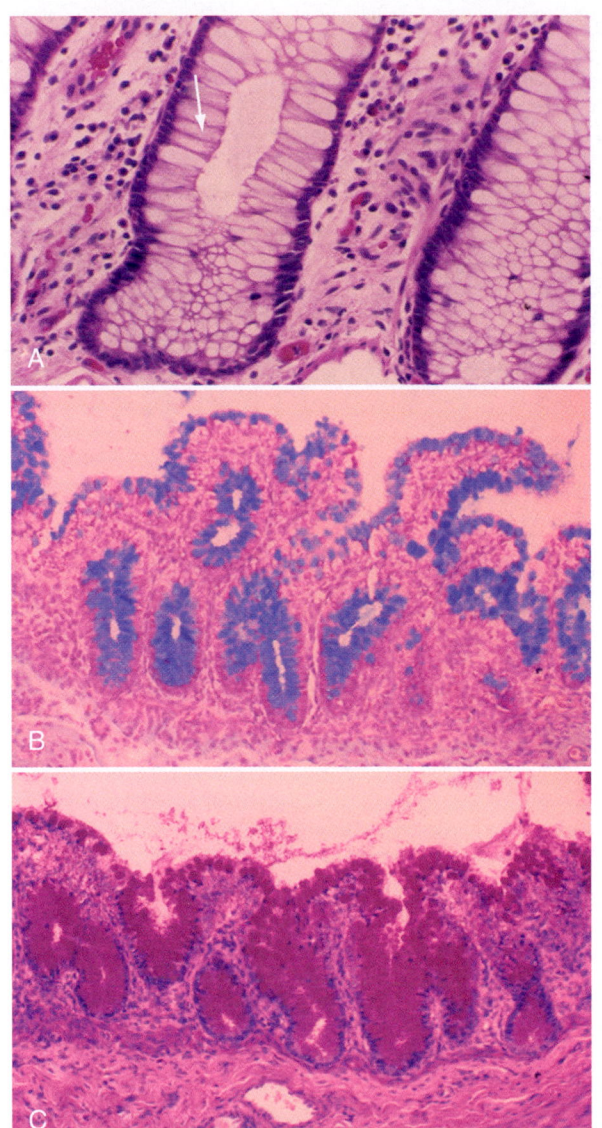

FIGURE 98-4. Photomicrographs of large and small intestine demonstrating goblet cells. *A,* Clear, empty-looking cytoplasm *(arrow)* and basal nuclei are seen with use of H&E, ×250. *B,* Metachromatic staining of the cytoplasm results with use of the alcian blue stain, ×150. *C,* The cells demonstrate red staining with use of periodic acid–Schiff stain, ×150.

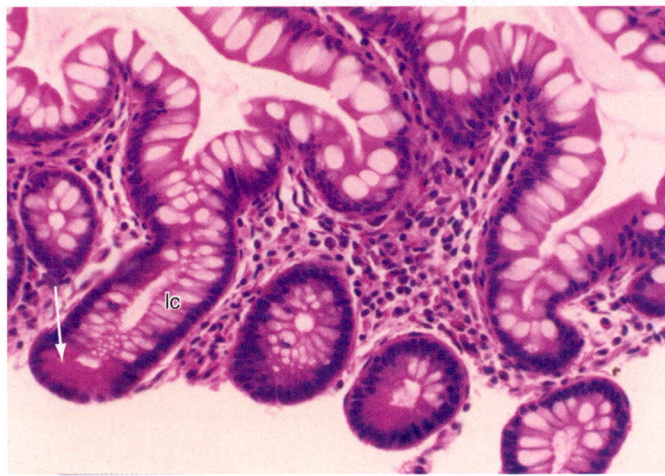

FIGURE 98-5. Photomicrograph of small intestinal mucosa demonstrating the crypts of Lieberkühn *(lc)* and Paneth cells *(arrow),* which are characterized by granular eosinophilic cytoplasm. (H&E, ×250.)

enterochromaffin cells and argyrophilic cells (i.e., granules reduce silver nitrate only in the presence of a chemical reducer). These chemical properties subdivide the cell types, but a unifying concept is derived from their common origin and functional capacity. The *a*mine *p*recursor, *u*ptake, and *d*ecarboxylation (APUD) concept characterizes the cells as having a common embryonic origin from the neural crest and displaying similar cytochemical and electron microscopic features.[2]

Ultrastructurally, enteroendocrine cells contain membrane-bound granules with variably sized electrodense cores (see Fig. 98-6B) that consist of large dense-core vesicles and smaller synaptic-type microvesicles. Neurosecretory granules can be demonstrated as dark granules with nonspecific agents (e.g., Grimelius stain [see Fig. 98-6C]), or more specific immunohistochemical stains can be used (e.g., neuron-specific enolase,

chromogranin, synaptophysin). Chromogranin enables visualization of the large dense-core vesicles, and synaptophysin targets the small synaptic-like microvesicles (see Fig. 98-6D).[2] With specific immunohistochemical staining agents, it is possible to identify the individual chemical and protein components of neuroendocrine cells. The differential expression of certain proteins also makes it possible to subdivide neuroendocrine cell populations. For example, vesicular monoamine transporter (VMAT) has 2 isoforms: VMAT1 is restricted to serotonin-producing enterochromaffin cells, and VMAT2 is expressed by histamine-producing cells, enterochromaffin-like cells, and pancreatic islet cells.[3]

The hormone products of these cells are discharged into the extracellular space on the basal and basolateral surfaces and have paracrine effects on absorption, secretion, motility, mucosal cell proliferation, possibly immunobarrier control, and even some endocrine effects upon systemic absorption.

The preferred designation of neuroendocrine cells is by their stored peptide. Serotonin-producing enterochromaffin cells, vasoactive intestinal polypeptide (VIP) cells, and somatostatin D cells are distributed throughout the small and large intestine. Cells that produce gastrin, ghrelin, gastric inhibitory peptide (GIP), secretin, and CCK are found predominantly in the stomach and proximal small intestine. Cells that secrete peptide YY, glucagon-like peptide (GLP)-1, GLP-2, and neurotensin are found in the ileum.[4]

M cells are specialized epithelial cells overlying lymphoid follicles and Peyer's patches in the small intestine and colon. M cells are an important site of luminal antigen sampling for immune processing by the mucosal lymphoid system. This process of sampling plays an important role in the development and maintenance of immune tolerance, host defense against pathogens, and intestinal homeostasis.

The interstitial cells of Cajal (ICC) are found in both the small intestine and colon and are located in the myenteric plexuses within the muscularis propria and the submucosa (Fig. 98-7 [see Chapters 99 and 100]). The ICC are important in the regulation of intestinal peristalsis and function as the pacemaker cells of the intestine. They influence the frequency of smooth muscle contraction, amplify neuronal signals, mediate neurotransmission from enteric motor neurons to smooth muscle cells, and set the smooth muscle membrane

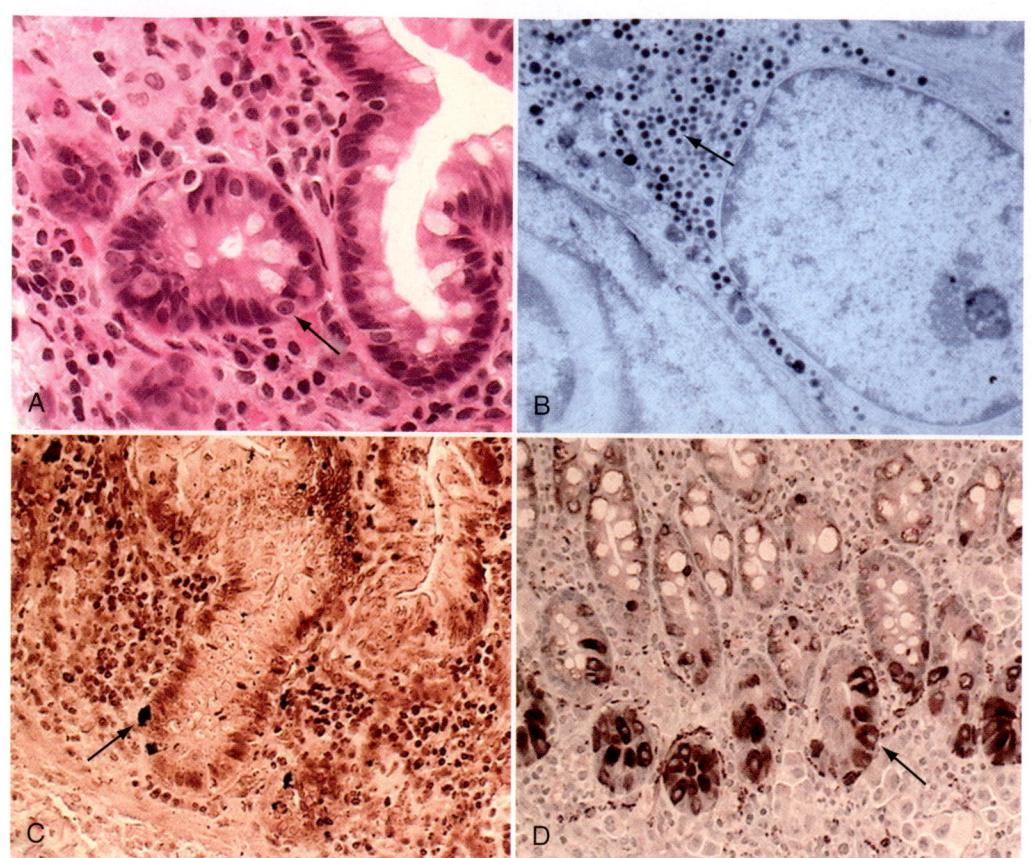

FIGURE 98-6. Microscopic characteristics of neuroendocrine cells of the small intestine. *A,* Features include clear cytoplasm and a round nucleus *(arrow).* (H&E, ×250.) *B,* Neurosecretory granules are seen as electron-dense, round black bodies *(arrow)* on electron microscopic examination, ×20,000. *C,* Granules in neuroendocrine cells are stained black with the Grimelius stain *(arrow),* ×150. *D,* Cells stained with synaptophysin have brown cytoplasm *(arrow),* ×250. *(B, Courtesy S. Teichberg, PhD.)*

TABLE 98-1 Enteroendocrine Cells of the Intestinal Tract: Cell Types and Products, Vesicle Markers, and Distribution

| Cell Type | Cell Product | Vesicle Markers | | Duod | Jej | Ileum | App | Colon | Rec |
		LDCV	SLMV						
P/D1	Ghrelin	CgA, VMAT2		f	f	f			
EC	5-HT	CgA, VMAT1	Syn	+	+	+	+	+	+
D	Somatostatin	CgA	Syn	+	+	f	f	f	f
L	GLI/PYY	SgII > CgA	Syn	f	+	+	+	+	+
PP	PP	CgA, SgII, VMAT2	Syn	e					
G	Gastrin	CgA	Syn	+					
CCK	Cholecystokinin			+	+	f			
S	Secretin, 5-HT	CgA		+	+				
GIP	GIP/Xenin	CgA		+	+	f			
M	Motilin			+	+	f			
N	Neurotensin	CgA		f	+	+			

App, appendix; CgA, chromogranin A; Duod, duodenum; e, presence of cells in fetus and newborn; EC, enterochromaffin cell; 5-HT, 5-hydroxytryptamine (serotonin); f, presence of few cells; GIP, gastric inhibitory polypeptide; GLI, glucagon-like immunoreactants (glicentin, glucagon-37, glucagon-29, GLP[glucagon-like peptide]-1, GLP-2); Jej, jejunum; LDCV, large dense-core vesicles; NESP55, neuroendocrine secretory protein 55; PP, pancreatic polypeptide; PYY, PP-like peptide with *N*-terminal tyrosine amide; Rec, rectum; SgII, secretogranin II (also known as *chromogranin C*); SLMV, synaptic-like microvesicles; Syn, synaptophysin; VMAT1, VMAT2, vesicular monoamine transporter 1, 2; +, presence of cells; >: heavier staining than.
Adapted from Solcia E, Capela C, Fiocca R, et al. Disorders of the endocrine system. In: Ming SC, Goldman H, editors. Pathology of the gastrointestinal tract. Philadelphia: Williams & Wilkins; 1998. p 295.

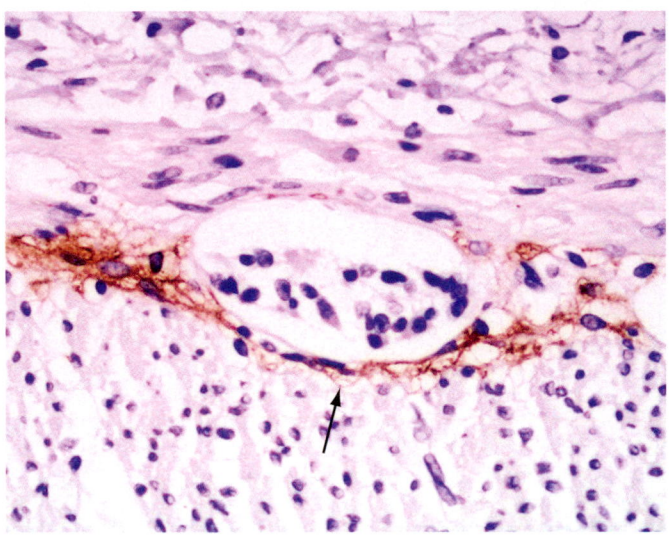

FIGURE 98-7. Photomicrograph showing interstitial cells of Cajal in the small intestine. Brown-staining, elongated cells are evident around the myenteric plexus *(arrow)*. (CD117 immunostain, ×250.)

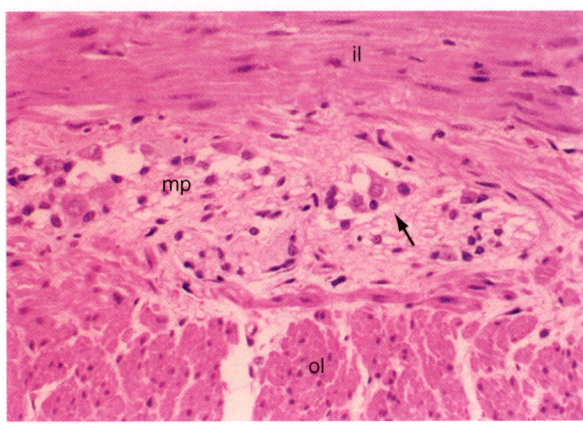

FIGURE 98-8. Photomicrograph of muscularis propria of small intestine. The myenteric plexus *(mp)* is seen as a pale area with ganglion cells between the inner and outer layers *(il, ol)* of the muscularis propria *(arrow)*. (H&E, ×250.)

potential gradient. The ICC are spindle-shaped or stellate cells with long, ramified processes and express c-kit (CD117), a tyrosine kinase receptor critical for their survival.[5]

Submucosa

The submucosa is a fibrous connective tissue layer that lies between the muscularis mucosae and the muscularis propria. It contains lymphocytes, fibroblasts, mast cells, blood and lymphatic vessels, and a nerve fiber plexus—Meissner's plexus—composed of nonmyelinated postganglionic sympathetic fibers and parasympathetic ganglion cells. The submucosa supports the mucosa in specialized functions of nutrient, fluid, and electrolyte absorption by conveying a rich network of blood vessels, lymphatics, and nerves that ensure efficient handling of absorbates.

Brunner's glands are submucosal glands (see Fig. 98-9B) found primarily in the first portion of the duodenum and in decreased numbers in the distal duodenum; in children, these glands may also be present in the proximal jejunum.

The function of Brunner's glands is to secrete a bicarbonate-rich alkaline secretion that helps neutralize gastric chyme, a mucinous secretion that helps lubricate the mucosa, epidermal growth factor, a variety of trefoil peptides, bactericidal factors, proteinase inhibitors, and surface-active lipids. The secretions that drain into the base of the duodenal crypts contribute to increased luminal pH by promoting pancreatic secretion and gallbladder contraction. The mucous layer protects the epithelial surface from peptic digestion; this protection is thought to be due to glycoprotein class III mucin glycoproteins.[6]

Muscularis Propria

The muscularis propria is mainly responsible for contractility and peristaltic movement of luminal contents through the GI tract. It consists of 2 layers of smooth muscle: an inner circular coat and an outer longitudinal coat arranged in a helicoidal pattern. A prominent nerve fiber plexus called the *myenteric* or *Auerbach's plexus* is located in the plane between these 2 muscle layers (Fig. 98-8). The ganglia in the myenteric plexus are more

prominent than their submucosal counterpart. Parasympathetic and postganglionic sympathetic fibers terminate in parasympathetic ganglion cells, and postganglionic parasympathetic fibers terminate in smooth muscle.

Serosa

The serosa is the outermost layer of the intestinal wall and is composed of a simple layer of mesothelial cells supported by connective tissue, the adventitia. It represents an extension of the visceral peritoneum and mesentery as it envelops the intestine.

Microscopic Organization

Small Intestine

The mucosa of the small intestine is characterized by folds (plicae circulares, or valves of Kerckring) and villi. The mucosal folds actually comprise mucosa and submucosa. Villi are mucosal folds that decrease in size from the proximal to distal small intestine and are of different shapes in the various segments of the small intestine. They may be broad, short, or leaf-like in the duodenum, tongue-like in the jejunum, and finger-like more distally (Fig. 98-9A). The villous pattern may vary in different ethnic groups; biopsy specimens from Africans, Indians, South Vietnamese, and Haitians have shorter and thicker villi, an increased number of leaf-shaped villi, and more mononuclear cells in comparison with specimens from North Americans. The implications of these changes with regard to subclinical GI infection are discussed in Chapter 108.

The height of the normal villus is 0.5 to 1.5 mm; villus height should be more than half the total thickness of the mucosa and 3 to 5 times the length of the crypts. Villi are lined by enterocytes, goblet cells, and enteroendocrine cells.

Enterocytes are tall columnar cells, each with a basally located, clear, oval-shaped nucleus and several nucleoli. The cells are tightly cemented to the basal lamina and adjoined to adjacent enterocytes at the apical pole by intracellular tight junctions. The luminal surface has microvilli that contain necessary enzymes for nutrient absorption; a central core cytoskeleton is made of actin, villin, fimbrin, brush border myosin, and spectrin. The apical surface of the epithelium carries brush border transporters, Na/H exchangers, and anion exchangers

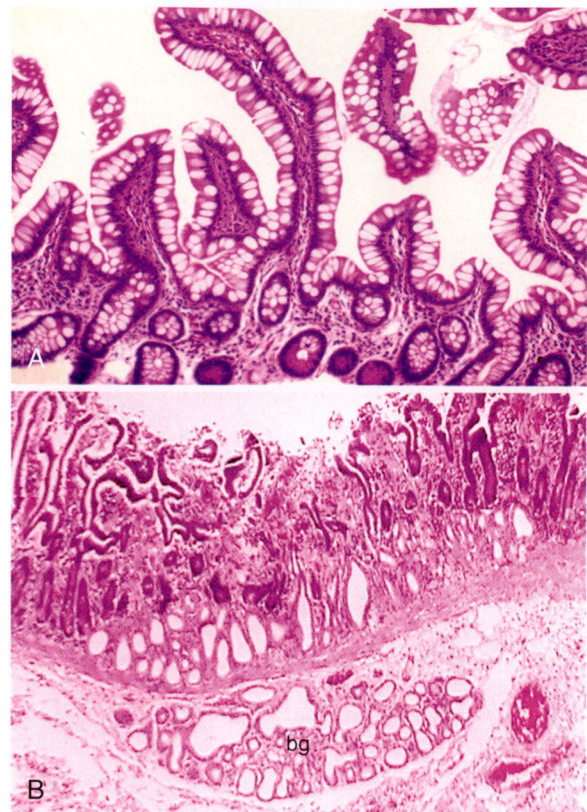

FIGURE 98-9. Photomicrographs of duodenal mucosa. *A*, Villi are seen as finger-like projections. *B*, Brunner glands *(bg)* are found below the mucosa. (H&E. *A*, ×250; *B*, ×150.)

(see Chapter 101). The junction complexes are made up of 3 components: the proximal tight junction (zonula occludens), the intermediate junction (zonula adherens), and the deep junction, which includes the spot desmosome and the macular adherens zone (see Chapter 101). Movement through junctions is by paracellular transport and is the dominant pathway for passive ion and fluid flow. Tight junctions consist of claudins, occludens, and junctional adhesion molecules that bind and prevent passage of molecules between them in a regulated manner. They are leakier and have a lower resistance in the proximal small intestine, and tighter in the distal intestine. The zonula adherens is less adherent and involved in cell signaling. Spot desmosomes are thought to augment transmembrane linkages spanning the intercellular gap and are involved in cell wall communications. The basolateral membrane is responsible for carriers to facilitate diffusion of organic solutes not coupled to ion movements. Gap junctions allow for communication and intercellular passage of ions and low molecular weight nutrients and intracellular messengers such as cyclic adenosine monophosphate (cAMP).[7,8]

Two types of glands are present in the small intestine: Brunner's glands (see above) and crypts of Lieberkühn (intestinal crypts). The crypts of Lieberkühn are tubular glands that extend to the muscularis mucosae (see Fig. 98-5); they are occupied mainly by undifferentiated cells and Paneth cells. Cells are generated at the crypt base and migrate up the villus. During this migration, these cells mature and differentiate into a secretory lineage (goblet cells, enteroendocrine cells) and enterocytes. The commitment of the stem cells to differentiate is acquired in the upper third of the crypt where cells lose their

ability to divide. The constant renewal of enterocytes is regulated by human acyl-coenzyme A synthetase.[9]

Paneth and columnar cells predominate in the base of the crypt. Above the base are absorptive cells and oligomucin cells; the latter originate from undifferentiated cells and differentiate into goblet cells. Goblet cells predominate in the upper half of the crypt. Enteroendocrine cells are admixed with goblet cells. A certain number of CD3+ intraepithelial T lymphocytes (up to 30 per 100 epithelial cells) are normally present in the villi. Smooth muscle is found in the lamina propria of the small intestinal villus, extending vertically up from the muscularis mucosae. Plasma cells containing primarily immunoglobulin (Ig)A, and mast cells are also present. Lymphoid tissue is prominent in the lamina propria as both solitary nodules and confluent masses—Peyer's patches—and is seen in the submucosa. Peyer's patches are distributed along the antimesenteric border and are most numerous in the terminal ileum; their numbers decrease with age.

Most types of enteroendocrine cells are present in the duodenum. Cells that produce ghrelin, gastrin, CCK, motilin, neurotensin, GIP, and secretin are restricted to the small intestine.[2]

The proportions of cells differ in the villi and crypts as well as in different segments of the intestine. Ninety percent of the villus epithelial cells are absorptive cells intermingled with goblet and enteroendocrine cells. The proportion of goblet to absorptive cells is increased in the ileum. The ICC are more abundant in the myenteric plexus of the small intestine than in the colon.[5]

Colon

The colonic walls are similar to those of the small intestine, both in the outer wall and mucosal layers. The outer layer forms the taenia coli, which run in parallel to the long axis of the colon throughout the entire colon. The width of the taeniae extends from 6 to 12 mm, and thickness gradually increases from the cecum to the sigmoid colon. The epithelial layer is smooth with crescentic folds corresponding to external sacculations. The surface epithelium is simple columnar type and is interspersed with vascular cells and goblet cells. The epithelial surface and upper third of the crypts are mostly lined with tall, slender absorptive columnar cells called *principal cells*. Goblet cells are the second most abundant cells on the surface of the colonic epithelium and produce mucin, which aids in the passage of feces. Colonic epithelial cells are generated from stem cells at the base of the crypts and migrate toward the intestinal lumen after 3 to 5 days on initiation of apoptosis. Most epithelial cells undergo apoptosis when they lose contact with the extracellular matrix and are shed into the lumen through caspase activation. Caspase activation is responsible for the cleavage of essential intracellular proteins that leads to apoptosis and therefore loss of anchorage.[10]

The colon can absorb a small amount of short-chain fatty acids produced by anaerobic bacteria upon fermentation of polysaccharides; these provide a source of energy for the colonic epithelium. The mucosa of the large intestine is characterized by the presence of crypts of Lieberkühn, associated predominantly with goblet cells intermixed with a few absorptive and enteroendocrine cells. The crypts of Lieberkühn dip to the muscularis mucosae and contain enteroendocrine cells and undifferentiated cells that are restricted to the lower third of the crypts. Glucagon-like immunoreactant (GLI) pancreatic polypeptide-like peptide (PYY) with *N*-terminal tyrosine amide–producing L cells predominate in the large intestine. Enterochromaffin, enterochromaffin-like, and pancreatic polypeptide-producing cells are also found. Paneth cells are scarce and normally are noted only in the proximal colon. The lamina propria of the large intestine contains solitary lymphoid follicles that extend into the submucosa. Lymphoid follicles are more developed in the rectum and decrease in number with age. Confluent lymphoid tissue is present in the appendix. Macrophages (muciphages) predominate in the subepithelial portion of the lamina propria, are weakly PAS positive, and are associated with stainable lipids.

Anal Canal

Microscopically, the anal canal is divided into 3 zones: proximal, intermediate or pectinate, and distal or anal skin. The proximal zone is lined by stratified cuboidal epithelium, and the transition with the rectal mucosa, which is lined by high columnar mucus-producing cells, is called the *anorectal histologic junction* (Fig. 98-10*A*). The intermediate or pectinate zone is lined by stratified squamous epithelium but without adnexae (e.g., hair, sebaceous glands) and is also referred to as *anoderm*. Its proximal margin, in contact with the proximal zone, is called the *dentate line*; its distal margin, in contact with the anal skin, constitutes the *pectinate line*, also referred to as the *mucocutaneous junction* (see Fig. 98-10*B*); some authors use the terms *pectinate line* and *dentate line* interchangeably.

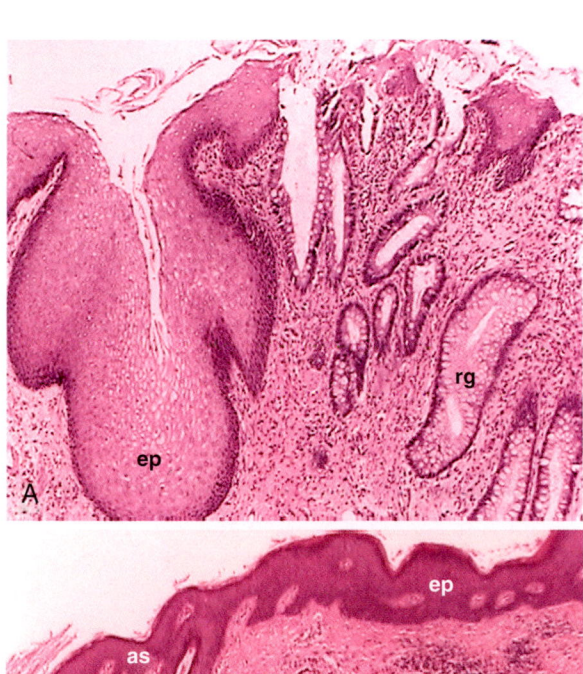

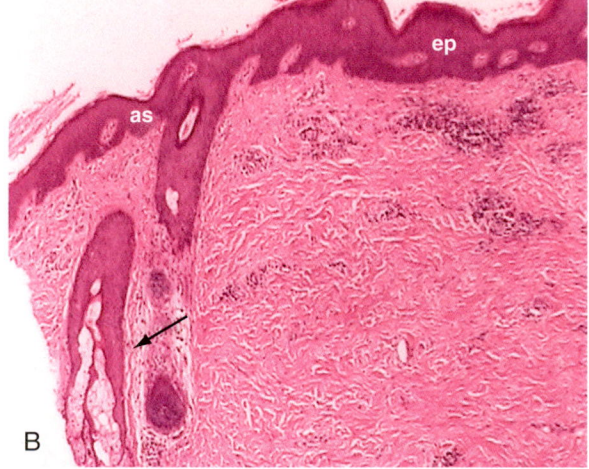

FIGURE 98-10. Photomicrograph of anal canal. *A,* Anorectal histologic junction. Transition from rectal glandular mucosa *(rg)* to proximal anal mucosa lined by stratified squamous epithelium *(ep)* is evident. *B,* Pectinate line is characterized by anal mucosa with stratified squamous epithelium *(ep)* and anal skin *(as)* containing adnexae *(arrow).* (*A* and *B,* H&E, ×150.)

The anal skin is lined by squamous stratified epithelium and contains hair and sebaceous glands.

Vasculature

Large arterial branches enter the muscularis propria and pass to the submucosa, where they branch to form large plexuses. In the small intestine, 2 types of branches arise from the submucosal plexuses: some arteries branch on the inner surface of the muscularis mucosae and break into a capillary network that surrounds the crypts of Lieberkühn. Other arteries are destined for villi, each villus receiving 1 or 2 arteries, and set up the anatomic arrangement that allows a countercurrent mechanism, thus aiding absorption. These vessels enter at the base of the villus and form a dense capillary network immediately underneath the epithelium of the entire villus structure. One or several veins originate at the tip of each villus from the superficial capillary plexus, anastomose with the glandular venous plexus, and then enter the submucosa to join the submucosal venous plexus.

In the colon, branches from the submucosal plexus extend to the surface, giving rise to capillaries that supply the submucosa, and there branch to form a capillary meshwork around the crypts of Lieberkühn. From the periglandular capillary meshwork, veins form a venous plexus between the base of the crypts and the muscularis mucosae. From this plexus, branches extend into the submucosa and form another venous plexus from which large veins follow the distribution of the arteries and pass through the muscularis propria into the serosa.

Lymph Vessels

The lymphatics of the small intestine are called *lacteals* and become filled with milky-white lymph called *chyle* after eating. Each villus contains 1 central lacteal, except in the duodenum, where 2 or more lacteals per villus may be present. The wall of the lacteal consists of endothelial cells, reticulum fibers, and smooth muscle cells. At the base of the villus, the central lacteals anastomose with the lymphatic capillaries between the crypts of Lieberkühn. They also form a plexus on the inner surface of the muscularis mucosae. Branches of this plexus extend through the muscularis mucosae to form a submucosal plexus. Branches from the submucosal plexus penetrate the muscularis propria, where they receive branches from plexuses between the inner and outer layers. Lymphatic vessels are absent in the colonic mucosa, but the distribution of lymphatics in the remaining colonic layers is similar to that in the small intestine.

Nerves

The intrinsic nervous system (enteric nervous system [ENS]) consists of subserosal, muscular, and submucosal plexuses. The subserosal plexus contains a network of thin nerve fibers without ganglia that connects the extrinsic nerves with the intrinsic plexus. The myenteric plexus, or Auerbach's plexus, is situated between the outer and inner layers of the muscularis propria (see Fig. 98-8); it consists of ganglia and bundles of unmyelinated axons that connect with the ganglia to form a meshwork. These axons originate from processes of the ganglion cells and extrinsic vagus and sympathetic ganglia. The deep muscular plexus is situated on the mucosal aspect of the circular muscular layer of the muscularis propria. It does not contain ganglia; it innervates the muscularis propria and connects with the myenteric plexus. The submucosal plexus, or Meissner's plexus, consists of ganglia and nerve bundles. The nerve fibers of this plexus innervate the muscularis mucosae and smooth muscle in the core of the villi. Fibers from this plexus also form a mucosal plexus that is situated in the lamina propria and provides branches to the intestinal crypts and villi. The ganglion cells of the submucosal plexus are distributed in 2 layers; 1 is adjacent to the circular muscular layer of the muscularis propria, and the other is contiguous to the muscularis mucosae. Ganglion cells are large cells, isolated or grouped in small clusters called *ganglia* (Fig. 98-11). Ganglion cells have an abundant basophilic cytoplasm, a large vesicular round nucleus, and a prominent nucleolus. Ganglion cells are scarce in the physiologically hypoganglionic segment 1 cm above the anal verge.

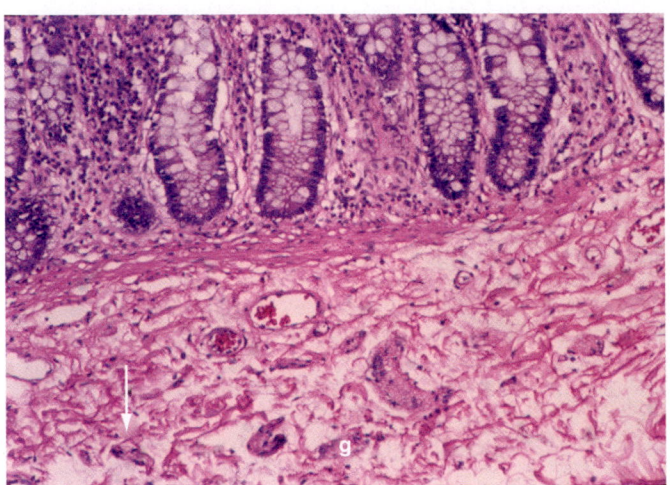

FIGURE 98-11. Photomicrograph showing a normal submucosal plexus of the colon. Ganglia *(g)* are identified by their oval structure, and nerve trunks are thin *(arrow)*. (H&E, ×150.)

EMBRYOLOGY

Intestinal Development

The embryo is a bilaminar germ disk at 3 weeks' gestation. Through a process called *gastrulation*, this disk becomes trilaminar and gives rise to the 3 primary germ layers: ectoderm, mesoderm, and endoderm. It also establishes bilateral symmetry, dorsal-ventral orientation, and anterior-posterior axis.

The surface facing the yolk sac becomes the definitive endoderm, the surface facing the amniotic sac becomes the ectoderm, and the middle layer is the mesoderm. The oral opening is marked by the buccopharyngeal membrane; the future openings of the urogenital and digestive tracts become identifiable as the cloacal membrane. At 4 weeks' gestation, the alimentary tract is divided into 3 parts: foregut, midgut, and hindgut, the endoderm connecting with the yolk sac.

These segments form a tube by growth and folding. The folding process brings together the endodermal, mesodermal, and ectodermal layers to the corresponding layers on the opposite side, converting the flat endodermal layer into the intestinal tube. Initially the foregut and hindgut are blind-ending tubes separated by a midgut that is open to the yolk sac. As the lateral edges of the midgut fuse to become a tube, there is a narrowing of the communication between the yolk sac and endoderm, producing the vitelline duct (Fig. 98-12). With folding of the embryo during week 4 of development, the mesodermal layer splits. The portion that adheres to endoderm forms the visceral peritoneum, whereas the part that adheres to ectoderm forms the parietal peritoneum. The space between the 2 layers becomes the peritoneal cavity.

The primitive intestine results from incorporation of the endoderm-lined yolk sac cavity into the embryo following embryonal cephalocaudal and lateral folding. The endoderm

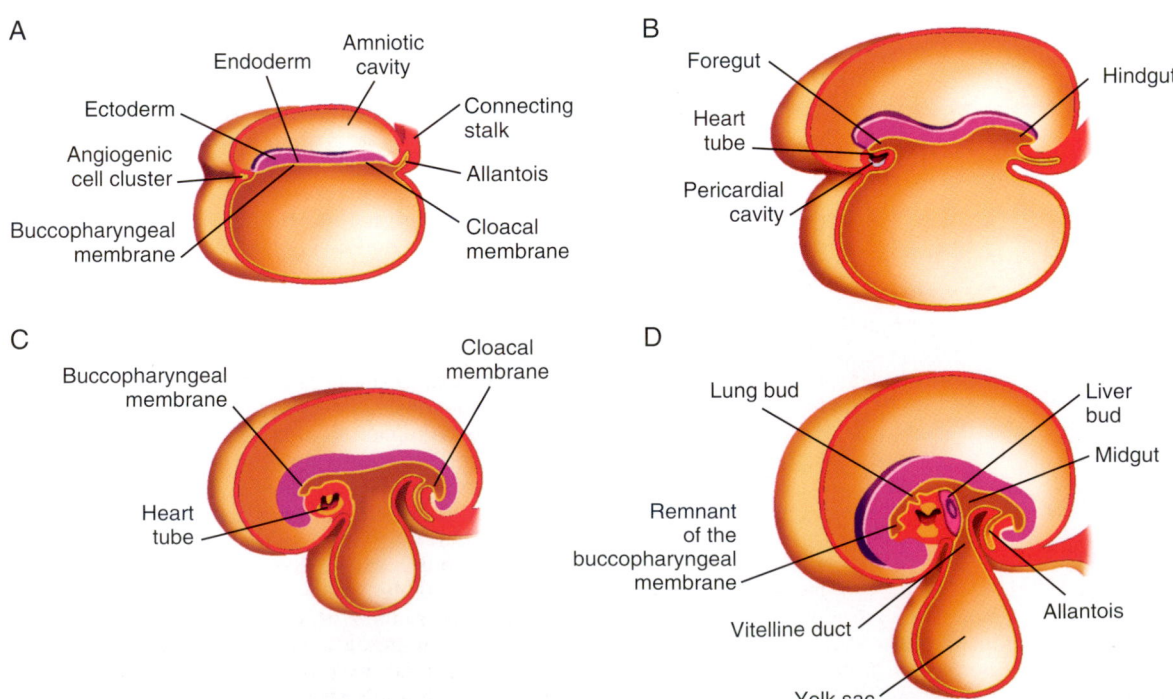

FIGURE 98-12. Formation of foregut, midgut, and hindgut (see text for details). *(From Sadler YW, editor. Langman's medical embryology. 10th ed. Philadelphia: Lippincott Williams & Wilkins; 2006.)*

gives rise to the epithelial lining of the GI tract; muscle, connective tissue, and peritoneum originate from the splanchnic mesoderm. During the 9th week of development, the epithelium begins to differentiate from the endoderm, with villus formation and differentiation of epithelial cell types. Organogenesis is complete by 12 weeks' gestation.

Initially the foregut, midgut, and hindgut are in broad contact with the mesenchyma of the posterior abdominal wall. The intraembryonic cavity is in open communication with the extraembryonic cavity. Subsequently the intraembryonic cavity loses its wide connection with the extraembryonic cavity. By week 5 of embryonic development, splanchnic mesoderm layers are fused in the midline and form a double-layered membrane, the dorsal mesentery, between the right and left halves of the body cavity. The mesoderm surrounds the intestinal tube and suspends it from the posterior body wall, allowing it to hang into the body cavity. The caudal portions of the foregut, midgut, and most of the hindgut are suspended from the abdominal wall by the dorsal mesentery, which extends from the duodenum to the cloaca. The dorsal mesentery forms the mesoduodenum in the region of the duodenum, the dorsal mesocolon in the region of the colon, and the mesentery proper in the region of the jejunum and ileum.[11]

Molecular Regulation of Intestinal Morphogenesis

Molecular regulation of intestine formation is a complex network of carefully orchestrated gene expression, activation of signal transduction pathways, and cell-cell interactions that works in a cooperative manner; the balance of signals often determines the developmental pathways that follow. Only selected molecular elements are presented here, but comprehensive reviews are available.[12-14]

Intestinal Tube Formation

Development of the intestinal tube requires simultaneous inductive and patterning steps. The transforming growth factor (TGF)-β superfamily member Nodal is required for the mesoderm and endoderm specification in all vertebrate species and plays a secondary role in anterior-posterior (A-P) patterning. Crosstalk and inductive cues exchanged between the mesoderm and endoderm are thought to play a critical role in gastrulation. The interruption of Fox factors (Fox A2, FoxH1), Gata factors, Sox17, Mixl1, or Smad signaling will result in a failure of tube formation, primarily by altering endoderm development and specification.[12-14] The Wnt signaling pathway also plays a critical role in intestinal tube formation.

Genes expressed during A-P patterning include *Hhex*, *FoxA2*, and *Sox2* in the anterior gut, while *Cdx* is expressed posteriorly. *Hox* genes play an important role in patterning of the mesoderm and ectoderm, while *Cdx2* is a critical gene in hindgut formation and intestinal specification and patterning, particularly in cecal development. Other genes and factors that play a role in A-P patterning of the endoderm include *FGF*, *Wnt*, *BMP*, and retinoic acid signaling. Gut elongation is also controlled by a number of genes. Deletion of *Wnt5a* results in an 80% reduction in small intestine and a 63% reduction in colonic length.[14] The absence of any 1 of a family of proteins that interact with Wnt5a (secreted frizzled related proteins) also adversely affect bowel length.[14]

Epithelial Cells and Villus Formation

The endoderm transitions from simple epithelium to columnar epithelium in a rostral-caudal (proximal-distal) manner,

including in the colon, which initially has villus-like structures until it undergoes reorganization. The mesenchyme invaginates to form longitudinal ridges that become epithelial folds. These folds evolve into villi, and crypt-shaped structures form as secondary lumina. This reorganization occurs through extensive crosstalk between the endoderm and mesoderm that involves TGF-β, PDGF, FGF, WNT, and EGF. BMPs also expressed in the mesenchyme influence endoderm-mesoderm interactions and epithelial development. A mutation in the receptor BMPR1a results in epithelial cell hyperproliferation and polyp formation, as seen in juvenile polyposis syndrome.[14]

Other important factors in the formation of the epithelium include the Hedgehog signals (Sonic [Shh] and Indian [Ihh]) and Gli transcription factors (Gli2, GLi3). The protein ezrin, which is required for polarization of the epithelium, and the transcription factor Elf3 interact with Crif1 to regulate epithelial differentiation and villus formation. The transcription factor HNF4α is expressed throughout the intestinal epithelium and, if deleted, causes the epithelium to develop into a colonic phenotype. Finally, beyond genes and transcription factors, global chromatin remodeling also has effects on intestinal epithelial development.

Proliferation and Differentiation of the Epithelium

The formation of villi occurs as epithelial cells proliferate and reorganize from a pseudostratified appearance to a simple columnar epithelium. As villi form, distinct epithelial cell types can be identified by morphology and the expression of specific markers. Unlike other aspects of intestinal development, proliferation and differentiation of the epithelium remain important processes that must be maintained throughout adult life. Two major signaling pathways involved in these processes are Wnt/β-catenin and Notch. The Wnt/β-catenin is important in crypt formation, maintaining the stem cell compartment, proliferation and differentiation in the embryonic and adult intestine, and Paneth cell maturation. Notch proteins are transmembrane receptors that are important in both proliferation and differentiation of the developing intestine. Evidence suggests that Notch activity regulates factors that influence whether undifferentiated cells will become absorptive or secretory epithelial cells. There also are factors downstream of Wnt/β-catenin and Notch that effect specific lineages: neurogenin[3] is required for the formation of enteroendocrine cells; SPDEF directs terminal differentiation of goblet cells; Sox9 regulates Paneth and goblet cell formation; Klf4 regulates colonic goblet cell differentiation.

Specific Structures and Systems

Duodenum

The duodenum originates from the terminal portion of the foregut and cephalic part of the midgut. Early during week 4 of gestation, the caudal foregut begins to expand to initiate formation of the stomach. The liver and pancreas arise at the junction of the midgut and foregut. With rotation of the stomach, the duodenum becomes C-shaped and rotates to the right; the fourth portion becomes fixed in the left upper abdominal cavity. The mesoduodenum fuses with the adjacent peritoneum; both layers disappear, and the duodenum becomes fixed in its retroperitoneal location. The lumen of the duodenum is obliterated during the second month of development by proliferation of its cells; this phenomenon is shortly followed by recanalization. Small intestinal villus and crypt formation occurs in a proximal-to-distal progression. The villi appear during week 8 of gestation, along with the microvillus enzymes. At 12 weeks' gestation, crypts are present and grow between the 10th and 14th week of gestation. At 14 weeks, the intestinal enzymes are at an adult level of activity.

Because the foregut is supplied by the celiac artery and the midgut by the SMA, the duodenum is supplied by both arteries and therefore is relatively protected from ischemic injury.[11]

Midgut

In a 5-week embryo, the midgut is suspended from the dorsal abdominal wall by a short mesentery and communicates with the yolk sac by way of the vitelline duct. The midgut gives rise to the duodenum distal to the ampulla, the entire small intestine, and the cecum, appendix, ascending colon, and proximal two thirds of the transverse colon. The midgut rapidly elongates with formation of the primary intestinal loop. Rapid growth of the midgut causes it to elongate, rotate, and begin to form a loop that protrudes into the umbilical cord. The cephalic portion of this loop, which communicates with the yolk sac by the narrow vitelline duct, gives rise to the distal portion of the duodenum, jejunum, and a portion of the ileum; the distal ileum, cecum, appendix, ascending colon, and proximal two thirds of the transverse colon originate from the caudal limb. During week 6 of embryonic development, the primary intestinal loop enters the umbilical cord (physiologic umbilical herniation) (Fig. 98-13). At 7 weeks' gestation, the small intestine begins to rotate counterclockwise around the axis of the SMA. At 9 weeks, growth of the intestine causes it to herniate further into the umbilical cord, where it continues to rotate and then return to the abdominal cavity. At 11 weeks' gestation, rotation continues to 270 degrees and retracts into the abdominal cavity. The jejunum returns first and fills the left half of the abdominal cavity ultimately taking its position in the upper left quadrant. The ileum returns next and fills the right half of the abdominal cavity ultimately assuming its final position in the right lower quadrant. The colon enters last, with fixation of the cecum close to the iliac crest and the

ascending and descending colon attaching to the posterior abdominal wall. Elongation of the bowel continues, and the jejunum and ileum form a number of coiled loops within the peritoneal cavity.[11]

The cecum originates as a small dilatation of the caudal limb of the primary intestinal loop by approximately 6 weeks of development. Initially it lies in the right upper quadrant, then it descends to the right iliac fossa, placing the ascending colon and hepatic flexure in the right side of the abdominal cavity. The appendix originates from the distal end of the cecal bud. Because the appendix develops during descent of the colon, its final position is frequently retrocecal or retrocolonic (Fig. 98-14).

Mesentery

As the caudal limb of the primitive intestine moves to the right side of the abdominal cavity, the dorsal mesentery twists around the origin of the SMA. After the ascending and descending portions of the colon reach their final destinations, their mesenteries fuse with the peritoneum of the posterior abdominal wall, and they become retroperitoneal organs. The appendix, cecum, and descending colon retain their free mesentery. The transverse mesocolon fuses with the posterior wall of the greater omentum. The mesentery of the jejunum and ileum is at first in continuity with the ascending mesocolon; after the ascending colon becomes retroperitoneal, the mesentery only extends from the duodenum to the ileocecal junction.[11]

Hindgut

The distal third of the transverse colon, the descending colon and sigmoid, the rectum, and the upper part of the anal canal originate from the hindgut. The fetal colon develops over 30 weeks in 3 stages. Primitive stratified epithelium similar to that in the small intestine appears between 8 and 10 weeks.

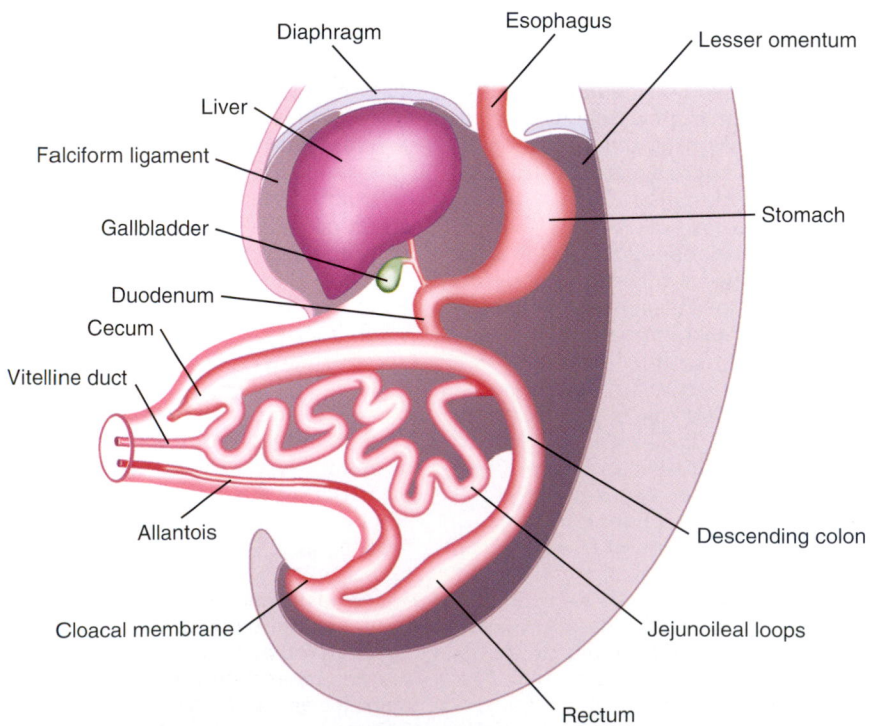

FIGURE 98-13. Physiologic umbilical herniation of the intestinal loop during normal development. Coiling of small intestinal loops and formation of cecum occur during herniation. The first 90 degrees of rotation occur during herniation; the remaining 180 degrees occur during return of intestine to abdominal cavity. *(From Sadler YW, editor. Langman's medical embryology. 10th ed. Philadelphia: Lippincott Williams & Wilkins; 2006, Fig. 14-26, p. 219.)*

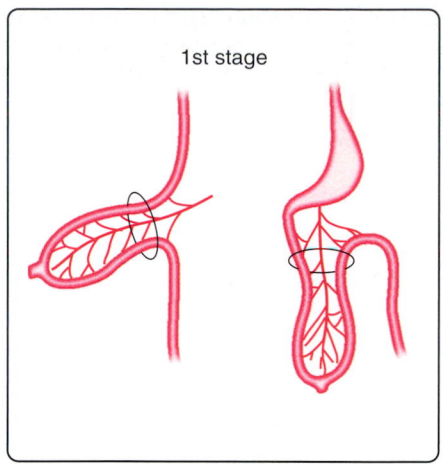
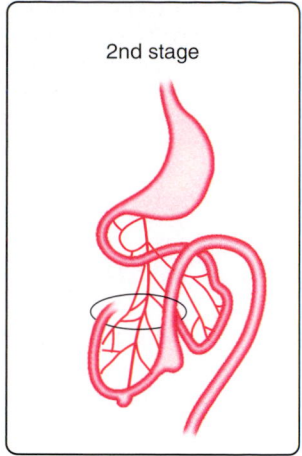
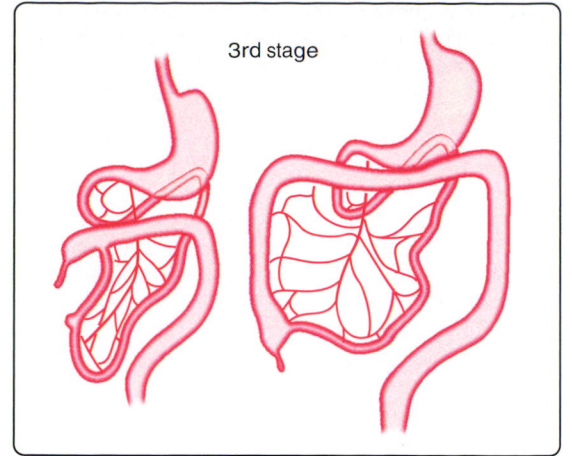

FIGURE 98-14. The 3 stages of normal intestinal rotation (see text for details). *(From Gosche JR, Touloukian RJ. Congenital anomalies of the midgut. In: Wyllie R, Hyams JS, editors. Pediatric gastrointestinal disease. Pathophysiology, diagnosis, management. 2nd ed. Philadelphia: WB Saunders; 1999.)*

Conversion to villus architecture with developing crypts occurs at 12 to 14 weeks. Remodeling to the adult-type crypt epithelium with loss of the villi occurs at 30 weeks. Initially the urinary, genital, and rectal tracts empty into a common channel, the cloaca. They become separated by the caudal descent of the urorectal septum into an anterior urogenital sinus and a posterior intestinal canal. The lateral fold of the cloaca moves to the midline, and the caudal extension of the urorectal septum develops into the perineal body. In a man, the lateral genital ridges coalesce to form the urethra and scrotum; in a woman, no fusion occurs, and the labia minora and majora evolve. The cloaca is lined by endoderm and covered anteriorly by ectoderm. The most distal portion of the hindgut enters into the posterior region of the cloaca, the primitive anorectal canal. The boundary between the endoderm and the ectoderm forms the cloacal membrane. This membrane ruptures by week 7 of embryonic development, creating the anal opening for the hindgut. The anal membrane separates the endoderm and ectodermal portions of the anorectal canal. The anal membrane marks the pectinate line. The pectinate line marks separation of vascular supply of the upper and lower parts of the anal canal. This portion is obliterated by ectoderm but recanalizes by week 9. Thus, the distal portion of the anal canal originates from ectoderm and is supplied by the inferior rectal artery, fed from the internal iliac artery; the proximal portion of the anal canal originates from endoderm and is supplied by the inferior mesenteric artery by way of the superior rectal artery. The inferior mesenteric ganglia and the pelvic splanchnic nerves innervate the superior portion of the anal canal. The inferior rectal nerve supplies the inferior rectal canal.

Arterial System

Vascular endothelial growth factor (VEGF)-A and its receptors, VEGFR-1 and VEGFR-2, are important for endothelial cell proliferation, migration, and sprouting. Angiopoietins and their receptors, Tie1 and Tie2, play a role in remodeling and maturation of the developing vasculature. For example, vascular dysmorphogenesis is seen with mutation in the Tie2 gene. Vascular malformation is briefly discussed in Chapter 37.

Arteries of the dorsal mesentery, originating from fusion of the vitelline arteries, give rise to the celiac, superior mesenteric, and inferior mesenteric arteries. Their branches supply the foregut, midgut, and hindgut, respectively.

Venous System

Vitelline veins give rise to a periduodenal plexus that develops into a single vessel, the portal vein. The SMV originates from the right vitelline vein, which receives blood from the primitive intestinal loop; the left vitelline vein disappears. The umbilical veins become connected to the hepatic sinusoids, after which the right umbilical vein disappears and the left umbilical vein joins the inferior vena cava; ultimately the umbilical vein is obliterated and forms the ligamentum teres. The cardinal veins and the proximal portion of the right vitelline vein are involved with forming the inferior vena cava.

Lymphatic System

Lymphatic vessels originate from endothelial budding of veins, after which the peripheral lymphatic system spreads by endothelial sprouting into the surrounding tissues and organs. Flt4 (also known as *VEGFR-3*), a receptor for VEGF, plays a role in development of the vascular as well as the lymphatic systems. Overexpression of VEGF-C, a ligand of Flt4, results in hyperplasia of lymphatic vessels in transgenic mice. Based on animal studies, the homeobox gene *Prox1* is essential for normal development of the lymphatic system. Homeobox genes contain a conserved sequence of 183 nucleotides. The proteins encoded by homeobox-containing genes act as regulatory molecules that control the expression of other genes. Several families of homeobox-containing genes are known, including the murine *Hox* family, which has been implicated in pattern formation during embryogenesis. Disruption of this gene in mice causes a chyle-filled intestine. Abnormalities in lymphatic system development can result in lymphangiectasia (see Chapter 30).

Enteric Nervous System

The ENS originates from vagal, truncal, and sacral neural crest cells. Most of the ENS cells derive from the vagal and truncal neural crest, enter the foregut mesenchyma, and colonize the developing intestine in a cephalocaudal direction. The truncal neural crest gives rise to ganglia of the proximal stomach, whereas the vagal neural crest supplies ganglia to the entire intestine, including the rectum; this colonization is complete by 13 weeks of embryonic development. A small component of the ENS originates from sacral neural crest cells. These cells form extraintestinal pelvic ganglia that colonize the hindgut mesenchyma before arrival of the vagal-derived neural crest cells.[15] Normal ENS development depends on the survival of cells derived from the neural crest and their proliferation, movement, and differentiation into neurons and glial cells. The prevertebral sympathetic ganglia develop next to the major branches of the descending aorta and innervate tissue supplied by the respective arteries. The vagus nerve and the pelvic splanchnic nerves provide preganglionic parasympathetic innervation to ganglia embedded in walls of visceral organs. Microenvironmental, genetic, or molecular mechanisms may intervene in these processes (see "Disturbance in the Enteric Nervous System").

Clinical Implications

Table 98-2 summarizes known congenital clinical entities that result from disturbances in embryologic development. GI malformations can be associated with extraintestinal defects when genes such as those that determine left-right asymmetry are involved. The *CFC1* gene plays a role in establishing the left-right axis. Mutations of this gene have been reported in extrahepatic biliary atresia, the polysplenia syndrome (inferior vena cava abnormalities, preduodenal portal vein, intestinal malrotation, and situs inversus), and right-sided stomach and congenital heart disease.[16,17]

ABNORMALITIES IN NORMAL EMBRYOLOGIC DEVELOPMENT

Abdominal Wall

Omphalocele

Current theories suggest that a teratogenic event during the first 3 weeks of gestation prevents return of the bowel to the abdomen and causes failure of lateral embryonic fold

TABLE 98-2 Abnormalities in Normal Embryologic Development

Body Wall	
Omphalocele	Failure of intestine to return to the abdominal cavity after its physiologic herniation
Gastroschisis	Weakening of abdominal wall
Mesentery	
Mobile cecum	Persistence of mesocolon
Volvulus	Failure of fusion of mesocolon with posterior abdominal wall
Vitelline Duct	
Meckel's diverticulum	Persistence of vitelline duct (see Fig. 98-17)
Omphalomesenteric cyst	Focal failure of vitelline duct obliteration
Patent omphalomesenteric duct	Complete failure of vitelline duct obliteration
Rotation	
Malrotation	Failure of rotation of the proximal midgut; distal midgut rotates 90 degrees clockwise
Nonrotation	Failure of stage 2 rotation (see Fig. 98-18)
Reverse rotation	Rotation of 90 degrees instead of 270 degrees
Proliferation	
Duplication	Abnormal proliferation of intestinal parenchyma
Intestinal Atresia and Stenosis	
"Apple-peel" atresia	Coiling of proximal jejunum distal to the atresia around the mesenteric remnant
Duodenum	Lack of recanalization
Small and large intestine	Vascular "accident"
Anorectum	Disturbance in hindgut development
Enteric Nervous System	
Hirschsprung's disease	Failure of migration of ganglion cells; microenvironment changes
Intestinal neuronal dysplasia	Controversial
Pseudo-obstruction	Multifactorial (see Chapter 124)
Miscellaneous	
Intestinal epithelial dysplasia	Abnormalities of the basement membrane
Microvillus inclusion disease	Defective protein trafficking and abnormal cytoskeletal and microfilament function
Other Genetic Defects	
Congenital chloride diarrhea	Abnormal Cl^--HCO_3^- exchange in ileum and colon (see Chapter 102)
Congenital glucose or galactose malabsorption	Absence of Na^+-glucose cotransporter for glucose and galactose (see Chapter 102)
Congenital lactase deficiency	Decrease in lactase-phlorizin hydrolase (see Chapter 102)
Congenital sodium diarrhea	Defective sodium-proton exchange
Congenital sucrase/isomaltase deficiency	Abnormal intracellular transport, aberrant processing, and defective function of sucrase or isomaltase (see Chapter 102)
CF	Defective CF transmembrane conductance regulator (see Chapter 57)

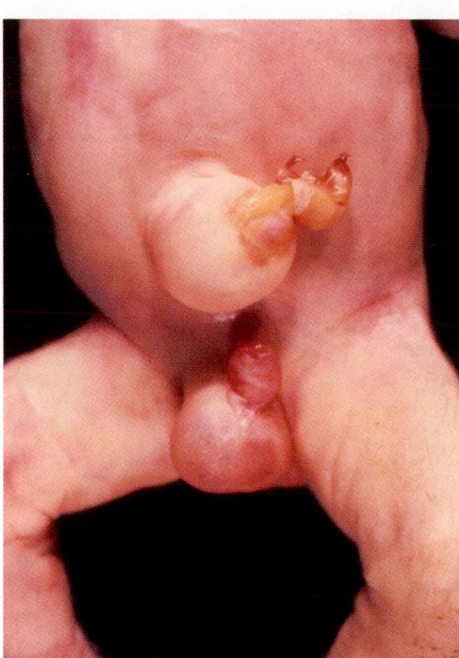

FIGURE 98-15. Newborn with omphalocele. Note the translucent sac-like structure with its attached umbilical cord.

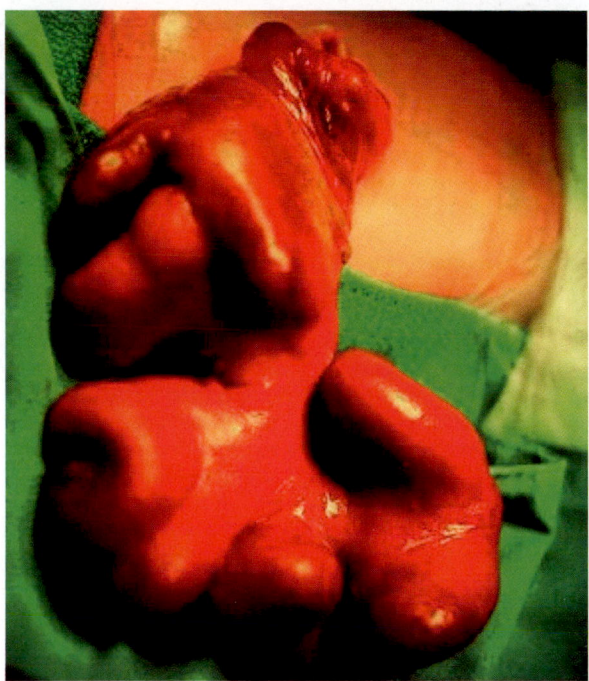

FIGURE 98-16. Gastroschisis. In this newborn, there are full-thickness disruption of the abdominal wall and protruding viscera without accompanying peritoneum. *(From Feldman's Online Gastro Atlas, Current Medicine.)*

development, with resultant omphalocele. Omphalocele, also known as *exomphalos*, occurs with a frequency of 1.5 to 3 in 10,000 births. Associated anomalies (e.g., sternal defects) result from failure of closure of the cephalic folds; failure of caudal fold development results in exstrophy of the bladder and, in extreme cases, exstrophy of the cloaca. Additional cranial fold abnormalities (i.e., anterior diaphragmatic hernia, sternal clefts, pericardial defects, and cardiac defects) in the setting of omphalocele is known as the *pentalogy of Cantrell*.[18]

Omphalocele is a congenital hernia involving the umbilicus. It is covered by an avascular sac composed of fused layers of amnion and peritoneum (Fig. 98-15). The umbilical cord is usually inserted into the apex of the sac, and the blood vessels radiate within the sac wall. Although a central defect is present in the skin and the linea alba, the remainder of the abdominal wall, including surrounding musculature, is intact. Because a small occult omphalocele may not be observed at birth, it is recommended that the umbilical cord be tied at least 5 cm from the abdominal wall at the time of delivery. Close inspection of the umbilical cord before clamping will avoid clamping an occult omphalocele.

With a large omphalocele, the liver and spleen are frequently outside the abdominal cavity. Associated anomalies occur in about 75% of children with omphalocele and include chromosomal abnormalities (e.g., trisomy 13 or 18), nonchromosomal syndromes like Beckwith-Wiedemann syndrome (mental retardation, hepatomegaly, large body stature, hypoglycemia), fetal valproate syndrome, exstrophy of the bladder or cloaca, and OEIS (*o*mphalocele, *e*xstrophy of the bladder, *i*mperforate anus, *s*pinal defect). Musculoskeletal, cardiovascular, and central nervous system malformations can also occur.[19,20]

Prenatally, increased levels of maternal serum alpha fetoprotein (AFP) suggest the possible presence of an omphalocele. Ultrasound examination during pregnancy allows the diagnosis of this abdominal wall defect in most infants. A fetus with omphalocele is at high risk for intrauterine growth restriction (IUGR), premature delivery, and fetal death.[21]

Fetal management, including possible termination of pregnancy, is determined by the physician in consultation with the family. If pregnancy is continued, mode of delivery and provision for care of a child with possibly coexisting anomalies should be considered before labor and delivery. Operative treatment is required in all patients with omphalocele. The size of the omphalocele determines whether a primary repair or delayed primary closure is selected. Escharification of the intact omphalocele sac has also been used for treatment. Reoperation is necessary in up to 25% of cases of omphalocele, either for reclosure of stomas or for subsequent bowel obstruction.

Gastroschisis

Gastroschisis is an abdominal wall defect most commonly located to the right of an intact umbilical cord (Fig. 98-16); rarely, the defect is to the left of the umbilical cord.[22] The incidence of gastroschisis is approximately 1 in 10,000 births overall but approaches 7 in 10,000 among mothers younger than age 20. Gastroschisis occurs more frequently in whites and in Hispanic infants than in other races or ethnicities. The cause of gastroschisis is unknown, although several theories have been proposed, including abnormal body wall folding, disruption of the right vitelline artery, and failure of mesoderm formation.[23] In gastroschisis, a sac is absent, and the extruded bowel is "padded" and thickened along its length from its extended exposure to amniotic fluid. Histologically, the bowel is usually normal. Some affected infants may have an inflammatory peel, or serositis, of the bowel that may make the bowel loops difficult to distinguish. Some 10% to 20% of infants with gastroschisis have associated anomalies (e.g., atresia) and almost all infants with gastroschisis also exhibit malrotation. Other congenital anomalies have been reported in a small number of patients.[19,20] Prematurity is more common in children born with gastroschisis than it is in children with omphalocele, and extraintestinal anomalies are much more common with omphalocele than they are with gastroschisis. Morbidity and mortality in patients with gastroschisis are largely related to intestinal atresia. Gastroschisis may be complicated by necrotizing enterocolitis, with all its attendant short- and long-term complications.

Increased maternal levels of AFP are suggestive of gastroschisis and omphalocele. IUGR is frequently observed. In the antenatally diagnosed fetus, serial ultrasound non-stress tests and delivery as close to term as possible are recommended.

In most children, the gastroschisis can be closed primarily, but for the child with significant intestinal atresia as an associated complication of gastroschisis, bowel exteriorization and secondary closure are often preferred. Most infants require special management and careful serial inspection of the bowel soon after delivery. Use of a spring-loaded silo to cover the bowel may assist with bowel decompression, as well as continuous inspection of blood flow.[24] It is crucial to conserve intestinal length in these children. Adhesive small bowel obstruction is a frequent and serious complication, especially in the first year of life.[25]

Omphalomesenteric (Vitelline) Duct Abnormalities

Between 5 and 7 weeks' gestation, the omphalomesenteric duct (which has connected the embryo to the yolk sac) attenuates, involutes, and separates from the intestine. Before this separation, the epithelium of the yolk sac develops an appearance similar to that of the gastric mucosa. Under normal circumstances the omphalomesenteric duct becomes a thin fibrous band that fragments and is absorbed spontaneously during the 5th to 10th week of gestation. Persistence of the ductal communication between the intestine and yolk sac beyond the embryonic stage may result in several anomalies of the omphalomesenteric (vitelline) duct (Fig. 98-17): (1) a blind omphalomesenteric duct, or Meckel's diverticulum; (2) a central cystic dilatation in which the duct is closed at both ends but patent in its center, an omphalomesenteric or vitelline cyst; (3) an umbilical-intestinal fistula (see Fig. 98-17*A*), resulting from the duct remaining patent throughout its length; and (4) complete obliteration of the duct, resulting in a fibrous cord or ligament that extends from the ileum to the umbilicus as an omphalomesenteric band.[26] In about 1% to 4%

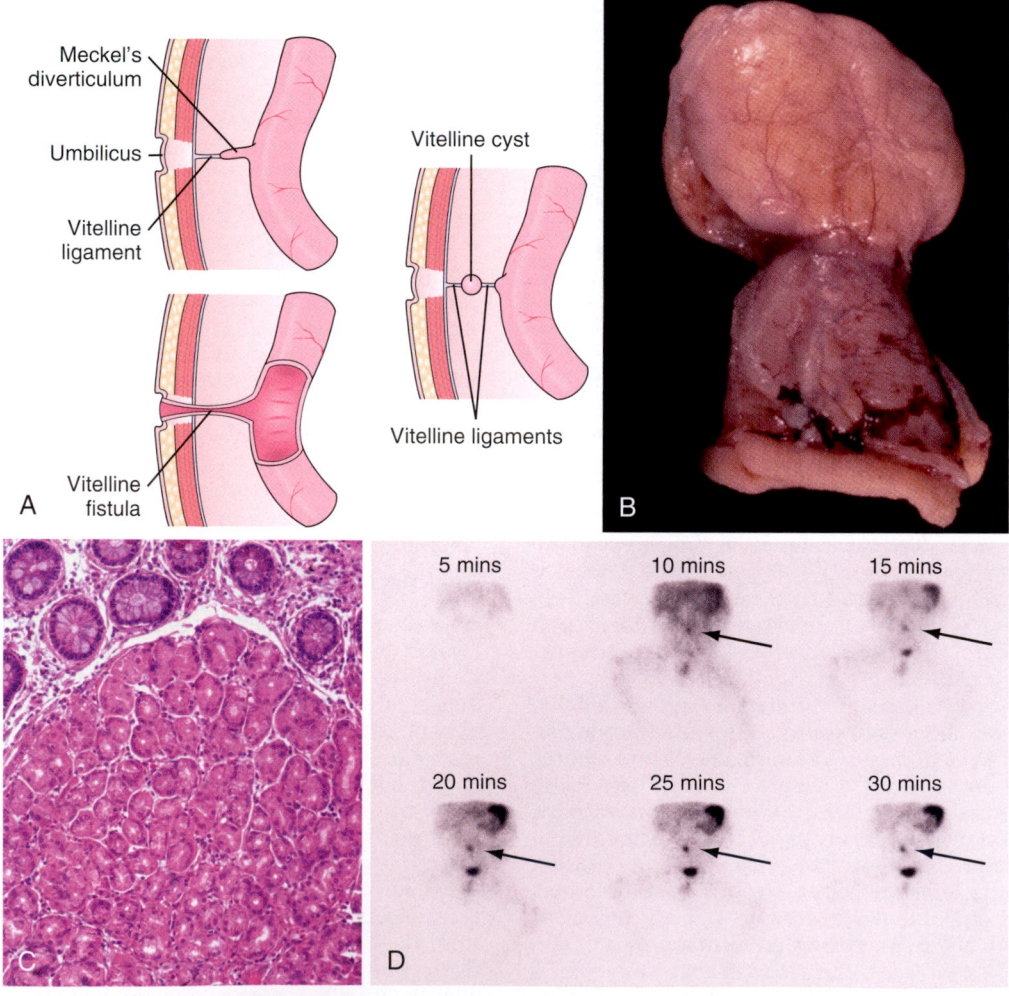

FIGURE 98-17. Vitelline duct abnormalities and features of Meckel's diverticulum. *A,* Schematic representations of a Meckel's diverticulum, vitelline cyst, and vitelline fistula. *B,* Surgical specimen revealing an outpouching of the ileum (Meckel's diverticulum). *C,* Photomicrograph showing replacement of small intestinal mucosa by ectopic oxyntic mucosa that lined a Meckel's diverticulum. (H&E, ×150.) *D,* Meckel's diverticulum scan demonstrating initial uptake of ⁹⁹ᵐtechnetium-pertechnetate *(arrows)* by the diverticulum at 10 minutes. (*D, Courtesy Dr. I. Zanzi.*)

of all infants, some remnant of the embryonic yolk sac is retained, making the omphalomesenteric or vitelline duct the most common site of congenital GI anomaly; lack of expression of the homeobox gene *CDX2* has been implicated in the pathogenesis of these anomalies.[27]

Meckel's Diverticulum

A Meckel's diverticulum is an antimesenteric outpouching of the ileum that is usually found some 2 feet from the ileocecal junction (see Fig. 98-17*B*). It occurs in 1.2% to 2% of the population and has a male-to-female ratio of 3:1.[28] Meckel's diverticula account for 67% of all omphalomesenteric duct remnants.[26] Length of the diverticulum varies (range, 1 to 10 cm). Ectopic GI mucosa—duodenal, gastric, biliary, colonic, or pancreatic tissue—is present in about 50% of Meckel's diverticula; most common is ectopic gastric mucosa, accounting for 80% to 85% of all Meckel's diverticula-associated ectopic tissue (see Fig. 98-17*C*).

Painless bleeding per rectum is the most common manifestation of a Meckel's diverticulum. Blood in the stool is usually maroon, even in patients with massive bleeding and hypovolemic shock. Bright red blood per rectum, as might be seen with bleeding from the left colon, is almost never encountered, but melena may be seen in patients with intermittent, less severe bleeding. The cause of bleeding is peptic ulceration secondary to acid production by the ectopic gastric mucosa within the Meckel's diverticulum. A "marginal" ulcer often develops at the junction of the gastric and ileal mucosae. Although *Helicobacter pylori* has been observed in the gastric mucosa within a Meckel's diverticulum, a relationship between bleeding from a Meckel's diverticulum and presence of this organism is unlikely. Despite massive bleeding, death seldom occurs in children because hypovolemia leads to contraction of the splanchnic blood vessels, causing the bleeding to diminish or cease. Also, children rarely have comorbid conditions that compromise their ability to compensate.

Intestinal obstruction is the next most common manifestation of a Meckel's diverticulum. This obstruction is caused either by intussusception with the diverticulum as the lead point or by herniation through or volvulus around a persistent fibrous cord remnant of the vestigial vitelline duct. In children older than age 4, intussusception is almost always secondary to a Meckel's diverticulum; however, Meckel's diverticulum–related intestinal obstruction may occur at almost any age. Volvulus around a vitelline cord has been described in the neonatal period. Bilious vomiting and abdominal distention are usually the initial signs of obstruction, and as with other causes of obstruction, intestinal ischemia and death may result.

Diverticulitis of a Meckel's diverticulum occurs as a result of acute inflammation. Most commonly, affected patients are diagnosed as having acute appendicitis, and the diagnosis of Meckel's diverticulitis is made at exploratory laparotomy. Perforation occurs in about a third of patients with Meckel's diverticulitis and may result from peptic ulceration.[29] A chronic form of Meckel's diverticulitis (Meckel's ileitis) may mimic Crohn's disease of the ileum. Rarely, Meckel's diverticulum can act as a predisposing factor to small intestinal malignancy.[30,31]

Meckel's diverticulum may be an incidental finding.[28] The presence of a Meckel's diverticulum should always be considered in an infant or child with significant painless rectal bleeding. However, standard abdominal plain films, barium contrast studies, and ultrasonographic imaging are rarely helpful in making the diagnosis. Because bleeding is almost always from ectopic gastric mucosa within the diverticulum, the Meckel's scan, which allows imaging of the gastric mucosa, should be the initial diagnostic study (see Fig. 98-17*D*). Uptake of ^{99m}Tc-pertechnetate is by the mucus-secreting cells of the gastric mucosa, not the parietal cells. The sensitivity and specificity of Meckel's diverticulum scintigraphy can be improved by administration of pentagastrin, glucagon, or pretreatment with an H_2-blocker. Pentagastrin increases the metabolism of mucus-producing cells, but because there is a risk of inducing perforation, this is not the preferred test. Glucagon enhances the study by inhibiting peristaltic dilution and washout of the radionuclide. H_2-blockers decrease peptic secretion but not radionuclide uptake, retarding the release of ^{99m}Tc-pertechnetate from the mucus-producing cells. Unfortunately, even an enhanced Meckel's study has only 85% sensitivity and 95% specificity, so a negative scan does not necessarily rule out a Meckel's diverticulum.

When the diagnosis of a bleeding Meckel's diverticulum is entertained and the Meckel's scan is negative, splanchnic angiography and ^{99m}Tc-labeled red blood cell studies may be used; diagnosis, however, is usually made at surgery. Small bowel wireless capsule endoscopy may detect a Meckel's diverticulum in some children with GI bleeding.[32] It is reasonable to perform EGD and colonoscopy to rule out other possible etiologic disorders.

Omphalomesenteric (Vitelline) Cyst

Omphalomesenteric (vitelline) cyst is more common in men and is characterized by a mucosa-lined intestinal cystic mass within the center of a fibrous cord.[26] The cyst may present as a palpable nodule within the umbilicus and be complicated by infection.

Patent Omphalomesenteric (Vitelline) Duct

Patent omphalomesenteric (vitelline) duct represents a persistent connection between the distal ileum and umbilicus. This fistula has a male-to-female ratio of 5:1 and accounts for 6% to 15% of omphalomesenteric duct remnants. Diagnosis is usually made in the first few weeks of life after separation of the umbilical cord from the newborn umbilicus. Foul-smelling discharge from the umbilicus is typical.[33] Common presenting symptoms include GI tract obstruction, acute abdomen, and umbilical abnormalities. Ectopic tissue is seen in a third of cases.[34] Examination of the umbilicus reveals either an opening or a polypoid mass resulting from limited prolapse of the patent omphalomesenteric duct. Definitive diagnosis can be made by fistulography. Complications of this type of fistula include prolapse of the patent duct or of the duct and the attached ileum through the umbilicus, which may lead to partial intestinal obstruction. Prolapse should not be mistaken for an umbilical polyp, because excision of involved tissue might result in perforation. Resection is warranted.[33]

Omphalomesenteric Band

In omphalomesenteric band, the solid cord connecting the ileum to the umbilicus remains intact. This cord may result in intestinal obstruction from an internal hernia or volvulus.

Vitelline Blood Vessel Remnants

Failure of involution of vitelline blood vessel remnants results in complications similar to those seen with a retained fibrous cord within the peritoneal cavity. Intestinal obstruction occurs when a portion of the small intestine wraps itself around the band. Treatment of all vitelline duct abnormalities is surgical.

Malrotations

Rotation defects result from errors in the normal embryonic development of the midgut, which gives rise to the distal duodenum, jejunum, ileum, cecum, and appendix, as well as the ascending colon and proximal two thirds of the transverse colon. Aberrations in midgut development may result in a variety of anatomic anomalies, including rotation and fixation, atresias and stenoses, duplications, and persistence of embryonic structures. Such congenital anomalies may cause symptoms not only in the newborn or neonatal period, but also later in childhood and adulthood. Therefore, congenital anomalies of the midgut are appropriate considerations in the differential diagnosis of intestinal obstruction and ischemia in patients of all ages.

Because anomalies of intestinal rotation may remain asymptomatic throughout life, their true incidence is unknown; a prevalence of 1 in 500 live births has been reported.[35] Symptoms usually manifest within the first month of life with bilious emesis and abdominal distention, but presentation may be delayed in mild cases to the fourth decade of life. Patients may have cramping abdominal pain, vomiting, diarrhea, abdominal tenderness, and blood or even mucosal tissue in the stool from ischemia. If ischemia is allowed to progress, peritonitis and hypovolemic shock may develop, potentially culminating in death. Delay in surgery in patients with ischemic injury may result in a short bowel, necessitating chronic TPN therapy and eventually small bowel transplantation, with or without liver transplantation. Most adult patients with anomalies of intestinal rotation have chronic symptoms for several months or years before diagnosis.

Classification

Anomalies of rotation are usually characterized by the stage in the rotational process at which normal embryonic development of the midgut has been interrupted. Most anomalies of midgut rotation occur during the second stage of rotation and have been characterized as nonrotation, reverse rotation, and malrotation (Fig. 98-18). Of these, nonrotation is most common and reflects complete failure of the second stage of rotation. With this anomaly, the intestinal tract occupies the same position in the abdomen as it does in an 8-week-old embryo; the small intestine is located to the right of the midline, and the colon is positioned to the left.

Defects in the first and third stages of rotation are uncommon. Abnormalities in the first stage are associated with extroversion of the cloaca; abnormalities of the third stage cause failure of cecal elongation, and the cecum remains in the right upper quadrant.

In adults, reverse rotation of the midgut loop is the most commonly diagnosed defect of the midgut. Reverse rotation of the midgut loop is rare, however, and accounts for only 4% of all rotational anomalies. In reverse rotation, the midgut rotates 180 degrees clockwise during the second stage of rotation, resulting in a net 90 degrees of clockwise rotation. This may produce either the retroarterial colon type, in which the colon is located behind the SMA, or the liver and entire colon are on the right side of the abdomen, a so-called ipsilateral type of reverse rotation.

Malrotation of the midgut loop, a developmental anomaly of intestinal fixation and rotation, occurs when the proximal midgut fails to rotate around the mesenteric vessels during the second stage of rotation. The distal midgut does rotate 90 degrees in a counterclockwise direction, however, with the result that the jejunum and ileum remain to the right of the SMA, and the cecum is situated in the subpyloric region. With the potential for the small intestine and cecum to twist around the SMA and each other, this is the rotation anomaly in adults most frequently associated with ischemic damage, therefore mandating surgical correction.

Associated Abnormalities

Associated anomalies are seen in 30% to 60% of patients with defects in intestinal rotation. Nonrotation of the midgut is a significant finding in patients with omphalocele, gastroschisis, and diaphragmatic hernia. Rotation defects are seen in about 30% to 50% of infants with duodenal or jejunal atresia and in 10% to 15% of children with intestinal pseudo-obstruction. They are also associated with a variety of other conditions, including Hirschsprung's disease, esophageal atresia, biliary atresia, annular pancreas, meconium ileus, intestinal duplications, mesenteric cysts, Meckel's diverticulum, urologic anomalies, and imperforate anus.[36]

Anomalies of rotation can cause acute or chronic intermittent obstruction due to volvulus (see Fig. 98-18D and E). Venous and lymphatic obstruction secondary to volvulus can lead to malabsorption and abnormalities in intestinal motility. Venous obstruction may lead to ischemic injury of the bowel. Patients may fail to thrive and present with chylous ascites and other symptoms and signs of lymphangiectasia resulting from chronic lymphatic obstruction.

Duodenal obstruction can be due to midgut volvulus and peritoneal bands between a malpositioned cecum in the subpyloric region and the peritoneum. These bands, called *Ladd's bands*, cross the second or third portion of the duodenum and cause obstruction by intestinal compression or kinking. Ladd's bands are an anomaly of peritoneal embryogenesis and persist throughout life.

Diagnosis and Management

If time allows, diagnosis can be made by upper GI contrast examination and delineation of the site of the duodenojejunal junction. Findings on ultrasonography may suggest malrotation if the SMV is seen located to the left of the SMA, in contradistinction to the normal anatomy. In the child with acute onset of bilious vomiting and peritoneal signs, no diagnostic studies should be performed if they delay surgical intervention. In the full-term infant with bilious emesis, anomalies of rotation should be considered first and foremost to avoid the morbidity and mortality associated with these lesions. Ladd's procedure, which consists of division of Ladd's bands, if present, widening of the mesentery, appendectomy, and fixation of the small intestine on the right and the colon on the left side of the abdomen, is the operation of choice.[37]

Proliferation

Enteric Duplication

Enteric duplications are rare, with an incidence of 1 in 4500 births. The term *duplication* was introduced by Ladd in 1937. Enteric duplications are either tubular or spherical; the tubular type communicates with the normal intestinal tract, whereas the spherical type does not. Tubular duplications may join the intestine at 1 or at both ends of the duplication. Except for duodenal duplications, duplications occur on the mesenteric side of the bowel, and a common blood supply and muscular coat are shared by the duplicated segment and the adjacent bowel. Duplication cysts may be completely isolated and have their own exclusive blood supply. Small intestinal duplications often contain ectopic pancreatic tissue or gastric mucosa; the latter can be diagnosed by ^{99m}Tc radioisotopic imaging.[38]

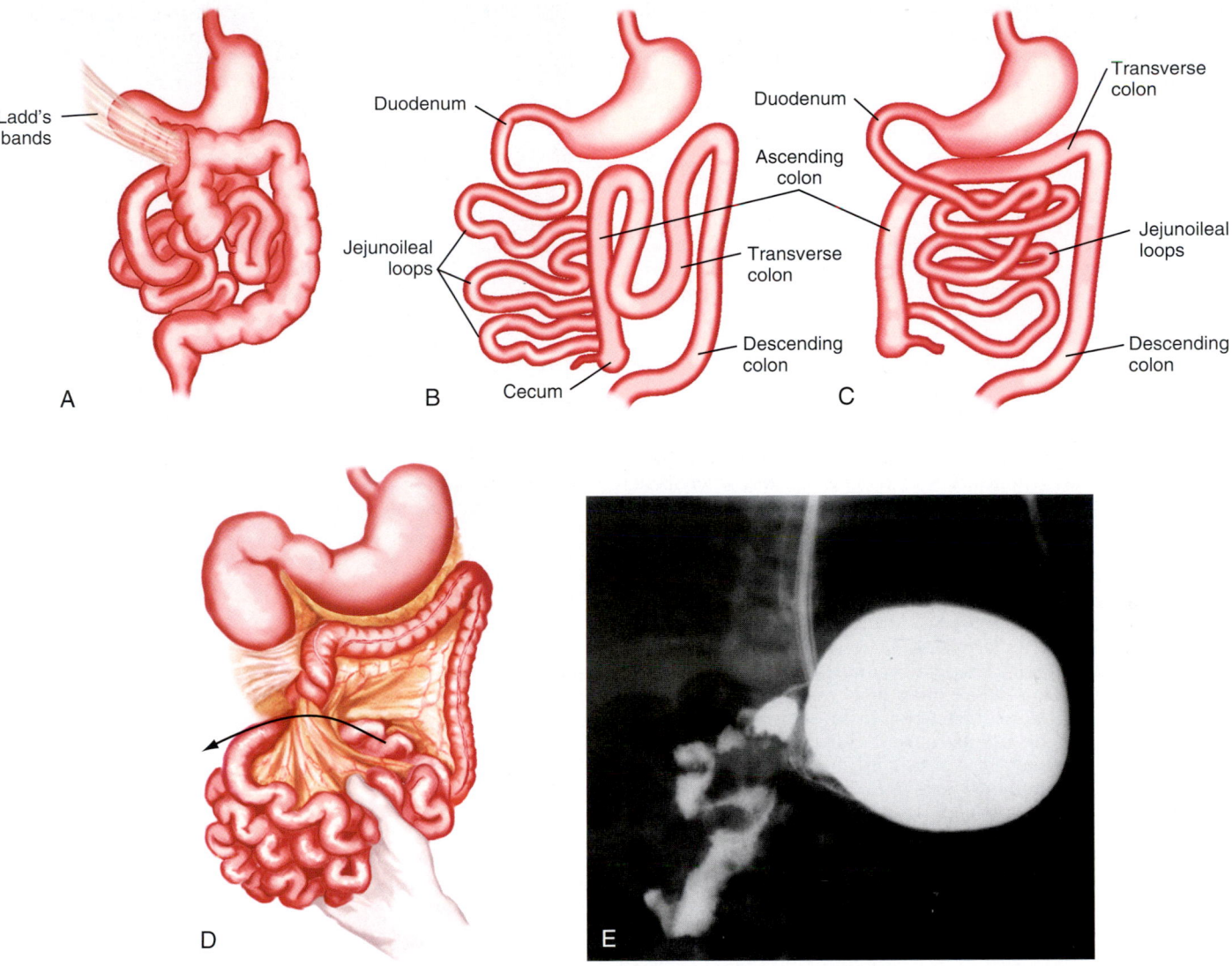

FIGURE 98-18. Rotation defects. *A* and *B,* Two examples of nonrotation. *A,* Ladd's bands are seen crossing the duodenum; some authors would refer to this as a "mixed rotation." *B,* In nonrotation, the small intestine is located to the right of the midline, and the colon is to the left of the midline. *C,* Reverse rotation. The transverse colon passes behind the duodenum. *D,* Malrotation with volvulus characterized by a clockwise twist of the mesentery and strangulation. *E,* Radiologic appearance of malrotation depicting the duodenum to the right of the spine, with a volvulus. (*A-C, From Gosche JR, Touloukian J. Congenital anomalies of the midgut. In: Wyllie R, Hyams JS, editors. Pediatric gastrointestinal disease. Pathophysiology, diagnosis, management. 2nd ed. Philadelphia: WB Saunders; 1999. D, Netter illustration from www.netterimages.com. © Elsevier Inc. All rights reserved. E, Courtesy Dr. J. Levenbrown.*)

The etiology of duplications is unclear but may involve a defect in intestinal recanalization. Enteric duplications occur throughout the GI tract but are most common in the ileum.[38] Gastric duplications occur least commonly. Depending on the site of the duplication and whether ectopic gastric mucosa is present (seen in ≈50% of cases), complications include intestinal hemorrhage, ulceration, perforation, intestinal obstruction, volvulus, intussusception, infection, pancreatitis, jaundice, hematobilia, and cutaneous enteric fistulas. Duplication of the rectum is the most common of large bowel duplications and may be associated with constipation or obstipation. Colonic duplications frequently involve the entire colon. Occasionally, large bowel duplications affect several segments of the colon, leaving "skip areas" of normal colon. A high percentage of children with duplications have associated malformations. Adenocarcinoma, neuroendocrine carcinoma, and squamous cell carcinoma have been documented with gastric, small bowel, and colonic duplications,[38,39] and carcinoid has been described in duplications of the rectum.

Neuroenteric cysts attach posteriorly to the spinal cord, are associated with asymptomatic hemivertebrae, and may occur at any level of the GI tract.

An intra-abdominal mass may be appreciated in a child with intestinal duplication, either by abdominal palpation or on rectal examination. Stool may contain occult blood from ulcerated ectopic gastric mucosa or ischemic damage. Other symptoms and signs include abdominal distention, constipation, vomiting, and respiratory distress.[40] Generalized peritonitis can be the first manifestation of a perforated duplication cyst. In adults, acute abdomen, intra-abdominal mass, symptoms of colonic diverticulitis, and chronic abdominal pain have been observed.[41]

Preoperative diagnosis by radiologic evaluation is problematic, but radioisotope studies may prove diagnostic if ectopic mucosa is present in sufficient quantities to yield a positive test.

Intestinal Atresia and Stenosis

Of all the congenital anomalies of the midgut, atresias and stenoses occur most frequently. *Intestinal atresia* refers to a congenital complete obstruction of the intestinal lumen, whereas *stenosis* indicates a partial or incomplete obstruction. Atresias occur more commonly than stenoses, and small bowel atresias have a reported incidence of 1 in 1500 live births.[42] Small bowel atresias are more common in black infants, low birth weight infants, and twins. Jejunoileal atresias are distributed equally throughout the jejunum and ileum, and multiple atresias are found in up to 20% of children. Colonic atresia occurs infrequently and accounts for less than 10% of all atresias.

In the duodenum, atresia results from failure of recanalization of the solid stage of duodenal development, whereas in the remaining small intestine and colon, atresia is the result of intestinal ischemia. Evidence of a vascular "accident" is noted in 30% to 40% of infants with atresia; proposed mechanisms include volvulus, constriction of the mesentery in a tight abdominal wall defect like gastroschisis, internal hernia, intussusception, and obstruction with perforation. Jejunoileal atresia may follow maternal use of ergotamine (in Cafergot) or cocaine taken during pregnancy and is also associated with congenital rubella. Atresias may also result from low-flow states and placental insufficiency[42]; in such cases, evidence of a vascular accident will be absent. Absence of fibroblastic growth factor 10 may also result in intestinal atresia.[43,44] In familial cases of jejunoileal atresia, there is probably a disruption of a normal embryonic pathway, making this type of atresia a true embryologic malformation rather than an acquired lesion.[45]

Duodenal obstruction may result from atresia (40% to 60%), stenosis (35% to 40%), or an intestinal web (5% to 15%); 80% of these atresias are contiguous with or distal to the ampulla of Vater, and virtually all webs are within a few millimeters of the ampulla. Atresias may be multiple. The incidence of duodenal obstruction varies, ranging from 1 in 10,000 to 20,000 live births. About 25% of patients with duodenal atresia are born preterm. Stenosis most often results from extrinsic duodenal obstruction from an annular pancreas. Other anomalies that may cause duodenal obstruction in children with malrotation are Ladd's bands, an anterior or preduodenal portal vein, or aberrant intramural pancreatic tissue.

Clinically, the presentation is that of a proximal intestinal obstruction with bilious vomiting on the first day of life, usually without abdominal distention. With gastric dilatation, the epigastrium may appear to be full by inspection and palpation. Excessive retention of gastric bile-stained fluid is typical. Duodenal obstruction is easily diagnosed by abdominal films revealing a typical "double bubble" sign with a paucity of small intestinal air (Fig. 98-19). Mothers of infants with duodenal obstruction often have polyhydramnios, and uterine ultrasonography may even demonstrate a double bubble in the unborn fetus. Vomiting, abdominal distention, delayed meconium passage, and jaundice are more frequent with jejunoileal than duodenal atresia.[46]

The classification system of Grosfeld and colleagues comprises 5 different types of jejunoileal and colonic atresias (Fig. 98-20).[47] In the "apple-peel" atresia or "Christmas tree" deformity (type IIIb), proximal atresia with wide separation of the bowel loops is associated with absence of the distal SMA. The distal ileum receives its blood supply by retrograde perfusion

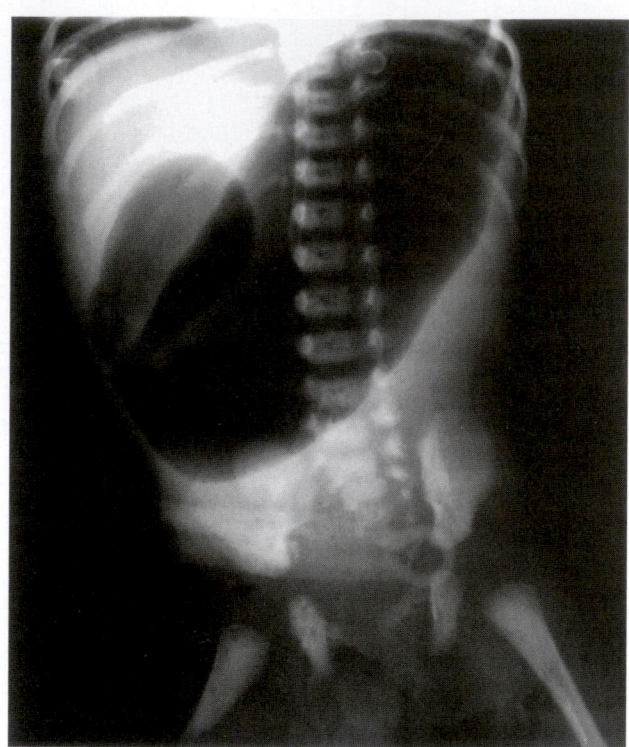

FIGURE 98-19. Plain film of the abdomen showing a "double bubble," typical of duodenal atresia. The larger bubble is the gastric bubble; the smaller is the duodenal bubble. *(Courtesy Dr. J. Levenbrown, Manhasset, New York)*

through the ileocolic artery. Type IIIb atresias account for less than 5% of all atresias. Atresias are far more common than stenoses, with a frequency ratio of 15:1. With the exception of multiple atresias and perhaps the apple-peel atresia, heredity appears to be of little significance in most cases.

Roughly 50% of children with duodenal atresia have associated malformations. Of this group, 30% have Down syndrome.[46] Major anomalies occur less frequently with jejunoileal atresias and colonic atresias than with duodenal atresia. The most common anomalies are malrotation, volvulus, and gastroschisis, all of which can cause intestinal ischemia in utero.[48] Extragastrointestinal anomalies associated with atresias include cardiovascular, pulmonary, and renal malformations, and skeletal deformities. Prematurity is common, ranging in incidence from 25% with ileal atresias to 40% with jejunal lesions; 50% percent of babies with multiple atresias are born prematurely. If the obstruction occurs beyond the ampulla of Vater, bilious or feculent vomiting with abdominal distention is seen. The presence of meconium in the colon is uncommon at surgery, but variable amounts may be noted. With distal obstruction, abdominal films may demonstrate multiple dilated air-filled bowel loops. If perforation has occurred in utero, extraluminal air and intraperitoneal calcifications or calcifications within the scrotal sac may be present, suggesting meconium peritonitis. A "soap-bubble" appearance of the ileum may suggest meconium ileus (cystic fibrosis). Air-fluid levels are rarely seen in meconium ileus. Prenatal ultrasonographic findings in jejunoileal atresia include dilated bowel and polyhydramnios.[49]

Considerations in the differential diagnosis of distal bowel obstruction include small intestinal and colonic atresias, meconium ileus, Hirschsprung's disease, and meconium plug with or without small left colon syndrome. In small left colon

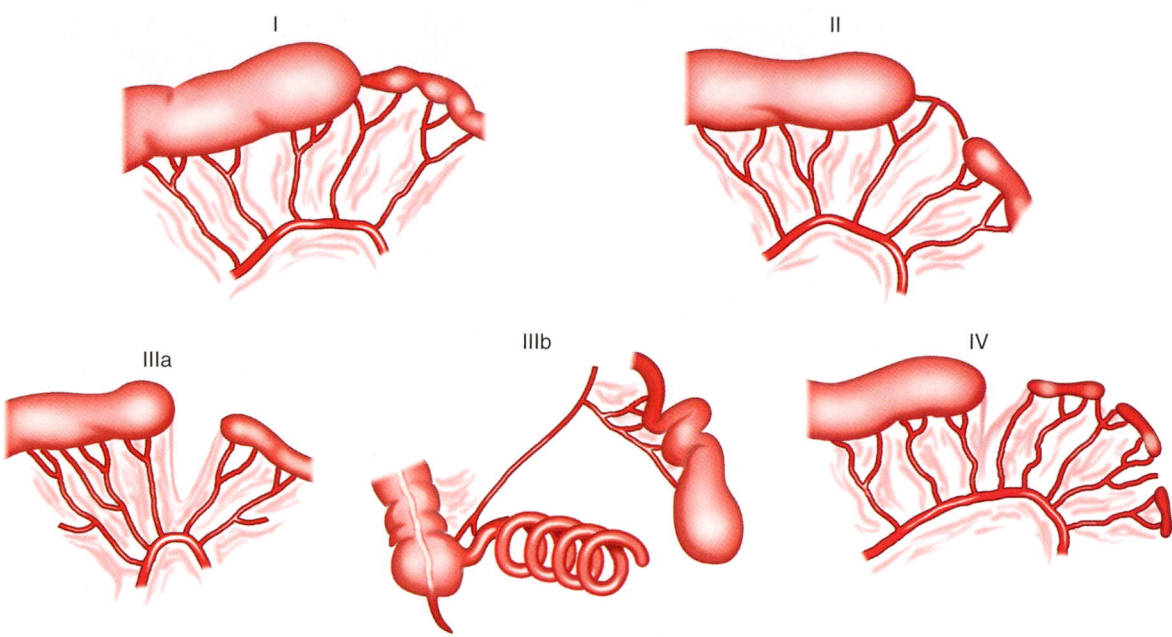

FIGURE 98-20. Classification of jejunoileal atresias. *Type I,* Mucosa and submucosa form a web or intraluminal diaphragm, resulting in obstruction. A defect in the mesentery is not present, and the intestine is not shortened. *Type II,* The dilated proximal intestine has a bulbous blind end connected by a short fibrous cord to the blind end of the distal intestine. The mesentery is intact, and the overall length of the small bowel is not usually shortened. *Type IIIa,* The defect in type IIIa is similar to that in type II in that both types have blind proximal and distal ends. In type IIIa, however, complete disconnection exists. In addition, a V-shaped mesenteric defect is present. The proximal blind end is usually markedly dilated and not peristaltic. The compromised intestine undergoes intrauterine absorption, and, as a result, the intestine is shortened. *Type IIIb,* In addition to a large defect of the mesentery, the intestine is significantly shortened. This lesion is also known as *Christmas tree deformity* because the bowel wraps around a single perfusing vessel like the tinsel coil wrapped around a Christmas tree; it is also called an *apple-peel deformity.* The distal ileum receives its blood supply from a single ileocolic or right colic artery, because most of the SMA is absent. *Type IV,* Multiple small intestinal atresias are present in any combination of types I to III. This defect often takes on the appearance of a string of sausages because of the multiple lesions. *(From Grosfeld JL, Ballantine TVN, Shoemaker R. Operative management of intestinal atresia and stenosis based on pathologic findings. J Pediatr Surg 1979; 14:368.)*

syndrome, the descending and sigmoid colon are narrowed, usually with a caliber transition at or near the splenic flexure. Typically, neonates with small left colon syndrome are born to mothers with gestational diabetes and may experience resolution of obstruction without operation. Contrast studies of the colon are helpful in making a proper diagnosis. An upper GI contrast study may provide additional important information.

Surgery is required to relieve the intestinal obstruction in the atretic or narrowed segment. Postoperative complications include fluid and electrolyte disorders, nutritional and feeding problems from diarrhea due to short bowel and small bowel failure, and failure to thrive.

Anorectum

Anorectal malformations comprise a wide spectrum of diseases that can involve the male and female anus and rectum as well as the urinary and genital tracts.[50] Anorectal malformations occur in 1 in 4000 to 5000 newborns and are more common among boys and in children with Down syndrome.[51]

During normal development, after appearance of the urorectal septum, migration of the primitive anus down the posterior wall of the cloaca may occur. Some experts postulate that a craniocaudal fusion of the lateral urorectal ridges occurs from the walls of the cloaca. Migration of the anus is completed when the urorectal septum reaches the perineum. Anorectal malformations during the 4th to 12th weeks of gestation are believed to result from failure of migration of the anus and excessive fusion. Vascular accidents, maternal diabetes, and maternal ingestion of thalidomide, phenytoin, and trimethadione have all been proposed causes. Defective development of the dorsal cloaca has also been implicated,[52] and distal 6q deletions have been reported in sacral or anorectal malformations.[53] Alteration in Shh signaling may also play a role in producing abnormal notochord development and sacral or anorectal malformations.[54,55] Anorectal malformations may occur with higher frequency in infants born after in vitro fertilization.[56]

Different types of anorectal malformations are illustrated in Figure 98-21. Anorectal malformations are divided into low (infra- or translevator), high (supralevator), and intermediate categories. A functional and practical classification of these malformations, the Wingspread classification, is summarized in Table 98-3A. The classification in Table 98-3B is designed, according to Pena,[57] to increase the physician's awareness of the possibility of the presence of these lesions, as well as to establish therapeutic priorities.

Anocutaneous Fistula

In anocutaneous (or perineal) fistula, the rectum traverses normally through most of the anal sphincter, but its lower portion

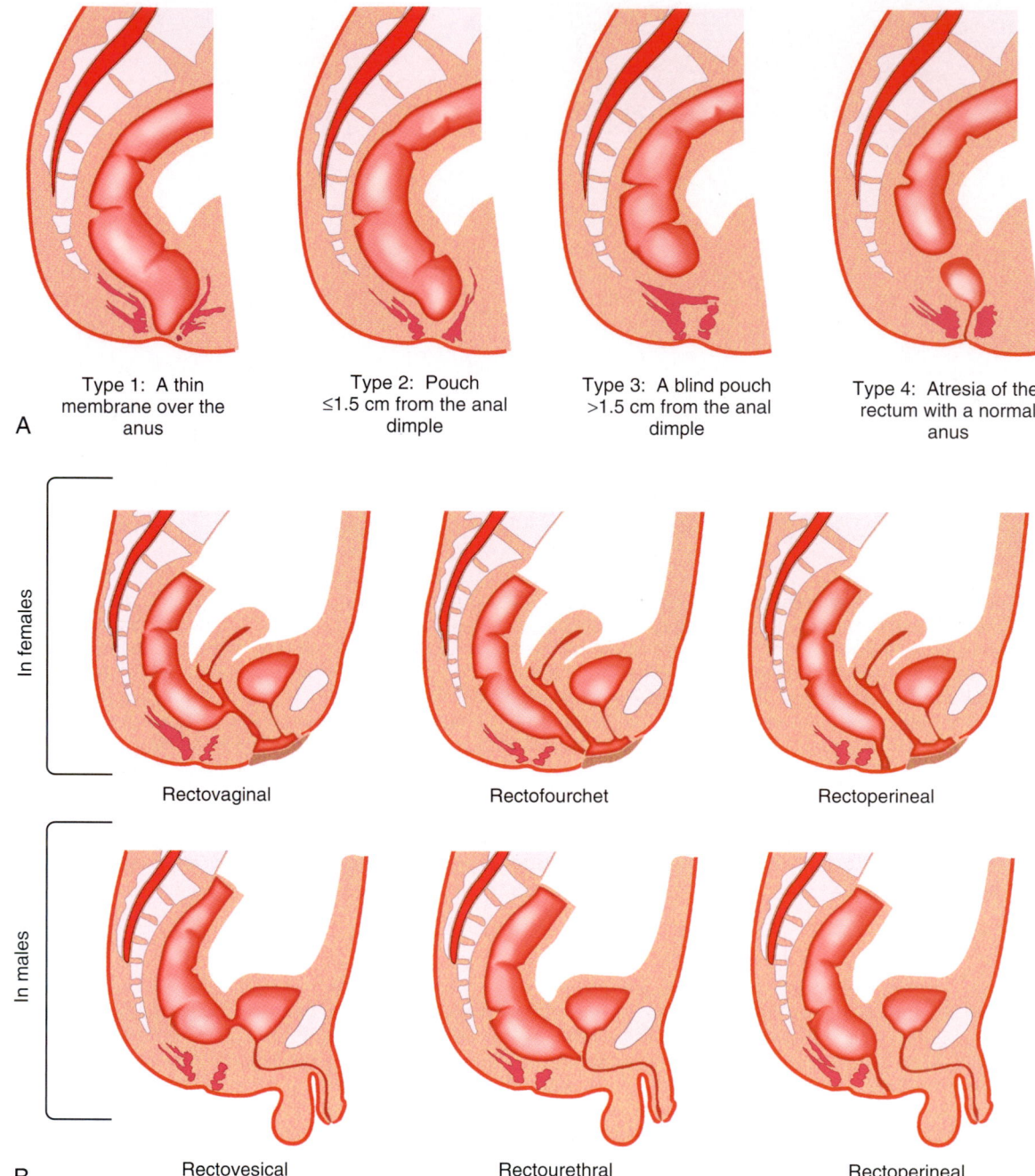

A

Type 1: A thin membrane over the anus

Type 2: Pouch ≤1.5 cm from the anal dimple

Type 3: A blind pouch >1.5 cm from the anal dimple

Type 4: Atresia of the rectum with a normal anus

In females

Rectovaginal

Rectofourchet

Rectoperineal

In males

Rectovesical

Rectourethral

Rectoperineal

B

FIGURE 98-21. Anorectal malformations. *A*, Types of imperforate anus. *B*, Types of associated fistulas. *(Netter illustration from www.netterimages.com. © Elsevier Inc. All rights reserved.)*

deviates anteriorly and ends as a perineal cutaneous fistula anterior to the center of the external anal sphincter. This anomaly is similar in the male and female child and is the least severe of all anorectal defects; associated urologic defects are uncommon (10%). All patients achieve bowel control after proper surgical treatment. Examination of the perineum may demonstrate features indicative of a perineal fistula, including a prominent midline skin ridge ("bucket-handle" malformation) and a subepithelial midline raphe fistula having the appearance of a black ribbon owing to its meconium content. Surgery consists of a simple anoplasty, usually done without a protective colostomy.

Rectourethral Fistula

In rectourethral fistula, by far the most frequent anorectal malformation in male children, the rectum descends through a portion of the pelvic floor musculature but focally deviates anteriorly and communicates with the posterior urethra. This fistula may end in either the lower posterior (bulbar) or upper posterior (prostatic) urethra.[57] Prenatal echogenic calcifications within the bowel (due to a mixture of meconium and urine) should suggest an anorectal malformation with rectourinary fistula and bladder outlet obstruction.[58] Children with prostatic urethral fistulas more commonly have sacral

TABLE 98-3 Classifications of Anorectal Malformations

A. Wingspread Classification

Male	Female
*Low**	
Anocutaneous fistula	Anovestibular fistula
Anal stenosis	Anal stenosis
	Anocutaneous fistula
Intermediate†	
Anal agenesis without fistula	Anal agenesis without fistula
Rectobulbar urethral fistula	Rectovaginal fistula
	Rectovestibular fistula
High‡	
Anorectal agenesis	Anorectal agenesis
With rectoprostatic urethral fistula	With rectovaginal fistula
Without fistula	Without fistula
Rectal agenesis	Cloaca

B. Classification Based on Need for Colostomy[57]

Male	Female
Colostomy Not Required	*Colostomy Not Required*
Perineal (cutaneous) fistula	Perineal (cutaneous) fistula
Colostomy Required	*Colostomy Required*
Rectourethral fistula	Vestibular fistula
Bulbar	
Prostatic	
Rectovesical fistula	Persistent cloaca
Imperforate anus without fistula	Imperforate anus without fistula
Rectal atresia	Rectal atresia

*Low: infra-, or translevator.
†Intermediate: between high and low.
‡High: supralevator.
B, From Pena A. Imperforate anus. In: Wyllie R, Hyams JS, editors. Pediatric gastrointestinal disease. Pathophysiology, diagnosis, management. 2nd ed. Philadelphia: WB Saunders; 1999. p 499.

and urologic defects (60%) than children with bulbar prostatic fistulas (30%). About 85% of children with rectourethral bulbar fistula achieve fecal continence after repair, compared with 60% of children with rectoprostatic fistula.

Rectovesical Fistula

In rectovesical fistula, the most proximal anorectal defect in male children, the rectum opens into the bladder neck. These malformations are associated with significant urologic defects (90%), and only 15% of children achieve bowel control after surgical repair.

Vestibular Fistula

In vestibular fistula, the most common anorectal defect of female children, the rectum opens into the vestibular bulb of the clitoris. The vestibular bulbs are erectile structures situated on either side of the vulvovaginal orifice. The rectum and vagina share a thin common wall. About 30% of affected children have associated urologic defects, and 90% of these achieve bowel control after surgery. In the case of vaginal fistula, the rectum opens in the lower or, less frequently, the upper half of the vagina.

Anorectal Agenesis (Imperforate Anus) Without Fistula

In anorectal agenesis, the rectum ends blindly without a fistula approximately 1 to 2 cm above the perineum. Sphincter function is usually preserved, with 80% of these patients achieving bowel control after surgery. Some 50% of children with imperforate anus have Down syndrome. Conversely, 95% of children with Down syndrome who have anorectal malformations will have this specific type of defect.

Rectal Agenesis (Atresia)

Rectal agenesis occurs more frequently in female than in male children, and consists of complete (atresia) or partial (stenosis) interruption of the rectal lumen between the anal canal and the rectum. On inspection of the perineum, the anus appears normal, but an obstruction can be found 1 to 2 cm above the mucocutaneous junction of the anus. Sphincter function is normal in these patients, and associated urologic defects are rare. Prognosis is excellent, with 100% achieving full bowel control after anorectoplasty.

Anal Stenosis

Anal stenosis, a fibrous ring located at the anal verge, causes constipation and gives the stool a ribbon-like appearance. Response to dilation or surgical disruption is excellent.

Persistent Cloaca

In the complex defect of persistent cloaca, the rectum, vagina, and urethra are fused into a single common channel that opens into 1 perineal orifice situated at the site of what should be the opening of the normal urethra. Prognosis depends on the intactness of the sacrum and the length of the common channel. Prognosis is better in children with a shorter common channel (<3 cm) than in those with a common channel longer than 3 cm; the latter have a higher incidence of urologic anomalies.[59] Associated urologic problems are an important consideration with persistent cloaca; urologic emergencies from obstructive uropathy are common, and hydrocolpos may compress the opening of the ureters, resulting in bilateral megaureters and massive vesicoureteral reflux.

Associated Abnormalities

Other associated abnormalities have been reported in 70% of children with anorectal malformation (Box 98-1).[50,51] Anorectal malformations occur in malformation syndromes and with chromosomal anomalies.[51,60]

The higher and more complex the anorectal defect, the greater the chance of severe urologic anomalies (72%); sacral abnormalities are also frequent. Children with a persistent cloaca or rectovesical fistula have a 99% chance of having an associated genitourinary anomaly, whereas fewer than 10% of children with a low fistula have such abnormalities. Overall, patients with additional anomalies are more likely to have high lesions than patients with isolated anorectal malformations.[51] Boys with low and high anorectal malformation have a high incidence of genital and GI anomalies, whereas urologic anomalies are more frequent in girls with high anorectal malformations.[61] Long-term bowel dysfunction occurs in a third of boys with perineal fistula.

In the first 24 hours of life, a decision should be made whether a child needs a colostomy or simple anoplasty. The presence of an associated defect, either urologic or cardiac, that might be life-threatening requires immediate evaluation. A cloaca with a common channel shorter than 3 cm can be

BOX 98-1 Common Abnormalities Associated with Anorectal Malformations

Cardiovascular
Atrial septal defect
Dextrocardia
Pulmonary stenosis
Tetralogy of Fallot
Ventricular septal defect

Central Nervous System
Aqueductal stenosis
Cerebral atrophy
Microcephaly
Myelomeningocele
Teratoma

Chromosomal Abnormalities
Trisomy 13
Trisomy 18
Trisomy 21

Craniofacial
Cleft palate
Epicanthal folds
Low-set ears
Potter facies
Simian creases

Gastrointestinal
Duodenal atresia
Esophageal atresia
Malrotation
Tracheoesophageal fistula

Genitourinary
Ambiguous genitalia
Cryptorchidism

Multicystic dysplastic kidney
Renal agenesis

Malformation Sequences
Caudal regression syndrome

Malformation Syndromes
Cat's-eye syndrome
Opitz syndrome
Potter syndrome type 1

Malformation Associations
VATER complex (vertebral defects, anal atresia, tracheoesophageal fistula with esophageal atresia, radial and renal anomalies)
VATERL complex (vertebral, anal, cardiac, tracheal, esophageal, renal, and limb anomalies)

Musculoskeletal
Abnormal rib number
Deformed or reduced number of sacral vertebrae
Dislocated hip
Hemisacrum
Hemivertebra
Micrognathia
Omphalocele
Polydactyly

Respiratory
Choanal atresia
Diaphragmatic hernia
Hypoplastic lungs
Subglottic stenosis

Data adapted from Cho S, Moore SP, Fangman T. One hundred three consecutive patients with anorectal malformations and their associated anomalies. Arch Pediatr Adolesc Med 2001; 155:587-91.

repaired by posterior sagittal intervention, whereas a common channel longer than 3 cm requires a laparotomy.[59]

Enteric Nervous System

Hirschsprung's Disease

Hirschsprung's disease (HD), first described by Harald Hirschprung in 1888, is due to a congenital absence of ganglion cells in both the submucosal (Meissner's) and myenteric (Auerbach's) plexuses. Aganglionosis extends continuously for a variable distance proximal to the internal sphincter. Short-segment HD is most common with a transition zone from aganglionic colon to ganglionic colon at the level of the sigmoid. In long-segment HD, the entire colon and even the small intestine may lack ganglia. With an incidence of 1 in 5000 live births, roughly 700 new cases of HD occur each year in the United States. The incidence is lowest in Hispanic and highest in Asian individuals. Some 10% of babies with Down syndrome have HD. Deletion of 17q21 and other chromosomal anomalies have also been reported.[62] Familial occurrence has been reported in about 7% of cases, and familial cases have a male predominance with an increased incidence of long-segment aganglionosis. Affected families carry a high risk of familial occurrence of long-segment HD.[63] Other genetic syndromes associated with HD include Waardenburg-Shah syndrome, Goldberg-Shprintzen syndrome, Mowat-Wilson syndrome, and Bardet-Biedl syndrome.[64] Known factors that influence familial recurrence include the occurrence of HD in a genetic syndrome, the presence of HD in 1 or more family members, and characteristics of the proband, including the length of involved GI segment, the proband's gender, and the gender of the at-risk baby. Four subcategories of HD are recognized: in 80% of individuals, aganglionosis is restricted to the rectosigmoid; in 15% to 20%, the aganglionosis extends proximal to the sigmoid; in 5%, aganglionosis affects the entire colon; and rarely, aganglionosis extends into the small bowel and sometimes even causes total intestinal aganglionosis.[65] HD is seen most commonly in full-term infants but on occasion does occur in premature births. In the short-segment type, a 4:1 male preponderance is observed, and in the long-segment type, the ratio is reduced to about 2:1. Short-segment HD accounts for nearly 90% of cases in childhood, long-segment HD accounting for the remainder. It is rare that ultrashort-segment HD manifests in the pediatric population, but it does explain certain cases of chronic constipation that come to attention in adulthood (Table 98-4).

Pathogenesis

Two pathogenetic mechanisms have been proposed for HD: failure of migration of neural cells, and alteration of the colonic microenvironment. Genetic, vascular, and infectious factors are invoked to explain these alterations.

Failure of Migration. Between the 5th and 12th weeks of gestation, premature arrest of the craniocaudal migration of vagal neural cells will result in HD.

TABLE 98-4 Genes Involved in Hirschsprung's Disease (HD)

Gene	Chromosome Location	Inheritance	Phenotype	Penetrance of HD Trait
RET	10q11.2	AD	HD	70% (male), 50% (female)
GDNF	5p13	AD	HD	Low
NTN	19p13	AD	HD	Low
SOX10	22q19	AD	WS4	80%
EDNRB	13q22	AR/AD	WS4/HD	Low
EDN3	20q13	AD	WS4/HD	5%
ECE1	1p36	AD	HD, CFD, CD	Low
ZFHX1B (SIP1)	2q22	AD	MCA-MR	60%
PHOX2B	4p12	AD	CCHS	20%
TCF4	18q21	AD	Epileptic encephalopathy	Low

AD, autosomal dominant; AR, autosomal recessive; CCHS, congenital central hypoventilation syndrome; CD, cardiac defect; CFD, craniofacial defect; MCA-MR, multiple congenital anomalies–mental retardation syndrome; WS4/HD, combination of Shah-Waardenburg syndrome with Hirschsprung's disease (see Box 98-2).
Data from Amiel J, Sproat-Emison E, Garcia-Barcelo M, et al. Hirschsprung disease, associated syndromes and genetics: a review. J Med Genet 2008; 45:1-14.

Colonic Microenvironment Changes. A basic defect in the microenvironment necessary for migration, development, and survival of ganglion cells has been postulated. Levels of various substances such as laminin, nicotinamide adenine dinucleotide phosphate (NADPH)-diaphorase, and neural cell adhesion molecules, as well as other polypeptides, have been shown to be reduced in the aganglionic segment. Some investigators have postulated that an alteration in the extracellular matrix with decreased concentrations of laminin and collagen IV constitutes a barrier to neutrophin 3, thereby impairing neuroblastic migration and colonization. Neutrophin 3 promotes survival of sympathetic and sensory neurons in vitro and supports growth and survival of differing subsets of neurons. Nitric oxide synthase is reduced in the aganglionic segment in HD, explaining the failure of relaxation of the affected colonic segment. Isolated case reports have linked the destruction of ganglion cells in segmental HD to cytomegalovirus infection and muscular hyperplasia of pericolonic vessels.

The genetics of HD have now been characterized.[15] Inheritance of the disease can be autosomal dominant, autosomal recessive, or polygenic. Penetration of mutations is generally low and depends on the extent of aganglionosis in affected family members. RET (re-arranged during transfection) and EDNRB (endothelin receptor type B) are 2 common genes that regulate survival, differentiation, migration, and proliferation of neural crest–derived cells and have been implicated in causation of HD.[65] RET mutation penetrance is incomplete and sex dependent. It appears that the mutation, although increasing the odds of a child's having HD, is not predictive of any specific abnormality. Alterations of several genes have been implicated.[66-69]

RET, a proto-oncogene that codes for a receptor tyrosine kinase protein, is a major susceptibility gene in HD and maps to chromosome 10q11.2. More than 100 mutations of this gene have been identified in patients with HD.[62] Identified gene mutations currently account for only about half of all cases of HD, but it is recommended that RET exon 10 mutation analysis be done in all children with HD[15]; germline RET mutations

can also cause multiple endocrine neoplasia type IIA (MEN-IIA). Although test results will be negative in the vast majority of cases, the significance of identifying MEN-IIA mutation carrier status for that individual and family appear to justify such testing.[62] Mutation of the RET gene has been noted in familial and sporadic HD.

Congenital birth defects are found in 5% to 33% of patients with HD.[62] Although HD usually occurs as an isolated event, in 30% of patients it may be part of a syndrome (Box 98-2).

Clinical Features

Most children with HD should be diagnosed in the newborn nursery. Any full-term infant who does not pass meconium within the first 48 hours of life should be suspected of having this disorder. Frequently, such infants will have abdominal distention and feeding difficulties. They also may have bilious emesis from partial bowel obstruction. Dilation of the empty rectum by the first examiner usually results in explosive expulsion of retained fecal material and decompression of the proximal normal bowel. HD-associated enterocolitis occurs more frequently in the first 3 months of life, in patients with delayed diagnosis, in children with trisomy 21, and with long-segment involvement; girls and children with a positive familial history are also more frequently affected. Enterocolitis due to ischemia from colonic distention proximal to the aganglionic segment may develop, with secondary infection from colonic bacteria; cases have also been reported of HD-associated enterocolitis in the aganglionic segment. *Clostridium difficile* has been isolated in children with this enterocolitis. Mortality rates of up to 30% have been reported for enterocolitis, which remains the major cause of death in HD. Colonic perforation, most frequently involving the cecum and rarely the appendix, may occur even in utero.

Most commonly, infants younger than 6 months of age with HD will continue to have variable but significant constipation, punctuated by recurrent obstructive crises or bouts of fecal impaction, often with failure to thrive. The abdomen may be distended with fecal masses, and peristaltic waves may be visible. Anemia and hypoalbuminemia are common. Blood-flecked diarrhea should suggest the presence of enterocolitis, and immediate evaluation should be undertaken. As the child with HD grows older, problems continue, and fecal soiling occasionally may occur. An infant with HD who is breast-fed may have fewer difficulties with defecation, because the high concentration of lactose in breast milk causes watery stools that are passed more easily. Once breast milk is discontinued, symptoms of HD may worsen.

Diagnosis

The child with symptomatic HD usually demonstrates signs and symptoms of bowel obstruction. The diagnosis may be made by 1 or a combination of the following tests: contrast enema, rectal biopsy, and anal manometry. Flexible sigmoidoscopy plays a complementary role in diagnosis.

A contrast enema performed on an unprepared colon will show the distal narrowed hypertonic segment of bowel (usually seen best in a lateral projection). The transition zone between the narrowed distal and dilated proximal intestine will be seen in the most common form of HD—the rectosigmoid form (Fig. 98-22A)—but may not be seen with long- or ultrashort-segment intestinal involvement. In ultrashort-segment HD, a radiologic picture indistinguishable from that of functional constipation with dilated bowel extending to the anus is usually seen. The transition zone may not be evident in rectosigmoid HD if the patient has undergone cleansing enemas or colonic irrigation before the study. Although it has

been suggested that the transition zone may not be evident in the first 6 weeks of life, it almost always is noted in the neonate with partial bowel obstruction.

Flexible sigmoidoscopy typically reveals a normal but empty rectum. The dilated proximal bowel, if within reach of the scope, is traversed easily unless there is abundant feces in the lumen; occasionally stercoral ulcers may be seen.

Anal manometry is the most reliable method by which the gastroenterologist can make the diagnosis of ultrashort-segment HD. The normal physiologic response to rectal distention is relaxation of the internal anal sphincter, which is smooth muscle. In HD, not only does rectal distention fail to induce internal sphincter relaxation, but a paradoxical rise in external sphincter pressure is often seen (see Fig. 98-22B). Sufficient volumes of air must be used to stimulate rectal distention for a reliable study. A false-positive result is most commonly due to a capacious rectum in a child with constipation or megacolon, in whom balloon distention may not stimulate the reflex. Up to 20% of normal children have a falsely absent reflex, especially if they are premature or of low birth weight. A positive response to rectal distention like internal sphincter relaxation is strong evidence against HD.

Suction biopsy of the rectal mucosa is the most reliable method of diagnosis, except in patients with ultrashort-segment HD. The biopsy capsule should be placed at least 2 cm above the mucocutaneous junction in infants and 3 cm above the junction in older children to avoid the physiologic hypoganglionic zone. To be certain of the absence of ganglion cells in the submucosal plexus, an experienced pathologist may need to review many serial sections. Hyperplastic sympathetic nerve fibers and proliferating Schwann cells are associated findings (see Fig. 98-22C) but can be absent in total aganglionosis.

Controversy exists regarding the type of stains necessary to make a diagnosis of HD. Because acetylcholinesterase (AChE) is increased in the muscularis mucosae and lamina propria in the aganglionic segment (see Fig. 98-22D), staining for this enzyme has been used for many years. This technique requires fresh, non–formalin-fixed tissue and technical expertise; at best, this stain is confirmatory. False-positive and false-negative reports have been documented in total colonic aganglionosis.[70] A variety of histochemical staining methods have been proposed for the identification of ganglion cells, but all are expensive, time-consuming, and unnecessary.

In the neonate, considerations in the differential diagnosis of HD include other causes of intestinal obstruction, such as meconium ileus, ileal atresia, meconium plug syndrome, and the microcolon seen in infants of diabetic mothers. When symptoms and signs of enterocolitis are present, diagnostic possibilities in the neonate also include primary necrotizing enterocolitis, HD-associated enterocolitis, milk protein–induced colitis (see Chapter 10), and sepsis with possible disseminated intravascular coagulation.

In the toddler or older child, HD must be differentiated from functional constipation (stool withholding, fecal retention). With fecal retention, history indicates that the child did pass meconium in the newborn nursery, and clinical problems did not arise until the child was usually at least 18 months old. Fecal impaction almost always is present in fecal retention, and fecal soiling is characteristic. Children with anterior displacement of the anus may be more prone to fecal retention. Idiopathic pseudo-obstruction and intestinal neuronal dysplasia can generally be distinguished from HD by rectal biopsy.

Management

Definitive treatment of HD is surgical. In all instances, biopsy of the muscularis propria of the bowel is indicated at the time

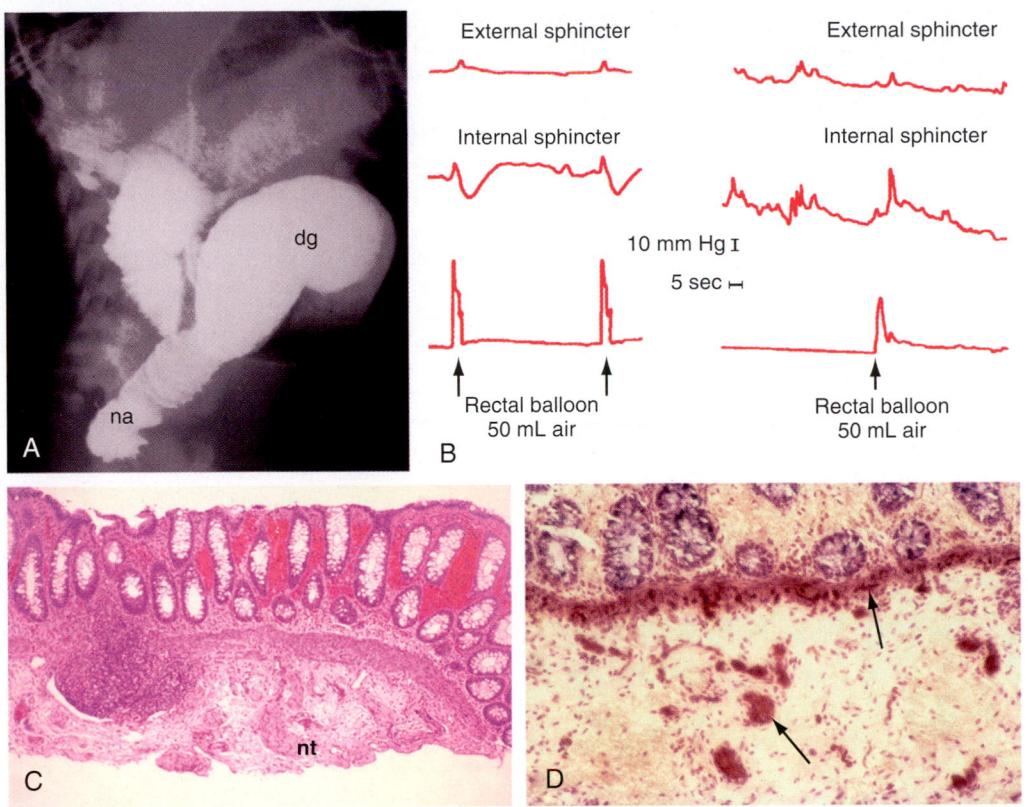

FIGURE 98-22. Hirschsprung's disease. *A*, Film from a barium enema examination showing transition zone between narrowed distal aganglionic segment *(na)* and proximal dilated ganglionic segment *(dg)*. *B*, Anal manometry. Left tracing illustrates normal function. In the right tracing, note lack of relaxation of the internal sphincter on rectal distention in a patient with Hirschsprung's disease. *C*, Photomicrograph of a rectal suction biopsy specimen showing the absence of ganglion cells and presence of thickened nerve trunks *(nt)* characteristic of Hirschsprung's disease. (H&E, ×125.) *D*, Acetylcholinesterase-positive fibers stained brown *(arrows)* in the muscularis mucosae and lamina propria, ×250. (*A*, *Courtesy Dr. J. Levenbrown.* B, *From Markowitz J. Gastrointestinal motility. In: Silverberg M, Daum F, editors. Textbook of pediatric gastroenterology. 2nd ed. Chicago: Year Book Medical Publishers; 1988.*)

of surgery to assess for the presence of ganglion cells in the myenteric plexus and to delineate the proximal extension of aganglionosis. All full-term babies with meconium plug in the newborn nursery should be evaluated for HD before discharge, because approximately 15% of children with HD have a history of meconium plug. Discharge of any newborn with undiagnosed HD and consequent delay in operative intervention may result in a greater frequency of enterocolitis, increased morbidity, and even mortality.

The specific method of surgery is operator dependent. Long-term prognosis varies and may depend on the length of the aganglionic segment. Even in the most common form of HD (short segment), it is usual to see older children continue to have defecatory issues, with fecal retention and encopresis. The exact reasons for these continuing problems remain unclear, but the mechanism may involve an intrinsic abnormality in what is described as normal colon or in the pacemaker system of the colon.

In the future, cell therapy using precursor cells from the developing human enteric system might prove to be a therapeutic option.[71]

Intestinal Neuronal Dysplasia

Intestinal neuronal dysplasia (IND) is a motility disorder that manifests with intestinal obstruction or severe chronic constipation and has a reported incidence of 1 in 7500 newborns.[72] Characteristic biopsy findings include an increased number of enlarged ganglia, neural hypertrophy (Fig. 98-23*A*),[73] and increased AChE activity in the lamina propria and muscularis mucosae. Full-thickness surgical biopsy is often necessary to diagnose IND. IND has been reported as an isolated lesion that especially affects premature infants or infants with a history of formula protein intolerance, ileal stenosis, or small left colon-meconium plug syndrome.

Three types of IND have been defined. IND type A usually manifests acutely in the neonatal period with severe constipation and enterocolitis. Biopsy features include mucosal inflammation (see Fig. 98-23*B*), ulceration with hyperplastic neural changes that are limited to the myenteric plexus, and increased AChE activity in the lamina propria and muscularis mucosae. The submucosal plexus in this type of intestinal neuronal dysplasia is histologically normal. IND type B usually is seen in children between 6 months and 6 years of age who have chronic constipation and megacolon. Histopathologic findings include hyperplastic submucosal ganglia with increased AChE-positive fibers in the muscularis mucosae and lamina propria. Ectopic ganglion cells in the muscularis mucosae and lamina propria have also been described. No changes are seen in the myenteric plexus. Some reports have speculated that some of the morphologic features described in type B are normal age-related phenomena. A third, mixed type of IND has an acute presentation and involves both the submucosal and the myenteric plexuses.

The pathogenesis of IND is controversial. In some patients it is a congenital malformation, whereas in others it is an

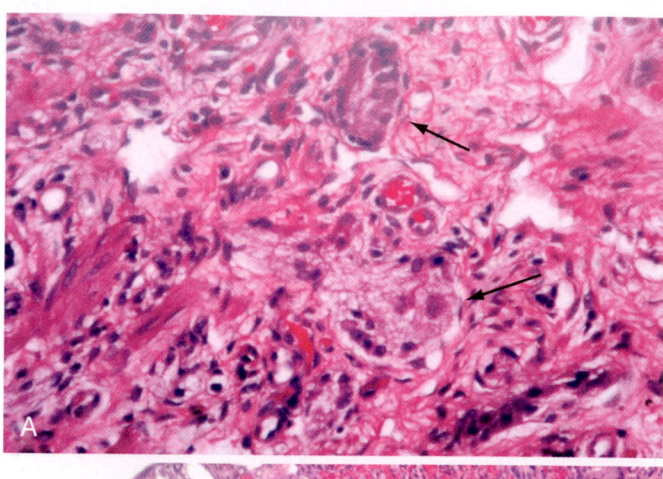

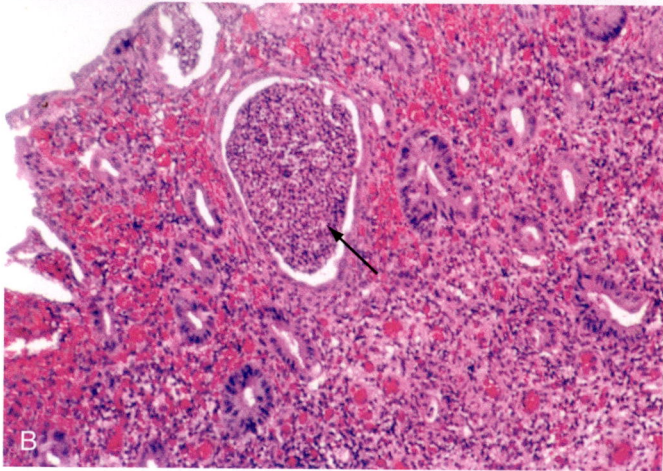

FIGURE 98-23. Photomicrographs of a rectal biopsy specimen from a patient with intestinal neuronal dysplasia. *A,* Increased number of enlarged ganglia *(arrows). B,* Active inflammation of rectal mucosa with a crypt abscess *(arrow). (A* and *B,* H&E, ×250.)

acquired phenomenon. IND is also seen in association with other syndromes such as neurofibromatosis or MEN-IIB, in proximal-segment HD, and with congenital anomalies, predominantly of the GI tract.[74] Other associated conditions include cystic fibrosis, microvillus inclusion disease, congenital anomalies, lipoblastomatosis, IBD, anorectal malformations, intestinal malrotation, megacystis-microcolon–intestinal hypoperistalsis syndrome (MMIHS, Berdon syndrome), congenital short bowel syndrome, hypertrophic pyloric stenosis, necrotizing enterocolitis, and Down syndrome.[73] In 1 series of patients, a de novo duplication has been detected on chromosome 12 in 1 patient. Therefore, IND may not represent a well-defined entity but rather a secondary phenomenon related to age, obstruction, or inflammation.[75] IND can resolve with age.

Chronic Intestinal Pseudo-obstruction

Congenital forms of neuropathic and myopathic pseudo-obstruction are rare and sporadic, perhaps representing new mutations (see Chapter 124). In these situations, a family history of pseudo-obstruction is lacking, as are any associated syndromes and evidence of other predisposing factors like toxins, infections, ischemia, or autoimmune disease. Children

with chromosomal abnormalities (e.g., Down syndrome), as well as those with MEN-III or Duchenne's muscular dystrophy, may suffer from pseudo-obstruction.

Miscellaneous and Genetic Defects

Microvillus Inclusion Disease

Congenital microvillus atrophy, also known as *microvillus inclusion disease* (MID), is an autosomal recessive disorder that may manifest with severe diarrhea shortly after birth and is characterized by atrophy of the intestinal villi, with characteristic electron microscopic findings (see later).[76] Although its prevalence is unknown, MID is reported to be the most common cause of familial intractable diarrhea.[77] A female gender predominance has been observed, and consanguinity is reported in 20% of cases. The incidence of MID may be higher among Navajo Indians and persons from the Middle East; in Navajo Indians, a mutation in MYO5B has been implicated.[78] Defective protein trafficking and abnormal cytoskeletal and microfilament function have been proposed as possible etiologies.[79] A blockage in the transport pathway from the Golgi apparatus leads to fusion of small vesicles into microvillus inclusions.[80] Secretory diarrhea is severe, with intolerance to oral feeding and unresponsiveness to most therapeutic modalities. Three variants of MID are recognized: congenital, the most frequent and severe, manifesting within the first week of life; late-onset, starting at 6 to 8 weeks; and atypical, with either early or late onset.

The wall of the small intestine is paper-thin in MID. The mucosa of the duodenum and small bowel is characterized by villus atrophy, hypoplastic or normal crypts, and normal or decreased cellularity of the lamina propria (Fig. 98-24*A*). Absence of the brush border membrane is demonstrated by lack of linear staining with PAS, carcinoembryonic antigen (CEA), Rab11, and CD10.[81,82] These stains also visualize the microvillus inclusions on light microscopy.

Evaluation by electron microscopy reveals characteristic ultrastructural abnormalities of the microvillus membrane, including disruption or absence of the brush border membrane, shortening and absence of the microvilli, and microvillus inclusions (see Fig. 98-24*B*). Although these lesions are most commonly noted in biopsies of the small intestine, microvillus inclusions may also be seen in specimens from the rectum and colon.

Total parenteral nutrition must be used to prolong survival. Secretory diarrhea persists but becomes less voluminous. Small bowel transplantation is the only hope to improve the quality of life and long-term prognosis in children with MID.[83,84]

Intestinal Epithelial Dysplasia

Intestinal epithelial dysplasia (IED), also known as *tufting enteropathy,* is a congenital enteropathy with early onset, severe intractable diarrhea, and characteristic microscopic findings.[85] In IED, there is a variable degree of villus atrophy. Surface epithelial cells are arranged in tufts with a round apex. Tufts can also be seen in the colonic mucosa. These epithelial cells have an abnormal expression of E-cadherin and do not contain inclusions on electron microscopic examination. In the basement membrane, heparin sulfate proteoglycan is increased and laminin is faint and irregular.[85]

The diarrhea is secretory, malabsorption is intractable, and growth is impaired. Several cases of IED have been associated with congenital anomalies.[85] Nonspecific punctate keratitis is observed in more than 60% of patients with IED. Most patients

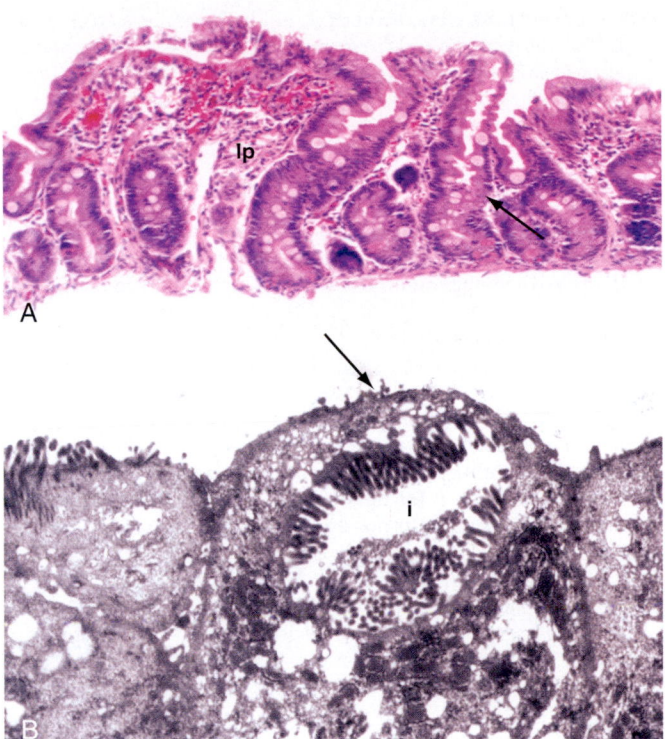

FIGURE 98-24. Photomicrographs of duodenum from a patient with microvillus inclusion disease. *A,* Villus atrophy with crypt hyperplasia *(arrow)* and decreased cellularity of the lamina propria *(lp).* (H&E, ×250.) *B,* On electron microscopy, lack of or shortened microvilli *(arrow)* and a cytoplasmic inclusion *(i)* composed of a vesicle lined by microvilli can be seen. (×15,000.) *(Courtesy S. Teichberg, PhD, Manhasset, New York)*

with IED have consanguineous parents or affected siblings. In the Middle East, IED is even more common than MID. IED is characterized by a basement membrane with abnormal distribution of 2 β_1-integrin adhesion molecules along the crypt-villus axis.[85] Tufts result from non-apoptotic epithelial cells that are no longer in contact with the basement membrane. Small bowel transplantation is required.

Congenital Glucose and Galactose Malabsorption

Familial glucose and galactose malabsorption, transmitted as an autosomal recessive trait and due to mutation in the *SGILT1* gene, is characterized by an absence of the active transport carrier protein (Na$^+$-glucose cotransporter) for glucose and galactose.[86] Ingestion of any formula that contains glucose or galactose in the newborn period results in severe life-threatening watery diarrhea. Stools are strongly positive for reducing substances. Neither blood nor white blood cells are present in the stool. Findings on biopsy of the small bowel and colon are normal. Discontinuation of formula containing glucose, galactose, or lactose (lactose is metabolized to glucose and galactose) and institution of a fructose-containing formula with resultant therapeutic benefit are usually sufficient to make a clinical diagnosis of glucose or galactose malabsorption. Diarrhea abruptly ceases and the newborn begins to thrive when fructose-containing formula feedings are instituted. Some reports indicate that the severity of the diarrhea from glucose or galactose malabsorption diminishes with age

because of the increased capacity of the intestinal flora to metabolize glucose.

Congenital Sucrase and Isomaltase Deficiency

Because sucrose is not a common dietary carbohydrate during the first 6 months of life, watery stools generally do not develop in children with this disorder until sucrose is administered in baby food. An exception to this rule is in the newborn receiving a formula (usually with soy protein or casein hydrolysate) with sucrose as the carbohydrate. Because sucrose itself is not a reducing substance, to make the diagnosis the stool must be hydrolyzed by boiling it with 1N hydrochloric acid for 20 minutes, thereby changing sucrose to glucose and fructose. Congenital sucrase or isomaltase deficiency, although extremely rare, is the most common congenital disaccharidase deficiency.

Congenital Lactase Deficiency

Congenital absence of lactase is extremely rare. Affected babies receiving a lactose-containing formula develop severe watery diarrhea, which resolves with the institution of a non–lactose-containing formula. Biopsy specimens of the small intestine are histologically normal, but assay for disaccharidases reveals diminished or absent lactase.

Congenital Chloride Diarrhea (Chloridorrhea)

Congenital chloride diarrhea is an autosomal recessive disorder of intestinal Cl-HCO$_3$ exchange caused by mutations of the *SLC26A3* gene.[87] The chloride-bicarbonate exchange mechanism in the ileum and colon is reversed, and chloride is actively secreted, resulting in a chloride-rich diarrhea (i.e., chloridorrhea). The baby with congenital chloride diarrhea is often premature and may present with an ileus or absence of meconium passage. Watery diarrhea with a high stool chloride content and low stool pH is lifelong; dehydration may result, and increased absorption of bicarbonate may lead to hypochloremic metabolic alkalemia, hyponatremia, and marked hypokalemia. The stool contains no blood, no white blood cells, and no reducing substances. Urinary chloride is low. Biopsy specimens of the small intestine and colon are normal. Treatment is fluid and electrolyte replacement. Acid reduction with proton pump inhibitors has been tried, with variable results.

Congenital Sodium Diarrhea

Congenital sodium diarrhea is caused by defective sodium or proton exchange.[88] Patients have acidemia and hyponatremia. The stool concentration of bicarbonate and sodium are increased.

Cystic Fibrosis

CF is an autosomal recessive disorder of cAMP chloride transport that is due to a defect in the cystic fibrosis transmembrane regulator (CFTR) (see Chapter 57).

About 10% to 15% of newborns with CF present with neonatal meconium ileus or its complications. Meconium plug syndrome may also occur, resulting in colonic obstruction rather than small bowel obstruction, as is seen with meconium ileus. Antenatally, small intestinal ischemia and perforation may occur, resulting in meconium cyst, intestinal atresia, or meconium peritonitis with intra-abdominal or scrotal calcifications.

KEY REFERENCES

Full references for this chapter can be found on www.expertconsult.com.

4. Schonhoff SE, Giel-Moloney M, Leiter AB. Minireview: Development and differentiation of gut endocrine cells. Endocrinology 2004; 145:2639-44.

19. Mastroiacovo P, Lisi A, Castilla EE, et al. Gastroschisis and associated defects: An international study. Am J Genet A 2007; 143:660-71.

20. Abdullah F, Arnold MA, Nabaweesi R, et al. Gastroschisis in the United States 1988-2003: Analysis and risk categorization of 4344 patients. J Perinatol 2007; 27:50-5.

36. Penco JM, Murillo JC, Hernandez A, et al. Anomalies of intestinal rotation and fixation: Consequences of late diagnosis beyond two years of age. Pediatr Surg Int 2007; 23:723-30.

40. Karnak I, Ocal T, Senocak ME, et al. Alimentary tract duplication in children: Report of 26 years' experience. Turk J Pediatr 2000; 42:118-25.

43. Fairbank TJ, Sala FG, Kanard R, et al. The fibroblast growth factor pathway serves a regulatory role in proliferation and apoptosis in the pathogenesis of intestinal atresia. J Pediatr Surg 2006; 41:132-6.

51. Cho S, Moore SP, Fangman T. One hundred three consecutive patients with anorectal malformations and their associated anomalies. Arch Pediatr Adolesc Med 2001; 155:587-91.

57. Pena A. Imperforate anus. In: Wyllie R, Hyams JS, editors. Pediatric gastrointestinal disease. Pathophysiology, diagnosis, management. 2nd ed. Philadelphia: WB Saunders; 1999. p 499.

62. Amiel J, Sproat-Emison E, Garcia-Barcelo M, et al. Hirschsprung disease, associated syndromes and genetics: A review. J Med Genet 2008; 45:1-14.

72. Meier-Ruge WA, Ammann K, Bruder E, et al. Updated results on intestinal neuronal dysplasia (INDB). Eur J Pediatr Surg 2004; 14:384-91.

85. Goulet O, Salomon J, Ruemmele F, et al. Intestinal epithelial dysplasia (tufting enteropathy). Orphanet J Rare Dis 2007; 2:20-9.

CHAPTER

99

Small Intestinal Motor and Sensory Function and Dysfunction

JANE M. ANDREWS, STUART M. BRIERLEY, AND L. ASHLEY BLACKSHAW

The most important goals of small intestinal motor and sensory function are efficient absorption of nutrients and maintenance of orderly aboral movement of chyme and indigestible residues along the small intestine. Small intestinal motility is also critically important in preventing SIBO. This is achieved by the net aboral flow of luminal contents during both the fed and fasting states, probably with the assistance of the gatekeeper function of the ileocecal junction, which prevents backflow of cecal contents.

Net movement of contents along the small intestine is antegrade, but retrograde flow also occurs normally over short distances. Optimal progression of luminal contents allows appropriate mixing of digested food with intestinal secretions and contact of contents with the epithelium; such contact is important for absorption and sensing of nutrients within the lumen. Both absorption and mucosal sensing of nutrients exert feedback control on gastric and small intestinal motor function, an interplay that optimizes the rate at which additional nutrients are presented to the absorptive epithelium, and minimizes the amount of nutrients lost to the colon. In association with nausea and preceding emesis, retrograde movement of small intestinal contents occurs over long distances, when a unique pattern of a strong zone of phasic small intestinal contractions travels in an orad direction over a large portion of the small intestine. These contractions deliver luminal contents back to the stomach for ejection into the esophagus during emesis. This coordinated motor pattern underscores the versatile modulation of small intestinal motility according to precise physiologic need.

The motor function of the small intestine depends directly on smooth muscle in the intestinal wall, which contains the basic control mechanisms that initiate contractions and regulate their frequency. Overlying these basic control mechanisms are the enteric nervous system (ENS) and the autonomic nervous system (ANS). In addition, a number of hormones modulate the frequency and patterning of small intestinal contractions. Each of these factors plays a role in the motility of the small intestine in health, and specific damage to each of these components in certain diseases has helped define their discrete roles.

ANATOMY

The small intestine is approximately 3 to 7 meters long and extends from the duodenal side of the pylorus to the ileocecal valve. It is divided into 3 regions—duodenum, jejunum, and ileum—based on structural and functional considerations. Although some structural and functional differences exist among these 3 regions, they exhibit similar motor characteristics. At each end of the small intestine, however, physiologic sphincters—the pylorus and ileocecal valve—have distinctly different motor patterns that give them the ability to act as controllers of flow between the antrum and duodenum and between the ileum and colon, respectively. The motor function of the pylorus and stomach are discussed in Chapter 49, the ileocecal region is discussed in Chapter 100, and general anatomy is discussed in Chapter 98. The duodenum is a fixed, largely retroperitoneal structure located in the upper abdomen, and the distal ileum generally is anchored in the right iliac fossa by its attachments to the cecum. Except for these regions, the small intestine is mobile within the peritoneal cavity.

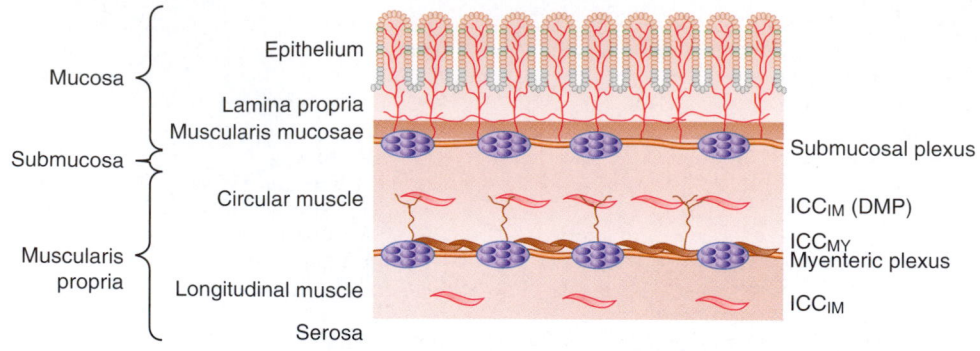

FIGURE 99-1. Diagram showing layers and components of the small intestinal wall. DMP, deep muscular plexus; ICC_{IM}, intramuscular interstitial cells of Cajal; ICC_{MY}, myenteric interstitial cells of Cajal. *(Advice from Dr. Elizabeth Beckett is acknowledged.)*

NORMAL SMALL INTESTINAL MOTOR AND SENSORY FUNCTION

Smooth Muscle

The wall of the small intestine comprises mucosa (which consists of the epithelium and lamina propria), submucosa, muscularis, and serosa (Fig. 99-1). The muscularis is composed of inner circular and outer longitudinal layers of smooth muscle that are present in continuity along the entire length of small intestine. Contractions within these layers are responsible for gross small intestinal motility. Another but much thinner muscular layer, the muscularis mucosae, is present between the mucosa and submucosa and plays a role in mucosal or villus motility.[1] The muscularis mucosae does not contribute to gross motility and is not considered further in this chapter.

The smooth muscle cells within each muscle layer form a syncytium. Myocytes communicate electrically with each other through physically specialized areas of cell-to-cell contact called *gap junctions*; these are visible by electron microscopy. This intimate contact between adjacent myocytes gives low-resistance electrical contact or coupling among them, enabling them to be excited as a unit. Mechanical connections among myocytes in each layer enable them to function as a contractile unit. At a cellular level, mechanical connections are provided by intermediate junctions, and at a tissue level, mechanical connections are provided by the dense extracellular stroma of collagen filaments between bundles of smooth muscle cells. Within each layer, the smooth muscle cell bodies are arranged in parallel, such that the circular muscle layer encircles the lumen, and the longitudinal layer extends axially along the small intestine. Each may be controlled independently, thus reducing luminal diameter or shortening small intestinal length, respectively, alone or in combination.

The myocytes themselves are spindle-shaped cells that derive their contractile properties from specialized cytoplasmic filaments (actin and myosin) and from the attachment of these filaments to cytoskeletal elements. On electron microscopy, condensations of electron-dense, amorphous material are noted around the inner aspect of the cell membrane (dense bands) and throughout the cytoplasm (dense bodies). The contractile are arranged in a fashion similar to that in skeletal muscle and insert onto the dense bands and bodies approximately in parallel with the long axis of the cell. Thus, when the contractile filaments are activated to slide over each other, cell shortening results. Most of the Ca^{2+} required for activating the contractile apparatus enters the cells via L-type Ca^{2+} channels (Fig. 99-2). Ca^{2+} entry also can be supplemented to a varying extent by release of Ca^{2+} from the sarcoplasmic

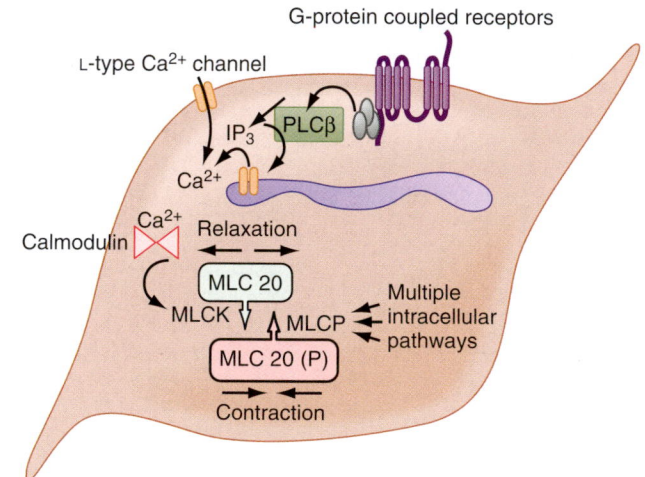

FIGURE 99-2. Diagram of a smooth muscle cell showing pathways that lead to contraction and relaxation. See text for details. MLC 20, 20-kd myosin light chain; MLCK, myosin light chain kinase; MLCP, myosin light chain phosphatase; (P), phosphorylated; PLC, phospholipase C. *(Modified from Sanders KM. Regulation of smooth muscle excitation and contraction. Neurogastroenterol Motil 2008; 20[Suppl 1]:39-53.)*

reticulum membrane via IP3 receptor-operated Ca^{2+} channels. IP3 is generated by phospholipase C, which in turn is activated by G proteins, coupled to receptors for excitatory transmitters (G protein-coupled receptors).

The increased cytoplasmic Ca^{2+} binds to the Ca^{2+} binding protein calmodulin, enabling it to activate myosin light chain kinase, which phosphorylates the 20-kd light chain of myosin (MLC20). Phosphorylation of MLC20 facilitates actin binding to myosin and initiates cross-bridge cycling and development of mechanical force. Phosphorylation of MLC20 is reduced by MLC phosphatase. Dephosphorylation of MLC20 reduces cross-bridge cycling and leads to muscle relaxation. The dephosphorylation process is under a complex system of hierarchical control, which is important in setting the gain of smooth muscle contractility.[2]

Interstitial Cells of Cajal

Interstitial cells of Cajal (ICC) are specialized cells within the smooth muscle layer that are vital for normal small intestinal motor function. ICC are pleomorphic mesenchymal cells that form an interconnecting network via long, tapering cytoplasmic processes. ICC lie in close proximity to both nerve axons and myocytes, with which they form electrical gap junctions.[3] ICC serve 2 roles in the control of small intestinal motility: First, they act as pacemakers and generate the electrical slow wave that determines the basic rhythmicity of small intestinal contractions.[4] Second, they transduce both inhibitory and excitatory neural signals to the myocytes[5] and thus can vary the myocyte membrane potential and, in turn, contractile activity; this transduction occurs because ICC are interposed functionally between nerve terminals and the smooth muscle that the nerves supply. The neuroeffector junctions of the small intestine are not just simple contacts between nerve terminals and smooth muscle cells; they are contacts between enteric nerve terminals and ICC, and from there with myocytes by means of electrical gap junctions. Thus, effective neurotransmission results from the activation of specific sets of receptors on ICC, rather than by direct action on smooth muscle cells.

At least 3 separate functional groups of ICC exist. They are the myenteric ICC (ICC_{MY}), intramuscular ICC (ICC_{IM}), and ICC in the deep muscular plexus (ICC_{DMP}).

Cells of the ICC_{MY} population form a dense, electrically coupled network within the intermuscular space at the level of the myenteric plexus between the circular and longitudinal muscle layers. ICC_{MY} are the pacemaker cells in the small intestine and trigger generation of slow waves in the smooth muscle. These cells possess a specialized mechanism that uses their oxidative metabolism to generate an inward (pacemaker) current resulting from the flow of cations through nonselective cation channels in the plasma membrane. A *primary pacemaker* initiates slow waves. This depolarization from the primary event then entrains the spontaneous activity of other ICC within the network. This sequence results in a propagation-like phenomenon by which slow waves spread, without decrement, through the ICC network by means of gap junctions. A specialized type of ICC_{MY} lines the septa (ICC_{SEP}) between circular muscle bundles; these cells form a crucial conduction pathway for spreading excitation deep into muscle bundles of the human jejunum, which is necessary for the motor patterns that underlie mixing.[6]

ICC_{IM}, the second main population of ICC, are distributed within the muscle layers. ICC_{IM} are innervated preferentially by intrinsic enteric motor neurons. In the small intestine, a third population, ICC_{DMP}, which may be a specialized type of ICC_{IM} in the small intestine, is concentrated at the inner surface of the circular muscle layer at the region of the deep muscular plexus; it also receives preferential innervation.

Both inhibitory and excitatory enteric motor nerve terminals selectively target intramuscular ICC. Their responses are transduced in turn to smooth muscle cells through gap junctions. Inputs from enteric excitatory motor neurons are mediated by muscarinic acetylcholine receptors (M_2 and M_3) and NK1 substance P-receptors that result in increased inward currents, thereby causing depolarization. When depolarization reaches the level of the smooth muscle, it increases the opening of L-type Ca^{2+} channels during slow waves. These conditions result in greater Ca^{2+} entry and more forceful phasic contractions. Inputs from inhibitory enteric motor neurons are mediated by neurotransmitters including nitric oxide (NO) and vasoactive intestinal polypeptide (VIP), which activate both receptor and non-receptor mechanisms in ICC_{IM}. The result of these inputs is an increased opening of K^+ channels that, in turn, has a stabilizing effect on membrane potential, reduces Ca^{2+} channel opening, and results in less forceful contractions of the smooth muscle. Therefore, the mechanical response of small intestinal muscle to the ongoing slow wave activity depends strongly upon regulation of its excitability by the enteric nervous system via ICC_{IM}.

ICC in general play broadly similar roles in the small intestine and colon (for colon, see Chapter 100, Fig. 100-2, and References 4, 5). Absence or inactivity of ICC has been implicated in a number of clinical disorders that manifest as disturbed intestinal motility (see Chapter 124).

Recent focus has also centered on involvement of "fibroblast-like cells," which have similar anatomic distributions as ICC, but represent a discrete separate population of cells. These fibroblast-like cells can be identified by staining with antibodies for platelet-derived growth factor receptor α (PDGFRα), which demonstrates that they are closely associated with both ICC and nerve varicosities. Myenteric and intramuscular PDGFRα-immunopositive cells express small-conductance Ca^{2+}activated K^+ (SK3) channels, which are a potential mediator of purinergic enteric inhibition. Because PDGFRα-immunopositive cells also form gap junctions with smooth muscle cells, fibroblast-like cells are also likely participants in motor neurotransmission and thus may contribute to the integrated motor responses of smooth muscle and possibly the frequency of phasic activity, such as peristalsis and segmentation.[3]

Neurons

The small intestine is richly innervated with both intrinsic and extrinsic neurons. Intrinsic neurons have their cell bodies located within the wall of the small intestine and constitute the ENS. The majority of these intrinsic enteric neurons have their peripheral terminals within the intestinal wall. However, a separate class of neurons termed *intestinofugal neurons* have cell bodies within the myenteric plexus, but have projections out of the intestinal wall, via extrinsic nerve trunks, to prevertebral ganglia (PVG). Intestinofugal neurons sense and receive information regarding mechanical distension of the intestine and transmit this information to postganglionic sympathetic neurons in the PVG. Overall, these various types of intrinsic neurons greatly outnumber the neurons of the extrinsic supply, which have their cell bodies outside the intestinal wall, but projections that end within the intestinal wall. Extrinsic neurons can be classified anatomically according to the location of their cell bodies (cranial or spinal ganglia) and the route along which their projections travel. Extrinsic motor neurons belong to the ANS and connect the central nervous system (CNS) with the ENS and, from there, the small intestinal smooth muscle through the ICC. Furthermore, some extrinsic motor neurons terminate directly in the muscle layers. Extrinsic *sensory* neurons from the small intestine do not belong to either the ANS or ENS and are classified as spinal or vagal in origin, depending on the whether they follow vagal or spinal nerve pathways en route to the CNS (Fig. 99-3).

Neurons that supply the intestine are designated either *afferent* or *efferent*, depending on the direction in which they conduct information. By convention, information is conducted centrally by *afferent* neurons and peripherally by *efferent* neurons. Thus, in regard to the neural supply, the term *afferent* is used to describe pathways conducting information that is detected in the intestine and transmitted to the CNS. It should be noted that in most texts the term *afferent* is interchangeable with *sensory*; however, most sensory information from the small intestine is not perceived at a conscious level. The sensory information that is perceived generally arises in the form of bloating, discomfort, and pain. The terms *efferent* and *motor* in regard to neural supply are used to describe pathways that conduct signals toward the "effector," in this case the small intestinal smooth muscle. Although the importance of motor innervation for motility is self-evident, the pivotal role of afferent function in determining motor

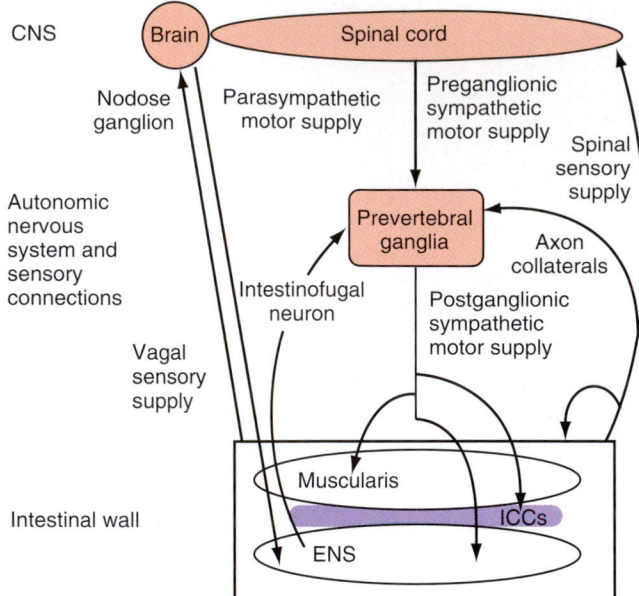

FIGURE 99-3. Schematic representation of relationships among components of small intestinal motor control system. For further details, see text. CNS, central nervous system; ENS, enteric nervous system; ICC, interstitial cells of Cajal.

responses has been less well appreciated. The importance of the extrinsic afferent innervation in sensory signaling is emphasized by the observation that at least 80% of vagal fibers are afferent rather than efferent.[7]

Intrinsic Neurons

ENS elements of the small intestine can be subdivided into 3 major functional groups: primary sensory (afferent) neurons, motor (efferent) neurons, and interneurons. The latter 2 groups can be further subdivided into excitatory and inhibitory motor neurons and ascending and descending interneurons, respectively. Together these 3 groups form complex networks that are responsible for coordinating intestinal motility. Within this network, specific ascending and descending circuits are synchronously activated in response to luminal contents. Contractions are the resultant process of ascending pathways, with ascending interneurons synapsing onto excitatory motor neurons, whereas relaxations result from descending interneuron activation of inhibitory motor neurons. Other categories of neurons, including secretomotor and vasomotor neurons and motor neurons to endocrine cells, are recognized but not considered further in this chapter. Additional distinct subgroups of enteric neurons are now well characterized both structurally and functionally and are reviewed in detail elsewhere.[8,9]

The cell bodies of ENS neurons are grouped together in the ganglia (clusters of cell bodies) of 2 main intramural plexi. These plexi lie in the submucosa (Meissner's submucosal plexus) and between the circular and longitudinal muscle layers (Auerbach's myenteric plexus). A deep plexus (Schabadasch's plexus) exists within the circular muscle but does not contain ganglia. The ganglia in the submucosal and myenteric plexuses are connected by interganglionic fascicles. These fascicles are composed predominantly of the axons of motor neurons and interneurons because sensory nerve processes do not often extend for any distance outside the ganglia.

The myenteric plexus consists of ganglia that are spaced at regular intervals and connected by a network of interganglionic fascicles; this major network is known as the *primary plexus*. Within this main structure, smaller branches of nerve bundles arise from the primary plexus and form the secondary plexus, and still smaller branches form the tertiary plexus.

The submucosal plexus has 2 layers, 1 close to the mucosa and another nearer to the circular muscle layer. These 2 layers are connected by interganglionic fascicles. The submucosal plexus does not have a hierarchy of subordinate plexuses.

Intrinsic Afferent Supply

The primary afferent neurons of the ENS are characterized morphologically as Dogiel type II neurons (neurons with numerous processes).[10] Intrinsic primary afferent neurons (IPANs) that respond to mucosal chemical stimuli have their cell bodies in the myenteric plexus, and they project axons toward the mucosa. The myenteric plexus also contains the cell bodies of intrinsic afferent neurons that discharge in response to mechanical stimulation of the muscle layer induced by muscle activity or stretch. Intrinsic afferent neurons that respond to mechanical stimulation of the mucosa also are believed to exist, based on enteric reflexes seen in extrinsically denervated preparations. The cell bodies and processes of these neurons have not yet been identified definitively, although available evidence is consistent with the presence of their cell bodies in the submucosal ganglia.[10]

Intrinsic sensory neurons synapse in the intramural plexuses with intrinsic motor neurons and interneurons, which they excite mainly by the release of acetylcholine and substance P. A more detailed account of the function and role of intrinsic afferent neurons can be found in a review by Furness and coworkers.[10]

Recent observations indicate that IPANs are not the only class of enteric neurons that respond to mechanosensory stimuli; for example, mechanical distortion of the myenteric ganglia, which occurs regularly during contraction or motility events, activates about 20% of all myenteric neurons in the ileum. These ileal myenteric neurons display rapidly adapting responses to mechanical stimulation, whereas colonic neurons display slowly adapting responses, which suggests these neurons can directly encode dynamic changes in force in response to phasic or tonic contractions. These findings also suggest that the ENS behaves as a global sensorimotor network rather than as separate individual components allowing for processing of sensory, integrative, and motor functions.[11]

Efferent Supply

The axons of the intrinsic motor neurons that supply small intestinal smooth muscle exit the intramural ganglia and enter either the circular or the longitudinal muscle layer, where they pass in close proximity to both the myocytes and ICC. Unlike skeletal muscle, no specific neuromuscular junctions are present in small intestinal smooth muscle, although multiple varicosities along the motor axons probably represent specialized areas of neurotransmission. The motor axons discharge along their length, potentially activating large numbers of myocytes through the ICC but possibly also directly activating them. The lack of exclusive specific neuromuscular junctions, the electrical gap junctions among myocytes, and the overlap of innervation of myocytes from more than 1 motor axon mean that functionally discrete motor units in the intestinal smooth muscle do not appear to exist, which is in contrast with that of skeletal muscle. The ENS motor supply itself is both inhibitory and excitatory, with intrinsic inhibitory and excitatory motor neurons generally containing both a fast and a slow neurotransmitter. The predominant excitatory transmitters are acetylcholine (fast) and substance P (slow), and the predominant inhibitory transmitters are NO (fast), VIP (slow), ATP (fast), and β-nicotinamide adenine dinucleotide (β-NAD) (fast).[12]

Interneurons

Interneurons connect ENS neurons of the same class or of different classes with one another. They permit local communication within limited lengths of intestinal wall (measured in millimeters or centimeters) and are implicated in simple local responses by means of release of acetylcholine or NO, respectively, depending on their oral or aboral direction of projection. Some evidence also suggests the presence of connections within the intestinal wall along greater distances, but these neural pathways are not well defined. These longer connections may be provided anatomically by the ENS or by connections between the ENS and ANS. Interneurons that play an additional sensory role have been identified, and respond directly to mechanical changes in muscle length, rather than muscle tone or tension.[13]

A special type of interneuron, the intestinofugal neuron, may be important for controlling local reflexes. Intestinofugal neurons have cell bodies within the myenteric plexus. These cell bodies receive input from several local enteric neurons and project to the prevertebral ganglia, where they synapse with sympathetic motor neurons (see Fig. 99-3).[8]

It is becoming clear that these various subtypes of ENS neurons have the potential to be modulated by enteric glia, a unique class of peripheral glial cells within the GI tract. Until recently, enteric glia were thought to be "silent" in the intestinal wall. Major populations of enteric glia are found in the myenteric and submucosal plexuses of the ENS and within the lamina propria of the mucosa and the circular muscle. Within ganglia, enteric glia are similar to the astrocytes of the CNS, in that they detect and integrate neural activity. Glia within the ENS can be activated by synaptic stimulation, which suggests they play an active role in synaptic transmission and actively modulate physiologic intestinal processes. This adds further complexity to an already complex regulatory system.[14]

Extrinsic Neurons

Afferent Supply

The small intestine is innervated by both vagal and spinal extrinsic afferents. The pathway of small intestinal vagal afferent innervation is relatively straightforward. The vagal afferent neurons have endings in the intestinal wall and cell bodies within the nodose and jugular ganglia, which deliver input directly to the brainstem. Spinal afferent fibers travel along perivascular nerves to the prevertebral ganglia, where neurons do not end but might give off axon collaterals that synapse on postganglionic sympathetic motor neurons; these fibers then pass into the thoracic spinal cord along the splanchnic nerves. Spinal afferent neurons have their cell bodies throughout the thoracic dorsal root ganglia and enter the spinal cord through the dorsal roots; they synapse mainly on neurons of the superficial laminae of the spinal gray matter.[15] These neurons in turn can send projections to numerous areas of the brain involved in sensation and pain control. Spinal afferent neurons can also give off axon collaterals closer to the intestinal wall that synapse on components of the ENS, blood vessels, smooth muscle, or secretory elements (Fig. 99-4). In general, vagal afferents have lower mechanical activation thresholds and display saturated responses at higher intensities, whereas

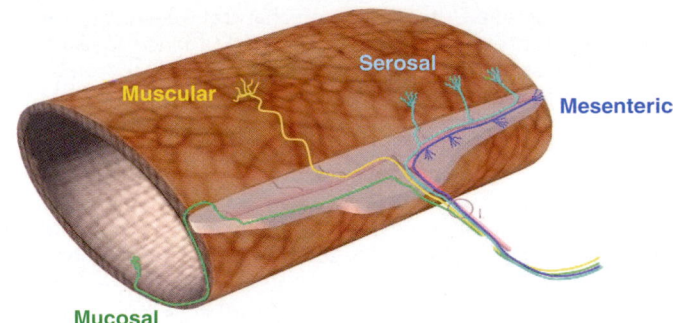

FIGURE 99-4. Schematic representation of various subtypes of extrinsic sensory afferent nerve fibers that innervate the small intestine via vagal and spinal nerve pathways. For further details, see text. *(Courtesy Dr. S.M. Brierley.)*

spinal afferents are activated at higher thresholds. These different stimulus response profiles of vagal and splanchnic mechanoreceptors are generally interpreted as evidence that vagal afferents subserve physiologic regulation such as fullness and satiety, whereas spinal afferents mediate discomfort, bloating, and pain.[15-17] Functionally, 3 distinct and characteristic patterns of terminal distribution can be identified within the intestinal wall. Extraluminal afferent fibers have responsive endings on blood vessels in the outer serosal layer and in the mesenteric connections.[18] Muscular afferents form endings either within the muscle layers or within the myenteric plexus.[15] Mucosal afferents form endings in the lamina propria, where they are positioned to detect substances that are absorbed across the mucosal epithelium or released from epithelial and subepithelial cells, including enterochromaffin and immunocompetent cells.[15] These 3 different populations of afferent endings have different sensory modalities, responding to both mechanical and chemical stimulation.[19,20] Serosal and mesenteric afferents are found mainly in the splanchnic innervation and are activated by distortion of the intestine and its attachments; they do not normally signal distention or contraction of the bowel wall unless it is strong enough to cause distortion of the outer layers.[15,21] Serosal and mesenteric receptors also commonly show evidence of chemosensitivity and express many algesic channels and receptors.[16,22] This observation hints at potential responsiveness to circulating or locally released factors like cytokines, proteases, histamine, and bradykinin, especially in view of the localization of these receptors on or near blood vessels.[15,16,22] Muscular afferents respond to distention and contraction with lower thresholds for activation, and they reach maximal responses within levels of distention that are encountered normally during digestion. Muscular afferents show maintained responses to distention of the small intestine and signal each contractile event, giving rise to the term *in-series tension receptors*.[23] Nerve tracing studies have identified vagal afferent terminals in the longitudinal and circular muscle layers that are described as intramuscular arrays (IMAs) and consist of several long (up to a few millimeters) and rather straight axons running parallel to the respective muscle layer and connected by oblique or right-angled short connecting branches.[24,25] IMAs were proposed to be the in-series tension receptor endings, possibly responding to both passive stretch and active contraction of the muscle, although direct evidence for this proposal is currently lacking.

Vagal afferent terminals that surround the myenteric plexus throughout the GI tract have been described as intraganglionic laminar endings (IGLEs). These endings are in intimate contact with the connective tissue capsule and enteric glial cells that surround the myenteric ganglia, and they have been hypothesized to detect mechanical shearing forces between the orthogonal muscle layers. Evidence for such a mechanosensory function of IGLEs has been elaborated by mapping the receptive field of vagal afferent endings in the esophagus, stomach, and large intestine, and showing morphologically that individual hot spots of mechanosensitivity correspond with single IGLEs.[26] Functional evidence exists for muscular afferents in both the vagal and the spinal innervation, but the anatomic appearance of spinal distention-sensitive afferents in the small intestine remains to be determined. Its structure and the receptors and channels it expresses, however, are likely to be distinct from those of vagal afferents, owing to spinal muscular afferents displaying higher activation thresholds to distention.[27]

Small intestinal mucosal afferents have been found in the vagal supply, but their existence in the spinal supply can be inferred only from the fact that they exist in the colon.[15,28] Mucosal afferents do not respond to distention or contraction but are exquisitely sensitive to mechanical deformation of the mucosa, as might occur with particulate material within the lumen.[17,29] In the rat duodenum and jejunum, vagal afferent fibers penetrate the circular muscle layer and submucosa to form networks of multiply branching axons within the lamina propria of both crypts and villi.[24] Terminal axons are in close contact with, but do not seem to penetrate, the basal lamina and thus are in an ideal position to detect substances including absorbed nutrients and mediators that are released from epithelial cells and other structures within the lamina propria.

Efferent Supply

The extrinsic efferent pathways to the small intestine are supplied by the parasympathetic and sympathetic divisions of the ANS. The small intestinal parasympathetic supply is cranial and cholinergic, whereas the sympathetic supply is spinal (thoracic) and adrenergic. These 2 motor pathways are not entirely separate, however, because postganglionic sympathetic fibers arising from cervical ganglia are sometimes found within the vagus nerve.

The parasympathetic motor neurons of the small intestine have cell bodies within the dorsal motor nuclei of the vagi in the medulla oblongata. Their axons extend through the vagi to the intestinal intramural plexuses, where they synapse with motor neurons of the ENS. The sympathetic motor supply is more complex. Primary motor neurons within the intermediolateral horn of the thoracic spinal cord synapse with second-order neurons in the prevertebral ganglia, which then synapse with ENS motor neurons within the intestinal intramural plexuses, directly with smooth muscle, or possibly with ICC.

Both excitatory and inhibitory extrinsic motor outputs to the small intestine have been identified. Excitatory outputs depolarize, whereas inhibitory outputs hyperpolarize the smooth muscle, thereby respectively facilitating and impeding the development of contractions. In general, the sympathetic motor supply is inhibitory to the ENS, and this ENS inhibition leads to decreased smooth muscle activity, with the opposite effect seen in sphincter regions. Direct sympathetic inhibitory and excitatory outputs to smooth muscle also exist. The parasympathetic motor output to the ENS is more diffuse, each primary motor neuron supplying a large area. Excitatory parasympathetic motor output occurs to either inhibitory or excitatory ENS motor neurons, through which parasympathetic efferents can selectively inhibit or excite smooth muscle.

Central Connections of Neural Control Elements

Centrally, the sensory and motor supplies to the small intestine are closely interrelated; the vagal sensory input and the parasympathetic motor output are closely located, as are the spinal sensory input and the sympathetic motor output. Both the vagal parasympathetic and the spinal sympathetic supplies have widespread connections to many other areas throughout the CNS that are implicated in feeding, arousal, mood, and other reflex behavior. The proximity of the CNS areas involved in small intestinal regulation, and their interconnections, makes it likely that the vagal parasympathetic and the spinal sympathetic control mechanisms are interconnected and might function less independently than has been previously thought.

The parasympathetic primary motor neurons are located bilaterally in the dorsal motor nuclei of the vagus in the medulla, which lie close to and receive substantial input from neurons of the nuclei tracti solitarii (NTS). The NTS is the site of terminals of vagal afferent fibers that enter through the tracti solitarii and have cell bodies in the nodose ganglia. Each NTS also has extensive connections to other CNS regions, and several of these regions have input to the dorsal motor nuclei of the vagus, thereby influencing vagal motor output to the intestine.[15]

The central connections of the spinal and sympathetic supply to the intestine are less well described. The spinal sensory neurons enter the spinal cord, where they synapse ipsilaterally on second-order sensory neurons and also provide direct feedback to sympathetic preganglionic motor neurons through axon collaterals. The second-order sensory neurons then ascend the spinal cord either contralaterally or ipsilaterally, after which they terminate in numerous areas,[30] including the raphe nuclei and periaqueductal gray matter in the brainstem and the thalamus. The thalamus has extensive ramifications throughout the CNS. The central influence on sympathetic motor output to the small intestine is complex and not well understood, but stress and arousal level play a role. These influences have their output through the brainstem and descending tracts to the sympathetic preganglionic motor neurons in the intermediolateral horn of the spinal cord, which send their axons to the prevertebral ganglia, whereupon they synapse with sympathetic postganglionic adrenergic nerves.[31]

Gastrointestinal Hormones

GI hormones are discussed in detail in Chapter 4, but it is important to emphasize here their vital role in modulating small intestinal motor and sensory function. GI hormones relevant to small intestinal function can act in either a humoral or paracrine fashion on both enteric neurons and myocytes, and generally they are released in response to the presence (or anticipation) of enteral nutrition. The best known of these hormones include CCK, somatostatin, VIP, glucagon-like peptide-1 (GLP-1), gastric inhibitory peptide (GIP), ghrelin, and motilin.[32] Most of the hormones released in response to the presence of food in the lumen lead to slowing of small intestinal transit, signals of satiety, and increased mixing or segmenting contractions (see later).

INTEGRATED CONTROL OF MOTILITY

When we consider how the structure and function of individual components of the neuromuscular apparatus of the small intestine operate together to produce known motility patterns, several gaps in our knowledge are revealed because the evidence for contribution of specific mechanisms is often circumstantial. Two important examples of motility patterns—peristalsis and the interdigestive motor cycle (IDMC)—illustrate the involvement of integrated hierarchical levels of control and our current level of understanding of the control systems.

Peristalsis

Peristalsis is the fundamental integrated motility pattern of the small intestine and can be coordinated entirely within the ENS and circular and longitudinal muscular layers. It may be initiated in response to a number of mechanical and chemical stimuli in the lumen and consists of progression of contractile activity usually, but not always, in an aboral direction. Therefore, both sensory and motor aspects to peristalsis are recognized.

The populations of IPANs described earlier probably are responsible for detection of luminal stimuli, either directly or following release of mediators from mucosal enteroendocrine cells. Their activation results in transmitter release onto neighboring interneurons and motor neurons, the activity of which is coordinated subsequently as a network to provide synchronous activation of circular and longitudinal muscles on 1 side of the bolus (usually the oral side) and synchronous inhibition of muscle on the other side (usually the aboral side). This networked activity normally travels aborally, but the mechanism of propagation is not yet understood. It might result from patterns of activity in interneurons that can project over distances of several millimeters and thus mediate a general descending excitation. The mechanism by which peristalsis is reversed—for example, in conditions of luminal toxicity, to generate emesis—is not known, but the fact that reverse peristalsis does occur in the small intestine illustrates that the pattern is not a totally polarized phenomenon.

Debate is ongoing about the precise interactions of transmitters and mediators in the normal function of peristalsis, but peristalsis is known to be affected by exogenous activation of several pre- and postsynaptic mechanisms, some of which also may be active endogenously. Of particular interest are serotoninergic mechanisms, which have been shown to have involvement in initiation of peristalsis and modulation of transmission between subclasses of enteric neurons.[33]

Interdigestive Motor Cycle

The IDMC serves to demonstrate the extraordinary integrative capacity of the ENS; other aspects of the IDMC are described later in this chapter. The IDMC is a complex series of periods of variable contractile activity with distinct phases that show different contractile amplitudes, propagation, and regularity. The pattern as a whole sweeps slowly down the small intestine in the fasting state and recurs at regular intervals. Although a number of candidate hormones are proposed to be involved in its initiation and recurrence, the switch between quiescent and active phases and their orderly migration along the bowel are functions of the ENS; this ENS autonomy is demonstrated by occurrence of the IDMC in extrinsically denervated or autotransplanted intestine. The ENS therefore is capable of controlling large segments of the small intestine independent of extrinsic input, probably by virtue of its extensive interneuronal connections and constant sensory feedback.

Although the ENS has this regulatory capacity, normal function is modulated by ANS efferent output, which in turn may be influenced by locally or centrally processed information gathered from primary spinal or vagal afferents. In particular, synapses outside the CNS in the prevertebral ganglia are capable of subserving inhibitory intestino-intestinal reflexes that are potentially important in the minute-to-minute regulatory control of motility.[31] Small intestinal neuromuscular function is also influenced by a number of hormones acting in either an endocrine or paracrine fashion.

Little direct information is available on the precise contribution of each extrinsic pathway to motor function of the small intestine in humans. Vagal reflexes generally are thought to make an important contribution in the integration of major homeostatic functions like motility, secretion, blood flow, and control of food and water intake.[17,30] The role of sympathetic reflexes is thought to be concerned primarily with inhibition of motility and other functions in response to noxious stimuli, rather than in digestive small intestinal functions.

ABNORMAL MOTOR AND SENSORY FUNCTION

Much of the evidence for the mechanisms involved in dysfunction of the small intestine is derived from animal models in which mucosal inflammation or infection has been induced, after which alterations in physiology, pharmacology, and anatomy of motor and sensory elements are assessed. These models provide some clues to the underlying mechanisms involved in motor abnormalities that are seen clinically; because many clinical manifestations are of unknown etiology, however, this approach is limited in the extent to which basic findings can be directly translated.

Infection and inflammation of the intestine can result in long-term changes in all elements, including myocytes, ICC, and in intrinsic and extrinsic neurons. Symptoms in functional GI diseases such as functional dyspepsia and IBS may be partly due to specific sensorimotor abnormalities occurring locally in the intestine, but they also are attributable to alterations in the extrinsic neural control system of the intestine and possibly to alterations in central perception, processing of afferent information, or both (see Chapters 14 and 122). Abnormalities in pain control systems in the brain and disordered processing of affective components of visceral sensations also have been described in these conditions[34] and can produce symptoms through the central connections described in the preceding sections. Some clinical scenarios in which discrete abnormalities have been identified or hypothesized in small intestinal motility are outlined in Table 99-1.

Smooth Muscle Dysfunction

It is often difficult to separate pathologic changes in the function of smooth muscle from those in neural control mechanisms, but a number of changes can be attributed directly to alterations in smooth muscle. Cytokines play an important role in the abnormal smooth muscle function associated with GI inflammation and infection. Different insults induce different cytokine patterns, which in turn determine the type of infiltrating immune or inflammatory cells, which in turn release specific mediators. Thus, the resultant effect on smooth muscle function depends on the origin of disease. For example, nematode infection induces mastocytosis and eosinophilia, which lead to activation of intracellular signaling pathways in smooth muscle by interleukin (IL)-4 and IL-13, ultimately resulting in hypercontractility of smooth muscle.[35] By contrast, chemically induced inflammation is characterized by the presence of neutrophils and macrophages among other cells. Inflammation and infection can lead to changes at sites in the small intestine distant from the affected site, and the functional effects of inflammation in smooth muscle can persist following recovery from the acute insult as is seen with postinfection IBS. Smooth muscle hyperresponsiveness may be characterized by enhanced responses to cholinergic and non-cholinergic excitation and are observable in human IBD.[36]

Intrinsic Neural Dysfunction

Several abnormalities of small intestinal intrinsic control are due to developmental dysfunction and are dealt with

TABLE 99-1 Disorders Associated with Abnormal Small Intestinal Motility

Disorder	Smooth Muscle Abnormalities	Neural Abnormalities	Sensory Abnormalities	Potential Outcomes
IBS	NaV1.5 mutation causes loss of function and increased reporting of pain	Postinfection and inflammatory changes (subset of patients)	Altered afferent function Increased visceral sensitivity	Heightened sensation Disordered motility
Acute severe illness	Decreased strength of contractions	Altered neurotransmission (? related to metabolic or electrolyte disturbances)	Heightened sensitivity to neurohumoral feedback loops	Delayed transit Ileus Decreased intestinal absorption
Pregnancy	Decreased strength of contractions	None identified	None identified	Slowed transit
Diabetes mellitus	Altered ICC function	Altered neurotransmission	Enhanced perception of GI stimuli	Abnormal patterning of contractions Slow or rapid transit
Metabolic disturbances*	Possible decreased strength of contractions	Altered neurotransmission	Nausea Altered sensory perception	Abnormal patterning of contractions Slow or rapid transit
Drugs†	Possible decreased strength of contractions	Altered neurotransmission	None identified	Ileus Slow or rapid transit Disordered contractions
Intestinal obstruction	Hypertrophy, if chronic	None identified	None identified	High-amplitude forceful contractions
Pseudo-obstruction syndromes	Myopathy of hollow viscera	Multiple neural abnormalities: neuron loss, plexus abnormalities, altered distribution of neurotransmitters	None identified	Feeble contractions Absent phase III of the IDMC Slow or failed transit
Scleroderma and other connective tissue disorders	Ischemia and fibrosis	Nerve loss in intestinal wall Extrinsic neural supply may also be damaged by vasculitis	None identified	Feeble contractions Thickening of bowel wall Slow transit
Neurologic syndromes‡	N/A	Neural absence or loss	Loss of afferent neurons with consequent loss of sensory information for reflux control	Disorganized IDMC Failure to convert to fed pattern Transit failure
Rare myopathies	Myocyte and mitochondrial abnormalities; inadequate contractile force	N/A	NaV1.7 mutation leading to rectal pain	Insufficient force for transit and mixing
Radiation enteritis	Fibrosis (? related to ischemia)	Increased muscarinic 3 receptors	None identified	Less mixing, disordered transit Stasis, bacterial overgrowth, diarrhea
Acromegaly	None identified	Postulated autonomic nerve dysfunction	None identified	Delayed orocecal transit time SIBO

*Examples include disturbances of potassium, calcium, and magnesium homeostasis, and renal and hepatic failure.
†Examples include antidepressants, calcium channel blockers, and beta blockers.
‡Examples include dysautonomia and Parkinson's disease.
ICC, interstitial cells of Cajal; IDMC, interdigestive motor cycle; N/A, not applicable.

separately in Chapter 98. Changes in the ENS also can occur after a bout of intestinal infection or inflammation. Many of these changes are centered on the IPANs. These neurons become more excitable because of changes in the expression of ion channels that initiate generation of action potentials and those that determine recovery of membrane potential after an action potential. Thus, the long after-hyperpolarization that distinguishes IPANs from other classes is shortened, and they are able to fire in longer trains. This ability directly affects the responses of other interneurons and motor neurons that receive inputs from these afferent neurons and that therefore are involved in intrinsic (ENS) reflexes. Changes in excitability may be observed during an acute phase of infection or inflammation[36,37] or for several weeks afterward,[38] at least in the large intestine. In some cases the hyperexcitability can be suppressed with acute exposure to blockers of histamine, adenylate cyclase, COX, or leukotriene pathways.[39] Acute inflammation also dramatically decreases the number of viscerofugal neurons, at least in animal models.[40] This loss is apparent 24 hours after the start of the inflammatory response, persists over several months, and only occurs in the area of inflammation.[40]

These longer-term changes are referred to as *plasticity* and might partly explain the occurrence of exaggerated motor responses to a given stimulus in the acute phase and after recovery of mucosal lesions. Changes can result from alterations in gene expression in enteric neurons that persist beyond the initial insult, from persisting increases in locally released mediators following alterations in mucosal cell types, or from both types of responses.[41]

In animal models of insulin-dependent diabetes mellitus, altered levels of neuropeptides may be seen, which might explain the disordered motility noted clinically in diabetes mellitus. The only reported neuroanatomic human study in a patient with type 1 diabetes mellitus showed that ICC were markedly decreased throughout the entire thickness of the jejunum. A decrease in neuronal NO synthase, VIP, pituitary adenylcyclase-activating peptide (PACAP), and tyrosine hydroxylase-immunopositive nerve fibers was observed in the circular muscle layer, and substance P immunoreactivity was increased.[42] Although patients with type 1 diabetes mellitus and sympathetic denervation have abnormally slow gastric emptying (see Chapter 49), their transit of a liquid meal through the distal small intestine is more rapid, which might play a part in causing diarrhea. Diabetic patients also show abnormal duodenal motility patterns, such as early recurrence of phase III after a meal (see later). No consistent correlation, however, has been found between changes in manometric parameters and the degree of cardiac autonomic neuropathy, nor has any correlation yet been established between changes in enteric neurotransmitters and manometric or transit observations. Recent studies, however, suggest that altered expression of Ano1, which is thought to underlie Ca^{2+}-activated Cl^- currents, reduces ICC function and directly contributes to diabetic gastroparesis in humans.[43] Other studies suggest that degeneration of the ICC itself may be associated with the pathogenesis of diabetic gastropathy in human diabetic patients, because ultrastructural changes (e.g., pre-apoptosis of the ICC) are accompanied by electrical dysrhythmia of slow waves in intestinal muscle.[44]

Extrinsic Afferent Dysfunction

Mechanisms that lead to extrinsic afferent dysfunction after infection or inflammation are similar to those involved in IPANs and smooth muscle dysfunction. It is well established that a wide range of chemical mediators can influence mechanosensitivity of extrinsic primary afferents, in addition to

evoking direct responses as detailed earlier.[16,45] These chemical mediators can be released in conditions of inflammation, injury, or ischemia from a variety of cell types, including platelets, neutrophils, lymphocytes, macrophages, mast cells, glial cells, fibroblasts, blood vessels, muscles, and neurons.[16,45] Each of these specific cells can release several modulating agents, some of which act directly on the sensory nerve terminal; others act indirectly, causing release of other agents from other cells in a series of cascades. The end result of these actions is that the response properties of extrinsic afferents, like their intrinsic counterparts, are subject to plasticity, usually resulting in an increased sensitivity of the afferent endings; this process is described as *peripheral sensitization*. Evidence supports involvement of algesic mediators, including prostaglandins, purines, cytokines, proteases, and histamine, in the changes leading to peripheral sensitization,[16,45,46] with effector channels such as the Transient Receptor Potential (TRP) family of ion channels contributing to the hypersensitive responses.[16,22,47] Other endogenous chemical mediators, including somatostatin,[27] can down-regulate small intestinal afferent sensitivity such that an imbalance in pro-sensitizing and anti-sensitizing mechanisms leads to a disordered sensory signal. A specific example of this balance between pro- and anti-sensitizing mechanisms is evident in the regulation of nociceptive afferents by products released from immune cells. Whereas TNF-α causes sensitization via TRPA1 channels, beta-endorphin causes inhibition via μ-opioid receptors, although the latter is manifested only in effects of healthy immune cell products, whereas the former is manifested only in the effects of immune cell products from diarrhea-predominant IBS patients.[22]

In animal models, it is clear that a bout of intestinal infection or inflammation causes afferent hypersensitivity, neuronal hyperexcitability, and correspondingly, hyperalgesia and allodynia.[16,45] It is also apparent that this hyperexcitability, hyperalgesia, and allodynia can persist for a period of weeks or months following healing of the initial injury.[15,21,45] For example, following *Trichinella spiralis* infection, both low- and high-threshold jejunal afferents display pronounced mechanical hypersensitivity 1 and 2 months following infection.[48] Development of this long-term mechanical hypersensitivity is dependent upon a $P2X_7$ receptor-dependent increase in immune cell IL-1β expression and release. Notably, deletion of $P2X_7R$ results in a clear attenuation of the innate inflammatory response and no postinfection mechanical hypersensitivity at any time point.[23] Taken together, these mechanisms are likely to be clinically relevant in patients with postinfection IBS and in those with ongoing GI symptoms with IBD despite mucosal healing in whom increased perception of mechanical and chemical stimulation is apparent. Moreover, because these afferents also serve to trigger reflex mechanisms that control and coordinate intestinal motor function, their sensitization can contribute to chronic dysmotility, resulting in a cycle of disordered sensory and motor function.

MEASUREMENT OF SMALL INTESTINAL MOTILITY

Basic Principles

Spatiotemporal Measurements

The outcomes of small intestinal motor activity depend on the patterning of small intestinal contractions in both space and time. Therefore, the question remains: Where and when do the contractions occur with respect to each other? Measurement methods must therefore gather functionally relevant information on the temporospatial organization of small intestinal motility. This presents substantial challenges, especially in humans, because of the length of the small intestine, the spatiotemporal complexity of motor events, and the long time frame (several hours) over which small intestinal motility determines the successful absorption and movement of each meal.

In health, the occurrence and patterning of a large number of individual motor events determine the outcomes of absorption and transit, so that whole-animal measures of small intestinal transit and absorption yield a gross, or summary, report. More detailed descriptions of small intestinal motility report great variability in the patterning of individual contractile events, depending in part on the technique used, the time frame over which motility is observed, and the temporospatial resolution of the measurement technique itself.

To understand the relationship between individual motor events and transport in the small intestine, the temporal resolution of the measurement technique must be greater than the duration of each discrete motor event. Based on similar principles, the spatial resolution of measurements is also an important parameter to consider if relationships between motor events and intraluminal flow(s) are to be defined. The importance of spatiotemporal resolution can be appreciated by considering Figure 99-5. Direct evaluation of small intestinal motility requires methods of measurement with a time resolution of at least 2 seconds so that contractions can be recognized as separate from one another, rather than as continuous or as an increase in basal pressure. In humans, the intrinsic frequency of duodenal contractions is up to 12 per minute (i.e., each must be completed [having started from a basal pressure and then resolved] within 5 sec); measurements must be performed at about half this time interval to be able to be sure of what is phasic as opposed to tonic (each contraction usually lasts 1 to 3 sec). The optimal spatial resolution for studies of small intestinal motor function has not been determined, but the spatial patterning of pressures is known to vary over relatively small distances,[49] with most propagating pressure wave sequences travelling less than 6 cm. Because of practical limitations of data handling and the number of sensors one can place in the small intestine, measurement techniques usually either achieve high temporospatial resolution over a short distance or low temporospatial resolution over a far greater distance. Realistically this means that data gained from different studies are usually interpreted alongside one another to provide more complete information.

Evaluation of Single Cell Functions

At the cellular level, a number of techniques can be used to yield insights into small intestinal motor physiology. Intracellular recordings of electrical potential can be obtained from a number of cell types within the small intestine and its extrinsic neural control system. These recordings give detailed information about the signals received and transmitted by individual cells, with excellent temporal resolution, but generally they cannot be applied concurrently over a significant length of intestine and therefore have limited real-time spatial resolution with regard to motor events.

A combined functional and neuroanatomic approach whereby imaging of specific neurons with intracellular or extracellular recordings and chemical coding using immunohistochemistry are performed concurrently has allowed important correlations to be made between structure and function. In particular, this approach has led to understanding of the function of IGLEs and IMAs (see "Extrinsic Afferent Supply" earlier).

Although electrophysiologic and anatomic methods provide information on structure, neurotransmitters used, and

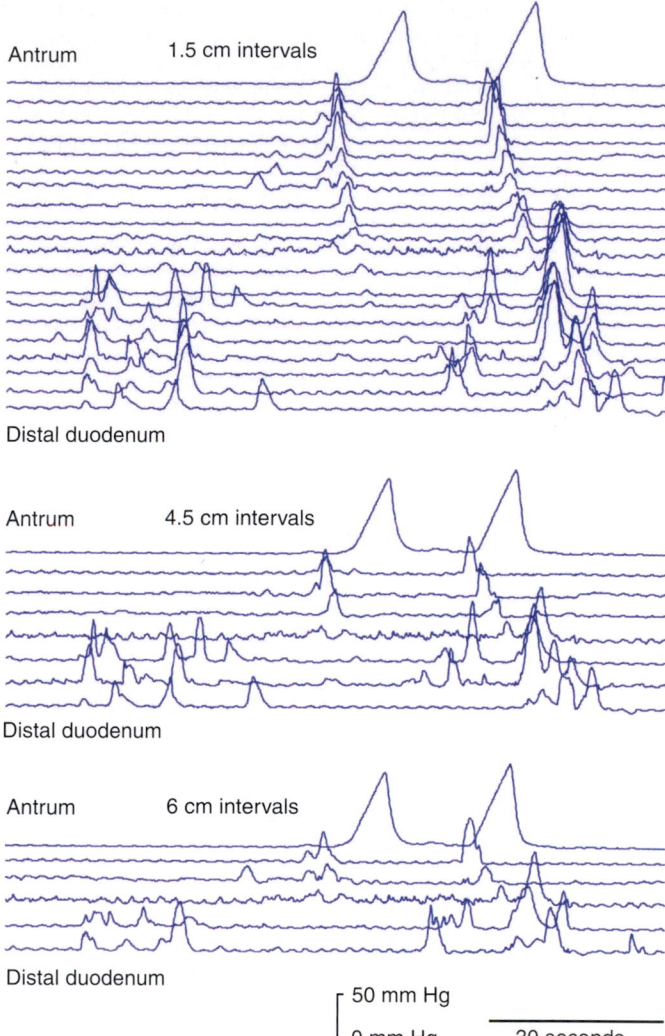

FIGURE 99-5. Multichannel manometric recordings of the human antrum and duodenum, with recording points placed at varied intervals: 1.5 cm *(top panel)*, 4.5 cm *(middle panel)*, and 6 cm *(bottom panel)*. These data demonstrate some of the limitations of varying the interval between recording points: As a phasic contraction travels along a section of intestine, the associated rise in pressure is detected only at each measurement point. If the interval between recording points is too wide, unrelated pressures may be judged to be related to the propagated pressure wave, or a propagated pressure wave sequence may be judged to be a limited phasic event. Spatial detail is lost as recording interval is widened. *(Courtesy of Dr. J.M. Andrews.)*

proximity to other elements, they cannot describe precisely how these relate to the actual resulting motility and its temporospatial organization. Although such single-cell techniques generally have been applied to animal tissues, the results also probably apply to humans, because a similar structural organization of control elements is seen in human tissue.

Recording of Muscle Contractions

Increased muscle tension generally is directly recorded with strain gauges; these can be used in muscle strips, isolated loops of intestine, and whole-organ preparations or even chronically implanted in animals. Strain gauges are capable of excellent temporal resolution of motor events, but spatial resolution is limited by the size and number of strain gauges that are used concurrently. Over short lengths of intestine, a spatial resolution of approximately 1 cm is possible. Unfortunately, strain gauges are not suitable for use in human subjects, although they have provided much valuable information on the organization of motor events in animals.[50]

Muscle contractions also can be measured by surrogate measurement techniques that record associated phenomena. One such approach is fluorescence measurement of calcium transients (rapid increases in free intracellular calcium) in smooth muscle.[51] Over short sections of intestine (1 to 2 mm), such measurements provide excellent temporospatial resolution and are helpful in elucidating neurophysiologic control rather than describing whole-organ function. Other measurement techniques that record phenomena resulting from contractions of smooth muscle include luminal manometry (reflecting intraluminal pressure increases), fluoroscopy (showing wall movement and movement of intraluminal contrast), and transit studies performed by a number of approaches.

Luminal manometry measures the change in intraluminal pressure that results mainly from lumen-occlusive or near lumen-occlusive contractions. Fortunately, because the small intestine is tubular with a relatively small diameter, a large portion of motor events are recognized as pressure rises. Researchers have hypothesized that contractions not resulting in a detectable change in intraluminal pressure are less important in determining flow, and therefore little mechanical information is lost by failure to detect them, but small changes in intraluminal pressure can be pivotal in producing flows in some regions of the small intestine.[52] Manometry can be applied in several settings, ranging from short isolated intestinal segments in the laboratory to clinical use in humans. Modern computer-based recording systems allow excellent temporal resolution ($\approx$10 Hz), and spatial resolution can be tailored to give either close spatial resolution (intervals of 1 to 2 cm) over 20 to 40 cm, or wider resolution, while still covering a longer segment of small intestine. Traditional manometric assemblies were either of the perfused side-hole or the solid-state sensor design and were capable of routinely recording at up to 22 sites. New fiberoptic high-resolution manometry assemblies allow recording of up to 72 sensor sites and are long enough to allow record pressure from the entire human colon.[53] This high-resolution manometry has allowed the amount of retrograde propagating activity to be determined, analysis that is lost with the traditional low-resolution recordings. A new, although highly invasive, electrode platform has recently been developed and validated based on flexible printed circuit board (PCB) technology. This technology allows high-resolution electrical mapping of human evaluate slow wave behavior in the GI tract.[53]

Wall Motion and Transit Studies

Contrast fluoroscopy is the most widely available wall motion study. It yields detailed information on the time and space patterning of motor events in vivo and useful insights into associated movements of luminal contents. When this technique is used in combination with other techniques (e.g., manometry, intraluminal impedance, strain gauges), useful correlations can be made between contractions or luminal pressures and transit of contents. These insights are likely to lead to improved understanding of pressure patterns, which in turn might enable us to better interpret less-intrusive techniques such as manometry and impedance in humans. Improving the interpretation of these other techniques is important because risks associated with radiation exposure

restrict the use of prolonged or recurrent fluoroscopy in humans.

Other in vivo imaging methods for assessing small intestinal wall motion and movement of intraluminal contents include MRI, US, and intraluminal impedance recording. These approaches are suitable for human use with good temporal resolution, although they have significant practical limitations. These limitations previously restricted their applications outside of research centers as an alternative to contrast fluoroscopy, but they are now gaining more widespread use.

MRI allows prolonged observation but, because of the anatomic complexity of the small intestine, difficulties with spatial resolution can limit views. Additionally, MRI is expensive, and not all centers have sufficient MRI capacity for it to become a routine clinical tool for this indication.

US also allows prolonged observation and repeat measurements, but only of short segments and with relatively poor spatial resolution. US is limited in many instances by patient factors, such as body habitus and intestinal gas, and it is operator dependent.

Multichannel intraluminal impedance (MII) is a technique for assessing intraluminal bolus transit rather than motility. The technique is based on the different conductivities of intraluminal air and liquids compared with those of opposed sections of bowel wall. Voltage is applied to a recording assembly along which several electrodes are sited. The current recorded between electrode pairs depends on the conductivity and thickness of any air or fluid bolus straddling the electrode pair. In this fashion, MII sequentially measures the transit of a conducting bolus between electrode pairs. Recordings in the small intestine can, therefore, depend on the state of its filling,[54] and motility in an empty bowel might not be assessed accurately.

Other transit and absorption measurements demonstrate whether mass transit occurs but give no information on the mechanical pattern by which the transport of contents is achieved. Methodology for transit studies includes breath tests and scintigraphy.

Breath tests are based on the exhalation of gases such as H_2 or CO_2 (labeled with ^{13}C or ^{14}C, which are liberated when a labeled test meal reaches the colon and undergoes bacterial degradation. Scintigraphic tests of small intestinal transit visually assess the arrival of a labeled meal at the cecum. These 2 transit techniques yield the lowest temporospatial resolution in assessing small intestinal motility but are clinically useful and are discussed later in this chapter.

In vitro techniques for detailed assessment of small intestinal wall movements reveal subtle motility patterns that cannot be detected with manometry or in vivo wall motion studies. For example, 1 technique using digitized video recording can measure changes in diameter and length of an immobilized segment of intestine[55] and has the unique capacity to appreciate discrete changes in the longitudinal and circular muscle layers.

Clinical Approach

The broader issues of measurement of small intestinal motor function were considered earlier, and the discussion that follows is limited to the clinically relevant techniques used to assess small intestinal motor function.

Small Intestinal Transit Studies

Small intestinal transit time can be measured with breath tests or scintigraphic observation of the movement of intraluminal contents. Unless the test substance is delivered beyond the pylorus by tube, these techniques also include gastric emptying (and thus gastric function) in their measurements; they are, therefore, imprecise about actual small intestinal transit time and are more accurately termed *tests of orocecal transit time*. Because each technique measures a different aspect of motility, results obtained from different techniques are not directly comparable.

The lactulose breath test is perhaps the best known and most widely used of these techniques. Lactulose is a nonabsorbable disaccharide that is fermented on reaching the bacteria-laden environment of the colon. The H_2 gas that is formed is rapidly absorbed and exhaled from the lungs. Samples of exhaled gases are taken at baseline and at regular intervals after the ingestion of lactulose. The orocecal transit time is taken as the time at which a sustained rise in exhaled H_2 is seen. An early rise, or a high baseline level, may be evidence of SIBO (Chapter 105), but this measure is relatively insensitive for SIBO. The administration of lactulose itself is known to hasten small intestinal transit and so the result is not directly comparable with other transit time measures.

Similar principles are used in ^{13}C or ^{14}C breath tests, which measure gastric emptying combined with the evaluation of small intestinal absorption of specific nutrients. Acetate, octanoic acid, and triolein have been used for this purpose. Acetate appears to be a good liquid marker, octanoic acid is better suited for solids, and triolein is useful in suspected cases of malabsorption. This nutrient-focused assessment of small intestinal function can be combined with the H_2 lactulose breath test to measure orocecal transit time as well.

The more familiar visual and anatomic scintigraphic measurement of small intestinal transit is also widely available. The major difficulty with these studies is the lack of a reliable anatomic landmark for the cecum. Either the cecum is defined arbitrarily as the right iliac fossa and a skin marker is used, or it is considered retrospectively as the area in which radioisotope accumulates. Two approaches are used to report the scintigraphic orocecal transit time: in the simpler approach, the time of first appearance of isotope in the cecum is given; in the other, the initial activity of the radiolabeled meal is quantified in the stomach, and the orocecal transit time is reported as the time taken for 50% of this initial gastric activity to reach the cecum. Values obtained vary depending on which of these methods is used, and each laboratory should set its own normal range.

Fluoroscopy

Contrast fluoroscopy is useful for detecting mural disease and fixed narrowings of the intestinal lumen that can induce secondary changes in motility, transit, and absorption. Fluoroscopy is insensitive for detecting abnormal nutrient absorption and measuring transit time. Clinical fluoroscopy is limited by the necessarily short observation times because of concern with radiation exposure; therefore, only gross disturbances of motor activity may be detected. Once a substantial amount of contrast has entered the small intestine, the usefulness of fluoroscopy is reduced further because overlying loops of bowel hinder interpretation of the movement of contrast.

Manometry

Manometry of the small intestine gives direct measurement of the forces that are applied to luminal contents as a result of motor function. Manometry can be performed over hours or even days and over long or short segments; it is capable of excellent spatial resolution, although it has major practical limitations. Manometric assemblies can be placed in any part of the human small intestine and are moderately well tolerated, although placement of such an assembly along the small intestine can be demanding even in healthy persons, and it is especially challenging in patients who have major abnormalities of motor function.

Manometry allows recognition of some abnormal patterns of pressure over time at individual recording points, but no studies have yet performed a critical evaluation of the best spacing of pressure recording points and of diagnostic criteria for abnormal pressure patterns to distinguish between health and disease. This lack of specific criteria reflects the limited understanding of the relationship between small intestinal intraluminal time-space pressure patterning and the achievement of mixing and propulsion within the small intestine.

Because of practical limitations, one must choose between high spatial resolution over a short segment and lower spatial resolution over a longer segment of intestine. Both approaches are likely to be necessary in achieving an accurate understanding of small intestinal motor physiology, perhaps in conjunction with a technique to assess wall motion or intraluminal flow.

Multiple Intraluminal Impedance

Recording assemblies can be used to measure impedance in humans in much the same fashion as manometry. Multiple intraluminal impedance (MII) can measure episodes of bolus transit in any tubular section of the upper intestine. MII gives good spatiotemporal resolution, but owing to technical limitations of how far apart the sensors can be spaced, it cannot give continuous cover age in measuring transit over long lengths of the intestine. MII is increasingly used for the clinical evaluation of esophageal motility, and in recent times it has been applied to the proximal small intestine with success.[54] In combination with manometry, MII has the potential to show real-time pressure-flow relationships.

Magnetic Resonance Imaging

MRI is capable of excellent spatiotemporal resolution of small intestinal wall motion and movement of intraluminal contents. Because the small intestine is not all within 1 plane, however, it cannot at present be viewed routinely all at once. MRI does not involve a radiation dose and thus is not time limited on this basis. Because it is also an anatomic imaging technique, it has a substantial advantage over other techniques of being able to offer additional information in the assessment of patients with suspected small intestinal motility problems. Wall thickening, fibrosis, inflammatory changes, and stenoses all can be revealed, and this information can help with directing diagnosis and even therapy.[56]

MRI has several disadvantages: it is expensive; some claustrophobic subjects find it too confining; patients who have older pacemakers or other metallic prostheses cannot be assessed with MRI. At present, use of MRI to assess small intestinal motility is restricted to units with a research interest in functional GI MRI.[57] Its use is increasing in clinical gastroenterology, however, especially for small intestinal Crohn's disease,[56] and it also has the potential to encompass clinical motility assessments.[58]

NORMAL IN VIVO SMALL INTESTINAL MOTILITY PATTERNS

Contractions at a Fixed Point

Increased smooth muscle tension that arises from muscular contractions can result in increased intraluminal pressure,

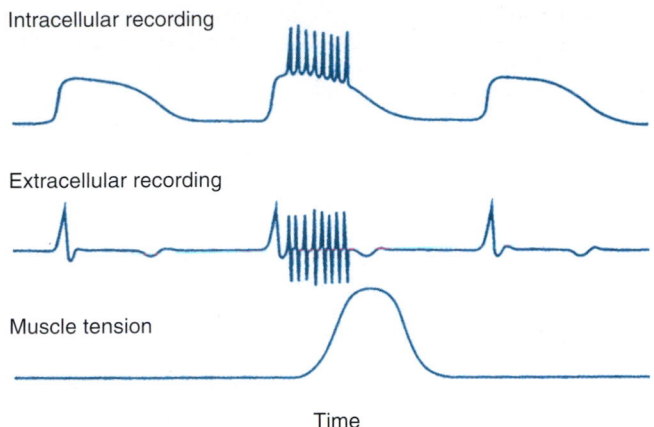

Intracellular recording

Extracellular recording

Muscle tension

Time

FIGURE 99-6. Schematic representation of the relationship among slow waves, spike bursts, and muscle contraction. *Top tracing* is from an intracellular electrode in the muscle; *middle tracing* is from an extracellular electrode; and *bottom tracing* shows muscle tension. The cyclical fluctuation in membrane potential in the top tracing is the slow wave. When spike bursts are superimposed on the peak of the slow wave, the muscle depolarizes, and contraction occurs. *(From Christensen J. Gastrointestinal motility. In: West JB, editor. Best and Taylor's physiologic basis for medical practice. Baltimore: Williams & Wilkins; 1990. p 614.)*

decreased intraluminal diameter, small intestinal shortening, or a combination of these effects. Smooth muscle contractions can be tonic or phasic, but common usage has labeled tonic contractions as tone and phasic motor events as contractions. Human phasic small intestinal contractions generally last from 0.8 to 6.0 seconds.

Small intestinal electrical recordings reveal continuous cyclical oscillations in electrical potential, referred to as the *slow wave, basic electrical rhythm,* or *pacesetter potential.* This slow wave is generated by the ICC (see earlier). In humans, the slow-wave frequency decreases from a peak of 12 per minute in the duodenum to approximately 7 per minute in the distal ileum. A small intestinal contraction arises when an electrical action potential, or spike burst, is superimposed on the slow wave (Fig. 99-6). Spike bursts may be caused by the intrinsic motor output from the ENS to the ICC and are likely also to be modulated by the extrinsic motor supply. Except during phase III of the IDMC (interdigestive migrating motor complex), not every slow wave leads to a phasic contraction. The region-specific frequency of the slow wave thus controls small intestinal rhythmicity by determining the timing and maximal frequency of contractions.

The rapid increases in free intracellular calcium, or calcium transients, that underlie smooth muscle contraction can be visualized with fluorescence techniques and appear to spread in a coordinated fashion over an area of smooth muscle and to extend over variable distances of the bowel wall. These calcium transients are extinguished by collision with each other or by encountering locally refractory regions.[51]

Contractions that Travel along the Small Intestine

The electrical slow wave migrates along the small intestine in an aboral direction so that each subsequent site along the intestine is depolarized sequentially. When a slow wave results in contraction, the propagation of the slow wave along the small intestine also leads to the contraction propagating along the small intestine. The propagation velocity of the slow wave thus determines the maximal rate at which contractions

can travel along the small intestine. Because not every slow wave leads to a contraction, however, contractions do not always travel at this maximal rate. The distance over which muscular excitation or inhibition spreads appears to be determined by ENS influences mediated through local inhibitory and excitatory circuits.[51]

Contraction sequences travel aborad (in an antegrade direction) or orad (in a retrograde direction). From animal data and some human studies at high spatial resolution, it is known that a large portion of contractions travel along the small intestine rather than remaining static, although most contractions are limited to only a few centimeters in extent.[59,60] Further data are needed to determine the contribution that these short contraction sequences make to overall transit compared with the less frequent longer sequences.

Patterned Motility

From isolated small intestinal segments, ascending excitation and descending inhibition are the simplest well-recognized patterns of motility. *Ascending excitation* refers to the contraction that occurs proximal (orad) to a stimulus, and *descending inhibition* refers to the inhibition of motor activity that occurs distal to a stimulus. These simple reflexes can be demonstrated in the absence of any extrinsic innervation and are thus entirely attributable to the ENS, although extrinsic influences can modulate their occurrence. These 2 patterns are thought to be responsible for peristalsis and retroperistalsis when they travel in a coordinated fashion along the intestine.

Recordings of human small intestinal motility show isolated (stationary) phasic contractions, but often, spatial patterns are more complex. The limited spatial resolution of many recording techniques can lead to over-reporting of the fraction of stationary contractions. Commonly, phasic motor activity consists of a recognizable group of contractions associated along the small intestine in space and time; phase III activity of the IDMC (see later) is a good example of this association. Several other types of grouped small intestinal contractions have been described and include contractions associated with emesis[61] and discrete clustered contractions, which are said to be common in IBS (see Chapter 122).[62] The most commonly observed motor patterns in the healthy small intestine, however, are described simply as the fed or postprandial pattern and the fasting (interdigestive) pattern, or IDMC (Fig. 99-7).

The motor pattern is determined by the presence or absence of a significant amount of nutrient within the small intestine. Despite a large number of studies on fasting motility, few studies have been performed on human postprandial small intestinal motility; this paucity probably exists because of the difficulty in knowing which aspects of postprandial motility to study, in contrast to fasting motility, which has an easily recognized cyclic pattern and thus easily studied parameters. The fed motor pattern ensures transit of small intestinal contents at a rate consistent with normal digestion and absorption. The fasting motor pattern is less involved with orderly luminal transport and is thought to serve important roles in clearing the upper intestine of solid residues, which otherwise can accumulate and form bezoars; in maintaining relative sterility of the small intestine by keeping it empty; and in preventing net orad migration of colonic bacteria.

Within 10 to 20 minutes of consumption of a meal, the IDMC that is in progress at the time of eating is interrupted.[63] The presence of intraluminal nutrients is sensed by mucosal nutrient contact, as evidenced by the fact that portal-venous or IV administration of nutrients does not have the same effects as those consumed orally.[64] Several neural and humoral signals result from mucosal nutrient contact and are

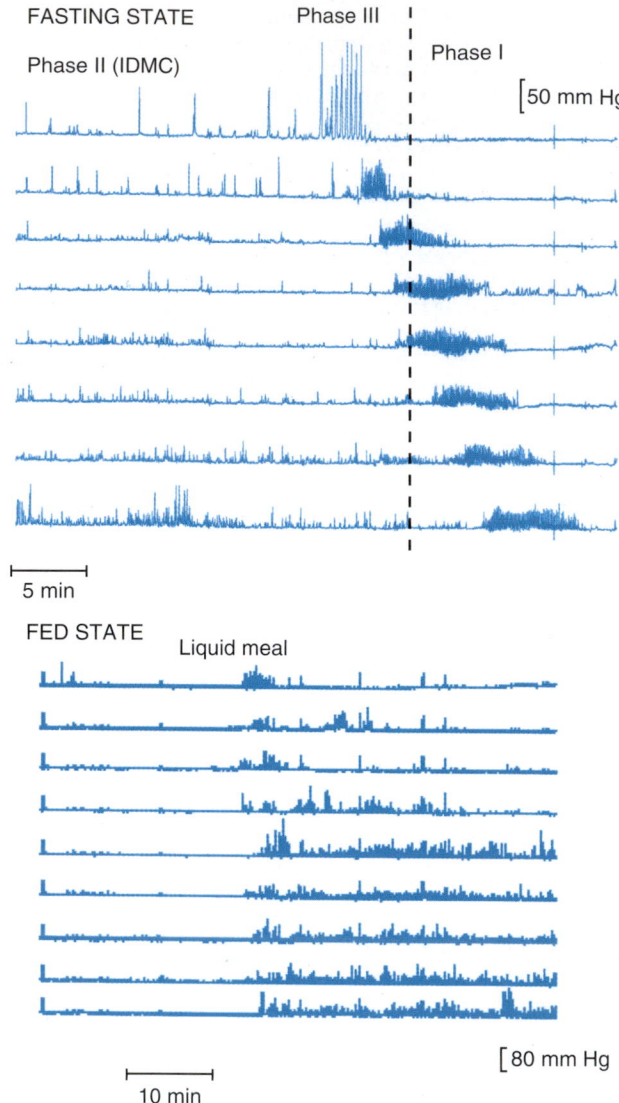

FASTING STATE   Phase III

Phase II (IDMC)   Phase I

[50 mm Hg

5 min

FED STATE

Liquid meal

[80 mm Hg

10 min

FIGURE 99-7. Manometric tracings that demonstrate small intestinal motility in fasting *(top)* and fed *(bottom)* state. The 3 phases of the interdigestive motor cycle (IDMC) and conversion to a fed motor pattern by infusing a liquid nutrient meal into small intestine are shown. In the *top* set of tracings, at a given time point *(dashed vertical line)*, all 3 phases of IDMC can be encountered at different points along the small intestine. The similarity of phase II and fed motor pattern can be appreciated by comparing the *top* (fasting) and *bottom* (fed) sets of tracings. *(Professor R.J. Fraser provided data for this figure.)*

implicated in the induction of the fed motor pattern, including vagal afferent signals, CCK, and GLP-1. Moreover, the sensing of intraluminal nutrients is relatively complex because different types of nutrients, or variable amounts of the same nutrient, generate recognizably different motor responses.[49,50,65,66] In general, the presence of unabsorbed small intestinal nutrients slows small intestine transit by decreasing the frequency and length of travel of phasic contractions, so that the rate at which a substance is absorbed limits its transit rate. In the absence of sufficient proximal small intestinal nutrient stimulation, the fasting motor pattern re-emerges 4 to 6 hours after a meal. In the absence of its interruption by intraluminal nutrients, the IDMC repeats continuously.

Distention, intraluminal pH changes, and hyperosmolar contents are capable of stimulating small intestinal motor activity. Hyperosmolar contents and pH changes probably are sensed by receptors in the mucosa, whereas distention is signaled by receptors in the muscle. In the normal course of events, these stimuli occur concurrently with the presence of nutrients, and the significance of their isolated effects in healthy subjects is unclear.

The small intestine also exerts negative feedback control on the rate of gastric emptying through neural and humoral means. This negative feedback is achieved by the release of neural signals and intestinal hormones that suppress phasic gastric motor activity, relax the gastric fundus, and increase tonic and phasic pyloric pressures subsequent to mucosal sensing of small intestinal nutrients.[67] This process indirectly also prolongs whole-meal small intestine transit time by slowing the input of chyme to the small intestinal. The small intestine, in particular the duodenum, is also thought to offer direct mechanical resistance to gastric emptying by acting as a capacitance resistor[68] and by re-augmenting gastric contents as a result of duodenogastric reflux.[69]

Fed Motor Pattern

Radiologic Observations

Early radiologic observations of the small intestine in animals described several different patterns of wall motion and transit of intestinal contents. Walter Cannon[61,70] observed both localized contractions over short segments of intestine in association with to-and-fro movement of contents and intermittent episodes of propulsion of contents over greater distances caused by aborally traveling waves of peristalsis. In the fed state, the most common pattern of wall motion consisted of localized circular contractions that recurrently divided and formed short columns of chyme into new aliquots by temporary local occlusion of the lumen over distances of less than 1 to 2 cm, this pattern being labeled *rhythmic segmentation*.[61,70] These contractions did not travel along the small intestine and did not result in much if any net oral movement of contents.[61,70]

Peristalsis also was commonly observed, often in combination with segmentation. During small intestinal nutrient loading, peristalsis was noted to have 2 forms: 1 was a slow advance of chyme over short distances in association with segmentation, and the other was a rapid transit of chyme over longer distances, sometimes several loops, of the small intestine. The "fast peristalsis" was often seen in the cat duodenum.[70] Similar observations have been made in other animal species[50,61] and correlate with some of the motor patterns seen during clinical radiologic studies in humans (although these studies usually are performed when the subject is fasting and show the rapid peristaltic pattern more than the segmenting postprandial activity).

Transit Time Observations

The small intestinal transit time for a meal varies greatly according to the amount and nature of what is consumed, because both caloric content and physical form of a meal determine the gastric emptying rate and the rate of transport along the intestine.[60,71-73] Depending on the test and parameter used, postprandial orocecal transit time usually is less than 6 hours. As assessed by lactulose breath testing, however, orocecal transit time can be as rapid as about 70 minutes with low nutrient loads. A systematic evaluation of the optimal conditions for nutrient loading is much needed to reveal abnormal small intestinal motor function, using transit studies.

Manometric Observations

Postprandial small intestinal motility is characterized by irregular phasic pressure waves without a discernible cyclical pattern. Most small intestinal motility data are quite limited in spatial resolution because of the length of the small intestine. Nevertheless, most phasic pressures (pressure wave sequences) are thought to travel only a short distance[49,50] and probably represent the mixing and segmenting contractions noted in earlier radiologic studies.[61,70] In animal studies, postprandial small intestinal motility is more segmenting than is fasting phase II activity, and phasic pressures occur less frequently and travel shorter distances along the bowel, resulting in slower transit of the contents.[50] A similar suppression in the frequency of pressure wave sequences now has been found in the human duodenum.[49] This segmenting motor pattern is thought to assist in mixing food with digestive enzymes and in maximizing the exposure of food to the mucosa to optimize absorption.

Fasting Motor Pattern

During fasting, small intestinal motor activity adopts a repetitive cyclic motor pattern, the IDMC. The IDMC is absent in a number of disease states, presumably because of a primary neuropathic process. This absence is associated clinically with stasis of small intestinal contents, malabsorption, and small intestinal bacterial overgrowth.[62,63]

Radiologic Observations

Contrast agents can stimulate small intestinal mucosal receptors sensitive to pH, caloric content, and osmolarity changes. It is possible, therefore, that radiologic studies of "fasting" motility do not truly represent the fasting state. In general, however, contrast agents appear to move more swiftly through the small intestine during fasting than during the postprandial state and to be associated with more episodes of peristalsis over 1 or more loops and fewer segmenting contractions. When the phase of the IDMC is assessed concurrently (see later), little net movement of small intestinal contents is seen during phase I, but residual luminal contents are swept through the small intestine and into the terminal ileum during late phase II and phase III of the IDMC. This finding is not surprising because, by definition, phase I is the absence of measurable phasic pressure waves, which are likely to be necessary to generate a sufficient intraluminal pressure gradient to cause intraluminal flow.

Transit Time Observations

Studies of transit time through the small intestine also probably do not represent a true assessment of fasting motor function, because most of the substrates used to measure transit also interact with small intestinal mucosal receptors. The lower the caloric content, the more closely fasting motility will be assessed (see earlier).

Manometric Observations

The IDMC is defined manometrically and comprises 3 main phases. Phase I is defined as motor quiescence (<3 pressure waves per 10 minutes at any 1 site); phase II is characterized by random pressure waves at less than the maximal rate; and phase III is characterized by pressure waves at the maximal rate (for the region) for longer than 2 minutes and, ideally, extending over a segment longer than 40 cm. Some authors also include a fourth phase (phase IV) as a transitional period

between phases III and I, although this approach is not universal. Phases I and III are quite distinctive and easily recognized, whereas phase II can be recognized reliably only when sandwiched between phases I and III, because it superficially resembles the fed pattern. The phases of the IDMC start proximally and migrate distally over variable distances; few phase IIIs reaching the ileum.[59] Phase III of each IDMC can start at any of a variety of locations; approximately one third of IDMCs have a gastroduodenal component, and most onsets of phase III occur near the proximal jejunum.[59] Because of the length of the small intestine and the velocity of travel of the IDMC, 1 part of the small intestine can be in phase I while other parts are in phase II or III (see Fig. 99-7). The normal periodicity of the IDMC varies greatly both within and between subjects; however, its median duration is 90 to 120 minutes.

CLINICAL CONSEQUENCES OF DISORDERED SMALL INTESTINAL MOTILITY

Most of the time, the overall outcome of small intestinal motility is achieved without conscious awareness, but a range of symptoms can arise when an optimal outcome is not attained. Fortunately, like other organs, the small intestine has a substantial reserve capacity and copes with many insults, including infection, resection, inflammation, and denervation, before clinical problems become manifest. In IBS, the most common clinical syndrome in which altered motility is implicated, the sufferer's physical well-being rarely is threatened even when symptoms are considerable. Infrequently, the motor disturbances are severe enough to disrupt a person's ability to maintain oral nutrition.

The most important diseases and clinical settings associated with abnormal small intestinal motility are listed in Table 99-1. Because these disorders are covered elsewhere in this book, they are mentioned here only with regard to their associated small intestinal motor disturbances.

In IBS, a number of abnormalities of visceral sensation have been documented (see Chapter 122). These sensory abnormalities probably also lead to disordered motility; however, whereas motor abnormalities have been documented in some patients with IBS, they are absent in others. Because it appears likely that IBS is an as-yet-undefined generalized enteric neuropathy or low-grade neuro-inflammatory/immune disorder,[22,74-76] failure to detect specific motor abnormalities might simply reflect our current poor understanding of normal small intestinal motor physiology and the relatively gross measures by which motility has been assessed in patients with IBS.

Small intestinal motility is severely disrupted in acutely ill persons and is increasingly recognized as an important factor to consider in postoperative and ICU patients. Such motility disturbances likely result from several factors, including sepsis and drugs, which disrupt the slow wave rhythm; abdominal trauma and surgery, which stimulate reflex motor responses; and inflammatory mediators and cytokines, which affect neurotransmission within the CNS, ANS, and ENS.[77,78]

Pregnancy is known to alter the function of the lower esophageal sphincter, to delay gastric emptying and disturb the frequency of gastric slow waves, and often to be associated with constipation. In view of these widespread findings related to altered intestinal motility, it is likely that small intestinal motor function also is altered. In guinea pigs, the strength of the contraction of intestinal circular smooth muscle has been shown to be impaired during pregnancy by down-regulation of $G\alpha q/11$ proteins (which mediate contraction) and up-regulation of G_s alpha protein (which mediates relaxation).[79] It is intriguing that G protein associations are now also being reported in functional GI disorders, suggesting a final common pathway for sensorimotor intestinal disturbances.[80]

Diabetes has widespread effects on GI motility. Acute effects result from changes in blood glucose levels, but they also can result from the autonomic neuropathy that develops in patients with long-standing disease. As indicated predominantly by studies of the stomach, hyperglycemia can alter the rhythm of the slow wave, modulate sensory signaling, lead to changes in the temporospatial pattern of phasic contractions, and even stimulate inappropriate phase III-like IDMC activity in the small intestine. In diabetic patients with fecal incontinence, impaired rectal sensory function is common, and it has been shown that experimental diabetes selectively affects sensory afferents that detect low-threshold physiologic rectal distention, such as that which might occur during rectal filling prior to defecation.[81] As such, loss of this sensory feedback may promote incontinence and disrupt motility patterns in the small intestine and colon.

Metabolic disturbances of potassium, magnesium, and calcium homeostasis are likely to impair small intestinal motor function, because these chemicals are vital for normal neuromuscular function. The effects of abnormal levels of these electrolytes on normal human small intestinal function have not been studied specifically, but in organ bath experiments, their alterations have caused gross disturbances in neural and muscular function. In addition, renal and hepatic failure are likely to alter small intestinal motility because of the multiple homeostatic inputs of the affected organs; altered motility, however, is not usually a prominent clinical feature in these conditions.

Many drugs affect small intestinal motility, especially those that alter ion transport (e.g., antidepressants, calcium channel blockers, beta blockers). Sedatives and narcotic analgesics also alter motility but usually do not cause clinically important small intestinal motor dysfunction except in critically ill patients or those with acute severe pain.

Pseudo-obstruction, scleroderma and other connective tissue diseases, dysautonomia, visceral myopathies, and other rare diseases in which abnormal small intestinal motor function occur are discussed in detail in other chapters. These diseases may be uncommon causes of disordered small intestinal motility, but they have increased our understanding of normal motility, because in some cases, the neural and myopathic processes are impaired separately. For example, a gain-of-function mutation in the voltage-gated sodium channel Nav1.7 (SCN9A) is linked to the human condition "familial rectal pain syndrome," now renamed "paroxysmal extreme pain disorder." As the name suggests, it is characterized by rectal and abdominal pain, commonly associated with defecation, and it is presumed that the hyperactive variety of NaV1.7 is expressed in sensory afferents in the colon or rectum which, when activated, triggers extreme pain.[82,83] In contrast, a related channel, NaV1.5 is expressed in ICC and smooth muscle in the circular layer of the human intestine. IBS patients with mutations in SCN5A (the gene encoding NaV1.5) are more likely to report GI symptoms, especially abdominal pain.[84]

APPROACH TO PATIENTS WITH POSSIBLE SMALL INTESTINAL MOTOR DYSFUNCTION

Taking a thorough history is a vital first step in approaching a patient who may have abnormal small intestinal motility. A review of exposures to drugs and toxins, family history, and

in the younger patient, milestones of growth and development are especially important to consider. Findings on physical examination in this setting often are unremarkable. First-line investigations generally are suggested by the history, physical examination, and age of the patient and may include a plain abdominal film (to look for dilated small intestinal loops, thickened bowel wall, or air-fluid levels), complete blood count with determination of red blood cell indices (to look for evidence of malabsorption), measurement of serum albumin and electrolyte levels, and random testing of blood glucose or glycosylated hemoglobin level. How much further to proceed with investigation depends on these results and on the severity of the patient's condition.

Special investigations may be indicated to answer particular questions. No standard approach has been recognized, however, and local interest and expertise often determine which investigations are available. Fluoroscopy is widely available and can help exclude medically or surgically treatable problems. Endoscopy with small intestinal biopsy or aspiration is useful if celiac sprue, SIBO, or intestinal infection is considered likely. Analysis of stool may be necessary to exclude malabsorptive or secretory causes of small intestinal diarrhea. Small intestinal manometry, if available, can help distinguish neuropathic from myopathic forms of disordered motility, although in many settings, the abnormalities associated with these 2 forms overlap (see Table 99-1). Manometry can show features typical of intestinal obstruction, although abdominal imaging by a variety of radiologic techniques is a better tool to identify an obstruction. In selected cases, full-thickness biopsy of the small intestine is necessary, but such biopsy should be performed only in centers with expertise in immunohistochemistry of intestinal neurons, because standard histologic approaches often yield little useful information.

Unfortunately, there are few therapies to date, beyond supportive measures, that can be offered to patients with disordered small intestinal motility. Nutritional status is of prime importance, and where patients can manage this independently, no further specific treatment may be needed. Symptomatic treatment approaches include modifications in diet (small frequent meals, lower fat intake), exercise (which is shown to improve bloating symptoms and expulsion of intestinal gas), antinausea agents, antispasmodics, and drugs to modulate sensory function.

Thus far, there are no clinically available agents that specifically modify visceral hypersensitivity, and simple analgesics, opiates, and antidepressants are all used. Apart from the tricyclic antidepressants and selective serotonin reuptake inhibitors, there is little proof that these offer significant benefit, and opiates can even worsen symptoms, leading to the narcotic bowel syndrome. Treatment of psychological comorbidities also is important because anxiety and depression can heighten the perception of, and distress caused by, intestinal symptoms. Prokinetic agents have been limited in their therapeutic benefit, and because of safety concerns, availability of several (e.g., cisapride, tegaserod) has been restricted. There is hope, however, that prokinetics and visceral-specific analgesics might offer a better balance between safety and efficacy in the future.

KEY REFERENCES

Full references for this chapter can be found on www.expertconsult.com.

2. Sanders KM. Regulation of smooth muscle excitation and contraction. Neurogastroenterol Motil 2008; 20(Suppl 1): 39-53.

4. Sanders KM, Koh SD, Ward SM. Interstitial cells of Cajal as pacemakers in the gastrointestinal tract. Annu Rev Physiol 2006; 68:307-43.

5. Ward SM, Sanders KM. Involvement of intramuscular interstitial cells of Cajal in neuroeffector transmission in the gastrointestinal tract. J Physiol 2006; 576:675-82.

8. Furness JB. Types of neurons in the enteric nervous system. J Auton Nerv Syst 2000; 81:87-96.

9. Wood JD. Enteric nervous system: Reflexes, pattern generators and motility. Curr Opin Gastroenterol 2008; 24:149-58.

14. Gulbransen BD, Sharkey KA. Novel functional roles for enteric glia in the gastrointestinal tract. Nat Rev Gastroenterol Hepatol 2012; 9:625-32.

15. Brierley SM, Hughes P, Harrington A, Blackshaw LA. Innervation of the gastrointestinal tract by spinal and vagal afferent nerves. In: Johnson LR, editor. Physiology of the gastrointestinal tract. 5th ed. Oxford: Academic Press; 2012. p 703.

26. Zagorodnyuk VP, Brookes SJ. Transduction sites of vagal mechanoreceptors in the guinea pig esophagus. J Neurosci 2000; 20:6249-55.

38. Krauter EM, Strong DS, Brooks EM, et al. Changes in colonic motility and the electrophysiological properties of myenteric neurons persist following recovery from trinitrobenzene sulfonic acid colitis in the guinea pig. Neurogastroenterol Motil 2007; 19:990-1000.

53. Dinning PG, Arkwright JW, Gregersen H, et al. Technical advances in monitoring human motility patterns. Neurogastroenterol Motil 2010; 22:366-80.

57. Schwizer W, Steingoetter A, Fox M. Magnetic resonance imaging for the assessment of gastrointestinal function. Scand J Gastroenterol 2006; 41:1245-60.

61. Cannon WB. The mechanical factors of digestion. London: Edward Arnold; 1911.

62. Husebye E. The patterns of small bowel motility: Physiology and implications in organic disease and functional disorders. Neurogastroenterol Motil 1999; 11:141-61.

72. Hunt JN, Smith JL, Jiang CL. Effect of meal volume and energy density on the gastric emptying of carbohydrates. Gastroenterology 1985; 89:1326-30.

CHAPTER OUTLINE

Each day, 1200 to 1500 mL of ileal effluent enter the colon, 200 to 400 mL of which are finally excreted as stool. The colon mixes its contents to facilitate transmural exchange of water, electrolytes, and short-chain fatty acids and, in doing so, stores stool for extended periods. The mixing process involves rhythmic to-and-fro motions, together with short stepwise movements of contents, resulting in an overall net aboral flow rate that averages 1 cm per hour. When dehydration threatens survival, such as with water deprivation or severe diarrhea, the ability of the colon to reabsorb fluids is of major physiologic significance; appropriate motility patterns are important in achieving this function. The colon has the capacity to increase its fluid absorption five-fold when required, but this ability is greatly impaired when transit is accelerated. Under normal circumstances, viscous contents are occasionally propelled aborally at a rapid rate, and if circumstances are appropriate, stool is evacuated under voluntary control. Thus, the colon is capable of showing a diverse range of motor patterns suited for particular physiologic functions. The generic term *motility* describes the range of motor patterns and the mechanisms that control them.

Common sensorimotor bowel symptoms (e.g., constipation, diarrhea, bloating, abdominal pain, rectal urgency) can arise from disturbances of ileocolonic delivery, colonic propulsion, or stool expulsion. Clearly these symptoms and dysmotility must be linked, although our current understanding of such linkages is limited, largely because of technical difficulties involved in studying the human colon. Because of differences among species, care is required in extrapolating data from animal studies to humans. For many years, intraluminal motility recordings in humans were obtained mainly from the rectum and sigmoid, but it is now clear that the motor activity of these distal regions is not representative of the colon as a whole. The contents of the colon become increasingly viscous distally, and this alteration complicates the relationship between propulsion and the contractile activity of the smooth muscle. Colonic movements are much less frequent and transit is considerably slower than in other regions of the GI tract. The highly propulsive stereotypical motor patterns associated with stool expulsion generally occur only once or twice daily. Hence, study of the motor patterns in the human cannot be achieved using contrast radiology. Prolonged recording techniques must be used to capture such infrequent motor patterns.

METHODS TO RECORD COLONIC MOTILITY

Recording of colonic intraluminal pressure across multiple sites simultaneously can only be achieved by manometry. Recent advances in fiberoptic technology have made it possible to record high-resolution pressure profiles throughout the entire length of the colon. Measurement of colonic wall tone using a barostat provides information on nonocclusive colonic wall movements, but it tells us nothing of the spatiotemporal patterning of motility. Smooth muscle electromyography provides insight into the patterning of muscle activity but generally requires access to the muscular wall of the colon, which is problematic in humans for ethical reasons. Scintigraphy recorded over prolonged periods, with suitably high frame rates, can resolve discrete movements of the contents within the colon, but it is time-consuming and suboptimal for measuring actual wall motion. The recent success of videocapsule imaging of the GI tract, along with the desire to avoid radiologic studies, has driven a move to ingestible telemetric (wireless) devices to assess GI motility and transit. In vitro study of the cellular basis of motility using isolated specimens of colon faces fewer technical and ethical limitations, but data obtained at the cellular level, often under rather nonphysiologic conditions, can be difficult to extrapolate to the more complex integrated responses of the entire organ in vivo. Although we recognize the intrinsic limitations of all these measurement techniques, in combination they have allowed us to piece together a number of concepts that have provided important insights into the relationships among muscle activity, wall motion, intraluminal pressure, and flow.

ANATOMY AND BASIC CONTROL MECHANISMS OF THE COLON AND ANORECTUM

Macroscopic Structure of the Colon

The human colon is just over 1 meter long and divided anatomically into the cecum; the ascending, transverse, descending, and sigmoid colon; and the rectum, which lies between the rectosigmoid junction and the anal canal. The outer longitudinal smooth muscle layer forms three thick, cord-like structures called the *teniae coli*, which are spaced evenly around the circumference of the colon. Between the teniae, the longitudinal smooth muscle is much thinner, allowing the wall to bulge noticeably.

Irregularly spaced circumferential constrictions pinch the colon into a series of pockets called *haustra* that give the colon a sacculated appearance for much of its length. Some *haustra* are fixed structures and can be readily seen during colonoscopy. Localized contractions of the circular muscle result in functional haustrations that move, disappear, and re-form during the propulsion of colonic contents. Myogenic activity alone, however, does not seem sufficient to explain haustration, and neural input likely contributes to their formation, especially during active propulsion of content.

The teniae fuse to form a continuous outer longitudinal smooth muscle layer at the rectosigmoid junction. The longitudinal layer then continues down to the distal margin of the anal canal, insinuating itself between the internal and external anal sphincters. Throughout the length of the colon, the circular smooth muscle layer consists of thick bundles of cells separated by connective tissue septa. The internal anal sphincter consists of a thickening of the circular muscle layer over the last 2 to 4 cm of the anal canal.

Gross anatomy of the colon and anorectum are discussed in Chapters 98 and 129, respectively.

Structure and Activity of Colonic Smooth Muscle

Structure

Smooth muscle cells in the human colon, as in other muscular organs, are spindle-shaped, nucleolated cells with tapered ends. The surface area of the smooth muscle cell membrane is increased greatly by numerous caveolae, or small pits. Individual smooth muscle cells are connected mechanically to neighboring cells by intermediate junctions and electrically by gap junctions that allow ions and small molecules—those with molecular weights up to about 1000 kD—to diffuse between the cells, thereby ensuring that the cells are functionally coupled to one another. Smooth muscle cells therefore do not contract as individual cells but together in a large coordinated assembly called a *syncytium.*

Spontaneous Activity

Like smooth muscle throughout the GI tract, colonic smooth muscle shows spontaneous oscillatory electrical activity even when all neural activity is blocked. Two types of rhythmic myoelectrical activity occur[1]: *slow waves* and *myenteric potential oscillations* (MPOs).

A major pacemaker region is located at the submucosal border of the circular muscle. This region produces larger-amplitude, slower myogenic oscillations in membrane potential called *slow waves*, which spread decrementally through the thickness of the circular smooth muscle by means of gap junctions. When slow waves reach a threshold for contractions, phasic pressure waves are often recorded by manometry. Slow waves occur throughout the human colon at a frequency of 2 to 4 per minute and propagate over short distances up or down the colon. Complex interactions occur as waves coming from different initiation sites collide, leading to mixing of contents with slow overall propulsion.

MPOs are small-amplitude rapid oscillations with a frequency of 12 to 20 per minute that originate in the plane of the myenteric plexus. These small oscillations spread by means of gap junctions into both the longitudinal and circular smooth muscle layers, where they summate with slow waves and often reach the threshold potential to generate smooth muscle action potentials.

The currents produced by pacemaker cells at the submucosal and myenteric borders decay as they spread through the thickness of the circular muscle layer. Cells in the middle of the circular smooth muscle layer display complex spontaneous electrical activity consisting of a mixture of MPOs and slow waves, with superimposed smooth muscle action potentials.

These myogenic patterns do not function in isolation. Enteric neural activity generates motor output that is superimposed on the myogenic activity, adding yet more variety to colonic motor patterns. Enteric neuronal output can simply augment the phasic myogenic contractions, bringing them to threshold level to drive simple rhythmic activity.

Alternatively, enteric neural circuits can generate powerful patterned contractions of much longer duration than those produced by slow waves. These contractions can propagate for long distances along the colon and are known as *propagating sequences* or *mass movements*.[2] These are understood to primarily be the result of activation of polarized enteric neural pathways, and thus represent a form of "neurogenic peristalsis."

The functions of the colon circular smooth muscle are quite well understood; in contrast, the role the longitudinal muscle layer plays in colonic motility, mixing, and propulsion is a matter of some controversy. The longitudinal muscle probably acts in synergy with the circular muscle, preventing excessive lengthening when the circular muscle contracts. It may also contribute to propulsion by pulling the colon over its contents so that circular muscle contractions gain more purchase.

Ion Channels in Colonic Smooth Muscle

The membrane of colonic smooth muscle cells contains a variety of ion channels, including several types of potassium, calcium, chloride, and nonselective cation channels.[3] Although the exact physiologic roles of many of these ion channels are unknown, the high-threshold voltage-operated calcium channels (L-type calcium channels) do play a crucial role in colonic muscle contractility. These channels open when the membrane potential of smooth muscle cells is depolarized beyond a voltage threshold, and they are responsible for the rapid upstroke of smooth muscle action potentials. The influx of calcium through L-type calcium channels during action potentials is a major trigger for activation of the contractile apparatus. It is therefore not surprising that pharmacologic blockade of L-type calcium channels by dihydropyridine drugs like nifedipine can substantially reduce the contractility of colonic smooth muscle. Release of calcium from intracellular stores, which is triggered by excitatory neurotransmitters, may also play a role in muscle contraction.

Interstitial Cells of Cajal

Since 1991, the interstitial cells of Cajal (ICC) have been shown to play at least two important roles in the control of GI motility: control of myogenic activity and mediating or amplifying the effects of motor neurons on the smooth muscle apparatus. ICC are non-neuronal in origin and are derived from common progenitors of smooth muscle cells. Mutant mice and rats deficient in ICC have profoundly disturbed intestinal motility, an observation that provides insight into the roles of ICC in the human GI tract.

In the human colon, three types of ICC are recognized, usually by their immunoreactivity for c-Kit (CD117). They are named according to their locations: ICC in the plane of the myenteric plexus (ICC$_{MY}$), ICC near the submucosal plexus (ICC$_{SM}$), and intramuscular ICC located between the circular and the longitudinal muscle layers (ICC$_{IM}$). ICC$_{MY}$ and ICC$_{SM}$ form extensive networks along the colon and are electrically coupled to one another and to the smooth muscle layers by gap junctions (Figs. 100-1 and 100-2). ICC$_{MY}$ are probably the pacemakers for the small, rapid (12 to 20/min) MPOs of longitudinal and circular smooth muscle layers. ICC$_{SM}$ are the pacemakers for the large-amplitude slow waves (2 to 4/min) that originate in the plane of the submucosal plexus; these slow waves have a powerful influence on the patterning of circular muscle contraction.

Although the exact ionic basis of rhythmicity in ICC$_{MY}$ and ICC$_{SM}$ that gives rise to MPOs and slow waves is not entirely clear, oscillations in membrane potential are an intrinsic property of both ICC$_{MY}$ and ICC$_{SM}$. ICC$_{IM}$ are a major target of

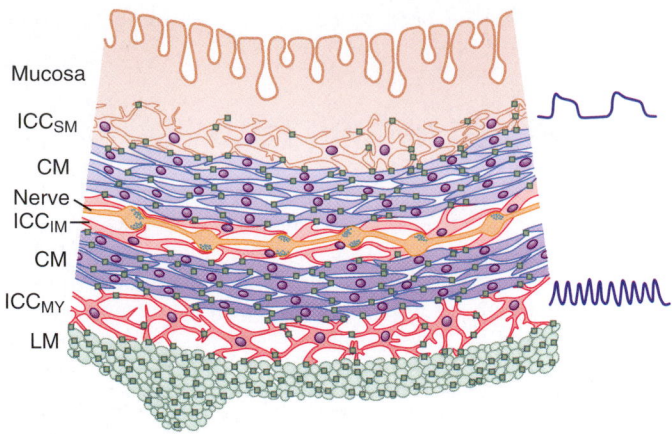

FIGURE 100-1. Schematic cross-section of the human colon. The outer longitudinal smooth muscle layer *(LM)* is thickened at the teniae. In the plane of the myenteric plexus is a network of interstitial cells of Cajal *(ICC)*, which generate a rapid myenteric potential oscillation (ICC$_{MY}$ [see lower waveform on right]). The circular muscle layer *(CM)* is innervated by axons of enteric motor neurons with transmitter release sites (clusters of clear vesicles) that are associated with specialized intramuscular ICC *(ICC$_{IM}$)*. At the inner border of the circular muscle is another network of submucosal ICC that generate slow waves (ICC$_{SM}$ [see upper waveform on right]). Also present are axons of motor neurons in the longitudinal muscles and ICC$_{IM}$. *Tiny green squares* represent gap junctions, which electrically couple cells.

neurotransmitters released from the axons of excitatory and inhibitory enteric motor neurons. Acetylcholine and nitric oxide (ACh and NO,) and probably several other motor neuron transmitters, evoke changes in the membrane potential of ICC$_{IM}$, which then spread through the smooth muscle by means of gap junctions. ICC$_{IM}$ may also be involved in amplifying the slow waves as they spread through the muscle layers. Thus, these cells appear to be key players in integrating non-neuronal pacemaker activity and neuronal inputs to smooth muscle.

Recently, another cell type that likely contributes to colonic motility control has been identified in the human colon. These "fibroblast-like cells" are characterized by immunoreactivity for platelet-derived growth factor receptor alpha (PDGFRα) but not for the prototypical marker of ICCs, c-Kit. They form plexuses within the longitudinal and smooth muscle layers and are closely intertwined with networks of ICCs. Like ICC$_{IM}$, they are also closely apposed to axons of enteric motor neurons within the muscle layers.[4] In animal models, these fibroblast-like cells are involved in inhibitory neurotransmission to the smooth muscle and appear to mediate the purinergic component due to ATP.

The discovery that cellular mechanisms long considered to be the properties of smooth muscle cells are actually mediated by ICC may have important clinical implications. In the distal bowel, reduced numbers of ICC or reduction in the total volume of ICC have been associated with anorectal malformations, colonic manifestations of Chagas' disease, normal aging, and possibly some cases of slow-transit constipation.[5] Some reports have suggested that the density of ICC may be reduced in the aganglionic segments of colon in Hirschsprung's disease and that this deficit might contribute to diminished propulsive activity; this finding, however, has not been consistent among studies.[5]

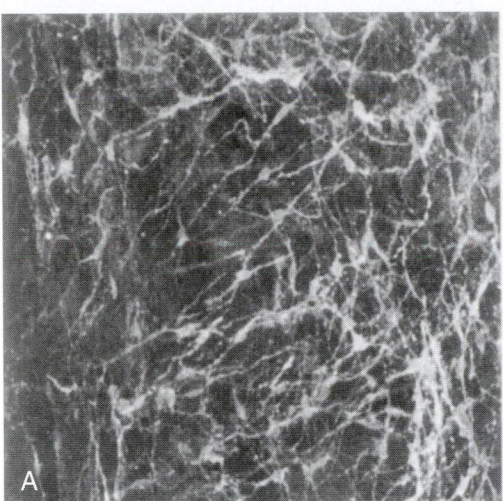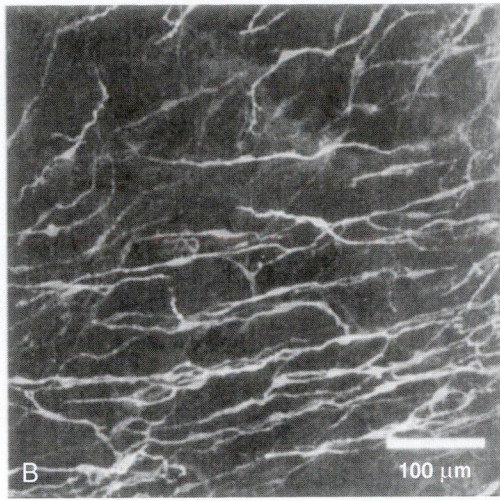

FIGURE 100-2. Micrographs of interstitial cells of Cajal (ICC) in the human colon, labeled by c-Kit immunohistochemistry. *A*, ICC in the plane of the myenteric plexus (ICC$_{MY}$) have an irregular shape, form a dense network of cells, and probably function as pacemakers. *B*, A different plane of focus of same region shows spindle-shaped intramuscular ICC (ICC$_{IM}$) in the overlying circular muscle layer. These cells probably are involved in neuromuscular transmission to smooth muscle. *(Courtesy Liz Murphy and David Wattchow, Adelaide, South Australia.)*

INNERVATION OF THE COLON

Enteric Nervous System

Direct neuronal control of colonic motility is mediated mostly by the enteric nervous system (ENS).[6] Although the ENS is capable of expressing a diverse repertoire of motor patterns, its functions are modulated by sympathetic, parasympathetic, and extrinsic afferent pathways (Fig. 100-3). In terms of numbers of nerve cells, the ENS is by far the largest component of the autonomic nervous system, with considerably more neurons than those of the parasympathetic and sympathetic divisions combined. The nerve cell bodies of the ENS are located in plexuses of myenteric ganglia (Auerbach's plexus) that lie between the longitudinal and the circular muscle layers of the muscularis externa, or in the submucosal ganglia that lie between the muscle and mucosa (Fig. 100-4).

The submucosal plexus is divisible into at least two networks: *Meissner's plexus*, which lies closer to the mucosa, and *Schabadasch's plexus*, which lies adjacent to the circular muscle. Some authors have identified an additional intermediate plexus. Internodal strands that contain hundreds of axons run within and between the different plexuses. Finer nerve trunks innervate the various target tissues of the intestinal wall, including the longitudinal muscle layer, circular muscle, muscularis mucosae, mucosal crypts, and mucosal epithelium. Within the ganglia of each plexus, different functional classes of enteric nerve cell bodies are intermingled, and differences in the proportions of cell types among the plexuses have been observed. It has become clear that an exquisite degree of organization is characteristic of the ENS, each class of nerve cell making highly specific and precise projections to its particular target.

The ENS uses many transmitters in addition to the major transmitters ACh and NO, including tachykinins, purines, numerous other modulatory peptides, and some amines. Many other substances released from neural and non-neural cells also modulate neuronal and muscular excitability, including gaseous mediators (NO, carbon monoxide, and hydrogen sulfide) and, in inflammation, prostanoids, cytokines, purines, bradykinin, H$^+$ ions, and neurotrophins.

Primary Afferent Neurons

Much of the motor and secretory activity of the intestine can be conceptualized as a series of reflexes evoked by mechanical or chemical stimuli. These reflexes involve activation of enteric primary afferent neurons, integration by interneurons, and execution of appropriate responses by motor neurons. The first neurons in these reflex circuits are primary afferent neurons (sometimes called "sensory" neurons, although they do not give rise to conscious sensation). These neurons are located in both myenteric and submucosal plexuses and characteristically have several long axonal processes. Some primary afferent neurons fire action potentials in response to stretch or tension in the bowel wall; others are activated by chemical or mechanical stimuli of the mucosa. These mucosal stimuli probably work at least in part by activating specialized enteroendocrine cells (e.g., serotonin-containing enterochromaffin cells) in the mucosal epithelium. The enteric primary afferent neurons then release synaptic transmitters, such as ACh or tachykinins or other peptides, to excite other classes of enteric neurons in nearby ganglia. Enteric primary afferent neurons also make excitatory synaptic contacts onto other neurons of their own class, so that they fire as coordinated assemblies.

Motor Neurons

Enteric motor neurons typically have smaller cell bodies than afferent neurons, with a few short dendrites and a single long axon. Separate populations of motor neurons innervate the circular and longitudinal muscle layers. *Excitatory motor neurons* synthesize ACh, which they release from their varicose axons in the smooth muscle layers; some also release the tachykinin peptides substance P and neurokinin A, which also excite smooth muscle. Typically, axons of excitatory motor neurons project either directly to the smooth muscle close to their cell bodies or orad for up to 10 mm.[7] Once in the smooth muscle layers, the axons turn and run parallel to the smooth muscle fibers for several millimeters; they branch extensively and form many small varicosities, or transmitter release sites, closely associated with ICC$_{IM}$ and fibroblast-like cells.

Inhibitory motor neurons are typically slightly larger than excitatory motor neurons, and there are fewer of them. They

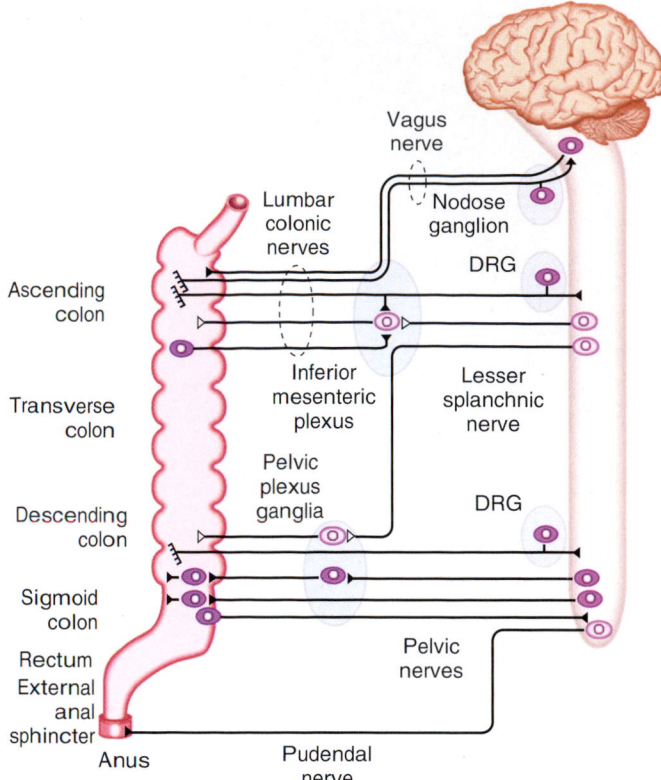

FIGURE 100-3. Extrinsic innervation of human colon. Parasympathetic efferent pathways *(filled cell bodies)* arise from the dorsal motor nucleus (of the vagus) in the brainstem and pass through the vagus nerve and prevertebral sympathetic ganglia, through the lumbar colonic nerves to the proximal colon. Parasympathetic pathways also extend from nuclei in the sacral spinal cord and run through the pelvic nerves to either synapse in the pelvic plexus ganglia or run directly into the bowel wall. Sympathetic pathways *(open cell bodies)* consist of preganglionic neurons in the thoracic spinal cord that synapse with sympathetic postganglionic neurons either in the inferior mesenteric plexus or pelvic plexus. Enteric nerve cell bodies in the colon receive input from both parasympathetic and sympathetic pathways. Viscerofugal enteric neurons project out of the bowel to the prevertebral ganglia. Afferent pathways consist of vagal afferent neurons from the proximal colon with cell bodies in the nodose ganglia. In addition, spinal afferent neurons with cell bodies in lumbar dorsal root ganglia *(DRG)* run through the lesser splanchnic and colonic nerves to the colon and mediate nociception. Another population of spinal afferents with cell bodies in the sacral DRG runs through the pelvic nerves and pelvic ganglia to the rectum; these include sensory neurons that transmit non-nociceptive information about rectal distention. The striated muscles of the pelvic floor (including the external anal sphincter) are supplied by motor neurons with cell bodies in the spinal cord and axons that run in the pudendal nerves. *Triangles* represent transmitter release sites; *combs* represent sensory transduction sites.

also have short dendrites and a single axon, but unlike excitatory motor neurons, they project aborally to the smooth muscle layer for distances of 1 to 15 mm in the human colon.[7] Once the axon reaches the smooth muscle, it branches extensively to form multiple varicose release sites. Inhibitory motor neurons release a cocktail of transmitters that inhibit smooth muscle cells, including NO, adenosine triphosphate (ATP or a related compound like NADH), and peptides like vasoactive intestinal polypeptide (VIP) and pituitary adenyl cyclase-activating peptide (PACAP). The varicose transmitter release sites of inhibitory motor neurons are also associated with ICC_{IM}, as are the release sites of excitatory motor neurons. Interstitial cells probably mediate a large component of the electrical effects on smooth muscle of neurotransmitters released by enteric motor neurons. Inhibitory motor neurons are usually tonically active, modulating the ongoing contractile activity of the colonic circular smooth muscle. Inhibitory motor neurons are particularly important in relaxing sphincteric muscles in the ileocecal junction and the internal anal sphincter.

Interneurons

When a region of colon is stimulated, such as by a bolus that distends it, enteric primary afferent neurons are activated. These neurons then activate excitatory and inhibitory motor neurons that, because of their polarized projections, cause contraction of the muscle orad to the bolus and relaxation aborally. These effects tend to propel the contents aborally. From the new position of the bolus, another set of polarized reflexes is triggered, and peristaltic propulsion results. The *ascending excitatory reflex* and the *descending inhibitory reflex* are sometimes called the "law of the intestine." These reflexes spread farther than is predicted by the projections of the excitatory and inhibitory motor neurons, because interneurons are also involved in these reflex pathways. Ascending cholinergic interneurons in the human colon have axons that project up to 40 mm orad and extend the spread of ascending excitatory reflex pathways. In addition, several classes of descending interneurons are present in the human colon, with axons that project 70 mm or further aborally. Some of these interneurons are involved in spreading descending inhibition along the colon, but others are likely to be involved in the propagation of migratory contractions. It is also likely that some interneurons are themselves stretch sensitive, thereby functioning as primary afferent neurons. In addition to the sensory neurons, interneurons, and motor neurons, viscerofugal nerve cells project to the sympathetic prevertebral ganglia, vasomotor neurons innervate blood vessels, and secretomotor neurons stimulate secretion from the colonic epithelium.

Sympathetic Innervation

The major sympathetic innervation of the proximal colon arises from the inferior mesenteric ganglion and projects through the lumbar colonic nerves to the ascending and transverse colon (see Fig. 100-3). A small number of sympathetic neurons in the celiac and superior mesenteric ganglia, in the paravertebral chain ganglia, and in the pelvic plexus ganglia also project to the colon (see Fig. 100-3). These neurons receive a powerful cholinergic drive from preganglionic nerve cell bodies in the intermediolateral column of the thoracolumbar spinal cord (principally segments L2-L5). This is a major pathway by which the central nervous system modifies bowel activity, such as during exercise. Sympathetic efferent neurons also receive input from the enteric viscerofugal neurons and from extrinsic spinal sensory neurons with cell bodies in the dorsal root ganglia, forming several reflex loops with the distal bowel.

Sympathetic nerve fibers from prevertebral ganglia cause vasoconstriction of the mucosal and submucosal blood vessels. Other sympathetic neurons project to the enteric ganglia, where they cause generalized presynaptic inhibition in the ENS and thus depress reflex motor activity. Another target for sympathetic axons is the circuitry of the submucosal plexus (largely Meissner's plexus) involved in controlling epithelial

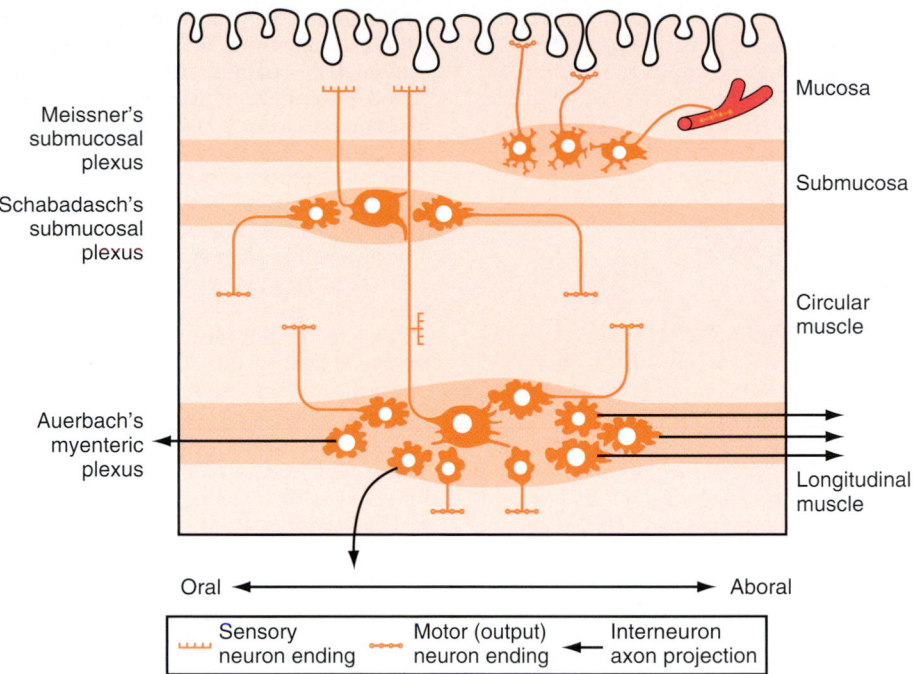

FIGURE 100-4. Diagram showing layers and components of the intestinal wall. The lumen is at the *top* and the longitudinal muscle layer is at the *bottom*. Auerbach's myenteric plexus and the submucosal plexuses (Meissner's and Schabadasch's plexuses) are shown, along with some of their major classes of enteric neurons. The networks of interstitial cells are shown in Figure 100-1.

secretion. Hence, these pathways inhibit colonic motor activity, reduce blood flow, and inhibit secretion to limit water loss from the body during times of sympathetic activation. In addition, some sympathetic axons innervate the smooth muscle directly, particularly the ileocecal junction and internal anal sphincter, where they cause contraction; these effects are also consistent with closing down enteric motor activity during sympathetic arousal.

Parasympathetic Innervation

The colon receives parasympathetic innervation from both the vagus nerve and pathways in the sacral spinal cord. Branches of the vagus nerve reach the prevertebral ganglia (superior hypogastric plexus) and then run with sympathetic axons to the cecum and the ascending and transverse colon. The distal colon is largely supplied by sacral parasympathetic axons via the pelvic nerves (pelvic splanchnic nerves). Some of these cholinergic spinal efferent neurons synapse first onto nerve cell bodies in the pelvic plexus (inferior hypogastric plexus), and others project directly to the colon. From their point of entry into the colon, many of the axons run in an orad direction and form thick trunks called *shunt fascicles*. Parasympathetic axons project to the enteric ganglia in the colon, where they make excitatory cholinergic synapses onto enteric nerve cell bodies. Sacral parasympathetic pathways play an important role in increasing the propulsive activity of the distal colon before defecation. They are probably also involved in triggering the sequences of propagating complexes that start in the transverse and ascending colon up to an hour before defecation.

Extrinsic Afferent Pathways

Sensation from the colon is mediated by primary afferent neurons with cell bodies outside the bowel wall. Vagal afferent neurons with nerve cell bodies located in the nodose ganglia project to the proximal colon and run with the vagal efferent parasympathetic pathways. Currently, their exact role in reflex control and sensation is not clear, but they are unlikely to be involved in the transmission of pain sensation from the colon.

The entire colon also is innervated by spinal primary afferent neurons with nerve cell bodies in the lumbar dorsal root ganglia. Lumbar spinal afferents project along the lumbar splanchnic nerves, through the prevertebral inferior mesenteric ganglion, and through the lumbar colonic nerves to the colon, where they terminate in sensory endings in the mesentery, muscular layers, and mucosa throughout the entire colon and rectum. In addition, a population of spinal afferents with cell bodies in the sacral dorsal root ganglia projects along the pelvic nerves to the colon and traverses the pelvic plexus en route. Evidence indicates that many sacral spinal afferent neurons comprise a functionally distinct population from the lumbar spinal afferents. Sacral afferents include many mechanoreceptors with low thresholds and wide dynamic ranges; these mechanoreceptors are probably responsible for graded sensations of rectal filling and activating defecatory reflexes.[8]

Lumbar spinal afferents, in contrast to spinal afferents, have much higher thresholds. These sensory neurons and some higher-threshold sacral afferents are responsible for generating pain sensations from all regions of the colon and rectum. They respond to gross distention of the bowel wall, traction on the mesenteric membranes, powerful colonic contractions, or chemical stimulation of the mucosa by bile acids, high osmolarity, and other stimuli. It is well established that the sensitivity of many spinal afferents is greatly increased by inflammation in the colon wall. In addition to their role in sensation, spinal afferents also have axon branches (collaterals) in enteric ganglia and prevertebral sympathetic ganglia and on mucosal blood vessels, where they might play a role in generating peripheral reflex responses to noxious stimuli.

In summary, sacral afferent and efferent (parasympathetic) pathways run in parallel and connect the distal bowel with neural circuitry in the sacral spinal cord via pelvic and rectal nerves. The important role of these pathways in both rectal sensation and generating the enhanced motility required for defecation is clearly demonstrated by the effects of nerve lesions at several levels. Thus, severing of peripheral nerves and distal spinal cord injury can lead to loss of rectal sensation and to severely impaired defecatory ability.

ANORECTAL ANATOMY AND INNERVATION

Although the rectum is in direct continuity with the colon, the longitudinal muscle layer within this region is not organized into teniae; rather, it forms a continuous outer layer, uniformly encircling the rectum and insinuating between the internal and external anal sphincters to the distal end of the anal canal. The narrowed distal rectum, or anorectal junction, is formed by the longitudinal muscle coat of the rectum, which is joined by the sling fibers of the puborectalis muscle, attachments of the levator ani muscles, and proximal margins of the internal and external anal sphincters.

The puborectalis and levator ani muscles have important roles in maintaining continence and in defecation. These striated muscles form part of the pelvic floor and are in a state of constant tone that serves to pull the rectum anteriorly and elevate it, thereby reducing the anorectal angle; this mechanical effect tends to prevent entry of stool into the upper anal canal.

The *internal anal sphincter* is a thickened band of smooth muscle with relatively high spontaneous tone that is in continuity with the circular smooth muscle of the rectum. By contrast, the *external anal sphincter* is a striated muscle and is located distal to but partly overlying the internal sphincter. The external sphincter also has a high resting tone, but unlike that of its internal counterpart, its tone can be influenced by voluntary efforts to help maintain continence.

As expected, the sources of innervation of the internal and external anal sphincters are different. The internal sphincter directly receives a powerful inhibitory innervation from intrinsic enteric inhibitory motor neurons and also extrinsic input from lumbar sympathetic and sacral parasympathetic nerves that project via the pelvic plexus ganglia. The external anal sphincter and other pelvic floor muscles are innervated through the pudendal nerve (S3-S4) by motor neurons with cell bodies in the spinal cord. The external sphincter and surrounding connective tissue also receive a sensory innervation via the pudendal nerves. In contrast, the rectum and proximal anal canal are richly supplied with sensory receptors of pelvic nerve origin that respond to rectal stretch and the composition of the intraluminal contents. These receptors are important for detecting rectal filling, triggering sensations of urgency, facilitating rectal accommodation, and differentiating the composition (stool or gas) of rectal content (see Chapters 98 and 129).

RELATIONSHIPS AMONG CELLULAR EVENTS, PRESSURE, AND FLOW

Layers of the intestinal wall that include the smooth muscle, mucosa, and connective tissue can collectively be regarded as a viscoelastic body. The mechanical properties of this body comprise a "contractile element" that generates tone or contraction, a "series elastic element," and a "parallel element" that corresponds to connective tissue.[9]

Under the combined influence of enteric neuronal and myogenic mechanisms, smooth muscle can generate both active contractions and active relaxations. Contractions result from the entry of Ca^{2+} ions via voltage-dependent channels (L-type Ca^{2+} channels), often in the form of smooth muscle action potentials. These propagate modestly across the gap junctions between muscle cells and lead to relatively localized nonpropagating areas of contraction.

The mechanical state of intestinal muscle is described by the plot of changes in stress against strain; the slope is referred to as *compliance*. When muscle is activated by either excitatory enteric neuronal input or depolarizing myogenic mechanisms, it tends to generate tension, shorten, or both. This means that the stress/strain relationship becomes steeper, and compliance is decreased. How much it can shorten is determined by the resistance of the contents. However, passive viscoelastic properties of the intestine, including stress relaxation, creep, and hysteresis, make this analysis complex.[10]

Changes in compliance reflect the extent to which the bowel wall can stretch to accommodate contents. A muscle that is very distensible, because of powerful inhibitory motor neuron activity, is said to have a high compliance. During muscular excitation, the resistance of the bowel wall to stretch increases and is said to have a low compliance for the time it is activated. If bowel contents are fluid and there is no downstream resistance to impede flow, activated smooth muscle will rapidly shorten. The contents will then be propelled, with a minimal increase in intraluminal pressure. By contrast, if resistance to forward flow of contents is high (e.g., by a lumen-occluding contraction distally), activated smooth muscle will not shorten and propulsion will not occur, but wall tension will increase, causing a rise in intraluminal pressure. From this brief consideration, it should be clear that deducing the relationships among intraluminal pressure, propulsion of content, and excitation of smooth muscle from any of the recording techniques listed above ("Methods to Record Colonic Motility") is more complex than is sometimes appreciated.

COLONIC AND ANORECTAL MOTOR PATTERNS

Nonpropagating Motor Patterns

Most published literature detailing colonic motor patterns describes an abundance of nonpropagating random phasic pressure waves. This activity is presumed to serve segmenting or mixing functions. The predominant frequency of nonpropagating colonic contractions in vivo is generally 2 to 4 cycles per minute, similar to the frequency of the spontaneous myogenic slow waves generated by ICC_{SM} at the submucosal border of the circular muscle.[6] With the recent development of high-resolution fiberoptic colonic manometry,[11] it has become apparent that a proportion of the "nonpropagating activity" actually consists of relatively low-amplitude contractions that propagate over short distances (<9 cm). These propagating motor patterns were often misclassified in previous studies of colonic manometry, because the sensors in the manometry catheters were spaced too far apart (7 to 12 cm) to identify their propagating nature (Fig. 100-5).[12] Despite the new insights provided by colonic high-resolution manometry, isolated nonpropagating contractions, usually of relatively low amplitude, are still seen throughout the colon (see Fig. 100-5).

Propagating Motor Patterns

When enteric excitatory motor neurons are strongly activated, powerful lumen-occlusive contractions often result. These can last longer than slow waves and can propagate substantial

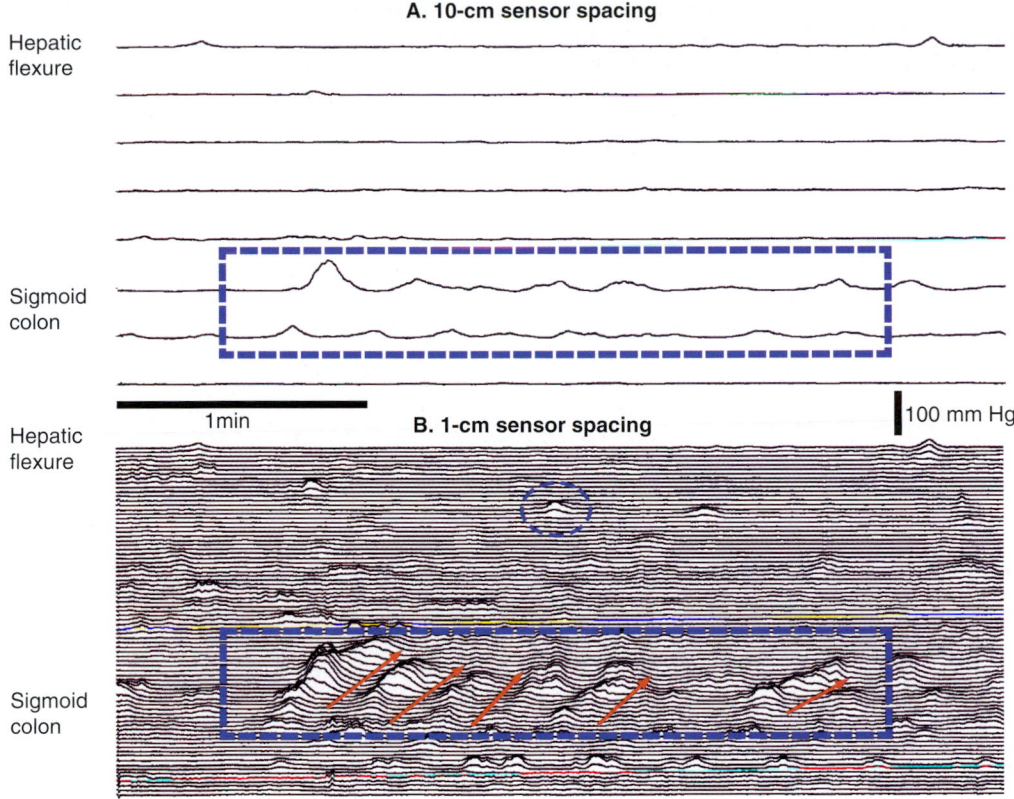

FIGURE 100-5. Section of a colonic manometry tracing recorded by a high-resolution fiberoptic manometry catheter in a healthy control subject. A subset of the data is displayed in *(A)*, in which data from every 10th sensor are shown. *Panel A* represents a traditional low-resolution manometry recording. Nonpropagating activity can be seen in the blue hatched box. In *(B)*, the complete data set is shown. Note that the nonpropagating activity shown in *(A)* actually consists of a series of retrograde-propagating contractions *(red arrows)* that travel a short distance along the colon. These motor patterns are not evident in the low-resolution recording. It is also apparent that even with high-resolution recording, there remain some episodes of nonpropagating activity *(blue hatched circle)*.

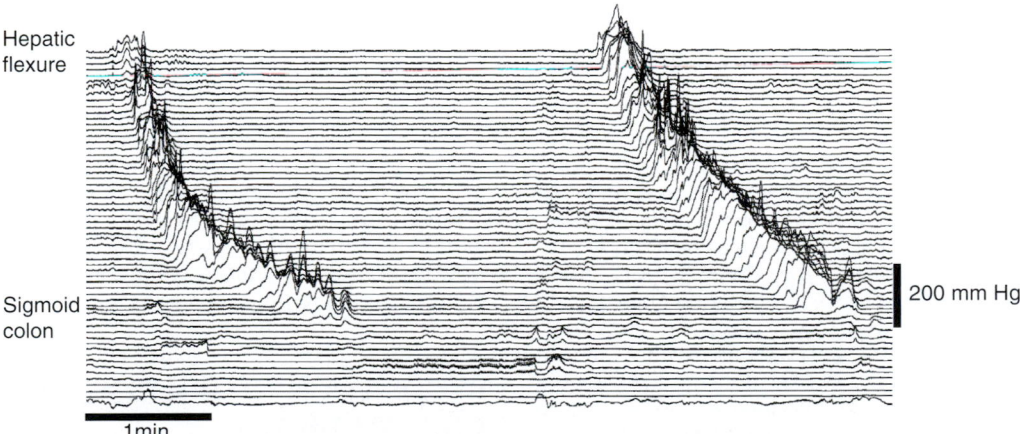

FIGURE 100-6. Two high-amplitude propagating sequences recorded in a healthy control subject. These motor patterns propagate in an anal direction and represent the manometric equivalets of colonic mass movement.

distances along the colon. These colonic motor patterns are readily identifiable and commonly referred to as *high-amplitude propagating sequences* (also termed *propagating contractions* or *high-amplitude propagating contractions* [HAPCs]). HAPCs propagate toward the anus (Fig. 100-6). Low-amplitude propagating sequences are also recorded in the colon and can

be further classified as *antegrade* (aboral) or *retrograde* (orad). Based on low-resolution manometric recordings, it was reported that in the healthy colon, antegrade propagating sequences are at least three-fold more abundant than retrograde propagating sequences.[13] High-resolution colonic manometry recordings, however, show that the converse is

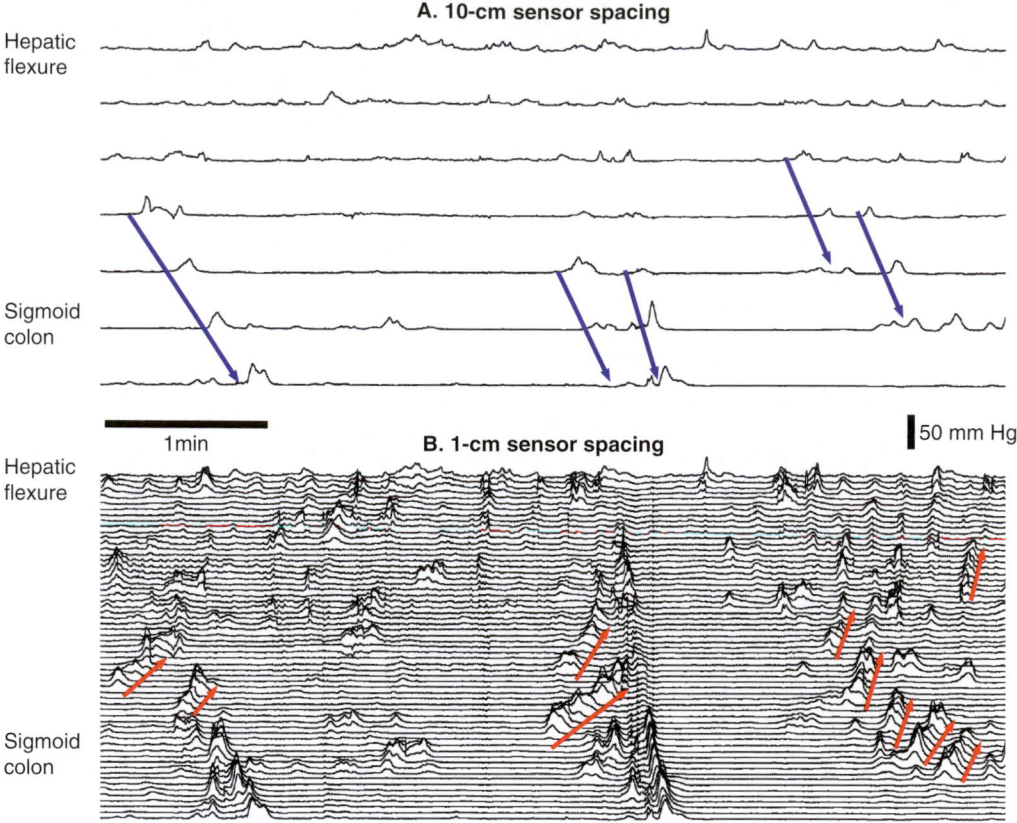

FIGURE 100-7. Section of a colonic manometry tracing recorded by a high-resolution fiberoptic manometry catheter in a healthy control subject. Data are displayed as *(A)* a low-resolution recording (10-cm spacing) and *(B)* high-resolution recording (1-cm spacing). In *(A)*, a series of apparent anally propagating motor patterns can be seen (antegrade propagating sequences *[blue arrows]*). However, when the complete data set is viewed, these propagating events can be seen to move in an oral direction (retrograde propagating sequences *[red arrows]*). A catheter with sensors spaced at 10-cm intervals does not provide sufficient resolution to record some of the propagating events that exist in the colon.

actually true.[12,14] Short-extent motor patterns that propagate in a retrograde direction are the predominant colonic activity in the descending and sigmoid colon (Fig. 100-7).

Rectal Motor Complexes

Periodic contractile activity predominates in the sigmoid colon and rectum. This activity is commonly termed the *rectal motor complex* (RMC) or *periodic rectal motor activity* (PRMA). The mean RMC amplitude ranges from 15 to 60 mm Hg, with the duration of complexes falling into the range of 3 to 30 minutes.[13] The RMC is reported to be more prevalent during sleep, which suggests that extrinsic neural input (sympathetic or parasympathetic) may partially suppress this pattern during the hours we are awake. The relationship between the RMC and flow is still incompletely understood. RMCs can be triggered by propagating pressure waves from the proximal colon and by the arrival of stool or gas from the sigmoid colon.[15] During defecation in both humans and animals, RMCs are inhibited, which suggests that RMCs provide a braking mechanism to keep the rectum empty. Consistent with this, recent high-resolution colonic recordings show that the RMCs can be composed of a series of the short-extent retrograde propagating events that probably retard flow (Fig. 100-8).[12] Motor patterns with similar characteristics of the RMCs have been recorded throughout the colon, which suggests that "rectal" motor complex may not be an accurate descriptor of this motor pattern.[2]

Regional Variation of Propagating Sequences

Contractile activity in the human colon demonstrates marked regional variation. For example, high-amplitude propagating sequences originate almost exclusively in the proximal colon and propagate up to or beyond the splenic flexure. The short-extent retrograde propagating pressure waves (previously mislabeled as "nonpropagating pressure waves") make up a higher proportion of activity in the distal colon.[13] Thus, motor activity in the distal colon may function to retard forward flow (see Relationships between Colonic Motor Patterns and Flow).

REGULATION OF COLONIC FILLING AND TRANSIT

Role of the Ileocecal Junction

In humans, the ileocecal junction regulates colonic filling and prevents coloileal reflux, thereby largely preventing contamination of the small bowel with colonic bacteria.[16] In the fasting state, cecal filling is slow and erratic, and chyme is retained in the distal ileum for prolonged periods.[17] The close physical link between the terminal ileum and the cecum by the ileocecal ligaments behaves functionally as a valve and is responsible in part for continence of the ileocecal junction. A specialized

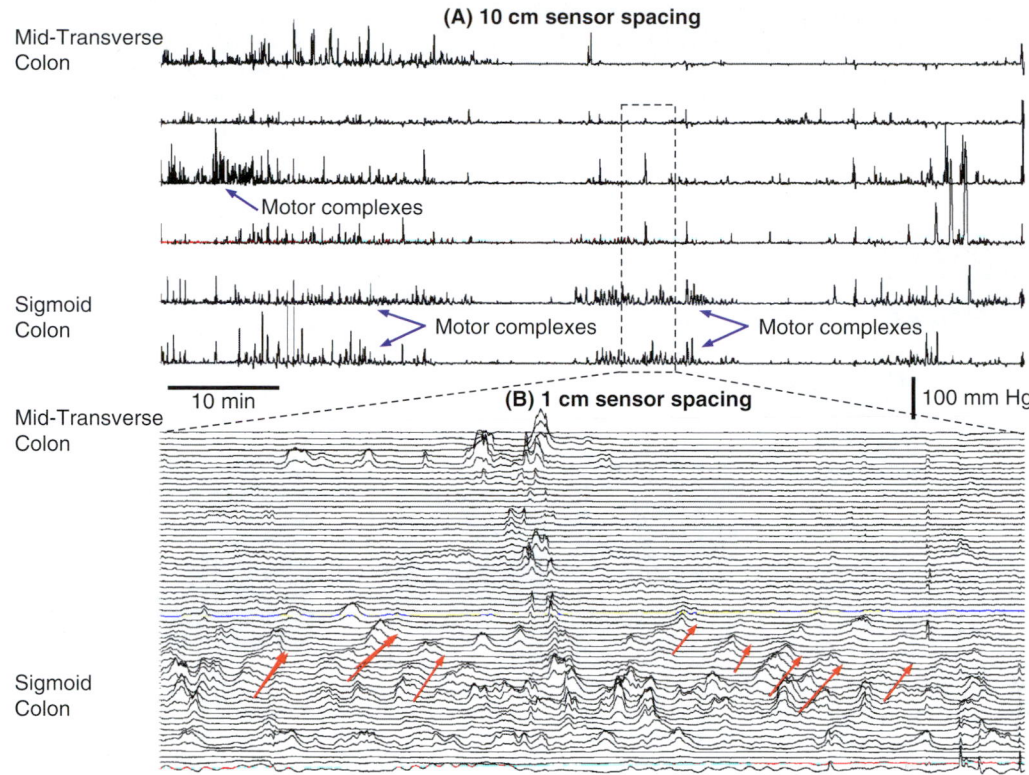

FIGURE 100-8. Section of a colonic manometry tracing recorded by a high-resolution fiberoptic manometry catheter in a healthy control subject. A compressed 90-minute section of tracing is shown in *(A)* at low-resolution recording (10-cm spacing). In this section of tracing, several motor complexes can be seen *(blue arrows)*. B, When a small section *(hatched black rectangle)* of the tracing in *(A)* is expanded and displayed at high resolution, the rectal motor complex can be seen to consist of a series of retrograde propagating sequences.

band of muscle forms a low-pressure tonic sphincter[18] and prominent 6 cycles-per-minute (cpm) phasic contractions contribute to the resistance of the ileocecal junction. Phasic and tonic activity are inhibited concurrently with episodic terminal ileal flow or distention of the ileum. Conversely, the tone of the ileocecal junction increases during cecal distention.[18]

Phase III of the interdigestive motor cycle (or migrating myoelectric-motor complex), a motor pattern that occurs every 90 to 120 minutes in the upper intestine during fasting (see Chapter 99), does not contribute to ileocecal transit because it rarely reaches the terminal ileum in humans. Ileal propagating contractions, synchronized with inhibition of phasic contractions of the ileocecal junction, account for most ileocecal propulsion, which occurs in a pulsatile fashion within 90 minutes of a meal. Prolonged studies that correlate ileocecal movement of isotope with intraluminal pressures show that 72% of episodes of ileocecal transport result from monophasic ileal propagating pressure waves.[16] Furthermore, 93% of cecal propagating pressure waves were temporally associated with episodes of cecal filling. This suggests that episodic cecal filling may be one of the triggers for proximal colonic high-amplitude propagating contractions (Fig. 100-9).[16]

The Colon as a Storage Organ

In 1902, Cannon[19] proposed that the proximal colon is the major site of storage and mixing, whereas the distal colon acts as a conduit for expulsion. His conclusions were based on radiologic observations. Subsequent studies, however, found no difference in the dwell time for radiopaque markers in the proximal, middle, and distal colon: roughly 11 hours in each.

Composition of the diet influences regional transit and probably accounts for some of the discrepancies between studies. With a liquid diet, the ascending colon empties rapidly, within 1 to 2 hours, whereas the transverse colon retains isotope for 20 to 40 hours.[20] A solid diet is associated with slower transit through the cecum and ascending colon. With a mixed diet, particulate matter and liquids are stored in both the ascending and transverse colon.[21]

Relationships between Colonic Motor Patterns and Flow

Emptying of the proximal colon accelerates when wall tone is increased (e.g., by intraluminal fatty acids) compared with when tone is low; volume and consistency of the contents also affect the rate of emptying. Isotonic fluid infused into the proximal colon stimulates proximal colonic emptying, which suggests that distention per se can activate propulsive motor patterns. However, irritant laxatives in the proximal colon (which act by stimulating mucosal receptors) trigger propagating contractions much more reliably than distention alone.[22] Hence, proximal colonic emptying depends on both increased wall tone and propagating contractions, probably under the influence of both chemical and mechanical factors.

Mass movements, first detected radiologically, are infrequent movements of stool over long distances. More often, movement of colonic content occurs in a stepwise manner over short distances and in both antegrade and retrograde directions.[23] By combining manometric and radiologic studies in animals, or with high frame-rate scintigraphy in humans, it has been shown that 93% of all propagating sequences in the

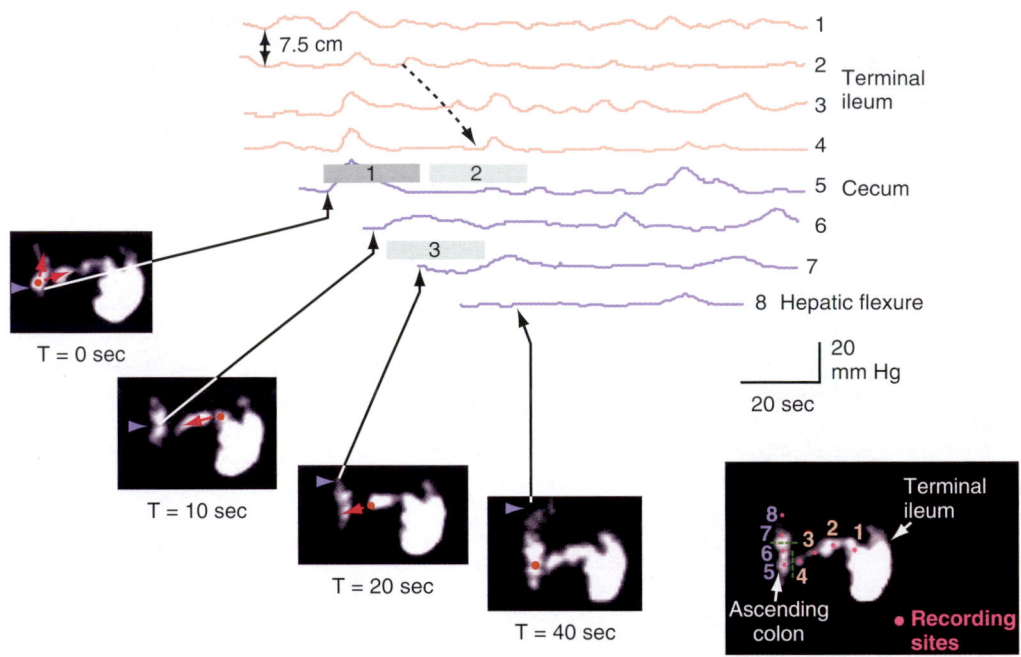

FIGURE 100-9. Propagating pressure wave sequences identified in the terminal ileum and proximal colon during prolonged combined scintigraphic and manometric recordings. *Bottom left corner of far right box* shows a scintigraphic image of technetium sulfur colloid in the terminal ileum and ascending colon of a healthy control subject. *Pink circles* indicate the location of the recording side holes, each spaced at 7.5 cm. *Green hatched lines* indicate the regions where luminal flow was recorded. Four scintigraphic images have been selected to indicate flow across the ileocolonic junction *(solid bars 1 and 2)* and mid-ascending colon *(solid bar 3)*. *Black arrows* correspond to the time (horizontal axis) of acquisition of each 10-second scintigraphic frame. *Small blue arrowheads* on scintiscans indicate the location of the manometric side hole from which the corresponding pressure tracing was recorded. Corresponding with the scintigraphic frame at T = 0, a cecal pressure wave is recorded. This cecal pressure wave initiates an ascending colonic propagating sequence that was temporally associated with coloileal reflux *(solid bar 1)* and flow across the mid-ascending colon *(solid bar 2)*. During the coloileal reflux, an ileal propagating sequence is initiated *(hatched black arrow)*, and this ileal propagating sequence is temporally associated with antegrade flow across the ileocolonic junction *(solid bar 3)*. *Red circle* on scintiscan images T = 0 to T = 40 follows the direction of retrograde flow from cecum to ileum (T = 0 and T =10 sec) and then antegrade flow from the ileum to cecum (T = 20 sec and T = 40 sec).

proximal colon, regardless of amplitude or polarity, are temporally associated with discrete movements of isotope-labeled colonic contents within the unprepared colon (Fig. 100-10).[23]

Previous studies attempting to correlate pressure and flow have shown that more than half of the antegrade movements of colonic content were attributed to repetitive nonpropagating pressure waves. As described earlier, it is likely many of these "nonpropagating" pressure waves do actually propagate over short distances (see Fig. 100-5), so it is not surprising that they propel content. Nonetheless, some movement of content cannot be attributed to identifiable changes in intraluminal pressure using current technology. As described in the section "Relationships among Cellular Events, Pressure, and Flow," some unexplained propulsion may be caused by muscle activity that does not generate significant intraluminal pressure. This may include longitudinal muscle shortening, some non–lumen-occluding circular muscle contractions, or alterations in regional wall tone, especially when downstream resistance to flow is low.

Retrograde movements occur frequently. About half of retrograde contractions follow immediately after an antegrade movement, indicating frequent reflux of content back into the region from which it had just moved. Some retrograde flow, particularly in the distal colon, is likely to be associated with short-extent retrograde propagating pressure waves.

Interesting insights into the propulsion of colonic content have come from ingestible capsule-based techniques. The Magnetic Tracking System (MTS [Motilis Medica SA,

Lausanne, Switzerland])[24] accurately tracks a magnet housed in an ingested capsule with an accuracy of less than 1 cm. Studies in healthy controls indicate that slow, retrograde movement from the transverse colon to the caecum can occur over 4 to 5 hours, before rapid forward propulsion to the descending colon (presumably associated with high-amplitude propagating events).

In summary, apart from the immediate pre-defecatory phase (see later), the distal colon displays a high frequency of short-extent retrograde propagating pressure waves. In contrast, the proximal colon displays more higher-amplitude propagating events. Thus, motor patterns of the proximal colon move content toward the distal colon. These propulsive antegrade motor patterns are often associated with motor complexes (short-extent retrograde propagating sequences) in the distal colon and rectum (see Rectal Motor Complexes above) that likely retard the flow of colonic contents, prevent rectal filling, and control challenges to continence. The relatively high frequency of short-extent retrograde propagating events probably also causes some mixing of content, which assists the colon in performing its critical function of absorption of water, salts, and electrolytes.

DEFECATION

The propagating motor activity in the distal colon as just described would limit or even prevent colonic contents

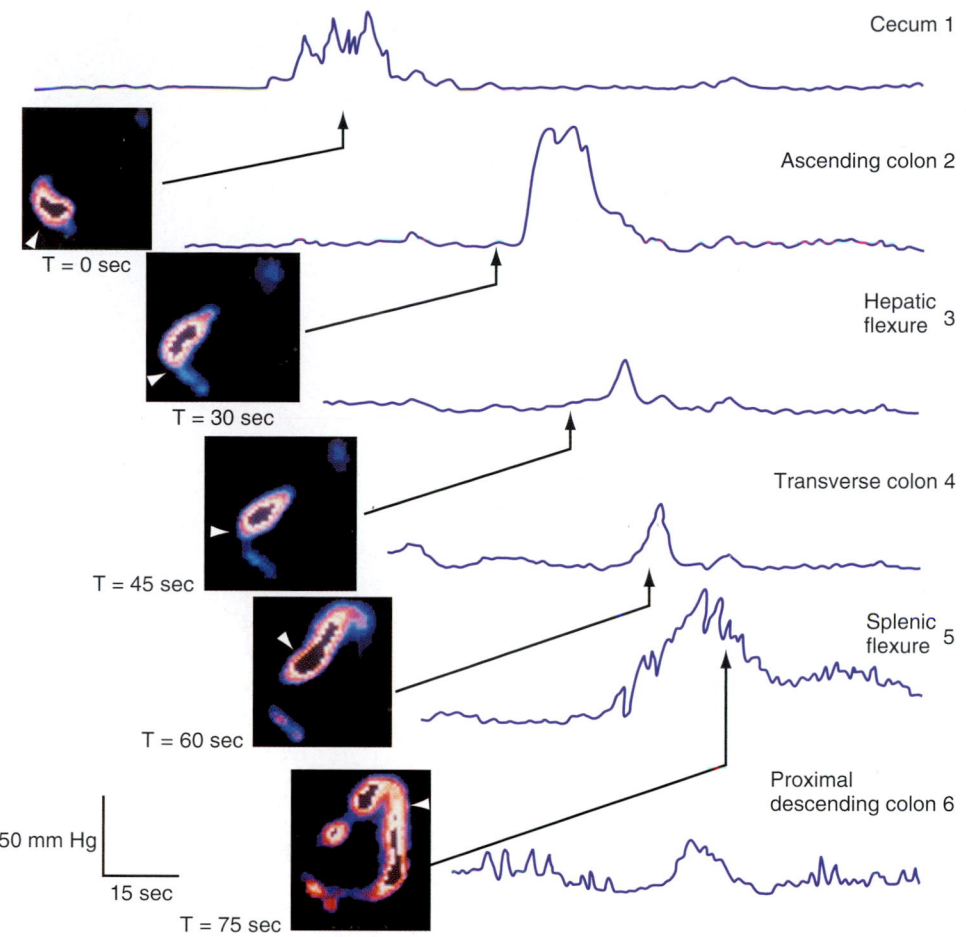

FIGURE 100-10. Intracolonic pressure measurements and corresponding scintiscans that show a clear correlation between a propagating pressure wave sequence and discrete movement of colonic contents from the cecum to the sigmoid colon. This particular movement of contents was not associated with defecation or sensation. *Oblique lines ending in vertical arrows* correspond to the time of acquisition of each 15-second scintigraphic frame. *Small arrowheads* on scintiscans indicate the location of the manometric side hole from which the corresponding pressure tracing was recorded. In the proximal colon and mid-colon *(channels 2, 3, and 4 from the top)*, a close temporal relationship exists between movement of the isotope and onset of the propagating pressure wave upstroke. When the pressure wave reaches the splenic flexure, however, the proximal descending colon is seen to expand to accommodate the isotope, consistent with loss of lumen occlusion at this region. The pressure waves in channels 5 and 6 do not appear to correspond to lumen-occluding contractions. Note also that propagating pressure-wave amplitudes in channels 3 and 4 are only 30 and 39 mm Hg, respectively, yet the motor pattern is clearly propulsive. *(From Cook IJ, Furukawa Y, Panagopoulos V, et al. Relationships between spatial patterns of colonic pressure and individual movements of content. Am J Physiol 2000; 278:G329.)*

from ever reaching the rectum and being expelled. Clearly, additional mechanisms must occur from time to time that lead to defecation. Traditionally, defecation was conceptualized as an exclusively anorectal function, although it is now clear that colonic activity is widely integrated in the defecatory sequence.

Radiopaque markers and scintigraphic recordings have shown that a large proportion of the entire colonic content is evacuated in some cases. Furthermore, pancolonic manometric studies have demonstrated that the preparatory phase of defecation may involve most of the colon's length; it can also commence up to 1 hour before stool expulsion.[25] In this predefecatory phase, the high-amplitude propagating pressure waves occur in a characteristic sequence. The first ones start in the proximal colon, with each successive sequence originating slightly more distal than the preceding one. These first priming sequences do not evoke conscious sensation but

successively propel content distally. In the 15 minutes leading up to defecation, a dramatic increase occurs in the frequency of these propagating sequences, which leads to a strong, conscious defecatory urge. During this late phase, propagating pressure waves originate in the distal colon, but each successive propagating sequence originates from a site *proximal* to the preceding one. Each sequence also tends to run for a slightly longer distance and has a higher amplitude than its predecessor (Fig. 100-11). These final sequences generate the forces necessary to fill and distend the rectum with semisolid fecal matter. As the distal sigmoid and rectum are distended, specialized low-threshold sacral spinal afferent mechanoreceptors are activated. These mechanoreceptors then give rise to the defecatory urge, prompting the expulsive phase in which the anorectum comes into play. This is assisted by activation of sacral parasympathetic pathways to the distal bowel.

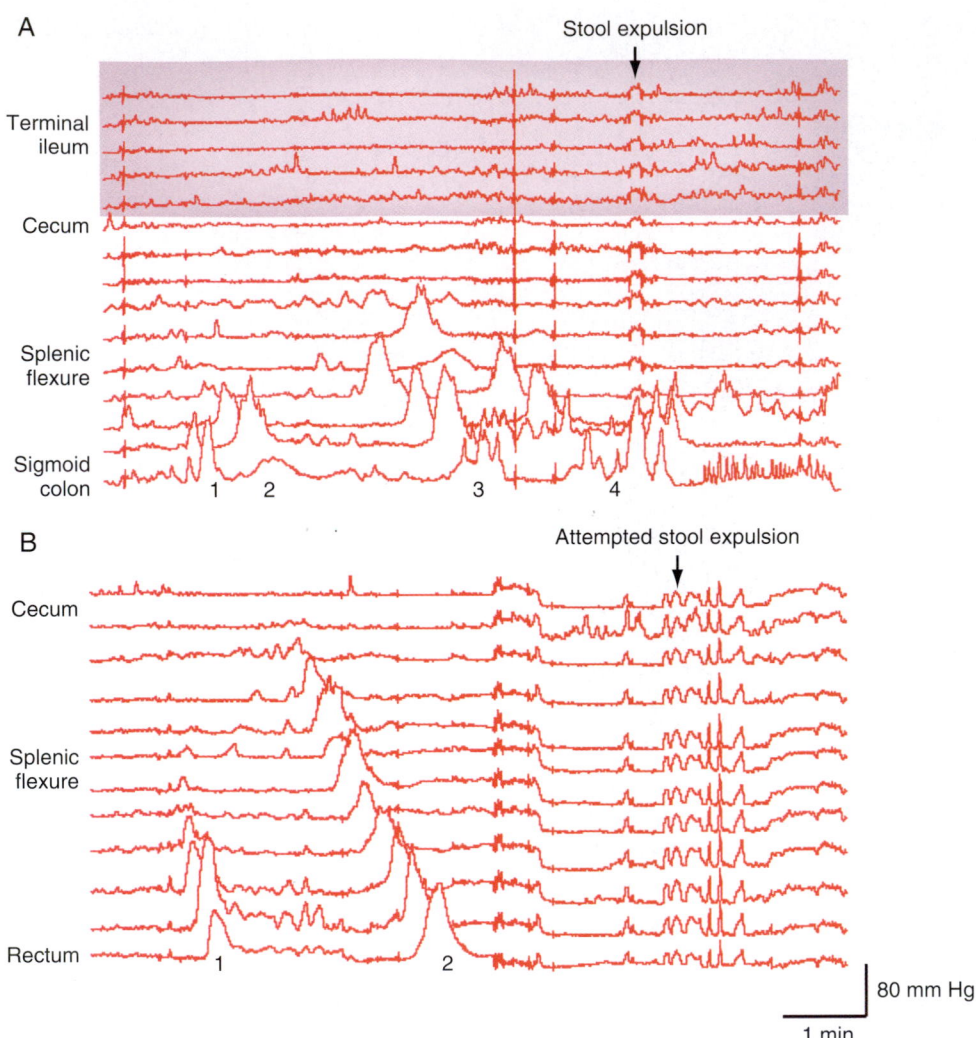

FIGURE 100-11. Intracolonic pressures leading to spontaneous defecation by the healthy human colon. Recordings were made with a perfused Silastic catheter passed transnasally to produce 15 recording sites at 7.5-cm intervals. *A,* Stool expulsion is preceded by four propagating sequences *(1-4)*, the last of which actually was associated with stool expulsion. Each propagating sequence originates from a site more proximal than the preceding sequence. Note also the increase in amplitude and slowing of propagation velocity with successive sequences leading to stool expulsion. *B,* Two propagating sequences *(1-2)* precede defecation; however, attempted stool expulsion is associated with straining only. *(From Bampton PA, Dinning PG, Kennedy ML, et al. Spatial and temporal organization of pressure patterns throughout the unprepared colon during spontaneous defecation. Am J Gastroenterol 2000; 98:1027.)*

Rectal Filling, Capacitance, Accommodation, and Motility

When stool or gas enters the rectum, the rectal wall is stretched, thereby activating an enteric descending inhibitory reflex that causes transient relaxation of the internal anal sphincter. Simultaneously, an extrinsic reflex pathway is activated, leading to a brief contraction of the external anal sphincter that preserves continence. The recto-anal inhibitory reflex can be demonstrated and tested by balloon distention of the rectum; its presence reflects the integrity of enteric neural pathways. Thus, the recto-anal inhibitory reflex is absent in Hirschsprung's disease, which is characterized by loss of enteric ganglia in the distal bowel. In health, this reflex permits entry of a small amount of content into the upper anal canal, but continence is maintained by the reflexive contraction of the external anal sphincter. This then allows sampling of content by sensory receptors in the proximal anal canal, allowing solid or liquid stool and gas to be distinguished. Sampling reflexes of this kind occur many times each day in response to small rectal distentions. These are generally not registered consciously and do not cause an urge to defecate.

A large-volume rectal distention causes an internal sphincter relaxation of longer duration that is registered consciously. Often an extra voluntary contraction of the external anal sphincter is needed to maintain continence while the person decides how best to deal with the intraluminal content (stool or gas). Suppression of the defecation urge at this time, together with receptive accommodation of the rectum (see later), results in temporary storage of content in the rectum. Typically this is followed by gradual retrograde propulsion back to the sigmoid colon. Although the rectum is usually empty, it has the capacity to temporarily store feces until evacuation is convenient. Rectal storage is facilitated by the ability of the rectum to accommodate an increasing volume without a corresponding increase in intrarectal pressure, in a manner

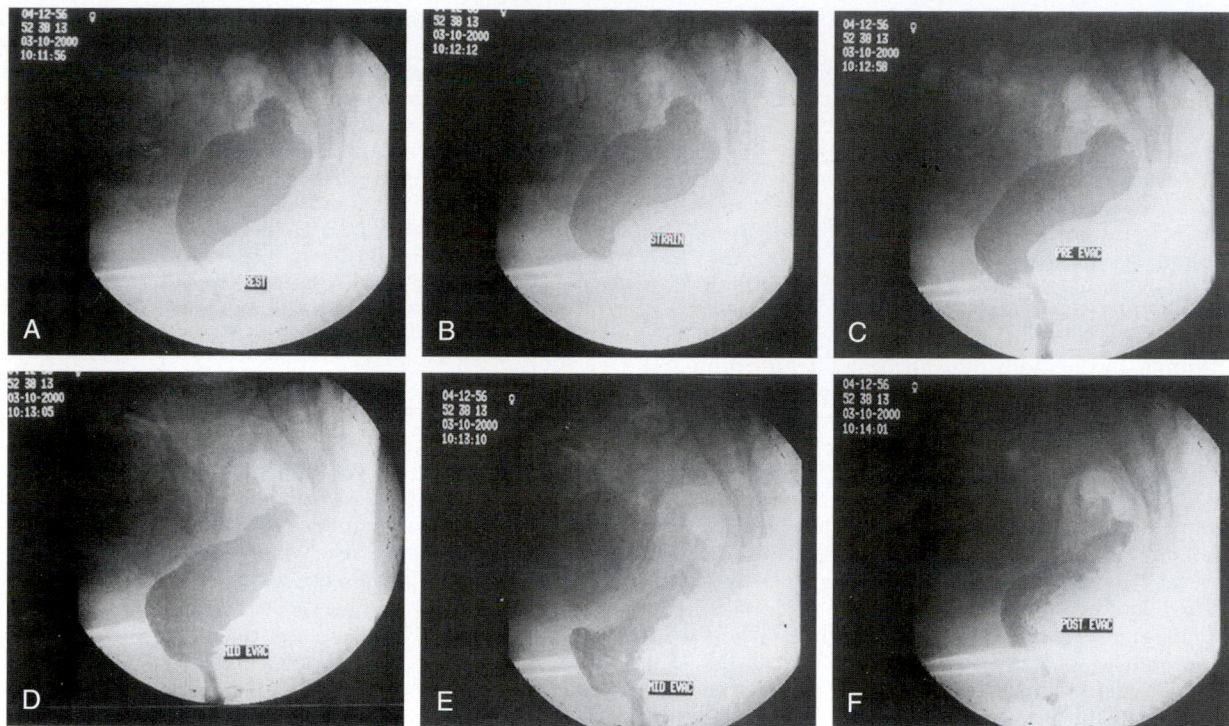

FIGURE 100-12. Some of the mechanical processes that facilitate stool expulsion, as illustrated by sequential films of a simulated defecation of thickened barium during defecation proctography. *A,* Rectum at rest, with a normal resting angle of approximately 90 degrees; anal canal is closed. *B,* On straining, as the anterior rectal wall begins to flatten, the proximal anal canal begins to funnel as barium contrast is forced into it. *C,* As more pressure is exerted, the anterior rectal wall flattens further, contrast fills the anal canal, and evacuation begins. At this time, the puborectalis muscle and external anal sphincter are relaxing, resulting in onset of descent of the rectoanal junction. At the same time, the levator ani muscles are activated and help control the descent of the rectoanal junction (note posterior indentation resulting from contraction of pubococcygeus muscle). *D,* Puborectalis is fully relaxed; this, in combination with vigorous straining, has resulted in nearly complete descent of the rectoanal junction. Note the position of rectoanal junction, which in this frame is well below the horizontal pale artifact (due to the water-filled toilet seat), compared with that in the previous frame, in which the junction is level with this artifact. This descent has now opened up the anorectal angle, thereby further reducing the resistance to outflow through the anal canal. *E,* Rectal emptying continues, and anterior rectal compression is more obvious. *F,* After evacuation, the anorectal junction has ascended to its original position, and the anorectal angle has returned to its more acute resting angle. *(Courtesy Prof. D.Z. Lubowski, Hurstville, New South Wales.)*

similar to gastric fundic relaxation.[26] This adaptive increase in rectal compliance, mediated by enteric inhibitory nerves, is important for maintaining continence, because it allows fecal storage without a constant urge to defecate. Such rectal distention also has negative feedback effects on the proximal bowel and inhibits gastric emptying, slows small bowel transit, reduces the frequency of proximal colonic propagating pressure waves, and delays colonic transit.[27] Typically, rectal tone is increased following a meal. Under some conditions, pathologic reduction of rectal compliance occurs (e.g., after pelvic radiotherapy). This increases the persistence of rectal urgency. Conversely, excessive compliance, as in megarectum, attenuates the urge to defecate. These findings are consistent with the features of the low-threshold rectal mechanoreceptors that are activated by intramural tension.

Anorectal Motility during Defecation

If the processes just described give rise to the urge to defecate and the social circumstances are appropriate, the full defecation process is activated. This involves a combination of pelvic reflexes coordinated in the medulla and pons. Rectal distention by stool stimulates complete relaxation of the internal anal sphincter via enteric reflexes, and the stool moves into the upper anal canal, heightening the sense of urge. Postural

changes and straining facilitate this process in several ways. Sitting or squatting causes descent of the anorectal junction, and straining produces further rectal descent. Both activities serve to increase the anorectal angle, thereby reducing resistance to outflow. At this point, if the person wishes to proceed to expel stool, the external anal sphincter is relaxed voluntarily. At the same time, the puborectalis muscle is relaxed (further increasing the anorectal angle), the levator ani muscles contract, the perineum descends further, and stool is funneled into the anal canal and expelled by increasing strain-induced intrarectal pressure (Fig. 100-12). Once the expulsion phase has commenced, evacuation of stool can proceed in some cases without further straining, as a consequence of colonic contractions propagating toward the anus (see Fig. 100-11).[25] Expulsion of stool is possible in response to strain alone without rectosigmoid contractions, although a contribution from increased rectal wall tone cannot be excluded.

MODULATORS OF COLONIC MOTILITY

Physiologic

Twenty-four hour recordings of either myoelectric activity or intraluminal pressure show that colonic tone and contractility are increased 1 to 2 hours after a meal (the "gastrocolic" response) and are markedly suppressed at night.[28] During stable sleep, colonic motility virtually ceases—except for the antipropulsive RMCs, which increase—thereby reducing the challenges to continence at a time when anal sphincter tone and awareness of colorectal sensations are minimal. If the subject shifts to a lighter level of sleep, even without actually awakening, an immediate increase occurs in both propagating and nonpropagating pressure waves. Forced awakening at night and spontaneous early-morning awakening both stimulate an immediate increase in colonic propagating pressure waves. This phenomenon is clearly linked with the readily identifiable habit of defecation soon after awakening in the morning and demonstrates the potential for profound modulation of colonic motor activity by the central nervous system.

The entire colon responds predictably to a meal, with an increase in colonic wall tone, migratory long spike-bursts, and propagating and segmenting contractile patterns. A minimum caloric load of approximately 300 kcal is required to generate the colonic response to a meal; a meal of 200 kcal only increases rectal muscle tone.[29] The meal response is highly dependent on the fat content of the caloric load. For example, 600 kcal of fat induces the response, whereas an equicaloric load of protein or carbohydrate does not. The mechanism of the colonic meal response remains unclear, although it is known that neither the stomach nor the spinal cord has to be intact to display the response. Non-nutrient gastric distention by balloon or water can also stimulate rectosigmoid motility, yielding a similar response to that following intraduodenal lipid infusion. Both of these responses are markedly attenuated by prior IV administration of the 5-hydroxytryptamine-3 (5-HT$_3$) receptor antagonist granisetron, which suggests that 5-HT$_3$ receptors on vagal afferents may be involved in the gastrocolic response.[30] Cholecystokinin (CCK), which is released by fats and fatty acids in the duodenum, can replicate the gastrocolic response, but only at doses exceeding those occurring postprandially. The CCK-A antagonist loxiglumide blocks the effects of CCK on the colon but does not abolish the gastrocolic response, thus making CCK an unlikely mediator of the response.

Stress and emotional factors have long been believed to influence colonic motility, but experimental evidence for this is conflicting, possibly because of a reliance on measurements from the distal colon, which might not be representative of the entire colon. In light of the profound waking response cited earlier, it is likely (but unproved) that stress does induce propagating pressure waves. Because of technical difficulties of recording physical activity and colonic motility simultaneously, data on the colonic response to physical activity are sparse. However, physical exercise, perhaps through increased sympathetic tone, decreases colonic motility.[31] The colonic response to stress and exercise highlight the importance of the autonomic nervous system in modulating colonic function. Similarly, autonomic dysfunction resulting from pelvic surgery, childbirth, or neural degradation has been implicated in several colonic disorders, including slow-transit constipation and IBS.[32]

Pharmacologic

Laxatives exert their diarrheal actions by increasing mucosal secretion or by stimulating colonic propulsive activity. For example, the irritant laxative bisacodyl and the bile acid chenodeoxycholic acid both stimulate high-amplitude colonic propagating pressure wave sequences, thereby leading to mass movements. Bisacodyl exerts its motor effect through mucosal afferent nerve fibers; the response can be blocked by

topical application of lidocaine to the mucosa.[22] In addition to the local response, these agents, when administered rectally, can stimulate motor activity in the proximal colon, thereby indicating the existence of long reflex pathways between the rectum and proximal colon.

Colchicine, a natural alkaloid, is well known to cause diarrhea. Colchicine increases the frequency of spontaneous bowel movements and accelerates colonic transit in patients with chronic constipation. The mode of action is not yet clear, but colchicine has been shown to increase prostaglandin synthesis and promote intestinal secretion, the latter mediated through cyclic adenosine monophosphate (cAMP). In the rat, colchicine given into the small intestine stimulates myoelectric activity.[33]

Lubiprostone, a type 2 chloride channel (ClC2) activator, is a member of a new class of compounds known as *prostones*. Activation of ClC2 increases intestinal chloride secretion and results in increased intraluminal fluid accumulation, which accelerates intestinal transit, softens stools, and increases spontaneous stool frequency in patients with constipation. In constipated patients, use of the drug has resulted in slight improvement over placebo, but there are notable side effects, including nausea and headache.[33,34]

Serotonin (5-HT) is an important mediator of bowel physiology, and both 5-HT$_3$ and 5-HT$_4$ receptors play a role in colonic peristalsis and transit. The 5-HT$_3$ receptor antagonists granisetron and ondansetron blunt the gastrocolic response and delay colonic transit, respectively. Alosetron, another antagonist of the 5-HT$_3$ receptor, exerts a significant constipating effect by slowing colonic transit. In contrast, 5-HT$_4$ agonists (e.g., tegaserod, prucalopride, renzapride) act on presynaptic receptors and facilitate release of ACh and other transmitters from enteric nerve terminals, thereby inducing colonic propagating contractions and accelerating colonic transit. Although this class of drug shows promise for the treatment of constipation, tegaserod was withdrawn from the market because of concerns about adverse cardiovascular events. Other highly selective 5-HT$_4$ agonists, such as prucalopride, might be attractive options because they do not interact with 5-HT$_3$ or 5-HT$_{1B}$ receptors, and prucalopride does improve stool frequency and symptoms in severe constipation.[35]

Opiates are well known to have an antidiarrheal effect, but their mechanism of action is less clear. In the human colon, morphine increases phasic segmenting activity, reduces colonic tone, and attenuates the bowel's response to a meal. Opiates are known to inhibit presynaptic and postsynaptic enteric neural circuitry. The reduction in neurally dependent propagating contractions and the enhancement of myogenic mixing movements and fluid absorption contribute to the constipating effect of the drug. Specific constipation syndromes like opiate-induced constipation or postsurgical ileus might respond to opiate antagonists such as methylnaltrexone and alvimopan (see Chapter 124).[36]

Nitric oxide is a potent endogenous inhibitor of colonic propulsive activity, and the human colon appears to be under a state of tonic nitrergic inhibition. For example, infusion of the NO synthase inhibitor L-NMMA (N^G-monomethyl L-arginine) is a potent stimulator of proximal colonic propagating contractions,[37] while sensitizing the distal colon to distention.[38]

Nonpharmacologic

Probiotics are living organisms that, when ingested in adequate amounts, are claimed to exert a health benefit to the host (see Chapter 130). Relatively few rigorously designed studies have been conducted with probiotics, but some strains have been shown to have a beneficial effect in IBS (see Chapter 122), UC (see Chapter 116), and diarrhea. In the colon, probiotics are likely to modulate the inflammatory response through activation of signals with the epithelium and immune system. Probiotics may well influence colonic motility, but this has not yet been systematically evaluated.[39]

Sacral nerve stimulation modulates the extrinsic nerves that innervate the pelvic floor and colon. Electrical stimulation of the S3 sacral root alters motor patterns in patients with slow transit constipation[40] and patients with fecal incontinence,[12] although the precise mode of actions remains unknown. The substantial latency between stimulus and pelvic floor or colonic contractile responses is longer than would be expected via a polysynaptic efferent pathway, which suggests possible involvement of extrinsic sensory pathways. An uncontrolled study utilizing sacral nerve stimulation in patients with constipation has shown some promise in alleviating symptoms.[41]

Acupuncture has significant effects upon upper GI tract disorders like nausea and vomiting (see Chapter 131). Acupuncture reportedly improved stool frequency in children, but these results were not replicated in adults; this warrants further study. Acupuncture is thought to activate neural, opioid, humoral, and serotoninergic pathways and therefore potentially has a clinical role in treating disorders like IBS. To date, however, no study has provided compelling evidence that acupuncture is superior to sham as a treatment for IBS.[42]

Biofeedback has been shown to improve stool frequency and rectal evacuation in patients with pelvic floor dyssynergia, and the technique has been shown to accelerate colonic transit in this subset of patients with constipation (see Chapter 19).[43] The mode of action of biofeedback is not fully understood, but evidence suggests that extrinsic autonomic efferent pathways mediate the response.[44]

DISORDERS OF COLONIC MOTILITY

Disorders due to disturbed colonic motor function are discussed elsewhere in this book (Chapter 124). It is useful, however, to consider how disturbances in the mechanisms of colonic motility described in this chapter might relate to symptoms or pathophysiologic phenomena.

Constipation

One would expect that constipation and diarrhea should be manifestations of hypomotility and hypermotility, respectively. Sometimes this is true, but in the distal colon at least, the converse may be true. An increase in nonpropagating (segmenting) contractions and myoelectrical short spike-bursts has been reported in the rectosigmoid region in constipated patients, which until recently has seemed paradoxical. As discussed earlier, much of this nonpropagating activity probably consists of short-extent retrograde-propagating pressure waves. If this motor pattern retards flow, then increased frequency may contribute to constipation in some patients. Conversely, patients with diarrhea have hypomotility in this region, indicating that a normal physiologic brake (retrograde propagating sequences) has been removed, allowing content to be propelled unheeded into the rectum.

In severe slow-transit constipation, prolonged manometric studies have confirmed a reduction in the overall number of high-amplitude propagating pressure waves,[45] but the overall number of propagating pressure waves of all magnitudes is often normal or increased. In the largest study to date examining the motor patterns of patients with slow-transit

constipation, 41% (of 80 patients) were diagnosed with "normal" motility patterns.[46] The underlying pathogenesis of severe slow-transit constipation is unclear, but changes in enteric excitatory motor innervation of the smooth muscle in patients with severe slow-transit constipation are likely to contribute to this disorder.[32] Constipation is fully discussed in Chapter 19.

Diarrhea

Detailed scintigraphic studies in patients with diarrhea have shown the dominant feature to be early and rapid transit through the ascending and transverse colon. Normally, propagating sequences are more frequent in these proximal regions than elsewhere. Manometric data from the entire colon in patients with diarrhea might help explain these observations but have not yet been reported. A relative lack of distal colonic segmenting activity, perhaps in combination with increased proximal colonic propagating pressure waves, might explain this preferential acceleration of proximal colonic transit, but proof of this hypothesis is awaited. Diarrhea is fully discussed in Chapter 16.

Irritable Bowel Syndrome

Although colonic transit generally is slower in constipation-predominant IBS and faster in diarrhea-predominant IBS, no colonic motor pattern is specific for IBS.[47] Exaggerated responses to stimuli such as meals, CCK, and mechanical stimuli have been reported, but a consistent disturbance has not emerged, probably because of the heterogeneity of the disease and the methodologies used for characterization. In addition, remarkably little study of proximal colon function in IBS has been conducted to date. At present, compelling evidence regarding the pathophysiology of IBS suggests a major contribution by afferent hypersensitivity, in addition to a variable alteration in colonic motor function. IBS is fully discussed in Chapter 122.

Colonic Motility Disturbances Secondary to Nonmotor Intestinal Disorders

Altered motility secondary to underlying inflammation or a hormonal disturbance can contribute to the colonic symptoms of a nonmotor disease. The diarrhea of idiopathic IBD, for example, results from a combination of enhanced secretion, reduced absorption, and altered colonic motor function. In UC, rectosigmoid segmenting nonpropagating pressure waves are diminished, whereas postprandial propagating pressure waves are increased.[21] Rectal compliance is also reduced, and together these effects can exacerbate diarrhea, as suggested by studies demonstrating rapid rectosigmoid transit in UC.[21] The motility of the healthy colon can also be perturbed by ileal diseases. For example, exposure of the healthy proximal colon to supranormal concentrations of bile salts, such as from terminal ileal disease or resection, not only stimulates net colonic secretion but also initiates high-amplitude propagating pressure waves, thereby accelerating colonic transit.[21]

KEY REFERENCES

Full references for this chapter can be found on www.expertconsult.com.

1. Rae MG, Khoyi MA, Keef KD. Modulation of cholinergic neuromuscular transmission by nitric oxide in canine colonic

circular smooth muscle. Am J Physiol Gastrointest Liver Physiol 1998; 275(6 Pt 1):G1324-32.

3. Farrugia G. Ionic conductances in gastrointestinal smooth muscles and interstitial cells of Cajal. Ann Rev Physiol 1999; 61:45-84.

6. Rae M, Fleming N, McGregor D, et al. Control of motility patterns in the human colonic circular muscle layer by pacemaker activity. J Physiol 1998; 510:309-20.

9. Hill AV. First and last experiments in muscle mechanics. Cambridge: University Press; 1970.

10. Costa M, Wiklendt L, Arkwright JW, et al. An experimental method to identify neurogenic and myogenic active mechanical states of intestinal motility. Front Syst Neurosci 2013; 7:7.

11. Arkwright JW, Underhill ID, Maunder SA, et al. Design of a high-sensor count fibre optic manometry catheter for in-vivo colonic diagnostics. Opt Express 2009; 17:22423-31.

12. Patton V, Arkwright JW, Lubowski DZ, Dinning PG. Sacral nerve stimulation alters distal colonic motility in patients with faecal incontinence. Br J Surg 2013; In Press.

13. Scott M. Manometric techniques for the evaluation of colonic motor activity: Current status. Neurogastroenterol Motil 2003; 15:483-513.

14. Dinning PG, Wiklendt L, Gibbins I, et al. Low-resolution colonic manometry leads to a gross mis-interpretation of the frequency and polarity of propagating sequences: Initial results from fibre-optic high-resolution manometry studies. Neurogastroenterol Motil 2013; 25:e640-e649.

22. Hardcastle JD, Mann CV. Study of large bowel peristalsis. Gut 1968; 9:512-20.

24. Hiroz P, Schlageter V, Givel JC, Kucera P. Colonic movements in healthy subjects as monitored by a Magnet Tracking System. Neurogastroenterol Motil 2009; 21:838-57.

25. Bampton P, Dinning P, Kennedy M, et al. Spatial and temporal organization of pressure patterns throughout the unprepared colon during spontaneous defecation. Am J Gastroenterol 2000; 95:1027-35.

32. Bharucha AE, Pemberton JH, Locke GR 3rd. American Gastroenterological Association technical review on constipation. Gastroenterology 2013; 144:218-38.

34. Dinning PG, Scott SM. Novel diagnostics and therapy of colonic motor disorders. Curr Opin Pharmacol 2011; 11:624-9.

35. Tack J. Current and future therapies for chronic constipation. Best Pract Res Clin Gastroenterol 2011; 25:151-8.

101

Intestinal Electrolyte Absorption and Secretion

MRINALINI C. RAO, JAYASHREE SARATHY, AND JOSEPH H. SELLIN

The GI tract processes 8 to 9 L of fluid daily that is derived from oral intake and endogenous exocrine secretions. Intestinal fluid absorption is a process that functions with 98% efficiency, allowing only 100 to 200 mL to be excreted each day. The intestine also extracts nutrients, vitamins, and minerals from ingested materials; excludes destructive antigens and microbes; and excretes waste (Fig. 101-1). This multitasking is achieved by the unique tissue, cellular, and molecular architecture of the small and large intestine in combination with a complex array of intricate regulatory mechanisms (Fig. 101-2). Regulation is accomplished by crosstalk between endocrine and paracrine hormones, neurotransmitters, immunomodulators, and luminal factors. Remarkably, this orchestration proceeds smoothly on a daily basis, but when the balance is perturbed, as occurs with an enteric infection, diarrhea ensues.

Over the past 4 decades, our understanding of intestinal ion transport processes has been revolutionized by elucidation of the molecular basis of 2 devastating diseases, cholera and cystic fibrosis (CF). Although the 2 diseases affect opposite ends of the physiologic spectrum—too much versus insufficient fluid secretion, respectively—examination of their underlying physiologic, regulatory, and genetic parameters have vastly advanced our knowledge. This increased insight of how the intestine transports fluid and electrolytes has had significant clinical impact, most notably in the development of oral rehydration therapy (ORT) for diarrheal diseases, a major health advance of the 20th century.

In this chapter, we review current understanding of the cellular and molecular underpinnings of ion and solute trafficking in different regions of the small and large intestine, and their regulation in health and disease states. The functional activities of intestinal transporters have long been recognized, but only recently has it become apparent that there are a plethora of transport proteins that carry out these specific functions. This understanding is critical for appreciating normal intestinal function, the pathophysiology of intestinal absorptive abnormalities, and the development of therapeutic strategies for specific diseases.

INTESTINAL ARCHITECTURE AND TRANSPORT

The structural and functional design of the intestine is optimally geared to absorb nutrients and transport fluids. In the small intestine, a 600-fold amplification of the absorptive surface is achieved by structural features like the circular folds of Kerckring (plicae circulares), villus-crypt architecture, and microvilli. Using a cylinder as the model, it has been estimated that the surface area of the small intestine is about $3300\ cm^2$; the plicae circulares, villi, and microvilli amplify the surface

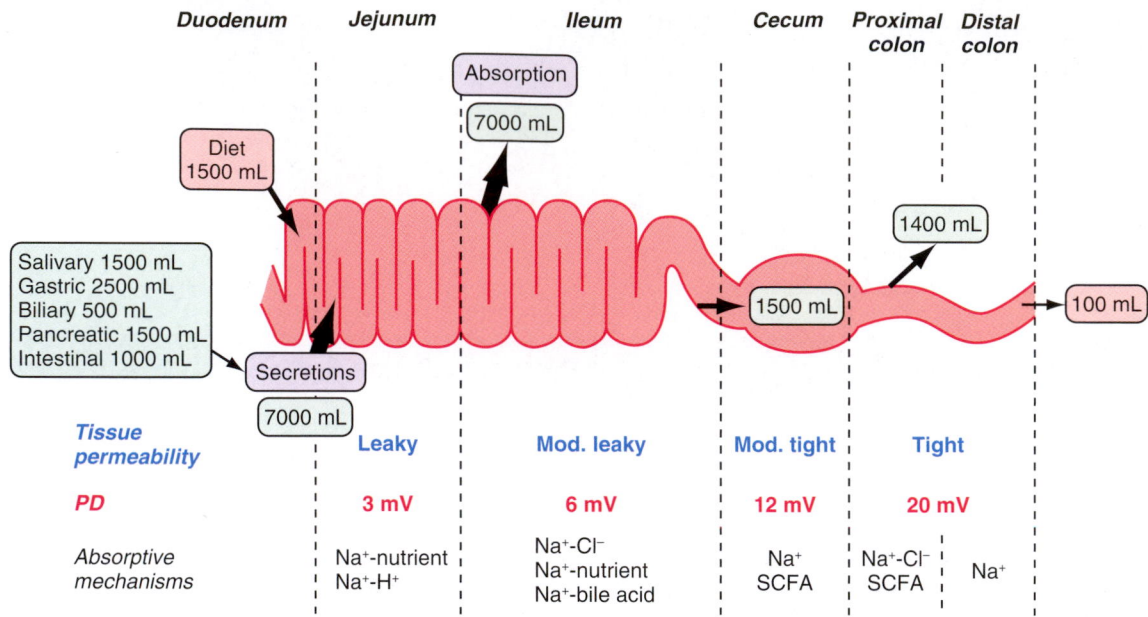

FIGURE 101-1. Overview of intestinal fluid balance. About 8.5 L of fluid flow into the intestine daily. Salivary, gastric, biliary, pancreatic, and intestinal secretions make up most of this amount. The bulk of this fluid is absorbed in the small intestine, and approximately 1500 mL cross the ileocecal valve. The colon efficiently reabsorbs most of this fluid, with only 100 to 200 mL lost in stool. Permeability can be viewed as a surrogate to conductance, which is a reciprocal of resistance. Ohm's law states that current = potential difference divided by resistance (I = PD/R). If I is a constant, PD increases as R increases. Permeability of the intestinal epithelium decreases down the length of the cephalocaudal axis, the distal colon having a relatively tight epithelium. Thus, the spontaneous PD demonstrates a corresponding rise with resistance along the cephalocaudal axis. Absorptive mechanisms differ in each segment of the intestine; chloride secretion is found throughout the intestine. SCFA, short-chain fatty acid.

area by factors of 3, 10, and 20, respectively, ultimately giving a surface area of about 2,000,000 cm². In the large intestine, the spatial separation of crypts and surface cells allows efficient reabsorption of fluid. The overall architecture of the intestinal musculature influences bulk fluid flow and transit time via changes in motility patterns (see Chapters 99 and 100), but the work of fluid transport occurs in the epithelia.

Most epithelia serve as semipermeable barriers. They act as the first line of defense between the mucosal (luminal) and serosal (blood-side) compartments and are capable of bulk transport of fluid from 1 compartment to the other. These epithelia, including those of the intestine, share common characteristics. One fundamental property of epithelia is cellular polarity, with molecularly distinct apical (luminal) and basolateral (serosal) membranes demarcated by intercellular tight junctions. Tight junction permeability varies from being relatively leaky in the small intestine to fairly tight in the large intestine, and these differences determine an individual epithelium's effectiveness as a barrier. A loss of tight junction integrity disrupts the barrier function and vectorial transport capabilities of the tissue.

BASIC EPITHELIAL CELL MODEL

All GI epithelial cells have 2 fundamental similarities: discrete apical and basolateral membranes with distinct biochemical and biophysical properties, separated by tight junctions; and a basolateral Na⁺ pump (ouabain-inhibitable Na⁺/K⁺-ATPase [adenosine triphosphatase]) that establishes a specific intracellular electrochemical environment with a low intracellular Na⁺ concentration ($[Na^+]_i$) and a negative intracellular voltage.

This basic cell model is modified by insertion of transporters into either the apical or basolateral membrane or by the characteristics of tight junctions that determine the unique qualities of a specific epithelial segment. A complex interaction of protein-sorting signals, cytoskeletal elements, and intracellular trafficking processes determines whether a newly synthesized protein is targeted to either the apical or basolateral membrane. Proteins with a glycosyl phosphatidyl inositol (GPI) anchor (e.g., alkaline phosphatase or carcinoembryonic antigen) are often associated with lipid rafts, and the GPI anchor serves to direct them toward the apical membrane.[1] Membrane proteins destined to be delivered to the basolateral membrane carry specific membrane-sorting signals (amino acid sequences) in their cytoplasmic tails. In contrast, other proteins can insert randomly into either an apical or basolateral domain, but they may be retained in the basolateral pole by specific components like ankyrin.[2]

Regulation of intracellular trafficking ensures delivery of the right protein to the right membrane and is critical for establishing epithelial polarization and vectorial transport. When tight junctions are disrupted in vitro, diffusion and intermingling of apical and basolateral proteins in the fluid phase of the membrane result in a loss of epithelial cell polarity.

The most prominent feature of epithelial cell polarity is targeting of the Na⁺/K⁺-ATPase pump to the basolateral membrane, for which expression of the β subunit of Na⁺/K⁺-ATPase is critical. The Na⁺ pump is electrogenic, extruding 3 Na⁺ ions in exchange for 2 K⁺ ions, and thereby maintaining relatively low intracellular Na⁺ and high intracellular K⁺ concentrations compared with concentrations of these electrolytes in the extracellular environment (see Fig. 101-2). There is also greater membrane permeability for K⁺ over Na⁺, which favors

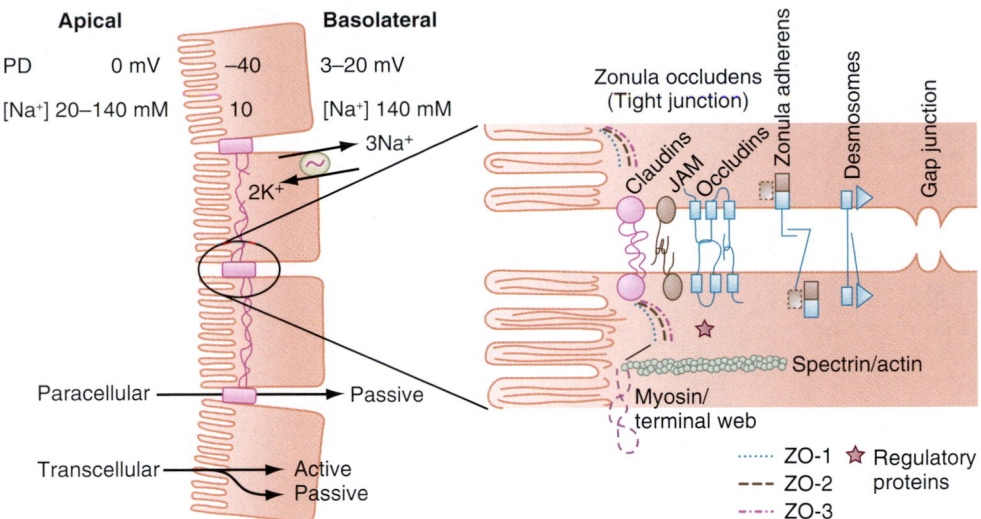

FIGURE 101-2. Architecture of intestinal epithelia. Intestinal epithelial cells are structurally and functionally geared for vectorial transport. The cell membrane is divided into distinct apical and basolateral domains by the tight junctions. Depending on the tissue, the apical membrane can have a more or less prominent brush border appearance due to the presence of numerous microvilli. Parallel actin filaments cross-linked by actin-bundling proteins, such as villin and fibrin, maintain the integrity of the microvilli. These actin bundles extend from the microvilli into the cell and are rooted in a filamentous structure running perpendicular to the microvilli and linked by proteins such as myosin and spectrin, termed the *terminal web*.[1] When contracted, the terminal web can lead to the spreading of the microvilli, thus increasing the surface area exposed to the lumen and aiding the absorption of glucose and water. Functionally, the epithelial cells are polarized with an asymmetrical distribution of transporters; the Na^+ pump on the basolateral membrane is integral to maintaining an electrochemical profile; this profile permits downhill entry of sodium from either the apical or basolateral side; and water and solutes can cross the epithelium either between the cell (paracellular) or through the cell (transcellular).

Transcellular transport across the membrane can be passive or active. The paracellular pathway is characterized by a series of structures defined by specific molecular distributions. The tight junction, or zonula occludens (ZO), is made up of a network of strands and grooves that consists of membrane proteins (e.g., occludins, claudins, and junctional adhesion molecules [JAMs]) that attach to a group of scaffolding proteins (zonula occludens proteins [ZO-1, ZO-2, ZO-3], multi-PDZ domain protein-1 [Mupp1]). These scaffolding proteins are then linked to the cytoskeleton via a number of proteins and kinases that regulate junctional assembly and also participate in vesicular transport via monomeric guanosine triphosphatase (GTPase) of the Ras superfamily. Cadherins span the paracellular pathway across the zonula adherens (ZA) and are responsible for cell-to-cell attachment and maintenance of cell polarity. Cadherins bind to catenins, which are linked to the actin cytoskeleton through an additional family of molecules, including radixin, vinculin, and α-actinin. Molecules associated with the ZA, including rab, src, and yes, are involved in intracellular signaling through second messengers. Desmosomes are cadherin-like molecules that are linked to intermediate filaments. Gap junctions, made by an assembly of membrane spanning proteins called *connexins*, allow the exchange of small molecules between neighboring cells. PD, potential difference.

diffusional exit of K^+ from the cell over diffusional cellular entry of Na^+. These features, in combination with the large number of intracellular proteins with fixed negative charges, lead to the characteristic negative intracellular potential difference compared with either the mucosal or serosal compartments.* Low [Na^+] and electronegativity establish a favorable electrochemical gradient for passive Na^+ entry into the cell. Functionally, the epithelial cell uses the energy of the favorable Na^+ gradient to transport not only Na^+ ions but also a variety of nutrients, vitamins, and electrolytes.[1]

These properties provide the basic mechanisms of ion and water transport that apply to all epithelia. In the intestine, differences in transport can be seen along its cephalocaudal length as well as along the surface-crypt axis within a particular segment of intestine. Tissue- and segment-specific nuances arise from structural-functional and regulatory differences of both intracellular and intercellular proteins.[3]

SEGMENTAL HETEROGENEITY OF TRANSPORT

All intestinal segments from the duodenum to the distal colon have mechanisms for transepithelial fluid movement and are supported by the varied array of transporters encountered within them. For example, the glucose- and amino acid-coupled transporters in the jejunum are well suited for absorption of large volumes of nutrients and water, but the cecum, proximal colon, and distal colon exhibit distinctly different transporters, with electrogenic Na^+ absorption in the distal colon accomplishing the necessary final fluid extraction to prepare feces.[4-7] Different transporter molecules have been identified in specific segments of the GI tract. What is not clear is why an individual transporter is located only in a specific segment of the intestine. Although anion exchange activity occurs throughout the intestine, the DRA (downregulated in adenoma) anion exchanger protein is predominantly expressed in the colon[8,9] (see discussion of bicarbonate transport).

There is also segmental heterogeneity along the crypt-villus axis. Stem cells near the base of the crypt differentiate and migrate upward to form villus enterocytes in the small

---
*There are several potential differences across the epithelium: across the apical membrane into the cell, from the cell interior across the basolateral membrane, across the epithelium, across the mucosa, and across the entire GI tract. By convention, the potential differences across the epithelium, mucosa, and entire GI tract are generally considered the same.

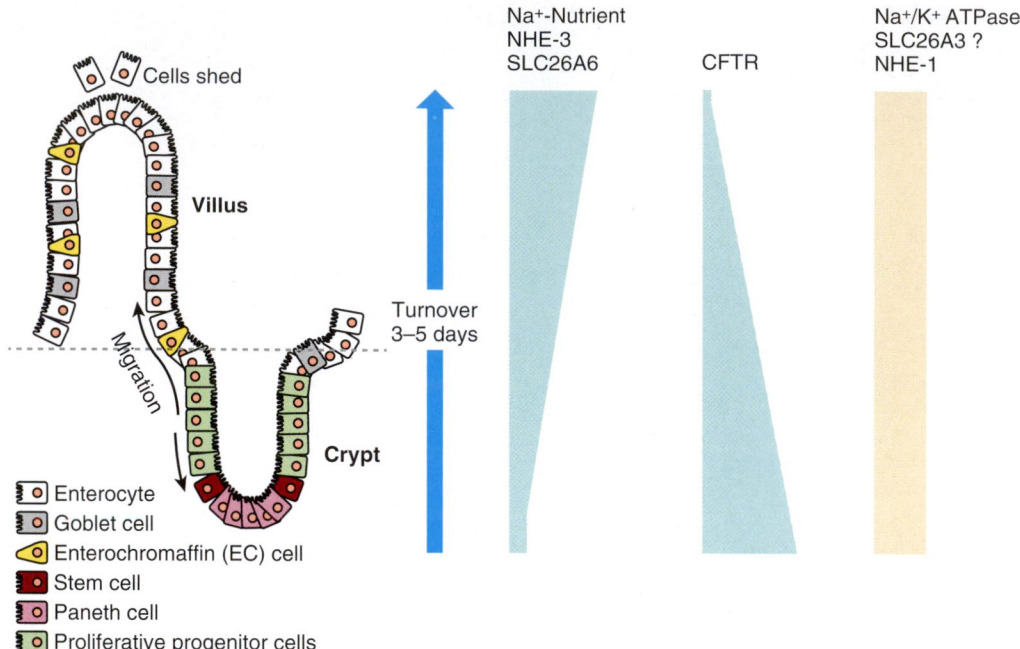

FIGURE 101-3. Types of epithelial cells of the intestinal mucosa and the relative distribution of transport proteins. The 4 major small intestinal cell types are enterocytes, endocrine cells, goblet cells, and Paneth cells. All of these originate from the stem cells located near the base of the crypt. Rapidly proliferating cells arise from the stem cells, move up the crypts, and begin to express differentiation markers for the 3 lineages—enterocytes, endocrine cells, and goblet cells—as they reach the crypt-villus junction.[143] The differentiated cells migrate up the villus axis as a band of cells, further mature, and eventually undergo apoptosis, sloughing off after 3 to 5 days at the tip of the villus. Some stem cells differentiate into Paneth cells that migrate to the bottom of the crypts, where they generate defensins, which are antimicrobial agents important in host defense. Each crypt is believed to be monoclonal, whereas multiple crypts contribute to a single villus, making the latter polyclonal. There is also significant spatial geometry of transport proteins along the crypt-villus axis. Some transport proteins are found at relatively constant concentrations along this axis, whereas some proteins exhibit a greater density in the base of the crypt, and others are denser toward the villus or surface. CFTR, cystic fibrosis transmembrane conductance regulator; SLC26A3, solute carrier 26A3 (also known as DRA [down-regulated in adenoma]); NHE, sodium-hydrogen exchanger; SLC26A6 (formerly known as PAT-1 [putative anion transporter]).

intestine or surface colonocytes in the large intestine while undergoing important changes in their transport and barrier properties (Figs. 101-3 and 101-4).[10,11] As epithelial cells migrate away from the proliferative zone, the complexity of their tight junctions increases, the microvillus architecture of their apical membrane becomes more pronounced, and underlying cytoskeleton and signaling molecules undergo change. There also is increased expression of Na^+ nutrient-coupled transporters, apical Na^+-H^+ exchangers, and brush border membrane hydrolases. In contrast, the levels of the Na^+ pumps remain relatively constant, and others (e.g., the signaling molecule adenylate cyclase and the cyclic adenosine monophosphate [cAMP]-associated Cl^- channel CFTR [cystic fibrosis transmembrane conductance regulator]) decrease in more mature villus cells.

This spatial distribution of transporters (see Figs. 101-3 and 101-4) is consistent with a model in which secretory function resides primarily in the crypts and absorption occurs in villus or surface cells. This segregation of absorptive and secretory functions might explain why, in diseases that selectively damage villi (e.g., celiac disease), secretion predominates. However, this dichotomy between absorptive surface and secretory crypt cells is not rigid and exhibits plasticity, varying with altered physiologic and pathophysiologic states. The underlying mechanisms range from altered localization of key transporters or their regulation by specific post-translational modifications and protein-protein interactions. There are examples where colonic crypts absorb Na^+ and fluid,

and small intestinal villus cells secrete Cl^- via CFTR.[12,13] In addition, depending on their relative position along the crypt-villus axis, the crosstalk between transporters and their signaling molecules can vary and fine-tune intestinal function.

MOVEMENT ACROSS THE INTESTINAL EPITHELIUM

Movement of ions and solutes across the epithelium is bidirectional and occurs via the transcellular and paracellular routes. Paracellular movement is largely passive in response to a variety of gradients, including concentration, electrical, osmotic, and hydrostatic; transcellular movement of ions and solutes occurs by active and passive transport mechanisms. Net transport is termed *absorptive* if the mucosal-to-serosal flux (J_{ms}) is greater than the serosal-to-mucosal (J_{sm}) flux and, and it is termed *secretory* if J_{sm} exceeds J_{ms}. Changes in either or both can alter the direction of net movement; for example, the ileum, which normally exhibits an absorptive flux, responds to cholera toxin with a decrease in J_{ms} and an increase in J_{sm} for Cl^-, resulting in massive fluid secretion. In contrast, increasing evidence points to a failure of Na^+ absorption as the major ion transport aberration associated with IBD.

Characteristics of the tight junctions (i.e., tight vs. leaky) vary along the length of the intestine and dictate the

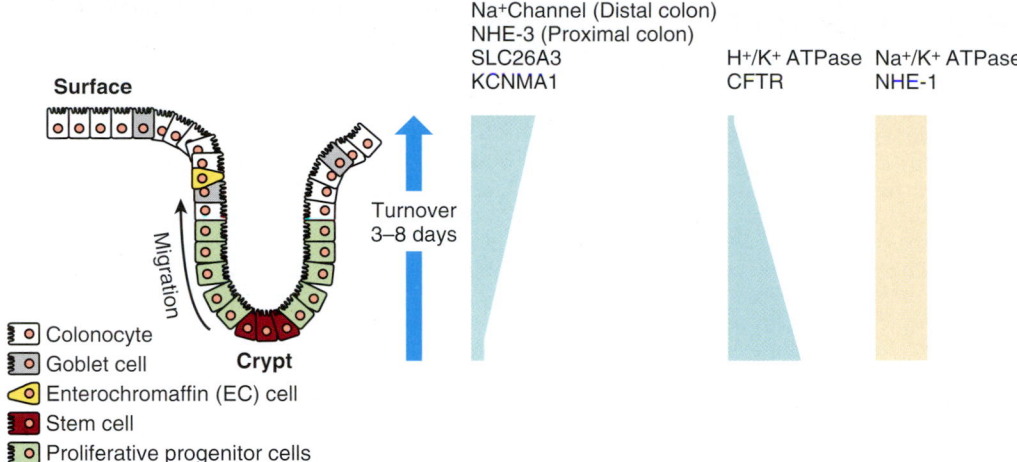

FIGURE 101-4. Types of epithelial cells of the colonic mucosa and the relative distribution of transport proteins. Colonic mucosa epithelium is composed of colonocytes, endocrine cells, and goblet cells. Unlike the small intestine, the colon does not normally have Paneth cells.[143] As in the small intestine, the various colonic cell lineages arise from stem cells. These are located at the base of the crypt and give rise to proliferative progenitor cells. These cells begin to express differentiation markers of the different cell lineages when they reach the upper third of the crypt in the colon and rectum. As they migrate up the crypt axis, they mature and eventually differentiate into surface cells. After 3 to 8 days, the mature surface cells undergo apoptosis and are sloughed off. There is also significant spatial geometry of transport proteins along the crypt-surface axis in the colon. Some transport proteins are found at relatively constant concentrations along this axis, whereas some proteins exhibit a greater density in the base of the crypt, and others are denser toward the surface. CFTR, cystic fibrosis transmembrane conductance regulator; SLC26A3, solute carrier 26A3 (also known as *DRA* [down-regulated in adenoma]); NHE, sodium-hydrogen exchanger; KCNMA1, large-conductance calcium-activated potassium channel, subfamily M, alpha member 1.

contribution of paracellular fluxes to overall transport. The effectiveness of a transepithelial gradient may be modified by series of physical barriers, including an unstirred layer created by the glycocalyx above the apical membrane, the lipid composition of the apical and basolateral membranes, the tight junctions, the geometry of the basolateral space between cells, and the basement membrane. Generally, movement of an uncharged particle is dictated solely by concentration gradients. In contrast, the transport of an ion is governed by the electrical potential and concentration differences (the electrochemical gradient) across the transported surface. *Solvent drag*, a nonspecific entraining of solutes along with the movement of water across paracellular pathways, is an absorptive mechanism that may be especially important in the small intestine, as seen in Na⁺-coupled solute absorption.

TIGHT AND LEAKY EPITHELIA

The paracellular space and junctional complexes between cells define the barrier function of epithelia. Epithelia with a low transepithelial voltage and low resistance are considered leaky, and those that exhibit a high transepithelial voltage and high resistance are considered tight. The tight junctions in villi have higher resistance than those in crypts, and transepithelial resistance increases in a cephalocaudal direction (see Fig. 101-1).[12]

Since the 1990s, the model of paracellular transport and tight junctions has rapidly evolved from a static rigid barrier to a finely regulated, dynamic complex structure (see Fig. 101-2). Movement through the space is exclusively passive, but it is influenced by electrical conductivity, charge selectivity, and its ability to be regulated. Cell-to-cell communications along the paracellular pathway occur in several discrete structures: the zonula occludens (ZO [tight junction]), zonula adherens

(ZA), desmosomes, and gap junctions. The ZO is composed of 50 or more families of proteins that determine its physical and biological properties. For example, claudins belong to a family of 24 membrane-spanning proteins (24 to 27 kd) that form pores by interactions of the extracellular domains of claudins of adjoining cells; homotypic adhesion claudins are important in determining the charge selectivity of the tight junction.[14-16]

Additional proteins in the tight junction include occludins, junctional adhesion molecules (JAMs), and scaffolding proteins such as the ZO proteins (ZO-1, ZO-2) and multi-PDZ domain protein-1 (Mupp-1). Scaffolding proteins serve to link membrane proteins to an array of protein kinases, phosphatases, and (via filamentous actin) myosin in the terminal web, thereby influencing paracellular permeability.[17,18] Disruption of tight junctions by enteropathogenic *Escherichia coli* is specifically associated with protein kinase Cζ activation.[19] Another junctional complex that allows cell-to-cell interaction is the ZA. In epithelia, the ZA is primarily made up of E-cadherins, 120-kd transmembrane glycoproteins with extracellular motifs that engage in calcium-dependent homotypic interaction with cadherins of adjoining cells. Intracellularly, cadherins bind to a family of adhesion molecules, the catenins, which in turn anchor to a dense actin-filament network. Alterations in cadherin-catenin distribution or function have been implicated in carcinogenesis.[20]

Desmosomes are junctional complexes that are structurally similar to ZA junctions, although instead of actin, they link to intermediate filaments through a dense plaque of intracellular anchor proteins. Gap junctions have a unique function. They bridge gaps between cells, allowing neighboring cells to exchange small molecules. They are made up of an assembly of connexins, a 4-pass membrane–spanning protein, 6 of which join to form a hemichannel. When these hemichannels in 2 adjoining cells are aligned, they form a continuous pore that connects the interior of the 2 cells.[1]

TRANSEPITHELIAL TRANSPORT

Our current understanding of the movement of ions, solutes, and fluid across epithelia is gleaned from a combination of in vitro studies using reductionist models of cell lines or isolated epithelial sheets, and from complex in vivo methodologies such as the triple-lumen perfusion technique. All these models underscore that transepithelial ion (largely Na^+) movement from the mucosa to the serosa drives fluid absorption, whereas net ion (largely Cl^-) movement in the reverse direction drives fluid secretion. Although different approaches help elucidate a complex mechanism, at times they give confounding results. For example, some in vitro studies report decreased Cl^- secretion and increased Na^+ absorption in the jejunum of CF patients, implying that the intestinal manifestations of the disease are due to hyperabsorption of water. In contrast, in vivo studies show decreases in both Cl^- secretion and passive Cl^- absorption, which suggests that rather than a hyperabsorption of fluid, the severity of the disease is reflected by decreased fluid absorption.[21]

The reductionist models allow us to focus on transport processes at the cellular and paracellular level. In the intact intestine, however, things are more complicated. The geometry of the intestinal wall and the unstirred layer influence the distance an individual molecule must traverse to reach the apical membrane. The extracellular glycosylated domains of apical membrane proteins make up the glycocalyx, which contributes to the thickness and permeability of the unstirred layer; this layer can be a diffusive barrier to the movement of large lipophilic molecules in a chiefly aqueous milieu. Physical parameters like the mixing of luminal contents by peristalsis, villus motility, and the finer movement of the microvilli influence this rate.

TRANSCELLULAR TRANSPORT

Transcellular transport of ions and solutes can be passive or active. Because of the semipermeable nature of the lipid membrane, movement through the cell requires deployment of specialized membrane proteins such as channels, carriers, and pumps. The negative intracellular potential favors cation entry into, and anion exit from, the cell. This leads to the curious situation in which ions can move passively against their concentration gradient. For example, although the chemical concentration of Cl^- in the cell is relatively low (≈ 35 mmol) compared with the outside concentration (≈ 110 mmol), the intracellular electronegativity creates a driving force for Cl^- exit out of the cell.

WATER MOVEMENT

The intestines are exposed to a constantly fluctuating external milieu that requires nuanced processes for moving water across the epithelium. Not surprisingly, the mechanism(s) of water transport in the intestine are still being delineated. Transepithelial water movement is inextricably linked to the movement of solutes; about 175 molecules of water can be transported per ion or molecule of solute.

Two processes are in play to transport water across epithelial cell membranes: osmosis, which is passive and governed by even small differences in the chemical potential of water and hydrostatic pressure[22]; and "active" processes, which are energized by and coupled to the movement of solutes with coupling ratios of solute/water molecules. Water movement across the epithelium can follow 4 routes: (1) diffusion through the lipid bilayer, or via proteins including (2) water channels, (3) uniporters, and (4) cotransporters.

Aquaporins (AQPs) are a family of at least 13 different water channel proteins; 8 have been localized to either the small or large intestine. Although considerable attention has been given to localization, regulation, and role of AQPs in the intestine,[23] AQP knockout studies have not identified a specific functional intestinal water channel. The absence of a clear role for AQPs in the intestine is not surprising, considering the milieu. AQPs are advantageous in that they can increase the rate of water transport and save metabolic cost. In the intestine, however, where a hyperosmotic lumen to cell gradient during digestion may serve to favor water loss rather than absorption, they play a less prominent role than in the proximal renal tubule, where fluctuations in osmolarity are smaller.[24] Water can also move via molecules known to transport ions and solutes, definitively establishing a role for membrane proteins as conduits for water transport.[25,26] These include the apical Na^+-glucose transporter (SGLT), the urea transporter, and the Na^+/K^+-$2Cl^-$ cotransporter 1 (NKCC1). Water transport can be strictly osmotically driven, as seen with AQPs and uniporters like the urea channel; strictly coupled to the functional turnover of the protein, as seen with the K^+-Cl^- cotransporter (KCC) on the basolateral membrane of absorptive epithelia and NKCC1 on the basolateral membrane of secretory epithelia; or a combination of both, as seen with the hexose transporters apical SGLT and the Na^+-independent uniporter glucose transporters, GLUT1 and GLUT2.

Ultimately, water movement across the intestine occurs under both isotonic conditions, when luminal and serosal osmolarity are 300 mOsm, and when the luminal osmolarity increases in the upper small intestine in response to a meal. Under isotonic conditions, water flux is maximal and decreases as luminal osmolarity increases; water flux ceases when luminal osmolarity is 250 to 300 mOsm greater than serosal osmolarity. Water movement through the paracellular pathway is governed by hydrostatic and osmotic gradients and tissue geometry. Cellular transport of water involves movement across the apical membrane, cytosol, and basolateral membranes. In response to a meal, water is most likely absorbed by passive water permeability in combination with transport through SGLT1 and amino acid transporters on the apical membrane and exits the basolateral membrane via GLUT2 and the K^+-Cl^- cotransporter. The latter energetically couples the efflux of 1 K^+:1 Cl^- with transport of 500 molecules of water. In secretory intestinal cells, the basolateral NKCC1 couples the influx of 1 Na^+:1 K^+:2 Cl^- to 590 molecules of water. While Cl^- exits the cell through apical channels and Na^+ moves paracellularly, it is not known how water exits the apical membrane in the intestine.[23]

The emerging picture that multiple mechanisms contribute to water movement in the intestine is not surprising, considering the complexity of the luminal milieu.

CHANNELS, CARRIERS, AND PUMPS

Small hydrophobic and uncharged molecules move across the lipid bilayer of the cell by diffusion, the rate of transport determined by the concentration gradients and diffusion coefficients (Fig. 101-5). Oxygen, carbon dioxide, fat-soluble vitamins, and unconjugated bile acids are examples of substances transported by diffusion. Because the majority of ions and solutes cannot cross the phospholipid membrane by diffusion, the cell employs an array of distinct integral membrane proteins, including channels, carriers, and pumps, to cross cell membranes (see Fig. 101-5).[1]

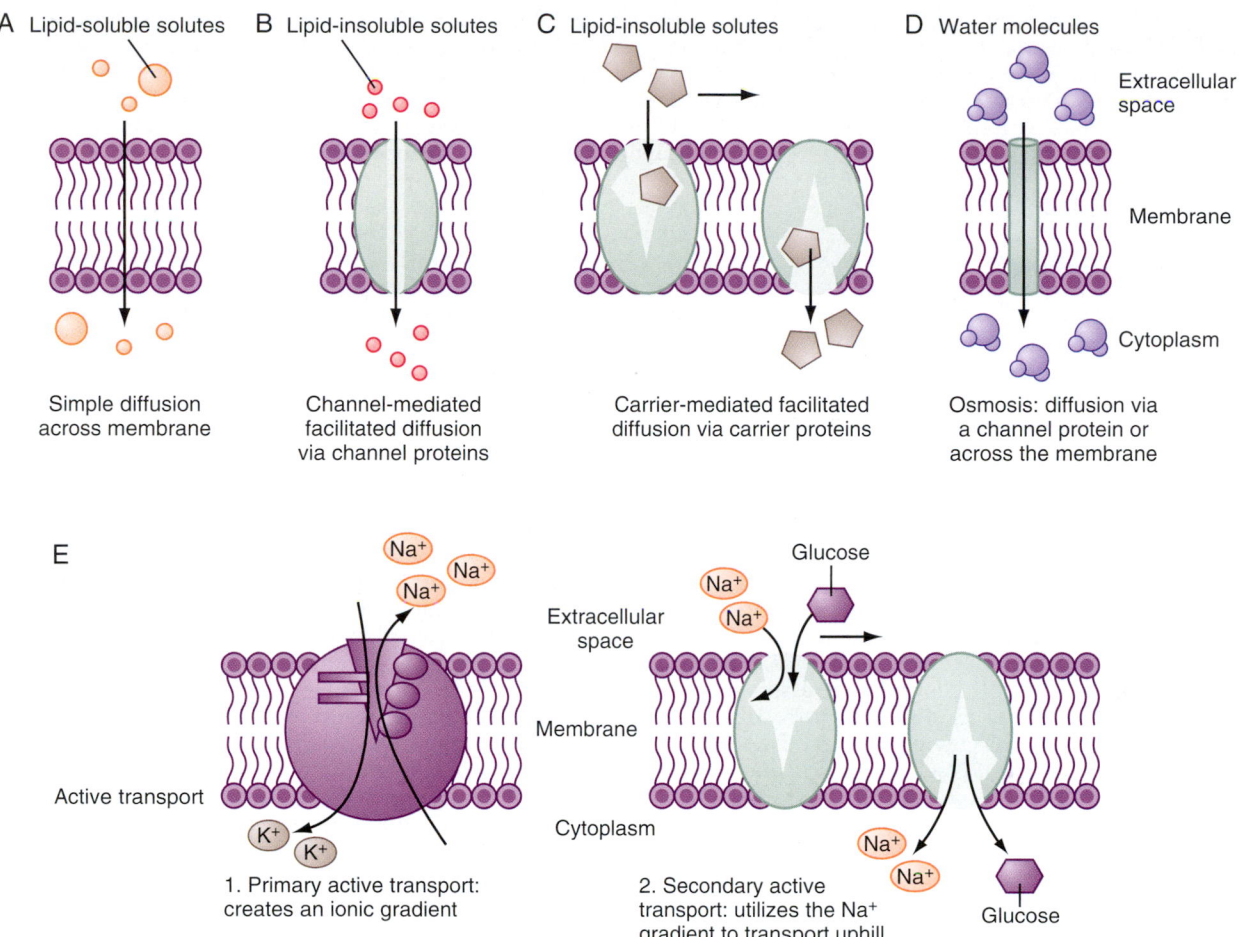

FIGURE 101-5. Channels, carriers, and pumps. Because only nonpolar solutes freely cross a lipid domain by simple diffusion (A), the transfer of ions and charged molecules necessitates specific transmembrane proteins to modulate entry and exit. Ion-specific channels mediate membrane transport by facilitated diffusion (B). Carriers permit facilitated diffusion and transfer specific solutes across the membrane by undergoing a conformational change (C). Transcellular transport of water molecules occurs via channel proteins or carrier proteins (D). Active transport occurs against an electrochemical gradient and can be driven by ATP (primary active transport [E1]) or an ionic gradient (secondary active transport [E2]).

Channels are pores that allow swift (>10^6 ions/sec) and controlled (by rapid opening and closing) transit of ions across the membrane, driven by an electrochemical gradient. The advent of molecular cloning techniques, patch clamp methodology (which allows measurement of function of single channels), and membrane protein crystallography have greatly advanced our knowledge of how these proteins function. Channels tend to be ion selective. For example, Na+ channels exclude K+ despite its same charge and smaller size. Selectivity is determined by the hydration radius of the ion and the physiochemical nature of the pore. Overall transport of a particular ion is determined by the electrochemical gradient, density of channels, and gating (open-close time) of the channel; gating may be modulated by voltage, ion concentration, or intracellular regulation. Mutations of critical residues in the channel protein can have dire functional consequences; in CF, specific mutations of the CFTR affect the ability to transport chloride and bicarbonate.[27,28]

Carriers are another class of integral membrane proteins responsible for transport of ions and solutes, but at rates several orders of magnitude lower than channels. Carrier-mediated transport exhibits substrate specificity, saturation, and inhibitory kinetics. Carriers undergo a series of sequential conformational changes to facilitate transport of substrates across a membrane. When concentration or electrochemical gradients drive carrier-mediated transport, the process is downhill and is termed *facilitated diffusion*. For example, fructose entry into the enterocyte via GLUT5 is by facilitated diffusion. The entering fructose is rapidly isomerized to glucose, maintaining the downhill gradient for fructose.

In contrast, other carriers harness the electrochemical energy established by the downhill movement of a second ion, usually Na+, to move a solute or another ion uphill. This process is termed *secondary active transport* because the specific gradient is indirectly created by a distinct energy-using process. For example, glucose uptake via apical membrane SGLT is driven by the Na+ gradient generated by the basolateral Na+/K+-ATPase. Carriers exhibit substrate specificity, so SGLT transports D-glucose but not L-glucose. Equally important, carriers can transport single or multiple substrates and perform the transport in different directions. *Uniporters,* such as GLUT2 in the basolateral membrane, transport 1 type of substrate, hexoses. *Symporters,* such as the Na+/K+-2Cl− cotransporter, move Na+/K+, and Cl− in the same direction, whereas *antiporters,* such as the Na+-H+ exchangers, move the 2 ions in opposite directions.

Pumps are the third class of integral membrane proteins and directly use energy, generally adenosine triphosphate

(ATP) hydrolysis, to move ions against an electrochemical gradient. This process is termed *primary active transport*. While the Na^+/K^+-ATPase is the quintessential pump, the luminal gastric and colonic H^+/K^+-ATPases and the basolateral Ca^{2+}-ATPases are also important in GI epithelial transport.

ION TRANSPORTERS

Apical Sodium Channel

In the GI tract, the surface epithelial cells of the distal colon and rectum exhibit electrogenic Na^+ absorption against a fairly steep concentration gradient. The downhill electrochemical gradient created by the Na^+ pump drives Na^+ entry via an apical membrane Na^+-specific ion channel (Fig. 101-6) that belongs to the family of epithelial Na^+ channels (ENaCs); members of the ENaC family are found in many epithelia.[29-31] They are multimeric proteins composed of α, β, and γ subunits, exhibit a high sensitivity to the diuretic amiloride, and are stimulated by mineralocorticoids and cAMP. Colonic ENaCs are inhibited by increases in intracellular Ca^{2+}. Unlike many other channels that regulate transport by gating, ENaCs modulate transport by varying the channel density in the cell membrane; this variation may be accomplished through increases or decreases in synthesis (e.g., aldosterone) or exocytosis (e.g., cAMP, vasopressin) of the channels. Aldosterone or cAMP further increase cell membrane ENaC by blocking the degradation pathway for ENaC.

Nutrient-Coupled Sodium Transport

Nutrient transporters are largely the purview of the small intestine. Transport of many hydrophilic nutrients including glucose, amino acids, and some vitamins occurs against their

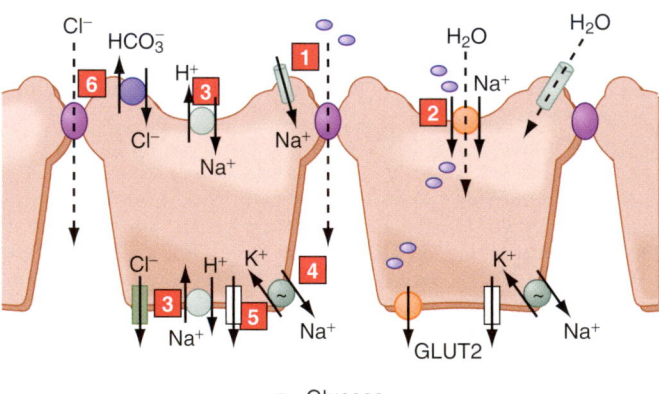

○ —Glucose

FIGURE 101-6. Apical sodium transporters. Sodium crosses the apical membrane of the epithelial cell down an electrochemical gradient. The mechanisms may be *(1)* an ion-specific channel that can be blocked by amiloride; *(2)* a carrier (e.g., SGLT1) that couples the movement of sodium and a nutrient like glucose; or *(3)* a carrier (e.g., antiport carrier [e.g., NHE3]) that allows electroneutral entry of sodium in exchange for intracellular hydrogen). The common exit pathway across the basolateral membrane is the Na^+ pump *(4)*. K^+ channels help maintain the electrochemical gradient *(5)*. Cl^- moves passively through the paracellular pathway or via cellular transporters *(6)*. Glucose exits the basolateral membrane via the facilitated diffusion hexose transporter GLUT2. NHE3, sodium-hydrogen exchanger 3; SGLT1, sodium-glucose cotransporter 1.

concentration gradients via secondary active transport at the apical membrane and facilitated diffusion across the basolateral membrane.

Glucose transport processes, elegantly elucidated by Wright and coworkers, provide a good example of nutrient transport.[32] Transport across SGLT1 is electrogenic (2 Na^+ to 1 glucose), stereospecific (D-isomer), and transports galactose but not fructose.[32] Glucose exit across the basolateral membrane occurs via a separate family of facilitated diffusion carriers, the glucose transporters (GLUT2) (see Fig. 101-6). Fructose enters the cell via another member of this family, GLUT5, and exits via GLUT2.

Although it is clear that Na^+ and glucose absorption stimulates water absorption, the mechanism is not fully delineated. The classic explanation is that basolateral exit of glucose creates a hypertonic compartment in the paracellular space, thereby generating an osmotic gradient for fluid entry from the lumen. Some enticing evidence suggests that secondary to transcellular transport via SGLT, passive processes triggers contraction of the actomyosin ring in the terminal web (described in Fig. 101-2), resulting in increased paracellular permeability to glucose and to water. Additionally, SGLT activation results in a protein kinase-dependent recruitment of GLUT2 to the apical membrane, which then serves as a high-capacity, low-affinity route for sugar entry during feeding.[33,34] As discussed under "Water Movement," SGLT can transport water (210 molecules/turnover) and could account for about 5 L of fluid reabsorption in the fed state.[35] How molecular regulation of transporters is translated into net nutrient absorption during feeding in vivo is a critical area of inquiry. For a description of similar advances made in our understanding of amino acid and vitamin transport, see Chapters 102 and 103.

Sodium-Hydrogen Exchangers

Exchange of extracellular Na^+ for intracellular H^+ is a process driven by the electrochemical gradient for Na^+ and by a pH gradient that results from a moderately acidic intracellular environment; this process occurs in almost every cell. In mammalian intestine, members of the Na^+-H^+ exchange (NHE) gene family play an important role in electroneutral sodium absorption. Electroneutral Na^+ absorption may be down-regulated during eating and increases postprandially after nutrient absorption.

Ten mammalian isoforms of NHE have been cloned. NHE1-4 and 6-9 exhibit species- and segment-specific distribution in the GI tract.[36-38] NHE1-5 are primarily found in the plasma membrane, NHE8 is found in brush border membranes of epithelial cells, and the rest are found in membranes of subcellular organelles.[39] NHE1 is a ubiquitous plasma membrane protein found in most cells. It is expressed on epithelial basolateral membranes and functions as the housekeeper regulator of intracellular pH, cell volume, and growth. NHE2 and NHE3 are apical membrane proteins restricted to epithelia and are the major conduits for electroneutral Na^+ absorption in the intestine (see Fig. 101-6). NHE2 is expressed throughout the GI tract, but maximal expression is predominantly in the proximal colon. NHE3 is considered a marker for the absorptive cells of the small intestine and colon; it is expressed only in the villus or surface cells, and not in the crypts. There are significant overall differences in the expression and function of NHE2 and NHE3 in the intestine, and studies done by knocking out these transporters have demonstrated a predominant role for NHE3 in small intestinal absorption.[40] NHE4 is located in the basolateral membrane, primarily in gastric parietal and chief cells, where it might have a role in acid secretion. NHE5 and NHE10 are not expressed in the GI tract, and the roles of NHE6, 7, and 9 remain to be determined. The luminal-membrane NHE8 may have an important role during intestinal epithelial development.[39,41] Epidermal growth factor (EGF) reduces basal transcription of NHE8 and might be critical in regulating NHE expression during intestinal maturation.[42] NHE activity is differentially modulated by neural, paracrine, or endocrine stimuli through intricate scaffolding complexes that include the exchanger itself, a family of NHE regulatory factors (NHERFs) that act as a bridge between the exchanger and a variety of kinases, phosphatases, and other transporters.[43,44] Different stimuli use differing scaffolding complexes to exert their effect. Glucocorticoids stimulate Na$^+$ absorption and up-regulate NHE3 and NHE8[45] but not NHE1, 2, or 4, consistent with their respective roles in vectorial transport and housekeeping. Glucocorticoids act via a serum- and glucocorticoid-inducible kinase, SGK1; SGK1 stimulates the activity of NHE3 by interacting directly with NHERF2.

Alternatively, increases in cAMP (as seen in cholera) inhibits NHE3 by activating protein kinase A (PKA), which is recruited to the C-terminus of NHE3 by NHERF1, NHERF2, and an additional cytoskeletal protein, ezrin. In this location, PKA induces its inhibitory effect by phosphorylating NHE3. Other modulators like *E. coli*-stable toxin A or guanylin activate brush border membrane guanylate cyclase C (GUCY2C) to increase cyclic guanosine monophosphate (cGMP); cGMP inhibits NHE3 activity by triggering the formation of a complex between cGMP-dependent protein kinase II (cGKII) and NHERF2 and the cGKII anchor protein (GKAP), all located in the brush border membrane (Fig. 101-7).[43] NHERF2 is critical to NHE3 regulation; it is involved in the stimulation of NHE3 by lysophosphatidic acid (LPA), and studies on NHERF2-null mice demonstrate that NHERF2 is necessary to maintain both basal NHE3 activity and its inhibition by cAMP, cGMP, and intracellular calcium ([Ca^{2+}]$_i$).

Electroneutral Sodium Chloride Absorption

Sodium absorption is coupled to the movement of Cl$^-$ through a Cl$^-$-HCO$_3^-$ anion exchanger, located specifically in the ileum and proximal colon. The rates of the transporters are similar and coordinated by cell pH and HCO$_3^-$. Alkalinization of the cell by NHE drives the exit of HCO$_3^-$ in exchange for Cl$^-$, resulting in electroneutral Na$^+$ and Cl$^-$ absorption, maintenance of cell pH, and luminal release of H$^+$ + HCO$_3^-$ (water and CO$_2$). Coupling of the 2 exchangers exhibits species and segmental variations; it is fairly tight in the ileum and proximal colon, whereas in other intestinal segments, although NHE is dependent on Cl$^-$ or HCO$_3^-$, the linkage between Na$^+$ and Cl$^-$ transport is variable.

Chloride (Anion) Absorption

The transepithelial lumen negative potential difference contributes to passive movement of Cl$^-$ and other anions via the paracellular pathway in the jejunum.[6] Cellular Cl$^-$ absorptive pathways are segment specific, involving multiple and distinct anion exchangers in the apical and basolateral membranes. Coupled Cl$^-$-HCO$_3^-$ and Na$^+$-H$^+$ exchangers govern electroneutral transport across the apical membrane in the ileum and proximal colon, whereas sodium-independent Cl$^-$-HCO$_3^-$ exchange occurs in the distal colon (see Fig. 101-6). Similarly, exit mechanisms for Cl$^-$ across the basolateral membrane involve both channels (e.g., ClC2) and anion exchangers (SLC4A family). Anion exchangers are discussed in detail later under "Bicarbonate Transport."

Chloride Secretion

The principal driving force for fluid secretion is the transcellular movement of Cl$^-$ from the serosal to the luminal compartment. Na$^+$ and water follow passively in response to the ensuing electrical and osmotic gradients (Fig. 101-8). The small and large intestine exhibit a basal rate of Cl$^-$ secretion that is maintained by the interplay of cell volume, [Cl$^-$]$_i$, and paracrine, autocrine, neuronal, endocrine, luminal, and immune modulators. Disruptions in the balance of these regulatory processes can lead to secretory diarrhea.

Several epithelia in the GI tract exhibit electrogenic Cl$^-$ secretion. Although there are some tissue-specific regulatory differences, the mechanisms underlying this secretion are remarkably similar. The Na$^+$ pump provides the driving force, and Cl$^-$ enters the cell across the basolateral membrane via an electroneutral cotransporter (NKCC1). The Human Genome Organization (HUGO) Gene Nomenclature Committee (HGNC) has classified the more than 360 identified solute carriers (SLC) into 52 families (SLC1-SLC52) and each solute carrier belongs to one of these families. In the superfamily of cation transporters, the NKCC (solute carrier family 12, member 2 [SLC12A2]) cotransporters are characterized by their selectivity to Cl$^-$ and Br$^-$ and their inhibition by the loop diuretics bumetanide and furosemide.[46-48] NKCC1 phosphorylation and activity are increased by a drop in cell volume or increases in [Cl$^-$]$_i$; it is also regulated by many phosphatases, actin-myosin interactions and kinases, including a unique proline-alanine–rich STE20-related kinase (PASK0; STE20 represents "sterile20", a super class of mitogen activated protein kinases (MAP4K) first identified in yeast from whence the name is derived). The NKCC1 cotransporter effectively couples the movement of 2Cl$^-$:1K$^+$ (and 590 molecules of H$_2$O) uphill for the expenditure of a single Na$^+$ ion. The Cl$^-$ leaves the cell via specific channels on the apical membrane; Na$^+$ entering the cell through NKCC1 exits via the Na$^+$ pump, and K$^+$ leaves via K$^+$ channels either on the apical or the basolateral membrane. This complex interplay of transporters is an elegant demonstration of cellular economy. The pump-to-leak relation between K$^+$ channels and the Na$^+$ pump helps maintain the interior of the cell as electronegative, providing the driving force for Cl$^-$ exit. Basolateral K$^+$ exit electrically balances the large Cl$^-$ flux across the apical membrane.

Chloride Channels

Three classes of Cl$^-$ channels belonging to separate protein families and with distinct electrophysiologic characteristics have been identified in secretory epithelia. There is increasing evidence, however, that the predominant Cl$^-$ channel in the intestine is the CFTR.

CFTR Chloride Channel

The CFTR protein is coded for by the gene that is defective in CF (see Chapter 57). The crucial role of this channel is underscored by the exocrine pathologies that are the hallmark of CF. In addition to abnormalities of the lungs, sweat glands, and pancreas, infants with CF often present with meconium ileus, and 15% of adults with CF exhibit distal intestinal obstructive syndrome. Interestingly, the major pathology of the CFTR-deficient mouse is meconium ileus, which results in early mortality unless treated with an osmotic laxative.

CFTR is present on the apical membrane of enterocytes and chiefly localized to intestinal and colonic crypts.[49] It is a membrane protein of 1480 amino acids that belongs to the superfamily of ATP-binding cassette proteins (Fig. 101-9).

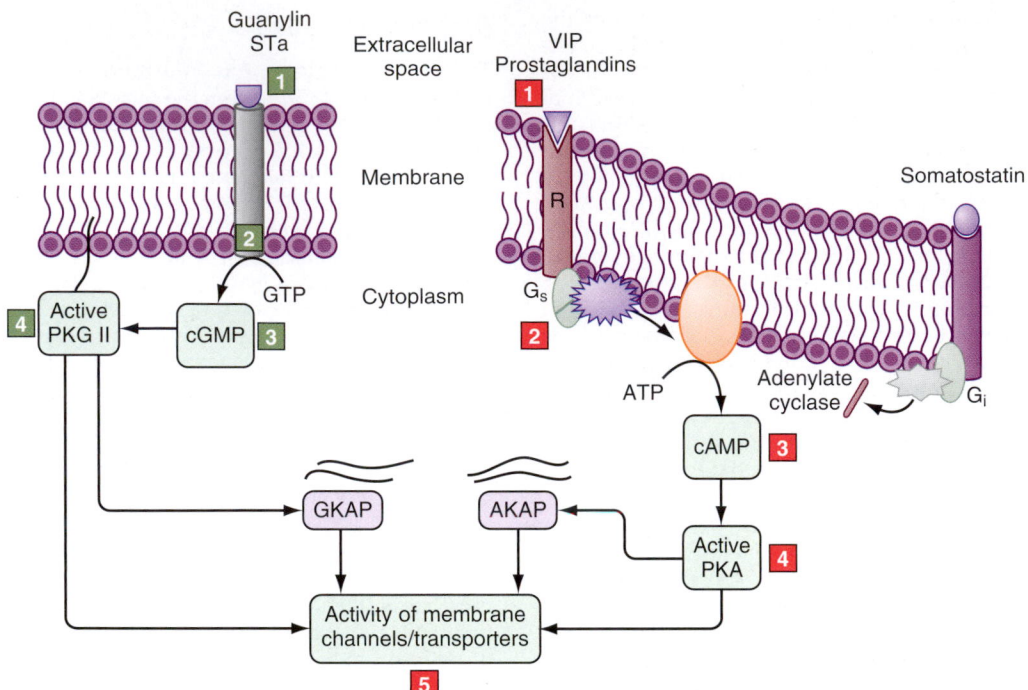

FIGURE 101-7. Second messengers: cAMP and cGMP. Five steps are involved in transduction of an external signal into a change in cellular function: *(1)* binding of either a stimulatory or an inhibitory agonist to an appropriate receptor of the membrane-bound adenylate cyclase or guanylate cyclase system; *(2)* binding of ligand to receptor modulates cyclase activity, either within the same molecule in the case of guanylate cyclase (GUCY2C) or by activating the corresponding membrane-bound heterotrimeric guanine nucleotide regulatory proteins (G proteins) in the case of adenylate cyclase; *(3)* an intracellular signal results from production of cAMP from ATP and cGMP from GTP; *(4)* an increase in $[cAMP]_i$ (intracellular cAMP concentration) activates protein kinases such as PKA, and an increase in $[cGMP]_i$ activates protein kinases such as PKG II, which is fixed to the membrane by myristoylation; involvement of kinase-anchoring proteins such as A kinase-anchoring proteins (AKAPs) and G kinase-anchoring proteins (GKAPs) has been demonstrated during the signaling; *(5)* protein kinase phosphorylation of specific target proteins results in a change in the activity of channels or transporters such as the cystic fibrosis transmembrane conductance regulator (CFTR) chloride channel or the Na^+-H^+ exchanger. (For easy explanation, steps 1 to 5 are drawn apart). In the intact cell, the molecules described in steps 1 to 5 (receptors, cyclase, kinase, anchoring protein, and target transporter) may be in close proximity, allowing for spatial and localized regulation.

In cAMP signaling, binding of stimulatory regulators (e.g., VIP, prostaglandins) to specific receptors causes activation. Activated receptors couple via G_s with adenylate cyclases to catalyze conversion of ATP to cAMP, which then activates specific cAMP kinases. An inherent GTPase returns G_s to its nascent state; cholera toxin prevents this occurrence by covalently modifying G_s, leaving enterocyte turnover as the only recourse to returning the tissue to its basal state. Other hormones, such as somatostatin, trigger the activation of inhibitory G proteins (G_i) to decrease cAMP. The adenylate cyclase cascade is localized to the basolateral membrane of epithelial cells.

In cGMP signaling, cGMP is generated by the activation of membrane or soluble guanylate cyclases (GCs). In contrast to the adenylate cyclases, membrane GCs are single-pass transmembrane proteins for which the extracellular domain serves as the receptor-binding domain and the intracellular domain catalyzes conversion of GTP to cGMP. Thus, the GCs are specific for their ligands, which include the endogenous atrial natriuretic peptides, guanylin, and uroguanylin, as well as enterotoxins such as the heat-stable enterotoxin of *E. coli*. The intestinal cGMP protein kinase is tethered to the membrane via a myristoylated N-terminal region. The soluble GCs are the target of nitric oxide activation; they are minimally expressed in the small intestinal epithelium, but they are present in colonic epithelia, subepithelial elements, and smooth muscle, where they cause muscular relaxation. ATP, adenosine triphosphate; cAMP, cyclic adenosine monophosphate; cGMP, cyclic guanosine monophosphate; G_i, inhibitory G protein; G_s, stimulatory G protein; GTP, guanosine triphosphate; PKA, protein kinase A; PKG, protein kinase G; STa, heat-stable toxin; VIP, vasoactive intestinal peptide.

CFTR is a small-conductance (8-10 pS) linear channel with an ion selectivity of $Br^- > Cl^- > I^- > F^-$ that can also transport HCO_3^- and ATP.[50,51] In secretory diarrheas such as cholera, cAMP increases channel activity and the number of channels in the apical membrane (see Fig. 101-9 and Fig. 101-10). The more than 1000 mutations of CFTR have been grouped into 6 classes: class I, truncated protein translation; class II, improper folding; class III, abnormal gating; class IV, decreased pore conductivity; class V, reduced surface expression; and class VI, reduced membrane residence time. However, some 70% of CF patients carry the same mutation, a single amino acid deletion ($\Delta F508$) that results in improper folding (class II mutation [Fig. 101-9]).

CFTR is pleiotropic and interacts with many other proteins, such as ENaC, NKCC, and anion exchangers. Some of this interaction occurs through crosstalk via shared scaffolding proteins; for example, the C-terminal of CFTR interacts with NHERF, a protein that also binds NHE3. CFTR can influence the expression, regulation, and modulation of other proteins by mechanisms that are not fully deciphered. Diminished intestinal fluid secretion in $CF^{-/-}$ mice is associated with goblet cell hyperplasia, increased crypt cell proliferation, Paneth cell abnormalities, and increased inflammation.[52] Whether all these changes are secondary to decreased fluid secretion or result from more direct effects of CFTR on other protein

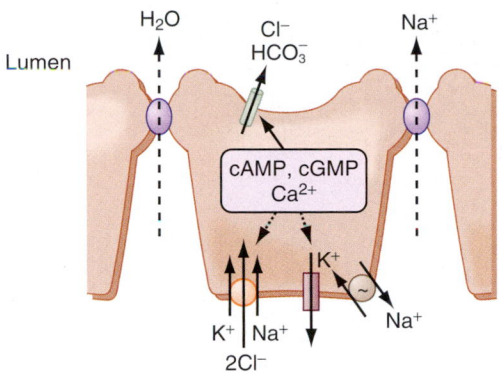

FIGURE 101-8. Intestinal chloride secretion. Discrete basolateral entry steps and apical exit steps are integral to chloride secretion across any secretory epithelium. The Na^+/K^+-$2Cl^-$ carrier (NKCC1) couples the movement of Na^+, K^+, and Cl^- in a 1:1:2 stoichiometric relationship and permits Cl^- to accumulate in the cell in a concentration greater than its electrochemical equilibrium. Cl^- then exits the cell across the apical membrane by means of a chloride channel; Na^+ and water follow passively. The Na^+ and K^+ that entered with the Cl^- are recycled by, respectively, the Na^+ pump and a basolateral K^+ channel, both of which are critical to maintaining the driving force. These transporters can be regulated by second messengers like Ca^{2+}, cAMP (cyclic adenosine monophosphate), and cGMP (cyclic guanosine monophosphate) (See Fig. 101-7). The molecular nature and isotypes of these key transporters may vary with the tissue and species. Thus, NKCC1 is the predominant isoform in secretory epithelia. The basolateral K^+ channels can either be the cAMP-activated KCNE3/KCNQ1 channels (potassium voltage-gated channels, Isk-related family, member 3/ KQT-like subfamily, member 1), or the Ca^{2+}-calmodulin-activated KCNN4 channels (potassium intermediate/small conductance calcium-activated channel, subfamily N, member 4). As described in the text, the apical membrane Cl^- channel is predominantly CFTR (cystic fibrosis transmembrane conductance regulator [see Figure 101-9 for further details]). There is some evidence, albeit controversial, that the apical membrane could also possess ClC-257 (a proposed target for lubiprostone) and the Ca^{2+}-activated transmembrane Cl^- channel, TMEM16a.[60-62] Other investigators suggest basolateral location for the ClC-2 and TMEM16a channels.[59]

functions remains to be determined (see later). Using combinatorial chemistry, compounds have been designed to specifically inhibit or stimulate CFTR, thereby serving as therapeutic strategies for secretory diarrhea or CF; many are in various phases of clinical trials.[53,54] Most exciting, in 2012, the U.S. Food and Drug Administration (FDA) approved an oral medication, Kalydeco, for CF patients older than age 6 who have the G551D (class III, non-ΔF508) mutation of CFTR. Patients with G551D have an apical membrane CFTR with lower than normal activity; the potentiator drug increases Cl^- conductance, improves lung function, and decreases pulmonary CF exacerbations. A side effect of Kalydeco is mild diarrhea (13%). Any effect to alleviatinge meconium ileus in the newborn cannot be tested because of FDA regulations.

ClC Family of Chloride Channels

The ClC chloride channel family,[55,56] especially the widely distributed plasma membrane ClC2, is involved in regulation of epithelial transport, intracellular pH, intracellular chloride and cell volume. ClC2 gained clinical interest as a potential alternative secretory pathway to CFTR because it is a target of lubiprostone, a novel prostaglandin-related laxative.[57] Although lubiprostone undoubtedly stimulates Cl^- secretion, the specific role of ClC2 in this process is controversial. Some studies show that lubiprostone activates ClC2 in the apical membrane of human colonic cell lines. Other studies using the same cell line demonstrate it activates CFTR, although it fails to rescue Cl^- secretion in intestinal tissues of CF patients or CFTR-deficient mice. In contrast to the apical membrane location of CFTR, ClC2 is localized to the basolateral membrane of murine surface colonocytes, and ClC2-deficient mice demonstrate impaired electroneutral NaCl and KCl absorption, not Cl^- secretion. The importance of ClC2 in human colonic function remains to be clarified.

Calcium-Activated Chloride Channels

The calcium-activated Cl^- (CLCA) channels may play a role in goblet cell function[58] and have been implicated in the diarrhea of rotaviral infection in intestines of young but not adult mammals (see "Microbiome and Microbial Pathogens" later). The molecular nature of the channel eluded precise identification until by using distinct molecular approaches, 3 separate laboratories identified TMEM-16A (1 of 10 anoctamins, a family of transmembrane proteins) as the epithelial Ca^{2+}-activated Cl^- channel. In the intestine, TMEM 16A plays a role in intestinal smooth muscle contraction. Its location in intestinal epithelia remains to be resolved; a strict basolateral role in cell volume regulation has been found by some,[59] whereas others provide evidence for an apical location.[60-62]

Potassium Transport

Many K^+ transport processes help the intestine cope with its need to balance fluid and electrolyte movement.[63,64] Potassium secretion and absorption occur along the length of the intestinal tract, although the specific pathways are segment specific. In the small intestine, the luminal negative potential difference drives the passive absorption of K^+. In contrast, K^+ absorption in the distal colon occurs by primary active transport via luminal membrane H^+/K^+-ATPase pumps in concert with basolateral K^+-Cl^- cotransporters and K^+ channels. These H^+/K^+-ATPase pumps are related to the gastric H^+/K^+-ATPase, and like the Na^+ pump are P-type ATPases, pumps that catalyze the phosphorylation (P) of a conserved aspartate residue during each turnover of the enzyme. At least 2 colonic isoforms have been identified: ouabain-sensitive isoform in the crypt cells and ouabain-insensitive isoform in the surface cells. Depletion of aldosterone and K^+ up-regulates the ouabain-insensitive H^+/K^+-ATPase and stimulates K^+ absorption.

Potassium channels are the largest group of ion channels in the human genome. Only a few K^+ channels localized to intestinal cells are mentioned here, using the HGNC nomenclature, which designates them as KCNxx and so forth (see http://www.genenames.org/genefamilies/m-p/). In addition to transepithelial transport, various K^+ channels are involved in differentiation, apoptosis, and carcinogenesis. K^+ channels are regulated by changes in membrane voltage, cytosolic calcium, pH, cell swelling, cell metabolism, and covalent post-translational protein modifications (e.g., addition or removal of phosphate groups [phosphorylation] or addition or detachment of small ubiquitin-like modifier [SUMO] proteins [sumoylation]). Found primarily on the basolateral membrane of epithelial cells, K^+ channels contribute significantly to intestinal electrolyte homeostasis through several mechanisms. Cell swelling activates K^+ channels, leading to a regulatory volume decrease, a function critical for intestinal cells that live in an environment with constant fluctuations in

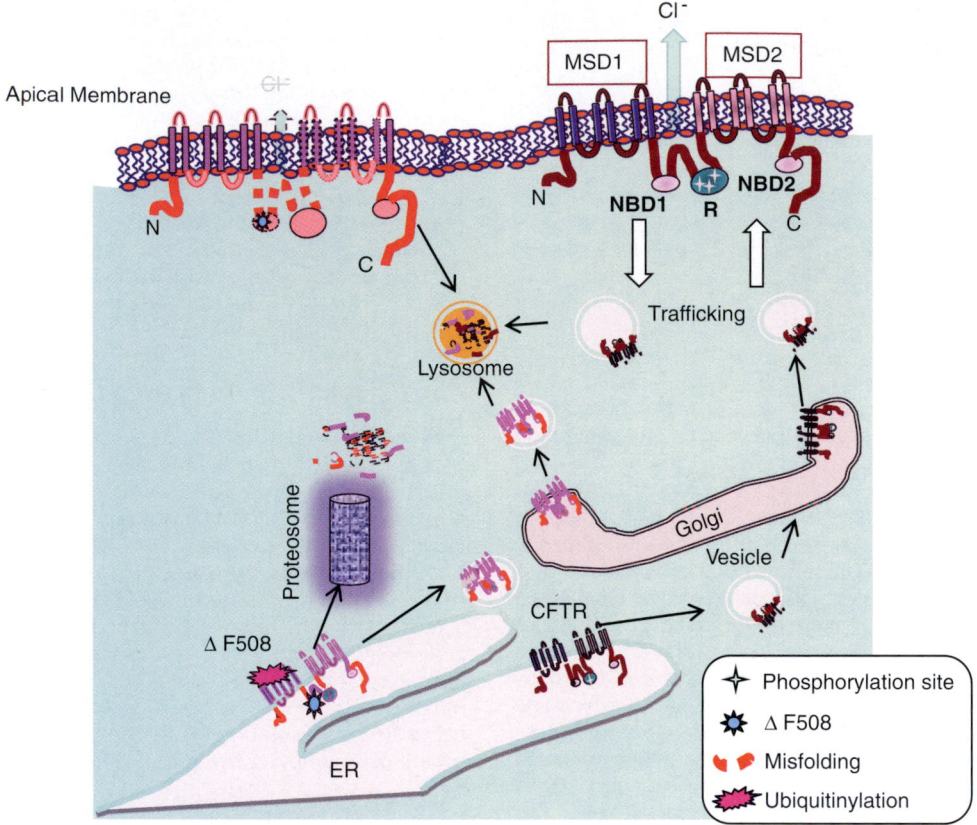

FIGURE 101-9. Structure and trafficking of cystic fibrosis transmembrane conductance regulator *(CFTR)*. CFTR is present on the apical membrane of enterocytes and chiefly in intestinal and colonic crypts. CFTR is a 1480 amino acid membrane protein synthesized in the endoplasmic reticulum *(ER)* and trafficked through the Golgi apparatus and endosomal compartments. It has 2 membrane-spanning domains *(MSD1, MSD2)*, 2 ATP-binding domains *(NBD1, NBD2)*, and a regulatory *(R)* domain that has many phosphorylation consensus sequences, specifically for PKA. Gating of the channel is regulated by sequential binding of ATP to the 2 domains and phosphorylation and dephosphorylation of the R domain. PKA activates the R domain to increase channel activity and stimulates the recruitment of CFTR-bearing endosomes to the apical membrane to increase channel numbers. There are 6 classes of CFTR mutations, but 70% of CF patients carry the ΔF508 mutation that results in improper folding and diversion of the majority of the protein to the proteasomes for degradation instead of apical membrane insertion. Misfolded or other mutant proteins that reach the apical membrane get targeted to the lysosome for degradation. ATP, adenosine triphosphate; MSD, membrane spanning domain; NBD, nucleotide (ATP) binding domain; PKA, protein kinase A.

osmolarity. K^+ channels modulate the hyperpolarization of the cell interior required for vectorial voltage-driven transport processes. In the basolateral membranes of the small and large intestine, the cAMP-activated KCNE3/KCNQ1 channels (potassium voltage-gated channels, Isk-related family, member 3/KQT-like subfamily, member 1; resulting in a slow-delayed rectifying K^+ current) and the Ca^{2+}-calmodulin–activated KCNN4 channels (potassium intermediate/small conductance calcium-activated channel, subfamily N, member 4) hyperpolarize the membrane and promote Cl^- secretion. Basolateral K^+ channels contribute to the transepithelial potential difference, which influences paracellular movement. The apical KCNMA1 (MaxiK; potassium large-conductance calcium-activated channel, subfamily M, alpha member 1) channels, regulated by calcium and mineralocorticoids, are primarily responsible for colonic K^+ secretion.

Bicarbonate Transport

Bicarbonate is a metabolic product and a critical anion in fluid homeostasis in the intestine. In clinically significant diarrhea,

bicarbonate is the major anion in the stool. It is secreted by electrogenic and electroneutral processes in the duodenum, ileum, and colon. Being a metabolic product, intracellular HCO_3^- can arise from intracellular metabolism, diffusion of CO_2, or the action of transporters such as the basolateral Na^+-HCO_3^- cotransporter. Electrogenic HCO_3^- secretion can occur via apical anion channels, including CFTR; the major mechanism for HCO_3^- secretion in the small and large intestine, however, is inexorably linked to the inward movement of Cl^- via apical Cl^--HCO_3^- exchangers.[65] It is postulated that electrogenic Cl^- secretion via CFTR provides luminal Cl^-, which is then recycled across the apical membrane in exchange for intracellular HCO_3^-. A separate HCO_3^- conductive pathway might mediate bicarbonate secretion into the duodenum. SCFA-dependent bicarbonate secretion has also been observed in surface cells of the colon.[66]

The bulk of HCO_3^- transport occurs via solute carriers. Although the prototype of anion exchangers, the red cell Cl^--HCO_3^- exchanger (AE1/SLC4A1), has been extensively studied, identification of intestinal exchangers is relatively recent. The SLC4A1, SLC4A2, and SLC4A3 exchangers are

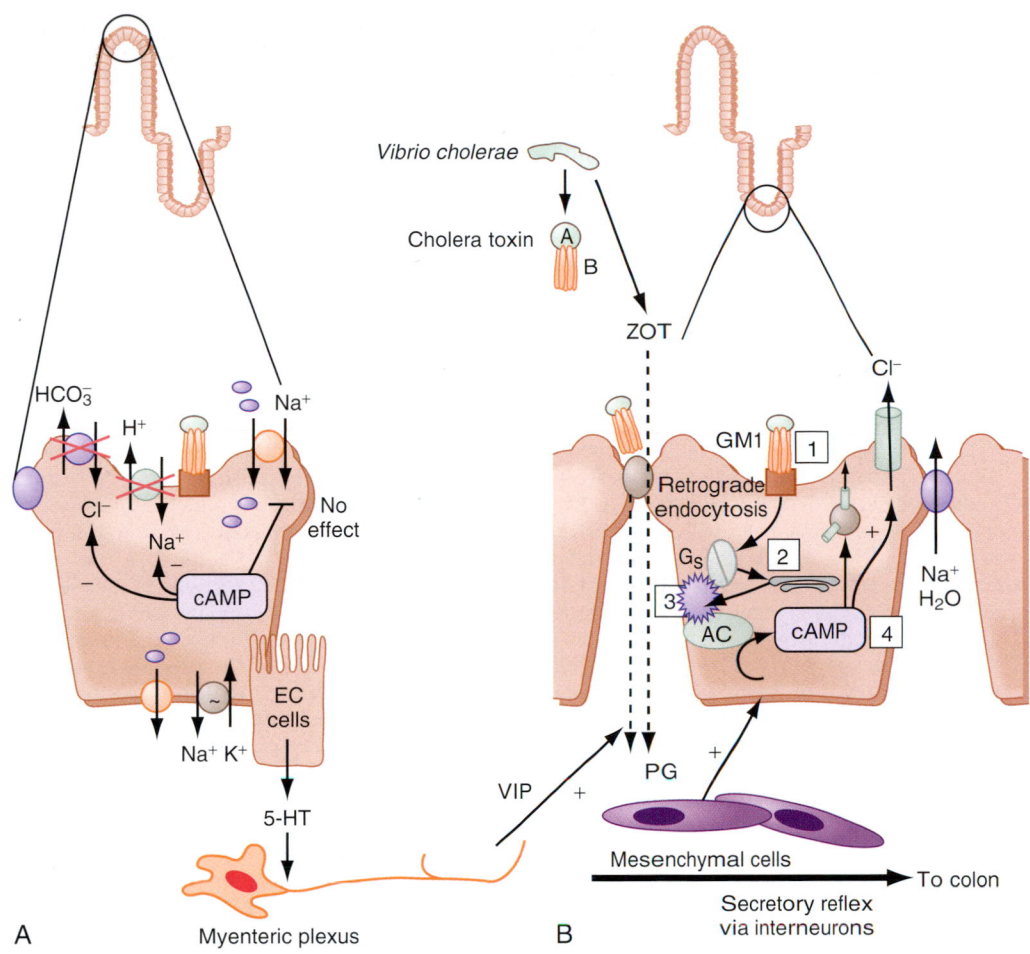

FIGURE 101-10. Mechanism of action of *Vibrio cholerae* enterotoxin. *V. cholerae* produces an enterotoxin, a zonula occludens toxin (ZOT) that disrupts tight junction permeability, and other toxins (not shown here) that are not fully identified. Cholera toxin (CT) induces diarrhea by inhibiting absorptive processes in the villus and surface epithelial cells *(A)* and by stimulating the secretory processes in the crypt epithelial cells *(B)*. As shown in *A*, a CT-mediated increase in cyclic adenosine monophosphate *(cAMP)* leads to inhibition of salt absorption (Na$^+$-H$^+$ and Cl$^-$-HCO$_3^-$ transporters) but does not affect Na$^+$-glucose transport. The events that follow enterotoxin binding that lead to cAMP generation are similar in villus and crypt cells. As shown in *B*, the enterotoxin binds to ubiquitous GM1 gangliosides via its B subunits on the intestinal brush border membrane *(1)* and, by capturing elaborate cellular processes, including lipid rafts, retrograde endocytosis, and endoplasmic reticular proteolysis *(2)*, transmits the A1 peptide of its A subunit to the basolateral membrane. At the basolateral membrane, A1 catalyzes the adenosine diphosphate ribosylation of G$_{\alpha s}$ (G$_s$). This permanently activates G$_s$ by covalently inhibiting the nascent GTPase and preventing activated G$_s$ from returning to its nascent state *(3)*. Activated G$_s$ then stimulates adenylate cyclase *(AC)* to produce an unregulated increase in cAMP *(4)*. Although the major pathophysiologic effects are attributed to the enterotoxin, *V. cholerae* also recruits multiple components of the ALPINES, including enteric neurons, enterochromaffin cells, prostaglandins, and serotonin (as shown at the bottom of the figure) that together contribute to the copious fluid output in the small intestine. In addition, interneurons between the small and large intestines underlie the ability of cholera toxin in the small intestine to trigger a reflex secretory response in the colon. cAMP, cyclic adenosine monophosphate; EC, enterochromaffin; GM1, monosialotetrahexosylganglioside; G$_s$, stimulatory G protein; 5-HT, serotonin; PG, prostaglandin; ALPINES, autocrine, luminal paracrine, immunologic, neural, and endocrine systems; VIP, vasoactive intestinal polypeptide.

Na$^+$ independent, whereas the Na$^+$-dependent forms are either electrogenic (SLC4A4 [NBC1, sodium bicarbonate cotransporter 1], SLC4A5 [NBC4]) or electroneutral (SLC4A7 [NBCn1, sodium bicarbonate electroneutral cotransporter 1]).[67] Using a combination of pharmacologic and gene knockout approaches, the Na$^+$-dependent exchangers SLC4A4 and SLC4A7 appear to play a role in basolateral HCO$_3^-$ entry into the enterocyte/colonocyte; SLC4A4 appears to be important in regulating systemic pH. In contrast, the Cl$^-$-HCO$_3^-$ exchanger SLC4A2's location on the basolateral membrane of surface/villus and crypt cells suggests a role in basolateral exit of Cl$^-$,

whereas SLC4A3 appears to be on both membranes. Clearly the precise intestinal roles of the SLC4A remain to be fully elucidated.[68-70]

Structurally distinct from the SLC4 bicarbonate transporter family and gaining a lot of attention is the SLC26 multifunctional anion exchange family. SLC26 exchangers can transport Cl$^-$, HCO$_3^-$, sulfate, formate, oxalate, hydroxyl ions, and other anions with differing affinities. Their varied distribution along the GI tract provides them with the flexibility to handle a variety of luminal anions. Two members of this family, SLC26A3 and SLC26A6, are of special interest.[9,71-73] SLC26A6, formerly known as *putative anion transporter 1* (PAT-1), is expressed abundantly in the apical membrane of villus enterocytes and less so in the colon. SLC26A6 transports more than $2HCO_3^-:1Cl^-$ ion. Mice lacking SLC26A6 do not exhibit a diarrheal phenotype. In contrast, mutations in SLC26A3, first identified as DRA (down-regulated in adenoma), cause congenital chloride diarrhea that manifests with volume depletion and metabolic alkalosis. DRA is expressed abundantly on the apical membranes of colonocytes, but not enterocytes. DRA also transports more than $2Cl^-:1HCO_3^-$ ion. DRA plays a pivotal role in electroneutral NaCl absorption. Mice deficient in DRA exhibit severe diarrhea, increased colonic proliferation, and compensatory increases in ion absorption. DRA is decreased in inflammation, including models of IBD; enteropathogenic *E. coli* and *Citrobacter rodentium* decrease DRA surface expression and its activity.[67]

A number of regulatory pathways strongly influence HCO_3^- secretion. Agents that inhibit NHE3 activity (e.g., cAMP, cGMP, $[Ca^{2+}]_i$) decrease DRA activity. DRA does not act in isolation; it interacts with scaffolding proteins like NHERF3 with NHE3 and with CFTR; DRA and CFTR mutually influence each other's expression, and anion exchange is downregulated in CF. Equally important, agents that promote absorption, ranging from neuropeptide Y to butyrate, lysophosphatidic acid, and probiotics such as *Lactobacillus acidophilus*, increase DRA activity by both short-term (trafficking) and long-term (protein expression) regulation. Interestingly, the effects are specific to DRA, and similar changes are not seen in SLC26A6, making DRA a popular therapeutic target.

In contrast to the apical NHE isoforms, anion exchangers are present on the apical membranes of crypt and surface cells. The physiologic implications of the spatial distribution and varied anion transporters in net HCO_3^- secretion remain to be elucidated.

Short-Chain Fatty Acid Transport

The 2- to 4-carbon short-chain fatty acids (SCFAs) (e.g., acetate, propionate, butyrate) are generated by bacterial fermentation of poorly absorbed carbohydrates. Unlike the small intestine, in which Cl^- and HCO_3^- predominate, the major luminal anions (60 to 150 mmol/kg) in the colon are SCFAs. The magnitude of the daily colonic load and absorption of SCFAs is comparable to that of colonic Na^+. SCFAs, especially butyrate, are a major source of metabolic fuel for the colonocytes, modulate epithelial growth and differentiation, and have been implicated in the pathogenesis of and therapy for several inflammatory diseases of the colon, such as bypass colitis.

SCFAs are rapidly absorbed in the colon and also greatly enhance Na^+ and fluid reabsorption through linked transport mechanisms and by up-regulating expression of NHE3 and DRA on the apical membrane of colonocytes.[67,74] SCFAs are weak electrolytes and can be ionized or protonated. Ionized SCFAs need specific carriers, whereas non-ionized protonated species can diffuse across the colonocyte membrane; at luminal colonic pH, SCFAs are 95% to 99% ionized.

The molecular basis of SCFA transport is beginning to emerge.[31,75] First, apical NHEs can create an acidic pH microclimate and thereby enhance diffusion of protonated SCFAs into the cell. Monocarboxylate transporters (MCTs), members of 2 different SLC families, are involved in electroneutral carrier-mediated SCFA transport. Members of the SLC16 family, specifically SLC16A1 (MCT1), transport $1H^+:1SCFA^-$ and require an ancillary protein for their function.[76] Inflammation and enteropathogenic *E. coli* reduce the expression of SLC16A1, whereas pectin, butyrate, and somatostatin increase MCT1 transcript or protein expression.[77-79] High-affinity (SLC5A8) and low-affinity (SLC5A12) Na^+-dependent MCTs

have been identified in the colon and intestine and may be luminal. Although their molecular identity is unclear, Cl^--butyrate exchangers and $SCFA^-$-HCO_3^- exchangers, functionally coupled to Na^+-H^+ exchange, might account for SCFA promotion of electroneutral Na^+ and Cl^- absorption.[66,80]

AUTOCRINE, LUMINAL, PARACRINE, AND IMMUNONEUROENDOCRINE SYSTEMS (ALPINES)

Extracellular factors, including autocrine, luminal, paracrine, immunologic, neural, and endocrine systems (ALPINES), regulate intestinal ion transport in a complex and coordinated manner. The borders separating members of ALPINES are arbitrary at best, because there is considerable overlap and crosstalk of the underlying factors, and patterns can be altered in different disease states (Fig. 101-11). The influence of the luminal microbiome in health and disease is huge (see later); in addition, luminal mechanical (stroking and stretch) or chemical (toxins) stimuli can activate mechanoreceptors and chemoreceptors, respectively, to in turn activate 1 or more arms of ALPINES. All these interactions are compounded by many of the factors acting through cell-specific multiple receptors and signaling pathways.

Within the subepithelium, structural elements of ALPINES, including blood vessels, are in close proximity (Fig. 101-11), so release of mast cell mediators can easily target neurons and vice versa; this proximity and interplay contribute to the minute-by-minute local regulation necessary in the intestine. Although it is possible to separate the specific effects of an individual component in vitro, clinically they are inextricably intertwined. For example, Verner-Morrison syndrome (pancreatic cholera) is classified as an endocrine-mediated diarrhea because pancreatic islet cell tumors in this syndrome produce large amounts of vasoactive intestinal peptide (VIP). In the healthy adult, however, VIP is not found in the pancreas but is a peptidergic neurotransmitter of the enteric nervous system that stimulates epithelial cell secretion and smooth muscle relaxation. Another example is that of a single agonist like cholera toxin that directly acts on epithelial cells while simultaneously stimulating neural, paracrine, and immune responses. In a third example, serotonin (5-hydroxytryptamine [5-HT]) released by mucosal enterochromaffin cells acts via distinct receptors on epithelial cells to directly stimulate secretion. It acts on myenteric neurons to release acetylcholine (ACh) and elicit migratory contractions, or it acts on submucosal neurons to release ACh and calcitonin gene-related peptide to stimulate peristalsis and secretory reflexes.

Fluid secretion is the major component in the production of diarrhea and the host's defensive response to intestinal challenge; motility, mucus secretion, and blood flow—all regulated by ALPINES—are important adjuncts to the process. The involvement of ALPINES in motility helps explain diarrhea associated with rapid intestinal transit (e.g., following gastrectomy), altered anorectal motility (e.g., small-volume diarrhea), or decreased motility (e.g., bacterial overgrowth). Decreased motility leads to bacterial increase in the small intestine, which causes diarrhea by a variety of mechanisms (see Chapters 16, 99, 100 and 105). Alternatively, inflammatory mediators (e.g., prostaglandins, bacterial enterotoxins) target both the epithelial and muscle layers to elicit a coordinated secretory response, whereas promoters of absorption (e.g., opiates, enkephalins) suppress motility and promote electrolyte absorption. Thus, ALPINES allow for a coordinated and integrated response to multiple extracellular signals.

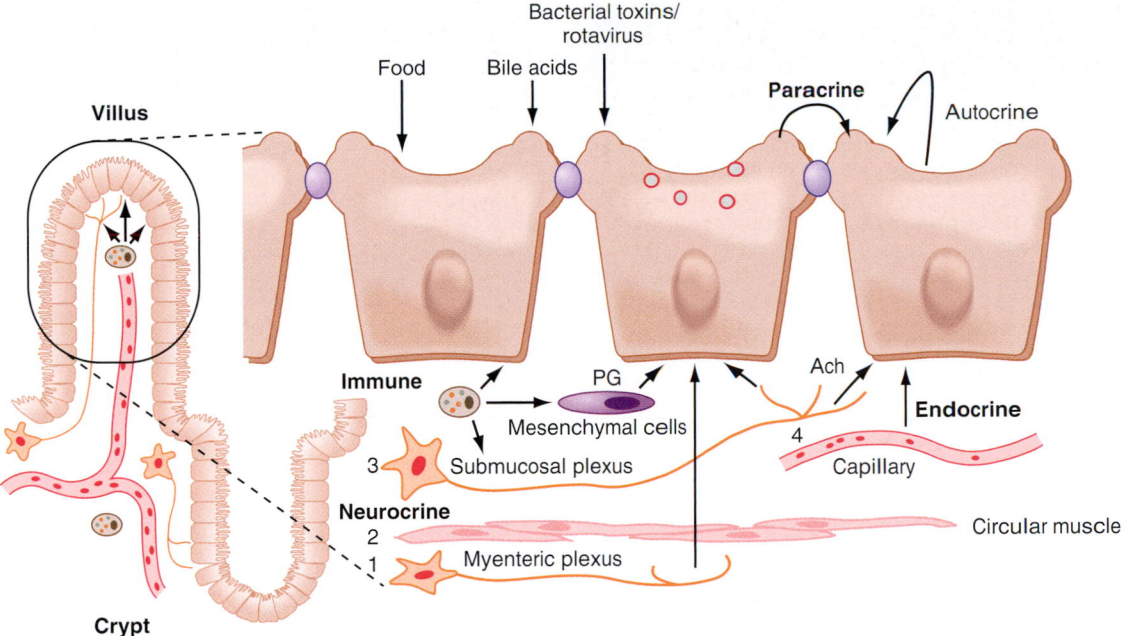

FIGURE 101-11. Model depicting the integral components of the complex systems that regulate intestinal ion transport. The components include *(1)* neurons responsive to intraluminal mechanical and chemical stimuli (e.g., food, bile acids, bacterial toxins, rotavirus); *(2)* interneurons in either the myenteric or submucosal plexuses; *(3)* secretory neurons that release acetylcholine *(ACh)*, which acts on epithelial cells; and *(4)* interactions among secretory neurons and blood vessels, immune cells, and paracrine cells. Immune responses arise from the gut-associated lymphoid tissue (GALT), cells that are often distinct from their systemic counterparts; in non-inflamed intestine, T lymphocytes account for 60% of GALT, with smaller numbers of B lymphocytes and plasma cells (25% to 30%), macrophages (8% to 10%), mast cells, and polymorphonuclear cells (2% to 5%) (usually eosinophils).[85] Intestinal cells can release an array of secretory factors that can act either directly on the epithelium or indirectly by stimulating the mesenchymal cells or enteric neurons to release prostaglandins *(PG)* or ACh. See text for details.

EXTRACELLULAR REGULATION

Tables 101-1, 101-2 and 101-3 list the major neurohumoral substances and toxins that modulate intestinal fluid transport. Agents that promote net fluid secretion generally inhibit Na+ absorption and stimulate Cl− secretion, whereas agents that promote net fluid absorption increase Na+ uptake and attenuate Cl− secretion. In a healthy person, net absorption prevails, and when this balance is disrupted, diarrhea can ensue. It is unclear if there is a corollary for a predominant absorptive pattern in a subset of patients with constipation.

AUTOCRINE, ENDOCRINE, PARACRINE, AND JUXTACRINE REGULATION

Intestinal transport is modulated by autocrine, classic endocrine, paracrine, and juxtacrine processes. Epithelial cells can self-regulate (autocrine) by secreting factors such as eicosanoids,[81] which act on epithelial cell receptors to alter function.[81] Intestinal endocrine cells are interspersed between epithelial cells and function as sensors that rapidly respond to changes in the luminal environment by releasing secretory granules containing biogenic amines and hormones; these mediators cross the basolateral membrane and the hormones can act either in a classic endocrine manner on distant target cells (via the circulation) or in a local (paracrine) manner by affecting neighboring cells in the intestinal wall. Juxtacrine mediators are those released from non-endocrine cells (e.g., neural and inflammatory cells), and they affect neighboring

cells. Intestinal mesenchymal cells, in particular myofibroblasts, are a rich source of cytokines, chemokines, eicosanoids, and growth factors that can alter intestinal transport.

Neural Regulation

Neural input is critical in the regulation of fluid and electrolyte transport (Fig. 101-11) and involves interactions of the parasympathetic and sympathetic divisions of the autonomic nervous system with the labyrinthine enteric nervous system (ENS) (see Chapters 4, 99, and 100). Cholinergic stimulation of secretion, predominantly through parasympathetic vagal input, and adrenergic stimulation of absorption through prevertebral and sympathetic ganglia have long been recognized as fundamental neural pathways affecting the intestinal epithelium. The ENS is the end-controller of neural activity in the intestinal wall, although it also independently integrates the regulation of epithelia, muscles, and blood vessels, with input and modification from the central nervous system (CNS). Like other neural networks, the ENS has reflexes that can have important clinical implications. Target cells for neurons include components of ALPINES, blood vessels, and epithelial cells. Sensory input into the ENS comes from changes in the luminal content (e.g., acidity, dietary content, pathogens) or volume (e.g., stretch). Thus, acid or distension can activate TRVP1 (transient receptor potential cation channel subfamily V member 1) vanilloid receptor on capsaicin-sensitive afferent nerves, which in turn evokes secretion by stimulating submucosal neurons and causes vasodilation by direct action on submucosal arterioles.[82,83] Endocrine, dendritic, and/or paracrine cells releasing serotonin, adenosine (see later), and other signals are implicated as auxiliary sensors. Primarily cholinergic,

TABLE 101-1 Agents That Stimulate Intestinal Absorption of Fluid and Electrolytes

Endogenous Absorbagogues	Intracellular Mechanism	Source
α-Adrenergic agonists	Decreases cAMP	Adrenal medulla
Aldosterone	Genomic and non-genomic, SGKI	Adrenal cortex
Angiotensin II	?	Endothelial cells
Enkephalins	Decreases cAMP	ENS; EC cells
Glucocorticoids	Genomic, non-genomic, SGKI	Adrenal cortex
Growth hormone	Tyrosine kinase	Pituitary gland
Neuropeptide Y	Decreases cAMP	ENS
Peptide YY	Decreases cAMP	EC cells
Prolactin	Tyrosine kinase	Pituitary gland
Short-chain fatty acids	?	Colonic lumen
Somatostatin	Decreases cAMP	ENS and EC cells

Pharmacologic Agents	Intracellular Mechanism
Berberine	?
Clonidine (α₂-agonist)	Decreases cAMP
Cyclooxygenase inhibitors	Inhibits prostaglandin production
Glucocorticoids	See above
Lithium	Decreases PIP_2 and Ca^{2+}
Mineralocorticoids	See above
Octreotide	Decreases cAMP
SST analog	
Opiates	Decrease cAMP
Propranolol (beta blocker)	Blocks cAMP production

cAMP, cyclic adenosine monophosphate; EC, enterochromaffin; ENS, enteric nervous system; PIP_2, phosphatidyl inositol bisphosphate; SGKI, serum- and glucocorticoid-inducible kinase I; SST, somatostatin.

TABLE 101-2 Endogenous Agonists of Intestinal Secretion

Agonist	Intracellular Mediator	Source
Acetylcholine	Ca^{2+}	ENS
Adenosine	cAMP	Immune cells
Arachidonic acid	cAMP	Immune cells, cell membranes
Atrial natriuretic peptide	cGMP	Heart
Bombesin	Ca^{2+}	??
Bradykinin	cAMP	Immune cells
Calcitonin, calcitonin gene-related peptide	Ca^{2+}, cAMP?	ENS
Galanin	Ca^{2+}	??
Gastric inhibitory polypeptide	?	??
Gastrin	Ca^{2+} (PKC/MAPK?)	Endocrine cells
Guanylin	cGMP	Goblet, epithelial cells
Histamine	Ca^{2+}	Immune cells
Leukotrienes	?	Immune cells
Motilin	Ca^{2+}	Endocrine M cells
Neurotensin	Ca^{2+}	ENS
Nitric oxide	cGMP	Immune cells, mesenchymal cells
Peptide histidine, isoleucine	cAMP	ENS
Platelet activating factor	cAMP	Immune cells
Prostaglandins	cAMP	Immune cells, mesenchymal cells
Reactive oxygen species	cAMP	Immune cells
Secretin	cAMP	Endocrine cells
Serotonin	Ca^{2+}	ENS
Substance P	Ca^{2+}	ENS
Vasoactive intestinal polypeptide	cAMP	ENS

cAMP, cyclic adenosine monophosphate; cGMP, cyclic guanosine monophosphate; ENS, enteric nervous system. PKC/MAPK?, Protein kinase C/mitogen-activated protein kinase?

interneurons are believed to underlie ENS-mediated regulation of colonic epithelial responses to distant small intestinal challenges. Motor neurons that innervate epithelial and submucosal cells can be cholinergic or VIPergic, each releasing additional neuroactive substances.

A basal cholinergic secretory drive is tempered by sympathetic tone; loss of adrenergic sympathetic innervation in diabetic neuropathy is associated with development of "diabetic diarrhea" and may be corrected by α₂-adrenergic agonists.[84] As in the brain, recognition of the number and variety of compounds that act as neuroactive agents has ballooned, adding to the complexity of our elucidation of underlying mechanisms. For example, neurons can release specific combinations of mediators such as VIP, cholecystokinin, gastrin-releasing peptide, and ATP, not just a single substance. Individual neurotransmitters can have biphasic effects that vary with concentration. Furthermore, agents can act as classic neurotransmitters and alternatively as neuromodulators, fine-tuning the neuronal circuits of presynaptic sites of neurons or as paracrine mediators (e.g., serotonin).

Immunologic and Inflammatory Regulation

The intestine is the first line of defense against the onslaught of foreign substances in the lumen. It is equipped with highly

TABLE 101-3 Luminal Agents That Stimulate Intestinal Secretion

Agent	Intracellular Mediator
Bacterial Enterotoxins	
Aeromonas spp.	cAMP
Campylobacter jejuni	cAMP
Clostridium difficile (toxin A)	Ca^{2+}
Clostridium perfringens	??
Escherichia coli (heat-labile toxin)	cAMP
Enteropathogenic *E. coli*	Ca^{2+}
Enteroadherent *E. coli*	cAMP
E. coli (heat-stable toxin)	cGMP
Rotavirus NSP4	Ca^{2+}
Salmonella spp.	cAMP
Vibrio cholerae	
Accessory cholera enterotoxin	??
Enterotoxin	cAMP
Zonula occludens toxin	??
Vibrio parahaemolyticus	Ca^{2+}
Yersinia enterocolitica	cGMP
Miscellaneous Agents	
Bile salts	cAMP/Ca^{2+}
Laxatives	??
Long-chain fatty acids	cAMP/Ca^{2+}

cAMP, cyclic adenosine monophosphate; cGMP, cyclic guanosine monophosphate; NSP, nonstructural protein.

regulated gut-associated lymphoid tissue (GALT), that has features distinct from its systemic counterpart.[85] The clinical correlation between intestinal inflammation and diarrhea is obvious (see Chapter 2), with ulceration, exudation of protein, changes in motility, and loss of absorptive surface area implicated as causing the fluid losses of (inflammatory) diarrheas. Immunocompetent cells of the intestine reside chiefly in the lamina propria and secrete a vast array of soluble products (chemokines, cytokines, eicosanoids, nucleotides, biogenic amines), actions of which are intimately intertwined with other elements of ALPINES. Intestinal inflammation increases the number of immunocytes, the cause of the inflammation determining the type of inflammatory cells. Acute bacterial infections increase polymorphonuclear leukocytes, whereas parasitic infections dramatically enlarge the mast cell population, and celiac disease is characterized by intraepithelial lymphocytes. In IBD, there is activation of all components of GALT, with an increase in immunoglobulin (Ig)G-secreting cells.[86,87] The innate immune system, a rapid-response team for the intestinal mucosa, has become increasingly recognized as an important factor in intestinal function (see Chapter 2). Thus, the cause of the inflammatory reaction can determine the types of immunocytes recruited, the range of cytokines released, and the specific effects on transport and motility.

Many inflammatory mediators are potent secretagogues, including peptides (e.g., cytokines, platelet-activating factor, substance P, interferon [IFN]-γ, kallikreins, and bradykinin), eicosanoids (e.g., arachidonic acid, leukotrienes, and prostaglandins), and oxidants (e.g., superoxides). These mediators either interact directly with epithelia to alter ion transport and barrier function or elicit these effects indirectly by activating other ALPINES elements (Fig. 101-11). Prostaglandins are central to the secretory response associated with inflammation, affecting various ALPINES components, such as enteric neurons, and with mediators such as bradykinin, which liberates arachidonic acid to stimulate prostaglandin production. In interpreting the effects of the inflammatory mediators in normal model systems, it is important to recognize that in vivo, cells damaged by the inflammatory process might not be able to function normally. With this caveat, a few examples are provided.

Mucosal mast cells are strategically located close to enteric neurons, blood vessels, and epithelial cells, and they are central to several inflammatory reactions. Mast cell mediators, including histamine, eicosanoids, and cytokines, elicit secretion by direct effects on the epithelial cells and by indirect neural stimulation and prostaglandin release.

The mechanisms of secretion resulting from polymorphonuclear infiltration of the mucosa have recently become better understood. Polymorphonuclear leukocytes, responding to chemoattractants (e.g., fMLP [formyl-Met-Leu-Phe]), uniquely present in the inflamed colon, leave the vasculature, and interact with epithelial cells.[88] The white blood cells burrow through the intercellular space of the colonic cells in a complex integrin-dependent process. The migrating leukocytes release 5-AMP, which is converted to adenosine by apical membrane enzymes. Adenosine is a potent secretagogue, and this adenosine-stimulated secretion might serve as a mechanism to cleanse the crypt lumen.[89] Thus, complex specific immunocyte–epithelial cell interactions are important in alterations of electrolyte secretion associated with mucosal inflammation. Anti-integrin targeted therapy may be effective in treating IBD (see Chapters 115, 116).

During inflammation, reactive oxygen species (ROS) like superoxides, oxygen free radicals, hydrogen peroxide, and hydroxyl radicals are released from neutrophils and stimulate Cl^- secretion; cytokines such as interleukin (IL)-1 and IL-3 also stimulate secretion.[90] ROS can also be released by epithelial cells under pathophysiologic conditions. In contrast, IFN-γ and tumor necrosis factor (TNF)-α can cause diarrhea more through an anti-absorptive effect by down-regulating particular transporters[91-93] or by altering permeability of tight junctions. Similarly, studies on colonic specimens from patients with IBD indicate that diarrhea in Crohn's disease and ulcerative colitis (UC) results not from stimulated secretion but from increased tissue permeability combined with decreased apical Na^+ channel and DRA expression, basolateral K^+ channel, and Na^+/K^+-ATPase expression, all of which lead to decreased NaCl absorptive capacity.[67,87] The multiplicity of transport malfunctions seen in IBD might reflect a sick-cell syndrome rather than specific alterations modulated by 1 or 2 unique cytokines.

SYSTEMIC EFFECTS

Acid-base balance modulates intestinal electrolyte transport in vivo and in vitro. Metabolic acidosis is a potent stimulator of electroneutral NaCl absorption, whereas metabolic alkalosis inhibits this process.[94,95] Intracellular bicarbonate concentrations can modulate basal Cl^- secretion; intracellular pH and Pco_2 can alter Na^+/H^+ exchange. Volume status and intestinal blood flow also alter ion transport. Any decrease in intravascular volume, such as with hemorrhage, elicits a series of responses that increase fluid absorption. These responses may be mediated by increased sympathetic input into the ENS, angiotensin II, antidiuretic hormone, and atrial natriuretic peptide.[96,97] Metabolic status is important because a well-fed intestine transports more effectively, with changes being observed even at 16 hours of fasting.[98] There are distinct segmental preferences for metabolic fuels. Although the entire intestinal tract uses glucose, the small bowel effectively uses glutamine, and the colon preferentially uses SCFAs, particularly butyrate, as sources of nutrients.[99,100]

OSMOTIC EFFECTS

Unlike the kidney, the intestinal epithelium cannot maintain an osmotic gradient. Under normal physiologic conditions, the duodenum and upper jejunum are subject to major fluid shifts as they adjust to dietary intake of hypertonic foods and liquids. Rapid equilibration is usually accomplished by movement of water into the intestinal lumen, and absorptive processes along the remainder of the intestine steadily decrease the luminal volume. The continued presence of a non-absorbable solute within the intestinal lumen, however, can negate functioning absorptive pathways in the distal intestine. This is the basis for osmotic diarrhea (see Chapter 16).

Carbohydrates, usually disaccharides, are a common source of non-absorbable solute. Disaccharides must be hydrolyzed to monosaccharides before they can cross the apical membrane of the small intestine (see Chapter 102). The most common clinical example of maldigestion is lactose intolerance, in which the glucose-galactose disaccharide cannot be broken down because of a deficiency of the specific disaccharidase, lactase. Because the human intestine does not possess lactulase, the disaccharide lactulose reliably increases small intestinal fluid because of luminal hyperosmolarity and bacterial fermentation of the disaccharide. The limited intestinal absorptive capacity for several sugars found in processed foods and drinks (e.g., fructose and sorbitol) can play important but often overlooked roles in osmotic diarrhea, bloating, abdominal pain, and IBS (see Chapter 122).

The physiology of carbohydrate-induced osmotic diarrhea is complicated by the fact that non-absorbable solutes in the small intestine can be converted into absorbable solutes by colonic bacteria. Almost all classes of carbohydrates not absorbed by the small intestine are rapidly converted to SCFAs once they cross the ileocecal valve and encounter colonic bacteria; these SCFAs are absorbed by and serve as metabolic fuel for the colon. Thus, depending on the rate of carbohydrate conversion to SCFAs by the intestinal microbiota and the colonic capacity for SCFA absorption, small intestinal fluid loss may be compensated by colonic fluid absorption. However, if the capacity of either of these colonic functions is exceeded, additional unmetabolized carbohydrates in the colon could exacerbate the osmotic effects of non-absorbable solute.[101]

Cations (e.g., magnesium) or anions (e.g., sulfate and phosphate) are poorly absorbed by the normal intestine, and their excessive intake easily leads to osmotic diarrhea, as seen with ingestion of magnesium-containing antacids or supplements. The colonic lavage preparations given prior to colonoscopy cleanse the colon by causing an osmotic diarrhea induced by non-absorbable molecules, including polyethylene glycol and sulfate.

In clinical situations in which there is malabsorption or a generalized destruction of the epithelium, solutes normally absorbed readily can remain in the intestinal lumen and thereby contribute an osmotic component to an inflammatory diarrhea or a malabsorptive state. Osmolality is an important factor in patients receiving enteral nutrition (see Chapters 6 and 106). Compared with simple sugars, complex carbohydrates provide a significant amount of calories with minimal osmolality. Absorption of dipeptides and tripeptides instead of amino acids reduces intestinal osmolality. This balance between calories and osmolality becomes clinically relevant in effectively designing appropriate tube-feeding regimens. Osmolality is also important in designing second-generation oral rehydration therapy (ORT) formulations; by replacing glucose with complex carbohydrates like rice, intestinal absorption is further stimulated by creating a hypotonic luminal environment, thereby enhancing water absorption. In addition to providing numerous sugar molecules per milliosmole, complex carbohydrates such as rice and amylase-resistant starches have another advantage when used in ORT: they are metabolized by commensal bacteria in the colon to release SCFAs, which in turn promote fluid absorption (see earlier discussion of SCFAs).[102]

SPECIFIC REGULATORY FACTORS

Absorptive Factors

Agents that stimulate intestinal absorption—absorbagogues—are listed in Table 101-1.

Mineralocorticoids (e.g., aldosterone) primarily influence electrogenic Na^+ absorption in the distal colon and have little effect on the small intestine, which exhibits electroneutral Na^+ absorption. Aldosterone increases the activity and numbers of the apical membrane ENaC (see earlier discussion of Na^+ channels) and stimulates activity of the Na^+/K^+ pump and SGK1 (see earlier discussion), resulting in an increase in Na^+ absorption. Aldosterone increases both K^+ absorption and K^+ secretion.[103] In contrast to adults, neonates exhibit enhanced colonic Na^+ absorption that can be correlated to high circulating levels of aldosterone.[23] Clinically, the physiologic role of aldosterone can be seen in the increased colonic Na^+ absorption after Na^+ depletion (aldosterone stimulation) or in the diarrhea associated with Addison's disease (aldosterone deficiency).

Glucocorticoids are also potent stimulators of Na^+ absorption in the small intestine and colon. At low concentrations, glucocorticoids stimulate electroneutral Na^+ absorption and suppress electrogenic Na^+ absorption, whereas at high concentrations they stimulate both processes. The actions of glucocorticoids are complex, species- and segment-specific, and may be directed at the level of apical Na^+ transporters and at the Na^+ pump. In the rabbit jejunum, ileum, and colon, glucocorticoid-stimulated increases in Na^+ absorption are associated with selective increases in NHE3, but not NHE2 or NHE1 mRNA and protein. Both glucocorticoids and aldosterone evoke rapid cellular responses that involve the SGK1 pathway as well as genomic transcriptional effects. These effects might account in part for the potent antidiarrheal action of glucocorticoids in a wide variety of clinical settings.[37]

Catecholamines, enkephalins, and somatostatin all stimulate electroneutral Na^+ absorption and often decrease HCO_3^- secretion with similar patterns of action. They bind to specific heptahelical membrane receptors and activate the $G\alpha_i$ cascade, which in turn suppresses the prosecretory cAMP signaling cascade. Of these absorbagogues, catecholamines such as dopamine and epinephrine act on α-adrenergic receptors to elicit similar absorptive properties. The theoretical basis for the use of clonidine as an antidiarrheal agent, particularly in diabetic diarrhea, is rooted in this adrenergic absorptive pathway.[104]

The use of plant opiates as antidiarrheal agents dates back 2 millennia to the early Egyptians, underscoring their effectiveness. Elucidating their therapeutic effect led to the characterization of the mammalian opioid peptides—enkephalins, endorphins, and dynorphins—a classic example of molecular mimicry.[105] Acting via 1 of 3 main opioid receptor subtypes—mu, delta, and kappa—the opiates and opioid peptides decrease secretion and promote non-propulsive motility patterns, thereby increasing intestinal transit time. They can act directly on epithelial and smooth muscle cells or modify the electrical and synaptic behavior of ENS neurons. The constipation associated with morphine intake can result from hyperpolarization of secretomotor neurons and suppression of secretion or to a centrally mediated stimulation of sympathetic noradrenergic discharge, or both. Direct activation of K^+ channels and inhibition of Ca^{2+} channels via a G protein-mediated mechanism underlie these effects. Chronic treatment with opiates leads to tolerance, and diarrhea ensues upon abrupt withdrawal. Management of constipation in patients receiving opiates as analgesics can be a clinical challenge.

The development of long-acting analogs of somatostatin has transformed this ubiquitously distributed hormone from a physiologically fascinating regulator to a clinically relevant pharmacologic agent (see Chapter 4). In the intestine, enterochromaffin D cells produce somatostatin, which stimulates salt and water absorption in the ileum and colon and blocks the effects of several secretagogues.[106,107] Somatostatin analogs such as octreotide are effective in treating several types of diarrheal diseases, particularly endocrine-related secretory diarrhea. Their therapeutic effect is due to a combination of inhibiting hormone release from tumors, slowing of intestinal transit, and a direct effect on epithelial cells. Paradoxically, elevated somatostatin levels, as encountered in somatostatinomas or with large pharmacologic doses of octreotide, can precipitate diarrhea secondary to steatorrhea.[104] Other peptide hormones, including peptide NPY, YY, angiotensin II, and insulin, have been implicated as proabsorptive agents, but their physiologic significance awaits full elucidation.

Secretory Factors

Endogenous agents that stimulate intestinal secretion are listed in Table 101-2. Many hormones and neurotransmitters have been shown to stimulate intestinal secretion and generally act to inhibit electroneutral NaCl absorption and stimulate Cl^- secretion. Interestingly, most of these agents also affect intestinal motility. They are classified by their mechanisms of action: ACh (via the muscarinic M3 receptor), serotonin, and neurotensin, which increase $[Ca^{2+}]_i$; VIP and related peptide hormones (e.g., secretin and peptide histidine leucine) that increase intracellular cAMP; and some prostaglandins that increase intracellular cAMP; and guanylin, which acts by increasing cell cGMP. Many agents have been demonstrated to act via multiple pathways; for example, calcitonin increases Cl^- secretion via a PKA- and Ca^{2+}-signaling pathway. Selected examples follow.

Eicosanoids

Although there are subtle differences in their biological actions, in general, eicosanoids (e.g., arachidonic acid, prostaglandins, leukotrienes) are secretagogues. As described in the section "Immunologic Regulation," prostaglandins from submucosal immunocytes have autocrine and juxtacrine effects on epithelial cells and enteric nerves, and alter intestinal motility and blood flow. Depending on the type of prostaglandin and receptor subtype, they act primarily via cAMP and, to a lesser extent, via $[Ca^{2+}]_i$. Prostaglandins contribute to the basal secretory tone of the epithelium, as demonstrated by cyclooxygenase inhibitors indomethacin or aspirin increasing basal rates of absorption.

Increased intestinal production of eicosanoids contribute to the diarrhea of IBD (see Chapters 115 and 116). Glucocorticoids can decrease prostaglandin synthesis. Although the 5-ASA (acetylsalicylic acid) class of medications, which are a mainstay of IBD treatment, target cyclooxygenase and decrease prostaglandin production, their clinical efficacy probably depends on additional mechanisms that involve other inflammatory pathways, including nuclear factor (NF)-κB and ROS.[108,109] Although their mechanisms are less well understood, leukotrienes contribute to fluid imbalance by activating secretomotor neurons in the subepithelium.

Serotonin and Adenosine

Serotonin plays a critical role in modulating intestinal motility, sensation, and secretion, and is responsible for the diarrhea associated with carcinoid tumors. About 95% of the body's serotonin is produced by enterochromaffin cells, and the remainder is produced by serotoninergic neurons of the myenteric plexus. Sensory receptors on enterochromaffin cells are activated by mechanical stimuli, acidity, invading pathogens, and dietary contents; for example, SGLT-like protein activates enterochromaffin cells, which serve as a glucose sensor to secrete serotonin (see Fig. 101-10).[110] Although not completely elucidated, this signaling involves a complex sequence of autocrine and paracrine actions: ATP is released and converted extracellularly to ADP, which in turn activates a purinergic (P2Y) receptor-mediated calcium signaling cascade in the enterochromaffin cell to release 5-HT.[110] 5-HT then acts in a paracrine manner to stimulate epithelial cells, intrinsic primary afferent neurons (IPANs), and extrinsic primary afferent neurons (EPANs). Specific 5-HT receptor subtypes on different IPANs modulate the secretory reflex. Thus, 5-HT$_{1P}$R on submucosal IPANs and amplifying presynaptic 5-HT$_4$ receptors cause the release of ACh and calcitonin gene-related peptide, which stimulate peristaltic and secretory reflexes. In contrast, 5-HT$_3$Rs on myenteric IPANs trigger the release of ACh to stimulate giant migrating contractions.[110-112] Serotonin stimulation of EPANs results in CNS-mediated responses of nausea and discomfort.

The major mechanism of serotonin inactivation is by a serotonin reuptake transporter (SERT) on enterocytes and neurons. Interestingly, SERT may be decreased in patients with diarrhea-predominant IBS (IBS-D) and with UC. There has been a concerted effort to alter intestinal function clinically by pharmacologic manipulation of specific serotonin receptors. Thus, 5-HT$_3$ receptor antagonists (e.g., alosetron) are used to treat IBS-D, and tegaserod, a partial 5-HT$_4$ agonist, can alleviate constipation associated with IBS-C. Unfortunately, significant side effects have limited the clinical use of alosetron, and tegaserod has been removed from the market (see Chapter 122).[104,112,113]

Adenosine and related purine nucleotides play unique and complex roles in modulating secretion in vivo. They can stimulate secretion directly or indirectly via release of 5-HT.[110] However, adenosine acting via P1 purinoreceptors has also been shown to attenuate secretion evoked by mechanical stimuli. Activation or inhibition of different populations of channels can underlie these seemingly opposite effects.

Guanylin and Nitric Oxide

The search for an endogenous activator of the receptor for *E. coli* heat-stable enterotoxin, STa, the causal agent of traveller's diarrhea, led to the discovery of the peptides guanylin and uroguanylin, chiefly synthesized in goblet and enterochromaffin cells, respectively. These peptides, like their molecular mimic STa, are small, have a secondary structure that is resistant to intestinal proteases, activate membrane GUCY2C to increase intracellular cGMP, and elicit fluid secretion. Several recent clinical observations corroborate the relevance of the GUCY2C/guanylin axis in intestinal homeostasis. A Norwegian familial diarrheal syndrome with increased susceptibility to IBD has been ascribed to a gain-in function mutation of GUCY2C. In contrast, a loss of function GUCY2C mutation in a Bedouin family has been associated with a high incidence of meconium ileus.[114] Evidence also suggests a novel role for

GUCY2C in the gut-brain axis, dysregulation of which leads to obesity and colorectal cancer. Development of a stable guanylin analog as a treatment for constipation and IBS-C may well have significant impact on management of these common clinical problems in gastroenterology.[115,116]

In contrast, nitric oxide, a neuroimmune regulator, stimulates soluble guanylate cyclase to increase cGMP.[117] This enzyme is far more prevalent in the subepithelium of the small intestine, but it is expressed in colonic epithelia. Activation of soluble guanylate cyclase in the subepithelium has been implicated in immunomodulation and in relaxation of smooth muscle, including vasodilation.

Microbiota and Microbial Pathogens

The mature human intestinal microbiota is made up of 9 divisions and 500 to more than 1000 species of bacteria the vast majority of which belong to the *Bacteroidetes* and *Firmicutes* phyla. The advent of pyrosequencing has led to an information explosion on the importance of the host-microbiome relationship in dictating almost all aspects of human function (see Chapter 3). As described earlier under bicarbonate and SCFA transport, the role of probiotic species in normal physiology to promote absorption and generate SCFA is pivotal, and their mechanisms are still being elucidated (also see later).

In contrast, microbial pathogens (bacteria, viruses, and fungi) can alter electrolyte transport, increase intestinal permeability, and trigger inflammation to elicit diarrhea. They do this by a variety of mechanisms, including attaching to epithelial cells to insert their own products and alter host cell machinery, and by elaborating enterotoxins, which may be cytotoxic or can capture cell-signaling mechanisms to elicit secretion or disrupt tight junctions (see Table 101-3 and Chapter 110).[118-122] In addition, the intestinal microbiota has been shown to influence host susceptibility to infectious colitis.[123,124] A few examples are provided here.

The archetypal enterotoxin-mediated diarrhea is cholera. *Vibrio cholerae* carries a virulence cassette that produces at least 3 different molecules: an enterotoxin, a zonula occludens toxin (ZOT) that disrupts tight junction permeability, and an accessory cholera toxin (ACE), a channel-like protein that remains to be characterized.[125] The enterotoxin causes an unregulated increase in cAMP, activates CFTR, and inhibits NHE3, resulting in copious fluid secretion (see Fig. 101-10 legend for details). Mice lacking CFTR do not respond to cholera toxin. Despite voluminous secretion, specific intestinal Na^+-coupled nutrient absorptive (Na^+-glucose, Na^+-amino acids) pathways are unaltered by the toxin, forming the physiologic basis for ORT. Bacteria such as *Salmonella* species, *Campylobacter jejuni*, and *E. coli* elaborate enterotoxins similar to cholera toxin, and likewise employ the cAMP machinery to elicit fluid secretion.

Strains of *E. coli* and *Yersinia enterocolitica* associated with traveler's diarrhea elaborate small molecular weight, heat-stable enterotoxins (STa), which increase cGMP to stimulate fluid secretion; signaling cascades distinct from cAMP and cGMP also activate CFTR and inhibit NHE3 (see the discussion of intracellular mediators). *Vibrio parahaemolyticus* elaborates a thermostable direct hemolysin (TDH) and is a major cause of gastroenteritis; its associated intestinal fluid secretion is attributed to an increase in $[Ca^{2+}]_i$ and activation of the Ca^{2+}-calmodulin and protein kinase C signaling pathways.[104,122] Thus, the secretory diarrheas associated with cholera and traveler's diarrhea result from noninvasive pathogens that elaborate enterotoxins that capture and turn on the secretory machinery of the epithelium.

Rotavirus, the major cause of infantile gastroenteritis, induces watery diarrhea. The virus predominantly infects the mature enterocyte of the villus and elaborates an enterotoxin, non-structural glycoprotein (NSP4).[126,127] NSP4 can inhibit brush border membrane disaccharidases and SGLT1 activity, thereby limiting Na^+-glucose and fluid absorption, with resultant diarrhea. NSP4 in vitro elicits Cl^- secretion via a calcium-phospholipase C pathway that stimulates Ca^{2+}-activated Cl^- channels, presumably transmembrane protein 16A (TMEM16A; listed as anoctamin 1, calcium activated chloride channel, ANO1 by HGNC). This transient secretion resembles the actions of carbachol. Unlike cholera toxin, NSP4 has no effect on crypt cell secretion, but under favorable electrochemical conditions, it stimulates secretion from villus cells. Paradoxically, NSP4 can also stimulate Cl^- absorption from villus cells. Efforts to define the role of NSP4 in vivo are stymied by the necessity to use non-human animal models and cell lines. Parallel to its pathogenic profile in humans, rotaviral NSP4's action on fluid secretion occurs in young (7 to 14 days) but not in adult murine models. NSP4 can stimulate secretion in isolated ileal and colonic crypts of CFTR-deficient, young but not adult mice, suggesting a non-CFTR mechanism.[128] Whether NSP4 acts via the TMEM16a Cl^- channel remains to be established; evidence[60] both for and against[59] such a role have been published.

In contrast to cholera toxin and STa, other bacteria release toxins that penetrate the enterocyte to affect function. For example, *Shigella* causes dysentery by release of Shiga cytotoxins that enter the epithelial cell, inhibit protein synthesis, impair absorption, and damage the mucosa.

Many bacterial pathogens use different signaling molecules (e.g., kinases, phosphatases) to perturb the delicate balance of tight junctional proteins and cytoskeletal elements, thus disrupting intestinal permeability. The anaerobic bacterium *Clostridium difficile*, which causes antibiotic-associated pseudomembranous colitis (see Chapter 112), and *Clostridium perfringens*, which is associated with food-borne illnesses (see Chapter 111), alter intestinal permeability by using 2 distinct processes. The *C. difficile* toxins A and B interact with the Rho family of cellular proteins to disrupt the perijunctional actin-myosin ring, whereas the tight-junction claudin proteins serve as receptors for *C. perfringens* enterotoxin (CPE), and binding results in a disruption of tight-junctional fibrils. Other bacteria, including *Bacteroides fragilis* and *V. cholerae*, elaborate proteases that attack junctional proteins (e.g., occludins, claudins, cadherin) to disrupt the integrity of tight junctions.[104,122]

Enteropathogenic (EPEC) and enterohemorrhagic (EHEC) *E. coli* decrease transepithelial resistance using different signaling cascades. EPEC strains use a fascinating arsenal to alter host cell responses. They adhere to intestinal cells and in the process recruit a complex network of host cytoskeletal elements and use a distinct "type III" secretion apparatus to insert effector molecules into the host cell, which then co-opt the cell machinery to cause changes in the actin-myosin network, alter tight-junction proteins, and decrease surface expression of DRA to decrease absorption and increase fluid accumulation.[119,121] Many bacterial strains, including EPEC, EHEC, ETEC, *Salmonella*, and *Shigella*, trigger a highly specialized cascade of cellular processes to stimulate ion secretion. These pathogens induce the expression of receptors for the peptide neurohormone galanin, whereas uninfected cells do not possess galanin receptors. Galanin in turn activates Cl^- secretion via Ca^{2+}-dependent signaling processes.[129-132] The ever-expanding spectrum of toxin-induced mechanisms underscores the importance of delineating the intrinsic regulatory processes and the molecular pathophysiology of infectious diarrhea, both to better treat diarrheal diseases and to unravel the molecular bases of mucosal defense and secretion.

The mouse pathogen equivalent of EPEC, *Citrobacter rodentium*, is very useful in elucidating how intestinal microbiota influence host susceptibility to infectious colitis.[123,124]

Protection of mice from lethal colitis was associated with higher levels of *Bacteroidetes* species,[123] again attesting to the increasingly appreciated role of the commensal microbiota in health and disease. C3H/HeOuJ mice demonstrate an inherent genetic susceptibility to *C. rodentium* infection with resultant mortality, whereas C57BL/6 mice develop a self-limiting acute colitis with little associated mortality after infection with the same organism. Infection-induced dehydration in C3H/HeOuJ is a consequence of defective expression of carbonic anhydrase isoforms I and IV and the colonic ion transporter DRA; expression of these genes was normalized, thus overcoming the innate susceptibility to colitis, after colonization of C3H/HeOuJ mice with the C57BL/6 microflora.

Dietary composition can alter the microbiome sufficient to cause dysbiosis. For example, a diet high in saturated fat given to colitis-susceptible mice leads to expansion of the pathobiont *Bilophila wadsworthii*, increased inflammation, and presumably alteration of underlying ion transport mechanisms.[133]

Further, as explained in the section on anion absorption, the antidiarrheal nature of probiotics like *L. acidophilus* (LA) is due to their increasing the expression and activity of DRA and NHE3, thereby promoting[134,135] intestinal electrolyte absorption. Some probiotics are also anti-inflammatory and counteract proinflammatory TNF-α effects by increasing expression of SMCT1 (sodium-coupled monocarboxylate transporter 1) and thereby stimulating butyrate absorption.[136]

Bile Acids and Long-Chain Fatty Acids

An increase in colonic bile acids secondary to ileal malabsorption or oral supplementation can cause diarrhea (see Chapters 16, 64).[12,13] Only 7α-dihydroxy bile acids (conjugated and unconjugated) such as chenodeoxycholic acid (3α, 7α), but not 7β-dihydroxy bile acids, are associated with diarrhea.[23] At high concentrations, bile acids act as a detergent and increase intestinal permeability. At more physiologic concentrations, bile salts indirectly increase cAMP and activate mast cells; more importantly, they stimulate colonic epithelial cell Cl⁻ secretion in a species specific manner either via the cAMP cascade[144] or via the Ca^{2+} and PKCδ cascade.[137,138] The ability of bile salts to stimulate Cl⁻ secretion appears to be developmentally regulated, occurring only in the adult animal and absent in the neonatal and weanling rabbit.[137]

Long-chain fatty acids are seen in increased concentration in the colonic lumen in conditions such as celiac disease, when long-chain triglycerides are digested by lipase but the fatty acids are malabsorbed within the small intestine (see Chapters 104 and 107). Hydroxylated fatty acids are more potent secretagogues than the corresponding long-chain fatty acids and arise from colonic bacterial metabolism; ricinoleic acid is the long-chain fatty acid that is derived from orally administered castor oil, which is a non-toxic oil before it is hydroxylated by intestinal bacteria. Specific fatty acid transporters have been identified in the intestine, and their mechanisms of action in electrolyte secretion are similar to those of bile acids.[139,140]

INTRACELLULAR MEDIATORS

The barrage of extracellular stimuli has to be translated into an intracellular language so the cell can regulate its transport machinery. The second messenger cascades of the cell include the cyclic nucleotides cAMP and cGMP, $[Ca^{2+}]_i$, and the inositol phosphate-diacyl glycerol and tyrosine kinases. These messenger systems are common to several organ systems, and many cell-specific and tissue-specific structural and functional nuances contribute to the net biological response. More detailed descriptions of second messenger systems can be found elsewhere, but an overview is provided here.[141]

Epithelial cells require rapid response cascades for turning on and turning off ion transport systems. For example, cyclases are poised to synthesize cyclic nucleotides, and phosphodiesterases are set to degrade them. The net biological response is governed by the relative contributions of the accentuating and attenuating processes. In addition to the burgeoning increase in new signaling molecules awaiting definition of their roles, there are other variables that compound the resulting net biological response.

The molecules at almost every step in the signal transduction cascade—from the activating hormone to the receptors, cyclases, kinases, phosphatases, and finally the transporters themselves—exist as multiple isoforms and variants (see Fig. 101-7). These isoforms exhibit differences in species, tissue, cell type, and subcellular distribution and are subject to regulation during their development as well as in response to routine physiologic demands.

The canonical sequence of stimulus → second messenger → kinase → response is an oversimplification; extensive crosstalk exists between different signaling pathways. Other post-translational modifications such as glycosylation, myristoylation, nitration, and sumoylation are increasingly recognized as important modulators. Within a signaling cascade, there are critical feed-forward and feedback regulatory steps.

Thus, protein kinases catalyze the transfer of the terminal phosphate from ATP to the hydroxyl group of a serine, threonine, or tyrosine of a target protein, leading to both conformational and functional changes, such as altered affinity for substrate. Protein kinases exhibit specificity in their activators and substrates, and their action is essentially irreversible in living cells. Phosphoproteins can only be dephosphorylated by protein phosphatases, which are a separate class of enzymes that also are subject to regulation. Phosphoproteins may be the transporters themselves or may be modulator proteins in the membrane or cytosol, or both. Protein phosphorylation is not synonymous with activation; the dephosphorylated protein may be the active form. In general, Ca^{2+}-specific and cyclic nucleotide-specific protein kinases are serine-threonine kinases, whereas tyrosine-specific protein kinases are associated with receptors of cytokines and hormones involved in growth (e.g., EGF). In addition to specific serine-threonine and tyrosine phosphatases, dual-specificity kinases and phosphatases add to the complexity of crosstalk.

Compartmentalization of components of the signaling cascade via cytoskeletal runners, anchoring domains, or sequestration in vesicles as a means of regulation is especially germane to the polarized enterocyte. Localizing transporters and their signaling systems into specific subcellular domains is the norm rather than the exception. This is a dynamic and highly regulatable process. Scaffolding proteins can promote docking of various proteins, kinases, and phosphatases by protein-protein interactions—to each other, to the cytoskeleton, and/or to the membrane (see Fig. 101-7). For example, GUCY2C and the intestinal protein kinase GII have cytoskeletal and membrane interacting domains that bring them in close proximity to CFTR in the brush border membrane (see Fig. 101-7). Cholesterol-rich membrane domains like lipid rafts influence membrane fluidity and anchor specific transporters and their regulators. It should come as no surprise that many anchoring domains serve as multienzyme signaling complexes. Finally, trafficking of transporters into and out of the membrane via endosomal vesicles is an effective way of rapidly altering the V_{max} of the transporter. For example, cAMP increases CFTR translocation to the membrane and NHE3 and DRA retrieval from the membrane, resulting in an increase in Cl⁻ secretion and a decrease in Na⁺Cl⁻ absorption

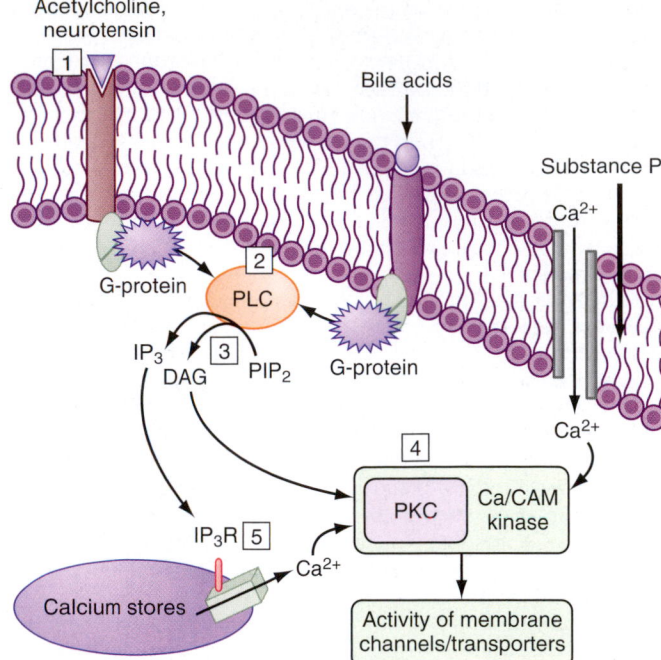

FIGURE 101-12. Calcium signaling in intestinal epithelial cells. Certain hormones and neurotransmitters (e.g., substance P, acetylcholine) activate secretion by increasing $[Ca^{2+}]_i$. Substance P can stimulate Ca^{2+} channel activity, and acetylcholine binds to M3 muscarinic heptahelical membrane-spanning (HHMS) receptors coupled to the Gaq class of G proteins *(1)*. Activated Gaq stimulates phospholipase C-β *(PLC)* *(2)* to hydrolyze PIP_2 to release DAG and inositol IP_3 *(3)*. DAG can also be produced from phosphatidic acid by the activation of phospholipase D by tyrosine kinase receptors. DAG is rapidly metabolized and does not increase $[Ca^{2+}]_i$; its major action is to stimulate PKC, a family of phosphatidyl serine-dependent enzymes that have far-reaching biological actions *(4)*. In contrast to DAG, IP_3 binds to specific receptors to release Ca^{2+} from intracellular compartments *(5)*. Intracellular free Ca^{2+} is tightly regulated and maintained at less than micromolar concentrations, in contrast to the 1 to 2 mmol/L in the plasma. Transient elevations in $[Ca^{2+}]_i$ are sufficient to elicit a host of biological responses, including ion transport. Calcium directly activates target proteins, such as Ca^{2+} channels, or binds to the ubiquitous Ca^{2+}-binding protein calmodulin to activate specific calcium-calmodulin protein kinases. Ca^{2+}-dependent secretagogues may be responsible for the minute-by-minute regulation needed in the intestine. This is underscored by the transient nature of Ca^{2+} signaling and its desensitization to Ca^{2+}-dependent secretagogues. Ca^{2+} is rapidly resequestered by Ca^{2+}-dependent adenosine triphosphatases on the endoplasmic reticulum or effluxed by Na^+-Ca^{2+} exchange on the plasma membrane. The transient receptor potential channels allow replenishment of intracellular Ca^{2+} from the extracellular compartment. PLC activation can concomitantly release polyinositol phosphates such as inositol 3,4,5,6-tetrakisphosphate, which function as ileal brakes and dampen Ca^{2+}-induced Cl^- secretion. Phenothiazines and loperamide can interfere with Ca^{2+} metabolism. CAM, calmodulin; DAG, diacylglycerol; IP_3, inositol triphosphate; IP_3R, inositol triphosphate receptor; PIP_2, phosphatidyl inositol bisphosphate; PKC, protein kinase C; PLC, phospholipase C.

(see Fig. 101-10). Thus, the cAMP-stimulated increases in Cl^- secretion and decreases in Na^+ absorption, respectively, result from an increase in CFTR translocation to, and NHE3 retrieval from, the membrane.

Although not associated with rapid responses, neurohumoral stimulation can cause changes at the transcriptional level, leading to the synthesis of new proteins (e.g., aldosterone), which increases ENaC synthesis in the distal colon. Diseases like cystic fibrosis underscore the importance of intracellular quality control in the cell machinery; thus ΔF508 CFTR, the most common mutation, is a misfolded protein and is tagged for degradation. All signal-transduction mechanisms have to be assessed with respect to their physiologic relevance in the intact intestine, because reductionist models, although a necessity, do not provide the complete picture. With these caveats, some common themes have emerged.

Generally, agents that elevate intracellular cAMP, cGMP, or Ca^{2+} increase fluid secretion (see Tables 101-2 and 101-3). They can activate 1 or more transporters associated with electrogenic Cl^- secretion: apical Cl^- and K^+ channels, basolateral K^+ conductances, and NKCC1; they also inhibit the apical NHEs, NHE2 and NHE3. Conversely, fluid absorption is associated with a decrease in these messengers or with activation of some tyrosine kinase pathways. An additional role of cAMP is to promote trafficking of transporter-bearing vesicles (CFTR in crypts and distal colonic Na^+ channels) to the apical membrane.[102,127]

The cAMP cascade is triggered by a hormone (e.g., VIP) that binds to a specific member of the superfamily of heptahelical membrane-spanning receptors (7TM-VPAC1 and VPAC2) (see Fig. 101-7).[142] Activation of membrane (GUCY2C) or soluble guanylate cyclases (sGCs) by peptides or nitric oxide, respectively, generates cGMP (see Fig. 101-7). The natriuretic peptides guanylin and uroguanylin share their receptor GUCY2C with the heat-stable enterotoxins (see discussion of guanylin). Hormones and neurotransmitters like substance P and ACh activate secretion by increasing $[Ca^{2+}]_i$ (see Fig. 101-12).

A number of growth factors, cytokines, and inflammatory mediators use entirely different signaling pathways that involve a combination of extracellular regulated kinases (ERKs), dual-specificity kinases, receptor kinases, and receptor-associated tyrosine kinases.

EPITHELIAL REGULATION IN CONTEXT

Given the vicissitudes in luminal content, mucosal environment, and systemic factors, intestinal epithelial cells must be prepared for large and rapid changes in the rates of ion and nutrient transport. What enters the cell on 1 side must exit the cell at the other end at a similar rate. If not, the cell will either shrink or explode, owing to a rapid change in ionic content and osmolality. The fact that this is accomplished so effectively is a testament to the finely tuned integration of multiple interrelated networks that modulate intestinal absorption and secretion.

KEY REFERENCES

Full references for this chapter can be found on www.expertconsult.com.

1. Alberts B, Johnson S, Lewis J, et al. Molecular biology of the cell. New York: Garland Science, Taylor & Francis Group; 2007.

3. Barrett KE, Seely SJ. Integrative physiology and pathophysiology of intestinal electrolyte transport. San Diego: Academic Press; 2006.

12. Field M. Intestinal ion transport and the pathophysiology of diarrhea. J Clin Invest 2003; 111:931-43.

15. Schneeberger EE, Lynch RD. The tight junction: A multifunctional complex. Am J Physiol 2004; 286:C1213-28.

16. Marchiando AM, Graham WV, Turner JR. Epithelial barriers in homeostasis and disease. Annu Rev Pathol 2010; 5:119-44.

23. Rao MC, Sarathy (nee Venkatasubramanian) J, Ao M. Intestinal water and electrolyte transport in health and disease colloquium series on integrated systems physiology: From molecule to function to disease. Lecture #31. Granger DN, Granger JP, series editors. Morgan and Claypool Life Sciences; 2012. Vol. 4, No. 1, pp. 1-105.

24. Zeuthen T. Water-transporting proteins. J Membr Biol 2010; 234:57-73.

32. Wright EM, Loo DD, Hirayama BA, Turk E. Surprising versatility of Na^+-glucose cotransporters: SLC5. Physiology (Bethesda) 2004; 19:370-76.

37. Zachos NC, Tse M, Donowitz M. Molecular physiology of intestinal Na^+/H^+ exchange. Annu Rev Physiol 2005; 67:411-43.

40. Kato A, Romero MF. Regulation of electroneutral NaCl absorption by the small intestine. Annu Rev Physiol 2011; 73:261-81.

56. Jentsch TJ, Neagoe I, Scheel O. ClC chloride channels and transporters. Curr Opin Neurobiol 2005; 15:319-25.

93. Weber CR, Turner JR. Inflammatory bowel disease: Is it really just another break in the wall? Gut 2007; 56:6-8.

102. Rao MC. Oral rehydration therapy: New explanations for an old remedy. Ann Rev Physiol 2004; 66:385-417.

112. Gershon M, Tack J. The serotonin signaling system: From basic understanding to drug development for functional GI disorders. Gastroenterology 2007; 132:397-414.

125. Thiagarajah JR, Verkman AS. New drug targets for cholera therapy. Trends Pharmacol Sci 2005; 26:172-5.

Digestion and Absorption of Dietary Fat, Carbohydrate, and Protein

NADA A. ABUMRAD, FATIHA NASSIR, AND AKIVA MARCUS

CHAPTER OUTLINE

Nutrient digestion and absorption are essential processes for the survival of an organism, making them among the most important tasks of the GI system. Most nutrients are absorbed with remarkable efficiency; less than 5% of ingested carbohydrate, fat, and protein is excreted in the stool of adults who consume a normal diet.[1] Even the 20 to 60 g of carbohydrates that escape digestion and absorption in the small intestine are absorbed from the colon as short-chain fatty acids (SCFAs) that are liberated by bacterial breakdown of fiber.[2,3] The intestinal tract of neonates is less efficient: infants fail to absorb 10% to 15% of their dietary fat, and in prematurity as much as 25% to 35% may be lost in the stool.[4,5] In old age, nutrient absorption remains highly efficient unless the intestine becomes diseased.

Despite considerable variations in types of food ingested and nutritional intake across national, racial, and ethnic groups, absorption remains efficient. Absorptive mechanisms adapt to the nature and amount of various nutrients presented to the GI tract. Such changes occur not only during early development[6] but throughout life, and also at times of specific need (e.g., during pregnancy).[7] In achieving the overall objective of nutrient absorption, the different parts of the GI tract act in a closely integrated and coordinated manner under the control of neural and humoral regulatory mechanisms.

The understanding of intestinal digestion and absorption at a molecular level has improved our knowledge of the integration and coordination of these functions within the GI tract. The pharmacokinetics and pharmacodynamics of several key carbohydrate, fat, peptide, amino acid, vitamin, and nutrient transporters are being increasingly understood. In this chapter, integration of intestinal function with the dietary intake, digestion, and absorption of major nutrients (carbohydrate, protein, fat) is discussed along with evolving genetic and molecular bases of these functions.

AN OVERVIEW OF GASTROINTESTINAL INTEGRATION

The cerebral phase of digestion, whether triggered by the sight, smell, or thought of food, initiates the digestive process.

Salivary and gastric secretory responses to these stimuli are mediated via the autonomic nervous system, and there is modest stimulation of pancreaticobiliary secretion via the vagus nerve.[8] The additional stimulus of nutrients in the mouth and upper GI tract markedly potentiates secretion by both humoral and local neural mechanisms (see Chapter 4).[9]

The rapidity with which food is normally chewed and swallowed affords little time for significant oral digestion of nutrients. Nonetheless, mastication and mixing of food with saliva initiates digestion of starch by salivary amylase. Gastric acid would soon switch off these enzymes were it not for the buffering capacity of food that allows some digestion to continue. The optimal pH for gastric lipases is 4.5 to 6.0, and it has been suggested that a considerable proportion of dietary triglyceride (TG) may be digested by these lipases.[10,11] Protein digestion begins in the stomach when gastric pepsinogens are converted to pepsins by gastric acid. Pepsins become increasingly active as intraluminal pH falls, and therefore the digestive action of pepsins on proteins is restricted to the stomach.

During ingestion of food, intragastric pressure rises little because of neurally mediated receptive relaxation. The mechanisms by which individuals perceive satiety and, therefore, cease eating are complex and explained only partly by the sensation of fullness. Although dozens of enzymes and hormones are secreted by the GI tract in response to intraluminal food, only a few are able to influence food intake directly. Satiety signals are relayed to the hindbrain, either indirectly via neural paths (e.g., vagus nerve) or directly via the blood, and most factors that influence how much food is eaten during individual meals act by changing sensitivity to these satiety signals.[12,13]

CCK, gastrin-releasing peptide, and apolipoprotein (apo) A-IV have all been implicated as messengers that transmit the satiety signal to the CNS[14-18]; they potentiate each other's actions and may act in combination. Additional peptides known as the *anorectic peptides*, including peptide tyrosine tyrosine (peptide YY, PYY), pancreatic polypeptide (PP), glucagon-like peptide 1 (GLP-1), and oxyntomodulin, also have been shown to decrease appetite and promote satiety in both animal and human models.[17,19]

Leptin, a hormone released from adipocytes, is an important peripheral signal from fat stores and acts on receptors in the arcuate nucleus and hypothalamus to diminish food intake.[20] Leptin deficiency and leptin receptor defects produce massive obesity. Only 1 GI signal, ghrelin, has been shown to increase appetite.[12,13]

The major digestive processes are initiated in the duodenum. Delivery of chyme from the stomach is regulated so it enters the duodenum at a controlled rate, thus allowing efficient mixing with pancreaticobiliary secretions. Control of gastric emptying is thus critical to ensure optimal digestion (see Chapter 49) and is determined by the consistency, pH, and osmolality, as well as the lipid and calorie content of the gastric contents.[21] The pylorus is selective in that it allows rapid passage of liquids while retaining solid particles with diameters of 2 mm or more.[22,23] The relatively large particles are progressively reduced in size by the gastric antral "mill," a process referred to as *trituration*. Trituration ensures particles will be small enough to allow them reasonably close apposition to digestive enzymes once the nutrient is allowed to enter the duodenum. Meals of high viscosity empty more slowly than do those of low viscosity.

Duodenal mucosal receptors for pH and osmolality trigger a delay in gastric emptying when the gastric effluent is acidic, hypertonic, or hypotonic.[24,25] When duodenal luminal contents are neutralized by pancreaticobiliary bicarbonate and osmolality is adjusted by water fluxes, gastric emptying is again

facilitated. This careful titration in the duodenal lumen ensures that nutrients are presented optimally to the pancreatic enzymes, which function best at neutral pH.

The total calorie content of meals also controls the rate of gastric emptying; on average, the human stomach delivers about 150 kcal/hr to the duodenum.[26] Receptors for FAs, amino acids, and carbohydrates in the duodenal mucosa are involved in this response, which probably is mediated by both neural and humoral feedback mechanisms.[27]

Gastric emptying additionally is controlled by a mechanism involving the ileum and colon. If much nutrient escapes digestion and absorption in the jejunum, its presence in the ileum and colon delays GI transit, thus providing more time for digestion and absorption.[28,29] This "ileal brake" acts to provide more time for digestion and absorption, and perhaps regulates the feeling of hunger.[30-34,74]

A number of secretory events coordinately regulate digestion across the GI tract, and some are triggered by FAs, involving FA receptors (e.g., GPR120, GPR40, CD36) on enteroendocrine cells (EECs).[52,76] GLP-1 and -2 are co-secreted by EECs in the small and large intestine in response to luminal fat and carbohydrate. GLP-1 decreases appetite, slows gastric emptying, and enhances glucose-induced insulin secretion. GLP-2 has effects on gastric acid secretion, gastric emptying, and nutrient absorption. GLP-2 regulates CD36 glycosylation, increasing its apical expression in the proximal intestine, which enhances fat absorption and chylomicron secretion.[77] Circulating levels of GLP-1 and GLP-2, low in the fasted state, increase rapidly after nutrient ingestion.[78]

CCK and secretin stimulate gallbladder contraction and pancreatic secretion and are released by nutrient interaction with receptors on I (CCK) and S (secretin) cells, mostly in the duodenum. CCK stimulates the pancreas by excitation of sensory nerves and by triggering of long vagovagal or enteropancreatic reflexes. Acetylcholine, nitric oxide, and neuropeptides such as gastrin-releasing peptide, generated by neurons of the ENS, regulate the exocrine pancreas. Vagal cholinergic pathways mediate CCK effects on pancreatic secretion. Human pancreatic acini lack functional CCK-A receptors, and a CCK infusion that produces plasma CCK levels similar to those seen postprandially stimulates pancreatic exocrine secretion by an atropine-sensitive pathway.[35]

Serotonin (5-HT) released from enterochromaffin cells in the intestinal mucosa and nerve terminals of the ENS and the intrapancreatic nerves may be involved in both stimulatory and inhibitory mechanisms through its various receptor subtypes; 5-HT also mediates the actions of secretin and CCK. Peptides that affect appetite and originate from the intestine (e.g., leptin and ghrelin) or from the pancreas (e.g., PP and neuropeptide Y [NPY]) appear to modulate the exocrine pancreas via hypothalamic centers.[37,38] Pancreatic juice provides both positive and negative feedback regulation of pancreatic secretion through mediation of both secretin- and CCK-releasing peptides. Pancreatic phospholipase A2 from pancreatic juice and intestinal secretions appears to function as a secretin-releasing peptide.[37,39,40]

The simultaneous release of bile salts, pancreatic enzymes, bicarbonate, and enteropeptidase (enterokinase) from duodenal mucosa provides optimal conditions for further nutrient digestion. Adequate lipid digestion is critically dependent on the presence of bile salts, pancreatic lipase, and co-lipase at nearly neutral pH,[41-43] whereas digestion of carbohydrate and protein depends on the combined sequential actions of intraluminal secreted enzymes and then enzymes situated on the brush border membrane (BBM) and within the intestinal mucosa. At the brush border, the close physical relationship between the sites for terminal digestion of protein and carbohydrate and the active absorption of digestive products provides a very efficient mechanism for dealing with these nutrients.

Two other simultaneous phenomena encourage efficient digestion and absorption. Ingestion of a meal stimulates salt and water secretion by the jejunal mucosa, thereby maintaining luminal contents in a sufficiently fluid state for proper mixing and digestion (see Chapter 101).[44] The other phenomenon is the motor response of the intestine (see Chapter 99). After feeding, the characteristic repetitive motility pattern that occurs during fasting is disrupted. Instead, a predictable different coordinated pattern is seen that, presumably, ensures nutrients are well mixed and brought into close contact with intestinal mucosa. There is close integration of the neurohumoral control mechanisms involving the motor and secretory responses of the intestine.[45] For rapidly absorbed molecules, intestinal blood flow may be the rate-limiting step.[46,47]

Efficient conservation and recycling mechanisms ensure that GI secretions are not entirely lost. Gastric acid secretion is balanced to a large extent by pancreaticobiliary bicarbonate secretion, so that overall acid-base balance is not disturbed. Although intact digestive enzymes are reabsorbed only in trace amounts, the nitrogen they contain is reabsorbed after their digestion. Finally, an efficient enterohepatic circulation recycles bile salts several times each day so they may be utilized approximately twice for each meal.[48] Although bile salts are passively reabsorbed throughout the small intestine, most reach the terminal ileum, where they are reabsorbed via specific active absorptive mechanisms. Thus, bile salts remain in the lumen where they are needed for lipid digestion, after which they are largely reabsorbed to avoid being lost by the colon (see Chapter 64).

Once intestinal chyme leaves the ileum and enters the colon, most nutrients have been digested and absorbed. Colonic function largely serves to dehydrate luminal contents through absorption of salt and water and to store the residuum. Dietary fiber may be digested by bacteria, with release of SCFAs, which are avidly absorbed. SCFAs are the major source of nutrition for colonocytes.[8] SCFAs have minor nutritional significance, except with high-fiber diets. The type of ingested fat can also influence the absorptive function of the intestinal mucosa for nutrients such as carbohydrate.[82]

DIETARY LIPIDS

The American Heart Association's (AHA) Nutrition Committee recommends that total fat intake not exceed 35% of ingested calories, with intake of saturated fats limited to less than 7% and the remainder consisting of monounsaturated and polyunsaturated fats. Cholesterol intake is recommended not to exceed 300 mg/day. In the United States, fat intake rose from approximately 34% of total energy consumed in the 1930s to around 40% in the late 1960s and 1970s. From 1971 to 2000, the percentage of energy contributed by fat decreased back to 33%, reflecting in part about a 25% increase in total energy intake. During the same period, the percentage of energy derived from carbohydrate increased from 40% to 50%, and these trends have since remained stable (Table 102-1).[49] Excessive intake of fat is linked to obesity because of its high energy content and to its property of increasing food palatability. In the past several decades, emphasis on importance of minimizing dietary fat to protect against obesity and coronary artery disease, combined with the increasing availability of processed carbohydrates and sugars, has led to increased consumption of low-fat, high-carbohydrate foods. The associated decline in fat consumption, however, correlated with an increase rather than a decrease in the prevalence of obesity, especially among children, a phenomenon referred to as the

TABLE 102-1 U.S. Trends in the Intake of Macronutrients for Children (≥Age 2 yr) and Adults from 1999-2000 and 2007-2008*

Intake	1999-2000	2007-2008
Total energy (Kcal)	2223	2091
Fat (%)	32.4	32.5
Protein (%)	13.7	14.6
Carbohydrates (%)	54.9	53.8

*Intake for each food group is expressed as percent of total caloric intake.
Data are from Centers for Disease Control and Prevention. Trends in intake of energy and macronutrients. 2004; 53:80-2; and from Alpers D. Digestion and absorption of carbohydrates and proteins. In: Johnson L, editor. Physiology of the gastrointestinal tract. 2nd ed. New York: Raven Press; 1987. p 1469.

"American paradox." A simple explanation of this paradox is that obesity is caused by a basic excess of energy intake over energy expenditure, and switching the type of dietary nutrient consumed without concern about total caloric intake or energy expenditure is wasted effort.[50] The national trends for an increase in total calorie intake combined with a more sedentary lifestyle are the major contributors to the current obesity epidemic (see Chapter 7). Added to these are the increased consumption of refined sugars and corn sweeteners and the dependence on processed food, which contains high concentrations of added sugar and fat.[49,51] Dietary fats consumed in moderation are an important nutrient essential for human health. They supply the body with essential FAs and fat-soluble vitamins and play an important role in regulating satiety and overall energy homeostasis.[52]

Dietary fat consists mainly of TGs (90% to 95%) but also of phospholipids (Fig. 102-1), sterols, and fat-soluble vitamins. The major sterols are cholesterol from animal fat and sitosterol from plants, which is not absorbed by the human intestine. Humans absorb 20% to 80% of cholesterol delivered to the intestine by intake (≈300 mg/day) or via the bile (≈1 g/day). In contrast, TG absorption is very efficient, and 95% of a 500-g fat load can be absorbed per day. Chain length of the FAs in TGs influences absorption, with medium-chain FAs being better absorbed than long-chain (LC)FAs. Position of the FA at the 1, 2, or 3 position on the glycerol backbone determines whether it is absorbed free (1 or 3 position) or as a constituent of 2-monoacylglycerol (2-MG). The major FAs of dietary TG are oleate, palmitate, stearate, and linoleate. Animal TGs contain mostly long-chained (>14 carbon chains) saturated FAs (Table 102-2). Polyunsaturated FAs (linoleic and linolenic acids) are derived from phospholipids of vegetable origin, and because they cannot be synthesized de novo, they are considered essential (see Fig. 102-1). Phospholipid ingestion is 2 to 8 g/day, and the most abundant dietary phospholipid is phosphatidyl choline (lecithin), enriched in linoleate and arachidonate. Phospholipids in the duodenal lumen (10 to 22 g/day) exceed intake as a result of contribution from endogenous sources, particularly bile. Commercial hydrogenation of unsaturated FAs raises their melting points, allowing the production of margarines and spreads of variable consistency. In addition to saturation, hydrogenation results in cis to trans isomerization of double bonds.[53] Because trans FAs were linked to risk of cerebrovascular disease[54] New York City and California passed regulations discouraging their use,[55] and the AHA's Nutrition Committee recommended limiting their intake to less than 2 g/day.

Lipids are efficiently absorbed by the small intestine, and only 5% of ingested lipid is excreted in the stool. By

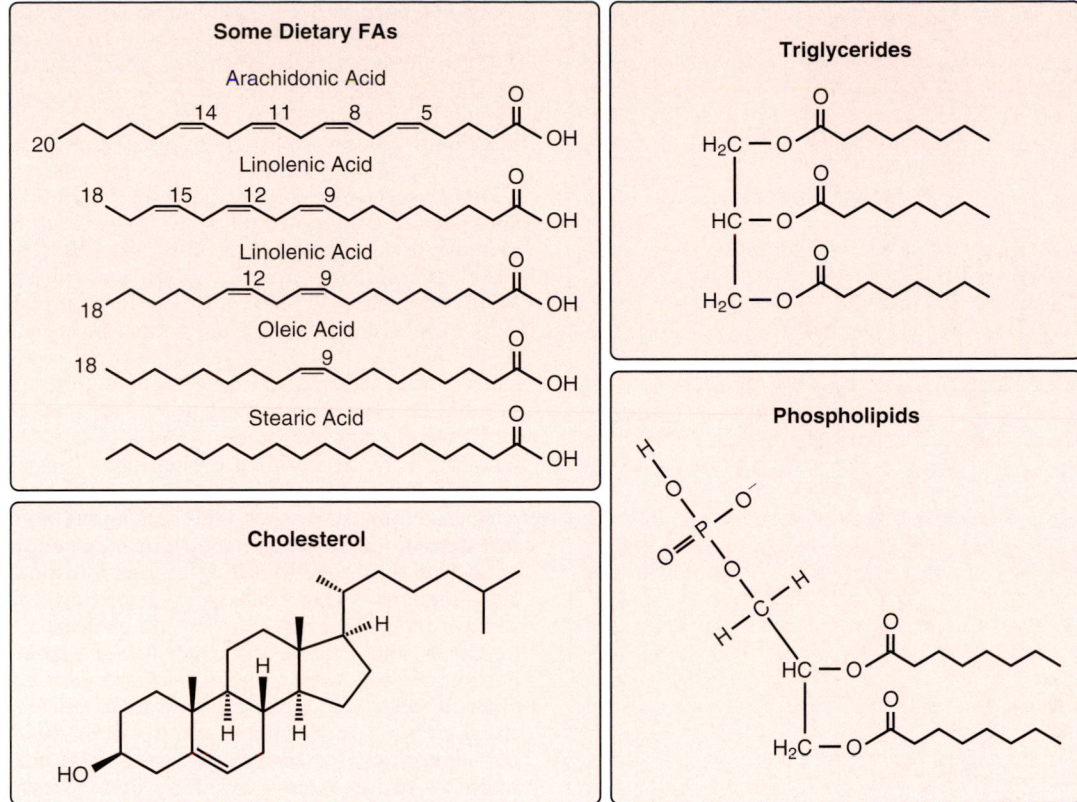

FIGURE 102-1. General molecular structure of fatty acids (FA; representative dietary FAs are shown), TGs, phospholipids, and cholesterol.

TABLE 102-2 Representative Dietary Fatty Acids (FAs), Showing Length of Carbon Chain and Number of Double Bonds	
Fatty Acid	**Carbon Double Bonds**
Saturated FAs	
Butyric	4:0
Caproic	6:0
Lauric	12:0
Myristic	14:0
Palmitic	16:0
Stearic	18:0
Mono-Unsaturated FAs	
Oleic	18:1
Palmitoleic	16:1
Polyunsaturated FAs	
Arachidonic*	20:4
Linoleic*	18:2
Linolenic*	18:3

*Essential fatty acid.

comparison, 10% to 15% and 25% to 35% of dietary fat is excreted by the intestines of neonates and premature infants, respectively. In neonates, this reflect limited capacity for digestion and absorption of FA released from intestinal hydrolysis of TGs.[56] Lipid absorption is regulated by neural and humoral factors that closely coordinate digestion across the different parts of the GI tract. Events that precede food intake, such as seeing, smelling, or thinking of food, induce salivary and gastric secretions via the autonomic nervous system and stimulate pancreatic and biliary secretions via the vagus nerve. These modest secretions are potentiated via humoral and local neural mechanisms when the nutrients are in the mouth and when they reach the upper GI tract.[52,57]

ORAL PERCEPTION OF DIETARY FAT

The orosensory properties of foods are usually perceived through a combination of taste, texture, and olfaction, which are then influenced by cognitive input to modulate the perceived reward value of the ingested food.[58] Individuals differ in their ability to experience the taste of various foods. According to the National Institutes of Health, approximately 25% of Americans are non-tasters, 50% are medium tasters, and 25% are supertasters. Great progress has been recently accomplished in the identification of taste receptors for various sensations such as sweet, salty, and bitter, enhancing our understanding of the interaction between heredity and the environment in determining food preferences and intake patterns. Humans display large variations in the orosensory detection thresholds for dietary fat.[59] Although gustatory detection of carbohydrates and proteins is well documented to involve taste receptors specific for these nutrients, this was not thought to apply to perception of dietary fat. Evidence in rodents and humans, however, now strongly supports involvement of fat taste receptors and of gustatory cues in fat perception[59-61] (Fig. 102-2). Dietary fat is composed mainly of TGs, but the nutrient sensed is LCFA, which has signal transduction capabilities and is generated from TG digestion by

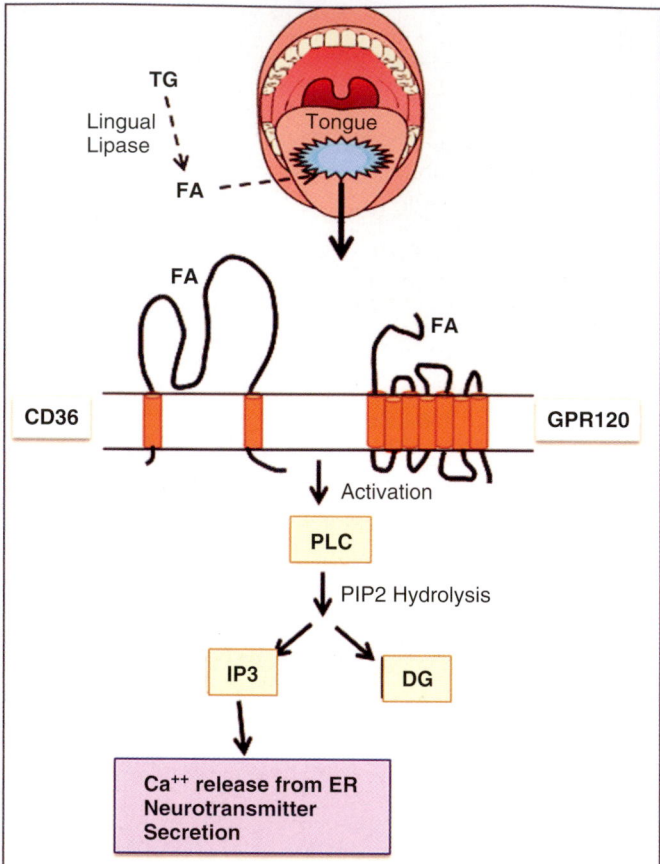

FIGURE 102-2. Oral perception of fat. Accumulating evidence supports gustatory cues in fat perception similar to those for the 5 basic tastes (salty, sour, umami, sweet, bitter). In the case of dietary fat, which is composed mainly of TGs, the nutrient sensed upon exposure of the tongue to fat is long-chain fatty acid (LCFA), which has signal transduction capabilities and is generated from TG digestion by lingual lipase in the mouth. The FA interacts with specific receptors (CD36 and GPR120) expressed on taste bud cells in the circumvallate and fungiform papillae (back and sides of the tongue, respectively) to induce intracellular calcium release from the endoplasmic reticulum. This in turn triggers calcium flux from membrane store-operated calcium channels, leading to neurotransmitter release. The 2 FA receptors identified on taste bud cells in rodents and humans are CD36 and GPR120 (see Table 102-4), and both were shown to impact sensitivity to oral perception of dietary fat. CD36, cluster of differentiation 36; DG, diacylglycerol; GPR120, G protein-coupled receptor 120; IP3, inositol trisphosphate or inositol 1,4,5-trisphosphate; PIP2, phosphatidyl inositol-bisphosphate; PLC, phospholipase C.

lingual lipase. Rodents have robust lingual lipase activity, and its inhibition reduces the spontaneous preference for TG.[62] Humans have low amounts of lingual lipase, but its activity is sufficient to mediate FA generation from TG in the mouth, because its inhibition by orlistat reduces sensitivity to oral perception of triolein but not to oleic acid.[60]

The FAs released by lingual lipase interact on taste bud cells with receptors (see Fig. 102-2) that include CD36[63] and the G protein-coupled receptors (GPRs).[64] CD36 is a heavily glycosylated membrane-spanning protein with high affinity for LCFAs[52]; it is expressed on taste bud cells of rodents, pigs, and humans and was shown to influence fat taste perception

and preference in mice[63] and humans.[60,65] CD36 gene deletion in mice abolishes spontaneous preference for FAs in the 2-bottle preference test and the cephalic phase of biliary and pancreatic secretions triggered by the tongue's exposure to FA. The GPRs that function in FA recognition are members of the large family of G-coupled receptors, usually with 7 transmembrane segments.[66] LCFAs are recognized by GPR120 and GPR40, which were shown, using the 2-bottle test, to influence spontaneous preference for fat in rodents.[64] Interaction of the FA with its taste bud cell receptor was shown in the case of CD36 to result in formation of tri-inositol phosphate (IP3), which interacts with its receptor on the endoplasmic reticulum (ER) to release calcium. This in turn induces store-operated membrane calcium flux, which further increases cytosolic calcium and leads to the release of neurotransmitters[63] (see Fig. 102-2). The pathways triggered by FA interaction with the GPR usually involve heterotrimeric G (G_s, G_i, G_q) proteins, resulting in production of cyclic adenosine monophosphate (cAMP) and IP3, as well as activation of MAP kinases and various cellular responses. GPR120[67] and GPR40[68] enhance the response of intracellular calcium to LCFA addition in enteroendocrine cells, resulting in release of intestinal peptides (see later sections). Their effects in taste bud cells might also involve the IP3 pathway for calcium release that is activated by CD36. The increase in intracellular calcium that mediates neurotransmitter release and fat perception also induces the cephalic phase of digestion, characterized by the release of small amounts of bile acids and by an increase in serum TG. Fat-induced cephalic-phase responses also include transient increases of intestinal CCK, PP, PYY, and insulin.[57] GPR120 and CD36 expression was examined in mouse taste buds during the day/night cycle and with dietary manipulations.[69] CD36 expression was down-regulated in the dark period during food intake and associated with a reduction in fat preference.[69] Thus CD36 sensing of dietary lipid might gradually decrease appetite for fat during a meal while GPR120 appears unresponsive to the ingested fat.[69]

The influence of oral fat perception on fat intake remains unclear. In humans, excessive dietary fat intake attenuates the nutrient-sensing response in the oral cavity, which could associate with changes in diet and weight.[70] In humans, common variants in the CD36 gene that influence CD36 protein levels[71] influence sensitivity to fat perception on the tongue[60] and the preference for added fat,[65] but the relationship to fat intake remains unexplored. CD36 variants' association to the BMI was reported in some but not all studies,[72] possibly reflecting interactions with dietary factors. The role of the GPR FA receptors in human fat taste perception remains unknown. GPR120, mRNA, and protein was detected in human taste buds as well as in surrounding epithelial cells, while GPR40 expression was not.[64] A rare non-synonymous variant in the GPR120 gene is associated with obesity.[73] The implications of oral fat taste perception with respect to fat intake, and possibly the etiology of obesity in humans, is an important area for future study.

FAT DIGESTION IN THE STOMACH AND SMALL INTESTINE[74-76]

Oral fat perception prepares the intestine and organism for food arrival and might result in mobilization of an intestinal pool of TG that contributes to early postprandial lipemia.[57] Fat digestion itself, however, begins in the stomach with the action of gastric lipases and continues through nutrient passage in the intestine. These processes are described in the preceding section on An Overview of Gastrointestinal Integration.

Emulsification

The insolubility of fat in water underlies the mechanisms that have evolved to accomplish its digestion and absorption.[83] The digestion products have to be transported across the bulk water phase in the lumen and then across the epithelial cell membrane. Within the cell, the fat is reconstituted into larger molecules, predominantly TG, which requires specialized processing for export from the cell. Despite these complex processes, most ingested fat is absorbed. Dietary fat is mostly TG, and liberation of FA from the glycerol backbone of TG (lipolysis) is achieved by lipases acting at the surface of

emulsified droplets (Fig. 102-3). Human gastric lipase, a 379–amino acid protein that does not share homology with pancreatic lipase, contributes 20% to 30% of intraluminal lipid digestion and does not hydrolyze phospholipids or cholesteryl esters.

The gastric milling of food produces an unstable emulsion, but formation of a stable emulsion in the duodenum is important for the close apposition of lipase and TG needed for efficient lipolysis (see Fig. 102-3). To stabilize the emulsion, the fat droplets are coated with dietary phospholipid. The ratio of ingested phospholipid to TG is about 1:30, and more is added in the duodenum from bile. Emulsification is enhanced

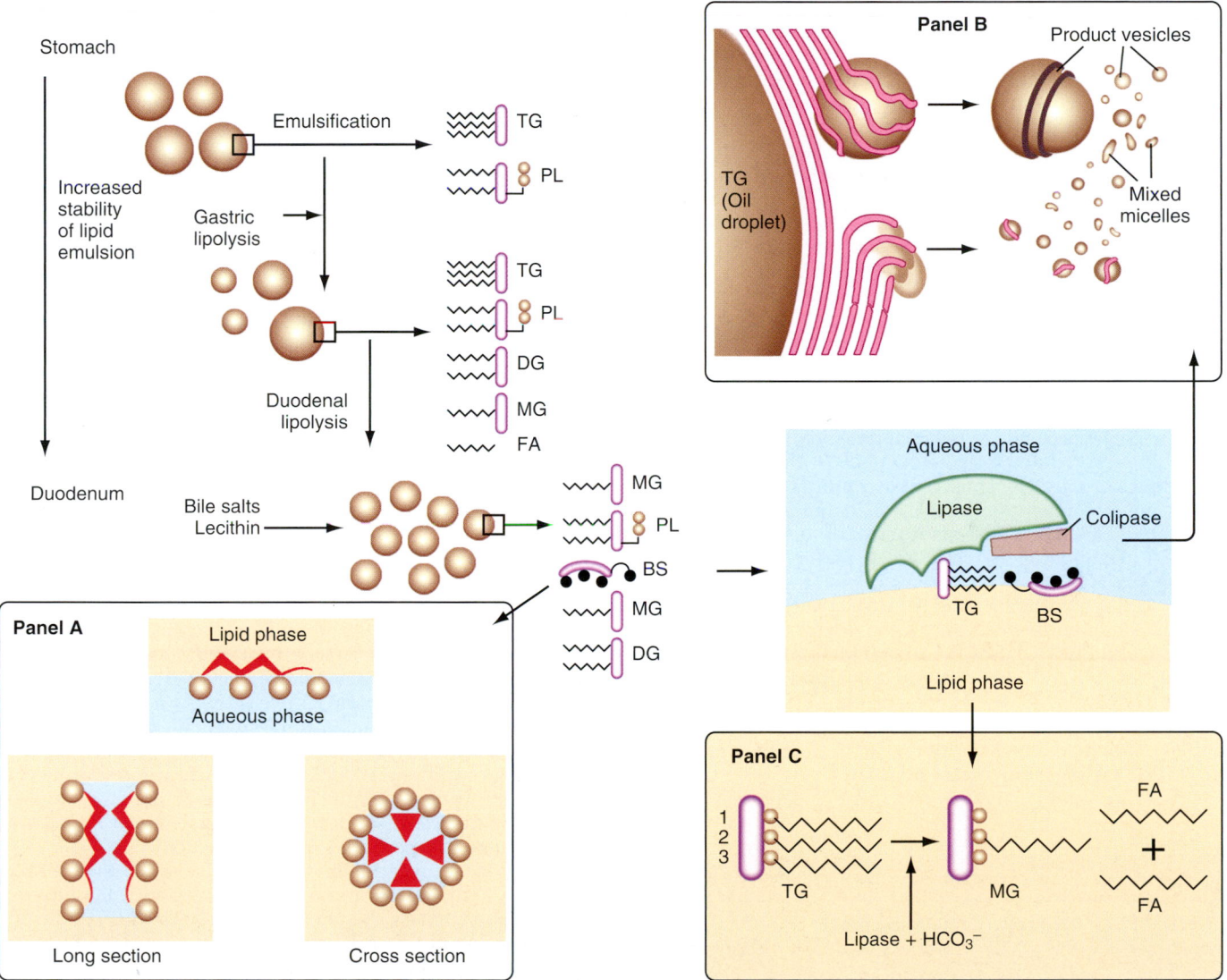

FIGURE 102-3. Steps in lipolysis of dietary fat. The initial step in lipolysis is to increase stability of the fatty emulsion. Gastric lipase acts on TGs to yield fatty acids (FAs) and diglyceride (diglyceride enhances emulsification). This step is enhanced in the duodenum by bile salts and phospholipid (lecithin), which enable lipase, in the presence of co-lipase, to act at the surface of the emulsion droplet to bring it close to the TG molecule, whereupon monoglyceride and FAs are released. Lipolysis in the duodenum yields FAs (from the 1 and 3 positions) and 2-monoglyceride and occurs in a rapid and efficient manner at nearly neutral pH. *Panel A*, Diagrammatic representations of bile salt molecules *(top)* oriented at an oil-water interface with its hydrophobic sterolic backbone in the oil phase, and its hydrophilic hydroxyl and either taurine or glycine conjugates in the aqueous phase. At above their critical micellar concentration, bile salts aggregate as simple micelles in water, with their hydrophilic groups facing into the aqueous phase *(bottom 2 diagrams). Panel B*, Dispersion of lipolytic products into lamellae at the surface of the oil phase, and from there into vesicles and micelles, is shown. *Panel C*, FAs and monoglycerides released from TGs by pancreatic lipase, assisted by co-lipase, transfer to bile salt to form mixed micelles. BS, bile salt; DG, diglyceride; MG, monoglyceride; PL, phospholipid.

by the FA liberated by intragastric lipolysis and by bile salts. The mixed emulsion formed in the duodenum consists predominantly of TGs together with cholesteryl esters and some diglycerides and is coated by phospholipids, partially ionized FAs, monoglycerides, and bile salts (see Fig. 102-3).

Lipases

Pancreatic TG lipase efficiently digests the stabilized lipid emulsion (see Fig. 102-3).[81] The lipolytic domain of the enzyme is hydrophobic, buried within the protein,[84] and is revealed upon close apposition to the lipid surface, a process that requires assistance of colipase, which is secreted by the pancreas in a 1:1 molar ratio with the lipase. Colipase attaches to the TG ester bond and binds the lipase (see Fig. 102-3). Colipase is secreted by the pancreas as pro-colipase that is activated in the small intestinal lumen by trypsin cleavage of an N-terminus pentapeptide (enterostatin), which is a fat ingestion-specific satiety signal.[85] The importance of colipase is illustrated by the finding that an arginine-to-cysteine polymorphism at position 92, which results in protein misfolding, associates with an increased risk of type 2 diabetes.[86] Phospholipase A2 digestion of the emulsion phospholipid coat, which requires calcium for activation, exposes the TG core and enhances colipase-dependent lipase anchoring. Bile salts further assist TG lipolysis by facilitating removal of lipolytic products (see Fig. 102-3). In the absence of colipase, bile salts on the surface of the emulsion inhibit lipase activity.

Pancreatic lipase is most active at neutral pH (Table 102-3), and secretion of bicarbonate by the pancreas and biliary tree is critical to neutralize gastric acid. In the jejunum, luminal pH is around 6; bile salts lower the optimal pH for lipase activity, which efficiently digests TG and cholesteryl esters.[81] Glycine-conjugated bile salts precipitate below pH 5, and FAs are in their protonated form below pH 6, with limited solubility in bile salt micelles. Thus, under conditions where intraluminal pH becomes more acidic, as in the Zollinger-Ellison syndrome, pancreatic lipase is inactive, bile acids precipitate, and FA partitioning in micelles is reduced, resulting in steatorrhea.

In addition to lipase and colipase, pancreatic acini synthesize the homologous pancreatic lipase-related proteins (PLRP-1 and PLRP-2). PLRP-1 has no known activity. PLRP-2 hydrolyzes TG and also phospholipids and galactolipids, 2 fats not hydrolyzed by pancreatic lipase. PLRP-2 mRNA appears before birth, whereas pancreatic lipase mRNA appears at the suckling-weaning transition, suggesting the importance of PLRP-2 for digesting breast-milk fat.[87]

TABLE 102-3 Characteristics of Lipase Activity

Source of Lipase	Optimal pH	Site of Lipase Activity	Other
Milk	7.0	α-1, -2, and -3 ester bonds	Stimulated by bile salts
Stomach	4.0-6.0	α-1 ester bond	Inhibited by pancreatic proteolysis
Pancreas	7.0	α-1 and -3 ester bonds	—

Modified from Farrell J. Digestion and absorption of nutrients and vitamins. In: Feldman M, Friedman LS, Brandt LJ, editors. Sleisenger and Fordtran's gastrointestinal and liver disease. 9th ed. Philadelphia: Saunders; 2010. p 1699.

Micelles

The transport of lipolytic products depends in part on formation of bile salt micelles (see Fig. 102-3). The concentration of bile salts in bile is approximately 35 mM and is diluted in the duodenum to 10 to 20 mM, which is above the critical micellar concentration (CMC). Mixed micelle formation depends on pH, presence or absence of lipids, and the types of bile salts present (see Chapter 64).[88] Bile salts are amphipathic, with water- and lipid-soluble portions, and act as emulsifying agents at an oil-water interface. Micelles are formed when bile salt levels exceed CMC and aggregate in disk-like particles, with their hydrophobic sterol backbones oriented toward each other and their hydrophilic groups facing the aqueous phase. Bile salt micelles can dissolve FA, monoglycerides, and cholesterol, but not TG.[89] The lipid is surrounded in the micelle by bile salts oriented with their hydrophilic groups facing outward. Mixed micelles are about 50 to 80 nm in diameter and, unlike emulsion droplets, are too small to scatter light; hence, micellar solutions are clear. The phospholipid secreted in bile enlarges the mixed micelles, enhancing capacity for fat dissolution.

Lipid-containing particles other than bile salt micelles might participate in mucosal transfer of lipid. As the emulsion shrinks during lipolysis, multilamellar or unilamellar vesicular structures form at its surface and can be seen under the electron microscope budding off occasionally close to the BBM[90] to possibly provide a physical phase of lipid transfer that is independent of bile salt micelles. This could explain how almost 50% of dietary TG can be absorbed in the absence of bile salts. These vesicles usually rapidly release their lipid to the micelles when adequate concentrations of bile salts are present, and micelles, normally much more common than lipid vesicles, are the major route for lipid traffic.

Unstirred Water Layer

An unstirred water layer (≈40 μm deep in humans) is present on the surface of the intestinal epithelium and rate-limits uptake of long-chain but not short- or medium-chain FAs. The microclimate next to the epithelium is slightly acidic (pH between 5 and 6), owing to activity of a BBM sodium-hydrogen (Na^+/H^+) exchanger. This acidic microclimate decreases micellar FA solubility to promote FA release close to the mucosa and increases the undissociated, protonated FA that can diffuse across the cell bilayer. The FA partitioning model proposes that these conditions yield the high FA concentration necessary for diffusion across the mucosal membrane.[91] Strong evidence, however, now supports a protein-facilitated component of FA uptake in enterocytes (see next section).

A surfactant-like material present close to the BBM is secreted by enterocytes and contains phosphatidylcholine and alkaline phosphatase. Alkaline phosphatase influences dietary fat absorption but its role in this process is unclear. Deletion of alkaline phosphatase in mice increases lipid absorption and accelerates weight gain.[92] It has been reported that CD36 (see next section) is dephosphorylated by alkaline phosphatase, which reduces fat absorption.[93]

Phosphatidylcholine, the major dietary phospholipid (see Fig. 102-1), is hydrolyzed by pancreatic phospholipase A2 (PLA2) to yield FA from the 2-position and lysophosphatidylcholine. Pancreatic PLA2 is activated in the small intestine by tryptic cleavage of an N-terminal heptapeptide and requires a 2:1 bile salt-to-phosphatidylcholine molar ratio for optimal activity. The bulk of intestinal PLA2 is derived from the pancreas, but there is some contribution from the intestinal mucosa, where PLA2 is concentrated in the brush border.[94]

The products of phospholipid and cholesterol hydrolysis follow the same route to the BBM as the FAs and monoglycerides from dietary TG. FAs and monoglycerides increase micelle cholesterol solubility, enhancing its absorption. Unabsorbed LCFAs that enter the colon undergo bacterial modification, principally hydroxylation. Normally, no undigested TG is found in the stool, and the fecal fat estimate of 7 g/day reflects the total excretion of saponification products (i.e., FA, mainly arising from bacteria and membrane phospholipid).

BRUSH BORDER TRANSPORT OF FATTY ACIDS

The hydrolysis products of TGs and cholesteryl esters, FAs, 2-monoglycerides, and free cholesterol, are taken up across the enterocyte BBM, and early studies argued against cellular uptake of whole micelles.[95] Although enterocyte uptake of digestion products was thought to occur by passive diffusion down a concentration gradient, recent work strongly suggests existence of a regulated protein-facilitated component of FA uptake.[52]

Small intestinal cells absorb LCFAs by passive diffusion[96] and protein-facilitated transfer.[52] Passive "flip-flop" of protonated FA across the BBM is favored by the acidic microclimate next to the mucosa. Transfer is proposed to be coordinated with intracellular FA trapping through binding to abundant cytosolic FA binding proteins and/or by conversion to the membrane-impermeable acyl-CoA derivatives.[97] However, a probable scenario for entry of LCFAs across the BBM is endocytosis within vesicles formed from lipid rafts that contain caveolin-1 and CD36 (Fig. 102-4). Signal transduction mediated by FA interaction with CD36 might promote formation and endocytosis of the transport vesicles.[52,98]

The protein facilitated component of FA uptake by isolated proximal enterocytes is evident at low nanomolar concentrations of monomeric FA[99] similar to those measured in other cell types. In the intestinal lumen, the FA released from TG digestion is incorporated into bile salt micelles that, like serum albumin, can solubilize millimolar FA concentrations. The FA dissociated from the micelle is the species important for cellular uptake,[95] and its concentration is estimated to be in the low micromolar range[100] compared with the nanomolar range of albumin-dissociated FA in the circulation. Enterocyte FA uptake is a saturable function of the FA monomer, and the cellular entry site (i.e., apical or basolateral) determines metabolic processing of the FA and monoacylglycerol.[101] These observations support a role for apical membrane proteins in FA transfer and metabolic targeting. Three apical membrane proteins, (1) the scavenger receptor CD36[102]; (2) FATP4, a member of the very long-chain acyl-CoA synthetases, also known as *fatty acid transport proteins* (FATPs)[103]; and (3) caveolin-1, a protein constituent of membrane caveolae, will be discussed.

CD36

The role of CD36, a platelet membrane protein receptor for thrombospondin-1, in lipid uptake was uncovered in 1993 when the protein was identified as important for uptake of LCFAs[104] and oxidized low-density lipoproteins (oxLDL).[105] CD36 (88-kd, 472 amino acids) is a heavily glycosylated transmembrane protein (Fig. 102-5) with broad ligand specificity[106,107]; it is abundant in tissues such as heart, skeletal muscle, adipose tissue, immune cells, and the intestine.[104] Lipid ligands of CD36 (LCFAs, oxLDLs, oxidized phospholipids) bind within a hydrophobic loop in the amino terminal half of the extracellular domain. The binding includes hydrophobic interaction that involves the alkyl chain as well as hydrostatic interactions with CD36 lysine 164.[107,108] The protein is subject to post-translational modifications, such as glycosylation, phosphorylation, palmitoylation, ubiquitination (attachment by specific ligases of ubiquitin tags that target the protein to degradation), and acetylation (see Fig. 102-5), and these modifications play a role in CD36 recruitment to the membrane and in its FA uptake and signaling functions. Studies in CD36-deficient mice and humans documented a defect in tissue FA uptake and abnormalities of FA metabolism. Polymorphisms in the *CD36* gene were linked to alterations in plasma FA, cholesterol, and TG levels and to metabolic syndrome susceptibility.[72] For recent reviews on the role of CD36 in FA transport and metabolic phenotypes, refer to references.[52,72,109,110]

CD36 is abundantly expressed in the digestive tract, where it plays a number of roles related to fat perception, regulation of food intake, and fat absorption. In the small intestine, *CD36* is most abundant in the most proximal third of the intestine, where it is detected on the BBMs of duodenal and jejunal villi.[111] *CD36* epithelial cell immunostaining is low in the ileum and colon of humans. This expression pattern is consistent with a function in lipid absorption. The molecular nature of this function is incompletely understood, but it is now established that *CD36* directs FA absorbed in the proximal intestine to chylomicron formation and export via the lymph (see later section). Primary enterocytes isolated from the proximal but not distal intestine of *CD36* null mice show a 50% reduction in FA and cholesterol uptake compared with those from wild-type mice. Intragastric administration of triolein also results in reduced oleic acid enrichment of mucosal lipids in the proximal intestine of *CD36* null mice and in more lipid reaching the distal small intestine. Oleic acid uptake by the mouse duodenum for formation of oleoylethanolamide (OEA), which plays a role in modulating satiety in response to lipid ingestion, is suppressed by CD36 deficiency.[112] Thus *CD36* appears to function in high-affinity (Km in the low nM) FA uptake in proximal enterocytes.[113] CD36 contribution to net intestinal FA absorption, however, appears small. It will be rapidly saturated at luminal FA levels, functioning only in early digestion stages. There is also evidence that FAs down-regulate levels of the CD36 protein by promoting its ubiquitination, and this regulation, which occurs in enterocytes, would tend to minimize CD36 contribution to absorption as digestion progresses. Furthermore, the proximal intestinal defect in FA uptake is compensated for by non-CD36-mediated FA uptake in distal segments.[52]

CD36 deficiency is rare in Caucasians but is relatively common (≈6%) in persons of Asian and African descent and associates with abnormalities of plasma lipids.[72] The abnormal plasma lipids in humans with *CD36* deficiency or with single nucleotide polymorphisms (SNPs) in the *CD36* gene reflect, in part, abnormal peripheral clearance of plasma FAs; impaired tissue FA uptake has been documented in humans with *CD36* deficiency. Contribution of defective lipid processing by the small intestine to the lipid abnormalities, however, is suggested by findings of postprandial lipemia and high *apoB*-48 levels in *CD36*-deficient subjects.[114,115]

Fatty Acid Transport Protein 4 (FATP4)

Among the candidate intestinal FA transporters, FATP4 is especially appealing by virtue of its high expression in mammalian villus enterocytes and because of its endogenous acyl-CoA synthetase (ACS) activity. These properties would provide FATP4 with the capacity to function not only in FA transport but also in the process of metabolic trapping of FA

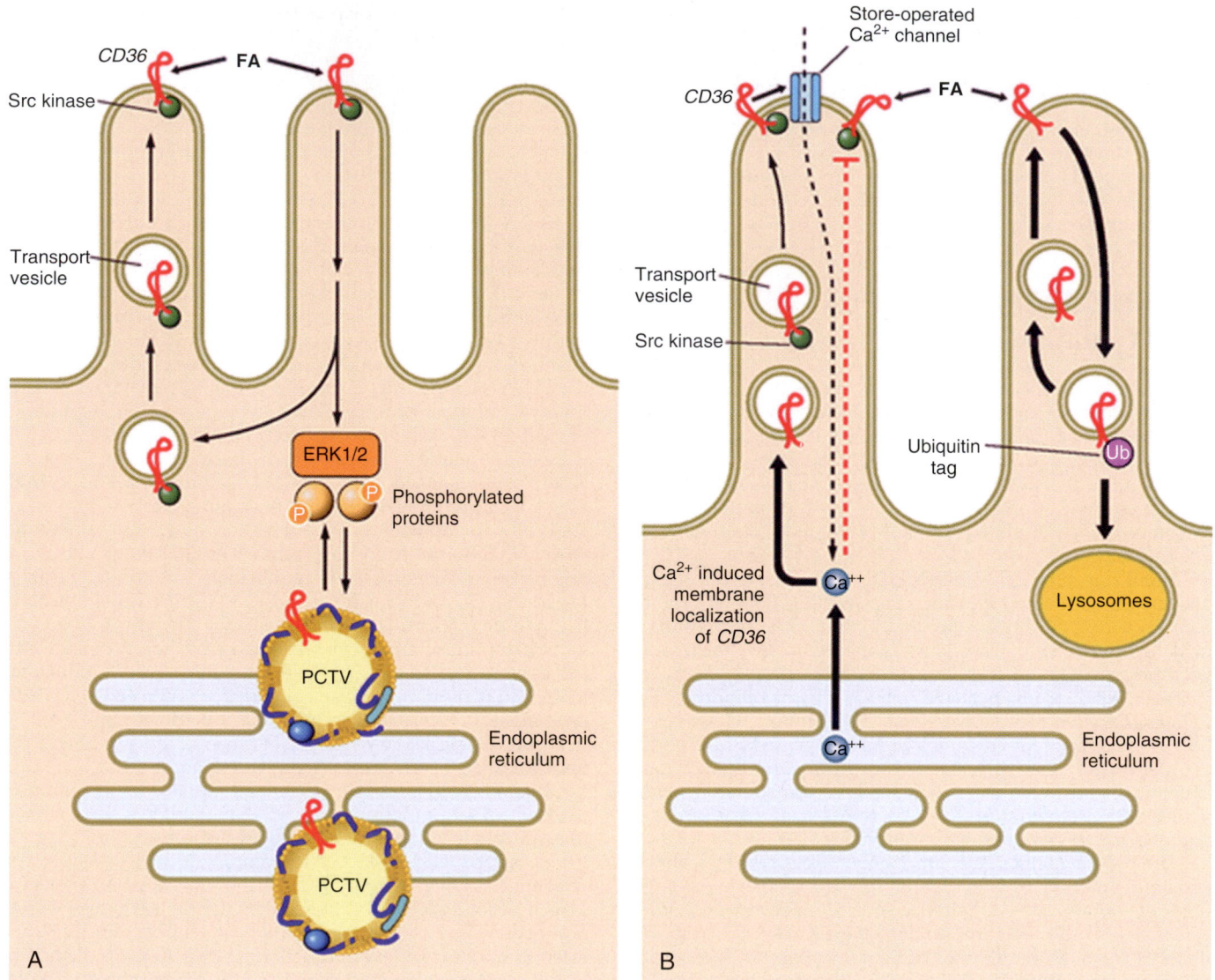

FIGURE 102-4. Working model showing the molecular steps that may be involved in how intestinal *CD36* facilitates fatty acid (FA) uptake and chylomicron formation in the small intestine. *A,* CD36 is highly expressed on the apical side of enterocytes of the proximal intestine, where it interacts with FA released from digestion of dietary TG. CD36 facilitates the uptake of FA, probably by internalizing the FA within vesicles derived from membrane lipid rafts where the protein localizes. CD36-mediated uptake likely occurs during the early phase of digestion when FA concentrations are relatively low and is saturated as digestion proceeds and FA levels increase. CD36-mediated FA uptake, however, associates with intracellular signaling to promote events that facilitate chylomicron assembly. CD36 signaling is initiated in most cases via the sarcoma (Src) kinases that associate with the C-terminus of CD36 *(green circle)* and downstream via extracellular regulated kinase (ERK1/2). This signaling pathway may be important for phosphorylating proteins required to coordinate endoplasmic reticulum (ER) processing of prechylomicron vesicles (PCTV). CD36 has also been identified in the protein complex required for formation of PCTV. *B,* CD36 signaling may be mediated by a rise in intracellular calcium via inositol triphosphate (IP3)-induced release of ER calcium (see Fig. 102-3). ER calcium release promotes membrane CD36 localization and also induces calcium influx via store-operated calcium channels. A sustained increase in intracellular calcium could influence multiple events related to lipid processing or secretion. Panel *B* also illustrates the concept that CD36 is down-regulated by FA that promote its ubiquitination (attachment by specific ligases of ubiquitin tags that target the protein to degradation) on its carboxyl terminus *(circle with Ub)*. This feedback loop may work to reduce CD36 function in the presence of excess FA supply. Inside enterocytes, a FA-induced decrease in CD36 associates with reduced activation of ERK1/2, which may serve to up-regulate an abundance of microsomal TG transfer protein (*MTTP*), initiating chylomicron assembly. *(Reproduced from Abumrad NA, Davidson NO. Role of the gut in in lipid homeostasis. Physiol Rev 2012; 92:1061-85.)*

through conversion to Co-A derivatives.[116] Unlike native LCFAs, which are freely diffusible, fatty acyl-CoA products are hydrophilic and undergo rapid metabolic conversion into various lipids (di- and TGs phospholipids, cholesteryl ester). Careful examination showed FATP4 to localize in the ER and

in subapical membranes, so its participation in FA uptake would be primarily mediated by its ACS activity, trapping the FA via acyl-CoA generation.[117] Deletion of FATP4 led either to embryonic lethality or perinatal death, mainly from skin abnormalities that restricted breathing and caused severe

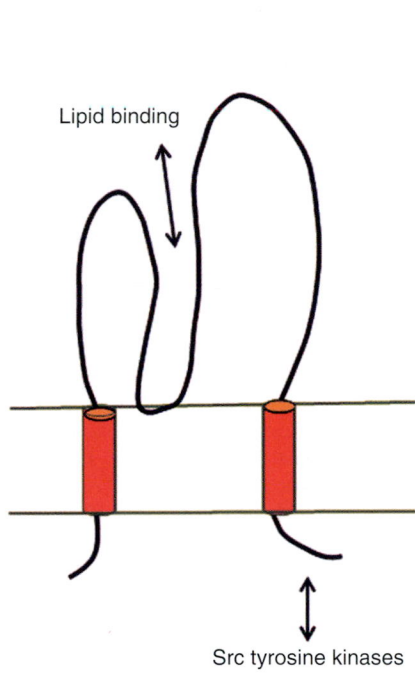

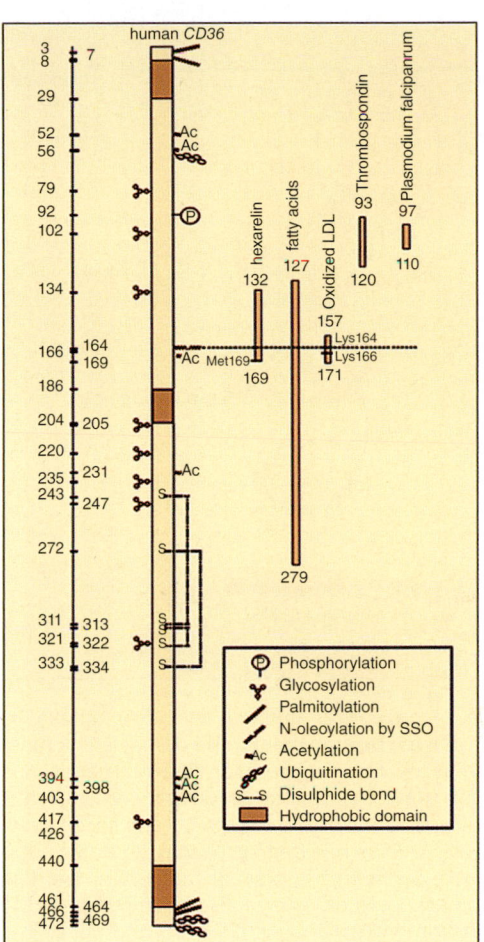

FIGURE 102-5. Schematic representation of CD36 structure, its binding domains, and post-translational modifications. CD36 has 2 short intracellular domains at both termini, 2 transmembrane segments, and a large extracellular domain with a hydrophobic sequence where lipid ligands bind. The C-terminus can associate with Src tyrosine kinases, which usually initiate most of CD36-mediated signal transduction. Post-translational modifications of the protein (*right panel*) include glycosylation, palmitoylation, ubiquitination, phosphorylation, and acetylation. Glycosylation has been shown to be important for CD36 membrane recruitment and is regulated by GLP-2. This regulation was proposed to mediate the effect of GLP-2 to enhance chylomicron production.[77] Dephosphorylation of CD36 accomplished by alkaline phosphatase is thought to reduce the uptake of fatty acids (FAs), and deletion of alkaline phosphatase enhances fat absorption.[93] Both N- and C-termini contain 2 palmitoylation sites that localize CD36 to membrane lipid rafts, which are important for FA uptake.[120] Binding sequences for CD36 ligands are aligned to the backbone of CD36, and the FA-binding site K164 is highlighted with a dotted line (for details, see Ref 107).

dehydration. Rescue of the perinatal lethality was accomplished by transgenic FATP4 expression in keratinocytes in the absence of small intestine FATP4 expression.[118] No detectable effect of intestinal FATP4 deletion on intestinal fat (cholesterol or TG) absorption and no protection from high fat diet–induced weight gain were observed in the transgenic mice. Thus FATP4 appears dispensable for intestinal FA uptake, and its role in mucosal lipid transport remains to be elucidated.

Caveolins and Lipid Rafts

Lipid rafts are membrane domains enriched in cholesterol and sphingomyelin that contribute to the lateral compartmentalization of surface proteins; they function as organizational centers in signal transduction and in the internalization of ligands and receptors. Caveolins 1-3 are proteins that associate with lipid rafts to form smooth invaginations of the plasma membrane or caveolae. Caveolae endocytosis has been implicated in cholesterol transport and is proposed to traffic

cholesterol between the plasma membrane and late endosomes and lysosomes.[119] Lipid rafts have been suggested to function in transport of LCFAs by adipocytes.[120] Caveolin-1 was also shown to influence FA uptake into cells.[121] Mice deficient in caveolin-1 are lean and protected from high fat diet–induced adiposity.[122] It has been suggested that caveolins might influence FA uptake by modulating CD36 localization to lipid rafts,[123] but CD36-independent effects of caveolin on FA uptake can be observed.[121] In the intestine, caveolin-1 is expressed on enterocyte BBMs, and the apically absorbed FA appears to be internalized by enterocytes in detergent-resistant and caveolin-1–containing vesicles that also contain alkaline phosphatase and CD36. In cell lysates, alkaline phosphatase, CD36, and caveolin-1 co-immunoprecipitate, consistent with functional interaction. In agreement with the in vitro data, caveolin-1 knockout mice displayed impaired FA absorption; more FA was recovered in the cecal contents of these mice.[98] In addition, these mice display metabolic inflexibility and reduced ability to perform the fuel switching necessary during fasting/feeding transitions,[124] a phenotype shared by CD36

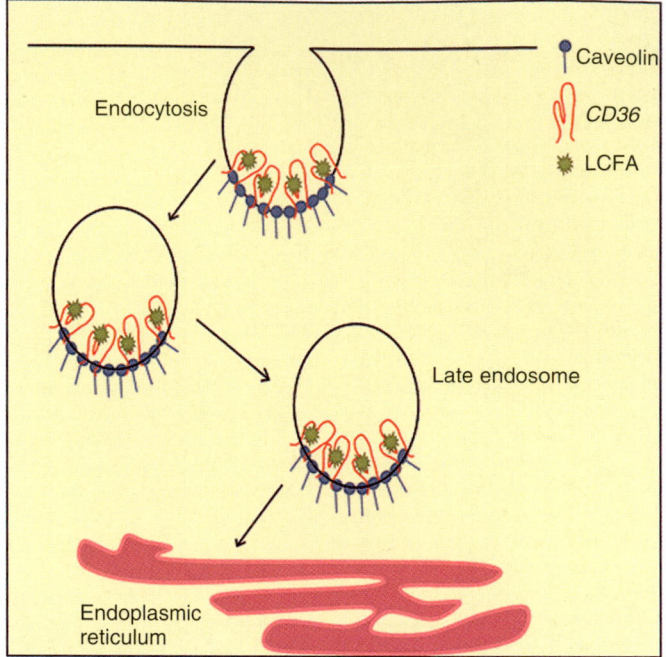

FIGURE 102-6. Role of caveolin-1 in fatty acid (FA) uptake by enterocytes. Lipid rafts are plasma membrane domains that function as organizational centers in internalization of ligands and receptors. Caveolins are proteins that associate with lipid rafts and form smooth invaginations of plasma membrane called *caveolae*. Endocytosis of caveolae has been proposed to traffic nutrients (e.g., cholesterol between the plasma membrane and late endosomes/lysosomes). Lipid rafts have also been suggested to function in transport of long-chain FAs (LCFAs), and caveolin-1 was shown to bind LCFA and influence their uptake into cells. In the intestine, caveolin-1 is expressed on enterocyte brush border membranes, and the apically absorbed FA appears to be internalized by enterocytes in detergent-resistant and caveolin 1–containing vesicles that also contain CD36 (and alkaline phosphatase, not shown). Co-immunoprecipitation of caveolin-1, CD36, and alkaline phosphatase is consistent with potentially functional interactions between the 3 proteins.[98]

null mice.[125] A simplified diagram in Figure 102-6 illustrates the potential role of caveolin-1 and CD36 in FA internalization by enterocytes.

Monoacylglycerol Uptake

Digestion of dietary TG within the intestinal lumen yields 2-MG together with unesterified FA. The few studies that examined 2-MG transport into Caco-2 cells as a model of enterocytes showed 2-MG uptake to be a saturable function of 2-MG concentration and to exhibit sensitivity to trypsin digestion, implying facilitation by a membrane protein.[100] 2-MG inhibited cellular uptake of LCFAs, but triolein (glyceryltriole-ate), glycerol, diacylglycerol, or mono-octanoate had no effect, suggesting that FA and 2-MG transport may be coordinated to optimize intracellular TG resynthesis. The metabolic fate of 2-MG in enterocytes, like that of FA, depends on the site of cellular entry.[126] The ratio of TG to phospholipid (TG:PL) formed from 2-MG was 10-fold higher for apical compared with basolateral delivery, findings that were qualitatively similar to those with FA. The role of the cytosolic FA binding protein L-FABP in binding and intracellular targeting of 2-MG in enterocytes helps explain some of the above observations

(see later under FABP); however, more studies are needed to identify the apical proteins that facilitate 2-MG uptake and how uptake might influence cellular processing.

BRUSH BORDER TRANSPORT OF CHOLESTEROL

Cholesterol is an essential component of mammalian cell membranes and plays a role in the biosynthesis of bile acids, vitamin D, and steroid hormones. Body cholesterol homeostasis is regulated by endogenous synthesis, intestinal absorption, and fecal excretion. In addition to dietary cholesterol, bile and the sloughing of intestinal epithelial cells contribute to luminal cholesterol levels. Absorption of cholesterol ($\approx$50% of intake) varies among individuals and takes place mostly in the duodenum and proximal jejunum. Digestion of dietary cholesteryl esters and solubilization of free cholesterol in bile/phospholipid micelles are followed by enterocyte uptake of free cholesterol via endocytosis into lipid raft vesicles that target the endocytic recycling compartment (ERC) as discussed later. Several apical proteins have been implicated in enterocyte cholesterol transport (Fig. 102-7), the major player being the Niemann-Pick C1-like 1 (NPC1L1) protein. *CD36* might contribute to the process, while the ATP-binding cassette transporter pair ABCG5/8 removes the excess cholesterol and plant sterols that are not processed by the esterifying enzyme acyl-cholesterol acyltransferase ACAT2. On the enterocyte basolateral side, ABCA1 removes unesterified cholesterol by effluxing it to HDL. The scavenger receptor class B type I (SR-B1) is present on both apical and basolateral membranes, but its function in cholesterol homeostasis by the small intestine remains elusive.

Niemann-Pick C1-Like 1 (NPC1L1)

NPC1L1 plays a crucial role in the absorption of dietary cholesterol, as well as in reabsorption of bile acid cholesterol (see Fig. 102-7). NPC1L1 is a homolog of NPC1, which is the defective gene ($\approx$95% of cases) in Niemann-Pick type C1 disease, a lysosomal storage disease characterized by abnormal accumulation of unesterified cholesterol.[127] NPC1 is a large transmembrane protein that binds cholesterol and oxysterols. NPC1 functions together with NPC2, a cytosolic cholesterol-binding protein[128] that extracts cholesterol from inner membranes of late endosomes, transferring it to NPC1 for export out of lysosomes.[128,129]

Like NPC1, the NPC1L1 protein has 13 transmembrane regions (5 of which constitute the sterol-sensing domain), 3 extracellular luminal loops, 6 short cytoplasmic loops, and a C-terminal cytoplasmic tail.[130] In humans, NPC1L1 is found on the apical membrane of enterocytes and also on hepatocytes, ovary, lung, and muscle cells, whereas in rodents, it is primarily expressed on enterocytes. NPC1L1 cycles between the enterocyte plasma membrane and endocytic compartments[131] (Fig. 102-8). In membranes, NPC1L1 forms cholesterol-rich microdomains with the lipid raft proteins flotillin 1 and 2 that facilitate cholesterol internalization to the ERC.[132] Depletion of ERC cholesterol initiates NPC1L1 recruitment to the plasma membrane to stimulate cholesterol uptake.[52] Ezetimibe reduces cholesterol absorption by blocking internalization of the NPC1L1 cholesterol complex.[133] Poor absorption of plant sterols (<5%) primarily reflects NPC1L1 specificity.[110]

ATP-Binding Cassette (ABC) Transporter G5/8

Beta-sitosterolemia is a condition characterized by hypercholesterolemia, xanthomatosis, and premature atherosclerosis.

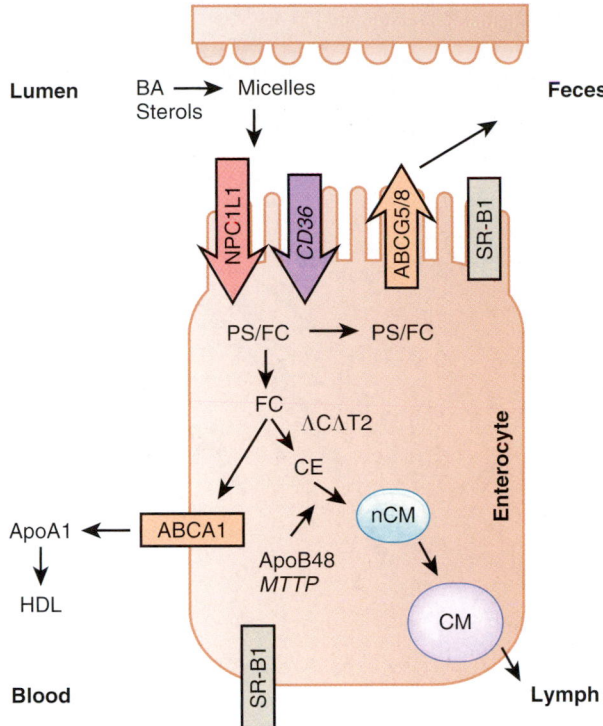

FIGURE 102-7. Intestinal absorption and secretion of cholesterol and plant sterols by enterocytes. Dietary sterols including free cholesterol (FC) and free plant sterols (PS) are mixed with bile acids to form micelles. FC and PS solubilized in mixed micelles are transported across the brush border membrane and into enterocytes mostly via a NPC1L1-dependent mechanism. CD36 also contributes to cholesterol uptake, but its role is unclear. FC is delivered to the endoplasmic reticulum for esterification with fatty acids to cholesteryl esters (CE) by ACAT2. Esterified cholesterol is packaged into nascent chylomicron particles that are further processed in the Golgi apparatus before secretion into lymph. FC that escapes ACAT2 esterification is directly transported to apoA-1 in nascent HDL through ABCA1 located at the basolateral membrane. FC and PS, which are poorly processed by ACAT2, are secreted back to the intestinal lumen by the apical transporter pair ABCG5/G8. ABCA1, ATP-binding cassette transporter A1; ABCG5/8, ATP-binding cassette transporters G5 and G8, which work as heterodimer; ACAT2, acyl cholesterol acyl-transferase 2; apoA-1, apoprotein A-1; *apoB*-48, apoprotein B-48; BA, bile acids; CM, chylomicron; HDL, high-density lipoproteins; *MTTP*, microsomal TG transfer protein; nCM, nascent chylomicrons; NPC1L1, Neiman-Pick 1-Like protein 1; SR-B1, scavenger receptor B1.

The condition reflects increased absorption of dietary plant sterols (20% to 30%, compared with 5% in healthy subjects)[134] because of mutations in 2 genes that encode 65-kd protein members of the ABC transporter family: ABCG5 (sterolin-1) and ABCG8 (sterolin-2). ABCG5/G8 proteins (see Fig. 102-7) work together as an obligate heterodimer on the apical membrane of enterocytes, where they function in efflux of cholesterol back into the lumen. In addition, the transporter pair secretes back into the intestinal lumen the sitosterols and sterols other than cholesterol that are poor substrates for esterification by ACAT2. Defects in ABCG5/G8 decreases biliary excretion of cholesterol and plant sterols, leading to 50- to 200-fold increases in plasma sitosterol,[135,136] while intestinal ABCG5/ABCG8 overexpression reduces cholesterol absorption by increasing its fecal excretion.[135]

ATP-Binding Cassette (ABC) Transporter 1

High-density lipoproteins (HDLs) mediate transport of cholesterol from various tissues to the liver for biliary excretion and elimination from the body; this process is referred to as *reverse cholesterol transport* (RCT). The ABC1 transporter transfers cellular cholesterol and phospholipids to apoA-1 in HDL,[137] mediating the rate-limiting step in RCT (see Fig. 102-7). Mutations in ABCA1 result in Tangier disease, characterized by low HDL.[138] ABCA1 promotes cholesterol efflux across the enterocyte basolateral membrane into the blood, so its role in cholesterol absorption is indirect. Absorption in mice lacking intestinal ABCA1 is unchanged.[139]

CD36 and Scavenger Receptor Class B Type I (SR-B1)

The role of CD36 in cholesterol uptake (see Fig. 102-7) was demonstrated using primary enterocytes from the proximal intestine of wild-type (WT) and *CD36* null mice.[52] In addition, in vivo studies demonstrated a 50% reduction in cholesterol output into the lymph of *CD36* null compared with WT mice. Similar to NPC1L1, *CD36* appears to function in cholesterol absorption for chylomicron assembly, but cholesterol absorption measured by 24-hour fecal excretion is unaltered in *CD36* null mice and in mice null for both SR-BI and *CD36*.[140] Thus, *CD36* does not have a primary role in cholesterol absorption but could optimize absorption targeted to chylomicrons along with NPC1L1.

SR-B1 (84 kd), a member of the class B scavenger receptor family, is expressed in the liver, intestine, adrenal gland, testis, and ovary[141] and plays an important role in RCT from peripheral tissues to the liver for input into bile. In the intestine, SR-B1 is found at both apical and basolateral enterocyte membranes[142] (see Fig. 102-7). In vitro BBM treatment with anti-SR-B1 blocking antibodies reduces cholesterol uptake, but studies in mice with SR-B1 deletion or overexpression did not alter intestinal cholesterol absorption.[143] SR-B1 overexpression in the intestine has little impact on cholesterol absorption.[143,144]

In addition to the classic RCT pathway involving SR-B1,[145] an alternate route for cholesterol disposal has been identified in enterocytes, the transintestinal cholesterol efflux (TICE), which involves cholesterol transfer from the basolateral to the apical membrane for its efflux to luminal bile micelles and excretion. SR-B1 was proposed to function in TICE at the apical membrane, but a recent study showed that intestinal overexpression of SR-B1 did not enhance TICE in a mouse model that preferentially uses TICE for cholesterol disposal (NPC1L1-LiverTg mouse).[143]

Additional Proteins That Regulate Cholesterol Absorption

Cholesterol absorption is influenced by transcription factors such as the nuclear hormone receptors that heterodimerize with retinoid X receptors (RXR). These include the oxysterol (LXR) and bile acid receptor (FXR), which regulate intestinal transporters, the cholesterol esterification enzyme ACAT-2, and bile acid biosynthetic enzymes.[146,147] Mice deficient in mucin, which forms the intestinal mucus layer, display 50% reduction in cholesterol absorption.[148] Deletion of ACAT2, which esterifies cholesterol, thereby facilitating its incorporation into chylomicrons by the microsomal TG transfer protein (MTTP), reduces cholesterol absorption in mice.[149] Intestinal cholesterol absorption is reduced in apoB or MTTP knockout mice.[150] Deletion of L-FABP also reduces cholesterol absorption.[151] The proprotein convertase subtilisin/Kexin type 9

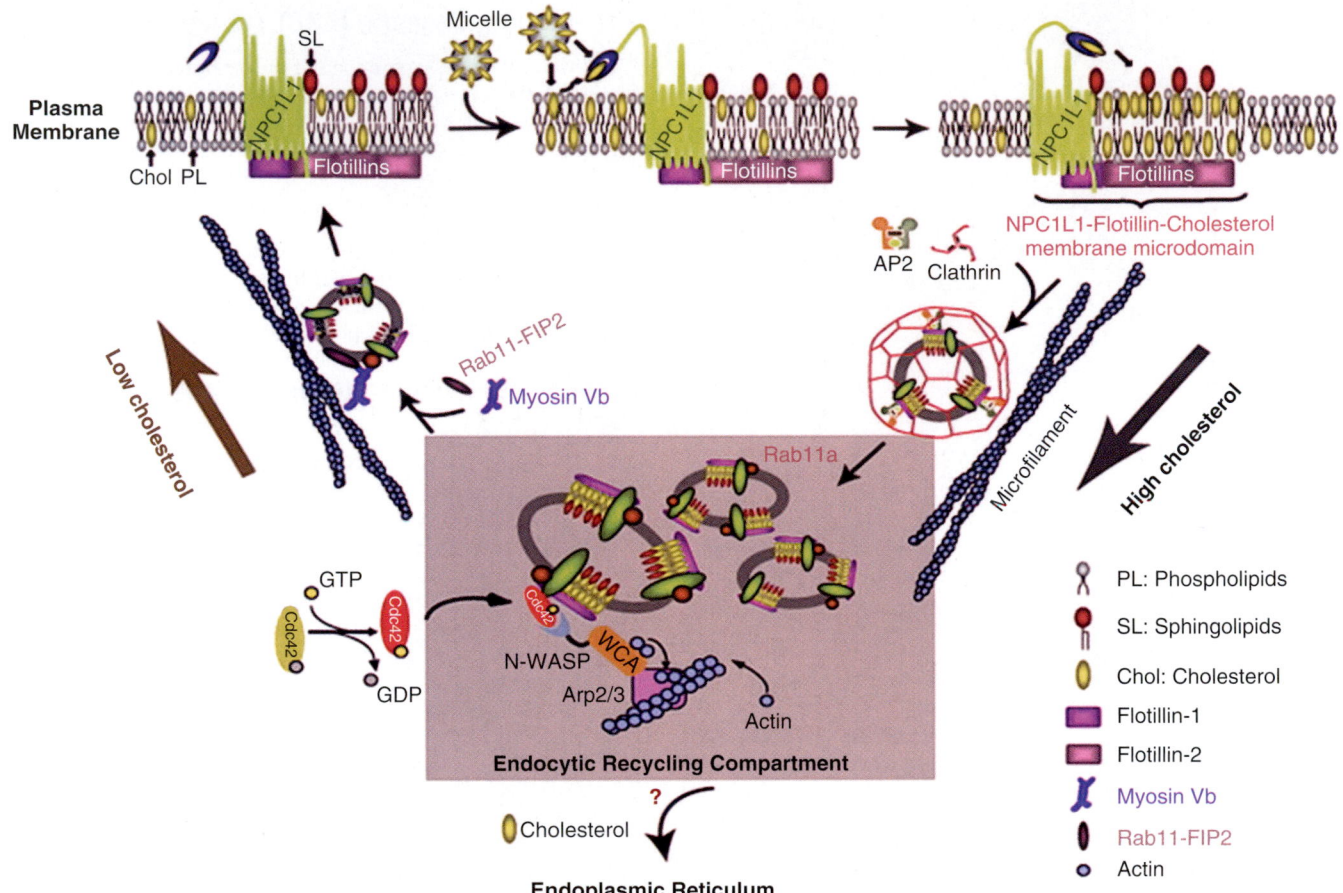

FIGURE 102-8. NPC1L1-mediated cholesterol uptake and intracellular trafficking. NPC1L1 and flotillin proteins associate in cholesterol-rich microdomains that are subsequently coated by clathrin/AP2 complex. These microdomains undergo endocytosis and the internalized vesicles are transported along microfilaments to the endocytotic recycling compartment (ERC). Cholesterol is released from ERC for transport to the endoplasmic reticulum via an unclear mechanism. When intracellular cholesterol level is low, Cdc42 is activated and binds to NPC1L1, promoting recruitment of Myosin Vb and actin. The Cdc42 downstream effectors N-WASP and Arp2/3 are activated and initiate actin polymerization and transport of NPC1L1-flotillin complex to the plasma membrane to enhance cholesterol uptake. Arp2/3, actin-related protein 2/3; Cd42, a member of the Rho family of small GTPases; NPC1L1, Neiman-Pick 1-like protein 1; N-WASP, neural Wiskott-Aldrich syndrome protein. *(Reproduced from Wang LJ, Song BL. Niemann-Pick C1-like 1 and cholesterol uptake. Biochim Biophys Acta 2012; 1821:964-72, with permission.)*

(PCSK9), a proteinase K serine endoprotease family member present in liver and intestine, influences degradation of the low-density lipoprotein receptor (LDLr).[152] It enhances cholesterol uptake in Caco2 cells via up-regulating NPC1L1 and *CD36*. PCSK9 was implicated in chylomicron secretion[152] and in TICE.[153]

CHYLOMICRON ASSEMBLY AND SECRETION

The products of fat digestion, FA, 2-MG, and cholesterol, are re-esterified inside enterocytes, assembled into large TG-rich lipoprotein particles called *chylomicrons*, and secreted into the lymph and then into the circulation (Fig. 102-9). In enterocytes, digestion products must travel to the ER to be resynthesized into complex lipids. Free FAs, which are toxic, are kept at low levels in the cell by binding to cytosolic FA binding proteins (FABPs), a family of abundant small (14 kd) proteins involved in intracellular trafficking of hydrophobic ligands.[154] All FABPs bind 1 FA, except for liver FABP (L-FABP), which

binds 2 FAs, and some FABPs bind other hydrophobic molecules such as eicosanoids and bile salts.[154] L-FABP and intestinal (I)-FABP are expressed by enterocytes in the proximal intestine, and ileal (IL)-FABP is expressed in the distal intestine. L-FABP and I-FABP have high affinity for FA, while IL-FABP binds bile acids and is involved in their apical and basolateral transport.[155] L-FABP might target absorbed FA to oxidation versus TG synthesis by I-FABP.[156] L-FABP null mice show reduced recovery of dietary monoolein in intestinal mucosal TG. L-FABP directs 2-MG to TG synthesis,[157] which could explain why L-FABP null mice have reduced secretion of intestinal lipid.[158] L-FABP also contributes to cellular pre-chylomicron trafficking (see the following section).

Enzymes for Synthesis of Triglycerides and Cholesteryl Esters

In the enterocyte, FA, 2-MG, and cholesterol are re-esterified to TG and cholesteryl esters. FA is activated by acyl-CoA synthases for LCFA (ACSL) to its CoA derivative before esterification by monoglycerol-acyltransferase (MGAT) and

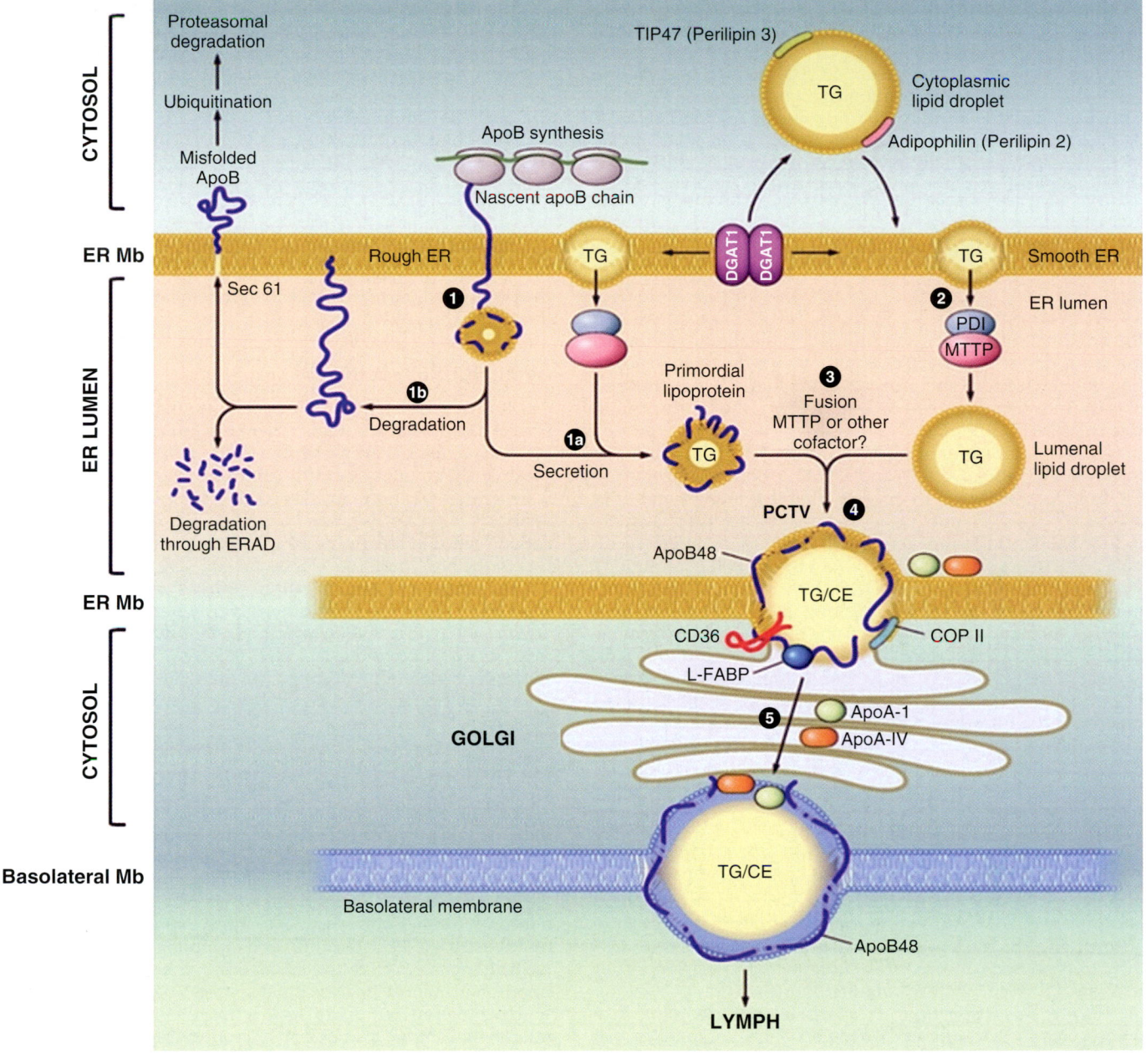

FIGURE 102-9. Assembly of intestinal chylomicrons. Nascent apoB polypeptide *(pictured in blue)* is cotranslationally translocated across rough endoplasmic reticulum (ER). When TG is available, the microsomal TG transfer protein (MTTP) *(pink oval)*, present as a heterodimeric complex with chaperone disulfide isomerase (PDI), interacts with the N-terminal domain of apoB to promote its optimal folding and initiate biogenesis of primordial lipoprotein particle (1a). MTTP can also promote mobilization of TG-rich lipid droplets from the membrane of adjacent smooth ER into ER lumen to generate luminal lipid droplets. Under conditions of low lipid availability or with defective MTTP, nascent apoB is misfolded (1b) and degraded either via ER-associated degradation pathways (ERAD) or proteasomal pathway. During the second step of chylomicron assembly, the primordial lipoprotein particle fuses with lumenal lipid, resulting in prechylomicron. After acquisition of key vesicular transport proteins, including COP II proteins, prechylomicron particles are incorporated into a vesicular complex that buds from the ER. In addition to MTTP and apoB, CD36 and L-FABP participate in PCTV formation and budding. PCTV fuses with Golgi membranes and acquires apoA-1 and apoA-IV apoproteins. Chylomicron particles are then secreted into pericellular spaces where they enter the lymphatic system. *(Reproduced from Abumrad NA, Davidson NO. Role of the gut in lipid homeostasis. Physiol Rev 2012; 92:1061-85.)*

diacylglycerol acyltransferase (DGAT). Cholesterol is converted into cholesteryl ester by acyl cholesterol acyltransferase (ACAT). The synthesized lipid is transferred to *apoB*-48 by *MTTP* to form primordial lipoprotein.

The diacylglycerol (DG) precursor for TG is formed by the monoglycerol (MG) or the glycerol phosphate (Kennedy) pathways. The MG pathway contributes 75% to 80% of TG resynthesis in the intestine and involves acylation of 2-MG.[159] The Kennedy pathway contributes less than 25% and involves acylation of 3-glycerol phosphate twice to generate phosphatidic acid that is dephosphorylated to yield DG, and it becomes the major route for TG formation during fasting.

During lipid absorption, 2-MG is high, and the MG pathway facilitates its esterification with FA to TG while the glycerol phosphate pathway is inhibited.

The acyl CoA synthetases for LCFAs (ACSL) catalyze the first reaction in FA esterification by converting the FA to its CoA ester. Of the 11 ACSL family members for LCFAs,[160] ACSL3 and ACSL5 are the major isoforms present[97] in the intestine, with a small amount of ACSL1. Specificity of intestinal ACSL remains unexplored, but in the liver ACSL3 delivers FA-CoA for phospholipid synthesis,[161] while ACLS5 was shown to increase TG production when expressed in McArdle-RH7777 hepatoma cells.[97]

MGAT forms diacylglycerol from monoacylglycerol and fatty acyl-CoA to generate DG. Of the known MGAT1-3, MGAT1 is expressed in the stomach, MGAT2 is expressed in the proximal intestine,[162] and MGAT3 in the ileum of humans but not rodents.[163] MGAT2 null mice have reduced lipid secretion into the blood[162] and are resistant to high-fat diet–induced obesity. Intestinal rescue of MGAT2 restores the fat absorption rate in MGAT2 null mice.[164]

DGAT is a rate-limiting enzyme for TG synthesis. The intestine expresses DGAT1 and DGAT2. Both localize to the ER, but DGAT2 also co-localizes with mitochondria and lipid droplets.[165] DGAT1 null mice are resistant to high fat diet–induced obesity[166] and have reduced chylomicron secretion[167,168] that is normalized by DGAT1 rescue in the intestine.[169] Pharmacologic inhibition of DGAT1 in mice reduced chylomicron secretion partly by delaying gastric emptying and resulted in lipid accumulation in the distal small intestine.[168,170] DGAT2 null mice die shortly after birth due to skin abnormalities.[171] DGAT1 does not compensate for loss of DGAT2, which is involved in TG synthesis in most tissues except for the intestine.[171] Recent studies implicate DGAT1 in the regulation of intestinal peptide production (GLP-1 and PYY).[172] Thus, DGAT1 is important in TG synthesis for chylomicrons, while DGAT2 contributes to TG synthesis in other tissues.

The free cholesterol in enterocytes is converted by ACAT to cholesteryl ester for chylomicron formation. Two mammalian ACATs have been identified.[173] ACAT-1 is ubiquitously expressed, while ACAT-2 is restricted to mainly liver and intestine.[173] ACAT2 is important for intestinal cholesterol absorption, which drops in ACAT2 null mice to 16% from 46% in wild-type mice and reduces chylomicron cholesteryl ester to about 1% from 12% of chylomicron mass.[174]

During fat absorption, TGs are temporarily stored in enterocytes as cytosolic lipid droplets (LDs), organelles that play a dynamic role in lipid storage and mobilization.[175] The LDs contain a core rich in TG and cholesteryl ester surrounded by a surface layer of phospholipids, cholesterol, and proteins, notably the perilipins (PLN). Intestinal LDs expand or are depleted depending on dietary intake.[176] Two perilipins, PLN2 (adipophilin) and PLN3 (TIP47), coat LDs in the intestine. Perilipin 3 levels are higher after an acute fat challenge, whereas those of PLN2 respond to sustained lipid intake. Thus PLN3 plays a role in the formation of LDs from newly made TG, and PLN2 stabilizes the TG pre-stored in the LDs.[128] Intestinal mucosal LDs harvested after acute intragastric lipid administration differ in size and composition. Analysis of LD content after separation into large (chylomicron-like), intermediate, and small or HDL-like droplets showed the presence of MGAT2 in all LDs. The largest LDs contained MTTP, ACAT1/2, and the lipases, hormone-sensitive lipase (HSL) and adipose TG lipase (ATGL). Thus, enterocyte LDs contain enzymes involved in the different steps of FA and cholesterol metabolism and function in the accumulation and possibly metabolic transformation of the absorbed lipids in coordination with the ER.[177]

Enterocytes package TGs, cholesterol, cholesteryl esters, and phospholipids for export in the form of chylomicrons or very-low-density lipoproteins (VLDLs). After a meal, chylomicrons predominate, whereas VLDLs are the major TG-rich lipoprotein during fasting. VLDL and chylomicron TGs have different FA composition that reflects different metabolic sources. The FAs derived from dietary TG are predominantly used for chylomicrons, whereas those from phospholipid are used for VLDL.[178] Chylomicron particles range between 75 and 450 nm[179] in diameter, with a core of TG and cholesteryl esters and a surface coat composed of phospholipids (80%) and apoproteins. Chylomicron assembly (see Fig. 102-9)[180] involves the coordinated functions of *MTTP* and *apoB* to form the primordial particle that is then transferred from the ER to the Golgi apparatus.

Apolipoprotein B (ApoB)

ApoB is a large hydrophobic protein required for the formation of TG-rich lipoproteins. There are 2 forms of *apoB*: *apoB*-100 and *apoB*-48.[181] Transcription of the *apoB* gene generates a 14-kb mRNA that yields a full-length *apoB* (*apoB*-100). ApoB-48 is generated when the mRNA editing complex (apobec-1 and apobec-1 complementation factor [ACF]) introduces a stop codon (cytidine to uridine RNA editing) resulting in translation of the N-terminal 48% of *apoB*-100.[182] ApoB-48 is the intestinally expressed form of *apoB* in rodents and humans. Only *apoB*-100 is expressed in human liver, whereas both *apoB*-48 and *apoB*-100 are expressed in the rodent liver.[182,183] Apobec-1 null mice, which synthesize only *apoB*-100, display slower TG secretion and retain more TG in their intestinal mucosa.[184] Transgenic rescue of apobec-1 in the intestine restored intestinal *apoB*-48 production.[185]

Microsomal Triglyceride Transfer Protein (*MTTP*)

MTTP is a 97-kd heterodimeric protein that transfers lipids to the newly synthesized *apoB*-48 during its translocation to the ER lumen to generate the primordial lipoprotein (see Fig. 102-9). Failure to transfer lipid to *apoB* leads to its misfolding, ubiquitination, and degradation by both proteosomal and non-proteosomal pathways.[186,187] ApoB can also be degraded by ER-associated degradation and autophagy. The primordial particle separates from the ER membrane to form the nascent lipoprotein, which fuses with absorbed lipid to generate the prechylomicron. Supply of *apoB* is not rate-limiting for chylomicron TG output. For example, *apoB* output into the lymph does not change after intraduodenal lipid infusion, even though lymphatic TG output increases 7- to 8-fold. In addition, *apoB*-48 synthetic rates are not increased by acute or chronic fat feeding, but they can be reduced by bile exclusion secondary to a loss of cholesterol.[52]

MTTP is present in the ER lumen of enterocytes (and hepatocytes) in a complex with the chaperone protein disulfide isomerase (PDI). *MTTP* transfers lipid (from membranes and lipid droplets) to nascent *apoB*[188] (see Fig. 102-9). It transfers TG, cholesterol, and phospholipids[189] to form either chylomicrons or VLDL.[190,191] Pharmacologic inhibition of *MTTP* blocks secretion of *apoB* and lipoproteins.[192] Deletion of *MTTP* in mice is embryonic lethal,[193] so its role has been examined using intestine targeted deletion or partial deficiency of *MTTP*. In both mice models, intestinal secretion of *apoB*-containing lipoproteins is reduced.[193-195] In humans, mutations in the *MTTP* gene result in abetalipoproteinemia, a rare disorder with low blood *apoB* lipoproteins and with LD accumulation in the small intestine and liver.[196] Genetic defects associated with abnormal *apoB* are mostly caused by nonsense and frameshift mutations in the *apoB* gene that result in C-terminal truncations.[197] The population frequency of APOB gene mutations causing truncated *apoB* proteins is about 1:3000. By clinical criteria, heterozygous familial hypobetalipoproteinemia (FHBL) may occur in 1:500 to 1:1000, while homozygous FHBL is rare. Homozygous hypobetalipoproteinemia associates with abnormally low serum lipids and *apoB*. Symptoms can include fat malabsorption, neurologic defects, red cell acanthocytosis, and nonalcoholic fatty liver disease.[198]

Intestinal *MTTP* is highly regulated, exhibiting diurnal regulation in response to visual and nutritional cues and in concert with plasma TG levels. This involves the circadian regulatory clock and nocturnin proteins and the transcriptional repressor SHP (short heterodimeric partner).[199,200] Leptin signaling regulates *MTTP*, involving the melanocortin-4 receptor.[201] ER stress increases intestinal *MTTP*[202] and augments chylomicron secretion.[203]

Transport of Prechylomicrons from the Endoplasmic Reticulum to the Golgi Apparatus

Because of the large size of these particles, transport requires the formation of prechylomicron transport vesicles (PCTV) (≈250 nm in diameter) (see Fig. 102-9). The PCTV consist of *apoB*-48, vesicle-associated membrane protein 7 (VAMP7), *CD36*, and L-FABP.[204] L-FABP is present within a multiprotein complex in the cytosol.[205] Phosphorylation of complex components by protein kinase C (PKCζ) dissociates L-FABP, allowing it to bind to the ER to initiate PCTV formation.[205] Budding of the PCTV from the ER involves L-FABP and *CD36* and is markedly reduced in enterocyte fractions derived from mice deficient in either protein.[204] Fusion of PCTV to the Golgi apparatus involves multiple proteins including SNARE (soluble *N*-ethylmaleimide-sensitive factor attachment protein receptor), VAMP7, and syntaxin-5.[206] The prechylomicron undergoes maturation in the Golgi apparatus with apoA-I addition, alteration of *apoB*-48 glycosylation, and more TG transfer by *MTTP*. The trans-Golgi–associated ADP-ribosylation factor–related protein 1 (ARFRP1) and its target GRIP domain protein (RAB2) play an essential role in the lipidation and maturation of chylomicrons in the Golgi apparatus, including addition of apoA-I.[207]

Golgi-derived chylomicrons are incorporated into the basolateral membrane and secreted by exocytosis into the lymphatic circulation (see Fig. 102-9). Plasma apoA-IV appears important for chylomicron secretion. ApoA-IV levels rise in response to fat intake,[208] with synthesis of the apolipoprotein increasing by about 5-fold.[209] ApoA-IV is part of the prechylomicron formed within the ER,[210] and its overexpression increases TG output into the lymph by increasing particle size. The C-terminus of apoA-IV (amino acids 344 to 354) is important for chylomicron TG output into the lymph.[211] ApoA-IV interaction with *apoB* in *apoB*-containing particles enhances particle expansion and TG secretion.[212] During absorption, lacteals distend and gaps open between endothelial cells, allowing chylomicron passage.[213]

Disorders of Chylomicron Production

Apolipoproteinemia is a rare genetic disorder in which the liver and intestine fail to make TG-rich lipoproteins.[214] The disorder results from mutations in the *MTTP*[215] that impair its lipid transfer activity leading to *apoB* degradation. Anderson's disease or chylomicron retention disorder is characterized by hypobetalipoproteinemia with selective absence of *apoB*-48 postprandially and the accumulation of lipid droplets in enterocytes.[216] The disease is caused by mutations affecting the Sar1B protein, a small GTPase involved in the vesicular ER to Golgi transport of proteins[217] shown to be required for fusion

of PCTV with the Golgi apparatus. *CD36* deficient humans have high levels of plasma TG, and *apoB*-48,[115] which was suggested to increase atherosclerotic risk by enhancing levels of lipoprotein remnants because of increased intestinal secretion of particles smaller than chylomicrons.[115]

FATTY ACID SENSING BY THE GUT AND ITS SIGNALING FUNCTIONS (Fig. 102-10)

The regulation of energy homeostasis involves afferent and efferent signals that connect metabolic organs to the hypothalamus and brainstem. The GI tract plays a role in this regulation through signals transmitted via the blood or vagal afferent fibers. Dietary fat reaching the intestine has pro-satiety effects. It suppresses secretion of ghrelin,[218] a hormone with positive effects on appetite. This suppression requires digestion, but it is unclear whether it is mediated by LCFAs. Dietary fat also stimulates secretion of a number of pro-satiety intestinal peptides (see Fig. 102-10 and following sections). Dysfunction of oral or intestinal fat-sensing or a blunting of the pro-satiety effects of dietary fat by other ingested nutrients might contribute to obesity.[61]

Intestinal Fatty Acid Sensing and Lipid Absorption

LCFAs are recognized on the surface of intestinal cells by membrane receptors that include *CD36* and a number of G protein-coupled receptors (GPRs). FA binding to *CD36* results in signal transduction involving sarcoma (Src) tyrosine kinases, phospholipases A2, and associates with increases in intracellular calcium and cAMP.[111,219] Ligand binding to the GPRs triggers a conformational change that leads to activation of intracellular heterotrimeric G proteins, which activate distinct signal transduction pathways dependent on the type of G-protein coupling.[76] Proteins that are involved downstream of the receptor include adenylyl or guanylyl cyclase, phospholipases A2 and C, phosphodiesterases, and phosphatidylinositol-3 kinases (PI3Ks). GPRs 40, 41, and 43 were identified as FA receptors in 2003.[220,221] The abundant dietary FAs and palmitic, stearic, and oleic acids were reported as GPR40 ligands and SCFA GPR41 and GPR43 ligands. GPR84, GPR119, and *GPR120* are activated, respectively, by medium-chain FAs, the oleic acid derivative OEA, and omega-3 FAs.[76] GPR40 mediates effects of FAs on insulin secretion[222] and *GPR120* that of FAs on intestinal incretin release.[76] The first site of lipid sensing in the GI tract involves FA perception via taste receptors within the oral cavity (See previous section on Oral Perception of Dietary Fat). This interaction also triggers the cephalic phase of digestion, which primes the intestine to optimize absorption. Fat-specific cephalic-phase responses include secretion of lipases, transient increases of intestinal CCK, PP, and PYY, and insulin release.[223]

In addition to the oral cavity, LCFA receptors are distributed throughout the GI tract, where they act to coordinate absorption with nutrient processing through the release of intestinal peptides (Table 102-4). In the duodenum and jejunum, LCFAs released from fat digestion in the lumen influence secretion of peptides that modulate the digestive process. EECs in the intestinal mucosa, which constitute less than 1% of the epithelial cell population, are the sensors and express the LCFA receptors GPR40, *GPR120*,[224,225] and *CD36*.[111] LCFAs stimulate CCK secretion[226] by I cells in the mucosa of the duodenum, jejunum, and proximal ileum. CCK helps optimize fat digestion by regulating gastric emptying, gallbladder contraction, pancreatic secretion, and intestinal motility.[227]

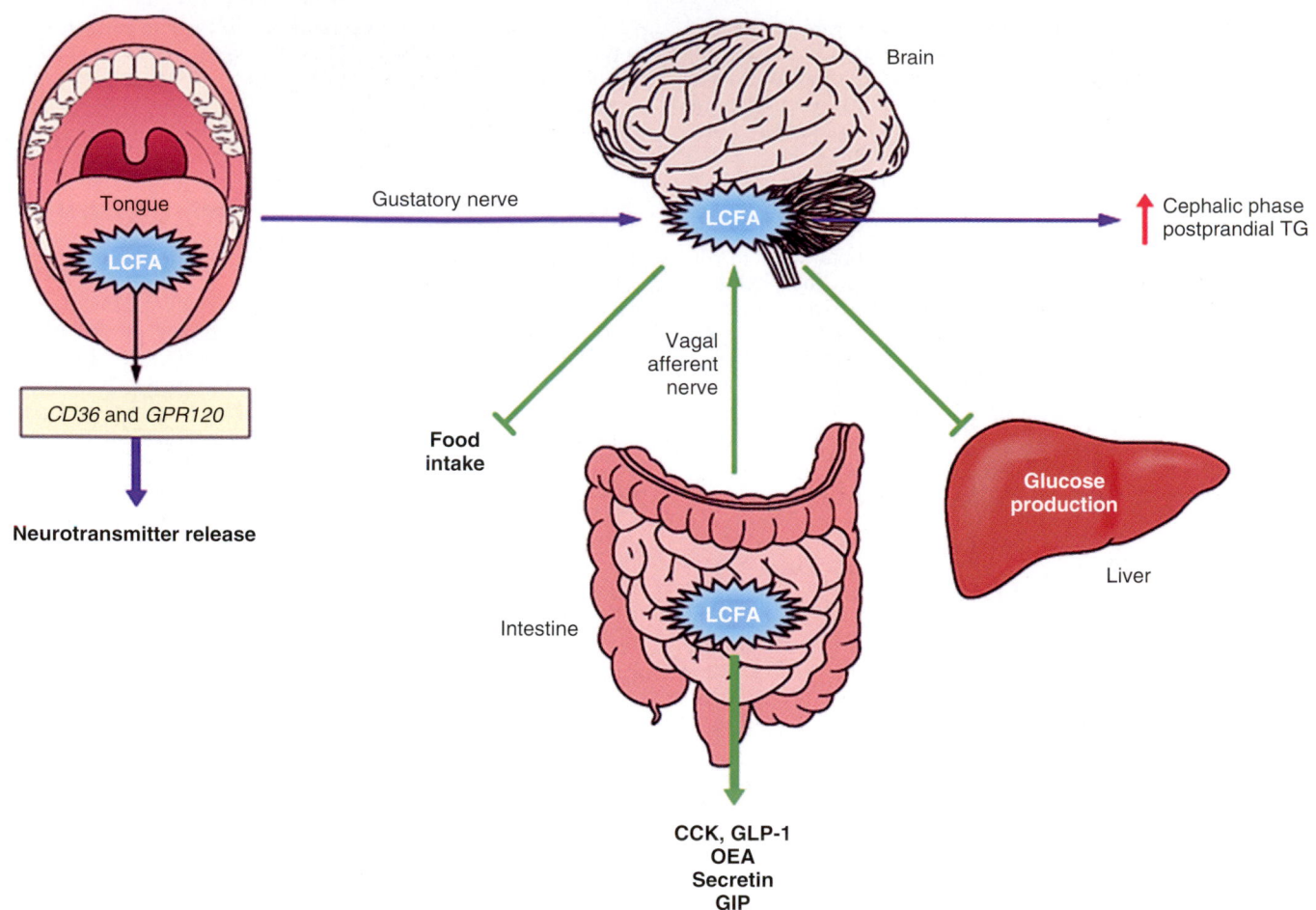

FIGURE 102-10. Signaling functions of intestinal long-chain fatty acids (LCFAs). Dietary TG hydrolysis during digestion releases LCFAs that have important signaling functions at various levels of the digestive tract. In the oral cavity, LCFA receptors (CD36, GPR120) present on apical surface of taste bud cells in the tongue[97,150] contribute to fat taste perception, which associates with secretion of neurotransmitters, signal transmission to brain centers, and induction of the early cephalic phase of digestion[150] *(blue arrows)*. In the intestinal lumen, dietary lipid has satiety effects *(green arrows)* mediated by LCFA signaling to release peptides with inhibitory effects on food intake (GLP-1, CCK, OEA). GLP-1 and CCK also delay gastric emptying and lipid absorption.[71] GLP-1 and GIP enhance insulin release from the pancreas and glucose metabolism.[229] Lipid sensing in the proximal intestine, mediated by accumulation of long-chain fatty acyl-CoA, also activates an intestine-brain-liver axis to inhibit glucose production by the liver.[233] During feeding, TG is resynthesized largely from absorbed FA and monoglyceride. During fasting, TG and phospholipid are synthesized from α-glycerophosphate derived from glucose entering across the basolateral membrane of the enterocyte, and from FA. Unsaturated FAs tend to form phospholipid. CoA, coenzyme A; GIP, gastric inhibitory polypeptide; GLP-1, glucagon-like peptide-1; OEA, oleoylethanolamide. *(Reproduced from Abumrad NA, Davidson NO. Role of the gut in lipid homeostasis. Physiol Rev 2012; 92:1061-85.)*

LCFAs induce S and K cells in the duodenum and jejunum to release, respectively, secretin and the glucose insulinotropic peptide (GIP). Secretin inhibits gastric emptying and synergizes with CCK to induce pancreatic secretions.[228] GIP has insulinotropic effects.[229] GPR40[68] and *CD36*[111] have been implicated in mediating the effect of FA on CCK. Isolated I cells that express GPR40 respond to linoleic acid with increases in intracellular calcium and CCK release. CCK secretion induced by oleic acid is reduced in GPR40 null mice.[68] The *CD36* null mouse displays a 50% reduction in release of CCK and secretin in response to gastric administration of oil. Diminished release in response to FA is also observed with CD36-deficient intestinal segments in vitro. In EECs that express CD36, release of CCK and secretin involves FA-induced increases in calcium and the second messenger cAMP.[111] GPR40 is present on EECs expressing GIP, GLP-1, and CCK, and its disruption reduces secretion of these peptides.[224]

GLP-1 is formed in intestinal L-cells in the jejunum, distal ileum, and colon from the post-translational processing of a proglucagon precursor.[230] GLP-1 influences gastric emptying and GI motility.[231] Release of GLP-1 is stimulated in vivo by FA reaching the distal intestine (or administered directly into it) and requires protein kinase C zeta.[232] GLP-1 release from the distal intestine by polyunsaturated FA involves GPR120.[76]

Satiation Effect of Intestinal Lipid

Dietary fat in the intestine inhibits food intake in rats and humans, an effect mediated by LCFA signaling to release several regulatory peptides (see Fig. 102-10). CCK has pro-satiety effects that are mediated by CCK receptors on vagal afferents in the duodenum, which signal to the brain nucleus of the tractus solitarius to reduce the feeling of hunger.[227] LCFAs induce production by the small intestine of OEA, a pro-satiety lipid and agonist of peroxisome proliferator activated receptor alpha (PPAR-alpha). OEA is generated from absorbed oleic acid and acts centrally to prolong

TABLE 102-4 Peptide Secretion Induced by Fatty Acids in The Taste Buds and Enteroendocrine Cells and The Membrane Fatty Acid Receptors Involved in Coordinating Absorption and Nutrient Processing

Taste Bud Cells	Peptide	Primary Site	Fat Type	FA Receptor
	GLP-1	Circumvallate*	LCFA	GPR120
	Serotonin	Circumvallate	LCFA	CD36
EEC				
K cells	GIP	Duodenum/jejunum	LCFA	GPR40,119, 120
S cells	Secretin	Duodenum/jejunum	LCFA	CD36
I cells	CCK	Duodenum/jejunum	LCFA	GPR40, CD36
L cells	PYY	Ileum/colon	SCFA	GPR41, 43
L cells	GLP-1	Ileum/colon	LCFA	GPR40,119, 120

Circumvallate refers to circumvallate papillae of the tongue.
CCK, cholecystokinin; CD36, cluster of differentiation 36; EEC, enteroendocrine cells; FA, fatty acid; GIP, gastric inhibitory polypeptide, also known as the *glucose-dependent insulinotropic peptide*; GLP-1, glucagon-like peptide 1; GPR, G protein–coupled receptor; LCFA, long-chain FA; PYY, peptide tyrosine tyrosine; SCFA; short-chain FA.

inter-meal intervals and reduce feeding frequency.[233] Generation of OEA is CD36 dependent, and disruption of CD36 or PPAR-alpha blunts fat-induced satiety. Effects of OEA on satiety may involve GLP-1 release by EECs after OEA binding to GPR119.[234] Fat intake promotes intestinal secretion of *N*-acylphosphatidyletholamine (NAPE)[235] and apo A-IV,[236] and SCFAs induce L cells to release PYY,[226] all shown to have central pro-satiety effects (see Table 100-4). The satiety-inducing property of fat, however, can be blunted by factors like simultaneous ingestion of carbohydrates and release of endocannabinoids by a palatable fat-sugar mix (as found in processed food).[237] Also, regulation of fat intake involves a number of factors with positive (e.g., ghrelin, galanin) effects on appetite.[85]

Intestinal Fatty Acid Sensing and Glucose Metabolism

FA sensing by the gut-brain axis regulates glucose metabolism (see Fig. 102-10), mainly via release of GIP and GLP-1, secreted by EECs in response to dietary fat and carbohydrates.[238] GIP and GLP-1 amplify glucose-dependent pancreatic insulin release (incretin effect). GIP has direct effects on adipose tissue to promote glucose uptake and energy storage. GLP-1 has an anti-hyperglycemic action that reflects its reduction of gastric emptying and meal-induced liver glucagon secretion. GLP-1-receptor agonists resistant to hydrolysis by dipeptidyl peptidase-4 are being used for treating type 2 diabetes.[229] Inhibition of gastric emptying by several intestinal peptides released by LCFAs reduces blood glucose.[239] Lipid sensing in the upper intestine also activates an intestine-brain-liver axis to inhibit hepatic glucose output (see Fig. 102-10), a pathway that becomes defective in fat-fed rodents.[240] In the brain, long-chain fatty acyl-coenzyme A accumulation and subsequent activation of PKC directly impact the centers that regulate glucose production and energy homeostasis.[241]

CARBOHYDRATES

Dietary Intake

Glucose plays a central role in energy metabolism. In Western civilization, carbohydrates make up some 40% to 45% of the total caloric intake of human beings. Ingested carbohydrates include simple sugars (e.g., glucose, galactose, fructose), disaccharides (e.g., lactose, sucrose) and complex carbohydrates (e.g., starch, glycogen).[242,243] Simple sugars, disaccharides, and complex carbohydrates account, respectively, for approximately 5% to 10%, 30% to 40%, and 45% to 60% of consumed dietary carbohydrates. In total, the amount of glucose produced by digestion is about 180 g/day (≈1 mol).[244]

Fructose had been increasingly added to our diets (frequently in excess of 50 g/day) through the widespread use of corn syrup as a sweetener.[245-247] All ingested glucose and galactose is absorbed normally, but the capacity to absorb fructose is limited in both young children and adults, as shown by a study of healthy young adults (medical students in the United States and the United Kingdom), 70% of whom developed abdominal pain, bloating, borborygmi, flatus, and a positive hydrogen breath test after ingestion of 50 g of fructose.[248] The increased intake of fructose over the last 4 decades, especially in soft drinks (2 12-oz cans of some popular soft drinks contain about 50 g of fructose in the form of corn syrup), has been associated with a multitude of disorders, including obesity, diabetes, and heart disease.[249-252]

About half of the digestible carbohydrate in an average Western diet is starch (the main storage form of carbohydrates), which is derived from cereals and plants. Starch, as either amylose or amylopectin, is made up of long chains of glucose molecules. Amylose, a linear polymer in which each glucose molecule is coupled to its neighbor by α-1–4 linkage, has a molecular weight of 10^6. Amylopectin, in contrast, is a branched-chain polymer in which α-1–6 links provide angulations between adjacent chains of α-1–4 linked glucose molecules (Fig. 102-11); it has a molecular weight greater than 10^9. Most starches contain more amylopectin than amylose, but the ratio varies widely. Although starches are relatively easily digested, food preparation can influence their biological utilization. Utilization also may be determined by proteins that are associated with the starch, particularly gluten.[1,23]

Other major sources of dietary carbohydrate include milk (lactose), fruits and vegetables (fructose, glucose, sucrose), or purified and cane or beet sources (sucrose). Processed foods form a major source of dietary sugars, particularly fructose and corn syrup; the latter contains not only fructose but also oligosaccharides and polysaccharides. The sugar alcohol sorbitol is used widely in the manufacture of "diabetic" sweets

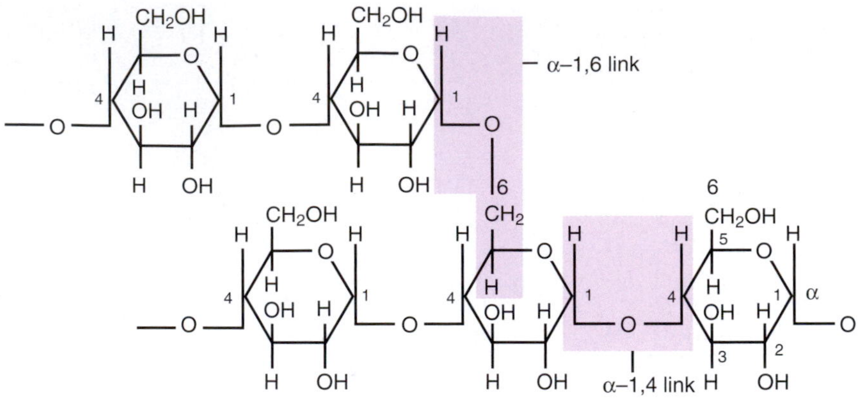

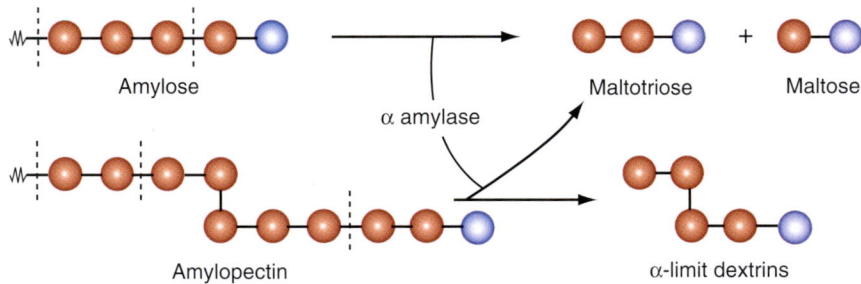

FIGURE 102-11. Part of an amylopectin molecule, indicating disposition of α1–4 and α1–6 linkages between glucose molecules.

FIGURE 102-12. Action of pancreatic α-amylase on amylose and amylopectin molecules. Because the α1–6 link in the latter is resistant to amylase, the products include α-limit dextrin. *Brown circles*, glucose units; *Blue circles*, reducing glucose units. *(From Gray GM. Carbohydrate absorption and malabsorption. In: Johnson LR, editor. Physiology of the gastrointestinal tract. New York: Raven Press; 1981. p 1064, fig. 42-1.)*

and preserves and is found naturally in apples, pears, peaches, and prunes.[253] Sorbitol is formed when the aldehyde group of glucose is hydrogenated to an alcohol group, slowing its rate of absorption and thus diminishing its effect on blood sugar concentrations.[254]

Glycogen is the major storage form of polysaccharides in animals, but the amounts ingested in a normal diet are small. The structure of glycogen is similar to that of amylose and composed of straight chains of α-1–4–linked glucose monomers.[242]

Non-starch polysaccharides form the majority of unavailable carbohydrates. The dietary fiber component of unavailable carbohydrate is found most abundantly in cereals, peas, beans, carrots, and peanuts. In the United States, 10 to 15 g of dietary fiber, consisting predominantly of celluloses and hemicelluloses, is consumed by each person every day.[255,256] Cellulose is made up of β-1–4-linked glucose molecules in straight chains, and hemicelluloses are pentose and hexose polymers with both straight and branched chains. Both forms are resistant to digestion in the small intestine, because the β-1–4 bond, unlike the α-bond in starch, is resistant to amylases. They are, however, broken down to some extent by colonic bacteria to yield SCFAs that are avidly absorbed by colonic mucosa.[3,257] The quantity of cellulose and hemicelluloses in vegetables and fruit varies markedly and depends on their age and ripeness.[258]

Other unavailable carbohydrates include pectins, gums, and alginates, which are only partially metabolized in the colon. Lignins, elaborated by plants in the process of becoming woody, are completely indigestible.[254,259]

It is well recognized that an increased intake of dietary fiber may ease constipation by increasing fecal bulk, mainly as a result of the increase in the mass of fecal flora. Dietary fiber has other roles, however, and also affects the absorption of other nutrients. For example, fiber delays absorption of sugars and fats and curtails the insulin response to a carbohydrate meal. Some fiber (e.g., lignins) may lower serum cholesterol values by binding bile salts.[260] It may be these effects that have led to the widespread recommendation of a high-fiber diet for management or prevention of diabetes mellitus and atherosclerosis. Satiety is achieved more rapidly from a diet rich in fiber than from a low-fiber diet, and it takes longer to ingest a high-fiber meal. The management of obesity takes advantage of this fact (see Chapter 7).

Intraluminal Digestion

Salivary and Pancreatic Amylase

Salivary and pancreatic α-amylases are endoenzymes—that is, they cleave the α-1–4 links internal to or at the second or third bond from the end of the polysaccharide chain. The products of amylase digestion, therefore, are short, linear oligosaccharides of maltotriose and maltose (Fig. 102-12). Because α-1–6 links and the adjacent α-1–4 bonds in the branched chains of amylopectin are not hydrolyzed by amylase, the products of amylopectin digestion include short, branched oligosaccharides termed *α-limit dextrins*. Amylase proteins are encoded by a clustered gene family located on chromosome 1 of the human genome.[261] In humans, the *AMY1* gene is expressed in the parotid gland, and the *AMY2* gene is expressed in the pancreas.[262] The sequences of the pancreatic and salivary complementary DNAs are 94% similar, encoding for polypeptides with the same number of amino acids.[263]

The initial digestion of complex carbohydrates begins in the mouth with salivary α-amylase, also known as *ptyalin*. This endoenzyme is secreted by the acinar cells of the parotid and submandibular glands and starts the digestion of starch and other complex carbohydrates before ingested food is even swallowed.[244] Salivary amylase depends for its effect on its proximity to the ingested starches and the time they spend within the mouth. Thus, careful, slow chewing affords a good start to digestion, whereas rapid swallowing of poorly chewed foods, often a problem for edentulous persons, may cause suboptimal salivary amylase action.[264] Salivary amylase is rapidly inactivated by gastric acid, but some activity may persist within the food bolus; short-chain oligosaccharides offer further protection for the enzyme against inactivation at acid pH. Approximately 30% to 40% of complex carbohydrate digestion takes place before the food reaches the small intestine, where luminal digestion is completed by pancreatic α-amylase.[242]

Pancreatic amylase is the major enzyme of starch digestion and, as with salivary amylase, produces short oligosaccharides, maltotriose, maltose, and α-limit dextrins; glucose monomer is not produced. Most of this hydrolysis occurs within the intestinal lumen, but because amylase also attaches itself to the BBM of enterocytes, some digestion may occur at this site as well. Amylase concentration becomes limiting for starch hydrolysis only in severe cases of pancreatic insufficiency when luminal enzyme activity levels are reduced to less than 10% of normal.[265] Human milk contains amylase activity, which may be important for carbohydrate digestion in infants.[266]

Brush Border Membrane Hydrolases

The terminal products of luminal starch digestion, together with the major disaccharides in the diet (sucrose and lactose), cannot be absorbed intact and are hydrolyzed by specific BBM hydrolases that are maximally expressed in the villi of the duodenum and jejunum. Several types have been identified.[244,267]

Lactase hydrolyzes lactose (the primary sugar in milk) to produce 1 molecule of glucose and 1 of galactose.

Sucrase-isomaltase (*SI*, sucrase-α-dextrinase) comprises 2 subunits of the same enzyme, each with distinct enzymatic activity. Both sucrase and isomaltase remove glucose molecules from the non-reducing end of α-limit dextrins. Sucrase hydrolyzes sucrose to yield 1 molecule each of glucose and fructose, whereas isomaltase ("debrancher" enzyme) hydrolyzes the 1-6 glycosidic linkages in α-limit dextrins. The concerted action of sucrase and isomaltase is to yield monomeric glucose molecules from sucrose and α-limit dextrins (Fig. 102-13).

In addition, 2 other carbohydrases participate in terminal hydrolysis of starch products: maltase-glucoamylase and α-limit dextrinase. Maltase-glucoamylase acts on 1-4–linked oligosaccharides containing as many as 9 glucose residues, to liberate glucose monomers. The human maltase-glucoamylase gene (*MGAM*) is located on chromosome 7 and has structural homology similar to the *SI* gene.[268] The maltase-glucoamylase enzyme does not undergo intracellular or extracellular proteolytic cleavage and is expressed in the BBM as a monomeric protein. Maltase-glucoamylase is expressed prenatally, with similar levels after birth and into adulthood.[269] It has been suggested that while isomaltase hydrolyzes the smallest α-limit dextrin, another enzyme, α-limit dextrinase, is responsible for rapid hydrolysis of penta- and hexa-α-limit dextrins.[270]

The combination of *SI*, maltase, and α-limit dextrinase serves to liberate glucose monomers very rapidly and close to

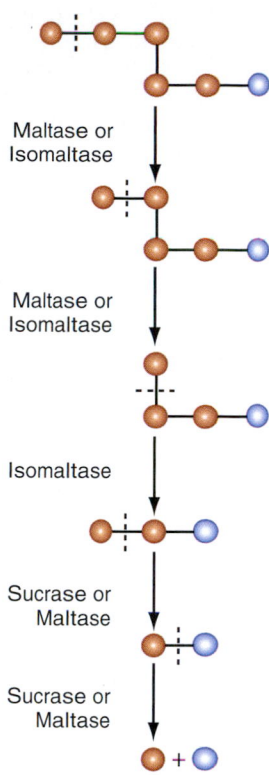

FIGURE 102-13. Actions of brush border membrane hydrolases. Combined actions of maltase, isomaltase, and sucrase yield glucose molecules from α-limit dextrins. Isomaltase is necessary to split α1–6 link. *Brown circles*, glucose units; *Blue circles*, reducing glucose units.

hexose carriers, thus encouraging efficient absorption. Because free hexoses are found in the intestinal lumen, it is likely that the transport process is the rate-limiting step for uptake of monomers into the epithelium, rather than the actions of the carbohydrases.

Trehalose is a disaccharide found predominantly in mushrooms, insects, algae, and other fungi, so it is an insignificant element of the normal diet; nevertheless, there is a specific brush border enzyme, trehalase, for its hydrolysis (α-1,1 linkage) to its 2 glucose molecules. If consumed by individuals with trehalase deficiency, trehalose may cause GI distress in the form of bloating, flatulence, and diarrhea.[271] Congenital trehalase deficiency is very rare in Caucasian Americans but has been reported in up to 8% of Greenland natives, resulting in severe diarrhea after ingestion of mushrooms.[269]

Disaccharidase Biosynthesis and Regulation

Much has been learned about the gene regulation, biosynthesis, and processing of the disaccharidases.[272-276] The human trehalase gene (*TREH*) is located on chromosome 11 and encodes a 583–amino acid protein with a molecular mass of about 75 kd. *SI* is encoded by a single gene in the human,[277] located on the human chromosome 3 at locus 3q-25-26.[278] The 5′ flanking region of the *SI* gene has a number of DNA regulatory regions that control initiation of gene transcription.[279,280] Using mouse genetics, all 4 epithelial cell types in the small intestinal mucosa have the transcriptional machinery to express the *SI* gene.[281,282] The elements necessary to direct intestinal epithelial cell-specific expression are embodied in a 201-nucleotide, evolutionary conserved, 5′ flanking region of the gene.[283] At least 3 types of transcriptional proteins are involved in *SI* promoter transcription, including hepatocyte nuclear factor 1 (HNF1),[284,285] GATA family members (GATA 4 and 5),[286] and caudal-related homeodomain proteins (Cdx).[287] The interaction of tissue-specific and tissue-restricted transcription factors facilitates the transcription of genes in a single cell type.[288]

Congenital *SI* deficiency (CSID) is an autosomal recessive intestinal disease that is characterized by the absence of the sucrase and most of the maltase digestive activity within the *SI* enzyme complex; the isomaltase activity varies from absent to normal. Clinically, the disease is manifested as an osmotic-fermentative diarrhea upon ingestion of disaccharides and oligosaccharides. Analysis of this disorder at the molecular and subcellular levels has unraveled a number of phenotypes of CSID, which are characterized by perturbations in the intracellular transport, polarized sorting, aberrant processing, and defective function of *SI*.[289-291]

Changes in diet have a marked effect on the expression of *SI*. Starvation leads to a decline in brush border proteins and *SI* activity; this decline in *SI* activity is restored rapidly after refeeding.[292] The type of carbohydrate ingested is important for regulation of *SI* expression. Starch and sucrose both induce *SI* activity, although sucrose is a more potent inducer.[293] Study of the intestinal cell line Caco-2 has shown that a promoter region of the human sucrase gene (nucleotides −370 to +30) can down-regulate *SI* transcription in the presence of glucose.[294]

The human lactase gene is approximately 55 kb long with 17 exons and is located on the long arm of chromosome 2.[295,296] Studies in intestinal cell lines have identified functional DNA elements in the lactase gene promoter that interact with nuclear transcription factors.[297] Cdx proteins and GATA 5, a member of the GATA-type zinc-finger transcription factor family, and HNF-1 alpha all have been shown to interact with the human lactase gene promoter and to activate transcription.[298]

Lactose intolerance is the most common manifestation of disaccharidase deficiency and results from an absence or drastically reduced level of lactase. In humans, lactase is expressed in fetal small intestine at a time in gestation just after the onset of expression of *SI*. Lactase expression is maintained throughout development and during childhood, although sometime during childhood, lactase activity declines to 5% to 10% of early childhood levels in most of the world's populations. This decline occurs at the same time that intestinal *SI* activity is increasing. Ingestion of milk or milk products by persons with diminished lactase activity leads to flatulence, abdominal cramping, and diarrhea. This pattern of reduction of lactase activity has been termed *late-onset lactase deficiency* or *adult-type hypolactasia*. Although initially it was thought that the regulation of lactase-phlorizin hydrolase (LPH) was post-translational and associated with altered structural features of the enzyme, it is now believed that the major mechanism of regulation of LPH is transcriptional.[299-301] Other forms of lactose intolerance include the rare congenital lactase deficiency and secondary forms, such as those caused by mucosal injury resulting from infectious gastroenteritis, parasitic infection, celiac disease, drug-induced enteritis, and Crohn's disease.[302]

Differential activation of both the lactase and the *SI* promoter is effected by multiple similar transcription factors, including GATA factors, HNF-1 alpha, and Cdx-2, alone and in combination. This synergistic activation may be a method to achieve higher levels of tissue-specific expression.[303]

Disaccharidase synthesis occurs within the ER, and the proenzymes then follow the path for secretory proteins through the Golgi complex before being inserted into the BBM. All are glycoproteins and all undergo extensive intracellular processing, with removal of redundant segments of the

molecule. In the case of *SI*, final processing occurs on insertion into the BBM after exposure to luminal pancreatic proteases (Fig. 102-14).[304] At this point, it is cleaved into its 2 active subunits; in contrast, lactase is already completely processed before its insertion.[305,306]

In their final active form, the carbohydrases project into the intestinal lumen, forming part of the glycocalyx, and they are attached to the membrane by a hydrophobic anchor that represents about 10% of the total mass of the molecule. Evidence suggests that MYO1A (brush border myosin I), a group of monomeric actin-based motors that are known to associate with membranes in intestinal villi, are involved in the retention of *SI* within the brush border.[307]

Disaccharidases are synthesized by both crypt and villus cells but are expressed only on the latter. Expression of these genes in the intestine exhibits a complex spatial pattern along the vertical (crypt-to-villus) and horizontal (proximal-to-distal) axes.[308] There is little *SI* activity in the crypts and villus tip cells, with maximal activity in lower- and mid-portions of the villus.[309] The major mechanism for regulating expression of the *SI* protein along the crypt-villus axis is the steady-state level of *SI* mRNA; however, post-transcriptional and post-translational regulation likely play a role in the expression of the functional *SI* protein along the intestinal crypt-villus axis.[310]

A functional difference also exists between the jejunum and distal ileum that reflects differences in the expression of different genes, or gradients of gene expression, along the proximal-distal axis of the intestine. For example, *SI* activity is 4- to 5-fold greater in the jejunum than in the ileum,[311] although *SI* mRNA appears to be similar in the 2 areas. Although there are minor differences in the pattern of glycosylation in the Golgi apparatus, the major difference in regulation between the jejunum and ileum appears to be at the level of mRNA translation.[312]

Pancreatic proteolytic enzymes shorten the half-life ($T_{1/2}$) of the carbohydrases.[313] After meals, *SI* $T_{1/2}$ may drop as low as 4.5 hours, compared with more than 20 hours during fasting. Presumably, proteolysis, as largely determined by meals, is responsible for the diurnal variation in carbohydrase activity.[254]

The levels of *SI* and other saccharidases also may decrease with infection and inflammation. In some cases, a decline in enzyme activity leads to malabsorption of carbohydrates, with resultant diarrhea, flatulence, and weight loss. In most disease processes, however, diminished levels of *SI* are associated with global dysfunction of the small intestinal mucosa.

Transport Across the Mucosa

The 3 major diet-derived monosaccharides—glucose, galactose and fructose—are absorbed by saturable carrier-mediated transport systems located in the BBM of enterocytes in the proximal and middle small intestine.[314] These transport proteins facilitate transport of D-isomers (but not L-isomers) of hexoses.[244]

Active transport of glucose and galactose is achieved by the sodium-coupled secondary active transport symporter, also known as the *sodium-glucose transporter* (primarily SGLT1 [see Chapter 101])[315]; active glucose transport is driven by the sodium gradient across the apical cell membrane. First, a low intracellular sodium concentration is generated by the sodium pump (sodium-potassium-adenosine triphosphatase [Na+, K+-ATPase]) located in the basolateral membrane of the enterocyte, which transports 3 Na+ out of the cell and 2 K+ into the cell, resulting in a low intracellular Na+ concentration. Then 2 Na+ ions bind to the outer face of the transporter, producing a conformational change that permits subsequent high-affinity

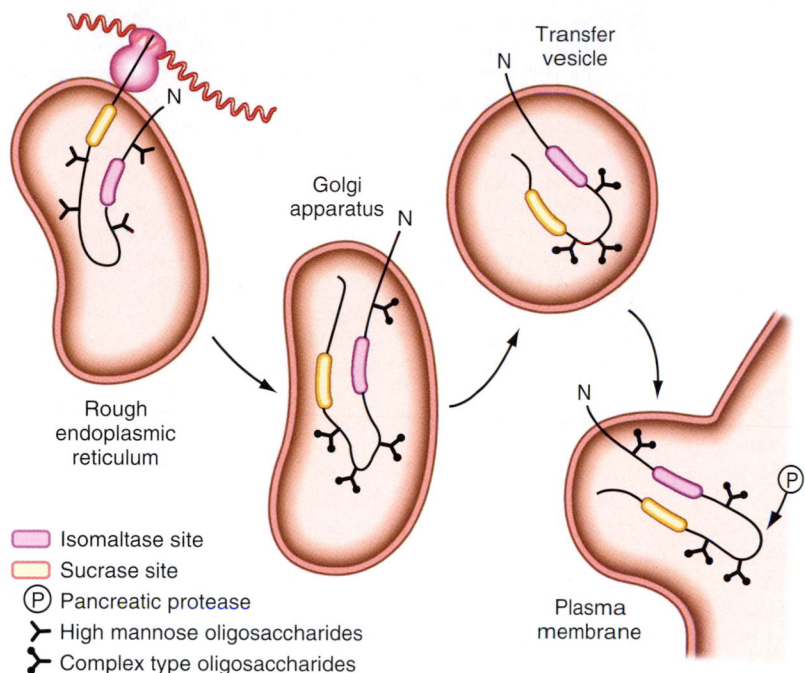

Isomaltase site
Sucrase site
(P) Pancreatic protease
High mannose oligosaccharides
Complex type oligosaccharides

FIGURE 102-14. Biosynthesis of sucrose isomaltase. Nascent polypeptide is translocated across the endoplasmic reticulum membrane after ribosomal mRNA translation. Oligosaccharide side chains join the polypeptide to be transferred to the Golgi apparatus for further processing. After incorporation in the plasma membrane, luminal proteases cleave the molecule into its active subunits. *(From Lloyd ML, Olsen WA. Intestinal carbohydrases. Viewpoints Dig Dis 1991; 3:13-8.)*

sugar binding, after which the 2 Na^+ ions and the glucose molecule are transferred to the cytoplasmic face of the membrane through another conformational change involving a coordinated rotation and/or tilt of transmembrane helices.[316] At the cytoplasmic surface, the 2 Na^+ ions dissociate from their binding sites, causing the transporter affinity for glucose to decrease, with subsequent release of the sugar into the cytosol and production of a ligand-free transporter. The low affinity of the cytosolic sites for glucose and Na^+, and the low intracellular Na^+ concentration relative to the extracellular concentration (10 vs. 140 mEq/L), promote these dissociations. The ligand-free transporter then relaxes to the outward-facing conformation to complete the cycle. The complete enzymatic turnover of the transporter occurs about 1000 times a second at 37°C.[244]

Although some of this glucose fuels cellular metabolism, a sizable fraction passes out of the cell across the basolateral membrane into the blood, either through facilitated glucose transporters/uniporters (GLUT2), exocytosis, or simple diffusion. GLUT 2 also has the capacity to transport fructose (see below), galactose, and mannose across the basolateral membrane.[317,318]

The net result of the above process is that for every glucose molecule transported across the brush border, Na^+ ions (and 2 accompanying anions) also are transported across the epithelium. This in turn draws about 1100 water molecules across the epithelium to maintain iso-osmolarity of the absorbate. Ion and nutrient absorption across the intestine do not increase the osmolarity of the fluid remaining in the intestinal lumen. The coupling between glucose, salt, and water absorption provides the explanation for the finding that water absorption across the upper and mid-intestine is glucose dependent, and is the rationale for the oral rehydration therapy (ORT) used so effectively to treat patients with secretory diarrhea, including cholera (see Chapter 110).[319,320]

The prevailing opinion is that there are 2 types of glucose transporters found across brush borders: 1 is a high-affinity Na^+-dependent, phlorizin-sensitive transporter (SGLT1), and the other is a low-affinity transporter that may be Na^+-dependent and phlorizin-sensitive; candidates for the latter role in humans include GLUT2, SGLT4, and SGLT6.[321]

SGLT1 has been characterized extensively.[322-324] Activity of this 73-kd co-transporter in the intestinal BBM rests with the presence of 4 independent, identical subunits arranged in a homotetramer. The sodium glucose co-transporter resides on chromosome 22 and has been cloned and sequenced. The cloned complementary (c)DNA encodes for transport activity with the same relative specificity as the previously characterized native transport system: D-glucose > α-methyl-D-glucose > D-galactose > 3-O-methyl-D-glucopyranose ≫ L-glucose.[325] The cDNA encodes a 662–amino acid protein with a predicted molecular weight that correlates well with the biochemically defined size. SGLT1 is predicted to have 14 membrane-spanning domains, with 1 asparagine-linked carbohydrate group on the third extracytoplasmic loop.[326]

Expression and activity of glucose transport in the intestinal brush border are regulated by both short-term and longer-term processes. In the short term, activity of glucose transport is increased by both protein kinase A- and C-dependent processes.[327] The mechanism of this enhanced activity is an increase in the number of membrane transporters, mediated by changes in exocytosis and endocytosis of membrane vesicles that contain the transport protein. Longer-term regulation of glucose transport is mediated by changes in the expression of SGLT1, which is controlled by changes in the nutrient environment.[328]

Glucose-galactose malabsorption is characterized by the neonatal onset of severe diarrhea.[329] Multiple distinct mutations in the SGLT1 gene have been identified, including missense, nonsense, frameshift, splice-site, and promoter mutations, most of which are responsible for defective passage of SGLT1 through the biosynthetic machinery from the ER, or poor trafficking from the Golgi apparatus to the BBM. Rarely do mutant SGLT1 proteins reach the brush border at a normal rate, in which case, the glucose transport is defective.[321,330]

Fructose absorption occurs by facilitated diffusion (i.e., transport that occurs not against a concentration gradient but with a carrier protein to achieve transport rates greater than one would expect from simple diffusion). This process is completely independent of glucose absorption. Studies in humans have shown that there is a saturable facilitative transport system for fructose in the intestinal epithelium that has a lower activity than that for transport of glucose and galactose. The protein responsible for most apical membrane fructose transport is a member of the facilitative monosaccharide transporter family called GLUT5[331] and encoded by the gene SLC2A5. In humans, this 501–amino acid protein has 12 membrane-spanning domains, as do other GLUT molecules, and transports fructose exclusively[332]; GLUT2 may assist in absorption of excess luminal fructose.[331] Little fructose is metabolized in the enterocytes, and fructose is transported across the basolateral membrane (by both GLUT2 and GLUT5), taken up, and metabolized rapidly by the liver, with resultant low postabsorptive blood levels of fructose. There may be more than 1 type of fructose transport system. Malabsorption of fructose in humans can be prevented by the simultaneous administration of glucose, suggesting that there maybe another, glucose-responsive, system present in the enterocytes. No inherited disorders of fructose transport (GLUT5) have been reported, and no mutations in the protein coding region of the SLC2A5 gene in patients with fructose malabsorption have been detected to date.[333,334] Overall, fructose is not as well absorbed as glucose, and high levels of dietary fructose may cause diarrhea, excessive intestinal gas, and recurrent abdominal pain. Fructose malabsorption has been associated with similar symptoms.[335]

Debate has developed over the mechanism of the passive or "diffusive" component of intestinal glucose absorption and, indeed, whether it exists.[336] Pappenheimer and colleagues proposed that paracellular solvent drag contributes a passive component, which, at high concentrations of sugars similar to those in the jejunal lumen immediately after a meal, is several-fold greater than the active component mediated by the Na^+-glucose cotransporter SGLT1.[337] Other investigators have argued that the kinetics of glucose absorption can be explained solely in terms of SGLT1, and that a passive or paracellular component play little if any part.[338,339] More recent data suggest that the passive component of glucose absorption exists, but that it is facilitated and mediated by the rapid glucose-dependent activation and recruitment of the facilitative glucose transporter GLUT2 to the BBM. This process is regulated through a protein kinase C-dependent pathway activated by glucose transport through SGLT1 and also involves mitogen-activated protein kinase (MAP kinase) signaling pathways.[340]

Exit from the Epithelium

Most hexoses are exported from the epithelial cell by way of the basolateral membrane, although small amounts are utilized for intracellular metabolism. Exit across the basolateral membrane depends on facilitated diffusion (not requiring energy) via a specific carrier. The 2 genes that encode these facilitative sugar transporters are SLC2A2 (which encodes GLUT2), a predominantly basolateral membrane-associated glucose transporter, and SLC2A5 (encodes GLUT5), an apical membrane fructose transporter.[341-344] GLUT 2 has molecular structural characteristics similar to those of the other members of this family of genes. The protein has approximately 500 amino acids with many hydrophobic residues that predict a total of 12 membrane-spanning domains. There is 1 long extracellular loop between membrane-spanning domains 1 and 2 that contains an asparagine that is N-glycosylated, and 1 long cytoplasmic loop between membrane spanning domains 6 and 7.[345,346] Once the hexoses have entered the interstitial space, they diffuse into the portal circulation.

A congenital defect in glucose transport by GLUT2 has been identified and named the *Fanconi-Bickel syndrome*. Because GLUT2 is normally expressed in the liver, pancreas, and kidney as well as in the intestine, defects in this transporter are expected to have a widespread effect on glucose homeostasis. Indeed, patients with the Fanconi-Bickel syndrome exhibit tubular nephropathy, fasting hypoglycemia, rickets, stunted growth, and hepatomegaly secondary to glycogen accumulation.[347,348]

The accepted dogma of intestinal glucose absorption at the basolateral membrane by glucose transporters has been challenged by studies of intestinal glucose absorption in GLUT2 null mice and in patients with GLUT2 deficiency; in both cases, glucose absorption was not impaired.[349,350] Additional work has suggested that there are 2 separate pathways for the exit of sugar from enterocytes: 1 that involves GLUT2 and another that requires glucose phosphorylation, the transfer of glucose-6-phosphate into the ER, and the release of free glucose into the blood. The release mechanism is unclear, but it has been proposed to involve vesicle trafficking. This postulate is supported by oral tolerance tests performed in a patient with congenital deficiency in glucose-6-phosphate translocase 1 in whom glucose absorption was impaired but not eliminated.[348]

Not all potentially digestible carbohydrate is absorbed in the small intestine. As much as 20% of dietary starch may escape into the colon, particularly that derived from cereals and potatoes.[2] Most of this unclaimed carbohydrate, however, is metabolized by colonic bacteria, and the SCFAs thus derived are readily absorbed. Hydrogen and methane also are generated and contribute to flatus production.[3]

PROTEINS

Dietary Intake

Proteins are essential for a vast array of enzymatic, immunologic, mechanical, and structural functions within living organisms. Dietary proteins are the major source of amino acids, and in the average Western diet provide about 10% to 15% of energy intake. Affluent populations ingest more protein than needed to maintain their normal protein balance. An average adult in a Western country consumes 70 to 100 g/day of dietary protein, whereas the poor in Asia and Africa consume 50 or fewer g/day.[242,244,254,351]

Almost half of all protein that enters the intestine is derived from endogenous sources. Of this, 20 to 30 g/day include enzymes, hormones, and immunoglobulins present in salivary, gastric, pancreatic, biliary, and jejunal secretions. Another 30 g/day of protein are provided by epithelial cells desquamated from the villus tips, and 2 g of plasma proteins are delivered into the intestinal lumen each day.[242,244,351]

Recommended dietary requirements vary from 0.75 to 1 g/kg of body weight per day, but deficiency states are rare, even with intakes of 0.5 g/kg/day or less.[351] Recent data from the National Health and Nutrition Examination Survey (NHANES) showed that 7.7% of adolescent females and about 8% of older adult women were not getting the minimum recommended amount of protein in their diets.[352] Little harm appears to occur in the unusual subgroups of society who consume very large amounts of protein, although renal function can be impaired by this dietary habit. The Masai tribes of Africa and the Gaucho of South America, who consume 250 to 300 g/day (largely of animal origin), suffer no obvious untoward effects.[254,353]

The variety of types of animal and plant proteins is enormous. Generally, plant proteins are less digestible than those derived from animals, but some fibrous animal proteins (e.g., keratin, collagen) are also relatively indigestible. High-proline proteins such as the glutenins are less thoroughly digested than are others. The quality of proteins depends largely on their amino acid composition; those proteins rich in essential amino acids are regarded as being of high quality. Proteins from animal sources have a high content of essential amino acids, unlike proteins from certain specific plant sources, which are said to be incomplete because they lack or contain certain essential amino acids.[354] Such deficiencies in essential amino acids typically are overcome in a mixed diet, although the relative contribution of dietary animal and plant protein varies according to geographic region. In developed countries like North America and Europe, animal protein contributes about 70% of the total protein, compared with developing nations in the Middle East and Africa where the animal protein contribution can be as low as 20%.

Food processing (e.g., by heat or alkaline treatment) may cause inter- and intramolecular bonding in the proteins to produce polymeric forms that are relatively resistant to hydrolysis.[1] Other constituents of the diet may also interfere with protein digestion; for example, starch and reducing sugars have the potential to impair digestion.[254,355] Despite these interferences, digestion and absorption of proteins are remarkably complete, and only about 3% to 5% of ingested nitrogen is lost in the stool, probably because of the resistance of some peptide bonds to hydrolysis.[1] A few selected proteins are resistant to proteolysis in the small intestine, including secretory IgA and intrinsic factor. Among the 20 common amino acids that form animal and plant proteins, 8 cannot be synthesized by animals: leucine, isoleucine, lysine, methionine, phenylalanine, threonine, tryptophan, and valine. These 8 "essential" amino acids have to be ingested, usually in plant-derived foods. Histidine also is required for growth in infants.

Intraluminal Digestion

Pepsins

For many years it was believed that proteins are completely hydrolyzed to free amino acids in the intestinal lumen and that their absorption is mediated by various amino acid transporters. In the 1970s, however, studies revealed that small peptides of 2 and 3 amino acids in length (i.e., di/tripeptides) are the main product of intestinal protein digestion.[356] Luminal digestion of proteins begins with gastric proteases, followed by pancreatic proteases, and unlike the digestive enzymes for carbohydrates and lipids, these proteases are secreted as proenzymes that require conversion to their active form for protein hydrolysis to occur.

Pepsins are a family of endoproteases that hydrolyze internal peptide bonds in proteins. They act preferentially on peptide bonds that are formed by the aromatic amino acids phenylalanine and tyrosine, and by the branched-chain amino acid leucine. There are 2 immunologically distinct groups of pepsins (groups 1 and 2), although 8 fractions are identified electrophoretically. Both of the immunologically separated species are secreted as inactive pepsinogens by chief cells, but group 2 isoforms also are present in the mucus cells in the oxyntic and pyloric areas of the stomach and in Brunner's glands of the duodenum. Their substrate specificities vary little, and their pH optima differ slightly (between 1.8 and 3.5); all are irreversibly inactivated in alkali. At neutral or alkaline pH, the pepsinogen amino-terminal region is folded in such a way as to mask the catalytic site. In the acidic environment of the stomach, the catalytic site is uncovered and then proceeds to remove the amino-terminal region, which consists of 40 amino acids, thereby generating the active form of the molecule, pepsin. Pepsinogen release from chief cells is stimulated by gastrin, histamine, and cholinergic stimulation, and closely mirrors acid secretion.[351,357]

Pepsins remain active at the acid pH of gastric contents to produce a mixture of peptides with a small portion of amino acids. Pepsin activity is therefore confined to the stomach and accounts for the digestion of 10% to 15% of dietary proteins. The completeness of intragastric proteolysis depends in part on the rate of gastric emptying, the pH of intragastric contents, and the types of protein ingested. Moreover, the products of protein digestion by pepsins in the stomach may further influence acid and pepsinogen secretion as well as gastric emptying. Subjects who are achlorhydric or have altered gastric emptying as a result of pyloroplasty or partial gastrectomy do not appear to have a problem with assimilation of protein, suggesting that gastric proteolysis is not an essential component of digestion.[244]

Pancreatic Proteases

Similar to pepsin, and in contradistinction to amylase and lipase, which are secreted in their active forms, each of the pancreatic proteases is secreted as a proenzyme (or zymogen) and, therefore, must be activated within the intestinal lumen. *Enteropeptidase*, also known as *enterokinase*, plays a key role in proteolysis. It is liberated from its superficial position in the BBM by the action of bile acids,[358] its action being to convert trypsinogen to trypsin by removing the hexapeptide of its NH_2 terminus. Trypsin in turn activates the other proteases and continues to split more trypsin from trypsinogen (Fig. 102-15).

Pancreatic proteases are classified as endo- and exopeptidases, according to the sites of the peptide bonds against which they are most active. Endopeptidases include trypsin, chymotrypsin, and elastase, and exopeptidases include carboxypeptidase A and B. Trypsin, chymotrypsin, and elastase split peptide bonds within the protein molecule to produce short-chain oligopeptides, in contrast to exopeptidases, which remove a single amino acid from the carboxyl terminal end of the peptide.[359] Trypsin is the most specific of the endopeptidases and cleaves internal peptide bonds at lysine and arginine residues; chymotrypsin cleaves bonds at aromatic or neutral amino acid residues, and elastase cleaves bonds at aliphatic amino acid residues. The resulting oligopeptides are further hydrolyzed by the exopeptidases carboxypeptidase A and B. Carboxypeptidase A cleaves aromatic amino acids, while carboxypeptidase B cleaves arginine or lysine peptides from the carboxy terminal end of proteins and peptides. The final products of intraluminal digestion thus are produced by cooperative activity of endo- and exopeptidases and consist of a number of neutral and basic amino acids together with peptides of 2 to 8 amino acids in length. About 30% of luminal amino nitrogen is found in amino acids and about 70% in oligopeptides.[360]

In addition to nutrient protein hydrolysis, pancreatic proteases have other functions: They split vitamin B_{12} from R protein, to which it is linked, so it can then bind intrinsic factor[361,362]; they increase the turnover of BBM hydrolytic enzymes and, as discussed above, initiate the final steps in

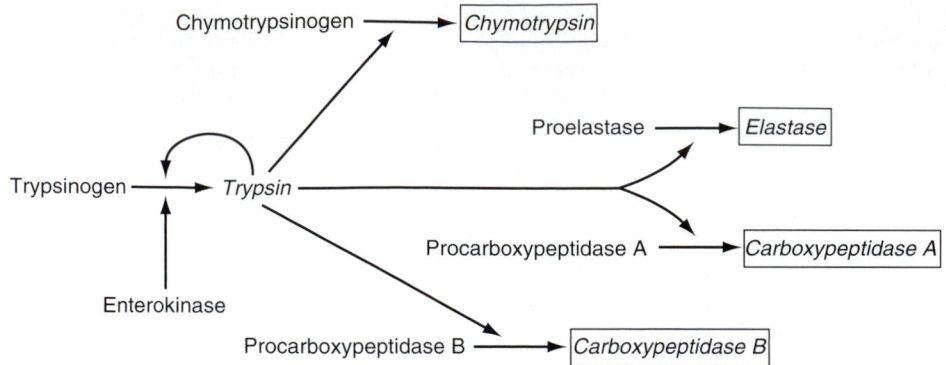

FIGURE 102-15. Activation of pancreatic proteolytic enzymes. Enterokinase (enteropeptidase) plays a critical role in activating trypsinogen to form trypsin. Trypsin in turn activates not only more trypsinogen but also other proteolytic enzyme precursors.

processing of the *SI* complex[304]; and finally, they may have a role in the inactivation of some microorganisms.[1]

Digestion at the Brush Border Membrane and in the Cytoplasm

In contrast to the absorption of carbohydrate, which is largely restricted to uptake of hexose monomers across the BBM, amino acids can be absorbed either as monomers or as di- or tripeptides.[363] Indeed, amino acid absorption is achieved more efficiently in the form of peptides than as single amino acids (Fig. 102-16).[364] The fact that the vast majority of the end-products of protein digestion that reach the portal circulation are amino acids, however, speaks strongly in favor of the presence of peptidases in the epithelium.

Patients with cystinuria and Hartnup disease, who have specific defects in the absorption of basic and neutral amino acids, respectively, do not develop protein-deficiency states, because the absorption of peptides in these patients is normal.[351] The discovery that di- and tripeptides are actively transported by the BBM of enterocytes has been in valuable in explaining this observation, and emphasizes the need for critical evaluation of the supposed nutritional advantage provided by elemental diets that consist only of free amino acids.

A range of peptidases are present on the brush border and in the cytoplasm of villus epithelial cells, in contrast to oligosaccharidases, which are found only at the brush border (Table 102-5). These peptidases account for the hydrolysis of oligopeptides up to about 8 amino acid residues in length.[351,365-367] The peptidases on the BBM differ in several important respects from those within the cytoplasm. About 90% of the dipeptidases are found in the cytoplasm and only about 10% in the brush border, whereas peptidases for pentapeptides and larger molecules are confined almost entirely to the BBM. Tripeptidases are the most variable in their distribution. Cytoplasmic enzymes are much more heat labile than those in the brush border, and there are differences in the electrophoretic mobility patterns for the 2 sets of enzymes.[368]

Most oligopeptidases appear to be aminopeptidases—that is, they act by removing residues from the amino terminus of the peptide. The chain length of the peptides is an important factor that determines not only whether the site at which hydrolysis occurs is at the brush border or within the cell but also its rate. Thus, rates of BBM hydrolysis for tripeptides are most rapid, and for dipeptides least rapid, while tetra- and pentapeptide hydrolysis rates occupy an intermediate position.[363,364,369]

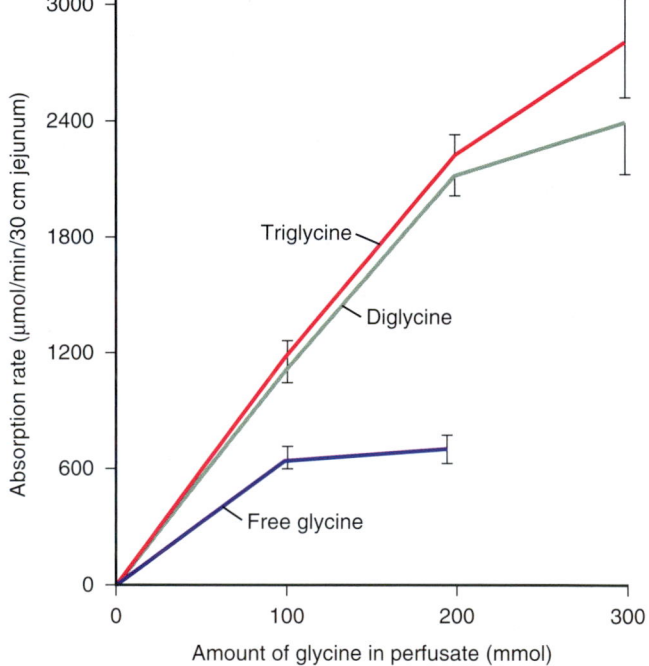

FIGURE 102-16. Rates of glycine absorption (mean ± standard error of mean) from perfusion solutions containing equivalent amounts of glycine in free or peptide form. Results are from studies in the jejunum of 4 normal humans. *(From Adibi SA, Morse EL, Masilamani SS, et al. Evidence for 2 different modes of tripeptide disappearance in human intestine. Uptake by peptide carrier systems and hydrolysis by peptide hydrolases. J Clin Invest 1975; 56:1355-63.)*

Distinct from the amino oligopeptidases are at least 3 other peptidases. Aminopeptidase A has specificity for peptides with acidic amino acids at their amino terminus. Aminopeptidases 1 and 3 (distinguished on electrophoretic mobility) have specificities for different substrates with different amino acid peptide bonds.[1,351,369]

Proline-containing oligopeptides are not readily hydrolyzed by most proteases, despite the fact that many proteins (e.g., collagen, gliadin, casein) are rich in proline. Two proline-specific carboxypeptidases, however, have been demonstrated in the BBM. They have slightly different substrate

TABLE 102-5 Peptidases Found on The Brush Border Membrane and in The Cytoplasm of Villus Epithelial Cells

Peptidase	Action	Products
Brush Border Membrane Peptidases		
Amino-oligopeptidases	Cleave amino acids from carboxy terminus of 3-8 amino acid peptides	Amino acids and dipeptides
Aminopeptidase A	Cleaves dipeptides with acidic amino acids at amino terminus	Amino acids
Dipeptidase I	Cleaves dipeptides containing methionine	Amino acids
Dipeptidase III	Cleaves glycine-containing dipeptides	Amino acids
Dipeptidyl aminopeptidase IV	Cleaves proline-containing peptides with free α-amino groups	Peptides and amino acids
Carboxypeptidase P	Cleaves proline-containing peptides with free carboxy terminus	Peptides and amino acids
GGTP	Cleaves gamma glutamyl bonds and transfers glutamine to amino acid or peptide acceptors	Gamma glutamyl amino acid or peptide
Folate conjugase	Cleaves pteroyl polyglutamates	Monoglutamate
Cytoplasmic Peptidases		
Dipeptidases (several types)	Cleave most dipeptides	Amino acids
Aminotripeptidase	Cleaves tripeptides	Amino acids
Proline dipeptidase	Cleaves proline-containing dipeptides	Proline and amino acids

specificities[370] and, together with a cytoplasmic proline dipeptidase, are likely to be responsible for hydrolysis of proline-rich peptides.

A number of other BBM peptidases merit mention. GGTP hydrolyzes gamma glutamyl peptide bonds, with the transfer of the gamma glutamyl group to another amino acid to form a gamma glutamyl amino acid or peptide derivative.[1] The role of this BBM in the intestine is not yet clear. Folate conjugase, an enzyme concerned with hydrolysis of dietary folate, will be considered later. Angiotensin I-converting enzyme (ACE) has now been demonstrated in intestinal mucosa, suggesting that it too may hydrolyze dietary peptides.[371] Indirect evidence suggests that endopeptidases also may be present on the BBM, because protein digestion occurs even in the complete absence of pancreatic function; these enzymes have yet to be isolated.

As with other proteins, synthesis of each specific peptidase occurs in the rough endoplasmic reticulum; following transfer to the Golgi apparatus, the proteins are transported to the BBM, where they are inserted by exocytic fusion.[372,373] They are attached to this membrane by short anchoring pieces in a manner analogous to the attachment of disaccharidases[374]; however, unlike the latter enzymes, there is little post-translational processing, either within the cytoplasm or by pancreatic enzymes on the brush border. These membrane-bound peptidases produce the most absorbable products of protein hydrolysis, including amino acids, dipeptides, and tripeptides. Although these peptidases are active throughout the small intestine, they appear to be most active in the ileum.[375]

The most abundant of the cytoplasmic dipeptidases appears to be one with broad specificity for neutral amino acid-containing dipeptides.[376] The cytoplasmic tripeptidase that has been isolated has broad specificity for amino-terminal residues and high specificity toward tripeptides containing proline as the amino-terminal residue, which distinguishes it from the BBM amino oligopeptidase. Other characteristics of a tripeptide that are required for rapid hydrolysis include a free alpha amino group, an alpha carboxyl group, and an L-configuration for the 2 amino acid residues.[377]

Absorption

Peptides

The small intestine is the primary site of protein absorption. Although protein digestion starts in the stomach (with pepsin), almost no absorption of protein products occurs at that site.[378] Substrate inhibition studies indicate that tri- and dipeptides inhibit uptake of each other from the lumen, but neither is affected by single amino acids. Such evidence suggests that small peptides use a separate transporter system from those utilized by single amino acids. By contrast, tetrapeptide absorption is inhibited by single amino acids but not by di- and tripeptides, suggesting that tetrapeptides are split before absorption.

The advantage of dipeptide absorption over single amino acid absorption has been largely demonstrated experimentally with single peptides containing a single amino acid, usually glycine.[364] Several studies, however, have demonstrated the kinetic advantage of peptides over amino acids, even in complex mixtures of partial digests of proteins.[379,380] Absorption was greater from tryptic hydrolysates of proteins than from a mixture of amino acids. Furthermore, the wide variation in rates of absorption seen with different individual amino acids was reduced when they were presented as a tryptic hydrolysate.

A number of other factors influence digestion and absorption. The presence of amino acids in the lumen inhibits peptide hydrolysis (product inhibition), whereas luminal glucose and luminal acidification each inhibit amino acid and peptide absorption.[364] There is good evidence to suggest that di- and tripeptides are taken up by a single type of transporter in the small intestine with some stereospecificity, because the length of the amino acid side chains on the di- or tripeptides is important; the longer the side chain on dipeptides, the more preferred the substrate for the absorption site.[381] For dipeptides, L-isomers of the amino acids are much preferred to the D-isomers, whereas the presence of acidic and basic amino acid residues in a dipeptide reduces its affinity for the transport system, compared with neutral amino acid residues. The tripeptide transporter is more specific for the D-isomer acidic or basic amino acids and for short side chains. Affinity is also greater for dipeptides than for tripeptides, at least in peptides that contain glycine. The transporter for peptides is not dependent on sodium, but co-transport with protons instead.[382]

While there are several specific amino acid transporters, the proton-coupled uptake of the more than 8000 different oligopeptides (specifically di/tri-peptides) is performed by the peptide transporter PEPT1.[383,384] The oligopeptide transport family includes PEPT1 (found primarily in the intestines and kidneys) and PEPT2 (found mainly in the kidneys).[385] PEPT1 is the major intestinal transporter of oligopeptides and also facilitates the absorption of numerous peptidomimetic drugs, including many antibiotics.[386,387] PEPT1 is encoded by the *SLC15A1* gene on chromosome 13 and is a member of a superfamily of H⁺-coupled peptide transporters. In humans it is expressed in the duodenum, jejunum, and ileum but not in the esophagus, stomach, or colon. In the small intestine, it is expressed only on absorptive epithelium. The human protein consists of 708 amino acids, with a predicted core molecular size of 79 kd that contains 12 transmembrane domains. It recognizes a variety of neutral, anionic, and cationic dipeptides as substrates, which explains the broad substrate specificity of the intestinal peptide transport system.[390-392]

A most interesting feature of this transport process is that it uses a transmembrane electrochemical H⁺ gradient rather than a transmembrane electrochemical Na⁺ gradient as its driving force.[393] There is an acid pH microclimate on the luminal surface of the intestinal BBM that creates a H⁺ gradient across the BBM in vivo. This acid pH microclimate is generated and maintained by the combined action of the Na⁺-H⁺ exchanger in the BBM and Na⁺, K⁺-ATPase in the basolateral membrane of the enterocyte. The mechanism of the transport process is a simultaneous translocation of H⁺ and peptide that involves a single H⁺ binding site on the protein (Fig. 102-17).[394,395] A multitude of well-established processes are involved in the absorption of peptides and include a Na⁺/H⁺ exchanger located in the BBM that maintains an intracellular alkaline pH; a Na⁺, K⁺-ATPase located in the basolateral membrane that maintains an inside negative membrane potential; and several cytoplasmic peptidases that prevent intracellular accumulation of absorbed peptides. These enzymes convert most of the absorbed oligopeptides to amino acids that are either used by the absorbing cells or are released into the portal circulation via the amino acid transporters located on the basolateral membrane of these cells. The oligopeptides that escape hydrolysis by the cytoplasmic peptidases are transported across the basolateral membrane into the portal circulation by a peptide transporter that appears to be different from the PEPT1 transporter. Oligopeptide transport could be regulated by alteration in the activity or abundance of PEPT1, Na⁺/H⁺ exchanger, Na⁺, K⁺-ATPase, cytoplasmic peptidases, and basolateral oligopeptide transporter.[244,396,397]

Studies of individual substrates and hormones in cell culture have shown that the membrane population of PEPT1 is increased by dipeptides, certain amino acids, insulin, and leptin, and decreased by EGF and triiodothyronine. In the case of dipeptides, EGF, and thyroid hormone, there are parallel changes in the gene expression brought about by alteration of transcription and/or stability of PEPT1 mRNA. In contrast, treatment with insulin and leptin does not induce any alteration in the expression of PEPT1. The apparent change in protein expression appears to be increased trafficking from a preformed cytoplasmic pool to the apical membrane.[396-399]

Amino Acids

Whereas there appears to be only 1 type of oligopeptide transporter in the BBM, there is a multiplicity of transport

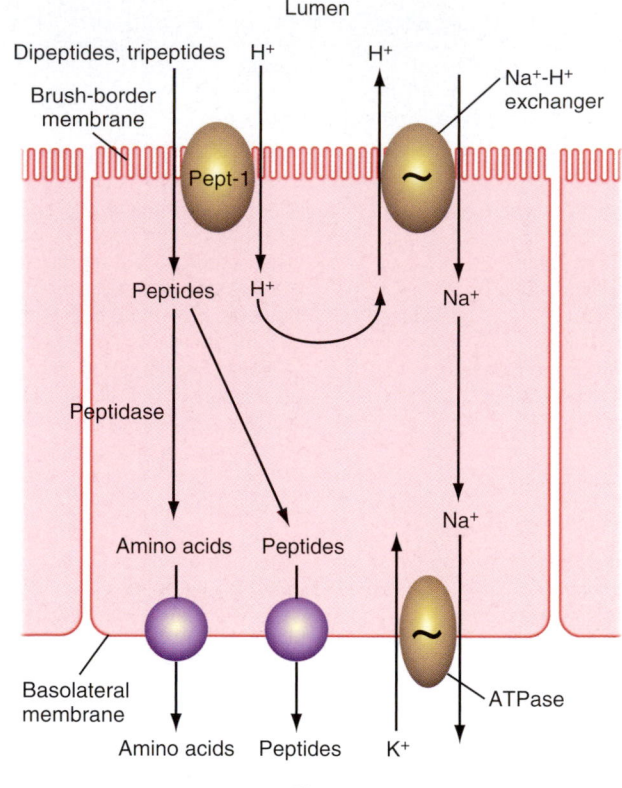

FIGURE 102-17. Peptide transport across the intestinal epithelium. The transport process uses a transmembrane H⁺ gradient rather than a transmembrane electrochemical Na⁺ gradient as the driving force. An acid pH microclimate on the luminal surface of the intestinal brush border membrane (BBM) is generated and maintained by the combined action of Na⁺/H⁺ exchanger in the BBM and Na⁺, K⁺-ATPase in the basolateral membrane of the enterocyte. The mechanism of the transport process is a simultaneous translocation of H⁺ and peptide substrate involving a single H⁺ binding site on the protein. Pept-1, Peptide transporter-1.

mechanisms for the 20 individual amino acids. In adults, these are situated on villus enterocytes and involve carrier-mediated active transport or facilitated diffusion processes, which are typically dependent on the Na⁺ gradient as the driving force; a small proportion may be absorbed by simple diffusion, independent of any ion gradient.

In addition to their stereospecificity (L-amino acids are preferentially transported), amino acid transporters exhibit broad/overlapping substrate specificity; consequently there has been some difficulty in defining the number and types of transporters. Several amino acids utilize a number of different transport systems (Table 102-6). On the basis of kinetic studies, at least 4 active processes for transport of neutral amino acids across the apical cell membrane have been identified. Each is electrogenic and sodium dependent: 1 has broad specificity for a number of neutral amino acids (NBB system or B⁰ system), a second provides another route for phenylalanine and methionine (PHE system), a third provides a mechanism for imino acid absorption (IMINO system), and the fourth transports beta amino acids. Separate sodium-dependent, active transport processes for basic and acidic amino acids also have been demonstrated, and there is some evidence to suggest that facilitated diffusion of these types of amino acids also occurs, although this is likely to be a minor pathway.[242,383,400,401]

TABLE 102-6 Major Amino Acid Transport Systems Detected in Intestinal Epithelial Cells	
Transport System	**Substrates**
Brush Border Membrane	
Neutral Amino Acids	
SLC6A19	Broad specificity for neutral amino acids
SLC36A1	Imino acids; proline, hydroxyproline
SLC6A20	Imino acids
SLC6A14	Neutral and cationic amino acids
SLC1A5	Ala, Ser, Cys, Gln, Asn
SLC7A9/SLC3A1	Neutral amino acids, cationic amino acids, cystine
Basic Amino Acids	Lysine, Cys, basic amino acids
Acidic Amino Acids	
SLC1A1 (X-GA⁻)	Glutamate, aspartate
Basolateral Membrane	
L	Broad selectivity
A	Broad selectivity
SLC1A5 (ASC)	Neutral amino acids, Ala, Ser, Cys
N	Glutamine, histidine, Asn

Ala, alanine; Asn, asparagine; Cys, cysteine; Gln, glycine; Ser, serine.

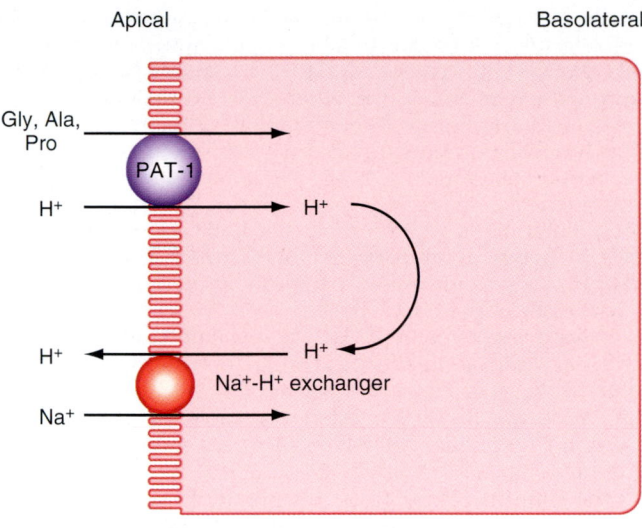

FIGURE 102-18. Intestinal amino acid transport. Human PAT-1 transporter is involved in absorption of small amino acids across the apical membrane. The acid microenvironment generated by the Na^+/H^+ exchanger provides an electrochemical proton gradient that drives amino acids to the cytosol. Ala, alanine; Gly, glycine; PAT-1, Proton-assisted amino acid transporter-1; Pro, proline. *(From Boll M, Daniel H, Gasnier B. The SLC36 family: Proton-coupled transporters for the absorption of selected amino acids from extracellular and intracellular proteolysis. Pflugers Arch 2004; 447:776-9.)*

Genomic advances have allowed most mammalian amino acid transport functions to be attributed to specific gene products: at least 52 amino acid transporter-related gene products are grouped within 12 solute carrier families, with their own new nomenclature.[402] The classic Na^+-dependent imino acid transporter has been identified as the human PAT1 (or human *proton-coupled amino acid transporter 1*) or solute carrier SLC36A1. This high-capacity imino acid carrier has been localized to the small intestinal luminal membrane and transports imino and amino acids (glycine, praline, alanine, taurine).[403,404] Human PAT1 mediates 1:1 symport of protons and small neutral amino acids. The acid microclimate of the BBM drives transport of amino acids into the cytosol. Transport activity is independent of Na^+ and Cl^- (Fig. 102-18). In addition, the IMINO system is a Na^+-dependent transporter with specificity toward the imino acids proline and hydroxyproline. The protein responsible for this transport activity is SIT1 (Na^+-coupled imino acid transporter 1).[405,406]

System $B^{0,+}$, also present on the BBM, mediates the Na^+- and Cl^--coupled electrogenic transport of neutral as well as cationic amino acids across the BBM. The gene encoding the protein responsible for this activity, *ATB^{0,+}* is located on human chromosome X. A separate Na^+-dependent transport system, X^-_{AG} (*SLC1A1*), is specific for the anionic amino acid aspartate and glutamate. The glutamate transporter expressed in the intestinal BBM is known as the EAAT3. This transporter is defective in the inherited amino acid transport defect known as *dicarboxylic aciduria*.[351]

Hartnup disease is a disorder of renal and GI neutral amino acid transport that is inherited as an autosomal recessive trait.[407] The gene causing Hartnup disease has been localized to chromosome 5p15 (it had previously been localized to chromosome 19), and the gene, *SLC6A19*, a Na^+-dependent and Cl^--independent neutral amino acid transporter, has been suggested as the defective gene by 2 separate groups.[408,409] This transporter has been shown to be expressed in the intestine and has properties of system B^0. *System B^0* refers to a broad range of amino acids with neutral (0) charge. SLC1A5 is the proposed ASC carrier for neutral amino acids: alanine, serine, and cysteine.[410] Whereas the *SLC1A1* carrier co-transports 3 Na^+ and 1 H^+ with countertransport of 1 K^+, the SLC1A5 transporter mediates Na^+-dependent transport.

The $B^{0,+}$ is a Na^+-independent transport system that recognizes neutral and cationic amino acids in addition to the disulfide amino acid cystine. It is a heterodimer consisting of a light and heavy chain, with the genes responsible for each chain found on chromosomes 2 and 19, respectively; this transporter is defective in cystinuria.[411,412]

Several hormones have been shown to alter the amino acid and peptide transport process in the intestine. Somatostatin and VIP decrease these transport processes, whereas EGF, neurotensin, CCK, and secretin enhance them.[413–415] Human PEPT1 appears to be inhibited by protein kinase C[416] and cAMP.[417] Expression of the intestinal peptide transporter is also modulated by dietary protein content.[418] Even though the peptide transporter is expressed along the entire small intestine, diet-induced changes in transporter expression are specific to certain regions. A high-protein diet increases the steady-state levels of the transporter-specific messenger RNA in the middle and distal regions of the small intestine. Expression of the brush border peptidases dipeptidylcarboxypeptidase and dipeptidylaminopeptidase IV, which releases dipeptides from oligopeptides, also is enhanced by a high-protein diet.[386] Recent evidence has also demonstrated the potential role the intestinal microbiota plays in the regulation of protein absorption, specifically with respect to enhancing PEPT1 expression.[419-422]

Exit from the Epithelium

Exit through the basolateral membrane operates via a number of different mechanisms that involves active transport and diffusion of both facilitated types.[351] Active Na^+-dependent processes exist at this membrane for the uptake of neutral amino acids, which presumably supply nutrients for crypt cells and for villus enterocytes during fasting when a luminal source is unavailable. Villus enterocytes normally receive the amino acids necessary for production of their own protein from luminal nutrients; crypt cells obtain their supply from the portal circulation. Of all the amino acids, glutamine appears to be a unique and major source of energy for enterocytes; ammonia is an important metabolic by-product of this process. Active uptake of glutamine at the basolateral membrane, as well as via apical membrane processes, is therefore of particular importance.[423,424]

It has been estimated that approximately 10% of amino acids are utilized in the production of enterocyte protein. Some of these proteins are secreted across the basolateral membrane, specifically by villus enterocytes, including apoA-1 and apo-IV, secretion of which increases many-fold after a fatty meal.[254]

The intestinal basolateral membrane possesses a set of amino acid transport systems that differ from those in the BBM. The amino acid transport systems in the basolateral membrane function to export amino acids from the enterocytes into the portal circulation during feeding. They also participate in the import of amino acids from the portal circulation into the enterocyte for cellular metabolism when amino acids are not available from the intestinal lumen, such as between meals. The intestinal basolateral membrane possesses a peptide transporter system that is probably identical to that in the BBM, and that facilitates the exit of hydrolysis-resistant small peptides from the enterocyte into the portal circulation.[351]

Several well-documented amino acid transport systems have been described in the basolateral membrane. System y$^+$L is the amino acid exchanger that permits Na$^+$-independent efflux of cationic amino acids from intestinal cells into the blood, coupled to the Na$^+$-dependent influx of neutral amino acids from the blood into intestinal cells. System A is a Na$^+$-coupled transport system for neutral amino acids, including glutamine, that plays a role in the entry of amino acids from the blood into intestinal cells for cellular metabolism. This Na$^+$-coupled neutral amino acid transporter (SNAT) consists of 3 subtypes, SNAT1, 2, and 4; SNAT2 is expressed in the small intestine.[425-427]

Whereas very small amounts of di- and tripeptides have been detected in the portal circulation after a meal, the great majority of absorbed products of protein digestion that reach the circulation are in the form of single amino acids. A somewhat surprising finding is that digestion of protein continues into the ileum, with about 40% of ingested protein undergoing transport in this segment of small intestine.[428]

KEY REFERENCES

Full references for this chapter can be found on www.expertconsult.com.

12. Woods SC. Gastrointestinal satiety signals I. An overview of gastrointestinal signals that influence food intake. Am J Physiol Gastrointest Liver Physiol 2004; 286:G7-13.
13. Hellström PM. Satiety signals and obesity. Curr Opin Gastroenterol 2013; 29:222-7.
35. Owyang C, Logsdon CD. New insights into neurohormonal regulation of pancreatic secretion. Gastroenterology 2004; 127:957-69.
52. Abumrad NA, Davidson NO. Role of the gut in lipid homeostasis. Physiol Rev 2012; 92:1061-85.
63. Khan NA, Besnard P. Oro-sensory perception of dietary lipids: New insights into the fat taste transduction. Biochim Biophys Acta 2009; 1791:149-55.
81. Brownlee IA, Forster DJ, Wilcox MD, et al. Physiological parameters governing the action of pancreatic lipase. Nutr Res Rev 2010; 23:146-54.
83. Mansbach CM, Siddiqi SA. The biogenesis of chylomicrons. Annu Rev Physiol 2010; 72:315-33.
180. Pan X, Hussain MM. Gut triglyceride production. Biochim Biophys Acta 2012; 1821:727-35.
241. Rasmussen BA, Breen DM, Lam TK. Lipid sensing in the gut, brain and liver. Trends Endocrinol Metab 2012; 23:49-55.
242. Goodman BE. Insights into digestion and absorption of major nutrients in humans. Adv Physiol Educ 2010; 34:44-53.
245. Havel PJ. Dietary fructose: Implications for dysregulation of energy homeostasis and lipid/carbohydrate metabolism. Nutr Rev 2005; 63:133-57.
288. Boudreau F, Rings EH, van Wering HM, et al. Hepatocyte nuclear factor-1 alpha, GATA-4, and caudal related homeodomain protein Cdx2 interact functionally to modulate intestinal gene transcription. Implication for the developmental regulation of the sucrase-isomaltase gene. J Biol Chem 2002; 277:31909-17.
348. Santer R, Hillebrand G, Steinmann B, Schaub J. Intestinal glucose transport: Evidence for a membrane traffic-based pathway in humans. Gastroenterology 2003; 124:34-9.
351. Ganapathy V. Protein digestion and absorption. In: Johnson L, editor. Physiology of the gastrointestinal tract. 5th ed. Amsterdam: Academic Press; 2012. p. 1595.
387. Zhang Y, Sun J, Sun Y, et al. Prodrug design targeting intestinal PepT1 for improved oral absorption: Design and performance. Curr Drug Metab 2013; 14:675-87.

103

Intestinal Digestion and Absorption of Micronutrients

HAMID M. SAID AND TIMOTHY M. TREBBLE

CHAPTER OUTLINE

WATER-SOLUBLE VITAMINS

Ascorbate (Vitamin C)

Metabolic Role and Effect of Deficiency

Ascorbate (vitamin C) exists in reduced (ascorbic acid [AA]) and oxidized (dehydro-l-ascorbic acid [DHAA]) forms. The physiologically important form is AA, and it acts as a cofactor in a variety of metabolic pathways, including maintenance of metal ions (e.g., iron, copper) in their reduced forms, scavenging of free radicals, synthesis of collagen (and other connective tissue proteins), and synthesis of catecholamine; it also plays a role in regulating cystic fibrosis transmembrane regulator (CFTR)-mediated chloride secretion in epithelial cells (see Chapter 101). Deficiency of vitamin C leads to a variety of clinical abnormalities, including scurvy, poor wound healing, vasomotor instability, and connective tissue disorders. DHAA is structurally similar to glucose and is converted back to AA intracellularly.

Sources and Recommended Daily Allowance (RDA)

Humans, other primates, and guinea pigs—in contrast to most mammals—cannot synthesize ascorbate because of a lack of the enzyme l-gulonolactone oxidase and must obtain the vitamin from dietary sources. Rich sources of vitamin C include fruits (citrus, cantaloupe, mango, strawberries, watermelon) and vegetables (cabbage, broccoli, cauliflower, potatoes, tomatoes). The RDA for AA for adults is between 90 and 120 mg/day.

Digestion and Absorption

Physiologic Aspects

Unlike a number of other water-soluble vitamins (see later) where 2 sources are available to the host (dietary and bacterial sources; the latter refers to vitamins produced by normal colonic microbiota), only the dietary source is available in the case of vitamin C.[1] Intestinal absorption of AA occurs via a concentrative, carrier-mediated, and Na^+-dependent mechanism that is localized at the apical brush border membrane (BBM) domain of the polarized enterocytes[2] (Fig. 103-1). Absorbed AA then leaves the absorptive cells across the basolateral membrane (BLM) via a carrier-mediated mechanism.[2] Intestinal absorption of dietary DHAA occurs via a Na^+-independent carrier-mediated process that is competitively inhibited by sugars (because of structural similarities among these compounds).[3] Internalized DHAA is then metabolized to AA by the action of the enzyme DHAA-reductase, a process that also insures low nontoxic levels of the compound.

Molecular Aspects

Two known AA transport systems have been identified in humans and other mammals: the sodium-dependent vitamin C transporter-1 (SVCT-1; product of the *SLC23A1* gene) and the sodium-dependent vitamin C transporter-2 (SVCT-2; product of the *SLC23A2* gene), both of which are expressed in the small intestine.[4] Neither SVCT-1 nor SVCT-2 can transport DHAA, but both can act as Na^+ uniporters in the absence of AA, allowing Na^+ to leak into cells.[4]

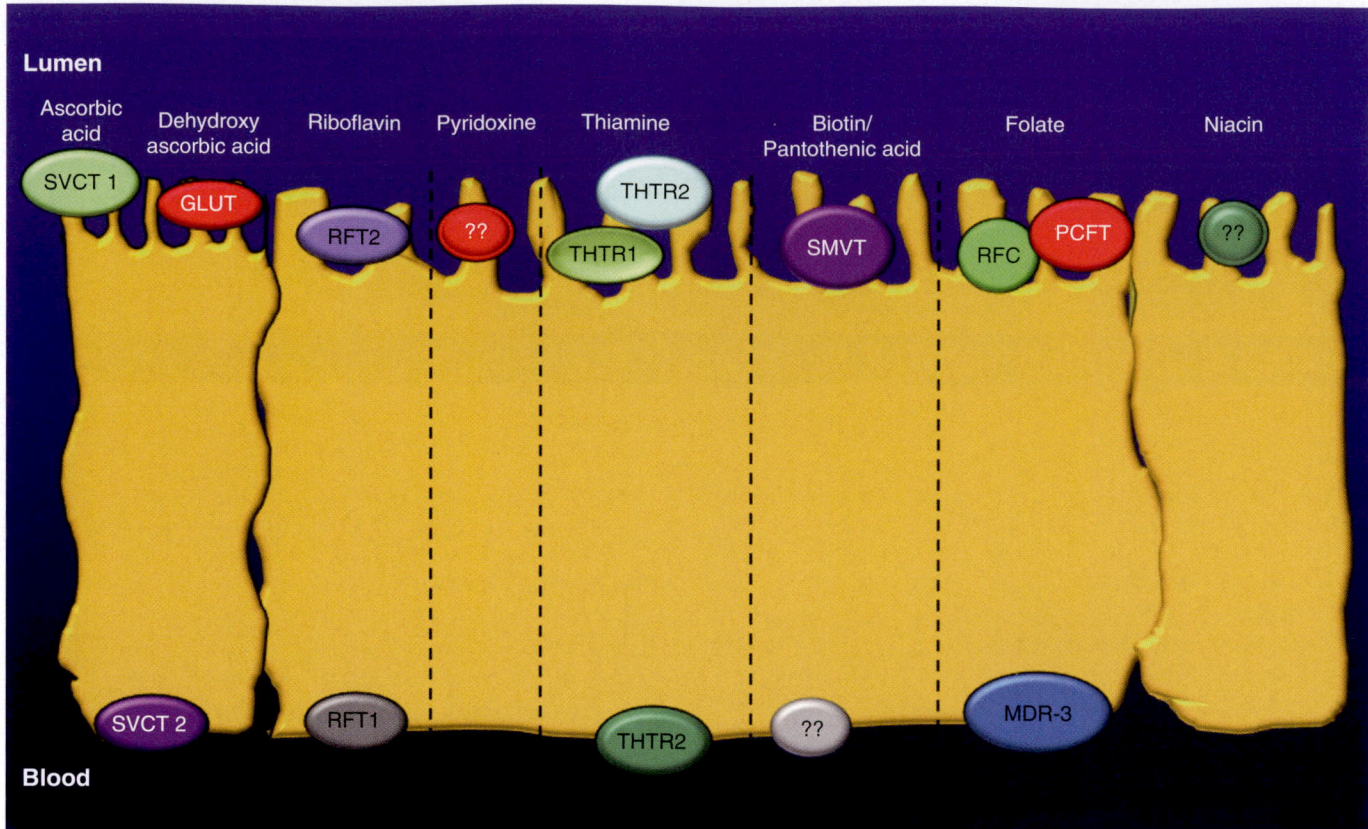

FIGURE 103-1. Membrane transporters involved in the absorption of dietary water-soluble vitamins in the small intestine. The diagram shows localization of transporters for water-soluble vitamins at the brush border and basolateral membrane domains of polarized enterocytes. GLUT, glucose transporter; MDR-3, multidrug-resistance protein-3; PCFT, proton-coupled folate transporter; RFC, reduced folate carrier; RFT-1, riboflavin transporter-1; RFT-2, riboflavin transporter-2; SMVT, sodium-dependent multivitamin transporter; SVCT-1, sodium-dependent vitamin C transporter-1; SVCT-2, sodium-dependent vitamin C transporter-2; THTR-1, thiamine transporter-1; THTR-2, thiamine transporter-2.

DHAA is absorbed by glucose transporters GLUT1, GLUT3, and GLUT4[2,3]; the latter transporters, however, cannot transport AA.

Cell Biology Aspects

Confocal imaging and video rate measurements using live human intestinal epithelial cells and human SVCT-1 fused to yellow fluorescent protein (hSVCT1-YFP) have shown that the hSVCT-1 protein is expressed at the apical membrane domain of these cells, with some localized to a heterogeneous population of intracellular structures (small vesicles, tubular-like structures, and large, hollow vesicular structures; all can be viewed at: http://www.jbc.org/cgi/content/full/M400876200/DC1). The molecular determinants that dictate targeting of the human sodium-dependent multivitamin transporter (hSMVT) protein to the apical membrane of intestinal epithelial cells are located in the cytoplasmic tail of the SMVT polypeptide.[5-7] Mobility of these structures depends on temperature and on existence of an intact intracellular microtubule network.[7] Studies involving co-localization, in vitro knockdown, and in vivo knockout approaches have also shown that Rab8a (a small recycling GTPase protein) is important for physiologic function and apical membrane delivery of hSVCT-1 in intestinal epithelial cells.[8] SVCT-2 protein appears to be expressed at the basolateral domain of the polarized intestinal epithelial cells.[9]

Regulatory Aspects

A variety of extracellular and intracellular factors/conditions regulate the intestinal ascorbate uptake process. Thus, changes in extracellular ascorbate levels lead to adaptive regulation in intestinal uptake of the vitamin. Supplementation of animals with AA or maintaining human intestinal epithelial cells in the presence of high levels of the vitamin leads to a down-regulation in intestinal AA absorption.[10,11] In the latter study, the decrease in AA uptake following supplementation with AA was associated with a decrease in expression of hSVCT-1 mRNA. Other studies have used senescence marker protein-30/gluconolactonase knockout mice (which are incapable of synthesizing AA in vivo) to show that feeding a vitamin C-deficient diet leads to induction of SVCT-1 mRNA expression in the intestine.[12] The intestinal AA uptake process also undergoes differentiation-dependent regulation as the cells move from the crypt to the villus area.[13]

Biotin (Vitamin H)

Metabolic Role and Effect of Deficiency

Biotin (vitamin H) acts as a cofactor (a carboxyl carrier) for 5 carboxylases that play critical roles in essential pathways of intermediate metabolism (e.g., fatty acid synthesis, fatty acid entry into mitochondria for beta oxidation, catabolism of odd-carbon fatty acids and branched-chain amino acids, gluconeogenesis). It also plays a role in regulating gene expression, intracellular cyclic guanosine monophosphate (cGMP) level, normal immune function, and cell proliferation. Biotin deficiency leads to growth retardation, neurologic disorders, and dermatologic abnormalities. Animal studies have shown that biotin deficiency during pregnancy leads to embryonic growth retardation, congenital malformation, and death.[14] Deficiency and suboptimal levels of biotin have been reported in a variety of conditions, including inborn errors of biotin metabolism, inflammatory bowel diseases, long-term therapy with anticonvulsant drugs, long-term parenteral nutrition, and chronic alcoholism.

Sources and RDA

Biotin is widely distributed in foodstuff, although at a lower level than that of other water-soluble vitamins; good sources of biotin include egg yolk, liver, nuts, legumes, and certain vegetables. Accurate data on human biotin requirements are not available, but the recommended safe and adequate daily oral intake of the vitamin in adults has been estimated to be between 30 and 35 µg.

Digestion

The human intestine is exposed to 2 sources of biotin: dietary and bacterial, the latter produced by normal colonic microbiota. Dietary biotin exists in free and protein-bound forms. The latter form cannot be absorbed and thus is first digested by GI proteases and peptidases to biocytin (biotinyl-L-lysine) and biotin-short peptides, conjugates that are then converted to free biotin by the action of the enzyme biotinidase. Human biotinidase has been cloned, and a number of clinical mutations have been identified in patients with "biotinidase deficiency."[15,16] Those affected by this autosomal recessive disorder display seizures, vision problems, alopecia, developmental delay, and hearing loss. Such individuals cannot convert biocytin and biotin-short peptides to free biotin, and thus fail to absorb dietary biotin; they also cannot recycle endogenous biocytin and biotin-short peptides that arise from catabolism of protein-bound biotin in cells to free biotin.[17]

Supplementation with high pharmacologic doses of free biotin brings about a favorable clinical outcome in patients affected by biotinidase deficiency.[16,17]

Intestinal Absorption

Physiologic Aspects

Intestinal absorption of free biotin (which carries a negative charge at physiologic pH) occurs via a carrier-mediated Na^+-dependent process.[18] In adults, absorption of biotin is higher in the proximal small intestine and decreases distally. Functional, immunologic, and confocal imaging studies have localized the Na^+-dependent carrier-mediated system to the apical BBM domain of the polarized intestinal epithelial cells (Fig. 103-2).[18] Exit of biotin out of the absorptive cells across the BLM also occurs via a carrier-mediated process, but this process is Na^+ independent.[18] One of the interesting features of the intestinal Na^+-dependent biotin uptake process is its ability to also transport 2 other functionally unrelated nutrients: pantothenic acid (another water-soluble vitamin) and lipoate (a potent intracellular and extracellular antioxidant). It is for this reason that the uptake system involved is referred to as the *sodium-dependent multivitamin transport system*, or SMVT.

A substantial portion of the biotin generated by the normal colonic microflora in the large intestine exists in the free form and is available for absorption.[1] Indeed, human colonocytes can absorb biotin via an efficient Na^+-dependent carrier-mediated mechanism that again involves SMVT. Demonstration of the existence of an efficient carrier-mediated process for biotin uptake in the large intestine, when considered in combination with the long residual time colonic luminal contents stay in that segment, suggest that microbiota-generated biotin contributes to host biotin, and especially to the cellular nutrition of the local colonocytes.

Molecular Aspects

The intestinal SMVT system has been cloned from a number of species, including human, and its functionality has been characterized following expression in a number of cellular

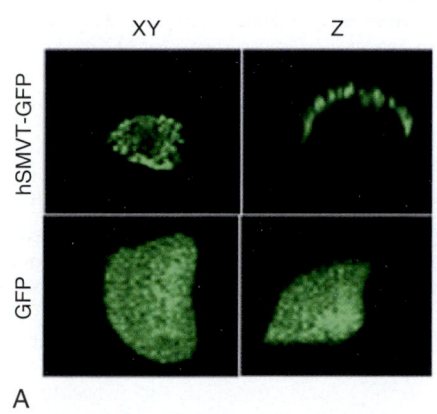
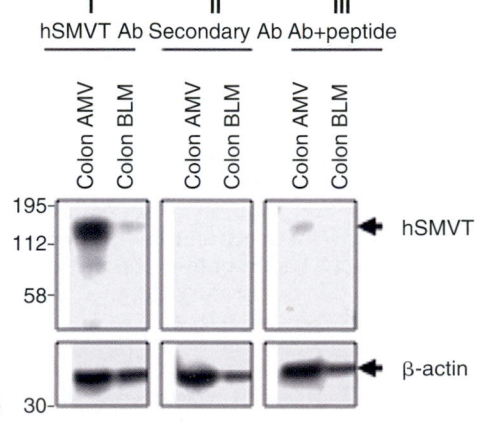

FIGURE 103-2. Distribution of human sodium-dependent multivitamin transporter (hSMVT [fused to green fluorescent protein, GFP]) in human intestinal epithelial Caco-2 cells, and expression of hSMVT protein in the apical membrane of native human colonocytes. *A*, XY and Z confocal image showing Caco-2 cell expressing hSMVT-GFP and dsRed (a cytoplasmic dye) 48 hours post transfection. *Lower panels* show the distribution of GFP alone. *B*, Western blot analysis showing expression of hSMVT protein at native human colonic apical (but not basolateral) membrane. Colonic tissue was obtained from organ donors. AMV, apical membrane vesicles; BLM, basolateral membrane. *(Adapted from Subramanian VS, Marchant JS, Boulware MJ, et al. Membrane targeting and intracellular trafficking of the human sodium-dependent multivitamin transporter in polarized epithelial cells. Am J Physiol 2009; 296:C663-71.)*

systems.[18] SMVT encodes a protein of 635 amino acids that is predicted to have 12 transmembrane domains (TMD) and is N-glycosylated at positions Asn 138 and Asn 489. Glycosylation appears to be important for the function of human SMVT (hSMVT).[19] In addition, a number of potential phosphorylation sites were predicted in the SMVT polypeptide, of which Thr286 has been experimentally shown to be involved in mediating the protein kinase C (PKC)-mediated regulation of intestinal biotin uptake.[19] The SMVT system is expressed along the length of the intestinal tract.

Although another potential biotin uptake system has been postulated to operate in nonintestinal cells (peripheral blood mononuclear cells and keratinocytes), the SMVT system appears to be the only biotin uptake system that operates in the intestine, a conclusion based on an intestinal-specific (conditional) SMVT knockout (KO) mouse model.[20] In the latter studies, a complete inhibition in intestinal biotin (and pantothenic acid) uptake was observed in the KO mice compared with their sex-matched wild-type littermates. Interesting phenotypes were also observed in these KO animals.[20] First, two thirds of the animals died prematurely before reaching the age of 2.5 months, the cause of death being acute peritonitis. Second, all KO mice showed severe growth retardation, decreased bone density and length, and decreased biotin status compared with same-sex control littermates. Third, histologic abnormalities were observed in the small intestine (shortened villi, dysplasia) and large intestine (chronic active inflammation, dysplasia) of the KO mice (Fig. 103-3). The mechanism(s) that mediates the intestinal inflammatory response seen in the KO mice is unclear, but it may be related to the role played by biotin in maintaining normal innate and adaptive immune functions.[21] Biotin, for example, is essential for activity of intestinal natural killer (NK) cells.[22] These cells play an important role in maintaining intestinal epithelial homeostasis and promoting antipathogen response.[23] Activity of these cells and biotin levels are both decreased in patients with Crohn's disease (see Chapter 115).[22-25]

Cell Biology Aspects

As mentioned earlier, the SMVT system is exclusively expressed at the apical membrane domain of the polarized intestinal epithelial cells,[18] and the molecular determinants that dictate the targeting of the hSMVT protein to the apical membrane are located in the cytoplasmic tail of the SMVT polypeptide.[26] Furthermore, distinct trafficking vesicles were found to be involved in intracellular movement of the hSMVT protein, and mobility of these vesicles depends on an intact microtubule network.[26]

Other studies have identified a PDZ-containing protein, PDZD11, that interacts with hSMVT at a sequence in the cytoplasmic tail of the latter[27] (Fig. 103-4); this interaction influences the function and cell biology of hSMVT. Co-expression of PDZD11 with hSMVT led to an increase in biotin uptake, whereas knocking down PDZD11 led to an inhibition in the vitamin uptake.[27]

Regulatory Aspects

A variety of extracellular and intracellular factors/conditions regulate the intestinal biotin uptake process. The *SLC5A6* gene encodes SMVT in human intestinal epithelial cells.[18,28] The intestinal biotin uptake process is adaptively regulated by extracellular biotin availability.[18,29] Biotin deficiency leads to a specific and significant up-regulation in intestinal carrier-mediated biotin uptake, and over-supplementation with high levels of biotin leads to a specific and significant down-regulation in uptake. This adaptive regulation in biotin uptake is associated with changes in level of expression of SMVT protein and mRNA. Thus, biotin deficiency up-regulates biotin uptake and causes an induction in the level of expression of hSMVT protein and mRNA, the latter because of an increase in the transcriptional activity of the *SLC5A6* gene in deficiency.[29] Studies have also identified the region in the *SLC5A6* promoter that responds to biotin deficiency and showed it to be in a 103-bp stretch that contains the cis-element gut-enriched Kruppel-like factor (GKLF). A role for the GKLF site in mediating the up-regulatory response in biotin deficiency has been established by mutational analysis.[29]

The intestinal biotin uptake process is also regulated during early life.[18,30] Studies in animal models have shown that the preferential site of biotin uptake during the suckling period is the ileum, but with maturation to adulthood it becomes the jejunum. This change is associated with parallel changes in the level of expression of the SMVT protein and mRNA, and in the transcriptional activity of the *SLC5A6* gene.[30]

Finally, the intestinal biotin uptake process is under the regulation of an intracellular PKC-mediated pathway that appears to affect the V_{max} of the uptake process (i.e., affects activity and/or number of carriers).[31] The PKC appears to act through Thr286 of the hSMVT polypeptide; mutation of this phosphorylation site leads to significant reduction in the PKC-mediated effect on hSMVT function.[19]

Pathophysiology of Intestinal Biotin Uptake

A significant reduction in plasma biotin levels is observed in chronic alcoholics.[32] Studies using animal models chronically fed alcohol have shown that this results, at least in part, from inhibition of intestinal biotin absorption.[33] This inhibition in intestinal biotin uptake is associated with a significant reduction in the level of expression of SMVT at the protein, mRNA, and heterogeneous nuclear RNA (hnRNA) levels, as well as a decrease in the activity of the *SLC5A6* promoter in transgenic mice that carry this human promoter.[33] Chronic alcohol feeding also caused a significant inhibition in colonic biotin uptake, which suggests impairment in uptake of bacterially generated biotin.[33] Similar findings were observed in studies using human intestinal epithelial cells that were chronically exposed to alcohol.[33] Chronic alcohol use also inhibits the renal biotin reabsorption process via a similar transcriptional mechanism(s).[34] Other factors that interfere with intestinal biotin uptake are anticonvulsant drugs like carbamazepine and primidone.

Cobalamin (Vitamin B$_{12}$)

Metabolic Role and Effect of Deficiency

Cobalamin (Cbl, vitamin B$_{12}$) refers to cyanocobalamin and all other forms of vitamin B$_{12}$ that have biological activity. Cbl in its active coenzyme forms (i.e., 5'-deoxy-adenosyl-Cbl [Ado-Cbl, the most abundant natural form of Cbl] and methyl-Cbl [Met-Cbl]) plays an essential role in catabolism of fatty acids in mitochondria and in the conversion of homocysteine to methionine (and thereby the production of S-adenosyl-methionine, the active methyl group donor) in the cytoplasm. Deficiency of Cbl leads to, among other things, megaloblastic anemia and neurologic disorders and, when prolonged, may lead to irreversible neurologic damage. Cbl deficiency is common and occurs in patients with pernicious anemia, atrophic gastritis, celiac disease, Crohn's disease, after GI surgery, as well as in individuals on strict vegetarian or vegan diets. In

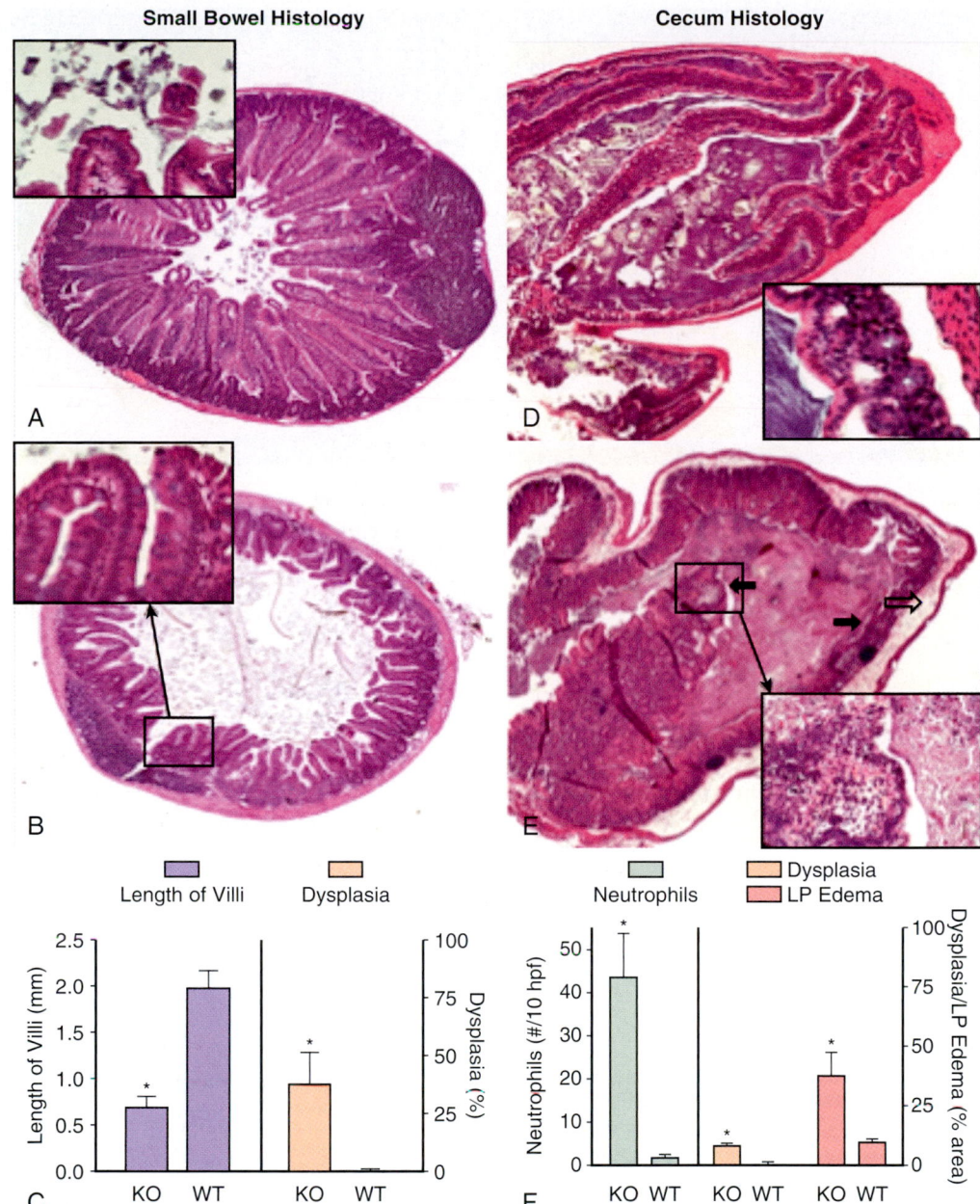

FIGURE 103-3. Histology of the small bowel *(A-C)* and cecum *(D-F)* of intestinal-specific (conditional) sodium-dependent multivitamin transporter knockout (KO) mice and their sex-matched wild-type (WT) littermates. *A,* Normal small intestinal morphology of WT littermates. *B,* Shortening of villi and focal dysplastic changes *(B insert). C,* Small intestinal villi length in mm *(left y-axis)* and total area of dysplasia as a percentage *(right y-axis).* (*$P < 0.01$, $n = 5$). *D,* Representative section of WT cecum. *E,* Small intestine of the KO mouse showing significant submucosal edema *(open arrow)* and acute inflammation involving surface *(closed arrows)* and crypts. *F,* Number of neutrophils in 10 high-power fields (×400) *(left y-axis),* and total area of dysplasia and submucosal edema as a percentage *(right y-axis).* (*$P < 0.01$, $n = 5$). LP, lamina propria. *(Adapted from Ghosal A, Lambrecht NW, Subramanya SB, et al. Conditional knockout of the Slc5a6 gene in mouse intestine impairs biotin absorption. Am J Physiol Gastrointest Liver Physiol 2013; 304:G64-71.)*

older adults, Cbl deficiency and suboptimal levels of Cbl are often due to intestinal malabsorption.[35] Treatment of Cbl deficiency in patients who are capable of absorbing the vitamin is via supplement with physiologic doses, whereas treatment of patients unable to do so requires lifelong injection therapy or oral administration of high pharmacologic doses of the vitamin.[36] Megadoses of hydroxy-Cbl (OH-Cbl) are used as an antidote to treat cyanide poisoning (cyanide displaces the

hydroxyl group from OH-Cbl, leading to the formation of CN-Cbl, which is then excreted in urine[37]).

Sources and RDA

Cbl is obtained from food of animal origin in which the vitamin was produced by intestinal bacteria, then absorbed and accumulated in the animal's tissues. Good sources of Cbl

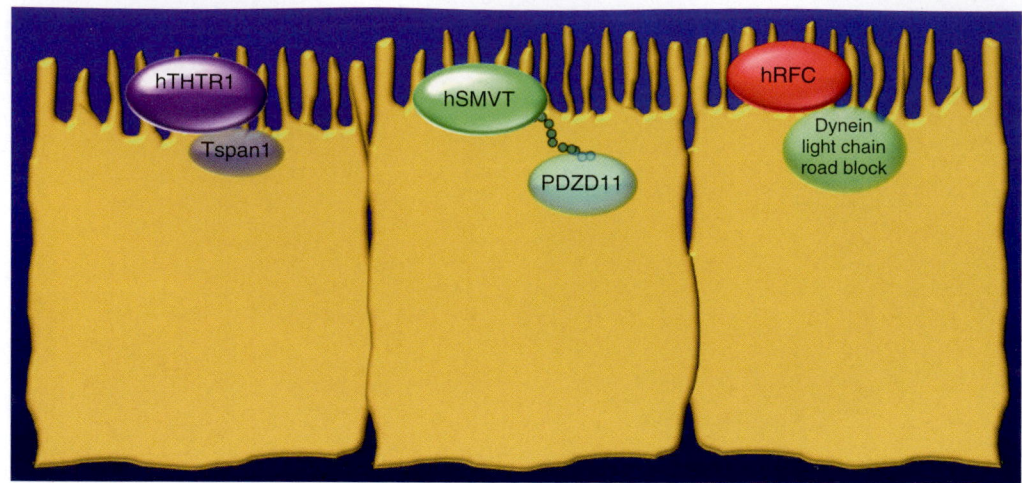

FIGURE 103-4. Identified accessory proteins that interact with human intestinal thiamine, biotin, and folate membrane transporters and affect their physiology and/or cell biology. Depicted are the interactions between recently identified accessary proteins and specific transporters of water-soluble vitamins in human intestinal epithelia. hRFC, human reduced folate carrier; hSMVT, human sodium-dependent multivitamin transporter; hTHTR-1, human thiamine transporter-1; PDZD11, PDZ-containing protein-11; Tspan1, tetraspanin protein-1.

include meat, poultry, eggs, and dairy products. Food of plant origin is virtually devoid of this vitamin, but fortified cereals are a good alternative. Some nutritional yeast products contain vitamin B_{12}. The RDA of Cbl is around 2.4, 2.6, and 2.8 µg, respectively, for adults, during pregnancy, and during lactation.

Digestion and Absorption

Physiologic Aspects

Dietary Cbl is bound to proteins. Part of the bound Cbl is hydrolyzed to free Cbl during food preparation, and the rest is liberated by the chewing of food and proteolytic action of pepsin at low gastric pH (Fig. 103-5). Liberated Cbl (and other inactive derivatives of the vitamin, called *cobalamins*) then binds in the stomach to the Cbl-binding protein haptocorrin (rapid binder, HC), a glycoprotein synthesized mainly by the salivary glands.[38] HC is resistant to acid and pepsin digestion, and these features protect the Cbl molecule while it passes through the stomach. Cbl is released from HC in the upper small intestine by pancreatic trypsin and chymotrypsin,[39] after which Cbl binds to intrinsic factor (IF) with high affinity (dissociation constant $>10^{-12}$ mol/L). IF is a glycoprotein that is synthesized by gastric parietal cells and is resistant to the effect of the digestive enzymes present in the upper GI tract[40]; it also has preference for Cbl over inactive cobalamins, thus insuring selective absorption of the bioactive molecule. Upon reaching the terminal ileum, IF-bound Cbl (IF-Cbl) binds to the specific receptor cubam located at the apical BBM domain of the ileal enterocytes; this is followed by endocytosis of the entire complex (Fig. 103-6).[41-43] Following internalization of the cubam-IF-Cbl complex, it goes to endosomes, where the receptor cubam is recycled back to the apical BBM, the IF-Cbl complex moves to the lysosomes where IF is degraded, and the released Cbl is transported out of the lysosomes (most likely via the lysosomal membrane protein LMBRD1).[44] Cbl is then exported out of the absorptive cells across the BLM via a process that involves, at least in part, the multidrug-resistance–associated protein-1 (MRP1) (see Fig. 103-6).[45] Circulatory transcobalamin II carries Cbl to the liver for utilization and storage.

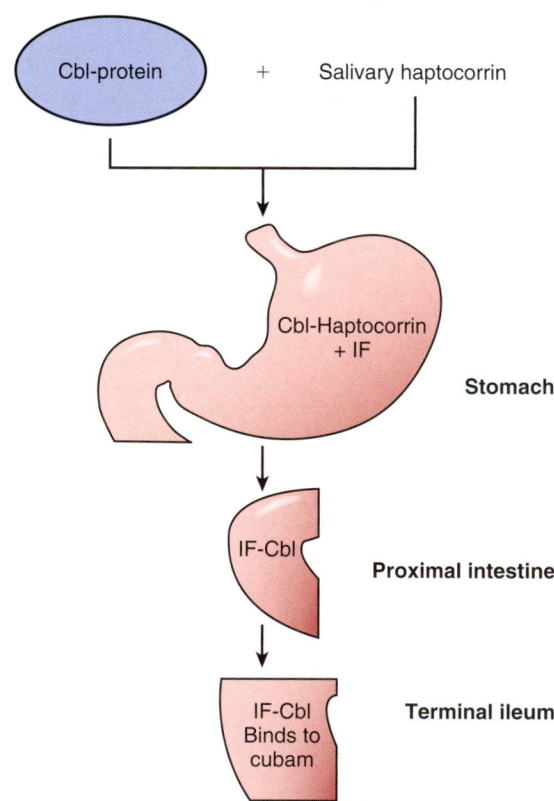

FIGURE 103-5. Digestion and luminal processing of dietary cobalamin (Cbl). Steps involved in processing protein-bound dietary Cbl in the GI tract. After liberating dietary protein-bound Cbl, the vitamin binds to haptocorrin (HC) secreted by salivary glands. HC is then enzymatically degraded in the upper small intestine with the liberated Cbl then binding to intrinsic factor (IF), which is derived from parietal cells in the gastric mucosa. The IF-Cbl complex then travels to the terminal ileum and is taken up by a specific receptor-mediated endocytosis.

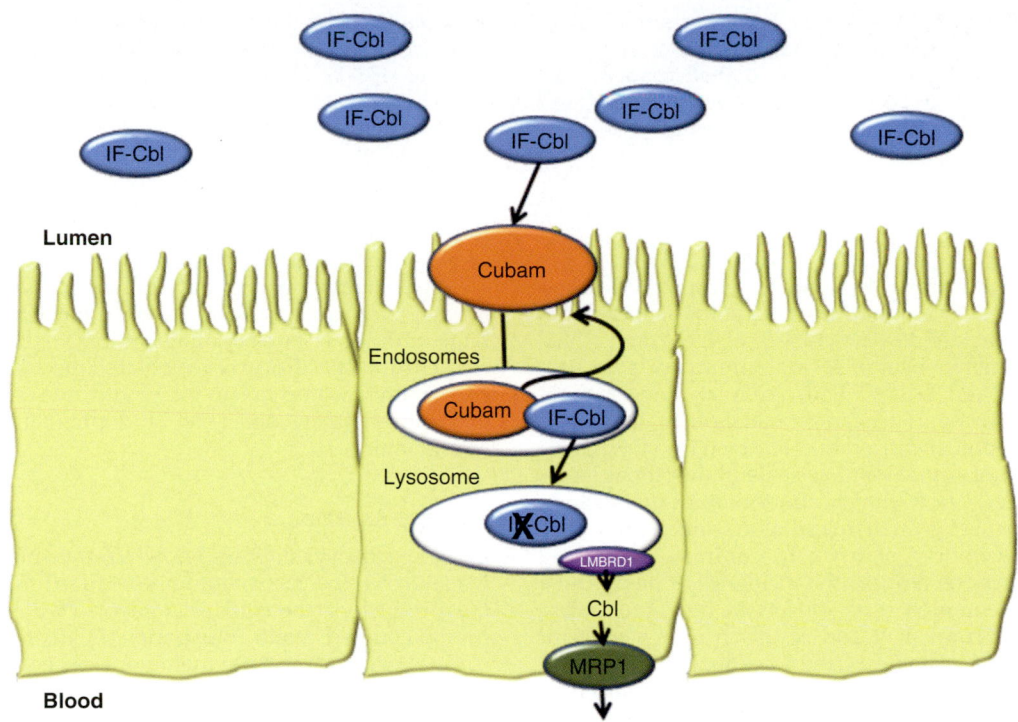

FIGURE 103-6. Uptake of intrinsic factor–cobalamin (IF-Cbl) by ileal enterocytes. IF-Cbl binds to cubam, and the complex then undergoes endocytosis. In the endosomes, cubam-IF-Cbl dissociates into cubam (which recycles back to the apical membrane) and IF-Cbl; the latter then enters into lysosomes where IF is degraded (shown by X), while Cbl is transported out of lysosomes by lysosomal membrane protein (LMBRD1). Cbl is transported out of the ileal enterocytes across the basolateral membrane via multidrug-resistance-associated protein-1 (MRP1).

Molecular Aspects

In humans, the IF gene is located in chromosome 11, and the protein has been cloned and characterized.[43,46] IF is a 417-amino acid protein that may disintegrate into 2 moieties, a 30-kd N-terminal portion and a 20-kd C-terminal portion. Each of these moieties can recognize Cbl, but when they exist together in solution, the joint moieties bind only to 1 Cbl molecule.[47] A 20- to 50-amino acid sequence in the C-terminal portion of the IF appears to be important for the high-affinity binding to Cbl.[48] Also, the IF is a glycoprotein, and the carbohydrate moiety plays a role in protecting the protein against enzymatic degradation.

The IF receptor cubam is a complex composed of 2 units: cubilin and amnionless. Cubilin is the unit that recognizes IF and is expressed in both ileal and renal proximal tubule epithelial cells. Cubulin consists of an N-terminal portion that does not span the membrane, followed by 8 epidermal growth factor repeats and 27 CUB domains.[49] The N-terminal portion of cubilin is responsible for recognizing the IF.[50] Amnionless is a transmembrane protein that provides membrane anchorage and endocytic capacity via 2 sequence signals within its cytosolic domain (phenylalanine-X-asparagine-proline-X-phenylalanine [FXNPXF]). These signals promote internalization of the entire complex via binding to the clathrin-associated sorting proteins disabled-2 (Dab2) and autosomal recessive hypercholesterolemia (ARH).[51] Mutations in amnionless have been identified in patients with Imerslund-Gräsbeck's disease, a disorder that usually clusters in Norway and Mediterranean regions and leads to Cbl malabsorption and proteinuria.[52] Amnionless is also believed to play a role in delivering cubilin to the cell membrane.[53,54]

Regulatory Aspects

Intestinal Cbl absorption seems to be under limited regulation compared with other water-soluble vitamins. The process appears to be dependent on the capacity of the intestinal IF-Cbl receptor, cubam. Thus, after administration of a dose of 2 to 4 μg of vitamin B$_{12}$, the intestine cannot absorb a second dose of the vitamin with equal efficiency until 4 to 6 hours later.[55] In healthy adults, fluctuation in the normal level of IF appears to have little effect on Cbl absorption, because the daily output of IF (≈20 nmol) is markedly higher than the few nanomoles needed to absorb ingested Cbl.[55] Finally, a role for thyroid hormone in regulating Cbl absorption (via an effect on expression of cubilin) has also been reported.[56]

Pathophysiology of Intestinal Cobalamin Absorption

Pernicious anemia (PA) is a well-recognized cause of Cbl malabsorption and deficiency and results from lack of IF due to an atrophic body gastritis caused by an autoimmune reaction (see Chapter 52). Although more common in older adults, PA also may occur in younger individuals who suffer from other autoimmune conditions like thyroid disease and diabetes.[57] Other conditions associated with lack/decreased levels of IF include patients who have undergone total gastrectomy,[58] those with *Helicobacter pylori* infection,[57] and those on long-term treatment with PPIs.[59]

Intestinal absorption of Cbl is also influenced by conditions that affect the cubam receptor. Although the inherited defects in the 2 units of this receptor (cubilin and amnionless) are rare conditions,[60] disorders like Crohn's disease, especially when there has been partial ileal resection, is a relatively common explanation for Cbl malabsorption.[61,62]

Finally, chronic use of metformin by diabetic patients has also been reported to reduce Cbl levels[63] via malabsorption[64] because of a reduction in the level of haptocorrin.[65]

Folate (Vitamin B₉)

Metabolic Role and Effect of Deficiency

Folate (vitamin B₉) is a term that refers to a group of 1-carbon derivatives of folic acid required for the synthesis of pyrimidine and purine nucleotides (precursors of DNA and RNA, respectively) and metabolism of several amino acids, including homocysteine and serine. Thus, cellular deficiency of folate leads to impairment in 1-carbon metabolism, DNA synthesis and methylation, incorporation of uracil into DNA, and in the metabolism of several amino acids. Suboptimal levels of folate lead to a variety of clinical abnormalities that include megaloblastic anemia, growth retardation, and neural tube defects in the developing embryo. In contrast, optimizing folate body homeostasis reduces the incidence of neural tube defects (the most common birth defects in humans). Folate deficiency is highly prevalent and results from a variety of causes, including impairment of the intestinal folate uptake system (e.g., hereditary folate malabsorption syndrome), intestinal diseases (e.g., celiac disease, tropical sprue), drug interactions (e.g., sulfasalazine, trimethoprim, pyrimethamine, diphenylhydantoin), and chronic alcohol use.

Sources and RDA

Folate is widely distributed in food. Rich sources of the vitamin include green vegetables, liver, beans, and lentils. Since 1998, cereal products in the United States and a number of other countries have been supplemented with folate and also represent a good source of the vitamin. The RDA for folate for adults is 400 µg; the same dose is recommended for women periconceptually to reduce the incidence of neural tube defects.

Digestion

The human intestine is exposed to 2 sources of folate: dietary and bacterial, the latter from folate generated by normal colonic microbiota.[1] Dietary folates exist in free (i.e., folate monoglutamate) and polyglutamate forms; the latter is the predominant form. Conjugated folate polyglutamates cannot be absorbed because of their size and multiple negative charges and must undergo progressive hydrolysis to free folate prior to absorption. This process is accomplished by the action of the enzyme folylpoly-γ-glutamate carboxypeptidase (also called *folate hydrolase*). There are 2 forms of this enzyme in intestinal absorptive cells: the first is expressed at the BBM domain of the cells, and the other is intracellular (localized in lysosomes).[66,67] The BBM form of folate hydrolase is expressed mainly in the proximal part of the small intestine, and the intracellular form is expressed uniformly along the length of the small intestine. The membrane form of the enzyme has been cloned,[68] and its activity appears to be adaptively up-regulated in folate deficiency[69] and during development.[70]

Intestinal Absorption

Physiologic Aspects

Intestinal absorption of the negatively charged folate (pKa values of the α and γ carboxyl groups of the folate molecule are 3.5 and 4.8, respectively) of dietary origin occurs in the proximal half of the small intestine and involves a specific acidic pH- (but not Na⁺-) dependent carrier-mediated process (see Fig. 103-1). In animal studies, resection of the proximal small intestine leads to a marked induction of carrier-mediated folate uptake in the ileum. The intestinal folate uptake process has similar affinities for reduced (e.g., 5-methyltetrahydrofolate and 5-formyltetrahydrofolate), oxidized (e.g., folic acid), and substituted (e.g., methotrexate) folate derivatives.[71,72] Absorbed folate leaves the enterocytes across the BLM via another carrier-mediated process.[73]

A substantial portion of the folate synthesized by the normal microbiota exists in the absorbable free form, and the large intestine is capable of absorbing free folate via a highly efficient and specific carrier-mediated mechanism.[74-76] Interferences with this mechanism may contribute to the development of localized folate deficiency and premalignant changes in colonic mucosa.[77,78]

Molecular Aspects

Three specific systems are known to transport folate in mammalian cells: the transmembrane reduced folate carrier (RFC, the product of the *SLC19A1* gene),[79,80] the transmembrane proton-coupled folate transporter (PCFT, the product of the *SLC46A1* gene),[81] and the membrane-anchored (via a glycosyl phosphatidyl-inositol linkage) folate receptor (FR).[82] The first 2 systems (RFC and PCFT) are both expressed and functional in the intestinal tract, but the third is neither expressed nor functional under normal physiologic conditions.[83]

The human RFC (hRFC) operates optimally at a neutral/alkaline pH of 7.0 to 7.4, and the hRFC polypeptide consists of 591 amino acids and is predicted to form 12 TMD. The hRFC shares a high degree of sequence homology with the RFC system of other mammals (e.g., rodents, chimpanzee).[84] RFC functions as an anion exchanger and moves the negatively charged folate molecule against its concentration gradient in exchange for downhill movement of an anion.[84] RFC mRNA is expressed along the length of the intestinal tract, with expression of the RFC protein at the apical membrane domain of the polarized small intestinal and colonic epithelia.[73,85]

The hPCFT system operates optimally at acidic pH (5.8 to 6.0), and the hPCFT polypeptide consists of 459 amino acids and is predicted to form 12 TMD.[81,86] Folate transport mediated by PCFT is electrogenic and involves the net movement of a positive charge (i.e., it functions as a folate⁻:H⁺ symporter[86] [see Chapter 101]). Folate is transported by this system against its concentration gradient using the energy generated by the downhill movement of protons. The inwardly directed proton gradient is provided by the intestinal surface acid microclimate, which has a pH of 5.8 to 6.0 at the proximal part of the small intestine. The hPCFT mRNA is expressed mainly in the proximal part of the human small intestine, with less expression in the distal small intestine and the large intestine.[81,84,87] Expression of hPCFT is restricted to the apical membrane domain of the intestinal epithelial cells.[88]

Both the PCFT and RFC systems contribute to overall intestinal assimilation of exogenous folates. PCFT appears to be the predominant folate uptake system in the proximal half of the small intestine, where the pH at the luminal surface is around 5.8 to 6.0.[89] This belief is supported by the identification of individuals with hereditary folate malabsorption syndrome, a condition caused by mutations in hPCFT.[74,81] The hRFC system appears to operate in the lower half of the small intestine and in the colon, where the pH at the luminal surface is near neutral.[89]

The folate transport system at the BLM domain of the intestinal absorptive epithelial cells is believed to be a member(s) of the MRPs.[86]

Knowledge about the structural features of the hPCFT and hRFC systems that are important for their function have also been emerging in recent years. The conserved histidine residues located at positions 247 and 281 of the hPCFT polypeptide appear to be critical for function of the transporter.[90] In addition, clinical mutations identified in hPCFT in patients with hereditary folate malabsorption syndrome have implied a role for the amino acid residues located at positions 65, 66, 113, 147, 318, 376, and 425 of the polypeptide.[86] These mutations were shown to lead to a spectrum of consequences that include an early stop codon and a frame shift (both of which lead to absence of hPCFT protein) or to a defective intracellular trafficking/membrane targeting of the protein and/or protein instability[86] (and references therein).

Amino acid residues located at positions 45, 46, 104, 105, 127, 130, 297, and 309 as well as the intracellular loop between transmembrane 6 and 7 of the polypeptide appear to be important for function of RFC.[84,91]

Cell Biology Aspects

The molecular determinants that dictate targeting of the hRFC protein to the cell membrane appear to reside within the hydrophobic backbone of the polypeptide and not within its N- or C-terminal domains.[92] Also, the integrity of the hRFC backbone is critical for exporting the polypeptide from the endoplasmic reticulum to the cell surface. Intracellular movement of RFC appears to involve trafficking vesicles whose mobility depends on an intact microtubule network (real-time movies can be viewed at: http://www.jbc.org/cgi/content/full/277/36/33325/DC1).[92] The hRFC also appears to have an interacting partner, dynein light-chain road block-1, which is located in intestinal epithelial cells and is important for the function of hRFC[93] (see Fig. 103-4).

A beta-turn sequence between the second and third TMD of hPCFT appears to be essential for its targeting to the apical membrane of intestinal epithelial cells; mutations in this sequence lead to retention of the protein in the endoplasmic reticulum. Again, cell surface delivery of the hPCFT polypeptide appears to involve trafficking vesicles whose mobility depends on an intact microtubule network.[88]

Regulatory Aspects

A variety of extracellular and intracellular factors/conditions regulate the intestinal folate uptake process. Globally, transcription of the SLC19A1 gene involves at least 6 alternative promoters and leads to generation of many distinct 5' untranslated regions, but with a common hRFC open reading frame. These promoters are regulated by both ubiquitous (SP, USF) and tissue-specific (e.g., AP1, C/EBP) nuclear factors and by methylation.[80,86,94] In the intestine, SLC19A1 promoter B appears to drive the transcription of hRFC.[79,94] The minimal region required for basal activity of the hRFC promoter B in intestinal epithelial cells is encoded in a sequence between −1088 and −1043.[95] The minimal promoter required for basal activity of SLC46A1 has been mapped to a region 157 bp upstream of the ATG and contains putative GC-box sites as well as enhancer elements (YY1 and AP1) that appear to be important for function.[96]

Intestinal folate uptake undergoes differentiation-dependent regulation.[97] Thus, a significant up-regulation in carrier-mediated folate uptake occurs as intestinal epithelial cells move from the undifferentiated stage to the differentiated stage. This increase in uptake with differentiation was associated with a marked increase in the level of expression of the hRFC and hPCFT at the protein, mRNA, and promoter levels.[97] The latter finding suggests that this mode of regulation in intestinal folate uptake is, at least in part, mediated via transcriptional mechanism(s).[97]

Intestinal folate uptake is also regulated by extracellular folate levels; folate deficiency leads to an induction in intestinal folate uptake via an increase in the level of expression of RFC and PCFT mRNA.[69,95,98,99] For the hRFC, this induction appears to be, at least in part, transcriptionally mediated, with the folate-deficient responsive region being encoded in a sequence between −2016 and −1431 of the hRFC promoter B.[95]

Intestinal folate uptake undergoes developmental regulation during the early stages of life.[100] A progressive decrease in folate uptake occurs with maturation (i.e., from suckling to weaning to adult). This is associated with a parallel decrease in the level of expression of RFC and in the transcription rate of the SLC19A1 gene (changes in level of PCFT were not examined in these studies).

Finally, intestinal folate uptake appears to be under the regulation of intracellular protein tyrosine kinase- and cAMP-mediated pathways[76,101] that function by affecting the V_{max} of the folate uptake process.

Intestinal folate digestion is also adaptively regulated by the substrate level in the diet, with significant induction in folylpoly-γ-glutamate carboxypeptidase activity occurring in folate deficiency.[69] Further, the folate digestive process undergoes developmental regulation during the early stages of life.[70]

Pathophysiology of Intestinal Folate Absorption

It is well recognized that chronic alcohol use is associated with folate deficiency. A variety of factors contribute to the development of this deficiency, including inhibition in intestinal absorption of the vitamin.[102,103] Chronic alcohol consumption affects both the initial hydrolysis of dietary folate polyglutamates to free folate and subsequent absorption of the generated free folate.[102-104] The latter is via inhibition in folate transport across the BBM and BLM domains of the absorptive epithelial cells and is associated with a marked reduction in level of expression of RFC.[105,106] Other investigations have reported impairment in the activity of the intestinal folylpoly-γ-glutamate carboxypeptidase (folate hydrolase) in disease conditions that affect the intestinal mucosa (e.g., celiac disease, tropical sprue[107-109]) and as a result of long-term use of sulfasalazine.[110-113]

Niacin (Vitamin B₃, Nicotinic Acid)

Metabolic Role and Effect of Deficiency

Niacin (nicotinic acid, nicotinamide, vitamin B₃) serves as a precursor for nicotinamide adenine dinucleotide (NAD) and nicotinamide adenine dinucleotide phosphate (NADP), cofactors that play important roles in energy metabolism (i.e., glycolysis and the pentose phosphate shunt). Nicotinic acid and nicotinamide have equal biological activity. Niacin deficiency leads to pellagra, a disease characterized by inflammation of mucous membranes, skin lesions, diarrhea, dementia, and general weakness; patients with pellagra also may develop colitis.[114-116] Niacin deficiency and suboptimal levels of the vitamin occur in chronic alcoholics, patients with Crohn's disease,[114-116] and in Hartnup's disease; individuals with the latter disease have mutations in the membrane transporter of the amino acid tryptophan, which is the endogenous precursor of niacin. Optimizing niacin body homeostasis, in contrast, may protect against Alzheimer's disease and also age-related cognitive decline. Pharmacologic doses of niacin have lipid-lowering effects.

Sources and RDA

Humans obtain niacin from endogenous and exogenous sources. The former source is provided via the metabolic conversion of tryptophan to niacin (each 60 mg of tryptophan yield ≈ 1 mg of niacin), and the latter source is the diet. Good dietary sources of niacin include meat, fish, bread, and yeast. There is also evidence that some niacin is generated by the normal colonic microbiota[117,118] and that the colon has an efficient uptake mechanism for this niacin (Said et al., unpublished observations). Establishing the RDA of niacin with accuracy has not been easy because of its endogenous synthesis, but the reference intake of the vitamin in adult humans ranges between 14 and 18 mg/day.

Intestinal Absorption

Intestinal uptake of physiologic concentrations of nicotinic acid involves a specific high-affinity (apparent K_m of 0.53 μM) acidic pH- (but not Na^+-) dependent carrier-mediated mechanism[119] (see Fig. 103-1). This mechanism appears to be regulated by an intracellular protein tyrosine kinase-mediated pathway. The molecular identity of the niacin uptake system has not been well defined, but a role for the human organic anion transporter-10 (hOAT-10) has been suggested.[120] Nothing is currently known about how niacin leaves the intestinal absorptive cells across the BLM.

Pantothenic Acid (Vitamin B₅)

Metabolic Role and Sources

Pantothenic acid (vitamin B_5) is the functional moiety of coenzyme A and plays a central role in energy-yielding metabolic reactions as well as in fat and protein metabolism. Because pantothenic acid has a ubiquitous distribution (Greek: *panto-then*, "from all sides, everywhere") in foodstuff, deficiency of this vitamin has not been unequivocally reported in humans. Requirements for pantothenic acid have not been established, but an adequate intake for adults of about 5 mg/day is recommended.

Intestinal Digestion and Absorption

Humans obtain pantothenic acid from 2 sources: dietary and bacterial, the latter produced by the normal colonic microbiota.[1] Both of these sources of pantothenic acid are bioavailable and contribute to host nutrition. Dietary pantothenic acid exists mainly in the form of coenzyme A, which is hydrolyzed to free pantothenic acid in the intestinal lumen.[121] Free pantothenic acid is then absorbed in the small intestine via a Na-dependent carrier-mediated process that involves SMVT.[18,20] The same process also operates in the large intestine to absorb the bacterially generated pantothenate. There is no information about how absorbed pantothenic acid leaves the intestinal epithelial cells across the BLM.

Pyridoxine (Vitamin B₆) and Derivatives

Metabolic Role and Effect of Deficiency

Vitamin B_6 refers to 3 compounds—pyridoxine, pyridoxal, and pyridoxamine—and their phosphorylated forms. The vitamin plays a central role in amino acid metabolism; it also plays a role in carbohydrate metabolism to modulate the action of steroid hormones, and to regulate gene expression. Pyridoxal 5'-phosphate is the most biologically active form of the vitamin. Deficiency of vitamin B_6 leads to a variety of clinical abnormalities (e.g., neurologic disorders, anemia) and occurs in chronic alcoholics, patients with diabetes mellitus, celiac disease, and those on long-term therapy with isoniazid and penicillamine. Patients with vitamin B_6-dependent seizure (an autosomal recessive disorder thought to result from impairment in vitamin B_6 transport into cells[122]) also display suboptimal levels of the vitamin.

Sources and RDA

Vitamin B_6 is widely distributed in foodstuff; rich sources include meat, fish, potatoes (and other starchy vegetables), and fruits (other than citrus). The RDA for vitamin B_6 is 1.5 to 2 mg/day for adults.

Intestinal Absorption

Physiologic Aspects

The human intestine encounters 2 sources of vitamin B_6: dietary and bacterial, the latter produced by the normal colonic microbiota. Both of these sources are bioavailable to the host, although their relative contribution to total body homeostasis of vitamin B_6 is not well defined. Dietary vitamin B_6 exists in free and phosphorylated forms; the latter is hydrolyzed by intestinal phosphatases to free forms prior to absorption.[122] Absorption of free vitamin B_6 in the small and large intestine occurs via a specific high-affinity, acidic pH-dependent, Na-independent, carrier-mediated mechanism that is sensitive to the diuretic amiloride[123,124] (see Fig. 103-1). Nothing is currently known about the molecular identity of the intestinal pyridoxine uptake system of any mammalian species, nor about how absorbed vitamin B_6 leaves the intestinal epithelial cells across the BLM.

Regulatory Aspects

Intestinal absorption of vitamin B_6 is regulated by extracellular and intracellular factors. Vitamin B_6 deficiency leads to a specific and significant up-regulation in vitamin uptake via what appears to be a transcriptional mechanism(s).[124] Intestinal uptake of vitamin B_6 appears to be under the regulation of an intracellular protein kinase A (PKA)-mediated pathway.[123]

Riboflavin (Vitamin B₂)

Metabolic Role and Effect of Deficiency

In its metabolically active coenzyme forms, flavin mononucleotide (FMN) and flavin adenosine dinucleotide (FAD), riboflavin (RF, vitamin B_2) plays an important role as an intermediary for the transfer of electrons in biological oxidation-reduction reactions. These reactions involve carbohydrate, amino acid, and lipid metabolism, as well as the conversion of folic acid and vitamin B_6 to their active forms. RF deficiency occurs for patients with IBD and in chronic alcoholics and leads to a variety of clinical abnormalities, including degenerative changes in the nervous system, endocrine dysfunction, skin disorders, and anemia. RF deficiency also occurs in patients with Brown-Vialetto-van Laere syndrome, a rare neurologic disorder associated with sensorineural deafness, bulbar palsy, and respiratory compromise, which is thought to be caused by a mutation in RF transporter-2.[125] Conversely, optimizing levels of RF has been reported to lead to a reduction in the risk of esophageal squamous cell carcinoma.[126]

Sources and RDA

RF is widely distributed in foodstuff, with good sources being dairy products, eggs, meat, green leafy vegetables, and legumes. The RDA of RF for adults ranges between 1.3 and 1.6 mg.

Intestinal Digestion and Absorption

Physiologic Aspects

As with other water-soluble vitamins, the human intestine is exposed to 2 sources of RF: dietary (which is digested and absorbed in the small intestine) and bacterial (the normal colonic microbiota producing the free form of the vitamin in quantities believed to be several-fold more than what is ingested in the diet[1]). The relative contribution of these 2 sources to overall body homeostasis of RF under normal and disease conditions is unclear. What is clear, however, is that the human large intestine can absorb luminal RF and that this occurs via a highly efficient uptake system (see later).[127,128]

Dietary RF exists in free and conjugated (FMN and FAD) forms; conjugated forms are broken down to free RF by intestinal phosphatases prior to absorption.[129] Absorption of free RF both in the small and large intestine occurs via an efficient and specific Na+-independent carrier-mediated mechanism located at the apical BBM domain of the polarized epithelial cells (see Fig. 103-1). Absorbed RF then leaves the cells across the BLM via another specific carrier-mediated mechanism.[18]

Molecular Aspects

Both of the recently cloned RF transporters (i.e., RF transporter [RFT]-1 and 2) are expressed in the small and large intestine.[130-132] These 2 transporters share 43% identity with each other. The human RFT-1 (hRFT-1) polypeptide consists of 448 amino acids and is predicted to form 10 TMD. The human RFT-2 (hRFT-2) polypeptide consists of 468 amino acids and is predicted to form 11 TMD. The level of expression of hRFT-2 and its activity as an RF transporter is significantly higher than that of hRFT-1. These findings imply a prominent role for hRFT-2 in intestinal RF uptake, a conclusion further supported by the severe inhibition in RF uptake by intestinal epithelial cells treated with gene-specific hRFT-2 siRNA.[132]

More than 10 different mutations have been found in RFT-2 in patients with Brown-Vialetto-van Laere Syndrome.[125,133,134] These mutations display different phenotypes when expressed in cellular systems.[135]

Cell Biology Aspects

Confocal live cell imaging studies have shown that the hRFT-1 protein is mainly expressed at the BLM domain of intestinal absorptive cells, while expression of hRFT-2 is exclusively confined to the apical membrane domain of these cells[132,136] (see Fig. 103-1). Also, an essential role for the COOH-terminal sequence of TFT-2 in dictating cell surface expression of the protein, with a specific role for the conserved cysteine residues (C463 and C467), has been demonstrated.[136] Furthermore, intracellular trafficking of hRFT2 was found to involve distinct vesicular structures whose motility is critically dependent on an intact microtubule network.[136]

Regulatory Aspects

A variety of extracellular and intracellular factors/conditions regulate the intestinal RF uptake process; it is adaptively regulated by the prevailing vitamin level.[137-139] Thus, RF deficiency leads to a significant up-regulation in intestinal RF uptake, whereas over-supplementation with RF leads to a significant down-regulation in the vitamin uptake. These adaptive changes in intestinal RF uptake by substrate levels appear to involve, at least in part, transcriptional regulatory mechanism(s). The intestinal RF uptake process also appears to be developmentally regulated during early stages of life, with a decrease in RF uptake occurring with maturation.[140] Finally, the intestinal RF uptake process appears to be under the regulation of an intracellular PKA- and Ca^{2+}/calmodulin-mediated signaling pathways.[141] In laboratory investigations, the intestinal RF uptake process appears to be sensitive to the inhibitory effect of the Na+/H+ exchanger amiloride and to the effect of the tricyclic phenothiazine drug chlorpromazine (which shares structural similarity with RF).[137,142,143] Whether these pharmacologic agents also affect intestinal RF absorption in vivo has not been tested.

Thiamine (Vitamin B$_1$)

Metabolic Role and Effect of Deficiency

Thiamine (vitamin B$_1$) is the first water-soluble vitamin to be described, with reference to effects of its deficiency (beriberi) suggested in Chinese medical literature dating back more than 4000 years. Thiamine in its pyrophosphate form (i.e., thiamine pyrophosphate [TPP], the most abundant form of the vitamin in mammals) is indispensable for oxidative energy (sugar) metabolism and ATP production in the mitochondria[144] via its role as a cofactor for multiple enzymes (transketolase, pyruvate dehydrogenase, α-ketoglutarate dehydrogenase, and branched-chain ketoacid dehydrogenase). The vitamin also plays an important role in reducing cellular oxidative stress by maintaining the normal cellular redox state.[144,145] Thus, low intracellular thiamine levels lead to impairment in oxidative energy metabolism (acute energy failure) and to a propensity for oxidative stress,[144,145] as well as impairment in mitochondrial structure and function.[146] Other forms of thiamine, like thiamine triphosphate (TTP), also appear to have biological function: TTP plays a role in regulating the function of membrane chloride channels and acts as a phosphate group donor to proteins. Thiamine deficiency in humans leads to 2 distinct types of abnormalities: beriberi and Wernicke's encephalopathy. Beriberi is recognized in 3 different forms: (1) dry beriberi, which is a symmetrical ascending peripheral neuritis that usually affects older individuals and may or may not be associated with cardiac involvement; (2) wet (or edematous) beriberi, which involves the heart and leads to lower extremity edema; and (3) acute "fulminating" beriberi (also called *shoshin beriberi*), which occurs mainly in infants and is associated with heart failure and metabolic abnormalities, with little evidence of peripheral neuritis. Wernicke's encephalopathy and Korsakoff's psychosis are associated with chronic alcoholism and can manifest synchronously as Wernicke-Korsakoff syndrome. Korsakoff's psychosis is associated with confusion and loss of recent memory. Wernicke's encephalopathy develops later and is associated with neurologic abnormalities (nystagmus, extraocular palsy, ataxia, confabulation, coma) and anatomic lesions (hemorrhagic lesions in the thalamus pontine tegmentum and mammillary body, with severe damage to astrocytes, neuronal dendrites, and myelin sheaths).

Thiamine deficiency is a significant nutritional problem in both underdeveloped/developing and developed countries. In underdeveloped and developing countries, the main cause of thiamine deficiency is poor dietary intake of the vitamin, whereas in developed countries, chronic alcoholism is probably the main cause[147,148]; deficiency also occurs in patients with diabetes mellitus,[149] IBD, celiac disease, renal diseases, and in patients on chronic diuretic therapy. Thiamine deficiency has also been reported in older adults, despite an average daily intake that exceeds their recommended requirement. Also recognized in recent years is the occurrence of localized (tissue-specific) thiamine deficiency disorders, which occur despite normal plasma levels of the vitamin. Examples of the latter situation are the autosomal recessive disorders thiamine-responsive megaloblastic anemia (TRMA) and thiamine-responsive Wernicke's-like encephalopathy. TRMA is characterized by megaloblastic anemia, sensorineural deafness, and non–type 1 diabetes mellitus[150] and is due to mutations in the human thiamine transporter-1 (hTHTR-1, a product of the *SLC19A2* gene).[151-153] Thiamine-responsive Wernicke's-like encephalopathy is characterized by seizures, ophthalmoplegia, nystagmus, and ataxia and is believed to be due to mutations in hTHTR-2, a product of the *SLC19A3* gene.[154] In both disorders, oral administration of pharmacologic doses of thiamine brings about significant improvements in many of the clinical symptoms.

Optimizing thiamine body homeostasis appears to have the potential of preventing diabetes-associated nephropathy, retinopathy, and tissue damage.[155]

Sources and RDA

Thiamine is widely distributed in foodstuff. Rich sources of the vitamin include dried baker's yeast, whole grain cereal, rice bran, nuts, and dried legumes; poor sources include highly refined foods like polished rice, oils, and refined sugar. Attention must to be paid to the existence of several dietary antagonists that affect thiamine levels: sulfite, a food preservative that can cleave the thiamine molecule; and heat-stable polyhydroxyphenolic compounds, which exist in certain food (e.g., ferns, blueberry, red chicory, red beetroot, black currant, brussels sprouts, and red cabbage). Certain foodstuff and microorganisms also contain thiamine-degrading enzymes (thiaminease I and II). Thiaminease I exists in a variety of microorganisms (e.g., *Bacillus thiamineolyticus*), plants (e.g., fern), fish (e.g., carp), and insects (e.g., African silkworm *Anaphe* spp.) and catalyzes a reaction between the thiamine molecule and a variety of bases. Such a reaction not only depletes thiamine but also leads to the generation of by-products that can act as thiamine antagonists. Thiaminease II is relatively rare and exists in a small number of microorganisms like the intestinal *B. thiamineolyticus* and *Clostridium thiamineolyticum*.

The RDA for thiamine is 1.4, 1.1, 1.5, 1.6 mg/day for men, women, and during pregnancy and lactation, respectively. Because the requirement for thiamine relates to total caloric intake (especially that from carbohydrate), consumption of an unbalanced (calorie-rich) diet may change the RDAs.

Intestinal Absorption

Physiologic Aspects

As with other water-soluble vitamins, there are 2 sources of thiamine: dietary and bacterial, the latter from the normal colonic microbiota.[1] Dietary thiamine from animal sources exists mostly in the phosphorylated form, while that from plant sources exists as a mixture of free and phosphorylated forms. Phosphorylated dietary thiamine is hydrolyzed to free thiamine by the action of intestinal phosphatases, which are abundantly expressed in the small intestine.[156] Free thiamine is then absorbed mainly in the proximal small intestine via a specific pH- (but not Na⁺-) dependent and electroneutral carrier-mediated mechanism[157,158] (see Fig. 103-1). This mechanism involves an exchange between the cationic thiamine molecule and H⁺. Absorbed thiamine leaves the enterocytes across the BLM by means of a specific carrier-mediated mechanism.[159]

The normal microbiota of the colon synthesizes considerable amounts of thiamine, which exists in both free and phosphorylated forms.[1,160,161] The human intestinal microbiome has been classified into 3 functionally different enterotypes—enterotypes 1, 2, and 3)—with enterotype 2 (with a predominance of *Prevotella* and *Desulfovibrio*) (see Chapter 3) being enriched in enzymes involved in the synthesis of TPP.[160] Studies have shown that human colonocytes possess a highly efficient and specific uptake mechanism for both free thiamine[161] and TPP.[162] Because colonocytes possess little or no alkaline phosphatase activity compared with epithelial cells of the small intestine,[163-165] identification of a TPP uptake system in these cells suggests that this form of thiamine is also bioavailable to humans. Collectively, the findings of efficient uptake mechanisms for free and phosphorylated thiamine suggest that the bacterially synthesized vitamin contributes to overall thiamine nutrition, and especially to the cellular nutrition of the local colonocytes.

Molecular Aspects

The 2 known thiamine transport systems that have been identified in humans (and other mammals), namely THTR-1 and THTR-2, are both expressed and functional in the small and large intestine.[151-154,166] Human THTR-1 encodes a protein of 497 amino acids, and hTHTR-2 encodes a protein of 496 amino acids; these proteins share 48% identity and 64% similarity with each other, and both polypeptides are predicted to form 12 TMD. The hTHTR-1 functions in the micromolar range, and hTHTR-2 functions in the nanomolar range.[167] The hTHTR-1 protein is expressed at both the apical and the BLM domains of polarized enterocytes, but expression of the hTHTR-2 protein is restricted to the apical BBM domain of absorptive cells (see Fig. 103-1).[168,169]

The relative contribution of the 2 uptake systems to intestinal carrier-mediated thiamine uptake has also been investigated using 2 approaches. The first is the selective gene-silencing approach in vitro, using gene-specific small interfering RNAs (siRNAs), and the other is gene knockout (KO) in vivo.[168,170] Results of the siRNA approach have suggested that both hTHTR-1 and hTHTR-2 are involved in intestinal thiamine uptake, and that together they account for total carrier-mediated thiamine uptake across the apical membrane domain of human absorptive cells.[168] Findings with the KO approach showed a significant and specific reduction in intestinal thiamine uptake and a significant reduction in blood thiamine levels in THTR-2 KO mice compared with sex-matched wild-type littermates.[170] In the THTR-1 KO mice, however, because of an induction in the level of expression of THTR-2 to compensate for the loss of THTR-1, no significant difference in intestinal thiamine uptake was observed between the KO mice and their sex-matched wild-type littermates, and blood thiamine level was similar in the 2 groups.[170] Thus, patients with TRMA (who have mutated and dysfunctional hTHTR-1) have normal plasma thiamine levels (probably as a result of induction in the level of intestinal expression of hTHTR-2 that leads to normalization in the amount of thiamin absorbed[170,171]).

More than 16 missense and nonsense mutations have been found in hTHTR-1 in patients with TRMA, which leads to impairment in the function of the protein via changes in its stability, membrane targeting, and/or transport activity.[172,173]

A number of mutations have also been found in hTHTR-2 in patients with thiamine-responsive Wernicke's-like encephalopathy that lead to functional impairment.[154] Other mutations in hTHTR2 have been reported in patients with biotin-responsive basal ganglia disease,[174] but it is unclear how mutations in a specific thiamine transporter lead to pathologic conditions that respond to biotin, because hTHTR-2 is not a biotin transporter.[175]

Cell Biology Aspects

Confocal imaging of live human intestinal epithelial cells has shown that the hTHTR-1 protein (fused to green fluorescent protein [GFP]) targets to both the apical and BLM domains of the polarized cells,[169,176] and that the signal(s) that dictate membrane targeting of the protein is(are) embedded within its N-terminal and backbone. Further, intracellular trafficking of hTHTR-1 was shown to involve numerous trafficking vesicles, and movement of these vesicles is temperature dependent and requires an intact microtubule network (real-time movies can be watched at: http://www.jcb.org/cgi/content/full/278/6/3976/DC1). Recent studies have also shown that hTHTR-1 interacts with a member of the tetraspanin family of proteins (Tspan-1) in intestinal epithelial cells, and this interaction is important for stability of the thiamine transporter[177] (see Fig. 103-4).

Live cell confocal imaging has shown that hTHTR-2 protein is expressed exclusively at the apical membrane domain of the polarized intestinal absorptive epithelial cells, and this membrane targeting is dictated by the transmembrane backbone of the protein.[176] Again, intracellular trafficking of the protein was found to be via trafficking vesicles, the mobility of which depend on existence of an intact microtubule network.[176]

Regulatory Aspects

The 5'-regulatory region (promoter) of the SLC19A2 gene has been cloned and characterized in the intestine both in vitro and in vivo.[178,179] The minimal promoter region required for basal activity of this gene was mapped to a sequence between −356 and −36.[34,39] A role for the cis-regulatory elements GKLF, NF-1, and SP-1 in promoter activity also has been documented.[179] Activation of the SLC19A2 promoter by the p53 tumor suppressor transcription factor was reported in murine erythroleukemia cells,[180] but a role for this factor in regulating the SLC19A2 promoter in intestinal epithelial cells has not been tested.

The SLC19A2 promoter has been cloned and its activity characterized in intestinal epithelial cells both in vitro and in vivo. The minimal promoter region required for basal activity of this gene was identified to be in sequences between −77 and +59; a critical role for the stimulating protein-1 (SP1)/GC-box binding site (located at position −48/−45 bp) in activity of this promoter has been documented.[181]

Intestinal thiamine uptake undergoes differentiation-dependent regulation.[182] Thus, a significant up-regulation in carrier-mediated thiamine uptake occurs as the intestinal epithelial cells move from the undifferentiated stage to the differentiated stage. This up-regulation is associated with a significant increase in the level of expression of hTHTR-1 and hTHTR-2 protein and mRNA, as well as in activity of the SLC19A2 and SLC19A3 promoters. The differentiation-responsive region in the SLC19A2 promoter was mapped to a sequence between −356 and −275 bp, and that for the SLC19A3 promoter was mapped to a sequence between −77 and −13 bp.[182] Critical and specific roles have been demonstrated for the cis-element NF1 (−348 to −345 bp) in the SLC19A2 promoter and for the SP1/GC-box (−48 to −45 bp) in the SLC19A3 promoter in the differentiation-dependent regulation of the intestinal thiamine uptake process.[182]

Intestinal thiamine uptake is adaptively regulated by the prevailing level of the substrate.[183,184] Thiamine deficiency in humans leads to an increase in intestinal thiamine uptake via changes in the V_{max} and the apparent K_m of the uptake process.[183] Similar adaptive up-regulation in intestinal thiamine uptake occurs in mice and is associated with a significant increase in the level of expression of THTR-2 (but not THTR-1) protein, mRNA, and activity of SLC19A3 promoter.[184] These data provide evidence that adaptive up-regulation in the intestinal thiamine uptake process in thiamine deficiency is mediated via an induction in the level of expression of THTR-2, and that induction is, at least in part, mediated via transcriptional mechanism(s).

Intestinal thiamine uptake undergoes developmental regulation during early stages of life.[185] Thus, the intestine absorbs more thiamine during the suckling period than adulthood, and this is associated with a higher level of expression of THTR-1 and THTR-2 and higher activity of their respective promoters in the former than in the latter periods.[185] This suggests the developmental regulation in intestinal thiamine uptake is again, at least in part, mediated via transcriptional mechanism(s).

Finally, intestinal thiamine uptake appears to be under the regulation of an intracellular Ca^{2+}/calmodulin (CaM)-mediated pathway.[162,186] The same pathway appears to regulate thiamin uptake in other cell types (e.g., pancreatic beta cells, renal epithelial cells, retinal pigment epithelial cells[187,188]) as well, suggesting the wide utility of this intracellular signaling pathway in the regulation of thiamin uptake.

Pathophysiology of Intestinal Thiamine Absorption

Chronic alcohol use leads to impaired intestinal thiamine absorption and thiamine deficiency.[189] Animals chronically fed alcohol develop significant inhibition of carrier-mediated thiamine transport across both the BBM and BLM domains of the polarized enterocytes, which is at least in part mediated via transcriptional mechanism(s)[185]; inhibition of intestinal thiamin uptake was noticeable as early as 2 weeks after initiation of alcohol feeding.[190] Chronic alcohol feeding also inhibited carrier-mediated thiamine uptake in the large intestine,[190] suggesting that absorption of bacterially synthesized thiamine is also impaired by chronic alcohol consumption.

Infection with the Gram-negative enteropathogenic Escherichia coli (EPEC), a food-borne pathogen (see Chapter 111), also appears to severely inhibit intestinal thiamine uptake.[167] Inhibition is not generalized; intestinal uptake of the water-soluble vitamins riboflavin and folate is not affected. Further, EPEC inhibition of thiamine uptake is associated with a significant decrease in membrane expression of hTHTR-1 and hTHTR-2, and in activity of the SLC19A2 and SLC19A3 promoters. These findings suggest that EPEC infection has a rapid onset of action to affect expression of the thiamine transporters at the enterocyte cell membrane, followed by a more prolonged effect that is mediated via inhibition of SLC19A2 and SLC19A3 transcriptional activities.

FAT-SOLUBLE VITAMINS

Vitamins A, D, E, and K are polar, non-swelling, insoluble lipids (Fig. 103-7). Their respective fat solubility influences their absorption following dietary intake, as well as aspects of their metabolism, excretion, and storage. There are considerable differences among these vitamins, however, and only vitamin E is an obligate dietary constituent, the bioavailability

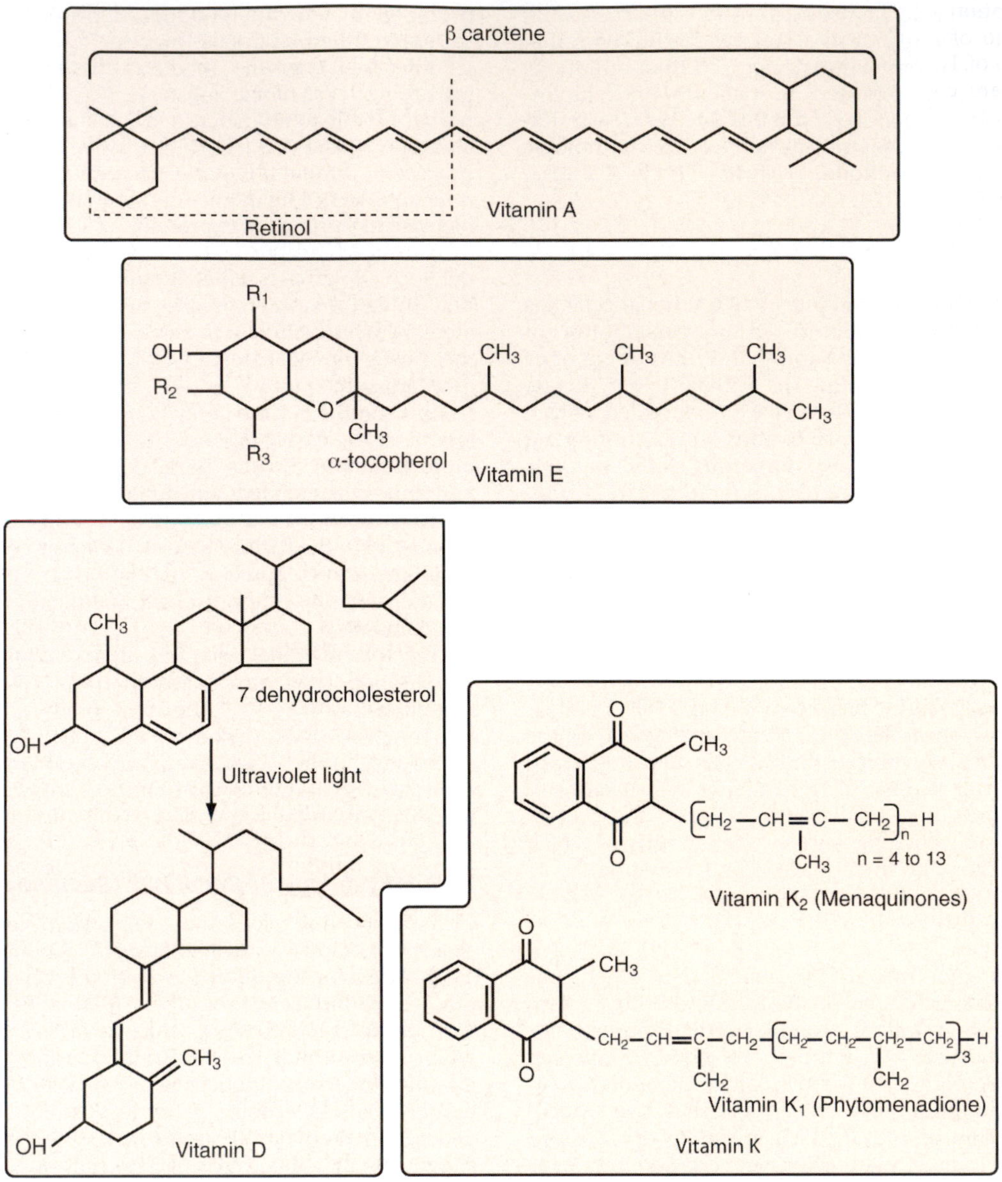

FIGURE 103-7. Chemical structures of fat-soluble vitamins A, D, E, and K.

of the other vitamins reflecting a variety of routes of intake and metabolism. Although their chemical structures are known, the retention of a letter to signify their individuality is useful because each consists of a number of closely related compounds with similar properties.[191]

Vitamin A

Although recognition of the functional role of a liver-derived nutrient was suggested by Hippocrates (466-377 BC), vitamin A was only confirmed as a dietary vitamin by Moore in 1957. The complexity surrounding its dietary sources, requirement, and availability reflects the existence of both retinyl esters ([preformed], previtamin A) and carotenoids (provitamin A), both of which require subsequent metabolism to active forms. This is further complicated by apparent differences in their properties, regulatory function, and potential clinical response.[192]

Metabolic Role and Effect of Deficiency

Preformed vitamin A is consumed from the diet in a number of forms, including retinol (vitamin A_1) and retinal (3-dehydroretinol [vitamin A_2]), predominantly as retinyl esters (principally as palmitate). The basic unit of activity is termed a *retinol equivalent*.

Provitamin A carotenoids are isoprenoid compounds containing up to 15 conjugated double bonds and are synthesized in plants and by certain fungi and bacteria.[192] Only about 50 of the 600 known carotenoids exist in the human diet, 10 of which have been identified in significant amounts in humans. Of these, only 3 are provitamin A precursors: α-carotene, β-carotene, and β-cryptoxanthin. Only β-carotene contains 2 β-ionone structures with the capacity to form 2 vitamin A_1 molecules, thus twice the activity of the other carotenes[193]; more recent data suggest that activity of other carotenoids may be higher than initially considered.[194] Taking into account its dietary absorption of roughly 17% from a mixed diet and a conversion ratio of 2:1, β-carotene results in a vitamin A equivalency ratio of 12:1 by weight.

Carotenoids are considered to have 2 primary roles in humans: as macula pigments and as natural precursors for vitamin A. Carotenoids include carotenes (with provitamin A capability) and others (without this capability) including lycopene, lutein, and zeaxanthnin.[195,196] Despite significant variation in the food sources of carotenoids globally, however, the evidence for populations being deficient in carotenoids is limited.

In contrast, retinoids are considered to have a critical role in the mammalian life cycle, with major consequences of vitamin A deficiency[192] for eyesight (xerophthalmia and blindness)[197] and immune function—in particular, with measles and diarrheal illness–associated mortality in children.[198] This may reflect its role in regulating differentiation of T cell-related immunity, maintaining intestinal mucosal integrity and immunoglobulin (Ig)A production. Deficiency of vitamin A differs between developing and developed worlds, reflecting the dependency on pro- and preformed vitamin A-containing foods.

Vitamin A toxicity can have serious consequences, particularly in the first trimester of pregnancy, when it is associated with severe teratogenesis. Vitamin A has a recognized role in embryogenesis,[199] and an adequate availability is required for normal development. Hunters in the Arctic regions know that to eat polar bear liver, with its rich content of vitamin A, can be fatal, a mortality shown to be due to acute vitamin A poisoning.

Sources and RDA

Vitamin A is preformed within dietary constituents such as meat and meat products, dairy, egg yolk, liver, and fish oils, and is fortified in margarine. Provitamin A is found in orange and green vegetables like spinach, carrots, mango, and papaya, with fortification through food coloring.[200] Of the carotenoids, β-carotene has the greatest biological activity compared with β-cryptoxanthin and α-carotene.[201] In western societies, provitamin A from plant sources provides less than 30% of vitamin A, with the remainder from animal sources; in developing countries, plant sources provide more than 70% as provitamin A.[202]

Historical studies suggest that signs of vitamin A deficiency rarely occur among populations subject to starvation, owing to the availability of carotenes in green plants and vegetables and, during food shortages, in herbs and grasses. Among Key's Minnesota experiments on healthy subjects given semistarvation vegetable diets, there was no evidence of vitamin A deficiency either biochemically, clinically, or on dietary analysis.[203] The RDA for vitamin A is age dependent and altered in pregnancy, lactation, and childhood. For adults, it is equivalent to 900 μg in males and 700 μg in females.[204]

The necessary intake of carotenoids remains unclear, but 2 and 4 mg/day is recommended, particularly where dietary intake of preformed vitamin A is considered insufficient.[200] Dietary intakes of vitamin A among the U.S. population recorded in the National Health and Nutrition Examination Survey (NHANES) was estimated at about 500 μg/day, the RDA commonly achieved through vitamin supplementation.[205]

Intestinal Absorption

Intestinal absorption of vitamin A reflects different processes for both provitamin and previtamin A, and in the fed and fasting state. Other confounding factors include the contrasting rates of absorption for different members of each form, differences in regulatory mechanisms, and the postabsorption activity and metabolism. Retinol and carotene are absorbed in the small intestine, carotene less so than retinol.[206,207] Preformed vitamin A is well absorbed.

Dietary retinal (vitamin A aldehyde) esters first are hydrolyzed to retinol in the intestinal lumen before absorption. Because vitamin A is a fat-soluble dietary constituent, it has increased absorption during stimulation of pancreobiliary secretions, with its inclusion within lipid micelles.[208] The mechanism of retinyl ester hydrolysis, which is required prior to absorption, remains uncertain. Diffusion and transport-dependent mechanisms have been noted, with co-consumption of fat leading to rapid uptake of retinol forms and secretion as retinyl esters in chylomicrons; in the absence of fat, retinol is absorbed via a non–lipoprotein-dependent mechanism with secretion across the intestinal cell. Thus, absorption of vitamin A may occur in the form of both retinyl esters and free retinol.

Absorption of carotenoids is variable and influenced by the complexity of the food matrix, food preparation, dose, co-consumption of preformed fiber, fat, and preformed vitamin A and other carotenoids, and possibly by the availability of micronutrients.[193] Like the retinyl esters, carotenoids are solubilized into micelles with other lipids and absorbed across the luminal interface, although there appears to be both concentration-dependent passive diffusion and a saturable active transporter mechanism, predominantly based on β-carotene. In the latter case, activity of the transporter mechanism may be dependent on the cis-transisomeric form that may compete for the transport mechanism.[208]

Following dietary consumption of previtamin A and release of retinyl esters, or ingestion of carotenoids that are converted to retinol in the enterocytes, retinol is re-esterified predominantly by lecithin, retinol acyltransferase, and with palmitic acid before incorporation into chylomicrons with other dietary lipids. Chylomicrons enter the systemic circulation via lymphatics, and other than a small proportion of retinyl ester that is removed by skeletal and cardiac muscle, adipose, and other tissues, the major proportion remains in the chylomicron remnant prior to apolipoprotein E-dependent internalization by hepatocytes in the liver parenchyma.[209] This results in intrahepatocyte hydrolysis and subsequent storage within the hepatic stellate cells, with a smaller proportion remaining in hepatocytes. Vitamin A is stored in hepatic stellate cells as retinyl esters (mainly palmitate), forming roughly 40% of the cell's lipid and accounting for the majority of the body's retinoid stores. It is released into the systemic circulation, depending on physiologic requirement, as retinol bound to retinol binding protein (RBP).

RBP, a 21-kd protein with a single retinol binding site, is produced in hepatocytes and other tissues and is responsible for carrying vitamin A to peripheral tissues from the liver. RBP is bound as a 1:1 complex with the thyroxine hormone carrier transthyretin. RBP levels are tightly regulated, therefore regulating the systemic bioavailability of retinol. RBP is a specific transport protein for retinol and other retinoids and is responsible for the "recycling" of retinol between hepatic stellate cells and the systemic circulation,[210,211] and probably transport within the liver itself. RBP accounts for over 95% of retinol in the plasma, with the remainder as retinyl esters in lipoproteins released from the liver.

Vitamin D

Vitamin D represents a family of secosterol compounds that is unique among vitamins because it can be endogenously produced through ultraviolet B wavelength sun exposure, becomes conditional where this is insufficient, and then risks deficiency in the absence of dietary supplementation. The vitamin D group includes vitamin D_3 (cholecalciferol) and D_2 (ergocalciferol), with the originally identified vitamin D_1 subsequently recognized as a mixture of different sterols.[212] Another unique aspect of vitamin D is its dependence on structural modification for activation to its active form, $1,25\alpha$-dihydroxycholecalciferol ($1,25\alpha$-[OH]$_2$D$_3$), through a series of organ-specific enzyme-dependent metabolic steps that require circulation through the human body.[213]

Metabolic Role and Effect of Deficiency

The principal function of vitamin D is traditionally related to its effect on calcium and phosphate homeostasis and its antirachitic properties, but there is increasing evidence of its importance in other areas like cellular proliferation, diabetes, and immunomodulation.

Vitamin D exerts its effects via the vitamin D receptor (VDR), a member of the steroid hormone superfamily, leading to transcriptional regulation of target genes,[214] including up-regulation of osteocalcin and RANKL and down-regulation of parathyroid hormone (PTH). VDR is noted in high levels in the intestinal epithelial cells, where it modulates calcium absorption; renal tubular epithelial cells and collecting ducts where calcium resorption occurs; bone tissue, including osteoblasts; and parathyroid tissue. VDR is also noted in high concentrations in pancreatic beta cells and immune cells, including activated T-lymphocytes, and the monocyte/macrophage line, where it influences differentiation.

Vitamin D as $1,25\alpha$-(OH)$_2$D$_3$ influences calcium absorption through both transcellular and paracellular transport mechanisms.[215] In the former, it is suggested that there are modulator effects on the TRPV6 calcium receptor, the calcium binding protein that facilitates cytosolic diffusion. It is also suggested, however, that such transport mechanisms are only critical during states of calcium deficiency and remain only 1 of a number of alternative mechanisms for transcellular calcium transport through the intestinal epithelium.

Paracellular transport of calcium is considered to occur by passive absorption, which may depend on the electrochemical gradient between lumen and extracellular environment and the integrity of the intercellular tight junctions; this mechanism may be influenced by $1,25\alpha$-(OH)$_2$D$_3$-induced expression of claudins to facilitate calcium transport and inhibit cadherin and aquaporin protein expression, thus modulating calcium transport. Finally, it is suggested that $1,25\alpha$-(OH)$_2$D$_3$ regulation of tight junction proteins may have a role in protecting against mucosal injury and maintaining the integrity of the bowel mucosa.[216] Limited animal model data suggest that the effect on expression of transporter proteins via a transcription effect may also extend to phosphate absorption (NaPi-IIb).[217]

$1,25\alpha$-(OH)$_2$D$_3$ exerts influence over calcium resorption in the kidney through a number of mechanisms,[218] including an indirect effect of increasing calcium absorption and release with increased calcium excretion, a synergistic effect with PTH to increase the efficiency of calcium resorption through increasing mRNA of both PTH and PTHrp receptors, enhancement of calcium absorption in the distal tubules consistent with localization of VDR,[214] and increased expression of the PMCa pump for calcium transportation at the BLM of distal tubular cells.

Vitamin D deficiency is associated with metabolic bone disease through altered calcium and phosphate regulation, an effect on PTH formation and release, and a direct effect on bone tissue. Rickets in children and osteomalacia in adults

develop as a consequence of impaired bone mineralization. It is now recognized that associated hypocalcemia and a resultant increase in PTH release with subsequent bone breakdown also leads to osteoporosis. This is associated with skeletal malformations in children and risks of fracture in all age groups. Vitamin D deficiency has a recognized association with a range of other conditions, including cardiovascular disease, immune deficiency, diabetes, arterial hypertension, and cancer.[219,220]

Sources and RDA

Vitamin D is present in food as a natural constituent and a fortificant. The richest sources of vitamin D are fatty fish including salmon, tuna, and mackerel, which themselves ingest vitamin D in plankton near the surface of the sea,[191] and from the oils of fatty fish (e.g., cod liver oil).[221] It is also found in eggs and liver. Human breast milk contains sufficient vitamin D to prevent rickets, but cow's milk is a poor source of vitamin D. Dairy products, orange juice, margarine, and cereals are fortified with vitamin D.[213]

Dietary intake is complementary to endogenous production of vitamin D through skin sun exposure with UVB light. It is suggested that for populations between 4 and 64 years of age, summer sunlight exposure is sufficient to provide adequate vitamin D,[222] though a reference RDA of 10 µg/day also has been recommended. The value of sunlight, however, is dependent on sun exposure time and the requirement for vitamin D, and is reduced by sunscreen and clothing.[223,224] There also may be an effect of skin color, with populations having fairer skin color gaining more vitamin D from sunlight exposure. A seasonal variation is noted in populations from temperate climates, with serum concentrations of vitamin D falling in winter and spring, but geographical location is also important.

RDA varies with age, but is 600 IU/day in adults, including pregnant and breastfeeding women[225]; it is suggested that higher intakes may be of value in maintaining bone health.[226]

Intestinal Absorption

Physiologic Aspects

As with vitamin A, vitamin D absorption occurs by simple passive diffusion in the small intestine.[227] Bile salts are unnecessary, but luminal pH influences absorption. Absorption is reduced at neutral pH and increased in an acidic milieu.[228] Most absorbed vitamin D passes into the lymphatics unchanged in chylomicrons.

Metabolic Aspects

The metabolic pathway for vitamin D is well defined. UVB exposure (290 to 320 nm) converts 7-dehydrocholesterol, a cholesterol-like compound in the skin, to the secosterol previtamin D_3 by opening the sterol B ring, that then rearranges to vitamin D_3, cholecalciferol. Vitamin D_3 is transported in the circulation by vitamin D binding protein (DBP) to the liver.[229]

Both vitamins D_2 and D_3 are converted in the liver to $25(OH)_2D_3$ through the P450 cytochrome vitamin D 25-hydroxylase, of which CYP2R1 may be the key.[230] Following transportation in the blood to the proximal renal tubule, further hydroxylation occurs to convert $25(OH)_2D_3$ to the hormonally active $1,25\alpha$-(OH)$_2$D$_3$ by renal 1α-hydroxylase, CYP27B1 that is limited predominantly to the kidney although also noted in some extra-renal tissues[231]; 1α-hydroxylase appears to be an essential step in the vitamin D pathway.[232]

Regulation

Regulation of the availability of active $1,25\alpha\text{-}(OH)_2D_3$ includes 2 key processes: (1) the production of competing low-activity forms through reduction in available precursor $25(OH)_2D_3$ to $24,25(OH)_2D_3$ by 24-hydroxylase or conversion of $1,25\alpha\text{-}(OH)_2D_3$ to $1,24,25(OH)_2D_3$; (2) though negative feedback loops involving inhibition of 1α-hydroxylase activity, transcription by PTH, and 24-hydroxylase transcription.[231] These negative feedback mechanisms work to modulate $1\alpha,25(OH)_2D_3$ function and availability to prevent overactivity and metabolic dysregulation of calcium.

Vitamin E

Vitamin E represents 2 families of natural antioxidants derived from plant chlorophyll and tyrosine[233]: the tocopherols have a chromanol ring with a saturated 15-carbon tail, and the tocotrienols with an unsaturated isoprenoid 16-carbon side chain. Each of these includes 4 isomers, α, β, γ, δ, depending on the position of a methyl group, and with effect on bioavailability and, therefore, biological activity. Interest in vitamin E has been principally with α-tocopherols, but there is increasing evidence that clinical benefits, particularly related to supplementation, are seen more with the tocotrienols (see Fig. 103-7).[234]

Metabolic Role and Effect of Deficiency

The principal role of vitamin E is as a lipid-soluble membrane-bound potent peroxyl radical scavenger that restricts the propagation of free radical breakdown of membrane lipids, specifically with respect to membrane polyunsaturated fatty acids, degradation of which can lead to further free radical release and self-propagating membrane injury.[235] Free radicals preferentially react with vitamin E as tocopherol,[236] leading to the formation of a tocopherol-free radical complex that is "recycled" by reducing agents (including vitamin C) and restored to its antioxidant activity. It is suggested from animal studies that tocotrienols may exhibit antioxidant activity through induction of antioxidant enzymes (e.g., superoxide dismutase and glutathione peroxidase).[237,238] The effectiveness vitamin E supplementation, however, may be dependent on in situ antioxidant availability. Furthermore, it is suggested that other mechanisms of clinical response may be present, such as interfering with vitamin K metabolism and an inhibitory effect on the clotting cascade.[235]

At a cellular level, tocotrienols are associated with transcriptional, translational, or post-translational effects and direct interaction, leading to a range of effects in addition to antioxidant effects.[239] Such targets include growth factors like transforming growth factor (TGF)-β, which modulates proliferative effects, caspase-8 and other signaling pathways involved in apoptosis, and suppression of angiogenesis through inhibition of vascular endothelial growth factor (VEGF) and receptor signaling.

Studies of the role of vitamin E in inflammation have produced contradictory results, possibly because the contrasting effects of the various isoforms of vitamin E may represent competing and opposing influences on the inflammatory pathway.[240] This is demonstrated by apparently stimulatory and inhibitory effects on the vascular adhesion molecule, VCAM-1, by α-tocopherol and γ-tocopherol, respectively, including VCAM-1–dependent lymphocyte transmigration, with demonstrated direct antagonizing effects following supplementation. The immunomodulatory effects of vitamin E extend to a range of other components in the inflammatory pathway. Tocopherols demonstrate modulation of signal transduction of protein inflammatory mediators including PKC, protein tyrosine kinases, and the regulatory enzymes in the eicosanoid pathways, including 5-, 12-, and 15-lipoxygenases, cyclooxygenase-2, phospholipase A2, and modulation of protein-membrane interaction.[241] There are conflicting reports of regulation of cytokine expression, including tocotrienol lead suppression of TNF-induced activation of nuclear factor (NF)-κB,[242] an effect not seen with α-tocopherol. Furthermore, tocopherol isomers have been shown to modulate inflammation in models of asthma, without an effect on cytokines or other inflammatory mediators.[243]

The clinical importance of vitamin E deficiency has been demonstrated in patients with deficiency due to dietary or inherited metabolic conditions. Neurologic consequences include cerebellar ataxia (assumed secondary to the effects of uncontrolled oxidative stress) and cellular membrane damage or function; these have been seen in patients with congenital metabolic deficiencies such as chylomicron retention disease[244] or deficiencies of α-tocopherol transfer protein through gene mutation.[245] Although dietary deficiencies of vitamin E are rare, vitamin E deficiency may result from fat malabsorption and have been reported to cause neurologic symptoms following bariatric surgery.[246] Clinical benefits of antioxidant and membrane-protective effects of vitamin E have produced conflicting results in studies of cardiovascular risk. Positive effects of tocotrienols on cardiovascular mortality have been postulated through multiple systems, including antioxidant effects, but also both antiproliferation and coagulation effects.[247] The role of vitamin E, particularly tocotrienols, also has been suggested as cancer preventive, through antiproliferative inhibitory effects on the cell cycle progression and apoptosis.[248] A potential benefit has been demonstrated in prostate cancer risk with α-tocopherol supplementation, but there was accompanying evidence of an increase of colorectal adenomas.

Sources and RDA

The RDA for vitamin E is 15 mg/day (22.4 IU), with lower levels recommended in childhood and increased levels recommended in lactation.[249] Vitamin E, mainly as α-tocopherol, is found in a range of lipid-rich plant seeds and oils and vegetables, including wheat germ, sunflower, almond, hazelnuts, peanuts, corn, and soya bean, in addition to broccoli, tomato, and spinach. Margarine is rich in vitamin E, and breast milk contains a higher level of vitamin E than cow's milk. Tocotrienols are high in palm oil and rice bran, coconut oil, and cocoa.[250]

Intestinal Absorption

Physiologic Aspects

Vitamin E is absorbed passively across the intestinal mucosa.[251] The ester form, in which many vitamin preparations are presented, is hydrolyzed by pancreatic and/or duodenal esterases before absorption, but the ester can be absorbed intact.[252] After incorporation into micelles, vitamin E is transported into enterocytes and incorporated into chylomicrons for transfer into lymphatics. The absorption of vitamin E is affected by concurrent dietary fat intake, and radiolabelled studies in healthy subjects suggest this applies to up to 33% of the total ingested.[253] Results comparing supplementation of the isoforms of both tocopherol and tocotrienols in healthy human subjects suggest that marked increases in plasma α-tocopherol levels occur after supplementation, with negligible increases in all others. Supplementation with supra-high levels of tocotrienol (e.g., up to 300 mg/day), however, lead to marked raised plasma levels,[254] suggesting a dose-dependent response.

The biological activity of α-tocopherol is based on a metabolic response and is not relative antioxidant potency. Activity appears to be secondary to a process of selective retention in the liver that is mediated by α-tocopherol transfer protein (α-TTP), which incorporates α-tocopherol into lipoproteins prior to its return to the circulation. Incorporation occurs at the expense of other forms of vitamin E that demonstrate lower levels of affinity for binding and are therefore degraded and excreted by comparison. Therefore, although the antioxidant properties are similar, the biological properties are highest for α-tocopherol.[255] Through this mechanism, the liver serves to regulate bioavailability of α-tocopherol, leading to its predominant role in the circulation. Radiolabelled studies suggest that the half life of natural α-tocopherol is less than 60 hours in the circulation, with lower rates for other isoforms,[256] rapid recirculation between liver and systemic circulation, and almost daily replacement of the vitamin E pool.[257] Tocopherols are metabolized by cytochrome P450 side-chain degradation and oxidation and are eliminated via biliary excretion.

Vitamin K

In common with the other fat-soluble vitamins, vitamin K is acquired from dietary sources as phylloquinone, K_1, and from endogenous sources as menaquinones, K_2, acquired from bacterial synthesis in the colon. These have structures similar to chlorophyll (from which phylloquinone is derived) but differ in the nature of their side-chain structure, with a 20-carbon isoprenoid alcohol in phylloquinone and repeated isoprene units from 1 to 14 for menaquinones (MK-1 to 14).[212] Menaquinones also may be absorbed in small quantities from the diet and (MK-4) can be converted from dietary phylloquinone in certain tissues.

The roles of vitamin K have been traditionally considered to center on the coagulation pathway, although wider systemic relevance has been increasingly noted, particularly for menaquinones.

Metabolic Role and Effect of Deficiency

The traditionally recognized function of vitamin K is vitamin K-dependent (VKD) protein carboxylation for intracellular activation of VKD proteins. VKD carboxylase is an endoplasmic reticulum membrane bifunctional enzyme[258] that catalyzes both the oxygenation of vitamin K hydroquinone to vitamin K epoxide and carboxylation of multiple glutamate residues to γ-carboxyglutamate (Gla) on VKD proteins, resulting in their activation[259]; this is an essential step in the synthesis of clotting factors II, VII, IX, and X within the liver. VKD carboxylase, however, has also been identified as being present in tissues other than the liver and therefore as having a wider role of VKD protein activation than hemostatic mechanisms alone. This includes matrix Gla protein and osteocalcin, which relate to bone calcification. The post-oxygenation vitamin K epoxide is reduced by vitamin K epoxide (VKOR) (the target of warfarin) and recirculated.

Deficiencies of vitamin K are rare and considered primarily a problem for neonates, reflecting poor transfer across the placenta.[260] Vitamin K deficiency in adults may occur with fat malabsorption and maldigestion and is associated with very high doses of vitamin E. In addition to coagulation disorders, chronically altered vitamin K bioavailability is associated with metabolic bone disease and increased risk of fracture; adequate vitamin K intake is required for bone health.[261]

Sources and RDA

Because it is derived from chlorophyll, vitamin K_1 (phylloquinone) is obtained from green leafy vegetables including broccoli, spinach, lettuce, herbs, and kale. Absorption and bioavailability is variable, however, and dependent on a range of factors, including the nature of the food matrix. Studies have suggested that absorption from raw vegetables is markedly low (<10%) compared with fortified oil.[262] Co-consumption of fat, and specifically polyunsaturated forms, facilitates digestion and absorption.

In addition to synthesis within the bowel by anaerobic bacteria, menaquinones (e.g., MK-4) may be consumed in small amounts in meat, eggs, and dairy foods.[263] Absorption of MK-4 and other forms, however, is considered to result in peak bioavailability of less than 20% of phylloquinone,[264] possibly because of greater rates of clearance or reduced absorption. Menaquinones contribute less to vitamin K status in humans than previously thought.[265]

Adequate vitamin K intakes are 120 µg/day for adult males and 90 µg/day for adult females. Lower levels are recommended for children.[260]

Intestinal Absorption

Phylloquinone is absorbed through the lipid pathway and is dependent on biliary and pancreatic enzymes. Enterocyte uptake of phylloquinone is achieved by a carrier-mediated process,[266] whereas K_2 absorption is entirely passive.[267] Following absorption, transport of vitamin K is by chylomicrons, with delivery to the liver in the chylomicron remnant. Available information relating to the uptake of vitamin K by the liver is limited, but there are differences in subsequent carriage, with phylloquinone in triglyceride-rich lipoproteins (TRL) and long-chain menaquinones mainly in low-density lipoproteins (LDL).[262]

MINERALS AND TRACE ELEMENTS

Calcium

Calcium is an abundant mineral in the human body, with a role in both structural and physiologic aspects of health. Its RDA in adolescents and adults is between 1000 mg/day and 1200 mg/day, reflecting gender, age, and growth.[268] Milk and other dairy products are the most valuable sources of calcium, accounting for up to 75% of dietary calcium intake; cereals, legumes, and other vegetables contribute lesser amounts. Phytic acid or oxalate in vegetables binds strongly to calcium, reducing its availability. Dietary fiber also binds calcium and can interfere with its absorption; by contrast, dietary lactose enhances its absorption.[269] Fractional, or true, absorption is only about 20% to 30% of total dietary calcium, the remainder being excreted in stool.

Absorption of calcium across the intestinal mucosa is achieved by 2 parallel processes: an active saturable transcellular transport process, which dominates with lower levels of calcium intake, and a passive non-saturable paracellular diffusive process, which becomes more important at higher levels of calcium intake (Fig. 103-8).[270-272] Under normal dietary conditions, the duodenum and proximal jejunum are the major sites of active calcium transport, whereas passive paracellular transfer occurs throughout the small intestine. Despite this localization of the active transport site, quantitatively more calcium may be absorbed in the jejunum and ileum than in the duodenum because of the relative amounts of time luminal contents spend in these regions of intestine. The human jejunum absorbs calcium faster than does the ileum, and absorption rates in both regions are increased by the total quantity of calcium consumed and certain physiologic states (e.g., pregnancy, lactation).[273] Calcium absorption across the intestine is markedly influenced by vitamin D status,[274] with

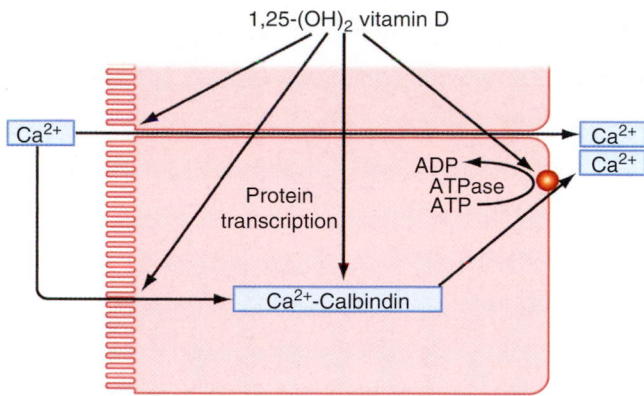

FIGURE 103-8. Mechanisms of intestinal calcium absorption. A paracellular route allows bidirectional flux. Transport into the epithelial cell occurs via specific channels down an electrochemical gradient. A critical step is binding to calbindin, which then presents calcium for export via a calcium-dependent adenosine triphosphatase (ATPase) on the basolateral membrane. Each of these processes appears to be influenced by 1,25-$(OH)_2$ vitamin D, although maximal effect is on the synthesis of fresh calbindin. ADP, adenosine diphosphate, ATP, adenosine triphosphate.

evidence from animal studies of a reduction of more than 75% in deficient states, resulting in inhibited transcellular transport and cellular trapping in the intestinal mucosa.[275]

The paracellular route (via the tight junctions) influences calcium transport, because passive transport increases in response to treatment with vitamin D.[276] Furthermore, there is evidence to suggest that tight-junctional permeability increases during sugar transport, and this might provide another mechanism for control of paracellular transport.[277]

The transcellular route, a process of facilitated diffusion, involves transport across the apical membrane, transfer across the cytoplasm, and exit across the BLM (see Fig. 103-8). Entry is mediated by TRPV6, a specific non–voltage-gated calcium channel[278] in the apical membrane and down the prevailing electrochemical gradient. Within the cytoplasm, binding to a calcium-binding protein, calbindin D9K (or calbindin 3), is a key step.[279] Maximal transport rates correlate closely with calbindin concentrations, a key step in calcium regulation and modulated by target genes calbindin D9k and D28k of vitamin D.[280] Calbindin D9K is present in concentrations of 0.1 to 0.2 mmol and must rapidly take up the calcium entering the cell, because intracellular free calcium concentrations are carefully maintained at very low values ($\approx 10^{-7}$ M). Transient rises in intracellular calcium act as key second-messenger signals for secretory responses in enterocytes. Absorbed calcium thus is presumably segregated from the calcium concerned with cell signaling, and calbindin D9K plays a vital role here by bringing calcium to the transporter at the BLM.[281]

Another calcium-binding protein, calbindin D28K (CALB1), is induced by vitamin D and binds 4 calcium ions, compared with calbindin D9K, which binds 2 calcium ions. An active mechanism utilizing calcium-dependent ATPase then drives calcium uphill against the electrochemical gradient.[279]

Calcium arrives at the basolateral pole bound to a site at the cytoplasmic aspect of the calcium-dependent ATPase that spans the BLM. There follows a phosphorylation-induced change in the conformation of the calcium-dependent ATPase, and the calcium ion is extruded through the channel formed by the transmembrane elements of the enzyme.[282]

The rate-limiting step in the intestinal absorption of calcium is the intracellular calbindin concentration, which is regulated by a metabolite of vitamin D, 1,25-dihydroxyvitamin

D (1,25α-$[OH]_2D_3$), produced in the kidneys from 25-hydroxyvitamin D (25-$[OH]_2D_3$).[271] The vitamin also has a modest effect on the calcium entry step and enhances activity of the basolateral calcium ATPase. Up-regulation of the calbindin gene in response to vitamin D occurs largely in villus cells.[283]

Some evidence supports colonic absorption of calcium, which also can be enhanced in response to vitamin D.[284] Although the colon normally accounts for only up to 7% of total calcium absorption, it becomes an important route for calcium absorption in patients with short bowel syndrome.[285]

Active duodenal calcium absorption is increased in calcium deficiency states and reduced in calcium repletion states. Increased production of the active 1,25α-$(OH)_2D_3$ metabolite in response to a small drop in plasma calcium concentration is responsible for increasing calcium absorption, and this change occurs within a day of changing from a high-calcium to a low-calcium diet.[286] This same mechanism is likely to be the cause of the enhanced calcium absorption seen during late pregnancy and lactation.

At birth, the active vitamin D-dependent absorptive mechanisms already are present in the human duodenum. Ingestion of large amounts of calcium with the lactose in breast milk ensures adequate intake at this critical stage of life. Calcium absorption declines with age, which might result in part from a lack of vitamin D or decreased responsiveness of the intestine to vitamin D.[269]

Magnesium

An average diet provides 300 to 500 mg of magnesium per day from a wide range of vegetables. Magnesium absorption has been less thoroughly investigated than that of calcium, but it seems likely that the mechanisms involved are different. In contrast to calcium absorption, magnesium absorption in the basal state is greater in the human ileum than in the duodenum or jejunum.[274] Jejunal absorption of magnesium is increased by vitamin D, whereas ileal absorption is not. Ileal transport involves both a paracellular diffusive pathway and a transcellular carrier-mediated saturable process.[287] There is some competition from calcium for the diffusive pathway but not for the saturable, presumably carrier-mediated, process.[288] Quantitatively, magnesium fluxes across ileal mucosa are several-fold greater than those for calcium, but the overall efficiency of magnesium absorption after normal dietary intake ranges from 21% to 27%.

Magnesium deficiency is associated with associated alterations in calcium, potassium, and sodium status, reflecting its role in electrolyte regulatory mechanisms.

Iron

Iron is a transition metal able to exist in a number of oxidative states, through which it provides a range of essential metabolic roles. Iron serves as a cofactor for both heme and non-heme proteins and enzymes, has a critical role in oxygen binding and transport, and metabolism and cellular respiration.[98]

Meat-eating affluent societies ingest about 20 to 30 mg of iron per day, largely as myoglobin or hemoglobin. Vegetarian societies in poor countries ingest much less than this in wheat and vegetables, and iron in these foods is less readily available for absorption. Furthermore, certain foods demonstrate an iron sequestration capacity, including phytates and tannins.[289]

Of the 3 to 5 grams of iron present in the human body, most is present within hemoglobin or myoglobin for oxygen carriage and muscle function, respectively, with transient or storage iron in spleen, liver, and bone marrow.[290] A careful balance of absorption and loss is maintained in normal adults; each is about 1 mg/day. Developing children and adolescents need to absorb about 0.5 mg/day more to build up total body iron to adult values. Iron is present in breast milk in the form of lactoferrin, for which a specific BBM receptor has been demonstrated[291,292] that facilitates iron absorption in neonates. During reproductive life, normal women need to compensate for menstrual losses, which are on the order of 5 to 50 mg per month and about 500 mg for each pregnancy.

Because dietary intake often markedly exceeds the body's need for iron, it is necessary to absorb only a small portion of that ingested. Overall, there is a positive and linear relationship between the amount ingested and that absorbed, but the fraction absorbed decreases as more is taken in.[293]

Total body iron content is regulated by controlling the level of iron absorbed from the diet. Under normal circumstances, only about 10% (1 to 2 mg/day) of dietary iron is absorbed. Most absorption occurs in the proximal small intestine, and the ferrous (Fe^{2+}) form is absorbed better than the ferric (Fe^{3+}) form. The latter is insoluble at pH values greater than 3, and gastric acid and some sugars and amino acids render it more available for absorption. The presence of some anions (e.g., oxalate, phosphate, phytate) precipitate iron out of solution and reduce its absorption. The presence of bile enhances absorption, but the mechanism of this enhancement is unclear.

Dietary iron is predominantly found in the ferric form, but Fe^{3+} is highly insoluble under physiologic conditions. Therefore, during uptake, Fe^{3+} is converted to the Fe^{2+} form at the apical cellular membrane before it attaches to an acceptor protein in the membrane. The intestinal mucosa reduces Fe^{3+} to Fe^{2+}[294] via duodenal cytochrome b, a membrane-associated ferrireductase[295] associated with apical transport via divalent metal transporter-1 (DMT1).[288] The reduction of Fe^3, however, is also a function of ascorbic acid which therefore facilitates iron absorption through co-consumption. Increased ferrireductase activity correlates with enhanced iron uptake induced by iron deficiency and hypoxia.[296,297]

Iron uptake occurs at 2 interfaces of the intestinal epithelium: the apical and basolateral plasma membranes (Fig. 103-9).[298] The apical plasma membrane of the differentiated enterocyte is specialized for transport of heme and ferrous iron into the cell. Three major pathways of iron transport across the apical membrane have been proposed. The best-characterized pathway is via the divalent metal transporter 1 (DMT1, also known as *Nramp2*),[299] which is located in the BBM, primarily in the villus tip cells. There are 2 splice variants of DMT1 that yield 2 messenger RNAs (mRNAs): 1 containing an iron-responsive element (IRE) termed *DMT1 (IRE) mRNA*, and another without an IRE designated *DMT1 (non-IRE) mRNA*. DMT1 is a proton symporter that transports ferrous iron and other divalent metals from the intestinal lumen into the enterocyte (see Fig. 103-9). It is up-regulated during iron deficiency and down-regulated in cases of iron excess.

In order of substrate preference, DMT1 can mediate import of Fe^{2+}, Zn^{2+}, Mn^{2+}, Co^{2+}, Cd^{2+}, Cu^{2+}, Ni^{2+}, and Pb^{2+}. The idea that the transporter responsible for dietary iron absorption recognizes other divalent cations agrees well with observations that Zn^{2+}, Mn^{2+}, Cd^{2+}, and Cu^{2+} all can inhibit this process. DMT1 mRNA is found in many different tissues, but the protein and its mRNA are most abundant in the proximal duodenum, with decreasing absorption along the distal axis, consistent with a function in intestinal iron absorption.[110] Iron depletion results in increased DMT1 mRNA levels in the intestine, which suggests that IREs in its 3′ untranslated region bind and stabilize the DMT1 mRNA.[110] Although the major route for dietary iron absorption likely is mediated by DMT1,

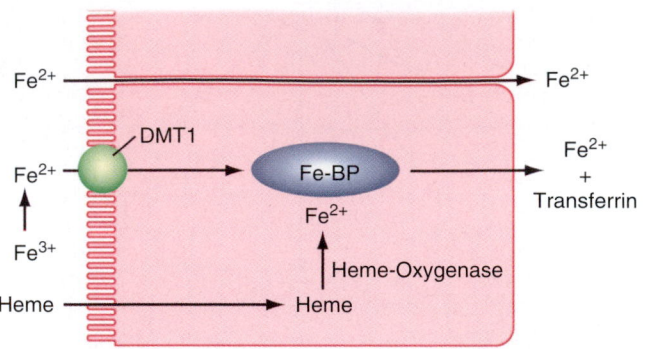

FIGURE 103-9. Mechanisms of intestinal iron absorption. A small amount of inorganic iron may pass through the paracellular route. Inorganic iron is converted into its ferrous form at the brush border membrane before transport into the cell. Heme iron is transported into the cell by a separate mechanism. Within the cell, 1 or more iron-binding proteins take up iron and transfer it to the basolateral membrane for delivery across the membrane and subsequent binding to transferrin. DMT1, divalent metal transporter-1; Fe-BP, iron-binding protein.

this transporter is found only in the apical surface of enterocytes. Thus, other factors must be involved in the transfer across the intestinal epithelium.

DMT1 may be involved in the pathogenesis of hereditary hemochromatosis (see Chapter 75). *HFE* is the gene responsible for hereditary hemochromatosis. HFE protein is found in the crypt cells of the duodenum associated with β_2-microglobulin and transferrin receptor. It is hypothesized that HFE protein facilitates transferrin receptor-dependent iron uptake into crypt cells and that mutant HFE protein might lose this ability, leading to a relative iron deficiency in duodenal crypt cells. In turn, this might lead to an increase in the expression of DMT1, resulting in increased iron absorption in hereditary hemochromatosis. Up-regulation of DMT1 expression has been confirmed in the HFE-knockout mouse and in humans with hereditary hemochromatosis.[300]

Iron can also be absorbed in the form of heme iron (in hemoglobin and myoglobin), which is readily transported across the brush border of the enterocytes as an intact heme moiety. It is the presence of globin that increases absorption of iron in this form. Heme-carrier protein 1 (HCP1) has been isolated from the mouse duodenum. This large hydrophobic transporter is present in the apical membrane during iron deficiency and in the cytoplasm during iron overload, making it a putative candidate for heme-iron transport.[301] Once within the cell, heme is broken down by heme oxygenase, and the iron is released into the non-heme pool for incorporation into intracellular ferritin and export out of the cell.[302,303]

Another iron absorptive pathway has been proposed that involves intestinal mucins, a 56-kd protein designated mobilferrin, an integrin, and a ferric reductase. This pathway is regulated and depends on metabolic energy, and it appears to be encouraged by nonessential fatty acids.[296,304,305] A small proportion of the iron crossing the mucosa uses a paracellular route by simple diffusion (see Fig. 103-9). Once within the enterocyte, expression of the iron-storage protein ferritin is regulated by the intracellular concentration of iron. Ferritin synthesis increases when iron is present in excess and decreases when iron level is low.

Iron transport across the basolateral plasma membrane of villus enterocytes involves at least 2 proteins: a ferroxidase called hephestin, which is associated with the BLM, and a basolateral iron transporter termed *ferroportin 1* (FPN1), *iron-regulated protein 1*, or *metal-transport protein 1*. These proteins may work in close conjunction with each other, with ferroportin 1 transporting ferrous iron out of the cell and hephestin oxidizing the ferrous iron to ferric iron, which permits the avid incorporation into circulating apotransferrin (apoTF).[298] The transferrin receptor, in combination with the hemochromatosis protein (HFE), allows the binding of apoTF-bound iron and its reuptake back into intestinal cells.[306] FPN1 is a membrane-bound protein containing IREs that is up-regulated during iron deficiency and down-regulated during iron excess. Hepcidin, a circulating peptide hormone[307] produced in the liver, might influence enterocyte iron transport by binding to FPN1, resulting in the internalization and degradation of FPN1 and thereby reducing iron absorption.[308]

The majority of the body's iron requirements are met by iron recycling from erythrocyte degradation and capture by reticuloendothelial macrophages.[309] Because of the limited requirement for additional daily iron and the absence of an effective system of iron removal from the body, total body iron status is matched to body requirements by tightly regulating iron absorption. This occurs in at least 3 ways. The long-standing concept of *mucosal block* is based on the observation that after a large oral iron dose, enterocytes do not absorb additional iron for several days. This may reflect the inhibition of FPN1 by hepcidin in response to increased iron stores, but a direct effect on DMT1 is also possible, although as yet unproved.[309] A second regulatory mechanism of iron absorption is termed the *stores regulator*. It acts on a pathway that facilitates a slow accumulation of non-heme dietary iron. The functioning of the stores regulator is of great physiologic importance because it prevents iron overload after ensuring iron needs are met. The exact molecular mechanism of the stores regulator has not been established, but it has been proposed to involve soluble factors such as transferrin-bound iron, serum ferritin, serum transferrin, or hepcidin. The *erythropoietic regulator* is a third regulatory mechanism that adjusts intestinal iron absorption in response to the demands of erythropoiesis, independent of body iron stores. This regulator must signal directly between the hematopoietic bone marrow and the duodenum. Although the erythropoietic regulator has been proposed to be a soluble component of the plasma, it is distinct from the stores regulator. This is evidenced by the rate of iron uptake in anemic persons that is much greater (20 to 40 mg/day) than could be produced by the stores regulator alone.

The stores and erythropoietic regulators are circulating factors that maintain iron homeostasis of the entire organism. Within individual cells, the iron regulatory proteins (IRPs) IRP-1 and IRP-2 act to control iron availability by translational control of the synthesis of proteins such as transferrin and ferritin. IRPs are cytoplasmic RNA-binding proteins that function on mRNAs that contain IREs. Functional IREs are present in the 3' untranslated region of mRNAs for transferring in 1 of the 2 isoforms of DMT1 (DMT1 IRE) and in the 5'-untranslated region of mRNAs for ferritin, ferroportin 1, mitochondrial aconitase, and the erythroid-specific form of δ-aminolevulinic acid synthase. IRPs functionally connect intracellular iron availability with cellular iron utilization; IRP function can also be altered by inflammation and oxidative stress.

Basolateral iron uptake from the plasma by cryptal enterocytes plays an important role in sensing body iron stores. There is considerable evidence that the iron concentration within the cryptal enterocyte is an important determinant of iron absorption. The mechanism by which the intracellular iron concentration can respond to body iron needs is poorly understood. It is clear, however, that cells in the crypts of Lieberkühn always express transferrin, and the endocytic mechanism imparts information about body iron storage based on plasma transferrin saturation. It is also well recognized that acute changes in body iron status, whether overload or deficiency, are not reflected by changes in iron absorption for a period of 2 to 3 days. This lag response time probably correlates with the migration time for proliferating cells in the crypts to differentiate and migrate into functional mature enterocytes of the villi. Thus, the luminal epithelial cells may be preprogrammed in the crypts based on body iron needs. This preprogramming would, in turn, initiate synthesis of iron transport proteins required for dietary iron uptake across the membranes of the villus enterocyte.

Zinc

Zinc is a nutrient of fundamental biologic importance, with ubiquitous presence in mammalian metabolism. It is frequently described as a type 2 nutrient, reflecting its varied roles in enzyme function as a catalyst, maintaining structure and regulation of gene expression via a metal-binding transcription factor (MTF) and a metal response element (MRE) in the promoter of the regulated gene.[310] Zinc is present in the body in about half the amount of iron (≈2 g) and largely in a wide variety of enzymes. Zinc status in humans, however, is vulnerable owing to a small endogenous pool that is dependent on regular dietary repletion and bioavailability; it demonstrates rapid depletion with insufficient dietary intake (often within weeks) and rapid response to improved availability.[311]

Zinc is found particularly in meat, shellfish, cereals, and legumes. Daily requirements are approximately 12 to 15 mg/day in adults. Persons who consume a low-energy diet might take in marginal amounts of zinc, and requirements are increased during pregnancy and lactation.

Absorption is impaired by phytates and oxalates in the diet through their chelating properties, and food processing can render zinc less available for absorption.[312] The protein content of a diet is positively correlated with zinc absorption, likely because of amino acids or small peptides that facilitate enterocyte uptake of zinc. Overall, the efficiency of zinc absorption from a regular diet is 15% to 35%.

There is enterohepatic circulation of zinc, and reabsorption appears to be maximal in the distal small intestine.[313] Studies with vesicles of porcine jejunal BBMs have identified 2 uptake processes: an active saturatable carrier-mediated process (which dominates at low or normal intake) and a non-saturatable diffusive process (which contributes more to absorption at higher intake).[314] The relative importance of each is unknown.

There are 9 members of the ZNT family of zinc transporters, with ZNT1, 2, and 4 occurring mainly in the villus.[315,316] ZNT1 is a ubiquitously expressed protein that is present in the villi of the proximal small intestine. ZNT1 expression in rats was increased in response to zinc supplementation but not to zinc restriction.[317] These and other observations have led to the consensus that ZNT1 functions mainly as a zinc exporter and might play a role in zinc homeostasis for zinc acquisition and elimination under conditions of excess zinc.[315] ZNT2 and ZNT4 are involved in intracellular transport of zinc by the enterocyte. Zinc kinetic studies suggest homeostasis is maintained by regulation of absorption through zinc transporter availability, a saturatable intracellular transportation mechanism, and by regulation of excretion.[318]

Zinc exists in a number of pools, including intracellularly in organelles and metallothionein bound, and in plasma, where it is principally albumin bound. Although zinc-dependent proteins are found throughout the cell, small quantities of zinc may be maintained as a reserve within the Golgi apparatus and endoplasmic reticulum. Intracellularly, zinc is regulated by a ZNT transporter mechanism.[319]

Metallothionein (MT) is an intracellular metal-binding protein associated with a number of metal nutrients but most commonly bound to zinc. MT has tissue-dependent isoforms, with MT-2a the most prevalent.[320] Up to 7 zinc molecules can bind to a single MT molecule. MT bioavailability reacts rapidly to zinc status, with high dietary levels leading to increased intestinal synthesis and sequestration and altered binding capacity[321]; therefore, MT may have roles both in storage of zinc and regulation.[310,322]

Clinical consequences of zinc deficiency are both anatomical (e.g., skin rashes) and metabolic (e.g., altered immune function and response to oxidative stress).[323] Homeostatic responses include a marked reduction in zinc excretion as a mechanism for maintaining bioavailability. Subjects on a low-zinc diet respond by decreasing their urinary excretion rate of zinc and by increasing its absorption rates.[313,324] Absorption increases in pregnancy and during lactation.[325] Expression of ZNT1 has been measured and found to be directly related to serum zinc levels but unaffected by MT levels.[326] Thus, MT might function in cellular responses to limit free zinc concentrations within narrow ranges and function as a zinc pool.[315,326]

Another transporter potentially involved in zinc and other metal uptake is DCT1, a transmembrane polypeptide found in the duodenum in the crypts and lower villi; it may be available for the uptake of several metal ions.[316] The ZIP (Zrt-, Irt-like protein) family of proteins are believed to be involved in zinc transport.[327] ZIP4 and ZIP5 likely exist on the apical side and BLM of the enterocyte, respectively, and may be responsible for zinc transport into the circulation.[328]

Copper

Copper is an essential nutrient with a metabolic importance that is disproportionate to total body availability in humans; total body levels are appropriately 10 μg, although this varies by organ, with highest levels in liver, brain, and kidney.[329] In common with other micronutrients, bioavailability and total body status of copper is closely regulated.[330]

Copper is found in green vegetables and fish, and the average Western diet provides 1 to 3 mg/day, which is adequate for a daily need of about 1 mg/day. Dietary copper is absorbed very efficiently from the stomach and small intestine, especially the duodenum. Although the precise mechanisms involved in copper absorption remain incompletely known, within physiologic ranges of intake, absorption is probably by active transport. Competition for absorption between copper and zinc or iron may be demonstrable with large doses of these elements but not with normal dietary intakes.[331] Copper uptake might increase in pregnancy.[332] Bioavailability differs depending on the food or animal source of copper,[333] and dietary levels predict efficiency of absorption, with higher absorption during deficiency states. In high-intake states, absorption can be as low as 12%,[334] and with the dependent variability in excretion[335] reflects a mechanism for regulation, homeostasis, and toxicity avoidance.

Active transport and passive diffusion are both responsible for copper absorption in humans. A putative high-affinity protein copper transport protein, denoted hCtr1, has been identified by functional complementation of the respiratory defect in yeast cells defective in copper transport due to inactivation of both the *CTR1* and *CTR3* genes.[336]

Human Ctr1 is a 190–amino acid protein with 3 TMDs and significant homology to yeast Ctr1 and Ctr3, which suggests that mammalian high-affinity copper transporters may have evolved from Ctr1 and Ctr3. RNA blotting analysis has demonstrated that that hCtr1 is expressed in all organs and tissues examined. Liver, heart, and pancreas exhibited the highest levels of expression, intestine had intermediate levels of expression, and expression in brain and muscle was low. Whether hCtrl1 plays an important role in copper uptake into intestinal mucosal cells has yet to be firmly established.[337,338]

Two putative low-affinity mammalian copper transporters, hCtrl2 and Nramp2, have also been identified. It is unclear what role hCtr2 plays in copper homeostasis, because its mRNA levels are highest in the placenta and very low in liver, intestine, and colon.[337,339] The Nramp2 protein has also been identified as a proton-coupled metal ion transporter that transports a broad range of metal ions.[340]

Acting as a permease or by endocytosis, Ctr1 delivers Cu^{2+} within cells.[341] The mechanism for reduction of copper ion before uptake remains unknown. If uncontrolled, this pool of cuprous ions could lead to generation of reactive oxygen species; however, very few, if any, free copper ions exist in the cytoplasm.

The delivery of copper to target cuproenzymes depends on an elegant metallochaperone system. Several cytoplasmic chaperones have been described (Atox1, CCS [copper chaperone for Cu, Zn superoxide dismutase], and Cox17) as well as membrane-associated copper-transporting ATPases (ATP7A and ATP7B).[341] The copper-transporting Menkes ATPase ATP7A (MNK) is responsible for copper export from the enterocyte and may be defective in patients with Menkes disease, in whom copper accumulates in intestinal cells.[342,343]

On entering the plasma, copper is bound with albumin and histidine in the portal blood and rapidly deposited in the liver, where hCtr1 may play a role in this process. The liver has a pivotal role in regulation of copper throughout the metabolism and total body status. Ceruloplasmin, a major copper-containing protein in plasma, is synthesized in the liver with incorporation of copper by the Wilson disease protein, which has a high homology with MNK and is defective in Wilson disease patients who suffer from copper accumulation in the liver (see Chapter 76).

Iodine

Iodine is present in varying amounts in a wide range of foods, depending on the soil content in the region where animals were reared and vegetation was grown. Seafood is particularly rich in iodine. Iodine is absorbed largely as inorganic iodide, but some iodine is transported as amino acid complexes.[344]

Selenium

Selenium is found predominantly in association with amino acids, and about 60% of dietary selenium is absorbed. Selenium deficiency states have been reported from China (Keshan disease), where there is very little selenium in soil and water,[345] but not in New Zealand, where intake is equally sparse.[346] Absorption of selenium occurs rapidly when it is associated with amino acids, as in selenomethionine, probably by active transport mechanisms operative for the amino acid.[347] Inorganic selenium is absorbed more slowly, possibly by simple diffusion.

Other Trace Elements

The mechanisms underlying the absorption of other trace elements, including manganese and chromium, are largely unknown.[344] Deficiencies of trace elements are rare in normal persons, even in those with poor protein and calorie intake. Exceptions occur when local geographic availability is suboptimal, as can occur with iodine and possibly with selenium.

KEY REFERENCES

Full references for this chapter can be found on www.expertconsult.com.

2. Liang WJ, Johnson D, Jarvis SM. Vitamin C transport systems of mammalian cells. Mol Membr Biol 2001; 18:87-95.

18. Said HM. Intestinal absorption of water-soluble vitamins in health and disease. Biochem J 2011; 437:357-72.

21. Mock DM. Biotin. In: Zempleni J, McCormick DB, Suttie JW, editors. Handbook of vitamins. New York: CRC Press; 2006. pp 361-77.

43. Quadros EV. Advances in the understanding of cobalamin assimilation and metabolism. Br J Haematol 2010; 148:195-204.

86. Zhao R, Matherly LH, Goldman ID. Membrane transporters and folate homeostasis: Intestinal absorption and transport into systemic compartments and tissues. Expert Rev Mol Med 2009; 11:1-27.

192. von Lintig J. Provitamin A metabolism and functions in mammalian biology. Am J Clin Nutr 2012; 96:S1234-44.

208. Harrison EH. Mechanisms involved in the intestinal absorption of dietary vitamin A and provitamin A carotenoids. Biochem Biophys Acta 2012; 1821:70-7.

215. Christakos S, Dhawan P, Porta A, et al. Vitamin D and intestinal calcium absorption. Mol Cell Endocrinol 2011; 347:25-9.

231. Christakos S, Ajibade DV, Dhawan P, et al. Vitamin D: Metabolism. Endocrinol Metab Clin North Am 2010; 39:243-53.

239. Aggarwal BB, Sundaram C, Prasad S, et al. Tocotrienols, the vitamin E of the 21st century: Its potential against cancer and other chronic diseases. Biochem Pharmacol 2010; 80:1613-31.

258. Dowd P, Ham SW, Naganathan S, et al. The mechanism of action of vitamin K. Annu Rev Nutr 1995; 15:419-40.

288. Pantopoulos K, Porwal SK, Tartakoff A, et al. Mechanisms of mammalian iron homeostasis. Biochem J 2012; 51:5705-24.

307. Nemeth E, Ganz T. The role of hepcidin in iron metabolism. Acta Haematol 2009; 122:78-86.

310. King JC. Zinc: An essential but elusive nutrient. Am J Clin Nutr 2011; 94:S679-84.

330. van den Berghe PV, Klomp LW. New developments in the regulation of intestinal copper absorption. Nutr Rev 2009; 67:658-72.

CHRISTOPH HÖGENAUER AND HEINZ F. HAMMER

In the past, it was believed that most malabsorptive diseases manifested with diarrhea, steatorrhea, or both. It is now recognized that many malabsorptive disorders, such as celiac disease, might have subtle clinical presentations (e.g., bloating, changes in bowel habits) or mainly extraintestinal manifestations (e.g., anemia, bone loss, menstrual disturbance) that lead to erroneous diagnoses. Awareness is also increasing that subtle malabsorption of single nutrients like calcium or vitamin B_{12} can, if unrecognized, lead to complications that may be difficult to reverse or that are even irreversible. The clinical challenge today is to recognize and treat malabsorption despite its subtle manifestations, a challenge made even more difficult by the restricted availability of tests for malabsorption, such as the 72-hour fecal fat determination.

Classically, *maldigestion* is defined as defective intraluminal hydrolysis of nutrients, and *malabsorption* is defined as defective mucosal absorption. Although this distinction may be useful on pathophysiologic grounds, the clinical presentation and complications of maldigestion and malabsorption are similar. Moreover, physiologic processes other than digestion

and absorption (e.g., solubilization, intestinal motility, hormone secretion) contribute to the normal absorption of nutrients, vitamins, and minerals, so the classic definitions of maldigestion and malabsorption do not cover the actual pathophysiologic spectrum of the malabsorption syndrome. In this chapter, the terms *digestion* and *absorption* or *maldigestion* and *malabsorption* are used separately only in the discussion of pathophysiology. When the distinction between these terms is not of clinical relevance, only the terms *absorption* and *malabsorption* are used.

Malabsorption can be caused by many diseases of the small intestine and also by diseases of the pancreas, liver, biliary tract, and stomach (Box 104-1). In some of these diseases, malabsorption may be the presenting feature; in others, malabsorption may be only a minor clinical problem or detected only as a laboratory abnormality.

This chapter provides an overview of basic pathophysiologic mechanisms that lead to symptoms or complications of maldigestion or malabsorption, reviews the clinical manifestations and complications of malabsorption, describes tests that

BOX 104-1 Diseases That Cause Nutrient Malabsorption

Gastric Diseases
Atrophic gastritis
Autoimmune gastritis (pernicious anemia)
Gastric resection or bypass surgery

Pancreatic Diseases
Congenital pancreatic enzyme deficiencies:
 Colipase deficiency
 Lipase deficiency
 Trypsinogen deficiency
Pancreatic insufficiency:
 Chronic pancreatitis
 Cystic fibrosis
 Johanson-Blizzard syndrome
 Pearson's marrow-pancreas syndrome
 Shwachman's syndrome
Pancreatic tumors

Liver Diseases
Inborn errors of bile acid biosynthesis and transport
Cirrhosis and other liver diseases
Portal hypertension

Obstructive Biliary Diseases
Biliary tumors
Primary and secondary sclerosing cholangitis

Intestinal Diseases
Amyloidosis
Autoimmune enteropathy
Celiac disease
Collagenous sprue
Congenital intestinal defects (see Table 104-10)
Crohn's disease
Enteroendocrine cell deficiency:
 Autoimmune polyglandular syndrome type 1
 Enteric anendocrinosis
Enterokinase deficiency
Eosinophilic gastroenteritis
Fistulas
Food allergy
Graft-versus-host disease
Hypolactasia
Ileal bile acid malabsorption
Intestinal infections:
 AIDS (HIV infection): cryptosporidiosis, *Mycobacterium avium*
  complex infection, viral infections

Giardiasis
Helminthic infections
Tuberculosis
Whipple's disease
Immunoproliferative small intestinal disease
Intestinal ischemia
Intestinal lymphoma
Intestinal resections or bypass
Mastocytosis
Nongranulomatous chronic idiopathic enterocolitis
Postinfection malabsorption
Primary immunodeficiency diseases
Radiation enteritis
Refractory sprue
Sarcoidosis
SIBO
Tropical sprue

Lymphatic Diseases
Primary intestinal lymphangiectasia
Secondary intestinal lymphangiectasia:
 Lymphoma
 Solid tumors
 Thoracic duct trauma, damage, or obstruction

Neuroendocrine Tumors
Carcinoid syndrome
Glucagonoma
Somatostatinoma
Zollinger-Ellison syndrome

Cardiac and Vascular Diseases
Constrictive pericarditis
Heart failure

Endocrine Causes
Addison's disease
Diabetes mellitus
Hyperthyroidism

Systemic Diseases
Cronkhite-Canada syndrome
Mixed connective tissue disease
Neurofibromatosis type 1
Protein-calorie malnutrition
Scleroderma
SLE

can be used clinically to evaluate digestive and absorptive function, provides a rational diagnostic approach to the individual patient, and discusses malabsorptive diseases and general measures in the treatment of malabsorption syndrome not covered in other chapters of this book.

ETIOLOGY AND PATHOPHYSIOLOGY

From a pathophysiologic point of view, mechanisms that cause malabsorption can be divided into premucosal (luminal), mucosal, and postmucosal (vascular and lymphatic) factors. For clinical purposes, this approach is of limited value because the various clinical pictures caused by malabsorption syndromes are determined mainly by the nature of the malabsorbed substrates. We therefore discuss the mechanisms causing malabsorption on the basis of the malabsorbed substrate. A separate section is devoted to the role of mechanisms that compensate for the consequences of malabsorption.

Normal uptake of nutrients, vitamins, and minerals by the gastrointestinal (GI) tract (see Chapters 102 and 103) requires several steps, each of which can be compromised in disease.

Solubilization is a prerequisite for absorption of such nutrients as fat or calcium. Fat and fat-soluble vitamins are solubilized by the formation of micelles, and calcium is solubilized through acidification in the GI lumen. Alternatively, increased solubilization of the components of intestinal chyme can contribute to the manifestations of GI diseases, such as increased absorption of oxalate, which can result in the development of kidney stones in patients with short bowel syndrome (see Chapter 106).

Digestion of macromolecular compounds like polysaccharides, triglycerides, and proteins to their molecular components—monosaccharides, fatty acids, and amino acids, respectively—is achieved by soluble or membrane-bound digestive enzymes. Absorption of undigested or partially digested macromolecular compounds occurs to a very minor degree in health and may be increased slightly in various

TABLE 104-1 Mechanisms of Malabsorption, Malabsorbed Substrates, and Representative Causes

Pathophysiologic Mechanism	Malabsorbed Substrate(s)	Representative Causes
Maldigestion		
Conjugated bile acid deficiency	Fat Fat-soluble vitamins Calcium Magnesium	Hepatic parenchymal disease Biliary obstruction SIBO with bile acid deconjugation Ileal bile acid malabsorption CCK deficiency
Pancreatic insufficiency	Fat Protein Carbohydrate Fat-soluble vitamins Vitamin B_{12} (cobalamin)	Congenital defects Chronic pancreatitis Pancreatic tumors Inactivation of pancreatic enzymes (e.g., ZES)
Reduced mucosal digestion	Carbohydrate Protein	Congenital defects (see Table 104-10) Acquired lactase deficiency Generalized mucosal disease (e.g., celiac disease, Crohn's disease)
Intraluminal consumption of nutrients	Vitamin B_{12} (cobalamin)	SIBO Helminthic infections (e.g., *Diphyllobothrium latum* infection)
Malabsorption		
Reduced mucosal absorption	Fat Protein Carbohydrate Vitamins Minerals	Congenital transport defects (see Table 104-10) Generalized mucosal diseases (e.g., celiac disease, Crohn's disease) Previous intestinal resection or bypass Infections Intestinal lymphoma

Decreased transport from the intestine	Fat
	Protein
		Intestinal lymphangiectasia
		  Primary
		  Secondary (e.g., solid tumors, Whipple's
		    disease, lymphomas)
		Venous stasis (e.g., from heart failure)

Other Mechanisms		
Decreased gastric acid and/or intrinsic factor secretion	Vitamin B_{12}	Pernicious anemia Atrophic gastritis Previous gastric resection
Decreased gastric mixing and/or rapid gastric emptying	Fat Calcium Protein	Previous gastric resection Autonomic neuropathy
Rapid intestinal transit	Fat	Autonomic neuropathy Hyperthyroidism

intestinal diseases. Although such absorption does not play a nutritive role, it may be important for the normal function of the immune system and the pathogenesis of diseases such as food allergy (see Chapter 10).

Liberation of substrate (e.g., vitamin B_{12}) from binding sites in food or, conversely, *binding* to factors like intrinsic factor allows absorption to take place.

Chemical changes to nutrients may be required for absorption, such as reducing the charge of iron from Fe^{+3} to Fe^{+2}.

Mucosal absorption can occur by active or passive carrier-mediated transport or simple or facilitated diffusion (see Chapter 101). *Postmucosal transport* of absorbed substrates occurs in blood vessels and lymphatic vessels.

Intestinal sensory and motor function permits detection of the presence of nutrients, facilitates adequate mixing of nutrients with intestinal secretions and delivery to absorptive sites, and provides adequate time for nutrient absorption (see Chapter 99).

Neural and hormonal functions are required to stimulate and coordinate digestive secretions, mucosal absorption, and intestinal motility (see Chapters 4 and 99).

An overview of pathophysiologic mechanisms of maldigestion and malabsorption is provided in Table 104-1. This table also shows the ingested substrates primarily affected by individual pathophysiologic mechanisms and lists examples of etiologic disorders for these mechanisms.

FATS

Defective Mixing

For sufficient digestion and absorption of lipids, dietary fat must adequately mix with digestive secretions. Gastric resections or GI motility disorders that result in rapid gastric emptying or rapid intestinal transit, such as autonomic

TABLE 104-2 Pathophysiologic Mechanisms That Result in Deficiency of Luminal Conjugated Bile Acids

Pathophysiologic Mechanism	Causes
Decreased synthesis and/or secretion of conjugated bile acids	Parenchymal liver diseases (e.g., cirrhosis, PBC) Biliary obstruction (e.g., tumors) Biliary fistulas Inborn errors of bile acid synthesis CCK deficiency
Intestinal loss of conjugated bile acids	Ileal resection Severe ileal mucosal disease Congenital defects of the ileal sodium-bile acid cotransporter
Luminal deconjugation of bile acids	SIBO
Binding of bile salts or insolubilization of bile salts as a result of low luminal pH	Cholestyramine (binding) ZES (low pH) Exocrine pancreatic insufficiency (low pH)

neuropathy due to diabetes mellitus or amyloidosis, can cause fat malabsorption consequent to impaired GI mixing of dietary fat.[1]

Reduced Solubilization of Fat

Fat malabsorption resulting from decreased formation of micelles occurs if the luminal concentrations of conjugated bile acids are lower than the critical concentration required for forming micelles.[2,3] Table 104-2[1,4] details the pathophysiologic mechanisms and representative diseases that cause luminal bile acid deficiency.

Decreased Lipolysis

If exocrine pancreatic function is severely reduced, impairment of pancreatic lipase and colipase secretion results in decreased luminal hydrolysis of dietary fat.[5] Chronic pancreatitis, cystic fibrosis, pancreatic duct obstruction by pancreatic and ampullary tumors, and pancreatic resection are the most common causes of pancreatic insufficiency.[1] Even when pancreatic enzyme concentrations are normal, reduced pancreatic lipase activity resulting from low luminal pH,[6] excessive calcium ingestion,[7] or ingestion of the specific lipase inhibitor orlistat[8] can cause pancreatic steatorrhea. Selective congenital lipase or colipase deficiency is a rare cause of pancreatic fat malabsorption.[9]

Decreased Mucosal Absorption and Chylomicron Formation

Generalized mucosal diseases like celiac disease are often associated with fat malabsorption. Defective uptake of free fatty acids and monoglycerides results from reduced mucosal surface area secondary to villus shortening, reduced enterocyte function, and mucosal inflammation.[1] Intestinal fat absorption is also impaired in diseases that result in disturbance of intracellular formation of chylomicrons and accumulation of lipids within the enterocytes, including abetalipoproteinemia, hypobetalipoproteinemia, and chylomicron retention disease.[10]

Defective Lymphatic Transport of Chylomicrons

Impairment of lymphatic transport of chylomicrons is a cause for postmucosal malabsorption of dietary fat. Decreased lymphatic transport can result from congenital diseases such as primary intestinal lymphangiectasia or from obstruction of lymphatic vessels as a result of metastatic solid tumors, lymphoma, Whipple's disease, retroperitoneal fibrosis, or trauma[6] (see Chapter 30). Usually, lymphatic vessels in the mucosa become dilated (lymphangiectasia), and chylomicrons are lost postprandially into the intestinal lumen and also in the fasting state[11]; steatorrhea in these situations usually is only mild to moderate.[1]

PROTEINS AND AMINO ACIDS

Defective digestion or absorption of dietary proteins has to be differentiated from excessive loss of serum proteins into the GI tract, which is termed *protein-losing enteropathy* (see Chapter 30).

Defective Intraluminal Proteolysis

Protein digestion may be impaired in patients who have undergone partial or total gastric resection, presumably as a result of poor mixing with digestive secretions, although gastric pepsin deficiency could be contributory. Impaired activation of pepsin due to acid inhibition by PPIs can result in an increased risk of food allergy like childhood asthma, owing to decreased gastric digestion of proteins (see Chapter 10).[12] Defective proteolysis also occurs with exocrine pancreatic insufficiency.[1,13,14] In congenital diseases, pancreatic proteolysis can be impaired by inborn errors in the synthesis of proteolytic enzymes (trypsinogen deficiency)[14] or by defective activation of pancreatic proenzymes resulting from congenital deficiency of intestinal enterokinase (see later).[15]

Defective Mucosal Hydrolysis of Peptides and Decreased Absorption of Oligopeptides and Amino Acids

Generalized mucosal diseases, such as celiac disease, result in global malabsorption, which includes malabsorption of oligopeptides and amino acids secondary to lack of mucosal hydrolysis of oligopeptides and defective mucosal absorption.[14] Reduction of intestinal absorptive surface, as in short bowel syndrome (See Chapter 106) or jejunoileal bypass, also results in protein and amino acid malabsorption.[14,16] Congenital defects of amino acid transporters on the enterocytes (e.g., Hartnup's disease, lysinuric protein intolerance) can lead to selective malabsorption of a subgroup of amino acids (see later).

CARBOHYDRATES

The pathophysiologic mechanisms and clinical role of carbohydrate malabsorption has been recently reviewed.[17]

Defective Intraluminal Hydrolysis of Carbohydrates

Pancreatic α-amylase is normally secreted in excess into the intestinal lumen. In mild forms of pancreatic insufficiency, carbohydrate digestion usually is at least partially preserved,[18] but severe pancreatic insufficiency results in clinically apparent carbohydrate malabsorption and diarrhea due to decreased luminal hydrolysis of ingested starch.[19]

Mucosal Defects of Carbohydrate Digestion and Absorption

The most common cause of carbohydrate malabsorption is late-onset lactose malabsorption due to decreased levels of the intestinal brush border enzyme lactase (adult-type hypolactasia, acquired primary lactase deficiency). Depending on ethnic background, lactase is present in less than 5% to more than 90% of the adult population; its deficiency results in a selective malabsorption of lactose. Acquired malabsorption of carbohydrates occurs commonly after extensive intestinal resections, in diffuse mucosal diseases like celiac or Crohn's disease, or temporarily after self-limited GI infections (postinfection carbohydrate malabsorption).[18,19] The pathophysiologic mechanisms of carbohydrate malabsorption are reduction of the intestinal mucosal surface area and reduced activity or expression of intestinal oligo- and disaccharidases or transport proteins for monosaccharides.[18] Congenital disaccharidase deficiencies (lactase, sucrase-isomaltase, trehalase)[20] and congenital deficiency or malfunction of transport molecules, as in congenital glucose-galactose malabsorption,[21] can cause early onset of malabsorption of mono- or disaccharides (see later). Intolerance of fructose is discussed in a subsequent section.

VITAMINS

Fat-Soluble Vitamins

Diseases that cause malabsorption of dietary fat commonly cause malabsorption of fat-soluble vitamins because they require similar absorptive mechanisms. This is especially important in diseases that result in impaired micelle formation due to bile salt deficiency.[22] Fat-soluble vitamins also are malabsorbed in diffuse diseases of the mucosal surface area, in diseases affecting chylomicron formation and transport,[23] and in exocrine pancreatic insufficiency.[24] Some authors have suggested that absorption of fat-soluble vitamins is less affected by exocrine pancreatic insufficiency than by small intestinal diseases with resultant steatorrhea.[24] Genetic defects of bile acid conjugation may also result in malabsorption of fat-soluble vitamins.[25]

Water-Soluble Vitamins

Vitamin B₁₂ (Cobalamin)

Decreased release of dietary vitamin B_{12} from food sources because of impaired pepsin and acid secretion, as in atrophic gastritis[26] or with use of PPIs,[27] usually results in only mild cobalamin malabsorption without clinical consequences. By contrast, deficiency of gastric intrinsic factor (IF) secretion, as occurs in pernicious anemia or after gastric resections, or secretion of an abnormal IF, as in some congenital diseases, results in severe vitamin B_{12} malabsorption with clinical consequences.[26]

Autoimmune gastritis of pernicious anemia is the most common cause of vitamin B_{12} malabsorption (see Chapter 52).[28] Cobalamin malabsorption in pernicious anemia is caused by decreased IF secretion, which results from parietal cell destruction and by the production of blocking autoantibodies that inhibit binding of IF to vitamin B_{12}.[28] Mild cobalamin

malabsorption may be found in patients with Zollinger-Ellison syndrome and in patients with pancreatic insufficiency, owing to decreased proteolytic release of vitamin B_{12} from its complex with R-binding protein[26,29] (see Chapters 33, 59, and 103).

In SIBO (see Chapter 105) or helminthic infection with *Diphyllobothrium latum* (see Chapter 114), dietary cobalamin is made unavailable to the host or consumed by the microorganisms or parasites in the intestinal lumen and is therefore unavailable for intestinal absorption.[28]

Diseases and conditions that affect the ileal mucosa (e.g., Crohn's disease, ileal resection) lead to a reduction of specific absorptive sites for the IF-vitamin B_{12} complex.[26] Ileal resections of more than 60 cm usually result in clinically significant vitamin B_{12} malabsorption.[30] Imerslund-Graesbeck syndrome, a disease of autosomal recessive inheritance due to abnormalities of the cubulin-amnionless complex, is characterized by selective ileal malabsorption of the IF-vitamin B_{12} complex despite normal ileal morphology (see Chapter 103).[26,31] Congenital diseases affecting transcobalamin II also result in malabsorption of cobalamin.[26,32]

In previously healthy persons it usually takes several years of vitamin B_{12} malabsorption before cobalamin deficiency develops, because hepatic stores contain large amounts of cobalamin and the daily requirement is relatively small.

Folate

Folate malabsorption occurs with mucosal diseases that affect the proximal small intestine, such as celiac disease and Whipple's disease.[33] Folate deficiency is common in chronic alcoholism, where it is postulated to be caused by decreased dietary intake as well as decreased intestinal absorption of folate.[34] As discussed later, several drugs result in impaired intestinal uptake of folate, and an inherited form of selective folate malabsorption has been described. In contrast to cobalamin, body stores of folate are small relative to daily requirements, so folate deficiency develops much faster (i.e., within weeks) than cobalamin deficiency in the setting of malabsorption. Increased serum folate levels resulting from bacterial production of tetrahydrofolate have been reported in SIBO.[35]

Other Water-Soluble Vitamins

Other water-soluble vitamins, such as ascorbic acid and the B-complex vitamins, are absorbed in the small intestine either by carrier-mediated transport or passive diffusion. Generalized malabsorption syndromes from intestinal causes impair the absorption of these vitamins, thereby leading to deficiency states.[36,37] Deficiency of water-soluble vitamins also occurs in chronic alcoholism, probably owing to decreased oral intake and reduced intestinal absorption.[34]

MINERALS

Calcium

Severe calcium malabsorption can occur in diseases that affect the small intestinal mucosa (e.g., celiac disease) and luminal malabsorption (e.g., exocrine pancreatic insufficiency), and has been shown to result in low-trauma fractures.[38] In these disease states, calcium absorption is impaired directly because of the reduction of the intestinal surface area (celiac disease) and indirectly because of formation of insoluble calcium soaps with malabsorbed long-chain fatty acids (pancreatic insufficiency). Diseases that cause malabsorption of long-chain fatty acids by other mechanisms, such as bile acid deficiency, can also result in calcium malabsorption.[23] In many of these diseases, malabsorption and deficiency of vitamin D further contribute to intestinal calcium malabsorption.[23] Selective intestinal malabsorption of calcium (i.e., without fat malabsorption) can occur in renal disease, hypoparathyroidism, and inborn defects in formation of 1α,25-dihydroxyvitamin D or in the intestinal vitamin D receptor.[23,39] Calcium malabsorption also commonly occurs after gastric resection (see "Malabsorption after Gastric Resection" [later]). Dosage of PPIs and duration of gastric acid suppression PPIs are associated with increased risk of hip fractures, presumably due in part to decreased or impaired absorption of dietary calcium, although both the magnitude and exact explanation of risk are controversial.[40]

Magnesium

In many generalized malabsorptive disorders, magnesium deficiency due to magnesium malabsorption results from a reduction in mucosal absorptive surface area and luminal binding of magnesium by malabsorbed fatty acids.[41] A congenital form of selective intestinal magnesium malabsorption has also been reported.[42]

Iron

Iron deficiency is common in patients with gastric resection or celiac disease. Reduction in the mucosal surface area of the small intestine as a result of diffuse mucosal disease, intestinal resection, or intestinal bypass can result in impaired iron absorption, potentially leading to iron deficiency.[43] A congenital form of iron malabsorption has also been described (see Table 104-10).[44] Intestinal loss of iron from chronic GI bleeding is, however, the most common GI cause of iron deficiency.[45] Worldwide, hookworm infection is the most common cause of iron deficiency.

Zinc

Zinc, like other minerals, is malabsorbed in generalized mucosal diseases of the small intestine.[46] A congenital selective defect of zinc absorption, acrodermatitis enteropathica, is caused by a defect in the zinc transport protein hZIP4 (See Table 104-10).[47]

Others

Generalized malabsorption can cause deficiency of copper and selenium.[48,49] In Menkes disease (kinky hair disease), an inherited disorder of cellular copper transport, selective intestinal copper malabsorption results (see later). It is uncertain whether malabsorptive diseases result in deficiencies of chromium and manganese.[46]

MECHANISMS THAT COMPENSATE FOR MALABSORPTION

Role of the Colon

The colon has the capacity to absorb a limited number but wide variety of substances and nutrients including sodium, chloride, water, oxalate, short-chain fatty acids, calcium, water-soluble vitamins (biotin, folate, pantothenic acid [B_5], pyridoxine [B_6], riboflavin [B_2], thiamine [B_1]), and vitamin K (see Chapter 103). Although colonic nutrient absorption plays a lesser role in health, the nutritive role of the colon in patients with severe malabsorption is clinically relevant.[50] Colonic

salvage of malabsorbed nutrients can also result in symptoms and complications[51] like colonic hyperabsorption of oxalate, which contributes to formation of renal stones (see later).

Colonic Salvage of Incompletely Absorbed Carbohydrates

In healthy people, between 2% and 20% of ingested starch escapes absorption in the small intestine[52]; pancreatic insufficiency or severe intestinal disorders further increases this amount.[19] Carbohydrates that reach the colon cannot be absorbed by the colonic mucosa but can be metabolized by colonic bacteria. Metabolism by anaerobic bacteria results in breakdown of oligosaccharides and polysaccharides to mono- and disaccharides, which are further metabolized to lactic acid, short-chain (C2 to C4) fatty acids (SCFAs; e.g., acetate, propionate, butyrate), and odorless gases (e.g., hydrogen, methane, carbon dioxide).[53]

Studies in normal subjects have suggested that bacterial metabolism of starch to small carbohydrate moieties is a rapid process in the normal colon. The rate-limiting step in the overall conversion of polysaccharides to SCFAs appears to be the conversion of monosaccharides to SCFAs.[19] Colonic absorption of SCFAs results in reduction of the osmotic load and, as a result, mitigation of osmotic diarrhea.[54] In normal subjects, more than 45 g of carbohydrates must reach the colon to cause diarrhea, and up to 80 g of carbohydrates per day can be metabolized by bacteria to SCFAs; approximately 90% of these SCFAs are absorbed by colonic mucosa[55] (Fig. 104-1). Chronic carbohydrate malabsorption causes adaptive changes in bacterial metabolic activity that result in even higher efficiency of the bacterial microbiota to digest carbohydrates,[56] but at the expense of increased flatus production (see later).

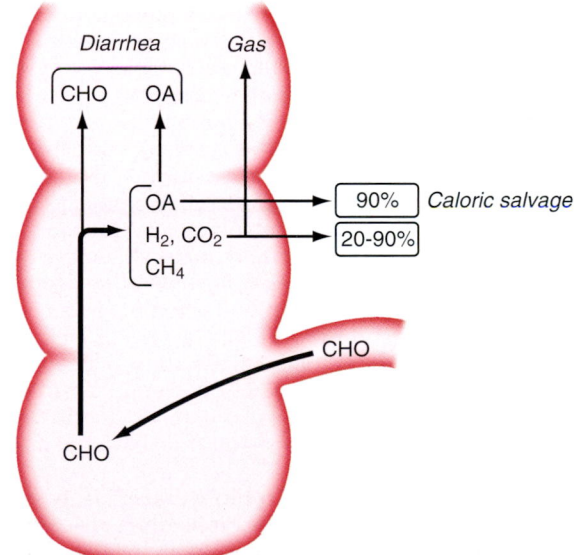

FIGURE 104-1. Carbohydrate metabolism and absorption of metabolic products in the colon. Up to 80 g of carbohydrate (*CHO*) that reaches the colon can be metabolized by colonic bacteria to organic acids (*OA*)–lactic acid and the SCFAs acetate, proprionate, and butyrate–and to hydrogen, carbon dioxide, and methane. Approximately 90% of the OA produced is absorbed by the colonic mucosa, which permits salvage of calories. Osmotic diarrhea results when OAs that escape absorption and CHO that escapes bacterial metabolism accumulate in the colon. Between 20% and 90% of gases produced in the colon is absorbed by the colonic mucosa; the remainder is excreted as flatus.

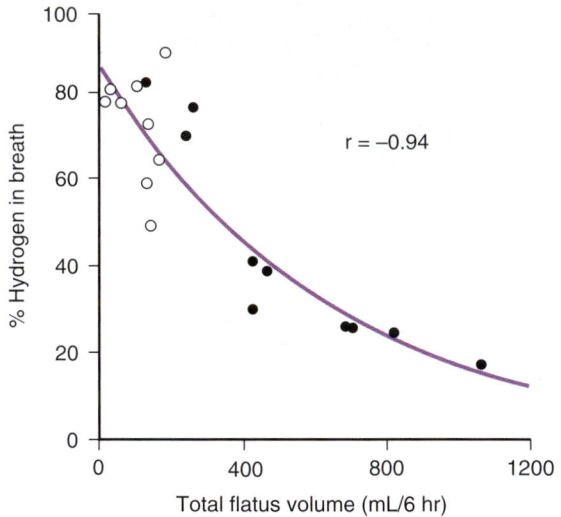

FIGURE 104-2. Relationship between flatus volume and colonic hydrogen absorption during fasting *(open circles)* and after ingestion of 12.5 g of lactose *(closed circles)*. At high flatus volumes, the fraction of hydrogen excreted in breath decreases to about 20% of total hydrogen excretion; the remaining 80% is excreted in flatus. *(From Hammer HF. Colonic hydrogen absorption: Quantification of its effect on hydrogen accumulation caused by bacterial fermentation of carbohydrates. Gut 1993; 34:818.)*

Because SCFAs have caloric values between 3.4 and 5.95 kcal/g,[57] their colonic absorption can contribute positively to overall calorie balance. In patients with short bowel syndrome, colonic salvage of malabsorbed carbohydrates can save up to 700 to 950 kcal/day, provided a substantial part of the colon remains in continuity with the small intestine.[58] Not all SCFAs are absorbed by the colon, and those not absorbed contribute to osmotic diarrhea (See Chapter 106).

The benefits of colonic bacterial carbohydrate metabolism may be offset by side effects due to gas production (see Chapter 17). Up to 10-fold differences in the volume of gas produced in the colon have been observed in normal persons.[59] The colon also can absorb gas, and if intracolonic gas volumes are low, up to 90% of the volume of intracolonic gas can be absorbed; if gas volumes are high, however, this proportion can decrease to 20%[59] (Fig. 104-2). Therefore, persons who have the disadvantage of producing more gas in their colons have an additional disadvantage of absorbing a smaller fraction of the gas. Gas produced from bacterial carbohydrate metabolism is odorless. The odor of flatus is due to volatile sulfur-containing substrates that result from bacterial metabolism of protein.[60]

Impaired colonic salvage of carbohydrates has been suggested to contribute to the diarrhea in Crohn's disease[61] and UC.[62] Bacterial carbohydrate metabolism may be lessened by antibiotic treatment.[63] In some patients, antibiotic-associated diarrhea may be the result of impaired colonic salvage of carbohydrates that are not normally absorbed or the result of dietary fiber that can accumulate in stool because of decreased bacterial fermentation.[64]

Role of the Colon in Fat Malabsorption

Long-chain triglycerides or fatty acids, which constitute most dietary fat, cannot be absorbed by the human colon. Long-chain fatty acids bind calcium in the colon, thereby increasing the amount of oxalate that is absorbed bound to sodium.[65]

Fatty acids with chain lengths longer than 12 carbons can cause diarrhea because they increase mucosal permeability and inhibit colonic absorption of fluid and electrolytes.[66] An increase in colonic permeability due to long-chain fatty acids also may be a contributing factor for the increased colonic oxalate absorption seen in patients with steatorrhea and hyperoxaluria.[67]

Patients with short bowel syndrome can gain caloric energy from colonic absorption of medium-chain fatty acids coming from medium-chain triglyceride supplementation if they have at least part of the colon in continuity with the remaining small intestine.[68] In the rat colon, absorption of octanoate is not affected by the simultaneous presence of other luminal substrates.[69]

Colonic Salvage of Calcium

Although most unabsorbed calcium is insoluble when it reaches the terminal ileum,[70] preservation of at least half of the colon in patients with extensive small bowel resection improves calcium absorption by about 40%, compared with calcium absorption in patients who have an ileostomy.[71] Absorption of calcium requires solubilization of calcium salts. Bacterial metabolism of dietary fiber or incompletely absorbed carbohydrates can help solubilize calcium by causing a decrease in the pH of luminal contents in the colon. Once calcium is solubilized, it can contact the cecal mucosa, which, in the rat, has the highest calcium absorption rate per surface area of intestine.[70] Calcium solubilization in the colon from bacterial fermentation of malabsorbed lactose can also occur in patients with lactose malabsorption; in this condition, the bioavailability of calcium from milk is greater than that from mineral water.[72] In addition to their effect on luminal pH, the SCFAs acetate and propionate, which are products of bacterial metabolism of lactose, have been shown to directly enhance calcium absorption in the human colon.[73]

Role of Intestinal Transit in the Salvage of Malabsorbed Nutrients

The lower parts of the GI tract do not normally contact nutrients, and when they do, intestinal transit time is prolonged.[74,75] This delay in transit could contribute to compensatory mechanisms in malabsorptive diseases, but nutritional salvage by this mechanism has not been quantitated. SCFAs prolong colonic transit time and thereby increase the contact time of liminal contents with the colonic mucosa.[76]

CLINICAL FEATURES AND EVALUATION

Malabsorption usually is suspected on the basis of the patient's history, signs and symptoms, or findings on routine laboratory evaluations. Malabsorption of an ingested nutrient or substrate can be confirmed by measuring its increased stool concentration or its decreased serum concentration or urinary excretion. Finding the cause of malabsorption often requires tests like endoscopy with small intestinal biopsy; under certain clinical circumstances, noninvasive tests or radiologic imaging are helpful in providing a specific diagnosis.

Suspecting and Confirming the Presence of Malabsorption

History and Physical Examination

Table 104-3 lists symptoms and signs suggestive of malabsorption, although virtually all can have causes other than

TABLE 104-3 Symptoms and Signs of Malabsorption and Relevant Pathophysiology

Symptom or Sign	Pathophysiologic Explanation
Gastrointestinal	
Diarrhea	Osmotic activity of carbohydrates or short-chain fatty acids
	Secretory effect of bile acids and fatty acids
	Decreased absorptive surface
	Intestinal loss of conjugated bile acids:
	Ileal resection
	Severe ileal mucosal disease
	Congenital defects of the ileal sodium-bile acid cotransporter
Abdominal distention, flatulence	Bacterial gas production from carbohydrates in colon, SIBO
Foul-smelling flatulence or stool	Malabsorption of proteins or intestinal protein loss
Pain	Gaseous distention of intestine
Ascites	Protein loss or malabsorption
Musculoskeletal	
Tetany, muscle weakness, paresthesias	Malabsorption of vitamin D, calcium, magnesium, and phosphate
Bone pain, osteomalacia, fractures	Protein, calcium, or vitamin D deficiency; secondary hyperparathyroidism
Cutaneous and Mucosal	
Easy bruisability, ecchymoses, petechiae	Vitamin K deficiency, vitamin C deficiency (scurvy)
Glossitis, cheilosis, stomatitis	Vitamin B complex, vitamin B_{12}, folate, or iron deficiency
Edema	Protein loss or malabsorption
Acrodermatitis, scaly dermatitis	Zinc and essential fatty acid deficiency
Follicular hyperkeratosis	Vitamin A deficiency
Hyperpigmented dermatitis	Niacin deficiency (pellagra)
Thin nails with spoon-shaped deformity	Iron deficiency
Perifollicular hemorrhage	Malabsorption of vitamin C
Spiral or curly hair	Malabsorption of vitamin C
Other	
Weight loss, hyperphagia	Nutrient malabsorption
Growth and weight retardation, infantilism	Nutrient malabsorption in childhood and adolescence
Anemia	Iron, folate, or vitamin B_{12} deficiency
Kidney stones	Increased colonic oxalate absorption
Amenorrhea, impotence, infertility	Multifactorial (including protein malabsorption, secondary hypopituitarism, anemia)
Night blindness, xerophthalmia	Vitamin A deficiency
Peripheral neuropathy	Vitamin B_{12} or thiamine deficiency
Fatigue, weakness	Calorie depletion, iron and folate deficiency, anemia
Neurologic symptoms, ataxia	Vitamin B_{12}, vitamin E, or folate deficiency

malabsorption. For example, greasy stools might indicate malabsorption, but a greasy appearance also can be caused by mucus in the stool. Floating of stool in the toilet water can be due to a high stool fat content, but it can also be caused by high gas content. Nevertheless, such symptoms and signs are helpful in raising the clinician's index of suspicion for malabsorption and in guiding the physician as to which specific laboratory tests, structural evaluations, or function tests should be ordered.

The current obesity epidemic has led to a changing picture of malabsorption; for example, few patients today with celiac disease are underweight at diagnosis, and some are even overweight. These patients have been reported to be less likely to present with classic features like diarrhea or anemia. In these patients, a further increase in weight after dietary gluten exclusion may be a cause of morbidity.[77]

Laboratory Findings

Certain blood tests might yield abnormal results in malabsorption, but with rare exceptions they are not specific for malabsorptive diseases. Blood tests also can be used as a screening tool to help the physician decide how vigorously to evaluate a patient for malabsorption. Table 104-4 lists blood tests in which abnormal results should raise the suspicion of malabsorption and stool tests that should be used to confirm that suspicion.

Quantitative fecal fat measurement followed by measurement of fecal chymotrypsin or elastase concentration may be helpful, both in establishing malabsorption and in differentiating between pancreatic and intestinal causes of malabsorption. Low levels of serum β-carotene, cholesterol, triglycerides, and calcium and a prolonged prothrombin time suggest malabsorption of fat and fat-soluble vitamins. Low levels of vitamin B_{12}, folate, iron, and albumin suggest malabsorption of water-soluble substances and therefore indicate intestinal disease rather than pancreatic or biliary disease. Severe deficiency of fat-soluble vitamins might indicate intestinal or biliary disorders. Low levels of plasma citrulline are associated with destructive small intestinal disease (e.g., celiac disease) or can follow intestinal resection,[78] although fasting plasma citrulline tests are poor predictors of enterocyte dysfunction in clinical practice. An oral citrulline generation test has been proposed to improve its predictive value.[79]

TABLE 104-4 Useful Laboratory Tests for Patients with Suspected Malabsorption and for Establishing Possible Nutrient Deficiencies

Test	Comment(s)
Blood Cell Count	
Hematocrit, hemoglobin	Decreased in iron, vitamin B_{12}, and folate malabsorption or with blood loss
Mean corpuscular hemoglobin or mean corpuscular volume	Decreased in iron malabsorption; increased in folate and vitamin B_{12} malabsorption
White blood cells, differential	Decreased in vitamin B_{12} and folate malabsorption; low lymphocyte count in lymphangiectasia
Biochemical Tests (Serum)	
TGs	Decreased in severe fat malabsorption
Cholesterol	Decreased in bile acid malabsorption or severe fat malabsorption
Albumin	Decreased in severe malnutrition, lymphangiectasia, protein-losing enteropathy
Alkaline phosphatase	Increased in calcium and vitamin D malabsorption (severe steatorrhea); decreased in zinc deficiency
Calcium, phosphorus, magnesium	Decreased in extensive small intestinal mucosal disease, after extensive intestinal resection, or in vitamin D deficiency
Zinc	Decreased in extensive small intestinal mucosal disease or intestinal resection
Iron, ferritin	Decreased in celiac disease, in other extensive small intestinal mucosal diseases, and with chronic blood loss
Other Serum Tests	
Prothrombin time	Prolonged in vitamin K malabsorption
β-Carotene	Decreased in fat malabsorption from hepatobiliary or intestinal diseases
Immunoglobulins	Decreased in lymphangiectasia, diffuse lymphoma
Folic acid	Decreased in extensive small intestinal mucosal diseases, with anticonvulsant use, in pregnancy; may be increased in SIBO
Vitamin B_{12}	Decreased after gastrectomy, in pernicious anemia, terminal ileal disease, SIBO, and infection with *Diphyllobothrium latum*
Methylmalonic acid	Markedly elevated in vitamin B_{12} deficiency
Homocysteine	Markedly elevated in vitamin B_{12} or folate deficiency
Citrulline	May be decreased in destructive small intestinal mucosal disease or intestinal resection
Stool Tests	
Fat	Qualitative or quantitative increase in fat malabsorption
Elastase, chymotrypsin	Decreased concentrations and output in exocrine pancreatic insufficiency
pH	Less than 5.5 in carbohydrate malabsorption

Diagnostic Approach

Clinical Clues to the Presence of Specific Diseases

Clinical clues (Table 104-5) or results of laboratory tests (Table 104-6)[80] can indicate the presence of a specific underlying disease or can help in the differential diagnosis. The following questions may be helpful and should be asked as part of the history before physical examination:
- Has the patient undergone previous surgery, such as gastric or small bowel resection or a GI bypass operation?
- Is there a family or childhood history of celiac disease?
- Is there a history of travel to underdeveloped countries or endemic areas of tropical sprue, giardiasis, or other GI infections?
- Is there excessive alcohol consumption?
- Does the patient have a history of chronic pancreatitis or symptoms suggesting a pancreatic tumor?
- Does the patient have clinical features of thyrotoxicosis, Addison's disease, Whipple's disease, biliary or liver disease, or diabetic neuropathy?
- Does the patient eat a diet high in poorly absorbable carbohydrates (sweeteners like sorbitol or fructose) or fat substitutes or an unbalanced diet that could result in malnutrition?
- Is there a likelihood of human immunodeficiency virus infection?
- Is the patient receiving treatment with a drug that can cause malabsorption?
- Does the patient have a history of stem cell or organ transplantation or abdominal radiation?
- Does the patient have a history of extraintestinal manifestations of inflammatory bowel disease, celiac disease, or Whipple's disease?

A rational approach to establishing the cause of malabsorption can require several diagnostic steps. Depending on the clinician's background, the availability of different tests, and the patient's preferences, different diagnostic approaches may be used. If time constraints are not a consideration, a stepwise approach may be used, starting with noninvasive evaluations that can guide further invasive procedures or even provide a diagnosis. In other instances, the physician may choose a more invasive test in the hope of reaching a diagnosis with the fewest possible tests and in the shortest possible time. Diagnostic approaches differ depending on the epidemiologic or ethnic background of an individual patient. For example, if parasitic infections are a likely possibility, stool examination

TABLE 104-5 Cardinal Clinical Features of Specific Malabsorptive Disorders

Disorder	Cardinal Clinical Features
Adrenal insufficiency	Skin darkening, hyponatremia, hyperkalemia
Amyloidosis	Renal disease, nephrotic syndrome, cardiomyopathy, neuropathy, carpal tunnel syndrome, macroglossia, hepatosplenomegaly
Bile acid deficiency	Ileal resection or disease, liver disease
Carcinoid syndrome	Flushing, cardiac murmur
Celiac disease	Variable symptoms: dermatitis herpetiformis, alopecia, aphthous mouth ulcers, arthropathy, neurologic symptoms, and (life-threatening) malnutrition; elevated liver biochemical test levels, mild iron deficiency
Crohn's disease	Arthritis, aphthous mouth ulcers, episcleritis, uveitis, pyoderma gangrenosum, erythema nodosum, abdominal mass, fistulas, perianal fistulae, primary sclerosing cholangitis (PSC), laboratory signs of inflammation
CF	Chronic sinopulmonary disease, meconium ileus, distal intestinal obstruction syndrome (DIOS), elevated sweat chloride
Cystinuria, Hartnup's disease	Kidney stones, dermatosis
Diabetes mellitus	Long history of diabetes and diabetic complications
Disaccharidase deficiency	Bloating and cramping, intermittent diarrhea
GI fistulas	Previous intestinal surgery or trauma, Crohn's disease
Glucagonoma	Migratory necrolytic erythema, enlarged gallbladder
Hyperthyroidism, hypothyroidism	Symptoms and signs of thyroid disease
Hypogammaglobulinemia	Recurrent infections
Intestinal ischemia	Other ischemic organ manifestations; abdominal pain with eating (chronic mesenteric ischemia)
Lymphoma	Enlarged mesenteric or retroperitoneal lymph nodes, abdominal mass, abdominal pain, fever
Mastocytosis	Urticaria pigmentosum, peptic ulcer
Mycobacterium avium complex infection	AIDS
Pancreatic insufficiency	History of pancreatitis, abdominal pain, or alcoholism; large-volume fatty, oily stools; passage of orange oil
Parasitic infection	History of travel to endemic areas
PBC	Jaundice, itching
Scleroderma	Dysphagia, inability to open the mouth widely, Raynaud's phenomenon, skin tightening
SIBO	Previous intestinal surgery, motility disorder (scleroderma, pseudo-obstruction), small intestinal diverticula, strictures
Tropical sprue	History of travel to endemic area
Tuberculosis	Specific history of exposure, living in or travel to endemic area, immunosuppression, abdominal mass or intestinal obstruction, ascites
Whipple's disease	Lymphadenopathy, fever, arthritis, cerebral symptoms, heart murmur (pulmonary valve), oculomasticatory myorhythmia
ZES	Peptic ulcers, diarrhea

TABLE 104-6 Useful Laboratory Tests in the Differential Diagnosis of Malabsorption

Test	Comment
Blood Cell Count	
Acanthocytes	Abetalipoproteinemia
Albumin	Low with protein-losing enteropathy, chronic inflammation (Crohn's disease)
Nuclear remnants in erythrocytes (Howell-Jolly bodies)	Splenic atrophy in celiac disease, IBD, radiation enteritis, amyloidosis
White blood cells, differential	Eosinophilia in eosinophilic gastroenteritis and parasitic disease
	Low lymphocyte count in lymphangiectasia, tuberculosis, protein-losing enteropathy
	Low CD4 count in AIDS
Platelets	Increased in inflammatory diseases
Other Tests	
ESR, C-reactive protein	Increased in Crohn's disease, Whipple's disease, lymphoma
Ferritin	Increased in inflammatory diseases, lymphoma; decreased in iron deficiency
Iron	Decreased in celiac disease, chronic occult intestinal bleeding, chronic inflammatory diseases
Liver biochemical tests	Increased in PBC and other liver diseases, celiac disease
Immunologic Markers	
Immunoglobulins	IgA deficiency, immunodeficiency syndromes; elevated IgM in PBC
Allergen-specific IgE	IgE-mediated hypersensitivity
Autoantibodies (e.g., ANA)	Connective tissue diseases
HLA-DQ2 or HLA-DQ8	Celiac disease, refractory sprue
Antimitochondrial autoantibodies	PBC
HIV-ELISA/Western blot	AIDS
Neuroendocrine Markers	
ACTH, cortisol	Abnormal values in Addison's disease
Chromogranin A	Elevated in neuroendocrine tumors
5-Hydroxyindoleacetic acid in urine	Elevated in carcinoid syndrome
Gastrin*	Elevated in ZES
Glucagon*	Elevated in glucagonoma
Serum TSH	Decreased in hyperthyroidism; increased in hypothyroidism
Somatostatin*	Elevated in somatostatinoma (normal in duodenal somatostatinoma)
Tissue transglutaminase antibodies, EMA	Celiac disease
Stool Tests	
Occult blood test	Erosive or ulcerative intestinal disease or tumor
Ova and parasites	Repeated samples may be needed to detect *Giardia lamblia*
Leukocytes, calprotectin	Present in some inflammatory diseases of the intestine

*Perform this test if there is a strong suspicion of an underlying neuroendocrine tumor.[341]
ANA, antinuclear antibodies; EMA, endomysial antibodies; ESR, erythrocyte sedimentation rate; Ig, immunoglobulin; TSH, thyroid-stimulating hormone.

can provide a rapid diagnosis by noninvasive testing. In populations with a very low prevalence of lactose intolerance, a secondary cause of lactose malabsorption is more likely than it would be in populations with a high prevalence of acquired primary lactase deficiency, so additional tests are appropriate.

The sequence of tests thus depends on the affected person's symptoms and history, as well as results of previous testing (Box 104-2). Tests that can detect the most common causes of malabsorption or are noninvasive or inexpensive usually should be performed initially (first-line tests). In some patients, testing for rarer causes of malabsorption and use of more invasive or more expensive tests may be necessary to establish the diagnosis (second-line tests). For unusually difficult cases, additional tests may be required that may be available only in specialized centers (third-line tests).

For some disorders (e.g., bile acid malabsorption, lactose malabsorption, SIBO) it may be difficult to establish a causal link between symptoms and the malabsorbed substrate. In these conditions, observation of the response to therapy may be critical in proving or disproving a causal relationship.

Anatomic Investigations

Endoscopic examination of the stomach, duodenum, or ileum and histologic examination of mucosal biopsy specimens can establish a diagnosis of some conditions causing malabsorption. The role of radiologic imaging examinations is limited mostly to answering questions about abdominal regions not easily accessible to endoscopy, such as parts of the small intestine, parenchymatous organs, the peritoneal cavity, the mesentery, or the retroperitoneum. Capsule endoscopy, balloon enteroscopy, and MRI are contributing to making these areas more accessible to diagnostic evaluation. Radiologic studies of the small intestine can show evidence of stasis, blind loops, diverticula, fistulas, rapid transit, and other abnormalities that can assist in diagnosis (see later).

BOX 104-2 Tests to Establish the Cause of Malabsorption Based on Main Symptoms

Weight Loss, Osteomalacia or Osteopenia, Diarrhea, Suspected Steatorrhea, or Deficiency of Fat-Soluble Vitamins
First-Line Tests
Abdominal and small intestinal US
Chymotrypsin or elastase concentration in stool
EGD with small intestinal biopsies
Endomysial or tissue transglutaminase antibodies
Laboratory tests (CBC, white blood cell differential, cholesterol, TGs, electrolytes, calcium, magnesium, serum ALT, AST, AP, bilirubin levels, prothrombin time, serum albumin level, erythrocyte sedimentation rate and C-reactive protein, TSH)
Ova, parasites, calprotectin and leukocytes in stool

Second-Line Tests
Abdominal CT, MRI
Endoscopic examination of the terminal ileum, including ileal biopsies
Enteroscopy, including biopsies
ERCP/MRCP
More extensive laboratory investigation (immunoglobulins, HIV ELISA, antinuclear antibodies, ferritin, food allergen–specific IgE, ACTH cortisol, chromogranin A, gastrin, urinary 5-HIAA)
Quantitative fecal fat
Quantitative small intestinal culture or breath tests for SIBO
Small bowel series/small bowel MRI
Special staining of small intestinal biopsies (e.g., Congo red for amyloid, PAS for Whipple's disease)
Therapeutic trial of pancreatic enzymes, antibiotics (tetracycline, metronidazole), cholestyramine, or a gluten-free diet
Video capsule endoscopy

Tests in Unusually Difficult Cases (Third-Line Tests)
Mesenteric angiography
Antienterocyte antibodies
EUS
MRA
PET
Serum or plasma glucagon, somatostatin
Somatostatin (octreotide) scan
Special tests of intestinal biopsies (e.g., flow cytometry of intraepithelial lymphocytes for lymphoma and refractory celiac disease, PCR for *Tropheryma whipplei* or other infective organisms, chromogranin A stain for enteroendocrine cells)

Spiral CT of the pancreas
Tests for bile acid malabsorption
Tube test for exocrine pancreatic secretion (secretin, CCK, or Lundh test)

Bloating, with or without Diarrhea
First-Line Tests
Fructose H_2 breath test
Lactose H_2 breath test
Lactose tolerance test

Second-Line Tests
Chymotrypsin or elastase concentration in stool
EGD with duodenal biopsies
Endomysial or tissue transglutaminase antibodies
Genetic testing for hypolactasia
Quantitative small intestinal culture or breath tests for SIBO
Stool pH (in patients with diarrhea)

Anemia and Suspected Malabsorption: Microcytic or hypochromic anemia (low MCV, MCH)
EGD with duodenal biopsies
Endomysial and tissue transglutaminase antibodies
Iron, ferritin, and transferrin in serum
Ova and parasites in stool
Video capsule endoscopy
Calprotectin
FOBT

Macrocytic anemia (high MCV, MCH)
First-Line Tests
Folic acid in serum or red blood cells
Vitamin B_{12} in serum

Second-Line Tests in Cases of Vitamin B_{12} Deficiency
CT, small bowel series, enteroclysis, video capsule endoscopy
EGD with gastric and duodenal biopsies
Endomysial and tissue transglutaminase antibodies
Evaluation of ileum (e.g., colonoscopy to ileum with biopsy, balloon enteroscopy with biopsy)
Ova and parasites in stool
Quantitative small intestinal culture or breath tests for SIBO
Calprotectin
Schilling test (with and without intrinsic factor)

Second-Line Tests in Cases of Folate Deficiency
EGD with duodenal biopsies
Endomysial or tissue transglutaminase antibodies

AP, alkaline phosphatase; CBC, complete blood cell count; FOBT, fecal occult blood test; 5-HIAA, 5-hydroxyindoleacetic acid; IgE, immunoglobulin E; MCH, mean corpuscular hemoglobin; MCV, mean corpuscular volume; PAS, periodic acid–Schiff; TSH, thyroid-stimulating hormone.

Endoscopy, Biopsy, and Duodenal Aspiration

Endoscopy

Endoscopic inspection of the duodenal mucosa can provide clues to some causes of malabsorption. Mosaic-like scalloping of duodenal folds (Fig. 104-3A) and reduction in the number of duodenal folds are highly suggestive of villus atrophy in celiac disease, although these abnormalities may be seen in other diseases (see Chapter 107).[81] The appearance of villus atrophy may be enhanced endoscopically using magnification endoscopy and chromoendoscopy with indigocarmine staining[82] or by virtual chromoendoscopy (narrow-band imaging [NBI], Flexible spectral Imaging Colour Enhancement [FICE]).[83,84] A normal duodenal fold pattern should not deter the endoscopist from taking multiple mucosal biopsy specimens. Aphthae suggest Crohn's disease, and small, diffuse, white-yellowish, punctate lesions can be seen in primary or secondary lymphangiectasia (Fig. 104-3B). Endocrine tumors causing malabsorption, such as duodenal gastrinomas or somatostatinomas or ampullary tumors that obstruct the pancreatic duct, can also be detected during endoscopy. If ileal disease is the suspected cause of malabsorption, visual examination and biopsy of the ileal mucosa may be required to establish a diagnosis; this can be accomplished by retrograde intubation of the ileum at colonoscopy or by single- or double-balloon endoscopy.

Biopsy

Examination of endoscopic biopsy specimens from the duodenum may be diagnostic or highly suggestive of a variety of

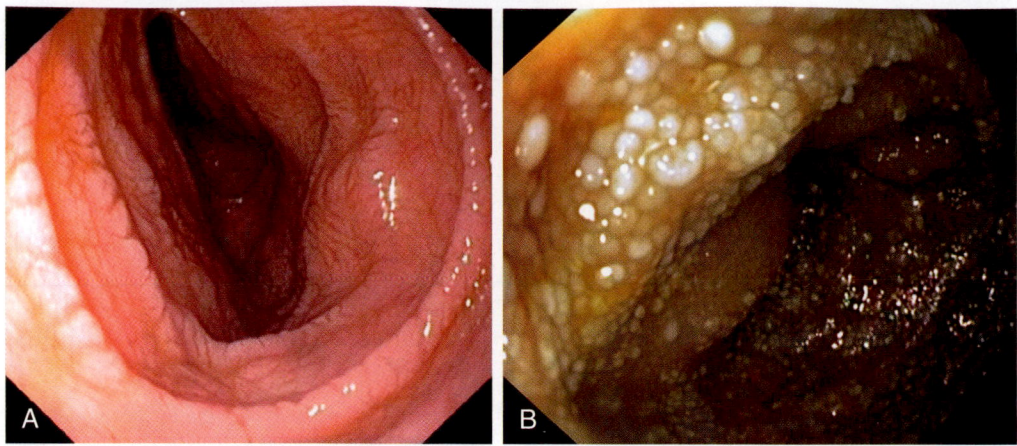

FIGURE 104-3. *A,* Endoscopic image showing scalloping of the duodenal folds in a patient with celiac disease. *B,* Endoscopic appearance of the ileum in a patient with primary intestinal lymphangiectasia; villi show a yellow-whitish studded appearance.

TABLE 104-7 Causes of Malabsorption That Can Be Diagnosed by Small Bowel Biopsy

Cause	Main Histologic Features
Generalized Histologic Abnormalities	
Abetalipoproteinemia, hypobetalipoproteinemia	Lipid accumulation and vacuolization of enterocytes
Collagenous sprue (Chapter 107)	Collagenous band below atrophic epithelium
Mycobacterium avium complex infection (Chapter 34)	Acid-fast bacilli, foam cells
Whipple's disease (Chapter 109)	Foamy macrophages with PAS-positive inclusion bodies
Patchy Histologic Abnormalities	
Amyloidosis	Congo red-stained deposits with apple-green birefringence in polarized light
Crohn's disease (Chapter 115)	Epithelioid granulomas and characteristic focal inflammation
Eosinophilic gastroenteritis (Chapter 29)	Eosinophilic infiltration
Lymphangiectasia (Chapter 30)	Ectatic lymph vessels
Lymphoma (Chapter 31)	Clonal expansion of lymphocytes
Mastocytosis (Chapter 36)	Diffuse infiltration with mast cells
Parasites and worms (*Giardia lamblia, Strongyloides stercoralis, coccidia*) (Chapters 113, 114)	Some parasites may be seen on histologic examination

PAS, periodic acid–Schiff.
Modified from Riddell RH. Small intestinal biopsy: Who? How? What are the findings? In: Barkin JS, Rogers AI, editors. Difficult decisions in digestive diseases. Chicago: Year Book; 1989. p 326.

small bowel disorders resulting in malabsorption (Table 104-7); follow-up small intestinal biopsy can be used to assess treatment effects. Duodenal biopsy specimens should be obtained from patients with atypical or nonspecific GI symptoms like abdominal pain, bloating, anemia, and weight loss and should not be limited only to patients with diarrhea.[85,86] The adequacy of mucosal biopsy specimens is a function of their size and the number obtained.[87] If large specimens are obtained using jumbo biopsy forceps, they can be oriented on a piece of filter paper before they are put into a fixing solution[88]; 2 or 3 jumbo biopsy specimens are usually sufficient to allow histologic sectioning parallel to the villi and crypts. Specimens may also be obtained with smaller forceps, although the number of specimens obtained must then be increased to 4 to 6.

The diagnostic yield of biopsy is influenced by the distribution of histologic abnormalities, which in some diseases is diffuse but in other diseases is patchy. Tropical diarrhea and an malabsorption syndrome (see Chapter 108), abetalipoproteinemia, and immunodeficiency usually result in a diffuse alteration of small intestinal mucosa. Thus, a normal duodenal biopsy specimen largely rules out these disorders. In contrast, primary lymphangiectasia has a patchy distribution, so a

single mucosal biopsy might not rule out the disorder (see Chapter 30). Patchy distribution has also been described for the histologic changes in some patients with celiac disease, especially when symptoms are subtle, although this disorder usually affects the small intestine diffusely.[82] Other possible sources of error and misdiagnosis include poorly oriented specimens and those obtained proximally, where confounding peptic injury can be the cause of mucosal alterations. Additional biopsy specimens from the stomach and duodenal bulb can help the pathologist establish the extent of peptic injuries in the upper GI tract and interpret inflammatory changes in the duodenum in relation to these lesions. Distortion of villus architecture over Brunner's glands or lymphoid aggregates, common in the duodenum, should be interpreted with caution.

Specific histologic features may be diagnostic for some rare causes of malabsorption (see Table 104-7)[89] like Whipple's disease (Fig. 104-4), abetalipoproteinemia or hypobetalipoproteinemia, intestinal lymphangiectasia, giardiasis (Fig. 104-5), lymphoma, or collagenous sprue. In most patients with small intestinal disorders, however, histologic examination is not diagnostic[89] (Box 104-3) and reveals a spectrum of mucosal responses ranging from infiltration by lymphocytes to a flat

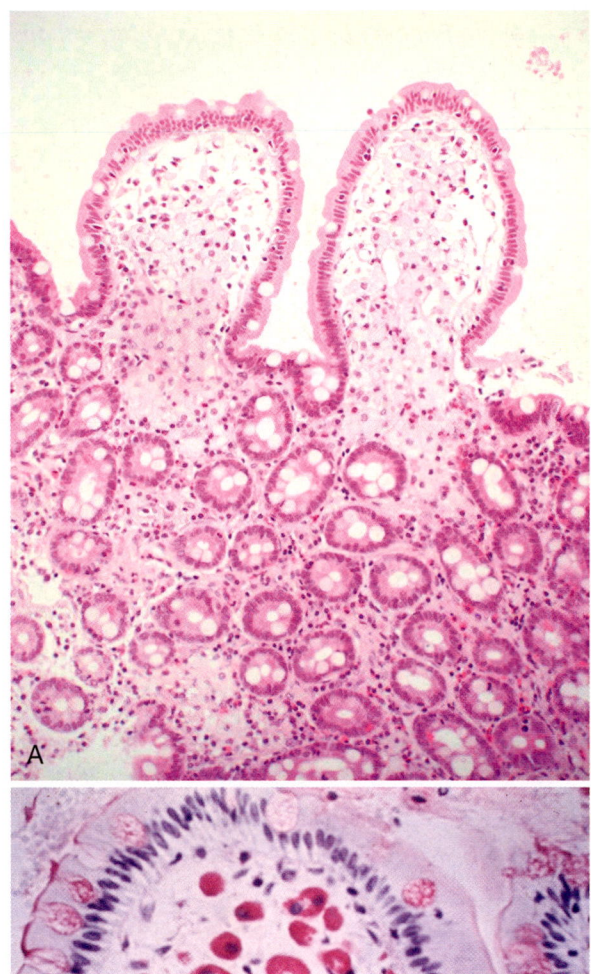

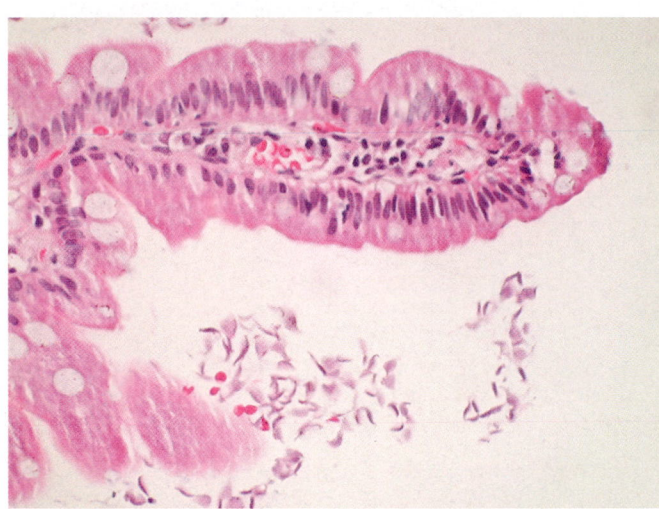

FIGURE 104-5. Small bowel biopsy specimen from an immunocompetent patient with giardiasis. A normal-appearing villus and adjacent pear-shaped organisms with red-staining nuclei are evident. *(Courtesy Cord Langner, MD.)*

FIGURE 104-4. Duodenal biopsy specimen from a patient with Whipple's disease. *A,* H&E staining shows villus blunting. Lamina propria is infiltrated with pale-staining foamy macrophages. *B,* High-power view demonstrates purple-red macrophages. (Periodic acid–Schiff stain.) *(A courtesy Cord Langner, MD. B courtesy Günter J. Krejs, MD, Graz, Austria.)*

mucosa with villus atrophy and crypt hyperplasia (Fig. 104-6). In many parts of the world, celiac disease is by far the most common cause of this type of histologic alteration, but a definite diagnosis of celiac disease cannot be established by mucosal biopsy alone (see Chapter 107).

Some disease states can be identified only with use of special histologic stains, such as Congo red (intestinal amyloidosis), periodic acid–Schiff (PAS) (Whipple's disease), or immunohistochemical techniques for detecting refractory celiac disease, small intestinal lymphoma, or enteroendocrine insufficiency (see later). Polymerase chain reaction (PCR) analysis of intestinal biopsy specimens for *Tropheryma whipplei* may be helpful in evaluating patients in whom Whipple's disease is suspected (see Chapter 109)[90]; the clinician specifically has

---

BOX 104-3 Malabsorptive Diseases with Abnormal but Nondiagnostic Small Intestinal Histologic Findings

Increased Lymphocyte Infiltration with or without Crypt Hyperplasia
AIDS enteropathy (Chapter 34)
Celiac disease (Chapter 107)
Infection (due to *Giardia lamblia, Cryptosporidium* [Chapter 113]; viral enteritis [Chapter 110])
Tropical sprue (Chapter 108)

Flat Lesion with or without Mucosal Inflammation
Celiac disease (Chapter 107)
Drug-induced enteropathy (NSAIDs, colchicine, neomycin (Chapter 119))
Food protein hypersensitivity (rye, barley, egg, fish, rice, poultry) (Chapters 10, 29)
Immunodeficiency (hypogammaglobulinemia) (Chapter 2)
Immunoproliferative small intestinal disease (IPSID) (Chapter 31)
Infection (due to *Giardia lamblia, Cryptosporidium*) (Chapter 113)
Intestinal transplantation (Chapter 106)
Lymphoma (Chapter 31)
Nongranulomatous chronic idiopathic enterocolitis (Chapter 107)
Autoimmune enteropathy (Chapter 98)
Prolonged folate or cobalamin deficiency
Protein-calorie malnutrition
Traumatic injury
Tropical sprue (Chapter 108)

Atrophic Lesion
Chronic radiation damage (Chapter 40)
Cicatrizing Crohn's disease (Chapter 115)
Diffuse lymphoma (Chapter 31)
Idiopathic diarrhea of infancy (microvillus inclusion disease) (Chapter 98)
Unresponsive gluten sensitivity (lymphoma or ulcerative jejunitis) (Chapter 107)

Modified from Riddell RH. Small intestinal biopsy: Who? How? What are the findings? In: Barkin JS, Rogers AI, editors. Difficult decisions in digestive diseases. Chicago: Year Book; 1989. p 326.

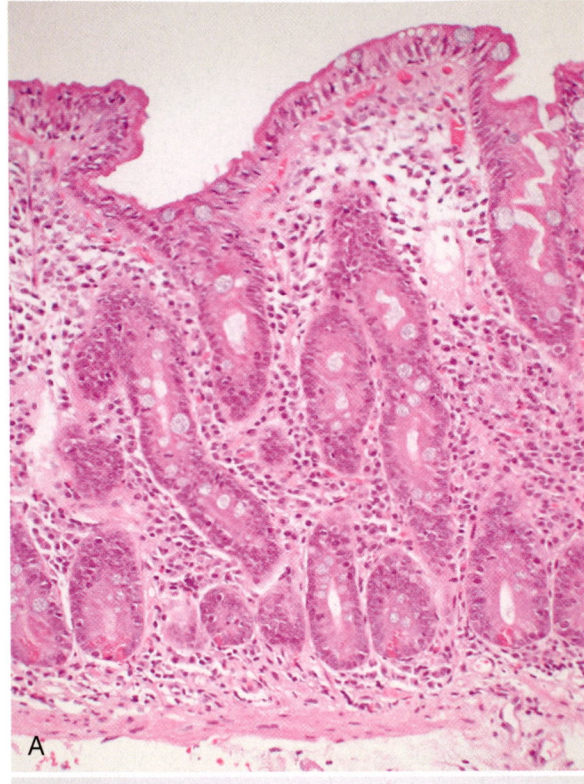

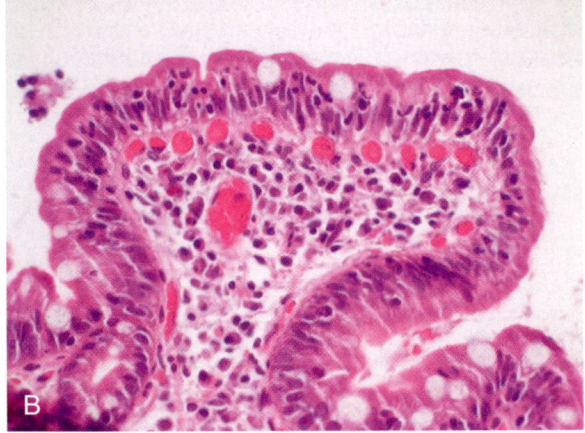

FIGURE 104-6. Duodenal biopsy specimen from a patient with untreated celiac disease. *A*, Subtotal villus atrophy, crypt elongation, and lymphoplasmacytic infiltration of lamina propria can be seen. *B*, High-power view demonstrates villus blunting with increased intraepithelial lymphocytes. (H&E stain.) *(Courtesy Cord Langner, MD.)*

to request these tests. Measurement of mucosal enzyme activities in a jejunal biopsy can be used to confirm disaccharidase deficiency, although this is not recommended for routine clinical use.

Aspiration

Fluid aspirated from the descending part of the duodenum may be examined microscopically for *Giardia lamblia* (see Chapter 113) or cultured to detect SIBO in patients with diffuse small intestinal motility disorders (see Chapters 99, 105, and 124).

Video Capsule Endoscopy and Balloon Enteroscopy

Video capsule endoscopy (VCE) is an increasingly popular technique for diagnosing diseases of the small intestine. VCE was initially introduced for evaluating suspected bleeding in the small intestine, but it has subsequently been used to diagnose a wider range of diseases such as Crohn's disease, celiac disease, and other malabsorptive disorders. In several studies, lesions suggesting Crohn's disease were detected by VCE when they had been missed by conventional diagnostic procedures.[91] These reports must be interpreted carefully because they lack biopsy specimens and there are no long-term evaluations to confirm diagnoses.

VCE appears to be superior to conventional radiologic imaging of the small intestine and CT enterography to detect subtle mucosal changes like aphthous or erosive lesions of the small intestine.[91] In celiac disease, detection of villus atrophy by VCE has a good correlation to villus atrophy seen in duodenal biopsy specimens,[92,93] but it is questionable whether this procedure can detect subtle changes, such as Marsh 1 and 2 lesions. Changes on VCE that suggest villus atrophy are scalloping, mosaic pattern, and fissuring. In a study of VCE in patients with celiac sprue, villus atrophy was seen in the duodenum and jejunum in 59% of cases, in the duodenum only in 32%, and in the jejunum only in 3%.[93]

In refractory celiac disease, VCE can detect changes such as ulcerations and strictures that suggest T-cell lymphoma but that are missed by conventional techniques.[94] This test may be used in patients with established malabsorption in whom no diagnosis has been established despite extensive diagnostic workup.

In some cases of malabsorption, balloon enteroscopy with biopsies of the jejunum and ileum can be helpful to establish the diagnosis. Compared with VCE, balloon enteroscopy has the advantage of being able to obtain biopsy specimens from altered mucosal areas, but it is time consuming and uncomfortable for the patient. In a series of 12 patients with malabsorption, diagnoses of various small intestinal diseases that would have been missed with duodenal biopsies were solely established by balloon enteroscopy in one third of patients.[95] Balloon enteroscopy with jejunal biopsy is reserved for patients with an elusive diagnosis; for celiac disease, endoscopically obtained jejunal biopsies are rarely helpful compared with duodenal biopsies.[96]

Abdominal Imaging

Small Bowel Follow-through and Small Bowel Enteroclysis

The principal role of small bowel radiologic series in evaluating malabsorption is to identify focal or diffuse abnormalities that predispose to SIBO, such as diverticula, stagnant loops of intestine, generalized intestinal hypomotility or dilatation, intestinal fistulas, and tumors.[97]

Small bowel enteroclysis is preferred to small bowel follow-through examination, because distention of the lumen results in better demonstration of the small bowel contour.[98] Double-contrast enteroclysis, in which the upper jejunum is intubated for direct instillation of contrast material, has a higher sensitivity than small bowel series for detecting mucosal changes, although it is less acceptable to the patient and can miss focal changes in the duodenum, such as diverticula. Use of an intravenous agent such as glucagon to reduce motility enables overlapping loops of small intestine to be separated and imaged more distinctly.

Alterations associated with diffuse, localized, or distal mucosal changes that might have been missed by more proximal mucosal biopsy also may be identified. A normal small bowel series does not exclude intestinal causes of malabsorption and should not dissuade the clinician from performing biopsy of the small intestine.

Ulcerations and strictures may be seen in various malabsorptive disorders, including Crohn's disease, radiation enteritis, celiac disease, intestinal lymphoma, and tuberculosis. Aphthous ulcers and cobblestoning of the mucosa, either alone or with thickened and distorted folds, are features of Crohn's disease but can also be present in other conditions. Reduced numbers of jejunal folds and an increased number of and thickening of ileal folds can suggest celiac disease.[97] Mass lesions can be found with intestinal lymphoma or, rarely, with hormone-producing tumors.

The disadvantage of conventional enteroclysis is that direct imaging of the bowel wall and surrounding structures is not possible, and overlapping bowel loops potentially impair complete evaluation of the whole small bowel—hence the rationale for combining enteroclysis with CT or MRI scanning.[99]

Abdominal CT

Abdominal CT for small bowel evaluation is performed after administration of oral or IV contrast agents.[100] Small intestinal CT scanning is useful to detect focal intestinal lesions, such as thickening of the small bowel wall in Crohn's disease or small intestinal lymphoma, intestinal fistula, and dilated bowel loops; however, mild mucosal changes like aphthae in Crohn's disease or villus atrophy from various causes are missed by this technique. Diffuse thickening of the small bowel may be seen in Whipple's disease and in graft-versus-host disease.[100] In some cases of celiac disease, reversal of the jejunoileal fold pattern is observed.[101] CT is a sensitive test to detect enlarged abdominal lymph nodes, which can be present in disorders such as Whipple's disease, small bowel lymphoma, or small intestinal inflammatory diseases like Crohn's disease. Evidence for pancreatic disease that may be detected on CT includes calcifications of the pancreas, dilatation of the pancreatic duct, and pancreatic atrophy. Tumors that obstruct the pancreatic duct or hormone-secreting neuroendocrine tumors can also be located by CT.

MRI of the Small Intestine

MRI may be used to image the small intestine, either with administration of oral contrast media or by enteroclysis. Segmental bowel wall thickening with inflammatory involvement of the mesentery, cobblestoning, and ulcerations may be seen in Crohn's disease; this method is very sensitive for demonstrating complications of Crohn's disease (e.g., intestinal fistula formation). In celiac disease, small bowel MRI with oral contrast can demonstrate small intestinal dilatation, mucosal thickening, and an increased number of folds in the ileum (ileal jejunization) with flattening of duodenal and jejunal folds reversal of pattern).[102,103] The extent of MRI findings suggestive of celiac disease depends on clinical presentation of celiac disease and are more extensive when classical symptoms are present than when celiac disease is silent.[103] Most signs of celiac disease are also found in other inflammatory diseases of the intestine, but the fold pattern abnormalities are most specific for celiac disease.[102] MRI enteroclysis also is very useful to detect changes suggesting complications like lymphoma or carcinoma[104] and has been shown helpful in distinguishing refractory celiac disease type II from uncomplicated

celiac disease. In refractory celiac disease type II, 2 or more of the following features were present on MRI: presence of less than 10 folds per 5 cm jejunum, mesenteric fat infiltration, and bowel wall thickening.[105] With MRI enteroclysis, subtle mucosal changes might be missed and be more evident on conventional small bowel enteroclysis[106] or capsule endoscopy.[91] Because MRI or CT imaging of the small intestine may not require tube placement and displays the whole intestinal wall, these techniques have largely replaced classic small bowel enteroclysis.

US Examination

Transabdominal US examination has the advantage of no radiation exposure and therefore can be used in pregnant patients. Ultrasound examination often is performed by the treating gastroenterologist and is therefore widely available without a substantial waiting period in many countries. Ultrasonography is often used to investigate the pancreas, although the sensitivity for detecting pancreatic tumors is lower than that of ERCP or CT. Nevertheless, obstruction of the biliary tract, pancreatic calcifications, dilatation of the pancreatic duct, or stones within the pancreatic duct may be demonstrated. Ultrasound examination of the small intestine has been used with increased frequency in recent years. Inflammatory diseases of the small intestine like celiac disease, Crohn's disease, mycobacterial infections, and Whipple's disease, as well as small intestinal lymphomas, can exhibit thickening of the small bowel wall, loss of the small bowel layers, and enlarged mesenteric lymph nodes on US.[107] In celiac disease, thickening of the small bowel wall (>3 mm) and dilatation of the bowel loops (>2.5 cm) have been suggested to be the most sensitive markers.[108] A hyperechoic appearance of the bowel wall may be suggestive for Whipple's disease (Fig. 104-7), AIDS enteropathy, or mycobacterial infections,[109] and the presence of intraluminal abscesses in the ileocecal region for intestinal tuberculosis.[110] Intravenous and oral contrast agents have been used for better differentiation of small intestinal alterations on US examination.[107]

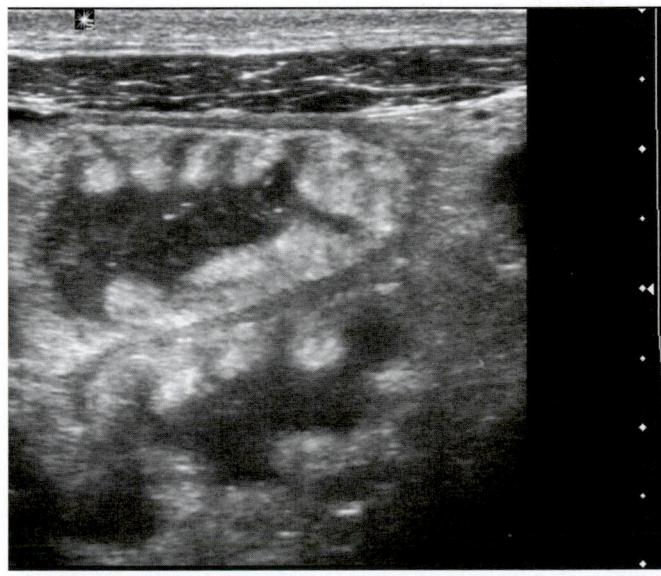

FIGURE 104-7. Ultrasound examination of a patient with Whipple's disease, showing hyperechoic wall thickening of small intestine, submucosal lymphatic prominence, and dilatation of intestinal loops. (*Courtesy Christina Genger, MD.*)

Other Studies

A plain film of the abdomen may be helpful to detect pancreatic calcifications if exocrine pancreatic insufficiency is suspected, although morphologic signs of chronic pancreatitis alone do not prove a pancreatic cause of malabsorption, because the function of the exocrine pancreas must be severely impaired before malabsorption becomes evident. A plain film of the abdomen can also document dilated loops of intestine; dilated loops predispose to SIBO or suggest the presence of an obstruction.

ERCP can help establish the cause of pancreatic insufficiency (see Chapter 59). It can also help distinguish chronic pancreatitis from pancreatic tumor and can document pancreatic duct stones. ERCP and EUS are the methods of choice for documenting various causes of biliary obstruction. MRCP is increasingly being used to replace diagnostic ERCP. If a neuroendocrine tumor (e.g., gastrinoma, somatostatinoma) is the suspected cause of malabsorption, an indium-111 octreotide scintigraphic scan, PET, or an EUS examination of the pancreas may be helpful to establish the diagnosis or demonstrate the extent of disease (see Chapter 33).

Noninvasive Evaluation of GI Digestive and Absorptive Function

Some conditions that cause malabsorption can be diagnosed by noninvasive testing, although, as illustrated in Table 104-8, diagnostic accuracy may be limited, and further tests may be necessary to identify underlying diseases or differentiate primary and secondary causes. Apart from providing a diagnosis, tests that evaluate GI absorptive and digestive function may be helpful in evaluating complex disease presentations. For most or all of the following tests, the potential benefits with regard to the costs of workup or to patient acceptability have not been established. Because test procedures and ana-

lytical methods can vary among laboratories,[111] each laboratory should establish its own reference values for these tests.

Fat Malabsorption

Quantitative Fecal Fat Analysis

The van de Kamer method is the quantitative titration of fatty acid equivalents in which results are expressed as fecal output of fat in grams per 24 hours. This method is considered the gold standard for fecal fat analysis.[112] Modifications in which the extracted fats are weighed rather than titrated[113] have an excellent correlation with the results of the van de Kamer method. Near-infrared reflectance analysis may be a less cumbersome method to quantify fecal fat output in stool collections,[114] because it requires less handling of stool by laboratory personnel, but it still requires a 48- to 72-hour collection to exclude the influence of day-to-day variability. The stool must be mixed before a sample is obtained for analysis.

Fecal fat excretion of less than 7 g/day with a fat intake of 100 g/day usually is considered normal. The volume effect of diarrhea by itself, however, may increase fecal fat output to levels of up to 14 g/day (secondary fat malabsorption)[115] (Fig 104-8). With significant diarrhea, a fecal fat excretion of 14 g/day should be used as the upper limit of normal. Diet is important in considering causes of steatorrhea; for example, elevated fecal fat values can be observed in patients consuming a diet rich in the fat substitute olestra.[113]

Quantitative fecal fat analysis is routinely available now in only a few centers. Reasons for its limited clinical use are: (1) If the main symptom of malabsorption is chronic diarrhea, measurement of fecal fat might not influence the subsequent evaluation, because the diagnostic tests performed to establish the etiology of diarrhea are similar to the tests for the workup of steatorrhea. (2) An elevated fecal fat level usually cannot differentiate among biliary, pancreatic, and enteric causes of

TABLE 104-8 Malabsorptive Diseases or Conditions in Which Noninvasive Tests Can Establish Malabsorption or Provide a Diagnosis

Disease or Condition	Diagnostic Test(s)*	Comment(s)
Lactose malabsorption	Lactose hydrogen breath test Lactose tolerance test	Tests do not differentiate between primary and secondary lactose malabsorption.
Incomplete fructose absorption	Fructose hydrogen breath test	
SIBO (see Chapter 105)	^{14}C-D-xylose breath test Glucose hydrogen breath test Schilling test with and without antibiotics	A predisposing factor should be sought if the result of any of the tests is positive.
Bile acid malabsorption	SeHCAT test, ^{14}C-TCA test	Does not differentiate between primary and secondary causes.
Exocrine pancreatic insufficiency	Quantitative fecal fat determination Fecal elastase or chymotrypsin, tubeless tests (see Chapters 56 and 59)	Used to establish malabsorption in chronic pancreatitis Variable sensitivity and specificity, depending on the type of test and stage of the disease.
Vitamin B$_{12}$ malabsorption	Schilling test	The test is performed without intrinsic factor and, depending on the result with intrinsic factor, with antibiotics or pancreatic enzymes (see text). Further tests are necessary if SIBO, terminal ileal disease, or pancreatic disease is suspected.

*See text for diagnostic accuracy of the different tests listed.
SeHCAT, selenium-75-homotaurocholic acid test; TCA, taurocholic acid.

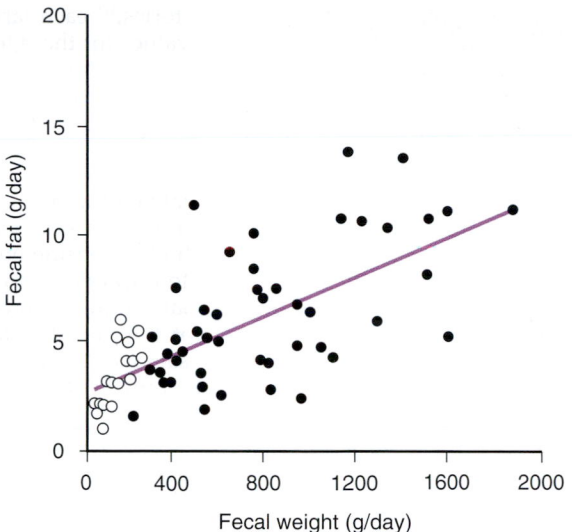

FIGURE 104-8. Graph showing fecal fat output (average of a 3-day stool collection) plotted as a function of fecal weight from normal subjects *(open circles)* and subjects with induced diarrhea *(closed circles)*. The washout effect of diarrhea increases fecal excretion of fat to levels above the upper limit of normal (7 g/day). With significant diarrhea, a fecal fat excretion of 14 g/day should be used as the upper limit of normal. *(From Fine KD, Fordtran JS. The effect of diarrhea on fecal fat excretion. Gastroenterology 1992; 12:1936-9.)*

malabsorption. (3) In many patients with severe steatorrhea, the stools have a very foul smell and a characteristic porridge-like appearance, and quantitative studies are not necessary to establish fat malabsorption. (4) Fat absorption may be normal despite malabsorption of other nutrients, so a normal fat balance does not imply normal absorptive function of the GI tract. (5) Finally, accuracy depends on quantitative stool collections for 48 to 72 hours, adherence to a diet that contains 80 to 100 g of fat daily, and a diet diary to determine fat intake. Science aside, quantitative fecal fat analysis has never been popular among patients, physicians, or laboratory personnel performing the test.

Despite the limitations of quantitative fecal fat analysis, it nevertheless is still useful in several clinical circumstances: to establish malabsorption and avoid nutritional deterioration[116] when overt features of intestinal or pancreatic disorders are lacking, as in some cases of osteoporosis, osteomalacia, anemia, or weight loss; to monitor treatment in patients with established malabsorptive disorders, such as exocrine pancreatic insufficiency or short bowel syndrome; to estimate fecal calorie loss in patients with severe malabsorption syndromes; and to quantitate fecal fat excretion in patients with diarrhea who have undergone ileal resection, thereby distinguishing steatorrhea due to bile acid deficiency from secretory diarrhea caused by bile acid loss.[117]

Semiquantitative Fat Analysis

For the acid steatocrit (AS) test,[118] a sample of stool is diluted 1:3 with distilled water in a test tube. The diluted stool is homogenized, and a 500-μL aliquot is pipetted into a tube. Then 100 mL of 5M $HClO_4$ is added to allow better fat extraction and separation of the lipid layer. An aliquot of the diluted stool-$HClO_4$ mixture is put into a non-heparinized microcapillary tube and sealed on one end. After centrifugation of this aliquot at 13,000 rpm for 15 minutes, the fatty layer (FL) and

the solid layer (SL) are measured, and the AS is determined according to the following equation:

$$AS\ (\%) = \left[\frac{FL}{(FL + SL)}\right] \times 100$$

An AS of less than 31% is normal. In a small study, the AS for random spot stool samples had a high sensitivity and specificity for detection of steatorrhea, compared with the van de Kamer method, which is performed on a 72-hour stool collection. A linear correlation was also found between results obtained with the AS and those of the van de Kamer method, although results were quite divergent in some patients.[118] Because quantitative fecal fat measurements are based on 48- to 72-hour stool collections (to minimize the effect of day-to-day variability in fecal fat excretion), the AS cannot be expected to replace quantitative measurement of fat output in borderline cases or cases where exact measurement of fecal fat loss is required.

Qualitative Fecal Fat Analysis

Although fat analysis by microscopic examination of random stool samples might provide a clue to the presence of steatorrhea, it cannot be used to exclude steatorrhea; its sole advantage is its ease of performance. A sample of stool is placed on a glass slide to which several drops of glacial acetic acid and Sudan III stain are added. Acidification of stool samples improves fat extraction and separation of the lipid layer.[118] The slide is held over a flame-burner, and the acidified mixture is heated to boiling then examined while still warm for the presence of orange fat globules. A count of up to 100 globules, each with a diameter less than 4 mm, per high-power field is normal.[6]

Results of qualitative fat analysis by this method and of quantitative fat analysis do not correlate very well.[119] In a small study, Sudan staining of spot stool samples had a sensitivity of 78% and a specificity of 70% for the detection of steatorrhea.[118] A quantitative microscopic method of counting and measuring fat globules using the Sudan stain has been shown to correlate well with chemically measured fecal fat output.[120]

Breath Tests for Fat Malabsorption

The principle of the ^{14}C-triolein breath test is to measure [14]CO_2 in the breath after ingestion of a triglyceride that has been radiolabeled with [14]C. Fat malabsorption results in decreased pulmonary excretion of [14]CO_2.[121] Because of erroneous results in a variety of metabolic and pulmonary diseases, lack of sensitivity in mild malabsorption, radiation exposure to the patient, cost of the substrate, and the need for expensive equipment, this test has not found widespread acceptance for clinical use. The nonradioactive isotope ^{13}C is used to label triglycerides instead (see later).

Serum Tests for Fat Malabsorption

The photometric measurement of β-carotene at 456 nm[122] has been suggested as a useful screening test for steatorrhea, although experience with this technique is limited. Values less than 100 mg per 100 mL suggest the presence of steatorrhea, and values less than 47 mg per 100 mL strongly indicate steatorrhea. Concentrations in excess of 100 mg per 100 mL do not exclude mild steatorrhea, although they make steatorrhea with fat losses in excess of 16 g/day very unlikely. Normal values also have been established in the pediatric population.[123] β-Carotene can be falsely low in patients with liver disease or in alcoholics who consume a diet deficient in β-carotene. Disorders in lipoproteins or intake of carotene-containing food additives can also influence results.

Carbohydrate Malabsorption

The hydrogen breath test is a noninvasive test that takes advantage of the fact that in most people, bacterial metabolism of carbohydrate results in accumulation of hydrogen, which then is absorbed by the colonic mucosa and excreted in the breath. Using different carbohydrates, such as lactose or fructose, the hydrogen breath test can be used to detect malabsorption of these carbohydrates. Measurement of breath hydrogen excretion after ingestion of lactulose has been used to assess orocecal transit time, and glucose has been used as a substrate to detect SIBO, although sensitivity and specificity are poor.[124] Unfortunately, up to 18% of people are hydrogen nonexcretors,[125] and in these persons, hydrogen breath test results may be falsely negative because hydrogen is further metabolized by bacteria to methane. Such limitations and pitfalls of breath hydrogen testing have to be taken into account when test results are interpreted.[126]

The diagnosis of lactose malabsorption is established if an increase in breath hydrogen concentration of greater than 20 parts per million over baseline occurs after ingestion of 20 to 50 grams of lactose. An increase within the first 30 minutes after ingestion of lactose has to be disregarded because it may be due to bacterial degradation of lactose in the oral cavity. Up to 4 hours may be required for the increase in breath hydrogen concentration to occur. Breath hydrogen measurements obtained before and at 30, 60, 90, 180, and 240 minutes after ingestion of 50 g of lactose provide the best diagnostic yield with the fewest possible measurements.[125]

The lactose hydrogen breath test is still performed by most clinicians for evaluating lactose malabsorption, but this test can miss the disorder in hydrogen nonexcretors. In these patients, a lactose tolerance test—measurement of blood glucose levels before and 30 minutes after ingestion of 50 g of lactose—can be used. An increase in glucose concentration of less than 20 mg/dL over baseline within 30 minutes of ingestion of 50 g of lactose indicates lactose malabsorption. The lactose tolerance test has a lower sensitivity than the lactose hydrogen breath test for diagnosing lactose malabsorption.[125]

Lactase deficiency in acquired primary lactase deficiency (adult-type hypolactasia) is not caused by mutations in the gene coding for intestinal lactase (LPH gene). It has been shown, however, that a single-nucleotide polymorphism (SNP), either the C or T nucleotide −13910 upstream of the LPH gene, is involved in regulating intestinal lactase expression.[127] A CC genotype at −13910 C/T is associated with acquired primary lactase deficiency (adult-type hypolactasia), whereas TC and TT genotypes are linked with lactase persistence.[128,129] This polymorphism can be used as a diagnostic test for adult-type hypolactasia.[129,130] This SNP is only associated with adult-type hypolactasia in whites; other SNPs are linked to adult-type hypolactasia or lactase persistence in Africans.[131] In patients with diarrhea, a stool test to detect a fecal pH lower than 5.5 can serve as a qualitative indicator of carbohydrate malabsorption.[132] In the research setting, fecal carbohydrates can be determined by the anthrone method, which measures carbohydrates on a weight basis.[133] By contrast, the reducing sugar method gives results on a molar basis and provides information about the osmotic activity of malabsorbed carbohydrates.[19] Total SCFAs and lactic acid, which are the products of bacterial carbohydrate metabolism, can be measured in stool by titration.[134] Individual SCFAs can be determined by gas chromatography.[135]

Protein Malabsorption

The classic test to quantify protein malabsorption, measurement of fecal nitrogen content in a quantitatively collected stool specimen,[13] is rarely used today. For research purposes, a combined ^{14}C-octanoic acid–^{13}C-egg white breath test, accompanied by measurement of the urinary output of phenol and p-cresol, has been used to assess the effect of gastric acid on protein digestion.[136] In this method, labeling of the ^{13}C-egg protein test meal with ^{14}C-octanoic acid allows simultaneous measurement of protein assimilation and gastric emptying rate. Phenol and p-cresol are the quantitatively most important phenolic compounds in feces and urine and are specific metabolites of tyrosine, produced by bacterial fermentation in the colon. They result from protein that has escaped digestion and absorption in the small intestine and are rapidly absorbed in the colon, detoxified, and excreted in urine. Recovery of higher amounts of urinary phenols observed after omeprazole treatment in the study of this test indicated an increased availability of protein in the colon.

Vitamin B₁₂ (Cobalamin) Malabsorption

Schilling Test

The Schilling test can be used clinically to distinguish between gastric and ileal causes of vitamin B_{12} deficiency but is rarely performed today. Because both IF and hydrochloric acid are produced by parietal cells in humans, alternative approaches to diagnosing pernicious anemia are to document atrophic gastritis by endoscopy and biopsy, to confirm achlorhydria by acid secretion analysis (also rarely performed today) and increased serum gastrin levels, and to look for antibodies in the serum directed against parietal cells or IF.[28,137] Because the IF used in the Schilling test is of bovine origin, the test is not commercially available in most countries.

The Schilling test is performed by administering a small oral dose of radiolabeled vitamin B_{12} and, simultaneously or within 1 or 2 hours, a large intramuscular flushing dose of nonradiolabeled vitamin B_{12}. The unlabeled B_{12} saturates vitamin B_{12} carriers, so any radioactive vitamin B_{12} absorbed by the intestine is excreted in the urine. If less than 7% to 10% of the administered dose is recovered in urine within 24 hours, vitamin B_{12} malabsorption is confirmed. To specify the site of vitamin B_{12} malabsorption, a second phase of the Schilling test is performed subsequently with oral administration of IF. In patients with pernicious anemia, the results of the Schilling test normalize after oral administration of IF.[26,137]

Patients with pancreatic exocrine insufficiency might have an abnormal result on the Schilling test, with or without added IF, but results normalize with addition of pancreatic enzymes (see Chapter 59). In SIBO, results of the Schilling test can improve after antibiotic therapy (see Chapter 105). In ileal disease or following ileal resection, abnormal results of the Schilling test persist despite IF. Schilling test results are normal in patients with dietary vitamin B_{12} deficiency, in protein-bound (food-bound) vitamin B_{12} malabsorption,[26] and sometimes in congenital transcobalamin II deficiency.[138] False-positive results on the Schilling test can result from renal dysfunction or inadequate urine collection.[137] The value of this test is diminished by the need for accurately timed urine collections. Results in the 5% to 10% excretion range often are difficult to interpret. A variation of the standard Schilling test is the dual-isotope or single-stage Schilling test, in which 2 different cobalamin isotopes are given simultaneously, 1 of them bound to IF. This makes it possible to perform the first 2 phases of the Schilling test in 1 day, but the results of this test are not as accurate as those obtained with the standard protocol.[26,137]

Serum Test for Vitamin B$_{12}$ and Folate Deficiency

Measurements of serum cobalamin and folate concentrations are commonly used to detect deficiency states of these vitamins. The sensitivity and specificity of these tests are unknown because no gold standard test has been established and because serum levels do not always correlate with body stores.[26,139] Furthermore, results of vitamin B$_{12}$ levels vary with different commercial tests.[140]

Several causes of misleading serum cobalamin levels have been established. Serum vitamin B$_{12}$ levels can be normal despite depleted body stores in SIBO (as a result of production of inactive cobalamin analogs by the bacteria), liver disease, myeloproliferative disorders, congenital transcobalamin II deficiency, and with high levels of IF antibodies. In contrast, oral contraceptives, pregnancy, and folate deficiency can cause low serum cobalamin levels despite normal body stores.[137] Therefore, if there is a high suspicion, especially for cobalamin deficiency, parenteral replacement with monitoring of the clinical response is recommended.[140] Measurement of methylmalonic acid, homocysteine, and holotranscobalamin are of limited clinical use in establishing vitamin B$_{12}$ deficiency.[140]

Serum folate concentrations decrease within a few days of dietary folate restriction even if tissue stores had been normal immediately prior to restriction. Feeding also influences serum folate levels; therefore, determination of folate in the fasting state is recommended. Measurement of red blood cell folate concentration has been considered a better estimate of folate tissue stores than serum folate levels by some authors.[137]

SIBO

Tests for the diagnosis of SIBO are covered in more detail in Chapter 105. Briefly, tests used to diagnose SIBO are the quantitative culture of a small intestinal aspirate (which is considered to be the gold standard diagnostic test), measurement of deconjugated bile acids or vitamin B$_{12}$ analogs in intestinal aspirates, measurement of serum folate, and several breath tests, including the ^{14}C-glycocholate breath test, the ^{14}C-D-xylose breath test, the lactulose hydrogen breath test, and the glucose hydrogen breath test. The rationale for the breath tests is the production by intraluminal bacteria of volatile metabolites (i.e., [14]CO$_2$ or H$_2$), from the administered substances, which can be measured in the exhaled breath.

Exocrine Pancreatic Insufficiency

Pancreatic function tests are discussed in detail in Chapters 56 and 59. Invasive pancreatic function tests require duodenal intubation and measurement of pancreatic enzyme, volume, and bicarbonate output after pancreatic stimulation by a liquid test meal (the Lundh test) or by injection of CCK or secretin. Noninvasive tests include measurement of fecal chymotrypsin or elastase concentration, the fluorescein dilaurate test, and the N-benzoyl-L-tyrosyl para-aminobenzoic acid (NBT-PABA) test. Elastase has a higher sensitivity than chymotrypsin for detecting exocrine pancreatic insufficiency,[141] but the specificity of elastase is low.[142]

Measurement of pancreatic enzymes and components of pancreatic fluid in duodenal aspirates obtained during endoscopy and after IV stimulation with secretin and CCK can have an excellent correlation with the more classic intubation tests for secretory function.[143] Secretin-enhanced MRCP has also been used to assess exocrine pancreatic function; its results correlate best with changes of severe pancreatitis, but this method is too insensitive for assessment of mild pancreatic insufficiency.[144]

Bile Salt Malabsorption

In patients with steatorrhea due to ileal disease or resection, bile salt malabsorption usually is present, but measurement of bile acid malabsorption is of limited clinical value. In patients with diarrhea and no steatorrhea, bile salt malabsorption may be present in the absence of overt ileal disease, and in such cases, measurement of bile salt absorption is helpful.

Measurement of Fecal Bile Acid Output

Elevated fecal bile acid concentrations or output can indicate intestinal bile acid malabsorption.[145] Under steady-state conditions, the increased fecal bile acid output reflects increased hepatic synthesis of bile acids.[146] In severe bile acid malabsorption, fecal bile acid output can be reduced if hepatic synthesis of bile acids becomes impaired. Measurement can be performed by enzymatic methods or by gas chromatography. This test requires a quantitative stool collection, and the analytic techniques are time consuming and require considerable expertise. Enzymatic methods may be unreliable in severe steatorrhea.[147]

[14]Carbon-Taurocholate Bile Acid Absorption Test

The ^{14}C-taurocholate bile acid absorption test requires a 72-hour stool collection after ingestion of radioactively labeled bile acid. The rate of intestinal bile acid absorption is calculated from the fecal recovery of ^{14}C-labeled taurocholic acid (^{14}C-TCA). Normal values for this test have been established in normal persons with laxative-induced diarrhea, because diarrhea by itself can increase fecal losses of bile acids,[146] presumably because of accelerated intestinal transit.[148] Clinical limitations of this test are that it requires substantial analytical work, access to a gamma camera, and a time-consuming stool collection.

Therapeutic Trial of Bile Acid-Binding Resins (Cholestyramine)

A therapeutic trial of cholestyramine or other bile acid-binding resins can be used to diagnose bile acid malabsorption as a cause of diarrhea. To what extent a clinical response to cholestyramine correlates with the presence of bile acid malabsorption is controversial; cholestyramine may have a nonspecific constipating effect in patients with diarrhea from other causes. Failure of diarrhea to remit within 3 days of initiation of cholestyramine makes bile acid malabsorption an unlikely cause of diarrhea; however, some patients with bile acid malabsorption respond only to large doses of cholestyramine.

In patients with established bile acid malabsorption in whom no improvement is obtained with bile acid-binding resins, it is very unlikely bile acid malabsorption is the cause of diarrhea. In these patients, bile acid malabsorption is considered a secondary phenomenon due to a washout effect.[146] In patients with severe bile acid malabsorption and resultant steatorrhea, cholestyramine might even aggravate fat malabsorption and diarrhea.[3] Therefore, without further testing for bile acid malabsorption, neither a positive nor a negative result of a therapeutic trial of cholestyramine constitutes proof of the presence or absence, respectively, of bile acid malabsorption.

Selenium-75-Labeled Homotaurocholic Acid Test (SeHCAT)

The radioactive taurocholic acid analog used for this test is resistant to bacterial deconjugation. After it has been administered orally, the patient undergoes serial gamma scintigraphy to measure whole-body bile acid retention or, as suggested by some authors, bile acid retention in the gallbladder.[149] Although this test is used commonly in some countries,[150] it has several limitations. First, normal values for bile acid retention, which are used to compare normal and abnormal bile acid absorption, were obtained for SeHCAT only in healthy persons without diarrhea[151]; secondary bile acid malabsorption, however, can be induced by diarrhea itself and is proportional to the stool weight, as demonstrated with the ^{14}C-TCA test.[146,148] For this test to be clinically useful, normal values have to be established for patients with diarrhea. Finally, this test is very time consuming because bile acid retention must be measured either 4 or 7 days (depending on the protocol) after the bile acid administration.

D-Xylose Test

Absorption of the pentose D-xylose is facilitated by passive diffusion. Approximately 50% of the absorbed D-xylose is metabolized, and the remainder is excreted in urine. After an overnight fast, a 25-g dose of D-xylose is ingested, and the patient is encouraged to drink sufficient volumes of fluid to maintain good urine output; urine is collected for the next 5 hours. As an alternative, 1 hour after ingestion of D-xylose, a venous sample may be obtained.[152] Less than 4 g (16% excretion) of D-xylose in the urine collection or a serum xylose concentration below 20 mg/dL indicates abnormal intestinal absorption. The traditional urine test appears to be more reliable than the 1-hour blood test.

False-positive results occur if the duration of urine collection is too short or if the patient is dehydrated or has renal dysfunction, significant ascites, delayed gastric emptying, or portal hypertension. D-Xylose absorption may be normal in patients with only mild impairment of mucosal function or with predominantly distal small intestinal disease. Because D-xylose is susceptible to bacterial metabolism, absorption is diminished in patients with SIBO, although the test has a poor sensitivity for detecting bacterial overgrowth.[153] The test is of limited clinical value today and mostly has been replaced by small intestinal biopsy.

Intestinal Permeability Tests

Intestinal permeability tests mostly are used in studies of the pathophysiology of intestinal disorders; they do not provide a specific diagnosis.[154]

Most current permeability tests are based on the differential absorption of mono- and disaccharides. Damage to the mucosa can result in increased permeability for disaccharides and oligosaccharides consequent to epithelial injury, and this can result in decreased permeability of monosaccharides secondary to reduction of mucosal surface area.[155] Absorption is measured by urinary excretion. Expression of results as the absorption ratio of the mono- and disaccharide minimizes the influences of gastric emptying, intestinal transit, renal and hepatic function, and variations in time of urine collections.[156]

Increased intestinal permeability has been shown to predict the development of Crohn's disease or relapse in patients with this disease.[157] In celiac disease, the finding of considerably increased permeability is a sensitive marker for advanced disease. Permeability tests have also been used to judge response to a gluten-free diet[158] or to screen

first-degree relatives for celiac disease. Elevated serum aminotransferase levels in patients with celiac disease correlate with increased intestinal permeability.[159] Disturbances of intestinal permeability have been documented in users of NSAIDs,[160] in inflammatory joint disease,[161] and in diabetic diarrhea.[162]

^{13}Carbon Breath Tests

The increasing availability of stable isotopes has raised interest in replacing radioactive ^{14}C with nonradioactive ^{13}C for breath tests.[124,163] In malabsorptive diseases, ^{13}C-labeled substrates have been evaluated in the diagnosis of steatorrhea,[164] SIBO and exocrine pancreatic insufficiency[165] and in the evaluation of the digestibility of egg protein. Because of concerns about diagnostic accuracy, cost, and limited availability, these tests have not gained widespread acceptance.

MALABSORPTION IN SPECIFIC SITUATIONS AND DISEASE STATES

Lactose Malabsorption

Deficiency of the intestinal brush border enzyme lactase can lead to lactose malabsorption, which can result in lactose intolerance. Unlike other intestinal disaccharidases, which develop early in fetal life, lactase levels remain low until the 34th week of gestation.[166] Transient lactase deficiency in premature infants can lead to symptoms of lactose malabsorption, such as diarrhea, until normal intestinal lactase activity develops. In rare cases, enzyme deficiency is manifest at the time of birth and is permanent, and congenital lactase deficiency (OMIM #223000)* is diagnosed. Reversible lactase deficiency can occur at all ages as a result of transient small intestinal injury associated with acute diarrheal illnesses.

Acquired primary lactase deficiency (adult-type hypolactasia, OMIM #223100) is the most common form of lactase deficiency worldwide. Most populations lose considerable lactase activity in adulthood.[167] The decline in lactase activity is a multifactorial process that is regulated at the gene transcription level[168] and leads to decreased biosynthesis, retardation of intracellular transport, or maturation of the enzyme lactase-phlorizin hydrolase.[169] In whites, a SNP −13910 T/C upstream of the gene that codes for lactase-phlorizin hydrolase (*LPH* gene) has been found to be involved in regulation of the enzyme.[127] The CC genotype of the SNP −13910 T/C upstream of the *LPH* gene is associated with adult-type hypolactasia; TC and TT genotypes are linked with lactase persistence.[128] In other populations (e.g., some African and sub-Saharan African populations), the SNP −13910*T polymorphism is not associated with lactase persistence.[131,170] Because it is present in most of the adult human population, this form of lactase deficiency has to be considered normal rather than abnormal.

Lactase deficiency usually produces symptoms only in adulthood, although lactase levels in affected persons start to decline during childhood.[171] Lactase activity persists in most adults of Western European heritage[172] (Box 104-4). Even in this group, however, the activity of lactase is only about half the activity of sucrase and less than 20% of the activity of

---

*The Online Mendelian Inheritance in Man (OMIM) system assigns numbers to specific diseases according to a continuously updated catalog of human genes and genetic disorders (http://www.ncbi.nlm.nih.gov/omim/).

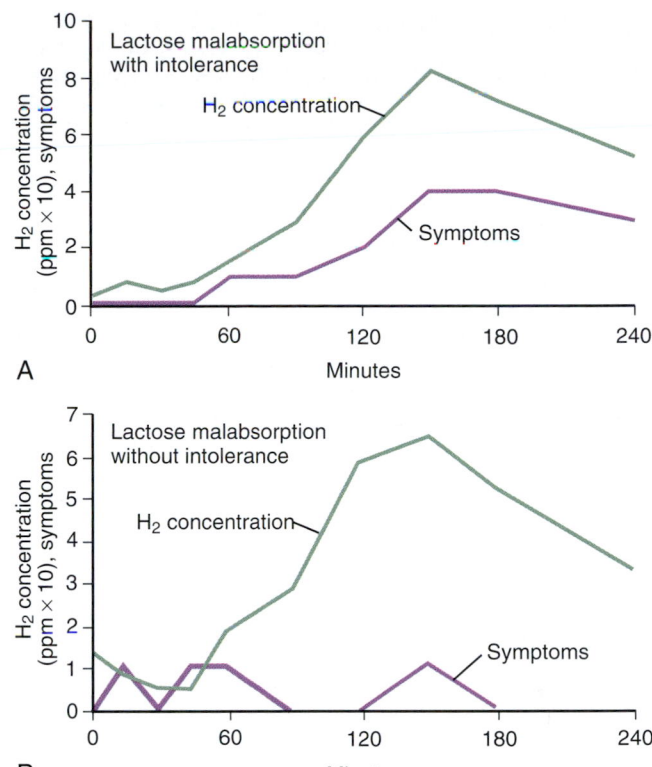

FIGURE 104-9. Graphs illustrating the role of symptoms in determining the clinical importance of lactose malabsorption. Assessment of the clinical relevance of an abnormal lactose hydrogen breath test is made by monitoring abdominal symptoms (bloating, cramps, pain) during the test. Breath hydrogen concentration in parts per million (ppm) and GI symptoms using an arbitrary scoring system for 2 different patients are plotted on the graphs. The patient in A has symptoms associated with an increase in breath hydrogen concentration and therefore can be considered to have lactose intolerance. The patient in B has no increase in symptoms, although the breath hydrogen concentration increases considerably, so the patient has lactose malabsorption without lactose intolerance.

maltase.[171] Accordingly, in these persons, lactase activity is much more susceptible to a reduction in function with acute or chronic GI illnesses.

In patients with lactose malabsorption, it may be unclear whether the condition results from acquired primary lactase deficiency or is a consequence of another small intestinal disorder. Therefore, in the individual lactose malabsorber, especially if there is an ethnic background associated with a low prevalence of acquired primary lactase deficiency, it may be necessary to exclude other malabsorptive disorders like celiac disease. The main symptoms of lactose intolerance are bloating, abdominal cramps, increased flatus, and diarrhea. Development of bloating and abdominal cramps is presumably associated with increased perception of luminal distention by gas,[173] because no clear relation has been observed between the amount of lactose ingested and the severity of symptoms.[174] Ingestion of as little as 3 g of lactose may be required to induce symptoms in persons with lactose malabsorption.[175] GI symptoms, including diarrhea, have been shown to be more severe in adults with shorter small intestinal transit time,[176] but no such relation between intestinal transit and symptoms is observed in children.[177] Also, in pregnant women and in thyrotoxic patients with Graves' disease, changes in intestinal motility play a role in the clinical manifestation of lactose malabsorption.[178,179] To make a diagnosis of lactose intolerance, and in view of the poor correlation between lactose malabsorption and lactose intolerance, it is very important to monitor symptoms during a lactose hydrogen breath test and to confirm that any symptoms experienced by the patient during the test are truly those the patient complains of and that they are associated with a significant increase in breath hydrogen levels (Fig. 104-9).

Adult-type hypolactasia may also be a risk factor for developing osteoporosis and bone fractures, either owing to patients' avoidance of dairy products[180] or interference with calcium absorption.[181]

Patients in whom a clear association can be established between symptoms and lactose malabsorption should be educated about lactose-reduced or lactose-free diets. Yogurt may be tolerated by such patients[182] and provides a good source of calcium. Consuming whole milk or chocolate milk rather than skim milk, and drinking milk with meals can reduce symptoms of lactose intolerance, presumably as a result of prolonged gastric emptying. Alternatively, supplementation

of dairy products with lactase of microbiological origin can be suggested.[183] Furthermore, because many carbohydrates other than lactose are incompletely absorbed by the normal small intestine,[52,184] and because dietary fiber also may be metabolized by colonic bacteria, persistence of some symptoms while the patient is on a lactose-free diet is not uncommon. It also must be kept in mind that symptoms arising after ingestion of dairy products may be due to milk protein allergy or fat intolerance rather than lactose intolerance.

Fructose Malabsorption

Fructose is found in modern diets either as a constituent of the disaccharide sucrose or as the monosaccharide, both of which are used as sweeteners in a variety of food items. The average daily intake of fructose varies from 11 to 54 g around the world.[185] Fructose as a constituent of sucrose is absorbed by a well-characterized absorptive system that integrates enzymatic hydrolysis of the disaccharide sucrose by sucrase and transfer of the resulting 2 monosaccharides, glucose and fructose, through the apical membrane of the epithelial cell. The absorptive capacity for fructose that is not accompanied by glucose, however, is relatively small[186] and dose dependent.[187] Healthy subjects have the capacity to absorb up to 25 g of fructose, but normal absorption of fructose also depends on other ingested nutrients and is not well understood; many individuals will have malabsorption and intolerance with intake of 50 g of fructose.[188]

Ingesting food that contains fructose in excess of glucose can result in symptoms such as abdominal bloating or diarrhea[189] and especially can provoke symptoms in patients with IBS.[190] It has been suggested that as little as 3 g of fructose can precipitate symptoms in patients with functional bowel disorders. Women might complain more often of fructose-associated symptoms and exhibit more fructose malabsorption than men; there is no adaptation to regular consumption of fructose.[191] Fructose malabsorption usually is identified by a positive result on a hydrogen breath test after ingestion of 25 or 50 g of fructose.[192] Because the fructose content in fruit and in soft drinks usually is less than 8 g per 100 g of fruit or drink, the amounts of fructose used in the hydrogen breath test are not physiologic, and no data are available on how many otherwise asymptomatic people would have a positive test result with these larger doses. Fructose contents of 30 to 40 g per 100 g are present in some chocolate, caramel, and praline products.[193]

In a group of patients with isolated fructose malabsorption, no defect of the gene that encodes the luminal fructose transporter (GLUT5) could be detected.[194] It is therefore unlikely that patients who present with GI symptoms have a true defect of intestinal fructose absorption. It is more likely that they belong to a subset of people in whom ingestion of fructose-rich foods provokes symptoms related to other disorders (e.g., IBS) or as a result of unique but not necessarily abnormal colonic bacterial activity. The latter is suggested by a study in asymptomatic and symptomatic persons with fructose malabsorption in whom it was demonstrated that the disappearance rate of fructose in anaerobic, but not aerobic, stool cultures was significantly elevated in the symptomatic group compared with the asymptomatic group.[195]

A placebo-controlled study on patients with incomplete fructose absorption has shown that ingestion of the enzyme xylose isomerise, which catalyzes the reversible isomerization of glucose and fructose, decreases pain, nausea, and the area under the breath hydrogen curve after ingestion of a watery fructose load.[196] Future studies will have to evaluate whether this effect is also present during ingestion of carbohydrate mixtures or food containing fructose and whether it persists over a lengthy observation period.

Testing for fructose malabsorption by the hydrogen breath test may be useful to identify patients in whom dietary restriction of foods with excessive fructose content may be beneficial in treating bloating and diarrhea. Symptoms in these persons are probably the result of ingestion of unphysiologic amounts of fructose and not the consequence of a defect in fructose absorption. In addition to fructose, other poorly absorbable and rapidly fermentable carbohydrates may contribute to symptoms.

Bile Acid Malabsorption

Bile acid malabsorption is usually present in patients who have undergone ileal resection or bypass operations or who have severe disease of the ileum, where specific bile acid transport proteins are located. The clinical consequences of bile acid malabsorption depend on whether bile acid loss can be compensated by increased hepatic synthesis.[197] Ileal resection of more than 100 cm usually results in severe bile acid malabsorption that cannot be compensated by increased hepatic synthesis; in such cases, steatorrhea results from impaired micelle formation due to decreased luminal concentrations of conjugated bile acids.[3,197] With ileal resections of less than 100 cm, bile acid malabsorption usually can be compensated by increased hepatic synthesis, and malabsorbed bile acids cause secretory diarrhea rather than steatorrhea.[3,197] Secretory diarrhea caused by or associated with bile acid malabsorption is discussed in detail in Chapter 16.

Knowledge of the differing pathophysiology of steatorrhea and of secretory diarrhea from bile acid malabsorption is important not only for understanding the clinical presentation but also for choosing the appropriate therapy. In patients with compensated bile acid malabsorption, binding of bile salts in the lumen of the intestine by cholestyramine reduces diarrhea. By contrast, in decompensated bile acid malabsorption, cholestyramine further depletes the bile acid pool, thereby worsening steatorrhea. In several cases of decompensated bile acid malabsorption after extensive ileal resections, intestinal fat absorption was improved markedly by oral administration of conjugated bile acids.[117,198,199] Cholylsarcosine in a dose of 2 to 3 g per meal has been reported to enhance fat absorption and nutritional status in patients with short bowel syndrome who have residual colon[117,199,200]; natural conjugated bile acids lessen severity of steatorrhea in such patients to a smaller extent.[200] Improved fat absorption was associated with decreased urinary oxalate excretion.[199]

A syndrome of primary bile acid malabsorption with normal ileal morphology has been reported in children who, at birth, develop severe diarrhea, severe steatorrhea, and failure to thrive and who have reduced plasma cholesterol levels.[201] In an index case, this type of bile acid malabsorption was shown to be caused by mutations in the ileal sodium-bile acid cotransporter gene (SLC10A2).[4] Adult-onset bile acid malabsorption is not caused by SLC10A2 mutations,[202] and although its exact pathophysiology is unknown, accelerated intestinal transit may be a causative factor.[203]

Amyloidosis

Malabsorption has been reported in AL-type amyloidosis, AA-type amyloidosis, and hereditary amyloidosis (see Chapter 36). Malabsorption occurs in 5% to 13% of patients with AL or AA amyloidosis[204,205] and was present in 58% of Swedish patients with familial amyloidosis.[206] Fecal fat excretion can reach levels of 60 g/day.[206] GI absorption of D-xylose and vitamin B_{12} can be reduced,[206,207] and protein-losing enteropathy can develop.[208] Amyloid deposits are found in the muscle layers, the stroma of the lamina propria and the submucosa, the wall of mucosal and submucosal blood vessels in the GI tract, and in enteric and extraenteric nerves.[209,210]

In many patients with amyloidosis who have diarrhea or malabsorption, or both, symptoms suggesting autonomic neuropathy are present.[148,206] Autonomic neuropathy can cause rapid intestinal transit, which in turn can lead to severe diarrhea and malabsorption despite normal transport capacity of the intestinal mucosa.[148] Other suggested mechanisms of malabsorption in amyloidosis are chronic mesenteric ischemia, decreased absorption from a physical barrier effect of amyloid deposits,[210] and SIBO, which also might be a consequence of autonomic neuropathy.[207]

Bile acid malabsorption is found in many patients with amyloidosis associated with autonomic neuropathy[211] and is caused by rapid intestinal transit rather than impaired absorptive transport in the terminal ileum.[148] Diarrhea in these patients usually fails to respond to bile acid-binding agents.[148]

Barium studies in patients with amyloidosis usually are normal but might show thickened folds, nodular lesions, filling defects, dilatation of bowel segments, or altered transit.[212] The endoscopic appearance of the GI mucosa may show a fine granular appearance, polypoid protrusions, erosions, ulcerations, atrophic changes, and mucosal friability, but in many patients, no macroscopic changes are evident.[210,212]

Histologic examination demonstrates amyloid deposits in 72% of esophageal, 75% to 95% of gastric, 83% to 100% of small intestinal, and 75% to 95% of colorectal biopsy specimens.[205,210] Subcutaneous fat pad aspiration or biopsy is another diagnostic approach. Amyloid deposits might not be seen with routine histologic stains and become more evident with Congo red staining.

Therapy of diarrhea in patients with amyloidosis includes attempts to prolong intestinal transit time with opioids or octreotide and to avoid further amyloid deposition in the tissue by treatment of the underlying disorder in AA amyloidosis, the plasma-cell dyscrasia in AL amyloidosis, and by administration of colchicine to patients with familial Mediterranean fever.

Drugs and Food Supplements

Table 104-9 lists drugs and food supplements reported to induce malabsorption of vitamins, minerals, or nutrients, as well as the suggested pathophysiologic mechanisms by which this occurs.[23,26,27,34,115,137,213-232]

Gastric Resection or Bariatric Surgery

Gastric Resection

Severe steatorrhea after total and partial gastric resections has been a long-observed complication of these operations. Fecal fat excretion rates after such operations usually are between 15 and 20 g/day,[1] but values of up to 60 g/day have been reported.[228] Suggested mechanisms for steatorrhea include defective mixing of nutrients with digestive secretions, lack of gastric acid and gastric lipase secretion, decreased small bowel transit time, SIBO, and pancreatic insufficiency.[1,233] However, studies have shown that pancreatic enzyme supplements[234] and antibiotic treatments[233] neither improve fat absorption nor relieve symptoms after gastric resection. Total and partial gastric resections also can result in significant protein malabsorption, whereas absorption of carbohydrates does not seem to be significantly impaired. Nutrient malabsorption in these

patients also can result in GI symptoms like diarrhea and severe weight loss.[235]

Vitamin E deficiency can occur if food does not pass through the duodenum. The differential diagnosis of neurologic symptoms in postgastrectomy patients should include hypovitaminosis E.[236]

Loss of parietal cells after total gastric resection results in diminished IF secretion, which in turn leads to malabsorption of vitamin B_{12} and, in approximately 30% of patients, vitamin B_{12} deficiency. SIBO and lack of release of food-bound cobalamin secondary to diminished gastric acid and pepsin secretion have been implicated as additional pathogenic factors.

Iron malabsorption with resultant iron deficiency anemia is also commonly present in patients who have undergone gastric resection, although the mechanisms for iron malabsorption are not fully established. Lack of acid secretion with resultant decreased solubilization of iron salts has been suggested as a possible cause.

Calcium absorption can be severely impaired in patients with gastric resections and result in reduced bone density.[237] The mechanisms for calcium malabsorption probably are several, including decreased solubilization of calcium salts due to loss of gastric acid secretion, rapid intestinal transit, low calcium intake secondary to milk intolerance, and malabsorption of vitamin D. Studies in rats after gastrectomy have suggested that diminished calcium absorption results mainly, if not entirely, from decreased calcium solubilization.[238] By contrast, studies in humans have shown that calcium absorption is normal in patients with atrophic gastritis and in persons in whom acid secretion was inhibited by acid-inhibiting drugs.[239]

Treatment for patients who have undergone gastric resection should include adequate supplementation of malabsorbed vitamins and minerals to prevent serious long-term complications.[240]

Bariatric Surgery

The number of patients undergoing bariatric surgery is increasing; indications for and procedural details of the various procedures are described in Chapter 8. These patients need to be monitored for long-term problems like changes in bone metabolism. Risks of malabsorption can increase beyond

TABLE 104-9 Drugs and Dietary Products That Cause Malabsorption

Substance	Substrate Malabsorbed	Suggested Mechanism	Reference(s)
Acarbose	Carbohydrate	Inhibition of α-glucosidase	213
Antacids	Phosphate, iron, vitamin A	Luminal binding of substrates	214
Azathioprine	Generalized malabsorption	Villus atrophy	215
Biguanide (metformin)	Cobalamin, folate, glucose	Reduced ileal absorption of intrinsic factor (IF)-cobalamin complex; inhibition of intestinal glucose or folate absorption	214, 216, 217
Carbamazepine	Folate	Inhibition of intestinal folate absorption	218
Cholestyramine	Fat, fat-soluble vitamins, bile acids	Binding of conjugated bile salts	214
Colchicine	Fat, xylose, nitrogen, cobalamin, carotene	Mucosal damage and villus atrophy at high doses (impaired processing of IF-cobalamin receptor [the cubilin-amnionless complex])	26, 214, 219

Continued

TABLE 104-9 Drugs and Dietary Products That Cause Malabsorption—cont'd

Substance	Substrate Malabsorbed	Suggested Mechanism	Reference(s)
Contraceptives, oral*	Folate	Inhibition of pteroylpolyglutamate hydrolase (folate conjugase)	214
Ethanol	Xylose, fat, glucose, nitrogen, thiamine, cobalamin, folate	Mucosal damage; decreased disaccharidase activity; decreased pancreatic exocrine function and bile secretion	34, 214
Fiber, phytates	Iron, calcium, magnesium, zinc	Chelation	220
Glucocorticoids	Calcium	Inhibition of calcium absorption	23
H2RAs	Cobalamin	Impaired release of food-bound B_{12} owing to reduced gastric acid and pepsin secretion (and reduced IF secretion)	221
Laxatives, irritant type (phenolphthalein, bisacodyl, anthraquinones)	Fat, glucose, xylose	Washout effect; toxic effect on mucosa	115, 214
Methotrexate	Folate, fat, cobalamin, xylose	Mucosal damage; inhibition of intestinal folate transport	214, 220
Methyldopa†	Generalized malabsorption	Mucosal damage	222
Neomycin	Fat, nitrogen, fat-soluble vitamins, cobalamin, mono- and disaccharides, iron	Mucosal damage; disruption of micelle formation	214, 220
Olestra*	Fat-soluble vitamins	Binding of fat-soluble vitamins	223, 232
Orlistat	Fat, fat-soluble vitamins	Inhibition of pancreatic lipase	213
Para-aminosalicylate	Fat, cobalamin, folate	Unknown	26, 214
Phenytoin	Folate, calcium	Inhibition of folate and calcium absorption owing to luminal alkalinization; impaired vitamin D metabolism	23, 220, 224
PPIs*	Cobalamin, calcium?, magnesium?	Impaired release of food-bound cobalamin by pepsin owing to reduced gastric acid secretion; SIBO	27
Pyrimethamine	Folate	Competitive inhibition of intestinal folate absorption	225
Somatostatin analogs (e.g., octreotide)	Fat	Inhibition of hepatobiliary bile acid secretion; inhibition of pancreatic enzyme secretion; inhibition of CCK release	226, 227
Sulfonamides and sulfasalazine	Folate	Inhibition of pteroylpolyglutamate hydrolase and folate transport	137, 220
Tetracycline	Calcium	Precipitation of luminal calcium	229
Thiazides	Calcium	Decreased 1,25 dihydroxyvitamin D synthesis	230
Triamterene*	Folate	Competitive inhibition of intestinal folate absorption	225, 231

*Malabsorption usually does not result in deficiency states.
†Findings in case reports.

those that might be expected from the procedure over time because of poor compliance with supplementation or inadequate intake.

Malabsorption plays only a minor role in reducing average net intestinal energy absorption after long-limb Roux-en-Y gastric bypass. In a study of 9 severely obese patients, gastric bypass reduced fat absorption in every patient, although the severity of malabsorption varied widely and was correlated with the length of the biliopancreatic limb. Bypass caused protein malabsorption in some patients but did not cause carbohydrate malabsorption in any patient. Intestinal absorption of combustible energy averaged 3505 kcal/day before bypass, 1318 kcal/day 5 months after bypass, and 1914 kcal/day 14 months after bypass. The vast majority of the reduction in energy absorption after bypass was explained by reduced intake rather than malabsorption (e.g., at 5 months, reduction in intestinal energy absorption by malabsorption was 135 kcal/day vs. 2052 kcal/day from reduced intake).[241]

Long-term GI problems from bariatric surgery depend on the type of surgical procedure performed. Restrictive procedures and Roux-en-Y gastric bypass have only a mild component of noncaloric malabsorption compared with other procedures like biliopancreatic diversion, which was used more extensively in the past, and which can result in severe malnutrition.[242] Roux-en-Y gastric bypass can result in deficiency of proteins, iron, calcium, folate, vitamin B_{12}, and vitamin D. Deficiencies in vitamin B_1 are rare but potentially serious.[243,244]

Iron deficiency after gastric bypass can develop for several reasons, such as intolerance to red meat, diminished gastric acid secretion, and exclusion of the duodenum. Menstruating or pregnant women may be particularly predisposed to iron deficiency after gastric bypass surgery. Postoperatively, oral iron and vitamin C supplementation should be prescribed because once iron deficiency has developed, it may be refractory to oral treatment.[245]

In Roux-en-Y gastric bypass, colonization of both gastric chambers with aerobic and anaerobic bacteria has been demonstrated, resulting in a positive hydrogen breath test in 41% of subjects; no clinical symptoms such as diarrhea, malabsorption, or pneumonia could be attributed to this bacterial overgrowth.[246]

It has been suggested that after bariatric surgery, patients should have yearly measurements of a basic metabolic panel, magnesium, complete blood cell count, iron studies, vitamin D, parathyroid hormone, and bone density.[242] Routine and lifelong use of multivitamins is considered necessary.[247]

Aging

Malabsorption in elderly persons should not be ascribed to the aging process; it should be evaluated just like malabsorption that occurs in younger patients. In healthy elderly persons, small bowel histologic features are normal despite a decline in cell turnover and continual cell renewal.[248,249] Malabsorption of fat has been described in chronic congestive heart failure[250] and chronic intestinal ischemia (see Chapter 118), but this is not due to aging per se. Elderly persons may be more susceptible to GI insult and subsequent decompensation of GI function.[251] Changes in pancreatic anatomy and secretion occur with advanced aging, but only rarely do they result in overt pancreatic insufficiency.[252]

Deficiencies of some nutrients, however, presumably caused by malabsorption, may be present in elderly persons with no overt GI disease. An increased risk of folate and vitamin B_{12} deficiency despite adequate intake of these vitamins has been reported in the elderly.[253] Malnutrition in the

elderly can contribute significantly to morbidity and mortality, although it may be difficult to ascertain whether weight loss results from altered appetite, increased catabolism, or malabsorption.

SIBO in elderly persons with gastric hypochlorhydria from atrophic gastritis or treatment with a PPI is usually not associated with clinically significant malabsorption,[254] but an improvement in nutritional status after antibiotic treatment has been described in some elderly patients.[255] An increased prevalence of lactose malabsorption in the elderly may be the result of clinically unapparent SIBO.[256]

Connective Tissue Diseases

PSS

The GI tract is involved to a variable degree in most patients with systemic sclerosis. Early pathologic changes are characterized by vasculopathy, which results in ischemia and progressive organ dysfunction.[257] Typical histologic findings include atrophy of the muscle layers with increased deposition of elastin and collagen in the submucosa and serosa and between smooth muscle bundles of the muscularis externa.[258] Small intestinal biopsy specimens might reveal an increased number of plasma cells within the lamina propria and collagen deposits around and between lobules of Brunner's glands in the submucosa of the duodenum.[259]

Malabsorption in scleroderma usually results from SIBO secondary to ineffective motility in the small intestine,[260] but other factors (e.g., decreased mucosal blood flow[261]) can also contribute. Malabsorption and SIBO are not limited to patients with diffuse disease; they can also occur in patients with long-standing limited cutaneous systemic sclerosis.[262] Elevated serum concentrations of motilin and CCK have been described in patients with systemic sclerosis and fat malabsorption, but they are thought to result from myogenic or neurogenic disturbances of intestinal or gallbladder contraction.[263] In addition to antibiotic treatment of SIBO, low doses of octreotide (50 μg subcutaneously every evening for 3 weeks) have been shown to induce intestinal migrating motor complexes, reduce bacterial overgrowth, and relieve abdominal symptoms.[260]

Lupus Erythematosus and Other Connective Tissue Diseases

Excessive fecal fat excretion associated with abnormalities of D-xylose breath testing may be found in some patients with lupus erythematosus; these findings may be accompanied by flattened and deformed villi with an inflammatory infiltrate seen on duodenal biopsy specimens.[264] Malabsorption that resolved after treatment with prednisolone has also been described in association with the hypereosinophilic syndrome in lupus erythematosus.[265] Malabsorption is an uncommon feature of mixed connective tissue disease and polymyositis.[266,267]

Congenital Defects

Table 104-10 lists congenital intestinal diseases that result in malabsorption of specific substrates or in a generalized malabsorption syndrome.

Amino Acid Transport Defects

Amino acids are absorbed by the enterocyte as oligopeptides, dipeptides, and free amino acids. In several inborn

Text continued on p. 1819

TABLE 104-10 Congenital Disorders of the GI Mucosa That Result in Malabsorption[342]

Disorder	Causative Gene	Suggested Mode of Inheritance	Malabsorbed Substrate(s)	Suggested Mechanism of Malabsorption	Clinical Features	Reference(s)
Malabsorption of Amino Acids						
Hartnup's disorder OMIM#234500	SLC6A19	AR	Neutral amino acids (tryptophan, leucine, methionine, phenylalanine, tyrosine, valine, ?histidine, ?lysine)	Decreased intestinal absorption of free neutral amino acids	Most patients are asymptomatic; some patients have photosensitive skin rash, intermittent ataxia, psychotic behavior, mental retardation, diarrhea	268
Cystinuria (types A, B, AB) OMIM#220100	Type A: SLC3A1 Type B: SLC7A9	AR (type A) and incomplete AR (type B)	Cystine and/or dibasic amino acids (lysine, ornithine, arginine)	Decreased intestinal absorption of specific free amino acids owing to a defective amino acid transporter at the brush border membrane Type A: no transport of cystine, lysine, or arginine Type B: reduced or normal cystine transport and reduced or no lysine and arginine transport	Aminoaciduria, cystine stones in the urinary tract	269
Lysinuric protein intolerance OMIM#222700	SLC7A7	AR	Dibasic amino acids (lysine, ornithine, arginine)	Defect of the basolateral transporter (y+LAT-1) for dibasic amino acids (also malabsorption of di- and oligopeptides)	Sparse hair, hyperammonemia, nausea, vomiting, diarrhea, protein malnutrition, failure to thrive, aversion to protein-rich food	271
Isolated lysinuria*	?	?	Lysine	Decreased intestinal absorption of lysine	Mental retardation, malnutrition, failure to thrive	271
Iminoglycinuria OMIM#242600	SLC6A20 SLC6A19 SLC36A2	AR	L-Proline	Impaired intestinal absorption of L-proline in a subgroup of subjects	Aminoaciduria; benign disorder	270
Blue diaper syndrome* OMIM#211000	?	AR	Tryptophan	Intestinal tryptophan absorption defect	Blue discoloration of diapers, failure to thrive, hypercalcemia, nephrocalcinosis	343

Disease	Gene	Inheritance	Substrate	Defect	Clinical Manifestations	Page
Methionine malabsorption syndrome* (Oasthouse syndrome) OMIM%250900	?	AR	Methionine	Intestinal methionine absorption defect	Mental retardation, convulsions, diarrhea, white hair, hyperpnea; urine has characteristic sweet smell of dried celery	344
Lowe oculocerebral syndrome OMIM#30900	OCRL1	XR	Lysine, arginine	Impaired intestinal lysine and arginine absorption	Aminoaciduria, mental retardation, cataracts, rickets, choreoathetosis, renal disease	345
Malabsorption of Carbohydrates						
Congenital lactase deficiency OMIM#22300	LCT	AR	Lactose	Permanent very low lactase activity	Diarrhea, bloating, and dehydration in the first days of life	272
Sucrase-isomaltase deficiency OMIM#2229000	SI	AR	Sucrose, starch	Sucrase activity is absent; isomaltase activity is absent or reduced; reduced maltase activity	Osmotic diarrhea after starch or sucrose ingestion; failure to thrive	272
Trehalase deficiency OMIM%612119	TREH	AR	Trehalose	Lack of intestinal trehalase activity	Diarrhea and/or vomiting after ingesting mushrooms	272
Glucose-galactose malabsorption OMIM#606824	SLC5A1	AR	Glucose, galactose	Defect of the brush border sodium-glucose cotransporter (SGLT1)	Neonatal onset of osmotic diarrhea, dehydration, intermittent or constant glycosuria	273
Malabsorption of Fat						
Abetalipoproteinemia OMIM#200100	MTP	AR	Fat, fat-soluble vitamins	Defective lipoprotein assembly owing to a lack of MTP, resulting in TG accumulation in the enterocyte and no chylomicron formation	Steatorrhea, diarrhea, neurologic symptoms, retinitis pigmentosa, failure to thrive, absence of chylomicrons and VLDL in the blood, acanthocytosis	10
Familial hypobetalipoproteinemia OMIM#615558	APOB	Incomplete AD	Fat, fat-soluble vitamins	TG accumulation in the enterocyte in homozygotes owing to formation of a truncated apolipoprotein B	Homozygotes: clinical manifestations as for abetalipoproteinemia Heterozygotes: fat absorption probably normal; hypolipidemia, neurologic manifestations	10

Continued

TABLE 104-10 Congenital Disorders of the GI Mucosa That Result in Malabsorption[342]—cont'd

Disorder	Causative Gene	Suggested Mode of Inheritance	Malabsorbed Substrate(s)	Suggested Mechanism of Malabsorption	Clinical Features	Reference(s)
Chylomicron retention disease Anderson's disease OMIM#246700	*SAR1B*	AR	Fat	Defective chylomicron formation and accumulation in the enterocyte	Steatorrhea, failure to thrive, absence of chylomicrons and reduced LDL levels in the blood; neurologic symptoms in some patients	10, 346
Wolman's disease, cholesteryl ester storage disease OMIM#278000	*LIPA*	AR	Fat	Deficient activity of hLAL, cholesteryl ester hydrolase, causing accumulation of cholesteryl esters and TGs in various body tissues; infiltration of intestinal mucosa with foamy cells, intestinal damage	Steatorrhea, hepatosplenomegaly, abdominal distention; failure to thrive, adrenal calcifications	347, 348
Malabsorption of Vitamins						
Congenital IF deficiency (congenital pernicious anemia) OMIM#261000	*GIF*	AR	Cobalamin (vitamin B$_{12}$)	Defective synthesis of IF or synthesis of an abnormal IF with either reduced affinity for cobalamin or for the ileal IF receptor, or increased susceptibility to proteolysis	Megaloblastic anemia, neurologic symptoms, delayed development	32, 138
Imerslund-Gräsbeck syndrome (ileal B$_{12}$ malabsorption, megaloblastic anemia type I) OMIM#261100	*CUBN* or *AMN*	AR	Cobalamin (vitamin B$_{12}$)	Impaired ileal absorption of IF-cobalamin complex owing to defects in the cubilin-AMN complex (IF-cobalamin receptor)	Megaloblastic anemia, neurologic symptoms, proteinuria	26, 31, 138
Transcobalamin II deficiency OMIM#275350	*TCN2*	AR	Cobalamin (vitamin B$_{12}$)	Defective transport of cobalamin out of enterocytes into the portal blood owing to absence or malfunction of transcobalamin II	Vomiting, diarrhea, failure to thrive, anemia, immunodeficiency, neurologic symptoms	32, 138
Hereditary folate malabsorption OMIM#229050	*SLC46A1*	AR	Folate	Defective folate transport across the intestinal mucosa	Megaloblastic anemia, diarrhea, neurologic symptoms	349

Malabsorption of Minerals

Disease	Gene	Inheritance	Mineral	Defect	Clinical Features	Ref
Acrodermatitis enteropathica OMIM#201100	SLC39A4	AR	Zinc	Defective zinc absorption in the small intestine owing to a defect in the zinc transport protein (hZIP4)	Diarrhea, scaling erythematous dermatitis, alopecia, neuropsychiatric symptoms; onset after weaning	47
Isolated magnesium malabsorption (hypomagnesemia with secondary hypocalcemia [HOMG]) OMIM#602014	TRPM6	AR	Magnesium	Selective defect in intestinal magnesium absorption	Tetany, convulsion, diarrhea, hypomagnesemia with secondary hypocalcemia	41
Menkes disease OMIM#309400	ATP7A	XR	Copper	General copper transport disorder; intestinal copper malabsorption with copper accumulation in the intestinal mucosa owing to a defective transmembrane copper-transporting ATPase (MNK)	Cerebral degeneration, diarrhea, abnormal hair, hypopigmentation, arterial rupture, thrombosis, hypothermia, bone changes	350
Occipital horn syndrome (X-linked cutis laxa) OMIM#304150	ATP7A	XR	Copper	Milder form of same defect as in Menkes disease; low levels of functional MNK	Inguinal hernias, bladder and ureteral diverticula, skin and joint laxity, chronic diarrhea, bone changes	350
Iron-refractory iron-deficient anemia 206200	TMPRSS6	AR	Iron	Intestinal iron transport disorder	Iron-deficient anemia that is unresponsive to oral iron supplementation	44
Hereditary selective deficiency of $1\alpha,25(OH)_2D$ (pseudo–vitamin D deficiency rickets) 264700	CYP27B1	AR	Calcium	Defective $25(OH)D$ 1α-hydroxylase, resulting in $1\alpha,25(OH)_2D$ deficiency and reduced intestinal calcium absorption	Bone pain, deformities and fractures, muscle weakness	351
Hereditary generalized resistance to $1\alpha,25(OH)_2D$ (vitamin D-resistant rickets) OMIM#277440	VDR	AR	Calcium	Malfunction of the vitamin D receptor owing to defective hormone binding, defective receptor translocation to nucleus, or defective receptor binding to DNA, resulting in malabsorption of calcium	Bone pain, deformities and fractures, muscle weakness, alopecia	351

Continued

TABLE 104-10 Congenital Disorders of the GI Mucosa That Result in Malabsorption[342]—cont'd

Disorder	Causative Gene	Suggested Mode of Inheritance	Malabsorbed Substrate(s)	Suggested Mechanism of Malabsorption	Clinical Features	Reference(s)
Other Defects						
Enterokinase deficiency 226200	PRSS7	AR	Protein, fat	Defective activation of pancreatic proenzymes owing to lack of intestinal enterokinase	Diarrhea, failure to thrive, hypoproteinemia, edema, anemia	15, 352
Congenital bile acid malabsorption OMIM#613291	SLC10A2	AR	Bile acids, fat	Defect of the ileal ASBT	Steatorrhea, diarrhea, failure to thrive	4
Microvillus inclusion disease OMIM#251850	MYO5B	AR	Carbohydrates, fat, cobalamin, electrolytes, water	Villus atrophy with microvillus inclusions in enterocytes, absent or shortened brush border microvilli	Severe watery diarrhea and steatorrhea requiring total parenteral nutrition	353
Hyperinsulinism, with enteropathy and deafness OMIM#606528	USH1C, ABCC8, or KCNJ11	AR	Generalized malabsorption	Enteropathy with villus atrophy and inflammation	Hyperinsulinism, profound congenital sensorineural deafness, enteropathy, renal tubular dysfunction	354
Immune dysregulation polyendocrinopathy and enteropathy, X-linked (IPEX) OMIM#304790	FOXP3	XR	Generalized malabsorption	Villus atrophy	Polyendocrinopathies, severe diarrhea, hemolytic anemia	286
Enteric anendocrinosis* OMIM#610370	NEUROG3	AR	Generalized malabsorption	Lack of enteroendocrine cells	Severe diarrhea, failure to thrive, type 1 diabetes mellitus	312
Congenital proprotein convertase 1/3 deficiency OMIM#600955	PCSK1	AR	Generalized malabsorption	Lack of functional hormone production by enteroendocrine cells	Severe diarrhea, polyendocrinopathies, failure to thrive, overweight in later age	313
Congenital tufting enteropathy OMIM#613217	EpCAM	AR	Generalized malabsorption	Intestinal epithelial cell dysplasia and villus atrophy	Severe diarrhea, failure to thrive	355

% sign (in place of #) means that the gene causing the disease is unknown in this case.
*Reported in only a few cases.
AD, autosomal dominant; AMN, amnionless; AR, autosomal recessive; ASBT, sodium bile acid cotransporter; CUBN, cubulin; hLAL, human lysosomal acid lipase; IF, intrinsic factor; LDL, low-density lipoprotein; MTP, microsomal TG transfer protein; 1α,25(OH)₂D, 1α,25-dihydroxyvitamin D; 25(OH)D, 25-hydroxyvitamin D; VLDL, very-low-density lipoprotein; XR, X-linked recessive.

inborn errors of metabolism, transport defects for different groups of amino acids have been identified in the intestine and kidney (see Table 104-10).

In iminoglycinuria, Hartnup's disorder, and cystinuria, the intestinal transport defect seems to be of no or only minor clinical significance, because the amino acids affected by the transporter defects still can be absorbed as oligopeptides and dipeptides, and protein malnutrition can be avoided.[268-270] Manifestations in these diseases, therefore, are mainly due to amino acid transport defects in the kidney. In Hartnup's disorder, oral administration of nicotinamide and a high-protein diet have been shown to relieve symptoms to some extent.[268]

In lysinuric protein intolerance, however, the transport defect is located on the basolateral membrane of the enterocyte and leads to malabsorption of cationic amino acids in both their monopeptide and dipeptide forms. Patients with lysinuric protein intolerance therefore cannot tolerate high-protein foods and are prone to develop protein malnutrition. Malabsorption of lysine with resultant deficiency of this essential amino acid is thought to be important to the development of several disease manifestations in these patients.[271] Treatment consists of protein restriction and supplementation with oral citrulline.

Disaccharidase Deficiency and Transport Defects for Monosaccharides

In sucrase-isomaltase deficiency, affected infants usually become symptomatic after weaning when starch and sucrose are introduced to the diet. Symptoms and signs include osmotic diarrhea, failure to thrive, excess flatus, and occasional vomiting. Diagnosis can be established by an oral sucrose absorption test. Treatment includes avoidance of dietary starch and sucrose.[272] In patients with this disease, symptoms tend to resolve spontaneously with age.

Patients with glucose-galactose malabsorption suffer from severe diarrhea that leads to dehydration in the first days of life. The diarrhea stops only if glucose and galactose are eliminated from the diet. Older children and adults tolerate the offending carbohydrates better, but the transport defect is lifelong. Diagnosis can be established with an oral glucose tolerance test or by in vitro glucose absorption tests performed on intestinal biopsy specimens. Therapy consists of a fructose-based diet free of glucose and galactose. After the age of 3 months, addition of foods containing low quantities of glucose or galactose such as vegetables, fruits, and cheese is considered safe.[273]

Congenital Disorders of Lipid Absorption

Abetalipoproteinemia is a disorder of autosomal recessive inheritance characterized by triglyceride accumulation in the enterocyte. This disease seems to be caused by mutations in the gene for microsomal triglyceride transfer protein (MTP), with resultant defective assembly of triglyceride-rich lipoproteins.[10]

Familial hypobetalipoproteinemia, a disorder of autosomal dominant inheritance, has clinical manifestations similar to those of abetalipoproteinemia when in the homozygous state. This disease seems to be caused by mutations of the apolipoprotein B gene in most cases.[10]

Chylomicron retention disease and Anderson's disease are caused by defective release of chylomicrons by enterocytes. The distinction between the 2 conditions derives from differences in the partitioning of lipid between membrane and cytoplasmic compartments, although both diseases are due to a defect in the same gene (SAR1B).

General treatment measures in abetalipoproteinemia, hypobetalipoproteinemia, chylomicron retention disease, and Anderson's disease include replacement of triglycerides that contain long-chain fatty acids with medium-chain triglycerides and dietary supplementation with tocopherol.[10]

Wolman's disease and the milder late-onset cholesteryl ester storage disease are seemingly caused by mutations in different parts of the *LIPA* gene, resulting in infiltration of intestinal mucosa with foam cells and intestinal damage.

Congenital Disorders of Cobalamin Absorption

Several congenital diseases can result in vitamin B_{12} malabsorption. Absence of IF synthesis is the most common cause of congenital cobalamin deficiency; abnormal results on Schilling tests normalize with the coadministration of IF.[26,138] In some patients, an abnormal (nonfunctional) IF is secreted that has decreased affinity for cobalamin, decreased affinity for the ileal IF-cobalamin receptor (cubilin-amnionless complex), or increased susceptibility to proteolysis.[26,138]

Imerslund-Graesbeck syndrome is a congenital disease characterized by malabsorption of the cobalamin-IF complex despite normal ileal morphology. This syndrome can be caused by mutations in either of 2 genes that code for the cubilin and AMN proteins, which are co-localized in the ileal mucosa and form the IF-cobalamin receptor.[31]

In transcobalamin II deficiency, serum levels of cobalamin commonly are normal, although in most patients intestinal cobalamin absorption is abnormal.[138] Diagnosis is established by demonstrating the absence of transcobalamin II in the plasma.[138] All congenital disorders of cobalamin absorption are treated by the parenteral administration of cobalamin, although high-dose oral cobalamin also might be effective.

Intestinal Enterokinase Deficiency

Enterokinase, an enzyme secreted by the intestinal mucosa, initiates activation of pancreatic proenzymes. Several patients have been reported to have an inborn deficiency of this enzyme, with resultant diarrhea, failure to thrive, and hypoproteinemia mainly from protein malabsorption. These patients respond well to pancreatic enzyme replacement, and some patients show a tendency to improve with age. Secondary enterokinase deficiency also has been reported in patients with villus atrophy, although patients with celiac disease seem not to be affected.[15]

Primary Immunodeficiency Diseases

Malabsorption commonly occurs in entities characterized by deficiencies in humoral or cellular immunity[274] (see Chapter 2). The immunodeficiency syndromes most commonly associated with malabsorption are selective immunoglobulin (Ig)A deficiency, common variable immunodeficiency (CVID), and severe combined immunodeficiency. The etiology of the malabsorption varies for the different syndromes.

Selective Immunoglobulin A Deficiency

Selective IgA deficiency is the most common primary immunodeficiency disorder and is characterized by a selective near-absence of secretory and serum IgA that renders one susceptible to respiratory, urogenital, and GI infections. Autoimmune and allergic diseases are also commonly seen in patients with this disorder. A 10- to 16-fold increased incidence of gluten-sensitive enteropathy has been reported in patients with IgA deficiency,[275] and a subgroup of patients with selective IgA deficiency have sprue-like small intestinal lesions that lead to severe diarrhea and malabsorption but are unresponsive to a gluten-free diet.[276] Improvement with immunosuppressive therapy has been described in one case report.[277] Pernicious anemia, giardiasis, and secondary disaccharidase deficiencies are also seen with increased frequency in patients with selective IgA deficiency.[276,278]

Common Variable Immunodeficiency

CVID, or CVID-acquired hypogammaglobulinemia, is a clinically and genetically heterogeneous group of immunodeficiency disorders characterized by decreased serum IgG levels and variably decreased serum levels of other immunoglobulin subclasses with T-cell defects. About 10% to 20% of CVID are familial forms, and most cases are sporadic. Onset of the disease usually is in adulthood and manifests with recurrent respiratory and GI infections. Affected patients are also at increased risk for autoimmune and neoplastic diseases. Malabsorption and diarrhea occur in 9% to 40% of patients with CVID[276]; malabsorption involves dietary fat, carbohydrates, vitamin B_{12}, and folate.[274,279]

Small intestinal biopsy specimens show either sprue-like features, including villus shortening with increased numbers of lymphocytes in the epithelium and lamina propria, or a pattern similar to that in graft-versus-host disease (see Chapter 35).[276,280] Some specific histologic features, such as a near-absence of plasma cells, are observed. The disease responds to a gluten-free diet in a minority of patients, and it appears that the sprue-like syndrome in CVID is a distinct entity,[279,281] sometimes referred to as "hypogammaglobulinemic sprue."[282] In some patients with CVID, foamy macrophages are present, as in Whipple's disease, but in contrast with Whipple's disease, the macrophages do not contain material that stains with PAS.[280] In addition, nodular lymphoid hyperplasia can be detected in the GI tract of a high proportion of CVID patients but does not correlate with the presence of malabsorption. The incidence of small bowel lymphoma is increased in CVID, and both disorders have to be considered as potential causes of malabsorption in these patients. *Giardia* organisms are often isolated from patients with CVID, and SIBO has been documented in a number of cases.

Unfortunately, only some patients with malabsorption associated with CVID respond to antimicrobial treatment.[280] Some patients with sprue-like intestinal changes have benefited from glucocorticoids,[278,281] but the value of IV immunoglobulins is questionable.[281] Improvement of enteropathy with infliximab has been described in case reports.[283] Patients with CVID have a higher prevalence of atrophic gastritis with cobalamin malabsorption, although antibodies against parietal cells and IF are absent.[276,279]

X-Linked Infantile Agammaglobulinemia (Bruton's Agammaglobulinemia)

X-linked infantile agammaglobulinemia (Bruton's agammaglobulinemia [OMIM #300755]) is an immunodeficiency disease characterized by lack of mature B lymphocytes and failure of Ig heavy chain rearrangement; it is caused by mutations in the gene for Bruton tyrosine kinase.[284] This disease usually manifests after the first 6 months of life and is characterized by recurrent severe bacterial infections. Severe GI problems like malabsorption and chronic diarrhea are less common than in CVID[280]; the prevalence of chronic gastroenteritis was 10% in one large series.[285] In affected patients, the possibility of giardiasis and SIBO must be considered.[280,285]

Immune Dysregulation-Polyendocrinopathy-Enteropathy–X-Linked Syndrome

Immune dysregulation-polyendocrinopathy-enteropathy-X-linked syndrome (IPEX [OMIM #304790]) is a disorder of early childhood characterized by protracted diarrhea, dermatitis, insulin-dependent diabetes mellitus, thyroiditis, thrombocytopenia, and hemolytic anemia. It is a disorder of X-linked recessive inheritance caused by mutations in the *FOXP3* gene.[286] Diarrhea and malabsorption are secondary to severe villus atrophy with inflammation. Anti-enterocyte antibodies are commonly present. The enteropathy usually does not respond to a gluten-free diet, but immunosuppressive therapy has been shown to be of some benefit. IPEX usually is fatal in childhood. Successful bone marrow transplantation with amelioration of enteropathy has been reported in some cases.[287]

Other Congenital Immunodeficiency Syndromes

In severe combined immunodeficiency (OMIM #300400), diarrhea and malabsorption are common. Symptoms are associated with stunting of intestinal villi or their complete absence. The pathophysiology of malabsorption is unknown, and the syndrome usually fails to respond to antimicrobial treatment.[276,278] Malabsorption also has been reported in DiGeorge's syndrome (thymic hypoplasia [OMIM #188400]) and chronic granulomatous disease of childhood (OMIM #306400), but little is known about its cause in these disorders.[276]

Neurofibromatosis Type 1 (von Recklinghausen's Disease)

Malabsorption can be an intestinal complication of neurofibromatosis type 1 (OMIM #162200). Mechanisms of malabsorption include periampullary duodenal tumors, which are mainly somatostatin-containing neuroendocrine tumors, and pancreatic carcinomas with resultant pancreatic duct obstruction; tumors can cause exocrine pancreatic insufficiency and biliary obstruction.[288] Duodenal somatostatinomas in von Recklinghausen's disease usually do not increase plasma somatostatin levels, although one case of somatostatinoma syndrome has been reported.[289] Infiltrating mesenteric plexiform neurofibromas and vascular damage caused by proliferation of nerves can cause lymphatic or vascular obstruction (or both), with resultant abdominal pain, protein-losing enteropathy, diarrhea, steatorrhea, and bowel ischemia.[290,291] In patients with von Recklinghausen's disease, an increased incidence of neuroendocrine tumors in other locations has been observed; gastrinomas with Zollinger-Ellison syndrome have also been reported in some of these patients (See Chapter 126).[292]

Nongranulomatous Chronic Idiopathic Enterocolitis and Autoimmune Enteropathy

Nongranulomatous chronic idiopathic enterocolitis is an entity that is distinct from refractory celiac disease and IBD.[293] The etiology of this disease is unknown, although chronic infection and an autoimmune cause have been suggested. Severe diarrhea and malabsorption occur as a result of diffuse villus atrophy, and ulcerations may be present in the small and large intestine. Small intestinal villus atrophy and neutrophilic inflammation of the mucosa with crypt abscesses may be seen in biopsy specimens from the small intestine and colon (Fig. 104-10); the number of intraepithelial lymphocytes is not increased.[293,294] Patients respond dramatically to glucocorticoids, and most require long-term low-dose maintenance therapy.[293,294] Improvement with cyclosporine and long-term

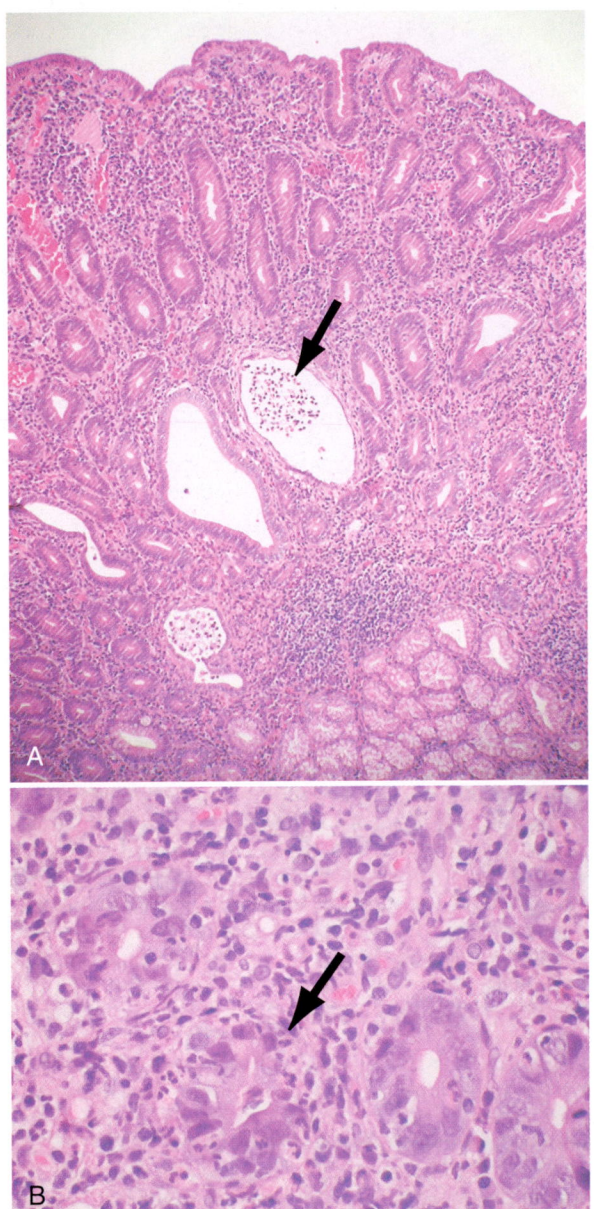

FIGURE 104-10. Duodenal biopsy specimen from a patient with nongranulomatous chronic idiopathic enterocolitis. *A,* Histopathologic features include villus atrophy, diffuse infiltration of lamina propria with inflammatory cells, and crypt abscesses *(arrow). B,* High-power view demonstrates crypt infiltration by neutrophils *(arrow).* (H&E stain.) *(Courtesy Cord Langner, MD.)*

and malabsorption; exclusion of other small intestinal diseases, such as celiac disease; histologic changes on intestinal biopsies such as partial or complete villus blunting, deep crypt lymphocytosis, increased crypt apoptotic bodies, and minimal intraepithelial lymphocytosis; and the presence of anti-enterocyte antibodies and anti-goblet cell antibodies. Absence of antibodies, however, does not exclude the diagnosis.[296] Therapy of autoimmune enteropathy is challenging, and some patients have been treated successfully with glucocorticoids and immunosuppressive drugs such as cyclosporine A and tacrolimus. Two patients with autoimmune enteropathy unresponsive to steroids have been reported to respond to infusion of mesenchymal stromal cells.[298]

Endocrine and Metabolic Disorders

Adrenal Insufficiency (Addison's Disease)

Some patients with adrenal insufficiency, independent of its etiology, have fat malabsorption, with fecal fat excretion of up to 30 g/day having been documented.[299] Fat malabsorption is also observed in rats after adrenalectomy.[300] The pathophysiologic mechanism of malabsorption in this disease is unknown, but fat absorption normalizes upon glucocorticoid replacement.

Isolated autoimmune Addison's disease has been associated with pernicious anemia[301] and celiac disease.[302] An increased incidence of celiac disease and pernicious anemia is also found in autoimmune polyglandular syndrome (APS) type 2 (Schmidt's syndrome), which is characterized by the association of autoimmune Addison's disease and other autoimmune endocrine disorders (except hypoparathyroidism).[303]

Enteroendocrine Deficiency (Autoimmune Polyglandular Syndrome Type 1 [Autoimmune Polyendocrinopathy, Candidiasis, Ectodermal Dystrophy (Apeced)], Enteric Anendocrinosis, and Congenital Proprotein Convertase 1/3 Deficiency)

Autoimmune polyglandular syndrome type 1 (APS 1 [OMIM #240300]) is characterized by multiple endocrine organ failure (especially hypoparathyroidism and adrenal insufficiency) due to autoimmune destruction, with ectodermal dystrophy and susceptibility to chronic *Candida* infections.[303] APS type 1 is inherited as an autosomal recessive disorder and is caused by mutations in the *AIRE* gene.[304] Severe malabsorption, which tends to be recurrent, develops in some 20% of patients with APS type 1. In one patient, malabsorption was caused by a transient and selective destruction of small intestinal enteroendocrine cells, leading to a temporary deficiency of enteroendocrine hormones (especially CCK)[305]; this has been confirmed by observations in subsequently reported patients.[306-308] These patients have autoantibodies to tryptophan hydroxylase, which are directed against enteroendocrine cells (including CCK-producing cells).[309] The long-known association of hypoparathyroidism or hypocalcemia and steatorrhea may be caused by the same mechanism, because in most reports of this association, patients fulfill the diagnostic criteria for APS type 1.[310,311]

Selective absence of small intestinal enteroendocrine cells can be diagnosed by special immunohistochemical stains for these cells (e.g., immunohistochemical stains for chromogranin A or CCK [Fig. 104-11]) or by measurements of postprandial serum levels of the affected hormones. Patients with APS type 1 also have an increased incidence of vitamin B_{12} malabsorption as a result of autoimmune gastritis.[303] Lack of enteroendocrine cells also results in congenital malabsorption

antibiotic therapy has been reported in one patient each.[295] The condition is associated with a high mortality rate.[293,294]

Nongranulomatous chronic idiopathic enterocolitis shares several clinical and histologic features with adult autoimmune enteropathy.[294,296] In many patients with adult autoimmune enteropathy, anti-enterocyte antibodies, anti-goblet cell antibodies, and alterations in regulatory T-cell function are present.[296,297] This entity has been reported in children as well as adults, and other autoimmune disorders are frequently present in these patients. Symptoms are chronic severe high-output diarrhea and malabsorption.[296] Diagnosis relies on a combination of clinical and histologic findings. Proposed diagnostic criteria require the presence of chronic diarrhea

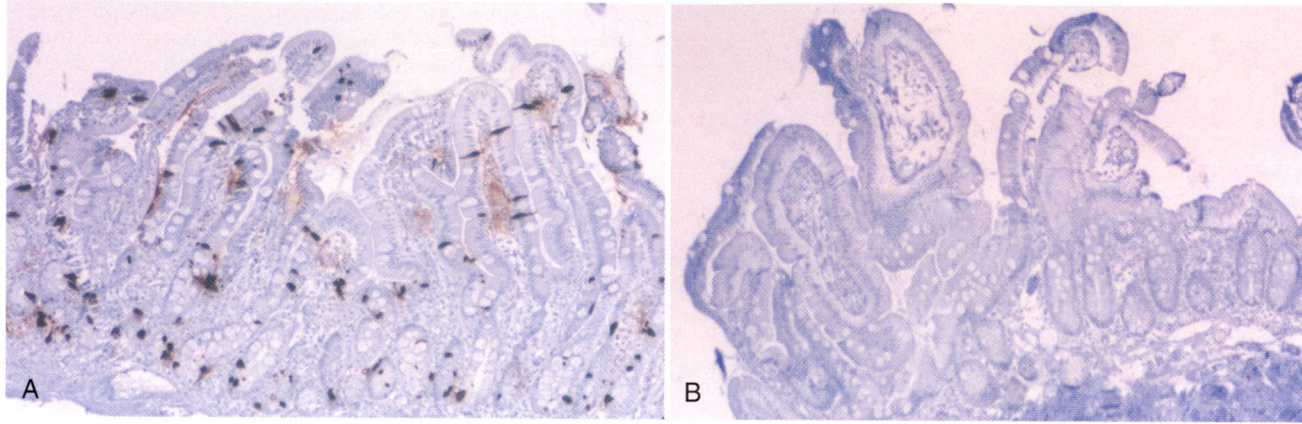

FIGURE 104-11. Chromogranin A immunohistochemical staining of enteroendocrine cells in duodenal biopsy specimens obtained from a normal subject (A) and from a patient with malabsorption associated with autoimmune polyglandular syndrome type 1 (B). In B, enteroendocrine cells are absent. See text for details.

in 2 newly described diseases resulting from mutations in the *NEUROG3* gene (diarrhea 4; enteric anendocrinosis [OMIM #610370]) and *PCSK1* gene (congenital proprotein convertase 1/3 deficiency [OMIM #600995]) (see Table 104-10).[312,313]

Hyperthyroidism and Autoimmune Thyroid Disease

Some reports suggest that up to 25% of hyperthyroid patients have at least some degree of fat malabsorption, but data from large series of patients are lacking. Fecal fat values in hyperthyroid patients can reach 35 g/day.[314] The mechanism of steatorrhea in hyperthyroidism has not been established. Motility studies in hyperthyroid patients (including patients with and without diarrhea) have demonstrated accelerated small intestinal and whole-gut transit times[315]; fecal fat values were not reported in these patients. It can be hypothesized that more pronounced disturbances of intestinal transit can lead to decreased mixing of food and digestive secretions and reduced intestinal absorption of nutrients. Some of the steatorrhea in hyperthyroid patients might result from hyperphagia with increased dietary intake of fat.[316]

An increased number of lymphocytes and plasma cells and some degree of edema in small intestinal biopsy specimens have been found in patients with steatorrhea and hyperthyroidism; villus architecture is normal.[314] Absorption of glucose and D-xylose is normal in hyperthyroid patients with and without malabsorption.[316] Fat malabsorption tends to normalize when patients attain a euthyroid state.[314,316]

In patients with autoimmune thyroid diseases, an increased prevalence of celiac disease[302] and PBC,[301] both of which can result in fat malabsorption, has been recognized. The prevalence of celiac disease in patients with autoimmune thyroid disease is approximately 2% to 4%.[302] Cobalamin malabsorption resulting from autoimmune gastritis is found in a considerable number of patients with autoimmune thyroid disease.[28,301]

Diabetes Mellitus

Chronic diarrhea is common in patients with diabetes mellitus, especially in those with long-standing diabetes mellitus type 1.[317] Mild steatorrhea often is present in patients with diabetic diarrhea and also in diabetic patients who do not complain of diarrhea.[318]

Although the pathophysiologic mechanism of malabsorption and diarrhea in patients with diabetes mellitus is unknown, poor glycemic control is an important cofactor.[319]

Most of these patients have signs of autonomic neuropathy, such as orthostatic hypotension, impotence, bladder dysfunction, incontinence, inappropriate heart rate variability, and abnormal sweating.[320] Therefore, in some patients, diarrhea and malabsorption has been attributed to rapid gastric emptying and rapid intestinal transit, causing impaired mixing of nutrients with digestive secretions and decreased contact time between nutrients and the intestinal mucosa.

The clinician has to be aware that certain treatable diseases, such as celiac disease,[321,322] SIBO,[320] and pancreatic insufficiency,[323] can be associated with diabetes mellitus. In patients with diabetes mellitus type 1, a high prevalence (3% to 8%) of celiac disease has been reported from screening studies, but most of these patients are asymptomatic.[324] Markedly reduced pancreatic exocrine function, as determined by fecal elastase measurement, has been reported in 30% of patients with type 1 diabetes and 17% with type 2 diabetes, compared with 5% of control subjects. In 40% of diabetic patients with reduced fecal elastase levels, fat malabsorption with fecal fat output of more than 10 g/day was detected.[325] GI symptoms and steatorrhea in these patients did not correlate with fecal elastase levels.[323,325] In addition, the unresolved specificity of elastase raises the possibility that not all of these patients truly had pancreatic insufficiency.[326] The presence of cobalamin malabsorption caused by autoimmune atrophic gastritis is increased 3- to 5-fold in patients with diabetes mellitus type 1 compared with the nondiabetic population.[327]

Ingested carbohydrates are malabsorbed in patients receiving acarbose as part of their diabetes treatment, which in turn can lead to symptoms of diarrhea and malabsorption. Foods recommended to diabetics because they contain poorly absorbable carbohydrates such as fructose or sorbitol can result in bloating and diarrhea.

Metabolic Bone Disease

Special consideration has to be given to osteoporosis and osteomalacia in malabsorptive diseases. Patients with these metabolic bone diseases usually do not present with suggestive symptoms or abnormalities either on physical examination or on routine laboratory examinations. Reduced bone mineral density is a common finding in patients with gastric resection,[328] celiac disease,[329] and lactose malabsorption.[180] Osteoporosis has been suggested to result from calcium malabsorption or reduced calcium intake, which leads to secondary hyperparathyroidism, which in turn increases bone turnover and cortical bone loss. Vitamin D malabsorption is probably of lesser importance. Although up to one half of patients on a gluten-free diet have osteoporosis,[330] some studies have shown significant improvement in bone mineral density 1 year after starting a gluten-free diet.[331] In Crohn's disease, which may be accompanied by malabsorption, other factors like glucocorticoid use or testosterone deficiency[332] may contribute to decreased bone mass.

In addition to treating the underlying cause of malabsorption, calcium supplementation is needed to ensure a daily intake of 1500 mg of calcium. Vitamin D deficiency also must be corrected. If osteoporosis is present, bisphosphonate treatment is suggested.[329] Nutritional management is discussed in more detail in Chapters 5 and 6.

GENERAL APPROACH TO MANAGEMENT

Treatment of malabsorptive diseases must be directed against the underlying condition if possible, and nutritional deficits must be corrected. The reader is referred to the relevant chapters of this book for discussion about treatment of specific diseases and their nutritional management. In patients with abdominal bloating and gas-related complaints due to sugar malabsorption, a diet with reduced content of poorly absorbable carbohydrates (e.g., fructose, sorbitol, fermentable dietary fibers) is an effective long-term therapy.[333] Interest has recently surrounded the potential role of Fermentable Oligosaccharides, Disaccharides, Monosaccharides, and Polyols (FODMAPs) in the treatment of patients with symptoms of IBS[334].

In pancreatic insufficiency, disorders of intestinal fat absorption, and short bowel syndrome, medium-chain triglycerides can be used as a source of dietary calories. In patients with short bowel syndrome and some remaining colon, colonic salvage capacity can be used to regain calories from carbohydrates[335]; these patients should consume a diet rich in carbohydrates and medium-chain triglycerides. Teduglutide, a glucagon-like peptide 2 analog, has been shown to reduce the need for parenteral volume supplementation and the amount of malabsorbed calories.[336] The suggested mechanisms for the proabsorptive effects of teduglutide are increased growth of intestinal mucosa, reduced gastric emptying and secretion, and prolonged intestinal transit time.[336,337]

In bile acid malabsorption after extensive ileal resections, intestinal fat absorption can be improved markedly by oral administration of natural conjugated bile acids[198] or synthetic cholylsarcosine.[117,199,200] Replacement of conjugated bile acids also reduces urinary oxalate excretion and therefore should protect against development of kidney stones.[199] Patients with cystic fibrosis or short bowel syndrome who are unable to absorb vitamin D from their diet may benefit from treatment with an ultraviolet lamp, which emits ultraviolet radiation similar to sunlight.[338]

In patients with malabsorption and an intact colon, fluid depletion must be avoided to prevent kidney stones associated with hyperoxaluria.[339] In patients with malabsorption syndrome, special care should be given to the replacement of vitamins, iron, calcium, and trace elements to avoid deficiency syndromes (see Chapters 5 and 6).

In patients with diarrhea, symptomatic treatment with opiates or loperamide can increase the time available for absorption of nutrients.

In patients with home parenteral nutrition, catheter-related bloodstream infections remain the major threat. A prevention strategy using taurolidine, which is a potent antimicrobial agent, has been shown to reduce the risk of these infections.[340]

KEY REFERENCES

Full references for this chapter can be found on www.expertconsult.com.

1. Wilson FA, Dietschy JM. Differential diagnostic approach to clinical problems of malabsorption. Gastroenterology 1971; 61:911-31.
3. Hofmann AF, Poley JR. Role of bile acid malabsorption in pathogenesis of diarrhea and steatorrhea in patients with ileal resection. Gastroenterology 1972; 62:918-34.
6. Ryan ME, Olsen WA. A diagnostic approach to malabsorption syndromes: A pathophysiological approach. Clin Gastroenterol 1983; 12:533-50.
17. Hammer HF, Hammer J. Diarrhea caused by carbohydrate malabsorption. Gastroenterol Clin North Am 2012; 41:611-27.
89. Riddell RH. Small intestinal biopsy: Who? How? What are the findings? In: Barkin JS, Rogers AI, editors. Difficult decisions in digestive diseases. Chicago: Year Book Medical Publishers; 1989. p 326-31.
100. Horton KM, Corl FM, Fishman EK. CT of nonneoplastic diseases of the small bowel: Spectrum of disease. J Comput Assist Tomogr 1999; 23:417-28.
106. Ryan ER, Heaslip IS. Magnetic resonance enteroclysis compared with conventional enteroclysis and computed tomography enteroclysis: A critically appraised topic. Abdom Imaging 2008; 33:34-7.
111. Fine KD, Schiller LR. AGA technical review on the evaluation and management of chronic diarrhea. Gastroenterology 1999; 116:1464-86.
115. Fine KD, Fordtran JS. The effect of diarrhea on fecal fat excretion. Gastroenterology 1992; 102:1936-9.
124. Romagnuolo J, Schiller D, Bailey RJ. Using breath tests wisely in a gastroenterology practice: An evidence-based review of indications and pitfalls in interpretation. Am J Gastroenterol 2002; 97:1113-26.
185. Gibson PR, Newnham E, Barrett JS, et al. Review article: Fructose malabsorption and the bigger picture. Aliment Pharmacol Ther 2007; 25:349-63.
214. Longstreth GF, Newcomer AD. Drug-induced malabsorption. Mayo Clin Proc 1975; 50:284-93.
243. Poitou Bernert C, Ciangura C, Coupaye M, et al. Nutritional deficiency after gastric bypass: Diagnosis, prevention and treatment. Diabetes Metab 2007; 33:13-24.
252. Holt PR. Intestinal malabsorption in the elderly. Dig Dis 2007; 25:144-50.
342. Online Mendelian Inheritance in Man. McKusick-Nathans Institute of Genetic Medicine, Baltimore: Johns Hopkins University; and Bethesda (Md.): National Center for Biotechnology Information, National Library of Medicine [2008 Sep 30]. Available from: http://www.ncbi.nlm.nih.gov/omim/.

The very term *bacterial overgrowth* succinctly conveys what those who coined this term sought to transmit: a situation where an increase in the numbers and/or change in the type of bacteria in the small intestine results in clinical consequences. The idea that an alteration in the bacterial contents of the small intestine and, specifically, the presence of bacterial species normally confined to the colon could lead to problems may date as far back as the late 19th century. The impact of such overgrowth, or "contamination," on a variety of intestinal functions and human nutrition was elegantly demonstrated in a series of classical studies performed during the 1950s through the 1970s.[1,2] Up until recently, the clinical context most typically linked with SIBO was malabsorption/maldigestion. Lately, however, SIBO has been incriminated in a host of other intestinal and extra-intestinal disorders, often on the basis of imprecise methodology and/or limited data. Such studies have generated considerable controversy and thrown the definition of SIBO into sharp relief.

DEFINITION

For the purpose of clarity, this discussion of SIBO will distinguish 2 potential clinical manifestations of SIBO:
1. SIBO as a cause of maldigestion/malabsorption. Here the clinical presentation can be related to effects of the contaminating organism on host morphology or function (Table 105-1), which in turn result in the clinical consequences typically associated with SIBO (e.g., steatorrhea, diarrhea, protein-losing enteropathy, and/or specific deficiency states).
2. SIBO associated with symptoms or clinical entities in the absence of evidence of maldigestion/malabsorption (e.g., SIBO in association with IBS) and where the pathophysiologic linkage with SIBO is less clearly defined.

In relation to the first of these clinical contexts, SIBO can be defined as "clinical and/or laboratory evidence of maldigestion/malabsorption related to qualitative and/or quantitative alterations in the small intestinal microbiota." Here the emphasis is on the clinical context, and SIBO is incriminated—firstly by documenting its presence and secondly by demonstrating a clinical response to its eradication. Here we are dealing with what could be regarded as "classical" SIBO.

The second scenario, the "expanded" version of SIBO, has proved much more problematic because much of the evidence advanced to support an association between SIBO and a given entity has been reliant on the performance characteristics of the test used to define it and, specifically, the ability of that test to distinguish health from disease. Typically, a response to SIBO eradication has not been reported, or if it has, its interpretation remains rather murky. Absent such evidence and lacking biochemical and/or pathologic findings that can be plausibly linked to SIBO, it has often been unclear in these situations whether SIBO is a cause, a consequence, or an epiphenomenon in relation to the other supposedly associated disorder.

PATHOGENESIS OF SYMPTOMS AND CLINICAL FINDINGS

The human GI microflora is a complex ecosystem comprising at least 400 bacterial species. Because the small intestine is the site of digestion and absorption of food, bacterial numbers are normally much lower there than in the colon to prevent unwanted competition with the host and abnormal entry of bacteria across the more permeable epithelium of the small intestine. In addition, gas production from bacterial fermentation of food is minimized.

TABLE 105-1 Pathophysiology of Symptoms and Clinical Consequences in SIBO

Process	Mechanisms of Action	Clinical Consequences
Mucosal injury induced by bacteria and/or their toxins or products	Loss of brush-border enzymes Injury to epithelial barrier leading to enhanced intestinal permeability Inflammatory response generating inflammatory cytokines	Carbohydrate maldigestion Protein-losing enteropathy; bacterial translocation and portal and systemic endotoxemia Liver injury and inflammation, systemic inflammatory responses
Luminal competition with the host for nutrients	Consumption of dietary protein Consumption of vitamin B_{12} Consumption of thiamine Consumption of nicotinamide	Hypoproteinemia, edema B_{12} deficiency, megaloblastic anemia, neurologic symptoms Thiamine deficiency Nicotinamide deficiency
Bacterial metabolism	Fermentation of unabsorbed carbohydrates Deconjugation of primary bile acids Synthesis of vitamin K Synthesis of folate Synthesis of D-lactic acid Synthesis of alcohol Synthesis of acetaldehyde	Bloating, distension, flatulence Diarrhea due to the effects of deconjugated bile acids in the colon; depletion of the bile acid pool leading to fat and fat-soluble vitamin malabsorption Interference with dosing of vitamin K antagonists (e.g., warfarin) High serum folate levels D-lactic acidosis Liver injury Liver injury

Although SIBO usually is defined in quantitative terms as the number of colony-forming units (CFU) per mL, interpretation of such definitions must be mindful of 2 facts: first, from where in the intestine the sample was obtained; and second, as revealed by molecular techniques such as genomics and metabolomics, that as much as 60% of the normal microbiota is not identified by culture-based methods. These reservations notwithstanding, SIBO is usually, and pending validation of a more accurate methodology based on molecular microbiology, defined as the presence of more than 10^5 CFU/mL of bacteria in the proximal small intestine.[3,4] Other authors have entertained the diagnosis of SIBO in the presence of lower colony counts (>10^3 CFU/mL), provided the species of bacteria isolated in the jejunal aspirate is one that normally colonizes the large bowel (e.g., Enterobacteriaceae, enterococci, *Pseudomonas* spp., *Bacteroides* spp.) or that the same species is absent from saliva and gastric juice.[5] This approach is supported by the identification of anaerobes in jejunal aspirates from patients with malabsorption and chronic diarrhea due to SIBO.[6] In the context of maldigestion/malabsorption, these definitions are based on rather firm foundations as bacterial numbers, and prevalent species have been linked not only to symptoms but also to various measures of digestive and absorptive function, as well as to changes in intestinal morphology.

The impact of SIBO on intestinal morphology and physiology was elegantly demonstrated in a series of classical clinical and laboratory studies performed during the latter half of the last century[1-4] and is summarized in Table 105-1.

Mucosal Injury

Mucosal injury in SIBO will contribute to symptoms by the loss of brush border enzymes (e.g., disaccharidases). This loss will result in the presentation of more unabsorbed carbohydrates to intestinal bacteria for fermentation and could also contribute to lactose intolerance.[7] Damage to the epithelial barrier will enhance permeability and, in the most severe cases, lead to a protein-losing enteropathy (see Chapter 30). Enterotoxins elaborated by some contaminating species will further exacerbate mucosal injury. Such injuries may also trigger an inflammatory response, with the generation of inflammatory cytokines such as TNF-α that may contribute to hepatic and systemic complications.

Luminal Competition with Host for Nutrients

Bacterial digestion of luminal protein will leave the affected individual susceptible to malnutrition and will also contribute to hypoproteinemia and edema. A number of phenomena combine to make SIBO an important cause of vitamin B_{12} deficiency (see Chapter 103). These include consumption of cobalamin by anaerobes, bacterial production of cobalamin analogs (with subsequent loss of the parent vitamin to the host), malabsorption of the vitamin at the ileal receptor as a result of competitive binding with cobalamins from bacterially generated metabolites of cobalamin, and in instances of more severe overgrowth, actual mucosal damage that involves the cubilin-amnionless binding site. Bacterial utilization of vitamins in SIBO also has been invoked in the development of thiamine[8] and nicotinamide deficiency.

Bacterial Metabolism

Deconjugation of bile acids and consequent depletion of the bile acid pool will lead to maldigestion of fat and fat-soluble vitamins. Here, there is 1 particular paradox: Bacterial production of vitamin K, combined with enhanced absorption of the vitamin—a result of greater intestinal permeability—may serve not only to sustain but even increase vitamin K levels to a degree that warfarin doses may have to be adjusted to maintain therapeutic anticoagulation.[9] Bacterial synthesis of folic acid may result in the rather unusual combination of high folate and low B_{12} levels in the circulation, which may be diagnostically suggestive of SIBO (see later).

Among individuals with short bowel syndrome, levels of overgrowth can be such as to lead to the generation of large amounts of D-lactic acid and result in an encephalopathic state.[10] It is interesting to note that bacteria involved in SIBO have also been documented to produce alcohol[11] and acetaldehyde, the latter potentially contributing to alcoholic liver disease.

The convergence of SIBO, enhanced intestinal permeability, and impaired immunity can lead to the translocation of bacteria or bacterial components into the portal circulation and has thereby been incriminated in the pathogenesis of systemic sepsis and SBP in liver disease,[5,12,13] as well as catheter-related infections in the patient with intestinal failure.[14]

The influence of SIBO on hepatic morphology and function was convincingly demonstrated some years ago in relation to individuals who had undergone jejunoileal bypass surgery for morbid obesity and developed florid nonalcoholic steatohepatitis (NASH),[15] sometimes leading to end-stage liver disease.[16] Similar mechanisms are now being invoked in general to explain the pathogenesis of NASH and related disorders (see later).

Immunologic reactions to the contaminating bacteria have been linked to a reactive arthropathy in SIBO,[17,18] while other "immune-mediated" disorders, including immune-mediated enteropathies, have been linked to long-standing SIBO.[19]

CAUSES

In health, the most important defensive factors against the development of SIBO are gastric acid and intestinal motor activity. In the stomach, acid kills and suppresses the growth of most organisms that enter from the oropharynx. In the small intestine, the cleansing action of aboral propulsive forces and especially phase III of the interdigestive migrating motor complex (MMC) limit the colonizing ability of bacteria.[20] Other protective factors are the integrity of the intestinal mucosa, including its protective mucus layer and intrinsic antibacterial mechanisms (e.g., defensins, immunoglobulins); the enzymatic activities and bacteriostatic properties of intestinal, pancreatic, and biliary secretions; the protective effects of the commensal flora; and the mechanical and physiologic properties of the ileocecal valve.[21]

Disorders leading to alterations in 1 or more of these defensive systems may be associated with SIBO (Box 105-1).

Dysmotility

Because dysmotility predisposes to an increase in colonic bacteria in the small intestine, diseases that result in impaired intestinal motility are likely to have SIBO as a complication; virtually every condition that has been linked to small intestinal dysmotility has been associated with SIBO.[22-30] Diabetic autonomic neuropathy and scleroderma are prominent examples of dysmotility-related SIBO. In a patient with diabetes who has diarrhea, especially the individual with long-standing type 1 diabetes,[22] SIBO should be sought as a potentially remediable cause. SIBO has been documented in 43% to 56% of scleroderma patients,[29,30] a prevalence linked with a higher global symptom score and, especially among scleroderma patients, with a high score for digestive symptoms. Other factors predictive of SIBO in scleroderma include the presence of diarrhea and constipation. Eradication of SIBO, which is successful in 52% to 73%, results in symptom improvement.[29,30] Intestinal pseudo-obstruction and jejunal diverticulosis are 2 less common examples of SIBO based on myogenic or neurogenic intestinal dysmotility. Morphologic studies suggest that disorders of intestinal motility such as PSS, visceral myopathies, and neuropathies play an important role in the formation of small bowel diverticula.[31] Diverticula in the jejunum occur in 0.07% to 2% of the population and tend to be large and multiple, whereas those in the ileum are small and single. These features explain the observation that symptoms and complications, such as SIBO, have been reported more frequently in association with jejunal than with ileal diverticula.

<table>
<tr><td colspan="1" style="background:#4B2354;color:#fff;">BOX 105-1 Diseases and Disorders Linked to SIBO Based on Pathophysiology</td></tr>
</table>

Dysmotility
Acromegaly
Amyloidosis
Chronic opiate use
Diabetic autonomic neuropathy
Gastroparesis
Hypothyroidism
Idiopathic intestinal pseudo-obstruction
Long-standing use of motility-suppressing drugs
Myotonic muscular dystrophy
Systemic sclerosis/scleroderma

Altered Anatomy
Blind loops
Gastrocolic or jejunocolic fistula
Ileocecal valve resection
Small intestinal diverticulosis
Strictures (Crohn's disease, radiation, surgery)
Surgically induced alterations in anatomy (Billroth II gastrectomy, end-to-side anastomosis)

Hypochlorhydria
Long-term acid suppression (?)
Postsurgical

Immune Deficiency
Acquired immune deficiency (e.g., AIDS, severe malnutrition)
Inherited immune deficiencies

Multifactorial Causes
Advanced age
Celiac disease
Chronic pancreatitis
Crohn's disease
Cystic fibrosis
End-stage kidney disease
Intestinal failure
Liver disease
Radiation enteropathy
Tropical sprue

Unclear or Undefined Relationship to SIBO
Erosive esophagitis
Interstitial cystitis
IBS
Parkinson's disease
Restless legs syndrome
Rosacea
Severe obesity

Jejunal diverticula are twice as frequent in men and are observed predominantly among those older than age 60.

Altered Anatomy

A variety of surgical procedures that alter GI anatomy have been associated with SIBO[8,32] and much of the original work on SIBO was performed on post-gastrectomy patients.[33] Here again, a number of pathophysiologic factors may be operative: hypochlorhydria, formation of blind loops (depending on the nature of the surgical procedure), lack of contact between chyme and bile and/or digestive enzymes, and disruption of intestinal motility. Stagnation and/or recirculation of intestinal contents resulting from strictures, fistulas, enterostomies, and anastomoses also predispose to SIBO, thus explaining the frequent association of SIBO with Crohn's disease, radiation enteropathy, and reconstructive surgery. Indeed, SIBO should be considered in the differential diagnosis of symptomatic relapse of Crohn's disease.[34]

Hypochlorhydria

Initially described in relation to surgical procedures that reduced gastric acid secretion, hypochlorhydria has more recently been invoked in the development of SIBO among individuals on long-term treatment with PPIs. Though some studies suggested that long-term PPI therapy was associated with SIBO,[35,36] others have failed to confirm this.[37] Furthermore, though their meta-analysis revealed a pooled odds ratio of 2.82 for SIBO among PPI users compared with non-users, Lo and Chan found that this association held true only for studies that employed intestinal culture rather than breath tests to diagnose SIBO.[33] Ratuapli and colleagues, who failed to identify a relationship between PPI use and SIBO, based their analysis on breath tests.[37] Though gastric acid secretion and immune responses may decrease in later life, small intestinal dysmotility, rather than fasting hypochlorhydria or immunodeficiency, is probably the major contributor to the relatively high prevalence of SIBO that has been reported among older adults. It also is worthwhile to emphasize that hypochlorhydria may be an important cofactor in the development of SIBO when it coexists with other predisposing factors.

Immune Deficiencies

SIBO has been described in association with inherited and acquired forms of hypogammaglobulinemia,[38] as well as with disorders of cellular immunity (e.g., HIV infection).

Multifactorial Causes

The cause of SIBO in chronic pancreatitis is multifactorial and includes loss of pancreatic enzymes, a decrease in intestinal motility as a result of the inflammatory process, the effects of narcotics on intestinal motility, and the presence in some instances of intestinal obstruction.

SIBO has long been regarded as a potential complication of celiac disease and 1 of the causes of a failure to respond to gluten withdrawal[39,40]; here again, a number of factors may be operative (e.g., dysmotility, impaired defenses against bacterial colonization, pancreatic insufficiency). Overall, SIBO is considered to be responsible for approximately 10% of nonresponsive celiac disease.[41,42] Those with coexistent SIBO have evidence of more severe malabsorption, although a more recent study failed to demonstrate any benefit from a course of rifaximin among a group of nonresponsive celiac patients.[43] This latter observation is similar to observations in tropical enteropathy that revealed no impact of rifaximin on symptoms, suggesting—contrary to prior opinion—that SIBO may not be a major factor in the pathogenesis of this disorder.[44] It is likely that multiple pathophysiologic factors contribute to SIBO reported in association with cystic fibrosis,[45,46] chronic kidney failure,[24] intestinal failure,[47,48] and liver disease.[49]

SIBO has been frequently documented in association with liver disease, and it is in this context that relationships between SIBO and systemic sepsis have been most extensively explored.[12] Risk factors for SIBO in liver disease have included the presence of cirrhosis and more advanced disease as evidenced by such features as portal hypertension,[50] ascites,[51,52] and jaundice.[51] SIBO also has been linked to systemic endotoxemia in patients with liver disease,[13,52] and in some[12] but not all[5] studies, to a greater risk of developing SBP. Intestinal bacteria clearly are fundamental to the causation of overt hepatic encephalopathy, and SIBO also has been linked to minimal hepatic encephalopathy.[53] SIBO and altered intestinal permeability, another common finding in liver disease, may, through the systemic effects of bacterial endotoxin, also play a role in the pathogenesis of what is now 1 of the most common liver disorders worldwide: nonalcoholic fatty liver disease (NAFLD).[54]

Unclear or Undefined Relationship to SIBO

SIBO has been linked with rosacea,[55] interstitial cystitis,[56] restless legs syndrome,[57] Parkinson's disease,[58,59] erosive esophagitis,[60] and severe obesity.[61] While plausible hypotheses have been proposed to suggest a role for SIBO in the pathogenesis of various manifestations of these disorders, their relationship with SIBO remains to be firmly established; in some instances, this is because SIBO was diagnosed using relatively inaccurate methods.

By far, the greatest controversy related to SIBO over the past 15 years or so has been the proposal that SIBO is linked to IBS. The initial reports from Pimentel and colleagues,[62,63] using the lactulose breath test for diagnosis, documented SIBO in 84% of their patients with IBS. Use of neomycin to normalize the lactulose breath test in this group resulted in a significant improvement in IBS symptoms. Though reports of high rates of positive lactulose breath tests continue to accumulate among both children (65%)[64] and adults (34% to 84%)[56,57,62,63,65-67] who have IBS (studies that employ the glucose breath test document lower rates of positivity [6% to 16%]),[67,68] significant concerns have been raised regarding the validity of this association.[69-73] In an important systematic review and meta-analysis of the link between SIBO and IBS, Ford and colleagues drew attention to the impact of the test modality on SIBO prevalence. The average prevalence of SIBO by breath testing was 54%, in sharp contrast to a mean prevalence of just 4% for jejunal aspirate cultures.[74] These authors also drew attention to the impact of diagnostic criteria, which varied considerably among studies, on study outcome.[74] To muddy the waters further, it has been suggested that the apparent link between SIBO and IBS may reflect the influence of PPI use that is so common in this patient population.[75] One can only conclude that although some patients with SIBO may present with IBS-type symptoms, SIBO is not a major contributor to the pathogenesis of IBS in general.[76] Furthermore, the modest improvement in IBS symptoms that has now been reported with some consistency in patients with IBS who have been treated with antibiotic therapy[77,78] may owe more to the effects of these agents on the colonic microbiota than on SIBO.

DIAGNOSIS

Clinical Features

The clinical manifestations of SIBO are protean and can range from detection of laboratory abnormalities, such as vitamin B_{12} or iron deficiency in an asymptomatic individual, to florid steatorrhea with protein-losing enteropathy. SIBO is an important cause of otherwise unexplained diarrhea in older adults and may also present with weight loss accompanied by relatively nonspecific symptoms like bloating, flatulence, and abdominal discomfort. The clinical presentation of SIBO is changing, and the classical features of SIBO are rarely seen nowadays, with the possible exception of individuals with short bowel syndrome (see Chapter 106).[47] This change is undoubtedly multifactorial and related to such factors as disappearance of the surgical procedures that accounted for many past instances of SIBO, earlier diagnosis and effective treatment of other predisposing disorders (e.g., Crohn's disease[79,80] and celiac disease),[39-43] and earlier recognition and treatment of SIBO per se. For all these reasons, SIBO is now primarily recognized as a cause of unexplained diarrhea[81] and occult malabsorption[82] in older adults. In a large retrospective series of patients who had duodenal aspirates performed, the main clinical factors predictive of the presence of SIBO were older age, steatorrhea, and narcotic use; significantly associated disorders were IBD, chronic pancreatitis, and jejunal diverticulosis, not IBS or PPI use.[83] The change in clinical presentation of SIBO is also reflected in recent surveys of small intestinal histology in SIBO, which have reported at most only relatively minor alterations in mucosal morphology. In 1 such study of 67 consecutive patients with SIBO (duodenal aspirate cultures with ≥10^5 CFU/mL) compared with 55 controls (duodenal aspirate cultures with <10^5 CFU/mL), villus blunting was the only feature more common in SIBO than in controls. More than half of biopsies from SIBO patients were histologically unremarkable. The authors therefore concluded that SIBO needs to be considered as a potential etiology for GI symptoms even when duodenal biopsies are found to be normal.[84] Furthermore, levels of fecal calprotectin have been found to be normal among both children[85] and adults[86] with SIBO, suggesting that SIBO is nowadays associated with at most a negligible inflammatory response and very little in the way of mucosal injury.

Aspiration and Culture

Traditionally, the direct aspiration and culture of jejunal fluid, with results expressed as CFU/mL of jejunal fluid, although invasive, was regarded as the gold standard for the diagnosis of SIBO.[87-90] Allowing presumably for a higher background level of bacterial contamination in the tropics, Bhat and colleagues defined SIBO among their patients in southern India as more than 10^7 CFU/mL.[91] This is an important observation and has implications for comparisons between disease states and control subjects in different geographic regions, as well as from varying socioeconomic and dietary backgrounds. The significance of jejunal aspirate bacterial counts that are higher than those of healthy controls but fall below the level of 10^5 CFU/mL, as described in a number of GI disorders, is unclear.[92] This dilemma was recently exemplified by the study of Posserud and colleagues among IBS patients.[93] Although the majority did not have bacterial counts over 10^5 CFU/mL, and the overall prevalence of SIBO so defined was not different from controls, bacterial counts were numerically higher in the IBS subjects, and if a lower cut-off of 10^4 had been used, the prevalence of SIBO would have been higher.[93] Choung and colleagues made similar observations in relation to PPI use,[83] which, though linked to higher numbers of bacteria in the duodenum, was not associated with SIBO when conventional criteria were employed. The significance of these subthreshold levels of bacterial contamination and of SIBO limited to the more distal reaches of the intestine is unknown at this time.

Numerous methods have been used to obtain bowel contents for culture, including the classic technique of jejunal intubation under fluoroscopic guidance, a variety of endoscopically guided aspiration methods,[92] mucosal brushings using a cytology brush,[94] and mucosal biopsies.[95] However, it is particularly important not to extrapolate diagnostic criteria from 1 technique to another, as is commonly done in the case of endoscopically derived aspirates where samples are derived from the second part of the duodenum and not the jejunum; the microbiota may differ both quantitatively and qualitatively in these locations. Though widely quoted and applied, it must be emphasized that while the so-called gold standard for the definition of SIBO based on aspirate and culture (i.e., >10^5 CFU/mL of bacteria in the proximal small bowel) correlates well with clinical features in "classical" SIBO,[33] its

application to the diagnosis of SIBO outside of this context has not been validated. In fact, Khoshini and coworkers concluded in their systematic review that no gold standard exists for the diagnosis of SIBO once one strays beyond the narrow confines of maldigestion/malabsorption, and that various proposed thresholds had not been validated in sufficiently large, diverse, and truly normal populations.[97] Thresholds based on duodenal aspirates are even more tenuous in terms of source and validation.

These considerable issues in relation to definition, technique, and patient selection notwithstanding, aspiration-based approaches also suffer from being invasive, time consuming, and costly. Moreover, this approach is vulnerable to contamination of the aspirate by oropharyngeal flora (which are mainly Gram-positive), the presence of which has not correlated well with SIBO-related symptoms. However, oropharyngeal floral contamination can be addressed by oral antisepsis or by the simultaneous culture of saliva and aspirate.[98] These observations also form the basis for the proposal by some investigators to restrict the range of organisms included in the definition of SIBO (whether >10^3 or >10^5 CFU/mL) to what would be regarded as colonic-type bacteria (i.e., Gram-negative organisms, anaerobes, enterococci), organisms that have been linked to SIBO symptoms and whose effects in the SIBO syndrome have a plausible pathogenetic basis. Indeed, a considerable body of evidence exists to link contamination of this degree (and with such organisms) to what might be referred to as the "classical" SIBO syndrome: diarrhea, steatorrhea, vitamin B_{12} deficiency, and hypoproteinemia.[1-4,33] The culture technique is also beset with potential problems, ranging from challenges inherent to maintaining anaerobic conditions during the collection, transport, and evaluation of samples to the enthusiasm and skill of the microbiologist; it is no wonder the reproducibility of this approach has been reported to be low.[47]

Of greatest concern is the revelation by methodologies based on genomics and metabolomics that only 5% to 40% of the intestinal microbiota has been identified employing conventional culture methods. Application of these molecular techniques to the study of small intestinal aspirates should ultimately prove to be the most precise methodology for the definition and diagnosis of SIBO.[99]

Breath Tests

Because of the pitfalls with direct aspiration of intestinal fluid, a variety of indirect tests have been developed. These tests are now widely employed as an alternative to direct aspiration, their attractiveness enhanced by being relatively noninvasive and less costly.[100]

The first breath test developed for the diagnosis of SIBO was the bile acid breath test.[101,102] Bile acids were radiolabelled with ^{14}C or ^{13}C, and when deconjugated by bacteria, $^*CO_2$ was ultimately released, absorbed, and excreted in breath samples.[103] In different studies, sensitivity and specificity have been quite variable, ranging from 30% to 70% and 33% to 90%, respectively.[104-107] False-positive test results may also occur with disease or resection of the terminal ileum, the site of bile acid absorption. When ^{14}C is used, the test also carries a radiation risk, especially problematic in children, pregnant women, or women of child-bearing potential.

The ^{14}C or ^{13}C-D-xylose breath test[108,109] depends on the capacity of intestinal bacteria to metabolize ^{14}C or ^{13}C xylose to release $^{14}CO_2$ or $^{13}CO_2$, which is then absorbed and ultimately eliminated in the breath where it can be quantified. Sensitivity and specificity of the ^{14}C xylose test has ranged from 14% to 95% and 40% to 94%, respectively.[110-114]

Hydrogen breath tests are based on the premise that carbohydrate fermentation by intestinal bacteria and, most notably, anaerobic bacteria in the colon is the body's only source of H_2 production. In the case of malabsorption, some of the ingested sugar reaches the colon and is the source of excess hydrogen production. The same principle applies when "colonic" bacteria have colonized the small intestine, as in SIBO; exposure of carbohydrate to bacteria in the small intestine produces a large and premature amount of hydrogen gas. H_2 produced in this manner diffuses into the systemic circulation and is excreted in the expired air via the lung; in all, about one fifth of the H_2 gas produced is exhaled.[115]

Hydrogen breath tests may employ simple sugars that should normally be absorbed in the small intestine or may involve the use of a nonabsorbable compound. The general principles of these hydrogen-based breath tests are as follows.[100,115,116] After a 12-hour overnight fast and a low-fiber diet for 1 day, subjects are asked to exhale into a tube that is connected to a sampling bag and syringe to obtain H_2 baseline values before intake of the substrate. Then the carbohydrate substrate is administered orally, and sequential end-expiratory breath samples are collected at timed intervals for 3 to 5 hours.

Tests based on excretion of hydrogen in the breath, because of their low cost and relative simplicity, have become the most commonly used of all breath tests in the diagnosis of SIBO, but are bedeviled by several problems in interpretation:

1. False-negative tests: Sequestration of the hydrogen produced during the fermentation process may occur in some instances consequent to the activity of 2 types of bacteria—methanogenic and sulfide-reducing—that convert hydrogen into methane and hydrogen sulfide, respectively.[117] If the intestine harbors methanogenic species, a hydrogen breath test may produce a false-negative result if only methane is produced, hence the need to measure both gases.
2. Alterations in intestinal motility: Results of hydrogen breath tests also can be significantly disrupted by altered transit, such as in gastroparesis or states of intestinal "hurry." The shorter the transit time, the greater the likelihood of a false-positive result.
3. States of carbohydrate malabsorption: False-positive test results will also occur among subjects who have carbohydrate malabsorption from conditions such as chronic pancreatitis or celiac disease, because the sugar is available to be fermented by the colonic flora.[118-120] It may be difficult to differentiate malabsorption and SIBO, because SIBO itself can result in false-positive lactose hydrogen breath tests.[120] It is recommended that SIBO first be sought before an evaluation for sugar malabsorption is performed.
4. Oral flora: The oral flora may contribute a confusing early peak, as will ingestion of a high-fiber diet on the day before the test.[121]
5. Diet, smoking, and exercise: Recent food ingestion may lead to an exaggeration, and smoking and exercise a suppression, of the H_2 response. Accordingly, the subject is requested to fast and avoid all fluids except water for 12 hours before the test, as well as to avoid smoking and exercise during the test.[122]

For all these reasons, the sensitivity and specificity of breath tests, in comparison to those of jejunal aspiration, as well as their inter-subject variability, have been of concern.[100,115,123,124]

The lactulose hydrogen breath test (LHBT) is based on the use of lactulose, a nonabsorbable substance, and is 1 of the most widely used hydrogen breath tests. The rise of hydrogen level after lactulose ingestion in SIBO was first reported by Bond and Levitt.[125] The colonic flora ferments lactulose, with the production of hydrogen and/or methane. After administration of 10 g of the sugar, breath samples are taken at 15-minute intervals for 3 hours.

Methane production upon ingestion of lactulose, and related to the activities of methanogenic species in the intestinal flora, has been estimated to occur in 36% to 50% of healthy subjects[117,126,127] and, among subjects with functional GI symptoms, has been associated with constipation.[62,70,128] However, the flat H_2 curve, characteristic of a methanogenic flora,[129] cannot be explained simply on the basis of an abundance of the methanogenic organism, *Methanobrevibacter smithii*, which accounts for only about 10% of all anaerobic bacteria in the healthy adult colon, in contrast to the Bacteroidetes and Firmicutes phyla (both H_2 producers), which together represent more than 90% of the flora.[130] The ability of methanogens to compete for hydrogen is a more plausible explanation.[131]

Criteria for the diagnosis of SIBO using the LHBT have generated controversy ever since its inception, and this test has, of all those employed in the diagnosis of SIBO, yielded the most conflicting data.[69,100] The proposed main criteria of the LHBT include:

1. A high basal level of H_2 related, it is thought, to the action of the bacterial flora on a previous meal or unabsorbed carbohydrate in the intestine. Some consider this finding alone as diagnostic.
2. A double peak on the breath hydrogen expiration graph has become an established criterion for the diagnosis of SIBO by LHBT. The first peak is due to H_2 production by the bacterial population in the small intestine, and the second results from the action of colonic flora on lactulose.[89,100,115,122,132] It may be difficult, however, to distinguish a double peak in many cases.
3. A rise in H_2 above baseline within 90 minutes and/or an absolute rise of greater than 20 ppm above the basal H_2 level within 180 min of lactulose ingestion.[62,70,93,133,134] A caveat that must accompany this definition of a positive test is the fact that the average orocecal transit time as assessed by LHBT is only slightly longer, so many apparently healthy subjects will appear to have SIBO. Rapid transit, as may occur in conditions like IBS, further compounds interpretation, especially because lactulose itself may accelerate intestinal transit. It has been proposed that rapid transit, rather than SIBO, may explain positive breath hydrogen tests in diarrhea-predominant IBS.[135]

After LHBT, the glucose hydrogen breath test (GHBT) is the next most commonly used test to diagnose SIBO.[115,136] Glucose is given in a dose of 50 to 75 g dissolved in water as a 10% solution, after which breath is sampled at baseline and every 15 minutes for 3 hours. Otherwise, the preparation for and conduct of the test follow the same guidelines as the hydrogen-based breath tests. A GHBT is considered positive if the basal H_2 level is greater than 12 ppm or rises more than 12 ppm above the baseline value within 2 hours of glucose ingestion.

Which is the better of the hydrogen breath tests? In terms of the 2 main substrates, lactulose, in general, seems to have a lower sensitivity and specificity than glucose.[69,89,124,132,137,138] Using culture as the standard, 1 study directly compared the sensitivity, specificity, positive and negative predictive values, and diagnostic accuracy of the LHBT and GHBT. The LHBT had greater specificity (86%) compared with the GHBT (80%) but lower sensitivity (21% vs. 44%) and accuracy (55% vs. 65%).[137] Others, however, have failed to identify any significant differences in sensitivity or specificity between the LHBT and GHBT.[93,139,140]

Other Tests

Apart from identifying anatomic causative factors (e.g., jejunal diverticulosis or stricture), imaging studies are of little value in the direct diagnosis of SIBO because small intestinal mucosal changes in SIBO are neither specific nor diagnostic, and mucosal injury and villus atrophy are evident only in the most severely affected individuals.

Cholyl-PABA, a synthetic compound created by conjugating cholic acid with para-aminobenzoic acid (PABA), is catabolized by bacterial hydrolase to release free PABA, which can then be detected in the urine. In fact, PABA provided a simple noninvasive method for detecting SIBO but could not distinguish between SIBO and other causes of malabsorption with any degree of reliability.[141] Though this test correlated well with results of ^{14}C xylose breath testing, it never gained widespread clinical application.

Urinary indican (indoxyl sulfate, a by-product of intestinal bacterial metabolism of tryptophan) levels also have been used to test for SIBO. Although the overall sensitivity of this urinary marker was promising at 80% to 90% in early studies,[142,143] no recent studies have been performed to support the validity of the test.

Various serum markers, including bile acids, folic acid, and cobalamin, have been proposed as biomarkers for SIBO, but none has sufficient diagnostic accuracy to be of value in the detection of SIBO.

The above tests, while indirect, are relatively noninvasive and have appeal for clinical practice. While abnormal results may support the diagnosis of SIBO, however, none has been adequately validated as a diagnostic test of SIBO. Some have not been extensively tested in humans, and those that have are less than optimal in terms of sensitivity and specificity.

Therapeutic Trial

Given the problems associated with all of the above-described tests for the diagnosis of SIBO, it should come as no surprise that clinicians have turned to therapeutic trials of antibiotics as an alternative diagnostic strategy. However, appealing as the therapeutic trial may seem, it currently lacks standardization with respect to choice of antibiotic, as well as the dose and duration of therapy or appropriate outcome measures. It is for now an entirely empirical approach.

The limitations of our currently available diagnostic methods were vividly illustrated in a study by Kerckhoffs and colleagues.[144] They performed both the LHBT and a jejunal aspirate on 11 healthy controls and 15 subjects predisposed to SIBO; breath testing was associated with a high false-positive rate and, disappointingly, the use of molecular methods did not increase the yield of aspirates.

TREATMENT

There are 3 components to the treatment of SIBO: (1) treating the underlying disease, (2) eradicating bacterial overgrowth, and (3) addressing any associated nutritional deficiencies. Clearly, the primary goal should be the treatment or correction of any underlying disease or defect when possible. Unfortunately, several of the clinical conditions associated with SIBO (e.g., visceral myopathies and multiple jejunal diverticula) are not readily reversible. It stands to reason that medications associated with intestinal stasis, such as drugs known to inhibit intestinal motility or gastric acid secretion, should be eliminated or substituted for by other agents whenever possible.

When surgical correction of the clinical condition associated with SIBO is not an option, management is with antimicrobials, and the goal of such treatment is not to eradicate the bacterial flora but to alter it in a way that leads to symptomatic improvement. Although ideally the choice of antimicrobial agents should reflect in vitro susceptibility testing, this is usually impractical because many bacterial species typically

---

BOX 105-2 Antibiotic Regimens for SIBO

Ciprofloxacin (250 mg twice daily)
Norfloxacin (800 mg once daily)
Metronidazole (250 mg 3 times daily)
Trimethoprim/sulfamethoxazole (160/800 mg twice daily)
Doxycycline (100 mg 2 times daily)
Amoxicillin-clavulanic acid (500 mg 3 times daily)
Tetracycline (250 mg 4 times daily)
Neomycin (500 mg 2 times daily)
Rifaximin (800-1200 mg once daily)

---

coexist, each with different antibiotic sensitivities. Antibiotic treatment remains, therefore, primarily empirical. Despite the volumes that have been written regarding the prevalence and causes of SIBO, the clinician faced with treating this condition has relatively few studies to guide therapy. Effective antibiotic therapy must cover both aerobic and anaerobic enteric bacteria, and different treatment schedules have been suggested (Box 105-2). In general, a single 7- to 10-day course of antibiotic may improve symptoms for up to several months in most (46% to 90%) patients with SIBO and render breath tests negative in 20% to 75% of cases.

In recent years, the more widespread availability of the poorly absorbed antibiotic rifaximin has led to a significant increase in the number of randomized trials of SIBO therapy. In controlled studies, rifaximin in doses that ranged from 800 mg/day for 4 weeks to 1200 mg/day for 7 days was effective in eradicating SIBO[145,146] and, in 1 trial at least, was superior to metronidazole.[145] These findings were supported by a retrospective review.[147]

Recurrence following 1 course of antibiotic therapy remains an issue (up to 44% at 9 months) and is more likely among older subjects, those who have undergone an appendectomy, and those with a history of chronic PPI use.[148] Because of recurrent symptoms, some patients will need either cyclical (e.g., the first 5 to 10 days out of every month) or continuous courses of antibiotic therapy. For the latter, rotating antibiotic regimens are recommended to prevent the development of resistance. Decisions on management should be individualized and consider such risks of long-term antibiotic therapy as diarrhea, *Clostridium difficile* infection, intolerance, bacterial resistance, and costs. Preferred options include use of antibiotics with less toxicity and lower systemic absorption and 7-day regimens incorporating norfloxacin, amoxicillin-clavulanic acid, metronidazole, or where available, rifaximin. It is not necessary to repeat diagnostic tests for SIBO following antibiotic therapy, should GI symptoms respond.

Although recent studies have reported some effects for probiotic and prebiotic supplements in the treatment and evolution of GI diseases such as IBD and IBS, results in SIBO have been inconclusive with the exception of 1 study that found addition of the prebiotic preparation guar gum enhanced the efficacy of rifaximin.[149] The value of adding prokinetic agents like cisapride and erythromycin is uncertain. Moreover, cisapride has been withdrawn in many countries, owing to cardiovascular side effects. Because octreotide stimulates propagative phase 3 activity in the small intestine, low doses (50 μg per day) have been advocated for patients who do not respond to antibiotics, cannot tolerate them, or develop antibiotic-related complications. Nonabsorbable purgative solutions may improve GI symptoms in children with short bowel syndrome and SIBO.

Nutritional support is an important component of the management of SIBO. Dietary modifications may include the institution of a lactose-free diet, replacement of vitamin deficiencies (especially fat-soluble vitamins), and correction of deficiencies in nutrients such as calcium, magnesium, and B_{12}. In severe cases, because mucosal damage may persist for some time even after complete eradication of bacterial overgrowth, nutritional support may be required over a prolonged period of time.

Two clinical scenarios may be encountered that may involve SIBO. The first scenario, which may be regarded as classical SIBO, refers to the situation where clinical features can be pathophysiologically linked with SIBO; affected patients typically present with symptoms and signs of malabsorption and/or maldigestion. In these instances, the diagnostic and therapeutic approaches have been rather well developed and, to some degree, validated. In this more restricted concept of SIBO, culture of jejunal fluid remains a valuable benchmark because abnormal results correlate well with such clinical and pathologic consequences as steatorrhea and anemia. The second scenario relates to the patient with no overt evidence of malabsorption/maldigestion in whom symptoms have been linked to SIBO. Here it is clear that we do not have validated criteria for the incrimination of SIBO, because the accuracy of all current tests in this context remains limited. When we extend the concept of SIBO into these areas, we are bereft of a gold standard, and issues such as the clinical implication of lower levels of contamination and distal overgrowth come into play; these dilemmas are unresolved. From a clinical perspective, only a full clinical response to a course of appropriate antibiotics can satisfy the clinician that SIBO is the villain, but here again, effects on the colonic flora may complicate interpretation. Modern genomic and metabolomic techniques offer much promise in defining true normality and then fully identifying alterations in the flora in disease states; we look forward to their applications in the diagnosis and management of SIBO.

KEY REFERENCES

Full references for this chapter can be found on www.expertconsult.com.

12. Almeida J, Galhenage S, Yu J, et al. Gut flora and bacterial translocation in chronic liver disease. World J Gastroenterol 2006; 12:1493-502.
30. Parodi A, Sessarego M, Greco A, et al. Small intestinal bacterial overgrowth in patients suffering from scleroderma: Clinical effectiveness of its eradication. Am J Gastroenterol 2008; 103:1257-62.
36. Lo WK, Chan WW. Proton pump inhibitor use and the risk of small intestinal bacterial overgrowth: A meta-analysis. Clin Gastroenterol Hepatol 2013; 11:483-90.
42. Dewar DH, Donnelly SC, McLaughlin SD, et al. Celiac disease: Management of persistent symptoms in patients on a gluten-free diet. World J Gastroenterol 2012; 18:1348-56.
49. Quigley EM, Stanton C, Murphy EF. The gut microbiota and the liver. Pathophysiological and clinical implications. J Hepatol 2013; 58:1020-7.
74. Ford AC, Spiegel BM, Talley NJ, Moayyedi P. Small intestinal bacterial overgrowth in irritable bowel syndrome: Systematic review and meta-analysis. Clin Gastroenterol Hepatol 2009; 7:1279-86.
81. Fan X, Sellin JH. Review article: Small intestinal bacterial overgrowth, bile acid malabsorption and gluten intolerance as possible causes of chronic watery diarrhoea. Aliment Pharmacol Ther 2009; 29:1069-77.
83. Choung RS, Ruff KC, Malhotra A, et al. Clinical predictors of small intestinal bacterial overgrowth by duodenal aspirate culture. Aliment Pharmacol Ther 2011; 33:1059-67.
84. Lappinga PJ, Abraham SC, Murray JA, et al. Small intestinal bacterial overgrowth: Histopathologic features and clinical correlates in an underrecognized entity. Arch Pathol Lab Med 2010; 134:264-70.
100. Simren M, Stotzer PO. Use and abuse of hydrogen breath tests. Gut 2006; 55:297-303.
122. Gasbarrini A, Corazza GR, Gasbarrini G, et al. Methodology and indications of H_2 breath testing in gastrointestinal diseases: The Rome Consensus Conference. Aliment Pharmacol Ther 2009; 29(Suppl 1):1-49.
135. Yu D, Cheesman F, Vanner S. Combined oro-cecal scintigraphy and lactulose hydrogen breath testing demonstrate that breath testing detects oro-cecal transit, not small intestinal bacterial overgrowth in patients with IBS. Gut 2011; 60:334-40.
144. Kerckhoffs AP, Visser MR, Samsom M, et al. Critical evaluation of diagnosing bacterial overgrowth in the proximal small intestine. J Clin Gastroenterol 2008; 42:1095-102.
147. Yang J, Lee HR, Low K, et al. Rifaximin versus other antibiotics in the primary treatment and retreatment of bacterial overgrowth in IBS. Dig Dis Sci 2008; 53:169-74.
149. Lauritano EC, Gabrielli M, Scarpellini E, et al. Small intestinal bacterial overgrowth recurrence after antibiotic therapy. Am J Gastroenterol 2008; 103:2031-5.

106
Short Bowel Syndrome

ALAN L. BUCHMAN

Short bowel syndrome (SBS) is characterized by malabsorption due to congenital absence or resection of large portions of the small intestine, typically leaving the adult with 150-200 cms of functional small intestine. Individuals that are left with SBS are left with an insufficient intestinal surface area such that they are unable to absorb sufficient fluid, macronutrients, micronutrients and micronutrients, and therebt lose nutritonal autonomy are defined as having *intestinal failure*. It is important to recognize that not all individuals with SBS have intestinal failure and that intestinal failure may be caused by conditions other than SBS that lead to a functional SBS (Box 106-1). The spectrum of SBS ranges from limited ileocolonic resections with moderate nutritional compromise to extensive small intestinal and colonic resections with duodenostomy, proximal jejunostomy, or jejunocolonic anastomosis and severe nutritional consequences.

ETIOLOGY

The major causes of SBS in adults are Crohn's disease for which multiple intestinal resections have been performed; mesenteric infarction from venous or arterial thrombosis, arterial embolism, or midgut volvulus; massive enterectomy performed to manage traumatic injuries or tumor resection; and radiation injury (Box 106-1). The causes of SBS in the pediatric population are congenital abnormalities (see Chapter 98), including gastroschisis, intestinal atresia, malrotation, aganglionosis, and necrotizing enterocolitis. More than 90% of infants now survive the extensive intestinal resections required for these conditions, and these patients need careful follow-up for their SBS as they mature to adulthood. Intestinal failure also can result from chronic intestinal pseudo-obstruction syndrome in both adults and children (see Chapter 124), as well

as from unclassified celiac disease in adults (see Chapter 107) and congenital villus atrophy in children.

INCIDENCE AND PREVALENCE

The incidence of SBS is difficult to assess in the United States because of lack of a national registry for affected persons and lack of prospective studies in defined populations of patients who have undergone extensive intestinal resections. The incidence of severe SBS necessitating long-term parenteral nutrition (PN) is estimated to be 2 to 4 cases per 1 million persons per year, based on multinational European data.[1] It is estimated that between 10,000 and 20,000 patients in the United States follow a home PN regimen for SBS. Approximately 50% to 70% of patients with SBS who initially require PN can be weaned from this therapy and therefore might not be reflected in the prevalence estimates.[2,3] Such patients often still require aggressive nutritional monitoring. The incidence and prevalence of SBS associated with Crohn's disease are decreasing now that infliximab and strictureplasty have become commonplace.

PATHOPHYSIOLOGY

The major consequence of extensive intestinal resection is loss of absorptive surface area, which results in malabsorption of macronutrients, micronutrients, electrolytes, and water.[4] The degree of malabsorption is determined by the length of the remnant intestine; the specific portions of small and large intestine resected, along with their site-specific transport processes and endocrine cells; and the adequacy of adaptive processes in the residual intestine over time. Three types

BOX 106-1 Causes of Short Bowel Syndrome (SBS) and Intestinal Failure in Adults and Children

Adults
Catastrophic vascular accidents:
- Superior mesenteric arterial embolism
- Superior mesenteric arterial thrombosis
- Superior mesenteric venous thrombosis

Chronic intestinal pseudo-obstruction*
Intestinal resection for tumor or trauma
Midgut volvulus
Multiple intestinal resections for Crohn's disease
Radiation enteritis*
Refractory sprue*
Scleroderma and mixed connective tissue disease*

Children
Congenital villus atrophy*
Extensive aganglionosis*
Gastroschisis
Jejunal or ileal atresia
Necrotizing enterocolitis

*Functional SBS can also occur in conditions associated with severe malabsorption and intact bowel length.

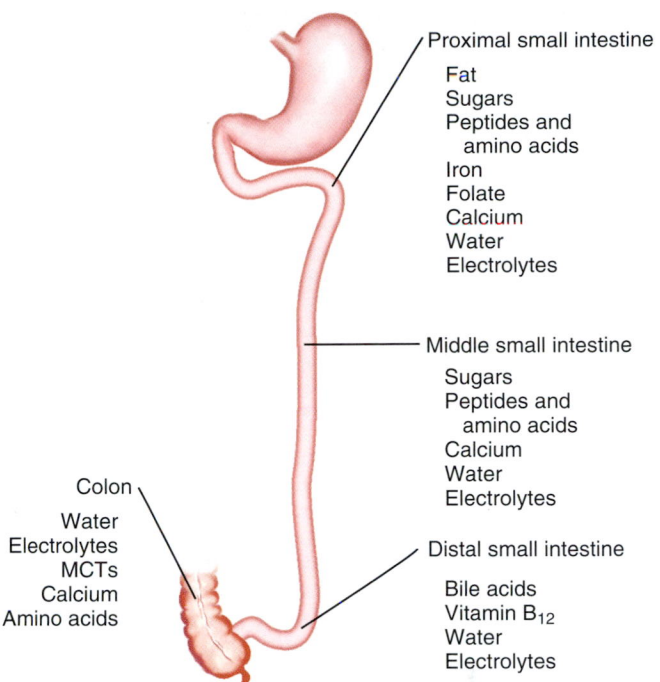

FIGURE 106-2. Specific areas of absorption of dietary constituents and secretions in the small intestine and colon. Macronutrients and micronutrients are absorbed predominantly in the proximal jejunum. Bile acids and vitamin B_{12} (cobalamin) are absorbed only in the ileum. Electrolytes and water are absorbed in both the small and large intestine. Medium-chain triglycerides (MCTs), calcium, and some amino acids can be absorbed in the colon.

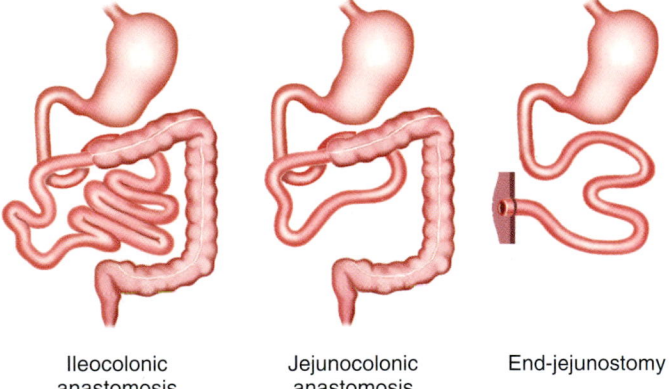

Ileocolonic anastomosis   Jejunocolonic anastomosis   End-jejunostomy

FIGURE 106-1. The 3 common types of intestinal resection and anastomosis observed in patients with Short Bowel Syndrome: ileocolonic anastomosis, jejunocolonic anastomosis, and end-jejunostomy.

of intestinal resections typically are encountered: limited ileal resection for Crohn's disease, often with cecectomy or right hemicolectomy; extensive ileal resection with or without partial colectomy and with jejunocolonic anastomosis; and extensive small intestinal resection and total colectomy resulting in proximal jejunostomy (Fig. 106-1). Patients in the 2 latter groups commonly suffer from Crohn's disease or have had mesenteric infarction.

Loss of Absorptive Surface Area

Nutrient Malabsorption

The length of the small intestine is estimated at 3 to 8 meters, and nutrient absorption is preserved until more than one half of the small intestine is resected.[5-9] Most macronutrients (carbohydrate, fat, and nitrogen) are absorbed in the proximal 100 to 150 cm of intestine.[10] Specific areas of absorption in the small intestine for nutrients, minerals, vitamins, electrolytes, and trace elements are discussed in Chapters 101 to 103 and

are illustrated in Figure 106-2. Enterocytes lining the small intestine appear uniform from the duodenum to the ileocecal valve, but a distinct proximal-to-distal gradient exists in both morphology and function.[11] Villi are taller and crypts are deeper in the jejunum than in the ileum, and the activity of microvillus enzymes and nutrient absorptive capacity per unit length of intestine are several-fold higher in the proximal than in the distal small intestine; loss of part of the jejunum initially compromises nutrient absorption more than does loss of an ileal segment of similar length because of these morphologic and functional differences. The ileum, however, eventually is able to compensate for jejunal loss, whereas the jejunum is unable to compensate for ileal absorption of bile salts and vitamin B_{12}.

Normal digestion and absorption depend on the gradual gastric emptying of partially digested nutrients, mixing of these nutrients with bile and pancreatic enzymes in the duodenum, and rapid digestion and absorption of the digestive products in the proximal small intestine. Patients with a proximal jejunostomy have rapid gastric emptying of liquids and rapid intestinal transit because of impaired release of GLP-1, GLP-2, and PYY (see later on), which can compromise the gastric phase of digestion and result in inadequate mixing with biliary and pancreatic secretions, insufficient enzymatic digestion, and nutrient maldigestion. Rapid intestinal transit decreases nutrient-enterocyte contact time, and therefore, segmental absorption is decreased. Patients with a proximal jejunostomy are net secretors of salt and fluid, because jejunal fluid secretion is stimulated by oral intake and subsequent gastric emptying of nutrients; these patients excrete more fluid than they ingest and absorb, and accordingly, their fluid management may be challenging.[12]

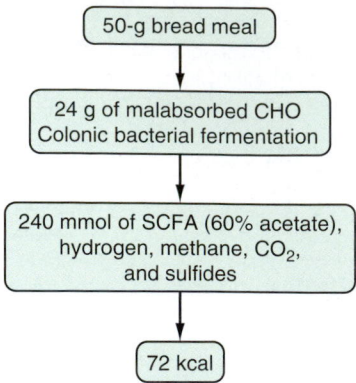

FIGURE 106-3. Colonic absorption of malabsorbed carbohydrate (CHO) following ingestion of a 50-g bread meal in a hypothetical patient with Short Bowel Syndrome. Unabsorbed CHO (≈24 g), non-starch polysaccharides, and soluble fiber are fermented by colonic bacterial flora to hydrogen, methane, CO_2, sulfides, and about 240 mmol SCFA, including acetate, butyrate, and propionate to generate 72 kcal. Normal persons absorb 220 to 720 mmol SCFA from fermentation of 30 to 60 g non-starch polysaccharides.

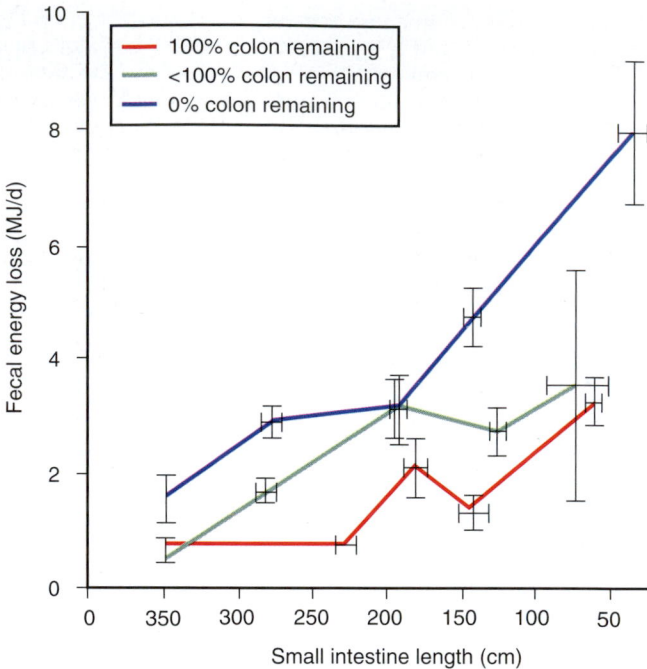

FIGURE 106-4. Role of the colon as an important digestive organ in patients with short bowel syndrome. Upwards of 1000 kcal/day (4.2 MJ) can be assimilated by means of metabolism of short chain fatty acids synthesized during carbohydrate fermentation; as more colon is sacrificed, more energy is lost in the stool. *(From Nordgaard I, Hansen BS, Mortensen PB. Colon as a digestive organ in patients with short bowel. Lancet 1994; 343:373-76.)*

Most patients whose jejunum is shorter than 100 cm and who have no colon require long-term PN. Preservation of even some colon at surgery is highly beneficial for nutrient absorption. Moreover, the ileocecal valve acts as a brake to slow intestinal transit, thereby increasing nutrient-enterocyte contact time and enhancing absorption. In addition, malabsorbed carbohydrates are fermented by bacterial enzymes in the colon to short-chain fatty acids (SCFAs), which are readily absorbed and used by colonocytes (Fig. 106-3). It has been estimated that this intracolonic digestive process can generate up to 1000 kcal (4.2 MJ) per day; in energy supply (Fig. 106-4), 1.0 MJ equals 238.8 kcal.[13-15] Small intestine should be anastomosed to colon as soon as the patient is stable.

Water and Electrolyte Malabsorption

Loss of intestinal absorptive surface area can result in significant stomal or fecal losses of electrolytes, water, minerals, and trace elements (Table 106-1). The proximal small bowel receives approximately 7 to 9 L daily of water and electrolytes from food and secretions each day, of which 6 to 8 L are reabsorbed (see Chapter 101). On unrestricted diets, patients with a proximal jejunostomy cannot reabsorb such large volumes, a consequence of which is that voluminous diarrhea develops, often complicated by hypovolemia, hyponatremia, and hypokalemia. For example, in 1 study,[12] the diarrheal volume in 6 jejunostomy patients with a mean jejunal length of 50 cm ranged from 3.2 to 8.3 L/day when they were allowed free access to food and water. All 6 patients were in negative sodium and water balance, 4 of the 6 were in negative potassium balance, and all 6 required PN with electrolyte replacement and restriction of oral intake of food and water to avoid unacceptable stomal losses. In the same study, 7 of 9 other jejunostomy patients who had a mean jejunal length of 120 cm were able to maintain positive water and sodium balance under the same conditions; absorption of water, sodium, and potassium in these 15 jejunostomy patients was correlated with jejunal length. At least 100 cm of intact jejunum is required to maintain positive water and electrolyte balance, similar to the length of jejunum required for nutrient absorption.

TABLE 106-1 Daily Stomal or Fecal Losses of Electrolytes, Minerals, and Trace Elements in Severe Short Bowel Syndrome*

Component	Amount Lost
Sodium	90-100 mEq/L
Potassium	10-20 mEq/L
Calcium	772 (591-950) mg/day
Magnesium	328 (263-419) mg/day
Iron	11 (7-15) mg/day
Zinc	12 (10-14) mg/day
Copper	1.5 (0.5-2.3) mg/day

*For sodium and potassium, the average concentration per liter of stomal effluent is given. Values for minerals and trace elements are mean 24-hour losses, with the range in parentheses. See text for details.

In general, patients with a proximal jejunostomy lose 90 to 100 mEq sodium and 10 to 20 mEq potassium per liter of stomal effluent (see Table 106-1).[16] Consequently, urine sodium loss decreases and plasma aldosterone concentration increases.[17] Some of these patients require long-term parenteral electrolyte and water supplements, often administered overnight, but others can maintain a positive balance by sipping a glucose-saline oral rehydration solution (ORS) throughout the day. The tight junctions of the jejunum are relatively leaky compared with the tight junctions of the ileum and colon, and therefore, a high NaCl concentration (>90 mmol/L) is required in the glucose-saline solution to achieve net sodium and water absorption.[18,19] Actively absorbed solutes (e.g., glucose, glucose polymers, galactose, oligopeptides, or L-amino acids) promote intestinal ion transport, although solutes also may be absorbed passively by means of solvent drag once active electrogenic Na^+ absorption occurs (see Chapter 101).

Water transport into the enterocyte is directly proportional to Na^+ transport. Na^+ also is absorbed by means of an active electrogenic mechanism coupled with Cl^- and H^+ exchange and solvent drag. Absorptive and secretory processes occur simultaneously. A mixture of 90 to 120 mmol/L NaCl and 50 mmol/L glucose is recommended, although such a solution might not be palatable. This mixture takes advantage of the coupled active transport of sodium with glucose and amino acids in the jejunum (see Chapter 101). Electrolyte and water absorption continue in the colon, and in normal humans only 100 to 150 mL of water is lost in the stool each day. The colon has a large reserve absorptive capacity for electrolytes and water, estimated to be 3 to 4 L of isotonic salt solution per day. Preservation of even part of the colon can reduce fecal electrolyte and water losses significantly in patients with SBS. A comparison of 2 groups of patients with similar jejunal length and jejunum that either ends in a jejunostomy or is anastomosed to colon showed that patients in the latter group were less likely to require oral or IV supplements.[20]

Loss of Site-Specific Transport Processes

Nutrient absorption potentially can take place at any level of the small intestine, albeit at different rates, owing to the proximal-to-distal gradient in functional activity of microvillus enzymes and transporters. Absorption of some compounds is restricted to certain areas of the small intestine (see Fig. 106-2), with calcium, magnesium, phosphorus, iron, and the water- and fat-soluble vitamins being absorbed predominantly in the duodenum and proximal jejunum (see Chapters 101-103).

Most patients with SBS have an intact duodenum and a variable length of jejunum, so the development of iron, phosphorus, or water-soluble vitamin deficiency, even in patients with a proximal jejunostomy, is relatively uncommon. Calcium absorption was found to be highly variable in a large study of patients with small intestinal resections.[21] The net absorption of calcium (intake minus fecal loss) ranged from +573 to −268 mg/day, with a median of +65 mg/day; 64% of the patients, however, were in a negative calcium balance (intake minus fecal and urinary loss). In a study of 25 patients with a mean jejunal length of 128 cm, large-volume diarrhea (2 to 6 L/day), and steatorrhea,[22] hypocalcemia, and hypomagnesemia developed in 13 and 18 patients, respectively, during a trial of enteral hyperalimentation—despite supplementation with calcium, magnesium, and vitamin D. Malabsorption of calcium and magnesium is a consequence of fat malabsorption, because these minerals are precipitated intraluminally by unabsorbed long-chain fatty acids. Calcium and magnesium absorption improve on a low-fat diet in patients with small intestinal resections.[23]

Active absorption of vitamin B_{12} and bile acids is restricted to the ileum. B_{12}-intrinsic factor complexes and bile acids are taken up by specific transport proteins in the ileal enterocytes (see Chapters 64 and 102). Most patients with SBS have lost part or all of the ileum, as a result of which vitamin B_{12} and bile acid malabsorption develop. The degree of malabsorption depends on the length of resected ileum. Vitamin B_{12} malabsorption usually is demonstrable when more than 60 cm of

ileum has been resected.[4] Resection of less than 100 cm of ileum causes moderate bile acid malabsorption and increased bile acid loss to the colon or in stomal effluents.[24] The increased loss of bile acids to the colon induces electrolyte and water secretion and can exacerbate diarrhea, a condition called *cholerrheic enteropathy*. More extensive ileal resections (>100 cm) cause severe bile acid malabsorption, which, if bile acid loss exceeds hepatic synthesis, can result in a reduced bile acid pool size, with insufficient micellar solubilization of lipolytic products and resultant steatorrhea. After extensive ileal resection, fat malabsorption develops, accompanied by fat-soluble vitamin deficiency; essential fatty acid (linoleic acid) deficiency is rare. Loss of unabsorbed long-chain fatty acids to the colon can exacerbate diarrhea if the fatty acids are hydroxylated by colonic bacteria, because hydroxylated fatty acids stimulate colonic electrolyte and water secretion.[25]

Loss of Site-Specific Enteroendocrine Cells and GI Hormones

Synthesis of GI hormones in the intestinal mucosa is distributed in a site-specific manner along the GI tract (see Chapter 4). Gastrin, CCK, secretin, gastric inhibitory polypeptide, and motilin are produced by endocrine cells in the proximal GI tract and regulate secretory processes and motility. The area within which these hormones are synthesized usually is intact in patients with SBS, and hormonal profiles are normal. In some 50% of patients with extensive intestinal resections, however, hypergastrinemia and increased gastric acid secretion temporarily develop in the early postoperative phase.[26,27] The cause of this postoperative hypergastrinemia is not known but could be loss of inhibitory signals, because it resolves spontaneously.

Glucagon-like peptides 1 and 2 (GLP-1 and GLP-2), neurotensin, and peptide YY (PYY) are produced in the ileum and proximal colon, and these intestinal segments are often lost in SBS patients.[28] GLP-1, GLP-2, and PYY are released by intraluminal fat and carbohydrates, cause a delay in gastric emptying, and slow intestinal transit (the ileal brake).[29,30] Jejunostomy patients demonstrate impaired release of these hormones in response to a meal, rapid gastric emptying, and rapid intestinal transit of liquids.[31,32] Patients with SBS and a preserved colon have increased GLP-1 and GLP-2 concentrations and demonstrate normal gastric emptying.[33] GLP-1 and GLP-2 and PYY also have been shown to inhibit gastric acid secretion and promote intestinal growth in animal models.

Loss of the Ileocecal Valve

The primary functions of the ileocecal valve are to separate ileal and colonic contents, thereby minimizing bacterial colonization of the small intestine, and to regulate emptying of ileal contents into the colon. The ileocecal valve is removed in most ileal resections, as a consequence of which intestinal transit time decreases, and bacterial overgrowth is risked if the ileum is anastomosed to the colon. Bacterial overgrowth can worsen nutrient and cobalamin malabsorption (see Chapters 102, 103, and 105) because bacteria compete with enterocytes for nutrient assimilation. Rapid intestinal transit in these patients, however, can diminish the risk of bacterial colonization. In patients with SBS, studies are lacking to document the role bacterial overgrowth plays in malabsorption.

INTESTINAL ADAPTATION TO RESECTION

Adaptive changes in the intestine that remains after intestinal resection have been studied extensively in animal models and to a limited extent in humans[34,35]; adaptive changes are more pronounced in the ileum than the jejunum. After jejunectomy and duodenoileal anastomosis, the ileum attains the morphologic characteristics of the jejunum, with taller villi and deeper crypts[36]; with time, an increase in ileal diameter and length also occurs. A prospective study of 7 patients with jejunoileal bypass operation (20 cm of jejunum anastomosed to 25 cm of ileum) showed an increase in the length and diameter of the jejunum (80% and 40%, respectively) and ileum (128% and 50%, respectively) after 18 months of observation.[37] An increase in absorptive capacity was demonstrated in another study of 41 patients with SBS (mean jejunal length, 119 cm) in whom the mean stool volume decreased from 2.5 to 0.9 L per day over a period of 3 months with continuous oral intake[38]; patients gained weight, and nitrogen balance increased from +3.2 g in the first month to +7.8 g in the second month postoperatively. The same study also demonstrated a gradual increase in intestinal transit time, which was most pronounced for ileal transit. The result of all of these changes is an increase in intestinal absorptive surface area, with an increase in microvillus enzyme activity and absorptive capacity per unit length of intestine.[39] An improvement in mineral absorption with time also has been observed in a series of 30 patients with SBS (mean jejunal length, 81 cm) in whom fractional calcium absorption was correlated with time after surgery.[40] Porcine studies have suggested that colonocytes also increase in number after massive small bowel resection.[41]

In humans, these adaptive changes can take 1 to 2 years to develop fully; the younger the patient, the more profound the adaptive response. Adaptive changes depend on the presence of food as well as biliary and pancreatic secretions in the intestinal lumen[42]; adaptive hyperplasia of the ileum failed to develop in jejunectomized animals fed only by parenteral alimentation.[43] To induce these adaptive processes, patients with SBS are encouraged to start oral intake as early as possible in the postoperative phase of recovery. Patients with SBS whose colon is in continuity demonstrate qualitative and quantitative changes in colonic flora that result in an increased capacity to metabolize carbohydrate and in an increased fecal bacterial mass.[44] Recent investigation has suggested increased prevalence of *Lactobacillus* species and a decreased prevalence of *Clostridium leptum*, *Clostridium coccoides*, and *Bacteroides* species.[45]

Adaptive hyperplasia is the result of an increase in crypt cell production rate, presumably mediated by growth factors released by the presence of food and secretions in the intestinal lumen. Vascular endothelial growth factor (VEGF), CCK, gastrin, insulin, neurotensin, GLP-2, platelet-derived growth factor (PDGF-α), and L-glutamine have been shown to stimulate intestinal growth in experimental animals[46-48,49]; studies in humans have not indicated any value of supplemental glutamine to enhance intestinal adaptation.[50,51] These extracellular growth factors stimulate polyamine synthesis in crypt cells, which in turn induces increased DNA synthesis and mitotic activity.[52] Inhibition of polyamine synthesis in jejunectomized animals prevents adaptive changes in the ileum.[53] Elucidation of the mediators that regulate enterocyte proliferation eventually can lead to development of pharmacologic interventions that can accelerate intestinal adaptation in patients with SBS. The presence of comorbid conditions and the health of the residual bowel and its blood flow are important prognostic factors for patients who have undergone massive enterectomy. Plasma citrulline concentration, an indicator of bowel mass, may be a useful predictor for nutrition autonomy. Individuals with a plasma citrulline concentration greater than 20 μmol/L had a 92% sensitivity and 90% specificity for distinguishing children who gained independence from PN.[54]

MEDICAL MANAGEMENT

Initial management of the patient with SBS consists of primarily supportive care designed to enhance survival potential. This care includes achievement of hemodynamic stability and appropriate fluid and electrolyte management. In the immediate postoperative phase, most patients with extensive intestinal resections are kept fasting and are supported with TPN. Weight and volume status are carefully monitored, and stomal, fecal, and urinary losses of water, sodium, and potassium are measured to ensure optimal electrolyte and water balance. H₂RAs or PPIs are given IV to suppress hypergastrinemia-induced gastric acid hypersecretion and limit volume losses.[55,56] Patients with jejunostomies have stomal effluents up to several liters per day in this early phase, with obligatory losses of sodium, potassium, and possibly magnesium. Enteral tube feeding, followed by oral feeding, is begun in the late postoperative phase once the patient is hemodynamically stable, adequate intestinal blood flow has been restored, and postoperative ileus has resolved. Patients with extensive resections should have a second-look operation performed at 24 to 48 hours to assess the healing of enteric anastomoses.

Limited Ileal Resection

Patients with a limited ileal resection (<100 cm), with or without right hemicolectomy, may resume intake of solid food in the late postoperative phase. The response to solid food is determined mainly by the length of ileum removed and whether or not the right colon was resected; patients can develop diarrhea or steatorrhea with consumption of a regular diet. Secretory diarrhea without steatorrhea is the typical finding in limited ileal resections. Treatment with a bile acid-binding resin, such as cholestyramine (2 to 4 g with meals) or colestipol (1 to 2 g with meals) often ameliorates diarrhea if bile acid malabsorption is the main cause. Colestipol, because it is odorless and tastes better, often is tolerated better than cholestyramine. The diarrhea of some patients with limited ileal resection and right hemicolectomy does not respond to cholestyramine or colestipol, despite documented bile acid malabsorption, presumably because the intestinal absorptive capacity for sodium chloride is lost.[57]

Patients with documented fat malabsorption on a regular diet might have less severe steatorrhea while on a low-fat (40 g), high-carbohydrate diet; however, oral energy intake also will be reduced because fat is calorically dense (9 kcal/g). Patients maintained on such a diet experience a decrease in diarrhea and steatorrhea and improve their net absorption of calcium, magnesium, and zinc.[4] If necessary, medium-chain triglycerides (MCTs), which do not require micellar solubilization, can be added as a source of fat calories. The possibility of vitamin B₁₂ malabsorption should be considered, although the Schilling test to document this is no longer available. Therefore, patients with ileal disease or resection who are at risk for vitamin B₁₂ malabsorption should be treated each month for life with parenteral B₁₂, usually in a dose of 1 mg intramuscularly.

Malabsorption of fat-soluble vitamins, calcium, and magnesium is a risk in patients with fat malabsorption. Fourteen of 27 patients with ileal resections of 50 to 150 cm and an intact colon were in negative calcium balance when studied on a fixed daily calcium intake of 800 mg supplemented with 400 to 800 IU of vitamin D daily.[22] Supplementation with vitamins, calcium, and possibly magnesium should be initiated before overt signs of vitamin deficiency or hypocalcemia and hypomagnesemia develop. Magnesium supplementation by mouth may be unrewarding because magnesium is a cathartic.

Although magnesium gluconate is water soluble and therefore may be the most readily absorbed magnesium salt, some patients still require periodic parenteral replacement. Magnesium deficiency can occur despite a normal serum concentration, because most Mg^{2+} is present in the intracellular space. Therefore, measurement of 24-hour urine Mg^{2+} concentration is prudent in patients who have suspected magnesium deficiency but normal serum Mg^{2+} concentration. Magnesium deficiency can result in calcium deficiency because release of parathyroid hormone is impaired in the presence of hypomagnesemia.[58]

Most patients with SBS already are in a negative calcium balance[59] and therefore oral supplementation of calcium at a daily dose of 800 to 1500 mg is recommended. Tests to assess vitamin and mineral balance and recommended dosages in patients with malabsorption are discussed in Chapters 5 and 103. Absorption of water-soluble vitamins, carbohydrates, and proteins is, in general, not compromised in patients with limited ileal resections.

Extensive Small Intestinal Resection and Partial Colectomy

Fluid and Electrolytes

Massive enterectomy is associated with gastric hypersecretion for about the first 6 months postoperatively. These patients benefit from IV H_2RAs or oral or IV PPIs; absorption of orally ingested medications may be impaired, and more than the usual doses of these agents may be required (Table 106-2). Rapid intestinal transit contributes to malabsorption and diarrhea, and use of antidiarrheal drugs is common (see Table 106-2). These medications should be taken 1 hour before meals, and their effect on volume of diarrhea should be evaluated before long-term treatment is recommended.

Use of anti-motility agents is important to control fluid losses; such agents include loperamide hydrochloride (4-6 mg 4 times daily) and diphenoxylate-atropine (2.5 to 5 mg 4 times daily), codeine (15 to 60 mg 2 to 4 times daily) tincture of opium 0.6 mL (2.5 mg) 2 to 4 times daily, and the somatostatin analog octreotide (50 to 100 μg 2 to 3 times daily). Most studies have shown that these agents reduce stomal output by up to 50%,[60,61] but a positive water and electrolyte balance rarely is achieved. Octreotide usually is not necessary except for some patients with a proximal jejunostomy. Octreotide can slow intestinal transit and increase sodium and water absorption,[62-65] but it also decreases splanchnic protein synthesis, thereby inhibiting post-resectional intestinal adaptation[64]; the risk of cholelithiasis also is increased with octreotide.[65] The α_2-adrenergic agonist clonidine also may be useful to decrease diarrhea by its effects on chloride absorption. Transdermal administration avoids the potential for medication malabsorption.[66] Glucose polymer-based ORSs should be provided to patients to improve hydration and thereby reduce TPN requirements.

Glucose and sodium are absorbed by the same active transport mechanism and stimulate absorption of each other. In addition, glucose promotes sodium and water absorption by means of solvent drag (see Chapter 101).[67] Therefore, because the jejunum is permeable to both sodium and chloride, passively absorbed solutions that have a high sodium chloride concentration are absorbed to a significant degree; sodium is not as readily absorbed from isotonic or hypotonic solutions. A simple solution developed by the WHO can be formulated by dissolving 2.5 g (1 tsp) of table salt, 1.5 g (1/4 tsp) of potassium chloride (KCl); requires a prescription), 2.5 g (1/2 tsp) of sodium bicarbonate ($NaHCO_3$), and 1.5 g (1/5 tsp) of table sugar (sucrose) in 1 L of water. This solution provides a sodium concentration of approximately 90 mmol/L. Additional salt may be added to increase the osmolarity as tolerated, to 100 to 120 mmol/L or more, which can increase effectiveness.[68] Sodium losses actually increase when solutions are consumed that contain less sodium than is in the small bowel effluent (90 mmol/L). The use of ORS is not as critical in patients in whom the colon is intact, provided that sufficient dietary sodium is present, because of the colon's ability to absorb sodium and water. For patients who have had significant jejunal resections, addition of glucose to the ORS is not helpful because glucose does not enhance ileal water absorption.[69] In addition to sodium losses, significant quantities of bicarbonate and magnesium are lost in feces.

Diet

Patients with SBS should be encouraged to eat substantially more than usual to compensate for malabsorption; they might need to consume 2 to 3 times as much energy as that normally ingested before their abdominal catastrophe. This may be the single most important dietary intervention to reduce PN requirements. It has been suggested that patients may counterbalance the discomfort associated with increased fecal volume by the satisfaction of recovering relatively normal eating habits and requiring less PN.[22] Patients also should be encouraged to eat small portions throughout the day rather than at defined meal times. Separation of liquid and solid portions of meals is impractical and not associated with decreased fecal wet weight loss.

Patients with SBS whose colon is in continuity with the remaining small intestine should be provided a high complex-carbohydrate diet that includes starch, non-starch polysaccharides, and soluble fiber (Table 106-3). These foodstuffs typically are not absorbed by the human small intestine[70]; however, when they pass undigested into the colon, colonic bacteria ferment them into SCFAs such as butyrate, acetate, and propionate. Butyrate is the preferred fuel for the colonocyte.[71] Approximately 75 mmol of SCFAs are produced from

TABLE 106-2 Therapeutic Agents Used to Decrease Intestinal Transit and Diarrheal Volume in Patients with Short Bowel Syndrome (SBS)

Agent	Dosage
Loperamide*	4-6 mg 4 times daily
Diphenoxylate-atropine*	2.5-5 mg 4 times daily
Codeine phosphate*	15-60 mg 2 to 4 times daily
Tincture of opium	0.6 mL (2.5 mg) 2 to 4 times daily
Ranitidine†	300 mg twice daily
Omeprazole‡	40 mg twice daily
Octreotide	50-100 μg SC twice daily
Clonidine	0.3 mg transcutaneous patch once weekly

*The antidiarrheal agents loperamide, diphenoxylate-atropine, and codeine phosphate are given 1 hour before meals and at bedtime. Dosages may be increased over those recommended because of incomplete absorption in patients with SBS.
†Cimetidine, famotidine, and nizatidine are alternatives.
‡Esomeprazole, lansoprazole, rabeprazole, and pantoprazole are alternatives.
SC, subcutaneously.

TABLE 106-3 Macronutrient Requirements in Patients with Short Bowel Syndrome

Colon Present	Colon Absent
Carbohydrate	
Complex carbohydrates/starches 30-35 kcal/kg/day Soluble fiber	Variable types 30-35 kcal/kg/day
Fat	
MCT/LCT 20%-30% of caloric intake	LCT 20%-30% of caloric intake
Protein	
Intact protein 1.0-1.5 g/kg/day	Intact protein 1.0-1.5 g/kg/day

LCT, long-chain triglycerides; MCT, medium-chain triglycerides.

10 g of unabsorbed carbohydrate (see Fig. 106-3). A person with an intact colon can absorb a wide range of up to 310 to 740 kcal (1.3 to 3.1 MJ) daily when fed a 60% carbohydrate diet.[15] Other studies have indicated that up to 525 to 1170 kcal (2.2 to 4.9 MJ) daily can be absorbed by an intact colon from fermentation of unabsorbed carbohydrate and soluble fiber.[13] The amount of energy absorbed is proportional to the amount of residual colon[15,20] (see Fig. 106-4) and can increase as part of the adaptive response to enterectomy.[46,72] During this adaptive period, colonic bacteria increase and β-galactosidase and other enzymes increase in concentration or activity.[44] Sodium and water absorption are stimulated by SCFAs as well, although decreased fecal fluid and sodium losses have not been documented clinically.[15]

When more than 100 cm of terminal ileum have been resected, fat maldigestion can develop because bile salt malabsorption leads to decreased micelle formation, which results in poor fat solubilization. Use of bile salt replacement therapy with ox bile or a synthetic conjugated bile acid (cholylsarcosine) has been reported only in a few patients,[73,74] decreasing fecal fat in most but leaving fecal volume either unchanged or increased. The bile acid-sequestering agent cholestyramine may be useful to decrease bile salt-related diarrhea in patients with less than 100 cm of terminal ileum resected, but it can worsen steatorrhea in patients who have undergone a more significant resection; because of its binding to dietary lipid,[75] fat-soluble vitamin deficiency can also develop. In addition, cholestyramine binds to many medications, including warfarin, antibiotics, beta-blockers, diuretics, oral hypoglycemia agents, and others.

Limited data are available to support the use of low-fat diets in patients with massive enterectomy,[76] although fat restriction often does lead to decreased steatorrhea in patients with limited terminal ileal resections. Because fat is concentrated energy, however, dietary fat restriction results in decreased energy intake and can worsen the patient's energy balance; a low-fat diet also may be unpalatable. Although a high-fat diet has greater energy content than that of a high-carbohydrate diet, it is associated with increased loss of divalent cations (Ca^{2+}, Mg^{2+}, and Zn^{2+}),[77] slows gastric emptying, and can induce early satiety, leading to reduced total energy intake. Diets high in fat can also lead to water secretion from the colon.

Because MCTs (C8 to C10, 8.3 kcal/g) can be absorbed in the colon, dietary supplementation with MCTs can lead to increased energy absorption.[78] MCT supplementation is of much more limited benefit in patients with an end-jejunostomy.

MCTs also do not supply essential fatty acids, and excessive MCT intake is associated with nausea, vomiting, and ketosis.

Experience with long-term PN mainly has been gained in patients with severe SBS (see Chapter 6). Despite the limited adaptive capacity of the jejunum, about 50% of patients on a home PN regimen can discontinue TPN and resume oral intake after 1 to 2 years.[79] The diet composition for patients with a jejunostomy who are taking food by mouth can be more liberal because the percentages of energy absorption are similar for a low-fat, high-carbohydrate and a high-fat, low-carbohydrate diet.[80,81] The average daily stomal losses of electrolytes, minerals, and trace elements in severe SBS are listed in Table 106-1.[23,77,80,82,83]

Water-soluble vitamins, except for vitamin B_{12}, are absorbed in the proximal jejunum, as are macronutrients (see Chapters 102 and 103). It is unusual for deficiencies of these vitamins to develop except in patients with a proximal jejunostomy or duodenostomy, and these patients invariably require TPN with vitamin supplementation. Loss of the ileum results in bile acid and vitamin B_{12} malabsorption, but patients who suffer such a loss, as well as those with extensive jejunal resection, also are at risk for more pronounced malabsorption of nutrients, minerals, vitamins, and electrolytes and water than is seen in patients with limited ileal resections, because of the greater loss of absorptive surface area and rapid intestinal transit. Fat-soluble vitamin (A, D, E, K) deficiency is encountered much more commonly as a result of concurrent fat malabsorption than as a result of absorptive surface area loss. Most of the human daily vitamin K requirement is synthesized by colonic bacterial flora,[84] so patients with any residual colon are at lower risk for developing vitamin K deficiency than are those whose colon has been resected (See Chapter 103). Conversely, patients who have received broad-spectrum antibiotics also are at risk for vitamin K deficiency. Zinc and selenium are lost in significant concentrations in the feces. The concentration of zinc is 12 mg/L in small bowel effluent and 16 mg/L in stool.[85] Oral supplementation of vitamins, minerals, and trace elements generally is required for patients who do not require TPN (Table 106-4).

Malabsorption of medication also occurs in patients with SBS.[86,87] Many medications are absorbed in the jejunum, but medication malabsorption still can occur in patients who have undergone ileal resections alone, because their intestinal transit time is decreased.

Loss of the ileocecal valve increases the risk of bacterial overgrowth in the small intestine, which can worsen nutrient absorption and make management more difficult. The ultimate goal is to ensure a stable condition in which all nutritional needs are met, preferably by oral intake alone. In a series of 38 patients whose jejunum was shorter than 200 cm and in continuity with the colon, all those with a jejunal length of more than 100 cm could be managed on oral intake alone.[20]

In the late postoperative phase, the liquid diet is replaced by solid food, and the absorptive capacity of the remaining intestine is assessed again by measurement of fecal fat, volume, weight, and electrolytes while the patient is on a known nutrient and liquid intake. In general, fat absorption is more compromised than is nitrogen or carbohydrate absorption in SBS patients. The optimal diet composition for patients with SBS has been debated, but a low-fat, high-carbohydrate diet is of documented advantage in patients whose colon is in continuity with the remaining small intestine.

Nitrogen is the least affected nutrient in SBS. Because absorption of dietary protein in the form of dipeptides and tripeptides occurs in the very proximal bowel, patients with only short segments of residual jejunum can benefit from the use of hydrolyzed protein or free amino acid-based enteral formulas. McIntyre and colleagues compared energy, nitrogen, and fat absorption in 7 patients, each of whom had

TABLE 106-4 Vitamin and Mineral Requirements* in Patients with Short Bowel Syndrome

Micronutrient	Requirement
Vitamin A	10,000-50,000 units daily*
Vitamin B$_{12}$	1000 µg SC monthly for patients with terminal ileal resection or disease
Vitamin C	200 mg daily
Vitamin D	50,000 units of 1,25(OH)$_2$-D$_3$ twice weekly to twice daily
Vitamin E	30 IU daily
Vitamin K	10 mg weekly
Calcium	1000-1500 mg daily
Magnesium	See text
Iron	As needed
Selenium	60-150 µg daily
Zinc	220-440 mg daily (sulfate or gluconate form)
Bicarbonate	As needed

NOTE: The table lists rough guidelines only. Vitamin and mineral supplementation must be monitored routinely and tailored to the individual patient, because relative absorption and requirements can vary. Supplements may be taken orally unless otherwise indicated.

*Use cautiously in patients with cholestatic liver disease because of the potential for liver toxicity.

IU, international units; SC, subcutaneously.

an end-jejunostomy, when they were provided with either a polymeric formula or a peptide-based formula. The length of residual jejunum in these patients ranged between 6 and 150 cm; no differences in nutrient absorption were observed.[80] Similar uncontrolled observations were reported by Levy and coworkers.[88] Contrary to these results, however, were those of Cosnes and associates, who reported modest improvement in nitrogen absorption in 6 end-jejunostomy patients (mean residual small bowel length, 90 to 150 cm) who received a peptide-based diet, although absorption of fats and calories was unaffected.[89] The patient populations in these studies were somewhat heterogeneous, and the peptide chain length and relative concentrations varied among formulas, making it difficult to compare the 3 studies. Lactose malabsorption that results from substantial loss of jejunal length can worsen diarrhea, but a study of 14 patients with SBS on either a lactose-free diet or a diet with 20 g of lactose per day showed no significant differences in stool volumes.[90] Patients with SBS whose colon is in continuity should receive an oxalate-restricted diet (see "Calcium Oxalate Kidney Stones" under "Complications") (Table 106-5).

HOME PARENTERAL NUTRITION

For the patient who requires long-term TPN, infusions typically are given on a continuous basis in the hospital until postoperative recovery has progressed and fluid needs and other metabolic issues have stabilized. Patients should be encouraged to adopt a hyperphagic diet while TPN volume and nutrient support are adjusted to maintain reasonable weight, fluid status, and nutrient sufficiency. As a patient gains weight or retains additional fluid, TPN fluid volume and nutrient composition can be decreased. It is important not to suppress the hypothalamic hunger center. Even if patients are unable to increase their oral intake significantly, they still should be encouraged to eat to stimulate normal gallbladder contraction (if the gallbladder is in situ) and prevent biliary complications (see later).

To prepare the patient for home TPN, the TPN regimen should be compressed gradually in 2- to 4-hour daily increments so the total volume can be infused over a 10- to 12-hour period, typically overnight. Some patients with hyperglycemia or renal or congestive heart failure require a more prolonged infusion. The TPN infusion generally is then tapered off over a 30- to 60-minute period to avoid hypoglycemia. Patients with a proximal jejunostomy might require additional fluid before or following completion of home TPN and, in some cases, during the day as well. TPN solutions are hypertonic and therefore must be infused into a central vein (e.g., superior or inferior vena cava) through a tunneled catheter to decrease the risks of infection and thrombosis.[91,92] Percutaneously inserted central catheters (PICCs) should be reserved for short-term use (<6 months). For the patient to qualify for Medicare benefits, home TPN must be required for at least 3 months, and fat malabsorption as well as failed enteral nutritional support must be documented.

The patient should be instructed about the indications for TPN, appropriate catheter care and dressing changes, the pump, preparation of TPN solutions, and acute complications of TPN, including air embolism, hypoglycemia, and catheter-related infections. Instruction on glucose self-monitoring should be included if hyperglycemia has been a problem or if insulin is required. The patient will need to add multivitamins, insulin, and possibly other additives to the TPN solution each night, because these other medications are not sufficiently stable to be added by the home TPN pharmacy. TPN solution typically is delivered in 1- to 2-week batches, so the patient will need a refrigerator dedicated to TPN.

The patient's home environment should be assessed. An appropriate location for setting up the TPN infusion and storing supplies, catheter cleaning, and hookup devices should be identified; this should not be a contaminated area such as a bathroom or kitchen.

Patients often find it helpful to contact a local support group of the Oley Foundation (1-800-776-OLEY or www.oley.org). This independent nonprofit organization includes patients and their families as well as health care providers, and provides information, outreach services, emotional support, and conference activities. Physicians caring for patients on a home TPN regimen also should be familiar with TPN- and catheter-related complications and their recognition and treatment. These topics are beyond the scope of this chapter but have been reviewed in Chapter 6 and elsewhere (Figs. 106-5 and 106-6).[93,94]

Patients in whom the frequency of TPN infusions can be reduced to fewer than 5 nights per week should have their micronutrient status monitored 2 to 3 times yearly to detect deficiencies. At the clinical visit, particular attention should be paid to the catheter exit site for evidence of erythema, purulent discharge, warmth, or tenderness. A catheter may remain in place indefinitely if it is properly maintained.[95]

COMPLICATIONS

Gallstones

Interruption of the enterohepatic circulation of bile acids by ileal resection results in decreased hepatic bile acid secretion

TABLE 106-5 Dietary Recommendations for Patients Who Require an Oxalate-Restricted Diet

Foods Classified by Oxalate Content

Little* or None (<2 mg per Serving) Eat as Desired	Moderate (2-10 mg per Serving) Limit: Two 1/2-cup Servings per day	High (>10 mg per Serving) Avoid Completely
Beverages		
Apple or pineapple juice	Cranberry juice (4 oz)	Cocoa
Bottled beer	Grape juice (4 oz)	Draft beer
Coffee	Nescafe powder	Juices containing berries
Colas (12-oz limit/day)		Lemonade or limeade
Distilled alcohol		Tea
Milk, yogurt		Tomato juice
Orange juice (4 oz)		
Tap water		
Wine (red, rosé)		
Meats, Fish		
Lean lamb, beef, pork	Sardines	
Poultry		
Seafood		
Vegetables		
Asparagus	Broccoli	Beans
Avocado	Cucumber	Beets
Brussels sprouts	Eggplant	Carrots
Cabbage	Green peas	Celery
Cauliflower	Lettuce	Chives
Mushrooms	Lima beans	Collards
Onions	Squash	Dandelion greens
Potatoes	Tomato, 1 small	Endive
Radishes	Turnips	Escarole
Sweet corn	Vegetable soup	French fried potatoes
		Kale
		Leeks
		Okra
		Parsnips
		Sweet potato
		Swiss chard
Fruits		
Bananas	Apples	Berries
Cherries, Bing	Apricots	Concord grapes
Grapefruit	Black currants	Red currants
Grapes, white	Cherries, red sour	Tangerines
Mangos	Fruit cocktail	
Melons	Orange	
Nectarines	Peaches	
Pears	Plums, red	
Pineapple	Prunes	
Plums, green/golden		
Bread, Pasta, Cereal		
Macaroni	Cornflakes	Bran cereal
Noodles	Spaghetti, canned in tomato sauce	Grits, white corn
Oatmeal	Sponge cake	Soybean crackers
Rice		Wheat germ
Spaghetti		
White bread		
Miscellaneous		
Butter	Chicken noodle soup, dehydrated	Chocolate
Cheese, cheddar	Fruitcake	Nuts
Eggs		Peanut butter
Jelly or preserves (made with allowed fruits)		Pepper (>1 tsp/day)
Mayonnaise		Pretzels
Salad dressing		Soybean curd (tofu)
Soups (made with allowed ingredients)		
Sugar		
Vegetable oils		

*For a low-oxalate diet, restrict oxalate to 40-50 mg daily.

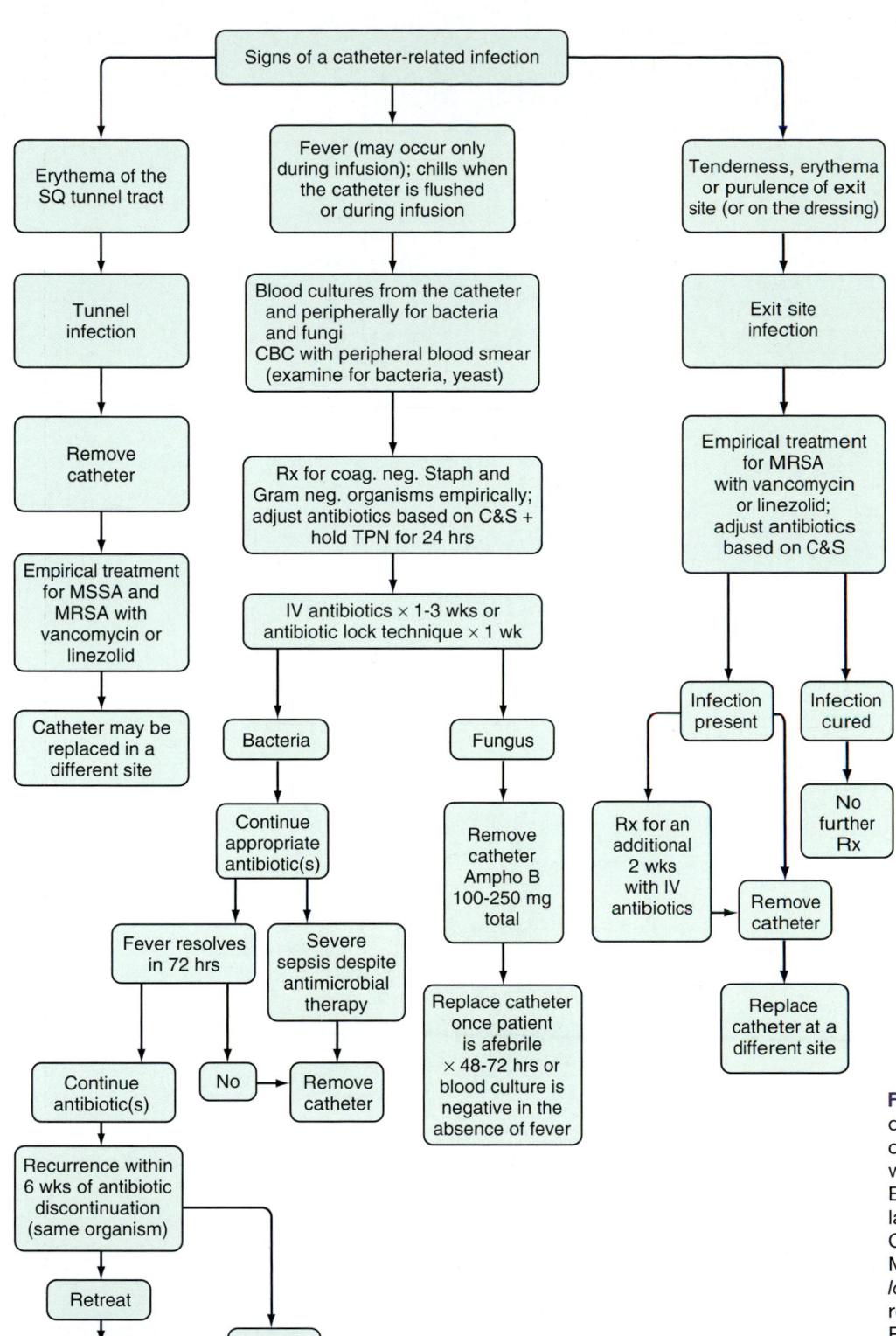

FIGURE 106-5. Algorithm for the diagnosis and management of catheter-related infection in a patient with short bowel syndrome. ampho B, amphotericin B; coag., coagulase; CBC, complete blood count; C&S, culture and sensitivity testing; MSSA, methicillin-sensitive *Staphylococcus aureus*; MRSA, methicillin-resistant *S. aureus*; neg., negative; Rx, treatment; SQ, subcutaneous; Staph, *Staphylococcus*; TPN, total parenteral nutrition.

and altered composition of hepatic bile in terms of its organic components: bile acid, cholesterol, and phospholipids (see Chapters 64 and 72). Hepatic bile becomes supersaturated with cholesterol, with subsequent formation of cholesterol crystals and gallstones in gallbladder bile (see Chapter 65). Most gallstones in patients with SBS, however, are composed of calcium bilirubinate, the pathophysiology of which is

unclear. Asymptomatic gallstones were found in 44% of 84 patients with severe SBS who required TPN.[20] Formation of biliary sludge and gallbladder hypomotility probably contributed to the high prevalence of these stones, because many of these patients were on long-term PN.[96] Postprandial CCK concentration is decreased in some patients with SBS,[97] and injections of CCK have been used experimentally to induce

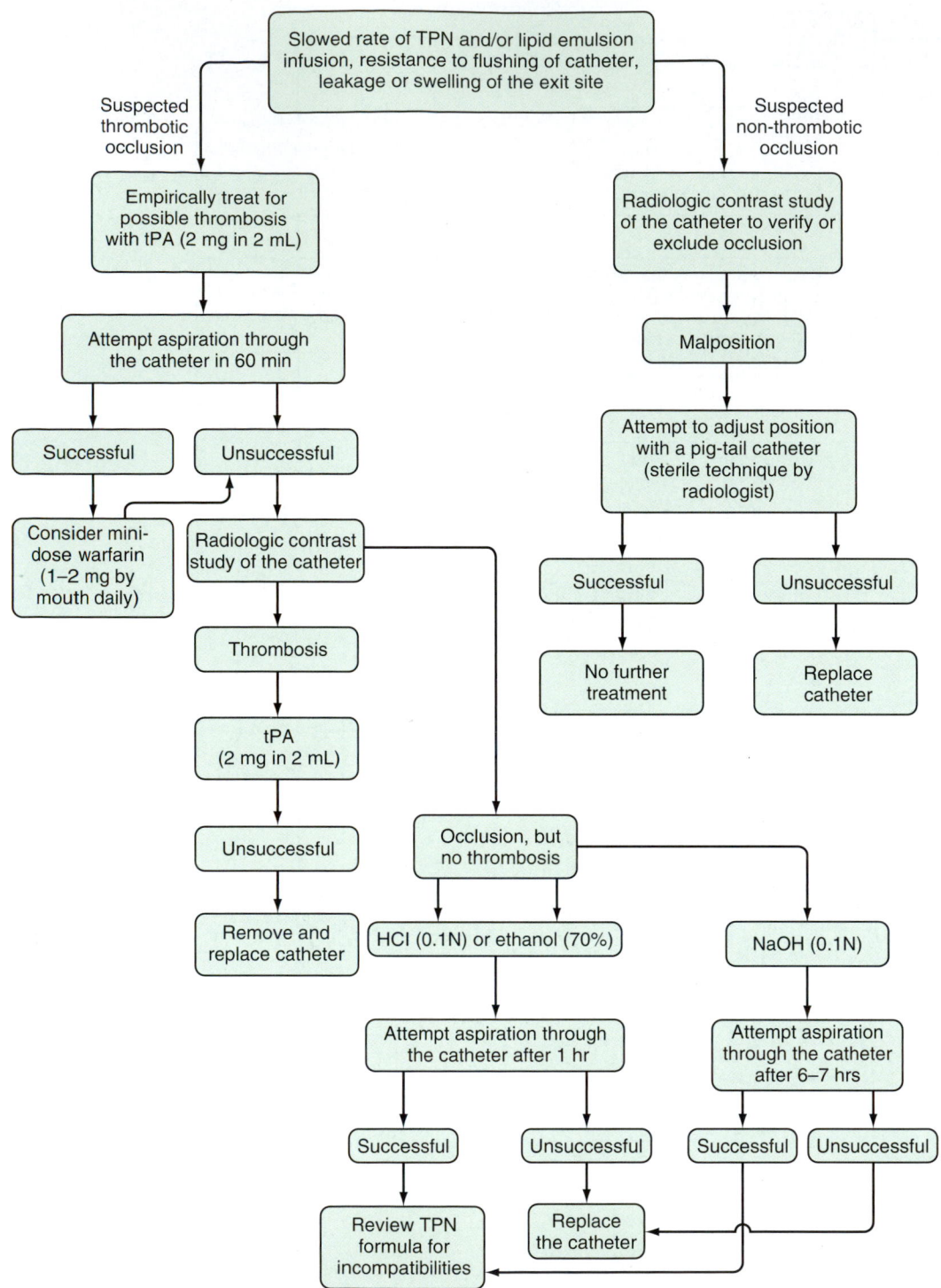

FIGURE 106-6. Algorithm for the diagnosis and management of thrombotic or nonthrombotic catheter-related occlusion. tPA, tissue plasminogen activator; HCl, hydrochloric acid; NaOH, sodium hydroxide.

gallbladder contraction, although this therapy is not always successful and may result in nausea, vomiting, and abdominal pain.[98,99]

Liver Disease

Liver disease often develops in patients who require long-term TPN. Formerly known as *parenteral nutrition–associated*

liver disease (PNALD), this complication is now known as *intestinal failure–associated liver disease* (IFALD). After 5 years of TPN, more than 50% of these patients will be found to have severe liver disease, defined as grade 2 fibrosis, cirrhosis, or 1 of the following: total serum bilirubin greater than 3.5 mg/dL for longer than 1 month, ascites, portal hypertension, hepatic encephalopathy, or liver failure with a factor V concentration less than 50% of normal.[100] Liver failure develops in approximately 15% of all TPN-dependent patients.[101] The incidence, prevalence, and severity of liver disease in young children and infants, in particular, are much greater than in adults.[102] The incidence and prevalence of liver disease and liver failure specifically in patients with SBS requiring TPN are unknown. Although these disorders often are referred to as "TPN-associated liver disease," the pathogenesis probably is related to malabsorption of nutrients such as choline[103] and to the route of nutrient assimilation rather than the portal circulation.[104] Patients with the least amount of residual intestine are at greatest risk for developing liver disease.[105,106]

Diagnosis of liver disease related to intestinal failure in the patient with SBS requires the exclusion of other potential causative disorders. SBS-related liver disease can manifest as cholestasis, steatosis, or steatohepatitis; cholestasis is more common in infants. Studies have suggested benefit from oral lecithin, although it is poorly absorbed, and from IV choline (investigational) and, to a lesser extent, ursodeoxycholic acid.[107-112] A recent uncontrolled case series of 18 infants described the substitution of a fish oil-based lipid emulsion for the conventional long chain triglyceride-based emulsion. Compared with historic controls from a different era, reversal of cholestasis occurred sooner (9.4 vs. 44.1 weeks) in the fish oil-supplemented group.[113] Dextrose overfeeding (>40 kcal/kg/day) and excessive fat emulsion infusion (2.5 g/kg/day, possibly only 1.0 g/kg/day) should be avoided.[100] A minimum of 2% to 4% of total calories, however, should be provided as linoleic fatty acid (50% of most lipid emulsions) to prevent essential fatty acid deficiency. Carnitine supplementation is not useful.[114]

Calcium Oxalate Kidney Stones

Fat malabsorption secondary to bile acid deficiency in patients with extensive ileal resection is associated with an increased risk of oxalate kidney stones if the colon is preserved. Oxalate in food usually precipitates as calcium oxalate in the intestinal lumen and is lost in the stool. Lipolysis in patients with SBS and fat malabsorption is normal, and unabsorbed long-chain fatty acids compete with oxalate for available luminal calcium. Consequently, a larger amount of free oxalate is lost to the colon, where it is absorbed and ultimately excreted by the kidney (Fig. 106-7), manifesting as just hyperoxaluria or with calcium oxalate stone formation. Patients with SBS who do not have a colon in continuity are not at increased risk. In 1 study, symptomatic kidney stones developed within 2 years of enterectomy in 9 of 38 patients (24%) with SBS and an intact colon.[20] Urinary oxalate excretion should be monitored regularly in these patients. Treatment of hyperoxaluria consists of restriction of oxalate-containing food products (see Table 106-5). If hyperoxaluria persists, then oral administration of calcium citrate should be tried; the extra calcium precipitates dietary oxalate, and the citrate prevents stone growth in the urine. A single case report describes the use of conjugated bile acid supplementation to reduce hyperoxaluria.[115] Hyperoxaluria also may be related to the metabolism of the vitamin C in TPN solution in the presence of light.[116]

D-Lactic Acidosis

D-Lactic acidosis is a rare complication of SBS and in this setting is observed only in patients with a preserved colon. The episodes of acidosis usually are precipitated by increased oral intake of refined carbohydrates and can be induced in the patient with SBS by carbohydrate overfeeding.[117] Malabsorbed carbohydrate is metabolized by colonic bacteria to SCFAs and lactate, which lower intracolonic pH. A lower pH inhibits growth of the predominant *Bacteroides* species and promotes

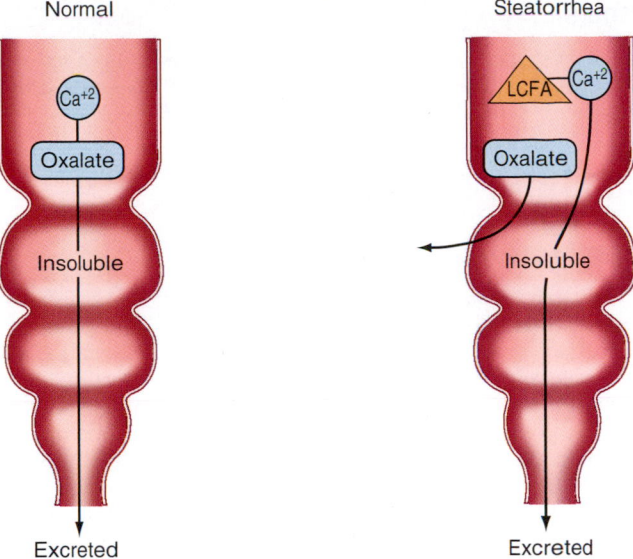

Normal Steatorrhea

FIGURE 106-7. Mechanism of oxalate hyperabsorption in patients with steatorrhea. Normally, oxalate in food is precipitated as calcium oxalate in the intestinal lumen and lost in the stool *(left)*. Lipolysis is normal in patients with Short Bowel Syndrome who have fat malabsorption *(right)*, and unabsorbed long-chain fatty acids (LCFA) compete with oxalate for available calcium. Consequently, a larger amount of free oxalate passes from the small intestine to the colon, where it is absorbed and ultimately excreted by the kidney, often resulting in hyperoxaluria.

growth of acid-resistant, Gram-positive anaerobes (*Bifidobacterium*, *Lactobacillus*, and *Eubacterium*) that have the capacity to produce D-lactate. D-Lactate is absorbed from the colon and is metabolized to only a limited extent in humans because of our lack of D-lactate dehydrogenase. The main excretory route for D-lactate is the kidney.[118]

Absorbed D-lactate results in development of metabolic acidosis and characteristic neurologic signs and symptoms of nystagmus, ophthalmoplegia, ataxia, confusion, and inappropriate behavior. Patients with D-lactate acidosis often are suspected of being inebriated, although their blood alcohol levels are normal. The constellation of specific neurologic symptoms and metabolic acidosis in a patient with SBS should raise the suspicion of possible D-lactic acidosis. Blood tests will confirm a metabolic acidosis and a normal lactate level; however, the clinical laboratory should be notified to quantify the D-lactic acid, if possible, rather than the L-lactic acid concentration, which is routinely assayed. The diagnosis is confirmed by measurement of whole-blood D-lactate concentration, which will be elevated significantly (to >3 mmol/L, compared with the normal level of <0.5 mmol/L).

Treatment consists of correcting the acidosis with sodium bicarbonate and stopping oral intake, which usually results in rapid abatement of neurologic symptoms. The potential benefit of antibiotic treatment to change the colonic microbiota is debated. Substitution of refined carbohydrates for starch has prevented recurrent D-lactic acidosis in a few patients.[119] The mediator of the neurologic symptoms still is unknown, and infusion of D-lactic acid in normal subjects to achieve blood levels commonly observed in patients with D-lactic acidosis does not cause any neurologic symptoms. The neurologic symptoms have a striking resemblance to those of Wernicke's encephalopathy, and in 1 patient with SBS, recurrent D-lactic acidosis was prevented by thiamine supplementation.[120]

Others

Renal dysfunction,[121] metabolic bone disease,[122] memory deficits,[123] and neurologic abnormalities[124] all have been described in patients with SBS who require long-term TPN.

SURGICAL MANAGEMENT

Intestinal Lengthening Procedures

The most important surgical procedure is reanastomosis of the residual small bowel to the residual colon. This procedure carries relatively low mortality and morbidity rates and allows enhanced energy absorption from SCFAs produced from the bacterial fermentation of unabsorbed carbohydrate. A number of other surgical procedures, such as tapering enteroplasty, construction of intestinal valves, creation of recirculating loops, reversal of a short intestinal segment, or colonic interposition, have been attempted to increase intestinal transit time. These procedures are considered experimental, the experience with each is limited, and outcomes generally are not optimal.[1] More recent data using the segmental bowel reversal procedure (10-cm reversed segment) suggested a modest improvement in macronutrient absorption (≈10%) and PN independence in adults.[125]

Longitudinal intestinal lengthening and tailoring (LILT, Bianchi procedure) (Fig. 106-8) may be useful in patients who have segmental dilation and nonfunctional intestine due to dysmotility and SIBO. In this procedure, the surgeon divides the dilated bowel, creates 2 hemiloops, and anastomoses the hemiloops in an end-to-end fashion, thereby doubling the bowel length (Fig. 106-9).[126] Although the surface area is not truly increased, bowel function can improve, allowing reduction or elimination of PN. Nearly all of the roughly 100 operations reported have been undertaken in children. This procedure should be attempted only as a last resort before intestinal transplantation, and it should be performed only in centers with significant experience in this area. To date, no studies have been conducted to compare medical and surgical therapies.

A less complex procedure, the serial transverse enteroplasty (STEP), developed by Kim, is a novel technique during which a linear surgical stapler is applied from alternating and opposite directions along the intestine's mesenteric border to incompletely staple and divide the dilated intestine (Fig. 106-10).[127] This procedure leads to tapering of the intestine in a zigzag pattern, which results in nutrients being channeled along a narrower but longer intestine. Rather than an intestinal lengthening procedure, this technique is better described as an intestinal tapering procedure. Results reported from an international registry comprising 111 patients from 50 centers (as of January 2010) have indicated the procedure increases intestinal length by almost 50%, and it has resulted in substantial increases in nutrient absorption, with enteral autonomy obtained in approximately 50% of patients after a median of 21 months.[128,129] These improvements in some patients, however, may have been due in part to increased segmental absorption, observed as part of the natural postenterectomy adaptation process. Nevertheless, the tapering of a dilated, essentially nonfunctional loop of bowel might decrease SIBO and improve nutrient absorption. Furthermore, STEP might have an advantage over the Bianchi procedure, because in addition to being less technically demanding, it may allow better preservation of the intestinal blood supply by avoiding intestinal transection.

Intestinal Transplantation

Intestinal transplantation is being performed in an increasing number of centers worldwide. The main indication for transplantation in children and adults is TPN-dependent SBS complicated by progressive liver disease. Combined intestine-liver transplantation is the only alternative for patients in whom end-stage liver disease has developed. Isolated intestinal transplantation may be considered for patients with clinically significant liver disease that has not yet progressed to cirrhosis.[130] Patients who have significant fluid losses and experience frequent episodes of severe dehydration despite appropriate medical management also may be candidates for isolated intestinal transplantation. Medicare has approved other indications, including 2-major-vessel thrombosis, a single episode of fungemia, a single episode of bacterial sepsis with shock, and 2 lifetime episodes of catheter sepsis, although the preponderance of evidence does not support these as appropriate indications for transplantation.

Survival has improved considerably since intestinal transplantation was initiated, with reported survival and nutritional autonomy of up to 18 years.[131] As of May 31, 2011 (most recent data from the International Small Bowel Transplant

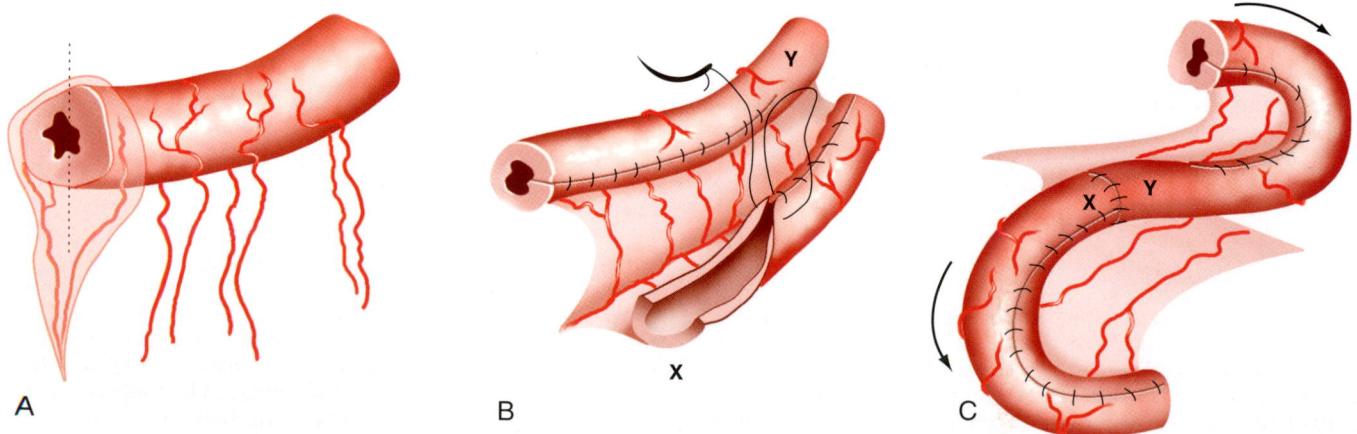

FIGURE 106-8. Schematic diagram showing the Bianchi procedure for intestinal lengthening. *A,* The bowel is split lengthwise (dashed line). *B,* Two hemiloops (X and Y) are thereby created as the bowel is closed. *C,* Hemiloops (X and Y) are anastomosed end to end.

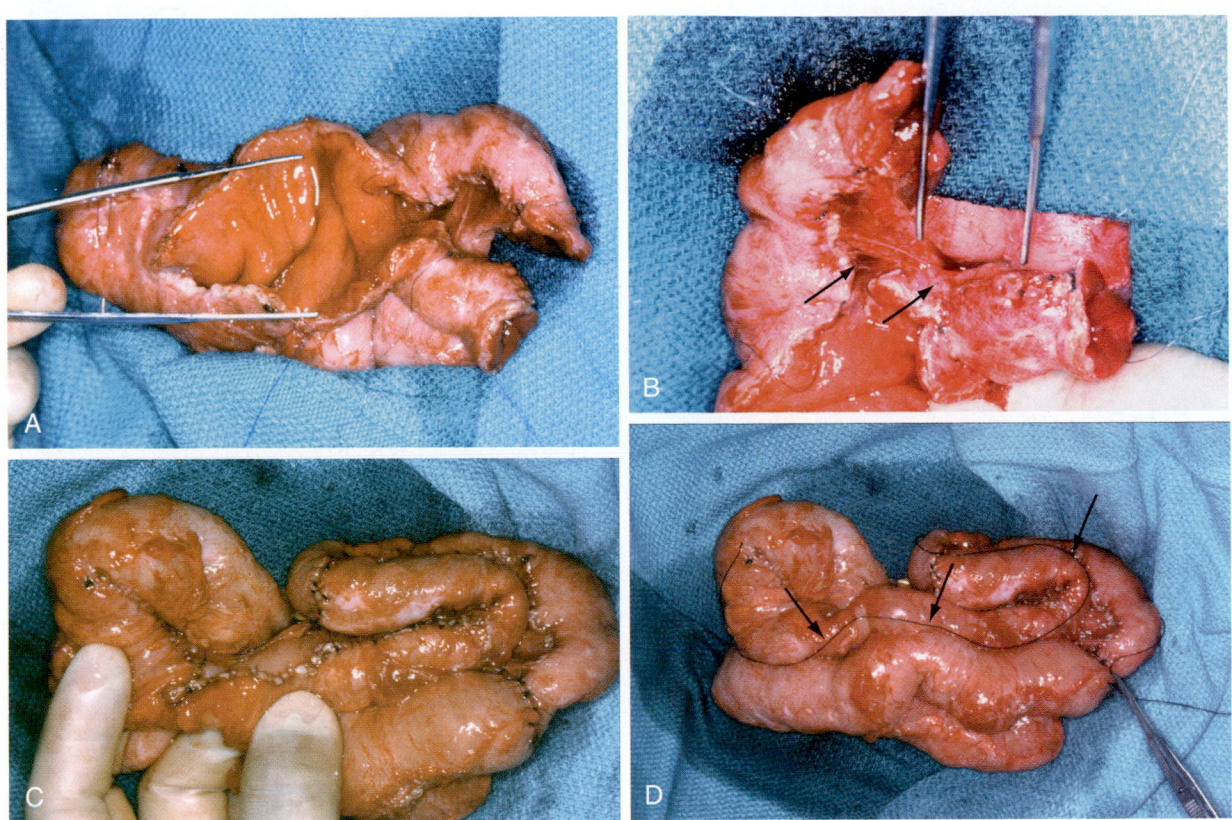

FIGURE 106-9. The Bianchi procedure shown in intraoperative photographs. *A,* The tips of the forceps are within the dilated loop of intestine, which has been opened; the beginning of each hemiloop is evident *(right side). B,* A blood vessel can be seen coursing towards the left hemiloop. *C,* The completed anastomosis. *D,* A suture (arrows) shows the gain in length of the intestine. The first hemiloop extends from the tip of the forceps to the first perpendicular suture line. The distance from that point to the end of thread represents gain in intestinal length (≈26 cm in this infant). *(Photographs kindly provided by Kishore R. Iyer, MD, New York, NY.)*

TABLE 106-6 Patient and Graft Survival Rates (%) for Transplants Performed for Short Bowel Syndrome from January 1988 to March 30, 2007 in the United States

Transplant Type	1 Year		3 Years		5 Years		10 Years	
	Patient	**Graft**	**Patient**	**Graft**	**Patient**	**Graft**	**Patient**	**Graft**
Isolated intestine (*n* = 662)	84.3	74.3	68.4	53.2	59.1	42.1	38.4	19.3
Intestine/liver (*n* = 443)	64.8	61.1	53.5	50.4	50.0	46.2	33.1	28.9
Multivisceral (*n* = 742)	71.1	68.2	58.4	54.9	53.7	49.2	N/A	N/A

Based on Organ Procurement and Transplantation Network (http://optn.transplant.hrsa.gov/) data as of January 18, 2013. This work was supported in part by Health Resources and Services Administration contract 234-2005-370011C.
N/A, not available.

Registry), 2569 transplantation procedures had been performed in 78 centers around the world, most of which were in North America, and 38 of which remain active. 1431 of the patients were still alive at the time of the report. This experience included 1114 isolated intestine, 841 intestine-liver, and 498 multivisceral transplants. Patients who have undergone transplantation more recently generally have had better survival because of improved technique and optimized immunosuppressive regimens. Mean hospitalization was 44 days for isolated intestine, 55 days for intestine-liver, and 49 days for

multivisceral transplant recipients. Some 90% of patients were successfully weaned from PN, although 5% to 10% required continued IV fluid and electrolytes. Additional information can be found on the International Intestinal Transplant Registry website, http://intestinaltransplant.org, which is updated every 2 years (last time, June 2013). Current patient and graft survival data for the United States are presented in Table 106-6.

The mortality rate for patients waiting for an intestinal-liver transplant is significantly greater than for those waiting

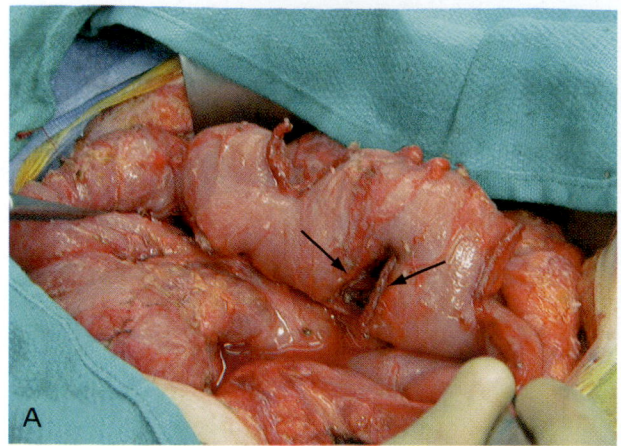

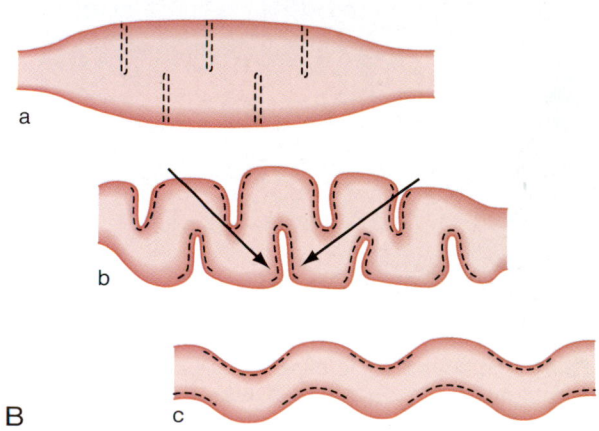

FIGURE 106-10. The serial transverse enteroplasty (STEP) procedure shown intraoperatively *(A)* and in line drawings *(B)*. STEP is a technique in which a linear surgical stapler is applied from alternating and opposite directions along the intestine's mesenteric border to incompletely staple and divide the dilated intestine. Arrows in *A* and *b* point to an invagination produced by the staples. Configuration after recovery is shown in *c*. *(Photograph kindly provided by Kishore R. Iyer, MD, New York, NY.)*

for an isolated liver transplant.[1] Therefore, early referral to an intestinal transplantation center at the first sign of liver disease is recommended even if a transplant does not ultimately become necessary. Intestinal and multiorgan transplantations are expensive and generally cost between $250,000 and $3 million per case. Post-transplantation complications and the most common causes of death afterward include acute rejection, chronic rejection, CMV infection, sepsis (often complicating rejection), and post-transplantation lymphoproliferative disease (PTLD).[132] Anti-rejection medications amount to another $10,000 yearly, in addition to repeated hospitalizations for infection and rejection. For patients who do well, however, nearly all are successfully weaned from TPN, although a few require some maintenance IV fluids. This expense compares with a charge of $100,000 to $150,000 per year for home TPN, in addition to the costs of hospitalization for complications; the actual costs of TPN (including pharmacists' time), however, are closer to $25 to $30 per day. Intestinal transplantation has reached a stage at which it is a feasible but not yet practical alternative to conservative treatment of the patient with SBS.

One of the greatest dilemmas facing intestinal transplantation is balancing the avoidance of premature transplantation with late referral for transplantation; the latter often requires addition of a liver graft and often results in a less optimal outcome.[133] High-risk patients likely to develop complications on home TPN need to be identified early, and every attempt must be made to enhance nutrient and fluid absorption and decrease the need for TPN. Both the MELD score and C-reactive protein (CRP) can be used to predict mortality in patients who require long-term TPN. In a study by Putchakayala and colleagues,[134] each point of increase in the MELD (to >15) was associated with an increased death risk of 12%, and MELD scores were significantly elevated up to 180 days before death, although they were less reliable when obtained 90 days or more before death in a group of 133 patients with intestinal failure; mortality was 50% at 328 days patients with a MELD score between 15 and 25. Increased CRP was also an independent predictor of death within 90 days before death, and a CRP of 4 or greater universally predicted mortality.[134] One unit increase in CRP was associated with a 20% increased risk of immediate death. Further evaluation of such predictors of poor outcome will be necessary, however, before they can be used reliably to support early intestinal transplantation. Although recipient survival rates have improved since the early days of intestinal transplantation, most notably 1-year survival, survival rates have plateaued and a significant drop-off in survival is seen after 5 years, often related to chronic organ rejection.

PHARMACOLOGIC ENHANCEMENT OF BOWEL ADAPTATION

The increasing knowledge about growth factors has stimulated several clinical studies in patients with SBS. The promising results with the use of growth hormone and dietary L-glutamine in a large uncontrolled study of TPN-dependent patients with SBS[135] raised hopes that intestinal mucosal growth could be enhanced beyond the adaptive period.[6] Two placebo-controlled studies of identical growth hormone and L-glutamine supplementation failed to show any beneficial effect on absorption,[50,51] however, and 2 other studies showed only marginal improvements in fluid and nutrient retention.[136,137]

GLP-2 is an intestinotropic enteric hormone that initially was evaluated in a small uncontrolled study of 8 patients with SBS, who received native GLP-2 400 mg subcutaneously twice a day for 35 days.[138] Treatment resulted in an increase in several absorptive parameters, body weight, and mucosal growth. Use of a synthetic analog of GLP-2 (teduglutide) was associated with increased villus height and increased fluid absorption, with more modest improvements in energy and nitrogen absorption that regressed once the medication was discontinued.[139] Double-blind randomized multicenter studies have indicated administration of this GLP-2 analog resulted in a significant decrease in the requirement for PN (generally 1 to 2 nights per week), although only a few subjects were able to be fully weaned[140,141]; patients most likely to be weaned successfully are those with relatively modest PN requirements. Teduglutide use was associated with increased plasma citrulline concentration. Increased fluid retention was associated with less chronic dehydration,[142] a primary factor in the development of nephropathy in patients who require long-term TPN.[143] GLP-2 also may enhance mesenteric blood flow.[144] Once teduglutide is discontinued, there is morphologic return towards baseline,[145] although clinical benefit may persist in some patients.[146] Teduglutide has now been approved

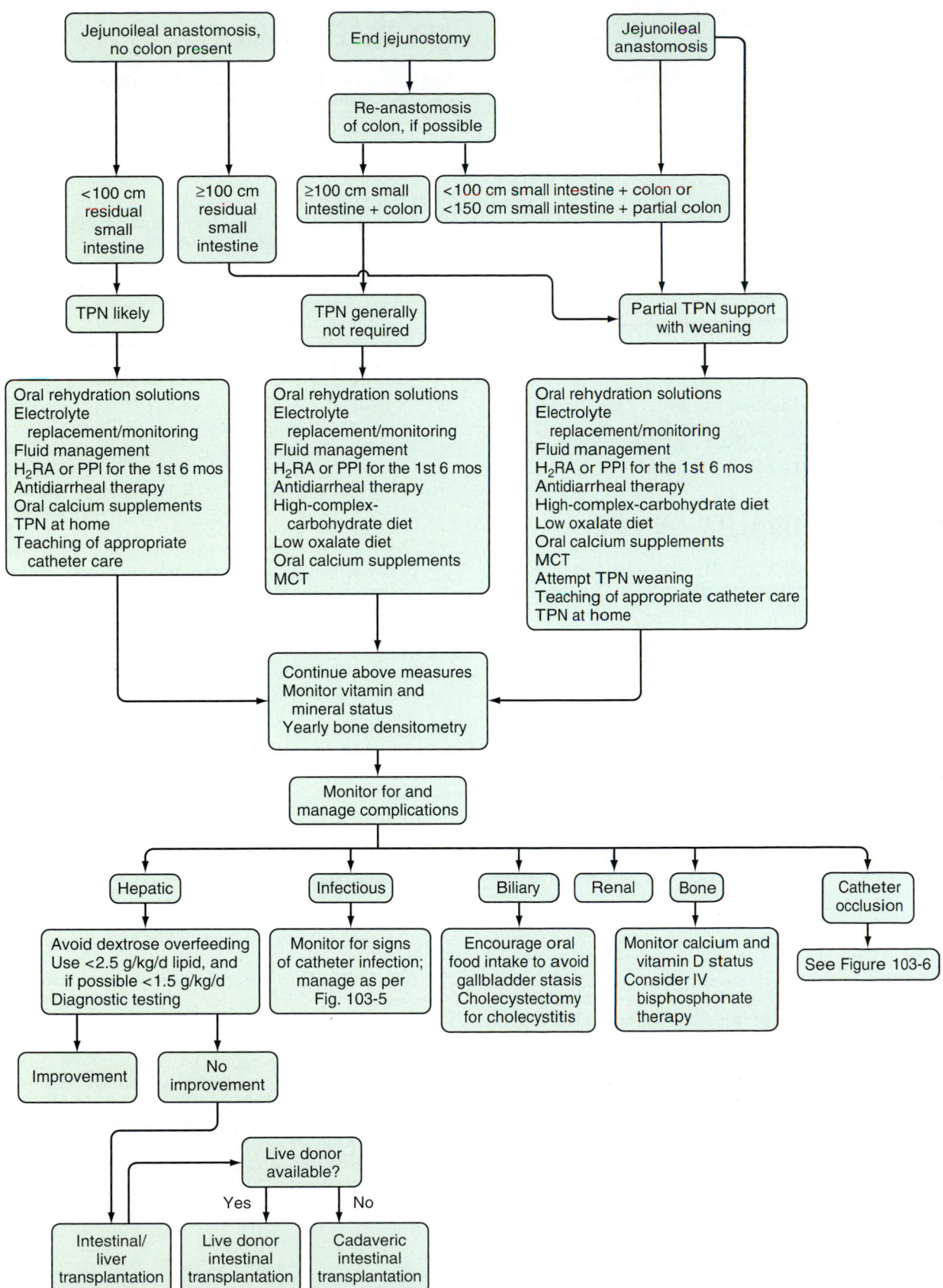

FIGURE 106-11. Algorithm for management of the patient with Short Bowel Syndrome. MCT, medium-chain triglycerides; tPA, tissue plasminogen activator.

for use for up to 24 weeks by the FDA, although long-term maintenance studies will have to be completed. The rapid advance in our knowledge of epithelial growth factors undoubtedly will lead to discovery of still other growth factors that can stimulate intestinal epithelial growth and thus benefit these patients.

A double-blind randomized controlled trial of growth hormone (0.1 mg/kg/day for 4 weeks) in 41 PN-dependent patients showed that PN requirements in treated patients could be reduced by an additional 2 L per week (or 1 night weekly) over the reduction with standard therapy described earlier in this chapter.[147] It is unclear whether these effects were related to improved absorption or appetite stimulation. This study led to FDA approval of growth hormone injections for treating PN-dependent SBS. The benefit from this therapy lasted nearly 4 months following completion of 3 weeks of daily growth hormone injections; it is unclear whether booster injections will be required. The benefits of this therapy must be weighed against the potential side effects, which include fluid retention, edema, arthralgias, and carpal tunnel syndrome. It also is unknown whether any of the potential growth factor therapies would be more effective if administered during the adaptive phase following enterectomy.

SURVIVAL AND QUALITY OF LIFE

The prognosis for patients with SBS is determined primarily by the type and extent of intestinal resection and by the underlying disease. Patients with limited small intestinal resections in general have an excellent prognosis with careful management of their specific malabsorptive defects. Patients with high jejunostomies and severe malabsorption present difficult management problems, and their long-term care poses a challenge for surgeons, gastroenterologists, and dietitians. The rate of survival, prognosis, and quality of life are, however, steadily improving even in this group of patients because of increasing experience with long-term PN and better methods to assess nutritional needs.

The probability of survival and PN dependence has been assessed in a prospective study of 124 patients with SBS.[79] Most of these patients had intestinal resection for either mesenteric infarction or radiation enteritis. The probability of survival was 86% at 2 years and 75% at 5 years. PN dependence rates were 49% at 2 years and 45% at 5 years, suggesting that most patients requiring long-term PN can be weaned successfully within 2 years using conventional techniques. In a multivariate analysis, survival was related negatively to high jejunostomy, small bowel length less than 50 cm, and mesenteric infarction as a cause for intestinal resection. PN dependence was related primarily to small bowel length. Remnant bowel length less than 100 cm was highly predictive of permanent intestinal failure and lifelong TPN dependence. Similar results were reported in a study of 225 patients from the Mayo Clinic.[148]

Most patients with SBS have a good quality of life and can work full time. Figure 106-11 depicts an algorithm for managing the patient with SBS.

KEY REFERENCES

Full references for this chapter can be found on www.expertconsult.com.

1. Buchman AL, Scolapio J, Fryer J. AGA technical review on SBS and intestinal transplantation. Gastroenterology 2003; 124:1111-34.
2. Messing B, Crenn P, Beau P, et al. Long-term survival and parenteral nutrition dependence in adult patients with SBS. Gastroenterology 1999; 117:1043-50.
13. Nordgaard I, Hansen BS, Mortensen PB. Importance of colonic support for energy absorption as small-bowel failure proceeds. Am J Clin Nutr 1996; 64:222-31.
32. Jeppesen PB, Hartmann B, Hansen BS, et al. Impaired meal stimulated glucagon-like peptide 2 response in ileal resected short bowel patients with intestinal failure. Gut 1999; 45:559-63.
50. Scolapio JS, Camilleri M, Fleming CR, et al. Effect of growth hormone, glutamine, and diet on adaptation in short-bowel syndrome: A randomized, controlled trial. Gastroenterology 1997; 113:1074-81.
76. Woolf GM, Miller C, Kurian R, Jeejeebhoy KN. Diet for patients with a short bowel: High fat or high carbohydrate? Gastroenterology 1983; 84:823-8.
93. Buchman AL. Complications of long-term home total parenteral nutrition: Their identification, prevention and treatment. Dig Dis Sci 2001; 46:1-18.
94. Buchman AL. Practical nutrition support techniques. Thorofare, NJ: Slack; 2003.
100. Cavicchi M, Beau P, Crenn P, et al. Prevalence of liver disease and contributing factors in patients receiving home parenteral nutrition for permanent intestinal failure. Ann Intern Med 2000; 132:525-32.
103. Buchman AL, Iyer K, Fryer J. Parenteral nutrition–associated liver disease and the role for isolated intestine and intestine/liver transplantation. Hepatology 2006; 43:9-19.
109. Buchman AL, Sohel M, Dubin M, et al. Choline deficiency causes reversible hepatic abnormalities in patients during parenteral nutrition: Proof of a human choline requirement; a placebo-controlled trial. JPEN J Parenter Enteral Nutr 2001; 25:260-8.
121. Buchman AL, Moukarzel A. Metabolic bone disease associated with total parenteral nutrition. Clin Nutr 2000; 19:217-31.
133. Fryer JP. Intestinal transplantation: Current status. Gastroenterol Clin N Am 2007; 36:145-59.
134. Putchakayala K, Polensky S, Fitzhugh J, et al. An evaluation of the model for end-stage liver disease and serum C-reactive protein as prognostic markers in intestinal failure patients on parenteral nutrition. JPEN J Parenter Enteral Nutr 2009; 33:55-61.
141. Jeppesen PB, Pertkiewicz M, Messing B, et al. Teduglutide reduces need for parenteral support among patients with short bowel syndrome with intestinal failure. Gastroenterology 2012; 143:1473-81.

CIARÁN P. KELLY

CHAPTER OUTLINE

DEFINITIONS

Celiac disease is a chronic, small intestinal, immune-mediated enteropathy that is precipitated by dietary gluten in genetically predisposed individuals.[1] *Gluten* is the commonly used term for the complex of water-insoluble proteins from wheat, rye, and barley that is harmful to patients with celiac disease. Celiac disease is characterized by villus atrophy of the small intestinal mucosa associated with malabsorption of nutrients, prompt clinical and subsequent histologic improvement after strict adherence to a gluten-free diet (GFD), and clinical and histologic relapse when gluten is reintroduced.[2] Other names used to describe celiac disease include *celiac sprue, gluten-sensitive enteropathy, nontropical sprue, celiac syndrome, adult celiac disease, idiopathic steatorrhea,* and *primary malabsorption.*

Celiac disease exhibits a wide spectrum of clinical presentations. In the past, *typical celiac disease* (also called *classical celiac disease*) denoted a clinical presentation with signs and symptoms of malabsorption such as diarrhea, steatorrhea, weight loss, and nutritional deficiencies. The term is now questionable, however, because in modern clinical practice, most patients do not present with these so-called typical manifestations. In contrast, presentations previously described as *atypical celiac disease* (e.g., anemia, fatigue, abdominal bloating and discomfort, osteoporosis, or infertility) are now more common. *Asymptomatic celiac disease* (also called *silent celiac disease*) is usually identified by screening using celiac-specific serology and is characterized by gluten-induced enteropathy in individuals who lack symptoms or signs of celiac disease. *Potential celiac disease* (also called *latent celiac disease*) denotes those with normal small intestinal histology who are at increased risk of developing celiac disease (usually identified by positive celiac-specific serology). *Nonresponsive celiac disease* is defined as ongoing or recurrent symptoms or signs that suggest active celiac disease despite a strict GFD for more than 6 to 12 months. *Refractory celiac disease* (a subset of nonresponsive celiac disease) is defined as symptomatic, severe small intestinal villus atrophy despite a strict GFD for more than 6 to 12 months. Refractory celiac disease is a diagnosis of exclusion that is not explained by inadvertent gluten ingestion, other causes of villus atrophy, or overt intestinal lymphoma.[2,3]

*The author gratefully acknowledges the important and valuable contributions of the authors of previous editions, Drs. Jerry S. Trier and Richard J. Farrell.

Celiac serology denotes serology tests that specifically identify untreated celiac disease and includes immunoglobulin (Ig)A or IgG tissue transglutaminase, IgA or IgG endomysium, and IgA or IgG deamidated gliadin peptide antibodies. IgA or IgG antigliadin antibodies are generally excluded because they are relatively nonspecific. *Non-celiac gluten sensitivity* refers to symptoms or signs that develop upon gluten ingestion in people in whom a diagnosis of celiac disease has been excluded. The Oslo definitions for celiac disease and related terms provides a more comprehensive elucidation of definitions currently used in celiac disease.[1]

HISTORY OF CELIAC DISEASE

Celiac disease was recognized as a clinical entity by Aretaeus the Cappadocian in the first century AD.[4] The name *sprue* was coined in the 18th century and is derived from the Dutch word *spruw*, which means "aphthous disease," so named because of the high prevalence of aphthous mouth ulcers in these patients. In 1888, Samuel Gee published his paper "On the Coeliac Affection," which described many of the clinical features of celiac disease in patients of all age groups and concluded, "If the patient can be cured at all it must be by means of the diet."[5] It was not until the middle of the 20th century, however, that the link between certain cereals and celiac disease was made by Willem Karel Dicke, a Dutch pediatrician. He became convinced that the consumption of wheat flour was directly responsible for the deterioration in patients suffering from this condition.[6] During World War II, cereals used to make bread were particularly scarce in the Netherlands, and during this time, children with celiac disease improved, only to relapse after the supply of cereal was reestablished at the end of the war. It was this serendipitous observation that led to the finding that wheat ingestion exacerbated celiac disease. Subsequent work by van de Kamer and coworkers showed that it was the water-insoluble portion, or gluten moiety, of wheat that produced intestinal injury in patients with celiac disease.[7]

In 1954, Paulley provided the first accurate description of the characteristic intestinal lesion in patients with celiac disease.[8] With the development of effective peroral suction biopsy instruments in the late 1950s, Rubin and coworkers demonstrated that celiac disease in children and idiopathic or nontropical sprue in adults were identical diseases with the same clinical and histopathologic features.[9]

Since the 1980s, we have seen substantial advances in our understanding of the genetic, immunologic, and molecular mechanisms fundamental to the pathogenesis of celiac disease. In 1986, Howell and associates observed that celiac disease was associated with specific HLA-DQ2 haplotypes.[10] In 1993, Lundin and colleagues demonstrated that HLA-DQ2 preferentially presents gluten-derived gliadin peptides to activate intestinal mucosal T cells in celiac patients.[11] Subsequently, the enzyme tTG (more specifically tTG type 2 [tTG2]) was identified as a celiac autoantigen, which led to more accurate serologic diagnostic tests.[12] In 1998, Molberg and colleagues reported that modification of gliadin by host tTG2 enhances gliadin-specific celiac disease T cell responses.[13] The identification of specific tTG-modified deamidated gliadin peptides (DGPs) as dominant α-gliadin T cell epitopes highlighted the pivotal role played by tTG2 in the pathogenesis of celiac disease.[14]

Epidemiologic studies using endomysial antibody (EMA) and tTG serology have substantially increased estimates of celiac disease prevalence in the United States as well as the breadth of celiac disease prevalence worldwide.[15] This in turn has led to renewed interest in potential non-dietary treatments including gluten detoxification, glutenase therapy, modifiers of small intestinal tight junction function, tTG2 inhibitors, and immune-based interventions including attempts to reverse intolerance to gluten.[16,17]

EPIDEMIOLOGY

Epidemiologic studies using specific celiac serology testing indicate that celiac disease has a wide geographic distribution and affects individuals from multiple and diverse ethnic and racial backgrounds. The overall prevalence of celiac disease in Europe has been estimated at 1%, with the highest reported prevalence of 2.4% in Finland.[18] Factors such as predominant HLA haplotype, timing of introduction of gluten into the diet, differences in the gliadin concentration of infant formulas, and interobserver variation in interpreting small intestinal biopsy findings might explain differences in prevalence.[19] Celiac disease is prevalent in the Bengal and Punjab provinces of northwest India, where wheat rather than rice has, for many generations, been a staple of the diet. The condition has been reported in blacks, Arabs, Hispanics, Israeli Jews, Sudanese of mixed Arab-black descent, and Cantonese and is particularly high among the Saharawi population in northwest Africa.[20] Peoples rarely affected include those of purely sub-Saharan African, African-Caribbean, or Southeast Asian (including Chinese or Japanese) descent. Some authors have noted a female-to-male ratio of 2:1, while others have reported ratios as low as 1.3:1, but still suggesting a slight female predominance.

Studies in the United States indicate that the prevalence is comparable with that in Europe. A large multicenter study by Fasano and coworkers[15] determined the prevalence of anti-endomysial antibodies in more than 13,000 at-risk and not-at-risk American subjects to be 1 in 22 and 1 in 39 among first-degree and second-degree relatives of subjects with celiac disease, respectively.[15] A prevalence of 1 in 56 was documented among patients with celiac-like GI symptoms or with associated disorders. Of most significance, these investigators found a prevalence of anti-endomysial antibodies of 1:133 among 4126 "not-at-risk" subjects.

The population prevalence of celiac disease appears to be increasing. In 1 U.S. study, tTG seropositivity was 0.2% among 9133 subjects whose blood samples were stored circa 1950 compared with 0.9% in comparable, modern-day sera, suggesting a substantial (4-fold) increase in celiac disease prevalence over time.[21] Interestingly, those positive for IgA-tTG showed a 4-fold increased risk of death over the intervening 45 years.[21] The estimated prevalence of celiac disease has also risen in Finland, from 1% in 1980 to 2% in 2000.[22]

Epidemiologic studies using celiac serology indicate that asymptomatic or minimally symptomatic celiac disease is more common than diagnosed or symptomatic disease.[23] More than 80% of cases were undiagnosed in 1 study in the United States.[24] A Finnish study of 3654 schoolchildren of ages 7 to 16 years, using 2 serologic screens with anti-endomysial and tTG antibodies, demonstrated that 1 in every 99 children had biopsy-proved celiac disease,[25] although only 10 of 56 subjects (18%) with a positive serology had overt symptoms of celiac disease. Two subjects with positive antibodies and HLA-DQ2 haplotype had normal mucosa consistent with potential celiac disease. Another study demonstrated fluctuations in tTG2 serology positivity over time in children with potential celiac disease.[26] In the latter study, 12 of 39 children (31%) with potential celiac disease developed villus atrophy over 3 years of follow-up. Thus, there appears to be individual variation in the natural history of celiac disease, at least in children, where tTG2 seropositivity and celiac enteropathy may fluctuate over time.

PATHOLOGY

Celiac disease affects the mucosa of the small intestine; the submucosa, muscularis propria, and serosa usually are not involved. The mucosal lesion can vary considerably in severity and in extent.[9] Examination under magnification of the small intestinal mucosal surface in severe untreated celiac disease reveals a flat mucosal surface with complete absence of normal intestinal villi. Histologic examination of tissue sections confirms this loss of normal villus structure (Fig. 107-1A). The intestinal crypts are markedly elongated and open onto a flat absorptive surface. The total thickness of the mucosa may be reduced only slightly, because crypt hyperplasia compensates for the absence or shortening of the villi. These architectural changes decrease the amount of epithelial surface available for digestion and absorption.[9]

The enterocytes, which appear columnar in normal biopsy specimens, are cuboidal or, at times, squamoid in celiac disease. Their cytoplasm is more basophilic (i.e., RNA rich), the basal polarity of the nuclei is disrupted, and the brush border is markedly attenuated. When viewed by electron microscopy, the microvilli of the absorptive cells appear shortened and often fused. The number of free ribosomes is increased, reflecting impaired differentiation and resulting in the increased cytoplasmic basophilia evident on histologic examination. Degenerative changes, including cytoplasmic and mitochondrial vacuolization and the presence of many large lysosomes, are also obvious.

Structural abnormalities of tight junctions between damaged absorptive cells provide a morphologic explanation for the increased permeability of the mucosal barrier in celiac disease.[27] The endoplasmic reticulum is sparse, explaining the low level of synthesis of digestive enzymes, including disaccharidases and peptidases. Thus, mature absorptive cells are reduced in number and functionally compromised.

Unlike the absorptive cells, undifferentiated crypt cells are markedly increased in number in patients with severe untreated celiac disease, and the crypts are therefore lengthened. Moreover, the number of mitoses in crypts is strikingly increased. Cytologic features and histochemistry of the crypt cells are normal by both light and electron microscopy. Studies of epithelial cell kinetics in untreated celiac disease suggest that "villus atrophy" is a misnomer because there is evidence for an actual increase in enteropoiesis in the crypts. Wright and colleagues[28] estimated that intestinal mucosa from patients with celiac disease produces 6 times as many cells per hour per crypt as does normal small intestine, and that the cell cycle time is halved, reflecting premature shedding. The experimental evidence suggests, therefore, that the central mechanism of villus shortening in celiac disease is a toxic effect on maturing enterocytes that results in their premature loss into the intestinal lumen and a compensatory increase in cryptal enterocyte replication. Such a mechanism would explain many of the histologic abnormalities described earlier.

The cellularity of the lamina propria is increased in involved small intestine. The cellular infiltrate consists largely of plasma cells and lymphocytes. The number of IgA-, IgM-, and IgG-producing cells is increased 2-fold to 6-fold, but, as in normal mucosa, IgA-producing cells predominate.[29] Polymorphonuclear leukocytes, eosinophils, and mast cells also can contribute substantially to this increased cellularity. The number of intraepithelial lymphocytes (IELs), often reported per 100 enterocytes, is increased in untreated celiac disease.[9] In normal small intestinal mucosa, lamina propria T cells are predominantly CD4+ (helper/inducer) cells, whereas the IELs are mainly CD8+ (cytotoxic/suppressor) cells. In untreated celiac disease, this distribution of lamina propria T cells is maintained, but the density of cells in both compartments is increased.

Marsh[30] pioneered the theory of sequential progression of the celiac lesion in the small intestinal mucosa. Starting with a normal, pre-infiltrative (stage 0) mucosa, the initial observed event is an increase in IELs, followed by infiltration of the lamina propria with lymphocytes (stage 1). Crypt hyperplasia (stage 2) precedes villus atrophy (stage 3) and is observed only in the presence of lamina propria lymphocytosis, suggesting that IELs are not sufficient to induce intestinal architectural changes in celiac disease. Finally, total mucosal atrophy (stage 4) develops and is characterized by complete loss of villi, enhanced apoptosis, and crypt hyperplasia.

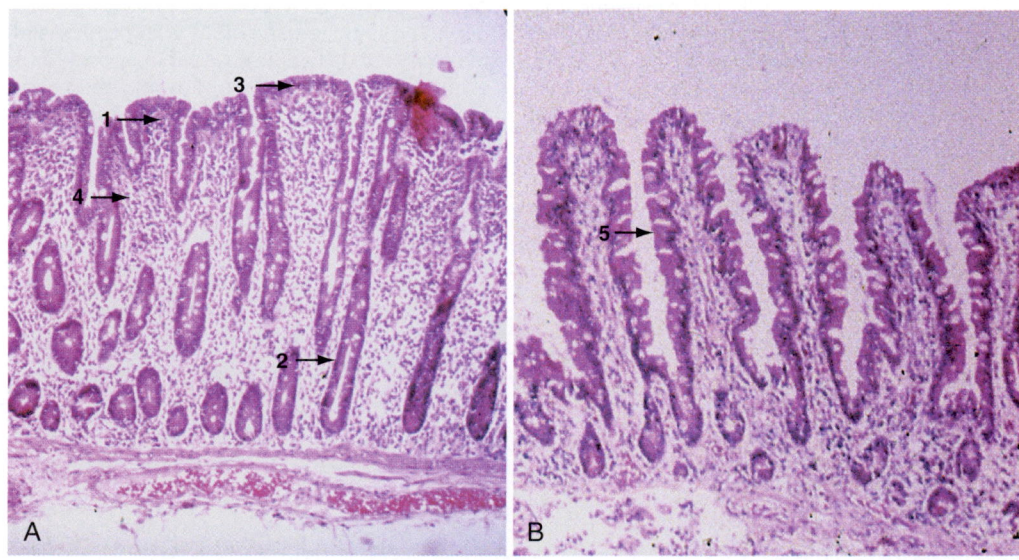

FIGURE 107-1. Mucosal pathology in celiac disease. *A*, Duodenal biopsy specimen of a patient with untreated celiac disease. The histologic features of severe villus atrophy *(arrow 1)*, crypt hyperplasia *(arrow 2)*, enterocyte disarray *(arrow 3)*, and intense inflammation of the lamina propria and epithelial cell layer *(arrow 4)* are evident. *B*, Repeat duodenal biopsy after 6 months on a strict gluten-free diet. There is marked improvement, with well-formed villi *(arrow 5)* and a return of the mucosal architecture toward normal.

In untreated patients, the length of small intestinal involvement by the celiac disease lesion varies among individual patients and correlates with the severity of clinical symptoms. When the intestinal lesion does not involve the entire length of small bowel, the proximal intestine is usually the most severely involved; sparing of proximal intestine with involvement of the distal small intestine can occur, but is uncommon.[9] An increase in IEL count alone is not sufficient for a histologic diagnosis of celiac disease. This finding is nonspecific and is seen in many other conditions including SIBO, peptic duodenitis, Hp infection, NSAID use, and in other autoimmune disorders. Thus, some shortening of the villi, crypt hyperplasia, cytologically abnormal surface cells, and increased lamina propria cellularity must be present to establish the diagnosis firmly.

Treatment with a GFD results in significant improvement in intestinal structure (see Fig. 107-1B). The cytologic appearance of the surface absorptive cells improves first, often within a few days. Tall, columnar absorptive cells with basal nuclei and well-developed brush borders replace the abnormal, immature cuboidal surface cells; the ratio of IELs to absorptive cells decreases. Subsequently, villus architecture reverts toward normal, with lengthening of the villi and shortening of the crypts; the lamina propria decreases in cellularity. The mucosa of the distal small intestine improves more rapidly than that of the more severely involved proximal bowel.[30,31] In some patients, months or even years of gluten withdrawal may be required before the mucosa reverts to normal; indeed, some residual abnormality, which may be striking or subtle, often persists, possibly because of inadvertent gluten ingestion.[32] Finally, the mucosal lesion of celiac disease can be histologically identical to the mucosal response to injury typical of a wide range of other enteropathies (see "Differential Diagnosis").

PATHOGENESIS

The interaction of the water-insoluble protein moiety (gluten) of certain cereal grains with the mucosa of the small intestine in susceptible persons is central to the pathogenesis of celiac disease. Celiac disease is considered an immune disorder that is triggered by an environmental agent (gliadin) in genetically predisposed persons. The wide spectrum of clinical manifestations is the result of a complex interplay of varying environmental, genetic, and immune factors. How these factors control the varied expression of celiac disease and passage from latent to overt disease remains unknown.

Environmental Factors

Celiac disease is a model for autoimmune diseases with a defined environmental trigger. Early work that involved physiologic digestion with pepsin and trypsin, followed by separation according to solubility properties, identified several wheat proteins as being responsible for the grain's toxicity in celiac disease. Wheat protein exists in a number of storage forms that can be categorized into 4 general groups based on solubility characteristics: prolamins (soluble in ethanol), glutenins (partially soluble in dilute acid or alkali solutions), globulins (soluble in 10% NaCl), and albumins (soluble in water). The term *gluten* encompasses both the prolamins and the glutenins. Although most toxicity studies have been performed with prolamins, there are data to indicate that glutenins also may damage the celiac intestinal mucosa.[33]

The prolamins of wheat are referred to as *gliadins*. Prolamins from other cereals also are considered to be gluten and are named according to their source (*secalins* from rye, *hordeins* from barley, *avenins* from oats, and *zeins* from corn). The taxonomic relationships of the major cereal grain families provide a framework on which their toxicities in celiac disease can be predicted (Fig. 107-2).[34] Wheat, rye, and barley belong to the tribe known as Triticeae, and oats belong to a neighboring tribe known as Aveneae. Avenin is genetically less similar to gliadin than gliadin is to secalin and hordein. Despite their genetic differences, however, prolamins from oats, barley, wheat, and rye still have immunologic cross-reactivity because of their common ancestry.[35] Grains that do not activate disease (rice, corn, sorghum, and millet) are separated still further from wheat, rye, and barley in terms of their derivation from the primitive grasses.

Gliadin can be separated electrophoretically into 4 major fractions that range in molecular weight from 20 to 75 kd and exist as single polypeptide chains. These have been designated α-, β-, γ-, and ω-gliadins, and all 4 fractions appear to be toxic to patients with celiac disease.[36] The complete amino acid sequences of several of the gliadins and related prolamins in grains other than wheat are known.[33] Anderson and colleagues[14] identified a partially deamidated peptide, consisting of amino acids 56 to 75 of α-gliadin as a dominant epitope, responsible for activation of T cells in celiac disease. The complexity and diversity of the gliadin-specific T cell response, however, is far greater than was previously appreciated, and persons with celiac disease can respond to a diverse repertoire of gluten peptides.[37] Furthermore, the release of intracellular tTG leads to the deamidation of gluten proteins and an enhancement of T cell responses to the resulting DGPs.[14]

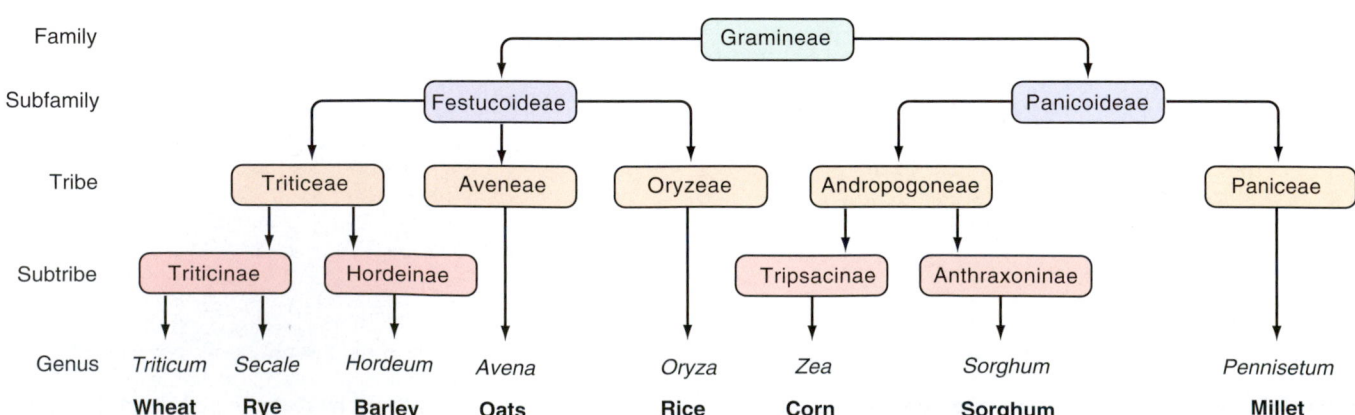

FIGURE 107-2. Taxonomic relationships of the major cereal grains. *(From Kasarda DD, Okita TW, Bernardin JE, et al. Nucleic acid [cDNA] and amino acid sequences of α-type gliadin from wheat [Triticum aestivum]. Proc Natl Acad Sci U S A 1984; 81:4712-5.)*

In organ cultures, a synthetic peptide that corresponds to amino acids 31 to 49 of α-gliadin has been shown to be toxic to intestinal mucosa and to induce epithelial lesions via recruitment of IELs. Peptide 31-49 does not activate intestinal CD4+ T cells from patients with celiac disease in vitro, but a related peptide corresponding to amino acids 31 to 43 is capable of activating peripheral CD4+ T cells isolated from patients with celiac disease and of inducing epithelial cell apoptosis and activating macrophages, thereby indicating a likely role for innate immune responses in disease pathogenesis.[38] Gianfrani and colleagues[39] reported that the α-gliadin-derived peptide corresponding to amino acids 123 to 132 is recognized by CD8+ T lymphocytes from patients with celiac disease and is associated with cytotoxic activity. By contrast, another peptide corresponding to amino acids 57 to 68 appears to function in adaptive immunity via stimulation of intestinal T cells in vivo but does not appear to be directly toxic to the intestinal mucosa of patients in vitro.[37]

The reason oats are tolerated by almost all patients with celiac disease is not obvious, because the prolamin fraction of oats contains the same amino acid sequences (QQQPF, where Q = glutamine, P = proline, and F = phenylalanine) that in wheat gliadin have been shown to be toxic.[40] A possible explanation for this paradox is that oats contain a relatively smaller proportion of this toxic prolamin moiety than do toxic gluten-containing cereals. Although a feature common to prolamins of wheat, rye, and barley is a high content of glutamine (≈30%) and proline (≈15%), the prolamins of oats have an intermediate content of these amino acids, and the nontoxic prolamins of rice, corn, and millet have an even lower content of them.[41] This hypothesis is supported by collectively considering the studies on oat challenge in patients with celiac disease; these studies suggest that tolerance to oats might depend at least in part on the total amount consumed.[42] Daily oats consumption of less than 40 to 60 g/day by patients whose celiac disease is in remission appears to be well tolerated.

The data on oats also highlight the important relationship between the amount of gluten consumed and the severity of disease manifestation. A 5- to 10-fold higher incidence of overt celiac disease in children from Sweden compared with Denmark (2 populations with similar genetic backgrounds) has long been cited as evidence of the importance of environmental over genetic factors in pathogenesis of celiac disease. Subsequent studies found as much as a 40-fold difference in the gliadin concentration of Swedish compared with Danish infant formula.[19] This finding suggests that early exposure of the immature immune system to significant amounts of gliadin may be an important cofactor for the development of overt celiac disease.

The age at which gluten is first introduced into an infant's diet also might play a pivotal role in facilitating gluten tolerance or intolerance. In 1 study, early exposure to dietary gluten (within 3 months of birth) was associated with a 5-fold increased risk for celiac disease compared with later gluten introduction (4 to 6 months).[43] In the same study, delaying gluten introduction (after 7 months of age) also was associated with a slightly increased risk for subsequent celiac disease (1.9-fold compared with the nadir for optimal introduction at 4 to 6 months).

Genetic Factors

Family studies that demonstrate frequent intrafamilial occurrence of celiac disease reflect the importance of genetic factors in its pathogenesis.[42] Concordance for celiac disease in first-degree relatives ranges between 8% and 18% and reaches 70% in monozygotic twins.[44] Our understanding of the nature of this genetic predisposition began with the observation

that celiac disease was associated with specific HLA-DQ2 haplotypes.[10] HLA class II molecules are glycosylated transmembrane heterodimers (α and β chains) that are organized into 3 related subregions—DQ, DR, and DP—and encoded within the HLA class II region of the major histocompatibility complex on chromosome 6p. An important link to a genetic predisposition was provided by the isolation of gliadin-specific HLA-DQ2-restricted T cell clones from celiac disease mucosa.[11,45]

The HLA class II molecule DQ2 is present in more than 90% of persons with celiac disease compared with approximately 35% of the general white population. DQ2 is a heterodimer composed of either α1*0501 (DQ2.5) or, less commonly, α1*0201 (DQ2.2) together with β1*02. The DQ α1*0301, β1*0302 heterodimer, known as HLA-DQ8, is found in almost all of the remaining patients with celiac disease.[46] Occasional cases of celiac disease have been reported in patients who are DQ2 and DQ8 negative but nonetheless carry a single DQ2 allele. Thus, in some cases, typing of individual celiac-associated alleles may be helpful in addition to determining DQ2 and DQ8 status. A gene dose-effect also has been identified, whereby persons who are homozygous for DQ2 are at greater risk than heterozygotes for developing celiac disease.

It is now known that after gluten is absorbed, lamina propria antigen-presenting cells (probably dendritic cells) that express HLA-DQ2 or HLA-DQ8, present gliadin peptides on their α/β heterodimer antigen-presenting grooves to sensitized T lymphocytes expressing the α/β T cell receptor (TCR). These lymphocytes then activate B lymphocytes to generate immunoglobulins and other T lymphocytes to secrete cytokines, including interferon (IFN)-γ, as well as interleukin (IL)-4, IL-5, IL-6, IL-10, TNF-α, and transforming growth factor (TGF)-β.[47] These cytokines induce not only enterocyte injury but also expression of aberrant HLA class II cell-surface antigens on the luminal surface of enterocytes, possibly facilitating additional direct antigen presentation by these cells to the sensitized lymphocytes (Fig. 107-3).

Only a minority of persons who express DQ2 actually develop celiac disease. HLA-DQ2 is expressed by approximately 35% of Europeans and their descendants, but it is rare in other populations (e.g., in sub-Saharan Africa or far eastern Asia). Thus, much of the genetic predisposition to celiac disease is conferred by genes other than those encoding HLA-DQ molecules. The search for other genes that confer susceptibility to celiac disease has revealed numerous loci of interest on several different chromosomes, some of which also are associated with susceptibility to type 1 diabetes.[48-51]

Immune Factors

There is substantial evidence implicating both humoral- and cell-mediated immune responses to gliadin and related prolamins in the pathogenesis of celiac disease. There is a 2- to 6-fold increase in the numbers of immunoglobulin-producing B cells in the lamina propria of the small intestine in untreated celiac disease patients.[28] In addition, IgA and IgG serum antibodies to purified gliadin, all major fractions of gliadin, and DGPs can be detected in the sera of most patients with untreated celiac disease.[14,52-55] Many normal persons have increased IgA or IgG antigliadin.[56] The frequency of elevated IgA or IgG DGP antibodies in healthy controls, however, is very low, possibly reflecting the antigenic potency of DGPs and their more central role in disease pathogenesis.[14,53-55] Many persons with celiac disease have increased levels of serum antibodies against other food proteins, such as β-lactoglobulin, casein, and ovalbumin.[57] It is unclear whether this reflects a general aberrant immune responsiveness to food antigens in

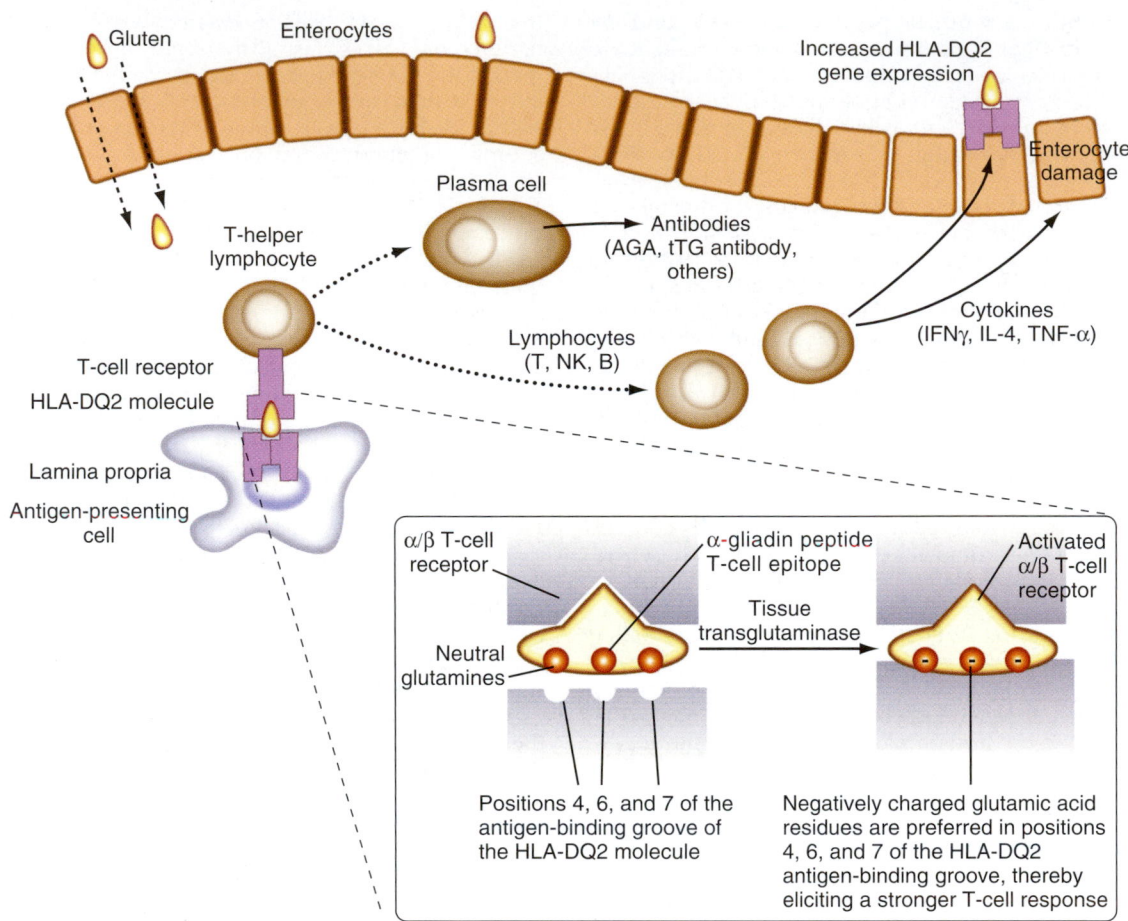

FIGURE 107-3. Proposed pathogenesis of celiac disease. Gluten is absorbed by the small intestinal mucosa into the lamina propria and presented in conjunction with HLA-DQ2 (or DQ8) cell-surface antigens by antigen-presenting cells, probably dendritic cells, to sensitized T lymphocytes that express the α/β T-cell receptor (afferent limb). Tissue transglutaminase (tTG) deamidates gliadin peptides, generating acidic, negatively charged glutamic acid residues from neutral glutamines (inset). Because negatively charged residues are preferred in positions 4, 6, and 7 of the antigen-binding groove of HLA-DQ2, deamidated gliadin elicits stronger T-lymphocyte responses. These T lymphocytes then activate other lymphocytes to generate immune products (cytokines) that damage the enterocytes, resulting in villus atrophy (efferent limb). Induction of aberrant HLA class II cell-surface antigens on the enterocytes can permit additional gluten antigen presentation by these cells to the sensitized lymphocytes. AGA, antigliadin antibodies; IFN-γ, interferon gamma; IL-4, interleukin-4; NK, natural killer.

patients with celiac disease or enhanced systemic exposure to these proteins because of increased small intestinal permeability. Gluten can be absorbed across normal epithelium, but it is unclear if this results in immune tolerance in persons who are not genetically predisposed to develop celiac disease.

The identification of more specific autoantibody responses has altered our understanding of the pathogenesis of celiac disease. IgA antibodies to endomysium, a connective tissue structure surrounding smooth muscle, are virtually pathognomonic for celiac disease and are found but rarely in the absence of disease.[58] It is now known that the target autoantigen contained within the endomysium is the enzyme tTG-2.[12] Gliadin is a preferred substrate for this ubiquitous calcium-dependent intracellular enzyme, and it has been shown that tTG deamidates key neutral glutamine residues in gliadin and converts them into negatively charged glutamic acid residues, which are preferred in positions 4, 6, and 7 of the nonpeptide antigen-binding groove of the HLA-DQ2 heterodimer (see Fig. 107-3),[13,14,59] thereby facilitating antigen presentation. Thus, tTG-mediated modification of gliadin to generate DGPs plays a pivotal role in eliciting a stronger proliferative response by gliadin-specific T cells.

With gliadin serving as the glutamine donor, tTG also can generate additional novel antigenic epitopes by cross-linking molecules of the extracellular matrix with gliadin or with tTG-gliadin complexes.[60] As evidence of the fundamental role of tTG in celiac disease pathogenesis, 1 of the dominant epitopes responsible for the T cell response contains a deamidated glutamine residue (Q65E) of α-gliadin.[14]

Given the marked infiltration of lymphocytes into the small intestinal mucosal epithelium and lamina propria in active disease, it is not surprising that cell-mediated immune responses also are important in the pathogenesis of celiac disease. Many findings support interplay between adaptive immunity, characterized by a specific and memory T-cell response to gluten peptides, and innate immunity, involving less specific mechanisms. Many of the T cells in the small intestinal mucosa are activated in untreated celiac disease and release potent proinflammatory mediators such as IFN-γ, TNF-α, IL-2, IL-6, and TGF-β.[47] Activated T lymphocytes, most of which are CD4+ cells, are abundant in the lamina propria of the small intestine.[61] In contrast, IELs, which are present in large numbers in untreated celiac disease, are predominantly CD8+ T cells.[62]

There is an influx of primed memory T cells, marked by high CD45RO expression, in the mucosa of untreated celiac disease patients.[63] In healthy persons, more than 90% of IELs express the α/β TCR, whereas expression of the γ/δ TCR by IELs in patients with untreated celiac disease is increased as much as 6-fold (to 35%) and is considered a hallmark of the disease.[64] These primitive lymphocytes recognize bacterial non-peptide antigens and unprocessed stress-related proteins. They appear to act as mucosal guardians and might protect the intestinal mucosa from chronic exposure to dietary gluten in gluten-tolerant persons by secreting IL-4, which dampens Th1 in favor of Th2 reactivity.[65] Their continuous presence in patients on a GFD might indicate inadvertent gluten ingestion. Patients with refractory celiac disease also have aberrant IELs with restricted γ/δ *TCR* gene rearrangements indicating oligoclonality. The pathogenetic role of these lymphocytes, compared with lamina propria lymphocytes, continues to evolve (see "Refractory Celiac Disease").[66]

Studies suggest that IL-15 may play a key role in bridging the innate and adaptive immune responses in the pathogenesis of celiac disease.[38,67,68] This enterocyte- and macrophage-derived proinflammatory cytokine is increased greatly in the mucosa of patients with active celiac disease and refractory celiac disease. Although mechanisms that lead to its overproduction remain unknown, IL-15 regulates IEL homeostasis by promoting migration, preventing apoptosis, and enhancing the capacity of dendritic cells to function as antigen-presenting cells.[38] In response to gliadin peptides, IL-15 triggers an adaptive CD4+ T-cell response in the lamina propria and also is capable of inducing direct epithelial cell injury by inducing IEL secretion of IFN-γ.[68]

CLINICAL FEATURES

Samuel Gee's classic description, with its evocative account, was concerned largely with the gross manifestations of the disorder.[5] This florid presentation, however, is now unusual in the Western world, constituting only the extreme tip of the celiac iceberg. Although some patients still present with severe illness, most have few, subtle, or no symptoms at diagnosis. Such cases may be identified by screening relatives of patients or from screening patients with associated disorders, such as type 1 diabetes mellitus, autoimmune thyroid disease, or Down syndrome. Incidental hematologic abnormalities (e.g., iron deficiency anemia) or biochemical abnormalities (e.g., elevated serum aminotransferase levels) also can lead to a diagnosis of celiac disease.

Childhood Presentation

The classic presentation of celiac disease in infancy is with diarrhea, steatorrhea, and occasional cramping abdominal pain that can occur any time after cereals are introduced into the diet, but especially in early childhood. Classically, the child fails to thrive, is apathetic and irritable, and has muscle wasting, hypotonia, and abdominal distention. Watery diarrhea, or occasionally constipation, may be reported. Diagnosis is more difficult when GI features are less prominent, and the possibility of gluten sensitivity should be considered in all children who present with short stature or failure to thrive, even when there are no other symptoms to suggest an enteropathy. Once a GFD is commenced, catch-up growth is well documented.[69] Nutritional deficiencies, particularly anemia, are another common mode of presentation, especially in older children. With earlier diagnosis, clinical rickets now is an uncommon complication but is seen occasionally, especially among Asian children with untreated celiac disease. Many

pediatric patients enjoy a temporary, spontaneous remission of symptoms during adolescence, and it is unusual for celiac disease to first manifest during the teens.

Considerable debate continues as to why celiac disease tends to be diagnosed later and with milder signs and symptoms than in the past. A number of studies suggest that breastfeeding can significantly delay the onset of symptoms,[70,71] but not all studies support this conclusion.[72] In 1 study of at-risk children, the introduction of gluten into the diet during the first 3 months of life or after 7 months of age was associated with a significantly increased risk for celiac disease compared with introduction at 4 to 6 months.[43]

Adulthood Presentation

In the past, celiac disease was perceived to be a pediatric disorder, but the diagnosis now is being made increasingly in adults; currently, the overall mean age at presentation is approximately 45 years. Symptoms also have changed during the past 50 years. Diarrhea now is reported less often, and many patients present with higher body mass indices. In 1 report, 21% of newly diagnosed adults were overweight, and an additional 12% were obese. The unmasking of asymptomatic disease by surgery that induces rapid gastric emptying (e.g., gastric resection, pyloroplasty) or the finding of the typical lesion in asymptomatic relatives of celiac disease patients suggests that adults can have silent celiac disease for some time. A proportion of these adult patients have short stature or give a history consistent with unrecognized celiac disease in childhood. In many, however, there is nothing to suggest previous disease, and it is possible that celiac disease can develop for the first time in adult life. Celiac disease also is being diagnosed increasingly in later life, with approximately 25% of cases diagnosed in patients older than 60 years.[73]

GI Features

Clinical manifestations of celiac disease vary tremendously from patient to patient. Because many of the symptoms result from intestinal malabsorption, they are not specific for celiac disease and resemble those seen in other malabsorptive disorders. Many adults present with GI symptoms including diarrhea, steatorrhea, abdominal bloating, flatulence, and weight loss similar to those seen in childhood celiac disease. Diarrhea often is episodic rather than continuous. Nocturnal, early morning, and postprandial diarrhea are common. Patients with extensive intestinal involvement can have more than 10 stools per day. Steatorrhea often is absent in patients with disease that is limited to the proximal small intestine.

Several factors contribute to the diarrhea associated with celiac disease. The stool volume and osmotic load delivered to the colon are increased by malabsorption.[74] In addition, the delivery of excessive dietary fat into the colon results in bacterial production of hydroxy fatty acids, which are potent cathartics. Electrolytes actually are secreted into, rather than absorbed from, the lumen of the severely damaged upper small intestine in symptomatic patients. This secretion further increases luminal fluid in an intestine with an already compromised absorptive capacity. There also is evidence that secretin and cholecystokinin release in response to a meal are impaired in celiac disease, thus diminishing delivery of bile and pancreatic secretions into the intestinal lumen and possibly compromising intraluminal digestion.[75] Alterations in the secretion of other intestinal peptides have been noted and can contribute to the observed diarrhea. Finally, if the disease extends to and involves the ileum, patients can experience the direct cathartic action of malabsorbed bile salts on the colon.[74]

The amount of weight loss in a patient with celiac disease depends on the severity and extent of the intestinal lesion and on the ability of the patient to compensate for the malabsorption by increasing dietary intake. Some celiac disease patients with substantial malabsorption have enormous appetites and lose little or no weight. Rarely, in severe disease, anorexia develops with associated rapid and severe weight loss. In such debilitated patients, some of the weight loss may be masked by fluid retention caused by hypoproteinemia. Malaise, lassitude, and fatigue also are common even when anemia is absent. Occasionally, severe hypokalemia resulting from fecal loss of potassium causes severe muscle weakness.

Vague abdominal discomfort and especially abdominal bloating are extremely common and can lead to a mistaken diagnosis of IBS. Because of the difficulty in distinguishing celiac disease with mild GI manifestations from symptomatic IBS, serologic testing of IgA EMAs or IgA tTG should be considered in patients with symptoms that suggest diarrhea-predominant IBS.[76] Severe abdominal pain can occur but is uncharacteristic in uncomplicated celiac disease; its occurrence can suggest the presence of complications such as intussusception, ulcerative jejunitis, or intestinal lymphoma. Abdominal distention with excessive amounts of malodorous flatus is a common complaint. Conversely, nausea and vomiting are uncommon in uncomplicated celiac disease. Symptoms of GERD may be significantly more common in untreated celiac disease and improve on a GFD.[77] Recurrent, severe, aphthous stomatitis affects many celiac patients, may be their sole presenting complaint and typically resolves on a GFD.[78]

Celiac crisis is a rare, life-threatening syndrome in which children or adults with untreated celiac disease present with profuse diarrhea that leads to severe dehydration, metabolic disturbances, renal dysfunction and, in some instances, hemodynamic instability.[79] Early diagnosis is important, and management includes IV fluids as well as glucocorticoids and/or parenteral nutrition where indicated. Patients eventually respond well to a GFD.

Extraintestinal Features

As patients with celiac disease get older, they tend to present with complaints not directly referable to the GI tract. These extraintestinal symptoms and clinical findings often result from nutrient malabsorption and can involve virtually all organ systems (Table 107-1).[80]

TABLE 107-1 Extraintestinal Manifestations of Celiac Disease

Manifestation	Probable Cause(s)
Cutaneous	
Ecchymoses and petechiae	Vitamin K deficiency; rarely, thrombocytopenia
Edema	Hypoproteinemia
Dermatitis herpetiformis	Epidermal (type 3) tTG autoimmunity
Follicular hyperkeratosis and dermatitis	Vitamin A malabsorption, vitamin B complex malabsorption
Endocrinologic	
Amenorrhea, infertility, impotence	Malnutrition, hypothalamic-pituitary dysfunction, immune dysfunction
Secondary hyperparathyroidism	Calcium and/or vitamin D malabsorption with hypocalcemia
Hematologic	
Anemia	Iron, folate, vitamin B_{12}, or pyridoxine deficiency
Hemorrhage	Vitamin K deficiency; rarely, thrombocytopenia due to folate deficiency
Thrombocytosis, Howell-Jolly bodies	Hyposplenism
Hepatic	
Elevated liver biochemical test levels	Lymphocytic hepatitis
Autoimmune hepatitis	Autoimmunity
Muscular	
Atrophy	Malnutrition due to malabsorption
Tetany	Calcium, vitamin D, and/or magnesium malabsorption
Weakness	Generalized muscle atrophy, hypokalemia
Neurologic	
Peripheral neuropathy	Deficiencies of vitamin B_{12} and thiamine; immune-based neurologic dysfunction
Ataxia	Cerebellar and posterior column damage
Demyelinating central nervous system lesions	Immune-based neurologic dysfunction
Seizures	Unknown
Skeletal	
Osteopenia, osteomalacia, and osteoporosis	Malabsorption of calcium and vitamin D, secondary hyperparathyroidism, chronic inflammation
Osteoarthropathy	Unknown
Pathologic fractures	Osteopenia and osteoporosis

tTG, tissue transglutaminase.

Anemia

Anemia is a common manifestation of celiac disease in children and adults and usually is caused by impaired iron or folate absorption from the proximal intestine; in severe disease with ileal involvement, vitamin B_{12} absorption also is impaired. Coagulopathy resulting from impaired intestinal absorption of fat-soluble vitamin K occurs rarely, and in such cases bleeding can aggravate preexisting anemia. Hyposplenism of unknown cause, with thrombocytosis, deformed erythrocytes, and splenic atrophy, occurs in up to 50% of adults with celiac disease but only rarely is seen in children.[81] Evidence of hyposplenism may disappear with elimination of gluten from the diet.[81]

Osteopenia

Osteopenia is a common complication of celiac disease, and its prevalence increases with age at diagnosis. More than 70% of patients with untreated celiac disease have osteopenia,[82] and osteoporosis occurs in more than one quarter of all celiac disease patients.[83] Osteopenia develops as a result of impaired calcium absorption (secondary to defective calcium transport by the diseased small intestine), vitamin D deficiency (caused by impaired absorption of this fat-soluble vitamin), and binding of intraluminal calcium and magnesium to unabsorbed dietary fatty acids (forming insoluble soaps, which are then excreted in the feces). Chronic intestinal inflammation also contributes to bone loss through release of inflammatory mediators.

Patients can present with bone pain, especially of the lower back, rib cage, and pelvis. Calcium and magnesium depletion can cause paresthesias, muscle cramps, and even tetany. With prolonged calcium malabsorption, patients may develop secondary hyperparathyroidism, resulting in mobilization of calcium from the bones, further exacerbating the osteopenia.

Osteopenia is less common in patients with silent celiac disease, in whom prevalence rates between 30% and 40% have been reported.[84] Whereas bone disease generally is more severe among patients with symptomatic disease, severe osteopenia has been reported in up to one third of symptom-free adults whose celiac disease was diagnosed during childhood and who resumed a normal diet during adolescence.[85]

A key unanswered question is the functional consequence of osteopenia. An increased risk of fractures was observed in patients with overt celiac disease in 1 study[84] but not in another.[86] The fracture risk among patients with silent celiac also remains unclear.

Neurologic Symptoms

Neurologic symptoms caused by lesions of the central or peripheral nervous system occasionally occur in patients with celiac disease and are poorly understood. Celiac disease often is found in patients who present with non-hereditary ataxia, and progressive gait and limb ataxia may be the sole manifestations of disease in some patients. These abnormalities, referred to as *gluten ataxia*, are believed to result from immunologic damage to the cerebellum, posterior columns of the spinal cord, and peripheral nerves.[87] Muscle weakness and paresthesias with sensory loss also are encountered occasionally, and pathologic evidence of peripheral neuropathy and patchy demyelinization of the spinal cord, cerebellar atrophy, and capillary proliferation suggestive of Wernicke's encephalopathy have been described rarely.

Although potential causative roles for specific vitamin deficiencies (including vitamin B_{12}, thiamine, riboflavin, and pyridoxine) have not been established, neurologic symptoms have been reported to improve in some patients who are given multivitamins, including vitamins A, B, and E, and calcium. Night blindness is a clear indication for vitamin A therapy. Peripheral neuropathy and ataxia, however, often appear unrelated to specific vitamin deficiency states and usually do not respond to gluten withdrawal.[88]

The associations of celiac disease and epilepsy, frequently complex partial seizures, and bilateral parieto-occipital cerebral calcification are well recognized.[89] In 1 series, epilepsy was reported in approximately 5% of children and young adults with celiac disease.[90] The cause remains unclear, and response of the epilepsy to a GFD is unpredictable.

The prevalence of psychiatric disorders such as anxiety or depression do not appear to be increased in patients with celiac disease in the United States.[91] Although most patients with celiac disease appear psychologically normal at presentation, many affected subjects report an improvement in mood and level of energy after commencing a GFD.[92]

Gynecologic and Fertility Problems

Gynecologic and obstetric problems are common in women with untreated celiac disease.[93] Amenorrhea occurs in one third of women of childbearing age, and menarche is often delayed, typically by 1 year, in untreated subjects. Women with untreated celiac disease can present with infertility, and it is common for infertile women with celiac disease to become pregnant shortly after commencing a GFD.[94]

A high prevalence of silent celiac disease has been reported in women with recurrent spontaneous abortions, intrauterine fetal growth retardation, and unfavorable outcomes of pregnancy, underlining the need to test for celiac disease in these situations.[95] Binding of anti-tTG antibodies to the trophoblast has been implicated as a mechanism whereby implantation and pregnancy outcomes are impaired in untreated celiac disease.[96]

Infertility secondary to impotence or an abnormally low sperm count can occur in men with untreated celiac disease.[97] Although malnutrition, including folate deficiency related to malabsorption, can contribute to male infertility, abnormalities in hypothalamic-pituitary regulation of gonadal function and gonadal androgen resistance that disappears on gluten withdrawal also have been incriminated.[97]

Physical Examination

Physical findings, like symptoms, vary considerably among patients with celiac disease. Patients with mild disease often have a completely normal physical examination. In more severe disease, physical abnormalities usually result from malabsorption and, therefore, are not specific for celiac disease.

Growth retardation commonly occurs in children, but when they commence a GFD before puberty, a compensatory growth spurt occurs so the effect on adult height potentially can be minimized. Persons with celiac disease are, on average, 3 inches shorter than their peers. Tall patients are seen, however, and a height of more than 6 feet does not preclude the diagnosis.

In patients with severe celiac disease, emaciation with evidence of weight loss, including loose skin folds and muscle wasting, may be prominent. It is common for adults with celiac disease to experience significant weight gain following institution of a GFD.[98]

Clubbing of the fingers occurs occasionally, and koilonychia may result from long-standing iron deficiency anemia. There may be pitting edema of the lower extremities secondary to hypoproteinemia. Hypotension may be related to fluid and electrolyte depletion, and the skin may be dry with poor turgor, if there is dehydration. Occasionally a low-grade fever associated with anemia is found in untreated celiac disease, but this finding might indicate a concurrent complication, such as infection or malignancy, particularly lymphoma. Increased skin pigmentation may be obvious in severely ill patients. In addition to dermatitis herpetiformis (DH) (see later), other dermatologic findings may include spontaneous ecchymoses related to hypoprothrombinemia, hyperkeratosis follicularis caused by vitamin A deficiency, and pallor caused by anemia.

Examination of the mouth may show aphthous stomatitis, angular cheilosis, and glossitis with decreased papillation of the tongue. Dental enamel defects are common.[99] In severe cases, the abdomen may be protuberant and tympanitic, with a characteristic doughy consistency, owing to distention of intestinal loops with fluid and gas. Hepatomegaly and abdominal tenderness are uncommon, but ascites may be detected in patients with significant hypoproteinemia. Peripheral lymphadenopathy is unusual in the absence of complicating lymphoma.

The extremities may reveal loss of various sensory modalities, including light touch, vibration, and position, usually resulting from peripheral neuropathy and, rarely, demyelinating spinal cord lesions. If neuropathy is severe, deep tendon reflexes are diminished or even absent. Hyperpathia may be present. A positive Chvostek or Trousseau sign may be elicited in patients with severe calcium or magnesium depletion. In such persons, bone tenderness related to osteoporosis may be elicited, especially if collapsed vertebrae or other fractures are present.

DIAGNOSIS

Laboratory findings in celiac disease, like the symptoms and signs, vary with the extent and severity of the intestinal lesion. Specific celiac serology tests (IgA EMA, IgA tTG, IgA or IgG DGP) and small intestinal biopsy are the most reliable diagnostic tests for celiac disease. Stool studies, hematologic and biochemical tests, and radiologic studies may be abnormal, but they seldom provide a specific diagnosis because similar abnormalities often are seen in patients with other malabsorptive diseases (see Chapter 104). Testing for HLA DQ2 and DQ8 may be useful to exclude celiac disease in specific clinical circumstances.[100,101]

Serology

In current clinical practice, there are many serologic studies to aid in the diagnosis of celiac disease; the single most useful test for diagnosis and for monitoring of celiac disease is IgA tTG assay. Both IgA EMA and IgA tTG are based on the target antigen tTG. Assays based on DGPs also show excellent diagnostic accuracy.[14,53-55] IgA and IgG AGAs, which are based on native gliadin as target antigen, are not specific and should be avoided.[101]

The approximate sensitivity and specificity of commonly used serum antibody tests are outlined in Table 107-2.[101-105] In addition to laboratory variation, the predictive values of these tests depend on the prevalence of the disease in the tested population and the severity of the disease. In 1 study of 101 patients with biopsy-proved celiac disease, the sensitivity of IgA EMA among patients with total villus atrophy was 100% compared with only 31% in those with partial villus atrophy.[106]

Immunoglobulin A Endomysial Antibody

Serum IgA EMA binds to connective tissue (endomysium), surrounding smooth muscle cells, producing a characteristic staining pattern that is identified by indirect immunofluorescence.[58] The target antigen has been identified as tTG. The test result is reported simply as positive or negative because even low titers of serum IgA EMA are highly specific for celiac disease. IgA EMA has a sensitivity of 90% or greater and a specificity approaching 100% in untreated celiac disease.[58,107] Antibody levels fall on a GFD, the test often becoming negative in treated patients.[108] IgA EMA testing is used less commonly than IgA tTG because indirect immunofluorescence is more labor intensive, requires more expertise, is more prone to laboratory variation in performance and interpretation, and is more expensive than the widely available enzyme immunoassays (EIAs) for IgA tTG.

Tissue Transglutaminase Antibodies

The epitope against which EMA is directed has been identified as type 2 tTG (tTG-2).[12] Type 1 tTG, which has different structure, enzymatic activities, and tissue distributions, is not implicated in celiac disease. Type 3 (epidermal) tTG plays a distinct role in DH (discussed later). Type 6 tTG has been implicated in neurological disorders associated with celiac disease.

TABLE 107-2 Sensitivity, Specificity, and Positive and Negative Predictive Values of Serologic Tests for Untreated Celiac Disease

Serologic Test	Sensitivity* (%)	Specificity* (%)	Positive Predictive Value (%)	Negative Predictive Value (%)
Immunoglobulin A Tissue Transglutaminase				
Endomysial antibody by indirect immunofluorescence assay	85-98	97-100	98-100	80-95
Guinea pig tTG[†] ELISA	95-98	94-95	91-95	96-98
Human tTG[‡] ELISA	95-100	97-100	80-95	100
Antigliadin Antibodies (AGAs)				
IgA	75-90	82-95	28-100	65-100
IgG	69-85	73-90	20-95	41-88

*Wide variations in test sensitivity and specificity rates are reported among different laboratories.[102]
†The guinea pig tTG antibodies data are based on 2 large studies.[232,233]
‡The human tTG antibodies data are based on 2 large studies.[109,110]
AGA, antigliadin antibodies; ELISA, enzyme-linked immunosorbent assay; Ig, immunoglobulin; tTG, tissue transglutaminase.

Enzyme-linked immunosorbent assays (ELISAs) that use human tTG are preferred above earlier assays based on guinea pig tTG because the human tTG assays are more specific.[109,110] IgA guinea pig tTG tests are prone to false-positive results in persons with autoimmune diseases, liver disease, congestive heart failure, and in patients with other inflammatory bowel diseases.[102] A false-positive IgA human tTG result is unlikely (especially at high titer), and in the setting of a normal biopsy might indicate potential celiac disease. Although IgG and IgM tTG assays are useful in patients with IgA deficiency, they are not as sensitive as the preferred IgG DGP testing.[111]

Deamidated Gliadin Antibodies

It is known that tTG-2 catalyzes the deamidation of gliadin peptides. This increases their binding to the antigen groove of DQ2, thereby increasing their toxicity.[14] Based on this knowledge, DGP serology has been developed using synthetic DGPs that replicate the structure of tTG-modified gliadin antigens. IgA and IgG DGP assays are available with sensitivities that approach those obtained using IgA tTG (see Table 107-2).[53-55,101,103-105] The specificity of a positive DGP test result is substantially greater than that of prior AGA assays, presumably indicating that celiac-associated AGAs recognize DGP, whereas AGAs in persons who do not have celiac disease recognize other epitopes less specific for the disease.

DGP testing is increasingly used, and potential applications include the confirmation or exclusion of celiac disease in persons who have small bowel biopsy findings consistent with celiac disease but a negative IgA-tTG test result (including those with IgA deficiency where DGP-IgG can be used) and in persons with positive AGA test results but a negative IgA-tTG.[101,111] DGP concentrations fall on a GFD in a similar fashion to AGA or anti-tTG concentrations.[53,112] A more controversial application of DGP testing is to use anti-tTG and anti-DGP assays in combination for diagnosis or exclusion of disease without small bowel biopsy.

Serum IgA and IgG AGA levels often are elevated in untreated celiac disease. Unfortunately, these tests have only moderate sensitivity, and their specificity is substantially lower than those of IgA EMA, IgA tTG, IgA DGP, or IgG DGP.[113] Thus, false-positive results are common, and hence testing for AGA no longer is recommended as a primary test for untreated celiac disease; IgA tTG testing is preferable.[101]

Clinical Application of Serologic Tests

Serologic tests are used to evaluate patients with suspected celiac disease, monitor adherence and response to a GFD, and potentially, screen asymptomatic persons for the disease.

An approach to diagnosing celiac disease is outlined in Figure 107-4.[101,114] When the index of suspicion is low—the pretest probability is less than 5%—a negative result for IgA tTG has a high negative predictive value and can obviate the need for small bowel biopsy. Falsely negative IgA tTG test results are more likely to occur in very young children (<2 years of age), those with mild celiac enteropathy, and, of course, in IgA deficiency. Because the specificity of IgA tTG tests are high, their positive predictive values are high even in low-risk populations.[107,115,116] If a second test is to be used, either total IgA (to evaluate for IgA deficiency) or an IgG DGP assay can be performed.

When the index of suspicion is moderate to high—the pretest probability is greater than 5%—the very high specificity of IgA tTG has led to debate as to whether a positive result in the appropriate clinical setting can be considered diagnostic

and eliminate the need for small bowel biopsy. We recommend that both IgA tTG *and* a small bowel biopsy be performed before dietary treatment is recommended, because this approach provides the best means of making a definitive diagnosis of celiac disease at the outset. If for some reason biopsy will not be performed, then combination IgA tTG and IgA or IgG DGP testing should be considered.

IgA tTG levels decrease in the months following a GFD and are useful in assessing dietary compliance and excluding inadvertent gluten ingestion.[52,53,112,117] Hence, a pretreatment antibody level should be determined at the time of diagnosis. A normal baseline value typically is reached within 3 to 12 months, depending on the pretreatment antibody concentration (IgA tTG concentrations fall with a half-life of approximately 6 to 8 weeks) and on the degree of success in avoiding gluten ingestion. If the levels do not fall as anticipated, the patient may be continuing to ingest gluten either intentionally or inadvertently.[118]

The advent of highly sensitive and specific serologic tests has changed the epidemiology of celiac disease radically by revealing the high incidence of silent celiac disease; this awareness in turn has led to debate on the merits of mass screening. To date, the benefit of screening for asymptomatic celiac disease, usually using IgA tTG or EMA, remains uncertain.[119] The potential advantages of screening for asymptomatic celiac disease are a reduction in risk for malignancy, including enteropathy-associated T cell lymphoma (EATL); a reversal of unrecognized nutritional deficiency states; resolution of mild or ignored intestinal symptoms; possible reduction in T-cell activation and "antigenic drift" to other autoantigens, thereby reducing the onset of other autoimmune disorders; and an improvement in general well-being.[120,121] All of these hypothetical benefits, however, depend on compliance with a burdensome dietary regimen, and asymptomatic patients may not be motivated sufficiently to adhere to a strict GFD.[122] There also may be adverse psychological effects when asymptomatic individuals are given the diagnosis of a chronic, incurable disease. Furthermore, the natural history of undetected celiac disease and the consequences of screening and treating silent celiac disease are unknown. For these reasons, mass screening of asymptomatic persons generally is not advocated at this time.[123]

The current standard of care is a case-finding approach that targets at-risk subjects such as patients with mild GI symptoms, iron deficiency anemia, or IBS-like symptoms, all instances in which the value of serologic testing for celiac disease is accepted widely. Simply by case finding among at-risk subjects in a primary care setting, Hin and colleagues[124] observed a 4-fold increase in the number of celiac disease diagnoses during a 1-year period. Thus, for now, increased awareness of the typical and atypical presentations of celiac disease, coupled with a low threshold for serologic testing in at-risk subjects, can uncover a substantial portion of the submerged celiac iceberg.

Genetic Testing for HLA DQ2/DQ8

As discussed earlier, almost all patients with celiac disease are positive for HLA DQ2 or DQ8. Approximately 35% of persons of European ancestry are DQ2 or DQ8 positive, however, so a positive result is of little diagnostic value.[101,113,125] Hence, HLA testing should not be used routinely for celiac disease diagnosis. HLA testing may be helpful in excluding celiac disease in specific clinical situations. One of the most important clinical indications for HLA DQ2/DQ8 testing is in patients already adhering to a GFD and with negative celiac serologies but without prior diagnostic serology or histopathlogy.[101] In this setting, a negative HLA DQ2/DQ8 test result will exclude

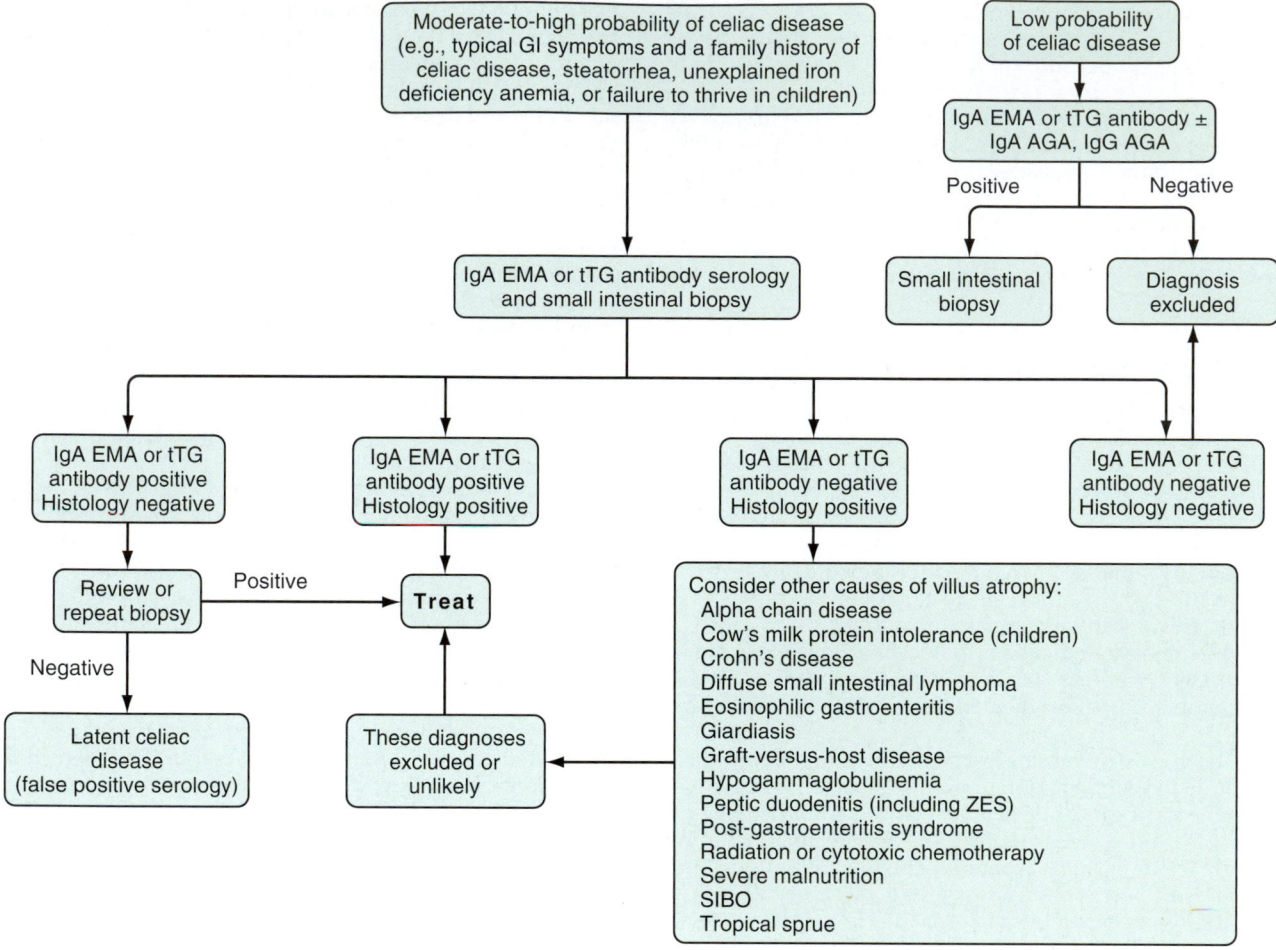

FIGURE 107-4. Diagnosis of celiac disease. A false-positive immunoglobulin (Ig)A EMA or tTG is rare; a false-negative IgA EMA and tTG can occur with mild enteropathy, in children younger than 2 years of age, and in patients with IgA deficiency. AGA, antigliadin antibodies; EMA, endomysial antibody; tTG, tissue transglutaminase. *(From Farrell RJ, Kelly CP. Diagnosis of celiac sprue. Am J Gastroenterol 2001; 96:3237-46.)*

celiac disease and so obviate the need for diagnostic gluten challenge (Fig. 107-5). Other indications for HLA DQ2/DQ8 testing include the evaluation of patients with celiac-like enteropathy but negative IgA tTG, EMA, and DGP serologies; patients with persisting villus atrophy despite a GFD where the initial diagnosis of celiac disease is uncertain; and perhaps for definitive exclusion of celiac disease in at-risk individuals, such as children with close relatives who have celiac disease or patients with Down syndrome.[100,101]

Small Intestinal Biopsy

Although the diagnosis of celiac disease may be suspected on clinical grounds or as a result of abnormal serologic tests, biopsy of the small intestine has remained the standard test to establish the diagnosis. Biopsies usually are performed during endoscopic examination of the upper GI tract, an examination that may be indicated for reasons related or unrelated to celiac disease (e.g., investigation of iron deficiency anemia or upper abdominal discomfort).[126] Multiple biopsies should be obtained (e.g., a total of 6 to 8 biopsies from the second and third parts of the duodenum). Biopsies taken from the duodenal bulb may increase diagnostic sensitivity, but can show mucosal architectural distortion produced by

Brunner's glands and inflammatory changes caused by peptic duodenitis, both of which can cause errors in histopathologic diagnosis.[9]

Scalloping or absence of duodenal folds has been noted in some patients with celiac disease (see Fig. 107-6).[127] Scalloping is not specific for celiac disease, however, and may be seen in eosinophilic enteritis, giardiasis, amyloidosis, tropical sprue, and HIV enteropathy.[128] Other endoscopic features include flattening of the duodenal folds, multiple fissures, or a mosaic-like appearance where the fissures circumscribe areas of mucosal nodularity in a manner similar to the grouting around a mosaic tile. The mucosa of celiac disease, however, often appears normal at endoscopy, and absence of the previously described macroscopic features does not obviate the need for biopsy and histologic examination if celiac disease is suspected, based on clinical grounds or serologic testing.

Capsule endoscopy and enteroscopy provide opportunities to examine the more distal small intestine, where the macroscopic features just described might also be evident. Because these features are not specific, however, capsule endoscopy cannot replace biopsy and histopathologic examination, and is not necessary for routine diagnosis and management. Capsule endoscopy may be valuable in patients with complicated or refractory celiac disease in whom ulcerative jejunitis or intestinal lymphoma may be found.

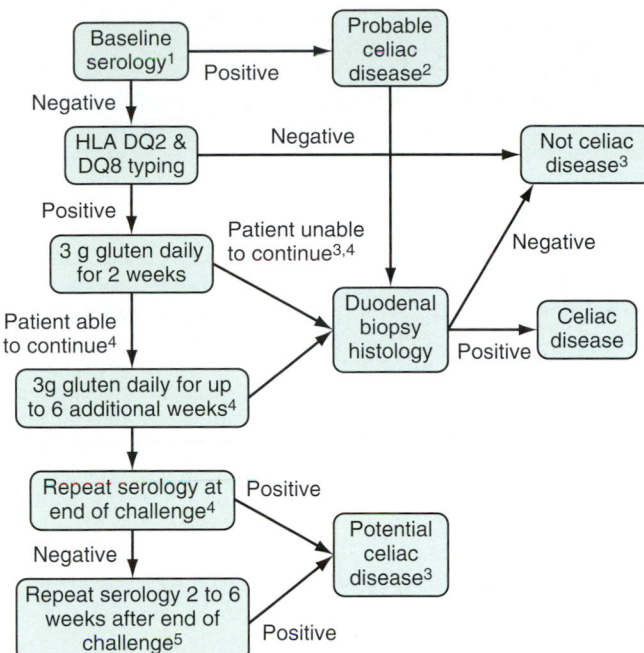

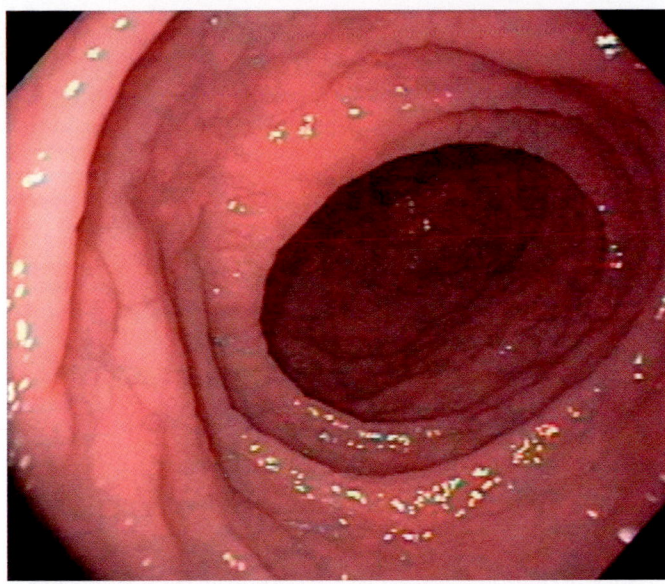

FIGURE 107-6. Endoscopic view of the duodenum showing scalloping of the folds in a patient with celiac disease; if present, this finding should alert the endoscopist to the possibility of this diagnosis. Scalloping, however, is not specific for celiac disease and has been seen in other conditions, including eosinophilic gastroenteritis, giardiasis, amyloidosis, tropical sprue, and HIV enteropathy. Other endoscopic features include flattening of the duodenal folds, nodularity, and multiple fissures leading to a mosaic-like appearance.

FIGURE 107-5. An approach to a gluten challenge for the diagnosis or exclusion of celiac disease in patients maintained on a GFD without prior definitive diagnostic testing. *Footnotes: 1,* tTG (tissue transglutaminase), endomysium, and/or DGP (deamidated gliadin peptide) antibody serology. *2,* Normal or nondiagnostic histology in a patient who has positive serologic test results for celiac disease while maintaining a GFD (gluten free diet) requires gluten challenge and repeat biopsy for definitive diagnosis or exclusion of celiac disease. *3,* Those with positive serologic test results for celiac disease but a normal biopsy result have potential celiac disease and should be evaluated and monitored further depending on their clinical circumstances. *4,* In a study of subjects who received a gluten challenge for 14 days, Marsh III histology was seen in 68%, positive celiac serologic test results in 75%, and either Marsh III histology or positive serologic testing in 90%. Thus, a 2-week gluten challenge may yield false-negative results in 10% of patients. The added diagnostic sensitivity of extending the challenge to 8 weeks is unknown. *5,* Celiac serologic antibody concentrations may continue to rise after a gluten challenge ends. In 1 study, positive tTG serology was seen in 25% of subjects, and positive DGP serology in 30% at the end of a 14-day gluten challenge; 50% had at least 1 positive serology on day 14. Positivity rates rose to 55% and 45%, respectively, 14 days later, despite the fact that subjects had resumed a GFD; 75% had at least 1 positive serology on day 28, 14 days after the gluten challenge ended. DGP, diamidated gliadin peptide; GFD, gluten-free diet. (*Adapted from Leffler D, Schuppan D, Pallav K, et al. Kinetics of the histological, serological and symptomatic responses to gluten challenge in adults with coeliac disease. Gut 2013; 62:996-1004; and Rubio-Tapia A, Hill ID, Kelly CP, et al. ACG clinical guidelines: Diagnosis and management of celiac disease. Am J Gastroenterol 2013; 108:656-76.*)

Gluten Challenge

In the past, gluten challenge—discontinuation of the GFD, followed by repeat biopsy of the small intestine—was considered a routine confirmatory step in the diagnosis of celiac disease. In current practice, however, gluten challenge is mainly reserved for patients in whom a diagnosis of celiac disease has not been confirmed but who are already adhering to a GFD. Symptom improvement on the GFD cannot reliably differentiate celiac disease from non-celiac gluten sensitivity.

One study from the United States found that most persons (89%) following a GFD did not have a confirmed diagnosis of celiac disease.[24] Gluten challenge also should be considered if a diagnosis of celiac disease was made during childhood based on small intestinal biopsy abnormalities in the absence of positive celiac serology (EMA, tTG, or DGP), because a number of transient childhood enteropathies can mimic the celiac lesion (see later). Gluten challenge is seldom necessary for patients who present with typical signs or symptoms of celiac disease and have documented abnormalities consistent with a celiac lesion on small bowel biopsy. A positive EMA, tTG, or DGP serology lends further support to the diagnosis of celiac disease and makes a later gluten challenge superfluous.

A recent guideline, based on a prospective trial of gluten challenge in celiac patients, highlights several important elements in performing gluten challenge (Fig. 107-6).[101,129] Patients who experience severe symptoms following gluten ingestion are unlikely to tolerate formal gluten challenge and might prefer to remain on a GFD despite diagnostic uncertainty. Serologic studies (IgA tTG, DGP) should be performed at baseline; positive serology results suggest that celiac disease is both present and active. HLA DQ2/DQ8 typing is often helpful because a negative result virtually excludes celiac disease and obviates the need for a formal gluten challenge. A baseline small bowel biopsy may be obtained also; if villus atrophy is found gluten challenge may become unnecessary.

Gluten challenge should be initiated with caution because occasionally patients are exquisitely sensitive to small amounts of gluten.[130] If a small amount of gluten, such as a small cracker or one quarter of a slice of bread, is tolerated, the amount can be doubled every 2 to 3 days until the patient is ingesting the equivalent of 1 to 2 slices of bread daily. This lower-dose gluten challenge (2 to 4 g daily) is as effective as higher doses in causing histologic and serologic changes but is less likely to cause intolerable symptoms.[129] Ideally, the challenge should be continued for 6 to 8 weeks at which time both celiac serologic tests (tTG +/− DGP) and small bowel biopsy should be performed. If the patient's symptoms are such that a longer challenge is intolerable, then biopsy performed as early as 2 weeks may be diagnostic.[129] If celiac serologic test results remain negative at the end of the challenge period, they should be repeated at 4 weeks after the challenge ends as antibody concentrations continue to rise.[129] If serologic tests and small bowel biopsy both are negative, the patient should be monitored for signs and symptoms of celiac disease on a normal diet for at least 6 months, after which serologic testing should be repeated.

Other Laboratory Studies

A variety of hematologic and biochemical abnormalities may be found in persons with untreated celiac disease, including deficiencies of iron, folic acid, vitamin B_{12}, vitamin D, and zinc. These abnormalities reflect nutritional deficiency states secondary to enteropathy-induced malabsorption. Iron deficiency anemia is common in both children and adults with celiac disease, and combined iron and folate deficiency is characteristic, especially in children. With the exception of pregnancy, severe anemia is uncommon, usually develops with extensive disease, and should raise the suspicion of a complication or dual cause. The peripheral blood film might reveal target cells, siderocytes, Heinz bodies, crenated red blood cells, and Howell-Jolly bodies, which suggest splenic atrophy.[81] Chronically elevated serum aminotransferase levels in the range of 1.5 to 2 times normal values occur in 27% of patients with untreated celiac disease, and in most patients, elevated levels resolve on a GFD. Conversely, undetected celiac disease is the cause of otherwise unexplained elevated serum aminotransferase levels in 3% to 4% of cases.[131]

If malabsorption is sufficient to produce significant steatorrhea, a watery or bulky, semi-formed, light tan or grayish, malodorous, greasy-appearing stool results. Microscopic evaluation of the fat content of a stool suspension stained with Sudan III or IV after hydrolysis with glacial acetic acid and heat is a helpful test. To document steatorrhea unequivocally, the amount of fat in a 3-day collection of stool may be determined quantitatively, using the reliable van de Kamer chemical method (See chapter 104).

Although relevant to patient evaluation and management, none of these hematologic or biochemical tests is sufficiently sensitive nor specific to serve as useful screening or diagnostic tools. Similarly, although an oral D-xylose test, lactulose-mannitol test, or fecal fat evaluation may be abnormal in untreated celiac disease, they, too, lack sensitivity and specificity and so are not useful as routine investigations in suspected celiac disease.

Radiology

Barium studies of the small intestine seldom are required in the evaluation of patients with suspected celiac disease. Abnormal roentgen findings include dilatation of the small intestine and a so-called reversal pattern in which jejunum resembles ileum (i.e., the normal delicate feathery mucosal pattern of the jejunum is replaced with either marked thickening or complete obliteration of the mucosal folds and straightening of the valvulae conniventes). With modern, less viscous barium preparations, the classic malabsorption pattern with flocculation, segmentation, and clumping of contrast is only occasionally seen in severe cases. In patients with mild or moderate disease, the distorted mucosal pattern usually is confined to the proximal small intestine, whereas patients with severe disease may have an abnormal mucosal pattern through the entire small intestine. Excessive secretion of fluid into the proximal small intestine, coupled with defective absorption of intraluminal contents, causes dilution of the barium, resulting in decreased contrast in the distal small intestine.

Small bowel studies are most useful in suggesting diagnoses other than celiac disease, including Crohn's disease, small bowel diverticulosis, scleroderma, or collagenous disease (bowel wall rigidity). Patients with mild celiac disease often have a normal small bowel barium study, and these studies are not as sensitive as small intestinal biopsy or serology in providing diagnostic information. Small bowel barium studies, CT enterography or MR enterography, or capsule endoscopy may be useful in identifying complications of celiac disease, such as lymphoma, carcinoma, ulcerative jejunoileitis, or stricture. Abdominal CT or MR may also reveal splenic atrophy, ascites, mesenteric lymphadenopathy, or cavitating mesenteric lymph nodes. It is important to note, however, that mesenteric lymphadenopathy is common in active celiac disease and does not, in and of itself, indicate a need for investigations to exclude lymphoma.

DIFFERENTIAL DIAGNOSIS

Celiac disease often presents with mild to moderate, sometimes intermittent, GI symptoms that include abdominal bloating, abdominal discomfort, and diarrhea. As such, IBS and lactose or fructose intolerance are prominent in the differential diagnosis. In current clinical practice, 1 of the most common issues in the differential diagnosis of celiac disease arises when patients report symptoms that respond to treatment with a GFD after several weeks or months of gluten avoidance when the serologic and histologic features of celiac disease, if ever present, may well have disappeared. Celiac disease and non-celiac gluten sensitivity usually cannot be differentiated based on history alone, and this differential is now the most common clinical indication for gluten challenge (see earlier and Fig. 107-6 for the recommended approach).[101]

The differential diagnosis of celiac disease also includes other causes of malabsorption and GI disorders that are associated with changes in proximal small intestinal morphology. In both children and adults, the high positive predictive value of a positive EMA, tTG, or DGP test result means that celiac disease usually can be diagnosed with a high degree of certainty from the outset, thereby avoiding the need for an in-depth evaluation of alternative diagnoses and for formal gluten challenge. Malabsorption and steatorrhea can result from pancreatic insufficiency, cholestatic liver disease, terminal ileal disease or resection, or SIBO. In some patients, microscopic colitis, SIBO, or pancreatic insufficiency may be present concurrently with celiac disease, and it is important to exclude these disorders in patients who do not respond to treatment with a GFD (see later).[132,133]

In adults, celiac disease is histologically distinguished easily from Whipple's disease and from malabsorption caused by infiltration of the mucosa with *Mycobacterium avium* complex. Changes in mucosal morphology can be seen in parasitic infections, including strongyloidiasis, coccidiosis, and hookworm disease, but with the exception of *Giardia* infection, these changes rarely include villus atrophy. Although villus atrophy is characteristic of untreated celiac disease, it is by no means pathognomonic and may be seen in varying degrees in a wide variety of other enteric disorders (see Fig. 107-1); villus atrophy on small intestinal biopsy is not in itself sufficient to diagnose celiac disease.[134]

Crypt cell activity, enterocyte characteristics, and the nature of the inflammatory infiltrate also must be examined and in some instances will point toward another diagnosis. For example, patients with hypogammaglobulinemia can have an architectural lesion that resembles celiac disease, but plasma cells may be absent or markedly diminished in the lamina propria—not increased as in celiac disease. Absence of the other histologic features of celiac disease often suggests an alternative diagnosis. After an acute viral gastroenteritis, the morphologic abnormalities may be indistinguishable from those of celiac disease.

In infants and young children, cow's milk or soy protein intolerance also can result in biopsy findings identical to those of celiac disease.[135,136] Soy protein often is used as a substitute for milk protein in cow's milk protein intolerance, but some children also develop mucosal abnormalities that resemble those of celiac disease after ingestion of soy protein.[136]

A rare condition that can cause diagnostic confusion is collagenous sprue. Patients with collagenous sprue might present initially with symptoms and biopsy findings consistent with celiac disease, but their symptoms fail to respond to gluten withdrawal, and with time, extensive deposition of collagen in the lamina propria develops just beneath the absorptive epithelium.[137] The relationship between celiac disease and both collagenous sprue and the microscopic colitides (lymphocytic and collagenous colitis) is discussed later.

Diseases Associated with Celiac Disease

A large number of diseases occur more commonly among patients with celiac disease and are delineated in Box 107-1.[138] In addition to an association with autoimmune disorders, some of the associated diseases also have similar HLA haplotype associations.

Dermatitis Herpetiformis

DH is a skin disease characterized by papulovesicular lesions that occur symmetrically over the extensor surfaces of the extremities and the buttocks, trunk, neck, and scalp. Unlike celiac disease, DH rarely is diagnosed in childhood and usually manifests in early or middle adult life. DH is slightly more common in men (3:2), but in patients younger than 20 years, women predominate (3:2).[139] The rash is intensely pruritic, and scratching off the vesicle relieves the itching; hence, intact vesicles might not be present except for the earliest lesions.

The diagnosis of DH requires demonstration by immunofluorescence of granular or speckled IgA deposits in an area of perilesional skin—that is, skin close to a lesion but not affected by blistering.[139] DH is associated with a mild patchy enteropathy indistinguishable from celiac disease, and because it has a non-uniform distribution, multiple intestinal biopsies may be required for diagnosis.[139] DH-associated enteropathy tends to be less severe than celiac disease, and only a minority of patients has intestinal symptoms. An increased risk of intestinal malignancy has been reported, however, as in celiac disease,[140,141] and in DH, most lymphomas occur in patients whose DH was not controlled by a strict GFD or in those who had been treated with a GFD for less than 5 years.[141,142]

Approximately 5% to 15% of patients with DH-like skin lesions have linear IgA deposits along the dermoepidermal junction. This condition has been termed *linear IgA disease* and is distinguished from DH on the basis of its unique immunofluorescent finding; the presence of circulating IgA antibasement membrane antibody, which binds to a 97-kd protein found in normal human skin[143]; the absence of circulating IgA EMA or tTG; different HLA susceptibility genes; and,

BOX 107-1 Disorders Associated with Celiac Disease

Definite Association
Bird-fancier's lung
Dermatitis herpetiformis
Diabetes mellitus type 1
Down syndrome
Epilepsy with cerebral calcification
Fibrosing alveolitis
Hypothyroidism or hyperthyroidism
Idiopathic pulmonary hemosiderosis
Immunoglobulin (Ig)A deficiency
IgA mesangial nephropathy
IBD
Microscopic colitis
Recurrent pericarditis
RA
Sarcoidosis

Negative Association
Diabetes mellitus type 2

Possible Association
Addison's disease
Autoimmune hemolytic anemia
Autoimmune liver diseases
Cavitary lung disease
Congenital heart disease
Cystic fibrosis
Immune thrombocytopenic purpura
Iridocyclitis or choroiditis
Macroamylasemia
Myasthenia gravis
Polymyositis
Schizophrenia
Sjögren's syndrome
Systemic and cutaneous vasculitides
SLE

Modified from Mulder CJ, Tytgat GN. Coeliac disease and related disorders. Neth J Med 1987; 31:286-99.

most important, the lack of any associated gluten-sensitive enteropathy.[58,144]

Sardy and colleagues shed light on the pathogenesis of DH by demonstrating that epidermal (type 3) transglutaminase (eTG) is the dominant autoantigen in DH (rather than the type 2 tTG autoantigen of celiac disease).[145] This helps explain why DH skin lesions appear in only a minority of patients having celiac disease. They also showed that the IgA precipitates in the papillary dermis of patients with DH, the defining manifestation of the disease, contain eTG but not tTG or keratinocyte transglutaminase. In DH, the prevalences of HLA-DQ2, circulating antigliadin, antireticulin, and EMA parallel those observed in patients with celiac disease without DH.[139] Although many patients with DH have elevated IgA tTG antibodies, confirming its pathogenic relationship with celiac disease, its prevalence in DH (75%) is lower than that found in celiac disease (95% to 98%).[146]

Thus, DH and celiac disease are 2 very closely related gluten-sensitive disorders but nonetheless distinct clinical disease entities. Most, if not all, patients with DH also have at least latent celiac disease, whereas less than 10% of patients with celiac disease have DH. Dapsone treatment at a dose of 1 to 2 mg/kg daily is effective and often diagnostic in its ability to heal the rash of DH and to relieve the pruritus rapidly, but the enteropathy associated with DH does not improve with dapsone. Six to 12 months of gluten withdrawal, however, usually reverses not only the intestinal but also the skin lesions in most patients with DH, and a strict GFD allows most patients to reduce or discontinue dapsone.[147] Iodine can also exacerbate DH and should be avoided, especially in refractory cases. Patients with DH, just like those with celiac disease, can include moderate amounts of oats in their GFD without deleterious effects to their skin or intestine.[148]

Other Disease Associations

Autoimmune disease is strongly associated with celiac disease and has a prevalence of approximately 20% in adult patients.[91] The strong association between celiac disease and type 1 diabetes mellitus (T1DM) reflects, in part, the increased frequency of the celiac-associated DQ alleles in patients with T1DM. The frequency of celiac disease in T1DM patients is approximately 5% (ranging from 3% to 8%),[149-151] and the frequency of T1DM in celiac disease is also approximately 5%.[152] Most patients with T1DM who have celiac disease are asymptomatic from the point of view of their celiac disease, but unexpected episodes of hypoglycemia or diarrhea in patients with T1DM should alert clinicians to the possibility of coexisting celiac disease. Control of diabetes in patients with celiac disease can be difficult because of varying nutrient absorption.

Recently, an inverse relationship between celiac disease and type 2 diabetes mellitus (T2DM) was identified whereby patients with known celiac disease are approximately 3 times less likely to develop T2DM (3.1% in celiac disease vs. 9.6% in age- and gender-matched controls).[153] The prevalence of metabolic syndrome was also significantly lower in patients with celiac disease compared with controls (3.5% vs. 12.7%). The mean BMI of patients with celiac disease was somewhat lower than that of controls (24.7 vs. 27.5); however, this alone does not explain the protection, because celiac disease was still associated with a substantially lower risk of T2DM, after controlling for BMI. Thus, the basis for this markedly lower prevalence of T2DM is unknown.

There also is a high prevalence of autoimmune thyroid disease among patients with celiac disease, hypothyroidism being more common than hyperthyroidism.[154] Celiac disease also can be associated with a variety of other autoimmune connective tissue diseases, including IBD, chronic hepatitis, sclerosing cholangitis, PBC, IgA nephropathy, interstitial lung disease (including chronic fibrosing alveolitis), idiopathic pulmonary hemosiderosis, SLE, Sjögren's syndrome, and polymyositis.[2,51,113,125,138,152-156]

Although the relationship between celiac disease and many autoimmune disorders has been explained by the sharing of a common genetic factor, Ventura and colleagues[157] suggested an increased incidence of autoimmune disease with increased age at diagnosis and lack of diet therapy. The role of a GFD to prevent subsequent development of autoimmune disease, however, has been challenged by other studies.[158]

Although many patients with celiac disease exhibit lactose and fructose intolerances at the time of diagnosis, only a small percentage has persistent disaccharidase deficiency after gluten withdrawal. These patients experience abdominal boating, discomfort, or diarrhea with disaccharide intake, and diagnosis can usually be made just by history or an appropriate hydrogen breath test. Should concomitant disaccharidase deficiency be present, the relevant disaccharide should be reduced or excluded from the diet.

Selective IgA deficiency occurs in approximately 2% of celiac disease patients (20 times the population prevalence). Hyposplenism and splenic atrophy have been noted frequently in patients with celiac disease; the incidence increases with advancing age, duration of exposure to dietary gluten, and disease activity.[81] The underlying mechanism is unknown, but affected patients may be at increased risk of developing bacterial infections[159] and might benefit from vaccination for pneumonia.

There is a well-established relationship of celiac disease with IBD (see Chapters 115 and 116) and the microscopic colitides (see Chapter 128).[160-162] Mild to moderate small intestinal lymphocytosis is common and partial (occasionally) or subtotal villus atrophy is seen in both lymphocytic and collagenous colitis.[161] Conversely, mild colonic lymphocytosis occurs in many patients with untreated celiac disease and usually improves on a GFD.[162,163] Rectal gluten challenge in patients with celiac disease has been shown to induce a mild lymphocytic proctitis.[164] Furthermore, a GFD may be an effective therapy in some patients with refractory collagenous colitis.[165] The demonstration that patients with celiac disease and microscopic colitis share a set of predisposing HLA-DQ genes[166] underscores the overlap between both diseases.

Confusion also can arise in patients with refractory celiac disease, who have a higher prevalence of colonic lymphocytosis than patients with responsive celiac disease. Colonic lymphocytosis can be difficult to distinguish from lymphocytic colitis, although most colonic IELs in lymphocytic colitis are CD8$^+$, whereas those in the colonic lymphocytosis of refractory celiac disease rarely are CD8$^+$.[133]

TREATMENT

Gluten-Free Diet

Removal of gluten from the diet is essential for treating patients with celiac disease (Box 107-2).[80] The importance of gluten withdrawal was established by Dicke's, van de Kamer's, and Weijers' astute studies in the early 1950s when the toxicity of wheat protein in children with celiac disease was demonstrated.[6,7] In 1962, Rubin and colleagues[31] showed that instillation of wheat, barley, and rye flour into the histologically normal small intestine of persons with treated celiac disease rapidly induced celiac-like symptoms, and that these symptoms were accompanied by the development of the typical celiac lesions in the exposed mucosa.

Because a GFD represents a lifetime commitment for patients with celiac disease, is more expensive than a normal diet, and carries a social liability, it should not be undertaken casually or as a therapeutic trial. In reality, complete dietary

---

BOX 107-2 Principles of Initial Dietary Therapy for Patients with Celiac Disease

Avoid all foods containing wheat, rye, and barley gluten (pure oats usually safe).
Avoid malt unless clearly labeled as derived from corn.
Use only rice, corn, maize, buckwheat, millet, amaranth, quinoa, sorghum, potato or potato starch, soybean, tapioca, and teff, bean, and nut flours.
Wheat starch and products containing wheat starch should only be used if they contain less than 20 ppm gluten and are marked "gluten free."
Read all labels and study ingredients of processed foods.
Beware of gluten in medications, supplements, food additives, emulsifiers, or stabilizers.
Limit milk and milk products initially if there is evidence of lactose intolerance.
Avoid all beers, lagers, ales, and stouts (unless labeled gluten free).
Wine, most liqueurs, ciders, and spirits, including whiskey and brandy, are allowed.

ppm, parts per million.
Modified from Trier JS. Celiac sprue and refractory sprue. In: Feldman M, Scharschmidt BF, Sleisenger MH, editors. Gastrointestinal and liver disease. 6th ed. Philadelphia: WB Saunders; 1997. p 1557.

BOX 107-3 Some Potential Sources of Hidden Gluten

Beers, ales, other fermented beverages (distilled beverages acceptable)
Bouillon and soups
Candy
Communion wafers
Drink mixes
Gravy and sauces
Herbal tea
Imitation meat and seafood
Lipstick and lip balms
Medications (pills and capsules)
Nutritional supplements
Play-Doh
Salad dressings and marinades
Self-basting turkeys
Soy sauce
Toothpaste

BOX 107-4 Key Elements in the Management of Celiac Disease

Consultation with a skilled dietitian
Education about the disease
Lifelong adherence to a gluten-free diet
Identification and treatment of nutritional deficiencies
Access to an advocacy group
Continuous long-term follow-up by a multidisciplinary team

From the National Institutes of Health Consensus Development Conference Statement on Celiac Disease, June 28-30, 2004. Gastroenterology 2005; 128:S1-9.

---

elimination of all gluten-containing cereal grains is a challenge for most patients to achieve and maintain. Hidden gluten is present in a wide variety of processed foods, because wheat flour is used widely in the food industry as a thickener and inexpensive filler for many commercial products, precooked meals, and convenience foods, including ice cream, pasta, sausages, fish sticks, cheese spreads, salad dressings, soups, sauces, mixed seasonings, mincemeat for mince pies, and even some medications[167] and vitamin preparations (Box 107-3). Furthermore, grains that are naturally gluten-free can become contaminated with wheat, barley, or rye in the field during harvesting or transport, or when mills use the same production lines and equipment to process both gluten-containing and gluten-free products. Beers, lagers, ales, and stout should be avoided (apart from the few available specifically gluten-free products), but wines, many liqueurs, and ciders as well as spirits, including brandy, malt, and scotch whiskey, can be consumed (unless gluten-containing flavorings have been added after distillation).

Helpful recipes as well as detailed instructions regarding GFDs have been published in excellent, inexpensive books that are of great value to patients with celiac disease.[168,169] National celiac societies in many countries publish regularly updated handbooks that list the available gluten-free products. Food lists are applicable for use only in the country in which they were compiled. Similar foods with well-known brand names may be made under franchise using slightly different recipes in different countries and may be gluten-free in one country and not in others. Consequently, patient education is crucial, and the institution of an effective GFD requires extensive and repeated instruction of the patient by the physician and dietitian, as well as a motivated and basically suspicious, label-reading patient. The importance of patient education and support by a multidisciplinary team of health care providers was emphasized in the National Institutes of Health consensus development conference statement (Box 107-4).[170]

There is considerable variation among patients with celiac disease in their ability to tolerate gluten. Some patients can ingest small amounts of gluten without developing symptoms. Others are exquisitely sensitive to ingestion of even minute amounts of gluten and can develop massive watery diarrhea within an hour or 2 of ingesting tiny amounts of gluten. Occasionally, the diarrhea is so severe that it can induce acute dehydration, an occurrence termed *gliadin shock* or *celiac crisis*.[79,130]

Patients with untreated celiac disease might have accompanying brush border lactase deficiency secondary to surface epithelial cell damage. Therefore, milk and dairy products should be avoided upon initiation of a GFD. After the disease responds to the diet, however, these products can be reintroduced, if they are tolerated.

It is now clear that moderate amounts of oats are not toxic to the vast majority of patients with celiac disease. In a carefully conducted randomized clinical trial, adults with celiac disease who consumed 50 to 70 g of oats per day for 6 to 12 months did not differ in regard to symptoms, nutritional status, or duodenal mucosal histology compared with patients maintained on an oat-restricted, gluten-free diet[171]; in a smaller follow-up study, the same investigators showed no harm in celiac disease patients from 5 years of oat ingestion.[172] Patients with DH also can include moderate amounts of oats in their GFD without deleterious effects to the skin or intestine,[140] and an open-labeled study showed that a 6-month trial of commercial oat breakfast cereal also was safe for children with newly diagnosed celiac disease who were beginning a GFD.[173] It should be stressed, however, that oat products obtained from the grocery store shelf can contain significant amounts of other grains, especially wheat, because of contamination in the field, during harvesting or transport, or at the mill. Consequently, oats often are avoided initially in patients with newly diagnosed celiac disease until remission is achieved on a GFD. Subsequently, up to 2 ounces of uncontaminated oats per day from a reliable source may be introduced and continued if tolerated.

A GFD can be rich in nutrition and conducive to excellent general health. Careful attention is needed, however, to avoid certain pitfalls of the GFD. The GFD often contains inadequate iron, calcium, vitamin D, and B vitamins.[174] Hence, nutritional counseling and monitoring, together with a daily gluten-free multivitamin supplement, is recommended to avoid deficiency states. Avoiding wheat, barley, and rye often leads to inadequate fiber intake and constipation unless steps are taken to replace these with other sources of dietary fiber. Some weight gain is common after starting a GFD as malabsorption resolves; however, excess weight gain or obesity can easily ensue, especially if fat- and calorie-rich gluten-free processed foods and snacks are consumed in excess.[98] Preparing meals using fresh ingredients including gluten-free grains and reducing the use of prepared or processed foods are often the keys to a healthful GFD.

After starting a GFD, most patients improve within a few weeks. In many, substantial symptomatic improvement is noticed within 48 hours, although it can take weeks or months to achieve full clinical, serologic, and histologic remission. Pink and Creamer[175] reported that 70% of patients with celiac disease who started a GFD returned quickly to normal health and reported improvement in their symptoms within 2 weeks.

Although an increase in enterocyte height may be evident within a week of gluten withdrawal, the return of villus architecture toward normal takes considerably longer and might not be evident on rebiopsy for several months. In some patients, histologic resolution can take up to 2 years; the main reason for this slow or partial recovery may be inadvertent exposure to gluten.[31] Although a return to normal is common in children, in approximately 50% of adults on a GFD, biopsies show only partial improvement; the less severely damaged distal intestine recovers more rapidly than the maximally damaged proximal intestine.[176] The investigation and management of patients who have celiac disease and whose symptoms or signs do not respond to dietary gluten avoidance are discussed later (see the discussions of nonresponsive and refractory celiac disease).

Dietary Supplements

In addition to a GFD, patients with newly diagnosed celiac disease should receive appropriate supplemental therapy to help correct nutritional deficiencies caused by malabsorption, iron deficiency being the most common. Deficiencies of vitamin D, vitamin B_{12}, or folic acid also occur. Patients with purpura, bruising, or other evidence of abnormal bleeding might have prolongation of their prothrombin time and require supplemental vitamin K. Patients with severe diarrhea and dehydration, and in particular those presenting in celiac crisis, require vigorous IV replacement of fluids and electrolytes. IV calcium gluconate (1 to 2 g) should be administered promptly to a patient who has tetany. If there is no response, the tetany may be caused by hypomagnesemia and require magnesium replacement.

The risks of osteopenia and osteoporosis should be explained to all patients with celiac disease, and general advice should be given about the benefit of weight-bearing exercises, supplemental dietary calcium and vitamin D intake, and the adverse effects of smoking and excessive alcohol consumption. There is compelling evidence that strict adherence to a GFD protects against further bone loss and initially is associated with an increase in bone mineral density (BMD).[177] A total daily calcium intake of 1500 mg should be ensured—a cup of skim milk provides 300 mg. If dietary calcium is inadequate, 500 to 1500 mg of supplemental calcium should be given. Vitamin D deficiency should be sought and treated (particularly in patients with significant steatorrhea) until the malabsorption has responded to gluten withdrawal to prevent mobilization of skeletal calcium.

One year of gluten withdrawal has been shown to reverse osteopenia in most patients, including postmenopausal women and patients with incomplete mucosal recovery,[178] but patients who have secondary hyperparathyroidism at the time celiac disease is diagnosed tend to have more refractory osteopenia, and their BMD might not normalize even after several years of gluten withdrawal.[179]

Clinicians often rely on serum calcium, phosphate, and alkaline phosphatase measurements, but osteomalacia still can exist even if these tests are normal. If these tests are normal and osteomalacia still is suspected, a serum 25-hydroxy vitamin D level can be determined, as well as a parathyroid hormone assay. A low-normal calcium and an elevated parathormone level indicates secondary hyperparathyroidism, and calcium (500 to 1000 mg daily) together with vitamin D (400 to 2000 units daily) should be given.[180]

All patients should have their BMD measured 1 year after diagnosis. Recent guidelines suggest that patients with treated celiac disease who have progressive osteoporosis despite correction of calcium and vitamin D deficiency should be offered oral biphosphonate or other therapy for osteoporosis and have their BMD checked every 1 to 2 years.[180]

Vitamin A, thiamine, riboflavin, niacin, pyridoxine, vitamin C, and vitamin E, all in the form of a multivitamin preparation, probably should be taken daily by all patients with celiac disease, in light of their predisposition to malabsorption and the risks for nutritional deficiencies associated with a GFD.[174] Some patients have reported symptomatic improvement with correction of magnesium, copper, and zinc deficiencies.[181]

Drugs, like nutrients, may be unpredictably absorbed by patients with severe celiac disease. Medications considered essential for the patient's well-being might need to be administered parenterally or monitored closely until absorption improves in response to treatment with a GFD.

Glucocorticoids

In vitro studies have shown that the addition of glucocorticoids prevented the harmful effects of gluten on biopsy specimens from patients with celiac disease.[182] Although celiac disease can be treated with glucocorticoids, with rapid improvement in symptoms, the effect rarely persists once treatment is stopped, and significant side effects are common.[183] Therefore, glucocorticoids are not indicated in the routine management of celiac disease, but are reserved for refractory celiac disease or for severely ill patients who present with acute celiac crisis manifested by severe diarrhea, dehydration, weight loss, acidosis, hypocalcemia, and hypoproteinemia.[184] These few patients usually benefit from a short course of glucocorticoids until the GFD takes effect. A brief course of glucocorticoids also may be used in the rare instances of gliadin shock that occurs occasionally in treated patients who are subject to gluten challenge.[130]

Monitoring of Patients on Treatment

Once a GFD is initiated, patients should be seen at intervals of 3 to 6 months during the first year of therapy to evaluate their symptom response, their adherence to the diet, to provide additional counseling, education, and support and to measure serum tTG (and/or DGP) antibody concentrations to determine if these are decreasing at the expected rate. If nutritional deficiencies were evident at diagnosis, these should be addressed and monitored until resolved. After 1 year of treatment, a BMD test is often recommended. Thereafter, annual follow-up should be provided to evaluate symptoms, to provide continued education on, and encourage continued adherence to, the GFD, and to ensure that nutritional deficiencies are avoided and that celiac serologic testing remains negative. A repeat biopsy to evaluate healing is often offered after 2 years of dietary therapy but is not mandatory. Unless nonresponsive celiac disease occurs, earlier biopsy is unwise because histologic healing often substantially lags symptom improvement and normalization of celiac serology.

NONRESPONSIVE CELIAC DISEASE (NRCD)

NRCD is a clinical diagnosis that is defined by the persistence of symptoms, signs, or laboratory abnormalities typical of celiac disease despite adherence to a GFD for at least 6 to 12 months.[131,185,186] About 10% of patients with celiac disease are nonresponsive either immediately after the initial diagnosis (primary NRCD) or following a period of response to a GFD (secondary NRCD).[185] An approach to the evaluation of NRCD that is based on the early identification and correction of common causes and that culminates in the diagnosis of refractory celiac disease (which affects 1% to 2% of patients with celiac disease) is outlined in Figure 107-7.[101,132,187]

The first step in evaluating NRCD is to carefully review the primary diagnostic studies, because if the diagnosis of

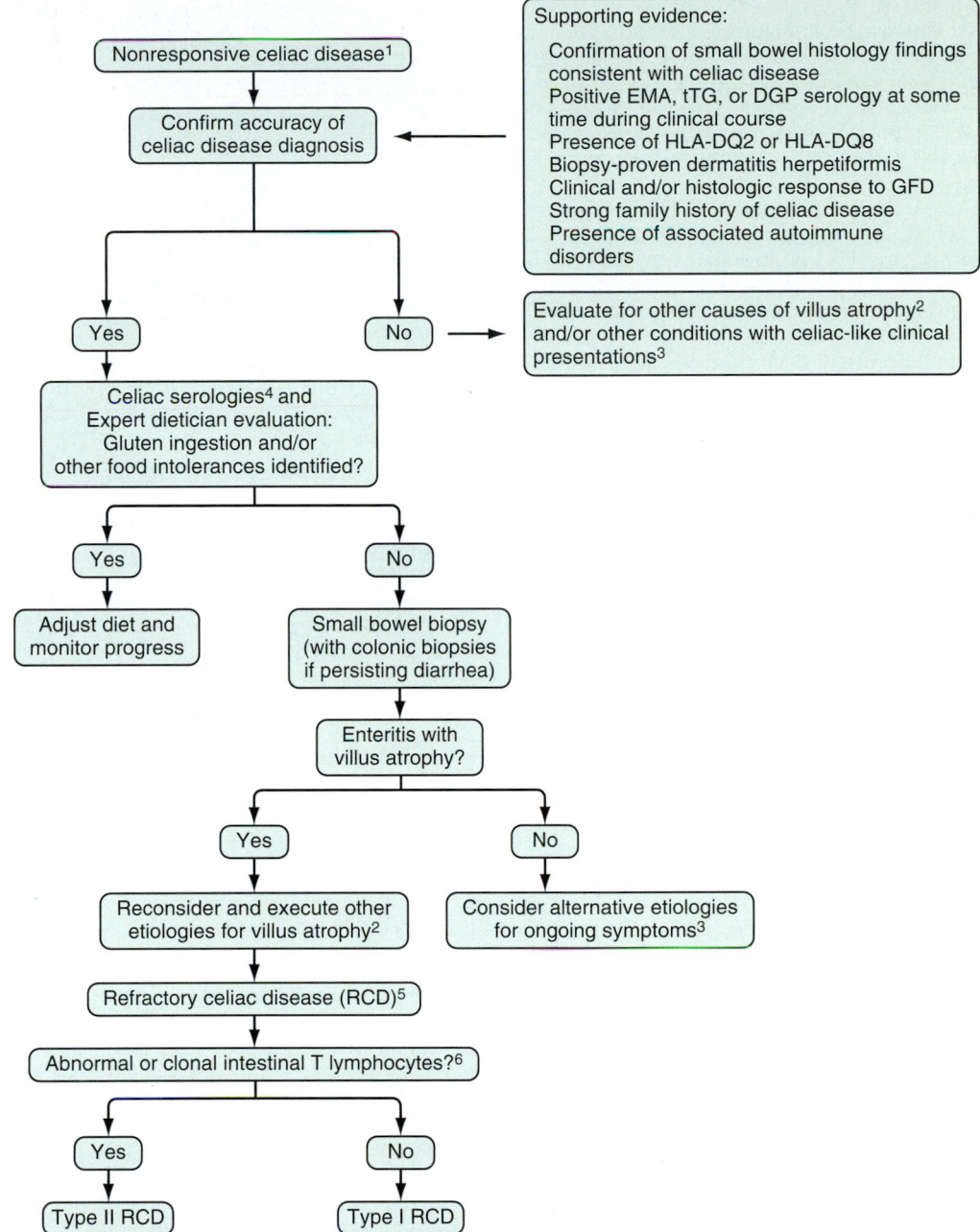

FIGURE 107-7. Diagnostic approach to patients with nonresponsive celiac disease. *Footnotes: 1, Nonresponsive celiac disease* may be defined as persistent symptoms, signs, or laboratory abnormalities typical of celiac disease despite 6 to 12 months of dietary gluten avoidance. *2,* Causes of non-celiac small intestinal villus atrophy that may be misdiagnosed as celiac disease include autoimmune enteropathy, tropical sprue, SIBO, hypogammaglobulinemia, combined variable immunodeficiency, collagenous sprue, eosinophilic enteritis, Crohn's disease, and peptic duodenitis. *3,* Conditions that present clinically in a fashion similar to celiac disease but where villus atrophy is not evident include IBS, food intolerances, SIBO, eosinophilic enteritis, Crohn's disease, and microscopic colitis. *4,* Positive serologic testing for celiac disease despite 12 months of treatment with a GFD suggest that there may be ongoing gluten ingestion. *5, Refractory celiac disease* (RCD) is defined as persistent or recurrent malabsorptive symptoms and signs, with small intestinal villus atrophy despite a strict GFD for more than 12 months and in the absence of other disorders including overt lymphoma. *6,* Abnormal intestinal lymphocytes may be identified by immunohistochemistry of intraepithelial lymphocytes or by flow cytometry showing an increased number of CD3-positive cells that lack CD8 or by the identification of clonal T-cell receptor gene rearrangement by molecular analysis. EMA, endomysial antibody; DGP, deamidated gliadin peptide; GFD, gluten-free diet; tTGA, tissue transglutaminase antibody. *(Adapted from Abdallah H, Leffler D, Dennis M, Kelly CP. Refractory celiac disease. Curr Gastroenterol Rep 2007; 9:401-5; and Rubio-Tapia A, Hill ID, Kelly CP, et al. ACG clinical guidelines: Diagnosis and management of celiac disease. Am J Gastroenterol 2013; 108:656-76.)*

celiac disease is mistaken, a sustained response to a GFD cannot be expected. This is especially the case for patients who test negative for anti-tTG at first presentation. In such circumstances, careful review of the biopsy pathology by an expert GI pathologist is warranted to seek alternative diagnoses. HLA DQ2 and DQ8 typing, testing for hypogammaglobulinemia and measurement of DGP antibodies also may be helpful.

The single most common cause for NRCD is continued gluten ingestion, which is often inadvertent and occult. A persisting elevation of anti-tTG is strongly associated with ongoing gluten exposure.[185] Intolerance to disaccharides (e.g., lactose, fructose) also is common, especially in primary NRCD. Thus, evaluation by an expert dietitian to seek ingestion of hidden gluten and intolerance of disaccharides is an essential next step.[132]

If no dietary causes can be identified, a small bowel biopsy should be repeated and the findings compared with the initial pretreatment biopsy. If the enteropathy has healed or is substantially improved, diagnostic considerations for ongoing symptoms and signs include IBS (22%), SIBO (6%), other food allergies and intolerances (1%), and pancreatic insufficiency.[185,186] If diarrhea is a prominent symptom, colonic biopsy also should be performed and examined for microscopic colitis (6%). If repeat intestinal biopsies show ongoing changes consistent with active celiac disease, refractory celiac disease becomes likely. Other causes of a celiac-like enteropathy, however, should again be considered, including SIBO, peptic duodenitis, hypogammaglobulinemia, tropical sprue, intestinal infections (e.g., giardiasis), Crohn's disease, and autoimmune enteropathy.[185,186] Patients with NRCD who show substantial weight loss are at a significantly greater risk for refractory celiac disease.[185]

REFRACTORY CELIAC DISEASE

Refractory celiac disease is defined as symptomatic, severe small intestinal villus atrophy that mimics celiac disease but does not respond to at least 6 to 12 months of a strict GFD and is not accounted for by other causes of villus atrophy or overt intestinal lymphoma.[2,3,113] It can be divided into type I and type II; the latter type is more aggressive and characterized by an abnormal, undifferentiated, oligoclonal mucosal T-cell population (as discussed later).[188] Refractory celiac disease is uncommon in adults (1% to 2% of those diagnosed with celiac disease), extremely rare in children, and largely a diagnosis of exclusion (see Fig. 107-7).[189] It is important to note that symptoms can persist in treated celiac disease patients for a variety of other reasons that are far more common than refractory celiac disease as described earlier in the section on nonresponsive celiac disease (see Fig. 107-7).[132,185,186,190]

Ulcerative Jejunoileitis

Ulcerative jejunoileitis, also known as *chronic, nongranulomatous ulcerative enterocolitis* or *non-granulomatous jejunitis*, is a rare but serious complication of celiac disease characterized by ulceration and strictures of the small intestine. Whether ulcerative jejunoileitis truly is a discrete entity has been questioned because lymphoma ultimately is diagnosed in many of these patients.[191] Indeed, ulcerative jejunoileitis in association with EATL previously was designated *malignant histiocytosis.*

Ulcerative jejunoileitis should be suspected in patients with celiac disease who present with weight loss, abdominal pain, and diarrhea that do not respond to a GFD. Areas of

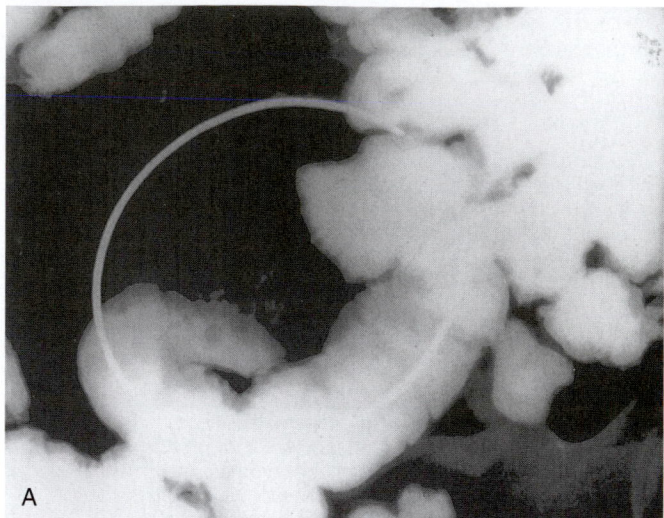

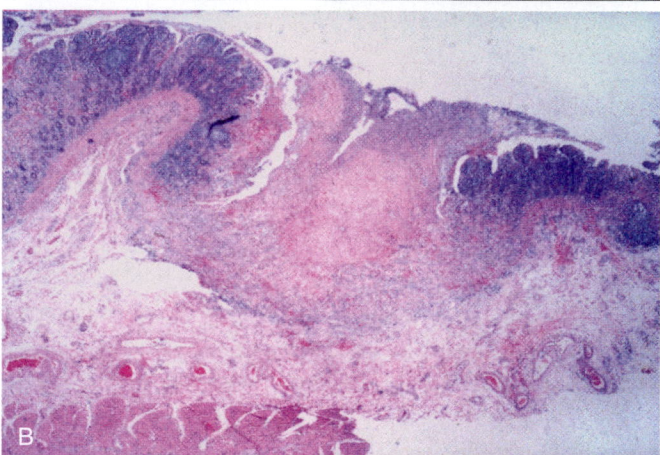

FIGURE 107-8. A small bowel barium contrast study and corresponding histopathology from a patient with ulcerative jejunoileitis complicating celiac disease. *A*, A segmental area of fixed narrowing with associated mucosal distortion and ulceration in the distal jejunum and proximal ileum is seen. *B*, Histopathology of a segment of resected small intestine showing ulcerated mucosa with adjacent diffuse villus atrophy and lymphocytic infiltration consistent with celiac disease. Lymphocytes within the epithelium and lamina propria were positive for T-cell antigen (CD3); no overt lymphoma was evident, but a Southern blot analysis revealed clonal T cell receptor gene rearrangements in both the involved and uninvolved small intestine and an adjacent mesenteric lymph node, consistent with cryptic enteropathy-associated T cell lymphoma.

intestinal ulceration and stricture formation typically cause hemorrhage and obstruction, respectively (Fig. 107-8); perforation with peritonitis also can occur. Diagnosis is made by enteroscopy, contrast studies of the small intestine, abdominal CT, capsule endoscopy, or laparotomy.

Some patients respond to a GFD, but surgical excision of the worst affected segments of small intestine so far has proved to be the most effective treatment. There is a high risk for transition to diffuse or multifocal EATL, but in a few patients with well-documented celiac disease and localized jejunoileitis, no evidence of malignant disease develops, and there is a response to either surgical resection or therapy with glucocorticoids and azathioprine.[192] Even in the absence of overt malignant transformation, however, the 5-year survival rate for patients with ulcerative jejunoileitis is less than 50%.

Collagenous Sprue

Collagenous disease is characterized by the development of a subepithelial collagen band thicker than 10 μm in the small intestine. Although collagenous disease has been regarded as an entity distinct from celiac disease,[137] deposition of collagen under the intestinal epithelial cells has been noted in up to 36% of patients with classic celiac disease.[193] Furthermore, there are several reports of patients with collagenous disease who have elevated tTG antibodies[194] or complications of refractory celiac disease, specifically ulcerative jejunoileitis[195] and lymphoma.[67]

Although collagenous disease often is refractory to therapy, the presence of subepithelial collagen does not, a priori, preclude a successful response to gluten withdrawal.[193,196] Collagenous sprue should be considered in the differential diagnosis of NRCD and must be distinguished from collagenous colitis (which rarely accompanies celiac disease).[165] Compared with both celiac disease and collagenous colitis, the prognosis in collagenous sprue is poor, and many patients die from the disease because of severe diarrhea, electrolyte abnormalities, and malnutrition.

Treatment

In patients with celiac disease and no demonstrable cause for lack of response to a GFD, a variety of treatments (based mostly on small, uncontrolled studies) have been described; these include glucocorticoids, immunosuppressive drugs, elimination diets, and dietary supplementation with zinc and copper.[197-201]

Evidence to support the use of glucocorticoid or other immunosuppressive therapy in the treatment of refractory celiac disease is anecdotal; to date, no controlled trials have been performed.[200] Enteric-coated (EC) budesonide is often effective in treating persisting symptoms in patients with refractory celiac disease and is preferable to systemic glucocorticoid therapy. In a study of patients with refractory celiac disease, 16 of 29 (55%) responded fully to treatment with oral EC budesonide (Entocort, 9 mg daily), and an additional 6 (21%) showed a partial response.[202] Improvements were evident in patients with and without coexisting microscopic colitis. Oral budesonide was well tolerated, and no serious side effects were reported. Because of its good side-effect profile, oral budesonide is fast becoming a drug of first choice for treatment of refractory celiac disease. Small intestine-release mesalamine has an excellent safety profile, is suitable for maintenance therapy, and may be effective, but appears to be less potent than EC budesonide.[203]

Systemic glucocorticoid treatment also may be necessary in patients with refractory celiac disease. Azathioprine or 6-mercaptopurine may be used as a glucocorticoid-sparing agent if a dose of 10 mg or more of prednisolone per day is required to keep the condition under control.[197] In 1 open pilot study, 13 adult patients with refractory celiac disease were treated for 2 months with oral cyclosporine in doses titrated to achieve serum levels of 100 to 200 ng/mL; small intestinal histology improved in 8 patients (61%), and villi normalized in 5 (38%).[201] Cyclosporine therapy has been reported to be life-saving in occasional patients with refractory celiac disease-like disease, and it can result in reversal of glucocorticoid resistance, but its efficacy remains unproved.[198] There also have been reports on the efficacy of infliximab, a chimeric antibody to TNF-α, in refractory celiac disease.[199]

Complications

It has long been appreciated that patients with refractory celiac disease are at high risk for developing fatal complications such as ulcerative jejunoileitis and lymphoma. Until recently, the precise link between refractory celiac disease and these complications, as well as between refractory celiac disease and celiac disease, remained controversial. The spectrum of autoimmune enteropathy was implicated in a handful of adult refractory celiac disease patients by the presence of anti-enterocyte antibodies.[204,205] It is now becoming clear, however, that refractory celiac disease, EATL, and ulcerative jejunoileitis represent a heterogeneous, but related, group of clinical conditions at the extreme end of the celiac disease spectrum. Moreover, there is now growing realization that many of these patients have a cryptic intestinal T-cell lymphoma, characterized by phenotypically abnormal IELs that have monoclonal rearrangements of the *TCRγ* gene.[67]

Early immunophenotypic studies demonstrated that the normal cell counterpart of EATL was the IEL.[206] It was not until 1995, however, that Murray and colleagues[207] made the remarkable observation that in patients with overt EATL, lymphocytes from adjacent non-lymphomatous mucosa contained the identical monoclonal *TCR* gene rearrangement as the overt lymphoma and coined the term *cryptic intestinal T-cell lymphoma*. Ashton-Key and colleagues[208] later confirmed this finding and showed that both the inflammatory ulcers and the intact (non-lymphomatous) mucosa in cases of ulcerative jejunoileitis harbored a monoclonal T-cell population and that the lymphomas developing in these patients consisted of the identical T-cell clone.

Cellier and colleagues[66] showed that the IELs in refractory celiac disease patients are abnormal in that they lack expression of mature T-cell markers such as CD8, which is consistently found on most normal or celiac disease IELs. Subsequent work confirmed this finding and showed that the abnormal IELs in ulcerative jejunoileitis and non-lymphomatous mucosa in EATL shared not only the genotype but also the immunophenotype of the lymphoma.[209] Cellier and colleagues[67] detected aberrant clonal IELs (similar to those in most cases of EATL) in 16 (84%) of 19 patients with refractory celiac disease (type II refractory celiac disease). Of these 19, 7 (37%) had collagenous disease, 6 (32%) had ulcerative jejunoileitis, 6 (32%) had mesenteric lymph node cavitation, and 3 (16%) developed overt EATL that was clonally identical to the IELs of the pre-existing refractory celiac disease. The 3 patients (16%) without aberrant clonal IELs (type I refractory celiac disease) all made a complete clinical and histologic recovery with glucocorticoid therapy plus a GFD.

Thus, the cumulative evidence now points to type II refractory celiac disease being a manifestation of an aberrant clonal IEL-mediated neoplastic process. These cells have destructive properties, possibly related to their cytotoxic phenotype,[210] which leads to mucosal ulceration and lymph node cavitation, and they sometimes, but not always, undergo further molecular and clinical progression to lymphoma. As noted earlier, the proinflammatory cytokine IL-15 is massively increased in the intestine of patients with refractory celiac disease. IL-15 induces IEL secretion of IFN-γ and increases IEL cytotoxicity against epithelial cells, thereby favoring the severe enteropathy characteristic of type II refractory celiac disease.[68] Increasing evidence suggests that IL-15, through its key role in modulating IEL homeostasis, ultimately might lead to lymphomatous transformation because IL-15 provides signals mandatory for the survival or expansion of the abnormal clonal IELs.

Based on this evidence, patients with suspected refractory celiac disease should have immunohistochemical studies performed to look for reduced CD8 expression in small intestinal IELs and/or evaluation of TCR clonality in their small intestinal biopsy samples. Those with aberrant, oligoclonal, small intestinal mucosal T cells (type II) carry a poor prognosis and often require aggressive management including parenteral nutrition, whereas those who lack such abnormal T cells (type I) have a good prognosis and typically respond to EC budesonide or other medications.[197-203]

CELIAC DISEASE AND MALIGNANCY

In the past, patients with celiac disease or DH had been reported to have a 10-fold increased risk for certain GI tract malignancies and a 40- to 70-fold increased risk for non-Hodgkin's lymphoma (NHL).[140,211] Recent studies, however, indicate that the increase in risk of malignancy, particularly lymphoma, is much less than initially believed. A large retrospective Swedish study followed almost 12,000 hospitalized patients who had either celiac disease or DH between 1964 and 1994, with a mean follow-up of 10 years.[141] The overall malignancy (cancer and lymphoma) risks were increased only modestly (standardized incidence ratio [SIR], 1.3; 95% CI: 1.2-1.5; and SIR, 5.9; 95% CI: 4.3-7.9, respectively). In a prospective Italian study, patients with celiac disease had a 3.1-fold increased risk of NHL.[212] Conversely, the prospective BioMed European Working Group on Celiac Disease and Malignancy, which reviewed data from 10 countries, reported that the prevalence of celiac disease was increased 2.6-fold in 1446 patients with NHL compared with 9659 control subjects.[213] The European study suggested that the risk of NHL is even less evident in silent celiac disease.

Small intestinal lymphoma, often multifocal and diffuse, accounts for one half to two thirds of the malignancies complicating celiac disease and typically occurs after 20 to 40 years of disease (see Chapters 31 and 125).[141,211] Whereas in the general population, most small intestinal lymphomas are of B-cell origin, intestinal lymphoma in celiac disease is typically of T-cell origin, and the term *EATL* (enteropathy-associated T-cell lymphoma) was coined to describe both the intestinal and extraintestinal lymphomas that complicate celiac disease. The European multicenter study indicated that intestinal T-cell lymphomas, chiefly EATL, are highly characteristic, occurring almost exclusively in those with celiac disease (odds ratio of 28 compared with population controls).

The clinical onset of EATL may be insidious, and its initial presentation and small bowel biopsy appearance can mimic those of untreated celiac disease. EATL commonly is accompanied by mucosal ulceration, as seen in ulcerative jejunoileitis, and these ulcers sometimes are the only endoscopic manifestation of lymphoma. Although some patients with EATL have a partial or temporary response to a strict GFD, most are eventually unresponsive to gluten withdrawal. In patients whose disease was previously controlled on a GFD, recurrence of GI symptoms (e.g., abdominal pain, weight loss, diarrhea) should raise the clinical suspicion of lymphoma. In some patients with lymphoma, mucosal histology adjacent to and distant from the lymphoma is indistinguishable from that of untreated celiac disease, yet the patient's symptoms do not respond to gluten withdrawal.[206] There is long-standing controversy whether such patients had latent celiac disease that became evident after lymphoma developed, refractory celiac disease complicated by lymphoma, or refractory enteropathy induced by primary intestinal T-cell lymphoma and indistinguishable by histologic criteria from celiac disease.[67]

Molecular and immunohistochemical studies that have advanced our understanding of the relationships among celiac disease, refractory celiac disease, and EATL are discussed in the earlier section on refractory celiac disease.

Other features that suggest lymphoma include intestinal obstruction, intestinal bleeding, fever, hypoalbuminemia, lymphadenopathy, and erythrophagocytosis evident in bone marrow or peripheral blood. Small intestinal radiology, enteroscopy with biopsy of the mucosa at multiple levels, capsule endoscopy, and CT or MRI may be diagnostically helpful. Mesenteric lymphadenopathy with central cavitation has been described in celiac disease, both with[214] and without[215] lymphoma. If the index of suspicion is high and studies are not diagnostic, full-thickness biopsy specimens of the small intestine should be obtained at laparoscopy or laparotomy with careful examination of the entire length of the small intestine and examination of mesenteric lymph nodes. Even with such an aggressive approach, EATL can be extremely difficult to diagnose.

EATL commonly is fatal: Overall 1-year and 5-year survival rates of 31% and 11%, respectively, were reported in 1 small series, with long-term survival almost exclusively confined to those treated with chemotherapy.[216]

Carcinomas, particularly of the oropharynx, esophagus, and small intestine, account for one third of the remaining malignancies that complicate celiac disease. The average patient so affected is older than 50 years. The Swedish study reported elevated risks for small intestinal cancer (SIR, 10), oropharyngeal cancer (SIR, 2.3), esophageal cancer (SIR, 4.2), and primary liver cancer (SIR, 2.7).[141] Patients with DH also had a slightly increased overall cancer risk (SIR, 1.2) owing to excesses of lymphoma and leukemia, but they had no increases in GI carcinomas.[141]

The mechanisms responsible for the increased prevalence of malignancy in celiac disease are unknown. Increased crypt mitotic activity, increased turnover of lymphoid cells within the mucosa, penetration of the damaged intestinal mucosa by carcinogens, infection with oncogenic viruses, and underlying abnormalities in the mucosal immune system and surface epithelium all are potential factors. In the Swedish study, the excess risk of malignancies, which was confined to adults, disappeared after a 10-year follow-up.[141] This declining risk of malignancies with increased duration of follow-up, and thus with the length of adherence to a GFD, supports the results of a previous study, which indicated that a strict GFD for 5 years reduced the risk of all malignancies, not just EATL, to that of the general population.[140]

PROGNOSIS

Celiac disease has an excellent prognosis if it is diagnosed early and the patient adheres to a lifelong GFD. Conversely, if it is not recognized and properly treated, patients can develop marked malnutrition and debilitation and can die of complications such as intercurrent infection or malignancy. Increased mortality has been reported in celiac disease (1.9-fold[217] and 3.4-fold[218]) but especially in patients who were not adhering to a GFD, as well as patients with refractory celiac disease and intestinal lymphoma. A study of 335 adults with celiac disease from Finland, at least 83% of whom adhered strictly to a GFD, showed that the 5-year survival was comparable with that of the general population.[152] Growth and development in infants and children with celiac disease proceed normally following gluten withdrawal. In adults, absorptive functions usually return, and many of the manifestations of disease disappear after a GFD is initiated. Certain complications, however, such as peripheral neuropathy, ataxia, or pathologic fractures secondary to severe osteopenic bone disease, particularly in the setting of secondary hyperparathyroidism, might not be completely reversible. The potential protective effects of a GFD against the development of other autoimmune diseases or on clinical outcomes in silent celiac disease remain unknown.

Several lines of evidence suggest that celiac disease is not always a lifelong condition. First, the long-term follow-up of children with proven celiac disease shows that 10% to 20% develop latent celiac disease and become tolerant (defined on clinical, biological, and histologic grounds) to gluten during adolescence. Second, it also has been shown, in individual cases, that the mucosal lesions typical of the disease can appear de novo during adulthood.[219] The factors leading to the appearance or disappearance of gluten-sensitive enteropathy, however, are still unknown. Although adolescent patients might stray from their GFD, often without apparent ill effects, their inability to tolerate gluten remains, and many asymptomatic adolescent patients can be shown to have persistent serologic, hematologic, biochemical, and morphologic abnormalities.[85,220] If gluten ingestion continues into adult life, most patients with celiac disease eventually develop recurrent clinical evidence of celiac disease. Therefore, patients with unequivocal evidence of celiac disease in childhood should be encouraged to remain on a GFD indefinitely if recurrent clinical disease is to be avoided during adult life.

FUTURE THERAPIES

Improved knowledge of celiac disease epidemiology and pathogenesis, the development of nonresponsive and refractory celiac disease and the burden of treatment associated with the GFD all encourage the search for alternative or adjunctive treatments.[17] Shan and colleagues[221] showed that treatment of gliadin peptides with a combination of digestive enzymes in conditions that mimic the in vivo situation, released a protease-resistant 33–amino acid peptide (33-mer) encompassing a cluster of 3 immunodominant T-cell epitopes. The resistance of this peptide to human digestive enzymes was ascribed to its high proline content. Rapid hydrolysis, however, was achieved in the presence of a bacterial prolyl-endopeptidase.[221] Oral glutenases from bacterial or cereal sources are now being studied for their potential therapeutic use in cleaving toxic gliadin peptides within the stomach and proximal small intestine, thereby potentially abrogating gluten toxicity.[222,223]

An increase in intestinal permeability is a well-documented feature of celiac disease and can facilitate the passage of gluten across the epithelial layer to be taken up by antigen-presenting cells and activate gliadin-specific T cells. Larazotide acetate is an octapeptide inhibitor of paracellular permeability, the structure of which is derived from a protein (zonula occludens toxin) secreted by Vibrio cholerae.[224] In early clinical trials, larazotide acetate showed promise in preventing symptoms and signs of celiac disease activity during gluten challenge.[224-226]

Genetic modification of wheat to delete toxic peptides has been proposed to prevent the activation of celiac disease. This approach is complicated by the large number of T-cell epitopes and by the complexity of wheat genetics. Furthermore, nature has already provided a wealth of nontoxic cereal alternatives. An alternative strategy might be to develop peptide analogs capable of interfering with HLA-DQ binding and T-cell activation to redirect the immune response toward tolerance. In mice, a vaccine based on the intranasal administration of whole gliadin or 1 of its isoforms partially inhibited the systemic T-cell response to parenteral challenge by whole gliadin.[227] Similar approaches, aimed toward inducing tolerance to gluten, are being pursued in humans.[228]

As mentioned earlier, tTG modification of gliadin peptides greatly increases their immunogenicity and toxicity in celiac disease.[229] Thus, tTG inhibitors are also being evaluated for their ability to reduce gluten toxicity.

Another strategy, suggested by Maiuri and colleagues,[38] is blockade of signals derived from the cytokine IL-15. This proposal may be premature for uncomplicated celiac disease in the absence of data concerning the consequences of IL-15 blockade in vivo in humans. Blocking IL-15 and its signals, however, may be useful in refractory celiac disease when patients have become unresponsive to the GFD and do not experience a response to conventional anti-inflammatory therapy.

Because celiac disease is, in most cases, a benign disease effectively treated by a safe, established diet, any alternative treatments that emerge must meet high standards of efficacy and safety. That stated, many patients with celiac disease would welcome the development of agents that could reduce the daily burden of strict gluten avoidance and also improve control of their disease.[230,231]

KEY REFERENCES

Full references for this chapter can be found on www.expertconsult.com.

6. Dicke W. Coeliac disease: Investigation of harmful effects of certain types of cereal on patients with coeliac disease. Utrecht: University of Utrecht; 1950.
12. Dieterich W, Ehnis T, Bauer M, et al. Identification of tissue transglutaminase as the autoantigen of celiac disease. Nat Med 1997; 3:797-801.
13. Molberg O, McAdam SN, Korner R, et al. Tissue transglutaminase selectively modifies gliadin peptides that are recognized by gut-derived T cells in celiac disease. Nat Med 1998; 4:713-7.
15. Fasano A, Berti I, Gerarduzzi T, et al. Prevalence of celiac disease in at-risk and not-at-risk groups in the United States: A large multicenter study. Arch Intern Med 2003; 163:286-92.
17. Mukherjee R, Kelly CP, Schuppan D. Nondietary therapies for celiac disease. Gastrointest Endosc Clin N Am 2012; 22:811-31.
21. Rubio-Tapia A, Kyle RA, Kaplan EL, et al. Increased prevalence and mortality in undiagnosed celiac disease. Gastroenterology 2009; 137:88-93.
45. Sollid L, Markussen G, Ek J, et al. Evidence for a primary association of celiac disease to a particular HLA-DQ alpha/beta heterodimer. J Exp Med 1989; 169:345-50.
59. van de Wal Y, Kooy Y, van Veelen P, et al. Selective deamidation by tissue transglutaminase strongly enhances gliadin-specific T cell reactivity. J Immunol 1998; 161:1585-8.
100. Green PH, Cellier C. Celiac disease. N Engl J Med 2007; 357:1731-43.
101. Rubio-Tapia A, Hill ID, Kelly CP, et al. ACG clinical guidelines: Diagnosis and management of celiac disease. Am J Gastroenterol 2013; 108:656-76.
105. Leffler DA, Schuppan D. Update on serologic testing in celiac disease. Am J Gastroenterol 2010; 105:2520-4.
141. Askling J, Linet M, Gridley G, et al. Cancer incidence in a population-based cohort of individuals hospitalized with celiac disease or dermatitis herpetiformis. Gastroenterology 2002; 123:1428-35.

170. National Institutes of Health Consensus Development Conference Statement on Celiac Disease, June 28-30, 2004. Gastroenterology 2005; 128:S1-9.

185. Leffler DA, Dennis M, Hyett B, et al. Etiologies and predictors of diagnosis in nonresponsive celiac disease. Clin Gastroenterol Hepatol 2007; 5:445-50.

188. Cellier C, Delabesse E, Helmer C, et al. Refractory sprue, coeliac disease, and enteropathy-associated T-cell lymphoma. French Coeliac Disease Study Group. Lancet 2000; 356:203-8.

Infection with enteric pathogens is very common and often asymptomatic in the indigenous population of tropical countries. In contrast, short-term visitors to the tropics tend to develop symptomatic infections with diarrhea of variable duration.[1,2] Cross-sectional studies show that significant proportions of the rural population in some tropical countries are infected by a variety of pathogens, including *Campylobacter, Cryptosporidium, Giardia,* and *Salmonella*.[3-5] Even though asymptomatic infections are common, many residents will develop diarrheal illnesses,[6,7] largely attributed to the heavy contamination of basic foodstuffs that is so common in these areas,[8,9] and which probably results from poor hygiene practices and a high ambient temperature that fosters proliferation of contaminating infectious organisms in food.

Malabsorption is not uncommon in long-term residents of the tropics, although the predominant cause varies with geographic location.[10-13] Tropical sprue continues to remain the major cause of malabsorption in adults in many tropical countries but is less common in children in whom a variety of other etiologies, including celiac disease and transient postinfection malabsorption, may be implicated; tropical enteropathy is a cause of significant morbidity and long-term consequences in children. Parasitic infections of the small intestine are probably the next most common cause of chronic diarrhea and malabsorption in tropical countries. Intestinal TB, SIBO, and tropical pancreatitis with pancreatic insufficiency are other significant causes of malabsorption in the tropics. This chapter deals mainly with tropical sprue and tropical enteropathy, but it discusses very briefly other specific causes of diarrhea and malabsorption in the tropics.

INFECTIOUS DIARRHEA IN THE TROPICS

Acute and chronic infectious diarrhea in the tropics is caused by a variety of bacterial, viral, and parasitic agents (Box 108-1). Although these pathogens affect the indigenous population of the tropics, many infected persons remain asymptomatic, probably because of immunity acquired by earlier exposures to the same or related infectious agents. The risk of diarrhea in visitors to the tropics ranges from 20% to 60%, depending on the specific travel destination.[14]

Cholera is the most dramatic form of acute diarrhea, and results in death from dehydration and electrolyte imbalance if untreated. Cholera is endemic in the Indian subcontinent, particularly in the southern and eastern parts; the Indonesian islands; the Philippines; and Latin America; it may also afflict Western travelers to these countries.[15,16] Epidemics of cholera occur intermittently in tropical developing countries, related to breakdown in sanitation that is very often related to economic reasons, but sometimes due to war or civil strife. Of 17,353 travelers returning from tropical countries, 22.2% developed acute diarrhea and 11.3% developed chronic diarrhea;[17] parasitic diarrhea (giardiasis and amebiasis) was most common, whereas bacterial diarrhea (*Campylobacter* > *Shigella* > non-typhoidal *Salmonella*) was more common in travelers to Southeast Asian countries. Diarrhea in travelers is often geographically determined, being caused, for example, by enterotoxin-producing *Escherichia coli* with travel to South America or to Mexico, by *Giardia lamblia* and *Cryptosporidium* in southern Central Asia, and by

---

BOX 108-1 Causes of Infectious Diarrhea in the Tropics

Bacteria
Aeromonas hydrophila
Arcobacter butzleri
Bacteroides fragilis, enterotoxigenic
Campylobacter jejuni
Escherichia coli: enterotoxigenic, enteroaggregative, enteroinvasive, enterohemorrhagic
Laribacter hongkongensis
Plesiomonas shigelloides
Salmonella, non-typhoidal
Shigella species: *S. dysenteriae, S. flexneri, S. sonnei, S. boydii*
Vibrio cholerae O1, O139, non-O1 non-O139
Vibrio parahemolyticus
Yersinia enterocolitica

Helminths
Paracapillaria philippinensis
Fasciolopsis buski
Heterophyiasis (*Metagonimus yokogawai, Haplorchis taichui*)
Schistosoma mansoni
Strongyloides stercoralis

Protozoa
Blastocystis hominis
Cryptosporidium parvum
Cyclospora cayetanensis
Encephalitozoon intestinalis
Enterocytozoon bieneusi
Giardia lamblia
Isospora belli
Leishmania donovani

Viruses
Astroviruses
Caliciviruses: Norovirus and Sapovirus
Enteric adenoviruses
HIV
Picornaviruses
Rotavirus

BOX 108-2 Causes of Malabsorption Syndrome in the Tropics

SIBO
Following ulcer surgery
Secondary to intestinal TB and Crohn's disease

Infections
Bacteria
Mycobacterium avium intracellulare complex
Mycobacterium tuberculosis

Helminths
Paracapillaria philippinensis
Strongyloides stercoralis

Protozoa
Cryptosporidium parvum
Cyclospora cayetanensis
Encephalitozoon intestinalis
Enterocytozoon bieneusi
Giardia lamblia
Isospora belli
Leishmania donovani

Lymphatic Obstruction
Intestinal lymphangiectasia

Mucosal Diseases
Autoimmune enteropathy
Celiac disease
Eosinophilic gastroenteritis
HIV enteropathy
Immunoproliferative small intestinal disease
Intestinal lymphoma
Primary immunodeficiencies
Tropical sprue

Neonatal Diseases
Microvillus inclusion disease
Tufting enteropathy

Pancreatic Insufficiency
Alcoholic pancreatitis
CF
Tropical pancreatitis

Specific Transport Disorders
Abetalipoproteinemia
Fructose malabsorption
Glucose-galactose malabsorption
Hypolactasia
Sucrose intolerance

Campylobacter in Southeast Asia.[17] *Arcobacter* species and Enterotoxin-producing *Bacteroides fragilis* have recently been recognized as important causes of diarrhea in travelers to tropical countries.[18] Infection with the coccidian parasites—*Cyclospora, Isospora*, and microsporidia—is a cause of persistent diarrhea in travelers who have returned from the tropics.[19] *Blastocystis hominis* is another opportunistic protozoan that occasionally causes acute or chronic diarrhea in travelers.[20] Noroviruses are another emerging cause of diarrhea associated with travel to tropical countries.[21]

TROPICAL SPRUE

Tropical sprue is a major cause of malabsorption in tropical countries. Despite much investigation, the etiology of this disease has never been satisfactorily elucidated. In recent times, tropical sprue appears to have become less common in several parts of the world and, in northern India, especially Delhi and Punjab, celiac disease has now become much more common than tropical sprue. There is anecdotal evidence that tropical sprue may be resurgent in individuals who return to temperate climates after prolonged stays in tropical developing countries.[22] Tropical sprue needs to be differentiated from a variety of other conditions that also cause malabsorption in residents of the tropics (Box 108-2).

Definition

Tropical sprue has been defined as a primary malabsorption syndrome that occurs in visitors to or residents of the tropics. Baker and Klipstein,[23] working in South India and Central America respectively, defined tropical sprue as an intestinal mucosal disease characterized by malabsorption of 2 or more unrelated nutrient groups (e.g., fat, carbohydrate, vitamins) for which other known causes of malabsorption had been excluded. Historically, this definition originated at a time when testing for intestinal absorption was commonplace. The availability of specific diagnostic tests for many of the diseases that cause malabsorption, such as abdominal imaging for chronic pancreatitis or anti-endomysial and anti-tissue transglutaminase antibody for celiac disease, led to a general decline in the use of traditional tests for absorption. In the developed world it is now uncommon to find laboratories that perform tests for absorption, particularly quantitative fecal fat estimation, which once was considered the gold standard for the diagnosis of steatorrhea.[24] The diagnosis of tropical sprue, however, continues to require the demonstration of malabsorption along with tests to exclude specific pathologies including celiac disease, chronic pancreatitis, and parasitic infections.

History

Modern medical history records the first description of tropical sprue from Barbados in the West Indies by William Hillary in 1759.[25] He described this disease (aphthoides chronica) as commencing with severe mouth ulcers and glossitis, followed sequentially by diarrhea, marasmus, and death. The word *sprue* probably originated from the Dutch term *sprouw* used to describe a condition characterized by severe aphthous ulceration of the mouth.[26] The Dutch used the term *Indische Sprouw* to describe what appeared to be the same condition occurring in their colonies in Southeast Asia. A similar illness was noted in Europeans who spent time in the Asian colonies of India, Indochina, and China and that went by many names including "chronic diarrhea of the tropics" before being named "sprue" by Manson in 1880.[26] Although these descriptions primarily concerned Westerners who had spent more than 3 months in the tropics, descriptions of a malabsorption syndrome in the indigenous population in India date back to the second century BC. The ancient Indian medical textbook *Charaka Samhita*[27] described an illness (*Grahani vyadhi*) characterized by glossitis, diarrhea, malabsorption-like stools, and wasting and ascribed it to a loss of the "digestive fire." Tropical sprue appears to have become much less common in recent years, but resurfaces sporadically.

Epidemiology

Tropical sprue has been described in South and Southeast Asia, Central America, South America, the Caribbean islands, parts of Africa and tropical Australia (Fig. 108-1). Tropical sprue is most often recognized in Western visitors who have spent at least a few months in the tropics before returning home,[22,28-30] although tropical sprue or tropical malabsorption also occurs in indigenous residents of the tropics.[31-34] In expatriates returning to Western developed countries, tropical sprue can sometimes be attributed to specific prolonged intestinal infections.[35]

Tropical sprue also has occurred in epidemic form, in soldiers and prisoners of war in Asia during the Second World War,[36,37] and also was reported in South India during the 1960s and 1970s.[38] Epidemic tropical sprue affected adults more often than it did children, and exposure during the first wave of an epidemic often conferred protection during the second wave; intrafamilial secondary transmission of disease also has been noted. In the early 1960s, epidemic sprue was responsible for the deaths of 30,000 to 40,000 people in South India alone. Seasonal occurrence of tropical sprue was noted in Puerto Rico, where it was common during the first 3 months of the year.[39]

Epidemic sprue is no longer reported from any part of the world; however, sporadic tropical sprue continues to account for a significant proportion of adult malabsorption and a smaller proportion of childhood malabsorption in South Asia.[11-13,32,33]

Etiology

The etiology of tropical sprue remains unknown despite extensive searching for etiologic agents in the past. Persistent infection of the small intestine with coliform organisms was postulated to cause the disease. Indeed, overgrowth of toxin-producing coliforms (*Klebsiella* spp., *Enterobacter cloacae*, or *E. coli*) in the small intestine, associated with feasting and ingesting excessive amounts of long-chain unsaturated fatty acids, has been implicated in the causation of malabsorption and tropical sprue in Haiti and Puerto Rico.[40,41] Bacterial overgrowth in the proximal small intestine in patients with tropical sprue has been noted variably in other parts of the world, and may be due to the slow small intestinal transit that is well known to characterize the disease.[42] The normal human jejunum contains up to 10^3 bacteria per milliliter of luminal

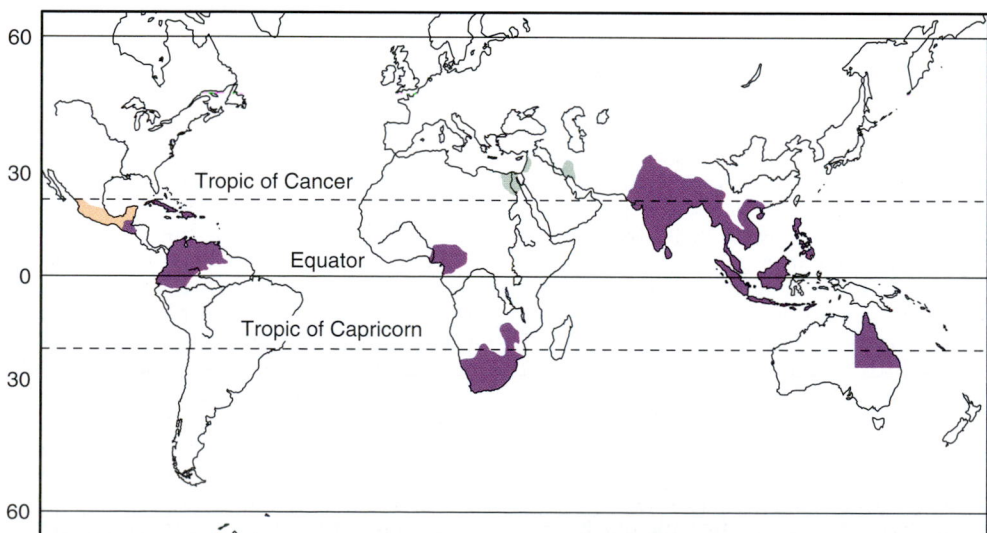

FIGURE 108-1. Geographic distribution of tropical malabsorption. *Purple* indicates areas where overt tropical sprue occurs; *yellow* indicates areas where a disorder resembling tropical sprue occurs. Green areas are where only subclinical abnormalities of small intestinal structure or function have been observed. Today, such subclinical abnormalities (tropical or environmental enteropathy) have been observed in most countries of South Asia, Southeast Asia, Africa, and South America that fall within the tropics. (*Modified from Klipstein FA. Tropical sprue in travelers and expatriates living abroad. Gastroenterology 1981; 80:590-600.*)

fluid in Western residents, and bacterial overgrowth is considered to occur when the concentration of bacteria exceeds 10^5/mL (see Chapters 3 and 105). Studies in South India, however, have demonstrated that bacterial counts in jejunal luminal fluid ranged up to 10^5/mL in healthy asymptomatic persons,[43] and were neither qualitatively nor quantitatively different from the bacteria and bacterial counts, respectively, in the proximal small intestine of patients with tropical sprue. Toxin-producing bacteria were not found in the intestines of patients with tropical sprue in South India.[44] Instillation of fat into the duodenum of patients with tropical sprue was associated with an increase in serum levels of peptide YY and neurotensin and slowing of small bowel transit,[45] leading investigators to propose that an exaggerated ileal brake in response to unabsorbed fat was responsible for SIBO in patients with tropical sprue.

Viral particles that resemble human enteric coronaviruses have been identified in the stool and jejunal enterocytes of patients with tropical sprue,[46] but they also may be present in apparently normal persons, so they have not been definitely implicated in the etiology of sprue. Acute and reversible flattening of the small intestinal mucosa identical to that seen with tropical sprue has been noted in the absence of gluten-sensitive enteropathy and ascribed to a probable viral etiology.[47]

The etiology of tropical sprue in visitors to the tropics may be quite different from that occurring in residents of tropical climates. Long-term visitors might experience 1 or more episodes of diarrhea, usually in response to enteric infection with pathogens such as enteropathogenic *E. coli*, *Giardia intestinalis*, or *Cyclospora* species; persistent intestinal inflammation following such infection has been blamed as the cause of tropical sprue in this setting. Although tropical sprue might very well occur following exposure to certain known pathogens, the possibility has never been examined that this disorder also might occur in response to otherwise harmless bacteria, namely to an overload of apparently nonpathogenic bacteria. In most cases, tropical diarrhea in visitors is short-lived and self-limited or is truncated by antibiotic use. Some persons, however, develop chronic diarrhea with evidence of malabsorption, and the intestinal mucosal biopsy specimens reveal villus atrophy and inflammatory infiltration in the lamina propria. Tropical sprue in visitors to tropical countries is thus sometimes termed *post-infection malabsorption*.

Figure 108-2 summarizes possible etiopathogenic pathways for the development of tropical sprue. The etiologic agents considered include toxins (bacterial or fungal) and viruses. Involvement of intestinal epithelial stem cells as the primary target is derived from electron microscopic studies.[48] Innate immune reactions probably are important, although they have not been investigated. Finally, mucosal damage and inflammation may be perpetuated by SIBO secondary to delayed transit. As investigation into the intestinal microbiota and microbiota-intestinal signaling becomes more widespread, our knowledge of the pathophysiology of tropical sprue will likely increase, just as it is beginning to grow for a wide variety of other GI diseases.

Clinical Features

Tropical sprue typically affects adults, although it is also known to occur in children. The typical presentation is with chronic diarrhea, soreness of the tongue, and weight loss (Table 108-1). The stool has features of steatorrhea, being pale, bulky, frothy, and foul smelling. Abdominal distension and borborygmi are very prominent features. In expatriates, and during epidemics, the illness often begins with fever and watery, or rarely, bloody diarrhea. These symptoms,

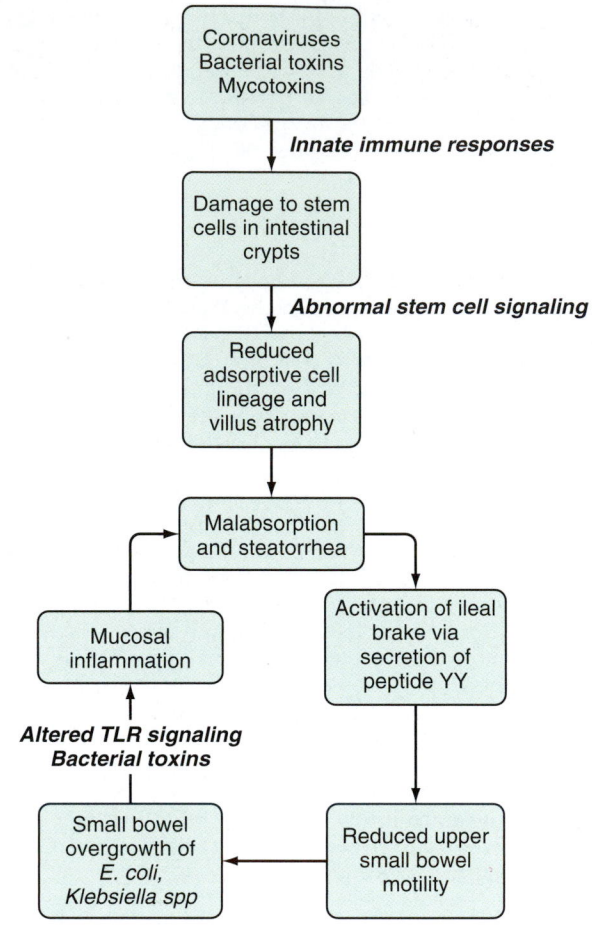

FIGURE 108-2. Etiopathogenesis of sprue. This figure summarizes our current understanding of how etiologic agents that target intestinal epithelial stem cells lead to mucosal damage and malabsorption that is perpetuated by small intestinal bacterial colonization because of ileal production of peptide YY, with resultant small bowel dysmotility. TLR, Toll-like receptor.

reminiscent of an infection, often resolve after a week or so to be followed by lingering diarrhea associated with weight loss.

Physical signs that may be found in affected patients (see Table 108-1) include pallor from iron and vitamin B deficiency; angular stomatitis, cheilitis, and glossitis from vitamin B deficiency; and peripheral edema and skin and hair changes secondary to hypoproteinemia. Glossitis is characterized by diffuse redness of the tongue; the aphthous ulceration associated with celiac disease is not common. Hyperpigmentation of the buccal mucosa, palms, and knuckles (Fig. 108-3) is often present in patients with the full-blown syndrome, but may occasionally be its only presenting symptom; such hyperpigmentation is ascribed to disturbed melanin metabolism secondary to vitamin B_{12} deficiency. Vitamin A deficiency with night blindness, Bitot's spots, and corneal xerosis are much rarer. Fever has been noted in a quarter of patients in South India. Patients are grossly emaciated in the later stages of untreated illness, with muscle weakness, particularly of the proximal muscles.

Peripheral neuropathy may be present, but subacute combined degeneration of the spinal cord from vitamin B_{12} deficiency, once noted in tropical sprue, is no longer found, perhaps because of earlier diagnosis and treatment. The presence of finger clubbing should suggest other illness such as immunoproliferative small intestinal disease, in which this

TABLE 108-1 Clinical Features of Tropical Malabsorption, Their Causes, and Their Mechanisms

Clinical Feature(s)	Cause(s)	Mechanism(s)
Diarrhea	Carbohydrate malabsorption Unabsorbed fatty and bile acids	Osmotic diarrhea Colonic water secretion
Pale, bulky stool	Fatty acid and bile malabsorption	Mucosal disease Pancreatic insufficiency
Foul-smelling stool	Fat and protein malabsorption	Oxidation of malabsorbed fatty acids Production of skatole from tryptophan
Borborygmi, abdominal fullness	Carbohydrate malabsorption	Bacterial fermentation of unabsorbed carbohydrate
Nocturia	Delayed water absorption	Small intestinal disease delays water absorption
Pedal edema, skin changes, leukonychia, muscle wasting	Hypoproteinemia and protein-losing enteropathy	Loss of mucosal surface Ulceration Functional pancreatic insufficiency
Pallor	Anemia due to vitamin B_{12}, folate, and/or iron deficiency	Mucosal disease in the duodenum (folate, iron) and ileum (B_{12})
Koilonychia	Iron deficiency	Mucosal disease in duodenum
Hyperpigmentation of palms, knuckles, mouth	Vitamin B_{12} deficiency	Disturbed metabolism of melanin
Angular stomatitis, glossitis	Vitamin B deficiency	Mucosal disease of small intestine
Night blindness, corneal xerosis, Bitot's spots	Vitamin A deficiency	Steatorrhea with malabsorption of vitamin A
Muscle weakness	Hypophosphatemia, hypokalemia, hypomagnesemia	Mucosal disease with malabsorption or secretion
Tetany, carpopedal spasm	Hypocalcemia	Steatorrhea
Hemorrhagic diathesis	Vitamin K deficiency	Steatorrhea with malabsorption of vitamin K
Lack of taste (ageusia)	Zinc deficiency	Increased zinc losses in stool
Metabolic bone disease	Vitamin D deficiency Hypoproteinemia	Malabsorption of fat-soluble vitamins Malabsorption of protein
Weight loss	Reduced calorie intake Increased fecal calorie loss	Anorexia secondary to folate and B_{12} deficiency Malabsorption
Ogilvie's syndrome	Colonic pseudo-obstruction Electrolyte disorders (e.g., hypokalemia, hypomagnesemia)	Gut neuro-immune-endocrine dysfunction

finding is characteristic (Fig. 108-4). Sprue coma, manifest by listlessness and apathy was described in the past and attributed to a deficiency of divalent cations, particularly magnesium. Rarely, a syndrome similar to the Ogilvie syndrome occurs (see Chapter 124), characterized by abdominal pain and distention with exaggerated bowel sounds secondary to colonic pseudo-obstruction.

Histopathology

Although tropical sprue typically is a disease of the small intestine, involvement of the stomach and colon has been reported. Many patients with sprue have reduced acid secretion detected by gastric secretory testing, and examination of biopsy specimens showed more than half of patients with

tropical sprue had atrophic gastritis.[49] These studies were performed before the recognition of Hp and, therefore, their true significance is unknown. Small intestinal biopsy specimens originally were taken using a peroral biopsy capsule, and today it is standard to obtain biopsies from the distal duodenum or proximal jejunum during upper GI endoscopy. Biopsies obtained using the capsule were examined with a hand lens or a dissecting microscope and showed characteristic blunting and fusion of the villi. The endoscopic parallel of this finding is scalloping of the duodenum.[50] Originally described in celiac disease, it is now appreciated that scalloping indicates villus atrophy and is a nonspecific finding.

Histologically, small intestinal biopsy specimens in tropical sprue show varying degrees of villus shortening (atrophy), and crypt elongation.[51-53] In addition to blunting, the villi

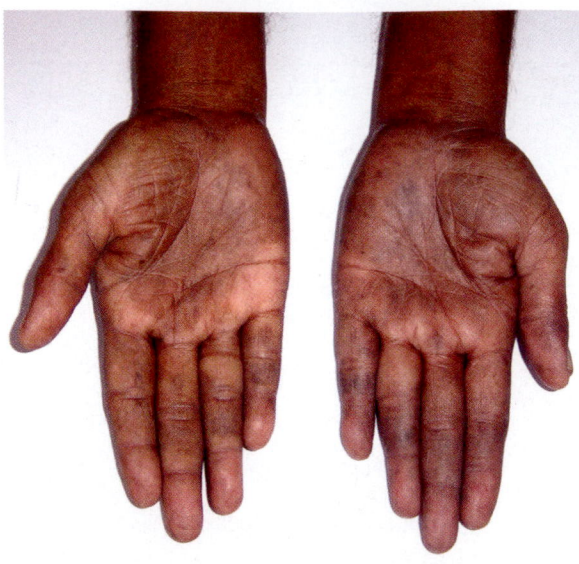

FIGURE 108-3. Hyperpigmentation of the palms in a patient with tropical sprue. This finding is often seen in patients with tropical sprue in southern India and has been ascribed to vitamin B_{12} deficiency.

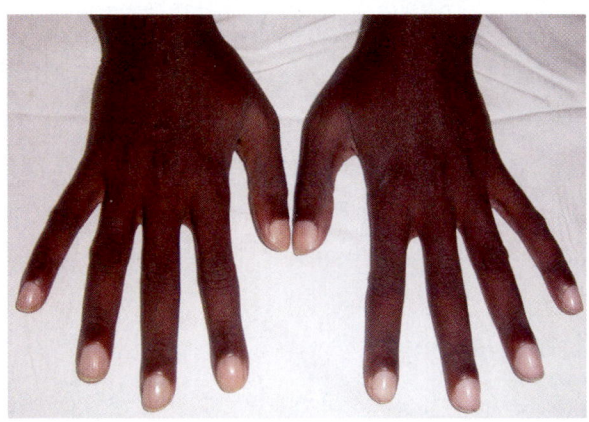

FIGURE 108-4. Finger clubbing in a patient with immunoproliferative small intestinal disease.

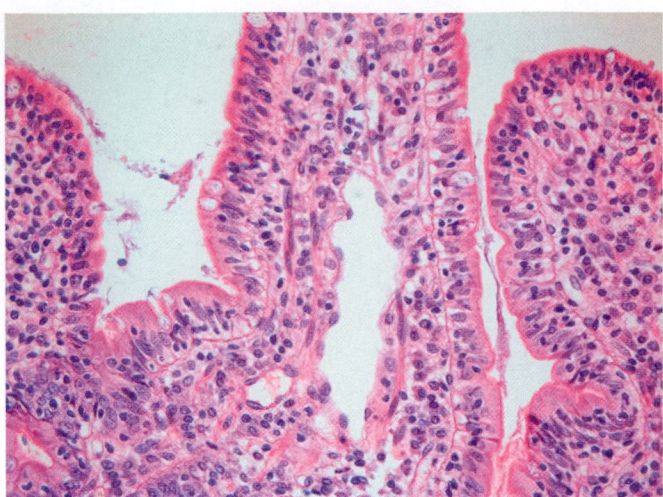

FIGURE 108-5. Small intestinal mucosal biopsy from a patient with tropical sprue showing an increase in intraepithelial lymphocytes.

sometimes show fusion. The normal villus-to-crypt ratio in the jejunal mucosa is 4:1 or 5:1; in the partial villus atrophy seen with tropical sprue this ratio is reduced to 2:1 or 1:1. Complete villus atrophy, noted in some patients with celiac disease, is not seen in tropical sprue. The lamina propria of the small intestine is infiltrated by lymphocytes, and there is an increase in intraepithelial lymphocytes. Increase in intraepithelial lymphocytes, however, is a nonspecific finding and, although characteristic of celiac disease, is also noted in tropical sprue (Fig. 108-5).[54] Baker and Mathan[48] graded the histologic changes in tropical sprue on a scale of 0 to III (Fig. 108-6), which is somewhat different from the Marsh scoring system that is widely used to score celiac disease biopsy specimens.

Electron microscopy reveals degenerating cells in the crypts of the small intestine,[48] a finding similar to that seen in radiation enteritis and in enteritis secondary to chemotherapy. In addition to changes noted in the stomach and the small intestine, an infiltration of the colonic mucosa by lymphocytes also is seen in tropical sprue,[55] similar to the lymphocytic colitis that may be seen in association with celiac disease.[56]

Pathophysiology

The characteristic finding in tropical sprue is villus atrophy accompanied by elongation of the crypts. Ultrastructural studies show the microvilli of the epithelial cells are distorted and grouped. These changes lead to a marked reduction in the total absorptive surface area of the small intestine, which is reflected by a reduced xylose absorption test.[57] In contrast to celiac disease, electron microscopy in tropical sprue reveals degenerating and dead cells in the basal region of the crypts, which suggests there is an intestinal stem cell defect in tropical sprue that prevents adequate restoration of absorptive surface area. Dead epithelial cells at the villus base are extruded more rapidly than normal, and this is compensated by increased crypt cell proliferation and enterocyte migration up the villus.[58] The marked reduction in absorptive enterocytes and the increase in crypt epithelial cells suggest that stem cell signaling pathways in the small intestinal epithelium are probably altered, but this has not been formally investigated.

Fat malabsorption in tropical sprue is secondary to small intestinal epithelial cell damage. It also has been shown that in tropical sprue, the pancreatic enzyme response to an indirect test such as the Lundh meal is impaired, although pancreatic response to secretin is normal. Such functional pancreatic insufficiency results from inadequate pancreatic stimulation as a consequence of mucosal disease and is reflected in an abnormal pancreolauryl test in more than 50% of patients with tropical sprue.[59] The fat in the stool is largely in the form of free fatty acids, both saturated and unsaturated, depending on the nature of the ingested dietary fat.[44]

Folate and iron deficiency in tropical sprue reflect proximal small intestinal involvement, whereas B_{12} malabsorption reflects involvement of the terminal ileum. The 3-stage Schilling test in tropical sprue evidences mucosal abnormality, because defective vitamin B_{12} absorption is not corrected either by intrinsic factor or by antibiotic therapy. Bile acid malabsorption also results from terminal ileal involvement and can contribute to diarrhea. Colonic malabsorption of water and electrolytes also plays a role in the diarrhea of tropical sprue and can result from the action of unabsorbed bile acids and free unsaturated fatty acids in the stool, which inhibit colonocyte Na^+, K^+-ATPase.[44,60]

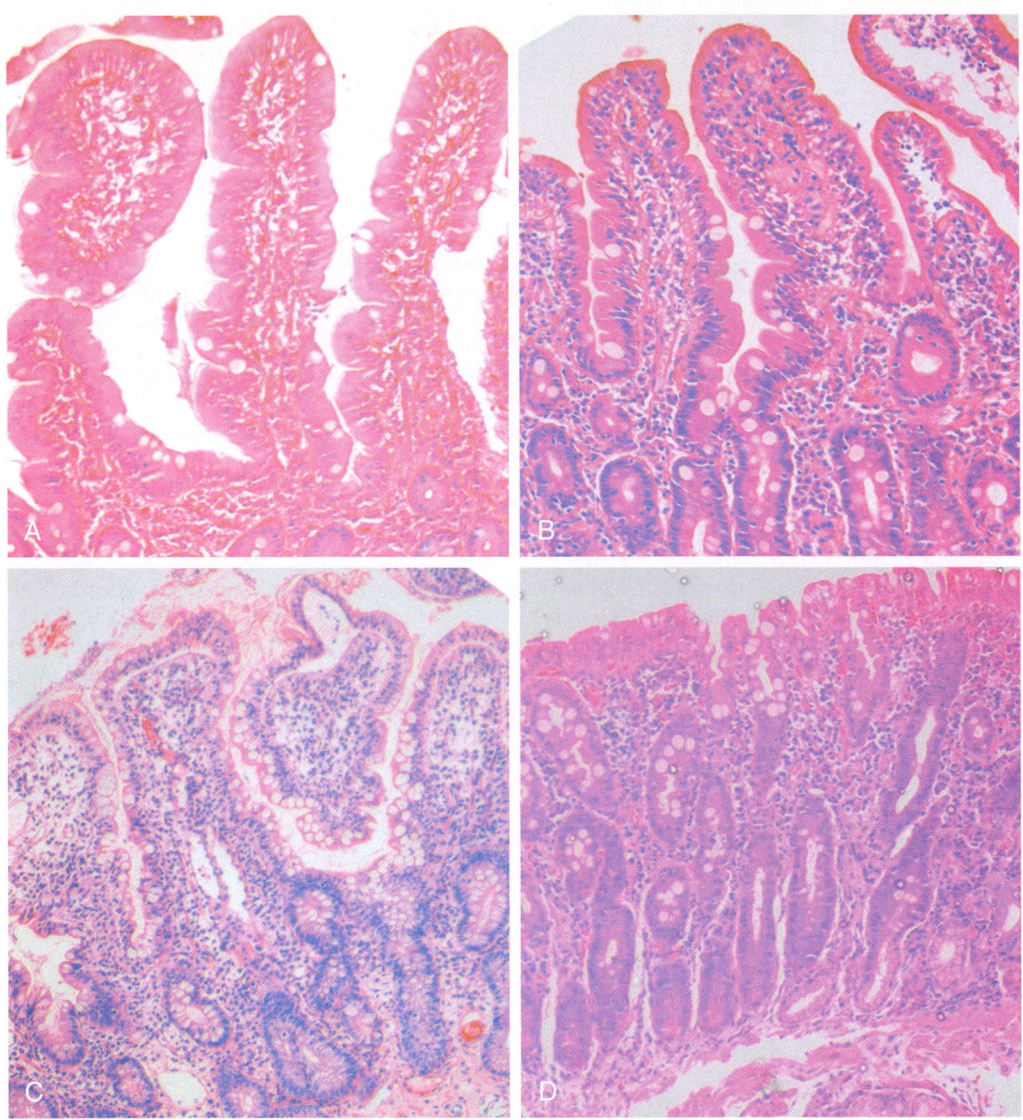

FIGURE 108-6. Histopathology of tropical sprue. Endoscopic duodenal biopsy specimens showing a gradation of mucosal histology according to the grading system of Baker and Mathan[41]: *A,* Grade 0: normal. *B,* Grade I: shortening of the villi, increase in the depth of the glandular layer, and increase in lymphocytic infiltration of the lamina propria and surface epithelial cells. *C,* Grade II: further increase in the depth of the glandular layer extending up to half the total distance from the crypt base to the villus tip with more cellular infiltration. *D,* Grade III: the glandular layer occupies more than half the distance from the crypt base to the villus, together with flattening of surface epithelial cells, disorganization of the brush border, and marked cellular infiltration of the lamina propria and surface epithelial cells. The completely flat mucosal surface that occurs in some cases of celiac disease is not seen in tropical sprue (see Fig. 107-1A).

Diagnosis

There is no single test to diagnose tropical sprue. Although electron microscopy of the jejunal mucosa of patients with tropical sprue in South India showed the presence of degenerating cells in the crypts, an apparently specific change, its expense and lack of widespread availability detracts from its use as a diagnostic test. In practice, tropical sprue continues to be diagnosed by establishing the presence of malabsorption, by excluding other known causes of malabsorption, and by demonstrating the characteristic alterations in small intestinal mucosal histology.

Malabsorption commonly is established by testing for fecal fat, measuring serum levels of vitamin B_{12} and folate, and testing for D-xylose absorption (see Chapter 104).

Two abnormal tests in the appropriate setting are consistent with tropical sprue in the absence of other causes of malabsorption.

The quantitative fecal fat estimation of van de Kamer[61] is the gold standard for establishing steatorrhea but is no longer available in most laboratories. Because of difficulties in performing this test, steatorrhea often is assessed qualitatively using Sudan staining of oil (TG) droplets in stool. The acid steatocrit, a test based on the separation of fat from nonfat components by centrifugation of acidified stool in a hematocrit tube, was developed as a simple test to evaluate the steatorrhea of pancreatic insufficiency, in which fecal fat is in the form of TGs.[62] In the steatorrhea of mucosal disease, however, excreted fat is in the form of free fatty acids and the validity of the steatocrit under these conditions has not been established.[63]

In tropical sprue in India, D-xylose malabsorption, steatorrhea, and vitamin B_{12} malabsorption are found in about 99%, 90%, and 60% to 90% of patients, respectively. Xylose absorption is tested either by measuring urinary excretion of the sugar over a 5-hour period after its ingestion, or by measuring the blood xylose level 1 hour after its ingestion. In the tropics, a 5-gram dose rather than the traditional 25-gram dose of D-xylose is used because the lower dose does not cause vomiting or diarrhea. Xylose absorption is a reflection of surface area of the small intestine, because this pentose sugar is absorbed by passive diffusion. It is a good, but nonspecific, indicator of reduced mucosal surface area in tropical sprue.

In contrast to celiac disease, in which involvement of the proximal small intestine predominates and, therefore, serum folate levels are low and vitamin B_{12} levels are normal, tropical sprue affects the distal small intestine and terminal ileum; as a result, serum folate levels are normal and vitamin B_{12} levels are low. Vitamin B_{12} deficiency is common in tropical sprue and is demonstrated best by the 3-stage Schilling test. Today, Schilling tests are not commonly done and vitamin B_{12} deficiency is diagnosed by elevations in serum methylmalonic acid. In tropical sprue, an increase of breath hydrogen after glucose or D-xylose ingestion has been interpreted as evidence of SIBO, whereas the abnormal lactulose breath hydrogen test suggests prolonged small bowel transit.

Fecal examination for occult blood and for parasites is essential. Protozoan parasites that cause diarrhea must be sought using special stains of the feces including modified acid-fast stains. In tropical sprue, characteristic changes observed on small bowel series include thickening of the mucosal folds of the jejunum, loss of the feathery mucosal pattern in the proximal jejunum, and delayed transit through the small intestine (Fig. 108-7). CT scanning of the abdomen is more commonly performed than small bowel series today and may show dilated, featureless, atonic loops of small intestine with dilution of oral contrast, that suggests a hypersecretory state. The main role of CT, however, is to exclude intestinal masses and lymphadenopathy within the mesentery and retroperitoneum, which are characteristic of other inflammatory and infectious diseases, such as TB, lymphoma, parasitic infestations, and eosinophilic enteritis. Videocapsule endoscopy of the small intestine is sometimes undertaken in patients with small bowel diarrhea after excluding the presence of strictures; however, double-balloon or single-balloon enteroscopy has the advantage of being able to biopsy all parts of the small intestine and is likely to become the standard for diagnosis in these patients, especially to exclude secondary causes of malabsorption.[64,65]

Mucosal biopsies of the small intestine are taken from the third or fourth part of the duodenum during upper GI endoscopy to exclude specific causes of malabsorption and to diagnose tropical sprue. Endoscopy can reveal a scalloped duodenal mucosa similar to that seen in celiac disease, and which results from mucosal atrophy and loss of the villus pattern (Fig. 108-8). A similar appearance of the jejunal mucosa also may be found during enteroscopy. Magnification endoscopy, enhanced by application of a 3% acetic acid spray, has been reported to increase the recognition of patchy villus atrophy and to allow targeted mucosal biopsies that can more likely provide a diagnosis in tropical sprue.[66] Narrowband imaging, coupled with magnification endoscopy, is available as standard on many current endoscopes, and can be used to detect patchy villus atrophy more reliably than white light imaging.[67] Several patterns of villus atrophy have been described on narrow-band imaging that correlate with the villus morphology seen with the handheld dissecting lens (Fig. 108-9). SIBO may be demonstrated by quantitative aerobic and anaerobic culture of the small intestinal contents aspirated either during endoscopy or by a jejunal tube. Fasting counts exceeding 10^5 bacteria/mL of jejunal fluid indicate bacterial overgrowth.

Treatment

Dehydration and electrolyte imbalance must be corrected with appropriate IV fluids (e.g., full-strength lactated Ringer's solution). Profound hypokalemia occurs in some patients with severe diarrhea and might need to be corrected under electrocardiographic monitoring. Deficiencies of magnesium and

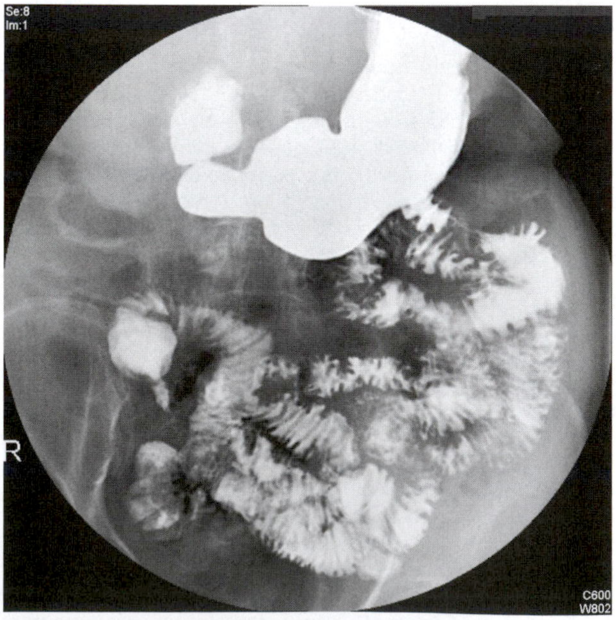

FIGURE 108-7. Film from a barium follow-through study of the small bowel in a patient with tropical sprue showing loss of the normal feathery mucosal pattern in the small bowel, with dilatation of jejunal loops and thickening of the mucosal folds.

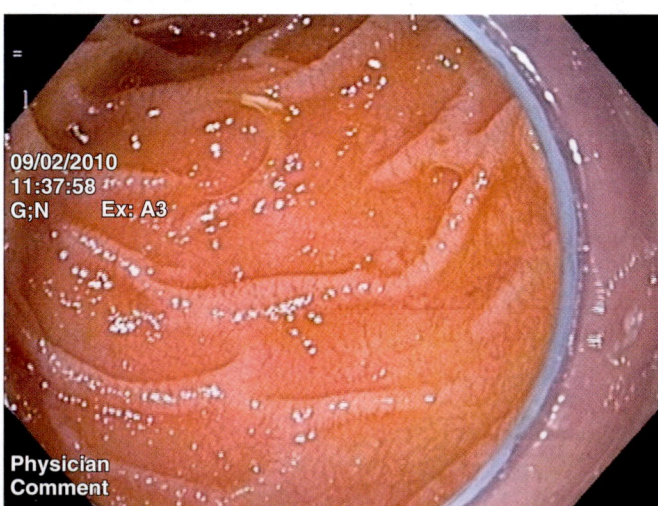

FIGURE 108-8. Endoscopic view of the second part of the duodenum in a patient with tropical sprue showing scalloping of the duodenal mucosa, a finding due to villus atrophy. *(Image courtesy Dr. Amit Kumar Dutta, Vellore, Tamil Nadu, India.)*

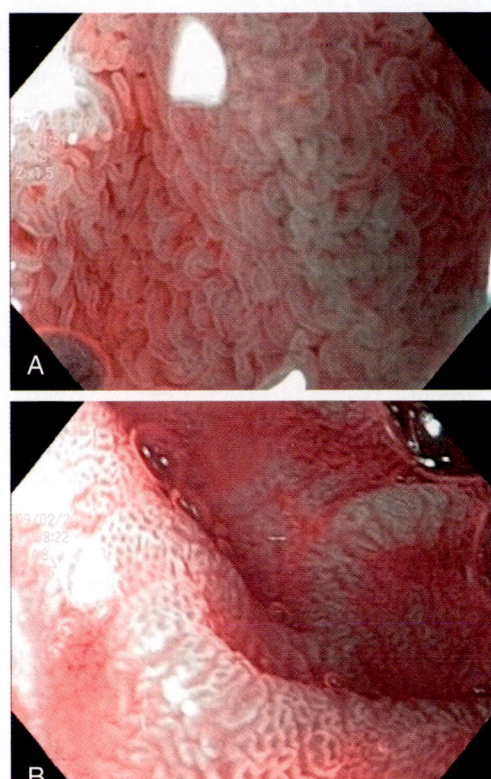

FIGURE 108-9. Endoscopic view of the second part of the duodenum using narrow band imaging. *A* shows normal finger-like villi, and *B* shows areas of atrophic villi interspersed with areas of absent villi in a patient with tropical sprue. *(Images courtesy Dr. Amit Kumar Dutta, Vellore, Tamil Nadu, India.)*

calcium need to be corrected with parenteral magnesium and calcium, respectively, in patients with long-standing illness.

Deficiency of vitamin D and calcium may be treated with oral supplements, but deficiency of vitamin A, indicated by corneal xerosis or symptoms of night blindness, should be corrected with parenteral administration of the vitamin. Vitamin B₁₂ given parenterally and folic acid given orally quickly lead to resolution of symptoms of anemia, glossitis, and anorexia and result in weight gain. Folate supplementation results in improvement of both macrocytic anemia and villus atrophy.

Tetracycline 250 mg 4 times daily (or doxycycline 100 mg once daily) for 3 to 6 months is prescribed as specific therapy for tropical sprue[68,69]; there is only anecdotal experience with other antibiotics. A high-calorie, high-protein, fat-restricted diet usually is given to these patients. Restriction of long-chain fatty acids in the diet, and its substitution by medium-chain TGs, is particularly useful in reducing diarrhea and steatorrhea. Colonic pseudo-obstruction, seen in the rare patient with tropical sprue, can require colonic decompression endoscopically but may also respond to IV metoclopramide (see Chapter 124). Relapses of disease after completion of therapy are uncommon, and recurrent symptoms require investigation to exclude other causes, especially intestinal lymphoma.

Tropical Enteropathy and Its Distinction from Tropical Sprue

The mucosa of the small intestine of residents of the tropics is structurally different from that of residents of temperate countries. This difference, believed to result from environmental

factors peculiar to the tropics, has been variously labeled *tropical enteropathy*, *environmental enteropathy*, and *subclinical tropical malabsorption*.

Tropical enteropathy was first appreciated when small intestinal biopsy, using a variety of biopsy capsules, became available in the 1960s. Typically in tropical enteropathy, intestinal villi are shorter than those of the residents of temperate climates, crypts are more elongated, and there are increased numbers of lymphocytes and plasma cells in the lamina propria. These changes lead to a significant reduction in the surface area of the intestine, which manifests with abnormal D-xylose absorption and increased intestinal permeability detectable by an altered urinary mannitol-to-lactulose ratio after an oral dose of these sugars. In contrast to persons with tropical sprue, individuals with tropical enteropathy are asymptomatic.

The issue of whether tropical enteropathy is a mild form (subclinical malabsorption) of tropical sprue remains controversial. Baker and Mathan[51] emphasized a clear distinction between tropical sprue and tropical enteropathy, the former causing symptomatic malabsorption and the latter being an asymptomatic condition with mild abnormalities of absorption. Menzies and coworkers found that 218 healthy volunteer residents of tropical areas had a higher mean lactulose-to-rhamnose ratio and lower mean 5-hour recoveries of 3-O-methyl-D-glucose, D-xylose, and L-rhamnose, indicating higher intestinal permeability, lower mucosal surface area, and lower absorptive capacity than 228 healthy volunteer residents of subtropical and temperate regions.[70] Investigation of visiting residents in subtropical and temperate climates suggested that differences in intestinal permeability and absorptive capacity were related to one's area of residence rather than area of origin.[70]

Histologic enteropathy continues to be observed even today in residents of tropical countries, with mucosal biopsy specimens that show blunting of villi and increased cellularity of the lamina propria in persons without overt intestinal disease. It has been postulated that tropical enteropathy might represent an adaptation of the intestine to frequent intestinal infection in childhood. There is some evidence that the mucosal damage of tropical enteropathy is mediated by T cells.[71]

In a large longitudinal study, Kelly and colleagues performed regular monthly bacteriologic and parasitologic examinations of the stool and annual endoscopic jejunal biopsy with morphometry on 238 asymptomatic adults in Zambia. The mean 5-hour urine xylose excretion was low (16.6 ± 6.9%) in 182 members of a cohort drawn from a township compared with that of 13 staff members undertaking the study (25.5 ± 4.4%), which in turn was significantly less than that of healthy volunteers in London (33.1 ± 0.7%).[3] The mucosal biopsies of those from the Zambian township showed an altered crypt-to-villus ratio of approximately 5:3. There were marked variations over time, including reduction in villus height (16%), reduction in xylose absorption (16%), and increase in intestinal permeability (28%) during the peak rainfall months of December and January, in association with an incidence of diarrhea that was higher than in other months.[3] Asymptomatic intestinal infections also were noted in approximately half of the participants, and enteropathy was more severe in persons who had been infected with *Citrobacter rodentium* or hookworm.

In Gambian infants, it has been postulated that increased intestinal permeability leads to absorption of endotoxins, systemic inflammation, and growth faltering.[72] Fecal neopterin excretion, however, which is a marker of inflammation, was associated with relative growth failure but did not correlate with intestinal permeability, a marker of tropical enteropathy.[73] Growth faltering, cognitive deficits, and reduced productivity have been reported in children who experienced repeated enteric infections in the first year of life, compared to their peers who did not have frequent enteric infections. These differences have been ascribed to the presence of enteropathy in the children with frequent enteric infections. Attempts to improve tropical enteropathy by oral administration of the probiotic bacterium *Lactobacillus* GG or by the administration of rifaximin, a non-absorbable oral antibiotic, in Malawian children did not reveal any effect of either probiotic or antibiotic treatment on mucosal function.[74,75] The association of cognitive deficits in children with repeated enteric infections in the first year of life is particularly interesting in view of recent work with the intestinal microbiota that has defined a brain-gut-microbiome axis (see Chapter 130).

Tropical enteropathy is not without clinical consequence. The reduced surface area implies that absorption of energy may be slightly diminished, which might explain a low BMI in many persons who live in the tropics. As an extension of the hygiene hypothesis that relates increased hygiene to an increased prevalence of auto-inflammatory diseases, it has been suggested that tropical enteropathy might protect against these inflammatory diseases through poorly understood immune and neuroendocrine mechanisms within the intestinal tract.[76] It also has been suggested that tropical enteropathy influences the severity of infectious gastroenteritis and that it has implications for the composition of oral rehydration solution, leading to the use of lower concentrations of sodium and glucose than in the original formulation that was isotonic with plasma.[77,78] Ongoing research also addresses the issue of whether tropical enteropathy has an impact on drug absorption, an issue particularly relevant to the management of a number of diseases including infection with HIV.

PROTOZOAN INFECTIONS THAT CAUSE MALABSORPTION

This topic is discussed in detail in Chapter 113.

Giardiasis

Infection with the protozoan parasite *G. lamblia* is most often asymptomatic in persons who live in the tropics.[10] Giardiasis can cause diarrhea in immunocompromised persons or in visitors from Western countries to the tropics, and it can cause self-limited illness in children. Diarrhea is associated with the presence of trophozoites in the stool, and the presence of cysts alone should be interpreted with caution. Decreased brush border surface area in the jejunum leads to carbohydrate malabsorption, and associated SIBO with consequent bile salt deconjugation leads to steatorrhea.

The diagnosis of giardiasis can be made by microscopic examination of fresh stool specimens using simple microscopy or by a direct fluorescence test. Examination of at least 3 fecal specimens is recommended because cysts and trophozoites are passed only intermittently. Examination of duodenal or jejunal biopsies does not increase the diagnostic yield over examination of diarrheal stool specimens. The parasites can be seen in the mucus layer overlying the epithelium, and the mucosa can show atrophy of villi and elongation of crypts with a mononuclear inflammatory cell infiltrate in the lamina propria. The most sensitive and specific test today to diagnose giardiasis is one that examines stool for *Giardia* antigen— either enzyme-linked immunosorbent assay (ELISA) or direct immunofluorescent antibody microscopy test.

Symptomatic giardiasis responds quickly to treatment with metronidazole, tinidazole, or other imidazoles.

Albendazole and nitazoxanide also have been used successfully (Table 108-2).

Other Protozoan Infections

Other protozoa associated with malabsorption include *Cryptosporidium parvum*, *Isospora belli*, *Cyclospora cayetanensis*, and the microsporidia *Enterocytozoon bieneusi* and *Encephalitozoon intestinalis*. Infection with these protozoa is widespread in tropical countries, and they may secondarily infect patients with a variety of causes of malabsorption, thereby exacerbating illness.[79] Most primarily infected persons are asymptomatic, but some develop self-limited diarrhea. Endoscopy with intestinal biopsy is helpful in diagnosis.[80]

Malabsorption that results from infection with these parasites occurs mainly in immunocompromised hosts, such as those with HIV infection, persons with primary immunodeficiency syndromes, and post-transplant immunosuppressed patients, as a consequence of epithelial cell infection. Cryptosporidiosis with malabsorption is treated with paromomycin and nitazoxanide. *Cyclospora* causes a malabsorption syndrome with villus atrophy and crypt hyperplasia. Infection with *Cyclospora* is treated with cotrimoxazole. Isosporiasis is treated with a 10-day course of cotrimoxazole followed by long-term low-dose cotrimoxazole in immunosuppressed patients. Microsporidiosis has been described in many countries in Asia, tropical Africa, and Central and South America, and its therapy in symptomatic persons depends on the infecting species. Visceral leishmaniasis, common in some tropical countries, is characterized by the presence of parasitized macrophages in the lamina propria of the small intestine with inflammatory cell infiltration; it can cause chronic diarrhea with malabsorption of vitamin A and D-xylose.

HELMINTHIC INFECTIONS THAT CAUSE MALABSORPTION

This topic is discussed in detail in Chapter 114.

Helminthic infections also can cause a malabsorption syndrome in the tropics. The most common helminthic infections are with *Strongyloides stercoralis* and *Paracapillaria philippinensis*. Infection with *S. stercoralis* can cause chronic diarrhea and malabsorption in immunocompetent persons, although immunosuppression, particularly with glucocorticoid use, predisposes to hyperinfection with this nematode. Infection with the human T-lymphotropic virus-1 (HTLV-1) is associated with persistent *Strongyloides* infection and chronic diarrhea. Diarrhea may be intermittent or persistent, and steatorrhea, anemia, and hypoproteinemia are common. Small bowel series can show changes suggesting mucosal infiltration and ulceration in the duodenum and jejunum. Diagnosis usually is made by examination of feces for the characteristic larvae, although occasionally the infection is only recognized upon small bowel biopsy. Treatment with thiabendazole, albendazole, or ivermectin is effective.

Intestinal capillariasis causes a malabsorption syndrome and is common in Southeast Asia, especially Thailand and the Philippines, but is now reported from other countries including Taiwan, Korea, India, Iran, and Egypt. Intestinal capillariasis is associated with protein-losing enteropathy as well as malabsorption of fat and D-xylose. It is usually treated with thiabendazole or albendazole.

HIV INFECTION AND AIDS

This topic is discussed in more detail in Chapter 34.

TABLE 108-2 Specific Therapy of Diseases that Cause Tropical Malabsorption

Disease	Specific Therapy	Duration
Capillariasis	Thiabendazole 25 mg/kg twice daily or Albendazole 400 mg twice daily	20-28 days 7-28 days
Celiac disease	Gluten-free diet	Lifelong
Common variable immunodeficiency	Human gamma globulin IV every 4 to 6 weeks Bone marrow transplantation	Lifelong
Cryptosporidiosis	Nitazoxanide 500 mg twice daily or Paromomycin 500 mg 3 or 4 times daily	3-7 days 14 days[a]
Cyclosporiasis	Trimethoprim/sulfamethoxazole 160 mg/800 mg twice daily or ciprofloxacin 500 mg twice daily Followed by trimethoprim/sulfamethoxazole 160 mg/800 mg every other day or 3 times a week, or ciprofloxacin 500 mg 3 times a week	7 days 10 weeks
Giardiasis	Metronidazole 250-400 mg 3 times daily or Tinidazole 500 mg twice daily or Albendazole 400 mg twice daily	7-14 days 7-14 days 7-14 days
Immunoproliferative small intestinal disease stage A	Tetracycline 250 mg 4 times daily	6 months to 2 years
Isosporiasis	Trimethoprim/sulfamethoxazole 160 mg/800 mg twice daily followed by 80/400 twice daily	10 days 3 weeks
Microsporidiosis due to *Encephalitozoon intestinalis*	Albendazole 400 mg twice daily	2-3 weeks
Microsporidiosis due to *Enterocytozoon bieuneusi*	Nitazoxanide 500 mg twice daily or Fumagillin 20 mg 3 times daily	3-7 days 60 days[b] 2 weeks
Strongyloidiasis	Thiabendazole 25 mg/kg twice daily or Albendazole 400 mg twice daily or Ivermectin 200 µg/kg	3 days 3-7 days 1-2 days
TB	Isoniazid, rifampicin, pyrazinamide, and ethambutol followed by 2-drug therapy with isoniazid and rifampicin	2 months 4-7 months
Tropical sprue	Tetracycline 250 mg 4 times daily	6 months

[a]For HIV-infected patients administer with anti-retroviral therapy.
[b]For HIV-infected patients with CD4 counts in the normal range.

Since the AIDS epidemic has spread throughout so many tropical countries, it has become necessary to exclude HIV infection in any patient with malabsorption syndrome or chronic diarrhea. Diarrhea and malabsorption lasting for longer than a month is an AIDS-defining condition, is associated with low CD4 counts, and usually is caused by infection of the small intestine with 1 of the protozoan pathogens mentioned earlier. Studies suggest, however, that chronic diarrhea is neither a very sensitive nor a specific indicator of AIDS in tropical countries, such as India.[81] Occurrence of pathogen-negative diarrhea and malabsorption in patients with AIDS has been attributed to possible direct viral (HIV) enteropathy, although this has not been proved. Diarrhea and malabsorption require specific therapy of the opportunistic infection as well as antiretroviral therapy.

INTESTINAL TUBERCULOSIS

Intestinal TB, comprising ulcerative, hypertrophic, and ulcero-hypertrophic varieties, is common in tropical countries. The ulcerative variety of TB commonly manifests with chronic diarrhea and malabsorption, whereas the hypertrophic variety more commonly causes abdominal pain and intestinal obstruction. In contrast to mucosal diseases such as tropical sprue, abdominal pain is a significant symptom and results from ulceration and partial obstruction of the small bowel. Biochemical evidence of malabsorption can be found in many patients with intestinal TB, even if the patient does not present with symptoms of malabsorption syndrome. Causes of malabsorption in TB include bacterial overgrowth in a stagnant loop, bile salt deconjugation, and diminished absorptive surface as a result of ulceration and lymphatic obstruction. The diagnosis is made in most cases by endoscopy with a combination of histology, culture, and PCR tests and complete resolution of the abnormalities detected at initial investigation needs to be documented (see Chapter 110).[82]

CROHN'S DISEASE

Crohn's disease is increasing in incidence in tropical countries and now is an important part of the differential diagnosis for any patient in whom TB is a possible diagnosis.[83] Malabsorption in Crohn's disease may be due to a number of factors. About a third of patients have small intestinal involvement, and this can reduce the absorptive surface area; extensive small bowel resections ultimately have the same effect. Terminal ileal disease or resections can lead to vitamin B_{12} deficiency and bile salt malabsorption, and ileocecal valve resections can result in SIBO with resultant malabsorption (see Chapter 115).

CELIAC DISEASE

Celiac disease (gluten-sensitive enteropathy), hitherto considered uncommon in the tropics, is increasingly described from northern India and selected areas of sub-Saharan Africa[84] and may be unmasked by intestinal infection. The disease often manifests in infancy around the time of weaning, but presentation at later ages, including adulthood, is not uncommon. Celiac disease is differentiated from tropical sprue by the presence of complete villus atrophy in mucosal biopsies. The diagnosis is confirmed by the presence of IgA anti-endomysial and anti-tissue transglutaminase antibodies, although these tests may be negative in persons with selective IgA deficiency. Clinical and histologic responses to gluten withdrawal are important in confirming the diagnosis (see Chapter 107).

PRIMARY IMMUNODEFICIENCY SYNDROMES

Common variable immunodeficiency (CVI) occurs sporadically in residents of the tropics and can manifest as a malabsorption syndrome.[85] Recurrent diarrhea, recurrent sinopulmonary infections, and recurrent meningitis are other manifestations of this disease. CVI first may be suspected when a small bowel biopsy shows reduced numbers of plasma cells in the lamina propria or by the finding of nodular lymphoid hyperplasia, which is occasionally associated with the disease. The most common intestinal infection in these patients is giardiasis. Other protozoa, such as *Isospora belli*, *Cryptosporidium parvum*, and microsporidia, also can colonize the small bowel and cause malabsorption. Selective IgA deficiency may be associated with a flat mucosa and giardiasis. Bacterial colonization of the upper small intestine occurs in some patients with primary immunodeficiency and causes malabsorption, but it responds quickly to treatment with tetracycline or other antibiotics. Periodic administration of IV gamma globulin is the major therapy for patients with CVI.

IMMUNOPROLIFERATIVE SMALL INTESTINAL DISEASE AND SMALL BOWEL LYMPHOMA

Immunoproliferative small intestinal disease (IPSID) and small bowel lymphoma, also termed *Mediterranean lymphoma*, is not uncommon in the tropics,[86] and usually affects socioeconomically disadvantaged persons.

Patients with IPSID present with chronic diarrhea and malabsorption in the second and third decades of life. Abdominal pain is usually a significant complaint, accompanied by weight loss and nutritional deficiencies. On physical examination, clubbing of the fingers may be noted and abdominal masses may be palpated (See Figure 108-4).

The disease is caused by a clonal proliferation of cells that produce an abnormal alpha heavy chain immunoglobulin, and can be diagnosed by immunoassay for the alpha heavy chain in the serum. It is suggested that the clonal expansion is driven by an infectious antigen, in a way similar to the link between Hp and mucosa-associated lymphoid tissue (MALT) lymphoma of the stomach. Indeed, *Campylobacter jejuni* infection has been causally associated with IPSID.[87] Mucosal biopsy of the small intestine reveals a dense cellular lymphoplasmacytic infiltrate in the lamina propria that results in crypt effacement.

The disease progresses over several years from a relatively benign infiltration of the entire small intestinal mucosa (stage A) to the development of lymphoplasmacytic and immunoblastic lymphoma (stage C). The disease is staged as other lymphomas by bone marrow examination, by looking for evidence of disease on either side of the diaphragm, and by CT of the abdomen. In patients with stage A disease diagnosed by mucosal biopsy, it is advisable to perform laparoscopy or laparotomy with full-thickness biopsy of the intestine to exclude transmural lymphoma before commencing antibiotic therapy. Areas of bulky tumor also are resected before chemotherapy and biopsy of enlarged mesenteric nodes is performed. In the premalignant stage A, long-term therapy with antibiotics such as tetracycline can cure the disease. In the more advanced stages of the disease (B and C), chemotherapy or total abdominal irradiation are utilized (see Chapter 31).

TROPICAL PANCREATITIS AND MALABSORPTION

Idiopathic chronic calcific pancreatitis or tropical pancreatitis is endemic in several tropical regions including the Indian subcontinent and southern Africa. Symptoms of recurrent abdominal pain typically develop in childhood or adolescence and often persist for 8 to 10 years. Exocrine pancreatic insufficiency, with a history of passing oil in the stool, eventually develops in more than 25%, and diabetes mellitus develops in more than 50% of affected patients. The fecal fat is grossly increased, and D-xylose absorption is normal. Vitamin B_{12} malabsorption is noted in some persons, resulting from lack of proteolytic cleavage of the R protein-vitamin B_{12} complex (see Chapter 104).

The disease is likely to be genetically determined, and both disease-inducing and disease-protective mutations have been noted. The most common mutation involves a serine protease (SPINK1) gene and occurs in about 40% of the patients.[88] Whether the association with diabetes mellitus in these patients requires a different or an additional mutation is controversial.

Diagnosis is made by detecting pancreatic calcification on plain films, CT scans, or US examination of the abdomen. The malabsorption is treated by restricting long-chain fats in the diet and substituting medium-chain TGs. Pancreatic enzymes with a high lipase content usually are administered with each meal and are most effective when ingested about halfway through the meal.

Therapy of the pain in this disease includes administration of pancreatic enzymes, celiac plexus block, endoscopic removal of calculi, and surgery with pancreatic drainage (see Chapter 59).[89]

APPROACH TO THE PATIENT WITH SUSPECTED MALABSORPTION

Patients presenting with chronic diarrhea and malabsorption in tropical countries first should be screened for infection with protozoa and helminths by obtaining 3 samples of stool for microscopy. Stool samples are examined by microscopy of wet smears, directly and after concentration (sedimentation and flotation) techniques for ova and cysts, and with special (trichrome and/or modified acid-fast) stains for coccidian parasites. Feces also is tested for occult blood to exclude ulcerative conditions of the GI tract. Testing for HIV infection after counseling is performed when indicated. Hematologic and biochemical evaluation is undertaken to establish the presence of specific nutrient deficiencies, including folate, vitamin B_{12}, and iron. Increasingly in specific populations, it is now necessary to evaluate serum immunoglobulin levels and to test for the IgA anti-tissue transglutaminase antibody to exclude celiac disease.

Because tropical sprue remains a major cause of malabsorption in the tropics and because there is no specific diagnostic test for this disease, it is necessary to establish the presence of steatorrhea by fecal fat estimation and to test for D-xylose absorption as an index of mucosal disease. If these tests are abnormal, endoscopy (using white light and, if possible, narrow-band imaging) with biopsies obtained from the third or fourth part of the duodenum or from the jejunum, may allow specific diagnosis of coccidian or helminthic infection, IPSID, and other infiltrative disorders, or it might show the villus flattening, crypt elongation, and inflammatory infiltration associated with tropical sprue. If duodenal biopsy does not provide a diagnosis, it is necessary to image the small bowel using barium or CT enteroclysis. At this stage, it is also appropriate to perform ileocolonoscopy and to take biopsies from the ileum and different segments of the colon. Double-balloon enteroscopy is sometimes necessary to obtain biopsies from areas suspected to be abnormal in the jejunum or ileum beyond the reach of the standard endoscopes. Rarely, a patient will require laparoscopy or laparotomy and enteroscopy with full-thickness biopsy to make a positive diagnosis of the small intestinal disease responsible for malabsorption in the tropics.

KEY REFERENCES

Full references for this chapter can be found on www.expertconsult.com.

2. Kendall ME, Crim S, Fullerton K, et al. Travel-associated enteric infections diagnosed after return to the United States, Foodborne Diseases Active Surveillance Network (FoodNet), 2004-2009. Clin Infect Dis 2012; 54(Suppl 5):S480-7.

7. Zaidi MB, Campos FD, Estrada-García T, et al. Burden and transmission of zoonotic foodborne disease in a rural community in Mexico. Clin Infect Dis 2012; 55:51-60.

9. Koo HL, Ajami NJ, Jiang ZD, et al. Noroviruses as a cause of diarrhea in travelers to Guatemala, India, and Mexico. J Clin Microbiol 2010; 48:1673-6.

11. Yadav P, Das P, Mirdha BR, et al. Current spectrum of malabsorption syndrome in adults in India. Indian J Gastroenterol 2011; 30:22-8.

12. Dutta AK, Balekuduru A, Chacko A. Spectrum of malabsorption in India—Tropical sprue is still the leader. J Assoc Physicians India 2011; 59:420-2.

13. Ghoshal UC, Mehrotra M, Kumar S, et al. Spectrum of malabsorption syndrome among adults and factors differentiating celiac disease and tropical malabsorption. Indian J Med Res 2012; 36:451-9.

18. Jiang ZD, Dupont HL, Brown EL, et al. Microbial etiology of travelers' diarrhea in Mexico, Guatemala, and India: Importance of enterotoxigenic *Bacteroides fragilis* and *Arcobacter* species. J Clin Microbiol 2010; 4:1417-9.

22. Batheja MJ, Leighton J, Azueta A, Heigh R. The face of tropical sprue in 2010. Case Rep Gastroenterol 2010; 4:168-72.

45. Ghoshal UC, Kumar S, Misra A, Choudhuri G. Pathogenesis of tropical sprue: Study of antroduodenal manometry, duodenocecal transit time and fat-induced ileal brake. Indian J Med Res 2013; 137:63-72.

53. Owens SR, Greenson JK. The pathology of malabsorption: Current concepts. Histopathology 2007; 50:64-82.

65. Fry LC, Bellutti M, Neumann H, et al. Utility of double-balloon enteroscopy for the evaluation of malabsorption. Dig Dis 2008; 26:134-9.

67. Singh R, Nind G, Tucker G, et al. Narrow-band imaging in the evaluation of villous morphology: A feasibility study assessing a simplified classification and observer agreement. Endoscopy 2010; 42:889-94.

79. Behera B, Mirdha BR, Makharia GK, et al. Parasites in patients with malabsorption syndrome: A clinical study in children and adults. Dig Dis Sci 2008; 53:672-9.

80. Wahnschaffe U, Ignatius R, Loddenkemper C, et al. Diagnostic value of endoscopy for the diagnosis of giardiasis and other intestinal diseases in patients with persistent diarrhea from tropical or subtropical areas. Scand J Gastroenterol 2007; 42:391-6.

83. Pulimood AB, Amarapurkar DN, Ghoshal U, et al. Differentiation of Crohn's disease from intestinal tuberculosis in India in 2010. World J Gastroenterol 2011; 17:433-43.

MATTHIAS MAIWALD, AXEL VON HERBAY, AND DAVID A. RELMAN

CHAPTER OUTLINE

Whipple's disease (WD) is a chronic systemic infection caused by a Gram-positive bacillus, *Tropheryma whipplei*. The small intestine is commonly affected, but a variety of other organs also may be involved, including the joints, central nervous system (CNS), and heart. Clinical symptoms and findings are protean and include weight loss, diarrhea, malabsorption, fever, arthralgias, skin hyperpigmentation, and dementia. WD was considered to be uniformly fatal in the pre-antibiotic era, but today, treatment with antibiotics usually leads to clinical remission. Many open questions still surround its pathogenesis, but host immunologic factors are presumed to influence susceptibility to the disease.

HISTORY

In 1907, the pathologist George Hoyt Whipple reported in detail the case of a 36-year-old male physician-missionary who died after a 5-year illness involving arthritis, chronic cough, weight loss, and chronic diarrhea.[1] At autopsy, Whipple found lipid deposits in the intestinal mucosa as well as in mesenteric and retroperitoneal lymph nodes. Microscopic examination further revealed a large number of macrophages with foamy cytoplasm in the lamina propria of the small intestine. Whipple suspected a disorder of fat metabolism and proposed the term *intestinal lipodystrophy* for the disease that subsequently came to bear his name.

In the following decades, only a few cases of WD were reported, and the diagnosis uniformly was made at autopsy. The first antemortem diagnosis was made in 1947 based on findings in a mesenteric lymph node removed at laparotomy,[2] and the first diagnosis by peroral intestinal biopsy was made in 1958.[3] In 1949, Black-Schaffer[4] introduced the periodic acid–Schiff (PAS) stain to the histopathologic diagnosis of WD and by demonstrating that inclusions within macrophages were PAS-positive (stained red), documented that the intracellular material was glycoprotein rather than lipid.

The first report of successful antibiotic treatment (using chloramphenicol) of WD was published in 1952.[5] In 1961, 2 groups independently showed bacteria in affected tissues by electron microscopy[6,7]; subsequent reports confirmed these observations. The organisms associated with WD are rod-shaped and of uniform size; also, consistent positive therapeutic effects were achieved with antibiotic treatment.[8] These findings and the positive PAS reaction[4] strongly suggested that WD was bacterial; however, prior to 2000, efforts to cultivate this bacterium failed to yield reproducible or consistent results.

The nature of the bacterium remained obscure until the early 1990s, when its 16S ribosomal DNA (rDNA) sequence was determined and phylogenetic analysis established its relationship to the actinomycetes.[9,10] The name *Tropheryma whippelii* was introduced,[10] and the novel 16S rDNA sequence provided the basis for sensitive diagnostic testing using PCR. In situ hybridization experiments showed that the unique bacterial 16S rRNA sequence co-localized with areas of pathology, thus supporting the relevance of the sequence and organism.[11] Further advancement came with successful propagation of the WD bacterium in co-culture with human fibroblast cells.[12] At that point, the bacterium formally was described as a new species, and its name was modified to *Tropheryma whipplei*.[13] With the availability of adequate amounts of purified genomic DNA, the complete genome sequences of 2 different bacterial isolates were determined and published in 2003.[14,15]

EPIDEMIOLOGY

WD is a rare disorder. The first comprehensive epidemiologic survey was performed by Dobbins in 1987,[8] compiling information on 696 patients and including 617 published and 79 unpublished cases recorded through 1986. According to his analysis, WD is a sporadic disorder with a predilection for middle-aged white men. Data on age and gender were available for 664 patients; 86% were male, and the mean age at diagnosis was 49 years. Most patients were white; only 10 were African, 1 was a Native American, 3 patients were from India, and 1 was Japanese. Most of the patients originated from Europe (373 patients) or from the United States (246 patients). Within Europe, Germany (114 patients) and France (91 patients) were strongly represented. Relatively few cases originated from South America (11 patients) and Australia (13 patients). A more recent review from 2010 estimated the total number of WD cases in the world literature at about 2000 or less.[16]

A small epidemiologic study from western Switzerland calculated the incidence of WD to be approximately 0.4 per million of the population per year.[17] A similar annual incidence of about 0.4 per million was estimated for Germany.[18] An epidemiologic analysis of 110 patients with WD in Germany, diagnosed between 1965 and 1995, noted the incidence of cases to be relatively stable over 3 decades and the geographic distribution of the patients' residences to be relatively even.[19]

In recent decades, several studies have indicated a statistically significant increase in the age of patients at diagnosis and an increasing percentage of female patients.[16,19-22] Currently, patients are first diagnosed at a mean age of about 56 years.[19,22] It has been speculated that the increasing use of antibiotics for unrelated complaints may be a contributing factor in delaying the age of onset of WD. In a cohort of 191 patients with a diagnosis of WD made between 1992 and 2007, 75% were male and 25% were female.[23] There are virtually no cases in children and young adults.

One remarkable epidemiologic feature in Dobbins' analysis[8] was the strong representation of patients with occupations in the farming and building trades, involving outdoor work or frequent contact with animals or soil. Thus, of 191 patients for whom data were available, 43 (22%) were farmers and 10 (5%) were carpenters; patients in all farming-related trades accounted for 34% of the total; by comparison, the fraction of farm workers among the total workforce in the analyzed countries was approximately 10%.

MICROBIOLOGY AND GENOMICS

After many unsuccessful attempts to cultivate the bacterium associated with WD, successful propagation of *T. whipplei* was reported in 2000, using infected heart valve tissue in co-culture with human fibroblasts.[12] The initial estimate of doubling time for the bacterium was 18 days, which represents extremely slow growth. Since the initial report, additional strains of *T. whipplei* have been isolated from various types of clinical specimens, including infected heart valves, duodenal biopsy specimens, ocular vitreous fluid, cerebrospinal fluid (CSF), synovial fluid, blood, mesenteric lymph node tissue, muscle tissue, and feces.[24-30] Methods to determine growth and identity of the bacterium in culture include immunofluorescence,[24,27] nucleic acid staining (Fig. 109-1),[28] endpoint PCR and sequencing,[24,27,28] quantitative PCR,[26,28] electron microscopy (Fig. 109-2),[28] and in situ hybridization.[28] Subsequent studies arrived at estimates of shorter bacterial doubling times between 28 hours and 4 days, but these doubling rates are still among the slowest recorded for any medically relevant bacterium in the laboratory.[26,28,31] A cell-free (axenic) medium has been designed using information from the genome sequence[31]; it consists of eukaryotic cell culture medium supplemented with extra amino acids. Despite these advancements, however, culture of *T. whipplei* at present is feasible only in specialized laboratories and is not suitable for routine diagnostic purposes.

Phylogenetic analysis of the *T. whipplei* 16S rDNA sequence, initially amplified by broad-range PCR from infected tissue, established that the bacterium is an actinomycete, a member of the class *Actinobacteria*.[9,10] A more detailed analysis placed the organism in an intermediate phylogenetic position

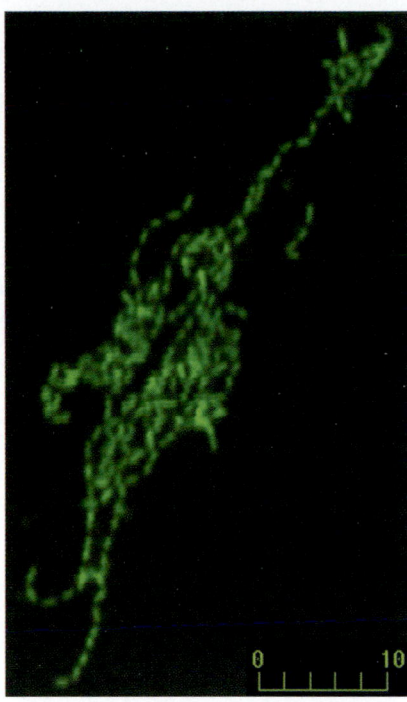

FIGURE 109-1. Photomicrograph of *Tropheryma whipplei* in a culture of cerebrospinal fluid from a patient with Whipple's disease. Bacteria were stained with YO-PRO-1 nucleic acid dye. Note the distinctive appearance of the small rods arranged in chains. (Scale bar represents micrometers.) *(From Maiwald M, von Herbay A, Fredricks DN, et al. Cultivation of* Tropheryma whipplei *from cerebrospinal fluid. J Infect Dis 2003; 188:801-8.)*

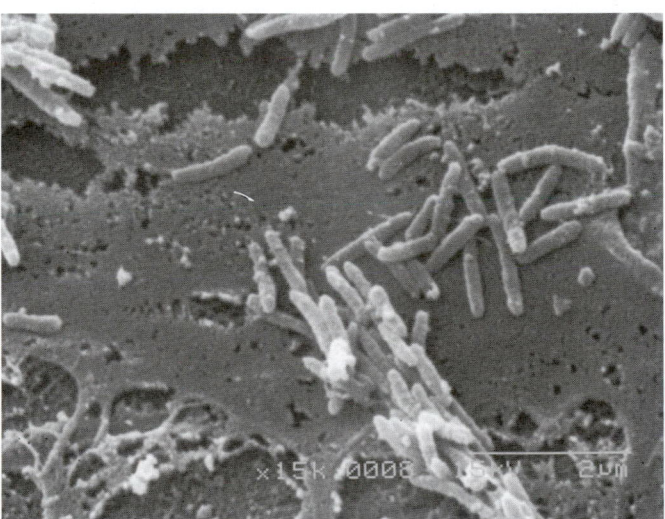

FIGURE 109-2. Scanning electron micrograph of *Tropheryma whipplei* from cerebrospinal fluid in fibroblast cell culture. Note the small rod-shaped bacteria outside of cells, arranged in cords. (Original magnification ×20,000.) *(From Maiwald M, von Herbay A, Fredricks DN, et al. Cultivation of* Tropheryma whipplei *from cerebrospinal fluid. J Infect Dis 2003; 188:801-8.)*

between the genus *Cellulomonas* (with the common group A peptidoglycan) and a rare group of actinomycetes (with group B peptidoglycan; i.e., a different linkage of cell wall components).[32] The relationships of *T. whipplei* to any of the other known actinomycetes, however, are quite distant.

Differences between strains of *T. whipplei* first were observed in the 16S-23S rDNA intergenic spacer sequence[33,34]; 7 different 16S-23S rRNA spacer sequence types have been described.[33-35] One study found the 2 most common spacer types (1 and 2) in a similar ratio ($\approx$1:2) among patients from the United States, Germany, and Switzerland.[33] When different samples from the same patient were investigated, the same spacer type was found in different anatomic compartments (e.g., intestine, blood, CSF[33]), which suggests systemic dissemination of a single bacterial strain in any given patient.

More recently, genome sequence information has been used to distinguish strains of *T. whipplei*. One study found that *T. whipplei* strains were quite heterogeneous when PCR-amplified sequences of 4 highly variable genomic loci were compared.[36] Another study, based on microarray hybridization of DNA from cultivated isolates, found that genomic divergence of strains is due mostly to differences in members of the novel WiSP (*T. whipplei* surface protein) family, but aside from these differences, genome content is relatively conserved.[30] Geographic variability in the occurrence of different strains has been noted, but so far there is no indication that different strain types are associated with different clinical manifestations.[37]

The genome of *T. whipplei* is quite small for a bacterium[14,15]; it consists of approximately 926,000 base pairs and is the smallest of all known actinomycete genomes. Its guanine + cytosine (G+C) content of 46% is unusually low for actinomycetes, which generally are organisms with high genomic G+C content. Genome size contraction is believed to have resulted from gene loss during the evolution of *T. whipplei* and is a general feature of bacteria that occupy a host-dependent ecological niche. *T. whipplei* lacks various metabolic capabilities in carbohydrate and energy metabolism and amino acid biosynthesis. Thus, the genome sequence suggests that the organism is highly dependent on nutrients from its host environment. The proposed extracellular location of the bacteria in patients with intestinal WD, in the villus tips below the intestinal basement membrane,[11] is a site with rich influx of nutrients, and would seem consistent with these requirements.

Two more features of the *T. whipplei* genome are quite remarkable. A relatively large fraction of its genes is dedicated to the biosynthesis of cell surface molecules, and features of the genome suggest multiple "built-in" mechanisms for antigenic variation involving the WiSP family. These mechanisms are believed to involve variable-number tandem repeat (VNTR) sequences, which, in other organisms, are known to be associated with antigenic phase variation. There also are 2 unusual, large genomic regions of non-coding repetitive DNA that are thought to contribute to genetic plasticity.[14] A comparative analysis revealed that the 2 sequenced strains are distinguished by inversion of a large segment ($\approx$57%) of the genome.[15] WiSP family protein genes at each end of the large segment serve as anchoring points for the inversion. Taken together, these features suggest that interaction of *T. whipplei* with its host and evasion of a host immune response are important components of the organism's lifestyle; these factors might contribute to its ability to sustain a chronic infection.

PATHOGENESIS AND IMMUNOLOGY

The natural occurrence, reservoirs, and routes of transmission of *T. whipplei* are topics of ongoing research.[37] Only humans seem to be affected by the disease, with outdoor workers more strongly represented than other professional groups.[8] *T. whipplei* DNA has been detected by PCR in sewage treatment plants in Germany, Austria, and France,[37-39] and initially, an environmental reservoir and mode of transmission were suspected. Several diagnostic PCR studies have yielded negative results with intestinal biopsy samples in persons without the histologic features of WD.[40-42] Several other studies, however, reported detection of *T. whipplei* DNA in saliva, gastric fluid, intestinal biopsies, and stool of asymptomatic persons,[39,43,44] although there is debate as to whether some studies overestimated the positivity rates.[45] Subsequent work reported similar findings for stool and saliva, albeit with lower positivity rates of 2% to 4% in stool and 0.2% in saliva of healthy adults, and 8% in stool and 2% in saliva of sewage workers.[46,47] Thus, it has been suggested that *T. whipplei* is a commensal bacterium of humans, that there is a healthy asymptomatic carrier state, and that WD occurs in only a small subset of such persons.[37,45] Reports of WD in relatives of persons with the disease are rare.[48,49]

The sequence of events leading to initiation of disease and pathology are still unclear. Earlier electron microscopic studies[50,51] would support the concept that *T. whipplei* has the capability to invade the mucosa of the proximal small intestine. Fluorescence in situ hybridization (FISH) demonstrates co-localization of *T. whipplei* 16S rRNA with areas of pathologic changes, and indicates that most viable *T. whipplei* in the intestinal mucosa are extracellular and located just below the epithelial basement membrane in the lamina propria.[11] From the intestinal mucosa, bacteria are thought to spread via lymphatics into mesenteric and mediastinal lymph nodes and into the systemic circulation.

Several abnormalities of immune function have been observed in patients with WD,[8,52,53] including both transient (i.e., during active disease) as well as persistent (i.e., after therapy) abnormalities; the persistent abnormalities are presumed to serve as predisposing factors for development of disease. Precisely defined immune defects, however, such as the physical or functional absence of specific cell types, mediators, or receptors, or particular genetic defects, have not yet been identified. Earlier case series[54,55] described an over-representation of the HLA-B27 haplotype in patients with WD, but this association was not supported by other series.[56,57] A more recent study has found the HLA alleles DRB1*13 and DQB1*06 to be more frequent among WD patients than among controls.[58]

During active disease, reduced CD4/CD8 T-cell ratios (both in the lamina propria and in peripheral blood), reduced proliferation of peripheral T cells to stimulating agents (e.g., phytohemagglutinin, concanavalin A), and reduced delayed-type hypersensitivity reactions to common antigens in skin tests have been observed.[52,54,59] This may be a consequence of malnutrition, however, rather than a preexisting immunologic abnormality. One study showed that the monocytes of a patient with WD exhibited an impaired ability to degrade bacterial antigens,[60] which is consistent with the prolonged persistence of bacterial remnants in intestinal macrophages after therapy that has been observed in histologic studies of WD.[8,61] Other immunologic abnormalities persist after therapy: reduced numbers of peripheral blood monocytes that express the alpha chain of complement receptor 3 (CD11b),[52] a reduced capability of peripheral blood monocytes to produce interleukin (IL)-12 on stimulation with bacterial antigens,[53] and a dysregulation of mononuclear cell function, such that the components of a Th1-type immune response are reduced and those of a Th2-type immune response are increased.[62] The latter observation was supported in a study with specific *T. whipplei* antigen from cultivated bacteria: duodenal lymphocytes and peripheral blood mononuclear cells from healthy people exhibited robust Th1-type immune reactivity, but those of patients with WD showed reduced or absent *T. whipplei*–specific Th1 responses.[63]

Macrophages from the duodenal tissue of 1 patient with WD exhibited a transcriptional pattern of M2/alternatively-activated macrophages, which is associated with a Th2-type immune response.[64] Similarly, peripheral monocytes and duodenal macrophages from patients with WD have a M2/alternative activation phenotype; studies in these patients have demonstrated reduced nitrite production by duodenal macrophages and a reduced oxidative burst in peripheral monocytes upon exposure to *T. whipplei*.[65] In addition, the *T. whipplei*–specific humoral immune response appears to be impaired: asymptomatic carriers have been found to exhibit a "paradoxically" higher IgG antibody response against the organism than did patients with WD.[66]

Another investigation showed that IL-16, a cytokine that is known to be constitutively expressed in T cells, mast cells, dendritic cells, and circulating monocytes, and to be released during apoptosis, was expressed at high levels and released by macrophages upon infection with *T. whipplei*.[67] Furthermore, IL-16, when added to the experimental model, promoted *T. whipplei* replication in both monocytes and macrophages.[67] Circulating blood levels of IL-16 and nucleosomes (a marker of apoptosis) also were found to be elevated in patients with active WD compared with patients with treated WD and controls.[68]

A few reports describe secondary or opportunistic infections in patients with WD.[61,69-71] Two case series described *Giardia lamblia* infection in 8% and 12% of patients, respectively.[61,71] Rare cases of infections with *Pneumocystis jiroveci*, *Cryptosporidium parvum*, *Nocardia* spp., *Mycobacterium tuberculosis*, *Serratia marcescens*, *Candida* spp., dermatophytes, and *Strongyloides stercoralis* also have been recorded. Conversely, there does not appear to be an increased incidence of WD in patients with primary immunodeficiencies or immunosuppression, apart from the fact that immunosuppressive therapy may hasten the onset of clinically apparent WD in patients with prodromal articular manifestations.[72] There is 1 case report that describes the detection of *T. whipplei* DNA by PCR in the duodenal biopsy of a patient with AIDS[73] and a more recent study showing that *T. whipplei* DNA is significantly more prevalent in bronchoalveolar lavage specimens from HIV-infected individuals than from non–HIV-infected persons.[74]

Based on observations of *T. whipplei* DNA in asymptomatic people[46] and also in some patients with acute, self-limited diseases, such as children with gastroenteritis,[75] some authors have suggested that *T. whipplei* may cause transient illnesses in a relatively large number of subjects but cause persistent infection and WD in a very small subset of these subjects who lack an adequate immune response[76,77]; this is still a hypothetical scenario that is awaiting to be confirmed by further research. In summary, all these clinical observations and laboratory findings suggest that host factors play an important part in facilitating the occurrence of WD.

CLINICAL FEATURES

WD is best known for its manifestations in the intestinal tract, which are largely responsible for the classic clinical features of the disease.[78,79] It is a systemic infection, however, and almost any organ system can be affected.[8] In many patients, arthralgias precede intestinal symptoms by several years (1 to 10 years; up to 30 years reported), although it is unclear whether joints are infected at those earlier time points; in some cases, low-grade intermittent fever also occurs for years before the diagnosis of WD.[21,80] Since the advent of PCR for *T. whipplei* in the early 1990s, the organism has increasingly been detected and implicated in a wider spectrum of clinical conditions and disease states, including "blood culture–negative endocarditis." Patients tend to have less advanced disease at the time of diagnosis, possibly as a result of earlier detection.[8,21]

Small Intestine and Lymphatic System

In classic intestinal WD, bacterial and macrophage-predominant inflammatory cell infiltration of the small intestinal mucosa and obstruction of mesenteric lymph nodes lead to a malabsorption syndrome with weight loss, diarrhea, and abdominal pain as the dominant signs and symptoms.[16,21,22,78-81] Weight loss of 5 to 20 kg occurs gradually, usually over a period of at least a year, sometimes resulting in severe cachexia in the terminal stage of untreated disease.[8,78,80] Diarrhea can consist of voluminous steatorrheic stools or may be watery.[78] Occult GI bleeding is not uncommon, and in some cases gross GI bleeding occurs.[8,78]

Abdominal (mesenteric and retroperitoneal) and peripheral lymphadenopathy are common,[16,21,22,78,80,81] and in some instances, enlarged abdominal lymph nodes have raised the suspicion of malignancy.[81] In rare instances, malignant lymphomas have occurred in patients with WD.[82,83]

Barium examination of the intestinal tract can reveal nonspecific abnormalities (e.g., prominent and edematous duodenal and jejunal folds and intestinal dilatation) that also are found in other malabsorption syndromes (Fig. 109-3).[8,80] CT (Fig. 109-4) or MRI can detect retroperitoneal or para-aortic lymphadenopathy.[80] Enlarged abdominal lymph nodes have a hypodense appearance on CT scans and are hyperechoic on US.[70,84]

Laboratory examinations in patients with intestinal WD often reveal an increased erythrocyte sedimentation rate, increased C-reactive protein, decreased serum carotene level, decreased serum iron concentration, anemia, decreased serum protein levels, proteinuria, and elevated stool fat content.[8,21,22,80]

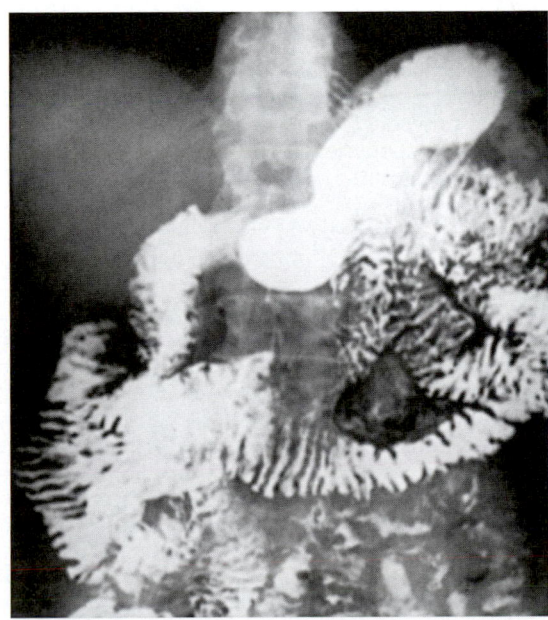

FIGURE 109-3. Film from a barium contrast study of the small intestine from a patient with Whipple's disease. There is marked thickening of the plicae circulares and a loss of the normal delicate mucosal relief pattern. The small intestine is slightly dilated. *(Courtesy Elihu Schimmel, MD, Boston, Mass.)*

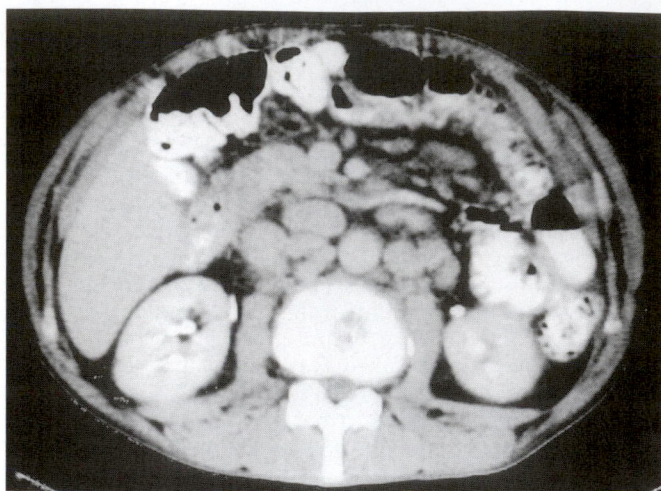

FIGURE 109-4. CT showing extensive retroperitoneal and mesenteric lymphadenopathy caused by Whipple's disease and simulating lymphoma. (*Courtesy Mark Feldman, MD, Dallas, Tex.*)

Central Nervous System

Symptomatic CNS manifestations have been reported in about 10% to 40% of patients with intestinal WD, with more recent series reporting lower rates.[16,21,22,78,80,81] Neurologic disease can occur concurrently with intestinal manifestations at the time of diagnosis, but it is more common upon clinical relapse, which can occur during or after treatment.[8,85] It is thought that *T. whipplei* enter the CNS early in the course of disease and that because most drugs do not penetrate the CNS well, the organisms persist during medical treatment. The result is the impression that intestinal disease enters remission initially and neurologic disease develops subsequently, even as antibiotics continue to be given. Relapses affecting the CNS are ominous because they tend to be refractory to renewed antibiotic treatment.[8,86] Although rare, instances of isolated primary neurologic WD have been reported in patients without intestinal or other manifestations.[87,88]

Two reviews summarized the neurologic findings of WD in 84 and 122 published cases, respectively.[89,90] Common findings are progressive dementia and cognitive changes (28% to 71%), supranuclear ophthalmoplegia (32% to 51%), and altered level of consciousness (27% to 50%); less common are psychiatric symptoms, hypothalamic manifestations (e.g., polydipsia, hyperphagia, insomnia),[91] cranial nerve abnormalities, nystagmus, seizures, and ataxia. Two signs that are indicative of CNS WD are oculomasticatory myorhythmia and oculofacial skeletal myorhythmia,[89] each consisting of slow rhythmic and synchronized contractions (≈1/sec) of ocular, facial, or other muscles; they occur in fewer than 20% of cases,[89,90] and they have not yet been documented in other CNS diseases.

Results of CT or MRI scanning may be normal or reveal mild to moderate brain atrophy or focal lesions without a predilection for specific sites.[89,90,92] These abnormalities are not specific for WD, but focal lesions may be used to guide stereotactic biopsies, which, in most cases, reveal characteristic histology[89]; MRI appears to be more sensitive than CT scan.[90] Results of standard CSF examinations usually are normal, although sometimes there is mild pleocytosis.[8,89] However, CSF cytology—when using cytocentrifugation followed by PAS staining—often reveals PAS-positive sickle-form particle-containing cells, and PCR often yields positive results for *T. whipplei* DNA, even in a considerable proportion of neurologically asymptomatic patients.[93]

Cardiovascular System

Cardiac manifestations of WD include endocarditis, myocarditis, and pericarditis.[8,21,22,94] Endocarditis may be encountered as part of intestinal or systemic WD, and it may occur in the setting of "blood culture-negative endocarditis" without detectable other organ involvement.[22,95,96] Autopsy series of classic WD from the 1960s[79] and 1970s[94] showed a high rate (53%) of valvular endocarditis with vegetations. In contrast, clinically apparent endocarditis was much less common (≤6%) in several more recent series of systemic or intestinal WD.[16,21,22] All valves may be affected, but the aortic and mitral valves are most commonly pathologically altered, and involvement of the aortic valve leads to the most significant symptoms[8,97]; some patients require valve replacement. PAS-positive macrophages and *T. whipplei* can be detected in native[98] and porcine prosthetic[99] valve tissue and in the myocardium[100] by histology and electron microscopy, respectively.

With the aid of broad-range and specific PCR testing of excised heart valve tissue, *T. whipplei* is increasingly implicated in blood culture-negative endocarditis, even in the absence of intestinal WD.[95,96,99,101-103] Data concerning the frequency of *T. whipplei* in suspected cases of endocarditis have become available from 2 large investigative series. One series from France[102] of 819 patients with suspected blood culture-negative endocarditis identified an etiologic agent in 476 patients, and this included *T. whipplei* in 19 cases (4% of identified agents). Another series from Germany[103] of 1135 patients with valve destruction found an etiologic agent in 255 patients, and identified *T. whipplei* in 16 cases (6%). In both series, *T. whipplei* was the fourth most commonly identified organism. Clinically, *T. whipplei* endocarditis is characterized by a relatively indolent course, frequent prodromal or concomitant articular symptoms, and frequent absence of fever and preexisting valvular disease.[22,95-97] The classical Duke criteria for diagnosing endocarditis are usually not met.[22,97]

Musculoskeletal System

Intermittent, migratory oligo- or poly- arthralgias or arthritis, usually involving the knees, wrists, ankles, elbows, or fingers, is a common complaint of patients with WD.[8,21,104] Rheumatoid factor usually is absent. Destructive joint changes or accumulation of synovial fluid are rare, but when present are accompanied by PAS-positive macrophages (by histology), bacteria (by electron microscopy), or DNA of *T. whipplei* (by PCR) in synovial tissue or joint fluid;[8,105,106] 1 synovial fluid specimen yielded *T. whipplei* in culture.[29] Sacroiliitis and spondylitis may occur, but ankylosing forms are rare, and there does not seem to be a strong association of these manifestations with HLA-B27.[8] Treatment of articular manifestations with immunosuppressive drugs may precipitate the onset of intestinal or other systemic illness.[72] Rare articular manifestations include infectious spondylodiskitis[107] and prosthetic joint infection.[108]

Other Clinical Manifestations

One common feature of WD is cutaneous hyperpigmentation, which has been found in 17% to 66% of patients.[16,21,78-81] This finding tends to occur in light-exposed areas of the skin. The pathophysiology of this hyperpigmentation is unknown, but appears to be unrelated to adrenal dysfunction or hyperbilirubinemia. PAS-positive cells or *T. whipplei* DNA may be detected in skin specimens, even in macroscopically healthy-appearing skin, and cultivation of *T. whipplei* isolate from 1 skin sample has been reported.[109]

Ocular manifestations of WD are diverse, but rare. These include uveitis, vitritis, retinitis, retrobulbar neuritis, and papilledema.[8] They usually are associated with CNS disease, and the majority of reported patients also had clinical or histologic evidence of intestinal involvement. PAS-positive macrophages, *T. whipplei* DNA, and visible bacteria may be detected in vitrectomy specimens.[110-112] One case of uveitis was reported in which the vitreous fluid and an intestinal biopsy specimen yielded positive PCR results, although intestinal histology was normal.[111] Another uveitis case yielded a positive culture.[25]

Chronic cough was a symptom in Whipple's original patient and was reported relatively frequently in earlier series[79] but infrequently since then.[21] Some patients have pleuritis with effusion or granulomatous pulmonary disease that resembles sarcoidosis.[8,22]

T. whipplei and its DNA are increasingly found in clinical settings and circumstances outside those of classic WD. Such findings include the detection of *T. whipplei* DNA in blood samples of patients with fever and cough in Senegal,[113] in stool samples of children with gastroenteritis in France,[75] and in bronchoalveolar lavage (BAL) samples of patients with pneumonia.[114] Remarkably, 1 of the patients with pneumonia was immunosuppressed and presented with community-acquired pneumonia leading to septic shock. *T. whipplei* DNA was abundant in the BAL specimen and was the only bacterial species detected in this specimen.[114] An interesting and related set of findings was reported from a comparison of the bacterial microbiota in BAL fluid from 82 HIV-infected compared with 77 non–HIV-infected individuals.[74] Here, *T. whipplei* DNA was more frequently found and more abundant in BAL specimens from HIV-infected than non–HIV-infected individuals, and in 11 HIV-infected individuals, *T. whipplei* sequences constituted more than 50% of all bacterial sequences detected. Antiretroviral treatment led to a significant reduction in the relative abundance of *T. whipplei* sequences. Most of these individuals did not report any serious lung problems. The pathogenetic role of *T. whipplei* in each of these scenarios is inherently difficult to establish,[114,115] yet these reports do suggest that the spectrum of illnesses with which *T. whipplei* is associated may be broader than currently appreciated.

PATHOLOGY

Small Intestine

On gross inspection, the mucosa of the distal duodenum and jejunum is abnormal in most patients with intestinal WD. Whitish-to-yellow plaque-like patches are observed in approximately three quarters of patients (Fig. 109-5); alternatively, the mucosa can appear pale yellow.[61,116] Abnormal villus structure and mild mucosal flattening become evident with magnifying optics.

The histopathologic features of intestinal WD are quite distinctive. Viewed with light microscopy, the visible patches reflect lipid deposits or lymphangiectasia, whereas villus distention results from infiltration by macrophages in the lamina propria (Fig. 109-6). The swollen cytoplasm of macrophages appears foamy when stained with H&E, but numerous granular particles become visible when the PAS stain is used (see Fig. 109-6). These particles correspond to phagolysosomes that are filled with numerous *T. whipplei*, and the positive reaction with PAS reflects the glycoprotein content of the bacterial cell walls. Single extracellular bacteria are barely visible with conventional light microscopy because of their small size, but they become evident in the mucosal stroma with high-resolution light microscopy and electron

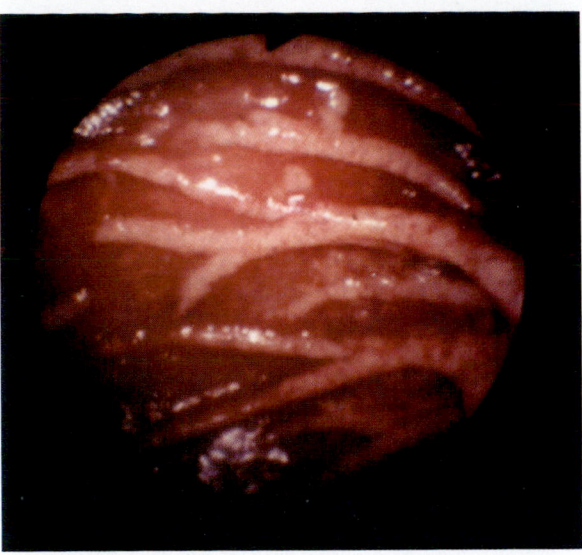

FIGURE 109-5. Endoscopic view of the distal duodenum in a patient with untreated Whipple's disease. The plicae circulares are swollen, and the mucosal surface is intact. Numerous whitish patches, reflecting lipid deposits, are present within the mucosa (see Fig. 109-6). *(Courtesy Hans Jörg Meier-Willersen, MD, Heidelberg, Germany.)*

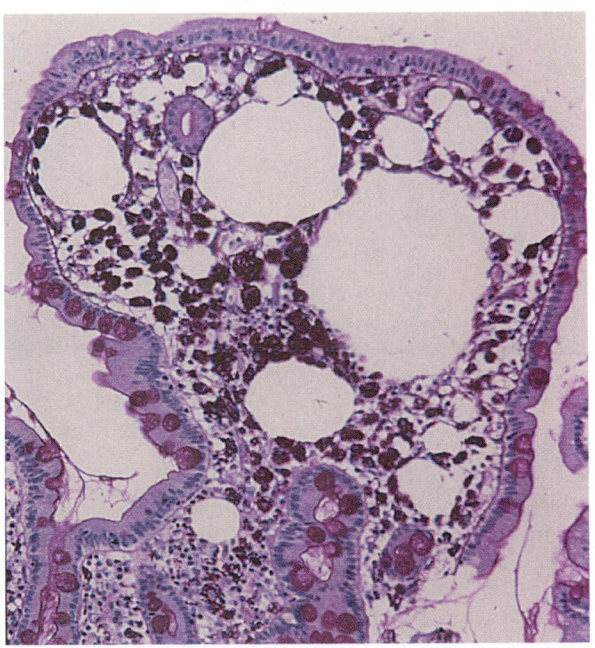

FIGURE 109-6. Histopathology of the small intestinal mucosa in the same patient as in Fig. 109-5. A villus is distended by an infiltrate of macrophages that contain periodic acid–Schiff–positive granular particles (type 1 cells) and by lipid droplets. The epithelial layer is intact. (Original magnification ×84.)

microscopy (Fig. 109-7). The number of bacteria varies greatly among patients.

Electron microscopy shows uniformity in size and shape of the bacteria, with an external diameter of 0.2 to 0.25 μm and a length of up to 2.5 μm.[51,117] There is an electron-dense outer layer that is not found in other bacteria, and which some

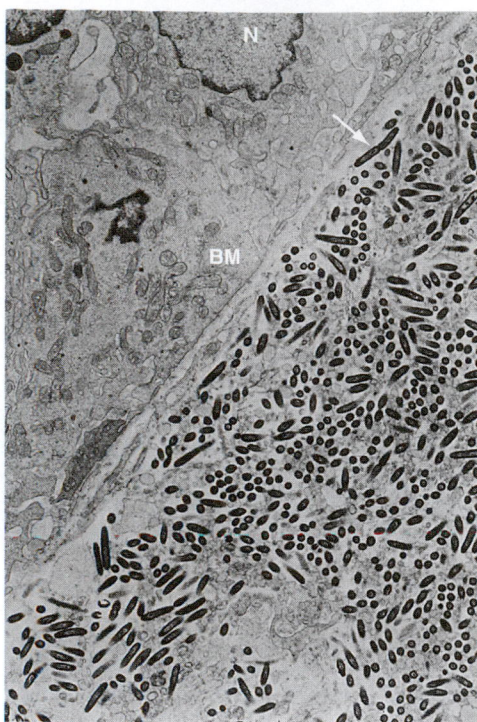

FIGURE 109-7. Electron microscopy of a small intestinal biopsy specimen in a patient with untreated Whipple's disease. Just beneath the epithelial basement membrane (BM), the lamina propria is densely infiltrated by extracellular rod-shaped bacteria. The bacteria are uniform in size and structure. Some of them are dividing *(arrow)*. N indicates the nucleus of an adjacent enterocyte.

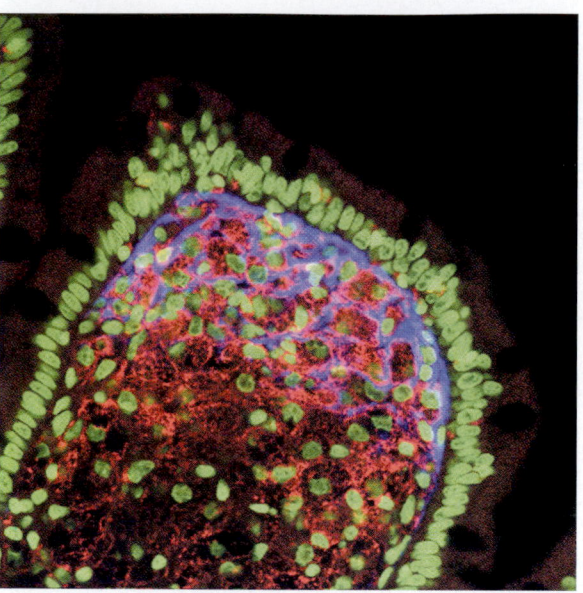

FIGURE 109-8. Fluorescent in situ hybridization of a small intestinal mucosal biopsy specimen in a patient with Whipple's disease. In this confocal micrograph of a single villus, nuclei of human cells are green, the intracellular cytoskeletal protein vimentin is red, and *Tropheryma whipplei* ribosomal RNA (rRNA) is blue. The *T. whipplei* rRNA signal is most intense in the extracellular spaces of the lamina propria, immediately subjacent to the basal membrane. (×200.) *(Courtesy David N. Fredricks, MD, Seattle, Wash.)*

authors have speculated may be of host origin.[117] Most of the structurally intact bacteria, including dividing forms, are found outside of host cells in the lamina propria (see Fig. 109-7).[8,117] In contrast, the intracellular bacteria in macrophages are often found in various stages of degradation. Findings based on FISH and using specific *T. whipplei* 16S rDNA probes support and extend the findings derived from electron microscopy[11]; the 16S rRNA signal from metabolically active bacteria is found in the intestinal lamina propria, just beneath the basement membrane, but it is absent from the PAS-positive macrophages (Fig. 109-8). Thus, *T. whipplei* appears to prefer extracellular environments within the host, despite its association with eukaryotic cells. Following the success of *T. whipplei* laboratory cultivation, antisera have been raised against *T. whipplei* isolates and have been used for testing small intestine, lymph node, heart, and brain tissue[12,118,119]; observed staining patterns are similar to those of PAS staining. These *T. whipplei*-specific antisera do not react with control bacteria and tissues affected by other diseases; however, immunohistology has not yet become widely available for routine diagnostic purposes.

Mucosal infiltration with PAS-positive cells usually is diffuse, but patchy lesions may be present. The cellular reaction generally is dominated by macrophages, while neutrophils, eosinophils, lymphocytes, and plasma cells are scarcer.[61,120] This cellular composition is unusual for an invasive bacterial infection, and suggests a disturbance of mobilization and chemotaxis of leukocytes.[61]

Variants of the usual histologic findings occur in some patients. These include rare cases with PAS-positive macrophages that are located exclusively in the submucosa, and rare cases with epithelioid granulomas in the affected

mucosa.[61] Taken together, the intestinal histopathology of WD demonstrates some heterogeneity. Although the characteristic lesions are almost invariably present in the proximal small intestine, they might extend continuously as far as to the terminal ileum.[79,121] Occasionally, the diagnosis of WD is first made with ileal biopsies obtained during colonoscopy.

During treatment, histologic findings in the intestinal mucosa change substantially but slowly, over several months or more.[50,61] Apart from a continuous decrease in the number of PAS-positive macrophages, the pattern of cellular infiltration of the mucosa changes from diffuse to patchy, necessitating multiple biopsies during follow-up endoscopic examinations. Mucosal infiltration shifts from the upper part of the mucosa (i.e., villi) to the lower part of the mucosa (i.e., pericryptal lamina propria) and submucosa. More significantly, the cytologic aspects of the PAS-positive macrophages undergo changes.[61] Before treatment, most macrophages have numerous granular particles in the cytoplasm that stain intensely red with PAS (type 1 macrophages; see Fig. 109-6). Within 1 to 6 months of treatment, the percentage of type 1 macrophages gradually decreases, and, in parallel, cells with only some coarse granular inclusions and a background of diffusely or finely granular, more faintly PAS-positive cytoplasm (type 2 macrophages) increase in number.

After 6 to 15 months, most macrophages that are still present have diffuse and faintly PAS-positive material in their cytoplasm, but lack granular inclusions (type 3 macrophages). Type 3 macrophages contain only filamentous remnants of bacteria.[61] Thus, their positive PAS reaction reflects the presence of glycoprotein residues of degraded bacterial cell walls. Even in adequately treated patients, some type 3 macrophages usually persist, occasionally for more than 10 years; in fact, the finding of type 3 macrophages alone is consistent with intestinal remission. Despite documented clinical remission of intestinal disease, however, some patients still harbor viable *T. whipplei* and can later develop extraintestinal WD. Thus, the prognostic value of intestinal histology during the follow-up of patients is limited.[61]

Extraintestinal Pathology

Autopsy reports of untreated patients with WD have revealed involvement of virtually any organ and tissue.[79] As with intestinal disease, the histologic hallmark of extraintestinal involvement is the presence of macrophages with intracellular PAS-positive granular particles. Because such PAS-positive findings are not specific for WD, however (see sections on diagnosis and differential diagnosis), their diagnostic significance in extraintestinal tissues is limited and additional evidence (e.g., positive findings on electron microscopy or PCR) is required for the diagnosis of WD. Rod-shaped bacteria of typical size and morphology for *T. whipplei* have been documented by electron microscopy in many extraintestinal organs, including liver, heart, lung, brain, eye, lymph nodes, bone marrow, and spleen[8]; these findings are consistent with direct involvement of *T. whipplei* in affected tissues.

Two different types of lymph node lesions are common in WD. Abdominal nodes generally contain lipid deposits that induce a granulomatous foreign body type of reaction.[1] Peripheral lymph nodes (inguinal, axillary, cervical) generally do not contain lipids but feature small clusters of epithelioid macrophages, some of which have PAS-positive particles that correspond to inclusions with *T. whipplei*. Rarely, and most commonly in the mediastinum, a third type of lymph node reaction may be observed that resembles sarcoidosis.

WD affects diverse regions of the brain. Most commonly, perivascular infiltrates of PAS-positive macrophages are present, as well as granulomas of variable size, consisting of glial cells with intensely PAS-positive granular particles.[8] Occasionally, granulomas in the ventricular system cause occlusive hydrocephalus. PAS-positive macrophages often can be detected free in the CSF, even in patients without neurologic or psychiatric symptoms.

DIAGNOSIS

The majority of patients with WD suffer from involvement of the intestinal tract, regardless of whether GI symptoms are present or absent.[21,22,80,81] Thus, the primary diagnostic approach to a patient with clinically suspected WD should be EGD (see Fig. 109-5) with mucosal biopsy. To avoid sampling errors in patients with patchy lesions, one should obtain approximately 5 biopsy specimens from regions as far distal as possible within the small intestine.[23] Histologic examination with routine H&E and PAS stains is usually sufficient to reach a working diagnosis (see earlier); however, it is recommended that PAS-positive histologic findings be confirmed with other methods when establishing the diagnosis of WD. Traditionally, electron microscopy has been used as the gold standard for this purpose by showing bacteria of characteristic size and shape[8]; more recently, PCR analysis has taken over the role as the preferred confirmatory test.[40,41]

Since the molecular characterization of *T. whipplei*, a number of PCR-based assays have been developed for diagnostic purposes.[10,34,40,41,122,123] These assays vary by their target DNA sequences and amplification strategy as well as by their degree of validation. Newer PCR tests increasingly use the real-time PCR platform.[99,123,124] In almost all patients with a histologic diagnosis of WD, well-designed and well-standardized PCR assays detect *T. whipplei* DNA in the intestinal mucosa.[40,41] PCR from intestinal biopsies is more useful

as a confirmatory or supplementary test than as a primary diagnostic approach, because WD only rarely is diagnosed by PCR in the setting of histologically negative intestinal biopsies,[40-42] and because *T. whipplei* DNA has been detected in asymptomatic control subjects.[43,44] In practical terms, normal intestinal histology in the absence of suggestive extraintestinal disease excludes the diagnosis of WD, provided that multiple biopsy specimens are examined.

Extraintestinal manifestations warrant the examination of specimens from affected sites. Histology and cytology with PAS staining, electron microscopy, and PCR all are useful for this purpose. A number of cases have been reported with positive PCR results in extraintestinal samples and intestinal histology that is negative for PAS-positive macrophages. Examples of such cases include febrile illness with erythrocyte-associated bacteria, and cases of uveitis, endocarditis, or neurologic disease.[95,96,99,101,111,123,125]

In an effort to distinguish between true WD and asymptomatic carriage, 1 study used quantitative real-time PCR with different sample types.[123] When both saliva and stool were positive, the sensitivity was 65% and the positive predictive value was 95% for detecting intestinal manifestations. The positive predictive value increased to 100% when the bacterial load was greater than 10^4 per gram of stool. When PCRs from both stool and saliva were negative, the negative predictive value for intestinal disease was 96% (1 of 23 intestinal cases was PCR-negative in both stool and saliva). The sensitivity for diagnosing extraintestinal disease was insufficient. Similarly, PCR from peripheral blood lacked sensitivity in this study, and its diagnostic value previously has been questioned.[126]

Considering the systemic nature of the disorder, it is important to evaluate commonly involved organ systems on a routine basis whenever a new diagnosis of WD has been established. US examination might reveal enlarged mesenteric lymph nodes that have unusually high echogenicity due to lipid deposits.[70] Neurologic examination is indicated, including the sampling of CSF.[93] Based on cytologic or PCR analysis of the spinal fluid, 70% of patients with intestinal WD in 1 study were found to have CNS infection with *T. whipplei*, even though they had no neurologic or psychiatric symptoms.[93] Imaging studies of the brain generally are not helpful in the absence of neurologic symptoms. In selected patients with WD and anemia, wireless capsule endoscopy (WCE) might detect a site of bleeding in the small intestine. In 1 case report of a patient with WD, WCE revealed diffuse disease and discrete areas of bleeding in the middle and distal portions of the jejunum, although the exact reason for the bleeding was not defined.[121]

During treatment, diagnostic assessments should be repeated at regular intervals. Endoscopic lesions usually resolve within months but can last for up to a year.[116] Intestinal histology improves within several months,[61] and PCR assays on intestinal biopsy tissues convert to negative within a time range of about 1 to 12 months after appropriate therapy has been instituted.[40] Some PAS-positive macrophages can persist for years,[61] even while the patient remains in clinical remission (see earlier). Enlarged abdominal lymph nodes can require more than a year to regress and can result in fibrosis. Follow-up examination of the CSF should include PCR analysis.[93] As has been documented in a culture-positive case, *T. whipplei* can persist in a viable state in the CNS despite prolonged administration of antibiotics.[28]

DIFFERENTIAL DIAGNOSIS

Almost all symptoms and findings of WD are nonspecific. The broad spectrum of possible clinical presentations generates a wide differential diagnosis, involving several subspecialties of medicine: gastroenterology, infectious diseases, rheumatology, cardiology, hematology, neurology, psychiatry, and ophthalmology.

Disorders that mimic the histology of WD are uncommon.[18] PAS-positive cells in intestinal biopsies can include mucosal smooth muscle cells that are rich in glycogen, or plasma cells that contain immunoglobulin (Russell bodies) in the setting of chronic duodenitis; other disorders include macroglobulinemia, intestinal xanthelasmas, and pseudomelanosis duodeni. Rarely, PAS-positive cells reflect infection with *Mycobacterium avium* complex or *Rhodococcus equi* (in HIV co-infected hosts), or *Histoplasma capsulatum*. Differentiation from WD usually is possible by means of histochemical stains (e.g., stains for acid-fast bacteria and use of diastase) and by immunocytochemistry.[18]

Sarcoid-like granulomas are rare in WD but can occur in the stomach,[127] small intestine,[61] liver,[128] and lymph nodes. A possible relationship between WD and sarcoidosis remains unresolved.[129] By means of PCR analysis, thoracic sarcoidosis[130] and intestinal sarcoidosis[131] tissues were both found to be negative for *T. whipplei* DNA.

Most patients with WD have enlarged abdominal lymph nodes.[82] Rare cases have been observed of WD associated with metachronous or synchronous malignant lymphomas,[82,83] but the relationship of *T. whipplei* infection to lymphoma, if any, remains unclear.

TREATMENT AND PROGNOSIS

The initial response of WD to antibiotic treatment usually is prompt.[132] Diarrhea often resolves within several days, arthralgias often resolve within a few weeks, and significant weight gain occurs within a few months.[78] In the 1970s and early 1980s, long-term tetracycline therapy usually was given,[21,81] but it became increasingly clear that patients treated in this manner often suffered relapses, many of which affected the CNS.[85] CNS relapses have a poor prognosis because they are often refractory to renewed treatment.[85] It therefore was suggested that the treatment of WD include antibiotics that cross the blood-brain barrier. Since the mid-1980s, trimethoprim/sulfamethoxazole has been used commonly.[85,133]

Sources of information concerning the choice of antibiotic treatment are numerous case reports,[8] several clinical series,[16,21,80,81] a few retrospective analyses of antibiotic regimens,[85,132] 1 randomized clinical trial,[134] and experimental susceptibility testing of cultivated isolates of *T. whipplei*.[135,136] In a retrospective analysis of 88 patients,[85] relapses were most common after monotherapy with tetracyclines, and this included relapses affecting the CNS. Only a small number of relapses, none of which affected the CNS, were observed after initial parenteral treatment with penicillin plus streptomycin, followed by long-term oral tetracycline (termed the "Duke regimen"). Tetracyclines were compared with trimethoprim/sulfamethoxazole (TMP/SMX) in another series of 30 patients.[132] TMP-SMX was superior to tetracyclines in inducing remission and was associated with a lower number of CNS relapses. However, despite its superior efficacy and ability to cross the blood-brain barrier, TMP/SMX treatment has been associated also with instances of treatment failure, including cases of CNS relapse as well as instances of acquired resistance by *T. whipplei*.[132,137-140] Some patients with treatment failure on oral antibiotics benefited from salvage therapy with courses of IV third-generation cephalosporins,[93,141] or from changes to other oral antibiotics, such as rifampin[138] or the oral third-generation cephalosporin, cefixime.[137]

An immune reconstitution inflammatory syndrome (IRIS), similar to that seen in the treatment of HIV infection, may complicate treatment of WD. It manifests as unexplained clinical deterioration starting from days up to a few months after the initiation of treatment. It was observed in roughly 10% of patients in 1 series and found to be more common in patients who received immunosuppressive treatment for articular manifestations preceding the diagnosis of WD.[142] IRIS often responds favorably to corticosteroid treatment.

The sole randomized clinical trial of treatment in WD[134] tested 2 weeks of IV induction therapy with ceftriaxone against 2 weeks of IV induction with meropenem, followed in both trial arms by 1 year of oral TMP/SMX, in 40 patients. No relapses were observed in either treatment group within a median follow-up period of 89 months; 1 death occurred in each group from unrelated causes; and 1 patient initially treated with ceftriaxone and retreated with meropenem experienced asymptomatic persistence of *T. whipplei* DNA in the CSF for 6.5 years that was eventually eradicated by a combination of minocycline and chloroquine.

Antibiotic susceptibility test results have become available from experiments with *T. whipplei* strains in culture, by way of assessing growth in the presence of the drugs with real-time PCR.[135,136] In co-culture with fibroblasts, the bacterium appears susceptible to doxycycline, macrolides, penicillins, rifampin, teicoplanin, and TMP/SMX; variably susceptible to imipenem; and only moderately susceptible or resistant to cephalosporins, fluoroquinolones, and vancomycin.[135] In axenic medium, the results were similar to those in cell culture, except that *T. whipplei* was susceptible to ceftriaxone and vancomycin.[136] Genome sequence analysis shows that *T. whipplei* lacks the gene for dihydrofolate reductase, which is the target for trimethoprim action,[143] so that the susceptibility to TMP/SMX most likely is based solely on its sulfamethoxazole component. Consistent with this, trimethoprim was found inactive in laboratory experiments.[136] Therefore, it has been proposed that the TMP/SMX combination should be replaced with single sulfonamide treatment, such as with sulfadiazine, which also has good CNS penetration.[97,144]

Another treatment regimen—doxycycline in combination with hydroxychloroquine—arose from in vitro experiments showing that this combination was bactericidal. Hydroxychloroquine raises the pH of intracellular vacuoles and thereby enhances the intracellular activity of doxycycline.[135] Initial clinical experience with this regimen (doxycycline 100 mg orally twice per day plus hydroxychloroquine 200 mg orally 3 times per day) in several patients with intestinal WD and *T. whipplei* endocarditis has been encouraging[97]; however, failure has also been reported in 1 patient.[145] Because of poor CNS penetration of doxycycline, it has been suggested that a sulfonamide be added to this regimen in patients with neurologic involvement.[97] One group of authors used a combination of minocycline and chloroquine—based on the fact that minocycline has better CNS penetration than other tetracyclines—to eradicate long-standing asymptomatic persistence of *T. whipplei* in the CSF of 1 patient.[146]

In summary, most treatment recommendations for WD include an induction phase of about 2 weeks using either penicillin G plus streptomycin, a third-generation cephalosporin (e.g., ceftriaxone), or a carbapenem (e.g., meropenem), followed by oral treatment, preferably with a drug that crosses the blood-brain barrier well (e.g., TMP-SMX or sulfadiazine) for at least 1 year, possibly longer. Initial results with the combination of doxycycline and hydroxychloroquine appear promising and await further clinical evaluation. An overview of antibiotic treatments, including suggested doses, is given in Table 109-1.

TABLE 109-1 Antibiotics Used to Treat Whipple's Disease

Drugs	Dose	Comments	Reference(s)
Ceftriaxone	2 g IV once or twice daily	Induction therapy (first 10-14 days) or salvage therapy	93,134
Meropenem	1 g IV 3 times daily	Induction therapy (first 10-14 days)	134
Penicillin G + streptomycin	6-24 million units IV daily (in divided doses) + 1 g IM once daily	Induction therapy (first 10-14 days)	8,78,85
TMP/SMX	160 mg/800 mg PO twice daily	Long-term therapy; first-line drug; good CNS penetration, but CNS relapses can occur	85,132
Sulfadiazine	1-1.5 g PO 4 times daily	Single sulfonamide for long-term therapy; limited experience	97,144
Penicillin VK	500 mg PO 4 times daily	Alternative for long-term therapy; limited experience	8,85
Doxycycline (or tetracycline)	100 mg PO twice daily (500 mg PO 4 times daily)	Long-term therapy, but relapses are a problem; may be combined with hydroxychloroquine	78,85,132
Minocycline	100 mg PO twice daily	Alternative to doxycycline with better CNS penetration; may be combined with hydroxychloroquine	146
Cefixime	400 mg PO twice daily	Alternative for long-term therapy; limited experience	137
Rifampin	600 mg PO once daily	Second-line drug; good CNS penetration	87,138
Chloramphenicol	500 mg PO 4 times daily	Second-line drug; worrisome side effects	5,8,87

CNS, central nervous system; IM, intramuscular; PO, oral; TMP/SMX, trimethoprim/sulfamethoxazole.

KEY REFERENCES

Full references for this chapter can be found on www.expertconsult.com.

8. Dobbins WO III. Whipple's disease. Springfield, Ill.: Charles C. Thomas; 1987.
10. Relman D, Schmidt T, MacDermott R, et al. Identification of the uncultured bacillus of Whipple's disease. N Engl J Med 1992; 327:293.
11. Fredricks D, Relman D. Localization of Tropheryma whippelii rRNA in tissues from patients with Whipple's disease. J Infect Dis 2001; 183:1229.
12. Raoult D, Birg M, LaScola B, et al. Cultivation of the bacillus of Whipple's disease. N Engl J Med 2000; 342:620.
13. La Scola B, Fenollar F, Fournier P, et al. Description of Tropheryma whipplei gen. nov., sp. nov., the Whipple's disease bacillus. Int J Syst Evol Microbiol 2001; 51:1471.
14. Bentley S, Maiwald M, Murphy L, et al. Sequencing and analysis of the genome of the Whipple's disease bacterium Tropheryma whipplei. Lancet 2003; 361:637.
15. Raoult D, Ogata H, Audic S, et al. Tropheryma whipplei Twist: A human pathogenic actinobacteria with a reduced genome. Genome Res 2003; 13:1800.

16. Ojeda E, Cosme A, Lapaza J, et al. Whipple's disease in Spain: A clinical review of 91 patients diagnosed between 1947 and 2001. Rev Esp Enferm Dig 2010; 102:108.
21. Vital Durand D, Lecomte C, Cathébras P, et al. Whipple disease: Clinical review of 52 cases. Medicine (Baltimore) 1997; 76:170.
22. Lagier JC, Lepidi H, Raoult D, et al. Systemic Tropheryma whipplei: Clinical presentation of 142 patients with infections diagnosed or confirmed in a reference center. Medicine (Baltimore) 2010; 89:337.
28. Maiwald M, von Herbay A, Fredricks D, et al. Cultivation of Tropheryma whipplei from cerebrospinal fluid. J Infect Dis 2003; 188:801.
45. Schneider T, Moos V, Loddenkemper C, et al. Whipple's disease: New aspects of pathogenesis and treatment. Lancet Infect Dis 2008; 8:179.
61. von Herbay A, Maiwald M, Ditton H, et al. Histology of intestinal Whipple's disease revisited: A study of 48 patients. Virchows Arch 1996; 429:335.
93. von Herbay A, Ditton H, Schuhmacher F, et al. Whipple's disease: Staging and monitoring by cytology and polymerase chain reaction analysis of cerebrospinal fluid. Gastroenterology 1997; 113:434.
97. Fenollar F, Puéchal X, Raoult D. Whipple's disease. N Engl J Med 2007; 356:55.

CHARLES F. HAINES AND CYNTHIA L. SEARS

CHAPTER OUTLINE

Infectious diarrhea is a major cause of illness throughout the world. Despite advances in oral rehydration therapies, vaccines, and sanitation, diarrhea remains a common cause of morbidity and mortality in developing countries, where its greatest impact is on infants and children. In 2010-2011, 1.7 billion episodes of diarrhea were estimated to occur globally in children younger than 5 years of age, with approximately 700,000 deaths.[1] Current estimates of the diarrheal disease burden in Western countries are limited. At least 70% of diarrheal illnesses are linked to food or water transmission, however, and a widely cited 1999 estimate for United States foodborne disease suggested that 76 million foodborne illnesses occur annually.[2] Thus, even in the United States, diarrheal disease accounts for a substantial health and economic burden due to loss of time from school or work.

This chapter focuses on bacterial and viral diarrhea and proctocolitis in adults. Disease due to many of the pathogens discussed is linked to ingestion of contaminated food or water (Table 110-1). Other key topics in enteric infectious disease are covered in Chapter 16 (persistent diarrhea), Chapter 34 (human immunodeficiency virus), Chapters 35 and 36 (immunocompromised patients), Chapter 111 (food poisoning syndromes), Chapter 112 (*Clostridium difficile*), and Chapters 113 and 114 (parasitic infections).

SUSCEPTIBILITY TO INTESTINAL INFECTION

Acquisition of an enteric infection is the result of the interaction of host factors that typically protect against infection and microbial virulence factors that function to overcome host defenses.

Host Defense Factors

Gastric acidity is a crucial first-line host defense that ingested pathogenic bacteria and other pathogens must survive to infect the small or large intestine.[3] In general, bacterial pathogens are highly susceptible to low pH, a pH below 4.0 being rapidly bactericidal, and achlorhydria facilitating bacterial survival during gastric passage. Consistent with the importance of gastric acid as a host defense, treatment with PPIs, and to a lesser degree with the shorter-acting and less potent H2RAs, is a risk factor for bacterial gastroenteritis, including *C. difficile* infection.[4]

The intestinal epithelium provides multiple components that contribute to protection of the host against potential enteric pathogens.[5] Within the intestine, commensal microbiota as well as potential enteric pathogens first encounter the mucus layer that coats the epithelium; this mucin complex is composed primarily of a secreted network of highly glycosylated MUC2 mucins. The outer loosely organized luminal mucus layer serves as a habitat for commensal microbiota in the colon, whereas the inner gel-like mucus layer largely excludes direct bacterial-epithelial cell contact. Bacteria that do penetrate this layer are thought to be cleared rapidly by the host mucosal immune system.[6]

Multiple cell types within the intestinal epithelium—including enterocytes, Paneth cells, goblet cells, and M cells—help protect the host against enterocolitis. Mechanisms of such protection include barrier formation via the tight junctions of enterocytes, enterocyte and Paneth cell secretion of

TABLE 110-1 Estimated Proportion of Infections with Common Enteric Pathogens That Are Foodborne and Travel Related

Pathogen	% Foodborne Illnesses	% Travel Related
Nontyphoidal salmonellae	94-95	11
Shigella spp	20-31	15
Campylobacter spp	80	20
STEC*	68-85	3.5-18
ETEC*	100	55
Yersinia spp	90	7
Non-cholera *Vibrio* spp	50-87 (depending on species)	10
Noroviruses	26-40	15

*ETEC, enterotoxigenic *Escherichia coli*; STEC, Shiga toxin-producing *E. coli*.
Data from Scallan et al. Emerg Infect Dis 2011; 17:7-15; Mead. Emerg Infect Dis 1999; 5:607-25; Dechet et al. Clin Infect Dis 2008; 46:970-6; and COVIS 2009 data.

antimicrobial molecules, goblet cell secretion of mucins, and M-cell presentation of antigens to the mucosal immune system, initiating, in many instances, a protective mucosal immune response. Specific molecules on cells of the intestinal epithelium also contribute to resistance to pathogens. Of particular importance are pattern recognition receptors (PRRs), which mediate recognition of microbes and lead to activation of innate and adaptive immune responses in the intestinal mucosa. The inflammatory responses that follow can serve to protect the host or, conversely, contribute to disease development.[7] Among key mechanisms protecting the host is the production of secretory immunoglobulin (Ig)A, which can be both nonspecific (e.g., through microbial agglutination) or specific, as part of a pathogen-specific adaptive immune response. Members of the commensal microbiota, as well as potential enteric pathogens, can initiate quite specific mucosal immune responses. Studies of these mucosal immune mechanisms have provided abundant and evolving insights into the complexity of host immune responses. Lastly, the enteric nervous system (ENS), which is involved with normal intestinal motility (see Chapters 99 and 100), also contributes to protect the host. Impaired intestinal motility in the setting of enteric infections, as well as hormones and molecules produced by the host, are known to influence disease severity.[8]

The luminal resident microbiota in the colon is composed of 10^{13} to 10^{14} bacteria per gram of stool and has increasingly been recognized as a powerful contributor to resistance to colonization and disease development with enteric pathogens. This is arguably best illustrated by the marked clinical responses of recurrent *C. difficile* colitis to fecal microbiota transplant therapy (see Chapter 130). Historical data as well as a recent controlled clinical trial demonstrate that approximately 80% to 90% of cases of this often recalcitrant condition respond to restoration of a healthy and diverse microbiota.[9]

Bacterial Factors

Bacterial pathogens have evolved various virulence factors and mechanisms that enable them to overcome host defenses, including adherence factors, enterotoxin and cytotoxin elaboration, and mucosal invasion among others.[10-13] The ability of bacteria to adhere to host mucosal cells is critical to the initial interaction of each enteric pathogen with the intestinal epithelium. Numerous adhesins that differ in morphologic features and receptor specificities have been identified and vary in their capacity to mediate colonization in human compared with animal hosts. The complexity of adherence mechanisms is enhanced by the observation that particular bacteria express and use more than 1 adhesin, a redundancy that likely enhances bacterial virulence. Many bacterial adhesins recognize oligosaccharide residues of glycoproteins or glycolipids displayed in the mucus or surface of intestinal epithelial cells.[13]

Enteropathogenic *Escherichia coli* (EPEC) cause disease, in part, because of tight intestinal epithelial adherence and serve as a classic model of the potential stages of adherence for enteric pathogens and their mechanistic complexity. EPEC initially exhibit non-intimate attachment to intestinal epithelial cells. This initial attachment is mediated by a bundle-forming pilus associated with a large plasmid common to EPEC isolates. Next, EPEC induces signal transduction events in the intestinal epithelial cells that lead to cytoskeletal changes in the enterocyte. Finally, intimate attachment of EPEC to the host cell membrane results and is mediated by an EPEC outer membrane protein called *intimin* that is encoded by the *eaeA* gene cluster on the EPEC chromosome.[14] This classic ultrastructural change, known as an *attaching-effacing lesion*, leads to elongation and destruction of microvilli, with classic pedestal formation (Fig. 110-1).[15] The role of the *eaeA* gene as a virulence factor that causes diarrhea in human EPEC infection has been confirmed in volunteer challenge studies.[16]

Non-intimate attachment using other adhesin molecules is typical of other noninvasive bacteria such as enterotoxigenic *E. coli* (ETEC), where molecular studies have demonstrated that non-intimate attachment through surface protein antigens known as *pili* or *fimbriae* (also referred to as *adherence-* or *colonization-factor antigens*) is required for a bacterium to colonize and be fully pathogenic. These adhesins bind to specific receptor sites on the surface of the intestinal cell via specific ligand-receptor interactions. Classic studies by Moon and coworkers, in which loss or gain of fimbriae by genetic manipulation resulted in the loss or gain of the ability to adhere to and colonize the intestine, identified that these colonization factors are important to the pathogenesis of *E. coli* diarrheal disease in animals.[17] Adherence not only permits colonization but also can facilitate delivery of enterotoxin to the epithelium.[17,18]

Production of toxins, usually proteins, by enteric pathogens is a key mechanism that contributes to the expression of diarrhea after infection. Nonetheless, asymptomatic colonization by enteric pathogens known to produce toxins and other virulence factors is common. Enteric toxins can be classified by their functional effect on the intestinal epithelium or by their precise molecular mechanism of action.[12] From a functional perspective, there are 2 major groups of enteric bacterial toxins: enterotoxins and cytotoxins. Classic enterotoxins such as cholera toxin or the enterotoxins of ETEC induce intestinal secretion without altering the morphology of the intestinal epithelium. The predominant site of action of most enterotoxins is thought to be the small intestine. In contrast, cytotoxins such as the *C. difficile* toxins or Shiga toxins of *Shigella dysenteriae* and *E. coli* (e.g., *E. coli* O157:H7 among others) often act in the colon, where morphologic changes in the intestinal epithelium result through a variety of mechanisms, such as by inducing epithelial cell injury or death, altering the cytoskeleton of the epithelial cells, and/or inducing an inflammatory response that results in injury to the epithelium. In addition, the actions of several enteric bacterial toxins, such as the *C. difficile* toxins, are known to be complemented by their

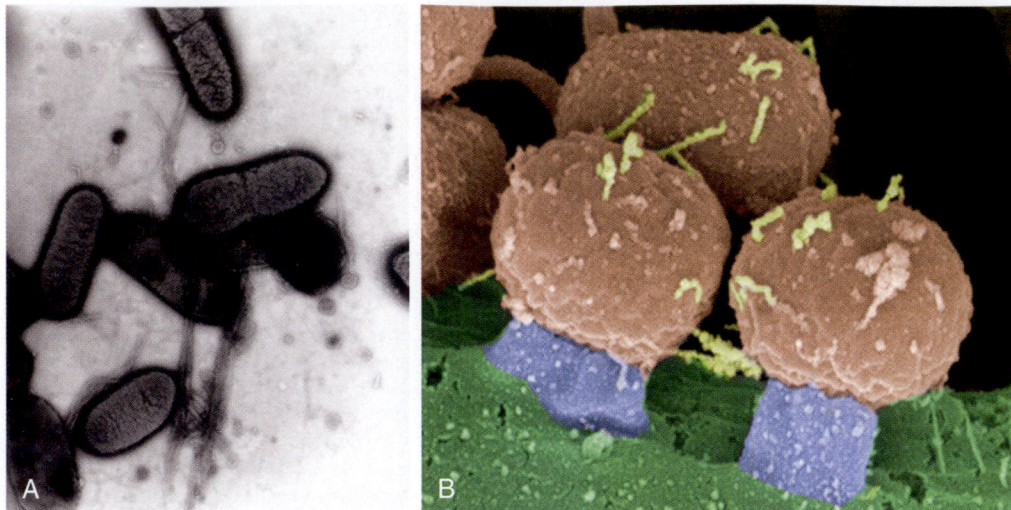

FIGURE 110-1. *A*, Electron micrograph of enteropathogenic *Escherichia coli* (EPEC) and the characteristic bundle-forming pilus. *B*, Electron micrograph of EPEC adherent to a cell and demonstrating the attaching and effacing lesion, also called *pedestal formation*. EPEC *(brown)*, pedestal *(blue)*, cell *(green)*. *(Micrographs courtesy Dr. Jorge A. Giron, Puebla, Mexico.)*

ability to alter enteric nervous system activity, also likely contributing to disease pathogenesis.

Although abundant descriptions of biological activity of many potential bacterial toxins identified in enteric bacteria exist, precise molecular mechanisms of action have been identified for but relatively few bacterial enteric toxins.[10,12] Classic mechanisms of action include alteration of intestinal epithelial cell cyclic nucleotide levels (e.g., cholera toxin, *E. coli* LT [heat-labile] or STa [heat-stable] toxins); inhibition of protein synthesis (e.g., Shiga toxins); modifications of actin cytoskeleton (e.g., *C. difficile* toxins [see Chapter 112]); and pore formation (e.g., *Clostridium perfringens* enterotoxin [see Chapter 111]). Other mechanisms likely contributing to induction of disease by enteric bacterial toxins include alteration of epithelial cell calcium signaling and changes in arachidonic acid metabolism among others. Ultimately, proof of the role of a particular enteric bacterial toxin in human disease is via volunteer studies and infrequent. Examples of enteric bacteria and their toxins studied in humans include *Vibrio cholerae*, *Shigella* spp., and pathotypes of *E. coli* among others.[12]

Disease induction by some enteric pathogens requires their ability to invade and multiply within intestinal epithelial cells, with resultant cell injury and possibly cell death that incites a mucosal inflammatory response. *Shigella* species, *Salmonella* species, *Campylobacter jejuni*, *Yersinia enterocolitica*, and some (enteroinvasive) strains of *E. coli* are classic examples of bacteria for which invasion contributes to disease pathogenesis. While the colon is most often the primary site of pathology with invasive enteric bacteria, non-*dysenteriae Shigella* spp. also produce enterotoxins that stimulate small bowel secretion and contribute to the first phase of watery diarrhea seen in shigellosis. Subsequent colon colonization and cellular invasion by non-*dysenteriae Shigella* spp. then results in colon inflammation with colitic symptoms and, occasionally, bloody diarrhea.

GENERAL PRINCIPLES OF INFECTIOUS ENTERITIS AND PROCTOCOLITIS

Evaluation

Only about 10% of patients who develop diarrheal disease present for medical consultation. The initial step in the diagnostic evaluation of a patient with acute diarrhea is a thorough history and physical examination, the goals of which are to identify patients who may be at risk of severe illness or susceptible to complications, and to identify risk factors for infection and those who will benefit from specific therapy. Most patients simply need rehydration therapy. Consideration of the patient's general health, severity and duration of illness, and the setting in which the illness was acquired should enable the clinician to determine who needs further evaluation (Fig. 110-2).

Patients who are debilitated, malnourished, or immunocompromised, and those who have severe comorbid illnesses, are at increased risk for complications of diarrhea and infection. The morbidity and mortality of infectious diarrheal diseases are highest in children younger than 5 years of age (particularly severe in those <2 years old[1]) and older adults. These high-risk patient groups may require hospitalization for diagnosis and treatment. Other patients who also require a more aggressive approach include those with systemic signs and evidence of inflammatory diarrhea, illnesses lasting more than 3 to 5 days, a history or physical examination suggesting specific pathogens that will benefit from specific therapy (Table 110-2), and infection with certain specific organisms (e.g., *V. cholerae*, *Salmonella* Typhi).[19] Bloody diarrhea can be considered a medical emergency and often requires hospitalization for diagnosis and management[20]; for example, Shiga toxin-producing *E. coli* (STEC) infection can present with bloody diarrhea, and early, aggressive fluid management may diminish complications (e.g., renal failure) of this infection.[21]

A traditional approach to help guide clinical diagnostic considerations has been the division of acute, presumably infectious, diarrheal disease into 2 broad clinical syndromes: a watery, non-inflammatory diarrheal syndrome and an inflammatory diarrheal syndrome (Table 110-3); a subgroup of the latter is the proctitis diarrheal syndrome. Classically, patients with non-inflammatory diarrhea present with watery stools without visible blood or pus, and sometimes complain of severe abdominal pain. These patients generally have few systemic signs or symptoms, and fever often is absent; abdominal cramping, nausea, and vomiting can occur. This syndrome is most frequent in individuals infected with enterotoxigenic pathogens or viruses (see later). Many pathogens that cause inflammatory disease, however, can mimic this

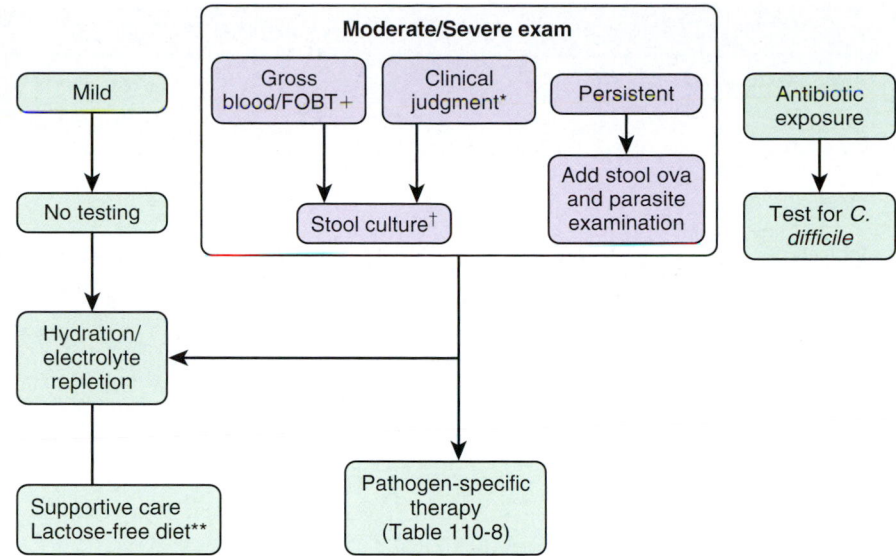

FIGURE 110-2. Algorithm for the diagnosis and treatment of infectious diarrhea. *Factors to be considered in assessing the diarrhea include whether it is community-associated and if the patient is immunocompromised, and the nature of the exposure (e.g., seafood, camping). **Avoid alcohol, caffeine, and lactose. Soft, easily digestible foods like soups, bananas, mashed potatoes, and rice are helpful. †Culture and sensitivities, Stx (Shiga-toxin) enzyme immunoassay (to detect all Shiga toxin–producing *Escherichia coli* [STEC]). *Clostridium difficile* toxin B testing is suggested when risk factors (most commonly antibiotic exposure and/or inpatient or outpatient health care exposure) are present. Additional, risk groups for *C. difficile* disease include postpartum women (because of exposure to colonized infants), patients with IBD, and young children (see Chapter 112). FOBT, fecal occult blood test.

TABLE 110-2 Clinical Findings That Suggest the Causative Organisms for Some Inflammatory Diarrheas

Finding	Causative Organisms
Hemolytic-uremic syndrome/thrombotic thrombocytopenic purpura	Shiga toxin-producing *Escherichia coli*; most common with *Shigella dysenteriae* among *Shigella* spp., but *S. dysenteriae* is not found in USA
Reactive arthritis*	*Salmonella* spp., *Shigella* spp., *Campylobacter* spp., *Yersinia* spp.
Bone marrow suppression	*Salmonella* serovars Typhi and Paratyphi
Guillain-Barré syndrome	*Campylobacter jejuni*
Toxic megacolon	*Shigella* spp., *Clostridium difficile*, *Salmonella* (rarely)
Aortitis/endovascular infection	Nontyphoidal salmonellae
Intestinal hemorrhage/perforation	*Salmonella* serovars Typhi and Paratyphi, TB enteritis
Right lower quadrant tenderness	*Yersinia* spp.
Cellulitis	*Vibrio vulnificus* and *alginolyticus* (see text)
Post infection IBS	All, including viral gastroenteritis; viruses typically yield less severe post infection IBS
Small bowel lymphoproliferative disease	*Campylobacter jejuni*

*Can occur with any enteric pathogen.

syndrome, particularly in the early phases of disease development (see later *Shigella* section).

Classically, patients with inflammatory diarrhea present with numerous small-volume stools that may be visibly mucoid, grossly bloody, or both. Such patients may appear toxic and usually are febrile. Abdominal cramping may be severe. Because of the small stool volumes, these patients are less likely to be dehydrated than those with non-inflammatory diarrhea. Organisms causing inflammatory diarrheas are typically invasive and usually affect the colon (see Invasive

Pathogens, later). Fecal leukocytes by microscopy (or positive stool lactoferrin test) and/or detection of fecal blood indicate an acute inflammatory process, and sheets of polymorphonuclear leukocytes (PMNs) usually indicate colitis. The acute inflammatory diarrheal syndrome also can have a noninfectious etiology, such as UC, Crohn's disease, radiation or ischemic colitis, and diverticulitis. Figure 110-3A-C shows the endoscopic appearance of selected inflammatory diarrheas.

Proctitis syndrome is characterized by frequent painful bowel movements that contain blood, pus, and mucus.

TABLE 110-3 Characteristics That Help Distinguish Inflammatory from Non-inflammatory Diarrhea

Characteristic	Inflammatory Diarrhea	Non-inflammatory Diarrhea
Clinical presentation	Bloody, small-volume diarrhea; lower quadrant abdominal cramps; patients may be febrile and toxic	Large-volume, watery diarrhea; patients may have nausea, vomiting, generalized abdominal cramps
Site of involvement	Colon	Small intestine
Diagnostic evaluation	Indicated	Indicated if the patient is severely volume depleted or appears ill
Fecal leukocytes	Frequently present	Small numbers often present
Causes	*Shigella* spp., *Salmonella* spp., *Entamoeba histolytica*, *Campylobacter* spp., *Yersinia* spp., invasive *Escherichia coli*, *Clostridium difficile*	Viruses, *Vibrio* spp., *Giardia lamblia*, enterotoxigenic *E. coli*, other enterotoxin-producing bacteria

Modified from Park SI, Giannella RA. Approach to the adult patient with acute diarrhea. Gastroenterol Clin North Am 1993; 22:483-97.

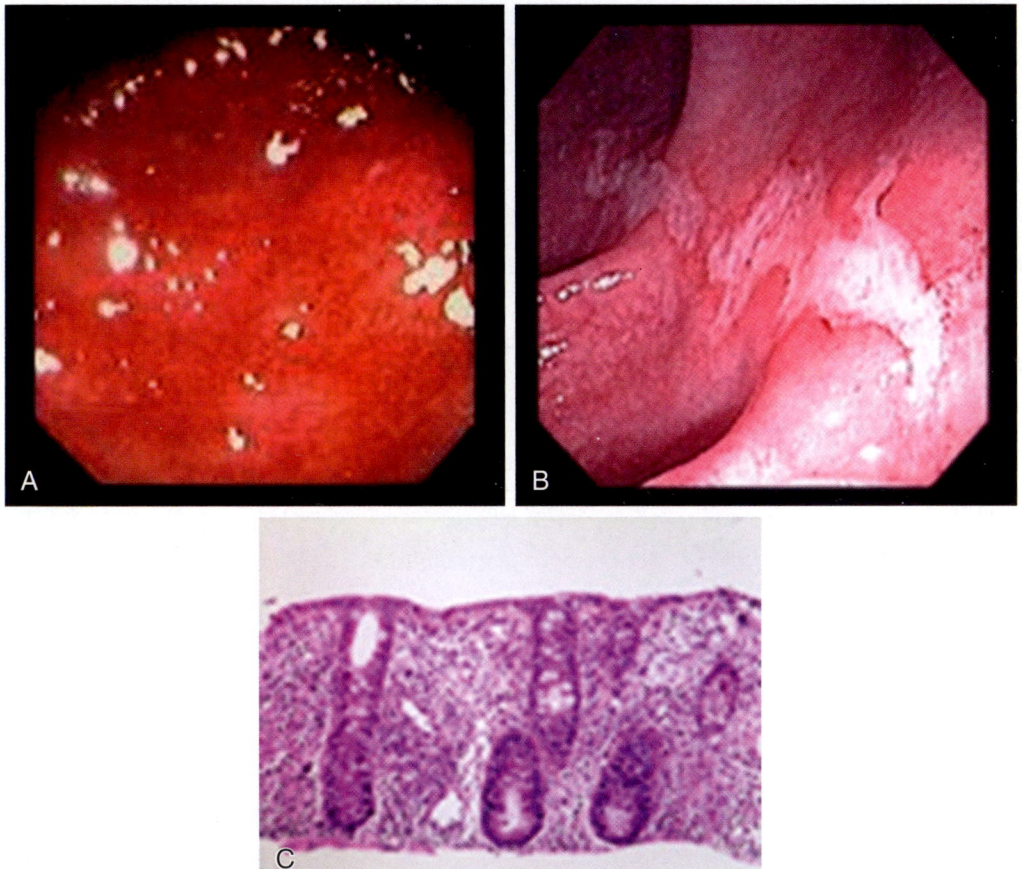

FIGURE 110-3. Sigmoidoscopy and histopathology of acute self-limited infectious colitis. A, a 24 year-old with bloody diarrhea in whom sigmoidoscopy revealed mucosal inflammation with erythema, edema, granularity, and loss of the normal vascular pattern. Stool culture grew Salmonella. The gross appearance resembles that of inflammatory bowel disease. B, a 58 year-old woman with bloody diarrhea in whom colonoscopy revealed mucosal inflammation with large, flat ulcers in the ascending colon. Stool culture grew *Campylobacter jejunii*. C, Histopathology of acute self-limited colitis, the cause of which could have been *Campylobacter*, *Salmonella* or any one of a number of other bacteria. The presence of inflammatory cells throughout the lamina propria and straight glands without architectural distortion or branching helps to differentiate acute from chronic colitis.

Tenesmus, often with rectal pain, usually is prominent. When acute, the most likely cause is 1 or more infectious agents (see Sexually Transmitted Infectious Proctitis, later). When a careful history reveals persistent, intermittent symptoms, non-infectious causes such as idiopathic ulcerative proctitis or Crohn's proctitis become diagnostic considerations.

Our growth in understanding the pathophysiology of infectious diarrheal diseases has led us to appreciate that inflammation is common to all infectious enterocolitides, with some infections (e.g., *S. dysenteriae* type 1) inducing dramatic colonic inflammation, and others (e.g., *V. cholerae*[22] and ETEC[23]) that induce more modest small bowel or colon inflammation. Thus, the classic division of enteric pathogens into those inducing non-inflammatory or inflammatory diarrhea is imperfect, and inflammation in response to enteric pathogens represents a continuum. Critical to the clinician, however, is identifying the patient at risk for morbidity or mortality due to infectious diarrheal disease. Most cases of watery diarrhea result in self-limited illnesses that require only advice on hydration maintenance and possibly diet. Evaluation of such patients with mild diarrhea for less than 3 to 5 days is typically unnecessary. By contrast, patients who often require diagnostic evaluation are those with particular risk factors such as extremes of age, 1 or more immunocompromising conditions, marked stool frequency, or dehydration. Thus, the clinician's assessment of the degree of illness, combined with the patient's history, are key contributors that guide clinical judgment regarding diagnostic evaluations in diarrheal disease. Frank clinical or fecal evidence of acute inflammatory diarrhea or bloody diarrhea always deserves a diagnostic evaluation, and diagnostic evaluations should always precede initiation of empirical antibiotic therapy of diarrheal disease.

Risk Factors

As already discussed, age is a primary determinant of diarrheal disease morbidity, with those at the extremes of age (i.e., <5 years and >65 years), particularly those living in long-term care facilities, at increased risk for poorer outcomes. Gastroenteritis outbreaks are common in nursing homes in high-income countries, with notable pathogens including norovirus, rotavirus, STEC, and *C. difficile* among others.[24-27] Enhanced risk of diarrheal disease in older adults is due to numerous factors, such as comorbid medical conditions, altered immunity with senescence, intestinal dysmotility, exposure to medications including antibiotics, and drug-induced or acquired hypochlorhydria.[4]

Immunocompromising conditions influence the risk of acquisition and disease severity for numerous enteric pathogens. Classic immunocompromising conditions include malignancy and its treatment, hemopoietic or solid organ transplantation, medications such as glucocorticoids or other immune modulators, and HIV infection. For example, lymphoproliferative diseases, glucocorticoid therapy, and HIV infection markedly increase the risk for salmonellosis. However, a number of other conditions, the immune effects of which are less well characterized, also enhance the risk of infection with enteric pathogens, including diabetes mellitus or liver disease (e.g., *Vibrio vulnificus*), hemolysis (e.g., salmonellosis), and iron overload (e.g., yersiniosis).

Food exposures or ingestion of contaminated water also constitute major risk factors for acquisition of enteric pathogens (see Table 110-1) (also see Chapter 111). Ingestion of undercooked or raw foods (e.g., meats such as hamburger or chicken, oysters, clams, other seafood) and unpasteurized milk or juices (e.g., apple cider) are of particular concern. Travel, largely because of exposure to contaminated food or water, is a classic risk factor for acquiring infectious diarrheal disease (see Traveler's Diarrhea, later). Animal exposures such as on farms or in petting zoos at county or state fairs (e.g., *Campylobacter*, *Salmonella*, STEC) or recreational exposures (e.g., camping or adventure tourism) also pose risk for enteric infections. Exposure to health care facilities, including hospitalization and treatment with antibiotics, increase the risk for *C. difficile* infection (see Chapter 112). Gastroenteritis and/or asymptomatic carriage of enteric pathogens is common in children in day care centers and serve as a source for infections in adults caring for the children.

Pregnancy and the peripartum period enhance risk for transmission of enteric pathogens. A pregnant woman may transmit enteric pathogens carried asymptomatically to the newborn child, who may then develop clinical disease. Conversely, neonates or infants can transmit infection, particularly *C. difficile*, to their mothers or caretakers, because *C. difficile* infection is typically asymptomatic in children under the age of 1 year. Ingestion of delicatessen foods by pregnant women may lead to bacteremia, septicemia, meningoencephalitis, fetal loss, or neonatal infection from *Listeria monocytogenes*. Onset of these serious illnesses may occur up to 30 days after the implicated food exposure.[28] Older adults and those with impaired immune systems are also at increased risk for invasive *L. monocytogenes* infection after contaminated food ingestion. In contrast, the immunocompetent host ingesting a food highly contaminated with *L. monocytogenes* develops abrupt but short-lived diarrheal illnesses with fever.[29]

Differentiating IBD and Infectious Diarrhea

The clinical distinction between infectious dysentery and UC can be difficult because diarrheal stools in both illnesses contain mucus and blood. Two features of infectious dysentery that distinguish it from UC are detection of a pathogen on diagnostic studies and a self-limited course that responds to antimicrobial therapy without relapse. Positive diagnostic tests for a pathogen in adults with diarrhea, however, are obtained in only about 50% of those studied.[30,31]

Longitudinal studies in the 1990s provided some guidance in differentiating acute infectious colitis and early-onset IBD.[32] Most patients with infectious colitis present early (within 1 week) to the physician and have early fever and a different histopathology upon biopsy (see later). In contrast, patients with IBD often have prior abdominal symptoms upon a careful history, less fever, and present later (>1 week after symptom onset). Travel may cause a patient to manifest either an acute exacerbation of IBD because chronic symptoms worsen as a result of travel-acquired enteric infection or de novo IBD that develops as a result of an altered intestinal microbiome superimposed on a genetic predisposition (see Chapters 115 and 116). Lastly, higher volume or frequency of diarrhea (especially >10 stools per day) is more commonly due to an infectious pathogen than IBD.

Histopathologic examination of colonic mucosa obtained by endoscopic biopsy can be helpful. Both the microbial form (dysentery) and idiopathic forms of acute colitis show edema, neutrophils throughout the lamina propria, and superficial cryptitis with preservation of the normal tubular crypt pattern (see Fig. 110-3D). Idiopathic UC, however, shows signs of chronicity (e.g., lymphoplasmacytosis) that typically involves the lower third of the lamina propria, and architectural crypt distortion (e.g., colonic glands with signs of regeneration such as branching). Resolving dysentery may have lymphocytes infiltrating the lamina propria, similar to UC, but crypt distortion and regeneration will not be present. Ultimately, there is no substitute for correlating clinical, endoscopic, and histopathologic features of disease to arrive at the proper diagnosis.[32,33]

Laboratory Diagnosis

Laboratory diagnosis of acute diarrheal disease should be pursued in any patient judged as moderately to severely ill by the clinician (e.g., fever, toxicity); in patients with risk factors (see earlier) including antibiotic exposure; in patients whose symptoms suggest inflammatory diarrhea or who have bloody diarrhea; and in patients with significant symptoms that persist beyond 3 to 5 days after disease onset. In general, most episodes of acute diarrheal illness in the United States are self-limited; diagnostic testing may be kept to a minimum, and treatment is aimed at preventing dehydration.

Recently published guidelines on utilization of the microbiology laboratory for the diagnosis of infectious diseases provide a comprehensive resource on fecal testing to identify enteric pathogens including bacterial, viral, and parasitic agents (http://cid.oxfordjournals.org/content/early/2013/06/24/cid.cit278.full.pdf).[34] Crucial points in diagnostic testing are: (1) Only diarrheal stools (i.e., those that take the form of the container) should be tested; (2) Rectal swabs are inferior to stool culture for testing in adults (and rejected by many clinical microbiology laboratories) but perform similarly in children; (3) Communication with the clinical microbiology laboratory is essential because the diagnostic testing capabilities of clinical microbiology laboratories vary. In particular, if the clinician is concerned about a particular organism(s), this should be communicated to the laboratory. Specific examples are STEC, *Vibrio*, and *Yersinia* testing, which may only be done on special request and/or require the assistance of public health authorities; (4) With improving technology and increasing use of molecular tests, single stool specimens in adults detect approximately 90% of enteric pathogens and, in children, 98%. Thus, 1 sample for children and a second for selected adult patients is reasonable for diagnosis. In patients with the proctitis syndrome, 1 sample is typically adequate for diagnosis. There are also published guidelines on the use of stool culture for enteric bacterial detection other than *C. difficile* in hospitalized adults.[35]

A range of tests are used to identify enteric pathogens, including bacterial and viral cultures, various pathogen-specific nucleic acid amplification tests (NAATs), and immunoassays (e.g., enzyme or fluorescent based; see later STEC

section), ova and parasite examinations, and certain specialized stains. Fecal examination for leukocytes, although a traditional approach to differentiate non-inflammatory and inflammatory diarrhea, is limited by the ability of most enteric pathogens to induce some inflammation and observations that even classic inflammatory pathogens (e.g., *Salmonella*, *Shigella*, *C. difficile*) often do not induce a marked fecal leukocyte response (Table 110-4). Further, the presence of sheets of PMNs is consistent with both infectious and non-infectious colitis. One commercial panel that can simultaneously detect 11 common viral, bacterial, and parasitic causes of infectious gastroenteritis from 1 stool sample received FDA clearance in 2013; published experience with this test, however, is limited.[36] Even with the use of several diagnostic tests, detection of the inciting cause of presumably infectious community-acquired diarrhea, even upon the patient's presentation to an emergency department for care, remains only about 50%.[30,31]

More invasive investigations, including flexible sigmoidoscopy with biopsies and upper GI endoscopy with duodenal aspirate and biopsies, are reserved for special situations like the immunocompromised host in whom stool examination has not yielded a diagnosis. Flexible sigmoidoscopy can be useful in evaluating patients with proctitis, tenesmus, or sexually transmitted diseases, or in identifying the pseudomembranes of *C. difficile* infection.

ENTEROTOXIGENIC PATHOGENS

The prototypical organisms in this group are *V. cholerae* and ETEC, both of which elaborate enterotoxins that cause dehydrating diarrhea. The salient characteristic of diarrhea caused by *V. cholerae* and ETEC is that disease primarily results from intestinal fluid loss, which is related to the action of the enterotoxin on the small intestinal epithelial cells. These organisms usually do not invade the mucosal surface, and thus, mucosal architecture remains intact. The fecal effluent is watery and often voluminous, producing clinical features of dehydration. Bacteremia is rarely a complication of toxigenic diarrhea.

Vibrio cholerae

Cholera, the prototypical toxigenic diarrhea, can cause dehydration and death within a few hours of onset.[37,38] Stool output can exceed 1 L/hr, with daily fecal outputs of 15 to 20 L if

TABLE 110-4 Variability in Clinical Presentation of Inflammatory Enteric Pathogens

Symptom/Sign/Test	STEC O157:H7	*Campylobacter* spp.	*Salmonella* spp.	*Shigella* spp.
		%		
Fever	41.4	50.9	69.4	56.6
Abdominal pain	72.0	45.4	28.8	33.5
Bloody stool	91.3	37.0	33.8	54.3
Gross blood	63.0	7.8	4.8	14.7
Occult blood	82.8	52.0	43.4	59.1
Fecal leukocytes	70.5	42.9	29.4	37.8
Peripheral leukocyte count >10,000/mm³	70.9	42.0	45.3	58.0

STEC, Shiga toxin-producing *E. coli*.
Adapted from Slutsker L, Ries AA, Greene KD, et al. *Escherichia coli O157:H7 diarrhea in the United States: Clinical and epidemiologic features. Ann Intern Med* 1997; 126:505-13.

parenteral fluid replacement keeps up with losses. The acutely ill patient typically has marked signs of dehydration: poor skin turgor, "washerwoman's" hands, absent pulses, reduced renal function, and hypovolemic shock.

More has been learned about pathophysiology—and normal intestinal function—from cholera than from any other intestinal disease.

Microbiology

First described in cholera stool by Filippo Pacini in 1854, *V. cholerae* is a Gram-negative, short, curved rod that looks like a comma. It is actively motile by means of a single polar flagellum. Vibrios are strongly aerobic and prefer alkaline and high-salt environments.

More than 200 serogroups of *V. cholerae* have been described, based on the O antigen, a cell wall lipopolysaccharide. Epidemic and pandemic disease are only caused by the O1 and O139 serogroups. *V. cholerae* strains that fail to agglutinate O1 or O139 antisera are referred to as *non-O1 non-O139 V. cholerae* and, in addition to diarrhea, occasionally cause severe extraintestinal infections, particularly in compromised hosts.[37]

The O1 serogroup is composed of 2 biotypes, classical and El Tor, which are differentiated on the basis of biochemical characteristics and/or biotype-specific genes. Further differentiation into 3 serotypes is based on type-specific O antigens (A, B, C: Ogawa [A, B]; Inaba [A, C]; Hikojima [A, B, C]).[39]

Toxigenic *V. cholerae* that agglutinates in O1 antiserum is the main cause of epidemic cholera. El Tor biotype *V. cholerae* is responsible for the current pandemic that began in 1961. El Tor vibrios are somewhat hardier than others in nature. Clinical disease is similar with both biotypes, although on average, El Tor infections are milder. The major serotypes associated with clinical disease are Inaba and Ogawa, and rarely Hikojima. The El Tor Inaba type was responsible for the 1991 outbreak in South America and a variant El Tor strain from South Asia for the 2010 Haitian cholera outbreak.[40]

In 1992, a toxigenic non-O1 strain, now designated *V. cholerae* O139 Bengal, was responsible for an epidemic that started in southern India and Bangladesh and spread rapidly to many countries in Southeast Asia.[41,42] This organism is closely related to *V. cholerae* O1 El Tor, with likely substitution of O139 for the O1 antigen via a genomic island.[38]

Cholera Toxin

Among the more than 200 serogroups that comprise the *V. cholerae* species, only serogroups O1 and O139 typically carry the cholera toxin genes. Cholera toxin (CT) is an 84-kd heterodimer composed of 5 B subunits that encircle a single A subunit. The B subunit is responsible for binding to the monoganglioside GM1 receptor on the intestinal epithelial cells. The A subunit is responsible for activation of adenylate cyclase located on the basolateral cellular membrane. The genetic material for CT is contained on a filamentous bacteriophage, CTXΦ, which can be integrated into a host chromosome or replicate as a plasmid.[43] *V. cholerae* also produces additional toxins that may contribute to disease, including the zonula occludens toxin (ZOT) that alters intestinal permeability by acting on intestinal epithelial cell tight junctions,[44] and the accessory cholera enterotoxin (ACE).[45]

Epidemiology

Seven cholera pandemics have occurred in the last 200 years. The seventh pandemic is ongoing and originated in Indonesia in 1961, spread through Asia, Africa, and South America, and is caused by the El Tor biotype. This biotype generally causes a milder disease with a higher frequency of inapparent infection compared with that caused by the classical biotype. In 2011, there were 589,584 cases and 7816 deaths reported to the WHO; most of these cases were from a large outbreak in Haiti following the devastating earthquake in 2010.[46] Cholera cases are underreported,[46] but a common estimate of the total disease burden is 3 to 5 million cases and 120,000 deaths annually.[47] In the United States, 42 cases were reported in 2011, of which 40 were imported.[46]

The clinical features of infection with the *V. cholerae* O139 strain are virtually indistinguishable from infection caused by *V. cholerae* O1.[48,49] To date, *V. cholerae* O139 has remained confined to Southeast Asia,[46] and the incidence has declined in most areas, save for pockets in China and Thailand.[50] In 1992, an El Tor variant emerged that produces the CT found previously only in classical O1 biotypes and is associated with more severe disease[51]; this variant El Tor strain also caused the 2010 Haitian outbreak described earlier.[40]

Cholera has both endemic and epidemic phases, with epidemics often superimposed on existing endemic cholera. The primary vehicle for spread of cholera is contaminated food and water, and a high inoculum dose ($\approx 10^8$ to 10^{11} organisms) is typically required for infection. There also is a complex aquatic environment reservoir, likely including copepods, zooplankton, aquatic vegetation, and water fowl, which maintains low levels of *V. cholerae*.[52] Cholera has marked seasonal variation and may emerge as a public health problem as a result of increased growth with warming of the environmental reservoir.[37,38] Spikes in aquatic *V. cholerae* counts are associated with human disease. Individuals with mild hypochlorhydria may represent a high-risk population.[52] Once cholera enters the human population, transmission will often become direct (human-to-human) via contact with feces or immediate contamination of food or water in the household. So-called rice water feces (see later) contains high concentrations of *V. cholerae* organisms, which are hyperinfectious for about 5 to 24 hours after passage. In epidemics, it appears that the majority of infections are due to direct transmission.[52] Locations with dense populations, poor sanitation, limited health infrastructure, and logistical issues, such as the conditions present in Haiti following the 2010 earthquake, all contribute to direct transmission.[38]

Pathogenesis

The clinical syndrome of cholera is caused by the action of the toxin on intestinal epithelial cells. Cholera toxin increases adenylate cyclase activity, resulting in elevated levels of cyclic adenosine monophosphate (cAMP) in the intestinal epithelial cells, and this in turn causes intestinal secretion. Fluid loss in cholera originates in the small intestine. The most sensitive areas are the upper intestine, particularly the duodenum and upper jejunum; the ileum is less affected, and the colon usually is in a state of absorption and is relatively insensitive to the toxin. Diarrhea results because the large volume of fluid produced in the upper intestine overwhelms the absorptive capacity of the colon.

Attachment of *V. cholerae* to the intestinal mucosa is mediated by various surface components, including a fimbrial colonization factor known as *toxin-coregulated pilus*. The toxin-coregulated pilus attachment protein might play an important role in producing naturally occurring protective antibodies against *V. cholerae*.[53]

Despite the derivation of the term *cholera* (Greek: *chole*, bile), the appearance of choleric stools resembles rice water; that is, the stool has lost all pigment and becomes a clear fluid with small flecks of mucus. The electrolyte composition

TABLE 110-5 Electrolyte Concentrations of Choleric and Nonspecific Fecal Fluid and of IV Fluids Used to Treat Infectious Diarrheas

Type of Fluid	Electrolyte Concentrations (mmol/L)			
	Sodium	Potassium	Chloride	Bicarbonate
Choleric Stool				
Adult	124	16	90	48
Child	101	27	92	32
Fecal fluid in Nonspecific Diarrhea (Child)	56	25	55	14
IV Therapy Solutions				
Lactated Ringer's	130	4	109	28*
5:4:1[†‡]	129	11	97	44
2:1[§]	141	—	94	47

*Equivalent concentration after lactate conversion to bicarbonate.
[†]Add glucose, 110 mmol/L (20 g/L).
[‡]IV solution that is 5 g of sodium chloride, 4 g of sodium bicarbonate, and 1 g of potassium chloride per liter.
[§]Solution that has a carbohydrate-to-sodium ratio of 2:1.

(Table 110-5) is isotonic with plasma, and the effluent has a low protein concentration. On microscopic examination of stool during *V. cholerae* O1 infection, there are typically few inflammatory cells and only small numbers of shed mucosal cells; *V. cholerae* O139, however, induces more intestinal inflammation.

Cholera vibrios (other than O139) do not invade the mucosal surface, and bacteremia is virtually unknown in this disease. A biopsy specimen taken from the mucosa during acute cholera largely shows normal architecture, in sharp contrast to the inflammatory and ulcerating lesions associated with *Salmonella* and *Shigella*.

Clinical Features

Like many other infectious diseases, there is a spectrum of clinical manifestations with *V. cholerae*, from an asymptomatic carrier state to a desperately ill patient with severe dehydration. Notably, in field situations, the clinical case rate is approximately 0.26%; that is, for every clinical case of cholera, there are approximately 400 asymptomatic people who have had contact with the organism, as demonstrated by an elevation in vibriocidal antibody titers. Thus, acquired immunity and genetic determinants (e.g., blood type) modulate disease expression. In clinical cholera, the initial stage is characterized by vomiting and abdominal distention and is followed rapidly by diarrhea that accelerates over the next few hours to frequent large volume rice-water stools. All the clinical symptoms and signs can be ascribed to fluid and electrolyte losses. Patients present with profound dehydration and hypovolemic shock, often leading to kidney failure. The stool is isotonic with plasma, although there is an inordinate loss of potassium and bicarbonate, with resultant hypokalemic acidosis (see Table 110-5). Mild fever may be present, but there are no signs of sepsis.

Treatment

Treatment of acute cholera is based on the physiologic principles of restoring fluid and electrolyte balance and maintaining intravascular volume. These objectives are accomplished with IV solutions or oral fluids that contain electrolytes in isotonic concentrations (see Table 110-5). Particular attention is paid to administration of bicarbonate and potassium, which are lost excessively in choleric stool. Various oral rehydration solutions (ORS) have been developed for treating mild to moderate cases (Table 110-6).[54]

The simple therapeutic principles of fluid replacement and antibiotic use saves many lives. This knowledge has been available only since approximately 1970; before then, the mortality rate for cholera was 50% to 75%. Application of these physiologic principles reduces the mortality rate in adults to less than 1%, as exemplified by such a mortality rate in the Peruvian epidemic in 1991. Children with cholera still have a mortality rate of 3% to 5% because fluid reserves are limited in young children.

Antimicrobial agents are useful ancillary measures to treat cholera, because their use reduces stool output, duration of diarrhea, fluid requirements, and *Vibrio* excretion. The CDC recommends doxycycline as a single oral dose of 300 mg for nonpregnant adults and 2 to 4 mg/kg for children (not to exceed 300 mg). A single oral dose of azithromycin 1 g is recommended for pregnant women.[55] Antimicrobial resistance to fluoroquinolone antibiotics, for example, is an increasing concern, but because of risk of direct transmission, antibiotics are indicated for moderate and severe cholera.[56] Antimicrobial therapy usage should be tailored to local *V. cholerae* susceptibility patterns when known. Zinc supplementation has been shown to reduce the duration and volume of diarrhea among children with cholera in Bangladesh and may be a useful adjunct to standard therapy.[57]

Vaccines

Currently, no vaccines for the prevention of cholera are available in the United States, nor is cholera vaccination recommended by the CDC for most travelers. The WHO has prequalified 2 oral killed cholera vaccines and currently recommends their use in endemic areas and areas at risk for outbreaks. Vaccination in response to outbreaks is indicated only for outbreaks during large humanitarian crises where high-priority prevention interventions cannot be delivered effectively.[46]

Other *Vibrio* Species

Non-O1/O139 Vibrio cholerae

In general, non-O1/O139 serogroups do not carry cholera toxin genes and cannot cause epidemic diarrheal disease, but

TABLE 110-6 Composition of Various Types of Oral Rehydration Solutions (ORS) and Commonly Used Beverages

ORS	Carbohydrate (g/L)	Sodium (mmol/L)	Potassium (mmol/L)	Chloride (mmol/L)	Base (mmol/L)[a]	Osmolarity (mOsm/L)
WHO (2002)	13.5	75	20	65	30	245
WHO (1975)	20	90	20	80	30	311
European Society of Pediatric Gastroenterology, Hepatology, and Nutrition	16	60	20	60	30	240
Enfalyte[b]	30	50	25	45	34	167
Pedialyte[c]	25	45	20	35	30	250
Naturalyte[d]	25	45	20	N/A	48	265
Pediatric Electrolyte[e]	25	45	20	N/A	30	250
CeraLyte[f]	40	50-90	20	N/A	30	220
Commonly Used Beverages (Not Appropriate for Diarrhea Treatment)						
Apple juice[g]	120	0.4	44	45	N/A	730
Coca-Cola classic[h]	112	1.6	N/A	N/A	13.4	650
Gatorade[i]	58.3	20	3.2	11	N/A	299
Gatorade carbohydrate energy formula[i]	222.5	43	11.5	N/A	N/A	1076

[a]Actual or potential bicarbonate (e.g., lactate, citrate, or acetate).
[b]Mead-Johnson Laboratories, Princeton, N.J. Additional information is available at http://www.mjn.com/app/iwp/HCP/Content2.do?dm=mjid=/HCP_Home/Product_Information/Product_Descriptions/Enfalyteiwpst=B2Cls=0csred=1r=342.
[c]Ross Laboratories, Abbott Laboratories, Columbus, Ohio. Data regarding flavored and Freezer Pop Pedialyte are identical. Additional information is available at http://www.pedialyte.com.
[d]Unico Holdings, Lake Worth, Fla. Additional information is available at http://www.unico-holdings.com.
[e]Nutramax Products, Gloucester, Mass. Additional information available at http://www.nutramax.com/.
[f]Cera Products, L.L.C., Jessup, Md. Additional information available at http://www.ceralyte.com/index.html.
[g]Meeting U.S. Department of Agriculture minimum requirements.
[h]Coca-Cola Corporation, Atlanta, Ga. Figures do not include electrolytes that might be present in local water used for bottling. Base=phosphate.
[i]Quaker Oats Company, Chicago, Ill. Additional information available at http://www.gatorade.com.
N/A, not applicable.
Adapted in part with permission from King et al. Managing acute gastroenteritis among children: Oral rehydration, maintenance, and nutritional therapy. MMWR Recomm Rep 2003; 52:1-16; and from Atia AN, Buchman AL. Oral rehydration solutions in non-cholera diarrhea: A review. Am J Gastroenterol 2009; 104:2596-604.

rather typically cause mild sporadic diarrheal illnesses. There are, however, examples of non-O1/O139 serogroups that do produce cholera toxin and have caused outbreaks of cholera-like illness in the United States.[58] Strains within the same species can produce different enterotoxins, cytotoxins, and hemolysins. The diversity of toxin production is matched by the diversity of clinical symptoms: diarrhea ranges from watery diarrhea to frank dysentery; some strains penetrate the intestinal mucosa, causing bacteremia or septicemia, sometimes with secondary end-organ involvement; others have been incriminated in wound or ear infections after exposure to ocean water or handling raw seafood.[59]

The most common antecedent history is consumption of raw oysters within the preceding 72 hours. Other seafood such as clams, mollusks, and crab all have been implicated in non-O1/O139 vibrio disease. In outbreaks, there is a high attack rate, with incubation periods that range from as short as 6 to 12 hours to as long as 3 days. Bacteremia can occur and is most common in patients with cirrhosis or who are otherwise immunocompromised. Over 90% of non-O1/O139 vibrios produce a polysaccharide capsule, and heavily encapsulated strains are associated with greater septicemia rate relative to unencapsulated strains.[60] Because the GI disease is typically self-limited and relatively benign in the United States, antibiotics are not recommended; however, septicemia, wound infections, and deep organ infections should be treated with appropriate antibiotics.

Vibrio parahaemolyticus

V. parahaemolyticus causes an acute diarrheal disease after consumption of contaminated raw fish or shellfish. Recognized as an important pathogen in Asia, *V. parahaemolyticus*

also has been isolated in the United States, although its exact prevalence is unknown. Strains of *V. parahaemolyticus* produce a number of distinct hemolysins, the most significant of which is responsible for the Kanagawa phenomenon (i.e., hemolysis of human red blood cells in Wagatsuma bacteriologic medium). Kanagawa-positive isolates are pathogenic for humans, whereas Kanagawa-negative strains are nonpathogenic members of the marine environment.

Epidemiology

Many outbreaks of *V. parahaemolyticus* gastroenteritis have been reported in Japan and the United States. According to the Cholera and Other Vibrio Illness (COVIS) Annual Summary, 2009, there were 386 reported cases of *V. parahaemolyticus* and 2 deaths.[61] Cases of all vibrio disease (excluding toxigenic *V. cholerae*) have been increasing in the United States since the mid-1990s, an increase that has been driven largely by increasing rates of *V. parahaemolyticus* disease. Cases tend to be clustered along coastal states where shellfish consumption and seawater exposure are common.[62] Rising seawater temperature has been proposed to promote outbreaks.[63]

The median attack rate of *V. parahaemolyticus* in foodborne outbreaks in the United States was 56% and varied from 3% to 100% of exposed persons. The median incubation period was 17 hours (range, 4 to 90 hours). Seafood, or cross-contamination with seafood, was the food vehicle in all outbreaks.[64]

Clinical Features

V. parahaemolyticus causes both foodborne and non-foodborne disease, and the clinical presentation may vary depending on the route of exposure. In the United States, non-foodborne *V. parahaemolyticus* infection represents only 11% of all *V. parahaemolyticus* infection, but constitutes 19% of all non-foodborne *Vibrio* spp. infections. Bacteria were most commonly isolated from wounds (79%), blood (10%), and the ear (6%). Cases tended to have fever (42%) and cellulitis (67%) and were often associated with swimming (61%), walking (49%), and boating (29%). Only 6 deaths (3%) among 216 *V. parahaemolyticus* infections were reported.[65]

Foodborne outbreaks in the United States are characterized by diarrhea with associated cramping, nausea, and vomiting. Outbreaks are most common between April and October. The median reported duration of illness was 2.4 days (range, 8 hours to 12 days). A single death was reported out of 1064 cases in outbreaks from 1973 to 1998.[64] In the United States from 1973-1998, 5% of sporadic *V. parahaemolyticus* infections presented as primary septicemia, of which over 90% had a history of recent oyster consumption; 29% of these septicemic patients died.[64] In Asia, *V. parahaemolyticus* infection has presented as a dysentery-like syndrome, but this is rarely reported in the United States.[60]

Treatment

The most important goal of *V. parahaemolyticus* gastroenteritis is repletion of fluid losses. The role of antimicrobial therapy is not clear because symptoms tend to be mild and self-limiting. Antibiotics can be considered in severe cases, based on organism sensitivity. In wound infection or septicemia, establishing control of local infection and systemic antibiotics are warranted.[60]

Additional Vibrio *Species*

V. vulnificus is perhaps the most important non-cholera *Vibrio* species in the United States because of its severity of illness, especially in patients with underlying liver disease, diabetes mellitus, or other compromising conditions. In 2009, COVIS reported 107 cases, of which 90% were hospitalized and 32% died.[61] *V. vulnificus* can be acquired as a wound infection, often with characteristic bullous, even hemorrhagic, necrotizing, skin lesions, through salt water exposure or by direct consumption of seafood, usually raw oysters; the mortality rate of resulting septicemia exceeds 50%. Because this infection can be fatal in patients with underlying liver disease, such persons should be warned to avoid eating raw seafood, especially oysters.[66] The recommended antimicrobial treatment of severe *V. vulnificus* infection (e.g., septicemia or necrotizing fasciitis) is a tetracycline plus a third-generation cephalosporin or a fluoroquinolone in conjunction with local débridement of infected tissue and supportive therapy for septicemia.[67]

In the United States, *Vibrio alginolyticus* is the second leading cause of wound infection and the leading cause of ear infections among *Vibrio* species; it is not commonly associated with foodborne vibriosis.[65] *Vibrio mimicus* acquires its name from its similarity to cholera vibrios, even in producing an enterotoxin that resembles CT, and is now believed to share a common ancestor with sixth pandemic *V. cholerae*.[68] The organism has been isolated from patients in the United States with diarrhea, septicemia, or wound infections. *Vibrio fluvialis* has a wide geographic distribution, although human disease is less common than from other *Vibrio* species.[69] Other pathogenic *Vibrio* species include *V. hollisae*, *V. furnissii*, *V. metschnikovii*, and *V. damsela*. Disease expression is similar to other non-O1/O139 vibrios and includes watery, even bloody, diarrhea, wound infections, and/or bacteremia/septicemia.

Aeromonas Species

Aeromonas species are ubiquitous environmental organisms found principally in fresh and brackish water, especially in the summer months. *Aeromonas* species are divided into 2 groups: psychrophilic (Greek: *psychros*, cold) aeromonads, which grow optimally at temperatures ranging from 22°C to 25°C, and mesophilic aeromonads, which grow best between 35°C and 37°C. Psychrophilic strains usually are isolated from environmental water sources and fish; *Aeromonas salmonicida* is the most common strain in this group. Based on their phenotypical features, the mesophilic aeromonads are grouped into 3 complexes: *Aeromonas hydrophila*, *Aeromonas caviae*, and *Aeromonas veronii*. All 3 of these *Aeromonas* species have been associated with human infection. In order to cause disease, aeromonads must adhere to and colonize the intestinal epithelium. *Aeromonas* strains produce an array of toxins, including heat-labile enterotoxin, hemolysin, and cytotoxin. There also may be some degree of invasion of the epithelial cells, with resultant dysentery or colitis.

Epidemiology

Aeromonas infections often are associated with drinking untreated water, such as well or spring water, or eating contaminated foods. Estimates of the disease burden vary widely and may differ by seasonal distribution and the predominant species. *Aeromonas* infection is not a reportable disease in the United States, so incidence data are limited. A study from California found an annual incidence of *Aeromonas* gastroenteritis of 8.6 infections/million population. Incidence was greatest in those younger than age 2 years and older than age 80 years. There was a seasonal pattern to the cases, which peaked around July and August[70]; studies in other countries have failed to demonstrate a seasonal pattern.[71] Although *Aeromonas* infection has been associated with diarrheal disease, other studies have found similar rates of aeromonad isolation from diarrhea cases and asymptomatic controls, leading some to question the pathogenicity of *Aeromonas*.[71]

Clinical Features

Aeromonas gastroenteritis can vary in clinical presentation from watery diarrhea to dysentery; diarrhea is seen in 75% to 89% of cases. Duration of diarrhea is typically 3 to 10 days, but chronic diarrhea for over 1 year has been reported; the frequency of chronic diarrhea is unknown. Fever and abdominal pain are variable.[70] Complications associated with *Aeromonas* gastroenteritis include segmental colitis, ischemic colitis, and hemolytic-uremic syndrome (HUS). *Aeromonas* septicemia may have a GI portal of entry with or without associated symptoms, particularly in immunocompromised patients, although up to 30% of septicemia cases have no underlying conditions. Furthermore, *Aeromonas* has long been recognized as a cause of wound infections after swimming in fresh or brackish water and of bacteremia or deep organ infections in immunocompromised hosts.

Treatment

Supportive care, particularly rehydration therapy, is sufficient intervention in many cases. The diarrhea is typically self-limiting and does not require antibiotics. In chronic diarrhea or in immunocompromised patients, there may be a role for antibiotics in reducing the duration of symptoms.[72] Aeromonads may carry several different β-lactamases and are consistently resistant to β-lactam antibiotics (e.g., penicillin, ampicillin, and first- or second-generation cephalosporins). Aeromonads tend to be sensitive to trimethoprim/sulfamethoxazole (TMP/SMX), third-generation cephalosporins, fluoroquinolones, tetracycline, chloramphenicol, and aminoglycosides. Given current susceptibility patterns, fluoroquinolones or third-generation cephalosporins are the preferred therapies. Carbapenems are also effective, but there have been reports of aeromonads expressing metallo-β-lactamases active against carbapenems.[72] Therapy should be altered based on antibiotic susceptibility data when available.

Plesiomonas shigelloides

Plesiomonas shigelloides is a motile Gram-negative rod, member of the family Enterobacteriaceae, and ubiquitous freshwater organism.[73] Most cases are associated with consumption of raw seafood, and the organism has been reported to cause outbreaks.[73] *P. shigelloides* also causes traveler's diarrhea and constitutes about 1% to 3% of such cases in Latin America and Africa and about 5% of such cases in Asia.[74] The pathogenesis of *P. shigelloides* infection is poorly understood. There is evidence that some degree of invasion of the colonic epithelium occurs and that several toxins also may be produced, including a cholera-like toxin.[73] Diarrhea ranges from mild and watery to severe colitis with visible blood. Abdominal pain often is prominent, and fever and vomiting are common. Extraintestinal manifestations, usually sepsis or meningitis, are rare and are more common in children and immunosuppressed patients.[73] The diarrhea is usually self-limiting, so antibiotics are likely of limited use. Chronic diarrhea and extraintestinal disease may benefit from antibiotic therapy.[73] *P. shigelloides* is commonly resistant to aminopenicillins and tetracyclines. Sporadic resistance to other antibiotics may occur. Potential effective treatment regimens are likely similar to those for other microbiological causes of dysentery and involve a fluoroquinolone, third-generation cephalosporin, or even carbapenems in severe or resistant infections, but little information is available on the efficacy of treatment.[73,75]

Escherichia coli Species

E. coli are common, but minority, commensal members of the microbiota in humans and animals. Although most strains are relatively harmless in the bowel, others possess virulence factors that cause diarrheal disease. At least 6 types of *E. coli* intestinal pathovars have been recognized (Table 110-7). Their virulence factors include toxin production, adherence to epithelial cells, and invasiveness, each of which is encoded by specific genetic elements (plasmids or chromosomal genes) that determine pathogenicity.

Enteropathogenic *Escherichia coli* (EPEC)

EPEC was initially recognized as causing severe neonatal diarrhea and remains a common cause of diarrheal illness and associated morbidity in children globally.[76] EPEC induces classic attaching and effacing lesions, in which bacteria attach to the intestinal cell membrane and cause effacement of the microvilli (see Fig. 110-1B). A common pathogenicity island (LEE, locus for enterocyte effacement) is responsible for these lesions and serves as the basis for molecular identification of EPEC.[77] EPEC is further divided into typical (tEPEC) and atypical (aEPEC). tEPEC produces bundle-forming pili, which causes a characteristic adherence pattern on cultured epithelial cells. aEPEC lacks the gene to produce bundle-forming pili and exhibit an atypical adherence pattern.[78] Once adherent, EPEC forms a pore and secretes multiple effector proteins directly into the enterocyte, which results in a complex cascade of changes within the cell. A diverse array of genes encode the effector proteins, but the functions of these proteins are not fully understood.[79] Some of the mechanisms described include disruption of tight junctions, stimulation of

TABLE 110-7 Diarrheagenic *Escherichia coli*

Strains	Pathogenic Mechanisms	Persons Affected	Clinical Features
DAEC	Diffuse adherence to Hep-2 cells	Children in developing countries	Watery diarrhea (acute) and persistent diarrhea
EAEC	Aggregative adherence to Hep-2 cells	Children in developing countries	Watery diarrhea (acute) and persistent diarrhea
STEC O157:H7 Non-O157:H7 O104:H4[a]	Shiga toxins 1 and 2	Children and adults Persons who ingest contaminated food, especially hamburger (outbreaks)	Watery diarrhea Bloody diarrhea (classic)
EIEC	Epithelial cell invasion	Children and adults	Watery diarrhea Dysentery

EPEC
  Typical
 	
  Atypical
	Attaching and effacing
	Bundle-forming pilus, attachment and effacement lesions or
	Atypical adherence pattern
		Children	Watery diarrhea (acute)
			Persistent diarrhea

ETEC	Heat-labile and/or heat-stable toxin Adherence	Children in developing countries; travelers	Watery diarrhea

DAEC, diffusely adhering *Escherichia coli*; EAEC, enteroaggregative *E. coli*; EIEC, enteroinvasive *E. coli*; EPEC, enteropathogenic *E. coli*; ETEC, enterotoxigenic *E. coli*; STEC, Shiga toxin-producing *E. coli*.
[a]EAEC that acquired Shiga toxin gene.

interleukin (IL)-8 release, stimulation of adenosine release, and inhibition of fluid resorption through disruption of NaCl transport mechanisms.[80]

EPEC has been reported as a major cause of diarrhea in children, particularly those younger than 1 year,[81] and in HIV-infected subjects.[82] In general, the burden of EPEC diarrheal disease has been declining in more recently published studies; this may be due to interventions such as breast-feeding, which is particularly effective against EPEC infection.[83] From 1990 to 2002, a systematic review of causes of pediatric diarrhea found that the median prevalence of EPEC diarrheal disease in community and inpatient settings was 8.8% and 15.6%, respectively.[76] Recent data suggest that aEPEC may be a more important pathogen than tEPEC,[84] but the proportion of diarrhea cases with aEPEC strains vary widely by both region and by studies within similar regions. Asymptomatic aEPEC colonization also may occur.[85]

Clinical presentation is characterized by acute diarrhea with vomiting and dehydration, but EPEC is also strongly associated with persistent diarrhea.[86] Although serogroup identification may suggest a diagnosis of EPEC infection, molecular methods to identify particular genes or culture methods to identify adherence patterns are superior for definitive identification of EPEC; these methods remain research procedures, and none are available for commercial use.[83,87] Little data exist on preferred antimicrobial treatment regimens. Most infections resolve spontaneously and require neither a definitive diagnosis nor antibiotics. Supportive care, notably rehydration, remains imperative in treating diarrhea, particularly in infants and children. The role of antibiotics in severe or persistent disease is unknown.[77]

Enterotoxigenic Escherichia coli (ETEC)

Inspired by the discoveries in cholera, investigators directed their attention to *E. coli* as a cause of acute toxigenic diarrheal disease. Originally in India, and thereafter in many parts of the world, strains of *E. coli* were found to elaborate an enterotoxin similar to that of *V. cholerae*.[88] ETEC is a group of *E. coli* distinct from EPEC serotypes. ETEC infections mostly are sporadic, but outbreaks of ETEC do occur.

Pathogenic Mechanisms

ETEC is acquired by consuming contaminated foods and liquids. Infection first requires adherence and then toxin production. Adherence is mediated primarily by colonization factors (CFs), which are carried on plasmids. More than 20 distinct CFs have been identified and are designated as CFA (colonization factor antigen) or CS (coli surface antigen), followed by a number. Worldwide, CFA/I, CFA/II, and CFA/IV are most common. ETEC colonizes the surface of small intestinal epithelium without penetrating the epithelial layer, and chromosomal loci *tia* and *tib* are believed to play a role in adherence to enterocytes.[89] As in cholera, there is neither mucosal damage nor bacteremia. Two types of enterotoxins are produced by ETEC.[14] The heat-labile toxin (LT) is an approximately 84-kd protein that is destroyed by heat and acid and, similar to cholera toxin, is composed of 1 A subunit and a pentameric ring of 5 B subunits. There are 2 groups of LT, LT-I and LT-II, that are differentiated on the basis of the target membrane receptor that binds the B subunit. Through its A subunit, LT acts pathophysiologically like cholera toxin by activating adenylate cyclase, thereby causing secretion of fluid and electrolytes into the small intestinal lumen.[89] The second ETEC toxin is heat stable (ST) and is able to withstand heating to 100°C. ST is a family of low molecular weight toxins with 2 primary classes, STa and STb. Only STa has

been associated with human disease; it is an approximately 2-kd peptide.[90] STa activates membrane-spanning guanylate cyclase; the resultant increase in cyclic guanosine monophosphate (cGMP) induces intestinal secretion from both the small and large intestine. ETEC strains may elaborate LT only, ST only, or both LT and ST.

Epidemiology

The major vehicles of infection appear to be contaminated foods and drinking water. In developing nations, infection occurs primarily in children younger than 2 years, and incidence declines between ages 5 and 15. Incidence then increases, and ETEC has been implicated in severe dehydrating diarrhea in adults.[91] In children younger than 5 years, there are an estimated 280 million ETEC cases in the developing world annually[92] and an estimated 380,000 deaths.[91] In a systematic review of the etiology of global diarrheal disease from 1990-2000, ETEC was the most common identified cause of community diarrhea (14.1%) and was associated with 9.5% of inpatient cases of diarrhea.[76] ETEC is also a common cause of traveler's diarrhea (~20% to 40% of cases).[91] Strains vary by country, and across the United States multiple ETEC outbreaks with varying strains have been reported since the mid-1970s; most are related to consumption of contaminated food or on cruise ships docking in U.S. ports.[93-96]

Clinical Features

In the endemic and outbreak setting, ETEC infection is typically a secretory diarrhea that can vary widely in severity but, like cholera, can cause severe dehydration. Associated vomiting is common, but fever is rare. Presentation is similar in adults and children. ST-producing ETEC may have higher risk for moderate or severe diarrhea than LT-producing ETEC in hospitalized children.[91] In a review of 17 ETEC outbreaks, 81% had a diarrhea/vomiting ratio of 2.5 or greater, which is higher than in viral gastroenteritis outbreaks, where vomiting tends to be a more prominent symptom.[93] The median incubation period was typically 24 to 50 hours and duration of illness more than 3 days.[93-96]

Immunity and Vaccines

Antibodies to the enterotoxins and colonization factors develop in persons infected with ETEC. It appears that people residing in areas at high risk for ETEC infection acquire some mucosal immunity over time.[14] Thus, for example, the risk that ETEC diarrhea would develop in students at a college in Mexico depended on their country of origin; those from South America had a relatively low risk of ETEC diarrhea, whereas those from North America had a high risk.[97] Vaccines have the potential to reduce the burden of ETEC disease. A recombinant inactivated whole cell (rCTB-CF ETEC) vaccine has shown some promise in American and European travelers to Africa, Asia, or Latin America, but failed to protect 6- to 18-month-old children in rural Egypt. Live-attenuated oral vaccines are under investigation.[91]

Diagnosis and Treatment

Molecular assays for diagnosis of ETEC are available, but often only in research settings. The stool electrolyte losses in ETEC diarrhea are similar to those in cholera, and fluid replacement should follow the same principles in both diseases. Studies of patients with acute traveler's diarrhea have demonstrated shortening of the duration of diarrhea when effective antimicrobial therapy is initiated early in the course of illness.[98,99] Although antibiotics are commonly used to treat traveler's diarrhea caused by ETEC, in endemic settings, because most episodes of ETEC diarrhea are self-limited or not specifically diagnosed, treatment with antibiotics generally is not necessary. Similar to other enteric pathogens, antibiotic resistance among ETEC strains is increasing.[98,100,101]

Enteroinvasive *Escherichia coli* (EIEC)

EIEC can be biochemically identified as *E. coli* but possesses the toxin and virulence factors of *Shigella*. Genetic analysis has demonstrated that the organisms traditionally considered to be in the *Shigella* genus should be reclassified as clones of *E. coli*.[102] Both *Shigella* and EIEC are believed to have evolved from noninvasive *E. coli*, but at different times (EIEC more recently than *Shigella*). Acquisition of the invasion plasmid (pINV) was likely the major event in the divergence of EIEC and *Shigella* from noninvasive *E. coli*. Ongoing evolution of these closely related species is predicted, such that in the future, EIEC and *Shigella* may be combined into an EIEC/*Shigella* pathovar.[103] Accordingly, the biology, epidemiology, presentation, diagnosis, and treatment will be discussed in more detail in the *Shigella* section.

Shiga Toxin-Producing *Escherichia coli*

In 1982, a new *E. coli* pathovar emerged as the cause of outbreaks of acute hemorrhagic colitis in Michigan and Ohio.[104] This new pathovar was characterized by Shiga toxin (verocytotoxin) production and was named the enterohemorrhagic *E. coli* (EHEC) pathovar, although it now is recognized by the broader term *Shiga toxin-producing* (STEC or VTEC) *pathovar*. STEC remains a major cause of foodborne diarrheal disease, particularly in the United States and Europe.

Epidemiology

STEC has become a foodborne pathogen of global importance since its emergence in 1982. In the United States, STEC is estimated to cause over 175,000 illnesses, 2000 hospitalizations, and 20 deaths annually.[105] STEC is typically classified as O157 and non-O157, with recent estimates attributing over 63,000 illnesses, nearly all of the 2000 STEC-related hospitalizations, and all 20 deaths to STEC O157.[105] A prospective study of patients presenting to emergency departments at 11 sites across the United States found that STEC was responsible for 2.6% of dysentery cases and was less common than *Campylobacter*, *Salmonella*, and *Shigella*.[106] 34 STEC outbreaks were reported to the CDC in 2010, of which 25 were O157 and 9, non-O157.[107] In 2011, FoodNet reported 463 cases of O157 and 521 cases of non-O157—again, fewer cases than *Campylobacter*, *Salmonella*, or *Shigella*; the incidence was highest among children aged 1 to 4 years. Forty-three percent of O157 cases and 18% of non-O157 cases were hospitalized, but only 2 O157 patients and 1 non-O157 patient died.[108] In 2011, Germany experienced the largest recorded outbreak of STEC, with 3842 cases. This outbreak was notable not only for its size but also a high proportion of adult patients with HUS that originated from an enteroaggregative *E. coli* (EAEC) strain that acquired the Shiga toxin gene *stx2a*.[109]

The leading vehicle of infection is hamburger meat, although outbreaks have been associated with fresh-pressed apple cider, produce, and unpasteurized milk.[110,111] Waterborne outbreaks have been associated with contaminated swimming pools and other recreational water bodies, well water, and municipal water systems.[14,111] Person-to-person transmission probably has played a role in outbreaks in day care centers, households, and nursing homes.[111,112] Infection

rates vary seasonally, and peak incidence is from June to September.

STEC strains are found in the fecal flora of a wide variety of animals, including cattle, sheep, pigs, goats, chickens, dogs, and cats. Many of these strains are of serotypes other than *E. coli* O157:H7. The most important reservoir of infection is cattle, hence, transmission via hamburger meat.

Pathogenic Mechanisms

In order to cause infection in humans, STEC must first adhere to the enterocytes. Most strains responsible for human disease cause attachment-effacement lesions as seen in EPEC and similarly carry the LEE pathogenicity island (see EPEC section).[90,113] STEC strains that lack LEE also are known to cause human disease, likely through other mechanisms.[114,115] Once attached, STEC produces many other effector molecules and a family of toxins called *Shiga toxin* (Stx). The Stx family has 2 members, Stx1 (differs from canonical Shiga tx produced by *S. dysenteriae* type 1 by 1 amino acid) and Stx2 (56% amino acid sequence identity with Stx1), each with multiple variants. Stx is composed of a homopentameric ring of 5 B subunits, responsible for receptor binding, and the A, enzymatically active, subunit. Stx toxins inhibit protein synthesis and activate numerous enterocyte signal transduction mechanisms, changing enterocytes into a proinflammatory state.[116] Transport of Stx toxins to the submucosa, with binding to endothelial cells, yields microvascular damage, platelet aggregation, microvascular fibrin thrombi, and a clinical and histologic picture that resembles ischemic colitis (See Chapter 118).[117-119] Further, Stx toxins bind to PMNs and circulate to other organs such as kidneys, where again, binding to endothelial cells initiates, in part, the cascade, resulting in HUS with renal failure.[10]

Clinical Features

After an incubation period of 1 to 14 days (mean, 3 to 4 days), watery non-bloody diarrhea begins, is associated with severe abdominal cramping, and often progresses to frankly bloody stools, especially if the infecting serovar is EHEC O157:H7. Other symptoms include nausea, vomiting, low-grade fever, and chills.

Colonoscopy demonstrates a segmental colitis with friable inflamed mucosa, patchy erythema, edema, and superficial ulcerations that is usually most evident in the ascending colon (see Fig. 110-3); virtually any part of the colon may be affected, just as with idiopathic ischemic colitis. Plain films of the abdomen might show subepithelial edema and hemorrhage (thumbprinting), usually in the ascending and transverse colon. Leukocytosis with a shift to the left usually is present, but anemia is uncommon unless infection is complicated by the development of HUS or thrombotic thrombocytopenic purpura (TTP).[117] Microscopic examination of the stool reveals red and white blood cells in low to moderate amounts. The median duration of diarrhea is 3 to 8 days, with longer durations in children and persons with bloody diarrhea.[117]

A striking association has been noted between intestinal infection with STEC and HUS. HUS is characterized by acute renal failure, microangiopathic hemolytic anemia, and thrombocytopenia. In Minnesota, the incidence of HUS increased progressively during the 1980s to the current rate of 2.0 cases per 100,000 child-years. *E. coli* O157:H7 was isolated in 46% of children presenting with HUS. Risk factors for HUS include age younger than 5 years, attendance at a large day care center, presence of bloody diarrhea, and a high WBC count.[120] The FoodNet 2011 report found that 76% of HUS cases had evidence of STEC or diarrhea.[108] A FoodNet study of STEC

O157 from 2000-2006 showed that HUS developed in 15% of children younger than age 5 years with STEC infection, and HUS developed in 6% of all STEC cases in the study.[121] In the 2011 German STEC outbreak, 855 cases of HUS (22% complication rate) were reported; 88% of cases were adults, 68% of whom were women, which differs markedly from prior reports.[122] This epidemiology was ascribed to food preferences, given the association of the outbreak with contaminated sprouts.[123]

Diagnosis

Several laboratory methods are used to diagnose STEC infections. Currently the CDC recommends a combination of culture for O157 STEC and a non-culture Shiga toxin assay.[124] Because most isolates of E. coli O157:H7 do not ferment sorbitol, screening for this pathogen usually is done with sorbitol–MacConkey agar (SMAC). Sorbitol-negative colonies can then be serotyped with commercially available O157:H7 antisera. Such colonies should be sent to a reference laboratory for confirmation.

The chances of obtaining a positive culture from stool depend on the time between the onset of symptoms and collection of the stool. Within 2 days of onset, virtually all stool specimens from O157-infected patients are positive, whereas after 7 days, only one third are positive.[125] In contrast, other studies have found that the median duration of excretion of STEC is 17 to 29 days, with some patients shedding the bacterium for as long as 124 days.[14,126,127]

Testing for Shiga toxin allows for detection of non-O157 STEC. A Shiga toxin enzyme immunoassay (EIA) has been available in the United States since 1995, and it is recommended the assay be performed on broth cultures incubated overnight, not directly on stool alone. The CDC recommends culture confirmation and strain serotyping by public health laboratories to confirm EIA-positive assays because of reports of false-positive EIA results.[124] PCR-based Shiga toxin tests have not been FDA approved, but many are used in public health departments or individual laboratories after internal validation and CLIA approval.[124]

Treatment

The desire to treat STEC infections is understandable because of the presence of bloody diarrhea and with the hope that treatment will decrease complications such as HUS; however, several reports have raised concern that the risk of HUS is increased by antimicrobial therapy. In a murine model, certain antibiotics, notably ciprofloxacin, caused enhanced STX production by E. coli O157:H7 in vitro via induction of bacteriophage encoded genes; this occurrence was associated with an increased death rate in antibiotic-treated mice.[128]

Antimicrobial therapy in humans does not appear to provide much benefit and might even be harmful. A randomized controlled trial (RCT) of TMP/SMX in children with E. coli O157:H7 enteritis found no effect of therapy on the duration of symptoms, pathogen excretion, or incidence of HUS.[129] One prospective cohort study identified 71 children with acute E. coli O157:H7 gastroenteritis, of whom only 9 had been treated with antibiotics; however, 5 of the 10 children in whom HUS developed had received either TMP/SMX or a cephalosporin.[130] In this study, antibiotic therapy was associated with a significantly increased risk of HUS, although this conclusion has been challenged by others.[131,132]

Because antibiotic use has not been shown to decrease morbidity resulting from STEC and might increase the risk of HUS, routine use of antibiotics is not recommended in the treatment of gastroenteritis if E. coli O157:H7 is the known or suspected cause. In cases of confirmed E. coli O157:H7 infection, patients should be followed closely for manifestations of HUS. A case-control study of adults with HUS in the 2011 Germany STEC outbreak demonstrated no benefit of plasmapheresis or eculizumab (a complement 5 inhibitor), although antibiotic treatment after HUS diagnosis was associated with earlier clearance of STEC and improved mortality while not affecting the HUS course.[133] Although these findings are encouraging, the applicability to other populations (pediatric) and other STEC strains is unknown. Additional studies are needed before recommendations enter routine practice.

Thorough cooking of ground beef, avoiding unpasteurized fruit juices, and hand hygiene if contact with farm animals occurs (e.g., state or county fairs) are important preventive measures.

Enteroaggregative Escherichia coli (EAEC)

Unlike the attaching and effacing adherence to cells seen with EPEC, some E. coli strains adhere in an aggregative motif, with the bacteria clumping to the cell surface in a stacked-brick pattern.[14] Although some investigations have implicated EAEC as a cause of acute and persistent diarrhea in children in developing countries,[14,134] other investigations have failed to find a significant association with diarrhea.[135-137] Up to one third of children infected with EAEC have grossly bloody diarrhea. EAEC has been associated with diarrhea in patients infected with HIV,[138] and EAEC has been shown to be a cause of traveler's diarrhea.[139]

Volunteer challenge studies with different strains of EAEC have yielded mixed results, suggesting that certain strains are more virulent than others.[139,140] As yet, there have been no studies documenting the need for or efficacy of treatment of EAEC infections. EAEC include numerous serogroups that largely are distinct from those of EPEC. Certain serotypes such as O44:H18 appear to be more pathogenic than others.

EAEC pathogenesis is complex but seems to have 3 major features: characteristic adherence, production of enterotoxins and cytotoxins, and mucosal inflammation. Adherence structures and genes in EAEC are highly diverse, with much variation among strains. EAEC toxin production is similarly diverse and variable. Some common toxins include enteroaggregative heat-stable toxin 1 (EAST1), shigella enterotoxin 1 (ShET1), and hemolysin. Most evidence suggests EAEC infection can cause mucosal inflammation through the IL-8 pathway. Several EAEC genes have been shown to affect IL-8 release.[141] In Europe during 2011, an EAEC strain that acquired Stx2a (E. coli O104:H4 [see also STEC section]) caused the largest known STEC outbreak. This outbreak was concentrated in adults and was notable for a high proportion of infections that resulted in HUS.[122]

There have been no RCTs of therapy for EAEC infections in children. One study of HIV-positive patients with diarrhea caused by EAEC found a 50% reduction in stool output, fewer intestinal symptoms, and microbiological eradication of the organism during treatment with ciprofloxacin.[142] Similarly, ciprofloxacin therapy of EAEC resulted in a reduction of the duration of diarrhea in patients with traveler's diarrhea.[139]

Diffusely Enteroadherent Escherichia coli (DAEC)

Another type of adherent E. coli is DAEC, which adheres to tissue culture cells in a diffuse pattern. DAEC constitute a heterogeneous group of organisms. The knowledge of the proteins and associated genes that mediate adherence is increasing, but the mechanism(s) of diarrhea pathogenesis remains largely unknown.[143] The role of these organisms in diarrheal disease is unclear, but they may be a cause of acute or persistent diarrhea in children.[113]

INVASIVE PATHOGENS

The principal pathogens in this group are *Salmonella*, *Shigella*, EIEC, *Campylobacter*, and *Yersinia*. There are important differences among these organisms, but they all share the property of mucosal invasion as their initiating event to cause disease resulting in endoscopic and histologic colon mucosal inflammation (see Fig. 110-3*A-D*). Three mechanisms are thought to contribute to the diarrhea caused by invasive pathogens: epithelial injury preventing fluid resorption from the intestinal lumen, induction of inflammatory mediators by organism invasion, and production of accessory virulence factors (including enterotoxins) by some invasive bacteria.

Shigella Species

Shigella organisms cause bacillary dysentery, a disease that has been described since early recorded history.[144] The inhabitants of Athens in the second year of the Peloponnesian War were ravaged by dysentery. In the American Civil War, more than 1,700,000 soldiers suffered from dysentery, with 44,500 deaths. World War I also produced a high incidence of dysentery: 371,000 total casualties in France and up to 486,000 casualties in East Africa. Although dysentery is a disease that becomes more prevalent in wartime, there is a constant endemic incidence in tropical countries and in temperate zones.

Microbiology

Shigella species are Gram-negative enteric organisms included in the family Enterobacteriaceae. Genetic evidence places *Shigella* as a member of *E. coli*, but for reasons of clinical and historical significance, it remains a separate genus (see the EIEC section).[90] Shigellae are highly adapted to the GI tract of humans and primates. The 4 major *Shigella* subgroups are *S. dysenteriae* (139 serotypes), *S. flexneri* (14 serotypes), *S. sonnei* (1 serotype), and *S. boydii* (18 serotypes)[145].

Unlike *E. coli*, shigellae are nonmotile, do not produce gas from glucose, and are generally lactose negative, except for *S. sonnei*. Group A (*S. dysenteriae* type 1), also known as the *Shiga bacillus*, produces the most severe form of dysentery. An outbreak in Central America in the late 1960s and early 1970s caused more than 10,000 deaths, mostly in young children.[146] This organism continues to cause outbreaks in many developing countries. By contrast, *S. sonnei* produces the mildest disease, most often nonspecific watery diarrhea.

Epidemiology

Shigellosis is a major diarrheal disease, estimated to cause over 165 million cases of diarrhea annually (114 million cases among children <5 years) and over 1 million deaths.[147] The epidemiology of *Shigella* has changed over time. Transmission is through fecal-oral contact. An inoculum of just 10 organisms has been shown to be capable of causing disease.[148] The ability of *Shigella* spp. to survive in acidic conditions might account for the small inoculum that can produce disease. Approximately 20% of persons in a household will acquire shigellosis after exposure to the index case.[148] Person-to-person transmission, facilitated by the low infective dose, accounts for rapid spread of *Shigella* in day care centers and among people living in conditions of poor hygiene. Secondary cases can occur in hospitals among other patients and hospital staff. Foodborne transmission, through raw foods likely contaminated by food handlers, can occur.[149] Shigellosis can also be sexually transmitted and men who have sex with men (MSM) are at increased risk.[150]

Patterns of shigellosis vary by time and region. Group A (*S. dysenteriae*) has been classically associated with epidemic disease since the late 1960s in much of the developing world. *S. dysenteriae* produces the most severe form of dysentery, with mortality rates of 5% to 15%.[151] Subsequently there was a shift towards group B (*S. flexneri*) and hyperendemic shigellosis in much of the developing world.[152] In industrialized nations, however, group D (*S. sonnei*) is the dominant species. *S. sonnei* is usually found in association with sporadic common source outbreaks.[144] The reasons for these temporal and regional changes are not known; however, as former developing nations undergo industrialization, the proportion of *S. flexneri* cases is declining and *S. sonnei* is increasing.[151,153] *S. boydii* infections remain relatively uncommon (about 6% of global reported cases) but have considerable geographic variation.[147]

It is estimated that there are 131,254 cases of shigellosis in the United States annually, with 1500 hospitalizations and 10 deaths.[105] Shigellosis in the United States is predominantly caused by *S. sonnei* (≈80%). *S. flexneri* is responsible for about 15% to 20% of cases. *S. boydii* and *S. dysenteriae* are responsible for 1% to 2% and fewer than 1% of cases, respectively. Both *S. boydii* and *S. dysenteriae* represent imported cases; *S. dysenteriae* is considered a bioterrorism threat. From 1998-2008, 110 foodborne outbreaks were reported, comprising less than 5% of total shigellosis cases reported over the same time; thus, foodborne disease is likely only a small contributor to the total disease burden.[149]

Pathogenic Mechanisms

All strains of *Shigella* may cause *dysentery*, a term that refers to a diarrheal stool that contains an inflammatory exudate composed of PMNs, mucus, and blood.

Shigella initially interacts little with enterocytes and instead triggers its uptake by M cells, after which it exits the basolateral side of the M cell into the submucosa. *Shigella* escapes resident macrophages by rapidly inducing apoptosis, which in turn elicits a robust immune response. The bacteria then invade the enterocytes via the basolateral side by macropinocytosis. Once phagocytosed, the bacteria lyse the phagosome and are released into the enterocyte cytoplasm. From there, enterocyte-to-enterocyte invasion occurs.[154]

Pathogenic *Shigella* all possess a large virulence plasmid, which has a 31-kb conserved region that encodes many virulence factors, most important of which are the invasion plasmid antigens (IpaA to IpaD) that facilitate organism entry into cells as well as escape from, for example, the phagosome. These virulence factors are injected into the enterocyte by a type III secretion system (T3SS) or injectosome, by which a needle-like protein apparatus found in some Gram-negative bacteria such as *Shigella*, but also EPIC and *Salmonella* spp., is used to inject toxin directly into a eukaryotic cell. Another virulence factor, intracellular spread protein (IcsA) catalyzes actin polymerization, which propels the bacteria forward until they reach the cell membrane. The membrane then protrudes and is endocytosed by a neighboring cell.[154]

The process of enterocyte invasion provokes a strong inflammatory response with release of IL-8 and recruitment of activated neutrophils, which effect much of the tissue damage and diarrhea. The bacteria may also release *Shigella* enterotoxin (ShET)1 and ShET2, thought to increase fluid secretion into the small intestinal lumen, contributing to the classic first phase of watery diarrhea often observed in shigellosis; the mechanisms of the ShET toxins, however, are not fully understood. Shiga toxin (Stx) is produced only by *S. dysenteriae* 1 and is related to Stx1 and Stx2 of STEC. Stx is cytotoxic and can also affect the kidneys and the central nervous system (CNS) (see STEC section).[154]

The major site of attack of *Shigella* is the colon, although scattered ulcerations can be seen in the terminal ileum as well. The stages of *Shigella* penetration of the mucosa and its cellular interactions eventuate in enterocyte death, focal ulcers, and mucosal inflammation. There is edema, formation of microabscesses (e.g., crypt abscesses), loss of goblet cells, and loss of tissue architecture (see Fig. 110-3). These events give rise to the characteristic clinical picture of bloody, mucopurulent diarrhea. Shigellae rarely penetrate beyond the intestinal mucosa and generally do not invade the bloodstream; however, bacteremia occurs in malnourished children and immunocompromised hosts.

Clinical Features

Classic *Shigella* dysentery is present in only a minority of patients, and clinical presentation varies considerably by *Shigella* spp. A volunteer study found that only 28% of subjects developed the classic symptom progression of fever (≈48 hours), abdominal pain, diarrhea (≈72 hours), and dysentery (≈120 to 144 hours).[155] Fever and abdominal pain may start within 24 hours after exposure but average 1.6 and 3.6 days, respectively. Diarrhea may begin after 24 hours and continue up to 2 weeks, but average onset is at 4 days. Dysentery may start as early as 3 days and as late as 17, but averages 7 days and may continue for more than a month.[155] Fever is present in up to 30%, diarrhea in 30% to 60%, stool mucus in 50% to 99%, and stool blood in 40% to 60%.[155-157] Dysentery is present in over 80% of patients with *S. dysenteriae* infection, and watery diarrhea in only 22%. In contrast, only 20% of patients with *S. sonnei* infection had bloody stool, and 10% had severe dehydration; most have watery diarrhea.[158]

Bacteremia is uncommon. Malnutrition, especially in young children, and infection with *S. dysenteriae* 1 are associated with a more severe course. Bacteremia may occur in young children, especially if they are malnourished. Among the intestinal complications of shigellosis are intestinal perforation and severe protein loss.

An extensive list of extraintestinal complications of various bacterial enterocolitides, including bacillary dysentery, is presented in Table 110-2.[159] Many patients complain of respiratory symptoms, such as cough and coryza, although pneumonia is rare. In young children, hypoglycemia can occur, and neurologic findings can dominate the clinical picture, even before the onset of diarrhea. Meningismus and seizures can occur with shigellosis, particularly in children (although there is no direct involvement of the CNS), and may be related to fever, metabolic derangements, and/or the effects of circulating Stx in cases of *S. dysenteriae*.[160] During the acute phase of disease, HUS may occur but is rare. *S. dysenteriae* is known to carry Stx and, on average, 13% of infections result in HUS. Risk of HUS with *S. dysenteriae* infection seems to be less when appropriate antibiotics are given within the first 4 days of symptoms. In general, early appropriate antibiotic therapy is beneficial.[161,162] Leukemoid reactions are associated with young age, *S. dysenteriae* infection, and increased mortality.[163] A rash (rose spots) can occur during the acute phase of shigellosis. Arthritis can develop 2 to 3 weeks after onset of dysentery. Joint pain or effusion usually is asymmetric and involves large joints. Arthralgias alone, not necessarily with other signs of reactive arthritis, occur, usually in patients who are positive for HLA-B27; autoantibodies to this antigen cross-react with *Shigella* proteins, thereby resulting in circulating antibody-antigen complexes.[164]

The course of shigellosis varies. Most children have mild infections, at least with non-*dysenteriae Shigella*, lasting no more than 1 to 3 days. The average length of symptoms in adults is approximately 7 days. In more severe cases, symptoms can persist for 3 to 4 weeks and often are associated with relapses. Untreated bacillary dysentery, particularly when the course is prolonged, can be confused with UC.

Deaths are rare in healthy persons, particularly adults, with bacillary dysentery; mortality usually is seen in young, often malnourished children.[152] Neurologic signs such as decreased level of consciousness and seizures are associated with a poor outcome in children.[160]

Chronic carriers of *Shigella* have been identified and can pass the organism in their feces for a year or more. Such carriers are distinctly uncommon and usually stop shedding the organism spontaneously. Carriers of *Shigella* are prone to intermittent attacks of the disease, in contrast to *Salmonella* carriers, who rarely become recurrently symptomatic with the strain they carry.

Diagnosis

Fecal specimens are required for diagnosis, because other microorganisms can also cause a dysentery syndrome (e.g., *Campylobacter*, *V. parahaemolyticus*, *Salmonella*); blood and urine rarely are positive. Because *Shigella* spp. are fastidious, stool specimens or rectal swabs should be inoculated promptly into appropriate media.

A subacute presentation of dysentery can masquerade as UC. When in doubt, treatment for shigellosis is recommended.

Treatment

The general principles for management of infectious diarrhea, most importantly rehydration, also apply to shigellosis (see Treatment, later). Antimotility agents are not recommended. Zinc supplementation (through complex actions including improving immune responses) and green bananas (by promoting production of short-chain fatty acids that serve as a metabolic energy source for colonocytes) have potential to decrease severity of shigellosis and associated morbidity.[165,166]

Antibiotic therapy reduces the duration of symptoms, duration of *Shigella* excretion in stool, and possibly complications.[167,168] No particular class of antibiotic has been shown to be superior to another, and empirical choices should be based on local susceptibility patterns.[167,168] Because of the highly contagious nature of shigellosis, antibiotic treatment is suggested for most patients with these infections, and certainly for all patients with moderate to severe disease. Antibiotic therapy is also suggested when the culture report returns positive for *Shigella*, even if the patient is now asymptomatic, to minimize shedding and transmission; this is, however, regarded as controversial by some. If shigellosis is deemed of concern by the clinician, empirical therapy should be considered—particularly if the patient is severely ill or hospitalized, immunocompromised, a health care worker, food handler, or an adult or child who is associated with day care. The value of eradicating this highly contagious infection is often compelling and generally outweighs the potential side effects of antibiotic therapy, or concerns about inducing antibiotic resistance.

Antibiotic resistance is a growing problem for *Shigella* treatment. FoodNet data in the United States from 2000-2010 found resistance to ampicillin and TMP/SMX in the majority of isolates. Travel-associated shigellosis was more likely to have resistance than domestically acquired shigellosis. Fluoroquinolone resistance was found in 0.5% of isolates.[169] If empirical treatment is indicated, a careful history focusing on regions of travel may help guide empirical antibiotic choices. In the United States, fluoroquinolones are a reasonable option for adults, whereas azithromycin or a third-generation cephalosporin is preferable in children. Recently, *S. sonnei* with decreased susceptibility to azithromycin was identified as causing an outbreak in California.[170] An older study suggested similar efficacy of azithromycin and ciprofloxacin in shigellosis, although *S. dysenteriae* type 1 exhibited higher treatment failure rates.[171] The 2005 WHO recommendations for shigellosis treatment list ciprofloxacin as the first-line regimen, followed by pivmecillinam, ceftriaxone, and azithromycin as second-line regimens. The guidelines also emphasize utilization of local resistance patterns when choosing an antibiotic.[172] Subsequent to the release of the WHO guidelines, there have been studies that showed increasing ciprofloxacin resistance, particularly in Asia, which serve to further emphasize the importance of local susceptibility patterns when empirically treating suspected shigellosis/dysentery.[173] It is important to be aware that amoxicillin, which is well absorbed and achieves higher serum levels than ampicillin, is not effective therapy for shigellosis even when the organism is sensitive to ampicillin/amoxicillin.[174] Ampicillin is the drug formulation preferred for treatment of sensitive *Shigella* strains.

Chronic carriers of *Shigella* are rare. Postinfection carriage generally lasts less than 3 or 4 weeks and rarely exceeds 3 to 4 months. In circumstances in which eradication of the carrier state is deemed necessary, choice of antibiotic should be guided by antibiotic sensitivity results.

Mild diarrhea and cramps can continue for days to weeks after treatment of bacillary dysentery, even when the organism is no longer present and the acute episode seems to have passed. These symptoms are not necessarily a cause for alarm and are presumed to result from slowly repairing bowel that has been injured by inflammation Approximately 10% of patients with shigellosis, however, may be left with symptoms of postinfection IBS.[175]

Shigellosis is highly contagious. Careful hand washing and stool precautions are important to prevent dissemination of this disease. No vaccine is currently available.

Nontyphoidal Salmonell Salmonella species

Nontyphoidal salmonellosis refers to disease caused by any serotype of the genus *Salmonella*, with the exception of *Salmonella* Typhi and *Salmonella* Paratyphi. In contrast to *S.* Typhi and *S.* Paratyphi, nontyphoidal *Salmonella* often have animal reservoirs, encounter humans, and cause disease.

Microbiology

Salmonellae are a group of predominantly motile Gram-negative bacilli comprising 2 species, *Salmonella bongori* and *Salmonella enterica*. *S. enterica* is divided into 6 subspecies, of which only subspecies *enterica* constitutes a major human pathogen (causing 99% of human salmonellosis). *Salmonella* are further divided into over 2500 serovars (serotypes) on the basis of O (somatic) and H (flagellar) antigen patterns, using the Kauffmann-White scheme.[176] For convenience, the *Salmonella* taxonomy can be abbreviated; for example, *S. enterica* subspecies *enterica typhi* can be written as *S.* Typhi. The *S. enterica* core genome differs from *E. coli* by about 10% and other *Salmonella* serovars by about 1%. The differences between *S. enterica* and *E. coli* suggest that these organisms diverged from a common ancestor about 100 million years ago.[177] These organisms are primarily intestinal pathogens, although some serovars have a propensity for invasion and dissemination; they are often isolated in sewage, river and sea water, and

certain foods. Most nontyphoidal *Salmonella* species have a wide range of hosts, whereas humans are the only reservoir for *S.* Typhi and *S.* Paratyphi A, B, C.

Epidemiology

The global burden of nontyphoidal salmonellosis is estimated at 93.8 million infections (80.3 million foodborne infections) and 155,000 deaths each year, using the WHO Global Salm-Surv data. In 2002, *S.* Enteriditis and *S.* Typhimurium were the 2 most commonly reported serovars, accounting for 65% and 12% of isolates, respectively. In Europe, *S.* Enteriditis accounted for over 80% of isolates. In North America, *S.* Typhimurium accounted for 29% of isolates, and *S.* Enteriditis for 21%. *S.* Enteriditis was the most common identified strain in Asia, Africa, and Latin America. Of note, developing countries were less likely to submit reports to the WHO Global Salm-Surv, potentially skewing the results.[178] In Canada from 2003-2009, a tripling of *S.* Enteriditis rates to 33% was observed; a similar increase was noted in chickens, which were implicated as a likely source, and 36% of cases were related to travel.[179] In the United States, nontyphoidal *Salmonella* are estimated to be the most common cause of bacterial foodborne illness, at just over 1 million cases annually.[105] Since 2003, the rates of *S.* Enteriditis have risen by 44%. Domestically produced chickens and shell eggs have been implicated as the likely cause of the increase. New FDA regulations are aimed at preventing *S.* Enteriditis contamination.[180]

Nearly 1750 foodborne *Salmonella* outbreaks were reported to the CDC from 1998 to 2010.[107] The sources of the outbreaks are highly variable; poultry (both live and processed), shell eggs, amphibian and reptile pets, raw vegetables, raw fruits, peanut butter, ground beef, dog food, and even pet hedgehogs have all been reported as the source of multistate *Salmonella* outbreaks.[181] In sub-Saharan Africa, nontyphoidal salmonellae are the most common cause of community-acquired bacterial bloodstream infection, often in HIV-infected hosts.[182]

Attack rates of *Salmonella* show a strong relationship to age. Children younger than 1 year have the highest attack rate, a susceptibility that may be related to immunologic immaturity. There also are high attack rates and increased mortality in older adults.

Salmonellae have a tendency to colonize domestic animals and are widely distributed in the animal kingdom. Reptiles are uniformly colonized with *Salmonella* and serve as a source for human infections and outbreaks. Among other animals, poultry has the highest incidence of *Salmonella* carriage; pigs and cattle also may be heavily contaminated. Vertical transmission via the transovarian route can occur in chickens, so even normal-appearing eggs can be contaminated with *Salmonella*. Many of these animals can cohabit peacefully with salmonellae and usually are asymptomatic.

Whereas livestock are considered the primary reservoirs for nontyphoidal salmonellae in developed countries, some studies suggest that person-to-person transmission may be important in developing countries. A study in Nairobi, Kenya, found that 6.9% of an asymptomatic population carried nontyphoidal salmonellae. Moreover, many of the recovered clones were related to isolates obtained from bacteremic patients. No clones related to bacteremic patients were recovered from livestock, suggesting that, at least in this setting, person-to-person transmission may be important.[183]

Pathogenic Mechanisms

Salmonellae attack the ileum and, to a lesser extent, the colon, causing mild mucosal ulcerations. The key events in salmonellosis are invasion of enterocytes and macrophages, intracellular replication and evasion of host defenses, and, in some hosts, systemic dissemination through lymph channels and the reticuloendothelial system (RES).[184]

Invasion of host enterocytes or macrophages occurs through a mechanism shared with other members of the Enterobacteriaceae family, the type III secretion system (T3SS). The T3SS injects effector proteins into the host cell. The T3SS and effector proteins have multiple functions important for host cell invasion, including the formation of the *Salmonella*-containing vacuole (SCV). The SCV helps *Salmonella* escape host cell defenses and replicate. For example, T3SS2, an effector protein, prevents trafficking of NADPH oxidase toward the SCV, thereby inhibiting the oxidative burst. After replication, the bacteria migrate into the lymphatic channels and lymphoid tissues where they are taken up by macrophages and dendritic cells and may spread systemically via the RES.[184]

A key host defense against nontyphoidal *Salmonella* is pattern recognition receptors such as Toll-like receptors and NOD-like receptors. Defects in these pathways and the associated effector T cells can lead to increased morbidity and mortality, such as in HIV infection, severe combined immunodeficiency, and chronic granulomatous disease.[184]

The genetic material containing the virulence factors is primarily located on the *Salmonella* pathogenicity islands (SPI). Twenty-one different SPIs have been identified. Many are shared, but some are found in only a single serovar. Genetic material is also carried on prophages and phage remnants.[184]

The infectivity of a specific strain is related to its serotype and the inoculum size. For example, 10^5 S. newport produce illness in some volunteers, whereas 10^{10} S. pullorum are unable to do so. The latter strain is poorly adapted to humans, as suggested by its rarity in clinical infections; it is well adapted to chickens, from which it is often isolated. A dose-response curve has been determined for certain strains of *Salmonella*; an approximately 50% infection rate is seen with 10^7 organisms, whereas the infectivity rate rises to 90% with 10^{10} organisms. Certain *Salmonella* serovars are known for bloodstream invasion (e.g., S. Choleraesuis and S. Dublin).

Predisposing Conditions

A number of conditions increase the risk of invasive salmonellosis. The relationship between sickle cell anemia and *Salmonella* osteomyelitis is well known. Indeed, several infectious causes of hemolytic anemia predispose to invasive *Salmonella* infection, including malaria and bartonellosis. The exact mechanism for this association is poorly understood and likely is a combination of diminished granulocyte oxidative burst and defects in macrophage microbicidal function from hemolysis; dysfunction of the RES; and, in the case of malaria, sequestration of infected erythrocytes in the intestinal microvasculature directly or indirectly (via inflammation) impairing the gut barrier and increasing bacterial translocation.[185-187] Patients with sickle cell anemia also have a decreased capacity to opsonize salmonellae because of defective activation of the alternative complement pathway.[188]

Immunosuppression resulting from HIV is a strong contributing factor to invasive salmonellosis. Interestingly, studies in rural Africa tend to have higher rates of nontyphoidal salmonellae bacteremia than S. Typhi, but this is reversed in the urban setting. In Asia, S. Typhi is more common than nontyphoidal salmonellae. These differences are likely due to the higher rates of HIV and *Plasmodium falciparum* malaria in rural Africa compared to the other settings.[189] Similarly a meta-analysis of community-acquired bloodstream infections found that 99% of North African S. *enterica* isolates were S. Typhi, in contrast to sub-Saharan African isolates of S. *enterica* that

ranged from 87% to 97% nontyphoidal salmonellae. Furthermore, HIV-infected subjects were over 8 times more likely to have a nontyphoidal salmonellae bacteremia than non–HIV-infected subjects.[182]

Genetic defects in the interferon (IFN)-γ and IL-12/23 pathways increase risk of invasive salmonellosis.[190] Neoplastic disease is associated with an increased risk of salmonellosis, and leukemia, lymphoma, and disseminated malignancy predispose patients to bloodstream invasion by this organism.[191] Use of glucocorticoids, chemotherapy, or radiation therapy is associated with *Salmonella* sepsis and schistosomiasis is associated with invasive salmonellosis.[192] UC also predisposes to *Salmonella* infection and the carrier state.[193] Just as with other enteric pathogens, gastric surgery and gastric hypoacidity can lead to increased risk for salmonellosis.[3]

Clinical Features

Clinical manifestations of nontyphoidal salmonellae can range from asymptomatic carriage, to enterocolitis, to bacteremia with distant foci of metastatic sites of infection. Rarely, toxic megacolon complicates salmonellosis similar to other bacterially induced inflammatory colitides. From the clinician's perspective, there are almost no definitive clues that a patient is suffering from salmonellosis. It is important to consider salmonellosis in the differential diagnosis and test appropriately. Of greater importance to the clinician is to be aware of the many clinical manifestations of salmonellosis.

Asymptomatic carriage is traditionally associated with S. Typhi (see Typhoid Fever, Carrier State) but can occur in nontyphoidal salmonellae, although usually for shorter periods of time. Shedding is thought to generally not persist for more than 1 year from infection in healthy patients, but cases of chronic fecal carriage have been reported.[194] The duration of shedding is not well known in immunocompromised hosts. Given the lack of a common persistent human carrier state, other reservoirs, typically livestock, are important in maintaining infection in developed countries. "Supershedders" have recently been identified among cattle and mice, but their importance in maintaining the transmission cycle is not fully understood.[195]

Enterocolitis is the most common clinical manifestation of salmonellosis, accounts for approximately 75% of infections, and is indistinct from that caused by other enteric pathogens. The incubation period varies by host and inoculum size, but typically ranges from 6 to 72 hours. Clinical manifestations are the acute onset of fever, diarrhea, and cramping, often preceded by nausea and vomiting.[196,197] *Salmonella* enterocolitis may present as dysentery, but watery diarrhea is a common prominent symptom and can vary from mild to cholera-like, particularly in patients who are hypochlorhydric.[3]

The most serious complication of salmonellosis is bacteremia and its sequelae. In developed countries, secondary nontyphoidal *Salmonella* bacteremia complicates approximately 5% of cases of enteritis and carries an attributable mortality of 1% to 5%. Enteritis and diarrhea need not precede *Salmonella* bacteremia. Primary nontyphoidal *Salmonella* bacteremia is most common in immunosuppressed adults and children (see Predisposing Conditions, earlier). Mortality in this patient population is also likely higher. The most feared complication of nontyphoidal *Salmonella* bacteremia is infectious endarteritis, classically involving the aorta, although metastatic infection at other sites can occur. Reports of the proportion of bacteremic patients who develop an endovascular infection vary widely, from 0.6% to 35%. The prognosis of infectious aortitis is grave, but with modern surgical techniques, survival has been reported to approach 80%.[196] Metastatic foci of disease can develop in practically any anatomic site;

osteomyelitis, septic arthritis, focal abscesses, and meningitis are all reported.

In developing nations, invasive nontyphoidal salmonellae infections have varied presentations. Diarrhea is frequently absent, and patients often present with a febrile systemic illness like that of enteric fever. Reported mortality rates are between 22% and 47% for African adults and children. As discussed above, malaria, HIV, and malnutrition are all thought to contribute to the increased risk of invasive disease. Nontyphoidal salmonellae are also a common cause of meningitis in sub-Saharan Africa, particularly among children. In Malawi, 15% of culture-proven meningitis was due to *S.* Typhimurium. Meningitis mortality is high, 52% among children and 80% among adults.[192]

Treatment

Although many antibiotics have been used to treat nontyphoidal *Salmonella* enteritis, all have failed to alter the rate of clinical recovery. A meta-analysis of 12 randomized trials found no differences in the duration of illness and diarrhea between patients treated with antibiotics and those treated with placebo. Risk of fecal carriage of the same serovar for 1 month after completion of antibiotics was nearly twice as high in the antibiotic treated groups compared with the placebo or no treatment groups.[198] Thus, antimicrobial therapy should not be used in most cases of *Salmonella* enterocolitis.

Despite this general rule, antibiotics should be used in conditions with high risk for extraintestinal spread, such as lymphoproliferative disorders, malignant disease, immunosuppressed states (AIDS and congenital or acquired immunodeficiencies), organ transplantation, known or suspected abnormalities of the cardiovascular system (e.g., prosthetic heart valves, vascular grafts, aneurysms, and rheumatic or congenital valvular heart disease), foreign bodies implanted in the skeletal system, hemolytic anemia, extreme ages of life, and pregnancy. In addition, patients with *Salmonella* enterocolitis should be treated with antibiotics when they exhibit findings of bacteremia/septicemia (e.g., high fever, rigors, hypotension, decreased kidney function, systemic toxicity).

Once a decision is made to initiate therapy, the choice of drug may be problematic because of high levels of antibiotic resistance; currently, a fluoroquinolone is the drug of first choice. Third generation cephalosporins are alternatives. For patients with strains sensitive to ampicillin or TMP/SMX, these agents can be used (Table 110-8). As might be expected, resistance to ciprofloxacin has been observed during therapy, and the U. S. Clinical Laboratory Standards Institute (CLSI) has recently raised the ciprofloxacin break points for *Salmonella* spp. to account for the increased resistance.[199] The U. S. National Antimicrobial Resistance Monitoring System data from 1996 to 2007 found no ciprofloxacin resistance to any invasive nontyphoidal *Salmonella* isolates, but 82% would have been classified as intermediate sensitivity by the revised CLSI guidelines. Ceftriaxone resistance was found in 2.5%.[200] As a consequence of the increasing levels of drug resistance, both domestically and internationally, empirical antimicrobial therapy of *Salmonella* infections must be limited to high-risk patients and, ultimately, should be based on sensitivity testing. Treatment of asymptomatic carriers is not recommended, because carriage is not eliminated faster, and resistance is more likely to develop.[201]

Salmonella bacteremia is a severe infection that can result in extraintestinal manifestations and death. In addition to appropriate antibiotic therapy, management should include an exploration for extraintestinal foci of infection through history and physical examination, with additional diagnostic workup as indicated. Some extraintestinal infections require

complicated management. For example, antibiotics alone may not be sufficient treatment for *Salmonella* aortitis, and urgent vascular surgery may be required. Likewise, endocarditis, meningitis, septic arthritis, osteomyelitis, and other complications can require a complicated treatment strategy. Consultation with an infectious diseases expert is recommended in any case where there is concern for systemic salmonellosis.

Prevention is centered around hygiene. Appropriate hand washing is needed when contacting high-risk carrier animals. Public health measures are important to reduce contamination and foodborne spread. Reduced antibiotic administration to livestock could help limit multidrug-resistant strains. No vaccine is available for nontyphoidal salmonellae.

Typhoid Fever

Typhoid (Greek *typhos*, "stupor" or "cloudy") fever is a febrile illness of prolonged duration, marked by hectic fever, delirium, persistent bloodstream infection, splenic enlargement, abdominal pain, and a variety of systemic manifestations. The illness caused by this pathogen differs from the nontyphoidal *Salmonella* infections in several respects. Typhoidal disease is not truly an intestinal disease and has more systemic than intestinal symptoms. *S.* Typhi is remarkably adapted to humans, who represent the only natural reservoir; the other salmonellae are associated with animals. Typhoid fever is an ancient companion of man; for centuries it plagued civilizations, killing more soldiers than did opposing armies. In 1914 at the dawning of World War I, Sir William Osler delivered an address to the Society of Tropical Medicine and Hygiene in which he recounted recent advances in scientific knowledge, including the discovery of the typhoid bacillus, its disease transmission, the typhoid carrier state, vaccination, and the importance of sanitation. He was hopeful that this knowledge would lead to fewer deaths.[202] A century later, much of his scientific and public health message remains true. Despite advances in sanitation and available vaccines, however, typhoid fever persists and is posing new challenges.

Although *S. enterica* serotype Typhi is the main cause of typhoid fever, other *Salmonella* serotypes occasionally produce a similar clinical picture, known variously as *typhoidal disease*, *enteric fever*, or *paratyphoid fever*. These serotypes are *S.* Paratyphi A, B, and C, as well as others, including *S.* Typhimurium. This section will focus on the common causes of enteric fever, *S.* Typhi and *S.* Paratyphi.

Microbiology

S. Typhi is biochemically similar to other *Salmonella* species and is distinguished primarily by its specific antigens. As a rule, this organism produces little or no gas from carbohydrates, elaborates only small amounts of hydrogen sulfide, and bears the Vi antigen on its surface. These markers should alert the laboratory to the possibility of this pathogen; confirmation of *S.* Typhi is accomplished by serotyping.

Pathogenic Mechanisms

The pathologic events of typhoid fever are initiated in the intestinal tract after oral ingestion of between 1000 and 1 million typhoid bacilli.[203] The organism penetrates the small intestinal mucosa and rapidly makes its way to the lymphatics, the mesenteric nodes, and the bloodstream. There is a paucity of local inflammatory findings, which explains the lack of intestinal symptoms at this early stage. This sequence of events is in marked contrast to that of other forms of salmonellosis and shigellosis, in which intestinal findings are prominent at the onset.

TABLE 110-8 Antibiotic Therapy for Nonsevere Infections with Common Bacterial Enteropathogens in Immunocompetent Adults

Organism	Recommended Antibiotic(s)	Alternative Antibiotic(s)
Shigella Species		
Shigella infection (non-dysenteriae; for Shigella dysenteriae type 1, see text)	Ciprofloxacin 500 mg twice daily (or levofloxacin 500 mg daily) × 3 days	Azithromycin 500 mg-1 g daily × 3-5 days TMP/SMX 160 mg/800 mg twice daily, if sensitive, × 3 days
Salmonella Species		
Enterocolitis, uncomplicated Typhoid and enteric fevers*	Not usually recommended (see text) Ciprofloxacin 500 mg twice daily (or ofloxacin 400 mg twice daily) × 7-14 days Ceftriaxone 2-3 g IV daily × 7-14 days	Can consider in areas of high fluoroquinolone quinolone resistance; Azithromycin 1 g daily × 5 days
Campylobacter Species		
Campylobacter jejuni	Not usually required Ciprofloxacin 500 mg twice daily × 3 days	Azithromycin 500 mg-1 g × 3-5 days
Yersinia enterocolitica		
Enterocolitis, uncomplicated	Not usually required	An aminoglycoside (parenteral) Tetracycline 500 mg 4 times daily × 5 days TMP/SMX 160 mg/800 mg twice daily × 5 days Ciprofloxacin 500 mg twice daily × 5 days Doxycycline 100 mg twice daily × 5 days
Escherichia coli†		
Enterotoxigenic	Endemic disease; Usually self-limited, supportive care (see text) Traveler's diarrhea: ciprofloxacin 500 mg twice daily × 3 days (see Table 110-9) Rifaximin 200 mg 3 times daily × 3 days	Azithromycin 500 mg-1 g daily × 3-5 days TMP/SMX 160 mg/800 mg twice daily, if sensitive, × 3 days
Shiga toxin-producing	Unclear if antibiotics are effective; may be harmful	
Vibrio Species		
Vibrio cholera	Doxycycline 300 mg × 1 dose	Ciprofloxacin 1 g × 1 dose Azithromycin 1 g × 1 dose Tetracycline 500 mg every 6 hours × 3 days
Vibrio parahaemolyticus	Usually not required; no controlled trials	As for V. cholerae

NOTE: All antibiotics are administered orally unless otherwise indicated. Recommendations are given for treatment of mild/moderate infections only. Treatments for complicated infections or severely ill, bacteremic, or immunocompromised patients are not listed above and may differ from treatments for mild disease.
*For severe typhoid fever, consider the addition of glucocorticoids (dexamethasone 3 mg/kg × 1, then 1 mg/kg every 6 hours × 48 hours) to parenteral antimicrobial therapy. Antimicrobial sensitivity testing is required. Fluoroquinolones (e.g., ciprofloxacin) should not be used as empiric therapy in Asia or other areas with high fluoroquinolone resistance.
†Enteropathogenic, enteroaggregative, and diffusely enteroadherent E. coli are omitted from this table because these types are defined in research laboratories and are not diagnosed in routine clinical practice. Enteroinvasive E. coli presenting as inflammatory diarrhea should be treated empirically as for Shigella spp.
TMP/SMX, trimethoprim/sulfamethoxazole.

After the initial bacteremia, the organism is sequestered in macrophages and monocytic cells of the RES. It undergoes multiplication and reemerges several days later in recurrent waves of bacteremia, an event that initiates the symptomatic phase of infection. Now in great numbers, the organism is spread throughout the host and infects many organ sites. The intestinal tract may be seeded by direct bacteremic spread to Peyer's patches in the terminal ileum or via drainage of contaminated bile from the gallbladder, which often harbors large numbers of organisms.

Hyperplasia of the RES, including lymph nodes, liver, and spleen, is characteristic of typhoid fever. The liver contains discrete micronodular areas of necrosis surrounded by macrophages and lymphocytes. Inflammation of the gallbladder is common and can lead to acute cholecystitis. Patients with preexisting gallbladder disease have a tendency to become carriers because the bacillus becomes intimately associated with the existing chronic disease and may be incorporated within gallstones. Lymphoid follicles in the intestine, such as in Peyer's patches, become hyperplastic. Subsequently, a follicle may ulcerate, penetrate through the submucosa to the intestinal lumen, and discharge large numbers of typhoid bacilli. As the bowel wall is progressively involved, it becomes paper-thin (most commonly in the terminal ileum) and is susceptible to perforation. Erosion into blood vessels can produce severe intestinal hemorrhage.

The polysaccharide capsule Vi antigen is 1 of the most important virulence factors for S. Typhi. No other Salmonella serovars carry the Vi antigen. Two regions, ViaA and ViaB, contain the genes for the Vi antigen and are located on SPI-7, a Salmonella pathogenicity island specific to S. Typhi. Three other SPIs are specific to S. Typhi: SPI-15, 17, and 18.[184] Vi antigen is believed to prevent innate immune response recognition through Toll-like receptors.[204] Neutrophils in the small intestine are not activated, facilitating systemic dissemination.[205] Vi-negative *S.* Typhi strains can still cause typhoid-like illness but are rare among clinical isolates. The low rate of Vi-negative typhoid fever is of importance because 1 vaccine uses purified Vi antigen to stimulate an immune response.[206]

Epidemiology

S. Typhi and *S.* Paratyphi are adapted specifically to the human host. Humans serve as a chronic reservoir, periodically shedding the organisms into the environment where they subsequently are ingested usually in contaminated food or water supplies. Endemic disease in many parts of the world likely persists where sanitation is poor but has largely been eliminated in the developed world.

A recent meta-analysis estimated the annual global burden of typhoid fever in 2010 to be 27.9 million episodes,[207] up from 21.6 million estimated annual episodes in 2000.[208] This increased incidence is likely driven by population growth, new data, and methodologic differences in burden estimation. No clear trend of increasing global typhoid fever incidence is known. Children younger than 5 years and older adults generally have the highest rates of disease. The paratyphoid fever burden was estimated at over 5 million cases annually in 2000, with 200,000 to 600,000 deaths from typhoid fever.[208] Asia is traditionally thought to be an area of particularly high typhoid fever incidence, but there is a large amount of regional variation.[207-209] Presumably because of HIV and malaria, sub-Saharan Africa is thought to have higher rates of nontyphoidal salmonellae infections than typhoid fever, rates of which are seemingly unaffected by HIV.[182] A recent study of a Kenyan urban slum found a typhoid fever incidence similar to that of urban slums in central Asia but much lower than in a rural area in Kenya.[210] Estimates of typhoid and paratyphoid fever burden are limited because of lack of population-level sampling data and diagnostic facilities, particularly in areas with poverty, high population density, and poor sanitation that may have a high incidence of disease.

From 2000-2010, the annual number of reported cases in the United States ranged from 300 to 500 and has changed little since 1980.[211] In 2006, 85% of the typhoid cases in the United States were travel related, and travelers returning from Asia and Africa had the highest typhoid fever rates. Multiple small domestic outbreaks have occurred in the United States, often associated with food.[212] In 2010, the largest domestic outbreak in over a decade, involving 12 cases, occurred in Nevada, California, and Oregon, with imported frozen mamey pulp as the implicated vehicle.[213]

Because *S.* Typhi cohabits exclusively with humans, the appearance of a case could indicate the presence of a carrier. An investigation by public health authorities should be instituted to determine the source and the presence of other cases. As they are discovered, chronic carriers are registered with the health authorities, and the particular microorganism is phage-typed so that it can be traced in the event of an outbreak. Treatment of carriers is discussed later.

Clinical Features

In its classic form and without treatment, typhoid fever lasts about 4 weeks and evolves in a manner consistent with the pathologic events. The illness is described traditionally as a series of 1-week stages, although variations in this pattern can be observed.[214] The incubation period generally is 7 to 14 days, with wide variations.

During the first week, high fever, headache, and abdominal pain are common. The pulse often is slower than would be expected for the degree of fever, a finding referred to as *Faget's sign*. Abdominal pain is localized to the right lower quadrant in most cases but can be diffuse. In approximately 50% of patients, there is no change in bowel habits; in fact, constipation is more common than diarrhea in children with typhoid fever. Near the end of the first week, enlargement of the spleen is noticeable, and an evanescent classic rash (rose spots) becomes manifest, most commonly on the chest.

During the second week, the fever becomes more continuous, and the patient looks sick and withdrawn. During the third week, the patient's illness evolves into the "typhoidal state," with disordered mentation and, in some cases, extreme toxemia. It is from this altered mental state that the term *typhoid* derives. In this period there is often intestinal involvement, manifested clinically by greenish pea-soup–like diarrhea and the dire complications of intestinal perforation and hemorrhage. The fourth week brings slackening of the fever and improvement in the clinical status, if the patient survives and recovers.

Typhoid fever is a less severe illness in previously healthy adults who seek medical attention for the earliest symptoms of fever, lassitude, and headache than it is in those whose care is delayed. Prompt diagnosis and appropriate therapy interrupt the classic 4-week scenario and produce an aborted illness consisting of little more than a few days of fever and malaise.

Because the typhoid bacillus is disseminated widely through recurrent waves of bacteremia, many organ sites can be involved. Patients with typhoid fever can have pneumonia, pyelonephritis, and metastatic infections of bone, large joints, and the brain. The gallbladder and liver are involved with inflammatory changes. Acute cholecystitis can occur during the initial 2 to 3 weeks, and jaundice, resulting from diffuse hepatic inflammation, has been observed in some patients.

The preeminent complications are intestinal hemorrhage and perforation.[215] These events are most likely to occur in the third week and during convalescence and are not related to the severity of the disease; they tend to occur in the same patient, with bleeding serving as a harbinger of possible perforation. Bleeding may be sudden and severe or a slow ooze. Before the availability of antibiotics, the incidence of hemorrhage was as high as 20%; it is less common since specific treatment has become available. Approximately 3% of patients with typhoid fever develop intestinal perforation, most commonly in the ileum.[216] Onset of perforation may be sudden, with signs of an acute abdomen, or there may be a leak of intraluminal contents to form an abscess in the lower quadrant or pelvis, producing a more insidious course.

After defervescence has occurred and the patient has apparently ridden through the storm, a potential for recurrence remains. Relapse generally occurs 8 to 10 days after cessation of drug therapy and consists of a reenactment of the major manifestations. The organism is the same as the one that caused the original infection, with the identical antimicrobial susceptibility pattern. The average mortality rate is about 1%, but has wide geographic variability, ranging up to 30% to 50% in some parts of the world. Failure to administer effective antibiotics is the most important contributor to poor outcomes.[217]

Carrier State

After 6 weeks, approximately 50% of typhoid victims still shed organisms in their feces. This figure declines progressively with time, and after 3 months only 5% to 10% are excreters; by 1 year the frequency is 1% to 6%.[218,219] The chronic carrier is identified by positive stool cultures for *S.* Typhi at least 1 year after the acute episode or, in some cases, positive stool cultures without a documented history of disease. The probability of spontaneously aborting the carrier state is highly unlikely after this time. Chronic carriers are more common in older age groups, women (a 3:1 ratio of women to men),[220] and persons with biliary disease. The organism usually is harbored in the gallbladder, although occasionally it is carried in the large intestine without involvement of the biliary tract.

Diagnosis

The diagnosis of typhoid fever is established by isolating the organism. Blood culture is the primary diagnostic test and is positive in 60% to 80% of patients, but declines closer to 40% outside of the study setting where many patients may have received prior antibiotic therapy. Bone marrow culture is considered the gold standard and has a yield of better than 90%, even in treated patients.[221] Stool cultures become positive in the second and third weeks. Sampling duodenal contents by a string test yields a positive culture in 70% of patients. By the third week, urine cultures reveal the organism in approximately 25% of patients. The titer of agglutinins against somatic (O) antigen (Widal test) rises during the second and third weeks of illness. Various titer thresholds for a positive result are used in different countries, but a 4-fold rise in convalescent titer is considered stronger evidence of typhoid fever. Problems with the Widal test include cross-reaction with other *Salmonella* strains causing false positives, and false negatives if the sample is collected too early in the disease course. PCR assays for the diagnosis of *S.* Typhi have been developed, but none are widespread in clinical use. Rapid, affordable, and accurate tests to address diagnostic deficiencies for typhoid are greatly needed, particularly in locations with endemic disease where current diagnostic methods are of limited implementation.[222,223]

S. Typhi carriers are traditionally difficult to identify, because bacterial shedding occurs intermittently. Repeated cultures are necessary to detect carriers, but this is cost-prohibitive as a public health intervention. Antibodies to the Vi antigen have been used in serologic testing for typhoid carriers, but its value in low prevalence settings is not clear, and this has not been widely adopted as a public health measure.[224]

Treatment

Therapy of both *S.* Typhi and *S.* Paratyphi is very similar, and most uncomplicated cases of enteric fever are treated with appropriate antibiotics and supportive care. The most important decision is to choose an antibiotic with activity against the particular infecting isolate. Empiric antibiotic decisions should be based on local drug susceptibility patterns and altered as soon as isolate-specific recommendations are available. Recommended treatment regimens are listed in Table 110-8.

For years, fluoroquinolones have been the drugs of choice.[217] Several meta-analyses have examined the role of these agents for treatment of typhoid fever and paratyphoid fever, and all studies concluded that fluoroquinolones performed at least as well as alternative regimens, if not better in certain settings; however, the available data limited further comparisons.[225,226] Strains of *S.* Typhi and *S.* Paratyphi resistant to chloramphenicol, ampicillin, and TMP-SMX have been circulating since the late 1980s and are known as *multidrug-resistant* (MDR) *strains*. This resistance is encoded on a plasmid and has been found over a wide geographic range, necessitat-

ing transition to fluoroquinolones as the first-line therapy.[227] Of great concern is the emergence of fluoroquinolone resistance that has occurred in Asia and is spreading worldwide, including to the United States.[228] Also worrisome is the emergence of strains with decreased ciprofloxacin susceptibility (DCS) that have been shown to increase the risk of therapy failure when fluoroquinolones are used.[229] These strains are also widespread, particularly in Asia and Africa. As a result of the increase in DCS and fluoroquinolone-resistant strains, the CLSI reduced the break point minimum inhibitory concentration (MIC), defining resistance to ciprofloxacin from 4 or more μg/mL to 2.0 or more μg/mL, and the intermediate range is now defined as 0.12 to 1.0 μg/mL. Naladixic acid testing may be used as a surrogate for the DCS phenotype but has a false-negative rate of 7% to 8%.[199] It is likely that intermediate or higher ciprofloxacin-resistant isolates are better treated with alternative antibiotics.

Azithromycin may hold promise as an alternative treatment for enteric fever. A meta-analysis concluded that azithromycin was equivalent to other treatments and may be an attractive alternative in DCS or fluoroquinolone-resistant strains.[230] Parenteral third-generation cephalosporins are a reasonable alternative therapy, but cefixime, an oral third-generation cephalosporin, had longer time to fever resolution and a higher rate of clinical failures than gatifloxacin.[231] Thus, cefixime may not be the best alternative therapy for uncomplicated enteric fever. It is interesting that the rates of resistance to traditional antibiotics used for enteric fever, such as chloramphenicol, ampicillin, and TMP-SMX, have declined in some areas, and these therapies should be viable alternatives if the infecting organism is susceptible.[232]

Severe disease, characterized by altered mental status, severe sepsis, or shock, requires hospitalization and treatment with a fluoroquinolone or third-generation cephalosporin. One clinical trial also demonstrated benefit to high-dose dexamethasone at an initial dose of 3 mg/kg, then 1 mg/kg every 6 hours for 48 hours.[233]

Intestinal perforation is 1 of the major complications of enteric fever and mandates surgical intervention. With surgical management and specific *S.* Typhi antibiotic therapy, mortality rates of 20% to 30% are reported. A large case series found that extremes of age and multiple perforations were risks for poorer outcomes. Improved surgical technique (2-layer closure) and addition of metronidazole and gentamicin reduced the mortality rate to 8%.[234] Addition of gentamicin and metronidazole provides broad-spectrum Gram-negative and anaerobic bacteria coverage needed for the intestinal spillage and resultant bacterial peritonitis/sepsis that may be missing from the specific *S.* Typhi antibiotic therapy chosen. Certain enteric fever treatment regimens, including fluoroquinolones and third-generation cephalosporins, have broad Gram-negative activity, but in the setting of intestinal perforation, metronidazole or another antibiotic with anaerobic activity should be added to the antibiotic regimen. Clindamycin may not have activity against *Bacteroides fragilis* and should not be used in this setting if better alternatives are available. Administration of appropriate antibiotics is important but serves only as an adjunct to surgical intervention.

Chronic Carriers

A chronic carrier who has been discharging *S.* Typhi for more than 1 year can be treated with antimicrobials in an attempt to eliminate the infection. The quinolone antibiotics, including ciprofloxacin and norfloxacin, have become the treatment of choice in eradicating the carrier state.[235] Reappearance of the carrier state after such treatment generally is associated with gallbladder disease. Cholecystectomy eliminates the carrier state in 85% of carriers with gallstones or chronic cholecystitis and is most clearly recommended for persons whose profession is incompatible with the typhoid carrier state, such as food handlers and health care providers. Decisions regarding cholecystectomy for other chronic carriers are made on an individual basis. Local health departments should be notified about S. Typhi carriers. Carriers will often be required to sign an agreement that they will not participate in food preparation or distribution or direct contact with young children, patients, or older adults until they are cleared of carriage.

Vaccines

The CDC and WHO currently recommend 2 typhoid vaccines: Ty21a, a live-attenuated orally administered S. Typhi strain; and a Vi capsular polysaccharide (ViCPS) vaccine, which is administered parenterally.[236,237] Both are about 50% to 80% effective, but ViCPS requires a booster every 2 years, and Ty21a requires a booster every 5 years. There are currently 212 countries for which the CDC recommends vaccination for travelers.[238]

Campylobacter Species

In 1906, Campylobacter was cultured for the first time and placed in the Vibrio genus before later being placed in its own genus. Not until 1970 was Campylobacter recognized as an enteric pathogen.[239] The taxonomy of Campylobacter has changed rapidly recently, and now there are 32 species with 13 subspecies, only several of which have been implicated in human disease. Campylobacter species are motile, comma-shaped, Gram-negative rods with a polar flagellum. The most important Campylobacter species found in human infections are C. jejuni, a major cause of diarrhea; C. fetus, which is generally found in immunocompromised patients and causes systemic disease; and C. coli, a rare cause of gastroenteritis. Other Campylobacter species that cause diarrhea on rare occasions are C. hyointestinalis, C. upsaliensis, and C. laridis. This section addresses either Campylobacter spp. in general or C. jejuni where indicated. A detailed description of each Campylobacter species is beyond the scope of this text.

Epidemiology

Campylobacter spp. are 1 of the most common causes of foodborne bacterial illness in the United States, estimated to result in over 1 million illnesses annually, 80% of which are foodborne.[105] The United States annual incidence is 13.6 cases/100,000 persons and has been stable since 2005 after trending down from 1996. Nearly 15% of cases are hospitalized, although mortality is reported in less than 0.1%. Children younger than 5 years are at the greatest risk for campylobacteriosis.[240]

Transmission to humans appears to occur most commonly from infected animals and their food products. The reservoir for Campylobacter is enormous because many animals can be infected, including cattle, sheep, swine, birds (poultry and others), and dogs. Most human infections are related to consumption of improperly cooked or contaminated foods.

The implicated transmission vehicles may differ by region, season, and setting (i.e., sporadic or common source outbreak). In the United States, the primary food vehicle for Campylobacter outbreaks was unpasteurized dairy products, followed by poultry.[241,242] Poultry is the most common vehicle for sporadic disease and outbreaks in Northern Europe and North America.[243] The incidence of sporadic campylobacteriosis increases in the summer, but outbreaks do not have a similar seasonal pattern. These differences in seasonality may be due to increased carriage or shedding in poultry during the summer months.[242] Raw produce and contamination of drinking water have also been implicated in outbreaks.[242] The burden of campylobacteriosis in the developing world is not thoroughly characterized, but the incidence is thought to be high in young children and to decline thereafter, perhaps as a result of immunity from repeated exposures.[244]

Pathogenic Mechanisms

The pathogenesis of Campylobacter infection seems to be mediated primarily through adhesion and invasion. A number of adhesion or binding factors that can vary according to the species have been identified. The mechanism of invasion by Campylobacter is unique. An adhesion factor, CadF, triggers a signaling process that leads to microtubule dependent internalization of the bacteria on the basolateral aspect of M cells. This invasion leads to early mucosal damage. Other bacterial factors are known, notably cytolethal distending toxin (CDT), which arrests the cell cycle and damages DNA to cause cell death.[245,246]

Clinical Features

The incubation period is 24 to 72 hours after organisms are ingested, but it can extend as long as 10 days. There is a wide spectrum of clinical illness, from frank dysentery to watery diarrhea to asymptomatic excretion.[247] Diarrhea is almost invariable (90%). Fever is present in 65% to 90% of cases.[248] Abdominal pain is usually present (70%), and the patient may note bloody stools (50%). Constitutional symptoms such as headache, myalgia, backache, malaise, anorexia, and vomiting are common. Stool examination suggests colitis on the basis of fecal leukocytes and/or occult blood.[247] Colonoscopy might reveal an inflammatory colitis (see Fig. 110-3). The duration of illness usually is less than 1 week, although symptoms can persist for 2 or more weeks, and relapses occur in as many as 25% of patients. Prolonged carriage of Campylobacter for 2 to 10 weeks after the onset of illness is reported in 16% of patients.[249]

Infections with Campylobacter rarely are complicated by GI hemorrhage, toxic megacolon, pancreatitis, cholecystitis, HUS, bacteremia, meningitis, and purulent arthritis.[247] Post-infection complications include reactive arthritis (0.7% to 2.6%), usually in patients with the HLA-B27 phenotype, Guillain-Barré syndrome (1 in 10,000)[250] and immunoproliferative small intestinal disease.[251] More recently, campylobacteriosis has been associated with both post-infection IBS and IBD. The mechanism for such associations is not known, and no studies have demonstrated a causal link.[252]

Diagnosis

The diagnosis of Campylobacter during acute gastroenteritis only can be established by stool culture. A selective isolation medium containing antibiotics must be used because Campylobacter organisms grow more slowly than do other enteric bacteria; the plates are grown at 42°C under CO_2 and reduced oxygen conditions. Dark-field or phase-contrast microscopy of fresh diarrheal stool may show the organism as a curved, highly motile rod, with darting corkscrew movements. Bacteremia with Campylobacter spp. occurs, particularly in immunocompromised hosts, and blood cultures are warranted in these hosts, as well as those severely or systemically ill with gastroenteritis. Development of the Guillain-Barré syndrome suggests an infection with *Campylobacter* rather than other pathogens in the previous few weeks.

Treatment

Mild *Campylobacter* enteritis is self-limiting with supportive care and does not typically require antibiotic treatment. A meta-analysis demonstrated that antibiotics shortened the duration of symptoms by 1.3 days if given within the first 3 days of diarrhea.[253] However, patients often do not present to the clinician until diarrhea persists for 5 or more days. Antibiotics should be administered in severe disease (i.e., patients with dysentery, extraintestinal infection, or prolonged duration of disease) and in patients at risk for severe disease, such as older adult or immunocompromised patients.

Treatment, when needed, is typically a fluoroquinolone or macrolide. A single dose of azithromycin has been shown to have higher cure rate and shorter duration of symptoms for traveler's diarrhea in a country with high levels of fluoroquinolone resistance.[254] Fluoroquinolone resistance has become widespread, with reports of 19% to 47% resistance in North American isolates, 17% to 99% in European isolates, and over 80% in Southeast Asian isolates. Macrolide resistance patterns vary with the particular *Campylobacter* species, bacterial reservoir, and region.[255]

In cases of severe disease with concern of resistance or systemic disease, other antimicrobials are available. *C. jejuni* can produce a β-lactamase, which causes resistance to ampicillin, amoxicillin, and ticarcillin, although combination with β-lactamase inhibitors improves susceptibility; imipenem is not affected by the β-lactamase.[256] Other options include aminoglycosides and tetracyclines, but not cephalosporins; resistance to these agents is common.[257]

Yersinia enterocolitica

Y. enterocolitica causes a spectrum of clinical illnesses from simple gastroenteritis to invasive ileitis and colitis. It is a non–lactose fermenting, urease-positive, Gram-negative rod. More than 60 serogroups and 6 biotypes have been identified, with varying pathogenicity and geographic distribution.[258]

Pathogenic Mechanisms

The pathogenesis of *Y. enterocolitica* is similar to other Enterobacteriaceae, involving adhesion to the intestinal epithelium, invasion of M cells, and entry into the submucosa. Once in the submucosa, *Y. enterocolitica* is phagocytosed by macrophages and delivered to the Peyer's patches or mesenteric lymph nodes, where microcolonies form.[259]

Virulence factors are located on the bacterial chromosome and a 70-kb virulence plasmid, pYV. Only strains carrying the pYV plasmid are virulent. Invasion is mediated by 3 proteins, Inv, YadA, and Ail. Ail, in particular, correlates with virulent isolates and has an additional role in intracellular survival. The pYV plasmid encodes a type III secretion system and corresponding effector proteins, which inhibits phagocyte defense mechanisms and inflammation. Expression of several genes are thermoregulated, notably flagellin transcription and several pYV plasmid genes. At body temperature (37°C), the bacteria are no longer motile and instead express genes related to invasion. The high-pathogenicity island (HPI) is a chromosomal region that contains multiple genes, most of which are involved in the production of the high-affinity siderophore yersiniabactin. The HPI is found exclusively in the high-pathogenicity biotype/serotype, 1B/O:8, and promotes bacterial replication within the host and systemic spread.[259]

Epidemiology

Transmission occurs primarily via the fecal-oral route, most commonly through contaminated food. Direct person-to-person transmission has not been clearly shown, although it may occur in some cases. Pigs are believed to be the major animal reservoir and lead to contamination during processing of the pork or pork products. Because most pork is cooked, transmission probably occurs through undercooked pork or improper food handling. Home-made sausage represents an often-reported disease vehicle. In Germany, sporadic *Y. enterocolitica* infections have been associated with the consumption of a spiced, raw, minced pork spread called "Mett" or "Hackepeter," particularly in young children.[260] *Y. enterocolitica* has been isolated from cows, sheep, and goats, and pets such as dogs or cats are potential reservoirs. In Japan, wild rodents have been shown to carry the same biotype of *Y. enterocolitica* that causes human disease.

Y. enterocolitica is generally found in cooler climates but shows regional variation by biotype. The high-virulence biotype 1B was traditionally the predominant strain isolated in North America but not elsewhere. More recently, biotype 1B has been declining in North America but has been found in Europe and Japan, although the primary biotypes in Europe and Japan are the low-pathogenicity biotypes 2 to 5.[258,261]

In the European Union, there were 6832 cases of yersiniosis in 2010 (91% *Y. enterocolitica*), for an incidence rate of 1.8 cases per 100,000 population. Lithuania and France have the highest rates at 12.9 and 9.8 cases per 100,000 population, respectively. There has been a decline in the incidence rate since 2006, although yersiniosis remains the third most common zoonosis in the European Union after campylobacteriosis and nontyphoidal salmonellosis.[262] Children younger than 5 years had an incidence rate 5 times higher than the average. Only 11 outbreaks were reported, affecting 84 people; sporadic infection represents the largest portion of the disease burden.[262] In the United States, *Y. enterocolitica* is estimated to cause about 100,000 infections and over 500 hospitalizations annually.[105] According to these estimates, *Y. enterocolitica* is the seventh most common cause of foodborne illness and costs an estimated $252 million annually in the United States.[263] *Y. enterocolitica* infection has also been associated with iron-overload states and blood transfusions, because iron likely promotes virulence of this organism. In China, *Y. enterocolitica* is most common in the colder regions, and the predominant sero/biotype distributions differ from those in Europe and North America.[264]

Clinical Features

Several clinical syndromes have been described with *Yersinia* and tend to vary with the age of the patient and the underlying disease state. Young children most often present with self-limiting diarrhea. Older children and adults typically present with fever, abdominal pain, diarrhea, and vomiting. Symptom onset occurs 24 to 48 hours after the exposure[261] and usually lasts 1 to 3 weeks. Microscopic examination of stool reveals leukocytes and red blood cells in most instances. Profuse watery diarrhea also can occur. Diarrhea can persist for several weeks and can raise the possibility of IBD. Radiologic findings, particularly in prolonged cases, are most intense in the terminal ileum and can resemble those of Crohn's disease[265]; most patients, however, have normal findings on endoscopy, intestinal biopsy, and barium studies.[266] In children older than 5 years, mesenteric adenitis and associated ileitis have been described. Accompanying symptoms include nausea, vomiting, and oral aphthous ulcers. Affected children often undergo a laparotomy, at which time enlarged mesenteric nodes and an ulcerated ileum are observed. Clinically, the condition may be confused with acute appendicitis, and ultrasonography can be useful in separating these processes.[267] *Yersinia* is less likely to cause severe disease in adults, in whom acute diarrhea may be followed 2 to 3 weeks later by joint symptoms and rash (erythema nodosum or erythema multiforme), reminiscent of reactive arthritis. Reactive polyarthritis occurs in 2% of patients with yersiniosis, and 80% are seropositive for HLA-B27. Studies have demonstrated that *Y. enterocolitica* interacts with HLA-B27 expression and affects T-lymphocyte function, which may lead to a reactive arthritis.[258]

Yersinia bacteremia is a relatively uncommon condition that is seen in patients with underlying diseases such as malignancy, diabetes mellitus, anemia, liver disease, iron overload (or treatment with an iron chelator), and blood transfusions. Metastatic foci can occur in bones, joints, and lungs.[258]

The diagnosis of yersiniosis is established by culture of stool or body fluids. Because organism identification can be difficult, the clinician should alert the laboratory that this infection is clinically suspected.

Treatment

Y. enterocolitica strains are susceptible to several antimicrobial agents, including tetracycline, TMP-SMX, fluoroquinolones, third-generation cephalosporins, and carbapenems, but they are resistant to penicillins and first-generation cephalosporins. Resistance to fluoroquinolones has increased in some regions, but no resistance has been reported to third-generation cephalosporins. Nevertheless, there are reports of clinical failures with third-generation cephalosporins. Tissue penetration is likely superior with fluoroquinolones, which are considered the first-line option.[259]

There is no substantial evidence that antibiotics alter the course of the GI infection,[258] and diagnosis often is established late in the course when the patient is already improving spontaneously. Antibiotics should be used in more severe intestinal infections, particularly those masquerading as appendicitis or in the immunocompromised host who is at high risk for systemic disease. While mortality in these patients has approached 50%, this has decreased with the use of third-generation cephalosporins and fluoroquinolones.[259] Antibiotic treatment is listed in Table 110-8.

SEXUALLY TRANSMITTED INFECTIOUS PROCTITIS

Many sexually transmitted infections are known to cause infectious *proctitis*, including *Neisseria gonorrhoeae*, *Chlamydia*, syphilis, and HSV-1 or 2. Infection typically occurs through receptive anal intercourse. The population at greatest risk is men who have sex with men (MSM), although infectious proctitis can occur in others. Rates of syphilis and gonorrhea infections have been increasing in the MSM population in the United States, but little national data are available on proctitis trends.[268] In San Francisco, rates of rectal chlamydia and gonorrhea have been steadily increasing among men, but may also be related to changes in screening.[269] Of the infectious causes of proctitis, *N. gonorrhoeae* is responsible for about 30%, *C. trachomatis* 19%, HSV 16%, and syphilis 2%[270]; *Lymphogranuloma venereum* (LGV) infections are less common (See Chapter 129.

Clinical presentation can vary depending on the organism, from asymptomatic disease to tenesmus, anorectal pain, ulcerations, inguinal lymphadenopathy, passage of blood and mucus per rectum, and fever. Symptoms can mimic IBD, and

clinical suspicion should prompt a diagnostic workup.[271] A sexual history is the first step in diagnosis. For *N. gonorrhoeae* and *C. trachomatis*, a nucleic acid amplification test (NAAT) of a rectal swab is preferred. For HSV, culture or PCR of an ulcer are the preferred methods of diagnosis. Syphilis is diagnosed using serologic testing, typically screening with nontreponemal–specific tests such as the rapid plasma reagin (RPR) or Venereal Disease Research Laboratory assay (VDRL), followed by a treponemal-specific test, such as a fluorescent treponemal antibody test. However, testing algorithms can vary.[272] Because co-infections with multiple STDs are common, the diagnostic approach is multi-pronged as per CDC guidelines.[272]

Current CDC treatment guidelines[272] do not differentiate between sites of genital infections, so the treatment for rectal infection is the same as for urethral, cervical, or other genital infection. Special considerations include testing for LGV, because the duration of antibiotics needed for LGV is longer than for uncomplicated *C. trachomatis* infection. HIV testing should be performed because its transmission is increased in the setting of proctitis. Finally, in the United States, the local health department should be notified of the infection, with the exception of HSV, which is not a notifiable disease. Sexual partners should also receive counseling.[272]

HPV is a common STD that can infect the anus (Chapter 129). Although HPV does not cause symptomatic inflammation or a proctitis syndrome, it causes anal warts and is highly associated with anal carcinoma. A meta-analysis found that 83.6% of all anal cancers were associated with HPV, and the most common infecting types were HPV16 (73.4%), HPV18 (5.2%), and HPV33 (4.8%).[273] Receptive anal intercourse is believed to be the most common risk for transmission but does not appear to be required for anal infection. Several studies have shown that HIV-infected MSM are at particularly high risk for HPV infection, with over 90% having anal HPV infection, often with multiple types. Studies of healthy women found that anal and cervical HPV infection rates are nearly identical.[274] Two vaccines, a quadrivalent and a bivalent vaccine, are available for the prevention of HPV infection; however, only the quadrivalent vaccine is currently FDA approved for the prevention of HPV-related anal cancer in both men and women.[275] Further discussion of prevention, screening, diagnosis, and treatment of anal cancer is beyond the scope of this chapter.

VIRAL PATHOGENS

Viruses are the leading cause of acute gastroenteritis in the United States and globally, accounting for the majority of diagnosed acute episodes of community-acquired diarrhea.[30,31,276] The leading human pathogens are rotavirus, caliciviruses (norovirus and sapovirus), enteric adenovirus, and astrovirus. Some picornaviruses (e.g., Aichi virus) likely cause gastroenteritis; other viral causes of gastroenteritis remain unproven.

Rotavirus

Discovered in 1963, rotavirus is a segmented double-stranded RNA virus with an icosahedral structure that resembles the spokes of a wheel, hence "rota" (Fig. 110-4). Seven rotavirus groups, A through G, have been identified, of which group A causes most human disease. Rotavirus infection is now recognized as a leading cause of infectious gastroenteritis worldwide and is extremely common in children, with the majority of cases occurring in those younger than age 5.[277]

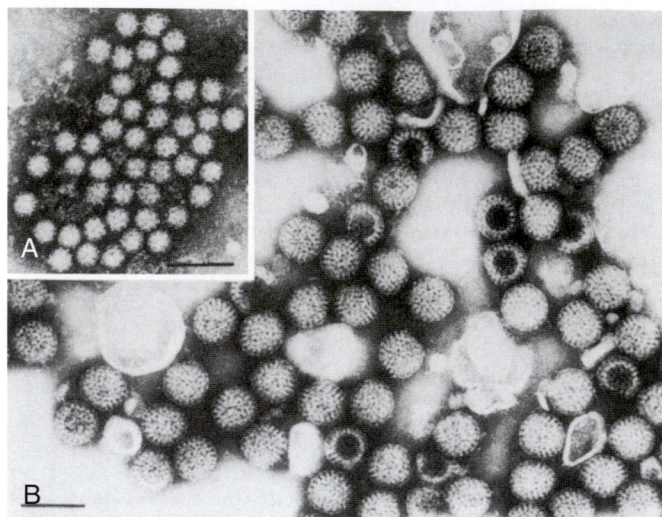

FIGURE 110-4. *A,* Electron micrograph of norovirus particles from the stool of a volunteer to whom the Norwalk agent was administered. *B,* Human rotavirus particles from the stool of an infant with gastroenteritis. The particles appear to have a double-shelled capsid. Occasional empty particles are seen. Bar = 100 nm. *(A and B courtesy A. Kapikian, MD, Bethesda, MD Previously published in Lennete EH, Schmidt NJ. Diagnostic procedures for viral, rickettsial, and chlamydial infections. 5th ed. New York: American Public Health Association; 1979. p 933.)*

Pathology and Pathogenesis

The pathophysiology of diarrhea with rotavirus is complex. Duodenal biopsy specimens of young children with rotavirus infection have demonstrated patchy abnormalities.[278] In its severe form, the infection can produce denuded villi and flattening of the epithelial surface that can persist for weeks, yielding reduced brush border levels of disaccharidases and malabsorption of carbohydrates, fats, and protein. Rotavirus also elaborates an enterotoxin, NSP4, that activates calcium signaling and the ENS, both of which stimulate intestinal secretion and diarrhea.[279]

Epidemiology

Rotavirus is nearly a ubiquitous infection among children younger than age 5 across the globe, with little difference in infection rates between the developing and developed world. Reinfections, although common, are typically less severe. Prior to vaccine development, rotavirus accounted for 30% to 70% of all hospital admissions in children with acute gastroenteritis. Thus, the clinical and economic impact of rotavirus is large and spurred vaccine development to prevent serious rotavirus disease. Disease tends to peak in the cooler months and winter. Secondary spread to adults is not infrequent (≈20%) and may be symptomatic; rotavirus causes outbreaks and morbidity in the older adult population.[24] Since introduction of live-attenuated rotavirus vaccines, cases and mortality are significantly reduced in both developing and developed countries. In the United States, with introduction of rotavirus vaccination, norovirus has become the leading cause of acute gastroenteritis in children seeking medical care, and accounts for a million health care visits annually (see later).[280]

Clinical Features

The infectious inoculum for rotavirus infection is small, estimated at 1 to 10 virions, and the incubation period is 1 to 3 days.[277] Rotavirus causes a range of clinical illness from asymptomatic carriage to severe dehydration and death.[281] Factors that can influence the severity of rotavirus infection include initial infection (with reinfections typically being less severe), malnutrition, immunocompromise, lack of maternal immunity (normally transmitted to the infant transplacentally or by breast milk), changes in the circulating community rotavirus serotype, and a large inoculum size. Vomiting often heralds the illness and is followed shortly by watery diarrhea, which often leads to dehydration. Fever is noted in about one third of children. The average duration of illness is 5 to 7 days, although chronic diarrhea has been noted. Asymptomatic excretion of virus for several weeks after infection occurs in approximately one third of infected children.[282]

Diagnosis

Although most cases are diagnosed clinically, rapid diagnostic tests are available for detection of rotavirus antigen in the feces using several commercial immunoassays (e.g., EIA, latex agglutination) or NAATs.[34]

Treatment and Vaccination

Because loss of fluids and electrolytes is the main pathophysiology of rotavirus infection, rehydration is the mainstay of therapy for this infection. Nutritional support complements fluid replacement therapy. A very small study suggested nitazoxanide may diminish symptoms in outpatients at least 12 years of age.[283]

Two rotavirus vaccines are commercially available in the United States and many other countries.[277,284] Both vaccines are live-attenuated vaccines that are administered orally. RotaTeq (Merck and Co, Inc, West Point, PA) is a pentavalent rotavirus vaccine (5 human reassortment human/bovine strains [RV5]), and Rotarix (GlaxoSmithKline, Philadelphia, PA) is a monovalent (RV1) vaccine. Both are recommended for administration in multiple doses beginning at 2 months of age (RotaTeq, 3 doses at 2, 4, and 6 months of age; Rotarix, 2 doses at 2 and 4 months of age). Both vaccines have been shown to be highly effective in preventing severe gastroenteritis, with reductions in diarrhea-related hospitalizations.[285] An earlier rotavirus vaccine was withdrawn from the market in 1999 owing to increased risk of intussusception associated with vaccination. Although a small excess risk of intussusception is possible with the current vaccines, the benefits of vaccination outweigh the risks as assessed by the Advisory Committee on Immunization Practices[277,286]; no excess risk of intussusception was identified in a Cochrane review.[285] Rotavirus vaccination is currently contraindicated in infants with a history of intussusception. WHO recommended inclusion of rotavirus vaccination in all global national vaccination programs in 2009.

Caliciviruses (Norovirus and Sapovirus)

Caliciviruses (Greek *kalyx,* the cup of a flower) are nonenveloped single-stranded RNA viruses composed of 2 genera of the Caliciviridae, norovirus and sapovirus. Noroviruses dominate as global pathogens (see Fig. 110-4); sapoviruses that induce an indistinguishable clinical disease are variably detected in both children and adults.[31,276] This section will focus on norovirus infections.

The canonical norovirus is the Norwalk agent identified in 1968 in Norwalk, Ohio, as the cause of an outbreak of "winter vomiting disease." Prior to viral sequencing, similar viruses were termed *Norwalk-like* and named for the location of discovery. Subsequently named *noroviruses,* this group of viruses exhibits error-prone replication, and their capacity for recombination has yielded 5 genogroups (GI and GII being key in human disease), 30 or more genotypes (e.g., GI.1, GII.4, etc.) and many variants (e.g., GII.4 Bristol/1993/UK, etc.).[287] The spectacular diversity and capacity for epochal evolution similar to influenza results in recurring peaks of illnesses as new norovirus genotypes emerge in communities. Most humans remain susceptible to repeated norovirus infections for life.

Epidemiology

Noroviruses are the most common cause of community-acquired diarrhea, gastroenteritis outbreaks, and foodborne disease in the United States and globally. Consistent with this high disease burden, recent incidence estimates for the United States indicate that norovirus causes up to 800 deaths, 71,000 hospitalizations, 400,000 emergency department visits, 1.9 million outpatient visits, and 21 million total illnesses annually.[288] These estimates are similar to the limited estimates available from other industrialized countries. In addition, introduction of rotavirus vaccination has resulted in norovirus emerging as the leading cause of medically attended acute gastroenteritis in children in the United States.[280] A number of epidemiologic networks now exist to identify and track the impact of norovirus disease globally including NORS (National Outbreak Reporting System, USA), CalciNET (USA), NoroNet (Europe), and ViroNet (Canada) among others. Norovirus infections are costly and in 2011 were estimated to result in $2 billion in costs for foodborne disease in the United States and $500 million in hospitalization costs. The cost of a single hospital outbreak was reported as approximately $650,000.[289]

Noroviruses may be the perfect infectious pathogen, contributing to their broad global epidemiologic impact.[290] These viruses are highly contagious (median infectious inoculum 18 to 1000 viral particles); use multiple transmission modes (person-to-person, food, water, airborne, fomites); are prolifically shed (≈100 billion particles/g feces, peak shedding); are environmentally stable (survive freezing, heating, multiple disinfectants); constantly evolve, yielding exposure of human populations to new variants; and induce limited, usually short-term host immunity. By being moderately virulent, noroviruses maintain a large pool of susceptible hosts.

Clinical Features

Clinically, most individuals of all ages are susceptible to norovirus infections, which occur year-round, although outbreaks may be more frequent in winter. The incubation period is 12 to 48 hours, and the resulting illnesses typically last 1 to 3 days; young children, older adults, and immunocompromised hosts may experience protracted illnesses.[287,291] There is a range of disease expression likely due to variability of the viral receptor and human blood group antigens that are expressed as oligosaccharides on the surface of intestinal epithelial cells.

Overall, about 10% of individuals are not susceptible to norovirus infection, whereas among the approximately 90% who acquire norovirus infection, 70% are symptomatic and 30% remain asymptomatic. Most symptomatic norovirus infections lead to nausea, vomiting, and diarrhea, with small subsets exhibiting only vomiting (children) or diarrhea (older adults). Low-grade fever is common (≈50%), as are systemic symptoms such as malaise. Disease expression is not linked to the norovirus type but is driven by the host's response to the infection. Viral shedding peaks at 1 to 3 days of disease, but median shedding can be protracted. In the healthy host, viral antigen (protein) is detected in stool for a median of 7 days, whereas median shedding is 28 days by viral nucleic acid testing (PCR).

Immunocompromised hosts can exhibit prolonged shedding or diarrhea, although transmissibility in these chronic infections is unclear.[291,292] In contrast, as noted earlier, acute symptomatic disease is associated with easy transmissibility to other individuals.[293] Mortality is low with appropriate fluid management. Similar to other diarrheal diseases, increased mortality may occur in young children or older adults. Recent data indicate that those older than 65 years are at greatest risk for norovirus-associated death, and children younger than 5 years have the highest rates of norovirus-associated medical care visits.[288] Mortality in older adults occurs early in dehydrating disease and has been linked to situations where the availability of health care personnel is limited.[25]

Diagnosis

The rapid diagnosis of noroviruses has been hampered by viral diversity and, thus, norovirus epidemics have traditionally been identified using Kaplan's criteria established in 1982: a norovirus outbreak is suspected if a short incubation period (1 to 2 days) is identified, the duration of illness is short (12 to 60 hours), over 50% of those affected exhibit vomiting, and stool cultures are negative.[294] These criteria have been found to be very sensitive (99%) but, as expected, not very specific (68%). Molecular methods for detection of norovirus are very sensitive and, thus, just as with testing for other enteric pathogens, should be used only on diarrheal stools obtained from symptomatic patients. No assays for norovirus are yet FDA approved. One norovirus antigen detection kit (RIDASCREEN NV) is approved by the FDA for outbreak evaluation. Although the cost/benefit of routine utilization of norovirus diagnostics is debated,[295] establishing that an illness is due to norovirus may assist the clinician in management and lead to less utilization of additional costly tests and procedures.

Treatment and Prevention

No specific therapy is available for norovirus infections, and maintenance of hydration is the cornerstone of care. In general, antimotility and antisecretory drugs appear safe to use in norovirus infections. A very small study suggested activity of nitazoxanide against norovirus, similar to rotavirus.[283] Decreasing or modifying immunosuppression may alter the disease course in immunocompromised hosts by augmenting host defenses. Prevention of norovirus infections is challenging, given the characteristics of the virus and its great potential for contagion.[296] Soap-and-water hand hygiene (washing for 20 seconds) is recommended because the virus is relatively resistant to alcohol-based hand sanitizers. Environmental cleaning with removal of visible material, followed by 1000 to 5000 ppm chlorine bleach solution cleaning is recommended. Ill individuals are to be excluded from work for 48 to 72 hours post illness, and individual rooms or cohorting is recommended for nosocomial infections. No vaccines are yet available to prevent norovirus infections, although a candidate norovirus vaccine is approaching a phase 3 efficacy trial.

Enteric Adenovirus and Astrovirus

Most adenoviruses cause upper respiratory infections, but a group of fastidious strains known as *serotypes 40 and 41*, which constitute subgenus F, are responsible for gastroenteritis in children, predominantly those younger than 2 years and in association with day care.[297-299] Nosocomial infections (e.g., in immunocompromised children) occur; disease in adults is uncommon. Unlike infection with rotavirus or norovirus, enteric adenovirus infection has a long incubation period of 8 to 10 days; the illness can be prolonged for up to 2 weeks.

Enteric adenoviruses are less infectious than rotavirus or norovirus and have an overall lower medical impact.[300] Diagnosis is typically by EIA or NAAT of stool.

Astrovirus causes endemic childhood diarrhea, diarrhea in day care centers, and nosocomial infections.[299,301,302] Unlike norovirus, astrovirus appears to be an infrequent cause of epidemic gastroenteritis but may cause outbreaks in institutionalized older adults. Immunocompromised patients, including those with AIDS and bone marrow transplants, appear to be at increased risk. Treatment is supportive and, similar to all viral gastroenteritis, emphasizes oral rehydration.

TRAVELER'S DIARRHEA

In 2011, an estimated 8% of 50 to 100 million travelers to developing countries sought medical care, of whom at least 25% to 50% had GI symptoms.[303] Diarrhea is considered the most common medical complaint of travelers. Fortunately, 90% of cases are brief and self-limited, but 5% to 10% of patients develop dysentery, and 1% to 2% of travelers have persistent diarrhea lasting at least 2 weeks; some develop post-infection IBS and have long-term, if not lifelong, irregular bowel habits thereafter.

Bacterial enteric pathogens, identified in 60% to 80% of cases, are the primary cause of traveler's diarrhea.[98,99] Most infections are acquired from food and drink. Although an array of pathogens has been found, the leading culprits are various forms of *E. coli*, particularly ETEC and EAEC, accounting for as many as 50% to 75% of cases overall (see Table 110-1). Regional differences in suspected etiologies of traveler's diarrhea exist. In a review of 51 studies,[74] ETEC, for example, was less common in Southeast Asia (7.2%) compared with other regions, and EAEC was uncommon in Africa (1.8%). Invasive infections (e.g., *Campylobacter* and *Salmonella*) were particularly common in Southeast Asia, whereas *Shigella* infections were most common in Africa and South Asia. Norovirus accounts for approximately 15% of traveler's diarrhea. The clinician should not forget the possibility of *C. difficile* in the traveler exposed to antibiotics. Parasitic causes, especially *Giardia, Entamoeba histolytica,* and *Cryptosporidium* (see Chapter 113) become more common etiologies of traveler's diarrhea as the duration of diarrhea increases, particularly once diarrhea is persistent (>14 days).

The risk of developing traveler's diarrhea depends on the host's susceptibility, travel and eating habits, length of stay, and destination. Risk of disease relates to levels of sanitation and water cleanliness. South Asia, sub-Saharan Africa, and South America exhibit the highest rates of disease, and North America, Japan, Australia, and Europe the lowest rates of traveler's diarrhea. The purpose of travel and the style of eating also influence the risk of developing disease. The greatest frequency of diarrhea occurs in people traveling as students or itinerant tourists, the lowest risk is in those visiting relatives, and an intermediate risk exists in business travelers.

Most traveler's diarrhea is watery and self-limited (1 to 3 days), and evaluation by a physician is not necessary. Evaluation is required in cases that are prolonged; accompanied by fever, systemic manifestations, or bloody stool; or that occur in immunocompromised persons (see Evaluation, earlier). The disease does not begin immediately after the traveler's arrival but generally has its onset 2 or 3 days later, consistent with the incubation period of the inciting enteric pathogen. If diarrhea persists more than 14 days and infectious causes have been excluded, the possibility of malabsorption or tropical sprue, as well potential unmasking of previously subclinical

---

BOX 110-1 Causes of Prolonged Diarrheal Illness after Travel

Infectious Etiologies
Persistent bacterial infection
Persistent protozoan infection
    Giardia lamblia
    Entamoeba histolytica
    Cryptosporidium hominis and parvis
    Cyclospora cayetanensis
    Isospora belli
Antibiotic-associated colitis

Post-infection IBS

Noninfectious Etiologies
Dietary intolerances
Disaccharidase deficiency
IBD
Celiac disease
Tropical sprue
Lymphocytic/collagenous colitis

From Chak A, Banwell JG. Traveler's diarrhea. Gastroenterol Clin North Am 1993; 22:549.

---

illnesses such as celiac disease, IBD, or lymphocytic colitis, should be considered. Prior GI infection is a risk factor for developing post-infection IBS. Box 110-1 lists causes of prolonged traveler's diarrhea.

As for all forms of diarrhea, treatment entails fluid replacement. Usually, ingestion of readily digestible foods (e.g., soups, saltines, bananas) is adequate. Milk and dairy products should be avoided because lactose intolerance is common. In mild cases, bismuth subsalicylate, which has antibacterial, antisecretory and anti-inflammatory properties, or loperamide as an antimotility agent alone may be effective.

Because of the high likelihood of a bacterial infection causing traveler's diarrhea, antibacterial therapy is highly effective to alleviate the distress of disrupted work or pleasure and is recommended in moderate to severe illness (Table 110-9). Three antibiotics are recommended: fluoroquinolones, rifaximin, and azithromycin.[98,99] Ciprofloxacin is often employed for empiric therapy of traveler's diarrhea, as either just 1 dose or, if there is not complete response, continuation with twice-daily dosing for 3 days. Concern exists about the potential for increasing tendinitis and tendon rupture, as well as a predisposition to *C. difficile* colitis, with use of fluoroquinolones. Additional concerns are increasing resistance of ETEC and *Campylobacter* to fluoroquinolones. In Southeast Asia, fluoroquinolone resistance of *Campylobacter* has exceeded 90%; in Nepal, where *Campylobacter* is the most frequent pathogen in traveler's diarrhea, resistance to ciprofloxacin is approximately 70%. Rifaximin is approved in the United States for the treatment of noninvasive, afebrile forms of traveler's diarrhea in patients older than 12 years. This drug has demonstrated minimal potential for development of bacterial resistance. Azithromycin is recommended for febrile or dysenteric traveler's diarrhea or as a rescue medication if failure of rifaximin or fluoroquinolones occurs. Recommended doses for therapy are found in Table 110-9. Azithromycin is active against invasive pathogens, including *Shigella* and *Campylobacter*. Trials have shown combination therapy with antibiotics and loperamide to be safe and effective, although a recent meta-analysis suggests benefit is limited to the first 24 to 48 hours of therapy.[304] A common approach is to arm a traveler going to a high-risk region with antibiotic and antimotility agents for self-therapy.[305] Development of probiotics as prevention or therapy for traveler's diarrhea is in progress, although data are as yet inadequate for

TABLE 110-9 Drugs Used for Prophylaxis and Treatment of Traveler's Diarrhea in Adults

Prophylaxis	Agent	Dose	Comments
Chemoprophylaxis is not indicated for most travelers.			
Nonantibiotic[a]	Bismuth subsalicylate (Pepto Bismol)	525 mg (1 ounce liquid or 2 tablets chewed of regular-strength preparation) 4 times daily	Avoid in persons taking salicylates or warfarin. Can interfere with the absorption of doxycycline used for malaria prevention, and can cause blackening of the tongue and stool.
Antibiotics[b]	Norfloxacin[c]	400 mg PO daily	Antibiotic prophylaxis should be reserved for highly selected persons (see text).
	Ciprofloxacin[c]	500 mg PO daily	
	Rifaximin	200 mg once or twice daily	

Treatment	Agent	Dosage	Comments
Medical care should be sought when there is volume depletion, severe abdominal pain, high fever, bloody stools, or persistent illness despite treatment.			
Hydration[d]	Specific oral rehydration salts or potable liquids ab libitum	Until thirst quenched	Hydration should be maintained in all forms of diarrhea.
Symptomatic[e]	Bismuth subsalicylate (Pepto Bismol)	525 mg (1 ounce liquid or 2 tablets chewed of regular-strength preparation) every half hour for 8 doses	Reduces the number of loose stools by ≈50%. Should not be taken by those with a salicylate allergy or who are taking salicylates or warfarin.
	Loperamide	4 mg PO then 2 mg after each loose stool, not to exceed 16 mg daily	More rapid onset of action compared with bismuth subsalicylate. Should not be used when there is a fever (temperature >38.5°C) or gross blood in the stool.
Antibiotics[f]	Fluoroquinolone Norfloxacin	800 mg PO once or 400 mg PO twice daily	A single dose can be given initially and then the response evaluated over the following 12-24 hr. If traveler's diarrhea is improved, the antibiotic can be discontinued; otherwise the antibiotic can be continued for up to 3 days (this applies to all fluoroquinolones listed).
	Ciprofloxacin	750 mg PO once or 500 mg PO twice daily	
	Ofloxacin	400 mg PO once or 200 mg PO twice daily	
	Levofloxacin	500 mg PO once or 500 mg PO twice daily	
	Azithromycin	500-1000 mg PO once or 500 mg daily × 3 days	Has better activity against fluoroquinolone-resistant *Campylobacter* that is an increased risk during travel to South and Southeast Asia. 1000-mg dose can cause nausea.
	Rifaximin	200 mg PO three times daily × 3 days	Can be used for the treatment of individuals ≥12 years of age with traveler's diarrhea caused by noninvasive strains of *Escherichia coli*.

[a]There is insufficient evidence for the efficacy of probiotic preparations in the prevention of traveler's diarrhea.
[b]Prophylaxis of traveler's diarrhea is generally not an approved use of antibiotics.
[c]Other fluoroquinolones are likely to be effective but have not been studied for prophylaxis against traveler's diarrhea.
[d]Hydration may be accomplished in healthy adults by drinking potable fluids ad libitum or in the young, older adults, or, those with chronic medical conditions, by drinking oral rehydration solutions (see text and table 110-6).
[e]Symptomatic therapy alone can be given to persons with mild to moderate traveler's diarrhea: 1 to 3 loose stools per 24 hours with or without mild enteric symptoms. PO, orally.
[f]Antibiotics can be given to persons with moderate to severe traveler's diarrhea: 3 or more loose stools within 24 hours, plus other enteric symptoms or diarrhea that has not responded to symptomatic treatment. In persons with traveler's diarrhea with no blood in the stool, combining an antibiotic with loperamide can lead to rapid relief of symptoms.
Adapted from Hill DR, Beeching NJ. Travelers' diarrhea. Curr Opin Infect Dis 2010; 23:481-7.

clear recommendations.[98] A Cochrane review supported use of probiotics to shorten acute diarrheal illnesses, although more research was needed to identify appropriate patient groups and products.[306]

The primary approach to prevent traveler's diarrhea is avoidance of unsafe foods and beverages. Bottled beverages generally are safe, although some epidemics have been associated with contaminated bottled drinks.[307] Carbonated beverages are safer than noncarbonated ones, owing to their low pH (generally 4.0 to 5.0), which has antibacterial properties. Beer or wine is generally safe, as is tea or coffee prepared with boiling water if consumed while still hot. Travelers are advised not to eat food from street vendors; it is recommended not to consume unpasteurized foods and unpeeled fruits.

The high incidence of bacterial pathogens as a cause of traveler's diarrhea makes the use of prophylactic antibiotics tempting; however, safe-eating and safe-drinking habits are the traveler's best methods of prophylaxis. Prophylaxis is recommended, however, for selected groups of travelers: those with severe kidney, liver, or heart disease; insulin-dependent diabetes; IBD; gastrectomy, achlorhydria; or ileostomies; also persons who are taking glucocorticoids or who have immunosuppressive illnesses. In addition, prophylaxis can be considered for people whose important business plans will be disrupted by illness. Bismuth subsalicylate, fluoroquinolones, or rifaximin are possible prophylactic agents (see Table 110-9). Pros and cons of use of these agents are discussed elsewhere.[99] The potential toxicity of antibiotics (e.g., rashes, photosensitivity, the rarer Stevens-Johnson syndrome, antibiotic-associated colitis, and vaginal candidiasis), as well as the development of antimicrobial resistance, should be considered.

TB OF THE INTESTINAL TRACT

Any region of the GI tract can be involved with TB. Intestinal TB accounts for 1% to 3% of TB worldwide. Among extrapulmonary tuberculous disease, intestinal involvement is less common than involvement of lymph nodes, the genitourinary tract, bone and joints, miliary disease, or meningeal disease. HIV infection, in particular among immunocompromising conditions, drives development of clinical TB disease globally, with up to 50% of TB in this population presenting with extrapulmonary TB. Other important risk factors for development of tuberculous enteritis include malignancies (especially lymphoma) and treatment with glucocorticoids or anti-TNF agents.[308,309]

Mycobacterium tuberculosis is the pathogen responsible for most cases of intestinal TB. *Mycobacterium bovis*, an organism found in contaminated dairy products, is responsible for some cases, although uncommon in Western countries. The usual route of infection is direct penetration of the intestinal mucosa by swallowed organisms, either in sputum or contaminated milk/food. In the past, intestinal TB was associated with active pulmonary infection and especially with active laryngeal involvement, but this is no longer true, and chest films are usually without evidence of primary disease or normal at the time of diagnosis of tuberculous enteritis. Alternatively, tuberculous enteritis results from direct extension from adjacent affected organs or military spread to the intestine.

TB can affect any region or multiple regions of the GI tract, although the ileum and cecum are the most common sites of intestinal involvement and are affected in 75% of cases. Both sides of the ileocecal valve usually are involved, leading to incompetence of the valve, a finding that helps distinguish TB from Crohn's disease.

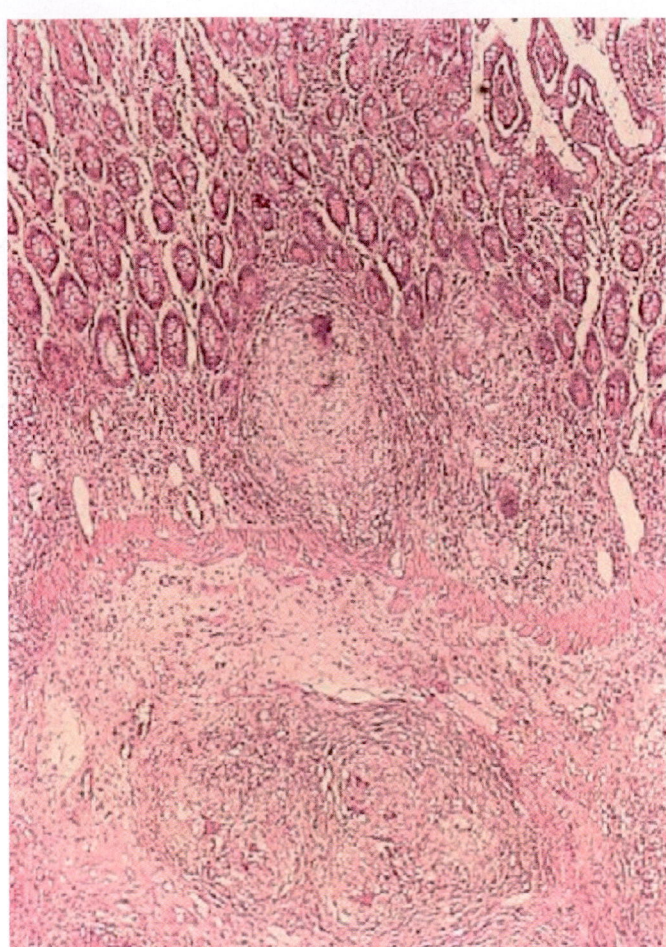

FIGURE 110-5. Photomicrograph of a colon biopsy specimen from a patient with intestinal TB, showing granulomas in the mucosa and submucosa. (H&E.)

The gross appearance of intestinal TB is divided into the following 3 categories: (1) ulcerative lesions (60% of patients) consisting of multiple superficial lesions confined largely to the epithelial surface; (2) hypertrophic lesions (10% of patients) manifesting as scarring, fibrosis, and heaped-up mass lesions that can mimic carcinoma; and (3) ulcerohypertrophic lesions (30% of patients) where mucosal ulcerations are combined with healing and scar formation.[310] Healing of ulcers results in fibrosis, causing stricture formation. Histologically, the distinguishing lesion is the granuloma, which is seen in 50% to 80% of tuberculous enteritis (Fig. 110-5); caseation is common but not always seen. TB bacilli are detected with an acid-fast stain in approximately 20% of mucosal samples; PCR is more sensitive (≈65%).[308]

TB is the great masquerader and can mimic almost any disease affecting the GI tract.[309] Presentation can be acute, chronic, or acute-on-chronic. Differentiating tuberculous enteritis from Crohn's disease can be difficult (see later). The most common complaint is nonspecific chronic abdominal pain, reported in 80% to 90% of patients. Accompanying symptoms can include weight loss, fever, diarrhea or constipation, and blood in the stool. A palpable right lower quadrant abdominal mass is found in approximately 25% to 50% of patients. Laboratory findings include mild anemia with a normal WBC count. Complications include intestinal hemorrhage, perforation, obstruction, fistula formation, and malabsorption. Perforation is uncommon but can occur even during treatment. Intestinal obstruction is a more common finding and typically results from segmental stenotic disease. Surgical intervention may be required to relieve obstruction, despite appropriate drug therapy. Malabsorption can occur when obstruction leads to proximal SIBO.

A presumptive diagnosis of intestinal TB can be established in a patient with active pulmonary TB and radiologic and clinical findings that suggest intestinal involvement. Colonoscopy with biopsy for histopathology, acid-fast bacilli staining/PCR, and culture (with drug sensitivities) is the most useful procedure for diagnosis. When TB is suspected, isolation masks are required in the endoscopy suite. A positive tuberculin skin test or, as an alternative test to detect *M. tuberculosis* infection, the interferon gamma release assay, is not very helpful because a positive test does not necessarily mean active disease. In addition, many patients, especially older persons and those with HIV infection, have a negative skin test in the face of active intestinal TB.

Similar to the clinical features, the radiologic appearance of TB enteritis is diverse.[311] Radiologic examination can reveal a thickened bowel wall with distortion of mucosal folds, ulcerations, varying degrees of bowel stenosis, and pseudopolyp formation (Fig. 110-6). CT can show thickening of the ileocecal valve, asymmetric bowel wall thickening, and

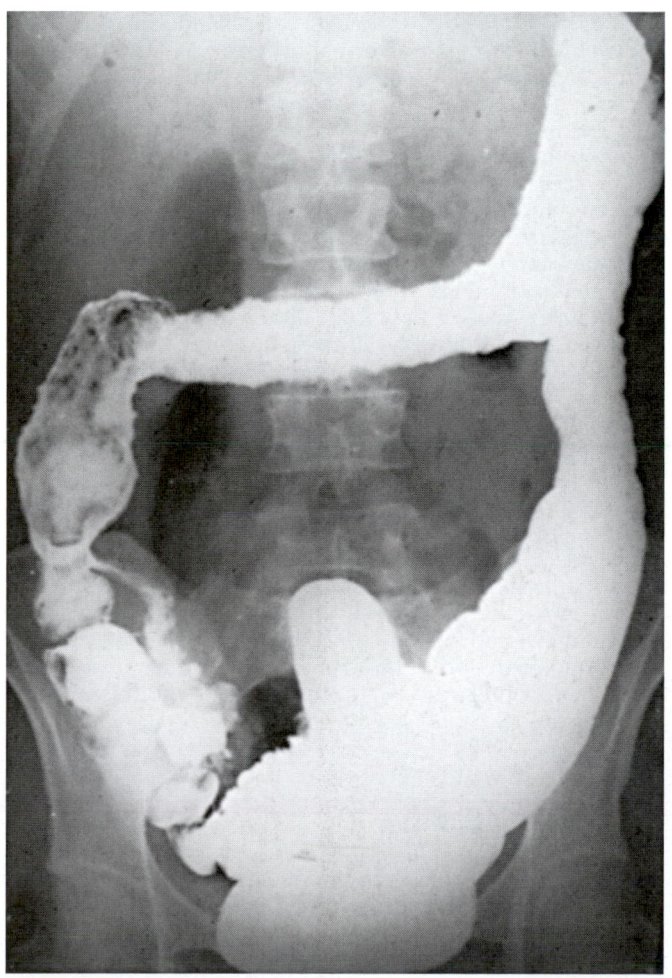

FIGURE 110-6. Film from a barium enema of a patient with colonic TB, showing extensive involvement of the cecum, ascending, and transverse colon. The ulcerated, narrowed ahaustral appearance is typical of colitis. *(Courtesy H.I. Goldberg, MD, San Francisco, Calif.)*

massive lymphadenopathy with central necrosis. The cecum is contracted with disease on both sides of the valve, and the valve itself often is distorted and incompetent; conification of the cecum, as seen on barium enema, is characteristic of TB and is referred to as *Stierlin's sign*. In the hypertrophic form, a mass may resemble a carcinoma. Calcified mesenteric lymph nodes and an abnormal chest film are other findings that aid in the diagnosis of intestinal TB.

Several diseases can resemble intestinal TB. Crohn's disease can manifest virtually all of the changes of intestinal TB except for the presence of the organism. Features of potential help in differentiating tuberculous enteritis from Crohn's disease include an inflammatory mass centered in the ileocecum; transverse, circumferential ulcers rather than linear ulcers along the bowel axis (the latter is seen in Crohn's disease); cecal valve incompetence with Stierlin's sign; and large, hypodense (necrotizing/caseous) mesenteric lymph nodes. Numerous infections can mimic tuberculous enteritis, including yersiniosis, histoplasmosis, actinomycosis, schistosomiasis, amebiasis, syphilis, and LGV. The abdominal masses of tuberculous enteritis can suggest malignancy. Colonoscopy with biopsy is critical in differentiating mimicking disorders.

TB is a reportable disease; if clinically suspected, public health authorities should be notified. A high index of suspicion warrants empirical anti-TB therapy pending the results of the diagnostic evaluation, including cultures and drug sensitivity testing. An expert in management of TB should be engaged to assist in therapeutic management. Tuberculous enteritis is generally treated similarly to pulmonary TB. If TB is the correct diagnosis, clinical responses to therapy often occur within 2 weeks, although the marked hyperplasia, masses, and stenosis of tuberculous enteritis respond more slowly. Occasionally an operative approach is still required for obstructive disease and/or if intestinal perforation or hemorrhage occur.

OVERVIEW OF TREATMENT

Fluid Therapy

Rehydration is the initial goal of therapy for all diarrheal illnesses. Oral rehydration solutions (ORS), used most widely in developing countries, can be used to rehydrate patients with moderate volume depletion and also can be used in patients with severe diarrhea after initial parenteral replacement of fluid.[312] Introduction of ORS in the 1950s proved to be a medical breakthrough, leading to substantial reductions in the morbidity and mortality of diarrheal illnesses globally.

The effectiveness of an ORS is a function of its electrolyte content, which is formulated to replace stool losses. ORS contain an actively transported substrate, commonly glucose. The use of ORS is based on the physiologic principle that glucose and other substrates enhance sodium absorption in the small intestine, even in the presence of secretory losses caused by infections (see Chapter 101). A variety of ORS formulations are available and effective (see Table 110-6).[312] Even in patients who are vomiting, small increments of ORS can be given effectively. Most studies of ORS have been conducted in children, but the results can be extrapolated to adults until evidence to the contrary for adults is available. In 2002, WHO recommended use of reduced-osmolarity ORS in children with acute non-cholera diarrhea (see Table 110-6). In general, studies of reduced-osmolarity ORS indicated that this ORS formulation resulted in a significant reduction in stool output and incidence of vomiting compared with standard WHO-ORS. Although there was initial concern, the risk of hyponatremia with reduced-osmolarity ORS is not increased, based on available data in studied populations that exceed 50,000 adults or children.[312] Polymer-based ORS is an alternative formulation in which typically rice (or other starch) is substituted for glucose. The concept for these formulations is that the polymers yield increased numbers of glucose molecules in the jejunum, as well as possibly short-chain fatty acids in the colon, thus enhancing sodium and water absorption. Patient acceptance of rice-based ORS is high, stool output is reduced, and cost may be less. Studies also suggest that polymer-based ORS is superior to standard WHO-ORS, but it is unclear whether it is superior to reduced-osmolarity ORS.

Diet

Eating during an acute diarrheal illness may be unpalatable. Although giving the bowel a rest may provide partial relief from symptoms, it is best to eat judiciously during an attack of diarrhea. In children, it is particularly important to restart feeding immediately after the child is able to accept oral intake. It is wise to avoid milk and dairy products during acute diarrhea because of the potential for secondary lactase deficiency. Caffeine in coffee, tea, cocoa, and cola soft drinks can potentiate abdominal cramps and diarrhea. Abstinence from alcohol is recommended. In addition to use of ORS (see Table 110-6), acceptable beverages for mildly dehydrated adults include fruit juices and some bottled soft drinks. Foods such as soups, saltine crackers, bananas, mashed potatoes, and rice are most acceptable to patients with acute diarrhea.

Antimicrobial Drugs

Only limited cases of acute infectious diarrhea benefit from treatment with antimicrobial drugs (see Table 110-8). Even when antibiotic therapy is prescribed, clinical impact on disease course is often modest, with older data suggesting that impact on symptom duration occurs primarily when treatment is initiated early (within 2 days) of symptom onset[313,314]; most patients do not seek medical care until later in the course of an acute diarrheal illness. Except in acute mild/moderate traveler's diarrhea, the decision to treat with antibiotics should be accompanied by obtaining a liquid stool sample for diagnostic testing. In clinically ill patients (e.g., febrile dysentery), blood cultures are also prudent to detect, for example, systemic salmonellosis. Specific diagnosis of ill patients with diarrhea is important, given rising rates of antibiotic resistance among enteric pathogens, overlap in the clinical presentation of enteric pathogens, and the inability to predict the offending pathogen at the bedside (see Table 110-4). Other concerns with use of antibiotics include the possibility of promoting an adverse outcome such as enhancing the risk of HUS with STEC infections (see STEC) or prolonging fecal excretion of *Salmonella*. Among bacterial pathogens, only *Shigella*, *C. difficile*, and *V. cholerae* are clear indications for antibacterial treatment of infectious diarrhea in the immunocompetent host.

Empiric therapy is clearly warranted in traveler's diarrhea[98,99,315] and in those who are severely ill with infectious diarrhea, such as those with high-volume diarrhea and evident clinical severity.[19,75,316] Therapy subsequently can be tailored based on the clinical course and/or the diagnostic evaluation, including results of in vitro antibiotic sensitivity testing for bacterial pathogens isolated in the microbiology laboratory. A fluoroquinolone is typically the drug of choice for adults, but these drugs are generally not recommended for children or pregnant women. Concerns with use of fluoroquinolones include GI disturbances, infrequent CNS toxicity, tendinitis, tendon rupture, hypersensitivity reactions, rarely disturbances of glucose metabolism, and drug interactions. Azithromycin is an alternative to fluoroquinolone treatment. Some authors,

however, consider azithromycin to be the drug of choice because of its activity against fluoroquinolone-resistant *Campylobacter* (common in Southeast Asia and Nepal/India) as well as its safety profile, including use in children and pregnant women. Concern about lethal arrhythmias due to QT-interval prolongation exists for both fluoroquinolones and azithromycin, particularly in those with underlying cardiovascular disease or potential drug-drug interactions.[317]

The optimal duration of antimicrobial therapy has not been defined with precision. Three to 5 days of antibiotic therapy is typical except when *C. difficile* is diagnosed (see Chapter 112). Five-day therapy with ciprofloxacin was superior to shorter durations of therapy for treatment of *S. dysenteriae* type 1.[318] In traveler's diarrhea and cholera, single doses of antibiotics may suffice. Additional details are contained in the individual sections on enteric pathogens in this chapter.

Nonspecific Therapy

Literally hundreds of antidiarrheal nostrums can be found in pharmacies and assorted medical establishments throughout the world. Many products contain a combination of drugs, most of which are therapeutically worthless and others potentially dangerous. A variety of over-the-counter and prescription preparations are available for symptomatic relief of diarrhea and abdominal cramping. Anticholinergic agents (e.g., dicyclomine, hyoscyamine) decrease intestinal motility and might provide relief of abdominal cramps but do not significantly alter diarrhea. Adsorbents such as kaolin, pectin, and activated charcoal decrease stool liquidity, but there is no evidence that these preparations decrease intestinal fluid loss or number of bowel movements.

The opiate derivatives loperamide and diphenoxylate-atropine are particularly useful in controlling moderate to severe diarrhea. Their overall effect is to enhance fluid transport, slow transit time, reduce fluid losses, and ameliorate abdominal cramping. Loperamide is arguably the best agent for acute, non-bloody, nonfebrile diarrhea, because it does not cross the blood-brain barrier, thereby reducing the risk for habituation or other CNS side effects. It also has the additional property of increasing anal sphincter tone. Treatment with loperamide tends to produce rapid improvement, often within the first day of therapy. The concern that an antimotility drug might exacerbate a case of dysentery[319] largely has been dispelled by clinical experience.[304] Nonetheless, these drugs are not recommended for use in patients with acute severe colitis, either infectious or noninfectious in origin.[315]

Bismuth subsalicylate is an antisecretory agent that has a low incidence of side effects and may help decrease stool liquidity and frequency (see Traveler's Diarrhea section). The drug possesses antimicrobial, antisecretory, and anti-inflammatory properties on the basis of its bismuth and salicylate moieties, respectively.

KEY REFERENCES

Full references for this chapter can be found on www.expertconsult.com.

5. Gill N, Wlodarska M, Finlay BB. Roadblocks in the gut: Barriers to enteric infection. Cell Microbiol 2011; 13:660-9.

14. Nataro J, Kaper J. Diarrheagenic *Escherichia coli*. Clin Microbiol Rev 1998; 11:142-201.

19. Pawlowski SW, Warren CA, Guerrant R. Diagnosis and treatment of acute or persistent diarrhea. Gastroenterology 2009; 136:1874-86.

31. Tam CC, Rodrigues LC, Viviani L, et al. Longitudinal study of infectious intestinal disease in the UK (IID2 study): Incidence in the community and presenting to general practice. Gut 2012; 61:69-77.

34. Baron EJ, Miller JM, Weinstein MP, et al. A guide to utilization of the microbiology laboratory for diagnosis of infectious diseases: 2013 recommendations by the Infectious Diseases Society of America (IDSA) and the American Society for Microbiology (ASM). Clin Infect Dis 2013; 57:e11-e121.

38. Harris JB, LaRocque RC, Qadri F, et al. Cholera. Lancet 2012; 379:2466-76.

75. Pfeiffer ML, DuPont HL, Ochoa TJ. The patient presenting with acute dysentery—A systematic review. J Infect 2012; 64:374-86.

99. Hill DR, Beeching NJ. Travelers' diarrhea. Curr Opin Infect Dis 2010; 23:481-7.

105. Scallan E, Hoekstra RM, Angulo FJ, et al. Foodborne illness acquired in the United States—Major pathogens. Emerg Infect Dis 2011; 17:7-15.

178. Majowicz SE, Musto J, Scallan E, et al. The global burden of nontyphoidal *Salmonella* gastroenteritis. Clin Infect Dis 2010; 50:882-9.

277. Cox E, Christenson JC. Rotavirus. Pediatr Rev 2012; 33:439-45; quiz 446-7.

287. Glass RI, Parashar UD, Estes MK. Norovirus gastroenteritis. N Engl J Med 2009; 361:1776-85.

312. Atia AN, Buchman AL. Oral rehydration solutions in non-cholera diarrhea: A review. Am J Gastroenterol 2009; 104:2596-604; quiz 2605.

316. Guerrant RL, Van Gilder T, Steiner TS, et al. Practice guidelines for the management of infectious diarrhea. Clin Infect Dis 2001; 32:331-51.

CHAPTER OUTLINE

BACTERIAL FOOD POISONING

Food poisoning is defined as an illness caused by the consumption of food contaminated with bacteria, bacterial toxins, parasites (e.g., trichinosis), viruses (e.g., hepatitis), or chemicals (e.g., amanitin with ingestion of mushrooms). Of food poisoning episodes for which an etiology can be determined, bacteria account for 75% of outbreaks and 86% of cases in the United States[1,2]; only 42% of outbreaks, however, fulfill microbiological standards for a confirmed etiology, and nonbacterial pathogens, while more common, are proved less often. Using data from surveillance networks, the Centers for Disease Control and Prevention (CDC) estimated that each year in the United States, 31 major pathogens cause 9.4 million episodes of foodborne illness. Most were caused by Norovirus, and only 39% were caused by bacteria, of which nontyphoidal *Salmonella* spp., *Clostridium perfringens*, and *Campylobacter* spp. accounted for the majority.[3] An additional 38.4 million episodes of domestically acquired foodborne gastroenteritis is caused by unspecified agents, including bacteria known to cause acute gastroenteritis, agents which may not be recognized as being transmitted in food (e.g., *Clostridium difficile*), and as yet undefined agents.[4]

A foodborne disease outbreak is defined by 2 criteria: similar illness, usually GI, in 2 or more persons; and epidemiologic or laboratory investigation that implicates food as the source. An extensive list of agents has been associated with foodborne illnesses (Table 111-1).[1,2,5] The major recognized causes of bacterial food poisoning are *C. perfringens*; *Staphylococcus aureus*; Vibrios, including *V. cholerae* and *V. parahaemolyticus*; *Bacillus cereus*; *Salmonella*; *Clostridium botulinum*; *Shigella*; *Escherichia coli* O157:H7; and certain species of *Campylobacter*, *Yersinia*, *Listeria*, and *Aeromonas*. Other bacteria, such as group A *Streptococcus* and *Listeria monocytogenes*, have been implicated in some outbreaks.

Salmonella and *Campylobacter* outbreaks predominate and constitute the majority of laboratory-confirmed cases of foodborne illness, in part because of their ease of recognition and the general awareness of physicians and the public about these organisms. *Shigella* is the next most commonly recognized cause of foodborne outbreaks, followed by Shiga toxin-producing *E. coli* and *C. perfringens*.[3] Several pathogens that rarely are reported, namely *B. cereus* and *V. parahaemolyticus*, have been well studied in certain parts of the world and their contribution to food-borne diarrheal illness in the United States has been recognized only recently. Vibrios occur naturally in estuarine or marine environments, and infection can occur from consumption of raw or undercooked seafood (e.g., oysters). The incidence of vibriosis has tripled from 1996 to 2010, most cases occurring during the summer months. The causes of this increase are not known, but may be a result of warming of coastal waters, which contributes to the growth and persistence of the organism.[6] Other new challenges have emerged. Globalization of the food trade, with centralized processing and wide distribution, provide opportunities for food-borne outbreaks to spread rapidly between countries, and indiscriminate use of antibiotics in the meat industry has led to increasing resistance of organisms to treatment.[7]

Approach to the Patient

A thorough history should provide clues to the etiology of the food-borne illness (Table 111-2). Details to be elicited should include the food ingested (Box 111-1); the time period between ingestion and onset of symptoms; the number of people who ingested the food and how many became ill; and the means of preparation and storage of the suspected food (e.g., picnic, home canning, restaurant).

Some foodborne illnesses are more common during certain seasons.[1,2] For example, during the summer months, illnesses due to bacteria such as *Salmonella*, *Shigella*, and *S. aureus* are prevalent. Disease from *Campylobacter jejuni* is more common in the spring and fall. *C. perfringens* outbreaks occur least often in the summer. Infections due to *B. cereus* and Norovirus occur year round.

In addition to considering the organism and its vector, one must also take into account the susceptibility of the host. Persons with liver disease have an annual rate of disease from *Vibrio vulnificus* 80 times greater and a death rate 200 times greater than those of adults without liver disease.[8,9] Patients

TABLE 111-1 Estimated Rates of Foodborne Illnesses and Associated Mortality in the United States, 2006

Pathogen	Estimated Total No. of Cases	Foodborne Transmission, %	No. of Deaths	Death Rate, %*
Bacteria				
Brucella	839	50	1	0.9
Campylobacter	845,024	80	76	0.1
Escherichia coli				
O157:H7 (EHEC)	63,153	68	20	0.5
Non-O157:H7 (non-EHEC)	112,752	82	0	0.3
Listeria monocytogenes	1591	99	255	15.9
Salmonella typhi	1821	96	0	0
Nontyphoidal Salmonella	1,027,561	94	378	0.5
Shigella	131,254	31	10	0.1
Vibrio parahaemolyticus	34,664	86	4	0.9
Vibrio vulnificus	96	47	36	34.8
Yersinia enterocolitica	97,656	90	29	2
Toxins				
Bacillus cereus	63,400	100	0	0
Clostridium botulinum (food botulism)	55	100	9	17.3
Clostridium perfringens	965,958	100	26	<0.1
Food Poisoning				
Staphylococcal	241,148	100	6	<0.1
Streptococcal	11,217	100	0	0
Parasites				
Cryptosporidium parvum	57,616	8	4	0.3
Cyclospora cayetanensis	11,407	99	0	0
Giardia lamblia	76,840	7	2	0.1
Toxoplasma gondii	86,686	50	327	0.2
Trichinella spiralis	156	100	0	0.2
Viruses				
Astrovirus	15,433	<1	0	<0.1
Norovirus and Norwalk-like viruses	5,461,731	26	149	<0.1
Rotavirus	15,433	<1	0	<0.1
Hepatitis A virus	1566	7	7	2.4
Sapovirus	15,433	<1	0	<0.1
TOTAL	9,388,075	—	1351	

*For laboratory-confirmed illnesses.
EHEC, enterohemorrhagic Escherichia coli.
From Scallan E, Hoekstra RM, Angulo FJ, et al. Foodborne illness acquired in the United States—Major pathogens. Emerg Infect Dis 2011; 17:7-15.

with compromised immune systems (e.g., chronic renal insufficiency, malignancy, diabetes, iron overload states and patients taking glucocorticoids) also probably are at increased risk for infection and death.[9] Gastric acidity is a natural defense mechanism against infection that may be compromised by prior gastric surgery or use of PPIs.

The presenting symptom complex also can give a clue to the etiologic organism. Symptom complexes may be classified as nausea and vomiting, non-inflammatory diarrhea, inflammatory diarrhea, neurologic symptoms, and systemic or miscellaneous symptoms.[1] Box 111-1 lists the characteristics of the more common types of bacterial food poisoning.

Staphylococcus aureus

Coagulase-positive S. aureus is a common cause of food poisoning in the United States; before 1973, it was the leading cause.

Microbiology

Five immunologically distinct enterotoxins have been associated with food-poisoning strains of S. aureus. These enterotoxins, termed A, B, C, D, and E, are heat-resistant polypeptides. When they are tested in a rat intestinal loop model, net secretion of water and electrolytes is observed.[10] Staphylococcal enterotoxins induce vomiting when fed to monkeys or human volunteers.

Epidemiology

Staphylococcal food poisoning has a short incubation period of about 3 hours, with a range of 1 to 6 hours. The disease usually is clustered within a family or group and has a high attack rate. Many foods have been implicated in this form of food poisoning; however, foods with a high-salt concentration (e.g., ham or canned meat) or high-sugar content (e.g., custard

TABLE 111-2 Features of Bacterial Food Poisoning

Organism	Common Vehicles	Median Incubation (hr) (range)	Primary Toxin	Clinical Features	Median Duration, days (range)	Secondary Attack Rate, %	Sources of Diagnostic Material
Bacillus cereus	Fried rice, vanilla sauce, cream, meatballs, boiled beef, barbecued chicken	2 (1-16) 9 (6-14)	Heat stable Heat labile	V, C, D D, C, V	0.4 (0.2-0.5) 1 (1-2)	0	Vomitus, stool, implicated food
Campylobacter jejuni	Milk, chicken, beef	48 (24-240)	Unknown	D, F, C, B, H, M, N, V	7 (2-30)	25	Stool, rectal swab
Clostridium perfringens	Beef, turkey, chicken	12 (8-22)	Heat labile	D, C (N, V, F rare)	1 (0.3-3)	0	Stool, rectal swab; food, food-contact surfaces
Escherichia coli spp.	Salads, beef	24 (8-44) 96 (24-120)	Heat labile Heat stable Verotoxin	D, C, N, H, F, M F, M, D, C B, C, F, hemolytic-uremic syndrome	3 (1-4)	0	Stool, rectal swab
Listeria monocytogenes	Milk, raw vegetables, cole slaw, dairy products, poultry, beef	?	Unknown	D, F, C, N, V, B	?	10	Stool, rectal swab
Salmonella spp.	Eggs, meat, poultry	24 (5-72)	Role of toxin unclear	D, C, N, V, F, H, B (rare), enteric fever	3 (0.5-14)	30-50	Stool, rectal swab from patients and food preparers; raw food
Shigella spp.	Milk, salads (potato, tuna, turkey)	24 (7-168)	Role of toxin unclear	C, F, D, B, H, N, V	3 (0.5-14)	40-60	Stool, rectal swab from patients, and food preparers; implicated food
Staphylococcus aureus	Ham, pork, canned beef, cream-filled pastry	3 (1-6)	Heat stable	V, N, C, D, F (rare)	1 (0.3-1.5)	0	Stool, vomitus; food or food-contact surfaces; nose, hands, purulent lesion on food preparer
Vibrio parahaemolyticus	Seafood (rarely saltwater) or salted vegetables	12 (2-48)	Role of toxin unclear	D, C, N, V, H, F, B (rare)	3 (2-10)	0	Stool, rectal swab; food, food-contact surfaces; seawater
Yersinia enterocolitica	Chocolate milk or raw milk, pork	72 (2-144)	Heat stable	F, C, D, V, pharyngitis, arthritis, mesenteric adenitis, rash	7 (2-30)	20	Stool from food preparer

B, bloody diarrhea; C, cramping abdominal pain; D, diarrhea; F, fever; H, headache; M, myalgias; N, nausea; V, vomiting.
From Snydman DR. Food poisoning. In: Gorbach SL, Bartlett JG, Blacklow NR, editors. Infectious diseases. Philadelphia: WB Saunders; 1992. p 771.

Beef and Pork
Salmonella spp.
Staphylococcus aureus
Clostridium perfringens
EHEC
Bacillus cereus
Yersinia enterocolitica
Listeria monocytogenes
Brucella spp.
Trichinella spiralis

Chinese Food
Bacillus cereus (in fried rice)
Monosodium glutamate poisoning

Eggs
Salmonella spp.
Staphylococcus aureus

Fish
Clostridium botulinum
Ciguatera poisoning
Scombroid poisoning
Diphyllobothrium latum
Anisakidosis

Honey
Clostridium botulinum

Milk and Cheese
Salmonella spp.
Campylobacter spp.
EIEC and EHEC
Yersinia enterocolitica
Group A streptococci
Brucella spp.
Listeria monocytogenes

Poultry
Salmonella spp.
Staphylococcus aureus
Campylobacter
Clostridium perfringens
Listeria monocytogenes

Shellfish
Vibrio parahaemolyticus
Vibrio cholerae (O1 and non-O1)
Hepatitis A
Norovirus and Norwalk-like viruses
Paralytic shellfish poisoning
Neurotoxic shellfish poisoning

Vegetables
Clostridium botulinum
Salmonella spp.
Shigella spp.
Bacillus cereus
Norovirus

EHEC, enterohemorrhagic E. coli; EIEC, enteroinvasive E. coli.
From Bishai WR, Sears CL. Food poisoning syndromes. Gastroenterol Clin North Am 1993; 22:579.

Pathogenic Mechanisms

There are 3 requisites for staphylococcal food poisoning: contamination of a food with enterotoxin-producing staphylococci, suitable growth requirements of the food for the organism, and suitable time and temperature for the organism to multiply. The emetic dose of enterotoxin A or B for humans has been estimated to be between 1 and 25 µg.

Clinical Features

Symptoms of staphylococcal food poisoning are primarily profuse vomiting, nausea, and abdominal cramps, often followed by diarrhea that occurs 1 to 4 hours after ingestion of a suspect meal. Vomiting is the dominant initial symptom and can lead to a severe metabolic alkalosis. Fever is unusual. Rarely, hypotension and marked prostration occur. Fatalities are unusual, and recovery is complete within 24 to 48 hours. Diagnosis is based on the typical presentation occurring a few hours following the ingestion of typical foods. Most people with staphylococcal food poisoning do not consult a physician, but more severe cases may require supportive care, particularly rehydration and correction of alkalosis. No specific therapy is available.

Clostridium perfringens

C. perfringens is a major foodborne pathogen that produces vomiting and diarrhea. The disease is caused by an enterotoxin elaborated by strains of C. perfringens type A. A more severe and often fatal foodborne illness, known variously as enteritis necroticans (Darmbrand) and pigbel, is caused by C. perfringens type C (see later).

Microbiology

Clostridia are Gram-positive, spore-forming, obligate anaerobes that can be found in the normal intestinal flora of humans and animals and in the soil. Although an anaerobe, C. perfringens is remarkably aerotolerant and survives exposure to oxygen for as long as 72 hours. C. perfringens produces several enterotoxins and 12 toxins that are mostly active in tissues. The food-poisoning syndrome is caused by a heat-labile protein enterotoxin, better termed a secretory cytotoxin, which is a structural component of the spore coat and is formed during sporulation; like other enterotoxins, it causes fluid accumulation in the rabbit ileal loop model, presumably by altering membrane ion permeability.[11,12] Unlike cholera and E. coli enterotoxins, clostridial enterotoxin has its maximum activity in the ileum, inhibits glucose transport, damages the intestinal epithelium, and causes intestinal protein loss.[12]

Epidemiology and Pathogenic Mechanisms

Epidemics of C. perfringens are characterized by high attack rates and a large number of affected persons, usually 40 to 50 per outbreak. The incubation period varies from 8 to 14 hours but can be as long as 22 hours. In almost every outbreak of clostridial food poisoning, poultry or roasted, boiled, stewed, or steamed meat is the vehicle of infection. Usually, the meat is cooked in bulk so that heat gain and internal pressure are insufficient to kill the spores. The implicated food invariably undergoes a period of inadequate cooling, which allows the spores to germinate. The organism proliferates rapidly at temperatures between 15°C and 50°C, and unless the food is reheated to a very high temperature, it will contain many viable organisms. Though largely preventable with proper food handling, large outbreaks, sometimes with fatal outcome,

and cream) selectively favor the growth of staphylococci. The major mode of transmission is from a food handler to the food product. Involved foods usually have been cut, sliced, grated, mixed, or ground by workers who are carriers of toxin-producing strains of S. aureus.

due to *C. perfringens* food poisoning unfortunately are still frequently reported.[13]

Clinical Features

C. perfringens type A food poisoning is characterized by watery diarrhea, severe cramping abdominal pain, and, often, vomiting that begins 8 to 24 hours after the incriminating meal. Fever, chills, headache, or other signs of infection usually are absent. The illness is of short duration, and usually lasts less than 24 hours. Rare fatalities have been recorded in debilitated or hospitalized patients and are usually caused by dehydration. No specific treatment is required.

Enteritis Necroticans

Enteritis necroticans is a disease that originally was described in post-World War II Germany, in an outbreak that affected more than 400 people who consumed rancid meat. Similar outbreaks, associated with the consumption of poorly cooked pork, have been described in Papua New Guinea and are referred to as *pigbel*.[14,15] Pigbel is caused by strains of *C. perfringens* type C that produce beta toxin. In malnourished patients, especially children, the toxin cannot be inactivated by the usual intestinal proteases and causes transmural intestinal wall necrosis; protease inactivation (e.g., by consuming large amounts of sweet potatoes, a food staple in Papua New Guinea) can facilitate the damage. Fibrin thrombi occluding superficial arteries and veins of the lamina propria and submucosa are characteristic of this condition, and animal studies suggest that vascular thrombosis is responsible for initiation of intestinal necrosis characteristic of type C infections.[16] Intestinal perforation, sepsis, and hemorrhage result in a 40% mortality rate. Fortunately, this disease is rare. In the uncomplicated case, treatment is symptomatic and supportive.

Outbreaks of pigbel have been related to consumption of pig in large native feasts. The pig is improperly cooked, and large quantities are consumed over 3 or 4 days. Other cases, most often in children younger than 10 years, occur in villages remote from the site of the cooking. Enteritis necroticans associated with the consumption of chitterlings (prepared pig intestine; a traditional African-American holiday food in the South) is encountered rarely in the United States.[15]

Listeria Species

Listeria are Gram-positive highly motile bacilli that are relatively heat resistant. They have been isolated from the intestinal tracts of humans and animals and from sewage and well water. Cases can occur as part of an outbreak or on a sporadic basis. In reported epidemics, the vehicles of infection have been raw and pasteurized milk, soft cheeses, cole slaw, shrimp, rice salad, pork dishes, and raw vegetables.[17,18] *Listeria* can be cultured from raw poultry, beef, or pork; prepackaged meat products; cheeses; and raw vegetables.[19]

Listeriosis usually is a systemic disease associated with bacteremia that can seed the meninges, heart valves, or body organs. Intestinal symptoms such as diarrhea and cramping often precede fever and bacteremia. Immunocompetent hosts occasionally develop gastroenteritis characterized by fever, headache, abdominal pain, nausea, and diarrhea; this form of listeriosis usually is not complicated by bacteremia.[20]

Listeria has been associated with high rates of hospitalization (estimated at 94%) and death (case-fatality rate of 16%). Indeed, *Listeria* accounts for 19% of all deaths from foodborne illness.[3] Neurologic sequelae can occur in a sizeable proportion of survivors of central nervous system listeriosis. The propensity of the organism to attack older adults, immunosuppressed persons, and pregnant women might account for

the apparent severity of the infection. The reason for this propensity is not known. Because anti–TNF-α drugs block the host's response against various microorganisms, particularly intracellular agents like *L. monocytogenes*, and increase the risk of disease, patients with IBD who are being treated with these agents should be aware of this risk and counseled on avoidance of high-risk foods.[21]

Bacillus cereus

B. cereus is an aerobic, spore-forming, Gram-positive rod that has been associated with 2 clinical types of food poisoning: a diarrheal syndrome and a vomiting syndrome.[22] Although associated with the same organism, the 2 syndromes are caused by different toxins and have different epidemiologies.

Diarrhea Syndrome

B. cereus diarrhea results from an enterotoxin that causes intestinal secretion by activation of adenylate cyclase in intestinal epithelial cells, an action similar to that of cholera toxin.

The median incubation period appears to be 9 hours, with a range of 6 to 14 hours. The clinical presentation is characterized by diarrhea (96%), generalized cramps (75%), and vomiting (23%).[22] Fever is uncommon. The duration of illness ranges from 20 to 36 hours, with a median of 24 hours. The original report of *B. cereus* as a cause of diarrheal disease was associated with consumption of contaminated meatballs, but strains of *B. cereus* associated with diarrhea have been found in approximately 25% of many foods sampled, including cream, pudding, meat, spices, dried potatoes, dried milk, vanilla sauces, and spaghetti sauces, all of which are contaminated before cooking.[23] If the food is prepared so that the temperature is maintained at 30°C to 50°C, vegetative growth is permitted. Spores can survive extreme temperatures, and when allowed to cool relatively slowly, they germinate, multiply, and elaborate toxin. There is no evidence that human carriage of the organism or other means of contamination plays a role in transmission.

Whether the diarrhea-causing heat-labile enterotoxin actually is ingested or produced in vivo is not known; however, the incubation of diarrheal illness is too long to be caused by preformed toxin, and a large inoculum is required to cause illness, observations that suggest intestinal colonization is necessary. Usually, no therapy is required because of the short duration of symptoms.

Vomiting Syndrome

Although the organism associated with the vomiting disease appears to be the same as the one causing diarrhea, a different type of toxin has been implicated.[24] *B. cereus* emetic syndrome results from ingestion of a preformed enterotoxin that is stable to heat. The emetic syndrome is more common than the diarrheal syndrome. When fed to rhesus monkeys, cell-free culture filtrates from these strains do not produce intestinal secretion and diarrhea, but rather vomiting.

The vomiting syndrome has a short incubation period of approximately 2 hours. Virtually all affected persons have vomiting and abdominal cramps. Diarrhea is present in only one third of patients. The duration of illness ranges from 8 to 10 hours, with a median of 9 hours; the illness usually is mild and self-limited, so no specific therapy is required. Nearly all reported cases involving the vomiting toxin have implicated fried rice as the vehicle.[22]

In England, almost 90% of uncooked rice was found to be colonized by *B. cereus*, although the number of organisms was relatively low.[25] The disease has been ascribed to the common practice in Chinese restaurants of allowing large portions of boiled rice to drain unrefrigerated to avoid clumping. Flash-frying during the final preparation of the fried rice does not produce enough heat to destroy apparently preformed heat-stable toxin. It appears that the emetic illness is caused by preformed toxin, because the incubation period is short, and there is an extremely high attack rate that approaches 100% in outbreaks.

Botulism

Botulism is a rare foodborne disease that results from exposure to neurotoxins secreted by strains of *Clostridium botulinum*. Between 1990 and 2000, there were 160 outbreaks of botulism in the United States, accounting for 263 cases and at least 11 deaths.[26] Although foodborne botulism is relatively uncommon, it is the most lethal of all the bacterial toxin-mediated foodborne diseases and the only one for which specific effective therapy is available.

Epidemiology

During the past few decades, foodborne botulism has become the least common form of botulism, trailing after wound and infant botulism. Foodborne botulism develops after the ingestion of preformed toxin in improperly preserved canned vegetables, salsas, meats, and fish. A disproportionate number of cases have occurred in the Pacific Northwest and Alaska, associated with Native American foods such as whale or seal that have been fermented or preserved with traditional methods. Outbreaks in the United States have been associated with baked potatoes, cheese sauce, beef stew, and garlic cooking oil,[5] with home-canned foods accounting for the majority of homemade food events.[26]

Infant botulism develops in infants whose GI tract becomes colonized with live *C. botulinum*, which then secrete small amounts of botulinum toxin. Absorption of low concentrations of the toxin leads to lethargy, poor feeding, constipation, diminished muscle tone, and a weak cry. The source of the botulinum toxin is not clear, but household dust, soil, and honey in feedings have been suggested as possible sources. It is recommended that honey not be given to infants.

Pathogenic Mechanisms

C. botulinum and closely related species of clostridia produce heat-resistant spores that are capable of surviving food preservation techniques that destroy non-sporulating organisms. There are 7 serologically distinct botulinum toxins designated by the letters A to G. Neutralization by type-specific serologic reagents is used to differentiate the serotypes. Types A, B, and E are responsible for most human cases of botulism.[27] Neurotoxin-producing strains of *Clostridium butyricum* and *Clostridium baratii* are less commonly responsible for human botulism. Toxin production occurs in the presence of anaerobic, low-solute, and low-acid conditions.

C. botulinum usually is unable to replicate in the mature human intestine, although the toxin is acid stable and traverses the stomach intact. After absorption, botulinum toxin binds irreversibly to presynaptic cholinergic nerve endings of the cranial and peripheral nerves, thereby resulting in inhibition of acetylcholine release and the characteristic clinical syndrome consequent to blockade of voluntary motor and autonomic cholinergic junctions.

Clinical Features

Ingestion of botulinum toxin initially results in GI symptoms, including nausea, vomiting, abdominal pain, and diarrhea, usually within 18 to 36 hours after toxin ingestion.[5] Once neurologic symptoms develop, constipation is common. Dry mouth, diplopia, and blurred vision are followed by dysarthria, dysphonia, dysphagia, and peripheral muscle weakness. The typical symmetrical descending paralysis starts with the cranial nerves and then affects the upper extremities, respiratory muscles, and, finally, lower extremities. Respiratory muscle paralysis can result in respiratory failure and death if mechanical ventilation is not instituted; higher cortical functions are unaffected.

Diagnosis

Botulism should be suspected in any patient with the acute onset of GI, autonomic nervous system, and cranial nerve dysfunction, especially if the patient recently has consumed home-canned foods. MRI or CT of the brain and results of lumbar puncture are normal in patients with botulism, but electromyography can show characteristic abnormalities. If foodborne botulism is suspected, stool, serum, and implicated foods should be tested for botulinum neurotoxin. These tests are performed at some state health department laboratories and the CDC.

Treatment

Supportive therapy with mechanical ventilation has helped to greatly reduce mortality rates from botulism. The diagnosis of botulism must be considered early in any case of unexplained paralysis, and antitoxin should be administered if the diagnosis is credible. The trivalent equine botulinum antitoxin is available only through the CDC, which maintains supplies of antitoxin at sites around the country for immediate release in case of an emergency. To obtain the antitoxin, physicians need to contact their state health department's emergency hotline or the CDC directly (telephone 800-232-4636).

Speed is of the essence because the antitoxin cannot displace the toxin once it has bound to the presynaptic nerve terminal; antitoxin only binds free circulating toxin. Once symptoms have developed, the usefulness of the antitoxin is greatly reduced. In a retrospective analysis of 134 cases of botulinum toxin A-mediated disease, patients who received antitoxin therapy early in the course had a mortality rate of 10%, as opposed to mortality rates of 15% in those who received the antitoxin more than 24 hours after the onset of symptoms and 46% in those who did not receive antitoxin at all.[28] Patients who received antitoxin stayed in the hospital an average of 10 days, compared with 56 days for the untreated group.

The current recommendation is to administer a single 10-mL dose of IV antitoxin to each exposed person. This recommendation is based on the calculation that each vial has enough neutralizing antibody (for types A, B, and E) to bind a titer of toxin that is 100 times greater than the highest titer documented to date by the CDC.

Bacillus anthracis

Although most anthrax infections are the result of cutaneous exposure to or inhalation of infected spores, ingestion of infected animal tissue can lead to GI disease.

Microbiology

B. anthracis is an aerobic, Gram-positive, spore-forming, non-motile bacillus that is found in soil. Endospores can remain dormant in soil for many years. Anthrax spores germinate in nutrient-rich environments. Vegetative anthrax bacilli elaborate an antiphagocytic polyglutamyl capsule and a toxin complex that is composed of protective antigen, lethal factor, and edema factor.[29] Protective antigen acts as the binding site for the lethal and edema factors. The lethal factor stimulates macrophages to release TNF-α and interleukin (IL)-1, which contribute to death from toxemia in anthrax infections characterized by high-grade bacteremia and multisystem organ failure.

Epidemiology

The consumption of endospore-contaminated meat from infected animals is the primary mode of transmission of GI anthrax. In 2005, an outbreak was identified in 3 Iranian family members who had consumed half-cooked meat from a sick sheep that was found to be contaminated with *B. anthracis*. Two of the cases presented with GI illness characterized by fever, abdominal pain, nausea, and vomiting, and the third was admitted with fever, sore throat, and painful neck swelling. One patient had *B. anthracis* identified in cerebrospinal fluid and blood cultures and died despite aggressive treatment. Fortunately, the other patients responded well to penicillin G and recovered.[30]

Pathogenic Mechanisms

Entry of endospores through the GI mucosa initiates infection. Macrophages phagocytose ingested endospores, which then germinate to form vegetative bacteria in mesenteric lymph nodes. The bacteria are then released from the macrophages, multiply in the local lymphatic systems, and enter the bloodstream. The release of the exotoxin complexes results in local tissue damage with massive edema, mucosal ulcerations, and the development of systemic toxemia.

Clinical Features

Approximately 1 to 7 days after the ingestion of raw or undercooked meat from infected animals, nausea, vomiting, abdominal pain, and fever develop. Patients often rapidly develop worsening symptoms characterized by bloody diarrhea, diffuse abdominal pain with rebound tenderness, and, occasionally, hematemesis. Ascites, which may be purulent, develops 2 to 4 days later. Ulceration of the bowel, usually in the region of the ileum and cecum is the primary manifestation of intestinal anthrax. *B. anthracis* has been isolated from human stool specimens; however, the organism is not often detected in stool cultures, and it is recommended that blood or ascitic fluid be collected for culture or PCR in patients with clinical symptoms that suggest anthrax.[31] More than 50% of episodes are fatal, with death occurring as a consequence of toxemia, intestinal perforation, or shock from hemorrhage and fluid losses.

Oropharyngeal anthrax is a less common form of infection that develops when spores are deposited in the oropharynx. Symptoms include fever, a severe sore throat, and dysphagia, which can progress to respiratory distress. Examination often reveals marked swelling of the neck, lymphadenitis, and pharyngeal ulcers that are covered by a pseudomembrane. Despite the relatively severe symptoms, this form of infection tends to be milder than the GI disease and rarely is fatal.

Treatment and Prevention

Because of the propensity of *B. anthracis* infection of the GI tract to progress to sepsis or death, it should be treated promptly and aggressively as a systemic disease.[31] Some strains of *B. anthracis* contain an inducible β-lactamase, and so initial therapy should consist of ciprofloxacin. Because there

is a higher risk of mortality in severe cases, the addition of rifampin or clindamycin, or both, is recommended in these situations. Penicillin and doxycycline are both highly active against *B. anthracis* in the absence of resistance. An anthrax vaccine, consisting of a sterile filtrate of an attenuated strain of the organism, is available to the U.S. military but not to civilians.

FISH POISONING

Food poisoning from marine toxins in fish is a common worldwide problem. The commonest of these are ciguatera and scombroid poisoning.[32,33]

Ciguatera

Ciguatera (Spanish: *cigua*, sea snail) poisoning manifests with a combination of GI and neurologic symptoms and findings. Though most common in the South Pacific and Caribbean, ciguatera poisoning has become a hazard to consumers in non-endemic regions because of expanding international trade in seafood from tropical fisheries.[34] It is the most common foodborne disease related to the consumption of finfish worldwide[35] and accounts for approximately half of fish-related outbreaks in the United States.

More than 400 species of fish have been associated with ciguatera poisoning, including grouper, red snapper, amberjack, and dolphin. The illness is caused by the consumption of fish that contain toxins produced by ingested dinoflagellates; toxin(s) are subsequently stored in the fish flesh and viscera. The toxin is concentrated up the food chain as small fish are consumed by larger fish. The fish are not affected by the toxins; they do not appear spoiled and they taste normal. The commonest toxin involved is ciguatoxin, a marine saponin, but a number of toxins can be involved.[36] Toxins are both heat- and acid-resistant and survive preservation (freezing) and preparation (cooking) procedures.

GI symptoms occur 3 to 6 hours after eating the contaminated fish and usually involve a combination of nausea, vomiting, abdominal cramps, and diarrhea. Sweating and headaches also can occur. A variety of neurologic symptoms occurs 3 to 72 hours after ingestion and include paresthesias, blurred vision, nerve palsies, and temperature-related dysesthesia (i.e., hot and cold reversal). Cardiovascular symptoms also can occur and include bradycardia, heart block, and hypotension. Variations in the symptom complex and in the severity of individual symptoms can occur depending on the type of fish eaten and presumably on the type and quantity of toxin or toxins consumed.

Diarrhea is the result of toxin-stimulated intestinal secretion mediated by changes in intracellular calcium. Neurologic symptoms are a consequence of alterations in voltage-dependent neural sodium channels. Illness can persist up to 1 month and, rarely, can last up to a year. Approximately 3% to 20% of patients have chronic effects, such as fatigue, myalgias, and headaches. Chronic symptoms may be aggravated or triggered by ingestion of caffeine or alcohol. Fatalities are rare and usually result from cardiovascular collapse.

The diagnosis is based on clinical suspicion and compatible signs and symptoms. There is no available confirmatory test and no specific treatment; treatment is supportive. IV mannitol may be helpful in severe cases.

Scombroid Poisoning

Scombroid (Greek: *scombros*, mackerel or tunny) poisoning is a common but underreported illness that often is misdiagnosed as a fish "allergy." It occurs after the consumption of fish that has been poorly refrigerated or improperly stored, allowing bacterial proliferation. Bacteria decarboxylate histidine in the muscle of fish, producing high levels of histamine. The fish do not appear spoiled but might taste peppery; histamine is not destroyed by cooking or freezing. The illness can occur after ingestion of either fresh or canned fish or consumption of foods such as tuna salad or tuna burgers. The most common fish involved are dark meat fish such as tuna, mackerel, and bonito, but scombroid poisoning can also occur with ingestion of mahi-mahi, bluefish, swordfish, or salmon.

The usual clinical presentation begins as soon as 1 hour after ingestion of the contaminated fish. Symptoms and signs include flushing, warmth, erythematous skin rash, pruritus, palpitations, and tachycardia. Patients also may experience headache, blurred vision, and respiratory distress. Occasionally, respiratory distress occurs from facial and lingual swelling. The illness usually resolves spontaneously within 12 hours without any sequelae. Diagnosis is a clinical one based on typical signs and symptoms. Plasma histamine levels, if measured acutely, may be elevated. Treatment mainly is supportive, and includes administration of antihistamines.

Tetrodotoxin Poisoning

Tetrodotoxin (TdT) poisoning is most commonly due to eating the flesh of the puffer fish (fugu), a sushi delicacy in Japan, although TdT also may be found in many other species of fish, and some mollusks, crabs, newts and frogs.[37] Fugu is prepared by specially trained chefs certified by the government to present the flesh free of the TdT-containing liver, gonads, and skin, and most poisonings occur after eating fish prepared by uncertified persons. TdT is thought to be synthesized by a bacterium or dinoflagellate associated with the puffer fish. It is a heat-stable, water-soluble molecule that acts on sodium channels in nerve tissue to prevent depolarization and propagation of action potentials in central and peripheral nerve cells. Symptoms usually occur 15 minutes to a few hours after ingestion and include lingual and circumoral paresthesias, followed by facial and extremity paresthesias and numbness, salivation, nausea, vomiting, and diarrhea with abdominal pain. Weakness, hypoventilation and difficulty speaking ensue, followed by respiratory muscle paralysis, cardiac arrhythmias, hypotension, seizures and coma. Mortality is estimated to approach 50% and care is supportive. Estimates Patients who survive the initial 24 hours of intoxication usually recover.

Shellfish-Poisoning Syndromes

Four distinct shellfish-poisoning syndromes have been identified: paralytic (PSP), neurologic (NSP), diarrheal (DSP), and amnestic (ASP).[38] All four share some common features and develop when contaminated shellfish, usually bivalve mollusks (e.g., mussels, clams, oysters, scallops), are ingested along with their contained toxins produced by dinoflagellates and diatoms.

Paralytic Shellfish Poisoning

PSP is the most severe of the shellfish poisonings. It occurs from June to October, especially in the colder coastal waters of the Pacific and New England, coasts, when mussels, clams, scallops, oysters, and lobsters become contaminated by the dinoflagellate *Gonyaulax* that is responsible for "red" tide. This dinoflagellate produces the neurotoxin saxitoxin, named after the butter clam (*Saxidomus giganteus*) in which it was first recognized. Saxitoxin blocks neuronal sodium channels producing a flaccid paralysis that leaves its victim calm and conscious through the progression of symptoms; patients may report having a "floating" sensation. The toxin is heat-resistant. Symptoms usually begin within 2 hours after eating the contaminated shellfish, and consist of circumoral paresthesias and tingling of the extremities, followed by nausea, vomiting, abdominal cramps, headache and then muscle weakness. In cases of severe poisoning, muscle paralysis and respiratory failure occur, and in these cases death may occur within 24 hours. Treatment is supportive; for survivors, recovery is usually complete.

Neurologic Shellfish Poisoning

Symptoms of NSP are milder than those of PSP, begin within 15 minutes to 18 hours after consumption of the contaminated shellfish and last up to 3 days. Symptoms include nausea, vomiting, abdominal pain and diarrhea; rectal burning; paresthesias of the face, trunk, and limbs; myalgias; dizziness and ataxia; and reversal of hot/cold sensation; less common are tremor and dysphagia. NSP is caused by brevetoxins which are polycyclic ethers made by the dinoflagellate *Karenia brevis*; like ciguatoxin, they bind to and stimulate sodium flux through voltage-gated sodium channels in nerve and muscle. Treatment is supportive.

Diarrheal Shellfish Poisoning

DSP manifests with nausea, vomiting, abdominal pain and diarrhea. DSP is caused by ingestion of shellfish that are contaminated with okadaic acid produced in dinoflagellates of the species *Dinophysis* and *Prorocentrum,* and which increases intestinal epithelial permeability. Treatment is supportive.

Amnesic Shellfish Poisoning

The only reported outbreak of ASP occurred in 1987 after ingestion of mussels harvested off Prince Edward Island, Canada. ASP is caused by ingestion of shellfish that are contaminated with domoic acid produced by the diatom *Nitzschia pungens*. Symptoms of gastroenteritis develop within 24 hours after ingestion and may be accompanied by dizziness, headache, disorientation, and permanent short-term memory loss. In severe poisoning, seizures, focal weakness or paralysis, and death may occur. Domoic acid causes neuronal depolarization and has been shown at autopsy to be associated with necrosis of the hippocampus and amygdala. Treatment is supportive.

KEY REFERENCES

Full references for this chapter can be found on www.expertconsult.com.

3. Scallan E, Hoekstra RM, Angulo FJ, et al. Foodborne illness acquired in the United States—Major pathogens. Emerg Infect Dis 2001; 17:7-15.
4. Scallan E, Griffin PM, Angulo FF, et al. Foodborne illness acquired in the United States—Unspecified agents. Emerg Infect Dis 2001; 17:16-22.
6. Newton A, Kendall M, Vugia DJ, et al. Increasing rates of vibriosis in the United States, 1996-2010: Review of surveillance data from 2 systems. Clin Infect Dis 2012; 54(Suppl 5):s391-404.
16. Uzal FA, McClane BA. Recent progress in understanding the pathogenesis of *Clostridium perfringens* type C infections. Vet Microbiol 2011; 153:37-43.

17. Schlech WF III. Foodborne listeriosis. Clin Infect Dis 2000; 31:770-5.

26. Sobel J, Tucker N, Sulka A. et al. Foodborne botulism in the United States, 1990-2000. Emerg Infect Dis 2004; 10:1606-11.

31. Beatty ME, Ashford DA, Griffin PM, et al. Gastrointestinal anthrax: Review of the literature. Arch Intern Med 2003; 163:2527-31.

34. Dickey RW, Plakas SM. Ciguatera: A public health perspective. Toxicon 2010; 56:123-36.

37. How CK, Chern CH, Huang YC, et al. Tetrodotoxin poisoning. Am J Emerg Med 2003; 21(1):51-4.

38. Sobel J, Painter J. Illnesses caused by marine toxins. Clin Infect Dis 2005; 41:1290-6.

ANTIBIOTIC-ASSOCIATED DIARRHEA

Etiology

Diarrhea is a common side effect of antibiotic use and can result from a variety of mechanisms.[1] The most common type of diarrhea, often called *simple antibiotic-associated diarrhea* (AAD), is believed to result from a disturbance of the normal colonic microflora that leads to alterations in bacterial degradation of non-absorbed carbohydrates and bile salts. Colonic bacteria normally ferment the complex carbohydrates in dietary fiber and other ingested carbohydrates that are not absorbed in the small intestine, and the fermentation products are then metabolized and absorbed in the colon. Disruption of this process by antibiotic therapy is believed to cause osmotic diarrhea. Some, but not all, bacteria can deconjugate bile salts, and unconjugated bile salts are known to stimulate fluid secretion by the colonic mucosa; another mechanism for AAD may be reduced bacterial degradation of bile salts within the colonic lumen. Bile salts increase intestinal permeability, increase cyclic-AMP, activate mast cells, and stimulate chloride secretion by the colon (see Chapter 101). Other mechanisms that can be responsible for AAD include stimulation of intestinal motility through the motilin-like effect of erythromycin, an allergic reaction, or infection with microorganisms other than *Clostridium difficile*, including *Clostridium perfringens* type A, *Staphylococcus aureus*, and *Salmonella enterica*.[2-4]

The genotype of *C. perfringens* that causes AAD appears to be distinct from those that induce food poisoning.[3,5] Type A strains isolated from patients with AAD carry the *C. perfringens enterotoxin (CPE)* gene in a plasmid, whereas those that cause food poisoning have a chromosomal *CPE* gene. *S. aureus* was identified as a cause of severe AAD and enterocolitis before *C. difficile* infection was identified.[2,6] Since the advent of sensitive and specific testing for *C. difficile*, however, very few cases of *S. aureus* AAD have been confirmed, and the true role played by this pathogen in AAD is unclear. Antibiotic-associated infection with *Klebsiella oxytoca* has been described in patients with right-sided hemorrhagic colitis. This rare pathogen releases several potent toxins, and it appears to colonize the bowel after the indigenous flora has been altered by exposure to antibiotics.[7]

AAD complicates 2% to 25% of antibiotic treatment courses, but the incidence varies depending on the antibiotic used; it is more common, for example, during therapy with ampicillin (5% to 10%), amoxicillin-clavulanate (10% to 25%), or cefixime (15% to 20%) and less common during therapy with fluoroquinolones (1% to 2%) or trimethoprim-sulfamethoxazole (<1%).[8]

Most cases of AAD are mild, self-limited, and unaccompanied by fever. Pseudomembranous colitis is absent, and significant complications are rare. *C. difficile* infection accounts for less than 10% of AAD cases but is an important pathogen to identify because it often requires specific antimicrobial therapy and can lead to life-threatening complications, as discussed in the following section. A comparison between the clinical features of AAD caused by *C. difficile* and AAD from other causes is presented in Table 112-1.[9]

Prevention and Treatment

Management of simple AAD consists of discontinuing the inciting antibiotic if possible and if symptoms are moderately severe or poorly tolerated. If necessary, antiperistaltic agents (e.g., loperamide) may be used to relieve symptoms; these are traditionally avoided for *C. difficile* infection because of concern for exacerbating toxin-mediated colonic mucosal injury or precipitating toxic megacolon.

Because AAD is believed to result from an alteration of the normal colonic microflora, a variety of probiotic agents has been evaluated for its treatment and prevention (see

TABLE 112-1 Differences between Antibiotic-Associated Diarrhea from *Clostridium difficile* Infection and from Other Causes

Characteristic	*C. difficile* Infection	Other Causes
Most commonly implicated antibiotics	Clindamycin, cephalosporins, penicillins, fluoroquinolones	Clindamycin, cephalosporins, ampicillin, or amoxicillin-clavulanic acid
History	Usually no history of antibiotic intolerance	History of diarrhea with antibiotic therapy is common
Clinical Features		
Epidemiologic pattern	May be epidemic or endemic in hospitals or long-term care facilities	Sporadic
Diarrhea	May be florid; evidence of colitis with cramps, fever, and fecal leukocytes is common	Usually mild-moderate in severity ("nuisance diarrhea") without evidence of colitis
Findings on CT or colonoscopy	Evidence of colitis is common; pseudomembranes often are present	Usually normal
Complications	Hypoalbuminemia, anasarca, toxic megacolon; relapse can occur after treatment with metronidazole or vancomycin	Usually none; occasional cases of volume depletion
Results of assay for *C. difficile* toxin	Positive	Negative
Treatment		
Withdrawal of implicated antibiotic	Condition can resolve but often persists or progresses	Condition usually resolves
Antiperistaltic agents	Contraindicated	Often useful
Oral metronidazole or vancomycin	Prompt response	Not indicated

From Bartlett JG. Clinical practice: Antibiotic-associated diarrhea. N Engl J Med 2002; 346:334.

Chapter 130). In a double-blind controlled clinical trial, oral capsules containing viable *Saccharomyces boulardii*, a nonpathogenic yeast, were coadministered with antibiotics; this combination treatment reduced the incidence of AAD in hospitalized patients from 22% in the placebo group to 9.5% in the *S. boulardii* group (P = 0.04).[10] Another randomized placebo-controlled trial, however, failed to demonstrate a beneficial effect for *S. boulardii* in an older adult population of antibiotic recipients.[11] *Lactobacillus* species, in particular *Lactobacillus rhamnosus* GG, also have been studied in clinical trials of AAD. In 1 study, *Lactobacillus* GG was effective in reducing the incidence of AAD to 5% in children being treated for respiratory tract infections compared with a 16% incidence in the placebo group[12]; other clinical trials of *Lactobacillus* GG have yielded negative results.[13]

A meta-analysis examined the results of randomized double-blind placebo-controlled trials of probiotic therapy for AAD published between 1966 and 2000.[14] Nine studies were analyzed, including 4 using *S. boulardii* and 4 using *Lactobacillus* GG. The combined odds ratio for AAD in the probiotic-treated groups was 0.37 compared with placebo (95% confidence interval [CI]: 0.26-0.53; P < 0.001). For *S. boulardii*, the odds ratio in favor of active treatment over placebo was 0.39 (95% CI: 0.25-0.62; P < 0.001) and for lactobacilli the odds ratio was 0.34 (95% CI: 0.19-0.61; P < 0.01). A second meta-analysis yielded similar results.[15] Thus, the weight of published evidence suggests that probiotic agents such as *S. boulardii* and lactobacilli, when used prophylactically in combination with antibiotics, reduce the risk for AAD. Such therapy may be especially advantageous in patients with a history of susceptibility to AAD.

PSEUDOMEMBRANOUS ENTEROCOLITIS

Pseudomembranous enterocolitis was a rare entity in the medical literature before the widespread use of antibiotics. In recent decades, pseudomembranous colitis emerged as a common complication of antibiotic use, and almost all cases are now caused by infection with toxin-producing strains of *C. difficile*.

A case report by Finney published in 1893 is considered to be the first description in the medical literature of pseudomembranous enterocolitis.[16,17] In that instance, fatal pseudomembranous inflammation of the small intestine followed surgery in a debilitated young woman with gastric outlet obstruction caused by peptic ulcer disease. The presence of an inflammatory pseudomembrane overlying intestinal mucosa characterizes pseudomembranous colitis (when the colon alone is involved) or pseudomembranous enterocolitis (when the small intestine also is involved).[17] The pseudomembrane consists of inflammatory and cellular debris and forms distinctive patches of yellow or gray exudate that obscure the mucosa underlying them. In early lesions, a 1- to 2-mm area of punctate ulceration may be visible. Grossly, pseudomembranes consist of ovoid plaques of 2 to 10 mm in diameter separated by areas of normal or hyperemic mucosa. Histologically, pseudomembranes can be seen to emanate from central areas of epithelial ulceration and erupt from the intestinal/colonic crypts in a "volcano-like" fashion. In more severe cases, the areas of ulceration and the overlying pseudomembranes can coalesce to cover large areas of mucosa, and even bear a resemblance to a coating of liquid stool.

Risk factors for the development of pseudomembranous enterocolitis in the absence of *C. difficile* infection include intestinal surgery, intestinal ischemia, and other enteric infections. During the 1940s to the 1970s, most reported cases of pseudomembranous enterocolitis occurred following abdominal or pelvic surgery.[18,19] Bartlett has identified descriptions of pseudomembranous enterocolitis in the medical literature associated with a wide variety of other intestinal disorders including *Shigella* infection, Crohn's disease, neonatal necrotizing enterocolitis, intestinal obstruction, Hirschsprung's disease, and colonic carcinoma.[17] Intestinal ischemia can result in histologic changes similar to those observed in severe *C. difficile* colitis, although classic pseudomembranes are uncommonly seen. Severe systemic insults including shock, advanced renal failure, spinal fracture, extensive burns, heavy metal poisoning, and hemolytic-uremic syndrome also have been associated with pseudomembranous enterocolitis. A potential common etiologic factor shared by many of these disorders is hypoperfusion of the intestinal mucosa with resultant ischemic necrosis and ulceration.

Other infectious agents have been implicated as causes of pseudomembranous colitis in the absence of *C. difficile* infection, most notably *S. aureus*.[2,3,6] Before *C. difficile* was identified as the most common cause of pseudomembranous colitis, *S. aureus* often was identified in stool cultures of patients with postoperative pseudomembranous enterocolitis, and oral vancomycin proved to be effective therapy.[6] In retrospect, it is difficult to ascertain whether the efficacy of vancomycin reflected its activity against staphylococcal infection or against unrecognized infection with *C. difficile*. Currently, 2% to 3% of patients with antibiotic-associated pseudomembranous colitis have negative stool tests for *C. difficile* and its toxins despite use of the most sensitive available assays; it remains unclear what proportion of these patients have false-negative tests for *C. difficile* or instead are infected with an unidentified infectious agent.

CLOSTRIDIUM DIFFICILE INFECTION

C. difficile, an anaerobic, Gram-positive, spore-forming, toxinogenic bacillus, was first isolated in 1935 from the fecal flora of healthy neonates.[20] The organism then passed into obscurity until 1978, when the association between toxins released by this organism and antibiotic-induced pseudomembranous colitis first was reported.[21,22] Since that time, the incidence of *C. difficile* infection (CDI) has increased dramatically, and the organism is now recognized as the primary cause of nosocomial infectious diarrhea in developed countries.[23-26]

The reported incidence of CDI has risen steadily over the past decade. For example, in the United States, the Agency for Healthcare Research and Quality identified 127,580 reported cases of CDI in hospitalized patients in 1997; by 2004 this had increased to 246,139 and by 2010 to 346,805.[27,28] Reported deaths from CDI in the United States rose from 793 in 1999 to 7483 in 2008.[29] Similarly, according to United Kingdom National Statistics, CDI as a primary or contributing cause of death rose from 13 per million population in 2001 to 83 per million in 2007. These observations prompted major efforts to reduce CDI in hospitals, and by 2011 the estimated number of *C. difficile*-related deaths in the United Kingdom had fallen dramatically to 19 per million population.

CDI also appears to be accompanied by heightened morbidity and mortality in the past decade, owing in part to the emergence of increasingly virulent strains. One such strain was initially identified in the 1980s by restriction endonuclease analysis and named BI, but is currently referred to as North American Pulsed Field type 1 (NAP-1) and PCR ribotype 027.[30,31] The NAP-1 strain has led to severe outbreaks of CDI with high mortality rates in both North America and Europe.[24,25,30,31] The NAP-1 strain also produces a third toxin called *binary toxin* (see below) and shows high level resistance to fluoroquinolones, making it more prevalent in patients receiving this class of antibiotics.[24,25,30-32]

Epidemiology

Intestinal carriage rates of *C. difficile* in healthy adults are low (0% to 3% in American and European populations) and might represent intestinal transit without true colonization. In contrast, hospital inpatients treated with antibiotics have reported colonization rates of 10% to 21%.[33-37] Acquisition from the hospital environment is a major source of CDI, not only from infected stool but also via environmental surfaces, soiled bedding, bedpans, and toilet seats. The hands and stethoscopes of health care workers are also potential sources of nosocomial CDI.[33] In 1 study, *C. difficile* was acquired, on average, in 3.2 days by patients who shared a room with an *C. difficile*-infected roommate compared with 18.9 days by patients in single rooms or with roommates whose stool cultures were culture negative for *C. difficile*.[35] In the same study, *C. difficile* was cultured from the hands of 59% of hospital workers caring for patients with positive *C. difficile* cultures. The organism also was frequently cultured from bedrails, toilets, floors, call buttons, and other surfaces in the rooms of infected patients.

Asymptomatic carriers rarely develop *C. difficile*-associated diarrhea, but they serve as an important reservoir of nosocomial infection.[33-35,37-38] In 1 study, 29% of environmental cultures taken from the hospital rooms of symptom-free carriers were positive for *C. difficile*, compared with only 8% of cultures from rooms of patients who were culture-negative for *C. difficile*.[35]

In antibiotic-treated animals, the infective dose of toxigenic *C. difficile* may be as low as 2 organisms.[22] If human susceptibility is similar, control of CDI in hospitals will continue to be a major challenge because up to 10^9 organisms per gram of stool are excreted in liquid feces.[39] Highly resistant spores of *C. difficile* can persist for many months in the hospital environment and can result in infection if ingested by a susceptible host.[39]

Although it is not possible to eradicate *C. difficile* and its spores from the hospital environment, certain control measures have been recommended to reduce the prevalence of *C. difficile*-associated diarrhea (Box 112-1).[26,40] Infected inpatients should be bedded in private rooms whenever possible to reduce patient-to-patient spread of *C. difficile*. Strict enteric precautions including use of gowns and gloves and regular hand washing after patient contact should be observed.[35,40,41] The use of alcohol-based hand gels may not be as effective as washing with soap and running water in removing *C. difficile* spores; hence, washing with soap and running water is recommended as an additional measure in an outbreak setting.[26,42] A controlled trial of using vinyl disposable gloves during patient contact also reduced the transmission of infection.[41] After discharge of infected patients, surface environmental disinfection is best performed with a cleaning agent (e.g., hypochlorite solution) that contains about 5000 ppm available chlorine (corresponding to a 1:10 dilution of household bleach).[26,42]

Hospital outbreaks of *C. difficile*-associated diarrhea are common and likely result from the close approximation of susceptible persons (elderly and infirm patients) who are taking antibiotics and who are then exposed to the pathogen either in the hospital environment or through direct person-to-person spread. Outbreaks of infection are seen with the emergence of virulent strains, which are highly toxinogenic and resistant to numerous antibiotics including fluoroquinolones.[30-32,25] Prophylactic therapy with metronidazole or vancomycin is not effective as a disease control measure,[43] and *C. difficile* diarrhea is prevented best by avoiding the unnecessary use of broad-spectrum antibiotics, especially in hospitalized patients, and by careful attention to hand hygiene and environmental cleaning.[26]

CDI may be hospital or community acquired. Hospital-acquired infections may have their onset of symptoms and signs of colitis in the hospital or after discharge to the

---

BOX 112-1 Proposed Checklist of Hospital Interventions to Decrease the Incidence and Mortality of Health Care–Associated *Clostridium difficile* Infection (CDI)

Clostridium difficile **Infection (CDI) Checklist**

Prevention Checklist

- **When an MD, PA, NP, or RN suspects a patient has CDI:**
Physician, Physician Assistant, or Nurse Practitioner:
  □ Initiate *Contact Precautions Plus*
  □ Order stool *C. difficile* toxin test
  □ Discontinue nonessential antimicrobials
  □ Discontinue all anti-peristaltic medications

RN:
  □ Obtain stool sample for *C. difficile* toxin test
  □ Place patient in single-patient room
  □ Place *Contact Precautions Plus* sign on patient's door
  □ Ensure that gloves and gowns are easily accessible from patient's room
  □ Place dedicated stethoscope in patient's room
  □ Remind staff to wash hands with soap and water following patient contact

Microbiology Laboratory Staff Person:
  □ Call relevant patient floor with positive *C. difficile* toxin test result
  □ Provide daily list of positive test results for Infection Control

Infection Control Practitioner:
  □ Check microbiology results daily for positive *C. difficile* toxin results
  □ Call relevant floor to confirm that patient with positive *C. difficile* toxin results is in a single-patient room and that the *Contact Precautions Plus* sign is on the patient's door
  □ Flag the patient's *C. difficile* status in the hospital's clinical information system or in the patient's paper chart
  □ Alert housekeeping that the patient is on *Contact Precautions Plus*

Environmental Services Staff Person:
  □ Prior to discharge cleaning, check for *Contact Precautions Plus* sign on the patient's door
  □ If *Contact Precautions Plus* sign is on the door, clean the room with a bleach-based cleaning agent
  □ Confirm for supervisor that bleach-based cleaning agent was used for discharge cleaning for every patient on *Contact Precautions Plus*

Treatment Checklist

- **When an MD, PA, or NP diagnoses mild CDI:** *All* of the following criteria must be present: diarrhea (<6 BM/day), no fever, WBC <15,000 cells/mm^3, no peritoneal signs, and no evidence of sepsis
Physician, Physician Assistant, or Nurse Practitioner:
  □ Initiate oral metronidazole at a dose of 500 mg every 8 hours
  □ If no clinical improvement occurs by 48-72 hours, treat the patient as if he/she have moderate CDI
  □ Continue therapy for at least 14 days total and at least 10 days after symptoms have abated

- **When an MD, PA, or NP diagnoses moderate CDI:** *At least one* of the following criteria must be present: diarrhea (6-12 BM/day), fever 37.5-38.5°C, WBC 15,000-25,000 cells/mm^3, or frankly visible stable lower GI bleeding
Physician, Physician Assistant, or Nurse Practitioner:
  □ Initiate oral vancomycin at a dose of 125 mg every 6 hours
  □ If no clinical improvement by 48 hours, add IV metronidazole at a dose of 500 mg every 8 hours
  □ Consider obtaining infectious disease consultation
  □ Consider obtaining abdominal CT scan
  □ Continue therapy for at least 14 days total and at least 10 days after symptoms have abated

- **When an MD, PA, or NP diagnoses severe CDI:** *At least one* of the following criteria must be present: diarrhea (>12 BM/day), fever >38.5°C, WBC >25,000 cells/mm^3, hemodynamic instability, marked and continuous abdominal pain, ileus, absence of bowel sounds, evidence of sepsis, or intensive care unit level of care is required
Physician, Physician Assistant, or Nurse Practitioner:
  □ Obtain immediate infectious disease consultation
  □ Obtain immediate surgical consultation to assess need for colectomy
  □ Obtain abdominal CT scan
  □ Initiate oral vancomycin at a dose of 250 mg every 6 hours together with IV metronidazole at a dose of 500 mg every 6 hours
  □ Consult a surgeon to assess the need for colectomy and consider rectal vancomycin

BM, bowel movement; MD, medical doctor; NP, nurse practitioner; PA, Physician Assistant; RN, registered nurse; WBC, white blood cell count.
Modified from Abbett SK, et al. Proposed checklist of hospital interventions to decrease the incidence of healthcare-associated Clostridium difficile *infection.* Infect Control Hosp Epidemiol 2009; 30:1062-9.

---

community.[26,44] The reported incidence of community-acquired CDI (8 to 12 cases per 100,000 person-years) is substantially lower than that of hospital-acquired CDI but has increased in recent years.[36] Community-acquired CDI often is diagnosed in patients who lack typical risk factors for the disease (e.g., recent antibiotic exposure).[44-45] In a recent population-based study, community-acquired CDI accounted for 41% of total cases; patients with community-acquired disease were more likely to be younger women with less comorbidity and likelihood of antibiotic exposure compared with individuals who had hospital-acquired disease.[46]

Pathogenesis

The pathogenesis of CDI requires the following conditions: alteration of the normal colonic microflora by antibiotics or, rarely, chemotherapeutic agents; oral ingestion of *C. difficile* or its spores with resultant colonization of the large intestine;

release of toxins A and B into the colonic lumen; binding and internalization of toxins by colonocytes and lamina propria inflammatory cells; and subsequent colonic damage (colitis). Several host factors, particularly the immune response to *C. difficile* toxins, determine whether a patient remains an asymptomatic carrier or develops colitis (Fig. 112-1).

Alteration of the Colonic Microbiota

As a consequence of antimicrobial therapy, the resident colonic microbiota (previously referred to as "microflora") is altered or perturbed in nearly all patients who develop CDI. The protective barrier provided by the intestinal microbiota often is referred to as *colonization resistance*; its impairment by antibiotics and subsequent infection with *C. difficile* can be demonstrated in animal models.[47-49] *C. difficile* also can colonize the intestines of germ-free mice but is eliminated after these animals are inoculated with feces from normal mice, clearly

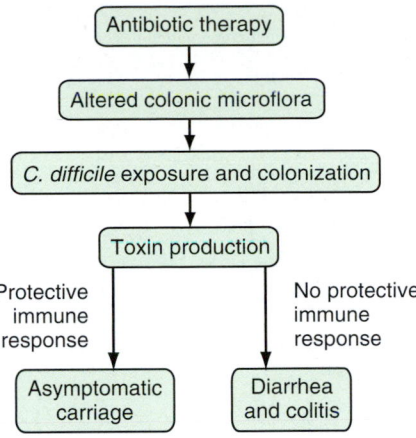

FIGURE 112-1. Pathogenesis of *Clostridium difficile*-associated diarrhea and colitis.

TABLE 112-2 Antimicrobial Agents That Predispose to *Clostridium difficile* Infection

Frequently	Sometimes	Rarely
Amoxicillin	Macrolides	Aminoglycosides
Ampicillin	Other penicillins	Bacitracin
Cephalosporins	Sulfonamides	Carbapenems
Clindamycin	Trimethoprim	Chloramphenicol
Fluoroquinolones	Trimethoprim ±	Daptomycin
	Sulfamethoxazole	Metronidazole
		Rifampin
		Rifaximin
		Teicoplanin
		Tetracyclines
		Tigecycline

Adapted from Kelly C, Lamont J. Treatment of Clostridium difficile *diarrhea and colitis. In: Wolfe MM, editor. Gastrointestinal pharmacotherapy. Philadelphia: WB Saunders; 1993. p 199.*

confirming the importance of the normal commensal organisms in preventing colonization and supporting the rationale for fecal microbiota transplantation (FMT) for prevention and treatment.[50]

Human neonates have poor colonization resistance because they have not yet developed a stable complex colonic microbiota.[20] Colonization rates with *C. difficile* of 25% to 80% have been reported in healthy infants and children up to 24 months of age, who, despite large concentrations of toxins in the feces, rarely develop *C. difficile*-associated diarrhea. Absence of toxin receptor expression on the immature colonic epithelium has been suggested as a mechanism to explain the symptomless carrier state in infants and children.[51]

Almost all antimicrobial agents can predispose to *C. difficile* diarrhea and colitis, including vancomycin and metronidazole,[52,53] but the precise risks associated with individual agents are difficult to establish. The frequency of association of specific antibiotics is related to their frequency of use, their route of administration, and their effect on the colonic microbiota.[54,55] Antibiotics commonly associated with CDI and diarrhea include clindamycin, second- and third-generation cephalosporins, ampicillin, amoxicillin, and (more recently) the fluoroquinolones (Table 112-2).[25,32,56,57] Cancer chemotherapeutic agents that possess antibacterial properties and bowel preparation regimens (e.g., before colonoscopy or colonic surgery) rarely can result in sufficient disturbance of the

intestinal microbiota to allow subsequent colonization with *C. difficile*.[58]

Clostridium difficile Toxins

Pathogenic strains of *C. difficile* produce 2 structurally similar protein exotoxins, toxin A and toxin B, which are the major known virulence factors. The genes encoding toxin A and toxin B reside in a 19.6-kb chromosomal region, the *C. difficile* pathogenicity locus, which contains the genes encoding toxin A (*tcdA*) and B (*tcdB*) as well as 2 putative regulatory genes (*tcdC* and *tcdD*, also called *tcdR*) (Fig. 112-2).[59,60] The *tcdD* gene product appears to up-regulate toxin transcription by complexing with RNA polymerase that binds to the toxin promoter regions. The *tcdC* gene is transcribed in the opposite direction to *tcdA*, *tcdB*, and *tcdD*, and its gene product appears to decrease toxin production.[59,60] The fifth gene of the pathogenicity locus, *tcdE*, encodes a protein with sequence similarity to bacteriophage pore-forming holin proteins and mediates the secretion of *C. difficile* toxins across the bacterial cell membrane and into the extracellular environment.[61]

Toxins A (308 kd) and B (220 kd) are members of the large clostridial cytotoxin family; they share a number of structural features, and are 49% identical at the amino acid level.[62-64] Both toxins carry an N-terminal enzymatic domain that mediates their toxic effects on mammalian cells, a central hydrophobic region that might act as a transmembrane domain to facilitate entry into the cytoplasm, and a C-terminal domain consisting of a series of repeated sequences that mediate toxin binding (Fig. 112-3).[25] More recently, a fourth domain has been identified, which encodes an intrinsic peptidase that releases the N-terminal enzymatic domain into the cytosol.[65]

Both toxins function as uridine diphosphate glucose (UDP-glucose) hydrolases and glucosyltransferases, a requirement for their cellular toxic effects. Following internalization into the host cell cytoplasm, the toxins catalyze the transfer and covalent attachment of a glucose residue from UDP-glucose to a conserved threonine amino acid on small (20 to 25 kd) guanosine triphosphate-binding rho proteins. Rho proteins are part of the Ras superfamily, are expressed in all eukaryotic cells, and act as intracellular signaling molecules to regulate cytoskeletal organization and gene expression. The rho proteins, RhoA, Rac, and Cdc42, are substrates for both toxins A and B, while Rap is a substrate for toxin A only.[iu,66,67] Glucosylation of rho proteins by the toxins leads to disordered cell signaling, disorganization of the cytoskeleton, disruption of protein synthesis, cell rounding, and cell death.[60,68] Both toxins also activate nuclear factor (NF)-κB, mitogen-activated protein (MAP) kinases, and COX-2 in target cells, leading to the release of proinflammatory cytokines including interleukin (IL)-1β, TNF-α, and IL-8.[68,69] These cellular proinflammatory effects contribute to the marked intestinal inflammatory response evident in *C. difficile*-associated diarrhea and pseudomembranous colitis.

Toxin A initially was thought to be the only enterotoxin based on studies in animals,[68,70,71] whereas toxin B, an extremely potent cytotoxin, appeared to have little independent enterotoxic activity in animals. This suggested that toxin B did not contribute to diarrhea and colitis in humans.[70,72] This view was challenged by studies on human colon showing that, in fact, toxin B is 10 times more potent than toxin A in inducing in vitro colon injury.[73,74] Furthermore, toxin A⁻/toxin B⁺ strains of *C. difficile* have been isolated from patients with diarrhea and pseudomembranous colitis,[75] confirming that toxin B is a major virulence factor in human disease.

A minority (≈15%) of *C. difficile* clinical isolates produce a third toxin—binary toxin—that is analogous to the iota toxin

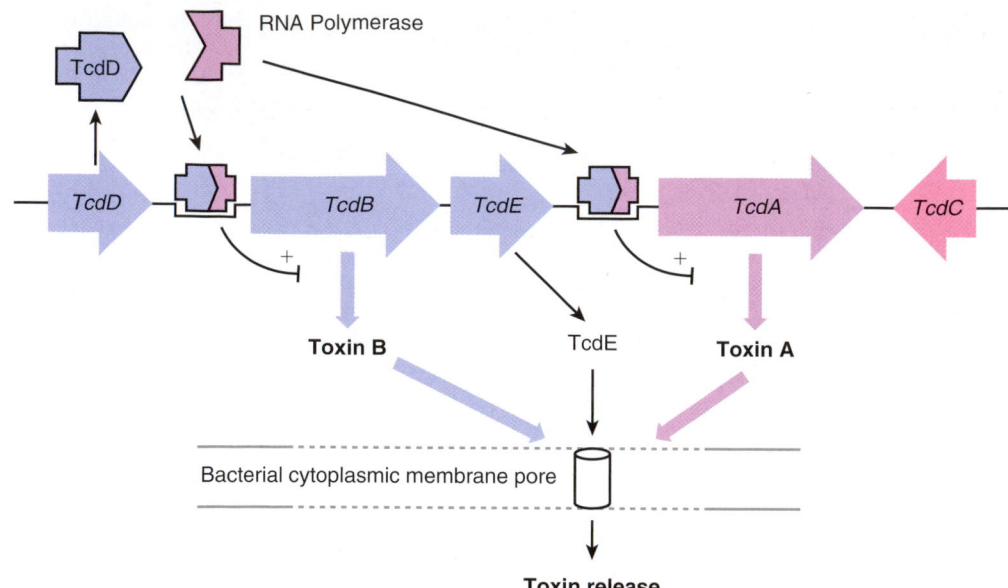

FIGURE 112-2. *Clostridium difficile* pathogenicity locus. The pathogenicity locus of *C. difficile* is a 19.6-kb segment that carries 5 genes (*TcdA-E*), including the genes encoding toxin A (*TcdA*) and toxin B (*TcdB*). *TcdD* (also called *TcdR*) appears to encode a positive regulator of toxin A and toxin B transcription. The TcdD gene product forms complexes with RNA polymerase that bind to the *TcdA* and *TcdB* promoter regions. *TcdC* appears to act as a negative regulator of toxin production. *TcdE* may mediate toxin release through its ability to form pores in the bacterial cytoplasmic membrane. *(Adapted from Warny M, Kelly C. Pathogenicity of* Clostridium difficile *toxins. In: Hecht G, editor. Microbial pathogenesis and the intestinal epithelial cell. Washington, D.C.: ASM Press; 2003. p 503.)*

of *C. perfringens* and is encoded at a site distant from the pathogenicity locus that encodes toxins A and B.[30,31] Binary toxin is composed of 2 parts: a 48-kd enzymatic protein and a 99-kd binding protein. Although binary toxin shows some enterotoxic activity in animal models, its role in the pathogenesis of *C. difficile*-associated diarrhea and colitis remains unclear. Most pathogenic strains of *C. difficile* lack binary toxin but nonetheless cause substantial colonic inflammation and injury. The NAP-1 strain is binary toxin positive, however, thereby raising renewed suspicion that this toxin might enhance the pathogenic effects of toxins A and B.[26,30]

Immune Response to Clostridium difficile

Serum IgG and IgA antibodies against *C. difficile* toxins are found in more than 50% of healthy children and adults.[76-80] Mucosal IgA antitoxin antibodies also are detectable in colonic secretions from more than 50% of humans and might inhibit receptor binding of toxin A.[78,80] Immunization against *C. difficile* toxins protects animals from *C. difficile* colitis but does not protect against colonization—a situation that may be similar to the asymptomatic carrier state in humans.[36,81]

High concentrations of IgG antitoxin A antibody in the serum are associated with protection against *C. difficile*–associated diarrhea and colitis,[82-84] and recurrent *C. difficile* diarrhea has been associated with low serum antitoxin antibody levels in children and adults.[76,80,85,86] In 1 study, adult inpatients with *C. difficile* diarrhea and a low level of serum IgG against toxin A had a 48-fold greater risk of recurrent disease after initial successful treatment compared with patients who had high antitoxin concentrations (Fig. 112-4).[36,87] High serum IgG antitoxin A concentrations also have been identified in asymptomatic carriers of toxinogenic *C. difficile*.[36] In a prospective study of nosocomially acquired *C. difficile*, 51% of infected patients who were asymptomatic carriers had serum IgG antitoxin A concentrations that were 3 times higher than those in patients with diarrhea (see Fig. 112-4).[36] The

immune response to toxin B has also been correlated with clinical outcomes, including risk of recurrence.[83,84,87]

Other Risk Factors for Clostridium difficile Infection

In addition to antimicrobial therapy and in-patient care, increasing age and increased comorbidity are important risk factors for CDI.[88] In 2009, the U.S. Agency for Healthcare Research and Quality reported an overall CDI rate in hospitalized patients of 110 per 100,000 population. Age was a major risk factor for infection, with rates of 1089 per 1,000,000 population in those aged 85 or older compared to 486 per 1,000,000 for those 65 to 84 years of age, 101 per 1,000,000 for those 45 to 64 years of age, and 28 per 1,000,000 for those 18 to 44 years of age. Older adults particularly are predisposed to infection with *C. difficile* because of increased nosocomial antibiotic exposure and reduced innate and adaptive immune function. In 1 study of antibiotic recipients, patients with severe underlying disease at the time of hospital admission were 8 times more likely to develop CDI compared with patients who were less severely ill.[36] Other reported risk factors for CDI include the use of an NG tube, GI procedures that are associated with bowel cleansing and/or ileus, ICU stay, and length of hospital stay.[54] The strengths of the associations of these risk factors with *C. difficile* vary from study to study. These factors often are markers of disease severity, older age, or both, and the significance of their association with *C. difficile* can decline or be lost after controlling for these confounding variables.[36,88,89]

There is a dose-dependent association between acid suppression and risk for *C. difficile*-associated diarrhea.[90,91] While many studies have confirmed this association, others have found that the initial apparent association was lost after adjusting for confounding variables, and meta-analyses disagree as to the strength of evidence for a primary association between PPI use and risk for CDI and whether or not a cause-effect relationship might exist.[92,93] Furthermore, the

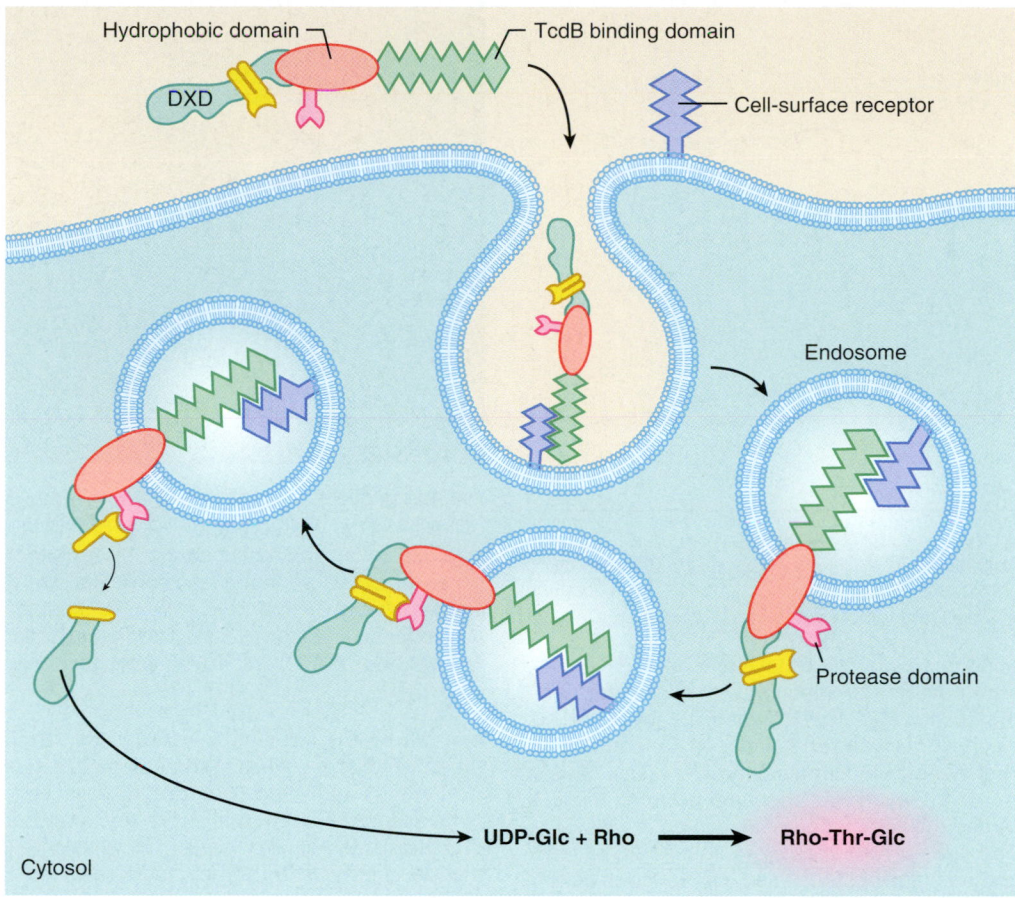

FIGURE 112-3. Structure and function of *Clostridium difficile* toxins: structure and function. Toxin A and toxin B share similar domains: a C-terminal binding domain *(green)* that is composed of contiguous repeating units also known as *clostridial repetitive oligopeptides* (CROPs); a central, major hydrophobic region *(red oval)* of 172 amino acids that is highly conserved and acts as a transmembrane domain; an intrinsic protease domain *(pink)*; and an N-terminal enzymatic domain *(light green)* that carries the consensus DXD (aspartate-any intervening amino acid-aspartate) glucosyltransferase domain and is responsible for cytotoxicity. Interaction of the toxin B binding domain *(green)* with cell-surface receptors *(dark blue)* induces receptor-mediated endocytosis. The acidic pH of the endosome triggers the first conformational change and results in pore formation by the hydrophobic, translocation domain *(red oval)*. Within the cytosol, a second conformational change activates intrinsic protease activity *(pink)*. Autocatalytic cleavage of toxin B releases the catalytic glucosyltransferase domain *(light blue)* into the cytosol. Glucosylation of the cytosolic target Rho GTPases at a conserved threonine residue (Thr) leads to disaggregation of the cytoskeleton and cell death (see text for greater detail). Glc, D-glucose; UDP, uridine diphosphate. *(Modified from Kelly CP, Lamont JT. Clostridium difficile—More difficult than ever. N Engl J Med 2008; 359:1932-40.)*

mechanism whereby a reduction in gastric acidity might facilitate CDI is not obvious because *C. difficile* spores are acid resistant.

Patients undergoing cytotoxic chemotherapy for malignancy are at risk for CDI because of frequent antibiotic use, nosocomial exposure to *C. difficile*, and severe comorbidity.[94,95] Even in the absence of antibiotic use, antineoplastic chemotherapy predisposes to CDI, reflecting the ability of these drugs to alter the colonic microbiota and reduce *C. difficile* colonization resistance.[62] *C. difficile*-associated diarrhea also has been reported in patients undergoing immunosuppressive therapy in the setting of solid organ or bone marrow transplantation.[96,97]

Patients with HIV infection are at risk for *C. difficile*-associated diarrhea because of multiple risk factors, including frequent prophylactic and therapeutic antibiotic use, hospitalization, and immunodeficiency.[98] *C. difficile* colitis behaves the same in HIV-infected patients as it does in control groups,[99] and testing for *C. difficile* should be a routine part of the diagnostic evaluation in these patients with diarrhea and a history of current or recent antibiotic treatment.

Patients with IBD are also at increased risk for *C. difficile* infection even in the absence of recent antibiotic treatment.[100-104] Infection with a broad range of enteric pathogens including *C. difficile*, *Campylobacter*, and *Salmonella* species can precipitate or mimic disease relapse in IBD. *C. difficile* is the most commonly identified specific pathogen in IBD patients in North America and Europe, however, and is present in as many as 5% to 19% of patients with relapse in some case series.[100-103] Many IBD patients with *C. difficile* infection do not have a history of recent antibiotic use, which suggests that IBD-related colitis itself can impair colonization resistance. The possibility of enteric infection with *C. difficile* or other pathogens should be considered in any patient with an increase in IBD disease activity. If CDI is identified in a patient with an IBD flare, antimicrobial therapy with metronidazole or vancomycin is indicated in addition to IBD treatment. In 1 study, IBD inpatients with coexisting CDI were more likely to have severe disease and to require colectomy than similar patients without coexisting infection.[103] Systemic glucocorticoid therapy has also been linked to increased mortality in hospitalized patients with CDI.[105]

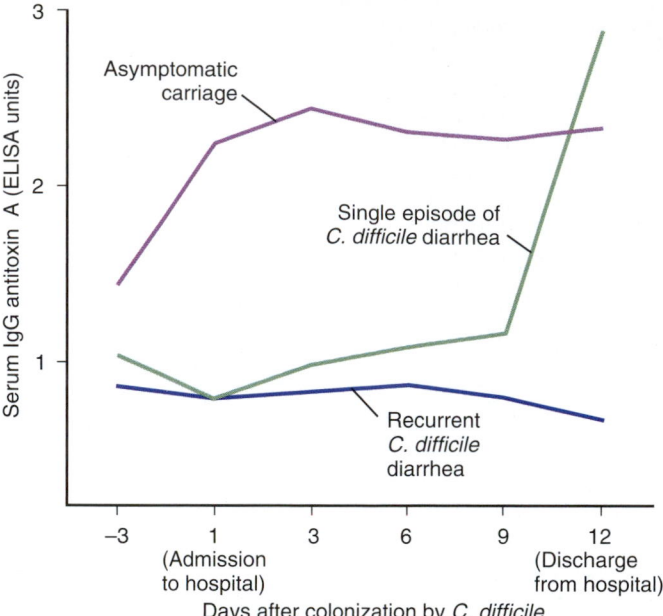

FIGURE 112-4. Serum immunoglobulin G (IgG) antitoxin A antibody response and clinical outcome of infection with *Clostridium difficile*. Patients with nosocomial *C. difficile* diarrhea were studied prospectively, and serum IgG antitoxin A antibody concentrations were measured by enzyme-linked immunosorbent assay (ELISA) at regular intervals. A correlation was observed between the IgG response to toxin A and the clinical outcome of infection. Asymptomatic carriers mounted an early memory immune response to toxin A. By contrast, no significant increase was found in serum IgG antitoxin A of patients who experienced recurrent *C. difficile* diarrhea. In those who had a single episode of diarrhea, IgG antitoxin A levels generally were increased on day 12 of their first episode. Thus, a serum antibody response to toxin A during *C. difficile* infection is associated with protection against symptoms and against recurrent diarrhea.[36,87]

Clinical Features

Clinical manifestations of CDI range from asymptomatic carriage to mild or moderate diarrhea to life-threatening pseudomembranous colitis with toxic megacolon. Asymptomatic carriage of *C. difficile* is common in hospitalized patients. Several large epidemiologic studies indicate that 10% to 21% of hospital inpatients receiving antibiotics in high-risk units are carriers.[27,35-37,106] Although most of the *C. difficile* isolates from carriers are toxin producing, carriers do not develop symptomatic disease, perhaps as a result of adaptive protective immunity.[27,35-37,106]

In patients who develop diarrhea with *C. difficile*, symptoms usually begin soon after colonization. The incubation period is usually less than a week, with a median time of onset of approximately 2 days.[27,35,36,107] Colonization can occur during or for up to 2 or even 3 months after antibiotic treatment.[108]

C. difficile diarrhea typically is associated with the frequent passage of loose or watery bowel movements. Some patients present with fever, leukocytosis, and cramping abdominal pain.[109] Mucus or occult blood may be present, but melena or hematochezia is uncommon and, if present, suggests IBD, colon cancer, or another source of bleeding. Because *C. difficile* is not an invasive pathogen, extraintestinal manifestations of CDI such as septic arthritis, bacteremia, or tissue abscess are extremely rare.[110-113] An oligoarticular, asymmetrical,

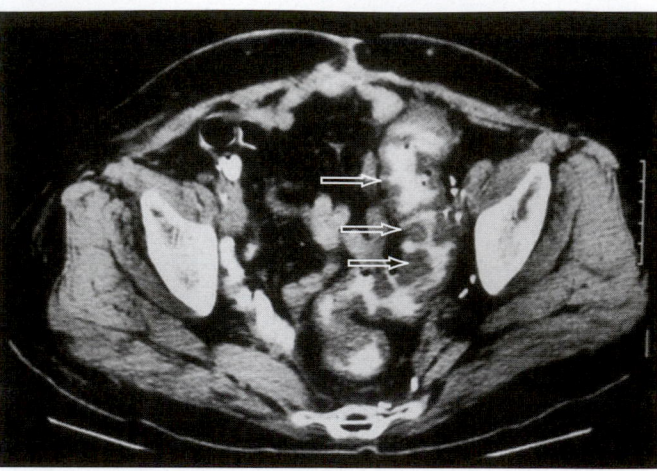

FIGURE 112-5. CT of the abdomen in a patient with *Clostridium difficile* colitis. Marked thickening of the colonic wall in the sigmoid colon and an accordion-like pattern, produced by a series of broad edematous colonic haustral folds, are evident (arrows). (*From Linevsky JK, Kelly CP. Clostridium difficile colitis. In: Lamont JT, editor. Gastrointestinal infections: Diagnosis and management. New York: Taylor & Francis Group; 1997. p 293.*)

non-deforming large-joint arthropathy, similar to that seen in other infectious colitides, sometimes is seen.[114]

Patients with more severe disease can develop colonic ileus or toxic dilatation and present with minimal or even no diarrhea.[109] In the absence of diarrhea, the only clues to the diagnosis may be high fever, moderate or marked (e.g., leukemoid) polymorphonuclear leukocytosis, lower or diffuse abdominal pain, tenderness, and distention.

Abdominal plain films might reveal a dilated colon (>7 cm in its greatest diameter), toxic megacolon, or small bowel ileus with air-fluid levels mimicking intestinal obstruction or ischemia. In such cases, a CT scan of the abdomen may reveal nonspecific features common to ischemic, infectious, and inflammatory colitides (Fig. 112-5).[115] Radiologic features of pseudomembranous colitis include mucosal edema, a thickened colonic wall, pancolitis, and pericolonic inflammation with or without ascites, and usually without small bowel involvement other than ileus; one notable exception is in patients with a mature ileostomy or ileal pouch where *C. difficile* can infect the colon-like altered ileal mucosa. Flexible sigmoidoscopy or colonoscopy is sometimes indicated to identify pseudomembranous colitis when the diagnosis remains unclear after initial evaluation (see later).

Complications of severe *C. difficile* colitis include dehydration, hypoalbuminemia, ascites, electrolyte disturbances, renal failure, hypotension, toxic megacolon, systemic inflammatory response syndrome, bowel perforation, and death.[26,109]

Diagnosis

The diagnosis of *C. difficile* diarrhea or colitis is based on the presence of diarrhea and other evidence of acute colitis, and demonstration in stools of *C. difficile* toxins or toxinogenic *C. difficile*.[23,25,26] Although a history of recent antibiotic use is common, it is not a requirement for diagnosis.[4,26,36]

Tests for Clostridium difficile *Infection*

The diagnosis of *C. difficile* diarrhea should be considered in any patient with acute diarrhea, especially if they had antibiotic exposure within the previous 2 to 3 months.[26] Most, but not all, cases occur during or after hospitalization. Approximately 40% of patients with *C. difficile* diarrhea at tertiary referral centers are symptomatic on admission to the hospital, and most have had a recent prior hospitalization.[35,36,116]

Testing of solid or formed stools for *C. difficile* toxin is not recommended because only patients with diarrhea require treatment.[26,35,36,43,106] Treatment of asymptomatic carriers with antimicrobial agents against *C. difficile* is not recommended because it might prolong the carrier state beyond the usual 2 to 6 weeks.[43] Follow-up stool testing to confirm cure also is not indicated in an asymptomatic patient, even in patients discharged to chronic care facilities, because asymptomatic carriage is already highly prevalent in these facilities. Stool carriage of *C. difficile* can persist for up to 6 weeks after cessation of symptoms and does not require therapy.[117] Because asymptomatic carriers can act as hidden reservoirs for CDI, especially in hospitals and nursing homes, universal precautions should be followed for all patients to reduce the likelihood of patient-to-patient spread of nosocomial infectious disease.

If *C. difficile* diarrhea is suspected, a freshly passed stool sample should be submitted immediately to the laboratory in a clean watertight container. Anaerobic storage or the use of transport media is not necessary, but storage at ambient temperatures can result in denaturation of fecal toxin or bacterial DNA; samples should therefore be tested immediately or refrigerated or frozen, pending later testing.[23,26]

A variety of laboratory tests are available to diagnose infection with toxinogenic *C. difficile*. Enzyme immunoassays (EIAs) to detect toxin antigens in stool currently are used most commonly (Table 112-3). These tests have the advantages of being relatively inexpensive, quick to perform (2 to 12 hours), and specific; however, their relatively low sensitivity can lead to false-negative results. Nucleic acid amplification tests (NAAT) such as PCR are now widely available and increasingly used because of their high sensitivity. The tissue culture cytotoxicity assay is also sensitive and has high diagnostic accuracy, but it is more resource intensive and time consuming (24 to 72 hours). Anaerobic culture followed by determination of toxin production is both sensitive and specific; however, it requires specialized resources and expertise, and results take several days to obtain, leading to its being used in epidemiology studies but seldom in clinical practice.

Enzyme-Linked Immunoassays

Commercially available EIAs are widely used to detect toxins A and B of *C. difficile* in stool specimens.[23,26,118] Toxin is detected by its interaction with either a monoclonal antibody or polyclonal antiserum that specifically recognizes toxin epitopes. EIAs are easier to perform than the cytotoxicity test, are relatively inexpensive, and are fast, with results in 1 to 6 hours. Although they have high specificity (83% to 98%), their main drawback is that they are less sensitive (75% to 95%) than the cytotoxicity test.[118,119] In addition, some EIA kits detect only toxin A, in which case diarrhea due to a toxin A$^-$/B$^+$ strain of *C. difficile* will have a falsely negative test result.[75,120] For this reason, assays that can detect both toxin A and toxin B are preferred.

Immunoassays also have been used to detect *C. difficile* common antigen (glutamate dehydrogenase [GDH]) in stool.[23,26,118] The initial latex agglutination assay method lacked diagnostic accuracy and is not recommended. More recent EIAs for fecal GDH have shown improved sensitivity (85% to 95%) and specificity (89% to 99%), are rapid, and are not expensive. These changes have led to the use of EIA for GDH as an initial screening test, with confirmation of positive results using another test such as a NAAT or the tissue culture cytotoxicity assay.[26,121]

Nucleic Acid Amplification Tests

PCR and other NAATs can detect toxinogenic *C. difficile* in clinical isolates. Recent systematic reviews of PCR assays indicate sensitivities and specificities in excess of 90% compared with toxinogenic culture or cytotoxicity assays and superior performance compared with toxin EIA.[118,122-124] Although NAATs are more expensive than EIA, this cost differential may be offset somewhat by the fact that clinicians may be more likely to rely on a single negative NAAT result, thereby avoiding the cost of duplicate or triplicate testing.[123] Two other phenomena are emerging regarding the widespread use of NAATs for *C. difficile* infection. First, introduction of NAATs in place of EIA may lead to an apparent increase in the incidence of positive test results because of greater sensitivity. Second, there is discussion as to whether NAATs may be "too sensitive" and detect tiny amounts of

TABLE 112-3 Stool Tests for the Diagnosis of *Clostridium difficile* Infection

Test	Target	Advantages	Disadvantages
Tissue culture cytotoxin	Toxin B (toxin A is 100- to 1000-fold less potent as a cytotoxin)	Traditional gold standard; highly sensitive and specific	Requires tissue culture facility; takes 24-48 hr
Enzyme immunoassay	Toxin A and/or B	Fast (2-6 hr); easy to perform; specific	Not as sensitive as the cytotoxin or NAATs nucleic acid amplification tests
	Glutamate dehydrogenase	Fast (2-6 hr); easy to perform; sensitive	Not specific; positive results must be confirmed by a more specific assay
Culture	Toxinogenic and non-toxinogenic *C. difficile*	Sensitive (current gold standard); allows strain typing in epidemics	Requires anaerobic culture; isolates must be tested for toxinogenicity; takes 2-5 days
PCR and other NAATs	Genes specific to toxinogenic *C. difficile*	Fast (1-4 hours); easy to perform; sensitive	More expensive; requires special equipment; may detect *C. difficile* genes in the absence of active infection and toxin production

C. difficile genes that are not associated with true colonization or infection. This highlights the importance of interpreting test results in clinical context.[125] Regardless of these issues, the use of NAATs to diagnose CDI is steadily increasing at the expense of EIAs.[122]

Tissue Culture Cytotoxicity Assay

The tissue culture cytotoxicity assay was the first clinical test to identify *C. difficile* toxins in stool.[21,22] Toxins A and B inactivate rho proteins, causing a disintegration of the actin cytoskeleton and a characteristic rounding of cells in the tissue culture. Despite its high sensitivity (67% to 100%) and specificity (85% to 100%) the test is seldom used currently because it requires 48 to 72 hours for completion, is expensive, and requires a tissue culture facility.

Clostridium difficile Culture

Culture of stool for *C. difficile* is sensitive (89% to 100%) but is not specific for toxin-producing strains of the bacterium. Therefore, cultured isolates then must be tested in vitro for toxin production to improve test specificity, but this is costly and time consuming. One advantage of culturing *C. difficile* is that it permits strain typing of individual isolates, and therefore it is useful in tracking hospital outbreaks for epidemiologic studies.[30,31,39,126]

Sigmoidoscopy and Colonoscopy

Neither sigmoidoscopy nor colonoscopy is required for diagnosis in most patients with *C. difficile* diarrhea.[26] Endoscopy is helpful, however, when the diagnosis is in doubt or when disease severity demands rapid diagnosis. Sigmoidoscopy may be normal in patients with mild diarrhea or might demonstrate nonspecific colitis in moderate cases. The finding of colonic pseudomembranes in a patient with AAD is virtually pathognomonic for *C. difficile* colitis (Fig. 112-6).[127,128] Pseudomembranes appear as yellow, gray, or white plaques 2 to 5 mm in diameter, and in some areas they can coalesce to cover large portions of the mucosal surface. Sigmoidoscopy might not be sufficient to identify all patients with pseudomembranous colitis, because approximately 15% to 20% only have pseudomembranes in the more proximal areas of the colon.[129] Other nonspecific endoscopic findings include erythema, edema, friability, small ulcerations, and erosions.

In mild disease, colonic mucosal biopsies may be normal or demonstrate only mild and nonspecific acute inflammatory changes with neutrophil infiltration. In more severe cases, colonic histology shows focal ulceration of the mucosa associated with the eruption of inflammatory cells and necrotic debris that covers the area of ulceration, the so-called summit or volcano lesion (Fig. 112-7).[127,130]

Miscellaneous Laboratory Tests

Many patients with acute *C. difficile* diarrhea develop a polymorphonuclear leukocytosis with a left shift. Occasionally a leukemoid reaction with an extremely high WBC count of more than 50,000 or even 100,000 cells/mm³ is seen. A peripheral WBC count of greater than 15,000 cells/mm³ is associated with negative clinical outcomes and a count of greater than 25,000 cells/mm³ is associated with an increased mortality risk.[131,132] Decreased serum albumin and elevated creatinine levels also are markers of severe disease. Patients with protein-losing colopathy and severe hypoalbuminemia can develop peripheral edema, ascites, or anasarca.

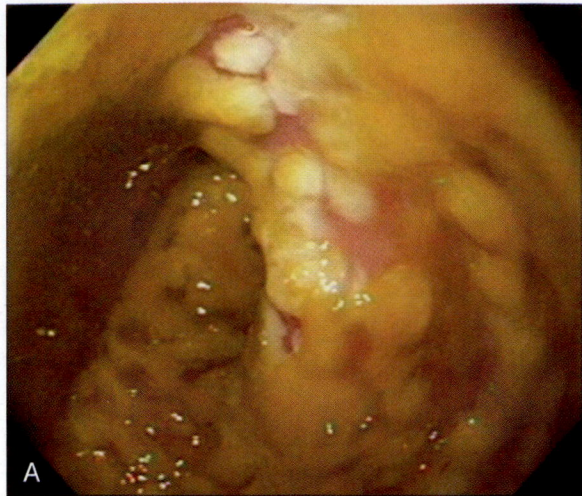

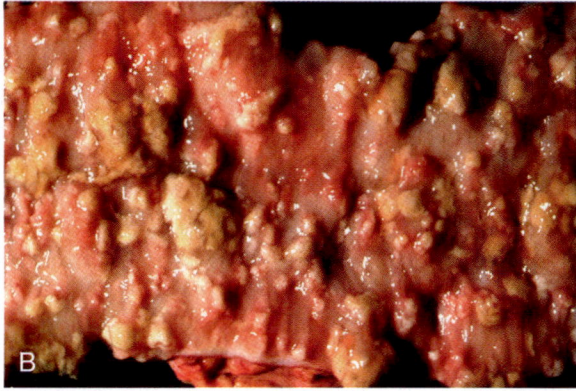

FIGURE 112-6. Colonoscopic appearance of pseudomembranous colitis *(A)* and a colon resection specimen from a patient with severe, refractory *Clostridium difficile* diarrhea and colitis *(B)*. Characteristic raised adherent yellow plaques that vary in size from 2 to 5 mm are visible on the colonic mucosa. In some areas, coalescing pseudomembranes are evident. There is some erythema of the colonic mucosa between the pseudomembranes, but the epithelium is intact. (A, *From Kwon JH, Kelly CP. Clostridium difficile and antibiotic-associated diarrhea. In: Bayless RM, Diehl AM, editors. Advanced therapy in gastroenterology and liver disease. 5th ed. Hamilton, Ontario: BC Decker; 2005. p 302; B, from Kelly CP, Pothoulakis C, Lamont JT. Clostridium difficile colitis. N Engl J Med 1994; 330:257-62.)*

Treatment

Mild to Moderately Severe Clostridium difficile-Associated Diarrhea and Colitis

The first step in the management of *C. difficile* diarrhea and colitis is to discontinue any precipitating antibiotics if possible (Box 112-2).[25,26,133,134] Concomitant treatment with antimicrobials other than those used to treat CDI is associated with poor outcomes of CDI therapy; in 1 study these included a lower and slower initial response to therapy (median time to resolution of diarrhea of 96 vs. 52 hours; P < 0.001), higher treatment failure rates after 10 days (16% vs. 7%; P < 0.001) and lower rates of sustained response without recurrence (66% vs. 75%; P = 0.005).[133]

If all antibiotics are discontinued, diarrhea resolves in approximately 15% to 25% of patients over 2 to 6 weeks without specific anti-*C. difficile* therapy.[108,135] Conservative therapy alone, however, is not appropriate in patients who

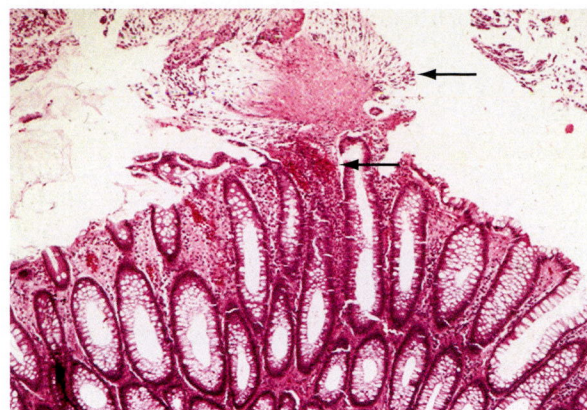

FIGURE 112-7. Histopathologic image of an endoscopic biopsy specimen from a patient with pseudomembranous colitis showing a summit or volcano lesion. Focal ulceration of the colonic mucosa is evident *(lower arrow)*, with exudation of a pseudomembrane made up of inflammatory cells, fibrin, and necrotic debris *(upper arrow)*. The adjoining mucosa is intact. *(From Kelly CP, Pothoulakis C, Lamont JT. Clostridium difficile colitis. N Engl J Med 1994; 330:257-62.)*

are severely ill or who have multiple other active medical problems and is seldom recommended in current hospital practice. In patients with active infections elsewhere (e.g., pneumonia and urinary tract infection) and in whom antibiotic therapy must be continued, the antibiotic regimen should be switched, if possible, to agents with a relatively low likelihood of exacerbating *C. difficile* diarrhea; for example, parenteral aminoglycosides, trimethoprim, or erythromycin (see Table 112-2). Antimotility agents such as diphenoxylate plus atropine (Lomotil), loperamide (Imodium), or narcotics often are avoided because of concern for impaired toxin clearance or precipitation of ileus and toxic dilatation, albeit the evidence supporting these concerns is limited and contradictory.[26,136,137]

Many antimicrobial agents show activity against *C. difficile* in vitro, and resistance to cephalosporins is so widespread that cefoxitin is used in selective media to culture *C. difficile*.[138,139] Clindamycin resistance is seen in some clinical isolates of *C. difficile* and has been associated with nosocomial outbreaks of CDI.[140] There is increasing evidence of fluoroquinolone resistance among nosocomial *C. difficile* isolates, and the NAP-1 strain that has caused several outbreaks shows high-level fluoroquinolone resistance.[24,25,30-32] Fortunately, resistance to metronidazole is rare, and resistance to vancomycin is essentially nonexistent. In 1 study of 186 clinical isolates of *C. difficile*, all were sensitive to both metronidazole and vancomycin, with minimum inhibitory concentrations (MICs) of 0.5 to 4 mg/mL.[139] In another series from Spain, 6% of 415 isolates showed intermediate sensitivity to metronidazole (MIC > 16 mg/mL), but this partial resistance pattern was not clonal and was not sustained in serial culture.[141] These findings suggest acquired tolerance rather than genetically determined metronidazole resistance.

Many antimicrobial agents, such as ampicillin or amoxicillin, which have in vitro activity against *C. difficile*, are common causes of *C. difficile*-associated diarrhea in clinical practice.[142,143] These observations illustrate the fact that in vitro sensitivity testing alone is a poor predictor of therapeutic efficacy in this disease. Specific antibiotic therapy to eradicate *C. difficile* is required in patients with severe symptoms or in those whose symptoms persist despite discontinuation of antibiotic treatment. The most effective antimicrobials for the treatment of *C.*

BOX 112-2 Treatment of *Clostridium difficile* Infection

Minimize use of concomitant antibiotics
Discontinue all other antimicrobial drugs whenever possible
If additional antimicrobials are required, change to those least likely to exacerbate *C. difficile* infection (see Table 112-2)

Initial Episode
Mild to Moderate Infection
Metronidazole (500 mg orally 3 times daily for 10-14 days)

Severe Infection or Unresponsiveness to or Intolerance of Metronidazole
Vancomycin (250 mg orally 4 times daily for 10-14 days)

Other Approved Therapy
Fidaxomicin (200 mg orally 2 times daily for 10 days)*

First Recurrence
Treat as for initial episode (see above)*

Second Recurrence[†]
Vancomycin in tapered and pulsed doses:
   125 mg daily 4 times daily for 14 days
   125 mg daily 2 times daily for 7 days
   125 mg once daily for 7 days
   125 mg once every 2 days for 8 days (4 doses)
   125 mg once every 3 days for 15 days (5 doses)
Fidaxomicin (200 mg orally 2 times daily for 10 days)*

Third Recurrence
Vancomycin in tapered and pulsed doses (see above)
Fidaxomicin (200 mg orally 2 times daily for 10 days)*
Vancomycin (125 mg orally 4 times daily for 14 days) followed by rifaximin (400 mg orally 3 times daily for 20 days)

Other Options for Recurrent Infection
Fecal microbiota transplantation[‡]
IV immune globulin (400 mg per kilogram of body weight every 3 weeks for a total of 2 or 3 doses)

---

*Fidaxomicin therapy is followed by fewer recurrences compared with vancomycin, both for an initial episode and for a first recurrence. The efficacy of fidaxomicin in second or subsequent recurrences is not yet known.
[†]A lactobacillus-containing probiotic or *Saccharomyces boulardii* may be added during the final 2 weeks of the vancomycin regimen and for 4 to 8 weeks thereafter. However, the efficacy of probiotics in preventing recurrent *C. difficile* infection is unclear.
[‡]Fecal microbial transplantation appears to be highly effective in preventing further episodes in patients with multiple recurrences (See Chapter 130).
Adapted from Kelly CP, Lamont JT. Clostridium difficile—More difficult than ever. N Engl J Med 2008; 18:1932-40.

---

difficile diarrhea are metronidazole (250 to 500 mg 3 or 4 times a day for 10 to 14 days), vancomycin (125 to 500 mg 4 times a day for 10 to 14 days), and fidaxomicin (200 mg 2 times daily for 10 days) (see Box 112-2).[26,144,145] Bacitracin, teicoplanin, nitazoxanide, rifaximin, and fusidic acid also have been used to treat acute infection but have few if any advantages over metronidazole, vancomycin, or fidaxomicin. The advantages and disadvantages of specific therapeutic agents are discussed in the sections that follow.

Metronidazole

Metronidazole generally is recommended as the drug of first choice for mild to moderately severe *C. difficile* diarrhea and colitis.[26,144] It is inexpensive and is usually effective. Several clinical studies before 2000 indicated that metronidazole therapy resulted in resolution of diarrhea and colitis in more than 95% of patients treated.[108,146,147] For example, in a prospective randomized trial of acute CDI, metronidazole (250 mg 4 times a day for 10 days) was as effective as vancomycin (500 mg 4 times daily for 10 days) in terms of response and recurrence rates.[135] Studies published after 2000, however, report an average failure rate of 19% for metronidazole (range, 7% to 38%) compared with only 4% for vancomycin (range, 3% to 6%).[25,148,149]

In 1 trial, subjects with acute CDI were stratified according to disease severity and then randomized to receive either metronidazole 250 mg or vancomycin 125 mg, each given 4 times per day. In mild disease, both treatments yielded similar response rates (90% and 98%; P = 0.36). In severe disease, however, metronidazole was less efficacious (76% vs. 97%; P = 0.02).[149] Thus, oral vancomycin should be used as the first-line agent in severe disease[26,122,144] and possibly also in mild to moderate disease in older adult patients with significant comorbidity.

Metronidazole, unlike vancomycin, is well absorbed in the upper intestine following oral administration. Fecal concentrations are low or absent in healthy persons or asymptomatic carriers of C. difficile, but higher fecal concentrations are observed in patients with C. difficile colitis, because metronidazole is secreted through the inflamed intestinal mucosa.[150] IV metronidazole (500 mg 4 times per day) may be used in patients who cannot tolerate oral medication, because it accumulates to reach bactericidal levels within the inflamed colon.[150]

Oral metronidazole therapy usually is well tolerated but can be associated with systemic side effects including nausea, a metallic taste, and a disulfiram-like reaction with alcohol.[150] A peripheral sensory neuropathy may occur with prolonged therapy—especially in older adults. Thus, metronidazole should not be administered for prolonged courses. Metronidazole can also potentiate the action of warfarin, resulting in prolongation of the prothrombin time.

Enigmatically, metronidazole has been identified as the antibiotic agent responsible for causing some cases of C. difficile diarrhea, demonstrating the importance of reduced colonization resistance in the pathophysiology of C. difficile-associated diarrhea.[53,151,152]

Vancomycin

Vancomycin was introduced for treating C. difficile-associated diarrhea and colitis in 1978,[153] and its pharmacokinetic properties make it an ideal agent for treating this infection. When given orally, vancomycin is neither absorbed nor metabolized significantly and, as a result, high concentrations in the colonic lumen are achieved. The efficacy of vancomycin in treating C. difficile colitis has been demonstrated in controlled trials.[135,145,148,149,153-156] Improvement in diarrhea usually is evident within 72 hours of initiating therapy, and complete resolution of symptoms occurs in most patients (96% overall) by the end of a 10-day treatment course.[135,145,148,149,153-156]

Fekety and coworkers[157] demonstrated that vancomycin at a dose of 125 mg 4 times a day is as effective as vancomycin 500 mg 4 times a day. The lower dose is recommended for patients with mild to moderate colitis, and the higher dose is recommended for patients with severe complicated disease (see below). Vancomycin may be administered by mouth, NG tube, or even by enema,[108,158] but it should not be given IV to treat CDI, because effective colonic luminal concentrations are not obtained with parenteral administration.[159,160]

Because oral vancomycin is not absorbed appreciably, systemic side effects are rare. Despite its many advantages, oral vancomycin is still considered a second-line agent for the treatment of mild to moderately severe CDI because of its higher cost and concerns regarding the spread of vancomycin-resistant enterococci.[161] Vancomycin therapy is recommended, however, for patients with severe infection and for patients who fail to respond to metronidazole, are intolerant of metronidazole, are pregnant, or are younger than 10 years.[26,122,144,158,161]

Fidaxomicin

Fidaxomicin, a novel macrocyclic antibiotic, is active in vitro against clinical isolates of C. difficile, has very little systemic absorption and hence few systemic side effects, and achieves high fecal concentrations, making it a promising candidate for treatment of CDI.[145,156,162] Furthermore, fidaxomicin shows more limited activity against other members of the intestinal microbiota, suggesting that it may be a more selective therapy against C. difficile and lead to fewer post-treatment recurrences.[145,163]

Clinical trials have compared fidaxomicin (200 mg twice daily) with vancomycin (125 mg 4 times daily) for treatment of CDI.[145,156] Initial response rates (i.e., resolution of diarrhea at the end of 10 days of treatment) were similar for both agents (88.2% for fidaxomicin, (n = 287) and 85.8% for vancomycin (n = 309) by modified ITT).[145] Recurrence rates over the subsequent 4 weeks were lower for fidaxomicin than for vancomycin (15.4% vs. 25.3%; P = 0.005). A sustained response to therapy (i.e., resolution of diarrhea without recurrence) was more common in the fidaxomicin group (74.6% vs. 64.1%; P = 0.006). These study findings have led to the approval of fidaxomicin for therapy of CDI in many countries, the first newly approved therapy since vancomycin 25 years earlier.

Although fidaxomicin was more effective than vancomycin overall, especially in achieving lower recurrence rates, this benefit was not seen for patients infected by NAP-1 strains. For the 36% of patients with the NAP-1 strain, rates of initial response and recurrence were the same as those with vancomycin. However, for the 64% of patients with other strain types, the recurrence rate was 7.8% with fidaxomicin versus 25.5% for vancomycin (P < 0.001).

The advantage of fidaxomicin over vancomycin in achieving lower recurrence rates was also demonstrated after combining patients who were treated for a first recurrence of CDI in 2 separate but similar clinical trials.[164] Second recurrences within 4 weeks of completing therapy developed in 13 of 66 patients treated with fidaxomicin and in 22 of 62 treated with vancomycin (19.7% vs. 35.5%; P = 0.045). In summary, fidaxomicin is as effective as vancomycin for initial treatment of CDI. It leads to fewer post-treatment recurrences in patients infected with non–NAP-1 strains of C. difficile. It also is associated with fewer subsequent recurrences in patients treated for a first recurrence of CDI. The place of fidaxomicin in CDI treatment algorithms is evolving as clinicians attempt to balance significantly higher sustained response rates against substantially higher costs of treatment.

Other Antimicrobial Agents

In randomized therapeutic trials, teicoplanin, 100 mg twice a day for 10 days, was as effective as vancomycin for treating C. difficile diarrhea.[165,166] Teicoplanin, however, is relatively expensive and is not available for oral administration in the United States. Nitazoxanide was compared with vancomycin for primary therapy of CDI in a small randomized trial. Response rates after 10 days of therapy were 17/22 for nitazoxanide and 20 of 27 for vancomycin (77% vs. 74%; 95% CI for non-inferiority, −24% to +28%).[167] There are limited published data on the use of rifaximin, 400 mg 3 times daily for 10 days, as primary therapy for CDI.[168] Bacitracin (25,000 units 4 times daily for 7 to 10 days) is less effective than metronidazole or vancomycin for treating C. difficile diarrhea, with an overall response rate of only 80% and a relapse rate of 30%.[155,169-171] Fusidic acid has been tested in a limited number of patients but appears to be less effective than metronidazole or vancomycin and is associated with a relapse rate of approximately 28%.[166,172] Treatment with colestipol, an ion exchange resin that binds toxins (10 g 4 times daily), is associated with a low response rate (36%) and is not recommended as primary therapy.[154]

Severe Clostridium difficile Infection

It has long been suspected that oral vancomycin may be superior to metronidazole for treatment of severe CDI.[127,158] Data to support this theory, however, were lacking prior to the publication of a study that stratified patients according to disease severity and then compared outcomes for those receiving vancomycin 125 mg 4 times daily with metronidazole 250 mg 4 times daily each for 10 days.[149] Response rates to vancomycin and metronidazole were similar in mild to moderate disease (98% and 90%, NS); in severe disease, however, vancomycin had higher response rates (97% vs. 76%; P = 0.02).

This study led to a change in many local and national guidelines whereby oral vancomycin 125 mg 4 times daily is now recommended as first-line therapy for treatment of severe CDI.[26,122,144] The best method to identify those at risk for severe disease at the time of choosing antimicrobial therapy, however, is not entirely clear. The study described above used an empirical scoring system whereby a score of 2 points or greater was considered severe. In that scheme, 1 point was assigned for age older than 60 years, temperature greater than 101°F (38.3°C), serum albumin less than 2.5 mg/dL, or peripheral WBC greater than 15,000 cells/mm^3, while 2 points were assigned for known pseudomembranous colitis at colonoscopy or a requirement for ICU-level care.[149] Others suggest using either an elevated peripheral WBC (>15,000 cells/mm^3) or an elevated creatinine (>1.5 times baseline) to indicate severe disease that requires treatment with oral vancomycin.[26]

Severe Complicated Clostridium difficile Infection

Severe complicated CDI occurs in less than 10% of patients but is associated with a high mortality rate.[113,173,174] Diarrhea may be minimal or absent because of ileus, and patients can present with abdominal pain, peritoneal signs, colonic dilatation, marked leukocytosis, and a clinical picture of progressive sepsis with hypotension (possibly requiring the use of a vasopressor), mental status changes, elevated serum lactate, or end-organ failure (e.g., renal, pulmonary).[26,71,122,135,175]

The first step is to discontinue non-*C. difficile* antibiotics whenever possible and to start therapy with high-dose oral vancomycin (500 mg 4 times per day), although there are no data to demonstrate that this higher dose is more effective than the standard dose.[122,158,176] IV metronidazole should be given in addition to oral vancomycin. In the presence of ileus, vancomycin (500 mg every 6 hours) may be administered via NG tube, with intermittent clamping of the tube.[108] Vancomycin may also be administered by enema (500 mg in 100 mL of normal saline).[108]

Fidaxomicin has proven efficacy in treating CDI, but its role in the management of severe complicated disease has not yet been examined. In patients not responding to combined treatment with vancomycin and metronidazole, salvage therapy with IV tigecycline (loading dose of 100 mg IV followed by 50 mg 2 times per day) or with pooled human immunoglobulin (400 mg/kg body weight) has been reported; the efficacy of these agents has not been evaluated in controlled clinical trials.[86,177-181] Failure of response to metronidazole and vancomycin are not related to acquisition of antibiotic resistance, which has not been documented in clinical isolates of *C. difficile*, but rather to host factors such as age, immune deficiency, comorbidity, or lack of compliance.

Surgery

Surgery sometimes is required in patients with severe colitis not responding to medical therapy, and a surgical consultation should be sought early in patients with severe disease.[174,175,179,182,183] Mortality in severe CDI usually is a result of a marked systemic inflammatory response leading to organ failure. Hence, colon perforation or toxic megacolon are not the sole indicators of a need for surgical intervention. In 1 study, colectomy appeared to be more beneficial in patients who were not immunosuppressed, were aged 65 years or older, had a leukocytosis of 20,000 or more cells/mm^3, or a lactate between 2.2 and 4.9 mmol/L.[184]

The standard operation has been a subtotal colectomy with temporary ileostomy, and surgical intervention in this setting is associated with a high perioperative mortality rate. Grundfest-Bronitowski and associates[183] reported an overall mortality rate of 42% in a series of patients who underwent surgery for fulminant, severe CDI. A recent study reported on a different surgical approach whereby a loop ileostomy was fashioned at laparoscopy, and intraoperative colonic lavage was then performed with 8 L of warmed polyethylene glycol colon preparation solution. Postoperatively, vancomycin solution (500 mg in 500 mL of lactated Ringers) was administered through the ileostomy into the colon every 8 hours for 10 days.[185] Of 42 patients with severe complicated CDI treated with this approach, only 7% required colectomy, and the mortality rate was 19% (compared with 50% in historic controls who underwent colectomy; odds ratio, 0.24; P = 0.006). This novel approach may carry several substantial advantages and clearly warrants further study.

Recurrent Clostridium difficile Infection

One of the most difficult clinical problems in treating patients with CDI is the high incidence of recurrences.[25,26,165] Approximately 25% of patients successfully treated with vancomycin or metronidazole suffer a recurrence after completing their initial antibiotic therapy.[26,134,145,186,187] Subsequent recurrence rates are higher (≈40%) in those treated for a first recurrence and exceed 50% in those treated for a second or subsequent recurrence.[87,164,188]

The clinical features of recurrence are similar to the initial attack, with watery diarrhea, cramping abdominal pain, or fever occurring 2 to 14 days after discontinuing therapy. Late recurrences are less common but can occur more than 2 months after stopping antibiotic treatment. The diagnosis of recurrent CDI is best confirmed by stool toxin assay whenever possible, or in rare instances by colonoscopy and biopsy. In patients with typical symptoms of recurrence, therapy can be reinstituted while awaiting stool assay results (see Box 112-2). Prompt therapy is especially important in patients whose initial attack of *C. difficile* diarrhea was severe, because they are more likely to suffer from severe recurrent disease, possibly because of their inadequate immune response to *C. difficile* toxins.[87,189]

Some patients with persistent symptoms after successful therapy of CDI develop diarrhea as a result of postinfection IBS.[190] Frequent watery diarrhea and cramping lower abdominal pain may be partially responsive to antibiotic therapy. Patients with post-*C. difficile* IBS have normal colonoscopy and biopsy, and their stools are usually negative on *C. difficile* testing. Other diarrheal conditions that require differentiation from recurrent CDI include IBD, microscopic colitis, celiac disease, and food (e.g., lactose) intolerance.

Bacteriologic typing studies demonstrate that symptomatic recurrence can result from relapse of infection with the same strain that caused the initial episode or a new infection with a different strain of C. difficile.[191,192] Resistance to metronidazole or to vancomycin is seldom if ever an important factor in recurrence. In some patients, C. difficile can be cultured from the stools during successful vancomycin therapy, and these patients may be more likely to relapse than those in whom eradication of the pathogen occurs during therapy[191]; however, C. difficile can also be cultured from the stools during and after successful antibiotic treatment in patients who do not relapse.[117]

Culture positivity during symptomatic improvement might reflect the persistence of antibiotic-resistant spores. In 1 study, 18 of 22 patients with recurrence were noted to have colonic diverticula, leading to the speculation that spores might survive in diverticula where they escape the normal cleansing action of diarrhea and might not be exposed to the high luminal concentration of antibiotics[193]; however, reinfection by bacterial spores through the usual fecal-oral route is a more likely mechanism of recurrence.[191,192] A recent study compared 128 patients with CDI who had diverticulosis to 137 patients with CDI who did not have diverticulosis and found no significant differences between the 2 groups in terms of risk for relapse or recurrence except perhaps for the small group of patients with diverticulosis of the ascending colon in whom the risk of relapse was increased.[194]

Conservative Therapy

In a report of 20 patients with clindamycin-associated pseudomembranous colitis, published before the discovery of vancomycin as effective therapy, all patients eventually recovered when clindamycin was stopped.[195] An important advantage to this form of management is that recurrence of diarrhea or colitis does not occur, probably because stopping all antimicrobial agents allows restoration of the colonic microbiota, which provides colonization resistance against C. difficile. Thus, some patients with mild symptoms of recurrence can be managed conservatively without specific antibiotic treatment, thereby avoiding subsequent recurrences. This approach may not be appropriate for older adults or infirm patients and is not advised for those with moderate or severe symptoms.

Standard Therapy with Vancomycin, Metronidazole or Fidaxomicin

Patients with recurrence typically are treated with a second 14-day course of the same antibiotic used to treat the initial attack; this has a success rate of about 40% after a first recurrence.[87,188] Fidaxomicin treatment of an initial episode of CDI is associated with fewer recurrences compared with vancomycin (15.4% vs. 25.3%; 39% reduction; P = 0.005).[145,156] The benefit of fidaxomicin over vancomycin in reducing subsequent recurrences is also evident in patients with recurrent CDI. In 1 study of patients treated for a first recurrence, fidaxomicin 200 mg twice daily for 10 days led to a recurrence rate of 19.7% compared with 35.5% for vancomycin 125 mg 4 times daily for 10 days (45% reduction; P = 0.045).[164]

Prolonged Tapering and Pulsed Vancomycin Therapy

Tedesco and colleagues[193] treated 22 patients who had multiple recurrences of C. difficile colitis with tapering doses of vancomycin for a 3-week period, followed by every-other-day therapy for 1 week and every-third-day therapy for an additional week. All patients responded symptomatically and remained well during a mean follow-up period of 6 months.

Although data from randomized, controlled trials are not available, 1 subsequent study that examined various physician-selected antibiotic regimens to treat recurrent CDI found that regimens incorporating prolonged or pulsed-dose oral vancomycin were the most effective.[196] Overall, 73 of 163 patients (45%) treated for recurrent CDI had a subsequent recurrence. Of all the regimens used, only those that incorporated prolonged-dose vancomycin (9 of 29 recurred [31%]; P = 0.01) or pulsed-dose vancomycin (1 of 7 recurred [14%]; P = 0.02) showed significantly lower recurrence rates. The mechanism whereby this treatment approach is effective is unknown and might simply reflect prolonged therapy.

Toxin production by C. difficile usually does not occur during the early exponential growth phase of the bacterium, but rather in the subsequent stationary phase.[197,198] Thus, after active C. difficile toxin-induced diarrhea and colitis have been controlled by treatment with vancomycin, a period of 24 to 72 hours is needed for the bacteria to reinitiate production and release of toxin. Thus, pulsed dosing might prevent toxin production and release, while also facilitating restoration of the normal colonic microbiota and hence C. difficile colonization resistance.

Binding Resins

Binding resins, which bind to toxins in the bowel lumen, have been proposed as a possible alternative to antimicrobial therapy. Clinical studies have been performed using colestipol, cholestyramine, and tolevamer. For colestipol, the symptomatic response in patients with acute C. difficile colitis was a disappointing 36%, compared with a placebo response rate of 22%.[147,154] Cholestyramine therapy yielded a somewhat better overall response rate of 68%,[147,154,199] but this still compares poorly with response rates of more than 90% with vancomycin or metronidazole. Therefore, binding resins are not used as primary therapy for C. difficile colitis but may be beneficial in treating recurrent CDI. Tedesco treated 11 patients who had relapsing C. difficile colitis with tapering doses of vancomycin plus colestipol 5 g every 12 hours.[200] Because anion-exchange resins bind vancomycin and other drugs, they must be taken at least 2 or 3 hours apart from the vancomycin, making such combination therapy cumbersome.

Tolevamer is a soluble anionic polymer specifically developed to bind C. difficile toxins. In a phase II human clinical trial, results with tolevamer were similar to those of vancomycin when used as primary treatment for mild or moderately severe infection.[201] In 2 larger phase III studies, however, response rates with tolevamer were substantially lower than with either vancomycin or metronidazole.[202] Interestingly, recurrence rates after successful tolevamer treatment were substantially lower than after antibiotic treatment with metronidazole or vancomycin, suggesting its potential use for primary or secondary disease prevention.[212] Tolevamer is not currently in any active trials and is not available for clinical use.

Probiotic Therapy

In contrast to treatment with antimicrobial agents that further delay recolonization by normal colonic bacteria, probiotic agents are an attractive addition to antibiotic therapy with metronidazole, vancomycin, or fidaxomycin for recurrent disease, because restoration of colonization resistance can lead to permanent eradication of C. difficile from the colon. In an open-label study, Lactobacillus strain GG was reported to be effective in preventing diarrhea in patients with recurrent C. difficile colitis.[203] Another placebo-controlled study of hospital patients receiving antibiotics used a probiotic drink mixture containing *Lactobacillus casei*, *Lactobacillus bulgaricus*, and *Streptococcus thermophilus* (DanActive) and found that simple AAD was reduced from 34% to 12% (placebo vs. active; P = 0.007), and CDI was reduced from 17% to 0% (placebo vs. active; P = 0.001).[204] Protection against AAD and against CDI also was reported with a probiotic mixture containing *Lactobacillus acidophilus* and *Lactobacillus casei*.[205] The reproducibility of these positive results using *Lactobacillus*-containing probiotic mixtures need to be confirmed in additional, multicenter controlled trials.

The yeast *S. boulardii* is used widely as a probiotic agent in continental Europe and is available in the United States without prescription.[10,206] In a double-blind controlled clinical trial, coadministration of oral capsules containing viable *S. boulardii* with antibiotics significantly reduced the incidence of AAD in hospitalized patients (from 22% on placebo to 9.5% in the *S. boulardii* group; P = 0.04).[10] In that study, however, few patients had *C. difficile*-associated diarrhea. A second randomized placebo-controlled trial examined the efficacy of *S. boulardii* in combination with either vancomycin or metronidazole in patients with *C. difficile* diarrhea.[188] Diarrhea recurrence rates were similar in subjects treated during their first episode of *C. difficile* diarrhea (19% in the *S. boulardii* group vs. 24% in the placebo group; P = 0.86). In contrast, patients with a history of recurrent *C. difficile* diarrhea who received *S. boulardii* had fewer recurrences than the placebo group (35% and 65%, respectively; P = 0.04). In a subsequent study, however, *S. boulardii* had no overall effect on recurrence rates (44% vs. 47% with placebo).[207] *S. boulardii* should not be administered to immunocompromised patients because of the risk of fungemia.

Another probiotic agent for CDI that is administered orally is a nontoxinogenic strain of *C. difficile*; this was reported to be effective in 2 patients with recurrent *C. difficile* diarrhea.[208] Clinical trials are under way using nontoxinogenic *C. difficile* to evaluate its safety and efficacy in preventing recurrence of CDI.[209]

Fecal Microbiota Transplantation

Fecal microbiota transplantation (FMT) was first described in the English language as an effective treatment for fulminant, antibiotic-associated, pseudomembranous colitis in 1958, 20 years before the etiologic role of toxinogenic CDI was identified.[210] This treatment is based on the recognition that alteration of the bacterial flora of the colon by antibiotics is the major predisposing cause of CDI, and that restoration of the normal microbiota can eliminate the pathogen. In recent years, FMT has been used mainly to prevent further episodes of CDI in patients in whom treatment for multiple recurrences has failed (see Chapter 130).[50] Typically, fresh feces are obtained from a screened donor, processed, and then administered via NG or nasoenteric tube, by enema, or during colonoscopy. The overall reported efficacy in uncontrolled studies is high: 81% for the gastric or small intestinal routes and 92% for the rectal or colonic routes.[211] In a recent randomized controlled trial, nasoduodenal infusion of donor feces was successful in preventing further episodes of recurrent CDI in 81% of patients compared with 31% who received vancomycin therapy (P < 0.001) and 23% who received vancomycin with bowel lavage (P < 0.001).[212] These results (81% efficacy) agree closely with the findings of a systematic review of uncontrolled case series in which gastric or small intestinal infusions were employed. Based on these data there is renewed interest in FMT for prevention and treatment of CDI. Steps are being taken to make this treatment approach more acceptable and more accessible to patients and their physicians through stool banking to provide already processed treatment units from prescreened donors and by the development of defined bacterial culture mixtures to replace human feces as the source material.[50,212-215]

Immunization against *Clostridium difficile* Toxins

As described earlier, there is considerable evidence that some persons have protective immunity against CDI and that protection is associated with higher antitoxin antibody concentrations in serum, intestinal secretions, or both.[36,80,82,85-87,189] Leung and coworkers reported on 6 children with multiple relapses of CDI who had low concentrations of serum IgG antibody to toxin A.[86] Five of these children were treated with IV normal immune globulin at a dose of 400 mg/kg, which contains high titers of IgG antitoxin A and antitoxin B. Symptoms resolved following treatment. Similar results have been reported by other investigators, but there are no reported controlled trials of normal immune globulin for treatment or prevention of CDI.[178,188] In a randomized controlled trial human antitoxin A and antitoxin B monoclonal antibodies were administered IV to patients receiving antibiotic therapy for acute CDI.[216] As expected, recurrent infection occurred in 25% of the placebo group following completion of anti-*C. difficile* antibiotic treatment. Conversely, only 7% of those who received the antitoxin antibodies suffered a recurrence (P < 0.001), clearly demonstrating the clinical potential for passive immunotherapy in CDI.

A *C. difficile* vaccine has been produced, which contains inactivated toxoid A and B. In early clinical trials, this vaccine was immunogenic,[217,218] and in a small case series, vaccination was associated with resolution of recurrent *C. difficile* diarrhea in 3 subjects.[219] Further studies are underway to determine whether passive or active immunization against *C. difficile* and its toxins can be effective in treating patients with refractory or recurrent disease. If effective, these therapeutic approaches also may be useful to prevent *C. difficile*-associated diarrhea in high-risk persons, such as older adults and infirm patients receiving antibiotic therapy in the hospital.

Overall Approach

The management of a first episode of recurrent *C. difficile*–associated diarrhea does not differ greatly from treatment of an initial episode (see Box 112-2).[26,122,144] Stool samples should be obtained to reconfirm infection with toxinogenic *C. difficile*. Patients with mild symptoms of recurrence may be managed conservatively without additional antibiotic treatment, just like patients with a primary episode. If symptoms persist or are severe, a standard course of metronidazole, vancomycin, or fidaxomicin should be administered. If a second recurrence occurs, other treatment approaches should be considered.

Fidaxomicin has the unique advantage of proven lower recurrence rates in randomized controlled trials both in primary therapy and in treatment of a first recurrence.[145,156,164] Tedesco and associates proposed a tapering and pulsed antibiotic regimen that is well tolerated and often successful.[193,195] Treatment with oral rifaximin 400 mg 3 times daily for 20 days after completion of a standard course of vancomycin or metronidazole may also be effective in reducing recurrence rates in patients with previous recurrences.[220,221] FMT has proven efficacy in patients with multiple previous recurrences of CDI and is quickly becoming a routine part of management.[5] A wide range of other approaches have been described, some of which are summarized in Box 112-2.

In some instances, multiple recurrences develop, and a variety of different regimens must be used before the organism is finally eradicated. In other cases, recurrences persist despite several different treatment approaches; in such cases, prolonged therapy with oral vancomycin (125 mg once or twice daily) is a pragmatic and effective means to prevent further recurrences. This approach is indicated in high-risk patients for whom other measures, including multiple antibiotic regimens, have failed and especially in those with severe underlying disease, a high likelihood of needing additional courses of antibiotic treatment, and where life expectancy is short.

KEY REFERENCES

Full references for this chapter can be found on www.expertconsult.com.

15. Cremonini F, Di Caro S, Nista EC, et al. Meta-analysis: The effect of probiotic administration on antibiotic-associated diarrhoea. Aliment Pharmacol Ther 2002; 16:1461-7.

21. Bartlett JG, Chang TW, Gurwith M, et al. Antibiotic-associated pseudomembranous colitis due to toxin-producing clostridia. N Engl J Med 1978; 298:531-4.

22. Larson HE, Price AB, Honour P, Boriello SP. *Clostridium difficile* and the aetiology of pseudomembranous colitis. Lancet 1978; 1:1063-6.

23. Crobach MJ, Dekkers OM, Wilcox MH, Kuijper EJ. European Society of Clinical Microbiology and Infectious Diseases (ESCMID): Data review and recommendations for diagnosing *Clostridium difficile* infection (CDI). Clin Microbiol Infect 2009; 15:1053-66.

25. Kelly CP, Lamont JT. *Clostridium difficile*—More difficult than ever. N Engl J Med 2008; 359:1932-40.

26. Cohen SH, Gerding DN, Johnson S, et al. Clinical practice guidelines for *Clostridium difficile* infection in adults: 2010 update by the Society for Healthcare Epidemiology of America (SHEA) and the Infectious Diseases Society of America (IDSA). Infect Control Hosp Epidemiol 2010; 31:431-55.

30. Loo VG, Poirier L, Miller MA, et al. A predominantly clonal multi-institutional outbreak of *Clostridium difficile*–associated diarrhea with high morbidity and mortality. N Engl J Med 2005; 353:2442-9.

31. McDonald LC, Kilgore GE, Thompson A, et al. An epidemic, toxin gene-variant strain of *Clostridium difficile*. N Engl J Med 2005; 353:2433-41.

36. Kyne L, Warny M, Qamar A, Kelly CP. Asymptomatic carriage of *Clostridium difficile* and serum levels of IgG antibody against toxin A. N Engl J Med 2000; 342:390-7.

102. Mylonaki M, Langmead L, Pantes A, et al. Enteric infection in relapse of inflammatory bowel disease: Importance of microbiological examination of stool. Eur J Gastroenterol Hepatol 2004; 16:775-8.

122. Surawicz CM, Brandt LJ, Binion DG, et al. Guidelines for diagnosis, treatment, and prevention of *Clostridium difficile* infections. Am J Gastroenterol 2013; 108:478-98.

124. O'Horo JC, Jones A, Sternke M, et al. Molecular techniques for diagnosis of *Clostridium difficile* infection: Systematic review and meta-analysis. Mayo Clin Proc 2012; 87:643-51.

145. Louie TJ, Miller MA, Mullane KM, et al. Fidaxomicin versus vancomycin for *Clostridium difficile* infection. N Engl J Med 2011; 364:422-31.

149. Zar FA, Bakkanagari SR, Moorthi KM, Davis MB. A comparison of vancomycin and metronidazole for the treatment of *Clostridium difficile*–associated diarrhea, stratified by disease severity. Clin Infect Dis 2007; 45:302-7.

212. van Nood E, Vrieze A, Nieuwdorp M, et al. Duodenal infusion of donor feces for recurrent *Clostridium difficile*. N Engl J Med 2013; 368:407-15.

CHAPTER 113

Intestinal Protozoa

CHRISTOPHER D. HUSTON

CHAPTER OUTLINE

Intestinal protozoa traditionally have been considered important pathogens in the developing world, where food and water hygiene are poor. A basic knowledge of the intestinal protozoa that cause human disease is of growing importance to physicians practicing medicine in the United States, Canada, and Europe, as a result of increasing world travel, globalization of the world's economy, and the growing number of chronically immunosuppressed people. For example, in patients throughout the world with AIDS and in organ transplant recipients, microsporidia, *Cryptosporidium* species, *Isospora belli*, and *Cyclospora cayetenensis* are the leading causes of chronic diarrhea. *Cryptosporidium* species, *I. belli*, and *C. cayetenensis* have been recognized as common pathogens in immunocompetent persons as well, and food- and water-borne outbreaks in the United States and Canada raise questions about the safety of our increasingly complex food and water supplies. Our understanding of the biology of these organisms often is still rudimentary, but is rapidly changing.

Examples include recent recognition that *Entamoeba histolytica*, the cause of amebic dysentery, and the nonpathogenic intestinal ameba *Entamoeba dispar* are distinct species; identification in 2012 of additional *Entamoeba* species of unclear pathologic potential that infect humans; reclassification in 2002 of the *Cryptosporidium* species of medical importance; and clarification of the population structure of *Giardia intestinalis* through genomic sequencing, which may shed light on the basis of variable clinical outcomes following human infection.

The emergence of these pathogens as major causes of disease in the developed world has stimulated a growing number of basic science studies of parasite biology and rapid development of new diagnostic tests, treatments, and attempts at vaccination. This chapter summarizes major recent advances in our understanding of the intestinal protozoa, with an emphasis on clinical epidemiology, disease characteristics, and optimal approaches to accurate diagnosis and treatment.

ENTAMOEBA HISTOLYTICA

Epidemiology

E. histolytica was first linked causally to amebic colitis and liver abscess by Lösch in 1875, and it was named by Schaudinn in 1903 for its ability to destroy host tissues. In 1925, Emil Brumpt proposed the existence of a second, morphologically identical but nonpathogenic *Entamoeba* species, E. dispar, to explain why only a minority of people infected with what was then termed E. histolytica developed invasive disease. Although Brumpt's hypothesis was not accepted during his lifetime, it is now clear that he was correct, and E. histolytica (Schaudinn, 1903) has been formally reclassified as 2 morphologically indistinguishable species: E. histolytica, the cause of invasive amebiasis, and E. dispar, a nonpathogenic intestinal commensal parasite (see later section).[1]

Entamoeba histolytica is a parasite of global distribution, but most of the morbidity and mortality from amebiasis occurs in Central and South America, Africa, and the Indian subcontinent.[2] Fortunately, most of the 500 million persons worldwide previously believed to be asymptomatic E. histolytica cyst passers are actually infected with E. dispar. The total burden of disease caused by E. histolytica is unknown, however, a recently reported multisite molecular epidemiologic study conducted in Africa and Asia indicates that it accounts for roughly 2% of life-threatening diarrhea in children ages 12 to 23 months of age.[3] In Dhaka, Bangladesh, where diarrheal diseases are the leading cause of childhood death, 80% of children studied prospectively were infected with E. histolytica at least once during 4 years of follow-up.[4] Furthermore, E. histolytica–associated diarrhea in these children was associated with significantly low weight and height for age.[5]

E. histolytica has a simple, 2-stage life cycle that consists of an infectious cyst and a motile trophozoite. The cyst form measures 5 to 20 μm in diameter and contains 4 or fewer nuclei. The ameboid trophozoite, which is responsible for tissue invasion, measures 10 to 60 μm and contains a single nucleus with a central karyosome (Fig. 113-1). The cysts are relatively resistant to chlorination and desiccation, and they can survive in a moist environment for several weeks.

Infection occurs following ingestion of cysts in fecally contaminated food or water. Within the lumen of the small intestine, the quadrinucleate cyst undergoes nuclear and then

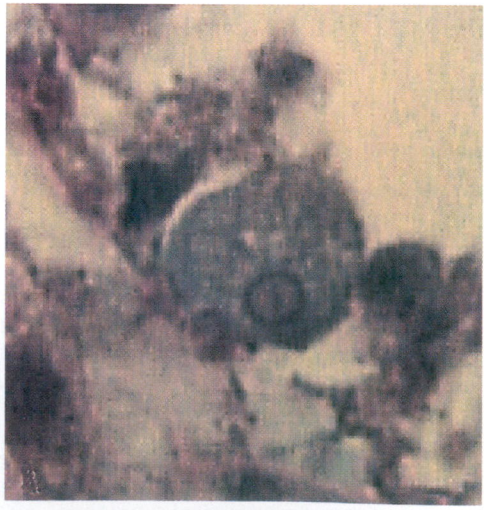

FIGURE 113-1. An *Entamoeba histolytica* trophozoite in a stool specimen. Note the nucleus with a prominent central karyosome. (H&E stain)

cytoplasmic division, giving rise to 8 trophozoites. Only about 10% to 20% of infected persons develop invasive disease, characterized by invasion of the colonic epithelium by trophozoites.[6] Trophozoites that gain access to the bloodstream can spread hematogenously to establish infection at distant sites (most commonly liver abscess, as discussed in Chapter 84). Why some persons develop invasive disease and others remain asymptomatic remains a mystery, but environmental, host, and parasite differences are all likely to be important.

A molecular epidemiologic study that used PCR to amplify a polymorphic region of the E. histolytica genome and assign a genotype to different clinical isolates has demonstrated a correlation between different E. histolytica strains and the outcome of infection.[7] The specific underlying genetic differences among strains that are responsible for altered virulence, however, remain unknown. On the host side, susceptibility to both intestinal and hepatic amebiasis is linked to HLA class II alleles, and a mutation in the leptin receptor that alters epithelial cell signaling is associated with E. histolytica infection in children and in a mouse model of colitis.[8-10]

Pathogenesis, Pathology, and Immunology

Both amebic factors and the host's inflammatory response contribute to tissue destruction during invasive amebiasis. Microscopy studies have defined a stepwise progression of disease (Fig. 113-2).[11] After excystation within the lumen of the small intestine, trophozoites adhere to colonic mucins and epithelial cells, largely via an amebic galactose/N-acetyl-D-galactosamine inhibitable surface lectin.[12-14] Secreted cysteine proteinases then facilitate tissue invasion by degrading human colonic mucus and extracellular matrix proteins.[15,16] Further disruption of the colonic epithelium results directly from contact-dependent apoptotic and necrotic cell killing of epithelial and immune cells, and from an acute epithelial cell inflammatory response with recruitment of neutrophils and immune-mediated tissue damage.[12,17-21] Cleavage and activation of pre–interleukin (IL)-1β by amebic cysteine proteinases cause additional inflammation and tissue damage.[19-21]

The cecum and ascending colon are affected most commonly, although in severe disease the entire colon may be involved. On gross examination, pathology can range from only mucosal thickening to multiple punctate ulcers with normal intervening tissue (Fig. 113-3) to frank necrosis. For unknown reasons, the downward invasion of amebic trophozoites often is halted at the level of the muscularis mucosa. Subsequent lateral spread of amebae undermines the overlying epithelium, resulting in the clean-based, flask-shaped ulcers so characteristic of classic amebic colitis.[22] Early in infection, an influx of neutrophils is typical, but in well-established ulcers, few inflammatory cells are seen.[22] Organisms may be seen ingesting red blood cells (erythrophagocytosis) (Fig. 113-4). At distant sites of infection (e.g., liver abscess), similar pathologic characteristics also include central liquefaction of tissue surrounded by a minimal mononuclear cell infiltrate.[22]

Because more than 90% of persons colonized with E. histolytica spontaneously clear the infection within a year, an effective immune response to amebiasis seems to develop.[23] Children with fecal anti-amebic lectin immunoglobulin (Ig)A have short-lived protection from subsequent intestinal infection.[4,24,25] The protective role of secretory IgA is not certain, however, and the contributions of humoral and cellular immunity to protection from amebiasis remain unknown. Nearly everyone with invasive amebiasis develops a systemic and a mucosal humoral immune response.[26-29] Antibodies alone are unable to clear established infection, however, because asymptomatic cyst passers remain infected for months

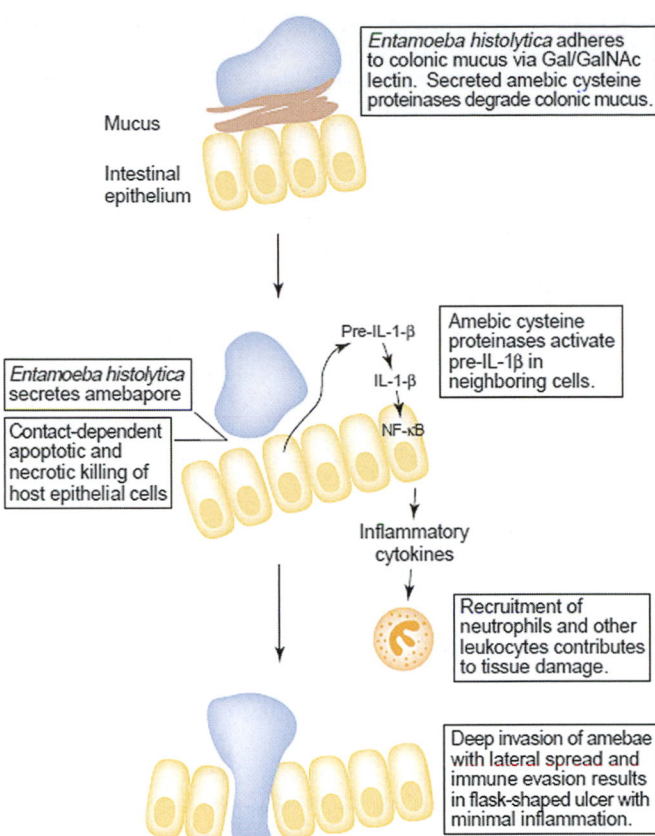

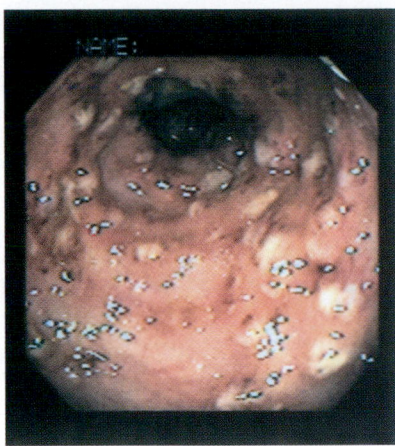

FIGURE 113-3. Colonoscopic findings in a patient with amebic colitis. Multiple punctate ulcers are visible.

FIGURE 113-2. Model for stepwise invasion of the colonic mucosa by *Entamoeba histolytica*. Following excystation, trophozoites (blue) adhere to colonic mucins, and degradation of mucus by amebic proteinases enables contact with the epithelium. Contact-dependent killing of epithelial cells and activation of an epithelial cell response marked by proinflammatory cytokine release follow. Amebapore is a protein that forms ion channels or pores in lipid membranes and depolarizes target cells thus contributing to the virulence of the trophozoite. Activation of pro–interleukin (IL)-1β by amebic cysteine proteinases, with resulting recruitment of neutrophils, further contributes to tissue damage. NFκβ, nuclear factor kappa beta *(From Huston CD. Parasite and host contributions to the pathogenesis of amebic colitis. Trends Parasitol 2004; 20:23-6.)*

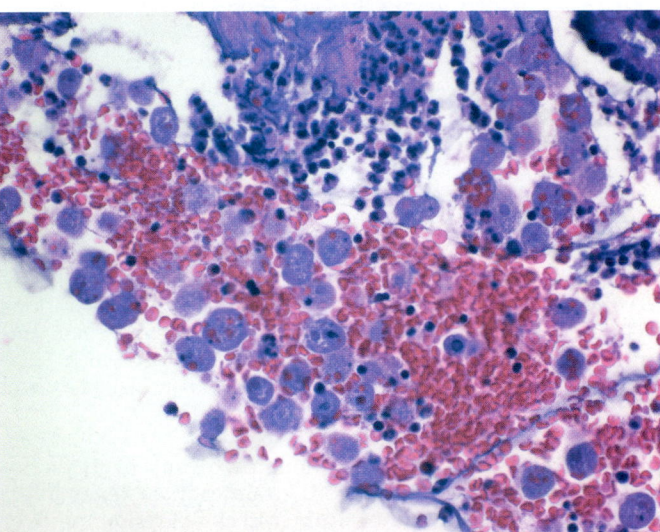

FIGURE 113-4. Amebic colitis. This high-power view of a colonic biopsy specimen shows acute inflammation, hemorrhage, and multiple amebic trophozoites, many of which have ingested red blood cells (erythrophagocytosis) (H&E stain). Nonpathogenic amebae do not exhibit erythrophagocytosis.

after anti-amebic antibodies develop.[23] Passive immunization experiments in a severe combined immunodeficient (SCID) mouse model of liver abscess do suggest an important role for pre-existing humoral immunity in protection from infection.[30] Reports that patients who are receiving glucocorticoids may be at increased risk for severe amebic colitis suggest that cellular immunity also plays an important role in control of *E. histolytica* infection.[31] Despite this concern, no increase in disease severity has been observed in patients with AIDS. In fact, in a mouse model of amebic colitis, disease was exacerbated by CD4+ T cells.[32]

Clinical Features

Infection with *E. histolytica* results in 1 of 3 outcomes. Approximately 80% to 90% of infected persons remain asymptomatic. The other 10% to 20% of infections result in invasive amebiasis characterized by dysentery (amebic colitis) or, in a minority of cases, extraintestinal disease (most commonly amebic liver abscess [see Chapter 84]).[1,23]

In the United States, immigrants from or travelers to endemic regions, male homosexuals, and institutionalized persons are at greatest risk for amebiasis. In addition, malnourished patients, infants, older adults, pregnant women, and patients receiving glucocorticoids may be at increased risk for fulminant disease.[2,31] When 1 or more of these epidemiologic risk factors are present, amebic dysentery should be considered in the differential diagnosis of occult or grossly bloody diarrhea.

The major diagnostic challenge for the clinician seeing a patient with amebic colitis is to distinguish the illness from other causes of bloody diarrhea. The differential diagnosis includes causes of bacterial dysentery, such as *Shigella*, *Salmonella*, *Campylobacter* species, and enteroinvasive or enterohemorrhagic *Escherichia coli*, and non-infectious diseases, including IBD and ischemic colitis.[2,33] In contrast to bacterial dysentery, which typically begins abruptly, amebic colitis begins gradually over 1 to several weeks (Table 113-1). Although more than 90% of patients with amebic colitis present with diarrhea, abdominal pain can occur without diarrhea; abdominal pain,

TABLE 113-1 Comparison of Amebic Colitis and Invasive Bacterial Dysentery

Feature	Amebic Colitis	Bacterial Dysentery*
Travel to or from an endemic area	Yes	Sometimes
Usual duration of symptoms (days)	>7	2-7
Diarrhea (%)	94-100	100
Fecal occult blood (%)	100	40
Abdominal pain (%)	12-80	≈50
Weight loss	Common	Unusual
Fever > 38°C	Minority	Majority

*See Chapters 107 and 110.
Adapted from Huston CD, Petri WA. Amebiasis. In: Rakel RE, Bope ET, editors. Conn's current therapy, 2001. Philadelphia: WB Saunders; 2001. pp 50-4.

tenesmus, and fever are highly variable. Weight loss is common because of the chronicity of the illness. Microscopic blood is present in the stool of most patients with amebic dysentery.[2,33,34]

The most feared complication of amebic dysentery, acute necrotizing colitis with toxic megacolon, occurs in 0.5% of cases. This complication manifests as an acute dilatation of the colon, and 40% of patients die from sepsis unless it is promptly recognized and treated surgically.[35] Unusual complications include the formation of enterocutaneous, rectovaginal, and enterovesicular fistulas and ameboma (a tumorous mass) due to intraluminal granulation tissue that can cause bowel obstruction and mimic carcinoma of the colon.[2,33]

Dysentery resolves prior to presentation in most patients with amebic liver abscesses, although a history of dysentery is common in these patients.[36-38] Extraintestinal sites of infection typically result either from direct extension of liver abscesses (e.g., amebic pericarditis or lung abscess) or from hematogenous spread of disease (e.g., brain abscess).[2]

Diagnosis

Because amebiasis patients erroneously treated for IBD with glucocorticoids can develop fulminant colitis, accurate initial diagnosis is critical.[31] The gold standard for diagnosis of amebic colitis remains colonoscopy with biopsy, and colonoscopy should be performed whenever infectious causes of bloody diarrhea are strong considerations in the differential diagnosis of UC. Because the cecum and ascending colon are affected most often, colonoscopy is preferred to sigmoidoscopy. Classically, multiple punctate ulcers measuring 2 to 10 mm are seen with essentially normal intervening tissue (see Fig. 113-3); however, the colonic epithelium might simply appear indurated with no visible ulcerations; appear like UC with a myriad of ulcerations and granular, friable mucosa; or, in severe cases where the ulcers have coalesced, the epithelium may appear necrotic. Histologic examination of a biopsy specimen taken from the edge of an ulcer reveals amebic trophozoites and a variable inflammatory infiltrate (see Fig. 113-4). Identification of amebae can be aided by periodic acid–Schiff staining of biopsy tissue, which stains trophozoites magenta.

Stool examination for ova and parasites, the traditional method for diagnosing amebiasis, should not be relied upon.

Although the presence of amebic trophozoites with ingested erythrocytes strongly correlates with E. histolytica infection, these rarely are present,[39] and in the absence of hematophagous trophozoites, microscopy cannot distinguish E. histolytica from E. dispar. Difficulty in distinguishing E. histolytica from nonpathogenic amebae (see later) and WBCs also limits the specificity of stool microscopy.[40] The sensitivity of microscopy for identification of amebae is at best 60%, and it may be reduced by delays in the processing of stool samples.[40,41] The primary utility of stool microscopy for ova and parasites in a patient with diarrhea, therefore, is to evaluate the stool for other parasitic causes of diarrhea.

Non-invasive methods to accurately differentiate E. histolytica from E. dispar include stool culture with isoenzyme analysis, serum amebic-antibody titers, PCR, and an enzyme-linked immunosorbent assay (ELISA) that detects the amebic lectin antigen in stool samples.[42-49] A multiplexed PCR kit that simultaneously detects 11 GI pathogens, including the parasites Giardia intestinalis and Cryptosporidium species, was recently approved for use in the United States and is likely to become widely available in the near future.[50] It is highly sensitive and specific for E. histolytica[50]; however, at present, the most specific clinically available test for diagnosis of amebiasis is a stool ELISA to detect the E. histolytica adherence lectin. Only 1 of the many ELISA tests developed thus far (the E. histolytica II test, TechLab, Blacksburg, Va.) accurately distinguishes E. histolytica from E. dispar.[41,47] This test's specificity, when compared with the gold standard of stool culture followed by isoenzyme analysis, was greater than 90%, and it was greater than 85% sensitive to diagnose intestinal amebiasis when fresh fecal samples were analyzed without delay.[47] In other studies, the sensitivity of this method has been less impressive, emphasizing the need for rapid processing of stool samples.[51,52] It also may be possible to use this antigen detection test to diagnose amebic liver abscess, because before treatment is initiated, amebic lectin antigen can be detected in the serum of greater than 90% of patients who have amebic liver abscess.[53]

Because serum antiamebic antibodies do not develop in patients infected with E. dispar, serologic tests for amebiasis accurately distinguish E. histolytica and E. dispar infection. From 75% to 85% of patients with acute amebic colitis have detectable anti-amebic antibodies on presentation, and convalescent titers develop in more than 90% of patients.[26,27,54] For amebic liver abscess, 70% to 80% of patients have detectable antibody titers on presentation, and convalescent titers develop in more than 90% of patients. Because antiamebic antibodies can persist for years, however, a positive result must be interpreted with caution.[26] For persons with known epidemiologic risks (e.g., emigration from or prior travel to an endemic region), a positive result might simply represent infection in the distant past. In the setting of recent travel to an endemic region and a positive antibody titer, diagnosis is confirmed by an appropriate symptomatic response to antiamebic treatment.

Treatment

Drugs for treatment of amebiasis are categorized as luminal or tissue amebicides on the basis of the location of their antiamebic activity (Table 113-2).

The luminal amebicides include iodoquinol, diloxanide furoate, and paromomycin.[55,56] Of these, paromomycin, a nonabsorbable aminoglycoside, is preferred because of its safety, short duration of required treatment, and superior efficacy. Its major side effect is diarrhea. Approximately 85% of asymptomatic patients are cured with 1 course of paromomycin, and, because it is nonabsorbable and has moderate

TABLE 113-2 Amebicidal Agents Currently Available in the USA

Amebicidal Agent	Advantages	Disadvantages
For Luminal Amebiasis		
Paromomycin	7-day treatment course; may be useful during pregnancy	Frequent GI side effects; rare ototoxicity and nephrotoxicity
Iodoquinol	Inexpensive and effective	20-day treatment course; contains iodine; rare optic neuritis and atrophy with prolonged use
Diloxanide furoate		Available in the USA only from the CDC; frequent GI side effects; rare diplopia
For Invasive Intestinal Disease Only		
Tetracyclines, erythromycin		Not effective for liver abscess; frequent GI side effects; tetracyclines should not be administered to children or pregnant women
For Both Invasive Intestinal and Extraintestinal Amebiasis		
Metronidazole	Drug of choice for amebic colitis and liver abscess	Anorexia, nausea, vomiting, and metallic taste in nearly one third of patients; disulfiram-like reaction with alcohol; rare seizures
Tinidazole	Alternative to metronidazole; once-daily dosing	Side effects are similar to those with metronidazole
Nitazoxanide	Useful alternative if the patient is intolerant of metronidazole or tinidazole	Limited clinical data for amebiasis; rare and reversible conjunctival icterus
For Extraintestinal Amebiasis Only		
Chloroquine	Useful only for amebic liver abscess	Occasional headache, pruritus, nausea, alopecia, and myalgias; rare heart block and irreversible retinal injury

CDC, Centers for Disease Control and Prevention.
Adapted from Huston CD, Petri WA. Amebiasis. In: Rakel RE, Bope ET, editors. Conn's current therapy, 2001. Philadelphia: WB Saunders; 2001. pp 50-4.

activity against trophozoites that have invaded the colonic mucosa, it might also be useful for single-drug treatment of mild invasive disease during pregnancy.[57,58]

The tissue amebicides include metronidazole, tinidazole, nitazoxanide, erythromycin, and chloroquine.[56,59] Of these, metronidazole and tinidazole are the drugs of choice, with cure rates greater than 90%.[60] Nitazoxanide, a new antiparasitic agent, appears to be efficacious, with similar cure rates in several randomized placebo-controlled trials.[59,61-63] Erythromycin has no activity against amebic liver disease, and chloroquine has no activity against intestinal disease.[64]

Because approximately 10% of asymptomatic cyst passers develop invasive amebiasis, E. histolytica carriers should be treated.[1,65] For non-invasive disease, treatment with a luminal agent alone is adequate (e.g., paromomycin 25 to 35 mg/kg/day in 3 divided doses for 7 days).[56] Patients with amebic colitis should first be treated with an oral nitroimidazole (either metronidazole [500-750 mg 3 times daily for 10 days] or tinidazole [2 g once daily for 3 to 5 days]) to eliminate invasive trophozoites. Metronidazole and tinidazole are believed to be less effective against organisms in the colonic lumen, and subsequent treatment with a luminal agent such as paromomycin is recommended to prevent recurrent disease.[56,60] It is also for this reason that the familiar tissue amebicides (e.g., metronidazole) are not recommended as first-line agents for treatment of asymptomatic infection. At the recommended doses of metronidazole and tinidazole, GI side effects including nausea and vomiting develop in approximately 30% of patients.[60] Because of severe GI side effects, simultaneous treatment with a nitroimidazole and a luminal agent generally is not recommended.

Most patients with colitis respond promptly with resolution of diarrhea in 2 to 5 days.[2]

Despite conflicting reports on the safety of the nitroimidazoles for the developing fetus during pregnancy, women with severe disease during pregnancy should probably be treated without delay. As discussed in Chapter 84, metronidazole (750 mg 3 times a day for 10 days) followed by a luminal agent is also the treatment of choice for amebic liver abscess.[56,64]

Control and Prevention

Prevention and control of E. histolytica infection depends on interruption of fecal-oral transmission. Water can be made safe for drinking and food preparation by boiling it for 1 minute, by halogenation (with chlorine or iodine), or by filtration.[66] In the United States and Europe, modern water treatment facilities effectively remove E. histolytica. The importance of safe drinking water is highlighted by an outbreak of amebiasis in Tblisi, Republic of Georgia, where there was a waterborne epidemic due to decay of the water treatment facilities following the demise of the Soviet Union.[67] In the vast majority of the developing world, however, no modern water treatment facilities exist, and none are likely to be constructed in the foreseeable future. Naturally acquired immunity to intestinal amebiasis provides short-lived protection against reinfection, giving hope that a vaccine may be feasible.[4,24,25] Because humans and some higher nonhuman primates are the only known hosts for E. histolytica, a vaccine that successfully prevents colonization might enable eradication of the disease.[68]

OTHER AMEBAE THAT INFECT THE HUMAN INTESTINE

Nine other ameba species commonly infect the human GI tract. These include *E. dispar*, *Entamoeba moshkovskii*, *Entamoeba bangladeshi*, *Entamoeba coli*, *Entamoeba hartmanni*, *Entamoeba gingivalis*, *Entamoeba polecki*, *Endolimax nana*, and *Iodamoeba butschlii*. *Dientamoeba fragilis* (discussed in the following section), previously thought to be an ameba, is more closely related to the flagellated protozoan *Trichomonas vaginalis* than to the true amebae.[66] With the exception of *E. gingivalis*, which has no known cyst stage, all of these true amebae have simple 2-stage life cycles, consisting of an infectious cyst form and a motile trophozoite form.[66] All but *E. dispar*, *E. moshkovskii*, and *E. bangladeshi* can be differentiated from *E. histolytica* using light microscopy based on characteristic features of the cyst and trophozoite forms. *E. dispar* must be differentiated from *E. histolytica* based on biochemical, antigenic, or genetic differences.[1]

E. dispar is a nonpathogenic protozoan parasite that is morphologically indistinguishable from *Entamoeba histolytica* by light microscopy.[1] An estimated 450 million people worldwide are infected with *E. dispar*, and infection with *E. dispar* is approximately 10 times more prevalent than *E. histolytica* infection.[1,65,69] Although *E. dispar* has been demonstrated to cause mucosal ulcerations in animal models, it has not been demonstrated to cause human disease and does not require treatment.[1] *Entamoeba moshkovskii*, which is primarily thought to be a free-living ameba, also has cysts and trophozoites indistinguishable from *E. dispar* and *E. histolytica* except that trophozoites of *E. histolytica* might show erythrophagocytosis. A high prevalence of human *E. moshkovskii* infection has been demonstrated in some studies, and, although its causation of human disease is still controversial, infection by *E. moshkovskii* is associated with diarrhea in infants.[70-73] *E. bangladeshi* is a recently described species that is also morphologically identical to *E. histolytica*. Based on its small rRNA gene sequence, *E. bangladeshi* is more closely related to *E. dispar* and *E. histolytica* than *E. moshkovskii*. Its pathogenic potential remains unknown.[74] There are currently no clinically available tests to identify *E. moshkovskii* and *E. bangladeshi*.

Besides *E. dispar*, *Entamoeba coli* is the intestinal commensal most commonly mistaken for *E. histolytica*. *Entamoeba coli* trophozoites contain a single nucleus with a prominent karyosome that usually is eccentric in location, distinguishing them from *E. histolytica* and *E. dispar* trophozoites, which have a centrally located karyosome. In addition, the cyst form of *Entamoeba coli* typically contains 5 to 8 nuclei. *Entamoeba coli* is nonpathogenic and requires no specific treatment; however, it is a valuable marker of fecal-oral exposure, and it can be found concurrently with *E. histolytica* in 10% to 30% of patients in endemic regions.[66]

E. hartmanni was classified as "small race" *E. histolytica* for many years. The trophozoites resemble those of *E. histolytica* except for their small size (<10 μm).[66] *Entamoeba hartmanni* now is recognized as a nonpathogen that does not require treatment.

E. gingivalis is the only ameba found in the oral cavity, where it lives in the anaerobic environment of the gingival crease. The trophozoite is identical in size to that of *E. histolytica* and contains a single nucleus with a prominent central karyosome. No cyst form of *E. gingivalis* has been identified, and oral-oral contact is believed to be its mode of transmission.[66,75] *E. gingivalis* is associated with poor dental hygiene and periodontal disease, but no causal relationship to periodontitis has been proved.[75] The increased frequency of colonization in this setting might simply reflect a hospitable host environment. *E. gingivalis* often is associated with periodontal disease in AIDS patients, however, and treatment with metronidazole has been reported to be effective.[76]

E. polecki, characterized by a uninucleated cyst, is primarily a parasite of pigs and monkeys that sometimes infects humans. It has been suggested that several distinct uninucleated cyst-producing *Entamoeba* species can infect humans, and it has been proposed that these organisms collectively be termed "*E. polecki*-like."[77] Infection with *E. polecki* is rare except in Papua New Guinea, where as many as 30% of children were found to be colonized in 1 study.[78] At present, specific treatment of *E. polecki*-like infections is not routinely recommended, but persons with heavy burdens of this parasite can develop nonspecific GI symptoms and might benefit from treatment. Good clinical responses to metronidazole and diloxanide furoate have been reported.[79]

Endolimax nana is a nonpathogenic intestinal ameba that often infects humans.[66] The distribution of *E. nana* is worldwide, but it is most common in the tropics, where 5% to 33% of persons are infected.[80,81] Infection requires no specific treatment, but it serves as a useful marker for fecal-oral exposure. *E. nana* trophozoites can be distinguished from *E. histolytica* by their vesiculate nucleus, large irregular karyosome, and relatively small size (8 to 12 μm).[66]

Iodamoeba butschlii is a nonpathogenic intestinal ameba passed by the fecal-oral route. Trophozoites of *I. butschlii* contain a single nucleus with a large karyosome (which is distinct from the punctate karyosome of *E. histolytica*); its cysts contain a single nucleus, and a large, eccentric glycogen mass that stains with iodine (hence the name *Iodamoeba*). *I. butschlii* infection requires no treatment.[66]

GIARDIA INTESTINALIS

Epidemiology

Giardia intestinalis (also called *G. lamblia* and *G. duodenalis*) is a ubiquitous flagellated intestinal protozoan. Van Leeuwenhoek accurately described its motile trophozoite form in his own stools in 1681, but it was not until 1915 that Stiles named the species.[66]

The life cycle of *Giardia* consists of an infectious cyst form and a motile trophozoite (Figure 113-5). The cyst is oval (8 to 12 μm long by 7 to 10 μm wide), contains 4 nuclei, and has a rigid outer wall that protects it from dehydration, extremes of temperature, and chlorination. *Giardia* cysts can survive in cold water for several weeks.[66,82] Ingestion of as few as 10 to 25 cysts can result in infection.[82] After ingestion, excystation occurs following exposure to stomach acid and intestinal proteases, each cyst giving rise to 2 trophozoites. Giardia trophozoites are pear-shaped (10 to 20 μm long by 7 to 10 μm wide), contain 2 nuclei, have 8 flagellae for locomotion, and replicate by binary fission. The trophozoites live in the duodenum, where they adhere to enterocytes. Eventually they encyst, following exposure to alkaline conditions or bile salts, and are excreted in the stool to complete their life cycle.[82]

G. intestinalis, which was defined originally as a species by morphology, is more accurately defined as a species complex with at least 7 major genotypes (assemblages A through G).[83] Of these, only assemblages A and B are known to infect humans. Both of these genotypes also commonly infect cats and dogs, highlighting the importance of these pets as reservoirs for human disease.[83] New data suggest that assemblage A isolates may be more virulent than assemblage B isolates.[84-86]

G. intestinalis is the most commonly identified intestinal parasite in the United States and was identified in 7.2% of stool samples examined by state health departments in

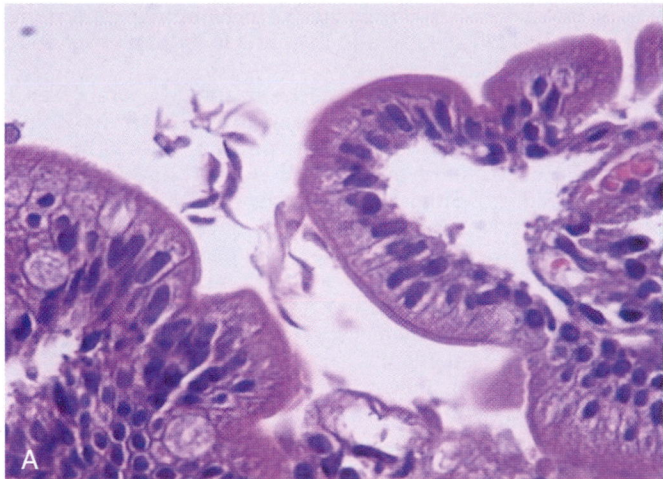

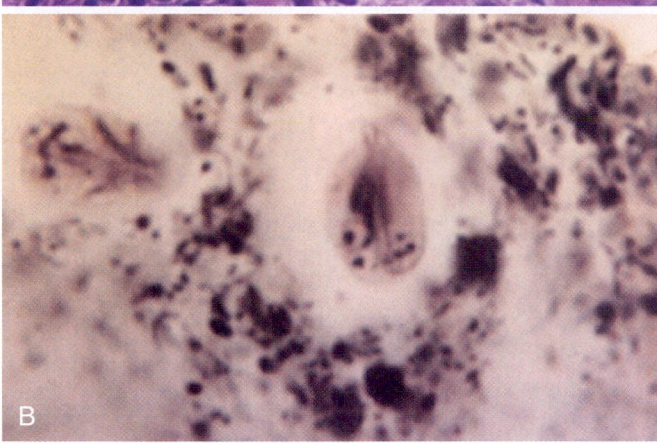

FIGURE 113-5. Giardiasis. A) High-power view of a duodenal biopsy specimen showing many trophozoites near the surface of the epithelium between villi. [Giemsa stain]; B) A *Giardia intestinalis* cyst in stool (original magnifcation 400×, Giemsa stain) *(Courtesy Carlo Denegri Foundation, Turin, Italy.)*

1987.[87] Giardiasis occurs in both endemic and epidemic forms via water-borne, food-borne, and person-to-person transmission.[88-94] Worldwide, *Giardia* infects infants more commonly than adults, and in highly endemic regions, essentially all children are infected by 2 to 3 years of age.[95,96] *Giardia* infection is associated with chronic diarrhea in children, but evidence that it causes acute diarrhea is controversial; some reports even suggest that it protects against acute diarrhea.[97-99] Nevertheless, even asymptomatic *Giardia* infection is associated with malnutrition and impaired growth.[95,100] In the United States, children in daycare and sexually active homosexual men have the greatest risk of infection.[87,101] During a year-long longitudinal study at a U.S. daycare center, *Giardia* cysts were identified at some time in the stool of more than 30% of children.[94] Additional risk factors for infection include drinking untreated surface water, a shallow well as a residential water source, swimming in any natural body of fresh water, and contact with a person who has giardiasis or contact with a child in daycare.[89]

Pathogenesis, Pathology, and Immunology

Giardia causes malabsorptive diarrhea by an unknown mechanism. Trophozoites adhere (perhaps by suction) to the epithelium of the upper small intestine using a disk structure located on their anterior ventral surface.[66,82] There is no evidence that trophozoites invade the mucosa,[102] but electron microscopy has shown they damage the mucosal brush border.[82,103] On biopsy, pathologic changes range from an entirely normal-appearing duodenal mucosa (except for adherent trophozoites), as was found in more than 96% of biopsy specimens in 1 large study, to severe villus atrophy with a mononuclear cell infiltrate that resembles celiac sprue.[102,104,105] The severity of diarrhea appears to correlate with the severity of the pathologic change.[82]

The host immune response plays a critical role in limiting the severity of giardiasis. When infected with *Giardia*, persons with common variable immunodeficiency develop severe, protracted diarrhea and malabsorption with sprue-like pathologic changes that resolve with treatment.[105] Both systemic and mucosal humoral immune responses can be measured consistently following *Giardia* infection. High titers of anti-*Giardia* IgM, IgG, and IgA can be detected in the serum, and anti-*Giardia* secretory IgA (sIgA) can be detected in the saliva and in breast milk of infected mothers.[106-108] Animal studies suggest that both early and late immune responses are important for control of *Giardia* infections. IL-6 is important in the early immune response to *Giardia* in mice, as are mast cells, which might function as IL-6 producers or via another mechanism.[109-111] In a B–cell-deficient transgenic mouse model, infection with *Giardia* does not resolve, confirming the importance of the humoral immune response for clearance of established infections.[112] In culture, *Giardia* trophozoites vary expression of a group of cysteine-rich surface proteins termed *variant surface proteins*, although their function has not yet been determined, and in experimental human infections, *G. intestinalis* isolates have been shown to undergo antigenic variation after approximately 2 weeks, roughly the time required to mount an initial antibody response.[113] Although the role of the variant surface proteins remains undetermined, antigenic variation might enable *Giardia* to evade the host immune response.[114]

The importance of a cellular immune response also is clear from animal studies. Athymic nude mice are unable to control *Giardia muris* infection, but reconstitution with immune spleen cells results in partial control. Upon immune reconstitution, however, severe inflammatory changes and villus atrophy develop in the intestine, suggesting that the immune response to infection also might contribute to pathologic findings.[115]

Clinical Features

The clinical manifestations of *Giardia* are highly variable, and range from asymptomatic infection to severe, chronic diarrhea with malabsorption. As noted earlier, *Giardia* infection in children is associated with chronic diarrhea, but epidemiologic evidence that it causes acute diarrhea in children in the developing world is limited.[97-99] In 1 large study of biopsy-proved giardiasis, only 32% of patients had diarrhea; most had nonspecific GI complaints.[102] Reported symptoms, in order of decreasing frequency, include diarrhea, fatigue, abdominal cramps, bloating, malodorous stool, flatulence, weight loss, fever, and vomiting (Table 113-3).[92,106] During a food-borne outbreak, the mean duration of diarrhea was 16 days, but symptoms resolved spontaneously in nearly half of infected patients after 7 to 8 days.[92] Many patients with clinically apparent giardiasis suffer from lactose intolerance, malabsorption, or both for months following cure of infection.[116]

As mentioned earlier, the severity of illness depends upon host and parasite factors. Different *Giardia* isolates have dramatically different abilities to cause disease during experimental human infections.[117] Furthermore, certain populations, including children younger than 2 years and patients with hypogammaglobulinemia, are more likely to develop serious

TABLE 113-3 Frequency of Symptoms in Patients with Giardiasis[92,102,106]

TABLE 113-3 Frequency of Symptoms in Patients with Giardiasis[92,102,106]

Symptom(s)	Frequency (%)
Diarrhea	32-100
Fatigue	22-97
Abdominal pain, cramps	75-83
Flatulence, bloating	58-79
Weight loss	60
Anorexia	45
Vomiting	17-26
Fever	12-21

disease.[95,105] Despite the importance of cellular immunity for controlling infection in animal models and the increased risk of *Giardia* infection among sexually active homosexual men, giardiasis is not more common, severe, or resistant to treatment in patients with AIDS,[118] except perhaps when AIDS is advanced.[119,120]

Diagnosis

Examination of concentrated, iodine-stained, wet stool preparations and modified-trichrome-stained permanent smears has been the conventional approach to identifying *Giardia* infections (see Fig. 113-5B). Because cysts and trophozoites are present only intermittently in the stool, however, the sensitivity of such testing is only about 50%, even with examination of multiple specimens.[104] With direct sampling of duodenal contents, such as duodenal aspiration or the string test, sensitivity can be improved to approximately 80%.[104] On small intestinal biopsy specimens, identification of trophozoites requires careful examination of multiple microscope fields to ensure accuracy (Fig. 113-5A).[102]

Numerous molecular tests based on ELISAs or direct immunofluorescent antibody (DFA) microscopy are now widely commercially available to diagnose giardiasis in stool samples.[121-123] These assay kits all work well and have sensitivities greater than 90% and specificities approaching 100%.[123] As noted earlier (under *E. histolytica*), a sensitive and specific multiplex PCR test was recently approved in the United States, but is not yet widely available.[50] The available molecular tests are all preferable to traditional microscopy and duodenal sampling as initial tests to evaluate for *Giardia* infection. The primary role of endoscopy is evaluation for other pathologic conditions.

Treatment

Metronidazole (250 mg orally 3 times a day for 5 days) is the preferred treatment for giardiasis.[56] At this relatively low dosage, metronidazole is generally well tolerated and is 80% to 95% effective at eradicating *Giardia*.[124] The most common side effects of metronidazole are nausea, a metallic taste, and a disulfiram-like reaction upon consuming alcohol.

Nitazoxanide appears to be at least as effective as metronidazole and has the advantage of being available in a liquid formulation for use in pediatric patients. The recommended dosage in children is 100 mg (ages 12 to 47 months) or 200 mg (age > 4 years) twice daily, and in adults is 500 mg twice daily for 3 days.[59,62,125]

Alternative regimens include tinidazole (2 g orally for 1 dose), quinacrine (2 mg/kg 3 times a day for 5 days; maximum 300 mg/day), furazolidone (100 mg orally 4 times a day for 7 to 10 days), or paromomycin (25 to 35 mg/kg/day in 3 divided doses for 7 days). Single-dose treatment with tinidazole has been used for years in Europe and the developing world and is approved by the FDA.[56] Because paromomycin is not absorbed and there have been conflicting reports regarding the safety of metronidazole and tinidazole for the developing fetus, paromomycin may be especially useful for treatment of giardiasis during pregnancy.[56]

As noted earlier, many patients have prolonged lactose intolerance following *Giardia* infection, which can mimic ongoing infection.[116] Therefore, the diagnosis should be reconfirmed before repeating therapy. For people in whom therapy fails, repeat therapy with the same drug (e.g., with higher doses of metronidazole) or combination therapy with metronidazole and quinacrine might work.[120,124] Nitazoxanide alone also may be effective.[126,127] Patients in whom treatment repeatedly fails should be evaluated for common variable immunodeficiency.[105,124]

Control and Prevention

Control of giardiasis relies on interruption of fecal-oral transmission. Water can be made safe for drinking and food preparation by boiling (for 1 minute), halogenation (with chlorine or iodine preparations), or filtration.[66,124] Because of the low infectious dose of *Giardia* cysts and the poor hygiene of infants and children, person-to-person spread in daycare centers is much more difficult to control. Temporarily removing infected ill children from daycare is ineffective, perhaps because many infected children remain asymptomatic and go unrecognized.[128] In the developing world, endemic giardiasis is unlikely to be controlled until facilities become available for adequate filtration of water and disposal of sewage.

A *Giardia* vaccine composed of killed *G. intestinalis* trophozoites has been licensed for use in cats and dogs, but there have been few studies that address human vaccination for giardiasis.[129] Reduced susceptibility of some people living in endemic areas suggests that vaccination may be possible.[130]

DIENTAMOEBA FRAGILIS

D. fragilis is a binucleate organism with an ameboid trophozoite that measures 4 to 12 μm in diameter. No cyst form has been identified. The organism initially was classified as an ameba, but it is more closely related to the flagellates (trichomonads) based on morphologic studies and phylogenetic analyses of small-subunit rRNA gene sequences. The mode of its transmission remains unknown. The absence of a cyst form makes direct fecal-oral transmission unlikely because the trophozoite is killed by gastric acid. Because of an association with *Enterobius vermicularis* (pinworm), some have hypothesized that it is carried in pinworm eggs.[131] *D. fragilis* infection is common throughout the world. *D. fragilis* was identified in 0.5% of all stool samples examined in a large U.S. study, and the prevalence is as high as 20% to 50% in selected populations.[87,132-135]

The role of *D. fragilis* as a pathogen was previously controversial because *D. fragilis* trophozoites do not invade tissue and many persons infected with *D. fragilis* are asymptomatic.[131] Furthermore, the organism often is identified in the presence of other intestinal parasites, making its role in disease unclear.[132,134,135] Several studies of patients infected only with *D. fragilis*, however, have found an association with diarrhea, abdominal pain, nausea, weight loss, anorexia, flatus, and malaise that resolved only after eradication.[133,136,137] Based on these studies, it now is believed that *D. fragilis* is pathogenic and should be treated. Treatment with metronidazole (500 mg to 750 mg 3 times a day for 10 days), paromomycin (25 to 35 mg/kg/day orally in 3 divided doses for 7 days), iodoquinol (650 mg orally 3 times a day for 20 days), or tetracycline (500 mg orally 4 times a day for 10 days) has been effective.[133,137-139]

BLASTOCYSTIS HOMINIS

Blastocystis hominis is an intestinal protozoan that commonly infects the human colon. It is of uncertain taxonomic classification. Diameter ranges from 3 to 30 μm. In culture, *B. hominis* has ameboid, vacuolated, granular,[66,140] and cystic forms.[141] The distribution of *B. hominis* is worldwide, but infection is most common in the tropics.[81,87,142-144] In a large study of intestinal parasitism in the United States, *B. hominis* was identified in 2.6% of stool specimens submitted to state health departments; more than 70% of positive samples were from California.[87] Among American travelers and expatriates, the prevalence often exceeds 30%.[81,144]

The significance of *B. hominis* as a pathogen remains controversial. Several studies have suggested an association with IBS, but neither cause nor effect has been established, and in most series, *B. hominis* infection is not more common among patients with GI complaints than among asymptomatic control subjects.[81,144-147] In addition, the parasite burden does not correlate with symptoms.[81,142] Nevertheless, multiple studies have used metronidazole (750 mg orally 3 times a day for 10 days) or iodoquinol (650 mg orally 3 times a day for 20 days) for treatment of symptomatic patients, with an overall improvement rate of about 50%.[80,148] Clinical improvement actually may be due to treatment of unrecognized infections with other organisms, because many people infected with *B. hominis* simultaneously harbor known pathogens.[132,149,150] In 1 series of patients with *B. hominis* infection, 84% of patients were found to have at least 1 recognized pathogen other than *B. hominis* (*E. histolytica*, *G. intestinalis*, or *D. fragilis*) when repeated stool examinations were obtained.[132]

CRYPTOSPORIDIUM SPECIES

Epidemiology

First recognized in 1907 by Tyzzer as a gastric infection in mice, *Cryptosporidium* species are tiny intracellular protozoan parasites (2 to 5 μm) that belong to the phylum Apicomplexa. Other medically important apicomplexan parasites include *Plasmodium* species, which cause malaria, and *Toxoplasma gondii*, which causes toxoplasmosis. *Cryptosporidium* species infect the GI epithelium of a wide range of vertebrates. Based on genetic and biological differences with other *Cryptosporidium*, *Cryptosporidium parvum* human genotype (genotype 1 or genotype H) was renamed *Cryptosporidium hominis* in 2002. The name *Cryptosporidium parvum* was retained for the bovine genotype (genotype 2). Together, *C. hominis* and *C. parvum* cause most human infections, but numerous other *Cryptosporidium* species occasionally infect humans.[151]

Cryptosporidium was brought to prominent medical attention in the early 1980s because of the devastating disease it caused in patients with advanced HIV infection. However, *Cryptosporidium* species increasingly are recognized as a cause of self-limited diarrhea, usually lasting 1 to 4 weeks, in immunocompetent persons.[152,153] In developing countries, children younger than 5 years are affected most frequently.[154] In a recent multisite epidemiologic study, *Cryptosporidium* ranked second to rotavirus as a worldwide cause of life-threatening diarrhea in children younger than age 1 a recent multisite epidemiologic study.[3] An inability to detect it reliably with non-molecular methods has likely contributed to delayed recognition of its importance. In industrialized countries, because *Cryptosporidium* oocysts are small and highly chlorine-resistant, cryptosporidiosis has been associated with water-borne epidemics, including numerous chlorinated swimming pool outbreaks, and it is the leading cause of diarrhea resulting from water-borne outbreaks in the United States.[155] A low infectious dose and ready person-to-person spread also has resulted in epidemics in hospitals and daycare centers.[156,157] In rural areas, zoonotic infections from direct contact with farm animals have been reported.[158] Asymptomatic infection is common, and infection appears to be more common in children who carry the DQB1*0301 HLA class II allele or the B*15 HLA class I allele.[159]

Pathogenesis, Pathology, and Immunology

Upon ingestion of an infectious dose that may be as low as 1 to 10 oocysts, excystation and release of sporozoa occur in the presence of bile salts in the small intestine. The sporozoites then attach to the intestinal epithelium, which triggers elongation of epithelial cell microvilli on either side of the point of attachment. Fusion of the elongated microvilli with one another encloses the sporozoite within a vacuole located just underneath the brush border inside the epithelial cell. The sporozoites then develop into merozoites, which replicate asexually. After several rounds of asexual replication, the merozoites exit the host cell and invade uninfected neighboring cells. In immunocompetent persons, second-generation merozoites undergo meiosis to yield the male and female micro- and macrogametocytes, respectively. The microgametocytes then divide, exit the cell, and fertilize the macrogametocytes, forming oocysts that are shed in the feces. Rarely, multiplication has been seen in biliary, respiratory, or even conjunctival epithelium in immunocompromised patients.[66]

Animal and human studies suggest that both humoral and cellular immune responses aid in the control of *Cryptosporidium* infections. Cryptosporidial diarrhea is clearly much more severe, and can be chronic, in patients with immunoglobulin deficiency, lymphocytic malignancies, or low CD4 counts associated with HIV infection.[153,160,161] For unknown reasons, many more rounds of asexual reproduction typically occur in immunocompromised persons before development of the merozoites into micro- and macrogametocytes, which at least in part explains the increased chronicity of infection that is seen in this context.

Clinical Features

Following a 1-week incubation period (range, 2 to 14 days), a watery, relatively non-inflammatory diarrheal illness typically lasts for 10 to 14 days in immunocompetent hosts. Nausea, vomiting, abdominal pain, and mild fever may also be seen. Rarely, respiratory symptoms, pancreatitis, and biliary tract involvement have been reported, the latter in HIV-infected patients (see Chapter 34). Brief recurrence of diarrhea may be seen after improvement.[162,163]

In immunocompromised patients, particularly those with very low CD4 lymphocyte counts, the diarrheal illness with cryptosporidial infection can be cholera-like, protracted (often for the duration of severe immune compromise), and fatal.[153]

Diagnosis

Because cryptosporidial infection usually is not identified in the laboratory except on specific request, the most important element in diagnosis is to consider it in patients with diarrhea that lasts longer than 5 to 7 days and to request the appropriate special fecal studies. Because *Cryptosporidium* is spread in water, it is reasonable to consider cryptosporidiosis whenever the diagnosis of giardiasis is considered. In addition, it should be considered as a cause of persistent diarrhea in immunocompromised patients.

Traditionally, cryptosporidial oocysts have been detected with a modified acid-fast stain of the stool (which can also detect *Cyclospora* and *Isospora*).[164] As with giardiasis, ELISA or direct fluorescence antibody tests of the stool have replaced microscopy as the diagnostic test of choice. Numerous commercial kits using either of these 2 methods have been developed that have sensitivities and specificities in excess of 90%.[123] The recently FDA-approved multiplexed PCR test discussed earlier for *E. histolytica* and *G. intestinalis* also detects *Cryptosporidium* in the feces and is likely to be widely available soon.[50] Occasionally, cryptosporidiosis is diagnosed with intestinal biopsy.

Serologic tests are helpful primarily in epidemiologic studies, especially because they may be negative at the time of initial clinical presentation and positivity persists after infection has resolved. Finally, abdominal US, CT scans, and ERCP may be helpful in diagnosis of cryptosporidial acalculous cholecystitis and cholangiopathies, especially in immunocompromised patients.

Treatment

A recent systematic review of the literature concluded that better treatments are urgently needed for cryptosporidiosis in children and immunocompromised individuals.[165] Nitazoxanide, an antiparasitic agent with broad-spectrum antiprotozoan and antihelminthic activity, is the only drug with demonstrated efficacy for treating cryptosporidiosis in immunocompetent adults.[59,61,166-168] Unfortunately, failure is common in young children and immunocompromised patients, such as those with advanced HIV infection, although some studies have shown benefit.[166,168] The recommended dosage in children is 100 mg (ages 12 to 47 months) or 200 mg (age > 4 years) twice daily, and in adults is 500 mg twice daily for 3 days. Nitazoxanide generally is well tolerated. It is converted to the active metabolite tizoxanide, which undergoes conjugation to tizoxanide glucuronide and is excreted in the urine, bile, and feces. Nitazoxanide and tizoxanide are yellow, resulting in yellow urine and, in some patients on prolonged therapy, in yellow discoloration of the eyes that resolves after the drug is discontinued. Paromomycin or paromomycin in combination with azithromycin have been suggested as additional treatment options, but most studies indicate that these are not effective.[165,169] Numerous groups are pursuing both cell-based and target-based approaches to identify more effective treatments, but all remain in early stages of development.[170-172]

Most important in treating HIV-infected patients with cryptosporidiosis is HAART, because ultimately, improvement of cryptosporidiosis depends on improvement in the immune compromise and the CD4 lymphocyte counts. Finally,

papillotomy may be required for biliary obstruction with papillary stenosis from cryptosporidiosis in patients with AIDS (see Chapter 34).

Control and Prevention

Most important in control and prevention of this difficult protozoan parasitic infection is education regarding boiling or careful filtration of water; filter pores must be less than 1 μm in diameter. In addition, scrupulous enteric precautions are required in institutions such as hospitals, daycare centers, or extended-care facilities for older adults. These precautions are especially important because chlorine is ineffective in reducing oocyst viability.

Other means for disinfection that are being studied include ultraviolet light and irradiation. In 1 study, 2.5% glutaraldehyde was effective at inactivating *Cryptosporidium* oocysts, but only when a relatively low number of oocysts (15,000) were present and after treatment for 10 hours. Because of the corrosiveness of glutaraldehyde, the need to immerse instruments with their contaminating oocysts for this length of time presents a challenge for endoscope sterilization.[173]

Finally, because of the potential substantial long-term impact of cryptosporidial infection on childhood growth and development, control of cryptosporidiosis is critical in developing areas and must receive appropriate high priority in programs directed at improved water and sanitation worldwide.[174,175]

CYCLOSPORA CAYETANENSIS

Epidemiology

Cyclospora was first reported as a cause of human disease by Ashford in 1979, who described infection of 3 patients in Papua, New Guinea by what was at that time an unnamed coccidian parasite.[176] This parasite came to wider attention when documented as a cause of protracted diarrhea in AIDS patients and persistent diarrhea in non-immunocompromised patients in New York City and the Caribbean, among expatriates in Nepal, and in an outbreak among house staff in a Chicago hospital.[177-179] Finally, in 1993, Ortega and colleagues at Cayetano Heredia University in Peru demonstrated formation of sporozoites (sporulation) within immature oocysts and excystation in vitro; they used electron microscopy to demonstrate that oocysts containing sporozoites also contained organelles characteristic of coccidians of the phylum Apicomplexa. They classified the organism as a member of the genus *Cyclospora*, and it has now been officially named *Cyclospora cayetanensis* to acknowledge this work.[180] Ribosomal DNA analysis of phylogenetic relationships suggest that *Cyclospora* is closely related to *Eimeria*.[181]

Like *Cryptosporidium*, *Cyclospora* is being increasingly recognized in immunocompetent as well as immunocompromised persons. The infection is usually highly seasonal (in summer or wet months) and is probably spread via fecal contamination of water and vegetables.[182,183] *Cyclospora* was brought to prominent attention throughout the United States and Canada after repeated outbreaks of diarrheal illnesses that occurred in more than 2000 patients every year from 1996 through 2000 in association with consumption of the late spring shipment of Guatemalan raspberries.[184,185]

Pathogenesis, Pathology, and Immunology

The pathogenesis, pathology, and immunology of *Cyclospora*, although not as thoroughly studied as for *Cryptosporidium*, appear to be similar for the 2 organisms. One important distinction, however, is that unlike *Cryptosporidium*, which is promptly infectious when it is excreted in the stool, *Cyclospora* requires development outside the host before it becomes infectious. Consequently, secondary person-to-person spread, which is very common with cryptosporidial infections, is not described with *Cyclospora* infections. Also, unlike the numerous mammalian hosts for the cryptosporidial infections that also can infect humans, animal reservoirs for *Cyclospora* are very poorly understood at present.

The histopathologic changes of *Cyclospora* infections are similar to those seen with cryptosporidiosis, with villus blunting and a mild inflammatory infiltrate in the lamina propria, predominantly in the small intestine.[186]

Clinical Features

The clinical presentation of *Cyclospora* infection is indistinguishable from that described with *Cryptosporidium* infections except perhaps for the more severe generalized fatigue and malaise with *Cyclospora* infections, even in immunocompetent patients. *Cyclospora* diarrhea typically lasts for 1 to 3 weeks and may be associated with significant weight loss. Also as seen with cryptosporidiosis, protracted diarrhea and acalculous cholecystitis can occur with *Cyclospora* infection in HIV-infected persons.

Diagnosis

As with *Cryptosporidium*, one must consider the diagnosis of *Cyclospora* in patients with protracted diarrhea. Diagnosis is best made at present with the acid-fast stain. *Cyclospora* oocysts measure 7 to 10 μm, nearly twice the size of those of *Cryptosporidium*, which are 4 to 5 μm.[187] *Cyclospora* exhibits striking blue-green autofluorescence when examined under fluorescence microscopy, a characteristic that might have contributed to its initial confusion with cyanobacteria.[188] Improved diagnostic methods using PCR have been developed, but they are not currently available for clinical use.[189]

Treatment

In contrast to *Cryptosporidium* infections, *Cyclospora* infections are readily treatable, even in immunocompromised patients. The drug of choice is trimethoprim/sulfamethoxazole at a dosage of 160/800 mg twice daily for 1 week. Treatment promptly eradicates the organism and relieves symptoms.[190,191] This treatment is similarly effective in patients with AIDS, although maintenance therapy with a single dose of trimethoprim/sulfamethoxazole 3 times per week may be needed to prevent relapse.[192] Recent data show that ciprofloxacin provides a reasonable alternative in patients unable to tolerate trimethoprim/sulfamethoxazole.[193] Nitazoxanide also appears to be effective.[61]

Control and Prevention

Although readily treatable, *Cyclospora* infections are extremely difficult to control or prevent because of our limited ability to detect low infectious doses (for humans) of oocysts, which can contaminate products such as raspberries, from which it is very difficult to eradicate. From limited studies, the organism also appears to be relatively chlorine-resistant and thus poses challenges to effective water treatment, much like *Cryptosporidium*. Elucidation of the reservoir of *Cyclospora* undoubtedly will enhance our ability to prevent and control the spread of this highly infectious parasite. For example, it remains unclear why it is only the spring rather than the fall shipment

of raspberries from Guatemala that has consistently posed problems with spread of *Cyclospora* infections. Whether this is related to migration of an avian reservoir has been questioned, but not proved.[194] Consistent with this, several studies have reported isolation of *Cyclospora* oocysts from chickens.[182,183]

ISOSPORA BELLI

Epidemiology

A relative of *Cyclospora* and *Eimeria*, *I. belli* is much larger, with elliptical oocysts measuring 20 to 30 μm long and containing 2 visible sporocysts that are acid-fast. Like *Cyclospora*, *Isospora* oocysts appear to require sporulation outside of the human host before they become infectious. There are no known non-human hosts for *I. belli*, and its distribution appears to be throughout tropical areas around the world. It is a less common cause of diarrhea in children who live in developing areas than is *Cryptosporidium*, and in North America it is typically seen in older children, institutionalized children, and immunocompromised patients.[195,196]

Pathogenesis, Pathology, and Immunology

The pathogenesis, pathology, and immunology of *Isospora* infections appear to be similar to that of *Cryptosporidium* and *Cyclospora* infections, although less thoroughly studied.

Clinical Features

Similar to *Cryptosporidium* and *Cyclospora* infections, *Isospora* characteristically produces a self-limiting diarrheal illness in immunocompetent persons and in travelers to tropical areas, with watery diarrhea and abdominal pain lasting 2 to 4 weeks. In immunocompromised patients, *Isospora* can produce a protracted sprue-like illness with malabsorption, weight loss, and prolonged diarrhea.[196] As with *Cryptosporidium* and *Cyclospora*, acalculous cholecystitis also has been reported in patients with AIDS and *Isospora* infections.

Diagnosis

The diagnosis of *Isospora* should be suspected in immunocompetent patients with diarrhea lasting longer than 5 to 7 days, especially following travel to tropical or developing areas, and in immunocompromised patients with persistent diarrhea. Unlike other protozoan infections, *Isospora* infections may be associated with peripheral eosinophilia and with Charcot-Leyden crystals in the stool. The diagnosis of *Isospora* relies on identification of the large, oval oocysts (20 to 30 μm by 10 to 19 μm) on microscopic examination of concentrated fecal specimens by acid-fast staining. Oocysts also may be seen in biopsy specimens from the small intestine. In contrast to *Cryptosporidium* and *Cyclospora* infections, *Isospora* organisms have been observed invading beyond the epithelium into the lamina propria.[151,197]

Treatment

As with *Cyclospora*, *Isospora* infections are readily treated with trimethoprim/sulfamethoxazole; the dosage is 160/800 mg orally 4 times a day for 10 days, and then 2 times a day for 3 weeks.[56] As previously described with *Cyclospora*, maintenance of suppressive therapy may be required in patients with AIDS.[191] Alternatives to trimethoprim/sulfamethoxazole may include ciprofloxacin.[193]

Control and Prevention

Prevention and control of *Isospora* infections will likely require improved sanitation in tropical areas.

MICROSPORIDIA

Microsporidia infections are also discussed in Chapter 34.

Epidemiology

Microsporidia, the nontaxonomic term for *Enterocytozoon bieneusi, Encephalitozoon* (old *Septata*) *intestinalis,* and several other nonintestinal members of the phylum Microspora, are important causes of diarrhea, primarily in patients with impaired cell-mediated immunity from AIDS or organ transplantation.[198,199] *E. bieneusi* causes approximately 90% of cases.[200] Microsporidia are identified in as many as 50% of AIDS patients with chronic diarrhea and are the most commonly identified pathogen in most series.[199] The prevalence of infection is strongly correlated with low CD4 T lymphocyte counts, although cases are not uncommon in persons with CD4 cell counts greater than 200 cells/mL.[153,200,201] Microsporidiosis is distinctly less common in immunocompetent persons. The reservoir and modes of transmission are not certain.[202-204] Epidemiologic data suggest that water-borne, person-to-person, and possibly sexual transmission occur.

Pathogenesis, Pathology, and Immunology

E. bieneusi enters only the cytoplasm of enterocytes, but *E. intestinalis* forms a parasitophorous vacuole in enterocytes, endothelial cells, fibroblasts, and macrophages, and it can disseminate to the kidney, prostate gland, and upper respiratory tract. Typically, intestinal pathology is marked by villus atrophy, crypt hyperplasia, and mild inflammation in the lamina propria.[198] The importance of cellular immunity in determining both infection and illness with intestinal microsporidia is indicated by its striking predominance in immunocompromised persons after organ transplantation or in those with AIDS.

Clinical Features

Although primarily limited to immunocompromised patients, microsporidia, regardless of one's immune status, can cause chronic watery, non-inflammatory diarrhea and weight loss, occasionally with abdominal pain, nausea, vomiting, fever, and acalculous cholecystitis or even sclerosing cholangitis.[198] *E. intestinalis* also can cause colitis and disseminate especially to the kidneys or less often to sinuses, bronchi, conjunctivae, or prostate.[205] Rarely, cases have been reported of self-limited diarrhea in travelers or health professionals.[202-204]

Diagnosis

Most laboratories use a modified trichrome stain to identify microsporidia in stool specimens.[206] This method requires considerable skill and has limited sensitivity because of the small size of the spores (*E. bieneusi* measures 1 by 1.5 μm; *E. intestinalis* is slightly larger). Sensitivity can be improved by initially screening samples with fluorescent chitin stains such as Fungi-Fluor chitin stain (Polysciences, Warrington, Pa.) or Uvitex 2B (Ciba Geigy, Rueil Malmaison, France), and then confirming positive results by modified trichrome staining.[207,208] In addition, Gram stain and electron microscopy can identify the organisms in intestinal biopsy specimens. Sensitive PCR methods have been developed that enable species differentiation, but use of these methods is currently limited to research applications.[204,209]

Treatment

E. intestinalis infections (≈10% of cases) respond well to albendazole, 400 mg twice daily for 3 weeks.[56] The response of *E. bieneusi* to albendazole is poor, but recent data indicate that oral fumagillin (20 mg 3 times daily for 2 weeks) may be effective for treatment of intestinal *E. bieneusi* infection in immunocompromised patients.[210] Side effects including neutropenia and thrombocytopenia are common, and fumagillin is not available in the United States. As with all opportunistic infections in patients with AIDS, effective HAART is essential for controlling microsporidial infections.

Control and Prevention

Because the reservoir and transmission of microsporidia remain unclear, control measures are primarily directed toward appropriate sanitary precautions and hand washing.

TRYPANOSOMA CRUZI (AMERICAN TRYPANOSOMIASIS OR CHAGAS' DISEASE)

Epidemiology

Although symptomatic Chagas' disease has been confined to South and Central America, at least 4 autochthonous (indigenous) cases, as well as occasional laboratory-acquired and imported cases of acute Chagas' disease, have occurred in the United States. Furthermore, increasing numbers of immigrants are presenting with chronic Chagas' disease and pose distinct risks for disease transmission via blood donation.[211] In patients surviving acute infection with *T. cruzi* in whom the chronic form of illness develops, myocardial disease is the most common manifestation. Megaesophagus and megacolon are the most common intestinal manifestations of American trypanosomiasis. Small intestinal dilatation and aperistalsis also are seen. At postmortem examination, even in patients with asymptomatic *T. cruzi* involvement of the intestine, the small intestine has a significant reduction in submucosal and myenteric autonomic plexuses.

American trypanosomiasis could prove to be a significant health problem in the United States because of the large reservoir of *T. cruzi* infection detected in animals in Arizona, California, New Mexico, Texas, Louisiana, Georgia, Florida, and Maryland. The epidemiologically important insects, the reduviid bugs of the Triatominae group, also have the same wide geographic distribution. Infection is transmitted when the reduviid bug infected with *T. cruzi* bites the victim. On biting, the arthropod discharges its feces, and the parasite is then introduced through the skin when the patient scratches the bite.

Pathogenesis, Pathology, and Immunology

Metacyclic trypanosomes, an extracellular, flagellated form of the parasite that develops in the triatomine bug's intestinal tract, are deposited with the feces of the bug during the time it is taking a blood meal. Characteristically, deposition occurs on or near mucous membranes, particularly on the outer canthus of the eye or around the nose or lips. The invading organisms are phagocytosed by histiocytes in the corium and invade the adipose and subcutaneous muscle cells. They then develop into the intracellular form, the amastigote, which replicates by binary fission within the host's cells. At variable intervals, the intracellular amastigotes differentiate into trypomastigotes, a flagellated form that emerges into the blood and lymphatic circulation. The trypomastigotes then either invade other cells in diverse areas of the body (where they transform back to amastigotes and multiply) or are taken up into another reduviid bug's midgut during a blood meal.

The signs and symptoms of Chagas' disease are caused by the intracellular amastigote forms. When the host cell ruptures, large numbers of amastigotes escape and temporarily enter the circulation as trypanosome forms. In the intestine, tissue injury can occur acutely or can trigger autoimmune damage to cardiac or nerve epitopes that cross-react with *T. cruzi* antigens to destroy the submucosal and the myenteric plexuses. The end result is enteromegaly, which at times may be massive. Immunosuppression as a consequence of chemotherapy or AIDS can reactivate chronic *T. cruzi* infection, causing acute disease or brain abscesses.

Clinical Features

Acute Chagas' disease occurs most often in children. It is characterized by high fever and marked edema, particularly with a periorbital distribution and often involving the entire body. In patients with acute Chagas' disease, the periorbital edema of 1 or both eyes is striking. The victim can appear to be suffering from myxedema. There usually is hepatosplenomegaly and enlargement of the thyroid gland, lymph nodes, and salivary glands. The acute stage lasts about 20 to 30 days.

Manifestations of chronic Chagas' disease depend on which major organ system is involved. Most commonly, symptoms are cardiac, manifested primarily as arrhythmias and congestive heart failure. With megaesophagus, the history, barium esophagogram, and esophageal motility tracing are indistinguishable from those of achalasia. With megacolon (Fig. 113-6), infrequent bowel movements and chronic constipation are the cardinal symptoms. With dilatation of the small intestine, diarrhea or constipation may occur. There also may be evidence of weight loss and abdominal distention caused by the markedly dilated bowel.

Diagnosis

Routine laboratory data provide no clue to the diagnosis of Chagas' disease. Diagnosis of acute disease depends on demonstration of the trypanosome forms on blood smears during periods when the amastigotes rupture cells. During febrile periods, if the blood smear results are negative, inoculation of a patient's blood into a guinea pig leads to proliferation of trypanosomes that often can be recovered and identified. Amastigote forms may be detected in bone marrow, the spleen, or enlarged lymph nodes.

Diagnosis of chronic Chagas' disease depends on the presence of a typical clinical and epidemiologic history and on serologic tests, because parasites are only rarely identifiable in the blood or on biopsies of affected organs. Serum antibodies to *T. cruzi* can be detected either by complement fixation or ELISA, and antibody testing can be requested from the CDC. Xenodiagnosis has been used but is relatively insensitive, identifying less than 50% of patients infected with chronic Chagas' disease. In this technique, trypanosome-free

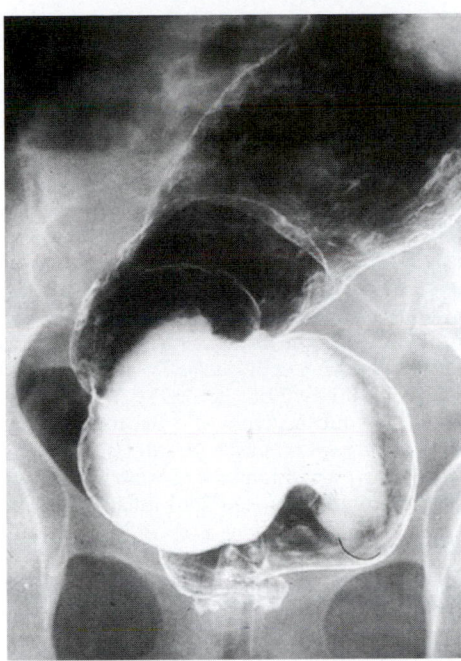

FIGURE 113-6. Film from a barium enema examination revealing megarectum and megasigmoid in a patient with Chagas' disease. This complication, caused by autoimmune destruction of the submucosal and myenteric nerve plexuses, is believed to be a consequence of a cross-reaction of nerve epitopes with an antigen from *Trypanosoma cruzi*.

laboratory reduviid bugs are allowed to bite suspected victims. The trypanosomes multiply rapidly in the intestinal tract of the insect, and examination of the intestine reveals flagellated trypanosomes in 10 to 30 days. Sensitive and specific PCR-based assays have been developed for diagnosis of acute and chronic Chagas' disease, but these assays are not available for clinical use.[212,213]

Treatment

Nifurtimox (8 to 10 mg/kg daily in 4 divided doses for 90 to 120 days) or benznidazole (5 to 7 mg/kg daily in 2 divided doses for 30 to 90 days) can be used for treatment of acute Chagas' disease.[56] Both are subject to availability problems, have limited efficacy, and are associated with significant side effects, including GI symptoms in 40% to 70% of patients (nausea, vomiting, abdominal pain, and anorexia) and frequent neurologic sequelae.[214] Treatment for the GI manifestations of chronic Chagas' disease only addresses the symptoms. Isosorbide dinitrate increases esophageal emptying in patients with achalasia resulting from Chagas' disease and might ameliorate dysphagia.[215,216] Most patients with Chagas achalasia are best treated with either balloon dilation of the esophagus or esophagomyotomy. Occasionally, aperistaltic segments of intestine that are responsible for symptoms need to be resected.

Control and Prevention

Control and prevention require improved housing, use of insecticides and netting, and screening of blood for antibody in endemic areas.

KEY REFERENCES

Full references for this chapter can be found on www.expertconsult.com.

2. Haque R, Mondal D, Duggal P, et al. *Entamoeba histolytica* infection in children and protection from subsequent amebiasis. Infect Immun 2006; 74:904-9.

7. Ali IKM, Mondal U, Roy S, et al. Evidence for a link between parasite genotype and outcome of infection with *Entamoeba histolytica*. J Clin Microbiol 2007; 45:285-9.

9. Duggal P, Guo X, Haque R, et al. A mutation in the leptin receptor is associated with *Entamoeba histolytica* infection in children. J Clin Invest 2011; 121:1191-8.

62. Rossignol JF, Ayoub A, Ayers MS. Treatment of diarrhea caused by *Giardia intestinalis* and *Entamoeba histolytica* or *Entamoeba dispar*: A randomized, double-blind placebo-controlled study of nitazoxanide. J Infect Dis 2002; 184:381-4.

83. Monis PT, Andrews RH, Mayrhofer G, Ey PL. Genetic diversity within the morphological species *Giardia intestinalis* and its relationship to host origin. Infect Gen Evol 2003; 3:29-38.

84. Haque R, Roy S, Kabir M, et al. *Giardia* assemblage A infection and diarrhea in Bangladesh. J Infect Dis 2005; 192:2171-3.

92. Osterholm MT, Forfang JC, Ristinen TL, et al. An outbreak of foodborne giardiasis. N Engl J Med 1981; 304:24-8.

97. Muhsen K, Levine MM. A systematic review and meta-analysis of the association between *Giardia lamblia* and endemic pediatric diarrhea in developing countries. Clin Infect Dis 2012; 55(Suppl 4):S271-93.

131. Johnson EH, Windsor JJ, Clark CG. Emerging from obscurity: Biological, clinical, and diagnostic aspects of *Dientamoeba fragilis*. Clin Microbiol Rev 2004; 17:553-70.

151. Xiao L, Fayer R, Ryan U, Upton SJ. *Cryptosporidium* taxonomy: Recent advances and implications for public health. Clin Microbiol Rev 2004; 17:72-97.

155. Hlavsa MC, Roberts VA, Anderson AR, et al. Surveillance for waterborne disease outbreaks and other health events associated with recreational water—United States, 2007-2008. MMWR Morb Mortal Wkly Rep 2011; 60:1-32.

162. Mac kenzie WR, Hoxie NJ, Proctor ME, et al. A massive outbreak in Milwaukee of *Cryptosporidium* infection transmitted through the public water supply. N Engl J Med 1994; 331:161-7.

167. Rossignol JF, Ayoub A, Ayers MS. Treatment of diarrhea caused by *Cryptosporidium parvum*: A prospective randomized, double-blind, placebo-controlled study of nitazoxanide. J Infect Dis 2001; 184:103-6.

168. Amadi B, Mwiya M, Musuku J, et al. Effect of nitazoxanide on morbidity and mortality in Zambian children with cryptosporidiosis: A randomised controlled trial. Lancet 2002; 360:1375-80.

193. Verdier RI, Fitzgerald DW, Johnson WD, Pape JW. Trimethoprim-sulfamethoxazole compared with ciprofloxacin for treatment and prophylaxis of *Isospora belli* and *Cyclospora cayetanensis* infection in HIV-infected patients. A randomized, controlled trial. Ann Intern Med 2000; 132:885-8.

DAVID E. ELLIOTT

Parasitic worms are found worldwide. Modern travel, emigration,[1,2] and consumption of "exotic" cuisines allow intestinal helminths to appear in any locale. People now acquire tropical helminths without leaving their industrialized temperate cities. Travel history is a critical, but often overlooked, aspect of the patient interview. Helminths may survive for decades within a host, so even a remote history of visits to or emigration from countries where helminths are endemic is important. Fresh food is flown around the world and often consumed raw, often at a great distance from its original point of origin.

Physicians need to remain alert to the possibility of infection with these organisms because some cause severe disease that requires years to develop or occurs only under special circumstances. For example, patients might have occult *Strongyloides stercoralis* until treatment with glucocorticoids causes fulminant disease, occult *Clonorchis sinensis* until they develop cholangiocarcinoma, or occult *Schistosoma mansoni* until they develop portal hypertension and bleeding from esophageal varices.

In developed countries, we usually diagnose an intestinal helminth because we stumble across it rather than because we actively pursue it. Helminths are complex organisms well adapted to their hosts; like quiet house guests, most cause no symptoms. Worms rarely cause diarrhea, but many medical laboratories do not assay formed stool routinely for parasite eggs. Physicians need to communicate their concerns of possible helminthic infection to laboratory personnel. A telephone call to the local laboratory before a sample is sent can improve diagnostic results dramatically. Occasionally, alarmed patients bring proglottids or whole worms that they passed with their stools. These specimens should be fixed in 5% aqueous formalin and sent for identification.[3] All specimens should be handled carefully with full precautions to avoid accidental exposure.

Some helminthic infections are difficult to diagnose, especially when the worm burden is light. Diagnosis can require serologic evaluation, analysis of multiple stools, or use of concentration techniques in addition to a high level of physician awareness. For example, *S. stercoralis* eggs do not appear in the stool, and diagnosis is best made serologically. *Ancylostoma caninum* causes eosinophilic enteritis but does not lay eggs when infecting people.

Some helminths can cause severe disease, but this is unusual. Most persons colonized with helminths have no symptoms or illness attributable to the parasites. Only with heavy or protracted infections does disease result. Well-adapted worms usually act more as commensals than as pathogens. It is even possible that exposure to helminths affords some protection against disease owing to robust immune reactions.[4] Helminths induce immune regulatory pathways.[5] Studies in mice and rats show that exposure to helminths can be used to prevent or treat colitis,[6] insulin-dependent diabetes,[7] and autoimmune encephalitis.[8] Studies in humans show that helminth exposure improves UC[9] and probably Crohn's disease[10,11] and that helminth eradication increases atopy[12] and worsens the course of multiple sclerosis.[13] Although it remains important to treat helminthic infections when they are discovered, further research on these organisms can enable discovery of new approaches to treat immune-mediated disease.

This chapter is divided into 3 sections: nematodes (roundworms), cestodes (tapeworms), and trematodes (flukes or flatworms). For the most part, each worm is addressed separately, noting its epidemiology, life cycle, clinical manifestations, diagnosis, and treatment.

NEMATODES

Ascaris lumbricoides

Ascaris lumbricoides is the largest of the nematode parasites that colonize humans. Females can grow to 49 cm (19 inches).[14] The name "lumbricoides" alludes to its resemblance to earth worms (*Lumbricus* sp.). The parasite is acquired by ingesting its eggs. *Ascaris* can cause intestinal obstruction and pancreaticobiliary symptoms. Treatment is albendazole.

Epidemiology

A. lumbricoides has a worldwide distribution, although these parasites are most numerous in less-developed countries and in areas with poor sanitation. About 1.2 billion people (25% of the world's population) harbor *A. lumbricoides*,[15,16] and 5.2 billion people are at risk of becoming infected.[17] Children acquire the parasite by playing in dirt contaminated with its eggs, whereas adults most often are infected by farming or eating raw vegetables from plants fertilized with untreated sewage. Pigs harbor *Ascaris suum*, which is very closely related to *A. lumbricoides*[18]; cross-infection can occur[19] but appears to be unusual.[20]

Life Cycle

Humans acquire the parasite by ingesting embryonated eggs that contain third-stage larvae. Freshly deposited fertilized eggs incubate in the soil for 10 to 15 days while the embryo develops and molts twice, after which the eggs become infective. The eggs are remarkably stable, can survive freezing, and can remain viable for 7 to 10 years. The eggs are resistant to most chemical treatments including pickling, but they rapidly die in boiling water.

Once ingested, eggs hatch in the duodenum and release their larvae, which penetrate the intestinal wall and enter the mesenteric venules and lymphatics. Larvae that migrate with portal blood pass to the liver, through the sinusoids to the hepatic veins, and then through the right side of the heart to enter the lungs. Larvae migrating via the lymphatics pass through mesenteric lymph nodes to the thoracic duct and enter the superior vena cava, also to arrive in the lungs. The larvae then lodge in the pulmonary capillaries and break into the alveoli, where they molt twice while growing to 1.5 mm in length. Larvae then ascend the tracheobronchial tree, arrive in the hypopharynx, are again swallowed, and pass into the small intestine, where they molt again and finally mature.

Mature male *A. lumbricoides* are smaller (10 to 30 cm) than females (20 to 49 cm). Worms mate in the small intestine, and females deposit about 200,000 eggs a day. Adult worms live for about 1 year (6 to 18 months). Because their eggs require incubation in the soil to become infective, *Ascaris* does not multiply in the host. Continued infestation requires repeat ingestion of embryonated eggs.

Clinical Features and Pathophysiology

A. lumbricoides produces no symptoms in most infected persons. Often, worms are found unexpectedly on endoscopy[21,22] (Video 114-1) or are seen on radiologic imaging,[23] or eggs are identified in stool specimens of patients with symptoms not directly attributable to the worms. Disease usually develops only in those with heavy worm burdens: pulmonary, intestinal, and hepatobiliary ascariasis are well described.

Pulmonary ascariasis (*Ascaris* pneumonia) develops 4 to 16 days after ingesting infective eggs. The larvae migrate into the alveoli and elicit an inflammatory response that can cause consolidation. The pneumonia usually is self-limited but can be life-threatening if larvae are numerous.

Large numbers of mature worms can cause severe intestinal symptoms including abdominal pain, distention, nausea, and vomiting. The most common complication of intestinal ascariasis is partial or complete small bowel obstruction; such patients often have a history of passing mature worms in their stool or vomitus. Patients with intestinal obstruction generally

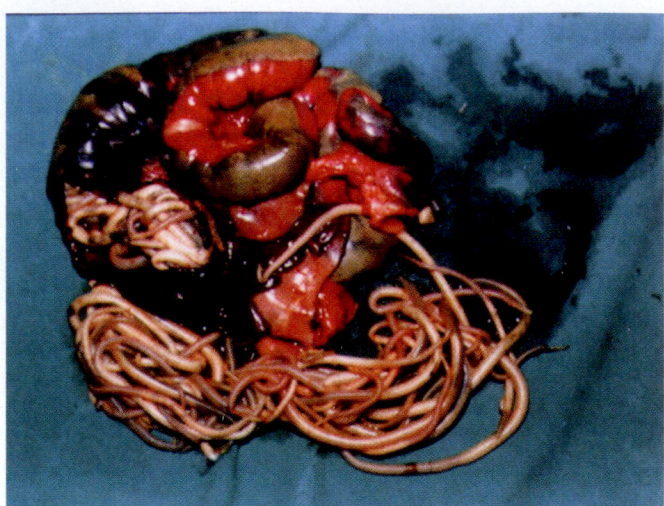

FIGURE 114-1. Surgical specimen showing small intestinal obstruction caused by *Ascaris lumbricoides*. *(From Wasadikar PP, Kulkarni AB. Intestinal obstruction due to ascariasis. Br J Surg 1997; 84:410-2.)*

have more than 60 worms,[24] and the rare patients with fatal disease often have more than 600 worms. Fatality results from intestinal necrosis caused by obstruction, intussusception, or volvulus (Fig. 114-1).[25] Most cases of intestinal obstruction, absent signs of peritonitis or perforation, can be managed conservatively.

A. lumbricoides is highly motile. Mature worms can enter the ampulla of Vater (Fig. 114-2) and migrate into the bile or pancreatic ducts, causing biliary colic, obstructive jaundice, ascending cholangitis, acalculous cholecystitis, or acute pancreatitis.[14] Pregnancy can promote biliary migration,[26] possibly because of relaxation of smooth muscle that is mediated by progesterone, although this has not been formally studied. *Ascaris* worms can move in and out of the papilla, producing intermittent symptoms and fluctuating laboratory tests. Recurrent ascending cholangitis or acute pancreatitis from ascariasis is rare in highly developed Western countries but can be fatal if the diagnosis is not entertained and treatment is delayed.[27]

Diagnosis

Often it is an alarmed patient who discovers *Ascaris* after passing a motile adult worm with a bowel movement. The worms, however, usually do not cause diarrhea. Most patients do not have specific symptoms or eosinophilia; eosinophilia is absent because the adult *Ascaris* lives in the intestinal lumen.

Ascaris eggs are visible in direct smears of stool (Fig. 114-3). The eggs begin to appear in the stool about 2 months after initial exposure. Fertilized eggs are 35 × 55 μm and have a thick shell and outer layer; females also lay unfertilized eggs that are larger (90 × 44 μm) and have a thin shell and outer layer. *Ascaris* eggs that lose their outer layer resemble the eggs of hookworms; the outer coating is not necessary for viability and can become easily separated.

Adults worms may be seen at endoscopy,[22] or identified on upper GI series as long, linear, filling defects within the small intestine.[23] The worms retain barium after it has cleared from the patient's GI tract, producing isolated linear opacities. Similar findings are seen on ERCP if a worm is within the bile or pancreatic duct (Fig. 114-4). *Ascaris* also has a characteristic appearance on US examination of the bile duct or pancreas, appearing as long, linear echogenic stripes that do not cast acoustic shadows.[23]

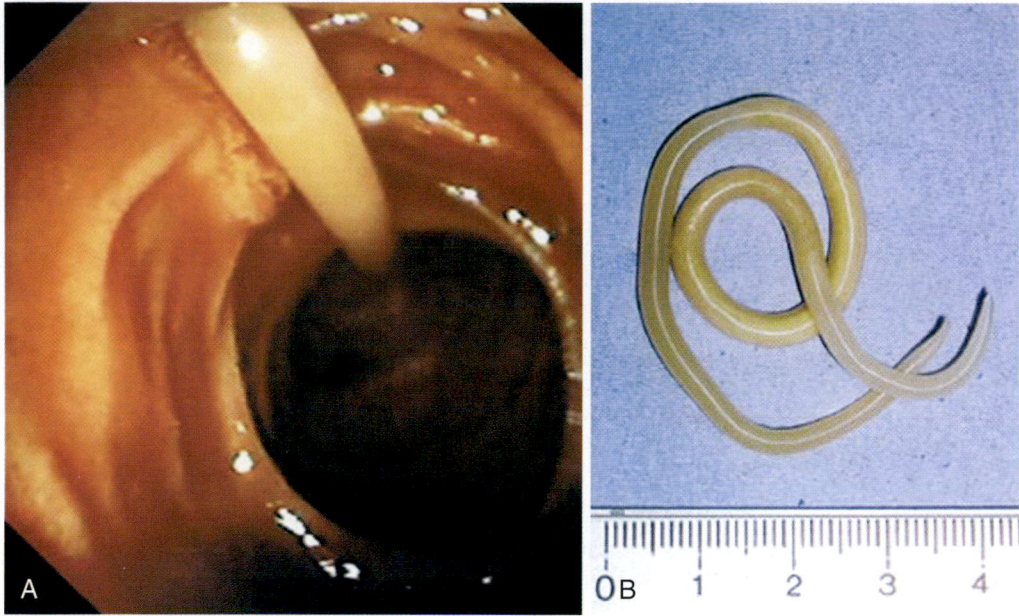

FIGURE 114-2. *A*, Endoscopic view of *Ascaris lumbricoides* partially within the ampulla of Vater. *B*, *A. lumbricoides* after removal. *(From Esser-Kochling BG, Hirsch FW. Images in clinical medicine.* Ascaris lumbricoides *blocking the common bile duct. N Engl J Med 2005; 352:e4.)*

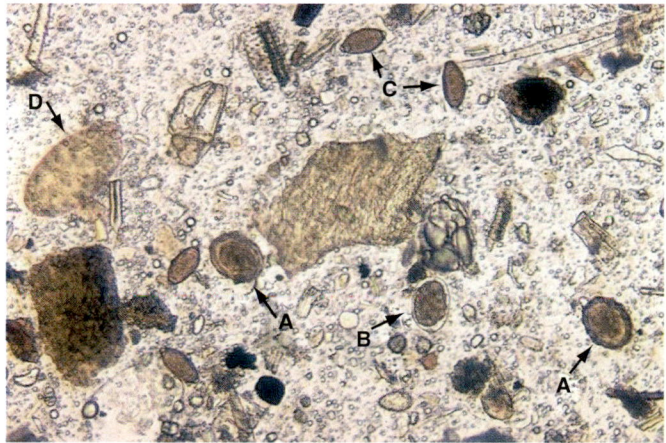

FIGURE 114-3. Wet prep of a stool specimen containing helminth eggs. *A, Ascaris lumbricoides. B,* Hookworm. *C, Trichuris trichiura. D, Fasciolopsis buski. (Courtesy Mae Melvin, MD, Atlanta, Ga.)*

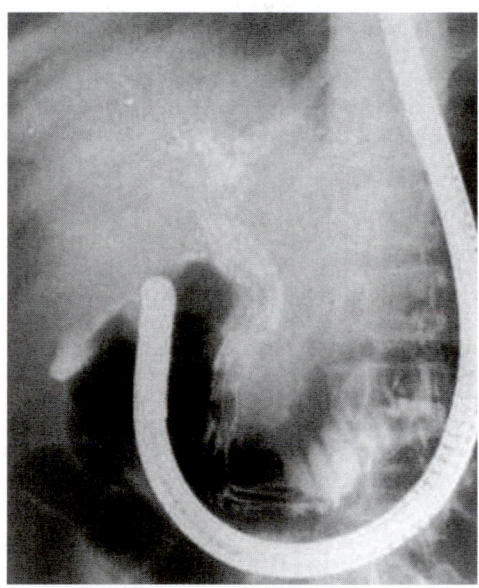

FIGURE 114-4. Film from an ERCP showing several *Ascaris lumbricoides* in the bile duct. *(From van den Bogaerde JB, Jordaan M. Intraductal administration of albendazole for biliary ascariasis. Am J Gastroenterol 1997; 92:1531-3.)*

Treatment

Asymptomatic colonization with *A. lumbricoides* is treated easily with a single 400-mg oral dose of albendazole.[28] Albendazole inhibits glucose uptake and microtubule formation, effectively paralyzing the worms. Albendazole is poorly absorbed but is still considered possibly teratogenic, and when possible, treatment of pregnant women with this agent should be delayed until after delivery. Previously, clinicians who work in endemic countries would avoid treatment of pregnant women; however, in areas where repeated pregnancy is common, this resulted in prolonged avoidance of potentially life-saving therapy. A recent study of 1257 women treated with albendazole showed no adverse effect of albendazole treatment on birth weight, perinatal mortality, or congenital anomaly compared with placebo.[29] Single-dose mebendazole also is efficacious for *Ascaris*.[30] A study of 1042 pregnant women in Peru found no adverse effect of a single 500-mg oral dose of mebendazole on birth outcomes.[31]

Patients with pulmonary ascariasis should be treated with glucocorticoids to reduce the pneumonitis and be given 2 400-mg doses of albendazole 1 month apart. Because albendazole is poorly absorbed, ascaricidal tissue concentrations are not achieved. The first dose kills mature worms that have finished their migration to the intestine, and the second dose kills worms that were in transit when the first dose was given. Albendazole is well tolerated, but can cause nausea, vomiting, and abdominal pain.

Intestinal ascariasis with obstruction often can be treated conservatively with fluid resuscitation, nasogastric decompression, antibiotics, and 1 dose of albendazole. Surgery is not required unless the patient develops signs of volvulus, intussusception, or peritonitis. If the bowel is viable, an enterotomy allows intraoperative removal of worms. Albendazole may be held until after the obstruction has resolved and then is used to eradicate any remaining organisms.

Hepatobiliary ascariasis also can be treated conservatively with fluid resuscitation, bowel rest, and antibiotics.[32] Worms in the bile duct are not effectively treated with albendazole because the drug is poorly absorbed and not concentrated in bile. This feature of albendazole is advantageous because were paralyzed worms within the duct unable to pass out through the sphincter of Oddi, they could become trapped in the bile duct. Patients with hepatobiliary ascariasis should be treated with albendazole each day for several days, because the worms only become susceptible to the drug after they migrate out of the bile duct.

Worms also can invade the pancreatic duct, and intrapancreatic *Ascaris* can be treated just as hepatobiliary ascariasis.[33] Ascending cholangitis, acute obstructive jaundice, or acute pancreatitis requires emergent ERCP with worm extraction from the ducts by balloon, basket, or forceps—preferably without sphincterotomy. Ampullary sphincterotomy permits worms easier access to the ducts and can increase the risk of recurrent pancreaticobiliary ascariasis.[34]

Strongyloides stercoralis

S. stercoralis is a free-living tropical and semitropical soil helminth, the filariform larvae of which can penetrate intact skin. As a parasite, *Strongyloides* lives in the intestine and lays eggs that hatch while still in the intestine. Filariform larvae develop within the intestine, migrate along defined paths, and mature to increase the number of adult parasites in the host; this results in prolonged infection that may extend to 75 years after one leaves an endemic area.[35] Immunosuppression and glucocorticoid treatment cause fulminant disease due to enhanced reproduction of parasites that can prove fatal. Treatment is ivermectin.

Epidemiology

S. stercoralis is endemic in tropical and semitropical regions, but it can also be acquired in the rural southeastern United States and northern Italy. *Strongyloides* exists as a free-living organism that does not require a host to replicate. Improved sanitation does not remove the risk of acquiring the parasite from soil. Patients from endemic areas, military veterans who served in Asia, and prisoners of war are at high risk for subclinical strongyloidiasis.

Life Cycle

Adult male and female *S. stercoralis* live in the soil and lay eggs that hatch rhabditiform larvae. Rhabditiform larvae develop in the soil into mature adults to complete the life cycle of this worm. Rhabditiform larvae (250 μm) also can develop into longer (500 μm) infective filariform larvae that can penetrate any area of skin that contacts soil, after which they migrate through the dermis to enter the cutaneous vasculature. The larvae circulate with the venous blood until they reach the lungs, where they break into the alveoli and ascend the bronchial tree. The worms then are swallowed with bronchial secretions and pass into the small intestine, where they embed in the jejunal mucosa and mature. Female *S. stercoralis* can lay fertile eggs by parthenogenesis and therefore do not require

males to reproduce. The eggs hatch within the small intestine, and rhabditiform larvae migrate into the lumen. Rhabditiform larvae, not eggs, are passed in the stool.

A critical feature of *S. stercoralis* infestation is that some rhabditiform larvae sporadically develop into infective filariform larvae within the intestine. Filariform larvae are able to reinfect (autoinfect) the patient, thereby increasing the parasite burden and permitting prolonged colonization so that subclinical strongyloidiasis can exist for many decades after the host has left an endemic area.

Clinical Features and Pathophysiology

Most patients with *S. stercoralis* infestation have no abdominal symptoms. Patients with autoinfection, however, might develop a serpiginous urticarial rash (larva currens) caused by the rapid (5 to 10 cm/hour) dermal migration of filariform larvae, usually on the buttocks and resulting from larvae that enter the perianal skin after they exit the anus. A study of prisoners of war found this creeping eruption to be a far more common symptom of chronic strongyloidiasis than were GI complaints.[36] Occasionally, patients have nausea, abdominal pain, or unexplained occult GI blood loss from *S. stercoralis*. The parasite also can cause colonic inflammation that resembles UC but is more right-sided and strongly eosinophilic.[37-39]

While the parasite burden remains balanced, symptoms are minimal or absent. Immunosuppression or glucocorticoid administration upsets this balance, with the result that previously asymptomatic, but chronically infested, patients develop fulminant, potentially fatal strongyloidiasis from massive autoinfection.[40] The mechanisms that permit massive autoinfection are unknown, but events that inhibit Th2-directed immune responses can release eosinophil-mediated control of the parasites. In addition, glucocorticoids can act directly on the parasites to increase the development of infective filariform larvae. Fulminant disseminated strongyloidiasis rarely complicates HIV and AIDS.[41]

Massive autoinfection produces disseminated fulminant strongyloidiasis. Migrating filariform larvae injure the intestinal mucosa and carry luminal bacteria into the bloodstream, resulting in polymicrobial sepsis with enteric organisms. *Streptococcus bovis* endocarditis or meningitis[42] also can result. Numerous larvae migrating through the lungs cause pneumonitis, and worms can arrive in unusual locations such as the brain. Fulminant strongyloidiasis often is fatal.

Diagnosis

A survey of U.S. physicians in training demonstrated very poor ability to identify or even consider strongyloidiasis in a Southeast Asian immigrant with new onset.[43] Patients with chronic strongyloidiasis often are asymptomatic. Peripheral blood eosinophils may be elevated, but a normal eosinophil count does not argue against infestation with this parasite. Currently, the best method for detecting previous exposure is enzyme-linked immunosorbent assay (ELISA) for immunoglobulin (Ig) G antibodies against *S. stercoralis*. This assay is performed by the CDC in the United States and is 95% sensitive,[44] sensitivity being highest for immigrants with prolonged exposure and lowest for returning visitors with lower-level recently acquired infestation.[45]

False-positive reactions can occur in patients that have been exposed to other helminthic parasites,[46] and serologic positivity can indicate prior exposure to *S. stercoralis*, not necessarily active infestation. Because chronic strongyloidiasis can remain subclinical and difficult to detect for decades, however, treatment of seropositive patients is warranted. Indeed, some argue that patients with only suspected strongyloidiasis, such as immigrants from endemic countries who have elevated eosinophil counts, should be treated empirically before they are treated with glucocorticoids.[40]

Active infestation can be diagnosed by finding rhabditiform larvae in direct smears of the stool, though this is an insensitive method. A 10-fold more sensitive technique is to spread stool on an agar plate and look for serpentine tracks left by migrating larvae.[47] Intestinal biopsy is also an insensitive means of diagnosis.

Treatment

Chronic strongyloidiasis is best treated with 1 dose of oral ivermectin (200 µg/kg); this dose is used in both adult and pediatric patients. Ivermectin is better tolerated than thiabendazole. Ivermectin paralyzes the intestinal adult worms but not the larvae migrating through tissue, and therefore patients can develop recurrent infestation from migrating larvae; a repeat dose after 2 weeks helps to prevent this outcome. Successful treatment causes a fall in antibody titer by 6 months in most (≈90%) patients.[44] Immunocompromised patients require repeat doses given 2, 15, and 16 days after the first dose.[48]

Capillaria (Paracapillaria) philippinensis

Capillariasis is acquired by eating raw fish infested with the parasite.[49] The nematode causing capillariasis has been renamed from *Capillaria philippinensis* to *Paracapillaria philippinensis*,[50] but by any name, it is deadly. The parasite replicates in the host, producing an ever-increasing number of intestinal worms. Patients develop protein-losing, sprue-like diarrhea with progressive emaciation and anasarca, which ultimately leads to death, absent treatment. Treatment is albendazole.

Epidemiology

The first known human case of capillariasis was reported in 1964, and it remains a rare but deadly parasitic infestation. From 1965 through 1968, an epidemic in the rural Philippines involved 229 cases, with an overall mortality rate of 30%.[51] As the name implies, *Paracapillaria philippinensis* is endemic to the Philippines, but it also is endemic in Thailand and recently has been reported in Egypt.[52] Cases also occur in Japan, Taiwan, and Iran. Modern travel transports cases worldwide.[53]

Life Cycle

Birds, not humans, are the natural hosts for *P. philippinensis*. In the avian small intestine, the larvae mature into adults. The adults are very small, measuring up to 3.9 mm for males and 5.3 mm for females. Adult worms mate and produce eggs are deposited in bird droppings into ponds and rivers and are swallowed by fish to complete the life cycle.

People become infested with the worm by eating raw or undercooked freshwater or brackish-water fish that contain the parasitic larvae. Some female adult *P. philippinensis* are larviparous and produce infective larvae instead of eggs, which then mature in the small intestine and increase the parasite burden. This pathway of autoinfection permits a massive increase in parasite numbers as shown by a rhesus monkey that originally was fed 27 larvae and had more than 30,000 worms by 162 days of infection.[54]

Clinical Features and Pathophysiology

Capillariasis produces a progressive sprue-like illness. Symptoms begin with vague abdominal pain and borborygmi. Two or 3 weeks after infection, patients begin to have diarrhea.

Initially intermittent, diarrhea becomes persistent and increasingly voluminous. Patients rapidly waste from escalating steatorrhea and protein-losing enteropathy. Eventually they manifest emaciation, anasarca, and hypotension; diarrhea produces severe hypokalemia. If untreated, patients die from cardiac failure or secondary bacterial sepsis, usually about 2 months after the initial onset of symptoms.

The progressive disease is believed to result from an ever-increasing number of poorly adapted intestinal parasites. In autopsy studies, the jejunal intestinal mucosa showed flattened, denuded villi with numerous plasma cells, lymphocytes, macrophages, and neutrophils infiltrating the lamina propria.[49]

Diagnosis

Diagnosis is made by finding eggs and larvae in stool specimens. No serologic tests for capillariasis are available. Symptomatic patients have detectable eggs in their stool. The eggs are easily confused with those of *Trichuris trichiura*, but *T. trichiura* eggs have prominent bipolar plugs that appear cut off in *P. phillipinensis*.[49]

Treatment

Capillariasis requires extended antihelminthic treatment with albendazole 200 mg orally twice daily for 10 days or mebendazole 200 mg orally twice daily for 20 days to prevent recurrence. Albendazole is better tolerated than mebendazole, though either can cause headache, diarrhea, and abdominal pain. Extended treatment is necessary because larvae are resistant to these agents.

Hookworms (*Necator americanus, Ancylostoma spp.*)

Worldwide, an estimated 740 million people are infested with hookworm,[15] usually by *Necator americanus, Ancylostoma duodenale*, or a mixture of the 2. Hookworm is acquired by skin contact with contaminated soil. Moderate infestation contributes to iron deficiency. Hookworm should be suspected in patients with eosinophilia and iron deficiency anemia. *Ancylostoma ceylanicum* has a broad host range including domestic pets and people. *Ancylostoma caninum* is a dog and cat parasite that is a cause of eosinophilic enteritis in humans. Treatment is albendazole.

Necator americanus *and* Ancylostoma duodenale

Epidemiology

The geographic distribution of *N. americanus* and *A. duodenale* extensively overlap, but *N. americanus* predominates in the Americas, South Pacific, Indonesia, southern India, and central Africa, whereas *A. duodenale* is more common in North Africa, the Middle East, Europe, Pakistan, and northern India. Hookworm infestation is acquired by contacting soil that has been contaminated with human waste. Hookworm is endemic in tropical to warm temperate areas that lack adequate sewage facilities. Indigenous hookworm infestation largely has been eradicated in the United States, although small pockets of transmission still exist.

Life Cycle

Infective third-stage hookworm larvae penetrate intact skin, typically between the toes while one is walking barefoot on contaminated ground. Larvae migrate through the dermis to

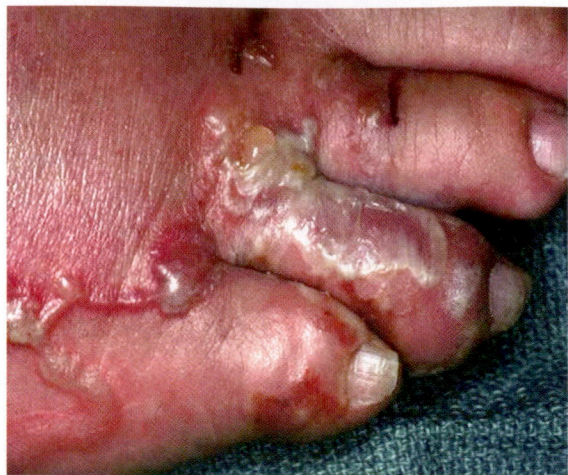

FIGURE 114-5. Serpiginous rash on the foot caused by hookworm larvae migrating through the dermis. *(Courtesy University of Iowa Department of Dermatology, Iowa City, Ia.)*

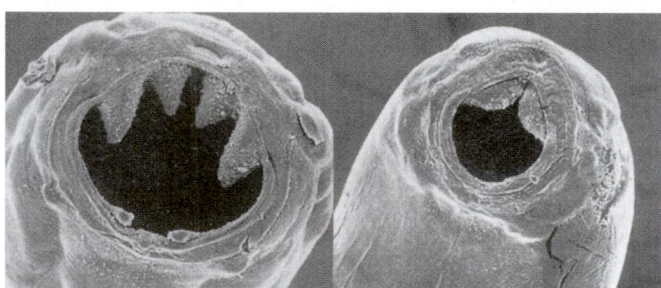

FIGURE 114-6. Scanning electron micrographic view of the buccal cavities of *Ancylostoma duodenale* (left) and *Necator americanus* (right). *(From Hotez PJ, Pritchard DI. Hookworm infection. Sci Am 1995; 272:70-4.)*

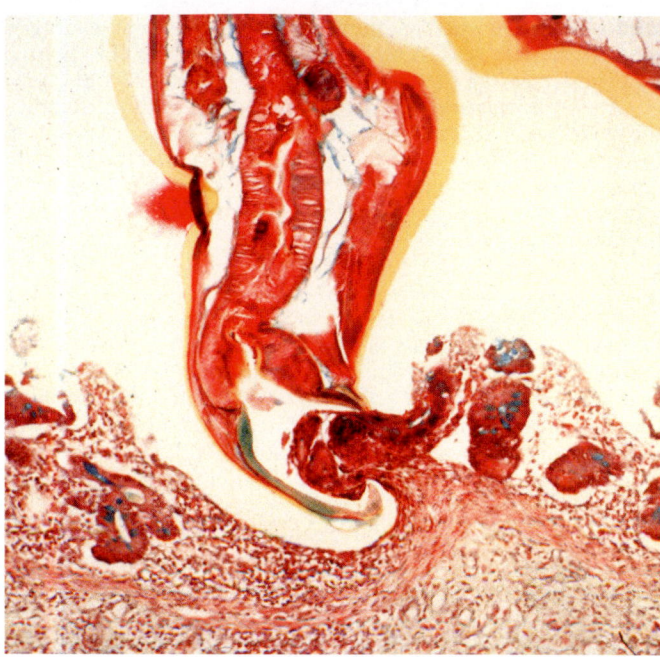

FIGURE 114-7. Longitudinal section of a hookworm grazing on intestinal mucosa. *(Courtesy Wayne M. Meyers, Washington, D.C.)*

TABLE 114-1 A Comparison of Daily Physiologic Iron Loss and Iron Loss Due to Hookworm Infection in Women*

Condition	Iron Loss (mg/day)
Physiologic Loss	
Menstruation	0.44
Pregnancy	2.14
Lactation	0.23
Loss Due to Hookworm Infection	
Necator americanus (60-200 worms)	1.10
Ancylostoma duodenale (20-100 worms)	2.30

*Losses shown are in addition to the basal iron loss of 0.72 mg/day.
Adapted from Stoltzfuss RJ, Dreyfuss ML, Chwaya HM, Albonico M. Hookworm control as a strategy to prevent iron deficiency. Nutr Rev 1997; 55:223-32.

reach blood vessels, a migration that can cause a pruritic, serpiginous rash, cutaneous larva migrans (Fig. 114-5). *Ancylostoma braziliense* normally infests dogs and cats, but it produces a similar rash during infective dermal wandering in humans and is the usual cause of cutaneous larva migrans. Larvae of *N. americanus* and *A. duodenale* enter blood vessels in the skin and migrate with venous flow through the right side of the heart to the lungs. *A. duodenale* larvae can arrest their migration and become dormant for many months before proceeding to the lungs.[55] Once in the lungs, larvae penetrate the alveoli and enter the air spaces, after which they migrate up the pulmonary tree, are swallowed with saliva, and pass into the small intestine, where they mature. Patients also can acquire *A. duodenale* by directly ingesting larvae crawling on contaminated fresh vegetables. Adult worms develop large buccal cavities and graze on the intestinal mucosa, ingesting epithelial cells and blood (Figs. 114-6 and 114-7). Adults are about 1 centimeter long and can live for up to 14 years. Mature worms mate and lay eggs. Each female *N. americanus* lays about 10,000 eggs a day, and each female *A. duodenale* lays about 20,000 eggs a day. Intensity of infection is usually measured by the eggs per gram of stool: light, fewer than 1999; moderate, 2000 to 3999; heavy, more than 4000. Eggs are deposited with feces in moist, shady soil, where they hatch to release larvae. The larvae molt twice, after which they move to the soil surface and await a suitable host.

Clinical Features and Pathophysiology

Light infestations with *N. americanus* and *A. duodenale* cause no symptoms.[56] The major consequence of moderate and heavy hookworm infestation is iron deficiency. Adult worms feed on intestinal epithelial cells and blood. The closely related *A. caninum* (see later) secretes anticoagulant peptides that inhibit clotting factors[57] and platelet aggregation,[58] thereby preventing hemostasis and permitting the hematophagous parasites to feed on host blood. Intestinal blood loss is estimated to be 0.01 to 0.04 mL/day per adult *N. americanus* and 0.05 to 0.3 mL/day per adult *A. duodenale.*[59] With a moderate number of worms, this blood loss becomes appreciable (Table 114-1). Iron deficiency results when iron loss outstrips iron absorption. The average North American diet is high in iron, so anemia might not develop, and men with a diet high in iron (>20 mg/day) can tolerate a burden of up to 800 adult hookworms without developing anemia.

Infestation with hookworm has been shown to modulate immune responses.[60] Clinical trials are underway or have recently been completed to determine if subclinical infestation

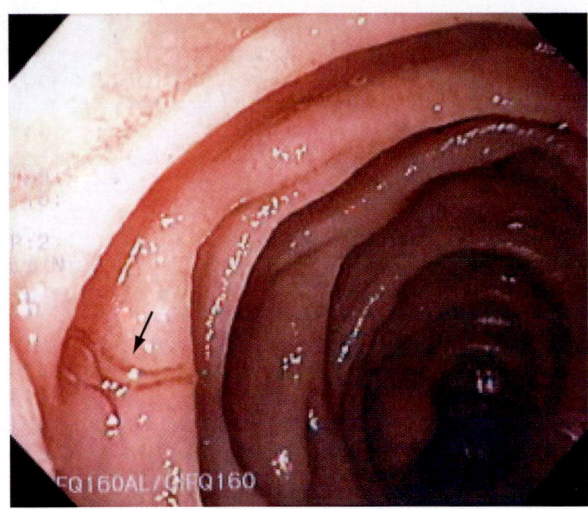

FIGURE 114-8. Endoscopic view of *Necator americanus* in the duodenum *(arrow). (From Reddy SC, Vega KJ. Endoscopic diagnosis of chronic severe upper GI bleeding due to helminthic infection. Gastrointest Endosc 2008; 67:990-2.)*

with hookworm inhibits immune-mediated disease such as Crohn's disease, asthma, and celiac disease. Dose-ranging studies in healthy volunteers suggested that low-level (light) hookworm infestation (10 larvae) is well tolerated.[61] Treatment in asthma was well tolerated but led to a non-significant reduction in airway responsiveness.[62] Although infection with *N. americanus* suppressed mucosal interferon (IFN)-γ and interleukin (IL)-17A production,[63] it did not suppress intestinal inflammation from gluten challenge in patients with celiac disease.[64]

Diagnosis

Hookworms can be visible endoscopically (Fig. 114-8),[65] including by videocapsule endoscopy,[66] but diagnosis is made by identifying eggs on direct smears of formalin-fixed stool (see Fig. 114-3). Evaluation of 3 stool specimens obtained on separate days should permit diagnosis of hookworm,[67] but light infestations can require concentration techniques. Eggs mature rapidly at room temperature and can hatch to release larvae. It is difficult to distinguish *N. americanus* eggs from those of *A. duodenale* simply by morphology.

Treatment

Albendazole 400 mg given orally as a single dose is adequate treatment for hookworm. Mebendazole 100 mg given orally twice daily for 3 days also is effective but not as well tolerated. *A. duodenale* larvae can remain in a dormant state for months before maturing and causing relapse, a situation that is treated with a repeat course of albendazole or mebendazole. Albendazole is an FDA pregnancy category C medication, though a recent study showed no treatment-associated fetal or maternal adverse effects.[29] There is a concerted effort to develop a vaccine for hookworm infections that would be used in endemic regions.[68]

Ancylostoma ceylanicum

Epidemiology, Life Cycle, and Clinical Features

A. ceylanicum is unusual in that it can establish productive infection in a broad range of hosts. Although infections with

human hookworm (*N. americanus* and *A. duodenale*) remain much more common, human infections with *A. ceylanicum* have been reported in West New Guinea, Philippines, Taiwan, Thailand, India, Laos, and Malaysia.[69] A study performed in remote West Malaysia used molecular techniques to identify hookworm eggs passed in feces. They found that 9% of villagers and 92% of their pets were infected with hookworm. In the villagers, 80% of the samples could be analyzed and showed that 23.4% of people with hookworm carried *A. ceylanicum* either alone or with *N. americanus* co-infection. In their pets, 52% carried *A. caninum* and 46% carried *A. ceylanicum*, suggesting that these animals could serve as reservoirs for the parasite.[69] Light infections with *A. ceylanicum* can be asymptomatic, but heavy infections can cause anemia.

Pathophysiology, Diagnosis, and Treatment

A. ceylanicum matures to adulthood in the human host and probably shares similar pathophysiology with *N. americanus* and *A. duodenale*. Like those strictly human hookworms, adult *A. ceylanicum* can be observed endoscopically.[70] Formal diagnosis is by identifying eggs in the stool, but the eggs of *A. ceylanicum* are not distinguishable from those of *N. americanus* and *A. duodenale* without resorting to molecular techniques. Treatment is with oral albendazole 400 mg given as a single dose. If the patient has close contacts with pets, the pets should be tested and treated if positive.

Ancylostoma caninum

Epidemiology and Life Cycle

A. caninum is a common hookworm of dogs and cats. It has worldwide distribution and is prevalent in the Northern Hemisphere. The parasite exists in areas with adequate sanitation because dogs and cats indiscriminately defecate in yards, parks, and sandboxes. The life cycle of *A. caninum* is similar to that of *A. duodenale*, and the worm can be acquired orally; however, *A. caninum* does not fully mature in the human host, so no eggs are produced, thereby making diagnosis difficult.

Clinical Features and Pathophysiology

A. caninum is a well-recognized cause of cutaneous larva migrans, a distinctive serpiginous rash caused by an abortive migration of the parasite in an unsupportive host.[71] *A. caninum* also can cause eosinophilic enteritis, although not all eosinophilic enteritis is caused by this parasite (see Chapter 29). Patients with eosinophilic enteritis from *A. caninum* often are dog owners and present with colicky mid-abdominal pain and peripheral eosinophilia,[72] but they do not recall having cutaneous larva migrans. Intestinal biopsies show high numbers (>45/high-power field) of mucosal eosinophils,[73] and eosinophilic inflammation is most prevalent in the distal small intestine. Unlike eosinophilic gastroenteritis, tissue eosinophilia is not present in the stomach. On endoscopy of the terminal ileum, patients may have scattered small superficial aphthous ulcers and mucosal hemorrhage.[74] Serologic evidence suggests that *A. caninum* also may be a cause of abdominal pain without eosinophilia or eosinophilic enteritis.[72]

Diagnosis

Diagnosis of *A. caninum* infestation is difficult. The parasite never fully matures, does not lay eggs, and is hard to detect. Serologic tests for *A. caninum* are research tools not routinely available. Therefore, treatment for *A. caninum* is empirical.

Treatment

Patients with distal small intestinal eosinophilic enteritis not attributable to another cause might benefit from empirical treatment for *A. caninum*. Albendazole 400 mg as a single oral dose or mebendazole 100 mg orally twice daily for 3 days is adequate to treat *A. caninum* infestation. Albendazole is an FDA pregnancy category C medication, though a recent study showed no treatment-associated fetal or maternal adverse effects.[29]

Whipworm *(Trichuris trichiura)*

T. trichiura, commonly called *whipworm*, has worldwide distribution. People acquire *Trichuris* by ingesting embryonated parasite eggs. Most persons have no symptoms, although heavy infestations are associated with a dysentery-like syndrome. Treatment is mebendazole.

Epidemiology

An estimated 800 million people harbor *T. trichiura*. It occurs in temperate and tropical countries and remains prevalent in areas with suboptimal sanitation. In 1 equatorial Cameroon province, 97% of the school-age children had *T. trichiura*.[75] Whipworm eggs are sensitive to desiccation, so prevalence is low in desert climates.

Life Cycle

T. trichiura has a simple life cycle. Colonization occurs by ingesting the parasite egg, each of which contains 1 developed larva. The eggs hatch in the intestine, and larvae migrate to the cecum, where they mature, mate, and lay eggs; this process takes about 8 to 12 weeks. Adult worms are approximately 3 centimeters long and have a thin tapered anterior region so that the worm resembles a whip (Fig. 114-9, Video 114-2).[76] A mature female worm lays about 20,000 eggs a day and can live for 3 years. Eggs are deposited with feces into the soil. Over the next 2 to 6 weeks, 1 larva develops within each egg, but the egg is not infective until it has fully embryonated. Therefore, *T. trichiura* does not multiply in the host and is not directly transmitted to other persons.

Clinical Features and Pathophysiology

Most persons with *T. trichiura* infestation have no symptoms attributable to the parasite. The majority of residents in an

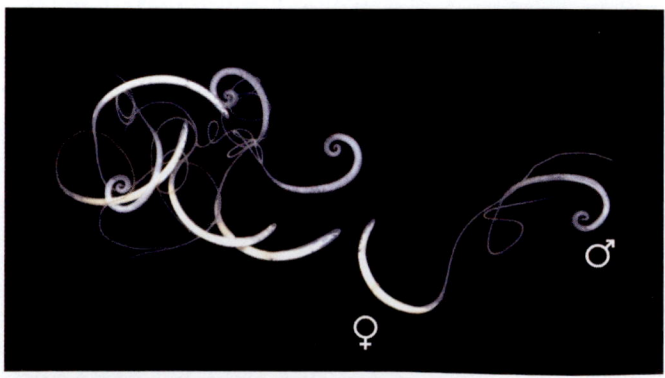

FIGURE 114-9. *Trichuris* species: Adult male (♂) and female (♀) whipworms.

endemic area are colonized by small numbers (<15) of worms and, for them, the parasite is a commensal organism rather than a pathogen. Some people harbor hundreds or even thousands of worms,[77] and they are the ones who develop symptoms[78]; this bimodal distribution of infestation persists after patients are treated and then become reinfected naturally, suggesting that unique host factors (genetic or behavioral) contribute to determining an individual patient's worm burden.

Rectal prolapse can occur in children with extremely high numbers of *T. trichiura* worms.[79] Some persons who harbor numerous worms have mucoid diarrhea and occasional bleeding, a combination of symptoms called the *Trichuris* dysentery syndrome (TDS). Children with this condition have growth retardation,[80] but studies attributing these symptoms to *T. trichiura* are complicated because persons with TDS often are socioeconomically deprived and may be co-infected with other pathogens. Colonic biopsy specimens from children with TDS show few or no abnormalities compared with healthy local children,[81] other than an increase in mast cells and in the number of cells that express TNF-α and calprotectin.[82]

A different but closely related species, *Trichuris muris*, infests mice. Mouse strains that react to the parasite with a strong Th2 response, characterized by production of IL-4, IL-5, and IL-13, are able to expel the worms, whereas strains that respond with a Th1 response (IFN-γ) have difficulty expelling the worms.[83] Blocking IL-4 makes resistant strains susceptible, and blocking IFN-γ makes susceptible strains resistant to chronic infestation with *T. muris*.[84] The type of immune response developed by inbred mice to *T. muris* is an important factor in determining length and intensity of infestation. A similar response in humans might explain why some people repeatedly acquire heavy infestations, whereas others carry only a few worms. Yet another closely related species is *Trichuris suis*, porcine whipworm. This organism is being evaluated in clinical trials to determine if it may be useful for treatment of chronic inflammatory conditions based on the immunologic responses it may engender.[85]

Diagnosis

Diagnosis is made by identifying *T. trichiura* eggs in stool specimens. *Trichuris* eggs are 23 μm × 50 μm and have characteristic plugs at each end (see Fig. 114-3).

Treatment

T. trichiura is treated with mebendazole 100 mg twice a day for 3 days; alternatively, patients can take albendazole 400 mg each day for 3 days. Heavily infested patients might require 7 days of treatment.[86] Single-dose treatment with albendazole is ineffective,[30] but 1 treatment with a combination of albendazole (400 mg) and ivermectin (200 μg/kg) appears quite effective, with cure rates of up to 80% and egg reduction rates of 94%.[87,88] Albendazole is an FDA pregnancy category C medication, though a recent study showed no treatment-associated fetal or maternal adverse effects.[29]

Pinworm *(Enterobius vermicularis)*

E. vermicularis, commonly called *pinworm*, is the most common helminthic parasite encountered by primary care providers in developed nations. It is acquired by ingesting parasite eggs, and most people remain asymptomatic after being colonized. Diagnosis is made by the cellophane tape test. Treatment is mebendazole for the affected patient and for all family members.

Epidemiology

E. vermicularis is a quintessential intestinal parasite with no geographic constraints. It is transmissible by close contact with colonized persons. People have had pinworm for thousands of years, and before modern sanitation, colonization by pinworm probably was universal. *E. vermicularis* eggs were identified in a 10,000-year-old human coprolite found in Utah.[89] The pinworm *Enterobius gregorii*, originally thought to be a separate species of pinworm,[90,91] actually may be just a young adult form of *E. vermicularis*.[92]

People of every socioeconomic group can acquire pinworm, and it remains quite prevalent. School-age children are most often colonized, compelling other household members to acquire the parasite. Crowding and institutionalization promotes acquisition. Eggs can survive in the environment for approximately 15 to 20 days and are resistant to chlorinated water (e.g., swimming pools).

Pinworm remains common in many areas, but it appears to be decreasing in prevalence because of increased hygiene. A survey of positive cellophane tape tests (see later) in New York City documented a sharp decline in positivity from 57 of 248 tests in 1971 to 17 of 165 in 1978 to 0 of 38 in 1986.[93] Similar trends are reported from California.

Life Cycle

E. vermicularis has a simple life cycle with a "hand-to-mouth" existence. The worm is acquired by ingesting parasite eggs. Most often these eggs are on the hands of the host; however, the small eggs also may become airborne, inhaled, and then swallowed.

Eggs hatch in the duodenum, releasing larvae that molt twice as they mature and migrate to the cecum and ascending colon (Fig. 114-10, Video 114-3).[94] The parasites are small: adult males measure 0.2 mm × 2 to 5 mm, and adult females measure 0.5 mm × 8 to 13 mm. After mating, gravid females migrate to the rectum. During the night, egg-laden females migrate out of the anal canal and onto the perianal skin, where each female deposits up to 17,000 eggs, which

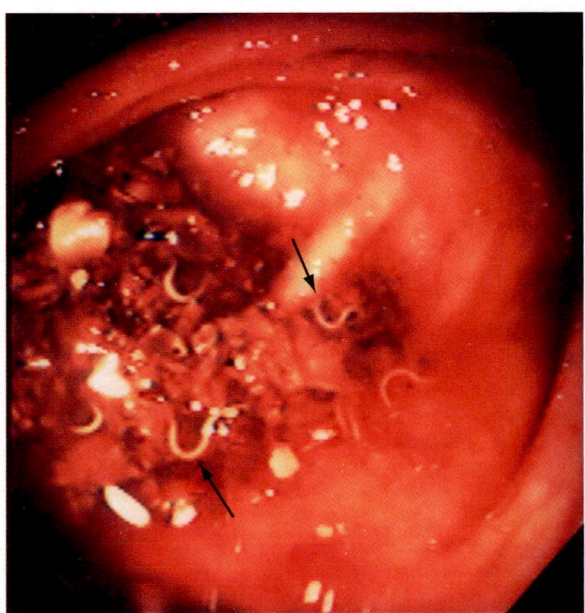

FIGURE 114-10. Pinworm *(Enterobius vermicularis; arrows)* found on screening colonoscopy of an institutionalized man.

mature rapidly, becoming infective within 6 hours. Pinworm infestation typically causes perianal itching, and scratching gathers eggs onto the hands, promoting reinfection and transmission to others.

Clinical Features and Pathophysiology

E. vermicularis is an extremely well adapted parasite that produces no specific symptoms in the vast majority of colonized persons. Most symptoms are minor, such as pruritus ani and restless sleeping. Rarely, pinworm causes eosinophilia or eosinophilic enteritis.[95] There are reports of *E. vermicularis* escaping into the peritoneum at the time of laparoscopic appendectomy.[96] This is treated with prompt disposal of the appendix, removal of identifiable free worms, and oral mebendazole administered postoperatively.

Vulvovaginitis is more common in girls with pinworm than in girls without this infection. Vulvovaginitis may be caused by migration of the worms into the introitus and the genital tract. Dead worms and eggs encased in granulomas have been found in the cervix, endometrium, fallopian tubes, and peritoneum, attesting to the migratory effort of female worms.[97] Ectopic enterobiasis is rare and causes no or very little overt pathology.

Infestation with *E. vermicularis* can influence mucosal immune responses. One case report described a 12-year-old girl with pinworm and apparently latent UC, who developed severe UC after treatment with pyrantel to remove the worms.[98] While she was colonized with *E. vermicularis*, intestinal biopsies showed increased expression of mRNA for IL-4, transforming growth factor (TGF)-β, IL-10, and *FOXP3* compared with biopsy specimens taken after anthelminthic treatment; these transcripts are associated with immune regulatory pathways that suppress inflammation.

Diagnosis

E. vermicularis eggs are not plentiful in stool, an observation that might explain the low prevalence rates found in studies that only use stool specimens for diagnosis. The NIH cellophane tape test is the classic diagnostic test for pinworm. A 2- to 3-inch piece of clear tape is applied serially to several perianal areas in the morning before washing. The tape is then applied to a glass slide. Microscopic evaluation demonstrates parasite eggs that measure 30 × 60 μm, have a thin shell, and appear flattened on 1 side. Three to 7 daily samples are needed to exclude pinworm infestation.

Treatment

Pinworm infestation actually requires no treatment unless the patient is symptomatic. It is highly transmittable, however, and for that reason should be expunged. *E. vermicularis* is readily treated with a single 100-mg oral dose of mebendazole or a 400-mg oral dose of albendazole. Reinfestation is common, and patients should receive a second treatment after 15 days. All members of the family should be treated, and clothes and bed linens should be washed. Albendazole and mebendazole are potentially teratogenic. Because *E. vermicularis* has very low pathogenicity, treatment of pregnant women should be postponed until after delivery.

Trichinella Species

Trichinosis is a systemic illness caused by any of the 8 closely related *Trichinella* species. People acquire the parasite by ingesting larvae that are present in raw or undercooked meat such as pork. Trichinosis has both intestinal and systemic phases characterized sequentially by nausea and diarrhea, fever, myalgia, and periorbital edema. Intense exposure can cause death due to severe myositis, neuritis, and thrombosis associated with tissue injury. Treatment is albendazole and glucocorticoids.

Epidemiology

Trichinosis is acquired by eating raw or undercooked meat that contains parasite larvae of *Trichinella* species. Worldwide, domestic pigs are the most common carriers. *Trichinella* species are divided into 2 groups[99]: 1 forms encapsulated muscle cysts and only infests mammals (*Trichinella spiralis*, *Trichinella britovi*, *Trichinella nelsoni*, *Trichinella native*, *Trichinella murrelli*); the other does not form encapsulated cysts and infests mammals and birds (*Trichinella pseudospiralis*) or mammals and reptiles (*Trichinella papuae*, *Trichinella zimbabwensis*). To date, only *T. zimbabwensis* has not been implicated in human disease.

Trichinella species all are closely related, morphologically nearly identical, and today are distinguished using molecular approaches. *Trichinella* has worldwide distribution, with *T. nativa* and *T. murrelli* in the Arctic and subarctic regions; *T. spiralis* and *T. pseudospiralis* in the Americas, Europe, and Russia; *T. britovi* in Europe, North Africa, the Middle East, and Asia; *T. nelsoni* in equatorial Africa; *T. zimbabwensis* in Zimbabwe, Ethiopia, and Mozambique; and *T. papuae* only in Papua New Guinea. Each of the *Trichinella* species can infect any mammal. Trichinosis was much more common in the United States than it is now. In the late 1940s, about 400 cases per year of symptomatic trichinosis were reported to various health agencies, and this number dropped to an average of 9 cases per year in the time period 2002-2007[100]; reports from Germany show a similar pattern.[101] This decrease is explained by 2 major factors: First is the strong admonition to thoroughly cook all pork products; second is a change in farming practice to now feed pigs only grain. Industrialized pig farms in North America have been free of trichinosis for more than 50 years, but trichinosis is a reemerging illness in eastern Europe, related to relaxed enforcement of regulations.[102]

Currently, most reported cases involve a discrete exposure. For example, a 1991 outbreak in Wisconsin involved 40 people who ate pork sausage from 1 shop. A 1995 outbreak in Idaho involved 10 people who ate cougar jerky.[103] A 2005 outbreak in Canada involved at least 14 people who ate frozen then stewed black bear meat.[104] A 2008 outbreak of *T. murrelli* in Northern California involved 30 people who ate raw or undercooked bear meat.[105] In France, several outbreaks have resulted from eating raw horse meat.[106] Outbreaks illustrate that all mammals—including herbivores—can transmit *Trichinella*.

Life Cycle

The same host harbors both the adult and larval form of *Trichinella*.[107] People acquire the parasite by eating raw or undercooked meat that contains encysted parasite larvae. Each cyst dissolves in the digestive tract, releasing 1 larva that invades the small intestinal mucosa and lives within the cytoplasm in a syncytium of about 45 villi (Fig. 114-11). Larvae mature rapidly and mate within 30 hours within the cells. Adults are minute: male worms measure 60 μm × 1.2 mm, and female worms measure 90 μm × 2.2 mm. Females are viviparous and begin releasing larvae into the epithelial cell compartment about 1 week after their initial ingestion. Adults are short-lived, producing larvae for only 4 weeks, by which time they are expelled by the host.

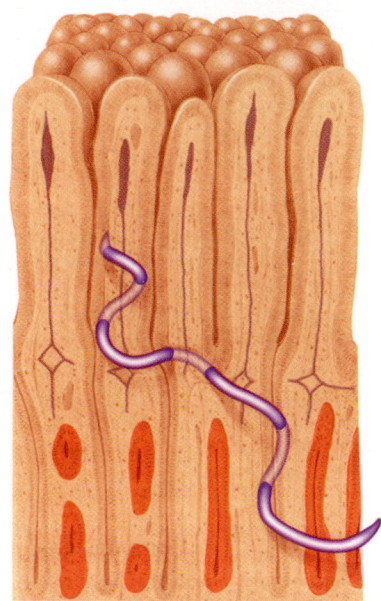

FIGURE 114-11. Illustration of *Trichinella spiralis* coiled through enterocytes in the small intestine. Each *Trichinella* larva lives within the cytoplasm of approximately 45 villus cells.

The larvae live much longer than the adult worms. Larvae measure 6 × 100 μm and enter the intestinal blood and lymphatic vessels. They are distributed by the circulatory system through the body but develop only within striated muscle. A larva enters a striated muscle fiber but does not kill the myocyte. Instead, it induces the cell to transform into a novel nurse cell that houses and feeds the parasite. The larva grows and develops into the infective stage in about 5 weeks. The coiled larva remains viable for many years awaiting ingestion by another animal.

Clinical Features and Pathophysiology

Although most infestations with *Trichinella* are asymptomatic, significant exposure produces illness and even death.[108] Clinical trichinosis has 2 phases caused by the enteral (adult) and parenteral (larval) stages of the parasite. Intestinal symptoms result from enteritis due to adult worms that have embedded themselves in the intestinal epithelium. Enteritis produces abdominal pain, nausea, vomiting, diarrhea, and low-grade fever. Intestinal symptoms begin about 2 days to 1 week and peak at 2 weeks after ingestion of contaminated meat. The timing and severity of symptoms vary with intensity of exposure. The intestinal phase of trichinosis often is misdiagnosed as viral gastroenteritis or food poisoning.

T. spiralis also infests mice and rats, permitting detailed study of the intestinal phase of infection.[109] Mice begin to expel adult worms about 2 weeks after initial infestation. Type 2 (Th2) cytokines (IL-4 and IL-5) promote worm expulsion, which results from focal immune attack, increased secretions, and enhanced intestinal motility; T lymphocytes, eosinophils, and mast cells assist this primary response. Rats previously exposed to *T. spiralis* rapidly expel the parasite upon rechallenge, a protection likely resulting from an immediate-type hypersensitivity response to the parasite triggered by IgE-armed mast cells.

The parenteral phase of trichinosis begins with the birth of migratory larvae about 1 week after ingestion of the contaminated meat. Larvae migrate into muscle and other organs such as the brain, spinal cord, and heart, evoking inflammatory responses; high fever, myalgia, periorbital edema, dysphagia, headache, and paresthesia result. Symptoms peak about 4 to 5 weeks after initial exposure and can take months to resolve. The severity and timing of symptoms vary with the intensity of exposure. Many patients develop systemic complaints without prior intestinal symptoms.

The inflammatory response to damaged cells and secretions deposited by migrating larvae produces myositis. Patients have eosinophilia and an elevated serum level of creatine phosphokinase (CPK). An intense exposure can cause fatal myocarditis, neuritis, and vasculitis or venous thrombosis. Patients are at highest risk of death between the third and sixth week after exposure. Because trichinosis is rare, index cases often are misdiagnosed initially. Numerous persons presenting in a narrow time frame and with similar symptoms compatible with trichinosis should prompt consideration of the diagnosis.

Diagnosis

Trichinella cannot by diagnosed by stool examination or intestinal biopsy. *Trichinella* species do not lay eggs, and no larvae are present in stool specimens. Even with heavy infestations, adult worms are too uncommon to be found by random biopsy. Diagnosis is made by muscle biopsy that demonstrates larvae within nurse cells. Diagnosis also can be made by serology. Acute and convalescent serum samples confirm a rise in anti-*Trichinella* antibody.

Treatment

Although adults are short-lived, treatment with albendazole 400 mg twice a day or mebendazole 5 mg/kg/day for 10 to 15 days[110] is warranted and abbreviates the production of larvae by adult worms. Addition of glucocorticoids reduces inflammation and systemic symptoms; however, glucocorticoids that are given in the absence of albendazole or mebendazole can prolong the intestinal phase, thereby increasing the number of larvae released.

Anisakis simplex

Anisakis simplex and another anisakid, *Pseudoterranova decipiens*, can infect people transiently, causing abdominal pain, hematemesis, or intestinal inflammation. *A. simplex* is also a potent allergen that might explain some cases of fish allergy. Anisakidosis is acquired by eating raw or undercooked fish. No treatment is usually required.

Epidemiology and Life Cycle

A. simplex and *P. decipiens* infest fish and marine mammals.[111] People become accidental hosts by eating raw or pickled fish. Anisakidosis has become more common with the increased popularity of eating raw fish (e.g., sashimi). Many species of saltwater fish harbor *A. simplex* larvae, including herring, mackerel, salmon, plaice, and squid. The parasite larvae initially infest crustaceans that are subsequently consumed by fish. The larvae migrate to the fish musculature and, if a parasitized fish is eaten by another fish, the larvae again migrate to the musculature of their new host. Eventually, a parasitized fish is eaten by a marine mammal that serves as the definitive host. In the intestine of the marine mammal, the parasite larvae matures into adult worms that lay eggs that are passed with feces. The eggs then hatch to release larvae that infest crustaceans, and the life cycle is thus renewed.

Clinical Features and Pathophysiology

A. simplex and *P. decipiens* cause transient infestations in humans. They do not reach full maturity in humans and therefore produce no eggs. The most common GI symptom is acute, severe stomach pain with nausea and hematemesis shortly after eating larva-infested raw fish. Endoscopy may demonstrate a small larva partially penetrating the gastric or intestinal wall.[112,113] Rarely, *A. simplex* can enter the intestinal wall and cause a strong inflammatory reaction that can mimic acute appendicitis[114] or Crohn's disease. Human infestations with either *A. simplex* or *P. decipiens* is termed *anisakidosis* after the family name (Anisakidae) for these parasites.

A. simplex is a potent allergen, and many cases of seafood (fish) allergy actually may be reactions to *A. simplex*,[115] including anaphylaxis from well-cooked marine fish.[116,117] In Spain, 12% to 22% of persons are seropositive for IgE against *A. simplex*.[118,119]

Diagnosis and Treatment

A history of recent (within 3 days) ingestion of raw fish suggests anisakidosis in the appropriately symptomatic patient. Diagnosis is made by finding the larvae on endoscopy or in surgically excised specimens. Gastric anisakidosis is diagnosed by endoscopy, and endoscopic removal of the anisakid alleviates symptoms. Intestinal anisakidosis can prompt surgery for patients presenting with symptoms of acute small bowel obstruction or peritonitis.[120] The latter results from either transmural inflammation or microperforation and peritonitis does not require surgical correction of a significant perforation. In either situation, surgery may be avoidable if a recent history of eating raw fish is elicited and conservative treatment is tolerated.[121]

A. simplex and *P. decipiens* infestations are transient because the parasites do not survive in humans. Therefore, treatment with an anthelminthic is not needed.

CESTODES

Diphyllobothrium Species

Fish tapeworm (*Diphyllobothrium* species) is the largest parasite of humans, reaching lengths of up to 40 feet (12 meters). People acquire the parasite by eating raw or undercooked freshwater fish. *Diphyllobothrium latum* absorbs dietary cobalamin and can cause vitamin B_{12} deficiency over time. Treatment is praziquantel or albendazole.

Epidemiology

D. latum is most common, but other *Diphyllobothrium* species (e.g., *Diphyllobothrium dendriticum*, *D. nihonkaiense*, *D. pacificum*) can colonize humans.[122] *D. latum* is endemic in northern Europe, Russia, and Alaska, but fish tapeworm has been reported in Africa, Japan, Taiwan, Australia, South America, North America, and Canada.[123] About 20 million people worldwide are infected with *Diphyllobothrium* species, and prevalence seems to be increasing in Russia, South Korea, Japan, and Brazil.[122]

Life Cycle

Some *Diphyllobothrium* species infect fresh-water fish (e.g., *D. latum*, *D. dendriticum*), others infect marine fish (e.g., *D. pacificum*, *D. cameroni*), and others infect anadromous (migrating

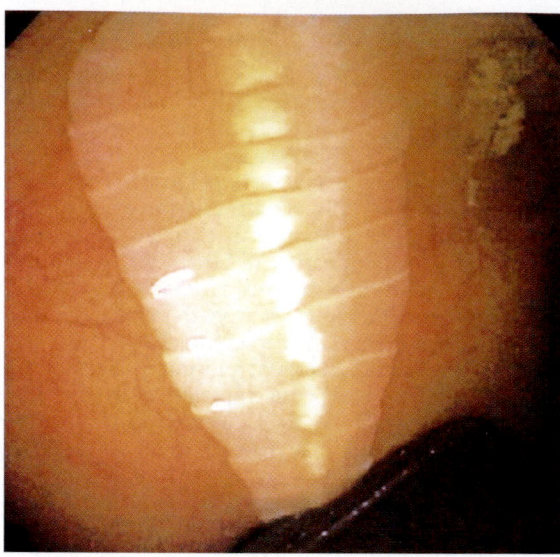

FIGURE 114-12. Endoscopic view of the cecum in a middle-aged woman with watery diarrhea after a fishing trip in Northern Canada during which she frequently ate sushi. Part of a fish tapeworm is seen, and the strobila with maturing proglottids is visible. The worm, which was several feet long, was residing in the small intestine and was retrieved by suction. She was treated successfully with praziquantel. *(Courtesy Dr. Roy Joseph, MD, Denton, Tex.)*

from sea to fresh water to breed) fish (e.g., *D. nihonkaiense*). Fish tapeworm has a complex life cycle with 2 intermediate hosts. Parasite eggs that reach water embryonate and then release free-swimming larvae called *coracidia*. Coracidia are ingested by water fleas (*Cyclops* and *Diaptomus*) and develop into procercoid larvae. Fish eat these small crustaceans, and the parasite changes into the infective plerocercoid form. The plerocercoid larva migrates to and embeds in fish muscle and various organs, growing to 2 centimeters in length. If an infected fish is consumed by another fish, the plerocercoid larva simply migrates into the flesh of the second fish.

Trout, salmon, pike, perch, and whitefish all can harbor *D. latum*. People acquire the parasite by eating raw or undercooked fish. *D. latum* also can colonize many other mammals, such as dogs, cats, bears, and seals. In mammals, the ingested plerocercoid larva attaches to the wall of the small intestine and matures into an adult worm. A long chain of proglottids, called a *strobila*, develops off of the scolex (Fig. 114-12). *D. latum* is the largest parasite of humans, reaching 12 meters (40 feet) in length. The proglottids release eggs into the lumen that pass with the feces.

Clinical Features and Pathophysiology

Fish tapeworm is not invasive and causes no direct symptoms. The worm obtains nutrients by absorbing luminal contents through its surface. *D. latum* produces a substance that splits B_{12} from intrinsic factor in the intestine,[124] thereby preventing host absorption of the vitamin (see Chapter 102). The tapeworm also avidly absorbs B_{12}, effectively competing with its host's use of the vitamin. *D. latum* is long-lived and, over time, can cause significant B_{12} deficiency in patients with limited dietary cobalamin. Rarely, B_{12} deficiency is severe enough to result in megaloblastic anemia and neurologic symptoms.

Diagnosis and Treatment

Fish tapeworm is diagnosed by identifying *D. latum* eggs in stool specimens. Occasionally, diagnosis is made because the patient passes proglottids and brings them in for identification, or the worm is seen on endoscopy.[125] Praziquantel is effective in a single oral dose of 10 mg/kg. Patients should be warned that they might pass a rather long worm 2 to 5 hours after taking the medication. Albendazole 400 mg each day for 3 days also kills the tapeworms. Albendazole is an FDA pregnancy category C medication, though a recent study showed no treatment-associated fetal or maternal adverse effects.[29]

Taenia spp.

An estimated 80 million people are colonized with beef (*Taenia saginata*) or pork (*Taenia solium, Taenia asiatica*) tapeworms. Colonization occurs by eating raw or undercooked meat infested with cysticerci. Taeniae usually cause no symptoms and can surprise an endoscopist who finds the unsuspected jejunal or colonic inhabitant (Videos 114-4 and 114-5).[126,127] Ingestion of *T. solium* eggs causes cysticercosis, a potentially fatal disease. Treatment is praziquantel or albendazole.

Epidemiology

Beef and pork tapeworm occur where livestock are exposed to untreated human waste and people eat raw or undercooked meat. *T. saginata* and *T. solium* have a worldwide distribution, although infestations originating in the United States and Europe are rare. Beef tapeworm is endemic in Africa, the Middle East, Eastern Europe, Asia, and Latin America. *T. solium* is endemic in Africa, India, China, Asia, and Latin America. *T. asiatica* is endemic in Korea, China, Taiwan, and Indonesia.[128] *T. solium* is rare in Muslim countries, where pork consumption is prohibited. *T. solium* is considered an eradicable parasite,[129] though progress in such eradication is hindered by socioeconomic barriers.[130]

Life Cycle

Adult tapeworms release gravid proglottids, each containing up to 100,000 eggs that are released when the proglottid degenerates. Proglottids and eggs are passed with the stool. Proglottids of *T. saginata* remain motile and can crawl out of the feces, alarming the patient. Untreated human waste used to fertilize fields allows cattle to eat infective eggs on vegetation. Free-ranging pigs are coprophagous and directly consume poorly disposed human waste.

Ingested eggs release an embryo (oncosphere) that penetrates the intestinal wall and enters the blood vessels or lymphatics. The oncospheres are carried to subcutaneous tissue, muscle, and organs, where they develop into cysticerci that can live for several years awaiting human consumption of infected meat or viscera. Once in the human intestine, the cysticercus evaginates to form a scolex that serves as the anterior attachment point of the tapeworm to the mucosa of the proximal jejunum. The worm develops over several months as proglottids form and mature in a chain referred to as the *strobila*, located behind the scolex. Beef tapeworms can reach 4 to 10 meters in length, and pork tapeworms attain lengths of 2 to 4 meters. Mature gravid proglottids break away from the distal end of the worm, pass with the stool, and rupture to release eggs to complete the life cycle. Adult tapeworms can live in the small intestine for 25 years.

Clinical Features and Pathophysiology

Most people colonized with adult *T. saginata* or *T. solium* are asymptomatic; those with symptoms complain of mild abdominal discomfort, loss of appetite, or change in stool pattern. Colonization usually is limited to 1 worm that obtains nutrients by absorbing luminal contents through its surface. Motile proglottids can crawl out of the anus or "swim" in the toilet, eliciting immediate concern. Rarely, acute biliary or pancreatic duct obstruction can occur if proglottids migrate into these sites.

The most feared complication of *T. solium* infestation is cysticercosis,[131] which occurs when people inadvertently consume *T. solium* eggs. Just as in pigs, the eggs release oncospheres that penetrate the intestinal wall, disseminate through the body, and form cysticerci. Cysticerci produce localized inflammation in the brain, spinal cord, eye, and heart, with dire consequences. Neurocysticercosis is a common cause of epilepsy in countries where *T. solium* is endemic. Worldwide, an estimated 50,000 people die of neurocysticercosis each year. In the United States, 221 people died from cysticercosis between 1990 and 2002,[132] and it remains a significant cause of morbidity.[133] In Los Angeles County, California, hospitalizations for neurocysticercosis averaged 219/year from 1991 to 2008.[134] Because the disease occurs after ingestion of parasite eggs, neurocysticercosis in a patient who has not visited or emigrated from an endemic country should prompt an effort to identify local carriers.

Diagnosis

Beef and pork tapeworm are diagnosed by identifying eggs or proglottids in stool specimens. The eggs of the 2 species are indistinguishable microscopically. The proglottids of *T. saginata* are 2 centimeters long and have more than 12 uterine branches; those of *T. solium* measure 1.2 cm and have fewer than 10 uterine branches. The proglottids of *T. asiatica* are 1 cm to 1.6 cm in length and have more than 16 uterine branches.[135] Egg and proglottid production can be sporadic, necessitating repeated stool tests. Cysticercosis usually is diagnosed by CT or MRI and may be aided by an enzyme-linked immunoblot transfer blot (EITB), which in the United States is available through the CDC.[136]

Treatment

Tapeworms can be killed either by praziquantel in a single oral dose of 10 mg/kg or albendazole 400 mg daily for 3 days. The worms usually break apart and are passed as sections of disintegrating strobila. Patients with cysticercosis should be treated with albendazole 7.5 mg/kg twice daily for 8 to 15 days to kill the cysticerci. Local inflammation transiently increases as cysticerci die. The addition of glucocorticoids prevents exacerbation of neurocysticercosis during therapy.

Hymenolepis spp.

Hymenolepis nana (dwarf tapeworm) is the smallest but most common tapeworm that colonizes people. It can be transmitted directly from person to person. Self-inoculation or internal autoinfection permits accumulation of a large number of worms that can cause anorexia, abdominal pain, and diarrhea. *Hymenolepis diminuta* (rodent tapeworm) is larger and rarely colonizes people. It is acquired by ingesting infested insects and usually causes no symptoms. Treatment is praziquantel.

Epidemiology

H. nana is the most common tapeworm of humans. Unlike other tapeworms, it can be transmitted from person to person without an intermediate host. Dwarf tapeworm has a worldwide distribution, with highest prevalence in warm and arid regions. A survey of Egyptian children found that 16% carried *H. nana*.[137] In the United States, a 1987 survey of state diagnostic laboratories found that 900 of 216,000 submitted stool specimens demonstrated *H. nana*, with 34 states reporting positive specimens.[138] *H. nana* also colonizes mice and rats; however, the strains that colonize people appear to differ from those of rodents.

Human colonization with *H. diminuta* is rare, but it too has worldwide distribution. Rats and mice are the parasite's usual hosts. People acquire rodent tapeworm by ingesting fleas, grain beetles, mealworms, or cockroaches infested with larval forms of the parasite. Most cases involve young children. The use of beetles in traditional oriental medications also permits transmission.[139]

Life Cycle

H. nana does not require an intermediate insect host. Ingested eggs release oncospheres that invade the mucosa of the small intestine. They lodge within the lymphatics of the villi and develop into cysticercoid larvae. Each cysticercoid larva then ruptures into the lumen and evaginates a scolex that attaches to the mucosa of the ileum. The worms mature, growing a strobila or chain of developing proglottids. Adult worms average 2 centimeters in length and have about 200 proglottids, each containing about 150 eggs. The most distal proglottids disintegrate to release eggs into the lumen. About 20 to 30 days after initial ingestion, the worm begins to shed eggs in the stool. *H. nana* adults live for only 4 to 6 weeks, but eggs shed in the stool are immediately infective. Self-inoculation or internal autoinfection allows colonization to persist for years. Ineffective sanitation or poor hand washing permits transmission to others.

Like other *Hymenolepis* species, *H. nana* can infest insects, forming cysticercoid larvae. Ingestion of infested fleas, beetles, mealworms, or cockroaches allows transmission of *H. nana*; however, acquisition by this pathway is rare, and most transmission is by direct ingestion of eggs.

H. diminuta requires intermediate insect hosts. Insects ingest eggs as they consume rodent droppings. The eggs release oncospheres that penetrate into the insect's viscera and form cysticercoid larvae. Rats and mice that eat infested insects acquire the tapeworm. People acquire rodent tapeworm the same way, by eating infested insects. Once in the intestine, the cysticercoid larva evaginates to form a scolex that attaches to the ileal mucosa. The worm matures, growing a strobila of proglottids and reaching a length of up to 90 cm. The distalmost proglottids disintegrate, releasing eggs into the intestinal lumen.

Clinical Features and Pathophysiology

Most people colonized with *H. nana* or *H. diminuta* have no symptoms, but self-inoculation or internal autoinfection can cause heavy infestations with *H. nana*, resulting in anorexia, abdominal pain, and diarrhea.

Because mice harbor *Hymenolepis*, the mechanisms that limit worm density can be investigated relatively easily. It appears that a Th1-mediated IFN-γ response provides protective immunity against cysticercoid larvae,[140] and a Th2 response involving IgE and mast cells assists in the expulsion of adult worms.[141,142] The mucosal immune response to the tapeworm can also alter intestinal inflammation elicited by other agents; for example, mice colonized with *H. diminuta* are protected from dinitrobenzene sulfonic acid (DNBS)-induced colitis[143] but are more susceptible to oxazalone-induced colitis.[144]

Diagnosis and Treatment

Dwarf and rodent tapeworm are diagnosed by finding parasite eggs in the stool. *H. nana* eggs measure 30 to 47 μm in diameter. The eggs of the much less prevalent *H. diminuta* are larger, measuring 56 to 86 μm in diameter. Examination of several stool specimens taken on different days is needed to identify low-level colonization. Adults of both parasites can be killed with a single oral dose of praziquantel at 25 mg/kg, although eggs escape this treatment. Therefore, patients with *H. nana* infestation should be retreated 1 week after initial treatment. Family members also should be examined and considered for treatment.

Dipylidium caninum

D. caninum (dog tapeworm) is a common parasite of household pets that rarely colonizes children. It is acquired by eating fleas that contain parasite cysticercoid larvae. Dog tapeworm causes no symptoms in humans, but parents who find proglottids crawling in their child's diaper understandably seek medical evaluation. Treatment is praziquantel.

Echinococcus species also are tapeworms of dogs. Ingestion of *Echinococcus granulosus*, *Echinococcus multilocularis*, or *Echinococcus vogeli* eggs causes severe disease due to formation of hydatid cysts (see Chapter 84).

Epidemiology

D. caninum is the most common tapeworm of domesticated dogs and cats, and it has a worldwide distribution. People acquire dog tapeworm by inadvertently ingesting fleas infested with the parasite. Most cases involve infants and young children who have close contact with their pets.

Life Cycle

Parasite eggs are ingested by the larval form of fleas that inhabit dogs or cats. Each egg releases an oncosphere that penetrates the intestinal wall and develops into a cysticercoid larva within the flea larva's viscera. The insect larva then develops into an adult flea that can distribute the cysticercoid larva to other animals. Dogs, cats, and occasionally children ingest infested adult fleas. Once in the mammalian intestine, the cysticercoid larva evaginates to form a scolex that attaches to the mucosa of the small intestine. The worm matures, forming a strobila or chain of developing proglottids that trails the scolex. The adult worm measures 10 to 70 cm in length. Gravid proglottids detach from the distal end of the worm and pass with the stool. The proglottids look like cucumber seeds (12 × 3 mm), are motile, and occasionally move out of the anus. They can be mistaken for maggots. As they dry, they release small packets, each of which contain 5 to 15 eggs.

Clinical Features and Pathophysiology

Because people don't often eat fleas, colonization is limited. Low numbers of dog tapeworms cause no symptoms. *D. caninum* is discovered when children or their parents find motile proglottids crawling in a diaper, underwear, or stool.

Diagnosis and Treatment

D. caninum is identified by its characteristic proglottid, which looks like a moving cucumber seed. Often the proglottids of *D. caninum* are mistaken for adult pinworms (*E. vermicularis*) because the latter is much more common than the former. Stool examination for egg packets usually is unrewarding.

D. caninum causes a self-limited colonization that spontaneously clears, and dog tapeworm requires no treatment. Most patients and their families, however, prefer that the parasite be expunged actively, and so treatment is given with a single oral dose of praziquantel 10 mg/kg.

TREMATODES

Intestinal Flukes

Most intestinal trematodes have a broad host range, and more than 50 different species are capable of colonizing humans.[145] Many of these are geographically restricted and are acquired because of specific indigenous dietary behavior. The more common intestinal trematodes are *Fasciolopsis buski*, *Heterophyes* species, and *Echinostoma* species. These parasites are acquired by ingesting larval metacercariae encysted on freshwater plants (*F. buski*) or in freshwater fish (*Heterophyes*, *Echinostoma*). The parasites usually cause no specific symptoms, but heavy infestations can cause diarrhea and abdominal pain. Treatment is with praziquantel.

Fasciolopsis buski

F. buski is the largest intestinal trematode that colonizes humans. Adults measure 7.5 cm long and 2 cm wide.

Epidemiology and Life Cycle

F. buski is endemic in Southeast Asia and Indonesia and is acquired by ingesting metacercariae encysted on freshwater plants.[146] The metacercariae excyst in the duodenum and attach to the small intestinal mucosa. Within 3 months, they mature to adult flatworms and begin to lay eggs. The eggs pass with feces and, if they are deposited into fresh water, they embryonate. Each egg releases a ciliated miracidium that seeks a suitable snail to infect. Each trematode species (and often strains) tend to infect specific species and strains of snails. Permissiveness of the snail to infection with the trematode is important because snail distributions influence geographic range of specific parasites and even help to preserve niches in areas where trematodes compete. The miracidium enters the snail, and in the foot process and/or "liver" of the snail, it develops into a sporocyst that asexually multiplies, releasing numerous cercariae. The cercariae swim to freshwater plants, and each encysts to form a metacercaria on the plant's surface, awaiting ingestion by a mammal.

Clinical Features and Pathophysiology

Adult *F. buski* live for about 1 year and cause no symptoms in most people.[147] Histology of jejunal biopsy specimens along with carbohydrate, fat, and protein absorption were normal in 1 study of patients harboring *F. buski*[148]; however, in 1952, a 15-year-old Thai girl, hospitalized for diarrhea and abdominal pain, died of anasarca with more than 470 adult worms in her small intestine.[149]

Diagnosis and Treatment

Diagnosis is by finding parasite eggs in the stool (see Fig. 114-3). Rarely the large flatworm is found on endoscopy (Video 114-6).[150,151] Treatment is 1 dose of praziquantel 15 mg/kg given orally.

Heterophyes Species

Heterophyes species and the closely-related *Metagonimus yokogawai* are small, flat worms that measure about 1.0 to 1.7 mm long × 0.3 to 0.6 mm wide.

Epidemiology and Life Cycle

Heterophyes heterophyes is endemic in West Africa, Egypt, Israel, Turkey, China, Japan, Taiwan, and the Philippines. *Heterophyes nocens* is endemic to Japan and Korea. *M. yokogawai* is endemic in Siberia, the Balkans, China, Korea, and Japan.

People acquire these parasites by eating raw or undercooked fish that contain metacercariae. In rural areas of northern Egypt, 32% of tilapia fish were infected with heterophyid metacercariae.[152] In the United States, a case of *H. heterophyes* involved a Pennsylvania woman who ate sushi that contained raw fish flown in from Asia.[153] The metacercariae ingested in raw fish excyst in the intestine, attach to the small intestinal mucosa, and develop into adults. The adults lay eggs that are deposited with feces. If passed into fresh or brackish water, the eggs release miracidia that swim in search of a suitable snail. A miracidium enters the snail and develops into a sporocyst that asexually multiplies, releasing numerous cercariae. The cercariae swim away from the snail in search of a fish to infect. Either freshwater fish or saltwater fish feeding in brackish outlets can become infected.

Clinical Features and Pathophysiology

These parasites produce no specific symptoms in most people. Occasional heavy infections cause mild abdominal pain and diarrhea. The worms attach at the villus crypts and produce a localized eosinophilic inflammation. Rarely, parasite eggs enter blood vessels and lymphatics, to produce distant granulomatous reactions.

Diagnosis and Treatment

Diagnosis is by finding eggs in the stool, which can require concentration techniques. The eggs of *Heterophyes* species appear similar to those of *M. yokogawai*. Treatment of the trematodes is a single 20-mg/kg oral dose of praziquantel.

Echinostoma Species

There are at least 16 species of *Echinostoma* that can colonize humans.[154] Adults are 2 to 6 mm long and 1 to 1.5 mm wide, depending on the species.

Epidemiology and Life Cycle

Echinostoma species are endemic in Taiwan, Korea, Thailand, Japan, Indonesia, and the Philippines. One outbreak of probable echinostomiasis involved 18 of 20 American travelers returning from Kenya.[155]

People acquire *Echinostoma* by eating raw or undercooked freshwater mollusks or fish infected with metacercariae. The ingested metacercariae excyst in the intestine, attach to the small intestinal mucosa, and develop into adults. The adults lay eggs that, if deposited into fresh water with feces, embryonate and hatch to release miracidia that swim in search of suitable snails. A miracidium enters a snail and develops into a sporocyst that asexually multiplies, releasing numerous cercariae. Depending on the species, the *Echinostoma* cercariae swim away from the snail in search of another mollusk or fish to infect.

Clinical Features and Pathophysiology

Echinostoma species produce no symptoms in most people, but can cause epigastric pain, abdominal cramps, and diarrhea.[155]

Diagnosis and Treatment

Diagnosis is by finding eggs in the stool or adults on endoscopy.[156] Echinostoma eggs resemble those of *F. buski* but are smaller. Treatment is 1 25-mg/kg dose of praziquantel given orally.

Liver Flukes

These trematodes reside in the bile ducts and are acquired by ingesting larval metacercariae encysted in freshwater fish (*Clonorchis sinensis, Opisthorchis*) or on freshwater plants (*Fasciola*). Most infections are asymptomatic, but these parasites can cause recurrent cholangitis. People chronically infected with *C. sinensis* or *Opisthorchis viverrini* may develop cholangiocarcinoma, and these flukes are considered carcinogens by the WHO International Agency for Research on Cancer (see Chapter 84).[157] *C. sinensis* or *Opisthorchis* infections are treated with praziquantel. *Fasciola* infections are treated with triclabendazole.

Clonorchis sinensis, Opisthorchis viverrini, and Opisthorchis felineus

C. sinensis and *Opisthorchis* species are closely related parasites that have similar life cycles and cause similar disease.

Epidemiology and Life Cycle

C. sinensis is endemic to China, Hong Kong, Taiwan, the Republic of Korea, and North Vietnam.[158] *O. viverrini* is endemic to Thailand, Lao People's Democratic Republic, and Cambodia.[159] *O. felineus* is endemic to Russia and the Ukraine. Infection with *C. sinensis* and other food-borne trematodes is increasing in prevalence, possibly because of fish farming.[160] People acquire these parasites by eating metacercariae present in raw or undercooked fish such as grass carp (*Ctenopharyngodon idellus*) or pond smelt (*Hypomesus olidus*). Studies in Korea show that at least 80 species of freshwater fish can harbor metacercariae.[161]

The metacercariae excyst in the stomach and duodenum as the meat is digested. The worms migrate along the mucosa to the ampulla of Vater and into the biliary tree, where they grow into adults. Leaf-shaped adult *C. sinensis* measure 5 mm wide × 2.5 cm long × 1 mm thick. *Opisthorchis* is smaller. The adult parasites lay eggs that pass with the bile into the intestinal lumen to be excreted. The excreted eggs are ingested by freshwater snails in which they hatch, releasing miracidia that develop into sporocysts. Each sporocyst asexually reproduces within the snail, eventually producing numerous cercariae. The cercariae exit the snail and swim in search of a suitable fish to invade. The parasites encyst as metacercariae in the muscles of the fish, awaiting ingestion by a mammalian host.

TABLE 114-2 Relative Risks of Cholangiocarcinoma in Patients with *Clonorchis* or *Opisthorchis* Infestation

Reference	Relative Risk	95% CI
Clonorchis sinensis		
146	3.1	0.13-8.4
147	6.5	3.7-12
148	6.0	2.8-13
Opisthorchis viverrini		
149	5.0	2.3-11.0
152*		
Light	1.7	0.2-16.3
Medium	3.2	0.4-30
Heavy	14.0	1.7-119

*Light, ≤1500 eggs/g stool; medium, 1501-6000 eggs/g stool; heavy, >6000 eggs/g stool.
CI, confidence interval.

Clinical Features and Pathophysiology

Most infections with *C. sinensis* or *Opisthorchis* are asymptomatic. With heavy exposures, patients develop fever, malaise, hepatic tenderness, and eosinophilia,[162] symptoms and signs that abate as the worms mature and begin laying eggs in the bile ducts (Video 114-7).[163] In a minority of patients, these parasites can cause relapsing cholangitis (see Chapter 84). The worms elicit a fibrotic and adenomatous reaction in the smaller branches of the biliary ducts, which can cause localized obstruction and hepatic abscess formation. The flukes also can migrate into the pancreatic duct and cause pancreatitis.

The most important complication of chronic infection with *C. sinensis* or *O. viverrini* is cholangiocarcinoma (see Chapter 69).[164] Infection with these parasites dramatically increases the risk of developing this otherwise rare cancer (Table 114-2)[165,166]: In the Khon Kaen province in Thailand, cholangiocarcinoma due to *O. viverrini* accounts for more than 85% of all cancers.[167] Parasites damage the bile duct, causing cellular desquamation followed by hyperplasia, adenomatous hyperplasia, periductal fibrosis, dysplasia, and finally cholangiocarcinoma. Cancer also can result from increased sensitivity to carcinogens. Hamsters infected with *O. viverrini* develop cholangiocarcinoma when treated with subcarcinogenic doses of dimethylnitrosamine.[168] *C. sinensis* and *O. viverrini* can sensitize patients to dietary or endogenously produced *N*-nitroso compounds and thereby increase the risk for DNA damage and cholangiocarcinoma.[169] Liver fluke–associated cholangiocarcinoma is also an important consideration in Western countries.[170] A 1977 study found that 26% of Chinese immigrants relocating to New York had *C. sinensis*.[171] Because of the increased cancer risk associated with these parasites, it is advisable to look for them in any patient from an endemic area.[172]

Diagnosis and Treatment

Diagnosis is by finding parasite eggs in the stool or duodenal aspirate. Symptomatic patients might have curvilinear lucencies in the biliary and pancreatic ducts on ERCP.[173] US findings include increased periductal echogenicity and floating echogenic foci in the gallbladder.[174] The recommended treatment is praziquantel 25 mg/kg every 8 hours for 3 doses.[160] Heavy infections may require 2 days of therapy. An alternative treatment is albendazole 10 mg/kg twice a day for 7 days.

Albendazole is an FDA pregnancy category C medication, though a recent study showed no treatment-associated fetal or maternal adverse effects.[29]

Fasciola hepatica *and* Fasciola gigantica

Epidemiology and Life Cycle

Fasciola hepatica has a worldwide distribution,[175] whereas *Fasciola gigantica* is endemic in Hawaii, Asia, India, the Middle East, and Africa. Both species infect sheep, goats, and cattle as their normal hosts.

Humans acquire these parasites by ingesting metacercariae encysted on freshwater plants such as watercress. Ingested metacercariae excyst in the small intestine, penetrate through the bowel wall, and enter the peritoneal cavity, where they migrate to the liver, penetrate the capsule, and travel through the hepatic parenchyma in search of a bile duct. They reside within the bile ducts, reaching maturity within 3 or 4 months, after which they lay eggs. Adult *F. hepatica* are 1.3 cm × 4.0 cm, and *F. gigantica* grow up to 7.0 cm in length. Adults of both species are only 1 millimeter thick and resemble leaves. *Fasciola* are long-lived; 1 documented infection persisted for 16 years. Adults lay eggs that pass with the bile into the intestinal lumen, from which they are excreted. Upon reaching fresh water, *Fasciola* eggs embryonate, hatch, and release miracidia that swim in search of a suitable snail. A miracidium enters a snail and develops into a sporocyst that asexually multiplies, eventually releasing numerous cercariae. The cercariae swim to a freshwater plant and encyst on the wall, awaiting ingestion by a mammal.

Clinical Features and Pathophysiology

Fasciola infestations usually are asymptomatic. In the acute phase, patients can have abdominal pain and hepatomegaly as the parasites penetrate the intestinal wall and hepatic capsule. Abdominal CT scan may show low-density areas in the periphery of the liver. Patients also develop symptoms from migration of the parasites to other sites such as subcutaneous fat.[176] Acute symptoms wane as the parasites enter the bile ducts. During the chronic phase of fascioliasis, patients can have symptoms of intermittent biliary obstruction and cholangitis. Rarely, patients develop pancreatitis.[177]

Diagnosis and Treatment

ERCP may show curvilinear lucencies in the bile duct (Fig. 114-13).[177,178] Diagnosis is by finding eggs in the stool. *Fasciola* release low numbers of eggs, however, making this test insensitive. Duodenal or bile aspirates also can demonstrate eggs. Commercial ELISAs are available but mostly are used to identify infections in sheep, goats, and cattle. The CDC will provide guidance on ELISA use but does not provide a serologic testing service like they do for other helminths. Unlike other trematodes, *Fasciola* are resistant to praziquantel. Triclabendazole is the drug of choice for fascioliasis. In 1 study, a single oral dose of triclabendazole (10 mg/kg) cured 79% of patients as measured by fecal egg counts and ELISA.[179]

Blood Flukes

Visceral (hepatosplenic and intestinal) schistosomiasis is caused by *Schistosoma mansoni*, *S. japonicum*, *S. mekongi*, and *S. intercalatum*. Schistosomes (including *S. hematobium*, which affects the urinary tract) infest more than 200 million people worldwide. People acquire the parasite through contact with contaminated water. Visceral schistosomiasis can cause colitis

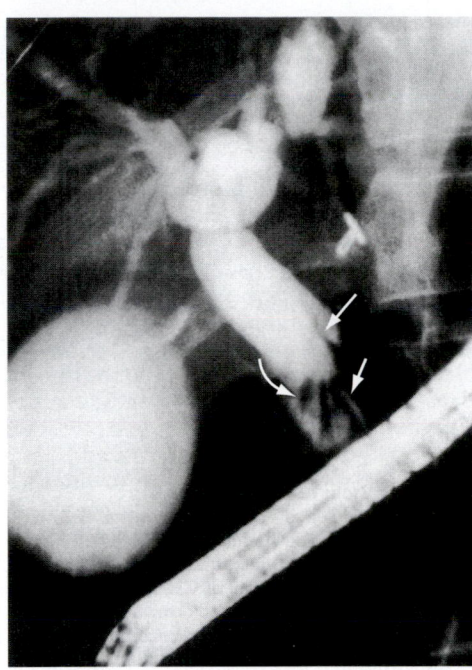

FIGURE 114-13. Film from an ERCP showing *Fasciola hepatica*, appearing as curvilinear lucencies *(arrows)* in the distal bile duct. A leaf-shaped fluke was extracted from the bile duct. *(From Veerappan A, Siegel JH, Podany J, et al. Fasciola hepatica pancreatitis: Endoscopic extraction of live parasites. Gastrointest Endosc 1991; 37:473-5.)*

and fibrosis of the portal venous system, producing portal hypertension. Treatment is praziquantel.

Epidemiology

Schistosomes are tropical parasites with a worldwide distribution.[180] *S. mansoni* is endemic in regions of Africa, the Middle East, Puerto Rico, the Dominican Republic, Central America, and South America. *S. japonicum* is endemic in China, Indonesia, the Philippines, and Thailand. *S. mekongi* is endemic in Laos and Cambodia. *S. intercalatum* is endemic in Africa. In most countries in which schistosomes are endemic, some regions have a high prevalence of infection; in other areas the parasite is absent. Schistosomes live in tropical snails for part of their life cycle. It is the distribution of these snails that helps define the geographic limits of schistosomes.

Construction of water reservoirs and irrigation canals has expanded the snail habitat in many countries, a practice that has increased the risk of acquiring schistosomiasis. Mice and other mammals also can harbor schistosomes and might allow spread of the parasite even were sanitation to be improved,[181] thereby making schistosomiasis difficult to eradicate. Nonetheless, *S. japonicum* was successfully eradicated in Japan and is coming under control in Indonesia,[182] while *S. mansoni* is vanishing from areas of Puerto Rico.[183]

Life Cycle

Schistosome worms are acquired by contacting fresh water that is infested with parasite cercariae. Cercariae are fork-tailed, microscopic larvae that swim through the water in search of a suitable mammalian host. Upon finding this host, they penetrate through intact skin, shed their tails, and transform into schistosomules that are covered with a double

lipid-bilayer tegument; this tegument thwarts most immunologic attacks (see later). Schistosomules migrate into blood vessels, where they are swept with the venous flow through the right side of the heart into the lungs. They migrate through the pulmonary capillaries, flow through the left side of the heart into the systemic circulation, and eventually reach the liver, where they mature, mate, and migrate against venous flow in the portal system. The 2-centimeter female is partly ensheathed by the shorter male, and the "couple" reside together within the mesenteric veins. *S. mansoni* and *S. intercalatum* prefer to dwell in the vessels drained by the inferior mesenteric vein, whereas *S. japonicum* and *S. mekongi* prefer the vessels drained by the superior mesenteric vein.

The worms remain in the mesenteric vessels, consuming blood and nutrients and depositing eggs. *S. mansoni* lays 250 eggs and *S. japonicum* lays 3500 eggs per worm pair each day. Many of the eggs pass through the intestinal wall and enter the lumen of the bowel. The eggs are excreted with the stool, and if deposited in fresh water, they hatch to release ciliated miracidia. Miracidia swim in search of a suitable tropical snail to infect. It is the distribution of snails that permits patent infection which determines the geographic foci of endemic schistosomiasis. For example, in Brazil, some strains of the snail *Biomphalaria tenagophila* are easily infected while other strains are completely resistant.[184] After penetrating into the snail's foot process, a miracidium transforms into a primary (mother) sporocyst. Secondary sporocysts bud off of the primary sporocyst, migrate to the snail's liver, and mature. Cercariae bud off the secondary sporocysts, exit the snail, and swim in search of a permissive mammalian host.

Clinical Features and Pathophysiology

Dermal invasion and migration by infecting cercariae usually produce no memorable symptoms. Patients with repeated contact can develop a mild papular rash, in contrast to the intensely pruritic papular rash that develops after exposure to avian schistosomes such as *Trichobilharzia ocellata*. These avian trematodes infect water fowl but are unable to live in mammals, and so the cercariae and schistosomules die in a person's skin, eliciting an immunologic response that produces swimmer's itch. Swimmer's itch is common in the Great Lakes region and has been found as far north as Iceland.[185] Swimmer's itch is not dangerous, but repetitive scratching can cause secondary cellulitis.

Schistosomules migrate through the body without producing symptoms. Juvenile and adult worms evade immune attack elegantly: Their tegument is coated with histocompatibility and blood group antigens derived from the host.[186] The tegument contains immunoglobulin receptors and proteases that might help cleave any bound antibody. Moreover, schistosomes produce several proteins that prevent complement, neutrophils, macrophages, or lymphocytes from injuring them.[186,187] Such immune evasion allows adult worms to survive in the blood vessels without causing much direct damage. The average life span of worms is thought to be about 6 to 10 years, but there are documented cases of adult worms surviving for more than 35 years after persons had left an endemic area.[188] Although the helminthes evade host responses, 2 specific functional polymorphisms in IL-13 (c.1-1111C>T, which influences transcription factor binding and R130Q which induces human PB monocyte STAT6 activation and B cell IgE switching) each provide protection against high-intensity infection, thus demonstrating some degree of immune system control.[189]

Schistosome worms release eggs each day throughout their long life, and it is the parasite's eggs that cause disease. Whereas the adult worms evade an immune response, the schistosome eggs invite one, exuding antigens that trigger a strong cell-mediated Th2 immune response.[190]

Katayama fever is the classic presentation of acute schistosomiasis. It results from a brisk early immune response to schistosome products that occurs within the first 2 to 13 weeks after contacting water that is heavily infested with cercariae.[191] Symptoms are caused by circulating immune complexes and resemble those of serum sickness. Patients have fever, malaise, arthralgia, myalgia, cough, and diarrhea, with the additional finding of marked eosinophilia. Serum aminotransferases are normal, and eggs usually are absent from the stool. *S. japonicum* causes the most intense acute schistosomiasis reaction, with fatality rates approaching 25%. Most people do not develop acute schistosomiasis, but in those who do and survive, symptoms resolve as the infection enters the chronic phase.

Each schistosome egg secretes antigens that provoke a focal granulomatous inflammatory reaction that helps move the egg from the inside of a capillary, through the intestinal wall, and out into the lumen.[190] Thus, inflammation actually benefits the parasite. Passage of eggs through the bowel wall causes intestinal schistosomiasis with guaiac-positive stools or even bloody diarrhea. Patients also can have tenesmus and tenderness over the sigmoid colon. Patients with *S. mansoni* can develop colitis with inflammatory pseudopolyps (Fig. 114-14) that contain numerous eosinophils and occasional eggs[192]— a picture that can resemble Crohn's disease or UC. *S. japonicum* prefers to dwell in veins drained by the superior mesenteric vein and lays thousands of eggs at a time. *S. japonicum* can produce upper abdominal pain unrelated to meals, gastric bleeding, and pyloric obstruction due to inflammation and fibrosis.

About half of the eggs pass out of the body; the other half lodge in the host's tissues and cause the pathology of chronic schistosomiasis. Eggs are carried by the portal flow, and some lodge in the liver. Other eggs lodge in the mesenteric and portal veins or remain in the intestinal wall. In these locations, the eggs elicit granulomatous inflammation with eosinophils, macrophages, lymphocytes, fibroblasts, and mast cells (Fig. 114-15). Eosinophils account for 50% of the schistosome egg granuloma cell population. When eosinophils degranulate, they deposit major basic protein that produces an eosinophilic halo around the eggs, termed the *Splendore-Hoeppli phenomenon*. This phenomenon is nonspecific and can be seen with bacterial, fungal, and parasitic infections. Eosinophils likely assist in killing the miracidia protected by the tough egg shell. After 1 or 2 weeks the miracidium dies, antigen release wanes, and the granuloma involutes to leave a fibrotic scar.

Over the years, the daily production of eggs, granulomas, and scars accumulates enough damage to produce disease. Eggs that lodge in the hepatic and portal vessels produce a unique pattern of scarring called Symmers' pipe stem fibrosis, in which the vessels become fibrotic and resemble clay pipe stems on cross section; this process causes the presinusoidal venous obstruction and portal hypertension characteristic of hepatosplenic schistosomiasis (see Chapter 84). Patients typically have an enlarged left hepatic lobe, splenomegaly, and thrombocytopenia due to platelet sequestration. Hepatocellular function remains normal because the blood supply to the liver is maintained by increased hepatic artery flow. Patients have normal serum aminotransferase levels and mildly elevated serum levels of alkaline phosphatase and GGTP. Patients with hepatosplenic schistosomiasis do not develop cirrhosis unless they are co-infected with hepatitis B or C, and so they lack stigmata of chronic liver disease. The classic presentation of decompensated hepatosplenic schistosomiasis is variceal hemorrhage.

Hepatosplenic schistosomiasis results from accumulated injury and requires prolonged, moderately intense infection.

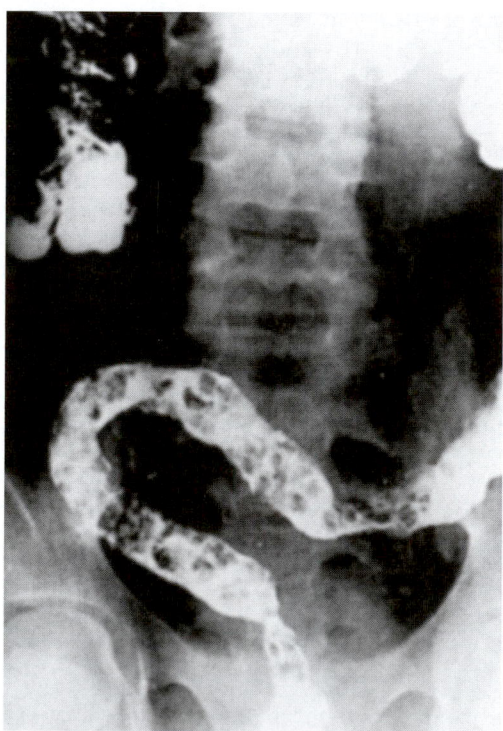

FIGURE 114-14. Film from a barium enema examination in a 20-year-old Egyptian man with bloody diarrhea and tenesmus. Multiple polypoid lesions due to *Schistosoma mansoni* are seen throughout the rectosigmoid colon, which is displaced out of the pelvis by a large pericolic abscess. *(From Reeder MM, Hamilton LC. Radiologic diagnosis of tropical diseases of the gastrointestinal tract. Radiol Clin North Am 1969; 7:57-81.)*

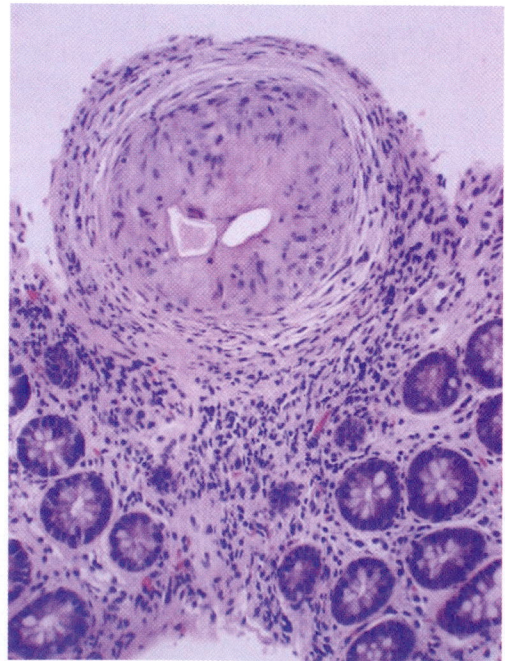

FIGURE 114-15. Histopathology of a colonic biopsy specimen from a patient with schistosomiasis. A schistosome egg granuloma is seen. (H&E)

Patients with hepatosplenic schistosomiasis typically range in age from adolescence to late 20s and have had schistosomiasis for 5 to 15 years. Compensated disease improves after schistosomes are killed by drug therapy, permitting the portal tributaries to heal and remodel.[193,194]

Schistosome eggs also can lodge in other sites besides the intestine, liver, spleen, and splanchnic venous circulation. Eggs can percolate through portocaval collateral vessels, lodge in the pulmonary capillaries, and over time cause pulmonary hypertension and cor pulmonale. Eggs can enter the vertebral venous plexus and embolize the spinal cord or brain. Granulomatous inflammation in the central nervous system can result in conus equinus syndrome, transverse myelitis, or schistosomal cerebritis.

Patients with schistosomiasis can present with recurrent bacteremia. Adult schistosome worms can ingest enteric bacteria transiently present in the portal circulation, harbor these bacteria, and serve as reservoirs for infection. Recurrent salmonella infection is particularly common in patients with schistosomiasis.[195]

Schistosomiasis can cause membranoproliferative glomerulonephritis or focal glomerulosclerosis with proteinuria, nephrotic syndrome, and end-stage renal disease. Schistosomal nephropathy results from deposition of immune complexes of parasite antigens and antibodies, and the renal disease can be progressive even if the parasites are killed with drug therapy.[196]

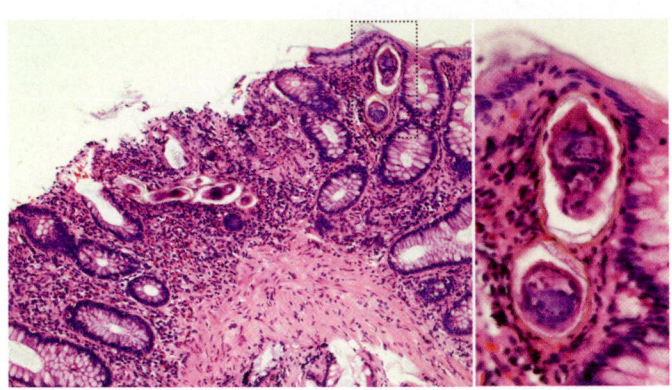

FIGURE 114-16. Histopathology of a colonic biopsy specimen showing *Schistosoma mansoni* eggs. A 20-year-old woman who had emigrated 5 years earlier from the Democratic Republic of the Congo was evaluated for persistent iron deficiency anemia. She had normal stool habits but occasional hematochezia. The mucosa was normal on colonoscopy except for some areas suggestive of neovascularization. Random biopsy specimens demonstrated viable *Schistosoma mansoni* eggs (H&E 20×; *inset,* 60×). She was treated with praziquantel, and the anemia resolved. *(Courtesy P. Kirby and F. Mitros, Iowa City, Ia.)*

Diagnosis

Schistosome eggs are present in stool, but not in high numbers. The classic method for detecting eggs is the Kato-Katz thick smear.[197] This technique is not performed as part of the standard ova and parasite test, and standard smear evaluation is not sensitive enough to find the relatively rare schistosome eggs. Even Kato-Katz thick smears are not highly sensitive and are unlikely to detect eggs at very low levels of infection. Formalin-ethyl acetate sedimentation can be used to identify schistosome eggs, but this technique is less sensitive than multiple Kato-Katz smears.[198]

The vast majority of patients with intestinal schistosomiasis are asymptomatic; patients come to medical attention during evaluation of mild anemia, positive fecal occult blood tests, or unexpected variceal hemorrhage. On endoscopy, a patient might have inflammatory polyps that contain eggs, but usually, the intestinal mucosa appears normal. Subtle changes in the vascular pattern can result from egg emboli that produce a terminal curling of small blood vessels.[199] Occasionally, histopathology of random biopsies of the colonic mucosa show schistosome eggs (Fig. 114-16), but this is an insensitive means of diagnosis. Biopsy of the rectum can demonstrate eggs, especially when the specimen is crushed between 2 glass slides and the whole biopsy specimen is surveyed microscopically. Evaluation of 6 crush biopsies is more sensitive than 2 Kato-Katz smears for *S. mansoni*.[200]

Although eggs lodge in the liver and cause portal hypertension, liver biopsy is an insensitive method for detecting schistosomiasis. Liver biopsy should not be used solely to test for schistosomiasis but rather to stage comorbid disease such as viral hepatitis B or C.

Present or past exposure to schistosomes is detectable by serology. Anti-schistosome antibodies are detected by ELISA using adult microsomal antigens. Sensitivity varies depending on whether the infecting schistosome is the same species as that used to prepare the antigens. The ELISA uses *S. mansoni* microsomal antigens, and immunoblot tests using antigens from *S. japonicum* and *S. hematobium* also can be performed.[201] The antibody assay also is useful to diagnose acute schistosomiasis (Katayama fever) because there are few or no eggs in the stool during the peak of the reaction. The ELISA does not distinguish active from prior infections, and therefore it is most useful for diagnosis in recent travelers rather than in expatriates. Because schistosomes can be long-lived, 1-time treatment of antibody-positive patients is reasonable.

Active infection can be demonstrated by detecting circulating schistosome gut-associated protein antigens CCA (circulating cathodic antigen) and CAA (circulating anodic antigen) in the patient's serum.[202] Serologic detection of CCA and CAA has an equivalent or higher sensitivity than the Kato-Katz thick smear, but each test misses some low-level infections.[203] Measurement of circulating antigens also can prove useful to document response to treatment,[204] but these tests are not commercially available in the United States.

Abdominal US is an important additional test in hepatosplenic schistosomiasis. US evaluation documents periportal fibrosis, splenomegaly, portal blood flow, and collateral vessels. Periportal fibrosis has a characteristic appearance: multiple echogenic areas, each with central echolucency that gives a fish-scale appearance.[205] A scoring system exists that uses a liver parenchyma and image pattern (IP), a portal thickening (PT), and a portal hypertension (PH) score to stage the disease (Table 114-3).[206,207]

Treatment

Praziquantel is the drug of choice to treat schistosomiasis. It is the safest schistosomicide in current use. Praziquantel administered orally in 3 doses of 20 mg/kg, each 4 hours apart (total dose, 60 mg/kg), gives the best cure rates of 60% to 98%, depending on the series. Eggs continue to be shed in the stool for up to 2 weeks after drug treatment, because eggs that were deposited before treatment can take this long to work through the intestinal wall. Patients who are not cured with a single course of praziquantel have a dramatic decrease in egg counts and respond to a second course of treatment. Periportal fibrosis improves after the worms are killed, halting the daily deluge of eggs and permitting the portal tributaries to heal and remodel.[193]

TABLE 114-3 WHO Criteria for Staging Hepatosplenic Schistosomiasis*

Liver Parenchymal Patterns on US and Image Pattern (IP) Scores

Pattern	Sonographic Appearance	IP Score
A	Normal structure	0
	Patterns Observed in Schistosomiasis†	
B	"Starry sky" (diffuse echogenic foci)	1
C	Highly echogenic "ring echoes," which correspond to the "pipe stems" seen in a scan perpendicular to the one in which rings are seen (see Fig. 84-4)	2
D	Highly echogenic "ruff" around the portal bifurcation and main stem	4
E	Highly echogenic "patches" extending from the main portal vein and branches into the parenchyma	6
F	Highly echogenic "bands" and "streaks" extending from the main portal vein and its bifurcation to the liver surface, where they retract the organ surface	8
	Patterns Indicating Pathology Different from Periportal Fibrosis (If these are present, no score is given.)	
X	Diffusely coarse liver texture, irregular liver surface, distorted hepatic veins, rounded caudal liver edge	—
Y	Diffusely increased liver echogenicity, loss of highly reflective edges of peripheral portal branches, possibly distal sound extinction, rounded caudal liver edge	—
Z	Other liver abnormalities	—

Periportal Thickening (PT) Score

If liver parenchyma shows indications of periportal fibrosis
  Assign a preliminary PT score of 1
  Continue the examination
Measure the thickness of the wall of the second order portal branches
  Calculate the mean wall thickness (both walls) for the 2 (or 3) vessels measured
  Adjust results for body height

Normal range	2 SD or less above mean	Score = 0
Increased	>2 SD but ≤4 SD above mean	Score = 3
Much increased	>4 SD above mean	Score = 7

  The result is an intermediate PT score
Calculate the final PT score
  Add the preliminary PT score to the intermediate PT score
  The result is a final PT score in the range 1 (1 + 0) to 8 (1 + 7)

Portal Hypertension (PH) Score

Portal vein diameter: Adjust the value for height

Normal	Increase 0 to ≤2 SD above the mean	Score = 0
Dilatation	Increase 2 to ≤4 SD above the mean	Score = 4
Marked dilatation	Increase >4 SD above the mean	Score = 6

Collateral veins

No collateral vessel detected	Score = 0
Collateral vessels detected	Score = 4

Ascites

None	Score = 0
Ascites present	Score = 3

Calculate the final PH score
  The result is the sum of the above 3 scores = PH score 0-13

Interpretation of the Final Score

IP score	PT score	PH score	Interpretation
0	0	0	No sign of periportal fibrosis
1	1	0	Incipient periportal fibrosis not excluded
2	1	0	Periportal fibrosis possible
4	1	0	Periportal fibrosis possible
2	4, 8	0	Periportal fibrosis
4	4, 8	0	Periportal fibrosis
6	1, 4, 8	0	Advanced periportal fibrosis
8	1, 4, 8	0	Advanced periportal fibrosis
4-8	1, 4, 8	3-13	Advanced periportal fibrosis + portal hypertension

*Staging is determined by assessing the degree of parenchymal changes, periportal thickening, and portal hypertension.
†Combined patterns can exist and are assigned an IP score corresponding to the highest IP score of the 2 or 3 patterns.
Adapted from Abdel-Wahab MF, Esmat G, Milad M, et al. Characteristic sonographic pattern of schistosomal hepatic fibrosis. *Am J Trop Med Hyg* 1989; 40:72-6.

KEY REFERENCES

Full references for this chapter can be found on
www.expertconsult.com.

14. Crompton DW. Ascaris and ascariasis. Adv Parasitol 2001;
48:285-375.
15. Bethony J, Brooker S, Albonico M, et al. Soil-transmitted
helminth infections: Ascariasis, trichuriasis, and hookworm.
Lancet 2006; 367:1521-32.
17. Pullan RL, Brooker SJ. The global limits and population at
risk of soil-transmitted helminth infections in 2010. Parasit
Vectors 2012; 5:81.
30. Keiser J, Utzinger J. Efficacy of current drugs against
soil-transmitted helminth infections: Systematic review and
meta-analysis. JAMA 2008; 299:1937-48.
40. Mejia R, Nutman TB. Screening, prevention, and treatment
for hyperinfection syndrome and disseminated infections
caused by *Strongyloides stercoralis*. Curr Opin Infect Dis
2012; 25:458-63.
60. Loukas A, Constant S, Bethony J. Immunobiology of
hookworm infection. FEMS Immunol Med Microbiol 2005;
43:115-24.
108. Capo V, Despommier D. Clinical aspects of infection with
Trichinella spp. Clin Microbiol Rev 1996; 9:47-54.
115. Pravettoni V, Primavesi L, Piantanida M. *Anisakis simplex*:
Current knowledge. Eur Ann Allergy Clin Immunol 2012;
44:150-6.
122. Scholz T, Garcia HH, Kuchta R, Wicht B. Update on the
human broad tapeworm (genus *Diphyllobothrium*),
including clinical relevance. Clin Microbiol Rev 2009;
22:146-60.
131. Nash TE, Garcia HH. Diagnosis and treatment of
neurocysticercosis. Nat Rev Neurol 2011; 7:584-94.
158. Hong ST, Fang Y. *Clonorchis sinensis* and clonorchiasis, an
update. Parasitol Int 2012; 61:17-24.
170. Fried B, Abruzzi A. Food-borne trematode infections of
humans in the United States of America. Parasitol Res 2010;
106:1263-80.
175. Furst T, Duthaler U, Sripa B, et al. Trematode infections:
Liver and lung flukes. Infect Dis Clin North Am 2012;
26:399-419.
180. Gryseels B. Schistosomiasis. Infect Dis Clin North Am 2012;
26:383-97.
207. Richter J. Ultrasound in schistosomiasis: A practical guide
to the standardized use of ultrasonography for the
assessment of schistosomiasis-related morbidity. Geneva:
World Health Organization; 2000.

115

Crohn's Disease

BRUCE E. SANDS AND COREY A. SIEGEL

CHAPTER OUTLINE

Idiopathic IBD comprises conditions characterized by chronic or relapsing immune activation and inflammation within the GI tract. Crohn's disease and UC are the 2 major forms of idiopathic IBD; less common, but increasingly recognized, are the microscopic colitides, primarily collagenous colitis and lymphocytic colitis (see Chapter 128). Other chronic inflammatory conditions of the intestine share some features of presentation and pathogenesis with idiopathic IBD, but they have identifiable etiologies; examples of these disorders include diversion colitis, bypass enteropathy, radiation colitis, and drug-induced colitides. The 2 major forms of IBD share many clinical and epidemiologic characteristics, suggesting that underlying causes may be similar. In approximately 10% of cases, Crohn's disease cannot be distinguished from UC on clinical grounds (see "Indeterminate Colitis" later), although the 2 diseases are distinct syndromes with divergent treatment and prognosis.

Crohn's disease is a chronic inflammatory disorder that may involve any part of the alimentary tract from mouth to anus, but with a propensity for the distal small intestine and proximal large bowel. Inflammation in Crohn's disease often is discontinuous along the longitudinal axis of the intestine and can involve all layers from mucosa to serosa. Affected persons usually experience diarrhea and abdominal pain, frequently accompanied by weight loss. Common complications include strictures and fistulas, which often necessitate surgery. Numerous extraintestinal manifestations also may be present. The etiology of Crohn's disease is incompletely understood, and therapy, although generally effective in alleviating the symptoms, is not curative.

EPIDEMIOLOGY

Accurate comparisons of epidemiologic data on the incidence and prevalence of Crohn's disease are hampered by a lack of gold-standard criteria for diagnosis and inconsistent case ascertainment. Moreover, the invasiveness and expense of diagnostic modalities ensures that diagnosed cases represent only a fraction of the diseased population. Finally, studies that rely on observations from large referral centers may be biased toward reporting more aggressive forms of the disease, thereby underestimating the true incidence of Crohn's disease.

Misclassification of disease is problematic. Historically, unidentified infections, later recognized by improved culture and diagnostic techniques, might have accounted for some portion of cases, particularly among persons with a single episode of disease. At times, differentiating Crohn's disease from UC may be difficult, especially at the time of diagnosis, and before the passage of time has allowed distinctive disease characteristics to become manifest. Reassignment of a diagnosis of Crohn's disease or UC may be as high as 9% in the first 2 years after diagnosis.[1]

Despite these methodologic limitations, distinct and reproducible geographic and temporal trends in incidence have been observed. A north-south gradient has reported in France[2] and the United States.[3] This observation has been linked to variations in exposure to sunlight,[4] with increasing levels of sunlight and vitamin D exposure inversely associated with epidemiologic and individual risk of Crohn's disease.[5] Incidence rates as high as 20.2 and 12.7 per 100,000 person-years have been reported in North America and Europe, respectively,[6] whereas in Asia, the incidence rate has remained low, with a mean estimated incidence of 0.54 per 100,000 person-years.[7] Incidence rates in Australia and New Zealand are comparable to those found in other parts of the developed world, at 29.3 and 16.5 per 100,000 person-years.[8,9] In all regions of the world where incidence has been recorded over time, the annual occurrence of new cases of Crohn's disease is rising,[6] including the United States. For example, in Olmsted County, Minnesota, rates had been steadily increasing from approximately 3 per 100,000 (1954-1963) to nearly 8 per 100,000 (1964-1973), although since the late 1970s these rates have not changed significantly.[10] Mortality trends for Crohn's disease in the United States have followed a similar pattern, with rising mortality until the mid-1970s and a stable rate since.[11] Although improved diagnostic capabilities might have played some role in the rising incidence leading up to the mid-1970s, the fact that Crohn's-related mortality was increasing in parallel argues against the theory that rising Crohn's diagnoses merely represented detection bias involving mild cases. There is a paucity of epidemiologic data from South America and Africa, and increasing access to health care may influence estimates from less affluent regions. Most recently, the prevalence of Crohn's disease in the United States was estimated to be 201 per 100,000 adults and 43 per 100,000 in children, adolescents, and adults younger than 20 years of age.[3]

Studies throughout the world have shown a small excess risk of Crohn's disease among women. Most reports show a female-to-male ratio in adult patients between unity and 1.3 : 1.[3,12,13] In the pediatric population this is reversed, with more boys having Crohn's disease than girls.[3] This slight difference in risk in adult-onset disease may be explained by hormonal or life-style factors and stands in contrast to the nearly equal or even slight male predominance seen in UC.

Crohn's disease is diagnosed most often among persons 15 to 30 years of age, although the age at diagnosis can range from early childhood throughout one's lifespan. Population-based studies have shown the median age of diagnosis to be approximately 30 years.[10,12] Conflicting information may be found regarding trends in the age of diagnosis. In Olmsted County, Minnesota, younger age groups have had a fairly stable incidence over the past 20 years, with rising rates in patients aged 60 and older.[10,12] These findings reflect diagnosis in a larger proportion of patients older than 60 years. Indeed, many[12] studies have shown a smaller second peak in incidence later in life, generally in the seventh decade. This second peak may be the result of ascertainment bias because of more frequent contact with medical care and more frequent evaluation of older patients. The pathologic findings in young and old patients are not different, although some studies have identified a greater proportion of colonic and distal disease among older patients,[14] compared with a predominance of ileocolonic disease in younger patients.[15]

ETIOLOGY AND PATHOGENESIS

Initiating Events

In light of the nature of the pathologic findings in Crohn's disease (see later) and UC, it long has been clear that IBD represents a state of sustained immune response. The question arises as to whether this is an appropriate response to an unrecognized pathogen or an inappropriate response to an innocuous stimulus. Many infectious agents have been proposed as the cause of Crohn's disease, including chlamydia, *Listeria monocytogenes*, cell-wall–deficient *Pseudomonas* species,

reovirus, and many others. A proposed association between early measles vaccination and Crohn's disease largely has been disproved.[16] Another suggestion has been that the commensal flora, although normal in speciation, possess more subtle virulence factors, such as enteroadherence, that cause or contribute to IBD.[17] Increasingly, evidence suggests that an intestinal dysbiosis exists in Crohn's disease, and which may precede the onset of disease. Primarily, there is a decrease in diversity of the microbial flora, with a notable reduction in *Firmicutes*.[18] In particular, *Faecalibacterium prausnitzii* has been shown to be depleted in the ileocolonic mucosa of patients with Crohn's disease.[18]

Among the most enduring hypotheses is that *Mycobacterium paratuberculosis* is the causative agent of Crohn's disease. This notion dates to Dalziel's observation in 1913 that idiopathic granulomatous enterocolitis in humans is similar to Johne's disease, a granulomatous bowel disease of ruminants caused by *M. paratuberculosis*.[19] *M. paratuberculosis* is extremely fastidious in its culture requirements, and some proponents of this hypothesis have speculated that the presence of *M. paratuberculosis* as a spheroplast may have confounded efforts to confirm this hypothesis by culture of the organism; to demonstrate it by immunohistochemistry, in situ hybridization, and PCR methodology; and to treat it empirically with antimycobacterial antibiotics (see "Medical Therapy," later). Most investigation in this area, to date, has been inconclusive, providing insufficient evidence to prove or reject the hypothesis.

In light of the diversity of substances and bacteria within the intestinal lumen, it is remarkable that the intestine is not perpetually inflamed. The presence of low-level physiologic inflammation within the healthy intestinal mucosa represents a state of preparedness to deal with potentially harmful agents. A more vigorous response would not be appropriate if directed toward the innocuous commensal flora of the intestine. Experiments in animal models of IBD suggest that in a genetically susceptible host, a classic pathogen is not necessary to cause IBD, but rather nonpathogenic commensal enteric flora are sufficient to induce an inappropriate chronic inflammatory response. In diverse models, animals raised under germ-free conditions show diminished or delayed expression of the IBD phenotype.[20] On introduction of defined bacterial flora, however, the expected phenotype of bowel inflammation becomes manifest.[20] Such models suggest that a diversity of genetic alterations, including those that affect intestinal barrier function and regulation of mucosal immunity, can result in intestinal inflammation. As in the animal models of IBD, evidence in patients with Crohn's disease also points to an over-responsiveness of mucosal T cells to the enteric flora, manifest in part by the presence of antibodies against an array of bacterial antigens. Patients with Crohn's disease who have disease-associated polymorphisms of the *NOD2* gene (see later) and their unaffected relatives have increased levels of antibodies against bacterial antigens such as *Escherichia coli* outer membrane porin C (OmpC) and flagellin.[21]

Genetics

The argument for a genetic predisposition to IBD begins with the observation that family members of affected persons are at greatly increased risk for developing IBD. The relative risk among first-degree relatives is 8 to 10 times higher than that of the general population.[22] Roughly 1 of 5 patients with Crohn's disease report having at least 1 affected relative. Many families have more than 1 affected member, and although there is a tendency within families for either UC or Crohn's disease to be present exclusively, mixed kindreds also occur; this suggests, and has recently been confirmed, the presence of some shared genetic traits as a basis for both diseases.

Ethnicity also plays a role. Eastern European (Ashkenazi) Jews are at a 2- to 4-fold higher risk of developing IBD than non-Jews of the same geographic location, and they are at greater risk of having multiple affected family members. Studies of monozygotic and dizygotic twins suggest that genetic composition is a more powerful determinant of disease for Crohn's disease than for UC. Thus, the concordance rate among monozygotic twins is as high as 67% for Crohn's disease but only 13% to 20% for UC, although a lower rate of concordance for Crohn's disease has been observed among monozygotic twins in a more recent study.[22,23] Most studies have suggested that concordance of disease location and disease behavior are higher than one would expect by chance. As noted before, some subclinical markers of Crohn's disease, including anti-OmpC antibodies, are more common among apparently healthy family members of Crohn's disease probands than among the general population.[24]

Only very rare forms of IBD are transmitted through Mendelian inheritance. These include autosomal recessive missense mutations of the interleukin (IL)-10 receptor gene, which cause severe disease through loss of function and, therefore, failure of IL-10 to down-regulate inflammation.[25] Risk for common Crohn's disease, however, is transmitted through non-Mendelian inheritance. Genome-wide association (GWA) studies have been more successful in IBD than in any other complex disease, and they have accelerated the pace of gene discovery, providing unexpected insights into pathogenesis.[26]

A landmark study provided deep insight into the genetic architecture and causation of IBD by combining data from more than 75,000 cases of Crohn's disease and UC, controls, and results from 15 GWA studies.[27] Among 163 IBD loci identified, 110 were associated with both diseases, 30 were classified as Crohn's disease–specific (Table 115-1), and 23 as UC-specific.[27] Identified loci include regions with key genes validated in functional studies, others with multiple potential coding regions, and still others with noncoding regions. The latter may control expression of distant coding regions and thereby influence functional biology. The notable overlap of genetic loci suggests that Crohn's disease and UC share many biological mechanisms. However, biological differences are also suggested by the observation that 2 risk loci, NOD2 and PTPN22, are protective for UC. Additionally, 113 of the 163 risk loci are common to other complex immune-mediated diseases, such as type 1 diabetes, ankylosing spondylitis, and psoriasis.[27] IBD loci also display enrichment for genetic loci associated with primary immunodeficiencies of Mendelian inheritance, in concordance with the observation that individuals with a variety of primary immunodeficiency syndromes have a higher than expected rate of Crohn's-like disease. GWA studies identify genes associated with susceptibility to mycobacterial infections, such as leprosy and Mycobacterium tuberculosis. The Mycobacterium tuberculosis susceptibility genes include VDR,[27] which encodes the vitamin D receptor, providing a possible link with epidemiologic data that associates risk of Crohn's disease with sunlight and vitamin D exposure, as previously noted.

The findings of GWA studies in Crohn's disease and IBD generally support a connection between disease susceptibility and host interactions with microbes. This is exemplified most strongly in the first described susceptibility locus for Crohn's disease. The NOD2 (Nucleotide-binding Oligomerization Domain containing 2) gene, also known as CARD15 (CAspase-Recruitment Domain 15) was identified in 2001.[28,29] The allelic variants most commonly associated with Crohn's disease in European and American populations include 1 frameshift

insertion leading to early truncation of the protein (Leu1007-fsinsC) and 2 missense mutations (Arg702Trp, Gly908Arg). Carriage of disease-associated allelic variants on both chromosomes confers an odds ratio for Crohn's disease of 17.1 (95% confidence interval [CI], 10.7 to 27.2), and heterozygous persons have an odds ratio of 2.5 (95% CI, 2.0 to 2.9) for the disease.[30] Genetic polymorphisms of NOD2/CARD15 have been associated with younger onset and ileal location of disease and increased likelihood of stricture formation.[30] It has been estimated that as many as 20% to 30% of patients with Crohn's disease bear abnormal NOD2/CARD15. Nevertheless, the penetrance of NOD2/CARD15 is not more than 5% of individuals bearing 2 copies of disease-associated polymorphisms, and roughly 0.5% in heterozygous persons.[31] This indicates that disease-related allelic variants of the gene may be found in a large number of persons who do not have Crohn's disease.

The discovery of the association of NOD2/CARD15 with Crohn's disease has opened a remarkable window into the pathogenesis of Crohn's disease. The gene product of NOD2/CARD15 is a cytosolic protein that functions as an intracellular sensor of bacteria. Specifically, the protein binds to muramyl dipeptide (MDP; MurNAc-L-Ala-D-isoGln), a component of bacterial peptidoglycan, found in Gram-positive and Gram-negative bacteria.[32] The NOD2/CARD15 protein is expressed in a wide diversity of cells, including macrophages, lymphocytes, fibroblasts, and intestinal epithelial cells, specifically Paneth cells,[22] which lie within the crypts and produce endogenous antimicrobial peptides called *defensins*. The NOD2/CARD15 gene consists of 2 CARD domains, a nucleotide binding domain (NBD), and 10 leucine-rich repeats (LRR). NOD2/CARD15 variants associated with Crohn's disease lie within the LRR and interfere with binding to MDP. In mononuclear cells, mutations in NOD2 result in decreased activation of nuclear factor (NF)-κB, whereas an excess of NF-κB expression is observed in tissue inflamed by Crohn's disease. This apparent paradox has yet to be unraveled completely, but it is clear that defects in NOD2 impair antibacterial responses, particularly to oral exposure to pathogens. Notably, production of β-defensins, which are antibacterial proteins produced by Paneth cells, is defective in Crohn's patients with variant NOD2.[33] These findings strongly implicate defects in innate immunity—the immediate and nonspecific immune responses to microbial infection—in a subset of patients with Crohn's disease, with subsequent chronic activation of adaptive immunity, the antigen-specific responses mediated by antigen-presenting cells (APCs) and T cells.

Beyond NOD2, multiple genetic defects in the autophagy pathway, which is implicated in the pathogenesis of Crohn's disease, also provide a link to defective host-microbe interactions.[34,35] Autophagy is an ancient cellular process, highly conserved in evolution, by which segments of cytoplasm are isolated within a membrane and delivered to lysosomes (or "inflammasomes") by mechanisms that do not involve transport through endocytic or vacuolar sorting pathways. This unique process plays a role in cellular homeostasis by clearing proteins that are long-lived, misfolded, or aggregated, and by clearing apoptotic bodies, which might otherwise trigger inflammation and autoimmunity. Autophagy has been shown to contribute directly to innate immunity through direct killing of pathogens, activation of Toll-like receptors and NOD-like receptors, which are pattern recognition receptors that activate the innate immune response, and elaboration of immunomodulatory cytokines such as interferon (IFN)-γ. Autophagy also stands at the interface of innate and adaptive immune responses, delivering antigen to HLA class II molecules in APCs for antigen-specific binding.[35]

GWA studies have identified variants that predispose to Crohn's disease in at least 2 autophagy-related genes. The

TABLE 115-1 Crohn's Disease–Specific Loci

Chr.	Position (Mb)	SNP	Key Genes (+no. of additional genes in locus)	Product and Description of Candidate Genes, if Known
1	78.62	rs17391694	(5)	
	114.3	rs6679677	PTPN22 (8)	Protein tyrosine phosphatase, nonreceptor type 22; gain-of-function variant confers reduced risk for Crohn's disease, while loss-of-function variants promote autoimmune disorders
	120.45	rs3897578	ADAM30 (5)	ADAM (A Disintegrin And Metalloprotease domain) metallopeptidase domain 30. Members of this family are membrane-anchored proteins implicated in a variety of biological processes involving cell-cell and cell-matrix interactions
	172.85	rs9286879	FASLG, TNFSF18 (0)	Fas ligand, causes apoptosis of some cell types, including lymphocytes Tumor necrosis factor (ligand) superfamily, member 18. Modulates T-lymphocyte survival in peripheral tissues, expressed in endothelial cells, and believed to be important for interaction between T lymphocytes and endothelial cells
2	27.63	rs1728918	UCN (23)	Urocortin, a ligand for corticotropin-releasing factor type 2 receptors
	62.55	rs10865331	(3)	
	231.09	rs6716753	SP140 (5)	SP140 nuclear body protein; in lymphocytes, implicated in the innate immune response to HIV1
	234.15	rs12994997	ATG16L1 (8)	Autophagy-related 16-like 1; involved in autophagy, by which there is clearance of some intracellular pathogens, as well as integration of innate and adaptive immune responses
4	48.36	rs6837335	(6)	
	102.86	rs13126505	(1)	
5	55.43	rs10065637	IL6ST, IL31RA (1)	Interleukin-6 signal transducer (gp130, oncostatin M receptor), a signal transducer shared by interleukin 6, ciliary neurotrophic factor, leukemia inhibitory factor, and oncostatin M, and activated when these cytokines bind their receptors Interleukin-31 receptor A; belongs to the type I cytokine receptor family, with homology to gp130. Expressed on monocytes, and involved in IL-31 signaling via activation of signal transducers and activators of transcription (STAT-3) and STAT-5
	72.54	rs7702331	(4)	
	173.34	rs17695092	CPEB4 (2)	Cytoplasmic polyadenylation element binding protein 4
6	21.42	rs12663356	(3)	
	31.27	rs9264942	(22)	
	127.45	rs9491697	(3)	
	128.24	rs13204742	(2)	
	159.49	rs212388	TAGAP (5)	T-cell activation Rho guanosine triphosphate (GTP) ase-activating protein; locus reported to be protective for perianal sepsis in Crohn's disease, and a shared risk locus with celiac disease
7	26.88	rs10486483	(2)	
	28.17	rs864745	CREB5, JAZF1 (1)	cAMP responsive element binding protein 5; binds to CRE as a homodimer or a heterodimer with c-Jun or CRE-BP1, and functions as a CRE-dependent trans-activator JAZF zinc finger 1; encodes a nuclear protein with 3 C2H2-type zinc fingers, and functions as a transcriptional repressor
8	90.87	rs7015630	RIPK2 (4)	Receptor-interacting serine-threonine kinase 2; a member of the receptor-interacting protein (RIP) family of serine/threonine protein kinases; contains a C-terminal caspase activation and recruitment domain (CARD). Implicated as a mediator of NOD2 signaling, and in susceptibility to leprosy
	129.56	rs6651252	0	
13	44.45	rs3764147	LACC1 (3)	Laccase (multicopper oxidoreductase) domain containing 1; implicated in susceptibility to leprosy

Continued

TABLE 115-1 Crohn's Disease–Specific Loci—cont'd

Chr.	Position (Mb)	SNP	Key Genes (+no. of additional genes in locus)	Product and Description of Candidate Genes, if Known
15	38.89	rs16967103	RASGRP1, SPRED1 (2)	Ras guanyl releasing protein 1 (calcium and DAG-regulated) activates the extracellular signal-regulated kinases (Erk)/mitogen-activated protein (MAP) kinase cascade and regulates T-cell and B-cell development, homeostasis, and differentiation Sprouty-related, Ena/VASP Homology 1 (EVH1) domain containing 1 is phosphorylated by tyrosine kinase in response to several growth factors, and can act as a homodimer or as a heterodimer with SPRED2 to regulate activation of the MAP kinase cascade
16	50.66	rs2066847	NOD2 (6)	**N**ucleotide-binding **O**ligomerization **D**omain containing 2's role in innate immune response is through binding of intracellular muramyl dipeptide, a component of bacterial cell walls
17	25.84	rs2945412	LGALS9, NOS2 (3)	Lectin, galactoside-binding, soluble, 9 is a S-type lectin, beta-galactoside-binding protein implicated in modulating cell-cell and cell-matrix interactions Nitric oxide synthase 2, inducible expressed in liver and is inducible by a combination of lipopolysaccharide and certain cytokines; the protein is a biologic mediator of antimicrobial and other processes
19	1.12	rs2024092	GPX4, HMHA1 (20)	Glutathione peroxidase 4 catalyzes the reduction of hydrogen peroxide, organic hydroperoxide, and lipid peroxides by reduced glutathione; it also protects mitochondria from oxidative damage in intestinal epithelial cells. Histocompatibility (minor) HA-1
	46.85 49.2	rs4802307 rs516246	(9) FUT2 (25)	Fucosyltransferase 2 is a Golgi stack membrane protein involved in creating a precursor of the H antigen, which is required for the final step in the soluble A and B antigen synthesis pathway
21	34.77	rs2284553	IFNGR2, IFNAR1 (10)	Interferon gamma receptor 2 (interferon gamma transducer 1) protein is the non-ligand-binding beta chain of the gamma interferon receptor. Human interferon-gamma receptor is a heterodimer of IFNGR1 and IFNGR2. Defects in IFNGR2 are a cause of Mendelian susceptibility to mycobacterial disease (MSMD) Interferon (alpha, beta and omega) receptor 1 forms one of the 2 chains of a receptor for interferons alpha and beta. Binding and activation of the receptor stimulates Janus protein kinases, which in turn phosphorylate several proteins, including STAT 1 and STAT2

From GWA studies as reported in Jostins L, Ripke S, Weersma RK, et al. Host-microbe interactions have shaped the genetic architecture of inflammatory bowel disease. Nature 2012; 491:119-24. Descriptions of gene products adapted from NCBI (National Center for Biotechnology Information, US National Library of Medicine) Gene database, http://www.ncbi.nlm.nih.gov/gene/. Accessed on June 30, 2013.

first, the autophagy-related 16-like 1 (ATG16L1) gene, was noted as having a disease-associated single nucleotide polymorphism (SNP) that encodes an amino acid substitution in exon 8, resulting in a change from alanine to threonine[34-36]; this minor allele is protective against Crohn's disease. ATG16L1 is expressed by intestinal epithelial cells, APCs, and various subsets of human T cells. The second autophagy gene associated with Crohn's disease is the IRGM (immunity-related GTPase [guanosine triphosphatase] family member M) gene on chromosome 5q33.1.[37] Careful study suggests that the disease-associated variants of this gene do not affect the amino acid sequence of its product, but they more likely alter its expression.[37] IRGM appears to be important in resistance to intracellular pathogens such as mycobacteria, Listeria monocytogenes, and Toxoplasma gondii.[35]

A third pathway associated with Crohn's disease is IL-23 and other gene products associated with this protein.[38] IL-23 is a heterodimeric cytokine comprising 2 linked subunits (p19 and p40). IL-23 is produced by many cell types, including dendritic cells and macrophages, in response to diverse microbial signals. Naïve CD4+ T cells up-regulate IL-23 receptor when exposed to IL-6 and transforming growth factor (TGF)-β, completing an autocrine loop in the generation of Th17 T cells, effector T cells that produce IL-17.[39,40] A rare variant of the IL23R gene leading to a glutamine at position 381 rather than an arginine is strongly protective for Crohn's disease, with an odds ratio of 0.26 to 0.45; other, more common SNPs are associated with increased risk for Crohn's disease and UC.[41] In the same pathway, variants of the IL12B gene, encoding the p40 subunit common to IL-12 and IL-23, and of the JAK2 and STAT3 genes, with roles in IL23R signaling, as well as in Th17 differentiation in the case of STAT3, also have been associated with Crohn's disease susceptibility.[42] Together, these findings support the pivotal role of this pathway in maintaining mucosal homeostasis in the normal intestine. As the functional alterations associated with the many other identified genetic risk loci are elucidated, it is certain that new insights into the causes of Crohn's disease will arise.

Environment

Even with notable progress in GWA studies, identified genetic risk factors account at best for only 25% of disease variance.[43] Additional, more rare genetic variants of new or already identified loci may yet be discovered, but it is clear that environmental factors also are important. As noted earlier, the rising incidence of Crohn's disease over many decades, and in developing countries, highly suggests an environmental contribution to the expression of disease. Epidemiologic studies have examined numerous risk factors for Crohn's disease. Most studies have found breast-feeding to be protective for IBD, presumably by playing a role in early programming of immune responses in the developing GI tract and in shaping the intestinal microbiome. Occupations associated with outdoor physical labor are relatively underrepresented among patients with Crohn's disease. Crohn's disease has been associated with higher socioeconomic status, presumably because of relative underexposure to diverse environmental antigens in the course of childhood—the hygiene hypothesis as it relates to intestinal mucosal immunity in IBD. Many, but not all,[5] studies have discerned an increased risk of Crohn's disease among women who use oral contraceptives. NSAIDs have been implicated not only in exacerbations of IBD but also as a potential precipitant of new cases, perhaps by increasing intestinal permeability. Increased intake of refined sugars and a paucity of fresh fruits and vegetables in the diet have been associated with the development of Crohn's disease. It is conceivable that this observation may be confounded by exacerbation of symptoms in patients with mild disease because of increased dietary fiber intake and subsequent avoidance of these food items before diagnosis.

Antibiotic use, particularly in childhood, has been observed to be associated with subsequent risk of IBD.[44-47] Such observations are plausibly connected to the etiology of Crohn's disease, given the role of the microbiome in shaping the developing immune system and host responses. However, caution should be maintained in assuming that such associations are causal, as an equally plausible explanation is that the genetic predisposition to Crohn's disease also confers increased susceptibility to a variety of infections.

A virtually unexplored area is the connection between environmental and genetic factors in the expression of disease. It is presumed that the most important environmental factors may be those that determine the composition of the intestinal flora, given its necessary role in the onset of IBD. Such factors might include breast-feeding, composition of the diet, hygiene, and many others.

Smoking is one of the more notable environmental factors for IBD. UC is largely a disease of ex-smokers and nonsmokers, whereas Crohn's disease is more prevalent among smokers. In addition, smokers have more surgery for their disease and a greater risk of relapse after resection. The reasons for the divergent effect of smoking on Crohn's disease and UC are poorly understood, but they might include effects on intestinal permeability, cytokine production, and clotting in the microvasculature. More recently, studies have focused on the role of carbon monoxide in stimulating immunosuppressive effects mediated by heme oxygenase-1.[48] Whether such biologic effects contribute to the different effects of smoking in Crohn's disease and UC is unknown.

Many patients report a correlation between disease exacerbations and stress. Although depression and anxiety are a common reaction to illness, Crohn's disease has not been shown to be caused by stress or by an anxious personality. The mind-body connection between emotional states or stress and intestinal inflammation in IBD is slowly being revealed, however, and studies indicate that stress may be associated with risk of relapse in Crohn's disease.[49]

Adaptive Immune Response and Inflammation

The interaction between effector T cells and APCs is critical to the pathogenesis of Crohn's disease (Fig. 115-1). The antigens that perpetuate the inflammatory response are taken up by APC. Degradation of antigen within proteasomes results in presentation of an epitope in the context of major histocompatibility complex (MHC) class II. Interaction between MHC class II and the T-cell receptor (CD3) results in antigen-specific interaction between the macrophage and the CD4[+] T cell. This event is necessary, but not sufficient, to activate the T cell. A second co-stimulatory signal is needed as well, because binding of CD3 to MHC class II without a co-stimulatory signal can result in anergy or apoptosis. Important co-stimulatory signals include binding of TNF to TNF receptor, CD40 to CD40 ligand, and B7 to CD28. Activation of T cells leads to production of IL-2, an important growth factor for T cells.

Inflammation normally is kept in check through an active process termed *immune tolerance.* The nature of the co-stimulatory signal, the type of APC, and the cytokine milieu influence the differentiation of T cells into populations of effector T cells, which are involved in harmful immune responses, and regulatory T cells, which ameliorate the immune response. Dendritic cells in the lamina propria actively sample the luminal contents and play a particularly vital role as key APCs capable of shaping the immune response.

As noted earlier, the p40 subunit is common to IL-12 and IL-23, each of which, in turn, is critical in shaping the Th1 and Th17 responses that characterize Crohn's disease. In addition to IL-23, the presence of TGF-β and IL-6 facilitate differentiation of naïve T cells into pathogenic Th17 cells.[39] Activated APCs further shape and amplify the immune response by producing the T-cell growth factor IL-2 and the proinflammatory cytokines IL-1 and TNF. Within mononuclear cells, the key nuclear transcription factor is NF-κB, which regulates the transcription of IL-1, IL-6, IL-8, TNF, and other peptides central to the inflammatory response.[50]

In addition to being essential to the formation of granulomas, TNF causes neutrophil activation and, along with IFN-γ, induces the expression of MHC class II on intestinal epithelial cells. Moreover, TNF and other proinflammatory cytokines contribute to the expression of adhesion molecules on the endothelial cells of the intestinal vasculature.

Expression of adhesion molecules is critical to amplify the immune response because the resident populations of granulocytes and mononuclear cells alone do not account for the vigorous inflammatory reaction characterizing IBD. Adhesion molecules on the leukocyte surface and their ligands on the endothelium of venules in the lamina propria interact in a coordinated multistep process that permits trafficking of inflammatory cells into the mucosa. First, a weak interaction between selectins on the leukocyte surface and the endothelium leads to rolling of the leukocytes along the endothelium. Second, in the presence of chemokines such as IL-8, activation occurs, and integrins are expressed on the leukocyte surface. Third, interactions between leukocyte integrins and immunoglobulin-like cellular adhesion molecules on the endothelial surface lead to spreading of the cell and diapedesis.[51] Specificity is conferred by the presence of tissue-specific cellular adhesion molecules. The integrins $\alpha_4\beta_7$ and $\alpha E\beta_7$ are of special importance in IBD, because the corresponding ligands—mucosal addressin cellular adhesion molecule and E-cadherin—are intestine specific. Mucosal addressin cellular adhesion molecule is expressed constitutively on the endothelium of venules in the lamina propria,[51] whereas

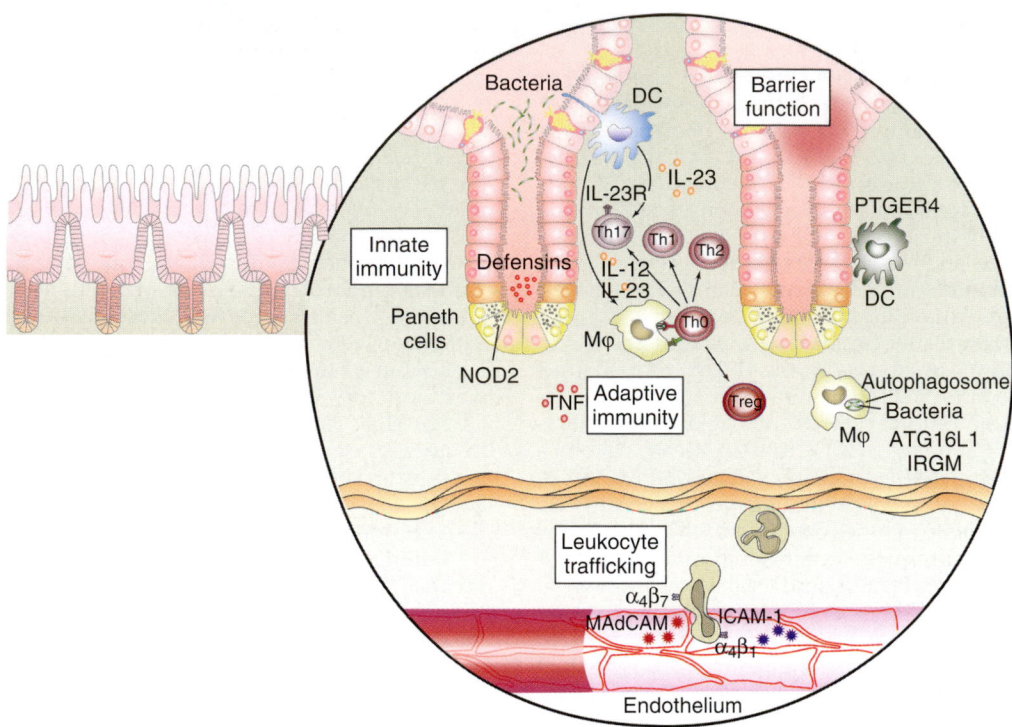

FIGURE 115-1. Pathogenesis of Crohn's disease. Animal models of IBD, studies of human genetics, and clinical trials with targeted therapeutic agents suggest that Crohn's disease is a complex, polygenic disease driven by disturbances in distinct physiologic pathways; however, not all defects or pathways appear to be aberrant in all patients. Thus, patients with allelic variants in *NOD2* have defective sensing of intracellular bacteria, as well as reduced production of defensins, which are natural antimicrobial products produced by Paneth cells in the base of the intestinal crypts. The net result is excessive activation of adaptive immune responses to compensate for defective innate immunity. Similarly, variant loci of the *ATG16L1* and *IRGM* genes are associated with defective autophagy, a process that is involved in defense against microbes and that stands at the interface of innate and adaptive immunity in the processing of intracellular pathogens and presentation of antigens to T cells. Adaptive immunity also may be deranged along the interleukin (IL)-12/IL-23 pathway, thereby shaping the expression of the helper T-cell response toward the spectrum of T helper Th17. Together, Th17 and Th1 responses, most closely associated with Crohn's disease, account for up-regulation of effector T-cell responses in Crohn's disease. Defects in regulatory T cells (Treg) of a few varieties also may be a factor in expression of disease. Dendritic cells (DCs) are active participants in maintaining immunologic tolerance within the intestine, continuously sampling luminal contents via podocytes extending through the epithelium. Activation of DCs and macrophages (Mφs) result in the expression of TNF within the mucosa. This pleiotropic cytokine has many downstream, proinflammatory effects that contribute to disease, and anti-TNF antibodies are effective in treating Crohn's disease. Antigen presenting cells (APCs), including Mφs and DCs, also lead to activation of T cells when antigen is presented to the T cell in the context of major histocompatibility complex (MHC) class II, along with a co-stimulatory signal. Defects in the barrier function of the intestinal mucosa (e.g., through variant PTGER4) can lead to increased microbial and antigenic penetration of the mucosa, also resulting in immune activation. Leukocyte trafficking is a necessary element in amplification of the mucosal immune response. Integrins are heterodimeric proteins that facilitate adhesion of leukocytes to the endothelium and recruitment into tissue. Integrins containing α4, such as α4β1 and α4β7, bind respectively to intercellular adhesion molecule 1 (ICAM-1) in the endothelium of inflamed tissues throughout the body and to mucosal addressin cellular adhesion molecule 1 (MAdCAM-1), which is specific to the intestinal endothelium. Blocking these interactions interferes with adhesion and recruitment of inflammatory cells, thereby disrupting inflammation.

binding of αEβ7 on intestinal lymphocytes to E-cadherin on intestinal epithelium permits localization of intraepithelial lymphocytes. Antibodies to the α4 subunit of integrin have proved to be therapeutic in Crohn's disease.[52]

Once recruited to the lamina propria, mononuclear cells and granulocytes elaborate a variety of injurious and proinflammatory substances that ultimately cause tissue destruction. These substances include prostaglandins, reactive oxygen metabolites, nitric oxide, leukotrienes, and proteases. Collagenase and matrix metalloproteinases play a pivotal role in the tissue destruction and complications, such as fistula and stricture, seen in Crohn's disease.[53] Counterbalancing these destructive substances are other substances that promote epithelial restitution and repair, including IL-11, trefoil peptides, and growth factors such as EGF and keratinocyte growth factor.

PATHOLOGY

Focal intestinal inflammation is the hallmark pathologic finding in Crohn's disease. This tendency for inflammation to be focal is evident in focal crypt inflammation, focal areas of marked chronic inflammation, the presence of aphthae and ulcers on a background of little or no chronic inflammation, and the interspersing of segments of involved bowel with segments of uninvolved bowel. Even within a single biopsy specimen, one can see a pronounced variability in the degree of inflammation. The presence of focally enhanced gastritis, characterized by a focal perifoveolar or periglandular lymphomonocytic infiltrate, is a common finding in patients with Crohn's disease. This finding underscores the focal nature of the inflammation, despite the strong potential for inflammation to occur anywhere along the entire longitudinal axis of the GI tract. To a certain extent, the nature of the findings and the depth of inflammatory changes depend on the chronicity of the inflammation.

Early Findings

Because of the variable and often long delay between the onset of the disease process and its diagnosis, it rarely is possible to observe the evolution of pathology from the earliest events. Studies of recurrent Crohn's disease after ileal resection have offered a window into the sequence of pathologic changes in the disease.[54]

Aphthous Ulcers

The earliest characteristic lesion of Crohn's disease is the aphthous ulcer. These superficial ulcers are minute, ranging in size from barely visible to 3 millimeters, and are surrounded by a halo of erythema. In the small intestine, aphthous ulcers arise most often over lymphoid aggregates, with destruction of the overlying M cells. In the colon, aphthae can occur without an endoscopically visible central erosion and may be associated with lymphoepithelial complexes. Crohn's aphthae typically occur in normal mucosa, although villus blunting may be seen in the surrounding small intestinal mucosa.

Aphthous ulcers represent focal areas of immune activation. The M cells and underlying lymphoid aggregates are primary locations for antigen sampling and antigen presentation, and HLA-DR is strongly expressed on the follicle-associated epithelium of the aphthous ulcer.[55] Contact with luminal contents is a key factor in the development of aphthous ulcers in Crohn's disease.

Aphthous ulcers heal in bowel excluded from the fecal stream by ileostomy, whereas reestablishing intestinal continuity leads to their recurrence[56]; these observations provide strong evidence for the role of luminal factors in the early pathogenesis of Crohn's disease.

Granulomas

The presence of granulomas (Fig. 115-2), while highly characteristic of Crohn's disease, is neither unique to Crohn's disease nor universally found.[57] Non-caseating granulomas, like aphthous lesions, are believed to be an early finding. Estimates of the prevalence of granulomas in Crohn's disease have varied greatly, ranging from 15% in endoscopic series to as high as 70% in surgical series. Whether granulomas are found appears to be, in part, a matter of how hard one looks and how much tissue is available to examine; the more tissue sampled, the larger the specimen, and the more levels taken for histopathology, the more likely granulomas will be found.

Granulomas may be discovered in involved and uninvolved bowel, in any layer of the intestine, and in mesenteric lymph nodes. Granulomas also may be found outside the GI tract—for example, in skin, eye, and liver—but extraintestinal granulomas are rare; occasionally, they may be recognized as millet seed–like nodules on the serosal surface of the bowel at laparotomy. The granulomas of Crohn's disease are sarcoid-like, consisting of collections of epithelioid histiocytes and a mixture of other inflammatory cells, including lymphocytes and eosinophils; giant cells occasionally are seen. The granulomas usually are sparse, scattered, and not well formed. In contrast to the granulomas of TB, there is little or no central necrosis, and acid-fast stains and mycobacterial cultures are negative. It also is important to distinguish the granulomas of Crohn's disease from those that can occur in association with

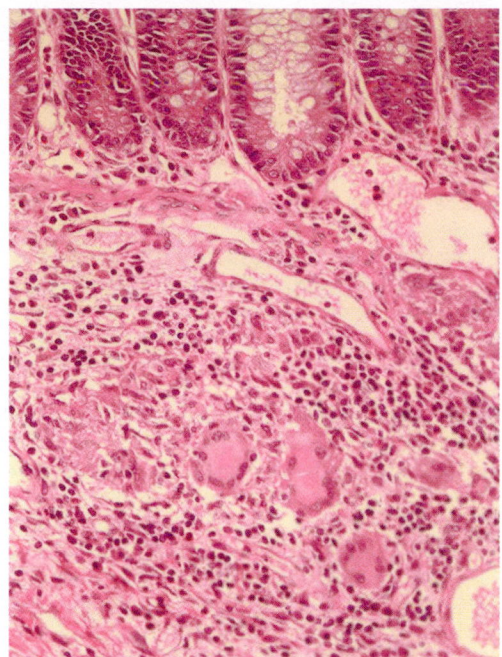

FIGURE 115-2. Photomicrograph of a typical Crohn's disease granuloma found in an endoscopic biopsy specimen. Note the loosely formed collection of cells, consisting of multinucleated giant cells (not always observed) and mononuclear cells, including T cells, and epithelioid macrophages. Central caseation is not noted. *(Courtesy Dr. Gregory Lauwers, Boston, Mass.)*

an injured crypt. The latter represent a response to mucin released from injured goblet cells and may be found in UC and other conditions.[57]

Regardless of whether granulomas are found, the granulomatous inflammation of Crohn's disease represents a particular process involving characteristic cell types and regulation by specific cytokines and adhesion molecules. TNF is the key cytokine in the formation of granulomas. Appreciation of this fact led to the concept of anti-TNF therapies as a treatment for Crohn's disease (see later).

Later Findings

Resected specimens of intestine may show localized foci of architectural distortion unaccompanied by chronic inflammation, an observation that suggests early superficial lesions such as aphthae may be transient and reversible. When the disease becomes chronic, however, aphthae can coalesce into larger ulcers with a stellate appearance. Linear or serpiginous ulcers can form when multiple ulcers fuse in a longitudinal direction. The classic cobblestoned appearance of Crohn's disease results when linear and transverse ulcers intersect and networks of ulcers surround areas of relatively normal mucosa and prominent submucosal edema. Ulcers also can extend down to the muscularis propria.

A prevailing generalization is that intestinal inflammation in Crohn's disease is a transmural process, in contrast to the more superficial inflammation of UC. The transmural nature of the inflammation, however, cannot be appreciated on superficial endoscopic biopsy specimens, and in resected specimens it tends to be focal. Transmural involvement is observed less commonly than is disease of the mucosa and submucosa, but to the extent that transmural disease is noted, it is highly consistent with a diagnosis of Crohn's disease. Dense lymphoid aggregates can enlarge the submucosa. At times, lymphoid aggregates also may be seen just outside the muscularis propria. The presence of lymphoid aggregates in the submucosa and external to the muscularis propria is a reliable sign of Crohn's disease even when granulomas are not seen. Lymphoid aggregates occasionally may be seen within the muscularis propria, most often adjacent to the myenteric plexus.

Large ulcers, sinus tracts, and strictures are late features of Crohn's disease. Sinuses and fistulas represent extensions of fissures; sinus tracts end blindly, and fistulas enter epithelial-lined organs, such as bowel, skin, bladder, or vagina. Intramural sinus tracts are recognized easily on barium studies. With penetration of inflammation to the serosa, serositis can occur, resulting in adhesion of bowel to loops of small intestine, colon, or other adjacent organs. As a result of the chronicity of the inflammatory process and adhesions, free perforation is much less common than walled-off or contained intra-abdominal abscesses or fistula formation. Fissures and fistulas are lined by neutrophils and surrounded by histiocytes and a mononuclear cell infiltrate; partial epithelialization also is often observed, perhaps reflecting incomplete healing.

Fibrosis is another transmural aspect of the disease. Fibrosis may be evident grossly as irregular thickening of the bowel wall and, along with hypertrophy of the muscularis mucosa, can contribute to the development of strictures. TGF-β is released locally in the presence of inflammation and is a cytokine that is critical for restitution and healing. In Crohn's disease, however, TGF-β may be a double-edged sword. Fibroblasts isolated from the lamina propria produce primarily type III collagen in response to TGF-β1, and in the inflamed tissues of Crohn's disease, significantly greater amounts of type III collagen are produced in response to this cytokine.[58] Thus, a cytokine essential to the healing process also is implicated in the fibrogenesis of Crohn's disease.

Other Findings

At the anatomic level, one of the most characteristic findings of Crohn's disease is the presence of *fat wrapping*, a term that refers to the creeping of mesenteric fat onto the serosal surface of the bowel. Surgeons have long taken fat wrapping as a reliable indicator of the presence of diseased tissue. Mesenteric adipose tissue hypertrophy and creeping fat are recognized early in the course of disease at laparotomy or laparoscopy. Locally, fat wrapping correlates with the presence of underlying acute and chronic inflammation, as well as transmural inflammation in the form of lymphoid aggregates. It is intriguing that patients with an increased ratio of visceral to subcutaneous fat are at significantly increased risk for complicated disease behavior.[59] Expression of peroxisome proliferator-activated receptor (PPAR)γ, a pivotal mediator in the regulation of adipose tissue homeostasis, is increased greatly in the tissues of patients with Crohn's disease.[60] In turn, adipocytes may participate in the inflammatory process of Crohn's disease by producing TNF and other inflammatory mediators.

At the microscopic level, the finding of pyloric metaplasia, normally a response to peptic ulcer disease when found in the duodenum, strongly suggests a diagnosis of Crohn's disease when found in the terminal ileum. Careful descriptive immunopathology of areas of pyloric metaplasia reveals the presence of an ulcer-associated cell lineage. Bud-like glandular structures arise adjacent to areas of ulceration and are distinguished by production of epidermal growth factor in acinar cells of the nascent gland and by trefoil proteins in the more superficial cells lining the tract. Epidermal growth factor and trefoil proteins, in turn, can promote restitution of the epithelium in adjacent mucosal ulceration.

CLINICAL FEATURES

Disease Location

Crohn's disease has a predilection for the distal small intestine and proximal colon. One third to one half of all patients have disease affecting both ileum and colon. Another one third have disease confined to the small intestine, primarily the terminal ileum, and there may be an increasing group with isolated colonic disease.[61,62] Isolated jejunal involvement is rare. Gross involvement of the esophagus, stomach, or duodenum also is rare and almost always is seen in association with disease of the distal small intestine or colon. Focally enhanced acute and chronic inflammation may be seen in gastric biopsy specimens of patients with Crohn's disease either with or without gross involvement of the stomach.[63] The discontinuous nature of the disease makes possible many variations in disease location, leading to considerable differences in clinical presentation. The disease usually stays confined to the segment in which it begins, but anatomic localization can vary over time, generally by involvement of additional segments of the alimentary tract, with a disease that has the potential to affect any segment of the GI tract.

Clinical Presentation

The presentation of Crohn's disease may be subtle and varies considerably. Factors contributing to this variability include the location of disease, the intensity of inflammation, and presence of specific intestinal and extraintestinal complications. Compared with UC, abdominal pain is a more frequent and persistent complaint. Pain is attributable to inflammation, abscess, or obstruction and may be intermittent and colicky or sustained and severe. Some patients experience symptoms that are mild but long-standing or that are atypical. Such patients are more likely to experience a delay in diagnosis that exceeds 1 year. Patients with Crohn's disease have a longer mean time to diagnosis than patients with UC, and as many as 25% of patients have a delay in diagnosis of over 2 years from onset of symptoms.[64] With improved diagnostic methods, and perhaps heightened awareness of the disease, more recent series have described typical delays of less than 1 year.[61] A prodromal period is common in Crohn's disease (not typically seen in UC) and might contribute to a delayed diagnosis, as does a prior diagnosis of IBS and older age at onset of symptoms.[65] Occasionally, radiologic and endoscopic findings are subtle, precluding definitive diagnosis even among patients with typical symptoms. Fecal occult blood may be found in approximately one half of patients, but in contrast to UC, gross rectal bleeding is uncommon, and acute hemorrhage is rare. Constitutional symptoms, particularly weight loss and fever, or growth retardation in children, may be prominent and occasionally are the sole presenting features of Crohn's disease.

Typical Presentations

Disease of the ileum, often accompanied by involvement of the cecum, can manifest insidiously. Some patients present with a small bowel obstruction, perhaps precipitated by impaction of indigestible foods, such as raw vegetables or fruit. Many years of subclinical inflammation can progress to fibrotic stenosis, with the subsequent onset of intermittent colicky pain, sometimes accompanied by nausea and vomiting. Physical examination can reveal fullness or a tender mass in the right hypogastrium, which may be more prominent during obstructive episodes. Patients with an active inflammatory component to their disease more often present with anorexia, loose or frequent stools, and weight loss; their examination might reveal fever or evidence of malnutrition. Occasionally, a patient presents with acute right lower quadrant pain, mimicking appendicitis.

Colonic disease can involve mainly the right colon or can extend distally to involve most or all of the colon (extensive or total colitis). In patients with Crohn's colitis, tenesmus is a less common complaint than in patients with UC, because the rectum often is not involved or may be less severely inflamed than other colonic segments. Nevertheless, proctitis may be the initial presentation in some cases, especially in older individuals (see later). The typical presenting symptom of colonic disease is diarrhea, occasionally with passage of obvious blood. The severity of the diarrhea tends to correlate with both the extent of colitis and the severity of inflammation, and the presentation may range from minimally altered bowel habits to fulminant colitis. Abdominal pain is often present to a greater extent than is seen in UC. Systemic manifestations such as weight loss and malaise also may be prominent.

Perianal disease is another common presentation of Crohn's disease. In as many as 24% of patients with Crohn's disease, perianal disease precedes intestinal manifestations, with a mean lead time of 4 years.[66] More often, however, perianal disease occurs concomitantly with or after the onset of symptoms of luminal disease. Perianal findings may be categorized as skin lesions, anal canal lesions, and perianal fistulas. Skin lesions include maceration, superficial ulcers, abscesses, and skin tags. Skin tags are generally of 2 types: type 1 ("elephant ears") are typically soft and painless and can be quite large; type 2, which often arise from healed fissures, ulcers or hemorrhoids, are typically edematous, hard, and tender.[67] Anal canal lesions include fissures, ulcers, and stenosis. The anal fissures of Crohn's disease tend to be located more eccentrically than the usual idiopathic fissures, which generally occur in the midline (see Chapter 129). In most cases, anal stricture is asymptomatic, but pain and occasionally obstruction occurs, particularly if stool consistency improves in the course of treatment. Deeper abscesses can arise secondary to fistulas, especially when the internal opening is located high in the rectum.

Unusual Presentations

Upper GI tract Crohn's disease is uncommon in the absence of disease beyond the ligament of Treitz. Approximately one third of patients with proximal Crohn's disease do not have evidence of distal Crohn's disease at the time of diagnosis, but virtually all develop distal disease in time. Patients with proximal Crohn's disease tend to be younger at the time of diagnosis and more often present with abdominal pain and malaise; they do not undergo surgery more often than do patients with lower tract disease alone, but the length of bowel that is resected tends to be greater.

Gastroduodenal Crohn's disease manifests as Hp-negative peptic ulcer disease, with dyspepsia or epigastric pain as the primary symptom. When outflow obstruction occurs because of stricture formation or edema, early satiety, nausea, vomiting, and weight loss can predominate.

Esophageal Crohn's disease is rare, occurring in less than 2% of patients. Presenting symptoms can include dysphagia, odynophagia, substernal chest pain, and heartburn. These symptoms may be progressive and lead to profound weight loss. Aphthous ulcers sometimes are found in the mouth and posterior pharynx. Esophageal stricture and even esophago-bronchial fistula can complicate the course of disease.

Crohn's disease that is confined solely to the jejunum and ileum is unusual and may be impossible to differentiate from ischemic jejunitis (See Chapter 118) ulcerative jejunoileitis, a distinct condition that occasionally responds to a gluten-free diet (see Chapters 107 and 119). Frank malabsorption and steatorrhea often occur. If the disease is confined to a short segment of intestine or has features consistent with Crohn's disease, initial management should be based on the presumed diagnosis of Crohn's disease.

Controversy continues to surround the diagnosis of Crohn's disease of the appendix. When idiopathic granulomatous inflammation is confined to the appendix, the presentation most often resembles that of acute appendicitis and occasionally periappendiceal abscess. The condition is rare, and the lack of disease in other locations of bowel portends a favorable prognosis, with a postoperative recurrence rate as low as 6%.[68]

Disease Behavior

Clinical observation suggests that disease behavior in Crohn's disease may be divided roughly into 2 categories: aggressive fistulizing disease and indolent cicatrizing disease; a third subset of patients appear to develop neither of these disease behaviors over long periods of observation. Moreover, these distinctions are not always neat. Both fistula and stricture can occur simultaneously in the same patient, such as in the patient with a fistula arising behind a terminal ileal stricture, or at different times.

Genetic factors are important in determining disease behavior, with *NOD2* variants being associated with stricturing or fistulizing disease, and hence, increased risk for surgery.[69] In addition, serologic antibody responses to microbial antigens and carbohydrates are associated with certain disease phenotypes.[70-72] Specifically, the presence of antiglycan antibodies to mannan (a constituent of the cell wall of baker's yeast anti-*Saccharomyces cerevisiae* antibody [ASCA]) correlates with small intestinal disease; identification of anti-CBir1 (anti-flagellin) is associated with internal penetrating and stricturing disease; and anti-*Escherichia coli* outer membrane porin C (anti-OmpC) predicts internal perforations. When perinuclear antineutrophil cytoplasmic antibodies (pANCA) are present in a patient with Crohn's disease, the phenotype is often that of an inflammatory "UC-like" Crohn's disease.

Fistula and Abscess

Fistulas are frequent manifestations of the transmural nature of Crohn's disease. Immune activation triggers the release of a variety of proteases and matrix metalloproteinases that can contribute directly to tissue destruction, sinus tract formation, and, finally, penetration to adjacent tissues. Perianal fistulas are common and are estimated to occur in 15% to 35% of patients (Fig. 115-3). When the fistula arises from an anal gland, a low-lying perianal fistula is the most common result. Such fistulas often are minimally symptomatic and can resolve with local care alone. Surprisingly, not all perianal fistulas occur in the setting of active rectal inflammation. In some cases, perianal fistulization may be extensive, forming a network of passages and extending to multiple openings that can include not only the perianal region but also the labia or scrotum, buttocks, or thighs.

Fistulas from 1 segment of the GI tract to another also occur commonly. Enteroenteric, enterocolonic, and colocolonic fistulas often are asymptomatic. Much more rarely, colonic disease penetrates normal duodenum or stomach to form a coloduodenal or cologastric fistula, respectively; affected patients might have feculent vomiting, or diarrhea from SIBO. If the fistula tracks posteriorly from the terminal ileum to the retroperitoneum, the ensuing phlegmon can ensnare the ureter (usually the right ureter), causing noncalculous

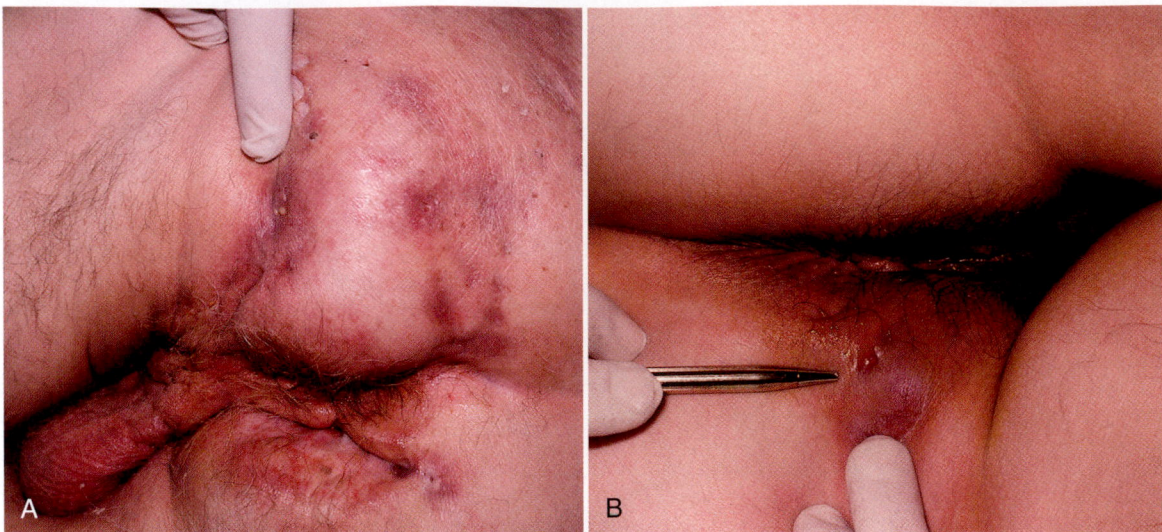

FIGURE 115-3. Perianal fistulas in Crohn's disease. *A,* Multiple complex fistulas in a man with Crohn's disease. Several are active and draining. The scrotum, perianal skin, and buttocks are discolored and hardened by healed fistulas and abscesses. *B,* A simple fistula in a woman with Crohn's disease. The purplish discoloration surrounding the fistula is from an abscess that drained spontaneously through the fistula. *(Courtesy Dr. Lawrence J. Brandt, Bronx, New York.)*

hydronephrosis; such patients often present with thigh pain or a limping gait. Deeper penetration yields the classic, but fortunately rare, psoas abscess. Affected patients typically present with right flank discomfort, fever, and a gait similar to those with ureteral entrapment.

Fistula to the vagina can occur with penetration from a severely inflamed rectal vault anteriorly (rectovaginal fistula) or from the small intestine. Rectovaginal fistulas tend to occur among women who have had a hysterectomy, permitting direct extension to the adjacent vaginal cuff without the interposing presence of a uterus. Patients present with foul, persistent vaginal discharge and occasionally with passage of flatus or frank stool per vagina. Patients also might complain of dyspareunia or perineal pain. The vaginal os of the fistula may be difficult to identify, but palpation might elicit tenderness of the posterior vaginal wall. Fistulas arising from terminal ileal disease often occur in the setting of an ileal stricture, back pressure and stasis perhaps contributing to the process. Enterovesicular or colovesicular fistulas can manifest as recurrent polymicrobial urinary tract infection or as frank pneumaturia and fecaluria. These fistulas are notoriously difficult to heal by nonsurgical means, although the resulting cystitis may be controlled with antibiotics. Enterocutaneous fistulas to the anterior abdomen, often occurring after surgery, may be especially troublesome. A classic presentation of Crohn's disease is the onset of an enterocutaneous fistula after appendectomy for what had been presumed to be appendicitis. Often the tract of the fistula follows the planes of dissection to the abdominal surface.

It has been estimated that as many as one fourth of all patients with Crohn's disease present with an intra-abdominal abscess at some time in their lives[73]; this figure is much less than one would imagine in light of the high incidence of fistulas. For the most part, inflamed serosal surfaces adhere to innocent serosa, thereby containing what would be an otherwise free perforation. Another common scenario is a perforation and abscess formation around the site of a surgical anastomosis. The classic presentation of an intra-abdominal abscess is that of a patient with spiking fevers and focal abdominal tenderness or localized peritoneal signs. Unfortunately, many of the patients at highest risk for perforation or

abscess also are taking glucocorticoids, which are notorious for suppressing peritoneal signs and fever and masking the presentations of infection; therefore, a high level of suspicion must be maintained. When free perforation and peritonitis occur, the situation is life-threatening.

Stricture

Stricture is another characteristic complication of Crohn's disease. Strictures represent long-standing inflammation and can occur in any segment of the GI tract in which inflammation has been active. Strictures do not develop in all patients with inflammatory disease, but are likely to recur, most often at the anastomosis, in patients who undergo bowel resection because of a stricture. These observations suggest that additional unidentified factors play a role in stricture formation. Strictures usually are silent until the luminal caliber is small enough to cause relative obstruction. Symptoms can include colicky, postprandial abdominal pain and bloating, punctuated by more severe episodes, and often culminating in complete obstruction.

Not all obstructive presentations, however, are caused by fibrotic strictures. The classic radiologic "string sign" of a markedly narrowed bowel segment amid widely spaced bowel loops (Fig. 115-4) is a result of spasm and edema associated with active inflammation rather than fibrostenosis; the typical string sign transiently resolves with administration of glucagon, which relieves smooth muscle spasm.

Short of demonstrating a clear response to anti-inflammatory therapy or reviewing a surgical specimen, the clinician may find it extremely difficult to differentiate a fibrostenotic from an inflammatory stricture. All strictures must be considered with suspicion, and biopsies of a stricture need to be pursued vigorously, because some strictures harbor cancer.

Classification of Disease

A major need in the clinical investigation of Crohn's disease is the ability to define subgroups of patients with distinctive, if not unique, characteristics. The ability to define such

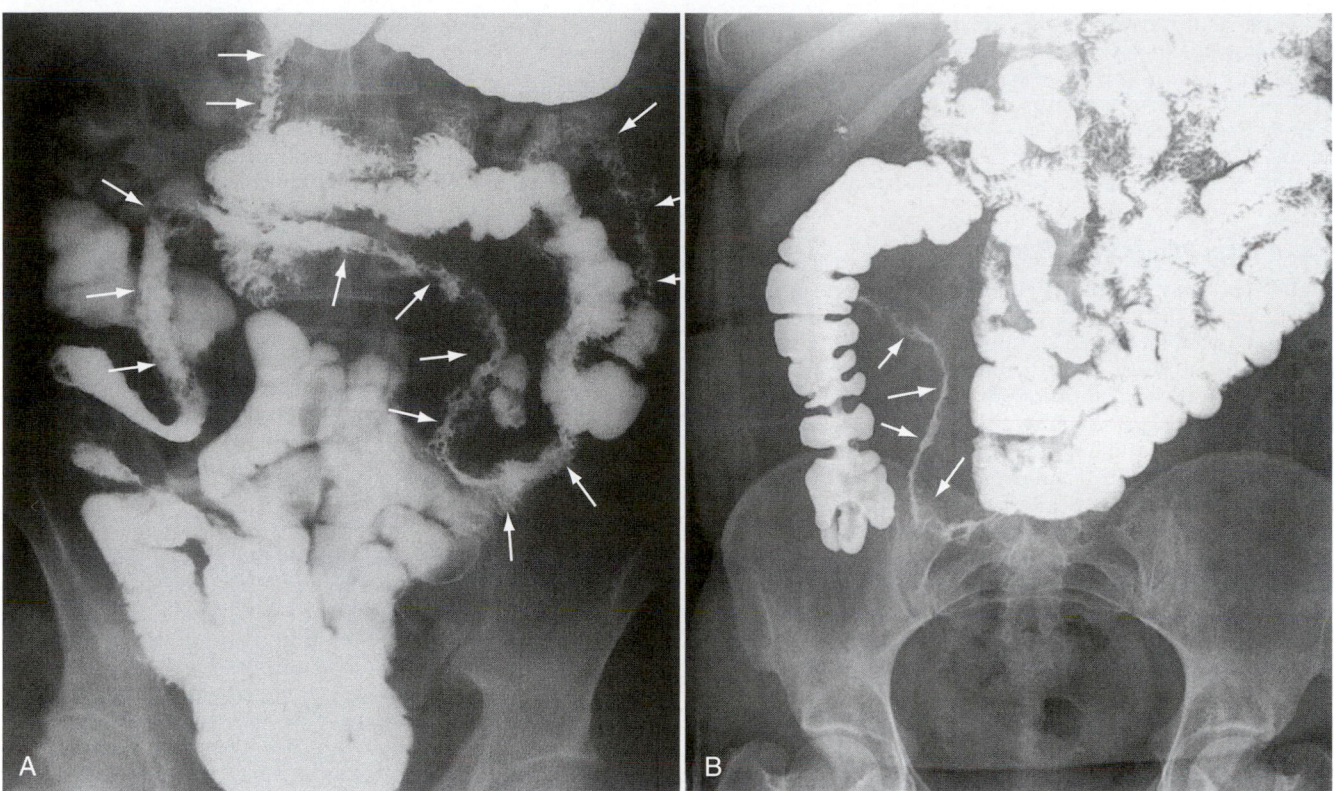

FIGURE 115-4. Films from an upper GI series and small bowel follow-through in a patient with Crohn's disease. *A*, Multiple areas of narrowed small bowel are evident *(arrows)*, with a classic cobblestoned appearance of the mucosa. Note also the separation of bowel loops. *B*, Small bowel follow-through that demonstrates a string sign in the right lower quadrant. The classic radiologic string sign *(arrows)* of a markedly narrowed bowel segment amidst widely spaced bowel loops is a result of spasm and edema associated with active inflammation rather than fibrostenosis; thus, the typical string sign transiently resolves with administration of glucagon, which relieves smooth muscle spasm. *(Courtesy Dr. Jack Wittenberg, Boston, Mass.)*

subgroups could add tremendous power to the investigation of new therapies and to genetic studies. In light of the wide heterogeneity of demographic, anatomic, and disease behavior characteristics, however, distilling the numerous possible phenotypes into simple categories is a formidable task.

The Montreal Classification of Crohn's Disease is 1 proposed scheme that incorporates the patient's age at diagnosis (A1, 16 years and younger; A2, 17 to 40 years; A3, >40 years), disease location (L1, ileal: L2, colonic; L3, ileocolonic), and disease behavior (B1, non-stricturing, non-penetrating; B2, stricturing; B3, penetrating).[74] In addition, modifiers for upper tract disease location (L4) and for perianal disease (p) may be added to the other categories. Increasingly, other associated characteristics such as serologic markers and genetic profiles may be used for their prognostic value in projecting outcomes in this heterogeneous disease.[75]

Pathophysiology of Common Symptoms and Signs

Diarrhea

Diarrhea is the most common complaint among patients with Crohn's disease. Increased stool frequency and decreased stool consistency arise through alterations in mucosal function and intestinal motility. In any given patient, multiple factors are likely to contribute to diarrhea. Altered fluid and electrolyte absorption and secretion can decrease stool consistency. Increased mucosal permeability from mucosal inflammation can result in exudation of protein and fluids. Increased production of prostaglandins, biogenic amines, cytokines, neuropeptides, and reactive oxygen metabolites all contribute to these alterations. An imbalance in the luminal concentration of bile salts relative to dietary fat can result in either bile salt–induced diarrhea or steatorrhea in the setting of ileal dysfunction or resection (see Chapter 102). Bacterial overgrowth can occur behind strictured bowel and contribute to malabsorption (see Chapter 105). Disordered colonic motility is seen in the setting of chronic inflammation and also contributes to diarrhea. Occasionally, medications used to treat Crohn's disease can exacerbate diarrhea. Thus, secretory diarrhea can occur with olsalazine, and any of the 5-aminosalicylates rarely can induce a paradoxical increase in diarrhea, usually a result of salicylate sensitivity.

Abdominal Pain

The pathophysiology of abdominal pain in Crohn's disease is not well understood. Numerous lines of investigation have provided tantalizing clues about the connection between the nervous system and Crohn's disease, although the relationship among the enteric nervous system, inflammation, and immune activation in Crohn's disease is quite complex. Stretch receptors in the intestinal wall may be stimulated as a food bolus passes through stenotic bowel, leading to abdominal pain and possibly vomiting. Visceral pain can result from serosal inflammation and local pain from abscess formation. The ganglia of the myenteric plexuses in the intestine in Crohn's disease are increased in size and number, possibly indicating neural dysfunction. Substance P binding can participate in the expression of pain, and substance P receptors have been found in increased numbers around lymphoid follicles, in the microvasculature, and on enteric neurons in Crohn's disease, even in locations distant from active inflammation; there also is increased binding of substance P to its receptors in the setting of an inflamed mucosa.[76,77]

Weight Loss and Malnutrition

Weight loss and malnutrition often are seen in patients with Crohn's disease and contribute to the complaints of weakness, irritability, malaise, and easy fatigability that are so common. In children, malnutrition can manifest as growth retardation. A host of specific nutritional deficiencies may be found even among patients whose disease has been in long-standing remission, including iron, folic acid, vitamin B_{12}, calcium, magnesium, zinc, and, particularly in the setting of malabsorption from small intestinal disease, fat-soluble vitamins. Potential contributing factors for these deficiencies are numerous and include inadequate intestinal absorption among patients with extensive small intestinal disease or resection and increased protein losses through exudation from inflamed intestine. Specific medications can cause absorption problems, including decreased calcium absorption with glucocorticoids; malabsorption of fat, fat-soluble vitamins, and calcium with cholestyramine; and folate malabsorption with sulfasalazine.

The catabolic state induced by intense inflammation can increase energy and protein requirements. Unrecognized infection can be a major contributing factor beyond the catabolism induced by the disease itself. Bypassing of small intestine by enteroenteric or enterocolonic fistulas also can contribute to undernutrition.

The most important factor in weight loss, however, is poor oral intake. Most often, poor intake results from fear of eating because of postprandial abdominal pain or diarrhea. This concern may be accentuated when in social situations, and it can contribute to a patient's lack of interest in being outside of the home. Decreased intake occasionally may be a consequence of unnecessarily restrictive diets imposed by the physician or the patient in an effort to control symptoms. Weight loss disproportionate to the burden of disease, however, should raise the suspicion of occult malignancy.

Anorexia, nausea, and vomiting also can contribute to weight loss and poor nutrition. As with other symptoms of Crohn's disease, diverse mechanisms may be contributory. TNF originally was discovered as a cytokine capable of inducing cachexia in patients with malignancy and sepsis. Indeed, serum levels of TNF in severely ill patients with Crohn's disease may be high enough to contribute to anorexia. Delayed gastric emptying of solids may be a causative factor for dyspepsia in individuals with Crohn's disease, even when the disease is inactive.[78,79] Finally, anorexia, nausea, or vomiting also may be caused by drugs used to treat the disease, including metronidazole, sulfasalazine, 6-mercaptopurine, azathioprine, and methotrexate.

Fever

Fever associated with active Crohn's disease usually is low grade and occasionally is the presenting complaint, especially in children; increased production of proinflammatory cytokines, including IL-1, IL-6, and TNF, likely are contributory. When spiking, high, or persistent fevers occur, the clinician needs to consider an infectious etiology and undertake an evaluation appropriate to the clinical picture. Rarely, such fever patterns are manifestations of Crohn's disease

activity alone without superimposed illness or even abscess formation.

Anemia

Anemia is found in one third of patients with Crohn's disease, primarily as a consequence of iron deficiency from blood loss. Macrocytic anemia can result from vitamin B_{12} deficiency because of ileal disease or resection, from SIBO or, less commonly, from folate deficiency because of proximal small intestinal disease or sulfasalazine therapy. Overproduction of IFN-γ, TNF, or IL-1 can inhibit erythropoietin production, contributing to anemia that is resistant to iron supplementation.[80]

Extraintestinal Manifestations

In addition to penetrating and cicatrizing complications that can arise in patients with Crohn's disease, numerous complications can occur distant from the bowel. Depending on the definition, it is estimated that between 6% and 25% of all patients with Crohn's disease have an extraintestinal manifestation (EIM) of IBD.[81] Many of these EIMs are common to Crohn's disease and UC and indeed to other non-idiopathic inflammatory conditions of the intestine. For example, patients with ileal Crohn's disease are at increased risk for cholelithiasis, but patients with extensive UC are at nearly the same risk. In Crohn's disease, however, the major risk factor for this complication appears to be the extent of ileal resections. In large series, EIMs are found to occur more often in Crohn's disease than in UC and are more common among patients with colonic involvement than in patients with no colonic inflammation. One fourth of those affected have more than 1 EIM.[82] Some EIMs occur as a direct result of the bowel disease (e.g., nephrolithiasis resulting from oxalate malabsorption). In the case of inflammatory mucocutaneous, joint, and ocular EIMs, the pathogenesis is an influx of mononuclear cells activated in the intestine but homing aberrantly to the involved extraintestinal organs.

Musculoskeletal

Among the most common EIMs are disorders of the bones and joints. Clubbing of the fingernails is a common and innocuous EIM. More consequential are arthritic manifestations, which are observed more commonly in patients with Crohn's disease than in those with UC. In a study of 976 patients with UC and 483 patients with Crohn's disease, pauciarticular arthropathy (type I, affecting ≤ 4 joints) occurred in 3.6% of patients with UC and in 6.0% of those with Crohn's disease.[83] In most patients, joint symptoms occurred in the setting of a relapse of intestinal symptoms. Polyarticular arthropathy (type II, ≥ 5 joints affected) occurred in 2.5% of patients with UC and 4.0% of those with Crohn's disease.[83] Among patients with Crohn's disease, nearly one half had joint symptoms in association with a relapse in intestinal disease.

Peripheral arthralgias occur in one fifth of patients with Crohn's disease, most strongly in association with colonic disease.[82] Patients tend to have waxing and waning joint pain and stiffness in association with flares of intestinal disease. Joints may be involved in an asymmetrical or migratory fashion. With rare exception, the disease is non-deforming and often is accompanied by skin (erythema nodosum) and eye (uveitis) complications. Rheumatoid factor typically is negative. Knee and ankle joints often are affected first, but elbows, wrists, proximal interphalangeal, metacarpophalangeal, and metatarsophalangeal joints may be involved subsequently. Patients who have undergone ileocecal resection for their disease tend to have fewer arthritic complications after their surgery.

Axial arthropathies are less common than peripheral arthropathies and occur in 3% to 10% of patients with IBD.[84] Spondylitis associated with IBD, like idiopathic ankylosing spondylitis, manifests as insidious low back pain and morning stiffness that is improved by exercise. As many as 75% of patients with Crohn's disease and spondylitis are positive for HLA-B27.[85] Iritis can occur in association with this manifestation. Bilateral symmetrical sacroiliitis without progression to spondylitis is more common than spondylitis and is reported to occur in 4% to 18% of patients.[86] In 1 study, sacroiliitis was found on MRI among 39% of patients, with two thirds reporting low back pain; 11% of patients with negative scans reported low back pain.[87]

Rarer rheumatologic complications include granulomatous vasculitis, periostitis, and amyloidosis. In addition, a septic joint, although a rare complication of Crohn's disease, should be kept in mind. A septic hip joint is a striking, devastating, and fortunately rare complication of a psoas abscess that extends directly to the acetabular capsule.

Glucocorticoids used to treat Crohn's disease may be a cause of joint pain. Withdrawal of glucocorticoids can lead to pseudoarthritis, with diffuse joint aches that gradually resolve; adrenal insufficiency should be considered in such patients. Aseptic necrosis of the hip and other joints can occur with or without the use of glucocorticoids and may be disabling. Osteomyelitis can occur as a result of direct extension by a fistula, usually to the pelvis, or it may be a recurrent problem distant to the site of inflammation, presumably through hematogenous spread of bacteria.

Metabolic bone disease is common in Crohn's disease; osteopenia (T score on dual energy x-ray absorptiometry between −2.49 and −1.0) or osteoporosis (T score −2.5 and lower) occurs in 30% to 60% of patients. Morbidity, as a consequence of increased susceptibility to bone fractures, includes debilitating and painful vertebral crush fractures, which can occur even in children with Crohn's disease. Although glucocorticoid use is the main risk factor for this metabolic bone disease in UC, low bone mineral density is a feature of Crohn's disease even upon diagnosis in both adults and children.[88,89] Contributing factors include malabsorption of calcium and vitamin D, smoking, and perhaps the effects of proinflammatory cytokines such as TNF.[90] Low BMI may be the most important risk factor for developing osteoporosis.[91] Sarcopenia (decreased muscle mass) is closely associated with decreased bone density and is seen in up to 60% of patients with Crohn's disease.[92]

Mucocutaneous

The most common skin lesions associated with IBD are pyoderma gangrenosum and erythema nodosum. Neither condition is found solely in IBD, and the finding of 1 or the other lesion is not specific for either major form of IBD.

Pyoderma gangrenosum (PG) appears first as a papule, pustule, or nodule. It can occur virtually anywhere on the body but most often it occurs on the leg or occasionally around a stoma, and progresses to an ulcer with undermined borders. The PG ulcer typically has a violaceous rim and crater-like holes pitting its base. The phenomenon of pathergy, or the development of large ulcers at the site of minor trauma, is characteristic of PG and also the skin lesions of Behçet's syndrome. Healing typically is associated with a cribriform, or pocked, scar. In Crohn's disease, PG often occurs without an associated flare of intestinal symptoms.

Erythema nodosum (EN) is seen much more commonly in women than in men. Like PG, many other diseases are associated with EN, including *Streptococcus* or *Yersinia* infection, TB, leprosy, fungal infections, Behçet's syndrome, and sarcoidosis. The classic appearance of EN is tender subcutaneous nodules with an erythematous or dusky appearance, most often on the pretibial region. There is a strong association of EN with arthropathy. EN often manifests during exacerbations of intestinal disease and tends to improve with treatment of the underlying bowel disease. Whenever possible, EN lesions should not be biopsied because biopsied lesions tend to scar; spontaneously resolving lesions heal without forming a scar.

Aphthous ulcers of the mouth are common among patients with Crohn's disease and UC but also are often seen among otherwise healthy persons. As the most cephalad part of the GI tract, the mouth rarely may be involved directly by the granulomatous inflammation of Crohn's disease. Features may include lip or facial swelling, angular cheilitis and oral mucosal cobblestoning.[93]

A rare EIM is metastatic Crohn's disease (i.e., granulomatous inflammation of the skin remote from the GI tract but histologically identical to the primary intestinal lesion).[94] Described cases have included lesions behind the ears, in the perineum, or on the feet, legs, penis, and vulva. Other rare skin manifestations of Crohn's disease include leukocytoclastic vasculitis, Sweet's syndrome (neutrophilic dermatosis), cutaneous polyarteritis nodosa, and epidermolysis bullosa acquisita. An increased occurrence of psoriasis among patients with Crohn's disease is in concordance with the reported genetic overlap between these diseases.[27,95]

Ocular

Ocular EIMs are estimated to occur in 6% of patients with Crohn's disease.[96] Episcleritis is more common in Crohn's disease than in UC, consists of injection of the sclera and conjunctiva, and does not affect visual acuity. Episodes tend to occur in association with active intestinal disease. Scleritis involves deeper layers of the eye, also occurs most often in parallel with active intestinal disease, and i can cause lasting damage if untreated. Uveitis usually manifests with headache, deep eye pain, lacrimation, blurred vision, and photophobia, as a consequence of iridospasm. Physical examination findings of uveitis include meiosis and ciliary flush. Visual acuity is preserved unless the posterior segment becomes involved. In contrast to the uveitis associated with ankylosing spondylitis, the presentation of uveitis in patients with IBD often is insidious, with bilateral involvement and extension to the posterior segment. Slit-lamp examination demonstrates an inflammatory flare in the anterior chamber. Of all the ocular EIMs, uveitis is the one that demands emergent ophthalmologic consultation. Other ocular complications of Crohn's disease include a particular corneal injury referred to as keratopathy and night blindness resulting from malabsorption of vitamin A.

Hepatobiliary

Gallstones occur in 14.35/1000 patient-years of follow-up among people with Crohn's disease, roughly twice the rate of the general population.[97] Asymptomatic and mild elevations of liver biochemical tests often are seen in Crohn's disease, but only few of these patients develop clinical evidence of cirrhosis. PSC more often is associated with UC, but it occurs in patients with Crohn's disease, and is more often small duct disease associated with colonic involvement.[98] Recent GWA studies in PSC indicated that 6 of 12 significant associations outside the human leukocyte antigen complex are more strongly associated with PSC than with IBD (rs7426056, 2q33,

CD28; rs5625822, 16q15*, *BACH2*; rs4147359, 10p15*, *IL2RA*; rs7937682, 11q23, *SIK2*; rs3184504, 12q24, *SH2B3*; rs60652743, 19q13*, *PRKD2*), despite the observation that nearly three quarters of PSC patients have comorbid IBD.[99] As the findings are more often confined to the small biliary radicals, the presentation is usually one of abnormal liver biochemical tests, pericholangitis on liver biopsy, and a normal cholangiogram. Other hepatobiliary complications of Crohn's disease include fatty liver and autoimmune hepatitis.

Renal and Genitourinary

In addition to the direct complications of perforating Crohn's disease with encroachment on the bladder and other genitourinary structures, and inflammatory entrapment of the ureter, uric acid and oxalate stones are common in patients with Crohn's disease.[100] In the setting of fat malabsorption resulting from intestinal resection or extensive small intestinal disease, the malabsorbed free fatty acids bind luminal calcium, thereby decreasing the calcium that is available to bind with and clear oxalate via intestinal excretion. Oxalate that remains in the intestinal lumen binds to sodium and as sodium oxalate has increased absorption compared with calcium oxalate, the result is hyperoxaluria and calcium oxalate stone formation. Uric acid stones are believed to result from volume depletion and a hypermetabolic state. Rare intrinsic renal complications include membranous nephropathy, glomerulonephritis, and renal amyloidosis. Interstitial nephritis has been associated with mesalamine use, but it is not clear if it is a direct result of the medication or of the disease itself. Penile and vulvar edema also have been reported, but the mechanism for these occurrences is unknown.

Vascular

A prothrombotic tendency has been noted in both UC and Crohn's disease. Patients might present with venous thromboembolism or, much less commonly, arterial thrombosis.[101] The incidence of venous thromboembolism increases with age, but a higher relative risk is observed in younger patients.[102] The hypercoagulable state can arise from many possible contributing causes: thrombocytosis, increased levels of fibrinogen, fibrinopeptide A, factor V, and factor VIII, antithrombin III deficiency, and free protein S deficiency, all related to active bowel inflammation. Circulating immune complexes, increased levels of plasminogen activator inhibitors, decreased levels of tissue plasminogen activator, and spontaneous platelet aggregation may be present independent of bowel inflammation. Defective methylenetetrahydrofolate reductase (MTHFR), along with folate and vitamin B_{12} deficiency, is linked to hyperhomocysteinemia, which in turn may predispose to thrombosis. Reports of increased prevalence of the factor V Leiden mutation and MTHFR have been observed by some but not other investigators.[103] In more than half of patients who experience thrombosis, no predisposing factor can be identified.

Other

Clinically significant disease of the lungs,[104] heart, pancreas, and nervous system[105] in association with Crohn's disease is unusual but reported. Subclinical lung involvement may be much more common than is apparent, perhaps reflecting the commonality of bronchus-associated lymphoid tissue and gut-associated lymphoid tissue.[104] Patients with IBD are more at risk to develop asthma, and there also may be an association with chronic obstructive pulmonary disease.[95,106] Cardiomyopathy can result from a variety of nutrient deficiencies in patients with marked malabsorption. Pleuropericarditis, myocarditis, and endocarditis occur rarely. Acute pancreatitis is uncommon, though may occur spontaneously or as a result of treatment with mesalamine or a thiopurine agent. Granulomatous pancreatitis and pancreatic insufficiency are rare.

DIFFERENTIAL DIAGNOSIS

Establishing a diagnosis of Crohn's disease usually is straightforward once it is considered. Nevertheless, a large number of alternative diagnoses may be considered during various stages of the evaluation. Reports are legion of other diseases mistakenly diagnosed as Crohn's disease and of Crohn's disease mistaken for other diseases. Misdiagnoses may be attributed to the protean presentations of Crohn's disease, which include considerable variation among patients with distinct anatomic distributions of disease, different degrees of inflammation, and the variable presence of intestinal complications and EIMs.

There are a number of clinical situations in which Crohn's disease should enter the differential diagnosis, including diarrhea or abdominal pain, especially when localized to the right lower quadrant; evidence of intestinal inflammation on radiologic or endoscopic studies; discovery of an intestinal stricture or fistula arising from the intestine; and evidence of inflammation or granulomas on intestinal histology. Categories of causation that overlap with Crohn's disease in clinical presentation include functional bowel disorders, primarily IBS; immune-mediated diseases, particularly other colitides and most importantly UC; medications, especially NSAIDs; vascular disorders, notably ischemic bowel disease and collagen vascular diseases; neoplasia, including carcinoma and lymphoma; infectious diarrheas, intestinal inflammation, or granulomas; and miscellaneous other diseases and syndromes, including diverticular disease. Once the presence of bowel inflammation has been confirmed, the differential diagnosis may focus on presentation according to the anatomic location of the findings (Box 115-1).

ESTABLISHING THE DIAGNOSIS AND EVALUATING DISEASE ACTIVITY

No single symptom, sign, or diagnostic test establishes the diagnosis of Crohn's disease. Rather the diagnosis is established through a total assessment of the clinical presentation with confirmatory evidence from radiologic, endoscopic, and, in most cases, pathologic findings.

Initial evaluation includes a thorough history-taking, physical examination, and basic laboratory tests. History-taking focuses on the key symptoms and their severity and duration. Specific points to be covered should include recent travel history, use of antibiotics and other medications, diet, and sexual preference and activity. A family history of IBD can raise the level of suspicion but does not guarantee the diagnosis. The review of systems should focus on eliciting EIMs and weight loss. Fever may be associated with the underlying disease or a suppurative complication. A careful examination of the abdomen for signs of obstruction, tenderness, or a mass should be undertaken. Thorough inspection of the perineum and a rectal examination might disclose findings highly suggestive of the underlying diagnosis or gross or occult blood.

Laboratory data may be normal. Anemic patients should undergo further evaluation to define the contributions of iron, folate, or vitamin B_{12} deficiencies. The WBC count may be

BOX 115-1 Differential Diagnosis of Crohn's Disease

Differential Diagnosis of Ileitis

Backwash ileitis in UC
Drug-related
Ectopic pregnancy
Endometriosis
Gynecologic disorders
Ileitis associated with spondyloarthropathy
Infection
  Actinomycosis israelii
  Anisakis simplex
  Cryptococcus neoformans
  Cytomegalovirus
  Histoplasma capsulatum
  Mycobacterium avium complex
  Mycobacterium tuberculosis
  Neutropenic enterocolitis
  Salmonella spp.
  Yersinia enterocolitica
  Yersinia pseudotuberculosis
Infiltrative disorders
  Amyloidosis
  Eosinophilic gastroenteritis
Lymphoid nodular hyperplasia
Neoplasms
  Carcinoid tumor
  Cecal or ileal adenocarcinoma
  Lymphoma
  Metastatic cancer
NSAID-related ulcer or stricture
Other inflammatory disorders
  Appendicitis/appendiceal abscess
  Cecal diverticulitis
Ovarian cyst or tumor
Ovarian torsion
Pelvic inflammatory disease
Radiation enteritis
Torsion of the appendiceal epiploica
Tubo-ovarian abscess
Vascular disorders
  Behçet's disease
  Intestinal ischemia: focal segmental ischemia: acute
    enteritis, chronic enteritis, stricture; chronic mesenteric
    ischemia; drug-induced (e.g., oral contraceptives,
    ergotamine, amphetamines, phenylephrine, cocaine)

Vasculitis: Henoch-Schönlein purpura, polyarteritis nodosa,
  eosinophilic granulomatosis with polyangiitis (EGPA,
  Churg-Strauss syndrome), SLE, Takayasu's arteritis,
  granulomatosis with polyangiitis, lymphomatoid
  granulomatosis, giant cell arteritis, rheumatoid
  vasculitis, thromboangiitis obliterans

Differential Diagnosis of Colitis

Acute self-limited colitis
Behçet's disease
Chronic granulomatous disease
Diversion colitis
Diverticulitis
Drug-induced colitis (NSAIDs, gold, penicillamine)
Eosinophilic gastroenteritis
Graft-versus-host disease
Indeterminate colitis
Infections
  Aeromonas spp.
  Campylobacter spp.
  Clostridium difficile
  Cytomegalovirus
  Entamoeba histolytica
  Escherichia coli (enterohemorrhagic, enteroinvasive)
  Mycobacterium tuberculosis
  Salmonella spp.
  Schistosoma mansoni
  Shigella spp.
  Strongyloides stercoralis
  Yersinia enterocolitica
Ischemic colitis
  Chronic ischemic colitis
  Ischemic stricture
  Ischemic colitis with toxic megacolon
  Transient ischemic colitis
Microscopic colitis
  Collagenous colitis
  Lymphocytic colitis
Radiation colitis
Sarcoidosis
Segmental colitis associated with diverticular disease
  (SCAD)
Solitary rectal ulcer syndrome
UC

From Sands BE. From symptom to diagnosis: Clinical distinctions among various forms of intestinal inflammation. Gastroenterology 2004; 126:1518-32, with permission.

normal or elevated; an increased number of band forms suggests the possibility of a pyogenic complication. In the patient with vague symptoms suggesting IBS, an elevated C-reactive protein or erythrocyte sedimentation rate, although not specific for IBD, can prompt further investigation. Stool studies should include culture, examination for ova and parasites, and testing for *Clostridium difficile* infection and should be performed before endoscopy or barium studies. Serology for *Entamoeba histolytica* should be considered in selected patients.

Ultimately, the diagnosis of Crohn's disease is confirmed by findings on imaging studies, endoscopy, and usually histopathology. Barium studies had been the mainstay of imaging Crohn's disease for many years, and they accurately define the anatomic location of disease and can reveal evidence of active inflammation (see Fig. 115-4). However, the small bowel follow-through study has largely been replaced at most centers with CT or MRI (see later). Fine details from barium studies are instructive in describing the anatomical findings of the disease, even if rarely used. Early findings include aphthous ulcers, a coarse villus mucosal pattern, and thickened folds.

Submucosal edema may be evident as thickening or flattening of the valvulae conniventes, whereas transmural edema manifests as widening of the separation between bowel loops. Ulcers most often occur on the mesenteric border, with consequent pseudosacculation of the antimesenteric border because of shortening of the mesenteric portion of bowel. Later findings include a cobblestone appearance resulting from edema and inflammation of relatively spared islands of mucosa separated by intersecting longitudinal and transverse knife-like clefts of ulceration. Still later, one can discern fistulas, sinus tracts, and fixed strictures; all but the finest and earliest details may now be seen with cross-sectional imaging modalities.

Standard CT studies do not demonstrate mucosal detail and often appear normal early in the course of disease. The advent of CT enterography, however, has allowed fine mucosal changes to be evaluated along with extraluminal features (and complications of Crohn's disease). CT enterography differs from routine CT by the use of a high-resolution multidetector scanner, IV contrast, and large volumes of oral contrast (either dilute barium or negative water-based contrast) to improve

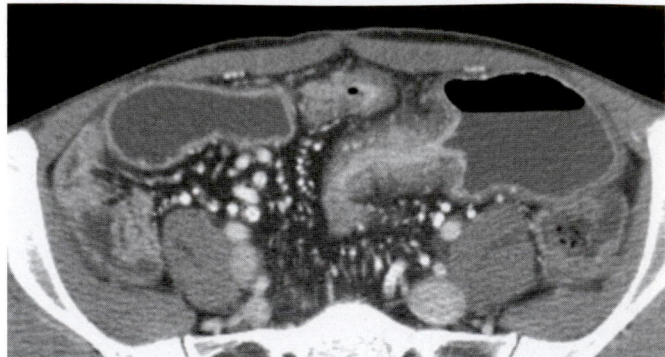

FIGURE 115-5. CT enterography in a patient with Crohn's disease showing an intestinal stricture with pre-stenotic dilatation. The stricture is partly inflammatory, with increased enhancement, mural thickening, and peri-enteric inflammation. *(Courtesy Dr. Edward Loftus and Dr. Joel Fletcher, Rochester, Minn.)*

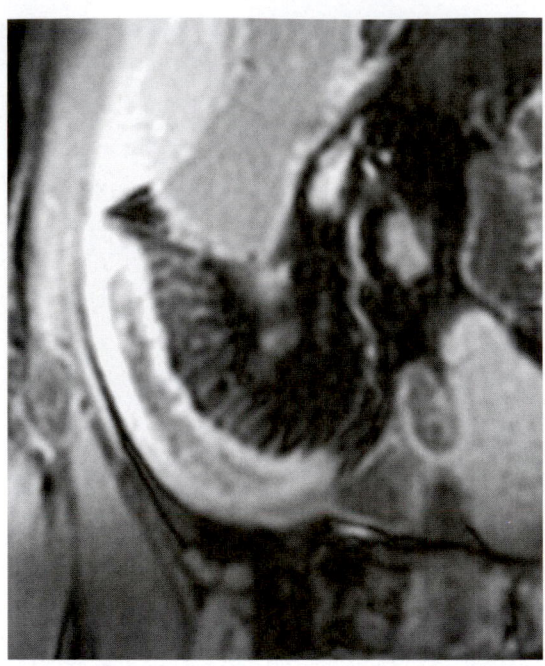

FIGURE 115-6. MR enterography with gadolinium contrast in a patient with Crohn's disease. This coronal view shows mural hyperenhancement, mural thickening, and the comb sign (engorged peri-enteric vasculature) involving the terminal ileum. The vessels are seen medial to the inflamed loop and resemble the teeth of a comb. *(Courtesy Dr. Edward Loftus and Dr. Jeffrey Fidler, Rochester, Minn.)*

visualization of the small intestinal wall and reveal luminal details (Fig. 115-5). Radiologic findings that are significantly correlated with endoscopic evidence of Crohn's activity include mural enhancement (segmental enhancement of all or part of the small intestinal wall); increased density of peri-enteric fat (focal increased inhomogeneous attenuation in the peri-enteric fat, compared with the appearance of subcutaneous or peri-enteric fat in adjacent non-inflamed intestinal loops); and the comb sign (segmental dilatation of the vasa recta involving an intestinal loop).[107] Mural enhancement may be the most useful finding and can be quantified in a semi-automated fashion using dedicated software.[107,108] When compared with a consensus diagnosis of Crohn's disease based on clinical presentation and 4 different imaging modalities, the sensitivity of CT enterography was 82%, specificity was 89%, and accuracy was 85%.[109] The safety of radiation exposure associated with the routine use of CT is a matter of much debate, and needs to be taken into careful consideration if this technology is to replace other diagnostic modalities, especially in children.[110,111]

As an alternative to CT, MRI is approaching equivalent image quality in evaluating the intestine. MR enterography has the advantages of providing high soft tissue contrast, obtaining static and dynamic images, and avoiding ionizing radiation.[112] Similar to CT enterography, patients drink an oral contrast agent before the procedure. Some European centers incorporate enteroclysis with nasoduodenal intubation to administer the contrast, which might increase the yield for subtle mucosal lesions but is likely to be less acceptable to most patients.[112] Findings of intestinal wall thickening, submucosal edema, vasa recta engorgement, and lymphadenopathy are signs of active disease (Fig. 115-6). Using dynamic FIESTA (fast imaging employing steady state acquisition), images can add information regarding the functional status of fibrotic segments. A scoring system was developed for assessing small intestinal Crohn's disease and gives higher scores for details such as increased wall thickness and contrast enhancement, stenosis and mucosal abnormalities, absence of peristalsis and distensibility, and extraintestinal findings.[113] Using these criteria, compared with the gold standard of ileocolonoscopy with biopsies, the MRI images yielded a diagnostic accuracy of 91%.

Other potentially useful diagnostic modalities include US and scintigraphy. Transabdominal US is used mainly to exclude other causes of abdominal pain (e.g., biliary and gynecologic disorders), but it can also be effective in evaluating disease activity of luminal Crohn's disease.[114] There has been

some interest in using EUS to differentiate Crohn's disease (transmural) from UC, but its major value is still to help evaluate and guide therapy of perianal disease.[115] Pelvic MRI, however, remains the preferred imaging modality to evaluate suspected pelvic, perirectal or perianal abscess or fistula. Doppler vascular flow studies to evaluate Crohn's disease activity have been investigated with mixed results.[116] US- and CT-guided percutaneous drainage of intra-abdominal abscesses is a safe and effective alternative to surgical drainage in well-selected patients.[117] Early findings suggest that US elasticity imaging may be useful to detect intestinal fibrosis in strictures.[118] 99mTc leukocyte scintigraphy has an accuracy of 84% compared with the gold standard of intraoperative findings,[119] although it is used seldom in clinical practice. Early data suggest a possible role for PET/CT scanning to help in evaluating the activity level and distribution of Crohn's disease.[120,121]

Because it allows direct inspection of the mucosa and permits biopsy for histopathology, endoscopy complements radiologic techniques. Typical mucosal features recognized on endoscopy include aphthous ulcers, stellate and other discrete ulcers, mucosal edema, cobblestoning, and luminal narrowing (Fig. 115-7). The visual impression of demarcated lesions on a background of normal mucosa is most easily recognized in early or mild disease. Rectal sparing is more specific before treatment has been initiated. The discontinuous segmental nature of the disease is an important clue to the diagnosis. Intubation and biopsy of the terminal ileum should be attempted in all patients having colonoscopy and greatly increase the sensitivity and specificity of the examination. In general, the diagnostic accuracy of colonoscopy and histologic interpretation is increased substantially by obtaining multiple biopsies from both involved and uninvolved sites. The use of jumbo forceps should be considered to improve submucosal

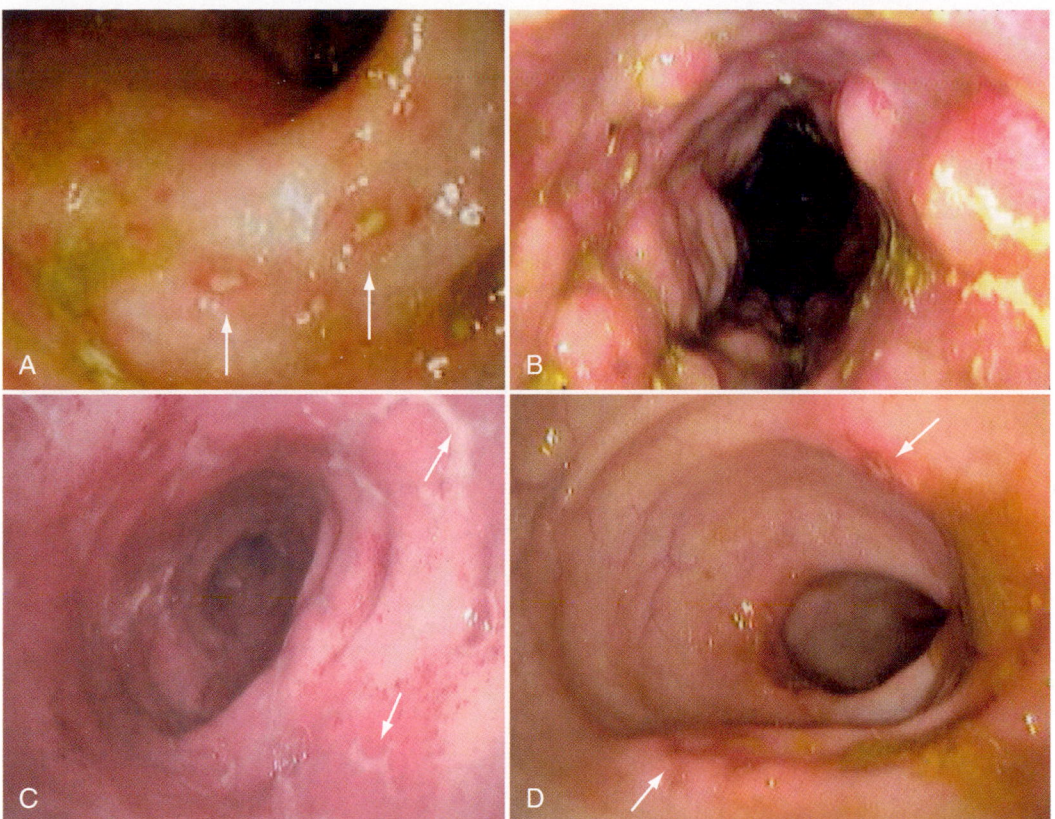

FIGURE 115-7. Endoscopic appearance of Crohn's disease. A wide variety of findings may be visualized on endoscopy, in part depending on the duration and severity of the inflammation. *A,* Typical aphthous ulcers *(arrows),* consisting of a central white depression surrounded by a slightly elevated, erythematous rim only a few millimeters in diameter. *B,* Findings more typical of advanced disease, with erythema, edema, and a cobblestoned appearance. *C,* Stellate ulcers *(arrows)* in the terminal ileum. *D,* Discrete ulcers *(arrows)* with normal intervening mucosa, typical of the patchy inflammation seen in Crohn's disease.

sampling. Balloon dilation of strictures is another application of endoscopy in Crohn's disease that might delay surgery or eliminate the need for it, but balloon dilation is associated with a measurable complication rate.

Video capsule endoscopy (VCE) has become routine for detecting the small intestinal lesions of Crohn's disease. Although VCE may be very sensitive in identifying lesions (even if standard endoscopy has been unrevealing),[122] its low specificity limits its use as a first-line study to diagnose small intestinal Crohn's disease.[109] The presence of significant bowel stricture should be excluded radiologically or by patency capsule[123,124] before attempting VCE, because capsule retention and obstruction may occur in 2.6% of patients.[125] Nonetheless, capsule retention can be clinically useful to localize occult strictures pre- and intraoperatively.[126] Increasingly, single- and double-balloon enteroscopy is being used to address jejunal and proximal ileal Crohn's disease,[127] allowing for biopsy and balloon dilation of strictures.

Differentiating Crohn's Disease from UC

When IBD is confined to the colon, the main diagnostic distinction is between Crohn's colitis and UC. As noted earlier, UC and Crohn's disease share many similarities in epidemiology, genetics, and clinical manifestations, and the distinction between them is becoming increasingly important with regard to choices of surgical and medical therapies. Patients with features of both diseases are said to have *indeterminate colitis* (also referred to as *IBD, unclassified*), a vague term applied in

various ways among different centers. As many as 10% of patients presenting with IBD are considered to have indeterminate colitis. A diagnosis of indeterminate colitis has particular implications for surgical therapy. Patients undergoing ileoanal pouch construction for indeterminate colitis have a relatively high likelihood of developing Crohn's-like complications of the pouch, although the rate of pouch failure is not significantly different from those with UC.[128] Histology, when applied without attention to clinical features, is highly likely to be unable to differentiate Crohn's disease from UC. Therefore, the entire clinical picture must be considered for accurate diagnosis (Table 115-2). Discriminating features for Crohn's disease include the presence of small intestinal disease, predominantly right-sided colonic disease, rectal sparing, fistulization (with the exception of rare rectovaginal or perianal fistulas in UC), major perineal complications, and granulomas. In cases initially labeled as indeterminate, the true diagnosis usually becomes clear with the passage of time.

With an incomplete understanding of the environmental and genetic determinants that produce a clinical phenotype of Crohn's disease or UC, the immunologic markers noted previously are being explored as a means of differentiating the 2 diseases. pANCA (perinuclear antineutrophil cytoplasmic antibodies) and ASCA (anti-*Saccharomyces cerevesiae* antibodies) were the first such markers shown to correlate with the diagnosis of UC and Crohn's disease, respectively. ASCA has relatively high specificity, above 95%, but sensitivity is less than 50%.[129] To improve the test characteristics, the prediction model has added anti-OmpC and anti-CBir1 to pANCA and

TABLE 115-2 Differentiation of Crohn's Colitis from UC

Feature	Crohn's Colitis	Ulcerative Colitis
Mucosal lesions	Aphthous ulcers are common in early disease; late disease is notable for stellate, rake, bear-claw, linear, or serpiginous ulcers and cobblestoning	Micro-ulcers are more common, but larger ulcers are seen Pseudopolyps are more common
Distribution	Often discontinuous and asymmetric, with skipped segments of normal intervening mucosa, especially in early disease	Continuous, symmetric, and diffuse, with granularity or ulceration found in the entirety of involved segments; however, peri-appendiceal inflammation (cecal patch) is common, even when the cecum is not involved
Rectum	Complete, or more often relative, rectal sparing	Typically involved with variable proximal distribution
Ileum	Often involved (≈75% of cases)	Not involved, except as backwash ileitis in panulcerative colitis
Depth of inflammation	Mucosal, submucosal, and transmural	Mucosal; transmural only in fulminant disease
Serosal findings	Marked erythema and creeping fat (the latter is virtually pathognomonic)	Absent except in severe colitis or toxic megacolon
Perianal complications	Often prominent, including large anal skin tags, deep fissures, perianal fistulas, that are often complex	Not prominent (fissure or fistula if present, should be uncomplicated)
Strictures	Often present	Rarely present; when present, suggests adenocarcinoma
Fistulas	Perianal, enterocutaneous, rectovaginal, enterovesicular, and other fistulas may be present	Absent, except for the rare occurrence of rectovaginal or perianal fistula
Histopathology	Granulomas are present in 15%-60% of patients (higher frequency in surgical specimens than in mucosal pinch biopsies) Crypt abscesses may be present Focally enhanced inflammation, often on a normal background, is the hallmark	Granulomas should not be present (microgranulomas may be associated with ruptured crypt abscess) Crypt abscesses and ulcers are the defining lesion Ulceration on a background of inflamed mucosa
Serology	pANCA in 20%-25%, ASCA in 41%-76%	pANCA in 60%-65%, ASCA in 5%

ASCA, anti-*Saccharomyces cerevisiae* antibody; pANCA, perinuclear antineutrophil cytoplasmic antibody.
From Sands BE. From symptom to diagnosis: Clinical distinctions among various forms of intestinal inflammation. Gastroenterology 2004; 126:1518-32, with permission.

ASCA.[72,130] Other antiglycan antibodies, such as antilaminaribioside (ALCA) and antichitobioside (ACCA) have also been associated with Crohn's disease.[131] Limited data are available to establish the predictive value of serologic markers in cases of indeterminate colitis observed over long periods of time.[132] Thus, serologic testing currently is an adjunct to diagnosis in selected cases—one additional piece of evidence to be considered but not definitive in establishing the diagnosis. Genetic research has led to great strides over the past few years, and *CARD15/NOD2* testing is available commercially. Owing to its low diagnostic accuracy, this test is not currently recommended as part of the diagnostic algorithm for Crohn's disease. Preliminary data suggest that models combining NOD2 genotyping with serologic biomarkers such as ASCA, anti-OmpC, anti-CBir1 pANCA and anti-I2, have acceptable receiver-operator characteristics for predicting complicated disease behavior such as stricture or fistula.[130]

Measuring Disease Activity

In daily practice, usually it is sufficient to follow the patient's symptoms and signs with treatment. Rarely is it necessary to subject the patient to repeated radiologic studies or colonoscopies to ascertain disease activity; disease location tends to be stable over time. Repeat studies are undertaken when symptoms have increased substantially or have changed and are suspected to arise not from persistent intestinal inflammation but from other causes, such as infection, complication, or a functional disorder. In clinical research, however, more quantitative evaluations are needed.

Composite scoring systems, most commonly the Crohn's Disease Activity Index (CDAI [Table 115-3]), are used in an attempt to integrate the many possible features of the disease. Other disease activity indices include the van Hees index,[133] the Cape Town index,[134] the Harvey-Bradshaw index,[135] the International Organization of IBD (or Oxford) index,[136] the St. Marks Crohn's index,[137] De Dombal's index,[138] the Talstad index,[139] and a Crohn's disease activity index for survey research.[140] Specialized indices also have been developed for use in children with Crohn's disease.[141,142] All these indices vary in the features included in the scoring system, but most include a combination of subjective symptoms and objective findings on examination and laboratory testing. A great deal of interobserver and methodological variation has been noted,

TABLE 115-3 Crohn's Disease Activity Index (CDAI)*

Variable	Scale	Weight
Liquid or very soft stools	Stool count summed daily for 7 days	2
Abdominal pain	Sum of 7 days of daily ratings as: 0 = none, 1 = mild, 2 = moderate, 3 = severe	5
General well-being	Sum of 7 days of daily ratings as: 0 = generally well, 1 = slightly below par, 2 = poor, 3 = very poor, 4 = terrible	7
Features of extraintestinal disease	Any of the following present during the 7 days of daily ratings: a. Arthritis or arthralgia b. Skin or mouth lesions, including pyoderma gangrenosum, erythema nodosum, aphthous stomatitis c. Iritis or uveitis d. Anal fissure, fistula, or perirectal abscess e. Other external fistula f. Fever > 100°F	20 each
Opiate use for diarrhea	0 = no, 1 = yes	30
Abdominal mass	0 = none, 2 = questionable, 5 = definite	10
Hematocrit value (%):	Males: 47 – hematocrit Females: 42 – hematocrit	6
% Body weight below standard	100 × [1 – (body weight/standard weight)]	1

*To calculate the CDAI, the scale is multiplied by the weighting factor for each variable, and then all 8 weighted variables are added.
From Best WR, Becktel JM, Singleton JW, et al. Development of a Crohn's disease activity index. National Cooperative Crohn's Disease Study. Gastroenterology 1976; 70:439-44, with permission.

even among experienced researchers,[143] and in fibrostenotic disease, indices that rely more heavily on subjective measurements can poorly reflect bowel inflammation as a cause of symptoms. Other approaches have included use of disease-activity indices that focus on a specific outcome, such as perianal disease,[144,145] endoscopic findings,[146,147] or achieving an individual goal of therapy.[148] Each of these approaches has advantages and disadvantages, but all have their application in research rather than in clinical practice.

Another approach with some merit is the measurement of biological markers of disease inflammation. The erythrocyte sedimentation rate and serum acute phase response proteins (e.g., C-reactive protein and orosomucoid) may be useful in tracking disease activity, but lack sensitivity and specificity. Direct measurements of intestinal immune activation in a mucosal sample could enhance sensitivity and specificity but are inconvenient, invasive, and, if dependent on biopsy, subject to variability and poor standardization. Fecal excretion of calprotectin (a calcium- and zinc-binding protein found in neutrophils) and of lactoferrin (an iron-binding glycoprotein secreted by most mucosal membranes) have been shown to be sensitive markers of intestinal inflammation[149] that also might correlate with relapse of quiescent disease and response to therapy with biologics.[129]

Ultimately, it is desirable to measure the patient's overall state of well being, or subjective health status. Health-related quality of life may be measured with generic instruments, which focus on various domains of health common to many disease states, or with disease-specific instruments, which focus on specific domains relevant to the disease of interest. The Inflammatory Bowel Disease Questionnaire is the most widely accepted disease-specific instrument and measures separate domains for bowel, social, systemic, and emotional function.[150]

TREATMENT

Goals

Because neither medical nor surgical therapy provides a cure for Crohn's disease, the primary goals of therapy are to induce and maintain remission. The definition of remission is evolving, and has moved beyond the CDAI and other subjective disease activity indices to include mucosal and histologic healing, which are more closely associated with improved long-term treatment goals and preventing bowel damage.[151,152] In achieving these goals, the intention is to ameliorate symptoms and improve the patient's quality of life. Therefore, it is essential to consider the adverse consequences of therapy, particularly with regard to any durable consequences of short-term treatment and adverse effects of maintenance therapy. Other goals may be specific to the individual patient, such as healing a fistula or achieving normal growth in a child. Maintaining adequate nutrition can at times be a challenge and is an important goal in all patients.

Medical Therapy

Aminosalicylates

In the United States, aminosalicylates (ASAs) are used in the treatment of UC and in mild to moderate Crohn's disease. Sulfasalazine, the parent compound of all ASAs used in IBD, was developed by the Swedish physician Nana Svartz in 1938-1939 as a treatment for RA. In 1941-1942 sulfasalazine was serendipitously found to improve the intestinal symptoms of patients with colitis who were being treated for associated arthropathy.

Most of the adverse effects of sulfasalazine are due to its sulfapyridine moiety, which serves as a carrier for the 5-ASA portion of the molecule. After a classic experiment by Azad Khan and colleagues implicated 5-aminosalicylate (5-ASA, mesalamine) rather than sulfapyridine as the therapeutic moiety of sulfasalazine,[153] other formulations were developed.

These delivery systems include enemas or suppositories, which provide the drug to the rectum and left colon; coating with protective materials that release the drug in a pH-dependent manner to achieve controlled (Pentasa) or delayed (Asacol and Lialda) delivery; and diazo-bonding the drug to a second 5-ASA molecule (olsalazine) or to an inert carrier (balsalazide).

Most studies have shown sulfasalazine to be superior to placebo in inducing remission in active Crohn's disease, when the colon is the primary site affected.[154,155] Efficacious doses, as used in the National Cooperative Crohn's Disease Study (NCCDS), are in the range of 4 to 6 g/day (1 g/15 kg body weight).[154] The European Cooperative Crohn's Disease Study (ECCDS) found sulfasalazine 3 g/day to provide no significant benefit in achieving remission.[156]

Early studies with controlled-release mesalamine (Pentasa) at doses less than 2 g/day failed to show efficacy in the treatment of mild to moderately active Crohn's disease.[157,158] A much larger study of 466 patients with mild to moderate Crohn's disease compared daily doses of 1, 2, and 4 g with placebo for 16 weeks. The 43% remission rate on 4 g mesalamine was statistically and clinically superior to the placebo response rate of 18%.[159] Notably, patients responding best to the 4 g/day dose were those with ileum-only disease, suggesting that mesalamine provides a potential benefit over sulfasalazine in treating this subgroup of patients. Subsequent trials of similar design, however, failed to show benefit over placebo; although the treatment effect was of similar magnitude, the placebo response was larger than the originally observed 18%. A meta-analysis failed to demonstrate a clinically significant benefit of Pentasa 4 g/day in patients with mild to moderate Crohn's disease.[160] Numerous studies with a variety of preparations have failed to demonstrate prevention of relapses of Crohn's disease with 5-ASA compounds.[155,161] Therefore, although maintenance therapy with mesalamine often is prescribed in Crohn's disease, little data justify the expense and inconvenience of this practice, and mesalamine-based products have been excluded from recent evidence-based treatment algorithms.[162]

In summary, sulfasalazine 4 to 6 g/day may be useful for inducing remission of mild to moderate colonic Crohn's disease, whereas the role of mesalamine is uncertain.[163] The small margin of benefit and relatively slow onset of effect (4 to 8 weeks) must be weighed against the excellent safety profile of these agents (Table 115-4).

Antibiotics

Antibiotics have a clear role in treating pyogenic complications of Crohn's disease. On the basis of relatively little evidence, antibiotics also are used to treat perineal disease, fistulas, and active luminal Crohn's disease. The largest reported experience has been with metronidazole and the anaerobic flora affected by metronidazole might have particular importance in the pathogenesis of Crohn's disease.[164]

Perhaps the clearest demonstration of this principle is a study of postsurgical prophylaxis after ileal resection. In this disease model, which in some ways might replicate the earliest events in the initiation of Crohn's disease, high-dose metronidazole (20 mg/kg/day for 3 months) demonstrated a prophylactic effect on endoscopic and clinical recurrence at 1 year, with numerical but not statistical advantages at 2 and 3 years of follow-up.[165] In this study, as in clinical use, side effects, including GI upset, nausea, dysgeusia, and peripheral neuropathy, were common. A study using ornidazole, also a nitroimidazole antibiotic, showed similar results.[166] Ornidizole might have fewer side effects than metronidazole, but toxicity was still a problem with this formulation. A meta-analysis concluded that nitroimidazole antibiotics are effective in the prevention of postoperative Crohn's disease, but that their side effect profile limits acceptability.[167]

Open-label experience suggests that metronidazole 20 mg/kg/day is beneficial in healing perineal fistulas.[168] Randomized controlled trial (RCT) data are limited, preventing further conclusions. Fistulas tend to recur with cessation of therapy, and long-term use is limited by side effects. Studies of metronidazole in active luminal Crohn's disease generally have not demonstrated benefit, but they have suggested better outcomes in subgroups of patients with colonic involvement.[169,170]

Ciprofloxacin is increasingly used to treat Crohn's disease. For perianal fistulas, ciprofloxacin may be similar in efficacy to metronidazole and with fewer side effects,[171] and its addition might improve the response to infliximab and adalimumab.[172,173] In the treatment of luminal disease, 1 study found ciprofloxacin 1 g/day to be equivalent to mesalamine 4 g/day in achieving remission of mild to moderately active Crohn's disease at week 6, with more than half of the patients in each group achieving remission.[174] In a longer-term study using ciprofloxacin 500 mg twice daily for 6 months in patients with moderately active disease, those who were given ciprofloxacin had a statistically significantly lower CDAI at 6 months compared with placebo ($P < 0.001$).[175] Another study compared the combined use of ciprofloxacin and metronidazole, 1 g each, against methylprednisolone for active Crohn's disease. The antibiotic combination was comparable with glucocorticoids in achieving remission over 12 weeks.[176] A more recent study failed to detect additional efficacy of the same dual antibiotic regimen over placebo when added to controlled ileal-release budesonide; however, a trend toward benefit was noted in the subgroup of patients with colonic disease.[177]

Preliminary evidence suggested that clarithromycin monotherapy was useful in treating active disease,[178] but a follow-up randomized trial did not confirm the open label experience.[179] Additional interest in clarithromycin is sparked by its role as part of a highly effective treatment regimen for atypical mycobacterial infection. As reviewed earlier, *M. paratuberculosis* has been the most extensively studied infectious agent thought to be important in the etiology of Crohn's disease. Studies of antimycobacterial therapy, however, have not shown consistent benefit. A large recent study of triple antibiotic therapy (clarithromycin, rifabutin, and clofazimine) combined with prednisolone showed an early clinical benefit, but when followed for 2 more years, this benefit was not sustained.[180] The authors concluded that the treatment regimen might have contributed to nonspecific antibacterial effects and improvement during the course of therapy, but the findings did not support a significant role for *M. paratuberculosis* in the pathogenesis of Crohn's disease.

Rifaximin is a nonabsorbable oral rifamycin antibiotic that is approved for the treatment of traveler's diarrhea, and it has shown success in the treatment of IBS. An RCT for treating mildly to moderately active Crohn's disease showed a numerical advantage for rifaximin 800 mg twice daily compared with once-daily dosing or placebo, but this difference was not statistically significant.[181] Treatment failures in the placebo group were significantly higher, and patients with an elevated

TABLE 115-4 Safety Profiles of Agents Used to Treat Crohn's Disease

Agent	Adverse Effects	Pregnancy*	Nursing*
5-Aminosalicylates (5-ASA)			
Sulfasalazine	Anorexia, dyspepsia, nausea and vomiting, hemolysis, neutropenia, agranulocytosis, folate deficiency, reversible male infertility, neuropathy; see also sulfa-free 5-ASAs	No evidence of teratogenicity; normal fetal growth; give with folic acid	Negligible amounts found in breast milk; safe for term neonates
Sulfa-free 5-ASAs (mesalamine, olsalazine, balsalazide)	Headache, drug fever, rash, paradoxical disease exacerbation, pancreatitis, hepatitis, pericarditis, pneumonitis, nephritis Secretory diarrhea (olsalazine)	No evidence of teratogenicity in humans, normal fetal growth Branded Asacol and Asacol HD with dibutyl phthalate coating is associated with teratogenicity in animals	Found in breast milk in low concentrations; rare watery diarrhea in breast-fed infants
Antibiotics			
Metronidazole	Anorexia, nausea and vomiting, dysgeusia, disulfiram-like effect, peripheral neuropathy, reversible neutropenia	Questionable teratogenicity, normal fetal growth	Found in breast milk; with rare exception, should not be used
Ciprofloxacin	Nausea and vomiting, headache, restlessness, rash, pseudomembranous colitis, elevated serum aminotransferase levels, spontaneous tendon rupture	Theoretical teratogenic potential; insufficient data in humans	Found in breast milk, should not be used
Glucocorticoids			
Classic	Sleep and mood disturbance, acne, striae, hirsutism, adrenal suppression, proximal myopathy, glucose intolerance, hypertension, narrow-angle glaucoma, cataracts, pseudotumor cerebri, infection, edema, impaired wound healing, growth retardation, bone loss, aseptic necrosis	No evidence of teratogenicity in humans, more frequent stillbirths and reduced fetal birth weight when used for other diseases; may be used as indicated by severity of disease	Safe for breast-feeding
Novel	Controlled ileal-release budesonide: adrenal suppression at doses of 9 mg daily and higher in 2 divided doses, but occurrence of classic glucocorticoid adverse effects are similar to placebo	Limited human data but probably low risk	No data available, probably safe for breast feeding
Immune Modulators			
6-Mercaptopurine, azathioprine	Nausea, drug fever, rash, arthralgias, leukopenia, thrombocytopenia, bone marrow suppression, pancreatitis, hepatitis, infection; lymphoma?	Teratogenic in animals, but large series in renal transplantation and other diseases do not show an increase in birth defects; evidence for fetal growth retardation and prematurity; isolated cases of neonatal immune and bone marrow suppression; outcomes appear favorable in limited series of patients with IBD; may be used when indicated because of disease severity	Small amounts excreted in breast milk; not recommended
Methotrexate	Anorexia, nausea and vomiting, leukopenia, megaloblastic anemia, alopecia, hepatic fibrosis, interstitial pneumonitis, neuropathy	Highly teratogenic, particularly in the first trimester; abortifacient	Small amounts excreted in breast milk; not recommended

Continued

TABLE 115-4 Safety Profiles of Agents Used to Treat Crohn's Disease—cont'd

Agent	Adverse Effects	Pregnancy*	Nursing*
Cyclosporine	Reversible or irreversible decrease in renal function, hypertension, tremor, headache, paresthesias, seizure, gingival hyperplasia, hypertrichosis, hepatotoxicity, infection, lymphoma	Significant levels in fetal circulation; does not appear to be teratogenic; intrauterine growth retardation and premature delivery are increased, especially at higher doses; little reported experience in IBD	Excreted in breast milk; not recommended
Biological Response Modifiers			
Anti-TNF antibodies (infliximab, adalimumab, certolizumab pegol)	Upper respiratory,tract and other infections, disseminated TB, increased risk of systemic fungal infection and other intracellular pathogens, acute or delayed hypersensitivity reactions, antinuclear antibodies, anti–double-stranded DNA antibodies, lupus-like reaction, demyelinating disease, lymphoma; contraindicated in heart failure because of increased mortality	Growing amount of evidence supporting safety, but still relatively limited data in humans. Infliximab and adalimumab can freely cross the placenta and lead to high levels in newborns, whereas certolizumab pegol only crosses the placenta in very limited quantities	Minimal levels in breast milk
Natalizumab	Headache, flushing, infections, progressive multifocal leukoencephalopathy, jaundice, liver failure	Teratogenic in animals	Unknown safety in nursing

*From Connell WR. Safety of drug therapy for inflammatory bowel disease in pregnant and nursing women. Inflamm Bowel Dis 1996; 2:33-47, with permission. Updated based on Ng S, Mahadevan U. Management of inflammatory bowel disease in pregnancy. Expert Rev Clin Immunol 2013; 9:161-73.
Adapted from Sands BE. Therapy of inflammatory bowel disease. Gastroenterology 2000; 118(2 Suppl 1):S72, with permission.

C-reactive protein did have a significantly better response. To follow up on these findings, an RCT was performed in over 400 patients with moderately active Crohn's disease. With the extended intestinal release formulation using 800 mg twice daily, significantly more subjects in the rifaximin group were in remission at 12 weeks compared with placebo (62% vs. 43%, P = 0.005).[182]

In summary, antibiotics can play an adjunctive role in the treatment of Crohn's disease and, in selected patients, they may be useful in treating perineal disease, enterocutaneous fistulas, or active colonic disease. As the antigenic determinants of the intestinal flora are elucidated further, more directed antibiotic approaches might be feasible.

Glucocorticoids

Glucocorticoids play a central yet vexing role in the treatment of Crohn's disease. Early favorable series of glucocorticoid treatment led to the validation of their short-term efficacy in the NCCDS (prednisone 0.5 to 0.75 mg/kg/day for initial treatment of active disease, with the dose adjusted according to CDAI)[154] and the ECCDS (6-methylprednisolone 48 mg/day in the first week, tapered to 12 mg by week 6, and held at 8 mg for remission up to 2 years).[156]

In usual practice, patients with mild to moderate disease that does not respond to primary therapy and patients with moderately severe symptoms are treated initially with 40 to 60 mg of prednisone, the dose then being tapered off over 6 to 12 weeks. Response rates are approximately 80% by 1 month.[183] When doses are pushed as high as 1 mg/kg/day for up to 7 weeks, 92% of patients can achieve clinical remission.[184] The onset of response is rapid, usually within the first 3 weeks of treatment. A Cochrane review of the use of corticosteroids for the induction of remission of Crohn's disease

supports this efficacy of traditional steroids over 5-ASA therapy and placebo.[185]

Patients with severely active disease usually respond to IV administration of glucocorticoids.[186] Options for IV glucocorticoid formulation include hydrocortisone (100 mg IV every 8 hours), prednisolone (30 mg IV twice daily), or methylprednisolone (16 to 20 mg IV every 8 hours). Hydrocortisone can cause slightly more salt retention and sodium wasting, but it is likely to be equally effective. In a randomized double-blind trial with UC patients, continuous infusion was no better than divided dosing for efficacy and safety.[187]

Unfortunately, the beneficial effects of glucocorticoids come at the expense of frequent and often severe adverse effects (see Table 115-4). The most common side effects are troubling neuropsychiatric symptoms, including mood disturbance and insomnia, and cosmetic effects, including acne, cushingoid appearance, hair loss, and hirsutism. Still more serious are metabolic consequences, including adrenocortical suppression, glucose intolerance, myopathy, and bone loss. The risk of infectious complications is increased, particularly at doses of prednisone higher than 40 mg; doses lower than 10 mg confer no appreciable increased risk of infection.[188] Among patients taking immunomodulators or infliximab, the concomitant use of prednisone appears to lead to more frequent serious infections and higher rates of mortality than when these agents are used alone.[189-191] The unfavorable risk profile of glucocorticoids makes their prolonged use hazardous.

Glucocorticoids are not effective as long-term therapy. A meta-analysis of maintenance glucocorticoid therapy in Crohn's disease failed to detect benefit in the prevention of relapse at 6, 12, or 24 months.[192] Conversely, once glucocorticoids are introduced, they cannot be discontinued without recurrent symptoms in many patients, even with gradual tapering; this problem is referred to as *glucocorticoid dependence*. Among patients with Crohn's disease who received glucocorticoids for the first time, no response (glucocorticoid resistance) was seen in 20% in the first 30 days.[183] Among the 80% who were complete or partial responders, 55% had a prolonged response, and 45% relapsed or could not have treatment tapered off within 1 year.[183] Similar results were seen in both adult and pediatric populations in a cohort from Olmsted County, Minnesota.[193,194] Clinical factors associated with glucocorticoid dependence include smoking, younger age at onset, colonic location, and non-fibrostenotic disease.[195] Mechanisms that can contribute to glucocorticoid resistance include up-regulation of the multidrug resistance *(mdr)* gene[196,197] and increased serum levels of glucocorticoid-binding globulin.[198] Moreover, only 29% of patients who achieve clinical remission on glucocorticoids also achieve endoscopic remission.[184] This finding suggests that the effect of glucocorticoid treatment in most patients is to suppress symptoms when given in doses above a threshold that can vary among patients and even in the same patient over time.

There are several principles of glucocorticoid use in Crohn's disease:

Use an effective dose. Underdosing at the start of therapy typically leads to dose escalation and prolonged dosing to achieve a response.

Do not overdose. Patients who do not benefit from 40 to 60 mg are unlikely to benefit from increased or prolonged oral dosing. Such patients require IV dosing or treatment with another rapidly acting agent, such as an anti-TNF agent (see later).

Do not treat for excessively short periods. Doses should not be tapered too quickly once symptoms have been controlled. Very brief courses of glucocorticoids (3 weeks or less) are likely to result in a rebound flare.

Do not treat for excessively long periods. Patients in whom a glucocorticoid taper fails should be considered candidates for glucocorticoid-sparing immune modulators. Glucocorticoids should not be begun without a strategy in mind for terminating treatment.

Anticipate side effects. Bone loss in particular may be anticipated with even short-term use. (See later, "Adjunctive Therapies.")

In an attempt to limit the unintended systemic effects of glucocorticoid therapy, novel glucocorticoids have been developed. Budesonide possesses glucocorticoid receptor affinity superior to that of traditional glucocorticoids and also takes advantage of enhanced first-pass metabolism by the liver to limit systemic exposure. A controlled ileal-release formulation of budesonide targets the terminal ileum and right colon. Studies have demonstrated that 9 mg/day of this preparation are superior to placebo and mesalamine and about 15% less effective than prednisolone in achieving remission, but with fewer side effects.[199] Pushing the dose higher results in better efficacy but at the expense of increasing adrenocortical suppression and side effects.[200] To evaluate the efficacy of budesonide for maintenance of remission, an RCT compared 6 mg to 9 mg at 12 months.[201] Both doses were associated with relatively low relapse rates (24% and 19%, respectively) that were not significantly different, but a placebo comparison group was not included, which limits the ability to understand the relevance of this study. Adverse events were not different in these 2 dosage groups, supporting the safety of the 9-mg dose over a 1-year period. A meta-analysis reviewed all studies that evaluated budesonide for the treatment of active luminal Crohn's disease, and concluded that budesonide was superior to placebo for inducing remission (RR = 0.73; 95% CI, 0.63 to 0.84) but not in preventing relapse (RR = 0.93; 95% CI, 0.82 to 1.04).[202] Therefore, lack of a

maintenance effect is consistent for both novel and traditional glucocorticoids.

In light of the superior response in comparison with mesalamine and its relative safety, budesonide may be considered as first-line therapy for patients with active ileal, ileocecal, or right colonic disease. In addition, some patients who are dependent upon conventional glucocorticoids may be switched successfully to budesonide, with the potential benefits of decreased systemic glucocorticoid exposure.[203]

In summary, glucocorticoids are effective for the short-term control of symptoms of Crohn's disease, but they are neither effective nor safe for long-term maintenance of response. In patients with disease that is refractory to or dependent on glucocorticoids, steroid-sparing strategies should be considered, including immune modulators or surgery.

Thiopurine Agents

The thiopurine antimetabolites azathioprine (AZA) and 6-mercaptopurine (6-MP) have been used to treat Crohn's disease since the initial report of Brooke and colleagues describing healing of fistulas with AZA.[204] Another decade would pass, however, before the efficacy of this class of drugs was demonstrated in an RCT by Present and colleagues[148]; earlier studies were marred by either insufficient power or incomplete understanding of adequate dosing and the slow onset of action of these agents.

A Cochrane meta-analysis of studies of AZA and 6-MP in Crohn's disease has provided the best summary of the effects of these drugs.[205] For active disease, thiopurine treatment produced a higher remission rate of 47% compared with a 37% placebo rate, but this corresponded to a non-significant relative risk of 1.23 (95% CI, 0.97 to 1.55). The outcome of remission or clinical response similarly yielded a higher but not statistically significant result compared with placebo (48% vs. 36%; RR 1.26; 95% CI, 0.98 to 1.62). The odds ratio for response increases after 17 weeks of therapy, suggesting the minimum duration for a trial of 6-MP or AZA. A steroid-sparing effect was significant (RR, 1.34; 95% CI, 1.02 to 1.77), and the number needed to treat (NNT) was about 6. Only 18 patients with fistulas were included, but a 54% rate of fistula response was noted, compared with a 29% healing rate on placebo; this, however, was not statistically significant (RR, 2.00; 95% CI, 0.67 to 5.93), most likely the result of a type II error. There is more convincing evidence of the benefit of thiopurines for maintenance of remission. The OR for maintenance of remission with AZA was 2.32 (95% CI, 1.55 to 3.49; NNT = 6) and with 6-MP 3.32 (95% CI, 1.40 to 7.87; NNT = 4).[206] The OR for AZA maintaining remission increased from 1.20 at 1 mg/kg up to 4.13 (95% CI, 1.59 to 10.71) at 2.5 mg/kg, demonstrating the importance of appropriate dosing.

Overall, approximately one half of patients may respond to thiopurine therapy, and once in remission about half to two thirds of patients will maintain that response. In earlier studies, mucosal healing was seen in approximately half of the patients who received thiopurines,[207] however, in a more recent large study, this was seen in only 16.5% of patients at 26 weeks.[208] In children, early administration of 6-MP soon after diagnosis was associated with steroid sparing and maintenance of remission.[209] However, this was not reproduced in adults in a recently published trial.[210]

In clinical practice, AZA and 6-MP are used virtually interchangeably, with the exception of dosing. AZA generally is used in doses of 2 to 2.5 mg/kg/day, and 6-MP is given in doses of 1 to 1.5 mg/kg/day. The introduction of thiopurine medications should be timed with their slow onset of action in mind; many patients require a tapering regimen of

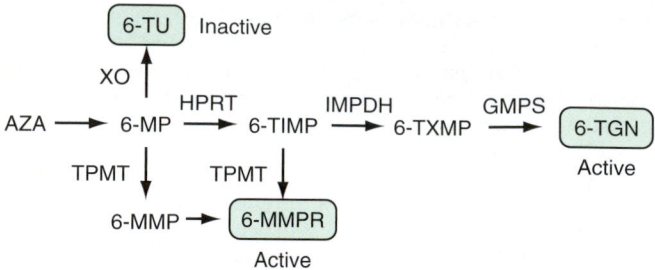

FIGURE 115-8. Metabolism of azathioprine (AZA) and 6-mercaptopurine (MP). 5-ASA, 5-aminosalicylate; 6-MMP, 6-methylmercaptopurine; 6-MMPR, 6-methylmercaptopurine ribonucleotides; 6-TGN, 6-thioguanine nucleotides; 6-TIMP, 6-thioinosine 5'-monophosphate; 6-TU, 6-thiouric acid; 6-TXMP, 6-thioxanthosine 5'-monophosphate; GMPS, guanosine monophosphate synthetase; HPRT, hypoxanthine phosphoribosyltransferase; IMPDH, inosine monophosphate dehydrogenase; TPMT, thiopurine methyltransferase; XO, xanthine oxidase.

glucocorticoids to bridge the time period until the thiopurines have taken effect. Thiopurine therapy also may be considered for the postsurgical prophylaxis of Crohn's disease,[211] although conflicting data exist about their efficacy.

Much is known about the metabolism of 6-MP and AZA (Fig. 115-8). AZA is a prodrug that is converted in part to 6-MP through non-enzymatic means and into a variety of other immunologically active and inert metabolites. Xanthine oxidase (XO) converts 6-MP to 6-thiouric acid, in competition with hypoxanthine phosphoribosyltransferase. The former enzymatic pathway accounts for an important drug reaction with allopurinol, a XO inhibitor (see later). Thiopurine methyltransferase (TPMT) plays a key role in the metabolic pathway. Persons who are homozygous for a recessive mutation that results in inactivation of TPMT ($\approx$1 in 300 persons) produce exceedingly high levels of 6-thioguanine (6-TG) nucleotides. These persons are unlikely to tolerate thiopurine agents and tend to develop profound leukopenia and other limiting adverse effects. In contrast, persons who are TPMT heterozygous ($\approx$10% of the population) are likely to have moderately high levels of 6-TG nucleotides.[212,213] They usually require lower doses of drug but are much more likely to respond. A steady state in the production of erythrocyte 6-TG nucleotides may be reached as early as 14 days after dosing,[214] but has recently been reported at a median time of 55 days in pediatric patients.[215]

There have been mixed results reported of the correlation between 6-TG nucleotide levels and response to therapy, but a meta-analysis of 6 studies did find an overall significant relationship.[216] A threshold of 230 to 260 pmol/8 $\times$ 10^10 red blood cells corresponded to a 62% rate of remission, compared with a rate of 36% in those with lower levels (OR, 3.27; 95% CI, 1.71 to 6.27) of 6-TG. Correlations between higher levels of 6-TG nucleotides and leukopenia, and between metabolite levels and response to therapy, might explain the clinical observation that patients who achieve mild leukopenia are more likely to respond to such therapy.[217] Conversely, however, leukopenia is not necessary to achieve a therapeutic response. It is not clear if routine measurement of thiopurine metabolite levels and directed dose adjustment would contribute to improved management of Crohn's disease, as opposed to the standard weight-based dose approach.

When a patient is not responding to thiopurine therapy after 3 to 4 months, it is useful to measure metabolite levels to identify patients who are noncompliant, under-dosed, or

shunting. *Shunting* refers to high TPMT activity that results in low 6-TG levels and high 6-methylmercaptopurine (MMP) levels (see Fig. 115-8); a 6-MMP:6-TG ratio of greater than 10 has been suggested as a profile of metabolism that is unlikely to lead to clinical benefit.[213,218] In these patients, it may be possible to add allopurinol and take advantage of the drug interaction noted earlier. A study testing this hypothesis showed that by decreasing the thiopurine dose to 25% to 50% of the original dose and adding a low dose of allopurinol, 6-TG levels rose significantly, with a coincident drop in 6-MMP levels and an improvement in clinical outcomes.[219] Although this strategy requires careful following of the WBC count, it has been shown to be well tolerated and safe in 1 study with a median follow-up period of 19 months.[220]

In a Cochrane analysis, adverse events severe enough to result in drug withdrawal were seen in 10% of patients.[205] Adverse events that lead to drug discontinuation typically occur soon after drug initiation, with a median time of 1 month.[221] Nausea within the first few weeks of treatment is reported in approximately 8% of patients, but typically will subside gradually. Allergic reactions consisting of fever, rash, or arthralgias are seen in 1% to 2% of patients, usually within a few weeks of introducing the drug. Pancreatitis, observed in 3% to 4%, is another idiosyncratic reaction and usually occurs in the first month of therapy. The presentation is typically classic with epigastric pain that radiates to the back, but may be atypical and subtle, with nausea and vague dyspepsia. When symptoms are recognized promptly, discontinuation of the drug leads to resolution of pancreatitis. Rechallenge with either drug should not be attempted, because recurrent pancreatitis is certain to occur. Elevated serum aminotransferase levels develop in approximately 3% of patients and have been correlated with the presence of very high levels of 6-MMP.[222] Mild elevations of liver tests can often revert to normal without any intervention, or with dose reduction. An exception is in the rare occurrence of cholestatic hepatitis or nodular regenerative hyperplasia (NRH), in which case thiopurine therapy should be withdrawn.

Bone marrow suppression is another concern with thiopurine agents. A 27-year, retrospective, single-center study of 739 IBD patients treated with AZA found 28 patients (3.8%) developed leukopenia (WBC < 3 $\times$ 10^9 cells/L [<3000 cells/mm^3]), 9 of whom (1.2%) had severe leukopenia (WBC count < 2 $\times$ 10^9 cells/L [<2000 cells/mm^3])[223]; 3 of these patients became pancytopenic, and 2 died of sepsis. A review of 66 studies that included over 8000 patients had a similar rate of myelotoxicity and, fortunately, a low risk (<0.1%) of death attributable to treatment.[224] Although leukopenia occurs early among patients with low TPMT activity, it might not be related solely to TPMT genotype and can occur at any time during therapy.[224] For this reason, it is advisable to continue monitoring the complete blood count every 1 to 3 months for the duration of therapy and more frequently (every 2 weeks if TPMT activity is normal, weekly if it is heterozygous) in the 8 to 12 weeks after introducing the drug or increasing dosage. Temporary cessation of therapy for a week or 2 and an adjustment in dose usually suffice to bring the leukocyte count back within normal range. Careful monitoring of the leukocyte count also should be performed during a tapering regimen of glucocorticoids. Concurrent treatment with glucocorticoids can raise the leukocyte count, but as the glucocorticoid is discontinued, leukopenia can develop.

Infections can occur in the setting of thiopurine therapy. Serious infections are reported to occur approximately 2% to 6% of the time, not necessarily in the setting of leukopenia.[208,221] Patients treated concurrently with glucocorticoids may be at greater risk of serious infection, including cytomegalovirus. Treatment should be interrupted when serious infections occur, although the effect of the drug will endure for weeks.

Malignancy associated with thiopurines has been a long-standing concern of patients and providers. Immunosuppressive regimens given to patients after organ transplantation and for other immune-mediated conditions are associated with an excess risk of malignancy, particularly non-Hodgkin's lymphoma (NHL). Such regimens have included AZA, often administered in higher doses than for IBD and in conjunction with other immunosuppressive agents. In IBD, there does appear to be an association between thiopurine exposure and lymphoma, specifically NHL. The rate of NHL is reported to be approximately 4 to 9 per 10,000 patient-years.[225,226] Data suggest that once stopping thiopurines, the risk of lymphoma returns to the patient's baseline risk. Non-melanoma skin cancer appears to have a clear association with thiopurine exposure, but not melanoma.[227,228] No other solid tumors have been found to be associated with thiopurines when used for the treatment of IBD.[229]

Once treatment with a thiopurine agent has proved to be effective, the question of how long to continue such therapy inevitably arises. One RCT demonstrated a clinical relapse rate of 21% 18 months after withdrawal of AZA in patients who had been in remission for at least 3.5 years on the drug,[230] compared with a relapse rate of only 8% in the group who continued AZA. The authors concluded, and most authorities agree, that AZA maintenance therapy should be continued longer than 3.5 years. The decision to withdraw thiopurine therapy should only be undertaken after discussion between doctor and patient of possible risks and benefits.

Methotrexate

Methotrexate (MTX) has long been used to treat psoriasis and RA. An RCT studied patients with chronically active Crohn's disease despite at least 3 months of prednisone (at least 12.5 mg/day) and with at least 1 failed attempt to taper off treatment.[231] All patients were brought to a 20 mg/day dose of prednisone to standardize therapy, with separate stratification for patients in whom the dose of prednisone was increased and for those in whom the dose had dropped to 20 mg before entry. Subjects then received either weekly injections of MTX 25 mg intramuscularly or placebo while executing a tapering prednisone regimen over 16 weeks. Overall, 39.4% of patients assigned to MTX achieved remission off prednisone compared with 19.1% of placebo-treated patients.[231] Most patients responded by the eighth week of treatment. Although the remission rates in the MTX-treated high- and low-prednisone group were nearly equal (39.0% and 40.0%, respectively), the remission rate for placebo-treated patients in the high-prednisone dose group was 10.0%, compared with 35.3% in the low-dose group.[231] This result often is misconstrued as showing that MTX works well for patients on high doses of prednisone but not for those on low doses of prednisone, but it merely shows an unexpectedly high placebo response rate among patients dependent on low doses of glucocorticoids.

MTX also is beneficial in maintaining remission. A follow-up study randomized patients who achieved remission by week 16 on MTX 25 mg intramuscularly once weekly to receive either weekly injections of placebo or MTX at a dose of 15 mg. At week 40, 65% of patients treated with MTX were still in remission, compared with 39% of placebo-treated patients (P = 0.04).[232] Treatment was well tolerated. Among patients who relapsed on the maintenance dose, more than half were able to achieve remission again with resuming a 25-mg dose. If the 16 weeks of induction therapy were included, the combined duration of therapy was nearly 1 year,

with some patients in selected practices treated successfully for over 4 years. Although 15-mg intramuscular dosing was studied for maintenance, many continue on 25 mg weekly without dose reduction. Pharmacokinetic studies in RA have shown equivalency for subcutaneous and intramuscular dosing, and therefore most gastroenterologists administer MTX subcutaneously.[233,234] Although oral dosing would be more convenient for long-term administration, a Cochrane review did not find evidence of efficacy when compared to placebo.[235] This may be explained by the variable intestinal absorption of MTX,[236] particularly in the presence of small intestinal disease.

Although MTX is a folate antagonist, the drug often is given with folic acid (1 to 2 mg/day) to prevent nausea and stomatitis, and so other modes of action are likely responsible for its efficacy. In addition to stomatitis and nausea, diarrhea, hair loss, and mild leukopenia can occur with MTX. Serum aminotransferase elevations sometimes occur, but correlate poorly with the complication of hepatic fibrosis. Liver biopsy is performed routinely in patients with psoriasis after cumulative doses of 1.5, 3, and 5 g have been administered, but these guidelines have not been widely adopted in patients with RA, in whom the risk of hepatic fibrosis appears to be lower. In 1 series of IBD patients who received a mean cumulative dose of methotrexate greater than 2.5 g and had liver biopsy, only minimal hepatic toxicity was evident.[237] Obesity, diabetes, and alcohol intake correlate with hepatic fibrosis. MTX interacts with sulfa medications and with AZA and 6-MP to cause severe leukopenia. Rare but potentially life-threatening interstitial pneumonitis can manifest as cough and dyspnea of insidious onset. Early detection, cessation of MTX, and prompt treatment with glucocorticoids is essential. MTX is toxic to sperm, and men should wait 3 months after stopping MTX before trying to conceive.[238] Finally, MTX is a potent abortifacient and is strongly teratogenic. Women of childbearing capacity must use MTX only with highly effective contraception.

MTX may be considered as an alternative to the thiopurine analogs, particularly among patients who do not tolerate these drugs. Studies comparing MTX to thiopurines in a head-to-head protocol have been too small to make definitive conclusions of superiority or equivalency.[235] Some patients who do not respond to 6-MP might respond to MTX.[239] In addition to its proved role as a glucocorticoid-sparing agent, MTX may be considered as a treatment for active disease, although its value for this indication is less clear.[240]

Other Immune Modulators

There appears to be little role for cyclosporine in Crohn's disease. Series of uncontrolled RCTs have shown high doses of cyclosporine to be efficacious in treating IBD and fistulas, but at an unacceptably high cost of adverse effects.[241] Moreover, lower doses, although somewhat safer, are not effective in maintaining remission.[242] One uncontrolled study suggested a benefit for hospitalized patients with Crohn's colitis, many of whom had been previously exposed to anti-TNF agents, but further data are required to understand its benefit to risk profile.[243] For virtually all Crohn's indications, equally effective and less hazardous medications are available.

Tacrolimus is absorbed more reliably from the intestine than is cyclosporine and has a similar mode of action via inhibition of calcineurin, thereby diminishing T-cell activation.[244] Preliminary data suggest that tacrolimus may be useful in treating glucocorticoid-resistant disease, and an RCT has demonstrated efficacy in healing fistulas.[245,246] The drug also may be effective as a topical agent for oral and perianal ulcerating disease[247,248]; long-term application of 0.1%

tacrolimus applied to broken skin and mucosa was safe and serum levels were undetectable.[249]

Thalidomide may have a role for some patients with Crohn's disease through the mechanism of down-regulation of TNF-α and inhibition of NFκB activity. It has been shown to be effective in small studies of patients naïve to biologics, and also in whom thiopurine, MTX, and anti-TNF therapy have failed.[250] The most frequent long-term toxicity is peripheral neuropathy, which is typically reversible, but not in all cases. Careful contraceptive measures are critical owing to well-known teratogenicity. Lenalidomide, an analog of thalidomide with similar immunomodulatory properties but with less toxicity (specifically neuropathy), was studied in an RCT, but did not show a response significantly different from placebo.[251]

Biological Therapy

Anti-TNF Agents

Infliximab is the first biological response modifier shown to be effective in Crohn's disease. This chimeric monoclonal TNF antibody had an unsuccessful history as an investigational antisepsis agent before its use in Crohn's disease was explored. Despite conflicting reports regarding the importance of TNF in IBD, the Dutch investigator van Deventer posited that in light of the critical role of TNF in granuloma formation, an anti-TNF agent might prove efficacious for granulomatous bowel disease. Open-label trials subsequently demonstrated rapid and prolonged improvement in disease activity, accompanied in many cases by mucosal healing.[252-254] An early short-term (12-week) RCT provided strong confirmation of the initial impression of efficacy.[255] Coincidental healing of enterocutaneous fistulas in some patients led to a separate successful RCT of infliximab for this indication.

Limited information regarding the efficacy of repeated dosing was available before the commercial release of infliximab in the United States. Maintenance dosing every 8 weeks at 5 mg/kg IV after a 0-, 2- and 6-week induction regimen was demonstrated to maintain response in patients with fistulizing and non-fistulizing disease.[256,257] In these studies, although significant differences were seen at the primary endpoints, the treatment effect was not as robust as with initial therapy. Approximately 60% of patients with luminal disease initially respond to therapy and 40% of those individuals maintain that response at 1 year. Other important observations from these studies included the steroid-sparing effect of infliximab, and sustained improvement in quality of life out to the 54-week duration of these trials.

Infliximab was approved for the treatment of moderate to severe pediatric Crohn's disease by the FDA in 2006. Fortunately, children had even higher response and remission rates than adults, which likely reflects the early nature of disease in children compared with adults and a different phenotype (e.g., inflammatory) at young age.

Since the success of infliximab, 2 additional anti-TNF agents have been approved for treating Crohn's disease. Adalimumab is a subcutaneously administered human immunoglobulin G1 (IgG1) monoclonal antibody that targets TNF. After success in RA, an early open-label study was performed of patients with Crohn's disease who had lost response to or become intolerant to infliximab. In this study, 59% responded to adalimumab therapy and 29% of patients were in remission at 12 weeks.[258] Importantly, no patients experienced acute or delayed hypersensitivity reactions to adalimumab. This paved the way to larger RCTs that showed efficacy for inducing remission[259] and maintenance at 1 year.[260] Based on results from these studies, the recommended adult dosing is 160 mg

subcutaneously at week 0, 80 mg at week 2, and then 40 mg every other week.

Certolizumab pegol, initially known as CDP870, is a polyethylene-glycolated Fab fragment of a humanized anti-TNF antibody. An exploratory study of a single dose in patients with Crohn's disease was promising[261] and led to a series of large RCTs. In the first, although clinical benefit clearly was evident, the primary endpoint of clinical response at 12 weeks missed statistical significance.[262] Post hoc analysis exposed a high placebo rate in subjects with low CRP levels, and subsequent recalculation limiting analysis to patients with an elevated CRP showed a significant difference. In 2 follow-up studies that stratified patients based on CRP levels, certolizumab pegol 400 mg, administered subcutaneously at weeks 0, 2, and 4 weeks and then every 4 weeks, proved to be effective to induce and maintain clinical response and remission out to 26 weeks.[263,264] Interestingly, patients responded equally regardless of their CRP status.

Infliximab, adalimumab, and certolizumab pegol are all effective for treating moderately to severely active Crohn's disease.[265] Although it is impossible to compare the response and remission rates of these agents because of different study designs and patient populations, all appear to have similar rates of initial response (≈60%) and maintenance of that response between 6 and 12 months (≈40% of the initial responders). Differences may be found over the longer term based on specific modes of action, pharmacokinetics, development of antibodies, and side effects. Although these 3 medications are similar, all anti-TNF agents are not equivalent, as illustrated by etanercept (a human soluble TNF receptor Fc fusion protein) and CDP571 (a humanized monoclonal antibody to TNF), both of which failed to show significant efficacy for Crohn's disease.[266,267]

The mode of action of anti-TNF agents is likely to be more involved than just its nominal binding of TNF. The antibody can bind and clear soluble TNF, but it also binds to cell-bound TNF. Through the latter mechanism, infliximab and adalimumab have been shown to induce apoptosis of cells expressing membrane TNF. Etanercept does not induce apoptosis, an observation thought to be the explanation for its lack of efficacy,[268,269] although neither does certolizumab pegol induce apoptosis,[270] and, as mentioned earlier, it has efficacy similar to that of these other agents. Therefore, the mechanism of action is most likely multifactorial, all pointing toward the ability to control the mucosal immune response.

Treatment with the anti-TNF agents usually is well tolerated. In the largest and longer-term clinical trials, between 4% and 16% of patients withdrew from study because of an adverse event.[257,271] Injection site and infusion reactions occur at variable rates. They are higher with infliximab than with adalimumab or certolizumab pegol.[272] Infusion reactions with infliximab typically are associated with antibodies to infliximab (ATI), also referred to as HACA (human anti-chimeric antibodies). ATI developed in 13% of infliximab-treated patients with Crohn's disease. Patients in whom ATI develop are more likely, although not uniformly so, to experience acute infusion reactions, which can consist of chest tightness, dyspnea, rash, and hypotension. ATI are less likely to develop in patients treated concomitantly with glucocorticoids or immune modulators, providing a justification for continuing MTX, AZA, or 6-MP, even when these treatments have failed.

Delayed hypersensitivity reactions, consisting of severe polyarthralgia, myalgia, facial edema, urticaria, or rash, are unusual complications that can occur 2 to 12 days after an infusion.[273] High ATI concentrations appear in such patients after the occurrence of such reactions, but they are not necessarily found before reinfusion. The major risk factor for delayed hypersensitivity appears to be a long delay (probably ≥ 6 months) between infusions, thereby priming an amnestic antibody response. Delayed hypersensitivity appears to be less common when a standard induction regimen is used and when an immune modulator is given concurrently.[274]

Antibody formation is not unique to infliximab. For adalimumab, human anti-human antibodies (HAHAs) can form. They were seen in only 2.6% of patients in a 1-year maintenance study of adalimumab in Crohn's disease[271] but in up to 17% in patients with RA.[275] Antibodies to certolizumab were seen in approximately 10% of patients in the induction and maintenance trials.[262,264] The clinical significance of the presence of anti-drug antibodies is a matter of debate, but data demonstrate an association with lower infliximab serum levels in the setting of episodic therapy, where ATI formation is highest,[276] and a decreased response rate to adalimumab among patients with HAHAs.[277]

Antinuclear antibodies are common and appear in approximately 50% of patients receiving infliximab after 2 years. Of patients who develop antinuclear antibodies, approximately 30% develop anti–double-stranded DNA.[276] Actual drug-induced lupus is rare but can occur. Treatment with certolizumab pegol has been observed to induce a lower rate of antinuclear antibodies than does infliximab or adalimumab, perhaps a result of this agent's inability to induce T-cell apoptosis. The clinical significance of these autoantibodies is unclear.

In clinical trials, infections were reported in up to 57% of anti-TNF treated patients, but typically the rate of infections seen with placebo is similar to those in the intervention groups.[271] Serious infections fortunately were unusual, occurring in only 2% to 4% of patients, which was consistent for all 3 anti-TNF agents.[256,260,263] In the course of treatment of patients with enterocutaneous fistulas, but especially with perineal disease, abscesses formation can arise from superficial healing and closure of an infected pocket. Any patient with a suspected pyogenic complication of Crohn's disease or any serious infection should undergo adequate drainage and treatment with antibiotics before starting or continuing infliximab. A systematic review found that sepsis had a mortality rate of 0.4% in anti–TNF–treated patients.[278] Patients with sepsis typically were older and had comorbidities. Primary contributing factors included the concomitant use of narcotics, prednisone, and other immune suppressing agents, which can independently increase the risk of serious infections and death.[190,279] Reactivation of TB has been observed with anti-TNF therapies, and has resulted in disseminated disease and death. The rate of occurrence of TB was estimated to be 0.2% in a recent meta-analysis of anti-TNF exposed patients with IBD.[280] All patients should be screened for pulmonary TB before starting anti-TNF therapy.

Since the early days of infliximab use, there has been concern of an increased risk of lymphoproliferative disorders, specifically non-Hodgkin's lymphoma. A meta-analysis of patients with Crohn's disease treated with anti-TNF agents reported the rate of NHL as 6.1 per 10,000 patient-years,[281] which compared with the background rate in the general population of 1.9 per 10,000 patient-years, corresponds to a standardized incidence ratio of 3.23 (95% CI, 1.5 to 6.9). Compared with the rate of NHL in Crohn's patients seen in the meta-analysis of immunomodulators noted earlier (4 to 9 per 10,000),[225] the standardized incidence ratio is 1.7 (95% CI, 0.5 to 7.1). Because most of the anti-TNF treated patients also were exposed to immunomodulators, however, it is not possible to determine the magnitude of risk contributed by the anti-TNF treatment alone. As described above, the absolute risk of lymphoma in IBD patients treated with thiopurines alone observed in the French CESAME cohort was 9 per 10,000 patient-years.[226]

A reasonable conclusion is that both immunomodulators and anti-TNF agents increase the absolute risk of NHL to a real but small extent. It is not clear if combination therapy increases this risk to any clinically meaningful extent.

Hepatosplenic T-cell lymphoma (HSTCL) has been described in patients with Crohn's disease who have been treated with anti-TNF agents in combination with immunomodulators and with immunomodulators alone (6-MP and AZA).[277] This nearly universally fatal form of NHL predominantly affects young men, but its incidence is unknown; fortunately it appears to be rare, and more often occurs in the setting of combination therapy. This, in addition to the uncertain magnitude of benefit of combination therapy for all patients, has led some authorities to recommend anti-TNF monotherapy, particularly in young male patients.[282] Because it appears that the risk of HSTCL does not begin until approximately 2 years of thiopurine exposure,[272] another approach to reduce risk would be to use combination therapy to induce and maintain remission, with plans to consider withdrawing the thiopurine if a stable remission is maintained.

Infliximab, adalimumab, and certolizumab pegol are class B agents for use in pregnancy. Most of the clinical data in Crohn's disease comes from experience with infliximab, but there are now similar data available for adalimumab and certolizumab. Infliximab and adalimumab cross the placenta in the third trimester and may be detectable in the infant up to 6 months after birth.[283] Certolizumab pegol can cross the placenta in the first trimester in low levels, but has the lowest level of placental transfer in the third trimester, leading to very low exposure to the newborn infant. The rate of birth defects does not appear to be elevated in pregnancies that have occurred while the mother is on anti-TNF therapy, but safety is not clearly established and use during pregnancy has not been routine.[284]

Optimizing Anti-TNF Response. Proper selection of patients is the key to using anti-TNF agents safely, effectively, and appropriately. Patients without objective findings of inflammation or with fibrostenotic disease are unlikely to benefit, and treating patients who have an undrained abscess is likely to be unsafe. In addition to proper patient selection, opportunities to optimize the response to anti-TNF treatment include dose modification, avoidance of smoking, using concomitant immunomodulators, administering early intensive therapy, and the use of drug and antibody levels to guide therapeutic decisions.

Dose intensification often is required to regain response. For infliximab, this means increasing the dose from 5 mg/kg to 10 mg/kg or increasing the maintenance frequency from every 8 weeks to every 6 weeks. This tactic works in the majority of patients and allows therapy to be continued after an attenuated response.[285] Increasing adalimumab dosing to 40 mg weekly (or 80 mg every 2 weeks) or giving an additional certolizumab pegol dose can yield similar results.[260,286] Because the response rate to a second anti-TNF agent is lower than the first, dose intensification is favored before moving on to a different anti-TNF drug. Smoking is a strong negative predictor of response to anti-TNF therapy, and all patients need to be informed of the poor initial and long-term outcomes associated with smoking.[287]

The value of the concomitant use of immunomodulators (6-MP, AZA, or MTX) to improve the anti-TNF initial response and maintenance effect is still somewhat controversial. As noted earlier, immunomodulators appear to decrease the production of anti-drug antibodies, thereby increasing serum drug levels, but the clinical significance of such increased levels is uncertain. A prospective study that addressed this question and used infliximab with or without MTX showed no difference in outcomes at the end of 1 year.[288] In support of this, post hoc analyses of RCTs also did not show a benefit of combination immunomodulator and anti-TNF therapy over anti-TNF therapy alone. Most of these patients, however, had already failed an immunomodulator to be entered into these studies. To evaluate the effect of AZA or infliximab monotherapy compared with combination therapy in patients without prior exposure to these agents, the Study of Biologic and Immunomodulator Naïve Patients with Crohn's Disease (SONIC) study was performed. SONIC found that 57% of patients receiving combination therapy were in steroid-free clinical remission at 6 months, compared with 44% receiving infliximab alone and 30% receiving azathioprine alone.[208] In addition, mucosal healing occurred more often in the combination therapy group. This landmark study has pushed the field to strongly consider combination therapy, particularly in immunomodulator and anti-TNF naïve patients. It is not clear if these results can be extrapolated to other anti-TNFs. The value of continuing immunomodulators after their use as monotherapy has failed is still uncertain; a recent meta-analysis showed that it may be important for infliximab, but not adalimumab or certolizumab pegol.[289] The decision to use anti-TNF mono- or combination therapy has to be made based on an individual patient basis, taking their expected benefits and risks into account.[290]

The strategy of early aggressive therapy for Crohn's disease has gained much attention because of the enthusiasm of this approach in RA, and favorable results have been reported in Crohn's disease.[291] In the study by D'Haens, 133 patients with recent-onset active Crohn's disease were randomized to receive early combined immunosuppression with AZA and infliximab (followed by maintenance AZA and on-demand infliximab) or conventional treatment with the sequential use of prednisone, AZA, and then infliximab.[291] At the end of 1 year, 62% of patients in the early-combination therapy group were in remission compared to 42% in the conventional group. By study design, all patients in the conventional group received glucocorticoids, but no patients in the early-combination group required glucocorticoids. Finally, at 2 years, 73% of patients in the early-combination group had complete mucosal healing, compared with 30% in the conventional group. The authors concluded that more intensive treatment early in the course of Crohn's disease could lead to better outcomes. There are significant limitations in this open-label study, including the lack of an arm of early immunomodulator treatment alone. Also, the use of episodic infliximab therapy is not standard of care, although it must be acknowledged that this strategy might yet prove effective in disease of recent onset. Despite these and other limitations, an important point is made that aggressive treatment early in the course of Crohn's disease can prevent the need for glucocorticoids and lead to a high rate of mucosal healing. *Post-hoc* studies of adalimumab and certolizumab clinical trials corroborate the premise of early aggressive therapy, showing increased response and remission rates in patients who received anti-TNF therapy within 2 years of diagnosis.[292] Although this work has highlighted the potential benefit of early aggressive therapy and intuitively makes sense to effectively treat an inflammatory condition before the onset of fibrosis and perforating disease, we still need to keep in mind that this paradigm shift is not yet supported by the strongest of evidence.

The newest tool in the armamentarium to optimize anti-TNF therapy is the ability to measure anti-TNF drug and antibody levels.[293] Previously, reliant on symptoms alone, empiric changes were made for drug dose or switch to another agent within class. Now, the availability of drug and antibody levels can guide our decision making. The most intuitive time to check drug levels is in the setting of loss of response. In this scenario, drug and antibody levels are checked at trough.[293,294]

Low or undetectable drug levels without antibody (or low-level antibody) present should lead to an increase in dose or shortening of the dosing interval. Low or undetectable drug levels with high antibody titer should prompt a change to a different anti-TNF agent. High drug levels should prompt an objective evaluation for disease activity. If there is no active disease, then an alternative explanation for symptoms should be sought. If there is active disease with circulating drug at trough, then there should be a consideration for switching to an agent with a different mechanism of action than anti-TNF. The other time to consider checking levels is to optimize dosing preemptively before infusion reactions or loss of response occurs. The hypothesis is that anti-drug antibodies form when there is no circulating drug, and these antibodies can lead to infusion reactions and/or increased drug clearance. Therefore, by optimizing the dose to prevent time without circulating drug, antibody formation can be suppressed, thereby leading to better and more sustained anti-TNF response.

Another emerging concept is that once antibodies develop, they may resolve.[295] If there are low levels of antibodies to the drug, dose optimization (to increase the trough level) and the addition of an immunomodulator if not already prescribed could be considered. This may salvage the current anti-TNF drug before having to move onto another agent in its class. High levels of antibodies to anti-TNF agents typically cannot be overcome and, if present, a switch to a different agent within class is recommended.

In addition to optimizing treatment, there is also an effort to better define the goals of therapy. There has been focus on mucosal healing, both as a treatment goal and a predictive factor for disease progression. The hypothesis is that persistent inflammatory change, even if not causing symptoms, will lead to structural damage of the bowel, and ultimately lead to complications of Crohn's disease. Data from the pre-biologic and biologic era support better long-term outcomes if mucosal healing is achieved.[292] Because we are unable to achieve complete healing in most patients, we need to understand how far to push the therapeutic regimen to achieve a possibly unattainable goal. It is hoped that new disease indices that look at cumulative bowel damage will help us understand how mucosal healing and other endpoints should be used in clinical trials and in practice.[152]

Natalizumab

Natalizumab is humanized monoclonal antibody against α_4-integrin that inhibits leukocyte adhesion and migration into inflamed tissue. Also used for the treatment of multiple sclerosis (MS), natalizumab is the first new class of drug approved for the treatment of Crohn's disease since approval of infliximab in 1998. It is administered IV at a dose of 300 mg every 4 weeks. The large RCTs, Efficacy of Natalizumab as Active Crohn's Therapy (ENACT)-1 and ENACT-2,[52] confirmed its efficacy in both induction and maintenance of remission in moderate to severely active disease.

Unfortunately, in the open-label extension portion of the ENACT studies, 1 patient died from progressive multifocal leukoencephalopathy (PML),[296] a progressive degenerative neurologic disease caused by infection with John Cunningham virus (JCV); it typically is seen in patients with AIDS. This information, together with 2 additional reports of PML in natalizumab-treated patients with MS led to a temporary withdrawal of natalizumab from the market for MS (for which it had already been approved) and suspension of further clinical studies in Crohn's disease. After careful scrutiny and follow-up of all treated patients,[297] natalizumab was returned for use in MS and approved by the FDA in 2008 for treating patients who have moderate to severe Crohn's disease with evidence of active inflammation refractory to prior treatment, including anti-TNF. A mandatory patient registry, Tysabri Outreach Unified Commitment to Health (TOUCH), tracks all treated patients in the United States. Since return to the market, additional cases of PML have been reported, almost all of whom had MS, but additional cases have been reported in patients Crohn's disease as well.

Progress had been made to understand who is at most risk for PML. Three risk factors were identified, including treatment beyond 2 years, prior exposure to immunosuppressants, and the presence of anti-JCV antibodies. Because all Crohn's disease patients receiving natalizumab have prior immunosuppressant exposure, the risk factors to consider in this patient population are anti-JCV status and duration of treatment. An anti-JCV virus assay is commercially available, and the recommendation is to perform this test before determining if natalizumab is an appropriate treatment for a particular patient. Data show that if a patient has all 3 risk factors listed above, the risk of developing PML is approximately 1 in 100.[298] Because this risk is higher than most patients and providers will tolerate, natalizumab is not recommended to patients with a positive anti-JCV antibody, unless under extraordinary circumstances. If anti-JCV antibody is negative, however, the PML risk may be close to zero, and, therefore, treatment with natalizumab may be considered, with repeat anti-JCV antibody testing every 6 months.

In addition to PML, severe hepatic toxicity that could lead to death or the need for liver transplantation has been reported, but this also appears to be very rare.[297,299] Typically, natalizumab is very well tolerated: approximately 10% of patients in the treatment arm of ENACT withdrew because of an adverse event, and serious infections were reported at a rate of 2% to 3%, which is no different from the rate in placebo-treated patients. The future of natalizumab for the treatment of Crohn's disease is uncertain. Although risk can be managed with the use of anti-JCV antibody testing, newer medications with a similar mechanism of action, but without PML risk may take its place (see vedolizumab below).

Adjunctive Therapies

Many other therapies are used to control the symptoms and adverse consequences of Crohn's disease. Antidiarrheal and anticholinergic agents can help to alleviate diarrhea and cramping. Patients with ileal disease or resection can require parenteral vitamin B_{12} supplementation or the addition of cholestyramine (1 to 4 g/day) or colesevelam (625 to 3800 mg/day) to control bile salt diarrhea. Iron supplementation also may be needed. Smoking cessation should be vigorously pursued as a means of improving long-term outcomes.[300]

Bone loss should be anticipated as a potentially serious complication in all patients.[301] Bone density should be checked at diagnosis and at regular intervals thereafter, with appropriate medical management of bone loss. Strategies to preserve bone density include smoking cessation and, at a minimum, daily supplementation of calcium and vitamin D; 1000 mg/day of elemental calcium is enough for younger men and premenopausal women, whereas men and women older than 50 years should have as a goal elemental calcium intake of 1500 mg/day. For most people, 400 to 800 IU of vitamin D daily is adequate. In patients at the highest risk and without contraindications, bisphosphonates should be considered at the time corticosteroids are initiated. One study showed that a single-dose of zoledronate could be effective to prevent bone loss when administered during a flare requiring corticosteroids.[302]

Aside from its role in preventing bone loss, vitamin D has also gained interested for its potential immunomodulatory role. As noted earlier, low vitamin D levels may be associated with an increased risk of developing Crohn's disease.[5] Taken a step further, there is some suggestion that replacing vitamin D can be helpful as an adjunctive therapy to decrease Crohn's disease activity level.[303] We still need to learn more about the importance of vitamin D and Crohn's disease, but a general recommendation is to keep vitamin D, specifically 24(OH)D3, above 32-40 ng/ml.

Novel Therapies

Progress in understanding the pathogenesis of Crohn's disease has borne fruit in the development of a wide variety of novel therapeutic agents. In addition to holding real promise for safer and more effective therapy in the future, clinical trials of novel therapeutics offer access to these agents for patients whose disease has exhausted approved therapies.

Promising agents under investigation include antibodies directed against the shared p40 subunit of IL-12 and IL-23. The human anti IL-12/23 monoclonal antibody ustekinumab was studied in a blinded crossover trial involving 104 patients with moderate to severe Crohn's disease.[304] Although the primary endpoint of clinical response at 8 weeks was not achieved, significant differences compared with placebo were seen at other time points, with the largest differences seen in patients who had previously received infliximab. This prompted an RCT of over 500 patients.[305] In this study, patients were treated with a single IV induction dose of 1 mg/kg, 3 mg/kg, 6 mg/kg, or placebo. The patients who had a response at 6 weeks were then randomized to a subcutaneous dose of either 90 mg or placebo. At the time of the primary endpoint at 6 weeks, 40% of patients had responded to therapy compared with 24% in the placebo group (P = 0.005). Of the responders, 42% were in remission at week 22 compared with 27% in the placebo group (P = 0.03). Treatment was well tolerated. Serious adverse events were rare and primarily related to active Crohn's disease.

Vedolizumab is an anti-integrin molecule similar to natalizumab, but in contrast to natalizumab, which targets both $\alpha4\beta1$ and $\alpha4\beta7$, vedolizumab only targets $\alpha4\beta7$. This is important because there are no $\alpha4\beta7$ receptors in the brain, and therefore PML theoretically is not a concern with vedolizumab; animal models and experience in humans have supported this claim. Vedolizumab was studied in patients with Crohn's disease using an IV dose of 300 mg given at baseline and again 2 weeks later.[306] There was a statistically significant rate of clinical remission at week 6 (15% treatment group vs. 7% placebo group, P = 0.02). Patients without prior failure to anti-TNF did better than those in whom anti-TNF therapy previously failed. Although the week 6 data were somewhat disappointing, the maintenance data were significantly better.[307] By week 52, there were statistically significant differences for treatment with vedolizumab (administered every 4 or 8 weeks) compared with placebo for the outcomes of clinical remission, clinical response, and corticosteroid-free remission. As was also seen in UC, vedolizumab may prove to be 1 of our most effective and durable maintenance medications for Crohn's disease. Based on these results, vedolizumab was approved in the United States for both Crohn's disease and ulcerative colitis in 2014.

Inhibition of Janus kinase (JAK) is another pathway showing promise for the treatment of Crohn's disease. When cytokines bind to the cell surface, receptors lead to polymerization and activation of JAK. Activated JAK in turn phosphorylates signal transducer and activator of transcription (STAT) protein, which dimerizes and moves to the cell nucleus to activate new gene transcription.[308] The oral JAK inhibitor tofacitinib is showing promise for both UC and Crohn's disease. In a phase 2 study of 139 patients with moderate to severe Crohn's disease, there was a dose-dependent treatment effect on CRP levels and on clinical response.[309] There was also a dose-dependent increase in LDL cholesterol, so this safety signal will have to be monitored in future trials of this agent.

Probiotic therapies have been examined as a safe means of modulating the intestinal immune response in IBD, but studies in pediatrics and in the setting of postoperative prophylaxis have been disappointing.[310,311]

Some novel agents defy conventional approaches to the treatment of Crohn's disease. Porcine whipworm (*Trichuris suis*) has been administered as a possible treatment for both Crohn's disease and UC, with promising effect and excellent safety and tolerability.[312] Theoretically, this iatrogenic helminthic infestation might prove effective through the induction of regulatory T cells.

Although the hypotheses underlying these unusual therapies have yet to be proved, the excitement over the novel mechanisms and how they inform us of the pathophysiology of Crohn's disease continue to stimulate enthusiasm.

Nutritional Therapy

Nutritional therapy in Crohn's disease conceivably has 2 purposes: repletion of nutrients and treatment of the primary disease (see Chapter 6). Specific deficits should be identified and corrected. Protein-calorie malnutrition should be addressed, preferably with enteral supplementation. Many, but not all, patients with Crohn's disease are lactose intolerant and may need increased calcium supplementation. TPN may be considered for patients with severe malnutrition before surgery or for selected patients with severe Crohn's disease as a primary therapy in combination with bowel rest. Patients with short bowel syndrome from numerous small bowel resections can require enteral nutrition with defined diets; rarely, patients with severe short bowel syndrome require lifelong TPN.

A meta-analysis has found defined enteral diets to be inferior to glucocorticoids in achieving clinical response,[313] but defined enteral or polymeric diets still may be useful in some children for whom glucocorticoids are undesirable.[314] Elemental diets do not appear to be superior to polymeric diets.[313] Children may be taught to receive nocturnal feedings after self-intubation with an NG tube. Long-term tolerance may be poor, however, and disease tends to recur when the patient's usual diet is reintroduced.

A number of dietary interventions have been evaluated. Most of the focus has been on elimination diets, dietary fiber including prebiotics, glutamine, fish oil, and carbohydrates. Although patients frequently report associations between diet and symptoms,[315] none of these interventions to date have consistently shown benefit in clinical trials.[316] Patients with a stricture might tolerate raw fruits and vegetables poorly or might experience complete intestinal obstruction.

A compelling newer avenue of research is to study the impact of diet on the intestinal microbiome. Because the microbiome may contribute to disease manifestations through host-microbe interactions, alteration of the microbiome with diet may be a strategy to prevent or manage Crohn's disease. Much work in this area is needed, but early data confirm a link between dietary patterns and intestinal microbial enterotype.[317]

Surgical Therapy

Surgery plays an integral role in the treatment of Crohn's disease to control symptoms and to treat complications. By the 20th year from the onset of symptoms, roughly 75% of patients have had some surgical procedure.[318] Depending on the prevalent medical culture in the country of study, the rate of surgery within 3 years of diagnosis varies from 25% to 45%. Approximately 30% of patients require a second surgery by 5 years after the first, and about one third of patients who need a second surgery eventually require a third.[319] These percentages stayed fairly stable from 1950-2000, but likely have decreased since the introduction of biologic agents.[318] Because of the high likelihood of recurrence after segmental resection, the guiding principle of surgery in Crohn's disease is preservation of intestinal length and function. Taking wide margins does not reduce the likelihood of recurrent disease and, with repeated resection, can contribute to short bowel syndrome and intestinal failure.

Indications for surgery include complications such as intra-abdominal abscess, medically intractable fistula, fibrotic stricture with obstructive symptoms, toxic megacolon, hemorrhage, and cancer. Patients with symptoms refractory to medical therapy also should be considered for surgery, particularly when they remain dependent on or refractory to glucocorticoids despite optimal medical therapy. Some patients prefer to consider a limited small bowel resection as opposed to a trial of immunomodulator or biologic therapy.[320] A well-timed bowel resection may be indicated for children with growth failure. In patients with indeterminate colitis for whom colectomy is required, ileal pouch–anal anastomosis (IPAA) can be considered, but pouch-related complications are seen at a higher rate than in patients with UC.[128] In patients with Crohn's disease, there is a high rate of pouch failure and IPAA typically is avoided. In selected patients with rectal sparing and lack of fistulizing disease, however, IPAA or ileorectal anastomosis may be considered (see Chapter 117).[321,322] Increasing facility with minimally invasive laparoscopic approaches and enhanced recovery pathways for Crohn's disease might reduce operative morbidity, reduce hospital stays, and improve outcomes.[323-326]

COSTS OF CARE

Substantial medical and societal costs are incurred in the course of Crohn's disease. One study estimated the total cost in the United States for patients with Crohn's disease exceeds $2 billion annually.[327] Studies from the United States and Canada estimate the average cost of hospitalization for a patient with Crohn's disease to be approximately $10,000 to $15,000 and annual costs of anti-TNF agents to be $25,000 to $30,000.[328,329] Despite the expense of the anti-TNF drugs, analyses have shown that these agents improve quality of life and are cost-effective because of prevention of hospitalizations and surgery.[330]

CROHN'S DISEASE IN THE LIFE CYCLE

Approximately 25% of new Crohn's disease diagnoses are made in persons younger than 20 years of age. In most respects, Crohn's disease has the same pathophysiology and clinical features in children as it does in adults. The special consequences of Crohn's disease in children and adolescents relate to the vulnerability of this population to disturbances in physical growth, sexual maturation, and psychosocial development.

Crohn's disease affects many persons in the peak of their reproductive years. Studies have varied in the assessment of female fertility in Crohn's disease, showing either no difference from the general population or a slight decrease. Studies that have detected diminished fertility generally have correlated this finding with increased disease activity. Contributing factors can include true infertility or a conscious decision to avoid childbearing. In men and women, decreased libido because of symptoms (e.g., diarrhea, abdominal pain, fatigue) are not uncommon; in women, dyspareunia and rectovaginal fistulas can play additional roles. Except for reversible sperm abnormalities caused by sulfasalazine and MTX, men with Crohn's disease have normal fertility.

The effect of pregnancy on the course of Crohn's disease depends on the status of the disease at conception.[331] Women with quiescent disease at conception have the same rate of relapse during pregnancy as nonpregnant women. Among women with active disease at conception, the one-third rule applies: one third improve, one third worsen, and one third have unchanged symptoms during their pregnancy.[332]

Most pregnancies carried by women with Crohn's disease are normal, but there appears to be an increased rate of adverse conception outcomes (i.e., spontaneous abortion), adverse pregnancy outcomes (e.g., preterm birth, child small for gestational age, stillbirth) and pregnancy-related complications.[333] Other than preterm birth, the contribution of disease activity to these outcomes may be lower than previously thought.[333,334] For a review of the safety of medical therapies in pregnancy and nursing, see Table 115-4.

Compared with younger patients who have Crohn's disease, older patients are more likely to have disease of the colon, particularly of the distal colon. As with children, the presentation may be subtle; extraintestinal symptoms can predominate, and diagnosis may be delayed. Medical management is essentially no different for the older patient, but the clinician more often must consider the variety of other conditions prevalent among older patients when choosing therapies. As expected, older IBD patients who are hospitalized have a higher morbidity and mortality than younger patients,[335] and are at a higher risk of adverse events from immune suppressive therapy.[336]

PROGNOSIS

Morbidity

The natural history of Crohn's disease is a moving target, continuously changing as therapeutic strategies improve.[318] The course of disease is highly variable and difficult to predict for a given patient. Population-based studies from Scandinavia provide the best information regarding the course of disease. In the first year after diagnosis, the cumulative relapse rate is high, approaching 50%, with 10% of patients having a chronic relapsing course.[337] Thereafter, patients generally are true to their own history: The rate of relapse in the first 2 years of the disease correlates with the risk of relapse in the ensuing 5 years.[338] Symptomatically active disease in the preceding year yields a high likelihood of active disease in the following year. Conversely, a year in which symptoms are quiescent has an 80% probability of being followed by another year without exacerbation.[338] Over a 4-year period, the same analysis has shown that 22% of patients remain in remission, 25% experience chronically active symptoms, and 53% have a course that fluctuates between active and inactive disease.[338] Although most persons continue to lead productive lives, the course of the disease may be punctuated by periods of poor productivity. Over time, approximately 10% of patients are disabled by their disease.

Increasingly, serologic markers are recognized as providing prognostic information. Pediatric patients with Crohn's disease who have higher immune responses to the microbial antigens ASCA, anti-CBir, and anti-OmpC have higher rates of complicated disease.[339] Furthermore, the highest antibody sum group has the most rapid disease progression. Similar results also have been seen in adults, and with other serologic antibody markers (antibodies to carbohydrates).[71,340,341] There have been mixed results regarding the utility of genetic polymorphisms in predicting the natural history of disease, perhaps reflecting our currently incomplete understanding of the genetic and environmental factors that shape disease expression.[339,342] In the future, predictive models will most likely use a combination of clinical, serologic, and genetic markers to help prognosticate disease severity and course.[343]

Cancer

The estimated risk of colorectal cancer (CRC) in Crohn's disease has varied widely, ranging from no more risk than that of the general population to an estimated standardized incidence ratio as high as 26.6 (see Chapter 127).[344] One meta-analysis estimated the absolute risk at 10, 20, and 30 years to be 2.9%, 5.6%, and 8.3%, respectively. For patients with Crohn's colitis, this was higher than expected in the general population, but not different from what was reported for patients with UC. For patients with isolated ileal disease, the relative risk of colon cancer was not statistically higher than those without IBD. The overall rate of colon cancer in Crohn's disease over the past 30 years may have decreased.[345]

The general recommendation for CRC surveillance for patients with Crohn's disease that involves the colon is to follow the same guidelines as for UC.[346] Segments of bowel excluded by diversion procedures are at greatly increased risk for developing CRC and present a great challenge to screening and surveillance.

Little controversy surrounds the increased risk of small bowel adenocarcinoma associated with long-standing disease or in bypassed loops of small intestine. Small intestinal cancers are rare in Crohn's disease, but in comparison to the extremely low incidence of this disease in the general population, there is a high associated relative risk.[345] The association between Hodgkin's and non-Hodgkin's lymphomas and Crohn's disease remains unclear. Studies relying on cases at referral centers have found an increased risk of lymphoma, whereas population-based studies have not.[229] The most likely explanations are either a referral bias or an increased risk confined to patients with more severe disease. Squamous cell carcinomas can arise in association with a chronic fistula to the skin and in anal Crohn's disease. Some studies also have found an association between Crohn's disease and respiratory cancers,[347] perhaps attributable to smoking behavior.

Mortality

Whether having Crohn's disease conveys an increased mortality is debated. Older population-based studies from the 1980s-1990s generally showed a modestly increased mortality rate in Crohn's disease. A U.S. population-based study reporting on the years 1996 to 2003 demonstrated a 40% increase in the standardized mortality rate among patients with Crohn's disease compared with controls, but the absolute difference in death rates was still small.[348] Specifically, the standardized mortality rate among Crohn's disease patients was 66.9 deaths per 10,000 person-years compared with 49.7 deaths per 10,000 person-years in the general population, and representing an excess of 17 deaths per 10,000 person-years attributable to Crohn's disease. More recently, European population-based studies did not show a difference in mortality compared with the general population.[349-351] A recent meta-analysis continues this debate, with the report of an increased mortality rate, driven by CRC, pulmonary disease and nonalcoholic steato-hepatitis.[352] These data are not conclusive, but a reasonable explanation is that Crohn's disease may be associated with a slightly higher mortality rate.

COPING WITH CROHN'S DISEASE

Although the old myths surrounding psychopathology as an underlying cause of IBD have long been debunked, coping with diarrhea, pain, malaise, and decreased energy takes a toll on all persons who suffer from Crohn's disease, as well as on their families. Depression and anxiety often diminish daily functioning that already may be impaired by the physical manifestations of the disease; psychosocial functioning, of course, has a large impact on the patient's quality of life, even in the absence of active disease.[353,354] Patients cite concerns about lack of energy, loss of control, body image, fear and isolation, feeling unclean, and not reaching their full potential.[355] The medical provider can help greatly in alleviating these concerns by providing accurate and plentiful information. Lay organizations such as the Crohn's and Colitis Foundation of America provide valuable resources in support of affected persons and their families (http://www.ccfa.org). An attitude of hopefulness is warranted because an astounding number of therapeutic innovations—and someday perhaps a cure—continue to unfold.

KEY REFERENCES

Full references for this chapter can be found on www.expertconsult.com.

22. Cho JH, Brant SR. Recent insights into the genetics of inflammatory bowel disease. Gastroenterology 2011; 140:1704-12.
43. Franke A, McGovern DPB, Barrett JC, et al. Genome-wide meta-analysis increases to 71 the number of confirmed Crohn's disease susceptibility loci. Nat Genet 2010; 42:1118-25.
54. Rutgeerts P, Geboes K, Vantrappen G, et al. Natural history of recurrent Crohn's disease at the ileocolonic anastomosis after curative surgery. Gut 1984; 25:665-72.
152. Pariente B, Cosnes J, Danese S, et al. Development of the Crohn's disease digestive damage score, the Lemann score. Inflamm Bowel Dis 2011; 17:1415-22.
161. Akobeng A, Gardener E. Oral 5-aminosalicylic acid for maintenance of medically induced remission in Crohn's Disease. Cochrane Database Syst Rev 2005; CD003715.
206. Prefontaine E, Sutherland LR, Macdonald JK, et al. Azathioprine or 6-mercaptopurine for maintenance of remission in Crohn's disease. Cochrane Database Syst Rev 2009; CD000067.
208. Colombel JF, Sandborn WJ, Reinisch W, et al. Infliximab, azathioprine, or combination therapy for Crohn's disease. N Engl J Med 2010; 362:1383-95.
226. Beaugerie L, Brousse N, Bouvier AM, et al. Lymphoproliferative disorders in patients receiving thiopurines for inflammatory bowel disease: A prospective observational cohort study. Lancet 2009; 374:1617-25.
281. Siegel C, Marden S, Persing S, et al. Risk of lymphoma associated with anti-TNF agents for the treatment of Crohn's disease: A meta-analysis. Gastroenterology 2008; 134:A14.
291. D'Haens G, Baert F, van Assche G, et al. Early combined immunosuppression or conventional management in patients with newly diagnosed Crohn's disease: An open randomised trial. Lancet 2008; 371:660-7.
293. Ordas I, Feagan BG, Sandborn WJ. Therapeutic drug monitoring of tumor necrosis factor antagonists in inflammatory bowel disease. Clin Gastroenterol Hepatol 2012; 10:1079-87; quiz e85-6.
318. Cosnes J, Gower-Rousseau C, Seksik P, et al. Epidemiology and natural history of inflammatory bowel diseases. Gastroenterology 2011; 140:1785-94.
331. Mahadevan U, Cucchiara S, Hyams JS, et al. The London Position Statement of the World Congress of Gastroenterology on Biological Therapy for IBD with the European Crohn's and Colitis Organisation: Pregnancy and pediatrics. Am J Gastroenterol 2011; 106:214-23; quiz 24.

CHAPTER OUTLINE

UC is a chronic idiopathic inflammatory disease of the GI tract that affects the large bowel and is a major disorder under the broad group of conditions termed *inflammatory bowel disease*, which also includes Crohn's disease (CD). Dr. Samuel Wilks is credited with being the first to describe UC in 1859 when he wrote on "idiopathic colitis" and recognized it as distinct from the then more common bacillary dysentery.[1] He also reported the pathologic finding of dilated and thinned colon with severe pancolonic inflammation in a patient with this condition.[2] In 1909, Hawkins described the chronic and relapsing nature of the disease course and the "stealthy hemorrhage" onset of distal disease, in which bleeding often occurred in the presence of constipation.[3] In that same year, Sir Arthur Hurst gave a more complete description of UC, including its sigmoidoscopic appearances and differentiation from bacillary dysentery.[4]

The etiology of UC remained controversial, however, and an infectious or psychosomatic origin was considered its primary cause. The discovery of the double-helix structure of DNA by Watson and Crick in the 1950s paved the way for the era of genetic research, and in the last several decades, immunology has taken the central stage of research in attempting to unravel the pathogenesis of UC. At present, the precise etiology of UC still is unknown, but it is thought to be multifactorial, involving genetic, immunologic, and environmental factors. It also is now evident that patients with UC can have a broad spectrum of clinical presentations and extraintestinal manifestations.

Although UC is not associated with an increased mortality compared with the general population, it can have substantial morbidity and can lead to sizable direct and indirect health care costs. Fortunately, significant advances have been made regarding management of UC and its associated complications, including medical therapies and surgical techniques.

EPIDEMIOLOGY

The incidence and prevalence of UC vary with geographic location and ethnicity. Rigorous epidemiologic studies have been limited by several potential issues: diagnosis of UC may be difficult because of its varied clinical manifestations and, in some regions, the common occurrence of infectious colitis that can mimic UC. Differences in health care systems also contribute to inaccurate estimation of cases, and reliable determination of the epidemiology of UC for a particular population might not be possible. With improved diagnostic techniques and increased awareness, UC is now recognized worldwide, although despite this increased recognition, most of the available epidemiologic data derive from population- or hospital-based studies conducted in North America and northern Europe.

It is currently estimated that there are approximately 800,000 people afflicted with UC in the United States and 1.4 million in Europe.[5] In general, there has been a distinct north-south gradient in risk. The areas with the highest rates of reported incidence and prevalence of UC include North America and northern Europe (Tables 116-1 and 116-2). In North America, incidence rates range from 7.6 to 19.5 cases per 100,000 person-years, and the prevalence ranges from 170 to 249 cases per 100,000 persons. In Europe, incidence rates range from 1.7 to 13.6 cases per 100,000 person-years, with a prevalence of 43 to 294 cases per 100,000 persons. The disease initially had been considered more common in northern Europe, although studies now suggest that the incidence of

UC in southern Europe is comparable to that in northern Europe.[6] In contrast, studies have reported significantly lower incidence rates of 0.3 to 5.8 per 100,000 person-years in other parts of the world, including Asia and Africa.[5]

A recent systematic review discovered that the incidence and prevalence of UC are increasing with time across the globe.[7] The authors performed time-trend analyses, which demonstrated that 60% of UC studies worldwide showed increasing incidence. The increasing incidence and prevalence of UC could be due to a number of factors. Industrialization has been postulated to lead to IBD, possibly owing to changes in microbial exposures, sanitation, pollution, diet, and medication exposures.[8] Other factors that could lead to the increasing incidence and prevalence of UC worldwide are heightened awareness of IBD by physicians and patients, improvements in diagnostic techniques (endoscopy and radiologic testing), increased utilization of these tests, and greater access to health care by the public.[7] With respect to the health care burden of UC in the United States, a recent study reported that hospital discharges for UC have increased 32% over the last decade, with over 37,000 discharges in 2009 accounting for more than 228,000 hospital days and an aggregate cost exceeding $408 million.[9]

There appears to be a marked ethnic variation in the incidence of UC. One ethnic group with high incidence of this disease is the Jewish population. Incidence rates of UC among Jews have been shown to be several-fold higher than in the non-Jewish population across various geographic regions. In the United States, for example, the annual incidence of UC among Jews is 13 cases per 100,000 person-years compared with 3.8 per 100,000 among non-Jewish whites.[10] Within Israel, Ashkenazi Jews have a higher incidence than do Sephardic Jews, but they have a lower incidence than in the United States and northern Europe, suggesting that environmental factors also play an etiologic role.

UC traditionally has been considered extremely uncommon in minority populations, but recent studies have challenged this notion. Early studies reported that UC was rare in blacks. Most of these studies, however, were conducted in regions with limited black populations, and more recent studies suggest an increasing incidence of UC among African Americans. By the late 1970s, incidence rates were comparable between whites and nonwhites in the United States.[11,12] An increase in the incidence of UC also has been observed among blacks in South Africa, although the incidence rate still remains lower than that for South African whites.[13]

In Asia, UC is generally is less common than in Western countries, although its incidence and prevalence appear to be on the rise.[7] Several studies have also demonstrated that South Asian immigrants in England are more likely to have UC than are European natives.[14-16] This changing epidemiology with a population emigrating from a low-risk to a high-risk geographic region supports the concept of environmental influences on development of disease.

UC can occur at any age, although diagnosis before the age of 5 years or after 75 years is uncommon. The peak incidence of UC occurs in the second and third decades of life. Studies have reported a second, smaller peak in older adults, between the ages of 60 and 70 years. This second peak of disease incidence is less pronounced than that for CD. Most studies have not shown any gender difference in the occurrence of UC, and a male-to-female ratio of nearly 1:1 applies to all age groups.

Certain lifestyle and socioeconomic factors have been associated with the development of UC. It is more common in industrialized than in less developed countries and among urban than rural populations. Within a defined population, there may be a slightly higher incidence of disease among those of higher socioeconomic status. As mentioned before,

TABLE 116-1 Incidence of UC in Various Geographic Regions

Region	Period of Study	Incidence (per 100,000 Person-Years)
North America		
Alberta	1981	19.5
Nova Scotia	1940-2000	7.6-8.8
Minnesota	1998-2000	14.3
Europe		
Germany	1980-2006	2.4-3.9
Hungary	1977-2001	1.7-11.0
Italy	1989-1992	3.8-9.6
Scandinavia	1958-2005	4.2-13.6
Spain	1991-2003	3.2-9.6
Asia		
Israel	1965-1994	0.9-5.8
Japan	1974-1991	0.5-1.9
South Korea	1986-2005	0.3-3.1
Africa		
South Africa	1980-1984	0.6-5.0

Adapted from Cosnes J, Gower-Rousseau C, Seksik P, et al. Epidemiology and natural history of inflammatory bowel diseases. Gastroenterology 2011;140:1785-9.

TABLE 116-2 Prevalence of UC in Various Geographic Regions

Region	Period of Study	Prevalence (per 100,000 Persons)
North America		
Alberta	1981	170
Minnesota	1940-2000	214-229
Nova Scotia	1998-2000	249
United States	1999-2003	191-238
Europe		
Denmark	2003-2005	294
Spain	1977	143
Italy	1989-1992	121
Hungary	1981-1988	43
Asia		
Israel	1965-1994	45
Japan	1991	18
South Korea	1986-2005	7.6-31

Adapted from Cosnes J, Gower-Rousseau C, Seksik P, et al. Epidemiology and natural history of inflammatory bowel diseases. Gastroenterology 2011; 140:1785-9.

studies of immigrants moving to high-risk geographic regions have shown increases in their incidence rates of UC compared with the incidence rate for the same ethnic groups living in their native countries. Together, these observations support the notion that environmental factors influence the development of UC.

ETIOLOGY AND PATHOGENESIS

The etiology of UC (and CD) is currently unknown but is likely multifactorial. The currently held paradigm involves a complex interaction of 3 elements: genetic susceptibility, host immunity, and environmental factors. Dysregulation of the enteric immune response in genetically predisposed persons leads to the development of acute and chronic inflammation and the pathologic feature of mucosal damage. The specific inciting antigens for the inflammatory process have yet to be identified, but several sources have been suggested, including pathogenic and commensal microorganisms, metabolic byproducts of these agents, and normal epithelial structures.

Genetics

Family History

Genetic factors have been linked to the development of UC, supported largely by the observation that family history is 1 of the most important risk factors for developing the disease. A familial incidence of UC has been recognized for many years, and although figures vary widely in different studies, about 10% to 20% of patients have at least 1 other affected family member.[17] Familial associations generally occur in first-degree relatives. The relative risk of the same disease in a sibling of a person with UC has been estimated to be between 7% and 17% based on North American and European studies. Second-degree relatives appear to be at a lower risk for developing UC than are first-degree relatives. Data from the United States suggest a preponderance of parent-sibling combinations, but in the United Kingdom, the disease is shared more commonly by siblings. Indeed, the strongest evidence of a genetic influence for UC is derived from twin studies. In 3 large European twin pair studies, approximately 6% to 16% of monozygotic twin pairs had concordant UC compared with 0% to 5% of dizygotic twin pairs.[18-20] These concordance rates are substantially lower than those for CD, suggesting that genetic determinants, although important, play a less significant role for UC than for CD. No twin pair demonstrated both UC and CD, further supporting the genetic basis of these disorders.

Familial association is greater in persons of Jewish descent, a heritage known to have a higher incidence of IBD. The lifetime risk of developing disease is 3-fold higher among first-degree relatives of Jewish patients compared with relatives of non-Jewish patients.[21] A similar increase in risk also has been observed in relatives of patients who had early onset of disease. This familial association contrasts with the low incidence of UC among spouses of patients with IBD in most series. Although reports of IBD in both spouses are rare, a study of 30 conjugal instances of IBD (17 of which were concordant for CD, 3 for UC, and 10 mixed) found that the majority of these couples developed IBD after cohabitation, thus suggesting a shared environmental exposure.[22]

For all affected first-degree relatives within a family, there is a high concordance for type of disease (UC vs. CD) and occurrence of extraintestinal manifestations.[23] In fact, epidemiologic studies in families with multiple affected members have demonstrated disease-type concordance rates of 75% to 80%, the other 20% to 25% of families being mixed (i.e., having members with both UC and CD).[24] The overlap in inheritance patterns among the mixed families suggests that a subset of genes associated with IBD confers susceptibility to both UC and CD, whereas others are specific to 1 disease or the other.

Numerous studies have examined the effect of family history on disease location. In UC, no consistent correlation has been observed in the studies that examined disease extent namely, left-sided colitis versus extensive colitis and family history of UC.[25]

Genetic Mutations

The inheritance of UC (and CD) cannot be described by a simple Mendelian genetics model. It is likely that multiple genes are involved and that different genes confer susceptibility, disease specificity, and phenotype. A recent genome-wide association study, which identified an additional 71 genetic loci associated with susceptibility to IBD, reported that there are now a total of 163 loci that may confer increased risk for the development of IBD.[26] These loci are thought to account for 7.5% of the disease variance of UC and 13.6% of the disease variance of CD. Twenty-three of these loci are specific to UC and 30 are specific to CD. Interestingly, 110 of these 163 loci are associated with both UC and CD, and 43 of the remaining 53 show the same direction of effect in the non-associated disease, thus implying that almost all biological mechanisms involved in 1 disease have the same role in the other disease. Even more fascinating is the finding that 113 of the 163 loci are associated with other autoimmune diseases, most strongly with psoriasis and ankylosing spondylitis as well as primary immunodeficiencies and mycobacterial infections. What these results may mean is that not only are UC and CD part of the same spectrum of disease, rather than being individual diseases, but also that many autoimmune diseases and even susceptibility to certain infections may all be part of a long continuum of disease.

UC-specific loci have been identified on chromosomes 1-7, 11, 15-17, 19 and 20.[26] The *NOD2/CARD15* gene mutations located on chromosome 16 associated with CD have not been associated with UC, although UC patients from families with a history of CD and UC might possess *NOD2* variants.[27] The CD autophagy gene *ATG16L1* on chromosome 2q37 (which encodes autophagy-related 16-like protein) is not seen in patients with UC, whereas another autophagy gene, *IRGM* on chromosome 5q33 (which encodes immunity-related GTPase [guanosine triphosphatase] family, M), is shared between diseases; both of these genes are involved in bacterial processing and the protection of cells from various bacterial pathogens and their toxins (i.e., autophagy). A number of CD loci or genes (or both) have been identified in UC, however, and include IL-23R on chromosome 1p31, which encodes the interleukin (IL)-23 receptor; chromosome 3p21, which encodes *MST1* and other potential genes of interest; IL-12β on chromosome 5q33, which encodes the IL-12 receptor β1 subunit (also known as p40) that constitutes part of both the IL-23 and IL-12 receptors; NKX2-3 on chromosome 10q24, which encodes NK2 transcription factor related, locus 3; and chromosome 17q21, which encodes *STAT3* and other potential genes of interest. With respect to the gene encoding IL-23R, several polymorphisms of this gene have been identified, most notably the Arg381Gln polymorphism.[28] Heterozygous carriage of the glutamine allele is associated with a 3-fold decreased risk of CD and a more modest reduction in the risk of UC in non-Jewish populations; this reduction is not seen in UC within the Jewish population. IL-23R is important because it plays a key role in the differentiation of a relatively newly discovered subset of T cells called *Th17 cells* (see later).

Environmental Factors

It is now almost universally accepted that the pathogenesis of IBD is a result of continuous antigenic stimulation by commensal enteric bacteria, fungi, or viruses, which leads to chronic inflammation in genetically susceptible hosts who have defects in mucosal barrier function, microbial killing, or immunoregulation. Several infectious organisms, including mycobacteria and viruses, have been implicated in the pathogenesis of IBD. No specific infective organism, however, has been isolated consistently from patients with UC, and therefore it is unlikely that the disease is caused by a single common infectious agent.

Numerous clinical and experimental observations have suggested involvement of intestinal bacterial microbiota in the pathogenesis of IBD. The most obvious observation perhaps is that CD and UC preferentially occur in regions of the bowel that contain the highest concentration of bacteria, namely, the terminal ileum and the colon, where bacterial concentrations approach 10^{12} organisms per gram of luminal contents. Interestingly, diverting the fecal stream in patients with CD can treat and even prevent disease, whereas reinfusion of ileostomy contents leads to new inflammatory changes within only 1 week.[29] Other human data have shown that antibiotics are useful in the treatment or postoperative prevention of CD and pouchitis. Finally, probiotics (discussed later in this chapter) have been shown to have efficacy in the primary and secondary prevention of pouchitis. The most glaring evidence of the necessary role of bacteria in the pathogenesis of IBD from rodent data is that genetically susceptible mice or rats in a gnotobiotic (germ-free) environment do not have intestinal inflammation; however, these same rodents rapidly develop intestinal inflammation after bacterial colonization.[30-33] Just as in humans, rodent gut inflammation can be treated and prevented with antibiotics and probiotics.[34,35]

With respect to the human GI microbiome, much has been learned in the last few years (see Chapter 3). Complex mathematical models have estimated that the human GI microbiome contains at least 1800 genera and between 15,000 and 36,000 species of bacteria[36-38]; 3 studies have identified more than 45,000 bacterial small-subunit (SSU) rRNA genes, a technique that captures at most only 50% of the predicted species-level biodiversity.[36-38] Of the bacterial genes identified to date, almost all (>98%) can be grouped into 4 phyla: Firmicutes accounts for 64% of the total and includes the family Lachnospiraceae (e.g., *Clostridium* groups XIVa and IV) and the subgroup *Bacillus* (e.g., Streptococcaceae and Lactobacillales). Bacteroidetes accounts for 23% of the total, Proteobacteria accounts for 8% of the total and includes the family Enterobacteriaceae (e.g., *Escherichia coli*), and Actinobacteria accounts for 3%.[38]

Four general mechanisms have been postulated to explain how components of the normal intestinal microbiome might initiate or contribute to the development of the chronic inflammatory state.[39] First, microbes can induce intestinal inflammation, either by adhering to or invading intestinal epithelial cells, thereby causing downstream proinflammatory cytokine production or by producing enterotoxins. Second, a breakdown in the balance between protective and harmful intestinal bacteria, termed *dysbiosis*, can lead to disease. Most studies comparing the intestinal microbiome in IBD with that in healthy controls show biodiversity in the IBD populations is decreased by 30% to 50%. One study found that this reduction in biodiversity was due to decreased concentrations of Firmicutes (specifically Lachnospiraceae) by 300-fold and Bacteroidetes by 50-fold.[38] The loss of these organisms is important because they are known to produce short-chain fatty acids, such as butyrate, which nourish colonocytes. As a result of

their decrease, the relative concentrations of Proteobacteria and Actinobacteria increase in IBD patients relative to controls, although quantitative PCR analysis showed that the absolute numbers of Enterobacteriaceae were not higher in IBD patients than in controls. Loss of protective bacteria, however, could set the stage for overgrowth of pathogenic bacteria. Another interesting finding in this study was that the microbiota of patients with CD and UC were similar to each other. In addition, the study did not identify any individual species that was particularly prevalent in grossly abnormal diseased tissue, and thus no active bacterial etiologic agent was suspected of causing or propagating disease. The third and fourth ways bacteria could play a role in the pathogenesis of IBD deal with the host itself. Genetic defects in host microbial killing or impaired mucosal barrier function can lead to immune hyper-responsiveness to intestinal bacteria, as the microbes have more exposure to epithelial cells and can trigger the production of high levels of proinflammatory cytokines. Finally, genetic defects in host immunoregulation can lead to a heightened immune response to even nonpathogenic bacteria, such as abnormal antigen processing or presentation, loss of tolerance, or overly aggressive T-cell responses.

In addition to infectious agents, several other environmental factors have been proposed as contributing etiologic factors of UC. The best characterized environmental factor associated with UC is cigarette smoking. Numerous studies have consistently shown that UC is more common among nonsmokers than among current smokers, with the relative risk of UC in nonsmokers ranging from 2 to 6[40]; this association is independent of genetic background and gender. Furthermore, there may be a dose-response relationship, with the disease more common in current light smokers than in heavy smokers. This relationship is consistent with observations that clinical improvement with nicotine therapy in patients with UC appears to be limited to those treated with high doses of nicotine and not those receiving lower doses. This risk of developing UC with smoking is particularly high for former smokers, especially within the first 2 years of smoking cessation. The rebound effect also is higher for former heavy smokers than for former light smokers.[41] Smokers also appear to have reduced rates of hospitalization for UC and reduced rates of pouchitis following colectomy.[42] Studies on the role of passive smoking in UC have yielded conflicting results. A recent meta-analysis of 10 studies examining this issue found no association between passive smoking and future development of UC.[43] Several mechanisms have been postulated to account for the apparent protective effect of active smoking on UC. These include modulation of cellular and humoral immunity, changes in cytokine levels, increased generation of free oxygen radicals, and modification of eicosanoid-mediated inflammation. Smoking also might have an effect on mucus production by the colonic mucosa, and might alter colonic mucosal blood flow and intestinal motility. No single mechanism, however, can explain the clinical observation of the beneficial influence of smoking on UC and its adverse effect on CD (see Chapter 115).

Other environmental risk factors that have been suggested to influence the development of UC include diet (wheat, maize, cow's milk, refined sugar, fruits and vegetables, alcohol), oral contraceptives, food additives (silicon dioxide), toothpaste, and breast-feeding; none, however, has been shown conclusively to be associated with UC. Studies have suggested an inverse relationship between appendectomy and the subsequent development of UC[44,45]; the mechanisms for this protective effect of appendectomy on UC are unknown. It is possible that removal of appendiceal-associated lymphoid tissues abrogates certain pathologic alterations in mucosal immune responses and therefore prevents the onset of UC.

Immune Factors

The prevailing theory of the pathogenesis of UC emphasizes the role of the enteric immune response. The physiologic state of the intestine is one of constant low-grade inflammation in response to environmental stimuli such as bacterial products or endogenous factors. Breaches in this well-regulated mucosal immune system lead to the chronic, uncontrolled mucosal inflammation observed in UC. In this regard, immunologic mechanisms in the pathogenesis of UC involve both humoral and cell-mediated responses.

Humoral Immunity

Histologic examination of the inflamed colon indicates a marked increase in the number of plasma cells. This increase is not uniform among cells producing different classes of immunoglobulins. The largest proportional increase occurs in immunoglobulin (Ig)G synthesis, which has the highest pathogenic potential among antibody classes. The increase in IgG synthesis in UC is most pronounced in the IgG_1 and IgG_3 subclasses, in contrast to CD, in which the increase in IgG_2 synthesis is more prominent.[46,47] This disparity in the local IgG subclass response likely reflects differences in antigenic stimuli or host immunoregulatory responses between the 2 groups of IBD patients. The increased IgG synthesis in IBD may represent polyclonal stimulation; patients with UC often have circulating antibodies to dietary, bacterial, and self-antigens that are mostly of the IgG isotype, usually the IgG_1 subclass. Many of these antibodies are thought to be epiphenomena because the serum antibody titers do not correlate with clinical features. Nevertheless, the known cross-reaction between enterobacterial antigens and colonic epithelial epitopes may be an important triggering event, even though, later in the course of the disease, the serum antibody titer to either the bacterial or the colonic antigen may be unimportant.

The concept that UC is an autoimmune disease is supported by its increased association with other autoimmune disorders, including thyroid disease, diabetes mellitus, and pernicious anemia.[48] Patients with UC have varying levels of autoantibodies to lymphocytes, RNA, smooth muscle, gastric parietal cell, and thyroid tissue; these are specific for neither tissue nor disease. Antibodies to epithelial cell-associated components, which specifically recognize intestinal antigen, also have been described.[48] The best-characterized intestinal autoantigen is a 40-kd epithelial antigen found in normal colonic epithelium.[49] This autoantigen is recognized by IgG eluted from the inflamed colonic mucosa of patients with UC and is a component of the tropomyosin family of cytoskeletal proteins.[50] The antibody response to this 40-kd protein appears to be unique to UC and is not found in CD or in other inflammatory conditions. This autoantigen shares an epitope with antigens found in the skin, bile duct, eyes, and joints, sites often involved in the extraintestinal manifestations of UC. The precise pathogenic significance of this autoantibody in UC, however, remains unclear at present.

An autoantibody that has received significant attention in UC patients is pANCA.[51] This autoantibody is present in 41% to 73% of patients with UC.[52] It is synthesized within the lamina propria and is of the IgG_1 subclass. The antigen to which the pANCA is directed has not yet been determined with certainty, and a variety of putative antigens have been proposed, including nuclear histone and nonhistone proteins. The most recent evidence suggests that the antigen is a 50-kd nuclear envelope protein that is specific to myeloid cells.[53] Just as with other autoantibodies found in patients with UC, the pathogenic relevance of pANCA in this disorder is unknown. In fact, the prevailing thought is that pANCA has no pathogenic role in UC, but that it might serve as a potential marker of susceptibility and genetically distinct subsets of UC. The level of pANCA titer does not correlate with disease activity, but it might decline in patients with long-standing remission or in patients who have had colectomy at least 10 years previously. Studies have suggested that pANCA may be associated with a more aggressive disease course[54] and with the development of pouchitis after ileal pouch-anal anastomosis (IPAA) in patients with UC.[55,56] Also of interest is that CD patients with colonic disease have higher rates of pANCA seroreactivity than those without colonic disease, suggesting a possible UC-like CD phenotype.[57]

Antibodies much more commonly seen in CD, including anti-*Saccharomyces cerevisiae* antibody (ASCA) and antibodies against bacterial antigens, including anti-CBir1 (antibody to flagellin from *Clostridium* species), anti-OmpC (antibody to outer membrane porin C of *E. coli*), and anti-I2 (antibody to *Pseudomonas*-associated sequence I2), can also be seen in UC patients.[52] The presence of these antibodies in CD may predict the development of complicated disease (strictures and/or fistulae).[58] In UC, the presence of anti-CBir1 and anti-OmpC has been associated with the development of pouchitis.[59,60]

Cellular Immunity

Immune dysregulation in UC (and CD) also involves cell-mediated immunity. Cell-mediated immunity consists of 2 components, innate immunity and adaptive immunity. The innate immune system, which involves largely monocyte-macrophages and dendritic cells, is nonspecific and untrained and acts as the first line of defense against foreign antigens, particularly bacterial antigens. Bacteria prompt immune responses largely through pattern-recognition receptors (PRRs), which include the 11 Toll-like receptors (TLRs) and 23 nucleotide-binding oligomerization domain (NOD)-like receptors (NLRs) that have been identified to date. Activation of the TLRs and NLRs results in downstream activation of nuclear factor (NF)-κB, which then stimulates the transcription of genes coding for various proinflammatory cytokines (including TNF, IL-1, IL-6, and IL-8), chemokines, adhesion molecules, and costimulatory molecules. In addition, activation of NF-κB stimulates the maturation of dendritic cells, which are involved in antigen presentation. Defects in any of the PRR pathways can lead to abnormal bacterial processing and possibly IBD.[61]

The adaptive immune system, which is governed by T cells and B cells, is specific. Mucosal lymphocytes often are divided into 2 groups based on location: lamina propria lymphocytes and intraepithelial lymphocytes (IELs). Lamina propria lymphocytes express surface adhesion molecules, α4β7, that provide a homing signal for peripheral immune cells to the mucosal sites.[62] Most investigators have found a similar distribution of T-cell subsets ($CD4^+$, $CD8^+$) within the lamina propria in patients with UC compared with that in controls.[63] Also, the absolute number of IELs is normal or reduced in UC, most of which are $CD8^+$ cell. The function of IELs has not been well characterized, but it has been suggested that they are cytotoxic and perhaps active in suppressing local immune response. Regardless of their functional status, mucosal T cells within the lamina propria and epithelium, as well as peripheral blood T cells, display a variety of activation markers, suggesting an activated memory phenotype.[64] Studies have suggested that the T cell receptor repertoire is altered in active IBD.[65]

Although T-cell–mediated immunity has attracted the most attention in the pathogenesis of UC, nonspecific cellular immunity also is altered. In patients with active disease, there is an overproduction of circulating monocytes as well as mucosal macrophages.[66] The inflamed mucosa of patients with UC also exhibits infiltration of substantial numbers of granulocytes.

Epithelial Cells

Intestinal epithelial cells serve barrier functions and play a role in enteric immunity. Colonocytes express class II major histocompatibility complex (MHC) antigens and can function as antigen-presenting cells.[67] In addition, they also express cytokine receptors, secrete various cytokines and chemokines, and express leukocyte adhesion molecules.[68-71] Thus, abnormalities in colonic epithelial cells can contribute to the development of UC. Patients with UC have an increased turnover rate of colonic epithelium[72] and other abnormalities of epithelial cells including reduced metabolism of short-chain fatty acids, especially butyrate, abnormal membrane permeability,[73] and altered composition of glycoprotein mucus produced by the colonic epithelium.[74] Specifically, the mucus layer in UC appears to be thinner than normal.[75] These and other abnormalities can lead to the finding of increased numbers of adherent bacteria, in both the mucus layer and even at the epithelial surface, in patients with UC.[76-78] The role of epithelial cells in the pathogenesis of IBD is supported further by animal models of colitis produced by disruption of colonic epithelium.[79]

Consequences of Immune Activation

Activation of macrophages, lymphocytes, and colonic epithelial cells leads to the release of a variety of cytokines and mediators that further amplify the immune and inflammatory response of UC and result in tissue damage. Based on the cytokines they produce, proinflammatory CD4+ T cells have been divided into 3 major immune phenotypes: T helper 1 (Th1), T helper 2 (Th2), and a more recently recognized subset called T helper 17 (Th17).

The Th1 response is characterized by cell-mediated immunity and is associated with the production of IL-2 and interferon (IFN)-γ. The differentiation of T cells along a Th1 pathway is stimulated by IL-12 generated in response to exposure to infectious agents. The Th2 response is characterized by the production of cytokines IL-4, IL-5, IL-10, and IL-13, which amplify the humoral immune response. Th1 and Th2 subsets reciprocally down-regulate each other through cytokine production.[80] Th1 and Th2 pathways can be regulated by unique regulatory T-cell (Treg) subsets that produce IL-10 and transforming growth factor (TGF)-β and down-regulate inflammation.[81]

Historically, the oversimplified view of adaptive immunity in IBD is that CD is mediated by Th1 cells, whereas UC is mediated by Th2 cells; there is considerable evidence that the story is much more complex. Macrophages in the inflamed colon of patients with active UC synthesize IL-1β, TNF, and IL-6, whereas lamina propria T cells probably produce IL-2 and IFN-γ. This immune response can be up-regulated further by presentation of antigen to CD4+ lymphocytes by colonic epithelial cells that express HLA class II antigens.[67] Studies have implicated a specialized type of T cell, the natural killer (NK) T cell, which seems to mediate the Th2 response in UC.[82,83] These NK T cells, which are not classical NK T cells in that they do not express the typical NK T cell receptors seen with classical NK T cells, secrete large amounts of IL-5 and IL-13, and are actually cytotoxic for intestinal epithelial cells.

A more recently recognized T-cell–mediated inflammatory pathway, which appears to be involved in the pathogenesis of CD and possibly UC, involves the Th17 cell lineage. Th17 cells have been shown to produce a variety of cytokines, most notably IL-6 and IL-17. IL-17 is a potent proinflammatory cytokine that not only facilitates T-cell activation but also stimulates a variety of cells, including fibroblasts, macrophages, epithelial cells, and endothelial cells, to produce an array of proinflammatory cytokines, including IL-1, IL-6, TNF-α, and chemokines.[84] Th17 cell development is inhibited by Th1 and Th2 cells but is promoted by IL-6, TGF-β, IL-21, and IL-23R.[85] IL-23R, which is highly expressed by activated Th17 cells, also is expressed by NK cells, NK T cells, other CD4+ T cells, and CD8+ T cells. The interaction of IL-23 with its receptor has been shown to have a central role in the development of inflammation in various mouse models of colitis.[86,87] Antibodies to IL-23 thus represent another potential therapeutic strategy for the treatment of IBD.

Release of these various cytokines from the T-cell inflammatory pathways also might lead to other abnormalities seen in UC, such as increased epithelial cell permeability and collagen synthesis. Alteration of endothelium by a variety of cytokines can result in local ischemia. Increased expression of endothelial adhesion molecules in response to inflammatory mediators recruits circulating granulocytes and monocytes to the inflamed tissues, thus further perpetuating the inflammatory response. Elevated cytokine levels within the mucosa also stimulate the release of metalloproteinase from fibroblasts with subsequent matrix degradation. Mucosal concentrations of many mediators have been shown to be elevated in patients with active UC, including leukotrienes, thromboxane, platelet-activating factor, nitric oxide, and reactive oxygen metabolites.[88] These mediators, which are mostly released from active macrophages and neutrophils, contribute to inflammation and mucosal injury and alter epithelial cell permeability, thereby further contributing to diarrhea. Diarrhea in UC also is caused by complement activation and the release of kinins and other inflammatory mediators from mast cells and eosinophils (see Chapter 2).

Psychogenic Factors

Psychosomatic factors first were implicated in the pathogenesis of UC in the 1930s,[89] but there is no good direct evidence to support this concept. Since the introduction of glucocorticoids for the treatment of patients with UC and the focus on immunologic aspects of the pathogenesis of the disease in the 1950s, this previously widely held notion has diminished in popularity.

Experimental studies have helped identify mechanisms of the proinflammatory potential of stress in animal models of colitis.[89] When rats are exposed to stress before proinflammatory stimuli are introduced, the severity of colonic inflammation is increased. This particular response has been shown not to be mediated by either vasopressin or corticotropin-releasing factor. In addition, stress has been shown to directly increase intestinal permeability in rats, an action mediated by cholinergic nerves, and to potentiate intestinal inflammation in this particular situation. There are indeed studies reporting that psychosocial stress increases the risk of relapse in patients with quiescent UC.[90,91] Conversely, many of the psychological features observed in patients with UC are likely secondary to this chronic disease process, a phenomenon physicians must be aware of when managing these patients.

PATHOLOGY

At the time of initial presentation, approximately 45% of patients with UC have disease limited to the rectosigmoid, 35% have disease extending beyond the sigmoid but not involving the entire colon, and 20% of patients have

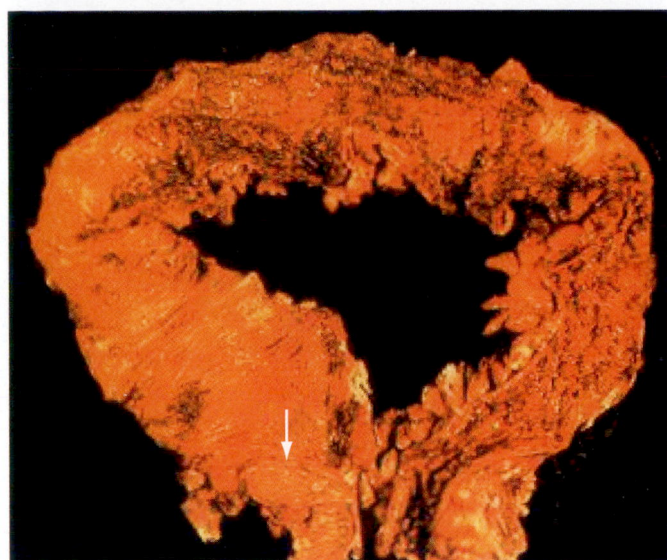

FIGURE 116-1. Total colectomy specimen from a patient with UC. The colon shows diffuse mucosal inflammation that extends proximally from the rectum without interruption to the transverse colon. The mucosa in the terminal ileum and cecum *(arrow)* is normal. The distal mucosa is erythematous and friable, with many ulcers and erosions. *(Courtesy Feldman M, Boland CR, editors. Slide atlas of gastroenterology and hepatology. Philadelphia: Current Medicine; 1996.)*

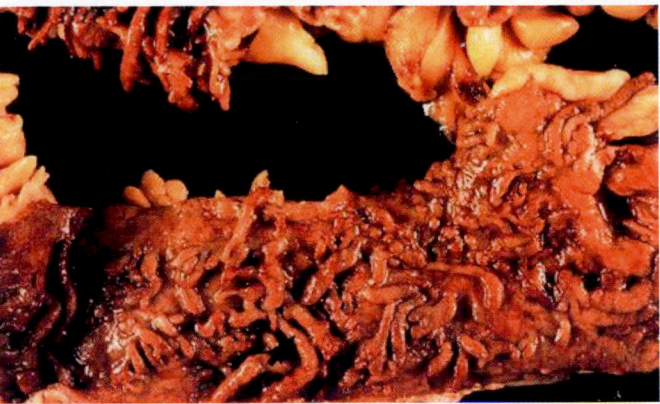

FIGURE 116-2. Surgical specimen of resected colon from a patient with severe UC showing numerous inflammatory polyps (pseudopolyposis). Pseudopolyps are most common in UC but also may be seen in Crohn's disease, ischemia, and other ulcerative conditions of the colon. These blunt or finger-like lesions develop as byproducts of ulcers that penetrate into the submucosa, leaving islands of adjacent regenerative mucosa. Although the intervening areas of colonic mucosa are ulcerated, pseudopolyps can persist even when inflammation has abated and the mucosa has healed. *(Courtesy Feldman M, Boland CR, editors. Slide atlas of gastroenterology and hepatology. Philadelphia: Current Medicine; 1996.)*

pancolitis.[92] The disease typically is most severe distally and progressively less severe more proximally. In contrast to CD, continuous and symmetric involvement is the hallmark of UC (Fig. 116-1), with a sharp transition between diseased and uninvolved segments of the colon.

There are a few exceptions to this general rule. First, medical therapy can result in areas of sparing. For example, topical enema therapy can lead to near-complete mucosal healing in the rectum and distal sigmoid colon. Second, up to 75% of patients with left-sided UC have periappendiceal inflammation in the colon and patchy inflammation in the cecum,[93] resembling the skip pattern characteristic of CD. These patterns of rectal sparing and skip lesions can lead to a misdiagnosis of CD.

Macroscopically, the mucosa in UC appears hyperemic, edematous, and granular in mild disease. As disease progresses, the mucosa becomes hemorrhagic, with visible punctate ulcers. These ulcers can enlarge and extend into the lamina propria. They often are irregular in shape with overhanging edges or may be linear along the line of the teniae coli. Epithelial regeneration with recurrent attacks results in the formation of pseudopolyps, which is typical of long-standing UC but which also may be seen in acute disease (Fig. 116-2). Another characteristic appearance of long-standing disease is atrophic and featureless colonic mucosa, associated with shortening and narrowing of the colon. Patients with severe disease can develop acute dilatation of the colon, also characterized by thin bowel wall and grossly ulcerated mucosa with only small fragments or islands of mucosa remaining. With perforation of the colon, a fibrinopurulent exudate may be seen on the serosal surface of the bowel.

Microscopically, the early stage of UC is marked by edema of the lamina propria and congestion of capillaries and venules, often with extravasation of red blood cells. This is followed by an acute inflammatory cell infiltrate of neutrophils, lymphocytes, plasma cells, and macrophages, often accompanied by increased numbers of eosinophils and mast cells. Neutrophilic infiltration of colonic crypts gives rise to cryptitis and ultimately to crypt abscesses with neutrophilic accumulations in crypt lumens. This migration of neutrophils from the circulation into the lamina propria occurs in response to a variety of chemoattractants, including chemotactic peptides of colonic bacteria, IL-8, activated complement, platelet-activating factor, and leukotriene B_4. The cryptitis is associated with discharge of mucus from goblet cells and increased epithelial cell turnover. Thus, the acute inflammatory infiltration results in the characteristic histopathology of goblet cell mucin depletion, formation of exudates, and epithelial cell necrosis. None of these histologic findings, however, is specific for UC.

Inflammation in UC characteristically is confined to the mucosa, in contrast to the transmural involvement of CD. The inflammatory changes typically end at the luminal aspect of the muscularis mucosa. With increasing inflammation, however, the surface epithelial cells become flattened, eventually ulcerate, and can become undermined if the ulcers are deep. At this stage of the disease, some inflammation and vascular congestion may be present in the submucosa, and ulceration can extend into the muscularis mucosa. This deeper involvement may be confused with CD, but it usually presents diffusely rather than with the segmental fissuring pattern of transmural inflammation that characterizes CD.

During the healing phase of UC, the inflammatory infiltrate subsides and epithelial regeneration takes place. Epithelial cells undergoing regenerative changes become cuboidal with eccentric, large nuclei, and prominent nucleoli. These features may be confused with dysplasia. Thus, a diagnosis of dysplasia in UC should be made with caution in the presence of acute inflammation. Accordingly, surveillance colonoscopy (see "Dysplasia and Colorectal Cancer") should be performed during a period of remission.

A classic histologic feature of chronic quiescent UC is crypt architectural distortion or actual dropout of glands (Fig. 116-3). Architectural changes include branching or bifid glands, wide separation among glands, and shortened glands that do

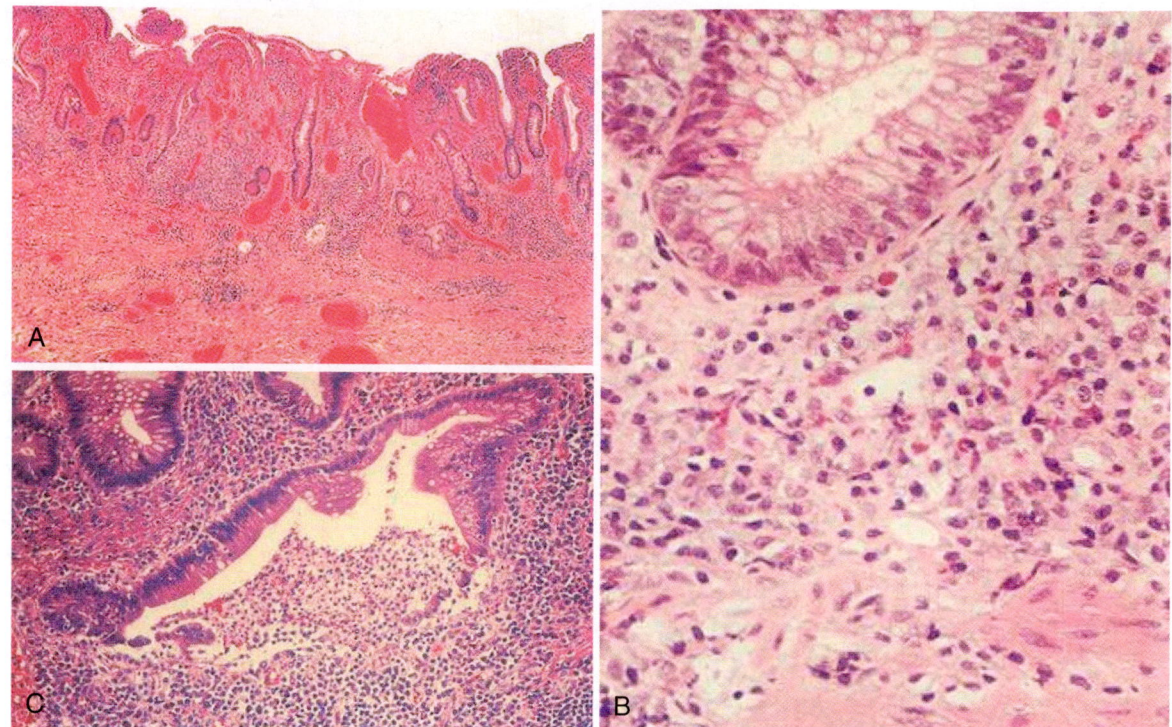

FIGURE 116-3. Photomicrographs of a colonic biopsy specimen showing the histology of UC. *A,* Diffuse chronic inflammation of the lamina propria and crypt distortion are present. These features are important in differentiating UC from acute self-limited colitis. *B,* The base of a single distorted colonic crypt. There are many plasma cells between the crypt and the muscularis mucosae, another important finding that helps differentiate acute from chronic colitis. *C,* A single crypt abscess. The bottom of this distorted crypt has been destroyed by an aggregate of polymorphonuclear neutrophils. This finding is not specific for UC and may be seen in Crohn's disease and other types of colitis. *(Courtesy Feldman M, Boland CR, editors. Slide atlas of gastroenterology and hepatology. Philadelphia: Current Medicine; 1996.)*

not extend down to the muscularis mucosa. Architectural alteration is a prominent feature of chronic quiescent UC, but the histologic abnormalities can revert to normal after mild flares early in the course of disease. Another characteristic feature of chronic quiescent UC is Paneth cell metaplasia, with Paneth cells located distal to the hepatic flexure, where they normally are absent. Other nonspecific chronic changes seen in UC include neuronal hypertrophy and fibromuscular hyperplasia of the muscularis mucosa. Varying degrees of acute or chronic inflammation of the lamina propria may be present in chronic quiescent disease. A thin band of predominantly lymphocytic inflammation occasionally may be seen deep to the muscularis mucosa, presenting diagnostic challenges.

Most of these pathologic findings are not specific for UC. Features that reflect chronicity and thus argue against a diagnosis of infectious or acute self-limited colitis include distorted crypt architecture, crypt atrophy, increased intercrypt spacing to fewer than 6 crypts per millimeter, an irregular mucosal surface, basal lymphoid aggregates, and a chronic inflammatory infiltrate.[94,95] The histologic severity of inflammation does not necessarily correlate with clinical disease activity in patients with UC, and patients may be relatively symptom free although histology reveals significant inflammation.

CLINICAL FEATURES

Patients with UC can present with a variety of symptoms. Common symptoms include diarrhea, rectal bleeding, passage of mucus, tenesmus, urgency, and abdominal pain. In more

severe cases, fever and weight loss may be prominent. The symptom complex tends to differ according to the extent of disease.[96] Patients with proctitis often have local symptoms of tenesmus, urgency, mucus, and bleeding, whereas patients with extensive colitis usually have more diarrhea, weight loss, fever, clinically significant blood loss, and abdominal pain. In general, the severity of the symptoms correlates with the severity of the disease; however, active disease may be found at colonoscopy in patients who are asymptomatic. Additionally, patients with known UC can have severe symptoms that are not necessarily due to UC, such as those caused by bacterial (e.g., *Clostridium difficile*) or viral (e.g., cytomegalovirus) infections or a host of other similar disorders.

The onset of UC typically is slow and insidious. Symptoms usually have been present for weeks or months by the time the typical patient seeks medical attention. The median interval between the onset of symptoms and diagnosis of UC is approximately 9 months.[97] Some patients with UC present much more acutely, with symptoms mimicking acute infectious colitis. Indeed, it is not uncommon to find a patient whose UC began after a documented GI infection, such as *Salmonella* or *C. difficile*. This observation raises the question whether the infection revealed preexisting but silent disease or whether it was actually the initiating factor.

Symptoms

Rectal Bleeding

Rectal bleeding is common in UC, and its characteristics are determined by the distribution of disease. Patients with proctitis usually complain of passing fresh blood, either separately from the stool or streaked on the surface of a normal or hard stool.[98] This symptom often is mistaken for bleeding from hemorrhoids. In contrast to hemorrhoidal bleeding, however, patients with ulcerative proctitis often pass a mixture of blood and mucus and might even be incontinent. Patients with proctitis also often complain of the frequent and urgent need to defecate, only to pass small quantities of blood and mucus without fecal matter. When the disease extends proximal to the rectum, blood usually is mixed with stool or there may be grossly bloody diarrhea. When disease activity is severe, patients typically pass liquid stool containing blood, pus, and fecal matter. This stool often is likened to anchovy sauce, and some patients with this symptom do not actually recognize that they are passing blood. Unless the patient has severe disease, passage of blood clots is unusual and suggests other diagnoses such as a tumor. Active UC that is sufficient to cause diarrhea almost always is associated with macroscopically evident blood. The diagnosis needs to be questioned if visible blood is absent.

Diarrhea

Diarrhea is common but not always present in patients with UC. Up to 30% of patients with proctitis or proctosigmoiditis complain of constipation and hard stools.[98] Most patients with active disease complain of frequent passage of loose or liquid stools and may have nocturnal diarrhea. Fecal urgency, a sensation of incomplete fecal evacuation, and fecal incontinence also are common, especially when the rectum is severely inflamed. Diarrhea in this setting often is accompanied by passage of large quantities of mucus, blood, and pus.

The pathophysiology of diarrhea in UC involves several mechanisms, but failure to absorb salt and water is the predominant factor[99] and results from reduced Na^+,K^+-ATPase pump activity, increased mucosal permeability, and altered membrane phospholipids. High mucosal concentrations of lipid inflammatory mediators, which are detected in UC, have been shown to stimulate chloride secretion in normal colon, and it is possible that these mediators also contribute to diarrhea by increasing mucosal permeability. Urgency and tenesmus, which are common symptoms when the rectum is inflamed, are caused by decreased rectal compliance and loss of the reservoir capacity of the inflamed rectum.[100] With severe inflammation, the urgency can be sufficiently acute to cause incontinence.

Colonic motility is altered by inflammation, and there is rapid transit through the inflamed colon. With left-sided disease, distal colonic transit is rapid, but there is actual slowing of proximal transit,[101] which might help explain the constipation that is commonly seen in patients with distal colitis. Prolonged transit in the small intestine also occurs in the presence of active colonic inflammation.[101]

Abdominal Pain

Many patients with UC complain of abdominal pain with active disease, although pain generally is not a prominent symptom unless disease activity is severe. Patients can experience vague lower abdominal discomfort, an ache in the left iliac fossa, or intermittent abdominal cramping that precedes bowel movements and often persists transiently after defecation. Severe cramping and abdominal pain can occur in association with severe attacks of the disease. The cause of the pain is unclear but might relate to increased tension within the inflamed colonic wall during muscular contraction. Patients with active proctitis also often complain of tenesmus and urgency associated with painful straining and passage of mucus and blood with only scanty stools.

Other Symptoms

Disease of moderate or severe activity often may be associated with systemic symptoms. Patients can develop anorexia and nausea and, in severe attacks, might actually vomit. These symptoms, as well as protein loss through inflamed mucosa, hypercatabolism, and down-regulation of albumin synthesis caused by the inflammation, account for weight loss and hypoalbuminemia that may be profound. Fever, an added catabolic factor, usually accompanies severe attacks but is typically moderate. Patients also might complain of symptoms from anemia and hypoalbuminemia, including fatigue, dyspnea, and peripheral edema. Patients can present with extraintestinal manifestations, including acute arthropathy, episcleritis, and erythema nodosum, that typically parallel the activity of colitis.

Signs

Patients with mild or even moderately severe disease exhibit few abnormal physical signs. These patients are usually well nourished and well appearing and show no signs of chronic disease. Caution should be exercised because these patients can appear deceptively well. Weight always should be recorded and, for children and adolescents, both height and weight should be plotted on developmental growth charts. The affected portion of the colon may be tender on abdominal palpation, but tenderness usually is mild and not associated with rebound or guarding. Bowel sounds are normal. Digital rectal examination also is often normal, but the rectal mucosa might feel velvety and edematous, the anal canal may be tender, and blood may be seen on withdrawal of the examining finger.

Patients with severe attacks also might appear well, but most are ill with tachycardia, fever, orthostasis, and weight loss. The abdomen typically is soft, with only mild tenderness over the diseased segment. Abdominal tenderness may become diffuse and moderate with more severe disease. Bowel sounds may be normal or hyperactive but diminish with disease progression. In fulminant colitis, the abdomen often becomes distended and firm, with absent bowel sounds and signs of peritoneal inflammation.

There may be aphthous ulceration of the oral mucosa. Clubbing of the fingernails is a manifestation of chronic disease. Peripheral edema can occur secondary to hypoalbuminemia. Minor perianal disease may be present but is never as severe as is seen in patients with CD. Signs of extraintestinal manifestations also may be present.

Laboratory Findings

Laboratory findings in UC are nonspecific and reflect the severity of the underlying disease. Patients with active proctitis and proctosigmoiditis often have normal laboratory test results. Patients with limited distal disease often pass visible blood in the stool, but the amount of blood loss typically is small and anemia, if present, is mild. Patients with active extensive disease or severe distal disease can demonstrate laboratory abnormalities. Hematologic changes, including anemia, leukocytosis, and thrombocytosis, reflect active disease. In contrast, patients with quiescent UC typically manifest no laboratory abnormalities. Iron deficiency anemia may be present because of chronic blood loss. Anemia also may be present secondary to bone marrow suppression resulting from chronic inflammation or medications, including azathioprine, 6-mercaptopurine (6-MP), and sulfasalazine.

Mild or moderate attacks rarely are associated with any biochemical disturbance. Hypokalemia, metabolic alkalosis, and elevated serum levels of blood urea nitrogen and creatinine may be present in severe flares of UC, reflecting volume depletion. Hypoalbuminemia may be seen with acute and chronic disease. Minor elevations in serum levels of aspartate aminotransferase or alkaline phosphatase also are commonly associated with severe disease, but these changes are transient and return to normal when the disease enters remission; these abnormalities probably reflect a combination of fatty liver, sepsis, and poor nutrition. Persistently elevated liver biochemical tests, especially serum alkaline phosphatase, are seen in about 3% of patients with UC and should lead to further investigation, particularly to exclude PSC (see Chapter 68).

Serum inflammatory markers including erythrocyte sedimentation rate (ESR) and C-reactive protein (CRP) may be elevated in active disease. These abnormalities are typically absent or minimal in patients with mildly to moderately active disease. Elevation in these inflammatory parameters is neither sensitive nor specific for UC; measuring them, however, may be useful in clinical practice to assess disease activity in individual patients, particularly if these values are normal during periods of inactive disease. For following clinical changes, CRP is more sensitive than ESR because of the shorter half-life of CRP.

A newly recognized and clinically useful inflammatory marker for UC disease activity is fecal calprotectin, which is a protein secreted by neutrophils in the feces and is therefore a marker of intestinal inflammation. Multiple studies have shown that fecal calprotectin is predictive of relapse in UC; values above 250 µg/g are often predictive of relapse, whereas levels below 50 µg/g are often predictive of remission. A recent meta-analysis of prospective studies reported a pooled sensitivity of 77% and specificity of 71% of fecal calprotectin for UC relapse.[102] In addition, fecal calprotectin was recently found to be a useful surrogate marker for endoscopic lesions in UC.[103]

NATURAL HISTORY AND PROGNOSIS

Most (80%) patients with UC have a disease course characterized by intermittent flares interposed between variable periods of remission. The duration of relapse-free periods varies greatly from patient to patient. More than 50% of patients present with mild disease at their first attack, and 6% to 19% of patients have severe disease at presentation.[104,105] Following the initial flare, 40% to 65% of patients have an intermittent course, and 5% to 10% of patients have a chronic continuous course.[106,107] Up to 10% of patients have a severe first attack ultimately requiring colectomy.[101] In population-based studies, the proportion of patients with active disease remains relatively constant over years, with approximately 50% of all patients being in remission at any time point during follow-up (Fig. 116-4).[92,106] Twenty-five years after the diagnosis of UC, 90% of patients still have a relapsing course (Fig. 116-5)[91]; however, disease activity in the preceding years predicts the subsequent chance of disease activity. The probability of remaining in remission for 1 year after a relapse has been estimated at 30%. After being in remission for 1 year, the risk of relapse decreases to 20% for the following year. Few patients (1%) with UC have only 1 attack followed by a relapse-free course,[106] and they likely have misdiagnosed infectious colitis.

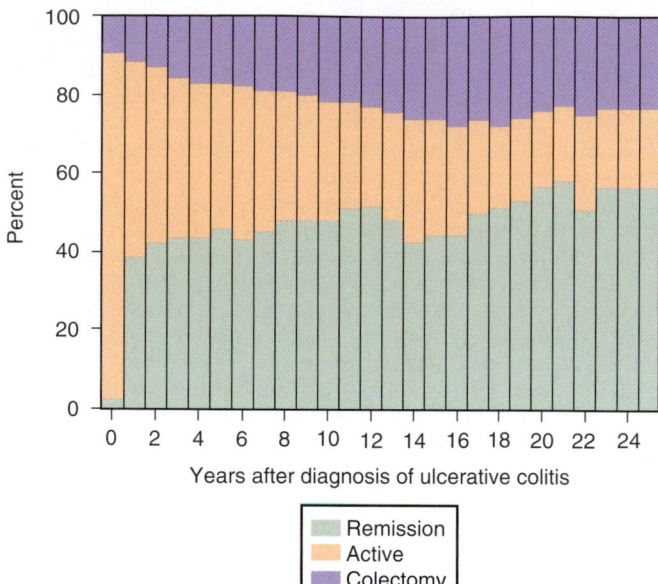

FIGURE 116-4. Percentage of patients with UC who were in remission, had active disease, or have had a colectomy each year after diagnosis. After a few years, the fraction of patients in remission remains relatively constant, with approximately 50% of all patients in remission at any time point during follow-up. The fraction of patients with active disease gradually decreases to about 30%, and approximately 20% of patients undergo colectomy within 25 years after diagnosis. (*Adapted from Langholz E, Munkholm P, Davidsen M, et al. Course of ulcerative colitis: Analysis of changes in disease activity over years. Gastroenterology 1994; 107:3-11.*)

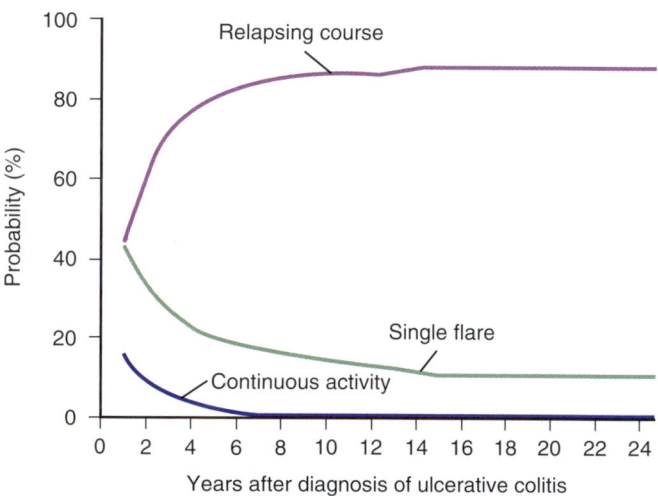

FIGURE 116-5. Cumulative probabilities of various disease courses after a diagnosis of UC. At 25 years after the diagnosis, 90% of patients had a course with multiple remissions and relapses. The cumulative probability of a completely relapse-free course (single flare) decreased rapidly with time to approximately 10% after 25 years. Similarly, the cumulative probability of a continuously active course was low: 1% after 5 years and 0.1% after 25 years. (*Adapted from Langholz E, Munkholm P, Davidsen M, et al. Course of ulcerative colitis: Analysis of changes in disease activity over years. Gastroenterology 1994; 107:3-11.*)

Factors influencing disease relapse and remission include bacterial and viral infections, the use of NSAIDs and antibiotics, smoking, seasonality, and psychosocial stress. Both the severity and extent of disease are important prognostic factors for the first attack of UC. In general, patients with disease that is limited to the distal colon do better than those with extensive colitis. UC diagnosed in older adults generally has been thought to manifest with more severe initial attacks, but this pattern has not been observed consistently. No one factor has been consistently identified as predicting future disease activity. In patients initially presenting with proctitis or proctosigmoiditis, disease extension occurs in approximately 10% to 30% of patients at 10 years after diagnosis.[104,107-109] Less commonly, extensive colitis regresses over time with treatment.

Colectomy rates vary in different studies, in part related to the different proportions of patients with extensive versus limited disease, but rates seem to be highest in the first year of diagnosis. In 1 Scandinavian study, the colectomy rate was 10% within the first year of diagnosis, 3% in the second year, and approximately 1% per year thereafter.[106] In general, the overall colectomy rate is 24% at 10 years and 30% at 25 years (see Fig. 116-4).[98] The probability of colectomy was higher in patients with extensive colitis. A more recent European study reported a lower colectomy rate of 9% at 10 years, with a 4-fold higher risk of colectomy in patients with extensive colitis.[110]

Despite the burden of a chronic illness, more than 90% of patients with UC are able to maintain capacity for work after 10 years of disease, and data suggest that the overall quality of life is not impaired significantly, including marital issues, physical activities, and social function.[92,105,111] The disease can affect the quality of life to some degree during acute flares, however, and even during periods of remission, patients might remain anxious for fear of relapse and alter their lifestyle accordingly.

Despite the morbidity of UC, mortality associated with the disease has dropped dramatically since the late 1950s and 1960s. The mortality rate for a severe attack of UC was approximately 35% before the introduction of glucocorticoid therapy and now is less than 2%. Long-term survival does not differ significantly from that expected for age-matched controls, even with the risk of colorectal cancer that attends long-standing colitis. It is now generally believed that patients with UC have life expectancies comparable to those of the general population, although studies have reached conflicting conclusions.[104,107,112-115] Mortality risk is greatest in older adults and in those with extensive colitis, mostly related to postoperative complications within the first 2 years of disease and to comorbidities.

DIAGNOSIS

Currently, there is no single test that allows the diagnosis of UC with acceptable sensitivity and specificity. Thus, diagnosis relies on a combination of compatible clinical features, endoscopic appearances, and histologic findings. Stool cultures should be obtained to exclude infection with routine bacterial pathogenic organisms; assay for toxins A and B of *C. difficile*, and examinations for ova and parasites also should be performed. Infection with *E. coli* O157:H7 should be considered and requires special stool cultures (or molecular probes). Similarly, special cultures for gonococcus or *Chlamydia* may be necessary in selected cases. In immunosuppressed patients, the possibility of opportunistic infection of the colon must be excluded (see "Differential Diagnosis"). The diagnosis of UC should be questioned if there is only a single episode of acute illness or if the histopathology findings are nonspecific and lack signs of chronicity.

Endoscopy

The diagnosis of UC can be strongly suggested by sigmoidoscopy in most cases. In patients presenting with their first attack of UC, sigmoidoscopy with biopsies usually is sufficient to confirm the diagnosis, thereby allowing initiation of therapy. In patients with active flares, sigmoidoscopy is best performed in unprepared bowel so that the earliest signs of UC can be detected without the hyperemia that is often present because of preparative enemas. Colonoscopy is not recommended in patients with severely active disease for fear of perforation; care must be taken to avoid excessive distention. After active disease has been controlled in a patient with newly diagnosed UC, colonoscopy should be performed to establish the extent of the disease and to exclude CD or other disease states that can complicate UC.

Multiple biopsy specimens should be taken from throughout the colon to map the histologic extent of disease and to confirm the diagnosis if there is concern about CD.[116] In addition, intubation and biopsy of the terminal ileum should be attempted to exclude the presence of CD or other disease states that can mimic IBD. In patients with an established diagnosis of UC who present with a typical flare, sigmoidoscopy usually is not necessary, although it may be indicated for patients suspected of having *C. difficile* infection. Pseudomembranes usually are absent in patients with UC and *C. difficile* infection, however, and are seen in only 0% to 13% of cases.[117] Sigmoidoscopy combined with histologic evaluation may be useful for assessing disease severity, particularly when therapeutic response is in question. Colonoscopy may be similarly useful, especially in patients whose symptoms seem out of proportion to the known extent of disease. Additionally, colonoscopy is essential for colorectal cancer surveillance (see below).

The hallmark of UC is symmetric and continuous inflammation that begins in the rectum and extends proximally without interruption for the entire extent of disease. The earliest endoscopic sign of UC is a decrease or loss of the normal vascular pattern, with mucosal erythema and edema (Fig. 116-6); distortion or loss of vascular markings may be the only endoscopic evidence of UC in patients with quiescent disease. As disease progresses, the mucosa becomes granular and friable. With more severe inflammation, the mucosa may be covered by yellow-brown mucopurulent exudates associated with mucosal ulcerations. In UC, mucosal ulcerations occur in areas of inflammation, vary in size from a few millimeters to several centimeters, and may be punctate, annular, linear, or serpiginous. Finally, severe UC is associated with mucosa that bleeds spontaneously, and, with diffuse colitis, there may be extensive areas of denuded mucosa from severe mucosal ulcerations (see Fig. 116-6). Marked edema can at times lead to narrowing of the lumen.

In patients with long-standing UC, pseudopolyps may be present. Inflammatory pseudopolyps develop in active disease and result from inflamed, regenerating epithelium that is interposed among ulcerations. These inflammatory pseudopolyps may give the colonic mucosa a cobblestoned appearance. With repeated inflammation that is followed by healing, these pseudopolyps remain during the quiescent phase of disease and usually do not regress with treatment. Endoscopically, pseudopolyps typically are small, soft, pale, fleshy, and glistening; however, they may be large, sessile, or pedunculated and may have surface ulcerations. Differentiation of these benign pseudopolyps from neoplastic polyps may be difficult and require histologic confirmation.

There is a loss of normal colonic architecture with long-standing inflammation that is characterized by muscular hypertrophy, loss of the normal haustral fold pattern,

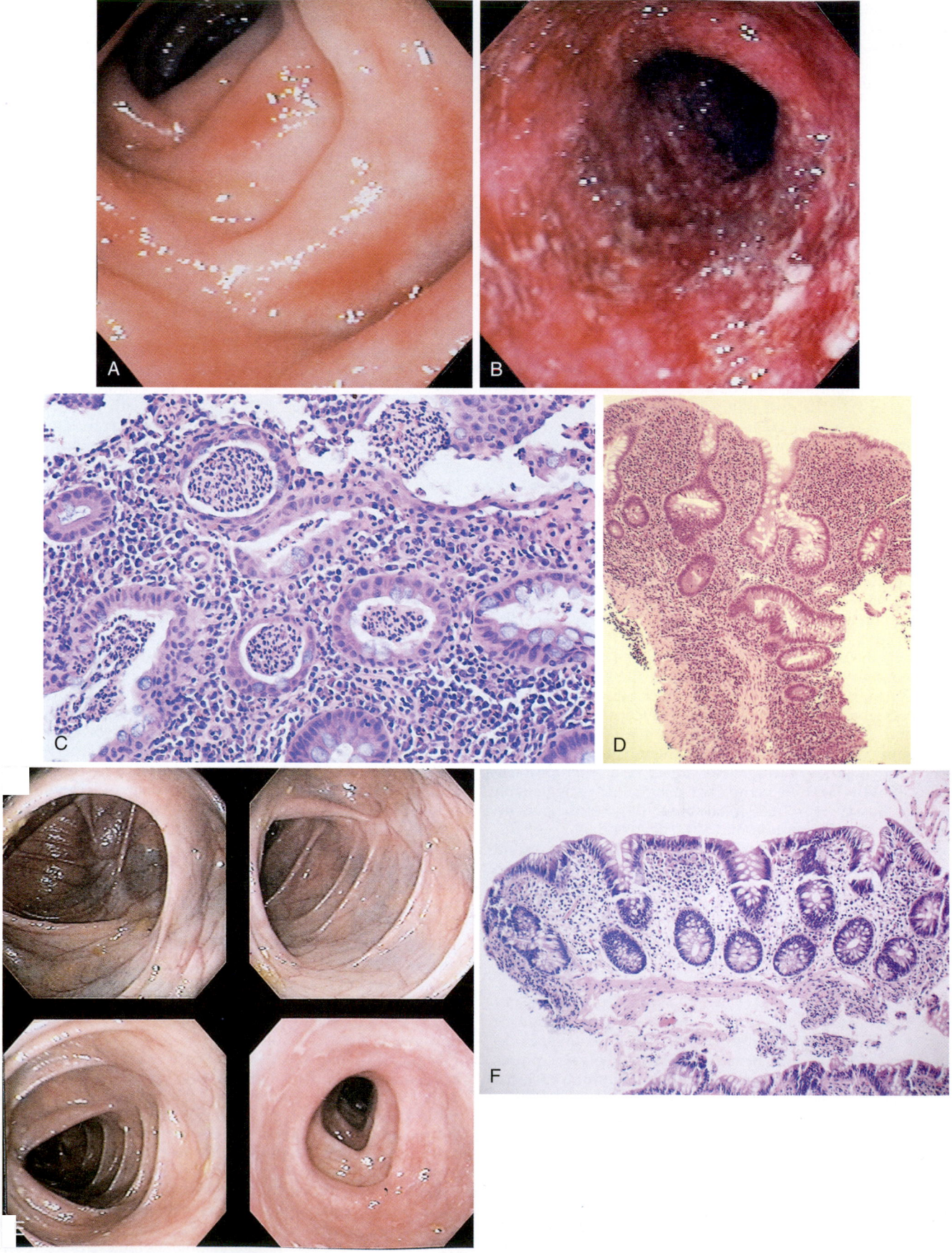

FIGURE 116-6. Spectrum of severity of UC. *A*, Colonoscopic findings in mild UC demonstrating edema, loss of vascularity, and patchy subepithelial hemorrhage. *B*, Colonoscopic findings in severe UC demonstrating loss of vascularity, hemorrhage, and mucopus. The mucosa is friable, with spontaneous bleeding as well as bleeding after the mucosa is touched by the endoscope. *C*, Histopathology showing a severe acute and chronic inflammatory process, with multiple crypt abscesses. *D*, Histopathology showing distortion of the colonic architecture with a loss of crypts and abnormal branching of the crypts. Recognition of disordered architecture is useful in differentiating acute from chronic colitis. *E*, Colonoscopy findings in a patient with chronic UC undergoing surveillance for colorectal cancer. The ascending colon *(top left)*, transverse colon *(top right)*, and descending colon *(bottom left)* are normal, but the sigmoid colon shows active inflammation *(bottom right)*. *F*, A biopsy specimen of the normal-appearing colon demonstrates abnormal architecture with shortened crypts but no active colitis.

decreased luminal diameter, and shortening of the colon; a resultant featureless appearance of the colon in chronic UC gives rise to the lead pipe appearance seen on barium enema. Strictures can occur in patients with chronic UC and result from focal muscular hypertrophy associated with inflammation. Malignancy must be excluded in patients with UC who have strictures, particularly long strictures without associated inflammation and strictures proximal to the splenic flexure (see later).

Radiology

Plain Films

Patients with a severe attack of UC should have a supine plain film of the abdomen. The presence of intraperitoneal air may be missed on plain abdominal films, however, and CT has demonstrated a better diagnostic yield than plain abdominal radiology for detecting disease complications and extent. In the presence of severe disease, the luminal margin of the colon—the interface between the colonic mucosa and the luminal gas—becomes edematous and irregular. Thickening of the colonic wall often is apparent on a plain film, and prognostic signs such as islands of residual mucosa surrounded by extensive deep ulcerations, distention of the small bowel, and dilatation of the colon can be detected (Fig. 116-7).

Plain films also are useful for detecting the presence of fecal material. Inflamed colons seldom contains feces, and no fecal material is present when the whole colon is involved. It is common, however, for a patient with left-sided disease to have proximal constipation (Fig. 116-8). Thus, a plain film can give considerable information with respect to the extent of disease. The presence of marked colonic dilatation suggests fulminant colitis or toxic megacolon. A plain abdominal film also can detect unsuspected free air and is especially useful in following the daily progress of a patient on high-dose glucocorticoid therapy in whom such a complication may be otherwise masked.

Barium Enema

With the advent of endoscopy, barium studies have been used less often in the care of patients with UC. Barium studies of the colon remain important, however, and may be superior to colonoscopy for certain specific scenarios, such as evaluation of colonic strictures; barium enema provides information on their location, length, and diameter and allows visualization of the entire colon when the presence of strictures precludes advancement of the colonoscope. Upper GI barium study and small bowel follow-through with air-contrast visualization of the terminal ileum should be performed to exclude CD.

The earliest radiologic change of UC seen on barium studies is fine mucosal granularity (Fig. 116-9). The mucosal line becomes irregular and is not as sharp as that of a normal colon. With increasing severity, the mucosal line becomes

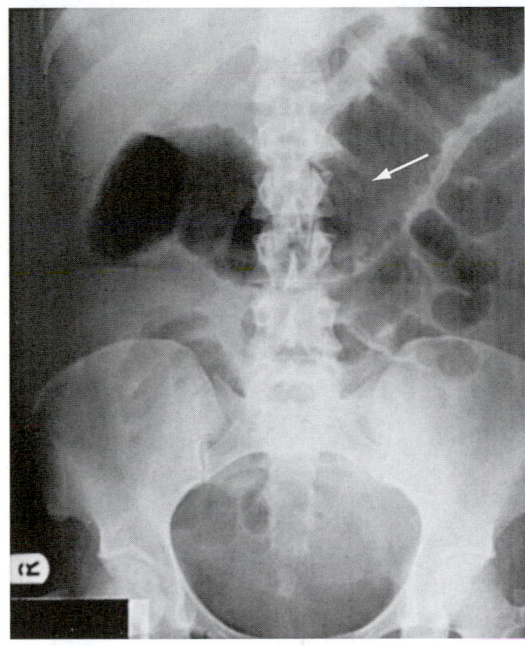

FIGURE 116-7. Plain abdominal film of a patient with severe UC. The transverse colon is dilated *(arrow)*, the colon wall is thickened, and mucosal islands are visible. In addition, distended loops of small bowel are apparent.

thickened and irregular, and superficial ulcers are well shown en face. Deep ulceration can appear as collar-stud or collar-button ulcers in tangent, which indicates that the ulceration has extended through the mucosa to the muscularis propria (Fig. 116-10).

Haustral folds may be normal in mild disease but become edematous and thickened as disease progresses. Loss of haustrations also can occur, especially in patients with long-standing disease (Fig. 116-11). Because the left colon may normally lack haustration, this sign is relevant for only the ascending and transverse colon. With long-standing disease, loss of haustration can lead to a featureless and tubular appearance of the colon.

Other chronic changes are shortening of the colon and widening of the presacral (retrorectal) space as seen on a lateral film of the rectum. Pseudopolyps may be present and can resemble a cobblestone pattern (see Fig. 116-11); pseudopolyps may also have a filiform appearance.

DIFFERENTIAL DIAGNOSIS

A variety of inflammatory and noninflammatory diseases of the colon can mimic UC and need to be considered in

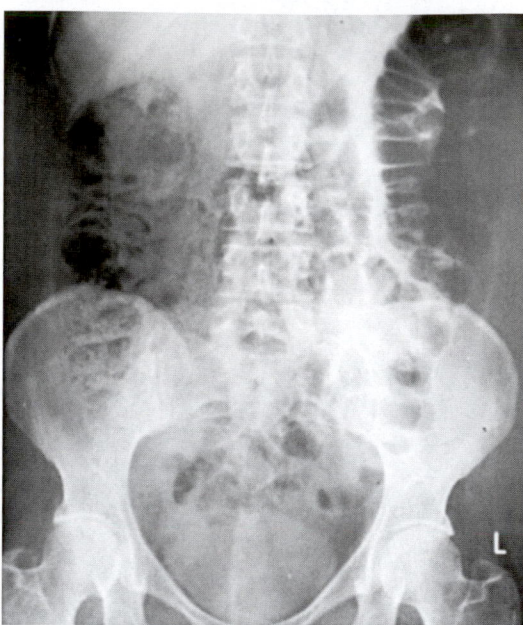

FIGURE 116-8. Plain abdominal film of a patient with mild left-sided UC showing a stool-filled proximal colon.

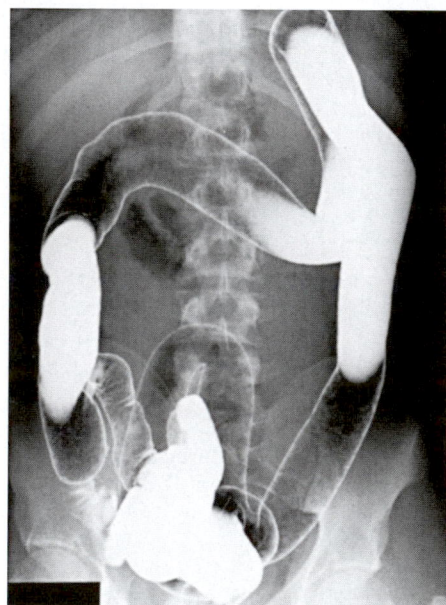

FIGURE 116-9. Film from a double-contrast barium enema examination in a patient with long-standing UC as indicated by a marked loss of haustration. The mucosa is finely granular throughout the colon, consistent with mildly active disease. The terminal ileum is normal.

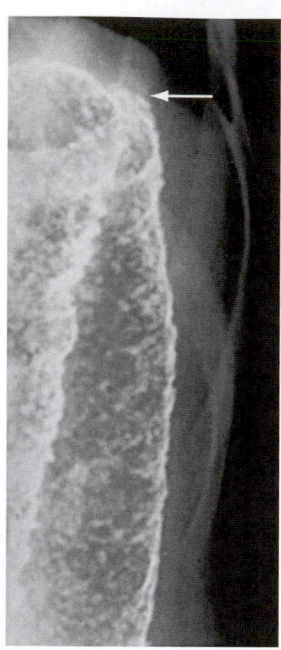

FIGURE 116-10. Film from a double-contrast barium enema examination in a patient with active UC. This localized view of the splenic flexure shows multiple ulcers. At the flexure itself there is deep ulceration appearing as a collar-button ulcer *(arrow)*.

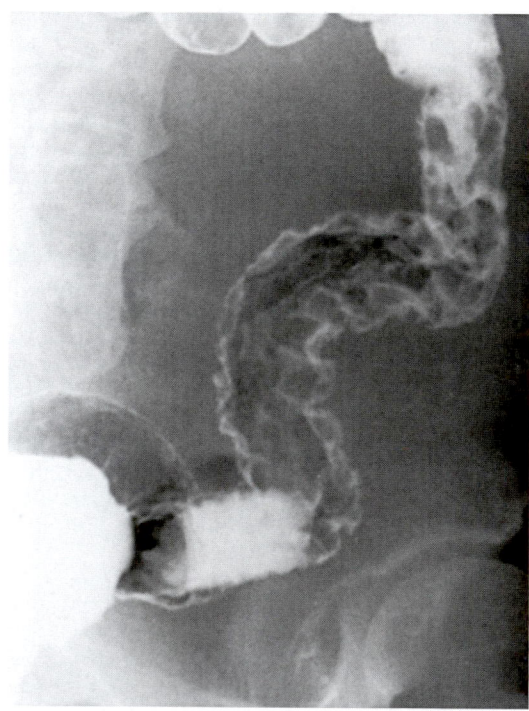

FIGURE 116-11. Film from a barium enema examination showing postinflammatory polyposis in a shortened sigmoid and descending colon in a patient with active UC.

establishing the correct diagnosis. This differential diagnosis can be grouped broadly into 3 categories: CD, infections, and noninfectious causes (Box 116-1).

Crohn's Disease

CD should be excluded in all patients given a diagnosis of UC, and colonoscopy with multiple biopsies is important in this regard. The presence of skip lesions or epithelioid granulomas supports the diagnosis of CD. It is important to recognize that

muciphage granulomas may be present in patients who do not have CD. Other endoscopic features distinguishing UC from CD are listed in Table 116-3.

It is not uncommon for patients with ileal CD also to have rectal involvement, and these patients might present with symptoms of proctitis rather than symptoms of small

TABLE 116-3 Endoscopic Differentiation of UC and Crohn's Disease

Feature	Ulcerative Colitis	Crohn's Disease
Distribution	Diffuse inflammation that extends proximally from the anorectal junction	Rectal sparing, frequent skip lesions
Inflammation	Diffuse erythema, early loss of vascular markings with mucosal granularity or friability	Focal and asymmetrical, cobblestoning; granularity and friability less commonly seen
Ulceration	Small ulcers in a diffusely inflamed mucosa; deep, ragged ulcers in severe disease	Aphthoid ulcers, linear or serpiginous ulceration; intervening mucosa is often normal
Colonic lumen	Often narrowed in long-standing chronic disease; tubular colon; strictures are rare	Strictures are common

BOX 116-1 Differential Diagnosis of UC

Infectious Causes
Aeromonas hydrophila
Campylobacter jejuni
Chlamydia spp.
Clostridium difficile
Cytomegalovirus
Entamoeba histolytica
Escherichia coli O157:H7, other EHEC
HSV
Listeria monocytogenes
Neisseria gonorrhoeae
Salmonella spp.
Schistosomiasis
Shigella spp.
Yersinia enterocolitica

Noninfectious Causes
Acute self-limited colitis
Behçet's disease
Crohn's disease
Diversion colitis
Diverticulitis
Drugs and toxins
   Chemotherapy
   Gold
   Penicillamine
Eosinophilic colitis
Graft-versus-host disease
Ischemic colitis
Microscopic colitis
   Collagenous
   Lymphocytic
Neutropenic colitis (typhlitis)
NSAIDs
Radiation colitis
Segmental colitis associated with diverticulosis (SCAD)
Solitary rectal ulcer syndrome

EHEC, enterohemorrhagic *Escherichia coli.*

intestinal involvement. In patients with proctitis or diffuse pancolitis, it may be impossible to differentiate UC and CD. Thus, it is advisable to obtain radiologic assessment of the small intestine in all patients with colonic disease, particularly in those with pancolitis or proctitis on colonoscopy and elevated inflammatory markers or hypoalbuminemia on laboratory testing. A definitive diagnosis of CD may not be able to be made until the development of small bowel disease or perianal complications.

IBD-unclassified (IBD-U), or formerly "indeterminate" colitis, is diagnosed in approximately 5% to 10% of adult patients and up to 30% of pediatric patients; this term is used when the distinction between CD and UC cannot be made.[118] The clinical course for most patients with IBD-U resembles UC, and, among pediatric patients, approximately 60% are ultimately reclassified as UC or CD, more commonly UC.[119] Thus, the management of these patients is similar to that of UC, unless the disease is reclassified as CD, in which case treatment modifications may be appropriate. The key points in the differential diagnosis between UC and CD are summarized in Tables 116-3 and 116-4.

Infection

Another major category of differential diagnosis for UC is infection (see Chapter 110). As mentioned previously, newly diagnosed UC can manifest as part of a well-documented episode of infectious colitis. It is unknown if the infection prompts the UC or simply unmasks underlying UC that previously had subclinical activity. Patients with documented UC in clinical remission also can develop acute infectious colitis and present with symptoms of a flare of UC. Thus, infections need to be excluded with each episode of disease exacerbation.

The most common organisms causing infectious colitis are *Salmonella, Shigella,* and *Campylobacter.* Patients with infectious colitides usually have a more acute onset of symptoms than do patients with a flare of UC, and they have a prominence of abdominal pain; they also might report diarrheal illness in 1 or more of their contacts. The sigmoidoscopic appearance of infectious colitis may be indistinguishable from that of UC, but the histologic appearance often is helpful in differentiating infectious acute colitis from a more chronic condition. The presence of a chronic inflammatory infiltrate, architectural disturbances, and basal lymphoid aggregates favors a diagnosis of UC, and these features distinguish infectious colitis from UC with a probability of 80%, albeit with considerable interobserver variation. One would not be able to identify bacterial superinfection on a background of chronic UC on histology, however, because the additional changes would be nonspecific; only viral (especially cytomegalovirus) or amebic superinfection would be readily identifiable on biopsy specimens by the presence of intranuclear inclusion bodies or the actual organisms themselves, respectively (see later).

Other bacterial infectious colitides include infection with *E. coli* O157:H7, which can occur in outbreaks or sporadically. Patients with this infection, particularly children and older adults, usually present with bloody diarrhea and can develop associated hemolytic-uremic syndrome or thrombotic thrombocytopenic purpura. Because the diagnosis requires a special culture medium and cannot be made on routine stool cultures, clinicians need to have a high index of suspicion and specifically request such a test. Development of molecular probes might facilitate the ability to establish this diagnosis.

Yersinia infections can cause enteritis, enterocolitis, or colitis and can last for several months before resolving spontaneously. The diagnosis is made on the basis of stool culture or a rising titer of serum antibody. Other, less common bacterial infections causing colitis include *Aeromonas hydrophila* and *Listeria monocytogenes*; the former is usually associated with drinking untreated water, and the latter is often associated with consumption of unpasteurized milk.

A history of antibiotic use suggests pseudomembranous colitis associated with *C. difficile* (see Chapter 112). This infectious colitis, which is among the most common infections in UC patients, manifests with diarrhea and may be

TABLE 116-4 Features That Distinguish UC from Other Diagnoses

Diagnosis	Clinical Features	Radiologic and Colonoscopic Features	Histologic Features
UC	Bloody diarrhea	Extends proximally from rectum; fine mucosal ulceration	Distortion of crypts; acute and chronic diffuse inflammatory cell infiltrate; goblet cell depletion; crypt abscesses; lymphoid aggregates
Crohn's colitis	Perianal lesions are common; may be associated with ileitis; frank bleeding is less common than in UC	Segmental disease; rectal sparing; strictures, fissures, ulcers, fistulas; small bowel involvement	Focal inflammation; submucosal involvement; granulomas; goblet cell preservation; transmural inflammation; fissuring
Ischemic colitis	Occurs in older adults; sudden onset, often painful; usually resolves spontaneously in several days	Segmental splenic flexure and sigmoid involvement are most common, with thumbprinting early and ulceration after 24-72 hr; rectal involvement is rare	Mucosal necrosis with ghost cells; congestion with red blood cells; hemosiderin-laden macrophages and fibrosis (when disease is chronic)
Microscopic colitis	Watery diarrhea; normal-appearing mucosa at colonoscopy	Usually normal	Chronic inflammatory infiltrate; increased intraepithelial lymphocytes (lymphocytic colitis) and/or subepithelial collagen band (collagenous colitis)
Infectious colitis	Sudden onset; identifiable source in some cases (e.g., *Salmonella* spp.); pain may predominate (e.g., *Campylobacter* spp.); pathogens are present in stool	Nonspecific findings	Crypt architecture is usually normal; edema, superficial neutrophilic infiltrate, crypt abscesses
Amebic colitis	History of travel to endemic area; amebae may be detected in a fresh stool specimen but ELISA for amebic lectin antigen is the preferable diagnostic test	Discrete ulcers; ameboma or strictures	Similar to UC; amebae present in lamina propria or in flask-shaped ulcers, identified by periodic acid–Schiff stain
Gonococcal proctitis	Rectal pain; pus	Granular changes in rectum	Intense polymorphonuclear neutrophil infiltration; purulent exudate; Gram-negative diplococci
Pseudomembranous colitis	Often a history of antibiotic use; characteristic pseudomembranes may be seen on sigmoidoscopy; *Clostridium difficile* toxin is detectable in stools	Edematous; shaggy outline of colon; pseudomembranes may be identified radiologically or seen at colonoscopy	May resemble acute ischemic colitis; summit lesions of fibrinopurulent exudate

ELISA, enzyme-linked immunosorbent assay.

superimposed on or even lead to a relapse of UC. *C. difficile* infection can occur in the absence of antibiotics, especially in older adults and in patients who are taking PPIs or who have had placement of a postpyloric tube. A recent study examining the health care burden of a number of GI diseases reported that hospital discharges for *C. difficile* infection have more than tripled over the last decade, with over 110,000 discharges in 2009, and that *C. difficile* infection now accounts for a proportion of inpatient mortality similar to that of GI hemorrhage.[9] In a national survey of hospitalized patients in the United States, the prevalence of *C. difficile* among UC patients was 8 times higher than that of either non-IBD gastroenterology patients or all hospital-discharge patients.[120] A more recent survey using the same database found that the prevalence of *C. difficile* infection in hospitalized UC patients increased from 2.4% in 1998 to 5.3% in 2007.[121] This infection can cause severe

colitis that may progress to toxic megacolon and bowel perforation. In fact, IBD patients hospitalized with *C. difficile* infection have a 3- to 4-fold increased risk of mortality and a 2.5-fold increased risk of colectomy compared with IBD patients who do not have *C. difficile* infection.[120,121] Thus, appropriate stool studies for toxin analysis are necessary to exclude superimposed *C. difficile* infection, even in patients with established UC who present with an exacerbation.

In patients from endemic areas, certain protozoan and parasitic infections need to be considered (see Chapters 113 and 114). Amebic colitis tends to have a more prolonged course than do most bacterial colitides, but and the appearance of amebic colitis can resemble that of UC, or CD, with uniform small ulcerations or larger discrete ulcers, respectively. Schistosomal colitis may be chronic and diffuse, exhibit pseudopolyps, and involve the rectum. The presence of characteristic ova in a biopsy specimen confirms the diagnosis.

Other infectious causes of a bloody diarrhea include opportunistic infections of the colon in immunosuppressed patients (see Chapters 34 and 35).

Cytomegalovirus (CMV) infection has been reported in patients with UC, typically those with long-standing disease who are being treated with glucocorticoids or immunosuppressants; the diagnosis of CMV infection should be considered whenever patients who have UC and are taking glucocorticoids either fail to respond as expected or lose their response to treatment. CMV colitis in steroid-naïve patients also has been described.[122] Patients with CMV colitis often present with abdominal pain and bloody diarrhea and have discrete deep ulcers on colonoscopy; however, CMV colitis can manifest with diffuse inflammation and resemble UC. Because the clinical presentation of CMV colitis may be indistinguishable from a flare of UC, a high index of suspicion is needed to make the diagnosis. Endoscopic biopsies should be obtained from both the ulcer bed and adjacent mucosa; careful histologic examination for giant cells with intranuclear inclusion bodies is important to confirm the diagnosis.

Mycobacterium avium complex usually causes patchy rather than diffuse inflammation.

Sexually transmitted causes of proctitis, including gonorrhea, *Chlamydia*, and lymphogranuloma venereum, usually do not cause diarrhea and are associated with large volumes of watery pus, especially gonorrhea. These diagnoses are suspected clinically and confirmed by appropriate cultures as well as histologic appearance on rectal biopsy specimens.

Other Diagnoses

Noninfectious causes of colitis that should be considered in the differential diagnosis of UC include diverticulitis, ischemia, radiation, collagenous colitis, lymphocytic colitis, and drug-induced colitis. Diverticulitis and ischemic colitis usually present acutely or (less commonly) subacutely, but most of the noninfectious colitides have prolonged presentations that can extend for several months.

Acute diverticulitis most commonly occurs in the sigmoid colon and does not involve the rectum (see Chapter 121). When the inflammation does extend to the rectum, it tends to be patchy and involves only the upper rectum. This appearance is more likely to be confused with CD than UC. Segmental Colitis Associated with Diverticulosis (SCAD) is another colitis that occurs in areas of the colon that bear diverticula. It may present with symptoms similar to those of UC, appear colonoscopically as erythema or superficial ulceration, and biopsy specimens may be compatible with UC, CD, ischemic colitis, nonspecific or normal.

Ischemic colitis usually occurs in older adults (see Chapter 118). The classic distribution is segmental involvement in the watershed areas around the splenic flexure or sigmoid colon but any area of the colon may be affected and isolated involvement of the right colon and ischemic proctitis also have been described.

Radiation colitis usually occurs in patients who have been given radiation therapy for uterine, cervical, or prostate cancer. The location of disease depends on the sites irradiated but typically involves the rectosigmoid. The onset of symptoms often temporally corresponds to the radiation therapy but can develop years afterward (see Chapter 40).

Microscopic colitis, including lymphocytic and collagenous colitis, manifests with diarrhea and should be distinguished readily from UC by lack of rectal bleeding, the normal endoscopic appearance, and characteristic histopathology (see Chapter 128).

A drug history must always be taken in a patient with colitis, because NSAIDs, gold, and penicillamine among many other drugs may induce colonic inflammation (see Chapter 128).

Patients with UC can present with symptoms similar to those of IBS (see Chapter 122), specifically diarrhea, abdominal pain, fatigue, and poor general well-being. Lack of rectal bleeding and laboratory markers of inflammation, as well as a normal endoscopic and histologic appearance, help to distinguish IBS from active UC. Patients with quiescent UC can have concomitant symptomatic IBS in the absence of active inflammation. The physician must be able to recognize these subtleties in order to provide appropriate management for the patient. Patients with UC also can present with symptoms mimicking colonic neoplasm (see Chapter 127), solitary rectal ulcer syndrome (see Chapter 128), diverticular disease (see Chapter 121), and factitious diarrhea (see Chapter 23). These diagnoses also do not give rise to diffuse inflammation in the colon and, therefore, should be distinguished easily from UC on colonoscopy.

ASSESSMENT OF DISEASE ACTIVITY

Assessment of disease activity is important for prognostication and therapeutic decision making. Unlike the case with CD (where there is 1 well-accepted and validated instrument to measure disease activity), there exist numerous instruments to measure disease activity for UC, some of which are purely clinical, endoscopic, or histologic, and others that combine clinical and endoscopic assessments. When evaluating these various activity indices, it is important to recognize that generally these measures are nonspecific, and thus patients with other disorders, such as IBS, could attain high scores even in the absence of any inflammation. Also, almost none of the outcome measures in UC have been prospectively validated. Moreover, the scores of the indices typically are derived by incorporating various signs and symptoms for which there are no standardized definitions. For these reasons, one should exercise appropriate caution when interpreting the results of a study of UC patients that uses an activity index.

Although none of these indices is accepted universally as standard, 1 of the most commonly used is that of Truelove and Witts.[123] This purely clinical classification categorizes disease as mild, moderate, or severe based on a combination of clinical findings and laboratory parameters, including frequency of bowel movements, rectal bleeding, fever, tachycardia, anemia, and elevated ESR (Box 116-2). The Truelove and Witts classification is reliable and simple to use in clinical practice, although it is most applicable for patients with extensive colitis and might not adequately reflect disease severity in patients with limited colitis.

A numerical disease activity instrument that has been used extensively in randomized controlled trials (RCTs) is the Mayo Score.[124] This index, which combines clinical and endoscopic assessments, is the sum of scores from 4 components: stool frequency, rectal bleeding, sigmoidoscopic findings, and physician's global assessment (Table 116-5). This disease activity index ranges from 0 to 12, with the higher total scores representing more severe disease. In general, a patient is considered to be in remission if the Mayo score is 2 or below and to have severe disease if the score is above 10. Clinical response is generally accepted when the score decreases 3 points from the patient's initial baseline score. A nearly identical index to the Mayo Score is the Ulcerative Colitis Disease Activity Index (UCDAI, also known as the Sutherland Index) which incorporates the same 4 components as the Mayo Score.[125]

TABLE 116-5 Mayo Score* for the Severity of UC

Score	Criteria
Stool Frequency	
0	Normal
1	1-2 stools/day more than normal
2	3-4 stools/day more than normal
3	5 or more stools/day more than normal
Rectal Bleeding	
0	None
1	Streaks of blood with stool less than half the time
2	Obvious blood with stool most of the time
3	Blood alone passed
Mucosal Appearance	
0	Normal
1	Mild disease (erythema, decreased vascular pattern, mild friability)
2	Moderate disease (marked erythema, absent vascular pattern, friability, erosions)
3	Severe disease (spontaneous bleeding, ulceration)
Physician Global Assessment	
0	Normal
1	Mild disease
2	Moderate disease
3	Severe disease

*Mayo Score: Range, 0-12.
From Schroeder K, Tremaine W, Ilstrup D. Coated oral 5-aminosalicylic acid therapy for mildly to moderately active ulcerative colitis: A randomized study. N Engl J Med 1987; 317:1625-9.

Other scales also have been developed, many of which are modifications of the Truelove and Witts classification and the UCDAI. None of these disease activity instruments has ever been formally validated. There also exist many endoscopic and histologic scales for grading the severity of colitis.[126,127] Endoscopic findings do not always correlate with clinical symptoms, and such correlations generally are more consistent within individuals. Thus, although therapeutic decisions are based primarily on clinical status, it may be useful to follow the sigmoidoscopic mucosal appearance over time in an individual patient if the clinical response to treatment is uncertain.

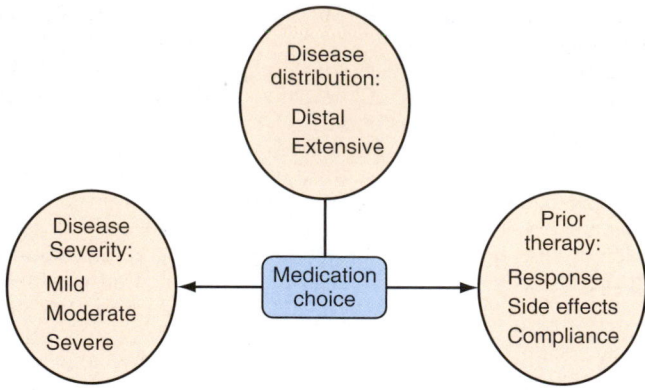

FIGURE 116-12. Factors that should be considered in the choice of medical therapies for UC.

In addition to the typical categorization of disease activity into mild, moderate, and severe, an important subgroup is fulminant colitis. Patients with severe colitis who appear toxic, with fever higher than 38.3°C (101°F), tachycardia, abdominal distention, signs of localized or generalized peritonitis, and leukocytosis, are considered to have fulminant colitis. Toxic megacolon is said to occur when there is radiologic evidence of transverse colon dilatation to greater than 6 cm in an acutely ill patient. Fulminant colitis and toxic megacolon are clinical diagnoses, and complete colonoscopic examination should be avoided in patients with severe or fulminant colitis because of the risk of inducing megacolon or perforation. In this patient population, a limited flexible sigmoidoscopy is appropriate to ensure that the etiology of the symptoms is UC itself and not other conditions.

TREATMENT

Medical Therapy

The goals of therapy of UC are to induce remission, to maintain remission, to maintain adequate nutrition, to minimize disease- and treatment-related complications, and to improve the patient's quality of life. Current management strategy focuses on using appropriate medical therapy and optimizing timing of surgery.

Several factors should be considered in determining optimal therapy for patients with UC (Fig. 116-12). Current therapeutic strategies can be classified broadly, based on disease activity, into those that treat active disease (induction therapy) (Box 116-3) and those that prevent recurrence of disease once remission is achieved (maintenance therapy) (Box 116-4). This concept of induction and maintenance of remission forms the basis of our evaluation of the efficacy of a specific therapy. The extent of disease is an important consideration that helps determine the route of administration of medication. Thus, for example, proctitis may be treated with suppositories or foam preparations as well as with oral therapy, and enema preparations may be used alone or in combination with systemic therapy for patients with left-sided disease. Other important factors to consider are a patient's prior response to or side effects from a specific medication and compliance with medication. These factors might favor or preclude the use of a specific agent. Given the chronic nature of UC, medications need to be efficacious and well accepted by patients from the standpoints of safety and ease of administration. The mainstay of medical therapy focuses on regimens that alter host response to decrease mucosal inflammation. Therapies that target other aspects of the systemic

BOX 116-3 Induction Therapy for UC Based on Disease Severity

Mild Disease
5-Aminosalicylates
  Topical (distal colitis)
  Oral (distal/extensive colitis)
  Combination

Moderate Disease
5-Aminosalicylates
  Topical (distal colitis)
  Oral (distal/extensive colitis)
  Combination
Glucocorticoids
  Topical (distal colitis)
  Oral (distal/extensive colitis)
  Combination
Azathioprine or 6-mercaptopurine
Infliximab or adalimumab

Severe Disease
IV glucocorticoids
Cyclosporine
Infliximab, adalimumab, or vedolizumab

BOX 116-4 Maintenance Therapy for UC

5-Aminosalicylates
  Topical (distal colitis)
  Oral (distal/extensive colitis)
  Combination
Azathioprine or 6-mercaptopurine
Infliximab or adalimumab

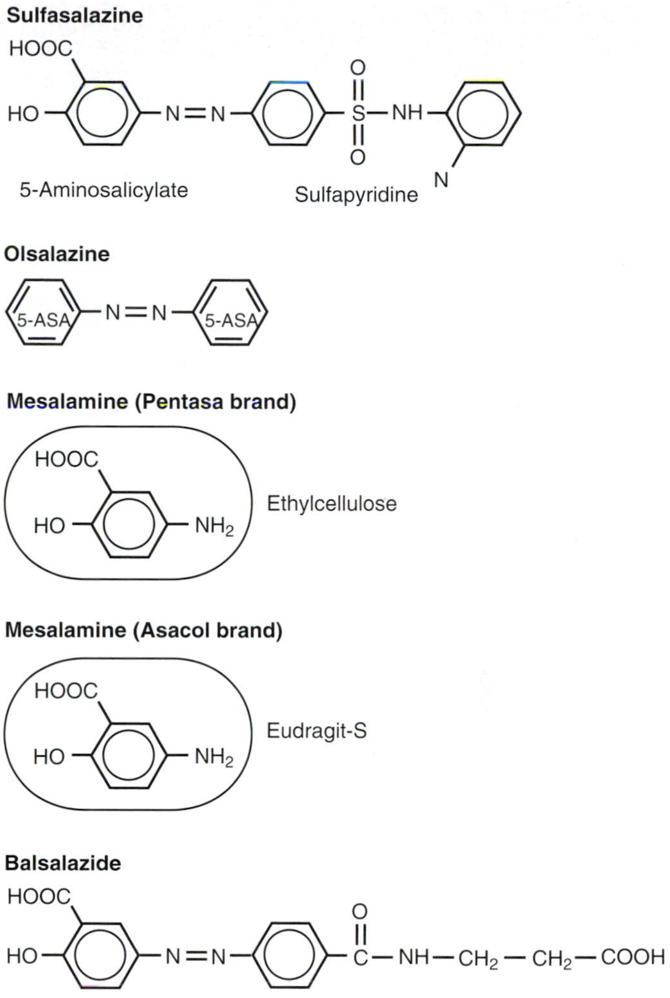

FIGURE 116-13. Molecular structures of 5-aminosalicylate (5-ASA) preparations.

inflammatory process or manipulate the enteric flora also have been developed to treat UC.

One important consideration when evaluating the efficacy of a particular medication (e.g., in an RCT that compares a novel therapy to placebo) is the placebo response rate. Even though placebos often are thought of as inert agents, they have been noted to lead to improvement in a variety of both subjective and objective outcome measures in a number of different medical conditions, such as anxiety, depression, insomnia, pain, asthma, obesity, hypertension, and even myocardial infarction.[128] In some of these disorders, placebo response rates of up to 40% have been reported. With respect to placebo response rates in UC, a meta-analysis of 40 randomized placebo-controlled trials, in which the most commonly used activity indices were the Mayo Score or the UCDAI, reported a pooled placebo response rate of 28% and remission rate of 13%.[129] Studies using less stringent outcome definitions were noted to have higher placebo response and remission rates. Univariate analysis suggested that longer follow-up duration, higher number of follow-up visits, longer disease duration, and lower disease severity at study entry were positively associated with the placebo remission rate.

Aminosalicylates

Oral

Sulfasalazine consists of an antibacterial component, sulfapyridine, bonded by an azo bond to a salicylate, 5-aminosalicylic acid (5-ASA, mesalamine) (Fig. 116-13).[130] The drug was synthesized by Nana Svartz in 1938-1939, and its benefit for the treatment of IBD was discovered serendipitously in 1941-1942 by her when patients with UC receiving this medication for a

presumed diagnosis of rheumatoid arthritis noted improvement in colitis symptoms[131]; in retrospect, these patients had peripheral arthropathy associated with their IBD, not rheumatoid arthritis. Research subsequently established that 5-ASA is the principal therapeutic moiety of sulfasalazine in IBD and that the sulfapyridine component of the parent drug serves as an inactive carrier, largely preventing absorption of 5-ASA in the small intestine and allowing it to be released in the colon.[132,133] Approximately 90% of sulfasalazine reaches the colon, and only a small amount is absorbed in the small intestine. On reaching the colon, the enzyme azoreductase, which is elaborated by anaerobic colonic bacteria, cleaves the azo bond to release the active constituent moiety, 5-ASA. After 5-ASA is absorbed from the colon, 20% of the compound undergoes hepatic acetylation, forming N-acetyl 5-ASA, and is excreted in the urine. Sulfasalazine is 1 of several agents in the class of 5-ASA compounds that is considered to be the first line of therapy for inducing remission in patients with mild to moderate UC.[130,134] Mesalamine derivatives have not been evaluated in a randomized, controlled fashion in patients with severely active disease. At a dose of 3 to 6 g/day, sulfasalazine induces remission in 39% to 62% of patients with mild to moderate UC, about twice the remission rate of placebo-treated patients.[135,136]

Various formulations and controlled-release systems (Table 116-6; see Fig. 116-13) have been developed to deliver 5-ASA to specific sites of the GI tract without the sulfapyridine moiety, which is thought to be responsible for most of the side

TABLE 116-6 Oral 5-Aminosalicylic Acid Preparations and Sites of Delivery in the GI Tract

Drug	Formulation	Site of Delivery
Prodrugs		
Sulfasalazine	Sulfapyridine + 5-ASA	Colon
Olsalazine	5-ASA dimer	Colon
Balsalazide	4-aminobenzoyl β-alanine + 5-ASA	Colon
Mesalamine Preparations		
Asacol, Claversal, Delzicol Salofalk/Apriso	pH sensitive, resin-coated; delayed release	Distal ileum, colon
Rowasa	Enema	Distal colon
Canasa	Suppository	Rectum
Pentasa	Ethylcellulose-coated microgranules; controlled release	Duodenum to colon
Lialda	pH sensitive, multi-matrix and polymethacrylate coated; delayed and slow release	Distal ileum, colon

5-ASA, 5-aminosalicylate.

effects. Olsalazine (Dipentum) is a 5-ASA dimer linked by an azo bond and is formulated in gelatin capsules. Balsalazide (Colazal) consists of a 5-ASA monomer linked to a biologically inactive carrier molecule, 4-aminobenzoyl-β-alanine. Similar to sulfasalazine, 5-ASA is released from olsalazine and balsalazide in the colon upon cleavage of the azo bond via the bacterial enzyme azoreductase. Approximately 99% of the drug is delivered intact to the colon, and its metabolites are cleared rapidly in the urine.

Four commonly used mesalamine preparations allow delivery of 5-ASA before the drug reaches the colon: Pentasa, Apriso, Asacol, and Lialda. Pentasa uses ethyl cellulose-coated microgranules that release mesalamine from the duodenum throughout the small bowel and the colon; about 50% of 5-ASA is released in the small intestine, and the remainder is released in the colon. Apriso uses a slightly different formulation of mesalamine granules with a delayed-release enteric coating that allows for the gradual release of mesalamine to the terminal ileum and throughout the colon at a pH of 6 or greater. Asacol is a Eudragit-S-100–coated mesalamine tablet that is released at a pH greater than 7, usually in the distal ileum and the colon. With Asacol, about 15% to 30% of mesalamine is released in the small intestine. Lialda (MMX mesalamine) is a novel mesalamine formulation that uses a multimatrix structure composed of an inner lipophilic matrix and an outer hydrophilic matrix. It is coated with a pH-dependent polymethacrylate film to allow the delayed release of mesalamine in the terminal ileum and colon at a pH greater than 7. This technology also allows mesalamine to be released slowly and in close proximity to the colonic mucosa.

These oral 5-ASA derivatives (mesalamines) have been shown to be superior to placebo for mildly to moderately active UC.[136-138] Meta-analyses have demonstrated that the mesalamines are as efficacious as sulfasalazine, and the various mesalamine preparations appear to be comparable in efficacy.[136,139] Balsalazide has been shown to have superior efficacy and a more rapid response compared with traditional mesalamine agents.[140,141] In a RCT, balsalazide 6.75 g/day, a dose equivalent to mesalamine 2.4 g daily, achieved higher rates of remission and had better tolerance compared with pH-dependent mesalamine 2.4 g/day.[140] It has been suggested that the greatest benefit of balsalazide is in patients with newly diagnosed left-sided UC.[141]

More important than the specific 5-ASA preparation is the dose-dependent response when 5-ASA is used as an induction therapy for active UC.[136,139] For this indication, mesalamine is not effective at doses lower than 2 g daily, and there may be an increased response at doses of 4 to 4.8 g daily for some

patients. For instance, the ASCEND I and II trials showed that mesalamine at doses of 2.4 and 4.8 g/day had similar efficacy for patients with mildly active disease, but that the higher dose (4.8 g/day) led to significantly higher response but not remission rates in patients with moderately active disease.[142,143] The ASCEND III trial reported that patients with moderate active UC treated with Asacol 4.8 g/day had significantly higher remission but not response rates than those treated with 2.4 g/day.[144] Also, data from ASCEND III and the Lialda trials found that the 4.8 g/day dosing was more effective than 2.4 g/day in patients previously treated with mesalamines or who did not achieve clinical remission after 8 weeks of therapy.[144,145] The 4.8 g/day dose of mesalamine is comparable to 12 g/day of sulfasalazine, which is impractical in clinical practice because of the high probability of intolerance. No RCT has evaluated the use of aminosalicylates for severely active UC, but these agents are generally thought not to be effective in severely active disease.

Once remission is achieved, sulfasalazine and other 5-aminosalicylates are effective in maintaining it.[146-149] This benefit appears to be dose dependent for sulfasalazine, with a dose of 2 g/day often used to balance efficacy and adverse side effects.[146] Such a dose-dependent response, however, has not been found with the other 5-ASA preparations, and at doses of 1.5 to 4.8 g/day, remission can be maintained in more than 50% of patients.[150] One meta-analysis has suggested that sulfasalazine might have a slight but statistically significant therapeutic superiority relative to the newer 5-ASAs in maintaining remission when considering trials of 6 months' duration; however, when these trials were combined with those of 12 months' duration, this statistically significant benefit was lost.[150] A double-blind RCT comparing 2 doses of balsalazide (1.5 g twice daily and 3 g twice daily) with mesalamine 0.5 g 3 times daily for 6 months reported a remission rate of 77.5% with the higher dose of balsalazide compared with remission rates of 56.8% and 43.8% with mesalamine and the lower dose of balsalazide, respectively.[151] In general, the same dose of 5-ASA derivative that induces remission is recommended for maintenance therapy, although this recommendation has not been formally tested in a randomized placebo-controlled fashion.

Common side effects of sulfasalazine include fever, rash, nausea, vomiting, and headache (Box 116-5). Other, less common but important side effects of sulfasalazine include hypersensitivity reactions, reversible sperm abnormalities, and impairment of folate absorption. Approximately 15% of patients taking sulfasalazine develop significant side effects that require discontinuing the medication. Up to 90% of

BOX 116-5 Side Effects of Sulfasalazine and 5-Aminosalicylates

Dose-Related
Alopecia
Anorexia
Back pain
Folate malabsorption (sulfasalazine)
Headache
Nausea, vomiting, dyspepsia

Non–Dose-Related
Agranulocytosis, aplastic anemia
Arthralgia
Acute kidney injury
Colitis
Fever
Fibrosing alveolitis, pulmonary eosinophilia
Hemolytic anemia (Heinz bodies)
Hepatitis
Hypersensitivity skin rashes (occasionally with photosensitivity)
Male infertility (sulfasalazine)
Pancreatitis
Pericarditis, myocarditis

patients who are intolerant to sulfasalazine, however, can tolerate mesalamine.[152] In clinical trials, the newer 5-ASA preparations and balsalazide have been shown to be better tolerated than sulfasalazine,[139,153,154] although the adverse event profiles during maintenance therapy appear to be similar for 5-ASA preparations and sulfasalazine.[150] Sulfasalazine can impair folate absorption (by competitively inhibiting the jejunal enzyme, folate conjugase) thereby contributing to anemia, and folate supplementation should be prescribed to patients receiving sulfasalazine. Olsalazine is associated with drug-induced diarrhea in up to 10% of patients, which often limits its use. It has been noted that if olsalazine is ingested with meals and is continued despite the diarrhea, the incidence of this side effect can be lessened substantially to 3%. A systematic review of oral 5-ASA for maintenance of remission in UC found olsalazine to be significantly inferior to sulfasalazine, and this reduced efficacy was related mostly to a significantly higher rate of withdrawals because of adverse events.[150] Oral mesalamine preparations do not appear to have significant dose-dependent toxicity. Oral mesalamine therapy also may place patients at very slightly increased risk of reversible acute kidney injury; for this reason, routine measurement of serum creatinine level is recommended for all patients receiving mesalamines.

Topical

Topical aminosalicylates can be administered in the form of 5-ASA enemas, 5-ASA suppositories, and, in Europe, 5-ASA foam. The use of enemas allows the medication to be delivered up to the level of the splenic flexure in about 95% of patients, and suppositories can be used to treat disease up to 15 to 20 cm from the anal verge.

Topical mesalamine derivatives may be used as an alternative monotherapy or as an adjunctive therapy to oral agents in patients with left-sided colitis or pancolitis. They are effective for inducing remission in patients with mildly to moderately active distal UC, without a clear dose-response effect[155,156] in nonrefractory patients. The standard dosing regimens used to induce remission are 1 to 4 g of 5-ASA in the form of an enema nightly, or mesalamine suppositories 1 to 1.5 g either nightly or in divided doses throughout the day. Mesalamine enemas have been shown to be comparable to oral sulfasalazine in the treatment of active distal UC, with fewer side effects.[154] Similar efficacies have been demonstrated for mesalamine enemas regardless of whether the 1-, 2-, or 4-g formulation is used for inducing remission in patients with mild to moderate left-sided UC not requiring concurrent glucocorticoids or immunomodulators. In fact, mesalamine enemas are perceived to be even more effective than topical glucocorticoid enemas in this setting.[156,157] A combination of topical and oral mesalamine also may be more effective than either agent alone in patients with left-sided colitis or pancolitis, suggesting a dose-response effect.[158,159] In patients with proctitis, mesalamine suppositories, 500 mg administered twice daily, have been shown to be beneficial for treating active disease.[160] Mesalamine foam has a more uniform distribution and longer persistence in the distal colon compared with mesalamine enemas. The foam preparation has been shown to have better patient acceptance than the enema preparation,[161] but mesalamine foams currently are not available in the United States.

Topical mesalamine preparations also are effective for maintaining remission in left-sided UC or proctitis.[155,156] The effective maintenance dosing interval ranges from nightly to every 3 days. Topical mesalamine is as effective as oral mesalamine,[162] and the combination of topical and oral mesalamine may be more effective than oral mesalamine alone as a maintenance regimen.[163]

Glucocorticoids

Systemic

At doses equivalent to 40 to 60 mg/day of oral prednisone, glucocorticoids are effective first-line therapy for moderate or severe flares of UC.[123,164,165] The use of doses higher than 60 mg/day is associated with increased side effects without appreciable clinical benefit and thus should be avoided. The addition of sulfasalazine to corticosteroids in moderately to severely active UC does not offer any incremental benefit. Although no study has directly compared the efficacy of oral and parenteral glucocorticoids, the latter commonly are used in severe disease.[166-168] No adequately designed controlled study has been performed to confirm the clinical impression that continuous infusion of parenteral glucocorticoids is superior to pulse therapy.

The use of adrenocorticotropin (ACTH) has been suggested as an alternative to conventional glucocorticoid therapy of active UC in small studies.[169] One double-blind RCT suggested that IV ACTH was more effective than IV hydrocortisone for the treatment of severely active UC only in steroid-naïve patients[170]; this observation has not been confirmed. Because most patients with severely active flares have been treated previously with glucocorticoids, ACTH rarely is used in clinical practice. A noteworthy complication of ACTH therapy is bilateral adrenal hemorrhage.

Glucocorticoids have no maintenance benefits in patients with UC. Steroid-dependent patients, or patients who are unable to taper off glucocorticoids without experiencing disease exacerbation, benefit from the addition of steroid-sparing agents. There has been no trial to date assessing mesalamine therapy and its efficacy in maintaining remission induced with glucocorticoids. The long-term remission rate in patients who require parenteral glucocorticoids for severe UC is approximately 50%.[171]

Immunomodulatory agents, as discussed, should be considered in patients who are dependent on steroids, who require 2 courses of glucocorticoids for induction of clinical response or remission within 1 year, or who require parenteral glucocorticoids to induce remission. In addition to the use of

---

BOX 116-6 Side Effects of Glucocorticoids

Cutaneous
Acne
Impaired wound healing
Purpura, ecchymoses, petechiae
Striae

Endocrine
Adrenal insufficiency
Cushingoid appearance

Gastrointestinal
Dyspepsia
Dysphagia/odynophagia (candidiasis)

Infectious Complications
Numerous pathogens

Metabolic
Electrolyte imbalance, hypokalemia
Fluid retention
Growth retardation
Hyperglycemia, secondary diabetes mellitus
Hyperlipidemia, altered fat distribution
Hypertension

Musculoskeletal
Myopathy
Osteonecrosis
Osteoporosis

Neuropsychiatric
Anxiety, mood swings
Depression
Insomnia
Psychosis

Ocular
Cataracts
Glaucoma

---

immunomodulatory agents, one should consider using inflix-imab for steroid-dependent patients.

Glucocorticoids are associated with many mild and serious side effects in patients with IBD (Box 116-6). These side effects occur commonly and involve nearly every organ system. Every effort should be made to minimize glucocorticoid use and exposure.

Budesonide is a glucocorticoid preparation that is structurally different from prednisone. The presence of 16α,17α-acetyl side chains allows enhanced topical anti-inflammatory activity and affinity for glucocorticoid receptors compared with prednisone.[172] In addition, budesonide has an approximately 90% first-pass metabolism in the liver and erythrocytes and is converted to metabolites that have little or no biological activity. The resultant low systemic bioavailability translates to significantly less toxicity compared with traditional glucocorticoids. Entocort is a controlled-ileal-release oral budesonide preparation consisting of Eudragit-L-100–coated microgranules with an internal ethyl cellulose component; it releases budesonide at pH greater than 5.5, and about 50% to 80% of budesonide is absorbed in the ileocecal region. Although a controlled study did not shown benefit of conventional oral budesonide for the treatment of active UC,[173] a new oral formulation of MMX budesonide (Uceris) that provides optimal release characteristics for the entire length of the colon was recently developed and has been shown to be efficacious for the induction of remission in mild to moderate active UC in the CORE I study.[174] Patients in this study were treated with MMX budesonide at doses of 9 mg or 6 mg once daily, Asacol

at 800 mg 3 times daily, or placebo, for 8 weeks, and the authors noted remission rates of 18%, 13%, 12%, and 7.4%, respectively (P = 0.014 for MMX budesonide 9 mg vs. placebo) at week 8. For this reason, the use of MMX budesonide at a dose of 9 mg daily for 8 weeks was recently approved by the FDA for the treatment of mild to moderate active UC.

Topical

Topical glucocorticoids in liquid and foam formulations are effective short-term therapy for active UC distal to the splenic flexure.[175,176] Foam preparations often are tolerated better by patients and may be easier to retain than liquid preparations. Topical glucocorticoids have been found to be less effective than topical mesalamine for inducing remission of distal UC[157]; however, the combination of topical corticosteroids and topical mesalamine has been more efficacious than either alone in the short-term treatment of distal UC.[177]

Whereas systemic absorption of glucocorticoids with topical therapy is significantly less than that with oral administration, prolonged treatment with topical glucocorticoids still may be associated with steroid-related side effects and should be avoided. As mentioned previously, budesonide is a potent corticosteroid with a rapid first-pass metabolism. Budesonide enemas, which currently are neither available nor approved in the United States, have been shown to be effective for the treatment of active distal UC in several controlled trials. In a double-blind RCT of patients with active distal UC, budesonide, 2 mg/100 mL for 6 weeks, resulted in a remission rate of 19% compared with 4% in patients receiving placebo therapy (P < 0.05).[178] Subsequent trials have shown budesonide enema to be as efficacious as or even superior to prednisolone enema without resultant depression of endogenous cortisol levels.[179-181]

Budesonide enema perhaps is inferior in efficacy to mesalamine enema,[182] but it clearly presents an alternative topical glucocorticoid for treatment of distal UC. The optimal dose for budesonide enema consistently has been shown to be 2 mg/100 mL once daily.[178,179,183] Budesonide in foam preparation also has been shown to have comparable efficacy with traditional hydrocortisone foam for the treatment of active proctosigmoiditis.[184] Additional studies are needed to determine the effect of longer-term topical budesonide use. As with other glucocorticoid preparations, budesonide enema is not effective for maintaining remission in UC.[183]

Immunomodulators

Azathioprine and 6-Mercaptopurine

Of the various immunomodulatory agents, the most widely used are azathioprine and 6-MP. These 2 agents are purine analogs that interfere with nucleic acid metabolism and cell growth and exert cytotoxic effects on lymphoid cells. They are inactive prodrugs with subtle structural differences. Azathioprine is nonenzymatically converted to 6-MP, which is then metabolized through a series of enzymatic pathways to active and inactive metabolites (see Fig. 115-8). The 2 primary classes of metabolites of 6-MP are 6-thioguanine nucleotides (6-TGNs) and 6-methylmercaptopurine ribonucleotides (6-MMPRs). The 6-TGN metabolites are thought be responsible for the immunomodulatory action of azathioprine and 6-MP and their bone marrow suppression property, whereas hepatotoxicity is thought to be related to 6-MP. One key enzyme involved in the biotransformation of 6-MP is thiopurine methyltransferase (TPMT), which converts 6-MP to its inactive metabolites, 6-MMP and 6-MMPRs.

There is a population polymorphism in the *TPMT* gene: 89% of the population have homozygous wild-type *TPMT*,

TABLE 116-7 Randomized Controlled Trials of Azathioprine (AZA) for UC

Reference	N	AZA Dose (mg/kg/day)	Duration of Therapy (Months)	Response (AZA)	Response (Control)	P-Value	Co-therapy
Induction							
186	80	2.5	1	78%	68%	NS	Glucocorticoids in all
187	20	2.5	3	60%	80%	NS	None; control = 5-ASA
188	44*	2-2.5	6	NR	NR	NS	None
189	72*	2	6	53%	19%	0.006	None; control = 5-ASA
Maintenance							
186	80	1.5-2.5	11	40%	23%	NS	Glucocorticoids for relapse
190	30*	1.5	6	NR	NR	NS	None
191	67	NR	12	64%	41%	0.039	5-ASA in most AZA withdrawal
192	25	2.5	18	42%	62%	NS	Glucocorticoid induction Control = 5-ASA

*All patients in this study were glucocorticoid-dependent.

5-ASA, 5-aminosalicylate; AZA, azathioprine; mo, months; N, number of patients; NR, not reported; NS, not significant.

and 11% and 0.3% of the population have heterozygous and homozygous mutations, respectively.[185] Individuals with heterozygous and homozygous *TPMT* mutations have decreased to absent enzyme activity. The clinical significance of this genetic polymorphism is that inherited differences in TPMT may be responsible for most of the variability in drug response observed among individual patients.

The efficacy of azathioprine in the treatment of UC is a matter of debate. Four RCTs have evaluated azathioprine for inducting remission in active UC (Table 116-7).[186-189] These 4 studies were small, heterogeneous in design, used different outcome definitions for response, and reached different conclusions. Two of the studies involved steroid-dependent patients,[188,189] 1 study used steroids for induction,[186] and 2 studies used 5-ASAs as a comparator group rather than placebo.[187,189] Only 1 study showed a significant benefit with azathioprine compared with 5-ASA for induction therapy in steroid-dependent disease.[189]

With respect to the use of azathioprine for maintenance of remission in UC, 4 RCTs have been performed (see Table 116-7).[186,190-192] Just as with studies of induction therapy, these 4 studies also had small sample sizes, used heterogeneous designs with different outcome definitions of response, allowed for various cotherapies, and again reached different conclusions. One of the studies was in steroid-dependent disease,[190] another allowed the use of steroids for relapse,[186] 1 study used 5-ASA as a comparator group rather than placebo,[192] and another included patients who were mostly taking 5-ASAs and was actually a study of azathioprine withdrawal.[191] Only this withdrawal study showed a benefit with continued azathioprine.

Thus, for the purpose of induction or maintenance therapy for UC, the use of azathioprine is largely based on its established efficacy in CD rather than any proved benefit in UC. One subset of patients, however, has been shown to obtain benefit with the use of azathioprine, specifically patients who have severely active UC and who are able to attain induction of remission with IV followed by oral cyclosporine. In these patients, maintenance therapy with azathioprine has been reported to decrease colectomy rates (see later).

The optimal dose of azathioprine or 6-MP for treating UC is unclear, and no formal dose-ranging study has been reported in the literature. The effective doses for 6-MP and azathioprine generally are 1 to 1.5 mg/kg/day and 2 to 3 mg/kg/day, respectively.[193] At these doses, however, there still may be nonresponders and, for them, higher doses may be necessary. Induction of leukopenia had been advocated for dose optimization,[194] but this practice was not supported by subsequent studies.[195-197] Monitoring metabolite levels may be beneficial in determining the optimal dose of azathioprine or 6-MP.

To date, at least 13 studies examining response in IBD with respect to 6-TGN level have been published. A meta-analysis of the first 12 of these studies found that the studies were similar in that they were retrospective and the majority of patients were adults with CD, but they were heterogeneous with respect to sample size, the proportion of patients in remission, and the activity indices used to assess response.[198] Of the 7 studies that reported data on 6-TGN threshold levels, a pooled analysis of the first 6 studies showed a 3-fold significantly higher rate of remission among patients with a 6-TGN level of greater than 230 to 260 pmol/8×10^8 red blood cells. Incorporation of 6-TGN metabolite measurement into the management regimen of patients receiving azathioprine or 6-MP therapy for IBD is helpful for identifying reasons for nonresponse to therapy and for suspected noncompliance. If used, metabolite levels should be determined at least 2 weeks following any dose adjustment to allow sufficient time for the metabolites to reach steady-state.

Currently, it is recommended in the package insert and by the FDA to determine *TPMT* genotype or phenotype before initiating therapy. The active metabolites, 6-TGNs, also are responsible for myelosuppression with therapy, and patients with *TPMT* mutation or decreased *TPMT* enzyme activity are more likely to experience this toxicity because of preferential shunting of 6-MP metabolism toward the excessive production of 6-TGN.[199] Thus, identifying *TPMT* polymorphism before initiating azathioprine or 6-MP therapy can decrease the risk of myelotoxicity. Patients with homozygous wild-type *TPMT* or normal (to high) *TPMT* enzyme activity level may receive these agents starting at the weight-based optimal dose of 2.5 mg/kg/day for azathioprine or 1.5 mg/kg/day for 6-MP. It has been suggested by some investigators that in patients with heterozygous *TPMT* mutation or intermediate enzyme activity level, 6-MP or azathioprine should be started at 50% of the weight-based optimal dose. Alternative therapy should be considered in patients with homozygous mutations for *TPMT*. Regardless of whether a patient's *TMPT* genotype or phenotype is known, continued frequent monitoring of complete blood counts remains necessary, because only 27% of all patients with leukopenia have *TPMT* mutations.[200] In addition, 2 studies have reported that TPMT testing may be cost-effective.[201,202]

Azathioprine and 6-MP therapy have a delayed onset of action. The mean time to clinical response with azathioprine or 6-MP therapy in patients with UC has been reported to be 3 to 4 months in uncontrolled studies,[203,204] a figure that is similar to the 17 weeks' response time to clinical benefit in placebo-controlled trials of azathioprine or 6-MP therapy for active CD.[205] IV loading of azathioprine at 40 mg/kg for 36 hours does not shorten the time required for a therapeutic response in patients with CD.[200] Such practice presumably would have the same results if attempted in patients with UC.

Because azathioprine or 6-MP therapy is associated with a number of potentially significant toxicities, its duration of therapy should be determined by weighing clinical benefit against these potential toxicities. The optimal duration of maintenance therapy with azathioprine or 6-MP currently is unknown in patients with UC. In patients with CD, the maintenance benefit of azathioprine or 6-MP can be observed for at least 5 years.[206,207] Based on these data in CD and the paucity of alternative maintenance therapies, in patients with UC in whom remission is maintained with azathioprine or 6-MP, treatment generally is continued indefinitely as long as there is no significant adverse side effect.

Common side effects of azathioprine and 6-MP therapy include nausea, vomiting, bone marrow suppression, pancreatitis, allergic reactions, and infections (Box 116-7).[208,209] Bone marrow suppression occurs in 2% to 5% of patients.[208,210] It is dose dependent and manifests primarily as leukopenia, although all 3 cell lines may be affected. This hematologic toxicity can increase with concurrent use of sulfasalazine or mesalamine compounds.[196,211-213] It is known that mesalamine can interact with the enzyme TPMT, leading to increased levels of 6-TGN, and that this interaction has been associated with leukopenia. Bone marrow suppression is managed by reducing the dosage of immunomodulator or withdrawing the medication. Routine monitoring of complete blood count with differentials is necessary for patients receiving azathioprine or 6-MP and should be continued for the entire duration of therapy. Allergic reactions to azathioprine or 6-MP usually manifest as fever, rash, and arthralgia and resolve following discontinuation of these medications.[210,214] Recurrence of similar reactions occurs with medication challenge, although patients who develop allergic reactions to 1 agent may be able to tolerate subsequent challenge with the other.[215] Pancreatitis also is idiosyncratic and independent of dosage.[210,216,217] It usually occurs during the first month of therapy and is reversible upon withdrawal of the drug.

Patients using azathioprine or 6-MP therapy can have abnormal liver biochemical tests, but these usually resolve following drug withdrawal.[218] Because liver biopsy is not performed routinely in these patients, their pattern of hepatic injury, if any, is unknown. Cholestasis with inflammation, nodular regenerative hyperplasia, and peliosis hepatis have been reported with azathioprine and 6-MP therapy.[210,218] As is the case for complete blood counts, routine monitoring of liver biochemical tests is recommended.

A 2- to 5-fold increased risk of lymphoma and non-melanoma skin cancer has been reported with thiopurine therapy.[219-221] The lymphoma that develops in patients who have IBD and receive these immunomodulatory agents is frequently non-Hodgkin's lymphoma associated with Epstein-Barr virus.[222] Patients receiving thiopurine therapy are encouraged to minimize sun exposure and have close dermatologic surveillance.

Cyclosporine

Cyclosporine A is a potent inhibitor of cell-mediated immunity. Its use in UC is primarily in patients with severe, steroid-refractory disease.

There has only been 1 randomized placebo-controlled trial evaluating the efficacy of IV cyclosporine in severe UC. In this study of 20 patients who did not respond to at least 7 days of IV hydrocortisone, 9 (82%) of the 11 patients receiving continuous IV infusion of cyclosporine at 4 mg/kg/day responded, compared with none of the 9 patients receiving placebo therapy.[223] The time to clinical response was rapid, at a mean of 7 days. After the IV route of therapy was converted to oral cyclosporine, 44% of those patients who responded initially required colectomy during the 6-month follow-up period.

IV cyclosporine monotherapy may be as effective as IV glucocorticoids in patients with severely active UC; its use thus potentially minimizes the toxicities of combination therapy.[224] The addition of azathioprine or 6-MP in patients who have responded to IV cyclosporine has been shown in other studies to reduce the rate of relapse or colectomy.[225,226] Thus, cyclosporine can be considered a bridge therapy to control active disease in patients with steroid-refractory UC while waiting for elective surgery or the onset of action of azathioprine or 6-MP.

With the addition of azathioprine, long-term remission at 1 year may be more likely in patients who initially respond to IV cyclosporine monotherapy than in those who respond to IV glucocorticoids. A European retrospective cohort study of 142 patients who were treated with cyclosporine, 118 of whom responded initially, reported the probability of avoiding colectomy to be 63% at 1 year, 41% at 4 years, and 12% at 7 years; overall, 54% of patients required colectomy at some point.[227] Patients who were already taking 6-MP or azathioprine at the time cyclosporine was initiated continued taking their current dose, and those who were naïve to 6-MP or azathioprine were started at target doses at the time of response to cyclosporine during their hospitalization. The authors found that 59% of patients previously taking 6-MP or azathioprine required eventual colectomy, compared with 31% for patients naïve to these drugs (P < 0.05).

Because most of the serious adverse effects associated with the use of cyclosporine are dose-dependent, IV doses lower than 4 mg/kg that still can achieve efficacy are desirable. One RCT has shown that a dose of 2 mg/kg is as effective as 4 mg/kg given IV in patients with severely active UC, judged by clinical response rates, time to response, and short-term colectomy rates.[228] The mean plasma cyclosporine levels were 237 ng/mL in patients receiving the 2 mg/kg dose and 332 ng/mL in patients receiving the 4 mg/kg dose. Thus, initiating therapy at 2 mg/kg may be reasonable, but regardless of the dose used, careful monitoring of plasma cyclosporine trough levels is necessary.

Cyclosporine has been associated with many adverse effects, including paresthesias, tremors, headache, hypertrichosis, and gingival hyperplasia (Box 116-8). Other potentially

---

BOX 116-7 Side Effects of Azathioprine and 6-Mercaptopurine

Abnormal liver biochemical test results
Bone marrow suppression
Hypersensitivity reactions (fever, rash, arthralgia)
Infections
Lymphoma, non-melanoma skin cancer
Nausea, abdominal pain, diarrhea
Pancreatitis

BOX 116-8 Side Effects of Cyclosporine

Anaphylaxis	Hypertension
Diarrhea	Infections
Electrolyte abnormalities	Nausea, vomiting
Gingival hyperplasia	Paresthesia
Headache	Renal insufficiency
Hepatotoxicity	Seizure
Hirsutism	Tremor

serious toxicities include hypertension, seizures, electrolyte and liver biochemistry abnormalities, nephrotoxicity, anaphylaxis, and opportunistic infections. These complications are mostly dose-dependent. Severe complications have been reported with cyclosporine in up to 12% of patients with UC,[229] and 2 large series have reported death rates of 1.8% to 2.8% with cyclosporine, more than half of which were due to infections acquired while taking the drug.[227,229]

Careful monitoring for adverse effects is critical during cyclosporine therapy. Baseline serum electrolytes, creatinine, cholesterol, and liver biochemical values should be measured. Cyclosporine therapy should be avoided in patients with an impaired creatinine clearance to minimize the risk of severe nephrotoxicity. Patients with serum cholesterol lower than 120 mg/dL should receive nutritional support to improve the level before initiating cyclosporine therapy, because a low cholesterol level is associated with an increased risk of seizures. During IV therapy, cyclosporine levels should be monitored daily, and the dose should be adjusted to achieve a trough concentration (measured 1 hour before dosing) between 200 and 400 ng/mL, determined by high-pressure liquid chromatography. Serum electrolytes and serum creatinine levels should be monitored daily or every other day. The dose of cyclosporine also should be decreased when the serum creatinine increases by 20% to 30% over baseline.

If patients respond to IV cyclosporine, the route of administration can be changed to oral therapy with 2 mg of oral agent for each 1 mg of IV cyclosporine. The drug can be administered in 2 divided doses daily. Drug monitoring during oral cyclosporine therapy includes weekly trough cyclosporine levels and weekly to biweekly electrolyte and creatinine levels. Oral cyclosporine should be continued for 3 to 6 months, while waiting for surgery or for azathioprine or 6-MP to take effect. Patients on long-term cyclosporine therapy should receive *Pneumocystis carinii* pneumonia prophylaxis with trimethoprim/sulfamethoxazole.

Methotrexate

Methotrexate is a folic acid antagonist and has antimetabolite and anti-inflammatory properties. Although early reports suggested potential benefit of methotrexate administered intramuscularly or orally in UC, the only randomized, placebo-controlled trial failed to demonstrate its efficacy for the treatment of active UC.[230] In this study of 67 patients with chronic active UC, oral methotrexate at 12.5 mg/wk for 9 months was comparable to placebo therapy in the rate of achieving first remission, time to first remission, relapse following remission, and the mean glucocorticoid dose. It is unknown if methotrexate at higher doses administered intramuscularly or subcutaneously may be beneficial in inducing or maintaining remission in UC, although 2 RCTs (one in France [METEOR] and the other in the United States [MERIT-UC]) are currently underway to investigate these questions. Until the results of these RCTs become available, methotrexate cannot be considered a standard therapy for UC.

Other Immunomodulators

Alternative immunomodulators have been explored for patients who do not tolerate or have not responded to the previously mentioned immunosuppressants. Mycophenolate mofetil has pharmacodynamic properties similar to those of azathioprine and 6-MP but a more rapid onset of action. A pilot study of patients with chronic active UC receiving concomitant prednisolone found azathioprine to be superior to mycophenolate mofetil throughout the 1-year study period, with remission rates at 1 year of 100% and 88%, respectively.[231] Uncontrolled studies reported less than 50% remission rates with mycophenolate mofetil therapy in patients with steroid-dependent UC,[232,233] and the intolerance rate was high.[232] A substantial number of patients developed adverse effects necessitating drug withdrawal, including recurrent upper respiratory tract infection, bacterial meningitis, depression, and migraine headache.[231,233]

Tacrolimus is another immunosuppressant with actions similar to those of cyclosporine. In contrast to cyclosporine, it has a 100-fold greater potency and a more rapid onset of action. A number of small uncontrolled studies have suggested benefit of oral or IV tacrolimus for the treatment of patients with refractory UC. The only randomized, placebo-controlled trial of tacrolimus in UC involved 63 Japanese patients with either steroid-dependent or steroid-refractory disease who were randomized to receive either initial oral tacrolimus at 0.05 mg/kg or placebo twice daily.[234] Patients in the high trough concentration (10 to 15 ng/mL) tacrolimus group had a significantly higher rate of response and nonsignificantly higher rate of remission than those in the placebo group at week 2, and a number of patients demonstrated response or remission (or both) after an additional 10 weeks of open-label therapy. As with cyclosporine, tacrolimus can result in a number of toxicities including nephrotoxicity, electrolyte abnormalities, nausea, diarrhea, headache, tremors, paresthesias, insomnia, alopecia, hirsutism, and gingival hyperplasia.[235,236] Thus, given the limited data and potential for harmful adverse events, the use of these alternative immunomodulators currently is not incorporated into standard practice.

Biological Therapy

Recent advances in our understanding of the pathogenesis of IBD have resulted in the development of therapies targeted at specific molecules or mediators involved in the inflammatory processes of these diseases.

Anti-TNF Antibodies

TNF is a key proinflammatory cytokine that has been demonstrated to play a role in several disease states, including IBD. Elevated TNF concentrations have been found in the inflamed intestine of patients with CD and UC, and stool and mucosal concentrations of TNF in patients with IBD have been shown to correlate with clinical disease activity. Infliximab (Remicade) and adalimumab (Humira) are monoclonal antibodies of IgG$_1$ subclass directed against human TNF-α, with infliximab being a chimera of 75% human and 25% murine components that is administered IV and adalimumab being fully human and administered subcutaneously. The efficacy of infliximab and adalimumab in CD are well established, and both are FDA approved for the treatment of patients with moderate to severe CD or UC. These antibodies are thought to operate in CD via a multitude of mechanisms, including antagonizing the activity of TNF-α,[237,238] initiating cytotoxicity on immune cells,[239] and inducing T-cell apoptosis.[240,241]

Results from 2 large, multicenter, randomized double-blind placebo-controlled trials (ACT 1 and 2) showed efficacy of infliximab therapy in UC.[242] In these 2 similarly designed trials, 728 patients with moderately to severely active UC who failed conventional therapy with glucocorticoids alone or in combination with thiopurines (ACT 1) or glucocorticoids alone or in combination with thiopurines and 5-aminosalicylates (ACT 2) were randomized to placebo, infliximab 5 mg/kg, or infliximab 10 mg/kg at weeks 0 and 2 and then every 8 weeks through week 46 (ACT 1) or week 22 (ACT 2). With respect to clinical response at week 8, in ACT 1 69% and 61% of patients receiving infliximab at 5 and 10 mg/kg, respectively, had a clinical response, compared with 37% of patients receiving placebo (P < 0.001 for both comparisons). In ACT 2 at week 8, 64% and 69% of patients receiving infliximab at 5 mg/kg and 10 mg/kg, respectively, had a clinical response, compared with 29% of patients receiving placebo (P < 0.001 for both comparisons). With respect to clinical remission at week 8 in ACT 1, 39% and 32% of patients receiving infliximab at 5 mg/kg and 10 mg/kg, respectively, attained remission, compared with 15% of patients receiving placebo (P < 0.003 for both comparisons). In ACT 2 at week 8, 34% and 28% of patients receiving infliximab at 5 mg/kg and 10 mg/kg, respectively, attained remission, compared with 6% of patients receiving placebo (P < 0.001 for both comparisons). The results for clinical remission at week 30 (ACT 1 and 2) and week 54 (ACT 1) were very similar for all groups, with highly significant greater than 2-fold higher remission rates for the infliximab-treated patients. The proportions of patients with a sustained clinical response or remission also were significantly higher in the infliximab groups. Treatment with infliximab also was shown to have steroid-sparing and mucosal healing properties.

A recent open-label RCT comparing infliximab to cyclosporine for the treatment of severe UC in 115 patients refractory to IV glucocorticoids found that these 2 drugs were comparable in efficacy.[243] Treatment failure was defined as the presence of any of the following at any time during follow-up: absence of clinical response at day 7, relapse between day 7 and 98, absence of steroid-free remission at day 98, severe adverse event leading to treatment interruption, colectomy, and death. The authors reported that treatment failure occurred in 54% of patients receiving infliximab and 60% of those receiving cyclosporine, with colectomy rates of 21% in the infliximab group and 17% in the cyclosporine group. Thus, for patients with severe steroid-refractory UC, the choice between infliximab and cyclosporine should be individualized.

With respect to adalimumab use in moderate-to-severe active UC, 2 large RCTs (ULTRA 1 and 2) have also been conducted.[244,245] In ULTRA 1, which was purely an induction trial in patients naïve to anti-TNF therapy, 390 patients were randomized to receive adalimumab 160 mg at week 0 and 80 mg at week 2 or 80 mg at week 0 and 40 mg at week 2 and then 40 mg at week 4 and 6, or placebo at week 0, 2, 4, and 6.[244] Remission rates were 18.5%, 10%, and 9.2%, respectively (P = 0.031 for adalimumab 160/80 mg group vs. placebo), and response rates were 55%, 52%, and 45%, respectively (P = NS for each adalimumab group vs. placebo) at week 8. In ULTRA 2, which examined induction and maintenance of remission but also allowed for inclusion of patients with prior anti-TNF exposure, 494 patients, stratified by prior anti-TNF exposure, were randomized to receive adalimumab 160 mg at week 0 and 80 mg at week 2 followed by 40 mg every other week starting week 4, or placebo, for up to 52 weeks.[245] Overall rates of remission and response were 16.5% vs. 9.3% (P = 0.019) and 50% vs. 35% (P < 0.005), respectively, at week 8 and 17.3% vs. 8.5% (P = 0.004) and 30% vs. 18% (P < 0.05) at week 52. However, in patients naïve to anti-TNF therapy, the differences were larger with remission and response rates of 21%

vs. 11% (P = 0.017) and 59% vs. 39% (P < 0.001), respectively, at week 8 and 22% vs. 12% (P = 0.029) and 37% vs. 24% (P = 0.019) at week 52.

Anti-TNF therapy is now accepted as part of the standard treatment options in patients with moderate to severe UC. Other anti-TNF agents include golimumab, for which a large RCT (PURSUIT) in active UC has recently been completed, and certolizumab pegol, which has shown efficacy for the induction and maintenance of remission in CD but has not yet been formally studied in patients with UC.

Combination therapy with infliximab and azathioprine for the treatment of moderate to severe UC has been preliminarily investigated in a 16-week trial (UC-SUCCESS) of biological-naïve patients who were failing glucocorticoids and were either naïve to azathioprine or had stopped azathioprine at least 3 months prior to the start of study.[246] The authors found that patients receiving combination therapy had higher rates of steroid-free remission (40%) compared to those receiving monotherapy (24% for azathioprine alone, 22% for infliximab alone). Rates of mucosal healing were also significantly higher in the combination group.

The most common adverse events with anti-TNF therapy include infusion or injection-site reactions, delayed-type hypersensitivity reactions, formation of autoantibodies (anti-nuclear and anti-dsDNA), and drug-induced lupus-like reactions.[247] Infliximab infusion reactions, which have an incidence of 4% to 16% in clinical trials, typically occur within 1 to 2 hours of administration and are characterized by symptoms of chest pain, shortness of breath, palpitations, fever or chills, urticaria, and hypotension. In addition, infectious complications are increased with anti-TNF agents, but serious infections, such as pneumonia, sepsis, reactivation of TB and HBV, and opportunistic infections, including listeriosis, aspergillosis, histoplasmosis, coccidiomycosis, and *Pneumocystis carinii* pneumonia, occur only rarely. For this reason, it is recommended that all patients be checked for active or latent TB, with a PPD skin test or quantiferon gold blood test and a chest x-ray, and for chronic hepatitis B, with a serum hepatitis B surface antigen, prior to the initiation of anti-TNF therapy. Anti-TNF therapy may also put patients at increased risk for lymphoma (including a very rare and highly aggressive hepatosplenic T-cell lymphoma when anti-TNF agents are combined with thiopurines) and skin cancer (including melanoma),[248-251] although the magnitude of these risk are unclear at the present time. Other rare adverse events associated with the use of anti-TNF drugs include demyelinating disease, peripheral neuropathy, worsening or new-onset heart failure, and hepatic necrosis.

Anti-Adhesion Molecules

Two agents directed at blocking small adhesion molecules have been evaluated for the treatment of UC. These molecules are glycoproteins expressed on the surfaces of endothelial cells and lymphocytes. Adhesion molecules are important in cellular trafficking in IBD and other diseases, in which immune and inflammatory cells from the periphery are recruited into sites of inflammation. Among these, natalizumab is a humanized IgG_4 monoclonal antibody against lymphocyte adhesion molecules, α_4 integrins. A pilot study of 10 patients with active UC suggested clinical benefit with a single infusion of 3 mg/kg of natalizumab.[252] Natalizumab, which is approved for treating patients with CD in whom anti-TNF therapy has failed, is associated with a risk of progressive multifocal leukoencephalopathy (PML), a highly morbid and often fatal brain disorder, as it also inhibits lymphocyte trafficking into the central nervous system. For this reason, a gut-selective anti-adhesion molecule, vedolizumab (previously known as

LDP-02, MLN02, and MLN0002), was developed. Vedolizumab, a humanized IgG$_1$ monoclonal antibody to $\alpha_4\beta_7$ integrin expressed on the surface of B and T cells, prevents the binding of these lymphocytes to mucosal addressin cell adhesion molecule-1 (MAdCAM-1), which is expressed primarily on gut vascular endothelium.[253] A recently completed RCT (GEMINI I) of vedolizumab for the treatment of moderate-to-severe UC, which included a 6-week induction phase and a separate maintenance phase for patients who underwent open-label induction therapy, reported that vedolizumab was significantly more effective than placebo for induction and that corticosteroid-free remission rates at week 52 were 45% and 42% for patients receiving IV infusions of vedolizumab every 4 and 8 weeks, respectively, versus 16% for patients receiving placebo.[254] Furthermore, in this trial vedolizumab had an impressive safety profile with no cases of opportunistic infections or PML. Vedolizumab was approved by the FDA in 2014.

Kinase Inhibitors

The Janus kinase (JAK) family of kinases, which include JAK1 and JAK3, mediate signal transduction for a variety of cytokines, including ILs 2, 4, 7, 9, 15, and 21, which are critical for lymphocyte proliferation, function, and activation.[255] Tofacitinib, a novel oral inhibitor of JAK1 and JAK3, was recently shown to be safe and effective for the treatment of moderate to severe active UC in a large phase 2 trial.[256] In this study, in which 194 patients were randomized to receive twice-daily tofacitinib at 0.5, 3, 10, or 15 mg, or placebo for 8 weeks, rates of response were 32% (P = 0.39), 48% (P = 0.55), 61% (P = 0.10), and 78% (P < 0.001) respectively versus 42% (placebo); rates of remission were 13% (P = 0.76), 33% (P = 0.01), 48% (P < 0.001), and 41% (P < 0.001) respectively versus 10% (placebo) at week 8. Potential toxicities of tofacitinib include elevation of both high- and low-density lipoprotein (HDL and LDL) and neutropenia, and possibly elevations of liver-associated enzymes and serum creatinine as well as anemia.

Other Biological Agents

Although historically considered more important in the inflammation of CD, as it is produced by Th1 cells, IL-2 also has been implicated in UC inflammation (see earlier). Two agents designed to block the binding of IL-2 to its receptor have been studied in UC but have been found not to be efficacious. Daclizumab, a humanized monoclonal antibody against the IL-2 receptor (CD25), was shown to be no better than placebo for inducing clinical remission or response in patients with active UC in a multicenter RCT of 159 patients.[257] Basiliximab, a chimeric monoclonal antibody to the IL-2 receptor, was found not to increase the efficacy of corticosteroids in an RCT of 149 patients with steroid-refractory UC.[258]

Along with the emphasis on T-cell–mediated immune response in the pathogenesis of UC, 2 other T-cell–directed drugs have been shown to lack efficacy in UC. Visilizumab, a humanized monoclonal antibody to CD3, was shown to be ineffective for inducing remission in an RCT of 127 patients with IV corticosteroid-refractory UC.[259] Abatacept, a recombinant fusion protein of the Fc domain of human IgG$_1$ and the extracellular domain of the human cytotoxic T-lymphocyte antigen 4, which inhibits T-cell costimulation, was found to lack efficacy for the induction or maintenance of remission in moderate to severe UC in a recent large RCT.[260]

Other biological therapies include agents targeted at tissue repair and restitution following mucosal injury. In this regard, EGF is a potent mitogenic peptide that stimulates cell proliferation in the GI tract. A preliminary study showed that EGF enemas at a dose of 5 μg daily for 2 weeks was effective in treating mild to moderate left-sided UC when administered along with oral mesalamine.[261] In contrast, another potent stimulant of intestinal epithelial cells, repifermin (keratinocyte growth factor 2) was not found to be more effective than placebo when administered IV in patients with active UC in a phase 2 dose-ranging study.[262] Further studies clearly are necessary to confirm some of these early promising findings.

Other Therapies

Antibiotics

Antibiotics have a limited role in the management of UC, and most controlled studies have not demonstrated their benefit either in active disease or maintenance of remission.[263-267] The most commonly used antibiotics in this setting are metronidazole and ciprofloxacin. One RCT found oral tobramycin to be superior to placebo as a short-term adjunctive therapy to glucocorticoids for active UC.[268] Another RCT reported a modest benefit for the addition of ciprofloxacin for 6 months in patients with UC refractory to mesalamine and corticosteroids.[269] At present, the data showing efficacy of antibiotics for treatment of patients with UC are not as convincing as are the data for antibiotic treatment of CD. Thus, at present the primary role of antibiotics in the treatment of UC is for its suppurative complications.

Probiotics, Prebiotics, and Synbiotics

Probiotics are living organisms in foods and dietary supplements that might beneficially affect the host in a number of ways, including improving its intestinal microbial balance, blocking adhesion sites on colonocytes (which might improve mucosal barrier function), and enhancing local immune response.[270] A probiotic can be a specific nonpathogenic strain of a bacterial species or a mixture of multiple species and strains, most commonly including *Lactobacillus* or *Bifidobacterium* species; sometimes they contain fungal antigens as well. An example of a common probiotic is VSL#3, which contains 4 strains of *Lactobacillus* (*Lactobacillus acidophilus*, *Lactobacillus delbrueckii* subspecies *bulgaricus*, *Lactobacillus plantarum*, and *Lactobacillus casei*), 3 strains of *Bifidobacterium* (*Bifidobacterium infantis*, *Bifidobacterium longum*, *Bifidobacterium breve*), and 1 strain of *Streptococcus* (*Streptococcus salivarius* subspecies *thermophilus*).

Prebiotics are nondigestible food ingredients that selectively stimulate the growth or activity of 1 or more organisms of the intestinal microbiota, such as *Lactobacillus* or *Bifidobacterium* species, thereby potentially conferring beneficial effects to the host.[271,272] The majority of prebiotics are nondigestible oligosaccharides, with galacto-oligosaccharide, fructo-oligosaccharide, lactulose, and inulin being the most commonly used agents. Because probiotics have the challenge of competing with indigenous microbiota for nutrients, scientists have developed synbiotics, which are combinations of probiotics and prebiotics, in the hope of facilitating the intestinal survival of probiotics.

With respect to the use of these agents for inducing remission in mildly to moderately active UC, 4 RCTs have been performed using different agents.[273-276] Two of 3 studies that measured rates of remission found no benefit of probiotics (VSL#3 in 1 study, fermented milk in the other) added to 5-aminosalicylates[273,274]; the third study found that *E. coli* Nissle 1917 combined with glucocorticoids had efficacy similar to that of mesalazine combined with glucocorticoids.[275] The fourth study, which used a synbiotic, reported a nonsignificant improvement in disease activity when the synbiotic was combined with standard therapy.[276] With respect to the use of these agents for the maintenance of remission in mildly to moderately active UC, 6 RCTs have been published.[275,277-281] Two of these studies reported significantly lower rates of relapse for patients receiving a probiotic (*Bifidobacterium* in 1 study, fermented milk in the other) after medically induced remission compared with those receiving placebo,[248,249] and the other 4 studies (using *E. coli* Nissle in 3 studies and *Lactobacillus rhamnosus* strain GG in the fourth) found no difference in rates of relapse.[276,279-281]

Nontraditional probiotic therapies that also have been evaluated include *Saccharomyces boulardii* and *Trichuris suis*.[282,283] A small, uncontrolled study of 24 patients with mild to moderate active UC suggested a potential benefit of *S. boulardii* when used in addition to mesalamine.[282] The use of helminths in active UC was investigated by Weinstock and colleagues, who randomized 54 patients with active disease to receive 2500 *T. suis* ova or placebo orally every 2 weeks for 12 weeks and reported that rates of improvement were significantly higher in the active treatment group at week 12 (43% vs. 17%; P = 0.04); significant improvement was seen as early as week 6.[283]

Fecal microbiota transplant (FMT), which can be considered an extreme form of probiotic treatment, has been reported in only a few patients with UC, albeit with good results. Clearly, this mode of therapy is in its infancy, and well-designed RCTs to evaluate efficacy and safety are needed before its use can be recommended.

In summary, at present, there is no convincing evidence to support the use of probiotics, prebiotics, or synbiotics for the treatment of UC. However, future large, well-designed RCTs are necessary to address this issue more definitively.

Nutritional Therapy

Short-chain fatty acids, especially butyrate, have been shown to be the main energy substrate for colonocytes. Butyrate metabolism accounts for approximately 70% of colonocyte oxygen use. The suggestion that there is an impairment of colonocyte oxidation of short-chain fatty acids in UC led to therapeutic investigations of this form of nutritional therapy. Indeed, placebo-controlled studies have found butyrate enemas to be beneficial in treating mildly active, left-sided colitis.[284-286]

Fish oil containing eicosapentaenoic acid has been found to attenuate colitis in animal models of colitis, probably by protecting the integrity of colonic mucosa, suppressing the inflammatory response, or both.[287-289] In a small, placebo-controlled, crossover study of patients with mild to moderate UC, treatment with fish oil resulted in a 56% reduction in disease activity compared with a 4% reduction in controls (P < 0.05).[290] This benefit has not been confirmed in other studies, and a benefit in maintaining remission has not been observed.[291-293] Furthermore, compliance is limited because of side effects and the odor of the fish oil preparation.

In contrast to CD, in which bowel rest and total parenteral nutrition can improve disease, multiple studies have not found total parenteral nutrition with or without bowel rest to have any therapeutic advantage in patients with UC.[294,295] Parenteral nutrition, however, can offer nutritional benefit in these patients. In general it is important to provide adequate nutrition to patients with UC who are about to undergo surgery. Nutrition is no more effective than placebo, however, for use as primary therapy of active UC.

Nicotine

Based on the observation that smoking is associated with a decreased risk of developing UC and that a former smoker with active colitis may gain clinical benefit on resuming smoking, nicotine has been used to treat patients with this disease. RCTs have shown some benefit of transdermal nicotine in the treatment of active UC.[296-299] When administered at the highest tolerated dosage of 22 mg/day or less for 4 weeks in patients with mildly to moderately active UC, transdermal nicotine resulted in clinical improvement in 39% of patients compared with 9% of patients who received placebo therapy (P = 0.007).[296] As a single therapy, however, transdermal nicotine was not as effective as low-dose prednisolone.[300] Common side effects included nausea, lightheadedness, itching, and tremor. Topical nicotine therapy has fewer side effects and may be an alternative. Pilot studies have shown topical nicotine to be beneficial in patients with distal UC, but no large RCT has been performed,[301,302] and transdermal nicotine has not been found to be effective as a maintenance therapy.[303] Thus, based on available data on clinical efficacy and the overall poor patient tolerability, nicotine cannot be considered part of the standard treatment for patients with UC.

Heparin

Heparin, a group of sulfated glycosaminoglycans, has anti-inflammatory and immunomodulatory properties in addition to its well-known anticoagulant activity. The exact mechanism whereby heparin might ameliorate UC remains uncertain. An anticoagulant benefit, however, might not be responsible, because similar efficacy has not been observed in patients with IBD when treated with warfarin.

Because of their negative charge, the glycosaminoglycans that constitute heparin have varied biological effects, including significant anti-inflammatory actions and augmentation of the peptide growth factors involved in intestinal mucosal repair and regeneration. Based on reports of fortuitous improvement in patients with UC receiving heparin for treatment of deep venous thromboses, pilot studies have suggested that unfractionated heparin may be effective for inducing remission in patients with severe, refractory UC.[304,305] Compared with glucocorticoids as a first-line therapy, however, small RCTs have reported conflicting results.[306,307]

IV heparin therapy has been associated with substantial bleeding complications. Low-molecular-weight heparin (LMWH) offers advantages over unfractionated heparin in its subcutaneous route of administration, and preliminary studies suggested a benefit of LMWH in the treatment of active UC.[308,309] Unfortunately, this finding was not confirmed in a large, placebo-controlled trial of patients with mildly to moderately active UC receiving LMWH for 6 weeks.[310] At this time, the use of either unfractionated heparin or LMWH cannot be advocated as primary therapy for patients with active UC.

Peroxisome Proliferator Receptor Agonists

Peroxisome proliferator-activated receptor (PPAR)-γ is a nuclear hormone receptor best known for its roles in regulating metabolism and adipocyte differentiation. It also has been shown to have immunomodulatory and anti-inflammatory properties in multiple sites, including the colon.[311-314] A randomized double-blind, placebo-controlled trial assessed the efficacy of a 12-week treatment with the PPAR-γ ligand rosiglitazone in 105 patients with mildly to moderately active UC.[315] The authors reported a significant benefit of rosiglitazone over placebo with respect to clinical response (44% vs. 23%; P = 0.04) and clinical remission (17% vs. 2%; P = 0.01) at 12 weeks based on the Mayo score. However, given the reports of a potential for increased risk of myocardial infarction and long-bone fractures with rosiglitazone (based on studies in diabetic patients, in whom this medication is mostly used), the use of rosiglitazone should be restricted to patients who have failed or cannot tolerate standard medical therapy.

Cytapharesis

Active UC is characterized by activation and infiltration of leukocytes in the colonic mucosa. Because leukocyte-derived inflammatory cytokines play an important role in initiating and perpetuating the inflammatory process, reduction of peripheral blood levels of leukocytes has been proposed as a therapeutic option for treating UC. Several methods of depleting peripheral blood leukocytes have been developed and have been shown to hold promise in the treatment of severely active UC in small controlled and uncontrolled studies.

Granulocyte/monocyte apheresis using the Adacolumn Apheresis System (JIMRO, Ltd., Takasaki, Japan) in patients with moderate to severe active UC was formally evaluated in a large, multicenter, randomized double-blind sham-controlled North American pivotal trial of 168 patients and a smaller identically designed companion trial of 47 patients in Europe and Japan.[316] In this study, patients were required to have active disease despite concomitant therapy with 5-aminosalicylates, glucocorticoids, or 6-MP and azathioprine. Neither the pivotal nor the companion study showed a difference in clinical remission or response rates (as defined by the Mayo score) at week 12 between the Adacolumn and sham treatment groups after a total of 10 apheresis sessions over a 9-week period. Thus, at this time, Adacolumn apheresis in similar patients cannot be recommended.

Algorithms for the Treatment of Ulcerative Colitis

An algorithm for treating patients with active UC of mild to moderate severity is outlined in Figure 116-14. The treatment of severely active UC is shown in Figure 116-15.

Surgical Therapy

Removal of the colon and rectum cures UC. Common indications for surgical therapy of UC are medically refractory disease, intractable disease with impaired quality of life, and unacceptable side effects from medical therapy (Box 116-9). Other indications include uncontrolled bleeding, toxic megacolon, perforation, dysplasia or carcinoma, systemic complications, and growth retardation. The goals of surgical treatment are to remove the entire diseased colon while preserving continence and sexual function. Elimination of the risk of colorectal cancer is also important. The role of prophylactic

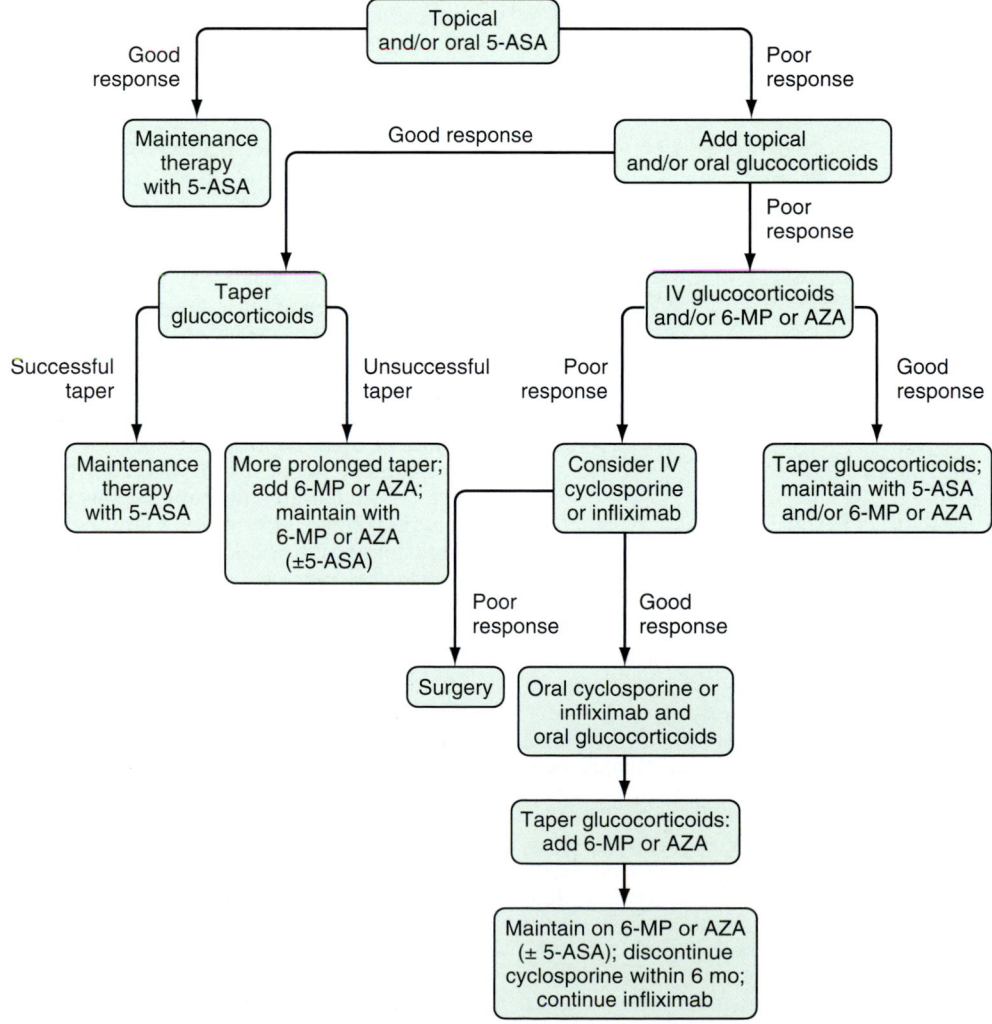

FIGURE 116-14. Algorithm for the management of mildly to moderately active UC. 5-ASA, 5-aminosalicylate; AZA, azathioprine; 6-MP, 6-mercaptopurine.

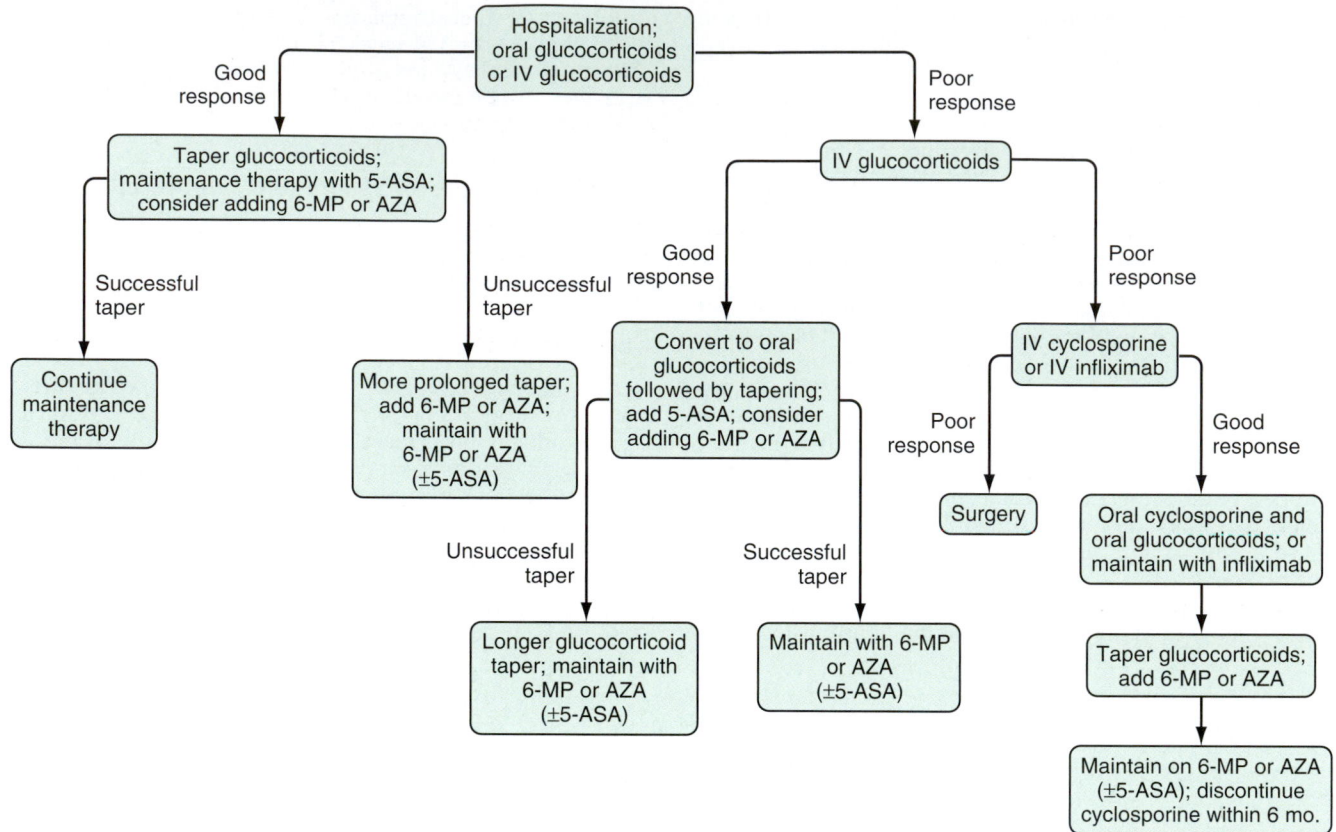

FIGURE 116-15. Algorithm for the management of severely active UC. 5-ASA, 5-aminosalicylate; AZA, azathioprine; 6-MP, 6-mercaptopurine.

BOX 116-9 Indications for Surgery in Patients with UC

Colonic dysplasia or carcinoma
Colonic perforation
Growth retardation
Intolerable or unacceptable side effects of medical therapy
Medically refractory disease
Systemic complications that are recurrent or unmanageable
Toxic megacolon
Uncontrollable colonic hemorrhage

---

proctocolectomy in patients with long-standing extensive UC is controversial. Whereas most clinicians do not routinely recommend proctocolectomy solely for the purpose of prophylaxis against colorectal cancer, patients should be informed of the limitations of our current colonoscopic surveillance program (see Chapter 127).

There are multiple surgical options for UC (see Chapter 117), including subtotal colectomy with ileostomy, colectomy with ileorectal anastomosis, proctocolectomy with Brooke ileostomy, proctocolectomy with continent ileostomy, restorative proctocolectomy with ileal pouch-anal anastomosis (IPAA), and proctocolectomy with ileal pouch-anal transition zone anastomosis (Fig. 116-16). The choice of operation is based on several factors, including the indication for and urgency of surgery, the age and general health of the patient, the status of the patient's anal function, and the patient's preference of functional outcome and lifestyle.

Colectomy

Subtotal colectomy with ileostomy is the least extensive of the operations for UC. Most of the colon is removed, a Hartman pouch or a mucus fistula is fashioned for the remaining colon, and an end-ileostomy is created. This surgery typically is performed in patients requiring emergent surgery for severe or fulminant colitis, and it has the advantage of allowing restorative surgery in the future. Colectomy with ileorectal anastomosis is similar to subtotal colectomy with ileostomy, but it maintains bowel continuity. Many patients continue to have attacks of proctitis and the retained rectal stump is at risk for developing colorectal cancer. Thus, lifelong endoscopic surveillance of the rectum is necessary for patients who elect this type of operation.

Total proctocolectomy with a permanent Brooke end-ileostomy was one of the earliest operations performed for UC. Removal of the entire colon and rectum eliminates any future disease and risk of colorectal cancer. The primary disadvantage of this operation is the presence of the permanent ileostomy, which might not be acceptable from the standpoint of quality of life for some patients. This is the operation of choice for older adult patients, those with anal dysfunction, and those who do not wish to have a restorative proctocolectomy. Proctocolectomy with continent ileostomy (Koch pouch) was developed as an alternative to the conventional end-ileostomy.[317] In this operation, loops of small bowel are used to create an intra-abdominal pouch with an intussuscepted (nipple) valve. This pouch allows storage of stool contents and is attached to the abdominal wall with a flush ostomy opening. The stool contents in the pouch are emptied by inserting a suction catheter through the stoma. Because of

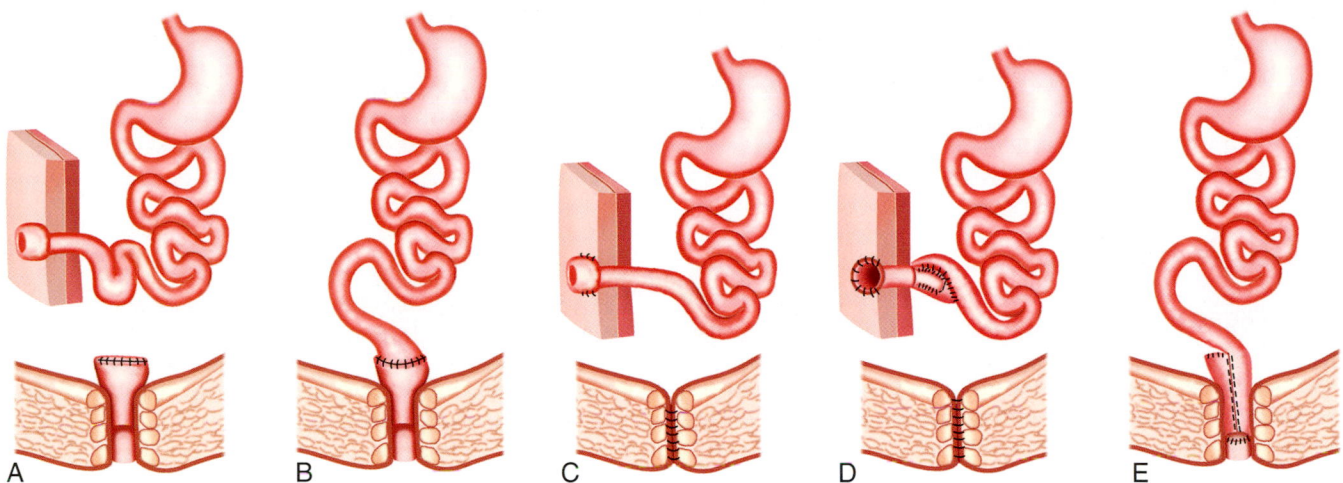

FIGURE 116-16. Schematic diagrams of various surgical options for the management of UC. *A,* Conventional (Brooke) ileostomy with a subtotal colectomy and a Hartman pouch. *B,* Subtotal colectomy with ileorectal anastomosis. *C,* Conventional (Brooke) ileostomy with a total proctocolectomy. *D,* Continent ileostomy (Koch pouch) with total proctocolectomy. *E,* Restorative proctocolectomy with ileal pouch-anal anastomosis (see Chapter 117). *(A-E, Adapted from Blumberg D, Beck DE. Surgery for ulcerative colitis. Gastroenterol Clin North Am 2002; 31:219-35.)*

technical challenges associated with this operation (e.g., slippage of the nipple valve) and the development of restorative procedures, proctocolectomy with continent ileostomy rarely is performed.

Proctocolectomy with Ileal Pouch-Anal Anastomosis

Restorative proctocolectomy with IPAA currently is the operation of choice for most patients with UC who require elective colectomy (see Chapter 117). In this procedure, the entire colon and rectum are removed, the anal sphincters are preserved, and a pouch is constructed from approximately 20 cm of the distal ileum (see Fig. 116-16). Bowel continuity is established by anastomosing this pouch with the anal canal. An IPAA usually is performed as a 2-stage operation, during the first stage of which a temporary diverting ileostomy is created to allow the ileal pouch to heal. This operation can be performed as a single-stage operation; however, there have been reports suggesting a higher rate of bowel obstruction and sepsis when this is done.[318] The ileostomy is reversed after approximately 2 to 4 months.

Proctocolectomy with IPAA presents technical challenges and might not be suitable or technically feasible for all patients. Most reports suggest satisfactory quality of life following IPAA surgery.[319] Mean stool frequency ranges from 4 to 9 bowel movements per day, including 1 or 2 nocturnal stools. Nocturnal seepage occurs in approximately 20% of patients in the early postoperative period but is infrequent after the first year.

Rates of complications following IPAA surgery vary widely. In a series from the Cleveland Clinic of more than 1000 patients undergoing restorative proctocolectomy and IPAA, most of whom had UC, the overall morbidity rate was 63% (early complications 28%, late complications 51%).[319] A larger case series from the Mayo Clinic included 1885 patients who had proctocolectomy with IPAA for UC and who were followed for up to 20 years (mean follow-up 11 years).[320] Pouch success rates were reported as 96.3%, 93.3%, 92.4%, and 92.1% by 5, 10, 15, and 20 years, respectively; however, complication rates also were high and included pouchitis (48% by 10 years, 70% by 20 years), small bowel obstruction (42% by 20 years), anastomotic stricture (39% by 20 years), abscess (16% by 20

years), and fistula (14% by 20 years), as well as pelvic sepsis. Other complications of proctocolectomy with IPAA are covered in Chapter 117 and include fecal incontinence and sexual and urinary dysfunction.

This surgery is best performed in centers with considerable experience with the operation and with managing pouch dysfunction. These high rates of complications will likely decrease over time as experience grows with this type of surgery.

A widely performed modification of proctocolectomy with IPAA is proctocolectomy with ileal pouch-anal transition zone anastomosis. This technically less complex surgery involves stapling the ileal pouch to the distal rectum in close proximity to the dentate line (1 to 4 cm), thereby eliminating the need to perform rectal mucosectomy. This type of surgery might carry a lower risk for fecal incontinence and may be performed as a single-stage operation without a temporary diverting ileostomy.

Laparoscopic approaches to the proctocolectomy with IPAA have become popular among both physicians and patients. Because this modality is relatively new, comparison data versus open proctocolectomy with IPAA are limited. A case-matched series from the Mayo Clinic, however, which included 100 consecutive laparoscopic IPAA case patients matched to 200 open IPAA control patients, reported that although the median operative time was significantly longer for the laparoscopic group by 103 minutes, laparoscopic patients had significantly improved recovery, as witnessed by lower median time to regular diet (3 vs. 5 days), time to ileostomy output (2 vs. 3 days), length of stay (4 vs. 7 days), and IV narcotic use (all P < 0.05).[321] In addition, postoperative morbidity and hospital readmission rates were similar between the 2 groups, and no mortalities were observed. Fewer patients required reoperation within 3 months with the laparoscopic approach (3% vs. 6.5%, P < 0.2). A follow-up survey in this same cohort of patients 1 year after operation showed that patients reported high cosmetic, body image, quality of life, and sexual function scores irrespective of the type of operation.[322]

A smaller randomized trial from Amsterdam of 60 patients who underwent laparoscopic or open IPAA found significantly higher operative time for the laparoscopic approach (by 77 minutes) but similar morbidity (20% vs. 17%), length of stay

(10 vs. 11 days), time to regular diet, narcotic requirement, and quality of life at 3 months after surgery in both groups.[323] Larger RCTs will need to be conducted before any definitive conclusions can be made regarding the superiority of 1 approach over another. The experience of the particular surgeon and surgical center is likely to be an important determinant of success rates irrespective of procedure.

COMPLICATIONS

Toxic Megacolon

Toxic megacolon is defined as acute colonic dilatation with a transverse colon diameter of greater than 6 cm (on radiologic examination) and loss of haustration in a patient with a severe attack of colitis.[324,325] Maximal colonic dilatation most commonly is observed in the transverse colon. This complication of UC results from extension of colonic inflammation beyond the mucosa to the underlying tissues, including the muscularis propria. Loss of contractility from the inflammatory reaction leads to the accumulation of gas and fluid within the lumen and subsequent colonic dilatation.

Toxic megacolon occurs in approximately 5% of severe flares of UC. It often is encountered early in the course of the disease and may be the initial presentation of UC. Nearly 50% of patients with toxic megacolon develop this complication within 3 months of their diagnosis.[326] Toxic megacolon usually occurs in patients with extensive colitis, but patients with disease limited to the left colon also can develop it. Precipitating factors for toxic megacolon include electrolyte imbalance (particularly hypokalemia), use of antimotility drugs including anticholinergic agents and narcotics, and procedures such as barium enema and colonoscopy performed during a severe attack.[327] These procedures should be avoided in the presence of a severe flare of UC. With clinical deterioration, patients can develop fever, tachycardia, hypotension, diffuse abdominal distention and tenderness, and decreased bowel sounds. Other laboratory parameters reflecting progressive severe systemic inflammation include marked leukocytosis, metabolic alkalosis, and electrolyte disturbances.

Medical management for toxic megacolon is directed at treating the underlying inflammation, restoring colonic motility, and preventing free colonic perforation. If colonic dilatation occurs during the initial presentation of UC, IV glucocorticoids and fluid replacement should be initiated and electrolyte abnormalities should be corrected. Reduction of fluid and air within the GI tract may be achieved through bowel rest and nasogastric decompression. Other conservative management approaches include maneuvers to reduce abdominal distention by allowing the redistribution or passage of colon gas. Gas tends to rise and fill the most superiorly located bowel segment, which is the transverse colon if the patient is in the supine position. Encouraging the patient to move about, rotating a patient who is bed-bound, using the knee-elbow position when the patient is prone, and inserting a rectal tube all have been suggested to be helpful in reducing bowel distention.[328,329]

Systemic antibiotics often are empirically administered, because mortality from toxic megacolon correlates with the development of sepsis.[330] Approximately 50% of acute dilatation resolves with medical therapy.[329,331] However, because the presence of colonic perforation is the most important predictor of mortality (44% in patients undergoing emergent colectomy after perforation compared with 2% in patients undergoing colectomy without perforation),[332] an important aspect of management is to determine the optimal time for surgical intervention. In general, patients who do not improve after 48

to 72 hours of medical therapy should undergo surgery.[329] Close clinical observation for signs of impending perforation is critical. Patients with progressive abdominal distention, development of rebound tenderness, or hemodynamic instability should undergo immediate colectomy.

For patients who achieve remission on medical therapy, subsequent management is controversial. In 1 series, nearly 50% of patients treated successfully for toxic megacolon eventually required colectomy for intractable disease.[333] Thus, some clinicians recommend elective colectomy following resolution of toxic megacolon.

Free perforation also can develop in the absence of colonic dilatation. This complication is rare, occurring in 1% of patients with UC without toxic megacolon.[331,334] Classic physical findings of peritonitis may be absent, largely because of the masking effect of administered glucocorticoids, but most patients have a marked deterioration in overall clinical condition after perforation. It is important to examine the abdomen for hepatic dullness every day in patients who have severe colitis and are taking high-dose glucocorticoids because they might have a free perforation and not have classic signs of peritonitis. A daily plain film of the abdomen also is recommended for the same purpose. As with toxic megacolon, patients with extensive colitis appear to be at greatest risk for this complication. The segment most at risk for free perforation is the sigmoid colon. The mortality associated with free perforation in UC patients without toxic megacolon has been reported to be more than 50%.[334] Thus, the possibility of free perforation must be considered in patients with fulminant UC, particularly if there is deterioration in general condition, even in the absence of colonic dilatation.

Strictures

Colonic strictures complicate UC in approximately 5% of patients, most commonly in those with extensive and long-standing colitis.[335] Patients with colonic strictures usually present with alterations in bowel habits, both constipation and diarrhea. Clinically significant obstruction is rare. Colonic strictures complicating UC typically are short (2 to 3 cm), occur distal to the splenic flexure, and represent hypertrophy and thickening of muscularis mucosa rather than fibrosis.[335]

There needs to be a high index of suspicion of malignancy in patients with colonic strictures associated with UC, especially when the strictures are located proximal to the splenic flexure.[336] One series reported malignancy in 24% of colonic strictures in patients with UC.[336] Moreover, in patients with UC, cancer associated with strictures tends to be more advanced than cancers not associated with strictures. Endoscopic appearance cannot reliably distinguish benign strictures from malignant strictures, and multiple biopsies are recommended at colonoscopy. Because carcinoma might not be detected on mucosal biopsies, surgical resection of the stricture is advised, particularly in patients with long-standing disease.

Dysplasia and Colorectal Cancer (CRC) (see Chapters 126 and 127)

Patients with UC have an increased risk of CRC. This risk depends on several factors, the most important being the duration and extent of the disease. Other risk factors include PSC, family history of CRC, age at diagnosis of disease, severity of inflammation, presence of pseudopolyps, and possibly backwash ileitis.[337-342] The incidence of CRC in UC varies depending primarily on the duration and extent of the disease and the patient population studied, but it has been estimated at approximately 7% to 10% at 20 years of disease and as high as 30% after 35 years of disease, translating to an increase of 0.5% to 1.0% per year after 8 to 10 years of disease in patients with extensive UC.[343] With respect to the cumulative risk of CRC for all UC patients (not just those with pancolitis), a recent meta-analysis of population-based cohort studies calculated a risk of less than 1% at 10 years, 0.4% to 2% at 15 years, and 1.1% to 2.5% at 20 years of follow-up; however, patients with extensive UC had a 5-fold increased risk of CRC compared with those with isolated proctitis or left-sided colitis.[344] The discovery of CRC in UC always warrants colectomy.

Although prophylactic colectomy can virtually eliminate the risk of CRC, patients often are unwilling to undergo surgery, particularly if there is no other indication for colectomy. Thus, colonoscopic surveillance programs have been developed in an effort to reduce the risk of CRC associated with UC. The primary goal of surveillance colonoscopy is to detect and potentially remove dysplasia, defined as unequivocal neoplastic epithelium, because currently it is the most important marker to detect concurrent or subsequent cancer.

Dysplasia is classified both histologically and endoscopically. Histologic assessment is classified as negative, indefinite, low-grade dysplasia (Fig. 116-17A), and high-grade dysplasia (see Fig. 116-17B). There are 2 major problems with the histologic assessment of dysplasia.[345] First, there are no gold standard criteria on how to diagnose or grade dysplasia (e.g., the number or proportion of cells or nuclei needed with

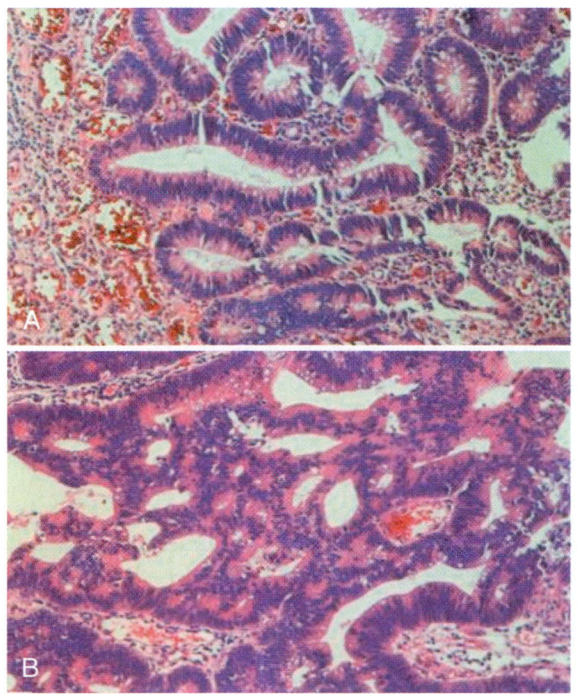

FIGURE 116-17. Photomicrograph of a colonic biopsy specimen showing the histologic features of dysplasia. *A,* Low-grade dysplasia is characterized by nuclear enlargement, crowding, and hyperchromasia in the colonic epithelial cells. Nuclei are stratified but remain in the basal half of the cells. There is some depletion of mucin. *B,* In high-grade dysplasia, the changes are more pronounced. Nuclei are stratified to the surface, and there is a marked increase in nuclear pleomorphism. Branching of the glands in a cribriform pattern and scattered cell necrosis are shown. No mucin-containing goblet cells are evident. *(Courtesy Feldman M, Boland CR, editors. Slide atlas of gastroenterology and hepatology. Philadelphia: Current Medicine; 1996.)*

certain characteristic abnormal appearances, how many crypts are needed to be involved). Second, a variety of confounding features on biopsy specimens can make the diagnosis of dysplasia challenging, including the presence of active inflammation (with its associated mucus depletion of epithelial cells and abnormal/dysplastic-appearing nuclei), serrated crypt patterns, rectal follicular inflammation, and processing issues (fixation, which enhances nuclear detail, and staining/sectioning artifacts). For these reasons, the diagnosis and grading of dysplasia by pathologists is inherently subjective, which gives rise to very low rates of interobserver agreement. This is especially true for indefinite for dysplasia and low-grade dysplasia, with overall interobserver agreement Kappa coefficients of 0.18 to 0.51 and pairwise Kappa coefficients as low as 0.06.[346-349] Even for high-grade dysplasia, interobserver agreement is low, with overall Kappa coefficients of 0.18 to 0.61.[346-348] This difficulty in diagnosing and grading dysplasia makes it very challenging to interpret studies that evaluate the risk of progression to cancer by grade of dysplasia, as the certainty of the underlying dysplasia diagnosis and grade must be called into question.

Endoscopically, dysplasia is best classified as invisible or visible. Invisible dysplasia is almost always characterized by flat lesions; visible dysplasia can manifest as a variety of forms, including raised lesions, such as polypoid lesions or masses, flat lesions, such as plaques, irregular mucosa, ulcers, or inverted lesions, or strictures.[350-352] Historically, it had been thought that flat dysplasia represented most of the dysplasia detected in patients with UC. However, 3 small retrospective case series have suggested that a surprising proportion of dysplastic or cancerous lesions may be visible on standard white-light colonoscopy.[350-352] In the past, visible dysplastic lesions in UC were distinguished based on whether they occurred in non-colitic mucosa (sporadic adenoma) or colitic mucosa (dyplasia-associated lesion or mass [DALM]). At one time, it was thought that the presence of DALMs was associated with higher risks of CRC and therefore, colectomy was recommended in patients with DALMs. Later, DALMs were classified as being adenoma-like (regular margins, easy to remove) or non-adenoma-like (irregular more sessile masses that were either difficult or unable to be removed endoscopically). Today, however, the most important issue regarding visible dysplasia is whether the lesion can be removed in its entirety endoscopically, irrespective of location (colitic vs. non-colitic mucosa) or appearance (irregular vs. regular margins, raised vs. sessile). Also, the term *DALM* has fallen out of favor given the historically heterogeneous group of dysplastic lesions that have been assigned that name.

A number of studies have demonstrated that if visible lesions can be removed safely, rates of subsequent CRC or high-grade dysplasia are very low and thus continued colonoscopic surveillance can be performed without need for colectomy.[353-357] A study from the United States of 34 patients with 38 adenoma-like DALMs or sporadic adenomas removed endoscopically with no coexistent invisible flat dysplasia reported that no patients subsequently developed invisible flat dyplasia or CRC after follow-up of 7 to 156 months.[353,354] A similar study that evaluated 48 patients with 70 adenoma-like DALMs or sporadic adenomas removed endoscopically with no coexistent invisible flat dysplasia reported that no patients subsequently developed invisible flat dyplasia or CRC after follow-up of 0.8 to 9.6 months.[355] A German study, in which 87 patients had endoscopic removal of adenoma-like DALMs or sporadic adenomas but 60 patients had these lesions left unremoved, observed a subsequent 5% rate of low-grade dysplasia and 2.3% rate of CRC in patients whose lesions were removed but a 23%, 13%, and 17% rate of low-grade dysplasia, high-grade dysplasia, and CRC, respectively, in patients whose visible lesions were not removed, thus suggesting that not only is endoscopic removal safe and can spare colectomy, but that it should be done whenever possible for visible lesions.[356] A study from the United Kingdom of 112 patients with 135 flat and raised DALMs revealed that flat/depressed lesions or large irregular sessile lesions, which accounted for 89 of the 135 lesions, if able to be removed endoscopically, did not warrant colectomy, as no patient developed further dysplasia after a follow-up of 3.6 to 5.1 years.[357] For patients with visible lesions that cannot be removed endoscopically, colectomy should be recommended.

With respect to invisible flat dysplasia, classification into high-grade dysplasia, multifocal low-grade dysplasia, and unifocal low-grade dysplasia is usually done for prognostic reasons that are useful. A systematic review of 10 surveillance studies of 1225 patients reported that 10 (42%) of 24 patients with high-grade dysplasia who underwent immediate colectomy had synchronous cancer, and 15 (32%) of 47 patients who were found to have high-grade dysplasia after an initially normal colonoscopy subsequently were found to have cancer.[358] Thus, the presence of high-grade dysplasia appears to be highly predictive of concurrent or subsequent CRC, and colectomy is recommended for these patients. For patients with multifocal low-grade dysplasia, colectomy is also typically recommended, although there is a paucity of data on this. A recent prospective study of 42 patients with low-grade dysplasia who were followed endoscopically observed that the presence of 3 or more biopsies with low-grade dysplasia was associated with a significant 6-fold increased risk of progression to high-grade dysplasia or CRC and that the risk of progression may increase with even 2 biopsies showing low-grade dysplasia, after a mean of 3.9 years of follow-up.[359]

Recommendations are much less clear for the case of invisible flat unifocal low-grade dysplasia, as the predictive value of low-grade dysplasia for the development of more advanced lesions varies widely among studies. To date, more than 20 studies evaluating the risk of CRC, high-grade dysplasia, or both, in patients with low-grade dysplasia have been performed and have reached different conclusions. A meta-analysis of 20 studies published through July 2005 included 508 patients with low-grade dysplasia out of more than 2677 patients with UC who were enrolled in a CRC surveillance program and calculated an incidence rates of 1.4% and 3% per person per year of CRC or any advanced lesion, respectively, after a diagnosis of low-grade dysplasia.[360] Even though the pooled rates of progression of low-grade dysplasia are low, some studies report very high rates of synchronous or subsequent high-grade dysplasia or cancer, while others demonstrate exceedingly low rates. For instance, a study from the United States found that in 46 UC patients with flat low-grade dysplasia on surveillance colonoscopy, unexpected advanced neoplasia occurred in 4 (24%) of 17 patients who underwent immediate colectomy, and 5 additional cases of cancer at stage II or higher occurred despite surveillance examinations.[361] These results are in great contrast to 2 European studies, 1 of which reported that 10% of patients with low-grade dysplasia developed subsequent CRC after a mean follow-up of 10 years,[349] while the other observed that only 3.3% of patients developed high-grade dysplasia and none developed CRC after a mean follow-up of 10 years.[362] Thus, the risk of progression to advanced neoplasia after finding low-grade dysplasia is uncertain, and both options of continued surveillance or colectomy are reasonable. Treating physicians should present these data to their patients so that the patients can make the best choice for themselves. Other factors that should be taken into consideration include age, duration of disease, severity and course of disease, coexistent PSC, family history of CRC, and presence of comorbidities.

When doing surveillance colonoscopy, most authorities recommend colonoscopy with biopsies every 1 to 3 years in patients who have UC extending beyond the rectum and who have had disease for 8 to 10 years.[363,364] Colonoscopic examination with biopsies should be performed during periods of inactive disease so as not to allow inflammation and reactive change to be potentially confused with dysplasia. Four-quadrant biopsies should be obtained every 10 cm throughout the colon, and targeted biopsies should be obtained from any raised or potentially dysplastic lesions. Thus, performing proper surveillance requires extensive biopsies. In fact, it has been estimated that 33 biopsies are required to achieve a 90% probability of identifying dysplasia or cancer if it is present, and 64 biopsies are necessary to exclude dysplasia or cancer with 95% certainty.[365] Unfortunately, data from questionnaire surveys show that many fewer biopsies are obtained in routine clinical practice.[366,367] For patients with unifocal invisible flat dysplasia who elect to pursue continued surveillance rather than colectomy, more frequent surveillance (at least yearly) is recommended, although the frequency has not been standardized (e.g., every 3 to 6 months for the first year).

Colonoscopic surveillance is fraught with many potential pitfalls, including sampling error, interobserver variability for determining dysplasia, and difficulty detecting and differentiating dysplastic lesions from other lesions. Thus, techniques have been developed to enhance the diagnostic accuracy of surveillance colonoscopy in patients with UC. These techniques include the use of magnifying colonoscopy combined with either chromoendoscopy, in which tissue stains are applied to the GI mucosal surface at endoscopy to better enhance or characterize specific findings,[368-370] or narrow band imaging (NBI), which uses short wavelengths of the Hgb absorption bands to enhance mucosal vasculature and surface contrast.[371,372] These techniques do not currently represent the standard of practice. The use of magnification and chromoendoscopy as an adjunct to conventional colonoscopy has been shown, in comparison with conventional colonoscopy, to increase the rate of detecting dysplasia with a sensitivity and specificity of 93% for differentiating neoplastic and non-neoplastic lesions.[368] The use of NBI for detecting dysplasia in UC is still in its preliminary stages because it is unclear exactly which vascular patterns are associated with dysplasia. It is also unclear whether these alternative techniques will prove to be superior to high-definition white light colonoscopy (which is the current standard of care for polyp detection) for the detection of dysplasia.

In addition, research has investigated the use of molecular, genetic, and immunohistochemical markers to enhance diagnostic accuracy of colitis-associated dysplasia. Although sporadic CRC and IBD-associated malignancy follow a similar pathway from dysplasia to carcinoma,[373] studies have shown differences in the prevalence and timing of certain molecular events between these 2 neoplastic groups. Some of these differences in colitis-associated dysplasia include infrequent and late mutations in the APC and β-catenin genes, more frequent and early abnormalities in the 3p (von Hippel-Lindau) gene locus, p53, and p16 loci, and higher prevalence of Sialyl-Tn antigen expression.[374-381]

Another potential strategy to reduce the risk of CRC in UC is medical chemoprevention. Three different medications have shown promise in this regard and include folic acid, 5-ASAs, and ursodeoxycholic acid. The results of 2 observational studies examining the effects of folate have been published, both of which showed that folate supplementation was associated with a nonsignificant reduction in risk of dysplasia or CRC[382,383]; 5-ASAs have been studied more extensively in this regard. A meta-analysis of 9 studies (3 cohort and 6 case-control studies) totaling 1932 patients, and including 334 cases of CRC and 140 cases of dysplasia, showed a significant protective effect of 5-ASAs for the prevention of CRC (pooled OR, 0.51; 95% CI, 0.37 to 0.69) and CRC or dysplasia (pooled OR, 0.51; 95% CI, 0.38 to 0.69).[384] Two studies have shown that ursodeoxycholic acid might have significant benefit for preventing neoplasia in patients with UC and PSC.[385,386]

Even though proctocolectomy with IPAA is the most efficient way to prevent dysplasia and CRC in UC, there is still a potential risk of dysplasia or cancer to develop in the rectal cuff-anal transition zone and even in the ileal pouch. Since 1990, there have been at least 14 reported cases of cancer arising in the anorectal mucosa and 9 cases of cancer in the pouch.[387,388] A recent systematic review of 23 uncontrolled observational studies (most of which were retrospective case series), including a total of 2040 patients in whom no cancers were found, reported a pooled prevalence rate of 1.13% for dysplasia in the anorectal mucosa or pouch, with roughly equal prevalence in the anorectal mucosa and the pouch.[387] The authors noticed that dysplasia and cancer identified preoperatively or during surgery were significant predictors of the development of dysplasia, whereas pouchitis and length of follow-up were not. Currently, no guidelines exist for endoscopic surveillance after IPAA, but given that dysplasia and/or cancer can occur in the residual anorectal mucosa and pouch, periodic endoscopy with biopsy should be considered, especially in patients with a prior history of colonic dysplasia or cancer.

Pouchitis

Pouchitis is the most common long-term complication of colectomy with IPAA for UC (see Chapter 117) but, curiously, it is rarely seen in patients undergoing the same surgery for familial adenomatous polyposis. Pouchitis is said to occur when there is nonspecific inflammation of the ileal reservoir, resulting in variable clinical symptoms resembling those of UC. Pouchitis occurs in 7% to 51% of patients undergoing restorative proctocolectomy for UC.[389,390] The incidence is highest during the first 6 months after loop ileostomy closure.

Pathophysiology

The pathophysiology of pouchitis is not well understood but is likely multifactorial. Several etiologic mechanisms have been postulated including fecal stasis with bacterial overgrowth, recurrent UC following colonic metaplasia of the ileal epithelial cells of the pouch, CD, mucosal ischemia, and viral infection; another postulated mechanism is an ongoing immune process that may be recurrent UC, misdiagnosed CD, or an overlap or other form of IBD.[391,392]

Symptoms and Signs

Characteristic symptoms of pouchitis include increased bowel frequency, rectal bleeding, abdominal cramping, rectal urgency, tenesmus, and fecal incontinence.[393] Other associated symptoms are fever, malaise, arthralgias, and erythema nodosum. Endoscopic evaluation, which is essential to distinguish pouchitis from cuffitis (continued rectal cuff inflammation due to UC), CD in the small bowel, or irritable pouch syndrome (a condition of increased small bowel motility in the absence of mucosal abnormalities), may reveal mucosal erythema, edema, granularity, friability, petechiae, loss of vascular pattern, erosions, and superficial ulcerations. Deep and irregularly shaped ulcers similar to those seen in CD may be present. Histologically, pouchitis is marked by an acute inflammatory infiltrate with mucosal ulceration and crypt abscesses in addition to chronic inflammation, villus atrophy, and crypt hyperplasia. Similar to UC, the diagnosis of pouchitis is based on a constellation of clinical symptoms, endoscopic appearances, and histologic features.[393,394]

There appear to be 2 distinct clinical forms of pouchitis, acute pouchitis and chronic pouchitis. Acute pouchitis is defined by symptom duration of less than 4 weeks and prompt response to antibiotics (also classified as antibiotic-responsive), and chronic pouchitis is defined by symptom duration more than 4 weeks and need for long-term antibiotics or other therapeutic agents (also classified as antibiotic-dependent or antibiotic-refractory).[392,394] More than 20% of patients have chronic continuous symptoms, but less than 10% have severe chronic pouchitis requiring long-term maintenance therapy.[390]

Risk Factors

A number of studies examining risk factors for pouchitis have been performed. Unfortunately, many of these studies were based in referral centers, were retrospective, and had relatively short follow-up periods; they also did not distinguish acute pouchitis and chronic pouchitis, which at present seem to be very different disease entities. As a result, it should not come as a surprise that these studies identified different risk factors for developing pouchitis, with only a few studies agreeing on the same risk factors. Among these studies, risk factors for pouchitis that have been variably identified include the presence of extraintestinal manifestations and especially PSC, smoking, use of NSAIDs, various serologic markers, and preoperative thrombocytosis.

Acute versus Chronic Pouchitis

There is growing evidence that acute pouchitis and chronic pouchitis are distinct disease entities. For instance, fecal stasis with bacterial overgrowth presumably occurs in the pouch after IPAA in all UC patients,[395,396] yet only some develop acute pouchitis or chronic pouchitis. Also, chronic pouchitis typically appears sooner after stoma closure than does acute pouchitis.[397,398] In addition, the serologic profiles associated with acute pouchitis and chronic pouchitis seem to be different.[56,398-400] Finally, patients with acute pouchitis appear to react to endoluminal antigens only transiently, whereas those with chronic pouchitis have more persistent inflammation.

Two prospective studies from Cedars-Sinai Medical Center have examined risk factors for acute pouchitis and chronic pouchitis separately in the same group of patients.[398,400] The first study, which examined clinical risk factors for developing pouchitis, found that preoperative use of glucocorticoids and smoking were independently associated with the development of acute pouchitis, whereas extraintestinal manifestations, preoperative thrombocytosis, and increased length of follow-up were independently associated with the development of chronic pouchitis on multivariate analysis.[398] Interestingly, smoking was found to be significantly protective against the development of chronic pouchitis on multivariate analysis, thus again supporting the concept that acute pouchitis and chronic pouchitis may be distinct disease entities.

The second study, with longer follow-up, followed 238 patients for a median of 47 months (range, 3 to 142 months) and reported incidence rates of acute pouchitis and chronic pouchitis of 18% and 12%, respectively.[400] Although the median time to the diagnosis of chronic pouchitis was shorter than that for acute pouchitis (6 vs. 9 months), these differences did not attain statistical significance. The second study also looked at serologic profiles, specifically the presence or absence of pANCA or anti-CBir1 antibodies and the risk of pouchitis, and found that both antibodies were seen significantly more often in patients who developed pouchitis.[398] In addition, because the authors previously had shown that high pANCA levels (>100 U/mL) were associated with the development of chronic pouchitis but not acute pouchitis, they stratified the pANCA+ patients into high-level and low-level pANCA+ groups and found that acute pouchitis occurred with the same frequency in patients with high-level versus low-level pANCA expression, whereas chronic pouchitis occurred significantly more often in patients with high-level pANCA seroreactivity, thus confirming the results from their prior study. They also observed that anti-CBir1 expression influenced the onset of acute pouchitis only in patients with low-level pANCA expression, and the onset of chronic pouchitis only in patients with high-level pANCA expression.

Treatment

The mainstay of therapy for pouchitis is antibiotics. In 1 of the few placebo-controlled trials of antibiotics for the treatment of chronic active pouchitis, metronidazole at 1200 mg/day for 1 week resulted in an overall response rate of 73% compared with 9% for placebo.[401] Ciprofloxacin at 1 g/day for 2 weeks also is effective for the treatment of acute pouchitis and has been shown to be superior to metronidazole in efficacy and tolerability in an RCT.[402] Alternative regimens include topical metronidazole, amoxicillin/clavulanic acid, and combinations of ciprofloxacin with metronidazole, rifaximin, and tinidazole.[403-407] For patients on chronic therapy, cycling of multiple antibiotics at weekly intervals might help overcome bacterial resistance.

The second-line options for treating pouchitis include topical and oral mesalamines,[394,408] although the use of these agents is based on uncontrolled studies and anecdotal experiences. Topical and systemic glucocorticoids, including topical and oral budesonide, can be used for patients with pouchitis who do not respond to antibiotics and mesalamines.[409,410] Immunosuppressive and biological therapies, including cyclosporine enemas, azathioprine, infliximab, and adalimumab, also have been reported to be beneficial and may be considered in patients whose pouchitis is refractory to conventional therapies.[411,412]

Probiotic therapy is another option. The majority of data regarding the use of probiotics for pouchitis involves VSL#3. Three randomized placebo-controlled trials of VSL#3 for either primary (one study) or secondary (2 studies) prophylaxis of pouchitis showed significant benefit with the probiotic.[413-415] An open-label study from the Cleveland Clinic, however, showed that VSL#3 was ineffective for secondary prophylaxis of pouchitis.[416] Thus, it remains unclear whether probiotics are beneficial in patients with pouchitis, and larger randomized studies are needed to help resolve this issue. Two small studies have suggested a possible benefit of prebiotics (inulin) or synbiotics (probiotic *L. rhamnosus* GG combined with prebiotic fructo-oligosaccharide) for managing pouchitis.[417,418] Larger randomized studies are needed before any recommendations can be made regarding the use of these agents in pouchitis.

Other nonconventional therapies include nutritional replacement using known energy substrates for the bowel and bismuth carbomer enema. Bismuth has been used to treat pouchitis with varying results. Although an open-label study reported benefit of bismuth carbomer enemas in patients with chronic pouchitis,[419] a placebo-controlled study failed to show benefit.[420] Another uncontrolled study reported improvement in patients with chronic pouchitis treated with chewable bismuth subsalicylate tablets,[421] but this finding has not been confirmed in controlled trials. In the only randomized comparison of glutamine and butyrate suppositories in patients with chronic pouchitis after withdrawal of all conventional therapies, 60% of patients treated with glutamine 1 g twice daily for 3 weeks entered remission compared with 33% of patients receiving butyrate 40 mmol twice daily.[422]

Surgical options such as ileal pouch excision or reconstruction should be considered in cases refractory to medical therapies or cases in which the frequency or chronicity of pouchitis compromises the patient's quality of life.[423]

EXTRAINTESTINAL MANIFESTATIONS

Patients with UC commonly present with a wide range of systemic and local problems that can add to the complexity of treatment. These extraintestinal manifestations can affect any organ system, but they most commonly involve the skin, eyes, mouth, joints, and liver (Box 116-10). These complications often are classified by their relations to the activity of the colitis, but they can occur before, during, or following exacerbations of bowel disease. Manifestations that parallel disease activity usually improve upon successful treatment of the colitis.

BOX 116-10 Common Extraintestinal Manifestations of UC

Cutaneous/Oral
Angular stomatitis
Aphthous stomatitis
Erythema nodosum
Oral ulcerations
Psoriasis
Pyoderma gangrenosum
Pyostomatitis vegetans
Sweet's syndrome (acute febrile neutrophilic dermatosis)

Ophthalmologic
Conjunctivitis
Episcleritis
Retinal vascular disease
Scleritis
Uveitis, iritis

Musculoskeletal
Ankylosing spondylitis
Osteomalacia
Osteonecrosis
Osteopenia
Osteoporosis
Peripheral arthropathy
Sacroiliitis

Hepatobiliary
Autoimmune hepatitis
Cholangiocarcinoma
Pericholangitis
PSC
Hepatic steatosis

Hematologic
Anemia of chronic disease
Autoimmune hemolytic anemia
Hypercoagulable state
Iron deficiency anemia
Leukocytosis or thrombocytosis
Leukopenia or thrombocytopenia

Cutaneous/Oral

The most common dermatologic manifestations of UC are complications of drug treatment. These include hypersensitivity, photosensitivity, and urticarial rashes related to sulfasalazine and less commonly to mesalamine. Patients receiving glucocorticoids often develop acne, which can be distressing cosmetically. Other common dermatologic manifestations associated with UC are erythema nodosum and pyoderma gangrenosum.

Erythema nodosum occurs in 2% to 4% of patients with UC. Its activity typically parallels the activity of the underlying bowel disease. Erythema nodosum also can occur as a drug reaction to the sulfapyridine component of sulfasalazine. It classically manifests as single or multiple tender, raised, erythematous nodules on the extensor surfaces of the lower extremities. If possible, the diagnosis should be made clinically without biopsy, because biopsy is associated with increased tendency to form scars. Erythema nodosum usually responds to treatment of the UC. Severe or refractory cases can require systemic glucocorticoids or immunosuppressive therapy.

Pyoderma gangrenosum is less common than erythema nodosum and occurs in 1% to 2% of patients. It usually is related to the activity of colitis but can manifest or persist despite inactive bowel disease. Lesions may be single or multiple and usually occur on the trunk or extremities but can develop on the face, breast, or sites of trauma, including stoma and IV sites.[424] The classic lesion begins as erythematous pustules or nodules that break down, ulcerate, and coalesce into a larger, tender, burrowing ulcer with irregular, violaceous edges.[425] Although the appearance can be dramatic, the ulcers are sterile. Histopathologically, pyoderma has the features of a sterile abscess with a marked neutrophilic infiltration. Pyoderma gangrenosum can resolve with treatment of the underlying colitis. Most cases usually respond to intralesional glucocorticoid injections or topical therapy with cromolyn sodium, mesalamine, glucocorticoids, or tacrolimus.[425-427] More severe cases can require systemic glucocorticoids, immunosuppressants (e.g., cyclosporine, azathioprine, methotrexate, and tacrolimus), dapsone, or anti-TNF therapy (e.g., infliximab).[428,429]

Less common skin manifestations associated with UC include Sweet's syndrome (acute febrile neutrophilic dermatosis), and pyodermite végétante of Hallopeau. The latter has a presentation similar to that of pyoderma gangrenosum but also involves the mouth.

At least 10% of patients with UC develop oral aphthous ulcers. These lesions usually occur with flares of colitis and resolve on control of the bowel disease. Angular stomatitis and a sore tongue may be seen in patients with deficiencies of iron, B vitamins, or other micronutrients (see Chapter 103). A rare oral lesion that may be seen in patients with UC is pyostomatitis (pyoderma) vegetans, which appears as a pustular eruption of the oral mucosa resulting in a cobblestone appearance.[430]

Ophthalmologic

The 2 most common ocular manifestations associated with UC are episcleritis and uveitis, occurring in 5% to 8% of patients. Episcleritis is characterized by painless hyperemia of the sclera and conjunctiva without loss of vision. It typically parallels the activity of bowel disease and usually responds to anti-inflammatory therapy. In contrast, uveitis presents as an acute or subacute painful eye with visual blurring often accompanied by photophobia and headache. Temporal correlation of uveitis with the activity of the colitis is less predictable than with episcleritis. Patients with uveitis should receive prompt ophthalmologic consultation and treatment with local glucocorticoid ocular drops to prevent progression to blindness. The occurrence of uveitis increases with the dose and duration of glucocorticoid use. Glucocorticoid therapy also can lead to posterior subcapsular cataracts. Thus, patients receiving glucocorticoid therapy should be advised to undergo annual ophthalmologic examination.

Musculoskeletal

Musculoskeletal abnormalities associated with UC can be grouped broadly into rheumatologic disorders and metabolic bone diseases.

Peripheral Arthropathy

Peripheral arthropathy occurs in 5% to 20% of patients with UC. The risk of arthropathy increases with the extent of colonic disease. Peripheral arthropathy can be classified into 2 distinct types (Table 116-8).[431] Type 1 is asymmetrical and pauciarticular, affecting fewer than 5 joints and typically involving the large joints (knees, elbows, ankles). It usually manifests with acute, self-limited episodes that parallel the underlying bowel disease activity. Type 2 arthropathy is symmetrical and polyarticular, affecting 5 or more joints and typically involving the small joints. This type manifests with persistent symptoms independent of the colitis activity. Both forms are nondeforming and seronegative. The involved joints are swollen, erythematous, and hot. Peripheral arthropathy usually responds to treatment of colitis. Rest, physical therapy, intra-articular glucocorticoid injection, and therapeutic arthrocentesis also can help control symptoms.

Axial Arthropathy

Axial arthropathy occurs less often than does peripheral arthropathy in patients with UC and includes sacroiliitis and spondylitis.

Isolated sacroiliitis occurs in 10% to 15% of patients, but the incidence may be higher based on MRI. It usually does not parallel the activity of the bowel disease. The typical symptom is low back pain, but some patients are asymptomatic. Most

TABLE 116-8 Types of Peripheral Arthropathy Associated with UC

Feature	Type 1 (Pauciarticular)	Type 2 (Polyarticular)
Characteristics		
Frequency	35%	24%
Duration of attacks	<10 wk (median, 5 wk)	Months to years (median, 3 yr)
Association with bowel disease activity	Parallel	Independent
Joints Affected		
Number	<5	≥5
Type	Mainly large joints	Mainly small joints
Prevalence	Knee > ankle > wrist > elbow > MCP > hip > shoulder	MCP > knee > PIP > wrist > ankle > elbow > shoulder

MCP, metacarpophalangeal joint; PIP, proximal interphalangeal joint.
Adapted from Su C, Judge TA, Lichtenstein GR. Extraintestinal manifestations of inflammatory bowel disease. Gastroenterol Clin North Am 2002; 31:307-27.

patients with sacroiliitis are HLA-B27 negative and do not progress to ankylosing spondylitis.

Ankylosing spondylitis occurs in 1% to 2% of patients with UC, and most of these patients are HLA-B27 positive. Symptoms of ankylosing spondylitis can appear long before or after the onset of the intestinal symptoms and are independent of the activity of colitis. Patients often experience onset of severe back pain at a young age, usually associated with morning stiffness and exacerbated by periods of rest. The course of ankylosing spondylitis is progressive, resulting in permanent skeletal damage. Radiologic films in early stages may be normal or show only minimal sclerosis. Advanced stages are characterized by a bamboo spine, with squaring of vertebral bodies, bony proliferation, and ankylosis.

Treatment of axial arthropathy is similar to that for peripheral arthropathy, except that control of the underlying colitis does not alter the progressive nature of ankylosing spondylitis. Clinical success with anti-TNF therapy has been reported, with significant improvements in pain scales, range of motion, physical function, and overall quality of life.[432]

Low Bone Mineral Density

Patients with UC can develop low bone mineral density owing to several factors, including glucocorticoid therapy, low physical activity, and possibly inflammatory cytokines. In general, patients with UC who have not been treated with glucocorticoids are not considered to be at increased risk for osteopenia or osteoporosis. Bone densitometry (dual-energy x-ray absorptiometry [DEXA] scan) at 1- to 2-year intervals is recommended for patients who have received glucocorticoids at high doses or for a long duration.

Osteonecrosis, also known as *avascular or aseptic necrosis of bone* or *osteochondritis dissecans,* is a less common but serious complication in patients with UC. Patients typically present with joint swelling and pain exacerbated by motion. Most cases involve the hips and are bilateral, but the knees and shoulders may be affected. The most important risk factor for osteonecrosis is glucocorticoid therapy, with 1 series reporting a 4% incidence of osteonecrosis within 6 months of glucocorticoid therapy in patients with IBD[433]; concurrent use of total parenteral nutrition is another risk factor. Early diagnosis by MRI or bone scan is essential for proper treatment, including medical management, cortical decompression, and arthroplasty.

Management of decreased bone density includes calcium (typically calcium citrate at 500 mg 3 times daily) and vitamin D supplementation (at 1000 IU daily) initially. It also is useful to check a 25-OH-D (vitamin D_2) level initially to determine if a higher dose of vitamin D is needed. The addition of bisphosphonates should be considered for worsening osteopenia or osteoporosis.

Hepatobiliary

A wide range of hepatobiliary complications is associated with UC. Mild elevations in serum aminotransferase and alkaline phosphatase levels are common in severe attacks of UC. In most cases, serum enzyme levels return to normal once remission is achieved. These abnormalities are thought to be related to a combination of factors, including malnutrition, sepsis, and fatty liver. An excess of fat in the hepatocytes is found in 60% of patients who undergo urgent colectomy for severe colitis.

The most important hepatobiliary complication associated with UC is PSC, which occurs in approximately 3% of patients (see Chapter 68). PSC is a chronic inflammatory disease of the biliary tree resulting in fibrosis and, eventually, cirrhosis and hepatic failure. Intrahepatic or extrahepatic ducts (or both) may be involved. PSC is characterized radiologically by beading, irregularity, and stricturing of the bile ducts. The diagnosis of PSC is made on either endoscopic retrograde cholangiography or MR cholangiography. A liver biopsy might support the diagnosis but rarely is diagnostic. The classic histopathology of PSC on liver biopsy is the onion skin pattern, with concentric fibrosis around the small bile ducts and, ultimately, obliteration of the ducts. The histologic appearance can be variable, however, ranging from chronic inflammatory infiltration in the portal tracts to cirrhosis.

PSC should be excluded in patients with UC who have persistently abnormal liver biochemical tests or evidence of chronic liver disease. PSC is independent of the underlying colitis, and it usually follows a progressive course after many years of stable disease. However, there appears to be an interesting interaction between UC and PSC in which UC patients with PSC tend to have a higher incidence of pancolitis and possibly rectal sparing and backwash ileitis than UC patients without PSC.[434-436] In addition, the presence of PSC seems to dampen the inflammation in UC such that patients with UC and PSC tend to have a more clinically quiescent colitis than do UC patients without PSC.[434-436] In fact, the course of UC seems to worsen after liver transplantation for PSC.[437,438] Furthermore, a recent study discovered that the severity of PSC modulates the UC inflammation such that patients with severe PSC who undergo liver transplantation had an even milder course of UC prior to transplantation than those whose PSC is less severe and not requiring liver transplantation.[439] However, even if the colitis is less severe in UC patients with PSC, they are at a significantly increased risk for colorectal dysplasia and cancer.[440] Also interesting is the observation that the presence of an inflamed colon is important for the development of PSC, as several studies have shown that UC patients who do not undergo colectomy have higher rates of PSC recurrence after liver transplantation than those who have a colectomy before or during liver transplantation.[441-443]

Unfortunately, no medical treatment has been shown definitively to be effective for PSC. Ursodeoxycholic acid does not slow disease progression. Patients with a dominant extrahepatic biliary stricture can benefit from endoscopic dilatation or stent placement. Patients who develop end-stage liver disease require liver transplantation. PSC also places patients at increased risk for cholangiocarcinoma.

Hematologic

Hypercoagulability

The occurrence of hypercoagulability is a well-recognized complication of UC. The incidence of thromboembolic events in patients with UC varies widely in different studies, but most commonly they manifest as deep venous thrombosis or pulmonary embolism. Renal artery thrombosis, cerebrovascular accidents, coronary artery thrombosis, and venous thrombosis of mesenteric, portal, and hepatic vessels all have been reported.[444-446]

The cause of the thromboembolism is multifactorial. Physiologically, microvascular activation of coagulation is present in the inflammatory states of colitis. A variety of coagulation and platelet abnormalities are present in patients with UC, particularly those with severe disease, and include thrombocytosis; increased levels of fibrinogen, coagulation factors V and VIII, and plasminogen activator inhibitor; and decreased levels of antithrombin III, proteins C and S, factor V Leiden, and tissue plasminogen activator. Although there is no increased incidence of specific coagulation abnormalities in patients with UC, there may be an increased incidence of factor V Leiden mutation in patients with thromboembolic complications associated with UC.[447-449]

Patients with these complications should be treated with anticoagulants, just as in other patient populations. Although there may be concerns of an increased risk of GI bleeding with anticoagulation, it generally is safe and rarely is complicated by colonic bleeding.

Anemia

Another common hematologic complication is anemia. The anemia in patients with UC may be a result of acute or chronic GI blood loss, chronic disease, folate deficiency from sulfasalazine therapy, or autoimmune hemolysis. Autoimmune hemolytic anemia, usually Coombs positive, may be related to sepsis or glucose-6-phosphate dehydrogenase deficiency in patients taking sulfasalazine.

Others

Secondary systemic amyloidosis is a rare but serious complication associated with UC.[450] Amyloidosis in these patients usually affects the kidney and manifests with proteinuria followed by the nephrotic syndrome and subsequent renal insufficiency. Diagnosis is made with a fat pad aspiration or alternatively, biopsies from the liver, rectum, stomach, or kidney. Pericarditis, pleuropericarditis, and constrictive pericarditis have been reported in patients with UC[451-454] and also may be related to mesalamine therapy.[455,456] The pathogenesis of these complications is unknown, and their true association with UC is uncertain. Patients with UC can also develop abnormalities in pulmonary function, including a decrease in functional reserve capacity and diffusion capacity.[457] Other pulmonary diseases that have been described in patients with UC include bronchiectasis, bronchiolitis, fibrosing alveolitis, pulmonary fibrosis, and pulmonary vasculitis.[458-460]

KEY REFERENCES

Full references for this chapter can be found on www.expertconsult.com.

5. Cosnes J, Gower-Rousseau C, Seksik P, et al. Epidemiology and natural history of inflammatory bowel diseases. Gastroenterology 2011; 140:1785-94.
7. Molodecky NA, Soon IS, Rabi DM, et al. Increasing incidence and prevalence of the inflammatory bowel disease with time, based on systematic review. Gastroenterology 2012; 142:46-54.
26. Jostins L, Ripke S, Weersma RK, et al. Host-microbe interactions have shaped the genetic architecture of inflammatory bowel disease. Nature 2012; 491:119-24.
38. Frank DN, St. Amand AL, Feldman RA, et al. Molecular-phylogenetic characterization of microbial community imbalances in human inflammatory bowel diseases. Proc Natl Acad Sci U S A 2007; 104:13780-5.
39. Sartor RB. Microbial influences in inflammatory bowel diseases. Gastroenterology 2008; 134:577-94.
52. Prideaux L, De Cruz P, Ng SC, et al. Serological antibodies in inflammatory bowel disease: A systematic review. Inflamm Bowel Dis 2012; 18:1340-55.
61. Shih DQ, Targan SR. Immunopathogenesis of inflammatory bowel disease. World J Gastroenterol 2008; 14:390-400.
139. Sutherland L, MacDonald JK. Oral 5-aminosalicylic acid for induction of remission in ulcerative colitis. Cochrane Database Syst Rev 2006; CD000543.
150. Sutherland L, Macdonald JK. Oral 5-aminosalicylic acid for maintenance of remission in ulcerative colitis. Cochrane Database Syst Rev 2006; CD000544.
219. Kandiel A, Fraser AG, Korelitz BI, et al. Increased risk of lymphoma among inflammatory bowel disease patients treated with azathioprine and 6-mercaptopurine. Gut 2005; 54:1121-5.
242. Rutgeerts P, Sandborn WJ, Feagan BG, et al. Infliximab for induction and maintenance therapy for ulcerative colitis. N Engl Med J 2005; 353:2462-76.
243. Laharie D, Bourreille A, Branche J, et al. Ciclosporin versus infliximab in patients with severe ulcerative colitis refractory to intravenous steroids: A parallel, open-label randomised controlled trial. Lancet 2012; 380:1909-15.
245. Sandborn WJ, van Assche G, Reinisch W, et al. Adalimumab induces and maintains clinical remission in patients with moderate-to-severe ulcerative colitis. Gastroenterology 2012; 142:257-65.
320. Hahnloser D, Pemberton JH, Wolff BG, et al. Results at up to 20 years after ileal pouch–anal anastomosis for chronic ulcerative colitis. Br J Surg 2007; 94:333-40.
360. Thomas T, Abrams KA, Robinson RJ, et al. Meta-analysis: Cancer risk of low-grade dysplasia in chronic ulcerative colitis. Aliment Pharmacol Ther 2007; 25:657-68.

117

Ileostomy, Colostomy, and Pouches*

FARSHID ARAGHIZADEH

Total proctocolectomy with permanent ileostomy is curative for patients with UC and returns most patients to excellent health while removing premalignant mucosa in patients with UC or familial adenomatous polyposis (FAP). Improvements in surgical techniques and a better understanding of stomal physiology, along with better stoma appliances and improved patient education, have eliminated many of the dangers and disadvantages previously associated with an ileostomy.[1]

Frequent mechanical complications secondary to ileostomy dysfunction (e.g., partial obstruction), as well as the metabolic consequences of ileal stomas, became apparent in the 1940s as ileostomies were increasingly constructed.[2,3] Before advances in postoperative fluid and electrolyte management and development of newer techniques in ileostomy construction, ileostomies were made by exteriorizing the intestine through the abdominal wall, and suturing the serosal surface of ileum to the skin. Exposure of the ileal serosa to the alkaline stomal effluent resulted in serositis and ileostomy dysfunction. Accustomed to being bathed in the alkaline succus entericus, ileal mucosa is not susceptible to inflammation; thus, everting the full thickness of the exteriorized ileum and suturing its mucosa to the adjacent dermis alleviated the problem of serositis. This technique of ileostomy eversion was described in 1952 by Bryan Brooke in the United Kingdom, and this ileostomy is commonly referred to as a *Brooke ileostomy* (Fig. 117-1).[1] Patients' resistance to having an ileostomy has been in large measure alleviated by emphasizing the beneficial aspects of this operation (e.g., curing the disease), as well as by the development of new stoma appliances that have led to excellent long-term results.[4] Introduction of enterostomal therapy as an additional allied health field, and development of stomal support societies (see later), have provided significant support to patients with stomas.

Brooke ileostomies are incontinent, and in 1969, Nils Kock, a Swedish surgeon, developed the first continent ileostomy.[5] The Kock pouch procedure featured an ileal pouch, a nipple valve, and an ileal conduit, which led to a cutaneous stoma (Figure 117-2). Given that this was a continent stoma and that no appliance was necessary, it could be made flush with the skin. In the 1980s, the Kock pouch was used in selected patients with UC and FAP, but enthusiasm for this operation was tempered by the frequent occurrence of complications.[6]

Driven by the overall poor acceptance of ileostomy among patients, with its ever-present external appliance, surgeons explored other alternatives to the incontinent Brooke ileostomy. The straight ileoanal pull-through operation, which was used primarily in children for the surgical treatment of Hirschsprung's disease, was reconsidered as an option for patients who required proctocolectomy. This operation, which was plagued with excessive liquid bowel movements, was undesirable for an adult patient attempting to be free of the diarrhea that is associated with colitis. Therefore, an important technical modification was proposed: creation of an ileal reservoir (pouch) to reduce the frequency of daily bowel activity.[7,8] This operation preserves the function of the anal sphincter complex and allows for the normal exit of feces via the anal canal. Because of increasing experience with this operation over the last 3 decades, the ileal pouch-anal anastomosis (IPAA) is now the procedure of choice in most patients who require proctocolectomy for chronic UC or FAP.

This chapter describes the pathophysiologic and clinical implications of colectomy and reviews the options and alternatives for the control of enteric output. Three surgical options are available to patients with chronic UC and FAP: total proctocolectomy with the end-Brooke ileostomy, total proctocolectomy with IPAA, and ileoproctostomy (i.e., ileorectal anastomosis). Both the Kock pouch and IPAA are

*The author gratefully acknowledges the important and valuable contributions of the authors of previous edition, Drs. Robert R. Cima and John H. Pemberton.

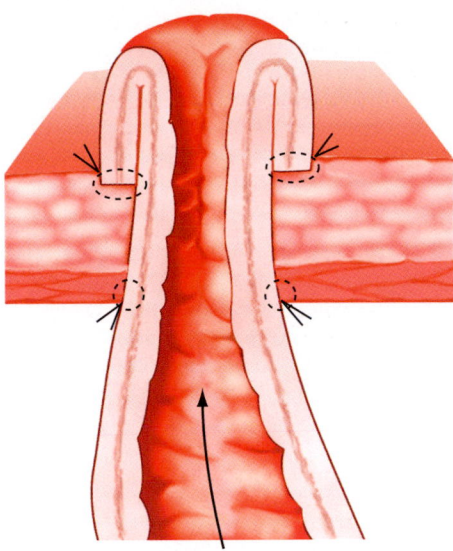

FIGURE 117-1. Anatomy of the Brooke ileostomy. The mucosa is everted and sewn to the skin. Therefore, no serosal surface is exposed to intestinal content, serositis is avoided, and the risk of ileostomy dysfunction is minimized.

Ileal flow

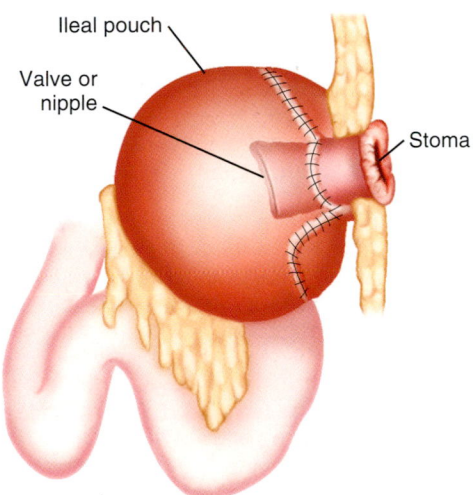

Ileal pouch

Valve or nipple

Stoma

FIGURE 117-2. The continent ileostomy. The pouch is formed from a loop of ileum, folded on itself as a U, and sutured along its antimesenteric borders. The 2 limbs that make up the pouch are then incised, exposing the mucosa, and the nipple valve is fashioned. The pouch is closed and positioned, as shown, underneath the abdominal wall. Note that the stoma is flush with the skin. (©Copyright 1991, Mayo Clinic, Rochester, Minn.)

contraindicated in patients with Crohn's disease, for whom segmental colectomy remains a viable option.

PATHOPHYSIOLOGIC CONSEQUENCES OF PROCTOCOLECTOMY

Fecal Output after Proctocolectomy

One of the physiologic functions of the colon is reabsorption of water and electrolytes, and its absence following a colectomy prevents this from occurring.[9] Although most patients do not suffer major pathophysiologic disturbances, some important principles must be noted. The normal colon absorbs at least 1000 to 1500 mL of water and 100 mEq of sodium chloride daily, and a healthy colon is able to increase this absorption to more than 5 L/day when presented with increased amounts of ileal effluent (see Chapter 101).[9-11]

Furthermore, during periods of salt depletion, the colon has a greater capacity for electrolyte conservation and reabsorption than does the small intestine. For example, under conditions of extremely low salt intake, sodium losses in normal stool can be reduced to 1 or 2 mEq/day, whereas patients with ileostomies have obligatory sodium losses of 30 to 40 mEq/day.[12-14] Most patients adapt to these daily losses through changes in salt and water intake and physiologic compensatory mechanisms.[15]

Well-functioning conventional (Brooke) ileostomies discharge 500 to 1200 g of material daily, 90% of which is water[13,14]; continent ileostomies and IPAAs contain similar volumes of effluent.[16] Ingestion of foods that contain significant amounts of unabsorbable residue increase the solid component of the ileostomy output. Although many anecdotes have described the effect of various foods on the volume and consistency of stomal effluents, the response to specific foods varies from 1 patient to another, and changes are usually insignificant.[17]

Functional Sequelae

When oral intakes of sodium, chloride, and fluid are adequate, patients with ileostomies do not become depleted in volume or electrolytes; negative sodium balance, however, can follow periods of diminished oral intake, vomiting, or excess perspiration.[18] In addition, chronic oliguria is to be anticipated, even in patients with established and well-functioning ileostomies, because normal stools contain approximately 100 mL of water, whereas ileostomies lose 500 to 600 mL/day.[15] Patients with ileostomies also have lower urinary Na^+/K^+ ratios because of compensatory renal conservation of sodium and water. These changes in urinary composition presumably contribute to the increased frequency of urolithiasis (about 5%) in patients with ileostomies, whose stones are predominantly composed of urate or calcium salts[19]; these patients have a relatively narrow tolerance for changes in their volume and electrolyte status, and even minor changes potentially result in life-threatening electrolyte disturbances.[20]

Following a major terminal ileal resection and construction of a proximal ileostomy, abnormalities in bile acid reabsorption and malabsorption of vitamin B_{12} (see Chapters 64, 103) develop. In addition, these patients suffer from steatorrhea, as well as excessive daily fluid losses (1 L/day). Such physiologic abnormalities usually do not occur after a colectomy performed for chronic UC or FAP, because the normal disease-free ileum is preserved. Colonic resection for Crohn's colitis may require removal of additional diseased ileum, with the possible consequences of malabsorption and even short bowel syndrome, depending on the length of small intestine removed, as well as the ability to preserve the ileocecal valve (see Chapters 101, 102, and 106).

Colectomy also reduces the exposure of bile acids to the metabolic effects of the fecal microbiota, and after ileostomy, secondary bile acids largely disappear from bile; no detrimental metabolic consequences have been noted in this situation.[21,22] The flora of ileostomy effluents have quantitative (10^4 to 10^7 colony-forming units [CFUs]/100 mL) and qualitative characteristics that are intermediate between those of feces and those of normal ileal contents, whereas the flora in an IPAA or Kock pouch are more similar to fecal microbiota.[23-25]

The principal pathophysiologic sequelae of colectomy with ileostomy are mainly the potential consequences of a salt-losing state; as such, liberal consumption of salt and increased fluid intake is recommended—especially at times of stress, in hot weather, and after vigorous exercise. A balanced salt solution such as Gatorade or Powerade is a good source of balanced electrolytes; patients with diabetes mellitus should consider Gatorade 2 (G2) as it contains less sugar than Gatorade. The limited ability of the small intestine to absorb sodium and water, however, means that stomal volumes also increase when the oral intake is increased.[14]

CLINICAL CONSEQUENCES OF PROCTOCOLECTOMY

After successful proctocolectomy, life expectancy is slightly below normal for the first few years owing to stomal complications and intestinal obstruction. After ileoproctostomy for UC, and especially for FAP, cancer may develop in the retained rectum. In general, however, the long-term mortality of patients after proctocolectomy and conventional ileostomy is the same as for an age-matched normal population.[26] Ninety percent of patients with conventional ileostomies who responded to a survey rated the results of their operation as excellent and claimed little inconvenience.[4] Overall, this study demonstrated no real difference in the reported quality of life (QoL) in patients with conventional ileostomies, continent ileostomies, or an ileal pouch.[27] Almost all such stoma or pouch patients are able to lead normal lives and enjoy normal sexual relationships; a few patients avoided certain strenuous physical activities.

The metabolic consequences of a proctocolectomy are the same regardless of whether a conventional ileostomy or an alternative procedure is performed. Patients in whom an ileostomy alternative achieves an excellent result may enjoy certain aspects of their QoL better than do patients with a stoma, because the former do not need to wear an ileostomy appliance. Pemberton and colleagues compared patients who had a Brooke ileostomy with those who had an IPAA and found that the latter experienced significant advantages in performing daily activities and enjoyed a better QoL.[28] There are certain unique complications of the newer operations, however, including incontinence or obstruction (Kock pouch), pelvic infections and sepsis, and pouchitis (IPAA), that must be considered; these are discussed later.

CONVENTIONAL BROOKE ILEOSTOMY

Major long-term complications of the Brooke ileostomy relate to dysfunction, prestomal ileitis, and irritation of the peristomal skin. An improperly constructed ileostomy, which is uncommon in today's surgical practice, may lead to obstruction. Patients with clinically significant stomal obstruction present with cramping abdominal pain, a paradoxically increased stomal output because of irritation and overflow of ileal effluent (up to 4 L/day), and fluid and electrolyte derangements. Excessive ileal output arises, at least in part, from increased intestinal secretion as a result of dilatation of the intestine proximal to the obstructed stoma. Stomal obstruction is usually demonstrated by examining the stoma with the little finger or by endoscopy with a small-caliber endoscope. Contrast studies of the intestine or CT scanning reveal a dilated ileum proximal to the point of obstruction. Most obstructed ileostomies require surgical revision, and at operation, ulcerations often are found in the resected specimen of terminal ileum; the etiology of such ulcers is unclear but is likely related in some way to the mechanical consequences of intestinal obstruction.

Prestomal ileitis is a much less common problem than stomal obstruction. Clinical features of this condition include signs and symptoms of mechanical bowel obstruction in addition to signs of systemic toxicity (e.g., fever, tachycardia, anemia).[29,30] In prestomal ileitis, the ileum exhibits numerous punched-out ulcers, sometimes extending to the serosa. It is not clear whether prestomal ileitis has a different pathogenesis from the changes that follow simple mechanical obstruction of the stoma; both complications involve ileum that was normal histologically at the time of colectomy. Backwash ileitis, seen typically in chronic UC, does not predispose to either prestomal ileitis or obstruction. Patients who have had colectomy and ileostomy for Crohn's disease experience problems with the ileal stoma more often than do patients with UC, perhaps because of transmural inflammation of the new terminal ileum. Whether stomal dysfunction is secondary to mechanical obstruction or recurrent Crohn's disease may be difficult to determine; this distinction may be elucidated with serum studies, endoscopy, or enterography.

Most people with an ileostomy lead a normal life and eat a normal diet; poorly digestible foods (e.g., nuts, corn, some fruits, lightly cooked vegetables) may obstruct the stoma and should be eaten in moderation and with careful chewing.[4] Some patients experience continuing difficulties managing their ileostomy. These problems vary in severity, some being minor inconveniences and others being significant drawbacks to the success of the operation. Mechanical difficulties because of a poorly fitting stomal appliance can cause excoriation of the skin around the ileostomy and can even erode the stoma to produce sinus tracts or a fistula. Some patients complain of unpleasant odors arising from the ileostomy bag, especially after eating certain foods such as onions and beans. Because most odor arises from bacterial action on the contents of the appliance, however, the problem may be alleviated by frequent emptying of the appliance or by adding sodium benzoate or chlorine tablets to the appliance. Oral bismuth subgallate also controls the odor, but its long-term use may be associated with neurotoxicity and encephalopathy.[31,32]

Studies of long-term outcomes associated with ostomies have demonstrated a high rate of complications. The most common problems related to ostomies are skin irritation and parastomal hernias, both of which contribute to difficulty with *appliance pouching,* a term used by enterostomal therapists that refers to the fitting of an ostomy device. Several risk factors predispose to development of parastomal hernias, including obesity, malnutrition, chronic respiratory disorders that are associated with increased intra-abdominal pressure, chronic use of glucocorticoids or other immunosuppressive agents, malignancy, advanced age, wound infection, and emergency operations.[33-37] Several techniques have been described for parastomal hernia repair, including primary fascial repair, stoma relocation, and mesh repair, of which mesh repair achieves the best outcomes.[34] The simplest approach, primary repair, is associated with very poor outcomes and nearly 100% recurrence rates. Stoma relocation may be an effective approach when the initial stoma site is unsatisfactory, but parastomal hernias occur at the new site in up to 76% of patients.[33,37,38] The use of prosthetic mesh for parastomal hernia repair has significantly improved outcomes, with recurrence rates reported as low as 10%.[39,40] To address concerns of possible mesh infection and erosion of mesh into the intestine with fistulization, the use of biological materials, such as human acellular dermal matrix (Alloderm), has been studied, with results that are comparable to synthetic mesh in small series.[41]

Trained enterostomal therapists and local ostomy societies can help patients with many aspects of ileostomy and colostomy postoperative care. Education of the patient is preferably begun before surgery; meetings with other ostomates and referral to specialized publications can allay many of patients' fears and uncertainties. The United Ostomy Associations of America (UOAA, P.O. Box 66, Fairview, TN 37062-0066; www.uoaa.org) publishes an excellent series of booklets dealing with all aspects of life for the ostomy patient. These materials also are of great help to patients and nursing staffs in the absence of a registered enterostomal therapist (wound ostomy and continence nurse [WOCN]). The location of a registered therapist can be obtained from the Wound Ostomy and Continence Nurses Society (WOCN Society National Office, 15000 Commerce Parkway, Suite C, Mt. Laurel, NJ 08054; www.wocn.org).

CONTINENT ILEOSTOMY (KOCK POUCH)

Clearly, 1 of the major (social) drawbacks to ileostomy could be eliminated if a continent stoma were possible. Nils Kock postulated that a pouch and nipple valve constructed of terminal ileum could store ileal content internally until emptied voluntarily by the patient's passing a large, soft catheter into the pouch several times daily, thereby obviating the need for an external appliance (See Fig. 117-2). In between catheter aspirations, the patient would simply cover the stomal opening with a Band-Aid. The first Kock pouch operation was reported in 1969, and the results were promising; however, the nipple valve sometimes failed, usually because it slipped out of the pouch, thereby resulting in incontinence.[5] Techniques gradually improved, and the most recent approaches have been more successful, providing continence in most patients. In 2 series, more than 90% of patients were continent for both gas and feces, never requiring an appliance.[36,42]

The high success rate of the Kock pouch, however, is achieved at the price of additional operations in most patients for nipple or pouch dysfunction, fistula, or stricture. Wasmuth and colleagues reported a 50% rate of reoperation by 14 years after continent ileostomy construction.[43] Furthermore, in a series of 96 patients with continent ileostomy reported by Lepisto, 24% of patients had it converted to a conventional stoma and 59% required reoperation, with a total of 85 pouch reconstructions being performed: 42 patients had 1 reconstruction, 9 had 2 reconstructions, 3 had 3 reconstructions, 1 had 4 reconstructions, and 2 had 6 reconstructions.[44] Others have reported similar findings: patients generally did well after initial continent ileostomy construction, but a sizable minority required repeated surgical intervention either to salvage pouch function or remove the pouch.[45,46]

Despite requiring numerous reoperations, the majority of Kock pouch patients are satisfied with the outcomes of their functioning pouch. In a recent comparative study on QoL in patients with standard ileostomies, ileal pouch, and Kock pouch, the Kock pouch patients did not fare significantly better or worse than those with a conventional ileostomy or IPAA; 56% of the continent ileostomy patients, however, did require reoperation to maintain function of their ileostomy.[27]

Patients' enthusiasm for the Kock pouch procedure is quite surprising given the numerous and frequent complications, which often require major surgical intervention. The Barnett Continent Ileostomy Reservoir (BCIR) was designed to reduce the incidence of valve slippage and fistula formation; however, no controlled data exist to suggest that this modification is superior to the original Kock pouch procedure.[47] Another continent ileostomy, the T pouch, has been developed to combat the problem of nipple valve slippage[48]; its design prevents slippage of the intussusceptive nipple valve constructed in the traditional Kock pouch. In the T pouch, the valve mechanism

is made by securing an isolated distal ileal segment into a serosal-lined trough formed by the base of 2 adjacent ileal segments. The high-volume/low-pressure reservoir is fashioned around this isolated valve segment. Once constructed, the distal end of the valve mechanism is brought up through the skin as a stoma. T pouches have been constructed in only a few patients, and the results are promising, but long-term follow-up studies to assess the structural integrity and clinical success of the new valve design are lacking. Given the success of the IPAA operation, continent ileostomy operations are rarely performed in modern-day surgical practice and are reserved for the few patients who desire enteric continence, whose Brook ileostomy has failed following a proctocolectomy, and for those individuals who are not candidates for IPAA because of rectal cancer or poor anal sphincter function. A patient who desires continence and whose occupation may preclude frequent visits to the toilet also may be a candidate for a continent ileostomy.

Before performance of a continent ileostomy operation, careful exclusion of Crohn's disease is mandatory (see Chapter 115). A detailed anorectal examination must also exclude the presence of fistula-in-ano. Construction of a continent ileostomy is contraindicated when Crohn's disease is suspected, since the risk of recurrent Crohn's disease is increased and future intestinal resections may render the patient with short bowel syndrome and dependent on parenteral nutrition.[49,50]

ILEAL POUCH-ANAL ANASTOMOSIS

IPAA is now the procedure of choice for most patients who require proctocolectomy for UC or FAP. IPAA is not considered suitable for patients with Crohn's disease, although this recommendation now is being reevaluated.[51,52] An ileal pouch has several major advantages: nearly all mucosal disease is removed—in contrast to ileoproctostomy, in which all of the rectal mucosa remains intact and is at continued risk for cancer; the normal route for fecal elimination is maintained, and a permanent stoma is not required; the anal sphincters are undisturbed; and the pelvic dissection, being less extensive than in cancer operations, should not endanger innervation of the sexual organs.

In 1947, Ravitch and Sabiston first described ileoanal anastomosis, an operation that was revived by the success of pediatric surgeons who used it in children with Hirschsprung's disease.[7] Initially, the operation was performed as a straight pull-through procedure, and the terminal ileum was sutured directly to the anal verge.[53] Although results in children were encouraging, excessive stool frequency and anal seepage were unacceptable sequelae to many adult patients. Subsequently, the operation was modified to include 1 of several forms of ileal pouch. The basic surgical steps are as follows: a proctocolectomy is performed; the distal rectum is divided at the top of the anal canal, which leaves a small cuff of residual rectal mucosa and all of the anal canal mucosa intact; an ileal pouch is fashioned from the terminal 15 to 20 cm of the ileum and then stapled or sutured to the cuff of remaining rectal and anal canal tissue. If a hand-sewn technique is used, a mucosal proctectomy is performed to remove all (or nearly all) of the mucosa to allow for an anastomosis between the mucosa of the ileal pouch and the dentate line. A diverting ileostomy is usually required for 2 or 3 months until the anastomosis heals completely. At a second operation 8 to 12 weeks later, the diverting ileostomy is closed.

The Mayo Clinic has acquired considerable experience with IPAA, having performed more than 2200 of these operations.[54-56] Although pouches of different configurations have been advocated by various surgical groups in the past,

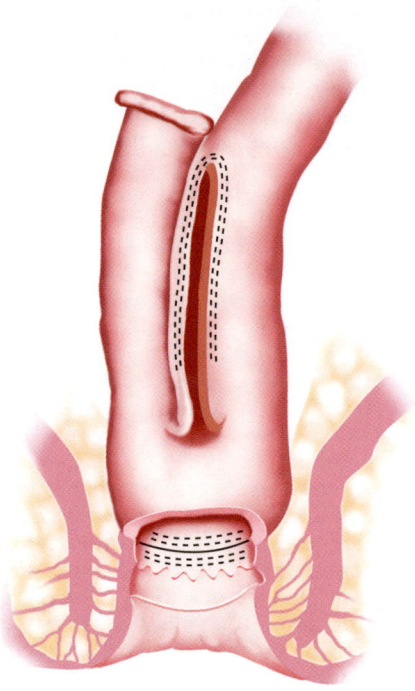

FIGURE 117-3. The anatomy of the most commonly used type of ileal pouch, the J-pouch. A pouch approximately 12 to 15 cm long is constructed by opening the common wall between the 2 limbs of the J formed from the distal terminal ileum. The apex is then anastomosed to the upper anal canal.

the pouch routinely used today is the J-pouch because of its ease of construction and reliable function (Fig. 117-3).

Clinical Results

Following IPAA, many centers report an average stool frequency of 6 stools during the day and 1 stool at night.[54-56,61] Daytime and nocturnal stool frequency and the ability to discriminate flatus from stool remain relatively stable over time, whereas the need for stool bulking and hypomotility agents declines. The lower stool frequencies 6 months after surgery, compared with the frequency in the early postoperative period, are likely attributable to a "settling in" of the pouch in the pelvis, increased pouch capacity, and pouch adaptation to the ileal effluent load and over time.

In the Mayo Clinic series, major fecal incontinence (>twice per week) occurs in 5% or less of patients during the day and 12% of patients during sleep.[56] In contrast, minor episodes of nocturnal incontinence (e.g., seepage) occur in up to 30% of patients at least 1 year after the operation. A pad must be worn by 28% of patients for protection against seepage. Minor perianal skin irritation is reported by two thirds of patients. Patients older than age 50 have a higher daytime stool frequency (8/day) than patients younger than 50 (6/day). Men and women have similar stool frequencies postoperatively, but women have more episodes of fecal soilage during the day and night; this is thought to be related to a shorter average anal canal length in women. Some 78% of patients report excellent continence 1 year after surgery (which remains unchanged at 10 years), 30% experience minor incontinence, and 2% have poor control. Of patients with minor incontinence at 1 year, 40% remain unchanged, 40% improve, and 20% worsen by 10 years.[58] Nocturnal fecal spotting increases only marginally during the 10-year period.

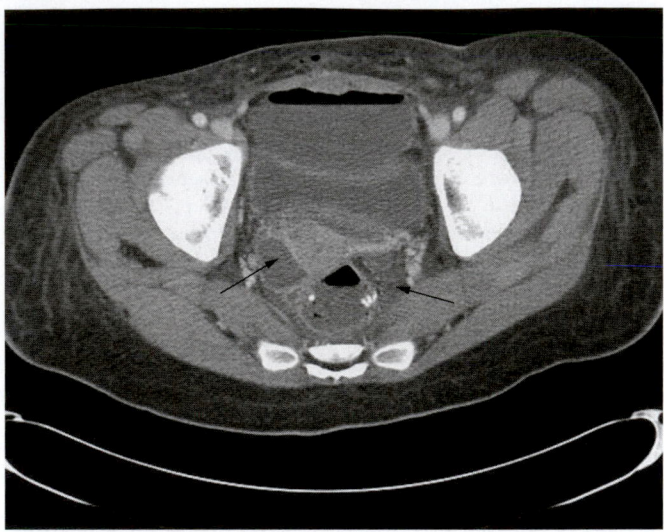

FIGURE 117-4. CT showing a peripouch abscess *(arrows)* identified 8 days after surgery. This complication is best managed by placement of a percutaneous drain under CT guidance.

Complications

Pelvic sepsis, an ominous development, occurs in 5% to 24% of patients after IPAA.[55,56,60,61] CT is useful for demonstrating pelvic fluid collections or phlegmon. Patients with pelvic phlegmon usually respond to nonoperative treatment with broad-spectrum IV antibiotics and bowel rest, whereas patients with a pelvic abscess ideally should undergo CT-guided drainage, if technically feasible, or laparotomy and drainage (Fig. 117-4). The most common risk factor for pelvic sepsis is chronic or high-dose glucocorticoid use in the perioperative period.[62] Anastomotic leak and pelvic sepsis may lead to pouch excision in the early postoperative period; fortunately, this is a rare occurrence. Compared with patients who did not experience pelvic sepsis, however, long-term functional results of the pouch in patients who had pelvic sepsis are worse, and there is a higher rate of pouch loss.[58]

A diverting temporary ileostomy, while minimizing the clinical impact of pelvic sepsis, is also associated with a number of complications, including intestinal obstruction and stoma-related complications, some of which may require surgical correction.[63] Closure of temporary ileostomies also may be associated with complications. Peritonitis and postoperative intestinal obstruction occurred in 4% and 12% of patients, respectively. Unrecognized intestinal serosal tears during mobilization of the stoma, in addition to anastomotic leaks, are important causes of peritonitis in patients undergoing ileostomy closure. During ileostomy closure, our practice is to resect all of the extraperitoneal intestine (afferent and efferent limbs and the stoma itself) to eliminate unrecognized intestinal perforation.

Almost all patients have a web-like stricture of the ileoanal anastomosis before ileostomy closure (Fig. 117-5). This stricture generally can be gently dilated digitally without difficulty, but narrowing can recur and is the most common indication for surgical intervention after IPAA.[64] If the pouch retracts under anastomotic tension, heavy scarring can result in a long, fibrotic stricture. This type of stricture manifests by increased straining to empty the pouch, a sensation of incomplete pouch evacuation, or a high stool frequency (>10 to 12 stools/day). Repeated anal dilation can prevent progression of the stricture. Occasionally, surgical revision of the ileoanal

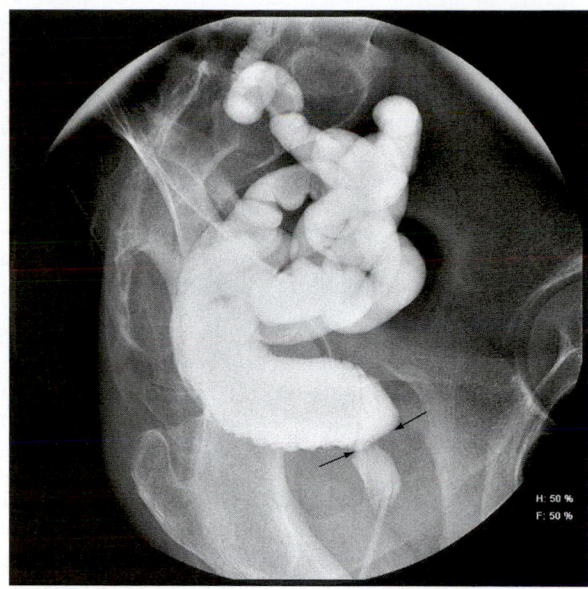

FIGURE 117-5. Film from a water-soluble radiocontrast enema performed before ileostomy closure and demonstrating a mild anastomotic narrowing (arrows). This stricture was dilated in the operating room before the ileostomy was closed.

anastomosis with a perineal only, or an abdominoperineal, approach may be required to treat the stricture.

Pouchitis and Cuffitis

Although a precise definition for pouchitis is lacking, it is generally agreed that pouchitis is an idiopathic, nonspecific acute inflammation of the ileal pouch. With a reported incidence that varies between 16% and 48%, it is 1 of the most common complications following restorative proctocolectomy with IPAA.[65] Furthermore, the incidence of pouchitis has been shown to increase with time after surgery, from approximately 40% of patients reporting at least 1 episode 10 years after IPAA construction, to up to 70% of patients with this complaint 20 years after surgery.[66-68]

Pouchitis may occur in patients with UC or FAP, although it is significantly more common in patients with UC, particularly those with sclerosing cholangitis.[69] An early experience demonstrated that IPAA patients who had preoperative extraintestinal manifestations of UC, especially those with sclerosing cholangitis, had significantly higher rates of pouchitis (39%) than did patients without such manifestations (26%). Although patients with a postoperative diagnosis of Crohn's disease have a higher incidence of pouchitis, this risk is less clear in patients with indeterminate colitis.[65] A study by Hoda and colleagues demonstrated that whereas extraintestinal manifestations might indicate a predisposition to episodes of acute pouchitis, they are not predictors of chronic pouchitis.[68] The patients at highest risk for chronic pouchitis suffered from postoperative complications, more specifically anastomotic and septic complications.[68]

Other investigators have suggested that there is a biological predisposition for pouchitis and that better risk stratification can be obtained by the preoperative use of serum markers of IBD.[70-72] In a study by Hui and colleagues, 63% of patients who went on to develop chronic pouchitis had a positive perinuclear-staining antineutrophil cytoplasmic antibody (pANCA) preoperatively, and only 17% had negative serologic results.[70] There remain questions about these findings, however, because not all authors have demonstrated such a relationship.[73] Furthermore, although such serologic information is scientifically intriguing, it is unclear whether it provides any information that would change surgical decision making before surgery, because the surgical options are limited.

More surgeons now prefer a double-stapled technique for the IPAA operation, as opposed to mucosectomy and handsewn anastomosis. This surgical technique leaves a cuff of distal rectal mucosa in situ, which is at risk for intermittent or chronic activity of the UC and is termed *cuffitis*.[74] The symptoms of cuffitis mimic those of pouchitis, and in a study of 61 IPAA patients with symptoms of pouchitis, 7% were found to have cuffitis.[75]

Diagnosis

The diagnosis of pouchitis is often based on clinical symptoms alone. Most patients with apparent pouchitis or cuffitis have intermittent symptoms and respond well to therapy. In a few, however, symptoms are severe and persistent enough to lead to surgical removal of the pouch. Patients present with lower abdominal cramps, increased volumes of fecal output (diarrhea), urgency, fatigue, malaise, bleeding, discomfort from the pouch, and general symptoms similar to those of the initial disease. Presenting symptoms are classified as acute (<4 weeks) or chronic (>4 weeks) and include cramping lower abdominal pain, increased volumes of fecal output (diarrhea), liquid consistency of stool, urgency, bleeding per anus, malaise, anorexia, and general symptoms similar to those of the initial disease. Low-grade fever, anemia, and dehydration as a result of diarrhea may be variably present; fecal incontinence also is common. Extraintestinal dermatologic and rheumatologic manifestations are seen occasionally, suggesting an ongoing systemic inflammatory response.[66]

Endoscopy in a patient with pouchitis shows the pouch mucosa to be reddened and swollen, with occasional ulcerations. The mucosa is friable and bleeds readily from the minor trauma of endoscopy; inflammatory changes usually are confined to the pouch but also can be seen in the adjacent ileum. Histologic examination of the pouch mucosa reveals a range of acute and chronic inflammatory changes depending on severity, including villus atrophy, distortion of crypt architecture, ulcerations, and polymorphonuclear leukocyte infiltration. The Pouchitis Disease Activity Index (PDAI), which combines clinical, endoscopic, and histologic features, has been developed to quantify and compare these findings (Table 117-1).[67] Exclusion of possible etiologies that may require specific treatment is essential before initiating treatment for pouchitis. It must be remembered that patients with ileal pouches are not immune to superimposed specific enteric infections and that stool culture and microscopy for parasites, as well as a *Clostridium difficile* toxin assay, are crucial to the evaluation of any patient with symptoms or findings of pouchitis or cuffitis.

Unsuspected Crohn's disease in the pouch is always a major concern. The clinical features of the underlying colitis that led to the operation should be reviewed carefully, including gross and histologic examination of the resected bowel. A small but definite proportion of colitis falls into an unclassifiable group (indeterminate colitis), and some patients with previously unrecognized Crohn's disease present with pouchitis that is actually a manifestation of (recurrent) Crohn's disease. Surgically treatable problems such as an anastomotic stricture resulting in partial pouch outflow obstruction need to be investigated carefully and treated with dilations (See before).

TABLE 117-1 Pouchitis Disease Activity Index*

Criteria	Score
Clinical	
Postoperative Stool Frequency	
Usual	0
1 or 2 stools/day more than usual	1
≥3 stools/day more than usual	2
Rectal Bleeding	
None or rare	0
Present daily	1
Fecal Urgency or Abdominal Cramps	
None	0
Occasional	1
Usual	2
Fever (>100°F)	
Absent	0
Present	1
Endoscopic	
Edema	1
Granularity	1
Friability	1
Loss of vascular pattern	1
Mucoid exudate	1
Ulceration	1
Histologic	
Polymorphonuclear Leukocyte Infiltration	
None	0
Mild	1
Moderate + crypt abscess	2
Severe + crypt abscess	3
Percent of Mucosa That Is Ulcerated per Low-Power Field (Average)	
<25	1
25-50	2
>50	3

*Pouchitis is defined as a total score of 7 or greater. The total score is the sum of the individual scores.
Adapted from Sandborn WJ, Tremaine WJ, Batts KP, et al. Pouchitis after ileal pouch-anal anastomosis: A pouchitis disease activity index. Mayo Clin Proc 1994; 69:409.

Pathogenesis

Acute, nonspecific inflammation of an ileal pouch apparently reflects the propensity of the patient for IBD. Thus, pouchitis is much more common in patients with IBD than it is in patients with FAP; however, patients operated on for FAP are not completely protected from pouchitis. In a meta-analysis performed by Lovegrove and colleagues, the risk of pouchitis was 30.1% for patients with chronic UC and 10% for those with FAP.[76] The etiology of pouchitis remains ambiguous and is likely to be multifactorial. Hoda and colleagues found that risk factors for development of pouchitis following IPAA included duration of UC, occurrence of postoperative complications, presence of extraintestinal manifestations of UC, fulminant colitis with a 2-stage operation, duration of diverting ileostomy following pouch formation, PSC, and the number of operations used to construct the IPAA.[68] The predominance

of pouchitis in chronic UC and rare occurrence in FAP suggests that the underlying immune dysregulation is instrumental in its development.[65]

Histopathologic evaluation of healthy and diseased pouches has shown that chronic inflammation is usual, even when the patient is asymptomatic.[77,78] Villus architecture is distorted, and colonic metaplasia is present in biopsy specimens from most pouches, even in the absence of severe acute inflammation. Thus, these changes are considered natural sequelae of the altered anatomy, just as the histologic changes of experimental and clinical blind-loop syndrome have been attributed to bacterial overgrowth.

Other possible causes of pouchitis have little supportive evidence in the literature, including damage by bile acids or their bacterial metabolites and lack of short-chain fatty acids (SCFAs).[67] Normal colonic mucosa uses SCFAs, primarily propionate and butyrate, as a source of nutrition, and some authors have proposed that IBD can result when the colon is deprived of SCFAs.[79] The clearest clinical experience that tests this hypothesis is diversion colitis. Harig and coworkers proposed that diversion colitis is caused by deprivation of SCFAs,[80] support for which is provided by the observation that diversion colitis improves in response to SCFA enemas. Ileal pouches contain high concentrations of SCFAs (≥100 mmol), however, and so a state of deprivation seems unlikely; moreover, pouchitis has been shown to become worse or shown no predictable response to SCFA enemas.[81] In a detailed evaluation of luminal factors, including fecal concentrations of bacteria, bile acids, and SCFAs, there were no differences between patient cohorts with or without pouchitis.[67] Alteration in butyrate metabolism has been linked to pouchitis.[82]

At present, there is no definitive cause for pouchitis, but it most likely does involve an interaction between the pouch microenvironment and the patient's underlying immune response to that environment. In the Mayo Clinic experience with patients who have had their IPAA for nearly 20 years, the rate of having at least 1 episode of pouchitis was 48% at 10 years, and it rose to 78% at 20 years.[58] In this cohort, less than 5% of patients developed chronic pouchitis, and only 2% required pouch removal or permanent diversion.

Treatment

If diarrhea alone is the major complaint, treatment with simple antidiarrheal measures may be all that is required. For more severely symptomatic patients, a variety of empirical treatments have emerged. Metronidazole (15 to 20 mg/kg/day or 500 mg twice daily for 14 to 28 days), is often used as a first line of treatment. Alternatively, ciprofloxacin (1000 mg/day) has been shown to be equally efficacious in the treatment of acute pouchitis,[83,84] although a recent Cochrane database report suggested ciprofloxacin is more effective than metronidazole at inducing remission.[85] Several randomized controlled trials (RCTs) have examined the effectiveness of other medications in the treatment of pouchitis, including budesonide,[86] rifaximin,[87] and probiotics (*Lactobacillus* GG[88] and VSL#3).[89] The Cochrane database, which included 11 RCTs, concluded that only budesonide and VSL#3 were more effective than placebo.[85] These studies do not support use of *Lactobacillus* GG, bismuth enemas, or butyrate and glutamine suppositories.[85]

Pouchitis usually responds dramatically to broad-spectrum antibiotics, but patients with recurrent or chronic pouchitis may require long-term maintenance therapy. Recurrence of pouchitis after initial therapy should be treated with a second course of the same therapy used for initial treatment. Combination antibiotic therapy has been recommended in patients whose pouchitis continues to recur, if they can tolerate the regimen. A combination of rifaximin (1 g twice daily) and ciprofloxacin (500 mg twice daily) for 15 days improved symptoms in 88% of patients, with a complete response rate of 33%.[90] Mimura and colleagues demonstrated that the combination of metronidazole (500 mg twice daily) and ciprofloxacin (500 mg twice daily) for 4 weeks resulted in a remission rate of 82%.[91] The use of 3 or more antibiotics (ciprofloxacin, metronidazole, amoxicillin/clavulanic acid, and erythromycin) in rotation at weekly intervals has also been suggested for patients with chronic pouchitis, but supporting evidence for such a regimen is limited.[92] Several studies have shown promising results with the use of VSL#3 in the treatment of patients with chronic pouchitis.[89]

If pouchitis fails to respond to antimicrobial therapy, exclusion of other etiologies such as *C. difficile* or cytomegalovirus (CMV) is essential. *C. difficile* may be treated with oral metronidazole, or oral vancomycin, if the patient has not responded to metronidazole. There is limited but favorable experience using fecal microbiota transplantation (FMT) to treat non-responsive pouchitis. CMV infection generally responds to treatment with ganciclovir. Irritable pouch syndrome, NSAID enteropathy, ischemic pouchitis, and other autoimmune disorders are conditions that should be considered.[65]

When antibiotics are ineffective, treatment should consist of regimens that are effective in IBD: glucocorticoid and/or mesalamine enemas, aminosalicylates, and even systemic glucocorticoids. In some cases of antibiotic resistant pouchitis, bismuth subsalicylate (Pepto-Bismol) 270 mg daily for 3 weeks is an effective treatment. Most patients unresponsive to antibiotics improve on 1 of these programs.

The risk of chronic active pouchitis is approximately 10% to 12% and is a leading cause of pouch failure and pouch explantation. Recalcitrant pouchitis may respond to rescue therapy with immunosuppressive agents such as azathioprine, 6-MP, or infliximab. In a recent retrospective, multicenter study of 31 patients with chronic refractory pouchitis, infliximab induced a complete response in 21% of patients, while 63% of patients experienced a partial clinical response.[93] Although these results and therapy with adalimumab[94] are promising, Crohn's disease should be excluded as the culprit for refractory pouchitis. Severe, recurrent, recalcitrant pouchitis or major extraintestinal symptoms may necessitate pouch explantation and permanent ileostomy.

Sequelae

Although the prevalence of chronic pouchitis is low, the potential consequences of chronic inflammation of the neorectum, especially dysplasia and malignant change, are of concern. Morphologic and biochemical changes occur in the ileal pouch mucosa, including villus atrophy and blunting, chronic inflammatory infiltrates, variable transition to production of a colonic type of mucus (sulfomucins), and increased cellular proliferation.[95] Observations based on long-term follow-up (mean, 6.3 years) reveal 3 patterns of mucosal metaplasia: approximately half of the patients showed mild villus atrophy and minimal inflammation; slightly fewer had transient moderate or severe atrophy and inflammation with intervals of recovery; and approximately 10% had permanent subtotal or total villus atrophy with chronic inflammation.[77] In this study, 3 of 8 patients developed low-grade dysplasia; in 1 patient it developed 2 years postoperatively. In patients having a double-stapled anastomosis, the remaining rectal cuff and anal canal transition zone tissue represent tissue at risk for malignant transformation. In 1 series of 225 patients who had a stapled IPAA, 238 rectal cuff and anal canal

biopsies were obtained; 202 (84.9%) had histologically confirmed chronic inflammation, 11 (4.6%) had acute inflammation, and 25 (10.5%) were read as normal.[96] Interestingly, 9 of the 11 patients with acute inflammation were asymptomatic.

Pouch Neoplasia

Following IPAA, dysplasia or carcinoma may occur in the residual rectal cuff (anal transition zone [ATZ]), or in the pouch itself. Only limited data are available to document the incidence and natural history of pouch neoplasia, with few studies reporting follow-up periods of over 10 years. Current evidence indicates that for both the ATZ and the pouch itself, the incidence of invasive carcinoma remains low. In a meta-analysis by Chambers and colleagues, 25 published reports were identified that described adenocarcinoma of the pouch or the ATZ. Of these 25 patients, cancer was noted in the pouch (11), at the anastomotic site (4), in the residual rectal cuff (4), in the anal canal (3), and in the afferent limb remnant of an excised pouch (1).[97,98]

Pouch Failure

The definition of pouch failure varies considerably although it is generally agreed that pouch failure implies the need for permanent defunctioning ileostomy (fecal diversion), or explantation of the pouch due to pouch specific complications. Large series have reported failure rates between 3% and 30%,[60,84,86,99-101] and in the Mayo Clinic series, 8% of patients ultimately required pouch excision or construction of a permanent ileostomy.[58,102] The most common causes of pouch failure, either alone or in combination, include anastomotic leak and pelvic sepsis, high stool volumes, Crohn's disease, and uncontrollable fecal incontinence; idiopathic pouchitis is the sole cause in only 2% of all patients with pouch failure. Pouch failure occurs within 1 year in 75%, by 2 years in 12%, and by 3 years in 12% in patients whose pouch fails. Fortunately, pouch failure is relatively uncommon. Early failures are almost always related to technical issues or complications related to the original operation, whereas late failures are more commonly related to chronic pouchitis or Crohn's disease in the pouch.

When surgery is considered for pouch failure, options include proximal diversion alone with creation of a loop ileostomy from the afferent limb of terminal ileum proximal to the pouch, or excision of the pouch with construction of an end-Brooke ileostomy or a continent stoma (i.e., Kock pouch). Pouch excision is a major operative procedure with significant associated perioperative morbidity. Data regarding outcomes after pouch excision are sparse. A small retrospective study by Karoui and colleagues reported outcomes for 68 patients who underwent pouch excision with creation of either an end-ileostomy (61 patients) or continent Kock ileostomy (7 patients). The study reported a 62.3% rate of early and late morbidity, and a 1.3% mortality. With a median follow-up of 30 months, the most common late complications included those related to the perineal wound (40.3%) and small bowel obstruction (14.9%). Perineal pain and sexual dysfunction were reported in 7% of patients.[103]

Given the high risks associated with pouch excision, an alternative procedure such as diverting loop ileostomy, leaving the pouch in situ, may be an attractive option. The advantages of this operation include avoiding the technically challenging pelvic dissection, with its potential for damage to pelvic organs and its associated risk for septic complications (i.e., pelvic abscess) and an unhealed perineal wound. The disadvantages of leaving the pouch in situ include persistent drainage from the pouch, as well as the risk of malignant transformation of the pouch mucosa or the ATZ; few studies have evaluated these 2 options. Kiran and colleagues from the Cleveland Clinic reported on 136 patients with pouch failure who underwent pouch excision (*n* = 105) or loop ileostomy with the pouch remaining in situ (*n* = 31). With a median follow-up of 9.8 years, the QoL parameters were significantly better in the patients who underwent pouch excision compared with those who had diverting ileostomy alone.[104] These findings are also consistent with other studies that report improved QoL after pouch excision compared with loop ileostomy.[105] Contemporary data, though limited, suggest that when feasible in appropriate-risk patients, pouch excision is superior to loop ileostomy alone. Patients who undergo pouch excision may have a better QoL compared with those who are permanently diverted with a loop ileostomy.

Sexual Dysfunction

Michelassi and colleagues have reported impotence and retrograde ejaculation rates in men of 1.5% and 4%, respectively. Dyspareunia developed in 7% of women postoperatively.[55,56] Early studies of IPAA focused on physiologic assessment, but recent studies have concentrated on more multidomain QoL assessments. A prospective evaluation of sexual function in patients with IPAA was performed using validated survey instruments, including the International Index of Erectile Function in men and the Female Sexual Function Index in women. Overall QoL was assessed using the Short IBD Questionnaire. Preoperative scores were compared with scores at 6 and 12 months postoperatively. Of the 59 patients who completed the study, male sexual function and erectile function scores remained high 12 months after surgery, and female sexual function improved 12 months after surgery. QoL significantly improved after IPAA in both men and women.[107] Others have reported similar improvements after IPAA.[108,109]

Quality of Life

Often, QoL is the deciding factor for patients choosing a particular operation for UC. Several studies that analyzed the outcome of surgery for UC have demonstrated that most patients are satisfied with the operation and have a normal lifestyle regardless of whether proctocolectomy with permanent end-ileostomy or restorative proctocolectomy has been performed. In a study of QoL by Pemberton and coworkers, patients were highly satisfied with either a Brooke ileostomy (93%) or an IPAA (95%) done for UC and FAP.[28] Daily activities such as sexual life, participation in sports, social interaction, work, recreation, family relationships, and travel, however, were more likely to be adversely affected with a Brooke ileostomy than by IPAA.

Fazio and colleagues prospectively evaluated long-term QoL and functional outcome after restorative proctocolectomy with IPAA using the Cleveland Global Quality of Life instrument. With a median follow-up of 5 years, results revealed an increase in QoL 2 years after surgery; this change may be related in part to the increased prevalence of perfect continence from 75.5% before surgery to 82.4% after surgery. Although there was some deterioration in continence over time, the change was not significant and continence remained improved, with 75% of patients reporting perfect continence 5 to 8 years after surgery. Based on this study, there was no deterioration in patient-reported function, QoL, or satisfaction over time; 98% of patients continued to recommend surgery to other patients at 5 years.[98,106]

Long-Term Results

Total proctocolectomy with IPAA is a complex operation, and complications occur frequently. The overall morbidity rate still ranges between 25% and 30% in multiple series.[55-57] Failure, however, is rare, even in those who suffer a postoperative complication.

In a comprehensive report from the Mayo Clinic, the overall pouch success rate was 92% in patients, some of whom had had their IPAA for up to 20 years.[58] In this series of 1885 IPAA operations performed for chronic UC over a 20-year period with a mean follow-up of 11 years, the overall rate of pouch success at 5, 10, 15, and 20 years was 96.3%, 93.3%, 92.4%, and 92.1%, respectively. Over time, the mean daytime stool frequency increased from 5.7 times at 1 year to 6.4 times at 20 years; nighttime stool frequency also increased from 1.5 to 2.0. This increase in stool frequency with long-term follow-up may be explained by an increased pouch size and pouch flaccidity that develops over decades, perhaps exacerbated in an aging patient whose sphincter may not function as well as it did previously. The incidence of frequent daytime fecal incontinence increased from 5% to 11% during the day and from 12% to 21% at night. This series demonstrated, however, that IPAA is a reliable surgical procedure for patients requiring proctocolectomy for UC and indeterminate colitis. Furthermore, it showed that the clinical and functional outcomes are excellent and durable.

The outcomes of IPAA are excellent when performed in centers that have experience with this operation[59]; also, these centers understand the potential complications and their management in IPAA patients. The key to a successful outcome is a surgeon who performs the operation comfortably; the operation struggled through is the one fraught with complications and sometimes with failure.

Controversies

Double-Stapled versus Hand-Sewn Anastomosis

The controversy over whether the anastomosis of the ileal pouch to the anal canal should be performed with a double-stapled technique or hand-sewn technique revolves around functional outcomes related to preservation of the ATZ mucosa. In non-randomized trials, a stapled anastomosis has been equated with better outcomes because of reduced stretch injury (dilation) to the anal sphincters, preservation of the ATZ and thus improved anal sensory discrimination, maintenance of the rectoanal inhibitory reflex (RAIR), and improved nocturnal continence.

In a randomized prospective study that compared the double-stapled IPAA (17 patients) to the hand-sewn technique (15 patients), Haray and colleagues demonstrated that stool frequency and incidence of daytime and nighttime fecal incontinence were similar in the 2 groups.[110] In the stapled cohort, 1.5 to 2.0 cm of ATZ was preserved, whereas complete mucosectomy was performed in the hand-sewn group. The overall complication rates were the same in the 2 groups; however, fewer patients treated with the double-stapled technique experienced nocturnal incontinence.

Similar findings have been reported by other groups.[111] In a meta-analysis of over 4000 patients, Silvestri and colleagues concluded that both techniques had similar early postoperative outcomes; stapled IPAA offered improved nocturnal continence, however, which was reflected in higher anorectal resting pressures as well as anal squeeze pressures.[76]

Role of Defunctioning Ileostomy

The most feared complication of IPAA is anastomotic failure and pelvic sepsis. Therefore, after pouch construction, a defunctioning (diverting) ileostomy is usually performed to divert ileal contents from the pouch and allow it to heal.[112] The reported rate of pelvic sepsis after IPAA ranges from 0% to 25% . In a series from the Mayo Clinic, the incidence of pelvic sepsis was relatively low (6%); however, when it occurred, it was responsible for a significant proportion of the failed pouches.[58,64] Ogunbiyi and colleagues identified pelvic sepsis as a major predictor of pouch failure in 27 patients who underwent IPAA salvage surgery, which accounted for 58% of pouch excisions.[113]

Proponents of diverting ileostomies argue that diverting stomas allow the pouch to fully heal and "settle" in the pelvis prior to use. Creation of a loop ileostomy does not completely protect the patient from pelvic sepsis; however, its presence minimizes the adverse clinical sequelae of a leak and makes it easier to manage a patient with this complication. Supporters of a 1-stage procedure (total proctocolectomy and IPAA without a diverting ileostomy) believe that an IPAA can be performed without increased risk of pelvic sepsis.[114-118] A 1-stage procedure avoids an ileostomy and a second hospitalization and operation, lowers the total cost, and results in a shorter hospital stay and perhaps a decreased incidence of small bowel obstruction.[112]

In the large single-surgeon study reported by Sugerman and associates, there were no differences in the complication rates and functional outcomes of patients who did not have a diverting ileostomy compared with those who had a diverting ileostomy; there also was no relationship to glucocorticoid use.[114,119] Whereas there might be no significant difference in the complication rate in patients without a defunctioning ileostomy, 1 study has suggested that the severity of complications was greater in patients without a protecting ileostomy.[120]

Although it is our practice to perform a diverting ileostomy in all patients undergoing IPAA, in properly selected patients who have an uncomplicated procedure performed by experienced surgeons, a 1-stage IPAA might be appropriate. The surgeon and patient care team must be attentive to the early signs of pelvic sepsis, aggressively investigate the possibility of a pouch leak, and intervene expeditiously if necessary.

Additional Issues

Risk of Cancer

Patients with chronic UC are at risk for developing adenocarcinoma of the colon and rectum, a risk that increases with the duration of disease and extent of colonic involvement (see Chapters 116 and 127). Figures suggest that the risk of colon cancer for people with IBD increases by 0.5% to 1.0% yearly, beginning 8 to 10 years after diagnosis.[121] Any operation that leaves behind diseased colonic mucosa puts the patient at risk for developing dysplasia or neoplasia in this residual tissue. The risk of developing a carcinoma in the residual mucosa may be directly related to the amount of residual mucosa remaining in situ. Complete excision of the rectal mucosa during IPAA substantially decreases the risk of dysplasia. With the more commonly used stapled IPAA, however, a small amount of residual rectal and anal canal tissue is retained.

Early studies by Tsunoda and colleagues demonstrated the presence of dysplasia in mucosectomy specimens, which they believed supports the use of a mucosectomy and hand-sewn anastomosis.[122] Even performing a mucosectomy, however, does not ensure that all rectal and at-risk anal canal mucosa is removed. In 1 study that evaluated anal canal specimens, islands of mucosa were present despite "complete" mucosal resection (i.e., mucosal proctectomy).[123] In a study with long-term follow-up, however, the risk of dysplasia was quite low in these patients.[124] A cohort of 289 patients with stapled IPAAs was followed and had multiple biopsies of the rectal cuff and ATZ performed over a 10-year period. Dysplasia was identified in 8 patients, including 4 with low-grade and 4 with high-grade dysplasia. No cancer in the ATZ was found during the study period. The authors concluded that ATZ dysplasia after stapled IPAA was infrequent and usually self-limiting. ATZ preservation did not lead to the development of cancer in the ATZ (with a minimum of 10 years of follow-up), although long-term surveillance was recommended to monitor dysplasia.

Detection of neoplastic change in the pouch itself is another reason to closely monitor patients with IPAA. A subgroup of patients has been identified in whom the mucosa of the pelvic pouch develops severe villus atrophy,[77] and these patients seem to have a significantly higher incidence of dysplasia compared with patients without villus atrophy (71% vs. 0%). The former group may be at greater risk for developing carcinoma and might require more intensive follow-up with regular pouch endoscopy and biopsy. Despite these findings, dysplasia in a pouch is a rare event. In group of 45 patients followed for a median of 6 years (1 to 28 years), dysplasia of any type was found in 4% of pouch biopsies, and there was no evidence of malignancy.[125]

To date, there have been only a small number of case reports of carcinoma arising in ileal pouches or in the region of the anastomosis.[126-129] Surprisingly, many of these cancers have arisen in patients who have undergone a complete mucosectomy with hand-sewn anastomosis. In a recent review, Branco and colleagues found the occurrence of adenocarcinoma after IPAA for UC to be an infrequent event.[130] They concluded that post-IPAA cancer can occur following mucosectomy or stapled anastomosis, and furthermore, that this malignancy can occur after IPAA performed for UC without colorectal cancer or when chronic UC is complicated by colorectal cancer prior to the IPAA operation, and that this complication is seen regardless of whether the initial cancer or dysplasia had involved the rectum. Given the known occurrence of dysplasia in pouch mucosa and the rare reports of cancers arising in pouches, yearly clinical and endoscopic surveillance should be performed in patients after their IPAA.

Fertility and Pregnancy

Many women with UC are in their childbearing years, and so it is important that women be informed of and consider the effect of IPAA on fertility and pregnancy when surgery for their UC becomes necessary. The majority of the relevant literature demonstrates a negative effect of IPAA on fertility,[131-133] and pregnancy may be at least 5 times less likely to occur compared with the general population. In a meta-analysis by Rajaratnam and colleagues, a statistically significant increase of 3.91 in the relative risk of infertility was demonstrated after IPAA surgery.[134] A number of studies have evaluated fertility and the course of a subsequent pregnancy after surgery.[135,136] Patients who have had a proctocolectomy and end-ileostomy or Kock pouch can expect to have a normal pregnancy and delivery; however, these women often have temporary stoma or Kock pouch dysfunction.[137] A similar disturbance of pouch function is seen in IPAA patients, in whom a slight increase in stool frequency, incontinence, and pad use is reported during the pregnancy.[135,136] Fortunately, this is temporary, and patients return to their baseline pouch function after the pregnancy. There is a reported higher rate of cesarean sections in IPAA patients, but there appears to be no contraindication to vaginal delivery, and the decision to proceed to a cesarean section should be based upon obstetric considerations.

Previous studies evaluated the course of pregnancies after IPAA, but the specific issue of fecundity after IPAA had not been considered. In 1999, however, a Swedish population-based study demonstrated a significant reduction in fecundity after IPAA.[132] More importantly, of the post-IPAA patients who became pregnant, 29% of pregnancies occurred only after in vitro fertilization (IVF) compared with the expected 1% of all pregnancies in Sweden during the study period. The cause of this decreased fertility is unknown, but the authors hypothesized that changes in pelvic anatomy resulting from removal of the rectum and dense adhesions from the pelvic dissection that resulted in scarring of the ovaries and fallopian tubes were major contributors to the problem. Various techniques have been attempted to reduce the effect of surgery on ovarian and tubal function. Interposition of an omental pedicle graft or placement of adhesion barrier products, such as Seprafilm (Genzyme Corporation, Cambridge, Mass.), may help reduce adhesions and thereby keep the ovaries out of the pelvis. Oophoropexy, a procedure involving suturing the ovaries to the pelvic brim, has also been attempted but may complicate the retrieval of the ova if IVF subsequently becomes necessary.[87,138]

A case-controlled study comparing women with IPAAs and female controls who had previous abdominal surgery found that women who had an IPAA had significantly more infertility evaluations and need for infertility treatments.[139] Analysis of infertility treatments for post-IPAA women demonstrated that they suffered a reduction in the probability of conception rather than complete infertility. This reduction in fecundity is not seen in women who have undergone ileorectal anastomosis (IRA) for FAP, which further the supports the idea that postoperative adhesions or altered pelvic anatomy contribute to this problem.[133]

Given the growing evidence that IPAA reduces a woman's fecundity, women need to be counseled regarding this prospect during the informed consent before IPAA. If this is a major concern in a young woman suffering from medically refractory UC, a subtotal colectomy and ileostomy to control the disease without disturbing the pelvic anatomy may be offered, with a planned completion proctectomy IPAA after childbearing is concluded. In rare circumstances, total abdominal colectomy with IRA (discussed later) may be chosen until childbearing is completed.

Patients with IPAA who wish to conceive postoperatively should be referred to a fertility specialist. The most common treatments in patients with IPAA who desire pregnancy are clomiphene and IVF. Olsen and colleagues compared the expected pregnancy and birth rates of a cohort of women with UC to age-matched women without UC in Sweden. There was no difference in the expected birthrate in women form the onset of UC to the time of proctocolectomy. However, there was a significant reduction of births after IPAA. More importantly, In the post-IPAA patients who became pregnant, 29% of pregnancies occurred after IVF compared with the expected 1% of all births in Sweden.[133] Success rates in fertility treatments are difficult to compare, given the variations between studies and fertility programs. Further investigations are necessary to determine the true success rates of fertility treatments following IPAA.[98,133]

Ileal Pouch-Anal Anastomosis and Indeterminate Colitis

Among 1519 consecutive patients with UC undergoing IPAA between January 1981 and December 1995, 82 patients (5%) had features of indeterminate colitis, including unusual distribution of inflammation, deep linear ulcers, neural proliferation, transmural inflammation, fissures, and creeping fat.[140] In a study from the Mayo Clinic, 12 (15%) of the 82 patients with indeterminate colitis eventually developed Crohn's disease during follow-up, compared with only 26 (2%) of 1437 patients diagnosed with UC. The probability of remaining free of Crohn's disease at 10 years was 98% in patients with UC and 81% in the indeterminate colitis patients. After IPAA, patients with indeterminate colitis who did not develop Crohn's disease experienced long-term outcomes nearly identical to those of patients with UC (i.e., nearly 85% had functioning pouches 10 years after the operation). Crohn's disease, however, regardless of whether it develops and is diagnosed after IPAA operations for UC or indeterminate colitis, is associated with poor long-term outcomes. Other institutions also have shown that although pouch complications are higher in patients with indeterminate colitis, the functional results after IPAA for indeterminate colitis are identical to those after UC, unless the patients develop Crohn's disease, in which case results are not as good. In a large retrospective study by Delaney and colleagues in 2002, a diagnosis of indeterminate colitis was found to be associated with a higher risk of developing perianal fistula and pelvic abscesses, suggesting a clinical picture more consistent with Crohn's disease; however, pouch failure rate was equivalent to those patients with UC.[88,141]

Impact of Biological Medical Therapy

The inclusion of newer biological therapies (e.g., infliximab) in the treatment of UC has raised concerns regarding their impact on the surgical outcomes after IPAA. In a study by Selvasekar and colleagues, 47 patients with UC received infliximab prior to restorative proctocolectomy and 254 did not.[142] Patients who received infliximab were statistically more likely to have postoperative infectious complications and pelvic abscesses. In this study, after multivariate adjustment for disease severity and other medication use, infliximab remained independently associated with an increased risk of ileal pouch-related and infectious complications. Another study of 85 patients with UC who received infliximab preoperatively found that they were at increased risk for postoperative septic complications as well as late complications compared with patients who did not receive infliximab.[143] The authors noted that patients who received infliximab were more likely to have undergone a 3-stage IPAA (total abdominal colectomy with end-ileostomy, followed by completion proctectomy and IPAA with loop ileostomy, followed by ileostomy closure), likely due to surgeon reluctance to perform an IPAA in the setting of preoperative infliximab administration.

Both of these studies are limited in their ability to allow any conclusion regarding the exact role of infliximab in the increased postoperative infection rate, owing to the retrospective nature of the analyses and possible selection bias. Most likely, patients who require infliximab for treatment of their UC represent a sicker and thus higher-risk group of patients at the time of surgery. Further prospective studies need to be performed to clarify this important issue.

As previously discussed, pelvic sepsis and abscess are devastating postoperative complications and are the leading risk factor for ileal pouch loss.[58] Given the uncertainty about a contributing role of biological therapy to this problem, or the possibility of much sicker patients presenting for surgery, a 3-stage approach in patients who have received preoperative infliximab may be considered.

ABDOMINAL COLECTOMY AND ILEORECTAL ANASTOMOSIS

The aim of a colectomy with an IRA is to extirpate most of the diseased colonic mucosa, thus reducing the risks of hemorrhage, malignant degeneration, and the possible development of fulminant or toxic colitis, while allowing the rectum to retain continence for stool and gas. The rationale for an IRA is that the operation avoids a permanent stoma, minimizes or eliminates injury to the pelvic splanchnic nerves (resulting in maintenance of bladder and sexual function), avoids a perineal wound and its associated complications, and is relatively easy to perform; other operations, if they become necessary, are not precluded.[144-147] The rationale against the operation, however, is nearly as convincing: subsequent proctectomy is required in nearly 40% of patients, poor results have been reported in up to 50% of patients, and the risk of developing carcinoma in the retained rectum approaches 17% after 27 years.[147,148]

In a study by Pastore and colleagues, who reviewed the course of 48 patients with UC and 42 patients with Crohn's disease who underwent IRA, 84% of the UC and 91% of the Crohn's disease patients reported an improvement in QoL.[149] One patient with UC developed carcinoma of the rectal stump 11.5 years after colectomy and IRA; the cumulative probability of remaining free of cancer was determined to be 85.7% at 12 years.

In patients with Crohn's disease and minimal or no rectal involvement, IRA with excision of the diseased colon is an appropriate operation. In addition, IRA, as a sphincter-saving procedure, continues to have a place in the surgical treatment of UC for high-risk or older patients who are not good candidates for IPAA and who have relatively mild disease. It is also important that patients who are considering IRA or have an IRA understand the need for continued surveillance of the rectum because of possible malignant degeneration of the retained rectal mucosa. The QoL after IRA has been reported to be very good; patient satisfaction is high, and an active, productive lifestyle can be preserved.[149,150]

Patient Selection

Patients are candidates for IRA if the rectum is distensible and only minimally involved with the disease (UC, Crohn's), and if patients are willing to undergo follow-up screening for rectal cancer. Although there is no maximum age that contraindicates ileoproctostomy, functional results related to poor sphincter function must be considered in older patients, especially in older female patients. Anorectal physiologic testing may be considered in older patients prior to abdominal colectomy with IRA in order to estimate postoperative physiologic function.

Complications

Operative mortality for elective IRA has been reported to vary between 2% and 8%.[150,151] In the series of UC patients reported by Leijonmarck and colleagues, complications occurred in 7 of 43 patients (16%) who underwent an elective 1-stage procedure.[150] There were 2 postoperative deaths (4%); 22 patients (43%) had a functioning IRA at the time of follow-up, with a mean follow up of 13 years. The cumulative probability of having the IRA functioning properly at 10 years was 51%. The causes of total excision were recurrent inflammation in the retained rectum ($N = 23$), dysplasia ($N = 3$), and postoperative complications ($N = 3$). No rectal carcinoma was noted in this study.

Physiology

The primary advantage of an IRA is that the major anatomic mechanisms responsible for maintaining continence are retained; the rectal reservoir, pelvic floor, and internal and external anal sphincters are preserved. The absorptive capacity of the proximal colon is lost, however, and ileal content is continually presented to the rectal remnant.

The rectum should be large and compliant to allow passive accommodation. Compliance depends on rectal wall elasticity, and in active inflammatory disease, compliant accommodation is impaired as a result of inflammation. Rectal compliance is inversely related to severity of inflammation. Thus, more inflammation (proctitis) leads to a less compliant rectum, which translates clinically to more stools per day (diarrhea); conversely, less inflammation leads to a more compliant rectum, which is associated with fewer stools per day. Sphincteric function in patients after IRA is similar to that of the general population. In patients with quiescent or minimal rectal disease following IRA, the rectal segment adapts to the influx of ileal effluent and begins to increasingly absorb sodium and water over a period of 3 to 6 months. Moreover, with quiescent disease, the rectum is capacious and distensible, resulting in low stool frequency and little or no incontinence. Conversely, an inflamed rectal mucosa leads to reduced distensibility and capacity, as well as impaired absorption of sodium and water, which results in greater fecal volume and in turn leads to increased stool frequency, urgency, and fecal incontinence.

QoL after IRA is very good; satisfaction is high and a productive lifestyle is achieved. Overall satisfaction is tempered, however, by the fact that patients often know they have not been cured and because they must undergo frequent follow-up examinations.

Colostomy in the Management of UC

In patients with UC, partial/segmental colectomy or colostomy has no role in management, either electively or emergently. Partial colectomy to remove left-sided colitis, leaving uninvolved proximal colon intact, often results in recurrent disease activity. Resection of the rectosigmoid, coloanal anastomosis, and cecoanal anastomosis are operations for UC mentioned here only to be condemned. Urgent or emergent surgical intervention for toxic or fulminating UC is best managed by abdominal colectomy, Brooke ileostomy, and either oversewing the rectal stump or establishing a rectal mucous fistula. Completion proctectomy with or without IPAA may be performed subsequently once the patient recovers and the physiologic and nutritional abnormalities have been corrected.

LAPAROSCOPIC APPROACH

The most important change in surgical practice related to all of these procedures is the application of laparoscopic techniques. Minimally invasive colon and rectal surgery began in the early 1990s; however, improvements in image technology and instrumentation have only recently facilitated complex

TABLE 117-2 Comparison of Surgical Options after Colectomy

Surgery	Stoma	Continence	Mortality, %	Overall Morbidity, %	Small Bowel Obstruction, %	Perineal Wound Complication, %	Stools per 24 hours	Failure, %	All Disease Removed?	Cancer Risk, %	Disease Indication
Brooke ileostomy	Yes	No	<1.0	19-70	15	33	N/A	—	Yes	0	CD, UC, FAP
Continent ileostomy	Yes	Yes	<1.0	15-60	7	35	3-5	50	Yes	†	UC, FAP
IPAA	No	Yes	<1.0	30-50	22	N/A	5-7	8	Yes*	*	UC, FAP
IRA	No	Yes	2.5-8.0	16-20	15	N/A	1-3	24-60	No	15 (30 yr)	CD, UC

Note: Maximum follow-up time is 13 years.
*10 instances of neoplasia in the cuff or pouch after IPAA have been reported in more than 12,000 cases.
†2 cancers in Kock pouches (continent ileostomies) have been reported.
CD, Crohn's disease; FAP, familial adenomatous polyposis; IPAA, ileal pouch-anal anastomosis; IRA, ileorectal anastomosis; N/A, not applicable.

colorectal procedures. Laparoscopic approaches for IPAA were developed to reduce the impact of surgery on patients who are already physiologically stressed, to decrease length of hospital stay, to reduce morbidity, and to improve cosmesis. The initial reports of laparoscopic IPAA were discouraging, however, because of very long operative times and few observed postoperative benefits.[152-154] Subsequent reports have clearly demonstrated the benefits of a minimally invasive approach in regard to postoperative decreases in length of stay, need for narcotics, overall morbidity, and return to normal function.[155-157] At our institution, the minimally invasive approach has become the preferred surgical operation for IPAA. Indications for operative intervention are not changed by the laparoscopic approach.

In a case-matched series from the Cleveland Clinic Foundation, 40 patients undergoing laparoscopic IPAA (LAP) were matched with open (laparotomy) controls for disease, age, gender, BMI, and date of operation. The LAP group exhibited significant benefits in time to ingesting clear liquids (1 vs. 3 days), eating a regular diet (3 vs. 4 days), and regaining bowel function (2 vs. 3 days).[124] Duration of narcotic use was shorter in the LAP group, and length of stay was reduced (4 vs. 7 days). LAP patients had longer operative times (270 vs. 192 minutes), but operative time decreased with experience and now averages 180 to 210 minutes. Subsequent studies in our institution have continued to demonstrate these short-term patient benefits.[158]

RISK-BENEFIT ANALYSIS

Conventional Ileostomy

The Brooke ileostomy is safe and reliable and has broad applicability to patients with IBD who require proctocolectomy. It is not, however, entirely free of complications (Table 117-2). Up to 30% of patients have a septic complication, 20% to 25% require revision of the stoma, 15% have recurrent small bowel obstruction, and stomal dysfunction can occur in up to 30% of cases.

Ileorectal Anastomosis

The primary benefit of an IRA is that the rectum is undisturbed by the operative dissection, the normal pathway of defecation is left in situ, and the incidence of bladder or

sexual problems is low. There also is no perineal wound (see Table 117-2). In many patients, the overall functional results are very good.

The major problem with IRA is that actual or potentially diseased mucosa is left in situ. In a few patients, inflammatory changes do resolve, but in most, the disease process continues unabated. The sequelae of leaving disease behind include poor anastomotic healing, which is responsible for the relatively higher mortality after IRA than after continent ileostomy and IPAA; continued need for anti-inflammatory therapy; continued bleeding and mucus discharge; incontinence and high stool frequency when inflammation flares up; and the possibility of malignant degeneration.

Continent Ileostomy

A major benefit of the Kock pouch is that although a stoma is constructed, discharge is controlled without the need for an external appliance. The principal problem with continent ileostomy is the high rate of complications, usually involving slippage of the nipple valve, with resultant incontinence or complete outflow obstruction; these complications, in turn, almost always require another operation. Continent ileostomy operations are rarely performed today because the success of IPAA has made this procedure obsolete.

Ileal Pouch-Anal Anastomosis

The major benefit of IPAA is that it successfully restores fecal continence in most patients; the major problem is the high complication rate (≈30%). Occasional incontinence appears early in nearly all patients after the operation, particularly at night. Major episodes of daytime incontinence affect approximately 10% of patients, but this frequency declines to almost zero after 4 years. Other complications include pelvic sepsis, anastomotic stricture, fistulas, sinus tracts, pouch leakage, and small bowel obstruction. As surgeons' experience with the operation have broadened, these surgical complications have decreased in frequency. Although nonspecific inflammation of the pouch (pouchitis) is the most important current drawback, in most patients it is treated effectively and simply with antibiotics. When severe and recurrent, pouchitis can lead to failure of the operation, but this is uncommon. Despite these problems, the benefits of IPAA are clear: all disease is removed, the patient avoids a stoma, and defecation is voluntary and controlled.

KEY REFERENCES

Full references for this chapter can be found on
www.expertconsult.com.

20. Weise WJ, Serrano FA, Fought Gennari FJ. Acute electrolyte and acid-base disorders in patients with ileostomies: A case series. Am J Kidney Dis 2008; 52:494-500.

28. Pemberton JH, Phillips SF, Ready RR, et al. Quality of life after Brooke ileostomy and ileal pouch-anal anastomosis. Ann Surg 1989; 209:620-6.

36. Israelsson LA. Preventing and treating parastomal hernia. World J Surg 2005; 29:1086-9.

56. Farouk R, Pemberton JH, Wolff BG, et al. Functional outcomes after ileal pouch-anal anastomosis for chronic ulcerative colitis. Ann Surg 2000; 231:919-26.

57. Hahnloser D, Pemberton JH, Wolff BG, et al. The effect of ageing on function and quality of life in ileal pouch patients: A single cohort experience of 409 patients with chronic ulcerative colitis. Ann Surg 2004; 240:615-21.

58. Hahnloser D, Pemberton JH, Wolff BG, et al. Results at up to 20 years after ileal pouch-anal anastomosis for chronic ulcerative colitis. Br J Surg 2007; 94:333-40.

62. Ziv Y, Church JM, Fazio VW, et al. Effect of systemic steroids on ileal pouch-anal anastomosis in patients with ulcerative colitis. Dis Colon Rectum 1996; 39:504-8.

74. Shen B, Fazio VW, Remzi FH, et al. Comprehensive evaluation of inflammatory and non-inflammatory sequelae of ileal pouch-anal anastomosis. Am J Gastroenterol 2005; 100:93-101.

124. Remzi FH, Fazio VW, Delaney CP, et al. Dysplasia of the anal transitional zone after ileal pouch-anal anastomosis: Results of prospective evaluation after a minimum of ten years. Dis Colon Rectum 2003; 46:6-13.

132. Olsen KO, Joelsson M, Laurberg S, et al. Fertility after ileal pouch-anal anastomosis in women with ulcerative colitis. Br J Surg 1999; 86:493-5.

142. Selvasekar CR, Cima RR, Larson DW, et al. Effect of infliximab on short-term complications in patients undergoing operation for chronic ulcerative colitis. J Am Coll Surg 2007; 204:956-62.

157. Larson DW, Cima RR, Dozois EJ, et al. Safety, feasibility, and short-term outcomes of laparoscopic ileal-pouch-anal anastomosis: A single institutional case-matched experience. Ann Surg 2006; 243:667-72.

Intestinal ischemia produces a broad spectrum of disorders, depending on the onset, duration, and cause of the injury; the area and length of bowel affected; the vessel involved; and the degree of collateral blood flow. Variability in these factors influences not only the presentation of the ischemic event but also its treatment and outcome. Ischemic injury may be acute or chronic. It may be caused by a disturbance in the arterial supply or venous drainage of the bowel and involve the small intestine, colon, or both.

Since the development and widespread use of colonoscopy, angiography, CT, and other imaging modalities, various types of ischemic injury to the GI tract have been recognized and increasingly appreciated (Table 118-1; also see Tables 118-2 and 118-3). In this chapter we describe the spectrum of ischemic damage to the GI tract and discuss the management of these conditions in light of recent advances.

ANATOMY OF THE SPLANCHNIC CIRCULATION

The celiac axis (CA), superior mesenteric artery (SMA), and inferior mesenteric artery (IMA) supply almost all of the blood flow to the digestive tract.[1] There is marked variability of vascular anatomy among individuals, but typical patterns have emerged from anatomic dissections and abdominal angiographic studies.

Celiac Axis

The CA (Fig. 118-1) arises from the anterior aorta and typically gives rise to 3 major branches: the left gastric artery, common hepatic artery, and splenic artery. The common hepatic artery gives rise to the gastroduodenal, right gastroepiploic, and anterior superior pancreaticoduodenal arterial branches. The splenic artery gives off pancreatic and left gastroepiploic arterial branches. The CA and its branches supply the stomach, duodenum, pancreas, and liver.

Superior Mesenteric Artery

The SMA (Fig. 118-2) has its origin from the anterior aorta near the neck of the pancreas. It gives rise to 5 major vessels: the anterior and posterior inferior pancreaticoduodenal vessels, middle colic, right colic, and ileocolic arteries, as well as to a series of jejunal and ileal branches, all of which supply their named portions of intestine. These intestinal branches typically form a series of arcades, and from the

TABLE 118-1 Types and Approximate Frequencies of Intestinal Ischemia

Type	Frequency (%)
Colon ischemia*	75
Acute mesenteric ischemia*	25
Focal segmental ischemia of the small intestine*	<5
Chronic mesenteric ischemia	<5

*Includes mesenteric venous thrombosis, which can manifest as colon ischemia, acute mesenteric ischemia, or focal segmental ischemia.

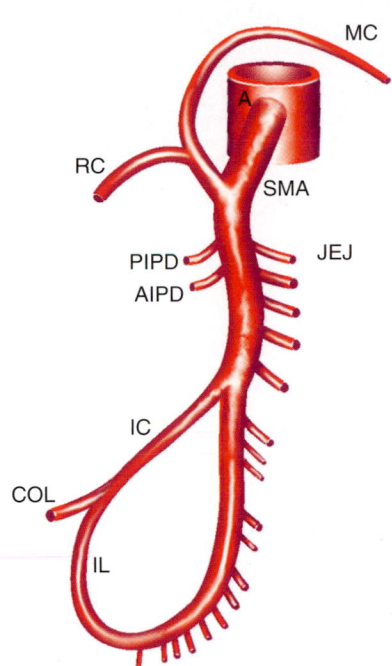

FIGURE 118-2. Diagram of typical superior mesenteric artery *(SMA)* anatomy. AIPD, anterior inferior pancreaticoduodenal artery; COL, colic branches; IL, ileal branches; IC, ileocolic artery; JEJ, jejunal branches; MC, middle colic artery; PIPD, posterior inferior pancreaticoduodenal artery; RC, right colic artery. *(From Nebesar RA, Kornblith PL, Pollard JJ, Michels NA. Celiac and superior mesenteric arteries: A correlation of angiograms and dissections. Boston: Little, Brown; 1969.)*

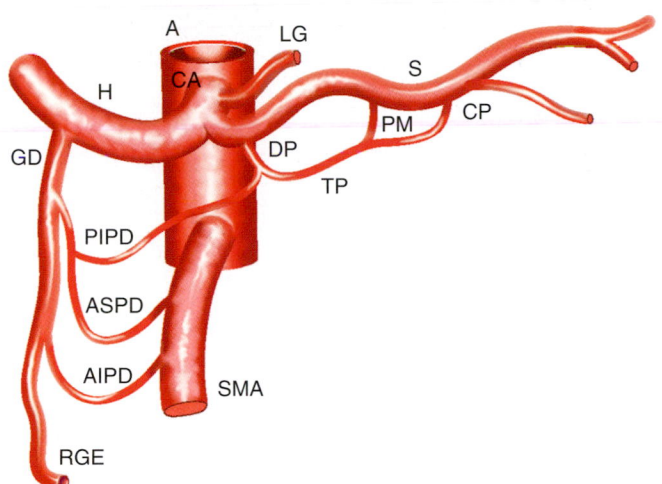

FIGURE 118-1. Diagram of typical celiac axis *(CA)* anatomy and its anastomoses with the superior mesenteric artery *(SMA)*. A, aorta; AIPD, anterior inferior pancreaticoduodenal artery; ASPD, anterior superior pancreaticoduodenal artery; CP, caudal pancreatic artery; DP, dorsal pancreatic artery; GD, gastroduodenal artery; H, common hepatic artery; LG, left gastric artery; PIPD, posterior inferior pancreaticoduodenal artery; PM, pancreata magna; RGE, right gastroepiploic artery; S, splenic artery; TP, transverse pancreatic artery. *(From Nebesar RA, Kornblith PL, Pollard JJ, Michels NA. Celiac and superior mesenteric arteries: A correlation of angiograms and dissections. Boston: Little, Brown; 1969.)*

terminal arcade, numerous straight vessels arise that enter the intestinal wall.

Inferior Mesenteric Artery

The IMA (Fig. 118-3) arises 3 to 4 cm above the aortic bifurcation close to the inferior border of the duodenum. It branches into the left colic artery, gives off multiple sigmoid branches, and terminates as the superior rectal artery. The IMA and its branches supply the large intestine from the distal transverse colon to the proximal rectum. The distal rectum is supplied by branches of the internal iliac (hypogastric) artery.

Collateral and Anastomotic Circulation

Abundant collateral circulation to the stomach, duodenum, and rectum accounts for the paucity of ischemic events in these areas. The major anastomosis between the CA and SMA is formed from the superior pancreaticoduodenal branch of the CA and the inferior pancreaticoduodenal branch of the

SMA. These vessels constitute the pancreaticoduodenal arcade and provide blood to the duodenum and pancreas. The splenic flexure and sigmoid colon have limited anastomoses, and ischemic damage is more common in these locations.

There are 3 potential paths of communication between the SMA and IMA: the marginal artery of Drummond, which is closest to and parallel with the wall of the intestine; the central anastomotic artery, a larger and more centrally placed vessel; and the arc of Riolan, an artery in the base of the mesentery. In the presence of SMA or IMA occlusion, a large collateral termed the *meandering artery* may be identified angiographically and represents a dilated central anastomotic artery or arc of Riolan (Fig. 118-4). It is critical to determine the direction of flow within a meandering artery before sacrificing the IMA, such as during aortic aneurysm surgery, lest the IMA be the main vessel supplying blood to the small bowel because of an occluded SMA.

PATHOPHYSIOLOGY AND PATHOLOGY

Ischemic injury of the intestine results from deprivation of oxygen and nutrients necessary for cellular integrity. Remarkably, the bowel can tolerate a 75% reduction of mesenteric blood flow and oxygen consumption for 12 hours with no changes on light microscopy, because only one fifth of the mesenteric capillaries are open at any time, and when oxygen delivery is decreased, the bowel adapts by increasing oxygen extraction.[2] Below a critical level of blood flow, however, these compensatory mechanisms are overwhelmed and no longer protective.

When a major vessel is occluded, collaterals open immediately in response to the drop in arterial pressure distal to

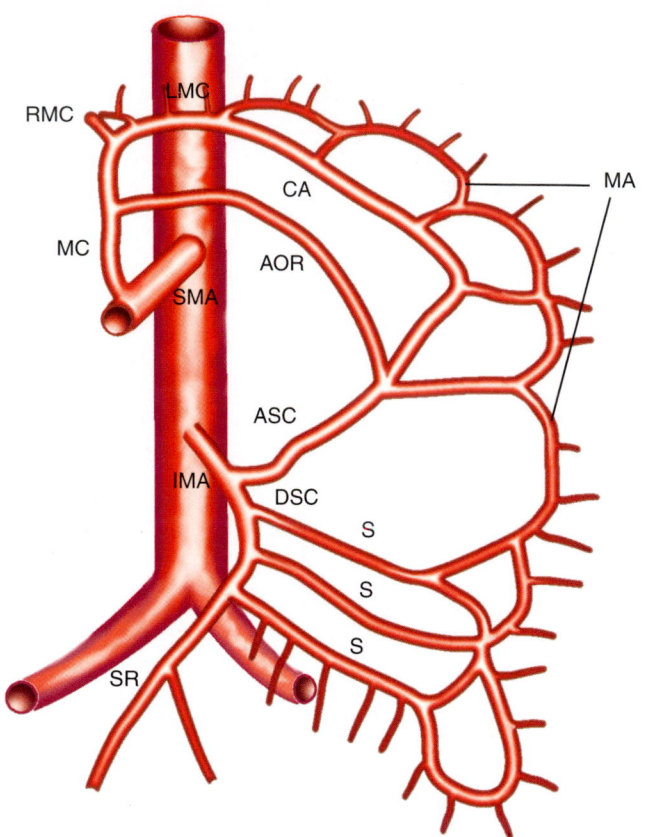

FIGURE 118-3. Diagram of typical inferior mesenteric artery *(IMA)* anatomy and its anastomoses with the superior mesenteric artery *(SMA)*. AOR, arc of Riolan; ASC, ascending branch of the left colic artery; CA, central artery; DSC, descending branch of the left colic artery; LMC, left branch of middle colic artery; MA, marginal artery; MC, middle colic artery; RMC, right branch of middle colic artery; S, sigmoid branches; SR, superior rectal artery. *(From Nebesar RA, Kornblith PL, Pollard JJ, Michels NA. Celiac and superior mesenteric arteries: A correlation of angiograms and dissections. Boston: Little, Brown; 1969.)*

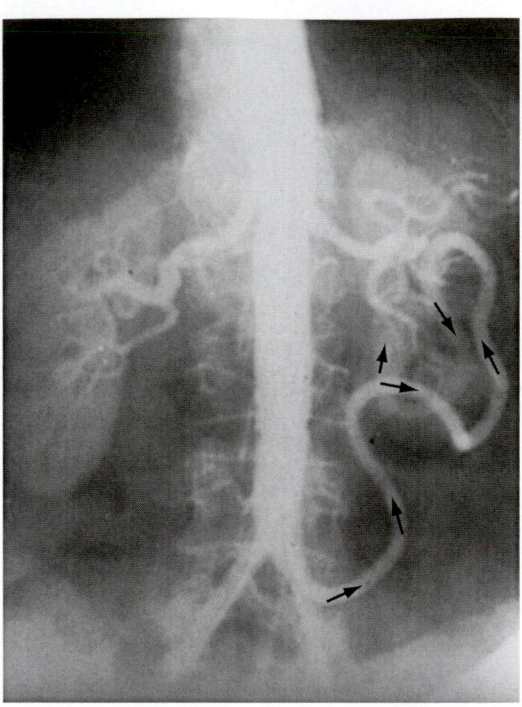

FIGURE 118-4. Film from a flush aortogram of a patient with superior mesenteric artery (SMA) occlusion. The presence of a prominent meandering artery indicates that collateral channels have been present for some time and occlusion is not acute. Arrows show direction of flow from inferior mesenteric artery to SMA. *(From Boley SJ, Brandt LJ, Veith FJ. Ischemic disorders of the intestines. Curr Probl Surg 1978; 15:29.)*

the obstruction and remain open as long as pressure in the vascular bed distal to the obstruction remains below systemic pressure. After several hours of ischemia, however, vasoconstriction develops in the obstructed bed, elevating its pressure and reducing collateral flow. If sustained for a prolonged period, the vasoconstriction can become irreversible and persist even after correction of the cause of the ischemic event. Such persistent vasoconstriction explains the operative findings of progressive bowel ischemia after cardiac function has been optimized and in the absence of arterial or venous obstruction.

Blood flow is affected by a variety of systemic, humoral, local, and neural influences. The sympathetic nervous system, mainly via α-adrenergic receptors, is of primary importance in maintaining resting splanchnic arteriolar tone; other vasoactive substances, including angiotensin II, vasopressin, and prostaglandins, have also been implicated in the pathogenesis of ischemic injury.

Ischemic damage results both from hypoxia during the period of ischemia and reperfusion injury when blood flow is reestablished. More reinjury from brief ischemia appears during reperfusion, but as the ischemic period lengthens, hypoxia becomes more detrimental than reperfusion[3]; the injury after 3 hours of ischemia and 1 hour of reperfusion is

more severe than that after 4 hours of ischemia. Reperfusion injury has been attributed to many factors, but particularly to reactive oxygen- and nitrogen-derived free radicals that can damage an array of molecules found in tissues, including nucleic acids, membrane lipids, enzymes, and receptors. Such widespread damage can result in the mucosal barrier being compromised through cell lysis, impaired cell function, and necrosis on reperfusion of ischemic tissues.[3]

A potent source of oxygen radicals in ischemic reperfused tissue is the enzyme xanthine oxidase (XO), the rate-limiting enzyme in nucleic acid degradation. In nonischemic tissue, this enzyme exists as a dehydrogenase (XDH) that uses nicotinamide adenine dinucleotide (NAD) rather than O_2 as the electron acceptor during purine oxidation; as a result, it does not produce oxygen radicals. During ischemia, XDH is converted to XO with production of reactive oxygen radicals. Inhibition of XO by allopurinol dramatically attenuates the epithelial cell necrosis and the increased microvascular permeability seen during reperfusion (see below).

Neutrophils are another source of reactive oxygen metabolites. During reperfusion, XO-derived oxidants initiate the production and release of leukotriene B_4 and platelet-activating factor, which lead to neutrophil adherence and migration. The adherent leukocytes mediate microvascular injury by release of proteases and physical disruption of the endothelial barrier. Oxygen radical scavengers (superoxide dismutase, dimethyl sulfoxide), XO inhibitors, and agents that inhibit leukocyte adherence and migration have been shown experimentally to protect various organs against reperfusion injury, but are not yet used clinically because, in large measure, they must be given before or coincident with the ischemic injury to have protective effects.[3]

TABLE 118-2 Causes and Approximate Frequencies of Acute Mesenteric Ischemia

Cause	Frequency (%)
SMA thrombosis	54-68
SMA embolus	26-32
Nonocclusive mesenteric ischemia	10
Mesenteric venous thrombosis	5
Focal segmental ischemia of the small intestine	5

SMA, superior mesenteric artery.

ACUTE MESENTERIC ISCHEMIA

Intestinal ischemia can be classified as acute or chronic and of venous or arterial origin. In the acute forms, intestinal viability is threatened, whereas in the chronic forms, blood flow is inadequate to support the functional demands of the intestine. Acute mesenteric ischemia (AMI) is much more common than the chronic type, and arterial disease is more common than venous disease. Arterial forms of AMI include SMA embolus (SMAE), nonocclusive mesenteric ischemia (NOMI), SMA thrombosis (SMAT), and focal segmental ischemia (FSI) (Table 118-2). Acute mesenteric venous thrombosis (MVT) and FSI are the venous forms of AMI.

AMI results from inadequate blood flow to all or part of the small intestine and can involve the right half of the colon because its blood supply is also from the SMA. Regardless of the cause of the ischemic insult, the end results are similar: a spectrum of bowel injury that ranges from transient alteration of bowel function to transmural gangrene. Clinical manifestations vary with the extent and severity of ischemic injury and, to a lesser degree, with its cause.

Incidence

AMI accounts for about 0.1% of admissions to our tertiary care center. This figure has risen over the last few decades owing to increased recognition of the disorder, an aging population, and the widespread use of intensive care units (ICUs) with the salvage of patients who previously would have died from cardiovascular conditions but who now survive to develop AMI as a delayed consequence of their primary disease. Most series of AMI reported in the late 1970s and early 1980s showed that SMAE was responsible for 40% to 50%, NOMI for 20% to 30%, and SMAT for 10% to 20% of cases. Retrospective studies that have addressed the etiology of AMI since then have shown SMAT to occur with the highest frequency (54% to 68%), followed by SMAE in 26% to 32%.[4,5] The incidence of SMAE and NOMI has now declined, likely because of advances in the management of risk factors for embolization; ICU monitoring enabling prompt correction of hypotension and blood volume deficits; effective management of cardiac arrhythmias; and the use of systemic vasodilators that serve to protect the vascular bed from spasm.

Clinical Features

Early identification of AMI requires a high index of suspicion, especially in patients older than 50 years who have long-standing congestive heart failure (particularly if the heart failure is poorly controlled), cardiac arrhythmias, recent myocardial infarction, or hypotension. The development of sudden abdominal pain in a patient with any of these risk factors should suggest the diagnosis of AMI. Younger patients, however, are not without risk of AMI, especially if they are taking vasoactive medications (e.g., phenylephrine, amphetamines, triptans), are using cocaine, or have underlying thrombophilia. Hence, unexplained, persistent, and severe abdominal pain should prompt consideration of AMI as an explanation for the pain. A history of postprandial abdominal pain in the weeks to months preceding the acute onset of severe abdominal pain is associated only with SMAT.

Most patients with AMI have acute abdominal pain.[4,5] Early in the course of disease, the pain of AMI is far more impressive than the physical findings. Initially, the pain is severe, but the abdomen usually is flat, soft, and sometimes not tender, or certainly less tender than expected based on the magnitude of the pain. The classic description of "pain out of proportion to abdominal findings" seems less accurate than previously believed, with only an estimated 29% of patients having this finding in the decade spanning from 2000 to 2010.[4] This decrease might reflect the shifting etiologies of AMI, since a more indolent and less striking onset typifies MVT, and with NOMI, appreciation of abdominal pain may be overshadowed by the precipitating acute disorders, such as hypotension, congestive heart failure, hypovolemia, or cardiac arrhythmias. SMAE, now seen less frequently, more commonly presents with sudden severe abdominal pain accompanied by rapid and often forceful bowel evacuation, especially with minimal or no abdominal signs.

Unexplained abdominal distention or GI bleeding may be the only indications of AMI when pain is absent, especially when AMI is due to NOMI. Distention, although absent early in the course of AMI, is often the first sign of intestinal infarction and is seen in approximately 25% of patients presenting with AMI. Right-sided abdominal pain and tenderness that may not occur together with passage of maroon or red blood in the stool characterizes isolated right colon ischemia and may be seen synchronously with AMI, because the blood supply to both the ascending colon and small intestine originates from the SMA. Rectal bleeding is seen in 13% to 16% of patients presenting with AMI.[4,5] Older adults with AMI have been reported to develop mental confusion acutely in as many as 30% of cases.[6] In patients who survive cardiopulmonary resuscitation and then develop recurrent bacteremia or sepsis, the suspected cause of sepsis should be NOMI that resulted in a segment of bowel that sustained subacute ischemic injury and is now acting as a portal for bacterial translocation.[7] Although episodes of sepsis may be treated successfully with antibiotics, the entire length of damaged bowel must be removed to prevent recurrent sepsis.

Although abdominal findings early in the course of intestinal ischemia may be minimal or absent, increasing tenderness, rebound tenderness, and muscle guarding reflect progressive loss of intestinal viability. Such abdominal findings strongly indicate the presence of infarcted bowel. The rate of progression from the onset of abdominal pain to intestinal infarction varies not with the specific cause of ischemia but with the severity of the ischemic insult; MVT generally has a more indolent course than arterial causes of AMI.

Laboratory Features and Diagnosis

On admission to the hospital, patients with AMI usually have a white blood cell (WBC) count greater than 15,000 cells/mm³.[3,4,5] A normal WBC count, however, cannot be used to exclude early AMI, just as a high WBC count does not make the diagnosis. Elevated levels of serum phosphate, L- and D-lactate,[8] amylase, and other enzymes have been noted, as have high peritoneal fluid amylase and intestinal alkaline phosphatase activity, but the sensitivity and specificity of these markers for intestinal ischemia have not been established.[9] D-dimer has been found to be the most sensitive early marker for AMI, but its specificity remains low.[9] More specific intestinal enzymes including diamine oxidase,[10] hexosaminidase, glutathione S-transferase,[11] and intestinal fatty acid-binding protein[12] also lack sufficient sensitivity and specificity to diagnose AMI. Moreover, serum markers, when elevated, usually indicate late-stage disease. There is no serum marker yet demonstrated to be reliable to diagnose *early* ischemic bowel injury.

Although they are poorly sensitive (30%) and nonspecific, plain films of the abdomen (or the initial scanning view of a CT scan) are still obtained in evaluating patients with suspected AMI. Plain films of the abdomen are usually normal in AMI before infarction. Later on, formless loops of small intestine, ileus, thumbprinting of the small bowel or ascending colon (Fig. 118-5), or still later, pneumatosis linearis and portal or mesenteric vascular gas (Fig. 118-6) may be seen. In one

study, the mortality rate of patients with normal plain film studies was 29%, whereas it was 78% in those with abnormal findings.[13] The primary purpose of plain films (or CT scans) is to exclude causes of abdominal pain other than ischemia that might mandate a different therapeutic approach.

Duplex scanning and Doppler flowmetry can be used to evaluate patients with suspected AMI, but these techniques are limited in their clinical use by the following factors:

- Only the proximal portions of the major splanchnic vessels can be studied reliably, not the peripheral aspect of the vasculature.
- Vascular occlusions are not diagnostic of intestinal ischemia, because complete occlusions can be seen in asymptomatic patients.
- Blood flow through the SMA is highly variable, which may make interpretation difficult.
- NOMI cannot be diagnosed reliably by US studies.

CT has largely replaced plain film study of the abdomen for diagnosis and is used to identify arterial and venous thromboses as well as ischemic bowel.[14-16] Findings on CT include colon dilatation, bowel wall thickening, abnormal bowel wall enhancement, lack of enhancement of arterial vasculature with timed intravenous contrast injections, arterial occlusion, venous thrombosis, engorgement of mesenteric veins, intramural gas and mesenteric or portal venous gas (Fig. 118-6), infarction of other organs, ascites, and signs perhaps related to the cause of the infarcted bowel, such as hernia.[14,16] Unfortunately, the early signs on CT are nonspecific, and the late signs reflect necrotic bowel.

In a study of 26 patients with AMI who had a preoperative multislice CT scan followed by exploratory laparotomy, CT scanning identified mesenteric arterial thrombosis in 16 of 17 patients and mesenteric vein thrombosis in 7 of 7 patients, all confirmed at operation. In this study, the sensitivity and specificity of CT scanning for occlusive AMI was 92% and 100%, respectively.[17] In a study of 94 patients who underwent exploratory surgery for acute abdominal pain, all 49 patients with AMI were diagnosed by CT scan prior to their surgery.[18] Relatively subtle CT findings are being increasingly appreciated as radiologists gain greater experience with CT imaging in patients with AMI. Mesenteric fat stranding and mesenteric ascites, although previously not recognized to be associated with AMI, appear to be indicative of early AMI; experimental

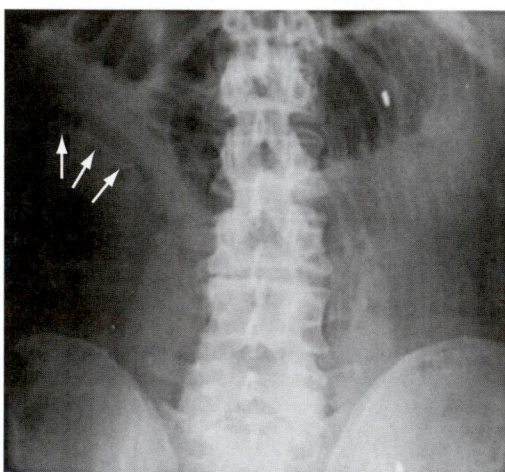

FIGURE 118-5. Plain film of the abdomen showing an ileus and a formless fixed loop of small intestine *(arrows)* in a patient with acute mesenteric ischemia from a superior mesenteric artery embolus.

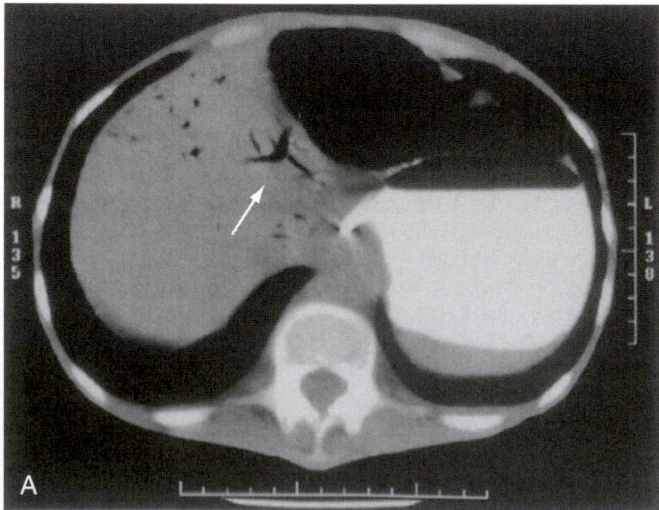
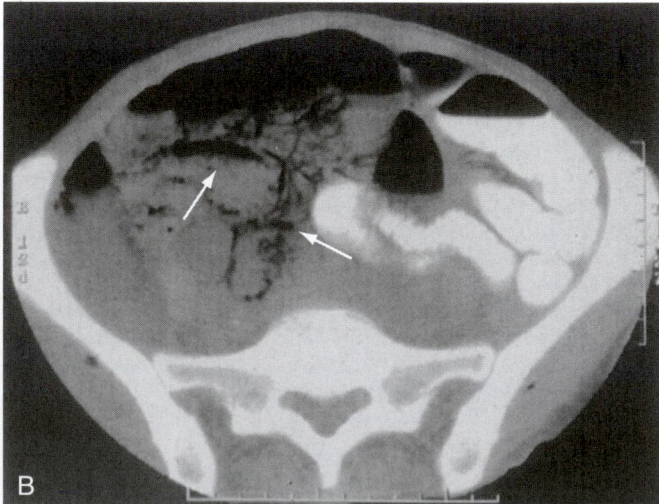

FIGURE 118-6. CT of a patient with acute mesenteric ischemia showing gas *(arrow)* in the portal veins *(A)* and gas *(arrows)* in the wall of the intestine as well as the mesentery and its vessels *(B)*. Pneumatosis intestinalis (linearis) is a late sign of ischemic injury, connotes bowel necrosis, and mandates explorative laparotomy.

models show that the mesentery is the first area to react to both arterial and venous compromise.[19] The predictive value of CT scanning in the community might not be as high as in these reports, because these studies involved only highly trained radiologists. Improved CT scanner technology, however, likely will yield higher detection rates than in the past.

CT angiography (CTA) has been shown to be the imaging modality of choice in the diagnosis of AMI. In 1 study, the added findings on CTA were believed to alter clinical management in 19% of 62 patients by making the diagnosis of AMI when CT alone did not.[20] When 91 patients with abdominal pain and suspected AMI underwent CTA, 18 of them had AMI diagnosed, with a diagnostic accuracy of 95.6%.[21] A separate study of 79 consecutive patients with abdominal pain found that 28 patients had confirmed AMI, 27 of whom were diagnosed via CTA (96.4%), with a sensitivity of 93% and specificity of 100%.[22] These promising findings for the increased use of CTA in patients with suspected AMI are somewhat tempered by other studies that showed up to 33% of findings typical for AMI (e.g., gas in the portal vein or gas in the bowel wall) were overlooked on initial CTA assessment.[23] Nonetheless, CTA is a highly accurate diagnostic tool for patients with suspected AMI.

Selective mesenteric angiography with papaverine infusion was previously the mainstay of diagnosis of both occlusive and nonocclusive forms of AMI. Sensitivity and specificity of mesenteric angiography for diagnosing AMI in most studies have been in the range of 90% to 100% and 100%, respectively.[24] Use of angiography as a diagnostic tool, however, has fallen out of favor given the ease of obtaining a CTA. CTA is highly accurate to detect occlusive disease of the SMA but not as reliable for NOMI. Selective mesenteric angiography is also an invasive procedure with attendant risks and might delay surgical intervention if not readily available. Regardless, early use of angiography for diagnosis and treatment of AMI before the onset of irreversible ischemic injury has been repeatedly shown to improve outcome in patients with AMI.

Magnetic resonance angiography (MRA) and venography (MRV) are imaging techniques that also can be used to diagnose AMI. Although this technique can accurately visualize the vasculature, its use in the diagnosis of AMI is limited by the time it takes to complete the study and so may result in delayed diagnosis and management. Prompt laparotomy is indicated for patients with suspected AMI if imaging of the vascular system, whether by angiography or CTA, cannot be performed expeditiously.

Laparoscopy may be useful, but it too can be misleading because early in ischemic injury, blood flow may be shunted to the serosa, giving it a normal appearance even when the mucosa is necrotic. Moreover, laparoscopy is potentially dangerous because SMA blood flow decreases when intraperitoneal pressure exceeds 20 mm Hg. One small study of patients treated for aortic dissection with suspected AMI showed that of the 9 patients who were assessed through diagnostic laparoscopy, 1 patient with AMI was identified on "first look" and 2 more patients during a "second-look" laparoscopy. A total of 9 "first-looks" and 3 "second-looks" were performed, and the outcomes and complication rates were similar to a cohort of 8 patients who did not undergo diagnostic laparoscopy. The authors concluded that diagnostic laparoscopy was feasible, was safe, and had low invasiveness.[25]

Treatment

Our approach to the management of AMI is based on several observations. First, if the diagnosis is not made before intestinal infarction, the mortality rate is unacceptably high at 70%

to 90%. Second, diagnosis of the occlusive and less so the nonocclusive forms of AMI can be made in most patients by a vascular imaging study, either CTA or angiography. Third, vasoconstriction, which can persist even after the cause of the ischemia is corrected, is the basis of NOMI and a contributing factor in the other forms of AMI. Finally, vasoconstriction can be relieved by vasodilators infused into the SMA. The cornerstones of our approach, therefore, are earlier and more liberal use of vascular imaging studies and incorporation of intraarterial papaverine whenever possible in the treatment of both occlusive AMI and NOMI. Duration of symptoms parallels mortality, so early diagnosis and treatment are paramount to increasing the chance for survival.[26]

AMI should be suspected in patients older than 50 years who have the risk factors previously described and in younger patients—especially those with atrial fibrillation, vasculitis, a coagulation disorder, and those on vasoactive medications—who seek medical attention for sudden severe abdominal pain that lasts longer than several hours. These patients should be managed according to the algorithm shown in Figure 118-7. Less absolute indications for inclusion into this protocol consist of unexplained acute abdominal distention, colonoscopic evidence of isolated right-sided colonic ischemia, and acidosis without an identifiable cause.

Initial management of patients with suspected AMI includes resuscitation and diagnostic imaging studies. Resuscitation includes relief of acute congestive heart failure and correction of hypotension, hypovolemia, and cardiac arrhythmias. Broad-spectrum antibiotics (e.g., levofloxacin, metronidazole, piperacillin-tazobactam) are given immediately because of the high incidence of positive blood cultures in AMI and because they have been shown to reduce the extent and severity of ischemic injury in experimental animals.[27] There are no randomized controlled trials showing the benefit of antibiotics in AMI, and it is unlikely such trials will ever be done. After resuscitation, plain films or CT scan of the abdomen are obtained, not to establish the diagnosis of AMI but rather to exclude other causes of abdominal pain; a normal plain film or CT scan does not exclude AMI. Ideally, patients are studied before (specific) radiologic signs appear, because these signs connote irreversibly damaged bowel. If no alternative diagnosis is made on these studies, one should consider CTA, with a low threshold for selective SMA angiography to be performed. Based on the angiographic findings and the presence or absence of peritoneal signs, the patient is treated according to the algorithm in Figure 118-7.

Even when the decision to operate has been based on clinical grounds, preoperative angiography should be performed, if possible, to manage the patient properly at and after laparotomy. When comparing surgical intervention alone with an approach that includes endovascular angiography prior to any surgery, angiography resulted in less frequent surgery, resection of shorter areas of necrotic bowel, lower rates of acute renal and pulmonary failure and, most important, a 90% risk reduction in mortality in patients with thrombotic causes of AMI.[28] A multidisciplinary approach is essential to the management of patients with AMI. One study assembled a team including gastroenterologists, vascular and abdominal surgeons, radiologists, and intensive care specialists, with a plan for all patients to undergo "medical management," including endovascular interventions. This multidisciplinary approach resulted in 95% survival at 30 days and 89% survival at 2 years.[29]

Relief of mesenteric vasoconstriction is essential to the treatment of emboli, thromboses, and the nonocclusive lowflow states. Infusion of the phosphodiesterase inhibitor papaverine through an angiography catheter in the SMA can be used to relieve mesenteric vasoconstriction preoperatively

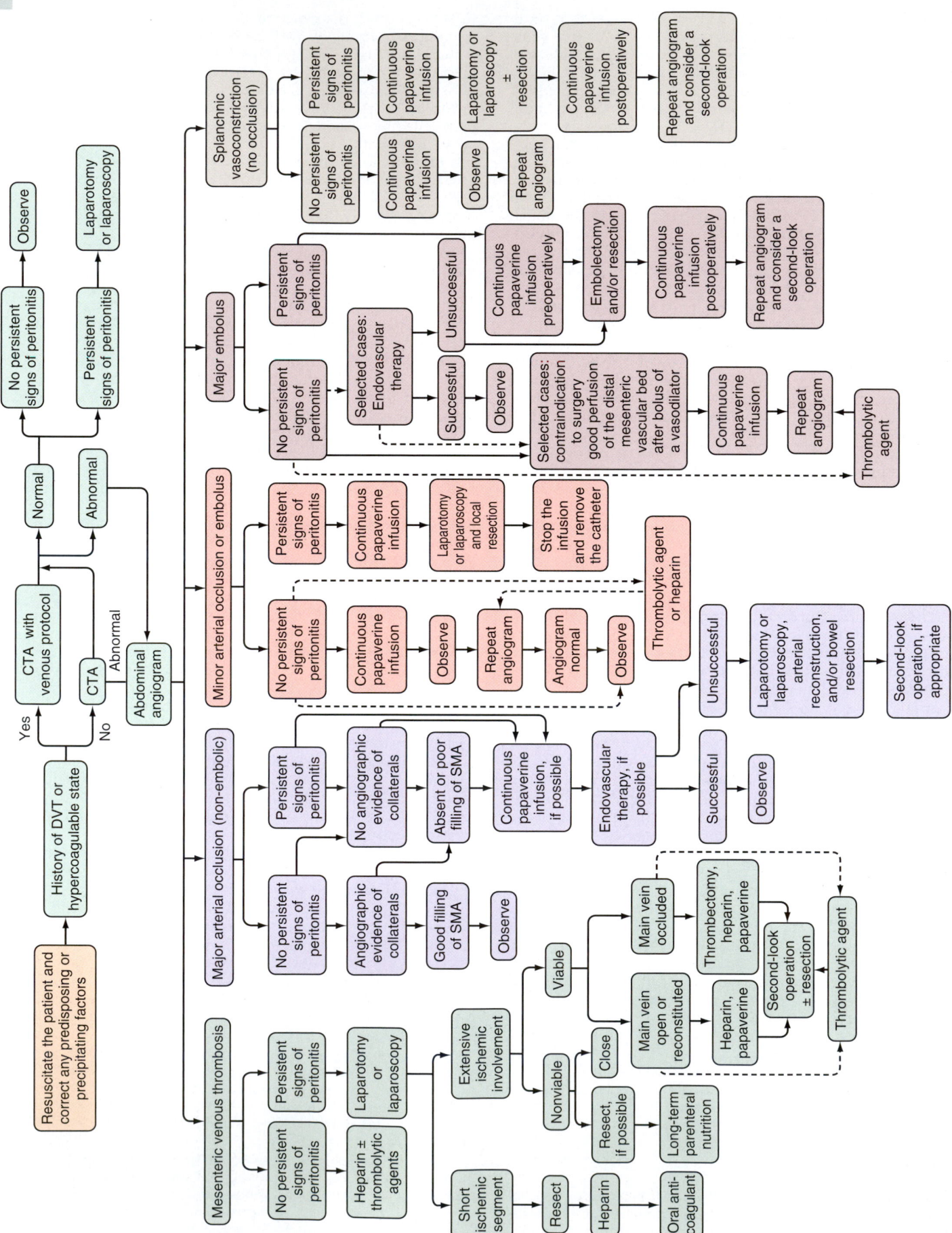

FIGURE 118-7. Algorithm for the diagnosis and treatment of intestinal ischemia. Solid lines show the conventional management plan; dotted lines show an alternative management plan. DVT, deep venous thrombosis; SMA, superior mesenteric artery. (*Modified from Brandt LJ, Boley SJ. AGA technical review on intestinal ischemia: American Gastrointestinal Association. Gastroenterology 2000; 118:954; corrected version in Gastroenterology 2000; 119:281.*)

and postoperatively. The papaverine is infused by pump at a constant rate of 30 to 60 mg/hr; papaverine concentrations may vary with the need for fluid restriction. If hypotension develops during SMA infusion of papaverine, the position of the catheter should be checked radiologically to ensure that it has not dislodged from the aorta.

Angiographers can also attempt to intervene on the vascular occlusion directly as a surgery-sparing measure; several small studies and case series have shown this approach to have excellent success.[28,30-32] Such endovascular techniques include aspiration embolectomy, SMA thrombolysis, and stenting of atherosclerotic occlusions. The methodology used is based on the mechanism of the ischemia, the length of the occlusion, and the appearance of the underlying and distal arteries.

Aspiration embolectomy is the angiographic procedure most commonly performed for proximal SMA emboli. Using an antegrade approach via the femoral artery, a guiding catheter is placed within the embolus, and a syringe is used to suction it simultaneously with sheath withdrawal; several passes are usually required to completely remove the embolus.[33]

SMA thrombolysis is rarely used as a solitary treatment, because there is usually insufficient time for complete treatment, given the risks of thrombus propagation and bowel necrosis and the risk of acute GI bleeding if the bowel is already necrotic. This technique is used as an adjunct when there is low suspicion for transmural intestinal infarction and most of the clot was able to be removed via aspiration embolectomy. Thrombolysis is performed by placing a multi-side-holed catheter within the proximal SMA. Tissue plasminogen activator is infused at a rate of 0.5 to 1 mg/hr, with reconfirmation of catheter location at 12-hour intervals.[33]

The primary angiographic therapy for underlying stenotic or occlusive lesions is percutaneous transluminal angioplasty (PTA) with subsequent vascular stenting using balloon expandable metal stents. The number of stents used depends on the size of the lesion, and following stent placement the pressure gradient across the lesion is measured. If the pressure gradient is greater than 12 mm Hg there is a high risk of restenosis, and further intervention is required.[34] In endovascular coronary interventions, filters and other protection devices are used to protect against propagation and embolization of thrombus as a result of the procedure. These protection devices are technically challenging to use during intervention within the SMA, and their safety and efficacy have not been reported.[33]

Laparotomy is performed in AMI to restore arterial flow obstructed by embolus or thrombosis, resect irreparably damaged bowel, or both. Embolectomy, thrombectomy, or arterial bypass precedes evaluation of intestinal viability, because bowel that initially appears infarcted can show surprising recovery after adequate blood flow has been restored. In the operating room, intestinal viability can be assessed clinically by any of several techniques, including Doppler US, pulse oximetry, and visible light spectrophotometry among others.[35] Animal models show that administration of intravenous glucagon, intravenous heparin-binding epidermal growth factor (HB-EGF)-like growth factor, or intraluminal nitroglycerin after revascularization of an acute arterial occlusion can improve mucosal viability and minimize reperfusion damage.[36,37]

In practice, glucagon is sometimes used because of its accessibility and anecdotally reported beneficial effects, despite lack of strong supporting data from human trials. Short segments of bowel that are nonviable or questionably viable after revascularization are resected, and a primary anastomosis is performed. If extensive portions of the bowel are of questionable viability, only the clearly necrotic bowel is resected, and re-exploration ("second look") is planned for within 12 to 24 hours. The interval between the first and second operations is used both to allow better demarcation between viable and nonviable bowel and to attempt to improve intestinal blood flow by using intra-arterial papaverine and maximizing cardiac output.

The use of anticoagulants in the management of AMI is controversial. Anticoagulation with heparin can cause intestinal or intraperitoneal hemorrhage and, except for MVT, should not be used routinely in the immediate postoperative period; 48 hours after embolectomy or arterial reconstruction, when thrombosis is common, anticoagulation is appropriate.

Specific Types of Acute Mesenteric Ischemia

Superior Mesenteric Artery Embolus

SMAE is responsible for about 30% of AMI episodes. Emboli usually originate from a left atrial or ventricular mural thrombus. Many patients with SMAE have had previous peripheral artery emboli, and roughly 20% have synchronous emboli. SMAEs lodge at points of normal anatomic narrowing, usually immediately distal to the origin of a major branch. Angiography typically reveals a rounded filling defect with nearly complete obstruction to flow. Mesenteric atherosclerosis is usually not as severe as in SMAT. Emboli proximal to the origin of the ileocolic artery are considered major emboli. Minor emboli are those that lodge in the SMA distal to the takeoff of the ileocolic artery or in the distal branches of the SMA (Fig. 118-8).

Various therapeutic approaches have been proposed for SMAE, depending on the presence or absence of peritoneal signs, whether the embolus is partially or completely occluding, and whether the embolus is above the origin of the ileocolic artery or more distal. Therapy for SMAE has included surgical revascularization, intra-arterial perfusion with vasodilators or thrombolytic agents, and anticoagulation.[24] In the absence of peritoneal signs, minor SMA emboli have been treated successfully with all these agents without the need for surgery. Exploration is usually performed in patients with major emboli after papaverine infusion is begun. The decision of whether to attempt endovascular treatment in patients with major emboli is dependent upon the skills of the endovascular interventionalist available at each medical center. In most centers, nonoperative therapy using only endovascular intervention is attempted when there are significant contraindications to surgery, no peritoneal signs, and adequate perfusion of the vascular bed distal to the embolus after a bolus of vasodilator into the SMA.

Exploratory laparotomy is mandatory when peritonitis is present; embolectomy and bowel resection are performed as necessary. If possible, intra-arterial papaverine is begun before surgery and continued during surgery. If no second-look operation is planned, infusion is continued for 12 to 24 hours postoperatively; persistent vasospasm is excluded by angiography before the catheter is removed (see Fig. 118-8). If a second operation is planned, the infusion is continued through the second procedure until angiography shows the vasoconstriction has ceased. Recognition of persistent vasoconstriction has prompted some authorities to recommend routine use of intra-arterial papaverine in all patients with SMAE; the best survival rates are seen in patients treated by this approach.[24]

Use of transcatheter aspiration embolectomy and/or thrombolytic therapy (e.g., tissue plasminogen activator) can be considered before exploratory laparotomy if the patient does not have signs of peritonitis. Case series have shown that aspiration thrombectomy alone[31] or in combination with

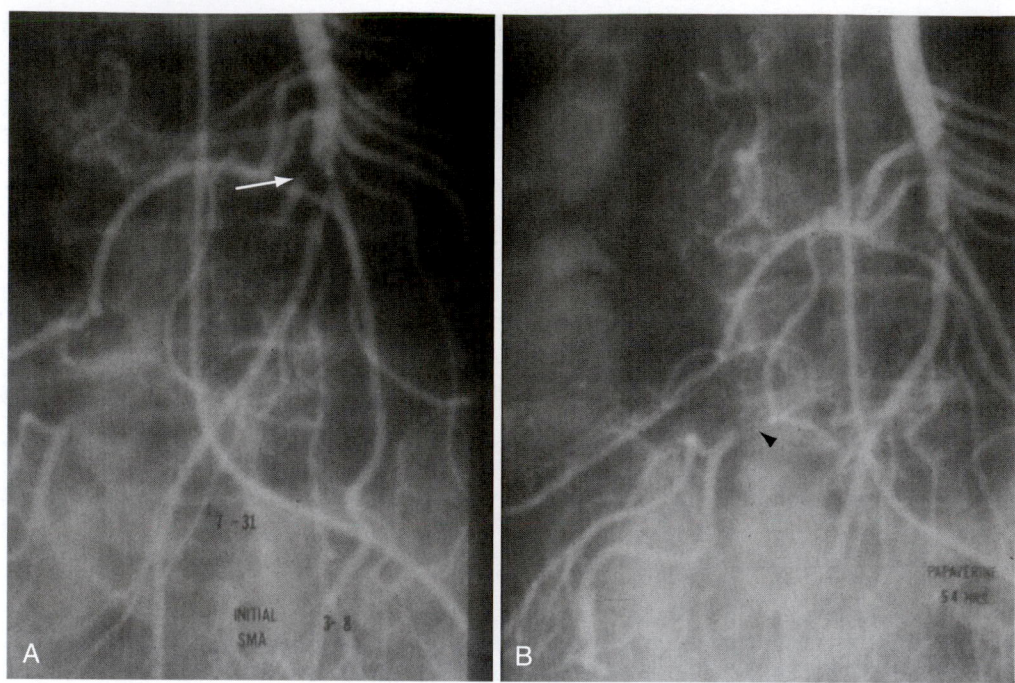

FIGURE 118-8. *A,* Superior mesenteric artery (SMA) angiogram in a 71-year-old man with abdominal pain, showing an embolus occluding the SMA at the level of the origin of the right colic artery *(arrow).* Mild vasoconstriction is noted distal to the embolus. *B,* A repeat angiogram done 54 hours after papaverine infusion into the SMA. Vasodilatation is seen, and all vessels are patent except for a distal jejunal branch, which contains a piece of the inciting embolus *(arrowhead)* that broke off during the course of vasodilator therapy because of endogenous thrombolysis. Papaverine protected the bowel within the distribution of the embolized vessel by enabling vasodilatation and maintenance of adequate blood flow. The patient was operated on after 54 hours of papaverine, and it was confirmed that all the bowel appeared healthy and free of ischemic necrosis.

thrombolytics[30] is a useful and safe surgery-sparing intervention. Prospective studies and meta-analyses have shown that thrombolysis may be effective in resolving thrombi, improving symptoms, and avoiding surgery in patients with lesions amenable to such therapy.[38,39] Thrombolytic therapy is most likely to be successful when the embolus is partially occluding or is minor and when the study is performed within 12 hours of the onset of symptoms.[40] A canine study showed that intra-arterial streptokinase was more effective than intra-arterial papaverine in lysing clots implanted into the SMA, although greater ischemic damage occurred with streptokinase than with papaverine because of papaverine's action to cause vasodilation and open collateral pathways for blood flow around the obstructing clot. When streptokinase and papaverine were administered simultaneously, neither medication functioned as well as it did alone, and intestinal damage was intensified.[41] There is increasing evidence that use of thrombolytic medications in patients with AMI might be helpful in appropriate circumstances (e.g., no evidence of bowel necrosis), especially when combined with other endovascular interventions as a surgery-sparing measure.

Nonocclusive Mesenteric Ischemia

NOMI is responsible for about 10% of AMI and is usually due to splanchnic vasoconstriction consequent to a preceding cardiovascular event. AMI can appear hours to days after the event, and vasoconstriction, which initially is reversible, can persist even after the precipitating event has been corrected. Precipitating causes for NOMI include acute myocardial infarction, congestive heart failure, arrhythmias, shock, cirrhosis, medications and drugs (e.g., sumatriptan, cocaine), cardiopulmonary bypass surgery, and chronic kidney disease, especially when patients are on either hemodialysis or peritoneal dialysis. When presenting with abdominal pain, patients on peritoneal dialysis may be thought to have peritonitis, thereby delaying the diagnosis of NOMI and resulting in a poor outcome.[42] Patients at risk for NOMI after elective cardiac surgery include those older than 70 years of age with preoperative renal insufficiency or being treated with diuretic therapy, whereas postoperative risk factors include the need for an intra-aortic balloon pump and serum lactate levels higher than 5 mmol/L.[43]

NOMI is diagnosed by angiography using 4 criteria: narrowing of the origins of SMA branches, irregularities in the intestinal branches, spasm of the arcades, and impaired filling of intramural vessels. Patients with these signs who are neither in shock nor on vasopressors and who do not have pancreatitis can be considered to have NOMI (Fig. 118-9). In recent years, given the advancements with noninvasive radiologic studies like CTA and the challenges in certain institutions of obtaining emergent angiography, criteria for the noninvasive early diagnosis of NOMI have been re-evaluated. In a 2-phase study that initially analyzed a series of 13 patients with early AMI, the most common clinical criteria found for NOMI were: (1) symptoms of ileus, including slow onset of abdominal discomfort or pain, (2) requirement for catecholamine administration, (3) an episode of hypotension, and (4) slow elevation of aminotransferase levels. The second portion of this study used these criteria to analyze 9 subsequent patients. Those who met 3 of the 4 criteria were referred for a multidetector-row CT (MDCT) instead of angiography. If the MDCT showed variable intestinal wall contrast uptake, spasm, or narrowing of the SMA, the patients were believed to have early NOMI and treated with prostaglandin E_1 (PGE$_1$) infusion. Eight of the 9 patients diagnosed using these criteria and treated with PGE$_1$ were able to avoid more severe acute-stage NOMI, although their outcomes were not compared with a control cohort.[44]

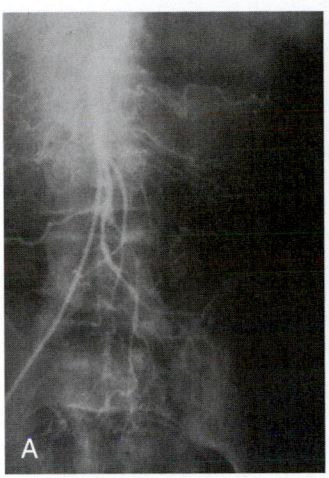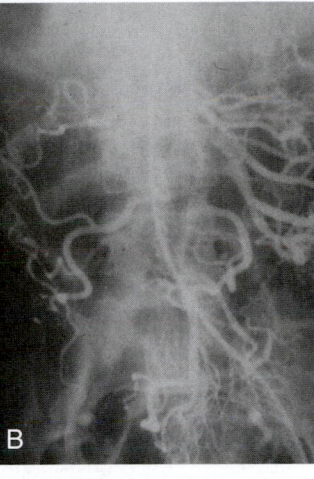

FIGURE 118-9. Superior mesenteric angiogram in a patient with nonocclusive mesenteric ischemia (NOMI) following a bout of GI hemorrhage and shock. *A,* Pretreatment film shows the diffuse vasoconstriction of NOMI. *B,* Marked vasodilatation is evident on repeat study after 48 hours of intra-arterial papaverine infusion. NOMI, nonocclusive mesenteric ischemia *(From Brandt LJ, Boley SJ. Ischemic intestinal syndromes. Adv Surg 1981; 15:1.)*

Although less invasive measures are being studied, the standard of care remains angiography with SMA infusion of papaverine as soon as the diagnosis of NOMI is made. Operation is performed if peritoneal signs are present, and the infusion is continued during and after exploration. Necrotic bowel is resected; it is better to leave bowel of questionable viability and perform a second-look operation than to perform massive enterectomy, because compromised but viable bowel often improves with supportive measures. The infusion is continued as for second-look operations following embolectomy.

When papaverine infusion is used as the only treatment for NOMI in patients without signs of peritonitis, it is continued for 24 hours, and repeat angiography is performed 30 minutes after changing the papaverine infusion to normal saline. Papaverine infusion is maintained and angiography repeated daily until there is no roentgenographic evidence of vasoconstriction and the patient's clinical findings resolve. Infusions, usually discontinued after 24 hours, have been given for as long as 5 days.

Acute Thrombosis of the Superior Mesenteric Artery

Acute SMAT occurs in areas of severe atherosclerotic narrowing, most often at the origin of the SMA. The acute ischemic episode may be superimposed on chronic mesenteric ischemia (CMI), and 20% to 50% of patients have a history of postprandial abdominal pain and weight loss during the weeks to months preceding the acute event. Evidence of coronary, cerebrovascular, or peripheral arterial insufficiency is common.

SMAT can be demonstrated on CTA in the presence of focal stenosis of the vessel with or without surrounding vascular calcification and on flush aortography, which usually shows occlusion of the SMA 1 to 2 cm from its origin. Some distal filling of the SMA via collaterals is common. Branches proximal and distal to the obstruction can show localized or diffuse vasoconstriction. In patients with abdominal pain, no abdominal tenderness, and complete occlusion of the SMA on aortography, it is important, though difficult, to distinguish between acute thrombosis and long-standing coincidental chronic occlusion. Prominent collaterals between the SMA and other

major splanchnic vessels indicate chronic SMA occlusion. If there is good filling of the SMA, the occlusion is considered chronic, and the abdominal pain is considered unrelated to mesenteric vascular disease (see Fig. 118-4). The absence of collateral vessels or the presence of collaterals with inadequate filling of the SMA indicates an acute occlusion and demands prompt intervention. If possible, an angiographic catheter is placed in the proximal SMA, and, when possible, attempts are made to perform thrombectomy with percutaneous transluminal angioplasty followed by stent placement. If this is unsuccessful, papaverine infusion is begun before surgery is undertaken. At surgery, necrotic bowel is resected, and the remaining bowel is revascularized. Papaverine infusion is continued throughout the operative period, and management is the same as for SMAE.

Complications

Complications of angiography and prolonged infusion of vasodilator drugs include transient acute tubular necrosis following angiography, local hematomas at the arterial puncture sites, catheter dislodgment, and fibrin clots on the arterial catheter. Infusion for more than 5 days has not had significant systemic effects.

Results

Although mortality rates of 70% to 90% were reported through the 1980s for patients whose AMI was diagnosed and treated conventionally, the approach described here can reduce these catastrophic figures. The best survival is reported in series in which there is a multidisciplinary approach to the patient, early diagnosis, and rapid use of CTA or angiography is routine.[29,45,46]

In our tertiary medical center, more than 50% of the patients with AMI treated according to our approach survived, and more than 75% have lost less than 1 meter of intestine. A study using an aggressive multidisciplinary approach including rapid angiography showed 95% survival at 30 days and 89% survival at 2 years in patients with occlusive AMI.[29] The importance of early diagnosis is emphasized by the survival of 90% of patients who had AMI but no signs of peritonitis, and who had angiography early in their course. Ideally, all patients with AMI should be studied when plain films of the abdomen and regular CT scanning are normal and before signs of an acute surgical abdomen and laboratory evidence of infarction appear.

Diagnosis before intestinal infarction occurs is the most important factor in improving survival of patients with AMI.

MESENTERIC VENOUS THROMBOSIS

MVT occurs as an acute, subacute, or chronic disorder. It is only since the development of recent imaging techniques that these various forms of MVT have been recognized; previously, only acute MVT was known, and diagnosis was made at laparotomy or autopsy.

Incidence

In early studies, MVT was believed to be the major cause of AMI, but most of these cases probably represented NOMI. Today, only 5% to 10% of patients with AMI have MVT. The mean age at presentation with MVT is in the mid-60s,[47] and a Swedish study showed that the highest incidence of MVT was 11.3 per 100,000 person years among those 70 to 79 years old.[48]

Predisposing Conditions

Previously, a cause of MVT was identified in fewer than half of patients. However, the discoveries of primary and secondary hypercoagulable states and the use of estrogens for contraception and hormone replacement have led to more frequent identification of cause. Risk factors for MVT can be broadly classified into heritable and acquired thrombophilias (e.g., antithrombin III, protein C deficiency, protein S deficiency), hypercoagulable (thrombophilic) states due to systemic disorders (e.g., nephrotic syndrome, malignancy), and local intra-abdominal processes (e.g., diverticulitis, trauma). Despite an extensive list of potential causes and risk factors, 21% to 49% of cases are still classified as idiopathic.[49] MVT has a similar frequency of associated thrombophilia (41.8%) compared with splenic vein thrombosis (45.5%) but a higher rate than either portal or hepatic vein thrombosis.[50] A list of predisposing conditions for MVT is given in Box 118-1.[49]

Pathophysiology

The location of the initial thrombus within the mesenteric venous circulation varies with its cause. MVT secondary to

---

BOX 118-1 **Conditions Associated with Mesenteric Venous Thrombosis**

Heritable Thrombophilias
Antithrombin III deficiency
Factor V Leiden mutation
Hereditary hemorrhagic telangiectasia
Hyperfibrinogenemia
JAK2 V617F mutation
Plasminogen deficiency
Protein C deficiency
Protein S deficiency
Prothrombin G20210A mutation
Sickle cell disease

Acquired Thrombophilias and Systemic Hypercoagulable States
Antiphospholipid antibodies:
   Anticardiolipin antibody
   Beta-2 glycoprotein-1 antibodies
Decompression sickness
DIC
Essential thrombocythemia
Heparin-induced thrombocytopenia
Hyperhomocysteinemia
Malignancy
Monoclonal gammopathy
Myeloproliferative disease
Nephrotic syndrome
Oral contraceptive agents and other medications
Paroxysmal nocturnal hemoglobinuria
Polycythemia vera
Pregnancy

Intra-abdominal Causes
Cirrhosis
Congenital venous anomaly
IBD
Intestinal volvulus
Intra-abdominal infection
Pancreatitis
Postoperative state
Trauma

Idiopathic

---

local factors (e.g., cirrhosis, neoplasm, operative injury) starts at the site of obstruction and extends peripherally, whereas the thrombosis of primary thrombophilic states begins in smaller branches and propagates into the major trunks. MVT is frequently associated with thrombosis of the portal and splenic veins but rarely of the inferior mesenteric vein (IMV),[51] perhaps because of the ease with which blood can be shunted through the internal iliac system via the rectal venous plexus.

The acuity of symptom onset and presentation is based on the nature of the thrombotic event. Intestinal infarction is rarely a consequence of acute MVT unless peripheral venous drainage is affected from the outset.[52] When there is sufficient venous occlusion to produce ischemia, but collateral vessels provide ample venous drainage to allow the possibility of recovery, a subacute form of MVT occurs.[53] When collateral circulation is inadequate and venous drainage from a segment of bowel is compromised, the affected intestine becomes congested, edematous, cyanotic, and thickened with intramural hemorrhage. Serosanguineous peritoneal fluid suggests hemorrhagic infarction. Arterial vasoconstriction can be marked in acute MVT, but arterial pulsations persist up to the bowel wall. Transmural infarction can make it impossible to differentiate venous from arterial occlusion.

Clinical Features

MVT can have an acute, subacute (weeks to months), or chronic onset. Clinical features are determined by the location and timing of thrombus formation within the mesenteric vasculature, as mentioned above. Except for late complications, chronic MVT is asymptomatic. As many as 60% of MVT patients have a history of peripheral vein thromboses.[54]

Acute MVT manifests with abdominal pain in more than 90% of patients and, as with acute arterial ischemia, the pain initially is out of proportion to the physical findings. The mean duration of pain before admission is 5 to 14 days but may be prolonged in as many as 25% of patients.[53] Other symptoms, including nausea and vomiting, occur in more than 50% of patients. Lower GI bleeding, bloody diarrhea, or hematemesis occur in approximately 15% of patients and indicate bowel infarction. Fecal occult blood is found in more than half of instances during the course of MVT. Initial physical findings vary at different stages and with different degrees of ischemic injury, but guarding and rebound tenderness develop as bowel infarction evolves. Most patients have a temperature higher than 38°C (100.4°F), and up to 25% may exhibit signs of septic shock.

Subacute MVT describes the condition in patients who have fluctuating abdominal pain for weeks to months but no intestinal infarction. Subacute MVT can be due either to extension of thrombosis at a rate rapid enough to cause pain but that allows collaterals to develop thus preventing infarction, or to acute thrombosis of venous drainage sufficient to permit recovery from ischemic injury. The diagnosis is usually made on imaging studies ordered to evaluate the cause of undiagnosed pain. Nonspecific abdominal pain usually is the only symptom of subacute MVT, and physical examination and laboratory tests are normal. Some patients who present with subacute MVT ultimately develop intestinal infarction; this blurs the distinction between the acute and subacute forms of MVT. At autopsy, coexistent new and old thromboses have been found in nearly half of the patients.

Chronic MVT is seen in patients who are asymptomatic at the time of thrombosis but who may develop GI bleeding from varices.[55] Most patients who bleed do so from gastroesophageal varices secondary to portal or splenic vein thrombosis, and they have physical findings of portal hypertension.

Laboratory studies may show secondary hypersplenism with pancytopenia or thrombocytopenia.

Diagnosis

Acute Mesenteric Venous Thrombosis

The absence of specific symptoms, signs, or laboratory results and the typical variability in the course of the disease has previously made it challenging to diagnose acute MVT. Today, advances in imaging technique and quality have allowed radiologic studies to substitute for emergency surgery or autopsy to diagnose MVT and have shortened the time from presentation to diagnosis from 1 week during 1978-1995 to approximately 1 day during 1995-2003.[48,56]

Abdominal plain film signs of MVT are similar to those of other forms of AMI and almost always reflect the presence of infarcted bowel. Barium enemas, although rarely done today, are of little diagnostic value because it is unusual for MVT to involve the colon. Characteristic findings on small bowel series include marked thickening of the bowel wall due to congestion and edema, with separation of loops and thumbprinting.

US, CT, and MRI have all been used to demonstrate thrombi in the SMV and portal vein.[57,58] Doppler US study is inexpensive, readily available, and non-invasive, but it has been limited by its inability to visualize smaller mesenteric vessels. It offers excellent specificity (≈100%) but mediocre sensitivity (70% to 90%).[49] CT with adequate portal venous phase contrast is highly sensitive and specific and has emerged as the most accessible and reliable diagnostic tool to diagnose MVT.[49] Specific findings of acute MVT include thickening and enhancement of the bowel wall greater than 3 mm in an adequately distended bowel segment, distended luminal diameter, thickened or hazy mesentery, indistinct bowel wall margins, the presence of new or unexplained ascites, enlargement of the SMV with a central lucency in the lumen of the vein (representing a thrombus), a sharply defined vein wall with a rim of increased density, and dilated collateral vessels in a thickened mesentery (Fig. 118-10).[49] The accuracy of these findings to diagnose MVT is higher than 90%.[59] CT is also very accurate in differentiating transmural infarction from non-transmural ischemia.[60] Magnetic resonance venography (MRV) is highly accurate for diagnosing MVT, with sensitivity and specificity of 100% and 98%, respectively.[61] MRV remains a diagnostic alternative to CT but is limited by availability, cost, and the extensive time required to complete the study. EGD and colonoscopy are rarely helpful, because the duodenum and colon are infrequently involved by MVT. As in other forms of AMI, laparoscopy may be useful either when other studies are contraindicated or in concert with imaging tests.[62]

Selective mesenteric arteriography, the diagnostic gold standard for MVT, can establish a definitive diagnosis before bowel infarction, differentiate venous thrombosis from arterial forms of ischemia, and provide access for vasodilator therapy. Angiographic findings of acute MVT include thrombus in the SMV with partial or complete occlusion, failure to visualize the SMV or portal vein, slow or absent filling of the mesenteric veins, arterial spasm, failure of the arterial arcades to empty, reflux of contrast medium into the artery, and prolonged blush in the involved segment.[63] When MVT is diagnosed on CT scanning, angiography might not be necessary, but in selected symptomatic patients it better delineates thrombosed veins and provides access for intra-arterial vasodilators. Indications for angiography include patients with thrombophilia who have either continuous or new abdominal symptoms and whose CT was normal/equivocal or patients who might be candidates for angiographic therapy.

At laparotomy, the hallmarks of MVT are serosanguineous peritoneal fluid, dark red to blue-black edematous bowel, thickening of the mesentery, good arterial pulsations in the involved segment, and thrombi in cut mesenteric veins. At this stage, some degree of intestinal infarction has invariably occurred.

Chronic Mesenteric Venous Thrombosis

Because chronic MVT is asymptomatic or manifests as GI bleeding, the diagnostic evaluation is directed toward determining the cause of the bleeding. Endoscopy and appropriate imaging studies should identify the cause and site of bleeding and the extent of thrombosis.

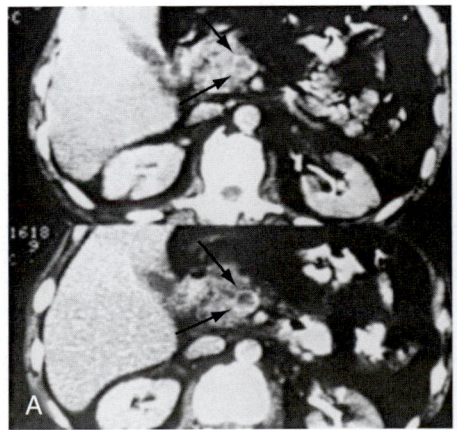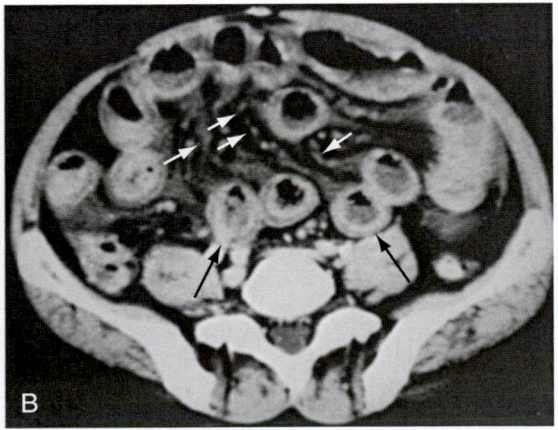

FIGURE 118-10. CT of superior mesenteric venous thrombosis. *A,* Abdominal CT with IV contrast demonstrating an enlarged superior mesenteric vein with a central lucency in the lumen, representing a thrombus. The wall of the vein is sharply defined, with a rim of increased density surrounding the thrombus *(arrows). B,* Abdominal CT with IV contrast showing thickening and persistent enhancement of the bowel wall *(black arrows)* and dilated collateral vessels within a thickened mesentery *(white arrows). (From Boley SJ, Brandt LJ. Ischemic disorders of the intestines. Surg Clin North Am 1992; 72:194.)*

Treatment

Acute Mesenteric Venous Thrombosis

Most patients with acute MVT initially are believed to have some form of AMI and are treated as discussed in earlier sections and as outlined in the algorithm of Figure 118-7. In asymptomatic persons in whom the diagnosis is made on a CT scan done for other than abdominal pain, either 3 to 6 months of anticoagulation or, in some cases, no therapy is reasonable. In symptomatic patients, treatment is determined by the presence or absence of peritoneal signs; signs of peritonitis mandate laparotomy and resection of infarcted bowel. If long segments of questionably viable bowel are found, papaverine is infused, and if arterial spasm is relieved and the SMV or portal vein is visualized, thrombectomy or a second look may be attempted to determine whether resection should be performed. Following surgery, heparin should be administered. Immediate heparinization for 7 to 10 days has been shown to diminish recurrence and progression of thrombosis and improve survival.[64-66] In the absence of peritoneal signs, immediate heparinization followed by a 3- to 6-month course of oral anticoagulation may be all that is needed. A comparison of patients who were treated surgically with those who were managed medically suggested that nonoperative management is a reasonable option provided the diagnosis on CT scan is certain and there is no transmural necrosis or perforation.[67] The use of thrombolytic agents, thrombectomy, or a combination of both has shown increasing promise for treatment of MVT, albeit only in small studies and case reports. The largest analysis using transcatheter thrombolytic therapy for acute MVT showed that 15 of 20 patients exhibited some degree of clot lysis and that none of the 15 patients required bowel resection or had recurrence after thrombolytic therapy. This technique decreased symptoms, mortality and the requirement for surgical intervention.[68] Despite a shortage of well-controlled studies to guide recommendations, aggressive intravascular therapy as an adjunct to anticoagulation should be considered in patients with acute MVT but without intestinal infarction or in those who are poor surgical candidates and who have intestinal infarction. Surgery might be considered for patients who are not good candidates for anticoagulation alone.

Current recommendations for the duration of anticoagulation are not supported by evidence-based data, but rather are based on conventional practice. If an underlying hypercoagulable state is found, lifelong anticoagulation therapy is advised. If no underlying thrombophilic state is documented, a 3- to 6-month course of therapy is thought to be sufficient.

Chronic Mesenteric Venous Thrombosis

Treatment of chronic MVT is aimed at controlling bleeding, usually from esophageal varices. Endoscopy (sclerotherapy, variceal banding), angiography (transjugular intrahepatic portosystemic procedures) and surgery (portosystemic shunts, devascularization procedures, and bowel resection) each have a place in treating selected patients. Use of beta blockers and anticoagulation was found to be associated with improved survival in these patients.[69] No treatment is indicated for patients with asymptomatic chronic MVT.

Mesenteric Phlebosclerosis

In patients without vasculitis, non-thrombotic stenosis of the mesenteric veins rarely causes intestinal ischemia, but when calcifications in the small mesenteric veins and their intraluminal branches result in abdominal pain, diarrhea, occult blood in the stool, and anemia, patients likely have mesenteric phlebosclerosis.[70] This rare entity has been reported in case series mostly out of Japan, and affected patients may also present with recurrent ischemic colitis. Endoscopic findings include edematous dark-colored mucosa with ulcerations. Biopsies of affected regions are characterized by thickening of venous walls with calcification, marked submucosal fibrosis, deposition of collagen in the mucosa, and foamy macrophages in the vessel walls.[70] Linear calcifications in and around the colon wall, stenosis in the right colon, and loss of haustral folds can be seen on abdominal plain films or CT scan in this entity.[71] The etiology of mesenteric phlebosclerosis remains a mystery. Mild symptoms usually are self-limited, whereas severe symptoms may require hemicolectomy.

Prognosis

Mortality associated with acute MVT is lower than that for other forms of AMI ($\approx$20%).[52] Intestinal infarction, not having a CT scan performed, and treatment on a nonsurgical ward all are associated with increased mortality.[48] Recurrence rates of 20% to 25% fall to about 15% if heparin therapy is begun promptly. The natural history of chronic MVT is not known, but from postmortem studies it appears that almost 50% of patients with MVT have no bowel infarction, and many have no symptoms.

FOCAL SEGMENTAL ISCHEMIA OF THE SMALL INTESTINE

Vascular insults to short segments of small intestine produce a broad spectrum of clinical features without the life-threatening complications associated with more extensive ischemia. The causes of focal segmental ischemia (FSI) include atheromatous emboli, strangulated hernias, immune complex disorders and vasculitis, blunt abdominal trauma, segmental venous thrombosis, radiation therapy, and oral contraceptives, among others.

With FSI there is usually adequate collateral circulation to prevent transmural infarction; the most common lesion is partial bowel wall necrosis with invasion by intestinal bacteria. FSI can manifest as acute enteritis, chronic enteritis, or a stricture. In the acute pattern, abdominal pain often simulates acute appendicitis. Physical findings are those of an acute abdomen, and an inflammatory mass may be palpated. The chronic enteritis pattern can resemble Crohn's disease, with cramping abdominal pain, diarrhea, fever, and weight loss.

Roentgenographic findings can also resemble those of Crohn's disease, except that FSI occurs anywhere in the small bowel, whereas Crohn's disease mainly affects the terminal ileum. The most common presentation is chronic small bowel obstruction from a stricture with intermittent abdominal pain, distention, and vomiting. Bacterial overgrowth in the dilated loop proximal to the obstruction can produce a blind loop syndrome. Radiologic studies typically reveal a smooth tapered stricture of variable length with an abrupt change to normal bowel distally and dilated bowel proximally.

Treatment of FSI is resection of the involved bowel.

COLON ISCHEMIA

Colon ischemia (CI) is a common disorder of the large bowel in older persons and is the most common form of intestinal

TABLE 118-3 Types and Approximate Frequencies of Colon Ischemia in Patients Seen at a Tertiary Referral Hospital

Type	Approximate Frequency (%)
Reversible colopathy and transient colitis	>50
Transient colitis	10
Chronic or recurring colitis	<20
Stricture	10
Gangrene	15
Fulminant universal colitis	<5

ischemic injury. It comprises a spectrum (Table 118-3) that includes reversible colopathy (subepithelial or intramural hemorrhage), transient colitis, recurrent or chronic colitis, stricture, gangrene, and fulminant universal colitis. The initial presentation usually is the same among these types and does not necessarily predict the course of disease, with the exception of ischemia involving the ascending colon. This latter pattern can simultaneously involve the small intestine, usually is caused by SMAE or NOMI, can have associated shock or sepsis, and carries a mortality rate of more than 50%.[72-74]

Incidence

The incidence of CI is underestimated because many patients suffer only mild or transient damage and do not seek medical attention. Also, CI is commonly misdiagnosed and confused with other disorders, notably IBD.

In our tertiary care hospital, CI accounts for approximately 1 in 2000 hospital admissions. Colonoscopy shows findings compatible with CI in roughly 22 per 100,000 procedures. A study using medical claims data from a large health care organization calculated a crude incidence rate of 7.2 cases per 100,000 person-years of observation in the general population. This study was prompted by the observation that patients with IBS treated with alosetron (see later) seemed to have a high incidence of CI and, in fact, the incidence for IBS patients was 42.8 cases per 100,000 person-years. After adjustment for age, sex, and calendar year, the incidence of CI in persons with IBS was 3.4 times higher than it was in those without it.[75] Other risk factors for CI in patients with IBS identified in a separate analysis include female gender, older age, and patients with chronic obstructive pulmonary disease (COPD).[76] Most studies assessing the incidence of CI address the disease in its most severe presentations and use colonoscopy to confirm the diagnosis. A study that looked at all presentations of acute lower GI bleeding found that CI accounts for 16% of cases.[77]

CI has female gender predilection, and more than 90% of patients with CI of non-iatrogenic causes are older than 60 years of age. CI affecting young persons is usually due to vasculitis, coagulation disorders, illicit use of cocaine, and a variety of iatrogenic causes, including a wide variety of medications such as estrogens, serotoninergic agonists and antagonists, sumatriptan, and methamphetamine. A comparison of risk factors between younger (20 to 45 years) and older (>45 years) patients with CI showed that smoking and hyperuricemia were more frequent in the younger population and were strongly associated with CI.[78]

Pathophysiology and Causes

CI can result from alterations in the systemic circulation or from anatomic or functional changes in the mesenteric vasculature, and it is thought to result from local hypoperfusion and reperfusion injury. In most cases, no specific cause for the ischemia is identified, and such episodes are viewed as localized nonocclusive ischemia, likely a result of small-vessel disease. An increasing variety of causes of CI is being defined, including hematologic disorders, thrombophilic states, and medications (see later) (Box 118-2).

Abnormalities on angiography rarely correlate with clinical manifestations of disease, and age-related abnormalities in the splanchnic vessels are common, including narrowing of small vessels and tortuosity of the long colic arteries. Fibromuscular dysplasia (FMD) of the superior rectal artery has been shown to contribute to CI. The colon is particularly susceptible to ischemia, perhaps owing to its relatively low blood flow, its unique decrease in blood flow during periods of functional activity, and its sensitivity to autonomic stimulation. What triggers the episode of CI, however, usually is not known.

Medications as a Cause of Colon Ischemia

Medications should always be considered as a possible etiology for CI.[79]

Antibiotics

Antibiotic-associated hemorrhagic colitis (AAHC) is believed to be mediated by CI. The penicillins and their derivatives, including amoxicillin and ampicillin, most commonly have been associated, although macrolides, cephalosporins, chloramphenicol, fluoroquinolones, and tetracyclines also are known precipitants. AAHC typically manifests 2 to 7 days after antibiotics are initiated, beginning with lower abdominal pain and loose stools and followed by hematochezia several hours later.[80] The exact mechanism of this side effect is unclear, but if AAHC is suspected, it is recommended that the antibiotic be stopped and an alternative regimen be started.

Chemotherapeutic Agents

When associated with chemotherapy, CI is usually seen with the alkaloid and taxane classes of chemotherapeutic agents (e.g., vinorelibine tartrate [alkaloid] and paclitaxel and docetaxel [taxanes]).[81] Although not proved, the mechanism of injury of CI with these compounds is believed to be either direct injury to the colonic epithelium or anti-angiogenic toxicity.[82] If patients develop CI while taking these medications, the clinician must reconsider the risks and benefits of their use.

Constipation-Inducing Agents

Patients taking medications that have constipation as a known adverse effect are potentially at increased risk for CI.[83] More than 250 different agents from a variety of medication classes fit this category.[79] One potential mechanism of CI caused by constipation-inducing agents is extrapolated from the observation that patients with idiopathic colonic slow transit have reduced baseline rectal and mucosal blood flow, possibly as a result of impaired efferent vagal cholinergic activity. Impaired cholinergic innervation is a side effect of many constipation-inducing medications, and the resultant unopposed sympathetic input leaves the colon susceptible to ischemic injury.

BOX 118-2 Causes of Colon Ischemia

Acute pancreatitis
Allergy
Amyloidosis
Heart failure or cardiac arrhythmias
Hematologic disorders and coagulopathies:
  Activated protein C resistance
  Antithrombin deficiency
  Factor V Leiden mutation
  Paroxysmal nocturnal hemoglobinuria
  Polycythemia vera
  Protein C and S deficiencies
  Prothrombin G20210A mutation
  Sickle cell disease
Infection:
  Bacteria (*Escherichia coli* O157:H7)
  Parasites (*Angiostrongylus costaricensis*)
  Viruses (HBV, HCV, cytomegalovirus)
Inferior mesenteric artery thrombosis
Long-distance running
Medications and toxins:
  Alosetron
  Cocaine
  Danazol
  Digitalis compounds
  Ergots
  Estrogens
  Flutamide
  Glycerin enema
  Gold salts
  Immunosuppressive agents
  Interferon-α
  Methamphetamine
  NSAIDs
  Penicillin
  Phenylephrine
  Polyethylene glycol 3350 colon lavage solutions

Pit viper toxin
Progestins
Pseudoephedrine
Psychotropic drugs
Saline laxatives
Sumatriptan
Tegaserod
Vasopressin
Pheochromocytoma
Ruptured ectopic pregnancy
Shock
Strangulated hernia
Surgery/procedures:
  Aortic aneurysmectomy
  Aortoiliac reconstruction
  Barium enema
  Colectomy with inferior mesenteric artery ligation
  Colon bypass
  Colonoscopy
  Exchange transfusions
  Gynecologic operations
  Lumbar aortography
Thromboembolism:
  Cholesterol (atheroembolism)
  Myxoma (left atrial)
Trauma (blunt or penetrating)
Vasculitis and vasculopathy:
  Buerger's disease
  Eosinophilic granulomatosis with angiitis
  Fibromuscular dysplasia
  Kawasaki's disease
  Polyarteritis nodosa
  Rheumatoid vasculitis
  SLE
  Takayasu's arteritis
Volvulus

Decongestants

Pseudoephedrine is used for relief of nasal congestion because its direct application to α_1-adrenergic receptors constricts vessels and relieves symptoms. The drug can be absorbed, however, and cause mesenteric vasoconstriction with resultant CI. Women are affected more often than men, and the splenic flexure watershed region seems to be most susceptible to injury by this agent. Patients with a history of CI or vasculitis or with a known thrombophilic state should be alerted to this potential complication.[79]

Diuretics

Diuretics like furosemide have been implicated in NOMI and CI. The presumed mechanism for CI with these agents is a decrease in extracellular fluid volume and reduction in peripheral resistance, which prompts a "steal" of blood from the intestine to the limbs.[84] Early correction of fluid balance is the preferred treatment.

Hormonal Therapies

Oral contraceptive pills (OCPs) are usually combinations of low-dose ethinyl estradiol and progestin, whereas hormone replacement therapy (HRT) often consists of ethinyl estradiol, with progestin added if the patient has an intact uterus. Young women taking OCPs are at a 6-fold greater risk of CI than an age-matched cohort not taking these agents.[85] In young, otherwise healthy women, the OCP is usually their only risk factor for CI,[86] although any woman who develops CI on OCPs should be evaluated for factor V Leiden deficiency. OCPs and HRT are known to result in a hypercoagulable state with ensuing microthromboembolic events and resultant CI. In any patient with other risk factors for CI, the use of OCPs or HRT, if clinically appropriate, should be monitored closely. Patients who experience CI while taking these medications should stop taking them and consider other options of birth control or seriously weigh the risks and benefits of continuing HRT.

Controlled or Illicit Pharmacologic Agents

Amphetamines are sympathomimetic vasoconstricting medications used for medicinal and recreational purposes. Significant increases in morbidity from a variety of ischemic insults attributed to their use have been reported, including myocardial ischemia and intestinal gangrene.[87] Amphetamine-induced CI is rare and usually manifests with hematochezia and mild to moderate abdominal pain. These medications tend to affect the ascending colon, possibly as a result of selective vasoconstriction of the SMA.[79]

Cocaine is known to induce CI.[88] The main mechanisms of injury with this agent include mesenteric vasoconstriction, a hypercoagulable state, and direct toxicity to the vasculature.[89] Twelve to 24 hours after intranasal or intravenous cocaine use, patients present with rectal bleeding with or without abdominal pain. Involvement of the descending colon, sigmoid colon, and occasionally the rectum are typical sites of cocaine-induced CI, which tends to occur in younger patients with a significantly higher mortality (26% vs. 7.7%) than CI from other causes.[90]

Interferon

The prevalence of CI during interferon-based therapies for treatment of hepatitis C virus (HCV) is 0.3 to 0.7%.[91] The advent of the protease inhibitors telapravir and bocepravir, which have greatly improved treatment efficacy for chronic HCV when combined with interferon and ribavirin, has significantly increased the number of people receiving interferon-based treatment, and HCV itself has been identified as a risk factor for poor outcome in CI.[92] Given this increased usage, CI will likely be seen more often, although there does not appear to be an association with any specific type of interferon. The descending colon is universally involved.[93] In 2 patients who developed CI while receiving interferon and ribavirin, it was found that stopping both medications for 1 week and restarting them for the full treatment course after resolution of symptoms did not result in a recurrence of CI, and sustained virologic response was achieved in both patients despite this break in therapy.[94] In 1 other patient receiving interferon and ribavirin for HCV, the therapy was permanently stopped after CI, and the patient had a virologic response for 3 months but a relapse within 1 year of stopping treatment.[93] If a patient develops CI while receiving interferon-based therapy, interferon should be stopped until there is resolution of symptoms, after which restarting the medication can be considered if the patient is highly motivated and close follow-up is assured.

Laxatives

Sodium polystyrene sulfonate (SPS, Kayexalate [Sanofi-Aventis, Bridgewater, N.J.]) is frequently used to treat hyperkalemia and has been reported to cause CI. In one report of a patient who experienced CI 10 days following administration of the medication, biopsies of the affected segment showed angular crystals and foreign bodies that were periodic acid–Schiff (PAS)-positive and non-polarizable, with surrounding fibrosis and inflammatory cells. These characteristics support SPS as the direct cause of the CI. CI due to SPS is usually self-limited, but other medications should be used to treat future episodes of hyperkalemia in these patients.[95] Case series have also shown that patients who have uremia and are given SPS are at increased risk for intestinal and colonic necrosis.[96] The proposed mechanisms are osmotic mucosal injury and NOMI induced by fluid shifts, elevated serum renin values, and angiotensin-mediated vasoconstriction. When using SPS, creatinine and urine output should be closely monitored.[79]

Magnesium citrate and sodium phosphate have been shown to cause CI,[97] which can manifest with abdominal pain and diarrhea as quickly as within 1 hour of taking the medication. It is believed that rapid fluid shifts from the mesenteric circulation to the colonic lumen results in transient hypoperfusion and ischemia. All reported cases have been self-limited.

Bisacodyl, a stimulant laxative, has been associated with CI in young, healthy patients.[98] It is believed that the mechanism of this disease is enhanced colonic motility resulting in decreased mucosal perfusion. Patients usually develop hematochezia and abdominal pain several hours after ingesting the drug. In patients with a history of CI, this medication is relatively contraindicated.

Glycerin enemas have been reported to cause hematochezia 6 hours after their use, with a flexible sigmoidoscopic appearance consistent with CI.[99] One possible mechanism of this insult is IMA spasm (seen on mesenteric angiography) resulting from increased colonic intraluminal pressure.

Nonsteroidal Anti-inflammatory Drugs

NSAID-induced colitis manifests with abdominal pain, diarrhea, and hematochezia, with occasional fevers and weight loss.[100] It is associated with an endoscopic and histologic appearance similar to CI. Injury induced by NSAIDs is more common with long-term use of the medication, and believed to result from a consequent decrease of vasodilating prostaglandins and increase of vasoconstricting leukotrienes (see Chapter 128).

Psychotropic Medications

First- and second-generation neuroleptic agents are associated with mild hypomotility of the digestive tract and also CI. The mechanism is believed to be similar to that proposed for constipation-inducing agents. The French Pharmacovigilence Database assessed first- and second-generation neuroleptic agents and found that between 1997 and 2006 there were 38 cases of CI associated with psychotropic medications. Clozapine, cyamemazine, levomepromazine, and haloperidol were the agents most frequently associated, and patients on more than 1 antipsychotic medication were at increased risk for CI.[101] Olanzapine, a commonly used second-generation neuroleptic medication used in the United States, has also been associated with CI.[102] These medications should be stopped or changed if a patient develops CI.

Serotonin Agonists and Antagonists

Serotonin (5-hydroxytryptamine [5-HT]) plays a critical role in modulating enteric neurotransmission and central nervous system signaling. The mechanisms for CI associated with serotonin agonists and antagonists are unproved, although several possibilities have been put forth, including cross-talk among 5-HT receptors and 5-HT_3-modulated neurotransmitter release, which possibly is aggravated in atherosclerosis.[103]

Sumatriptan, a 5-HT_1 serotonin receptor agonist used to treat migraine headaches, is an uncommon cause of CI. Its primary mechanism of action is intracranial vasoconstriction, but in patients with CI, it is believed to cause vasoconstriction of the colonic vascular bed as well.[104,105] Women are more commonly affected than men and typically present with abrupt-onset abdominal pain and hematochezia approximately 2 days after starting the medication. If CI is suspected, the medication should be discontinued.

Alosetron, a 5-HT_3 antagonist used to treat diarrhea-predominant IBS in women, was removed from the U.S. market in 2000 as a result of its observed association with CI. The drug was reintroduced in 2002 for use in patients with IBS-D who had not responded to conventional therapies. Since its reissuance, the estimated incidence rate of CI during alosetron treatment is 1.53 cases per 1000 patient-years.[106] Alosetron-induced CI is usually reversible and rarely has caused stricture or gangrene.[106]

Because of the association between serotoninergic medications and CI, these medications should not be used in any patient at an increased risk of CI or in women with a history of an ischemic event in any vascular bed. Relative contraindications to its use include a history of hyperactive vascular disorders (migraine headaches) and history of deep vein thrombosis.

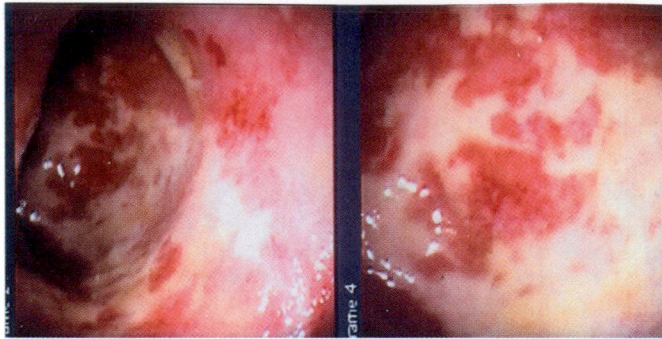

FIGURE 118-11. Colonoscopic views of deep ulcerations in a patient with colon ischemia whose illness was misdiagnosed as Crohn's disease.

Pathology

Morphologic changes after CI vary with the duration and severity of the injury. The mildest injury is mucosal and submucosal hemorrhage and edema, with or without partial necrosis and ulceration of the mucosa. With more severe injury, chronic ulcerations, crypt abscesses, and pseudopolyps develop, changes that can mimic IBD (Fig. 118-11).[107] Pseudomembranes may also be seen. Iron-laden macrophages and submucosal fibrosis are characteristic of ischemic injury. With severe ischemia, the muscularis propria is replaced by fibrous tissue, forming a stricture. The most severe form of ischemic damage causes transmural infarction.

Clinical Features and Diagnosis

CI usually manifests with sudden cramping, mild left lower abdominal pain, an urgent desire to defecate, and passage within 24 hours of bright red or maroon blood or bloody diarrhea. Mild to moderate abdominal tenderness is usually present over the involved segment of colon. Bleeding is not usually sufficient to require transfusion, but one prospective cohort study showed that 11.8% of patients presenting with severe hematochezia had CI.[108] Severe bleeding was seen more frequently in women, patients with severe lung disease, higher creatinine and glucose levels, and those on anticoagulation. Thirty-day outcomes for rebleeding, surgical intervention, and mean number of hospital days were worse for those with CI than those with other etiologies of lower GI bleeding.[108] Patients with ischemia isolated to the right side of the colon more often present with lower abdominal pain than with rectal bleeding or bloody diarrhea.[74]

A large retrospective study of patients with biopsy-proved CI showed that no region of the colon is spared from involvement. A segmental pattern of involvement is seen most commonly, and the left colon is affected most often (32.6%), followed by the distal colon (24.6%), right colon (25.2%), and entire colon (7.3%).[110] Although no specific etiology was associated with any specific anatomic distribution, pancolitis and isolated right-sided colonic disease were seen frequently in patients with sepsis.[111] In another study, there were no differences in clinical characteristics of presentation, cardiovascular risk factors or the presence of diabetes mellitus when comparing right- and left-sided CI. Those with isolated right-sided disease were more likely to have renal failure and a worse outcome.[112] In older reports, certain causes were believed to affect particular segments: local nonocclusive ischemic injuries, the watershed areas (splenic flexure and rectosigmoid), and ligation of the IMA, the sigmoid. The length of affected bowel can depend on the cause of CI: atheromatous

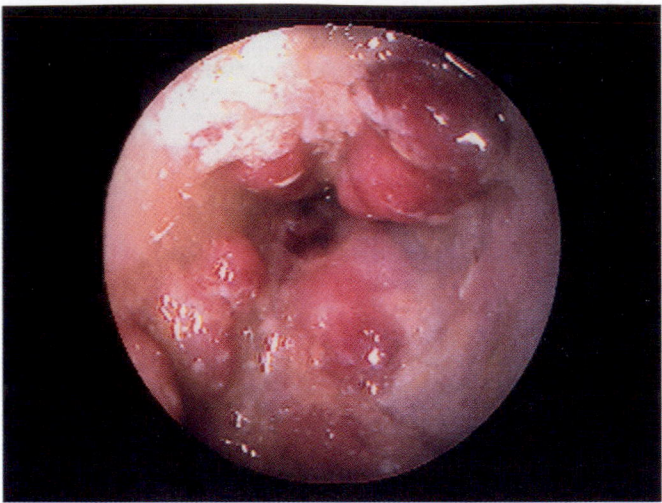

FIGURE 118-12. Colonoscopic equivalent of a radiologic thumbprint due to subepithelial hemorrhage and edema in a patient with colon ischemia.

emboli involve short segments, and nonocclusive injuries involve longer portions of colon.

If CI is suspected, CT scanning might support the clinical suspicion and also diagnose potential complications.[113] If the CT scan shows only nonspecific findings like a thickened segment of colon, or if the abdominal plain film appears normal, other attempts should be made to confirm or exclude the diagnosis of CI. Barium enema might provide insight into disease distribution and show the classic "thumbprinting" appearance of subepithelial hemorrhage, but it is now used infrequently because colonoscopy has become so widely available. One small study looked at the use of CT colonography as a way of assessing non-colorectal cancer conditions and found that CI could be detected by this technique.[114] MRI also shows promise as a diagnostic tool for patients with CI. A mouse model showed that the early phases and different levels of severity of CI might be well delineated by MRI.[115] At this time, colonoscopy is the best test for further assessment of CI and should be performed within 48 hours of symptom onset on the unprepared colon. During colonoscopy, care should be taken to not overdistend the colon, because high intraluminal pressure diminishes intestinal blood flow and can aggravate ischemic damage, particularly in patients with vasculitis.[116] Carbon dioxide is the preferred insufflation agent of choice over room air in patients with suspected or proved CI because it increases blood flow, in contrast to room air which decreases colon blood flow with increasing intraluminal pressure and because it is rapidly absorbed, thereby minimizing distention.[109] It is not necessary to advance proximal to the most distal extent of ischemic mucosa. Extent of disease can be determined by CT scan or other radiologic imaging tests.[109]

Colonoscopy is now the best test to diagnose CI because it enables direct observation of the affected tissue and provides a means to obtain biopsy specimens to confirm the diagnosis or even (rarely) establish causation.[109] Hemorrhagic nodules seen at colonoscopy represent bleeding into the subepithelial tissues and are equivalent to thumbprints seen on barium enema studies (Fig. 118-12). Segmental distribution of these findings, with or without ulceration, is highly suggestive of CI, but the diagnosis of CI cannot be made conclusively on the basis of a single examination unless mucosal gangrene is seen (Fig. 118-13). A colonoscopic finding called the *colon single-stripe sign* has been described in patients with CI, referring to a single line of erythema with erosion or ulceration oriented along the longitudinal axis of the colon. It had a 75% histopathologic yield in making the diagnosis of ischemic injury and signified a milder course than a circumferential ulcer.[117] When performing colonoscopy on a patient with suspected CI, the colon should be insufflated minimally with carbon dioxide if available, rather than with room air. Limited colonoscopy is appropriate to confirm the nature of CI suspected because of CT abnormality. However, there is no need to pass the instrument to the cecum and it is recommended that passage be halted once the distal most extent of disease is seen.

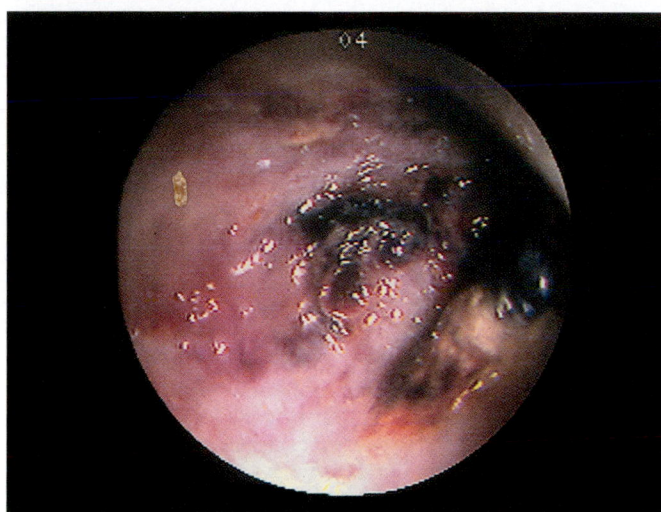

FIGURE 118-13. Colonoscopic view of mucosal gangrene in a patient with colon ischemia. Necrotic epithelium appears black against relatively healthier tissue. Biopsies probably should not be taken from areas of gangrene.[109]

Biopsies should be taken in most cases, except in cases of gangrene.[109] Segmental disease, rectal sparing, and rapid spontaneous evolution usually resulting in resolution of disease are characteristics of CI. In one study, colonoscopic findings of CI were retrospectively classified as either mild (e.g., redness and erosions) or severe (e.g., longitudinal or circumferential ulceration) and then compared. Patients with findings of severe disease presented more frequently with abdominal pain and had higher C-reactive protein levels and a longer average length of stay. Ischemic heart disease and connective tissue disease were independent predictors of colonoscopic findings consistent with severe disease.[118] The initial diagnostic study should be performed within 48 hours because thumbprinting disappears within days as the subepithelial hemorrhages are resorbed or the overlying mucosa sloughs. Studies performed 1 week after the initial study should reflect evolution of the injury—either normalization of the colon or replacement of the thumbprints with a segmental colitis-type pattern (Fig. 118-14). Universal colonic involvement, however, favors true UC, whereas fistula formation suggests Crohn's disease. Occasionally an abundant inflammatory response can produce heaping up of mucosa and submucosa that resembles a stricture or neoplasm (Fig. 118-15).

At the time of symptom onset, colon blood flow has typically returned to normal, so mesenteric angiography is not usually indicated. Two exceptions to this rule are when the clinical presentation does not allow a clear distinction to be made between CI and AMI, and perhaps when only the ascending colon is involved. Administration of air by enema or during flexible sigmoidoscopy or a limited colonoscopy can be used to reveal thumbprinting not otherwise visible on abdominal plain films; thumbprints stand out as relatively radiodense nodules against the radiolucency of the administered air. Nodules in the left colon or throughout the colon imply CI, whereas nodules isolated to the ascending colon suggest the possibility of otherwise silent SMA disease and the need to evaluate the mesenteric vasculature.

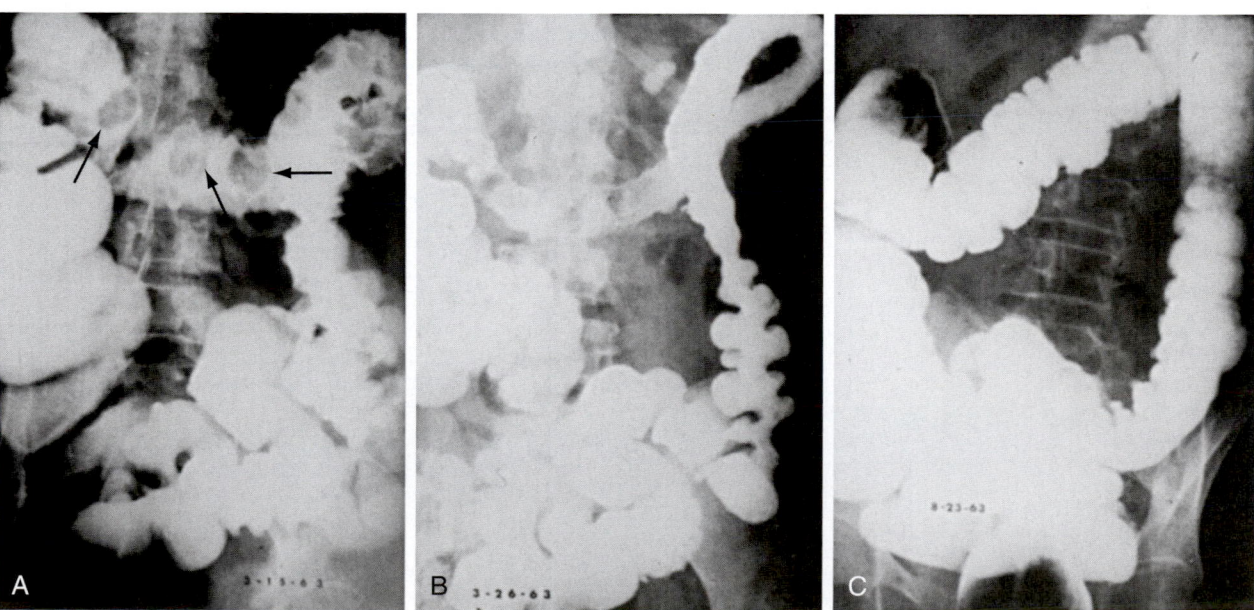

FIGURE 118-14. Films from serial barium enema examinations in a patient with reversible ischemic damage to the transverse colon and splenic flexure. *A*, The initial study shows dramatic thumbprints *(arrows)* throughout area of involvement. *B*, Eleven days later, thumbprints have resolved, and the involved colon has the appearance of a segmental colitis. *C*, Five months after onset, the colon has returned to normal. The patient was asymptomatic by 3 weeks after onset of her illness. *(From Boley SJ, Schwartz SS. Colonic ischemia: Reversible ischemic lesions. In: Boley SJ, Schwartz SS, Williams LF, editors. Vascular disorders of the intestines. New York: Appleton-Century-Crofts; 1971. p 589.)*

Clinical Course and Treatment

When CI is diagnosed and physical examination does not suggest gangrene or perforation, the patient is treated expectantly. Parenteral fluids are administered, and the bowel is placed at rest (Fig. 118-16). In experimental models, antibiotics reduce the extent and severity of bowel damage, so broad-spectrum antibiotics are given to "cover" the fecal flora. However, no randomized controlled blinded trials have been done to prove the validity of this recommendation. An electrocardiogram, Holter monitoring, and transthoracic echocardiogram should be obtained to exclude or confirm a cardiac source of embolism. Compared with other patients with CI, patients with segmental non-gangrenous CI who undergo such evaluation are 2.5 times more likely to have their cardiac risk factor identified.[119] Cardiac failure and arrhythmias are treated, and medications that may cause mesenteric vasoconstriction are withdrawn. If the colon appears distended, it is decompressed with a rectal tube. Serial imaging tests or endoscopic evaluations of the colon and continued monitoring of the hemoglobin level, WBC count, and electrolyte levels are indicated until the patient's condition stabilizes.

Increasing abdominal tenderness, guarding, rebound tenderness, rising temperature, and paralytic ileus indicate colonic infarction and demand immediate laparotomy and colon resection if appropriate Fig. 118-16. At operation, mucosal injury may be extensive despite normal-looking serosa, so the extent of resection should be guided by the distribution of disease as seen on preoperative studies rather than on the appearance of the serosal surface of the colon at the time of operation.

In more than half of patients with CI, the disease is reversible. Generally the symptoms of CI resolve within 48 to 72 hours, and the colon heals in 1 to 2 weeks. With severe injury, it may take 1 to 6 months for the colon to heal, but during this time the patient is usually asymptomatic.

Symptoms that persist for more than 2 weeks are also associated with a higher incidence of acute complications and irreversible disease: gangrene and perforation, segmental ulcerating colitis, or stricture.

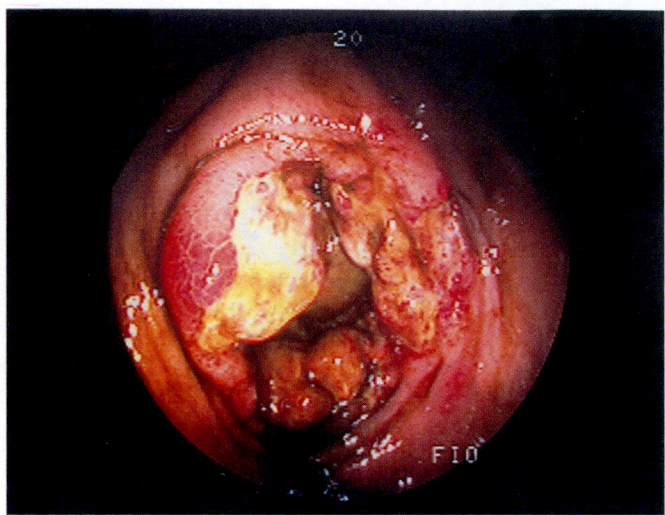

FIGURE 118-15. Colonoscopic view of colon ischemia resembling neoplasia in patient with metastatic cancer treated with interleukin-2 and interferon-α. The inflamed edematous mass was thought to be a cecal neoplasm. The lesion resolved spontaneously after just 5 days. *(From Sparano JA, Dutcher JP, Kaleya R, et al. Colonic ischemia complicating immunotherapy with interleukin-2 and interferon-α. Cancer 1991; 68:1538.)*

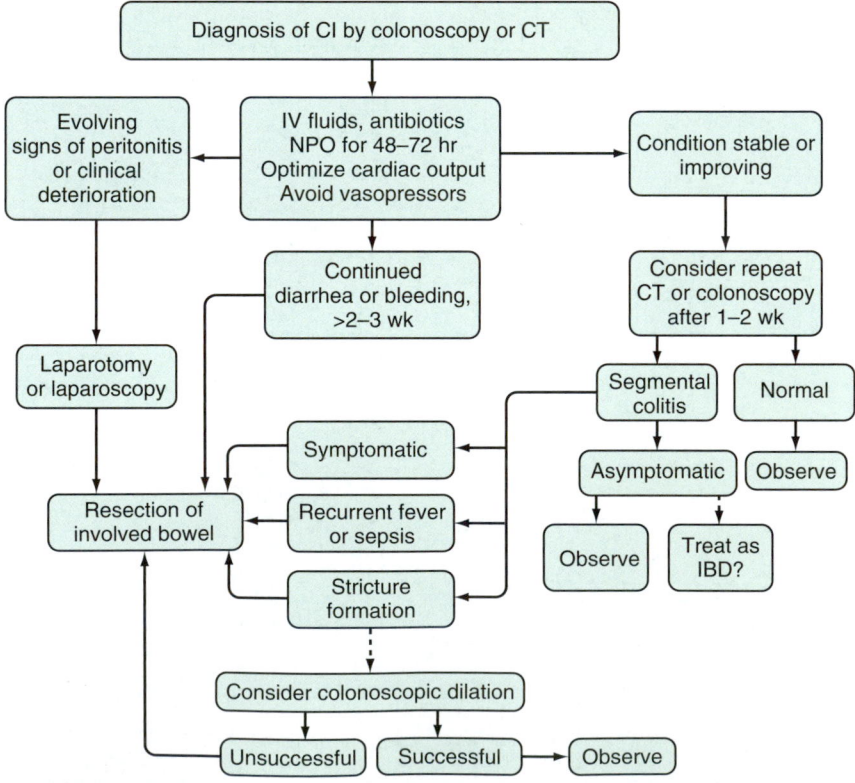

FIGURE 118-16. Algorithm for the management of colon ischemia (CI). Solid lines indicate a conventional management plan; dashed line indicates an alternative management plan. IV, intravenous; NPO, nothing by mouth. *(Modified from Brandt LJ, Boley SJ. AGA technical review on intestinal ischemia: American Gastrointestinal Association. Gastroenterology 2000; 118:954.)*

Gangrene

Abdominal tenderness with fever and signs of peritonitis suggests infarction and the need for emergent laparotomy.

Segmental Colitis

Segmental colitis may be seen with any of the following clinical patterns: recurrent fevers and sepsis, continuing or recurrent bloody diarrhea, and persistent or chronic diarrhea with protein-losing colopathy. Patients who are asymptomatic or minimally symptomatic but have endoscopic evidence of persistent disease should undergo follow-up colonoscopy to determine whether the colitis is healing, becoming chronic, or forming a stricture. Recurrent fever, leukocytosis, and septicemia suggest unhealed segmental colitis that is providing a portal of entry for colonic bacteria and, if found, mandates elective resection of the ischemic segment of bowel. Patients with persistent diarrhea, bleeding, or protein-losing colopathy of more than 2 weeks' duration are at high risk for perforation, and resection is indicated. Patients who present with segmental colitis are frequently misdiagnosed as having IBD. Response to oral glucocorticoid therapy is usually poor and may be associated with an increased incidence of perforation. Success has been achieved with fatty acid enemas and glucocorticoids given per rectum (Dr. L. Brandt, personal observation). Patients whose symptoms cannot be controlled medically should have a segmental resection, which usually is curative. At present there is no known prophylaxis to protect against recurrent CI, absent correction of a thrombophilic state or anatomic variant that predisposes to recurrence.

Ischemic Stricture

Ischemic strictures that produce no symptoms can be observed. Some resolve over 12 to 24 months with no therapy, but resection is required for those that cause obstruction. Despite the limited number of studies and small case series looking at dilation and stent placement as a temporizing measure or bridge to a surgical procedure, these techniques seem to show promise for the treatment of benign ischemic strictures.[120,121]

Universal Fulminant Colitis

Sudden onset of a toxic universal colitis picture with signs of peritonitis and a rapidly progressive course are typical of universal fulminant colitis, a rare variant of CI. Total abdominal colectomy with ileostomy usually is required.

Outcome Associations

Risk factors associated with poor outcome in patients with CI are essential to help the clinician decide on an appropriate course of treatment. Certain patterns of disease distribution, medical comorbidities, physical examination findings, serologic abnormalities, and radiologic imaging findings characterize CI that demands a lower threshold for more aggressive treatment and intervention.

A retrospective Korean study showed that CI in patients who have renal failure and are on hemodialysis tends to involve the right side of the colon and to have poor outcome, again confirming that patients with isolated right CI are at increased risk of short-term mortality.[111]

In addition to isolated right-sided CI, other factors are associated with poor outcome. Hyperthyroidism, history of stroke, and COPD were associated with increased risk of mortality in a series of 313 patients with biopsy-proved CI.[110]

Another study that used pathology to diagnose CI and excluded patients with IBD showed that those who presented with tachycardia on admission, experienced shock within 24 hours of admission, or had endoscopic evidence of ulceration were more likely to have severe illness (e.g., persistent symptoms of CI for >2 weeks, requirement of any surgical intervention for complicated or unresponsive CI, or mortality). If they had all 3 of these clinical factors, patients were 74 times more likely to have severe illness.[122] Abdominal guarding on physical examination at presentation, lack of bleeding per rectum, and chronic constipation were prognostic of severe disease and required surgical management in a cohort of patients with CI that was unassociated with recent vascular surgery or colonic tumors.[123] When 253 patients with CI were retrospectively assessed, 48 patients required surgical management either initially or more than 12 hours after admission. In this study, intraperitoneal fluid on CT and the absence of bleeding per rectum were strongly associated with need for surgery.[124] Patients' ages, leukocyte counts, blood lactate dehydrogenase (LDH) and lactate levels, and absence of vascular flow to the colonic wall on abdominal Doppler US study were independent predictors of complicated CI in a separate analysis; only absence of arterial flow was a significant predictor of complicated disease when confounding for other factors.[125] Disease severity can be predicted serologically by elevations in white blood cell count, blood urea nitrogen (BUN), and lactate dehydrogenase (LDH), or decreases in albumin, Hgb, sodium or bicarbonate.[109]

When focusing on patients 65 and older, a retrospective study of biopsy-proved CI showed that hematochezia was associated with a positive outcome that did not require surgical intervention, whereas malignancy, HCV infection, presence of peritoneal signs on initial presentation, isolated right colon involvement, and elevated serum LDH levels were associated with poor outcome as defined by colectomy or mortality.[92]

Special Clinical Problems

Isolated Ischemia of the Right Colon

Ischemia that only involves the right side of the colon (IRCI) has been shown to occur in roughly 25% of cases, an incidence more than twice the conventionally accepted incidence of 8% to 10%. This pattern is more likely to be associated with coronary artery disease and chronic kidney disease requiring hemodialysis.[110] Documenting such a pattern of involvement is important because these patients require surgery four times as often as and have a mortality rate twice that of patients with involvement of other areas of the colon, including those in whom the right side is involved synchronously with other segments (surgery: 44.3% vs. 11.5%; 30-day mortality 20.3% vs. 9.0%).[110] Because the SMA supplies blood to the right side of the colon—as well as to the small intestine—and because patients with IRCI may have it as the heralding presentation of otherwise silent SMA obstructive disease, we recommend evaluating the splanchnic vasculature in these patients. CTA will identify patients at risk for AMI, and if an SMA occlusion is found, revascularization should be strongly considered. IRCI is an *exception* to our general practice of not evaluating the splanchnic vascular system in a patient with CI.

Colon Ischemia in Patients with Carcinoma of the Colon and Other Potentially Obstructive Lesions

Less than 5% of patients with CI have a distal and potentially obstructing lesion or disorder of the colon, including carcinoma, diverticulitis, volvulus, fecal impaction, postoperative

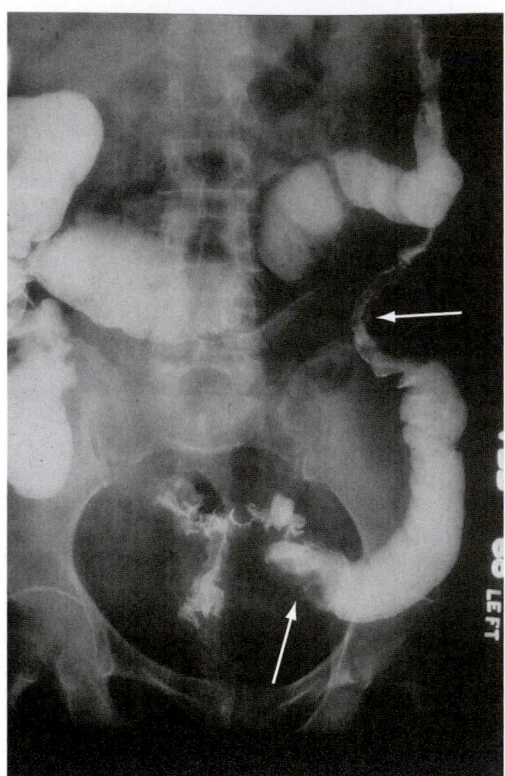

FIGURE 118-17. Film from a barium enema examination demonstrating a narrowed segment of colon ischemia *(upper arrow)* proximal to a carcinoma in the distal sigmoid *(lower arrow)*. The area of colon between the carcinoma and ischemic segment is normal. *(From Boley SJ, Brandt LJ, Veith FJ. Ischemic disorders of the intestines. Curr Probl Surg 1978; 15:1.)*

stricture, prior ischemic stenosis, or radiation stricture. Typically the associated lesion is distal, and there is a segment of normal colon between the distal lesion and the proximal colitis (Fig. 118-17). The mechanism of this association may involve increased intracolonic pressure proximal to the lesion, with resultant decreased colon blood flow and mucosal-to-serosal shunting of blood.

Colon Ischemia in Irritable Bowel Syndrome

CI occurs 2.75 to 11 times more frequently in the presence of IBS than without it.[126] Although some authors believe that patients with IBS visit their doctor more frequently and therefore are more likely to have CI diagnosed than the general population, others hypothesize there is a common pathophysiology in patients with IBS, such as hypersensitivity of the colonic vasculature, autonomic hyper-responsiveness, or differences in the sensitivity of serotonin receptors.[127] Clinical studies and experimental models have shown that alosetron increases risk for CI (see earlier discussion[104,128,129]). The incidence of CI, however, has been shown to be higher in IBS patients regardless of therapy used.[130] More studies, better data, and a greater understanding of the mechanisms of actions of serotoninergic agents are needed to further elucidate any such association.

Colon Ischemia Complicating Aortic Surgery

CI complicates elective aortic surgery in up to 7% of cases, and surgery for ruptured abdominal aortic aneurysms in up to

60% of cases.[131] CI is responsible for some 10% of deaths after aortic replacement. Preoperative hypotension, prolonged cross-clamp time, intraoperative ischemia, and postoperative acidosis all were associated with postoperative ischemia in one study,[132] and improper management of the IMA during aneurysmectomy has also been implicated as a cause of postoperative CI. Tonometric determination of intramural pH of the sigmoid before and after cross-clamping the aorta has been used successfully to predict which patients will develop CI after aneurysmectomy.[133] When looking at patients who had an infrarenal aortic repair, one study found that the incidence of postoperative CI requiring surgical intervention was 2.5%, with a mortality rate in this surgically treated group of 58.8%. The use of postoperative vasopressors and diagnosis in the ICU were associated with the necessity for surgical intervention.[134]

Because postoperative CI is serious and difficult to diagnose early, colonoscopy should be performed within 2 to 3 days after surgery for a ruptured abdominal aortic aneurysm or in patients with a prolonged cross-clamping time, a patent IMA on preoperative aortography, non-pulsatile flow in the hypogastric arteries during surgery, or postoperative diarrhea.[135] If CI is identified, oral feeding and liquids are stopped and antibiotic therapy is begun. Clinical deterioration requires reoperation. At surgery, all ischemic colon must be resected.

Advances in surgical technique allow some patients to have a less invasive endovascular repair of their aorta. Although a less frequent consequence of this type of surgery, CI is still seen in up to 23% of cases when colonoscopy was performed after repair in 36 of 39 patients who survived longer than 24 hours. In this study, 3 patients required exploratory laparotomy with bowel resection.[136] When colonoscopy was not performed post procedure, the incidence of CI was estimated to be as low as 1.4%.[137] It is recommended that flexible sigmoidoscopy be performed on each patient within 24 to 48 hours of the endovascular repair to detect subtle findings of CI, given the potentially high incidence of CI and the management changes that should occur in those who do have CI.[136]

CHRONIC MESENTERIC ISCHEMIA (INTESTINAL ANGINA)

CMI is uncommon and accounts for less than 5% of intestinal ischemic diseases; it almost always is caused by mesenteric atherosclerosis, although rare causes like collagen vascular disease and inflammatory vasculopathy are known. The presence of mesenteric artery stenosis (MAS) does not imply that abdominal pain or other symptoms are due to CMI. Because atherosclerosis is so common in the aged population, and numerous collateral pathways are available to maintain flow—especially with chronic occlusion—diagnosis of CMI is challenging. One study that addressed the prevalence of MAS in an older-adult population (mean age, 77.2 ± 4.9 years) found that 17.5% had MAS defined by visceral duplex ultrasonography, of which 86% had isolated celiac artery (CA) stenosis, 7% combined celiac and SMA stenosis, and 5% isolated SMA stenosis; 2% had all 3 vessels occluded. Renal artery stenosis and elevated high-density lipoproteins were associated with MAS, and there were no differences in age, race, gender, or body mass index between those with and without MAS.[138] In another review of CMI, 91% of patients had occlusion of at least 2 vessels, and 55% had involvement of all 3; 7% and 2% had isolated occlusion of the SMA and CA, respectively.[139] It is unclear why the distributions of disease differ extensively in these studies, but further well-controlled trials might clarify the observed differences.

There is no specific association of CMI and smoking, although 75% of patients with CMI have a history of smoking.[139] Abdominal pain, the most typical symptom of CMI, is likely caused by ischemia in the small intestine as blood is stolen from this organ to meet the increased demand for gastric blood flow as food enters the stomach.[140] This rationale for why the pain occurs so soon after eating, when food still remains in the stomach, is preferable to the traditional explanation that a fixed and limited blood supply is incapable of meeting the increased metabolic demands of the small intestine during digestion. Experimentally, at least under acute conditions, vascular "steals" within the splanchnic circulation are unlikely unless flow through both the CA and mesenteric arteries is compromised.[141]

Clinical Features

The cardinal clinical feature of CMI is abdominal cramping or discomfort that usually occurs within 30 minutes after eating, gradually increases in severity, and then slowly resolves over 1 to 3 hours. Although mild initially, abdominal pain progressively increases in severity over weeks to months. The association of pain with meals leads to fear of eating (sitophobia), with resultant weight loss. Nausea, bloating, episodic diarrhea, and malabsorption or constipation can occur, but it is the weight loss and intimate relation of the abdominal pain to the meals that characterize this syndrome. Early in the course of disease, if patients do not eat, they remain pain free; pain occurs only after eating or during a meal. Later, pain can become continuous, and this portends intestinal infarction. One study found that 100% of patients with CMI presented with some abdominal pain, 78% of which was postprandial; 68% had weight loss (mean, 23 ± 12 pounds); 13% had nausea and vomiting; 13% had constipation or diarrhea; and 8% presented with lower GI bleeding.[142] Uncommon presentations of CMI include antral ulcerations that are unassociated with *Helicobacter pylori* and do not heal on therapy with PPIs, gastroparesis (that resolves after revascularization), and acalculous cholecystitis. About one third to one half of patients have evidence of cardiac, cerebral, or peripheral vascular disease. Physical findings are usually limited, but patients with advanced disease can appear cachectic. The abdomen typically remains soft and nontender even during painful episodes, although distention may be appreciated. An abdominal bruit is common but nonspecific.

Diagnosis

Diagnosis of CMI is difficult because of the vague nature of the complaints and the lack of a specific diagnostic test. Abdominal plain films and CT scans are usually normal, although vascular calcification may be present. Endoscopic inspection of the GI tract usually reveals it to be normal, and random biopsies of the upper tract show only nonspecific abnormalities. Barium studies are normal or show nonspecific evidence of either malabsorption or a motility disturbance. Rarely, radionuclear emptying tests might show delayed gastric emptying.

US studies, MRA, and even traditional mesenteric angiography only reveal morphologic abnormalities and anatomic limitations to splanchnic blood flow; they do not establish the presence or absence of intestinal ischemia. Duplex US can be used to identify splanchnic artery stenoses but not to establish the diagnosis of CMI.[143] Elevated peak systolic velocity in the CA and SMA of 200 and 275 cm/sec, respectively, is a reliable sign of at least 70% stenosis of these vessels.[144] Duplex US and phase contrast cine MRI of the CA and SMA have been used to measure the effect of eating on mesenteric blood flow, based on the principle that under normal conditions, eating increases blood flow to the small intestine, whereas in CMI, this fails to occur. However, postprandial studies are no better than fasting examinations at lesser degrees of vascular stenosis.[144]

Gastric tonometry exercise testing (GTET) uses a NG tube and peripheral arterial catheter to obtain gastric juice and arterial blood, respectively, from a fasting patient who has been pretreated with acid-suppression medication and then undergoes a standard exercise protocol. Determination is made of the gastric-arterial PCO_2 gradient before, during, and after exercise. An increase in the gradient after exercise is an indicator of GI ischemia. In a study of diagnostic accuracy for CMI, GTET and duplex US, alone and in combination, were compared with the gold standard, angiography. Combined GTET and duplex US would not have missed any patients with symptomatic CMI, so it is currently believed to constitute the best diagnostic workup strategy, although the technique is not widely available.[145] GTET showed a diagnostic accuracy of 87% compared with angiography.[146] In another study, 24-hour tonometry using catheters in both the stomach and jejunum with standardized food intake was compared with GTET and predicted CMI in 13 of 17 patients and the absence of ischemia in 15 of 16 patients.[147] Yet another assessment looked at the most common ways to diagnose CMI, including history, imaging (e.g., CT, MRI, and angiography), and GTET. Each patient underwent all 3 diagnostic tests, and results showed that clinical features provided limited diagnostic yield on their own, whereas mucosal perfusion analysis with tonometry provides the greatest diagnostic ability. Overall, the combination of history, radiologic imaging and tonometry was most accurate in diagnosing CMI.[148]

Despite GTET being a very useful method to diagnose CMI, this technique is not available at most centers. Leukocyte counts, LDH levels, and C-reactive protein levels do not differ in those with and without CMI, but postprandial values of serum L-lactate and D-dimer are significantly elevated in patients with CMI.[149] When positive, these serologic tests favor a diagnosis of CMI, but further assessment is necessary to identify their reliability to diagnosis CMI.

In the absence of any widely available specific, reliable diagnostic test, the diagnosis of CMI is based on clinical symptoms in combination with radiologic demonstration of an occlusive process of the splanchnic vessels and, to a great measure, exclusion of other GI disorders. Angiography should show occlusion of 2 or more splanchnic arteries to support the diagnosis of CMI, but such occlusions (even of all 3 vessels) do not by themselves make the diagnosis, because they may be present with no corresponding clinical symptoms (see earlier). In most patients with CMI, at least 2 of the 3 splanchnic vessels are either completely obstructed or severely stenotic.

Treatment

CMI is not considered to require urgent therapy, although acute complete occlusion of the GI blood supply can occur if thrombosis is superimposed on already narrowed arteries. A patient with the typical pain of CMI and unexplained weight loss whose diagnostic evaluation has excluded other GI disease and whose angiogram shows occlusive involvement of at least 2 of the 3 major arteries should undergo revascularization (Fig. 118-18).

Surgical revascularization has been the traditional method of therapy for patients with CMI, but percutaneous transluminal mesenteric angioplasty (PTMA) alone or with stent insertion is now used as primary or secondary therapy as well. The results of surgical revascularization for CMI vary in different reports, depending on the nature of the operations used, the

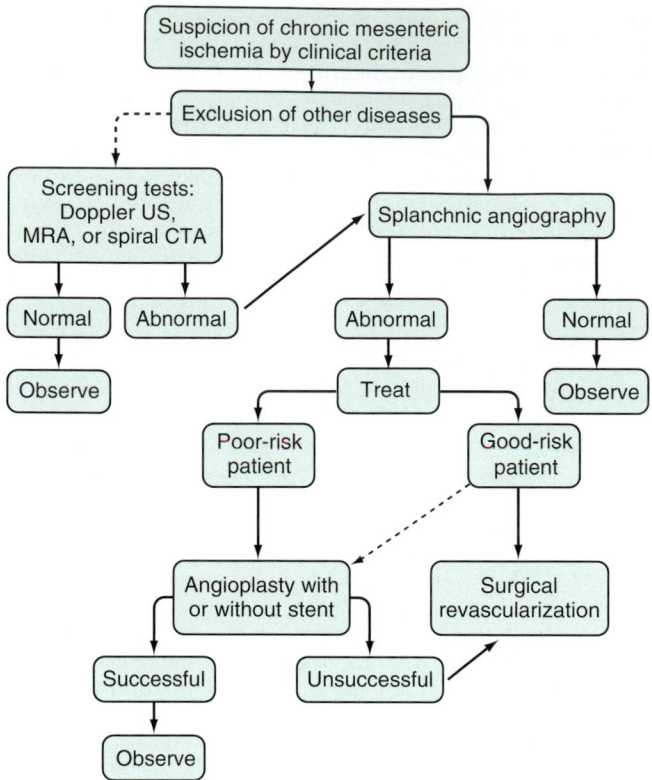

FIGURE 118-18. Algorithm for the management of chronic mesenteric ischemia. Solid lines indicate the conventional management plan; dashed lines indicate an alternative management plan. *(Modified from Brandt LJ, Boley SJ. AGA technical review on intestinal ischemia: American Gastrointestinal Association. Gastroenterology 2000; 118:954.)*

number of vessels revascularized, and whether concurrent operations like aortic reconstruction are performed.

The true efficacy of surgical revascularization and PTMA is difficult to determine because of the varied criteria used by different investigators to define a successful outcome. Some authors use graft or vessel patency rates, whereas others define success by relief of symptoms, recurrence rates, or long-term survival. When success is defined by relief of symptoms, surgical revascularization is successful in 84% to 94% of patients, with recurrence rates of 7% to 14%.[150] A retrospective study that looked at the United States Nationwide Inpatient Sample Database from 2000 through 2006 showed that surgical intervention for CMI was performed with morbidity and mortality rates of 38% and 13%, respectively, in 2128 patients. The major complications of surgical revascularization included acute renal failure (11%), bowel infarction requiring resection (8%), cardiac arrest (6%), respiratory complications (5%), myocardial infarction (5%), and GI hemorrhage (3%).[151] Most series have reported mortality rates less than 10%, success rates of more than 90%, and recurrence rates less than 10%.[24] Several long-term studies have shown that patients who survive surgical revascularization have cumulative 5-year survival rates of 80% to 90%.[24]

The rates of success for PTMA are similar to those for surgical revascularization. Complete vascular occlusion was believed to be a contraindication to PTMA in the past, but now the safety and feasibility of PTMA have been confirmed in selected cases when the thrombus is less than 2 cm in length.[150] Primary technical success in patients undergoing PTMA is very high (90% to 100%), with symptom relief in 73% to 99%. Relapse rates because of restenosis are estimated to be as high as 28%; these patients require repeat endovascular interventions.[150] Morbidity rates associated with PTMA were estimated to be 20%, while mortality rates were 3.7% in a large retrospective analysis.[151] The main complications from endovascular interventions occur at the vascular access points and include thrombosis, dissection, and hemorrhage. Complications from treatment of the primary thrombosis are less frequently seen, with dissection and distal embolization being most common. Overall, these complications are estimated to occur in 2% to 13% of patients. Acute renal failure (6.0%), infarction requiring bowel resection (3.0%) and acute myocardial infarction (3.0%) are the most common systemic complications observed.[151] Following stent placement, patients usually require clopidogrel and aspirin for 1 to 3 months to allow for endothelialization of the endovascular stent. There are currently no well-controlled studies that assess optimal anticoagulation times for patients who underwent PTMA with stent placement.

The decision of whether a patient should undergo surgical revascularization or percutaneous endovascular intervention is an important consideration for clinicians. A review of 43 articles including 1795 patients over the last 25 years showed that perioperative length of hospital stay, morbidity, and mortality were lower in the those who underwent endovascular therapy. No difference in survival was demonstrated, but patency rates were higher and recurrence of symptoms lower after open-operative intervention than after PTMA.[152] When the United States Nationwide Inpatient Sample Database was reviewed from 1988 through 2006, PTMA was seen to be increasingly used, having passed surgical intervention by 2002. When looking at the years 2000 to 2006, the mortality rate was significantly higher for patients who underwent surgery compared with PTMA (13% vs. 3.7%), and bowel resection was more common after surgical intervention (7% vs. 3%).[151] Patients who undergo PTMA were previously those with high-risk medical comorbidities, or it was used as a bridge to surgery, but with advances in surgical technique and increased usage, patients who previously would have only been considered for PTMA would now be candidates for surgical revascularization. Patients currently selected for surgery are more likely to have higher-risk lesions and more complicated disease, which probably explains part of the increased mortality rate in this group. To date, no head-to-head prospective trials of patients randomized to either PTMA or surgical intervention have been published. Patients with CMI who are younger and otherwise relatively healthy should be considered for surgical intervention as first-line therapy, given the decreased frequency of restenosis and better long-term patency rates. Initial treatment should be based on the patient's age, medical comorbidities, and the expertise of the center where treatment will be provided.

VASCULITIS AND ANGIOPATHY OF THE SPLANCHNIC CIRCULATION

Inflammation and necrosis can affect splanchnic blood vessels of all sizes: arteries, veins, the vasa recta, arterioles, and venules.[153] Symptoms depend on the size of the involved vessel and may be indistinguishable from AMI caused by emboli or thrombosis. Associated systemic features like renal failure, cutaneous nodules, and pulmonary infiltrates suggest a systemic disorder.

The vasa rectae, arterioles, and arteries may be affected in systemic vasculitides. With vasculitis, the ischemic injury typically involves short segments of the intestine. Abdominal pain, fever, GI bleeding, diarrhea, and intestinal obstruction are common with vasculitis, as are ulceration and stricture formation. With small-vessel involvement, perforation is less common than it is with larger-vessel involvement.

Typically, vasculitis is caused by immune complex deposition in the walls of the vessels, which leads to activation of the complement system and an inflammatory reaction. Aneurysm formation, vessel rupture and bleeding, vascular occlusion, thrombosis, or fibrosis can ensue.

One retrospective study of 62 consecutive patients presenting between 1981 and 2002 with vasculitis of the GI tract detailed 46 men and 16 women who were affected; their mean age was 48 ± 18 years. Most noted were polyarteritis nodosa (38 patients [21 hepatitis B-related]), eosinophilic granulomatosis with polyangiitis (Churg-Strauss syndrome) (11), granulomatosis with polyangiitis (6), microscopic polyangiitis (4), and rheumatoid arthritis (3). The most common presenting symptoms in descending order of frequency were abdominal pain, nausea or vomiting, diarrhea, hematochezia or melena, and hematemesis.[154] A variety of vasculitides that have been associated with intestinal ischemia are discussed briefly in the following sections.

Behçet's Disease

Behçet's disease (see Chapter 36) is characterized by oral and genital ulcers, recurrent iritis or chorioretinitis, and skin lesions; it is most often seen in Eastern Mediterranean men and is strongly associated with the *B51* allele. Small-vessel vasculitis accounts for much of the damage, but large-vessel involvement of arteries and veins is common. GI disease, present in 50% of patients, typically involves the ileocecal area, although involvement of the esophagus and small intestine has been reported.[155] Attacks are recurrent and usually self-limited except for the uveitis, which may be chronic. The most common GI symptoms are abdominal pain, diarrhea, and bleeding. Deep ulcers are responsible for the most common intestinal complications: severe bleeding and perforation. Mortality is low in Behçet's disease, but intestinal perforation is one of the common causes of death. Age less than 25 at diagnosis, history of prior laparotomy, and volcano-shaped ulcers are all independent risk factors for bowel perforation in these patients.[156] Surgical resection of the affected region is associated with a 58.3% recurrence rate; 30.6% of patients need reoperation during long-term follow-up. Intestinal perforation, volcano-shaped ulcers, and C-reactive protein above 4.4 mg/dL at the time of initial operation are associated with the need for long-term repeat surgical interventions.[157] Therapy with glucocorticoids, immunosuppressive agents, and colchicine has been tried, with varying success.

Buerger's Disease

Also called *thromboangiitis obliterans,* Buerger's disease involves medium-sized and small peripheral arteries and veins, especially the infrapopliteal vessels; foot claudication and rubor are its most common symptoms. Buerger's disease is largely a disease of men, especially those who have smoked cigarettes beginning from an early age, and typically has its onset before the age of 50 years. There is a distinct absence of other atherosclerotic risk factors in patients with Buerger's disease. Intestinal involvement is unusual, but most common is involvement of the vessels supplying the small intestine.[158] In the acute lesion, inflammation spreads outward from the thrombus-endothelium interface through the vessel wall. Later, microabscesses, necrotizing granulomas, and multinucleated giant cells occur in the thrombus, after which the thrombus organizes and becomes occlusive. Intestinal involvement usually requires resection.[159]

Cogan's Syndrome

Cogan's syndrome is a rare disorder of young people characterized by vasculitis of the conjunctiva, cornea, and cochlea.[160] Although this vasculitis usually is localized, it is considered to be a hypersensitivity reaction to an unknown viral agent, and the disease can become disseminated. Some 3% to 10% of patients develop GI symptoms, with diarrhea and bloody stools. High-dose glucocorticoids and occasionally cytotoxic agents are required. Vascular surgery may be needed after inflammation is controlled.

Eosinophilic Granulomatosis with Eosinophilia (Churg-Strauss Syndrome)

Allergic granulomatous angiitis is a disorder typified by asthma, glomerulonephritis, eosinophilia, and granulomatous inflammation associated with antineutrophil cytoplasmic autoantibodies.[161] Such necrotizing vasculitis affects small and medium-sized vessels and involves the GI tract in almost half the patients. As in other vasculitides, abdominal pain and bleeding secondary to ischemia are the usual manifestations. One study showed that patients with Churg-Strauss syndrome who have GI involvement are at increased risk of overall disease relapse.[162] Glucocorticoid therapy usually is effective.

Fibromuscular Dysplasia

Fibromuscular dysplasia (FMD) is a rare angiopathy related to neither atherosclerosis nor inflammation.[163] Its cause is unknown, although genetic factors might play a role, and there is an association with cigarette smoking and hypertension. There are several types of FMD depending on which arterial layer is involved: intima, media, or adventitia. The renal arteries are most commonly involved, followed by the carotid and vertebral arteries and then other vasculature including the mesenteric arteries. Splanchnic involvement can manifest with symptoms of acute or chronic mesenteric ischemia.[164] FMD has also been shown to mimic other chronic GI diseases like Crohn's disease.[165] Diagnosis is based on the same techniques used to image other vascular disorders; the classic "string-of-beads" appearance on angiography is typical of only the medial type of FMD, whereas aneurysms and dissection may complicate all types. Therapy consists of percutaneous transluminal angioplasty, surgical revascularization, and resection of necrotic bowel as indicated.

Henoch-Schönlein Purpura

Henoch-Schönlein purpura (see Chapter 36) typically affects children aged 4 to 7 years. It is characterized by immunoglobulin (Ig)A immune complexes deposited within the small vessels of the skin, GI tract, joints, and kidneys and is often preceded by an upper respiratory infection. The classic clinical triad consists of palpable purpura (usually below the waist), arthritis (knees and ankles), and abdominal pain; the GI tract is involved in up to 75% of patients.[166] Abdominal pain and GI bleeding are the most common GI symptoms and are caused by mucosal and submucosal hemorrhage; a submucosal hematoma may be the lead point of an intussusception. NOMI has been reported as a cause of death in a patient with Henoch-Schönlein purpura.[167] GI involvement may be documented by endoscopy[168] or CT study.[169] The disease is usually self-limited, but the outlook may be less favorable in adults, in large measure owing to development of renal failure.

Hypersensitivity Vasculitis

Hypersensitivity vasculitis uncommonly involves the splanchnic vasculature and affects mainly the postcapillary venules, in contrast to necrotizing vasculitis, which involves arteries. A large variety of causes are known to trigger this disorder, including infections (*Streptococcus, Staphylococcus,* hepatitis B virus, influenza virus, cytomegalovirus, mycobacteria, and rickettsiae), drugs, and chemicals.

Kawasaki's Disease

Kawasaki's disease, also called *infantile febrile mucocutaneous lymph node syndrome,* is a necrotizing vasculitis of medium-sized arteries.[170] It manifests as fever, rash on the palms and soles, desquamation, conjunctival congestion, strawberry tongue, and cervical lymphadenopathy in infants and children. Affected patients have nausea, vomiting, abdominal pain, and diarrhea and can suffer ileus, small bowel obstruction, bleeding, and perforation. Death may result from coronary artery aneurysms and myocardial infarction. Treatment standards include aspirin for the acute phase and large intravenous doses of gamma globulin for the prevention of coronary artery aneurysms. Alternative treatments (e.g., glucocorticoids, infliximab) are being evaluated.[171]

Köhlmeier-Degos Disease (Malignant Atrophic Papulosis)

Köhlmeier-Degos disease is a rare form of progressive occlusive vascular disease of young men that affects the small and medium-sized arteries, mainly those of the skin and intestine.[172] Typically, skin lesions of porcelain-white punctate scars with erythematous borders are found on the trunk and upper extremities. The rash is followed, within months to years, by the development of abdominal pain and spontaneous intestinal perforation, which may be recurrent.[173] Thrombosis of small and medium-sized vessels is found, without inflammatory cell infiltration. There is no known therapy for this disease, and it is generally fatal.

Polyarteritis Nodosa

Polyarteritis nodosa (see Chapter 36) is a necrotizing vasculitis of medium-sized and small arteries that is characterized by aneurysms at branch points. Abdominal symptoms are reported in up to half of patients with the disorder, the most common of which is abdominal pain, usually from ischemia.[174] Involvement of the small intestine is most common, followed by lesions of colon, liver, and pancreas. Diagnosis is suggested by angiographic findings of aneurysms up to 1 cm in diameter in the renal, mesenteric, and hepatic vasculature.[175] Treatment with glucocorticoids and cyclophosphamide or azathioprine has greatly improved survival.

Vasculitis resembling polyarteritis is also associated with hepatitis B and C virus infections.[176,177] Fifty percent of patients with classic polyarteritis are hepatitis B surface antigen positive, and in contrast to classic polyarteritis, only small arteries are involved. Patients develop a polyarteritis picture following the viral infection, presumably from deposition of antigen-associated immune complexes in the vessel wall.

Rheumatoid Vasculitis

Rheumatoid vasculitis affects the GI tract in 10% to 38% of patients, usually those who have subcutaneous nodules and are seropositive for rheumatoid factor.[178] As with all vasculitides, ischemia manifests with abdominal pain, bleeding, perforation, and gangrene. Rheumatoid vasculitis, although rare, is often catastrophic and may be associated with ischemic ulcers, bowel infarction, and a pancolitis.[178] Other diseases have been noted in association with rheumatoid arthritis, including atrophic gastritis, gastric antral vascular ectasia, IBD, collagenous colitis, and amyloidosis.

Systemic Lupus Erythematosus

Systemic lupus erythematosus (see Chapter 36) affects the GI system in about half of cases and can involve any of the hollow and solid GI organs.[153] The most common symptoms are nausea, vomiting, and abdominal pain, but diarrhea, malabsorption, pseudo-obstruction, peritonitis, pancreatitis, protein-losing enteropathy, and ascites are also well-known occurrences.[179] The systemic nature of the disorder makes differential diagnosis complicated, but vasculitis-induced ischemia underlies many of the presentations. The vasculitis typically involves small vessels and causes FSI and GI bleeding, both of which are associated with high mortality rates if not diagnosed promptly. Diagnosis can be supported by CT scans to evaluate the bowel wall and vasculature. Symptoms respond well to glucocorticoids and immunosuppressive agents.[179]

Takayasu's Disease

Takayasu's disease (pulseless disease) is an idiopathic chronic inflammatory disorder that most often affects the aorta and its branches in young women of Asian heritage. Involvement of splanchnic vessels is unusual.[180] Fibrotic occlusion of the involved vessels is the end result of the inflammatory process. Takayasu's disease rarely has been associated with Crohn's disease and UC, and in the serum of some of these patients, antibodies to colonic mucosa and aorta have been detected.[181] Treatment is large doses of glucocorticoids before reconstructive surgery. The 5-year survival rate is higher than 90%.

ACKNOWLEDGMENT

We are indebted to Dr. Scott J. Boley, who for decades worked to lay the groundwork for this chapter and who played a critical role in preparing earlier editions.

KEY REFERENCES

Full references for this chapter can be found on www.expertconsult.com.

5. Alhan E, Usta A, Çekiç A, et al. A study on 107 patients with acute mesenteric ischemia over 30 years. Int J Surg 2012; 10:510-13.
29. Corcos O, Castier Y, Sibert A, et al. Effects of a multimodal management strategy for acute mesenteric ischemia on survival and intestinal failure. Clin Gastroenterol Hepatol 2012; 11:158-65.e2.
33. Resch TA, Acosta S, Sonesson B. Endovascular techniques in acute arterial mesenteric ischemia. Semin Vasc Surg 2010; 23:29-35.
49. Harnik IG, Brandt LJ. Mesenteric venous thrombosis. Vasc Med 2010; 15:407-18.
70. Iwashita A, Yao T, Schlemper RJ, et al. Mesenteric phlebosclerosis: A new disease entity causing ischemic colitis. Dis Colon Rectum 2003; 46:209-20.

79. Hass DJ, Kozuch P, Brandt LJ. Pharmacologically mediated colon ischemia. Am J Gastroenterol 2007; 102:1765-80.

109. Brandt LJ, Feuerstadt P, Longstreth GF, Boley SJ. Guidelines for Diagnosis and Treatment of Colon Ischemia. Am J Gastroenterol 2014 (to be published).

110. Brandt LJ, Feuerstadt P, Blaszka MC. Anatomic patterns, patient characteristics, and clinical outcomes in ischemic colitis: A study of 313 cases supported by histology. Am J Gastroenterol 2010; 105:2245-52; quiz 2253.

145. Otte JA, Geelkerken RH, Huisman AB, Kolkman JJ. What is the best diagnostic approach for chronic gastrointestinal ischemia? Am J Gastroenterol 2007; 102:2005-10.

151. Schermerhorn ML, Giles KA, Hamdan AD, et al. Mesenteric revascularization: Management and outcomes in the United States, 1988-2006. J Vasc Surg 2009; 50:341-348.e1.

152. Pecoraro F, Rancic Z, Lachat M, et al. Chronic mesenteric ischemia: Critical review and guidelines for management. Ann Vasc Surg 2013; 27:113-22.

154. Pagnoux C, Mahr A, Cohen P, Guillevin L. Presentation and outcome of gastrointestinal involvement in systemic necrotizing vasculitides: Analysis of 62 patients with polyarteritis nodosa, microscopic polyangiitis, Wegener granulomatosis, Churg-Strauss syndrome, or rheumatoid arthritis-associated vasculitis. Medicine (Baltimore) 2005; 84:115-28.

175. Hokama A, Kishimoto K, Ihama Y, et al. Endoscopic and radiographic features of GI involvement in vasculitis. World J Gastrointest Endosc 2012; 4:50-6.

119

Intestinal Ulcerations

LAUREL FISHER AND JAMES M. SCHEIMAN

CHAPTER OUTLINE

Before the routine use of endoscopic imaging with capsule endoscopy (CE) and deep enteroscopy, discrete ulcers of the small and large intestine were thought to be rare, and associated with a broad spectrum of diseases. Similarly, the classic literature on these ulcers has emphasized symptomatic presentations, typically of diseases not confined to the small or large intestine alone. Our current ability to image the small intestine, and more importantly biopsy ulcerative lesions, has opened a new chapter in the approach to intestinal ulceration. Similar to its history in the upper GI tract, medication-induced injury in the small intestine, mainly from NSAIDs but attributable to other noxious mediations as well, is now recognized and appreciated to be common (Fig. 119-1). Clinical presentations associated with intestinal ulceration vary widely with location and degree of intestinal involvement, ranging from anemia and hypoproteinemia to abdominal pain, hemorrhage, obstruction, and perforation.

This chapter is divided into 2 sections. The first section covers isolated idiopathic small intestinal ulcers, and ulcerations induced by NSAIDs. The second section provides a contemporary approach to suspected and identified small intestinal ulcers, recognizing that many ulcerative conditions are discussed in greater detail in other chapters of this textbook: solitary rectal ulcer and stercoral ulcerations (see Chapter 128), diffuse ulcerations associated with refractory sprue (see Chapter 107), and other diffuse ulcerative diseases with such lymphoma (see Chapter 31).

NONSPECIFIC OR IDIOPATHIC SMALL INTESTINAL ULCERATION

Solitary ulcers of the small intestine result from a wide variety of causes (Box 119-1). Solitary ulcers beyond the duodenum that cannot be explained on the basis of any known etiology are referred to as *nonspecific* or *idiopathic* intestinal ulcers. Solitary nonspecific ulcers are rare and have been reported to occur at a rate of 4 per 100,000, although this estimated frequency antedates current imaging paradigms.[1]

Clinical Features

Patients with nonspecific ulcers of the small intestine can present with acute or chronic GI bleeding, symptoms of small bowel obstruction, abdominal pain, or perforation. Symptoms may be present from a few days to many years before diagnosis. A retrospective surgical case series reported in 1981 from the Mayo Clinic described 59 patients who were treated over a 22-year period for small intestinal ulcers, 89.8% of which had no identifiable cause.[1] The nature of a retrospective design is such, however, that medication exposure or development of other diseases after tertiary referral cannot be identified. For example, medications such as thiazide diuretics, potassium preparations (since removed from the market), and perhaps other medications not yet clearly recognized to cause intestinal ulcers, were not considered in this 1981 report. Patients ranged in age from 17 to 77 years, with most presenting in the fifth and sixth decades of life; no gender predominance was found. The most common presenting symptom was intermittent small bowel obstruction (63%). Physical findings ranged from nonspecific abdominal tenderness and distention to an acute abdomen resulting from intestinal perforation. Laboratory evaluation was notable only for anemia in one half of the patients. Radiologic studies localized the ulcer in a minority of patients.

More recently, reports from Japan and Europe have identified a similar, presumably idiopathic, small intestinal ulcerative condition that resembles NSAID enteropathy in many ways, but without apparent NSAID or offending medication exposure and without features of Crohn's disease or other identifiable illness.[2,3]

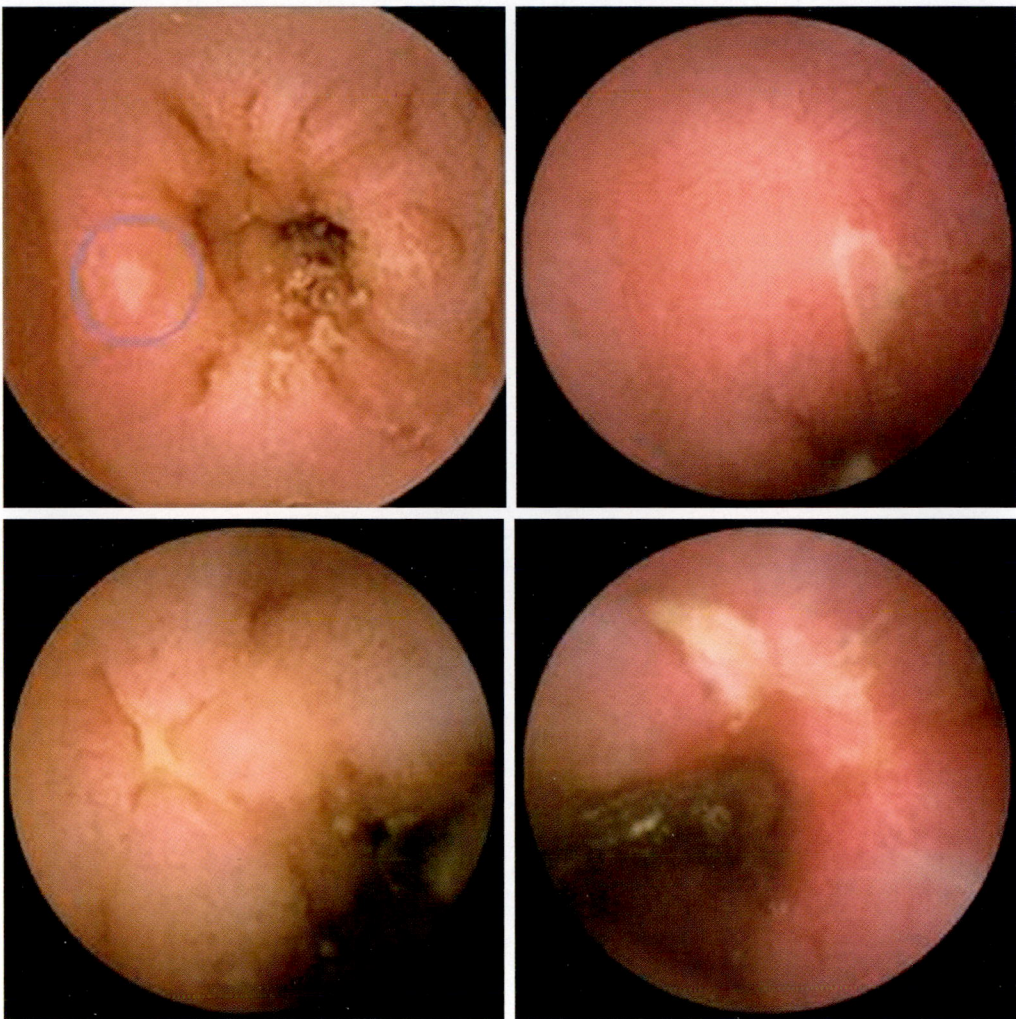

FIGURE 119-1. Examples of small intestinal ulcerations found on capsule endoscopy. *(Courtesy Dr. Laurel Fisher, University of Michigan.)*

Pathology

In the previously cited series of 59 patients from the Mayo Clinic with nonspecific small bowel ulceration, the ileum was the most common location of nonspecific ulceration (78%), while perforation (22%) occurred most commonly in the jejunum (78%).[1] Diagnosis was rarely made preoperatively, and at surgery, 41 patients were found to have solitary ulcers, 5 patients had 2 ulcers, and 6 patients had more than 3 ulcers. Ulcer size varied between 0.3 and 5 cm. On pathologic examination, ulcers were located predominantly on the anti-mesenteric border of the small intestine and, in some cases, were associated with a fibrous scar that narrowed the lumen. Microscopy revealed only nonspecific chronic inflammation that ended abruptly at the ulcer edge; intervening bowel and vasculature were normal. More contemporary series report similar distribution of disease and pathology, and have referred to this condition as either chronic nonspecific multiple ulcers of the small intestine (CNSU) or cryptogenic multifocal ulcerous stenosing enteritis (CMUSE).[2,3] Revised clinical criteria for this diagnosis have been proposed by Japanese investigators[4]: (1) Persistent and occult blood loss from the GI tract (except during bowel rest or postoperatively); and (2) Confirmation of characteristic small intestinal lesions by macroscopy, radiography, or enteroscopy: circular or oblique in alignment, sharply demarcated from surrounding normal mucosa, geographic or linear in shape, multiplicity in number with less than 4-cm distance from each other, ulcers not reaching the muscularis propria layer, including scarred ulcers presumed to be the healing stage in cases treated by bowel rest. These ulcerations often have thin overlying exudates and may be accompanied by stenosis that resembles NSAID diaphragm disease. Comparison with NSAID ulcers reveals a similar nonspecific histology, but suggests a distinction with regard to the site and stage of ulceration, perhaps related to the duration of illness, and which is reported to be more chronic with CNSU. In a small cohort of 9 patients, those with NSAID ulcers had involvement of both proximal and distal small intestine, whereas the location of CNSU ulcerations was exclusively ileal.[5] A report from France suggested a potential role for vasculitis in CNSU, but this was not a universal pathologic finding in all cases.[3]

A recent study has identified a patient with idiopathic small bowel ulceration who was found to have a novel inherited deficiency of cytosolic phospholipase A_2, an enzyme important in prostaglandin production, which lead to a global reduction in intestinal eicosanoid levels.[6] There likely are other rare genetic predispositions to ulceration linked to prostaglandins and other trophic factors that are critical in maintaining small intestinal integrity, and which may explain the so-called "idiopathic small bowel ulcer." Given the rarity of symptomatic yet unexplained small intestinal ulcers and a

---

BOX 119-1 Systemic Diseases Associated with Small Intestinal Ulceration

Acid-Related Disorders
Heterotopic gastric mucosa
ZES

Celiac Disease
Refractory celiac disease
Ulcerative enteritis

Collagen-Vascular and Other Immunologic Diseases
Autoimmune enteropathy
Eosinophilic granulomatosis with polyangiitis (Churg-Strauss syndrome)
Giant cell arteritis
Henoch-Schönlein purpura
Mixed connective tissue disease
Polyarteritis nodosa
Polymyositis-dermatomyositis
Reactive arthritis
Sjögren's syndrome (microscopic polyangiitis)
SLE
Thrombotic thrombocytopenic purpura
Vasculitis

Congenital
Duplications
Stenoses

Drugs
Antibiotics
Antimetabolites
Aspirin and other NSAIDs
Bacillus Calmette-Guérin (BCG)
Chemotherapeutic agents
Slow-release (enteric-coated) potassium

Hypersensitivity
Food allergies

Hypogammaglobulinemia
Infections
Bacteria
Fungi
Parasites

Protozoa
Viruses
Helminths

Inflammatory Diseases
Behçet's syndrome
Crohn's disease
Cryptogenic multifocal ulcerous stenosing enteritis
Eosinophilic gastroenteritis
Granulomatous enteritis
Lymphocytic enterocolitis
Nongranulomatous chronic idiopathic enterocolitis
Sarcoidosis
Tropical sprue

Ischemia
Incarcerated hernia
Intussusception
Mesenteric ischemia
Vascular abnormalities

Metabolic Disorders
Malnutrition
Uremia

Neoplasms
Angiocentric lymphoma
T-cell lymphoma
Enteropathy-associated T-cell lymphoma
Primary neoplasms
Metastatic neoplasms

Radiation
Accidental
Therapeutic

Toxins
Heavy metal poisoning

Trauma and Mechanical Injury
Foreign body ingestion
Stomal ulceration

---

literature that is limited to retrospective case series, it is very difficult to know if these lesions represent multiple conditions, or are atypical presentations of medication toxicity or commonly seen disorders such as Crohn's disease. Similar to earlier reports of "idiopathic" foregut peptic ulcer disease, 1 study evaluated 76 patients referred for CE to evaluate suspected small bowel pathology. Biochemical analysis confirmed that 13.6% of patients had evidence of unreported NSAID exposure and 1 patient underwent surgery for small intestinal ulceration, histopathology of which was consistent with NSAID-related injury.[7] This finding echoes earlier reports of patients who underwent terminal ileal evaluation at colonoscopy for possible Crohn's disease and who were found to have ileitis attributed to NSAID exposure.[8]

Treatment

All patients in the Mayo series were treated with segmental intestinal resection; only 2 patients had recurrent ulceration, 2 and 10 years after initial diagnosis and resection.[1] The French CMUSE series reported success with glucocorticoids but an inability to taper them because of symptomatic relapse, thus supporting the inflammatory and possibly vasculitic nature of the injury.[3] Ischemia, central nervous system disease,

infection, trauma, and hormonal influences all have been put forth as possible causes of primary nonspecific ulcerations, but the cause or causes still remains unknown.

ULCERATION INDUCED BY NSAIDS

NSAIDs are among the most frequently administered drugs in the world, and their adverse effects involve not only the esophagus, stomach, and duodenum but also the more distal portions of the small intestine and colon. Gastroduodenal risks of NSAIDs are well known, but lower GI tract risks of NSAIDs are being increasingly recognized.[9,10] The esophageal and gastroduodenal effects of NSAIDs are discussed in Chapters 46, 52, and 53.

Clinical Features

NSAIDs induce small intestinal and colonic injury with a wide spectrum of manifestations from clinically silent mucosal injury to significant ulceration with overt bleeding, intestinal obstruction, or perforation.[10,11] Injury secondary to NSAIDs can cause subtle changes known as NSAID enteropathy, in which there is increased intestinal permeability,

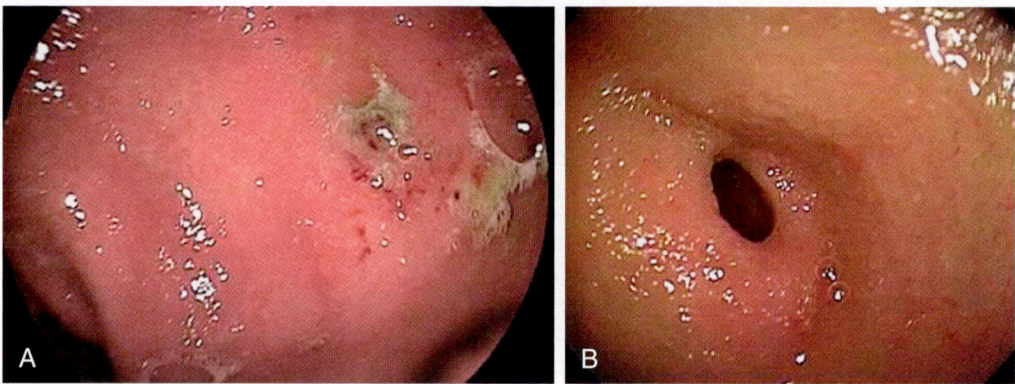

FIGURE 119-2. *A,* Endoscopic view of NSAID-associated ulcerations of the small intestine in a patient who presented with GI bleeding. *B,* Adjacent NSAID stricture.

inflammation, and chronic low level blood loss; macroscopic injury may not be evident. The clinical picture often is silent and undiagnosed unless it progresses to manifest with anemia and hypoalbuminemia. Less common presentations may include weight loss, anemia, diarrhea, overt bleeding, and perforation. Symptoms of partial small bowel obstruction such as vomiting and colicky abdominal pain may be seen secondary to development of diaphragm-like strictures (see below).[12] Laboratory evaluation often is notable for unexplained hypoalbuminemia and iron deficiency anemia. When studied by CE, evidence of mucosal injury, defined as a spectrum from petechiae and reddened folds to mucosal breaks and stricture, are seen in up to 70% of NSAID users[13,14] (Fig. 119-2*A* and *B*).

Pathology

Autopsy findings of NSAID users established that ulcerations of the small intestine distal to the duodenum are prevalent.[12] Of 713 consecutive autopsy patients who died in a hospital in Glasgow, NSAIDs had been prescribed to 249 in the 6 months before death; 8.4% of the NSAID users had ulcerations of the small intestine compared with only 0.6% of the NSAID nonusers. Although no information was available regarding morbidity caused by NSAIDs during life, 3 of the NSAID users in that series died of small intestinal perforation.[12]

The pathologic appearance of NSAID-induced ulceration is nonspecific: Ulcerations can be single or multiple and range from tiny punched-out ulcers to confluent areas of deep ulcer with stricture formation. CE has shown abnormalities ranging from reddening of the mucosa to erosions, ulcers, and active bleeding (see Fig. 119-2*A*),[15] with normal intervening mucosa. NSAID ulcers may not always be distinguishable from other medication or disease-related injury on the basis of their gross or microscopic pathologic appearance and must be distinguished from Crohn's disease. Ulcerations may rarely be associated with diaphragm-like strictures in patients with long-standing NSAID use, an association referred to as *diaphragm disease.* NSAID-diaphragms are thin (2- to 4-mm) septae that present as concentric strictures made up of mucosa and submucosa with or without submucosal fibrosis (see Fig. 119-2*B*). It is thought these lesions may be more common with drugs that undergo extensive enterohepatic recirculation because of prolongation of exposure. Direct pill-induced injury may contribute to ulcerations in the areas of narrowing, further contributing to fibrosis and narrowing.

Pathogenesis (Fig. 119-3)

Mechanisms of NSAID-induced injury to the small intestine remain under investigation, but clearly involve both systemic and local injury.[11] Just as with injury to the upper GI tract, concomitant inhibition of COX-1 and COX-2 plays an important role in intestinal mucosal injury; however, both animal studies and CE studies in man have confirmed that COX-2 inhibition alone can lead to mucosal damage.[16] COX-2 knockout mice have altered intestinal permeability and develop ileocecal perforation upon exposure to NSAIDs, thus supporting the etiologic role of COX-2 in NSAID injury.[17]

Although the role of COX-1 and COX-2 has not been clearly defined in NSAID-induced injury to the small intestine, there is evidence that COX-2 inhibitors cause less deleterious clinical effects on the small intestine than do dual COX inhibitors. Using CE, Goldstein and colleagues found significantly less small intestinal injury in healthy subjects taking a selective COX-2 inhibitor (celecoxib) than in those who were taking ibuprofen plus omeprazole.[18] Not surprisingly, multiple agents can synergize to worsen small intestinal injury, such as the addition of an antiplatelet drug to aspirin. The combination of a thienopyridine to low-dose aspirin also has been shown to exacerbate small bowel injury as quantified by CE, evidence which supports clinical experience of an increased overall bleeding risk for patients who take this combination and undergoing cardiac stenting.[19]

NSAIDs appear to cause a disturbance in the microcirculation, which results in a loss of epithelial cells.[20,21] Blood flow is compromised in the capillaries at the villus tips, endothelial cells become vacuolated, vascular stasis intensifies, and the overlying epithelial cells slough.[20]

The topical effects of NSAIDs appear to require prolonged mucosal exposure to the drug, and enterohepatic circulation of certain NSAIDs may thereby exacerbate injury. The initial insult progresses to mucosal barrier dysfunction. Indeed, Bjarnason demonstrated that NSAIDs cause increased intestinal permeability in humans by showing loss of chromium-51–labeled proteins into the intestinal lumen.[22] In another study, 33 of 49 (67%) patients taking oral NSAIDs were found to have intestinal inflammation, as documented by scintigraphic assessment of accumulation of indium-111–labeled white blood cells in the small intestine and by fecal excretion of indium-111.[23] Nineteen of 32 patients who also underwent simultaneous scanning with ^{99m}Tc-labeled red blood cells showed blood loss at sites identical to where intestinal

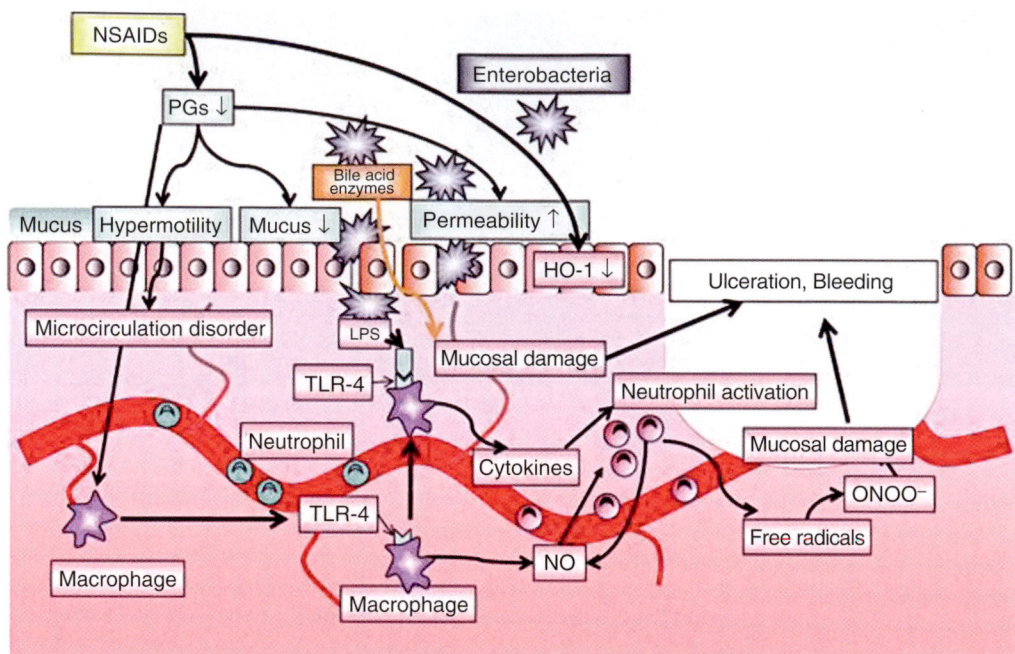

FIGURE 119-3. Mechanisms of NSAID-induced small bowel injury. NSAIDs decrease mucosal endogenous prostaglandins (PGs) and reduce mucus production; microcirculatory disturbances accompany abnormally increased intestinal motility, and the disruption of intercellular junctions leads to increased mucosal permeability. Mucosal injury can be intensified secondarily by bile acids, proteolytic enzymes, and intestinal bacteria. At the same time, inflammatory cytokines are induced and neutrophil infiltration occurs. *HO-1*, Heme oxygenase-1; *LPS*, lipopolysaccharide; *NO*, nitric oxide; *ONOO⁻*, peroxynitrite; *TLR4*, toll-like receptor 4. (*Modified from Higuchi K, Umegaki E, Watanabe T, et al. Present status and strategy of NSAIDs-induced small bowel injury. J Gastroenterol 2009; 44:879-88.*)

inflammation was demonstrated. Loss of mucosal integrity allows luminal contents, including bile acids, pancreatic secretions, bacteria, and food antigens, to enter the mucosa and exacerbate injury. This process results in neutrophil chemotaxis with nonspecific inflammation and ulceration in response to the initial injury. The observation by Wallace and colleagues,[24] that the intestinal microbiota may be altered and NSAID toxicity in the small intestine worsened in animals treated with PPI co-therapy, supports a potential etiogenic role for microbiota-associated injury. These data suggest that while PPIs are quite effective in reducing gastric and duodenal NSAID ulcers, small intestinal injury could actually be worsened. Clinical studies to further explore this possibility are awaited.

Diagnosis

Despite the widespread use of EGD, colonoscopy, and barium contrast studies, no source of blood loss is found in as many as one half of patients with iron deficiency anemia who are taking NSAIDs. CE and double balloon enteroscopy, however, have dramatically changed the diagnosis and management of small intestine ulceration and diaphragm disease. Tibble and associates demonstrated that fecal excretion of calprotectin, a non-degraded neutrophil cytosolic protein, can be used to assess intestinal inflammation, and therefore that this test might be a practical noninvasive means to diagnose NSAID enteropathy. Fecal calprotectin levels correlate with fecal excretion of indium-111.[25] Maiden showed that after 2 weeks of diclofenac, 75% of volunteers had increased fecal calprotectin levels and 68% showed injury on CE.[15] Thus, even short-term use of NSAIDs can cause injury and ulceration throughout the GI tract and therefore must be discontinued before extensive evaluation of patients with obscure GI bleeding because

of the likelihood that these agents are responsible for the blood loss.

Treatment

Discontinuation of NSAIDs is the most effective management option. A key practical consideration is whether NSAID-associated small intestinal injury is clinically relevant when choosing selective or nonselective NSAID formulations for the patient who requires anti-inflammatory therapy. To address this question, a randomized trial was performed comparing the nonselective NSAID Diclofenac SR + omeprazole (to reduce gastric and duodenal ulcers) with celecoxib therapy.[26]

The results of this large, randomized trial, known by the acronym CONDOR, confirmed a low rate of symptomatic and complicated ulcers in both study groups. However, when the endpoint included side effects beyond upper tract ulcers and bleeding, such as presumed small intestinal blood loss, there was a highly significant difference that favored the COX-2 inhibitor treatment. The hazard ratio for reaching this "comprehensive GI" primary endpoint was 4.3-fold higher in the NSAID + PPI compared with the COX-2 group, which supports the concept that, in some patients, selection of therapy should consider the risk and relevance of NSAID enteropathy.

A variety of potential therapeutic agents to reduce small intestinal NSAID injury have been evaluated using CE assessment of macroscopic injury. Misoprostol co-therapy has been shown to reduce damage in short-term studies in both NSAID and aspirin users. These pilot studies showed significant reductions in endoscopic injury, in some cases to baseline levels.[27-29] Other agents not available in the United States, rebamipide and geranygeranylacetone, have shown some efficacy in short-term endoscopy studies as well.[30,31] It is unclear if these studies, performed in healthy volunteers, with CE endpoints of macroscopic injury, are predictive of clinical outcomes, so definitive recommendations on use of any of these treatments cannot be made.[31] Metronidazole therapy given to 13 patients with NSAID enteropathy reduced inflammation and occult blood loss while preserving intestinal permeability; this study supports the role of secondary bacterial injury in exacerbation of the epithelial damage.[32] Sulfasalazine also has been shown to reduce intestinal inflammation, as measured by fecal indium-labeled neutrophil excretion, suggesting that active mediators of inflammation as well as bacteria normally found in the small intestine might play a role in the pathogenesis of NSAID enteropathy.[33] A variety of nutritional products (recombinant human lactoferrin, fish hydrolysate, glutamine, and bovine colostrum) have undergone preliminary studies with encouraging results in experimental animal and human models of NSAID enteropathy, and additional studies are awaited.[31] Recommendations on the use of antibiotics or any other agents to treat patients with NSAID-induced enteropathy have not been formalized, given the paucity of research and few long-term human studies.

NSAID Colopathy

The term *NSAID colopathy* has been used to refer to the nonspecific colonic injury that has been seen at colonoscopy in patients who are using NSAIDs (including low-dose aspirin) and that ranges from erosions to ulcers with or without strictures. NSAID colopathy does not have the protean manifestations of NSAID enteropathy. Resolution of these findings with cessation of NSAID exposure has supported their etiologic role, but proof by disease recurrence upon rechallenge has not been clearly demonstrated in most cases. Diaphragm disease of the colon may be considered diagnostic for NSAID-induced colon injury, although only a relatively small number of such cases have been reported (Fig. 119-4).[34] The presence of diaphragms with ulcers distinguishes these lesions from other nonspecific ulcers.

The pathogenesis of NSAID colopathy is thought to be similar to that of NSAID enteropathy, with a role for both topical and systemic injury initiated by NSAIDs. Diclofenac extended-release formulations have been frequently implicated, supporting a role for high local drug concentrations due to enterohepatic recirculation The colonic lesions, like the NSAID-associated lesions in the small intestine, are thought to result from the scarring that follows ulceration. Strictures are concentric and may present with a pinhole-size lumen. The mucosa between diaphragms is normal; the pathologic findings are also similar to those of NSAID enteropathy.

The most common clinical presentations of NSAID colopathy include occult blood in the stool, iron deficiency anemia, or frank bleeding, with or without abdominal pain or a change in bowel habits. Other findings can include intermittent obstructive symptoms or diarrhea. Colonoscopy is currently the diagnostic test of choice: the presence of characteristic diaphragmatic webs with normal intervening mucosa in a setting of NSAID use distinguishes the NSAID ulcer from other colonic ulcers. For non-stricturing NSAID lesions, discontinuing the NSAID often is curative and is essential to management; obstructive symptoms associated with stricture formation, however, require more aggressive management. For strictures that are easily accessible, endoscopic dilation with a through-the-scope (TTS) balloon has been reported to be safe and effective (see Fig. 119-4).[34] If endoscopic dilation is not possible, the area should be tattooed because there may be no serosal abnormalities or palpable areas of transition to guide resection. Surgery also is indicated for significant bleeding or perforation and when carcinoma cannot be excluded with confidence.

ULCERATIONS ASSOCIATED WITH OTHER DISEASES

Ulcers may involve the small intestine in a variety of other clinical conditions and may be distributed segmentally or diffusely throughout the small intestine, or in a more limited fashion with few or multiple, solitary, ulcerated lesions. Rarely are these lesions the initial manifestation of disease, but rather they are discovered during investigation of other symptoms of the primary disorders.

Specific Disease Associations

Diffuse small intestinal ulcerations are well described in Crohn's disease and can complicate celiac disease or be present in patients with sprue-like symptoms, who have either flat or normal intervening intestinal mucosa and who are refractory to gluten withdrawal. Ulcerative enteritis that is specifically associated with IBD is discussed more fully in the chapter on

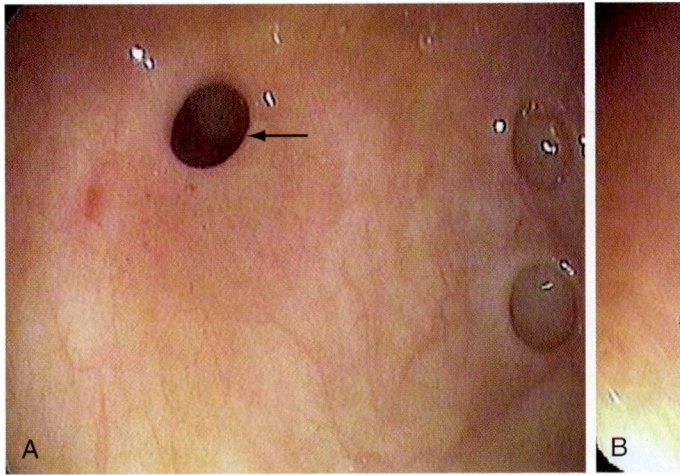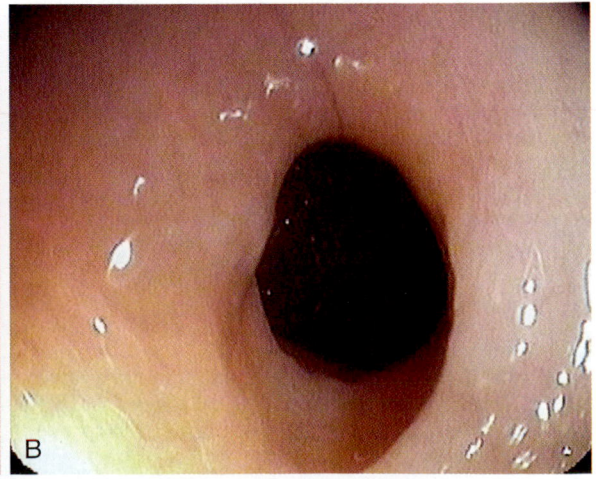

FIGURE 119-4. *A,* Colonoscopic view of a diaphragmatic stricture *(arrow)* associated with chronic use of NSAIDs. *B,* After balloon dilation there is no residual stricture. *(Courtesy Deepak Gopal, MD, Madison, Wis.)*

Crohn's disease (see Chapter 115). Ulcerations accompanying celiac disease (see Chapter 107) are much less common, and have been reported primarily as complications (e.g., ulcerative jejunitis in patients with severe or nonresponsive disease).[35,36] In a study that compared the clinical and biological characteristics of 57 patients with refractory celiac disease (RCD), ulcerative jejunitis was significantly more common in patients with the more serious RCD II (29/43; 67.4%) than in those with RCD I (4/14; 28.6%), and ulcerations larger than 1 cm in diameter were present only in patients with RCD II (P < 0.001).[37] In a second study of 38 celiac and 45 control patients who underwent CE, a greater number of ulcerations (>5) and more distal locations of lesions were reported in patients with celiac disease (23% and 32%) compared with non-celiac patients (0% and 6%) (P = 0.005 and 0.003, respectively). Extensive lesions in the ileum and distal jejunum were seen more often in RCD II patients (54%) compared with those with RCD I (9%) (P < 0.02).[38] Histology of these ulcerations is nonspecific,[39] and therefore sheds little light on etiology, but the presence of intestinal ulcerations associated with celiac disease appears to accompany severe or refractory disease, and reports of such ulcerative disease in simple celiac disease that is responsive to gluten withdrawal are lacking.

Other Diffuse Ulcerative Processes

Findings of diffuse small intestinal mucosal injury without specific disease associations are recognized more frequently today because of improved small bowel imaging. Many of these findings may eventually be categorized as Crohn's disease, complicated celiac disease, or NSAID enteropathy. However, occurrences of intestinal ulceration, reported primarily in case series, have been described in a variety of other settings such as ischemia, infection, or autoimmune states. Because the endoscopic appearance of small bowel ulcerations is without distinctive features, it is not clear whether these ulcers represent a discrete group previously referred to as nonspecific, or whether they are newly recognized forms of established clinical processes.

Ischemic Damage

Diffuse ulcerations seen in ischemic enteritis associated with small vessel vasculitides have been reported in SLE,[40] Churg-Strauss syndrome, and Behçet's disease,[41] although ulcers associated with these conditions are often focal and localized most frequently to the distal small bowel.[42] Although the most common GI complication in Henoch-Schönlein purpura (HSP) is intussusception, which may per se result in ischemic changes, it has been suggested that ulcerative duodenitis seen in HSP is related to vasculitis-induced mucosal ischemia.[43] Vasculitides involving medium-sized vessels have also been implicated in small bowel injury. One study that assessed patients with protein-losing enteropathy reported not only chronic nonspecific multiple ulcers (CMUSE) in 5 patients, but also 1 patient with distal ileal ulceration attributed to polyarteritis nodosa.[44] In a pediatric study of 42 patients with CF who underwent CE, small bowel findings showed diffuse inflammation characterized by edema, erythema, mucosal breaks, and ulcerations.[45] Vascular damage and multiple small bowel ulcers have been documented with the use of medications such as chemotherapeutic agents. The recurrent small intestinal ulcers seen with rechallenge of the interleukin (IL)-6 antagonist tocilizumab in RA patients[46] was attributed to possible inhibition of the mucosal wound healing properties of the cytokine. The obliterative arteritis seen in radiation enteritis (see Chapter 40) may progress to ulceration, stricture, fistula formation, or fibrosis. Additionally, mechanical forces

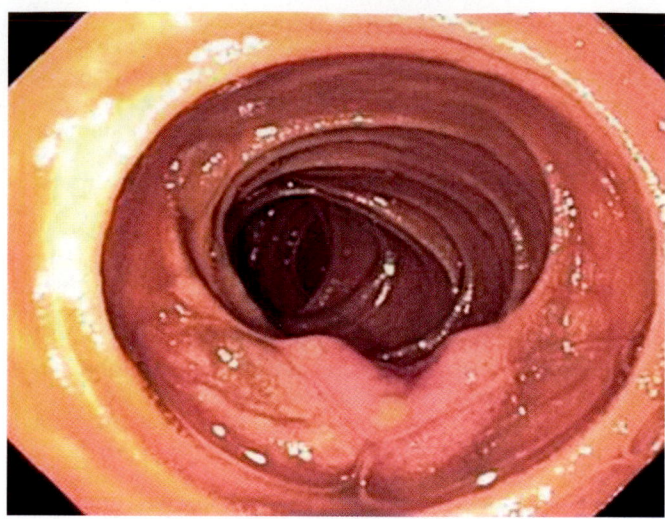

FIGURE 119-5. Endoscopic view of an ulcerated small bowel GIST. *(Courtesy Dr. Laurel Fisher, University of Michigan.)*

or intussusceptions that avulse the mesentery may result in ischemia and small bowel ulceration. There are no known histologic markers to distinguish these ulcers etiologically.

Other Associations

Infections with cytomegalovirus, cryptosporidium, or TB, particularly in the immunocompromised host, have been reported to cause ulcerative enteritis.[47] Ulcerated neoplasms such as sarcoma, metastatic lung carcinoma, carcinoid, or solitary GIST tumors are often first detected because of GI bleeding (Fig. 119-5). The ulcerative process in graft-versus-host disease (GVHD) commonly affects the small intestine, with nonspecific histologic features of gland destruction, ulceration, and submucosal fibrosis.[48] One study evaluated 11 allogeneic hematopoietic stem cell transplantation patients who presented with nausea, diarrhea abdominal pain, diarrhea and hematochezia, absence of skin lesions, and negative evaluations for infections. Nine underwent upper and lower tract endoscopy with biopsy, and all patients underwent CE. Ten of the 11 patients had jejunal or ileal ulcers or erosions on CE. In 7 of 9 patients who had upper and lower endoscopy studies and evidence of GVHD on biopsy, the small bowel lesions were judged to be more severe, prompting escalation of the disease severity grading scale.[49] Gastric acid hypersecretion is responsible for jejunal ulcerations in ZE and possibly in Meckel's associated ileal ulcers (Fig. 119-6). Intestinal ulceration in all these clinical settings likely represents mucosal injury as an extension of the underlying disease process.

APPROACH TO THE DETECTION AND DIAGNOSIS OF SMALL INTESTINAL ULCERS

While detection of small intestinal mucosal injury is facilitated by advances in endoscopic technologies, our understanding of the causes, characteristics, and mechanisms is still incomplete. Historically, investigation of the small intestine was difficult and progress limited because of inadequate diagnostic techniques to assess mucosal damage distal to the duodenum. More than a decade ago, with the advent of CE technology, the ability to visualize the small intestine was dramatically

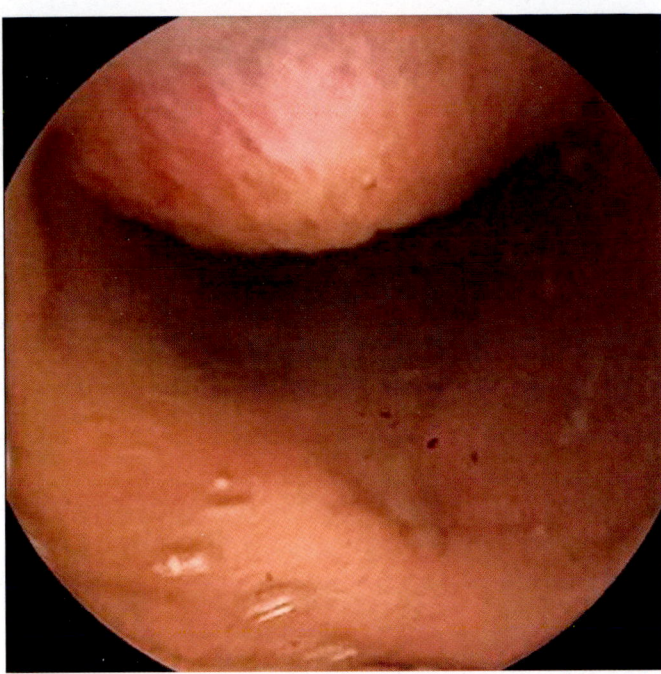

FIGURE 119-6. Capsule endoscopic view of a Meckel's diverticulum with associated mucosal ulceration.

enhanced and a new age in recognition and understanding of small intestinal disease began. The purely diagnostic nature of CE, however, prompted the development of therapeutic deep enteroscopy technologies including double balloon enteroscopy (DBE), single balloon enteroscopy (SBE), and spiral enteroscopy, all capable of biopsy, dilation, and hemostatic maneuvers. Because the opportunity to perform rigorous investigation and treatment of small intestinal disease is relatively recent, the approach to patients with suspected or confirmed ulcers of the small intestine is evolving. Improved diagnostics will help to demystify small intestinal ulcerative disease but must be interpreted in the context of appropriate clinical data by efforts to identify a cause.

There are currently several diagnostic options for investigating small intestinal mucosal injury.

Capsule Endoscopy (CE)

CE is the standard first-line diagnostic tool for evaluation of the small intestine. Currently, there are 3 FDA-approved small bowel capsules available in the United States.[50] In comparison studies, GIVEN Imaging's PillCam SB and Olympus' EndoCam have similar efficacy.[51] The more recent MiroCam has similar diagnostic yield, complication rate, and moderate concordance with EndoCam,[52] is concordant with PillCam SB for the diagnosis of obscure GI bleeding, and has[53] higher diagnostic yield than PillCam in detecting duodenal papillae.[54] All current CE devices capture more than 50,000 digital images of small intestinal mucosa with a resolution <0.1 mm and a field of view greater than 156 degrees; new designs have fields of view up to 360 degrees.[55]

Detection of Small Bowel Ulcerations

Visual Inspection

Clinical studies that evaluate the sensitivity of CE for detection of small intestinal ulceration outside of Crohn's disease are limited. In its early years, CE showed a great ability to detect ulcers missed by other modalities such as radiologic contrast studies of the small intestine,[42] and an early pooled data analysis asserted that the CE miss rate for ulcers in the small intestine was as low as 1%.[56] A lack of standardization in description of ulcers and other small bowel lesions, however, led to the development of the Lewis Score, which was based on villus appearance, stenosis, and ulcers, defined as "mucosal breaks with white or yellow bases surrounded by red or pink collars." Ulcer size was established by the percentage of the capsule image involved by the ulcerated lesion.[57] This scale is included in the PillCam SB software but is not uniformly used in descriptions of small intestinal capsule findings, and the recognition of ulcers and interpretation of CE images remains reader dependent.

Optical Enhancements

Recent optical enhancements in capsule devices have been introduced to facilitate lesion detection. The CE Blue Mode, which eliminates red light in image viewing, was designed to enhance mucosal detail, but, in 1 study, was judged to provide no benefit over white light in calculating the Lewis Score.[58] FICE (Fuji Intelligent Chromo Endoscopy) technology, which offers selection of 3 variable color wavelength settings using red, green, and blue light to enhance small intestinal mucosal lesions, has been incorporated into the PillCam SB capsule software. One study found that the use of FICE mode 1 (red 595 nm; green 540 nm; blue 535 nm) and mode 2 (red 420 nm; green 520 nm; blue 530 nm) during CE readings improved visualization of erosions/ulcers by 77.8% and 55.5%, respectively.[59] Others have shown that FICE improved detection rates of all small intestinal lesions by experienced readers[60] and trainees, possibly because of reduction in bile pigment effect[61]; 1 pilot study found improvements only in angioectasia detection and not ulcer recognition.[62]

Computer-Aided Technology

Other computer-aided technologies under development provide software platforms for existing CE systems which can distinguish mucosal ulceration from other lesions or normal tissue. One primary focus in this high-technology area is on textural features that are analyzed with multilayer neural networks using shape discrimination, "curvelet transformation" which represents images at different scales and angles, or data-mining techniques.[63] Other innovative models using color analysis and image processing algorithms have shown high accuracy in distinguishing healthy from ulcerative tissue. While these software platforms are not yet incorporated into existing CE systems, the ultimate goals are to create automatic CE image analysis[64] and to provide more rapid, objective ulcer detection.

Determination of Etiology

Currently, CE has limited capacity for detailed analysis of a recognized ulcer, and small intestinal ulcerations lack specific characteristics to allow determination of etiology, even in a highly suggestive clinical setting. There is clinical expert consensus about certain findings, such as large, deep, serpiginous ulcerations which more likely suggest the transmural injury seen in Crohn's disease than the superficial damage from NSAID exposure, although biopsies remain critical for definitive diagnosis. Advanced biotechnology consortia currently are working on nano-based molecular optical biopsy and recognition of cancer cells by small intestinal pill cameras, and there is the potential for maneuverable, tissue sampling

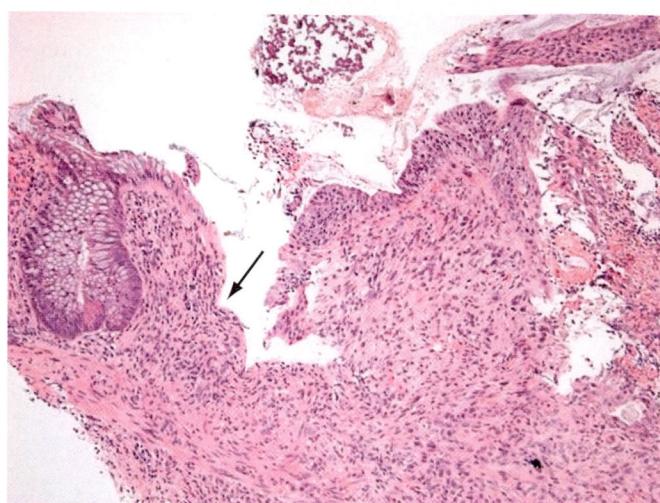

FIGURE 119-7. Histopathology of nonspecific small bowel ulceration (arrow) with regeneration at ulcer edge. *(Courtesy Dr. Henry Appelman, Department of Pathology, University of Michigan.)*

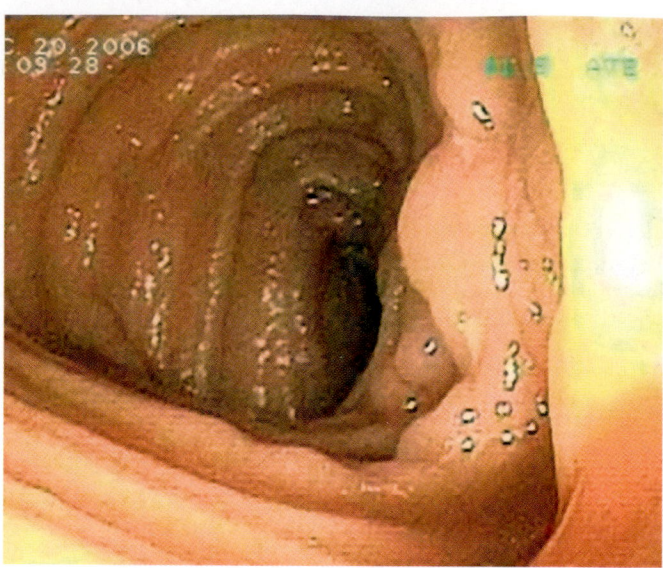

FIGURE 119-8. Endoscopic view of the nonspecific appearance of small bowel ulceration. Histopathology of this lesion obtained by double-balloon enteroscopy showed patchy lamina propria hypercellularity, villus flattening, a focus of pyloric metaplasia, and a tiny granuloma. While nonspecific, these features may be seen in Crohn's disease. This patient was treated with 5-aminosalicylic acid and budesonide with clinical response.

capsule devices to become standard therapeutic technology in the future.[65] When CE studies confirm the presence of small intestinal ulcerations, the decision should be made to perform deep enteroscopy with biopsy if there is no obvious clinical explanation for the bowel injury and if nonspecific histology, which is the likely finding, would influence therapy, such as medication selection (Fig. 119-7).

Device-Assisted Deep Enteroscopy

Small bowel enteroscopy with standard endoscopes have traditionally allowed limited therapeutic access for biopsy of the small intestine. The deep enteroscopy systems, first introduced by Yamamoto and colleagues in Japan in 2004, opened the entire jejunum and ileum to the endoscopist.[66,67]

Currently there are 3 deep enteroscopy systems: Fuji Double Balloon Enteroscopy (DBE); Olympus Single Balloon Enteroscopy (SBE); and Spirus Spiral Enteroscopy (SE). The balloon-assisted devices allow advancement of the endoscope by pleating the bowel over an overtube, whereas the spiral technique uses a screw-type clockwise rotation of the overtube for progression. One review found DBE and SBE to be similar with respect to depth of insertion, diagnostic yield, complications, therapeutic interventions and duration of procedure and sedation.[68] The spiral device was noted to have a lower diagnostic yield, but shorter procedure time. In a randomized prospective study, Messner and colleagues compared the rate of complete enteroscopies in 26 patients with suspected mid-gut disorders who were randomly assigned to DBE or SE.[69] Success rate for panenteroscopy using antegrade and retrograde approaches was 12 times greater (92% compared with 8%; P = 0.002) for DBE than for SE, although the effect on diagnostic yield, which is critical, was no different. Overall, antegrade enteroscopy has a higher diagnostic yield than retrograde enteroscopy (63.7% vs. 39.7%),[70] possibly because angioectasias are more frequently located in the proximal small bowel. The therapeutic ability of DBE includes hemostasis techniques, such as argon plasma coagulation (APC), injection of vasoconstrictors or sclerosing agents, or hemostatic clipping; dilation of inflammatory or fibrotic strictures; resection of polypoid lesions; and tissue sampling for histologic diagnosis. In a systematic review of 12,823 procedures, the major complication rate was 0.72%,[71] although the complication rate attending therapeutic procedures may be as high as 5%.[72]

Although we emphasize the diagnostic importance of biopsies obtained by device-assisted enteroscopy, the accuracy of histologic interpretation depends on the pathologist's acumen and is limited by the nonspecific nature of most specimens. Only in select clinical settings such as malignancy where identifiable cancer cells are present, or in Crohn's disease where characteristic granulomas are visible, can a biopsy be considered highly specific for diagnosis. In other contexts, studies identifying disease specific histology or markers are lacking, possibly because of a current lack of sophisticated probes, or possibly because no truly distinguishing findings exist. Diagnoses may be made with reasonable confidence when histology supports clinical and endoscopic findings, and when response to therapy in the setting of chronicity is documented (Fig. 119-8).

Cross-Sectional Imaging

CT and MR enterography (CTE, MRE) are important imaging modalities to assess small intestinal wall thickness and mucosal abnormalities, and are well described in the context of small intestinal Crohn's disease. MRE eliminates the high risk of radiation exposure with CTE, and the 2 techniques have similar accuracy in patients with suspected Crohn's disease[73] and comparable sensitivities for evaluating inflammation and stenosis in symptomatic IBD patients.[74] The use of cross-sectional imaging in other small intestinal diseases is less well documented and, currently, there are no CTE/MRE studies dedicated exclusively to the description and evaluation of noninflammatory ulcers in the small intestine.

Other Radiologic Studies

Because of the superficial nature of most small intestinal ulcerations, traditional imaging studies such as plain films and barium studies have no significant role in evaluation of small bowel ulcers.

New and enhanced technologies for visualization of the small intestine have revolutionized our ability to detect small bowel injury. Because the endoscopic appearance of a lesion is rarely diagnostic, our clinical judgments must rely on a careful history, a search for concomitant illness or medication exposure, and tissue sampling in cases where the diagnosis is in question. Although pathology also may be inconclusive, it can redirect the clinician toward a more focused differential diagnosis, and toward medical or procedural intervention in patients with an established diagnosis or significant disease. Intestinal ulcerations remain markers of small intestinal mucosal injury that is best managed after the underlying etiology has been determined.

KEY REFERENCES

Full references for this chapter can be found on www.expertconsult.com.

1. Boydstun JS Jr, Gaffey TA, Bartholomew LG. Clinicopathologic study of nonspecific ulcers of the small intestine. Dig Dis Sci 1981; 26:911-6.
4. Matsumoto T, Iida M, Matsui T, Yao T. Chronic nonspecific multiple ulcers of small intestine: A proposal of the entity from Japanese gastroenterologists to Western enteroscopists. Gastrointest Endosc 2007; 66(3 Suppl):S99-107.
7. Sidhu R, Brunt LK, Morley SR, et al. Undisclosed use of nonsteroidal anti-inflammatory drugs may underlie small-bowel injury observed by capsule endoscopy. Clin Gastroenterol Hepatol 2010; 8:992-5.
11. Higuchi K, Umegaki E, Watanabe T, et al. Present status and strategy of NSAIDs-induced small bowel injury. J Gastroenterol 2009; 44:879-88.
12. Allison MC, Howatson AG, Torrance CJ, et al. Gastrointestinal damage associated with the use of nonsteroidal antiinflammatory drugs. N Engl J Med 1992; 327:749-54.
13. Graham DY, Opekun AR, Willingham FF, Qureshi WA. Visible small-intestinal mucosal injury in chronic NSAID users. Clin Gastroenterol Hepatol 2005; 3:55-9.
34. Smith JA, Pineau BC. Endoscopic therapy of NSAID-induced colonic diaphragm disease: Two cases and a review of published reports. Gastrointest Endosc 2000; 52:120-5.
36. Kurien M, Evans KE, Aziz I, et al. Capsule endoscopy in adult celiac disease: A potential role in equivocal cases of celiac disease? Gastrointest Endosc 2013; 77:227-32.
37. Malamut G, Afchain P, Verkarre V, et al. Presentation and long-term follow-up of refractory celiac disease: Comparison of type I with type II. Gastroenterology 2009; 136:81-90.
50. Fisher LR, Hasler WL. New vision in video capsule endoscopy: Current status and future directions. Nat Rev Gastroenterol Hepatol 2012; 9:392-405.
57. Gralnek IM, Defranchis R, Seidman E, et al. Development of a capsule endoscopy scoring index for small bowel mucosal inflammatory change. Aliment Pharmacol Ther 2008; 27:146-54.
60. Imagawa H, Oka S, Tanaka S, et al. Improved detectability of small-bowel lesions via capsule endoscopy with computed virtual chromoendoscopy: A pilot study. Scand J Gastroenterol 2011; 46:1133-7.
66. Yamamoto H, Kita H, Sunada K, et al. Clinical outcomes of double-balloon endoscopy for the diagnosis and treatment of small-intestinal diseases. Clin Gastroenterol Hepatol 2004; 2:1010-6.
69. Messer I, May A, Manner H, Ell C. Prospective, randomized, single-center trial comparing double-balloon enteroscopy and spiral enteroscopy in patients with suspected small-bowel disorders. Gastrointest Endosc 2013; 77:241-9.
74. Jensen MD, Kjeldsen J, Rafaelsen SR, Nathan T. Diagnostic accuracies of MR enterography and CT enterography in symptomatic Crohn's disease. Scand J Gastroenterol 2011; 46:449-57.

HISTORICAL PERSPECTIVE

The first anatomic mention of the appendix was made by Leonardo da Vinci in the early 15th century. The first case report of clearly recognizable appendicitis was recorded in 1711 by the German surgeon Lorenz Heister,[1] but it was not until 25 years later that the first inflamed appendix was removed by Claudius Amyand, a Sergeant Surgeon to Queen Ann, King George I, and King George II. Amyand operated on an 11-year-old boy who had a perforated appendix within a scrotal hernia that he was able to excise and repair, respectively.[2] Throughout the 18th and 19th centuries, the prevailing medical opinion was that acute abdominal pain and right lower quadrant inflammation was a consequence of inflammation of the cecum or its surrounding tissues. The modern description of the pathophysiology of appendicitis and the role of the appendix in acute abdominal syndromes dates to 1886, the year Reginald Fitz presented a paper to the Massachusetts Medical Society in which he coined the term *appendicitis* and espoused early surgical intervention as its appropriate treatment.[1]

The first now-customary appendectomy for classic acute appendicitis actually had been performed by Lawson Tait in 1880, but it was not reported until 1889 when Charles McBurney, one of the great contributors to our understanding of appendicitis, published his recommendation for early laparotomy for the treatment of appendicitis.[3] It is in this paper that what subsequently became known as *McBurney's point* is described as the point of "maximum tenderness, one half to 2 inches inside the right anterior spinous process of the ilium on a line drawn from the umbilicus."[2,4]

Almost a century later, the first laparoscopic approach to appendectomy was described by Kurt Semm,[3] and with development of natural orifice transluminal endoscopic surgery (NOTES), the first successful transvaginal appendectomy was reported by Santiago Horgan and Mark A. Talamini in early 2009.[5]

EPIDEMIOLOGY

Appendicitis is the most common acute abdominal emergency seen in developed countries. The crude incidence rate of appendicitis in the United States for all age groups is 11/10,000 persons per year,[6] and similar rates are noted in other developed countries. Inexplicably, the rates of appendicitis are as much as 10 times lower in many less developed African countries.[7] The incidence rate of the disease peaks between 15 and 19 years of age at 48.1/10,000 population per year and falls to about 5/10,000 population per year by age 45 years, after which it remains constant.[6] Men are at greater risk than women, with a case ratio in most series of 1.4 : 1. The lifetime risk of appendicitis has been estimated at 8.6% in men and 6.7% in women.[6]

Approximately 250,000 appendectomies are performed each year in the United States; data from most European countries suggest that the incidence of appendicitis is decreasing. Between 1989 and 2000, a 15% decrease in the overall incidence of appendicitis was noted in an English study[8]; similar temporal trends have been noted in Greece and Finland.[9,10] However, multiple studies from the United States suggest that the number of appendectomies performed for acute appendicitis has been increasing since 1995.[11,12] Regardless of the direction of the epidemiologic trend, appendicitis remains the most common indication for emergency abdominal surgery.

*The author would like to acknowledge the significant contributions of Richard H. Turnage, MD, and Kfir Ben-David, MD, to this chapter in prior editions.

ANATOMY AND EMBRYOLOGY

The vermiform appendix and the cecum are best thought of as a single anatomic unit. Developmentally part of the midgut, the appendix and cecum form between the 8th and 12th weeks of gestation as a bud arising from the midgut loop, before the ascending colon has become delineated. Congenital malformations of the appendix such as agenesis and duplication are very rare. With an average length of 9 cm,[13] the origin of the appendix varies and the appendix may assume any of the positions of a clock hand, with the center considered the appendiceal origin.

Unlike the rest of the colon, the appendix has a complete longitudinal muscle layer. The blood supply of the appendix is found in a separate mesentery, the mesoappendix, and consists of an appendicular branch of the ileocolic branch of the superior mesenteric artery. The lymphatic drainage of the appendix is to the ileocolic lymph nodes, which are shared with the terminal ileum and right colon.

Although the right colon is fixed in the retroperitoneum, the appendix and cecum have a more variable position within the abdomen. The position of the appendix depends upon a number of factors: the degree of cecal descent and peritoneal fixation, the configuration of the cecum, appendiceal length, associated adhesions, and the habitus of the person.[14] Typically, the location of the appendix is described as retrocecal, pelvic, subcecal, or para-ileal (Fig. 120-1). The position of the appendix has important clinical implications: thus for example, because as many as 60% of people have a retrocecal or pelvic-positioned appendix, the clinical presentation of acute appendicitis is often atypical, with right upper quadrant abdominal or suprapubic pain.

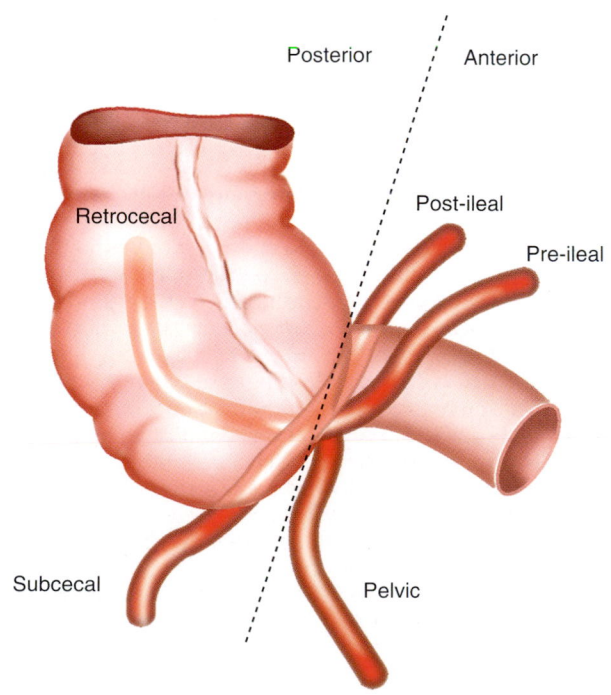

FIGURE 120-1. Positions of the appendix. Five different positions of the appendix are illustrated; variations in position can affect the clinical presentation of appendicitis (see text). *(From Buschard K, Kjaeldgaard A. Investigation and analysis of the position, fixation, length, and embryology of the vermiform appendix. Acta Chir Scand 1973; 139:293.)*

The classic surface anatomy of the appendix was described by McBurney in 1889 and, as mentioned earlier, McBurney's point is located at the junction of the lateral and middle thirds of a line drawn from the right anterior superior iliac spine to the umbilicus.[3] Classically, this surface marking has been important in both the diagnosis and treatment of acute appendicitis; however, investigators have shown that the appendix is located within 5 cm of McBurney's point in less than 50% of cases.[15] This anatomic finding helps explain why pain or tenderness located at McBurney's point is not found in all cases of appendicitis.

PATHOLOGY

Acute appendicitis is classified as acute, gangrenous, or perforated. The earliest gross findings of acute appendicitis are injection of the serosal blood vessels and edema of the appendiceal wall. In more advanced cases, the serosal surface appears dull and is covered by fibrinopurulent exudates. Over time, focal areas of gangrene develop, marked by greenish and black discoloration of the wall; with perforation, focal necrosis of the appendiceal wall develops and adjacent abscesses form.[16]

Microscopically, each of these forms of appendicitis has distinctive characteristics. In acute or suppurative appendicitis, a neutrophilic infiltrate involves the muscularis propria layer circumferentially, accompanied by acute inflammation, ulceration of the mucosa with edema and microabscesses in the appendicular wall, and vascular thrombosis. The hallmarks of gangrenous appendicitis are transmural inflammation of the appendix with focal areas of mural necrosis. Vascular thrombosis is more prominent in gangrenous than in suppurative appendicitis. The presence of mucosal inflammation alone ("catarrhal" inflammation) is more characteristic of infectious enteritis or colitis and is not considered evidence of acute appendicitis; for the microscopic diagnosis of appendicitis to be made, inflammation must extend to the muscularis propria.[16]

PATHOGENESIS

Despite more than 100 years of study, there still is no single explanation for all cases of appendicitis. The classic hypothesis is that obstruction of the appendiceal lumen by either a fecalith or lymphoid hyperplasia produces an increase in intraluminal pressure, which in turn results in venous hypertension, ischemia of the appendiceal wall, and subsequent bacterial invasion of the appendix with necrosis and perforation. Experimental evidence in animal models exists to support this hypothesis of the etiology of acute appendicitis.[17] This hypothesis, however, does not explain all cases of appendicitis. Careful review of pathologic series shows that luminal obstruction is found in a minority of cases. Fecaliths are present in only 3.6% to 27% of cases of acute appendicitis, with most series at the lower end of the range,[16,18] and lymphoid hyperplasia is more common in non-inflamed appendices than in acute appendicitis.[19] Other causes of luminal obstruction such as foreign bodies, tumors, and fibrous bands are uncommon. Direct measurement of intraluminal pressure at appendectomy for appendicitis reveals an elevated pressure in only a minority of cases.[20]

An alternative hypothesis for the etiology of appendicitis is based on the concept that either bacterial or viral enteric infection leads to mucosal ulceration of the appendix and subsequent bacterial invasion from the normal colonic flora. The finding that up to 75% of cases of appendicitis demonstrate well-defined superficial mucosal ulceration supports this theory. Furthermore, mucosal ulceration is a more consistent finding than dilatation of the appendix or fecaliths and is found earlier in the course of appendicitis.[21] One report found human cytomegalovirus (HCMV) early antigen expression in 64% of cases with acute appendicitis and no HCMV antigens in normal appendices, suggesting that in some cases, CMV infection might produce mucosal ulcerations and lead to acute appendicitis.[22]

Additional support for the role of infection in the etiology of appendicitis is found in 2 lines of epidemiologic evidence. The first is based in the hygiene theory of appendicitis advocated by Barker in the mid-1980s.[23] According to this hypothesis, changes in sanitation tied to the Industrial Revolution resulted in a decrease in enteric infections in infants, with subsequent decreased immunity to these infections in childhood and young adulthood. Acquisition of these infections later in life was believed to predispose people to appendicitis, explaining the rise in incidence rates of appendicitis in the first half of the 20th century. The decrease in the overall rate of enteric infections during the last half of the 20th century explains the overall decline in appendicitis. The second line of epidemiologic evidence supporting the role of infection in the etiology of appendicitis is the seasonal variance in incidence of appendicitis and the occurrence of temporal and spatial clusters of appendicitis, both hallmarks of infectious diseases.[24,25] It is important to recognize, however, that no specific infectious agent has been linked with all cases of appendicitis, suggesting that infection is not the complete story.

A decrease in dietary fiber intake (the fiber hypothesis) also has been proposed as a cause of appendicitis. According to this hypothesis, decreased dietary fiber causes firm stool and an increased enteric transit time, resulting in more fecaliths and more appendicitis. This hypothesis was felt to explain both the rise in appendicitis rates in the early 20th century and the marked differences in appendicitis rates between more developed Western countries and less developed African countries. Doubt has been cast upon this hypothesis, however, for several reasons. First, although dietary fiber ingestion has been falling in urban Africans, appendicitis rates have not risen markedly,[26] and a prospective series from Africa demonstrated continued high fiber intake even in patients with appendicitis.[27] Second, rates of appendicitis in the Western world have fallen without changes in dietary fiber intake.

It is likely that any 1 of several different inciting events (e.g., luminal obstruction, infection, or trauma) can initiate breakdown of the appendiceal mucosa, resulting in bacterial invasion; the end result is appendicitis.

CLINICAL FEATURES

A detailed history and careful physical examination remain cornerstones of the diagnosis of acute appendicitis. Although no single item of the history, in isolation, allows the diagnosis to be made reliably, combination of the classic symptoms and the typical progression of symptoms coupled with right lower quadrant tenderness allows good diagnostic accuracy. In the classic presentation of acute appendicitis, patients first note vague, poorly localized epigastric or periumbilical discomfort, which typically is not severe and often is attributed to "gastric upset." Patients commonly report feeling that a bowel movement should make the pain better, a sensation known as the *downward urge*.[28]

Diarrhea sometimes is seen early on with appendicitis, but this is not common. Within 4 to 12 hours of the onset of pain, most patients note nausea, anorexia, vomiting, or some combination of these 3 symptoms. The nausea usually is mild to moderate, and most patients have only a few episodes of emesis. If vomiting is the major symptom, the diagnosis of appendicitis should be questioned. Likewise, emesis that occurs before the onset of pain should suggest other diagnoses.[29] Many patients report mild fever or chills; high fevers or significant rigors are uncommon. The patient's abdominal pain typically increases in intensity, and a characteristic shift in pain to the right lower quadrant occurs over 12 to 24 hours. The character of the pain becomes achy and more localized. Localization of the pain to the right lower quadrant is a valuable finding when present and occurs in over 80% of patients with appendicitis.[29]

On physical examination, most patients appear slightly ill. Tachycardia is uncommon with simple appendicitis, but it may be seen with complicated appendicitis. Most patients with simple appendicitis have a temperature below 100.5°F; temperature above 100.5°F is most often associated with perforated or gangrenous appendicitis.[30] Patients with appendicitis, like other patients with peritonitis, tend to lie still rather than move about. Right lower quadrant tenderness and rigidity, both voluntary and involuntary, are common findings. Localized right lower quadrant tenderness is an important finding when present, but its absence does not rule out appendicitis. A variety of methods exist to elicit localized right lower quadrant peritonitis, including the cough sign (the presence of point tenderness with a cough), percussion tenderness, and formal elicitation of rebound tenderness. Although all of these techniques are reasonably sensitive, 1 small study showed rebound tenderness to be the most accurate predictor of the localized peritonitis associated with appendicitis.[31]

Additional findings that may be helpful in diagnosing appendicitis include the psoas sign, the obturator sign, Rovsing's sign, and rectal tenderness. The *psoas sign* is sought by having a supine patient actively flex the right hip against resistance, or by the examiner flexing and extending the patient's right hip with the patient in the left lateral decubitus position. Pain with either of these maneuvers is thought to result from irritation of the underlying psoas muscle by an inflamed retroperitoneal appendix. The *obturator sign* is elicited by internally and externally rotating the flexed right hip. Pain is thought to arise when the inflamed pelvic appendix irritates the adjacent obturator internus muscle. *Rovsing's sign* is the finding of right lower quadrant pain during palpation of the left side of the abdomen or when left-sided rebound tenderness is elicited. Rectal tenderness may be elicited when the examining finger reaches the wall of rectum adjacent to the inflamed appendix. All of these findings are valuable when present, but their absence does not exclude appendicitis.[29]

Appendicitis can be easy to diagnose when the presentation is typical, but a typical presentation is encountered in only 50% to 60% of cases. An atypical presentation of appendicitis occurs for a variety of reasons. The classic migration of periumbilical pain to the right lower quadrant is thought to occur when the parietal peritoneum in the right lower quadrant becomes irritated by the inflamed appendix. In cases of retrocecal or pelvic appendicitis, this site might not become irritated. Atypical presentations of appendicitis are particularly common in patients who are at the extremes of age, pregnant, or immunosuppressed, including those with AIDS and a low CD4 cell count.

Appendicitis in infants and young children remains a problematic diagnostic challenge because of difficulties in obtaining an accurate history. In young children, the characteristic history of pain is difficult to elicit, right lower quadrant pain is a less common finding, and nonspecific findings of vomiting, lethargy, and irritability tend to predominate.[32] Physical examination is difficult to perform because of poor patient cooperation and because localized right lower quadrant tenderness is found in fewer than 50% of patients.[33] In addition, the characteristic laboratory findings often are not present and leukopenia is as common as leukocytosis in young infants.[34] As a result, errors in diagnosis are common, and the frequency of complicated appendicitis is as high as 40% to 70%.[35]

The diagnosis of appendicitis in older adult patients also may be a challenge. In older adults, the classic pattern of pain migration, right lower quadrant tenderness, fever, and leukocytosis are observed in only 15% to 30% of cases.[34,36] Older patients also tend to present to medical attention in a delayed time frame relative to younger patients. For all of these reasons, the complication and perforation rates can be as high as 63% in patients older than 50 years of age.[37]

The presentation of appendicitis during pregnancy also is associated with an atypical clinical presentation, particularly in the later stages of pregnancy. In 1 series, only 57% of pregnant women with appendicitis had the classic progression of pain.[38] Nausea and vomiting tend to be more common in pregnant women with appendicitis, but they also are common occurrences during normal pregnancy. Fever and leukocytosis are less commonly seen in pregnant woman than in other patient groups, and the value of leukocytosis is obscured by the physiologic leukocytosis of pregnancy. Although right-sided abdominal pain and tenderness are found in more than 80% of pregnant women with appendicitis, pain is located in the right lower quadrant only 60% of the time.[39]

Immunocompromised patients in general, and patients with AIDS in particular, represent a challenging group in which to diagnose appendicitis. Abdominal pain is reported in 12% to 45% of AIDS patients with appendicitis. The range of diagnoses responsible for this pain is significantly greater than in patients without HIV and includes opportunistic infections and malignancies, although in most cases, the pain is related to a diagnosis not associated with HIV.[40] Research suggests that appendicitis occurs more often in HIV-infected patients than in HIV-negative patients, with as much as a 4-fold increase in incidence.[41] Although patients with AIDS usually present with the classic symptoms of appendicitis, there often is a history of chronic abdominal pain. Diarrhea also is a more common presenting symptom of appendicitis in HIV-positive patients, and leukocytosis is relatively uncommon. Declining CD4 counts are associated with delays in presentation for medical attention and increased perforation rates.[42] Despite the challenges of diagnosing appendicitis in patients with HIV, surgical outcomes with appropriate treatment are quite good; the largest series to date had no mortalities and a 13% complication rate, which is comparable to outcomes in patients without HIV.[42]

DIAGNOSIS

Diagnosis of appendicitis remains a significant clinical challenge because of the many different entities that manifest with acute abdominal pain and the relatively nonspecific initial presentation of the disease. Because the natural history of appendicitis is thought of as a time-dependent progression to perforation, there is some urgency in making a prompt and accurate diagnosis. Not all causes of acute abdominal pain, however, require surgical intervention, and a negative appendectomy carries some risks for the patient, including adhesion formation, infection, and postoperative disability. Table 120-1 illustrates common diagnoses that can mimic acute appendicitis. Compounding this diagnostic challenge, there is no single symptom, finding, or laboratory test that is completely sensitive or specific for appendicitis.[29]

Laboratory Studies

Laboratory findings in acute appendicitis include a variety of markers of acute inflammation. An elevated WBC in the range of 11,000 to 17,000/mm^3 is seen in approximately 80% of patients, but the specificity of this finding for acute appendicitis versus other causes of acute abdominal pain is poor.[43] An elevated proportion of granulocytes in the total WBC or an elevated total neutrophil count (left shift) also is seen in the vast majority of patients with appendicitis, but is not specific for appendicitis.[43] C-reactive protein (CRP), an acute phase reactant synthesized by the liver, is thought to rise within 12 hours of the development of an acute inflammatory process. Although CRP is elevated in 50% to 90% of cases of appendicitis, CRP is nonspecific when cutoff values of 5 to 25 mg/L are used.[44] A urinalysis often is obtained in patients with acute appendicitis to exclude urinary tract infections, but mild abnormalities, either pyuria or hematuria, are present in about 50% of cases of appendicitis.[45]

The value of laboratory investigations in diagnosing acute appendicitis has been a matter of some debate. In patients with a classic presentation by history and physical examination, many authors think that little additional information is obtained from laboratory studies. When all cases of appendicitis are considered, however, adding laboratory studies such as WBC, left shift, and CRP has been shown to improve diagnostic accuracy.[46] When clinical findings are compared with inflammatory markers, inflammatory markers are stronger predictors of appendicitis than individual history or physical findings. Direct comparison of WBC and CRP suggests that total WBC or total granulocyte count is more sensitive and accurate than CRP for detecting acute appendicitis.[44,46] The diagnostic performance of inflammatory markers is even better in identifying patients with perforated appendicitis.

All patients with suspected acute appendicitis should have a CBC. A pregnancy test should be obtained in women of childbearing age. The value of other laboratory tests such as amylase, liver biochemical tests, or urinalysis lies in helping to exclude other diagnoses that can mimic acute appendicitis (see Table 120-1).

Imaging Studies

Traditionally, there has been little role for routine imaging studies in patients with suspected acute appendicitis. As is stated in the classic surgical textbook, *Cope's Early Diagnosis of the Acute Abdomen*, "Over reliance on laboratory tests and radiological evaluations will very often mislead the clinician, especially if the history and physical examination are less than diligent and complete."[29,31] In 50% to 60% of cases, the diagnosis of appendicitis requires no imaging studies and can be made on clinical grounds alone.[47,48] When diagnosis is less certain, a variety of imaging tests has been used to help confirm or exclude the diagnosis of acute appendicitis: plain abdominal films, abdominal US, radionuclide scans, and abdominal and pelvic CT.

Plain Abdominal Films

Plain films of the abdomen often are the initial imaging test for patients with acute abdominal pain. Findings on plain films of the abdomen consistent with appendicitis include a radiopaque right lower quadrant coprolith, focal right lower quadrant ileus or a sentinel loop, loss of the right psoas shadow, and a right lower quadrant soft tissue mass. All of these findings are suggestive of but not definitive for appendicitis. In a prospective study in which plain

TABLE 120-1 Differential Diagnosis of Appendicitis

Diagnosis	Findings That Help Differentiate Entity from Appendicitis
Bacterial or viral enteritis	Nausea, vomiting, and diarrhea are severe; pain usually develops after vomiting
Epiploic appendagitis	Focal abdominal pain and tenderness without migration or progression of the pain; patients have a paucity of other GI symptoms such as anorexia or nausea. Laboratory findings are usually normal
Mesenteric adenitis	Duration of symptoms is longer; fever is uncommon; RLQ physical findings are less marked; WBC count is usually normal
Pyelonephritis	Pain is more likely to be felt in the right flank; high fever and rigors are common; marked pyuria or bacteriuria and urinary symptoms are present; abdominal rigidity is less marked
Renal colic	Pain radiates to the right groin; significant hematuria; character of the pain is clearly colicky
Acute pancreatitis	Pain and vomiting are more severe; tenderness is less well localized; serum amylase and lipase levels are elevated
Crohn's disease	History of recurrent similar attacks; diarrhea is more common; palpable mass is more common; extraintestinal manifestations may have occurred or be present
Cholecystitis	History of prior attacks is common; pain and tenderness are greater; radiation of pain is to the right shoulder; nausea is more marked; liver biochemical tests are more likely to be abnormal
Meckel's diverticulitis	Nearly impossible to distinguish preoperatively from appendicitis
Cecal diverticulitis	Difficult to distinguish preoperatively from appendicitis; symptoms are milder and of longer duration; CT is helpful; patients are usually older
Sigmoid diverticulitis	Usually occurs in older patients; changes in bowel habits are more common; radiation of the pain is to the suprapubic area, not RLQ; fever and WBC count are higher
Small bowel obstruction	History of abdominal surgery; pain is colicky; vomiting and distention are more marked; RLQ localization is uncommon
Ectopic pregnancy	History of menstrual irregularities; characteristic progression of symptoms is absent; syncope; positive pregnancy test
Ruptured ovarian cyst	Occurs in the middle of the menstrual cycle; pain is of sudden onset; nausea and vomiting are less common; WBC count is normal
Ovarian torsion	Vomiting is more marked and occurs at the same time as the pain; progression of symptoms is absent; abdominal or pelvic mass often is palpable
Acute salpingitis or tubo-ovarian abscess	Longer duration of symptoms; pain begins in the lower abdomen; often there is a history of STDs; vaginal discharge and marked cervical tenderness often are present

RLQ, right lower quadrant; STD, sexually transmitted disease.

abdominal films were ordered on all patients with suspected appendicitis, the films altered clinical management in only 6% of cases.[49]

Plain abdominal films should be used in the evaluation of acute appendicitis only when bowel obstruction or perforation is thought to be likely; their role in the routine evaluation of appendicitis should be discouraged.

US

Abdominal US has been used to image the acute abdomen since the 1980s. Although US is considered the imaging test of choice for biliary and gynecologic diseases, its precise role in the diagnosis of acute appendicitis remains unsettled.

The US characteristics of appendicitis are well defined. Using a 5- or 7.5-MHz transducer, the technique of graded compression is used to displace the mobile loops of bowel in the right lower quadrant of the abdomen. The diagnosis of appendicitis can be made with confidence if a 7-mm or thicker non-compressible blind-ended loop of bowel is identified (Fig. 120-2). The findings of a shadowing appendicolith, pericecal inflammation, or a localized pericecal fluid collection all support the diagnosis of appendicitis.[50] Recent work examining US in pediatric appendicitis suggests that the finding of inflamed periappendiceal fat may be the best predictor of appendicitis, and that focusing on findings of inflammation rather than anatomic features of the appendix may improve the accuracy of diagnosis.[51] Appendicitis is excluded during US study by demonstration of a normal appendix. A normal appendix, however, is demonstrated in fewer than 50% of adults even by experienced sonographers, thus reducing the value of a "negative" US study.[52]

In a collected review, the reported sensitivity of US examination in the diagnosis of appendicitis in adults was 86% and its specificity was 81%.[53] In contrast, US examination appears to be more sensitive and specific in children than in adults,

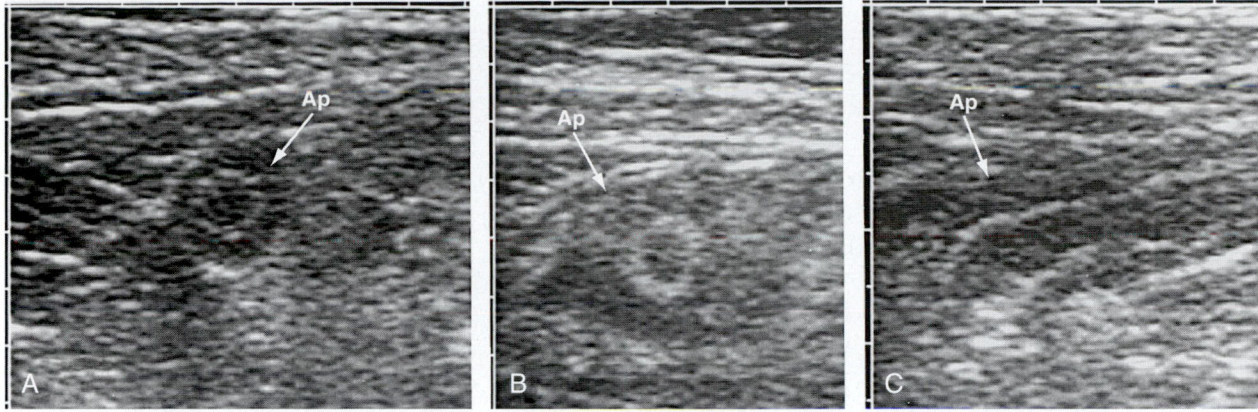

FIGURE 120-2. Transverse *(A and B)* and longitudinal *(C)* US of the right lower quadrant demonstrating a swollen, noncompressible appendix (Ap) proved at operation to be acute appendicitis. *(Courtesy Roy A. Filly, MD. San Francisco, CA.)*

with sensitivity and specificity better than 90% in most series and detection of a normal appendix in up to 90% of children.[54,55] There are some important limitations to the usefulness of US in the diagnosis of appendicitis. All US-based techniques are operator dependent. The excellent results just mentioned were achieved in dedicated trials performed by interested and experienced ultrasonographers. In 1 multicenter trial focused on diagnosis of the acute abdomen, the real-world sensitivity of US fell to 55%.[56] Recent work has also focused on the role of surgeon-performed bedside US in the diagnosis of appendicitis. A recent systematic review suggested that the accuracy of surgeon-performed US could approach that of radiologist-performed US, but there was considerable heterogeneity in this finding.[57] US study also is less sensitive in patients with a BMI over 25 and in those with perforated appendicitis.[58] Finally, US examination is more useful in confirming than in excluding the diagnosis of appendicitis, reducing its clinical utility in patients with a low pretest probability of appendicitis.

Radionuclide Scanning

Radionuclide scanning has been advocated when the diagnosis of appendicitis is uncertain. Two major techniques are used: either HMPAO (^{99m}Tc-hexamethylpropyleneamine oxime)-labeling of the patient's leukocytes, or ^{99}Tc-labeled antigranulocyte antibodies. In both of these techniques, an accumulation of the radionuclide in the right lower quadrant is considered positive for appendicitis. The reported sensitivity of radionuclide scanning is 91% to 94%, with specificities in the 82% to 94% range.[59] Limitations of these techniques remain their lack of availability in all hospitals, the relatively long time required to perform them, and operator dependence in their interpretation.

CT

Abdominal CT scans are considered the imaging study of choice in non-classic cases of appendicitis. With the development of rapid helical and multidetector CT scanners, CT imaging is used increasingly to evaluate patients with acute abdominal pain. CT has long been considered valuable in making the diagnosis of appendiceal abscess, and CT-based therapy of these abscesses has become common.[60] Since the 1990s, a number of authors have advocated broadening the use of CT scans to assist in the diagnosis of atypical appendicitis. A wide variety of techniques has been used for

appendiceal-protocol CT scans, which differ in terms of the amount of the abdomen scanned, the thickness of the individual cuts, and the types of contrast used. Several conclusions have emerged from these studies: thin (5-mm) cuts are better than thick (10-mm) cuts,[61] and use of IV and/or enteric contrast improves accuracy.

CT findings consistent with appendicitis include an inflamed, distended (>6 mm) appendix that fails to fill with contrast or air (Fig. 120-3), often accompanied by an appendicolith or appendiceal wall thickening; periappendiceal inflammation, cecal apical thickening, and pericecal fluid collections are associated findings in appendicitis.[62] Identification of a normal appendix or the finding of alternative intra-abdominal pathology constitutes a negative study.

The performance of CT scanning for appendicitis has been impressive, with sensitivity rates of 94% and specificity rates of 95% in 1 collected review of multiple studies.[53] The best results occur when enteric contrast is administered both by mouth and by rectum and contrast opacification of the cecum occurs. Limitations of CT scanning for appendicitis include the time required for enteric contrast to fill the bowel, decreased sensitivity in patients with low body fat, allergic reactions to IV contrast agents, exposure to ionizing radiation, and cost.

Overall Approach to Imaging

What constitutes the best imaging study has not been conclusively determined for all patients in whom a diagnosis of appendicitis cannot be made confidently after clinical history, physical examination, and review of laboratory findings. Based on current evidence, however, it would appear that CT scanning is more sensitive, more specific, and less operator dependent than US in adults.[63,64] In pregnant women and in very thin patients, especially in institutions with experienced ultrasonographers, abdominal US is probably an alternative first imaging study in atypical cases of appendicitis. In pregnant patients with equivocal findings on US study, follow-up imaging with MRI has been shown to be as accurate as CT scanning and should be the next study to confirm the diagnosis of appendicitis.[65] In pediatric patients, when the diagnosis of appendicitis cannot be made confidently after evaluation by a pediatric surgeon, US should be the first imaging test selected. This recommendation is based on the increased sensitivity of US study in children and on the theoretical 10-fold increase in lifetime cancer risk engendered by exposure of children to ionizing radiation.[66] In patients of any age, the

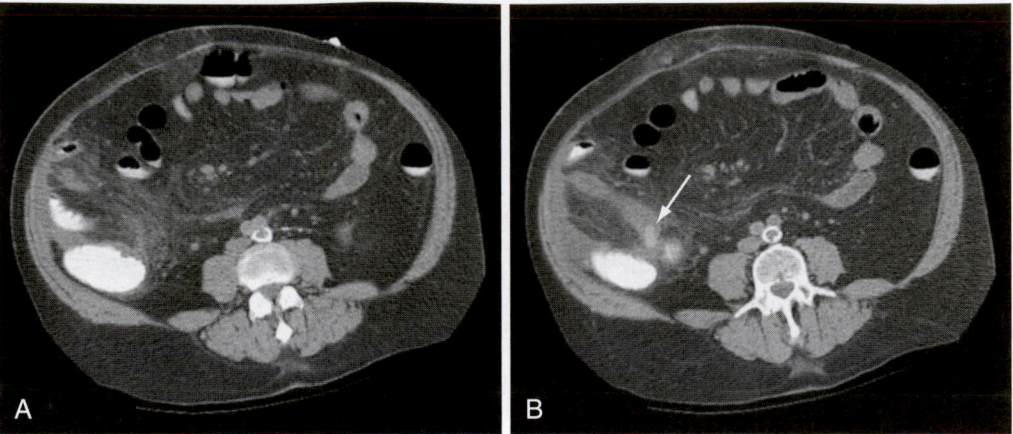

FIGURE 120-3. CT showing diagnostic findings of acute appendicitis. *A,* Diffuse inflammatory changes in the mesentery surrounding the distal ileum and cecum are seen in a patient with appendicitis. *B,* A fecalith is shown in the appendiceal lumen *(arrow). (Courtesy William R. Brugge, MD, Boston, Mass.)*

initial step in evaluating patients with suspected acute appendicitis should be evaluation of the patient by an experienced surgeon, because this diagnostic evaluation is at least as accurate as any imaging study.[67]

Clinical Scoring Systems and Computer-Aided Diagnosis

Based upon data suggesting that examiner experience improves diagnostic accuracy in acute appendicitis, a variety of scoring systems has been devised since the 1990s to aid in the diagnosis of appendicitis. Most of these scoring systems assign numerical weights to findings from history, physical examination, and laboratory values in an attempt to predict the probability of appendicitis. More than 10 different scoring systems have been published, all of which purport to reduce errors in diagnosis and negative appendectomy rates. In an examination of the performance of multiple published scoring systems on a single, well-defined patient data set, the ability of all scoring systems to predict appendicitis was disappointing.[68]

The ability of scoring systems to perform well when applied to patient populations other than the population for which they had been developed remains a problem; other studies have reported similar results looking at individual scores.[69] At this point there is no universally applicable scoring system for the diagnosis of acute appendicitis.

Laparoscopy

Laparoscopy has been proposed to assist in diagnosing equivocal cases of acute appendicitis. Inserting a laparoscope into the abdomen allows direct inspection of the appendix without appendectomy, if the appendix is found to be normal. The appeal of this approach is greatest in woman of childbearing age in whom gynecologic causes of acute abdominal pain can cloud diagnosis and who often are amenable to laparoscopic treatment. Two prospective studies of diagnostic laparoscopy in cases of possible appendicitis revealed gynecologic causes of pain in 48% to 73% of women with a normal appendix.[70,71] Because there is some, albeit weak, evidence to suggest appendectomy might predispose women to tubal infertility,[72] avoidance of unnecessary appendectomies is desirable in women of childbearing age. Diagnostic laparoscopy has been used in 2 prospective series to nearly eliminate negative appendectomies in women of childbearing age.[70,71]

Despite these promising results, some cautionary notes must be sounded. Most studies of diagnostic laparoscopy report examinations performed under general anesthesia, making this a resource-intensive test compared with radiologic imaging studies. Although diagnostic laparoscopy can be performed under local anesthesia, inherent technical constraints reduce its success rate. For example, gynecologic pelvic laparoscopy performed under local anesthesia fails to obtain complete visualization of the pelvis in up to 15% of cases[73]; this incomplete examination rate compares poorly with CT scanning. Currently, diagnostic laparoscopy cannot be recommended over appendiceal-protocol CT scanning as an initial test, but it probably should be used as a supplement to CT or US evaluations in which the results of these tests are equivocal.

Diagnostic Accuracy

The concept of diagnostic accuracy refers to the observation that not all patients with a preoperative diagnosis of appendicitis are found to have acute appendicitis at operation. Because of the time-dependent risk of appendiceal perforation, with its resultant increase in complications, it is important to make the diagnosis of appendicitis as quickly as possible.[74] As a result, treatment decisions often are made in the presence of incomplete clinical information. An appendectomy is termed "negative" when a normal appendix is found at exploration for acute appendicitis.

Traditionally, an inverse relationship has been found between the frequency of negative appendectomies and the frequency of perforation at operation. Studies have shown that an increased diagnostic accuracy at operation carries an increased perforation rate,[75] a tradeoff believed to be a consequence of the increased time required to confirm the etiology of acute abdominal pain in the absence of any specific test for appendicitis. In the interests of avoiding complications, standard teaching has been to accept a certain negative appendectomy rate to improve patient outcomes. Without diagnostic imaging, a negative appendectomy rate of 10% to 30% with a perforation rate of 10% to 25% is felt to represent a "good" balance[6,30,47]; in these series, the negative appendectomy rate was higher in women than men.

In recent years, the use of imaging studies has improved the diagnostic accuracy for appendicitis without concomitant increases in perforation risk. In multiple single-institution series in which imaging was used selectively or universally in cases of presumed appendicitis, negative appendectomy rates have been reduced to between 2% and 8% without an increase in perforation rates.[47,48,76-79] This improvement in diagnostic accuracy has been observed in all patient groups, but most notably in women and children. More significantly, data from the Washington State Surgical Care Outcomes and Assessment Program (SCOAP) has shown at a statewide level that the use of imaging to confirm the diagnosis of appendicitis decreased the negative appendectomy rate from 15.4% to 4.5%. With increased use of imaging statewide over the period 2006-2010, the negative appendectomy rate fell from 12% to 4.5% with no change in perforation rate.[80] These results suggest that with diagnostic imaging, it is possible to increase diagnostic certainty without exposing patients to an increased risk of perforation. Whether a policy of increased use of imaging studies in the diagnosis of appendicitis will prove to be cost-effective is not yet clear, but early data suggest it might be, if enough negative explorations can be avoided.[81]

As a result of all of these recent diagnostic modalities, a new approach is emerging to the patient with acute abdominal pain and suspected appendicitis (Fig. 120-4). The goal of this new approach relies on imaging techniques and laparoscopy to eliminate in-hospital observation as a tool to improve diagnostic accuracy, thereby reducing the time required to increase diagnostic certainty and decreasing the likelihood of time-dependent complications.

A strong incentive exists for avoiding negative appendectomies beyond diagnostic pride. Data from Sweden reveals that patients who undergo negative appendectomy have a higher Standardized Mortality Ratio (SMR) at 30 days than even patients with perforated appendicitis. The leading causes of mortality in patients with negative appendectomy are cardiovascular disease and infectious causes.[82] This increase in the SMR persists for 5 years, suggesting that the consequences of negative appendectomy have long-term health effects.[83] In addition, complication rates of 5% to 15% have been reported with removal of a normal appendix, the majority of which are infectious, including wound, pulmonary, and urinary tract infections. A 2.8% risk of small bowel obstruction is reported after appendectomy, but in cases with a negative appendectomy (i.e., appendectomy with a normal appendix), a higher risk of obstruction has been observed.[84] Of patients found to have a normal appendix at operation, only about 30% are found to have intra-abdominal findings that can explain their symptoms.

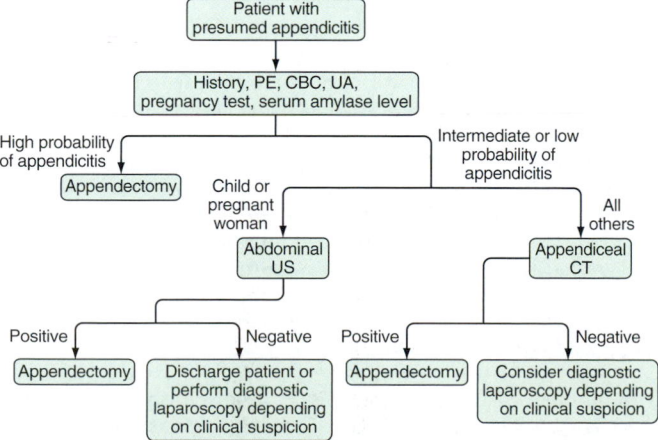

FIGURE 120-4. Algorithm for managing the patient with presumed appendicitis. CBC, complete blood count; PE, physical examination; UA, urinalysis.

COMPLICATIONS

The major complication of untreated appendicitis is perforation, with resultant peritonitis, abscess, and pylephlebitis. Overall, the perforation rate in most series is between 10% and 30%, but the rate of perforation varies widely with age; perforation is most common at the extremes of age. Perforation rates as high as 90% have been reported in children younger than 2 years,[33] and patients older than 70 years have perforation rates between 50% and 70%.[37,85] Patients between the ages of 10 and 30 years have the lowest perforation rates, generally between 10% and 20%.

The risk of perforation appears to increase as the duration of illness increases, particularly after 24 hours. Perforation of the appendix is classically thought of as a consequence of delay in diagnosis, and several studies have shown that patients with perforation have symptoms that average 30 hours longer than do patients with simple appendicitis.[74] Much of this delay appears to be a result of delays in presentation to medical attention rather than delays in medical decision making, but patients with perforation often have atypical presentations of their appendicitis, resulting in prolonged diagnostic times.

Patients with perforation are more likely to have significant fever, leukocytosis, and physical findings of peritonitis than are patients with uncomplicated appendicitis. Although perforation often can be predicted preoperatively based on the presence of these findings, not all patients with these findings have perforation.[86] Free perforation into the peritoneal cavity results in findings of diffuse peritonitis and can be associated with free intraperitoneal air on abdominal plain films. Patients with generalized peritonitis from appendicitis are difficult to distinguish preoperatively from patients with other causes of diffuse peritonitis.

An abscess will develop after perforation if the perforated appendix is walled off from the remainder of the peritoneal cavity because of its retroperitoneal location or if it is walled off by loops of small intestine or omentum. A localized collection of inflammatory tissue (phlegmon) initially forms, and subsequently a true abscess develops. On physical examination, patients with an abscess resulting from appendicitis often have a palpable right lower quadrant abdominal mass.

The most severe complication of appendiceal perforation is septic thrombophlebitis of the portal vein, also known as *pylephlebitis*. Pylephlebitis was more common early in the 20th century; today, diverticulitis is the most common cause. This rare complication should be considered in a patient with appendicitis who presents with high fever and mild jaundice. Treatment of pylephlebitis is control of the inciting infection and long-term (4 to 6 weeks) antibiotic therapy. The major organisms causing pylephlebitis are Gram-negative enteric aerobes and anaerobes. Even with aggressive therapy, the incidence of hepatic abscesses following pylephlebitis is 50%, and mortality rates are 30% to 50%.[87] A long-term complication of pylephlebitis is portal vein thrombosis with cavernous transformation of the portal vein and esophagogastric varices.

TREATMENT

Treatment of acute appendicitis is and remains appendectomy, despite the advent of sophisticated diagnostic and therapeutic modalities. Little has changed since Fitz and McBurney advocated early operative treatment of appendicitis in the late 19th century. Appendectomy is recommended, even though some cases of appendicitis resolve spontaneously. Although small studies have demonstrated that the vast majority of cases will improve with IV antibiotics alone, a recent meta-analysis of 5 randomized controlled trials that compared antibiotics and appendectomy demonstrated a treatment failure rate of 40% for antibiotics, mostly due to recurrent appendicitis.[88] We currently lack the ability to identify self-limited cases prospectively, however, and to wait for resolution places patients at risk for perforation with its resultant life-threatening complications. Thus, appendectomy is a surgical urgency, not a true emergency. Patients with appendicitis should be given appropriate IV fluids to correct volume depletion and electrolyte imbalances, and IV antibiotics to decrease wound infection rates; they should be taken to the operating room when they are stable. Brief periods of time may be taken to optimize the patient's concomitant medical conditions before operation, but long delays increase the rate of perforation and compromise outcome.

Two standard operative approaches exist for performing an appendectomy, either open appendectomy or laparoscopic appendectomy. Open appendectomy is performed though a muscle-splitting right lower quadrant incision; either an oblique or a transverse skin incision may be used. The appendix is identified and removed even if it is found to be normal. If normal, it is removed primarily to prevent future diagnostic confusion, and an exploration is carried out to identify other intra-abdominal causes of the patient's symptoms. If other surgical pathology is found at exploration, the initial incision may be extended or a separate incision performed to address the problem. In advanced cases with severe inflammation, cecectomy may be required.[89] Any abscesses are drained, and the abdomen is irrigated and closed.

The other common approach to appendectomy is the laparoscopic appendectomy. First described by Semm in 1983,[3] this procedure has been the subject of considerable study since that time. The technique of laparoscopic appendectomy has become standardized, and typically it is performed via a 3-trocar technique. After gaining access to the abdomen, the appendix and then the entire abdomen are inspected. If the appendix is inflamed, an appendectomy is performed. If other intra-abdominal surgical pathology is found, it can be treated laparoscopically, or an appropriate open surgical procedure can be performed. A new modification of laparoscopic appendectomy, single-incision laparoscopic surgery (SILS), is currently being studied, but the few studies to date have only shown equivalent results to conventional laparoscopic appendectomy.[90]

The general consensus from the published literature is that in patients for whom laparoscopy is feasible, laparoscopic appendectomy offers many advantages over open appendectomy. In a recent Cochrane meta-analysis of more than 50 studies comparing the 2 procedures, it was concluded that procedures are safe and effective in the treatment of non-perforated appendicitis.[91] After laparoscopic appendectomy, however, patients require less pain medication and return to normal activity sooner than after open appendectomy. The superficial wound infection rate is 50% lower with laparoscopic appendectomy than after open appendectomy, but there is an increased rate of intra-abdominal abscess formation. The hospital course after laparoscopic appendectomy is 1.1 days shorter, and patients resume a normal diet at about the same time as after open appendectomy. Laparoscopic appendectomy takes more time to perform, and is associated with higher in hospital costs, while total care costs are comparable.

At this point, it is not possible to say that 1 procedure is superior to another for all patients, but currently more than 75% of the appendectomies performed in the United States use the laparoscopic approach.[92] For some patient groups, laparoscopic appendectomy is preferable, especially young women,

employed patients who need to return to work as soon as possible, and those with an uncertain diagnosis.[91] Additionally, many consider laparoscopic appendectomy the procedure of choice for the treatment of acute appendicitis in the morbidly obese population, because it has been associated with shorter length of stay and lower morbidity.[93,94]

An exception to the statement that all patients with appendicitis require urgent appendectomy is the patient with perforation and a palpable right lower quadrant mass. These patients usually have extensive periappendiceal inflammation or abscess formation. In patients with a palpable mass who do not have diffuse peritonitis or toxicity, initial management can be operative or nonoperative. Although data quality is poor, 1 meta-analysis comparing early operation with conservative management showed that early operative intervention may be associated with a higher complication rate.[95] With initial non-operative management, patients are placed on bowel rest and given IV fluids and antibiotics, and a CT scan of the abdomen is obtained. If a single abscess 3 cm or larger is discovered, percutaneous drainage of the abscess under CT guidance is performed. If multiple abscesses are found or the patient does not improve within 24 to 48 hours of conservative therapy, operative drainage is performed. Success rates of 88% to 95% have been reported with initial nonoperative management.[96,97] Following resolution of the acute illness in older patients in whom a perforated cecal cancer is a possibility, colonoscopy, barium enema, or virtual colonography should be performed because the incidence of appendiceal or cecal cancer in patients older than 60 years who present with acute appendicitis can exceed 20%.[98] Some authors recommend interval appendectomy when the acute inflammation has resolved (6 to 12 weeks later), but the role of interval appendectomy remains controversial because the rate of recurrent appendicitis is less than 20% at 1 year.[99]

Natural orifice transluminal endoscopic surgery (NOTES) is an emerging field in minimally invasive surgery that is driving the development of new technology and techniques for procedures such as transluminal appendectomy. Although mostly investigational, NOTES procedures are performed using a transgastric, transcolonic, or transvaginal access point to the peritoneum. In 2004, Kalloo and his colleagues were able to demonstrate that natural orifices provide a port of entry via the GI tract to the peritoneal cavity. This approach requires the creation of a transluminal (e.g., per-oral transgastric) perforation into the peritoneal cavity using conventional endoscopes.[100] Theoretically, this approach could reduce postoperative abdominal wall pain, wound infection, hernia formation, and adhesions. A number of case reports describing the removal of the appendix using a NOTES technique has been reported in registries established by the Natural Orifice Surgery Consortium for Assessment and Research (NOSCAR) or other organized groups such as EuroNOTES and the Brazilian Registry. To date, no controlled trials have compared NOTES appendectomy to conventional or laparoscopic appendectomy, and the procedure should be considered investigational. As experience accumulates and instrumentation improves, NOTES may play an integral role in the future of abdominal surgery, including transluminal appendectomy.

OUTCOMES

The modern treatment of simple acute appendicitis is associated with excellent outcomes. Factors responsible for these outcomes are advances in anesthesia, antibiotics, IV fluids, and blood products. The mortality rate from acute appendicitis in 1 recent large series was 0.09% with a complication rate of 5.5%.[101] Older series have reported mortality rates of 0.2%

with a complication rate of 6%.[6] Patients typically are hospitalized for 24 to 48 hours after open appendectomy and 24 to 36 hours after laparoscopic appendectomy. Patients usually return to full activity 2 weeks after laparoscopic appendectomy and 3 weeks after open appendectomy.[102]

Morbidity and mortality attributable to appendicitis increase markedly with complicated appendicitis and in particular with perforation. Mortality rates of 1% to 4% and complication rates of 12% to 25% have been reported for perforated appendicitis.[96] In patients older than 70 years of age, in whom perforation and significant medical comorbidity are common, mortality has been reported to be as high as 32%.[37] Death in these circumstances usually is attributable to uncontrolled Gram-negative sepsis or peritonitis, and patients with perforated appendicitis often have a stormy postoperative course, with intra-abdominal abscesses and need for operative or percutaneous abscess drainage. Wound infection and dehiscence also are common in patients who have had open appendectomy, but these often promptly respond to wound drainage and antibiotics. These complications are minimized when a laparoscopic approach is chosen.

SPECIAL TOPICS

The Appendix and UC

A number of epidemiologic studies suggest that appendectomy protects against the development of UC,[103] particularly when performed for appendicitis; a similar relationship is not seen with Crohn's disease. A meta-analysis of 17 case-control studies suggests that the relative risk of developing UC after appendectomy is about 0.3 times that of controls.[104] Although these data come from case-control studies and questions can be raised about the appropriateness of the controls, this conclusion has been supported in 1 of the 2 large cohort studies performed.[105] Some researchers have suggested that appendectomy also attenuates the course of active UC[106,107] and UC has been reported to improve after appendectomy, especially in young patients.[108] In a mouse model of autoimmune colitis similar to UC, removal of the appendix early in life prompted significant attenuation of colonic inflammation.[109] Although these findings are far from conclusive, they provide potential insights into both UC and the potential normal function of the appendix.

Crohn's Disease of the Appendix

Although the appendix is often involved in patients with Crohn's disease of the ileum or colon, isolated Crohn's disease of the appendix is quite rare.[110] Crohn's appendicitis is difficult to distinguish from acute appendicitis preoperatively, although patients with Crohn's appendicitis commonly have a longer history of pain. The treatment of appendiceal Crohn's disease is appendectomy, which has a low rate of postoperative fistula formation.[111] The clinical course of Crohn's disease isolated to the appendix appears to be much more benign than that of typical Crohn's disease. Because isolated Crohn's disease of the appendix is quite rare, any patient found to have Crohn's appendicitis should undergo evaluation of the remainder of the GI tract for evidence of Crohn's disease.

Recurrent and Chronic Appendicitis

Recurrent appendicitis is the clinical scenario in which a patient with pathologically confirmed acute appendicitis relates 1 or more prior episodes with identical symptoms, which resolved without surgical intervention. This diagnosis remains somewhat controversial but has been documented in clinical series.[112] The diagnosis of recurrent appendicitis presupposes that some cases of appendicitis can resolve without medical intervention. Series of such cases exist in the radiologic literature, where patients with imaging findings consistent with appendicitis had rapid resolution of their symptoms without treatment. The percentage of cases of appendicitis that resolve spontaneously is unknown, but it is estimated at 6% to 8%. In small series of patients with spontaneous resolution of appendicitis, the recurrence rate is approximately 40%.[113] No prospective means of identifying spontaneously resolving appendicitis have been identified, and therefore all cases of appendicitis should be treated surgically. The existence of recurrent appendicitis serves as a reminder not to discount the diagnosis of appendicitis in patients just because of prior episodes of similar abdominal pain.

Chronic appendicitis is diagnosed when pathologic findings of fibrosis and chronic inflammation are found with a clinical syndrome consistent with appendicitis. Many of these patients report previous episodes of pain and relief of their symptoms after appendectomy.[114] This is not a common problem, and caution should be used in applying this diagnosis to patients with poorly characterized chronic abdominal pain, because many of these patients are unlikely to improve with appendectomy.

Diverticulitis of the Appendix

Diverticula of the appendix are uncommon, with a reported incidence in appendectomy specimens between 0.004% and 2.1%.[115] Two forms of diverticula exist: congenital and acquired. True congenital diverticula are quite rare, but acquired diverticula are found in 1% to 2% of appendectomy specimens.[116] Although the etiology of acquired appendiceal diverticula is unclear, they are thought to be pulsion diverticula, like colonic diverticula. Appendiceal diverticula typically are diagnosed incidentally on barium enema or CT scan or at surgical exploration.[117] Acute inflammation of appendiceal diverticula (diverticulitis) produces a clinical picture that mimics acute appendicitis, making diverticulitis of the appendix difficult to diagnose preoperatively. Appendiceal diverticulitis, however, typically occurs in patients in the fourth decade of life rather than in the first or second decades, and it tends to manifest with a more insidious course, with many days of pain before presentation.[118] CT scan can readily make the diagnosis. Appendiceal diverticulitis is more likely to be complicated by perforation than is the usual case of appendicitis, making surgery, rather than nonoperative management, the treatment of choice.

Epithelial Malignancies of the Appendix

Tumors of the appendix are rare and are found in approximately 1% of appendix specimens submitted for pathologic examination. The vast majority of appendiceal tumors are carcinoid, but this tumor is a rare cause of appendicitis because it usually arises in the tip of the appendix, not the base (see Chapter 33). The incidence of epithelial malignancies of the appendix has been estimated to be 0.12 per 1 million persons per year.[119]

There are 2 types of epithelial malignancies of the appendix: mucinous adenocarcinoma or cystadenocarcinoma and colonic type (non-mucinous) adenocarcinoma. Mucin-producing tumors are roughly twice as common as non–mucin-producing tumors.[120] Non–mucin-producing tumors of the appendix typically manifest with a clinical picture indistinguishable from that of acute appendicitis, with acute right lower quadrant pain and tenderness. On CT scan, findings of a soft tissue mass or an appendix larger than 15 mm in diameter should raise the suspicion of an appendiceal cancer.[121] In contrast, less than one third of mucinous appendiceal adenocarcinomas manifest as acute appendicitis. More commonly these lesions are found incidentally on imaging studies as a cystic right lower quadrant mass or in a patient with increasing abdominal girth secondary to pseudomyxoma peritonei.

The optimal treatment of all adenocarcinomas of the appendix is right hemicolectomy, either as a primary operation or as a secondary operation after adenocarcinoma of the appendix is noted on pathologic examination of an appendectomy specimen. Additionally, patients with appendiceal adenocarcinoma have a significant risk of synchronous and metachronous neoplasms, which often originate from the GI tract.[119] Overall survival of patients with adenocarcinoma of the appendix is roughly 60% at 5 years and is a function of tumor stage at presentation.

Appendiceal lymphoma is extremely uncommon, and primary lymphoma of the appendix accounts for 1% to 3% of all GI lymphomas (see Chapter 31).[122] Patients with appendiceal lymphoma usually present with acute appendicitis and an appendiceal diameter greater than 2.5 cm, with surrounding soft tissue thickening. Management of appendiceal lymphoma is appendectomy; right hemicolectomy is indicated only if there is extension of tumor beyond the appendix into the mesentery or cecum.[123]

Appendiceal mucoceles are uncommon entities arising from a variety of different pathologic processes, of which only a small subset are associated with development of pseudomyxoma peritonei. Hence, the pathologic diagnosis determines further management.[124] Perforation of a mucocele results in intraperitoneal dissemination of mucoid material, which can be acellular or can contain cells with varying degrees of dysplasia; cellular spread to the peritoneal surfaces leads to pseudomyxoma peritonei. These tumors usually are less aggressive than colorectal cancer, however, and they rarely manifest with lymph node or liver metastasis.[125] The combination of surgery and complete cytoreduction should be followed by intraperitoneal rather than IV chemotherapy, because the mainstay goal is prevention of locoregional recurrence, not prevention of systemic spread of disease.

Incidental or Prophylactic Appendectomy

The lifetime risk of appendicitis at birth is about 1 in 12, and declines to 1 in 35 by age 35 years. The greatest risk of appendicitis in a given year occurs over the second decade of life with a risk of about 0.25% per year.[6] Although appendicitis is the most common cause of emergent abdominal surgery, given the low lifetime risk of appendicitis, elective prophylactic appendectomy cannot be recommended. Incidental appendectomy, the removal of a normal appendix at the time of other abdominal surgery was, at 1 time, the leading cause of appendectomy in women. In light of the falling incidence of appendicitis, enthusiasm for incidental appendectomy has declined. In operations where it will not add morbidity, however, a case may exist for incidental appendectomy in patients younger than 30 years. In older patients, the low residual lifetime risk of appendicitis makes incidental appendectomy difficult to defend.

Epiploic Appendagitis

Epiploic appendagitis (EA) refers to self-limited inflammation of the epiploic appendices, and is important because it may mimic appendicitis, diverticulitis and other causes of localized abdominal pain. The epiploic appendages are fat-filled sacs that are covered by serosa, project outward from the colon wall toward the peritoneal cavity and are located throughout the colon although they are more numerous and larger in the transverse and sigmoid colon. They vary in size but usually are about 3 cm in length. They become acutely inflamed as a result of torsion or spontaneous thrombosis of a draining vein. EA is more common in men and usually occurs in the second to fifth decades of life. The major symptom of EA is nonmigrating, localized abdominal pain that typically is worse with defecation or urination. Appetite and bowel function are usually unchanged and nausea or vomiting are rare.

On physical examination patients with EA usually are afebrile, and have localized pain in the affected area, Rebound tenderness is usually not present. The white blood count and erythrocyte sedimentation rate are usually normal. EA is best diagnosed by CT scan although abdominal US is also useful in thin patients.

Most patients respond to treatment with NSAIDs in 4 to 7 days with laparoscopic removal of the inflamed appendage reserved primarily for patients who fail to respond to this conservative treatment.[126]

KEY REFERENCES

Full references for this chapter can be found on www.expertconsult.com.

1. Golden RL, Reginald H. Fitz, appendicitis, and the Osler connection—A discursive review. Surgery 1995; 118:504-9.
6. Addiss DG, Shaffer N, Fowler BS, Tauxe RV. The epidemiology of appendicitis and appendectomy in the United States. Am J Epidemiol 1990; 132:910-25.
13. Schumpelick V, Dreuw B, Ophoff K, Prescher A. Appendix and cecum. Embryology, anatomy, and surgical applications. Surg Clin North Am 2000; 80:295-318.
16. Carr NJ. The pathology of acute appendicitis. Ann Diagn Pathol 2000; 4:46-58.
29. Wagner JM, McKinney WP, Carpenter JL. Does this patient have appendicitis? JAMA 1996; 276:1589-94.
33. Rothrock SG, Pagane J. Acute appendicitis in children: Emergency department diagnosis and management. Ann Emerg Med 2000; 36:39-51.
46. Andersson RE. Meta-analysis of the clinical and laboratory diagnosis of appendicitis. Br J Surg 2004; 91:28-37.
63. Rosen MP, Ding A, Blake MA, et al. ACR Appropriateness Criteria(R) right lower quadrant pain—Suspected appendicitis. J Am Coll Radiol 2011; 8:749-55.
64. van Randen A, Bipat S, Zwinderman AH, et al. Acute appendicitis: Meta-analysis of diagnostic performance of CT and graded compression US related to prevalence of disease. Radiology 2008; 249:97-106.
74. Ditillo MF, Dziura JD, Rabinovici R. Is it safe to delay appendectomy in adults with acute appendicitis? Ann Surg 2006; 244:656-60.
80. Drake FT, Florence MG, Johnson MG, et al. Progress in the diagnosis of appendicitis: A report from Washington State's Surgical Care and Outcomes Assessment Program. Ann Surg 2012; 256:586-94.
91. Sauerland S, Jaschinski T, Neugebauer EA. Laparoscopic versus open surgery for suspected appendicitis. Cochrane Database Syst Rev 2010; CD001546.

Diverticular Disease of the Colon

TAFT P. BHUKET AND NEIL H. STOLLMAN

Historically, descriptions and investigations of diverticular disease of the colon are a relatively modern phenomenon. The French pathologist Jean Cruveilhier is widely credited with providing the first clear pathologic description in 1849: "…we not infrequently find between the bands of longitudinal muscle fibers in the sigmoid, a series of small, dark, pear-shaped tumours, which are formed by herniae of the mucous membrane through the gaps in the muscle coat."[1] In the 50 years subsequent to this description, there was relatively little mention of colonic diverticula or their clinical implication, highlighting the relative unimportance of the condition during this time span. In 1899, however, the German surgeon Ernst Graser described what we now consider to be the most common clinical manifestation of this condition: diverticulitis of the sigmoid colon.[2]

Graser's work was a prelude to our understanding and increasing appreciation of diverticular disease of the colon as a "modern disease." The early 20th century began with notable contributions by W.J. Mayo and colleagues, who reported the first surgical resection for diverticulitis in 1907,[3] and J.T. Case, who introduced the term *diverticulosis* in a radiologic case series in 1914.[4] In the subsequent 100 years, we have come to appreciate diverticular disease of the colon as one of the most common, burdensome, and yet incompletely understood GI disorders.

EPIDEMIOLOGY

The epidemiology of diverticulosis has changed markedly since its descriptions in the 19th and early 20th centuries. Clinical reports during this time were uncommon, and autopsy studies were used to estimate prevalence. At present, diverticulosis is considered one of the most common GI disorders, and trends suggest an increasing incidence of associated complications and health care costs.[5-9]

Because most persons with diverticulosis are asymptomatic and may never be identified, the true incidence and prevalence of this condition are still not known. Regardless, diverticulosis is a common condition, and medical literature suggests that approximately two thirds of adults will develop it by their ninth decade of life.[10,11] Our increasing use of colonoscopy further supports this notion and has helped refine our understanding of its prevalence. Diverticulosis is the most frequently reported abnormality found on colonoscopy, described in 42.8% of all colonoscopies and in 71.4% of patients older than 80 years of age.[6]

Two features dominate the epidemiologic profile of diverticulosis: geography and age. Prevalence clearly increases with age, ranging from less than 10% in those younger than 40 years of age to an estimated 66% in patients 80 years of age and older.[6,10-12] With regard to geographic association, diverticulosis has long been considered a disease of Western civilization. The classic observation holds that the disorder has the highest prevalence rates in Western and industrialized countries (e.g., the United States, Europe, and Australia) and is rare in rural Africa and Asia.[12] One long-standing explanation for this geographic variance is that the fiber-poor diet of Western countries plays a critical etiologic role.[13] Taken further, it was hypothesized that as immigrants acculturate to Western diets, prevalence patterns may shift. For example, in 1 study of non-Western immigrants (including those from Asia, Africa, and the Middle East), it was found that they began to have increasing rates of diverticular-related hospitalizations within 10 years of moving to Sweden.[14] In another report, Japanese-born persons who migrated to and lived in Hawaii had diverticulosis at autopsy in 52% of cases—much higher than the described prevalence of diverticulosis in Japan at that time.[15] The current idea of a Western-dominant prevalence of diverticulosis is well supported by the medical literature; however, it is intriguing to ponder the future effects of globalization and increasing access to colonic imaging on the disease's epidemiology. Reports from countries such as Israel, Japan, Kenya, Korea, Singapore, and Uganda[16-21] suggest a greater and growing prevalence of diverticulosis in these non-Western countries than previously appreciated.

The clinical impact of diverticulosis is remarkable and underscores its position as one of the "most burdensome" of GI disorders. In 2009, diverticular disease accounted for significant health care utilization in both the outpatient and inpatient settings: it was ranked as the number 1 GI cause for hospitalization (when combining diverticulitis and

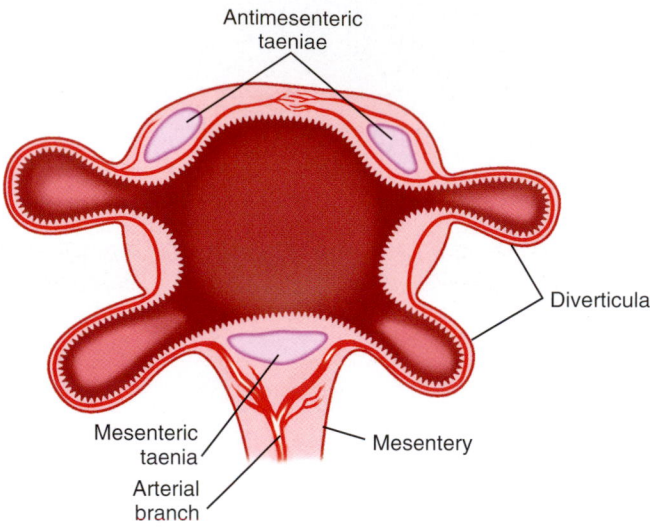

FIGURE 121-1. Diagram showing colonic diverticula and their relationship to the taeniae coli.

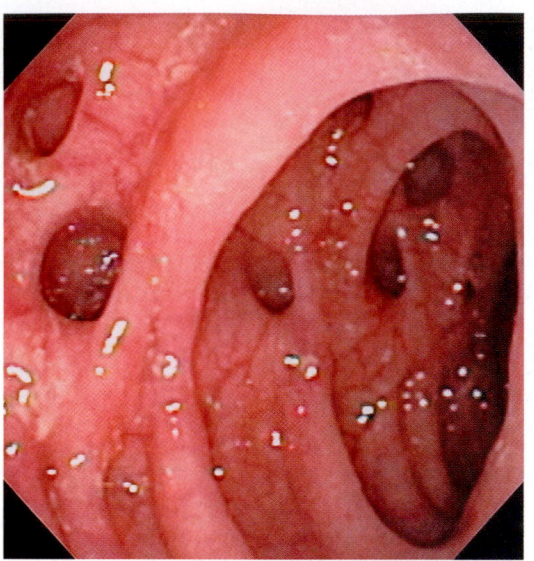

FIGURE 121-2. Colonoscopic view of sigmoid diverticulosis.

diverticular hemorrhage), accounting for approximately 283,000 admissions and $2.7 billion in costs. It was also the sixth leading GI diagnosis in the ambulatory setting, with approximately 2.7 million office visits.[7] In the United States in 2004, $100 million was spent on outpatient pharmacotherapy for diverticular disease.[22]

PATHOLOGY

Technically speaking, our almost daily use of the term *diverticula* is incorrect. True diverticula contain all layers of the bowel wall. Most diverticula in the colon are actually pseudodiverticula, consisting of herniations of the mucosa and submucosa through the muscular coat of the colon. In this chapter, the technically incorrect, but traditionally accepted, terms *diverticulum* (singular) and *diverticula* (plural) are used.

The outer longitudinal muscle fibers of the colon form 3 distinct long bands of smooth muscle known as the *taeniae coli* (also teniae coli). The 2 antimesenteric taeniae (the omental taenia and the free taenia) and the single mesenteric taenia flank the rows in which diverticula form. Diverticula do not arise randomly around the circumference of the colon. Rather, they originate in 4 distinct rows that correspond to the 4 sites of penetration of the bowel wall by the major branches of the vasa recta: on either side of the mesenteric taenia and on the mesenteric sides of the omental taenia and free taenia (Fig. 121-1). The diverticula point to the mesenteric border, and no bona fide diverticula arise from the antimesenteric intertaenial area. Diverticula maintain this fixed anatomic relationship to the taenia and are conspicuously absent from the portion of colon between the 2 antimesenteric taenia.

Diverticula can vary in number from 1 to literally hundreds (Fig. 121-2). The typical size of a diverticulum is 3 to 10 mm in diameter, but they can be much larger. Giant colonic diverticula have been defined as over 4 cm in diameter, and sizes up to 25 cm have been described. They are rare, with fewer than 200 cases described in the literature, but have been associated with complication rates approaching 30%.[23] Occasionally, a diverticulum can invert, where a diverticular dome protrudes into the lumen instead of out from it. These inversions often resemble polyps endoscopically, although they may be distinguished by their normal overlying mucosa,

broad base, surrounding circular folds, and location within a bed or row of diverticula. They are soft-appearing when probed with the endoscope tip or a biopsy forceps (pillow sign) and may be reduced by air insufflation, biopsy forceps, or water jet.[24-26] When inverted diverticula are encountered, their removal should be avoided because of a theoretically increased risk of perforation. It is notable, however, that inadvertent colonoscopic diverticulectomy has been reported, and these patients had uneventful recoveries with conservative therapy.[27]

Geography seems to be an anatomic determinant of where diverticula are found within the colon. In Western countries, a left-sided predominance has been described, with approximately 90% of patients having diverticulosis of this side of the colon.[28,29] In contrast, individuals from Asian countries tend to have a 75% to 85% right-sided predominance of diverticulosis.[17,30-32] Emerging data suggest that right-sided diverticulosis in Western countries has been previously underestimated, with some described rates between 20% and 33% of cases.[33,34] Although the precise factors causing such segmental predominance of left-colon and right-colon involvement in the West and East, respectively, are not known, environmental (e.g., dietary) and genetic factors are believed to play roles.

PATHOGENESIS

The pathogenesis of diverticulosis is multifactorial and incompletely understood. Investigation has focused on anatomic features intrinsic to the wall, alterations in the colonic wall with aging, abnormal motility, environmental factors, and heritable factors. The exact role of each of these influences and, perhaps more importantly, their inter-relation in the pathogenesis of diverticulosis is uncertain and merits continuing investigation.

Colonic Wall Structure

In colons with diverticula, both the longitudinal (taenia) and the circular muscle layers can appear markedly thickened, with shortening of the taeniae and a resultant accordion-like pleating of the folds. This appearance, called *myochosis* (Greek: *myo*, "muscle," and *chosis*, "a heaping up"), is corroborated by the colonoscopic appearance in which markedly thickened and rounded folds with luminal narrowing can be seen. Histologically, however, neither muscle hyperplasia nor hypertrophy is seen,[35] and thickening of the wall is attributed to elastin deposition within the muscle fibers.[36,37] Electron microscopic studies confirm that the colonic walls in patients with diverticulosis have structurally normal muscle cells, but compared with controls, they contain a greater than 200% increase in elastin deposition between the muscle cells in the taenia.[36] Elastin is laid down in a contracted form, resulting in shortening of the taenia and bunching of the circular muscle. An increase in type III collagen synthesis in patients with diverticulosis also has been described, raising the possibility that age-related changes in collagen composition also play an etiologic role.[36] In addition to an overall increase in the collagen content, an overexpression of a tissue inhibitor of metalloproteinases has been identified in colons with diverticula.[38,39] Because matrix metalloproteinases are believed to regulate deposition of extracellular matrix proteins, an increase in their regulatory molecule (i.e., tissue inhibitor) might explain the increase in elastin and collagen deposition found in diverticular colons. The importance of intestinal wall connective tissue also is underscored by the higher rate of diverticulosis reported in patients with connective tissue disorders, such as Ehlers-Danlos syndrome, Marfan syndrome, and scleroderma.[5]

Motility

Early investigations using colonic manometry demonstrated higher resting, postprandial, and neostigmine-stimulated luminal pressures in patients with diverticulosis compared with controls.[40,41] Based on simultaneous manometry and cineradiography, Painter proposed a theory of segmentation, postulating that contraction of the colon at haustral folds caused the colon to act not as a continuous tube, but as a series of discrete "little bladders" that led to excessively high pressures within each segment.[13,41] He further suggested that the Western diet, with its deficiency in fiber, may allow augmented hypersegmentation, thereby increasing the tendency to form diverticula. More recently, using flexible endoscopy to accurately place manometric catheters within the sigmoid colon, the previously described motility abnormalities have been confirmed.[42] Further, patients with symptomatic diverticular disease have been reported to have higher motility indices than either asymptomatic patients or normals.[43] In addition to increased contraction amplitude, retropropagation of contractile waves in diverticular segments of colon has been documented, indicating that motility in these patients may be abnormal in both magnitude and direction.[44]

The physiologic basis for the abnormal motility and elevated intraluminal pressures in the diverticular colon is not well understood. Ion transport across the epithelial membrane of diverticular colons is the same as in controls.[45] The number of myenteric and submucosal plexus neurons in diverticular colons are normal, but the number of interstitial cells of Cajal (enteric "pacemaker" cells) is reduced.[46] An increased activity of excitatory cholinergic nerves and a decreased activity of nonadrenergic, non-cholinergic inhibitory nerves have been demonstrated in diverticular colons compared with control colons.[47] The magnitude of electrically stimulated contraction in diverticulosis-affected sigmoid colon is markedly reduced by antagonists of cholinergic and tachykinin neurotransmitters.[48] In contrast, a study of the tachykinin neurotransmitter system showed a decreased contractility of circular muscle induced by substance P in diverticular colons compared with normal ones.[49] Though the exact details of the neurochemical derangements underlying diverticulosis still need to be clarified, there does appear to be an imbalance in the normal excitatory and inhibitory influences that results in the increased tonicity observed in colons with diverticulosis. The abnormal pressures and tonicity may contribute to both formation of diverticula and bowel dysfunction in patients with diverticulosis.

Environmental Factors

Environmental factors are thought to influence the presence of diverticulosis and/or its complications.[49a] A growing number of influences not previously appreciated now include: diets low in fiber and high in red meat,[12,50-55] obesity,[56-58] smoking,[17,58-61] physical inactivity,[62-64] alcohol,[17,61,65,66] and NSAIDs.[67,68] A recent series of 347 patients hospitalized with acute diverticulitis demonstrated that surgery for diverticulitis after at least 1 medically managed hospital admission for diverticulitis was more frequent in African Americans and less frequent in Hispanics. Caucasians were less likely than other races/ethnicities to suffer a recurrence of diverticulitis.[69]

These are summarized in Box 121-1. Of these, fiber has long held a special position. Specifically, greatest consideration has been given to the theory that low dietary fiber is central to the pathogenesis of diverticulosis. Burkitt and Painter were early proponents of this theory, labeling diverticulosis a "deficiency disease" of fiber.[12] They subsequently described markedly slower transit times and decreased stool weights in persons from the United Kingdom (with "low-fiber" diets) compared with those of a rural Ugandan (with "high-fiber" diets).[51] They asserted that longer intestinal transit times and smaller-volume stools seen in "low-fiber" diets resulted in increased intraluminal pressure, thus predisposing to diverticular herniation; bulkier stools, in contrast, were associated with less colonic contraction and lower wall pressures.

While low dietary fiber has been epidemiologically associated with increased risk of diverticulosis,[70-72] other data to substantiate this relationship has been both limited and conflicting, thus calling into question this classic dogma.[73] Thus, in the United States, fiber intake decreased by 28% from 1909 to 1975,[71] a period of dramatic increase in the prevalence of

---

BOX 121-1 Factors Associated with Diverticulosis or Its Complications

Increased Risk*
Alcohol
Aspirin and other NSAIDs
Diets high in red meat
Genetics
Increasing age
Low Dietary fiber intake
Obesity
Physical inactivity
Residence in Western countries (e.g., United States, Western Europe, Australia)
Smoking

Decreased Risk*
Dietary fiber intake
Residence in predominantly rural Asian or African countries (e.g., Kenya, Jordan, Thailand)

Equivocal or Normal Risk
Colorectal cancer
Gender

*African-American race may increase the risk and Hispanic or Caucasian risk may decrease the risk of diverticulosis or its complications.

diverticular disease. In a British study, a group of vegetarians on a high-fiber diet had a lower prevalence of diverticulosis than did non-vegetarians (12% vs. 33%).[70] Finally, dietary influences for diverticulosis may have different effects on the right and left sides of the colon. Right-sided diverticular disease was shown in an Asian study to have no association with intake of fruits and vegetables or supplemental fiber, but to be strongly associated with meat consumption.[54] Whether these associations apply to Westerners with right-sided diverticulosis is not known. A study by Peery and colleagues directly challenged the long-standing belief that fiber is protective against diverticulosis, concluding that a high-fiber diet is associated with a greater, not lower, prevalence of asymptomatic diverticulosis[74]; only recent dietary history was evaluated, suggesting that recall bias may be confounding. Nonetheless, fiber is still considered a mainstay of treatment for diverticulosis and its complications and is addressed later in this chapter.

Heritable Factors

The role of heritable risk factors is still being defined. There is no conclusive evidence that diverticular disease is associated with colorectal cancer.[75] Diverticulosis appears to be just as common in men and women,[76] although men may have a higher incidence of diverticular bleeding, and women may have more episodes of diverticulitis.[8,77] Genetic influence in diverticular disease is an area needing investigation. One notable study by Strate and coworkers, using the Danish National Registry, found that diverticulosis and its complications aggregate strongly in families. Specifically, siblings of index cases were 3 times more likely to develop diverticular disease than the general population.[78] Another recent investigation, utilizing the Swedish Twin and Inpatient Registries, reported an odds ratio of 7.15 for developing diverticular disease if a monozygotic twin was affected, and estimated the hereditable component of diverticular disease as approximately 40%.[79] Findings such as these challenge the existing paradigm of our environment's central influence on this condition.

CLINICAL PRESENTATIONS

Approximately 80% of patients with diverticulosis remain asymptomatic throughout their lifetimes. When diverticulosis does manifest, however, it typically presents in 1 of 3 distinct patterns: symptomatic uncomplicated diverticular disease (SUDD), diverticulitis, or diverticular bleeding. A newer, poorly understood, and increasingly diagnosed entity called *segmental colitis associated with diverticular disease (SCAD)* has also been described. The clinical presentations associated with diverticulosis are described below and outlined in Figure 121-3.

Asymptomatic Diverticulosis

Asymptomatic diverticulosis is usually an incidental finding in patients undergoing evaluation for other indications, such as occult blood loss or colon cancer screening. With increasing use of both colonoscopy and CT, it is likely that more such asymptomatic patients will be found. As previously noted, diverticulosis is the most common abnormality on colonoscopy.[6]

There is no clear indication for any specific therapy or special follow-up for the patients with asymptomatic diverticulosis, and whether the mere presence of diverticulosis in an aging population is even a disease or just a

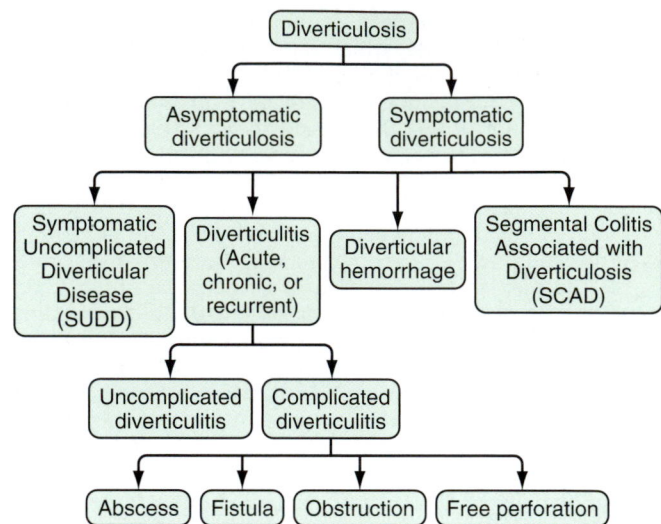

FIGURE 121-3. Overview of diverticulosis and its clinical presentations.

senescence-associated physiologic variant can be debated. With regard to dietary recommendations, a possible prophylactic benefit of a high-fiber diet has been suggested in 2 publications comprising 47,888 male health professionals who were followed over 4 years and in whom only 385 (0.75%) new cases of symptomatic diverticular disease were identified.[50,52] A dietary review found an inverse association between dietary fiber intake and the risk of subsequently developing clinically evident diverticular disease. Although these studies are provocative, there is a notable lack of supporting prospective randomized trials. As such, one can assert that there are no definitive data to support a recommendation for increased fiber intake in patients with asymptomatic diverticulosis for the sole purpose of preventing symptoms. That said, increased fiber intake might be considered as part of a sensible lifestyle change that might offer other salutary health benefits.

The long-held "old wives' tale" that patients with diverticulosis avoid nuts and seeds also has been challenged. Strate's group reported on nearly 47,000 men (from the aforementioned study) without known diverticular disease for a nearly 2-decade period. They reported that consumption of nuts, corn, popcorn or seeded fruit (strawberries or blueberries) did not increase the risk of diverticulosis or its complications. Further, men who consumed nuts or popcorn at least 2 times a week were at lower risk for diverticular complications.[80] Although there probably is not enough evidence to warrant actively encouraging patients with diverticulosis to eat large quantities of nuts, popcorn, or seeds, neither should these foods be categorically avoided.

Symptomatic Uncomplicated Diverticular Disease (SUDD)

Some patients come to clinical attention because of nonspecific abdominal complaints and are found to have diverticulosis. If the clinical features are thought to arise from a diverticular source and there is no evidence of complications of diverticular disease (i.e., diverticulitis and its complications, diverticular bleeding), the disease may be defined as symptomatic uncomplicated diverticular disease, or SUDD.

The true prevalence of SUDD is unknown, in large part the result of a body of natural history literature that has primarily focused on diverticulitis and diverticular hemorrhage. Further, clinical similarities between SUDD and IBS confound our ability to epidemiologically distinguish the 2. Like IBS, however, it is commonly held that SUDD typically runs a long-term, benign course. SUDD is also associated with a very low incidence of complications. Salem and colleagues reported in a prospective study of SUDD patients that 97% had few or no symptoms at median follow-up of 66 months: 1.7% had had episodes of acute diverticulitis, and 0.8% had required surgery.[81]

Pathophysiology

The pathophysiology of SUDD is not well defined. Some authorities have postulated that diverticula are, in fact, a late consequence of IBS. In a Danish cohort of IBS patients, one third of whom had diverticula, no difference in symptoms or prognosis was detected between those with diverticula and those without diverticula over more than 5 years of follow-up.[82] This finding led the investigators to assert that there is no basis to consider SUDD as a separate entity from IBS. Further highlighting this consideration, Ritchie reported that there was a similarity of pain sensation from rectal balloon distention in patients with IBS and those with diverticulosis.[83]

There are growing data to suggest an epidemiologic overlap between SUDD and IBS,[84] which points to an important direction of study. This suggested relationship also brings forth consideration of a shared pathophysiology and challenges us to evolve our understanding of diverticular disease.[85] As in the IBS literature, multiple factors are postulated to play contributing roles: visceral hypersensitivity, altered colonic motility, low-grade chronic inflammation, and most recently, an altered intestinal microbiota. The role of each of these is reviewed elsewhere,[85] but this insight into pathophysiologic mechanisms provides potential targets for therapy.

Clinical Features

A causal relationship between diverticulosis and abdominal symptoms often is difficult to establish. The presenting symptoms of SUDD overlap considerably with those of IBS. Most patients with SUDD present with left lower quadrant (LLQ) abdominal pain. The pain often is exacerbated by eating and is diminished by defecation or the passage of flatus. The British refer to this as *painful diverticular disease*, and there is the suggestion that such discomfort may be related to associated myochosis (see earlier). Patients may also report other symptoms of colonic dysfunction, including bloating, constipation, diarrhea, or the passage of mucus per rectum. Physical examination is typically normal, but abdominal fullness and mild tenderness in the LLQ can be seen. Frank rebound or guarding is absent.

Diagnosis

Although barium enema (or, increasingly, CT colography) may remain useful in certain cases (i.e., when colonoscopy cannot be performed safely or completely), endoscopic evaluation (see Fig. 121-2) has assumed a primary role in the evaluation of most patients, particularly to exclude neoplasia. It was once believed that performing colonoscopy in patients with diverticulosis was unsafe because of an increased risk of perforation; however, 1 manometric study showed that burst pressures for diverticula far exceed the usual pressures encountered during routine sigmoidoscopy or colonoscopy, even with the endoscope pressing against the wall or with heavy air insufflations.[86] These data and many years of clinical experience have demonstrated the relative safety of using colonoscopy to evaluate patients with diverticulosis who have a variety of abdominal symptoms.

The diverticula-laden colon can be challenging for the endoscopist to navigate because of spasm, luminal narrowing, fixation from prior inflammation and fibrosis, or confusion between luminal and diverticular openings. A number of solutions have been proposed to alleviate this problem. The use of a smaller-diameter pediatric colonoscope can be useful for difficult colons. One group has reported a success rate of more than 90% with a pediatric colonoscope when an adult colonoscope could not be passed through the sigmoid; 44% of these patients had diverticulosis.[87] A technique involving distention of the lumen with 100 to 300 mL of water, called the *sigmoid floatation maneuver*, was said to have facilitated colonoscopy in 6 technically difficult cases of severe diverticular disease.[88] A recent systematic review suggests that water-assisted colonoscopy may decrease discomfort and increase polyp detection.[89] In all patients with dense diverticulosis, air insufflation should be minimized and excessive force in advancing the colonoscope should be avoided.

In patients with SUDD, general laboratory diagnostic evaluation should be normal. There are, however, data to suggest a potential role for certain biomarkers in diverticular disease.[90] Specifically, in 1 small case-control study, fecal calprotectin was shown to be higher in patients with SUDD compared with normal controls and patients with IBS.[91] This intriguing finding offers 1 area of potential investigation for the diagnosis of SUDD. Because rates of occult bleeding in diverticulosis are similar to those in healthy controls, a positive fecal occult blood test *never* should be attributed to diverticulosis.[92]

Treatment

The suggestion of shared pathophysiologic paradigms for SUDD and IBS provides the basis for treatment options. Whether these 2 disorders are distinct entities is unknown and probably not clinically important, because both are treated in a similar nonspecific fashion with equally good prognoses.

For decades, fiber has been a mainstay of treatment for SUDD. It is important to note, however, that this practice is based on weak evidence that is old, largely observational, uncontrolled, and limited by high placebo response rates.[93-95] The limited double-blind randomized controlled data that do exist also have limitations that challenge their role as definitive substantiation for use of fiber: limited study size (18 to 30 patients),[96,97] significant time until benefit of fiber (3 months),[96] and no significant difference in pain scores or general symptom scores.[98] Further, the literature provides little guidance as to the type and quantity of fiber needed. It is notable that bran fiber can increase flatulence and actually worsen symptoms in some patients. Data from the IBS literature suggest that soluble fiber (psyllium) is superior to insoluble fiber (bran) in improving symptoms.[99] In sum, it is important to be aware of the lack of significantly convincing data when considering the use of fiber in these patients. The treatment of diverticular disease, in general, relies mainly on data from uncontrolled studies.[99a]

5-Aminosalicylic Acid (5-ASA)

Additional medical therapies for SUDD have been studied for more than a decade, drawing on approaches that are effective in other colonic diseases such as IBD and IBS. 5-ASA compounds, a well-established and first-line therapy for UC and Crohn's disease, have been evaluated as a potential treatment for SUDD. Although patients with SUDD by definition lack severe or overt inflammation, in some patients, subtle inflammation is suspected even without gross signs of diverticulitis; it is these patients whom the anti-inflammatory properties of 5-ASA might benefit. For example, in 1 case series of over 900 Mayo Clinic patients undergoing surgery for SUDD,

76% of cases had evidence of acute or chronic inflammatory changes.[100] Additionally, patients with SUDD, compared to controls, have been demonstrated to have increased expression of inflammatory modulators including TNF,[91,101] galanin and tachykinins,[101,102] and fecal calprotectin.[91] Prior uncontrolled studies that have examined the role of 5-ASA randomized patients to either daily or cycled (e.g., 10 days per month) 5-ASA and showed a significantly reduced symptom score relative to pretreatment scores; the lack of a control arm and the known high placebo-response rates in functional bowel syndromes make the results difficult to interpret. More recent controlled data are emerging, although not yet conclusive. The DIVA study, a randomized trial comparing 12 weeks of mesalamine 2.4 g/day with placebo after CT-confirmation of acute diverticulitis, demonstrated a consistent trend towards decreased SUDD symptoms, but was underpowered to detect differences in recurrent diverticulitis.[103] Another randomized trial compared 3 g of mesalamine daily with placebo; it did not meet its primary endpoint, likely in part to underpowering, but it too showed a consistent trend towards decreased symptoms.[104] These results, combined with the relative safety of this medication class, make 5-ASAs a promising therapy for SUDD, although further high-quality placebo-controlled trials supporting its efficacy will be needed before widespread use can be recommended.

Antibiotics and Probiotics

The role of pathogenic and nonpathogenic bacteria in intestinal disease is being increasingly scrutinized. Some have postulated that disturbances in the intestinal microbiota might predispose to inflammation.[105] Using this rationale, rifaximin, a nonabsorbable antibiotic with broad-spectrum activity, has been studied in SUDD with optimistic results, including reduction in frequency and severity of symptoms.[106,107] In a meta-analysis of 4 randomized controlled trials studying patients with SUDD, the combination of rifaximin with fiber was 29% more effective than placebo in obtaining symptom relief at 1 year. The number needed to treat (NNT) for this benefit was 3.[108] These are compelling data that will drive further studies considering rifaximin as a potential therapy for SUDD.

Based on the assumption that diverticular disease may reflect, at least in part, a dysbiosis, probiotics are also being increasingly studied in SUDD,[109-112] although specific data on microbiome alterations in diverticular disease are still unavailable. Some benefit has been shown in trials involving bacterial strains such as *Escherichia coli*, *Lactobacillus casei*, *Bifidobacterium infantis*, and combination products such as VSL#3, but such trials are generally small and lack a placebo group. Although higher-quality evidence needs to be produced to support this approach, the microbiota may become an important target for therapy in SUDD in coming years.

Anticholinergics and Antispasmodics

Hypermotility of the colon in diverticulosis suggests that anticholinergic or antispasmodic medications such as dicyclomine or hyoscyamine might improve symptoms by diminishing muscular contraction. Nonetheless, there are no adequately controlled therapeutic trials documenting such a benefit. IV glucagon has been reported to offer short-term relief of pain, presumably as a result of smooth muscle relaxation. There is no rationale for the use of narcotic analgesics in uncomplicated diverticular disease.

Role of Surgery

Surgical intervention generally is not considered for patients with uncomplicated diverticulosis, because the risks of surgery outweigh its benefits in most cases. Some patients with subclinical or smoldering diverticulitis present with pain characteristic of diverticulitis but show no signs of systemic inflammation, such as fever or leukocytosis. In the previously mentioned cohort of over 900 Mayo Clinic SUDD patients who underwent sigmoid resection with primary anastomosis for their symptoms, 76.5% had complete resolution of their symptoms, with 88% of patients being pain free after 1 or more years of follow-up.[113] This finding underscores the importance of clinical follow-up and an open mind regarding patients with apparently uncomplicated disease whose symptoms do not improve with conservative treatment.

Diverticulitis

Diverticulitis is defined as inflammation and/or infection of a diverticulum. Clinically, it presents as either an acute or chronic process; the absence or presence of subsequent complications helps us to define diverticulitis as either uncomplicated diverticulitis or complicated diverticulitis. *Complicated diverticulitis* refers to cases associated with abscesses, fistula, obstruction, or free perforation.

Diverticulitis is the most common complication of diverticulosis, occurring in approximately 10% to 25% of patients[28] and seems to be increasing. Etzioni's group analyzed The Nationwide Inpatient Sample (NIS), which is the largest all-payer inpatient care database in the United States, and found a 26% increase in hospitalizations for acute diverticulitis and a 38% increase in elective operations between 1998 and 2005.[9] Interestingly, subgroup analysis showed that younger patients (aged 18 to 44) were much more likely than older patients (aged 45 to 74) to be hospitalized for diverticulitis. These dynamic trends will certainly prompt continued investigation into our evolving understanding of the epidemiology and treatment of this disease.

Pathophysiology

The process by which a diverticulum becomes inflamed has been likened to that causing appendicitis, in which the diverticular sac becomes obstructed by inspissated stool in its neck; the fecalith abrades the mucosa of the sac, causing low-grade inflammation and further blocking drainage. Histologically, one of the earliest signs of inflammation is hyperplasia of the mucosal lymphoid tissue, with lymphoid tissue aggregation at the apex of the involved sac The obstructed diverticulum predisposes to an increase of the normal bacterial flora, diminished venous outflow with localized ischemia, and altered mucosal defense mechanisms. One such alteration is a defective CD2 pathway–induced apoptosis, which has been found in lamina propria lymphocytes in patients with diverticulitis, possibly leading to an up-regulation of the local immune response in these patients similar to that seen in patients with IBD.[114] Recent evidence also suggests that cytomegalovirus (CMV) reactivation may contribute to local inflammatory activity, because active CMV replication was found in tissue from the affected bowel segments of over two thirds of patients with diverticulitis.[115] The cascade of events initiated by fecalith obstruction, and possibly enhanced by underlying innate or acquired abnormalities, allows bacteria to breach the mucosa and extend the process transmurally, ultimately leading to perforation.[116] The extent and localization of the perforation determine its clinical behavior. Microperforations may remain very well localized, contained by the pericolic fat and mesentery, and cause small pericolic abscesses. A larger perforation can allow a more extensive abscess to form, which may track longitudinally around the bowel wall. This process can lead to a large inflammatory mass, fibrosis, extension to other organs, or fistula formation. Free perforation into the

TABLE 121-1 Hinchey Classification of Colonic Diverticular Perforation

Stage	Definition
I	Confined pericolic abscess
II	Distant abscess (retroperitoneal or pelvic)
III	Generalized peritonitis caused by rupture of a pericolic or pelvic abscess (not communicating with the colonic lumen because of inflammatory obliteration of the diverticular neck)
IV	Fecal peritonitis caused by free perforation of a diverticulum (communicating with the colonic lumen)

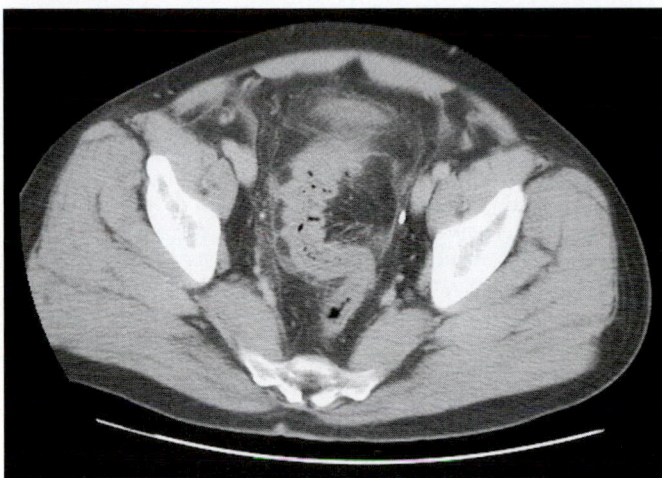

FIGURE 121-4. CT of a patient with acute uncomplicated diverticulitis showing colon wall thickening and stranding of the pericolic fat.

peritoneum with resultant frank bacterial or fecal peritonitis can be life threatening, but fortunately is uncommon, with a population incidence of 4 cases per 100,000 population per year.[8,117] Hinchey and colleagues have described a staged grading system that reflects the severity of perforation (Table 121-1) and which is useful to stratify patient management.[118]

Uncomplicated Diverticulitis

Uncomplicated diverticulitis is characterized by the presence of localized colonic inflammation with or without small abscess formation that is confined to the colonic wall.[94] It is the most common manifestation of diverticulitis, and occurs in approximately 80% patients admitted with a first attack.[119]

Clinical Features

Patients with uncomplicated diverticulitis typically present with LLQ abdominal pain, reflecting the propensity for this disorder to occur in the sigmoid colon in Western countries; a redundant sigmoid colon, however, may manifest with suprapubic or right-sided pain. In contrast, Asian patients with diverticulitis have predominantly right-sided symptoms, corresponding to the more typical location of their diverticula.[120] The pain may be intermittent or constant and frequently is associated with a change in bowel habits, either diarrhea or constipation. Anorexia, nausea, and vomiting also can occur. Dysuria and urinary frequency can result from bladder irritation caused by the adjacent inflamed sigmoid colon, a condition often referred to as a "sympathetic cystitis." The risk of recurrent symptoms following an attack of acute diverticulitis has been reported to range from 7% to 45%,[28,71] with half of second attacks occurring within 1 year.

Physical examination usually discloses localized tenderness, generally in the LLQ; however, as noted, right-sided signs do not preclude the possibility of diverticulitis. Guarding and rebound tenderness may be present, as may a tender, cylindrical, palpable mass. Bowel sounds typically are depressed but may be normal in mild cases or increased in the presence of obstruction. Rectal examination can disclose tenderness or a mass, particularly with a low-lying pelvic abscess. Fever is present in most patients, whereas hypotension and shock are unusual.

The differential diagnosis for diverticulitis is extensive. Acute appendicitis is the misdiagnosis most often made in patients with diverticulitis, particularly with right-sided disease. In Hong Kong, where awareness of the predominance of right-sided diverticulosis presumably is high, 34 of 35 patients with right-sided diverticulitis initially were believed to have acute appendicitis.[120] Other common diagnoses that need to be considered include IBD, other forms of colitis (infectious or ischemic), colorectal cancer, and gynecologic conditions such as pelvic inflammatory disease, ovarian cyst rupture, and ovarian torsion.

Diagnosis

It is held that a diagnosis of diverticulitis can often be made on the basis of history and physical examination alone.[121] The constellation of LLQ pain, fever, and leukocytosis are common and nonspecific, and 1 study has reported a normal WBC count with no left shift in 46% of patients.[122] Despite a "classic presentation," clinical diagnosis can be inaccurate, with misdiagnosis rates as high as 34% to 68%.[123] A number of investigators have, therefore, worked to develop diagnostic decision systems for diverticulitis and have identified a possible emerging role for biomarkers in diagnosis.[90] Specifically, C-reactive protein (CRP) in excess of 50 mg/L has been used as a key indicator in 2 separate studies. In 1 study, accurate diagnosis was made in 24% of patients who had 3 features: LLQ tenderness, absence of vomiting, and an elevated CRP (>50 mg/L).[124] In the other study,[123] 7 features (age, number of episodes, LLQ symptom localization, pain on movement, absence of vomiting, LLQ tenderness, and elevated CRP > 50 mg/L) were found to be independent predictors of acute left-sided diverticulitis. A nomogram constructed from these predictors gave a diagnostic accuracy of 86%.

In the setting of clinical uncertainty, radiologic evaluation can play a pivotal role in aiding diagnosis, identifying complications, guiding management, and even offering therapy. **CT.** CT scanning of the abdomen and pelvis has become the radiologic test of choice in patients with suspected diverticulitis (Fig. 121-4). Ideally, it is performed with water-soluble contrast, given both orally and rectally, and with IV contrast when it is not contraindicated. The main advantages of CT include its general availability, high test performance profile, and ability to identify complications. Sensitivity, specificity, and positive and negative predictive values have all been described at values greater than 97%.[125] Representative findings include bowel wall thickening, stranding of pericolic fat, pericolic fluid, and small abscesses confined to the colonic wall as well as extravasated contrast (i.e., intramural sinus tracts and fistula formation).

Other Imaging Studies. Plain films should be considered in the evaluation of any patient who presents with acute abdominal pain to exclude perforation or obstruction; however, because of limited sensitivity and specificity, they have little role in the diagnosis of diverticulitis.

Contrast barium enema once was the diagnostic standard for diverticulitis, but it has been supplanted by CT. Contrast enema has been shown to have a sensitivity of 62% to 94% for detecting acute diverticulitis, with false-negative results in 2% to 15%.[126,127] It can be considered in cases where CT is not feasible. In cases of suspected diverticulitis, only water-soluble contrast enemas should be used, because the use of barium in the setting of perforation carries the risk of barium peritonitis.

US has been advocated as a potentially useful diagnostic modality in diverticulitis, with relatively low cost, great convenience, and no risk of ionizing radiation. US has a reported sensitivity of 84% to 98% and a specificity of 80% to 93% for diverticulitis.[128,129] One meta-analysis has shown that graded compression US and CT are similarly accurate in the diagnosis of acute diverticulitis,[130] and another has shown that CT and US have similar positive predictive values for this diagnosis.[131] Despite these encouraging data, US for this purpose remains highly operator dependent, and CT provides greater accuracy for alternative diagnoses.[130] As such, US has not surpassed CT as the modality of choice in most medical centers.

MRI may have an emerging role in the diagnosis of acute diverticulitis; however, there is limited literature to demonstrating its utility in this regard. In 1 small study of 15 patients with acute diverticulitis, MRI was reported to have a sensitivity and specificity of 100%.[132] Concerns of limited resolution secondary to motion artifact in such patients may be overcome by technological advances in MRI scanners. MRI has significant potential as a radiation-free imaging test for the diagnosis of acute diverticulitis.

Endoscopy. Endoscopy generally should be avoided in patients with suspected acute diverticulitis because of the risk of perforation. In unclear cases, however, a limited sigmoidoscopy (with minimal air insufflation) may be considered to exclude alternative diagnoses, such as IBD, carcinoma, or ischemic colitis. Because CT findings in acute diverticulitis can mimic those of colon cancer, the American Society of Colon and Rectal Surgeons (ASCRS) and the ACG recommend that patients have a colonoscopy to exclude colorectal cancer 1 to 3 months after an acute episode of presumptive diverticulitis.[94,121] These recommendations, however, are based on limited data. To examine the possible relation of diverticulitis to colon cancer, Sai and coworkers performed a systematic review of studies in which patients with acute diverticulitis underwent surgery, colonoscopy, or barium enema within 24 weeks of presentation.[133] They found that the pooled prevalence of colorectal cancer in these patients was only "slightly higher" than the calculated prevalence in a population of similar age (2.1% vs. 0.68%). These data bring to question the clinical utility and cost-effectiveness of the current recommendations. More such studies are needed to validate or refute this widely recommended practice.

Treatment

An important initial consideration in the management of a patient with diverticulitis is the decision to initiate treatment as an outpatient or an inpatient. The ASCRS suggests that inability to tolerate oral intake, peritonitis, excessive vomiting, fever, or failure to improve with outpatient therapy should prompt one to consider hospitalization.[121] Absence of these features in combination with establishment of appropriate follow-up should allow consideration for outpatient management.

Outpatient management of diverticulitis has success rates described in the 94% to 97% range.[134] Aside from bowel rest and liquid intake, standard recommendations and practice have included oral antibiotic therapy directed at colonic bacteria, especially Gram-negative rods and anaerobic bacteria.[121] Prior studies have found that either single-drug or multiple-drug regimens are equally effective as long as both groups of organisms are covered.[135] No antibiotic regimen has been shown to have definitive superiority over the other.[136] Commonly used regimens in the United States include a quinolone or sulfa agent in combination with metronidazole (or clindamycin, if patient is intolerant of metronidazole), or amoxicillin-clavulanate as a single agent, typically for approximately 10 days. Interestingly, this standard antibiotic practice has previously been questioned,[137,138] and more recently, a multicenter randomized trial of 632 patients with acute, uncomplicated diverticulitis randomized to treatment with antibiotics or no antibiotics was reported. In this study by Chabok's group,[139] no clinical difference was found between the 2 groups in hospital stay (3 days in both arms) and recurrent diverticulitis, which occurred in 16% of patients in each arm. There was a non-significant difference in complications such as perforation or obstruction (1.0% vs. 1.9%). Relief of pain was not reported, and patients were without complications on entry, suggesting that close observation without antibiotics might be appropriate for selected patients with uncomplicated diverticulitis; this thought-provoking finding will require confirmation.

Inpatient treatment follows the basic principles of outpatient therapy, except that IV antibiotics and fluids should be used, and surgical consultation is more often relied upon. Symptomatic improvement with decreasing fever and leukocytosis should be observed within 2 to 4 days, at which point diet may be advanced. If improvement continues, patients may be discharged, but they should complete a 7- to 10-day course of oral antibiotics. Failure to improve with conservative medical therapy warrants a diligent search for complications, consideration of alternative diagnoses, and repeat surgical consultation. Etzioni and coworkers published a retrospective cohort study of 639 patients admitted for a first episode of diverticulitis and found that 57.6% of patients required only "minimal hospitalization," defined as a hospital stay 3 or fewer days, had no procedure performed, and had no readmission for diverticulitis within 30 days.[9] This interesting study questions whether more patients are suitable for outpatient management than our present practice patterns show.

Most patients hospitalized with acute diverticulitis respond to conservative medical therapy, have short stays, and will not require surgery. It has been estimated that only 15% to 30% of patients hospitalized with acute diverticulitis require surgery during their admission.[28,71,126] The parameters guiding the decision for surgical management of uncomplicated diverticulitis have evolved. In 2000, the ASCRS recommended consideration of surgery after 2 episodes of uncomplicated diverticulitis or 1 episode of complicated diverticulitis.[140] Subsequently, studies such as the 13-year experience of the Mayo Clinic reported that there is no significant difference in morbidity and mortality between those with multiple episodes of diverticulitis and with those who have had only 1 or 2 episodes.[141] A more recent decision analysis predicted that performing colectomy after the fourth attack of diverticulitis rather than after the second attack would result in fewer deaths and colostomies while having a superior cost-effectiveness.[142] Recognizing this trend, the updated guidelines from the ASCRS are now advocating evaluation on a case-by-case basis rather than empirically performing elective surgery after the second attack.[121]

Since the 1980s, a 2-staged surgical approach (colonic resection plus colostomy, followed by colostomy takedown) has been the standard[9]; however, there is ongoing dialogue within the surgical community as to whether a shift towards primary anastomosis might be more beneficial.[9,143] Using The Nationwide Inpatient Sample data from 1998-2005, Etzioni's group reported that there is no evidence that primary anastomosis is becoming more commonly used.[9] If the choice to operate is made, most patients will have a good functional outcome and low rates of recurrent disease after elective resection for diverticulitis.[144] It should be noted that despite the general intent for subsequent colostomy reversal, this only occurs approximately 50% of the time, and even less in older adults, which is likely a result of increased morbidity in this population.[145]

Complicated Diverticulitis

Approximately 15% to 20% of all patients with diverticulitis will develop significant complications.[146] Complicated diverticulitis is characterized by the presence of abscess, fistula, obstruction, or free perforation.

Abscess

Approximately 15% of patients with acute diverticulitis will develop pericolic or intramesenteric abscess.[147,148] When perforation of a colonic diverticulum occurs, the ability of the pericolic tissues to control the spread of the inflammatory process determines the subsequent clinical course of disease and its treatment. A localized phlegmon initially develops with limited spread. Further spread can lead to the formation of larger local (Hinchey stage I) or distant abscesses (Hinchey stage II). Generalized peritonitis from abscess rupture (Hinchey stage III) and fecal peritonitis from free perforation (Hinchey stage IV) also may occur and lead to sepsis and death if the patient does not undergo urgent surgical intervention (see Table 121-1). Clinical signs that suggest abscess formation include a tender abdomen, a tender mass on physical examination, persistent fever, and persistent leukocytosis despite an adequate trial of appropriate IV antibiotics. Once an abscess is suspected, radiologic evaluation with a CT scan is the best modality for confirming the diagnosis and following its course over time (Fig. 121-5).

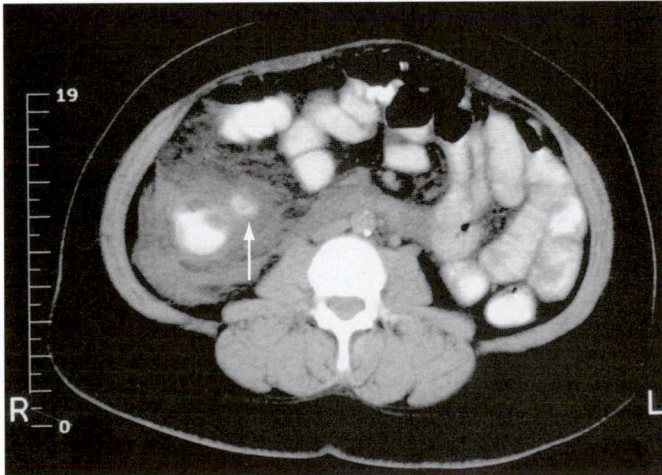

FIGURE 121-5. CT of a patient with a right lower quadrant abscess (*arrow*). The differential diagnosis of this finding includes right-sided colonic diverticulitis and appendicitis.

Small pericolic abscesses (Hinchey stage I) often can be treated conservatively with broad-spectrum antibiotics and bowel rest.[140] Abscesses less than 2 to 3 cm in diameter may resolve with antibiotics alone,[121,149] and continued noninvasive management of abscesses can be cautiously considered in stable patients who demonstrate unequivocal improvement in pain, fever, tenderness, and leukocytosis over the first few days of therapy.

CT-guided percutaneous drainage of abdominal abscesses has assumed a prominent complementary role to surgery (Fig. 121-6). The immediate advantage of percutaneous catheter drainage is rapid control of sepsis and patient stabilization without the need for general anesthesia. It often eliminates the need for a multiple-stage surgical procedure with colostomy,[150] instead allowing temporary palliative drainage and subsequent single-stage resection in 3 to 4 weeks. Success rates of CT-guided drainage for stabilizing patients and safely allowing subsequent single-stage procedures range from 74% to 80%.[151,152] An urgent surgical procedure is required in the 20% to 25% of patients in whom the abscess is multiloculated, anatomically inaccessible, or not resolving with percutaneous drainage. Elective resection generally is recommended if an episode of complicated diverticulitis is treated nonoperatively.[121]

As noted previously, both 2-stage surgery and primary anastomosis are the current surgical approaches. Regardless of approach, however, surgery for complicated diverticulitis has evolved into a relatively safe procedure with 1 of the highest success rates of any of the common GI surgical procedures.[153] Laparoscopic techniques represent a new frontier in the surgical approach to diverticular disease. A systematic review by Gaertner and colleagues reported that elective laparoscopic colectomy is associated with decreased hospital stay and fewer costs compared to open colectomy,[154] and others have reported laparoscopic approaches as the standard of care for all cases of diverticular disease.[155]

Fistula

When a diverticular phlegmon or abscess extends or ruptures into an adjacent organ, a fistula results. Fistulas are believed to develop in fewer than 5% of patients with diverticulitis but are present in about 20% of those who require surgery for diverticulitis.[156]

Presumably secondary to the left-sided predominance of diverticular disease and the adjacency of the bladder, colovesicular fistulae are the most common type of fistula to complicate diverticulitis. In a Cleveland Clinic review of 26 years' experience with diverticulitis-associated fistulae, 65% were colovesicular.[157] Women were half as likely as men to have colovesicular fistulae, ostensibly because the bladder is protected by the uterus. Cystoscopy, cystography, and barium enema can be useful to diagnose the fistula, although its actual demonstration often is difficult. In 1 series, pneumaturia was present in 57% and fecaluria in 42%.[158] Fecaluria is pathognomonic for colovesicular fistula. Surgical management is indicated, and single-stage operative resection with fistula closure and primary anastomosis was the procedure performed in 75% of patients in 1 case series,[157] with a less than 4% mortality.

Colovaginal fistulas are the next most common, representing approximately 25% of all cases.[157] The passage of stool or flatus per vagina is pathognomonic. Frequent vaginal infections or copious or feculent vaginal discharge should prompt consideration of this complication. Many patients who develop a colovaginal fistula have undergone a previous hysterectomy. Treatment is surgical resection of the diseased segment of colon with repair of the contiguous organ, which generally

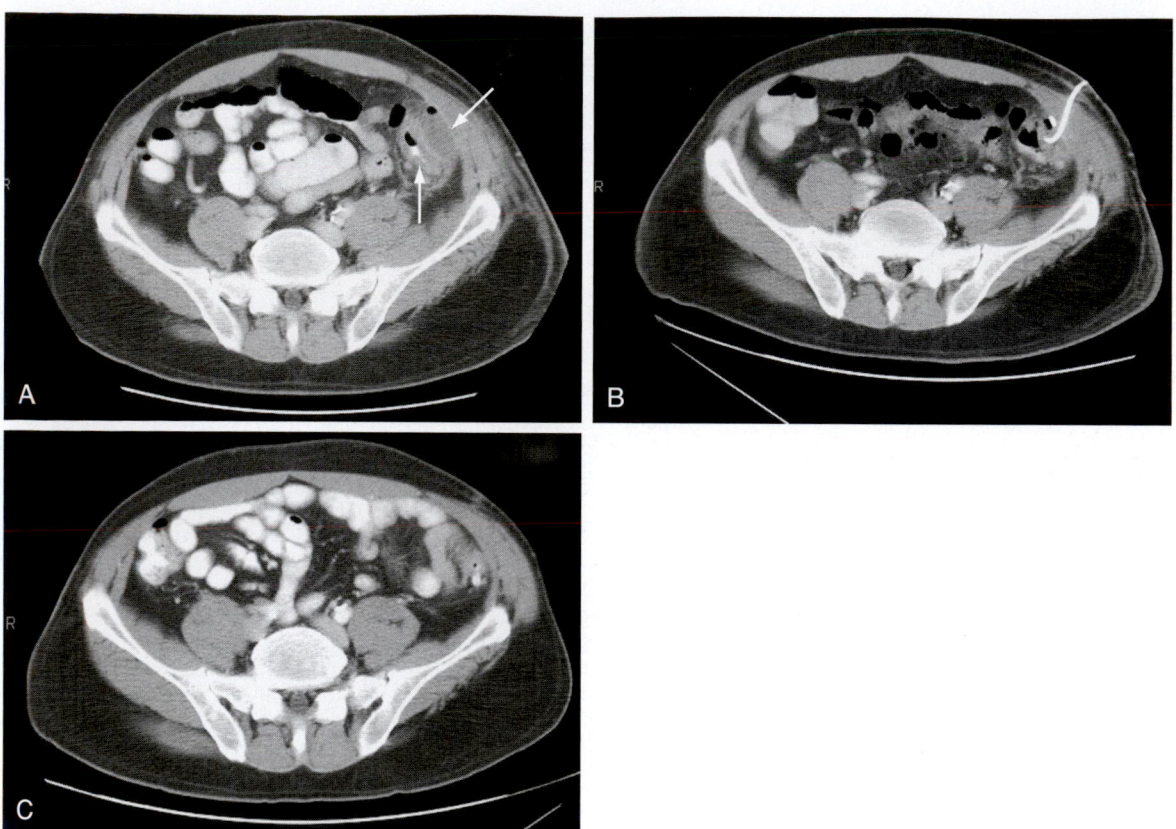

FIGURE 121-6. CT-guided percutaneous drainage of an abdominal abscess complicating acute diverticulitis. *A, Arrows* point to the abscess arising from the sigmoid colon. *B,* A drainage catheter has been inserted into the abscess. The patient also was treated with IV antibiotics. *C,* The catheter has been removed, and the abscess has resolved.

can be performed as a single-stage procedure.[140] A recent series of primary repair of both colovesicular and colovaginal fistula repairs reported an 8% mortality rate.[159]

Other fistulae, including coloenteric, colouterine, colo-ureteral, and colocutaneous, occur much less commonly. Although diverticular disease is a common cause of fistulae from the colon to adjacent organs, other conditions, including IBD, pancreatitis, radiation enteritis and colitis, infectious colitis, and malignancy, also can cause fistulas, and these diagnoses must be considered when a fistula involving the colon is discovered.

Obstruction

Obstruction can complicate diverticular disease either acutely or chronically. During an attack of acute diverticulitis, partial colonic obstruction can occur because of luminal narrowing from the pericolic inflammation, compression from abscess formation, or both. A CT scan with oral and rectal contrast can give useful information about diverticular obstruction while also assessing for extraluminal disease. Complete obstruction is unusual. Colonic ileus or pseudo-obstruction also can occur, as can small bowel obstruction if a loop of small intestine becomes incorporated into the inflammatory mass. These conditions usually improve with effective medical therapy including antibiotics, bowel rest, and NG suction.

Surgical intervention may be required for persistent obstruction from acute diverticulitis that does not respond to medical therapy. Ideally, a modified bowel preparation with gentle irrigation enemas or low-dose oral laxatives given over

a period of a few days can be performed preoperatively,[156] thereby allowing the possibility of primary anastomosis in some cases. In cases where bowel preparation is not possible, a Hartmann procedure usually is performed.

Recurrent attacks of diverticulitis, which may be subclinical, can initiate chronic stricturing of the colonic wall without ongoing inflammation. In such cases, high-grade or complete obstruction can occur. Colonoscopy can play an important diagnostic role, and 1 group that reported on the investigation of strictures with colonoscopy was able to distinguish a benign from malignant etiology in 67% of patients.[160] CT and water-soluble contrast enema also can be helpful in distinguishing benign stricture from neoplasm. Strictures in which malignancy cannot be excluded, despite colonoscopic and radiologic examinations, should be treated by surgical resection.

A trial of endoscopic dilation therapy can reasonably be attempted in patients in whom neoplasm is believed to be sufficiently excluded and in whom acute diverticulitis is not a concern. Success rates for balloon dilation of benign colonic strictures have been reported in 67% to 79% of patients.[161,162] Colonic self-expanding metal stents (SEMS) also have been used to provide temporary decompression in treating obstruction that complicates diverticular disease, allowing bowel preparation and subsequent single-stage resection without diversion.[163] In 1 case series, Small and coworkers used SEMS in 23 cases of benign obstructive colonic disease, of which 16 cases were diverticular or inflammatory in origin. SEMS placement was successful and obstruction was relieved in 95% of cases, but major complications (i.e., stent migration, re-obstruction, perforation) occurred in 38%. The authors concluded that medium-term relief was obtainable with SEMS, but at the cost of a high complication rate; they also recommended that if surgery was to be performed, it should be done within 7 days of stent placement.[164]

Free Perforation

Fecal peritonitis caused by free perforation (Hinchey stage IV) is a surgical emergency and requires urgent operative intervention. Fortunately, it is uncommon, with a population incidence of 4 cases per 100,000 population per year.[8,117] Although uncommon in the antibiotic era, mortality from generalized peritonitis associated with diverticulitis has been reported in the 12% to 26% range.[165] Early identification of free perforation is critical. CT scan can confirm the diagnosis in ambiguous cases, but an abdominal plain-film series showing free intraperitoneal air plus high clinical suspicion is sufficient to justify surgical exploration. Broad-spectrum IV antibiotics should be instituted immediately.

Practically, the decision of whether to perform a primary anastomosis or 2-stage approach is made intraoperatively based on the extent of disease, the difficulty of bowel mobilization, the degree of peritoneal contamination, and the surgeon's expertise. In most cases of free perforation, at least 2 separate operations are necessary regardless of whether primary or secondary resection is performed. In many cases, reanastomosis is not possible, and the colostomy is left indefinitely. Some cases with peritonitis also require pelvic drainage, clearance of the rectum of fecal material when possible, and mobilization of the splenic flexure to perform a tension-free anastomosis. With the increasing use of the laparoscopic approach to uncomplicated diverticular disease, some centers have extended this approach to perforated disease, with promising results.[166,167]

Special Topics Related to Diverticulitis

The Young Patient

Diverticulitis is relatively uncommon in patients younger than 40 years of age (2% to 5% of all patients with diverticulitis[168,169]), but the incidence in this age group may be rising.[170] Nevertheless, because diverticulitis is uncommon in the young, it is often missed or mistaken for other diagnoses, such as appendicitis or IBD. Like diverticulitis in older patients, the disease is mainly sigmoid in location, but in contrast, there seems to be a significant male predominance in young patients.[168,171] Attacks often are more severe, and 40% to 88% of younger patients require urgent surgery during their initial attack; recurrence and complication rates are also higher than in older patients.[168,171,172]

When patients with acute diverticulitis are managed nonoperatively, youth is an independent risk factor for poor outcome,[173] possibly due to delay in diagnosis. For these reasons, some authors have advocated elective segmental colectomy in a healthy young person after 1 well-documented episode of diverticulitis[94,126,173]; others have questioned this approach.[140,174,175] In the largest series to date of young patients with diverticulitis, the authors suggested that the higher incidence of surgical management in these patients relative to their older counterparts was not due to increased complication rates but rather to a higher rate of elective procedures done to prevent the expected poor outcomes.[170] Thus, the latest surgical guidelines are advocating more of a case-by-case approach to elective resections for all patients with diverticulitis.[121]

The Older Adult Patient

Because diverticular disease becomes more prevalent with aging, diverticulitis in older adults warrants special mention. Diverticulitis can manifest with more subtle symptoms and signs in older adults, making the diagnosis more challenging. Distinguishing diverticulitis from colorectal cancer becomes a much more important issue in older patients, because the incidence of colorectal cancer also increases with age. Though the risk of a severe initial attack of diverticulitis may be lower in older patients than in younger ones, the risk of death when diverticulitis results in perforation is more than 3 times higher in older adults.[176] It appears, however, that the number of comorbidities is a stronger predictor of mortality from perforated diverticulitis than age itself.[177] Because subsequent complicated disease is uncommon if the initial attack was mild,[173] and because older patients are less likely than younger patients to have recurrent disease after nonoperative management,[178] surgery is often delayed or set aside in older patients. Not only is surgery more risky in older adults, but colostomy reversal is also less often performed[179] and, when attempted, tends to have a higher rate of morbidity and mortality than in younger patients.[145]

The Immunocompromised Patient

Diverticulitis can manifest more subtly in immunocompromised patients and represents a more difficult diagnostic challenge than in those with a normal immune system. Although diverticulitis in such patients is not more common, it appears to have graver consequences. One study reported that 24% of immunocompetent patients needed surgery for diverticulitis, compared with 100% of immunosuppressed individuals.[180] Immunocompromised patients have a higher rate of free perforation (43% vs. 14%), need for surgery (58% vs. 33%), and postoperative mortality (39% vs. 2%) than do non-compromised patients.[181] In solid organ (e.g., heart, lung, kidney) transplant populations, mortality from diverticulitis has been found to be extremely high, ranging from 25% to 100%.[182-184] Because of this high risk, many authorities advocate elective resection after an initial episode of diverticulitis in an immunosuppressed patient.[94,185]

Right-Sided Diverticulitis

In Western countries, diverticulitis of the ascending colon or cecum is uncommon, in large part because of the relatively low prevalence of diverticula in these portions of the colon. Nonetheless, right-sided diverticulitis should be part of the differential diagnosis for any patient with right-sided abdominal symptoms.

In Asia, right-sided diverticulitis is the predominant form of diverticulitis. Especially in younger patients, the diagnosis of right-sided diverticulitis is more difficult to make than is left-sided disease and is virtually clinically indistinguishable from acute appendicitis. Clinical factors that might be helpful to distinguish diverticulitis from appendicitis in a person of Asian ethnicity are that patients with diverticulitis tend to be older and have a lower frequency of nausea and vomiting than do patients with appendicitis; the characteristic progression of symptoms seen with appendicitis is also absent.[186]

Radiologically, right-sided diverticulitis and appendicitis also are easily confused, especially when a local abscess is present. There is an estimated preoperative misdiagnosis rate in right-sided colon inflammatory conditions of 40% to 92%.[186,187] Even with excellent imaging, the diagnosis of right-sided diverticulitis often is made at laparotomy.

When the proper diagnosis is made preoperatively, treatment of right-sided disease is the same as for left-sided diverticulitis. One study has suggested better overall responsiveness of right-sided diverticulitis to medical therapy alone, even after multiple attacks.[188] The much more common complication associated with right-sided colonic diverticula is hemorrhage, discussed later in this chapter.

Segmental Colitis Associated with Diverticulosis (SCAD)

SCAD is now increasingly recognized as a distinct but poorly understood manifestation of diverticular disease.[158,189,190] SCAD was initially thought to be a rare form of Crohn's disease in a segment of colon that contained diverticula. It is now recognized, however, as a distinct entity seen in a very small subset of patients with diverticulosis. The prevalence of SCAD in patients with diverticulosis has been described as 0.3% to 1.3%, with 58.7% of patients being male, and with a mean age of 63.6 years.[191]

SCAD can mimic the clinical presentation of IBD and primarily affects the sigmoid colon. Presenting symptoms generally are LLQ cramping pain, diarrhea, and rectal bleeding. Endoscopically, the sigmoid colonic mucosa shows erythema, friability of varying degrees, and mucosal erosions, only within the segment of colon bearing the diverticula. The remaining segments of colon, including the rectum, are neither visibly nor histologically involved. Biopsy specimens can show chronic lymphocytic infiltration, cryptitis, crypt abscesses, and even granulomas; many cases are histologically indistinguishable from IBD or ischemic colitis.[192] In fact, a subset of patients when followed endoscopically over time appear to evolve into a picture similar to ulcerative proctosigmoiditis or Crohn's colitis. This observation should prompt a low threshold for endoscopic reevaluation if a patient with presumed SCAD develops persistent or progressive symptoms.

Patients with SCAD generally are responsive to 5-ASA compounds, with 1 series reporting that over 80% of treated patients achieved clinical remission.[189] In most cases, the clinical course tends to be benign and self-limited,[193] although there are reports of patients who required sigmoid colectomy for bleeding or stricture complications.[194] There does not appear to be a higher risk of diverticulitis or colon cancer in patients with SCAD.[189]

Diverticular Hemorrhage

Diverticular hemorrhage is arguably the most common cause of significant lower GI bleeding (LGIB) in adults and accounts for approximately 30% to 66% of such cases.[195-197] Because a culprit diverticulum is not frequently identified, diverticular hemorrhage is often a diagnosis of presumption and exclusion framed by the presence of diverticulosis, evidence of LGIB, and the absence of other identifiable sources. This circumstance challenges clarity of epidemiologic data. Jensen and his CURE Hemostasis Research Group, therefore, promote specific classification of a patient with diverticulosis and severe hematochezia as having either *presumptive diverticular hemorrhage* (i.e., no other source found besides diverticulosis after urgent colonoscopy, anoscopy, push enteroscopy, and capsule endoscopy), *incidental diverticulosis* (i.e., some other non-diverticular colonic, anorectal, upper GI or small-bowel source identified as the cause of the bleeding), or *definitive diverticular hemorrhage*.[198] Using this classification system, Jensen's group reported the following in a prospective study of 340 LGIB patients: incidental diverticulosis in 46%, presumptive diverticular hemorrhage in 34%, and definitive diverticular hemorrhage in 20%.[198] Bleeding is estimated to occur in approximately

10% to 15% of patients with significant diverticulosis, and severe hemorrhage to occur in 3% to 5% of patients.[199,200] Although most diverticula are in the left colon in Western patients, the site of bleeding diverticula has been believed to be in the proximal colon in more than one half of patients.[201-203] A large series of 180 Asian patients with diverticular hemorrhage reported a higher bleeding rate and greater need for surgery with right-sided than with left-sided disease.[203] Patients with pancolonic diverticulosis appear to have a higher hemorrhage rate than those with diverticula on only 1 side of the colon.[204]

Pathophysiology

The pathophysiology of diverticular bleeding is not well understood. It is thought to be related to intimal thickening and medial thinning of the vasa recta, which leads to weakening of the vessel.[205] As a diverticulum herniates, the supplying vessel (vas rectum) is draped over the dome of the diverticulum, with only the mucosal layer of the colon separating it from the colonic lumen. The combination of increased exposure and weakening of the vessel is thought to predispose to rupture. What predisposes to this arterial change and what precipitates its rupture are unknown. NSAIDs including aspirin, however, have been associated with an increased risk of diverticular bleeding in multiple studies, with reported odds ratios of 3 to 15.[67,204,206-208]

Clinical Features

Diverticular hemorrhage typically manifests as abrupt, painless, and self-limited hematochezia. The volume of blood is usually moderate or large, owing to the fact that the bleeding vessel is an arteriole. Patients often pass red or maroon clots, and melena is unusual. Because diverticular bleeding is overt, neither a positive fecal occult blood test nor iron deficiency anemia should be attributed to diverticular hemorrhage. Natural history studies report that bleeding ceases spontaneously in 70% to 80% of patients; 30-day rebleeding rates have been reported as high as 53%, and emergency surgery rates are as high as 35%.[200,202,203,209]

Diagnosis and Treatment

The initial evaluation of a patient with suspected diverticular hemorrhage should include an assessment of hemodynamic stability and initiation of resuscitation. Concurrent to this, the clinician should attempt to clarify the suspected diagnosis and to localize the site of bleeding. A high pretest probability for diverticular hemorrhage can be supported by classic clinical manifestations (noted earlier) in an older adult patient; however, other lower GI sources (e.g., angioectasias, hemorrhoids, colitis, colorectal cancer) also need to be considered in the differential diagnosis. Because a brisk upper GI bleed can present as massive hematochezia, NG lavage or EGD should be considered when clinically appropriate. Diagnostic modalities include colonoscopy, nuclear scintigraphy, and angiography. Therapeutic modalities include colonoscopy, angiography, and surgery.[153] The diagnosis and treatment of patients with LGIB in general have been reviewed comprehensively elsewhere (see Chapter 20).[197,209,210] The algorithm in Figure 121-7 summarizes the management of patients with diverticular hemorrhage.

Colonoscopy

Urgent colonoscopy (defined as within 12 to 48 hours of admission) affords the gastroenterologist the opportunity to

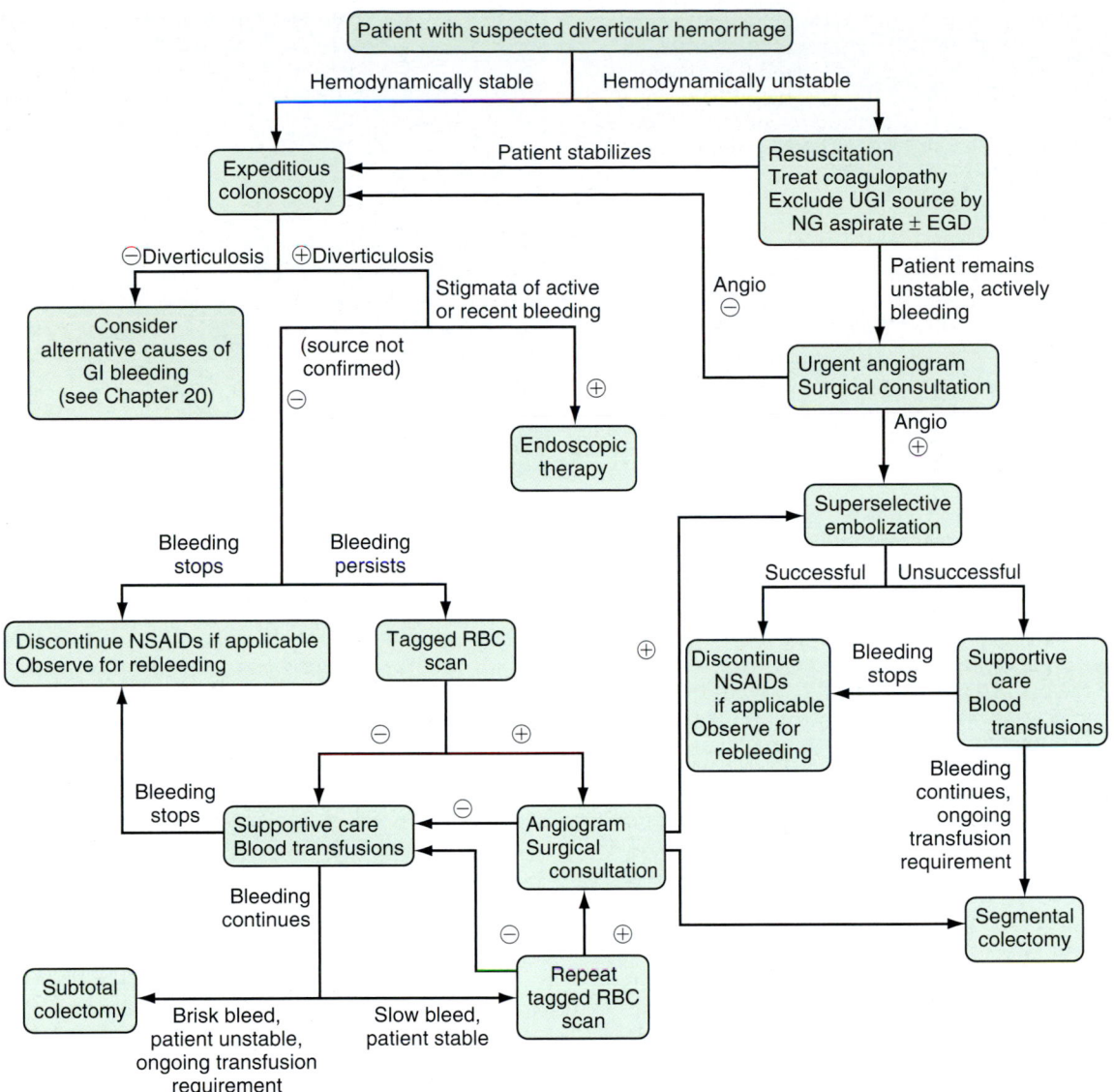

FIGURE 121-7. Algorithm for the management of patients with suspected diverticular hemorrhage. Angio, angiogram; RBC, red blood cell; UGI, upper GI.

diagnose, localize, and offer therapeutic intervention to patients with diverticular bleeding.[197] Endoscopic identification of active bleeding or stigmata of recent hemorrhage (e.g., visible vessel or adherent clot within a diverticulum) at a specific site (Fig. 121-8) is evident in about 10% to 20% of colonoscopic examinations for diverticular bleeding. Identification of a bleeding site allows endoscopic therapy to be applied[198]: epinephrine injection alone[211] or in combination with other therapies such as heater probe coagulation,[212] bipolar coagulation,[213,214] endoclips (see Fig. 121-8),[215-217] fibrin sealant,[218] and band ligation[219] all have been shown in small case series to achieve hemostasis safely in patients with diverticular bleeding.

Nuclear Scintigraphy, Angiography, and CT

When active bleeding is present but colonoscopy fails to allow localization or treatment of a bleeding source, further evaluation with nuclear scintigraphy (tagged red blood cell scan) or angiography can be undertaken, taking into account local availability and expertise. Nuclear scintigraphy (Fig. 121-9)

has many theoretical advantages in the evaluation of LGIB[220]: it is noninvasive, technically simple, and relatively inexpensive, and can detect bleeding rates as low as 0.1 mL/min. Scintigraphy, however, can identify only the site, not the etiology of the bleeding, and it has no therapeutic potential. Furthermore, some studies have questioned its accuracy[221] and have underscored a lack of proven impact on mortality, transfusion requirement, and eventual need for surgery.[222] Given its sensitivity and relative simplicity, however, many centers use scintigraphy as a "gateway" to angiography to minimize the chance of a negative angiogram and to help select a specific artery for injection of contrast.[223]

Angiography is not as sensitive as nuclear scintigraphy for LGIB but detects rates of bleeding in the range of 0.5 mL/min. The primary advantage of angiography is accurate identification of the bleeding site to direct segmental surgical resection or angiographic intervention via superselective embolization (Fig. 121-10) or embolization of distal arterial branches, both of which have been demonstrated to be effective (67% to 100% with lasting hemostasis) and relatively safe (ischemia rates < 20%).[224-227] Arterial embolization is increasingly becoming the

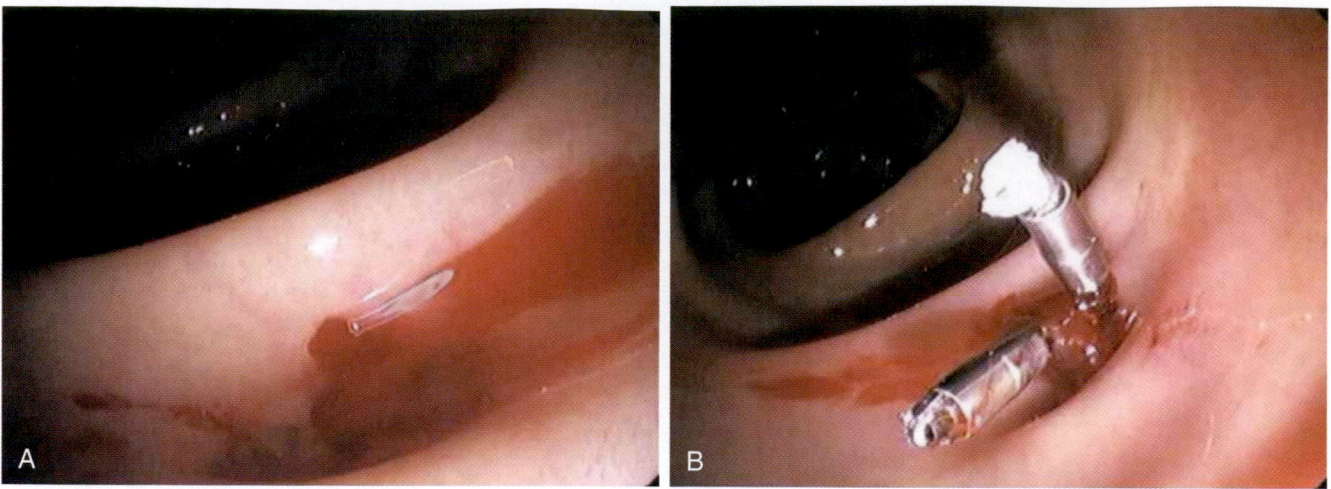

FIGURE 121-8. Colonoscopy in a patient with lower intestinal bleeding from a diverticulum in whom a site of active bleeding was identified *(A)* and treated successfully with placement of 2 endoclips *(B)*. *(Courtesy Janak Shah, MD. San Francisco, CA.)*

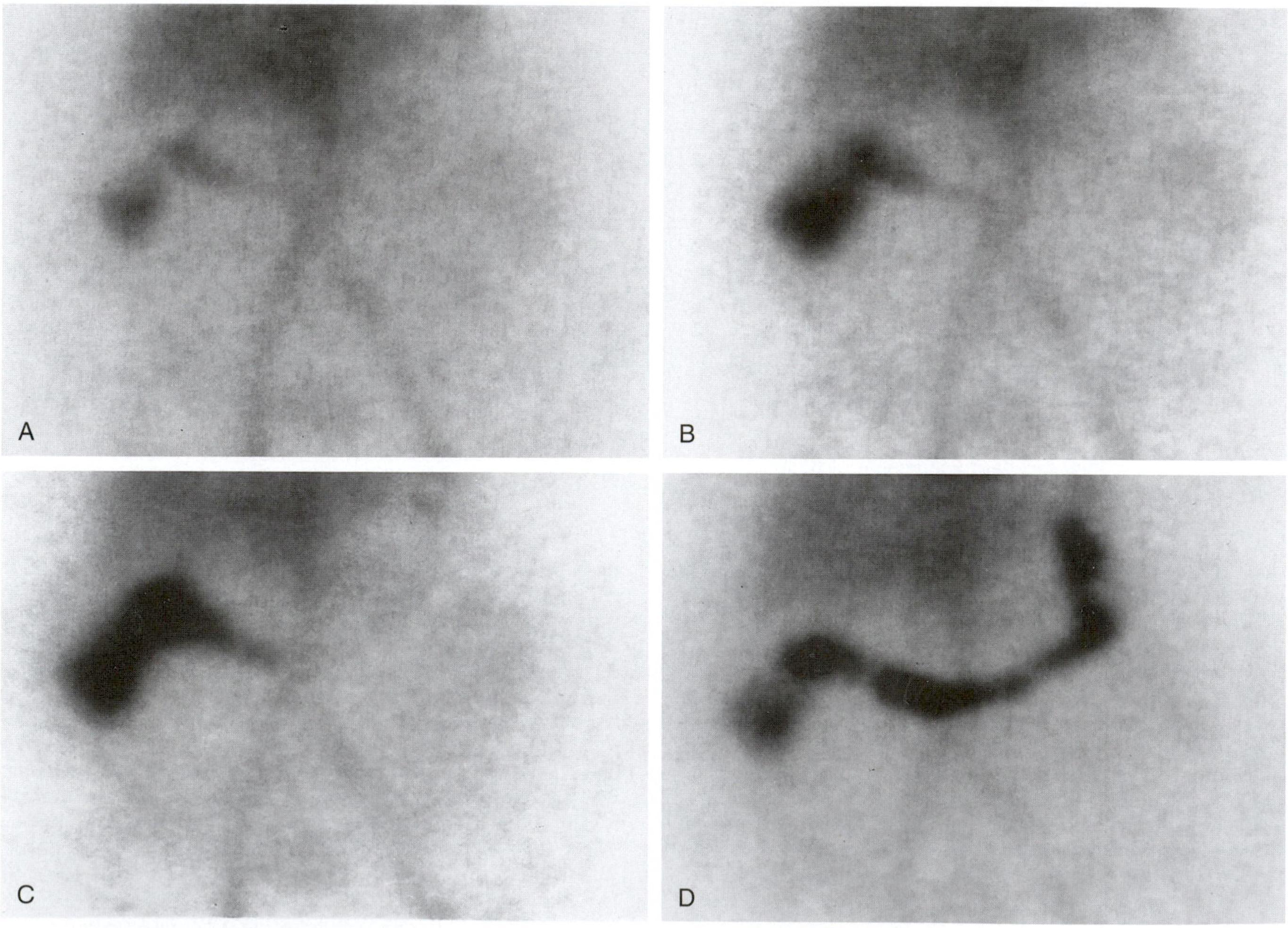

FIGURE 121-9. Nuclear scintigraphy using tagged RBCs in a patient with lower intestinal bleeding from right-sided diverticulosis. *A,* The early scan (anterior view) shows pooling of radiolabeled RBCs in the right upper quadrant corresponding to a bleeding site in the hepatic flexure. *B-D,* The subsequent images show radiolabeled RBCs progressing through the transverse colon over time. RBC, red blood cell.

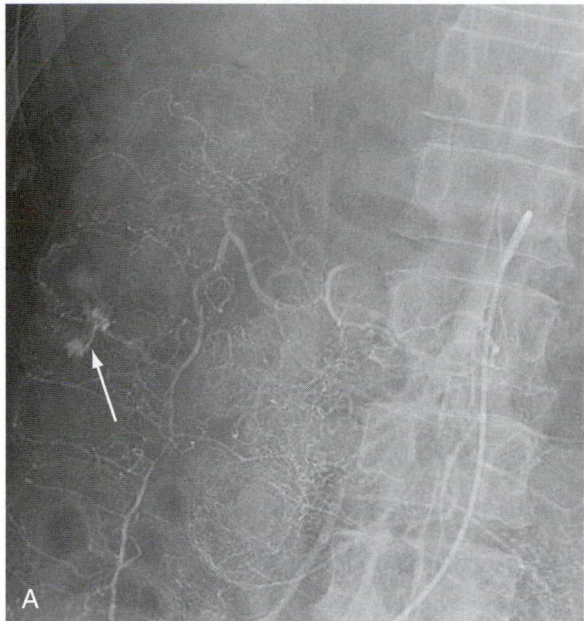 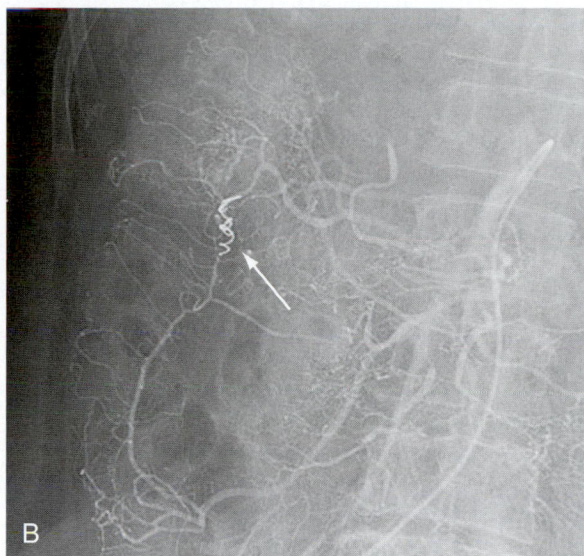

FIGURE 121-10. Selective angiography of the superior mesenteric artery in a patient with lower intestinal bleeding from diverticulosis. *A*, The bleeding site is identified in the ascending colon by a "blush" of contrast material *(arrow)*. *B*, The bleeding site has been embolized with microcoils, which are seen in the bleeding vessel *(arrow)*, and the extravasation of contrast material has stopped.

nonsurgical therapy of choice when endoscopic control of bleeding is not possible.

A third radiologic option, enhanced CT, also has shown promise for identifying active LGIB sources, although its role has yet to be defined, and it has no therapeutic potential.[228,229]

Surgery

Surgery for LGIB usually is avoided unless endoscopic or angiographic therapies are unavailable or fail. Because diverticular bleeding stops spontaneously in most instances, surgical management is required infrequently. The primary indications for operative management are large transfusion requirements, recurrent or continuing hemorrhage that is refractory or not amenable to therapy, or hemodynamic instability unresponsive to resuscitation. When surgery is necessary, a partial colectomy is preferred to a subtotal colectomy whenever possible. Segmental resection can be performed if the bleeding site is clearly identified from a therapeutically unsuccessful angiographic or endoscopic procedure, or when the extent of diverticulosis is confined to a specific segment of the colon. In patients with persistent, life-threatening bleeding and no identification of a likely bleeding site, a subtotal or "blind" colectomy may be required as a last resort. These patients have had an extremely high morbidity and mortality,[230] possibly because of the multiple invasive tests leading to that end and the resultant delay in definitive management. Additionally, a blind colectomy runs the risk of not resecting the bleeding lesion when the source is more proximal; 1 study reported an 18% recurrent bleeding rate, compared with a 4% rebleeding rate after a total colonic resection.[231] More recent literature, however, has shown morbidity and mortality rates of subtotal colectomy not to differ from those of blind hemicolectomy when the site of the bleeding is not identified.[231,232] A close collaborative relationship between the gastroenterologist and the surgeon is paramount in managing such patients.

ACKNOWLEDGMENT

The authors would like to acknowledge the contributions of the previous authors of this chapter, with particular note to Dr. Jeffrey Fox who co-authored the prior edition's chapter. We would also like to acknowledge the administrative support of Ms. Lynda Wilson.

KEY REFERENCES

Full references for this chapter can be found on www.expertconsult.com.

6. Everhart JE, Ruhl CE. Burden of digestive diseases in the United States part II: Lower gastrointestinal diseases. Gastroenterology 2009; 136:741-54.
9. Etzioni DA, Mack TM, Beart RW Jr, Kaiser AM. Diverticulitis in the United States: 1998-2005: Changing patterns of disease and treatment. Ann Surg 2009; 249:210-7.
49a. Strate LL. Lifestyle factors and the course of diverticular disease. Dig Dis 2012; 30(1):35-45.
73. Strate LL. Diverticulosis and dietary fiber: Rethinking the relationship. Gastroenterology 2012; 142:205-7.
74. Peery AF, Barrett PR, Park D, et al. A high-fiber diet does not protect against asymptomatic diverticulosis. Gastroenterology 2012; 142:266-72 e1.
76. Jun S, Stollman N. Epidemiology of diverticular disease. Best Pract Res Clin Gastroenterol 2002; 16:529-42.
85. Strate LL, Modi R, Cohen E, Spiegel BM. Diverticular disease as a chronic illness: Evolving epidemiologic and clinical insights. Am J Gastroenterol 2012; 107:1486-93.
90. Tursi A. Biomarkers in diverticular diseases of the colon. Dig Dis 2012; 30:12-8.
99a. Maconi G, Barbara G, Bosetti C, et al. Treatment of diverticular disease of the colon and prevention of acute

diverticulitis: A systematic review. Dis Colon Rectum 2011; 54:1326-38.

121. Rafferty J, Shellito P, Hyman NH, et al. Practice parameters for sigmoid diverticulitis. Dis Colon Rectum 2006; 49:939-44.

133. Sai VF, Velayos F, Neuhaus J, Westphalen AC. Colonoscopy after CT diagnosis of diverticulitis to exclude colon cancer: A systematic literature review. Radiology 2012; 263:383-90.

134. Abbas MA, Cannom RR, Chiu VY, et al. Triage of patients with acute diverticulitis: Are some inpatients candidates for outpatient treatment? Colorectal Dis 2012; 15:451-7.

138. Shabanzadeh DM, Wille-Jorgensen P. Antibiotics for uncomplicated diverticulitis. Cochrane Database Syst Rev 2012; 11:CD009092.

191. Mann NS, Hoda KK. Segmental colitis associated with diverticulosis: Systematic evaluation of 486 cases with meta-analysis. Hepatogastroenterology 2012; 59:2119-21.

198. Jensen DM. The ins and outs of diverticular bleeding. Gastrointest Endosc 2012; 75:388-91.

Irritable Bowel Syndrome

ALEXANDER C. FORD AND NICHOLAS J. TALLEY

CHAPTER OUTLINE

IBS is an important disease entity because of its high prevalence, substantial morbidity, and enormous costs.[1,2] In the United States, approximately 12% of patients seen by primary care physicians have IBS, but it is likely that this frequency is an underestimate.[3-5] In GI practices, more than one third of patients have functional GI disorders, IBS being the most common diagnosis.[6] Because a substantial proportion of gastroenterology practice comprises patients with IBS or other functional GI disorders, it is essential that clinicians develop expertise in their diagnosis and treatment. The diagnosis of IBS rests on a careful history and physical examination; that diagnostic tests often are not needed represents an important conceptual advance.[7] There is increasing evidence that at least a subset of IBS has an organic basis in the GI tract.[8] Nonetheless, only symptom-directed therapy rather than disease-modifying treatments are available; the evidence base for current therapy has strengthened considerably with the publication of well-performed meta-analyses. In this chapter, current knowledge of the epidemiology and pathophysiology of IBS is reviewed to provide a rational basis for its diagnosis and therapy.

DEFINITIONS

IBS is characterized by the presence of abdominal discomfort or pain associated with disturbed defecation.[1] Bloating is often present, but this is not considered an essential symptom for diagnosis.[1] Individual symptoms are neither sensitive nor specific enough on their own to diagnose IBS.[9]

Manning and associates first reported that 6 symptoms were more common in patients in whom IBS was subsequently documented (Box 122-1), although only 4 were statistically significant (abdominal distension, relief of abdominal pain after a bowel movement, looser stools with the onset of abdominal pain, and more frequent bowel movements with the onset of abdominal pain).[10] Later studies showed that these symptoms were specific, but not sensitive, for identifying IBS and were of greater diagnostic value in women.[9,11] The Kruis scoring system, which is based on the presence and duration of symptoms, negative physical examination findings, and normal simple laboratory tests, has modest diagnostic utility (see Box 122-1).[12]

In an effort to build on the diagnostic utility of the Manning and Kruis criteria, the Rome (I, II, and III) criteria were created following a formal consensus process to provide a standard for clinical research (see Box 122-1).[1] The Rome criteria are useful in clinical practice and can be used to make a positive clinical diagnosis.[1,2] The sensitivity and specificity of the Rome I criteria have been reported to be 71% and 85%, respectively,[13] and although adequate validation data for Rome III are lacking, the main criteria for Rome III are very similar to those of Rome I.[9] Comparisons have shown that Rome I and II criteria are specific and identify similar patient populations, although compared with Rome I criteria, the Rome II criteria identify fewer cases.[14-16] The Manning criteria identify

Manning Criteria*
Abdominal pain eased after bowel movement
Looser stools at onset of abdominal pain
More frequent bowel movements at onset of abdominal pain
Abdominal distention
Mucus per rectum
Feeling of incomplete emptying

Kruis Criteria
Patient's History
Abdominal pain
Flatulence
Irregularity of bowel movements
Symptoms for more than 2 years
Mixed diarrhea and constipation
Pellet-like stools or mucus

Physician's Assessment[†]
Abnormal physical findings
Erythrocyte sedimentation rate > 20 mm/2 hr
Leukocytosis (>10,000 cm^3)
Hemoglobin (female < 12 g/dL; male < 14 g/dL)
History of blood in stool

Rome III Criteria[‡]
Recurrent abdominal pain or discomfort[§] at least 3 days/month in the last 3 months associated with *2 or more* of the following:
   Improvement with defecation
   Onset associated with a change in frequency of stool
   Onset associated with a change in form (appearance) of stool

*Diagnostic cut-off: 3 or more of the 6 symptoms listed.
[†]IBS is excluded if any physical finding or any of the laboratory parameters assessed by the physician is abnormal.
[‡]Criteria fulfilled for the previous 3 months, with symptom onset at least 6 months before diagnosis.
[§]"Discomfort" means an uncomfortable sensation not described as pain. In pathophysiology research and clinical trials, a pain or discomfort frequency of at least 2 days a week during a screening evaluation is recommended for subject eligibility.
Manning criteria adapted from Manning AP, Thompson WG, Heaton KW, Morris AF. Towards positive diagnosis of the irritable bowel. BMJ 1978; 2:653-4.
Kruis criteria adapted from Kruis W, Thieme C, Weinzierl M, et al. A diagnostic score for the irritable bowel syndrome. Its value in the exclusion of organic disease. Gastroenterology 1984; 87:1-7.
Rome III criteria from Longstreth GF, Thompson WG, Chey WD, et al. Functional bowel disorders. In: Drossman DA, editor. Rome III: The functional gastrointestinal disorders. 3rd ed. McLean, Va.: Dagnon Associates; 2006. p 491. Used with permission from the Rome Foundation.

additional patients with IBS-like symptoms who do not fulfill any of the Rome criteria, but arguably also should be classified as having true IBS.[14-16]

CLINICAL FEATURES

History

Abdominal Discomfort or Pain

IBS should not be diagnosed in the absence of abdominal discomfort or pain.[1] The discomfort/pain in IBS typically is relieved by defecation, or its onset is associated with an increase or decrease in stool frequency, or with looser or harder stools. The pain often is poorly localized, waxes and wanes, may be aggravated by eating, and can occur in any part of the abdomen, although it more typically is located in the lower abdomen; it may be referred to different areas in the abdomen or to the chest or back. Exacerbation of pain by life events or difficult life situations is common. Abdominal discomfort/pain that is continuous or unrelated to defecation or that is induced by menstruation, urination, or physical activity is unlikely to be explained by IBS.

Constipation and Diarrhea

Patients with IBS experience constipation, diarrhea, or a mixture of these symptoms.[1] Symptom predominance has led some authors to attempt to classify IBS patients by their predominant symptom: constipation (IBS-C), diarrhea (IBS-D), and mixed (IBS-M), although these symptoms often are variable and intermittent, and patients can change from one stool pattern to another (see later). An irregular stool consistency (abnormal stool form) is characteristic.

The terms "constipation" and "diarrhea" can reflect a wide variety of different symptom experiences to different patients, and so whenever a patient uses these terms, an exploration of their meaning is required.[17] Stool form can be measured objectively and graded by patient or physician; the Bristol stool form scale (Fig. 122-1) is now used routinely in clinical trials, and changes in stool form (at the extreme ends of the scale) roughly correlate with colonic transit time (r value of .07).[18]

Bloating and Visible Distention

A feeling of bloating is very common in patients with IBS, and its site can be difficult for the patient to localize. Visible abdominal distention is characteristic, particularly in women, but less common than bloating[19]; it can be objectively measured and usually is not imagined.[20] Gas can mean excess bloating, belching, flatus, or even reflux symptoms to the patient, and so it is important to ask patients to explain the meaning of the terms they are using to describe their symptoms.

Noncolonic Symptoms

Other clinical features can help support the diagnosis of IBS but in themselves are not diagnostic. The odds of subjects with IBS having epigastric discomfort or pain (dyspepsia) is 8-fold that of individuals without IBS.[21] Symptoms compatible with GERD also occur more commonly in IBS patients, with a 4-fold increase in odds they will have such symptoms compared with individuals who do not have IBS.[22] Extraintestinal symptoms including headache (and migraine), backache, impaired sleep, chronic fatigue, increased urinary frequency or urgency, pelvic pain, and dyspareunia are more common in patients with IBS but have no accepted diagnostic value.[2,23] Musculoskeletal pain syndromes including fibromyalgia[24] and temporomandibular joint disorder also are associated with IBS.[24,25]

IBD and IBS

Typical IBS symptoms are common in patients with documented IBD in remission. In 1 meta-analysis of observational studies, 31% of patients with UC and 41% of patients with Crohn's disease reported symptoms compatible with IBS, and the prevalence of such symptoms was significantly higher among patients with Crohn's disease than in those with UC.[26] Clinically, IBS and IBD may, in some cases, share symptoms and be difficult to distinguish. IBS symptoms appear to be more prevalent before a diagnosis of IBD is made.[27]

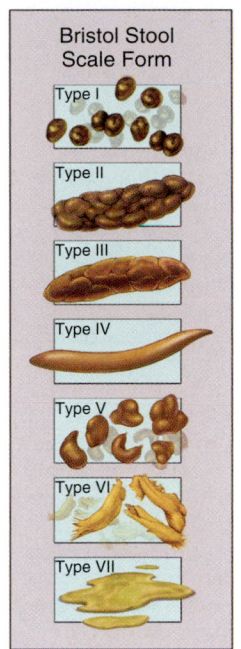

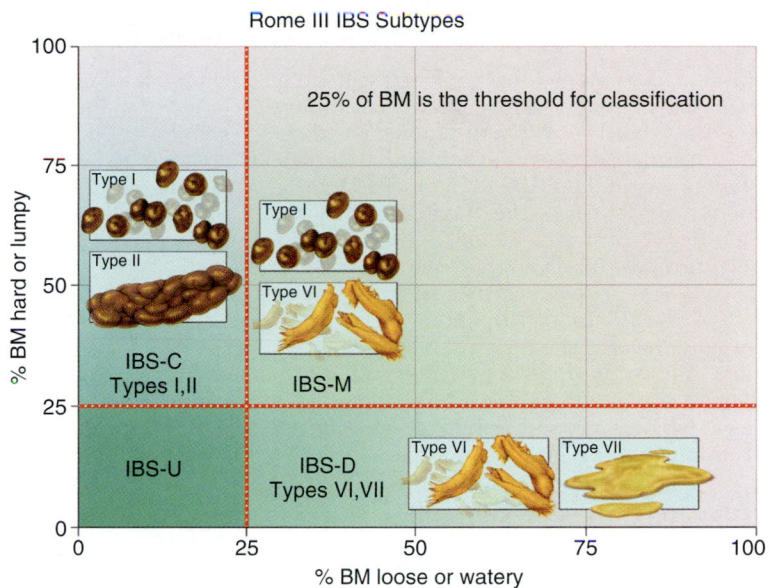

FIGURE 122-1. The Bristol stool form scale and classification of subtypes of IBS. BM, bowel movement; C, constipation; D, diarrhea; IBS, irritable bowel syndrome; M, mixed; U, unsubtyped. *(Adapted from Longstreth GF, Thompson WG, Chey WD, et al. Functional bowel disorders. In: Drossman DA, editor. Rome III: The functional gastrointestinal disorders. 3rd ed. McLean, Va.: Dagnon Associates; 2006. p 492. Used with permission from the Rome Foundation.)*

Chronicity

For a confident diagnosis of IBS, symptoms should have been present for at least 6 months[1]; IBS may accompany other chronic disorders. For example, IBS is present in up to one third of patients with celiac disease, even after institution of a gluten-free diet.[28] A number of different conditions can cause transient bowel symptoms including pregnancy, dietary indiscretion, food poisoning, traveler's diarrhea, bed rest, weight loss, and acute stress (nervous diarrhea); these must be distinguished from the chronic, recurrent symptoms of IBS.

Physical Examination

Physical examination in patients with IBS is usually normal, although deep tenderness over the colon may be appreciated.[9] Abdominal wall pain should be excluded clinically. Tensing the abdominal wall by flexing the chin on the chest or sitting up partially lessens tenderness that is caused by an intra-abdominal process. If tensing the abdominal wall muscles increases abdominal tenderness, a point of localized abdominal wall tenderness should be sought with a probing finger (Carnett's test); identification of such a point might enable the tenderness to be treated with an injection of lidocaine and triamcinolone.[29,30] The painful rib syndrome (point tenderness on springing the rib cage) also may be confused with IBS pain.[31] Ovarian cancer needs to be considered in any middle-aged or older woman presenting with new-onset IBS-like symptoms, particularly if abdominal distension is present.[32] A pelvic examination then may be required to exclude an irregular, fixed pelvic mass.

EPIDEMIOLOGY

IBS is a common disorder, with up to 1 in 10 individuals worldwide affected.[33] Epidemiologic studies have defined the prevalence of, and identified potential risk factors for, IBS.

Prevalence

Prevalence estimates for IBS have varied anywhere from 1% to 45% worldwide.[33] Prevalence, however, is influenced substantially by the definition applied. For example, in Olmsted County, Minnesota, the prevalence of IBS varied from 8% to 22% depending on the criteria used.[34] People in the community under 50 years of age have a higher prevalence of IBS.[33] Generally, it is believed that IBS is uncommon in the elderly, but population-based studies indicate that IBS, in fact, increases with advancing age. Thus, for example, using 3 or more of the Manning criteria to define IBS, the prevalence of IBS in Olmsted County ranged from 8% in those 65 to 74 years of age to more than 12% in those older than 85 years.[35] Obviously, organic disease is more prevalent in elderly persons and could account for some of the reported IBS-like symptoms, but it seems likely that IBS in the elderly is often underdiagnosed or misdiagnosed, for example, as diverticular disease.[36]

Gender and Race

Gender-specific prevalence rates for IBS are higher in women compared with men, with an odds ratio of 1.67 in a recent meta-analysis, although this was not observed in South Asia or South America.[37] In the United States, women with IBS outnumber men, which is partly explained by increased health care-seeking behavior among women. In contrast, data from India indicate more men than women present for care of IBS.[38] Healthy women have greater rectal sensitivity, slower colonic transit, and smaller stool outputs than do men, which might explain why certain symptoms, such as straining and passage of hard stools, seem to be more common in women.[39,40] The prevalence of IBS generally is similar in whites and blacks, although some data have suggested it may be lower in Hispanics than in non-Hispanic whites in the United States.[41,42]

Subgroups

The Rome III definition uses stool form to subclassify IBS, but definitions of IBS subgroups remain arbitrary, and different definitions have been used in different studies (see Fig. 122-1).[1] Data from 1 meta-analysis of community-based studies suggest that 22% of sufferers have IBS-C, 23% IBS-D, 24% IBS-M, and that the remainder cannot be classified (IBS-U).[33] Subgroups seem to differ according to gender, with men who have IBS more likely to report IBS-D and women more likely to report IBS-C.[37] It is unclear, however, if those with 1 predominant symptom—diarrhea or constipation—if followed long enough, eventually develop the other, namely, constipation in patients with IBS-D or diarrhea in patients with IBS-C. Recent data support this contention, with only 35% of patients being considered as a stable subgroup during a 2-week period of reported observation.[43]

Incidence and Disappearance of Symptoms

The onset rate of IBS was 67 per 1000 person-years by applying the Manning criteria to a cohort in Olmsted County that was surveyed at a 12- to 20-month interval.[44] This study did not exclude people with a past history of IBS, however, and hence this is not the true incidence.[44] Another study reported that the incidence of a clinical diagnosis of IBS in Olmsted County was 0.2% per year, but this figure reflects the lower end of the incidence rate, because people with IBS symptoms who did not seek consultation could not be included in this calculation.[45] Over a 12-year follow-up, 9% of community subjects who were symptom-free at baseline developed IBS.[46]

In a follow-up study in Olmsted County, 38% of subjects meeting the definition of IBS at entry did not meet these criteria 12 to 20 months later[44]; they lost their symptoms. The actual prevalence of IBS did not change from year to year, however, because the disappearance of symptoms in some patients with IBS was balanced by others who developed IBS. Among those in the community who lose their IBS, symptoms evolve to reflect another functional GI disorder in up to 50%[47-49]; hence IBS usually is a chronic disorder, although symptoms often are variable.

RISK FACTORS

The best-accepted risk factor for IBS is bacterial gastroenteritis.[50-53] The risk of postinfection IBS has been reported to be increased with depression,[54] adverse life events and hypochondriasis,[55] female gender, younger age, and prolonged duration of diarrhea following the initial attack.[56] Bacterial virulence factors also may be important,[57] but IBS also can follow non-bacterial enteritis, including viral gastroenteritis,[58] and infection with *Trichinella*,[59] or *Giardia*.[60]

Other risk factors for IBS include an affluent childhood environment,[61] premenopausal and postmenopausal estrogen use,[62] recent antibiotic use,[63] food intolerance,[64,65] extraintestinal somatic symptoms,[65] and poor quality of life (QOL).[66] IBS runs in families,[67] and low birth weight is also a risk factor for IBS, even after controlling for genetic influences.[68] In contrast, oral glucocorticoid users may be at a lower risk for IBS.[69] IBS is associated with an approximately 3-fold increased risk of ischemic colitis[70]; however, a cause-and-effect relationship has not been established, and the absolute risk remains very small (43 per 100,000 person-years). There may be decreased risk of

colorectal cancer in the 1 to 10 years after a diagnosis of IBS is made.[71]

Health Care Seeking

Understanding why a patient presents for care is important in terms of planning appropriate management strategies. There were in excess of 1.5 million physician visits for IBS in the United States in 2009.[72] The rate of health care seeking for IBS may, in part, be affected by health care access; consulting rates in the United States have varied between 25% and 46%, but up to 40% of patients do not have easy access to health care in this country.[73] In Australia, where health care access essentially is universal, consulting rates have been 73%.[73]

What drives health care seeking remains poorly documented.[73] The severity and chronicity of symptoms, especially abdominal pain, partly promote health care seeking.[74,75] IBS patients who consult a physician are more concerned about their health and more fearful of illness than those who do not seek consultation, which suggests that anxiety about illness may be another factor.[73] Children of a parent with IBS may see physicians more often than those who do not have a parent with IBS.[76] As adults, these individuals also are more likely to report poorer health in childhood, and to have received greater parental attention and gifts or rewards for being ill, which suggests early childhood programming of abnormal illness behavior.[77] Those who seek medical attention tend to be more disturbed psychologically than those who do not seek such consultation,[78-81] and those who consult for IBS also are more likely to consult about relatively minor complaints, as well as other non-GI somatic symptoms.[73] There remain other unknown factors that must be important, however, because these psychological factors still seem to poorly explain observed health care-seeking rates.[73]

Excess Abdominal Surgery

There is evidence that patients with IBS are at risk for undergoing excess surgery.[82-84] In a large health maintenance organization study, patients with IBS, compared with controls, reported having had more cholecystectomies (12% vs. 4%), appendectomies (21% vs. 12%), and hysterectomies (33% vs. 17%); IBS was independently associated with these operations.[82] A full explanation for these findings is uncertain, but presumably, some of this excess surgery reflects misdiagnosis and inappropriate intervention.[85] It also is possible that IBS could predispose to an excess of certain diseases that lead to surgery. For example, constipation is associated with an increased risk of gallstones,[86] but whether this association applies to IBS-C is uncertain. Alternatively, a history of a biliary event—identification of gallstones or a cholecystectomy—may be associated with an increased risk of new-onset IBS.[87] Some surgeons continue to believe that patients with IBS-type symptoms respond favorably to intra-abdominal surgery, although IBS patients who undergo cholecystectomy for gallstones show less improvement in QOL than those without IBS.[88]

Impact on Quality of Life and Costs

A systematic review concluded that there was good evidence for a decrease in health-related QOL in patients with moderate to severe IBS,[89] to a degree comparable with other chronic disorders, such as depression or GERD. Rather than IBS causing impaired QOL, an alternative explanation for this association is the converse (i.e., that poor QOL predisposes to a higher risk of IBS), and there is some evidence to support this contention.[66] Regardless, the presence of impaired QOL indicates that IBS deserves serious attention and therapeutic intervention.[89]

IBS is associated with substantial costs because of days lost from work, excess physician visits, diagnostic testing, and use of medications.[90-92] Patients with IBS miss 3 times as many days from work as do those without bowel symptoms.[93] IBS is the sixth leading physician diagnosis in outpatients in the United States, and this is likely an underestimate.[94] A comprehensive burden-of-illness study in the United States estimated that IBS cost almost $1 billion in direct costs and another $50 million in indirect costs.[95] Moreover, patients with IBS consume over 50% more health care resources than do matched controls without IBS.[90]

PATHOPHYSIOLOGY

A number of different mechanisms have been implicated in the pathogenesis of IBS, including abnormal motility, visceral hypersensitivity, low-grade inflammation, and stress.[2,7,96,97]

Genetic factors could modulate the processing of GI signals centrally and the inflammatory and immune responses locally, possibly predisposing to IBS. It seems reasonable to postulate that for IBS to manifest, several abnormalities— multiple hits—might need to occur (Fig. 122-2).

Altered Colonic and Small Bowel Motility

In IBS, diarrhea can result from multiple colonic mechanisms including increased high-amplitude propagated contractions (HAPCs), an enhanced gastrocolic response (prolonged rectosigmoid motor activity in response to a meal), or rectal hypersensitivity.[98-100] Constipation may be secondary to increased segmental (non-propulsive) contractions, decreased HAPCs, or reduced rectal sensation.[101-103] Colonic and small bowel transit has been documented to be delayed in IBS-C, and accelerated in IBS-D.[103]

Abdominal pain in IBS also may be associated with HAPCs.[104] A greater increase in phasic contractions in the terminal ileum and colon has been observed following distention, fatty meals, and CCK in patients with IBS (Fig. 122-3A).[105] Discrete clusters of jejunal contractions also have been noted with increased frequency and duration in IBS (see Fig. 122-3B), and they have been associated with pain in limited numbers of patients with IBS.[105]

Colonic motility in IBS can be increased by stress, anger, or instillation of deoxycholic acid, but this increase, although greater than in controls, is not specific for IBS.[2] A greater increase in colonic phasic contractions has been observed after administration of corticotropin-releasing hormone (CRH),[106]

and is reduced by a CRH antagonist.[107] Patients with IBS have greater small intestinal motor stimulation than controls after CCK infusion, a fatty meal, or ileal distention.[108] Autonomic dysfunction also has been reported in IBS patients with sympathetic adrenergic dysfunction associated with diarrhea and vagal dysfunction with constipation.[109]

Unfortunately, none of these motility parameters can be used as a diagnostic marker for IBS, and there remains no consensus on the exact patterns of motor derangement that actually induce constipation or diarrhea. It is possible that the motor abnormalities observed in IBS are secondary rather than primary phenomena.

Visceral Hypersensitivity

In the 1970s, balloon distention in the rectum was shown to induce pain at lower volumes in patients with IBS.[110] This has been confirmed in multiple studies that used a barostat balloon to control for changes in compliance, leading to the suggestion that colonic hypersensitivity is a useful biological marker of IBS.[111,112] Visceral hypersensitivity might explain the fact that IBS patients seem more likely than controls to be aware of the presence of gas or intestinal contractions after meals or stress. Visceral hypersensitivity probably is confined to the intestine because somatic pain thresholds are normal, although not all studies agree on this.[113-115]

Visceral hypersensitivity is not a universal finding in patients with IBS and affects about 60% of patients (Fig. 122-4).[116] In contrast to control subjects, patients with IBS and normal baseline visceral hypersensitivity might develop rectal hypersensitivity that is induced by repeated distention of the sigmoid colon.[117] This observation suggests that in IBS there is abnormal sensitization within the dorsal horn of the spinal cord or higher up in the central nervous system.

Putative neurotransmitters that are of relevance to visceral hypersensitivity include serotonin, neurokinins, and calcitonin gene-related peptide.[118] The capsaicin (red pepper) receptor on nerve fibers, also called *transient receptor potential vanilloid-1* (TRPV1), appears to be increased in the rectosigmoid colon in IBS and might mediate visceral pain.[119] The N-methyl-D-aspartate (NMDA) receptor also may be important because it modulates central (spinal cord) neuronal excitability.[120] Visceral sensitivity, at least in the esophagus, can be reduced by an NMDA receptor antagonist.[120]

Serine proteases are thought to act as signaling molecules via the activation of proteinase-activated receptors (PARs). Extracts derived from colonic mucosal biopsy specimens of patients with IBS (but not controls) have been observed to sensitize murine nerves in culture; this was blocked by a serine protease inhibitor.[121] A significant increase in serine

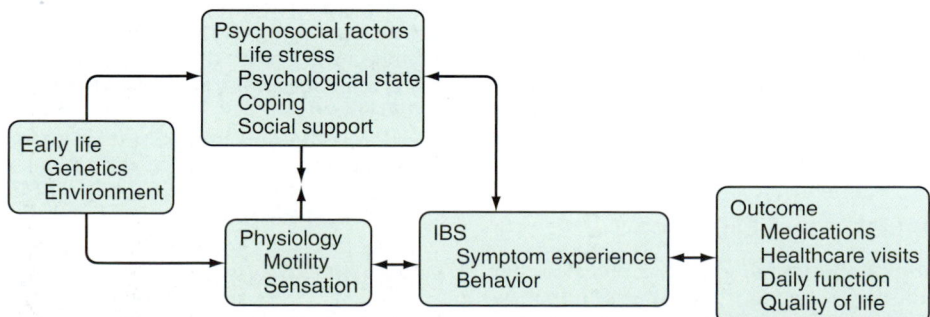

FIGURE 122-2. A conceptual model depicting the relationship between early life, psychosocial factors, physiology, symptom experience, behavior, and outcome. *(Adapted from Drossman D, Camilleri M, Mayer E, Whitehead W. AGA technical review on irritable bowel syndrome. Gastroenterology 2002; 123:2108-31.)*

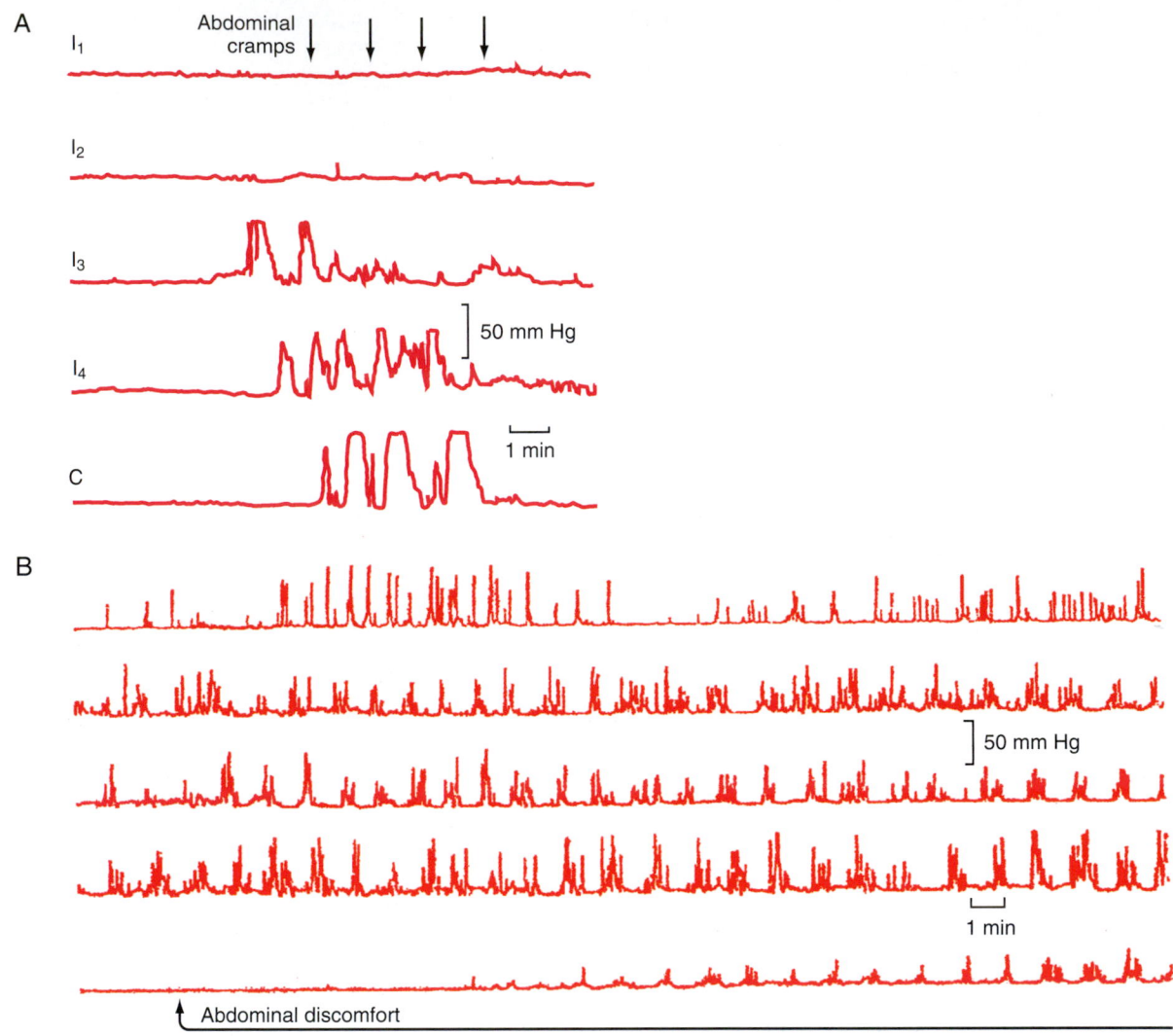

FIGURE 122-3. *A,* Motility recording from 4 sites between the terminal ileum (I_1 to I_4) and the cecum (C) in a patient with IBS. Note the coincidence of abdominal cramps with high-pressure peristaltic waves propagated from the ileum to the colon. *B,* Fasting small intestinal motility recordings from 4 separate sites in a patient with IBS. Note the clusters of contractions (minute rhythm) associated with abdominal discomfort; this pattern is seen more frequently in patients with IBS than in control subjects. *(From Kellow JE, Phillips SF. Altered small bowel motility in irritable bowel syndrome is correlated with symptoms. Gastroenterology 1987; 92:1885-93.)*

proteases has been observed in the stools of patients with IBS-D.[122] Serine proteases could potentially damage tight junctions and increase intestinal permeability via PAR activation.[123] The origin of stool serine proteases is uncertain, but they might derive from mast cells or the fecal microbiota.[123]

It is possible that inflammation is responsible for the sensitization in a subset of patients with IBS, as discussed later; however, numbers of mucosal immune cells were not associated with visceral hypersensitivity in a recent study.[124]

Abnormal Gas Propulsion and Expulsion

Ambulatory monitoring of abdominal girth has revealed that the abdomen normally swells during the day, peaking in the late evening, but decreasing on lying down; this phenomenon, the cause of which is unclear, often is exaggerated in IBS.[125] Retention of gas following its infusion into the small intestine is greater in patients with IBS than it is in healthy controls, and is associated with concomitant sensory dysfunction.[126]

Furthermore, in those with IBS, intestinal gas infusion induces more discomfort than it does in controls when subjects are asked to voluntarily suppress passing the gas.[126] During gas infusion, IBS patients, in contrast to healthy controls, involuntarily suppress their abdominal wall muscle contraction[127] and exhibit paradoxical diaphragmatic contraction, which suggests that abnormal accommodation is implicated in their distension.[128]

IV neostigmine has been demonstrated to clear retained intestinal gas and to reduce abdominal symptoms in patients with IBS and functional bloating.[129] Physical activity might also enhance gas transit,[130] and thus is to be encouraged.

Local Inflammation

The normal intestine is chronically in a state of low-grade, controlled inflammation, which results from interaction between commensal enteric organisms and the host immune system. Inflammatory cells, including mast cells, and activated T lymphocytes are increased above normal in the

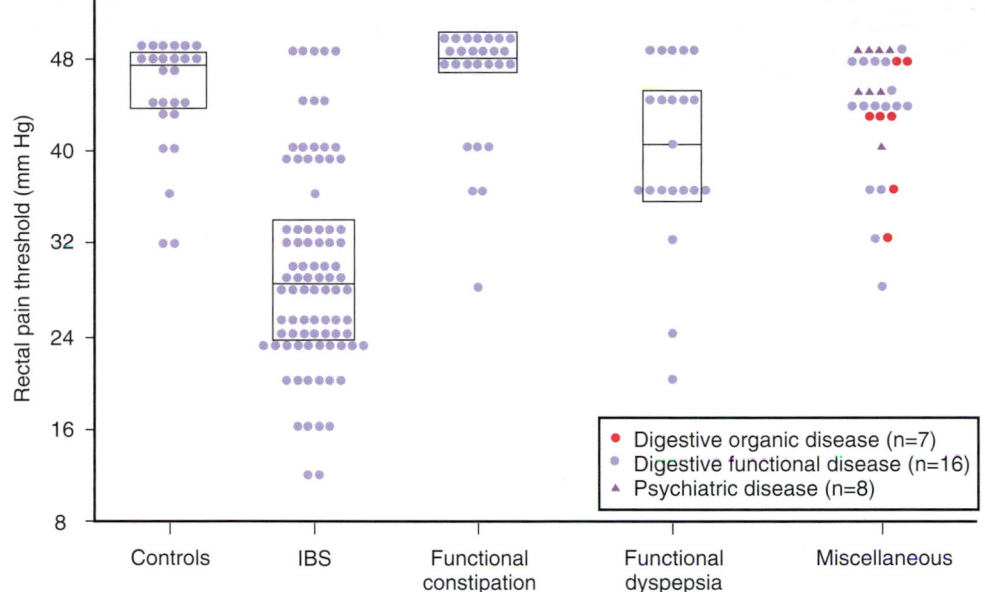

FIGURE 122-4. Distribution of rectal pain thresholds (distention pressure [mm Hg] that induce pain) for each subject in the following groups: asymptomatic controls, patients with IBS, patients with functional constipation, patients with functional dyspepsia, and a miscellaneous group as defined in the key. *Black bars and boxes* represent median ± 25% of pain thresholds and interquartile ranges. At the level of 40 mm Hg, the sensitivity of the rectal barostat for separating IBS patients from normal subjects and non-IBS patients was 95%, and the specificity was 71.8%. *(From Bouin M, Plourde V, Boivin M, et al. Rectal distention testing in patients with irritable bowel syndrome: Sensitivity, specificity, and predictive values of pain sensory thresholds. Gastroenterology 2002; 122:1771-7.)*

mucosa in a subset of patients with IBS,[131] suggesting that a low-grade IBD may be present. Furthermore, lymphocytic infiltration of the myenteric plexus that is associated with neuron degeneration has been observed in severe IBS,[132] as have increased mast cells in the muscularis externa.[133] Increased expression of Toll-like receptors, which are involved in pathogen-recognition, has been demonstrated in mucosal biopsy specimens from IBS patients, suggesting that the intestinal microbiota is engaging with the innate immune system.[134]

From 7% to 30% of patients who have recovered from a proved episode of bacterial enteritis develop IBS.[50-52,54,56,57] One study, however, has suggested that those with preexisting IBS who develop gastroenteritis may be more likely to seek medical consultation, thereby inflating the apparent risk estimates of this group.[135] If the illness lasts more than 3 weeks or there are organisms involved that are toxigenic, then the risk of postinfection IBS is increased[57]; those with psychological distress might have a further increased risk of postinfection IBS (Fig 122-5).[51,54,55] In those who develop postinfection IBS, there are increases in CD3, CD4, and CD8 T lymphocytes, macrophages, and enteroendocrine (enterochromaffin) cells (see Fig. 122-5).[54,136] Increased small intestinal permeability, as demonstrated by the lactulose-mannitol test, also has been reported to occur in postinfection IBS.[57,136] This test is confounded by intestinal transit and bacterial overgrowth, and whether abnormal intestinal permeability occurs remains speculative, although some investigators have demonstrated molecular alterations in tight junction signaling in IBS-D patients.[137]

Mast cells may play a central role in IBS. Activated mast cells release tryptase and histamine and have been observed to lie in close proximity to colonic nerves in patients with IBS; this finding has been correlated with abdominal pain (Fig. 122-6).[138] Supernatants prepared from colonic mucosal biopsies of patients with IBS have been shown to excite rat nociceptive visceral sensory nerves, which suggests that mast cell

mediators, including tryptase, histamine, and prostaglandin E_2, might represent another mechanism inducing visceral hypersensitivity in IBS.[139]

Colonic inflammation is associated with the production of a number of important mediators including 5-hydroxytryptamine (5-HT), prostaglandins, bradykinins, adenosine, and nerve growth factors.[7] Abnormal release of 5-HT might have a central role in the manifestations of IBS.[140] More than 95% of 5-HT is located in the enteroendocrine cells of the intestine, and 5-HT is released from these cells following stroking or increased pressure, such as after a meal; 5-HT then acts on primary intrinsic afferent neurons to initiate the peristaltic reflex via ascending excitation and descending inhibition.[7,141] 5-HT is taken up again by a specific serotonin transporter (SERT) that is expressed in enterocytes. In 1 study, 5-HT reuptake was reduced in IBS compared with controls, although 5-HT release was unaffected and the numbers of enteroendocrine cells were unchanged.[142] The findings were similar in IBS patients with constipation or diarrhea, leading to the hypothesis that in IBS there is increased availability of mucosal 5-HT that can induce diarrhea, but if there is desensitization of 5-HT receptors, this leads to constipation or an alternating bowel pattern[142]; confirmatory data currently are not available.[143] There is some evidence that an exaggerated release of 5-HT in IBS can occur after a meal.[144]

Role of Food

Many patients with IBS attribute their symptoms to certain foods, with wheat, dairy products, citrus fruits, potatoes, onions, and chocolate most commonly implicated.[145,146]

Wheat Intolerance or Allergy

Substantial amounts of wheat are eaten in Western countries, 10% to 15% of which is not digested by human enzymes.[7]

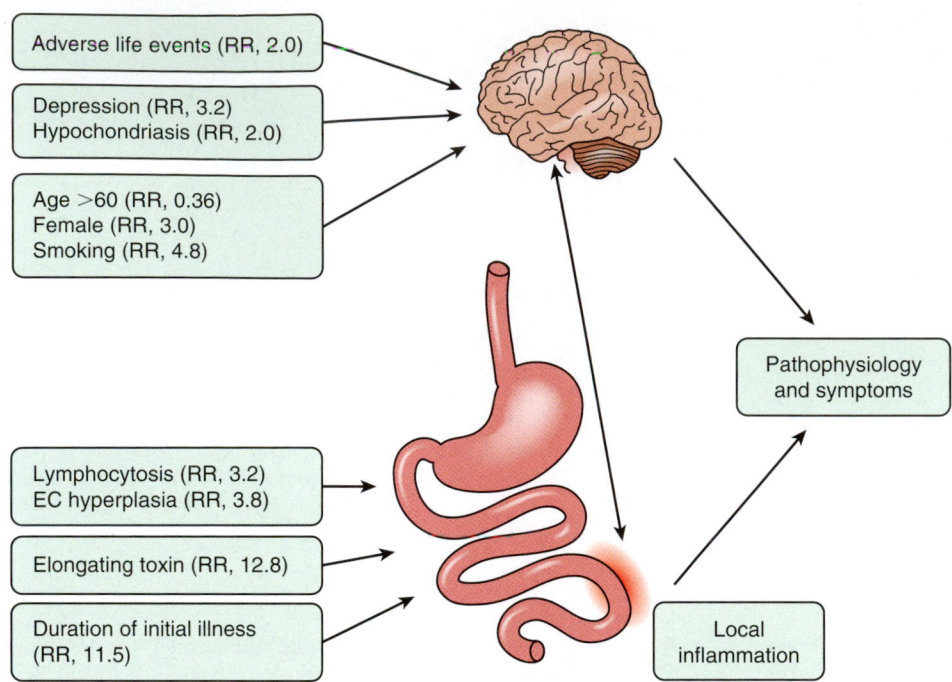

FIGURE 122-5. Postinfection IBS: A summary of established risk factors. EC, enterochromaffin cell; RR, relative risk. (*Adapted from Spiller R, Lam C. An update on post-infectious irritable bowel syndrome: Role of genetics, immune activation, serotonin and altered microbiome. J Neurogastroenterol Motil 2012; 18:258-68.*)

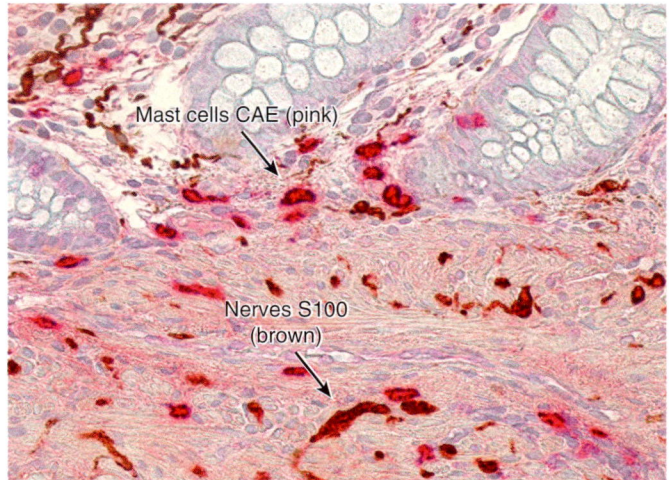

FIGURE 122-6. Rectal mucosal biopsy specimen from an IBS-diarrhea (IBS-D) patient. Note that mast cells (chloroacetate esterase reaction) lie in close proximity to nerves (S100 immunostaining). (*Image courtesy Drs. Suresh Ladva and Marjorie Walker, Newcastle, Australia.*)

There is growing evidence for the existence of non-celiac wheat intolerance as a distinct clinical entity.[147] In a double-blind placebo-controlled trial conducted among IBS sufferers in whom celiac disease had been excluded, a gluten-free diet led to a significant improvement in symptoms, compared with those who continued to ingest gluten.[148]

Sugar Malabsorption

Symptoms of IBS can be confused with those of lactose intolerance.[149] Prevalence of lactose intolerance depends on one's ethnic group and is seen in 10% of populations of northern European descent, 40% to 60% of persons of Asian descent, 90% of Chinese, and 60% to 80% of Africans (see Chapter 104). In acquired hypolactasia, there is some residual ability to digest small amounts of lactose, and because most people do not ingest more than 12.5 g of lactose a day, they do not suffer from such ingestion.[150] Unless a lactose-intolerant patient regularly ingests substantial amounts of lactose, lactose intolerance cannot explain the symptoms of IBS.[151]

Fructose and sorbitol malabsorption might contribute to IBS symptoms in some patients; however, fructose and sorbitol malabsorption, with a prevalence of 30% in those with IBS, may be no more common than in the background population.[152-155] In a double-blind rechallenge trial, 25 IBS patients who responded to fructose withdrawal were challenged with fructose or fructans; nearly 80% developed symptoms compared with less than 15% who were given glucose.[154]

Abnormal Colonic Flora and SIBO

It has been suggested that the colonic flora could be abnormal in a subset of patients with IBS, resulting in increased colonic fermentation, production of excess gas, and development of symptoms.[156] Global and deep molecular analysis of fecal samples from IBS patients demonstrate that the intestinal microbiota are significantly different from that of controls[157]; there are increased *Dorea, Ruminococcus,* and *Clostridium* species, and reduced *Bacteroidetes, Bifidobacterium,* and *Faecalibacterium,* leading to conjecture that in the future, it may be possible to diagnose IBS based on fecal microbiota patterns;[158] this observation has led to interest in the use of pre- and probiotic therapy and fecal microbiota transplantation to modulate the intestinal microbiota of patients with IBS.

SIBO has been speculated to contribute to bloating in IBS, but this is not established with certainty.[159,160] Although modest increases of bacteria have been documented in the proximal small intestine of patients with IBS,[161] a meta-analysis demonstrated that SIBO rates studied by a variety of different tests, including positive lactulose breath testing as a surrogate marker of SIBO, do not differ between patients with IBS and controls.[162] In addition, the abnormal rise in hydrogen during breath testing in a subset of IBS patients actually may have resulted from accelerated orocecal transit.[163]

Bile Acids

Escape of bile acids into the colon leads to secretory diarrhea. Excessive synthesis of bile acids has been implicated in the pathogenesis of IBS-D, with higher concentrations of bile acids in the stool of patients with IBS-D compared with those who have IBS-C.[164] This may occur because of increased bile acid synthesis and excretion that results from impaired negative feedback of bile acid reabsorption in the terminal ileum, via the effect of fibroblast growth factor 19 on hepatic synthesis.

Central Dysregulation

Visceral afferent signals from the intestine reach the brainstem and thalamus and are consciously perceived only occasionally, although there may be some subliminal registration of low-intensity signals.[1] Abnormal modulation of visceral afferent signals can occur at multiple levels in visceral, spinal, and central regions of the nervous system. Based on cerebral blood flow changes, functional brain imaging studies (functional MRI or PET) have suggested alterations in the brain response to visceral stimuli in IBS. Consistent activation of areas associated with emotional arousal, such as the cingulate cortex and amygdala, and the midbrain cluster, which modulates endogenous pain, has been reported following rectal distention.[165] These observations could explain why anxiety or stress can enhance perception of visceral pain, whereas relaxation or distraction decreases pain in IBS. Sex differences in brain networks concerned with anti-nociceptive and autonomic responses following rectal distention in IBS also have been observed.[166]

Psychological Factors (see Chapter 22)

Depression, anxiety, and somatization are the most common psychiatric conditions that coexist in IBS; in referral practice, 40% to 94% of patients with IBS are so affected.[167] Some have suggested that consultation (referral) bias explains the higher rates of psychological and psychiatric comorbidity in IBS patients compared with controls,[2,79-81,168-170] but other data suggest the association is real.[168-170] In patients with IBS, a history of sexual, physical, or emotional abuse also is reported more often than in those without IBS.[171-173] Abuse has not been shown to alter rectal sensation,[174] but it might modulate central responses to pain.[175,176] Patients with IBS are more likely to report greater lifetime and daily stressful events than those with organic disease or healthy controls, and may be more susceptible to stress-altering GI function.[2]

Childhood stress may be particularly important.[96] Gastric suction at birth was associated with a subsequent 3-fold increased risk of having a hospital admission for unexplained abdominal pain (or GI symptoms) compared with sibling controls who had not undergone gastric suction.[177] In rats, maternal separation in the perinatal period induces an anxiety state and is associated with visceral hypersensitivity.[96] Furthermore, in rats, moderately severe stress leads to the release of CRH and acceleration of colonic transit.[178] Stress in healthy volunteers changes intestinal secretion and permeability responses.[179] Sustained stress could, therefore, be important in both the onset and persistence of IBS.

Anxiety and depression, rather than being a primary problem, might occur secondary to production of proinflammatory cytokines.[180] Among community subjects who were free of anxiety or depression at baseline, the presence of IBS predicted new-onset anxiety or depression 12 years later.[46] Immune activation of the intestine has been linked to elevated TNF-α levels and anxiety, suggesting that anxiety in IBS might occur secondary to intestinal inflammation in some cases.[181]

Genetic Factors

Limited, but increasing, evidence points to at least a small hereditary component of IBS. There is clustering of IBS in families.[67,182,183] Twin studies generally have shown that there is a greater concordance of IBS in monozygotic compared with dizygotic twins, which suggests a modest genetic component, although the environmental component probably is much greater.[68,184-187]

Potential candidate genes have been reported to be associated with IBS, but further confirmatory evidence is required, and their functional significance must be unraveled.[188] A specific sodium channel mutation has been identified in IBS (SCN5A).[189] Patients with IBS have been reported to have significantly lower frequencies of the high-producer genotypes of interleukin (IL)-10. A lower amount of this anti-inflammatory cytokine might predispose to greater inflammation in response to an infectious insult in IBS,[190] and this is supported by a meta-analysis.[191] Associations with polymorphisms of the promoter region of the serotonin transporter gene in IBS have not been consistent,[189,192,193] although a functional variant in the serotonin type III receptor gene may be associated with IBS-D in women.[194]

Gene-environment interactions are likely to be more important, with emerging data to suggest, for example, that in the setting of a GNβ3 polymorphism, GI infection predisposes to the development of IBS.[195] Other data potentially implicate certain genes that are involved in the epithelial cell barrier and in the immune response to intestinal bacteria.[196]

DIAGNOSIS

Patients presenting with IBS-like symptoms who also report alarm features (or "red flags") warrant prompt investigation. Alarm features include any history of bleeding or unexplained weight loss, evidence of anemia, unexplained vomiting, progressive dysphagia, a family history of malignancy, and new-onset symptoms in older age (Box 122-2).[149,197,198] Traditional alarm features, however, have poor diagnostic utility.[2] For example, night-time symptoms are common in IBS and do not discriminate IBS from organic disease,[198] although most physicians would investigate patients awakened in the middle of the night by pain, or those with nocturnal diarrhea. While a negative colonoscopy is not required to diagnose IBS, any patient 50 years of age or older requires a colonoscopy, if one has not been performed previously, to exclude other disease, particularly colon cancer. Although older persons can develop IBS, risk of organic disease increases with advancing age.

Patients who meet the Rome criteria for IBS and who have no alarm features are unlikely to have a cause for their presentation other than IBS. For example, among 98 patients who met the Rome I criteria and had no alarm features, 50% of whom had been referred because of diagnostic uncertainty, the Rome I criteria had a positive predictive value of up to 100%, although their sensitivity was only 65%.[199]

Systematic reviews have evaluated the yield of diagnostic tests in IBS.[8] The results, based on limited numbers of referred patients, suggest that IBS patients do not have an increased risk of most organic diseases, compared with non-IBS controls. Extensive investigations to exclude the usual diseases are expensive, and carry the danger of potentially reinforcing abnormal illness behavior. There also is the risk of uncovering findings that are irrelevant to the diagnosis, but that may precipitate more expensive, and even dangerous, investigations.

Traditional screening tests that have low yields in IBS patients include a full blood count, renal and liver biochemical testing, thyroid function testing, and evaluation of 3 fresh stool samples for parasites; these are inexpensive tests, and they can be reassuring for both patient and physician if they are negative or normal.[7] An elevated C-reactive protein, although nonspecific, can indicate the presence of undiagnosed Crohn's disease, albeit only in a minority of cases. Fecal calprotectin has been shown to discriminate IBS from Crohn's disease with excellent sensitivity and specificity, although it is important to know that false-positive testing occurs with NSAID use.[13,200] Evaluation of the small intestine either radiologically or via capsule endoscopy has a very low yield in the setting of typical IBS symptoms without alarm features. Hydrogen breath testing to identify lactose intolerance or SIBO cannot be endorsed routinely.[162] Bile salt malabsorption, detected by seleno-25-homo-tauro-cholic acid (SeHCAT) scan has been proposed to explain IBS-D symptoms in up to 30% of patients, although many of the studies examining this issue have been retrospective, and so routine testing for bile salt malabsorption cannot be recommended at this time.[201] If diarrhea is persistent, colonoscopy with biopsy may be considered because microscopic colitis can mimic IBS-D symptoms,[202] although in a recent study the yield of colonic biopsy was only 1.5%.[203] In a setting of severe constipation, exclusion of pelvic outlet obstruction with anorectal manometry, including balloon expulsion testing, should be considered because the result might alter management.[2,7,25]

Routine testing for celiac disease is now recommended in patients with typical symptoms of IBS-D.[2] Data from a meta-analysis have shown a 4-fold increased odds of celiac disease in patients with IBS,[204] but rates in the United States appear lower.[205] Decision analysis suggests that testing is cost-effective unless the prevalence of celiac disease falls to less than 1% in the population with IBS-like symptoms.[206] A screening test (tissue transglutaminase antibody) in individuals who are consuming a normal diet, followed by duodenal biopsies in those with a positive test, should therefore be considered. Latent celiac disease (antibody positive, biopsy normal) might respond to a gluten-free diet, but its prevalence in IBS is unclear.[207]

Objective tests for positively identifying IBS are under active investigation using multiple serum (e.g., cytokines) or stool markers (e.g., fecal chromogranins and secretogranins),[208,209] but their diagnostic utility in this circumstance is yet to be established.

In summary, the diagnosis of IBS can be made by history (with particular attention to presence or absence of the Rome criteria) if there is an absence of any red flags. In this setting, the patient who responds to an empiric trial of therapy for IBS does not require any further diagnostic evaluation other than celiac serology (Fig. 122-7).[197] Those who fail to respond should undergo more extensive evaluation, depending on the predominant symptoms.

TREATMENT

Education and Support

IBS tends to be a life-long disorder, and establishment of a strong physician-patient relationship is key to providing the best clinical care.[7,210] Patients with IBS often perceive their physician as having a highly negative medical belief about the disorder, and this perception itself impedes best care.[211,212] A good physician-patient relationship has been associated with reduced use of medical services.[213]

It is important to discover why the patient has decided to visit the health care provider at the time he or she did. The reasons can vary: new life stressors, exacerbating factors in the diet or changes in medications, increased fear of serious disease, and the development of treatable psychiatric comorbidity. A hidden agenda, however, such as seeking disability or new narcotic abuse sometimes explains the consulting behavior. In terms of providing optimal reassurance, it is important first to educate patients and then to actively reassure them. Patients typically want to understand why their symptoms have occurred; they also want to obtain validation that their symptoms are real. Specific education classes appear to be useful therapeutic interventions,[214,215] and their benefit is supported by randomized controlled trials (RCTs).[216]

A stepped-care approach depending on the severity of the presenting symptoms provides a useful guide for considering therapies (Table 122-1).[217]

Diet and Lifestyle

The standard of care for IBS typically has been a high-fiber diet.[218,219] Data from a meta-analysis of RCTs indicate that soluble fiber, such as ispaghula (psyllium hydrophilic mucilloid; ispaghula husk), is of global benefit, with a number needed to treat (NNT) of 6 (Table 122-2), but insoluble fiber is no better than placebo.[220] NNT is used to assess the effectiveness of a health care intervention and is the number of patients who need to be treated to achieve 1 additional beneficial outcome. Fiber is not helpful for pain, but can benefit constipation and can sometimes firm up loose stools.

Fiber supplements should begin at a low dose and be increased very slowly in order to reduce the bloating, gas, and pain that typically are aggravated by their use. If the goal is

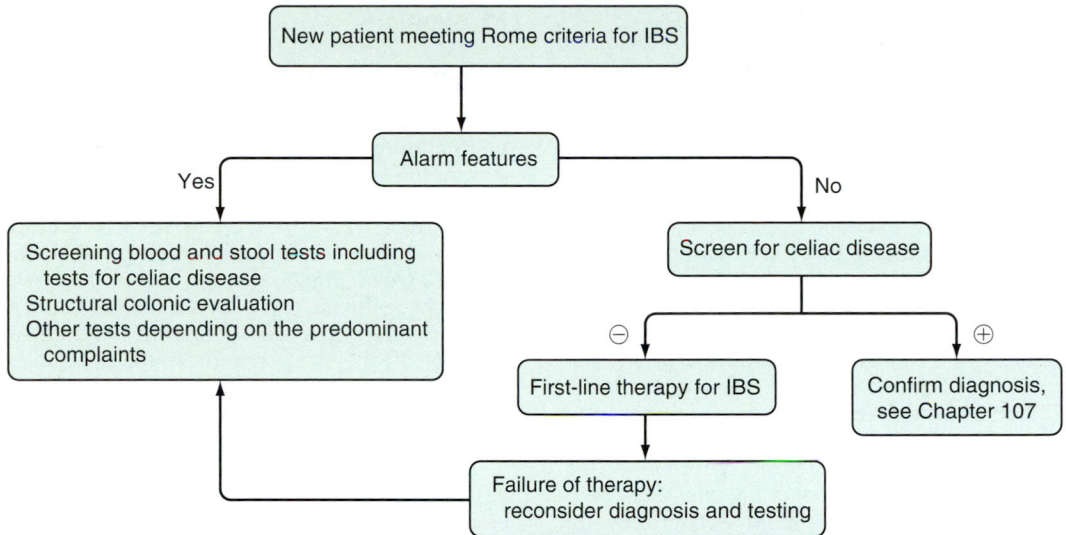

FIGURE 122-7. Algorithm for diagnostic testing in patients with possible IBS according to the Rome criteria. *(Adapted from Cash BD, Chey WD. Irritable bowel syndrome: An evidence-based approach to diagnosis. Aliment Pharmacol Ther 2004; 19:1235-45.)*

TABLE 122-1 Suggested Sequence of Treatment of IBS

Predominant Symptom	First Step	Second Step
Bloating	Adjust diet Treat constipation	Probiotic (e.g., containing *Bifidobacteria infantis*) Nonabsorbable antibiotic (e.g., rifaximin) Tricyclic antidepressant, SSRI
Constipation	Fiber supplement (e.g., ispaghula) Polyethylene glycol	Lubiprostone, linaclotide
Diarrhea	Loperamide	5-HT$_3$ antagonist (e.g., alosetron)
Abdominal pain	Antispasmodic, peppermint oil	Tricyclic antidepressant, SSRI Psychological therapy

5-HT, 5-hydroxytryptamine; SSRIs, selective serotonin reuptake inhibitors.

TABLE 122-2 Efficacy of Selected Non-pharmacologic Treatments for IBS

Non-pharmacologic Treatment	Number Needed to Treat	Adverse Effects	Comments
Hypnotherapy	2-3	No reports of adverse events in published randomized trials	Several controlled trials in different settings and populations support long-term efficacy
Cognitive behavioral therapy	3	No reports of adverse events in published randomized trials	Can be delivered effectively using the Internet
Soluble fiber	6	74% (any individual adverse effect)	No serious/life-threatening adverse event have been reported
Low FODMAP diet	4-5	No adverse effects reported	Small trials only
Exercise	6-7	No adverse effects reported	Single controlled trial only; results are only statistically significant for preventing a clinically important increase in symptoms
Probiotics	4	Adverse event rate similar to placebo	Magnitude of the benefit and the most effective species and doses remain uncertain

FODMAP, Fermentable oligo-di-mono-saccharides, and polyols.
Adapted from Halland M, Talley NJ. New treatments for IBS. Nat Rev Gastroenterol Hepatol 2012; 10:13-23.

to supplement approximately 10 to 15 g of fiber in total, the amount should be increased by 3 g every 1 to 2 weeks; for example, a tablespoon of most of the powder fiber supplements contains about 6 g of fiber.

Many patients with IBS suspect that food intolerance may be relevant to their symptoms. It is useful to determine the amounts of milk and milk products being consumed to decide whether lactose intolerance testing should be considered. Clinical experience suggests that even in the setting of a diagnosis of lactose intolerance and typical IBS symptoms, more often than not, IBS symptoms persist despite withdrawal of all lactose in the diet, indicating a chance overlap of common conditions.

Exclusion diets can be useful in some patients. One randomized trial measured immunoglobulin (Ig)G antibodies to foods and allocated subjects to an elimination diet based on the results, or sham diet.[221] Symptom scores were significantly lower among individuals who received an elimination diet. Recent interest has surrounded the potential role of fermentable oligosaccharides, disaccharides, monosaccharides, and polyols (FODMAPs) in generating symptoms in IBS, via their fermentation and osmotic effects. High FODMAP-containing foods include fruits (e.g., apples, cherries, peaches), artificial sweeteners, legumes, and green vegetables such as broccoli, sprouts, cabbage, and peas. In a trial that switched IBS patients between diets that were either low or high in FODMAPs, symptoms were significantly worse during the high-FODMAP diet (see Table 122-2).[222] Wheat intolerance may also be involved, and a recent trial conducted among IBS patients without confirmed celiac disease demonstrated that a gluten-free diet led to adequate control of symptoms in 60%.[148] A gluten-containing diet has been shown to increase small intestinal permeability, especially in HLA-DQ2/8 positive IBS patients with diarrhea,[223] which may allow luminal intestinal bacteria to activate an immune response in the GI mucosa.

Exercise has been shown to improve symptoms in IBS. Trial participants allocated to increased physical exercise demonstrated significant improvements in symptom severity scores compared with their scores at baseline, whereas those told to maintain current activity levels were more likely to experience worsening of symptoms (see Table 122-2).[224]

Medication

Anticholinergic and Antispasmodic Agents

In the United States, anticholinergic agents (dicyclomine, propantheline, belladonna, and hyoscyamine) continue to be used commonly for IBS.[220,225] A meta-analysis of RCTs concluded that antispasmodics were superior to placebo in the treatment of IBS (Table 122-3).[220] Overall, there was an improvement of abdominal pain and IBS global symptoms in the pooled analyses[220]; however, the quality of most of these trials was low, the results were mixed, and publication bias could not be excluded. Moreover, only the anticholinergic antispasmodic agents are available in the United States.[2] Non-anticholinergic antispasmodics, unavailable in the United States, that appear to be efficacious include otilonium (imetropium) and certain selective calcium channel blockers (e.g., pinaverium).[220]

Anticholinergic agents clinically seem most useful for patients with postprandial pain when taken 30 minutes before eating. No advantage of sublingual or suppository forms over oral anticholinergic preparations has been documented in patients with IBS. Peppermint oil is efficacious in IBS for abdominal pain, and is usually well tolerated; the NNT is 2.5 (see Table 122-3).[220] The usual dose of peppermint oil is 0.2 mL (4 drops) 3 times a day 30 minutes before meals (swallowed not chewed); adverse effects can include heartburn, perianal burning, and rarely interstitial nephritis.

Laxatives

The efficacy of this class of drugs for IBS-C is uncertain. In 1 RCT conducted among adolescents with IBS-C, polyethylene glycol, an osmotic laxative, significantly increased stool frequency, but had no effect on abdominal pain.[226] Stimulant laxatives are probably safer than has been appreciated, but they often induce abdominal cramping or pain and generally seem unsatisfactory for patients with IBS.[227]

Lubiprostone and linaclotide are drugs that act on chloride channels and guanylate cyclase receptors in the intestinal enterocyte, respectively, thereby stimulating intestinal fluid secretion (see Table 122-3). For women with IBS-C, a lower

---

TABLE 122-3 Efficacy of Selected Pharmacologic Treatments for IBS

Pharmacologic Treatment	Number Needed to Treat	Approximate Number Needed to Harm or Adverse Effects	Comments
Treatments for IBS-C			
Chloride channel activators (lubiprostone)	13	N/A	Up to 25% were reported to suffer nausea; no serious adverse events Long-term data, report less nausea than previously
Guanylate cyclase agonists (linaclotide)	7-8	20	Diarrhea is the most common adverse effect, occurring in ≈5%
Selective serotonin reuptake inhibitors	3-4	18	None
Treatments for IBS-D			
Rifaximin	11	8971	None
5-HT$_3$ receptor antagonists (e.g., alosetron)	8	19	Rare reports of ischemic colitis; use currently restricted to women under a risk-management strategy
Tricyclic antidepressants	8	18	None
Antispasmodics	5	17-18	Most common adverse events are dry mouth, dizziness, and blurred vision Efficacy of anticholinergics is not established
Peppermint oil	2-3	N/A	Adverse event rate is comparable to placebo

Adapted from Halland M, Talley NJ. New treatments for IBS. Nat Rev Gastroenterol Hepatol 2012; 10:13-23.

dose of lubiprostone currently is FDA approved (8 µg twice daily) than is used for chronic constipation (24 µg twice daily); the global benefit over placebo in IBS-C, however, is modest.[228] Linaclotide has been studied at a dose of 290 µg once daily in 2 large phase III trials in IBS-C, with NNTs of 7 or 8 versus placebo. Linaclotide is FDA approved for IBS-C.[229,230]

Antidiarrheal Agents

Loperamide is efficacious based on RCTs in IBS-D, but it does not improve abdominal pain or bloating.[231,232] It is most effective when taken prophylactically, rather than being taken after diarrhea has occurred; doses of loperamide range from 2 to 16 mg/day, and high doses seem safe. Diphenoxylate has not been tested in IBS, but may be similarly efficacious. Codeine phosphate, because of its side effects (dizziness, nausea, sedation) and high risk of inducing dependence, should be avoided in IBS. Bismuth subsalicylate anecdotally is also useful for control of diarrhea in IBS but must be used intermittently because of concerns about bismuth toxicity.

Serotonin-Receptor Drugs

Alosetron is a 5-HT$_3$ antagonist that is efficacious in women with severe IBS-D. The NNT is 8 (see Table 122-3),[233] and the drug has been shown to improve QOL.[234] The starting dose is 0.5 to 1 mg daily. In the United States, it is available only via a restricted prescribing program because of concerns about ischemic colitis and severe constipation.[235] The dose can be increased to 1 mg twice daily after 4 weeks if symptoms are not controlled and there have been no adverse effects. Ischemic colitis occurs in 0.1% of alosetron-treated patients and is drug related but dose independent; the ischemia is usually transient and without irreversible consequence, although up to 50% of patients with alosetron-associated ischemic colitis required hospitalization.[236] Constipation occurs in one third of alosetron-treated patients. The prescription of the drug is absolutely contraindicated in IBS patients with any history of constipation, thrombotic tendency, or ischemic colitis.

Antidepressants and Anxiolytics

The tricyclic antidepressants (TCAs) appear to be efficacious in IBS but might improve global well-being more than symptoms.[237] A meta-analysis reported the NNT to be 4 (see Table 122-3), although there were a number of low-quality trials.[238] A large, high-quality randomized placebo-controlled trial of desipramine (at a dose of 50 to 150 mg) in female patients showed that 60% were responders to the TCA versus 47% to placebo; this difference failed to reach significance in the intention-to-treat analysis but was significant in the per-protocol analysis.[239]

When using a TCA in IBS, it is recommended to start it at a low dose (e.g., 10 to 25 mg of desipramine or nortriptyline) and increase the dose by 10 to 25 mg weekly, aiming for a dose of 50 mg initially. Many patients do not require full antidepressant dosing unless comorbid depression is present. TCAs tend to be constipating, and therefore they may be of most benefit in IBS-D, although data to support this postulate are lacking. Adverse events with TCAs are a problem. Approximately 1 in 3 treated patients develops adverse effects, including drowsiness, dizziness, and dry mouth, with 1 in 22 adverse effects being potentially serious; up to 40% discontinue use or change therapy because of intolerance.[240]

The selective serotonin reuptake inhibitors (SSRIs) cause fewer side effects than the TCAs, and a meta-analysis of RCTs in IBS has reported a global benefit of SSRIs, with an NNT of

3.5 (see Table 122-3).[238] Findings among individual studies were inconsistent, however, and a recent trial conducted among non-depressed IBS patients reported no benefit.[241] It is possible that SSRIs may be more beneficial in IBS-C because they accelerate small intestinal transit.[242]

Benzodiazepines might have a small benefit over placebo in IBS, but the evidence for this observation is very weak.[243] Because of habituation, this class of drugs generally should be avoided.

Antibiotics

The nonabsorbable antibiotic rifaximin was superior to placebo in non-constipated patients with IBS in 2 large short-term treatment trials, for both global symptoms and bloating[244]; treatment effect was modest, however, with an NNT of 11 (see Table 122-3). The dose used was 550 mg 3 times daily for 14 days. The benefit seemed durable up to 10 weeks post therapy, but treatment of a recurrence of IBS symptoms with another course of rifaximin is not currently recommended, although uncontrolled data suggest patients will respond.[245]

Probiotics

It has been suggested that abnormal colonic microbiota could be relevant in the pathogenesis of IBS, which has led to great interest in using probiotics to try to naturally alter commensal organisms. Some initial small trials produced promising results with *Bifidobacterium infantis* and combination products.[246,247] A meta-analysis reported that the NNT with probiotics was 4,[248] although with considerable heterogeneity among studies, and different strains and species being used, so it was difficult to ascertain which, if any, were of particular benefit (see Table 122-2).

Drugs Acting on Pain Receptors

Pregabalin and gabapentin, drugs believed to inhibit pain via calcium channels, have been studied in small randomized trials. Pregabalin demonstrated a trend toward an improvement in average daily pain scores compared with placebo.[249] IBS patients treated with gabapentin demonstrated significantly increased rectal compliance, as well as higher sensory thresholds for bloating, discomfort, and pain.[250] Either of these could therefore be considered in patients with particularly troublesome pain or bloating (Table 122-4).

Emerging Drugs

AST-120, a carbon-based substance that can adsorb histamine, serotonin, and other substances implicated in IBS has been tested, but results at 8 weeks were disappointing.[251] LX1031 is another agent that interferes with serotonin, via inhibition of tryptophan hydroxylase. In a phase II study in non-constipated IBS, the drug led to a significant improvement in pain and discomfort at week 1, but the effect attenuated with time (see Table 122-4).[252]

Asimadoline, an agonist at the κ-opioid receptor, appeared promising in a small crossover trial,[253] although larger randomized trials have been disappointing.[254,255] Dextofisopam, a benzodiazepine receptor modulator, has been tested in non-constipated IBS. Although an improvement in bowel consistency was observed, more patients randomized to dextofisopam experienced worsening of abdominal pain.[256]

Inhibition of cholecystokinin (CCK) or corticotropin releasing hormone (CRH) may improve symptoms of IBS. Dexloxiglumide, a CCK antagonist, has been studied in female IBS-C patients, and the proportion with satisfactory relief of

TABLE 122-4 Selected Emerging and Possible Future Pharmacologic Treatments for IBS

Drug Class	Example of Drug	Comments
Drugs Acting on Pain Receptors		
Calcium channel inhibitors	Pregabalin and gabapentin	Improved pain scores, increased rectal compliance, and higher thresholds for pain, discomfort, and bloating
Drugs Targeting Visceral Hypersensitivity		
Serotonin synthesis inhibitors	LX1031	Positive phase II trial data, including a favorable adverse event profile, although the effect is attenuated with time
Peripheral opioid receptor agonists	Asimadoline/ JN-38488502	Promising findings from animal data have not been replicated in human studies
CCK-1 antagonists	Dexloxiglumide	Satisfactory relief of symptoms is higher than with placebo in females with IBS-C
Drugs Targeting Motility		
Corticotrophin-releasing factor antagonists	Pexacerfont	No effect on stool frequency, consistency, or IBS symptoms
$5HT_4$ agonists	Velusetrag, prucalopride, naronapride	Prucalopride is effective in chronic constipation; data from trials in IBS patients are awaited
Drugs Targeting Inflammation		
Mast cell stabilizers	Ketotifen	Promising data from a small controlled trial
5-ASA	Mesalazine	Well-designed trials in IBS patients are ongoing
Centrally Acting Drugs		
Benzodiazepine receptor modulators	Dextofisopam	Improved bowel consistency in a small trial, but concerns have been raised about higher rates of abdominal pain compared with placebo
Bile Acid Modulators		
Bile acid sequestrants	Colesevelam	Case reports of efficacy and limited trial data
Bile acid transporter inhibitor	A3309	Promising data from patients with chronic constipation
Bile acid	Chenodeoxycholate	Healthy volunteer data have demonstrated accelerated colonic transit

Adapted from Halland M, Talley NJ. New treatments for IBS. Nat Rev Gastroenterol Hepatol 2012; 10:13-23.

symptoms was higher than with placebo, although this was not statistically significant.[257] Pexacerfont, a CRH antagonist, has been evaluated in women with IBS-D, but had no effect on stool frequency or consistency, or subjective IBS symptoms, including pain and bloating.[258]

Targeting mast cells may be beneficial, with 1 small trial that demonstrated a trend towards a higher rate of relief of symptoms with ketotifen, compared with placebo (20% vs. 10%).[259] Mesalamine may also inhibit mast cells in IBS,[260] and a rigorous randomized trial is ongoing.[261] Other therapies include bile acid sequestrants, such as colesevelam, bile acid transporter inhibitors, and pancreatic enzyme supplements, all of which are under investigation.[262-264]

Placebo

The placebo response rate in IBS is high, estimated at 40% in a meta-analysis.[265] A recent trial randomized IBS patients to either open-label placebo, which they were told had "beneficial effects through mind-body self-healing processes," or no treatment.[266] Almost 50% of patients assigned to placebo reported adequate relief of symptoms, which was significantly higher than with no treatment.

Psychological Treatments

Psychotherapy, hypnotherapy, and cognitive behavioral therapy (CBT) have been proposed as useful treatments for IBS.[2] A systematic review concluded that these therapies were superior to wait-list controls (who are followed similarly, but are not treated) (see Table 122-2).[238] Hypnotherapy can improve cognition in IBS.[267] Excellent efficacy data exist for CBT,[268,269] albeit not in all controlled trials.[270] Mindfulness training, a technique involving focusing on present-moment experience and nonjudgmental awareness of body sensations, has been shown to be more effective, in terms of improvement in symptom severity, than a support group.[271]

There are no head-to-head studies that compare the different psychological interventions or combination therapies. Based on the available literature, IBS patients with abdominal pain, diarrhea, and psychological distress appear most likely to have a beneficial response to such intervention, particularly if the symptoms have been of short duration and have waxed and waned.[2] Patients with constant abdominal pain do poorly with psychological treatment.[2] Indeed, symptoms tend not to improve; rather, the ability to cope with IBS seems to drive any global benefit. The major advantage of psychological treatment is that despite the initial expense, long-term benefits might offset the cost.[272]

Alternative Treatments

Many different alternative remedies are used by patients with IBS.[273,274] In 1 high-quality RCT, Chinese herbal medicine (comprising a combination of 20 herbs) was superior to placebo, although this requires confirmation,[275] and the risks of using multiple herbal concoctions continue to be of concern.[276] Iberogast, also known as STW 5, which is a combination of various plant extracts, and St. John's wort, have also been the subject of placebo-controlled trials in IBS.[277,278] STW 5 was superior to placebo, but St. John's wort had no benefit. A meta-analysis reported that acupuncture was superior to pharmacologic therapy in several Chinese studies, but it was no more effective, in terms of symptom improvement, than sham acupuncture control.[279]

PROGNOSIS

There is no evidence for even a small increase in mortality in IBS,[280] despite referrals for invasive testing, excess abdominal and other surgery rates, and a link to ischemic colitis.[281] In clinical practice, once a diagnosis of IBS has been made, it usually requires no revision despite prolonged follow-up. Among IBS patients followed for a median of 29 years, survival was not different from expected, although 9% developed organic disease a median of 15 years after diagnosis.[213] Among 75 patients with a clinical diagnosis of IBS followed up for 10 to 13 years, none had another explanation uncovered for their symptoms, yet symptoms did not resolve in 92%, and 47% had undergone a repeat structural colonic evaluation to no avail.[282] Some IBS patients have spontaneous improvement over time, but IBS usually is a relapsing disorder. The presence of excessive psychological distress or anxiety, as well as a long duration of complaints, tends to indicate a poorer prognosis.[2]

KEY REFERENCES

Full references for this chapter can be found on www.expertconsult.com.

1. Drossman D, Corrazziari E, Delvaux M, et al. Rome III: the functional Gastrointestinal Disorders. 3rd ed. McLean, VA: Degnon Associates; 2006.
2. American College of Gastroenterology Task Force on Irritable Bowel Syndrome, Brandt LJ, Chey WD, Foxx-Orenstein AE, et al. An evidence-based position statement on the management of irritable bowel syndrome. Am J Gastroenterol 2009; 104(Suppl 1):S1-35.
33. Lovell RM, Ford AC. Global prevalence of and risk factors for irritable bowel syndrome: A meta-analysis. Clin Gastroenterol Hepatol 2012; 10:712-21.
46. Koloski NA, Jones M, Kalantar J, et al. The brain-gut pathway in functional gastrointestinal disorders is bidirectional: A 12-year prospective population-based study. Gut 2012; 61:1284-90.
72. Peery AF, Dellon ES, Lund J, et al. Burden of gastrointestinal disease in the United States: 2012 update. Gastroenterology 2012; 143:1179-87.
124. Braak B, Klooker TK, Wouters MM, et al. Mucosal immune cell numbers and visceral sensitivity in patients with irritable bowel syndrome: Is there any relationship? Am J Gastroenterol 2012; 107:715-26.
131. Ford AC, Talley NJ. Mucosal inflammation as a potential etiological factor in irritable bowel syndrome: A systematic review. J Gastroenterol 2011; 46:421-31.
134. Brint EK, MacSharry J, Fanning A, et al. Differential expression of Toll-like receptors in patients with irritable bowel syndrome. Am J Gastroenterol 2011; 106:329-36.
147. Carroccio A, Mansueto P, Iacono G, et al. Non-celiac wheat sensitivity diagnosed by double-blind placebo-controlled challenge: Exploring a new clinical entity. Am J Gastroenterol 2012; 107:1898-906.
148. Biesiekierski JR, Newnham ED, Irving PM, et al. Gluten causes gastrointestinal symptoms in subjects without celiac disease: A double-blind randomized placebo-controlled trial. Am J Gastroenterol 2011; 106:508-14.
157. Rajilic-Stojanovic M, Biagi E, Heilig HG, et al. Global and deep molecular analysis of microbiota signatures in fecal samples from patients with irritable bowel syndrome. Gastroenterology 2011; 141:1792-801.
216. Labus J, Gupta A, Gill HK, et al. Randomised clinical trial: Symptoms of the irritable bowel syndrome are improved by a psycho-education group intervention. Aliment Pharmacol Ther 2013; 37:304-15.
222. Ong DK, Mitchell SB, Barrett JS, et al. Manipulation of dietary short chain carbohydrates alters the pattern of gas production and genesis of symptoms in irritable bowel syndrome. J Gastroenterol Hepatol 2010; 25:1366-73.
224. Johannesson E, Simren M, Strid H, et al. Physical activity improves symptoms in irritable bowel syndrome: A randomized controlled trial. Am J Gastroenterol 2011; 106:915-22.
229. Chey WD, Lembo AJ, Lavins BJ, et al. Linaclotide for irritable bowel syndrome with constipation: A 26-week, randomized, double-blind, placebo-controlled trial to evaluate efficacy and safety. Am J Gastroenterol 2012; 107:1702-12.
230. Rao S, Lembo AJ, Shiff SJ, et al. A 12-week, randomized, controlled trial with a 4-week randomized withdrawal period to evaluate the efficacy and safety of linaclotide in irritable bowel syndrome with constipation. Am J Gastroenterol 2012; 107:1714-24.
244. Pimentel M, Lembo A, Chey WD, et al. Rifaximin therapy for patients with irritable bowel syndrome without constipation. N Engl J Med 2011; 364:22-32.

CHAPTER OUTLINE

Impairment to the aboral passage of intestinal contents can result from either a mechanical obstruction of the bowel or failure of normal intestinal motility in the absence of an obstructing lesion (ileus). Several categories have been used to classify differences in the various presentations of intestinal obstruction: degree of obstruction to flow (partial or complete), site of obstruction (small bowel or large bowel), and absence or presence of intestinal ischemia (simple or strangulated). Partial obstruction can be further divided into low grade (intestinal contrast passage not delayed) or high grade (intestinal contrast passage delayed), as defined by Shrake and associates.[1] Clinically, a partial obstruction would manifest as constipation with intolerance to oral intake, whereas patients with a complete obstruction are obstipated. A closed-loop obstruction is a mechanical obstruction in which both the proximal and distal parts of the involved bowel are occluded. These distinctions have important prognostic and therapeutic relevance. For example, partial small bowel obstruction (SBO) usually can be managed successfully without laparotomy, whereas strangulated and closed loop obstructions require urgent operative management.

SMALL BOWEL OBSTRUCTION

Epidemiology

SBO is a common problem with significant social and financial impacts. Based on National Hospital Discharge Survey data, there are between 224,015 and 344,080 hospitalizations for SBO each year.[2] Total cost for hospital and surgical expenditures is estimated to be approximately $1.3 billion yearly.[3] Despite advances in surgical treatment, these rates have not decreased over the last 20 years.[2]

Etiology

The most common cause of SBO is intra-abdominal adhesions following laparotomy; this accounts for approximately 60% to 85% of all cases. Additional causes are Crohn's disease (5% to 7%), neoplasia (2% to 5%), hernia (2% to 3%), radiation (1%), and miscellaneous causes such as volvulus, bezoars, Meckel's diverticulum, diverticulitis, and gallstone ileus (11%).[4-6] The "ABC" mnemonic—Adhesions, Bulge, Cancer/Crohn's—is a useful tool to remember this. A comprehensive list of causes of intestinal obstruction is shown in Box 123-1.

Adhesions

When the peritoneum is damaged, a complex process ensues that involves several cell types, cytokines, coagulation factors, fibrinolysis, and proteases all acting together to restore tissue integrity. It is widely accepted that the fibrinolytic system plays a central role in postoperative peritoneal healing. If fibrinolysis does not occur within 5 to 7 days of the peritoneal injury, the temporary fibrin matrix that persists gradually becomes more organized and leads to adhesion formation.[7]

It is estimated that patients have a 90% chance of developing intraperitoneal adhesions after abdominal surgery, and several factors contribute to the degree to which adhesions develop.[8] The most significant determining factor is the degree of damage to the peritoneum as evidenced by the observation that, with the exception of laparoscopic appendectomy, laparoscopic procedures are associated with lower risks of readmission because of SBO.[9] Additionally, location plays a role because lower abdominal or pelvic operations have a higher risk of adhesive SBO than do upper abdominal surgical procedures, such as cholecystectomy. The density and extent of adhesions can be further exacerbated by intra-abdominal infection, multiplicity of laparotomies, omental resection, external beam radiation, penetrating abdominal trauma, and the presence of foreign material, such as sutures. Risk of adhesive obstruction after appendectomy is approximately 1% at 30 years of follow-up and is greater for patients with

*Dr. Maureen Heldmann contributed to this chapter in previous editions of the textbook.

BOX 123-1 Causes of Intestinal Obstruction

Intrinsic Bowel Lesions
Congenital atresia or stenosis
Inflammatory causes
    Diverticulitis
    IBD (e.g., Crohn's disease)
    Ischemic injury
    Radiation injury
Intussusception
Obturation
    Bezoars
    Feces
    Foreign bodies
    Gallstones
    Polypoid neoplasms

Neoplastic strictures
Surgical anastomosis

Extrinsic Bowel Lesions
Abscess
Adhesions
Carcinomatosis
Congenital bands
Endometriosis
Hernias
Volvulus

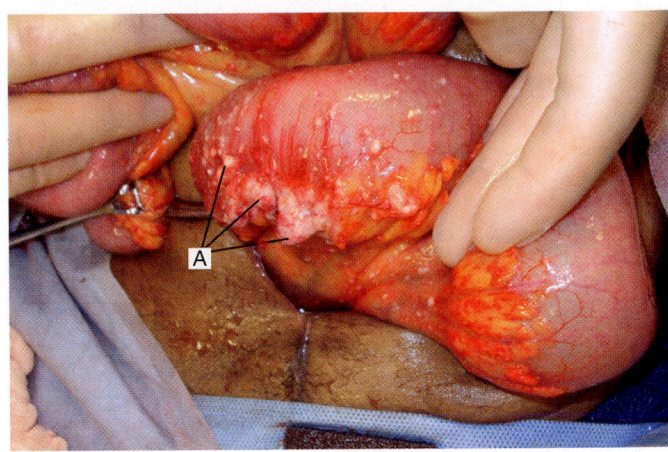

FIGURE 123-1. Bowel obstruction from metastatic colon cancer. Note the whitish-appearing tumor implants (A) on the external surface of the bowel.

perforated appendicitis (2.76% at 30 years) than non-perforated appendicitis (0.75% at 30 years).[10] This risk is in contrast to that after total proctocolectomy with ileal pouch-anal anastomosis, which has an 18% risk at 1 year.[11] Although SBO can occur any time after laparotomy, the risk is greatest in the first year.[12] Using Medicare data, Beck and colleagues found that the incidence of adhesive obstruction after intestinal resection and anastomosis was 14.3% within 2 years.[13]

Hernias

Although hernias account for a smaller percentage of obstructions than adhesions, up to 30% of patients who require an operation for SBO have an incarcerated hernia as the etiology of their obstruction.[4] Intestinal obstruction caused by a hernia has a particularly high risk of strangulation, failure to resolve spontaneously, and recurrence when it is not surgically corrected. In 1 study of 877 patients, three fourths of patients who presented with incarcerated hernias and SBO had ischemic bowel at the time of operation; the bowel was necrotic in 27%.[4] In contrast, only 29% of patients presenting with SBO due to adhesions had a strangulated obstruction, and of these, nonviable bowel was found in 11%.[4] The increased risk of obstruction and strangulation is due, at least in part, to the rigid fascial defect through which the herniated intestine passes. Femoral hernias, in particular, pose a high risk of intestinal strangulation (20% to 40%).[14] Although SBO from a groin hernia can occur at any age, it is particularly prevalent in older adults; advanced age, concomitant chronic illnesses, and treatment delay are associated with unfavorable outcomes in this subset of patients who present with SBO.[15]

Significant variability is noted in the individual etiologies of hernias; therefore, presentation, surgical treatment, and associated risks also vary widely. Abdominal wall hernias, incisional hernias, inguinal, and femoral hernias are much more common causes of SBO than internal or intra-abdominal hernias (e.g., paraduodenal hernias). Internal hernias may be congenital (e.g., paraduodenal) or acquired (e.g., hernias through mesenteric defects created in the performance of intestinal anastomoses). The 3% incidence of internal herniation of the Roux limb after gastric bypass for weight loss is a particularly important example of an internal hernia, given the frequency with which this procedure is performed today.[16] Congenital and acquired internal hernias are discussed in greater detail in Chapter 26.

The incidence of trocar site hernias after laparoscopic procedures is 1% to 2%, but the associated incidence of intestinal obstruction is significantly less common.[17] In these instances, the hernias usually occur at 10-mm port sites that are positioned at or close to the midline.[18] Intestinal obstruction after laparoscopic transabdominal preperitoneal herniorrhaphy usually results from herniation of the bowel through a defect in the peritoneal closure. In these instances, the bowel is tethered by adhesions between the partially peritoneal-covered prosthesis and the intestine, with formation of a kink or a point of torsion.

Crohn's Disease

In patients without previous abdominal surgery, Crohn's disease usually presents with a slower more chronic form of bowel obstruction due to progressive fibrosis over time. In acute exacerbations of Crohn's disease, however, obstruction can occur as a result of inflammation of the affected portion of bowel (see Chapter 115). Patients with Crohn's disease who have had previous bowel resections also can have adhesive obstructions just like patients without Crohn's disease.

Neoplasms

Neoplasms are a relatively unusual cause of SBO, accounting for less than 10% of cases.[5,19] In more than 90% of such neoplastic SBO, the small intestine becomes obstructed by extrinsic compression or by local invasion, usually from advanced GI or gynecologic malignancies (Fig. 123-1), of which colorectal cancer and ovarian adenocarcinoma are the 2 most common neoplasms, respectively. Hematogenous metastases from breast cancer, melanoma, or Kaposi's sarcoma also can involve the small intestine, with subsequent obstruction. Primary neoplasms of the small intestine, of which adenocarcinoma and carcinoid tumors are most common, are the cause of SBO in less than 3% of cases; this is in contrast to the colon, where primary adenocarcinoma accounts for more than 50% of instances of obstruction that result from neoplasms (see Chapters 125 and 127).

Pathophysiology

The duration and degree of obstruction and the presence and severity of ischemia determine the local and systemic consequences of intestinal obstruction. The intestinal mucosa is an important and early site of injury in both simple and strangulated intestinal obstruction. Microscopic evidence of epithelial injury occurs within the first 4 to 6 hours of intestinal obstruction and progresses to focal epithelial necrosis within 8 to 12 hours.[20] Strangulated obstruction exacerbates the injury, causing extensive mucosal necrosis and sloughing.

Intestinal obstruction causes the profound accumulation of fluid, swallowed air, and gas within the intestinal lumen proximal to the site of obstruction. Fluid accumulates because of impaired water and electrolyte absorption and also from enhanced secretion. This results in the net movement of isotonic fluid from the intravascular space into the intestinal lumen. The accumulation of swallowed air, and to a lesser extent gases generated by bacteria within the obstructed bowel (e.g., hydrogen, carbon dioxide, and methane), contribute to intestinal distention.

Failure of normal intestinal motility because of ischemia results in SIBO and loss of the normally increasing concentration gradient of bacteria from the jejunum to the ileum. Disruption of the ecologic balance of the normal enteric microbiota is associated with the translocation of bacteria to mesenteric lymph nodes and systemic organs. In a study by Deitch, enteric bacteria, particularly *Escherichia coli*, were cultured from mesenteric lymph nodes in nearly 60% of patients with simple intestinal obstruction, compared with only 4% of controls.[21] These observations are consistent with experimental studies that described the translocation of bacteria into the submucosa within 36 minutes of simple SBO.[22] Together, these data are consistent with the hypothesis that translocation of enteric bacteria contributes to the septic consequences of SBO.

The systemic manifestations of SBO are related to hypovolemia and the inflammatory response incited by bacterial translocation, with or without the influence of ischemic or gangrenous intestine. Hypovolemia primarily results from the loss of fluid into the intestinal lumen, the bowel wall, and the peritoneal cavity. When combined with anorexia and vomiting, a marked reduction in intravascular volume results. Intestinal ischemia markedly exacerbates loss of intravascular fluid locally into the intestine as well as systemically through a generalized microvascular leak. The generation and activation of proinflammatory mediators, including neutrophils, complement, cytokines, eicosanoids, and oxygen-derived free radicals, has been linked to remote organ failure and mortality caused by intestinal ischemia and reperfusion injury (see Chapter 118).

Clinical Features

History

Patients with SBO classically present with the acute onset of cramping mid-abdominal pain, vomiting, abdominal distention, and constipation or obstipation depending on the degree of obstruction. The magnitude of symptoms depends upon the degree (complete or partial), site, and duration of the obstruction. Typically, patients describe paroxysms of periumbilical pain that occur at 4- to 5-minute intervals for proximal obstructions and less frequently for more distal obstructions. With prolonged obstruction, the cramping pain subsides as motility in the distended intestine decreases. Patients with proximal intestinal obstruction have profuse vomiting, more frequent pain, and minimal abdominal distention, whereas patients with distal obstruction present with less frequent vomiting and much more abdominal distention. The emesis of patients with SBO is often feculent because of the increased bacterial count that occurs with stasis in the obstructed intestine. Patients with partial obstruction may continue to pass flatus and stool. Even patients with complete SBO can continue to pass gas and stool for a time as they evacuate the bowel contents distal to the obstruction. Continuous severe pain, particularly when localized, strongly suggests the presence of strangulated obstruction. Closed-loop obstructions are associated with the sudden onset of severe unremitting abdominal pain.

Physical Examination

In general, patients with simple SBO appear to be acutely ill, with abdominal distention and systemic evidence of intravascular volume depletion. Auscultation of the abdomen reveals periods of increased bowel sounds separated by intervals of relative quiet. The quality of the bowel sounds usually is described as high-pitched or musical. *Borborygmi* are pronounced rumbling bowel sounds that correspond with paroxysms of cramping abdominal pain. In the setting of prolonged obstruction, bowel sounds disappear as intestinal motility decreases. As alluded to earlier, the abdomen generally is distended and only minimally tender. Abdominal tenderness with guarding or other evidence of peritonitis suggests strangulation of the obstruction and necessitates urgent laparotomy. Patients with proximal SBO can have minimal abdominal distention if they have been vomiting. Patients with closed-loop obstructions can present with pain out of proportion to the physical findings, much like that of other causes of acute mesenteric ischemia, such as embolus in the superior mesenteric artery (SMA) (see Chapter 118). The presence of a tender mass at the site of an inguinal, femoral, incisional, or umbilical hernia strongly suggests strangulation or closed-loop obstruction as the etiology of the obstruction.

Diagnosis

Laboratory Findings

Patients with suspected SBO should have a complete blood cell count (CBC) and serum electrolyte and creatinine concentrations. The CBC in patients with simple intestinal obstruction often reveals a slight leukocytosis as well as evidence of hemoconcentration. Significant neutrophilia and immature WBC forms suggest strangulated obstruction, although the predictive value of this parameter is too low to be useful as a sole determinant of strangulation. Vomiting and the profound loss of fluid and electrolytes from the intravascular space that accompanies SBO cause hemoconcentration, increased blood urea nitrogen and serum creatinine concentration, and abnormalities of serum sodium, potassium, and chloride concentrations. The presence of a metabolic acidosis suggests severe intravascular volume depletion with or without intestinal ischemia.

Radiologic Findings

Abdominal Plain Films

After history and physical examination, plain abdominal films are an inexpensive and reasonable first step in the evaluation of patients with suspected intestinal obstruction. Films taken with the patient in supine and upright positions may confirm the diagnosis of intestinal obstruction, localize the obstruction to the small intestine or colon, provide evidence of the degree of obstruction (partial or complete), and, if the upright image includes the diaphragm, detect pneumoperitoneum, which, if present, suggests intestinal perforation.

Classically, the abdominal films of patients with SBO demonstrate multiple dilated gas- or fluid-filled loops of small intestine with a decompressed colon (Fig. 123-2). The finding of dilated small bowel loops containing air-fluid levels is insufficient to distinguish SBO from ileus; however, when combined with an absence of colonic gas, the diagnosis of SBO becomes very likely. When dilated small bowel loops are

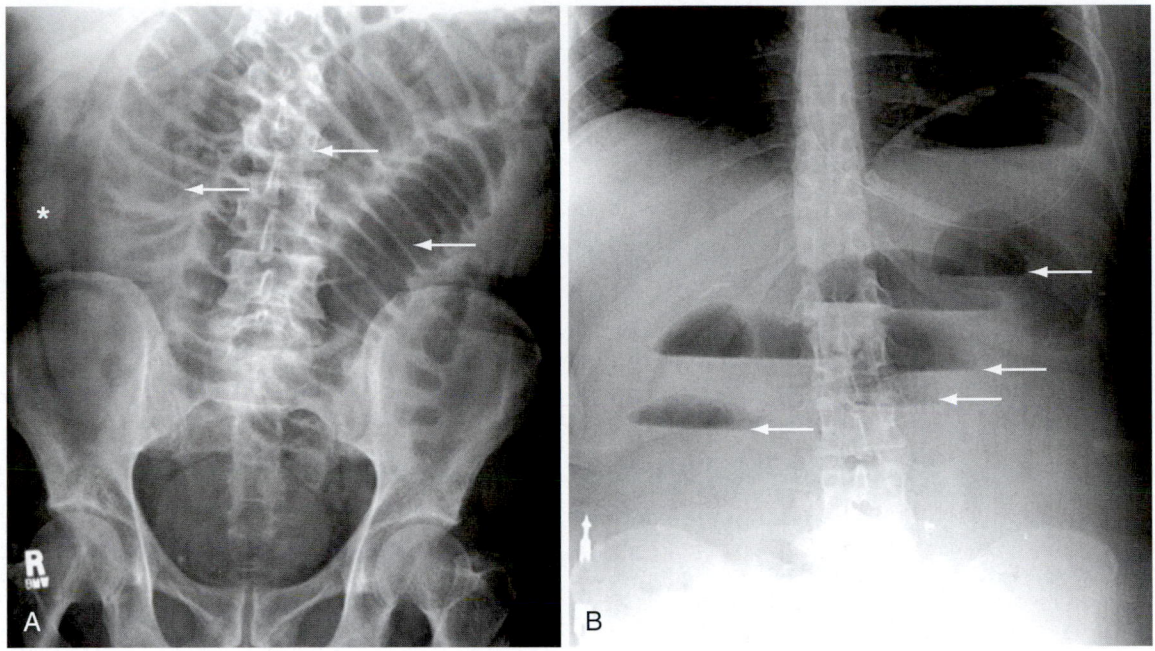

FIGURE 123-2. Supine *(A)* and erect *(B)* abdominal plain films in 2 patients with adhesive small bowel obstruction (SBO). *A,* Air-filled distended small bowel loops *(arrows)* with collapsed colon *(asterisk)*. Note that the small bowel folds (valvulae conniventes) typically extend completely across the intestinal loops. *B,* Multiple air-fluid levels in dilated small bowel loops *(arrows)* in the context of non-distended colon.

accompanied by colonic distention, ileus or large bowel obstruction become more likely (Fig. 123-3). A gasless abdomen may be seen in patients with a very proximal SBO or those in whom the intestine is filled with fluid (Fig. 123-4).

Lappas and colleagues reviewed 12 radiologic findings associated with SBO and found that the combination of air-fluid levels of different heights in the same bowel loop and a mean air-fluid level diameter of 2.5 cm were most predictive of a high-grade partial or complete SBO.[23] Thompson and coworkers corroborated the predictive value of these types of air-fluid levels and reported their sensitivity for SBO to be 59% to 93%.[24] The limitations of abdominal plain films in determining the presence of intestinal obstruction are well recognized: 20% to 30% of patients with proved SBO have equivocal or normal studies.[1,25] False-negative plain films are most likely to occur with low-grade, proximal, or closed-loop obstructions, and in such cases further imaging may be diagnostic (see Fig. 123-4).

CT

Many studies support the use of abdominal CT to evaluate patients with suspected intestinal obstruction.[26,27] Advances in CT hardware and software provide high-resolution reconstructed images in any plane, thus enhancing image resolution and diagnostic confidence.[28,29] Overall, CT is 90% to 95% sensitive, 96% specific, and 95% accurate in determining the presence of complete or high-grade SBO, and it provides important information regarding the site of obstruction and etiology in up to 95% of instances.

CT findings of mechanical SBO are listed in Box 123-2 and illustrated in Figures 123-4 to 123-8. The demonstration of dilated, fluid- or gas-filled loops of proximal bowel and collapsed loops of distal bowel supports the diagnosis of intestinal obstruction. A transition point between bowel loops with disparate calibers may be identified (see Figs. 123-4B and 123-5A). The degree of obstruction may also be determined by

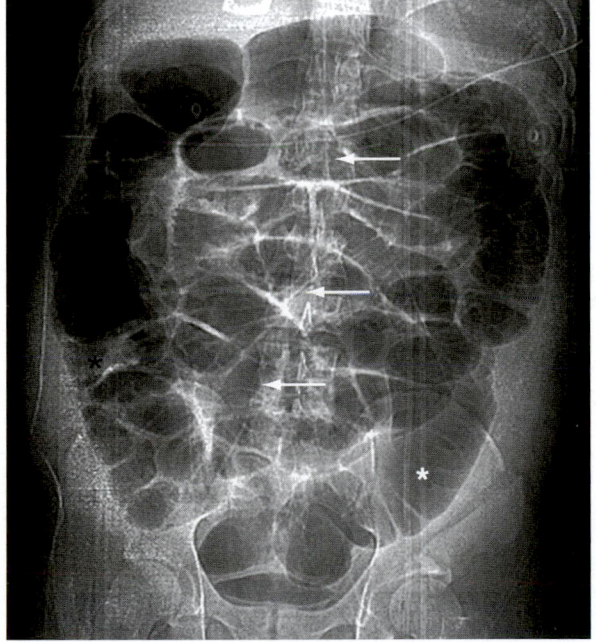

FIGURE 123-3. Supine abdominal plain film in a patient with an ileus. The small intestine *(arrows)* and the colon *(asterisk)* are significantly distended.

the amount of enteral contrast passing through the obstruction. Tapered bowel at the transition point can form a beak (see Fig. 123-5A), and a thorough search of this area may suggest the cause of obstruction. The *small bowel feces sign* refers to the presence of a mottled admixture of particulate matter and gas reassembling stool within the dilated bowel proximal to a low-grade obstruction or in the setting

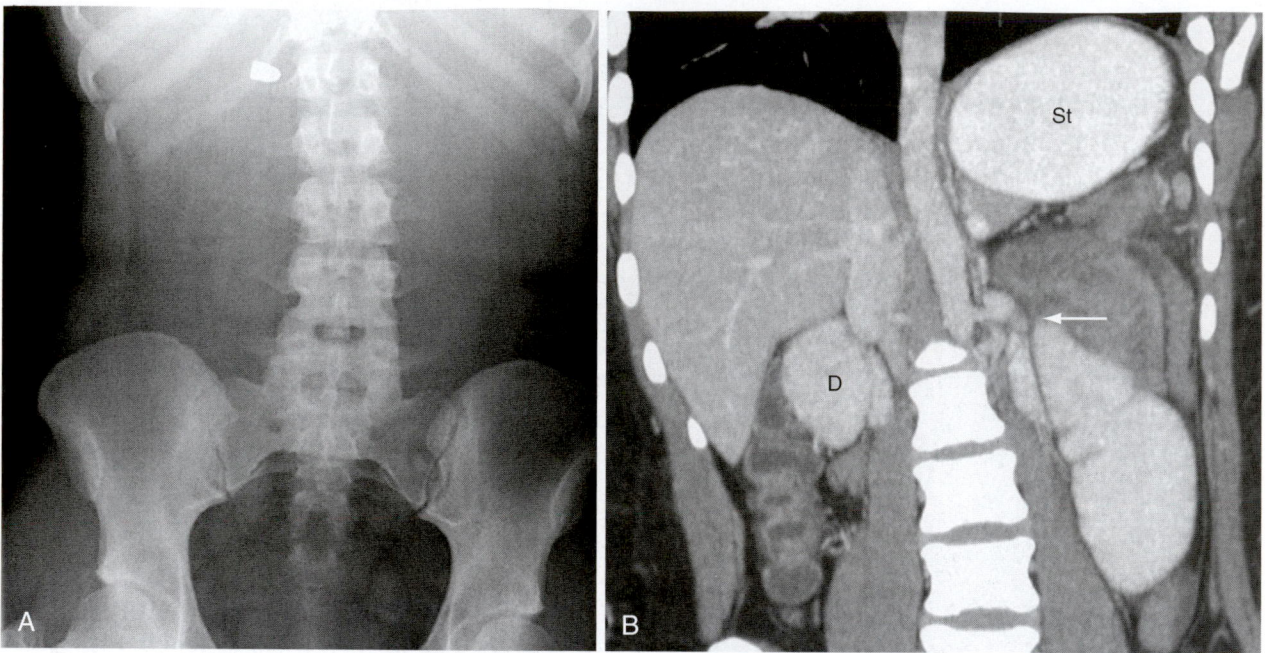

FIGURE 123-4. Supine abdominal plain film *(A)* and coronal CT image *(B)* in a patient with recalcitrant vomiting, obstipation, and a remote history of laparotomy for a gunshot wound to the abdomen. In this case, the abdominal plain film demonstrates a gasless abdomen; the bullet is seen near the midline to the right of the first lumbar vertebral body. CT demonstrates proximal jejunal dilatation, with an abrupt caliber change *(arrow)* and no passage of contrast beyond the obstruction. Proximal small bowel obstruction was relieved by adhesiolysis. D, duodenum; St, stomach.

BOX 123-2 CT Findings in Patients with Small Bowel Obstruction

Simple Complete Bowel Obstruction
Proximal bowel dilatation; discrete transition zone, with collapsed distal small bowel and no passage of oral contrast beyond the transition zone
Colon with little gas or fluid
Small bowel feces sign

Closed-Loop Obstruction
Bowel Wall Changes
U-shaped, distended, fluid-filled bowel loop
Whirl sign: tightly twisted mesentery around a collapsed bowel segment
Beak sign: fusiform tapering in the longitudinal section of bowel at the site of obstruction
Two adjacent collapsed round, oval, or triangular loops of bowel at the site of obstruction

Mesenteric Changes
Fixed radial distribution of several dilated bowel loops with stretched and thickened mesenteric vessels converging toward the point of obstruction

Strangulated Bowel Obstruction
Bowel Wall Changes
Bowel wall thickening with increased attenuation on unenhanced images
Target or halo sign: concentric rings of slightly different densities
Pneumatosis intestinalis linearis
Poor enhancement or lack of enhancement of the bowel wall with IV contrast
Serrated beak configuration of the obstructed bowel loop

Mesenteric Changes
A spectrum ranging from haziness and blurring of the mesenteric vessels to obliteration of the fatty mesentery and its vessels caused by mesenteric congestion and hemorrhage
Diffuse engorgement of the mesenteric vasculature
Unusual course of the mesenteric vasculature

Other Changes
Large amount of ascites
High-density ascites

---

of intestinal ischemia (see Fig. 123-6C).[30,31] A closed-loop obstruction or small bowel volvulus is suggested by U- or C-shaped dilated bowel loops and a radial distribution of stretched mesenteric vessels that converge toward a point of torsion (see Fig. 123-5B).[32] The *whirl sign*[33] also suggests intestinal torsion or volvulus and refers to a swirled mass of soft tissue and fat density that results when the bowel rotates on its mesentery (see Fig. 123-6B). Although peritoneal adhesions are not usually seen on imaging studies, the presence of a transition point without another identifiable cause strongly favors adhesive obstruction.

Many classic CT signs have been proposed to distinguish simple from strangulated SBO (see Box 123-2)[30-36]; these include circumferential bowel wall thickening and edema (see Fig. 123-5B), intraabdominal fluid (see Fig. 123-6D), mesenteric engorgement, abnormal vessel course (see Fig. 123-6A), altered enhancement of the bowel wall (see Fig. 123-7), and a bowel configuration suggesting a closed-loop obstruction or volvulus (see Fig. 123-5B). Decreased bowel wall enhancement is the most specific finding of intestinal ischemia (see Fig. 123-7), but its sensitivity is relatively low in most series (34% to 56%).[30,34,36] Portomesenteric venous gas, pneumoperitoneum,

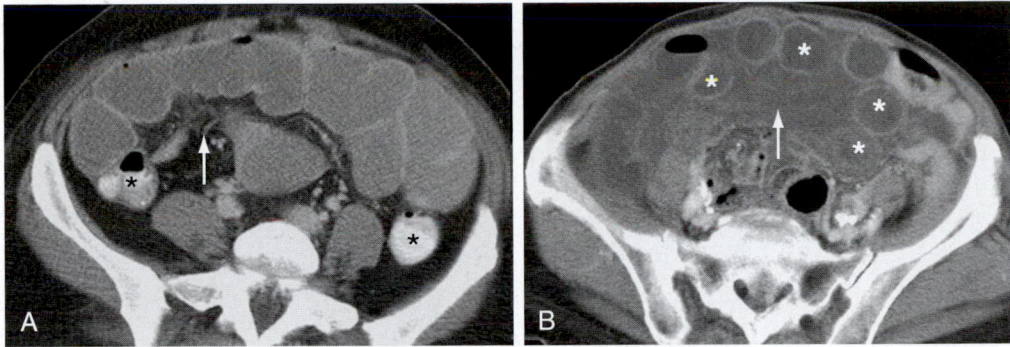

FIGURE 123-5. Axial CT images of simple *(A)* and closed loop *(B)* small bowel obstructions. *A,* The small bowel is dilated proximal to a transition point *(arrow)* and collapsed distally. Rectal contrast identifies the colon *(asterisks.)* *B,* Dilated, fluid-filled small bowel loops *(asterisks)* are radially arranged, and several demonstrate concentric rings of wall thickening and submucosal edema. There is complete loss of mesenteric fat *(arrow).* Infarcted ileum was resected at surgery.

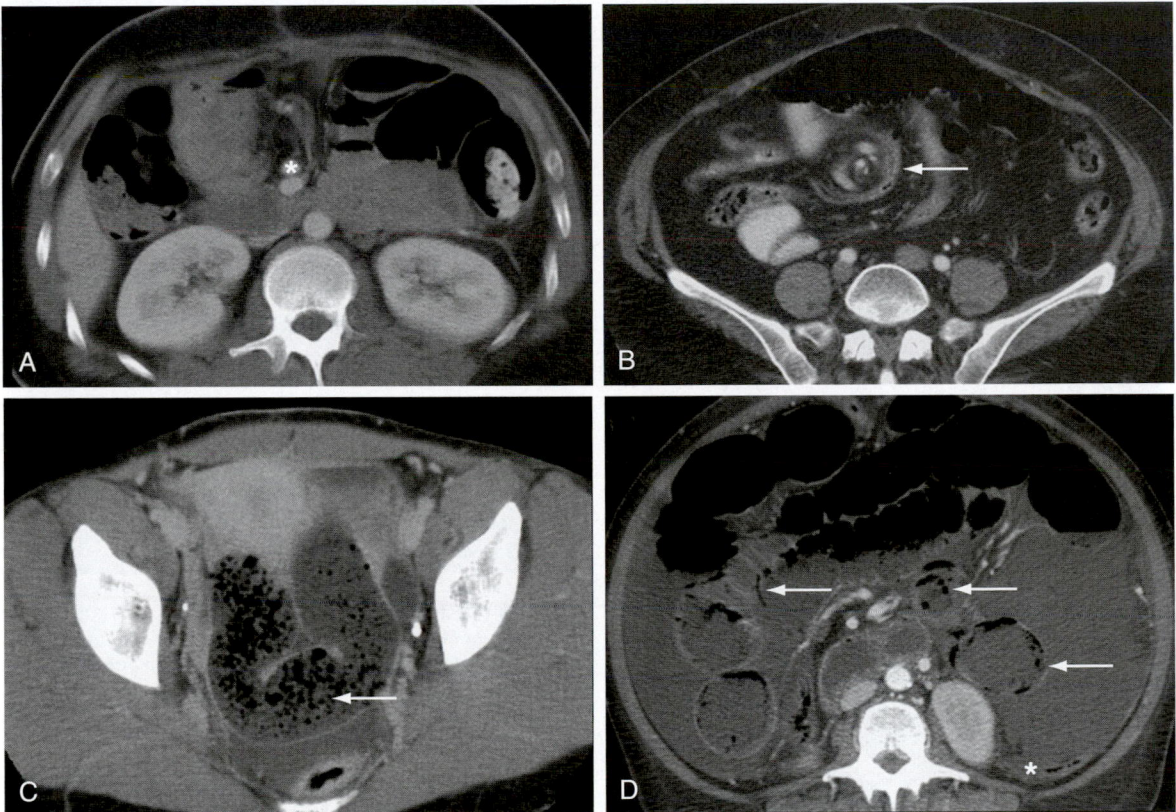

FIGURE 123-6. CT in small bowel obstruction. *A,* Abnormal position of mesenteric vessels: the superior mesenteric artery *(asterisk)* is anterior to the superior mesenteric vein. *B,* Whirl sign *(arrow).* *C,* Small bowel feces sign *(arrow).* *D,* Pneumatosis *(arrow)* and large-volume ascites. The colon *(asterisk)* is collapsed (see Box 123-2).

and pneumatosis intestinalis linearis (see Fig. 123-6D) may be seen very late in the natural history of strangulated obstruction and suggest the presence of extensive intestinal necrosis. Despite these many signs, early diagnosis of strangulated SBO remains a challenge, with reported sensitivity, specificity, and accuracy of these various criteria to detect strangulated obstruction ranging from 14% to 95%.[30]

Detection of low-grade or intermittent bowel obstruction may be extremely difficult using standard radiologic and CT approaches; diagnostic accuracy varies from 48% to 66%.[37] CT enteroclysis (see Fig. 123-8), which combines the advantages of active luminal distention with the mural and extra-enteric evaluation of cross-sectional imaging, has been shown to have

a sensitivity of 89% and a specificity of 100% in patients suspected of having SBO, and even greater accuracy when a history of abdominal malignancy was known or suspected.[38,39] CT enterography is especially useful in patients with SBO due to IBD. MRI also has been used to detect SBO and to characterize benign and malignant causation,[40] although its greater cost, lower spatial resolution, and lack of incremental diagnostic gain over CT has limited its widespread implementation.[41]

Barium and Water-Soluble Small Bowel Contrast Studies

Fluoroscopic studies of the GI tract with enteral contrast agents (barium sulfate or Gastrografin) have long been used

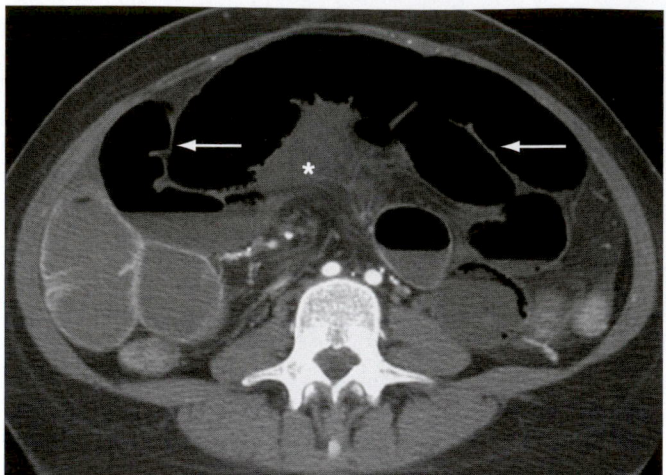

FIGURE 123-7. CT image revealing a strangulated obstruction of the small intestine. A long segment of obstructed small bowel wall does not enhance *(arrows)* after IV contrast, indicating poor perfusion. Note the high-density mesenteric fluid *(asterisk)*. Small bowel volvulus and impaired perfusion were found at surgery.

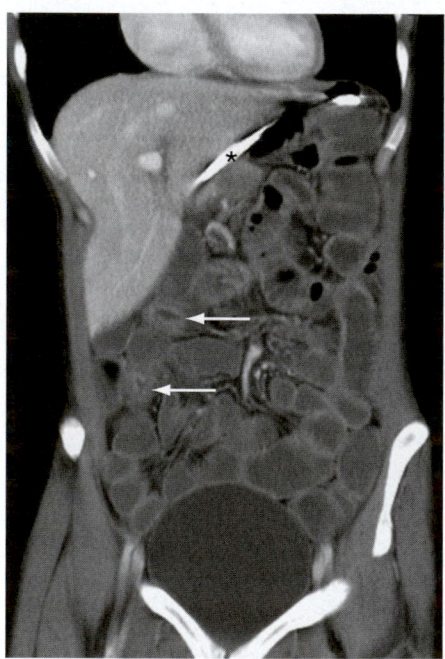

FIGURE 123-8. Image from coronal CT enteroclysis with oral and IV contrast. Neutral enteral contrast instilled via a transduodenal tube *(asterisk)* aids in the detection of active mucosal hyperemia *(arrow)* and lower grades of luminal narrowing in this patient with Crohn's disease.

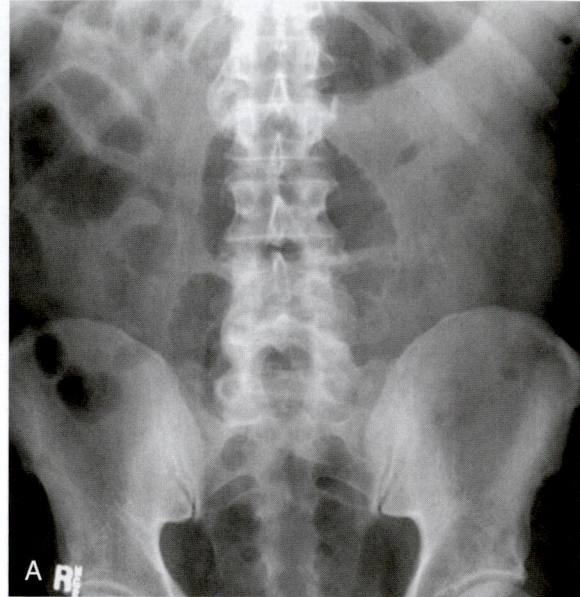

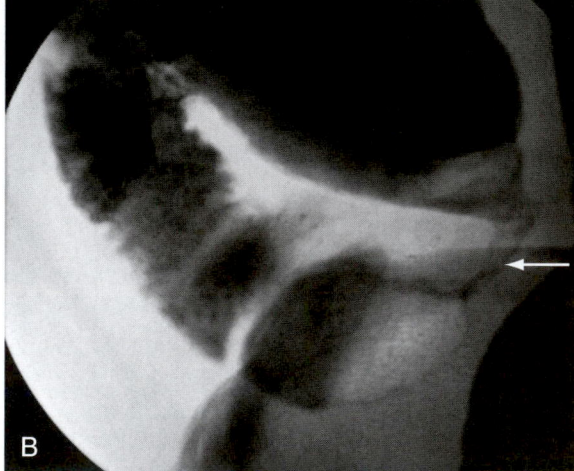

FIGURE 123-9. Nonadhesive small bowel obstruction. An abnormal but nonspecific bowel gas pattern on plain film *(A)* is confirmed to be from a chronic ischemic stricture *(arrow)* when further evaluated by tube enteroclysis *(B)*.

to evaluate patients with suspected SBO, particularly when the clinical presentation is atypical, abdominal plain films are nondiagnostic, and lower grades of bowel obstruction are suspected. Contrast study with barium sulfate has been shown to provide useful information—definite diagnosis, no obstruction, high-grade or complete obstruction—in 50% to 80% of patients examined,[42] and several studies suggest that passage of orally administered Gastrografin into the colon within 6 to 24 hours can identify patients most likely to respond to nonoperative management.[43-45] The disadvantages of fluoroscopic luminal studies, including prolonged examination times, the need to ingest large volumes of contrast agent, and limited visibility of mucosa at transition point, have caused these studies to fall out of favor and be largely replaced with CT or CT enteroclysis.

In patients with chronic partial SBO, fluoroscopic imaging of the site of obstruction may be facilitated by barium enteroclysis, which can characterize the site of obstruction accurately in 86% to 100% of instances (Fig. 123-9).[1] After intubating the duodenum or proximal jejunum, contrast material is delivered directly into the small intestine, and the small bowel then is evaluated for distensibility, stenoses, masses, and inflammatory changes. The degree of intestinal obstruction may be determined by challenging luminal distention and by identifying the arrival and passage of contrast through an area of narrowing. This study is, of course, contraindicated in patients who present acutely with obstructive symptoms or evidence of a complete or high-grade SBO. In patients with combined small bowel and colonic distention, a Gastrografin-contrast enema or CT with rectal contrast may be used to distinguish ileus from a distal large bowel obstruction.

Treatment

Medical Management

The initial step in the management of patients with SBO is the restoration of intravascular volume by the infusion of isotonic fluid. A Foley catheter should be placed to facilitate assessment of the patient's functional intravascular volume status and hence the adequacy of resuscitation. Abnormalities of serum electrolyte concentrations must be corrected as rapidly as possible, and metabolic acidosis should be treated by the restoration of normal intravascular volume. Persistent acidosis suggests the presence of ischemic bowel and hence strangulated obstruction. An NG tube should be placed to decompress the stomach and minimize further intestinal distention. In addition to reducing the discomfort associated with gastric and intestinal distention, NG decompression also can reduce the risk of aspiration. Little data exist to suggest that placement of a long tube into the small intestine compared with a standard NG tube for decompression improves the likelihood of successful nonoperative management.

Although there are no data to support the use of systemic antibiotics in the nonoperative management of patients with simple SBO, patients who are to undergo laparotomy should receive broad-spectrum antibiotics directed toward Gram-negative aerobes and anaerobes. Second-generation cephalosporins such as cefoxitin are used commonly. More recently, ertapenem is used because of its prolonged duration (24 hr) of clinical effectiveness, thus reducing the need for repeated dosing in long surgical cases.

In the absence of clinical evidence to suggest strangulated obstruction or an incarcerated hernia, 64% to 73% of patients with partial SBO can be managed successfully with fluid and electrolyte resuscitation and NG aspiration.[46,47] Foster and colleagues reported that 76% of 32,583 patients with SBO admitted to acute care hospitals in California in 1997 were managed without operation.[46] In contrast, less than half of patients presenting with a complete SBO are managed successfully nonoperatively.[47]

Most patients who can be successfully managed nonoperatively have substantial improvement within the first 48 hours of treatment. Clinical deterioration mandates urgent operation. Of patients in whom nonoperative management fails, almost 20% have strangulated obstruction.[47] As alluded to earlier, patients whose SBO is most likely to resolve without operation may be identified by the appearance of oral contrast within the cecum on abdominal films within 4 to 24 hours of administration (sensitivity, 0.96; specificity, 0.96).[48] CT, with enteral and parenteral contrast, can provide the same prognostic information with regard to the passage of oral contrast into the cecum; in addition, this modality also can provide radiologic evidence of ischemic bowel (see above and Box 123-2).

The data on whether orally administered Gastrografin enhances the likelihood of successful nonoperative management of SBO are conflicting. A Cochrane review by Abbas in 2007 showed that water-soluble contrast agents did not reduce the need for surgery, although they did reduce the duration of hospital stay.[45,48] A meta-analysis by Branco and coworkers in 2010, however, included 3 additional randomized controlled trials, and the result was a significant reduction in the need for surgery (29.6%-20.8%) and hospital stay (1.87 days).[49]

Surgical Management

Operative management of adhesive SBO requires dividing the obstructing adhesions and resecting any gangrenous bowel. The point of obstruction often can be identified as a transition

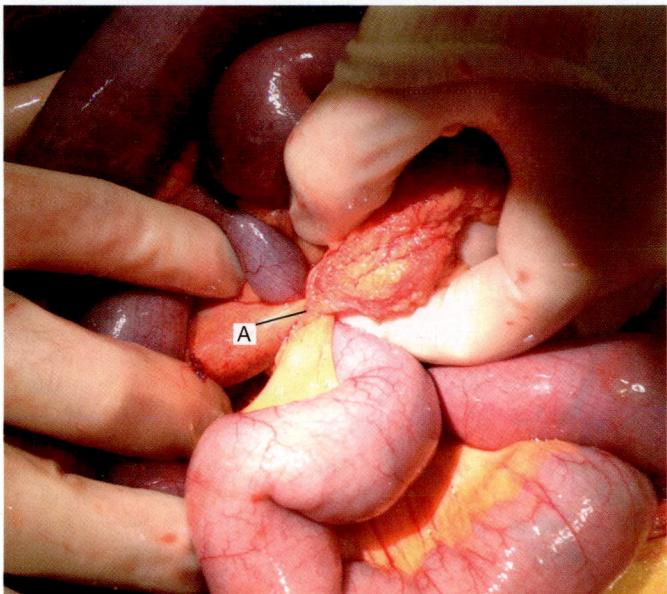

FIGURE 123-10. Small bowel obstruction caused by adhesions. Note the single band of omentum (A) tethered over the small bowel causing ischemic, but still viable, bowel distally.

zone of dilated intestine proximal to the point of obstruction and decompressed bowel distal to it (Fig. 123-10). All adhesions are usually not divided, because they will reform after surgery is completed. In the absence of frankly necrotic intestine, viability should be assessed several minutes after release of the obstruction. Return of normal color and peristalsis and return of arterial pulsation in the vasa recta suggest that the involved segment is viable. Detection of blood flow at the antimesenteric surface with a Doppler flowmeter and inspection of the bowel with a Wood's lamp following IV injection of fluorescein are other useful techniques to assess the viability of a segment of obstructed intestine.

Although laparoscopy has revolutionized the management of many GI diseases, its use for patients with SBO, first reported in 1991, has not been implemented as widely as for other conditions. There are no randomized controlled trials that show superiority of laparoscopy over open laparotomy for SBO. Several case series, observational studies, and retrospective controlled trials have shown that laparoscopy leads to a quicker resolution of postoperative ileus, a reduction in the length of hospital stay, and less morbidity and mortality than laparotomy.[50-52] Laparoscopic treatment of SBO, however, is limited by the technical difficulties associated with exploring the abdomen because of the presence of markedly distended loops of small intestine and the heightened risk of injury to the distended and thin-walled bowel.

In experienced hands, laparoscopic treatment of SBO is successful in about one half to two thirds of patients.[50,51,53] It may be especially useful when there has been only 1 or 2 previous abdominal operations and if the antecedent procedure was an appendectomy. Patients who present to the hospital relatively early after the onset of symptoms and are operated on within 24 hours of admission do better than those who have a longer trial of nonoperative management. The most common reasons for conversion to laparotomy are the presence of dense adhesions,[50] the need for intestinal resection, an iatric injury to the bowel, or an inability to identify the site of the obstruction.[53]

The morbidity and mortality rates associated with laparoscopic management of patients with SBO compare favorably with those of open approaches. In a systematic review of 29 studies that included over 2000 patients, O'Connor and Winter reported that morbidity was 14.8% and mortality was 1.5%; the enterotomy rate was 6.6% and the conversion rate to open laparotomy was 29%. Overall, laparoscopy was associated with reduced morbidity and length of stay.[6] The risk of intra-operative bowel injury can be mitigated by using endoscopic scissors rather than monopolar electrocautery to lyse adhesions; beginning bowel exploration from the cecum and collapsed distal small bowel loops, and working proximally toward the transition zone and dilated intestine; dividing only those adhesions relevant to the obstruction; gently manipulating the dilated bowel using atraumatic intestinal clamps placed on the mesentery instead of the intestinal wall; and using an open Hasson technique by which entry into the peritoneal cavity is performed under direct visualization, entering the abdomen at a site remote from any previous incisions.

For SBO due to a hernia, surgical repair of the hernia is indicated in nearly all cases. In most instances, this involves repair of the hernia defect with prosthesis. If the bowel is not viable, it is resected; usually a primary anastomosis can be performed.

In the case of obstruction from a primary malignancy, the area of obstruction usually can be resected, with either an anastomosis or proximal stoma, depending on the quality of the bowel proximal to the obstruction. If the obstruction results from metastatic disease, this may be treated by either resecting the site of obstruction or by bypassing the obstructed segment of bowel (see Special Considerations, later).

Prognosis

Outcome of patients with SBO may be considered in terms of immediate risk of morbidity and mortality and long-term risk of recurrent obstruction. Risk of death associated with intestinal obstruction ranges from 2% to 8% in studies published since 2000 (Table 123-1).[46,47,54-56] The most commonly cited risk factors for increased risk of death are advanced age and American Society of Anesthesiologists (ASA) class 3 or higher. Chronic illness, strangulated obstruction, and treatment delay also have been associated with an increased mortality risk.[4,55,56] The incidence of major complications after operative treatment of SBO ranges from 12% to 47% depending upon the procedure performed; bowel resection poses a greater risk of complications than does simple lysis of adhesions. The most common medical complications include pneumonia and respiratory failure, pulmonary embolism, cardiac complications, and prolonged ileus. The most common surgical complications are wound infections, intra-abdominal infections, intra-abdominal bleeding, and intestinal necrosis and perforation.[4,54-56]

Once a patient has developed adhesive SBO, the rate of recurrent obstruction is high. In 1 retrospective study of 500 patients who underwent operative treatment of SBO, the rate of recurrent obstruction was 18% with 10 years of follow-up and 29% at 30 years.[57] These figures are similar to those of Miller and coworkers, who found that one third of 410 patients presenting to the hospital with adhesive SBO were readmitted subsequently with recurrent obstruction.[58]

TABLE 123-1 Morbidity and Mortality in Patients with Small Bowel Obstruction (SBO)

Reference	Study Population	Years Studied	Mortality Rate	Study Design	Complication Rate	Outcomes and Risk Factors for Poor Outcomes
4	877 patients who underwent surgery	1961-1995	5%	Retrospective chart review	25.6%	Patient's age Premorbid illness Nonviable strangulation Treatment delay >24 hr
46	32,583 patients managed operatively (7935) and nonoperatively (24,648)	1997	Entire group: 7% Operated group: 5% Nonoperated group: 8%	Longitudinal, population-based	—	Patients managed nonoperatively had a greater mortality rate (8%) than those managed operatively (5%)
54	166 patients with SBO	1994-1995	Entire group: 4% Those with partial SBO: 1% Those with complete SBO: 5%	Prospective	12%	—
55	2002 patients who underwent surgery	1991-2002	7.7%	NSQIP database	37% of patients having lysis of adhesions and 47% of patients having bowel resection had >1 complication	Dirty or infected wounds ASA ≥ 4 Age > 80 years Dyspnea at rest
56	286 patients who underwent surgery	1997-2001	3%	Prospective, multicenter	14%	Age > 75 years ASA ≥ 3

ASA, American Society of Anesthesiologists class; NSQIP, National Surgical Quality Improvement Program; ref, reference.

Similarly, Foster and colleagues reported that 18% of 32,583 patients admitted to California hospitals in 1997 with a diagnosis of SBO had a subsequent admission for the same diagnosis within 5 years.[46]

Although obstruction can recur at any time in the patient's life, most (50% in Fevang's study[57]) occur within the first 5 years after the index operation for obstruction.[57] Evidence suggests that operative treatment of adhesive SBO is associated with a lower rate of recurrent obstruction[57] and a longer interval between admissions than is nonoperative management.[46,58] Miller and coworkers related the pattern of peritoneal adhesions to the likelihood of recurrent obstruction: a single adhesive band was associated with a 25% risk of recurrence, whereas when adhesions were dense and matted, the incidence of recurrent obstruction was 49%.[58]

Special Considerations

Early Postoperative Obstruction

The most important clinical feature that differentiates early postoperative SBO from postoperative ileus is the occurrence of obstructive symptoms after an initial return of bowel function and resumption of oral intake. Generally, patients with early postoperative SBO develop nausea and vomiting, abdominal distention, and abdominal pain as early as the fourth to eighth postoperative day. Plain films of the abdomen usually demonstrate dilated loops of small intestine with air-fluid levels and a paucity of gas in the colon. In contrast, abdominal plain films of patients with an uncomplicated postoperative ileus often have gas in both the large and small intestine. CT confirms the presence of a partial SBO and can provide important evidence of an internal hernia, volvulus, or strangulated obstruction. Furthermore, CT can identify other complications of the index operation that may be related to the occurrence of the obstruction, such as intra-abdominal abscess.

As with other patients with SBO, initial management of postoperative SBO begins with intravascular volume resuscitation and NG aspiration. In 1 series, 20 of 23 such cases resolved with nonoperative management alone, all within 6 days of treatment.[59] Although strangulated postoperative SBO is unusual, evidence of clinical deterioration with the development of severe abdominal pain, hemodynamic instability, or evidence of peritonitis suggests strangulation and mandates immediate laparotomy. In patients who develop SBO early after laparoscopy, the surgeon must suspect that a portion of the intestine herniated through a trocar site, and urgent operative relief of the obstruction is required.

Small Bowel Obstruction in Patients with Malignancies

Peritoneal spread of GI (colorectal cancer) and gynecologic (ovarian adenocarcinoma) malignancies is an important cause of SBO. In both colorectal and ovarian cancer, the risk of developing malignant obstruction is strongly linked to the initial stage of the disease. For example, Ellis and colleagues found that only 18% of patients who developed SBO after undergoing colectomy for early-stage colon cancer had recurrent cancer as the cause of their obstruction, whereas carcinomatosis was the cause of obstruction in 82% of patients with more advanced disease.[60] Similarly, Tunca and colleagues found that only 15% of patients with stage 1 ovarian cancer eventually developed malignant SBO, compared with 35% of patients with more advanced disease.[61] In the absence of recurrent malignancy, intestinal obstruction may be due to postoperative intraperitoneal adhesions or fibrosis from radiation therapy. Gadolinium-enhanced MRI and PET can assist in differentiating malignant from benign causes of intestinal obstruction in patients with a history of malignancy.

Because most instances of SBO from recurrent malignancy represent incurable disease, the goal of treatment is to improve the quality of life over the remainder of the patient's limited life expectancy. In such instances, the purpose of surgery is to relieve the symptoms of obstruction. Factors to consider in planning operative therapy include the chance of successful palliation, the risk of repeat obstruction, the quality of life for the patient after surgery, the ability to administer future chemotherapy, and the risk of operative morbidity and mortality. Surgical options include resection with reanastomosis, surgical bypass with an enteroenterostomy, and a diverting ileostomy. As a last resort in patients for whom no surgical options exist to facilitate passage of enteric contents, a gastrostomy tube is appropriate to decompress the stomach and prevent repeated episodes of emesis. In many instances, though, symptoms can be temporarily palliated by an operation.[62,63] In 1 retrospective study of 64 patients with recurrent ovarian cancer, the obstruction was relieved surgically in 84% of cases, and 71% of patients were able to tolerate a diet for at least 60 days postoperatively[64]; the median survival of those patients in whom the obstruction was relieved was about 12 months. CT scan has been shown in several studies to help predict which patients are most likely to benefit from surgical procedures.[65,66] Unfortunately, the incidence of operative and postoperative complications is high for patients undergoing an operative approach to malignant intestinal obstruction.[62]

Intussusception

Intussusception is the invagination of a proximal segment of bowel (intussusceptum) into an adjacent distal segment (intussuscipiens) (Figs. 123-11 and 123-12). Although more often recognized as a cause of SBO in children, about 5% of cases occur in adults. In contrast to children, in whom there is a pathologic lead point in the intestine approximately 5% of the time,[67] small bowel intussusception in adults is associated with an underlying pathologic process in 80% to 90% of cases. Benign tumors are the most common lead point in the small intestine, whereas adenocarcinoma is the most common lead point for ileocolic and colocolic intussusceptions.

The incidence of intussusception peaks in children between the ages of 4 and 7 months, with the majority of cases occurring before the child is 1 year of age. Most children present with the acute onset of vomiting, bloody stools, and abdominal pain; only about 20% have all 3 of these classic symptoms. In 1 study of 244 children with intussusception, only 6% had all 3 of these symptoms and an abdominal mass on examination.[68] Adults with intussusception present with cramping abdominal pain and symptoms of intestinal obstruction that often are several weeks in duration. An abdominal mass and evidence of GI bleeding or anemia are present in a minority of cases.[69-71]

In most medical centers, US is the initial procedure of choice to diagnose intussusception in the pediatric population. The accuracy of this technique is greater than 90% in experienced hands,[72] and its noninvasive nature and lack of ionizing radiation represent significant advantages over contrast enemas.[73] Most practices reserve the air or liquid enema for reduction of intussusceptions found by US in suitable candidates.

In nonpregnant adults, the procedure of choice for diagnosing intussusception is CT. CT and US can detect intussuscepted bowel along with variable amounts of mesenteric fat (see Fig. 123-11). Concentric rings of inner and outer bowel appear hypoechoic on US (intermediate density on CT), with the characteristic hyperechoic fat (low density on CT) between

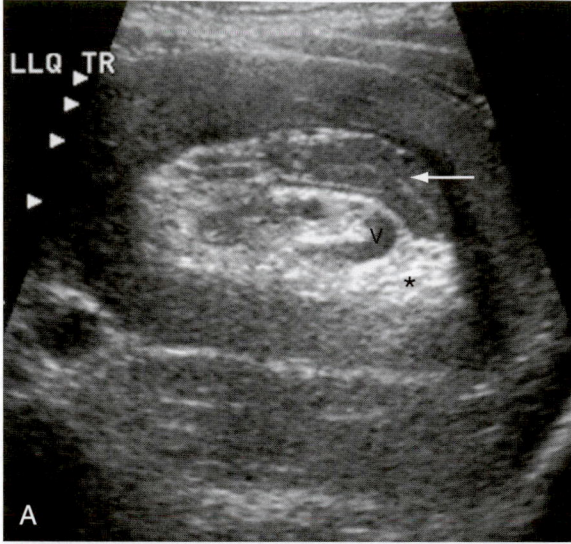

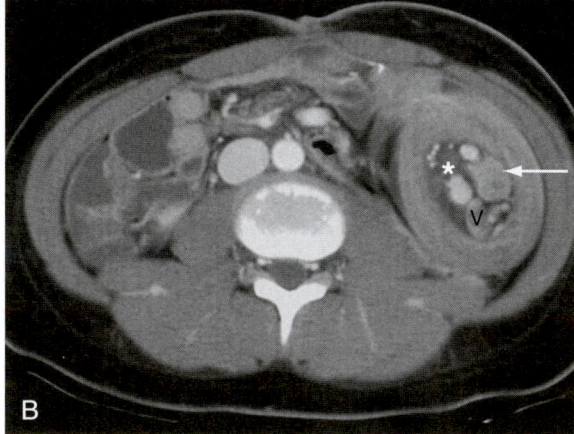

FIGURE 123-11. Abdominal US *(A)* and axial CT *(B)* images in a patient with intussusception. The intussuscepted bowel, or intussusceptum *(arrow)*, is collapsed and carries mesenteric fat *(asterisk)* and vasculature into the dilated intussuscipiens. Note the dilated mesenteric vessels (V).

the intussusceptum and intussuscipiens. Images obtained in long axis or obliquity might appear kidney (reniform)- or sausage-shaped. Most pediatric ileocolic intussusceptions occur in the subhepatic region.

Some 70% to 80% of intussusceptions in the pediatric population may be successfully managed nonoperatively by reduction with air- or liquid-contrast enemas under fluoroscopic or US guidance (see Fig. 123-12). The successful reduction of pediatric intussusception is equal between air-contrast enemas and liquid enemas,[67] but the success of these techniques diminishes substantially as the duration of symptoms exceeds 24 hours.[74] The overall rate of bowel perforation is low, and recurrent intussusception occurs in about 10% of cases.[73] Obvious contraindications to enema reduction include peritonitis, shock, sepsis, or pneumoperitoneum.

In adults, the association of neoplasms and other intestinal pathology with intussusception mandates resection of the involved bowel and makes hydrostatic or pneumatic reduction unreasonable. Primary resection *without* attempting reduction is the preferred treatment for colonic intussusception, including ileocecal intussusception. For lesions involving the right colon, a right hemicolectomy is performed. When the intussusception involves only the small bowel, resection is the preferred operative approach, although manual reduction of the intussusception with careful palpation of the intestinal wall might allow the surgeon to limit the amount of bowel resected.

Gallstone Ileus

Gallstone ileus is an unusual cause of intestinal obstruction, accounting for about 1% to 4% of all cases (see Chapters 65 and 66).[75] This complication of cholelithiasis is more common in older adults, with most patients presenting in the seventh or eighth decade of life. The term "gallstone ileus" is a misnomer because this condition represents a true mechanical obstruction of the intestine by a gallstone or gallstones within the lumen of the bowel. Most commonly, gallstones large enough to cause obstruction enter the bowel via a cholecystoduodenal fistula. As the stone migrates through the intestinal tract, it produces intermittent obstruction, with resultant waxing and waning of symptoms, thereby confounding early diagnosis. The most common site of obstruction is the ileum

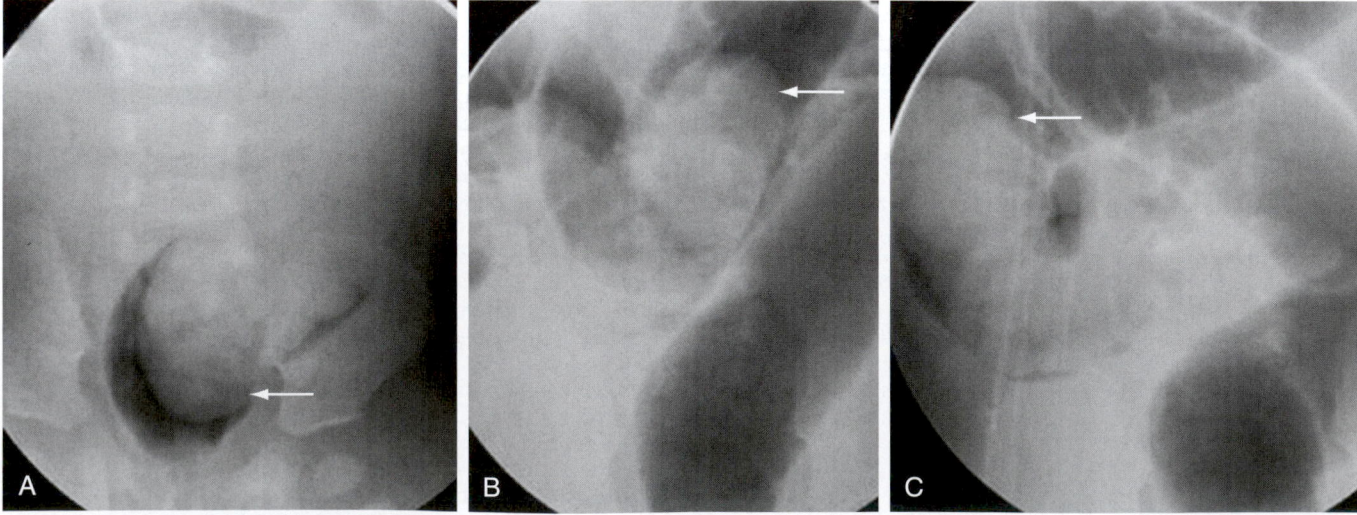

FIGURE 123-12. Air reduction of an ileocolic intussusception in a child. Retrograde instillation of gas with close monitoring of pressure and time may be successful in progressively reducing *(A through C)* the intussusceptum *(arrows)*. To ensure complete reduction, the goal of the procedure is reflux of air into the ileum.

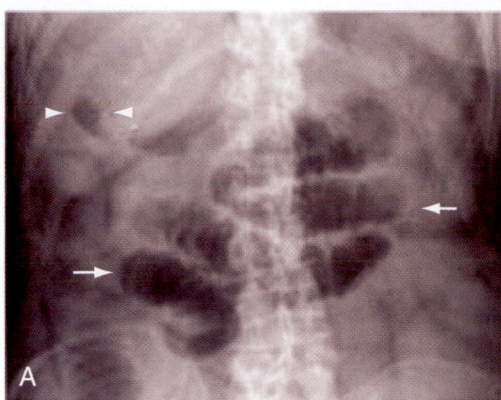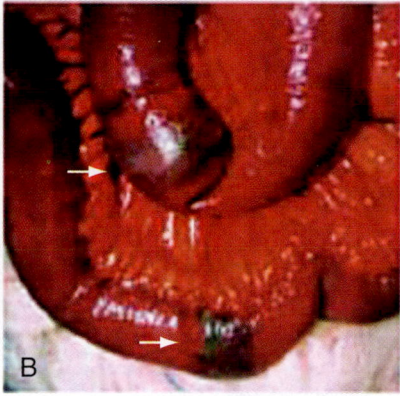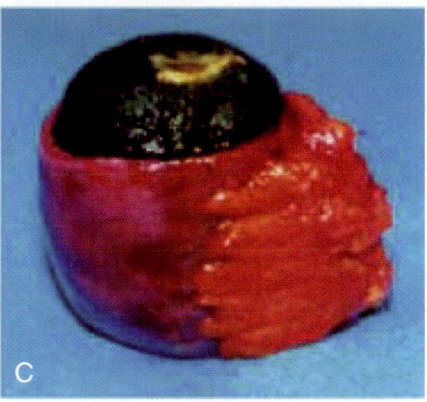

FIGURE 123-13. Gallstone ileus in a 78-year-old woman with a 2-week history of nausea and vomiting. *A,* Plain film of the abdomen revealing characteristic features of gallstone ileus, including air in the biliary tract *(arrowheads)* and dilated loops of small intestine *(arrows);* an obstructing stone was not seen on this plain film examination. *B,* At exploratory laparotomy, two obstructing gallstones *(arrows)* were identified in the jejunum, with adjacent perforations and fecal contamination of the peritoneal cavity. *C,* The stones were removed via enterotomy, and then segmental resection of the jejunum was performed. In addition, the cholecystoduodenal fistula was repaired and cholecystectomy was performed. *(From Besselink MG, Kroeze J. Gallstone ileus. Mayo Clin Proc 2005; 80:699.)*

(≈60% of cases), followed by the jejunum (15%), stomach (15%), and colon (5%). In the absence of an intestinal stricture, a gallstone of at least 2 cm is required to cause intestinal obstruction (Fig. 123-13).

The diagnosis of gallstone ileus is delayed in up to half of the patients because of nonspecific and inconsistent symptoms. Only 50% to 70% of patients have clinical features of SBO. The classic radiologic features of gallstone ileus include pneumobilia, intestinal obstruction, aberrant gallstone location (Rigler's triad), and a change in the location of a previously observed stone. Only about 10% of gallstones are sufficiently calcified to be identified on abdominal plain films, although the increasing use of radiologic imaging in the emergency department has led to descriptions of gallstone ileus on CT, MR, and US. In 2005, Lassandro and colleagues reported on the use of CT in 40 patients with surgically proved gallstone ileus. Pneumobilia and the biliary-enteric fistula were identified in nearly 90% and 12% of cases, respectively.[76]

Treatment of gallstone ileus is focused on removing the obstructing stone, usually by operative enterolithotomy; endoscopic removal of the stone with or without lithotripsy also has been reported. In general, enterolithotomy alone is the appropriate initial treatment, given the emergent nature of this procedure, the advanced age of many of these patients, and the common presence of a complex right upper quadrant mass that contains the cholecystoenteric fistula. Together, these factors argue against identification and repair of the fistula at the time of emergent laparotomy for intestinal obstruction. Elective cholecystectomy with repair of the fistula generally is performed after the patient has recovered from the initial operation, because up to 17% of patients develop recurrent gallstone ileus or other biliary complications after enterolithotomy alone.[77] Lobo and coworkers, however, reported 11 older adult patients who presented with gallstone ileus and were treated with enterolithotomy alone; none of these patients developed subsequent biliary symptoms with nearly 4 years of follow-up.[75]

Midgut Volvulus

Midgut volvulus resulting from intestinal rotational anomalies is an important cause of intestinal obstruction, particularly in neonates. The anatomy and embryology that underlies the development of duodenal obstruction from Ladd's bands and

midgut volvulus is discussed in Chapter 98. It is worth reiterating, however, that the most common anomaly associated with midgut volvulus is non-rotation, in which there is inadequate counterclockwise rotation of the midgut loop around the SMA. This limited rotation results in the duodenojejunal junction and the entire small intestine being located to the right of the midline, while the colon resides in the left abdomen and the cecum is positioned near the midline. The narrow mesenteric pedicle predisposes the patient to midgut volvulus, and the peritoneal attachments (Ladd's bands) that extend anterior and lateral to the duodenum to fix the cecum to the posterior body wall can obstruct the duodenum.

From 50% to 75% of malrotations are detected during the first month of life, and more than 90% are discovered within the first year. Infants with duodenal obstruction from Ladd's bands present with the clinical signs and symptoms of gastric and proximal duodenal obstruction, including bilious vomiting with minimal abdominal distention. Midgut volvulus also presents with obstructive symptoms and symptoms of intestinal ischemia. Occult bleeding is common, and if transmural necrosis develops, acidosis, thrombocytopenia, and frank sepsis can ensue.

The high risk of intestinal ischemia and necrosis from midgut volvulus and the associated very high mortality rate mandates early diagnosis and aggressive management of neonatal intestinal obstruction. An abdominal plain film that demonstrates a distended stomach and proximal duodenum with a paucity of small bowel gas suggests obstruction, which can obviate further radiologic evaluation. A normal plain film does not exclude malrotation, however, and direct imaging of the stomach and small intestine with an upper GI series (UGIS) is needed to confirm or exclude mechanical causes of bilious vomiting. A diagnostic UGIS demonstrates duodenojejunal junction malposition and can illustrate a characteristic corkscrew or coiled appearance of the duodenum and proximal jejunum when malrotation is complicated by midgut volvulus (Fig. 123-14). The use of a contrast enema to demonstrate malrotation is less direct than UGIS and can have false-positive and false-negative rates of 15% and 20%, respectively.

Treatment of intestinal malrotation, whether manifested by duodenal obstruction from Ladd's bands or midgut volvulus, is operative. Diagnosis of midgut volvulus, should be followed immediately by laparotomy because a delay of even hours could mean the difference between viable or infarcted

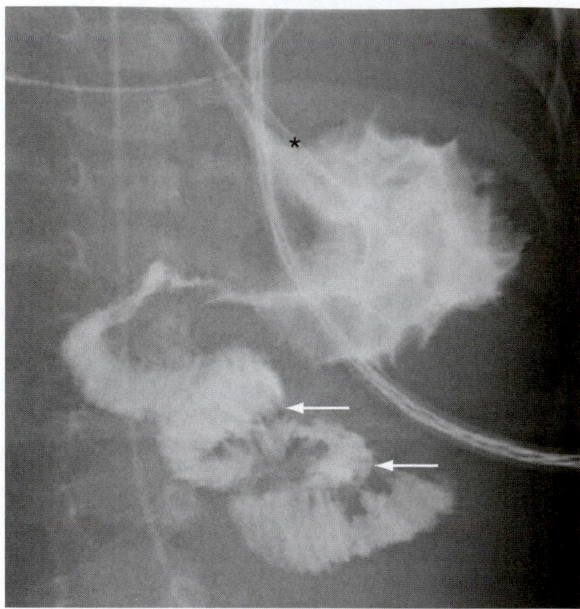

FIGURE 123-14. Upper GI series via NG tube *(asterisk)* in a patient with midgut volvulus. The third and fourth portions of the duodenum are abnormally vertical, and the intestine spirals around the superior mesenteric artery axis to produce a corkscrew sign *(arrows)*.

intestine. Operative repair of malrotation is achieved by the performance of the Ladd procedure. The first part of the Ladd procedure consists of relieving the midgut volvulus and dividing the peritoneal bands that tether the cecum, small bowel mesentery, mesocolon, and duodenum around the base of the SMA. This maneuver allows the mesenteric leaves to open widely but is associated with a 3% to 7% incidence of recurrent volvulus.[78] Then Ladd's peritoneal bands are divided to relieve the extrinsic compression and obstruction of the distal duodenum. This is accomplished by meticulous and complete mobilization of the entire duodenum, with division of all anterior, lateral, and posterior attachments. Finally, the bowel is repositioned and fixed, with the small intestine on the right side and the colon on the left side of the abdomen.

COLONIC OBSTRUCTION

Epidemiology

Although the exact incidence is difficult to determine, large bowel obstruction is approximately 3 to 4 times less likely than SBO. The incidence and etiology vary among various ages and patient populations because of diet, risk factors for malignancy, cultural factors, and genetic factors.

Etiology

In general, the 3 most common causes are adenocarcinoma of the colon and rectum (see Chapter 127), volvulus (see Chapter 123), and benign stricture from diverticulitis (see Chapter 121). These 3 conditions account for about 90% of cases of colorectal obstructions. Adenocarcinoma causes more than half of all cases of colonic obstruction. About 20% of patients with colorectal cancer present with obstruction, half of whom require emergency treatment. Most obstructing colon cancers occur distal to the splenic flexure, where the

colon diameter is relatively small and the stool is relatively solid. Cancers that occur in the right colon also can cause obstruction when they reach a size that occludes the lumen or by acting as the lead point of an intussusception.

Colonic volvulus is the axial twisting of the colon on its vascular pedicle. The anatomic factors necessary for the development of volvulus include a redundant segment of bowel that is freely movable within the peritoneal cavity, a long movable mesocolon, and close approximation of 2 points of fixation of the colon. Typically, a closed-loop obstruction is produced that causes ischemia of the bowel wall due to twisting of the vascular pedicle and increased wall tension from colonic distention. The sigmoid colon and cecum are the most common sites of colonic volvulus, accounting for about 75% and 22% of all cases, respectively. Rarely, volvulus occurs at the transverse colon (2%) or the splenic flexure (1%). Although colonic volvulus causes only 15% of colonic obstructions in the United States and other western countries, it is a significantly more common cause of colonic obstruction in parts of Africa and the Middle East.

Less than 10% of cases of colonic obstruction are due to a fibrotic inflammatory stricture caused by acute diverticulitis. The complications of diverticulitis are discussed further in Chapter 121.

Pathophysiology

The competency of the ileocecal valve is of great importance in the pathophysiology of colonic obstruction. The obstructed colon cannot decompress fluid and gas distally because of the blockage in the colon, and when the ileocecal valve is competent, neither can the colon decompress its contents proximally into the small intestine. A closed-loop obstruction results, which ultimately leads to colonic ischemia and perforation. In the setting of colonic obstruction, the cecum is most susceptible to ischemia because of the direct relationship between wall tension and radius as defined by Laplace's law ($T = P \times R$, where T is wall tension, P is pressure, and R is radius). The cecum has a greater diameter than any other segment of colon, as a result of which, as intraluminal pressure and the diameter of the obstructed colon increase, wall tension increases significantly. When wall tension exceeds capillary perfusion pressure, the bowel wall becomes ischemic. Generally, acute dilatation of the cecum to 10 cm suggests colonic wall ischemia, and a diameter greater than 13 cm implies imminent perforation.

Clinical Features

Many of the clinical manifestations of colonic obstruction are similar regardless of etiology. Periumbilical or hypogastric pain and abdominal distention are the 2 most common presenting features. The pain varies from a vague discomfort to the excruciating pain of peritonitis. Severe unremitting pain suggests gangrenous bowel and mandates urgent laparotomy. Patients can experience either diarrhea (reflecting the passage of liquid stool around an obstructing lesion) or obstipation, depending upon the degree and location of the obstruction.

Patients with left-sided colonic tumors or benign fibrotic strictures often note a change in stool caliber over recent months. Blood in the stool or an iron deficiency anemia are highly suggestive of carcinoma, as is the occurrence of weakness, weight loss, and anorexia. Vomiting, when present, is usually a late finding. Symptoms of malignant and diverticula-associated obstruction often are insidious, with a median duration of 3 months. In 1 study, 25% of patients with obstruction from colorectal cancer had symptoms for 6 to 24 months before diagnosis.[79]

Patients with sigmoid volvulus are usually in their sixth to eighth decades of life and often have concomitant chronic illnesses. Acute abdominal distention is the most common presentation of colonic volvulus and occurs in about two thirds of patients. About 20% of patients have abdominal pain, nausea, vomiting, and constipation. The duration of symptoms with colonic volvulus is significantly less than with a malignant or diverticular stricture. In 1 series of 228 patients with colonic volvulus, the average duration of symptoms before presentation was 73 hours.[80] Abdominal tenderness is present in less than one third of patients with volvulus, and peritonitis suggests impending or actual colonic necrosis and perforation.

Patients with cecal volvulus tend to be younger than patients with sigmoid volvulus and often have a history of prior abdominal operations. Most studies report occurrence predominantly in women. One third to one half of these patients have a concomitant partially obstructing lesion located more distal in the colon. A history of chronic constipation and laxative use is also common in patients with cecal volvulus.

Diagnosis

The initial diagnostic approach to patients with suspected colonic obstruction is similar to that of patients with SBO. Plain abdominal films in the supine and upright positions should be obtained to determine the site of the obstruction and whether the obstruction is partial or complete. As alluded to earlier, small bowel distention may or may not be present in patients with colonic obstruction, depending upon the competency of the ileocecal valve (Fig. 123-15). Abdominal plain films also may be diagnostic, or at least highly suggestive, of sigmoid and cecal volvulus. As described by Agrez and Cameron,[81] the standard radiologic feature of sigmoid volvulus is a distended ahaustral sigmoid loop—a bent inner-tube appearance—the apex of which is directed toward the right shoulder (Fig. 123-16A). Radiologic features of cecal volvulus include a massively dilated cecum located in the epigastrium or left upper quadrant, a distended kidney bean-shaped cecum, distended loops of small bowel suggesting SBO, and a single long air-fluid level present on upright or decubitus films (see Fig. 123-16B). Although these classic radiologic findings of colonic volvulus are seen in only 40% to 60% of cases, the diagnosis of colonic volvulus can be made with abdominal films alone in up to 85% of cases.

Performance of further diagnostic studies in patients with suspected colonic obstruction is predicated on the presence or absence of peritonitis and the degree of obstruction (partial or complete). Patients with peritonitis should undergo resuscitation and urgent laparotomy without additional diagnostic procedures. In contrast, patients whose abdominal plain film suggests a distal obstruction and who do not have evidence of peritonitis or strangulated obstruction should undergo a water-soluble contrast enema or CT with rectal contrast to confirm and localize the site of obstruction (Figs. 123-17 and 123-18). In patients with suspected sigmoid or cecal volvulus, a water-soluble contrast enema may be helpful by demonstrating a point of torsion (a mucosal spiral pattern or beak sign) while avoiding the risk of barium peritonitis in the case of unrecognized perforation (Fig. 123-19). Colonoscopy also can be used to assist with diagnosis, but caution must be used with insufflation so as not to further compromise the already distended bowel.

Treatment

Initial management of patients with colonic obstruction consists of fluid and electrolyte resuscitation and NG aspiration. As alluded to earlier, clinical evidence of peritonitis or strangulated obstruction mandates emergent laparotomy. In the absence of these findings, the therapeutic goals for managing

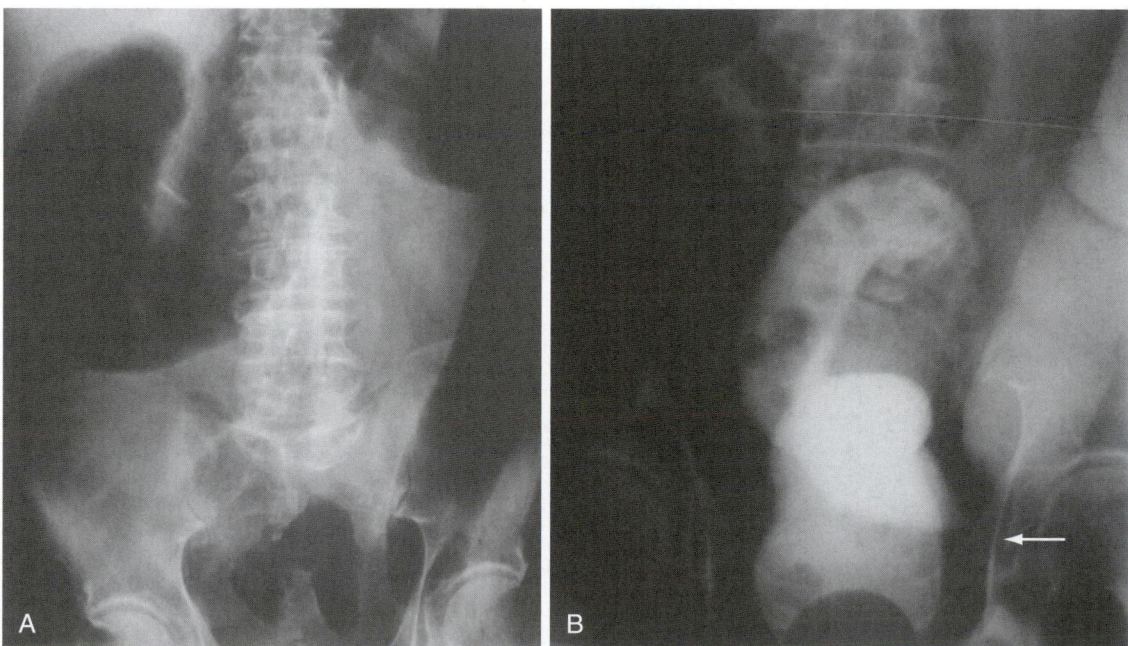

FIGURE 123-15. Abdominal plain film in a patient with a high-grade colonic obstruction and competent ileocecal valve. *A,* Note the markedly distended, gas-filled colon without dilatation or gas in the small intestine. The etiology of the patient's colonic obstruction was a left inguinal hernia, which is demonstrated on the water-soluble contrast enema *(B).* Although a common cause of small intestinal obstruction, inguinal hernias rarely obstruct the colon. The *arrow* demonstrates the point of obstruction of the sigmoid colon as it traverses the inguinal canal.

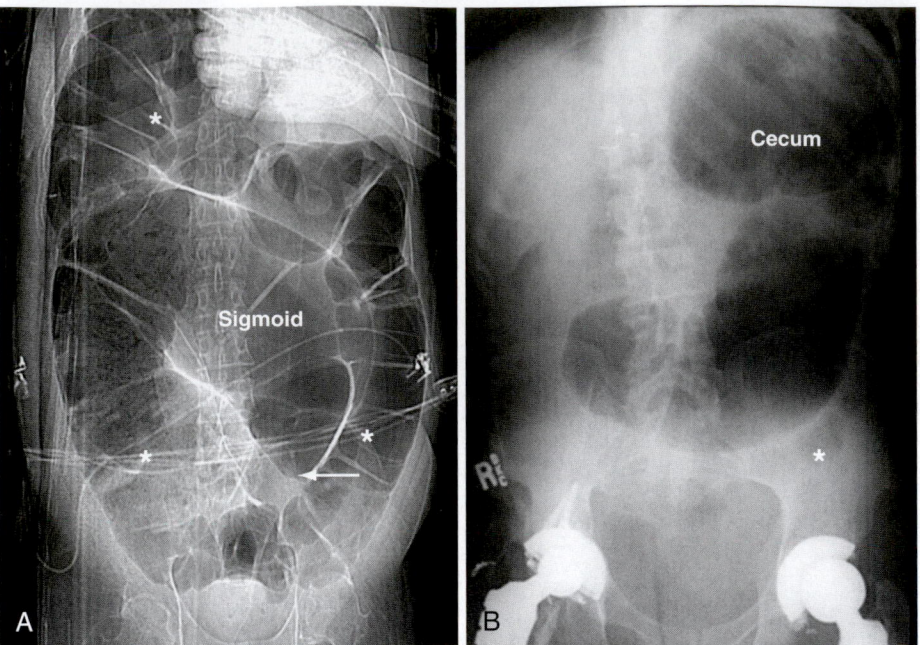

FIGURE 123-16. Abdominal plain films of sigmoid volvulus *(A)* and cecal *(B)* volvulus. *A,* In sigmoid volvulus, the right, transverse, and left colon are distended *(asterisks)* upstream from the point of sigmoid obstruction *(arrow)*. *B,* In cecal volvulus, note the bean shape and left upper quadrant location of the dilated twisted cecum and the collapsed distal colon *(asterisk)*.

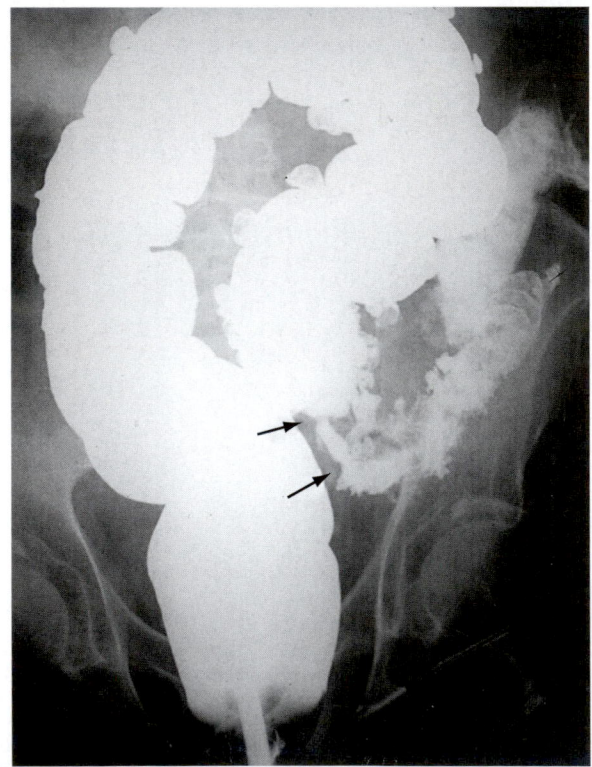

FIGURE 123-17. Representative film from a contrast enema in a patient with high-grade sigmoid obstruction from a stricture *(arrows* identify the proximal and distal extent of the stricture). Although this patient has multiple diverticula within the sigmoid colon, differentiation of this benign diverticular stricture from a malignant stricture is not possible on the basis of this study alone.

patients with colonic obstruction are prompt decompression of the obstructed colon, definitive treatment of the obstructing lesion, and reestablishment of intestinal continuity.

Benign and Malignant Colonic Strictures

Endoscopic balloon dilation of strictures has been shown to be effective in a variety of etiologies such as diverticulitis, anastomotic strictures, and IBD. Self-expanding metal stents also have recently been shown in numerous studies to relieve benign and malignant colonic obstruction before definitive resection, or to palliate obstructive symptoms in patients with advanced disease. Successful management has been shown in up to 80% to 90% of patients in whom colonoscopic stent placement has been attempted.[82-84] This approach allows for elective colonoscopy to clear the colon of additional lesions, and subsequent partial colectomy including the obstructing lesion with primary anastomosis by either laparoscopic or open operative techniques; significant concomitant medical illnesses is treated concurrently.[82] In Khot's systematic review of 262 cases in which colonic stents were used as a bridge to definitive resection, 223 were successful (85%).[84] Other authors have placed self-expanding colonic metallic stents in patients with obstructing colon cancers and unresectable metastases, allowing earlier administration of chemotherapy[85] and earlier discharge from the hospital.[86] Complications occur with stent placement in approximately 30% of cases and are related to perforation, stent migration, and recurrent obstruction.[87]

If colonic stenting is unsuccessful, patients should undergo the appropriate segmental colectomy with either an ostomy or primary anastomosis. The classic operative approach to patients with a distal tumor is often a left or sigmoid colectomy with an end colostomy and Hartmann's pouch because of the colonic distension and compromised bowel that is often present (Fig. 123-20). Numerous investigators, however, have reported on the safety of a primary anastomosis after emergent left colectomy for obstructing colorectal cancer and diverticular strictures[88-90] or sigmoid volvulus.[91] These studies have

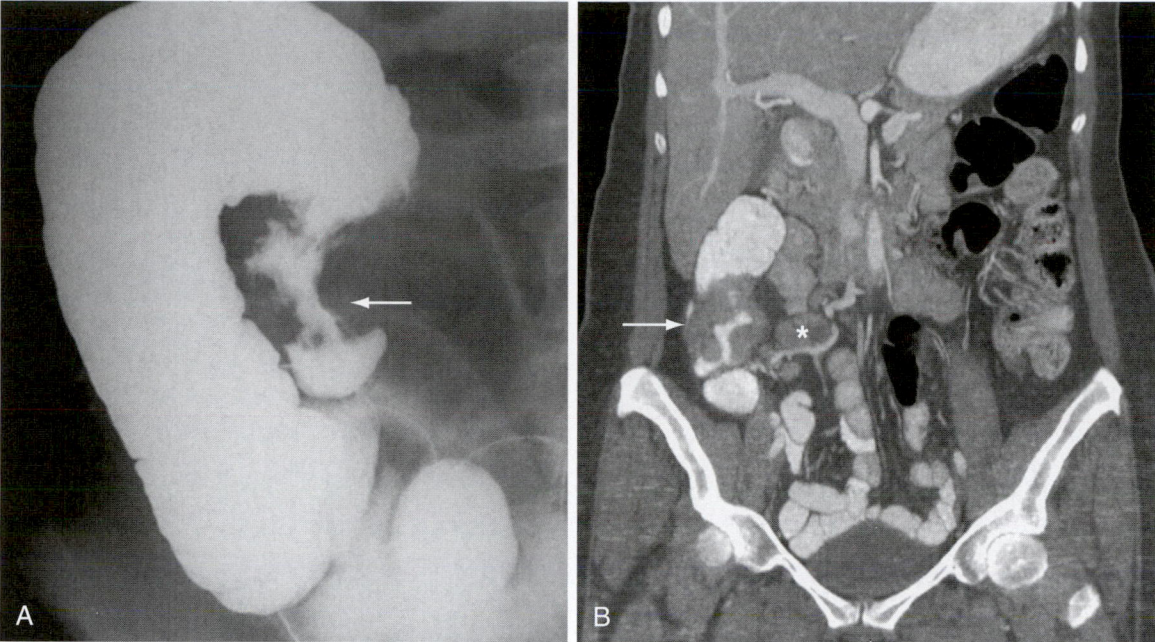

FIGURE 123-18. Carcinoma of the ascending colon. The contrast enema *(A)* demonstrates the typical apple-core lesion *(arrow)*, and the coronal CT with antegrade GI contrast *(B)* further shows the irregular luminal narrowing and mucosal disruption *(arrow)*. Ileocolic nodal tumor spread *(asterisk)* is noted on this staging CT.

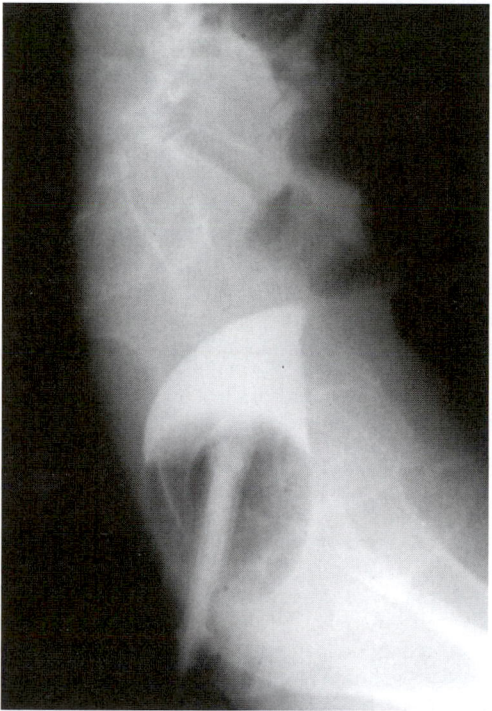

FIGURE 123-19. Contrast enema in a patient with a sigmoid volvulus demonstrating a characteristic bird's beak obstruction at the junction between the sigmoid colon and the rectum.

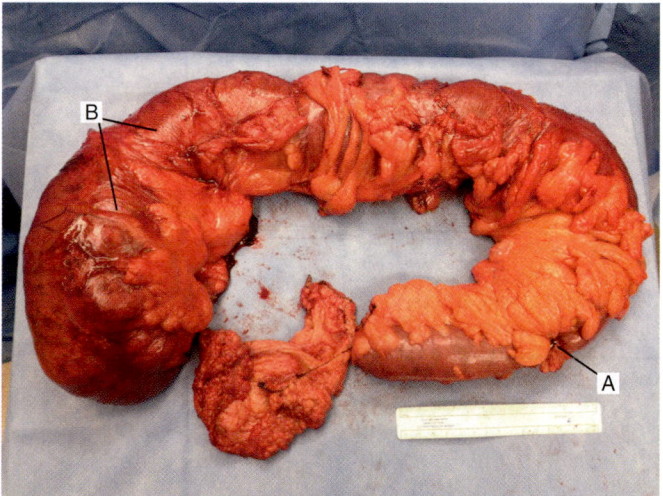

FIGURE 123-20. Colonic obstruction caused by an obstructing primary colon cancer (A) that narrowed the bowel lumen. Proximally, the colon is dilated and congested with splitting of the serosa and impending perforation (B).

shown rates of anastomotic leakage (1%-8%), wound infection (5%-16%), and mortality (1%-6%) comparable to earlier data with resection and end colostomy.[79] Lim and colleagues compared manual decompression and primary anastomosis with intraoperative colonic irrigation and found that intraoperative irrigation offered no improvement in outcome compared with manual decompression alone.[89]

Colonic obstructions located proximal to the splenic flexure are most often adenocarcinomas and are treated with partial colectomy and primary ileocolic anastomosis in all but the most unfit patients. The presence of nonviable colon necessitates resection in even the most severely compromised patient. In such an instance, resection with end ileostomy and distal mucous fistula obviates the risk of performing an anastomosis in a grossly contaminated field or in a critically ill patient in whom the risk of anastomotic dehiscence may be particularly high. Colonoscopically placed self-expanding metal stents also have been used with good results in the management of patients with obstructing proximal colon cancers.[92]

Volvulus

Decompression of a sigmoid volvulus may be accomplished with a flexible or rigid sigmoidoscope and the placement of a rectal tube. In a classic study, Ballantyne compiled 19 American series totaling 595 patients and found that sigmoidoscopy, either alone or combined with a rectal tube, successfully reduced the volvulus in 70% to 80% of attempts[93]; placement of a rectal tube for 48 hours can minimize the possibility of early recurrence. Endoscopic reduction of sigmoid volvulus alone is associated with a recurrence rate of 25% to 50%,[80,93] and therefore, sigmoid resection and coloproctostomy or, in medically compromised patients, end colostomy, should follow endoscopic decompression of the bowel; recurrence rates with this approach are 3% to 6%.[80,93] Patients who require emergent laparotomy for strangulated sigmoid volvulus should have sigmoid resection with end colostomy and a Hartmann's pouch or primary anastomosis as discussed earlier.[91] Right hemicolectomy with primary ileocolic anastomosis is the procedure of choice for cecal volvulus.

Prognosis

Regardless of the approach, emergent operations to relieve colonic obstruction are associated with significantly greater morbidity and mortality risks than those performed electively. Grossmann and colleagues found that the mortality rate was 24% for patients undergoing emergency operation for sigmoid volvulus compared with 6% for those undergoing elective resection.[80] Similarly, Sjo and coworkers reported that the early postoperative mortality rate was 19% after emergency operation for colorectal cancer compared with 3.5% for patients undergoing elective resection.[94] Emergency operation, ASA class 3 or 4, necrotic bowel, and advanced tumor stage have been consistently identified as independent predictors of early postoperative mortality.[80,94-96]

The long-term outlook for patients who present with obstructing colon cancers is significantly worse than that for patients without obstruction. Wang and coworkers found that despite similar tumor stages, patients who presented with obstructing right-sided colon cancers had significantly higher rates of tumor recurrence than did patients who presented without obstruction (49% vs. 22%, respectively). Similarly, the 5-year survival was worse for patients presenting with obstruction than for patients without obstruction (36% vs. 77%, respectively).[97] Even in the setting of a potentially curative resection, the cancer-specific survival at 5 years was 75% for patients without obstruction compared with 52% for patients presenting with obstruction.[98] For patients in whom procedures are done to palliate incurable disease, the results are much worse.[63]

KEY REFERENCES

Full references for this chapter can be found on www.expertconsult.com.

4. Fevang BT, Fevang J, Stangeland L, et al. Complications and death after surgical treatment of small bowel obstruction. A 35-year institutional experience. Ann Surg 2000; 231:529-37.
6. O'Connor DB, Winter DC. The role of laparoscopy in the management of acute small-bowel obstruction: A review of over 2,000 cases. Surg Endosc 2012; 26:12-7.
9. Schnüriger B, Barmparas G, Branco BC, et al. Prevention of postoperative peritoneal adhesions: A review of the literature. Am J Surg 2011; 201:111-21.
46. Foster NM, McGory ML, Zingmond DS, Ko CY. Small bowel obstruction: A population-based appraisal. J Am Coll Surg 2006; 203:170-6.
49. Branco BC, Barmparas G, Schnuriger B, et al. Systematic review and meta-analysis of the diagnostic and therapeutic role of water-soluble contrast agent in adhesive small bowel obstruction. Br J Surg 2010; 97:470-8.
50. Levard H, Boudet M-J, Msika S, et al. Laparoscopic treatment of acute small bowel obstruction: A multicentre retrospective study. ANZ J Surg 2001; 71:641-46.
55. Margenthaler JA, Longo WE, Virgo KS, et al. Risk factors for adverse outcomes following surgery for small bowel obstruction. Ann Surg 2006; 243:456-64.
57. Fevang B-T, Fevang J, Lie SA, et al. Long-term prognosis after operation for adhesive small bowel obstruction. Ann Surg 2004; 240:193-201.
63. Miner TJ, Brennan MF, Jaques DP. A prospective, symptom related, outcomes analysis of 1022 palliative procedures for advanced cancer. Ann Surg 2004; 240:719.
68. Kaiser AD, Applegate KE, Ladd AP. Current success in the treatment of intussusception in children. Surgery 2007; 142:469-77.
80. Grossman EM, Longo WE, Stratton MD, et al. Sigmoid volvulus in Department of Veterans Affairs Medical Centers. Dis Colon Rectum 2000; 43:414-8.
84. Khot UP, Lang AW, Murali K, Parker MC. Systematic review of the efficacy and safety of colorectal stents. Br J Surg 2002; 89:1096-102.
98. McArdle CS, McMillan DC, Hole DJ. The impact of blood loss, obstruction, and perforation on survival in patients undergoing curative resection for colon cancer. Br J Surg 2006; 93:483-8.

Ileus and *pseudo-obstruction* refer to intestinal dysmotility syndromes that have signs, symptoms, and the radiologic appearance of obstruction in the absence of a mechanical cause. Ileus occurs when the contents of the small intestine are acutely unable to transit because of impermanent neural or muscular inadequacy. Sudden and severe pain, nausea, vomiting, abdominal distention, and inability to tolerate a diet or to pass stools typically accompany ileus, but ultimately the condition resolves completely. Abdominal surgery is by far the most common cause of ileus. *Pseudo-obstruction* describes a chronic, severe neuromuscular condition of delayed intestinal transit that is characterized by disabling and life-threatening complications over time. This intestinal paralysis, or intestinoparesis, affects the small intestine, although the stomach (gastroparesis) and colon (colonoparesis) may be similarly affected. The disease can go unrecognized for years; it is often mistaken for acute small bowel obstruction, with patients undergoing needless operations that can further compromise a fragile nutritional balance.

Acute colonic pseudo-obstruction, or Ogilvie's syndrome, occurs most often in elderly patients with severe underlying disorders that may be responsible for the acuteness of the situation. Acute colonic pseudo-obstruction is characterized by massive dilatation of the cecum and right colon, with simultaneous, yet less severe, dilatation of the left colon and distal small intestine, without evidence of mechanical obstruction. With early aggressive treatment, the massive dilatation usually resolves and intestinal function returns to normal.

Megarectum and *megacolon* are terms applied to radiologic images or the intraoperative appearance of a chronically dilated rectum or colon that can develop as a result of pseudo-obstruction, inflammation, infection, spinal trauma, and metabolic or congenital disorders. The most common cause of congenital megarectum and megacolon is Hirschsprung's disease.

The GI tract has a unique and extensive intrinsic nervous system, the enteric nervous system (ENS; Fig. 124-1); unlike any other peripheral organ, it can function without direct input from the central nervous system (CNS). Neuronal control of GI function is regulated through the integrated activities of local enteric reflexes, reflexes that pass through sympathetic ganglia, and reflexes that pass from the intestine to the CNS. The ENS consists of visceral sensory afferents in the vagus, thoracic, and pelvic splanchnic nerves (see Fig. 124-1) and visceral motor efferents of the autonomic nervous system (ANS). These extrinsic neurons synapse with the ENS and connect it to the CNS.

The small intestine and colon transport contents over long distances by the action of propulsive and nonpropulsive motor activity, and they display divergent fasting and fed patterns of absorption, motility, and transit (see Chapters 99 and 100). Between meals, the migrating motor complex (MMC) propels food distally in a characteristic sequence that cycles every 1 to 2 hours. There are 4 phases to this intercibal fasting pattern: (1) oscillations of the smooth muscle without contractions, (2) intermittent smooth muscle contractions, (3) continuous sweeping contractions increasing to a maximum rate (11/min in the duodenum), and (4) a quiescent phase with cessation of all contractions. Feeding interrupts the MMC and is immediately followed by the fed pattern, which consists of continuous, low, varying-amplitude, ungrouped phasic contractions, the activity of which depends on the quantity and composition of the ingested food. The small intestinal motor activity facilitates gastric emptying; mixes chyme with digestive enzymes, bile, and intestinal secretions; propels material distally; helps absorb nutrients and resorb fluids; and delivers residue to the colon by the action of intermittent, giant phase 3 contractions. Discontinuous emptying from the ileum ensures time for nutrient exposure and salvage of remaining nutrients in the small intestine. The small intestine uses

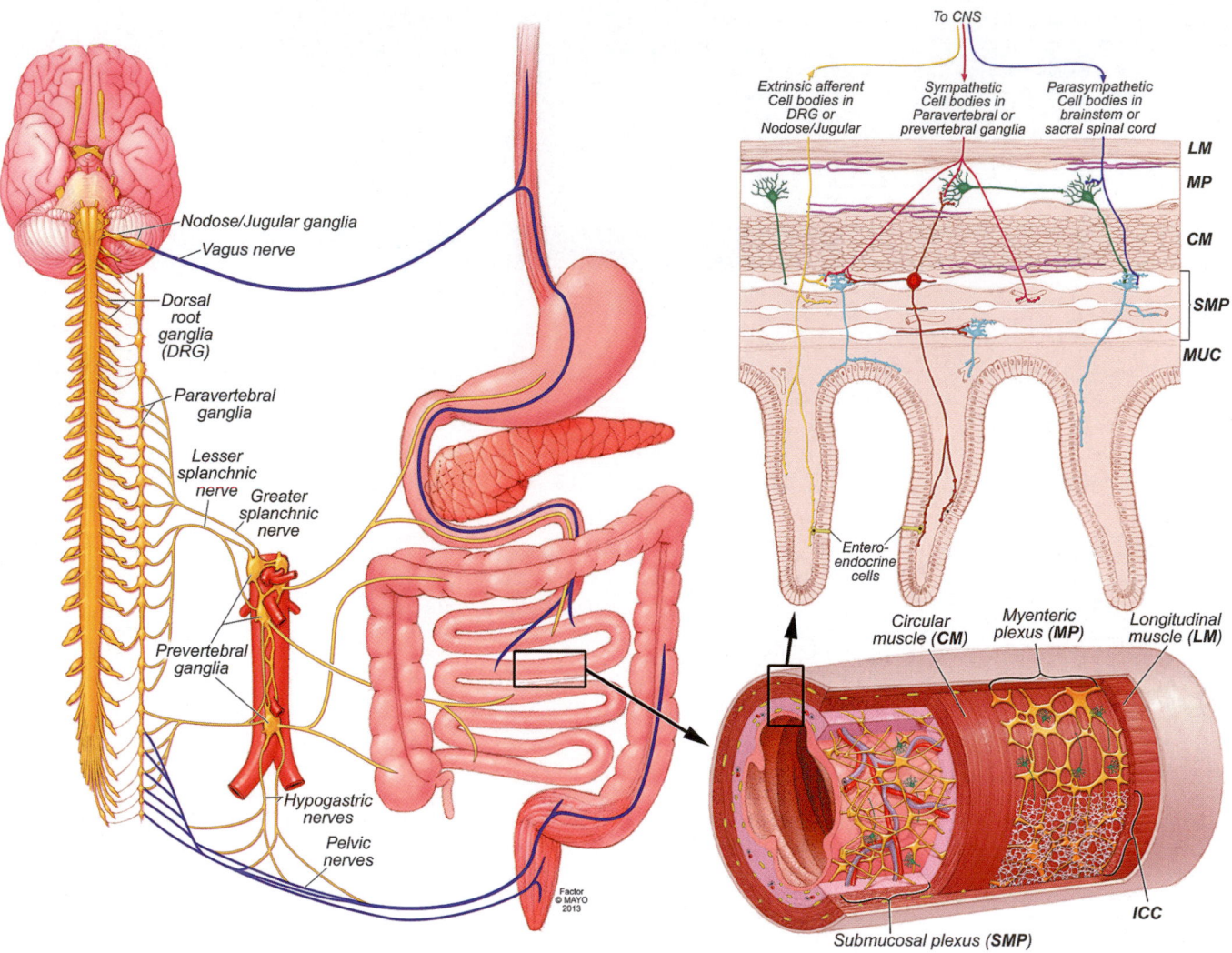

FIGURE 124-1. The autonomic and enteric nervous systems. Divisions of the autonomic nervous system (ANS) *(left)*, showing the para-sympathetic craniosacral *(blue)* and sympathetic *(yellow)* systems and their organ innervation. The enteric nervous system (ENS) is often considered a subdivision of the ANS. Cutaway/cross-sectional diagram *(right lower)* of the wall of the small intestine showing the myenteric and submucosal plexuses of the ENS with interstitial cells of Cajal (ICC) *(light purple)* and interneurons *(green)*. Cross-sectional diagram *(right upper)* of an interconnected network of nerve circuits including intrinsic primary afferent neurons (IPANs) *(red)*, interneurons *(green)*, secretory and vasomotor neurons *(blue)*, and ICC *(light purple)*. CNS, Central nervous system; MUC, mucosa. *(By permission of Mayo Foundation for Medical Education and Research. All rights reserved.)*

luminal sensing in transmitting feedback inhibitory reflexes, including the duodenal and ileal brake that delay functions such as gastric emptying and intestinal secretion while influencing the digestive process and ingestive behavior. These negative-feedback mechanisms include hormones (e.g., serotonin and CCK), neural mediators, and food constituents such as fat.

Colonic motor activity exhibits 2 primary components: propulsive and segmental. Propulsive activity includes (1) stimulus-invoked high-amplitude propagated contractions (HAPC) that are responsible for the mass movements that follow waking and eating and commonly precede bowel movements and (2) reiterative low-amplitude propagated contractions (LAPC) that move along fluid and flatus. Segmental activity is the main motor response to eating; it results in more gradual displacement of intraluminal contents, thereby allowing optimal absorption of fluid, nutrients, microbial metabolites, and substrates within the intestinal medium. The colon facilitates emptying of the small intestine into a microbial-rich environment; serves as a reservoir; absorbs

water and limited nutrients; propels intestinal contents distally via coordinated sensorimotor activity; and stores and expels intestinal residue.

This chapter focuses on the acute and chronic forms of intestinal dysmotility including ileus, acute colonic pseudo-obstruction, chronic intestinal pseudo-obstruction, and isolated megacolon and megarectum.

EPIDEMIOLOGY

The prevalence of intestinal dysmotility varies according to the underlying pathology and pathophysiology. Postoperative ileus (POI) is an unavoidable adverse response to abdominal or retroperitoneal surgery and accounts for delayed refeeding, prolonged hospitalization, and high health care costs. As such, it is a predictor of hospital resource utilization.[1] The economic impact of POI in the United States is estimated to be $750 million annually, not including lost work expense.[2] Acute colonic pseudo-obstruction is estimated to occur in 1%

of surgical patients hospitalized for orthopedic procedures[3] and 0.3% of critically ill patients with burn injury.[4] More than 95% of patients with acute colonic pseudo-obstruction have factors that predispose them to develop the condition,[5] including nonsurgical trauma, pelvic or hip surgery, cardiovascular disease, or infection.[6] As a result of multiple comorbidities and delayed diagnosis, acute colonic pseudo-obstruction is responsible for considerable morbidity, with a mortality rate of 25% to 31% overall, 40% to 50% of which is attributed to ischemia or perforation.[4]

Chronic intestinal pseudo-obstruction (CIP) occurs in association with systemic neurologic, metabolic, autonomic, connective tissue, and malignant causes, and when no cause is identified, it is referred to as *chronic idiopathic intestinal pseudo-obstruction* (CIIPO).[7] The majority of CIIPO cases in adults are sporadic. Despite advances in the field, the pathogenesis of CIIPO remains poorly understood. Defects or injury to ENS nerves and networks, smooth muscle cells, interstitial cells of Cajal (ICC), the ANS, and to the CNS are responsible for disturbances in intestinal motor patterns and fluid movement, which then dictate severity of disease. CIP generally has high morbidity and mortality rates, with patients experiencing marked impairment in quality of life and often life-threatening nutritional compromise.[7]

THE ROLE OF THE ENTERIC NERVOUS SYSTEM IN SMALL BOWEL AND COLONIC MOTILITY

The ENS consists of nerve cells, enteric ganglia, extensive submucosal ganglionic plexuses that lie within and supply intestinal muscle and other effector tissues, epithelial lining, intrinsic blood vessels, and gastroenteropancreatic endocrine cells.[8] In association with the muscle layers, the networks of the ICC are recognized as pacemakers that activate neuromuscular function. There are approximately 600 million neurons in the ENS, which is roughly equal to the number of neurons in the spinal cord. Neuronal control of intestinal function is the result of the integration of local enteric reflexes, reflexes that pass through sympathetic ganglia, and reflexes that emanate from the intestine and pass to the CNS.[8]

Intestinal muscle is responsible for the mixing and propulsion of food, storage, and expulsion of waste and noxious elements. The ENS and CNS are essential for coordination of intestinal muscle function; the extent that the systems are engaged differs depending on the region and physiologic circumstance. From brainstem circuitry located within the medulla oblongata, the CNS dominates muscle activity of the esophagus, whereas the ENS has a collateral role. Through brainstem circuits, and esophagogastric and gastrogastric reflexes, the CNS controls gastric volume, acid secretion, and strength of contractions; the propulsive movements of the stomach are largely myogenic.[8] The ENS governs the patterns of movement of the small and large intestine through reflex pathways, regulates fluid transport across epithelial cells, changes local blood flow, modifies nutrient handling, and interacts with immune and endocrine systems of the intestine[8]; defecation pathways are an exception, and the CNS controls bowel evacuation through defecation centers in the lumbosacral spinal cord.[9]

ILEUS

Ileus refers to the inhibition of GI propulsion that occurs in the absence of mechanical obstruction. Factors that contribute to

BOX 124-1 Factors That Contribute to Ileus

Infection
Abscess
Infected ascites
Pneumonia
Sepsis

Inflammation
Local tissue trauma
Pancreatitis
Peritonitis
Retroperitoneal hemorrhage

Metabolic
Hypercalcemia
Hyperphosphatemia
Hypocalcemia
Hypokalemia
Hypomagnesemia
Hyponatremia

Neurohumoral
Endogenous opiates
Nitric oxide
Vasoactive intestinal peptide

Pharmacologic
Anticholinergic agents
General anesthetic agents

Opioids
Tricyclic antidepressants

Surgery
Cardiothoracic
Colorectal surgery
Hip and knee arthroscopy
Genitourinary
Gynecologic
Laparoscopy
Laparotomy
Neurosurgical
Orthopedic
Spinal
Total hip or total knee repair
Transperitoneal approach

Miscellaneous
Anxiety
Excessive perioperative hydration
Immobility
Myocardial infarction
Pain

ileus are listed in Box 124-1, and include surgery (abdominal and nonabdominal), infection, inflammation, severe pain, medications, general anesthesia, and electrolyte abnormalities among many others. Abdominal or retroperitoneal surgery is the most common cause of ileus, which develops in essentially all such cases,[10,105] and is the focus of this section. The magnitude of POI can vary from merely a delay in the passage of flatus to severe paralytic ileus. POI is associated with significant patient morbidity and mortality, prolonged hospitalization, and high resource utilization, and it represents a substantial socioeconomic burden. POI is a predictor of the duration of hospital stay and health care costs for patients undergoing colectomy,[11] and the costs of managing POI are similar to those of managing other major postoperative complications such as wound infections, pulmonary embolus, and deep venous thrombosis (DVT).[12] At a time when health care costs are generally rising, optimization of patient care and costs is essential, particularly with colectomy where complications occur at a rate that exceeds most other operative procedures.[13] In fact, colectomy accounts for approximately 25% of all operative complications, but only about 10% of all operations.[14]

POI is defined as the time from surgery until the passage of flatus or stool along with adequate oral intake that has been maintained for 24 hours[15]; the usual range is 2 to 4 days for conventional procedures, but can be less than 2 days with laparoscopy (Chapter 123).[16] Uncomplicated, or primary, POI resolves in a predictable fashion: the small intestine resumes activity within 24 hours, the stomach within 24 to 48 hours, and the colon from 48 to 72 hours; the latter is often the rate-limiting factor in POI.[17] POI that extends beyond 7 days (secondary, prolonged, complicated) is defined by the same parameters as primary POI, though it is triggered by an operative complication such as abscess or peritonitis. Secondary POI occurs in fewer than 10% of all abdominal operations, although that number increases to 25% in hemicolectomy cases.[18] The pathophysiology and treatment of secondary POI will not be addressed in this section.

Pathophysiology

Incising the peritoneal cavity and manipulating the intestine is now recognized as the primary mechanism of POI, although many other factors play a role.

The primary cause of POI is the surgical procedure itself, with the nature and intensity of the applied stimuli serving as important determinants of the duration and severity of ileus.[15] There are 2 phases of ileus that have independent physiologic mechanisms and have been studied extensively in animal (rodent) models, although such data may not fully explain the human situation because of species differences, diverse neurohumoral elements, and unique transmitter and receptor expression.[15,16] The first phase is a brief one that is neurogenically mediated and involves spinal reflexes that are activated from the first abdominal incision to just after the surgery is completed (Fig. 124-2A). The second phase is sustained, inflammatory, begins during surgery, and continues for a variable time after surgery (see Fig. 124-2B); the second phase is more germane to clinical management.

Early Neurogenic Phase

Incising the skin briefly interrupts intestinal motility, which is neurogenically mediated through adrenergic pathways.[19] The mechanism involves a spinal reflex loop with afferent splanchnic nerves synapsing in the spinal cord and efferent nerves relaying signal back to the intestine (see Fig. 124-2A).[15] With a stronger stimulus such as mechanical handling of the intestine, there is prolonged inhibition of motility that is only partially blocked by adrenergic agonists; this inhibition involves high-threshold supraspinal pathways that activate specific nuclei located within the CNS, such as the paraventricular and supraoptic nucleus of the hypothalamus and the nucleus tractus solitarii[20] (see Fig. 124-2B). Corticotropin-releasing factor (CRF) probably has a key role in this pathway, and its release stimulates neurons in the supraoptic nucleus of the hypothalamus that relays information to the spinal cord, and to sympathetic preganglionic neurons, thereupon releasing noradrenaline[21]; these nerves then inhibit motility of the entire GI tract. In addition to this adrenergic inhibitory pathway, intense stimulation of splanchnic afferents triggers a vagally mediated pathway, which synapses to inhibitory nitric oxide (NO) and vasoactive intestinal peptide (VIP)-containing neurons located within the intestinal wall.[22] Activation of the neural pathways, various nociceptors, and mechanoreceptors stimulated during abdominal surgery ceases once the incision is closed.

Late Inflammatory Phase

Approximately 3 to 4 hours after abdominal surgery, a second phase of prolonged inhibition begins, the duration of which depends on the nature of the surgery; this is caused by inflammation of the intestinal musculature[23] and results from intestinal manipulation. There normally is a layer of resident macrophages residing at the level of the myenteric plexus between the circular and longitudinal muscle layers and on the serosal side of the intestine.[24] Beginning 3 to 4 hours after surgery, activation of these resident macrophages results in the release of cytokines and chemokines, followed by a massive extravasation of leukocytes, mostly polymorphonuclear leukocytes, into the muscularis.[23] Intercellular adhesion molecule-1 (ICAM-1) is a molecule that plays a central role in the recruitment of leukocyte populations in inflammation.

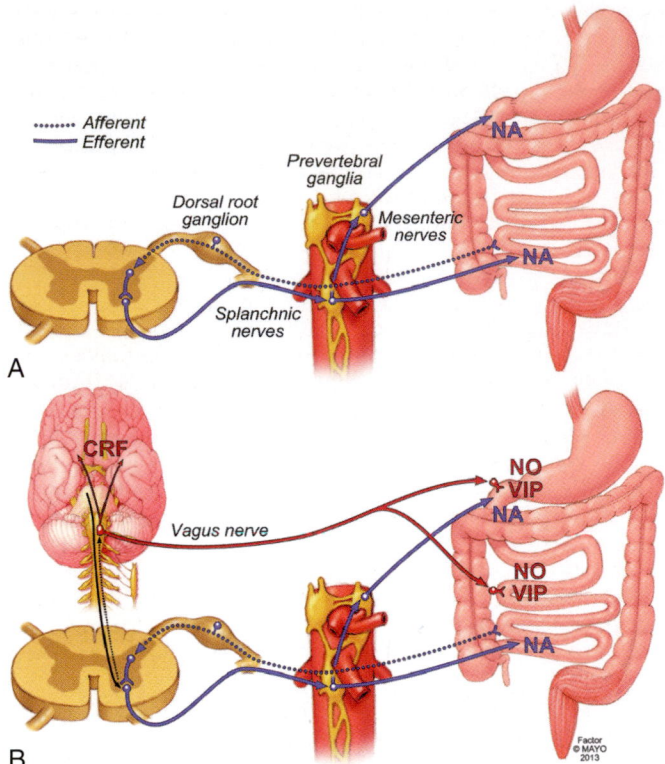

FIGURE 124-2. Schematic representation of two neural pathways triggered by abdominal surgery. The intensity and nature of nociceptive stimuli determine the severity and duration of ileus. Simple laparotomy activates spinal afferents that synapse in the spinal cord where they activate an inhibitory pathway involving prevertebral adrenergic neurons that stops intestinal motility briefly (A). Intestinal manipulation activates additional pathways. Afferent signals are transmitted to the brainstem where they trigger increased autonomic output to the neurons of the intermediolateral column of the thoracic cord, where sympathetic preganglionic neurons that release noradrenaline (NA) are located. Activation of these nerves inhibits the entire GI tract (B). In addition to this adrenergic inhibitory pathway, intense stimulation of splanchnic afferents triggers a vagally mediated pathway that synapses to inhibitory nitric oxide (NO) and vasoactive intestinal peptide (VIP)-containing neurons. Corticotrophin-releasing factor (CRF) seems to play a central role in this pathway. *(By permission of Mayo Foundation for Medical Education and Research. All rights reserved.)*

Blocking ICAM-1 by pretreatment with antibodies or antisense oligonucleotides against ICAM-1 prevents the influx of leukocytes and preserves the normal neuromuscular response.[25]

Mechanisms Involved in the Inflammatory Response of Postoperative Ileus

Our innate immune system, as well as host defense, plays a critical role in initiating inflammatory responses.[15] The innate immune system recognizes 2 large classes of macromolecules: those released in response to pathogens (pathogen-associated molecular patterns [PAMPs]) and those released in response to cell damage (damage-associated molecular patterns [DAMPs]).[26] Lipopolysaccharide (LPS), a component of Gram-negative cell walls, is the prototype for PAMP; there are many other PAMP types, including bacterial flagellin and peptidoglycan. Intracellular ATP, uric acid, and heat shock proteins, also known as "alarmins," are examples of DAMPs. PAMPs and DAMPs are identified through pattern recognition by Toll-like receptors (TLR) and receptors for advanced glycation end-products (RAGE). By example, when an LPS molecule is recognized by TLR4, the binding results in activation of immune cells expressing the TLR4 receptor.[15] DAMPs can lead to the activation of many inflammatory receptors, including a multiprotein complex called an "inflammasome" that is required for the synthesis of interleukin (IL)-1 and IL-8.[27]

Activation of Mast Cells

There is significant evidence to support an essential role for mast cells and resident macrophages of the innate immune system in the inflammatory response to intestinal manipulation. Even gentle fingering of the intestine at the beginning of surgery triggers DAMPs and the release of mast cell mediators, such as histamine and proteases, into the peritoneal cavity. This step may be a key step in the inflammatory cascade leading to enhanced permeability with translocation of bacterial products and intraluminal bacteria.[15,25]

Mast cells are located near blood vessels in the intestinal serosa and mesentery before they enter the intestinal wall and are especially close to afferent nerve fibers.[28] Mast cells, while essential to adaptive immunity, are also vital for the recruitment of neutrophils and the purging of bacteria from the peritoneal cavity[29]; mast cells serve as sentries of the peritoneal cavity, providing protection against latent threats.[15] Activation of mast cells is considered an essential event for the activation of resident macrophages, another stage of the inflammatory cascade.

Activation of Resident Macrophages

The intestinal mucosa, submucosa, and muscularis externa hold large numbers and various subsets of resident macrophages and antigen-presenting cells (APCs).[30] Resident macrophages are normally located in a layer at the intestinal myenteric plexus and at the serosa; most are phagocytic and are activated by LPS and other PAMPs. Following surgical manipulation, several mechanisms trigger the activity of resident macrophages: (1) intestinal handling causes release of DAMPs, which are potent activators of muscle macrophages and other phagocytes[31]; (2) PAMPS, such as LPS or cytokines entering the systemic circulation, activate resident macrophages, causing up-regulation of macrophage inducible nitric oxide synthase (iNOS) and COX-2; iNOS then stimulates NO, and COX-2 stimulates prostaglandin production, which inhibits smooth muscle contraction[32]; (3) evidence points to intestinal permeability and translocation of bacteria and bacterial products (e.g., LPS) occurring with intestinal handling and release of macrophages.[29] In addition, activation of resident macrophages results in the release of proteases, proinflammatory cytokines (e.g., TNF-α, IL-1β, and IL-6), and monocyte chemoattractant protein-1, which recruit circulating monocytes and neutrophils to subdue intestinal motor function[33]; the inflammatory response is reduced and smooth muscle contractility sustained by preoperative intestinal decontamination with polymyxin B and neomycin.[34]

Evidence in Humans

The and colleagues showed that mast cell mediators are detected in peritoneal lavage solution very early during surgery.[35] Even gentle handling of the intestine early during abdominal hysterectomy resulted in the instantaneous release of tryptase (mast cell-specific protease), followed by increased IL-6 and IL-8 levels. Three hours later, macrophage inflammatory proteins, TNF-α, IL-6, and IL-8 were detected, which in turn enhanced the expression of ICAM-1, recruitment of leukocytes, and inflammation. Interestingly, none of these mediators were increased during minimally invasive surgery or vaginal hysterectomy, except for a slight increase in IL-8 during laparoscopy. In intestinal specimens removed at surgery, inflammatory cells and leukocytes were increased. Leukocytes were located mainly around blood vessels in both the serosa and the muscularis propria, partly adhering to the endothelial lining and marking the ongoing recruitment during this stage of inflammation.

The degree of intestinal manipulation during surgery clearly influences mast cell activation, release of inflammatory mediators, and inflammation. The results may explain faster recovery after minimally invasive surgery.

Pharmacologic Mechanisms

Anesthesia

All anesthetic agents have an inhibitory effect on intestinal motility that is generally short lived, although the technique of administration can significantly influence the duration of POI. There is not sufficient evidence to direct the choice of anesthetic agents; however, the use of short-acting agents (e.g., propofol) rather than long-acting agents (e.g., bupivacaine) is a proactive measure that can hasten the return of GI function. In addition, short-acting inhalational agents may be an alternative to IV anesthesia.[36] Mid-thoracic (T6-T8) catheter placement to administer epidural analgesia and produce sympathetic blockade is frequently used as an adjunct to general anesthesia in abdominal operations and substantially reduces the severity and incidence of POI.[37] If initiated prior to the operation, epidural analgesia simultaneously blocks stress hormone release and attenuates postoperative hormone resistance.[36,38]

Opiates

The use of opiates for pain management in the postoperative period has improved patient comfort, although with their use comes a delay in the return of GI function. Exogenous and endogenous opioids contribute significantly to the development of POI.[39] Of the 3 main classes of opiate receptors (μ,κ,δ) located in the CNS and GI tract, CNS μ receptors mostly modulate analgesia within the brain and spinal cord. Endogenous opioids released from neurons within the submucosal and myenteric plexuses of the intestinal tract modulate peristalsis and sphincteric activity in a coordinated fashion.[40] Activation of μ receptors suppresses the release of acetylcholine from cholinergic neurons, resulting in delayed intestinal motility.[41]

Exogenous opioids increase gastric antral and proximal duodenal tone, with an overall inhibitory effect on motility. The effect of morphine on the small intestine is biphasic, initially stimulating MMC activity, followed by atony, which impedes propulsion and delays intestinal transit.[42] In the colon, morphine increases the tone and amplitude of nonpropagating contractions, thus reducing propulsive activity and slowing transit. The overall effect of opiates is to suppress intestinal motility.

Perioperative Fluid Excess

IV fluid excess during or after surgery can delay recovery of GI function and is associated with poor survival and complications. In randomized controlled trials (RCTs), goal-directed fluid management was shown to reduce surgical morbidity, largely in major abdominal surgery.[43] Goal-directed fluid therapy should be integrated with awareness of total fluid demands; it is 1 component of enhanced recovery programs (ERPs) that uses a multimodal approach to reduce morbidity and improve perioperative care.[44]

Clinical Features

Typical symptoms of ileus include poorly localized abdominal pain, abdominal distention, inability to tolerate solid food, and obstipation; nausea and vomiting also may occur. Physical examination reveals reduced bowel sounds. Symptoms range from mild to severe; some patients resume daily activities within 1 or 2 days, whereas others require prolonged, intensive monitoring, hydration, and pain management. Abdominal plain films show air-filled small intestine, often with air-fluid levels at various points that raise the question of bowel obstruction. Distention often extends up to the stomach and down to the colon. Abdominal CT will confirm unobstructed distension or identify mechanical obstruction and its various causes. Importantly, ileus in the early postoperative period does not require diagnostic evaluation. Prolonged POI exceeds 7 days' duration and is independently associated with perioperative blood loss and total narcotic dose.

Early postoperative bowel obstruction has a similar presentation to POI, although the consequences can be more serious. It is a complication of surgery that affects 0.7% to 10% of surgical patients,[45] with a mortality rate that exceeds 17%. Postoperative bowel obstruction is diagnosed if, within 30 days of surgery after resolution of POI and return of normal bowel function, abdominal pain, vomiting, and radiologic evidence consistent with small bowel obstruction are present.[46] CT can distinguish POI from early postoperative small bowel obstruction and identifies other complications.

Treatment

Historically, treatment for POI has included bowel rest, NG tube decompression, and IV fluid therapy. These interventions were thought to shorten recovery time by lowering the incidence of complications and improving outcomes. Critical review of the evidence, however, does not support such conclusions. Bowel rest neither shortens the time to first bowel movement nor decreases the time to oral intake.[47] Carbohydrate loading prior to surgery and early postoperative feeding are now used to hasten recovery. Regular use of NG tube decompression beyond surgery and abdominal drains is no longer recommended; similarly, urinary catheters are discontinued within 24 to 48 hours, because their use does not hasten recovery.

The advent of laparoscopic surgery, regional anesthesia, opioid-sparing analgesics, and several evidence-based treatments that hasten recovery from ileus has led to improved care of patients who undergo abdominal surgery. First described in the 1990s, ERPs (Enhanced Recovery Programs/ Pathways), fast-track surgery methods combine treatment modalities that individually improve outcome following major surgery.[48] An overarching goal of fast-track surgery is to lower rates of organ dysfunction, thereby reducing morbidity, hastening recovery, and shortening hospital stay.[49] Some benefits of ERPs are listed in Box 124-2. The concept has proved valid across all surgical specialties, but the most physiologic data are available for colonic surgery. Fast-track surgery has been shown to enhance recovery from POI. The majority of patients have a normal oral intake and defecate within 48 hours, and have a hospital stay of 2 to 4 days (reduced from 5 to 10 days) after uncomplicated open colonic surgery.[13,50]

BOX 124-2 Benefits of Enhanced Recovery Pathways for Colorectal Surgery

Accelerated recovery
Cost containment
Improved resource utilization
Low morbidity
Low readmission rate
Safe reduction in length of stay
Standardized health practice

BOX 124-3 Risk Factors for Postoperative Nausea and Vomiting (PONV)

Female gender
History of motion sickness
General anesthesia
   Long-acting agents
   Volatile agents (nitrous oxide)
Major abdominal surgery
   Blood loss
   Long duration
Non-smoker status
Opioids
Previous history of PONV

Modified from Gan TJ, Meyer TA, Apfel CC, et al. Society for Ambulatory Anesthesia guidelines for the management of postoperative nausea and vomiting. Anesth Analg 2007; 105:1615-28.

Prevention

Preoperative

Nutrition. Preoperative enteral carbohydrate loading has been shown to reduce preoperative patient stress and discomfort, postoperative insulin resistance, postoperative nausea and vomiting, and also to improve muscle mass. Carbohydrate loading with solid food or a liquid carbohydrate solution is recommended within 6 hours and up to 2 hours, respectively, before surgery.[50] This also enhances recovery and reduces duration of stay.

Reducing the Stress Response. Pre- and early postoperative nutritional support, epidural anesthesia, adequate analgesia including nonopioid pain management with NSAIDs and acetaminophen, and use of ERPs reduce the stress response to surgery, which has been associated with prolonged POI, delayed wound healing, fatigue, wound infections, and longer suppression of immune function.[50]

Mechanical Bowel Preparation. A systematic review that evaluated mechanical bowel preparation prior to elective surgery showed no statistical evidence of its benefit in anastomotic leak rate, reoperation, surgical site infection, or mortality with or without mechanical bowel preparation.[51]

Prophylaxis of Postoperative Nausea and Vomiting (PONV). PONV can be more stressful than pain. Risk factors are listed in Box 124-3 and include anesthesia, opioids, major surgery, and female gender.[52,53] At-risk individuals can receive PONV prophylaxis with dexamethasone sodium phosphate at induction, or a serotonin receptor antagonist at closure; general anesthesia with propofol and remifentanil along with prophylaxis can reduce symptoms.[54]

Intraoperative

Nature of Surgery. Minimally invasive surgery has smaller incisions, lower total analgesic doses, less inflammation and pain, faster return of GI function, shorter hospital stay, and lower cost compared with open surgery[55]; for example, laparoscopy reduces the inflammatory response, abdominal pain, and catabolism in colorectal surgery compared with open surgery.[36,56] A meta-analysis showed consistent improvement in short-term outcomes with laparoscopy, including lower short-term wound morbidity, time to first bowel movement, and earlier discharge.[36,56] Additionally, many RCTs that evaluated surgical technique have shown that compared with laparotomy, laparoscopy lowered blood loss by 50% and reduced major morbidity.[55]

Anesthesia. Regional anesthesia largely prevents the neuroendocrine stress response to surgery by preventing afferent neural transmission from reaching the CNS and by blocking efferent activation of the sympathetic nervous system; its use preserves immune function while reducing the need for opiates.[57] Epidural anesthesia and analgesia is recommended for open colorectal surgery, and for laparoscopy if patients have significant respiratory disease[58]; it also has been shown to enhance colonic blood flow and improve return of GI function.[59]

Hemodynamic Management. Several large trials have shown that excessive hydration in the perioperative period increases morbidity.[60] Fluid excess, which can cause bowel edema[61] and pulmonary compromise, is linked to prolonged POI and extended hospital stay.[62] Fluid management by perioperative optimization of hemodynamic function, known as goal-directed therapy, maximizes cardiac stroke volume by using small fluid challenges[63,64] and has been shown to improve patient outcome. Avoiding fluid overload by using goal-directed therapy can reduce postoperative complications and facilitate rapid functional GI recovery.[63]

Postoperative

Nasogastric Tubes, Drains, and Catheters. Routine use of NG tubes and abdominal drains increases morbidity from infectious and GI causes without providing benefit for patients[50]; their avoidance can lead to earlier recovery from POI.[55] Urinary catheters should be removed within 24 to 48 hours of surgery.[13]

Gum Chewing and Laxative Use. Chewing promotes peristalsis by increasing GI motility and secretion of fluids via neural and hormonal mechanisms.[50] GI recovery is significantly accelerated by liberal gum chewing in the postoperative period.[55] There is evidence to support the use of osmotic and stimulant laxatives to prompt early bowel evacuation and shorten the duration of POI. Small trials have examined the effect of bisacodyl suppository alone,[65] bisacodyl in combination with milk of magnesia,[66] and magnesium oxide combined with disodium phosphate,[67] the latter used in a fast-track rehabilitation protocol following abdominal hysterectomy. No significant adverse events have been reported with any agent, but high-quality prospective trials are needed.

Early Oral Intake and Nutrition. Liquids are started immediately in the postoperative period with no restrictions on dietary intake starting 24 hours after laparotomy and laparoscopic surgery.[13] Early enteral nutrition preserves a positive nitrogen balance and improves intestinal barrier function, lowers hyperglycemia and insulin resistance, improves anastomotic healing, and reduces the incidence of infections[50] compared with nothing by mouth. In combination with epidural analgesia and forced early mobilization, early enteral nutrition significantly improved nutrient uptake after colorectal surgery.[69]

Postoperative Pain Management. Opioid-sparing analgesia (including thoracic epidural analgesia) provides the best analgesia postoperatively.[70] Additional effective postoperative pain relief methods include patient-controlled analgesia, intrathecal analgesia, wound infusion and infiltration, systemic lidocaine infusion, and transversus abdominis plane block.[50,70] NSAIDs and acetaminophen are often used to achieve multimodal analgesia; however, there are reports of an increased risk of anastomotic leakage with use of COX-2 inhibitors.[71]

Early Mobilization. Effective pain management is key to early mobilization, as has been shown with ambulatory epidural analgesia.[72] Ambulation improves pulmonary function and tissue oxygenation; it also reduces insulin resistance, risk of pulmonary embolism, and muscle loss while improving muscle strength.[36] In 1 regimen, patients are advised to ambulate out of their room 5 times on the day of surgery and sit in a chair for 6 hours a day.[13] Nursing and physical therapy support is helpful.

Preset Discharge Criteria. ERPs include standardized discharge criteria: patients must be able to tolerate solid food for 3 consecutive meals, have passed gas or stool, have adequate analgesia with a low pain score on a visual analog scale, and also feel ready for discharge with adequate social support.[14]

Postoperative Nausea and Vomiting. PONV occurs in 30% of low-risk surgical patients and in up to 80% of high-risk surgical patients.[53] General anesthesia increases the risk of PONV 9-fold more than does the use of regional anesthesia.[73] Reducing risk factors (Table 124-1) when possible and using prophylactic agents in patients at high risk for PONV can shorten the duration of ileus; low-risk patients are less likely to receive benefit. Randomized trials have confirmed the efficacy of glucocorticoids, 5-HT^3 antagonists, and droperidol alone or in combination for prophylaxis of PONV,[74] and are recommended routinely in high-risk patients.[55]

The main components of ERPs are listed in Table 124-1.

TABLE 124-1 Evidence-Based Components of Enhanced Recovery Pathways (ERPs)

Preoperative	Intraoperative	Postoperative
Preoperative assessment; verbal explanation and written material provided on ERP; preset criteria for discharge and readmission reviewed	Goal-directed fluid therapy	Avoidance of NG tubes and drains; removal of urinary catheter within 24 hr
	Laparoscopy, or midline or transverse laparotomy incision	Early mobilization and ambulation
Carbohydrate loading by solution or solids up to 2 to 6 hours respectfully before surgery	C6-8 epidural anesthesia	Continuous epidural low-dose local anesthetic and opioid-sparing combinations or IV patient-controlled analgesia; NSAID and/or acetaminophen use as baseline analgesic
	Opioid-sparing anesthesia and analgesia	
Avoidance of mechanical colon preparation		Early enteral feeding
Prophylaxis of postoperative nausea and vomiting (PONV)		Early withdrawal of IV fluid
Reduction of the stress response		Use of chewing gum
		Use of laxatives
		Early scheduled follow-up

Drug Therapy

Opioid-Sparing Analgesia

NSAIDs are prostaglandin inhibitors used extensively in postoperative pain management, frequently in combination with other agents such as acetaminophen, to avoid opioid-related complications and to reduce PONV. There is some concern of increased anastomotic leakage with COX-2 inhibitors.[71] IV ketorolac alone or ketorolac in combination with IV morphine showed consistent opioid-sparing benefits compared with IV morphine alone.[75,76] IV lidocaine has been shown to improve analgesia and to reduce POI duration and hospital stay after colonic surgery.[47] Because of its safety, efficacy, and low cost, lidocaine is often included as a component of multimodal postoperative analgesia care.

Opioid Antagonists

Stimulation of μ-opioid receptors in the brain and intestine by morphine and other opiates imparts a potent central analgesic effect plus a dose-dependent inhibition of intestinal motility. Alvimopan is a peripherally acting μ-opioid receptor antagonist that ameliorates the inhibitory intestinal motor effect of opioids without compromising pain relief.[77] In patients undergoing open colonic resection, postoperative administration of alvimopan (12 mg) reduced the duration of POI by 15 to 18 hours, hospital stay by 1 day,[78] and the incidence of prolonged hospital stay (>7 days) from 6.8% to 2.1% by lowering POI-related morbidity.[79] Although alvimopan was FDA approved in 2008, its use has been associated with an increased risk of myocardial infarction, limiting its clinical application.[11,77] Trials are needed to determine if its reduced hospital stay and cost-saving potential are effective and safe in patients undergoing laparoscopic surgery.

Prokinetic Agents

There are no available effective prokinetic agents for the treatment of POI, and meta-analysis found that routine administration of prokinetics, including dopamine antagonists, erythromycin, cisapride, propranolol, vasopressin, and cholecystokinin-like drugs is not recommended.[80] These agents may not be as effective as originally predicted, because the surgical-inflammatory response (see earlier) strongly inhibits intestinal smooth muscle and transit. Neostigmine requires additional studies with clinically relevant outcomes to prove treatment effectiveness.[80]

Drug Therapies in Clinical Trials

IV lidocaine, in addition to its analgesic properties, can stimulate intestinal motility by blocking afferent and efferent inhibitory sympathetic spinal and prevertebral reflexes that contribute to ileus.[11] In most clinical trials, IV lidocaine infusion reduced the duration of POI by 1 day and reduced hospital stay, although the type of surgery and surgical approach influenced outcomes; for example, lidocaine therapy had an insignificant benefit in laparoscopic cholecystectomy.[81]

Methylnaltrexone is a peripherally acting μ-opioid receptor antagonist that preserves central analgesia while facilitating intestinal motility; it can reverse morphine-induced delay in orocecal transit time in healthy subjects.[82] In a phase II clinical trial of patients who underwent segmental colectomy, methylnaltrexone reduced POI and reduced hospital stay by 1 day compared with placebo.[83] In 2 phase III placebo-controlled trials of patients undergoing open colectomy, however, 2 doses of methylnaltrexone (12 mg and 24 mg) failed to show improvement in POI or discharge parameters.[84]

Ghrelin is an orexigenic and prokinetic hormone[11] that stimulates the MMC and gastric motility and emptying and coordinates patterns of smooth muscle propulsive activity.[85] Ghrelin mimetics are being evaluated in clinical trials as potential prokinetic agents, but they also activate an anti-inflammatory pathway that may be of additional benefit.[86] ZP-101 is a potent ghrelin agonist under evaluation as a treatment for POI; 2 phase IIb studies showed a decrease in the time to first bowel movement and shortened hospital stay.[87,88] TZP-101 is now being evaluated in phase III trials.

5-Hydroxytryptamine receptor⁴ (5-HT⁴) agonists are potent prokinetic agents that promote enhanced intestinal contractility in the upper and lower GI tract. Cisapride improved POI but was removed from the market because of cardiovascular adverse events.[11] Prucalopride is a high-affinity 5-HT⁴ molecule used as a treatment for chronic constipation. Patients with POI who had undergone partial colectomy and received 4 mg prucalopride once daily for 3 days had faster return of GI function than did patients who had received placebo[89]; phase III trials are planned. Mosapride citrate improved POI in patients undergoing colectomy,[90] and in a preclinical trial it improved ileus and caused a reduced surgery-evoked inflammatory response mediated by activation of myenteric neurons, with resultant suppression of resident macrophages.[91]

Intestinal Inflammation: Implications for the Treatment of Postoperative Ileus

The inflammatory phase of POI is most clinically relevant and, therefore, its prevention or reduction should be a primary goal of POI treatment. Minimal handling of the intestine and use of epidural anesthesia to block adrenergic and splanchnic nerve stimulation can reduce POI in minimally invasive surgery and simple laparotomy. Once the inflammatory cascade is activated, adhesion molecules such as ICAM-1, mast cells, and resident macrophages orchestrate the next cascade of events. Targeting these immune cells with antibodies and antisense molecules to ICAM-1, mast cell stabilizers, and drugs to inactivate or pharmacologically deplete resident macrophages has shown promise in in vitro and in some human trials.[15,23,92]

ACUTE COLONIC PSEUDO-OBSTRUCTION

Acute colonic pseudo-obstruction, also known as *Ogilvie's syndrome*,[93] is characterized by acute massive colon dilatation that involves primarily the right side of the colon and is unexplained by mechanical cause. It is most often diagnosed in hospitalized, debilitated, medical or surgical patients with a wide array of medical conditions (Table 124-2). Ogilvie's syndrome is estimated to occur in 0.1% of all surgical patients,[5] and patient outcome depends on the severity of underlying illness, the person's age, maximum diameter of the cecum, delay until colonic decompression, and the presence of colonic ischemia.[4]

Pathophysiology

Disruption of ANS activity is considered a key factor in the pathogenesis of acute colonic pseudo-obstruction. Parasympathetic (excitatory, causing contraction) innervation of the colon is from the vagus nerve, which supplies the right colon and extends to the splenic flexure; parasympathetic innervation of the distal colon and rectum is via the spinal supply off the sacral plexus. Sympathetic (inhibitory, causing relaxation)

TABLE 124-2 Conditions Associated with Acute Colonic Pseudo-obstruction (400 cases)

Health Condition (Most Common)	% of Cases
Trauma (nonoperative)	11.3
Infection (pneumonia, sepsis)	10.0
Cardiac (myocardial infarction, heart failure)	10.0
Gynecologic surgery	9.8
Abdominal/pelvic surgery	9.3
Neurologic (Parkinson's disease, spinal cord, multiple sclerosis, Alzheimer's disease)	9.3
Orthopedic surgery	7.3
Miscellaneous medical conditions (metabolic, cancer, respiratory failure, kidney failure)	32
Miscellaneous surgical conditions (urologic, thoracic, neurosurgical)	11.8

Originally reported by Vanek VW, Al-Salti M. Acute pseudo-obstruction of the colon (Ogilvie's syndrome): An analysis of 400 cases. Dis Colon Rectum 1986; 29:203-10. Modified from: Saunders MD, Kimmey MB. Systematic review: Acute colonic pseudo-obstruction. Aliment Pharmacol Ther 2005; 22:917-25.

BOX 124-4 Proposed Mechanisms for Acute Colonic Pseudo-obstruction

Intestine Fails to Contract
Excess sympathetic motor input
Decreased parasympathetic motor input
Stimulation of peripheral μ-opioid receptors (endogenous or exogenous)
Reflex motor inhibition through splanchnic afferents

Intestine Fails to Relax
Excess parasympathetic motor input
Inhibition of nitric oxide release

Modified from Delgado-Aros S, Camilleri M. Pseudo-obstruction in the critically ill. In: Scholmerich J, editor. Bailliere's best practice & research in clinical gastroenterology: Gastrointestinal disorders in the critically ill, vol. 17. London: Elsevier Science; 2003. pp. 427-44.

innervation of the colon is from the celiac and mesenteric ganglia (see Fig. 124-1). The proposed mechanisms of acute colonic pseudo-obstruction are summarized in Box 124-4.

Local stimuli effect an inhibitory reflex that results in dilatation of the colon, for which the splanchnic nerves provide both the afferent and efferent pathways. Local stimuli, including peritoneal inflammation, infection, and handling of the colon, result in the release of mast cells, leukocytes, and monocytes.[94-96] Inflammatory mediators such as ICAM-1, MCP-1, iNOS, and COX-2 are up-regulated during the first 18 hours after abdominal surgery, and the degree of postoperative intestinal impairment correlates with the intestinal inflammatory response.

The release of endogenous opioids after surgery has been related to the inflammation and impaired motor activity that characterizes the physiologic response to surgery. Administration of antidepressant, phenothiazine, antiparkinsonian, or

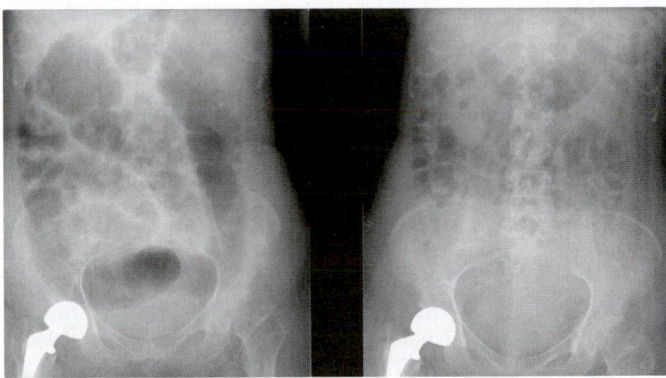

FIGURE 124-3. Plain abdominal films in a patient with acute colonic pseudo-obstruction. *Left,* Upright film of the abdomen revealing diffuse, but predominantly right, colonic distention (with a cecal diameter of 13 cm) that developed after placement of a right hip prosthesis for a fractured femur. *Right,* Colonic distention resolved shortly after administration of IV neostigmine. *(From Bharucha AE, Camilleri M. Common large intestinal disorders. In: Hazzard WR, Blass JP, Halter JB, et al, editors. Principles of geriatric medicine and gerontology. New York: McGraw-Hill; 2003. p 652.)*

narcotic medications can induce acute colonic pseudo-obstruction.[97] Opioids inhibit release of NO from inhibitory motor neurons in vitro and delay transit in vivo.

Clinical Features

Acute colonic pseudo-obstruction typically occurs in older (mean age, 60 years) men who are hospitalized or institutionalized (60%) with severe underlying medical or surgical conditions (see Table 124-2).

Symptoms and Signs

The most characteristic feature of acute colonic pseudo-obstruction is abdominal distention, which can develop gradually over 3 to 7 days or more acutely within 24 hours. About 60% of patients experience nausea and vomiting. Abdominal pain (80%) tends to be mild and constant, with occasional slight rebound tenderness and painless distention.[98] Low-grade fever may also be present. Disturbances of electrolyte levels occur, notably hypokalemia, hypocalcemia, hyponatremia, and hypomagnesemia. New abdominal pain or tenderness, increasing fever, and increasing WBC count are features of ischemia or perforation. About 90% of patients have abnormal bowel sounds, which vary from absent to hyperactive. In many cases, the abnormal bowel sounds are high-pitched and suggest mechanical obstruction.[99]

Imaging

The most distinctive feature of acute colonic pseudo-obstruction on a plain abdominal film is dilatation of the colon that preferentially affects the right side. The maximal diameter of the cecum typically ranges from 9 to 25 cm, often with a cutoff sign at the hepatic or splenic flexure (Fig. 124-3). The left colon, including the rectosigmoid, and the small intestine also may be dilated. Air-fluid levels can be seen in the small intestine but usually do not occur in the colon. Haustral folds often are seen despite severe distention.

Air throughout all colonic segments helps differentiate this condition from mechanical obstruction. Free air is usually a radiologic sign of intestinal perforation, although when free air accompanies pneumatosis intestinalis, it might not be associated with perforation. A water-soluble contrast enema or CT scan can exclude mechanical obstruction if gas and distention are seen throughout all colonic segments, including the rectum and sigmoid colon.

Differential Diagnosis

The differential diagnosis of acute colonic pseudo-obstruction includes mechanical obstruction, toxic megacolon, and ischemic colitis. Frequent clinical evaluation including WBC count and plain abdominal radiography are vital to identifying bowel perforation.

Prognosis

The mortality rate of patients with acute colonic pseudo-obstruction varies from 0% to 32% and is partly determined by accompanying comorbidities.[5,100] Older patients, poor clinical condition, and surgical treatment for acute colonic pseudo-obstruction are associated with an increased risk of mortality. There are no RCTs comparing surgical and medical treatment to clarify whether surgery itself or selection bias influences mortality associated with surgical treatment. Intestinal ischemia or perforation, which complicates approximately 1 in 7 cases, is associated with a 40% increase in the risk of death.[5]

The diameter of the colon is also a risk factor for mortality. When surgical decompression is used in patients with a mechanical obstruction and a cecal diameter greater than 9 cm, there is a dramatic reduction in mortality,[101] which is the basis for the 9-cm cutoff as a sign of impending perforation in patients with acute colonic pseudo-obstruction. In 1 study, perforation rates for cecal diameters less than 12 cm, 12 to 14 cm, or more than 14 cm were 0%, 7%, and 23%, respectively.[5] Mortality also was associated with delay in decompression: 15% in those decompressed less than 4 days after onset of dilatation, 27% when the decompression occurred after 4 to 7 days, and 73% after day 7.

Prevention

Minimally invasive surgery, thoracic epidural anesthesia, and nominal use of opioid analgesia have led to improved care of surgical patients. ERPs (see section on Ileus) combine modalities that individually have a lower morbidity compared with standard treatment.[13] Components of ERP are listed in Box 124-2. Studies have shown ERPs can reduce the duration of ileus and the costs and duration of hospital stay while decreasing cardiopulmonary morbidity and postoperative convalescence.

Treatment

The goal of management is to achieve colonic decompression. With correction of reversible potential causes or associated imbalances (e.g., infection, hypovolemia, hypoxemia, electrolyte levels) and discontinuation of medications that can induce ileus (e.g., anticholinergic agents, opiates), ileus resolves by day 6 in 83% to 96% of patients.[5] IV saline and glucose solutions suffice for hydration because of the usually short-lived and reversible nature of the dysfunction; in patients with prolonged acute colonic pseudo-obstruction, parenteral or enteral nutrition may be necessary.[102] NG aspiration is often ineffective because the functional obstruction affects the colon. Rectal tubes may be useful if the sigmoid colon is markedly dilated.

Enemas might "cleanse" the colon, but only Gastrografin enemas have shown efficacy, and these reports were anecdotal; also, enema use has been complicated by colonic perforation.[103] When the diameter of the cecum is greater than 9 cm and has not responded to treatment within the first 72 hours after diagnosis, decompression should be performed to reduce the risk of ischemia, perforation, and death.[5] A treatment algorithm is shown in Figure 124-4.

Medical Decompression

Adrenergic blockers and the acetylcholinesterase inhibitor neostigmine have been tested in open-label studies. Only neostigmine has been tested in RCTs and has an effective initial treatment response rate of 60% to 90%.[4,104]

Abdominal cramping with passage of gas and colonic decompression occurs promptly after administration of neostigmine, but such volume decompression has not been shown to reduce the risk of perforation and mortality in these patients. Nonetheless, if there are no contraindications to its use, neostigmine is a safe choice in patients whose cecal diameter is greater than 9 cm for 72 hours. Contraindications to neostigmine include bradycardia, hypotension, active bronchospasm, serum creatinine concentration over 3 mg/dL, mechanical obstruction of the GI or genitourinary tract, and peritonitis. Adverse events described after IV administration of 2 to 2.5 mg of neostigmine include abdominal cramps (17%), excessive salivation (13%), sweating (4%), nausea or vomiting (4%), and transient bradycardia (6%); a starting dose of 1 mg rather than 2 mg reduces the likelihood of bradycardia. A second dose of neostigmine should be considered if there is partial or no response to the first trial or if ileus recurs after an initial response.

5-HT$_4$ receptor agonists, motilin receptor agonists, and muscarinic receptor agonists have been the subject of anecdotal reports, but none have been formally tested in the setting of acute colonic pseudo-obstruction.[4] Metoclopramide has shown very small or insignificant benefit in the treatment of POI.[80] The peripherally acting μ-opioid receptor antagonist alvimopan significantly shortens the duration of POI, but neither metoclopramide nor alvimopan has been sufficiently tested as treatment for acute colonic pseudo-obstruction.[78-80]

Endoscopic Decompression

RCTs of endoscopic decompression are lacking. Colonoscopic decompression can be achieved technically in 80% of patients with acute colonic pseudo-obstruction, albeit with a risk of cecal perforation of 3% and a complication rate that ranges from 1% to 5%.[4,5,103] Colonic decompression has not been shown to improve the outcome of these patients. Acute colonic pseudo-obstruction has a high recurrence rate and colonoscopy in unprepared bowel can result in even greater distention with perforation.[5] Placement of a decompression tube into either the right or transverse colon has a technical success rate similar to that of colonic decompression.[100] Endoscopic decompression should be considered in patients with a high risk of cecal perforation when conservative and pharmacologic maneuvers have failed.

Percutaneous Cecostomy

In view of the high rate of recurrence of colonic dilatation after endoscopic decompression, alternative techniques to decompress the colon have been proposed to avoid surgery. Percutaneous cecostomy has been reported to be successful in case reports and 1 small case series, but it is associated with significant morbidity and generally is not recommended.

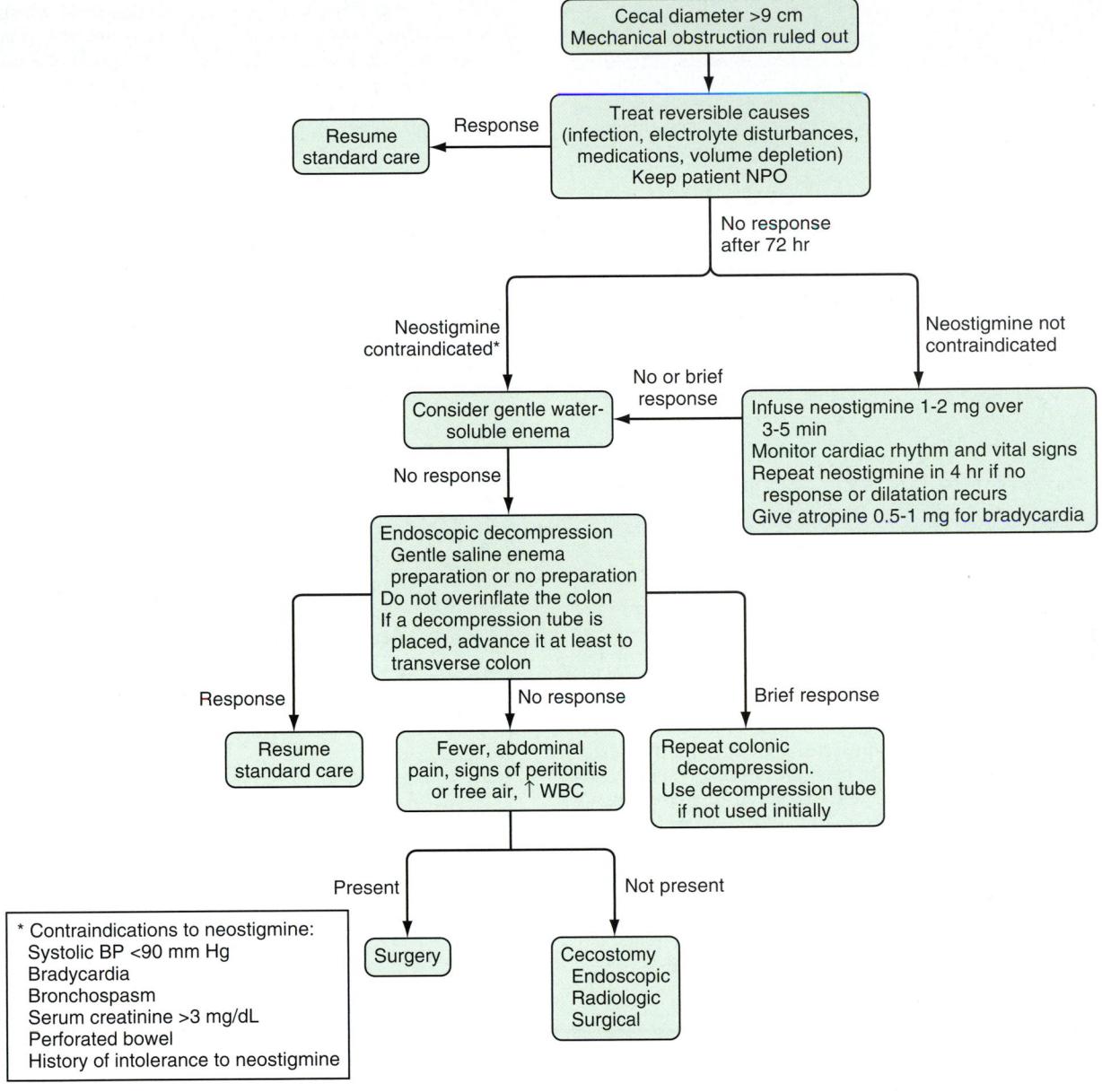

FIGURE 124-4. Algorithm for the treatment of acute colonic pseudo-obstruction.

Percutaneous cecostomy can be performed endoscopically, radiologically, or surgically.[106,107]

Surgical Decompression

Surgical decompression, which includes cecostomy, colostomy, or resection, is associated with a 6% morbidity and a 30% overall mortality rate.[6] It is used for patients with more-severe disease who have failed to respond to conservative or other measures. In cases of ischemia or perforation, segmental or subtotal colectomy is indicated.[106]

CHRONIC INTESTINAL PSEUDO-OBSTRUCTION

Chronic intestinal pseudo-obstruction is a syndrome that manifests insidiously with symptoms of intestinal obstruction in the absence of an anatomic lesion obstructing the flow of intestinal contents; its course is marked by subacute episodes.

This intestinal paralysis (intestinoparesis) is primarily a disorder of the small intestine but can involve more than 1 region of the GI tract. Rare familial and some secondary causes of chronic intestinal pseudo-obstruction can have characteristic extraintestinal manifestations (see later). The clinical presentation is variable but is characterized by progressively disabling GI symptoms that eventually persist, even between subacute episodes; there is difficulty in maintaining adequate oral nutrition and normal body weight, and quality of life suffers. A few studies have examined predictors of outcomes in chronic intestinal pseudo-obstruction, which are summarized in Table 124-3.[7] Having a high index of suspicion for this disorder is important to reduce complications and avoid potentially harmful surgical procedures.

Pathophysiology

Causes of chronic pseudo-obstruction are classified as primary or secondary; in most cases a cause is never determined and the term "idiopathic, non-familial, sporadic" is used. A

TABLE 124-3 Predictors of Better and Worse Outcomes in Chronic Intestinal Pseudo-obstruction

Better	Worse
Inflammatory (early)	Dilated intestine
Male gender	Early or acute onset
Motor response to neostigmine	Familial etiology
Motor response to octreotide	Female gender
Neuropathic cause	Malrotation
Normal bowel diameter	Myopathic cause
Absence of vagal dysfunction	Psychological disorder
Small bowel manometry: Presence of MMCs	Short bowel syndrome
Solid food tolerance	Small bowel manometry: Absence of activity fronts, Absence of MMCs, Bursts, Inadequate response to a meal
Sympathetic dysfunction	Surgery
	TPN
	Urinary tract involvement

Modified from Stranghellini V, Cogliandro RF, De Giorgio R, et al. Natural history of intestinal failure induced by chronic idiopathic intestinal pseudoobstruction. Transplant Proc 2010; 42:15-8. MMC, Migrating motor complex.

classification of CIP according to etiology is listed in Box 124-5.[108] When a cause is found, it most often is from an underlying condition affecting the intrinsic or extrinsic enteric neural pathways (neuropathies), the ICC (mesenchymopathies), the intestinal smooth muscle cells (myopathies), the mitochondria (mitochondrial myopathies), or the CNS. Overlap, such as neuropathy with features of myopathy or neuropathy plus mesenchymopathy, can occur. Familial causes are rare and far outnumbered by secondary causes. When a thorough diagnostic evaluation fails to reveal a cause, obtaining a full-thickness tissue specimen by laparoscopy with subsequent specific pathologic testing, including detailed light microscopic evaluation and ultrastructural analysis, will sometimes aid in making a diagnosis (Table 124-4).[109]

Enteric Neuropathies

Inflammatory neuropathies that cause CIP may be primary or secondary to a variety of infectious, paraneoplastic, and neurologic disorders. Enteric neuropathies and their estimated lifetime prevalences are listed in Table 124-5. Inflammatory neuropathies are characterized by an intense inflammatory infiltrate of CD4 and CD8 lymphocytes that are CD3 positive and confined to the myenteric plexus.[110,111] The juxtaposition of lymphocytes that are CD3 positive with myenteric neurons is the foundation by which immunologic interactions affect ganglion cell structure and survival.[109,112] In the GI tract, inflammation and immune activity have been shown to significantly influence the morphology and function of the enteric nerves.

Many patients with intestinal dysfunction secondary to paraneoplastic visceral neuropathy exhibit circulating antineuronal autoantibodies, such as anti-Hu antineuronal antibodies; autoantibodies reinforce a contributing role for the immune system in neuronal dysfunction.[107] Experimentally, these autoantibodies can elicit neuronal hyperexcitability[113] and modify the ascending reflex pathway of peristalsis.[108] When incubated with a primary culture of myenteric neurons, anti-Hu neuronal antibodies have been shown to trigger activity of caspase-3 and apaf-1 together with apoptosis,[114] which implies that anti-Hu antibodies contribute in a direct way to

BOX 124-5 Classification of Chronic Intestinal Pseudo-obstruction According to Etiology

Primary Chronic Intestinal Pseudo-obstruction
Familial
Familial autonomic dysfunction
Familial mitochondrial myopathies
Familial visceral myopathies
Familial visceral neuropathies

Sporadic
Visceral myopathies
Visceral neuropathies

Secondary Chronic Intestinal Pseudo-obstruction (Acquired)
Amyloidosis (Primary and Secondary)

Connective Tissue Disorders
Dermatomyositis
Polymyositis
PSS
SLE

Endocrine Disorders
Diabetes mellitus
Hypoparathyroidism
Hypothyroidism

Idiopathic Myenteric Ganglionitis

Infections
Trypanosoma cruzi (Chagas' disease)
Viral (cytomegalovirus, EBV)

Medications
Anticholinergic agents
Antiparkinsonian medications
Opiates
Tricyclic antidepressants

Neuromuscular Disorders
Muscular dystrophy (myotonic, Duchenne's, and oculopharyngeal muscular dystrophies)
Paraneoplastic syndrome
Parkinson's disease

Pheochromocytoma

Celiac Disease

Diffuse Lymphoid Infiltration

Acute and Chronic Irradiation

Psychiatric disorders (Anorexia Nervosa, Bulimia)

Modified from Sutton DH, Harrell SP, Wo JM. Diagnosis and management of adult patients with chronic intestinal pseudoobstruction. Nutr Clin Pract 2006; 21:16-22.

the lymphocytic infiltrate in ENS dysfunction and degeneration observed in patients with inflammatory neuropathy. Indication of viral infection, such as herpesvirus DNA, has been isolated deep in the myenteric plexus of some patients with severe neuropathic intestinal dysmotility, lending evidence to viral infectious agents as a cause of inflammatory ganglionitis.[115] Eosinophilic ganglionitis has been recognized in some pediatric patients with pseudo-obstruction,[116] although in these cases, eosinophilic ganglionitis did not appear to cause neuronal deterioration or loss.[108] Also, mast cell ganglionitis has been described in patients with severe intestinal dysfunction[117] and is associated with a reduced NOS expression, suggesting impaired inhibitory innervation of the ENS.

TABLE 124-4 Markers for and Targets of Intestinal Neuropathy

Markers	Cell Targets and Sites	Description
PGP9.5, NSE, MAP-2 NFs, tubulins, Hu C/D	Neurons: membrane and cytoplasm	Identification of the general structure of the ENS
B-S-100, GFAP	Glial cells: cytoplasm	Detection of enteroglial cells
C-Kit	ICC: membrane and cytoplasm	Different ICC networks
Substance P, VIP, PACAP, CGRP, neuropeptide Y, galanin, 5-HT, NOS, ChAT, somatostatin, calbindin, NeuN; NK1, NK2, NK3	Subclasses of enteric neurons; ICC: membrane and cytoplasm	Characterization of neurochemical coding and enteric neuron subclasses; subsets of ICC
Bcl-2, TUNEL, caspase-3, caspase-8, APAF1	Apoptosis and related mechanisms: nucleus and cytoplasm	Assessment of apoptosis and related pathways
Actin, myosin, desmin, smoothelin	Smooth muscle cells: cytoplasm	Assessment of smooth muscle integrity
CD3, CD4, CD8, CD79α, CD68; MIP-1α, TNF-α, IFN-γ	Immune cells, chemokines, and cytokines: membrane and cytoplasm	Evaluation of B (CD79α) and T lymphocytes (CD3), T-helper (CD4) cells, T-suppressor (CD8) cells, macrophages (CD68) in enteric ganglionitis; MIP-1α is a chemokine; TNF-α and IFN-γ are inflammatory cytokines

APAF1, apoptotic peptidase activating factor 1; Bcl-2, B cell lymphoma-2 protein; ChAT, choline acetyltransferase; ENS, enteric nervous system; CGRP, calcitonin gene-related peptide; GFAP, glial fibrillary acidic protein; 5-HT, 5-hydroxytryptamine (serotonin); Hu C/D, Hu C/D molecular antigen; ICC, interstitial cells of Cajal; IFN-γ, interferon γ; MAP-2, microtubule associated protein-2; MIP1-α, macrophage inflammatory protein 1-α; NeuN, neuronal-specific nuclear protein; NF, neurofilament; NK, neurokinin; NOS, nitric oxide synthase; NSE, neuron-specific enolase; PACAP, pituitary adenylate cyclase activating polypeptide; PGP9.5, protein gene product 9.5; TUNEL, terminal deoxynucleotidyl transferase–mediated doxyuridine triphosphate nick-end labeling; VIP, vasoactive intestinal polypeptide.
From Antonucci A, Fronzoni L, Cogliandro L, et al. Chronic intestinal pseudo-obstruction. World J Gastroenterol 2008; 14:2953-61.

TABLE 124-5 Enteric Neuropathies with Estimated Lifetime Prevalence

Enteric Neuropathy	Estimated Prevalence
Primary	
Chronic constipation	1 in 50-100
Congenital CIPO	1 in 10-20,000
Acquired CIPO	<1 in 2000
Idiopathic gastroparesis	1 in 4000
Idiopathic megacolon/rectum	1 in 4000
Hirschsprung's disease	1 in 5000
Idiopathic achalasia	1 in 10,000
Secondary	
Chagas' disease (GI involvement)	10% disease carriers
Diabetes mellitus	1 in 20
Crohn's disease	1 in 400
Parkinson's disease	1 in 500
Inflammatory (e.g., SLE)	1 in 1000
NF1	1 in 4000
MEN-2B	1 in 35,000
Paraneoplastic gut syndrome	<1 in 50,000

CIPO, chronic intestinal pseudo-obstruction; NF1, neurofibromatosis type 1.
Modified from Knowles CH, Lindberg G, Panza E, De Giorgio R. New perspectives in the diagnosis and management of enteric neuropathies. Nat Rev Gastroenterol Hepatol 2013; 10:206-18.

Noninflammatory (degenerative) neuropathies may be familial or sporadic and the result of dysfunctional mitochondria, altered calcium signaling, and accumulation of free radicals that leads to eventual degeneration and loss of neurons.[118] Sporadic cases can be primary or secondary to a wide range of conditions including radiation, diabetes mellitus, amyloidosis, myxedema, and drug toxicity.[108] Two predominant pathologic patterns have emerged in visceral neuropathy from degenerative sporadic causes. One pattern shows a reduction in the number of intramural cells that occur in relation to swollen processes and nerve cell bodies, an increase in glial cells, and fragmentation and loss of axons. In the second pattern, absent dendritic swelling or glial proliferation, there is a loss of the normal staining that occurs in subsets of enteric neurons.[108,109,119] Severe forms of idiopathic intestinal intrinsic neuropathy have been associated with a decreased expression of the protein encoded by *Bcl-2*, a gene related to one of the intracellular pathways leading to apoptosis.[120-122]

Enteric Mesenchymopathies

ICC are derived from mesenchymal cells that express c-Kit. ICC form network patterns that are important for pacing electrical slow-wave activity and for GI motor contractions.[123,124] (see Fig. 124-1; Chapters 99 and 100) Four morphologically distinct network patterns have been observed: periganglionic ICC-MY that connect with ICC-LM and ICC-CM, plexuses of ICC-LM within longitudinal muscle that extend toward the serosa, repetitive and organized ICC-CM layers that run parallel to the circular muscle axis and extend towards the submucosa, and a condensed ICC-SM layer that lines the submucosal border.[125] The division of morphologically distinct classes of ICC within different layers of the GI musculature suggests that different ICC can perform discrete physiologic roles in intestinal motility.[126]

ICC are closely apposed to nerve terminals and electrically coupled via gap junctions to neighboring smooth muscle cells. Studies indicate they play a fundamental role in the reception and transduction of both inhibitory and excitatory enteric motor neurotransmission.[127] Confocal electron microscopy shows abnormalities of ICC in patients with CIP that include irregular cell surface markings,[128] damaged intracellular organelles and cytoskeleton, and decreased ICC density.[108,129] As a result, it has been proposed that ICC involved in pacemaker activity and neurotransmission to smooth muscle can contribute to the enteric motility abnormalities detectable in patients with CIP.

Enteric Myopathies

Smooth muscle fibrosis and vacuolization are histologic abnormalities that have been observed in the circular and longitudinal muscle layers of some patients with primary visceral myopathies.[119,130] In a large series of well-characterized patients with CIP, a deficiency of 1 isoform of the cytoskeletal smooth muscle protein actin, α-actin, was described in approximately 25% of patients with the myopathic phenotype.[131] The authors proposed that a selective decrease or absence of α-actin staining in the circular muscle of the small intestinal wall could be a biological marker of CIP,[131] although controlled studies have not yet been done.

Primary Causes

Sporadic Visceral Neuropathy

Also known as *chronic idiopathic intestinal pseudo-obstruction* (CIIPO), sporadic, nonfamilial visceral neuropathy can result from injury to the myenteric plexus from various causes including drug toxicity, ischemia, radiation, or viral infections such as CMV, EBV, and HSV.[132] CIIPO is the most common diagnosis given to cases of intestinal pseudo-obstruction, followed by various secondary causes that are discussed later. Delayed gastric emptying and intestinal dysmotility have been observed in patients after viral gastroenteritis, which is associated with permanent damage to the myenteric plexus in some patients. Kamm and colleagues have documented such a syndrome in association with herpes viral elements in the myenteric plexus of patients with pseudo-obstruction.[115]

Patients with CIIPO often have disturbed motility of the entire GI tract. The intestine is rarely dilated. Histologic examination of the myenteric plexus may reveal a reduction in the number or an abnormal morphology of neurons, which may be enlarged with thick, irregular, clubbed processes. Hypertrophy of 1 or both muscle layers of the muscularis propria has been described. Intestinal phasic pressure studies are abnormal, but routine histology findings often were normal in patients whose tissue was available for analysis.[133]

Familial Intestinal Pseudo-obstruction

Primary familial cases of intestinal pseudo-obstruction result from abnormalities of smooth muscle cells of the muscularis propria (familial visceral myopathies) or abnormalities of the enteric neuronal structures (familial visceral enteropathies). These are rare genetic disorders with autosomal dominant, autosomal recessive, or X-linked transmission.[110] Abnormal genes and loci have been recognized in various syndromic forms of CIIPO, including the DNA polymerase gamma gene *(POLG)* on chromosome 21 (21q17), the transcription factor SOX10 on chromosome 22 (22p12), and a locus on chromosome 8.[108,110,111,126] X-linked recessive forms of CIIPO have been mapped to Xq28I, and a large cytoskeletal protein filamin A has been identified as vital for proper enteric neuron development.[132] Some familial disorders have been well characterized based on the pattern of inheritance and predominant abnormalities.

Familial Visceral Myopathies (FVMs)

FVMs are uncommon genetic disorders that cause CIP and are characterized by degeneration and fibrosis of GI smooth muscle; 1 type also involves urinary smooth muscle. There are at least 2 phenotypes.

Type I is autosomal dominant and usually is diagnosed after the first decade of life, with esophageal dilatation, megaduodenum, megacystis, and mydriasis. Patients respond favorably to regional resection or bypass of affected tissue segments, and the prognosis generally is good.

Type II, called MNGIE (mitochondrial DNA neurogastrointestinal encephalopathy), is the best-characterized myopathic phenotype, although the pathogenetic mechanisms causing its intestinal dysmotility remain unclear. It is an autosomal recessive mitochondrial encephalopathy that can lead to CIP because of dysfunction of the mitochondrial respiratory chain.[134] MNGIE is characterized by exacerbations with severe symptoms on a background of CIP with mildly dilated small intestine and stomach, lactic acidosis, ptosis, ophthalmic paralysis, peripheral neuropathy, alterations in the white matter on MRI of the brain, skeletal muscle ragged red fibers (Fig. 124-5), and specific mitochondrial changes at the ultrastructural level.[134,135] Patients manifest skeletal muscle pain and cramps and lactic acidosis with elevated circulating muscle enzyme levels, including creatine phosphokinase (CPK), ALT, and aldolase. Small intestinal diverticulosis complicated by inflammation and perforation is the cause of death in most of these patients during early adulthood.[134]

MNGIE syndrome results from mutations in the thymidine phosphorylase gene, which leads to markedly reduced

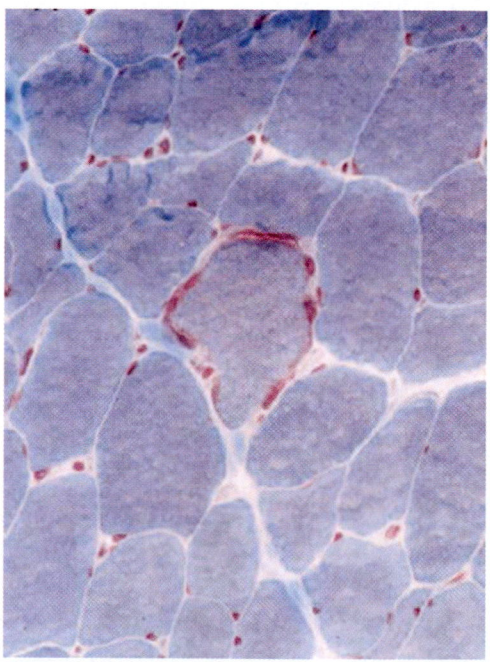

FIGURE 124-5. Histologic section of a biopsy specimen taken from skeletal muscle in a patient with MNGIE (mitochondrial DNA neurogastrointestinal encephalopathy) showing ragged red fibers *(center)* that contain subsarcolemmal accumulations of mitochondria. Most fibers are morphologically normal. *(Used with permission from Mueller LA, Camilleri M, Emslie-Smith AM. Mitochondrial neurogastrointestinal encephalopathy: Manometric and diagnostic features. Gastroenterology 1999; 116:959-63.)*

thymidine phosphorylase activity that, in turn, results in accumulation of thymidine (dThd) and deoxyuridine (dUrd) in blood and tissues.[136] High levels of dThd and dUrd lead to nucleoside pool imbalances that cause abnormalities in DNA including depletion, point mutations, and multiple deletions.[136,137] A link has been established between DNA depletion and myopathic changes involving the external layer of the muscularis propria.[134] Screening tests for MNGIE include measurements of serum lactic acid, circulating muscle enzymes, and thymidine phosphorylase levels in circulating leukocytes.[138]

Familial Visceral Neuropathies (FVNs)

FVNs are rare genetic diseases that are characterized by degeneration of the neural structures of the myenteric plexus. There are at least 2 distinct phenotypes of FVN.[139] Type I is autosomal dominant; results in segmental dilatation of varying lengths of the small intestine, megacolon, and gastroparesis; and has its onset of GI symptoms at any age. More than 75% of patients with FVN type I have GI symptoms. Histology demonstrates degeneration of argyrophilic neurons and reduced numbers of nerve fibers. Type II FVN is autosomal recessive and its findings include hypertrophic pyloric stenosis, malrotation of the small intestine, and short and dilated small intestine; CNS malformation and patent ductus arteriosus are seen in some cases. Onset of symptoms is in infancy, and histologically there is a deficiency of argyrophilic neurons and increased numbers of neuroblasts. There is no effective medical or surgical treatment for type II FVN, and prognosis is poor.

Several syndromic congenital neuropathies exist that can be classified broadly[140] as: (1) disorders of colonization by migrating neural crest-derived neurons (e.g., Hirschsprung's disease) related to abnormalities in the *RET* gene (the gene for tyrosine kinase) and GDNF (glial-derived neurotrophic factor), or the disorder of ET-3 (endothelin-3) and its receptor, ETB (endothelin B receptor); (2) disorders of differentiation of enteric nerves (e.g., intestinal ganglioneuromatosis) related to a specific germline point mutation in *RET* at codon 918 of exon 16 (M918T) or codon 883 (A883F) in MEN-IIB syndrome; and (3) disorders of the survival or maintenance of enteric nerves (e.g., hypoganglionosis and possibly congenital achalasia) related to 1 of several derangements of ligands (e.g., 5-HT or neurotrophin-3) and their receptors (e.g., 5-HT$_{2B}$ and tyrosine kinase C) or transcription factors (e.g., SOX10).

Disturbances in these mechanisms result in syndromic dysmotilities such as Hirschsprung's disease, Waardenburg-Shah syndrome, MEN type IIA or B, and idiopathic hypertrophic pyloric stenosis.

Hirschsprung's disease, perhaps the most common congenital neuropathy, occurs in 1 in 5000 live births (see Chapter 98). It is often associated with chromosomal abnormalities, the most frequent being trisomy 21 (Down syndrome), in whom it affects 2% to 10% of patients. Mutations may involve gene-encoding receptors or ligands, such as GDNF-Ret or ET-3-ETB, although the receptors are much more commonly affected. Different mechanisms can cause the terminal colon to become aganglionic: a deficiency of GDNF-Ret that is less severe and does not cause the entire bowel to become aganglionic; a deficiency of ET-3-ETB in which neural crest-derived cells differentiate prematurely and precursors cease dividing prematurely, leaving the last segment uncolonized; and other syndromes that result from mutations of transcription factors.

Waardenburg syndrome (WS) is an autosomal dominant familial disorder that affects body pigments and has a sensorineural hearing loss.[141] It occurs with an incidence of 1 in 50,000 live births and accounts for 2% to 5% of congenital hearing loss. There are at least 4 types of the syndrome, and 4 genes have been identified in this condition: *PAX3*, *MITF*, *EDNRB*, and *EDN3*. The combination of Hirschsprung's disease with WS defines the WS4 type.[142] Patients with a Sox10 mutation and WS4 can present with ataxia, central and peripheral demyelinating neuropathies, and megacolon.[143]

MEN type IIB syndrome is a severe congenital familial neuropathic condition transmitted as an autosomal dominant trait and characterized by medullary carcinoma and tumor development in the neuroendocrine system (see Chapter 126). Presenting symptoms include severe constipation or megacolon, diarrhea (when associated with enterocolitis), or obstruction, typically occurring shortly after birth.[140] External stigmata of MEN-IIB include a characteristic facies with "blubbery" lips due to mucosal neuromas that involve the lips, tongue, face, and eyelids[144]; marfanoid habitus; medullated corneal nerve fibers; and medullary thyroid carcinoma. Biopsy specimens characteristically show findings of transmural ganglioneuromatosis with massive proliferation of neural tissue, including neurons, and supporting cells; nerve fibers appear as thickened nerve trunks among mature nerve cells.

Childhood Visceral Myopathies (CVMs)

CVMs have been recognized as 2 distinctive forms of disease that differ from FVM in their mode of inheritance and clinical presentations (Table 124-6). Degeneration and fibrosis of GI and urinary smooth muscle can be detected in both types of CVM and result in obstructive symptoms, bowel dilatation, and hydroureteronephrosis or megacystis, the latter resulting from degeneration of bladder muscle.[145]

Secondary Causes

PSS

Systemic sclerosis (SSc) is a generalized disorder of the microvasculature and connective tissue that results in increased deposition of collagen and other matrix elements, leading to thickening and fibrosis of the skin, with involvement of synovia and fibrosis of intestinal organs. The highest incidence of SSc occurs between 45 and 55 years of age. The GI tract is the second most common target organ after the skin, and the esophagus is the most commonly affected GI organ, followed by the small intestine.[146] Small bowel dysmotility leads to bacterial overgrowth with resultant steatorrhea, malabsorption, and weight loss.

There are 2 forms of SSc, diffuse cutaneous and limited cutaneous. GI symptoms are associated with diffuse cutaneous SSc and occur along with other manifestations of systemic involvement, including interstitial lung disease, kidney failure associated with malignant hypertension crisis, and myocardial disease.

Intestinal and gastric involvement can be identified radiologically in up to 40% of patients. Contrast studies can reveal dilatation of the duodenum and jejunum, along with fixed, narrow, tightly packed valvulae conniventes, despite bowel dilatation, producing an accordion appearance or so-called "hide-bound" appearance (Fig. 124-6).[147] Wide-necked diverticula are seen more often in the colon than in the small intestine.

Disturbances of intestinal motility[148,149] result in delayed gastric or small bowel transit[150] and include absence or hypomotility of the interdigestive MMC, low-amplitude clusters of propagated and nonpropagated contractions, a prolonged MMC cycle, diminished activity of phase III,[149] and antral

TABLE 124-6 Classification of Childhood Visceral Myopathies

Characteristic(s)	Type I	Type II*
Mode of transmission	Autosomal recessive (?)	Autosomal recessive (?)

Clinical features
  Age of onset
  Gender
  Symptoms
	Infancy and young childhood
	Both
	Constipation, distention ± chronic pseudo-obstruction
		Infancy
		Predominantly female
		Obstipation, intestinal pseudo-obstruction

Extraluminal features	Megacystis and megaureter	Megacystis and megaureter
Gross lesions	Dilatation of entire GI tract	Short, malrotated small intestine and malfixation of microcolon
Histopathologic changes	Degeneration and fibrosis of GI and urinary smooth muscle cells	Vacuolar degeneration of GI and urinary smooth muscle cells
Treatment, prognosis	No effective Rx; poor prognosis	No effective Rx; poor prognosis

*Megacystis-microcolon-intestinal hypoperistalsis.
Rx, treatment.
From Camilleri M. Acute and chronic pseudo-obstruction. In: Feldman M, Friedman LS, Brandt LJ, editors. Sleisenger and Fordtran's gastrointestinal and liver disease: Pathophysiology, diagnosis, management. 8th ed. Philadelphia: Saunders Elsevier; 2006. pp 2679-702.

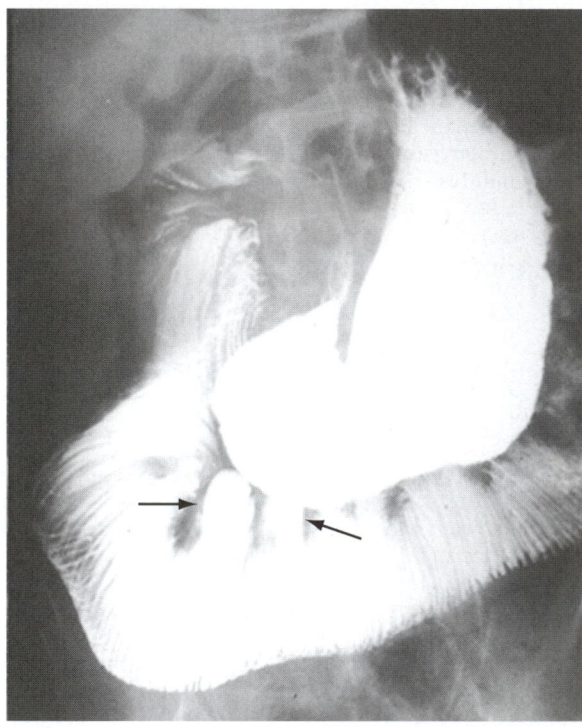

FIGURE 124-6. Select view from an upper GI series in a patient with systemic sclerosis, showing a markedly dilated duodenum and proximal jejunum, with an increased number of small bowel folds crowded together (despite luminal distention), producing a "hide-bound" appearance. Also note multiple outpouchings *(arrows)* due to asymmetrical fibrosis, with sacculation of the opposite bowel wall. *(Used with permission from Levine MS, Rubesin SE, Laufer I. Pattern approach for diseases of mesenteric small bowel on barium studies. Radiology 2008; 249:451-60.)*

hypomotility (characterized by low-amplitude contractions, typically < 40 mm Hg). Intestinal involvement usually causes fasting and postprandial contractile amplitude to fall below 10 mm Hg.[151] Gastric emptying may be delayed by resistance to flow in the hypomotile small intestine, even if the stomach

itself is unaffected. SSc patients without GI involvement demonstrate normal small bowel manometry[151] and normal intestinal transit time.

Dermatomyositis and Polymyositis

The GI tract is involved in half of the cases of dermatomyositis and polymyositis. Dysphagia is often the presenting symptom, associated with weakness and atrophy of esophageal striated muscles. Megaduodenum and delayed intestinal transit are prominent features accompanying CIP. Histopathology demonstrates atrophy and fibrosis of intestinal smooth muscle, most consistent with a visceral myopathy.[151]

SLE

Every system and organ can be affected by SLE,[152] which is an autoimmune condition characterized by a variety of auto-antibodies and immune complex formation; no specific auto-antibody has been associated with SLE gastroenteropathy. Abdominal pain is the most common GI complaint, which occurs in up to 20% of patients. Autopsy studies reveal a 65% prevalence of peritoneal inflammation, although documented cases of serositis as a cause of abdominal pain are rare. Smooth muscle dysfunction related to ischemia can lead to dilatation of the small intestine. Diarrhea occurs in 10% of patients with SLE. CIP can occur as the presenting symptom and is potentially reversible with early treatment.[153]

Lupus mesenteric vasculitis (mesenteric arteritis, lupus enteritis) is the term used to describe the bowel changes in this disease that result from vasculitis of small blood vessels. There is an acute illness that involves mainly the small intestine, and a chronic form with many ulcers in the colon.[152] Ischemia leads to intestinal mucosal ulceration, edema, and hemorrhage. Because the primary lesions are from an inflammatory ischemic vasculitis, prompt and aggressive immunosuppressive anti-inflammatory therapy should be initiated. If methylprednisolone and complete bowel rest does not yield an adequate response, IV cyclophosphamide may be added.[152]

The diagnosis often can be made radiologically, and small bowel changes include dilatation, thick folds, and thumbprinting related to subepithelial edema and hemorrhage. Unusual intestinal manifestations can cause diagnostic difficulties. Thus, SLE can simulate Crohn's ileitis or can cause a severe protein-losing enteropathy in association with vasculitis and basement membrane thickening that may be diagnosed on full-thickness jejunal biopsy.

Diabetes Mellitus

Patients with diabetes mellitus often have diarrhea, which may be due to SIBO, pancreatic exocrine insufficiency, bile salt malabsorption, impaired absorption or secretion, loss of adrenergic sympathetic innervation, or disturbed motility. In patients presenting with symptoms of gastroparesis, the small intestine also may be affected, and such involvement can be documented by prolonged transit,[150] by manometry,[154] or sometimes by evidence of a dilated intestine.

Motility studies of the small intestine in patients with diabetes have varied significantly. Normal MMCs are found in many patients with documented gastroparesis, but absence of intestinal phase III has been demonstrated in some. Other abnormalities include MMCs that originate in the distal duodenum or jejunum as uncoordinated bursts of nonpropagated contractions (Fig. 124-7).[155] The clinical relevance of these abnormal findings is uncertain. Demyelination of the proximal vagus nerve and sympathetic nerves supplying the bowel occurs in patients with long-standing diabetes. The intrinsic nervous system of the intestine does not appear to be affected, because no morphologic abnormalities of the myenteric or submucosal plexuses have been observed; however, animal models and a single case report of a patient requiring transplantation of the pancreas and kidneys showed ICC degeneration.[154] Although thickening of the small bowel muscle layers and eosinophilic hyaline bodies in smooth muscle cells have been observed,[156] most authorities believe that myopathy is not a cause of GI dysmotility in diabetic patients.

Parkinson's Disease

Patients with Parkinson's disease often have symptoms of GI dysfunction. Proximal dysphagia, bloating, constipation, and difficulty with evacuation of stool occur commonly.[157] Dilatation of the small intestine may be seen radiologically,[158] and small intestinal dysmotility does occur, but its frequency is not known, and the contribution of these abnormalities to symptoms is not clear. Compared with controls, manometric studies in patients with Parkinson's disease reveal infrequent or absent MMCs, hypomotility in the fed state, and an increased incidence of retrograde and tonic contractions.[159]

The pathogenesis of small intestinal dysmotility in Parkinson's disease has not been determined. Lewy bodies are neurons containing cytoplasmic hyaline inclusions that originally were identified in the brain of patients with Parkinson's disease. They have not yet been reported in the small intestine but have been found in the myenteric plexus of the esophagus and colon.[160] Dopaminergic neurons are reported to be deficient in colons from patients with Parkinson's disease with constipation.[161]

Spinal Cord Injury

Spinal cord injury usually produces only mild and probably insignificant dysmotility in the small intestine. The only documented changes in manometric studies performed in a group of patients with spinal cord injury were a greater number of phase III contractions that began in the duodenum rather than in the antrum in patients with high spinal cord lesions.[162] Patients with injury to the lower spinal cord demonstrated no abnormalities, a finding consistent with the preservation of innervation to the intestine from the vagus nerve and third thoracic sympathetic levels. One report described a woman with cervical spinal stenosis and paraplegia who displayed normal MMCs but a 2- to 3-fold prolonged interval between MMCs.

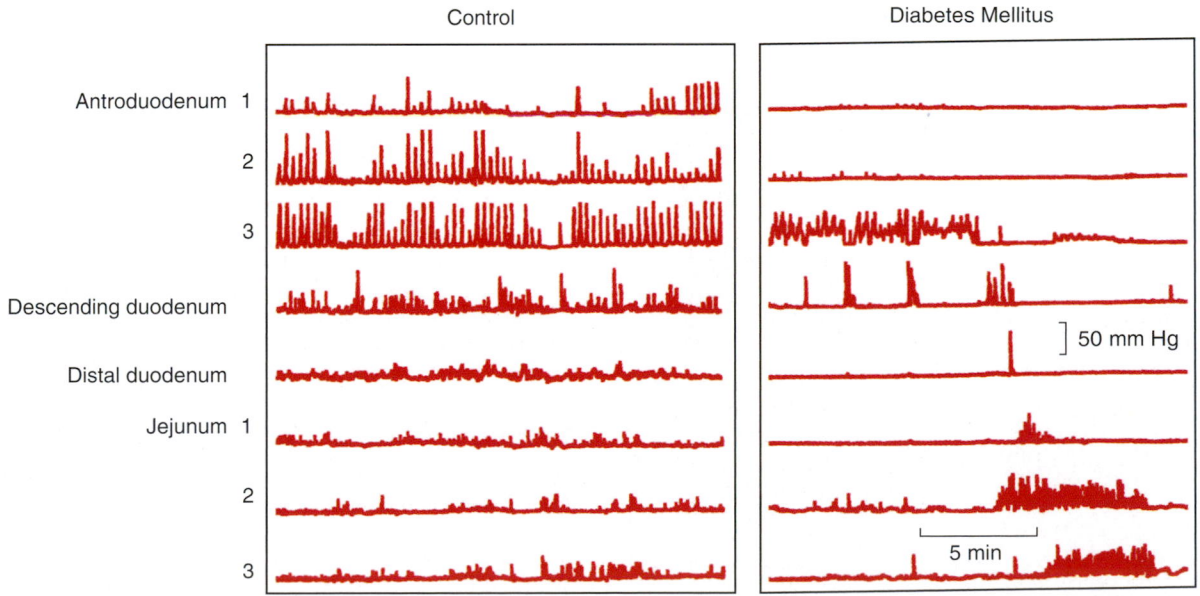

FIGURE 124-7. Gastroduodenal motility tracings in a healthy control subject and in a patient with diabetes mellitus. These postprandial tracings show normal amplitude and irregular contractility in the healthy control and a paucity of antral contractions, tonic contractions at the pylorus (third tracing), and development of a fasting-like migrating motor complex pattern in the small intestine in a patient with diabetes mellitus. (*Adapted from Camilleri M. Acute and chronic pseudo-obstruction. In: Feldman M, Friedman LS, Brandt LJ, editors. Sleisenger and Fordtran's gastrointestinal and liver disease: Pathophysiology, diagnosis, management. 8th ed. Philadelphia: Saunders Elsevier; 2006. p 2687.*)

Immediately after spinal cord injury, a state of spinal shock develops in which there is complete loss of all sensory, motor, and reflex function below the level of injury. Paralytic ileus with abdominal distention follows and usually resolves in a few days. In the long term, however, postprandial abdominal distention and discomfort occur in more than 40% of patients with spinal cord injuries; these symptoms are likely due to the more significant problem of constipation. Many stable patients with spinal cord injury exhibit increased amounts of gas in the small and large intestine on routine abdominal plain films.

Colonic dysmotility is well recognized and is responsible for the common problems of constipation and difficulty of evacuation in patients with spinal cord injury.[163] Spinal cord injury decreases colonic motility; though the postprandial colonic response is present, it is suboptimal and confined to the descending colon.[164] In these patients, rectal compliance and resting anal sphincter pressures are lower than normal values, and ramp rectal inflation demonstrates patterns of sphincter activity similar to those recorded in these patients' cystometrograms. There is no definite relationship of bowel function to the findings on anorectal manometry in patients with spinal cord injury.

Rehabilitation goals include continence of stool, simple voluntary independent defecation, and prevention of GI complications. Individualized person-centered bowel care includes diet, laxatives, enemas, suppositories, and scheduling of bowel care to initiate defecation and accomplish fecal evacuation. Digital rectal stimulation is a technique used during bowel care of patients with spinal cord injury to open the anal sphincter and facilitate reflex peristalsis.[165]

Neurofibromatosis (von Recklinghausen's Disease)

GI involvement in neurofibromatosis is estimated to occur in 11% to 25% of patients.[166] Small bowel dysmotility and intestinal pseudo-obstruction due to neurofibromatosis, however, are rare. Involvement of the intestine occurs in 3 principal forms: hyperplasia of the submucosal and myenteric nerve plexuses with mucosal ganglioneuromatosis, which can lead to disordered intestinal motility and CIP; GIST tumors that show varying degrees of neural or smooth muscle differentiation and typically manifest with bleeding; and a glandular, somatostatin-rich carcinoid of the periampullary region of the duodenum, which also has been associated with pheochromocytoma.[167]

Paraneoplastic Visceral Neuropathies

Paraneoplastic neurologic syndrome is a remote effect of cancer that results in visceral neuropathy. It is not caused by the tumor mass per se or metastases, nor is it caused by infection, ischemia, or metabolic disruptions.[168] Paraneoplastic neurologic syndrome is caused by autoimmune processes triggered by the cancer and is directed against antigens common to both the cancer and the nervous system, designated as onconeural antigens.[68] Paraneoplastic neurologic syndrome is rare, occurring in less than 0.01% of patients with cancer[169]; the Lambert-Eaton myasthenic syndrome is more common, occurring in nearly 1% of patients with small cell lung cancer (SCLC).[170] Less than 50% of patients have detectable antibodies, and up to 10% have an atypical antibody, albeit one that is not well characterized.[168] Paraneoplastic neurologic syndrome is considered to be mediated by the immune system, so suppression of the immune response represents a potential treatment approach.[168] Associated neoplasms include SCLC, thymoma, gynecologic and breast tumors, Hodgkin's lymphoma, multiple myeloma, and colon cancer.

The most commonly associated tumor is SCLC, and the most common antibodies are Hu-Ab or CV2-Ab.[168] Experimental evidence suggests that anti-Hu antibodies can exert a direct pathogenic role or can contribute, in association with the lymphocytic infiltrate, to ENS dysfunction in patients with CIP related to an inflammatory neuropathy.[108] Some patients with subacute parasympathetic and sympathetic autonomic failure and prominent GI dysfunction also have antibodies directed against the neuronal autonomic ganglion type of acetylcholine receptors (nAchR antibodies); in these cases, the main associated tumors are thymoma and SCLC.

Patients with paraneoplastic neurologic syndrome can experience weight loss, persistent bloating, and abdominal distention from damage to the neurons of the enteric plexuses.[168] Some patients present with dysphagia, nausea, and vomiting due to esophageal dysmotility or gastroparesis, or, more commonly, they present with severe constipation. Radiologic studies can show dilatation of the small intestine, colon, or stomach.[168] Esophageal manometry can reveal spasm or achalasia.

These inflammatory neuropathies are characterized by a dense inflammatory infiltrate with CD3-positive CD4 and CD8 lymphocytes that almost invariably are confined to the myenteric plexus.[110,111,126]

Myotonic Dystrophy

Myotonic muscular dystrophy is a slowly progressive disease characterized by myotonia, or difficulty in muscle relaxation. Diarrhea and abdominal cramping occur in up to one third of affected persons, malabsorption and steatorrhea have been reported in a few cases, and constipation is frequent and can alternate with diarrhea. The small intestine can demonstrate abnormal but nonspecific radiologic changes, including dilatation, diminished motility, and delayed transit.[171]

Dysmotility of the small intestine can play a significant role in causation of intestinal symptoms. Manometric findings included low-amplitude contractions in fasting and fed states, retrograde propagation of phase III waves, interruption of phase III, and increased incidence of tonic contractions.[172] Spontaneous pneumoperitoneum, megacolon, and low-amplitude small intestinal contractions have been reported.

Histologically, smooth muscle cells in the small intestine show changes similar to those found in dystrophic skeletal muscle: cells may be swollen, partially destroyed, decreased in size, or replaced by fat. Using silver stain, degenerative changes of the myenteric plexus of the colon were found in a patient with megacolon,[173] indicating that intestinal dysmotility may be caused by smooth muscle as well as enteric nerve dysfunction. In most patients, the predominant cause of dysmotility appears to be smooth muscle damage.

Duchenne's Muscular Dystrophy

Duchenne's muscular dystrophy is the most common of the inherited muscular dystrophies. A sex-linked disease, it affects 1 in 3500 boys; without respiratory support, death can occur before age 25 years. It is caused by mutations in the gene for dystrophin, a protein that helps stabilizes muscle cell membrane.[174] In some cases, the mutations lead to an aberrant messenger RNA and result in a highly truncated dystrophin or no protein at all. Without functional dystrophin, muscle cell membranes leak, followed by muscle fiber necrosis and degeneration, and progressive replacement of muscle by fibrosis and fat. The muscles steadily waste away, and paralysis eventually occurs.[174,175]

In a milder form with onset in the teens or early adulthood (Becker's muscular dystrophy), the muscle cells produce insufficient dystrophin, with resultant instability in the structure of the muscle cell membrane. As with Duchenne's, muscle weakness begins in the hips and pelvic girdle. The rate of degeneration is variable in Becker's muscular dystrophy with many patients living to old age.

GI symptoms usually are related to esophageal and gastric dysmotility, which are more severely affected than is the small intestine. Dysphagia is the predominant GI symptom (36% in 1 series), followed by vomiting, diarrhea, and constipation.[176] Delayed gastric emptying and acute GI dilatation characterize the clinical course.[177] Orocecal transit time can be normal in asymptomatic subjects, although severe bowel dysmotility can occur.

Amyloidosis

Amyloidosis is a mixed group of disorders characterized by extracellular deposits of abnormal protein fibrils with a β-sheet fibrillar structure. The abnormal structure can be identified by x-ray diffraction studies and visualized with electron microscopy, but clinically, amyloid is identified by viewing the intestine with polarized light after staining it with Congo red.[178]

In patients with amyloidosis, diarrhea and constipation often are present for years and are followed or accompanied by a myriad of disparate problems including GI bleeding, steatorrhea, protein loss, perforation, obstruction, intussusception, ischemia, pneumatosis, and pseudo-obstruction.[179] A variety of mechanisms might explain the diarrhea: delayed motility and SIBO,[180] bile salt diarrhea,[181] a sprue-like condition with amyloid deposition in the tips of the villi,[182] and rapid orocecal transit.[183]

The severity of GI dysmotility is correlated to the quantity and distribution of deposited amyloid. Amyloid is slowly deposited between muscle fibers, causing pressure atrophy of adjacent fibers so that eventually, the whole muscle layer is replaced by amyloid.[179] Neuromuscular infiltration initially affects the intrinsic nervous system and results in a neuropathic process[184] characterized by contractions that have normal amplitude but are uncoordinated.[179,185] At a later stage, tissue wall infiltration results in a myopathic process with low-amplitude contractions that typically are associated with prolonged transit as in other systemic disorders, such as scleroderma. The vasculature often is involved, with amyloid deposition in the subintima or adventitia, and often involving the submucosa. When the vessel wall thickens, the lumen of the vessel narrows and eventually closes, resulting in ischemia, infarction, and perforation.[186] Mucosal architecture remains normal until massive deposits of amyloid destroy the mucosal structures.

There are several forms of amyloidosis: primary (AL), secondary (AA), hemodialysis-related (Aβ₂MG), hereditary (ATTR), senile, and localized. AL is most common and has the most significant GI involvement. AL amyloid reflects a generalized deposition of excess light chains associated with plasma cell dyscrasia, and 15% of patients with AL have multiple myeloma.[187] Amyloid protein is deposited in the small intestine in all forms of amyloidosis.[188]

Secondary (AA) amyloidosis with acute-phase reactant serum amyloid A protein (A) is associated with infectious, inflammatory, or (rarely) neoplastic disorders.[179,189] The incidence of amyloidosis in patients with RA ranges from 7% to 21%, the highest prevalence derived from an autopsy study.[179] Other disorders associated with AA are Crohn's disease, ankylosing spondylitis, arthritis urethritica (previously called Reiter's syndrome), psoriasis, PSS, PBC, and SLE.

Inherited forms of amyloidogenic proteins are rare. The most common of this type is with variant transthyretin (TTR), which is produced by the liver,[179,180] and the resulting amyloidosis (ATTR) is called familial amyloidotic polyneuropathy. Besides familial amyloidotic polyneuropathy, there are hereditary non-neuropathic systemic amyloidoses associated with mutations in genes for apolipoprotein AI, lysozyme, and fibrinogen α chain.

Senile amyloidosis is found in 10% to 36% of patients older than 80 years of age and mainly involves the heart, but it also can be seen throughout the GI tract. Amyloid has been observed in the subserosal veins of the large and small intestine in 41% to 44% of elderly patients.[190]

Chagas' Disease

In nearly one third of patients, the late phase of infection with *Trypanosoma cruzi* leads to destruction of the submucosal and myenteric plexuses along the length of the GI tract, resulting in dilatation (see Chapter 113). Megacolon and megaesophagus are the most common presentations, although megaduodenum and megajejunum also can occur. Swallowing difficulties may be the first symptom of digestive disturbances and can lead to malnutrition. Some patients are entirely asymptomatic despite significant destruction of neurons. The early phase of gastric emptying of liquids is accelerated in patients who have Chagas' disease and megaduodenum, suggesting that increased duodenal receptivity has a significant effect on the gastroduodenal transfer of liquids.[191]

Thyroid Disease

The earliest and only manifestation of a thyroid disorder might be GI dysfunction. Hypothyroid patients often complain of constipation, and their gastric emptying time may be significantly delayed.[192] Intestinal dysmotility (associated with change in the frequency of the slow wave oscillations of smooth muscle electrical potential) results from the altered thyroid state and has been considered to be the cause of symptoms. In hypothyroidism, small intestinal transit is significantly slowed.[193] Many hypothyroid patients develop constipation, which may be the result of colonic dysmotility. In 1 patient, manometry revealed decreased amplitude of small intestinal contractions and an overall decreased motility index.[194] With severe hypothyroidism (myxedema), paralytic ileus and intestinal pseudo-obstruction can occur. These abnormalities return to normal after the thyroid disorder is corrected.

Hypoparathyroidism

Pseudo-obstruction and malabsorption have been observed in patients with hypoparathyroidism, although the mechanism is not known. Calcium is essential for smooth muscle contraction, and hypocalcemia can impair intestinal contractile activity. Symptoms improve with administration of calcium.

Medications

Many drugs profoundly affect GI motility.[195] Although the colon is considered the principal target organ for drug-induced dysmotility, the small intestine often is similarly affected. Tricyclic antidepressants are noted for causing ileus and constipation. Phenothiazines and some antiparkinsonian drugs decrease small intestinal and colonic motility and can cause adynamic ileus as well as constipation and colonic pseudo-obstruction. The anticholinergic agents atropine and scopolamine and related belladonna alkaloids decrease intestinal tone along with the amplitude and frequency of peristaltic contractions.

Opiate analgesics act on µ-opiate receptors throughout the intestinal tract to suppress motility; this effect is most pronounced in the colon. Loperamide, a predominantly peripheral opioid antagonist, causes chronic pseudo-obstruction by this antikinetic mechanism.[195] Morphine enhances the amplitude of nonpropulsive small intestinal contractions and markedly decreases propulsive contractions. The duodenum and jejunum are more prone to these effects than the ileum, and the overall effect is a delay in transit through the small intestine.

Calcium channel antagonists, particularly verapamil, by their direct stimulation of smooth muscle relaxation, cause constipation in up to 20% of patients and can also cause chronic pseudo-obstruction.[196] Small intestinal transit time in subjects taking verapamil was unchanged from pretreatment values, although transit through the colon was slowed and this effect likely accounts for the constipation seen with this drug.

Celiac Disease (see Chapter 107)

Intestinal pseudo-obstruction has been documented in association with celiac disease,[197] but the mechanism is unclear. Dilated loops of small intestine with delayed transport of barium can be observed radiologically. In 1 patient who underwent exploratory laparotomy with full-thickness jejunal biopsy, the nerves and muscle cells appeared normal on both light and electron microscopy.[197]

Jejunal Diverticulosis

Diverticula can occur anywhere in the small intestine (see Chapter 25), but diverticulosis is most common in the jejunum. Like their counterparts in the colon, diverticula represent herniations through the mesenteric side of the bowel and usually are acquired. Jejunal diverticulosis is associated with many diseases, including scleroderma, celiac disease, MNGIE cytopathy, and Cronkhite-Canada syndrome.[198] Patients can present with symptoms of SIBO, including diarrhea, steatorrhea, weight loss, and megaloblastic anemia. Local complications of diverticula also can occur, such as diverticulitis, bleeding, and perforation.

Acute and Chronic Irradiation

Ionizing radiation results in damage to all structures of the small intestine, including the mucosa, blood vessels, connective tissue, enteric nerves, and smooth muscle (see Chapter 40). Radiation damage to the intestine can be separated into acute and chronic injury.

Acute radiation injury is associated with symptoms of nausea, vomiting, abdominal pain, and diarrhea, which subside soon after exposure is discontinued. Small intestinal dysmotility can play a significant role in acute radiation enteropathy. Changes in small intestinal absorption are considered the main cause of diarrhea. Delayed fasting and fed intestinal motility patterns can persist up to 4 weeks following the last exposure.[199,200] One study has shown accelerated small intestinal transit in a group of patients undergoing abdominopelvic irradiation compared with their pretreatment values,[201] more than 75% of whom exhibited diarrhea during treatment.

Chronic radiation injury can cause GI complications decades after the initial exposure. The neuropathic and myopathic injury results in intestinal dysmotility that leads to SIBO, diarrhea, and malabsorption. Contrast studies often show dilated, thickened loops of bowel with air-fluid levels. Atrophy and fibrosis of smooth muscle fibers is a characteristic histologic finding, and proliferation of submucosal neurons

of the myenteric plexus with extension into the circular muscle coat has been observed.[202]

Diffuse Lymphoid Infiltration

Diffuse lymphoid infiltration is a rare cause of CIP and is characterized by a diffuse infiltration of small lymphocytes mixed with mature polyclonal plasma cells that reflects a pseudolymphoma rather than a true neoplasm.[176] It is a form of CIP that appears to be histologically distinct from visceral myopathies and neuropathies, perhaps related to diffuse immunoproliferative diseases.[176,203] Diffuse lymphoid infiltration affects all the layers of the intestinal wall[203] and is associated with extensive damage to the submucosal and myenteric nerve plexus.[176] Transient improvement may occur with use of antibiotics or cyclophosphamide and prednisone, though symptoms of CIP persist.[176]

Idiopathic Myenteric Ganglionitis

Ganglionitis refers to an inflammatory neuropathy characterized by a dense lymphoplasmacytic infiltrate of the myenteric plexus[130,202] and a marked reduction in the number of ganglia. Other cases have shown an eosinophil-predominant infiltrate, and neurons in the myenteric ganglia expressed the potent eosinophil chemoattractant IL-5.[116,176] Ganglionitis is typically associated with paraneoplastic, infectious, or neurologic disorders, although some cases remain idiopathic. The diagnosis of enteric ganglionitis is supported by detecting circulating antineuronal antibodies against certain targets, such as Hu and Yo proteins, neurotransmitter receptors, and ion channels.[130] A brief course of glucocorticoids or other immunosuppressive agent has been shown to be beneficial in some cases, thus reinforcing the value of establishing a correct diagnosis in the early stages of the disease process.[130,204]

Anorexia Nervosa and Bulimia

Delayed gastric emptying of solids and prolonged orocecal transit are well-established abnormalities in patients with anorexia or bulimia (see Chapter 9).[205] Electrolyte abnormalities (e.g., hypokalemia) may be responsible in some cases and be related to nutritional deficiencies or concomitant diuretic abuse. Typically, the motility disorder is less significant than the underlying psychological and nutritional manifestations of the disease, although debilitating pseudo-obstruction can ensue.

Clinical Features

Patients can experience cramping, generalized and epigastric abdominal pain or discomfort, bloating and distention, anorexia, early satiety, nausea and vomiting, and weight loss. Symptoms typically are aggravated by eating. Diarrhea can occur in patients as a result of SIBO and malabsorption. A history of repeated abdominal operations without evidence of mechanical obstruction is common; no surgeon wants to miss a true obstruction. Depression can develop as a result of chronic disabling digestive symptoms, deconditioning, and poor quality of life.

Physical findings vary according to the severity of symptoms and associated or causative disorders. In less symptomatic patients, physical examination may be normal. Patients with more severe symptoms may be dehydrated, cachectic, and malnourished because they are unable to take in adequate fluid or nutrients, or they might have malabsorption from SIBO, which leads to weight loss. The abdomen may be distended and mildly tender. Borborygmi (loud sounds of fluid and gas transfer) may be audible. During an acute obstructive episode of CIP, abdominal examination may be indistinguishable from that in true mechanical obstruction, which is why these patients' abdomens often have multiple surgical scars.

Dilatation of the small intestine or of isolated GI segments is not a consistent finding in CIP.[119] During acute exacerbation, abdominal plain films can show air-fluid levels and dilatation of the small intestine. A chronically dilated, atonic intestine and SIBO are more common in the CIP of intestinal myopathy and less likely in cases of neuropathic origin. Patients with intestinal dilatation often have malabsorption and steatorrhea, which causes additional weight loss. The prevalence and severity of recurrent obstructive episodes varies from patient to patient and from episode to episode in the same patient.

Extraintestinal features can occur, depending on the underlying disease. Megacystis and megaureter are commonly seen, along with megaduodenum in type I FVM; these patients can have urinary retention and frequent infections. Type II FVM (MNGIE), discussed earlier, is defined clinically by 2 or more of the following extraintestinal conditions: progressive external ophthalmoplegia, ptosis, polyneuropathy, leukoencephalopathy, or a family history with no other known cause of CIP.[206] MNGIE also is associated with hearing loss. Type III FVM is notable for marked dilatation of the entire GI tract without extraintestinal features.

In secondary CIP, patients may or may not have systemic manifestations of the underlying condition. Polymyositis and dermatomyositis are characterized by proximal muscle weakness; scleroderma is often associated with skin changes. Cardiac problems (e.g., cardiomyopathy) are common in patients with Chagas' disease. Causes of paraneoplastic syndrome include lung, breast, and ovarian cancer, Hodgkin's disease, and multiple myeloma. In patients in whom an underlying diagnosis has not been determined, extraintestinal symptoms and findings can provide important clinical clues. A careful review of systems is essential in all patients.

Complications

Malnutrition

Malnutrition occurs in patients with severe dysmotility of the small intestine as a result of insufficient food intake, vomiting, SIBO, diarrhea, and malabsorption. Anemia can occur due to deficiencies of iron, folate, and vitamin B_{12}. Serum cholesterol, calcium, and albumin levels may be low, especially in patients with malabsorption secondary to SIBO. In severe cases, especially in patients with intestinal dysfunction caused by myopathy, long-term enteral tube feeding or TPN may be necessary to provide sufficient nutrients.

TPN-Related Disorders

Patients with disabling GI symptoms and irreversible intestinal failure often require TPN (see Chapter 6). These patients are at risk for developing complications such as catheter-related sepsis, venous thrombosis, loss of venous access, and liver failure. Long-term TPN may be complicated by progressive cholestatic liver disease that can become irreversible. The onset of hepatic dysfunction in a patient who has intestinal failure and is on chronic TPN is an indication for transplantation of intestine, in isolation or combined with a liver graft.[207]

SIBO

Common in CIP, SIBO syndrome is a condition associated with the proliferation of colon-type bacteria within the small intestine (see Chapter 105). The syndrome is characterized by steatorrhea, flatulence, abdominal discomfort, and bloating, with symptoms of macrocytic anemia, malabsorption of nutrients and vitamins, and weight loss; some patients have no symptoms.[208] Direct quantitative cultures of jejunal contents was the diagnostic gold standard,[209] although it is clear that culture-independent techniques (e.g., gene sequencing) is redefining our knowledge in this area. In the clinical setting, noninvasive hydrogen breath tests are much more commonly used than routine cultures.[208]

Pneumatosis Cystoides Intestinalis (PCI)

PCI is a rare condition characterized by multiple gas-filled cysts in the submucosa or subserosa of the colon and, less often, the small intestine (see Chapter 128).[210] The mechanism is thought to involve increased gas production by intestinal bacteria, thereby altering the partial pressure of nitrogen in the intestinal wall.[211] PCI is more common in patients with COPD, but it occurs in cases of SSc and has been described in patients with polymyositis, diabetes, duodenal and gastric ulceration, regional enteritis, and GI malignancy. Intestinal peristaltic hypofunction associated with CIP leads to raised intraluminal pressure, allowing the gas to pass into the intestinal mucosa through breaks in mucosal integrity, forming pneumocysts. This condition can be diagnosed radiologically and endoscopically (Fig. 124-8). Subserosal pneumocysts, in particular, are liable to rupture, releasing free gas into the peritoneal cavity (pneumoperitoneum), making it important to distinguish this condition from bowel perforation. Pneumoperitoneum from rupture of pneumatosis cysts does not per se mandate operation, and is not complicated by peritonitis.

Natural History

CIP is a severely debilitating and progressive disorder. Familial cases have their onset at birth or typically in the first few years of life.[8] Childhood onset is characterized by a particularly severe course with high mortality rates.[212,213] The first obstructive episode in adults is often preceded by years of nonspecific and progressive digestive complaints. The diagnosis is made a median of 8.8 years after the initial onset of symptoms, and 88% of adults undergo a mean of 2.96 unnecessary operations[214] before the diagnosis is established.[108] The principal causes of death relate to complications of surgery, parenteral nutrition, transplantation, and septic shock of GI origin. Intestinal myopathy and intestinal hypomotility predict poor outcome. MNGIE has a particularly poor prognosis, with death occurring at about age 40 years.[108]

Diagnosis

The diagnosis of CIP is based primarily on clinical symptoms and is supported by radiologic, manometric, laboratory, histopathologic, and endoscopic investigations.

Radiologic Studies

Plain abdominal films are very useful in patients who complain of abdominal distention and bloating, because they might show gaseous distention of the areas affected by severe dysmotility; dilatation is greater in cases of CIP related to myopathy than when the cause is neuropathic dysmotility. Enteroclysis can be useful for detecting lesions in the small intestine and excluding mechanical obstruction. CT enteroclysis allows simultaneous internal and external views of the intestinal wall. Abdominal CT and MR scans are important in investigating possible causes of bowel compression, and MRA can noninvasively identify congenital or acquired vascular

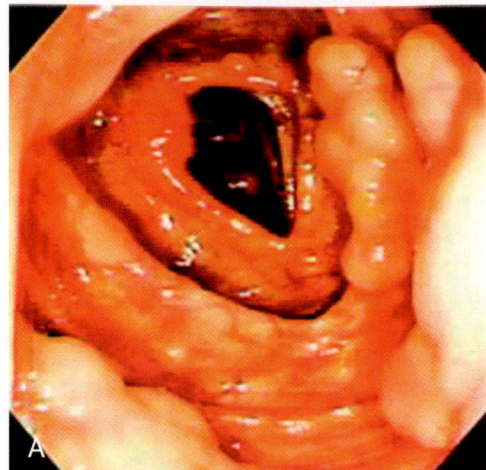

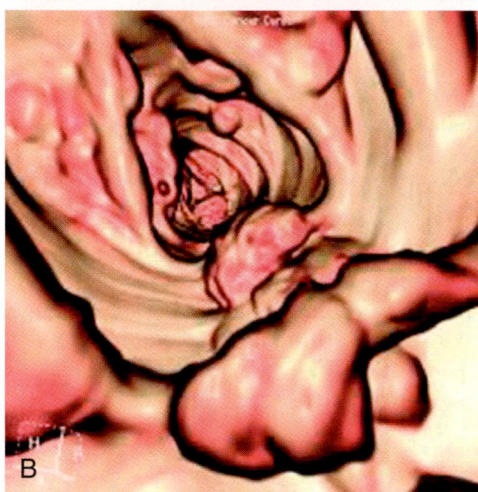

FIGURE 124-8. Pneumatosis cystoides intestinalis. *A,* Endoscopic view showing multiple cystic lesions with an overlying normal mucosal layer in the right colon. *B,* CT colonography image of the same patient showing multiple air-containing polypoid lesions in the ascending colon. *(From Kim BN, Jeong JY, Sohn KD, et al. Pneumatosis cystoides coli of the ascending colon: Colonoscopic and CT colonoscopic features. Endoscopy 2007; 39:E73-4.)*

abnormalities. Excretory urograms should be performed in patients with urinary symptoms.[108]

Radiopaque polyethylene motility markers are used to evaluate whole-gut transit. They are bead- or ring-shaped and ingested in a capsule containing 20 to 50 markers that move with the intestinal and colonic contents. More than 1 method has been suggested to measure transit. The single capsule method involves ingestion of 1 capsule followed by daily abdominal plain films that are obtained until all of the markers have passed. This is time consuming and has greater radiation exposure than the multiple-capsule technique.[215] By this method, 1 capsule is taken daily at the same time each day for 3 days, followed by abdominal plain films taken at the same time on days 4 and 7 only, or only on day 7.[216] The method works on the assumption that a 24-hour sampling interval approximates continuous observation. Rapid transit can cause all the markers to be lost in the feces before filming on the fourth day; conversely, in slow transit, all 72 markers may be present on the single plain film, in which case a film on day 7 provides more information.

Laboratory Tests

A complete blood count can reveal anemia and macrocytosis as a result of malnutrition and SIBO (see Chapters 104 and 105). Blood chemistries also reflect malnutrition and malabsorption. Diabetic patients have hyperglycemia, and hypoparathyroid patients can have hypocalcemia. Patients with connective tissue disease can have a positive antinuclear antibody or SCL-70. Patients with thyroid disease may have changes in serum T_3, T_4, and TSH levels. Muscular dystrophy or mitochondrial cytopathy patients can have elevated CPK and isoenzymes. Hemagglutination and complement fixation for Chagas' disease may be positive in patients who have lived in Central or South America.

Anti-neuronal nuclear antibody (ANNA), SCLC, and anti-Hu and anti-CV_2 antibodies should be sought in patients with an acute presentation of symptoms to exclude a paraneoplastic cause of pseudo-obstruction. Blood lactate, pyruvate (signs of acidosis), CPK, ALT (muscle damage), and leukocyte thymidine phosphorylase levels are screening tests for mitochondrial cytopathy.

Endoscopy

The main indication for upper endoscopy is to obtain biopsies from the small intestine in patients with malabsorption to exclude celiac disease and mucosal abnormalities, and to examine for signs of mechanical obstruction including gastric bezoar, pyloric stricture, dilated intestine and poor motility. Colonoscopy can be used to decompress the colon (see earlier).

Surgery

Full-thickness biopsies should be obtained from dilated and nondilated areas of the intestinal tract in all patients with suspected CIP who undergo surgery for unexplained intestinal obstruction; biopsy should be considered in patients with acute symptoms. Biopsies should be processed by traditional staining and by specialized immunohistochemistry techniques in dedicated laboratories with a specific interest in this area.[120]

Manometry

Small intestine manometry lacks the specificity to diagnose the underlying disease but can provide information about the pathophysiologic process (see below).

Myopathic Pattern

In patients with myopathy, manometry demonstrates low-amplitude contractions in the affected segment; this pattern generally is found during both fasting and fed periods. During fasting, the MMC usually is present but is diminished in amplitude. The fed pattern also is associated with reduced frequency of contractions. The poorly developed intestinal fed pattern is in part a result of reduced gastric emptying. Weston and associates showed that in myopathic disorders, antral amplitudes are usually less than 40 mm Hg and duodenal amplitudes are less than 10 mm Hg.[148]

Neuropathic Pattern

Neurologic disorders tend to produce uncoordinated bursts of intense contractions of variable duration but normal amplitude. The MMC often is absent or abnormal in these patients. An abnormal rate of migration and retrograde propagation of the activity front (phase III) also may be noted. Activity fronts can appear to be normal proximally, and then arrest or disappear in the more distal segments of the small intestine. In neuropathic disorders, the normal fed pattern might not replace the fasted pattern, MMC-like activity persists postprandially (normally, the MMC activity should be abolished for 1 hour per 200 kcal ingested), and the frequency of antral contractions in the first hour is typically less than 1 per minute, in contrast to the average 2 (range, 1 to 3) per minute in healthy controls.[151] These abnormalities reflect dysregulation by the enteric or extrinsic nervous system.

Mechanical Obstruction

The manometric pattern of mechanical obstruction (as opposed to pseudo-obstruction) is characterized by giant propagated or nonpropagated contractions lasting at least 10 seconds, or clustered contractions lasting 1 to 5 seconds followed by over 1 minute of absent motor activity.[119] Manometry is not the usual way to establish the diagnosis of mechanical obstruction, but it should alert the physician to the possibility of mechanical obstruction and mandate careful radiologic examination (e.g., enteroclysis).

Anorectal manometry is important to exclude Hirschsprung's disease, particularly in patients with intractable constipation and marked distention of the large intestine.

Wireless Motility Capsule Small Intestinal Transit

Small intestinal transit can also be measured with a wireless motility capsule that contains sensors to measure pH, pressure, and temperature.[217] It measures regional (gastric, small intestinal, and colonic) transit and whole-gut transit time, and can characterize pressure patterns and motility indices in the different regions of the GI tract. The transit of the capsule in the small intestine is presumed to depend upon phase II and phase III activity of the interdigestive motor complex, although the evidence supporting this is limited. Ileal prolonged propagated contractions may ultimately expel the capsule from the small bowel into the colon.[218]

Treatment

Treatment of CIP is suboptimal. Disabling digestive symptoms combined with dysfunction of the alimentary tract commonly lead to weight loss and malnutrition. Anemia can result from deficiencies of iron, folate, or vitamin B_{12}, and low serum cholesterol, calcium, and albumin levels can be seen, especially in patients with malabsorption secondary to SIBO. Therapies are primarily aimed at correcting the underlying processes when possible, preventing malnutrition and controlling symptoms.

Secondary Causes

A few types of secondary small intestine dysmotility—hypothyroidism, celiac disease, hyperglycemia associated with diabetes, and drug-induced dysmotility—can be treated with thyroid replacement, a gluten-free diet, improving glycemic control, and discontinuing the offending drugs, respectively. There are no specific treatments for most of the secondary causes of small intestine dysmotility.

Pain

Long-term narcotic use should be discouraged because patients can become addicted to narcotics, and narcotics can further disturb GI motility. Tramadol, gabapentin, and pregabalin sometimes are prescribed for such pain, but these too can retard intestinal transit. Unfortunately, there are conflicting data on transit effects of these medications in otherwise healthy people and virtually no such data in patients with CIP.[219-221]

Constipation

Constipation is common in patients who also have colon involvement. It is important to make certain that these patients have a good bowel movement at least once every few days, because constipation tends to increase symptoms of intestinal dysmotility. Milk of magnesia can be effective in doses of 30 to 60 mL per day (or 2 tablets 3 times daily). Enemas may be useful if patients have had no bowel movement for 3 days. Bulk-forming laxatives should be avoided in patients with severe small intestinal dysmotility, because they often exacerbate GI symptoms.

Acute Subocclusive Episodes

Acute episodes of pseudo-obstruction are treated similarly to acute mechanical obstruction. Fluid, electrolyte, and caloric support should be given IV. NG decompression may be beneficial for nausea and vomiting; rectal tubes often are ineffective, but placement of a colonoscopic decompression tube or cecostomy can be attempted for acute refractory dilation (see earlier). Pharmacotherapy using prokinetic agents can be used to reduce duration of the acute episode (see earlier). Prolonged subocclusive episodes necessitate appropriate nutritional support and IV or poorly absorbable antibiotics to prevent SIBO.

Nutrition Management

In patients with GI dysmotility, abdominal pain, bloating, nausea, and vomiting often are related to eating. Symptoms usually can be minimized by manipulating the amount, constituents, and frequency of meals. Patients need sufficient calories without overloading the inefficient bowel. A useful general rule is 25 kcal/kg of the patient's ideal body weight per day taken in small, equal-sized feedings 4 to 6 times daily. Multivitamins and salt supplementation generally is recommended. Because a liquid meal empties faster from the stomach and probably progresses more readily through the small intestine than a solid meal does, the liquid meal or perhaps an emulsified solid meal may be better tolerated than a solid meal. Supplemental formulas contain the daily vitamin and nutrient requirements, and many are lactose free. There is no advantage to using elemental formulas. Hypercaloric solutions are available, although generally formulas that have a lower caloric content (1 kcal/mL) are better tolerated than those with greater caloric density. Parenteral nutrition may be required to meet caloric and nutritional needs, but oral intake should continue as tolerated. TPN-related complications including catheter-related sepsis or thrombosis, hepatic insufficiency, pancreatitis, and glomerulonephritis[108] significantly increase the morbidity associated with CIP.

Pharmacotherapy

The aim of treatment is to reduce digestive symptoms and lower the risk of complications. Disordered motility of the small intestine leads to SIBO and malnutrition. Poorly absorbed antibiotics, such as rifaximin, are the preferred treatment for SIBO. Cycled treatments using metronidazole, ciprofloxacin, and doxycycline can limit resistance. Antiemetics and antispasmodic agents should be tried, although their benefit may be short lived. Improving intestinal motor function is another means of reducing symptoms. Two controlled trials showed cisapride improved symptoms and enhanced emptying in patients with chronic intestinal dysmotility.[222-224] The positive effect of cisapride is not as apparent in patients with vagal dysfunction (e.g., diabetes and following vagotomy).[224]

Other prokinetic agents, including erythromycin, metoclopramide, domperidone, neostigmine, and bethanechol, have been used to treat CIP, but results are anecdotal and high-quality studies are lacking. Domperidone is not FDA approved and is unavailable in the United States. In a small, short-term study, the somatostatin analog octreotide stimulated intestinal motility, possibly reduced SIBO, and improved abdominal symptoms in patients with scleroderma.[148] Other open-labeled studies confirmed the long-term effectiveness of octreotide with erythromycin in the treatment of chronic pseudo-obstruction. Some data show that octreotide retards gastric[225] and small intestinal transit in health, and many use the drug (50-μg dose) to induce MMC-like contractions at least 2 hours after the last meal of the day to sweep residue out of the small intestine toward the colon and prevent SIBO.[226] Oral pyridostigmine in pill or liquid form may be effective in reducing symptoms of bloating and constipation, but clinical trials with this agent are needed.

Treatment of inflammatory neuropathies should start early and be centered on the use of immunosuppressive therapies. The diagnosis should be suspected because of the presence of circulating antibodies and proved through specialized tissue analysis, if available.[119] An occult malignancy should be sought because treatment may also be directed at the tumor. When a diagnosis of an enteric ganglionitis or inflammatory neuropathy has been established, glucocorticoids, such as prednisolone (60 to 100 mg/day), methylprednisolone (up to 600 mg/day), or beclomethasone (200 μg 3 times daily), alone or in combination with other immunosuppressive treatments such as azathioprine, cyclophosphamide, and methotrexate, have been associated with significant clinical improvement, although firm evidence of benefit has not been proved.[130]

Surgical Therapy

Traditional surgical procedures are unable to correct the underlying disorder in most cases. In carefully selected patients, such as those with megaduodenum, resection or bypass of dysfunctional segments can have a good prognosis.[227] Venting gastrostomy and enterostomy may be used to reduce abdominal distention and vomiting, which can have a positive effect on conveying intestinal contents through the GI tract.[108] Because CIP tends to be a progressive disorder, surgery might provide only temporary benefit. Unnecessary surgery should be avoided because it can cause formation of adhesions and create future additional difficulties.

When all other treatment options have failed, small intestine and multi-organ transplantation can be considered.[225] (See Chapter 106) Indications for small bowel or multi-organ transplant include life-threatening complications from TPN, lack of venous access for TPN, intestinal failure with high mortality risk, and disease-related poor quality of life despite TPN.[8,228] Isolated intestinal transplant is technically less complex than transplantation of combined or multi-organ grafts, and it is preferred in cases of liver disease associated with intestinal failure, because the liver failure often reverses if transplantation is successful.[229] Organ rejection, repeat laparotomies, long-term TPN, and recurrent bacterial infections are frequent complications of intestinal transplantation for intestinal failure, with a 50% mortality rate at 5 years. In addition, there is a long-term risk of developing postoperative lymphoproliferative disorders.[8]

Immunosuppressive management (e.g., tacrolimus) represents a landmark in the treatment of patients undergoing transplantation for intestinal failure. Advances in immunosuppressive protocols, including induction therapy with monoclonal antibodies (daclizumab, alemtuzumab, or thymoglobulin), has lowered immunosuppressive requirements and reduced the risk of renal failure and sepsis. Advances in surgical techniques and graft monitoring via graft ileoendoscopy and intestinal biopsy have led to improved graft and patient survival rates.[229] In 1 series of isolated intestinal transplants in adult patients, survival rates were similar to those for other solid organ transplantations.[229] Three-year patient survival rates of 70% for isolated intestinal transplantations and 41% for multivisceral transplantations are reported, with mortality rates of 32.5% from sepsis (63%) or rejection.[229]

MEGACOLON AND MEGARECTUM

Megacolon and *megarectum* are descriptive terms without etiologic or pathophysiologic implications. Megacolon has been defined by a diameter of the rectosigmoid region or descending colon on abdominal plain film of greater than 6.5 cm; an ascending colon diameter of greater than 8 cm; or a cecal diameter greater than 12 cm. Megacolon can be caused by aganglionosis (Hirschsprung's disease), can be idiopathic (complicating chronic constipation of any cause), or may be a manifestation of a generalized GI dysmotility (intestinoparesis).

In congenital megacolon (Hirschsprung's disease), a congenital absence of the intramural neural plexus that mediates relaxation (aganglionosis) causes narrowing (most often of the rectum) of a variable distance proximally and results in functional obstruction (see Chapter 98). Short segment involvement (rectum or rectosigmoid) is most common, although an ultrashort segment of aganglionosis involving only the internal anal sphincter or long segment involvement (<20% of patients) can occur. Physiologic testing may be necessary to define ultrashort segment Hirschsprung's disease; radiologic confirmation of the diagnosis may be difficult. Hirschsprung's disease is detected more commonly in children than in adults, but ultrashort segment disease is usually not diagnosed until adulthood.[230]

Acquired megacolon describes any of the disparate causes of constipation that are associated with colonic dilatation not present at some earlier examination. A common background for acquired megacolon is colonic inertia, which can occur at both extremes of life. In children, this form can be confused with the congenital condition. Infection with *Trypanosoma cruzi* (Chagas' disease) is the most common cause of acquired megacolon worldwide.

KEY REFERENCES

Full references for this chapter can be found on www.expertconsult.com.

4. De Giorgio R, Knowles CH. Acute colonic pseudoobstruction. Br J Surg 2009; 96:229-39.
5. Vanek V, Al-Salti M. Acute pseudo-obstruction of the colon (Ogilvie's syndrome). An analysis of 400 cases. Dis Colon Rectum 1986; 29:203-10.
7. Stranghellini V, Cogliandro RF, De Giorgio R, et al. Natural history of intestinal failure induced by chronic intestinal pseudo-obstruction. Transplant Proc 2010; 42:15-28.
8. Furness JB. The enteric nervous system and neurogastroenterology. Nat Rev Gastroenterol Hepatol 2012; 9:286-94.

9. de Groat WC, Nadelhaft I, Milne RJ, et al. Organization of the sacral parasympathetic reflex pathways to the urinary bladder and large intestine. J Auton Nerv Syst 1981; 3:135-60.

11. van Bree SHW, Nemethova A, Cailotto C, et al. New therapeutic strategies for postoperative ileus. Nat Rev Gastroenterol Hepatol 2012; 9:675-83.

12. Asgeirsson T, El-Badowi KI, Mahmood A, et al. Postoperative ileus: It costs more than you expect. J Am Coll Surg 2010; 210:228-31.

13. Adamina M, Kehlet H, Tomlinson GA, et al. Enhanced recovery pathways optimize health outcomes and resource utilization: A meta-analysis of randomized controlled trials in colorectal surgery. Surgery 2011; 149:830-40.

15. Boeckxstaens GE, Jonge WJ. Neuroimmune mechanisms in postoperative ileus. Gut 2009; 58:1300-11.

23. Kalff JC, Carlos TM, Schraut WH, et al. Surgically induced leukocytic infiltrates within the rat intestinal muscularis mediate postoperative ileus. Gastroenterology 1999; 117:378-87.

33. Bauer AJ, Boeckxstaens GE. Mechanisms of postoperative ileus. Neurogastroenterol Motil 2004; 16(Suppl 2): 54-60.

50. Patel S, Lutz JM, Panchagnula U, Bansal S. Anesthesia and perioperative management of colorectal surgical patients—A clinical review. J Anesthesiol Clin Pharmacol 2012; 28:162-71.

55. Kehlet H. Postoperative ileus—An update on preventative techniques. Nat Clin Pract Gastroenterol Hepatol 2008; 5:552-8.

108. Antonucci A, Fronzoni L, Cogliandro L, et al. Chronic intestinal pseudo-obstruction. World J Gastroenterol 2008; 14:2953-61.

130. De Giorgio R, Guerrini S, Barbara G, et al. Inflammatory neuropathies of the enteric nervous system. Gastroenterology 2004; 126:1872-83.

CHAPTER OUTLINE

Small intestinal (SI) tumors (tumors of the duodenum, jejunum, and ileum) are uncommon in comparison with those occurring elsewhere in the GI tract. The SI is approximately 20 ft long, comprising 75% of the length of the GI tract and 90% of its mucosal surface area, but less than 2% of malignant GI tumors are derived from this organ. SI tumors are diverse in nature (≈40 different histologic types of SI tumors have been described) because they are derived from both epithelial and mesenchymal components of the SI (Box 125-1). The most frequent primary histologic types of SI malignant tumors include adenocarcinomas, carcinoids, lymphomas, and sarcomas (most are now classified as GISTs). Approximately 8800 new cases of primary SI cancer were estimated to occur in the United States in 2013 (equally distributed between men and women), with 1170 estimated cancer deaths.[1] The diverse nature of SI tumors makes it difficult to make generalizations about the group as a whole; some tumors represent distinct entities, whereas others share overlapping features.

EPIDEMIOLOGY

The frequency of SI tumors varies among different populations.[1-6] An average age-adjusted incidence of primary SI cancers of 1.9% per 100,000 men and 1.4 per 100,000 women has been reported in the United States[5]; Global incidence ranges between 0.3 and 2.0 per 100,000 when age-standardized. Small but significant increases in the incidence of SI adenocarcinomas and carcinoids have been noted since the 1970s,[4-6] with a slight male predominance. The incidence of SI cancers rises with age, beginning at 30 years, with a mean age of diagnosis of approximately 60 years.[7] Incidence rates for SI adenocarcinomas and malignant carcinoids are higher in African Americans than in whites.[5]

The relative frequency of primary tumors in the SI ranges in the literature, with adenocarcinoma (24% to 52%), malignant carcinoid (17% to 41%), lymphoma (12% to 29%), and sarcomas (11% to 20%) most frequently reported. Studies of changing patterns over time suggest that the overall frequency of SI tumors has increased over the last 20 years in the United States, mostly due to an increase in carcinoid tumors.[5,6] A recent study of trends over time based on the National Cancer Database and the Surveillance Epidemiology and End Results (SEER) database indicates an almost equal proportion of SI adenocarcinomas and carcinoids at this time (37%), with 8.4% stromal cell tumors and 17.3% lymphomas.[6] The pattern of distribution of tumors in the SI is dependent on histologic type. In Western countries, SI adenocarcinomas are more commonly found in the duodenum (3.0 per 1,000,000) than in the jejunum (1.2 per 1,000,000) and ileum (0.9 per 1,000,000).[5] In the setting of Crohn's disease, adenocarcinomas occur distally in the ileum. Carcinoids and primary lymphomas occur predominantly in the ileum, whereas sarcomas are more evenly distributed. Metastases to the SI from adenocarcinomas and sarcomas account for approximately 50% of all SI tumors.

Several hypotheses have been proposed to explain why SI tumors are relatively rare, but objective data are mostly lacking. Hypotheses include the following: (1) Rapid transit time and liquid lumenal contents reduce mucosal contact with putative carcinogens, while mucosal enzymes (e.g., benzpyrene hydroxylase) detoxify them. (2) Bacterial enzymes have been postulated to play a role in colonic carcinogenesis. When bacterial flora is altered, as in SIBO, SI carcinomas develop with a higher frequency than expected. The SI, however, has low bacterial counts (the upper two thirds of the SI contain low concentrations of aerophilic Gram-positive bacteria such as lactobacilli and enterococci), with an absence of anaerobes under normal conditions (see Chapters 3 and 105). (3) Stem cells located at the crypt base lie deeper in the SI than in the colon, perhaps reducing contact with lumenal carcinogens. The rapid differentiation of stem cells into mature, non-proliferating enterocytes and goblet cells may also protect against factors that deregulate cell growth and promote cancer development. (4) Apoptosis involving damaged cells and potentially tumorigenic clones differs between the small and large intestine. (5) Lymphoid tissue in the lamina propria and Peyer's patches of the ileum may provide immune surveillance against neoplastic cells through immunoglobulin (Ig)A-rich secretions.

Benign Epithelial Tumors
Brunner gland lesions[†]
Benign intestinal epithelial polyps
    Adenomas
    Hamartomas (Peutz-Jeghers syndrome, Cronkhite-Canada
        syndrome, juvenile polyposis, Cowden disease,
        Bannayan-Riley-Ruvalcaba syndrome)

Malignant Epithelial Lesions
Primary adenocarcinomas
Secondary carcinomas (metastases)
Carcinoid tumors (neuroendocrine tumors)

Lymphoproliferative Disorders
B cell
    Diffuse large-cell lymphoma
    Follicular lymphoma
    Marginal B cell lymphoma (MALT type cell lymphoma)
    Mantle cell lymphoma (multiple lymphomatous polyposis)
    Immunoproliferative small intestinal disease
T cell
    Enteropathy-associated T cell lymphoma

Mesenchymal Tumors[‡]
GISTs (benign and malignant)
Fatty tumors (lipoma, liposarcoma)
Neural tumors (intestinal autonomic tumors, schwannomas,
    neurofibromas, ganglioneuromas, granular cell tumors)
Paragangliomas
Smooth muscle tumors (leiomyoma, leiomyosarcoma)
Vascular tumors (hemangioma, angiosarcoma, lymphangioma,
    Kaposi's sarcoma)

*This is a partial list of tumors found in the small intestine. Although the overall incidence of small intestinal tumors is low, many different benign and malignant lesions have been described in this organ.
[†]It is unclear whether these lesions should be classified as hyperplasias, neoplasia, hamartomas, or adenomatous proliferations.
[‡]Some mesenchymal tumors represent clear-cut diagnostic entities, whereas many are more difficult to classify into any specific cell lineage. The latter are designated GISTs.

Although adenocarcinomas of the colon and SI often occur in the same populations, the limited descriptive epidemiology of SI tumors has not provided strong evidence for environmental influences on tumor formation similar to that of the large intestine. A recent prospective study of risk factors for adenocarcinomas and malignant carcinoids of the SI (the 2 most common tumor types) indicated that age 65 years or older was the only significant risk factor for adenocarcinomas, whereas male gender, BMI, and current menopausal hormone therapy use were positively associated with malignant carcinoids.[4] Race, education, diabetes, smoking, physical activity, and alcohol intake were not associated with either histologic subtype. These findings differ to some extent from previous publications in which modestly increased odds ratios for cigarette smoking and for heavy alcohol intake have been reported for adenocarcinomas and carcinoids in some but not all studies.[5,8] Several studies report a link between obesity and SI cancer, but again, this is not universal. Studies based on retrospective medical record review often do not take into account the amount and duration of exposures, dose-response trends, or adjust for other influences that may explain these differences. Weekly or more frequent consumption of red meat or salt-cured foods, frequent intake of foods rich in heterocyclic amines (fried bacon, ham, barbecued or smoked meat and fish), high sugar intake, intake of bread, pasta, and rice have all been associated with an increased risk of SI adenocarcinoma in small older studies, with reports of an inverse relationship with coffee, fish, vegetables, and fruit.

BIOLOGY AND BIOCHEMICAL CHANGES

In comparison with colorectal cancer (CRC), relatively little is known about the molecular genetic events associated with the evolution of SI tumors. Descriptive associations have been reported, but except for familial syndromes such as familial adenomatous polyposis (FAP) and Lynch syndrome, where germline associations in the adenomatous polyposis coli gene (APC) and mismatch repair genes, respectively, have been reported for adenocarcinomas, definitive data are lacking for most tumor types. Periampullary duodenal carcinomas and some ampullary carcinomas that arise from intestinal epithelium may have different molecular pathogeneses from ampullary tumors arising from the pancreaticobiliary ducts (see Chapters 60 and 69) and may influence treatment options.[9] Important molecular profiling studies that influence prognosis and therapy have been reported for GISTs (see later).

Cellular proto-oncogenes are evolutionarily conserved human genes that play a role in signal transduction and normal regulation of cell growth. Human *ras* genes encode guanine nucleotide binding proteins that regulate intracellular signaling pathways. Point mutations in *K-ras*, especially at codon 12, have been reported in 14% to 53% of primary SI adenocarcinomas[10,11] but not in carcinoids. *K-ras* mutations were common in 1 representative study in sporadic and Crohn's disease-associated adenocarcinomas of the SI.[12] *K-ras* mutations were present in all 4 sporadic carcinomas with contiguous adenomas, in 2 of 11 (18%) without adenomas, and in 4 of 7 (43%) of Crohn's disease-associated carcinomas.

Allelic losses involving tumor suppressor genes play major roles in the genesis of SI tumors. The *APC* gene on the long arm of chromosome 5 (5q21) is mutated in the germline of patients with FAP, and somatic mutations of *APC* occur in 60% to 80% of sporadic CRCs and adenomas (see Chapters 126 and 127). Mutation of the mouse homolog of *APC* (*Apc*) by chemical carcinogenesis or by genetic manipulation[13] results in development of colonic and small intestinal polyps. SI and periampullary adenomas and carcinomas are common in patients with FAP. *APC* mutations have also been reported in sporadic SI adenocarcinoma,[11] but they appear to occur at a much lower frequency than in sporadic CRC.

Deletions of chromosome 17p involve the *p53* tumor suppressor gene, whose product normally prevents cells with damaged DNA from progressing from the G_1 phase to the S phase in the cell cycle and regulates apoptosis. Mutations in *p53* were found in 27% of SI adenocarcinomas in 1 series,[11] whereas alterations in the p53 gene product and allelic loss of chromosome 17p were present in 47% of sporadic SI adenocarcinomas, 33% of contiguous adenomas, and 71% of Crohn's disease-associated carcinomas in a second series.[12]

Candidate tumor suppressor genes on chromosome 18q include *DPC4 (SMAD4)*. *DPC4* belongs to the SMAD gene family involved in signal transduction pathways that are activated through the transforming growth factor (TGF) β family receptors. Loss of 18q has been reported in SI tumors from the Apc 1638N mouse model,[13] but rarely in human SI adenocarcinomas.[12] Chromosome 18 deletions appear to be common events, however, in classical midgut carcinoids of the SI.[14,15]

Alterations in genes that help to maintain DNA fidelity during replication (mismatch repair, or MMR genes) are characteristic of patients with hereditary nonpolyposis CRC (HNPCC). Mismatch repair gene mutations in *hMLH1* and *hMSH2* were present in 15 of 42 (36%) of HNPCC-associated SI carcinomas in 1 series.[16] Pathogenic germline mutations in genes including *MLH1*, *MSH2*, and *MSH6* were identified in 81% of individuals with HNPCC and SI tumors, with loss of MMR protein expression in 89% of cases in another large series.[17] DNA replication errors characterized by microsatellite instability were also reported in 13% of sporadic SI carcinomas.[12] More recently, loss of MMR proteins was reported in 35% of a group of relatively young patients with primary SI adenocarcinomas.[18] A high percentage of patients in this study also had tumors that expressed abnormalities in expression of EGF receptor (EGFR) and vascular epidermal growth factor receptor (VEGFR). In another study, loss of E-cadherin expression or aberrant expression of β-catenin were observed in approximately 40% of SI adenocarcinomas.[19] SI neuroendocrine tumors (SI-NETs) are now 1 of the 2 most common malignancies of the SI. A recent study used massively parallel ("nextgen") DNA sequencing to examine 48 SI-NETs.[20] Frequently altered mechanisms of carcinogenesis included abnormalities in chromatin remodeling, DNA damage, RAS signaling, and axon guidance. Alterations with potential therapeutic relevance were found in *SRC*, *SMAD*, *AURKA*, *EGFR*, *HSP90*, and *PDGFR* genes. Alterations in *AKT1* or *AKT2* were common in patients with alterations of PI3K/Akt/mTOR signaling (often targeted in clinical trials of therapy for SI-NETs).

GISTs contain gain-of-function mutations that affect 2 receptor tyrosine kinase genes, *KIT* and *PDGFRA*.[21,22] *Kit* mutations are detected in 75% to 85% and *PDGFRA* mutations in 10% to 15% of GISTs. KIT mutations are most frequently found in exon 11 (70% to 75%), followed by exons 9 17 and 17, whereas PDGFRA mutations are most frequent in exon 18, followed by exon 12, and rarely exon 14. *KIT* activation is a crucial oncogenic mechanism in sporadic and familial GISTs. Mutations in *KIT* or *PDGFRA* predict prognosis and response to therapy with tyrosine kinase inhibitors (see below and Chapter 32). GISTs that carry *KIT* exon 11 mutations, for example, respond better to targeted treatment than tumors with wild-type *KIT* and *PDFGRA*, whereas both primary and secondary (acquired) mutations affecting the tyrosine kinase domain do not generally respond to imatinib.

RISK FACTORS AND ASSOCIATED CONDITIONS

Numerous risk factors and associated conditions have been described with relation to tumors of the SI (Box 125-2). Duodenal adenomas and adenocarcinomas occur in individuals with FAP (see also Chapters 126 and 127).[23-27] Periampullary duodenal carcinoma is the most common extracolonic malignant tumor in patients with FAP. A relative risk (RR) for duodenal adenocarcinoma of 331, and an RR of 124 for ampullary carcinoma, have been reported in patients with FAP compared with the general population.[23] Mean ages of diagnosis were 53 years for duodenal carcinoma and 49 years for ampullary carcinoma. Duodenal adenomas are common in patients with FAP and have been reported in up to 100% of such patients. A prospective study in 5 Nordic countries and the Netherlands demonstrated that at first endoscopy, 65% of individuals with FAP had duodenal adenomas at a median age of 38 years.[27] The cumulative incidence of adenomatosis at 70 years was 90%. The cumulative incidence of cancer was 4.5% at age 57 years. SI adenomas elsewhere in the bowel have also been reported in recent studies using capsule endoscopy.[24] Inactivation of 1 of the BER genes (*MYH* or *MUTYH*) is a cause of an autosomal recessive form of FAP (MUTYH-associated polyposis, or MAP). Duodenal cancers have been reported sporadically in MAP, but periodic screening of the proximal SI is recommended in a manner similar to FAP (see

---

BOX 125-2 Conditions Associated with an Increased Risk of Primary Small Intestinal Neoplasia

Adenocarcinoma
Celiac disease
Crohn's disease
Duplication cysts and Meckel's diverticula
Familial adenomatous polyposis
Ileal loop conduits, ileal pouches, ileal cystoplasty
Juvenile polyposis syndrome
Long-standing ileostomy (especially with Crohn's disease)
Lynch syndrome (hereditary nonpolyposis colorectal cancer)
Peutz-Jeghers syndrome
Previous history of cholecystectomy

Non-Hodgkin's B Cell Lymphoma
AIDS
Crohn's disease
Infectious agents (e.g., *Campylobacter jejuni* [immunoproliferative small intestinal disease])
Nodular lymphoid hyperplasia

Enteropathy-Type Intestinal T Cell Lymphoma
Celiac disease

GIST
Germline mutations in succinyl dehydrogenase genes
Type 1 neurofibromatosis (von Recklinghausen's neurofibromatosis)

---

later).[28] Lynch syndrome is an inherited disease in which colon cancers arise in discrete adenomas, but polyposis (i.e., hundreds of polyps) does not occur (see Chapters 126 and 127). SI cancer is part of the tumor spectrum of Lynch syndrome, with an estimated lifetime risk of 4%.[29] Patients with Lynch syndrome generally present with SI cancer 10 to 20 years earlier than the general population, and SI cancer may be the first manifestation. Tumors in Lynch syndrome may be distributed throughout the SI. In 1 analysis of kindreds with Lynch syndrome, 42 members of 40 families developed 42 primary and 7 metachronous SI tumors.[16] There were 46 adenocarcinomas and 3 carcinoid tumors. The median age at diagnosis of the index SI tumor was 49 years, and the SI was the first site of carcinoma in 24 (57%) patients. In another study of 32 individuals with SI carcinoma in the setting of Lynch syndrome, the median age at diagnosis was 39 years[17]; 50% of tumors were located in the duodenum. The relative risks of SI cancer in families that fulfilled the Amsterdam II and Bethesda criteria (see Chapters 126 and 127) were 36.1 and 5.75, respectively, in a recent report from a Swedish registry.[30] More recent data from the Colon Cancer Family Registry for 764 carriers of MMR gene mutations who had previous CRC indicates that the 10-year risk of developing SI cancer in these individuals is 1% (standardized incidence ratio compared with the general population, 72.68).[31]

Hamartomatous polyposis syndromes are a group of disorders marked by the finding of multiple hamartomatous polyps in the GI tract (see Chapter 126). The Peutz-Jeghers syndrome is an autosomal dominant disease, which in most families has been mapped to chromosome 19p13.3 and the *STK11* (serine threonine kinase 11) gene. Extracolonic cancers are common, occurring in 50% to 90% of patients (SI, stomach, pancreas, esophagus, ovary, lung, uterus, breast); the relative risk (RR) for all cancers is 15.2 compared with the general population.[32,33] The SI represents the most frequent site of cancer development, with an RR of development of adenocarcinoma of 520 compared with the general population. Patients often present with obstructive symptoms and may develop SI intussusception.

Juvenile polyposis syndrome is an autosomal dominant disease in which hamartomatous polyps may be limited to the colon, be limited to the stomach, or occur throughout the GI tract. Mixed juvenile and adenomatous polyps have been reported. The RR for SI cancer is unclear, but cancers of the duodenum have been reported. Patients may present with bleeding, intussusception, and SBO. A life-threatening protein-losing enteropathy has been reported in some patients. Germline mutations in the *SMAD4* (chromosome 18q21.1) and *PTEN* (chromosome 10q23) genes have been reported in separate kindreds with juvenile polyposis syndrome.[33]

An increased incidence of both SI adenocarcinoma and lymphoma has been reported to occur in Crohn's disease (see Chapter 115).[34-37] A dysplasia-carcinoma sequence occurs in the SI in Crohn's disease similar to that of the colon and rectum. Crohn's disease-associated SI carcinomas and dysplasias are accompanied by frequent genetic alterations in *K-ras* and *p53*. The RR of SI carcinoma in Crohn's disease (mostly ileal) has been estimated to be 60 to 100 times that of the general population, but a recent population-based case-control study found that although there was a strong association between Crohn's disease and SI cancer in patients older than 67 years (odds ratio, 12), the prevalence of Crohn's disease in individuals with SI cancer is low (1.6%).[35] SI (ileal) resection and prolonged salicylate use may be protective against SI adenocarcinoma in the setting of Crohn's disease.[37]

Diversion of bile to the lower SI either surgically or by feeding cholestyramine increases the yield of SI carcinomas in carcinogen-treated animals. Indeed, patients who underwent cholecystectomy had an increased risk of adenocarcinoma of the SI (RR, 1.71) and the right side of the colon.[38]

An increased risk of both SI adenocarcinoma and non-Hodgkin's lymphoma has been reported to be associated with celiac disease (see Chapter 107).[39] The overall incidence of malignant disease in this condition has been reported to be 11% to 13%, with an incidence of SI lymphomas of 4% to 7%. In some reported cases, it is not clear whether the primary diagnosis is actually celiac sprue or whether the histologic changes are secondary to lymphoma per se. Lymphomas in the setting of celiac disease are usually of T cell origin (enteropathy-associated T-cell lymphomas [EATLs]). Adenocarcinomas may arise in focal areas of dysplasia.

Other conditions may carry an increased relative risk for SI neoplasia (see Box 125-2), but they are relatively rare. Patients with urinary diversion to the SI (ileal loop conduits) appear to have an increased risk of carcinoma. Adenocarcinomas arise in the mucosa of ileostomies and ileal pouches in patients with IBD and FAP,[40] although this event is probably rare. Type 1 neurofibromatosis has been associated with development of SI GISTs.

CLINICAL FEATURES

The clinical signs and symptoms of SI neoplasms may have some common features, but for the most part they depend on the individual tumor type (Table 125-1). Abdominal pain may result from partial or complete SI obstruction (SBO), intussusception, or ischemia. SBO may be the result of the physical bulk of the tumor, infiltration, or annular constriction. An intense desmoplastic reaction by carcinoids causes intestinal buckling or kinking. Intussusception may occur with benign polypoid lesions, accounting for half of adult intussusception, and is common in patients with GISTs. Occult GI blood loss is another common feature of benign and malignant SI tumors. Bleeding may be acute and brisk, however, with ulcerated GISTs. Weight loss is especially common and pronounced in patients with SI lymphoma.

ADENOCARCINOMA

Adenocarcinoma is 1 of the most common primary malignant diseases of the SI, accounting for ≈37% of SI malignancies, which is similar to the incidence of carcinoid tumors.[6] Outside the setting of IBD, the majority of tumors occur in the

TABLE 125-1 Clinical Features of Small Bowel Tumors

Symptom	Benign	Malignant
Abdominal pain	Most frequent symptom	Most frequent symptom; one third of patients develop partial or complete small bowel obstruction
Intussusception	Most common cause of intussusception in adults, lipomas are the leading cause	Rare
Occult blood loss	25%-50% of cases	Up to 50% of cases
Frank bleeding	Rare	Rare; GIST is the most likely tumor to account for frank bleeding
Weight loss	Very rare	Up to 50% of cases; most severe with lymphoma
Palpable abdominal mass	Rare	40% of cases
Perforation	Very rare	About 10% of cases, almost all of which are lymphomas or GISTs
Jaundice	Rare occurrence with benign periampullary tumor	Occurs with about 80% of malignant periampullary tumors
Flushing	Metastatic spread of carcinoid tumor is required for carcinoid syndrome to occur	Occurs in a few cases of metastatic carcinoid tumor
Diarrhea	Very rare	Common with lymphoma and can occur with carcinoid syndrome

duodenum. The epidemiology of SI adenocarcinoma was discussed earlier.

Adenocarcinomas arise from adenomas or dysplastic changes of the SI (see Pathology, Natural History, and Staging). Adenomas and adenocarcinomas of the SI, and especially of the duodenum and ampulla of Vater, are most frequently encountered in the setting of FAP (see Chapter 125). There is no clear association between site of the mutation in the *APC* gene and severity of duodenal polyposis. A number of classifications describe the severity of duodenal polyposis; the most commonly used is the Spigelman classification, which takes into account size, histology, and severity of dysplasia of polyps.[25] Prospective studies of surveillance of the duodenum in individuals with FAP have demonstrated slow progression to carcinoma, with risk related to the Spigelman classification of severity.[25-27,41,42] The cumulative risk of duodenal cancer at age 57 was 4.5% in 1 large Scandinavian-Dutch study.[27]

Pathology, Natural History, and Staging

Adenocarcinomas of the SI arise in discrete adenomatous polyps, in adenomatous change involving the ampulla of Vater, or in dysplasia associated with IBD.[43] In hamartomatous polyposis syndromes, carcinomas may arise from discrete adenomas or mixed polyps containing adenomatous components. Dysplasia is associated with familial juvenile polyps, but not with solitary sporadic juvenile polyps. Dysplastic polyps contain markers suggesting a loss of proliferative control within the epithelium and mutations in *APC*.

Adenomas in the SI display the same gross and microscopic features as those in the large intestine (Fig. 125-1). They may be pedunculated or sessile. Tubular adenomas tend to be small, whereas those with villous architecture tend to be larger. The presence of multiple duodenal adenomas or adenomatous changes in the ampulla of Vater suggests the diagnosis of FAP. Tubular adenomas contain tall columnar, pseudostratified epithelial cells. Villous adenomas contain fingerlike villous or papillary processes similar to those in the colon. SI adenomas exhibit a spectrum of dysplasia ranging from mild dysplasia to intramucosal carcinoma and invasive cancer. Glandular crowding ("back-to-back" glands), loss of epithelial polarity, an increased nucleus-to-cytoplasm ratio, and increased mitoses characterize high-grade dysplasia. These changes, accompanied by invasion into the lamina propria, define intramucosal carcinoma.

Invasive carcinoma may be found in one fourth to one half of resected villous adenomas in the setting of FAP, but most duodenal adenomas appear to progress slowly to carcinoma, and the actual risk of malignant degeneration is probably considerably lower.[25-27,41,42] Progression to carcinoma appears to be related to number and size of duodenal adenomas, with dysplasia a harbinger of malignant degeneration. An adenoma-to-carcinoma sequence also appears to be characteristic of the development of adenocarcinoma in the setting of Lynch syndrome.[29] Adenomatous polyps of the SI do occur outside the setting of familial cancer, but even less is known about their natural history.

SI adenocarcinomas may appear grossly as flat, stenosing, ulcerative, infiltrating, or polypoid lesions (Fig. 125-2). Most are moderately differentiated tumors with gland formation and variable degrees of mucin secretion (see Fig. 125-2E and F). Poorly differentiated tumors occur in approximately 20% of cases. The presence of signet cells, in which a large vacuole of mucin displaces the nucleus to 1 side, is a feature of some of these tumors. Rare adenosquamous carcinomas of the duodenum have been reported.

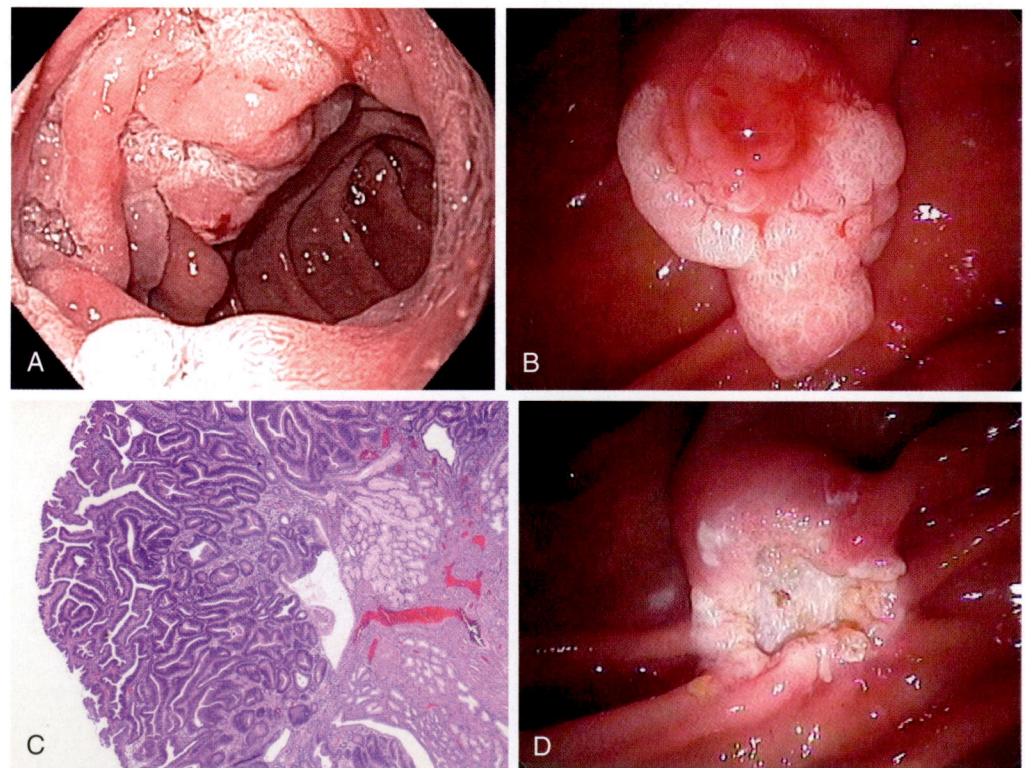

FIGURE 125-1. Small intestinal adenomas. *A,* Endoscopic view demonstrating a large adenoma involving the duodenal mucosa. *B,* Duodenal adenoma involving the ampulla of Vater seen with a side-viewing endoscope. *C,* Histopathology of duodenal adenoma showing branching dysplastic glands and hyperchromatic nuclei. *D,* Polypectomy site after endoscopic mucosal resection of the lesion seen in *B.*

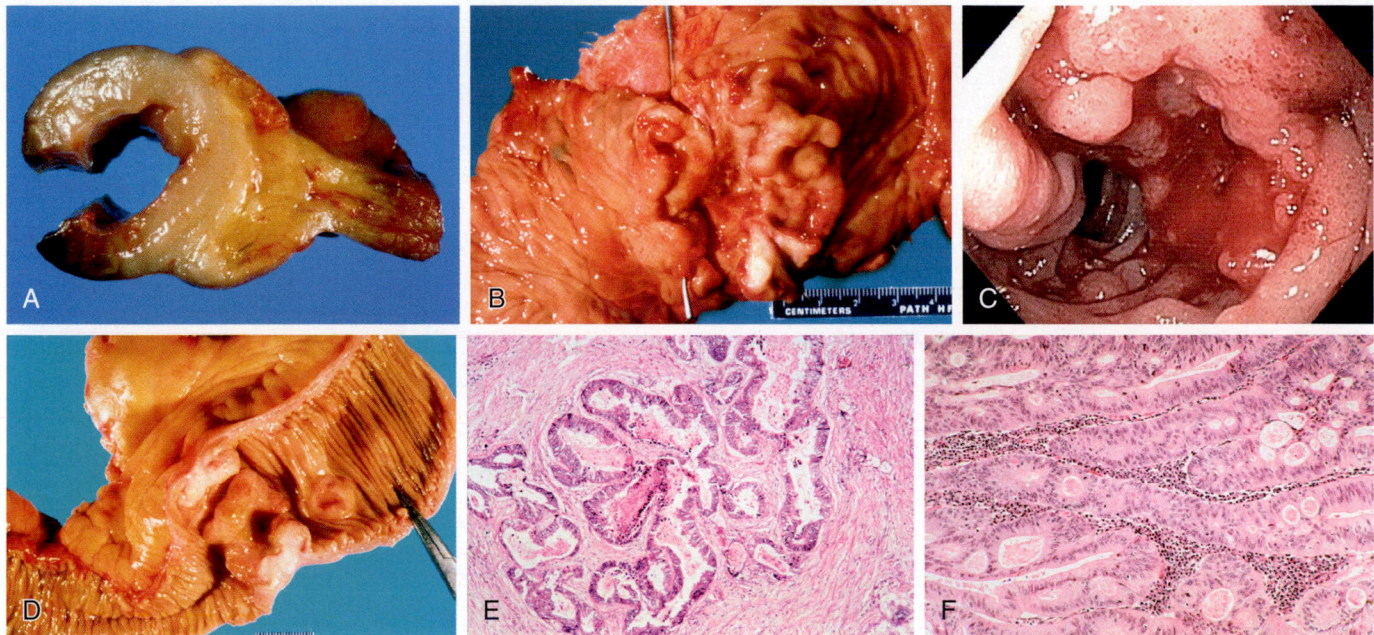

FIGURE 125-2. Adenocarcinomas of the small intestine. *A,* Gross specimen of annular small bowel carcinoma. *B,* Gross specimen with the opened section of the duodenum demonstrating a stenosing, infiltrating lesion. *C,* Endoscopic view demonstrating a circumferential lesion with active bleeding. *D,* Gross specimen of periampullary carcinoma of the duodenum. *E,* Histologic section demonstrating typical gland formation in a moderately well-differentiated adenocarcinoma. *F,* Histology of well-differentiated periampullary carcinoma.

Adenocarcinomas are staged according to the American Joint Committee on Cancer (AJCC) TNM classification, which denotes the extent of the primary tumor (T), the status of regional lymph nodes (N), and the presence or absence of distant metastases (M). Cases are assigned the highest value of TNM that describes the full extent of disease and are grouped into 5 stages (0 through IV) depending on the extent of bowel wall invasion, the presence or absence of invasion into adjacent structures, and the presence or absence of lymph node or distant metastases (Table 125-2).[44] The 7th edition of the *AJCC Cancer Staging Manual* includes a number of modifications of the SI cancer staging system designed to facilitate comparison with other GI sites, and to more accurately reflect the relationship between the extent of tumor invasion and the number of affected lymph nodes.[44]

The prognosis of patients with SI adenocarcinomas is poor. Almost one third of patients present with metastatic disease, and many patients with earlier-stage disease are not candidates for curative resection. In 1 report, the overall 5-year disease–specific survival in the United States was 30.5%, with a median survival of 19.7 months.[45] A more recent analysis of survival trends over 20 years indicated a 5-year survival rate of 39.9%.[6] Five-year survival rates approximate 65% for stage I, 48% for stage II, 35% for stage III, and 4% for stage IV tumors (Fig. 125-3; see Table 125-2 for staging definitions).[6,45-48] Factors significantly correlated with overall survival include tumor stage (depth of invasion and lymph node status), age (poorer prognosis for patients > 75 years old), tumor site (duodenum worse than jejunum or ileum), whether cancer-directed surgery was performed, and history of Crohn's disease (poorer prognosis).[49,50] In multivariate analyses, however, the most important independent prognostic factors have been curative (R0) resection, lymph node status, and ratio of positive to negative lymph nodes.[51] Poor prognosis after potentially curative resection has been associated with patients who were male, older (age > 55 years), black, and had duodenal, ileal, or diffuse tumors (compared with jejunal tumors), T4 lesions,

nodal or distant metastases, poorly differentiated tumors, or involved margins.[6] Adenocarcinomas arising in the setting of HNPCC have a better prognosis than those occurring in FAP or in the general population.[16] Patients with tumors arising at or near the ampulla of Vater may do better than those with more distal tumors, perhaps because they become symptomatic earlier. Five-year survival rates approaching 50% have been reported for patients with lymph node-negative cancers of the ampulla after radical resection.

Clinical Features

The mean age of presentation for SI adenocarcinoma is approximately 65 years, with a wide range of age at presentation. Less than 1% of tumors occur before age 30 years, and approximately 85% occur after age 50 years. Symptoms relate to tumor size, location, and blood supply. Small tumors are asymptomatic or may present with anemia secondary to chronic blood loss, but for the most part they are indolent and difficult to diagnose. Abdominal pain and other obstructive symptoms such as nausea and vomiting are common late symptoms as tumors obstruct from infiltration with luminal narrowing or mass effect. Anorexia and weight loss are also common symptoms. Ileal tumors uncommonly may present with intussusception. Tumors located in the periampullary duodenum or ampulla of Vater may cause obstruction of the bile duct, presenting with jaundice and other signs of biliary obstruction.

Diagnosis

Endoscopy with forward- and side-viewing instruments should be used to examine the duodenum when a lesion is suspected or in families with FAP. Screening for duodenal adenomas and ampullary tumors, and surveillance after endoscopic removal of adenomas, should be performed in persons who exhibit the FAP phenotype or in family members in

TABLE 125-2 TNM and American Joint Committee on Cancer (AJCC)/International Union Against Cancer (UICC) Staging Systems for Small Intestinal Adenocarcinomas

TNM Stage	Criteria
Tx	Primary tumor cannot be assessed
T0	No evidence of primary tumor
Tis	Carcinoma in situ
T1a	Tumor invades lamina propria
T1b	Tumor invades submucosa
T2	Tumor invades muscularis propria
T3	Tumor invades through the muscularis propria into the subserosa or into the non-peritonealized perimuscular tissue (mesentery or retroperitoneum) with extension of ≤2 cm*
T4	Tumor perforates the visceral peritoneum or directly invades other organs or structures (i.e., other loops of small intestine, mesentery or retroperitoneum >2 cm, abdominal wall, pancreas, or bile duct)
Nx	Regional lymph nodes cannot be assessed
N0	No regional lymph node metastases
N1	Metastases in 1-3 regional lymph nodes
N2	Metastases in ≥4 regional lymph nodes
M0	No distant metastases
M1	Distant metastases

AJCC/UICC Stage	Tumor	Node	Metastasis
0	Tis	N0	M0
I	T1	N0	M0
	T2	N0	M0
II A	T3	N0	M0
II B	T4	N0	M0
III A	Any T	N1	M0
III B	Any T	N2	M0
IV	Any T	Any N	M1

*The non-peritonealized perimuscular tissue is, for the jejunum and ileum, part of the mesentery, and for the duodenum, in areas where serosa is lacking, part of the interface with the pancreas. T1 lesions have been divided into T1a (invasion of the lamina propria) and T1b (invasion of the submucosa) to facilitate comparison with tumors of other GI sites; stage II has been divided into stage IIA and stage IIB; the N1 category has been changed to N1 (1-3 positive lymph nodes) and N2 (≥4 positive lymph nodes), leading to division of stage III into stage IIIA and stage IIIB. Adapted from American Joint Committee on Cancer. Chapter 12: Small intestine. In: AJCC cancer staging manual. 7th ed. New York: Springer-Verlag; 2010.

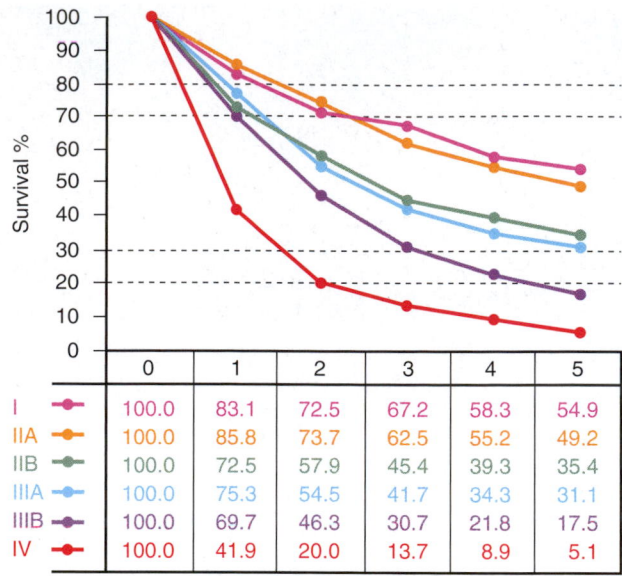

	0	1	2	3	4	5
I	100.0	83.1	72.5	67.2	58.3	54.9
IIA	100.0	85.8	73.7	62.5	55.2	49.2
IIB	100.0	72.5	57.9	45.4	39.3	35.4
IIIA	100.0	75.3	54.5	41.7	34.3	31.1
IIIB	100.0	69.7	46.3	30.7	21.8	17.5
IV	100.0	41.9	20.0	13.7	8.9	5.1

Years from diagnosis

FIGURE 125-3. Observed survival by stage of 3086 individuals with adenocarcinoma of the small intestine. (Data from Howe JR, Karnell LH, Menck HR, Scott-Conner C. The American College of Surgeons Commission on Cancer and the American Cancer Society. Adenocarcinoma of the small bowel: Review of the National Cancer Database, 1985-1995. Cancer 1999; 86:2693-706.)

whom genetic testing is positive for mutations in the *APC* gene. Individual polyps may be examined by biopsy or (if possible) removed by snare cautery, and the ampulla examined by biopsy as necessary. There is a high incidence of adenomatous change in the papilla, even if its appearance is normal (see Fig. 125-1*B* and *C*). It has been suggested that the slow evolution of duodenal and papillary lesions justifies endoscopic surveillance at an interval determined by their Spigelman classification.[25]

The age to begin surveillance has been debated, but surveillance beginning at 25 to 30 years has been suggested because diagnosis of duodenal cancer at an earlier age is rare.[25] Biopsies should be taken of any suspicious lesions and of the ampulla, even if normal appearing. Screening for SI neoplasia has also been suggested for individuals with Lynch syndrome, but no data exist from well-designed prospective studies.[29,52] Push enteroscopy is of use in identifying and biopsying SI lesions seen on imaging studies during evaluation of occult GI bleeding, and in surveillance of patients with Peutz-Jeghers syndrome, in whom polyps occur throughout the GI tract.[53] Although double balloon enteroscopy and other deep enteroscopy techniques have a diagnostic yield similar to videocapsule endoscopy (VCE) in evaluation of SI disease (see later), their use as an initial screening tool is limited by the labor-intensive nature of the exams.[54] Colonoscopy with intubation of the terminal ileum may be helpful in examining this area in patients with Crohn's disease or in biopsy of suspicious lesions suggested by radiologic procedures. EUS is helpful in staging duodenal and ampullary lesions (Fig. 125-4).

VCE has been shown to be effective in diagnosing SI adenocarcinomas and other tumors in patients with obscure GI bleeding (Fig. 125-5).[52-56] The overall frequency of SI tumors (adenocarcinoma, carcinoid, lymphoma, sarcoma) is reported to be 6% to 12% in patients undergoing VCE, most commonly for obscure GI bleeding. It has been suggested that the ability of VCE to visualize the entire SI makes it especially suitable for screening or surveillance in familial cancer syndromes in which individuals are prone to develop SI adenomas (e.g., FAP and Lynch syndrome).

Small bowel follow-through is 60% to 80% accurate for detection of duodenal lesions, and accuracy can be improved by the use of hypotonic duodenography. Barium studies, however, are not as accurate in detecting more distal tumors, and have for the most part of been supplanted by other techniques in many centers.[53,56] The tumor detection rate of enteroclysis is greater than that of upper GI series with small bowel follow-through, but is mostly used in the setting of Crohn's disease. The radiologic appearances of SI adenocarcinomas are similar to those of the colon and include annular narrowing or stricture formation (see Fig. 125-4*A*) and filling defects that may be polypoid or ulcerated masses: 70% of tumors in the duodenum are polypoid, large duodenal lesions are ulcerative in 20% of cases, and adenocarcinomas of the jejunum are primarily annular-constricting lesions (75%) and may be

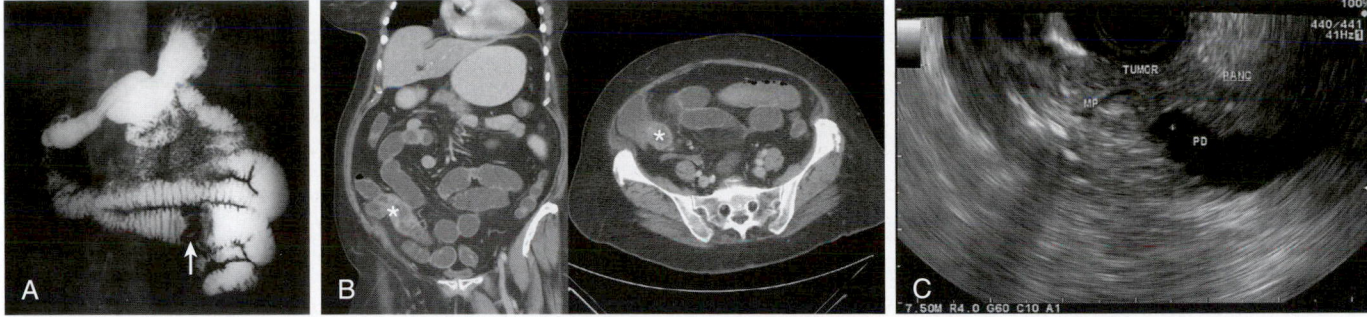

FIGURE 125-4. Imaging of small bowel adenocarcinomas. *A,* Upper GI barium study demonstrating annular constricting lesion of the jejunum. *B,* CT enterography with coronal reconstruction and axial CT images after IV and GI contrast, showing a proximal ileal mass (primary adenocarcinoma) with enhancement *(asterisks)* causing small bowel obstruction. *C,* EUS demonstrating adenocarcinoma of the duodenum invading the pancreas. *(B, Courtesy Raghu Vikram, MD Anderson Cancer Center, Houston, Tex.; C, courtesy Manoop Bhutani, MD, MD Anderson Cancer Center, Houston, Tex.)*

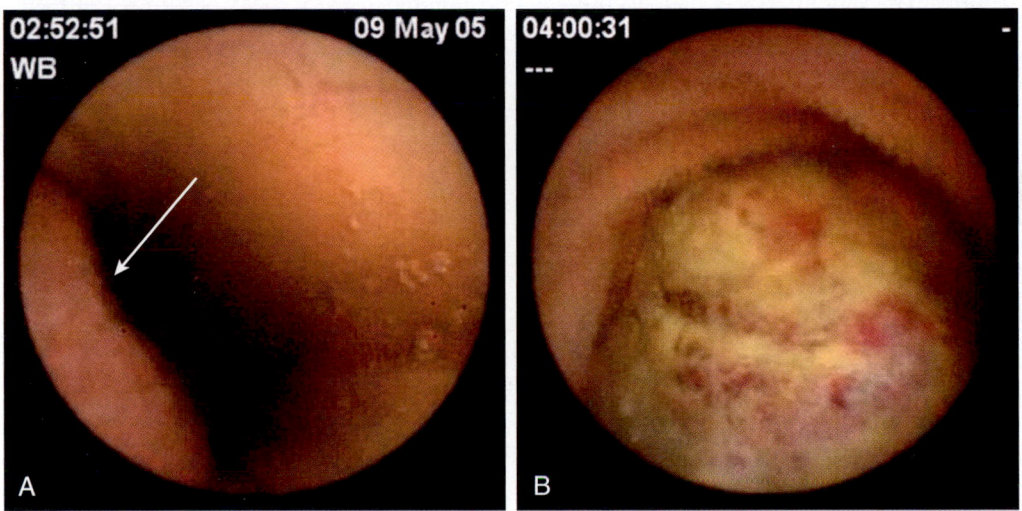

FIGURE 125-5. Capsule endoscopy. Small adenocarcinoma of the small intestine *(arrow)* demonstrating abnormal mucosal color, distortion of the villous pattern, and tumor bulge in the lumen. *B,* Pigmented lesion of the small intestine representing metastatic melanoma.

partially ulcerated or fungating. Differentiation of the infiltrating form of adenocarcinoma from stenosing Crohn's disease may be difficult.

Advances in multidetector CT and the introduction of neutral density enteric contrast have made CT enterography (CTE) an effective imaging modality for evaluating the SI (see Fig. 125-4B).[53,57,58] Cross-sectional imaging of the SI has advantages compared with fluoroscopic barium examination, including the ability to adequately visualize the entire SI through the availability of multiplanar imaging. Similar imaging of the SI may be obtained with magnetic resonance enterography (MRE). In a recent study, MRE was more specific than VCE, but both had the same sensitivity in detecting SI lesions, including tumors.[58] CTE and MRE are particularly useful in combination with IV enhancement for detection of hypervascular SI masses.

Treatment

Chemoprevention

Chemoprevention with aspirin and other NSAIDs may be useful in the care of patients with FAP. Whereas several short-term studies demonstrated the ability of these agents to reduce the size and number of colonic polyps in FAP, data concerning SI tumors are scant.[59]

Endoscopic Therapy

Several case series indicate that endoscopic mucosal resection (EMR) is feasible for treatment of sporadic SI adenomas and adenomas in high-risk patients. Complete resection has been reported in up to 98%, with recurrence rates of up to 37% in patients treated for sporadic adenomas and 100% in FAP patients.[60-65] The overall complication rate of EMR is 5% to 10%.[66,67] Intraprocedural and delayed bleeding and perforation are the most common complications, with rates of up to 10% and 6%, respectively[63,68,69]; lesions more than 1 to 2 cm in diameter are associated with higher complication rates.[68,70] EMR of benign tumors of the duodenal papilla with and without intraductal growth may be performed in some cases (see Fig. 125-1). Several case reports and case series describe successful resection of early-stage SI tumors, including adenocarcinomas and carcinoids.[71-79] The majority of patients with SI malignancies, however, present with late-stage disease, and the role of endoscopic treatment for SI malignancies remains ill defined in the absence of RCTs comparing long-term outcomes of endoscopic and surgical resection.

Surgery

The treatment of choice for SI adenocarcinoma is surgical resection. The type and extent of surgery depends on the location of the tumor. Adenocarcinomas located in the first and second portion of the duodenum are treated with pancreaticoduodenectomy (Whipple procedure). Tumors of the third and fourth portion of the duodenum, the jejunum, and the proximal ileum are preferentially resected by en bloc segmental resection with a 5-cm tumor-free margin and concomitant resection of the mesentery and regional lymphadenectomy. Similarly, carcinomas of the jejunum and the proximal ileum are preferentially resected by segmental resection. Adenocarcinomas of the terminal ileum are preferentially resected by terminal ileal resection with right hemicolectomy. The rate of R0 (curative) resection of SI adenocarcinomas is 40% to 65%.[65,80,81] Unfortunately, up to 53% of patients present at stages III and IV when outcomes are, in general, unsatisfactory.[65,81] Advanced disease prevents 25% to 50% of patients from being surgical candidates at the time of presentation.[48,65] Some 16% to 23% of patients undergoing surgery do not achieve R0 resection, and up to 44% to 66% of patients experience tumor relapse following R0 resection.[47,51,65,81,82] Five-year survival after R0 resection is 36% to 65%, and after R1 resection 12% to 30%.[51,65,82-84] Postsurgical histologic analysis has shown T3 and T4 tumors in up to 80% of resected specimens, and associated regional lymph node metastases were identified in 38% to 56%.[65,81,83] Patients with multiple or more distal tumors have worse 5-year survival rates.[82,83,85] Distal tumors have higher rates of retroperitoneal metastases (13.5% vs. 1.8%), whereas proximal tumors have higher rates of pancreatic invasion.[82] In up to 22% of patients, resection of an adjacent organ is necessary.[81] Postoperative mortality is 1.2% to 3.6%.[65,81,83] Outcomes differ significantly between curative and non-curative resection, with 5-year survival rates of up to 65% after R0 resection but only 13% with R1 resection; median survival of unresectable patients, however, is 6.9 months with 0% 5-year survival.[65,82,83,85,86] Prognostic factors associated with better survival on univariate analysis include R0 resection, T stage, and N stage. Five-year survival of patients with T1/T2 tumors was 57% to 82% versus 32% to 58% in patients with T3/T4 tumors.[51,65,82] Patients with N0 stage had a 5-year survival of 48% to 67% versus 21% to 29% in N1-stage patients.[65,81,82,87] Single studies reported anemia and weight loss to be positive prognostic factors.[49,85] The only consistently found independent negative prognostic factors include R1 resection and lymph node metastases.[47,51,65,82,88]

Chemotherapy

The use of adjuvant therapy after R0 resection for SI adenocarcinomas has increased throughout the last 3 decades in the United States.[6] However, there are no prospective RCTs at the current time to support this practice. Multiple studies—predominantly retrospective analyses—have assessed the benefit of adjuvant chemotherapy,[87,89] none of which was able to show a statistically significant survival benefit of adjuvant therapy in regard to disease-free or overall survival. Adjuvant chemoradiation or radiation therapy has shown to provide none to statistically non-significant moderate survival benefits.[47,82,84] Hence, at the current time there is no evidence supporting adjuvant therapy for SI adenocarcinoma.[90]

Most studies evaluating the benefits of chemotherapy in advanced SI adenocarcinoma are retrospective; many are single-arm studies, and most include only small patient numbers. In contrast to the lack of evidence for the benefit of adjuvant chemotherapy, there is increasing evidence of chemotherapy-associated benefits in patients with advanced SI adenocarcinoma.[64] Although single-agent 5-fluorouracil (5-FU) therapy does not seem to provide a significant survival benefit, its combination with platinum compounds does improve outcome. Several studies, both multicenter retrospective and prospective studies, showed response rates of 21% to 61% using 5-FU combined with platinum compounds, in particular oxaliplatin, compared with 13% to 17% response rates using other 5-FU-based or non–5-FU-based combination therapies.[91-94] Specifically, progression-free survival was improved by 4.8 months with 5-FU/platinum combined with other chemotherapy regimens; a trend toward improved overall survival (2.8 to 5.2 months) has been described with this combination versus no treatment.[64,91] In other non-RCTs, median survival of up to 22 months has been described with combination treatment with 5-FU (or its derivative capecitabine) combined with oxaliplatin.[92,93] The National Comprehensive Cancer Network (NCCN) currently recommends the use of their colon carcinoma therapy algorithm for SI cancer. Chemotherapeutic regimens such as FOLFOX (leucovorin, 5-FU, oxaliplatin) and FOLFIRI (leucovorin, 5-FU, irinotecan) have been assessed as first- and second-line chemotherapy in a few clinical trials in SI adenocarcinoma. Their use as second-line chemotherapy has shown partial response rates of 20% and stable disease rates of 22%.[94]

Molecular targeted agents have not been sufficiently evaluated in SI adenocarcinoma. VEGF-A EGFR were found to be overexpressed in 96% and 71% of SI adenocarcinomas.[18] Successful inhibition of the VEGF receptor with bevacizumab for treatment of SI adenocarcinoma, however, has only been reported in case studies.[94,95] Given the paucity of data, currently there is no role for use of molecularly targeted agents in this disease.

In summary, given the dismal prognosis of advanced-stage disease, and the increasing evidence of the treatment benefits of 5-FU or capecitabine in combination with oxaliplatin, this combination is a reasonable first-line treatment choice for unresectable SI adenocarcinomas.[96,97] Larger prospective RCTs, however, are needed for a conclusive assessment of survival benefit and the identification of the best chemotherapeutic regimen.

OTHER PRIMARY TUMORS OF THE SMALL INTESTINE

In addition to adenocarcinoma, the most common primary tumors of the SI include carcinoid tumors (see Chapter 33), GIST tumors (see Chapter 32), and lymphomas (see Chapter 31). Because these tumors are discussed elsewhere in chapters that broadly cover these tumor types, discussion will only highlight relevant issues specific to the SI.

Small Intestinal Neuroendocrine Tumors (Carcinoid Tumors) (see Chapter 33)

SI neuroendocrine tumors (carcinoid tumors) are now the most common malignancy of the SI, representing approximately 37% of SI tumors. From 1973 to 2004, the incidence of SI carcinoid tumors increased 4-fold. Indeed, most of the clinically significant carcinoid tumors are located in the SI, and 90% of SI carcinoids are found in the distal ileum. The median age at diagnosis is 60 years, but carcinoids have been detected from ages 22 to 84 years. In the United States, the incidence of SI carcinoids is somewhat higher in men and in African Americans.

Pathology, Natural History, and Staging

Carcinoid tumors are malignant, despite the indolent course associated with some tumors. SI carcinoids, in particular, are associated with locoregional spread or metastases at the time of diagnosis. The tumors are usually intramucosal, and they rarely extend to the lumen of the bowel. SI carcinoid tumors spread locally, and when serosal breach occurs, an intense local fibroblastic reaction commonly is seen, which is responsible for many of the clinical findings in these patients. Another characteristic feature of SI carcinoids is multicentricity. At the time of diagnosis, approximately one third of patients will have more than 1 tumor in the SI. Tumor size varies in several series, but most are 2 cm or less in diameter. Only 6% of SI carcinoids smaller than 1 cm have been associated with metastases, whereas 80% of patients with tumors larger than 2 cm will have metastases on presentation. Microscopically, sheets of uniform cells with hyperchromatic nuclei are arranged in characteristic clumps (Fig. 125-6). Light microscopy of metastases to the liver cannot differentiate the source as carcinoid or islet cell tumor.

Carcinoid tumors can be classified in terms of the substances they secrete, and over 40 different secretory products have been identified. "Typical" SI (midgut) carcinoids secrete serotonin (5-HT) and contain the enzyme dopa decarboxylase, which converts 5-hydroxytryptophan (5-HPT) to 5-HT. 5-HT is further metabolized and is excreted in the urine as the metabolite 5-hydroxyindoleacetic acid (5-HIAA). "Atypical" carcinoids (mostly foregut and hindgut) lack dopa decarboxylase and do not secrete 5-HT. 5-HPT is released into the blood and can be measured in platelets and urine. Some 5-HPT is decarboxylated in the kidney before excretion, and 5-HT can be detected in the urine.

In the 7th edition of the AJCC/UICC staging manual, SI neuroendocrine carcinomas are grouped with gastric, ampullary, and colorectal neuroendocrine tumors, but have distinct T-staging criteria (Table 125-3). Most authors describe SI carcinoids in terms of size, degree of bowel wall invasion, presence or absence of lymph node involvement, and presence or absence of distant metastases. In a recent study evaluating prognostic factors specific for SI carcinoids and using data of 6380 patients from 1977-2004 in the SEER database, tumor size greater than 2 cm, invasion depth beyond the muscularis propria, and age were found to be significant prognostic factors on multivariate analysis.[98] Using these parameters, a modified staging system was developed that differs from the AJCC/UICC staging system in terms of a cutoff point of 2 cm (rather than 1 cm for stages T1-3) and the absence of a T4 stage. Survival analysis showed 5-year survival rates of 96%, 86%, 68%, and 43% for stages I through VI; however, this system needs further validation in prospective clinical trials.

The natural history of SI carcinoids is more favorable than that of adenocarcinomas of comparable stage and shows overall 5-year survival rates of 60%.[6] However, the 25-year survival of patients with regional spread is reported to be less than 20%. Patients with liver metastases and carcinoid syndrome have a prognosis similar to that of patients with

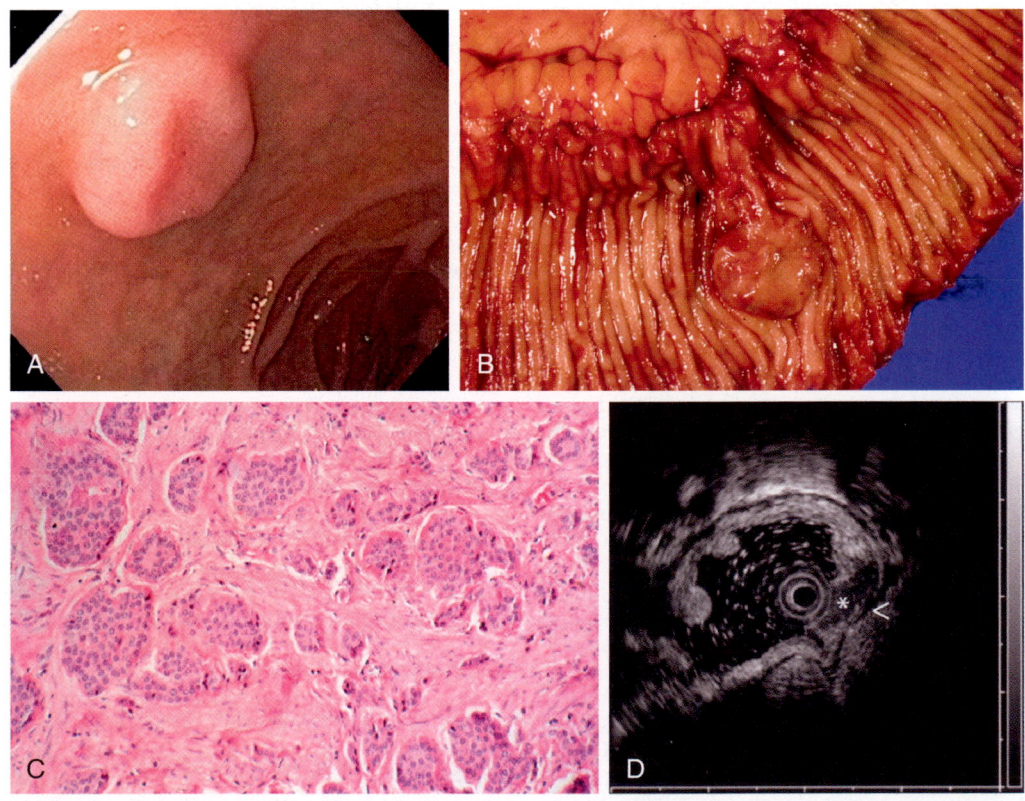

FIGURE 125-6. Carcinoid tumors of the small intestine. *A,* A nodular protuberance typical of small bowel carcinoid seen at endoscopy. *B,* Gross specimen of a small nodular carcinoid seen in an unfixed resected ileal specimen. *C,* A histologic section showing a small intestinal carcinoid tumor characterized by closely packed round, regular, monomorphous cell masses, buds, and islands. *D,* EUS showing a carcinoid tumor *(asterisk)* invading the submucosa but not the muscularis propria (T1 lesion). *(Courtesy Manoop Bhutani, MD, MD Anderson Cancer Center, Houston, Tex.)*

TABLE 125-3 TNM and American Joint Committee on Cancer (AJCC)/International Union Against Cancer (UICC) Staging Systems for Small Intestinal Neuroendocrine Carcinomas

TNM Stage	Criteria
Tx	Primary tumor cannot be assessed
T0	No evidence of primary tumor
Tis	Carcinoma in situ/dysplasia (tumor size < 0.5 cm), confined to mucosa
T1	Tumor invades lamina propria or submucosa, and ≤1 cm in size
T2	Tumor invades muscularis propria, or >1 cm in size
T3	Tumor penetrates subserosa
T4	Tumor invades visceral peritoneum (serosal) or other organs or adjacent structures
m	For any T, add "m" for multiple tumors
Nx	Regional lymph nodes cannot be assessed
N0	No regional lymph node metastases
N1	Regional lymph nodes metastasis
M0	No distant metastases
M1	Distant metastases

AJCC/UICC Stage	Tumor	Node	Metastasis
0	Tis	N0	M0
I	T1	N0	M0
II A	T2	N0	M0
II B	T3	N0	M0
III A	T4	N0	M0
III B	Any T	N1	M0
IV	Any T	Any N	M1

Adapted from American Joint Committee on Cancer. Chapter 12: Small intestine. In: AJCC cancer staging manual. 7th ed. New York: Springer-Verlag; 2010.

metastases who do not have the syndrome, but survival is lower for patients with carcinoid heart disease who develop valvular dysfunction.

Clinical Features

Patients with SI carcinoids can present with nonspecific GI symptoms, SBO, intestinal ischemia, intussusception, GI hemorrhage, hepatomegaly, or symptoms of the carcinoid syndrome. Many of the signs and symptoms of SI carcinoids result from the intense desmoplastic reaction of the mesentery in proximity to the tumor, leading to partial SBOs, weight loss, and intermittent cramping abdominal pain. Approximately 50% of patients with metastatic carcinoid initially present with SBO that requires surgery. Nodal involvement may cause compression of the main mesenteric arteries, leading to SI infarction. Regional vascular thickening of medium-sized arteries has been described with carcinoid, and this may act synergistically toward producing bowel ischemia. GI hemorrhage and intussusception are uncommon presentations of SI carcinoids. Asymptomatic hepatomegaly from metastases is more common with carcinoids and islet cell tumors than with neoplasms of epithelial origin, and aminotransferase levels may not be elevated despite hepatomegaly and a large tumor burden.

The most common clinical scenario is a prolonged history of nonspecific abdominal pain that did not much alter the patient's lifestyle. The median time from onset of symptoms to diagnosis is reported to be 2 years, but may be as long as 20 years. Investigation is not always sought by the patient, or has a low yield, thus prolonging the interval to diagnosis and treatment.

Patients with liver metastases from carcinoid may exhibit symptoms and signs of the carcinoid syndrome, which is caused by a variety of mediators (see Chapter 33). Overall, 10% to 18% of patients with SI carcinoid will present initially with the carcinoid syndrome. Diarrhea is seen in 75% of patients and manifests as intermittent episodes of explosive, watery diarrhea resulting from intestinal hypermotility; steatorrhea is rare. Abdominal cramping may accompany the diarrhea episodes about 50% of the time. Dyspnea can result from advanced carcinoid heart disease or, less frequently, from pulmonary fibrosis, bronchoconstriction, and asthma. Two thirds of patients with carcinoid syndrome will present with a large liver or an abdominal mass; 40% will have auscultable heart valve abnormalities at presentation. Other less common signs include cyanosis (25%), peripheral edema, arthritis, and pellagra (2% to 7%).

Diagnosis

Carcinoid tumors of the SI frequently do not manifest clinically until regional spread has occurred or metastatic disease is present. Small, localized tumors are most often diagnosed incidentally during endoscopic (see Fig. 125-6A) or radiologic examinations performed for unrelated reasons, or at the time of surgery for other abdominal disorders.

Biochemical Markers

Most SI carcinoids secrete 5-HT, and urinary 5-HIAA is subsequently high. Urinary 5-HIAA, platelet 5-HT, and urinary 5-HT levels are elevated in most, if not all, patients with SI carcinoids. Chromogranin A is another useful serologic marker of carcinoid tumors that is produced by most neuroendocrine tumors, and has a very high sensitivity for all types of neuroendocrine tumors. The sensitivity of chromogranin A for carcinoid tumors approaches 80%, and it can be used to monitor treatment response and recurrence or for diagnostic purposes in patients who do not have elevated 5-HIAA urine measurements. Other biochemical markers (e.g., bradykinin, substance P, neurotensin, neuropeptide PP, neuropeptide K, HCG) have been described, but none are as specific or predictive as chromogranin A or 5-HIAA.

Radiologic Imaging

Conventional barium studies of the SI, CT, or MRI may identify primary lesions as smooth, semilunar filling defects in the lumen or, more often, as wall thickening, lumen angulation, and nonspecific mass effect. When confined to the SI, small carcinoid tumors are difficult to detect using these modalities. Helical CT enteroclysis and CTE are generally more successful than conventional SI barium studies.[99-101] Both techniques can be performed with 3-dimensional imaging, which is useful for determining the full extent of the associated mesenteric mass and its relationship to blood vessels. Radiologic findings include mass lesions as well as calcification and fibrosis. Radiating strands of fibrosis and spiculation of the intestine are characteristic. Mesenteric lymph node metastases are seen on CT in 91% of cases. CT scans are also useful to detect hepatic metastases but are somewhat less sensitive than MRI owing to better soft tissue contrast with the latter modality. Somatostatin receptor imaging (SRI) can be accomplished using gamma-camera imaging (^{111}In-labelled octreotide) or with positron PET in combination with ^{68}Ga-labelled somatostatin analogs.[101] Hybrid imaging with PET/CT in combination with

^{68}Ga-DOTATATE (tetraazacyclododecane-tetra-acetic acid-Dph1,Tyr3-octreotide) also may be useful.

Endoscopy

SI carcinoids have been detected endoscopically in the duodenum, proximal jejunum, and terminal ileum. The tumors generally appear as nodular submucosal protuberances that are yellowish and shiny (see Fig. 125-6A); ulcerated lesions and pedunculated lesions also have been reported. Endoscopic biopsies of lesions are often unrevealing because the tumors are frequently subepithelial. Snare polypectomy or endoscopic mucosal resection of the lesion is much more successful for obtaining a histologic diagnosis. Duodenal carcinoids as small as 2 to 3 mm in size can also be diagnosed by EUS. Small, noninvasive lesions usually arise from the deep mucosa or submucosa, and at endosonography they appear as moderately hypoechoic masses in the second or third echo layers. Determination of invasion with EUS can be useful for staging purposes and to gauge the appropriateness of endoscopic resection as a therapeutic measure (see Fig. 125-6D). VCE has been shown to have utility in surveying the SI for carcinoid tumors and has superseded enteroscopy in this role.[53,55]

Treatment

Localized Tumors

Resection is the only curative therapy for SI carcinoids. For non-metastatic duodenal carcinoid tumors, the NCCN recommends endoscopic resection, local transduodenal excision with or without lymph node sampling, or pancreatoduodenectomy; for ileal and jejunal carcinoids, bowel resection with lymphadenectomy is recommended.[102] Localized SI tumors should be resected and removed completely. Duodenal carcinoids are less likely to metastasize, and they can often be removed endoscopically, preferably after EUS verification that there is no deep tumor invasion. Pedunculated carcinoids can be removed by snare polypectomy, but subepithelial sessile growths require endoscopic mucosal resection. In 1 small study that retrospectively evaluated the outcome of 21 patients in whom duodenal carcinoids less than 1 cm in diameter were treated endoscopically by snare polypectomy or endoscopic mucosal resection, complete resection without recurrence was described in all patients. In this study, evaluation of polypoid carcinoid tumors included EUS, restricting polypectomy to patients with polyps not invading the muscularis propria.[103] Similarly, case reports have described endoscopic excision of carcinoids of the ampulla of Vater, but given the paucity of data, surgical resection has been recommended for ampullary carcinoids larger than 2 cm in size.[104]

Tumors with Regional Spread

Duodenal carcinoids that show regional spread beyond the submucosa and carcinoids of the jejunum or ileum should undergo surgical resection. Surgery is effective for both local tumor manifestations (e.g., SBO, bleeding) and symptoms caused by secretory agents.

For patients who are undergoing surgical excision, the rate of R0 (curative) resection of SI adenocarcinomas is 50% to 65%.[65,81] Postsurgical histologic analysis has shown T3 and T4 tumors in up to 55%, and associated regional lymph node metastases were found in 38% to 67%[65,81]; liver metastases are found in up to 30%.[81] In particular, SI carcinoids larger than 1.5 cm in diameter are frequently associated with metastases.[105] Following surgical resection, 5-year survival rates of up to 76% after R0 resection have been reported. Following R1

resection, 5-year survival rates are 46% to 59.5% compared with 50% in unresectable patients.[65,81] Following curative resection, patients need to be monitored up to 10 years with testing for chromogranin A, 5-HIAA, CT or MRI imaging, and EGD.

Given the improved long-term survival rates with modern therapies, resection of the primary SI tumor in patients with metastatic disease is recommended to prevent mesenteric vascular ischemia, recurrent SBO, or mesenteric lymph node metastases.[105] Surgical resection, however, should also aim at preservation of SI length and also the ileocecal valve in order to decrease diarrhea-associated morbidity.[105] Up to 35% of patients with advanced carcinoid present with SBO and/or ischemia. In this setting, emergent resection is acceptable. In patients with partial SBO and/or mesenteric ischemia secondary to bulky mesenteric disease, surgical referral for mesenteric vascular resection and decompression is recommended; though technically challenging, up to 80% successful debulking rates have been described, along with symptomatic improvement.[105] Thorough examination of the remaining bowel during surgery is necessary because the incidence rates of synchronous lesions is 15% to 30%. In patients in whom octreotide treatment is anticipated, prophylactic cholecystectomy is recommended because of increased gallstone development with this therapy.

In patients for whom surgical resection of carcinoids tumors is planned, perioperative management aiming at prevention of carcinoid crises is extremely important.[105] Even with minor procedures, patients can develop carcinoid crises, with hypotension/hypertension, flushing, bradycardia/tachycardia, bronchospasm, and complete vasomotor collapse. The risk for carcinoid crisis is particularly high in patients with continuous flushing and those in whom there is manipulation of large, bulky serotonin-producing tumors.[105] For prevention of carcinoid crises, premedication with 250 to 500 µg octreotide is recommended, with subsequent intraoperative continuous octreotide infusion at a rate of 50 to 500 µg/hr. Postoperatively, octreotide can be decreased at a rate of 50% daily until it is deemed safe to discontinue octreotide treatment.[105]

Distant Metastases

Some 44% of patients develop hepatic metastases in the course of their disease, and 5-year survival rates without treatment in these patients is 13% to 54%. The approach to patients with metastatic SI carcinoids is multimodal. Goals of therapy are to suppress the symptoms of carcinoid syndrome, improve quality of life, and, if possible, prolong survival.

Patients with symptomatic SBO can undergo segmental bowel resection or enteroenteric bypass and, if possible, surgical debulking of tumor deposits to decrease symptoms related to tumor burden. Targeted scintigraphic therapies may be more successful when the tumor burden is small. Wedge resection or lobectomy of liver metastases can reduce symptoms and possibly improve survival.

Hepatic artery occlusion (ligation, embolization) has been shown to decrease symptoms of carcinoid syndrome and produce tumor regression in 50% to 65% of patients.[106] The intense vascularity of neuroendocrine tumors renders them particularly sensitive to embolic therapies. Various particulate and occlusive materials such as polyvinyl alcohol, Gelfoam, and trisacryl gelatin microspheres have been used for this purpose. Embolization combined with sequential cytotoxic chemotherapy such as doxorubicin or cisplatin also has been successful, with a reduction in tumor size noted in over three quarters of subjects. Cryosurgical debulking and radiofrequency ablation of hepatic metastases have been described for patients with limited numbers of hepatic metastases, but most data derive from small retrospective series.

Receptor-targeted therapy with radiolabeled somatostatin analogs (peptide receptor radiotherapy [PRRT]) enables delivery of radioisotopes to somatostatin receptor-expressing tumors. The newest generation of radiolabeled somatostatin analogs uses lutetium-177, a medium-energy beta emitter. The most commonly used peptide-isotope compound is ^{177}Lu-DOTA-Tyr3-octreotate (^{177}Lu-DOTATATE).[106]

Patients with unresectable disease but low tumor burden or absence of symptoms can be monitored at 3- to 12-month intervals. For patients with unresectable disease but large tumor burden and/or carcinoid syndrome, medical therapy is the first-line treatment. The mainstays of treatment in these patients are somatostatin analogs (e.g., octreotide, lanreotide) because they have significantly longer half-lives than somatostatin (half-life < 2 minutes). In general, these drugs are administered as long-acting formulations (LAR), which allows monthly dosing. These drugs function as agonists of inhibitory somatostatin receptors, thereby preventing hormone release. Somatostatin analogs also have antiproliferative effects. Octreotide significantly alleviates symptoms of carcinoid syndrome, with decrease in defecation frequency in 42%, reduction in flushing in 84%, and complete or partial symptom control in 66%. In addition, there is evidence of octreotide-mediated stabilization of disease. 5-HIAA serum concentrations were shown to decrease with octreotide treatment, and in the recent randomized controlled phase IIIb trial PROMID, octreotide LAR (30 mg/month) treatment more than doubled the time to tumor progression compared with placebo.[107] Octreotide is also used for the treatment of carcinoid crises that can develop following surgery, chemotherapy, or after exposure to certain medications (anesthesia used during surgery, epinephrine, pressors, ethanol) as a consequence of overwhelming hormone release (see previously). Pasireotide is a novel cyclohexapeptide somatostatin analog with high binding affinity for somatostatin receptors, and is in clinical development.[108]

Interferon (IFN)α-2a has been evaluated as a therapeutic agent in carcinoid patients. Although it has been shown to improve carcinoid syndrome-associated symptoms, in particular flushing, and stabilize tumor progression in up to 35% of patients, data on its combination with octreotide are inconsistent and require further study.[108,109]

Systemic cytotoxic chemotherapy (platinum combined with etoposide or irinotecan regimens) may be useful in the management of metastatic poorly differentiated high-grade carcinoids (response rates > 50%), but well-differentiated carcinoids tend to be resistant to these drugs, with response rates below 10%.[108] The use of chemotherapy for metastatic carcinoid, and use of targeted agents such as mTOR inhibitors (rapamycin) and angiogenesis inhibitors (bevacizumab, tyrosine kinase inhibitors [e.g., sunitinib]) are discussed in more detail in Chapter 33.

Mesenchymal Tumors (see Chapter 32 for GISTs)

Some mesenchymal tumors represent clear-cut pathologic entities (e.g., lipoma, ganglioneuroma), but most are more difficult to classify into any specific cell lineage. Tumors may share overlapping features of several diagnostic entities, or they may be histologically heterogeneous, so the general term *GIST* was coined to describe the group. Electron microscopy and immunostains indicate that most GISTs are not true smooth muscle tumors, and it has been suggested that up to 94% of so-called smooth muscle tumors in the older literature

actually are not of muscle origin and today would be classified as GISTs. Approximately 20% to 30% of GISTs occur in the SI, and the remaining tumors are scattered in the esophagus, colon, and mesentery. GISTs that exhibit benign behavior are 3 to 4 times more common than GISTs that exhibit malignant behavior. GISTs are gut-specific sarcomas and represented 8.4% to 11% of all SI malignant tumors in a recent series, with an age-adjusted incidence for SI GISTs of 1.9 cases per million persons (compared with 7 cases per million for all GISTs in the United States and Europe).[6,21] Malignant GISTs are somewhat more common in male than in female patients, and they can be found in all ages, but the most common age range at the time of diagnosis is 50 to 60 years. The majority of GISTs appear to be sporadic, although an association exists between GISTs and type 1 neurofibromatosis; this subset of GISTs is most common in the SI and rarely metastasizes.

Kaposi's sarcoma is thought to result from a herpes-type virus (see Chapter 34). SI schwannomas can be seen in patients with neurofibromatosis. SI ganglioneuromas have been reported in association with the MEN type II syndrome (see Chapter 33).

Pathology

GISTs of the SI occur most frequently in the jejunum, followed by the ileum, and then the duodenum. GISTs mostly arise from the muscularis propria and generally grow extramurally, although "benign" duodenal GISTs are more likely to grow intraluminally or intramurally. GISTs have a different histologic appearance than true leiomyomas, leiomyosarcomas, and schwannomas, with more cellularity and less cytoplasmic eosinophilia. SI GISTs generally have a spindle cell-like appearance, but infrequently they can appear epithelioid (Fig. 125-7). GISTs can be classified by ultrastructural characteristics as myoid, neural, or ganglionic phenotypes, but the frequent presence of several different ultrastructural phenotypes suggests a common origin to all subtypes.

Some 95% of GISTs express KIT or CD117, the product of the *KIT* proto-oncogene, a transmembrane receptor for the stem cell growth factor, and 60% to 70% of GISTs express CD34, the human progenitor cell antigen. DOG1 (discovered on GIST1), is a marker that is typically coexpressed with KIT, and may be useful in diagnosing cases of KIT-negative GIST.[115,116] Less frequently, GISTs stain positive for actin and desmin (implying myogenic differentiation), but seldom are they S100 positive (a protein found in neuron-differentiated cells). True leiomyomas and leiomyosarcomas are positive for actin and desmin but do not express CD117 or CD34, and schwannomas express S100 but not CD117 or CD34. When spindle cell tumors are excised, immunohistochemical markers should be used to determine whether or not the neoplasm is a GIST.

Natural History and Prognosis

GISTs of the SI tend to invade locally, and they frequently present with peritoneal seeding or direct invasion to adjacent organs. Lymph node metastases are uncommon, but 31% to 41% of patients with SI GISTs will present with liver metastases.

Overall, 5-year survival rates are variable, but a recent review suggested an observed survival rate of 39.9% for all SI GISTs.[6] Survival is favorable for patients without extraluminal tumor invasion or metastases and for tumors smaller than 2 cm (very low risk of recurrence after surgery) to 5 cm.[21]

Many factors have been suggested as prognostic indicators for GISTs (Table 125-4). Unfortunately, except for tumor size

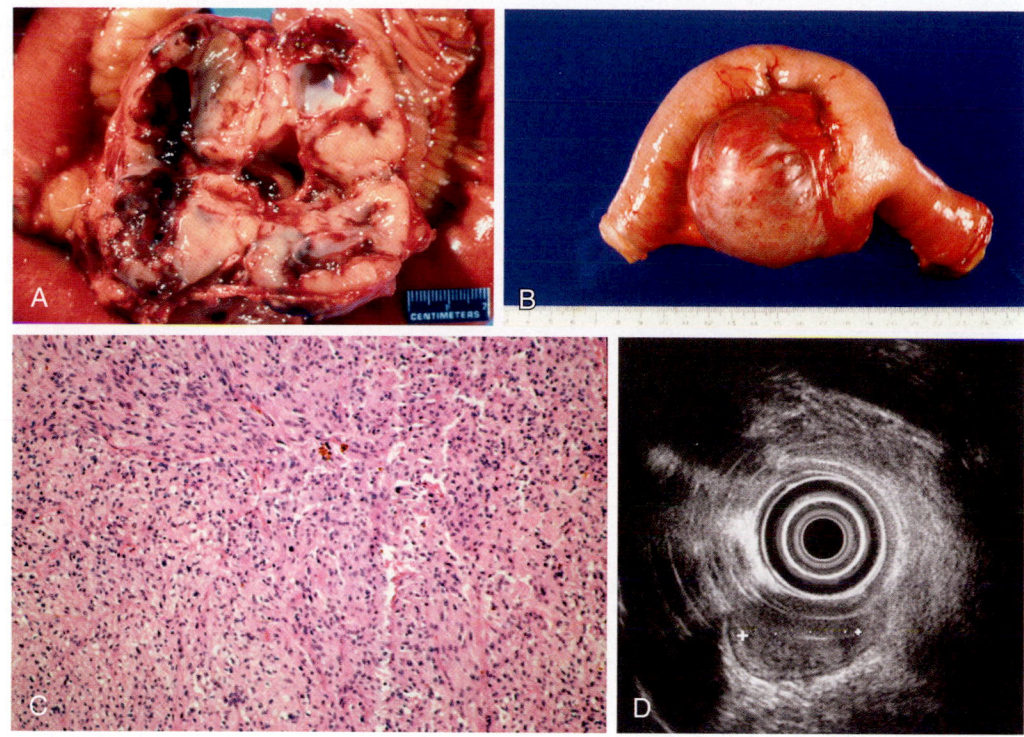

FIGURE 125-7. GIST of the small intestine. *A*, Cut surface of the tumor, demonstrating areas of hemorrhage and necrosis. *B*, Firm, rubbery mass protruding from the wall of the small intestine. *C*, Histopathology showing spindle cell appearance and several mitoses. *D*, EUS showing that the GIST arises from the fourth echo layer (muscularis propria) of the duodenum.

TABLE 125-4 GISTs: Prognostic Factors*

Factor	Risk of Malignancy	
	Low	**High**
Size	<2 cm	>5 cm
Mitosis	0-1 per 30-50/ high-power field	>5 per 10-50/ high-power field
Cellularity	Low	High
Necrosis	Absent	Present
KIT exon 11 deletion*	Absent	Present
Anatomic site	Rectum	Jejunum
Infiltration into lamina propria†	Absent	Present
Cystic spaces†	Absent	Present
Irregular borders†	Absent	Present

*Size and mitosis are the only consistently reported prognostic factors. Clinical variables negatively associated with outcome in GISTs include tumor rupture and performance status. Patients whose tumors contain exon 11 *KIT* mutations are more likely to respond to imatinib mesylate compared to those with *KIT* exon 9 mutations or wild-type *KIT*.
†EUS criteria.

and the number of mitotic figures, most of these factors are not found consistently. The most useful indicators of survival and the risk of metastases are the size of the tumor at presentation, the mitotic index (the number of mitotic figures per 50: high-power fields), and histologic evidence of tumor invasion into the lamina propria. Tumors that have ruptured are associated with a poor prognosis. GISTs should not be classified as benign or malignant, but rather by the risk for malignant behavior.

There is no specific staging system for SI GISTs. In the 7th edition of AJCC/UICC staging classification, SI GISTs are grouped with esophageal, colorectal, retroperitoneal, and omental GISTs.[110] This staging system uses tumor size, regional lymph node and distant metastases, and mitotic rate as staging criteria. In a recent analysis of 300 patients with non-gastric GIST, 5-year disease-free survival was 92% for stage I tumors (T1 or T2, N0, M0, low mitotic rate), 66% for stage II tumors (T3, N0, M0, low mitotic rate), 28% for IIIA tumors (T1, N0, M0, high mitotic rate; or T4, N0, M0, low mitotic rate) and 16% for IIIB tumors (T2, T3 or T4, N0, M0, high mitotic rate) (see Chapter 32 and Reference 110 for further definition of staging for GIST).[111]

Clinical Features and Diagnosis

Most GISTs smaller than 5 cm in diameter are often discovered incidentally at endoscopy, or in GI specimens resected for other reasons. GISTs may also be discovered in individuals undergoing VCE or device-assisted endoscopy for occult bleeding.[112] Small tumors are generally asymptomatic. In contrast, at least 80% of patients with larger tumors will have symptoms related to the GIST. More than 50% of patients with tumors larger than 5 cm will have either a palpable abdominal mass or GI hemorrhage. Bleeding from ulcerated SI GISTs is usually acute and may be brisk. From 30% to 40% of patients with SI GISTs will present with abdominal pain, nausea and vomiting, or weight loss, and 40% of patients with ileal tumors may present with intussusception.

CTE and MRE may be useful in the diagnosis of small GISTs; neutral-density enteric contrast combined with IV enhancement facilitates detection of hypervascular SI masses.[53] Endoscopic diagnosis of SI GISTs is difficult because most tumors are submucosal. If ulceration is present, biopsies can identify the tumor as a GIST. GISTs appear by EUS as hypoechoic masses arising from the fourth echo layer (muscularis propria). Putative EUS criteria to differentiate benign from malignant GISTs include tumor size over 4 cm, irregular extraluminal margins, and cystic spaces.[113] The positive predictive value for malignancy approaches 100% when any 2 of these findings are present.

Immunohistochemical staining should be performed on resected spindle cell tumors and biopsies of tumors suspected to be GISTs. CD117 positivity confirms that the tumor is a GIST in the majority of cases, and may be supplemented by staining for DOG1 if necessary.

Response to targeted therapies (see later) may be monitored with CT or fluorodeoxyglucose (FDG)-PET.

Treatment

Segmental bowel resection with complete resection of macroscopic tumor and documentation of negative margins is the standard treatment for primary resectable SI GISTs. Aggressive resection of organ segments that have been invaded with tumor and of hepatic metastases appears to confer some improvement in survival. Despite complete resection with negative margins, 44% to 80% of patients will suffer local or peritoneal recurrence; most recurrences will occur within 2 years, but lag times of 10 years have been reported. Imatinib mesylate is an inhibitor of the KIT, ABL, BCR-ABL, and PDGFR tyrosine kinases. Imatinib blocks KIT/PDGFRA signaling by binding the ATP-binding pocket required for phosphorylation and activation of the receptor. Neoadjuvant therapy for those with resectable disease is not recommended, but preoperative imatinib may be considered for those with marginally resectable tumors. The FDA has approved imatinib for patients with completely resected GISTS 3 cm or larger, based on a phase III trial of adjuvant imatinib after operative resection of primary GIST.[114]

Chemotherapy and radiation therapy for advanced GIST are highly ineffective for treatment of patients with unresectable metastases and for patients with tumor recurrence. Imatinib and several newer tyrosine kinase inhibitors (TKIs) that target KIT and PDGFR, however, are effective in the control of metastatic GISTs. Based on a large multinational randomized phase II trial in which nearly half of patients with metastatic disease who were treated with imatinib survived more than 5 years, the FDA approved imatinib for the treatment of advanced GIST.[115] Specific mutations in the *KIT* gene may affect prognosis and response to targeted therapy. Patients with exon 11 mutations are more likely to respond to imatinib than those with exon 9 mutations or wild-type *KIT*. Other TKIs with activity against GIST have been developed recently.[21,116] Sunitinib is a multitargeted TKI and is available for imatinib-refractory GISTs. The FDA recently approved the multikinase inhibitor regorafenib for treatment of unresectable GIST that no longer responds to imatinib or sunitinib.

Lymphomas (see Chapter 31)

Primary SI lymphoma (PSIL) is characterized by (1) absence of palpable peripheral lymphadenopathy, (2) a normal peripheral leukocyte count and differential, (3) no mediastinal lymphadenopathy on chest film, (4) involvement of only the organs of the GI tract and proximal regional lymph nodes, and (5) no involvement of the liver or spleen, unless by direct extension from the primary GI tumor.

Extranodal lymphomas of the SI can be classified according to cell lineage or according to clinical characteristics (Table 125-5). With the exception of EATL, most PSILs are B-cell derived. These include marginal zone B cell lymphoma of the MALT type, diffuse large B cell lymphoma, mantle cell lymphoma (multiple lymphomatous polyposis), follicular lymphoma, and Burkitt's lymphoma.[117] SI lymphomas are often categorized clinically into either PSILs, which tend to be focal, or immunoproliferative small intestinal disease (IPSID), which is diffuse.

SI lymphomas represent approximately 17% of all SI tumors, with an incidence of 4.4 cases per million.[6] PSILs occur most often in the ileum, followed by the jejunum, and then the duodenum. They are generally localized to one segment of the bowel, except in the case of mantle cell lymphoma, otherwise known as *multiple lymphoid polyposis* (MLP). The tumors have many different appearances (Fig. 125-8): large exophytic masses, polyp-like, ulcer-like, or nodular masses. Tumor growth and extension are frequently intramural for a prolonged period. Involvement of regional lymph nodes is present in approximately 50% of patients with most types of PSIL, except low-grade MALT lymphomas, in which lymph nodes are involved in only 30% of patients. IPSID tends to be a diffuse jejunal disease, affecting a significant portion of the intestine in a contiguous fashion; gross findings range from thickened folds to discrete masses. This feature probably explains the different clinical presentations of IPSID and PSIL; PSIL usually has normal mural architecture in unaffected bowel segments.

Clinical Features and Diagnosis

Symptoms of PSIL are usually nonspecific and may continue for 4 to 18 months before the diagnosis is made. Abdominal pain (often described as cramping) and weight loss are reported in 65% to 87% and about 50%, respectively, of patients with PSIL. Other symptoms are present in less than 30% of patients and include GI hemorrhage, malaise, night sweats, fatigue, and an acute abdomen resulting from perforation. SBO is the presentation in 5% to 12% of patients. Diarrhea and malabsorption are common in EATL and patients with celiac disease who become unresponsive to a gluten-free diet should be investigated for SI lymphoma (see Chapter 107). The most common physical finding is a palpable abdominal mass, present in 30% to 50% of patients.

Symptoms of IPSID differ from those of PSIL. Nearly all patients with IPSID have diarrhea, weight loss, anorexia, and abdominal pain; emesis and fever occur in 50% of IPSID patients. Physical examination in IPSID reveals clubbing of the fingers and ankle edema in 50% to 75% of patients. Later in the disease, ascites, hepatomegaly, and a palpable mass may be present. Up to 70% of patients will have the α–heavy chain paraprotein in the serum.

Because SI lymphomas are heterogeneous in appearance (polypoid, infiltrating, nodular, ulcerated, exophytic) and vary to some extent with type, findings on contrast studies are nonspecific. Enteroclysis, CTE, and MRE have all been reported to detect SI lymphomas, but comprehensive data are lacking to show which is the optimal modality.[53,99,117] Cross-sectional imaging is helpful for staging when an SI mass is suspected on VCE. Overtube-assisted deep enteroscopy can assist in obtaining tissue for diagnosis, which should be sent both in formalin for standard studies and in saline for flow cytometry analysis. Characteristic findings at EUS of an irregular

TABLE 125-5 Features of the Major Small Intestinal Lymphomas

Type	Histopathology	Immunohistochemistry	Genotype
Diffuse large B cell lymphoma	Diffuse growth of large lymphoma cells, often with necrosis	B-cell markers (B1), +sIG	Ig gene rearranged
Burkitt's lymphoma	Medium-sized cells with many mitoses; "starry sky" appearance from histiocytes	B-cell markers, +sIG, CD10+	Chromosomal translocation involving c-myc
Follicular lymphoma	Small cleaved lymphocytes or centrocytes with admixture of large cells	B-cell markers, sIG+, CD10+, bcl2+, CD5−, cyclin D1−	t(14:18) t(11:18), t(14:18), t(1:14), t(3:14) possible
Marginal B cell (MALT) lymphoma	Centrocyte-like cells with formation of lymphoepithelial lesions	B markers, CD5−, CD10- CD23−, cyclin D1−	
Mantle cell lymphoma (multiple lymphoid polyposis)	Monotonous small cells with irregular nuclei; epithelial invasion uncommon	B-cell markers, CD5+, CD23−, cyclin D1+, often IgM+ IgD+	t(11:114) Translocation with implication of bcl-1 oncogene
T cell lymphoma (predominantly enteropathy-associated T cell lymphoma)	Large cells with intense surrounding inflammation; adjacent atrophic mucosa	T-cell markers, CD103+, HML-1, CD4−, CD8−	T-cell receptor genes rearranged
IPSID (alpha chain disease)	Early: superficial plasma cells Late: atypical large lymphoma cells with bowel wall invasion	B-cell markers, KB61+, α−heavy chain paraprotein	

IPSID, immunoproliferative small intestinal disease; MALT, mucosa-associated lymphoid tissue; sIG, secretory immunoglobulin.

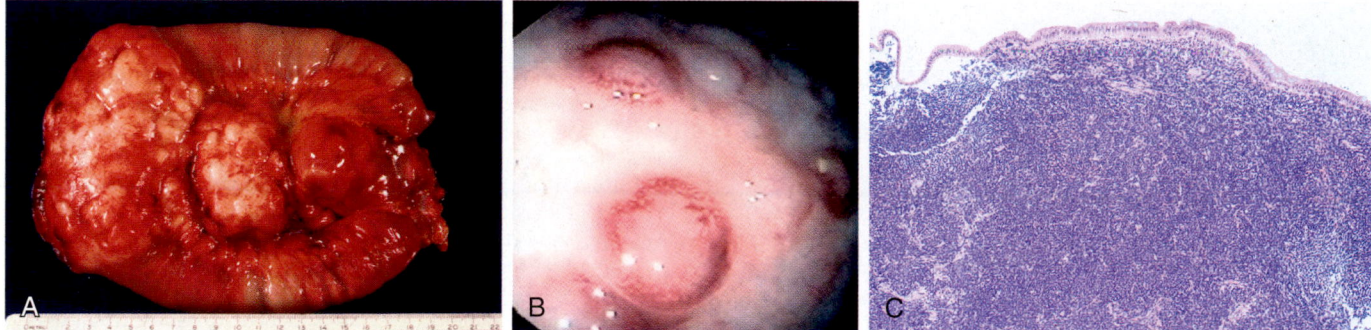

FIGURE 125-8. Primary lymphoma of the small intestine. *A,* Gross specimen of primary lymphoma extensively involving the small intestine. *B,* Lymphomatous polyposis characteristic of mantle cell lymphoma of the intestine. *C,* Low-power microscopic view of the tumor in *B.*

hypoechoic mass that disrupts the normal echo architecture may suggest the presence of a PSIL despite normal mucosal biopsies. Unlike primary gastric lymphomas (especially MALT lymphoma), the role of EUS in staging of duodenal lymphomas is not clear. Laparotomy for a diagnosis of lymphoma should be considered if the suspicion for IPSID is high despite normal endoscopic biopsies.

Secondary Tumors

Metastatic tumors represent the most common tumors involving the SI in many series. Grossly, secondary tumors often present as submucosal nodules or plaques, and they may grow to form intramural masses that cause obstruction, intussusception, or perforation. Often, tumors present as stenotic lesions or infiltrative lesions simulating Crohn's disease. Metastases from melanoma and from carcinomas of the lung, testes, adrenal, ovary, stomach, large intestine, uterus, cervix, liver, and kidney to the SI are well described. Metastatic melanoma accounts for one third of SI metastases. Lesions are typically multiple and present as polypoid lesions that may cause obstruction or intussusception (Fig. 125-9). Tumors of the pancreas, stomach, colon, or mesentery also may involve the SI by contiguous spread.

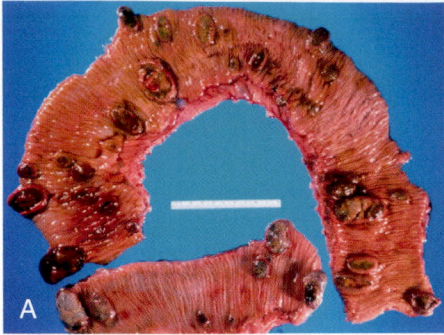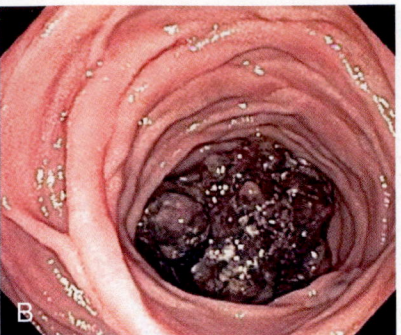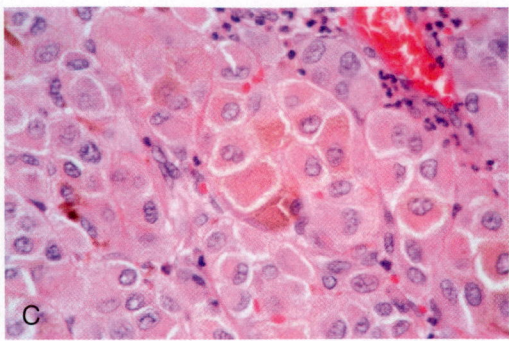

FIGURE 125-9. Melanoma metastatic to the small intestine. *A,* Multiple metastases appear as plaques and nodules with a target-like appearance caused by central necrosis. *B,* Metastatic melanoma of the jejunum seen at enteroscopy. *C,* Histopathology showing pleomorphic pigmented metastatic neoplastic cells accounting for the black gross appearance seen in *A, B,* and in Figure 125-5*B.*

KEY REFERENCES

Full references for this chapter can be found on www.expertconsult.com.

4. Cross AJ, Hollenbeck AR, Park Y. A large prospective study of risk factors for adenocarcinomas and malignant carcinoid tumors of the small intestine. Cancer Causes Control 2013; 24:1737-46.
6. Bilimoria KY, Bentrem DJ, Wayne JD, et al. Small bowel cancer in the United States: Changes in epidemiology, treatment, and survival over the last 20 years. Ann Surg 2009; 249:63-71.
18. Overman MJ, Pozadzides J, Kopetz S, et al. Immunophenotype and molecular characterisation of adenocarcinoma of the small intestine. Br J Cancer 2010; 102:144-50.
20. Banck MS, Kanwar R, Kulkarni AA, et al. The genomic landscape of small intestine neuroendocrine tumors. J Clin Invest 2013; 123:2502-8.
21. Joensuu H, Hohenberger P, Corless CL. Gastrointestinal stromal tumour. Lancet 2013; 382:973-83.
53. Dye CE, Gaffney RR, Dykes TM, et al. Endoscopic and radiographic evaluation of the small bowel in 2012. Am J Med 2012; 125:1228e1-1228e12.
55. Fisher LR, Hasler WL. New vision in video capsule endoscopy: Current status and future directions. Nat Rev Gastroenterol Hepatol 2012; 9:392-405.

82. Chang HK, Yu E, Kim J, et al. Adenocarcinoma of the small intestine: A multi-institutional study of 197 surgically resected cases. Hum Pathol 2010; 41:1087-96.
96. Halfdanarson TR, Grothey A. Establishing a standard of care for small bowel adenocarcinomas: Challenges and lessons learned. Oncologist 2012; 17:1133-4.
97. Overman MJ. Recent advances in the management of adenocarcinoma of the small intestine. Gastrointest Cancer Res 2009; 3:90-6.
99. Soyer P, Boudiaf M, Fishman EK, et al. Imaging of malignant neoplasms of the mesenteric small bowel: New trends and perspectives. Crit Rev Oncol Hematol 2011; 80:10-30.
106. Strosberg J. Evolving treatment strategies for management of carcinoid tumors. Curr Treat Options Oncol 2013; 14:374-88.
107. Rinke A, Muller HH, Schade-Brittinger C, et al. Placebo-controlled, double-blind, prospective, randomized study on the effect of octreotide LAR in the control of tumor growth in patients with metastatic neuroendocrine midgut tumors: A report from the PROMID Study Group. J Clin Oncol 2009; 27:4656-63.
113. Mullady DK, Tan BR. A multidisciplinary approach to the diagnosis and treatment of gastrointestinal stromal tumor. J Clin Gastroenterol 2013; 47:578-85.
114. Dematteo RP, Ballman KV, Antonescu CR, et al. Adjuvant imatinib mesylate after resection of localised, primary gastrointestinal stromal tumour: A randomised, double-blind, placebo-controlled trial. Lancet 2009; 373:1097-104.

Colonic Polyps and Polyposis Syndromes

STEVEN H. ITZKOWITZ AND JONATHAN POTACK

A GI polyp is a discrete mass of tissue that protrudes into the lumen of the bowel. A polyp may be characterized by its gross appearance and overall size, whether or not it has a stalk, and whether it is 1 of multiple similar masses occurring elsewhere in the GI tract. Regardless of these features, however, specific definition rests on histologic characteristics.

Because of their protrusion into the bowel lumen and the stresses of the fecal stream to which they are exposed, polyps can cause symptoms. They can ulcerate and bleed; abdominal pain can result when a peristaltic wave propels a polyp downstream, thereby stretching its blood supply and nerve fibers and occasionally producing intussusception; and large polyps rarely may even obstruct the intestine. Symptoms from polyps are uncommon, however, and the greatest concern with polyps is their silent potential to become malignant. The bulk of evidence supports the hypothesis that most colonic cancers arise within previously benign adenomatous polyps. Only a small percentage of all colonic adenomas progress to carcinoma, however, and because colonic polyps are so common in the industrialized world, universal detection and removal pose practical and economic problems. Sessile serrated polyps have recently been recognized as important precursors to colon cancer. To manage colonic polyps appropriately, the physician must understand the differences in pathogenesis and natural history of the distinct pathologic categories of these lesions.

COLONIC POLYPS

Colonic polyps may be divided into 2 major groups: neoplastic (adenomas and carcinomas) and non-neoplastic (Box 126-1). The adenomas and carcinomas share a characteristic—cellular dysplasia—but they may be subdivided according to the relative prominence of certain microscopic features. The increased realization that serrated polyps also have malignant potential now permits classifying them as neoplastic polyps, although hyperplastic polyps (considered to be the early part of this spectrum) are still considered non-neoplastic. Other non-neoplastic polyps may be further grouped into several distinct categories: juvenile polyps, Peutz-Jeghers polyps,

inflammatory polyps, "mucosal polyps," and others. Submucosal lesions also can impart a polypoid appearance to the overlying mucosa and therefore are briefly mentioned even though they are not true polyps.

Neoplastic Polyps

Pathology

Histologic Features

Adenomatous polyps are tumors of benign neoplastic epithelium that either can be pedunculated (i.e., attached by a stalk) or sessile (i.e., attached by a broad base with little or no stalk). The neoplastic nature of adenomas is apparent by histologic examination of their glandular architecture. Tubular adenomas are the most common subgroup and are characterized by a complex network of branching adenomatous glands (Fig. 126-1A). In villous adenomas, the adenomatous glands extend straight up from the center of the polyp to its surface, thereby creating long, finger-like projections (see Fig. 126-1B). Tubulovillous (villoglandular) adenomas manifest a combination of these 2 histologic types.

A polyp is assigned a histologic type on the basis of its predominant glandular pattern and, in practice, pure villous adenomas are quite rare. According to the World Health Organization (WHO), adenomas are classified as *tubular* if at least 80% of the glands are of the branching tubule type, and as *villous* if at least 80% of the glands are villiform.[1] Of all adenomatous polyps, tubular adenomas account for 80% to 86%, tubulovillous for 8% to 16%, and villous adenomas for 3% to 16%.[2,3] Tubular adenomas usually are small and exhibit mild dysplasia, whereas villous architecture is more often encountered in large adenomas and tends to be associated with more severe degrees of dysplasia (Table 126-1).

By definition, all colorectal adenomas are dysplastic. Adenomatous epithelium is characterized by abnormal cellular differentiation and renewal, resulting in hypercellularity of colonic crypts, with cells that possess variable amounts of mucin and are hyperchromatic with elongated nuclei arranged in a picket-fence pattern. These cytologic alterations confer

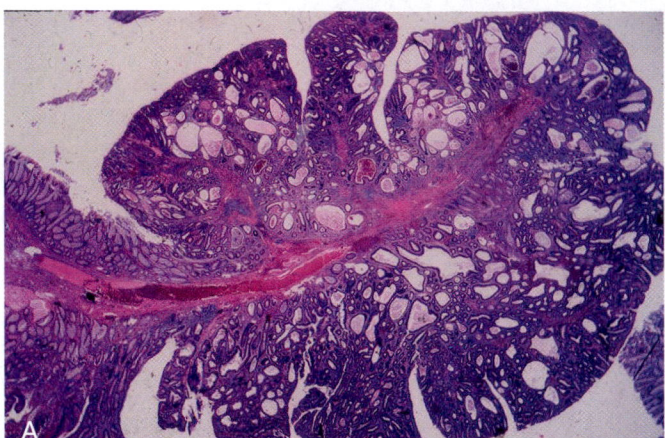
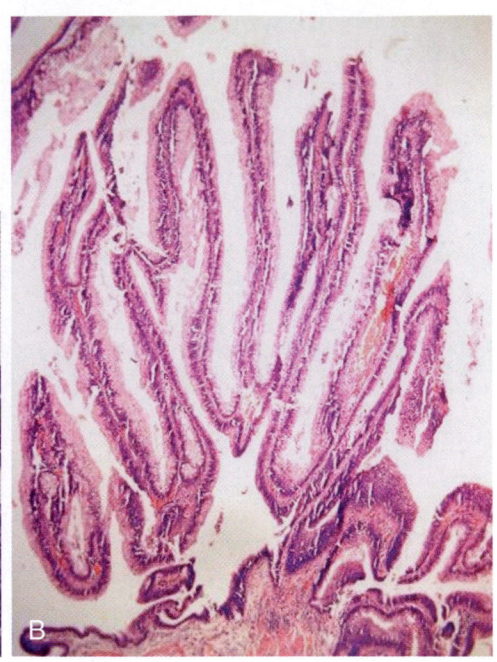

FIGURE 126-1. Comparison of tubular and villous histology. *A,* Tubular adenomas consist of branched, crowded glands arranged in a complex cerebriform pattern. *B,* Villous adenomas consist of glands that are long, finger-like fronds typically projecting from the polyp stroma to the surface without much branching. *(Courtesy of Noam Harpaz, MD, PhD, New York.)*

BOX 126-1 Classification of Colorectal Polyps

Neoplastic Mucosal Polyps
Benign (Adenoma)
Tubular adenoma
Tubulovillous adenoma
Villous adenoma

Malignant (Carcinoma)
Noninvasive carcinoma
    Carcinoma in situ
    Intramucosal carcinoma
Invasive carcinoma (through muscularis mucosae)

Serrated Polyps
Sessile serrated polyp/adenoma
Traditional serrated adenoma

Non-neoplastic Mucosal Polyps
Hyperplastic polyp
Juvenile polyp
Peutz-Jeghers polyp
Inflammatory polyp
Mucosal polyp (normal mucosa in a polypoid configuration)

Submucosal Lesions
Colitis cystica profunda
Pneumatosis cystoides coli
Lymphoid polyps (benign and malignant)
Lipoma
Carcinoid
Metastatic neoplasms
Other rare lesions

---

melanocytes. On cross-section, the inner contour of an adenomatous gland lumen usually is smooth, in contrast to the serrated appearance of a hyperplastic gland lumen (see later).

The dysplasia exhibited by all adenomas can be graded subjectively on the basis of certain cytologic and architectural features into 3 categories: mild, moderate, and severe. Some polyps contain the entire spectrum from mild to severe dysplasia, but in all cases, the adenoma is classified according to its most dysplastic focus. In cells that exhibit mild dysplasia, the nuclei maintain their basal polarity but are hyperchromatic, slightly enlarged, and elongated, yet uniform in size, without prominent nucleoli (Fig. 126-2*A*). There often is loss of goblet cell mucin. Architecturally, the glands manifest branching and budding and become more crowded. With moderate dysplasia, nuclei become stratified and pleomorphic, with prominent nucleoli, along with further loss of goblet cell mucin and increased glandular crowding. Severe dysplasia (see Fig. 126-2*B*) is characterized by further stratification and pleomorphism of nuclei, more numerous and prominent nucleoli, increased nucleus-to-cytoplasm ratios, and extreme glandular crowding. With further cell proliferation within the crypt, cells pile up, lose polarity, and create glands within glands, giving a disorderly cribriform appearance termed *carcinoma in situ* (see Fig. 126-2*B*). Most pathologists group severe dysplasia and carcinoma in situ, considering them both high-grade dysplasia[2]; the reason for this grouping is to avoid using the term "carcinoma" for these lesions because they often can be managed endoscopically rather than surgically (see later).

It is now common practice to categorize dysplasia in colorectal adenomas into only 2 grades: low-grade dysplasia, which includes mild and moderate dysplasia, and high-grade dysplasia, which comprises severe dysplasia and carcinoma in situ. Carcinoma in situ is characterized by intracryptal cell proliferation that leaves intact the basement membrane surrounding the gland. If a focus of neoplastic cells grows beyond the basement membrane and into the lamina propria of the

an increased basophilic appearance to the adenomatous epithelium on conventional H&E staining. Although the predominant cell type is an immature goblet cell or columnar cell, adenomas can contain other cell types, such as neuroendocrine cells, Paneth cells, squamous morules, and, rarely,

TABLE 126-1 Histologic Types of Adenomas and Their Features

Type of Adenoma	Size of Adenoma* (%)			Degree of Dysplasia† (%)		
	<1 cm	1-2 cm	>2 cm	Mild	Moderate	Severe
Tubular	77	20	4	88	8	4
Tubulovillous	25	47	29	58	26	16
Villous	14	26	60	41	38	21

*Adapted from Muto T, Bussey HJR, Morson BC. The evolution of cancer of the colon and rectum. Cancer 1975; 36:2251-70.
†Adapted from Konishi F, Morson BC. Pathology of colorectal adenomas: A colonoscopic survey. J Clin Pathol 1989; 35:830-41.

mucosa, the lesion is termed *intramucosal carcinoma* (see Fig. 126-2*B*). Both carcinoma in situ and intramucosal carcinoma are noninvasive lesions without metastatic potential, because lymphatics are not present in the colonic mucosa above the level of the muscularis mucosae.[4] Because clinical confusion often arises on encountering these 2 entities, it has been suggested that both carcinoma in situ and intramucosal carcinoma be reported as "noninvasive carcinoma" to avoid unnecessarily aggressive management. Only when a focus of neoplastic cells has spread through the muscularis mucosae is the lesion considered invasive carcinoma (Fig. 126-3). An adenoma that contains a focus of invasive carcinoma commonly is referred to as a *malignant polyp* (see later).

Of all adenomatous polyps, mild dysplasia is found in 70% to 86%, moderate dysplasia in 18% to 20%, severe dysplasia (carcinoma in situ) in 5% to 10%, and invasive carcinoma in 5% to 7%.[3,5,6] Higher grades of dysplasia are more common in adenomas of larger size and greater villous content,[2] and adenomas with severe dysplasia are more likely to contain foci of invasive cancer.

Adenoma Size

Adenomas are often categorized into 3 size groups: smaller than 1 cm, 1 to 2 cm, and larger than 2 cm.[5] Overall, most adenomas are smaller than 1 cm, but the size distribution of adenomas can vary greatly among studies depending on study design, age of the study population, and location of the adenomas within the colon. Thus, in autopsy series, which describe a presumably asymptomatic population dying of other causes, only 13% to 16% of adenomas are larger than 1 cm,[7,8] whereas surgical and colonoscopic series that include symptomatic or higher-risk patients report a higher prevalence (26% to 40%) of adenomas larger than 1 cm.[2,3,5] In countries where the prevalence of colon cancer is high, adenomas tend to be larger than in low-prevalence countries.[9,10] Adenoma size increases as a function of age,[8,11,12] even in low-prevalence countries,[10] and larger adenomas are more common in distal colonic segments.[2,5,8]

Diminutive Polyps

Diminutive polyps measure 5 mm or less in diameter and are commonly encountered during endoscopy. An earlier concept that these lesions were almost always non-neoplastic has been revised based on several flexible sigmoidoscopic and colonoscopic studies in which 30% to 50% of diminutive polyps were found to be adenomatous[13,14]; despite the frequency of adenomatous change, however, they represent little if any threat of cancer. Earlier studies found that less than 1% of diminutive polyps were villous or contained a focus of severe dysplasia and that they almost never harbored invasive carcinoma.[13,14]

An analysis of 2381 diminutive (<5 mm) and small (5 to 10 mm) polyps found a rate of advanced histology of 0.5% in diminutive polyps and 1.5% in small polyps.[15] Prospective colonoscopic studies confirm only a 24% to 34% prevalence of proximal adenomas in asymptomatic patients with distal diminutive polyps (of all histologic types)[16,17]; the likelihood of finding proximal adenomas is greater when the distal polyp is larger than 5 mm.[16] Diminutive adenomas manifest little, if any, appreciable growth over time.[18] A population-based study that involved fulgurating small polyps (even those up to 1 cm) without obtaining initial histologic identification reported that the subsequent risk for colorectal cancer and overall survival was no worse than in the general population.[19]

Taken together, these observations indicate that diminutive polyps, even when they prove to be adenomas, have little biological or clinical significance. Nonetheless, the fact that these tiny polyps often are missed by CT colonography (or virtual colonoscopy [see later]) has provided some fuel to the debate over the safety of leaving these lesions undetected. Recent appreciation that serrated polyps often go undetected, even at colonoscopy, adds additional concern, but even these polyps tend to enlarge before becoming dysplastic. Yet despite these recent concerns, there is a growing interest in a strategy of "resect and discard" for diminutive polyps in order to reduce pathology costs associated with polyp removal. It is still unclear if advanced imaging techniques (e.g., chromoendoscopy, narrow band imaging [NBI], or confocal endomicroscopy) will assist in this strategy. An important exception to the rule of the innocuous nature of diminutive adenomas is in the setting of Lynch syndrome, in which even small adenomas can display advanced pathologic features such as villous histology or high-grade dysplasia (see later).

Malignant Potential of Adenomatous Polyps

The 3 principal features that correlate with malignant potential for an adenomatous polyp are size, histologic type, and degree of dysplasia (Table 126-2). Although higher rates of malignant transformation are found when the source of the pathologic material is mainly from surgical polypectomies[5] rather than colonoscopic polypectomies,[6] the malignant potential is correlated directly with larger adenoma size, more villous histology, and higher degrees of dysplasia. These 3 histopathologic criteria usually are interdependent, so it is difficult to assign a primary premalignant role to any 1 of them. For example, although only 1.3% of all adenomas smaller than 1 cm harbor a cancer (see Table 126-2), if these small lesions have a predominant villous component or contain a focus of severe dysplasia, the cancer rate rises to 10% or 27%, respectively (Table 126-3). A small (<1 cm), tubular, mildly dysplastic adenoma is highly unlikely to harbor a focus

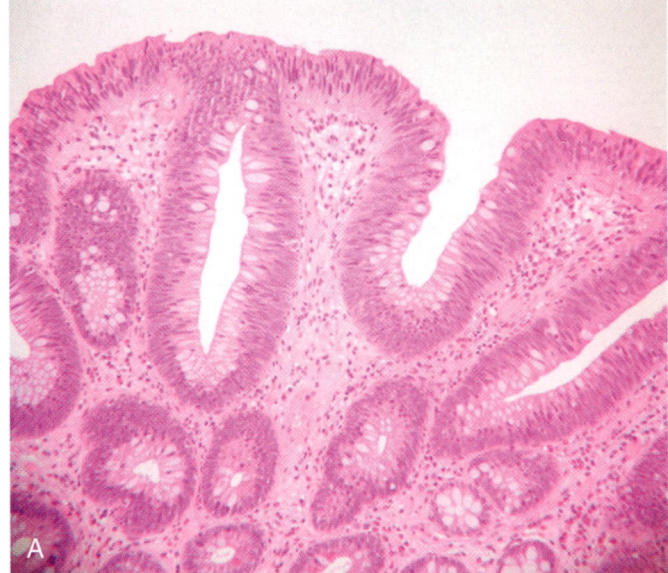

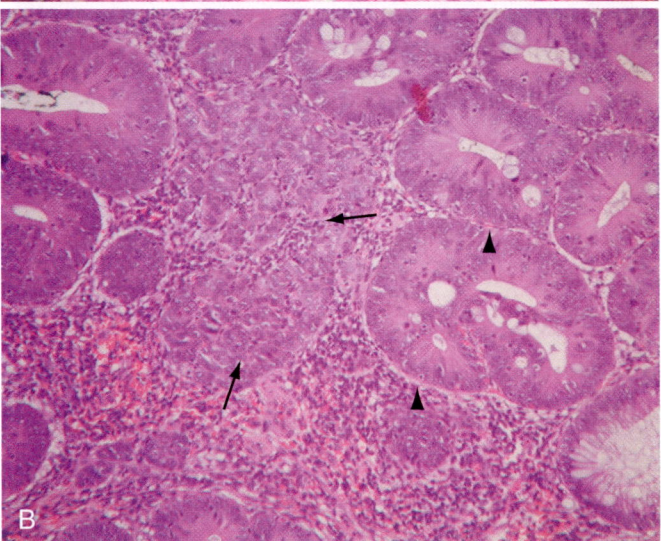

FIGURE 126-2. Histopathologic comparison of low-grade dysplasia (LGD) and high-grade dysplasia (HGD). *A,* LGD is characterized by branching crypts lined by cells with long, thin nuclei that begin to stratify, resulting in an increased nucleus-to-cytoplasm ratio and a loss of normal goblet cells. These changes occupy the entire crypt, including the surface epithelium. *B,* Adenoma with HGD and intramucosal carcinoma. This photomicrograph shows a section of adenoma with crypts demonstrating HGD *(right, arrowheads).* There is nuclear pleomorphism and abnormal cellular polarity, resulting in a cribriform appearance (i.e., glands within glands). A focus of intramucosal carcinoma is seen in the center *(arrows)* and is characterized by cells with pleomorphic nuclei and poor gland formation that are located in the lamina propria. *(Courtesy Noam Harpaz, MD, PhD, New York.)*

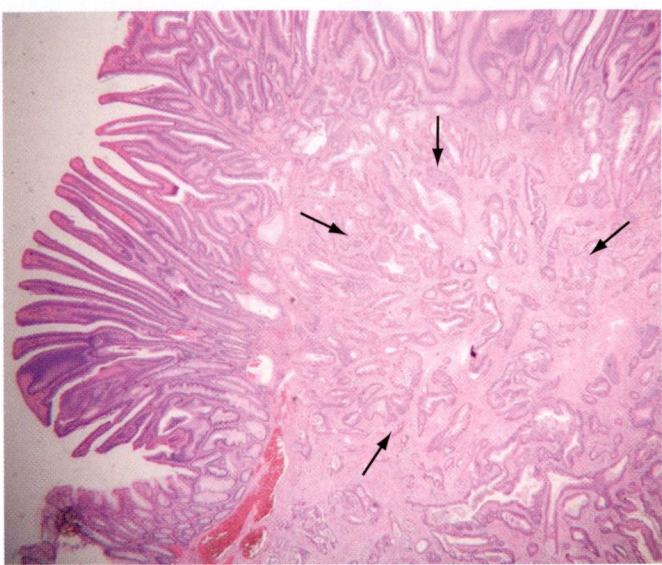

FIGURE 126-3. Histopathology of a malignant polyp. This pedunculated adenoma demonstrates tubulovillous histology on the surface. The entire stalk of the polyp *(center, arrows)* contains numerous malignant glands representing well-differentiated adenocarcinoma. Unlike the adenomatous glands on the surface, many of the invasive glands demonstrate sharply angulated edges. *(Courtesy of Noam Harpaz, MD, PhD, New York.)*

Flat Adenomas

A subset of adenomas, termed *flat adenomas* by Muto and coworkers,[20] has received increasing attention as potentially important lesions. Macroscopically, a flat adenoma is either completely flat or slightly raised, and can contain a central depression. By definition of the Japanese Society for Cancer of the Colon and Rectum, the diameter of this polyp is more than twice its thickness. Typically less than 1 cm in diameter, these lesions can be easily missed at endoscopy. This potential risk has prompted investigators, particularly in Japan, to adapt better methods of detection that involve dye-spraying (chromoendoscopy) to generate a contrast relief-map image of the mucosa, or magnification colonoscopy, for enhanced visualization.[21] In studies without such specialized endoscopic techniques, flat adenomas accounted for 8.5% to 12% of all adenomas and could be multiple.[22]

Prospective studies of Western populations aided by the use of chromoendoscopy found that 6.8% to 36% of all detected adenomas were flat. Compared with lesions that were polypoid, these flat polyps tended to be smaller and to have increased rates of high-grade dysplasia and early cancer.[23-25] A large study of more than 1800 veterans undergoing colonoscopy found a prevalence for flat or nonpolypoid neoplasms of 9.4%. These lesions were 10 times more likely to harbor a carcinoma, although the rate of carcinoma was quite low.[26] Indeed, it has been suggested that flat adenomas can have distinct biological and chromosomal profiles.[24,27] In contrast, reevaluation of adenomas removed during the National Polyp Study found no increased risk of high-grade dysplasia in polyps classified as flat, based on histologic features.[28] A more recent Austrian database study of over 17,000 colonoscopies found that the presence of high-grade dysplasia was more closely related to polyp size rather than morphology.[29] Future studies might help define whether broader acceptance of advanced endoscopic techniques such as chromoendoscopy or NBI by endoscopists in Western countries will result in higher

of invasive cancer. Nonetheless, although this type of lesion is innocuous in itself, once removed, it often is considered a marker of a person who is at (low) risk for developing a recurrent adenoma (discussed later). Because adenomas that are larger than 1 cm, have villous architecture, or manifest high-grade dysplasia or carcinoma represent a more biologically hazardous group, the term *adenoma with advanced pathology* (AAP) often is applied to adenomas that display any of these features.

TABLE 126-2 Malignant Potential of Adenomatous Polyps Removed Surgically or Colonoscopically

Variable	Surgical Polypectomies*		Colonoscopic Polypectomies†	
	Total No.	No. with Carcinoma (%)	Total No.	No. with Carcinoma (%)
Adenoma Size				
<1 cm	1479	19 (1.3)	1661	8 (0.5)
1-2 cm	580	55 (9.5)	2738	125 (4.6)
>2 cm	430	198 (46.0)	1387	150 (10.8)
Histologic Type				
Tubular	1880	90 (4.8)	3725	104 (2.8)
Tubulovillous	383	86 (22.5)	1542	130 (8.4)
Villous	243	99 (40.7)	519	49 (9.5)
Degree of Dysplasia‡				
Mild	1734	99 (5.7)	N/A	N/A
Moderate	549	99 (18.0)	N/A	N/A
Severe	223	77 (34.5)	N/A	N/A

*Adapted from Muto T, Bussey HJR, Morson BC. The evolution of cancer of the colon and rectum. Cancer 1975; 36:2251-70.
†Adapted from Shinya H, Wolff VI. Morphology, anatomic distribution and cancer potential of colonic polyps. Ann Surg 1979; 190:679-83.
‡This category refers to the most extensive degree of dysplasia outside the area of carcinoma but within the polyp. By convention, however, because an adenoma is classified according to the most severe grade of dysplasia, if carcinoma is present, the polyp is considered malignant regardless of the degree of surrounding dysplasia. N/A, not available.

TABLE 126-3 Relation of Adenoma, Histology, and Degree of Dysplasia to the Incidence of Invasive Carcinoma, by Adenoma Size

Adenoma Size (cm)	Histology (% with Invasive Carcinoma)			Degree of Dysplasia (% with Invasive Carcinoma)		
	Tubular	Tubulovillous	Villous	Mild	Moderate	Severe
<1	1	4	10	0.3	2	27
1-2	10	7	10	3	14	24
>2	35	46	53	42	50	48

Adapted from Muto T, Bussey HJR, Morson BC. The evolution of cancer of the colon and rectum. Cancer 1975; 36:2251-70.

detection rates of flat adenomas, lower colorectal cancer (CRC) incidence, or both following colonoscopy.[30]

The natural history of flat adenomas is not known. It is possible that they give rise to typical polypoid adenomas. Alternatively, the facts that residual flat adenoma tissue can be found adjacent to flat carcinomas, that some studies have observed a substantial incidence of high-grade dysplasia in these small lesions, and that flat adenomas have a lower incidence of K-ras mutations compared with polypoid adenomas, suggest that malignant progression from flat adenomas might not necessarily involve a polypoid phase.[31] Indeed, a recent study has shown that flat adenomas have lower rates of APC mutations than polypoid adenomas.[32]

Pathogenesis

Histogenesis

Adenomatous polyps are thought to arise from a failure in a step, or steps, of the normal process of cell proliferation and cell death (apoptosis). The initial aberration appears to arise in a single colonic crypt in which the proliferative compartment, instead of being confined to the crypt base, is expanded throughout the entire crypt. This disturbance results in a unicryptal adenoma. The DNA-synthesizing cells at the surface are not sloughed into the lumen, as normally occurs, and they accumulate in a downward infolding manner, interposing themselves between normal preexisting crypts. New adenomatous glands then are created either by further infolding or by branching. Thus, the unicryptal adenoma is believed to arise from a monoclonal expansion of an abnormal cell, and as the adenoma enlarges, the adenomatous cell population becomes polyclonal. Evidence for this concept comes from studying intestinal tissues from a patient with familial adenomatous polyposis (FAP) who was an XO/XY mosaic.[33] Analysis of Y chromosome expression in the intestinal mucosa of this patient revealed that normal crypts of the small and large intestine and even unicryptal adenomas were monoclonal (either XO or XY), whereas at least 76% of very small microadenomas were polyclonal. An analysis of the methylation diversity of cells within individual crypts is consistent with the hypothesis that each crypt contains a number of stem cells that compete with each other for their place in the crypt.[34] Moreover, it seems that most adenomatous crypts are produced at about the same time, early in tumor formation, followed by a period of relative stasis before clonal expansion.

Adenoma-Carcinoma Hypothesis

It is generally accepted that most colon cancers originate within previously benign adenomas, and to a lesser extent, serrated polyps. Older studies suggested that colon cancers can develop de novo in apparently flat, nonadenomatous epithelium although, as noted earlier, even these lesions might conceivably arise from preexisting flat adenomas or serrated polyps. Evidence in support of the adenoma-carcinoma sequence comes from epidemiologic, clinical, pathologic, and molecular studies.

Epidemiologic Evidence. The prevalence of adenomas within a population, and the prevalence of people with multiple adenomas, geographically parallel the prevalence of colon cancer.[9] Indeed, adenoma prevalence increases in migrants from low-risk to high-risk colon cancer regions (see Chapter 127). The prevalence rates for both adenomatous polyps and cancer increase with age, and age distribution curves indicate that the development of adenomas precedes that of carcinomas by 5 to 10 years.[5,35]

Clinicopathologic Evidence. The most compelling evidence for the adenoma-carcinoma sequence is the fact that in patients with FAP who have hundreds to thousands of adenomas, the development of CRC is inevitable. For persons in the general population without an inherited predisposition to colon cancer, perhaps the best evidence that adenomas give rise to carcinomas comes from endoscopic intervention studies. The National Polyp Study (see later) demonstrated that colonoscopic removal of adenomas results in a much lower than expected incidence of subsequent CRC.[36] In addition, 3 large, prospective, controlled studies of sigmoidoscopy from Italy,[37] United Kingdom,[38] and the USA[39] showed that sigmoidoscopy offered 21% to 31% reduction in incidence and 26% to 38% reduction in mortality from CRC. Pathology-based studies often describe the presence of remnant adenoma tissue within colon cancers. Conversely, small foci of cancer are extremely rare in normal mucosa but commonly are found in adenomas, particularly in those that are larger, more dysplastic, and more highly composed of villous elements (see Tables 126-2 and 126-3). Furthermore, the site distribution within the colon is similar for large adenomas and colon cancers. In addition, adenomatous polyps are found in one third of surgical specimens that contain a single colon cancer and in more than two thirds of specimens that contain more than 1 synchronous cancer.

Molecular Genetic Evidence. Molecular genetic studies provide some of the strongest experimental support for the adenoma-carcinoma hypothesis. The progression from adenoma to carcinoma results from an accumulation of molecular genetic alterations involving, among other changes, activation of oncogenes, and inactivation of tumor suppressor genes (see Chapter 127). The *K-ras* oncogene commonly undergoes point mutations at particular sites within the gene, thereby endowing it with the ability to transform cells. Only 9% of small adenomas exhibit *K-ras* gene mutations, compared with 58% of adenomas larger than 1 cm and 47% of colon cancers[40]; therefore, *K-ras* activation can act at an intermediate stage in tumorigenesis, perhaps contributing to a polypoid growth pattern. The fact that a large number of adenomas and cancers do not have *K-ras* gene mutations indicates that other genetic events also must play a role.

Tumor suppressor genes that normally function to suppress tumor development commonly are inactivated in colorectal neoplasms by mutation or allelic deletion, thereby promoting tumorigenesis. The loss of function of tumor suppressor genes on chromosomes 5q, 18q, and 17p is critical for colorectal tumorigenesis. The *APC* (adenomatous polyposis coli) gene on the long arm of chromosome 5 is considered the "gatekeeper" for the process of colon carcinogenesis. Mutation or loss of this gene is believed to be the crucial first step that confers susceptibility to colonic adenomas in patients with FAP as well as in people with sporadic adenomas. The APC protein plays an important role in colonic epithelial cell homeostasis (see later). Other tumor suppressor genes are located on chromosome 18q, in a region where the *DCC* (deleted in colon cancer) gene resides. Loss of function of *DCC*, or other nearby tumor suppressor genes, seems to contribute to later stages of adenoma progression, because allelic deletion at this locus occurs in only 11% to 13% of small tubular or tubulovillous adenomas, but increases to 47% of adenomas with foci of cancer and 73% of frank colon cancers.[41] Allelic deletion of chromosome 17p, at the locus that contains the *TP53* gene, is the most common region of allelic loss in CRCs. Because adenomas seldom manifest 17p deletion,[41] this alteration probably occurs as a late step in the adenoma-carcinoma progression. Perhaps the most compelling molecular evidence that colon carcinomas arise from previous adenomas is that when cancer cells arise in a malignant adenoma, their pattern of molecular alterations is identical to that of the neighboring adenoma cells, but in addition, they have acquired further mutations that are presumably critical for malignant behavior.[41]

Oncogenes and tumor suppressor genes enhance the adenoma-carcinoma process by directly stimulating cell proliferation and inhibiting cell death; however, stability genes, or "caretakers," normally keep genetic alterations to a minimum and, thus, when they are inactivated by mutation or loss, they permit mutations in other target genes to occur at a higher rate. Examples of stability genes include the DNA mismatch repair (MMR) and base-excision repair (BER) genes responsible for repairing subtle mistakes that are made during DNA replication. Germline mutations of DNA MMR genes (e.g., *hMLH1*, *hMSH2*, *hMSH6*) occur in persons with Lynch syndrome, whereas inheritance of a mutated BER gene (e.g., *MUTYH*, also known as *MYH*) is responsible for a type of attenuated adenomatous polyposis (see later).

Pathways of Colon Carcinogenesis

It is useful to consider the process of colon carcinogenesis in 2 general stages: the formation of the adenoma, termed *tumor initiation*, and the progression of the adenoma to carcinoma, termed *tumor progression* (Fig. 126-4). It is believed that most, if not all, adenomas arise from an initial loss of *APC* gene function, and for that to happen, epithelial cells must lose the function of both *APC* alleles (2 "hits"). In patients with FAP, 1 *APC* allele is inherited in a mutated form (germline mutation) from the affected parent. Adenomas arise when the second, normal copy of the *APC* gene from the unaffected parent either is lost or mutated (somatic mutation). Because persons with FAP are born with the first hit, they develop polyps at a much younger age and in much greater number than does the general population; thus, FAP can be considered a condition of accelerated tumor initiation. Despite this abnormal initiation rate, once adenomas form in patients with FAP, it is believed that each adenoma tends to display a normal progression to carcinoma. Thus, the inevitable progression to cancer in FAP is more a consequence of the numerous polyps than of any increased premalignant potential of the individual adenoma. In the general population, sporadic adenomas arise as a consequence of 2 acquired somatic mutations of the *APC* gene. Because 2 acquired hits are statistically less likely than 1 acquired hit, sporadic adenomas tend to occur later in life and to be fewer than the polyps in patients with FAP.

Another major molecular pathway for colon carcinogenesis involves mutations in DNA MMR genes (see Chapter 127);

this is the predominant pathway in patients with Lynch syndrome. Mutations in these enzymes result in a characteristic molecular phenotype termed *microsatellite instability* (MSI), a phenomenon that is observable in colon cancer cells from approximately 85% of Lynch syndrome colon cancers but in only 15% of sporadic colon cancers. It is believed that the numbers of adenomas that occur in patients with Lynch syndrome are similar to those in the general population but that Lynch syndrome is marked by an accelerated tumor progression stage, so the few adenomas that do arise often manifest advanced pathology (villous features, high-grade dysplasia) even at small sizes.[42] Indeed, adenomas in patients with Lynch syndrome often manifest MSI[43] even in their earliest stages of formation. Because these adenomas tend to progress more

rapidly to carcinoma,[44] surveillance intervals for colonoscopy following removal of adenomas in Lynch syndrome patients should be shortened (see later; see also Chapter 127).

Epidemiology and Etiology

Prevalence

The prevalence of adenomatous polyps is affected by 4 major factors: the inherent risk for colon cancer in the population, age, sex, and family history of CRC. The frequency of colon adenomas varies widely among populations, but it tends to be higher in populations at greater risk for colon cancer.[9] One illustrative example is the very high adenoma prevalence rate in Japanese living in Hawaii (a very high risk area for colon cancer) compared with the much lower adenoma prevalence rate in Japanese who still reside in Japan, an area of much lower risk. Even within Japan itself, adenoma prevalence correlates quite well with colon cancer prevalence in different prefectures of the country. Data from autopsy series provide an approximation of adenoma prevalence. In populations at low risk for colon cancer, adenoma prevalence rates are lower than 12%, whereas in most intermediate- and high-risk populations, adenomas are found in 30% to 40% of the population, and rates as high as 50% to 60% have been observed.[7,45] One half to two thirds of people older than 65 years in high-risk areas can harbor colonic adenomas.[7,45]

The prevalence rate of adenomatous polyps within an asymptomatic population has also been elucidated by studies of screening colonoscopy in average-risk, healthy persons without GI symptoms. These studies have mainly included individuals who are age 50 or older, because screening is not recommended at younger ages. Approximately 27% to 32% of such individuals will have an adenoma, and 6% to 10% will have an AAP (Table 126-4).[46-49] By comparison, colonoscopic screening of asymptomatic persons between 40 and 49 years of age revealed prevalence rates of only 8.7% for tubular adenomas and 3.5% for AAP or cancer.[50] Colonoscopic series indicate that men have a 1.5 relative risk of adenomas compared

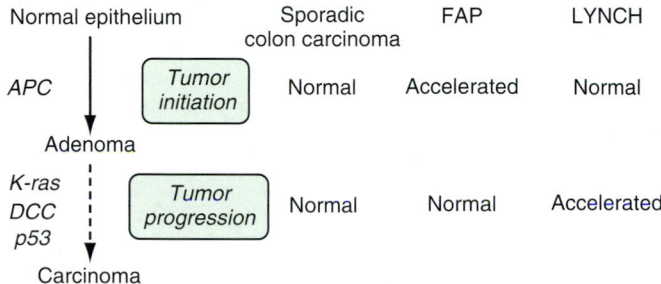

FIGURE 126-4. Pathways of colon carcinogenesis. Adenomas develop as a consequence of factors involved in initiating tumors, and they progress to carcinomas because of factors that act as tumor promoters. A simplified theory comparing the two hereditary colon cancer syndromes suggests that the adenoma initiation phase is accelerated in patients with familial adenomatous polyposis (FAP), accounting for numerous polyps. In contrast, the adenoma progression phase is accelerated in patients with Lynch syndrome (hereditary nonpolyposis colorectal cancer syndrome), accounting for the often rapid progression of adenomas to carcinoma. *APC*, adenomatous polyposis coli; *DCC*, deleted in colon cancer.

TABLE 126-4 Prevalence of Adenomas and Cancer in Asymptomatic Persons Older Than 50 Years of Age

	Screening Method			
	Colonoscopy		CT Colonography	Fecal DNA or FOBT*
Features	*Ref 46*	*Ref 47*	*Ref 48*	*Ref 49*
No. of patients	3121	1994	1233	4404
Mean age, year	62.9	59.8	57.8	68.8
Male gender (%)	96.8	58.9	59	44.6
Family history of CRC (%)	13.9	—	2.6	14
Adenomas (%)				
Any	31.9	—	13.6[†]	27
Advanced pathology	9.6	6.1	—	9.7
High-grade dysplasia	1.6		—	0.9
≥10 mm	4.9	2.5	3.9	5.2
Villous	2.9		—	3.2
Cancer (%)	1	0.6	0.2	0.7

*Patients with positive results were evaluated by colonoscopy.
†Includes only adenomas ≥ 6 mm.
CRC, colorectal cancer; FOBT, fecal occult blood test.

with age-matched women,[50,51] thus confirming earlier observations in autopsy series.[8,10] Men also have higher rates of AAPs than do women, with a relative risk of approximately 1.5.[52] A large database study found a higher rate of polyps larger than 9 mm in African Americans undergoing screening colonoscopy compared with age-matched whites.[53] Other data suggest that African Americans and Hispanics each had a higher incidence of adenomas and proximal adenomas than Caucasians.[54] More recently, a similar database study found no difference in the rate of adenomatous polyps larger than 10 mm in Hispanics compared with Caucasians.[55] The prevalence of adenomas is higher in older people, particularly those older than 60 years. In fact, age is the single most important independent determinant of adenoma prevalence[7,10,11,45,50,51] in high-risk and low-risk regions of the world. Not only is advancing age associated with a higher prevalence rate of adenomas, but it also correlates with a greater likelihood for multiple polyps, adenomas with more severe degrees of dysplasia, and, in some studies, larger adenomas. Adenoma prevalence is higher in persons with a family history of CRC and adenomas,[56] particularly if more than 1 relative is affected with CRC and if the affected relative is young.

Incidence

Estimating the incidence of new adenomas requires examining the colon at more than 1 point in time. Two types of endoscopic studies lend themselves to this analysis: surveillance studies following polypectomy (or following cancer resection) and interval examinations in persons who initially had a negative colonoscopic examination. Of course, for both types of studies, the small but measurable miss rate of adenomas can influence the rate of apparent incident adenomas (see "Detection," later). For the purposes of this discussion, adenomas found in persons after polypectomy are considered recurrences (see "Postpolypectomy Management"), whereas those found in persons after an initial negative colonoscopy are considered incident adenomas.

The incidence of new adenomas varies from 24% to 41%.[51] In 1 study, patients underwent colonoscopy twice on the same day to clear the colon of all potentially missed adenomas, and 38% were found to have new adenomas at colonoscopy 2 years later.[57] Three-year follow-up sigmoidoscopy after an initial negative examination in the Prostate, Lung, Colorectal, and Ovarian (PLCO) Cancer Screening Trial found a 3.1% incidence of all adenomas and 0.8% incidence of advanced adenomas or cancer.[58] Updated data from the PLCO study that analyzed combined results at 3- and 5-year follow-up sigmoidoscopy after a negative baseline examination showed a nonadvanced adenoma rate of 4.6% and advanced adenoma rate of 1.6%.[59] A large surveillance study looked at findings on follow-up colonoscopy performed within 5.5 years of the index colonoscopy. Patients who had 1 or 2 tubular adenomas smaller than 10 mm were no more likely to have advanced neoplasia than patients with negative baseline colonoscopies. In average-risk, asymptomatic persons with no adenomas at baseline colonoscopy, repeat colonoscopy within 5 years detects an adenoma in approximately 16% to 27%[60,61] and an AAP in approximately 1% to 2.4%.[60-62] Of individuals who underwent 3 colonoscopies at roughly 3-year intervals in a chemoprevention study, 10.3% had high-risk findings (≥3 adenomas or ≥1 advanced adenoma) at the third study colonoscopy. If the second colonoscopy showed high-risk findings, the results of the first exam added no significant information, whereas if the second colonoscopy was negative, the probability of high-risk findings on the third exam was significantly higher (12.3%) if the first exam showed high-risk findings compared with only 4.9% if the first colonoscopy showed low risk findings.[63]

Anatomic Distribution

The distribution of adenomatous polyps within the colon differs depending on the method of investigation (Table 126-5). In autopsy series in which the normal distribution is approximated in presumably asymptomatic subjects, adenomas are distributed uniformly throughout the colorectum; this even distribution has been confirmed in colonoscopic investigations of asymptomatic subjects.[18,45] Large adenomas in autopsy series have a distal predominance, in the region where most colon cancers arise, thereby supporting the adenoma-carcinoma hypothesis. Likewise, adenomas detected in surgical and colonoscopic studies of symptomatic people also display a left-sided predominance, indicating that distal adenomas are more likely to come to clinical attention. In older persons, particularly those older than 60, distribution of adenomas demonstrates a shift toward more proximal colonic locations. This phenomenon, which is based on autopsy[10,11] and on colonoscopic studies of symptomatic[64] and asymptomatic[17,46,47] subjects, has importance for choosing appropriate colon cancer screening approaches (see Chapter 127). Some data suggest that African Americans have a greater proportion

---

TABLE 126-5 Anatomic Distribution of Colorectal Adenomas Based on Autopsy and Colonoscopy Studies

Series Type	Anatomic Site of Colorectal Polyps (%)				
	Cecum and Ascending Colon	Transverse Colon	Descending Colon	Sigmoid	Rectum
Autopsy					
All adenomas[*,†]	34	26	10	19	10
Adenomas >1 cm[*]	34	11	14	16	21
Colonoscopy					
Asymptomatic[‡]	23	24	24	24	5
Symptomatic[§]	8	14	19	47	12

[*]Data from Rickert RR, Auerbach O, Garfinkel L, et al. Adenomatous lesions of the large bowel: An autopsy survey. Cancer 1979; 43:1847-57.
[†]Data from Arminski TC, McLean DW. Incidence and distribution of adenomatous polyps of the colon and rectum based on 1,000 autopsy examinations. Dis Colon Rectum 1964; 7:249-61.
[‡]Data from Johnson DA, Gurney MS, Volpe RJ, et al. A prospective study of the prevalence of colonic neoplasms in asymptomatic patients with an age-related risk. Am J Gastroenterol 1990; 85:969-74.
[§]Data from Konishi F, Morson BCJ: Pathology of colorectal adenomas: A colonoscopic survey. J Clin Pathol 1982; 35:830-41.

of proximal adenomas compared with whites, especially in persons older than 60 years.[53] Likewise, African Americans undergoing screening colonoscopy have demonstrated higher rates of AAPs and proximal AAPs than Caucasians.[65] Hispanics also have been found to have higher rates of proximal adenomas than Caucasians.[54]

Risk Factors for Susceptibility to Adenomas

Heredity and environment contribute to susceptibility to colonic adenomas. Indeed, the interplay between genetic predisposition and environmental factors supports a hypothesis proposed by Hill many years ago concerning adenoma causation, which was based mainly on epidemiologic and histopathologic observations.[66] He postulated that genetic susceptibility to colonic adenomas is extremely common throughout the world. For adenomas to form and then progress to cancer, several environmental factors, presumably dietary, must act in concert. One factor would be responsible for the initial development of adenomas, another would enhance the growth of adenomas, and 1 or more carcinogens or tumor promoters would finally give rise to cancer.

Inherited Susceptibility

There is a strong genetic component to the well-defined hereditary polyposis (FAP) and Lynch colon cancer syndromes that exhibit a mendelian pattern of inheritance (see later); however, 95% of common (sporadic) adenomas and carcinomas arise in people who do not have these syndromes. In the past, this observation was interpreted to mean that genetic predisposition played only a minor role in most colonic neoplasms. Epidemiologic studies, however, have revealed a 2- to 3-fold increased risk for colon cancer in probands who have a first-degree relative affected by colonic cancer or adenoma[67]; a similarly increased risk also has been found for adenomas in first-degree relatives of people with adenomas.[67] Moreover, data from the National Polyp Study indicate that siblings and parents of patients with adenomatous polyps are at an increased risk for colon cancer, particularly when the adenoma proband was younger than age 60 at diagnosis.[68] There is even a suggestion that adenomas in patients with a family history of CRC have faster growth rates.[69] Of patients with Lynch syndrome, 11% were found to have at least 1 adenoma on first colonoscopy; 5% had at least 1 hyperplastic polyp; and the frequency of adenomas, but not hyperplastic polyps, increased with older age.[70]

It is now estimated that as much as 10% to 30% of colon cancers are familial, implying the possibility of susceptibility genes that give rise to common colon cancers. Despite epidemiologic data to suggest an increased risk in patients with family members who have colon cancer or adenomas, however, it has been difficult to fully elucidate the causative genetic basis. Several genes have been identified that can contribute to common familial risk; these include a germline mutation in the *APC* gene at codon 1307 (I1307K) that appears to predispose Ashkenazi Jewish populations to colon cancer, mutations of the DNA MMR gene *hMSH6*, a type I transforming growth factor (TGF)-β receptor allele TbR-I(6A), and polymorphisms of certain genes involved in the metabolism of nutrients and environmental agents (e.g., methylenetetrahydrofolate reductase [MTHFR] and N-acetyltransferase-1 and -2).[67,71] A specific mutation in MTHFR has been found to be protective against colon cancer risk.[72] Germline mutations of *APC* and other genes involved in the APC pathway, such as β-*catenin* and *AXIN1*, as well as the DNA mismatch repair genes *hMLH1* and *hMSH2*, have been implicated in the predisposition to multiple adenomas.[73] The identification of genes

responsible for common susceptibility to colonic adenoma and carcinoma, particularly using polymorphisms of candidate genes, is an area of considerable research.

Dietary and Lifestyle Risk Factors

Although genetic predisposition clearly plays a role in colorectal carcinogenesis, diet and life-style factors also contribute. It is estimated that as much as a third to a half of colon cancer risk and a fourth to a third of distal colon adenoma risk might be avoidable by modification of dietary and lifestyle habits.[74] For the most part, dietary factors that correlate with a predisposition to colon cancer (see Chapter 127) also are associated with a risk for colonic adenomas.[74] Factors that have each been correlated with an increased adenoma risk include excess dietary fat, excess alcohol intake, obesity, and cigarette smoking.[75] Curiously, low calcium intake, despite being associated with increased risk for colon cancer, does not appear to confer risk for adenoma (although as discussed later, calcium supplementation does seem to lower adenoma recurrences). Among obese patients, a central distribution of obesity and increased visceral fat confers a higher risk of colorectal adenomas.[76] Patients with higher levels of insulin and C peptide have been found to have an increased risk of adenomas.[77]

Factors that have shown the most consistent protective effect against adenomas in epidemiologic studies include dietary fiber, plant foods, and carbohydrate. Indeed, analysis of dietary questionnaires from patients in the prospective PLCO trial found that those with the highest fiber intake had a 27% lower risk of adenomas compared with those who had the lowest fiber intake.[78] Other protective measures include increased physical activity, increased intake of calcium, and high intake of folate. An analysis of an asymptomatic, predominantly male veteran population undergoing screening colonoscopy found that smoking and moderate to heavy alcohol use increased risk, whereas cereal fiber intake, vitamin D intake, and use of NSAIDs decreased risk for advanced colonic neoplasia (AAPs and colon cancer).[79]

Unfortunately, the rather attractive hypothesis that "proper" diets would reduce colon cancer risk has not been substantiated when tested in prospective interventional studies.[80] Dietary changes maintained over 2 to 4 years have failed to significantly reduce recurrent or incident adenomas in several studies that tested reductions in fat with increases in fiber, fruits, and vegetables; combinations of low-fat with wheat bran or beta-carotene supplements, or both; supplements of wheat bran fiber with vitamins C and E; and a complex supplement of calcium, vitamin C, vitamin E, and selenium.

Unlike these null studies, 4 classes of chemopreventive compounds have shown protective effects against colon adenomas or cancers: NSAIDs, calcium, hormone replacement therapy (HRT), and selenium; of these, NSAIDs, including aspirin, are most well established. Over 90% of the more than 110 studies of various animal models and over 35 epidemiologic studies confirm a significant reduction in colorectal adenomas, cancers, and cancer-associated mortality among users of aspirin or NSAIDs.[80] For example, the Nurses' Health Study, a prospective cohort study of 27,077 nurses, found that regular use of aspirin was associated with a lower risk of developing colorectal adenomas.[81]

Three prospective randomized trials that investigated the use of aspirin to prevent colorectal adenomas have shown decreased rates of adenoma recurrence in the study groups compared with placebo. In 1 trial, which was terminated early because of significant results, 635 patients with a history of curative resection of CRC and randomized to 325 mg/day of aspirin (or placebo) were found to have a significant reduction in incident adenomas after a mean of 12.8 months.[82] Another trial in patients with prior colorectal adenomas compared 81 mg/day or 325 mg/day of aspirin with placebo and found that the 81 mg dose reduced the relative risk of developing adenomas and advanced adenomas by 19% and 41%, respectively, with a similar, but not significant, trend found with the higher dose.[83] The 1-year results of a trial comparing 2 doses of lysine acetylsalicylate with placebo found a significant reduction in recurrence of adenomas larger than 5 mm in both treatment groups, but a greater effect with the higher dose.[84] In contrast, in the Physicians' Health Study, administration of aspirin 325 mg every other day over 5 years showed no reduction compared with placebo in advanced adenomas or colon cancers.[85] A meta-analysis pooled data from 4 randomized trials of aspirin at doses from 81 mg to 325 mg daily compared with placebo. More than 2900 patients with a history of an adenoma were included. At a median follow-up of 33 months, the rate of recurrent adenoma was 37% in the placebo group and 33% in the aspirin group. The absolute risk reduction with aspirin use was 6.7%.[86]

NSAIDs act by inhibiting COX-1 and COX-2 enzymes, which thereby reduces cellular proliferation, enhances apoptosis, and reduces angiogenesis; other COX-independent effects also are operative. Based on these observations as well as studies that show selective COX-2 inhibition reduces the number of adenomas in patients with FAP (see later), 3 large-scale prospective studies of COX-2 inhibitors (celecoxib and rofecoxib) have been undertaken.[87] The APPROVe, APC, and PreSap trials randomized more than 5000 patients with a history of adenomas to treatment with celecoxib or rofecoxib or placebo. In all 3 studies, celecoxib or rofecoxib was superior to placebo in preventing recurrent adenomas and, specifically, AAPs; enthusiasm for these agents was tempered by the finding of increased cardiovascular adverse events in the COX-2 arms. The APPROVe study was terminated early and rofecoxib was withdrawn from the market, but the studies illustrated proof of principle that COX-2 inhibition leads to decreased polyp burden.[88]

Calcium supplements have been shown in 2 randomized placebo-controlled phase III studies to reduce adenoma recurrence by approximately 19% to 34%, with effects noticed even after 1 year of supplementation.[89,90] It has been suggested that calcium supplements might have a more pronounced effect on AAPs.[91] The mechanism for this protective effect likely is multifactorial, because calcium has been shown to decrease proliferation of colonic epithelial cells and to inhibit mucosal injury induced by bile acids and carcinogens in the fecal stream. Calcium may act by neutralizing the mutagenic effects of bile acids on the colonic mucosa or by directly inhibiting epithelial cell proliferation. Data suggest that the benefit of calcium in reducing the adenoma burden is maintained for at least 5 years after stopping calcium therapy.[92]

In a study investigating chemoprevention of skin cancer, selenium supplements were associated with a 58% reduction in colon cancer incidence as a secondary end-point.[80] This result has prompted additional trials to evaluate the effects of selenium on recurrent formation of adenoma. HRT has been associated in many studies with an approximately 20% reduction in colon cancer risk and a protective effect against colonic adenomas.[80] As with NSAIDs, the adverse side effects of HRT often outweigh the beneficial chemopreventive effects of these agents. A randomized placebo-controlled trial in patients with a history of adenomas found that use of ursodeoxycholic acid at a dose of 8 to 10 mg/kg over 3 years did not lead to a statistically significant decrease in recurrent adenomas; however, there was a statistically significant 39% decrease in adenomas with high-grade dysplasia.[93] Initial evidence from multiple cohort studies, including the Nurses' Health Study and Canadian National Breast Cancer Screening study, suggested a 40% lower risk of colorectal adenomas in women with the highest levels of folate intake. A randomized controlled trial of folate alone or in combination with aspirin, however, did not show a decreased risk of polyps or advanced neoplasia in the folate arms.[88] Currently, it is unclear if folate has a true benefit in reducing polyp burden.

Difluoromethylornithine (DFMO) suppresses polyamine levels in rectal mucosa likely by modulating ornithine decarboxylase, which can be abnormally expressed in the presence of an *APC* mutation. DFMO in combination with sulindac has been compared with placebo in patients with a history of an adenoma. At the 3-year colonoscopic follow-up, the rate of adenomas was 41% in the placebo group and 12% in the treatment group. The rate of AAP was 8% in the placebo group and 0.7% in the treatment group.[94] DFMO is relatively well tolerated, although ototoxicity is a concern at higher doses. Further work is needed to confirm the efficacy of this agent.

Other agents that continue to be examined as chemoprevention agents include 3-hydroxy-3-methylglutaryl-coenzyme A reductase inhibitors, vitamin E, metformin, and mesalamine compounds. Overall, given the need for long-term therapy and the potential adverse events associated with many of these agents, they are likely best studied in patients at high risk for colorectal neoplasia.

Diet and dietary supplements can affect the intestinal microbiota. Recent advances in the analysis of the microbiome are beginning to suggest a possible association between the microbiota and adenomas. Adenoma patients have demonstrated higher concentrations of *Dorea* spp. and *Faecalibacterium* spp., with lower concentrations of *Bacteroides* spp. than nonadenoma patients.[95] Other studies have noted increased microbial richness[96] and increased abundance of *Fusobacterium*[97] in normal rectal mucosa of individuals with adenomas, even after controlling for other adenoma risk factors. It has been postulated that an altered microbiota plays a role in colonocyte inflammation and tumorigenesis, although clear mechanisms have not been elucidated. It is not known if altering the intestinal microbiome by probiotics or antibiotics can affect risk of adenoma development or recurrence.

Conditions Associated with Adenomatous Polyps

A variety of clinical circumstances have been associated with adenomatous polyps. Of the conditions discussed here, the predisposition to have or to develop adenomas is strongest for ureterosigmoidostomy, acromegaly, and *Streptococcus bovis* bacteremia. Patients with any of these 3 conditions should undergo a thorough colorectal examination and, in the former 2 conditions, periodic surveillance should be considered (although the frequency of such examinations is not well defined). As for the other conditions, either data are conflicting or the risk is not strong enough to recommend a policy of surveillance.

Ureterosigmoidostomy Sites. Patients who have undergone a urinary diversion procedure with implantation of the ureters into the sigmoid colon are at particularly high risk for developing neoplastic lesions at the ureterosigmoidostomy sites.[98] At least 29% of such patients develop colonic neoplasms, usually close to the stoma, after this procedure. Adenomatous polyps and carcinomas have been found after mean latent periods of 20 and 26 years, respectively. Lesions that resemble juvenile polyps and inflammatory polyps also have been reported at ureterosigmoidostomy sites. It has been suggested that these lesions are produced by the generation of

N-nitrosamines from urinary amines in the presence of fecal flora. In view of the extremely high frequency of neoplasia in this setting, these patients should undergo lifelong colonoscopic surveillance, recognizing the long latent period between the implantation of the ureters and the subsequent development of colonic neoplasia.

Acromegaly. Patients with acromegaly have an increased tendency to develop colon cancers and adenomas.[99,100] Although these studies involved few subjects, consistently high prevalence rates of 5% to 25% for colon cancer and 14% to 35% for adenomatous polyps have been observed in patients with acromegaly. A meta-analysis found the pooled odds ratio for adenomas was 2.4 and for colorectal cancers was 4.3 in patients with acromegaly compared with controls.[101] The risk for colonic neoplasia may be higher in younger acromegalics[99] and in those with a family history of colon cancer,[102] multiple skin tags (acrochordons),[102] or previous colorectal adenomas.[103] The mechanism for enhanced colonic neoplasia in this disease is not clear but probably relates to increased growth hormone and/or insulin-like growth factor (IGF)-1 levels. In patients with acromegaly, high serum IGF-1 levels have been correlated with increased epithelial cell proliferation[104] and increased recurrence rates of colorectal adenomas.[103] Other studies in acromegalics, however, have not found that blood levels of growth hormone or IGF-1 correlated with the presence of neoplasms[100] and that the risk of neoplasia actually was greater in cured acromegalics than in those with active disease.[102]

Streptococcus bovis Bacteremia and JC Virus. Bacteremia and endocarditis caused by *S. bovis* have been associated with CRC, adenomatous polyps, and even FAP.[105,106] The fecal carriage rate of this organism is higher in persons with adenomas or carcinomas than in those with benign colon diseases or in normal controls.[107] It has been suggested that patients with *S. bovis* bacteremia undergo thorough colonic examination to exclude a neoplasm. Endocarditis caused by *Streptococcus agalactiae* (an organism that seldom is pathogenic in adults) has been reported in 2 patients, each of whom had a rectal villous adenoma with foci of carcinoma.[108] JC virus, an oncogenic polyomavirus that blocks tumor suppressor genes, also has been associated with colonic adenomas and carcinomas.[107]

Cholecystectomy. In some studies, cholecystectomy has been associated with an increased risk for colon cancer, although this increase is only modest and applies mainly to women and to lesions in the proximal colon.[109] It is postulated that in the absence of the gallbladder, there is enhanced delivery of bile acids to the colon and possibly a shift from primary to secondary bile acids that enhances the proliferative activity of the colonic mucosa. In general, however, case-control studies have not found an increased risk for adenomatous polyps among patients who have had cholecystectomy,[110] nor was this a risk factor for AAPs or colon cancer among asymptomatic male veterans.[79]

Clinical Features

Most patients with colonic polyps either have no symptoms referable to the GI tract or have nonspecific intestinal symptoms. In persons with symptoms that can be attributed to colonic polyps, the most common presenting symptom is occult or overt rectal bleeding. Histopathologic observations suggest that in contrast to colonic carcinomas, which exhibit considerable surface erosion, the generally less rigid adenomas maintain the integrity of their surface epithelium but can bleed into the polyp stroma.[111] These findings help explain the clinical impression that bleeding from polyps is intermittent and usually does not cause fecal occult blood loss or anemia.

Other symptoms that have been attributed to colonic polyps are constipation, diarrhea, and flatulence. Constipation or decreased stool caliber is more likely to be caused by bulky lesions in the distal colon. Large colonic polyps may be associated with cramping lower abdominal pain from intermittent intussusception. Unless these widely prevalent symptoms disappear with the removal of the polyp, they must be attributed to other causes.

A syndrome of secretory diarrhea with considerable and sometimes life-threatening water and electrolyte depletion occasionally has been observed in patients with villous adenomas.[112] Tumors that produce this syndrome are typically over 3 to 4 cm in diameter and are almost always located in the rectum or rectosigmoid, with little surface area distal to the tumor for reabsorption of fluid and electrolytes. In contrast to the absorption of water and sodium and secretion of potassium exhibited by normal colonic mucosa, secretory villous adenomas have a net secretion of water and sodium and an exaggerated secretion of potassium.[113]

Detection

Colorectal polyps usually are clinically silent. They typically are detected either in asymptomatic people being screened for colorectal neoplasia or incidentally during investigation for symptoms ostensibly referable to the colon or evaluation of unexplained iron deficiency anemia. A more complete discussion of CRC screening can be found in Chapter 127. This section addresses the issue of adenoma detection using the available screening modalities.

Fecal Occult Blood Testing

The actual frequency of bleeding from adenomas is difficult to determine. A significant adenoma (i.e., >1 cm or carcinoma in situ) is the cause in less than 10% of people who report frank rectal bleeding.[114] In general, polyps smaller than 1 cm do not bleed. This dictum is supported by quantitative measurements of fecal blood loss in people with known adenomas; these measurements indicate that only patients with adenomas larger than 1.5 to 2 cm lose more than the usual amounts of blood, regardless of the location of the polyp within the colon.[115] Thus, less than 40% of patients with known adenomas show positive fecal occult blood test (FOBT) results, and the higher rates occur primarily in patients with larger and distal polyps.[115]

When asymptomatic persons older than 40 undergo colon cancer screening with guaiac-based FOBTs, about 1% to 3% will have a positive result.[116] Upon colonoscopic evaluation, less than half of these people will have a colorectal neoplasm, and among the lesions found, adenomas outnumber carcinomas by 3:1. Thus the proportions of all positive guaiac tests attributable to colonic neoplasms (i.e., positive predictive values) are 30% to 35% for adenomas and 8% to 12% for cancer.[117] Despite the predominance of adenomas among lesions detected, 75% of adenomas still may be missed by guaiac testing (i.e., false-negative values) unless they are large or located in the distal portion of the colon. Positive test results for occult blood 1 to 2 years after a negative search will detect some of these missed polyps. Because small polyps seldom bleed and their rate of detection by occult blood testing is low, sigmoidoscopy or colonoscopy has been recommended to complement FOBTs.

CT Testing

Guaiac-based testing relies on a peroxidase reaction; false positives can occur if the patient recently had ingested vegetable peroxidases or rare red meat, and false negatives can occur if they had ingested high doses of antioxidants such as vitamin C. To avoid some of these drawbacks, fecal immunochemical testing (FIT) was developed using an immunoassay to detect human globin in stool. The advantages of FIT are that it has greater specificity for human blood than does guaiac-based testing; it does not require dietary restrictions; and it can be quantitative.

Two types of FIT studies have been performed: comparison studies to FOBT in which all patients received a colonoscopy, and in vitro studies to determine at what level FIT can detect blood in various samples. For a given lesion (i.e., adenoma or cancer), FIT, like the guaiac-based FOBT, detects more cancers than adenomas because cancers are more likely to bleed. Most studies report sensitivities of 30% to 60% for detecting either cancer or advanced neoplasia.[118,119] Few studies have looked at the sensitivity for only adenomas. One large study analyzed 7 different FIT tests in a screening population of over 1300 patients. FITs were better than guaiac-based FOBTs.[120] The 2 best-performing assays had sensitivities of 25% to 27% for AAPs. Specificity was high (97% for all adenomas and 93% for AAPs). When quantitative FIT tests were set at detecting 50 ng Hgb/mL in stool, the sensitivity for AAPs was 55%, and higher rates of detection correlated with larger polyps and multiple adenomas.[121] At present, although FIT is an improvement over guaiac-based FOBT, it remains inadequate for adenoma screening and is best used as a screening test primarily for CRC.

Sigmoidoscopy

For several decades, sigmoidoscopy was the mainstay of endoscopic CRC screening. Rigid sigmoidoscopy would detect polyps (of all histologic types) in about 7% of asymptomatic persons older than 40 years,[122] whereas the flexible sigmoidoscope would find polyps in 10% to 15%, principally because a greater length of bowel could be examined.[123] Screening sigmoidoscopy reduced mortality from distal rectosigmoid cancers by as much as 60% to 75%, in several retrospective case-control studies.[56] Conclusions from 3 large-scale prospective studies of screening sigmoidoscopy now show reductions in CRC mortality from 21% to 38%.[37-39] Increasing use of colonoscopy in the United States has resulted in a marked reduction in screening sigmoidoscopy examinations.

Barium Enema

Detecting adenomas by barium enema depends on their size. In the National Polyp Study, the detection rates of adenomas smaller than 6 mm, 6 to 10 mm, and larger than 10 mm were 32%, 53%, and 48%, respectively.[124] Common sources of error include inadequate cleansing of the colon, which contributes to the 5% to 10% false-positive rate, and diagnostic difficulty caused by the presence of diverticulosis, redundant bowel, or poor mucosal coating, which results in a 10% false-negative rate. Because of these issues, as well as the fact that barium enema never has been formally tested as a colon cancer screening tool, the use of barium enema for colon cancer screening has all but been abandoned in favor of colonoscopy or CT colonography (see later).

Colonoscopy

Colonoscopy is preferred to double-contrast barium enema examination for detecting adenomas because it has enhanced diagnostic accuracy as well as therapeutic capability. This diagnostic superiority has been demonstrated in studies of patients with known polyps[124] as well as in symptomatic patients who have negative findings on proctosigmoidoscopic and barium enema examinations.[125] Colonoscopy has become the preferred colon cancer screening test in many settings.[126] Despite its reputation as the gold standard for detecting adenomas, colonoscopy does have some limitations.[127] Colonoscopy fails to reach the cecum in up to 10% of cases, it usually requires sedating the patient, and it carries a higher cost than FOBT, FIT, or sigmoidoscopy. Colonoscopy also can miss neoplasms, especially those located at flexures or behind folds. In general, adenomas that are missed tend to be small. Studies using a tandem colonoscopy design demonstrate adenoma miss rates of 0% to 6%, 12% to 13%, and 15% to 27% for adenomas larger than 1 cm, 6 to 9 mm, and smaller than 6 mm, respectively.[127] CT colonography reveals that colonoscopy can miss 12% to 17% of adenomas larger than 1 cm.[127]

Given the concern about polyp miss rates, there has been increasing attention to quality measures for colonoscopy. Key measures of high-quality colonoscopy include adequacy of preparation, cecal intubation rate, withdrawal time, and adenoma detection rate. Inadequate preparation contributes to prolonged procedure times, decreased detection of lesions, and the need for repeat colonoscopy before recommended surveillance intervals.[128] Colonoscopy is not considered complete unless cecal intubation is accomplished. The majority of screening colonoscopy studies report a cecal intubation rate over 95%. Current guidelines suggest that cecal intubation rates should be over 90% for all colonoscopies and over 95% in screening colonoscopies.[128] Most screening colonoscopy studies report adenoma detection rates of 25% to 40%. Men have been consistently found to have a higher burden of adenomas than women. Current guidelines suggest that adenoma detection rates should be at least 15% in women and 25% in men.[128] In a large screening colonoscopy study, higher adenoma detection rates were associated with lower interval colon cancer rates.[129]

A key factor in adenoma detection rate is colonoscopic withdrawal time. A large study examined the effect of withdrawal time in more than 7800 colonoscopies performed by 12 endoscopists. The adenoma detection rate was 28.3% among endoscopists with a withdrawal time of 6 or more minutes compared with 11.8% when the withdrawal time was less than 6 minutes. The respective detection rates for AAPs were 6.4% and 2.6%[130]; slower withdrawal time has been validated by the same investigators in a follow-up study of over 2300 colonoscopies.[131] Current recommendations suggest that a withdrawal time of ≥6 minutes is necessary to maximize detection of adenomas. Continued emphasis on adhering to quality measures and detailed elucidation of the reasons lesions are missed can serve to improve colonoscopy further.

Several advanced imaging modalities have been developed in an attempt to detect small polyps by colonoscopy. Many studies using chromoendoscopy (dye-spraying the colonic mucosa) have shown only a small increase in adenoma detection rate over conventional colonoscopy. The procedure times are generally longer, and more non-neoplastic polyps are detected. A meta-analysis of randomized trials using NBI did not show an improvement in adenoma detection rate over high definition white-light endoscopy.[132] Other forms of "digital" chromoendoscopy (without dye spray) have offered no advantage over conventional colonoscopy.[133,134] In general, these advanced imaging techniques are not recommended for colonoscopic screening in an average risk population.

CT Colonography

Also known as virtual colonoscopy, CT colonography involves scanning the colon with a helical or spiral CT scanner to produce both 2-dimensional and 3-dimensional images of the colon and rectum. Patients typically undergo a standard bowel preparation, and the colon is distended with air or carbon dioxide while images are taken with the patient in the supine and prone positions without sedation.

A number of studies have compared the performance characteristics of CT colonography with standard optical colonoscopy for detecting polyps.[135] Factors affecting detection rates include the polyp prevalence rate in the population being studied, the experience of the radiologist, and technical aspects including bowel preparation techniques, software, and the use of single-row or multi-row scanners. In high-prevalence populations that included symptomatic patients, the sensitivity for detecting polyps ranged from 29% to 59% for small polyps, 47% to 82% for medium polyps, and 63% to 92% for large polyps (Fig. 126-5). Studies of cohorts with a low polyp prevalence fared less well, with sensitivities of 32% to 58% and specificities of 90% for polyps larger than 6 mm in diameter.

In the first large study to involve a pure asymptomatic screening population, CT colonography had a sensitivity of 86% for polyps 5 to 9 mm and 92% for polyps larger than 10 mm in the hands of highly skilled radiologists and with patients ingesting oral contrast prior to the study (fecal tagging) to facilitate distinguishing stool from mucosal

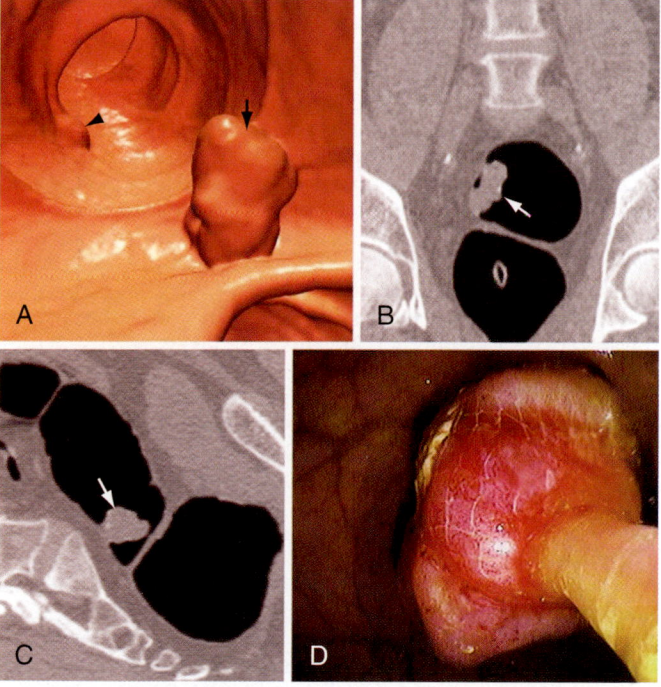

FIGURE 126-5. Findings on CT colonography (CTC) in a man at average risk for colorectal cancer. *A,* An endoluminal 3-dimensional CTC and colonoscopy image shows a 33-mm lobulated rectal polyp *(arrow)* and a 13-mm polyp *(arrowhead)* near the rectosigmoid junction. *B* and *C,* Two-dimensional coronal *(B)* and sagittal *(C)* CTC images confirm the presence and soft tissue composition of the larger polyp *(arrows)*. *D,* A digital photograph from same-day optical colonoscopy shows the endoscopic capture of the polyp immediately before resection. Pathologic evaluation revealed a large benign tubulovillous adenoma with high-grade dysplasia. The second lesion also had benign tubulovillous histologic characteristics but without high-grade dysplasia. *(From Kim DH, Pickhardt PJ, Taylor AJ, et al. CT colonography versus colonoscopy for the detection of advanced neoplasia. N Engl J Med 2007; 357:1403-12, with permission.)*

abnormalities[48]; a subsequent meta-analysis found very similar results.[136] A large multicenter study described a sensitivity of 90% for polyps larger than 10 mm and 78% for polyps 6 to 9 mm.[137] In all studies, the detection of polyps smaller than 5 mm by CT colonography has been consistently low. Updated data from the National CT Colonography trial of over 2600 patients reported similar sensitivity of 92% for polyps 1 cm or larger in patients younger than 65 years, and 82% for patients older than 65.[138]

An advance in CTC is the use of digital subtraction software that can "electronically cleanse" the colon. This allows for CTC to be performed without a bowel purgative. A study of 605 patients reported a sensitivity of 91% and 70% for adenomas larger than 1 cm and 8 mm, respectively.[139] Additional studies are needed to substantiate the efficacy of purgative-free CTC.

Several important questions remain unanswered regarding CT colonography. The management of polyps smaller than 10 mm is debated. The sensitivity of CT colonography for polyps smaller than 5 mm is quite low, and even if polyps of this size are detected, they are often not reported. Various strategies have been proposed for polyps 6 to 9 mm, including referral for polypectomy and CT colonography surveillance. There is a small but definite risk of advanced neoplasia in these polyps. Given the paucity of natural history data on polyps of this size, the safety of CT colonography surveillance of these polyps is unclear.

Concerns have been raised about radiation exposure in healthy screening populations. It has been estimated that the lifetime risk of cancer in any organ associated with a screening CT at age 50 years is 0.14%.[126] Given that CT colonography images the entire abdomen, incidental extracolonic findings are often encountered; the rate is as high as 70%, and up to 11% of these incidental findings are clinically significant.[126] These incidental findings can prompt additional testing, cost, and anxiety. Lastly, questions remain about the frequency of CT colonography surveillance intervals.

Newer Methods

Based on our knowledge of molecular genetic alterations in colon carcinogenesis, a noninvasive method for detecting altered human DNA in stool has been developed. In a large multicenter study of average-risk, asymptomatic persons older than 50 years, the sensitivity for colon cancer was 52% and specificity was 95%.[49] This study demonstrated that stool DNA analysis was 3 to 4 times more sensitive than guaiac-based FOBT for detecting invasive cancers and adenomas with high-grade dysplasia. Like other noninvasive FOBTs, stool DNA tests have traditionally shown a low rate of adenoma detection. New technology, however, detects 54% of adenomas larger than 1 cm, rising to 92% of those larger than 4 cm.[140] Unlike FOBTs, which are better for detecting neoplasms (adenomas and carcinomas) in the distal colorectum, stool DNA tests detect proximal and distal neoplasms equally well.

Treatment

Proper management of the patient with adenomatous polyps requires an understanding of the natural history of untreated adenomas, the relationship between multiple adenomas and carcinomas, and the course of patients after treatment (polypectomy).

Natural History without Treatment

Little is known about adenoma growth rate, primarily because polyps are removed readily at endoscopy, thereby interrupting the natural history of their growth. Thus, our limited knowledge about polyp growth rate has been pieced together from 2 main types of studies: older longitudinal follow-up studies on patients with nonresected (i.e., untreated) polyps and studies that compare the age distribution of people with adenomas with that of people with carcinomas.

The Untreated Adenoma. Longitudinal studies of people with untreated adenomas afford the most direct picture of the natural history of adenomas. In general, however, studies of this kind have been retrospective and either involved few patients or suffered from a lack of histologic confirmation of the index polyp. Despite these drawbacks, it appears that the adenoma-to-carcinoma progression is rather slow, requiring several years to unfold. Muto and associates reported that in 14 persons with nonresected polyps, it took at least 5 years and often over 10 years for histologically proved adenomas to progress to cancer.[5] The size of the index polyp affects the interval to carcinoma, because larger adenomas are more likely than smaller ones to develop, or already contain, a focus of cancer. But even starting with a 1-cm polypoid tumor of unknown histology, serial barium enema measurements have suggested that it can take 2 to 5 years for cancer to develop[141] and that the cumulative risk of cancer at the polyp site is 2.5% at 5 years, 8% at 10 years, and 24% at 20 years after diagnosis.[142] Other radiologic studies indicate that in adenomas with growth rates that are as rapid as those of cancer, doubling times are still longer than 4 to 6 months.[143]

Smaller polyps are likely to require even more time to progress to cancer, and even after several years, many adenomas do not enlarge. For example, in a study that involved 213 asymptomatic people with rectal polyps of unknown histology ranging in size from 0.2 to 1.5 cm, serial rigid sigmoidoscopies over 3 to 5 years detected only 2 cancers, and only 4% of the polyps grew larger; the other 96% of polyps remained unchanged, got smaller, or disappeared.[144] Also, over a 3-year period, adenomas smaller than 1 cm did not significantly change size, and those that were 5 to 9 mm actually showed slight regression.[145] In another endoscopic study, histologically proved diminutive adenomas were left in place for 2 years, after which time only half of them enlarged, but none grew to over 0.5 cm or developed severe dysplasia or cancer.[18] By contrast, other investigators reported that of 30 rectosigmoid polyps 3 to 9 mm that were left in place but measured every 6 months for 2 years, none regressed in size, although only 3 showed a fast growth rate (2 to 4 mm/yr).[146]

A mathematical model, using assumptions based on doubling-time calculations from serial barium enemas, predicts that a diminutive polyp (<0.5 cm) requires 2 to 3 years to reach 1-cm size.[147] A computational analysis of data from the National Polyp Study, where initial adenoma rates were high but incidence rates were low, also supports the notion that adenomas can regress.[148] A more recent CT colonography study followed 306 patients with polyps smaller than 9 mm over a mean of 2.3 years. They reported 22% of polyps grew in size, 50% remained stable, and 28% regressed, including 10% that showed complete regression.[149] Despite evidence of polyp regression or slow growth rates, from a clinical management standpoint, any polyp that is detected should be removed.

Age Distribution Studies. Additional, albeit indirect, support of the rather slow growth of adenomas comes from studies that have compared the mean age of people with adenomas with that of people with carcinomas. For instance, studies from St. Mark's Hospital in London and from the National Polyp Study in the United States indicate that the mean age of people with a single adenoma is about 4 to 5 years younger than those with a colon cancer.[5,150] A similar analysis in FAP patients has shown that patients with adenomas are about 12 years younger

than those with colon cancer.[5] The mean age of male veterans with AAP or colon cancer found by screening colonoscopy was 65.1 years, compared with 62.7 years for those without any polyps.[79] Kozuka and colleagues estimated that the transition period for adenomas with mild dysplasia to cancer is 8 years, whereas the time for adenomas with severe dysplasia to become malignant is 3.6 years.[35] Finally, Eide calculated that over a 10-year period, there is only a 2.5% risk that an adenoma-bearing person will develop colon cancer, but this risk would be greater if the adenoma were large or villous.[151]

Multiple Adenomas and Carcinomas. For proper management of patients and design of cancer screening and surveillance programs, it is important to know the frequency with which adenomas coexist with other adenomas or carcinomas. The term *multiple adenomas* (or carcinoma) simply means 2 or more neoplasms and should not be confused with the *multiple adenomatous polyposis syndromes* that are characterized by tens to hundreds of polyps (see later). An adenoma or carcinoma that is diagnosed at the same time as an index colorectal neoplasm is called a *synchronous lesion*, whereas one that is diagnosed at least 6 months later (a somewhat arbitrary limit) is considered *metachronous*.

The adenomatous polyp itself commonly is regarded as a marker of a neoplasm-prone colon. Indeed, 30% to 50% of colons with 1 adenoma contain at least 1 other synchronous adenoma, especially in the older age groups.[5,11,13] The risks of colon cancer and of high-grade dysplasia both rise with the number of adenomas present (Table 126-6) and approach 100% in people with FAP.

A synchronous adenoma can be found in 30% of colons that harbor a carcinoma[5,152-154] and in 50% to 85% of those that harbor 2 or more synchronous cancers.[5,152] If the synchronous adenoma is diagnosed preoperatively and is distant from the carcinoma, the surgical approach might have to be adapted to the particular circumstances.[152] For this reason, before surgical resection of any CRC, a thorough examination of the colon by preoperative colonoscopy or CT colonography is strongly recommended. Moreover, the presence of a synchronous adenoma in a patient with colon cancer increases the risk for developing subsequent colon cancer.[5,153] Likewise, a synchronous adenoma in a patient with a colonic polyp places that person at greater risk for developing metachronous polyps[155] and cancer.[155,156]

Initial Treatment

If a polyp is detected by barium enema or CT colonography, a colonoscopy is recommended to afford the simultaneous opportunities to remove the polyp and search for synchronous neoplasms. There is some debate as to whether rectosigmoid adenomas found at sigmoidoscopy are markers for proximal colonic neoplasia and thereby prompt the need for a full colonoscopy. This controversy applies particularly to patients who have only a single small tubular adenoma with low-grade dysplasia. Some studies indicate that in this subset of patients, colonoscopy does not discover a substantial number of proximal AAPs or cancers,[157-159] nor is there a subsequent risk of developing proximal cancer among those who do not undergo colonoscopy.[160] In contrast, 2 screening colonoscopy studies suggest that the odds of finding advanced proximal neoplasia, even with a single small tubular adenoma, are 2.6-fold to 4-fold that of finding no distal pathology (Table 126-7).[46,161]

Some authors have estimated that by not doing colonoscopy for a distal nonadvanced adenoma, 36% of advanced proximal neoplasms would be missed.[162] Furthermore, 52% of patients with advanced proximal neoplasia have no distal adenoma,[46] and 70% of proximal colon cancers lack a distal marker lesion.[163] These observations support the use of

TABLE 126-6 Correlation between the Number of Adenomas per Patient and Associated Carcinomas or High-Grade Dysplasia in Two Landmark Studies

No. of Adenomas per Patient	St. Mark's Hospital[5]		National Polyp Study[2]	
	No. of Patients	% of Patients with Carcinoma	No. of Patients	% of Patients with High-Grade Dysplasia
1	1331	30	1093	7
2	296	52	430	10
3	83	57	166	19
4	40	50	83	17
5	13	77	40	20
≥6	25	80	55	20

TABLE 126-7 Frequency of Advanced Proximal Neoplasia Related to Findings in the Distal Colon

Findings in Distal Colon	Frequency of Advanced Proximal Neoplasia					
	Ref 46*		Ref 47*		Ref 161[†]	
	%	Odds Ratio (95% CI)	%	Relative Risk (95% CI)	%	Odds Ratio (95% CI)
No distal polyps	2.7	1.0	1.5	1.0	5.3	1.0
Distal hyperplastic polyp	2.8	1.1 (0.6-2.1)	4.0	2.6 (1.1-5.9)	—	—
Distal adenoma	6.8	2.6 (1.7-4.1)	7.1	4.0 (1.9-8.3)	5.0	1.26 (0.81-1.98)
Distal advanced neoplasm			11.5	6.7 (3.2-16.6)		
Tubular adenoma >1 cm	8.6	3.2 (1.5-6.8)	—	—	4.5	1.66 (1.10-2.52)
Villous features	12.5	4.7 (2.1-10.4)	—	—	12.1	2.46 (1.60-3.77)
High-grade dysplasia	11.4	4.5 (1.5-13.4)	—	—	—	—
Invasive cancer	25.0	9.8 (3.6-26.4)	—	—	—	—

*Screening colonoscopy study.
[†]Screening sigmoidoscopy followed by colonoscopy study.
CI, confidence interval.

colonoscopy as a primary screening modality. Because risk factors for finding advanced proximal neoplasia are increasing age,[46,47,161] a positive family history of CRC,[46,161] and male gender,[47] performing colonoscopy in these persons on the basis of finding a distal small tubular adenoma would seem prudent. A risk index that stratified patients into low, intermediate, or high risk based on the type and size of distal colonic polyps as well as patient age and male sex was able to predict the risk of proximal advanced colonic neoplasia.[164]

There is little debate that if sigmoidoscopy reveals more than 1 adenoma or a distal AAP, a full colonoscopy is warranted because of the higher likelihood of finding synchronous proximal advanced neoplasms (see Table 126-7). Because negative biopsy results from a fractional sample of a polyp cannot possibly rule out cancer, total excision of a polyp is the only method of providing a thorough and accurate histologic diagnosis. For larger polyps, this can require piecemeal excision; for sessile growths, injection of saline into the polyp base can assist with complete endoscopic resection.

After apparent complete removal of a large adenoma, it is advisable to repeat the colonoscopy in 3 to 6 months to document the completeness of the excision. If a polyp cannot be completely excised after 2 or 3 endoscopic sessions, surgical therapy is recommended.

Based on reasons listed in the previous discussion, colonoscopy has gained acceptance in the United States as a primary screening tool for CRC (see Chapter 127), although many other countries with more limited resources do not yet subscribe to this philosophy. The PLCO trial suggested that an additional 15% of cancers could have been detected if colonoscopy rather than sigmoidoscopy were used for screening.[165]

Management of the Malignant Polyp

The term *malignant polyp* refers to an adenoma in which a focus of carcinoma has invaded beyond the muscularis mucosae into the submucosa (see earlier). This term is not applied to adenomas that contain either carcinoma in situ or intramucosal carcinoma, because these lesions are not invasive and carry no metastatic potential. Rarely, polyps consist entirely of carcinoma. These "polypoid carcinomas" usually are considered a subset of malignant polyps, and they most likely represent a previous adenoma that has been completely replaced by carcinoma. Sometimes islands of benign adenomatous epithelium are found beneath the muscularis mucosae, and care must be taken not to mistake such pseudocarcinomatous invasion for true invasive carcinoma; this important distinction may be particularly difficult in the rare instance when the ectopic benign epithelium exhibits features of high-grade dysplasia. Ectopic benign epithelium is seen more often in larger pedunculated polyps, especially in the sigmoid colon. Because the distinction between carcinoma in situ and invasive carcinoma influences both management and prognosis, it is crucial that tissue be properly oriented for pathologic examination and that close communication takes place among endoscopist, surgeon, and pathologist.

Endoscopic removal of the vast majority of colorectal polyps raises 2 central and related questions: Is endoscopic polypectomy alone adequate therapy for the malignant polyp? If not, what features of the polyp can predict the presence of residual disease or subsequent recurrence? The answers are vital because they determine the decision for subsequent surgical resection of bowel.

Complete endoscopic removal of an adenoma with noninvasive carcinoma is curative. The decision regarding therapy becomes more difficult when polyps contain invasive carcinoma. Although most of these lesions are treated adequately by endoscopic polypectomy, up to 10% of patients experience an adverse outcome, defined as residual cancer in the bowel wall or in lymph nodes, either at the time of polypectomy or on follow-up examination.[166] This rate of failure is comparable to that of the pre-colonoscopy era when adenomas were larger and patients underwent more complete surgical resections. Because malignant polyps account for only 5% of all adenomas, and because not all patients who have had colonoscopic removal of malignant polyps have had surgical resection or are available for follow-up, conclusions often are based on small numbers.

Notwithstanding these limitations, combined experience has identified certain favorable and unfavorable histopathologic features of a colonoscopically resected malignant polyp that can be used to classify a patient as being at low or high risk for an adverse outcome (see later) (Table 126-8). If none of these unfavorable risk factors is found, the patient is considered to have been cured by the endoscopic polypectomy. This principle applies even to endoscopically removed polypoid carcinomas, which have been associated with a surprisingly good outcome when not complicated by any unfavorable

histopathologic features. If 1 or more unfavorable features is found in a malignant polyp, the chance of an adverse outcome rises to about 10% to 25%, but can be as high as 45% to 50% depending upon the number of unfavorable features.[166] In such cases, surgical resection usually should be performed, taking into account the risk of operative mortality in older adult patients with comorbid illnesses.

Several aspects of defining these risk factors demand close collaboration between endoscopists and pathologists. First, some malignant polyps contain only a small focus of poorly differentiated carcinoma, and therefore meticulous pathologic analysis is essential. Second, identification of vessel invasion by cancer cells in malignant polyps may be difficult, in which case special stains of vascular endothelium can be used for clarification. Third, although the polypectomy margin may be found on microscopy to contain cancer cells, some studies suggest that if the endoscopist believes that a complete excision was achieved, surgical resection might not be necessary because the electrocautery might have effectively destroyed residual tumor in the bowel wall. Finally, when judging the adequacy of endoscopic polypectomy, the issue of submucosal invasion is important. When the leading edge of the cancerous component invades into the upper third (SM1), middle third (SM2), or lower third (SM3) of the submucosa in a sessile malignant polyp, the risk of lymph node metastasis increases from 0% for SM1 lesions to 14% for SM3 lesions.[166]

A pedunculated polyp differs anatomically from a sessile polyp in that the submucosa of the former projects up into the stalk, whereas the submucosa of the latter is in direct continuity with the bowel wall proper (Fig. 126-6). If cancer in a pedunculated polyp is confined to the submucosa of the stalk and all other histologic features are favorable, surgery is not indicated because the chance of an adverse outcome from endoscopic polypectomy is less than the operative mortality. Once the submucosa of the bowel wall is involved with cancer (a situation that occurs more readily in sessile polyps), the chance of an adverse outcome often outweighs the operative mortality, thereby justifying surgical resection. Furthermore, because endoscopic technique purposely avoids cutting deeply into the bowel wall submucosa, there are few published examples of sessile lesions that have been completely excised endoscopically with clear margins and no other unfavorable features.

Deciding on the optimal plan of management after polypectomy involves weighing the risks of morbidity and mortality from potential residual or recurrent cancer against the risks of morbidity and mortality from a surgical attempt to cure any such residual disease or lymph node metastasis. A few general recommendations, however, can be offered. If endoscopic excision of an adenoma is complete, endoscopic polypectomy alone is adequate therapy for adenomas that contain carcinoma in situ, pedunculated adenomas that harbor well-differentiated or moderately differentiated invasive carcinoma, and polypoid carcinomas. Resectional surgery is indicated for malignant polyps in which the invasive carcinoma is poorly differentiated, involves endothelium-lined channels (lymphatics, blood vessels), extends to or within 2 mm of the polypectomy margin, or involves the submucosa of the colonic wall (includes all sessile adenomas). Studies have examined the depth of submucosal invasion as a predictor of lymph node metastasis. Two studies found the rate of lymph node metastasis was zero when depth of submucosal invasion was less than 1 mm in 1 study and 2 mm in the other.[167]

Clearly, the ultimate plan of therapy must be individualized according to each patient's medical condition. For most patients with malignant polyps, polypectomy without surgical resection seems adequate, with the caveat that the polyp was deemed to be completely resected endoscopically, and

TABLE 126-8 Favorable and Unfavorable Features for Adverse Outcomes in Patients with Malignant Polyps

Feature	Favorable	Unfavorable
Degree of differentiation	Well or moderate	Poor
Invasion of veins or lymphatics	Absent	Present
Polypectomy margin	Clear or >2-mm margin	Involved
Invasion of submucosa of bowel wall	Absent	Present

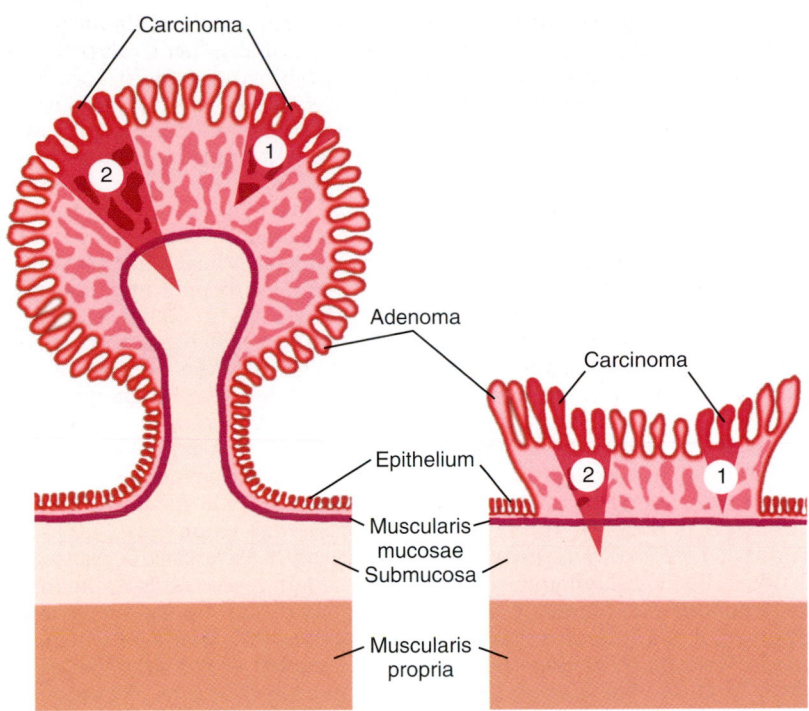

FIGURE 126-6. Comparison of carcinoma in situ and invasive cancer. Carcinoma is considered intramucosal or carcinoma in situ, as indicated by the area labeled "1," either in a pedunculated adenoma *(left)* or in a sessile adenoma *(right)* when there is not a breach of the muscularis mucosae. This lesion, as a rule, does not metastasize. Carcinoma in an adenomatous polyp is considered invasive when it breaches the muscularis mucosae, as indicated by the areas labeled "2." Invasive cancer in a pedunculated polyp *(left)* is unlikely to metastasize, and it is managed differently from invasive cancer in a sessile polyp *(right)*, which often requires surgical resection.

that postpolypectomy endoscopic surveillance will be incorporated into the patient's health care regimen.

Postpolypectomy Management

Polyp Recurrence Rates. Although patients in whom a colorectal adenoma has been excised completely are likely to develop subsequent (metachronous) neoplasms, the frequency and time course of these occurrences are not well understood. In long-term retrospective studies, the cumulative risk of adenoma recurrence is nearly linear, being 20% at 5 years after polypectomy and rising to 50% after 15 years (Fig. 126-7).[168] Information on this subject is inexact because earlier studies were primarily retrospective, involved short follow-up periods, and differed in endoscopic indications. Moreover, recurrence rates tend to be somewhat inflated because lesions missed during the index colonoscopy might be considered recurrences. With these caveats in mind, it is estimated that one third of people who have undergone polypectomy develop recurrent adenomas.[169-171] The recurrence rate at 1 year is as low as 5% to 15%[168,171] but ranges up to 30% to 45% based on prospective colonoscopy studies.[169,172,173] In the National Polyp Study, the overall adenoma recurrence rate was 42% for patients who underwent surveillance colonoscopy at 1 and 3 years after index polypectomy compared with 32% in the group that was examined only at 3 years.[36] There is general consensus that recurrent adenomas typically are smaller and less likely to harbor advanced pathology than are index adenomas.

Can histopathologic features of adenomas at the time of the index polypectomy be used to help predict recurrence of adenomas? Virtually all studies agree that the presence of multiple index adenomas is an important predictor of

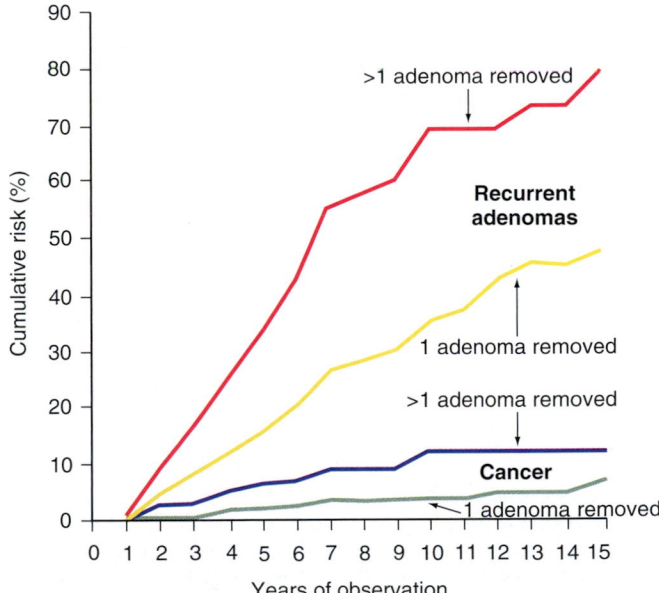

FIGURE 126-7. Risk of recurrent adenomas and of colon cancers after removal of adenomas. The risk of developing recurrent adenomas *(red, yellow)* or cancer *(blue, green)* is higher in patients who initially underwent removal of multiple (>1) adenomas *(red, blue)* than removal of a single adenoma *(yellow, green)*. (Modified from Morson BC, Bussey HJR. Magnitude of risk for cancer in patients with colorectal adenomas. Br J Surg 1985; 72[Suppl]:S23-5.)

subsequent recurrence of adenoma (and carcinoma) (see Fig. 126-7).[168,169,171,174,175] This dictum applies despite negative findings on colonoscopy 1 year after polypectomy. Some studies suggest that polyp size over 1 cm,[170,171,175] severe dysplasia,[176] villous histology,[171,174] and older age[169,171] also are risk factors for adenoma recurrence, but the independent relative importance of each of these factors is uncertain.

It can be argued that the most clinically important recurrence is an AAP. Some studies have reported a 6.3% to 7.0% recurrence rate for AAP over a 4-year follow-up period.[172] In the National Polyp Study, the recurrence rate of advanced adenomas was 3.3%, regardless of whether patients underwent colonoscopy at 1 and 3 years, or only 3 years, after polypectomy. The cumulative incidence of AAP was 4% at 3 years and 8% at 6 years of follow-up. Independent predictors for AAP at follow-up included more than 3 adenomas at the index colonoscopy, and age older than 60 at the time of adenoma diagnosis in a parent who had colorectal cancer CRC.[177] In the presence of these 2 risk factors, cumulative AAP recurrence rates rose to 10% at 3 years and 20% at 6 years of follow-up. The persons at lowest risk for developing AAP were those with a single adenoma diagnosed when they were younger than 60. Another colonoscopic follow-up study reported that multiple adenomas at the index colonoscopy increased the risk of AAP, but it also found that adenoma size larger than 1 cm and proximal location were additional risk factors.[175] A pooled analysis of 8 prospective trials with over 9000 patients found that more than 5 adenomas, size larger than 20 mm, proximal location, and the presence of villous features were the strongest predictors of recurrent AAPs.[178] Interestingly, the presence of high-grade dysplasia was not associated with recurrent adenomas, and neither was the site of the adenoma or AAP[179] or race.[180]

Effect of Polypectomy on Colorectal Cancer Incidence.

If adenomas are the precursor to colon cancer, then removing them should decrease the subsequent incidence of CRC. Indeed, studies strongly suggest that distal CRCs can be prevented and mortality reduced by screening proctosigmoidoscopy.[37-39] Retrospective studies found that removing adenomas by polypectomy was associated with an increased incidence of colon cancer.[181-183] Because these retrospective studies did not establish a polyp-free colon (or always consider adenoma size and histology), however, the higher colon cancer rate might have reflected malignant progression of other adenomas that had not been removed; 2 studies from the Mayo Clinic also did not establish a polyp-free colon at the time of polypectomy.[19,156] Despite these observations, if the removed polyps were small (<1 cm), there was no greater risk for subsequently developing colon cancer. In contrast, removal of large adenomas was associated with a greater risk of subsequent CRC, again supporting the concept that advanced neoplasms at index polypectomy are predictors of subsequent neoplasia. Important observations also come from the St. Mark's Hospital study, in which rectal adenomas were removed without any subsequent examinations.[160] If the index polyp was a small, tubular adenoma, there was no greater risk of subsequent cancer anywhere in the colon, whereas the risk was significantly increased if the index adenoma was large or contained villous elements. Other studies have shown a marked reduction in colon cancer incidence related to polypectomy.[184]

The most valid study design to address this issue is a prospective colonoscopic study in which an adenoma-free colon is established and patients are followed for subsequent development of colonic neoplasms. The National Polyp Study is a landmark study in this regard. This was a prospective multicenter randomized trial in which a cohort of 1418 patients underwent a clearing colonoscopy to remove 1 or more adenomas; patients were then followed at specific intervals for a

mean of 5.9 years. During the follow-up period, 5 early asymptomatic cancers were detected, representing only 10% to 24% of the expected incidence compared with 3 historical reference groups.[36] Two other studies (from Norway and Italy) confirm that colonoscopic polypectomy was associated with a 75% to 80% reduction in subsequent CRC incidence.[185,186] In a smaller study, the Funen Adenoma Follow-up Study, it was found that although the incidence of subsequent colon cancers was not reduced by polypectomy, the mortality was reduced.[187] In summary, these studies indicate that the adenoma is a marker of a neoplasm-prone colon, and that colonoscopic clearing of all adenomas is of considerable benefit. However, the data are heterogeneous in describing both the level and duration of protection following a clearing colonoscopy. Furthermore, the number, size, and location of removed polyps play a role in determining the level of protection afforded by a clearing colonoscopy. The uneven benefit in preventing subsequent CRCs afforded by colonoscopy is a major impetus in the drive to enhance the quality of colonoscopic examinations.

Frequency of Surveillance Colonoscopy.

The National Polyp Study has taught us that performing follow-up colonoscopy at 1 year is a low-yield proposition, as others have observed using sigmoidoscopy.[184] It also is worth realizing that an endoscopic examination of the colorectum can afford protection against colon cancer for 6 to 10 years.[37-39] Moreover, it has been proposed that a single lifetime sigmoidoscopy at about age 55 to 60 years could be standard policy for CRC screening, with referral of patients for colonoscopy and subsequent surveillance only if the sigmoidoscopy discloses a distal adenoma with advanced features.[123]

A consensus statement for postpolypectomy surveillance guidelines has been generated by the U.S. Multi-Society Task Force on Colorectal Cancer and the American Cancer Society (Table 126-9).[188] A complete colonoscopy should be performed at the time of polypectomy, clearing the colon of all existing adenomas; this can take more than 1 colonoscopy session for large or multiple polyps. The interval before the

TABLE 126-9 Surveillance Recommendations after Polypectomy

Findings on Colonoscopy	Next Colonoscopy (Years)
No polyps	10
Small (<10 mm) hyperplastic polyps in rectum or sigmoid	10
1-2 small (<10 mm) tubular adenomas	5-10
3-10 tubular adenomas	3
1 or more tubular adenomas >10 mm	3
1 or more villous adenomas	3
Adenoma with HGD	1
>10 adenomas	<3
Serrated Lesions	
Sessile serrated polyp(s) <10 mm with no dysplasia	5
Sessile serrated polyp(s) >10 mm	3
Sessile serrated polyp with dysplasia	3
Traditional serrated adenoma	3
Serrated polyposis syndrome	1

Modified from Lieberman DA, Rex DK, Winawer SJ, et al. Guidelines for colonoscopy surveillance after screening and polypectomy: A consensus update by the US Multi-Society Task Force on Colorectal Cancer. Gastroenterology. 2012; 143:844-57.

next surveillance colonoscopy is based on the patient's category of recurrent adenoma risk and features of the adenomatous polyps.

Serrated Polyps

Serrated polyps are the most common nonadenomatous polyps. Evidence is mounting to support the concept of a distinct serrated neoplasia pathway.[189] Serrated polyps are classified histologically into 3 distinct types: hyperplastic polyps (HPs), sessile serrated polyp/adenomas (SSP/As), and traditional serrated adenomas (TSAs) (Table 126-10). The terms *sessile serrated polyp* and *sessile serrated adenoma* are considered synonymous. HPs are generally believed to have no malignant potential and are therefore discussed later in the section "Non-neoplastic Polyps." In contrast, SSP/As and TSAs (Fig. 126-8) represent more clinically significant lesions.

Sessile Serrated Polyps/Adenomas and Traditional Serrated Adenomas

SSP/As are considered the precursor lesions for the large hyperplastic polyps found in the proximal colon of patients with hyperplastic polyposis (now termed *serrated polyposis*). When sporadic, SSP/As are found more commonly in the proximal colon. By contrast, TSAs look and behave like conventional adenomas: They are often pedunculated, have unequivocal adenomatous dysplasia with branching and budding crypts (albeit with crypt serration), and are found more often in the distal colon (see Table 126-10).

At the molecular level, most SSP/As appear to progress to CRC via a distinct molecular pathway that involves increased methylation of CpG islands. The CpG island methylation pathway (CIMP) results in decreased expression of genes, including DNA mismatch repair genes, which can lead to microsatellite instability (MSI). SSP/As often have *BRAF*

TABLE 126-10 Features of Serrated Polyps

Features	Hyperplastic Polyp	Sessile Serrated Polyp/Adenoma	Traditional Serrated Adenoma
Endoscopic appearance	Small, pale	Mucus cap, obscures submucosal vessels	Lobular
Most frequent colon site	Distal	Proximal	Distal
Shape	Sessile	Sessile	Pedunculated
Average size (mm)	<5	>5	>5
Irregular crypt bases	−	+	−
Gene mutations			
BRAF mutation	+/−	+	+/−
K-ras mutation	+/−	−	+/−
Malignant potential	−	+ (when dysplasia is present)	+

Modified from Limketkai BN, Lam-Himlin D, Arnold MA, Arnold CA. The cutting edge of serrated polyps: A practical guide to approaching and managing serrated colon polyps. Gastrointest Endosc 2013; 77:360-75.

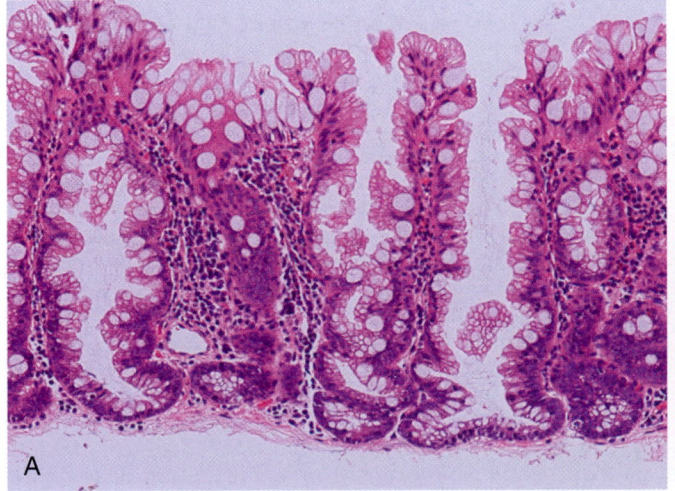
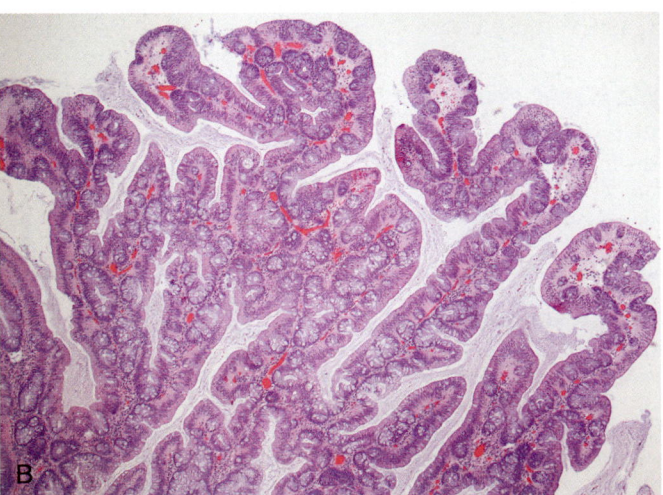

FIGURE 126-8. *A,* Histopathology of a sessile serrated polyp (sessile serrated adenoma). The crypts at the base of the polyp are broad and flattened, with nuclear pleomorphism and prominent nucleoli. The mid and upper portion of the same crypts show maturation toward more normal-appearing nuclei but with a serrated appearance on the luminal surface and dystrophic goblet cells. *B,* Traditional serrated adenoma. The long fronds of this adenoma are lined by dysplastic epithelial cells characterized by nuclear pleomorphism interspersed with cells that have dystrophic goblet cell vacuoles. *(Courtesy Noam Harpaz, MD, PhD, New York.)*

mutations and extensive DNA methylation, whereas TSAs usually have *K-ras* instead of *BRAF* mutations, and have only infrequent mutations of *APC*, *TP53*, and *MSI*.[189]

Epidemiology and Detection. SSP/As are much less common than HPs, accounting for less than 1% of all polyps and between 1% and 11% of adenomas.[190] The prevalence of high-grade dysplasia and cancer in these lesions, however, may be as high as 5% to 16%.[190] Compared with HP, most SSP/As are located in the right side of the colon. In general, risk factors for SSP/A and TSA are similar to risk factors for adenomas. Some patients will harbor both a traditional adenoma and an SSP/A. These patients tend to have larger and more advanced adenomas and SSP/As.[191] The risk of CRC may be as high as 1 in 17 in a patient with a proximal SSA. SSP/As have been associated with both synchronous and metachronous cancers as well as MSI cancers.[192,193]

SSP/As are typically flat, located in the right colon, and covered with a mucus cap. They may be hard to detect with conventional white light colonoscopy. It is not known if advanced imaging techniques such as chromoendoscopy or NBI reliably increase detection rates of SSP/A. Miss rates for detection of SSP/A have not been calculated but may exceed miss rates for conventional adenomas, given how subtle these lesions may be. Some studies have suggested adenoma detection rates correlate well with detection of SSP/A.[189]

Management. It is recommended that all serrated polyps be removed when detected. This is because it may not be possible to distinguish SSP/A or TSA from an HP, and SSP/As and TSAs have a significant risk of progression to invasive carcinoma. Diminutive SSP/As can be removed by biopsy forceps, but larger polyps should be removed by snare polypectomy. The general principles of adenomatous polypectomy apply to SSP/A and TSA. Recommendations addressing postpolypectomy surveillance of SSP/A and TSA are shown in Table 126-9.[189] In general, SSP/A and TSA surveillance is equivalent to surveillance of conventional adenomas.

Non-neoplastic Polyps

HPs are the most common non-neoplastic polyps, but have a close relationship to the SSP/A and TSA discussed earlier. Other non-neoplastic polyps fall into several distinct and unrelated groups: juvenile polyps, Peutz-Jeghers polyps, inflammatory polyps, and many other submucosal lesions (see Box 126-1).

Hyperplastic Polyps

HPs typically are small sessile lesions that may be grossly indistinguishable from small adenomatous polyps. Microscopically, the colonic crypts are elongated and the epithelial cells assume a characteristic papillary configuration (Fig. 126-9). The epithelium is made up of well-differentiated goblet and absorptive cells. The cytologic atypia that is characteristic of adenomatous polyps is not seen. Mitoses and DNA synthesis are limited to the base of the crypts, and orderly cell maturation is preserved. The epithelial cell and attendant pericryptal sheath fibroblast make up an epithelial-mesenchymal unit that migrates up the colonic crypt. In contrast to adenomatous polyps, in which the epithelium and fibroblast appear to be immature, this tissue is more differentiated, and abundant collagen is synthesized in the basement membrane.[194] It is thought that the migration of epithelial cells up the colonic crypt is slow and that HPs develop from the failure of mature cells to detach normally.

For the most part, true sporadic HPs are considered to have little if any intrinsic malignant potential; however, it is important to consider that HPs and neoplastic lesions can

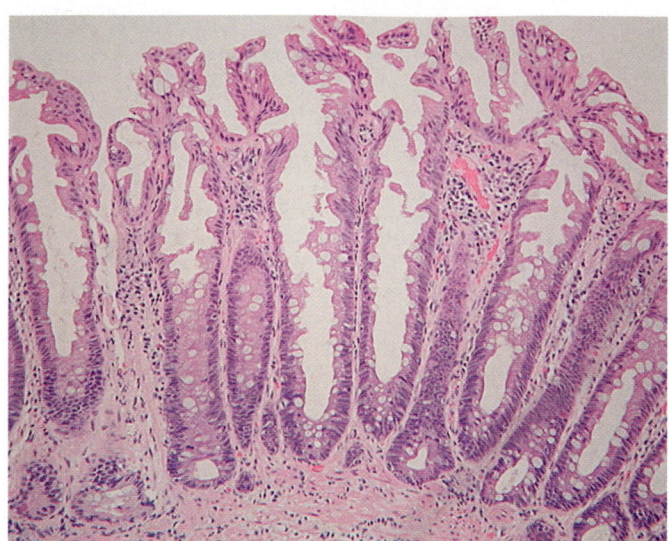

FIGURE 126-9. Histopathology of a hyperplastic polyp. This high-power photomicrograph demonstrates the crypts of a hyperplastic polyp, consisting of elongated epithelial cells with nuclei that retain their basal orientation and demonstrate no atypia. The surface of the crypts assumes a serrated appearance. *(Courtesy Noam Harpaz, MD, PhD, New York.)*

appear in the same colon, suggesting that the 2 may be pathogenetically related. Indeed, in one patient, a germline mutation of the *APC* gene has been associated with an unusually large number of colorectal HPs in association with adenomas.[195] Coexisting hyperplastic and adenomatous polyps also are common in the setting of a strong family history of CRC, including Lynch syndrome.[196] It appears, however, that in patients with sporadic adenomas, the coexistence of HPs does not confer an increased risk of recurrent adenomas during a 3-year follow-up period.[197]

Prevalence

The prevalence of HPs is not known with precision, but these growths are common. In colonoscopic examinations of asymptomatic patients aged older than 50 years, HPs were found in 9% to 10%,[198] although this frequency was higher (30% to 31%) among male veterans.[199] Sigmoidoscopic screening of asymptomatic relatives of adenoma-prone kindreds revealed 26% with HPs, a prevalence that was essentially identical (28%) to that of asymptomatic spouse controls.[200] Autopsy data report a prevalence rate of 20% to 35%.[8,11]

The incidence of HPs depends largely on the site of the colon being examined and on the age of the patient. Autopsy studies repeatedly observe a distal predominance of HPs.[8,10,11] Of course, sigmoidoscopic studies, which focus on the distal colon and rectum, find many HPs, but even screening colonoscopy studies detect more HPs in the distal than in the proximal colon.[62] Among all diminutive polyps (<5 mm) removed during colonoscopy, HPs outnumber adenomatous polyps in the rectum and sigmoid, and adenomas predominate in the remainder of the colon.[201] The prevalence of HPs increases with age.[9,42] There also is an association between prevalences of HPs and colon cancer, although this correlation is not as firm as the association between adenomas and colon cancers, nor does it necessarily imply any premalignant potential of the HP itself. Data suggest that current smoking is a risk factor for HPs.[79]

Treatment

HPs remain small, usually are sessile, and seldom, if ever, cause symptoms. Inasmuch as they are not likely to give rise to cancer, little is gained by removing them, but because they often cannot be distinguished from neoplastic or serrated polyps simply by gross examination, they usually are removed. Given their usual predominance in the distal colorectum, finding HPs in this location is not an alarming finding, particularly in older adults. Because sigmoidoscopic findings sometimes are used to decide the need for a full colonoscopy, the importance of the distal HP as a marker of proximal neoplasia has been questioned. A systematic review of the subject found that in asymptomatic persons, a distal HP is associated with a 21% to 25% risk for any proximal neoplasia and a 4% to 5% risk of advanced proximal neoplasia, thus justifying colonoscopy.[202] Although most patients with a distal HP likely will undergo colonoscopy, current guidelines suggest that if no adenomas are found, such patients can subsequently be followed at intervals similar to those without any polyps.[188]

Juvenile Polyps

Juvenile polyps (Fig. 126-10) are mucosal tumors that consist primarily of an excess of lamina propria and dilated cystic glands, rather than an overabundance of epithelial cells as seen in adenomatous and HPs; therefore, they are classified as hamartomas. The appearance of distended, mucus-filled glands, inflammatory cells, and edematous lamina propria has prompted some observers to call these lesions *retention polyps*.

Juvenile polyps appear to be acquired lesions because they seldom are seen in the first year of life and are most common from ages 1 to 7 years; occasionally they are found in adults. Juvenile polyps more often are single than multiple, usually are pedunculated, and tend to range in size from 3 mm to 2 cm. Because these polyps tend to be in the rectum and to develop a stalk, they can prolapse during defecation and even slough. In addition, their stroma contains a generous vascular supply, which explains the considerable blood loss suffered by some patients with juvenile polyps. Because of the high likelihood of bleeding and prolapse, removal of juvenile polyps is suggested.

Juvenile polyps have essentially no malignant potential when single,[203] and they tend not to recur. Although approximately 20% of individual juvenile polyps in the rectum may be associated with proximal polyps, proximal adenomas are rare, and the subsequent rate of dying of or developing CRC is no greater than these rates for the general population, even without specific surveillance.[203] When juvenile polyps are multiple (see "Juvenile Polyposis Syndrome," later), however, the risk of developing cancer is present, either because adenomatous epithelium may be present in some juvenile polyps or because of a coexistent adenoma.

Peutz-Jeghers Polyps

The Peutz-Jeghers polyp is a unique hamartomatous lesion characterized by glandular epithelium supported by an arborizing framework of well-developed smooth muscle that is contiguous with the muscularis mucosae (Fig. 126-11). The smooth muscle bands fan out into the head of the polyp and become progressively thinner as they project toward its surface. A Peutz-Jeghers polyp differs from a juvenile polyp in that the lamina propria is normal, and the characteristic architecture of the lesion derives chiefly from its abnormal smooth muscle tissue. These polyps almost always are multiple, and their distinctive appearance, in association with the extraintestinal manifestations, makes Peutz-Jeghers syndrome easily identifiable. This type of polyp seldom is found in the colon in the absence of generalized polyposis (see later).

Inflammatory Polyps (Pseudopolyps)

Inflammatory polyps are found in the regenerative and healing phases of inflammation. They usually are formed by full-thickness ulceration of epithelium followed by a regenerative process that leaves the mucosa in bizarre polypoid configurations. Less commonly, inflammatory polyps represent relatively normal mucosa sitting amidst reepithelialized ulcerations. Inflammatory polyps may be large and solitary, mimicking a neoplastic mass, or they can form mucosal bridges that span the lumen. Multiple lesions can mimic a polyposis syndrome. The term *pseudopolyp* is used to distinguish them from neoplastic lesions, but in reality these are true polypoid protuberances. Histologically, inflammation and exuberant granulation tissue may be seen in the early postinflammatory period, but later the polyp surface can resemble that of normal mucosa.

Any form of severe colitis, including chronic IBD (UC, Crohn's disease),[204] amebic colitis,[205] ischemic colitis, or bacterial dysentery, can give rise to inflammatory polyps. In chronic schistosomiasis, multiple inflammatory polyps that contain granulation tissue, eggs, or adult worms commonly are seen.[206] The significance of these polyps, which have no intrinsic neoplastic potential, is that they often appear in diseased colons that are at high risk for developing colon cancer (UC, schistosomiasis); therefore, they must be distinguished from neoplastic lesions that do carry premalignant potential. Giant or grouped pseudopolyps can cause colonic obstruction.

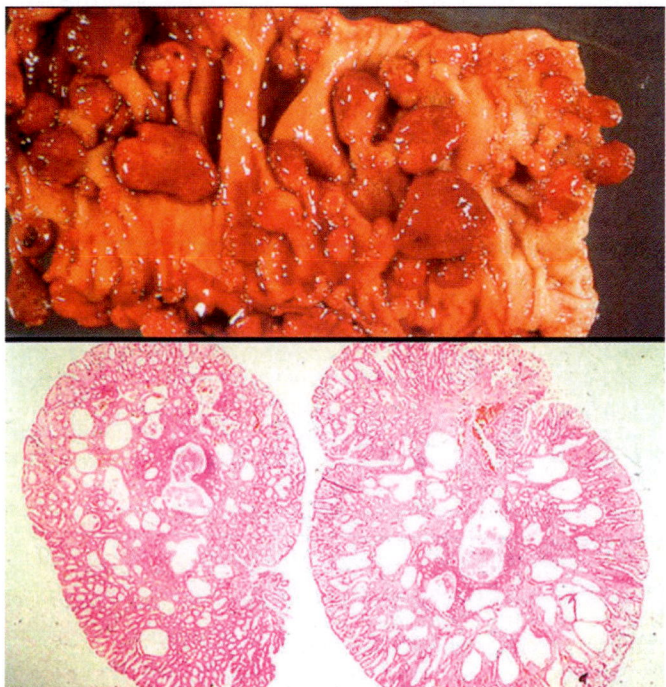

FIGURE 126-10. Juvenile polyps. *Top,* Resection specimen of a colon harboring multiple juvenile polyps. *Bottom,* Histopathology revealing the characteristic large cystic spaces of this lesion. *(From Demetris AJ, Finkelstein SD, Nalensnik MA, et al. Slide carousel of GI pathology course for medical students. Available at: http://www.pathology.pitt.edu/lectures/gi/. Copyright © Department of Pathology, University of Pittsburgh School of Medicine.)*

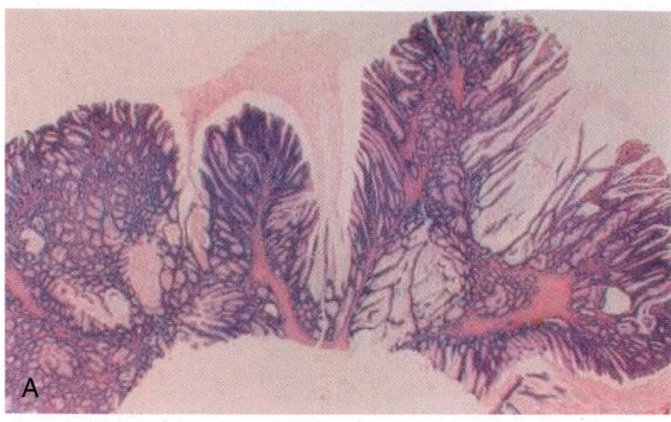
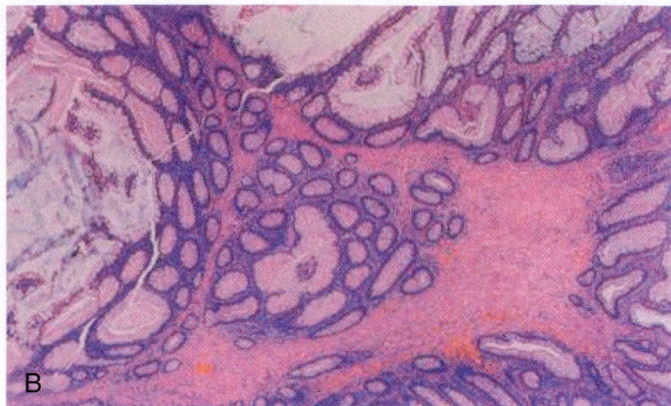

FIGURE 126-11. Low-power *(A)* and high-power *(B)* histopathology of a Peutz-Jeghers polyp. In this type of polyp, the glandular epithelium is supported by an arborizing framework of well-developed smooth muscle that is contiguous with the muscularis mucosae. *(From Boland CR. The colon, rectum, and anus. In: Feldman M, editor. Gastroenterology and hepatology: The comprehensive visual reference. Philadelphia: Churchill Livingstone; 1996.)*

Rare cases of multiple and recurrent inflammatory GI polyps that produce pain and obstruction have been reported on a sporadic and even a familial basis.[207] These lesions are found primarily in the ileum, may be very large, and can even cause intussusception. Cap polyposis is another rare condition characterized by inflammatory polyps with elongated crypts, a mixed inflammatory infiltrate in the lamina propria, and a surface cap of fibrinopurulent exudate.[208] Cap polyposis may be confused endoscopically with pseudopolyps in IBD. Mucosal prolapse has been suggested as a possible underlying etiology.

Mucosal Polyps

The colon commonly harbors excrescences or mammillations of tissue that histologically are normal mucosa. In these instances, the submucosa has elevated the normal tissue overlying it. These lesions may be termed *mucosal polyps*, and their presence has no clinical significance. Mucosal polyps almost always are small and can constitute 8% to 20% of the material recovered in a collection of colonoscopic biopsies.

Submucosal Lesions

Colitis Cystica Profunda

Colitis cystica profunda is a rare lesion consisting of dilated, mucus-filled glands in the submucosa that can form solitary or multiple polyps (see Chapter 128). The typical lesion is a solitary polyp smaller than 3 cm that most commonly is found in the rectum in the setting of chronic inflammation. Prior surgical procedures and ulcerative proctitis have been linked to the pathogenesis of this abnormality. The involved epithelium shows no evidence of dysplasia. The primary significance of this lesion is that it must be recognized and distinguished from colloid carcinoma, which can look similar histologically, because a mistaken diagnosis of colloid carcinoma could lead to inappropriate radical surgery.[209] The lesion is presumably caused by displacement of normal colonic glands to beneath the epithelium during the healing of a surgical wound or inflammation. Rarely, the polyps become large or recur and can even obstruct the colon. It has been suggested that the pathologic picture and clinical presentation of colitis cystica profunda are similar to those of solitary rectal ulcer and that both may be produced by rectal prolapse.[209]

Pneumatosis Cystoides Coli

Multiple gas-filled cysts are occasionally encountered within the submucosa of the colon (and small intestine) and can produce a polypoid appearance (see Chapter 128). The diagnosis of pneumatosis cystoides intestinalis may be made on full-thickness pathologic sections or by the characteristic radiologic or endoscopic appearance of the intramural gas-filled cysts. The diagnosis is substantiated at endoscopy if the cysts collapse after puncture/aspiration with a sclerotherapy needle or by unroofing them with a biopsy forceps. This condition can produce a variety of symptoms, some of which suggest colitis, but it also may be associated with vague symptoms or can remain asymptomatic.[210]

Two forms of pneumatosis intestinalis have been recognized. One type (pneumatosis linearis) may be associated with a fulminant mucosal process, such as inflammatory or ischemic bowel disease in adults or necrotizing enterocolitis in children. In these fulminant settings, in which the condition often is fatal, it is thought that the gas dissects through the bowel wall in a linear fashion and results from invasion of the submucosa by gas-forming bacteria. The more common type, pneumatosis cystoides intestinalis, is seen in adults and is more typically a chronic or incidental finding; it even may be associated with asymptomatic pneumoperitoneum. Pneumatosis cystoides intestinalis is associated with chronic obstructive pulmonary disease and may be seen in patients with scleroderma. The genesis of the gas-filled cysts in these benign settings is incompletely understood, but it has been demonstrated that gas within the bowel lumen diffuses into the cysts, which can contribute to their maintenance. Oxygen therapy results in the resolution of these cysts,[211] but the pathophysiologic basis of this response is by no means clear. The natural history can be deduced from only a small number of cases, but the disease can persist for months.[210-212] A single course of oxygen therapy (often as little as 5 to 6 L/min of oxygen) can result in resolution of symptoms for a long time. Antibiotic treatment is of no benefit.

Others

Any lesion beneath the colon mucosa can elevate the overlying epithelium to produce a polypoid appearance. Lymphoid tissue is present throughout the colon, and hypertrophied follicles may be mistaken for a pathologic mucosal process.

Benign lymphoid polyps can grow large enough to produce symptoms (pain, bleeding) or can become pedunculated. Multiple benign lymphoid polyps may be found as normal variants, particularly in children. The principal importance of benign lymphoid polyps is in their distinction from malignant lymphoid lesions. Malignant lymphoma[213] and chronic lymphocytic leukemia[214] can manifest as multiple colonic polyposis.

The colon is the most common GI site for lipomas, which tend to be solitary but may be multiple submucosal lesions. Lipomas usually are asymptomatic and detected incidentally. The low density of fat can give the lesions a characteristic radiologic appearance, and their soft, deformable nature and yellowish color are helpful to the colonoscopist in making the diagnosis grossly. Colonic lipomas are most common in the right colon and tend to occur on or near the ileocecal valve.[215] Removal of these lesions usually is not necessary.

Important tumors such as carcinoids, metastatic neoplasms (especially melanoma), and other rare cancers can produce submucosal lesions without distinctive identifying characteristics. Other submucosal lesions may be detected incidentally, including fibromas, neurofibromas, leiomyomas, granular cell tumors, hemangiomas, and endometriosis.

GASTROINTESTINAL POLYPOSIS SYNDROMES

GI polyposis refers to the presence of numerous polypoid lesions throughout the GI tract. The polyposis syndromes are distinct entities clinically and pathologically, and they have been sorted into recognizable categories over the past century (Box 126-2). Most of these syndromes are inherited, and most are associated with an increased colon cancer risk, but all are classified on the basis of the histologic type of polyp and the clinical presentation. Advances in genetics have permitted a more accurate understanding of the relationships among these syndromes, while the genes responsible for these conditions, particularly the adenomatous polyposis syndromes, have provided insight into the genetic basis of sporadically occurring colon cancer.

Inherited Polyposis Syndromes

The inherited adenomatous polyposis syndromes include several entities that are characterized by large numbers of adenomatous polyps in the colon. The identification of the *APC* gene set the stage for understanding how colon cancers arise, and permitted proper classification of Gardner's syndrome, attenuated familial adenomatous polyposis (AFAP), and many cases of Turcot's syndrome as variants of classic FAP (Table 126-11). The *MUTYH* (also known as *MYH*) base-excision repair gene also has been identified as an important cause of multiple colonic adenomas.

Familial Adenomatous Polyposis

Genetics

FAP is the most common adenomatous polyposis syndrome. It is inherited as an autosomal dominant disease with 80% to 100% penetrance and has an estimated prevalence of 1 in 5000 to 7500.[216] In this condition, 1 mutated *APC* allele is inherited as a germline mutation from the affected parent, and adenomas develop when the second allele (from the unaffected parent) becomes mutated or lost. Identification of the gene responsible for FAP began in 1986 with investigation of a patient who had multiple congenital malformations and a deleted portion of the long arm of chromosome 5 that was identified cytogenetically.[217] Genetic mapping studies and restriction fragment length polymorphism (RFLP) analysis in 1987 led to the localization of the gene responsible for FAP in the 5q21-q22 region.[218,219] At the same time, RFLP analysis suggested that 1 of the 2 alleles for this gene often was lost in sporadically occurring CRCs. The fact that a lost gene might contribute to tumor progression suggested that the FAP locus might encode for a tumor suppressor gene.[220]

In 1991, the *APC* gene responsible for FAP was cloned by 2 collaborating groups and reported simultaneously.[221-223] The large size of this gene (encoding 2844 amino acids) might account for the relatively high frequency of new mutations. Germline mutations are found in patients with FAP and Gardner's syndrome, and in most instances, the mutations create a stop codon resulting in a truncated protein. The germline mutations are dispersed throughout the 5′ half of the gene, whereas somatic mutations of *APC* tend to accumulate in the mutation cluster region near the center of the gene (Fig. 126-12).[224]

The APC protein is a multifaceted regulator of colonic epithelial cell homeostasis and participates in processes of cell proliferation, migration, differentiation, apoptosis, and chromosomal segregation.[225] The proximal portion of the APC protein contains regions that enable oligomerization as well as binding to proteins that regulate the actin cytoskeleton, thereby affecting cell morphology, polarity, and migration. In its central portion, the APC protein binds β-catenin, a protein that normally maintains cell-cell junctions by anchoring a cell surface adhesion molecule, E-cadherin. In normal cells, APC forms a complex with other proteins (axin, conductin, and the GSK3b serine-threonine kinase) to bind β-catenin. This binding results in phosphorylation of β-catenin, which subsequently undergoes down-regulation in the cytoplasm. If mutations

---

BOX 126-2 Classification of GI Polyposis Syndromes

Inherited Polyposis Syndromes
Adenomatous Polyposis Syndromes
Familial adenomatous polyposis
Variants of familial adenomatous polyposis
    Gardner's syndrome
    Turcot's syndrome
    Attenuated adenomatous polyposis coli
Familial tooth agenesis syndrome
Bloom's syndrome
MUTYH polyposis (*MYH* polyposis)

Hamartomatous Polyposis Syndromes
Peutz-Jeghers syndrome
Juvenile polyposis
PTEN hamartoma tumor syndromes
    Cowden's disease
    Bannayan-Ruvalcaba-Riley syndrome
Rare hamartomatous polyposis syndromes
    Hereditary mixed polyposis syndrome
    Intestinal ganglioneuromatosis and neurofibromatosis
    Devon family syndrome
    Basal cell nevus syndrome

Noninherited Polyposis Syndromes
Cronkhite-Canada syndrome
Serrated polyposis syndrome
Lymphomatous polyposis
Nodular lymphoid hyperplasia

MUTYH (mutY homolog [*E. coli*]); *PTEN* (phosphatase and tensin homolog) (see text for details).

TABLE 126-11 Adenomatous Polyposis Syndromes

Syndrome	Gene Mutation	Polyps	Extraintestinal Abnormalities
Classic FAP	APC (usually truncated protein)	Colonic adenomas (thousands) Duodenal, periampullary adenomas Gastric fundic gland polyps Jejunal and ileal adenomas Ileal lymphoid polyps	Mandibular osteomas Dental abnormalities
Gardner variant of FAP	APC	Same as FAP	Osteomas (mandible, skull, long bones) CHRPE Desmoid tumors Epidermoid and sebaceous cysts Fibromas, lipomas Thyroid, adrenal tumors
Turcot variant of FAP	APC DNA MMR*	Colonic adenomas (sometimes fewer than in classic FAP)	Medulloblastoma Glioblastoma multiforme CHRPE
Attenuated FAP	APC 5′ and 3′ regions	Colonic adenomas (<100; proximal colon) Duodenal, periampullary adenomas Gastric fundic gland polyps	Mandibular osteomas (rare)
Familial tooth agenesis	Axin2 (APC pathway)	Colonic adenomas Hyperplastic polyps	Agenesis of teeth
Bloom's syndrome	BLM	Colonic adenomas	Small stature Facial erythema/telangiectasia Male sterility Adenocarcinomas, leukemia, lymphoma
MUTYH polyposis	MUTYH (MYH)	Colonic adenomas (5-100) Duodenal polyposis Gastric cancer	CHRPE Osteomas

*May be more appropriately classified under hereditary nonpolyposis colon cancer (HNPCC) (see Chapter 127).
APC, adenomatous polyposis coli; CHRPE, congenital hypertrophy of the retinal pigment epithelium; FAP, familial adenomatous polyposis; MMR, mismatch repair; MUTYH (mutY homolog [E. coli]).

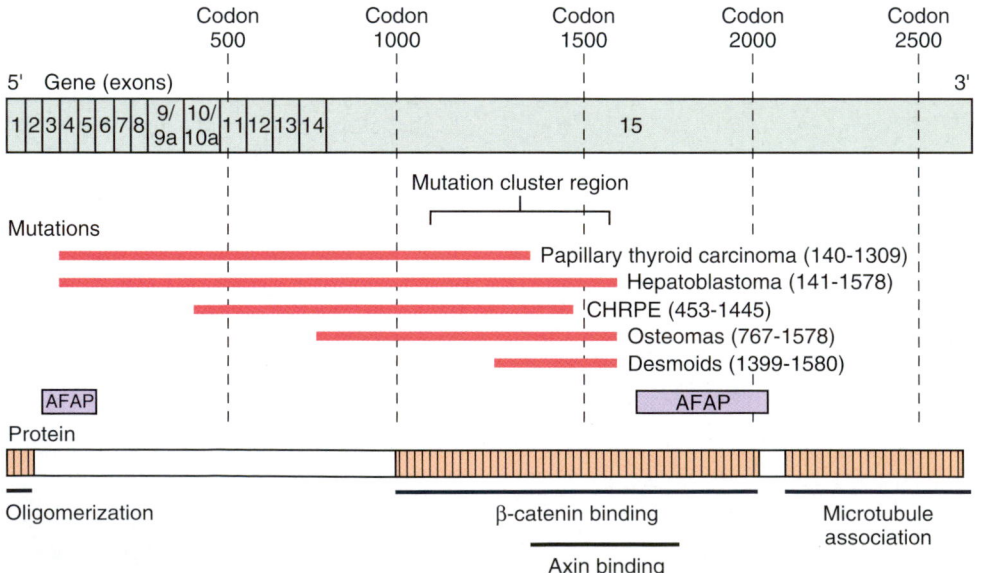

FIGURE 126-12. Schematic diagram of the *APC* gene, its mutations, and functional domains of the protein. The gene consists of 15 exons. Mutations associated with attenuated familial adenomatous polyposis (AFAP) occur in the 5′ and 3′ regions of the gene. Congenital hypertrophy of the retinal pigment epithelium (CHRPE) lesions are seen only with mutations downstream of exon 9. The mutation cluster region is in the center of the gene, where most mutations give rise to florid polyposis. Papillary thyroid carcinoma, hepatoblastoma, osteomas, and desmoid tumors are associated with the codon regions shown. Domains of the APC protein responsible for oligomerization, β-catenin binding, and microtubule association are shown along the bottom. *(Modified from Goss KH, Groden J. Biology of the adenomatous polyposis coli tumor suppressor. J Clin Oncol 2000; 18:1967; and Groen EJ, Roos A, Muntinghe FL, et al. Extra-intestinal manifestations of familial adenomatous polyposis. Ann Surg Oncol 2008; 15:2439-50.)*

occur in the β-catenin–binding region, however, β-catenin no longer is down-regulated, allowing it to enter the nucleus, where it acts in conjunction with other transcription factors to up-regulate target genes that then promote formation of adenomas. Similarly, germline mutations of axin were discovered to cause a multiple colonic adenoma phenotype (see later). The carboxy-terminal portion of APC contains a domain that contributes to proper chromosomal segregation and cytoskeleton regulation. Because the vast majority of *APC* mutations truncate the protein, this has the dual effect of disrupting the constitutive breakdown of β-catenin, leading to activation of cancer-associated genes and creating abnormal chromosomal segregation with resultant chromosomal instability.

Clinical Features

Colonic Findings. Classic FAP is characterized by the progressive development of hundreds to thousands of adenomatous polyps in the large intestine. A patient who inherits an *APC* mutation usually does not develop adenomas until approximately 10 to 12 years of age; rarely, however, polyps appear in the first decade of life. In 1 early series of FAP cases, the average age at onset of polyps was 25 years, but symptoms did not appear until the age of 33. The average age for the diagnosis of adenomas was 36 years, for cancer 39 years, and for death from cancer, 42 years; 90% of FAP cases have been diagnosed by the time the patient is 50.[226] A study that focused on early screening reported that 50% of FAP gene carriers have polyps at sigmoidoscopy by approximately 15 years of age.[227]

FAP begins with a small number of polyps, and the number increases progressively until the colon becomes studded with adenomas. All varieties of adenomatous polyps may be seen, including tubular, tubulovillous, and villous adenomas. The number of macroscopic polyps in a colectomy specimen averages 1000 but may be tens of thousands. Germline mutations of *APC* gene between codons 1250 and 1464 have been associated with more profuse carpeting of the colon (Fig. 126-13), whereas mutations elsewhere in the gene result in fewer

colorectal polyps (Fig. 126-14).[228] Histologic examination of the colon reveals numerous microscopic adenomas as well, the smallest of which can involve a single colonic crypt. The size and number of polyps correspond to the latent period between the onset of clinical disease and the time of detection; tumors tend to be more numerous in symptomatic probands than in asymptomatic younger relatives discovered by screening. Most polyps are small (<1 cm), and, individually, these polyps are identical to adenomatous polyps found in the general population.

CRC should be considered an inevitable consequence in the natural history of FAP, appearing approximately 10 to 15

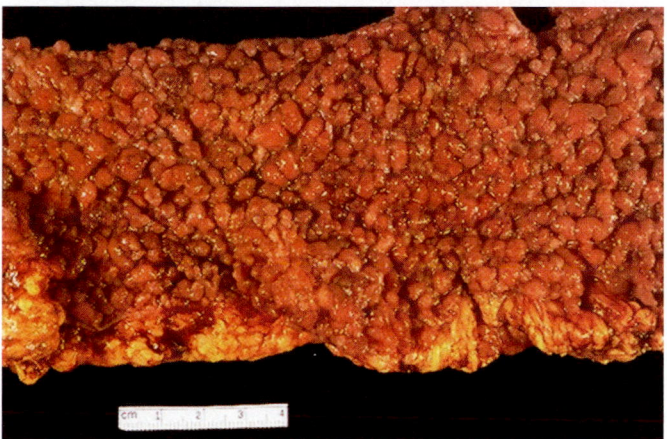

FIGURE 126-13. Surgical resection specimen from a patient with familial adenomatous polyposis (FAP). Patients with FAP have multiple adenomatous polyps that often carpet the colon, as demonstrated in this specimen. This close-up view demonstrates the presence of innumerable polyps, all of which are adenomas that can contain villous elements or carcinoma. A total proctocolectomy is the only reasonable management in this situation. (*Courtesy Arnold Markowitz, MD, New York.*)

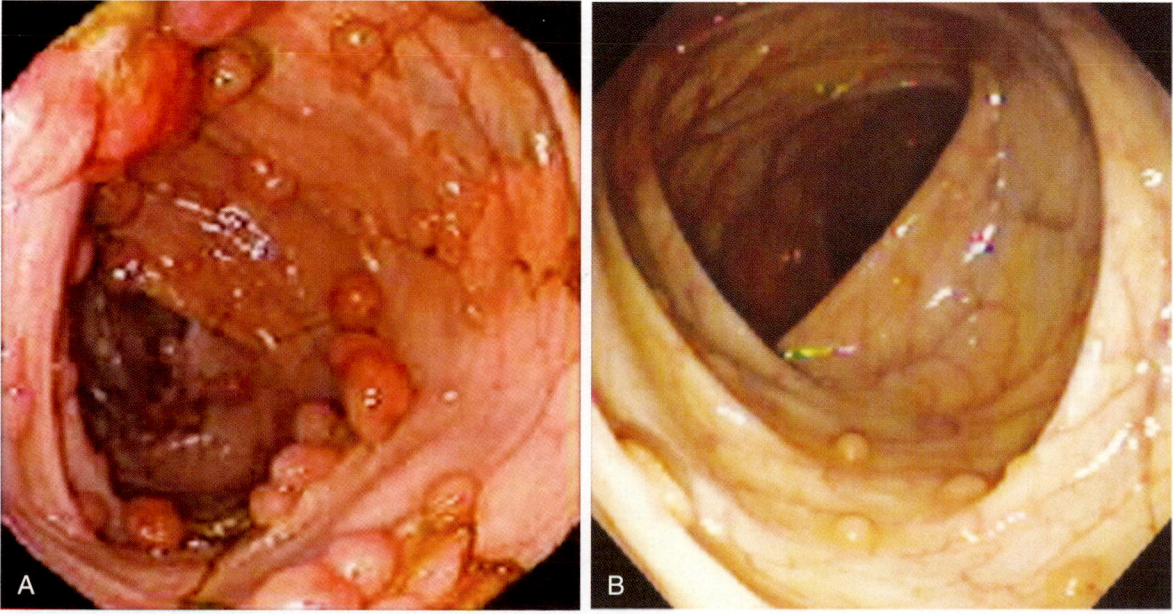

FIGURE 126-14. Colonoscopic views of familial adenomatous polyposis (FAP) (A) and attenuated FAP (B). *A,* In this patient with classic FAP, there were hundreds of polyps in the colon. *B,* In this patient with attenuated FAP, the polyps are fewer and smaller than in classic FAP. (*Courtesy Arnold Markowitz, MD, New York.*)

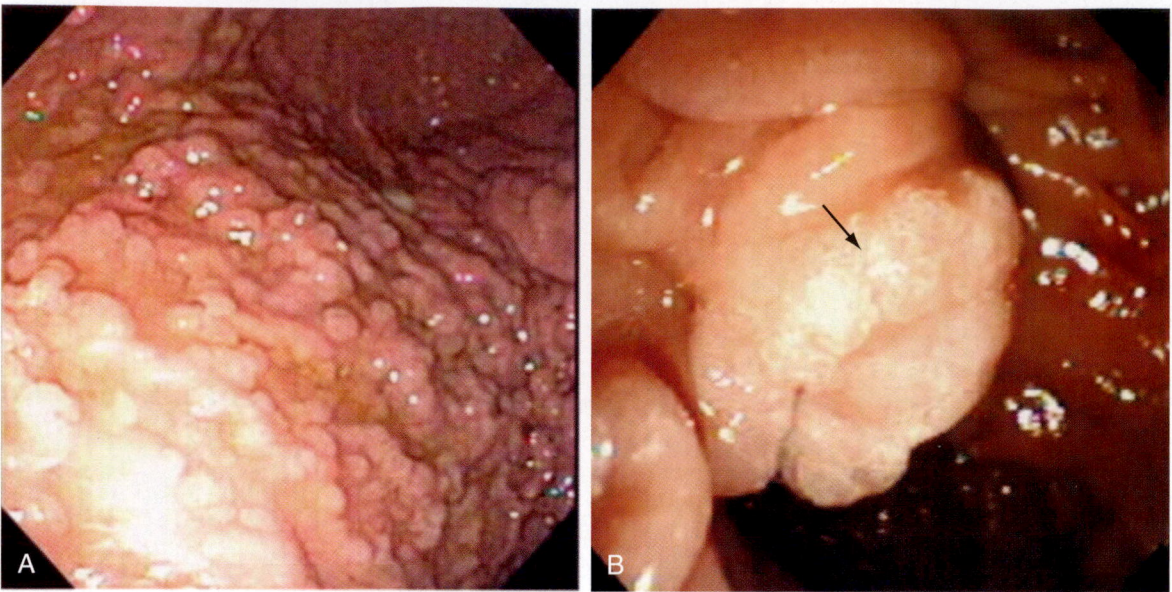

FIGURE 126-15. Endoscopic appearance of upper GI polyps in a patient with familial adenomatous polyposis. *A,* Gastric fundic gland polyposis with numerous small polyps distributed diffusely throughout the stomach. *B,* Adenomatous change of the papilla of Vater *(arrow).* These lesions may be subtle and require biopsy confirmation. *(Courtesy Arnold Markowitz, MD, New York.)*

years after the onset of polyposis. CRC is unusual in adolescence, but it has been diagnosed as early as 9 years of age.[229] The cancers have the same pathologic grades of malignancy and the same distribution within the colon as are seen in the general population, except that multiple simultaneous cancers are much more frequent (48% of cases).[226] Despite attention to screening and surveillance, as many as 25% of patients with FAP have CRC at the time of colectomy.[230]

Upper GI Lesions. Because FAP patients are born with a germline *APC* mutation in all cells of the body, tumors often develop in other organs besides the colon. For example, polyps in the stomach and small intestine are present in almost all FAP patients (Fig. 126-15).[231]

Gastric polyps occur in 30% to 100% of patients, and curiously, most polyps in the stomach are non-neoplastic fundic gland polyps. These polyps are typically 1- to 5-mm sessile growths characterized microscopically by hyperplasia of fundic glands and microcysts. They can appear in the first decade of life, even before other GI adenomas develop. Fundic gland polyps can be found in persons without FAP, especially those treated with PPIs for prolonged periods, but such growths are rarely dysplastic. By contrast, in patients with FAP, epithelial dysplasia can be seen in approximately 25% to 41% of fundic gland polyps and results from mutations of the *APC* gene.[232,233] Dysplasia in FAP-associated fundic gland polyps has been directly associated with larger polyp size, increased severity of duodenal polyposis, and antral gastritis, and it is inversely associated with use of acid-suppressive therapy and the presence of *Helicobacter pylori*.[233]

Gastric adenomas are uncommon and occur in approximately 5% of FAP patients, usually in the gastric antrum. The development of gastric adenocarcinoma in FAP patients is still rare in the USA[232,234] but is more common in Japan, where the gastric cancer rate in the general population also is higher.[235] In FAP registries, the prolonged life expectancy for FAP patients after preventive proctocolectomy has been associated with an increased incidence of gastric cancer (0.6% to 4.2%).[236,237] Microcarcinoids also may be found in the stomach of patients with FAP.[238]

A newly described autosomal dominant syndrome termed *gastric adenocarcinoma with proximal polyposis of the stomach* (GAPPS) may mimic the FAP phenotype in the stomach in that there are numerous fundic gland polyps in the proximal stomach that often harbor dysplasia.[239] Unlike FAP, patients with GAPPS are at very high risk of gastric adenocarcinoma and typically have no duodenal polyps and few if any colonic adenomas.

Duodenal adenomas occur in 60% to 90% of FAP patients, and their incidence increases with age.[240] There is a propensity for adenomas to involve the periampullary region and even to obstruct the pancreatic or biliary ductal system, rarely resulting in acute pancreatitis. As many as 50% to 85% of FAP patients manifest adenomatous change of the papilla of Vater (see Fig. 126-15).[231,240] As a consequence, a 4% to 12% lifetime incidence of duodenal cancer (usually periampullary) has been reported,[237] with relative risks of 124 to 331.[240,241] Collectively, these adenocarcinomas are the major cause of cancer death after prophylactic colectomy in FAP patients. The risk estimates for duodenal adenocarcinoma may be somewhat inflated by older prevalence studies, because under endoscopic surveillance a rather low rate of duodenal and ampullary adenoma progression to carcinoma has been observed.[242] Regardless, it is advisable to perform screening and surveillance of the stomach and duodenum. Development of duodenal carcinoma is extremely rare before age 30.[243]

The Spigelman Classification for duodenal polyposis classifies patients with duodenal polyposis into various stages depending upon polyp number, size, histology, and severity of dysplasia.[243] Patients with stage III and IV duodenal polyposis are more likely to progress to duodenal adenocarcinoma than those with earlier-stage disease. Although firm screening guidelines are not established, a suggested approach based on the Spigelman score has been proposed by a European consortium and is outlined in Table 126-12.

Jejunal adenomas have been detected in 40% and ileal adenomas in 20% of FAP patients. Fortunately, malignant transformation at these sites is rare,[231] but clinical vigilance is warranted and imaging with small bowel series, capsule

TABLE 126-12 Cancer Risks and Screening Recommendations in the Hereditary Polyposis Syndromes

Syndrome	Lifetime Risk	Screening Recommendations
Familial Adenomatous Polyposis		
Colon cancer	Near 100%	Sigmoidoscopy annually; start at age 10-12 yr*
Duodenal or periampullary cancer	5%-12%	EGD with side-viewing endoscope; start at age 25-30
		Spigelman stages 0 and 1: every 5 yr; stage II: every 3 yr; stage III: every 1-2 yr; stage IV (see text): consider surgery
Gastric cancer	≈0.5%	EGD every 1-2 yr if numerous FGPs (with or without LGD); every 6-9 months if HGD
In Families of an Affected Member		
Pancreatic cancer	≈2%	Possibly periodic abdominal US after age 20
Thyroid cancer	≈2%	Annual thyroid examination; start at age 10-12 yr
CNS cancer	<1%	Annual physical examination; periodic head CT or MRI
Hepatoblastoma	1.6%	Annual physical examination, hepatic US, serum AFP for first decade of life
Peutz-Jeghers Syndrome		
All GI cancers	2%-13%	Colonoscopy at symptom onset, or late teens if the patient is asymptomatic; interval is determined by the number of polyps, but is at least every 3 yr
		Upper GI endoscopy every 2 yr; start at age 10 yr
Small intestine	RR, 13	Annual Hgb; small bowel series or capsule endoscopy every 2 yr; start at age 10 yr
Pancreatic cancer	RR, 100	Endoscopic or abdominal US every 1-2 yr; start at age 30 yr
Breast cancer	RR, 8.8	Annual breast examination; mammogram every 2-3 yr; start at age 25 yr
Uterine cancer; ovarian cancer	RR, 8.0; 13	Annual pelvic examination, Pap smear, pelvic US; start at age 20 yr
Sertoli cell tumor (testicular)	Uncommon	Annual testicular examination beginning at age 10 yr; testis US if feminizing features are present
Juvenile Polyposis		
Colon cancer	<50%	Colonoscopy: start at symptom onset or early teens if no symptoms; interval is determined by the number of polyps, but is performed at least every 3 yr
Gastric, duodenal cancer	Rare	Upper GI endoscopy every 3 yr; start in early teens
Cowden's Syndrome		
Colon cancer	Little to none	No recommendations given
Thyroid cancer	3%-10%	Annual thyroid examination; start in teens
Breast cancer	25%-50%	Annual breast examination at age 25 yr; annual mammogram at age 30 yr
Uterine and ovarian cancer	Increased?	No recommendations given

*Sigmoidoscopy is used to identify a child with the FAP phenotype (i.e., polyps). If polyps are detected, colonoscopy usually is then performed to exclude proximal neoplasia.
AFP, alpha fetoprotein; CNS, central nervous system; FGP, fundic gland polyp; HGD, high grade dysplasia; LGP, low grade dysplasia; FAP, familial adenomatous polyposis; Pap, Papanicolaou; RR, relative risk.
Adapted from Burt RW. Colon cancer screening. Gastroenterology 2000; 119:837; and Vasen HF, Möslein G, Alonso A, et al. Guidelines for the clinical management of familial adenomatous polyposis (FAP). Gut 2008; 57:704-13.

endoscopy, or double balloon enteroscopy should be considered to examine the entire small intestine.[241,244] After subtotal colectomy or total proctocolectomy with ileal pouch-anal anastomosis, attention should be given to surveillance of the distal ileum for developing neoplasia. Lymphoid hyperplasia may be present in the ileum in FAP patients and can be distinguished from adenomatous polyps by biopsy.

Extraintestinal Features. Gardner's syndrome is a familial disease consisting of GI polyposis and osteomas associated with a variety of benign soft tissue tumors and other extraintestinal manifestations (see Table 126-11). Both FAP and Gardner's syndrome are variable manifestations of a disease caused by mutations of the *APC* gene. Bone abnormalities include osteomas of the mandible, skull, and long bones; exostoses; and various dental abnormalities including mandibular cysts, impacted teeth, and supernumerary teeth. When carefully sought, mandibular osteomas can be seen in up to 90% of patients with FAP even without other stigmata of Gardner's syndrome.[245] Radiologic examination of the mandible is a simple and noninvasive means to screen for young carriers of the FAP gene, but it is crucial to distinguish

nonspecific sclerotic lesions in the mandible from true osteomas. Mandibular osteomas in FAP tend to be multiple, whereas nonspecific sclerotic bony lesions usually are single and located close to a diseased tooth. Osteomas can occur in children before they develop colonic polyposis. Because osteomas have no malignant potential, they are removed only for symptomatic or cosmetic reasons.

Congenital hypertrophy of the retinal pigmented epithelium (CHRPE) has been reported in some families with FAP or Gardner's syndrome.[246,247] More than 90% of patients with Gardner's syndrome have pigmented lesions of the ocular fundus compared with 5% of controls. CHRPE lesions are likely to be multiple (63% have ≥ 4 lesions) and are bilateral in 87% of those affected.[246] Pigmented ocular fundus lesions are found in approximately half of the unaffected but at-risk first-degree relatives and have been identified in infants as young as 3 months old, suggesting that they are probably congenital. The presence of multiple bilateral lesions appears to be a reliable marker for gene carriage in FAP, and their absence predicts lack of carriage if carrier relatives show CHRPE.[247] CHRPE lesions are asymptomatic curiosities that

TABLE 126-13 Staging and Prognosis of Desmoid Tumors in Familial Adenomatous Polyposis

Stage	Definition	No. of Patients	Time from Colectomy to Desmoid (yr)	Rapid Growth	Death from Desmoid
I	Asymptomatic; <10 cm maximum diameter, and not growing	21	7.5	0	0
II	Mildly symptomatic; <10 cm maximum diameter, and not growing	36	5.8	3 (8%)	0
III	Moderately symptomatic or with bowel or ureteral obstruction; or 10-20 cm, or slowly growing	26	2.4	3 (12%)	4 (15%)
IV	Severely symptomatic; or >20 cm, or rapidly growing	18	1.4	6 (33%)	8 (44%)

From Church J, Lynch C, Neary P, et al. A desmoid tumor-staging system separates patients with intra-abdominal, familial adenomatous polyposis–associated desmoid disease by behavior and prognosis. Dis Colon Rectum 2008; 51:897-901.

need not be sought in patients with an established diagnosis of FAP. CHRPE perhaps reflects the most accurate genotype-phenotype correlation in FAP patients; these lesions occur in patients with *APC* gene mutations distal to exon 9 up through the proximal portion of exon 15 (see Fig. 126-12).[248]

A particularly serious complication of the adenomatous polyposis syndromes is the development of diffuse mesenteric fibromatosis, also called *desmoid tumors.* Desmoid tumors are reported in 4% to 32% of patients and rank second, after metastatic carcinoma, among lethal complications of the disease.[249] The absolute risk of desmoids in FAP patients has been estimated at 2.56/1000 person-years, which is 825 times the risk in the general population.[250] Desmoid tumors often display familial aggregation; FAP patients who are first-degree relatives of a patient with FAP and a desmoid have a 2.5-fold greater risk for developing desmoid tumors than patients with FAP in general.[249] Because a strong family history poses an increased risk of desmoids,[250] in this subset of patients it would be prudent to incorporate abdominal imaging studies into their overall surveillance regimen, even though firm guidelines for desmoid tumor surveillance are not yet established.

Desmoids occur when the disease-causing mutation is distal to codon 1444 (or in some studies, codon 1399) of the *APC* gene (see Fig. 126-12). Curiously, recurrent desmoid tumors can manifest a somatic mutation of *APC* gene that is different from that of the initial tumor.[224] Commonly, desmoid tumors result from progressive growth of mesenteric fibroblasts that occurs after laparotomy (e.g., after prophylactic proctocolectomy), but they occasionally appear spontaneously. The morbidity associated with desmoids that develop after a restorative proctocolectomy seems to be similar to morbidity with those developing after ileorectal anastomosis.[251] A large international cohort study demonstrated that significant risk factors for developing desmoid tumors included a positive family history of desmoids, abdominal surgery, and APC mutation site (distal to codon 1444).[252]

The fact that desmoids seem to occur more often in women than men and more often after early colectomy (<18 years) has prompted some experts to suggest considering delaying colectomy for some young female FAP patients.[253] Desmoids cause GI obstruction; constrict arteries, veins, and ureters; and are associated with a 10% to 50% mortality rate. Additional operative procedures usually are of no avail in this condition. Desmoid tumors can respond to radiation when localized and accessible.[254] Unfortunately, most tumors involve the mesentery in these patients, making radiation therapy impractical. Attempts at medical therapy have had some modestly encouraging results. The NSAID sulindac, which can often cause regression of colonic adenomas in FAP (see later), has resulted in partial tumor shrinkage in some patients but no response in others.[255,256] The anti-estrogen drug tamoxifen has been effective in a few patients, as has progesterone[257,258]; a combination of sulindac and tamoxifen is commonly used.[249]

A staging system for FAP-associated desmoid tumors has been proposed that should help with medical decision making (Table 126-13).[259] It appears that patients with early-stage desmoid disease have had a longer colectomy-to-desmoid interval, a somewhat reduced polyp burden, a higher likelihood that their desmoid will remain stable or disappear, and a much better prognosis. Multimodality therapy, including chemotherapy,[260] seems appropriate for stage III and IV disease because of the more aggressive course of these tumors. A scoring system that factors the use of pain medicines, desmoid tumor size larger than 10 cm, and the need for TPN, has been shown in 1 study to help predict mortality in stage III and IV disease.[261] For desmoids that significantly compromise the small bowel mesentery, small intestinal transplantation should be considered.

In addition to desmoid tumors, other soft tissue tumors are well described in FAP and Gardner's syndrome, including epidermoid cysts, fibromas, and lipomas. The epidermoid cysts, also called *inclusion cysts*, have erroneously been referred to as sebaceous cysts in the past. Epidermoid cysts are lined with normal epithelium and contain no sebaceous glands. When multiple epidermoid cysts appear before puberty in these kindreds, it is a harbinger of polyposis. Neoplasms of the biliary tree, liver, and adrenal glands also occur in these syndromes, and papillary carcinoma of the thyroid occurs in 1% of patients with FAP, predominantly in female patients.[262] Hepatoblastoma is rare and can affect very young children in FAP families. The extraintestinal manifestations of FAP have been reviewed in detail elsewhere.[262]

Genotype-Phenotype Correlations

Drawing precise genotype-phenotype correlations in FAP often is difficult because the identical *APC* gene mutation can give rise either to isolated colonic polyposis or to extracolonic manifestations.[222] Moreover, an identical *APC* gene mutation can manifest quite different colonic and extracolonic phenotypic features among unrelated families.[263] Even within a single family, the disease can express itself variably in different persons, including skipped generations and discordance in identical twins.[264] There are even some families that appear phenotypically to have FAP but do not have mutations of the *APC* gene.[265] While some of these may be due to *MUTYH* mutations (see below), other genetic or environmental disease-modifying factors appear to be responsible for generating phenotypic variation.

Despite the discrepancies in genotype-phenotype correlations, some general patterns have emerged (see Fig. 126-12). Profuse polyposis is found in the mid-portion of the gene (between codons 1250 and 1464, but especially around codon 1300), whereas a mild colonic phenotype is observed for mutations that affect the extreme proximal (5′) and distal (3′) ends of the *APC* gene responsible for attenuated FAP (see later). Desmoid tumors often, but not always, are seen with mutations just distal to the profuse polyposis region. CHRPE lesions are present with mutations distal to exon 9. Papillary carcinoma of the thyroid is associated with mutations proximal to the mutation cluster region.

Genetic Testing and Counseling

Genetic testing is an important component of the overall care of patients with FAP and their families, not so much for the management of the affected person but to detect mutant gene carriers.[266] Approximately 20% of patients with FAP have a negative family history and represent new mutations at the *APC* locus.[226] Genetic testing is performed by extracting DNA from peripheral blood leukocytes. Sequencing offers the best sensitivity for mutations of the *APC* gene, but it might detect variants of unknown clinical significance. Because most mutations of the *APC* gene result in a truncated protein product, the in vitro protein truncation test offers a useful method for detecting gene carriers. This assay is successful in about 80% of families tested and has the advantage of only requiring 1 affected person. If it is successful in 1 family member, this test is nearly 100% accurate for identifying other gene carriers in that family. New technology has made *APC* gene sequencing more feasible and affordable.

An affected person is tested first. Absence of a mutation in the affected person suggests that genetic testing of at-risk relatives is not likely to yield clinically useful information and that the family should be screened by clinical tests. A positive gene test allows at-risk relatives to be tested in a more focused manner. It is recommended that testing at-risk children be delayed until age 10 to 12 years, when clinical screening usually begins. Genetic testing of other family members is performed best within the context of a comprehensive genetic counseling program because it raises complex issues such as psychological denial, survivor guilt, premature worrying if testing is performed at too young an age, intrafamily strife, employment discrimination, and medical insurability.[267]

Diagnosis and Screening

Patients with FAP can present with nonspecific symptoms such as hematochezia, diarrhea, and abdominal pain. The key to the diagnosis and management of this disease, however, is to identify the presymptomatic person, and this objective is achieved by the assiduous pursuit of the diagnosis in the relatives of affected patients. The diagnosis is made easily by sigmoidoscopy, given the often diffuse distribution of polyps, but colonoscopy is preferred so that the full phenotype can be appreciated while excluding the presence of carcinoma elsewhere in the colon. The presence of more than 100 polyps and the confirmation that these are adenomas establish the phenotypic diagnosis of FAP.

Studies from St. Mark's Hospital in London on the natural history of FAP suggest that approximately 10 years elapses between the appearance of polyps and the development of cancer[226]; however, it is not advisable to delay surgery once the diagnosis is made, even in presymptomatic patients, except in persons who have not completed puberty. Performing genetic testing at approximately age 10 to 12 years for at-risk persons helps to streamline the clinical evaluation. In a family with a known mutation, children who test positive can then undergo a screening sigmoidoscopy to determine the status of their disease. If the gene test is negative, the child can be spared sigmoidoscopy, although it still might be prudent to perform sigmoidoscopy after adolescence just to offset the rare possibility of laboratory error.

Treatment

Surgery. Surgery is the only reasonable management option for colonic polyposis in FAP. The timing and extent of surgery are the major clinical considerations. Because any rectal mucosa that is left behind is at risk for developing carcinoma, the optimal treatment is to perform total proctocolectomy either with a conventional ileostomy or as a restorative proctocolectomy with ileal pouch-anal anastomosis. For the most part, the latter operation in skilled hands is associated with little morbidity and is preferred by patients, who must nonetheless be advised about the risk of decreased fecundity among women undergoing this procedure.[268] After restorative proctocolectomy, the ileal pouch needs to be monitored for the future development of adenomas and, very rarely, carcinoma.[269] For some patients, total proctocolectomy with conventional ileostomy is unacceptable, and they also do not want to risk the complications of an ileal pouch. In such cases, the decision to perform a subtotal colectomy with ileorectal anastomosis (IRA) can be considered, bearing in mind that the rectal segment will remain at risk for carcinoma, and the patient will have to comply with periodic surveillance examinations. A meta-analysis concluded that compared with restorative proctocolectomy, IRA was associated with less bowel frequency, nocturnal defecation, and use of incontinence pads, but more fecal urgency.[270] The 2 types of operation demonstrated comparable rates of sexual dysfunction, dietary restriction, and postoperative complications.

In contrast to older patients who undergo IRA, about one fifth of younger patients (median age, 35 years) with many rectal polyps develop cancer in 5 to 23 years. According to the Mayo Clinic experience of patients who are followed for over 20 years, about three fifths develop carcinoma in the rectal segment despite semiannual sigmoidoscopic surveillance and fulguration of all polyps.[271] The prognosis in patients who develop rectal cancers in this setting is quite poor; the 5-year disease-free survival rate has been reported to be 25%. In patients with IRA, the risk of subsequent rectal cancer was higher in patients who had an *APC* mutation between codons 1250 and 1464, a finding that awaits confirmation in other studies.[272] These data provide a strong case for total proctocolectomy for FAP patients.

In spite of this ominous warning, others have advocated rectum-sparing operations and have achieved reasonable degrees of success. The Memorial Sloan-Kettering group in New York has asserted that a subtotal colectomy is safe for patients whose rectums are free of polyps. They also spare the rectum in patients with rectal polyps, carefully follow the patients, and perform additional surgery as soon as malignant change is found.[273] The St. Mark's group in London reports satisfaction with rectum-sparing procedures for all patients with FAP and fulgurates only adenomas 5 mm or larger in diameter at 3- to 6-month intervals. This group reported that 11 of 173 of their patients developed carcinoma in the rectum, but that only 3 of the 11 died of rectal cancer.[274] The Cleveland Clinic has advocated the use of colectomy with IRA and reported an actuarial survivorship rate of 80% in 133 patients after 20 years, despite the presence of rectal polyps.[275] Other groups in the USA and Europe also prefer subtotal colectomy and IRA, but approximately one quarter of patients treated this way have required a total proctectomy at a later date for cancer or intractable benign polyps.[276]

It appears, therefore, that patients might elect the more limited procedure if they are willing to comply with rigorous follow-up (sigmoidoscopy every 3 to 6 months) and accept a risk of malignancy in the rectum of approximately 1% per year. Because of decreased fecundity rates associated with restorative proctocolectomy, young women with FAP might elect to undergo primary subtotal colectomy with IRA, with plans to convert to a restorative proctocolectomy after they are finished with child-bearing. However, they should be aware that desmoid tumors arising after the first operation might prevent secondary restorative proctocolectomy in a substantial minority of them.[277] Medical therapy has provided some options for the surgical management of FAP, but as discussed in the next section, rectal cancer can still occur despite adenoma regression.

Medical Treatment. Spontaneous regression of rectal polyps has been reported after subtotal colectomy and IRA for FAP,[278] and this must be taken into account when one is evaluating the response of a rectal-sparing surgical procedure or medical treatment for this disease. Because of its antioxidant characteristics and its effects in experimental colon cancer, ascorbic acid (vitamin C, 3 g/day) was tried in patients with FAP who had undergone subtotal colectomy with IRA at least 1 year earlier. A modest effect was observed, but it was neither consistent nor strong enough to advocate for general use.[279] Supplemental dietary calcium also was ineffective in polyposis patients.[280] A more ambitious trial has been reported in which 58 patients with FAP were treated with ascorbic acid (4 g/day), alpha-tocopherol (vitamin E, 400 mg/day), and supplemental fiber (22.5 g/day); a modest effect was seen after 2 years of therapy.[281]

A higher degree of enthusiasm has been generated for the use of NSAIDs in the treatment of colorectal polyps in FAP.[282] Sulindac has been shown in both uncontrolled and controlled trials to decrease the number and size of colorectal adenomas in patients with FAP[282] who had intact colons, as well as those with subtotal colectomy and IRA. Unfortunately, maintaining these patients on sulindac does not protect them from developing rectal cancer, and the drug's effect on reducing adenomas is reversible on its discontinuation. Sulindac is less successful for controlling upper GI neoplasia, and it does not appear to prevent the initial onset of adenomas in children who are genotypically affected with FAP.[283]

The mechanism by which sulindac causes colorectal adenoma regression in patients with FAP might relate in part to its ability to inhibit COX (prostaglandin synthase) activity and thereby to interfere with arachidonic acid metabolism. Because colorectal tumors (but not normal colonocytes) have high levels of COX-2 expression, it is possible that COX-2 inhibition by sulindac is responsible for adenoma regression.[284] Sulindac also is capable of restoring the deficient apoptosis seen in colonocytes of patients with FAP, even without affecting colonocyte proliferation.[285] The sulfone derivative of sulindac has no inhibitory effect on either COX-1 or COX-2 enzymes, yet it too has been shown to cause regression of rectal adenoma in FAP patients.[286] FAP patients with rectal adenomas treated with celecoxib, a selective COX-2 inhibitor, also demonstrated a significant reduction in the number and size of adenomas.[287] Likewise, in children, celecoxib at a dose corresponding to an adult dose of 400 mg twice daily was associated with a 44% reduction in the number of colorectal polyps.[286] Celecoxib reduced the number of duodenal adenomas in 1 study,[282] but further confirmation of this effect is awaited. Aspirin at a dose of 600 mg/day showed a trend toward lower polyp count and size in the CAPP1 Study (Colorectal Adenoma/Carcinoma Prevention Programme),[288] but whether lower doses of aspirin might be helpful is not known.

Screening of Extracolonic Organs

Upper GI screening should be performed at the time colonic adenomas are diagnosed or at least by age 25 years (see Table 126-12). A full evaluation of the entire small intestine should be performed at baseline. This can be done by small bowel series, capsule endoscopy, double balloon enteroscopy, or, if necessary, by performing intraoperative enteroscopy at the time of initial proctocolectomy. Upper GI polyps are rare before the onset of colonic disease, but side-viewing upper endoscopy should be performed in addition to conventional forward-viewing endoscopy because of its better visualization of the duodenal ampulla.

The overall approach to upper GI polyps is one of conservatism. Gastric polyps should be sampled to see if they are adenomas or fundic gland polyps with dysplasia. In the duodenum, villous adenomas, adenomas with high-grade dysplasia, large adenomas, and symptomatic adenomas, regardless of histology, should be removed if possible. Endoscopic ablation of periampullary adenomas can be performed relatively safely by endoscopists skilled in this procedure, but regrowth of adenomatous tissue is common.[279] If duodenal polyps are small or few, surveillance can be performed every 1 to 3 years. The presence of worrisome duodenal adenomas or adenomatous change of the duodenal papilla warrants endoscopic inspection at more frequent intervals. Surgical resection of the duodenum, whether by local excision or pancreaticoduodenectomy, may be required in selected patients. Screening of other organs at risk for cancer is summarized in Table 126-12.

Variant Familial Adenomatous Polyposis Syndromes

Turcot's Syndrome (Glioma-Polyposis)

The term *Turcot's syndrome* applies to a syndrome of familial colonic polyposis with primary tumors of the central nervous system (see Table 126-11).[289,290] The phenotypic spectrum is broad, with colonic manifestations that range from a single adenoma to profuse adenomatosis coli and brain tumors of different histopathologic types. Controversy exists as to whether this syndrome is inherited in an autosomal dominant or autosomal recessive manner.

A comprehensive molecular diagnostic study of 14 Turcot's syndrome families has clarified that Turcot's syndrome kindreds fall into 2 groups based on their types of brain tumor and particular genetic alteration.[291] The more common group has germline mutations of the *APC* gene, and these patients tend to have medulloblastomas. In several cases, the brain tumor preceded the diagnosis of polyposis. The *APC* mutations were heterogeneous, with no association between specific mutations and the development of brain tumors. The inactivation of both *APC* alleles in brain tumor tissue implicates the *APC* gene in the pathogenesis of these neoplasms. The risk of cerebellar medulloblastoma in FAP was calculated to be 92 times that of the general population. In contrast, the second group of patients, including the family originally described by Turcot, had glioblastoma multiforme tumors. These persons were found to have germline mutations in DNA MMR genes typical of Lynch syndrome.

Thus, Turcot's syndrome can be considered a true variant of FAP, although, as with Gardner's syndrome, maintaining a separate designation may be superfluous. Because of familial clustering, once a person with Turcot's syndrome has been identified, screening for affected family members should include colonoscopy as well as imaging studies of the brain (see Table 126-12).

Attenuated Adenomatous Polyposis Syndromes

Patients with classic FAP syndromes typically have tens to thousands of colonic adenomas; however, an attenuated form of FAP (AFAP) has been identified in which persons manifest fewer adenomas that often have a flat rather than polypoid growth pattern and tend to cluster in the proximal colon.[292] AFAP is associated with germline mutations of the very proximal and distal portions of the *APC* gene.[293] Like classic FAP, patients with AFAP are prone to develop multiple gastric fundic gland polyps, duodenal and gastric adenomas, and even periampullary carcinoma[294]; however, CRCs arise at a later age (≈55 years) in AFAP patients than in those with classic FAP. In AFAP patients, colonoscopic surveillance is recommended every 2 years starting at age 18 to 20 years.[243]

It is becoming increasingly clear that germline mutations, not only in the *APC* gene but in other genes of the *APC* pathway, such as for β-catenin and axin, can give rise to a multiple adenomatous polyposis phenotype. Multiple colonic adenomas, CRC, and even HPs have been described in a Finnish family with familial tooth agenesis as a result of a germline mutation of *Axin2*.[295] Even more intriguing is the observation that germline defects in genes involved in DNA repair also can result in a phenotype that mimics AFAP. For example, numerous colonic adenomas have been described in a patient with Bloom's syndrome, a condition characterized by growth retardation, male sterility, facial erythema, and multiple cancers resulting from increased chromosomal breakage.[296] It appears that the genomic instability induced by mutations in the causative *BLM* gene affects the *APC* gene, thereby resulting in the polyposis phenotype.

Mutations of the *MUTYH* (also called *MYH*) gene are a common cause of the multiple colorectal adenoma phenotype.[297] Among patients with 15 to 100 adenomas, up to 30% have germline (usually biallelic) *MUTYH* mutations.[243] Normally, when DNA is damaged, MUTYH acts in concert with other DNA base-excision repair enzymes to prevent mutations from occurring (Fig. 126-16). When *MUTYH* is defective, G:C → T:A transversions occur. Because the *APC* gene is a major target of MUTYH-induced mutations, the resulting loss of APC function gives rise to multiple adenomas. Colon cancers that occur are usually microsatellite stable.

Clinical features of MUTYH polyposis include multiple adenomas (usually 5 to 100, rarely a florid polyposis), frequent development of CRC, and even some HPs. The phenotype occurs at a later age than does FAP. Gastric cancer, duodenal adenoma, osteoma, and CHRPE lesions have been described in patients with *MUTYH* mutations, but unlike FAP, MUTYH polyposis is an autosomal recessive disorder. Thus, genetic testing and counseling is directed more toward siblings and spouses than to parents or children. It is recommended that patients with more than 10 adenomas should be tested for *MUTYH* gene mutations.[243] The most common mutations are Y179C and G396D (formerly called Y165C and G382D).[298] Biallelic, but not monoallelic, *MUTYH* mutations have been associated with increased risk of CRC. Approximately 1% of the general population is heterozygous for an *MUTYH* mutation. Like AFAP patients, colonoscopic surveillance of patients with biallelic *MUTYH* mutations is recommended every 2 years starting at age 18 to 20 years.[243]

It was recently recognized that *MLH1* and *KRAS* can also be targets of defective *MUTYH* gene function, resulting in a phenotype that may mimic Lynch syndrome or serrated polyposis, respectively. It has therefore been suggested that

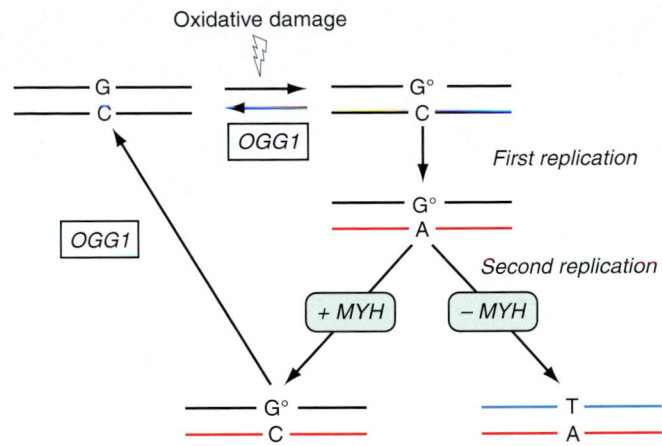

FIGURE 126-16. Function of the *MYH* gene in DNA base excision repair. Oxidative damage gives rise to 8-oxoguanine triphosphate, which is incorporated into DNA (G°). With the next DNA replication, DNA polymerase will preferentially insert adenine (A) instead of cytosine (C) opposite G°, giving rise to G°:A mispairs, with G° in the template strand. In the presence of normal *MYH* gene function (+MYH), with the subsequent replication, adenine is removed and base-excision repair will convert G°:A to G°:C, which can then be repaired by 8-oxoguanine glycolase 1 (OGG1) to GC. In the absence of *MYH* function (−MYH), G°:A mispairs remain uncorrected, giving rise to G:C → T:A transversion mutations.

the term "MYH-associated neoplasia" (MAN) should replace the term "MYH-associated polyposis" (MAP).[299]

Hamartomatous Polyposis Syndromes

Several familial syndromes have been described that are characterized by multiple hamartomatous polyps of the GI tract. These include Peutz-Jeghers syndrome, juvenile polyposis syndrome, *PTEN* (phosphatase and tensin homolog) hamartoma tumor syndromes (Cowden's syndrome and Bannayan-Riley-Ruvalcaba syndrome), and other rare syndromes (Table 126-14). Most of these syndromes are associated with an increased risk of CRC. The progression of these polyps to cancer is not well understood but represents a different mechanism than that seen with adenomatous polyposis. This mechanism has been called the "landscaper phenomenon" because changes that predominantly affect the lamina propria are what lead to the epithelial cancers.

Peutz-Jeghers Syndrome

Peutz in 1921 and Jeghers in 1949 described the familial syndrome consisting of mucocutaneous pigmentation and GI polyposis that now bears their names. Peutz-Jeghers syndrome appears to be inherited as a single pleiotropic autosomal dominant gene with variable and incomplete penetrance.[300,301] Germline mutations of the *STK11/LKB1*, a serine-threonine kinase gene on chromosome 19p, cause this syndrome,[302,303] but not all families with Peutz-Jeghers syndrome are linked to this gene locus, suggesting genetic heterogeneity.

Early in infancy, the characteristic mucocutaneous pigmentation of Peutz-Jeghers syndrome may be noted. These deposits of melanin, which develop in 95% of affected individuals, are found most commonly around the mouth, nose, lips, buccal mucosa, hands, and feet, and they also can occur in the perianal and genital regions (Fig. 126-17). The macular

TABLE 126-14 Familial Hamartomatous Polyposis Syndromes

Syndrome	Mutated Gene	Polyps	Location of GI Polyps	Other Features
Peutz-Jeghers syndrome	STK11/LKB1	Hamartomas with bands of smooth muscle in the lamina propria	Small intestine Stomach Colon	Pigmented lesions (mouth, hands, feet) Ovarian sex cord tumors Sertoli tumors of the testes Airway polyps Pancreatic cancer Breast cancer Colon and esophageal cancer
Juvenile polyposis	MADH4, BMPR1A, ENG	Juvenile polyps; also adenomas and hyperplastic polyps	Colon Small intestine Stomach	Colon cancer in some families Congenital abnormalities
Cowden's disease	PTEN	Hamartomas with disorganized muscularis mucosae	Stomach Colon	Trichilemmomas and papillomas Other hamartomas Benign and malignant breast disease Benign and malignant thyroid disease
Bannayan-Ruvalcaba-Riley syndrome	PTEN	Juvenile polyps	Colon	Macroencephaly; developmental delay
Neurofibromatosis	NF1 RET	Neurofibromas	Small intestine Stomach Colon	von Recklinghausen's disease MEN IIB

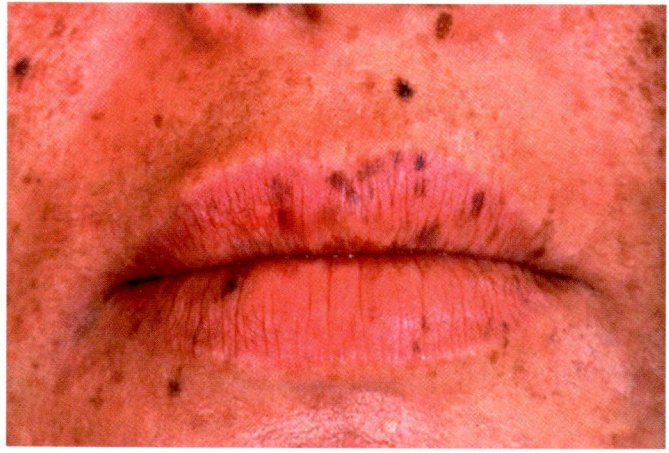

FIGURE 126-17. Mucocutaneous pigmentation of Peutz-Jeghers syndrome.

lesions are brown to greenish-black, are smooth and hairless, and, except for the buccal pigmentation, tend to fade at puberty. The clinician must distinguish these melanin deposits from ordinary freckles. Freckles are sparse near the nostrils and mouth, are absent at birth (but can occur in infancy), and never appear on the buccal mucosa. The presence of this pigmentation should alert the clinician to this syndrome, but the skin lesions and intestinal lesions occasionally are inherited separately.

Peutz-Jeghers polyps can increase in size progressively and cause small intestinal obstruction or intussusception that can occur as early as infancy. The polyps may be found in the stomach, small intestine, or colon, but they tend to be most prominent in the small intestine. Acute upper GI bleeding and chronic fecal blood loss can complicate the disease. The

average age of diagnosis is 23 to 26 years. Carcinomas of the colon, duodenum, jejunum, and ileum have been reported, and although it has been assumed that these cancers arise from rare foci of adenomatous epithelium that can develop within the Peutz-Jeghers polyps, evidence for loss of STK11/LKB1 expression in Peutz-Jeghers polyps even without dysplastic epithelium raises the possibility that the STK11/LKB1 gene itself might be the gatekeeper to carcinogenesis in this syndrome, much like APC is the gatekeeper in FAP.[304,305] Colon polyps should be removed for histologic examination, but the relative inaccessibility of small intestinal polyps and the unpredictability of neoplastic complications make it difficult to have a routine surveillance program for small intestinal cancer.

Cancers throughout the GI tract and other organs are quite common in familial Peutz-Jeghers syndrome (see Table 126-14).[306] The mean age of diagnosis of cancer is approximately 40 to 50 years, with a 93% overall cumulative risk of developing cancer between 15 and 64 years of age. The most common cancers include breast (54%), colon (39%), pancreas (36%), stomach (29%), ovary (21%), and small intestine (13%). Ovarian cysts and distinctive ovarian sex cord tumors are seen in 5% to 12% of female patients with this syndrome.[307] The ovarian tumors are histologically unique and can occur in young patients. Hormonally active Sertoli cell testicular tumors with feminizing features can occur in young boys with Peutz-Jeghers syndrome.[308] Breast cancers may be found in young women and may be bilateral,[309] and the magnitude of breast cancer risk in this syndrome is similar to that for other hereditary forms of breast cancer caused by germline mutations of BRCA1 and BRCA2. Other tumors that can occur in this syndrome include pancreatic cancers in young patients and polyps or cancers of the biliary tree and gallbladder.[310] Thus, Peutz-Jeghers syndrome confers an increased risk for cancer in a number of GI and nonintestinal organs. Neither the severity of polyposis, nor the presence of pigmentation, correlate with the risk of cancer.[298]

Guidelines for screening are difficult to make but should be directed toward at-risk organs for which early detection and treatment are reasonable, such as the entire GI tract, gonads (in both sexes), and breasts (in women). Video capsule endoscopy often reveals more polyps than do barium studies.[244,311] COX-2 inhibition can reduce the polyp burden in Peutz-Jeghers syndrome patients,[312] and rapamycin seems to reduce the polyp burden in an animal model of Peutz-Jeghers syndrome[313]; the role of these agents in clinical practice is not yet defined. With respect to the luminal GI tract, it is recommended that colonoscopy and small bowel imaging (by capsule or enteroscopy) be considered at age 8 and repeated every 2 years. Endoscopic polypectomy is the mainstay of treatment. Double balloon enteroscopy, or intraoperative endoscopy of the entire GI tract, should be considered. Surgery is reserved for large, difficult to remove, or recurrent polyps; attention is focused on polypectomy while trying to avoid bowel resection as much as possible.

Tuberous Sclerosis

Tuberous sclerosis is characterized by the presence of hamartomatous lesions, with the classic triad of mental retardation, epilepsy, and adenoma sebaceum, a misnamed lesion that are angiofibromas, and which occur in the skin of the central part of the face.[314] Hamartomatous polyps resembling Peutz-Jeghers polyps, as well as adenomatous polyps, can occur in this disease and often are located in the distal colon.

Juvenile Polyposis Syndrome

Juvenile polyps are distinctive hamartomas that usually are solitary and are located principally in the rectums of children and occasionally in adults. They have a smooth surface and are covered by normal colonic epithelium. Juvenile polyposis (i.e., the presence of multiple juvenile polyps) is a diagnosis of exclusion. The *PTEN* hamartoma syndromes, which also can be associated with juvenile polyps (e.g., Cowden's disease and Bannayan-Ruvalcaba-Riley syndrome) should be excluded (see next section). Once that is done, juvenile polyposis syndrome can be defined by any 1 of the following criteria: 5 or more juvenile polyps of the colon and rectum, juvenile polyps throughout the GI tract, or any number of juvenile polyps in the GI tract with a family history of juvenile polyps.[315] Extracolonic manifestations can affect the central nervous system (macrocephaly, hydrocephalus), thorax (coarctation of aorta, atrial septal defects, tetralogy of Fallot), urogenital tract (undescended testes, bifid uterus and vagina, unilateral renal agenesis), and GI tract (Meckel's diverticulum, malrotation).[315]

Juvenile polyposis typically causes GI bleeding, intussusception, and obstruction. The clinical presentations of juvenile polyposis syndrome and FAP differ. Juvenile polyps produce symptoms in childhood, whereas the adenomatosis syndromes rarely manifest in childhood and usually become evident in early adult life. The average age of a patient with juvenile polyposis syndrome is 4.5 years in the nonfamilial form and 9.5 years in the familial form.[316] The risk of colon and upper GI cancer is increased in familial juvenile polyposis.[315] In a large Iowa kindred, 38% of affected persons developed colon cancer and 21% developed upper GI cancer.[317] Others report a somewhat lower risk estimate of 17% incidence of GI malignancy.[318] Although juvenile polyps per se are not considered neoplastic, the synchronous adenomatous polyps and mixed juvenile-adenomatous polyps of these patients are what give rise to concern.[319,320] Thus, these polyps must be scrutinized by the pathologist for evidence of a mixed adenomatous appearance, coexisting adenomas must be excluded, and kindreds with CRC should be subjected to careful colonoscopic surveillance.

Juvenile polyposis syndrome manifests autosomal dominant inheritance. Approximately 20% to 25% of cases have a germline mutation of *MADH4 (SMAD4)*, a tumor suppressor gene involved in TGF-β signaling.[321] Another 20% of cases are caused by germline mutations of bone morphogenetic protein receptor 1A *(BMPR1A)*, another member of the TGF-β superfamily that depends on MADH4 for signal transduction. Mutations of *ENG* (endoglin) are associated with very early-onset juvenile polyposis.[298] Mutations in *ENG* are more common in hereditary hemorrhagic telangiectasia (HHT), and a syndrome of combined HHT and juvenile polyposis has been seen in up to 20% of individuals with *SMAD4* mutations, as well as with *ENG* mutations. A family history of juvenile polyposis syndrome occurs in 33% of cases (the other 66% are sporadic juvenile polyposis syndrome).

The diagnosis of juvenile polyposis syndrome is made by endoscopy (see Table 126-12). Screening colonoscopy and upper endoscopy usually begins after 15 years of age if symptoms have not occurred already. The cumulative risk of colorectal CRC and gastric cancer is approximately 50% and 21%, respectively. Asymptomatic relatives also should be screened. Identification of a *MADH4*, *BMPR1A*, or *ENG* mutation in a family member helps guide screening, analogous to *APC* mutation testing.

In general, juvenile polyps should be removed because of their tendency to bleed and obstruct. With a small number of polyps, periodic endoscopic polypectomy may be adequate. It has been suggested that surveillance endoscopy with polypectomy of the upper and lower GI tracts be performed yearly until the patient is polyp free, and then every 3 years.[315] For persons with numerous juvenile polyps, colectomy should be considered. If subtotal colectomy with IRA is chosen, the rectal segment must remain under surveillance.

Family history must be defined in patients with multiple juvenile polyps to determine the sites of involvement and the history of neoplastic lesions. Gastric polyposis can be quite diffuse and cause anemia, posing a difficult management problem. The risk of gastric cancer may be as high as 21%.[315]

PTEN Hamartoma Tumor Syndromes

Germline mutations of *PTEN*, a tyrosine phosphatase protein that functions as a tumor suppressor, account for 81% and 57% of Cowden's disease and Bannayan-Ruvalcaba-Riley syndrome cases, respectively.[315]

Cowden's Disease. Although reported in only a very small number of families, Cowden's disease, or the multiple hamartoma syndrome, consists of hamartomatous polyps of the stomach, small intestine, and colon along with extraintestinal manifestations that include orocutaneous hamartomas, fibrocystic disease and cancer of the breast, nontoxic goiter, and thyroid cancer.[315] The hallmark of this autosomal dominant condition is the presence of multiple facial trichilemmomas, which arise from follicular epithelium and typically occur around the eyes, nose, and mouth. GI symptoms and CRC are uncommon. The colorectal polyps in Cowden's disease are distinctive lesions characterized by disorganization and proliferation of the muscularis mucosae, with nearly normal overlying colonic epithelium.[322]

Ganglioneuromatosis of the colon and glycogenic acanthosis of the esophagus have been reported in association with Cowden's disease.[323] There does not appear to be an increased risk of GI cancer and, therefore, there are no specific screening recommendations for the colon; the major complication is cancer of the breast, uterus, and thyroid.

Bannayan-Ruvalcaba-Riley Syndrome. A rare autosomal dominant syndrome, Bannayan-Ruvalcaba-Riley syndrome consists of hamartomatous GI polyposis with macrocephaly, developmental delay and other developmental abnormalities, and pigmented spots on the penis.[324,325] Thyroiditis also has been described.

Rare Inherited Hamartomatous Polyposis Syndromes

Hereditary Mixed Polyposis Syndrome. A large kindred with a tendency to develop colonic polyps of mixed histologic types has been identified.[326] The disease appears to be inherited in an autosomal dominant fashion and is confined to the colon. The earliest age of onset of polyps was 23 years, the median age of symptoms was 40 years, and the median age of colon cancer diagnosis was 47 years. The characteristic polyp was an atypical juvenile polyp, although some persons had polyps of mixed histology, and others had more than 1 histologic type of polyp, including serrated adenomas. Linkage to chromosome 15q14-q22 has been described in a region that overlaps with a possible colonic cancer gene, CRAC1.[327,328] A gene duplication leading to increased and ectopic expression of GREM1 has been associated with this syndrome.[329] Colon cancer risk is increased, supporting the recommendation of surveillance colonoscopy every 1 to 2 years.[315]

Intestinal Ganglioneuromatosis and Neurofibromatosis. Approximately 25% of patients with von Recklinghausen's syndrome (caused by NF1 gene mutations) have neurofibromatosis involving the upper digestive tract, with multiple submucosal neurofibromas or, less commonly, ganglioneuromas that can cause dyspepsia, abdominal pain, or hemorrhage.[330] GI involvement usually is incidental and asymptomatic. Severe, uncontrolled symptoms have required surgical treatment in a few cases. Multiple intestinal ganglioneuromas also have been observed in families and individual cases unrelated to von Recklinghausen's disease.[331] Ganglioneuromas throughout the GI tract can occur in patients with MEN type IIB, related to mutations of the RET gene.[332]

Devon Family Syndrome. Multiple and recurrent inflammatory fibroid polyps of the stomach and intestine have been reported in a family.[333] These lesions, histologically distinct from juvenile polyps, can cause GI obstruction, with symptoms beginning in adult life.

Basal Cell Nevus Syndrome. Basal cell nevus syndrome is another syndrome that has been associated with multiple gastric hamartomatous polyps[334]; however, several kindreds have been reported without mention of GI lesions.

Noninherited Polyposis Syndromes

Serrated Polyposis Syndrome

Serrated polyposis syndrome (SPS) is characterized by multiple serrated polyps in the colon. SPS was previously called *hyperplastic polyposis syndrome* when HPs were the only known histologically serrated polyps in the colon. Patients with SPS often demonstrate the full spectrum of serrated polyps (HPs, SSP/As with or without dysplasia, traditional serrated adenomas) and even conventional adenomas. The WHO definition of SPS is: (1) at least 5 histologically diagnosed serrated polyps proximal to the sigmoid colon, with at least 2 larger than 10 mm; or (2) any number of serrated polyps occurring proximal to the sigmoid colon in a person who has a first-degree relative with SPS; or (3) more than 20 serrated polyps of any size distributed throughout the colon.[335] Others have categorized SPS into 3 phenotypes: (1) large SSP/As in the proximal colon with a high risk of

(CRC), (2) many small HPs throughout the colorectum with a lower risk of CRC, and (3) many small left-sided serrated polyps.[336]

A germline mutation that might explain this syndrome has not yet been identified. Although most cases of SPS are considered sporadic, hallmarks suggestive of an inherited syndrome include multiple lesions, younger age of onset of lesions, family history of SPS, and CRC. In fact, nearly half of SPS patients have a family history of CRC and also an elevated risk of SPS, suggesting there may well be an underlying genetic cause.[189] The median age at diagnosis is 44 to 62 years, with near equal gender distribution. There seems to be an absence of gastroduodenal polyps in this syndrome.[337] The risk of CRC is not well defined. Case series report rates of synchronous CRC at diagnosis of 25% to 50%, and the cumulative risk of CRC at 5 years for patients under surveillance was 7% in a retrospective series.[189] Surgery is recommended when CRC is diagnosed or when the size and/or number of polyps does not permit endoscopic control. Removal of colonic segments with cancer and those with large polyps is recommended, and usually the rectum is retained. Practically all patients with a retained rectum will demonstrate polyps on subsequent endoscopy, at least half of which are SSP/A or adenomas.[337] Colonoscopic surveillance of any residual colon or rectum is recommended annually, with attempts to clear all polyps or at least those larger than 5 mm. It is also suggested that first-degree relatives of patients with SPS begin their screening colonoscopy at age 40, or 10 years younger than the youngest affected relative.[189]

Cronkhite-Canada Syndrome

In 1955, Cronkhite and Canada reported the first examples of an acquired nonfamilial syndrome that now bears their names.[338] It is characterized by the presence of diffuse GI polyposis, dystrophic changes in the fingernails, alopecia, cutaneous hyperpigmentation, diarrhea, weight loss, abdominal pain, and complications of malnutrition.[339] Patients typically are middle-aged or older (average, 62 years) and present fairly acutely with a rapidly progressive illness consisting of chronic diarrhea and protein-losing enteropathy with the associated integumentary abnormalities. The diarrhea is attributable primarily to diffuse small intestinal mucosal injury, but bacterial overgrowth may be contributory. GI polyps are found in 52% to 96% of patients and range in location from the stomach to the rectum.[339] These polyps are hamartomas similar to the juvenile (retention) type, but unlike juvenile polyposis, the mucosa between polyps is histologically abnormal, with edema, congestion, and inflammation. As is the case with juvenile polyps, there may be foci of adenomatous epithelium that can confer a risk of carcinoma. It is estimated that the risk of colon cancer is approximately 9%, and the risk of adenomas or adenomatous change is 40%.[315] Gastric cancer risk is also increased. Thus, screening of the colon and stomach should be considered.

The malabsorption syndrome is progressive in most patients, and the prognosis is poor because there is no specific therapy. It has been suggested that complete symptomatic remission occasionally may be achieved with supportive management. In some cases, a variety of medical and surgical measures have been employed, making it difficult to identify the essential therapeutic modality(s). Glucocorticoids, anabolic steroids, antibiotics, and surgical resections have been tried in many of the patients in whom remissions have been reported. Despite this therapeutic dilemma, aggressive nutritional support appears to be the most important factor in effecting a favorable outcome. Enteral feeding (if possible) or parenteral feeding (if necessary) with sources of calories, nitrogen, and lipids, in addition to appropriate fluids, electrolytes, vitamins, and minerals, has resulted in complete symptomatic remissions with resolution of all the ectodermal aberrations. Antibiotics may be beneficial when SIBO contributes to the malabsorption. Although glucocorticoids have been used in some of the cases of symptomatic remission, the evidence to support their use is weak. Surgical therapy offers less and is risky in these malnourished patients.

One case of complete remission has been reported in a patient managed only with enteral administration of a nutritionally balanced complete liquid diet.[340] Attention should be paid to the possibility of secondary lactose or other disaccharide intolerance or protein-losing enteropathy in patients with diffuse small intestinal disease. Specific management awaits a better understanding of this perplexing syndrome.

Lymphomatous Polyposis

Lymphoma can manifest as multiple lymphomatous polyps of the GI tract.[341] A variety of pathologic variants of Hodgkin's and non-Hodgkin's lymphomas can manifest this way, including immunoproliferative small intestinal disease. One variant worthy of mention is the mantle zone lymphoma (MZL), which can produce nodular collections of proliferating lymphocytes in wide mantles that surround benign-appearing germinal centers.[342] The MZL has a characteristic histologic appearance and can have an indolent clinical course. These lesions are important because they require an adequate biopsy to distinguish them from true epithelial polyps and because of the possibility that MZL can have a prolonged clinical course.

Nodular Lymphoid Hyperplasia

Nodular lymphoid hyperplasia is a rare lymphoproliferative condition that is not related to a specific disease. It can be seen in healthy children and also has been described in the terminal ileum of some patients with Gardner's syndrome and in some immunodeficiency syndromes, particularly IgA deficiency. These polyps, which are more common in the small intestine and measure approximately 3 to 6 mm, typically do not cause symptoms.

KEY REFERENCES

Full references for this chapter can be found on www.expertconsult.com.

21. Kudo S, Lambert R, Allen JI, et al. Nonpolypoid neoplastic lesions of the colorectal mucosa. Gastrointest Endosc 2008; 68(4 Suppl):S3-47.
75. Kahi CJ, Rex DK, Imperiale TF. Screening, surveillance, and primary prevention for colorectal cancer: A review of the recent literature. Gastroenterology 2008; 135:380-99.
88. Arber N, Levin B. Chemoprevention of colorectal neoplasia: The potential for personalized medicine. Gastroenterology 2008; 134:1224-37.
126. Levin B, Lieberman DA, McFarland B, et al. Screening and surveillance for the early detection of colorectal cancer and adenomatous polyps, 2008: A joint guideline from the American Cancer Society, the US Multi-Society Task Force on Colorectal Cancer, and the American College of Radiology. Gastroenterology 2008; 134:1570-95.
166. Williams JG, Pullan RD, Hill J, et al. Management of the malignant colorectal polyp: ACPGBI position statement. Colorectal Dis 2013; 15:1-38.
188. Lieberman DA, Rex DK, Winawer SJ, et al. Guidelines for colonoscopy surveillance after screening and polypectomy: A consensus update by the US Multi-Society Task Force on Colorectal Cancer. Gastroenterology 2012; 143:844-57.
189. Rex DK, Ahnen DJ, Baron JA, et al. Serrated lesions of the colorectum: Review and recommendations from an expert panel. Am J Gastroenterol 2012; 107:1315-29.
243. Vasen HF, Möslein G, Alonso A, et al. Guidelines for the clinical management of familial adenomatous polyposis (FAP). Gut 2008; 57:704-13.
282. Kim B, Giardiello GM. Chemoprevention in familial adenomatous polyposis. Best Pract Res Clin Gastroenterol 2011; 25:607-22.
298. Shah N, Lindor NM. Lower gastrointestinal tract cancer predisposition syndromes. Hematol Oncol Clin N Am 2010; 24:1229-52.
315. Calva D, Howe JR. Hamartomatous polyposis syndromes. Surg Clin North Am 2008; 88:779-817.

CHAPTER OUTLINE

Cancer of the colon and rectum (colorectal cancer [CRC]) is a major cause of cancer-associated morbidity and mortality in North America, Europe, and other regions with similar lifestyles and dietary habits. CRC is the fourth most common newly diagnosed internal cancer overall in the USA, after cancers of the prostate, breast, and lung, and currently constitutes 9% of new cancers in men and women. In 2014, there will be an estimated 136,830 new CRC cases in the USA and 51,520 deaths.[1] CRC accounts for more than half of all GI cancer in the USA, and is the leading cause of GI-related mortality.[2] In the USA, CRC incidence rates in men and women are similar, although there appears to be a male predominance worldwide. Approximately 5% of the American population eventually will develop invasive colon or rectal cancer, and more than 6 million Americans who are alive today will die of the disease; the lifetime risk of dying from CRC in the USA is 2.5%.[3] Globally, CRC is the third most common cancer in men and the second most common in women, with mortality paralleling incidence. 1.2 million new CRC cases and 608,700 related deaths were estimated to have occurred worldwide in 2008.[4] Despite evidence that 5-year survival is 90% when CRC is diagnosed at an early stage, less than 40% of cases are diagnosed when the cancer is still localized.

Rapid growth of knowledge about the molecular and biological characteristics of CRC has provided useful insights into the pathogenesis of these neoplasms and cancer in general. New insights also have been gained in regard to primary prevention. Because CRC arises over long periods as a result of interactions between genetic predisposition and environmental insults, it has become possible to identify preneoplastic and early neoplastic lesions better and to improve survival rates. Rapidly evolving knowledge of CRC pathogenesis, especially in high-risk groups, is allowing the development of new tools to identify those who will benefit most from cancer surveillance and from adjuvant therapy following potentially curative surgery. After decades with limited options for treating advanced disease, new options for chemotherapy are now available.

EPIDEMIOLOGY

The frequency of CRC varies remarkably among different populations (Fig. 127-1).[4,5] Incidence rates are highest in developed countries in North America, Europe, Australia, and New Zealand; and lowest in South Central Asia, and sub-Saharan Africa. Internationally, the incidence of colon cancer in men

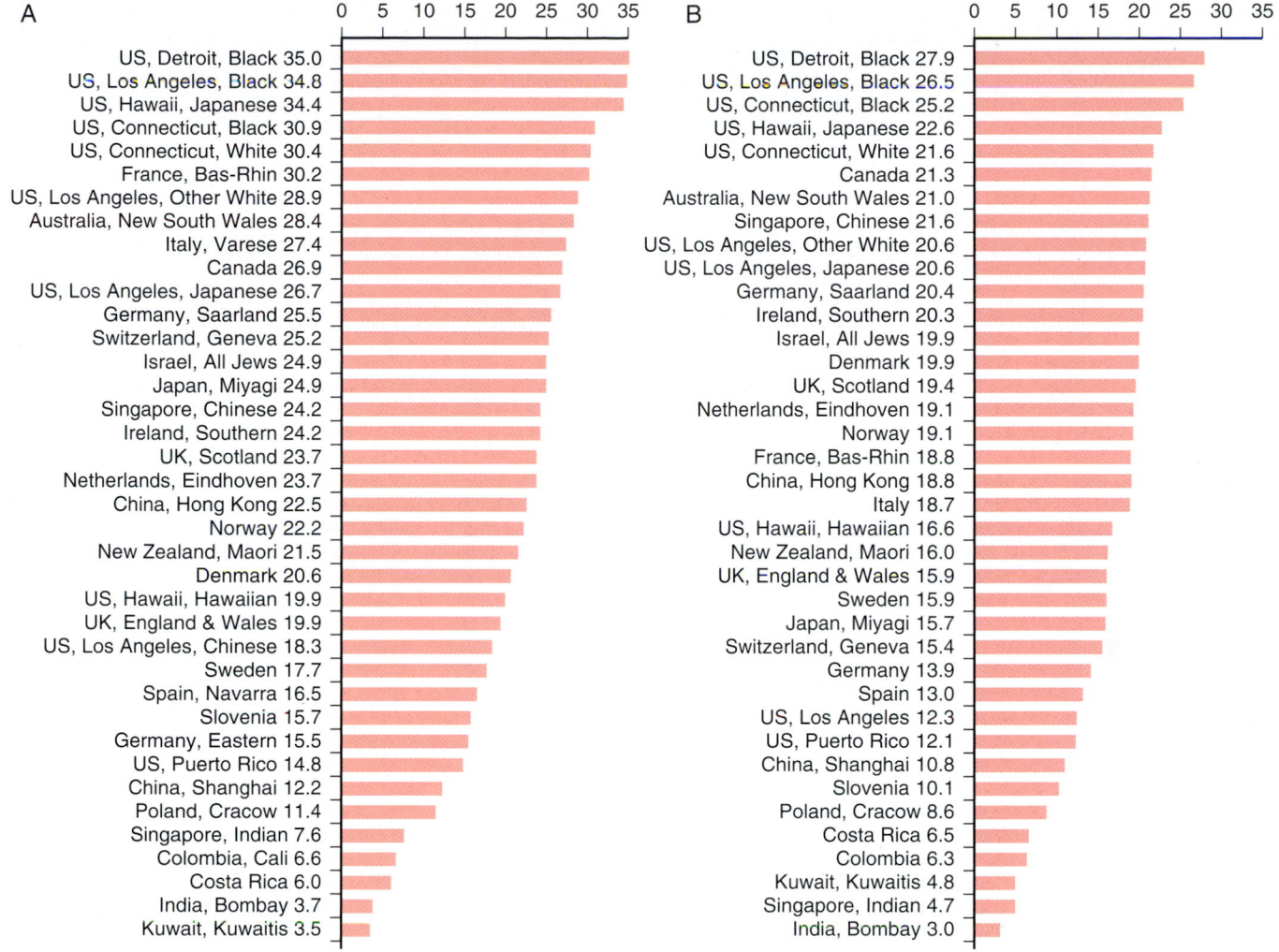

FIGURE 127-1. Age-standardized incidence of colon cancer per 100,000 population in various populations for men *(A)* and women *(B)*. *(Data from Parkin DM, Whelen SL, Ferlay J, et al. Cancer incidence in 5 continents. [IARC Sci. Publ. No. 143]. Lyon: International Agency for Research on Cancer; 1997; and Curado MP, Edwards SB, Shin HR, et al. Cancer incidence in 5 continents, vol. IX [IARC Sci. Publ. No. 160]. Lyon: International Agency for Research on Cancer; 2007.)*

differs by a factor of almost 90 between areas with the extreme lowest and highest rates; the incidence of rectal cancer differs by a factor of 13. CRC incidence also differs within countries, depending on region and population (Fig. 127-2). These differences most likely are explained by differences in environmental factors, including dietary patterns (discussed later).

Although the incidences of colon and rectal cancer overall are parallel, geographic variation is more pronounced for colon than for rectal cancer. High ratios of colon to rectal cancer (≥2:1) prevail in high-risk areas such as North America, whereas ratios below unity are often found in low-risk Asian and African populations. There is a steeper rise in the incidence of colon cancer for each unit increase in the incidence of rectal cancer in women compared with men, suggesting that colon and rectal cancer have related, but not identical, causes.

In the USA, the incidence of CRC also varies regionally. In general, rates in the southern and western United States (except the San Francisco Bay area, Hawaii, and Nevada) are lower than the U.S. average, whereas rates are highest in the northeastern and north central states. CRC incidence rates also are moderately higher for urban residents, although socioeconomic status is not a consistent risk factor for CRC in studies

of the U.S. population. These regional differences in the USA seem to be fading now, perhaps because of the increasing homogeneity of dietary patterns across the country.

Between 1950 and the mid-1980s, the incidence of colon cancer in the USA rose in the white population, whereas that of rectal cancer remained fairly stable. Mortality rates from CRC were stable among white men but decreased in white women. Both incidence and mortality rates for CRC increased substantially among African Americans during this period. CRC incidence and mortality have declined since 1985 in American adults at an average annual rate of 1.6% and 1.8%, respectively; these trends are more evident in whites than blacks. Overall death rates from CRC declined between 1990 and 2004 by almost 30% in men and 25% in women. While rates have been declining among adults 50 years of age and older, recently there appears to be an increase in cancers of the distal colon and rectum among younger individuals, perhaps reflecting dietary patterns in children and young adults. Currently, incidence and mortality rates for CRC are higher in the African American population compared with the white population; in the U.S. Latin American population, these rates are slightly lower.[6,7] The risk of CRC rises rapidly in populations that migrate from areas of low risk to areas of high risk. This

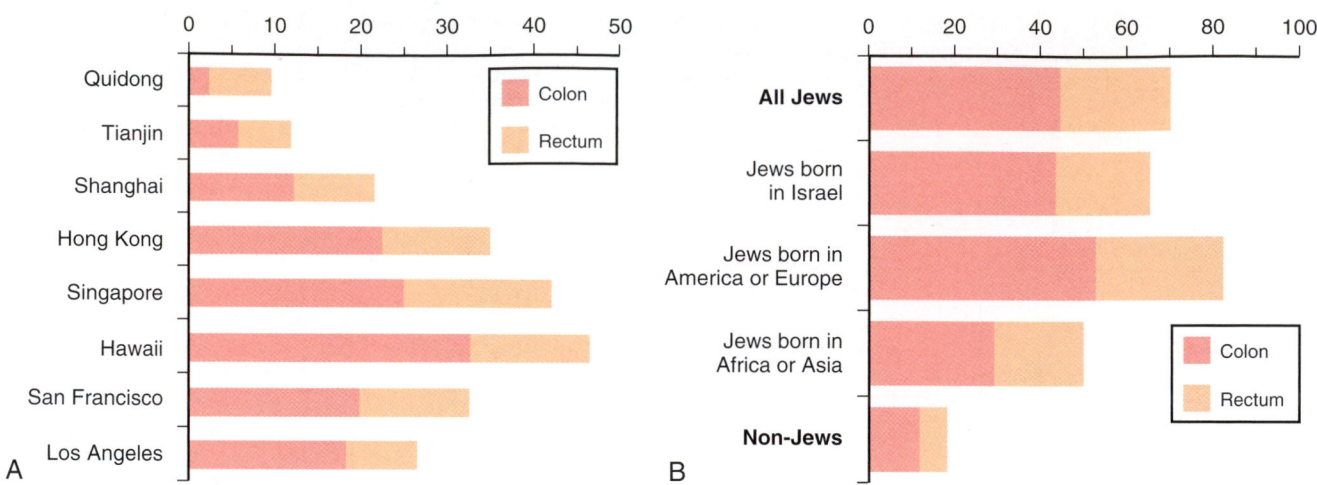

FIGURE 127-2. Age-standardized incidence of colon and rectal cancers per 100,000 (1988-1992) in ethnic Chinese *(A)* and populations in Israel *(B)*. Colorectal cancer incidence differs considerably within countries, depending on region and population, and in ethnic groups that migrate to areas with different diets and lifestyles. *(Data from Parkin DM, Whelen SL, Ferlay J, et al. Cancer incidence in five continents. [IARC Sci. Publ. No. 143]. Lyon: International Agency for Research on Cancer; 1997.)*

pattern was demonstrated clearly in Japanese immigrants to Hawaii and to the continental USA during the 1950s and 1960s. Cancer rates for Issei (the migrating generation) rose over a short period to exceed those of native Japanese living in Japan, and the incidence rates for Nissei (their U.S.-born offspring) rose progressively to approximate those of the native white population. A similar upward displacement of CRC risk was noted in Europeans who migrated to Australia after World War II and in Jews who migrated to Israel from low-risk areas in Yemen and North Africa. Longitudinal studies reveal that in many countries where CRC incidence and mortality rates were low before 1950, rates have increased sharply (including Spain and a number of countries within East Asia and Eastern Europe), whereas in countries where rates were high or moderate, they have decreased, stabilized, or increased slightly. Such trends likely reflect changes in dietary patterns, obesity, and prevalence of smoking. Japan is a good example of this change. Once a low-risk region for colon cancer, incidence rates have risen to exceed those in North America and Australia.[4] The USA is the only country with significantly decreasing incidence rates of CRC, perhaps reflecting detection and removal of early neoplastic lesions through screening (see later).

Studies of temporal trends by subsite location of large bowel cancer demonstrate that for both sexes, incidence rates have increased for cancers of the cecum, ascending colon, and sigmoid colon and have decreased for cancers of the rectum; this change might reflect differing susceptibilities to neoplastic transformation in the proximal and distal colon. Currently in the USA, the prevalence of CRCs in whites is higher in the cecum and ascending colon (22% in men, 27% in women) and in the sigmoid colon (25% in men, 23% in women) than elsewhere in the large bowel (Fig. 127-3).

ETIOLOGY

Inter-regional differences in the incidence of CRC, including differences among population groups living in geographic proximity but with different lifestyles, strongly suggest that environment plays a role in the development of this disease. Migrant studies and rapid changes in incidence in countries assimilating Western practices support this concept. Strong

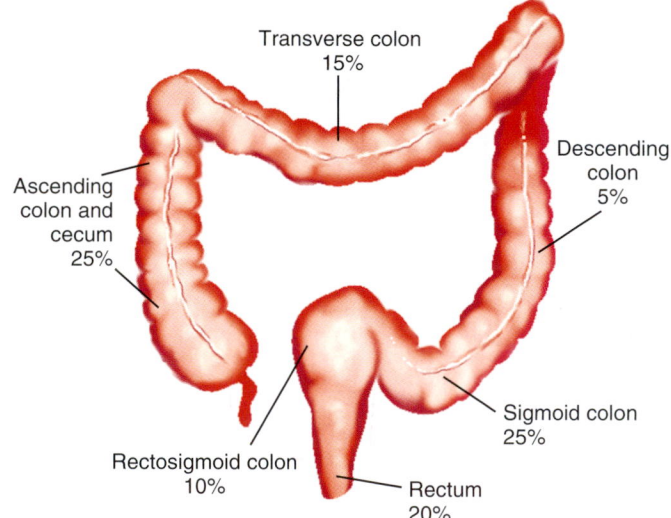

FIGURE 127-3. Distribution of colorectal cancers within the colon.

circumstantial evidence exists for a link between diet and CRC. Population studies and animal studies have attempted to delineate the effects of various fats and proteins, carbohydrates, vegetable and fiber components, and micronutrients on the genesis of cancer of the large bowel (Box 127-1).

Fat, Bile Acids, and Bacteria

Several lines of evidence suggest that diets containing large percentages of fat predispose to CRC, especially of the descending and sigmoid colon. Colon cancer rates are higher in populations whose total fat intake is high and are lower in those who consume less fat. On average, fat constitutes 40% to 45% of total calorie intake in Western countries with high rates of CRC, whereas in low-risk populations, fat accounts for only 10% to 15% of dietary calories. Results from case-control and cohort studies support the correlation of dietary fat with incidence and mortality rates from colon and, to a lesser degree, rectal cancer.

A prospective study assessed the relationship of meat, fat, and fiber intake among 88,751 women aged 34 to 59 years. After adjustment for total energy intake, intake of animal fat was significantly correlated with the risk of colon cancer. The intake ratio of red meat to chicken and fish was strongly associated with increased incidence of colon cancer. Similar findings have been reported that correlate the intake of saturated fat and the ratios of red meat to chicken and fish intake with both the incidence and recurrence of colorectal adenomas in women. Cohort studies and a combined analysis of 13 case-control studies that adjusted for total energy intake, however, failed to provide clear-cut evidence for the association between dietary fat and CRC observed in earlier studies. Studies that specifically examine the association between intake of saturated or animal fat and CRC suggest a stronger association than with total fat.

Animal studies lend additional support for the role of dietary fat in the development of colon cancer. These studies usually involve the injection of carcinogens such as 1,2-dimethylhydrazine (DMH) or azoxymethane into rodents fed various diets. Animals fed a variety of polyunsaturated and saturated fats develop greater numbers of carcinogen-induced colonic adenocarcinomas than do those on low-fat diets. The amount and source of dietary fat might affect tumor development in such studies; fatty acids derived from polyunsaturated fish oils (omega-3 polyunsaturated fatty acids or PUFAs) and monosaturated olive oil might not promote tumors to the extent that other polyunsaturated fats do, or may even reduce the risk of CRC. Intake of omega-3 PUFAs (eicosapentaenoic acid [EPA] and docosahexaenoic acid [DHA]) is associated with reduced CRC risk in epidemiologic and preclinical studies, and affects molecular pathways associated with mucosal epithelial proliferation and inflammation (discussed later).

It has been proposed that dietary fat enhances hepatic cholesterol and bile acid synthesis, thereby increasing the amounts of these sterols in the colon. Colonic bacteria convert these compounds to secondary bile acids, cholesterol metabolites, and other potentially toxic metabolic compounds. Population studies demonstrate increased excretion of sterol metabolites and fecal bile acids in groups that consume a high-fat, low-fiber Western diet compared with other groups, and high fecal bile acid levels are found in some patients with CRC. Dietary fat also has been shown to increase the excretion of secondary bile acids in carcinogen-treated rats; secondary bile acids do not act as primary carcinogens but as potent promoters of colon carcinogenesis in such animal models. Little is known about how lipid and sterol metabolites promote tumors, but both bile acids and free fatty acids have been shown to damage the colonic mucosa and increase the proliferative activity of its epithelium. Dietary consumption of high amounts of corn oil and beef fat increase colonic ornithine decarboxylase levels, which are associated with rapidly proliferating mucosa. Activation of protein kinase C (PKC) by bile acids in colonic mucosa also might represent an important intracellular event by which bile acids provoke a proliferative response. Mucin alterations are a common feature of colonic neoplasia, and alterations in MUC2 mucin have been associated with tumor progression in the colon. Bile acids induce mucin expression in human colon carcinoma cells by increasing MUC2 transcription through a process involving mitogen-activated protein (MAP) kinase-independent, PKC-dependent activation of the transcription factor AP-1.[8] Bile acids can, in addition, induce release of arachidonate and conversion of arachidonic acid to prostaglandins in the mucosa, which can enhance cell proliferation. Preclinical and clinical evidence indicate that NSAIDs, which reduce prostaglandin synthesis, reduce the incidence of large bowel cancer (discussed later); inhibition of the inducible enzyme COX-2 may be particularly important in this regard.

Certain fatty acids could promote carcinogenesis by altering membrane fluidity after being incorporated into cell membranes. Bacterial enzymes such as 7α-dehydroxylase (which converts cholic to deoxycholic acid), β-glucuronidase, nitroreductase, and azoreductase may be induced by a high-fat diet and also could convert ingested dietary compounds to active carcinogens (see later).

An inverse relationship has been reported between physical activity and risk for colon adenomas and CRC, especially in men. While moderate activity on a regular basis lowers the risk of CRC, vigorous activity may have an even greater benefit. Obesity is associated with elevated risk of CRC in both men and women. Studies examining body fat distribution and CRC consistently demonstrate that larger waist circumference or higher waist-to-hip circumference is associated with CRC risk.[9,10] Serum cholesterol and β-lipoprotein levels have been positively correlated with the development of colorectal adenomas and CRC, but this association has not been demonstrated consistently, and serum cholesterol levels can decline before the development of colon cancer. Adiponectin is a hormone secreted by adipose tissue, serum levels of which are inversely correlated with obesity and hyperinsulinemia. Variants of adiponectin and adiponectin receptor genes have been correlated with differences in CRC risk.[11]

It is now recognized that the human microbiota, consisting of as many as 100 trillion commensal organisms that inhabit the adult GI tract, are essential partners that benefit overall host physiology, metabolism, development, and immune homeostasis (see Chapter 3). A growing body of literature indicates that microbial "dysbiosis" may be etiologic for

CRC.[12-14] Factors such as antibiotic use, dietary fiber intake, and other host factors that modify the luminal microbe environment could contribute to bacterial dysbiosis. Metabolism of dietary substrates by selected bacterial groups of intestinal microbiota may lead to the production of mutagens (fecapentaenes, diacylglycerols, sulfide, secondary bile acids, and reactive oxygen species) that promote DNA damage. Microbial status modulates the development of colitis-associated CRC in susceptible mice. In turn, inflammation may create an environment that supports carcinogenesis through its effects on the microbiota.[15]

Fiber

Epidemiologic, case-control, and animal studies suggest that dietary fiber protects against the development of colon cancer. Dietary fiber is plant material that resists digestion and is composed of a heterogeneous mix of carbohydrates (e.g., cellulose, hemicellulose, pectin) and noncarbohydrates (e.g., lignin). Although the protective role of fiber is not completely clear, epidemiologic studies correlate high-fiber intake with a lower incidence of colorectal neoplasia.[16] The majority of observational, epidemiologic, and case-control studies support the protective effect of fiber-rich diets, but do not define the relationship between fiber-rich food and the nonfiber vegetable components, nutrients, and micronutrients in fruits and vegetables. The effect of fiber components on different portions of the large bowel also can vary, which might explain, in part, the inability of fiber supplementation to prevent adenoma recurrence in several randomized controlled trials (RCTs).[17,18]

Large prospective observational studies, including 1 from the Prostate, Lung, Colon, and Ovarian Cancer Trial (PLCO), found that increased fiber intake is significantly associated with reduced risk of colorectal neoplasia. Analysis of 13 prospective cohort studies included in the Pooling Project of Prospective Studies of Diet and Cancer demonstrated that dietary fiber intake was inversely associated with risk of CRC in age-adjusted analyses, but that after accounting for other dietary factors, high intake of dietary fiber was not associated with a reduced risk of CRC.[19]

Overall, diets rich in vegetables, fruits, and whole grains are associated with a decrease in CRC risk. Investigators postulate that fibers such as cereal bran exert their protective role by increasing stool bulk, thereby diluting carcinogens and carcinogenesis promoters, enhancing their elimination, and minimizing their duration of mucosal contact by decreasing intestinal transit time. Increased fiber intake in the form of whole wheat and rye bread also reduces the concentration of fecal secondary bile acids and fecal mutagens in healthy subjects. Animal studies also have demonstrated a decreased incidence of colonic tumors in DMH-treated rats fed diets high in fiber and fiber components (e.g., wheat bran, cellulose, hemicellulose). Cellulose and hemicellulose decrease the levels of bacterial metabolic enzymes, such as β-glucuronidase, in experimental animals and can diminish the activation of carcinogens or co-carcinogens. Furthermore, some fiber components can bind to toxic or carcinogenic substances, thus perhaps decreasing their contact with the colonic mucosa. Fiber components also are fermented by fecal flora to short-chain fatty acids, thereby decreasing colonic pH and potentially inhibiting carcinogenesis.

Carcinogens and Fecal Mutagens, Vitamins, and Micronutrients

The possibility that specific genotoxic carcinogens might play a role in the genesis of CRC was raised when it was noted that the stools of certain persons exhibited mutagenic activity for bacteria in vitro. Mutagenic activity often is present in the feces of populations at high risk for colon cancer and is low or absent in low-risk populations. Fecapentaenes, a specific group of highly unsaturated reactive compounds synthesized by colonic bacteria, might play a role in colon carcinogenesis. Numerous case-control and cohort studies have provided evidence that consumption of red meat is associated with CRC risk (see earlier). A recent meta-analysis of cohort studies estimated that daily consumption of approximately 100 g of red meat or 50 g of processed meat increases the risk of CRC by 15% to 20%[20]; some of this effect may be due to fat consumption. It also has been recognized that "charbroiled" and, to a lesser extent, fried foods contain mutagenic compounds such as heterocyclic amines and polycyclic aromatic hydrocarbons. In addition, the heme in red meat may act as a catalyst to nitrosamine formation, generating free radicals that may damage DNA. Furthermore, there is an association of an increased CRC risk with increased alcohol intake, especially among men. Consumption of more than 3 alcoholic beverages per day is associated with a 1.4-fold risk of CRC. A possible association between rectal cancer and beer- and ale-drinking also has been noted. A 2- to 3-fold increase in CRC also has been observed in automotive pattern and model makers, but the specific carcinogenic agent in this industrial environment has not yet been identified.

The exact nature of genotoxic carcinogens that might act in the human colon remains speculative, but the identification of such compounds could provide a basis for intervention and primary prevention of CRC. Limited data suggest that foods rich in carotene (vitamin A) and vitamin C could act as antioxidants and be used in the chemoprevention of colon cancer, but prospective trials have failed to demonstrate such an effect. Other areas that merit further exploration in the prevention of CRC include the role of yellow-green cruciferous vegetables and the role of micronutrients including selenium salts, vitamin E, folic acid, and calcium (see below).

Calcium and Vitamin D

Epidemiologic, clinical, and laboratory evidence suggest that calcium intake might protect against carcinogenesis in the colon. Calcium has numerous biological effects that could reduce colon carcinogenesis, including actions on the cell cycle, cyclic adenosine monophosphate (cAMP), calmodulin, tyrosine kinases, ornithine decarboxylase, and E-cadherin. The calcium-sensing receptor that is expressed in the intestine senses extracellular calcium, with resultant effects on differentiation and proliferation. Dietary calcium supplementation in the form of low-fat dairy foods can affect a variety of intermediate biomarkers thought to be associated with tumor progression in the colon, and supplemental calcium plus vitamin D alters preneoplastic features of colorectal adenomas.[21] Although the relationship between increased calcium intake and a lower incidence of colonic adenomas and carcinomas has not been uniformly demonstrated, overall, observational studies suggest a protective effect. A pooling project of 10 cohort studies strongly suggested that calcium intake is inversely related to the risk of CRC.[22]

Further support for the beneficial effect of calcium in preventing colonic cancer comes from numerous animal studies. The increase in colonocyte proliferation stimulated by intrarectal instillation of deoxycholate and free fatty acids or by dietary supplementation with cholic acid may be ameliorated by oral calcium supplementation in laboratory animals. Rodents that were fed high-fat diets also demonstrated a reduction in the number of carcinogen-induced tumors, especially tumors that showed K-ras mutations, when their diet was supplemented with calcium. Ornithine decarboxylase, an enzyme involved in polyamine biosynthesis and elevated in preneoplastic states, is reduced in rat colonic mucosa incubated with calcium in vitro, and supplemental calcium suppresses elevated levels of this enzyme in the mucosa of older adult patients with adenomatous polyps. It has been suggested that dietary calcium binds to ionized fatty acids and bile acids in the intestine, converting them to insoluble calcium compounds that are incapable of stimulating epithelial proliferation. Calcium increases fecal excretion of both phosphate and bile acids and modifies the amounts of bile acids in bile. In addition, calcium in milk products is capable of precipitating luminal cytotoxic surfactants, thereby inhibiting their effects on colonic mucosa. These potential beneficial effects of calcium have not been observed uniformly, however, and studies of the effects of calcium on rectal mucosa have not always demonstrated a reduction in the proliferation rates. In other studies, calcium supplementation normalized the distribution of proliferating cells in the colonic crypt without affecting the rate of proliferation in colorectal mucosa.

Vitamin D_3 metabolites and analogs have been shown to play an important role in the regulation of a number of important cellular processes, including proliferation, differentiation, and apoptosis, in addition to their established role in mineral homeostasis. These steroid compounds have rapid effects that do not involve gene transcription or protein synthesis, as well as genomic effects that involve the vitamin D receptor and other transcription factors. Vitamin D modulates more than 200 genes involved in cell cycle regulation, growth factor signaling, protection against oxidative stress, bile acid and xenobiotic metabolism, cell adhesion, DNA repair, angiogenesis, inflammation, and immune function. Effects of vitamin D and its metabolites have been demonstrated in normal and malignant colonocytes, and several potential mechanisms have been suggested by which these compounds might prevent carcinogenesis in the colon. Dietary supplementation with calcium and vitamin D in rodents fed colon tumor-inducing Western diets significantly reduced tumor incidence and multiplicity in addition to altering expression of a variety of genes linked to initiating formation of colon tumors.[23]

Arachidonic Acid, Eicosanoids, and COX-2

Clinical case-control and cohort studies have shown a 40% to 50% reduction in CRC-related mortality in persons who take aspirin and other NSAIDs on a regular basis compared with those not taking these agents. The exact mechanism for cancer protection with these agents is unknown, but it might relate to altered synthesis of arachidonic acid metabolites (eicosanoids) including prostaglandins, thromboxanes, leukotrienes, and hydroxy-eicosatetraenoic acids. These compounds modulate a number of signal transduction pathways that affect cellular adhesion, growth, and differentiation. COX (or prostaglandin-endoperoxide synthase) oxidizes arachidonic acid to prostaglandin G_2, reduces prostaglandin G_2 to prostaglandin H_2, and is the key enzyme responsible for production of prostaglandins and other eicosanoids.

COX exists in 2 isoforms: COX-1 and COX-2. COX-1, the constitutive form of the enzyme, is present in most tissues and is involved in the physiologic production of prostaglandins to maintain normal homeostasis. COX-2 is induced by cytokines, mitogens, and growth factors, and its level is elevated in both murine and human CRCs.[24,25] Expression of COX-2 is increased markedly in 85% to 95% of CRCs and in experimental models of CRC. COX-2 inhibition prevents cancer from developing during the initiation, promotion, and progression stages of carcinogenesis. Knockout of COX-2 results in suppression of intestinal polyposis in animal models of familial adenomatous polyposis (FAP). 15-Hydroxyprostaglandin dehydrogenase (15-PGDH) is a prostaglandin-degrading enzyme that is lost in human colon cancers and has been shown to be a physiologic antagonist of the prostaglandin-synthesizing activity of COX-2.[26] It has been speculated that NSAIDs might reduce formation of colon tumors by inhibiting prostaglandin-mediated proliferation, but other evidence suggests that part of their effect might result from inducing apoptosis. Overexpression of COX-2 has been demonstrated to decrease apoptosis, whereas inhibition of COX-2 leads to an increase in apoptosis.

NSAIDs potentially can induce apoptosis through elevation of the prostaglandin precursor arachidonic acid, which stimulates conversion of sphingomyelin to ceramide, a mediator of apoptosis. NSAIDs also might inhibit the activation of genes by the nuclear hormone receptor peroxisome proliferator-activated receptor δ (PPARδ) by disrupting the ability of this receptor to bind DNA. PPARδ expression is elevated in CRCs and repressed by the APC gene product, which is altered in CRC cells. Inhibition of PPARδ function enhances the ability of NSAIDs to induce apoptosis in colon cancer cells. PPARδ activates a variety of genes, including those involved in cellular growth and differentiation after exposure to a variety of ligands, such as eicosanoids. COX-2 inhibition could prevent production of these ligands and thereby prevent activation of PPARδ.

Other potential mechanisms by which COX-2 inhibition might affect tumor formation include alterations of cell adhesion to extracellular matrix proteins, inhibition of tumor neovascularization (angiogenesis), and reduction in carcinogen activation. A study using the $Apc^{\Delta716}$ mouse, an animal model of FAP, demonstrated that treatment with the COX-2-specific inhibitor rofecoxib (Vioxx) was associated with a significant dose-dependent reduction in size and number of polyps as well as alterations in polyp morphology. COX-2 inhibition was associated with decreased levels of vascular endothelial growth factor (VEGF) and with lower rates of DNA replication.[24] Environment and diet might affect the genesis of CRC, but their exact roles remain unclear. Their complex nature renders definition of the influence of individual environmental and dietary components difficult. Nonetheless, the American Cancer Society and other agencies have set forth guidelines on nutrition and physical activity for cancer prevention, including prevention of CRC.[9]

Chemoprevention

Chemoprevention refers to the use of natural or synthetic agents to reverse, suppress, or prevent progression or recurrence of cancer[27]; this is a cornerstone of primary prevention. Data on CRC chemoprevention come from studies in laboratory animals (see earlier), observational epidemiologic studies, case-control studies, and RCTs. Because the natural history of CRC is protracted, clinical RCTs often have concentrated on preventing colorectal adenomas, which represent a form of intraepithelial neoplasia and are the precursors to carcinoma. The duration of the studies and sample sizes required, cost, and ethical considerations make the use of cancer an impractical end point. This difficulty has led to an increasing use of surrogate biomarkers to study CRC chemoprevention.[28] To be valid, however, such biomarkers need to accurately represent the events involved in carcinogenesis, and there should be a clear relationship among the chemopreventive agent, modulation of the biomarker, and the development of cancer.

There has been interest in the use of magnifying endoscopy to study aberrant crypt foci of the colon as possible markers in chemoprevention trials.[29] Aberrant crypt foci

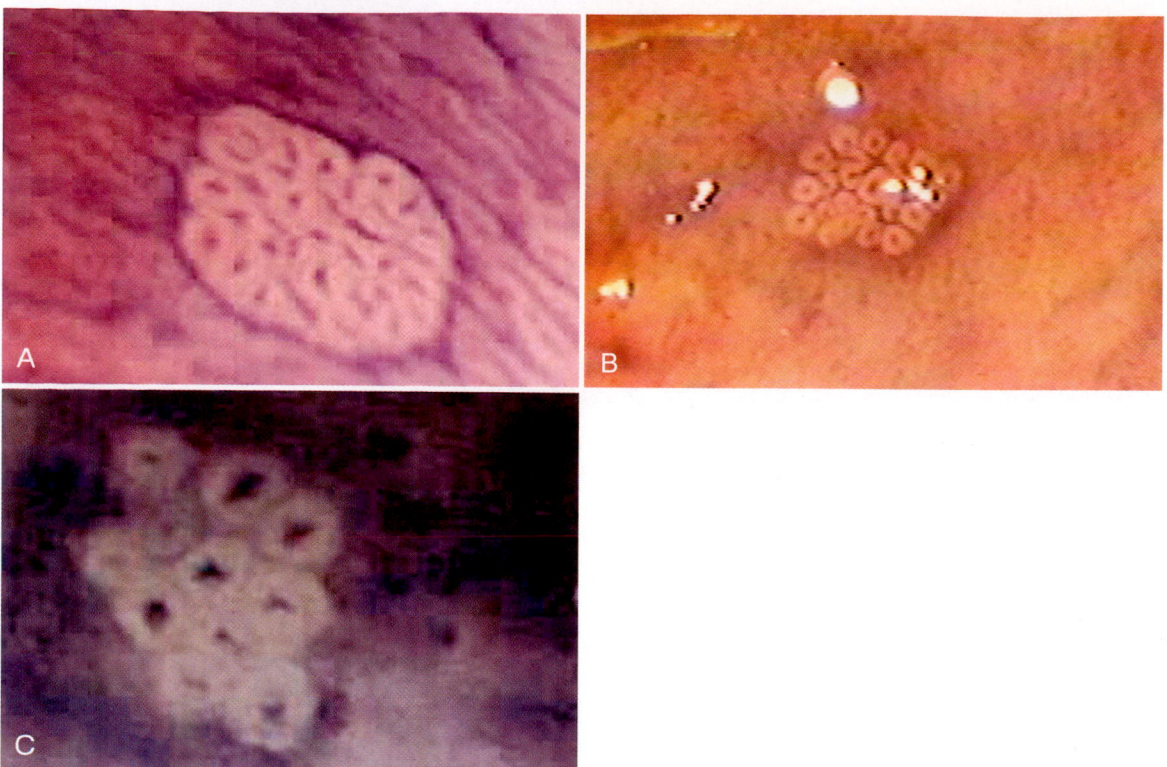

FIGURE 127-4. *A-C,* Three views of aberrant crypt foci at different magnifications. Aberrant crypt foci consist of large thick crypts and are thought to be precursors of adenomas in the colon.

consist of large, thick crypts with dysplastic features; they can be detected by chromoendoscopy using agents such as methylene blue or indigo carmine (Fig. 127-4) and are thought to be precursors of adenomas in the colon. It is unclear, however, whether these lesions, which appear to be precursors to neoplasia in animal models, play a similar role in the human colon,[27] and studies suggest that the majority of aberrant crypt foci in the human colon may be hyperplastic rather than dysplastic (see Chapter 126).

The potential benefit of low-fat, high-fiber diets based on descriptive epidemiology and case-control studies already has been discussed, but current data from prospective human trials are thus far equivocal or negative. Two large RCTs examined the effects of fiber supplementation on recurrence of adenomas. The Polyp Prevention Trial[18] randomized 2079 subjects with a history of colorectal adenomas to receive counseling together with a low-fat, high-fiber diet rich in fruits and vegetables or to receive their usual diet alone. The incidence of recurrent adenomas at 1 and 4 years, as determined by colonoscopy, was similar in both groups. In a study conducted by the Phoenix Colon Cancer Prevention Physicians' Network,[17] 1429 patients with a history of colorectal adenoma were randomized to receive 2 g or 13.5 g of supplemental wheat bran per day. Colonoscopy failed to show a difference in the incidence of recurrent adenomas at a median follow-up of 34 to 36 months.

A large body of observational and laboratory studies suggests a role for dietary calcium supplementation in chemoprevention. A prospective double-blind placebo-controlled trial showed that supplemental calcium (3000 mg of calcium carbonate per day, equivalent to 1200 mg of elemental calcium) reduced the incidence and number of recurrent adenomas in subjects chosen for a recent history of such lesions.[30] The effect of calcium was modest: 19% reduction in recurrence of adenomas and 24% reduction in the number of adenomas over 3 years, independent of age, sex, or dietary intake of calcium, fat, or fiber. The protective effect of calcium supplementation on the risk of colorectal adenoma recurrence extended up to 5 years after cessation of active treatment, even in the absence of continued supplementation.[31] Analysis of subjects' serum vitamin D status suggested that calcium supplementation and vitamin D status appear to act together to reduce the risk of adenoma recurrence.[32] The results of a Japanese study, the Fukuoka Colorectal Cancer Study,[33] support the joint action of calcium and vitamin D in preventing CRC.[34] A large prospective randomized trial aimed at delineating the individual and combined effects of calcium carbonate and vitamin D_3 supplementation (the Vitamin D/Calcium Polyp Prevention Study) on adenoma occurrence in susceptible individuals will soon be completed. This study also examines whether the effect of supplementation with vitamin D_3 is modified by variation in the vitamin D receptor (VDR) gene and other genes that code for proteins that control vitamin D and calcium signaling. Human trials using antioxidant vitamins A, C, and E have provided equivocal results, and current data do not support their routine use for CRC prevention in average-risk persons.

Folic acid and its metabolites play an important role in DNA synthesis, strand integrity, and methylation. Epidemiologic studies have found a lower incidence of CRC among those with high compared with low dietary intake of folate. This protective effect also was suggested by the Nurses' Health Study, in which high doses of folate (as part of multivitamin supplementation) given over several years were protective against CRC. A large prospective RCT[35,36] failed, however, to demonstrate a protective effect of 1 mg/day of folate supplementation on recurrence of adenoma compared with placebo, and suggested that folate supplementation in persons with prior adenomas actually might increase adenoma risk. Analysis of baseline dietary and serum folate levels in these subjects supports the idea that although moderate doses of folate may be protective compared with deficiency, at some point of sufficiency, supplementation provides no additional benefit.[37] Lack of folate (0.5 mg/day) supplementation to prevent adenoma recurrence also was found in another RCT.[38]

Epidemiologic, case-control, and prospective cohort trials suggest a protective effect against the development of CRC in women who take hormone (estrogen) replacement therapy. It has been postulated that estrogen might protect against colon cancer by decreasing production of secondary bile acids, by decreasing levels of insulin-like growth factor (IGF)-1, or through as yet undetermined direct effects on colonic mucosal epithelial cells. Data from the Women's Health Initiative demonstrated that short-term use of estrogen plus progestin was associated with a decreased risk of CRC; however, CRCs in women who took estrogen plus progestin were diagnosed at a more advanced stage than those in women who took placebo.[39] Cigarette smoking has been associated with incidence of and mortality from CRC in observational studies,[40] but the long-term effects of smoking cessation on CRC have not been studied.

The most promising results for CRC prevention come from trials using aspirin and NSAIDs. Case-control and cohort studies suggested that the risk for adenoma and carcinoma may be reduced 40% to 50% among aspirin and NSAID users compared with controls.[41] A prospective cohort study among male health professionals demonstrated that persons who take aspirin more than twice per week were at lower risk for CRC (relative risk [RR], 0.68) than were controls. An RCT that assessed the effect of low-dose aspirin in an average-risk population demonstrated no significant reduction in the number of CRC cases during the first 6 years of follow-up, and suggested that longer follow-up may be necessary to demonstrate a significant effect of aspirin on development of cancer. The Nurses' Health Study demonstrated that the benefits of aspirin might not be evident until after at least a decade of regular aspirin consumption. One analysis assessed the effects of aspirin on long-term incidence and mortality of CRC in relation to dose, duration of treatment, and tumor site.[42] This study established the effects of aspirin on CRC risk over 20 years by analysis of pooled data from 4 randomized trials of aspirin used for primary and secondary prevention of cardiovascular disease. Allocation of aspirin reduced the 20-year risk (24%) and mortality (35%) of colon cancer, but not rectal cancer. Benefit increased with scheduled duration of treatment such that aspirin use for at least 5 years reduced the risk of proximal cancer by about 70%, and the risk of rectal cancer by 42%. There was no increase in benefit at doses of aspirin greater than 75 mg daily. Part of aspirin's effect on mortality may result from a reduction in metastatic disease. Several prospective adenoma prevention trials (see later) now provide compelling evidence that aspirin use reduces the risk of colorectal adenoma in persons with a history of adenoma or carcinoma.[42-45]

Given the long natural history of CRC, prevention of adenoma recurrence after endoscopic removal often is used as an intermediate or surrogate end point in chemoprevention trials.[27] In FAP, chemoprevention trials often use reductions of the number and size of adenomas as end points in short-term studies. Such trials have suggested a potential role for NSAIDs as chemopreventive agents in this setting. Indeed, there is a significant decrease in the mean number and size of polyps in patients treated with the NSAID sulindac. In a small, double-blind RCT of 22 patients with FAP, treatment with sulindac reduced the number and mean diameter of colorectal polyps by 44% and 35% of respective baseline values after 9 months; 3 months after treatment was stopped, however, the number and size of polyps increased. A subsequent prospective cohort study[46] confirmed that long-term use of sulindac is effective in reducing the number of adenomas in patients with FAP. A 76% reduction in the number of polyps was seen at 1 year and was sustained (74% reduction) through 63 months of follow-up. Sulindac might not be effective, however, for primary prevention of adenomas in genetically disposed persons with FAP who have not yet developed macroscopic adenomas.[47]

A double-blind RCT studied the effects of celecoxib (Celebrex), a selective COX-2 inhibitor, on colorectal polyps in patients with FAP.[48] Treatment with high doses of celecoxib for 6 months was associated with a significant reduction (28%) in the number of colorectal polyps compared with placebo (4.5%). This drug is now approved in the USA as an adjunct to standard therapy in patients with FAP.

Data are now available on the role of nonselective NSAIDs and COX-2 inhibitors as chemopreventive agents for preventing sporadic adenomas. Four published trials have demonstrated a reduction in adenoma recurrence in chemoprevention trials that involve aspirin. An RCT of aspirin versus placebo[44] demonstrated that daily use of 81 mg of aspirin was associated with a 19% reduction in occurrence of adenoma and a 41% reduction in occurrence of advanced neoplasms (adenomas measuring at least 1 cm or with tubulovillous or villous features, severe dysplasia, or invasive cancer) compared with results of placebo treatment 3 years after removal of an index sporadic adenoma. In a similar trial, aspirin (300 mg/day) was associated with a 21% overall risk reduction for all adenomas and a 37% reduction in advanced adenomas at 3 years.[38] A prospective RCT in a higher-risk group for adenoma recurrence, those with a previous history of sporadic CRC, demonstrated a 45% risk reduction in those taking 325 mg of aspirin daily compared with those taking placebo, with a mean follow-up of almost 3 years.[43]

Given biological plausibility, preclinical in vitro and animal data, and data on regression of adenoma in patients with FAP, 3 randomized trials were undertaken to examine the effect of COX-2 selective inhibitors on formation of new adenomas in patents with a history of sporadic adenomas. The Adenoma Prevention with Celecoxib (APC) trial[49] randomized 2035 subjects to celecoxib at a dose of 200 mg or 400 mg twice daily. Use of celecoxib was associated with a dose-dependent 33% to 45% reduction in the development of new adenomas by 3 years, with a 57% to 66% reduction in the number of patients developing advanced adenomas. The Prevention of Sporadic Adenomatous Polyps (PreSAP) trial[50] randomized 1561 patients to receive 400 mg celecoxib once daily or placebo. Use of celecoxib was associated with a 36% overall reduction in formation of new adenomas and a 51% reduction in advanced adenomas over 3 years. The Adenomatous Polyp Prevention on Vioxx (APPROVe) Trial[51,52] was a double-blind RCT of the efficacy of oral rofecoxib, 25 mg daily, to prevent colorectal adenomas in 2587 subjects. The risk of adenoma recurrence over 3 years was lower for subjects on rofecoxib than on placebo, with a 24% overall reduction and a 30% reduction in advanced adenomas. The effect of drug was more pronounced in the first year (RR, 0.65; 95% confidence interval [CI]: 0.57-0.73) than in the subsequent 2 years.

Thus, 3 well-conducted prospective RCTs demonstrated a significant reduction in formation of new adenomas with the use of a COX-2 selective inhibitor in those with a history of colorectal adenomas. Unfortunately, adverse thrombotic cardiovascular events were associated with COX-2 inhibition in at least 2 of these trials.[48,49] Data now indicate that an increased risk of cardiovascular events is associated with most NSAIDs, and not just COX-2 inhibitors.

TABLE 127-1 Efficacy of Chemoprotective Agents for Colorectal Neoplasia

Agent	Observational Studies of Colon Cancer Incidence			Randomized Human Trials		
	Animal Studies	Case Control Studies	Cohort Studies	Reduction in Mucosal Proliferation	Reduced Number of Polyps in Patients with FAP	Reduced Number of Sporadic Adenomas
Aspirin or other NSAIDs	+	+	+	N/A	+	+
COX-2 inhibitors	+	N/A	N/A	+	+	+
Vitamins A, C, E	+	+	+	+	~	~
Folate	~	+	+	+	N/A	–
Calcium	+	+	+	~	N/A	+
Fiber	+	+	+	+	~	–
Selenium	+	+	~	N/A	–	N/A
Fish oil (omega-3 polyunsaturated fatty acids)	+	+	N/A	+	+	N/A
Organosulfur	+	N/A	N/A	N/A	N/A	N/A
Difluoromethylornithine	+	N/A	N/A	+	+	+*
Statins	+	+	~	+	N/A	N/A

*In combination with sulindac.
+, Most studies are positive for efficacy; –, most studies are negative for efficacy; ~, studies are equivocal for efficacy; FAP, familial adenomatous polyposis; N/A, not available.

"Essential" fatty acids are required for biological processes but cannot be synthesized by humans and must be obtained from dietary sources. The main PUFAs (DHA [$22:6^{\Delta 4,7,10,13,16,19}$] and EPA [$20:5^{\Delta 5,8,11,14,17}$]) are considered essential and are obtained predominantly from cold water oily fish such as mackerel and salmon. There is a growing body of experimental, epidemiologic, and preclinical evidence that indicates fish oil-containing diets rich in n-3 PUFAs are protective against colon tumorigenesis, especially in men. n-3 PUFAs derived from fish oils have been demonstrated to not only affect pathways related to colorectal carcinogenesis in animal models and in human subjects, but to be safe and well tolerated in humans.[53-55] A recent randomized trial in subjects with FAP demonstrated that an enteric coated formulation of EPA has chemopreventive efficacy in reducing rectal polyp burden to a degree similar to that previously observed with selective COX-2 inhibitors.[55] The role for N-3 PUFAs in "sporadic" colorectal adenoma prevention is currently being evaluated.

Other agents currently undergoing study for chemoprevention of colorectal neoplasia include the ornithine decarboxylase inhibitor difluoromethylornithine (DFMO), the bile acid ursodiol, 3-hydroxy-3-methylglutaryl-coenzyme A (HMG-CoA) reductase inhibitors (statins such as pravastatin and lovastatin), EGF receptor (EGFR) inhibitors, and matrix metalloproteinase (MMP) inhibitors.[27] Data will also soon be available from a phase III randomized trial of celecoxib and selenium for the prevention of colorectal adenomas.[56] An RCT to assess the efficacy of DFMO and sulindac to prevent sporadic adenoma recurrence in 375 subjects showed this combination was associated with a 70% reduction in new adenomas at 3 years compared with placebo.[57] Larger studies are needed to confirm this result and are ongoing. Statins modulate a number of processes such as cell growth, apoptosis, and inflammation and a population-based case-control study of persons with CRC and matched controls demonstrated a 47% relative reduction of CRC associated with statin use.[58] Evidence of such benefit of statins is equivocal and mostly from observational clinical studies. Further investigation is needed, such as the statin polyp prevention trial being performed by the National Surgical Adjuvant Breast and Bowel Project (NSABP) in patients with resected colon cancer.[59] Curcumin, the major constituent of turmeric, decreases inflammation and expression of COX-2 and endogenous DNA damage in adenoma tissue, and has been shown to have chemopreventive activity in murine models of FAP when given orally. Table 127-1 and Figure 127-5 summarize current studies that examine the effect of chemopreventive agents on colorectal neoplasia.

BIOLOGY

It has been suggested that carcinogens introduced into the bowel act in concert with other luminal factors (e.g., bile acid and other tumor promoters) to affect colonic epithelial cells. Carcinogenesis is a multistage process, however, and cells must be genetically primed (through either hereditary disposition or genotoxic events) and induced to proliferate, after which they must pass through a series of stages en route to immortalization and uncontrolled growth (see Chapter 1).

Abnormal Cellular Proliferation

Abnormal cellular proliferation is a hallmark of neoplasia (see Chapter 1). Actively proliferating cells are more susceptible to initiators of carcinogenesis (primary carcinogens) and genetic alterations than are resting cells. In the normal colon, DNA synthesis occurs and cells divide and proliferate only in the

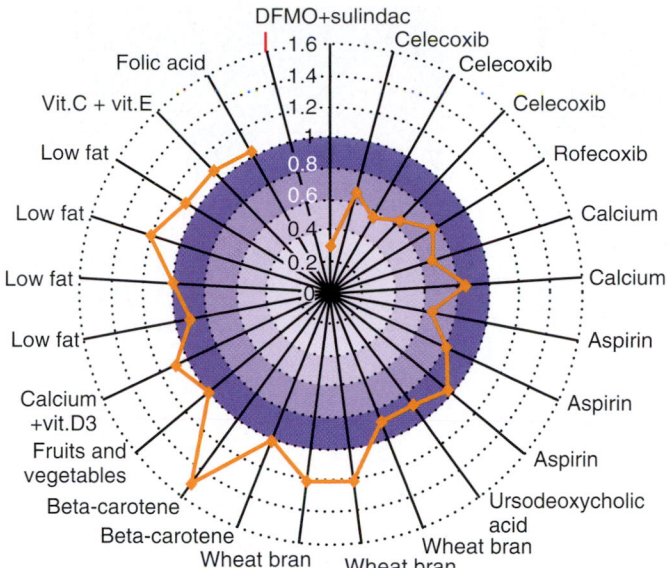

FIGURE 127-5. Diagram depicting the relative risk of colorectal adenoma recurrence after a clearing colonoscopy in different colorectal adenoma prevention studies using various potential chemopreventive agents. DFMO, difluoromethylornithine; vit., vitamin. *(Courtesy Asad Umar, DVM, PhD, Bethesda, Md.)*

lower and middle regions of the crypts. Normally, as cells migrate upward from deeper in the crypt, the number of cells that continue to proliferate decreases, and, on reaching the upper crypt region, cells become terminally differentiated and can no longer divide; this sequence of events is disordered during the evolution of neoplastic lesions in the colon. Increased proliferative activity and characteristic differences in the distribution of proliferating cells within the colonic crypts distinguish at-risk and affected members of kindreds with FAP and nonpolyposis inherited colon cancer from lower-risk groups. Correlations of rectal mucosal proliferation with clinical and pathologic features of nonfamilial colorectal neoplasia also have been demonstrated. Conversely, populations at low risk for developing colon cancer have relatively quiescent proliferative activity in their colonic mucosa. Disordered proliferative activity can be found in the colonic mucosa of rodents treated with a variety of chemical carcinogens, and increased proliferative activity is seen in animals whose colonic or rectal mucosa is exposed to tumor promoters such as secondary bile acids. Colonic epithelial cells also fail to repress DNA synthesis during epithelial renewal in UC, a condition associated with an increased risk of CRC. Ornithine decarboxylase, an enzyme marker of rapid cellular proliferation, is present at high levels in the mucosa of members of familial polyposis kindreds, and levels increase in the colonic mucosa during chemically induced colonic carcinogenesis in rats. Ornithine decarboxylase increases in the colonic mucosa with age and is elevated in older adult patients with colonic adenomas. Experimental evidence also suggests that PKC may be involved in the stimulation of colonic epithelial cell proliferation by tumor promoters. These findings have led to speculation that inhibitors of cellular proliferation might prove useful as anticancer drugs. NSAIDs and COX-2 inhibitors, for example, decrease proliferation and increase apoptosis (see earlier).

An explosion of knowledge in molecular genetics has demonstrated how the accumulation of genetic alterations (gene mutations and amplifications in proto-oncogenes and tumor suppressor genes) and epigenetic alterations (aberrant DNA

methylation, chromatin modifications) lead to disruption of mechanisms that regulate the normal cell cycle and cell proliferation. In some cases, such as FAP, the cell is predisposed to abnormal proliferation because of germline mutations, whereas in others, somatic mutations result from complex interactions with environmental factors, as detailed earlier.

Molecular Genetics and Biochemical Abnormalities

Molecular Genetics

Tumor cells in the colon, as elsewhere, are characterized by heritable phenotypic changes that are the result of quantitative or qualitative alterations in gene expression (see Chapters 1 and 126). A large body of evidence demonstrates that CRCs are associated with an accumulation of such genetic alterations (Fig. 127-6; Table 127-2). Genetic changes that lead to the development of CRC traditionally have been categorized into 3 major classes: alterations in proto-oncogenes, loss of tumor suppressor gene activity, and abnormalities in genes involved in DNA mismatch repair (MMR).[60,61] Adenomas and carcinomas arise in the context of genomic instability, by which epithelial cells acquire the number of mutations needed to attain a neoplastic state. Destabilization of the genome is a prerequisite to tumor formation and most commonly involves chromosomal instability (CIN), which is found in 80% to 85% of colorectal tumors with subsequent allelic loss, or chromosomal amplifications and translocations. Increased rates of intragenic mutation in tandemly repeated DNA sequences known as *microsatellites* (microsatellite instability [MSI]) are characteristic of about 15% of sporadic cancers. MSI-CRCs are characterized by the presence of at least 30% unstable loci in a panel of loci consisting of mono- and dinucleotide tracts (see later).[60]

Cellular proto-oncogenes are evolutionarily conserved human genes that contain DNA sequences homologous to those of acute transforming retroviruses. Many of these genes play a role in signal transduction and the normal regulation of cell growth. Inappropriate activation of these genes leads to abnormal transmission of regulatory messages from the cell surface to the nucleus that results in abnormal proliferation and, eventually, tumor formation. Three human *ras* genes—*K-ras*, *N-ras*, and *H-ras*—encode guanine nucleotide-binding proteins that regulate intracellular signaling pathways. Approximately 65% of sporadic CRCs have activating point mutations in a *ras* gene, most in *K-ras*. Most *ras* mutations appear to occur during intermediate stages of adenoma growth (see Chapter 126). *Ras* gene mutations occur in 47% of carcinomas (58% of adenomas > 1 cm, but only 10% of adenomas < 1 cm), suggesting that earlier events must contribute to formation of neoplasms. Alterations in signal transduction might lead to abnormal cell growth and thus participate in neoplastic transformation, but activation of *ras* alone is not sufficient for progression to carcinoma. The exact functional relationship between *ras* mutations and carcinogenesis remains to be established, but understanding the role of *ras* mutations to stimulate proliferation might lead to development of antitumor therapies aimed at interrupting signals that alter tumor cell growth.

Abundant evidence has shown that allelic losses, particularly at chromosome locations 5q, 17p, and 18q, play major etiologic roles for colon tumors.[60,61] A deletion within chromosome 5 in patients with FAP led to the identification of the *APC* gene on the long arm of this chromosome (5q21). Positional cloning identified a single tumor suppressor gene, which is mutated in both the germline of FAP patients and in sporadic colorectal tumors. The protein encoded by *APC* consists of 2843 amino acids and is located at the

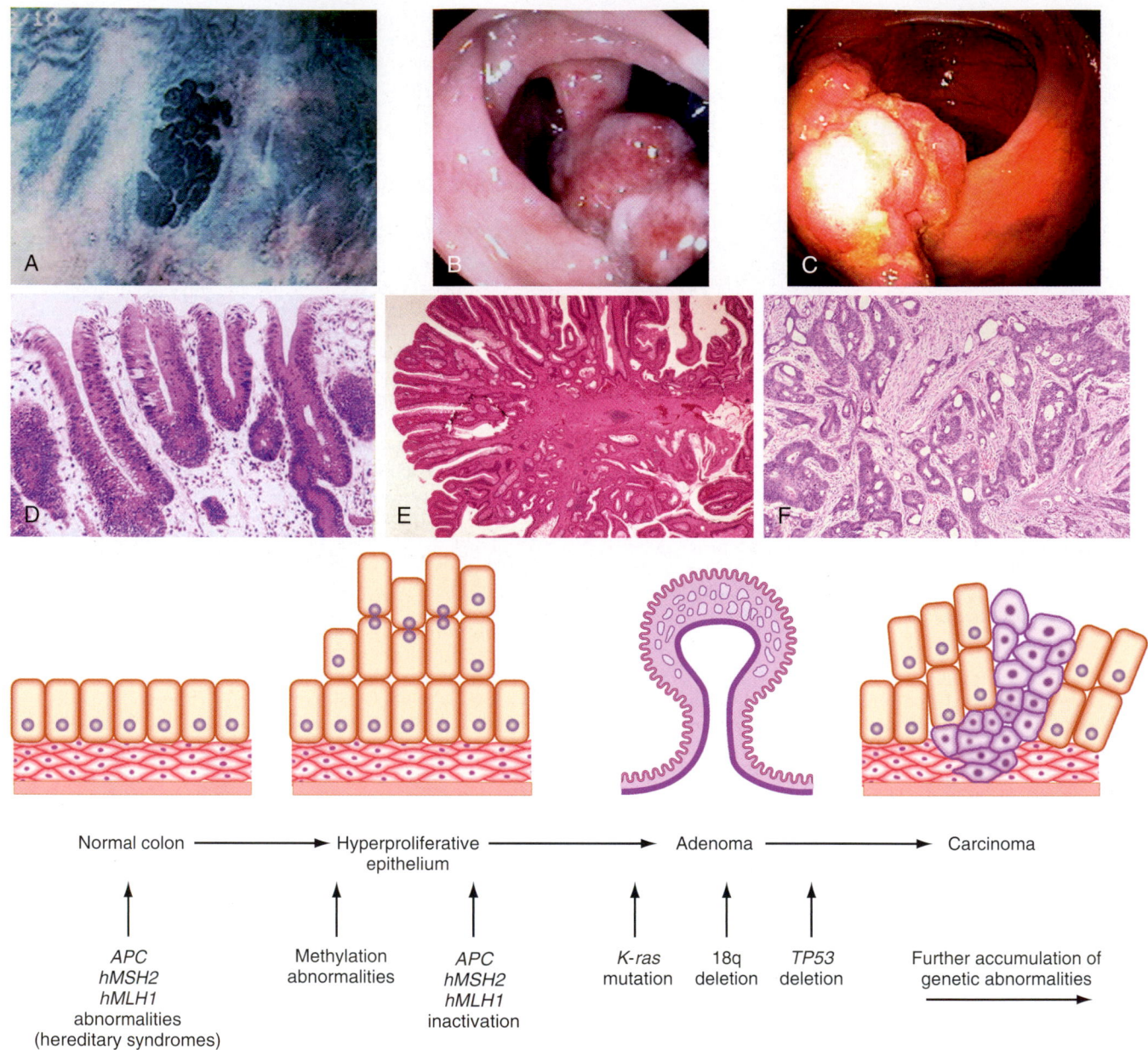

FIGURE 127-6. Proposed sequence of molecular genetic events in the evolution of colon cancer. Carcinomas arise from an accumulation of events, many of which have been defined. Alterations in *APC* or DNA mismatch repair genes may be inherited in the germline (familial adenomatous polyposis or Lynch syndrome, respectively) or may be acquired after birth (somatic mutations). Colorectal carcinomas (CRCs) may also arise as the result of different pathways involving genomic and epigenetic instability. These include chromosomal instability (CIN), microsatellite instability (MSI), CpG island methylator phenotype (CIMP), and global hypomethylation. These are distinct pathways by which CRCs arise and are associated with unique molecular features (see also Fig. 127-8). Images in this figure depict the traditional sequence of adenoma to carcinoma. An alternative "serrated pathway" involves gene silencing through a combination of epigenomic gene silencing and gene mutation. *Top row (A-C)* shows colonoscopic photographs, and *bottom row (D-F)* shows relevant histology. *Left to right,* Dysplastic aberrant crypt focus *(A and D),* adenomatous polyp *(B and E),* and invasive carcinoma *(C and F).* *(A,* methylene blue stain; *D, E,* and *F,* H&E stain.)

basolateral membrane of colorectal epithelial cells; expression is increasingly pronounced as cells migrate up through the colonic crypt.

Somatic mutations of the *APC* gene occur in 60% to 80% of sporadic CRCs and adenomas, including the smallest dysplastic lesions. These mutations result in truncation of the APC protein in more than 98% of cases, a finding that has led to the development of clinically useful tests for genetic screening of FAP families. Inactivation of both copies of the *APC*

gene appears to be the gatekeeping event for the initiation of colorectal neoplasia. The *APC* gene product interacts with at least 6 other proteins, including cytoplasmic glycogen synthetase 3β (GSK-3β) and axin. Inactivation of this gene is required for net cellular proliferation and initiation of colonic neoplasia.

APC functions to modulate extracellular signals that are transmitted to the nucleus through the cytoskeletal protein β-catenin, as part of the Wnt signaling pathway (Fig. 127-7).

TABLE 127-2 Genes Altered in Sporadic Colorectal Cancer

Gene	Chromosome	Frequency of Tumors with Gene Alterations (%)	Gene Class	Function of Gene Product
K-ras	12	50	Proto-oncogene	Encodes guanine nucleotide-binding protein that regulates intracellular signaling
APC	5	70	Tumor suppressor	Regulation of β-catenin that is involved in activation of WnT/TcF signaling (activates c-myc, cyclin D1)*; regulation of proliferation and apoptosis; interaction with E-cadherin (cell adhesion?)
DCC	18	70	Tumor suppressor?	Netrin-1 receptor; caspase substrate in apoptosis; cell adhesion
SMAD4 (DPC4, MADH4)	18	?	Tumor suppressor	Nuclear transcriptase factor in transforming growth factor (TGF)-β1 signaling; regulation of angiogenesis; regulator of WAF1 promoter; downstream mediator of SMAD2
TP53	17	75	Tumor suppressor	Transcription factor; regulates cell cycle progression after cellular stress; regulates apoptosis, gene expression, and DNA repair
hMSH2	2	†	DNA mismatch repair	Maintains fidelity of DNA replication
hMLH1	3	†	DNA mismatch repair	Maintains fidelity of DNA replication
hMSH6	2	†	DNA mismatch repair	Maintains fidelity of DNA replication
TGF-β1 RII	3	‡	Tumor suppressor	Receptor for signaling in the TGF-β1 pathway; inhibitor of colonic epithelial proliferation, often mutated in tumors with MSI

*β-Catenin mutations (downstream of APC) are found in 16%-25% of MSI colon cancers but not in MSS cancers.
†Approximately 15% of sporadic CRCs demonstrate MSI associated with alterations in mismatch repair genes (principally hMSH2 and hMLH1 but also hMSH3, hMSH6, hPMS1, and hPMS2).
‡Mutated in 73%-90% of MSI colon cancers. Up to 55% of MSS colon cancer cell lines demonstrate a TGF-β signaling blockage distal to TGF-β1 RII.
MSI, microsatellite instability; MSS, microsatellite stable; RII, type II receptor.

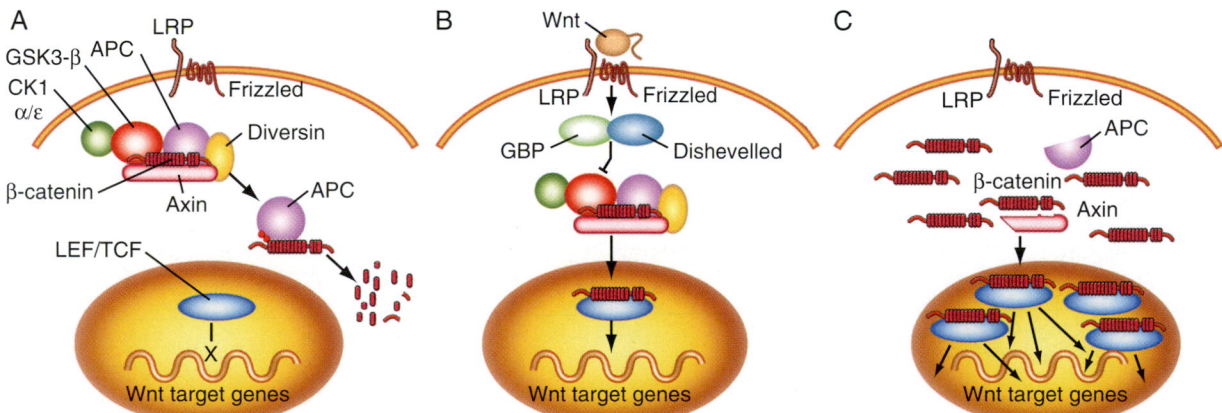

FIGURE 127-7. A model of Wnt signaling in normal (A and B) and cancer (C) cells. A, In the absence of Wnt signaling, APC, axin, and GSK3-β form a complex that results in β-catenin phosphorylation and degradation by a ubiquitin-dependent mechanism. B, Binding of Wnt to its cell surface receptor results in stabilization of β-catenin. Unphosphorylated β-catenin is able to translocate to the nucleus to form a complex with members of the LEF/TCF (lymphoid enhancer factor/T-cell factor) family and activates Wnt target genes. Frizzled and Dishevelled refer to gene products that participate in this pathway. C, Loss or mutation of APC results in lack of β-catenin degradation and high levels of this protein in the cytoplasm and nucleus. Strong evidence exists that misregulation of Wnt target gene expression is crucial to the transformation in colon cells. Many factors influence Wnt signaling, but evidence supports its importance in the evolution of most forms of colorectal cancer. GBP, glycogen synthase kinase-3 binding protein; LRP, lipoprotein receptor-related protein.

Nuclear β-catenin binds to transcription factors in the nucleus that are members of the lymphoid enhancer factor/T-cell factor (LEF/TCF) family, including Tcf-4, which in turn activate various target genes (e.g., *c-myc*, cyclin D$_1$)[62] that affect cell cycling and growth. *APC* is a tumor suppressor gene that binds to β-catenin and causes its degradation through phosphorylation. Loss of *APC* function, therefore, leads to accumulation of β-catenin and unopposed stimulation through the Wnt-Tcf signaling pathway, which in turn leads to increased and unregulated proliferation and decreased programmed cell death (apoptosis). *APC* gene abnormalities also might lead to disruption of normal cell-cell adhesion through altered association with the cellular adhesion molecule E-cadherin. Disruption of *APC*-mediated regulation of transcriptional activation is critical for colorectal tumorigenesis and is achieved most commonly through inactivating mutations of both *APC* alleles; disruption also can occur through dominant mutations of the β-catenin gene that render β-catenin Tcf-regulated transcription insensitive to the regulatory effects of normal wild-type *APC*.

Other genetic changes occur later in the adenoma-to-carcinoma sequence. Stepwise tumor progression is associated in more than 75% of cases with loss of tumor suppressor gene activity located on chromosome 18q. Several candidate genes are present on this chromosome, and loss of chromosome 18 is associated with a poor prognosis.[63] One gene, *DCC* (deleted in CRC), originally was thought to be important because its loss from a stage II (Dukes B) cancer was associated with a worse prognosis in some studies; more recently, its role as an important tumor suppressor gene has been questioned.

DPC4 (SMAD4) is another candidate tumor suppressor gene, inactivation of which might play a role in development of CRC. *DPC4* belongs to the SMAD gene family, which is involved in signal transduction pathways activated through the transforming growth factor (TGF)-β family receptors. Experimental inactivation of the homologue *Dpc4* in a mouse model of adenomatous polyposis coli results in malignant progression of intestinal and colonic polyps initiated by loss of the *Apc* gene (the mouse homologue of *APC*). Mutations in *SMAD4* and a related gene, *SMAD2*, have been reported in some sporadic CRCs. Deletions of chromosome 17p involve the *p53* tumor suppressor gene, the product of which normally prevents cells with damaged DNA from progressing from the G$_1$ to the S phase in the cell cycle. Deletions within chromosome 17p are present in approximately 75% of CRCs.

Loss of *TP53* also may be associated with reduced apoptosis of damaged cells. Inactivation of the *TP53* gene mediates the conversion from adenoma to carcinoma, a late and important event in colon carcinogenesis. Distant metastases from CRCs are associated with high fractional allelic loss and deletions of 17p and 18q. A distinct set of metastasis-suppressor genes also has been postulated.

Genomic instability creates a permissive state in which a cell acquires sufficient mutations to be transformed to a cancer cell; this is a common mechanism central to the development of most, if not all, colon cancers.[60,61] Several forms of genomic instability are common in colon cancer, including chromosome instability (CIN) and chromosome translocations, and MSI, in which subtle sequence changes, including base substitutions, deletions, or insertions, lead to a hypermutable state (Fig. 127-8). CIN may be produced by genes responsible for the human mitotic spindle checkpoint (*hBUB1* and *hBUBR1*), genes involved in the DNA damage checkpoint (*ATM, BRCA1* and *BRCA2, TP53,* and *hRad17*), and genes that control

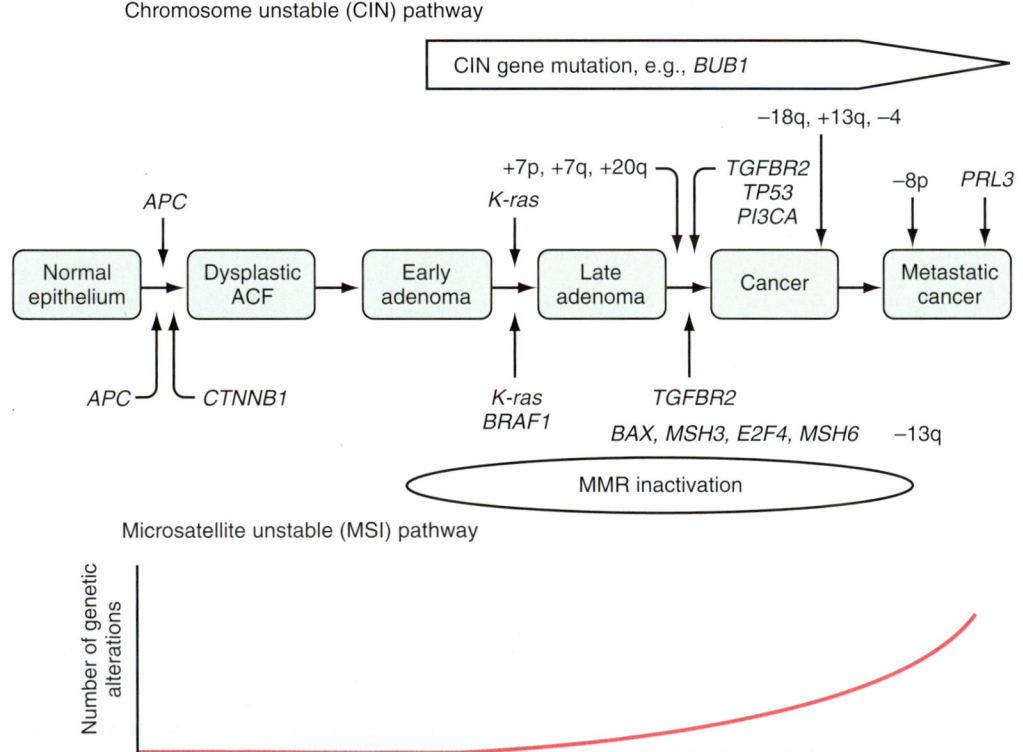

FIGURE 127-8. Model of colon cancer formation in tumors that progress through the adenoma-carcinoma sequence along pathways marked by chromosomal instability (CIN) or microsatellite instability. ACF, aberrant crypt focus; MMR, mismatch repair; TGF, transforming growth factor. *(Modified from Grady WM. Genomic instability and colon cancer. Cancer Metast Rev 2004; 23:11.)* (See text for details)

centrosome number. The CIN pathway is characterized by classic tubular adenoma histology, early acquisition of *APC* mutations, frequent early activation of *KRAS* mutations, loss of heterozygosity (LOH) in late adenomas, and *TP53* mutations that facilitate malignant transformation. Inactivation of genes involved in base excision repair (BER) resulting from oxidative damage are found in a subset of CRCs. Inactivation of 1 of the BER genes *(MYH)* is a cause of an autosomal recessive form of FAP. Although tumors that arise as the result of *MYH* germline mutations demonstrate chromosomal instability, they appear to have a unique pathogenesis compared with sporadic CRC.

The pathogenic significance of genomic instability became evident with the discovery of MSI in colon cancers associated with hereditary nonpolyposis CRC (HNPCC [Lynch syndrome]). Alterations in genes that help maintain DNA fidelity during replication are characteristic of HNPCC.[60,61] Alterations in MMR genes designated *hMLH1, hPMS1, hPMS2, hMSH2, hMSH3,* and *hMSH6* might lead to the inability to repair base pair mismatches and result in DNA replication errors or MSI. Inactivation of the MMR system causes genomic instability by increasing the rate of polymerase-generated replication errors and degrading the fidelity of DNA replication, particularly at microsatellite repeat sequences. MSI involves mutations or instability in short, tandemly repeated DNA sequences such as $(A)^n$, $(CA)^n$, and $(GATA)^n$. Such DNA sequences are found in several key genes that are important to maintain normal cellular function (Table 127-3). The receptor for TGF-β (TGF-βRII), for example, often is mutated as the result of MSI. Tumors with MSI frequently acquire *BRAF* mutations and are not associated with 18qLOH or *TP53* mutations. Sporadic MSI cancers often arise through the serrated neoplasia pathway.

Multiple lines of evidence suggest that the TGF-β pathway is an important tumor-suppressing pathway in the colon and that alterations in this pathway lead to tumor development. Less frequently targeted genes include the IGF-2 receptor; Bax and caspase 5, which are proteins that regulate apoptosis; E2F4, a transcription factor; and MSH3 and MSH6, DNA MMR proteins. β-Catenin mutations are present in up to 25% of MSI colon cancers. MSI, therefore, leads to accumulation of mutations in vulnerable genes, eventually resulting in the acquisition of the malignant phenotype. Although a high frequency of MSI (instability at >30% of microsatellite loci) is characteristic of HNPCC, similar alterations can be found in about 15% of sporadic CRCs and also in premalignant lesions. MSI tumors remain diploid. Patients whose tumors demonstrate MSI might have a better prognosis and respond differently to chemotherapy[60,64,65] than those whose tumors are characterized by CIN. Most patients with MSI colon cancers do not possess mutations in the known MMR genes, and evidence indicates that MSI in these tumors might arise through epigenetic mechanisms (i.e., clonal changes in gene expression without accompanying changes in DNA coding sequences).

The EGFR, which regulates cell growth and differentiation, is overexpressed in up to 82% of CRCs. Ras/Raf/MAPK and PI3K pathways are stimulated by EGFR. Monoclonal antibody therapies (e.g., cetuximab, panitumumab) that target the EGFR are used in treatment of advanced CRC (see later), but appear to only be effective in individuals whose tumors contain mutant *KRAS* (codons 12 and 13).

Epigenetic silencing is recognized now as an important mechanism in the evolution of a subgroup of CRCs.[66] DNA methylation within promoters and alterations in histone modifications appear to be primary mediators of epigenetic inheritance in cancer cells, and hypermethylation of the *hMLH1* promoter has been reported in up to 70% of sporadic MSI tumors. In the colon, aberrant methylation may be an important early event in the age-related field defect observed in

TABLE 127-3 Frequency of Some Target Gene Mutations in Colon Cancers with Microsatellite Instability (MSI)

Target Gene	Normal Function of Gene Product	Frequency of Mutation in Colon Cancers with MSI (%)
TGF-βR2	TGF-β signaling	90
ACVR2	Activin signaling	86
IGFIIR	IGF and TGF-β signaling	10
BAX	Apoptosis	50
hMSH 3	DNA mismatch repair	50
hMSH 6	DNA mismatch repair	33
E2F-4	Cell cycle control	65
PTEN	Growth regulation	19-34
MBD4 (MED1)	DNA repair and binding to methylated DNA	40
TCF4	Growth regulation	39
CHK1	G2 cell cycle checkpoint	10
STK11 (LKB1)	Signal transduction	<2
BLM	Chromosome stability, DNA repair; helicase	<18
Caspase 5 (ICErel-III)	Apoptosis	62
CDX2	Homeobox protein	<2
TPB	TATA binding protein	83
RIZ	Interacts with RB	26
hRAD50	DNA repair	31
SEC63	ER chaperone protein	49
AIM2	Interferon-inducible protein	48

NOTE: Most mutations cause frame shifts that prematurely truncate the protein, leading to inactivation of the affected allele.
ER, endoplasmic reticulum; IGF, insulin-like growth factor; RB, retinoblastoma protein; TGF, transforming growth factor.
Modified from Grady WM, Carethers J. Genomic and epigenetic instability in colorectal cancer progression. Gastroenterology 2008; 135:1079-99.

sporadic colorectal neoplasia. Aberrant methylation also contributes to tumor progression through a hypermethylator phenotype (CPG island methylator phenotype [CIMP]) that is responsible for most cases of MSI related to *hMLH1* inactivation (associated with about 15% of sporadic CRCs).[60,66,67] The hallmark of CIMP is abnormal methylation of several tumor promoters. In 1 model, hyperplastic aberrant crypt foci may be the initial lesions in a pathway leading to the development of serrated adenomas (see Chapter 126). Methylated promoters of the *MGMT, EVL, HLTF, SFRP1* and *SFRP2, SLC5A8, RUX3, CRBP1,* and *MINT1* and *MINT31* genes (MINTs are not genes per se, but loci found to be "methylated in tumor") develop during tumor initiation, and *hMLH1* promoter hypermethylation corresponds to the development of a serrated adenoma, with methylated *TSP1* and *TIMP3* helping to drive tumor progression.[60,61] DNA methylation and histone H3 lysine 9 hypoacetylation and methylation appear to form a mutually reinforcing loop that contributes to tumor suppressor gene inactivation in CRCs. A large number of additional genes are commonly methylated and silenced in CRC.[66]

The *BRAF* gene, encoding a downstream component of the *RAS/RAF/MAPK* pathway, is often mutated in sporadic MSI tumors, but not in tumors from patients with HNPCC (see later). Sporadic MSI tumors frequently carry *BRAF V600E* mutations. The presence of a *BRAF* mutation in an MSI tumor effectively eliminates the possibility that it arose in the setting of Lynch syndrome.

MicroRNAs are 18- to 25-nucleotide noncoding RNA molecules that regulate translation of many genes. MicroRNAs function in most cases to repress the activity of specific messenger (mRNA) molecules, either by promoting their degradation or preventing their translation into proteins. Expression patterns of microRNAs are altered in colon cancers, and they may be associated with survival and therapeutic outcome.[68,69]

Biochemical and Other Changes (see also Chapter 1)

Alterations in cell surface and secreted proteins and glycoproteins, including a number of important cell adhesion molecules, are characteristic of CRC.[70] Interactions between tumor cells or between tumor cells and their environment may be homotypic (involving like molecules) or heterotypic (involving different adhesion molecules). Homotypic interactions often maintain the integrity of primary tumors by fostering adhesion between neighboring tumor cells, whereas heterotypic interactions might occur among tumor cells and platelets, lymphocytes, vascular endothelial cells, and components of the basement membrane matrix. Most tumor-associated molecules represent quantitatively or qualitatively altered molecules found either on normal tissues or during development, such as oncofetal antigens (e.g., CEA). Many of these molecules appear to play a role in maintaining normal tissue homeostasis or targeting blood-borne cells to specific sites. Altered expression, therefore, might contribute to tumor invasion and metastasis.

MMPs (matrix metalloproteinases) are a family of enzymes that degrade extracellular matrix. Overexpression of MMP-1, -2, -3, -7, -9, and -13 and MT1-MMP has been demonstrated in human CRCs. The degree of overexpression of some MMPs correlates with stage of disease, prognosis, or both.[71]

Metastasis is a multistage process by which tumor cells escape the primary tumor and establish secondary foci at distant sites (Fig. 127-9). Cells in the primary tumor must become vascularized (angiogenesis via VEGFs). Then they must escape the primary tumor by overcoming adhesive interactions (e.g., loss of E-cadherin) and by disrupting basement membranes (metalloproteinases such as type IV collagenase, matrilysin, loss of tissue inhibitors of collagenase). Finally

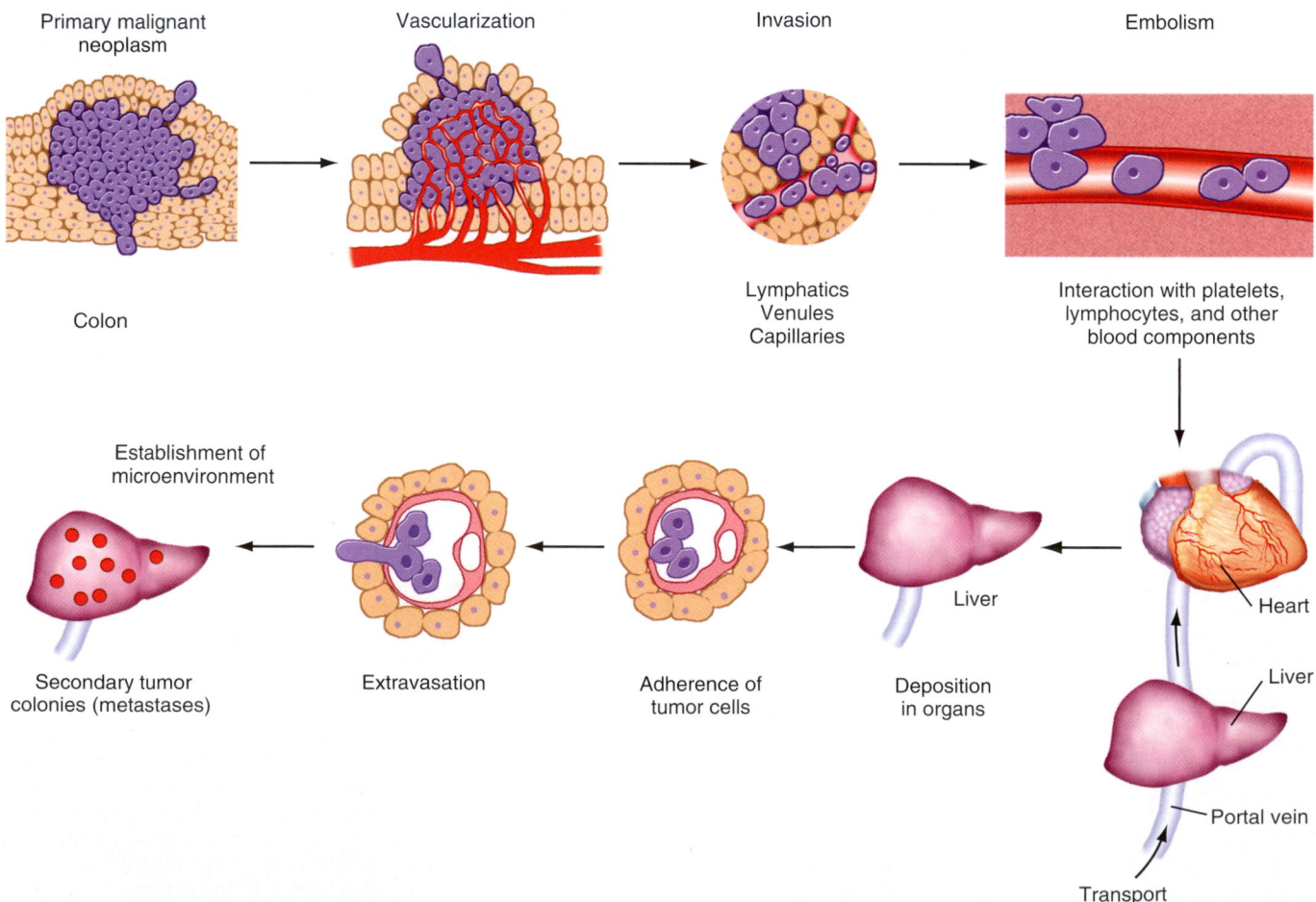

FIGURE 127-9. Multistage process of colon cancer metastasis. Cancer cells metastasize through a complex multistage process. For tumor cells to form metastatic foci at distant sites, they must complete all stages of this process.

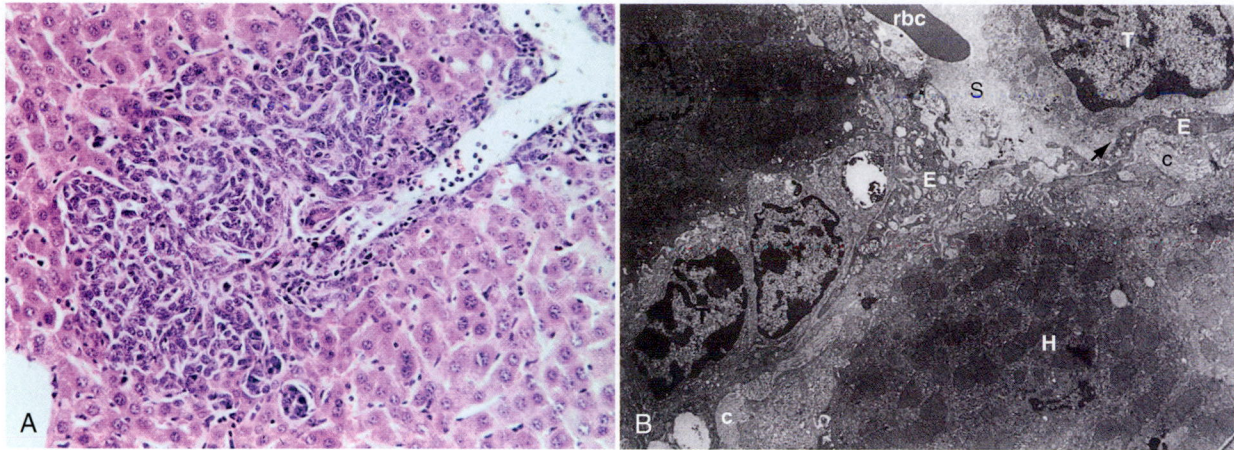

FIGURE 127-10. Colon cancer metastasis. On reaching the liver, colon cancer cells adhere to the sinusoidal endothelium through specific interactions and then invade the parenchyma. *A*, Photomicrograph showing tumor cells invading the liver after extravasation from a blood vessel. (H&E stain.) *B*, Electron micrograph showing collagen bundles (c) and tumor cells (T) adherent to sinusoidal endothelium (E) and invading between hepatocytes (H). rbc, red blood cell; S, sinusoid.

they must enter lymphatics, the circulation, or both. In the bloodstream, they must survive interactions with blood components and the immune system and be transported to distant organ sites (principally the liver). At distant sites, tumor cells adhere to target endothelia via specific interactions (e.g., tumor-associated sialoglycoproteins and endothelial selectins) (Fig. 127-10), extravasate, interact with the microenvironment (e.g., growth factors), and establish secondary tumor foci.

Tumor cell subpopulations with different metastatic potentials exist within the same primary tumor, and metastases result from the selective dissemination of tumor cells that possess the ability to participate in all stages of this complex process. Several carbohydrate antigens have been studied in relation to their potential usefulness as markers of metastatic potential and for their possible role in determining prognosis.[70-73]

FAMILIAL COLORECTAL CANCER

Genetic predisposition plays a role in a substantial number of CRCs. Although it is convenient to categorize CRCs into hereditary (or familial) and nonhereditary (or sporadic) types, it is more appropriate to assume that all cancers have genetic components that may be inherited or acquired to varying degrees. Accordingly, persons with familial CRC are born with an altered genome, and the environment might contribute additional genotoxic events, leading to the malignant phenotype. In the case of sporadic cancers, multiple somatic mutations are contributed by the environment (see Chapter 1).

The role of heredity in the genesis of colon cancer is manifested most obviously in those with the heritable polyposis syndromes (see Chapter 126). These syndromes are inherited in an autosomal dominant manner and are characterized by the presence of hundreds to thousands of colonic adenomas, with or without extracolonic tumors. Adenomas develop approximately a decade before the appearance of cancer, and virtually all affected persons eventually develop colon cancer if the colon is not removed. Nevertheless, these dramatic syndromes account for less than 1% of all cases of CRC.

Lynch syndrome (HNPCC) is an inherited disease in which colon cancers arise in discrete adenomas, but polyposis—hundreds of polyps—does not occur.[74,75] HNPCC

BOX 127-2 Amsterdam II Criteria for Hereditary Nonpolyposis Colorectal Cancer (Lynch Syndrome)

At least 3 relatives with CRC (one must be a first-degree relative of the other two) or a Lynch syndrome–associated cancer*
CRC involving at least 2 successive generations
One or more cancer cases before age 50 years
Familial adenomatous polyposis should be excluded
Tumors should be verified by histologic examination

*Endometrium, ovary, stomach, ureter/renal pelvis, pancreas, brain, hepatobiliary tract, small intestine, and multiple sebaceous adenomas and carcinomas and keratoacanthomas in the Muir-Torre variant of Lynch syndrome.
CRC, colorectal cancer.
Criteria defined by the International Collaborative Group on Hereditary Nonpolyposis Colorectal Cancer.

---

accounts for approximately 6% of colonic adenocarcinoma and is an autosomal dominant disorder with high penetration; approximately 80% are caused by germline mutations in genes that are responsible for repair of DNA errors (i.e., mismatches) that occur during DNA replication when DNA polymerase creates single base-pair mismatches, with resultant structural abnormalities (loop-outs) involving unpaired bases. These errors tend to occur at repetitive DNA sequences termed *microsatellites,* and they are repaired by enzymes coded for by MMR genes. The majority of reported germline mutations in DNA MMR genes have been associated with the *hMSH2* gene on chromosome 2 (40% to 50%) and the *hMLH1* gene on chromosome 3 (20% to 30%). Mutations in *hMSH6, hPMS1,* and *hPMS2* also have been reported in a small number of patients with HNPCC; no locus has been identified, however, for many HNPCC families.

HNPCC was most strictly defined by the International Collaborative Group on Hereditary Non-Polyposis Colorectal Cancer by the Amsterdam criteria (Box 127-2): at least 3 relatives with histologically verified CRC, 1 of them a first-degree relative of the other 2 (FAP excluded); at least 2 successive generations affected; and, in 1 of the individuals, diagnosis of CRC before age 50 years. Because these criteria do not account for the frequent occurrence of extracolonic cancers in such families or for small kindreds, broader clinical criteria were developed, such as the Bethesda Guidelines and Revised Bethesda Guidelines published by a National Cancer

Institute-sponsored workshop on HNPCC (Box 127-3).[75,76] HNPCC families include members whose heritable cancer is limited to the colon and rectum (site-specific HNPCC, HNPCC type a, Lynch's syndrome I) and families whose members also are prone to cancer of the female genital tract and other sites (cancer family syndrome, HNPCC type b, Lynch's syndrome II) (Fig. 127-11). In HNPCC syndromes, discrete polyps, but not polyposis, may be seen to antedate the cancers. Adenomas in the proximal colon often are flat or slightly raised lesions with foci of adenomatous change that are confined to the upper half of crypts (flat adenomas). HNPCC tumors have a tendency to involve the proximal colon and to be multiple (synchronous and metachronous), with a higher incidence of mucinous carcinomas (Table 127-4). These CRCs usually appear at age 40 to 50 years, 2 decades earlier than CRC in the general population. HNPCC accounts for 4% to 6% of CRCs.

Patients with Lynch syndrome and some unaffected family members have biological markers that resemble those in patients with FAP syndromes, including abnormal proliferative activity of colonic crypt cells, increased tetraploidy (twice the normal DNA content) in skin fibroblasts cultured in vitro, decreased degradation of fecal cholesterol, and cell-mediated immune defects in vitro that might interfere with the recognition of killing of incipient tumor cells in vivo. The

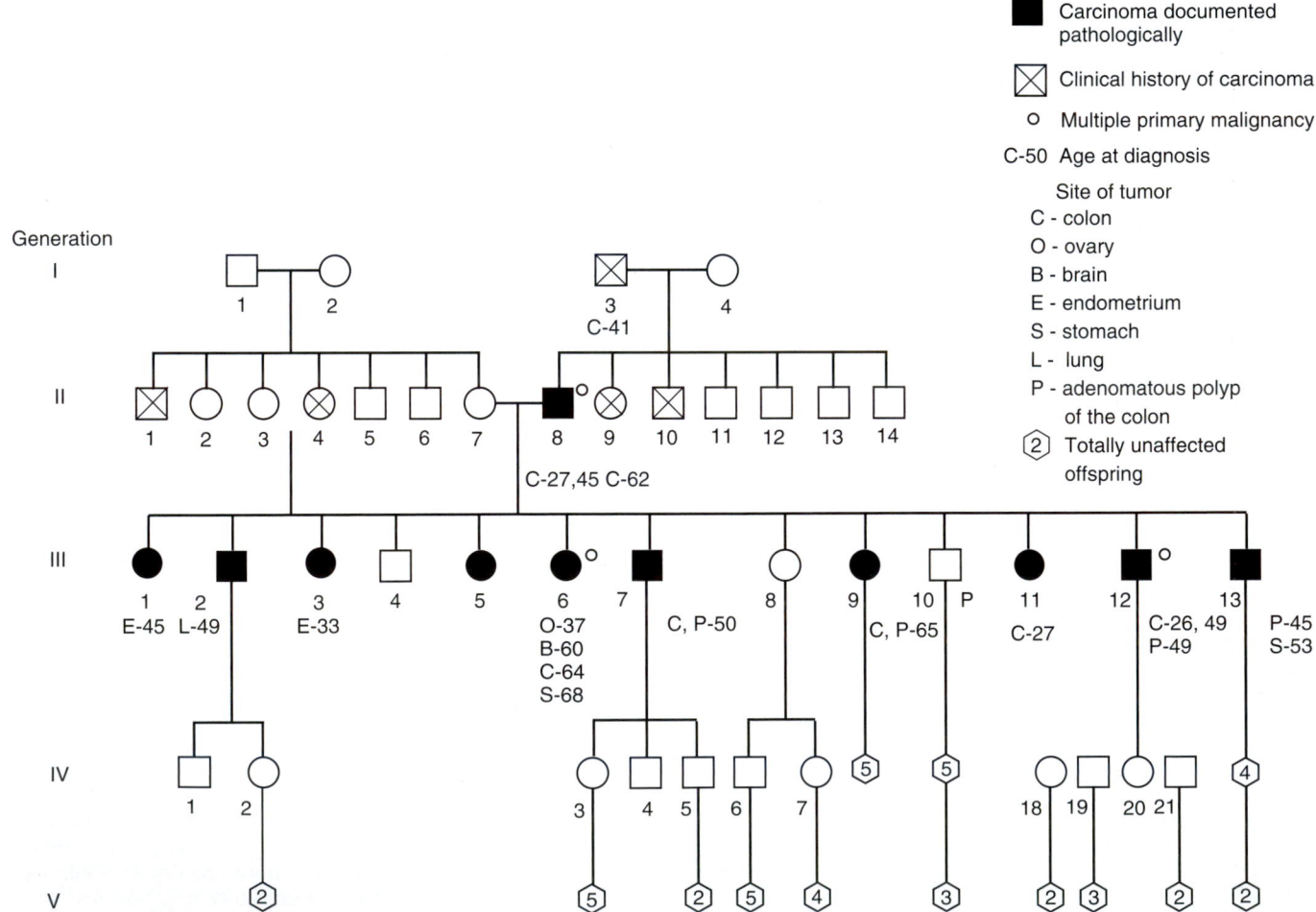

FIGURE 127-11. Pattern of inheritance of cancer in a familial aggregate with Lynch syndrome. Affected members were found in generations I, II, and III; members of generations IV and V were still young and at risk for developing carcinomas when the pedigree was obtained. *(From Boland CR. Familial colonic cancer syndromes. West J Med 1983; 139:351.)*

TABLE 127-4 Comparison of Clinical Features in Lynch Syndrome and Sporadic Colorectal Cancer

Clinical Feature	Lynch Syndrome	Sporadic Colorectal Cancer
Mean age at diagnosis (years)	45	67
Multiple colon cancers	35%	4%-11%
Synchronous colon cancers	18%	3%-6%
Metachronous colon cancers	24%	1%-5%
Proximal location of the initial cancer*	72%	35%
Increased risk of malignant tumors at other sites	Yes	No
Mucinous and poorly differentiated colon cancers	Common	Infrequent
Prognosis	Favorable[†]	Variable

*Proximal to the splenic flexure.
[†]Patients whose tumors demonstrate microsatellite instability have a more favorable prognosis than those with microsatellite-stable tumors.

BOX 127-4 Categories for Risk for Developing Colorectal Cancer (CRC)

Average Risk
Individuals ≥ 50 years of age with:
    No family history of colorectal neoplasia (adenoma, cancer)
    No personal history of adenoma or CRC
    No personal history of IBD

Increased Risk
Personal history of CRC
Personal history of adenoma*
Family history of sporadic CRC[†]
Family history of sporadic adenoma[†]

High Risk
Hereditary nonpolyposis CRC (Lynch syndrome)
Polyposis syndromes:
    Familial adenomatous polyposis (FAP)
    Attenuated FAP
    MYH-associated polyposis
    Peutz-Jeghers syndrome
    Turcot's syndrome
    Muir-Torre syndrome
    Juvenile polyposis syndrome
    Hyperplastic polyposis syndrome
IBD (UC, Crohn's disease)[‡]

*The risk of developing CRC in individuals with a personal history of adenoma varies according to the size, histology, and multiplicity of index lesions.
[†]The risk of developing CRC in those with a family history of sporadic adenoma or CRC depends on the number and degree (first degree, second degree, etc.) of affected relatives and the age at which neoplasia occurred in these individuals.
[‡]Individuals with IBD have been categorized as "increased risk" or "high risk" according to different guidelines. Risk is high in individuals with high-grade dysplasia or dysplasia-associated mass lesions.

genetic defect in HNPCC, however, results from loss of the *hMSH2*, *hMLH1*, and other genes, leading to increased susceptibility to mutation from failure to repair base-pair mismatches.[77]

Although CRC syndromes with apparent patterns of inheritance currently account for only a small portion of total colon cancer cases, hereditary factors may be present in a larger proportion of cases. Genetic susceptibility to CRC in the general population is suggested by the 2- to 3-fold increase in CRC in first-degree relatives of patients with sporadic adenomas and CRCs. The relative risk is even stronger when cancer occurs in family members younger than 50 years of age. The precise role of genetic factors in this group and their interaction with the environment in the evolution of CRC remains to be defined. Identification of susceptibility genes in this group is of great interest and has been aided by genome-wide scanning techniques in sibling pairs with colorectal neoplasia.[78]

PREDISPOSING FACTORS

The risk of developing CRC depends on a number of demographic factors (Box 127-4) including diet and other environmental factors (see Box 127-1, Table 127-1, and Fig. 127-5), age, personal history of adenoma or of carcinoma, existence of predisposing diseases (particularly IBD), and family history. It has been proposed that risk scores may be developed to aid in identifying and treating susceptible persons.[79]

Age

The risk of developing CRC rises sharply after age 40 in the general population; 90% of cancers occur in persons aged 50 years and older (Fig. 127-12). A 50-year-old person has about a 5% chance of developing CRC if he or she survives to age

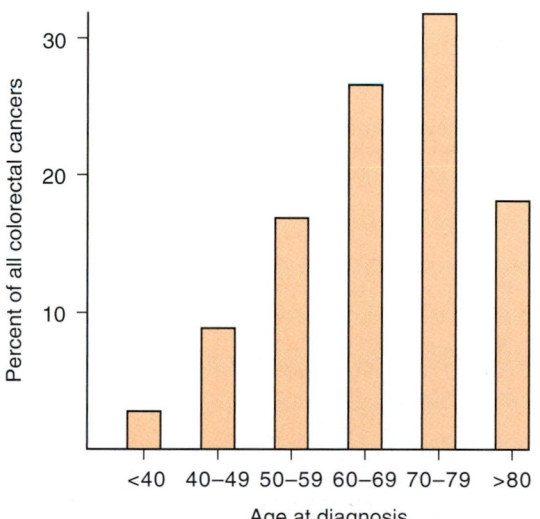

FIGURE 127-12. Frequency of colorectal cancers (CRCs) by age at diagnosis in the USA; 90% of CRCs occur after age 50 years.

80 years, and a 2.5% risk of dying from the disease; this has important implications for screening (see later). Sporadic CRCs arise in other age groups, however, and the diagnosis must be considered in younger persons with typical signs and symptoms, especially if they have a family history of colorectal neoplasia.

Prior Adenoma and Carcinoma

Adenoma

Present evidence strongly indicates that most CRCs arise from preexisting adenomas (see Chapter 126). The risk of CRC increases with the number of adenomas, the most extreme example being the familial polyposis syndromes. Clinical and morphologic evidence suggest that as adenomas grow larger, they progressively dedifferentiate, become dysplastic, and then become malignant. With increasing size or increasing villous architecture, the incidence of nuclear atypia, dysplasia, and in situ or invasive carcinoma increases. Despite the potential for adenomas to evolve to carcinomas, however, the actual risk of this phenomenon is unknown.

Adenomatous polyps are common, especially after age 50 years, in populations that consume a Western diet, but the prevalence of adenomas is high compared with the incidence of cancer. It has been estimated that 29% of the living population older than age 35 in Norway have colorectal adenomas, with an annual conversion rate of adenomas to carcinoma of 0.25. The malignancy rate is higher in advanced adenomas (i.e., large adenomas, adenomas with villous architecture, and adenomas with cytologic nuclear atypia or dysplasia). The estimated annual rate of conversion to invasive cancer in persons with adenomas larger than 1 cm, villous components, or severe dysplasias has been reported to be 3%, 17%, and 37%, respectively. Data from a national colonoscopy data base in Germany suggested that the annual transition rates from advanced adenoma to cancer also increase with age.[80]

Carcinoma

People with CRC have an increased risk of harboring a second carcinoma (synchronous carcinomas) or of developing another one subsequently (metachronous carcinomas). The frequency of more than 1 carcinoma in the same person ranges between 2% and 6% (0.7% to 7.6% for synchronous cancers and 1.1% to 4.7% for metachronous ones). Most patients with simultaneous cancers have 1 in the proximal colon and the other in the distal colon; in the minority of patients with synchronous cancers, the 2 lesions are located in the same colonic segment. The degree of invasiveness of synchronous cancers often differs, and prognosis depends on the worst-stage lesion. Five-year survival rates for patients with synchronous cancers whose cancers have been resected are similar to those with single lesions. The interval between an initial cancer and a metachronous one may be considerable (lesions separated by as long as 23 years have been reported), but several studies note that 50% of metachronous cancers arise within 5 to 7 years of the index lesion. Second cancers often occur at a site remote from the initial lesion.

Family History

The risk of CRC in first-degree relatives of those with sporadic CRC is increased 2- to 3-fold. The risk is higher when adenoma or carcinoma has occurred in a relative at an early age or when more than 1 relative has had carcinoma. These factors have been taken into account in screening guidelines that stratify patients according to potential cancer risk.[81-83] The inherited polyposis syndromes and their cancer risks, including FAP and its variants and the hamartomatous polyposis syndromes,[84,85] are discussed in Chapter 126.

IBD

Patients with idiopathic IBD (UC, Crohn's disease) are at increased risk for developing CRC (see Chapters 115 and 116).

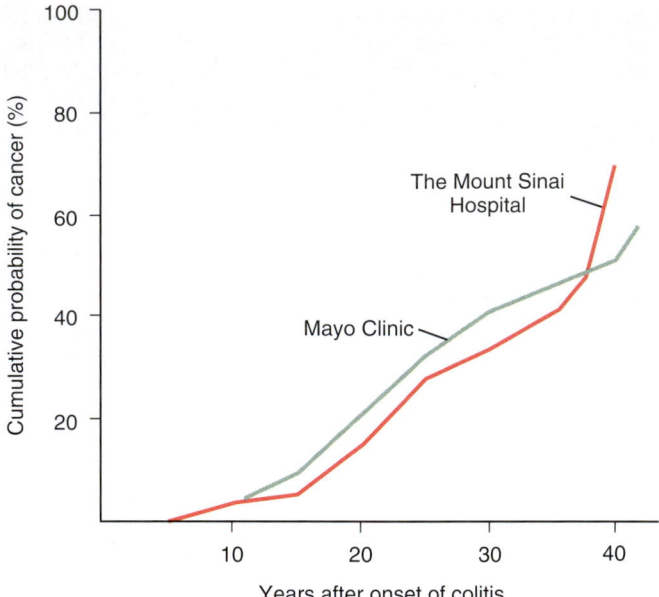

FIGURE 127-13. Cumulative probability of developing colorectal cancer in patients with UC seen at 2 tertiary referral centers. Data from primary care settings indicate a similar pattern but lower incidence rates.

Actuarially derived (life table) cumulative cancer incidences from tertiary referral centers (Fig. 127-13) agree that the risk of cancer in patients with UC begins after a disease duration of 7 years and rises about 10% per decade, reaching as high as 34% at 30 years. Nonetheless, difficulties related to sources of referral, sampling, recognition and characterization of disease, differences in follow-up procedures, and methods used to detect neoplastic disease cloud many such studies. More recent data indicate a CRC risk at 30 years of 15.8% to 18%,[86] with lower risks suggested in several smaller studies, including those from the primary care setting.

The risk of CRC for patients with UC correlates most closely with duration of disease. In a large group of patients with extensive disease who were followed prospectively, the risk of carcinoma per patient-year was zero before 10 years and 1 in 86 after 20 years; risk is greatest with universal colitis. It has been reported that the risk of cancer in left-sided disease (i.e., distal to the splenic flexure) begins approximately a decade later than with universal colitis, but at least 1 surveillance study found no difference between these groups in the temporal development of preneoplastic dysplasia. The risk for patients with ulcerative proctitis is only slightly increased compared with that in the general population.

The risk of cancer is not related to severity of the initial attack of colitis or age at onset of colitis, independent of disease duration. The relationship to disease activity per se is unclear, although chronic inflammation is a common theme in epithelial carcinogenesis. CRC in persons with UC is a risk factor for CRC in their relatives without colitis, and CRC in relatives without UC is a risk factor for those with colitis. There is an association of backwash ileitis with CRC in patients with UC who undergo proctocolectomy. Cancer that arises in the setting of UC traditionally has been thought to be a highly malignant lesion with a poor prognosis, but studies using matched controls from colon cancer populations without colitis have failed to show a significant difference in survival between the 2 groups.

The increased risk for CRC in patients with Crohn's disease or ileocolitis has been reported to be as much as 4 to 20 times that in the general population, although 1 cohort study failed to confirm an increased incidence of colon cancer in these patients. Cancer can arise at an earlier age in these patients than in the general population. Many of these cancers are mucinous carcinomas, and they often occur in surgically bypassed or strictured segments of colon.

Carcinomas do not develop de novo from normal mucosa but rather from mucosa that has undergone a sequence of morphologic changes that culminate in invasive carcinoma. As in precancerous adenomas, dysplasia is a precursor to carcinoma in IBD. Dysplasia comprises abnormalities in crypt architecture and cytologic detail (Figs. 127-14 and 127-15). Epithelial crypts are reduced in number, irregularly branched, and crowded together to give a pattern of so-called back-to-back glands. Cell nuclei may be enlarged and hyperchromatic, may have increased numbers of mitoses, and may be located at different levels in the cell, producing a picket-fence appearance (pseudostratification). Dysplasia is classified by grade as mild (or low grade) to severe (or high grade).

Retrospective analyses report that 90% of resected colons from patients with UC and cancer contain dysplastic mucosa somewhere in the colon and that 30% of patients with severe rectal or colonic dysplasia on resection or biopsy have coexisting carcinoma. Colonoscopic studies suggest that 25% of colons that demonstrate high-grade dysplasia on biopsy harbor a carcinoma. Dysplasia often is patchy, and it may be present in the colon but absent from the rectum.

Because the lack of uniformity of the definition of dysplasia can make interpretation of such data difficult, in 1983 the multidisciplinary Inflammatory Bowel Disease Dysplasia Morphology Study Group developed a standardized classification for dysplasia arising in the setting of IBD that is still used today in the USA despite attempts at alternative classification systems.[86] Biopsy specimens are classified as negative, indefinite, or positive for dysplasia (low and high grade). Several large prospective studies have attempted to determine the true risk of cancer in patients with colonic dysplasia and UC and the impact of screening programs for dysplasia.

Results suggest that biopsy surveillance programs can be effective in helping control the risk of carcinoma in patients with long-standing UC. The risk of cancer appears highest in those with high-grade dysplasia that arises in visible plaques or masses (dysplasia-associated lesion or mass [DALM], as illustrated in Fig. 127-15). A computer cohort decision analysis suggested that surveillance should increase life expectancy for patients with UC. Most investigators believe that patients who have UC for more than 7 to 8 years should undergo annual colonoscopy with multiple mucosal biopsies to identify areas of dysplasia; they advocate colectomy for severe dysplasia or DALM. Because the significance of low-grade or moderate dysplasia is less clear, immediate resection for patients with these levels of dysplasia is controversial. Prophylactic colectomy also has been recommended as an option for those with disease of at least 10 years' duration. Studies employing flow cytometry have detected aneuploid cell populations in colons resected for UC with dysplasia or early cancer. Chromosomal and molecular alterations, such as overexpression of p53 and relative loss of 18q, and findings of high MSI can occur early in UC-related neoplastic progression and appear to precede the histologic development of dysplasia.[86] Both dysplasia and increased risk of colon carcinoma have been reported in patients with Crohn's disease. As in UC, dysplasia appears in diseased colon segments, and its presence correlates with duration of disease.[86]

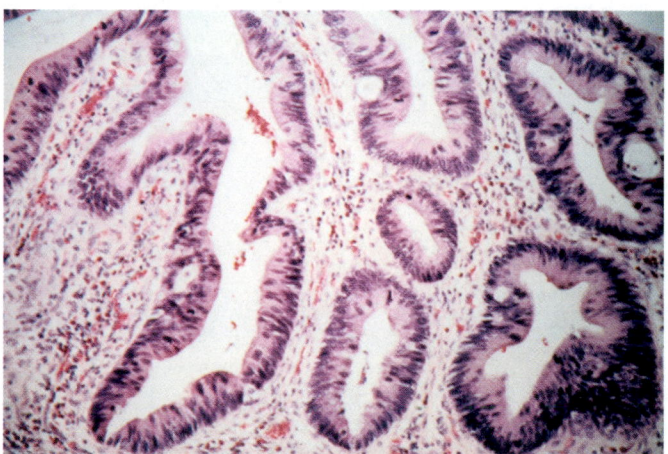

FIGURE 127-14. Histopathology of dysplasia in the setting of UC. The number of goblet cells is decreased. Glands are branched, irregular, and crowded together. Cell nuclei are hyperchromatic and occur at different levels, producing a pseudopalisading or picket-fence appearance. (H&E stain.)

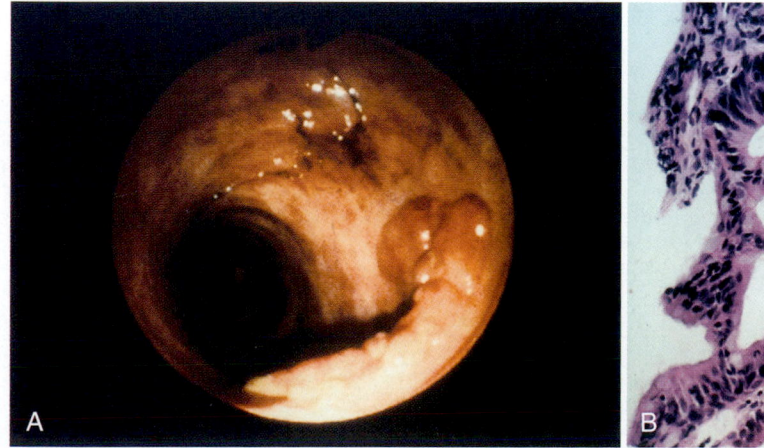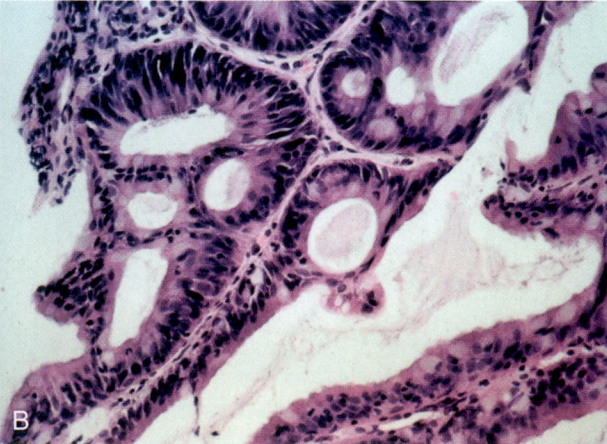

FIGURE 127-15. Plaque-like dysplasia-associated lesion or mass in a patient with long-standing UC. *A,* Colonoscopic view of the lesion. *B,* Histopathology of a biopsy specimen revealing high-grade dysplasia. (H&E stain.)

Other Associations

Diverting bile and bile acids to the lower small intestine, either surgically or by administration of cholestyramine, increases the yield of proximal colon tumors in carcinogen-treated animals. There is no evidence in humans, however, that chronic use of cholestyramine is associated with an increased risk of colon cancer. The possibility of an increase in colon cancer following cholecystectomy has been raised, although the clinical evidence for such an association is contradictory. Increased proliferative activity in the distal colonic mucosa has been demonstrated in patients who have undergone cholecystectomy, and an increased incidence of tubular adenomas has been observed in patients older than 60 years with a postcholecystectomy interval of more than 10 years; an increased risk of colon cancer for these patients has been both supported and refuted. A retrospective population-based cohort study that used the Swedish Inpatient Register evaluated almost 23,000 persons who had had cholecystectomy up to 31 years previously.[87] Patients having had cholecystectomy had an increased risk of proximal intestinal adenocarcinoma, which declined with increasing distance from the common bile duct. The risk was significantly increased for adenocarcinoma of the small bowel and ascending colon but not the remaining colon or rectum.

Diabetes mellitus has been associated with CRC. It has been suggested that insulin resistance and hyperin-sulinemia contribute to colorectal carcinogenesis. Although hypergastrinemia has been associated with CRC risk in animal models, there is less compelling evidence that this is clinically significant in humans.

PATHOLOGY

Gross Pathology

The gross morphologic features of CRC depend on the tumor's site. Carcinomas of the proximal colon, particularly those of the cecum and ascending colon, tend to be large and bulky, often outgrowing their blood supply and undergoing necrosis (Fig. 127-16); this polypoid configuration, however, also may be found elsewhere in the colon and rectum. In the more distal colon and rectum, tumors more commonly involve a greater circumference of the bowel and produce an annular constriction or napkin-ring appearance (Fig. 127-17). The fibrous stroma of these tumors accounts for the constriction and narrowing of the colon lumen, whereas the circular arrangement of colonic lymphatics is responsible for their annular growth. These tumors also can ulcerate, and occasionally they have a flatter appearance with predominantly intramural spread (Fig. 127-18); the latter are seen most often in the setting of IBD. Morphologic features of CRCs have clinical, diagnostic, and prognostic implications.

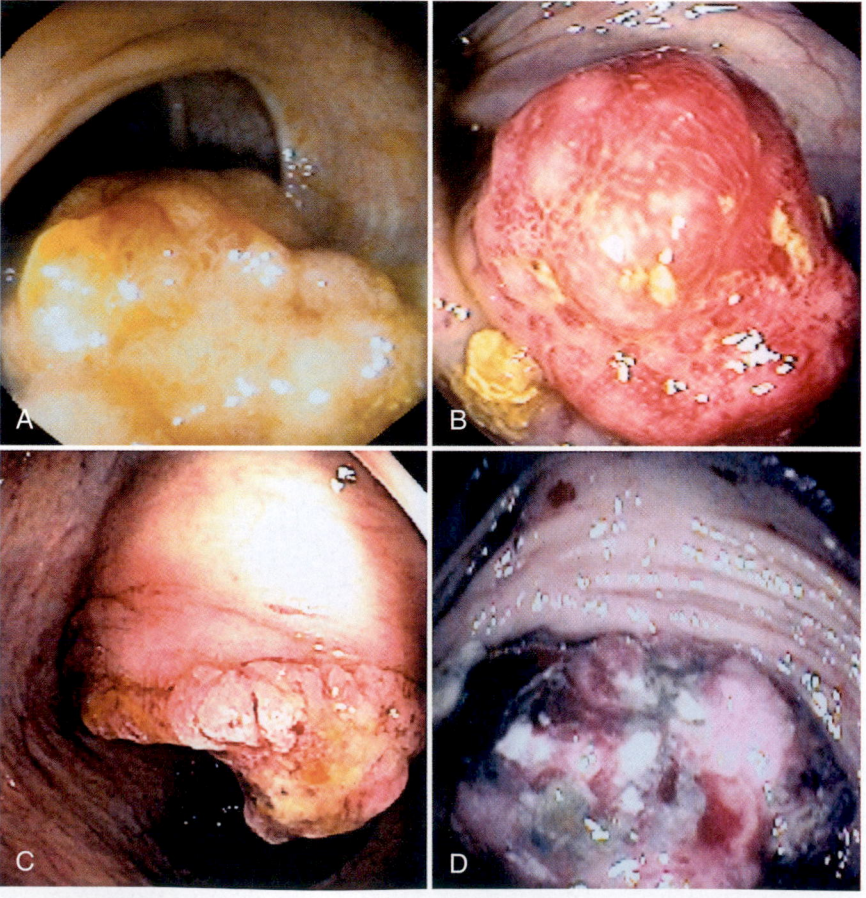

FIGURE 127-16. Carcinomas of the cecum seen at colonoscopy. Carcinomas of the proximal colon are often large and bulky polypoid lesions (A and B), may involve the ileocecal valve (C), and can outgrow their blood supply and become necrotic (D).

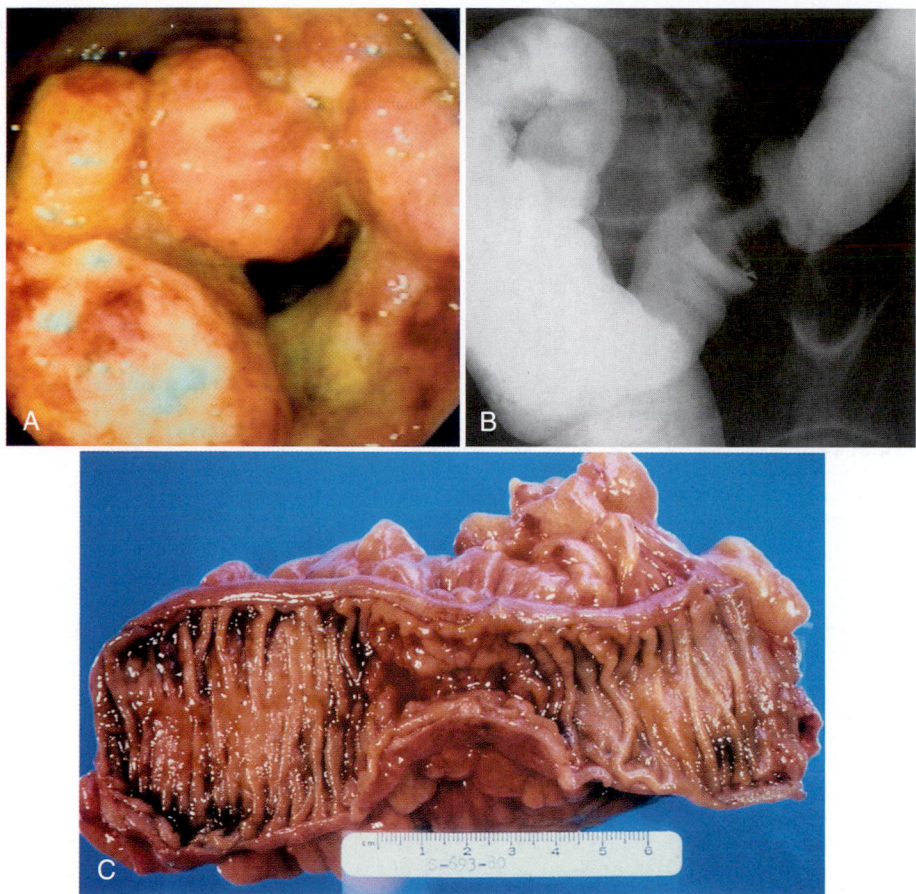

FIGURE 127-17. Obstructing carcinoma of the sigmoid colon. *A*, Colonoscopic view. *B*, Apple-core lesion seen on barium enema examination. *C*, Surgical specimen demonstrating an annular constriction or napkin-ring appearance.

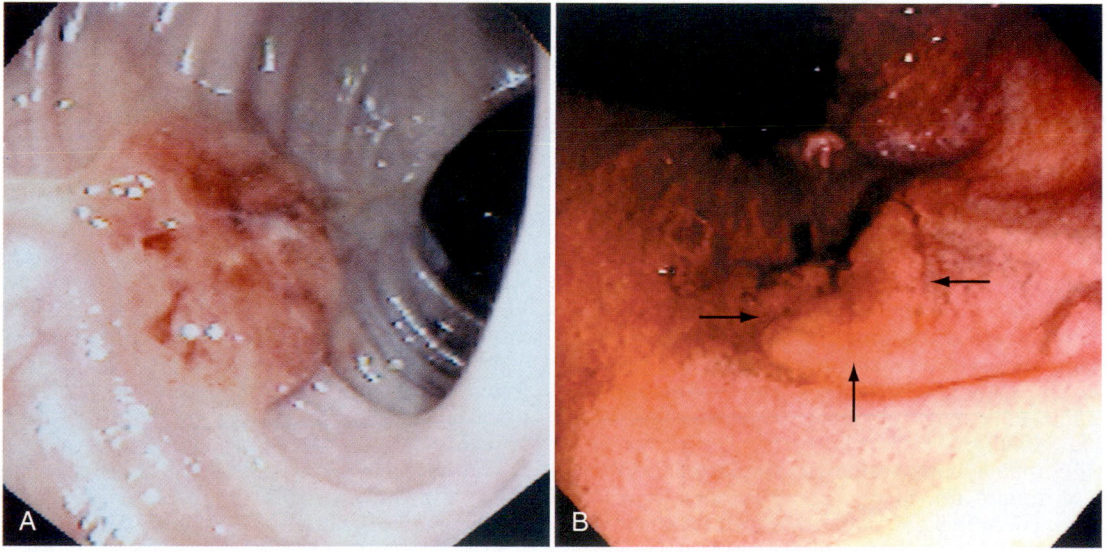

FIGURE 127-18. Colonoscopic view of flat, plaque-like carcinomas of the colon *(A)* and rectum *(B, arrows)* in patients with IBD.

Histopathology

Carcinomas of the colon characteristically are adenocarcinomas that form moderately differentiated to well-differentiated glands and secrete variable amounts of mucin (Fig. 127-19). Mucin, a high-molecular-weight glycoprotein, is the major product secreted by both normal and neoplastic glands of the colon and may be seen best with histochemical stains such as periodic acid–Schiff (PAS). In poorly differentiated tumors (see Fig. 127-19), gland formation and mucin production are present but less prominent. Signet ring cells, in which a large vacuole of mucin displaces the nucleus to 1 side, are a feature

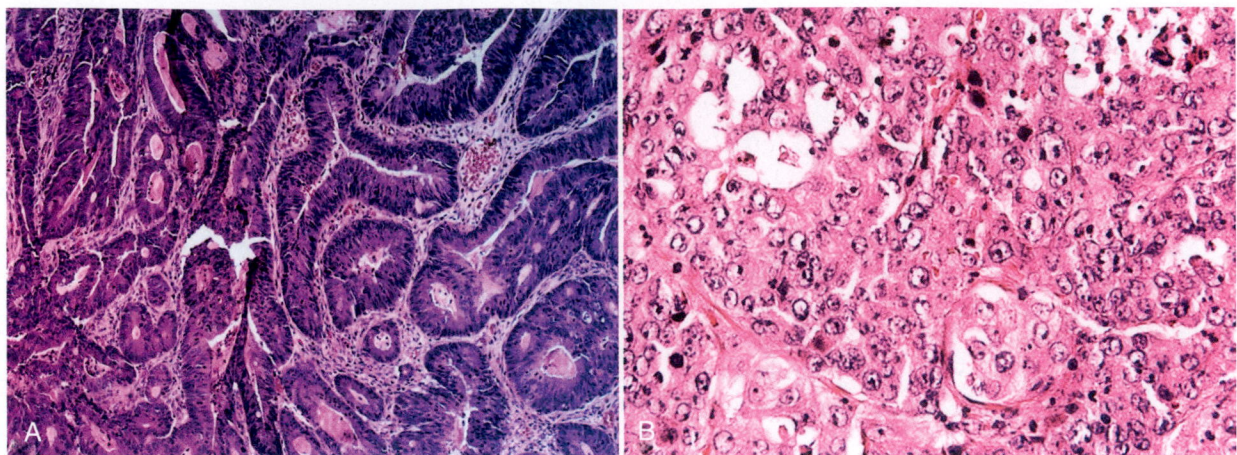

FIGURE 127-19. Histopathology of adenocarcinoma of the colon. *A,* Well-differentiated adenocarcinoma. Sections stained with H&E demonstrate crowded neoplastic glands containing variable amounts of mucin. *B,* Poorly differentiated adenocarcinoma.

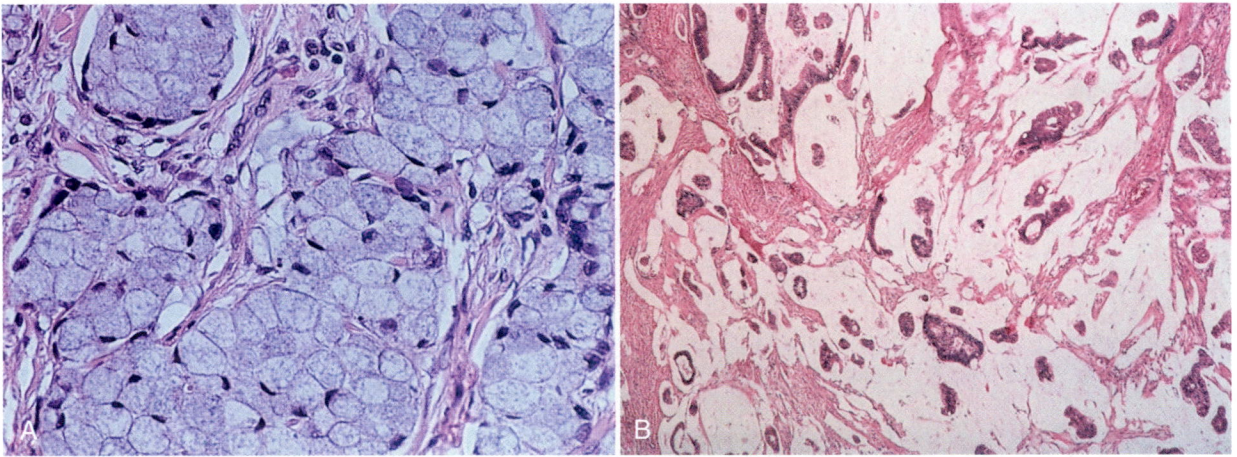

FIGURE 127-20. Histopathology of mucinous carcinomas of the colon. Histologic types include signet ring cell carcinoma in which a large vacuole of mucin displaces the nucleus *(A)* and colloid carcinoma with scattered nests of tumor cells floating in lakes of mucin *(B).* (H&E stain.)

of some tumors (Fig. 127-20*A*). In approximately 15% of tumors, large lakes of mucin contain scattered collections of tumor cells (see Fig. 127-20*B*). Such mucinous or colloid carcinomas are most common in patients with Lynch syndrome or UC and in patients whose carcinomas occur at an early age. Scirrhous carcinomas are uncommon and are characterized by sparse gland formation, with marked desmoplasia and fibrous tissue surrounding glandular structures. Sometimes tumors demonstrate a mixed histologic picture, with glands of varying degrees of differentiation.

Cancers other than adenocarcinomas account for less than 5% of malignant tumors of the large bowel. Tumors arising at the anorectal junction include squamous cell carcinomas, cloacogenic or transitional cell carcinomas, and melanomas (see Chapter 129). Primary lymphomas and carcinoid tumors of the large bowel account for less than 0.1% of all colon neoplasms (see Chapters 31 and 33).

NATURAL HISTORY AND STAGING

CRCs begin as intramucosal epithelial lesions, usually arising in adenomatous polyps or glands. As cancers grow they become invasive, penetrate the muscularis mucosae of the bowel, and invade lymphatic and vascular channels to involve regional lymph nodes, adjacent structures, and distant sites. Although CRCs grow at varying rates, they most often have long periods of silent growth before producing bowel symptoms. The mean doubling time of colon cancers determined radiologically in 1 older study was 620 days. Comparative lesion sequencing using modern molecular techniques combined with clinical observation suggests that it can take approximately 17 years for a large benign tumor to evolve to advanced cancer but less than 2 years for cells within that cancer to acquire the ability to metastasize.[88] Patterns of spread depend on the anatomy of the individual bowel segment as well as its lymph and blood supplies.

Cancers of the rectum advance locally by progressive penetration of the bowel wall. Extension of the primary tumor intramurally and parallel to the long axis of the bowel most often is limited, and lymphatic and hematogenous spread is unusual before penetration of the muscularis mucosae. Exceptions appear to be poorly differentiated tumors, which can metastasize via lymphatics or hematogenously before completely penetrating the bowel. Because the rectum is relatively immobile and lacks a serosal covering, rectal cancers tend to spread contiguously to progressively involve local structures. Transrectal US is useful to stage the depth of rectal cancers. Because of the dual blood supply of the lower third of the rectum, tumors arising here can metastasize hematogenously via the superior hemorrhoidal vein and portal system to the liver or by way of the middle hemorrhoidal vein and inferior vena cava to the lungs. The veins of the upper and middle thirds of the rectum drain into the portal system, and tumors in these segments first spread hematogenously to the liver. Occasionally, lumbar and thoracic vertebral metastases result from hematogenous spread via portal-vertebral communications (i.e., Batson's vertebral venous plexuses).

Colon cancers can invade transmurally and involve regional lymphatics and then distant nodes; lymphatic drainage generally parallels the arterial supply to a given bowel segment. The liver is the most common site of hematogenous spread (via the portal venous system) from colon tumors, and pulmonary metastases from colon cancer result, in general, from hepatic metastases.

In 1929, Cuthbert Dukes proposed a staging classification for cancers of the rectum and colon; it has since been modified many times to increase its prognostic value. The most commonly employed modification of the Dukes system is that of Astler and Coller (Table 127-5). This classification uses the following designations:

A: Tumors limited to the mucosa

B1: Tumors extending into, but not through, the muscularis propria

B2: Tumors penetrating the muscularis propria but without lymph node involvement

C: Tumors with regional lymph node involvement

TABLE 127-5 Dukes Staging of Carcinoma of the Rectum and Its Modifications for Colorectal Carcinoma

Stage	Dukes, 1932 (Rectum)	Gabriel, Dukes, Bussey, 1935 (Rectum)	Kirklin et al., 1949 (Rectum + Sigmoid)	Astler-Coller, 1954 (Rectum + Colon)	Turnbull et al., 1967 (Colon)	Modified Astler-Coller (Gunderson, Sosin), 1974 (Rectum + Colon)	Gitsg, 1975 (Rectum + Colon)
A	Limited to bowel wall	Limited to bowel wall	Limited to mucosa	Limited to mucosa	Limited to mucosa	Limited to mucosa	Limited to mucosa
B	Through bowel wall	Through bowel wall	—	—	Tumor extension into pericolic fat	—	—
B1	—	—	Into muscularis propria	Into muscularis propria	—	Into muscularis propria	Into muscularis propria
B2	—	—	Through muscularis propria	Through muscularis propria (and serosa)	—	Through serosa (m = microscopic; m + g = gross)	Through serosa
B3	—	—	—	—	—	Adherent to or invading adjacent structures	—
C	Regional nodal metastases	—	Regional nodal metastases	—	Regional nodal metastases	—	—
C1	—	Regional nodal metastases near primary lesion	—	Same as B1 + regional nodal metastases	—	Same as B1 + regional nodal metastases	1-4 regional nodes positive
C2	—	Proximal node involved at point of ligation	—	Same as B2 + regional nodal metastases	—	Same as B2 + regional nodal metastases	>4 regional nodes positive
C3	—	—	—	—	—	Same as B3 + regional nodal metastases	—
D	—	—	—	—	Distant metastases (liver, lung, bone) or parietal peritoneum or adjacent organ invasion	—	—

GITSG, Gastrointestinal Tumor Study Group.

Stage C tumors are divided further into primary tumors limited to the bowel wall (C1) and those that penetrate the bowel wall (C2). By contrast, in the system proposed by the Gastrointestinal Tumor Study Group (GITSG), C1 lesions are those in which 1 to 4 regional lymph nodes contain tumor, and C2 lesions are those in which more than 4 lymph nodes contain tumor (see Table 127-5). Another modification, by Turnbull and associates, added a D category referring to distant metastases.

The American Joint Committee on Cancer (AJCC) introduced the TNM classification for CRC,[89] which classifies the extent of the primary tumor (T), the status of regional lymph nodes (N), and the presence or absence of distant metastases (M). Cases are assigned the highest value of TNM that describes the full extent of disease and are grouped into 5 stages (0 through IV). The 5 stages have become important in uniformly randomizing patients for therapeutic trials (Table 127-6) and have, in most cases, replaced the Dukes classification for CRC. The seventh edition of the *AJCC Cancer Staging Manual* includes a number of modifications of the colon cancer staging system designed to more accurately reflect the relationship between the extent of tumor invasion and the number of affected lymph nodes.[90] Stage II tumors are now subdivided based on patterns of invasion (into pericolorectal tissues, visceral peritoneum, or adherent to other organs or structures), as this influences prognosis. Stage III nodal disease also is further subdivided based on the number of involved lymph nodes and includes N1a (1 positive regional node), N1b (2 to 3 positive nodes), N2a (4 to 6 positive nodes) and N2b (7 or more positive nodes). Satellite nodules without regional lymph node metastases are classified as N1c. Metastatic disease has been subdivided into disease with 1 metastatic site (M1a) or multiple metastatic sites (M1b).

PROGNOSIS

Clinical and pathologic variables that can affect the prognosis of patients with CRC are outlined in Table 127-7 and are important not only in predicting clinical outcome but in designing optimal strategies for treatment and follow-up. Their identification has led to a progressive modification of the staging classifications for CRC. The roles of histologic differentiation; tumor size, location, configuration, and degree of invasion; and lymph node status must be evaluated on the basis of prospective analyses of patients who undergo curative resections for CRC.

Surgical-Pathologic Staging

The depth of transmural tumor penetration and the extent of regional lymph node spread are the most important determinants of CRC prognosis (Fig. 127-21). The degree of bowel wall penetration affects prognosis, independent of lymph node status, and correlates with the number of involved nodes as well as with the incidence of local recurrence after surgical resection. The number of involved regional lymph nodes also correlates independently with outcome.

Tumor Morphology and Histology

The TNM classification (see Table 127-6) is based in part on the observation that for most cancers, tumor size correlates with local and distant spread and, thus, indirectly with prognosis. Numerous studies suggest that CRC is an exception, however, and that the size of the primary tumor per se does not correlate with prognosis. In fact, patients with exophytic

TABLE 127-6 AJCC TNM Staging of Colorectal Cancer	
Stage*	**Criteria†**
0	Carcinoma in situ: intraepithelial or invasion of lamina propria‡ (Tis N0 M0)
I	Tumor invades submucosa (T1 N0 M0) [Dukes A] Tumor invades muscularis propria (T2 N0 M0) [Dukes A]
II	Tumor invades through the muscularis propria into pericolorectal tissues (T3 N0 M0) [Dukes B] Tumor penetrates the surface of the visceral peritoneum (T4a N0 M0) [Dukes B] Tumor directly invades or is adherent to other organs and structures (T4b N0 M0) [Dukes B]
III	Any degree of bowel wall penetration with regional lymph node metastasis N1: metastasis in 1-3 regional lymph nodes N1a: metastasis in 1 regional lymph node N1b: metastasis in 2-3 regional lymph nodes N1c: tumor deposit(s) in the subserosa, mesentery, or nonperitonealized pericolic or perirectal tissues without regional nodal metastases N2: metastasis in ≥4 regional lymph nodes N2a: metastasis in 4-6 regional lymph nodes N2b: metastasis in 7 or more regional lymph nodes Any T N1 M0 [Dukes C] Any T N2 M0 [Dukes C]
IV	Any invasion of the bowel wall with or without lymph node metastasis, but with evidence of distant metastasis Any T Any N M1a: metastasis confined to 1 organ or site (liver, lung, ovary, nonregional node) Ant T Any N M1b: metastasis in more than 1 organ/site or the peritoneum

*Stage II is subdivided into IIA (for T3 tumors), IIB (for T4a tumors), and IIC (for T4b tumors). Stage III is subdivided into IIIA (T1-T2 N1/N1c or N2a M0), IIIB (T3-T4a N1/N1c M0) or (T2-T3N2aM0 or (T4bN1-N2M0), and IIIC (T4aN2aM0) or T3-T4aN2aM0) or (T4bN1-N2M0). Stage IV is divided into IVA (Any T Any N M1a) and IVB (Any T Any N M1b). N1 lesions have 1-3 positive nodes and are subdivided into N1a (one positive regional lymph node), N1b (2-3 positive regional lymph nodes), and N1c (tumor deposits in the subserosa, mesentery, or nonperitonealized pericoloic or perirectal tissues without regional nodal metastases); N2 tumors have ≥ 4 positive nodes and are divided into N2a (metastasis in 4-6 regional lymph nodes) and N2b (metastasis in 7 or more regional lymph nodes). This reflects the influence of the number of nodes on prognosis, and the importance of satellite tumor deposits now defined by site-specific factors that describes their texture and number. M1 has been divided into M1a for single metastatic site and M1b for multiple metastatic sites.
†Dukes B, which corresponds to stage II, is a composite of better (T3 N0 M0) and worse (T4 N0 M0) prognostic groups, as is Dukes C, which corresponds to stage III (any T N1 M0 and any T N2 M0).
‡Tis includes cancer cells confined within the glandular basement membrane (intraepithelial) or lamina propria (intramucosal) with no extension through the muscularis mucosae into the submucosa.
AJCC, American Joint Committee on Cancer; M0, no distant metastasis; M1, distant metastasis; N0, no regional lymph node metastasis (7th ed. includes several changes as compared to 6th ed.).
Based on the American Joint Committee on Cancer. AJCC cancer staging manual: Colon and rectum. 7th ed. New York: Springer-Verlag; 2010.

or polypoid tumors appear to have a better prognosis than those with ulcerating or infiltrating tumors.

Tumor prognosis correlates with histologic grade: poor differentiation confers a worse prognosis than does a high degree of differentiation. Mucinous and scirrhous carcinomas appear to be biologically more aggressive, and patients with

TABLE 127-7 Pathologic, Molecular, and Clinical Features That May Affect Prognosis in Patients with Colorectal Cancer

Feature or Marker	Effect on Prognosis	Feature or Marker	Effect on Prognosis
Pathologic		**Molecular**	
Surgical-Pathologic Stage		Loss of heterozygosity at chromosome 18q (*DCC, DPC4*)	Diminishes prognosis
Depth of colon wall penetration	Increased penetration diminishes prognosis		
Number of regional nodes involved by tumor	Greater number of involved nodes diminishes prognosis	Loss of heterozygosity at chromosome 17p (*TP53*)	Diminishes prognosis
Positive circumferential resection margin	Diminishes prognosis	Loss of heterozygosity at chromosome 8p	Diminishes prognosis
Residual tumor after resection	Diminishes prognosis	Increased labeling index for p21WAF/CIP1 protein	Improves prognosis
Isolated microscopic tumor cells in regional lymph nodes	May diminish prognosis	Microsatellite instability	Improves prognosis
		Mutation in *BAX* gene	Diminishes prognosis
Tumor Morphology and Histology		Mutation in *K-ras* codon 12 or 13	Lack of response to anti-EGFR therapy
Degree of differentiation	Well-differentiated tumors have a better prognosis than poorly differentiated lesions	**Clinical**	
		Diagnosis in asymptomatic patients	May improve prognosis
Mucinous (colloid) or signet ring cell histology	Diminishes prognosis	Duration of symptoms	No demonstrated effect
Scirrhous histology	Diminishes prognosis	Rectal bleeding as a presenting symptom	Improves prognosis
Invasion		Colon obstruction	Diminishes prognosis
Venous	Diminishes prognosis	Colon perforation	Diminishes prognosis
Lymphatic	Diminishes prognosis	Tumor location	Prognosis may be better for colonic than for rectal tumors
Perineural	Diminishes prognosis		Prognosis may be better for left colonic than right colonic tumors
Other Features			
Local inflammation and immunologic reaction	Improves prognosis		
Tumor morphology	Polypoid or exophytic tumors have a better prognosis than ulcerating or infiltrating lesions	Age < 30 yr	Diminishes prognosis
		High preoperative CEA level	Diminishes prognosis
		Distant metastases	Markedly diminishes prognosis
Tumor DNA content	Increased DNA content (aneuploidy) diminishes prognosis	Tumor regression grade	Complete eradication of tumor after preoperative therapy may improve prognosis
Tumor size	No effect in most studies		

these tumors do not survive as long as those who have other types of adenocarcinoma. Mucin-associated antigens might play a role in tumor progression and metastasis of colon cancer cells. Signet ring carcinomas have been reported to present at an advanced stage and to be highly invasive tumors.

Vascular invasion by CRC (Fig. 127-22*B*) usually correlates with local recurrence after resection, visceral metastases, and decreased survival, but it might not have independent prognostic value for tumors confined to the bowel wall. Although lymphatic invasion (Fig. 127-22*A*) is associated with decreased survival, it is not clear whether this variable is independent of depth of tumor invasion and regional nodal metastasis. Perineural invasion also is linked to increased local recurrence and decreased survival. Extranodal or peritumoral deposits (satellite nodules) are located in the pericolic or perirectal fat, with no evidence of residual lymph node tissue; most of these are thought to be due to lymphovascular or perineural invasion and carry a poor prognosis. An increased inflammatory response and immune (lymphocytic) reaction appear to confer a better prognosis. Prognosis may be related to the DNA content of the primary tumor, because survival is shorter for patients with non-diploid or aneuploid tumors than for those whose tumor cells have normal or diploid DNA content. Although DNA content of the primary tumor might correlate

with the potential for recurrence after primary resection, the value of routine flow cytometric measurements or image analysis of the DNA content of tumor cells to assess clinical prognosis and plan treatment remains to be determined. Deletions in chromosomes 18q and 17p (*TP53*) may be important indicators of prognosis, independent of stage. As indicated in Table 127-7, a growing number of other molecular markers also might predict prognosis or response to therapy.

Clinical Predictors of Prognosis

Data from recent case-control and prospective screening programs for CRC suggest that tumors diagnosed in asymptomatic patients are less advanced and are associated with a better prognosis than symptomatic tumors. Duration of symptoms may not correlate directly with prognosis, and some presenting symptoms, such as rectal bleeding, may be associated with better rates of survival. Bowel obstruction or perforation has been linked with poor prognosis. Patients who present with obstructing lesions might not be candidates for curative surgery and have higher rates of operative morbidity and mortality. Recurrence following "curative" surgery also is higher in patients who present with obstruction or perforation.

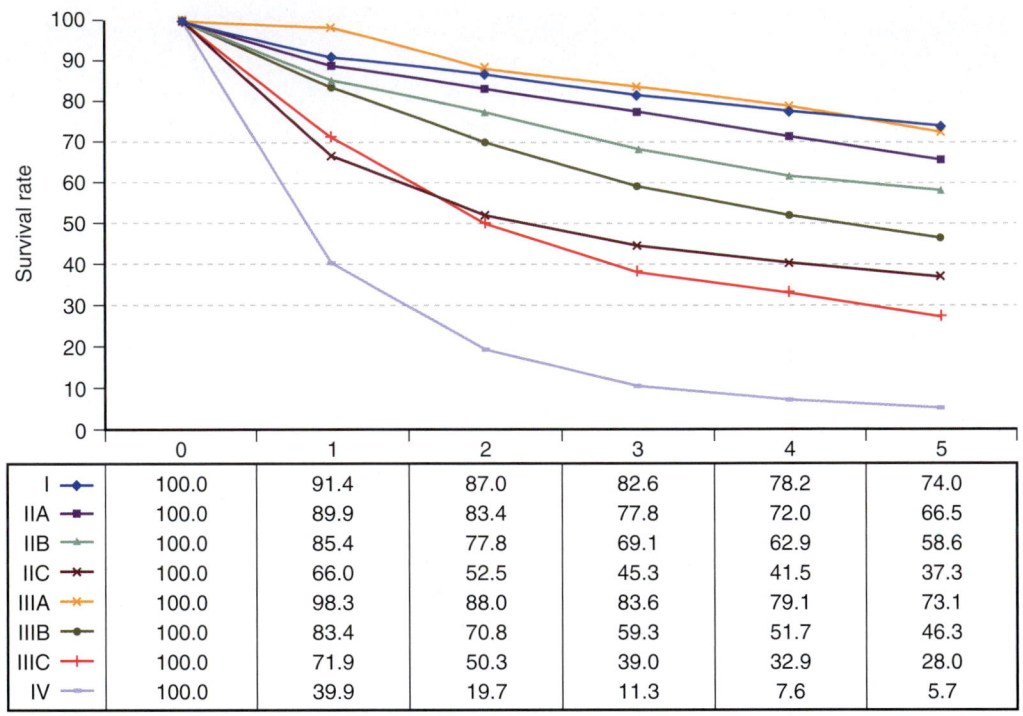

		0	1	2	3	4	5
I		100.0	91.4	87.0	82.6	78.2	74.0
IIA		100.0	89.9	83.4	77.8	72.0	66.5
IIB		100.0	85.4	77.8	69.1	62.9	58.6
IIC		100.0	66.0	52.5	45.3	41.5	37.3
IIIA		100.0	98.3	88.0	83.6	79.1	73.1
IIIB		100.0	83.4	70.8	59.3	51.7	46.3
IIIC		100.0	71.9	50.3	39.0	32.9	28.0
IV		100.0	39.9	19.7	11.3	7.6	5.7

Years from diagnosis

FIGURE 127-21. Observed survival rates by stage for 28,491 cases with adenocarcinoma of the colon. Data from the SEER 1973-2005 Public Use File diagnosed in years 1998-2000. Stage I: 7417; Stage IIA: 9956; Stage IIB: 997; Stage IIC: 725; Stage IIIA: 868; Stage IIIB: 1492; Stage IIIC: 2000; and Stage IV: 5036. Figure demonstrates the interaction among T and N classifications and number of positive lymph nodes. *(From American Joint Committee on Cancer. AJCC cancer staging handbook. 7th ed. New York: AJCC; 2010.)*

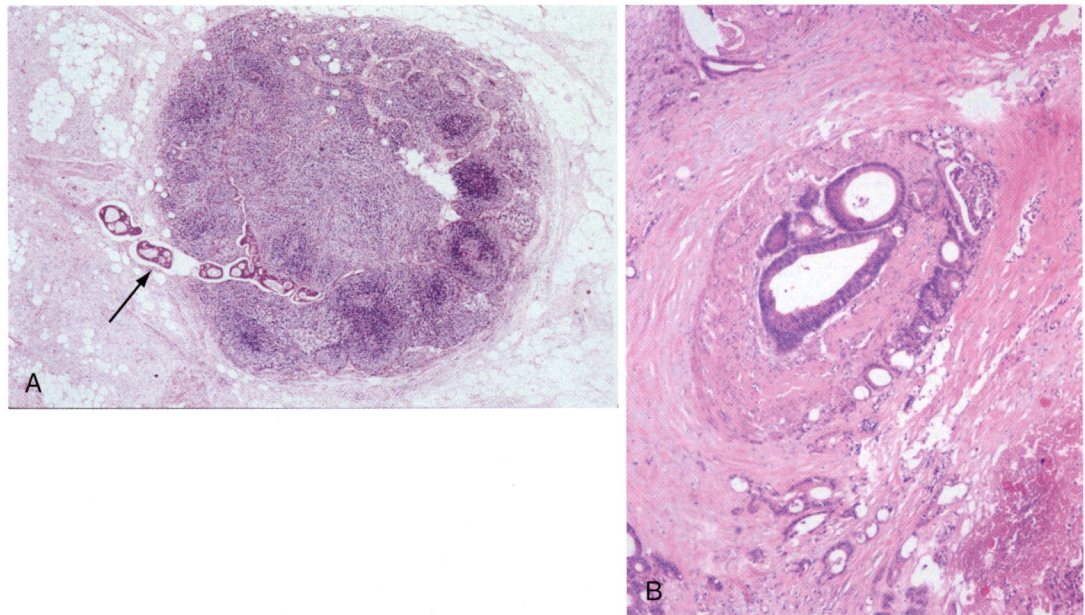

FIGURE 127-22. Pathologic features that can adversely influence prognosis include lymph node invasion *(A)* and vascular invasion *(B)*. The *arrow* in *A* points to a lymphatic vessel containing tumor cells. In *B*, high-magnification microscopy demonstrates an artery that contains adenocarcinoma cells. (H&E stain.)

Location of the primary tumor can influence outcome. Disease-free survival at 3 years appears to be 2% to 14% higher after surgery for tumors of the left than of the right colon. Some studies also suggest a survival advantage for patients with colon compared with rectal cancers.

As many as 3% of CRCs develop before 30 years of age, and only 11% of such persons have a predisposing condition such as FAP or UC. The prognosis is worse for this group than for older patients and is particularly poor in the pediatric age range. Poor prognosis may be related to a higher percentage

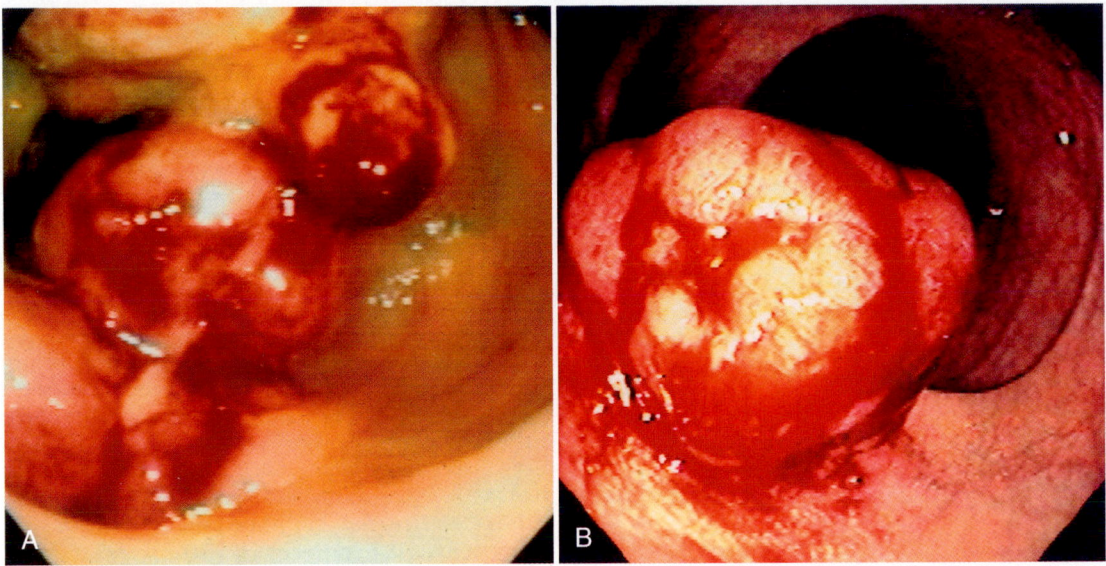

FIGURE 127-23. Colonoscopic view of bleeding carcinomas of the sigmoid colon *(A)* and cecum *(B)*. Carcinomas of the colon often bleed intermittently. Patients can present with evidence of microcytic anemia, hematochezia, or both, depending on the tumor site and the pattern of bleeding.

of more advanced cancers and mucinous adenocarcinomas in these young patients. Alternatively, patients with tumors that demonstrate MSI appear to have a better prognosis irrespective of age.[60] Thus, whereas CRCs occur at a younger age in those with Lynch syndrome, these patients have a better prognosis than those with microsatellite-stable cancers.

Outcome also is related to preoperative serum CEA levels. Tumor recurrence is higher, and the estimated mean time to recurrence is shorter, in patients with Dukes B (stage II) and C (stage III) cancers who have high preoperative CEA levels. The preoperative CEA level may be of prognostic value only in patients with Dukes C CRCs who also have 4 or more involved lymph nodes (stage C2), but not in patients with Dukes A (stage I) and B lesions or Dukes C lesions with fewer than 4 nodes involved. Expression of mucin-associated carbohydrate antigens other than CEA, such as sialyl Lewis[x], also can correlate with prognosis. Expression of the carbohydrate-binding protein galectin-3 correlates with tumor progression in the colon and may confer a poor prognosis.

Approximately one fourth of patients with CRC exhibit clinical evidence of hematogenous spread when seen initially, and one half of patients with CRC eventually develop metastases to a distant site, usually the liver; such metastases carry a poor prognosis at all times. The most important determinant of survival time for patients who present with liver metastases is the extent of hepatic involvement by tumor.

CLINICAL FEATURES

CRCs grow slowly and may be present for as long as 5 years before symptoms appear. Asymptomatic persons with cancer often have occult blood loss from their tumors, and bleeding rates increase with tumor size and degree of ulceration (Fig. 127-23). Symptoms depend to some extent on the site of the primary tumor. Cancers of the proximal colon usually grow larger than those of the left colon and rectum before they produce symptoms. Constitutional symptoms (e.g., fatigue,

shortness of breath, angina) from microcytic hypochromic anemia may be the principal presentation of right colon tumors. Less often, blood from right colon cancers is admixed with stool and appears as mahogany-colored feces. As a tumor grows, it can produce vague abdominal discomfort or manifest as a palpable mass. Obstruction is uncommon with right-sided tumors because of the large diameter of the cecum and ascending colon, although cecal cancers can block the ileocecal valve and cause small bowel obstruction.

The left colon has a narrower lumen than does the proximal colon, and cancers of the descending and sigmoid colon often involve the bowel circumferentially and cause obstructive symptoms. Patients can present with colicky abdominal pain, particularly after meals, and a change in bowel habits. Constipation can alternate with increased frequency of defecation as small amounts of retained stool move beyond the obstructing lesion. Hematochezia is seen more often with distal than proximal lesions, and bright red blood passed per rectum or coating the surface of the stool is common with cancers of the left colon and rectum. Rectal cancers also cause obstruction and changes in bowel habits, including constipation, diarrhea, and tenesmus. Rectal cancers can invade the bladder, vaginal wall, or surrounding nerves, resulting in perineal or sacral pain, but this is a late occurrence.

CRC is often misdiagnosed in symptomatic patients. Symptoms are ascribed to benign conditions such as diverticular disease (abdominal pain, bleeding, change in stool caliber), IBS (abdominal pain, change in bowel habits), or hemorrhoids (rectal bleeding) (Box 127-5). CRC should be considered when a patient, especially one older than 40 years, presents with hypochromic microcytic anemia or rectal bleeding. Too often, anemia in older adults is ascribed to "chronic disease," only to be diagnosed later as a sign of advanced CRC. Abdominal pain and bleeding of any type also merit evaluation for cancer in this age group. CRC can affect younger patients, particularly those with IBD or a strong family history for CRC and other cancers. When the history and clinical presentation suggest CRC, evaluation is warranted despite young age.

Mass Lesion
Benign tumor (mucosal and submucosal)
Endometriosis
Inflammatory mass
    Diverticulitis
    Infections (TB, amebiasis, fungi)
    IBD
    Ischemic colitis
    Solitary rectal ulcer

Stricture
Crohn's colitis
Ischemia
Radiation (late sequela)

Rectal Bleeding
Diverticulosis
Hemorrhoids
IBD
Infectious colitis
Ischemic colitis
Solitary rectal ulcer

Abdominal Pain
Diverticulitis
IBD
IBS
Ischemic colitis

Change in Bowel Habits
Infectious diarrhea
IBD
IBS
Medications

*This list includes common clinical situations that initially may be confused with symptoms or signs of colorectal cancer, but it is not meant to be all inclusive.

DIAGNOSIS AND SCREENING

Tests When Colorectal Cancer Is Suspected

When CRC is suspected because of clinical signs, symptoms, or positive screening tests (discussed later), prompt endoscopic or radiologic evaluation should be undertaken (Fig. 127-24). Air contrast barium enema (ACBE) traditionally had been performed in conjunction with flexible sigmoidoscopy, but given the low sensitivity of ACBE, CT colonography ("virtual colonoscopy") has, in most U.S. centers, replaced it for patients who cannot undergo colonoscopy (see later).

If a carcinoma is detected radiologically or by sigmoidoscopy, a full colonoscopic examination should be done because of the high incidence of synchronous lesions and possible implications of the colonoscopic findings for the surgical treatment plan. As many as half of the patients with proved CRC harbor additional lesions, and for almost 10%, the operative plan has to be modified as a result of preoperative colonoscopy.

Principles of Screening

Cancer prevention may be categorized as primary or secondary. *Primary prevention* refers to identifying genetic, biological, and environmental factors that are etiologic or pathogenetic and subsequently altering their effects on tumor development. Although several areas of study have been identified that can lead to primary prevention of colon cancer, available data do not yet provide a firm basis for the practical application of primary preventive measures. The goal of *secondary prevention* is to identify existing preneoplastic and early neoplastic lesions and to treat them thoroughly and expeditiously. The assumption is that early detection improves prognosis. Screening is an example of secondary prevention.

In symptomatic patients it is important to minimize diagnostic delay. If the clinical setting suggests CRC (e.g., iron deficiency anemia in an older adult patient), prompt diagnostic evaluation should be undertaken; this approach pertains to

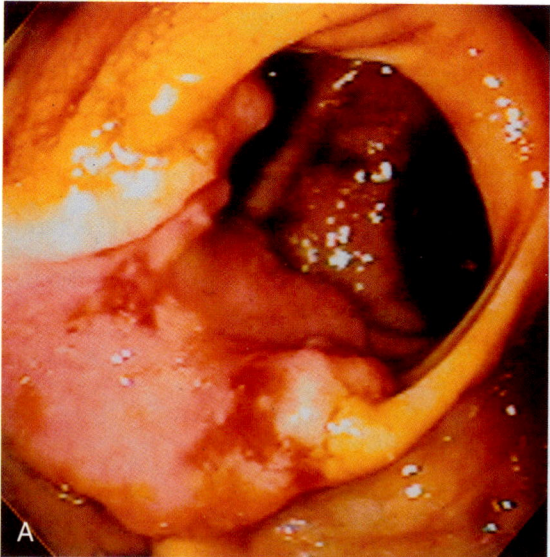
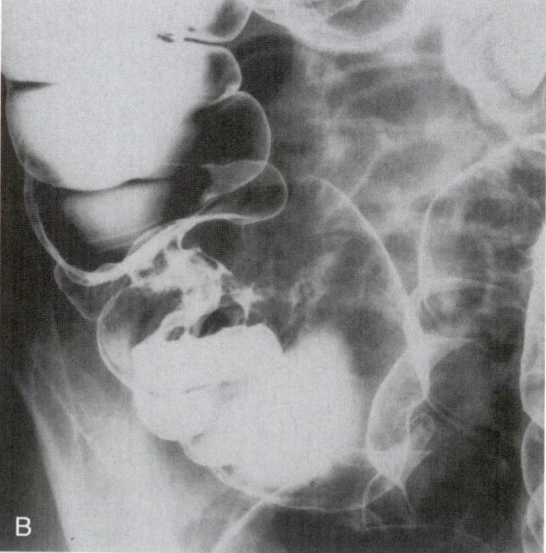

FIGURE 127-24. Carcinoma of the cecum. The tumor is seen infiltrating a cecal fold at colonoscopy *(A)* and on air-contrast barium enema *(B)*.

individual patients and small groups of patients seen in daily practice and is known as *case finding*. *Screening* pertains to large populations. Screening an asymptomatic population for any disease is worthwhile if the disease represents a major health problem, effective therapy is available, a sensitive and specific screening test is available that is readily acceptable to patients and physicians, and the screening test is cost-effective. CRC fulfills all these conditions. Furthermore, the prolonged natural history of CRC affords time to detect and eliminate early neoplastic lesions before they reach an advanced, incurable stage. The challenge that remains is to develop effective, easily administered, and cost-effective screening tests for the disease. Current evidence indicates that screening for CRC reduces related mortality and that there also is a reduction in CRC-related mortality from fecal occult blood testing (FOBT) and flexible sigmoidoscopy (see later). This finding has resulted in a recommendation by the U.S. Preventive Services Task Force (USPSTF) that screening for CRC should be performed in all persons aged 50 to 75 years.[91] Almost all major health-related agencies have endorsed screening for CRC (Table 127-8), but the key questions of who, how, and how often remain a source of debate.

In 2001, the American Cancer Society updated its recommendations on CRC screening to offer a broader set of screening choices for different levels of CRC risk, thereby allowing greater flexibility in achieving screening goals. This change was deemed necessary because evidence showed little progress in improving CRC screening rates. Screening options included annual FOBT, flexible sigmoidoscopy every 5 years, annual FOBT plus flexible sigmoidoscopy every 5 years, ACBE every 5 years, or colonoscopy every 10 years. These recommendations were modified slightly in 2002 with the addition of immunochemical FOBTs.

In 2008, a joint guideline on screening and surveillance for early detection of CRC and adenomatous polyps was issued jointly by the American Cancer Society, the U.S. Multi-Society Task Force on Colorectal Cancer, and the American College of Radiology (see Table 127-8).[81] This update of previous guidelines is notable in that it grouped screening tests into those that primarily detect cancer (annual FOBT including those that are guaiac-based or immunochemical tests, and stool DNA tests [interval not specified]), and those that can detect early cancer and adenomatous polyps (flexible sigmoidoscopy every 5 years, colonoscopy every 10 years, ACBE every 5 years, or CT colonography every 5 years). In November 2008, the USPSTF also issued updated guidelines (see Table 127-8).[91] Based on a targeted evidence-based review and a decision analytic modeling analysis, the USPSTF recommended screening of average-risk persons aged 50 to 75 years with high-sensitivity FOBT annually, sigmoidoscopy every 5 years plus FOBT every 3 years, or colonoscopy every 10 years. Notably, the USPSTF indicated that although the benefits of screening outweigh its potential harms for persons aged 50 to 75 years, the likelihood that detection and early intervention will yield a mortality benefit declines after age 75 because of the long average time between adenoma development and cancer diagnosis. Routine screening was therefore not recommended for adults 76 to 85 years of age, and screening was not recommended at all for adults older than 85. A recently published guidance statement from the American College of Physicians also recommends that clinicians stop screening for CRC in adults older than age 75 or in adults with a life expectancy of less than 10 years.[92] These guidelines also indicated that for all populations, there is insufficient evidence to assess the benefits and harms of screening with CT colonography or fecal DNA testing. The ACG Guidelines for Colorectal Cancer Screening also group options into cancer prevention tests (colonoscopy every 10 years, flexible sigmoidoscopy every 5 to 10 years, and CT colonography every 5 years) and cancer detection tests (annual FOBT with fecal immunochemical tests, fecal DNA testing every 3 years).[93] Colonoscopy is considered the preferred choice overall. The ACG also recommends that screening in African Americans begin at age 45 instead of age 50 for average-risk individuals, and that CT colonography replace double-contrast barium enema as a radiologic option. The *European Guidelines for Quality Assurance in Colorectal Screening and Diagnosis* is a 386-page document authored by 90 authors from 32 countries that provides an evidence-based review of existing data on CRC screening that stresses quality measures and cost-effectiveness.[89]

TABLE 127-8 Guidelines for Screening Average-Risk Persons for Colorectal Cancer

Screening Tool	U.S. Preventive Services Task Force*	American Cancer Society, U.S. Multi-Society Task Force, and American College of Radiology Joint Guidelines†
High-sensitivity FOBT (guaiac-based or immunochemical)	Recommended annually as an option	Recommended annually as an option
Flexible sigmoidoscopy	Recommended every 5 yr + high-sensitivity FOBT every 3 yr as an option	Recommended every 5 yr as an option
Colonoscopy	Recommended every 10 yr as an option	Recommended every 10 yr as an option
Double-contrast barium enema	Not recommended	Recommended every 5 yr as an option
CT colonography	Not recommended	Recommended every 5 yr as an option
Stool DNA testing	Not recommended	Recommended (interval uncertain)

*The U.S. Preventive Services Task Force recommends screening for adults aged 50 to 75 years. Screening for adults aged 76 to 85 years is not routinely recommended, and for adults older than 85 years, screening is not recommended.
†Testing options are divided into those that detect adenomatous polyps and cancer (flexible sigmoidoscopy, colonoscopy, double-contrast barium enema, CT colonography) and those that primarily detect cancer (FOBT, stool DNA testing).
FOBT, fecal occult blood test.
From Levin B, Lieberman DA, McFarland B, et al. Screening and surveillance for the early detection of colorectal cancer and adenomatous polyps 2008: A joint guideline from the American Cancer Society, the U.S. Multi-Society Task Force on Colorectal Cancer, and the American College of Radiology. CA Cancer J Clin 2008; 58:130-60; and U.S. Preventive Services Task Force. Screening for colorectal cancer: U.S. Preventive Services Task Force recommendation statement. Ann Intern Med 2008; 149:627-37.

TABLE 127-9 Best Case Values for Screening Procedures for Colorectal Polyps and Cancers*

Test	Reach	Specificity (%)	Sensitivity				Mortality Rate[†]
			Adenomas ≤ 5 mm (%)	Adenomas 6-9 mm (%)	Adenomas ≥ 10 mm (%)	Cancer (%)	
Hemoccult II	Whole colorectum	98.0	2.0	5.0	12.0	40.0	0
Hemoccult Sensa	Whole colorectum	92.5	7.5	12.4	23.9	70.0	0
Fecal immunochemical test	Whole colorectum	95.0	5.0	10.0	22.0	70.0	0
Flexible sigmoidoscopy (within reach)	To splenic flexure	92.0	75.0	85.0	95.0	95.0	0
Colonoscopy	To cecum	90.0	75.0	85.0	95.0	95.0	1/10,000

*Best case value assumes 100% adherence to screening tests, follow-up of positive findings, and surveillance of persons found to have adenomas.
[†]Mortality from the test itself.
Data from Zauber AG, Landsdorp-Vogelaar I, Knudsen AB, et al. Evaluating test strategies for colorectal cancer screening: A decision analysis for the U.S. Preventive Services Task Force. Ann Intern Med 2008; 149:659-69.

Numerous international CRC screening programs have been initiated as evidence grows for an impact of CRC screening on mortality.[94]

Although each of the test choices for CRC screening has inherent characteristics related to accuracy, prevention, potential costs, and risks, the concept has long been that any 1 of the tests is better than no test at all. Multiple options can be confusing, however, to both patients and physicians. Furthermore, the test options are not of equal efficacy, and such guidelines might lead to coverage of suboptimal testing by third-party payers.

The willingness of patients and physicians to comply with recommendations for screening programs has a major impact on the effectiveness of CRC screening. Compliance by potential screenees and physicians historically has been poor, and interventions to increase screening adherence have been disappointing. Adherence to recommended follow-up testing after an initial positive FOBT result also may be lower in the community setting than in larger screening trials. Up to one third of people who test positive might not respond to requests for follow-up. An analysis of diagnostic testing after a positive FOBT result in Medicare recipients indicated that not only was compliance poor, but follow-up diagnostic testing often was inadequate or improper. Unfortunately, compliance is often poorer among older adults, who are at greatest risk for CRC, and among minorities, in whom mortality is high. Despite the widespread availability of flexible sigmoidoscopy and colonoscopy, most older adults are reluctant to have these tests because of cost, discomfort, and fear.

Although most physicians agree in principle with guidelines for screening, many do not follow them with all patients. Reluctance to perform what is perceived as an uncomfortable and invasive procedure in asymptomatic persons, requirements for training, and limitations of time and resources contribute to reluctance on the part of primary care physicians. Compliance also is extremely important in any determination of cost-effectiveness. Compliance with CRC screening has a major impact on the cost-effectiveness of such programs. In 1 model, the cost per death prevented as the result of performing guaiac-based FOBTs increased from $225,000 to $331,000 as compliance decreased from 100% to 50%.[95] The FOBT is

TABLE 127-10 Costs of Screening Tests for Colorectal Cancer

Procedure	Institutional Charges (U.S. $)*	Medicare Payments (U.S. $)*
Fecal occult blood test	19.00	4.50
Flexible sigmoidoscopy	660.00	386.00
Colonoscopy	1991.00	634.87
Colonoscopy with polypectomy	2258.00	635.00
Air-contrast barium enema	573.00	113.00
CT colonography	1642.00	273.00

*Costs are based on institutional charges and Medicare payments in 2013 at the University of Texas MD Anderson Cancer Center and may vary by institution.

especially sensitive to the impact of compliance compared with other tests.[96]

In the absence of firm clinical data indicating which screening strategy provides the best balance of sensitivity, specificity, logistic feasibility, and cost, various mathematical models have been employed to examine this issue.[95,96] A decision analysis commissioned by the USPSTF used microsimulation models from the Cancer Intervention and Surveillance Modeling Network to assess life-years gained and colonoscopy requirements for screening strategies.[95] This group concluded that their findings support CRC screening with colonoscopy every 10 years, annual screening with a sensitive FOBT, or flexible sigmoidoscopy every 5 years with a mid-interval FOBT for patients aged 50 to 75 years. This was part of the basis for modifications to the USPSTF guidelines.

The use of screening modalities for detecting adenomatous polyps is discussed in Chapter 126. Table 127-9 presents some of the characteristics of tests used to screen for colorectal neoplasms. Table 127-10 lists the costs of these tests.

Screening Techniques

Fecal Occult Blood Testing (FOBT)

Qualitative chromogen tests, which rely on the oxidative conversion of a colorless compound to a colored one in the presence of the pseudoperoxidase activity of Hgb, have been standardized using guaiac-impregnated paper and developing solutions (hydrogen peroxide in denatured alcohol). These solutions (e.g., Hemoccult, Hemoccult II) have been widely studied and are available commercially, convenient to use, and inexpensive. Their effectiveness in detecting occult blood in the stool, however, depends on many factors that can either enhance (cause false-positive tests) or inhibit (cause false-negative tests) oxidation of the indicator dye, such as the degree of fecal hydration (increases sensitivity), amount of Hgb degradation during storage or by focal flora (decreases sensitivity), and the presence or absence of interfering substances (e.g., ascorbic acid). Any foodstuff that contains compounds with peroxidase or pseudoperoxidase activity (red meat, broccoli, turnips, cauliflower, radishes, cantaloupe) can produce a positive FOBT reaction and should be avoided for 3 days before and during testing, as should potentially interfering medications (e.g., iron supplements, vitamin C, aspirin and other NSAIDs). For these reasons, fecal immunochemical testing (FIT) is gradually replacing guaiac-based FOBT.

CRCs and adenomas bleed intermittently, and detecting fecal occult blood by Hemoccult testing depends on the degree of blood loss. In general, 2 mL of blood in the stool is necessary to produce a positive result. Sampling multiple stool specimens, therefore, is likely to result in fewer false-negative evaluations. Sampling 1 specimen yields a 40% to 50% false-negative rate, which improves progressively as more stools are sampled. Two samples of each of 3 consecutive (daily) stools should be tested, and testing should be performed within 4 to 6 days of sampling.

Location of the lesion also affects the ability to detect a cancer by Hemoccult testing. Right-sided cancers produce fewer false-negative tests than cancers elsewhere in the colon, because large bulky tumors bleed frequently. Potential blind spots of the Hemoccult test with high false-negative rates are the transverse and descending colon.

The value of a positive FOBT result performed on stool obtained by digital rectal examination has been disputed, and this FOBT method is not recommended, largely because a single examination done in this way is not nearly as sensitive as the recommended method in which 3 consecutive spontaneously passed stools are tested.[97] There also will be some false-positive results because digital rectal exam usually is not done in conjunction with dietary restrictions.

Rehydration of Hemoccult cards increases sensitivity but reduces specificity, and is not recommended for screening.

In studies that have examined the potential benefit of FOBTs for detecting colorectal neoplasms in large populations, compliance has been in the range of 50% to 70%, although older adult patients—those at substantial risk for colon cancer—tend to be less compliant.[81] The overall positivity rate ranges from 2% to 6% of those tested, and the positive predictive value is about 20% for adenomas and 5% to 10% for cancers. Most studies report that a large percentage of detected cancers are Dukes A and B (stages I and II) lesions.

Large controlled studies of Hemoccult testing of asymptomatic patients in the general population have been reported from the USA,[98,99] Great Britain,[100] Scandinavia, and France (Table 127-11).[101] These studies cite a rate of test positivity of 1% to 2.6% on first screen for nonhydrated slides and a predictive value for colonic neoplasms (adenomas plus carcinomas) of 22% to 58%. The positive predictive value for carcinomas alone is substantially less (5.6% to 18% for nonhydrated slides). Rehydration of slides with a drop of water before processing results in increased positivity and sensitivity but decreased specificity and positive predictive value. An 18-year follow-up in the Minnesota trial[99] demonstrated a marked reduction in Dukes stage D cancers in the screened groups compared with the control group. Long-term follow-up of patients tested with Hemoccult in a large group practice setting (Kaiser-Permanente) yielded similar results. The predictive value of a positive test for CRC was 8% at 1 year, 10% at 2 years, and 11% at 4 years. Predictive value depends on what group is screened, and it may be increased in older age groups.

Mortality data are available from the Minnesota Study, an RCT that has provided the best evidence for the effectiveness of screening with FOBT.[98,99] After 13 years of follow-up, data indicated a 33% reduction in CRC-associated mortality with annual screening, but an insignificant reduction of only approximately 5% with biannual screening.[98] Approximately 80% of samples were rehydrated, yielding a high positivity rate of 9.8% (compared with 2.4% for nonhydrated slides). These findings resulted in a 38% rate of colonoscopy, leading some to suggest that a substantial portion of the mortality reduction resulted from chance detection through colonoscopy of nonbleeding cancers. This challenge has been refuted by the investigators, who found that only 6% to 11% of the mortality reduction was explained by chance detection.

Results of 18 years of follow-up also have been reported,[99] and cumulative 18-year CRC mortality remains 33% lower in the annually screened group than in the control group. The group tested with biennial screening now demonstrates a 21% lower CRC mortality than did the control group. Other RCTs reported similar results. Data from Funen, Denmark, suggest an 18% decrease in CRC mortality during a 10-year study period, and data from Nottingham, England, indicate a 15% reduction in mortality at 7.8 years' follow-up.[100] Data from New York suggest a 43% reduction in mortality in the screened group at 10 years. A randomized French trial[101] also demonstrated a reduction in CRC mortality with biennial FOBT screening compared with a control population (mortality ratio, 0.84; 95% CI, 0.71-0.99) at 11 years of follow-up; reduction in mortality was more pronounced in compliant patients (mortality ratio, 0.67; 95% CI, 0.56-0.81).

Methods that can decrease the false-positive FOBT rates while maintaining or increasing sensitivity currently are being refined and compared for efficiency with Hemoccult-type slide tests. FITs are designed to detect human globin and are not affected by diet or drugs. Multiple FITs are now available world-wide, and FIT is likely to eventually replace guaiac-based FOBT. FITs have good performance characteristics compared with standard heme-based FOBT tests, and may have superior sensitivity and specificity for detecting colonic neoplasms.[102-105] Issues that remain to be resolved regarding FIT include the optimal number of samples to be tested, requirements for storage and shipping (e.g., effect of temperature), and the relative benefit of quantitative (positive or negative) versus qualitative reporting, including the optimal "cut off" for a positive test. The quantitative immunochemical FOBT has been shown to have good sensitivity and specificity for detection of clinically significant neoplasia in studies of asymptomatic and symptomatic patients, but test performance in prospective screening programs has been less well studied. Two recent studies suggested the effectiveness of FIT for programmatic screening.[104,105] FITs have now been included as the preferred form of FOBT in screening guidelines.

TABLE 127-11 Controlled Trials of Fecal Occult Blood Testing in Screening Asymptomatic Persons for Colorectal Cancer (CRC)

Variable	Trials				
	Minnesota[99]	Nottingham[98]	Goteborg	Funen	New York
Size of study population	46,000	152,850	28,000	61,933	22,000
Age range (yrs)	50-80	50-74	60-64	45-74	≥40
Study design	Randomized: annual vs. biennial control	Randomized	Randomized	Randomized: biennial vs. control	Allocation by month assigned
Rehydration of test cards*	Yes, most	No	Yes, most	No	No
Adherence (%)	Annual 75; biennial 78	50	—	56	—
Positivity rate (%)	2.4 (nonhydrated) 9.8 (rehydrated)	1st screen: 2.1 2nd screen: 1.2	1st screen: 1.9 (nonhydrated) 5.8 (rehydrated) 2nd screen: 4.8 (prev. rehydrated), 8.0 (prev. nonhydrated)	1st screen: 1.0 2nd screen: 0.8 3rd screen: 0.9 4th screen: 1.3 5th screen: 1.8	Regular attendees: 1.4 1st screen: 2.6
PPV for CRC (%)	2.2 (rehydrated) 5.6 (nonhydrated)	1st screen: 9.9 2nd screen: 11.9	1st screen: 5.0 (nonhydrated) 2nd screen: 4.2 (rehydrated)	1st screen: 17.7 2nd screen: 8.4	10.7
CRC mortality†	18-yr follow-up: 33% reduction for the annual group, 21% reduction for biennial group Mortality ratio: Annual: 0.67 Biennial: 0.79	7- to 8-yr follow-up: 15% reduction in cumulative CRC mortality Mortality ratio: 0.85	Not yet available	10-yr follow-up: 18% reduction in CRC mortality in the screened group Mortality ratio: 0.82	10-yr follow-up: 43% reduction in CRC mortality in the screened group

*Hemoccult test cards were used, rehydrated or nonhydrated.
†Reductions in mortality are relative risk reductions. A French trial[107] using biennial FOBTs yielded a 16% reduction in CRC-related mortality in the screened group. The mortality ratio was 0.84 (95% confidence interval, 0.71-0.99) after 11 years of follow-up.
PPV, positive predictive value; prev., previously.

Proctosigmoidoscopy

The benefit of proctosigmoidoscopy in screening programs for CRC was suggested by several uncontrolled studies that used rigid proctosigmoidoscopy. Those studies suggested that proctosigmoidoscopy in asymptomatic average-risk persons might detect early-stage cancers, and that detection and removal of adenomas could result in a lower-than-expected frequency of rectosigmoid cancers in the screened population.

Two case-control studies provided strong evidence that sigmoidoscopy can reduce CRC mortality. A study from the Kaiser-Permanente Medical Care Program[106] compared 261 members who died of cancer of the rectum or distal colon with 868 age- and sex-matched control subjects. Only 8.8% of case subjects had undergone screening by rigid sigmoidoscopy, compared with 24.2% of controls; rigid sigmoidoscopy had no effect on mortality in another group with lesions beyond the reach of the sigmoidoscope. Furthermore, the beneficial effect

of sigmoidoscopy extended 10 years. This and a second case-control study indicate that sigmoidoscopy can result in a 70% to 80% reduction in mortality from cancers within reach of the sigmoidoscope. Because approximately 50% of all CRCs can be detected using the 60-cm flexible sigmoidoscope or a gastroscope (see Fig. 127-3), these data suggest that periodic sigmoidoscopic screening could reduce overall CRC-related mortality by about one third.

Because the flexible sigmoidoscope is superior to rigid instruments in detecting lesions, flexible sigmoidoscopy using a gastroscope has replaced rigid sigmoidoscopy for CRC screening. Flexible sigmoidoscopy can be learned by nonphysicians and has been used successfully in screening programs that employ nurse practitioners; wide variations in adenoma detection rates were observed, however, in the U.K. Flexible Sigmoidoscopy Screening Trial.[107]

Three prospective randomized trials have now shown that programmatic screening with flexible sigmoidoscopy can have an impact on CRC-related incidence and mortality.[107-109]

The U.K. Flexible Sigmoidoscopy Screening Trial is a randomized trial that tested the hypothesis that a single flexible sigmoidoscopy screening examination offered at approximately 60 years of age can lower the incidence and mortality of CRC.[107] In per-protocol analyses, CRC incidence and mortality were reduced by 33% and 43%, respectively (23% and 31%, respectively, based on intention-to-treat analysis); incidence of cancer of the rectum and sigmoid was reduced by 50%. The Prostate, Lung, Colorectal, and Ovarian Cancer Screening Trial (PLCO) enrolled 154,900 subjects aged 55 to 74 years in a prospective randomized trial that compared flexible sigmoidoscopy with repeat screening at 3 or 5 years to a usual-care control group.[108] Flexible sigmoidoscopy reduced CRC incidence by 21%, with a benefit observed in both the proximal and distal colon, and reduced overall mortality by 26% (intention-to-treat analyses). Mortality from distal CRC (distal to the splenic flexure) was reduced by 50%, whereas mortality from proximal CRC was unaffected. The Italian Randomized Controlled Trial (SCORE) demonstrated that once-only sigmoidoscopy significantly reduced CRC incidence by 18% and insignificantly reduced mortality by 22% in intention-to-treat analyses; in per-protocol analyses, incidence and mortality were reduced 31% and 38%, respectively, both significant.[109] These data have resulted in once-in-a-lifetime flexible sigmoidoscopy being included as an option in the U.K. National Health Service Bowel Cancer Screening Programme (FOBT is the other option).

Colonoscopy, Barium Enema, CT Colonography, and Colon Capsule Endoscopy

Colonoscopy may well be the most effective tool for CRC screening, but data from prospective trials are lacking to firmly support this conclusion; a large prospective Veterans Administration screening trial is underway in the USA, and several other trials are ongoing in Europe to address this question). The National Polyp Study, on polypectomy and surveillance, strongly suggested a reduction in CRC mortality as the result of removing adenomatous polyps compared with historic reference populations. A recent update of this trial, with median follow-up of 15.8 years, indicated that colonoscopic polypectomy is associated with a 53% reduction in mortality from CRC compared with the expected incidence-based mortality from CRC in the general population.[110] A Canadian population-based study compared the risk of developing CRC after a negative colonoscopy in all Ontario residents who had a history of a complete negative colonoscopy with controls that consisted of the Ontario population without a history of colonoscopy.[111] In the negative colonoscopy cohort, the relative risk of distal CRC was significantly lower than the control group in each of the 14 years of follow-up, and the relative risk for proximal CRC was significantly lower, mainly during the last 7 years of follow-up. A second Canadian case-control study demonstrated that complete colonoscopy also was associated with fewer deaths from left-sided CRC but not from right-sided cancer.[112] Several other population-based analyses and analyses of individual screening programs in the USA, Canada, and Europe also suggest that increased use of colonoscopy is associated with mortality reduction from CRC, but that this reduction varies by site of the cancer.[113-117] A large case-control study using SEER-Medicare data demonstrated that colonoscopy was associated with a 60% decreased risk of CRC-related death, but the association was stronger for distal (OR, 0.24; 95% CI, 0.21-0.27) than proximal (OR, 0.58; 95% CI, 0.53-0.64) CRC, consistent with European and Canadian studies.[116]

These findings are of interest in light of arguments against the superiority of colonoscopy to sigmoidoscopy, because there may be a substantial incidence of proximal colonic cancers and advanced adenomas beyond the reach of the sigmoidoscope. Some of these persons might not have had distal findings on sigmoidoscopy that would have triggered a subsequent colonoscopy. Two trials[118,119] showed that approximately 50% of persons with advanced proximal neoplasms had no distal neoplasms, whereas less than 2% of those who did not have distal neoplasms had an advanced proximal lesion.[118]

Given the need for colonoscopic follow-up should FOBT or sigmoidoscopy be positive, colonoscopy also might be cost-effective. A decision analysis commissioned by the USPSTF supports colonoscopy every 10 years as a screening option measured in life-years gained.

High-contrast endoscopy using dye or stain solutions combined with colonoscopy (chromoendoscopy) or high-resolution optical methods (e.g., narrow-band imaging, laser confocal endoscopy) has been suggested as a means of identifying lesions in high-risk groups or as an adjunct to colonoscopy when flat lesions (flat adenomas) are suspected. Evidence suggests that flat or depressed neoplasms are more common than previously appreciated and that they carry a high relative risk of containing in situ or invasive carcinoma.[120] Chromoendoscopy detects more adenomas than colonoscopy using intensive inspection, but its usefulness in routine practice has not been established.[121]

ACBE has been included as an option in a variety of screening guidelines. No studies, however, have directly addressed the effectiveness of barium enema for CRC screening. Several studies have indicated that the sensitivity of ACBE is far less than that of colonoscopy, especially for detecting lesions smaller than 1 cm. A population-based study[122] suggested that if a cancer is present, there is approximately a 1 in 5 chance that it will be missed by ACBE.

CT colonography (CTC), or virtual colonoscopy, uses helical CT to generate high-resolution, 2-dimensional images of the abdomen and pelvis. Three-dimensional images of the colon can be reconstructed by computer generation offline (Figs. 127-25 and 127-26) and has the potential advantage of being a rapid and safe method of providing full structural evaluation of the entire colon. Recognition of the importance of CRC screening has raised concerns over the ability of existing resources to handle the ensuing volume of expected procedures such as colonoscopy. Colonography using CT or MRI could represent an alternate method with promise for the future.

The accuracy and potential of CTC as a screening tool for colorectal neoplasia has been debated because initial studies yielded a wide range of sensitivities. Two large multicenter trials fueled this controversy. One trial included 1273 asymptomatic persons who underwent same-day virtual and optical colonoscopy.[123,124] This study employed multidetector CT scanners, 3-dimensional endoluminal displays, and solid stool tagging and opacification of luminal fluid (optical cleansing). CTC demonstrated sufficiently high sensitivity (89% to 94%) and specificity (80% to 96%) to detect polyps across a broad range of sizes (>6 to >10 mm) to warrant its serious consideration as an option for screening. A second study of 600 subjects[125] reported a sensitivity for detecting even large polyps (55%) far below that of optical colonoscopy, but it used different technology and methods of analysis compared with the first study. Two other trials provide evidence that CTC may be a valid alternative for primary CRC screening. The National CT Colonography Trial[126] directed by the American College of Radiology Imaging Network (ACRIN) was a multicenter study that employed CTC and same-day colonoscopy using a standard matching protocol in 2600 asymptomatic persons. Per-patient sensitivity of CTC for adenomas larger than 10 mm

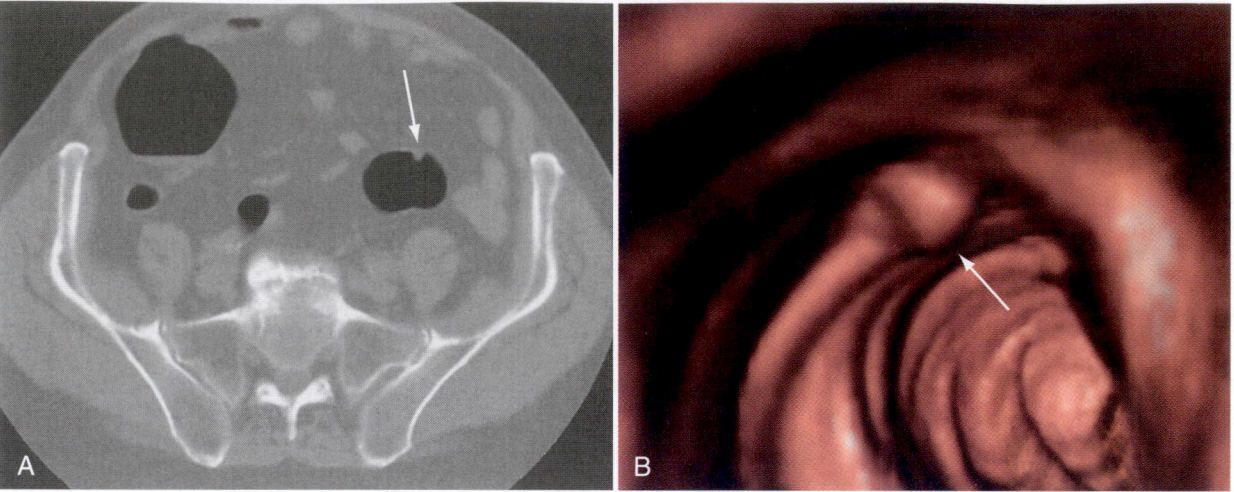

FIGURE 127-25. CT colonography (virtual colonoscopy). An 8-mm sigmoid polyp identified on an axial 2-dimensional CT image of the colon (*A, arrow*) and on an endoluminal 3-dimensional reconstruction (*B, arrow*).

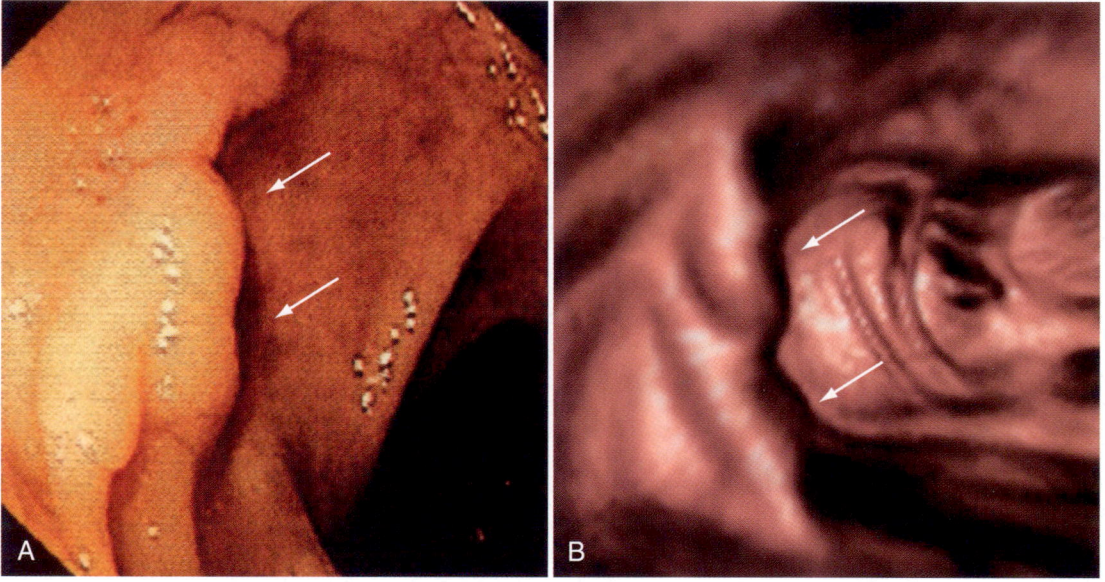

FIGURE 127-26. Representative views of a 2-cm sessile colonic lesion (*arrows*) seen on a fold. Lesion seen at colonoscopy (*A*) and on 3-dimensional reconstruction CT colonography (*B*).

was 90%, with a negative predictive value of 99%. A second trial[127] compared CTC and optical colonoscopy in parallel screening cohorts and demonstrated similar rates of detection of advanced neoplasia in both groups.

Several key issues need to be addressed as the use of CTC becomes more widespread, principal among which is determination of the size cut-off of a detected lesion that will necessitate follow-up colonoscopy. Other issues include the need for bowel preparation, the logistics of same-day colonoscopy, the ability to detect flat lesions, the significance of extracolonic lesions detected by CTC, the impact on compliance, and cost-effectiveness. Methodologies that employ CTC without need for cathartic preparation and with fecal tagging might make this a more attractive option for screening. The diagnostic accuracy of laxative-free CTC for the detection of adenomatous polyps in asymptomatic adults was recently studied. This method was accurate in detecting adenomas 10 mm or larger, but less so for smaller lesions.[124] CTC also might aid in detecting lesions located behind folds or near the

anal verge.[128] The Centers for Medicare and Medicaid Services (CMS) has, to date, denied coverage for CTC screening for CRC, in large part because of the USPSTF decision not to include CTC in their screening guidelines. Other societies such as the American Cancer Society, however, include CTC in their guidelines.

Pillcam colon capsule endoscopy employs an ingested capsule that allows imaging of the colon without the need for sedation or gas insufflation (analogous to the small bowel Pillcam), although a bowel preparation is required. The technique is available in Europe and other countries, but clinical indications and reporting measures have not been standardized.[129] There is a lack of specific studies based in the screening setting.

MR colonography is a radiation-free, IV contrast-enhanced examination of the abdomen with high resolution. There have been limited studies, to date, that have examined this modality for CRC screening, but recent data indicate that this modality can detect colorectal adenomas 6 mm or larger and advanced neoplasia with high levels of sensitivity and specificity, albeit with lower levels of sensitivity than colonoscopy.

Plasma- and Serum-Based Tumor Markers

A variety of proteins, glycoproteins, and cellular and humoral substances have been studied as potential tumor markers, but none has been found specific for CRC. Potential tumor markers may get into the blood by a variety of mechanisms. Some molecules may be released from the tumor cell surface by proteolytic cleavage. For example, CEA may be released through the action of phosphatidylinositol-specific phospholipase C (PI-PLC). Membrane-bound mucins also may be released by proteolytic cleavage or after engagement by specific ligands, whereas other molecules may be actively secreted. Tumor-associated molecules also may reach the blood in shed vesicles as exosomes, after outward budding of the plasma membrane and release into the extracellular space. Exosomes may contain tumor-derived proteins and may transport oncogenes and onco–micro RNAs (miRNAs). Other membrane vesicles include apoptotic bodies, which are created via bleb formation of the membrane of dying cells.

CEA may be useful in the preoperative staging and postoperative follow-up of patients with colon cancer, but it has a low predictive value for diagnosis in asymptomatic patients. Sensitivities for CEA alone and CEA-related cell adhesion molecule (CEACAM), for example, have ranged between 32% and 69% and are highly dependent upon tumor stage. The relatively low sensitivity and specificity of CEA combine to make it unsuitable for screening large asymptomatic populations. Several new protein and carbohydrate antigens are being examined and hold some promise in terms of specificity for preneoplastic and early neoplastic lesions in the colon[70,73,130-136]; their effectiveness for screening, however, remains to be determined. MicroRNAs are short noncoding RNAs that play important roles in various physiologic and developmental processes. Circulating microRNAs represent new potential biomarkers for diagnosis and prognosis in digestive tract cancers.[136]

The development of sensitive and specific markers that can be used for early detection of cancer is the focus of the National Cancer Institute-sponsored Early Detection Research Network (EDRN). Promising approaches using genomic or proteomic techniques applied to biomarker discovery are being pursued that might result in practical clinical tests. One such approach involves the study of candidate genes or proteins assembled into panels of markers. Another discovery-based approach uses high-throughput techniques that allow simultaneous assessment of tens of thousands of genes or proteins.[137] Multicenter prospective studies involving large numbers of patients will be required to define the impact of these and other tests on population screening.

Fecal DNA and Genetic Testing

A great deal of knowledge has been accumulated about genetic alterations that occur during colon carcinogenesis (see earlier), but specific genetic tests are not yet available for most patients at risk for sporadic CRC. A molecular approach to CRC screening is attractive because it targets biological changes that are fundamental to the neoplastic process. The feasibility of detecting altered DNA in stool has been demonstrated using a multi-target assay panel of molecular markers. One multicenter study compared fecal DNA testing using such a panel with FOBT and colonoscopy. The fecal DNA panel consisted of 21 mutations: 3 in the *K-ras* gene, 10 in the *APC* gene, 8 in the *TP53* gene, the MSI marker BAT-26, and a marker of long DNA thought to reflect disordered apoptosis

of cancer cells sloughed into the colonic lumen. Although most of the lesions identified by colonoscopy were not detected by either of the fecal tests, multi-targeted fecal DNA testing detected a higher proportion of important lesions compared with Hemoccult. A second study[138] compared stool DNA and FOBT for detecting screen-relevant neoplasia (curable-stage cancer, high-grade dysplasia, or adenomas > 1 cm). This blinded, multicenter cross-sectional study used 2 different methodologies for detecting alterations in stool DNA: a 23-marker panel and a new test targeting 3 broadly informative markers (point mutations on *K-ras*, a scanned mutator cluster region of *APC*, and methylated vimentin). Although the multi-panel test provided no improvement over FOBT (Hemoccult Sensa) for detecting screen-relevant neoplasms, the new test showed promise by detecting significantly more neoplasms than FOBT. A next-generation stool DNA test using quantitative allele-specific real-time target and signal amplification plus quantitative Hgb analysis shows promise for detection of early-stage CRC and large adenomas throughout the colon and rectum, with high levels of accuracy.[139] Recently the DeeP-C study of stool DNA testing for CRC in almost 10,000 average-risk individuals was completed. The sensitivity of a panel which included several DNA markers plus FIT for detecting CRC was 92.3% compared with 73.8% for FIT alone (with colonoscopy as the standard). The sensitivity for detecting advanced precancerous lesions (advanced adenomas or sessile serrated adenomas ≥1 cm) was 42.4% for the panel compared with 23.8% for FIT alone. Specificities with DNA and FIT were 86.6% and 94.9% respectively, among participants with nonadvanced or negative finding on colonoscopy.[140]

Genetic testing is now a reality for families with FAP and other hereditary polyposis and is discussed in detail in Chapter 126. It is important that proper genetic counseling is incorporated into the screening process.

Approach to Screening

Screening and case-finding approaches are different for patients in average-risk and high-risk groups. The former group consists of patients older than 50 years, and the latter group includes patients with long-standing UC, previous CRC, previous adenomas, female genital cancer, familial polyposis, HNPCC, and familial colon cancer. Data on the risk of CRC in women with a history of breast cancer are too limited at present to draw firm conclusions regarding appropriate screening intervals.

Average-Risk Group

Patients who are registered in a health care system should be categorized according to risk, so that appropriate CRC screening can be added to their proper medical evaluation. Relative risk should be assessed by family and personal history. A variety of options are available for screening average-risk patients (≈50 years old with no personal or family history of colorectal adenoma or CRC and no personal history of IBD). These have been discussed previously, including guidelines from various health care agencies (see Table 127-8). Although yearly FOBTs or flexible sigmoidoscopy every 5 years is an individual option, it has been suggested that combining the 2 tests can increase the benefits of either test alone. The tests are complementary because the FOBT has the potential for detecting occult blood from a lesion anywhere in the colon, whereas flexible sigmoidoscopy can detect bleeding and nonbleeding lesions distal to the splenic flexure.

Colonoscopy every 10 years has the advantages of examining the entire colon and rectum and providing the opportunity to biopsy or remove lesions should they be found.

A study of participants in a German colonoscopy screening program confirmed the low risk of CRC and advanced adenomas after a negative colonoscopy and supports this interval in average-risk individuals.[137] Growing evidence indicates that colonoscopy is a cost-effective option with an acceptable risk profile. Several trials are underway to examine colonoscopy for average-risk screening. A diagnostic evaluation is indicated for persons with a positive FOBT or distal neoplasm (adenoma, carcinoma) found at sigmoidoscopy. Colonoscopy is the diagnostic modality of choice. If colonoscopy is unavailable, not feasible, or not desired by the patient, CT colonography is an acceptable alternative to evaluate a positive FOBT result.

Screening should be accompanied by programs that educate patients and heighten physicians' awareness of the concepts and technologies involved in screening, diagnosis, treatment, and follow-up. The popular misconceptions that CRC is an incurable disease and that surgical intervention invariably leads to an impaired life-style, owing to a colostomy, must be discredited.

High-Risk Groups

Familial Adenomatous Polyposis, Nonpolyposis Syndromes, and Familial Cancer

Screening of family members in kindreds with familial polyposis is discussed in Chapter 126, and guidelines are available.[75,141,142]

Algorithmic approaches to screening and surveillance of families with Lynch syndrome or those suspected of having Lynch syndrome have been adopted by professional societies with clinical practice guidelines for genetic testing and risk assessment for patients and families.[75,143] Genetic testing and counseling is an essential part of quality care in families with known MMR gene mutations or those who meet the modified Bethesda criteria (see Box 127-3).[59,69] Because 70% to 80% of CRCs in the setting of Lynch syndrome are proximal to the splenic flexure, colonoscopy is the mandated screening modality for the colon. Most guidelines suggest that screening begin at age 20 to 25, or 10 years before the youngest case in the immediate family, and repeated every 1 to 2 years in at-risk individuals with MMR gene mutations.

CRCs occurring in the setting of Lynch syndrome are often right-sided, and precursor adenomas are commonly "flat." This has led to the common use of "red-flag" techniques such as chromoendoscopy in an attempt to better detect these lesions. High-magnification colonoscopy with chromoendoscopy using indigo carmine or methylene blue may improve the detection of neoplastic lesions in the colon of individuals with Lynch syndrome.

In approximately 30% of families that meet Amsterdam I criteria for Lynch syndrome, MSI testing and testing for MMR germline mutations is negative. These individuals develop CRC at a more advanced age and have fewer cancers than those with Lynch syndrome. In families without MMR deficiency, a less intensive surveillance protocol is recommended, with colonoscopy at 3- to 5-year intervals, starting at 5 to 10 years before the first diagnosis of CRC or at 45 years of age. Individuals in Lynch syndrome families who test negative for a known mutation and who are asymptomatic should undergo routine screening as recommended for individuals with a family history of CRC.

The approach to patients with a suggestive family history (e.g., 1 first-degree relative with colon cancer) is not firmly established, but existing data suggest that these patients should be monitored more rigorously than average-risk persons. The joint guidelines from the ACS and U.S. Multi-Society Task Force on Colorectal Cancer recommend that if CRC or adenomatous polyps occurred in any first-degree relative before age 60 years, or in 2 or more first-degree relatives at any age, then colonoscopy should be performed every 5 years, beginning at age 40 years or beginning 10 years before the youngest case in the immediate family.[81] If either CRC or adenomatous polyps occurred in a first-degree relative 60 years of age or older, or if CRC occurred in 2 second-degree relatives, then screening should begin at age 40 years using screening options recommended for average-risk persons. In those with more than 2 affected first-degree relatives, special care should be taken to exclude Lynch syndrome, and periodic colonoscopy is advised.

Prior Adenomas or Colon Cancer

Table 127-12 lists the ACS-Multi-Society-ACR guidelines for screening, surveillance, and early detection of colorectal adenomas and cancer for persons at increased risk or at high risk of disease. These guidelines suggest that those whose index lesion consists of 1 or 2 small tubular adenomas with low-grade dysplasia should have a follow-up colonoscopy 5 to 10 years after the initial polypectomy. The precise timing within this interval should be based on clinical factors such as prior findings, family history, and patient and physician preferences. A recent update of guidelines for colonoscopy surveillance after screening and polypectomy by the U.S. Multi-Society Task Force on CRC further supports this approach.[144]

One study examined the relative risk for advanced neoplasia within 5.5 years of a baseline colonoscopy.[145] There was a strong association between the results of baseline screening colonoscopy and the rate of serious incident lesions during surveillance. This study confirmed that patients with 1 or 2 small tubular adenomas represent a low-risk group compared with other patients with colorectal neoplasia. This conclusion was confirmed in a prospective study of surveillance colonoscopy performed in Korea.[146] In patients with a large (>1 cm) adenoma, multiple (3 to 10) adenomas, or adenomas with high-grade dysplasia or villous change, colonoscopy should be repeated within 3 years of the initial polypectomy. Although the risk for recurrence of advanced adenomas at this follow-up interval is greater in patients with high-risk adenomas than those with low-risk adenomas, the incremental risk is small.[147] If repeat examination is normal or shows only 1 or 2 small tubular adenomas with low-grade dysplasia, then the interval for the subsequent examination should be 5 years. Patients with more than 10 adenomas on a single examination should have a follow-up colonoscopy less than 3 years after the initial polypectomy, and the existence of an underlying familial syndrome should be considered. Patients with sessile adenomas that are removed in a piecemeal fashion should have follow-up colonoscopy in 2 to 6 months to verify complete removal. Guidelines of the British Society of Gastroenterology and the Association of Coloproctology for Great Britain and Ireland stratify patients into risk groups based on the number and size of adenomas, without consideration of histologic features. One key difference between U.S. and U.K. guidelines is that U.K. criteria recommend a single clearing colonoscopy at 1 year for individuals classified as high risk (those with ≥ 5 small adenomas or ≥ 3 adenomas, at least 1 of which is ≥ 1 cm).[148]

Patients with colon or rectal cancer should have high-quality perioperative clearing. Colonoscopy should be performed preoperatively, intraoperatively, or within 3 to 6 months after cancer resection. Those who have had a colon cancer resected should have colonoscopy performed 1 year after surgery or the original clearing colonoscopy. If the

TABLE 127-12 Surveillance Guidelines for Persons at Increased or High Risk of Colorectal Cancer (CRC)

Risk Category	Time or Age to Begin Surveillance	Recommended Test(s)	Comment
Persons with Adenomas at Colonoscopy			
Persons with 1 or 2 small tubular adenomas with low-grade dysplasia	5-10 yr after initial polypectomy	Colonoscopy	Precise timing is based on clinical factors and on patient and physician preferences
Persons with 3 to 10 adenomas or 1 adenoma >1 cm or any adenoma with villous features or high-grade dysplasia	3 yr after initial polypectomy	Colonoscopy	If the follow-up examination is normal or shows 1 or 2 small tubular adenomas, subsequent examination at 5 yr
Persons with >10 adenomas on a single examination	<3 yr after initial polypectomy	Colonoscopy	Consider familial syndrome
Persons with sessile adenomas that are removed piecemeal	2 to 6 months after initial colonoscopy	Colonoscopy	Surveillance individualized based on endoscopist's judgment
Persons with CRC			
Persons undergoing curative resection for CRC	Intraoperatively or 3 to 6 months after cancer resection	Colonoscopy	Persons with CRC should undergo high-quality perioperative clearing of the colon. For nonobstructing tumors, examination can be done preoperatively; for obstructing cancer, CTC or DCBE can be used to detect proximal neoplasms
	1 year after resection (or 1 year after clearing colonoscopy)	Colonoscopy	If the examination at 1 year is normal, perform the next examination at 3 yr. If that examination is normal, then perform the next examination at 5 yr. Periodic exam of the rectum (3- to 6-month intervals for the first 2-3 yr) may be considered after low anterior resection of rectal cancer
Persons with a Family History of CRC			
CRC or adenomatous polyps in a first-degree relative before age 60 yr or in 2 or more first-degree relatives at any age	Age 40 yr, or 10 yr before the youngest case in the immediate family	Colonoscopy	Every 5 yr
Either CRC or adenomatous polyps in a first-degree relative ≥ age 60 yr or in 2 second-degree relatives with CRC	Age 40 yr	Screening options at intervals recommended for average-risk persons	Screening should begin at an earlier age, but patients may be screened with any recommended form of testing
Persons at High Risk			
Genetic diagnosis of FAP or suspected FAP without genetic testing evidence	Age 10 to 12 yr	Annual FSIG to determine if the patient is expressing the genetic abnormality and counseling to consider genetic testing	If the genetic test is positive, colectomy should be considered
Genetic or clinical diagnosis of Lynch syndrome or persons at increased risk of Lynch syndrome	Age 20 to 25 yr or 10 yr before the youngest case in the immediate family	Colonoscopy every 1 to 2 yr and counseling to consider genetic testing (see Chapter 126)	Genetic testing for Lynch syndrome should be offered to first-degree relatives of persons with a known inherited DNA MMR gene mutation; it should also be offered when the family mutation is not known but when 1 or more of the first 3 of the modified Bethesda Criteria (see Box 127-3) is present
IBD (UC and Crohn's colitis)	8 yr after the onset of pancolitis or 12-15 yr after the onset of left-sided colitis	Colonoscopy with biopsies for dysplasia (see Chapters 115 and 116)	Every 1-2 yr

CTC, CT colonography; DCBE, double-contrast barium enema; FAP, familial adenomatous polyposis; FSIG, flexible sigmoidoscopy; MMR, mismatch repair.
Derived from Levin B, Lieberman DA, McFarland B, et al. Screening and surveillance for the early detection of colorectal cancer and adenomatous polyps 2008: A joint guideline from the American Cancer Society, the Multi-Society Task Force on Colorectal Cancer and the American College of Radiology. CA Cancer J Clin 2008; 58:130-60.

examination performed at 1 year is normal, then the interval before the next colonoscopy should be 3 years; if that examination is normal, the next colonoscopy should be at 5 years (see Table 127-12). Periodic examination of the rectum to identify local recurrence usually is performed at 3- to 6-month intervals for the first 2 or 3 years after low anterior resection for rectal cancer. Serum CEA levels should be measured at regular intervals because postoperative CEA determinations may be cost-effective for detecting recurrent cancers. How long an asymptomatic patient who has had multiple negative examinations should be tested by various modalities is at present unclear. It should be noted that these recommendations are, to some extent, educated guesses, and not all are based on prospective randomized trials.

IBD

Colonoscopic surveillance in patients with UC is discussed in Chapter 116 and in patients with Crohn's colitis in Chapter 115. Algorithms for screening and surveillance in patients with IBD can be found in references 75, 86, and 149.

Insurance Coverage for Screening

Based on evidence from several randomized trials, the Health Care Financing Administration (HCFA) decided to provide coverage for colon cancer screening procedures to Medicare beneficiaries beginning January 1, 1998. After intense lobbying by several groups, Medicare provided coverage for screening colonoscopy in average-risk persons every 10 years or at an interval 4 years from a previous sigmoidoscopy. This bill was signed December 21, 2000, and coverage was initiated July 1, 2001. The Affordable Care Act requires private health insurers to cover recommended preventive services, including CRC screening.[150] The requirement took effect for new plans sold or renewed on or after September 23, 2010. In some cases, however, insurers were reclassifying what appeared to be screening colonoscopies from preventive to diagnostic services. The methodology of how private insurers approached cost sharing for CRC varied substantially depending on how each provider considered scenarios wherein a polyp was detected and removed during screening, when a colonoscopy was performed as part of a 2-step process following a positive FOBT, and when individuals at increased risk required more frequent screening compared with average-risk individuals.[150] This approach often resulted in unexpected charges to consumers. Some of the confusion resulted from differences in coding by providers. Recently the Department of Health and Human Services released a statement indicating that "polyp removal is an integral part of colonoscopy" and should be considered part of screening. Under previous Medicare rules, cost sharing was waived for screening colonoscopy only when no polyp was removed.

The American Gastroenterological Association and the Entertainment Industry Foundation's National CRC Research Alliance issued the 2004 CRC Screening Legislation Report Card that analyzed the varied and complex state laws governing insurance for preventive CRC screening. The frequency of screenings complies with current Medicare CRC screening regulations. Data suggest that expansion of Medicare reimbursement to cover CRC screening was associated with an increased use of colonoscopy for Medicare beneficiaries and for those who received diagnoses of colon cancer, and that it was associated with an increased probability of diagnosis at an early stage.[151-154] National and regional CRC screening programs have been adopted by several countries including Canada (Ontario 2008), New Zealand, the United Kingdom, and other countries in the European Union. The primary

modality for screening varies among countries but usually entails a 2-step approach with FOBT as the initial test, followed by colonoscopy when FOBT is positive. These programs often stress that they consist of organized (as opposed to "opportunistic") screening with specified age categories, methods and intervals for testing, defined target populations, health care teams for decisions and care, and quality assurance structures. A report describing results of the first 2 years of the Cancer Care Ontario ColonCancerCheck program has recently been published.[154]

Screening Capacity, Screening in Underserved Populations, and Quality Assurance

It has been estimated that only half of the eligible U.S. population has been screened for CRC according to recommended guidelines. Efforts to increase compliance and screening recommendations should take into account the capacity to use various tests for screening and surveillance. Healthy People 2020 sets national objectives for use of recommended screening tests and identifies the National Health Interview Survey (NHIS) as a means to measure this progress. Data from the 2010 NHIS indicated an overall CRC screening rate in the USA of 58.6% (2020 target is 70.5%), with significantly lower rates in blacks or Asians than whites.[152] Hispanics were less likely to report being up to date with screening than non-Hispanics. Colonoscopy rates have increased every year since the introduction of CRC screening, while test rates for all other test modalities have steadily decreased.[153]

A forecasting model[155] using data from the U.S. Census Bureau and CDC survey indicated that capacity currently exists for widespread screening with the FOBT. The capacity for screening flexible sigmoidoscopy or colonoscopy depends on the proportion of available capacity used for CRC screening. Surveillance colonoscopy needs to be used appropriately as the availability of endoscopic resources decreases. A national survey of colorectal surveillance after polypectomy suggests that resources are being taxed by inappropriate surveillance practices that do not conform to current guidelines.[156] Risk stratification will become increasingly necessary as resources become limited. Alternative screening modalities such as CT colonography might reduce demand for endoscopic procedures when used to screen low-risk groups, but they will result in increased demand for persons trained in these techniques. The ability of CT colonography to reduce the demand for colonoscopy will also depend on the polyp size that generates a follow-up colonoscopy. Fecal DNA testing could increase compliance and reduce the need for screening colonoscopy if tests were sensitive and specific.

African Americans in the USA have a higher rate of CRC incidence and mortality compared with the non-Hispanic white population.[157-161] Compared with white persons, black men and women undergoing screening colonoscopy have a higher risk of larger polyps.[158] African Americans who have first-degree relatives with colon cancer are less likely to undergo colonoscopy screening compared with whites who have affected relatives.[159] Multiple explanations for these findings have been proposed including lack of access to care, cost, patient preference, physician recommendations (all of which affect screening rates), behavioral and environmental influences, and biological and genetic predisposition. Adherence to screening guidelines in urban minority populations may be aided by programs that assist in access and navigation through the health care system.[162,163]

Colonoscopy is now the most common endoscopic procedure performed in the USA. Although colonoscopic polypectomy is considered effective for preventing CRC, cancers may be discovered in intervals between planned screening or surveillance exams.[164] Such post-colonoscopy CRCs or "interval" cancers may result from missed lesions or arise de novo in high-risk groups. Whereas the precise definition of what constitutes an interval cancer varies among studies, approximately 7% to 9% of CRCs occur within 6 to 36 months following a screening colonoscopy and have been considered interval cancers.[165] As the number of colonoscopies (and colonoscopists) increases, quality-assurance measures will need to be adopted. One measure of quality assurance relates to adequate visualization of the colonic mucosa. One study from a community-based practice[166] suggested that detection of overall and advanced neoplasia may be related to withdrawal time during colonoscopy. After implementing a protocol of inspection during a minimum withdrawal time of 8 minutes, greater rates of detection were observed. Others, while agreeing that adequate visualization of the mucosa is an important quality-assurance parameter, have suggested that adequate examination relates more to the experience and quality of the endoscopist than to the withdrawal time per se. Adenoma detection rate (ADR) is defined by the percentage of screening or surveillance colonoscopies of average risk with at least 1 adenoma, and is the most commonly used quality measure in practice. Benchmarks for adequate ADRs have been suggested as at least 15% for women and 25% for men (20% overall). The ADR is considered by the ASGE/ACG Task Force on Quality in Endoscopy to be the best neoplasia-related indicator of quality performance for screening colonoscopy. The ADR has been demonstrated to be an independent predictor of the risk of interval CRC after screening colonoscopy.[167] Endoscopist characteristics (volume, polypectomy and completion rate, specialization and setting) derived from administrative data are associated with the development of post-colonoscopy CRC, and have potential use as quality indicators.[168] Other quality measures include quality of bowel preparation and completeness of polyp resection. The incomplete resection rate in the recently published Complete Adenoma Resection (CARE) study was 10.1% overall, and varied broadly among endoscopists.[169] A physician performance measurement set for endoscopy and surveillance has been proposed in a joint document by the ASGE, the AGA, the Physician Consortium for Performance Improvement, and the National Committee for Quality Assurance. Quality measures also have been stressed by European quality control programs.

TREATMENT

Surgery

Surgical resection is the treatment of choice for patients with invasive nonmetastatic CRC. Preoperative colonoscopy should be performed, if possible, to rule out synchronous lesions (see earlier), and serum CEA should be measured for staging and informed postoperative follow-up. Preoperative CT of the chest, abdomen, and pelvis can be valuable for evaluating focal hepatic and pulmonary metastases if partial hepatectomy, pulmonary resection, or chemotherapy is contemplated. PET/CT is not routinely recommended for baseline evaluation of follow-up. It has become standard practice in most centers to provide a trial of systemic chemotherapy in patients with hepatic metastases before resecting the primary tumor, because if there is no response, colonic resection will not be curative. CT also is useful for postoperative detection of pelvic recurrence in patients with rectosigmoid tumors. Transrectal EUS or MRI is of value in the preoperative assessment of patients with rectal cancer, and is now routinely recommended for clinical evaluation and staging. EUS and MRI both have high sensitivities for evaluating the depth of tumor penetration into the muscularis propria ($\approx$94%), although EUS is more specific than MRI for local tumor invasion (86% vs. 69%). CT, EUS, and MRI are comparable in evaluating lymph node involvement; however, only CT and MRI can evaluate iliac and mesenteric or retroperitoneal nodes.

The goal of surgery is wide resection of the involved segment of colon, together with removal of its lymphatic drainage (Fig. 127-27). The extent of resection is determined by the blood supply and distribution of regional lymph nodes. The resection should include a segment of colon at least 5 cm on either side of the tumor, although wider margins often are included because of obligatory ligation of the arterial blood supply. The number of lymph nodes recovered during colon cancer surgery has been identified as an important measure of quality cancer care. An analysis of 17 studies suggested that the number of lymph nodes evaluated after surgical resection is positively associated with survival of patients with stage II and stage III colon cancer.[170] The AJCC and American College of Pathologists recommend examination of a minimum of 12 lymph nodes to accurately identify stage II disease (i.e., no lymph node involvement is present).[171] Sentinel lymph node mapping by dye injection during surgery has not been shown to improve staging accuracy for colon cancer. Minimally invasive laparoscopically assisted surgery may be an acceptable alternative to open surgery for colon cancer in selected patients.

The approach toward rectal cancers depends on the location of the lesion.[171] Transanal excision may be performed for selected T1, N0 early-stage cancers where the cancer is within 8 cm of the anal verge, small (<3 cm), limited to 30% of the rectal circumference, moderately to well differentiated, and with no demonstrated lymph node involvement. Others should be treated with transabdominal total mesorectal excision. For lesions of the rectosigmoid and upper rectum, low anterior resection can be performed through an abdominal incision, and primary anastomosis can be accomplished (see Fig. 127-27F). Surgical treatment of rectal cancer should employ total mesorectal excision. This technique involves sharp dissection to create an avascular plane between the rectum, and mesorectum (tissue surrounding the rectum that contains lymphatics and vascular structures), and the pelvic side wall. Using sharp dissection, the rectum and mesorectum can be delivered as a single unit. Mesorectal excision is associated with a lower local recurrence rate compared with blunt dissection of the rectum away from surrounding structures.

Even for low rectal lesions, a sphincter-saving resection can be performed safely if a distal margin of at least 2 cm of normal bowel can be resected below the lesion, a goal now facilitated by end-to-end stapling devices. Tumor recurrence and survival for rectal cancer are similar after sphincter-saving resections and abdominoperineal resection (APR) if a 2-cm distal margin can be preserved in the former. The inability to obtain an adequate distal margin, the presence of a large, bulky tumor deep within the pelvis, and extensive local spread of rectal cancer all dictate the need for APR, by which the distal sigmoid, rectum, and anus are removed through a combined abdominal and perineal approach and a permanent sigmoid colostomy established.

In a patient with CRC, the primary tumor traditionally has been resected, even in the presence of distant metastases, to prevent obstruction or bleeding. More recently, a trial of chemotherapy has been recommended prior to resection in individuals with metastatic disease in order to determine response and to eliminate potentially unnecessary surgery. In patients with advanced disease and multiple medical problems, repeated palliative fulguration of rectal tumors may be preferable to surgery, and laser photoablation, argon plasma

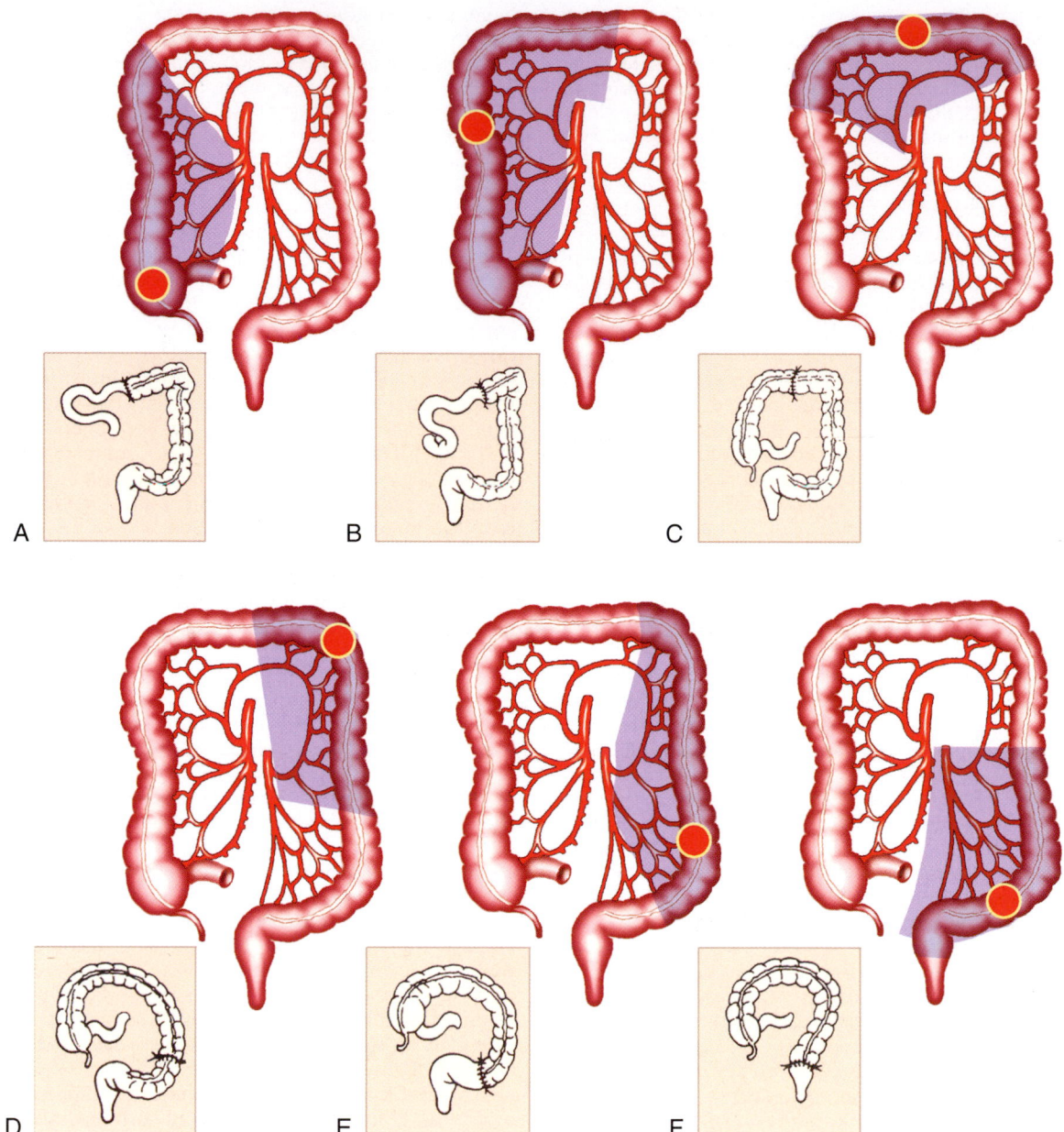

FIGURE 127-27. *A-F*, Surgical resection *(purple wedges)* of colorectal cancer based on location of the primary tumor *(circles)*, blood supply, and lymphatic drainage. *Insets* show anatomy after resection of the tumor and anastomosis.

coagulation, or endoscopic placement of expandable stents represent alternative means of palliation. Polypoid carcinomas may be removed endoscopically by snare polypectomy techniques (endoluminal resection).

Several studies indicate that although the age and physiologic status of a patient can affect operative mortality, advanced age per se does not affect tumor-associated mortality after surgery. Therefore, resection of cancer should not be limited or denied on the basis of age alone.

Follow-up

The incidence of recurrent colon cancer after surgical resection is high in persons who have serosal penetration or lymph node involvement by tumor; the incidence of metachronous CRC is 1.1% to 4.7%. Optimal strategies for surveillance after curative-intent surgery remain uncertain. It is not clear how often, or by what means, a patient should be evaluated following an apparently successful resection for cure. Colonoscopy is beneficial for detecting and removing synchronous and metachronous adenomatous polyps in high-risk groups.

History and physical examination, combined with CEA determinations at regular intervals, can provide a cost-effective means to detect recurrent cancers. The sensitivity for detecting early recurrences is about 61% using either CT or CEA, but CT can be especially useful in examining the pelvis for recurrence after resection of rectosigmoid tumors. CT portography is an accurate method for detecting liver metastases. Immunoscintigraphy after administration of radiolabeled monoclonal antibodies raised against various tumor antigens, including CEA, might provide clinically significant information in staging patients before surgery or in detecting recurrent disease, but use of this modality has not been standardized.

The role of PET currently is being evaluated. MRI ultimately might produce the clearest delineation of hepatic metastases. Intraoperative US (IOUS) now is being used to increase the ability to detect small and deep hepatic lesions that are not palpable during surgery.

Serial CEA determinations have been used to direct second-look surgical procedures. Measuring CEA levels at least every 2 months for the first 2 years after resection, and then every 4 months for the next 3 years, yields a small percentage of patients (<5%) for whom CEA-directed second-look operations for recurrent carcinoma may be indicated. Survival after second-look procedures is high when surgeons have specialized training in oncologic surgery, but other surgeons have had more limited success; long-term survival data are lacking. The concept of CEA-directed second-look laparotomy has been applied to resection of localized hepatic metastases.

Guidelines for CRC surveillance after primary surgery with curative intent have been produced by a number of agencies. All emphasize the importance of bowel surveillance with colonoscopy preoperatively, perioperatively, and at subsequent intervals.

Resection of Hepatic Metastases

The liver is the most common site of distant metastases from CRC. Synchronous metastases to the liver are evident at initial presentation in 10% to 25% of patients with colon cancer, and 40% to 70% of those whose cancers disseminate have hepatic involvement; 70% to 80% of hepatic metastases appear within 2 years after primary resection. The uniformly poor prognosis for patients with untreated hepatic metastases underlies an aggressive treatment approach. Hepatic resection is recommended for patients whose primary tumor has been resected with curative intent and in whom there is no evidence of extrahepatic disease. The extent of liver involvement that is deemed resectable varies from tumor that involves 1 lobe of the liver to focal disease in multiple lobes. The percentage of resectable liver metastases, therefore, varies in different series from 4.5% to 11% (5% to 6% in most series).

Modern techniques of anatomic dissection and hemostasis have resulted in an operative mortality of about 2% in highly trained hands. Dissections along nonanatomic lines have permitted the resection of multiple lesions that previously might have been considered unresectable. Improved preoperative imaging, routine use of IOUS, application of new surgical techniques, and improved perioperative care have increased the number of patients undergoing successful hepatic resections for isolated hepatic metastases. Overall 5-year survival rates range from 20% to 45% in selected patients. The literature is difficult to interpret, however, because staging often is not uniform, and prospective controls are lacking. Furthermore, reported 2- and 3-year survival rates may not be valid, because data suggest that patients with unresected solitary liver lesions live at least 3 years.

Long-term survival for those who undergo surgical resection of hepatic metastases depends on the absence of extrahepatic disease and the ability to achieve adequate surgical margins. In some series, the stage of the primary lesion also is a significant prognostic variable. It is not evident whether patients with a solitary focus of metastasis live longer after resection than those who undergo resection of multiple metastases in the same lobe. It is clear, however, that patients with bilobar metastases are at increased risk for recurrence of metastasis in the liver after resection, and that resection should not be attempted when more than 4 hepatic lesions are present. In patients whose tumor recurs after hepatic resection, the liver is the initial site of recurrence in about 35%. Repeat

hepatic resection for isolated metastases can result in long-term survival in selected patients.

Improved survival after resection of pulmonary metastases from CRC also has been reported. Patients with up to 3 nodules in the lung who are surgical candidates should have resection considered. Combined pulmonary and hepatic resection of metastatic disease has been used in selected cases.

Cryotherapy is a technique by which rapid freezing results in crystal formation with significant cellular damage and cell death. Tumors are frozen rapidly by means of a probe with IOUS guidance, so that malignant lesions can be ablated while the remaining liver tissue is preserved. Radiofrequency ablation employs radiofrequency energy to produce tissue destruction and often is performed during an open surgical procedure using US-guided needle electrodes that are inserted into the tumor. Cryotherapy and radiofrequency ablation are alternative approaches to treatment in patients whose liver metastases are unsuitable for surgical resection.

In patients with normal hepatic parenchyma, preservation of a perfused segment of liver that accounts for 25% of total hepatic volume is considered sufficient to prevent postoperative hepatic insufficiency. Preoperative portal vein embolization has been proposed as a means of initiating hypertrophy in segments of liver that would remain following a major liver resection and is under investigation.[172]

Chemotherapy

Adjuvant Chemotherapy

Adjuvant therapy refers to the use of chemotherapy or radiation in addition to surgery, whereas the term *neoadjuvant therapy* refers to the use of chemotherapeutic agents or radiation therapy before surgery in patients with advanced but locally confined malignancy. The prognosis for patients with CRC who undergo potentially curative surgery is correlated strongly with the stage of the primary tumor at surgery. Despite resection of all macroscopic tumor, patients whose primary tumor has penetrated the serosa or is associated with regional lymph node metastases at the time of surgery have high recurrence rates (see Tables 127-5 and 127-6). The risk of relapse after surgery ranges from 20% to 30% for stage II disease to 50% to 80% for stage III disease. Patients who undergo aggressive surgical resection of isolated hepatic or pulmonary metastases also have high tumor recurrence rates in the liver, lung, and elsewhere. An effective adjuvant program to eradicate microscopic tumor foci is needed for such high-risk patients, who number 35,000 to 40,000 each year in the USA and 200,000 worldwide.[173] The principle behind such adjuvant therapy is that treatment is most effective when tumor burden is minimal and cell kinetics are optimal. Data from numerous studies have now demonstrated delays in tumor recurrence and increases in survival for specific groups of patients with CRC who have received adjuvant therapy within 8 weeks of surgery.

Current recommendations for adjuvant therapy after surgical treatment of individuals with stage III CRC include 5-flurouracil (5-FU)/leucovorin (LV)/oxaliplatin (mFOLFOX6) as standard of care; bolus 5-FU/LV/oxaliplatin (FLOX), capecitabine/oxaliplatin (CapeOx), single-agent capecitabine, or 5-FU/LV are used in patients for whom oxaliplatin therapy is considered inappropriate.[170] Use of bevacizumab, cetuximab, panitumumab, or irinotecan in adjuvant therapy for nonmetastatic disease is not currently recommended outside of a clinical trial. A systematic review and meta-analysis indicated that each 4-week delay in initiating adjuvant chemotherapy results in a 14% decrease in overall survival, suggesting that adjuvant therapy should be initiated as soon after surgery as the patient is medically able.[174] Comparison of 5-FU plus levamisole and 5-FU plus leucovorin for the adjuvant treatment of CRC in RCTs indicated an advantage in disease-free and overall survival in favor of 5-FU plus leucovorin. Review of the combined data suggests that 5-FU plus levamisole given for 1 year is an effective regimen, but 5-FU plus leucovorin given for 6 months after curative surgery is superior with regard to convenience and efficacy.

The European MOSAIC trial[175] documented significant improvement in 3-year disease-free survival when oxaliplatin was added to infused 5-FU plus leucovorin in the FOLFOX regimen for patients with stage II and III colon cancer; 6-year follow-up data are now available that demonstrate significant overall survival in patients with stage III disease (72.9% vs. 68.7%; hazard ratio = 0.80). Similar results have been obtained by the Surgical Adjuvant Breast and Bowel Project (NSABP) using bolus 5-FU and leucovorin. These results have led to recommendations favoring combinations of oxaliplatin with IV 5-FU and leucovorin as optimal adjuvant therapy.[170] A randomized phase III trial compared FLOX (bolus 5-FU/LV/oxaliplatin) with bolus 5FU/LV in patients with stage II or III CRC[175,176]; 4-year disease-free survival rates suggested a 19% reduction associated with FLOX, but 7-year overall survival data were less convincing.

Capecitabine, an oral fluoropyrimidine, was approved in 2001 for treatment of metastatic disease (see later). This drug as a single agent was also studied as an alternative to bolus 5-FU plus leucovorin in the adjuvant setting . This trial demonstrated that disease-free survival was at least equivalent with the 2 regimens.[177] Capecitabine in combination with oxaliplatin (CapeOx) is associated with increased 3-year disease-free survival compared with 5-FU/LV (66.5% vs. 70.9%).

It is not clear whether patients with stage II node-negative colon cancer should receive adjuvant chemotherapy, because the risk-to-benefit ratio in this case has not been established. The Quasar study suggested that adjuvant chemotherapy with 5-FU and leucovorin could improve survival in patients with stage II colon cancer, but the benefit was small.[178] Most analyses suggest that the majority of benefit from adjuvant therapy is seen in patients with stage III disease. Currently, the standard of care is to treat all patients with stage III disease and high-risk patients with stage II disease (poorly differentiated histology, lymphatic or lymphovascular invasion, perineural invasion, bowel obstruction, localized perforation, positive margins, few lymph nodes analyzed after surgery) with adjuvant therapy, although such treatment of the latter group is controversial.

Other anatomic or biological features could, in the future, define subsets of patients with stage II colon cancer who will benefit from adjuvant therapy. Such features might include colloid, signet ring, or poorly differentiated cancers; high preoperative CEA cell levels; aneuploid DNA content or high S phase; alterations in molecular markers; and the expression of certain tumor-associated antigens (e.g., sialyl-Tn, sialyl Lewis^x) or other genetic determinants. One analysis[63] indicated that retention of 18q alleles in microsatellite-stable cancers and mutation of the gene for TGF-β1 in cancers with high levels of MSI indicate a favorable outcome after adjuvant therapy with 5-FU–based regimens in patients with stage III colon cancer (Fig. 127-28). Tumor MSI status also has been shown to predict benefit from 5-FU–based adjuvant therapy for colon cancer.[65] Stage II MSI-H patients may have a good prognosis and do not appear to benefit from 5-FU adjuvant therapy. Patients with poorly differentiated tumors that are also MSI-H may not be considered high risk.

Patients who undergo resection of isolated liver or lung metastases also should be offered neoadjuvant or adjuvant

chemotherapy.[171] It is now recommended that these individuals receive approximately 6 months of perioperative treatment. A recent meta-analysis suggested a survival advantage for surgery plus systemic therapy over surgery alone. Portal infusion of chemotherapeutic agents as adjuvant therapy reduces liver metastasis, but this approach has been limited to investigational use.

Rectal cancer is defined as cancer that is located within 12 cm of the anal verge (originally defined by rigid proctoscopy). Adjuvant therapy for individuals with stage II (T3-4 node-negative disease with tumor penetration through the muscle wall) or stage III (node-positive disease without distant metastases) rectal cancer should be considered separate from that for colon cancer, because patterns of failure are different, with a high risk of locoregional recurrence.[179,180] Local recurrence for stage II rectal cancer after primary resection approaches 25% to 30%, with a 50% or greater local recurrence rate in those with stage III tumors. Local recurrence is associated with significant morbidity, and patients with locally invasive rectal cancer are at high risk for systemic relapse. Surgery for rectal cancers usually includes complete pelvic extirpation with total mesenteric excision (TME). Studies since the 1980s have shown a significant decrease in local recurrence of rectal cancer in patients who receive moderate to high doses of preoperative and/or postoperative radiation (40 to 50 Gy in 25 to 28 fractions to the pelvis) but little impact on systemic recurrence and survival.

Combined adjuvant radiation and chemotherapy has been used to address this potential for local and systemic recurrence, and a number of RCTs have demonstrated that overall survival and disease-free survival are improved with the addition of postoperative 5-FU–based therapy. This was recently echoed in a recent meta-analysis of almost 10,000 patients with rectal cancer from 21 randomized trials conducted from 1975 to 2011.[181] Combined-modality therapy consisting of surgery, radiation therapy (preoperative preferred), and chemotherapy is therefore currently recommended for the majority of individuals with stage II or stage III rectal cancer. Current guidelines recommend concurrent fluoropyrimidine-based chemotherapy with ionizing radiation to the pelvis preoperatively (infusional 5-FU/RT or capecitabine/RT are preferred) and chemotherapy postoperatively.[180] A total of 6 months of perioperative (total pre- and postoperative) chemotherapy is preferred. Oral capecitabine appears equivalent to infusional 5-FU in the perioperative chemotherapy of individuals with rectal cancer. Current guidelines recommend the use of FOLFOX or capecitabine as postoperative adjuvant chemotherapy in rectal cancer, and, for the most part, are based on data available for colon cancer. The addition of oxaliplatin to preoperative neoadjuvant chemoradiation, however, is not recommended at this time. Accurate endorectal US and MRI staging has allowed the appropriate use of preoperative therapy, enabling the exclusion of patients with early-stage disease. Neoadjuvant therapy allows radiation to be delivered in a nonoperated abdomen, thereby reducing the chance of postoperative complications (e.g., adhesions, bowel damage), and higher doses of preoperative (vs. postoperative) radiation can be delivered. Approximately 50% to 60% of patients are downstaged following neoadjuvant therapy, with 20% showing a complete pathologic response. The most recent College of American Pathologists guidelines and the seventh edition of the *AJCC Cancer Staging Manual* require comments on treatment effect after neoadjuvant therapy.[90,171] Studies from Europe and the USA have suggested less toxicity from preoperative radiation therapy compared to postoperative radiation. A prospective randomized European trial[178] that compared preoperative and postoperative combined-modality therapy demonstrated a significant reduction in local tumor

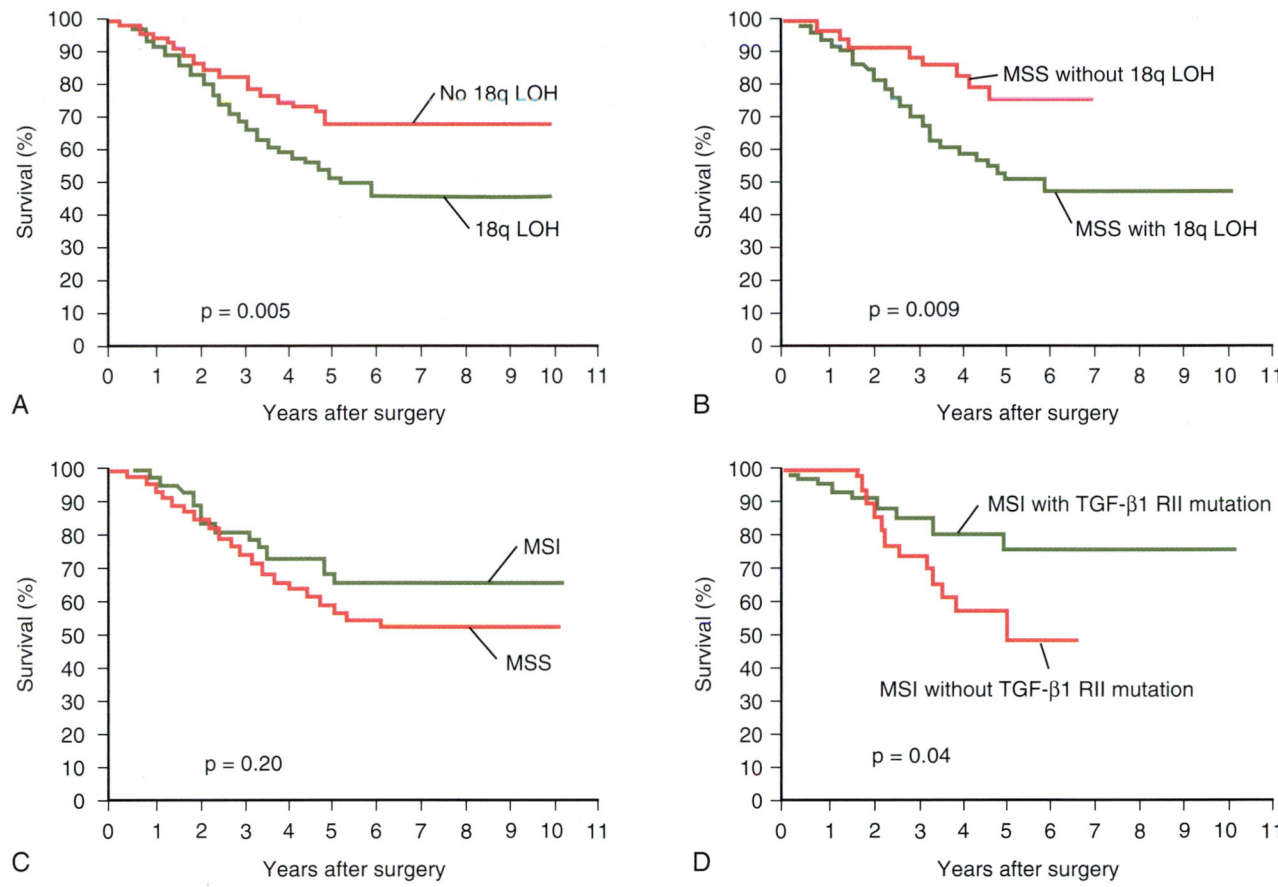

FIGURE 127-28. Molecular markers that influence survival of patients with colorectal cancer after adjuvant chemotherapy with 5-FU-based regimens. LOH, loss of heterozygosity; MSI, microsatellite instability; MSS, microsatellite stability; TGF-β1 RII, transforming growth factor-β1 receptor II. *(From Watanabe T, Wu T-T, Catalano PJ, et al. Molecular predictors of survival after adjuvant chemotherapy for colon cancer. N Engl J Med 2001; 344:1196-206.)*

relapse and less toxicity from preoperative combined-modality therapy compared with similar treatment given postoperatively. Preoperative combined chemoradiation was compared with radiation alone in a prospective randomized trial from the European Organization for Research and Treatment of Cancer (EORTC). Combined preoperative therapy was associated with a better pathologic response and a higher rate of conservative surgery compared with radiation alone, but there was no difference in disease-free or overall survival.

Patients with T4 and/or locally resectable disease are treated with preoperative infusional 5-FU/RT or bolus 5-FU with leucovorin/RT or capecitabine RT in an attempt to convert to a resectable tumor. Intraoperative radiotherapy (IORT) should be considered in patients with T4 tumors or if margins are very close or positive.

Chemotherapy for Advanced Disease

Patients who present with operable CRCs have benefited from improvements in surgical techniques and advances in adjuvant chemotherapy. Approximately 30% to 40% of patients with CRC, however, have locoregionally advanced or metastatic disease on presentation (20% to 34% present with synchronous liver metastases). Overall, about 50% to 60% of individuals diagnosed with CRC will eventually develop metastases, and 80% to 90% of these individuals have unresectable liver metastases. Furthermore, the 5-year survival rates for patients with stages II and III CRC (82% and 57%,

respectively) indicate that a significant portion of these patients will have postsurgical recurrences and related mortality. Systemic chemotherapy therefore is required for a large number of patients with advanced CRC.

5-FU is a fluoropyrimidine that, since the 1970s, has remained the mainstay of systemic chemotherapy for advanced CRC. 5-FU interacts with thymidylate synthetase to inhibit the methylation of deoxyuridylic to thymidylic acid, thereby inhibiting DNA synthesis. It has been administered orally, IV in bolus doses or by continuous infusion, and, when used as a single agent, is associated with response rates of 15% to 20% in most studies. Responses, however, are often short-lived (4 to 5 months) and have not been associated with long-term survival. Toxicity of 5-FU includes myelosuppression, vomiting, diarrhea, and stomatitis, and varies according to dose and mode of administration.

Despite the approval of a number of new drugs for treatment of metastatic CRC, 5-FU remains a component of most regimens. Various regimens combine 5-FU with high-dose leucovorin (tetrahydrofolate) because leucovorin potentiates the binding of 5-FU to thymidylate synthetase, and the combination is more effective than 5-FU alone. Combined data from numerous trials indicate a 2-fold increase in tumor response rates with 5-FU plus leucovorin compared with 5-FU alone (23% vs. 12%), and a small increase in survival. The optimal doses of 5-FU and leucovorin and the optimal mode of administration (bolus vs. infusion) are unclear, but continuous-infusion 5-FU appears to be superior to bolus

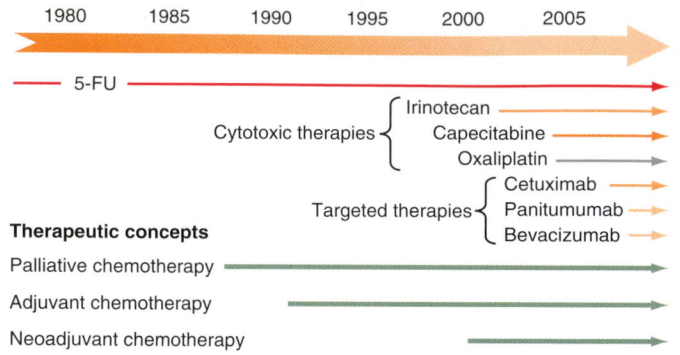

FIGURE 127-29. Historical timeline for advances in chemotherapy for colorectal cancer. 5-FU, 5-fluorouracil.

regimens in terms of response rates, toxicity, and survival.[182] There currently is a shortage of leucovorin in the USA, which may lead temporarily to adjustments in dosing or use of levoleucovorin, a compound commonly used in Europe. Capecitabine is an oral fluoropyrimidine that is converted to 5-FU in tumor tissues. Two large phase III trials that compared capecitabine with bolus 5-FU suggest similar efficacy but fewer side effects with the oral agent.[183,183a] UFT, an oral 5-FU prodrug composed of a 1:4 fixed molar ratio of tegafur and uracil, currently is not approved for use in the USA.

The advent of a variety of agents such as irinotecan (Camptosar), oxaliplatin (Eloxatin), and capecitabine, and molecular-targeted agents/small molecule inhibitors, such as cetuximab (Erbitux), panitumumab, bevacizumab, ziv-afliberecpt, and most recently regorafenib, has led to a rapid evolution in the systemic treatment of CRC (Figs. 127-29 and 127-30). Second-line and even third-line chemotherapy also has become standard for appropriate patients in whom first-line therapies have failed. The choice of therapy is individualized based on performance status, the type and timing of prior therapy, the differing toxicity profiles of the drugs to be used in various regimens, and in some cases the molecular characteristics of the tumor. For example, cetuximab or panitumumab should be used only in patients whose tumors are wild-type for K-ras.

Oxaliplatin is a diaminocyclohexane platinum that, unlike other platinum compounds, does not cause nephrotoxicity and has activity against CRC. Several different combinations of biweekly bolus and infusional 5-FU, leucovorin, and oxaliplatin, collectively called FOLFOX, have been shown to be effective for treatment of advanced CRC. Various FOLFOX regimens have evolved, the most recent being modified (m) FOLFOX 6. Infusional 5-FU regimens appear to be less toxic than bolus regimens, and bolus 5-FU should not be used with oxaliplatin or irinotecan (see later). A recent European phase III trial demonstrated that perioperative FOLFOX improves progression-free survival when chemotherapy in conjunction with surgery was compared with surgery alone.[184] Use of oxaliplatin is associated with an increased incidence of peripheral sensory neuropathy, which may require adjustments in dosing.

Irinotecan (CPT-11) is a potent inhibitor of topoisomerase 1, a nuclear enzyme involved in the unwinding of DNA during replication. Weekly treatment with irinotecan and 5-FU plus leucovorin was shown to be superior to the widely used regimen of 5-FU plus leucovorin for stage IV metastatic colon cancer in terms of response rate (39% vs. 21%), progression-free survival (7 vs. 4.3 months), and overall survival (14.4 vs. 12 months).[185] A second phase III trial confirmed these results,[186] and the combination of irinotecan, 5-FU, and leucovorin (IFL) was approved as first-line treatment for

advanced CRC. This regimen is associated with significant side effects because those of irinotecan (diarrhea, dehydration, neutropenia) and 5-FU (nausea, diarrhea, hematologic toxicity) overlap and may be especially severe with bolus 5-FU. The bimonthly regimen that combines leucovorin, 5-FU, and high-dose infusional irinotecan (FOLFIRI) has replaced IFL (no longer recommended) as a first-line therapy option for advanced or metastatic disease. FOLFOX and FOLFIRI appear to be equally efficacious as first-line treatment of metastatic CRC. A randomized study designed to determine the effect of using alternate regimens following first progression of disease showed that results with respect to progression-free and overall survival were similar with FOLFIRI and FOLFOX6.[187]

Bevacizumab is a recombinant humanized monoclonal immunoglobulin (Ig)G1 antibody that acts by binding all isoforms of circulating vascular endothelial growth factor-A (VEGF-A), thus decreasing VEGF-A–mediated angiogenesis and vascular permeability. A phase III trial compared IFL with IFL plus bevacizumab and showed that the regimen containing bevacizumab increased overall response rate from 35% to 45% and extended median survival from 15.6 to 20.3 months. Bevacizumab currently is approved for use in combination with IV 5-FU–based chemotherapy as first-line treatment of patients with metastatic CRC. Use of bevacizumab is associated with an increased risk of stroke, GI perforation, and decreased wound healing. An interval of at least 6 weeks between the last dose of bevacizumab and elective surgery is recommended. Ziv-aflibercept is a recombinant protein that has part of the human VEGF receptors 1 and 2 fused to the Fc portion of human IgG1. Ziv-aflibercept has been shown to be associated with a clinically modest but significant improvement in overall survival when given in conjunction with FOLFIRI in FOLFIRI-naïve patients, and has been approved by the FDA for this purpose.[188] Adverse events associated with ziv-aflibercept treatment include asthenia/fatigue, infections, diarrhea, hypertension, and venous thromboembolic events.

Cetuximab is a chimeric antibody directed against EGFR, an important molecule involved with cell cycling, survival, invasion, and metastasis. It has been used primarily in combination with irinotecan in irinotecan-refractory patients. In an analysis of tumor samples from patients with advanced CRC who were randomized to receive cetuximab plus best supportive care or best supportive care alone, cetuximab was found to be of benefit in patients whose tumors expressed wild-type K-ras but not in those whose tumors expressed mutated K-ras[189] (Fig. 127-31). Results suggesting that EGFR inhibition is only effective in treating CRCs containing wild-type K-ras also have been reported in studies using panitumumab, a humanized monoclonal antibody directed against EGFR. Genotyping of tumor tissue with respect to K-ras is recommended in all patients with metastatic CRC.

The National Comprehensive Cancer Network (NCCN) Colon cancer panel currently suggest a choice of 5 chemotherapy regimens for those who can tolerate intensive treatment: FOLFOX (mFOLFOX6), FOLFIRI, CapeOx, infusional 5FU/LV or capecitabine, or FOLFOXIRI (infusional 5FU/LV, oxaloplatin, and irinotecan). Biological agents used as part of initial combination therapy include bevacizumab, cetuximab, or panitumumab.[171,180]

Regorafenib is a small molecule inhibitor of multiple kinases (including VEGF receptors, fibroblast growth factor receptors, platelet-derived growth factor [PDGF] receptors, BRAF, KIT, and RET) that are involved with various processes, including tumor growth and angiogenesis. In the CORRECT trial, 760 patients who progressed on standard therapy were randomized to best supportive care with placebo or regorafenib.[190] The trial met its primary end point of overall survival (6.4 months for regorafenib vs. 5.0 months for

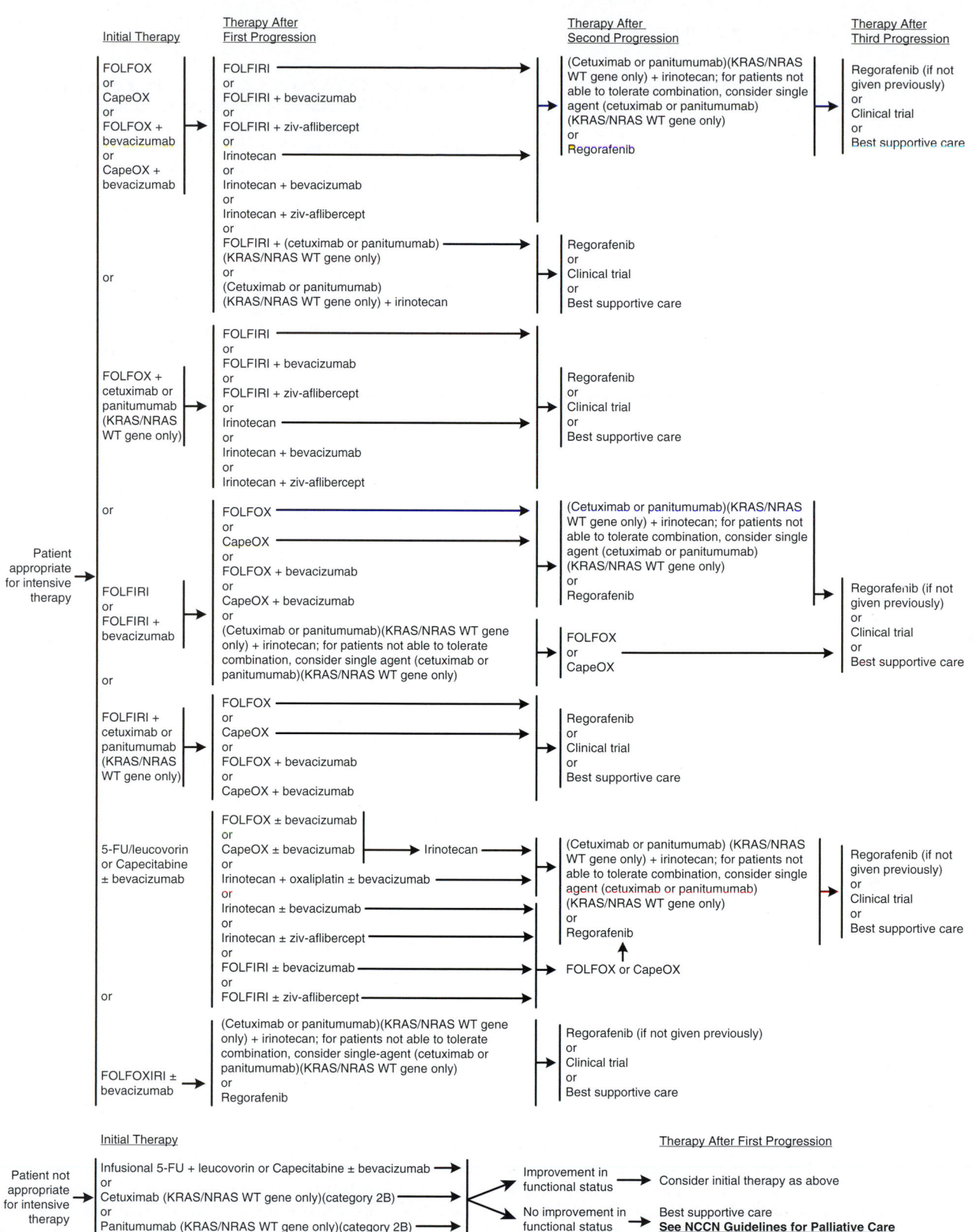

FIGURE 127-30. Options for chemotherapy for advanced or metastatic colon cancer. NOTE: Regimens containing cetuximab or panitumumab should be used *only* in individuals whose tumors express wild-type *K-ras*. Top, Therapeutic options in patients appropriate for intensive therapy. Bottom, Options in patients not appropriate for intensive therapy. CapeOX, capecitabine, oxaliplatin; FOLFOX, folinic acid (leukovorin), fluorouracil, (5-FU), oxaliplatin; FOLFIRI, folinic acid (leukovorin), fluorouracil, (5-FU), irinotecan, FOLFOXIRI, folinic acid (leukovorin), fluorouracil, (5-FU), oxaliplatin, irinotecan. *(Adapted with permission from the NCCN Clinical Practice Guidelines in Oncology (NCCN Guidelines®) for Colon Cancer V.1.2015. © 2014 National Comprehensive Cancer Network, Inc. All rights reserved. The NCCN Guidelines® and illustrations herein may not be reproduced in any form for any purpose without the express written permission of the NCCN. To view the most recent and complete version of the NCCN Guidelines, go online to NCCN.org. NATIONAL COMPREHENSIVE CANCER NETWORK®, NCCN®, NCCN GUIDELINES®, and all other NCCN Content are trademarks owned by the National Comprehensive Cancer Network, Inc.)*
NOTE: *For associated footnotes, regimens and references, please see the complete version of the NCCN Clinical Practice Guidelines In Oncology (NCCN Guidelines®) for Colon Cancer.*

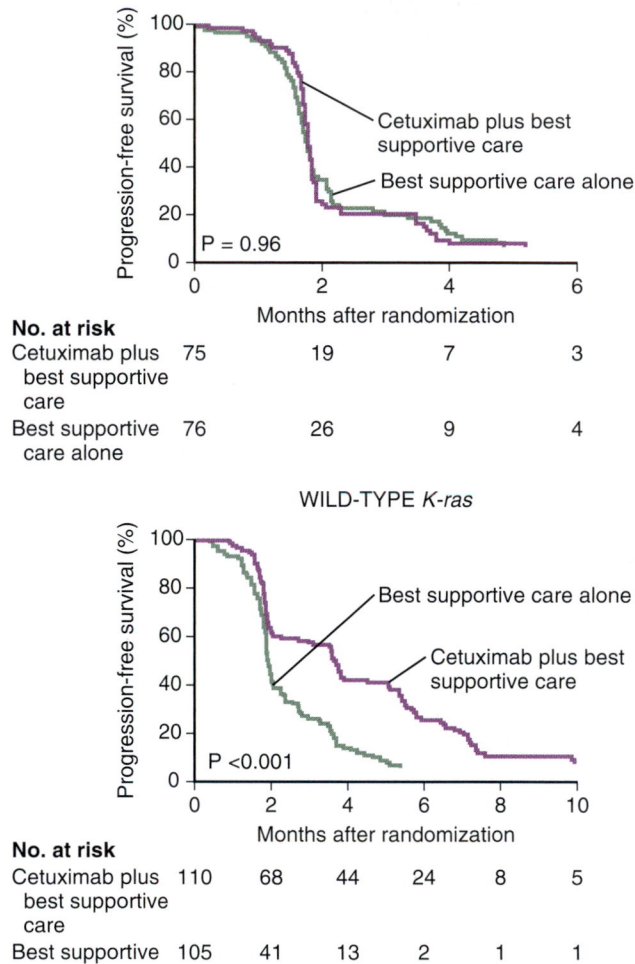

FIGURE 127-31. Kaplan-Meier curves of progression-free survival in patients with metastatic colon cancer treated with cetuximab plus best supportive care or best supportive care alone, stratified according to mutation status of the *K-ras* gene. *(From Karpetis CS, Khambata-Ford S, Jonker DJ, et al. K-ras mutations and benefit of cetuximab in advanced colorectal cancer. N Engl J Med 2008; 359:1757-65.)*

placebo). Progression-free survival was also significantly but modestly improved (1.9 vs. 1.7 months). Regorafenib has shown activity only in patients who have experienced progression on all standard therapies, and it has been recently approved by the FDA for this purpose. Adverse events associated with regorafenib include hand-foot skin reactions, fatigue, hypertension, diarrhea, and rash/desquamation. Severe and fatal liver toxicity occurred in 0.3% of 1100 patients treated with regorafenib across all trials.

Selective infusion of chemotherapeutic agents into the hepatic arterial system may be used to treat hepatic metastases. This method delivers more concentrated drug into the tumor capillary bed than do conventional means of delivery. The infusion catheter usually is implanted in the common hepatic artery (via the gastroduodenal artery) at the time of laparotomy. The development of implantable infusion pumps has led to increasing use of such therapy in major centers. Fluorinated pyrimidines, such as 5-FU and floxuridine (FUDR), have high hepatic extraction (80% to 95%), and it is

thought that high concentrations of these drugs can be delivered with low systemic toxicity by direct hepatic arterial infusion. FUDR has received the most attention, and its continuous hepatic arterial infusion to treat hepatic metastases from CRC in patients not previously treated can achieve response rates of 54% to 83%. Criteria for response vary, however, and it is still unclear if survival will be increased.

RCTs of systemic versus intrahepatic infusion of FUDR in patients with liver metastasis have shown significantly higher response rates for intrahepatic therapy but, again, the impact on survival remains unclear. Complications of the procedure, including arterial occlusion, local infection, and catheter leak, occur in a small number of patients. Morbidity of treatment consists of GI tract inflammation and ulceration, hepatic injury with elevation in serum bilirubin and aminotransferases, and biliary ductal sclerosis, all of which may be substantial. It has been suggested that alternating hepatic intra-arterial FUDR and 5-FU may produce less toxicity than FUDR alone. Some investigators have combined hepatic artery occlusion or embolization with chemotherapeutic agents (chemoembolization) in an attempt to achieve better response rates in patients with extensive hepatic tumor.

Immunotargeted Therapy and Immunotherapy

Use of monoclonal antibodies designed to modulate biological processes key to tumor growth and behavior, such as bevacizumab (directed against circulating VEGF) and cetuximab (directed against EGFR), already have been discussed. Both agents have been approved for treatment of advanced CRC.

Advances in immunology, molecular biology, and imaging have led to the development of radiolabeled monoclonal antibodies that can be used to detect CRC metastases (radioimmunodetection). These same antibodies can be linked to cytotoxic agents such as the A subunit of the plant toxin ricin, the toxin A chain of diphtheria, lymphokine-activated killer cells, and chemotherapeutic agents for immune-targeted therapy. Liposomes that contain chemotherapeutic agents can be linked to monoclonal antibodies and delivered in a similar fashion. Most patients treated thus far with such therapy have had advanced disease, and further studies using these agents in adjuvant therapy are needed.

Attempts to modulate the immune system of patients with metastatic disease also have been reported. A large body of preclinical and clinical evidence has suggested that the immune system can be stimulated against malignant cells by means of active specific immunotherapy strategies. These approaches, including experimental cancer vaccine strategies, currently are limited to clinical trials but might hold promise for the future.

Radiotherapy

Patients with rectal cancers whose tumors have penetrated the bowel wall or who have regional lymph node involvement are at 40% to 50% risk for local recurrence following resection of the primary tumor. Radiation therapy is used preoperatively or postoperatively to decrease local recurrence in those with high-risk rectal and rectosigmoid cancers (stages II and III lesions) or in a combined preoperative and postoperative "sandwich" approach. This approach also is used to convert unresectable large tumors and those fixed to pelvic organs to resectable lesions. Radiation therapy also is occasionally useful for palliation of bleeding and pain resulting from advanced rectal disease. The possible advantages of radiation therapy must be balanced against its potential complications of radiation proctitis and small bowel damage (see Chapter 40).

Preoperative radiation alone reduces local recurrence in patients with rectal and rectosigmoid cancers, but there is no convincing evidence that it improves survival. Postoperative radiation therapy generally is restricted to patients at high risk for local recurrence of rectal cancer. Prospective, but nonrandomized, series show a substantial reduction in local recurrence for those receiving postoperative radiation therapy (6% to 8% for those receiving radiation vs. 40% to 50% for those receiving surgery alone).[180] A randomized study also demonstrated results favoring radiation (an overall reduction in locoregional recurrence from 25% to 16%). Distant metastases remain a problem, however, and it is not clear whether survival is altered substantially. Given the demonstration of decreased recurrence and increased survival in patients with rectal cancer who received combined preoperative or postoperative radiation and combination chemotherapy, this should be considered the treatment of choice for high-risk patients with transmural tumor extension or lymph node metastases.

Endoscopic Therapy

Endoscopic therapy using the Nd:YAG laser or argon plasma coagulation (APC) has been used to recanalize the rectum as palliative therapy in patients with obstructing rectal cancers who are poor surgical risks or who have advanced stages of malignant disease; such palliation generally has been satisfactory.[191] Reported complications are bleeding and perforation, but they are fewer than would be anticipated after surgery in these high-risk patients. Electrofulguration using a heater probe device has been reported under similar circumstances. Endoscopy with the use of snare cautery also may be used to remove polypoid lesions (Fig. 127-32), often in a piecemeal fashion.

Photodynamic therapy (PDT) has been used to treat patients who are poor surgical risks. PDT involves the use of a photosensitizer that is taken up by the tumor and administered before photoradiation using a tunable dye laser delivered through a flexible optical fiber. The photosensitizer,

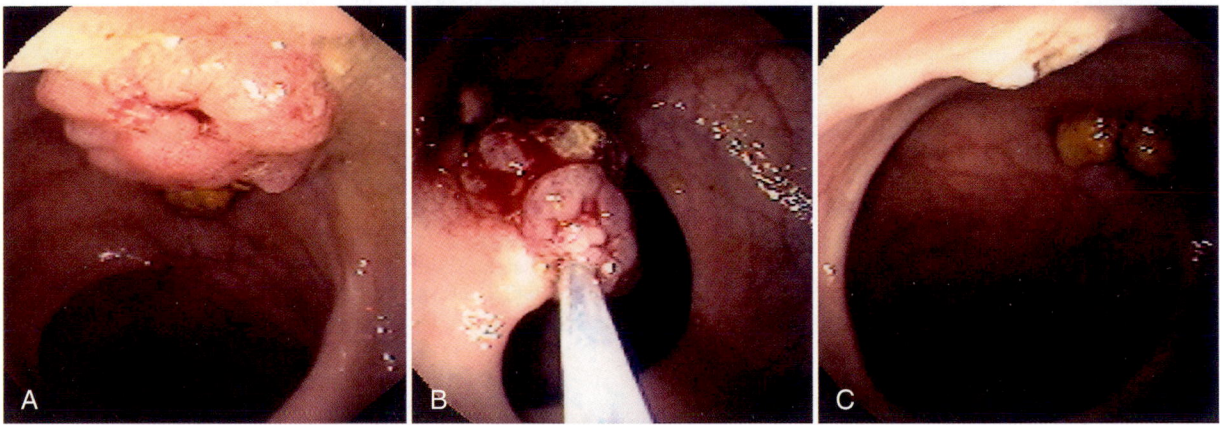

FIGURE 127-32. Colonoscopic views demonstrating removal of a polypoid carcinoma by snare cautery in a patient at high operative risk because of intercurrent illness. *A,* Polypoid carcinoma. *B,* Piecemeal removal by snare cautery. *C,* Site of lesion after removal.

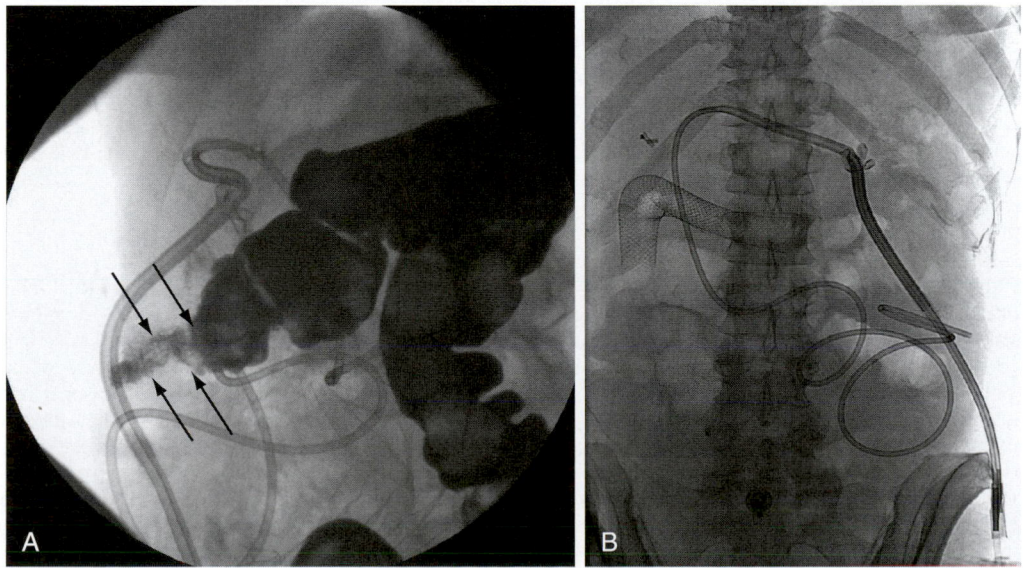

FIGURE 127-33. Expandable metal stent placed as palliative therapy in a patient with a lesion near the hepatic flexure. *A,* Obstructing lesion near the hepatic flexure seen on contrast exam *(arrows). B,* Expandable metal stent placed across the obstructing lesion. A long decompression tube is also seen in place.

porfimer sodium (Photofrin), has been approved by the FDA for palliation of esophageal cancers, but its use for rectal cancers has been more limited, given other available options. Limitations of PDT include cost and skin photosensitization; the availability of newer porphyrin derivatives associated with shorter periods of photosensitivity could lead to greater use of this modality. Although strictures occur commonly after PDT for esophageal lesions, it is unclear how common strictures are seen after treatment of rectal lesions.

Palliation of obstruction from colorectal lesions also may be accomplished by the use of expandable metal stents (Fig 127-33).[192] Intraluminal stents are being used with increasing frequency for palliation and for relieving colorectal obstruction preoperatively, because repetitive treatments as required for ablative therapies such as APC and PDT are obviated.[192]

OTHER MALIGNANT COLONIC TUMORS

Malignant tumors other than adenocarcinomas rarely originate in the large bowel but include lymphomas, carcinoids, GISTs, and leiomyosarcomas. In addition, lymphomas, leiomyosarcomas, malignant melanomas, and cancers of the breast, ovary, prostate, lung, stomach, and other organs can metastasize to the colon. Lymphomas, GISTs, and carcinoid tumors are discussed in Chapters 31, 32, and 33, respectively; carcinomas of the anal canal are discussed in Chapter 129.

KEY REFERENCES

Full references for this chapter can be found on www.expertconsult.com.

10. Norat T, Chan D, Lau R, et al. The associations between food, nutrition and physical activity and the risk of colorectal cancer. WCRF/AICR Systematic Literature Review Continuous Update Project Report. London: World Cancer Research Fund/American Institute for Cancer Research; 2010.
61. Pritchard CC, Grady WM. Colorectal cancer molecular biology moves into clinical practice. Gut 2011; 60:116-29.
80. Brenner H, Hoffmeister M, Volker A, et al. Protection from right-and left-sided colorectal neoplasms after colonoscopy: Population-based study. J Natl Cancer Inst 2010; 102:89-95.
83. Kahi CJ, Anderson JC, Rex DK. Screening for colorectal cancer: State of the art. Gastrointest Endosc 2013; 77:335-50.
89. Segnan N, Patrick J, von Karsa L, editors. European guidelines for quality assurance in colorectal cancer screening and diagnosis. Luxembourg: International Agency for Research on Cancer; 2010. pp 1-386.
108. Schoen RE, Pinsky PF, Weissfeld JL, et al. Colorectal cancer incidence and mortality with screening flexible sigmoidoscopy. N Engl J Med 2012; 366:2345-57.
110. Zauber AG, Winawer SJ, O'Brien MJ, et al. Colonoscopic polypectomy and long-term prevention of colorectal cancer deaths. N Engl J Med 2012; 366:687-96.
137. Brenner H, Haug U, Arrndt V, et al. Low risk of colorectal cancer and advanced adenomas more than 10 years after negative colonoscopy. Gastroenterology 2010; 138:870-6.
139. Ahlquist DA, Zou H, Domanico M, et al. Next-generation stool DNA test accurately detects colorectal cancer and large adenomas. Gastroenterology 2012; 142:248-56.
144. Lieberman DA, Rex DK, Winawer SJ, et al. Guidelines for colonoscopy surveillance after screening and polypectomy: A consensus update by the US Multi-Society Task Force on Colorectal Cancer. Gastroenterology 2012; 143:844-57.
148. Martinez ME, Thompson P, Messe K, et al. One-year risk for advanced colorectal neoplasia: U.S. versus U.K. risk-stratification guidelines. Ann Intern Med 2012; 157:856-64.
169. Pohl H, Srivastava A, Nensen SP, et al. Incomplete polyp resection during colonoscopy—Results of the Complete Adenoma Resection (CARE) Study. Gastroenterology 2013; 144:74-80.
171. National Comprehensive Cancer Network. Clinical practice guidelines in oncology. Colon Cancer, V.3.2013. Available from: www.NCCN.ORG.
188. Benson AB 3rd, Bekaii-Saab T, Chan E, et al. Metastatic colon cancer, Version 3.2013: Featured updates to the NCCN guidelines. J Natl Compr Canc Netw 2013; 11:141-52.
190. Grothey A, van Cutsem E, Sobrero A, et al. Regorafenib monotherapy for previously treated metastatic colorectal cancer (CORRECT): An international, multicentre, randomised, placebo-controlled, phase 3 trial. Lancet 2013; 381:303-12.

CHAPTER OUTLINE

LYMPHOCYTIC AND COLLAGENOUS COLITIS

Lymphocytic colitis (LC) and collagenous colitis (CC) are uncommon disorders characterized by chronic watery diarrhea and histologic evidence of chronic mucosal inflammation in the absence of endoscopic or radiologic abnormalities of the colon. The 2 disorders are distinct histologically but have been grouped under the term *microscopic colitis*. They differ principally by the presence or absence of a thickened collagenous band, which is located in the colonic subepithelium in collagenous colitis.

The term *collagenous colitis* was used first in 1976 by Lindstrom to describe a middle-aged woman in whom evaluation for chronic diarrhea was normal except for colonic biopsies that showed a thickened band of subepithelial collagen and increased lymphocytes in the lamina propria.[1] Histologically, the subepithelial collagen deposits resembled those in the small intestinal mucosa of patients with collagenous sprue. The term *microscopic colitis* was first used in 1980 by Read and associates, who described a group of patients with chronic diarrhea of unknown origin, a subset of whom had a normal colonoscopy but abnormal histopathology on biopsy specimens of the colon.[2] Subsequent review showed that most of these patients had CC, but that some had increased lymphocytes in the lamina propria in the absence of a thickened collagen band. The term *lymphocytic colitis* was proposed in 1989 by Lazenby and associates[3] as a more specific histopathologic diagnosis to distinguish this entity from patterns of microscopic colitis in which other cellular elements such as eosinophils, mast cells, or neutrophils predominate. The present consensus is that LC and CC represent 2 ends of the spectrum of a single disorder, and that their clinical presentations, evaluations, and treatments are similar.

Epidemiology

Both LC and CC occur most commonly between ages 50 and 70 years, with a strong female predominance and frequent association with arthritis, celiac disease, and autoimmune disorders. In a large population-based study in Spain, the demographic features of both LC and CC were similar: microscopic colitis was found in 9.5 of every 100 patients with chronic watery diarrhea and normal-appearing mucosa on colonoscopy; the incidence rate of LC was 3 times higher than that of CC.[4] This last observation contrasts strikingly with published reports that comprise more than 400 cases of CC compared with more than 60 cases of LC, a finding that suggests that there may be a publication bias. The overall mean annual incidence of both colitides was 4.2 per 100,000 inhabitants in Spain,[4] similar to the rates from an epidemiologic study conducted in Sweden.[5] More recent studies, however, indicate that the incidence of microscopic colitis has risen to 12 to 19/100,000 per year, comparable to that of macroscopic IBD.[6] Although incidence is clearly higher in older age groups, both LC and CC have been reported in children and teenagers, in whom the clinical presentation is similar to that of adults.

Pathology

In both LC and CC, there is a modest increase of mononuclear cells within the lamina propria and between crypt epithelial cells that consists mainly of CD8+ T lymphocytes, plasma cells, and macrophages.[3] There may be flattening of the surface epithelial cells, a mild decrease in the number of goblet cells, Paneth cell hyperplasia, and an increased number of intraepithelial lymphocytes (Fig. 128-1). Neutrophils are not prominent, and cryptitis and crypt distortion are unusual.

In CC, there is a thickened subepithelial collagen layer that may be continuous or patchy (Fig. 128-2). In normal colon, the width of this collagen band is less than 4 to 5 mm, whereas in CC, it is greater than 10 mm and usually ranges from 20 to 60 mm.[7] In normal colon, the subepithelial collagen band consists predominantly of type IV collagen, whereas in CC, the band is composed of type VI collagen, tenascin, and lesser amounts of types I and III collagen. Tenascin is a glycoprotein that is a marker of matrix remodeling and a product of intestinal subepithelial myofibroblasts.[8] These changes are absent in LC and suggest that the 2 main forms of microscopic colitis should be considered as different representations of the same disease. Although inflammatory changes occur diffusely throughout the colon, the characteristic collagen band thickening is highly variable; it occurs in the cecum and transverse colon in over 80% of cases and in the rectum in less than 30% of cases. Involvement of the left colon appears to be less intense than involvement of the right colon; nevertheless, multiple biopsies of the left colon above the rectosigmoid during flexible sigmoidoscopy are sufficient to make the diagnosis in approximately 90% of cases.[7] It is essential to emphasize that

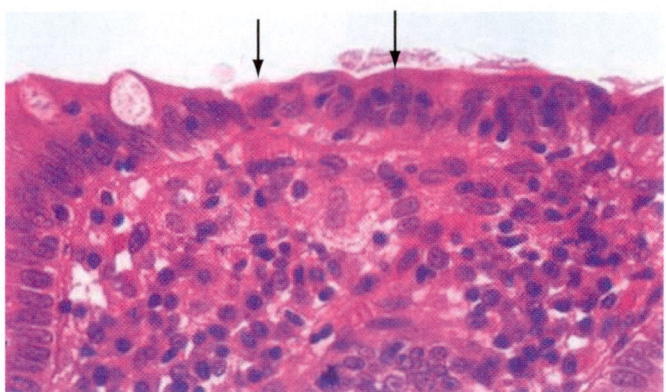

FIGURE 128-1. Histopathology of lymphocytic colitis. The *arrows* point to surface epithelial damage with increased numbers of intraepithelial lymphocytes. In addition, there is a superficial plasmacytosis without crypt distortion. Although a few intraepithelial neutrophils may be seen, widespread cryptitis is not a feature of lymphocytic colitis. (H&E). *(From Feldman M, Boland CR, editors. Slide atlas of gastroenterology and hepatology. Philadelphia: Current Medicine; 1996.)*

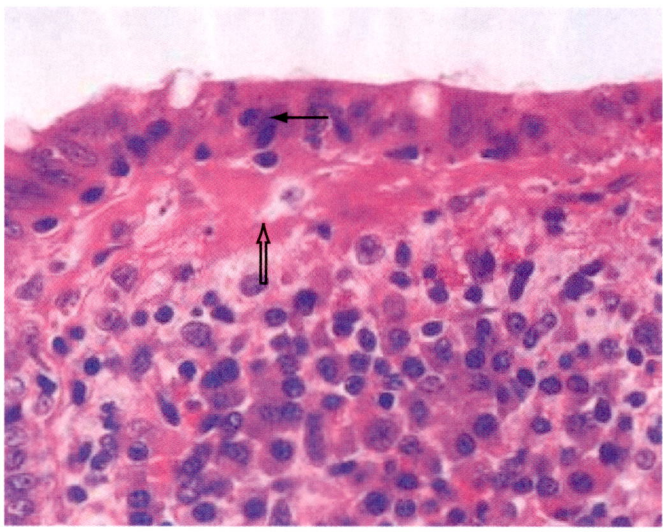

FIGURE 128-2. Histopathology of collagenous colitis. A thickened irregular subepithelial collagen table *(open arrow)* with patchy surface epithelial damage is shown. The surface epithelium also contains increased numbers of intraepithelial lymphocytes *(closed arrow)*. In addition, there is a superficial plasmacytosis with prominent numbers of eosinophils. Crypt distortion and crypt abscesses are not usually seen in collagenous colitis. (H&E). *(From Feldman M, Boland CR, editors. Slide atlas of gastroenterology and hepatology. Philadelphia: Current Medicine; 1996.)*

the diagnosis of CC requires both mucosal inflammation and a thickened collagen band, and that artifact resulting from poor orientation may give the mistaken appearance of a thickened basement membrane. It has been suggested that tenascin immunohistochemistry be used as a routine test in the diagnosis of microscopic colitis.[8]

Etiology and Pathogenesis

The cause of LC and CC is unknown. The most widely held hypothesis is that they are inflammatory disorders arising from epithelial immune responses to intraluminal dietary or nonbacterial contents. This hypothesis is supported by the regression of inflammation following diversion of the fecal stream and recurrence of inflammation following restoration of intestinal continuity in 3 patients.[9] The identity of the inciting antigenic factors is uncertain, although medications, bile salts, toxins, and infectious agents[10] have been postulated.

The strong association of rheumatologic diseases with microscopic colitis has raised the possibility that NSAIDs may play an etiologic role. One postulated mechanism by which NSAIDs may damage the colon is by increasing colonic permeability, thereby allowing luminal antigens to enter the lamina propria and promote inflammation. Because many patients with LC or CC have not used NSAIDs and because NSAID use in older adults is common but these disorders are uncommon, other causes have been invoked, including genetic susceptibility; genetic susceptibility is supported by the finding that 12% of patients with microscopic colitis had a family history of IBD. Studies now have observed independent associations with current smoking, lansoprazole, omeprazole, angiotensin 2 receptor antagonists, beta blockers, and sertraline.[11] Approximately 20% to 30% of patients with celiac disease have been reported to have LC, raising the possibility of similar pathogenetic mechanisms for these disorders.[12] In 40% of patients with CC in 1 study, small intestinal biopsies were compatible with celiac disease,[13] although in another study the frequency of celiac disease was only 2% of 45 patients with CC and 9% of 199 patients with LC.[10] Furthermore, patients with microscopic colitis do not respond to a gluten-free diet, and neither LC not CC is associated with HLAs B8 or DR3, as is celiac disease. Finally, CD8+ T intraepithelial cells are predominant in microscopic colitis, in contrast to celiac disease, in which CD3 and CD8 predominate.

Because autoimmune disorders such as arthritis and thyroid abnormalities[10] have been described in patients with LC and CC, there have been continued efforts to associate microscopic colitis with various autoimmune HLA haplotypes and serum markers. One small study showed that HLA-A1 antigens were expressed with increased frequency in LC but not CC,[14] whereas another study showed similar abnormal expressions of HLA-DR antigens by mucosal epithelial cells in both conditions. Whether such abnormalities are the cause or the result of these disorders is unknown. Another study found similarities in HLA-DQ loci between patients with celiac disease and patients with either LC or CC.[15] Although gluten is not the inciting antigen in microscopic colitis, similar, but as of yet unidentified, immune mechanisms may be involved in celiac disease and microscopic colitis.

The pathogenesis of the increased collagen band in CC is also unclear. It initially had been assumed that collagen synthesis is increased,[1] but colonic biopsies from patients with the disease showed decreased levels of interstitial collagenase, which suggests that reduced matrix degradation may contribute to the accumulation of matrix proteins.[16]

The mechanism of diarrhea in microscopic colitis is related to the severity of inflammation and not the extent or thickness of the collagen band. Perfusion studies have demonstrated defective active and passive absorption of sodium and chloride and reduced chloride-bicarbonate exchange in the colon[17]; 2 of 6 subjects had coexisting abnormalities of small intestinal fluid and electrolyte absorption. Other investigators have correlated colonic fluid absorption with the severity of inflammation.[18,19] A potential role for soluble mediators is suggested by a report that diarrhea was resolved by a histamine H_1 antagonist in a patient with microscopic colitis characterized by increased numbers of mast cells.[20] It has been

suggested that bile acid malabsorption may contribute to diarrhea in patients with CC, and that treatment with a bile acid-binding resin such as cholestyramine may lead to a reduction in diarrhea. Bile acids are unlikely to cause the histologic changes observed in CC, however, and reduction in diarrhea was not associated with a decrease in colitis. Hormonal studies, including serum gastrin, vasoactive intestinal polypeptide, and urine 5-hydroxyindoleacetic acid levels, have been normal in microscopic colitis.

Clinical and Laboratory Features

Patients with LC and CC usually complain of chronic watery diarrhea, with an average of 8 stools each day that range in volume from 300 to 1700 g/24 hours, and are associated with occasional fecal incontinence and abdominal cramps. Symptoms decrease with fasting.[5] Nausea, weight loss, and fecal urgency are variably present. Diarrhea generally is longstanding, lasting from months to years, with a fluctuating course of remissions and exacerbations. In 1 series of 172 patients, the median time from the onset of symptoms to diagnosis was 11 months, whereas in another smaller series, the median time to diagnosis was 5.4 years. Physical examination is usually unremarkable, and blood is not detected in the stool. Routine laboratory studies also are normal.

Examination of fresh stools showed fecal leukocytes in 55% of 116 patients with CC. In 2 smaller studies, fecal calprotectin was detected in 62% to 75% of patients with active microscopic colitis and, in the latter study, was diagnostically superior to fecal lactoferrin.[21,22] Mild steatorrhea, mild anemia, low serum vitamin B_{12} levels, and hypoalbuminemia have been reported in varying numbers of patients but are not characteristic. Autoimmune markers that have been identified in patients with CC include antinuclear antibodies (in up to 50%), perinuclear antineutrophil cytoplasmic antibodies (pANCA) (in 14%), rheumatoid factor, and increased C_3 and C_4 complement levels,[18] but none of these markers is of diagnostic value.

Colonoscopic examination is usually normal. Nonspecific abnormalities including patchy edema, erythema, friability, and an abnormal vascular pattern were reported in 1 study,[23] but the specificity or reproducibility of such findings is uncertain.

Differential Diagnosis

Infectious agents should be excluded by testing the stool for enteric pathogens, ova and parasites, and *Clostridium difficile* toxin. Many patients are incorrectly diagnosed with IBS, a disorder that can be excluded by a careful history, the finding of increased stool volume (which is atypical for IBS), and abnormal colonic biopsies.

Other diseases can produce colitis but should be distinguishable from microscopic colitis on histologic grounds. Acute infectious colitis is characterized by neutrophilic inflammation and decreased intraepithelial lymphocytes. Eosinophilic enterocolitis of the mucosal type is characterized by eosinophilic infiltration, shortened crypts, inflammation of the deeper parts of the lamina propria, and absence of increased intraepithelial lymphocytes. Amyloidosis has been mistaken for CC, but its distribution includes the basement membranes of the crypts and blood vessels as well as the epithelium; confirmation can be made by histochemical staining (see Chapter 36). Mild cases of UC and Crohn's disease should present no diagnostic confusion in view of the characteristic endoscopic and histologic findings. Hormone-producing tumors, surreptitious laxative abuse, and hyperthyroidism can be excluded on clinical and biochemical grounds.

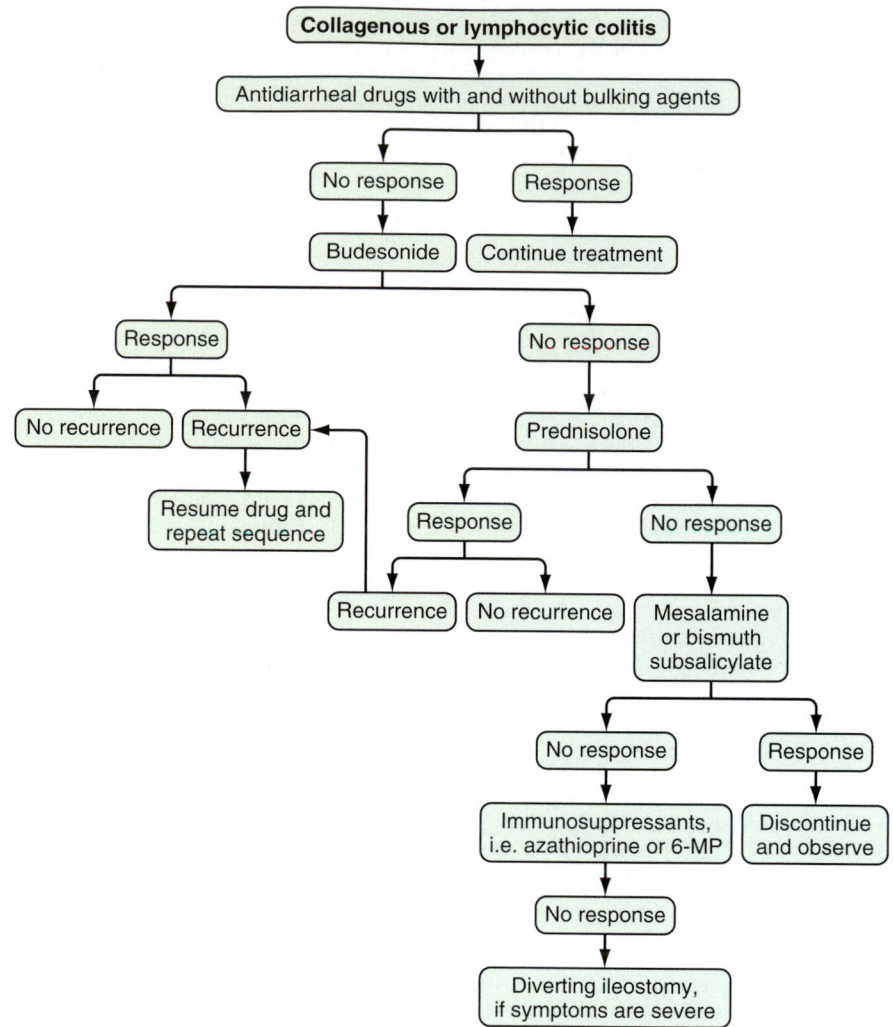

FIGURE 128-3. Algorithm for the treatment of collagenous or lymphocytic colitis.

Treatment

There have been few controlled trials for either LC or CC, and therapy is largely empirical (Fig. 128-3). Evaluation of therapy is difficult because both disorders usually exhibit a relapsing and remitting course over many years. No single agent works in all cases.[24]

About one third of patients respond to antidiarrheal agents, such as loperamide or diphenoxylate with atropine, as well as bulking agents such as psyllium or methylcellulose; clinical response is not associated with improvement of inflammation or collagen thickness.

Budesonide is a topically acting synthetic corticosteroid with both a high receptor-binding affinity in the mucosa and a high first-pass effect in the liver. Budesonide has been reported to be highly effective in 7 placebo-controlled trials in patients with microscopic colitis.[25] It was superior to placebo for both short-term and long-term clinical response and was associated with histologic improvement. In contrast, prednisolone was not superior to placebo for short-term clinical response. Symptom relapse occurred in 46% to 80% of patients within 6 months of cessation of budesonide treatment.[26]

The above findings were reinforced by a recent historical cohort study of 80 patients with microscopic colitis (40 with LC, 40 with CC) who were treated with glucocorticoids.[27]

Patients with microscopic colitis more often responded to budesonide than to prednisolone (complete response: 82.5% vs. 52.9%; odds ratio, 4.18; 95% CI, 1.3-13.5) and had lower recurrence rates (hazard ratio, 0.38; 95% CI, 0.18-0.85). Nevertheless, 64.4% required maintenance with glucocorticoids. In view of its proved efficacy, budesonide should be considered as first-line therapy in patients who do not respond to antidiarrheal agents.

In an open-label trial of bismuth subsalicylate (8 chewable tablets per day for 8 weeks) in 12 patients, diarrhea resolved and stool weight was reduced within 2 weeks; in 9 patients, colitis resolved along with disappearance of collagen band thickening.[28] Over a 7- to 28-month follow-up, 9 patients remained well, 2 were well but required retreatment, and 1 had persistent diarrhea. Both LC and CC responded similarly, and there were no side effects of treatment; a controlled trial by the same investigators published only in abstract form confirmed these findings. Although the basis for its potential efficacy is unknown, bismuth subsalicylate possesses antidiarrheal, antibacterial, and anti-inflammatory properties; bismuth enemas also have been reported effective in UC and chronic pouchitis.

Other treatment trials for LC and CC have studied 5-aminosalicylate (mesalamine) compounds, glucocorticoids, and bile acid resins, alone or in combination; these agents appear to improve diarrhea and inflammation in some, but certainly not all, patients.[25] Although glucocorticoids given by either the oral or rectal route provide symptomatic improvement and decrease inflammation in more than 80% of cases, relapse usually occurs quickly after the drug is stopped.[5,24] Moreover, long-term use of glucocorticoids has undesirable effects, especially in older patients. The effectiveness of other immunosuppressants, such as azathioprine and 6-mercaptopurine, has been reported, but there are no sizable studies using these agents.[25]

The only report of surgery for CC involved 9 patients who underwent ileostomy for disabling refractory disease, after which all had symptomatic and histologic remission.[29] In patients in whom intestinal continuity was restored, the disease recurred, and of 3 patients who underwent procto-colectomy with ileal pouch-anal anastomosis, problematic diarrhea occurred. Ileostomy should be considered only as a last resort but appears to be effective in patients with disabling and refractory symptoms.

DIVERSION COLITIS

Epidemiology

Diversion colitis is an inflammatory process that occurs in diverted segments of the colon and rectum after surgical diversion of the fecal stream. The entity was first reported in 1981 by Glotzer and associates in 10 patients who had undergone ileostomy or colostomy for various indications other than IBD.[30] Since then, diversion colitis has been found in patients who have undergone surgical diversion for many indications, although diversion colitis has been reported to occur more commonly in patients with IBD (87%) than in those with noninflammatory conditions (28%).[31] The prevalence of diversion colitis has been underestimated because many patients are asymptomatic; however, histologic changes are likely to occur in diverted segments of the colon within months of surgical diversion.

Pathology

A spectrum of histologic changes has been described in diversion colitis, ranging from lymphoid follicular hyperplasia and mixed mononuclear and neutrophilic infiltration to severe inflammation with crypt abscesses, mucin granulomas, and Paneth cell metaplasia[32,33]; large ulcers and transmural changes are absent, and crypt architecture generally is preserved. Endoscopic findings include erythema, friability, nodularity, edema, aphthous ulcerations, exudates, and frank bleeding, as in idiopathic IBD. After extended periods following diversion, inflammatory pseudopolyps and strictures may develop.

Pathogenesis

Diversion colitis is believed to result from mucosal nutrient deficiency in the region of the colon that has been removed from exposure to the fecal stream. The principal nutrient substrates of colonic epithelium are luminal short-chain fatty acids (SCFAs), which are metabolic products of carbohydrate and peptide fermentation by anaerobic bacteria.[34,35] Roediger demonstrated that SCFAs are the major and preferred energy source for colonic epithelium and that the distal colon is more dependent on SCFAs for its metabolic needs than is the proximal colon.[36] Butyrate supplies the bulk of oxidative energy to the distal colon, whereas acetate, glutamine, and ketones provide alternative sources of energy. Harig and associates demonstrated that excluded segments of colon contain

negligible amounts of SCFAs and that infusion of glucose results in no appreciable anaerobic fermentation.[37] The number of obligate anaerobes is reduced in the excluded colon, consistent with reduced SCFA production.[38] Instillation of enemas containing SCFAs resulted in disappearance of endoscopic changes within 4 to 6 weeks in 4 patients, although resolution of histologic abnormalities was slower and incomplete.[37]

Although SCFA deficiency has been widely accepted as the cause of diversion colitis, other observations suggest that SCFA deficiency may not be the entire etiologic explanation. First, studies in children indicate that SCFA enemas are not universally successful in treating diversion colitis. Second, in germ-free rodents with surgical diversion and in patients receiving long-term parenteral nutrition or elimination diets (circumstances in which luminal SCFA concentrations are low), mucosal atrophy occurs rather than inflammation.[39] Third, inflammation does not occur in urinary colon conduits, from which the fecal stream has been diverted, and urine does not contain measurable SCFAs.[40] Finally, in a prospective randomized double-blind study of 13 patients with diversion colitis, butyrate enemas given for 14 days provided no improvement in either endoscopic or histologic parameters.[41] In a subsequent study by the same group, administration of SCFAs did not affect the bacterial population in the excluded colon.[42] Other luminal elements besides SCFA deficiency must play a role, but the nature of such factors is unknown.

Diagnosis

The diagnosis of diversion colitis is based on the clinical picture and endoscopic and histologic findings. Diagnosis is relatively straightforward in a patient without preexisting IBD, but radiation colitis and ischemia should be considered in the appropriate clinical setting. Stool specimens for *C. difficile* toxin, ova and parasites, and cultures usually are adequate to exclude common infectious etiologies.

In patients with a preoperative diagnosis of Crohn's disease, diversion colitis must be distinguished from recurrent IBD. Colonoscopic findings such as linear ulcers and possibly strictures are said to favor Crohn's disease, as do transmural inflammation, marked crypt architectural abnormalities, and epithelioid granulomas. Lymphoid hyperplasia occurs in both disorders but tends to be more prominent in diversion colitis.[43] If rectal involvement with Crohn's disease is absent prior to diversion, rectal inflammation is more likely to be caused by diversion than by Crohn's disease.

Treatment

The preferred treatment of diversion colitis is surgical restoration of colonic continuity; this rapidly reverses symptoms and histologic changes. If symptoms are moderate to severe and reanastomosis is not feasible, SCFA enemas containing a mixture of 40 mmol of butyrate, 60 mmol of acetate, and 30 mmol of propionate, with 22 mmol of sodium chloride per liter are administered through the anus or mucous fistula twice daily for 4 weeks and then once or twice weekly.[43] Such preparations are not commercially available and must be formulated by compounding pharmacies, making it the most expensive of the nonsurgical options.[44] There are anecdotal reports that 5-aminosalicylate and hydrocortisone retention enemas are effective as well.[45] Because they are available commercially, these agents are considered to be first-line therapies for most patients. One report suggested that intraluminal irrigation with soluble and insoluble fiber solutions improved endoscopic and histologic abnormalities and might be useful to reduce inflammation prior to surgical restoration of bowel continuity.[46]

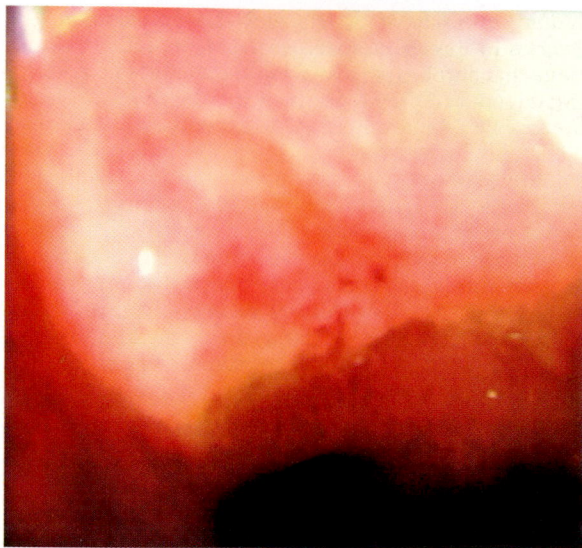

FIGURE 128-4. Endoscopic appearance of a nonspecific ulcer of the colon.

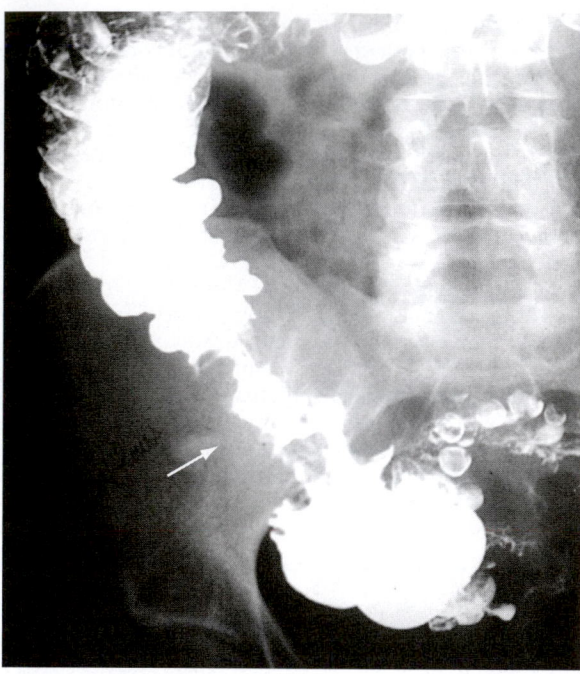

FIGURE 128-5. Barium enema examination showing the nonspecific ulcer of the colon in Figure 128-4 *(arrow)*. The initial interpretation was carcinoma of the ascending colon.

NONSPECIFIC COLONIC ULCERS

Benign nonspecific ulcers of the colon are uncommon, and their causes remain unknown. A large review of the literature encompassed 127 patients and indicated that colonic ulcers occur at any age, with a peak incidence in the fourth and fifth decades and a slight female predominance. Most such ulcers occur in the proximal colon, virtually all are solitary and located on the antimesenteric side of the colon, and most are round and sharply demarcated from relatively normal surrounding mucosa (Fig. 128-4).[47] Histologically, there is nonspecific acute and chronic inflammation.

Pathogenesis

The causes of nonspecific colonic ulcers are unknown. Hypotheses that have been advanced, but with little or no supporting evidence, include ischemia, cecal diverticulosis, and acid-peptic disease. Correlations with the use of drugs such as glucocorticoids, NSAIDs,[48,49] oral contraceptives, oxyphenbutazone, and most recently nicorandil, a coronary and peripheral vasodilator,[50] have been suggested, but these drugs have not been implicated in most of the reported cases of nonspecific colon ulcers. It is likely that no single causative agent explains all cases. There have been reports of associations of nonspecific colon ulcers with chronic renal failure and renal transplantation, Churg-Strauss syndrome, granulomatosis with polyangiitis (Wegener's), Behçet's disease, essential mixed cryoglobulinemia, and SLE. Perhaps a mechanism common to all exists, but none has been identified.

Clinical Features

The most frequent presenting symptoms are abdominal pain and bleeding. More than one half of patients with nonspecific colon ulcers present with acute or chronic abdominal pain, often in the right lower abdomen and mimicking appendicitis. One third have lower GI bleeding with hematochezia, and 16% present with an abdominal mass, most often when the ulcer is located in the left or sigmoid colon. A cecal ulcer should be suspected in a patient with GI bleeding associated with a clinical picture consistent with appendicitis or in a patient with symptoms suggestive of pelvic inflammatory disease, ovarian disease, or Crohn's disease when these diseases are not evident.

Diagnosis

Historically, nonspecific colonic ulcers usually were diagnosed at laparotomy after complications occurred. With the advent of endoscopy, many colonic ulcers are now diagnosed preoperatively and, in some cases, managed conservatively.

Colonoscopy is currently the diagnostic test of choice.[47] Flexible sigmoidoscopy is inadequate because most colonic ulcers are proximal to the splenic flexure. Abnormalities have been described in up to 75% of air-contrast barium enemas and include mucosal irregularities, intraluminal filling defects or narrowing, a mass effect, or localized colonic spasm (Fig. 128-5). Roentgen findings are nonspecific, however, and diagnostically inferior to direct inspection by colonoscopy. CT scans are most helpful in the presence of perforation or associated abscess formation.

The key to the diagnosis of nonspecific ulcers is exclusion of diseases that are associated with ulceration; these include Crohn's disease, infections (e.g., TB, *Entamoeba histolytica*, cytomegalovirus, *Salmonella typhi*), stercoral ulcers, and solitary rectal ulcer syndrome. Amyloidosis and neoplastic causes (e.g., carcinoma, lymphoma) are distinguished on histologic grounds but may not be distinguishable from nonspecific colonic ulcers on the basis of endoscopic appearance alone.

Treatment

Surgery is recommended for patients with ulcers complicated by perforation, significant GI or intra-abdominal bleeding, and for those with persistent symptoms and failure of the symptomatic ulcer to heal. In uncomplicated cases, however, an expectant approach has been advocated, with colonoscopy every 6 weeks to monitor healing. The most common surgical procedures are local excision of the ulcer, oversewing of the ulcer if there is significant bleeding, and occasionally more extensive resections of the affected colon.

DIEULAFOY-TYPE COLONIC ULCERATION

In 1897, Georges Dieulafoy first described massive GI bleeding from a relatively enlarged ("persistent calibre") submucosal artery by way of a minute mucosal ulcer at the most superficial point of the vessel; he called the lesion "exulceratio simplex."[51] Although originally described in the stomach and most commonly occurring in the gastric fundus, identical lesions have been described in other GI organs, including the colon and rectum. In the colon, Dieulafoy-type lesions appear to have a strong male predominance and have been reported in all age groups.[52]

Histologically, colonic Dieulafoy-type lesions are identical to those found elsewhere in the GI tract. The submucosal artery is tortuous and hypertrophic, curving toward the mucosa with persistence of caliber. Inflammation is absent, and the solitary mucosal ulceration extends no deeper than the upper submucosal layer of colon.

The clinical picture is one of acute and massive bleeding. Colonoscopy can identify the lesion in some cases[52] but is often difficult or impossible, especially when bleeding continues or thorough cleansing of the colon cannot be accomplished. Selective mesenteric angiography is the diagnostic study of choice, and surgical resection has been the principal form of therapy. Even after angiographic detection of the bleeding site, precise localization of the lesion is frequently difficult, and more extended resection often is required. In some cases, colonic lesions appear as pseudopolyps, and successful treatment with sclerotherapy, electrocautery, or hemoclipping may obviate the need for surgery.[53] Successful endovascular coil ablation of colonic Dieulafoy lesions has also been reported.[53a]

CATHARTIC COLON

Cathartic colon is an infrequent and severe manifestation of chronic irritant laxative abuse. In 1943, Heilbrun first described radiologic abnormalities of the colon and terminal ileum associated with prolonged abuse of irritant cathartics.[54] Fewer than 50 cases have been reported in the literature, all in women with duration of laxative abuse ranging from 10 to 70 years. It is important to emphasize that the term *cathartic colon* is based on barium enema characteristics and is not synonymous with prolonged use of laxatives or with laxative abuse. Indeed, misapplication of the term *cathartic colon* has led to inappropriate concerns over the chronic use of laxatives that, when used appropriately, is not associated with structural or functional damage to the colon. Cathartic colon is not the inevitable consequence of chronic laxative abuse, which may be associated with a variety of reversible symptoms as well as fluid and electrolyte abnormalities. In a review of 240 cases of chronic laxative abuse published in more than 70 reports, no case of cathartic colon was demonstrated.[55]

Radiologic and Pathologic Features

Heilbrun described the following characteristics in his original case report: loss of haustrations, pseudostrictures, dilated colon and terminal ileum, and gaping of the ileocecal valve[54]; similarities to the radiologic appearance of chronic UC were noted in this and subsequent studies. Characteristic changes are not always found throughout the colon, and there is a predilection for involvement of the ascending colon. Pathologic changes in resected specimens of cathartic colon have included mucosal atrophy, chronic inflammation with thickening of the muscularis mucosae, submucosal fatty infiltration, and mild fibrosis. Irreversible strictures and degenerative changes in intestinal neurons are absent. Neuronal changes have been found in patients with chronic laxative abuse, but these patients did not exhibit cathartic colon as defined here.

Effects of Laxatives on the Colon

The original suggestion that irritant laxatives, predominantly anthraquinones, damage the colon was based on studies in laboratory animals and in colons resected from laxative abusers.[56] Although mucosal atrophy and abnormalities of the enteric nervous system were described, detailed identities of the laxatives were not documented, nor was there information concerning preexisting conditions that might have prompted chronic use of laxatives.

Subsequent studies have reported changes in colonic epithelial cells and in the submucosa of patients with long-term laxative abuse, and both anthraquinones and bisacodyl have been implicated; however, the unclear nature and duration of laxative use and the inability to exclude preexisting conditions make the significance of these observations uncertain. Studies in rodents and in chronically constipated women do not support a deleterious effect of anthraquinones on the ultrastructure of colonic nerves,[57] nor is there evidence to suggest that sennosides, bisacodyl, or related substances cause significant morphologic damage to the colonic enteric nervous system in either experimental animals or humans. Perhaps 1 or more laxatives that are no longer in use (e.g., podophyllin) may have accounted for cases of cathartic colon, because no case of cathartic colon has been reported in persons who began to use or abuse irritant laxatives after 1960.[55]

Clinical Features

Habitual laxative users and abusers often complain of abdominal discomfort, bloating, fullness, or inability to defecate completely without using laxatives. In the more severe cases, electrolyte and fluid abnormalities such as hypokalemia and hypovolemia are associated with excessive thirst and weakness. Uncommonly, protein-losing enteropathy has been reported. All symptoms are reversible on withdrawal of laxatives or conversion to a more appropriate regimen of laxative use if there is no underlying diagnosis such as IBS.

Treatment

Treatment of cathartic colon and symptoms of chronic laxative use is focused on reducing or eliminating irritant laxatives, substituting bulking or osmotic agents, and retraining the bowel. Although often thought to be irreversible, there is evidence that cathartic colon can partially or completely reverse after withdrawal of laxatives. In severe or refractory cases, subtotal colectomy or proctocolectomy has been effective.

The cathartic colon is of historic interest and is unlikely to be identified in current clinical practice. There is no evidence that currently used laxatives can produce this entity. The term *cathartic colon* should not be confused with "chronic laxative abuse syndrome," nor should the term imply that current laxatives are dangerous if used chronically but appropriately.

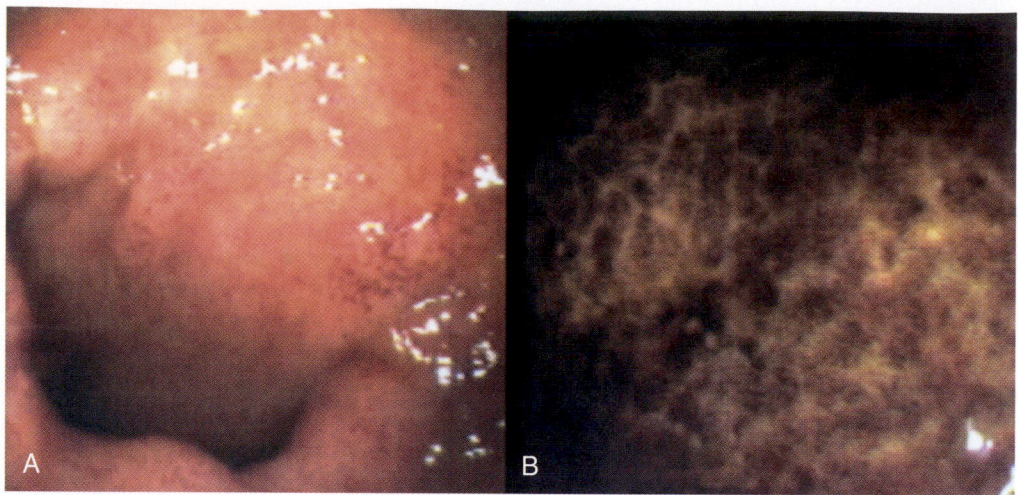

FIGURE 128-6. A colonoscopic view of pseudomelanosis coli associated with the chronic use of senna laxatives in a patient with ulcerative proctitis. There is little or no pseudomelanin pigment (lipofuscin) in the distal 30 cm of colon where there is active mild colitis *(left)*, in contrast to the heavy pigmentation in the remaining colon *(right)*. *(Courtesy Miguel Regueiro, MD, Pittsburgh, Pa.)*

PSEUDOMELANOSIS COLI

Melanosis coli is a brownish discoloration of the colonic mucosa caused by the accumulation of pigment in macrophages within the lamina propria (Fig. 128-6). First described in the early 19th century, the term *melanosis coli* was coined by Virchow in 1857 because the pigment was considered to be melanin or a melanin-like substance. Subsequently, histochemical and ultrastructural analysis proved the pigment to be not melanin, but lipofuscin, a "wear-and-tear" pigment that is composed of lipid-containing residues of lysosomal digestion.[58,59] The term *pseudomelanosis coli*, though more accurate, has not been adopted widely.

The association between pseudomelanosis coli and chronic use of anthraquinone laxatives is established firmly and is supported further by the development of characteristic pigmentation in laboratory animals after administration of anthraquinones.[60] Pseudomelanosis develops in more than 70% of persons who use anthraquinone laxatives (cascara, aloe, senna, rhubarb, and frangula), often within 4 months of use, but with an average of 9 months. The condition is widely regarded as benign and reversible, and disappearance of the pigment generally occurs within a year of stopping laxatives.[61] Pseudomelanosis can result from other factors or exposure to other laxatives, however, and is not pathognomonic for anthraquinone use.

The pigment in pseudomelanosis coli is now thought to originate from either macrophages or organelles within epithelial cells after damage by anthraquinone laxatives, which causes cells to die by apoptosis. Such a sequence of damage has been demonstrated in guinea pigs exposed to anthraquinones.[62] Histologically, the number and size of macrophages within the lamina propria are increased, and the greatest amount of pigment is found in macrophages farthest from the lumen. Abnormalities of colonic epithelial cells are noted on electron microscopy but not on light microscopy.[63]

Concern about a possible relationship between pseudomelanosis coli and the development of colonic neoplasms[64] has not been substantiated.[65] Other confounding factors such as chronic constipation or diet may account for an increased risk of colon cancer suggested by earlier studies.[66,67] Colonic neoplasms lack pigment-containing macrophages and therefore are identified easily in patients with pseudomelanosis coli

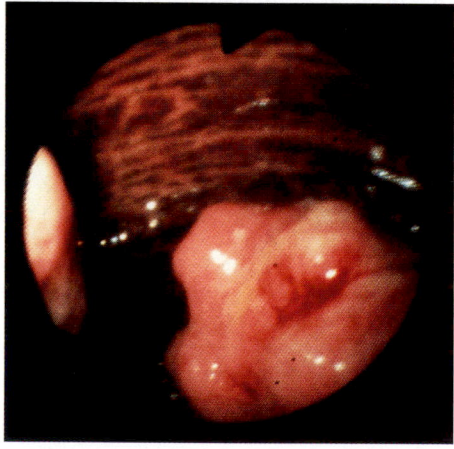

FIGURE 128-7. Colonoscopic view of a colonic cancer that is pale and thus easily seen in contrast against the dark background of pseudomelanosis. The neoplasm is pale because it lacks pigment-containing macrophages. *(Courtesy Juergen Nord, MD, Tampa, Fla.)*

(Fig. 128-7).[68] Biopsy specimens should be taken of any nonpigmented area of the colon in a patient with pseudomelanosis coli who undergoes colonoscopy.

CHEMICAL COLITIS

Damage to the colon has been reported after exposure to a number of rectally administered agents (Box 128-1), the better known of which are soaps and detergents used as "cleansing" enemas.[69,70] Other offending substances include hydrogen peroxide,[71] water-soluble contrast agents such as sodium diatrizoate (Hypaque, Gastrografin), vinegar, potassium permanganate, herbal medications, glutaraldehyde,[72] formalin,[73] and alcohol.[74] Milder damage to the mucosa occurs after use of monobasic or dibasic sodium phosphate enemas[75] and bisacodyl suppositories. Colonic damage presumably occurs from a detergent, hypertonic, or direct toxic effect on the

BOX 128-1 Chemical Agents Associated with Colitis

Acetic acid
Alcohol
Ammonia
Caustic soda (sodium hydroxide)
Chloro-m-xylenol (Dettol)
Ergotamine
Formalin
Glutaraldehyde
Herbal medicines
Hydrofluoric acid
Hydrogen peroxide
Lye
Potassium permanganate
Radiocontrast agents (Hypaque, Renografin-76)
Soap
Sulfuric acid
Vinegar

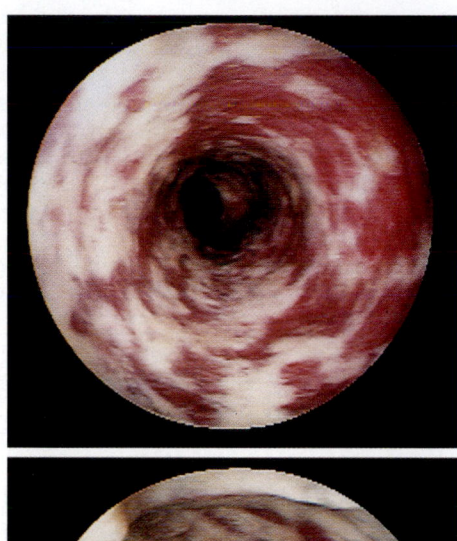

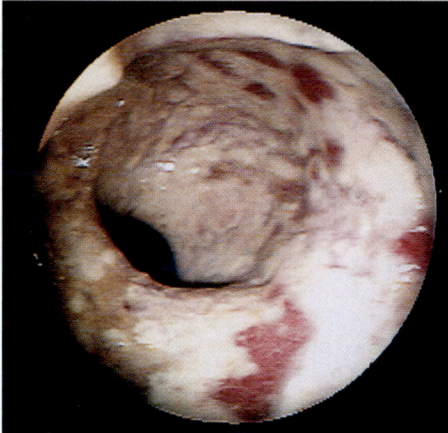

FIGURE 128-8. Colonoscopic view of hydrogen peroxide colitis in a patient to whom hydrogen peroxide was given to help remove a fecal impaction. Both panels show the so-called snow-white sign, referring to the appearance of the stark white necrotic mucosa. *(Courtesy Lawrence J. Brandt, MD, Bronx, N.Y.)*

mucosa. The severity of the reaction depends on the type and concentration of the substance, the duration and extent of its contact with the mucosa, and perhaps the presence of underlying colonic disease.[76]

Soaps consist of a number of substances, including strong alkali, potash, phenol, and sodium and potassium salts of long-chain fatty acids. These agents produce liquefaction necrosis with mild to severe inflammation and saponification of the layers of the colon wall. Acute histologic changes include necrosis, leading, in more severe cases, to ulceration and formation of granulation tissue. Acute colitis may heal without residua or with fibrosis and scarring or progress to transmural necrosis and perforation. The severity of damage probably is related to the concentration of soap and duration of mucosal contact. Endoscopic findings have ranged from loss of the normal mucosal vascular pattern to aphthae to mucosal sloughing and ulceration.

Hydrogen peroxide enemas are no longer frequently used, but at one time they were employed to relieve meconium ileus and to remove fecal impactions. There are reports of severe damage associated with use of hydrogen peroxide, including severe colitis, pneumatosis coli, perforation, sepsis, and death.[71] Within minutes of contact, diffuse mucosal emphysema occurs, and after about an hour, the colon may become ischemic and eventually ulcerate (Fig. 128-8). Acute colitis also has been reported after using glutaraldehyde to disinfect a colonoscope and then not sufficiently washing the agent off the instrument prior to its reuse (Fig. 128-9).[72]

Colitis has been reported following the use of several hyperosmolar water-soluble contrast materials that often are employed to opacify the colon in cases of partial obstruction and to treat fecal impaction in adults. Damage is believed to occur because of the hypertonicity of these agents, but the addition of Tween 80 to hyperosmolar agents to improve mucosal contrast may have contributed to mucosal damage because of its detergent properties. Most reports of injury have occurred in the colon proximal to an obstruction and mainly in the right colon, which suggests that prolonged contact with these agents predisposes to mucosal injury.

Prevention and Treatment

Proper cleaning and rinsing of endoscopes are required to minimize exposure of the patient to injurious disinfecting chemicals. Protocols require strict adherence to proper maintenance and adjustments in the rinse cycle of disinfecting

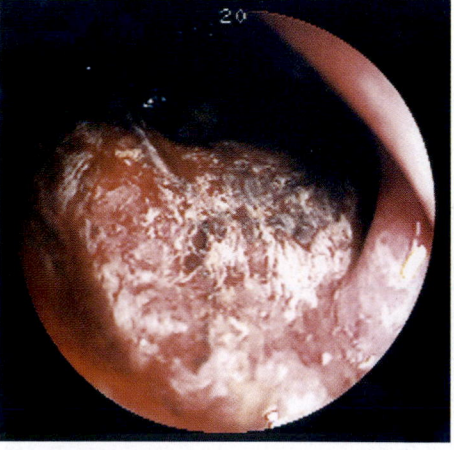

FIGURE 128-9. Endoscopic view of glutaraldehyde colitis in a young man who had had a normal colonoscopy 3 hours before this photograph was taken. The colitis was caused by glutaraldehyde that had been used to disinfect the flexible sigmoidoscope after its previous use but had not been sufficiently cleansed from the instrument. He complained of "agonizing" pain during the sigmoidoscopic examination and began to pass bright red blood 2 hours later. *(Courtesy Lawrence J. Brandt, MD, Bronx, N.Y.)*

machines. Forced-air drying and rinsing of endoscope channels and the exterior of the instrument should ensure a chemical-free procedure.

Patients and health care professionals should be cautioned that soapsuds enemas should not be used. Rectal instillation of substances for medicinal or ritualistic activities other than commercially available enemas should be discouraged.

Treatment of chemical colitis is largely supportive, with IV fluids and broad-spectrum antibiotics. Surgery may be indicated in severe cases of bowel necrosis leading to gangrene or perforation. Most patients will recover completely 4 to 6 weeks after injury.

PNEUMATOSIS COLI (PNEUMATOSIS CYSTOIDES INTESTINALIS)

The term *pneumatosis coli* is synonymous with *pneumatosis cystoides intestinalis* (PCI) when the disorder is limited to the colon. This uncommon disorder is characterized by multiple gas-filled cysts that are located in the submucosa and subserosa of the intestine. PCI must be distinguished from pneumatosis linearis, or gas within the wall of the bowel, which usually is associated with bowel necrosis, signifies loss of bowel viability, and mandates surgery. In AIDS, pneumatosis linearis may be associated with opportunistic infections of the colon and may resolve without surgery if the infection is treated successfully.[77]

Most cases of PCI occur in the jejunum and ileum, and only 6% of cases involve the colon, with a propensity for left-sided involvement. Numerous conditions have been associated with pneumatosis coli, including appendicitis, Crohn's disease, UC, diverticular disease, necrotizing enterocolitis, pseudomembranous colitis,[78] ileus,[79] and sigmoid volvulus. PCI also has been associated with non-GI conditions, including emphysema, collagen vascular diseases,[79] transplantation, AIDS,[77] glucocorticoid use, chemotherapy,[79] and certain medications including intestinal α-glucosidase inhibitors used as hypoglycemic agents; PCI resolved completely when the drugs were withdrawn.[80] In approximately 20% of cases, there are no associated medical conditions and PCI is considered primary.[81]

Etiology

Several theories have been suggested to explain the large and varied number of conditions associated with PCI, the most plausible of which are the mechanical theory and the bacterial theory.

According to the mechanical theory, intraluminal gas enters the bowel wall under pressure through a defect or potential defect in the intestinal mucosa. The mucosal defect may result from direct trauma or increased intraluminal pressure. This hypothesis could account for reports of PCI after colonoscopy and sigmoidoscopy without biopsy, in cases of colitis, perforated duodenal ulcers, and jejunal diverticula and after intestinal anastomoses. The plausibility of this theory, however, is diminished by the absence of a connection between the mucosa and the cysts and the presence of elevated levels of hydrogen gas in the cysts.[82]

The bacterial theory suggests that the cystic gas collections are the by-products of bacteria, specifically those that produce hydrogen. This theory has been supported by clinical observations and laboratory experiments. In laboratory animals, PCI can be induced by injecting gas-forming bacteria into the bowel wall. In addition to local invasion of the intestinal wall, bacteria may produce gas cysts by manufacturing large amounts of hydrogen gas as a result of carbohydrate fermenta-

tion. Levitt and Olsson theorized that the high hydrogen tension in the colonic lumen leads to rapid diffusion into an intramural gas bubble and may cause N_2, O_2, and CO_2 to diffuse from the circulation into the gas bubble.[83] According to their theory, the gas bubble enlarges if there is continued diffusion of hydrogen into it. Indeed, high hydrogen content in the cysts has been documented,[84] and cysts regress in patients fed an elemental diet to decrease the carbohydrate substrate for colonic bacteria. Two major observations argue against the bacterial theory of PCI: (1) that bacteria are not cultured from cysts; and (2) with cyst rupture and pneumoperitoneum, peritonitis is not seen.

It has been hypothesized that gas cysts form by counterperfusion supersaturation of H_2 gas by which super H_2 production by colonic bacteria provides the condition for H_2 tension in the colonic lumen to approach the level of N_2 tension in the blood.[85] One such mechanism is exposure to drugs, such as chloral hydrate, that inhibit the growth of H_2-consuming methanogenic bacteria in the colon, thereby increasing net H_2 production.[85] Another possible etiologic setting is the administration of a nonabsorbable carbohydrate such as lactulose, which increases colonic hydrogen production in a setting where bacteria that metabolize H_2 are deficient.[86] Successful treatment with antibiotics[84,86] and colonic washouts also supports a bacterial etiology for PCI. In 1 study, stools from patients with pneumatosis coli were demonstrated to lack 2 major species of hydrogen-consuming bacteria.[82] Because hydrogen normally is produced only in the colon and not in the small intestine, pneumatosis coli may differ from pneumatosis intestinalis with respect to pathogenic mechanisms.

Clinical Features and Diagnosis

The frequency of pneumatosis coli is highest in the sixth decade, with equal frequency in men and women.[81] In most cases, pneumatosis is an unexpected finding on abdominal plain films. The most common symptoms are diarrhea (68%), mucus discharge (68%), rectal bleeding (60%), and constipation (48%).[81] Approximately 3% of patients present with a complication of pneumatosis coli, including pneumoperitoneum, tension pneumoperitoneum, volvulus, intestinal obstruction, intussusception, and intestinal perforation. Physical examination may reveal an abdominal mass, and careful rectal examination may enable palpation of the cystic lesions. A plain abdominal film may identify radiolucent clusters or streaks along the bowel wall with pneumoperitoneum, if a cyst has ruptured. A markedly redundant sigmoid colon as well as the outline of the cysts or linear streaks may be seen on barium enema (Fig. 128-10).[81] Endoscopic examination with biopsy is necessary for definitive diagnosis, to exclude carcinoma, and to differentiate pneumatosis from familial adenomatosis polyposis and from the thumbprinting of colon ischemia. The endoscopic appearance is of multiple cysts, which vary in size from a few millimeters to several centimeters (Fig. 128-11) and which rapidly deflate on puncture with a needle or biopsy forceps. EUS also has been used to establish the diagnosis.[87]

Pathology

The cysts of PCI resemble soap bubbles. They usually are thin-walled, unilocular, and can occur separately or in clusters. They do not communicate with the intestinal lumen or with each other and have a spongy consistency that pops like a balloon when compressed. On cross-section they appear shiny and honeycombed, and range in size from a few millimeters to several centimeters. Microscopically, the cysts have an endothelial lining that tends to gather and coalesce, forming

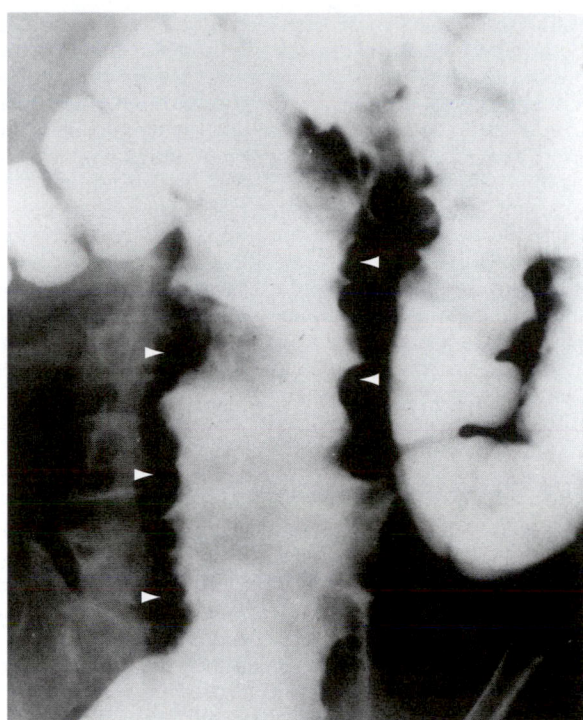

FIGURE 128-10. Single-contrast barium enema demonstrating the presence of gas-filled cysts in the wall of the colon *(arrowheads)* characteristic of pneumatosis coli. *(From Feldman M, Boland CR, editors. Slide atlas of gastroenterology and hepatology. Philadelphia: Current Medicine; 1996.)*

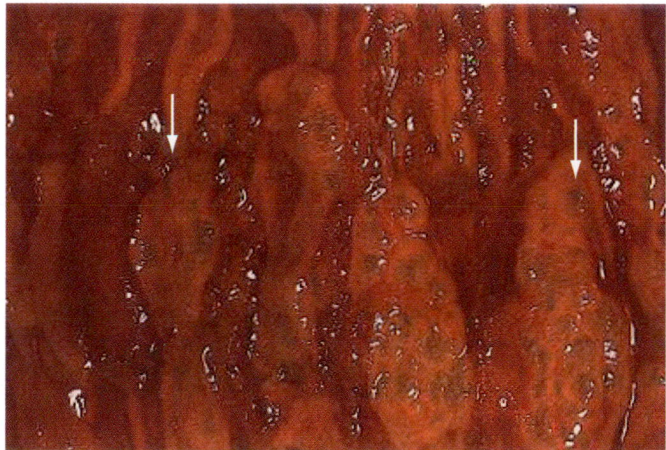

FIGURE 128-11. A colonic resection specimen with pneumatosis coli. Numerous gas-filled cysts are seen in this surface view of the mucosa *(arrows)*. *(From Feldman M, Boland CR, editors. Slide atlas of gastroenterology and hepatology. Philadelphia: Current Medicine; 1996.)*

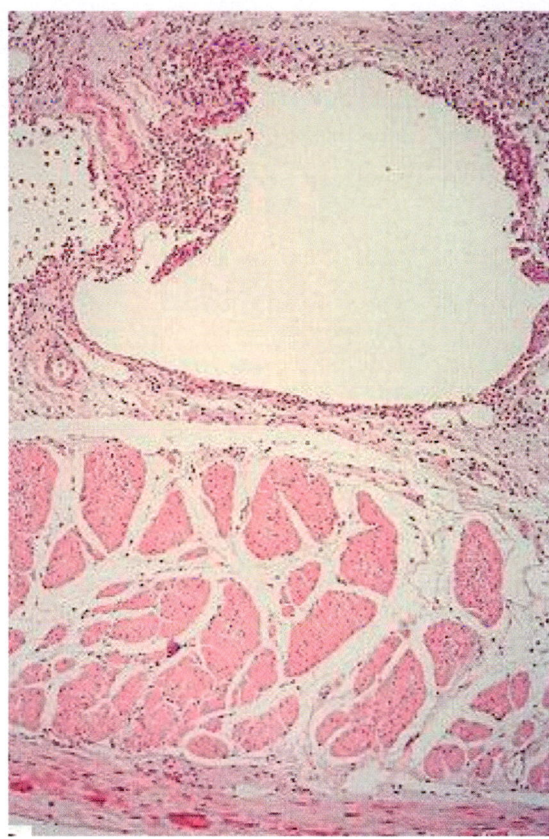

FIGURE 128-12. Histopathology of a large gas-filled cyst in the submucosa of the colon from a patient with pneumatosis coli. These cysts are usually lined by histiocytes and multinucleated giant cells. Cysts also may be present in the subserosa. (H&E). *(From Feldman M, Boland CR, editors. Slide atlas of gastroenterology and hepatology. Philadelphia: Current Medicine; 1996.)*

multinucleate giant cells that increase in number as the cysts collapse, undergo fibrosis (Fig. 128-12), and are eventually sloughed, leaving the cysts without a lining. Progressive fibrosis leads to a decrease in the size of the cysts and ultimately to their obliteration. The connective tissue surrounding the cysts may show a granulomatous inflammatory reaction made up of eosinophils, lymphocytes, macrophages, and plasma cells. Subserosal cysts are surrounded by fibrous connective tissue and can produce adhesion of adjacent bowel loops. The mucosa in PCI may be normal or thinned, and with or without ulcerations and inflammation where it is stretched over a cyst. Mucosal changes vary from mild focal abnormalities to extensive changes including granulomas, abnormal crypts with branching, shortening, cryptitis and abscesses, dilatation, and rupture.

Treatment

Because the natural history of PCI is one of spontaneous regression in up to 50% of cases, and because cysts may reappear after surgery, specific treatment is not recommended in asymptomatic individuals. Symptomatic patients may be treated successfully by breathing high-flow oxygen for several days or by use of hyperbaric oxygen, especially in resistant cases[87]; high oxygen levels lead to replacement of hydrogen by oxygen within the cysts and a corresponding reduction in their size. Because cysts may recur after oxygen therapy, a minimum of 48 hours of oxygen therapy is recommended to maximize the success rate. Metronidazole also has been used to treat pneumatosis coli, an observation that suggests that anaerobic bacteria play a role in the genesis of the disorder. Because cysts have been reported to recur after short courses of metronidazole, treatment should continue until complete resolution of the cysts is seen. In general, colonic resection is reserved for patients with complications such as intestinal obstruction and massive bleeding.

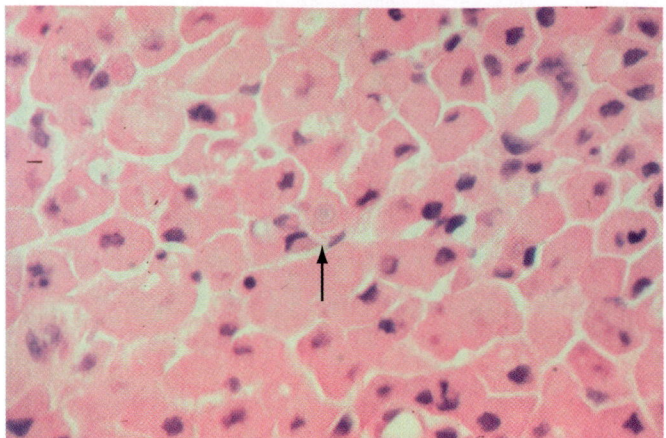

FIGURE 128-13. Histopathology of malakoplakia. Sheets of large pale cells characterize the histologic changes in malakoplakia. One of the histiocytes shows the characteristic ring-like Michaelis-Gutmann body *(arrow)*, consisting of a central core of partially digested bacteria coated with iron and calcium phosphate. (H&E). *(Courtesy Lawrence J. Brandt, MD, Bronx, N.Y.)*

MALAKOPLAKIA

Malakoplakia is a rare chronic granulomatous disease first described by von Hansemann in 1901[88] and reported by Michaelis and Gutmann in 1902.[89] The term *malakoplakia* is derived from the Greek "malakos" (soft) and "plakos" (plaque) and reflects its usual appearance as a friable, yellow mucosal lesion. Microscopically, coliform bacteria are located in the cytoplasm of macrophages (von Hansemann histiocytes), and laminated intracytoplasmic inclusion bodies (Michaelis-Gutmann bodies) are considered the diagnostic features of this disorder (Fig. 128-13).[89]

Malakoplakia may affect many organs, including lung, brain, adrenal glands, pancreas, bone, and the genitourinary tract. The GI tract is the second most common site of involvement (after the urinary tract). The most common sites of colonic involvement are the rectum, sigmoid, and right colon, in descending order of frequency.[90]

Etiology

The pathogenesis of malakoplakia is unknown. Proposed etiologies are infection, immunosuppression, systemic illness, neoplasia, and a genetic disorder. Evidence for an infectious etiology is based on the finding that some patients with malakoplakia have associated chronic infections.[91] This was first described in patients with urologic malakoplakia, more than 75% of whom were infected with *Escherichia coli*. This finding led to the belief that *E. coli* might be a primary cause of malakoplakia; however, other organisms also have been isolated, including *Klebsiella*, *Proteus*, *Mycobacterium*, *Staphylococcus*, and fungi,[92] suggesting that 1 infection is not the primary cause of the disease.

Other evidence points to a defect in macrophage killing as the cause of malakoplakia. Nondigested microorganisms are found within the lysosomes of macrophages in affected persons. Macrophages from these patients show a decrease in cyclic guanosine monophosphate, resulting in impaired bactericidal activity.[93] Peripheral blood monocytes also are found to have decreased bactericidal activity in malakoplakia. The defect in macrophage dysfunction may be reversed with the addition of a cholinergic agonist, both in vitro and in vivo (see later).[94]

Malakoplakia has been reported in patients receiving chemotherapy and immunosuppressive therapy for organ transplantation. Reversal of both macrophage abnormalities and clinical symptoms occurred after discontinuation of glucocorticoids and azathioprine.[95] Malakoplakia also has been reported in various immune deficiency states (e.g., primary hypogammaglobulinemia, AIDS) and has been associated with chronic systemic diseases (e.g., SLE, UC, sarcoidosis).[91]

There have been a substantial number of cases to support a neoplastic etiology for 1 form of malakoplakia.[96,97] In 1996, Bates and colleagues identified 19 cases of colorectal adenocarcinoma associated with malakoplakia,[97] which was present only in a focal area adjacent to the tumor, in contrast to cases not associated with a neoplasm, in which multiple organs may be affected. A possible genetic etiology was suggested by 1 report of colonic malakoplakia that clustered in a family.

Clinical Features and Diagnosis

Patients with malakoplakia usually present with abdominal pain, diarrhea, hematochezia, and fever.[90] Physical findings include a palpable rectal mass, abdominal mass, and weight loss. Diagnosis is by colonoscopy and biopsy, which generally reveal the following 3 patterns of the disease:

1. Isolated rectosigmoid involvement, in which lesions appear as yellowish plaques that may be sessile, polypoid, and ulcerated; the colonic lumen may be strictured, and intestinal fistulas may occur, suggesting a diagnosis of cancer or Crohn's disease
2. Diffuse colonic involvement, which is characteristic of immunosuppressed patients
3. Focal lesions, which may be associated with an adenomatous polyp or cancer

Biopsy is essential to confirm the diagnosis and to exclude an underlying colonic malignancy (see Fig. 128-13). Histology reveals the characteristic macrophages with voluminous cytoplasm that contains the classic von Hansemann histiocytes (intracellular organisms) and Michaelis-Gutmann bodies (intracytoplasmic concentric laminated inclusion bodies). The histiocytes (also termed *von Hansemann cells*) must be distinguished from those found in fungal disease, leprosy, Whipple's disease, reticulum cell sarcoma, and macrophages harboring *Mycobacterium avium* complex.

Treatment

Patients with newly diagnosed malakoplakia should undergo a thorough medical history and physical examination to determine if they are taking immunosuppressive medications or have coexisting medical illnesses or malnutrition. Tests of immune function and screening for associated bladder malakoplakia and colorectal cancer are prudent. Patients who are receiving immunosuppressive medications may improve after these medications are discontinued. Antibiotics such as trimethoprim/sulfamethoxazole and ciprofloxacin have been successful in treating malakoplakia.[98] Both antibiotics appear to kill the bacteria associated with malakoplakia and can penetrate the defective host macrophages. Cholinergic agents also may be useful in treating children with malakoplakia.[94] Surgical resection of the involved colon is recommended for cases associated with carcinoma or severe bleeding.

COLITIS CYSTICA PROFUNDA

Colitis cystica profunda (CCP) is a rare disease characterized by mucin-filled cysts located in the submucosa of the colon (Fig. 128-14). The disease was first described in 1766 by Stark,

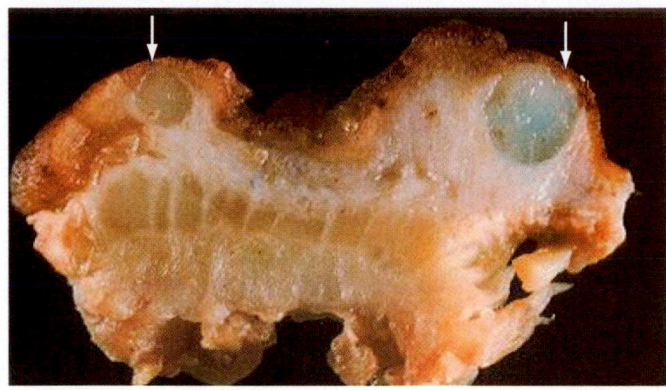

FIGURE 128-14. Resection specimen of colitis cystica profunda. Several submucosal cysts are filled with mucinous material *(arrows)*. This entity occurs in the setting of chronic IBD as well as the solitary rectal ulcer syndrome. These lesions have been confused with mucinous carcinomas, which also may be seen in chronic IBD. *(From Feldman M, Boland CR, editors. Slide atlas of gastroenterology and hepatology. Philadelphia: Current Medicine; 1996.)*

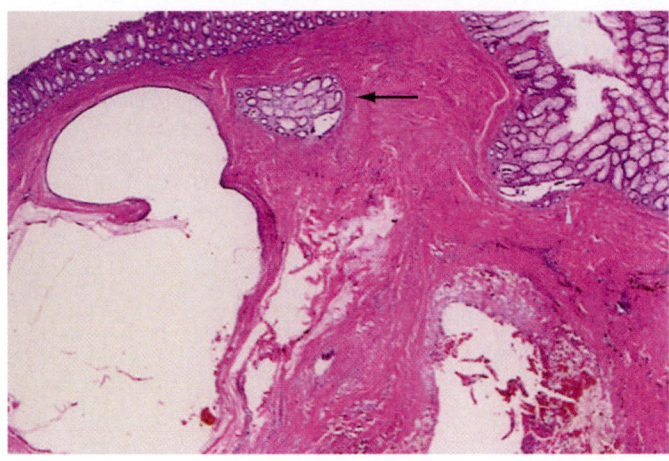

FIGURE 128-15. Histopathology of colitis cystica profunda showing the mucus-filled cysts and misplaced epithelium below the muscularis mucosae *(arrow)*. (H&E, ×5.) *(From Mitros FA, editor. Atlas of gastrointestinal pathology. New York: Gower Medical Publishers; 1988.)*

who reported 2 cases associated with dysentery.[99] CCP manifests in 3 patterns: (1) localized, with a polypoid lesion; (2) diffuse, with multiple polypoid lesions; and (3) diffuse, with a confluent sheet of cysts.

Etiology

The etiology of CCP is unknown, but several theories have been proposed. A possible congenital etiology is supported by several findings. In embryologic examinations, submucosal cysts have been found in multiple GI locations. The occurrence of CCP in children and its association with other congenital conditions such as Peutz-Jeghers syndrome also support a congenital origin for this disease. Absence of submucosal cysts in large autopsy series of infants and children, however, reduces the plausibility of this etiology.

CCP has been associated with several acquired diseases that predispose to mucosal ulceration and inflammation, including UC, Crohn's disease,[100] and infectious colitis.[101] Submucosal cysts also have been reported in areas exposed to local trauma, such as an intestinal anastomosis or colostomy. Proctitis cystica profunda developed in rats treated with irradiation[102] and at the site of small bowel stomas also created in rats.[137]

CCP has been found in association with adenocarcinoma of the colon, and several cases of adenocarcinoma of the stomach have been reported with gastritis cystica profunda, suggesting a somewhat undefined relationship with neoplasia[102a]. In some reports, there is strong evidence of a causal link between cancer and CCP, because the submucosal cysts are often found adjacent to the adenocarcinoma, whereas adjacent benign mucosa is devoid of submucosal cysts.

The localized form of CCP is associated with rectal prolapse and solitary rectal ulcer syndrome (SRUS).[99] Mucosal prolapse has been found in more than 50% of patients with the localized form of the disease, and it is thought that trauma or ischemia caused by chronic traction on the mucosa and intramural vessels may play a role in development of the submucosal cysts. Microscopic features of the localized form of the disease often include fibrosis of the lamina propria and hypertrophic muscle fibers, changes that are characteristic of SRUS.

Clinical Features and Diagnosis

CCP affects men and women equally. The most common symptoms are rectal bleeding, mucus discharge, and diarrhea[99]; less common are tenesmus, abdominal pain, and rectal pain. Rarely, the patient may present with intestinal obstruction that is caused by the cysts. At endoscopy, most lesions are located on the anterior rectal wall 6 to 7 cm from the anal verge. The lesions appear as polyps with overlying mucosa that may be normal, inflamed, or ulcerated. Endoscopy may disclose an associated rectal prolapse in some cases. The endoscopic appearance of the lesions may be indistinguishable from a variety of lesions, including adenocarcinomas, adenomatous polyps, submucosal lipomas, neurofibromas, inflammatory pseudopolyps, pneumatosis coli, and endometriosis.[99] Barium enema may reveal radiolucent filling defects. Transrectal US may be useful in differentiating this disease from cancer and reveals hypoechoic cysts that may be surrounded by intact submucosa, unlike invasive cancer.[103] Biopsy is necessary to differentiate this lesion from a variety of inflammatory, neoplastic, and infectious conditions. On biopsy, the submucosa is seen to be thickened by the presence of the mucus-filled cysts (Fig. 128-15). The cysts usually communicate with the lumen through small openings in the mucosa. Although usually confined to the submucosa, cysts that involve the muscularis propria and serosa have been reported. Glandular epithelium may be displaced into the submucosa (See Fig. 128-15), and care must be taken not to confuse these displaced glands with invasive carcinoma. The surrounding connective tissue often shows chronic inflammation, and there may be extensive replacement of the lamina propria by fibroblasts.

Treatment

A high-fiber diet and bowel retraining to avoid straining have led to regression of this disease in a few cases.[103] If fiber is not effective, polyethylene glycol solutions may be tried.[104] Glucocorticoid enemas also have been used with some success.[99] Most patients have been treated with surgery. In patients who have associated rectal prolapse, repair of the prolapse alone may treat the CCP successfully, whereas for disease localized to the rectum, and in the absence of procidentia, local excision through a transanal approach is efficacious.[104] When the disease is localized to the rectum but is circumferential, total excision may be accomplished by mucosal sleeve resection and coloanal pull-through.[104] More diffuse lesions have been removed by segmental resection. Segmental resection also may be necessary for large obstructing lesions and for lesions that cause hypokalemia, hypoalbuminemia, and severe anemia from chronic blood loss. A diverting colostomy may lead to regression of this disease and may be the best option for a patient with significant comorbidities.

NEUTROPENIC ENTEROCOLITIS (TYPHLITIS)

Neutropenic enterocolitis (typhlitis) is a potentially life-threatening condition, usually associated with neutropenia that is related to chemotherapy, although it also has been described after organ transplantation, with AIDS, and in patients who have leukemia treated with cytosine arabinoside, and those with solid tumors treated with combination chemotherapy.[105,106] The entity was described initially in 1970 by Wagner in children who were undergoing chemotherapy for leukemia.[107] The disease commonly affects the ileum and cecum and may result in intestinal perforation. The frequency of neutropenic enterocolitis in persons at risk varies from 1% to 46%.[108]

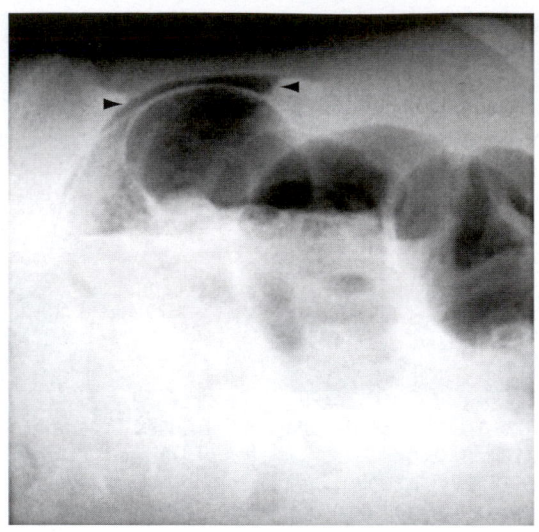

FIGURE 128-16. Left lateral decubitus plain film in a patient with neutropenic enterocolitis. The colon is dilated, with a prominent intraluminal gas-fluid interface and free peritoneal air *(arrowheads)* resulting from cecal perforation. *(From Hunger TB, Bjelland UJC. Gastrointestinal complications of leukemia and its treatment. AJR Am J Roentgenol 1984; 142:513-8.)*

Etiology

The cause of neutropenic enterocolitis may be multifactorial. The initial injury is an ulceration of the bowel mucosa, with no associated inflammatory response. Mucosal injury may occur from leukemic infiltration, stasis of bowel contents, or mucosal ischemia from splanchnic vasoconstriction resulting from sepsis.[108] Certain drugs also may contribute to mucosal damage. Cytosine arabinoside can cause necrosis and delayed regeneration of intestinal glandular epithelium. Vinca alkaloids used to treat leukemia also may contribute to cecal distention by damaging the myenteric plexus of the intestine. With mucosal injury in the setting of impaired host defenses, infectious colitis subsequently occurs. The infection is often polymicrobial; causative bacteria include *E. coli*, *Staphylococcus aureus*, *Clostridia septicum*, and *Klebsiella* species[109]; fungal organisms such as *Aspergillus* and *Candida* also have been isolated.[109] In addition to transmural infection of the intestine, the cecum may become gangrenous and perforate as a result of increased distention and ischemia. The process may involve the ileum alone or both the ileum and cecum.[109]

Clinical Features and Diagnosis

The most common presentation of neutropenic enterocolitis is with fever, diarrhea, nausea, vomiting, and abdominal pain in a patient who is receiving antineoplastic drugs. Abdominal tenderness typically is localized to the right lower quadrant of the abdomen, but may be absent or masked by drugs such as prednisone; localized tenderness may progress rapidly to diffuse signs of peritonitis as a result of intestinal perforation. Shock may occur as a result of bacteremia or intestinal perforation. On occasion, the sigmoid colon may be affected, further complicating the diagnosis. Neutropenia is universal, and blood cultures are positive in up to 50% of cases.[109] Differential diagnosis includes appendicitis, pseudomembranous colitis, ischemic colitis, volvulus, diverticulitis, and drug-induced diarrhea.

The diagnostic workup should include a radiologic evaluation to exclude other diseases, confirm the diagnosis, and determine the severity of disease. Abdominal films may demonstrate dilated loops of small bowel with decreased air in the right lower quadrant and free intraperitoneal air if intestinal perforation has occurred (Fig. 128-16). CT scans are most sensitive for establishing the diagnosis and help to exclude other conditions such as appendicitis and diverticulitis. The CT scan may reveal a thickened bowel wall, pneumatosis intestinalis, ascites, and free air. Barium enema should be avoided because of the potential risk of perforation. Stool assay for *C. difficile* toxin should be performed routinely.

Treatment

Management of neutropenic enterocolitis has varied. Approaches have included supportive measures alone, aggressive initial surgical resection, and combined medical and surgical treatment; successes and failures have been documented with all these approaches. In 2 studies, all patients treated medically recovered, whereas in another similar series, all patients managed medically died. Clearly, successful management of patients with neutropenic enterocolitis needs to be individualized to optimize outcome.

In general, medical management includes broad-spectrum antibiotics, NG suction, and bowel rest. Fluid resuscitation with isotonic solutions is critical to maintain renal perfusion in the face of decreased systemic vascular resistance from sepsis and intra-abdominal fluid sequestration. Close observation and serial abdominal and radiologic examinations are necessary to monitor the response to medical treatment. Antibiotics should have activity against enteric Gram-negative organisms, Gram-positive organisms, and anaerobes. Causative microorganisms include *Pseudomonas*, *S. aureus*, *E. coli*, and group A *Streptococcus*.[109] For patients who do not respond to antibacterial agents, amphotericin should be considered because coexisting fungemia is common.[109] Blood transfusions may be necessary because the diarrhea is often bloody. Granulocyte-macrophage colony-stimulating factor to correct the neutropenia is a useful adjunct to medical therapy.[110] Early surgical intervention has been recommended in persons with a rapidly deteriorating course despite maximal medical therapy. Two series have shown a decreased mortality rate in patients with severe disease who are treated surgically compared with those treated medically.[111] For patients with complications such as gangrene, intestinal perforation, and shock despite vasopressor support, surgical intervention is mandatory.

Controversy surrounds the choice of operation. Gangrenous or perforated bowel should be resected. When the bowel is edematous with no vascular compromise and no signs of perforation, successful management has included no resection, intestinal diversion with no resection, and resection of the involved bowel.[112] If resection is performed, construction of an ileostomy and mucous fistula may be the safest option because intestinal anastomoses may be prone to breakdown in the presence of neutropenia. Because recurrences of neutropenic enterocolitis are common when chemotherapy is restarted, right hemicolectomy is recommended before chemotherapy is resumed.[112]

ENDOMETRIOSIS

Endometriosis, defined as the presence of endometrial tissue outside the uterine cavity and musculature, was first described by von Rokitansky in 1860. Most often, these ectopic tissues lie in the vicinity of the uterus. Endometriosis occurs in up to 15% of menstruating women and up to 30% of infertile women. The initial description of nonpigmented endometriosis in 1986 resulted in increased recognition and a much higher prevalence of this disorder than appreciated previously.[113] In contrast to endometrial involvement of the female reproductive organs, GI involvement is less common, usually asymptomatic, and clinically less important. The most frequent GI organs involved are the rectosigmoid colon (96%), appendix (10%), and ileum (5%), with other organs involved less commonly. Intestinal endometriosis can mimic a wide variety of inflammatory, infectious, and neoplastic digestive disorders.[114]

Etiology and Pathogenesis

Several hypotheses have been advanced to explain the ectopic location of endometrial tissue. The most commonly accepted explanation is that of retrograde passage of endometrial tissue, which then implants and grows on pelvic organs and the peritoneum. From these sites, more distant implants arise via hematogenous or lymphatic dissemination; further dissemination may occur during surgical interventions. A less accepted hypothesis, which has fewer supporting data, is that of endometrial metaplasia, in which multipotential peritoneal mesothelial cells are induced by unknown factors to undergo metaplastic transformation to endometrial tissue.

Once implanted, endometrial tissue still appears to be regulated by hormonal influences, so that estrogen promotes and progesterone inhibits growth. These repetitive cycles of growth and sloughing of tissue can lead to serosal irritation and progressive invasion of intestinal muscle with fibrosis and muscle hypertrophy. Thus, pain may arise from nerve impingement or serosal inflammation, whereas obstruction may result from luminal narrowing or intestinal kinking.

Clinical Features

Endometriosis is found almost exclusively, but not always, in women of childbearing age, with clinical onset usually between the ages of 20 and 45 years. Women who experience symptoms or who undergo surgery for endometriosis beyond

menopause presumably have chronic fibrosis or exacerbations induced by exogenous estrogens.

Although most women with endometrial implants on intestinal structures have no symptoms, those with serosal implants may complain of localized tenderness, low backache, or abdominal pain. Penetration of endometrial tissue into the bowel wall may produce constipation, diarrhea, and partial obstruction that results in intermittent abdominal pain. Contrary to popular thinking, symptoms are not always cyclical and may not fluctuate with hormonal levels; nor are GI symptoms necessarily associated with gynecologic symptoms. Rarely, hematochezia occurs when endometrial implants penetrate to the mucosa or when severe colonic fibrosis results in ischemia. Less common presentations occur with more proximal colonic or small intestinal involvement and include acute appendicitis caused by an obstructing endometrioma, small bowel intussusception, and volvulus.[114,115] Actually, endometriosis is the most common cause of appendiceal intussusception in adults, followed by mucocele, adenoma, and carcinoid.

Diagnosis

The clinical diagnosis of intestinal endometriosis may be difficult because symptoms often are nonspecific and there may not be a close relationship between the symptoms and the menstrual cycle. Endometriosis should always be considered in women with recurrent abdominal pain and bowel symptoms, especially if they are in their reproductive years and have gynecologic complaints. Diagnosis is especially difficult because IBS is so common in women.

An important component of the evaluation is a careful pelvic examination that includes combined rectovaginal palpation. Finding tender nodules or irregularities in the cul-de-sac is highly suggestive of endometriosis. Because findings may vary considerably during the menstrual cycle, the pelvic examination should be performed immediately before and again after menstruation if no abnormalities were found initially.

It is rare to see endometrial implants on the colonic mucosa except when there is hematochezia. Thus, colonoscopy is often normal except for areas of extrinsic compression or strictures with intact mucosa.[116] More helpful is an air-contrast barium enema that demonstrates submucosal polypoid masses or areas of noncircumferential narrowing of the lumen (Fig. 128-17). Diagnostic yield and accuracy may be enhanced by performance of these tests just before the onset of menses. CT scan (Fig. 128-18), US, and MRI all have been reported to assist with the diagnosis or assessment of the extent of endometrial involvement. High-resolution transvaginal and transrectal US also may be useful to detect small endometrial implants, particularly in the retroperitoneal pelvis.[117]

Definitive diagnosis of endometriosis often is made by laparoscopy or laparotomy with biopsy and is especially useful in patients with intestinal implants without pelvic involvement. The appreciation that endometrial tissue may be nonpigmented has increased the yield of these procedures considerably.[113]

The differential diagnosis of intestinal endometriosis includes inflammatory disorders such as Crohn's disease and UC with stricture, diverticulitis, infectious diseases such as ileocolonic tuberculosis and schistosomiasis, benign and malignant neoplastic disorders, and colon ischemia.[114] It is important to emphasize that no radiologic or imaging finding is pathognomonic of endometriosis, that mucosal abnormalities permitting diagnosis by biopsy are rare, and that tissue for a definitive diagnosis is usually obtained only at laparotomy (Fig. 128-19).

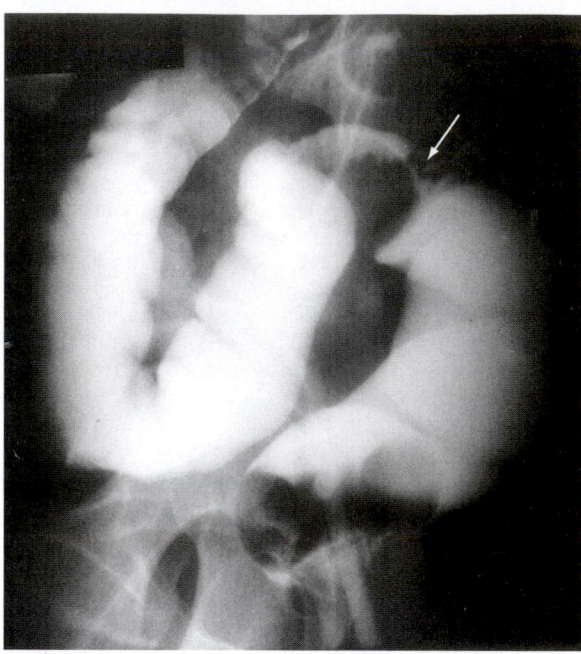

FIGURE 128-17. Single-contrast barium enema demonstrating a large, nodular, partially obstructing endometrioma in the rectosigmoid colon *(arrow)*. *(Courtesy Mark Peterson, MD, Pittsburgh, Pa.)*

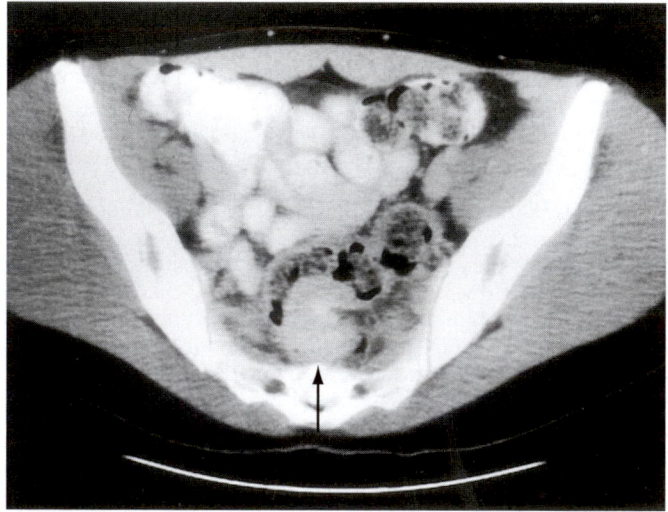

FIGURE 128-18. CT scan of the same patient as in Figure 128-17 showing the endometrial mass in the cul-de-sac *(arrow)* extending into the colon. *(Courtesy Mark Peterson, MD, Pittsburgh, Pa.)*

Treatment

In general, when a diagnosis of serosal intestinal endometriosis is made, hormonal therapy is often the first therapeutic option, similar to the standard approach to pelvic endometriosis.[118,119] Low-dose estrogen-progestin compounds cause a pseudopregnancy state that results in decidualization of endometrial tissue, often with relief of dysmenorrhea. Their use in more severe disease is questionable, however, and they generally are not recommended for symptomatic intestinal disease.

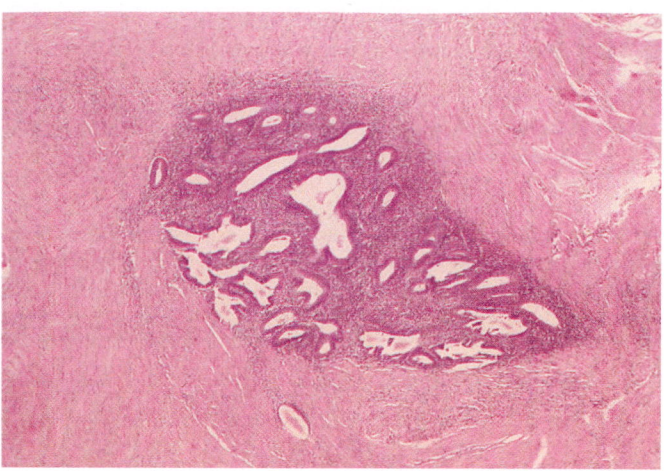

FIGURE 128-19. Histolpathology of endometriosis. Endometrial stoma is seen around the glandular structures in the muscularis propria of the colon in a woman presenting with obstructive symptoms. The diagnosis of endometriosis was proved at surgery. (H&E, ×10.) *(From Mitros FA, editor. Atlas of gastrointestinal pathology. New York: Gower Medical Publishers; 1988.)*

The most effective agents currently available are the synthetic androgen danazol and the gonadotropin-releasing hormone agonists.[120] Both act to decrease ovarian steroid synthesis by inhibiting pituitary release of follicle-stimulating hormone and luteinizing hormone. Although both are effective in decreasing pelvic pain associated with endometriosis and appear to decrease the size of endometrial implants, there are no studies of these agents in endometriosis-associated intestinal disease, and there is some concern that treatment may result in increased fibrosis and inadequate symptom resolution.[121] Ablation of endometrial implants on surfaces that can be visualized laparoscopically can be accomplished using a carbon dioxide laser.

For endometriosis that causes partial obstruction of the colon or small intestine, segmental resection of the involved area provides the best results and also serves to exclude an underlying carcinoma.[122,123] Resection can be performed by laparoscopic technique or by open surgery, according to available expertise. If the patient is postmenopausal or if future pregnancies are not wanted, hysterectomy and bilateral salpingo-oophorectomy can be done at the time of resectional surgery to minimize the risk of symptomatic disease in the future. Similar surgery also can be performed in premenopausal women who, despite medical therapy, have intractable symptoms.

SOLITARY RECTAL ULCER SYNDROME

First described by the French anatomist Jean Cruveilhier in 1839,[124] solitary rectal ulcer syndrome (SRUS) is an uncommon or underreported disorder of defecation that affects patients of all ages. SRUS became more widely recognized after a published review of 68 cases by Madigan and Morson in 1969.[125] The term is really a misnomer; patients can present with hyperemic mucosa only, a solitary ulcer, multiple ulcers, or even a polypoid lesion resembling carcinoma.[126]

Regardless of appearance, the histology of SRUS is characteristic, showing fibromuscular obliteration of the lamina propria and smooth muscle fibers that extend from a hypertrophied muscularis mucosa up toward the lumen.[126] The diagnosis of SRUS often is delayed because of its varied endoscopic appearance and a lack of awareness of the disorder.

Pathogenesis

SRUS is considered to be a disorder of defecation, but its pathogenesis is uncertain, and it has a spectrum of disease presentations. A large subgroup of patients with SRUS strain excessively during defecation, and some have a behavioral disorder. Occult or overt rectal prolapse with paradoxical contraction of the pelvic floor during defecation appears to be involved in many patients,[127] and evidence of inappropriate pelvic floor contraction has been shown in electromyographic and video-proctographic studies.[128] It has been suggested that the rectal mucosa can be traumatized from the pressure of being prolapsed against a closed anal canal and additional trauma to the apex of the prolapse, may result from manual attempts by the patient to reduce the prolapse digitally.[129] Alternatively, straining during defecation results in high fecal voiding pressures that reduce local blood flow, causing ischemia and ulceration. The mucosa of the anterior rectal wall 7 to 10 cm above the anal verge is the most common area of such prolapse into the anal canal, and this corresponds to the usual location of ulceration in SRUS. The association of SRUS and rectal prolapse, however, is not universal, and the prevalence of associated rectal prolapse varies from 13% to 94%.[126]

SRUS also has been associated with the use of ergotamine suppositories and is well known to occur after radiotherapy, further supporting a pathogenic role for ischemia.[130,131] Successful treatment of SRUS using biofeedback has been associated with an increase in local blood flow, which also suggests that SRUS may be associated with reduced rectal blood flow from impaired extrinsic autonomic cholinergic nerve activity.[132]

Du Boulay and colleagues have shown that the histology of the rectal mucosa in patients with SRUS is similar to that seen at other sites of mucosal prolapse, which suggests that prolapse of the mucosa alone rather than the entire rectal wall is important in SRUS pathogenesis.[133] Ischemia results in fibromuscular obliteration of the lamina propria and the formation of an ulcer. Once the ulcer is formed, it can further intensify the urge to defecate; this urge combined with straining and changes in local blood flow causes persistent symptoms and chronic ulceration.

Most patients with SRUS typically complain of passage of mucus and blood with defecation.[125,134] Some also complain of tenesmus, straining, altered bowel habits, or a sensation of incomplete evacuation. Although men and women are affected equally, the usual onset is a decade earlier in men. On average, the duration of symptoms ranges from 3 months to 30 years.[126,135] A retrospective analysis showed that 26% of patients with SRUS are misdiagnosed initially and treated for IBD.[135]

Diagnosis and Pathology

Diagnosis of SRUS is based on clinical symptoms, physical examination, endoscopic findings, and typical histology. On digital rectal examination, there may be reduced anal sphincter tone, and an indurated area or thickened folds may be palpated. Overt rectal prolapse may be demonstrated by having the patient assume a squatting position and straining as if to have a bowel movement. Sigmoidoscopy may demonstrate single or multiple ulcers or a patch of erythematous mucosa on the anterior rectal wall within 10 cm of the anal verge.[125] The lesion has a polypoid appearance (Fig. 128-20) in 25% to 44% of patients.[126] Differential diagnosis includes IBD, malignancy, ischemic colitis, stercoral ulcer, medication-

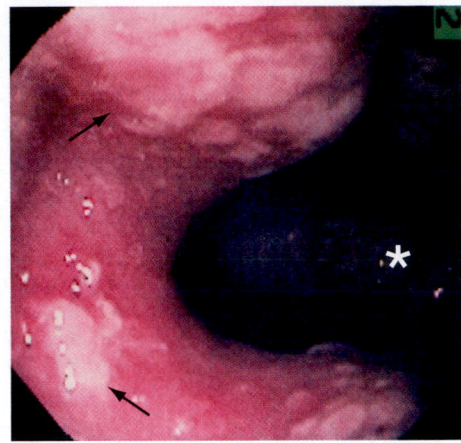

FIGURE 128-20. Photograph obtained during colonoscopy in a 40-year-old patient with solitary rectal ulcer syndrome. A large (4 × 3 cm) ulcer is seen in the distal rectum 3 cm above the anal verge. The ulcer margins have a polypoid appearance. *Black arrows* show exudative material amid the nodularity of the ulcer; the *white asterisk* is the colon lumen.

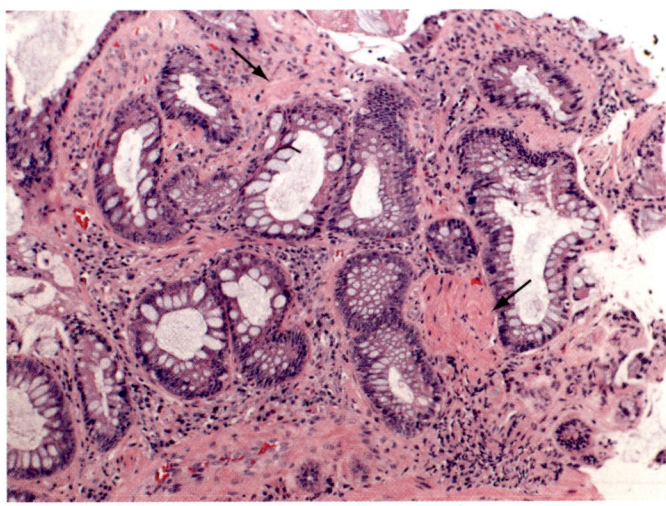

FIGURE 128-21. Histopathology of solitary rectal ulcer syndrome. The findings include disorganized crypts with reactive epithelium, mild lamina propria inflammation, and smooth muscle fibers abnormally present in the mucosa *(arrows)*. The smooth muscle fibers represent hyperplasia of the muscularis mucosae, a common histologic finding in this condition. (H&E). *(Courtesy Marie E. Robert, MD, New Haven, Conn.)*

induced ulceration, trauma, and infections, including amebiasis and secondary syphilis.

Biopsy specimens always should be taken from the ulcer margin and from any abnormal-appearing mucosa. In 1969, Madigan and Morson[125] were the first to describe the histologic features of SRUS. There is fibromuscular obliteration of the lamina propria by collagen from fibroblasts and smooth muscle fibers derived from the muscularis mucosae. The muscularis mucosae is often hypertrophied, and its fibers are in continuity with those in the lamina propria. There is no significant increase in the number of inflammatory cells. The polypoid variant is similar to the ulcerative variant except for regenerative hyperplastic changes such as cystic dilation and mucus production. Epithelial elements and lamina propria can be displaced into the submucosa (Fig. 128-21). This displaced tissue can then undergo cystic dilatation because of mucus retention. The misplaced and dysplastic-appearing glands may be misdiagnosed as adenocarcinoma, especially when the histologic and macroscopic features of SRUS are not recognized; at times, SRUS is present in association with a carcinoma, further confusing the issue.[136]

Although not required in most patients, defecography may be useful to shed light on the pathophysiology of SRUS, especially if surgery is being considered. Defecography is used to demonstrate mucosal prolapse, intussusception, rectal prolapse, a nonrelaxing puborectalis muscle, and incomplete or delayed evacuation.[128] Endorectal US can demonstrate the presence and components of rectal wall thickening, particularly the muscularis propria, and may be useful to distinguish SRUS from other conditions such as invasive cancer.[137]

Treatment

Asymptomatic patients might not require any treatment, and in some patients, SRUS resolves spontaneously. Treatment includes improving bowel habits; consuming a high-fiber diet; using bulk laxatives, local agents, and biofeedback; and undergoing surgery. Use of fiber as a bulking agent, along with bowel habit training to reduce straining, can improve symptoms in patients with mild disease. Local agents such as topical glucocorticoids and aminosalicylates are not effective. Sucralfate enemas and human fibrin sealant have been effective in small studies.[138] Argon plasma coagulation (APC) has been used to treat hemorrhage from SRUS; continued treatment with APC has been associated with symptomatic and endoscopic improvement.[139]

Biofeedback or instrument-assisted muscle retraining has been advocated as first-line therapy for those who fail conservative measures and have more severe symptoms.[132] This recommendation is based on uncontrolled studies and largely from a series of studies from the same institution. The most recent report suggested clinical improvement in 75% of patients, healing of the ulcer in 31%, and significant improvement in rectal mucosal blood flow in subjects who felt subjectively better after biofeedback.[132] The mechanism by which biofeedback works is unclear; an earlier study from the same institution indicated that the presence of dyssynergic defecation did not predict outcome.[140]

A number of surgical procedures have been reported in patients with SRUS, but the most appropriate procedure depends upon the assessment of each patient and is based upon the underlying anatomic pathology.[141] Surgical procedures include excision of the ulcer, low anterior resection, anterior resection with rectopexy, colostomy, and nonresectional laparoscopic ventral mesh rectopexy.[142] Unfortunately, there is a lack of well-controlled randomized studies, and it is difficult to compare surgical procedures because of the small numbers of patients in surgical series and the heterogeneous nature of the anatomic pathology that underlies SRUS.[143]

STERCORAL ULCERS OF THE COLON

Stercoral ulcers result from pressure necrosis of the mucosa that is a direct effect of an adjacent hard fecal mass (scybalum). Over time, the pressure of the scybalum results in local ischemic necrosis and ulceration and can lead to perforation. These ulcers are rare and usually asymptomatic until they manifest with lower GI bleeding or colonic perforation. Fecal disimpaction occasionally precipitates rectal hemorrhage when the scybalum is removed along with an adherent blood vessel in the subjacent ulcer crater. Maurer and coworkers

observed that 3.2% of colonic perforations in their series were caused by stercoral ulcers.[144]

Pathogenesis

The pathogenesis of stercoral ulcers is multifactorial. Chronic constipation is the major risk factor for stercoral ulceration; although described in patients of all ages, it is more common among older adult patients with clinical features that may be associated with constipation. Although constipation and fecal impaction are observed commonly, complications of stercoral ulceration are relatively uncommon.[145] Factors that increase constipation and formation of a scybalum, such as antacids containing aluminum hydroxide, use of opiate analgesics, constipating sedatives and psychiatric medications, and chronic renal failure, were noted in patients who developed stercoral ulceration.[146] Why a stercoral ulcer develops is unclear, although implicated factors predisposing the left colon to ulceration include dehydrated and hard feces, a narrow-diameter colon with high pressure, and relatively poor blood supply.

Diagnosis and Pathology

Patients with perforated ulcers usually present with peritonitis and findings of an acute abdomen.[145] The scybalum sometimes is palpable as an abdominal mass. Plain films of the abdomen might demonstrate pneumoperitoneum, fecal loading, or calcified scybala (Fig. 128-22). Nonperforating ulcers can manifest with lower GI bleeding. Caution must be used when performing disimpaction in patients with hard

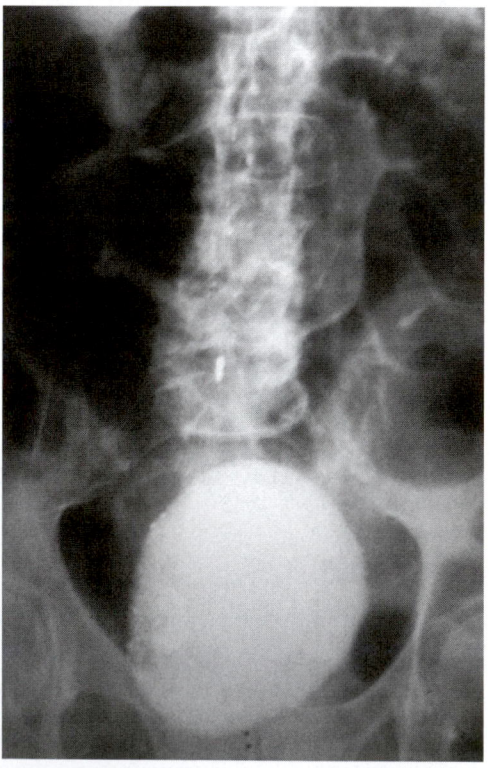

FIGURE 128-22. Plain film of the abdomen showing a calcified fecaloma in an older adult man with a history of prolonged confinement to bed. He presented with abdominal distention and ultimately had the mass removed at surgery. *(Courtesy Lawrence J. Brandt, MD, Bronx, N.Y.)*

fecal masses in the rectum, because removing the mass can result in severe hemorrhage if the underlying blood vessel in the ulcer base is torn during removal.

The antimesenteric border of the colon is most commonly involved, usually in the sigmoid or proximal rectum. Ulcers usually are large, irregular, and sharply demarcated and may be single or multiple. Ulcers conform to the contour of the impacted scybala as a result of ischemic pressure necrosis. A rounded or ovoid perforation may be seen in the center of the ulcer. Necrotic colonic mucosa with acute and chronic inflammation is noted on histology.[144] Differential diagnosis includes spontaneous colonic perforation, malignancy, ischemia, and infection.

Treatment

Perforated stercoral ulcers require emergency laparotomy with resection of the affected colonic segment. A Hartmann's operation is the preferred procedure and, along with extensive peritoneal lavage, it is associated with a lower mortality than other surgical procedures.[144,145] Nonperforating stercoral ulcers might respond to antibiotics and aggressive treatment of constipation, although surgical resection remains the only definitive treatment.

KEY REFERENCES

Full references for this chapter can be found on www.expertconsult.com.

6. Corti-Hoekstra LR, van den Brande JMH, Peppelenbosch MP. Report from the Falk workshop on microscopic colitis: Creating awareness for an underappreciated disease. Gastroenterology 2012; 143:e1-3.
22. Wildt S, Nordgaard-Lassen I, Bendtsen F, Rumessen JJ. Metabolic and inflammatory fecal markers in collagenous colitis. Eur J Gastroenterol Hepatol 2007; 19:567-74.
25. Chande N, MacDonald JK, McDonald JW. Interventions for treating microscopic colitis: A Cochrane Inflammatory Bowel Disease and Functional Bowel Disorders Review Group systematic review of randomized trials. Am J Gastroenterol 2009; 104:235-41.
26. Stewart MJ, Seow CH, Storr MA. Prednisolone and budesonide for short- and long-term treatment of microscopic colitis: Systematic review and meta-analysis. Clin Gastroenterol Hepatol 2011; 9:881-90.
35. Mortensen PB, Clausen MR. Short-chain fatty acids in the human colon: Relation to gastrointestinal health and disease. Scand J Gastroenterol 1996; 216:132-48.
44. Eggenberger JC, Farid A. Diversion colitis. Curr Treat Options Gastroenterol 2001; 4:255-9.
48. Masannat YA, Harron M, Harinath G. Nonsteroidal anti-inflammatory drugs-associated colopathy. ANZ J Surg 2010; 80:96-9.
57. Wald A. Is chronic use of stimulant laxatives harmful to the colon? J Clin Gastroenterol 2003; 36:386-9.
76. Cappell MS. Colonic toxicity of administered drugs and chemicals. Am J Gastroenterol 2004; 99:1175-90.
79. Knetchle S, Davidoff A, Rice R. Pneumatosis intestinalis: Clinical management and surgical outcome. Ann Surg 1990; 212:160-5.
87. Shimada M, Ina K, Takahashi H, et al. Pneumatosis cystoides intestinalis treated with hyperbaric oxygen therapy: Usefulness of an endoscopic ultrasonic catheter probe for diagnosis. Intern Med 2001; 40:896-900.
104. Beck DE. Surgical treatment for colitis cystica profunda and solitary rectal syndrome. Curr Treat Options Gastroenterol 2002; 5:231-7.
112. Davila ML. Neutropenic enterocolitis. Curr Opin Gastroenterol 2006; 22:44-7.
118. Olive DL, Pritts EA. Treatment of endometriosis. N Engl J Med 2001; 345:266-75.
119. Streuli I, de Zeigler D, Santulli P, et al. An update on the pharmacological management of endometriosis. Expert Opin Pharmacother 2013; 14:291-305.
125. Madigan MR, Morson BC. Solitary ulcer of the rectum. Gut 1969; 10:871-81.
144. Maurer CA, Renzulli P, Mazzucchelli L, et al. Use of accurate diagnostic criteria may increase incidence of stercoral perforation of the colon. Dis Colon Rectum 2000; 43:991-8.

CHAPTER

129

Diseases of the Anorectum

ABIER ABDELNABY AND J. MARCUS DOWNS

CHAPTER OUTLINE

ANATOMY

The anal canal, about 4 cm long in adults, is the terminal and most inferior part of the large intestine. It begins where the rectal ampulla narrows abruptly below the level of the U-shaped sling formed by the puborectalis muscle, and ends at the anus, the external outlet of the GI tract. The anus normally is contracted and forms an anteroposterior slit, except during defecation. The anal canal, surrounded by the internal and external anal sphincters, descends posteroinferiorly between the anococcygeal ligament and the perineal body. It is also surrounded by the levator ani muscles, which form the main part of the pelvic diaphragm. Because the anal canal slopes posteroinferiorly, the examining finger or instrument should be directed toward the umbilicus when introduced into the anal canal.[1]

The lining of the anal canal consists of an upper mucosal (endoderm) segment and a lower cutaneous (ectoderm) segment. The dentate (pectinate) line is the "saw-toothed" junction between these 2 distinct origins of venous and lymphatic drainage, nerve supply, and epithelial lining (Fig. 129-1). Above this level, the intestine is innervated by the sympathetic and parasympathetic systems. The arterial supply and venous drainage relate to the internal iliac vessels. The

lymphatics accompany these vessels and drain into the internal iliac nodes. Distal to the dentate line, the anal canal is innervated by the somatic nervous system, with blood supply and drainage from the inferior hemorrhoidal system.[2] These differences are important when the classification and treatment of hemorrhoids are concerned (see later).

Embryologically, the dentate line represents the junction between endoderm and ectoderm. Proximal to the dentate line, there is sympathetic and parasympathetic innervation. Distally, the nerve supply is somatic. Therefore, above the dentate line, pain sensation is negligible and biopsy can be done painlessly without local analgesia. Below the dentate line, however, the anoderm is highly sensitive, an important point to note when examining the anal canal or applying hemorrhoidal bands.

Above the dentate line, the mucosa appears to have 6 to 14 pleats called the *columns of Morgagni*. This configuration represents the funneling of the rectum as it narrows into the anal canal. Located at the base of the columns of Morgagni are anal crypts that lead to small, rudimentary anal glands. When compressed by feces, the anal glands exude mucus, which aids in evacuation of stool through the anal canal.[3] These glands extend through the internal anal sphincter, and if their ducts become blocked, an anal canal abscess or fistula can develop.

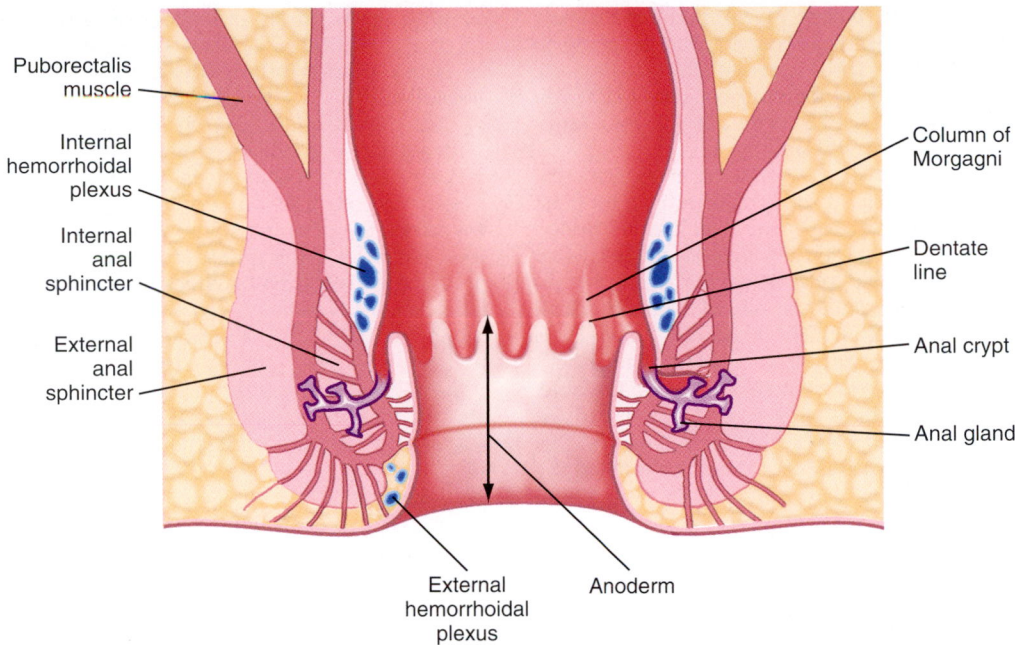

FIGURE 129-1. Schematic depiction of the anatomy of the anal region. The *vertical line with arrowheads* denotes the transition zone that extends from the anal verge proximally for 1 to 1.5 cm to the dentate line.

The cutaneous part of the anal canal consists of modified squamous epithelium that is thin, smooth, delicate, pale, stretched, and devoid of hair and glands. This is known as the *anoderm*. At the level of the anal verge, the epithelium becomes thicker and hair follicles begin to be seen.

The arterial blood supply of the anus and rectum is from the superior, middle, and inferior hemorrhoidal/rectal arteries, which are continuations of the inferior mesenteric, hypogastric, and internal pudendal arteries, respectively. Klosterhalfen and coworkers performed postmortem angiographic, manual, and histologic evaluations to show that in 85% of cases, the posterior aspect of the anal canal was less well perfused than other sections of the anal canal.[4] In a pathogenetic model of primary anal fissure, this diminished blood supply could result in relative ischemia at the posterior commissure,[5] which explains not only why anal fissure at this location may become chronic, but also why it can then can be healed by smooth muscle relaxants that act as vasodilators (e.g., nitroglycerin and diltiazem) and result in increased blood supply. The venous drainage from the anal canal is by both the systemic and portal systems. The internal hemorrhoidal plexus drains into the superior rectal veins, which drain into the inferior mesenteric vein and then into the portal vein. The distal part of the anal canal drains via the external hemorrhoidal plexus through the middle rectal and pudendal veins into the internal iliac vein (i.e., the systemic circulation).[5]

Lymph from the upper two thirds of the rectum drains exclusively upward to the inferior mesenteric nodes and then to the para-aortic nodes. Lymphatic drainage from the lower third of the rectum occurs not only cephalad, along the superior hemorrhoidal and inferior mesenteric arteries, but also laterally, along the middle hemorrhoidal vessels to the internal iliac nodes. In the anal canal, the dentate line is the landmark for 2 different systems of lymphatic drainage: above, to the systemic drainage system, and below, to the inguinal drainage basin. Therefore, inguinal adenopathy can be seen with malignant disease below the dentate line, whereas with more proximal lesions, the enlarged nodes are within the pelvis and not palpable.

The internal anal sphincter is an involuntary sphincter surrounding the superior two thirds of the anal canal. It is formed by a thickening of the circular smooth muscle layer of the intestine, and it is innervated by the pelvic splanchnic nerves (parasympathetic). This sphincter reacts to the pressure of feces in the rectal ampulla and is important for anal canal resting tonicity and passive continence.[5]

The external anal sphincter is a relatively large voluntary muscle that surrounds the inferior two thirds of the anal canal. It forms a broad band on each side of the anal canal and consists of subcutaneous, superficial, and deep parts. The external anal sphincter partly overlaps the inferior part of the internal anal sphincter. It is composed of skeletal muscle and contributes to our conscious control of defecation. The external anal sphincter assists in voluntarily closing the anal canal and anus. The puborectalis is the deepest component of the external anal sphincter, and its contraction draws the canal anteriorly, thereby increasing the anorectal angle to help facilitate evacuation. The innervation of the external anal sphincter is the inferior rectal nerve and the perineal branch of S4.

EXAMINATION OF THE ANUS AND RECTUM

All routine adult physical examinations should include a digital examination of the anorectum. When patients present with problems focused on the anorectal region or colon, a more comprehensive examination is indicated.

Examination begins with a thorough history. Active listening allows the patient to explain his or her symptoms and the physician to develop rapport with the patient. The patient's history will usually permit the physician either to identify the likely diagnosis or narrow the number of possibilities considerably. Such conversation also allows time for the patient's anxiety to abate. Very often patients with anorectal problems delay seeking medical care out of fear and embarrassment. During the anorectal examination, it is important to explain each step before it is done, let patients feel you touch them before you approach a sensitive area, and remember that any surprising contact will increase the anxiety you are trying to minimize. It is important to avoid causing pain during the examination. A calm voice and gentle touch are essential. Even so, there are times when the patient is so tender that the examination must be done under anesthesia.

Patients can be examined in the office in any of several positions, including the left lateral (the position used by most gastroenterologists), knee-chest, or prone jackknife. In the prone jackknife position, the patient is face-down, on his or her knees, with the arms folded and the shoulders and head on the examining table; some patients may be more comfortable resting on the left shoulder. The examiner may use a special hydraulic table that has a shelf upon which the patient may kneel and then drape his or her chest over the main table. The table then is raised and its head is tipped down, propelling the buttocks forward and elevating them. This position allows the buttocks to be splayed apart for a clear view of the anus. Appropriate illumination is critical.

Inspection

The examination begins with inspection of the skin. In some cases, looking at the patient's underwear will give a clue to the presence and character of anal drainage or whether there is stool incontinence. As the buttocks are gently retracted, scars, skin abnormalities, stool, discharge of blood or pus, anal tags, warts, hemorrhoids, or lesions adjacent to or prolapsing from the anal canal are noted. The anus is inspected for asymmetry, gaping, or scars.

The patient is then asked to squeeze the anus to evaluate movement of the anal muscles. There should be concentric movement of the anus and perianal skin. This maneuver is important when assessing for fecal continence. Next, the patient should be asked to strain so that the anal area can be examined for abnormal descent (>4 cm) below its resting level (perineal descent syndrome). Prolapse of the vagina or rectum,

bulging hemorrhoids, or leakage of urine also should be noted during straining. In some instances, rectal prolapse may be seen only if the patient is asked to strain when sitting on the toilet.

Traction applied laterally to each side of the anal orifice with a gauze pad allows eversion of the distal anus for further inspection. This technique is particularly helpful in viewing a fissure without causing undue pain (Fig. 129-2). Some examiners stroke the perianal skin with a cotton-tipped applicator to look for reflex contraction of the anal muscles (anal "wink", anocutaneous reflex) or check perianal sensation with a pinprick; these maneuvers give a crude determination of sphincter innervation and are important in evaluating for sensory neuropathies. The nearby skin of the buttocks, perivaginal region, base of the scrotum, and up to the tip of the coccyx should be viewed. Inguinal lymph nodes also should be assessed, especially if infection or neoplasia is suspected.

Palpation

Using a gloved and lubricated index finger, the examiner palpates the anal canal and perianal skin. Slow insertion and gentle pressure are appropriate. Anal tone is assessed in the resting state and when the patient contracts his or her anus. The index finger is then swept all around the anal canal, noting scars, masses, or tenderness. Internal hemorrhoids are not palpable unless they are thrombosed. If insertion of the index finger is too painful, pressure should be applied with the examining finger on the wall opposite the area of tenderness, which might allow insertion and palpation. If the examination is still too painful, use of sedation or anesthesia may be warranted. Approximately 80% of the resting anal canal pressure is contributed by the internal anal sphincter. The external sphincter is evaluated by having the patient voluntarily squeeze the anus around the examining finger; the external anal sphincter contributes about 20% of resting anal canal pressure.

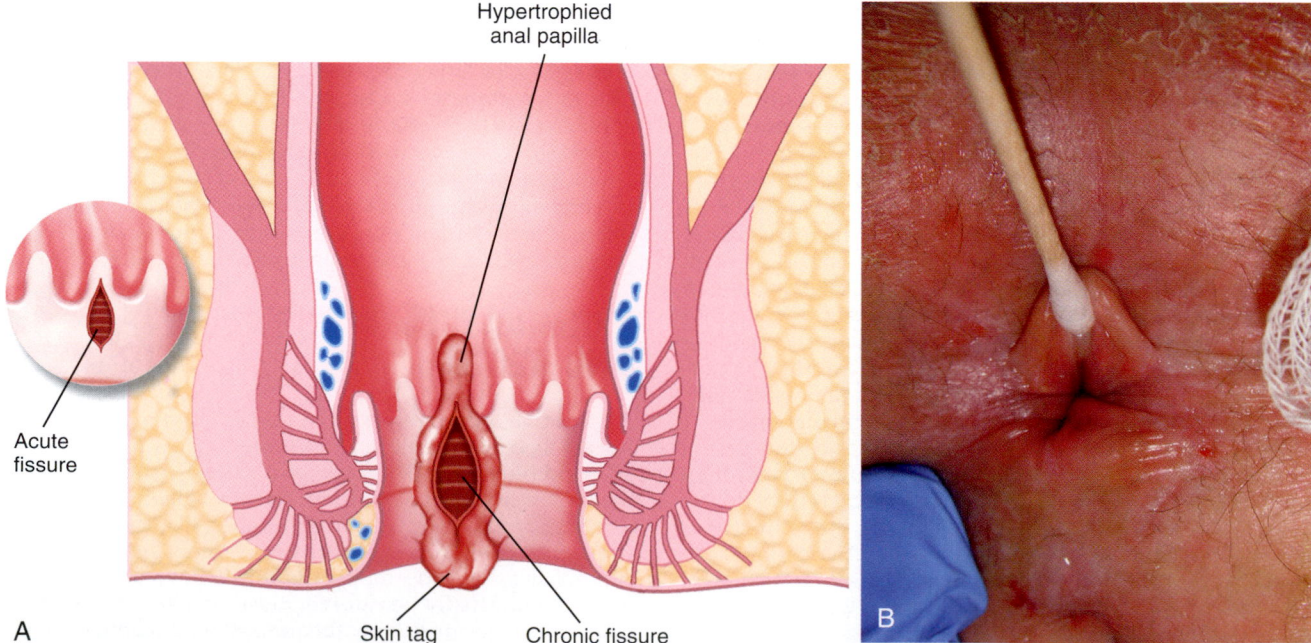

FIGURE 129-2. *A,* Schematic depiction of acute and chronic anal fissures. An acute fissure is depicted in the *inset on the left* as simply a split in the anoderm. A chronic fissure can show signs of chronicity with rolled edges, fibrosis, a hypertrophied anal papilla proximally, a tender distal skin tag, and exposed internal anal musculature. *B,* Inspection of an acute anal fissure with a cotton-tip swab. Once an acute fissure is identified, no internal examination is needed until the fissure is healed.

Abnormalities sometimes appreciated in the anal canal include fistula tracts, which feel like a cord or linear induration; the internal opening of a fistula, which may be appreciated as a knob of tissue in an otherwise smooth area of mucosa; cancers, which may be firm and hard; and ulcers, which feel uneven and craterous. Palpation anteriorly in a woman may reveal a rectocele or anterior defect in the sphincter complex.

Palpation of the distal rectum allows the detection of mass lesions, including polyps and cancers. Attention should be directed to the exact location of the lesion (anterior, posterior, right, left) and its size, mobility, and character (soft, ulcerated, hard, or pedunculated). Lesions outside the rectal wall also may be appreciated. The cervix can be felt through the anterior rectal wall in women, and the prostate should be examined in men. The character of the prostate should be noted, along with any hard nodularity that could represent cancer. The rectal mucosa should be assessed for its texture; in patients with proctitis, for example, the mucosa can feel rough and gritty; in patients with severe hypoalbuminemia, it can feel wet and slippery.

The levator muscles should be palpated. In some patients, especially women with unexplained anorectal pain, these muscles may be in spasm and tender (the levator ani syndrome). Similarly, the coccyx should be palpated between the examining internal index finger and the index finger of the opposite hand pressed over the external skin at the level of the coccyx. This maneuver is done to look for pain with motion (coccygodynia), as might be present with a coccygeal fracture.

The contents of the rectum should be assessed regarding the character and amount of stool. When the index finger is removed, any stool, blood, pus, or mucus on the glove should be noted.

Endoscopy

The decision to perform endoscopy depends on the findings on history and physical examination. Endoscopy usually is necessary for the evaluation and exclusion of organic disease in patients with fecal incontinence, constipation, unexplained anal pain,[6] anemia, diarrhea, and rectal bleeding.

Anoscopy

Anoscopy allows visualization of the anal canal, dentate line, internal hemorrhoids, and distal rectum. This is the best method of viewing the anal canal. The anoscope is a short metal or plastic tubular device, usually with a beveled end. Most adult anoscopes have a 2-cm diameter, but smaller ones are available. A fiberoptic light attachment provides optimal illumination; however, external lighting is used with some models.

The lubricated anoscope is inserted slowly as the examiner applies gentle pressure on the end of the obturator until the instrument has been fully advanced. An anoscope should *never* be inserted or turned without the obturator in place. The obturator is then removed, and the entire anal canal region is examined. This includes the distal rectum, followed by the upper anal canal, down to the anoderm. To reinsert the scope and view another area, the obturator must be replaced. Internal hemorrhoids can be seen bulging above the dentate line or prolapsing downward. Internal fistulous openings may be viewed, particularly along the dentate line. When the external skin is compressed, pus may be seen to bubble from the internal opening of a fistula. Rarely, the anoscope is needed to remove a low rectal polyp that cannot be removed by flexible endoscopy.

Rigid Proctoscopy

Rigid proctosigmoidoscopy is performed mainly by colorectal surgeons today. The rigid proctoscope is 25 cm long and 11 to 20 mL in diameter. It requires fiberoptic light for visualization.

In the modern era of video sigmoidoscopes, there are still some instances when a rigid proctoscope is advantageous. The proctoscope can be used to measure the exact distance of a rectal tumor from the anal verge. It also can give the precise location of a lesion on the wall of the rectum, whereas flexible scopes cannot easily discern anatomic left, right, anterior, and posterior—all information essential to operative planning. The rigid proctoscope is sometimes quicker and easier to use than a flexible instrument when evaluating the rectum, doing a biopsy, or aspirating fecal contents. The biopsy forceps used with flexible endoscopes also can be used through the rigid proctoscope, although typically a rigid alligator-toothed forceps is preferred.

Flexible Sigmoidoscopy

The flexible sigmoidoscope is simply a shorter version of a colonoscope, measuring 60 cm in length. Most endoscopists use a gastroscope for sigmoidoscopy because it is thinner, better tolerated by the patient than a sigmoidoscope or colonoscope, and easier to maneuver. One to 2 enemas are given before the examination, and sedation typically is not used, which is the reason patients who have undergone both colonoscopy and flexible sigmoidoscopy report that the latter was more difficult.[7] The goal is to examine the left colon, which should be reached at least 80% of the time.[8] Lesions can be biopsied and polyps removed, although the presence of polyps mandates full colonoscopy after a bowel preparation to exclude synchronous polyps or cancer. The use of electrocautery and argon plasma coagulation should be avoided during sigmoidoscopy, even if enemas have just been given and the preparation appears optimal, because intracolonic bowel explosions have occurred from ignition of bowel gas that has passed from the stool-containing proximal colon distally to the operative site.[9]

Flexible sigmoidoscopy can be used to enhance the diagnostic capability of barium enema, which at times fails to visualize the distal rectum optimally because of the obscuring effect of the balloon needed to distend the colon. Lesions of the rectum and sigmoid seen on radiologic studies also can be evaluated by flexible sigmoidoscopy. Flexible sigmoidoscopy permits serial examinations and treatments of diseases located in the rectosigmoid and left colon, such as proctosigmoiditis and radiation proctitis.

HEMORRHOIDS

Physicians face several unique problems when evaluating a patient complaining of hemorrhoids. First among these is that patients often attribute all anal symptoms to hemorrhoids.[10] In our practice, the majority of patients whose chief complaint is "hemorrhoids" have some other explanation for their symptom (e.g., fissure, pruritus ani, warts). Second is that hemorrhoids are a normal part of anatomy[11,12]; their presence does not imply a disease state. The corollary to this is that hemorrhoids can be expected to coexist with other anal pathology. Third is the multitude of treatment options available for treating hemorrhoids ensure there is no 1 treatment appropriate to every patient. Lastly, patients are fearful of hemorrhoid surgery, having usually heard "horror" stories related to hemorrhoidectomy.

Hemorrhoids are dilated vascular channels between the anal mucosa and underlying internal anal sphincter. They typically occur in the left lateral, right posterior, and right anterior positions. The presence of abnormalities that appear to be hemorrhoidal but are found in atypical locations of the anus may suggest their nature is other than hemorrhoidal (e.g., carcinoma, lymphoma, infectious masses). Internal hemorrhoids originate above the dentate line and are covered by columnar or transitional mucosa. External hemorrhoids are distal to the dentate line and are covered by squamous epithelium. Hemorrhoid complaints are common, accounting for between 1.9 and 3.5 million visits to physicians annually in the United States.[13] Common symptoms attributable to hemorrhoids include bleeding, prolapse, and swelling. Pain usually occurs only with thrombosis.

Hemorrhoid treatments have been recorded throughout human history. It is sobering to realize how closely today's treatments resemble those used for millennia: the Edwin Smith Papyrus (1700 BC) describes an infusion of acacia leaves, which is similar to witch hazel used today. Cautery was applied by Hippocrates (400 BC), and ligation was described by Celsus (25 BC-14 AD).[14]

Internal Hemorrhoids

Internal hemorrhoid symptoms probably occur because of loss of connective tissue support and resulting prolapse, rendering the vascular tissue more susceptible to trauma from straining or the passage of hard stools.[15] They are more likely to cause symptoms in patients with constipation, loose stools, or in those who sit on the toilet for prolonged periods of time.[16] Bleeding is painless and may be on the tissue or in the toilet. It may also be described as dripping and bright red. Less commonly it can accumulate in the rectum and be passed as dark blood or clots.[12] Prolapse can be graded as follows: grade I hemorrhoids may bleed but do not prolapse; grade II hemorrhoids protrude with defecation and reduce spontaneously; grade III hemorrhoids prolapse and can require manual reduction; grade IV hemorrhoids remain prolapsed.[12] Prolapsed hemorrhoids may cause blood or mucus on the patient's underwear. Perianal moisture can cause itching.[11] Although the exact incidence of hemorrhoidal disease is unknown, it is thought to be present in 10% to 25% of the adult population.

Evaluation

The diagnosis of internal hemorrhoids is best made with physical examination augmented by anoscopy using a beveled or slotted anoscope. Gentle eversion of the anal margin may reveal prolapsing hemorrhoidal tissue. Internal hemorrhoids also may be seen with flexible endoscopy on retrograde view. Anoscopy allows visualization of the degree of protrusion. In between symptomatic periods the exam may be normal.

Treatment

The initial treatment of symptomatic internal hemorrhoids is usually medical and consists of adequate fluid intake (6 to 8 glasses of nonalcoholic, noncaffeinated beverage daily), a high-fiber diet or fiber supplement (20 to 30 g daily), and recommendation to avoid straining and prolonged time on the toilet.[17,18] Patients may keep a diet diary to assess their usual fiber intake, then either alter their diet or add supplemental fiber. If stools remain hard, stool softeners such as docusate sodium can be added. Laxative and enemas are rarely needed.[19] These measures are also useful in preventing hemorrhoidal recurrence. Transient improvement may be obtained with some over-the-counter products. Hard stools or constipation symptoms may be treated with polyethylene glycol 3350 or docusate when fiber therapy alone is insufficient. Topical creams such as phenyleph-min oil-petrolatum or glucocorticoid-based creams may temporarily improve pain or itching. Glycerin suppositories have little if any role in treating hemorrhoids.

Phlebotonics are a heterogeneous class of drugs including plant extracts or flavonoids. They are known to improve venous tone and to stabilize capillary permeability. They are useful in alleviating bleeding from hemorrhoids and have an excellent safety profile.[20] Diosmiplex (Vasculera, Ferndale Laboratories) is 1 such product we usually add in the treatment of grade I and II hemorrhoids that have failed to resolve with fiber therapy and counseling.

When medical treatment is insufficient, more aggressive treatment may be needed. Nonsurgical treatment is usually tried unless the patient has grade IV hemorrhoids or has a large external component causing symptoms. Most nonoperative treatments are designed to affix the vascular cushion to the underlying sphincter. Options to achieve such fixation include rubber band ligation, sclerotherapy, cryotherapy, infrared photocoagulation, and ligation.

Rubber Band Ligation

Rubber band ligation (RBL) is the most common office procedure for the treatment of hemorrhoids[21] and is usually applied to grade II and III hemorrhoids. In addition to creating a scar and fixing the hemorrhoid to the underlying tissue, a small amount of hemorrhoidal tissue is actually removed when the RBL-entrapped hemorrhoid sloughs. Grade I hemorrhoids may be too small to be trapped by the band, and grade IV hemorrhoids are poorly treated with this technique.[22]

Rubber bands are usually applied by a colorectal surgeon via a slotted anoscope and by a gastroenterologist using a flexible gastroscope, usually in the retroview position. No bowel preparation is routinely used unless visualization is impaired, in which case a single sodium biphosphate and sodium phosphate enema may be used. Antibiotics are not used. Bands are placed just proximal to the internal anal cushion, above the dentate line. Distal placement that entraps squamous mucosa results in pain, and the band must be removed; bands should not be placed distal to the dentate line and are not used for external hemorrhoids. The number of bands placed at 1 sitting is controversial. Although studies have shown that multiple bands can be safely placed during a single procedure,[21,23] we generally band only 1 site per office visit in order to minimize pain. The patient is reassessed in 3 to 4 weeks, and repeat banding performed if needed. Most patients can be managed with 3 or fewer procedures. Often the offending column is easily seen and dealt with in a single visit.

Patients sometimes experience pain after RBL. They are advised to soak in a warm tub and use acetaminophen for pain. Narcotics are sometimes required. Immediate, severe pain usually signals too distal band placement, and the band should be removed. Symptoms vary from patient to patient. Most experience a feeling of rectal fullness or urge to defecate, which can last a day or 2; some experience no symptoms at all. Fiber and water are continued as described earlier. RBL is successful in 75% of patients with grade I and II hemorrhoids and in 65% of those with grade III hemorrhoids. Recurrence occurs in about 20% of hemorrhoids treated.

Major complications from RBL include bleeding, sepsis, cellulitis, and death. Some bleeding is common 4 to 7 days after the procedure when the band is usually sloughed. About 1% of patients develop severe bleeding requiring treatment,[23] although bleeding sometimes ceases with no intervention needed. Bleeding may be controlled with injection of epinephrine, suture ligation, or tamponade with a large-caliber Foley catheter balloon placed in the rectum. Severe bleeding mandates observation because quantification of blood loss is difficult, patients may become hypotensive, and rebleeding may occur.

A more serious complication is sepsis, which can be life threatening.[24] This is usually seen 2 to 8 days after banding. This complication should be considered in patients with worsening pain, difficulty urinating, and fever; these symptoms should be asked about when patients call with concerns after RBL. Patients at greatest risk for sepsis are those who are immunocompromised or have hematologic malignancies. Suture ligation should be used in immunocompromised patients. There is no demonstrated efficacy for prophylactic antibiotics in this population. Treatment is surgical débridement and IV antibiotics.

A relatively new technique for RBL, the CRH-O'Regan disposable hemorrhoid banding system, is a highly effective, minimally invasive and painless procedure that is performed in the office setting and can be completed in just a few minutes. Using a plastic anoscope and a gentle suction device, a small rubber band is placed around the rectal tissue just above the internal hemorrhoid, where there are a few pain-sensitive nerve endings. The procedure works by interrupting the blood supply to the hemorrhoid, causing the hemorrhoid to shrink and fall off, typically within a day or so. The resulting small ulcer usually heals within one to five days. Osborn and colleagues reported 257 internal hemorrhoidal banding events in 113 patients with a 94% rate of resolution of initial symptoms and a complication rate of about 1% each for pain and thrombosis and close to 2% for urinary hesitancy. Symptom resolution or improvement was reported via questionnaire to persist in more than 80% of patients at a 3-month follow-up.[24a]

RBL should not be electively performed on patients who are being treated with anticoagulants or antiplatelet agents. In such cases, either suture ligation may be performed, or if a short period off these agents is considered safe, they should be discontinued and not rebegun until a week after RBL.

Sclerosing Agents

Injection therapy for hemorrhoids has been practiced for more than 100 years. The goal is to inject an irritant into the submucosa above the internal hemorrhoid at the anorectal ring (this area does not have somatic innervation) to create fibrosis, tack down the hemorrhoid tissue, and prevent prolapse.[25] Usually 3 to 5 mL of sclerosant is injected at the apex of the hemorrhoid column.[5] The most common sclerosant is 5% phenol in an oil base. This is most successful in grade I and II hemorrhoids.

Sclerotherapy can produce a dull pain for up to 2 days after injection. Sepsis can rarely occur. Symptoms of sepsis usually occur 3 to 5 days after treatment and may be accompanied by perianal pain or swelling, watery anal discharge, fever, and leukocytosis. Prompt surgical intervention and IV antibiotics are mandatory.[24,25]

Patients with AIDS are often offered sclerotherapy because of their increased risk of complications with RBL.[26]

Cryotherapy

Cryotherapy uses liquid nitrogen to freeze tissue, thereby destroying the hemorrhoidal plexus. It has fallen out of favor because of difficulty in controlling the amount of tissue destroyed, the time it takes to perform the procedure, and the foul-smelling discharge resulting from tissue necrosis.[27]

Infrared Photocoagulation

Infrared photocoagulation uses infrared radiation to coagulate the tissue, leading to fibrosis. It is applied for 1.5 seconds to 2 or 3 sites proximal to the hemorrhoidal plexus. Multiple hemorrhoids can be treated at 1 visit. For grade I and II hemorrhoids, reported results are as good as those obtained with RBL or sclerotherapy,[22] although our experience tends to favor RBL. Larger hemorrhoids do less well with this treatment. Pain and other complications are rare with this procedure. We often use it on patients with small, bleeding, internal hemorrhoids and on patients who cannot tolerate RBL.

Surgical Therapy

Patients with hemorrhoids have increased anal canal pressure.[28] Anal dilation and sphincterotomy to reduce pressure were performed in the past but have no role in the treatment of hemorrhoids today.[29] Sphincterotomy is sometimes performed at the time of hemorrhoidectomy in patients with concomitant anal fissure.

Hemorrhoidectomy is the procedure of choice for patients with grade III hemorrhoids unresponsive to other measures, for most patients with grade IV disease, and for those who have symptomatic external hemorrhoids. This can be done under local, regional, or general anesthesia and is usually done as a day-surgery procedure. The wounds may be left open or closed and the excision performed with scalpel, cautery, or other energy device.[17,30,31] Long-term follow-up reveals a 26% recurrence rate at a median of 17 years, with 11% requiring an additional procedure.[29]

The most significant drawback to surgery for hemorrhoids is pain. Essentially every alternative to surgery mentioned, as well as every technical variation discussed, represents an attempt to minimize pain while alleviating the symptoms troubling the patient. Many adjuncts have been shown to decrease pain after hemorrhoidectomy, including topical agents such as glyceryl trinitrate,[32] anesthetic cream,[33] sucralfate,[34] and metronidazole.[35] A long-acting local anesthetic of liposome bupivacaine has been shown to reduce pain after hemorrhoidectomy and is routinely used today.

Two other surgical procedures deserve mention here because they are widely used and provide symptom relief similar to hemorrhoidectomy in selected patients, although with decreased pain. These are the procedure for prolapsing hemorrhoids (PPH) and Doppler-guided hemorrhoid artery ligation.

The PPH, also called *hemorrhoidopexy*, was introduced in 1998 by Longo[36] and uses a circular stapling device that excises a circumferential ring of mucosa just above the anorectal ring, interrupting the vascular supply to the cushions and restoring them to their correct positions (Fig. 129-3). It is used primarily for grade III and IV hemorrhoids. Results of randomized multicenter experience in the United States compared the PPH with excisional hemorrhoidectomy and showed that PPH-treated patients experienced significantly less pain.[37] Another study comparing PPH with RBL found patients reported more pain and an increased risk of postoperative bleeding with PPH; however, more patients in the RBL group required subsequent hemorrhoidectomy for persistent symptoms.[38]

PPH can have significant postoperative complications, of which bleeding and urinary retention are most common.[37] Severe, persistent postoperative pain occurs in one third of patients and may be related to placing the staple line too close to the dentate line.[39] The frequency of this complication has made us less likely to use this technique. Additionally, defecation urgency can be persistent in up to 28% of patients. Perhaps the most feared complication is pelvic sepsis leading

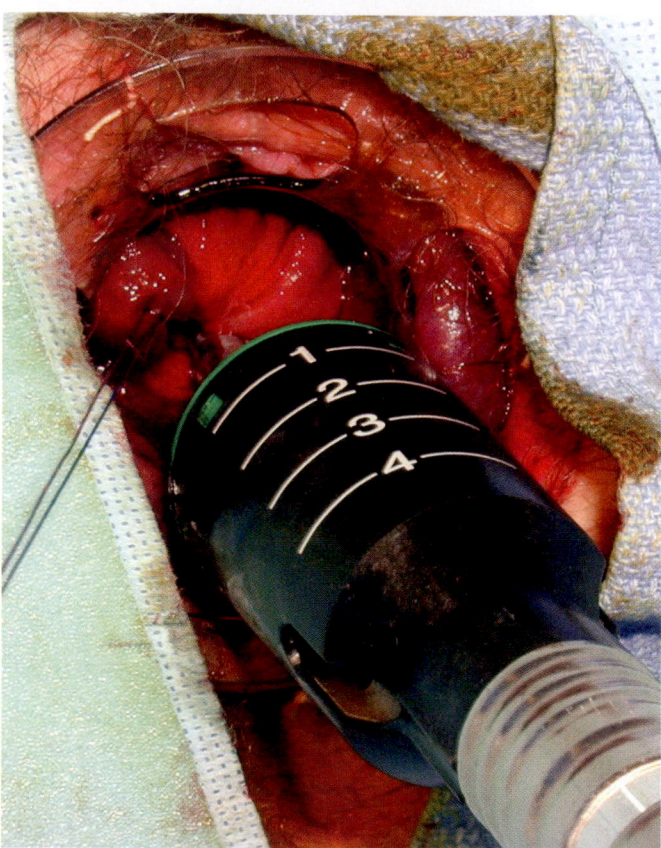

FIGURE 129-3. Stapled hemorrhoidopexy procedure. A purse-string suture is placed at the top of the hemorrhoidal column, around which a circular stapler is applied to resect the upper hemorrhoidal tissue, disrupt the hemorrhoidal blood supply, and restore the prolapsing distal hemorrhoidal tissue back into the anal canal.

to death.[40] Long-term results from prospective randomized studies comparing hemorrhoidectomy and PPH suggest a higher rate of recurrent symptoms in the PPH group.[41,42]

Doppler-guided hemorrhoidal artery ligation was described in 1995[43] and allows the Doppler probe to guide suture ligation in the lower rectum to interrupt blood flow to the anal canal. It is reported to have a recurrence rate of 9.0% for prolapse, and 7.8% for bleeding at 1 year.[44] A recent study showed similar results using ligation with and without the Doppler, suggesting the efficacy of the procedure was related to extensive ligation.[45]

Both PPH and ligation will control symptoms related to internal hemorrhoids, although neither specifically address the symptom related to external hemorrhoids, which should be excised at the time of surgery if symptomatic.

Table 129-1 summarizes the treatment options for internal hemorrhoids.

External Hemorrhoids and Anal Tags

Symptoms and Signs

External hemorrhoids are visible at the anal verge and actually represent residual redundant skin from previous episodes of external hemorrhoid inflammation, edema, and thrombosis. These skin tags typically occur in young and middle-aged adults and are easily seen on inspection. They usually cause no symptoms and do not bleed. Some patients complain of difficult hygiene related to the redundant folds of tissue, and of itching and irritation.

External hemorrhoids can manifest with acute symptoms related to thrombosis.[15] The level of pain is variable, ranging from none to severe disabling pain. Thrombosed hemorrhoids are easily diagnosed on physical exam. The overlying skin is taut, and bluish discoloration related to the underlying blood clot is usually evident. The overlying skin may ulcerate and bleed; such bleeding usually lasts 1 or 2 days and may alleviate pain.

Treatment

Treatment of external hemorrhoids is usually reassurance and proper anal hygiene, including delicate washing of the anal area and avoidance of aggressive wiping with harsh tissue. Excision can be performed, although wound healing in this area is often accompanied by skin tag formation, which can cause the same symptoms the patient sought to alleviate. When surgical excision is undertaken for internal hemorrhoids, as discussed earlier, any significant external component is excised at the same time.

Treatment of thrombosed external hemorrhoids depends on associated symptoms, specifically pain. When painless, the patient can be reassured that the swelling will subside over the next several weeks. When painful, excision may be helpful. We offer excision to patients with significant pain and in whom symptoms have been occurring for less than 3 days. Untreated, the pain typically subsides in 4 to 7 days, so excision at this point is not helpful. The outcome at 2 months is the same whether or not excision is performed. For severe pain, the clot is removed under local anesthesia. Because of the high rate of recurrent symptoms with simple incision, most surgeons recommend enucleation of the entire thrombosis along with excision of an ellipse of overlying skin. This procedure is done in the office with scissors and local anesthesia (Fig. 129-4).[46] The edges are usually left open to heal by secondary intention, but may be closed. If surgery is not performed, the patient is treated with sitz baths, analgesics, and a topical astringent such as witch hazel.

Topical nifedipine as a 0.3% cream has been used successfully.[47] It is speculated that this medication reduces pain both from its anti-inflammatory and smooth muscle-relaxing properties. It can reduce the need for excision.

Special Considerations

Crohn's disease commonly has anal manifestations (see Chapter 115), 1 of which may be large, edematous, shiny perianal skin tags (Fig. 129-5). They can have a waxy, bluish discoloration and may be described as "funny looking" or as "elephant ears". Also, the hemorrhoid-mimicking lesions of Crohn's disease often are found in atypical locations, not the usual location of hemorrhoids in the left lateral, right anterior, and right posterior positions. Careful history taking for symptoms of Crohn's disease is indicated. If suspected, colonoscopy with inspection of the terminal ileum is indicated. Excision of anal skin tags in Crohn's disease is to be avoided because of the risk of ulceration and nonhealing wounds.

Patients who are infected with HIV are treated as other patients as long as their immune status in not significantly compromised. Sclerotherapy in this group was previously mentioned. Patients with CD4 counts above $420/mm^3$ have been treated with RBL with good results.[48] Patients with CD4 counts below 200 may have poor wound healing, and surgery should be approached cautiously.

TABLE 129-1 Treatment Options for Internal Hemorrhoids

Type of Treatment	Hemorrhoid Grades	Success Rate	Comments
General			
Diet (increase in fiber and fluids) and bowel habit modification	1-4	Unknown	Patients with all grades of hemorrhoids should use these measures (see text) Patients with high grades of hemorrhoids will need additional therapy
Endoscopic			
Sclerosing agent	1-4	75%	May be the favored treatment of patients with AIDS (successful results even with grade 3 and 4 hemorrhoids) Life-threatening sepsis rarely complicates therapy
Rubber band ligation	2 and 3	65%-75%	Grade 1 hemorrhoids are too small, and grade 4 hemorrhoids are usually too large for this procedure The most commonly performed office procedure for hemorrhoids Life-threatening sepsis rarely complicates therapy; 1% risk of severe hemorrhage when band sloughs
Infrared coagulation	1 and 2	Less than for rubber band ligation	Equipment for the procedure is expensive Rare complications
Surgical			
Excisional hemorrhoidectomy	3 and 4	>85% on 10-year follow-up	External tags may be removed at the time of the surgical procedure Postoperative pain is pronounced
Procedure for prolapsing hemorrhoids (PPH)*	3 and 4	>75%; several studies show higher long-term recurrence rates than with excisional hemorrhoidectomy	Newer procedure Overall, significantly less postoperative pain than with excisional hemorrhoidectomy, but some patients experience severe, persistent postoperative pain or defecation urgency Pelvic sepsis and death have been reported after this procedure

*Also called *stapled hemorrhoidopexy.*

Pregnant women often have symptomatic hemorrhoids. These should be treated medically with fiber, fluid, and stool softeners. Topical medications may be used. Surgery is reserved for severe complications, such as acute prolapsed hemorrhoids with strangulation.

Patients on anticoagulation represent a unique challenge because they are more likely to bleed as a result of their medication and as a result of their procedure. There is no standard approach for these patients. For elective excision, the anticoagulants are managed as with any other surgical procedure. For patients with acutely bleeding hemorrhoids, RBL may be cautiously performed with the knowledge that they are at increased risk of bleeding when the band sloughs off in 4 to 7 days. Hemorrhoidectomy offers this group of patients the advantage that definitive therapy can be carried out as a single procedure, thereby minimizing the time off anticoagulation.

ANAL FISSURE

An anal fissure is a linear tear of the anoderm (see Fig. 129-2). Anal fissures typically occur after passage of a large, hard bowel movement, but they may also occur with diarrhea, IBD, or for unknown reasons. Patients experience intense pain that most often manifests with (or is greatly exacerbated by) the passage of stool. Pain may be associated with bright red blood. More than 90% of anal fissures are located in the posterior midline of the anus; 10% are anterior.[5] Any fissure not located in the anterior or posterior position or one that does not heal should alert the physician to the possibility of other diagnoses (e.g., Crohn's disease, TB, syphilis, squamous cell cancer of the anus, a leukemic ulcer, or an HIV-related ulcer).[5]

Etiology

The exact etiology of an anal fissure is unknown; however, reduced anodermal blood flow associated with hypertonicity of the internal anal sphincter is the most common accompanying physiology. Cadaveric and manometric studies have respectively revealed decreased blood supply to the posterior midline and elevated resting anal canal pressures in patients with fissure-in-ano.[5] Therefore, the main strategies for treatment of anal fissure are aimed at reducing resting intra-anal pressure and increasing anodermal blood flow.

Symptoms, Signs, and Diagnosis

Fissures are exquisitely tender, and the act of defecation is reported by patients to feel like passing "razor blades" or "cut glass." The classic history is severe pain during defecation, but patients can experience continued pain or burning after defecation for several hours. On examination, a tender edematous skin tag may be seen distal to the fissure; simply spreading the buttocks will allow its visualization. At this point in the exam, one should stop so as not to subject the patient to

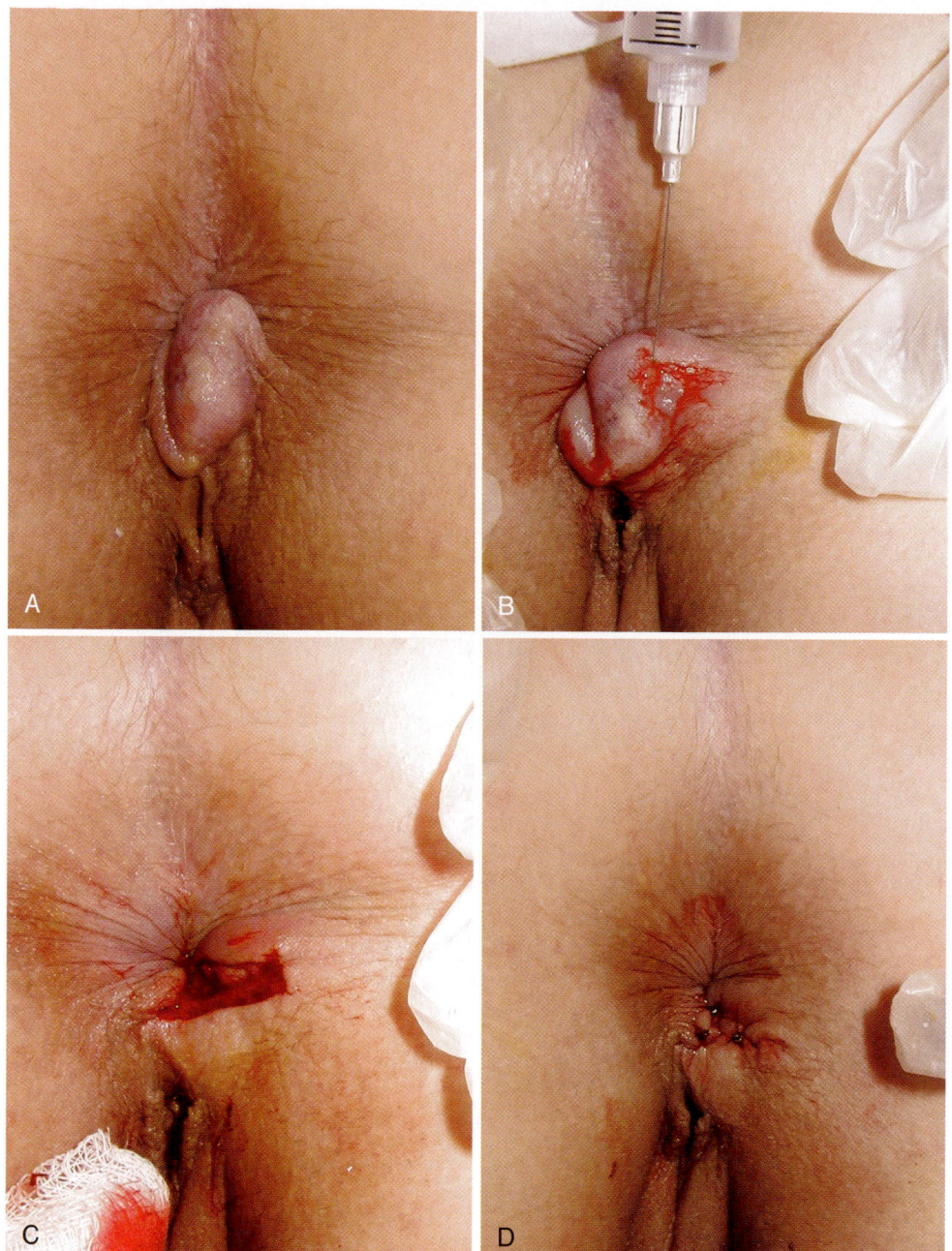

FIGURE 129-4. Office excision of a thrombosed external hemorrhoid. *A*, Thrombosed right anterior external hemorrhoid. *B*, Injection of 1% lidocaine with epinephrine. *C*, Excision of external component. *D*, Closure with 2 or 3 interrupted absorbable sutures.

unnecessary and severe pain. If the anal canal can be visualized, a hypertrophied papilla may be seen in patients with a chronic fissure. The fissure, hypertrophied papilla, and sentinel skin tag represent the hallmark triad of features associated with a chronic anal fissure (see Fig. 129-2).

Fissures can be acute or chronic. Acute fissures are a split in the anoderm without exposed internal sphincter fibers. Chronic fissures show fibrotic edges and deep ulceration with exposure of the underlying internal sphincter muscle.

Treatment (Table 129-2)

Most acute anal fissures will resolve with increased fiber and water intake as well as hygiene and comfort measures. Initial management begins with correcting any abnormalities in stool

consistency. A fiber supplement, either in powder or pill form, with appropriate amounts of fluid is generally more rapid than dietary measures in restoring stool consistency. A high-fiber regimen consisting of 20 to 35 g/day was shown to achieve healing in 87% of acute fissures. Furthermore, the use of unprocessed bran in the diet prevents fissure recurrence after initial healing and should be continued long term.[1,49,50]

Medical Therapy

Medical therapies are very successful in treating fissure-in-ano, particularly acute fissures (i.e., those presenting within 3 to 6 weeks of symptom onset). The traditional first-line therapy for acute fissures is warm sitz baths and bran bulking agents, with reported healing rates of 87%.[3] Improvement of dietary

TABLE 129-2 Treatment of Acute and Chronic Anal Fissures

Treatment	Comments
Acute	
Increase oral fluids, high-fiber diet, fiber supplements, sitz baths, and stool softeners if needed	Avoid digital rectal examination until the fissure is healed unless the diagnosis is in doubt (then perform the examination in the operating room)
	Usually responds to these measures
Chronic	
As for acute, usually with the addition of one of the following:	Avoid digital examination unless the diagnosis is in doubt
0.2-0.4% nitroglycerin ointment applied to the anal area	Headache is a common side effect
	Long-term success has been questioned
Calcium channel blockers (topical nifedipine or topical 2% diltiazem cream) applied to the anal area	Seem promising, but long-term success has been questioned
	Side effects (especially headache) may be less common than with nitroglycerin ointment
Botulinum toxin A injected into the anal muscle	Dose and optimal injection site are not clear
	Expensive
	Long-term success is unknown
Lateral internal sphincterotomy	Standard treatment
	Best results, with >90% long-term healing rate
	Durable
	Can lead to fecal incontinence

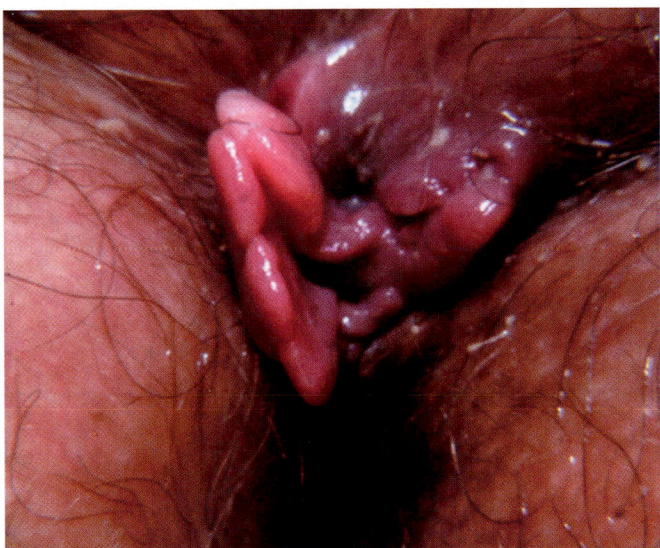

FIGURE 129-5. Anal skin tags associated with perianal Crohn's disease. Note the waxy bluish appearance of the tags. These are often referred to as "elephant ears".

and bowel evacuation habits of patients is a good long-term strategy and can help reduce the risk of fissures. Counseling on proper diet and institution of commercial bulking agents (e.g., psyllium seeds) are always indicated.

Patients with chronic fissures should be started on the acute fissure regimen, but are typically also started on other medical therapies as well. Nitroglycerin and calcium channel blockers are common medical modalities offered for treatment of fissures. Nitric oxide was reported to be the neurotransmitter mediating relaxation of the internal anal sphincter in the early 1990s. Since then, development and topical application of 0.2% glyceryl trinitrate ointment (GTN) has been found to relax the anal sphincter (see earlier), theoretically producing "reversible chemical sphincterotomy." For GTN, the limiting

side effects are headaches and tachyphylaxis; headache can be reduced by instructing the patient to rest lying down while applying the ointment and for shortly thereafter. Patients are also advised not to drive until they have seen the effects of the medication. Headaches may be reduced by using a finger cot or glove for application. Topical diltiazem (2%) produces similar efficacy with fewer side effects than GTN. Fissure healing can be anticipated in about 70% of patients with chronic fissures using GTN or diltiazem.[3]

The concept of reversible chemical sphincterotomy has also been applied to the use of internal sphincter injection of botulinum toxin (Botox), a technique that transiently produces striated muscle denervation leading to muscle paralysis and relaxation. In the treatment of chronic anal fissure, such relaxation of the internal anal sphincter is thought to promote increased blood flow to the affected perianal skin, allowing the fissure to heal;[3] however, a Cochrane review of the literature on nonsurgical therapies for anal fissure demonstrated no convincing evidence that botulinum injections were any more effective than placebo.[51] The most common side effect associated with botulinum toxin injections is temporary incontinence to flatus in up to 10% of patients. Two meta-analyses comparing Botox with lateral internal sphincterotomy (LIS) demonstrated that long-term healing was better with surgery, but that side effects and complications were far less frequent with Botox injection.[3]

Surgical Therapy

The standard treatment of chronic anal fissures has been LIS, and it remains the standard by which all other treatments must be measured. LIS can be performed using open or closed technique. Although the open technique allows clear visualization of the internal sphincter muscle, review of the literature does not support better healing rates for the open technique and generally describe a greater frequency of complications.[52] When open and closed sphincterotomy are considered together, large series confirm high success rates, with rates of fissure nonhealing and recurrence as low as 0% to 10%. Early and late complications can occur after LIS, including

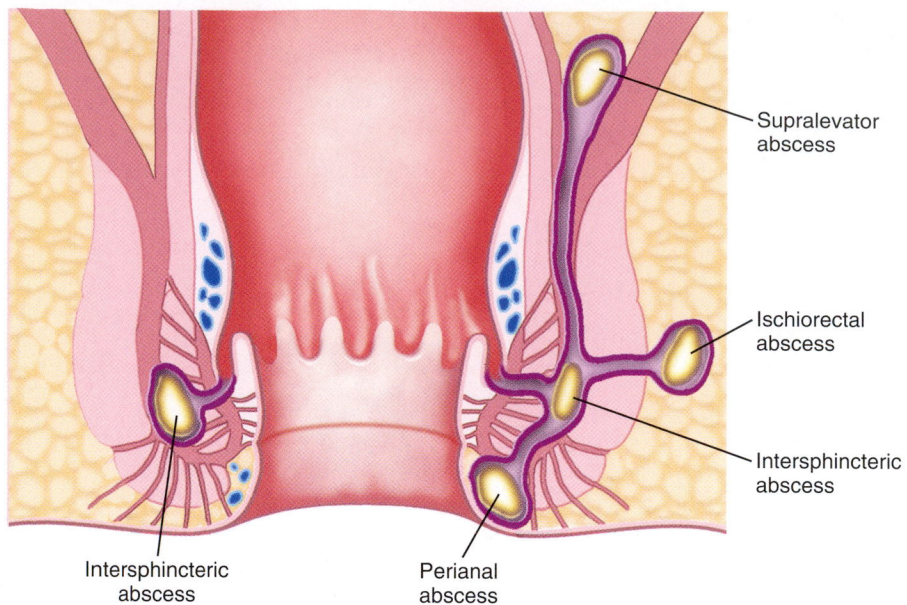

FIGURE 129-6. Schematic depiction of the classification of abscesses of the anal region based on their locations.

urinary retention, bleeding, and abscess or fistula formation, as well as seepage and (rarely) incontinence.[53]

ABSCESSES AND FISTULAS

Anorectal suppuration may have several causes, but by far the most common is a nonspecific infection of cryptoglandular origin. Other causes of infection are Crohn's disease, TB, actinomycosis, trauma, foreign bodies, anal surgery, pilonidal sinus, hidradenitis suppurativa, Bartholin's gland abscesses, carcinoma, and lymphoma. Infection originates in the intersphincteric plane, most likely in one of the anal glands. The most widely recognized cause is described in the cryptoglandular theory, which suggests that an anal gland becomes obstructed with inspissated debris and leads to infection.[54] These glands penetrate the anal sphincter complex to varying degrees, and the suppuration tends to follow the path of least resistance.

Abscesses

The abscess collects in whichever anatomic space the gland terminates, or wherever the path of least resistance leads. Anorectal abscesses are classified based on their location (Fig. 129-6). Four types of anorectal abscesses are commonly described: perianal (superficial), ischiorectal (perirectal), intersphincteric, and supralevator. Perianal is the most common type and is the simplest to treat. Collections are located in the superficial perianal tissues and typically are located close to the anal verge. Ischiorectal abscesses are located more deeply in the ischiorectal fossa and may extend to the contralateral side via the deep postanal space; this would be a classic example of a horseshoe abscess. Intersphincteric abscesses often are difficult to diagnose because they may reside completely within the anal canal. They are located in the intersphincteric space between the internal and external sphincter muscles. Patients affected by abscesses in this location complain of severe anal pain and often cannot tolerate an examination without anesthesia. The fluctuant collection may be found only by performing a digital rectal examination or anoscopy. Supralevator abscesses are rare and are typically diagnosed

through radiologic studies.[54] A patient presenting with this condition might complain of pelvic and rectal pain with tenesmus, but also of abdominal pain or symptoms of a urinary tract infection, because the abscess may extend superiorly in the abdomen. The abscess can sometimes be palpated by digital rectal examination performed by an experienced examiner. These abscesses are often related to perforated diverticular disease, IBD, or rarely neoplastic disease in the pelvis.

Treatment of a perineal abscess is incision and drainage; antibiotics alone are not adequate. Failure to drain an abscess promptly can result in spread to adjacent spaces, and some necrotizing infections can be mutilating and life threatening. Small abscesses can be drained in the office. The external opening should be made as close to the anal sphincter complex as possible without injuring it. Therefore, if a fistula develops, its tract will be short. The incision should be large enough or made in a cruciate fashion so that it will not close over before the inflammatory process has resolved.[54] Packing is used at the discretion of the surgeon. Large or high abscesses require drainage in the operating room. Hospitalization and IV antibiotics are reserved for patients who are immunocompromised or diabetic or who have signs of systemic infection. Patients should be closely followed to ensure that the process resolves.

Fistula-In-Ano

A fistula-in-ano is a tunnel that connects an internal opening, usually at an anal crypt at the base of the columns of Morgagni, with an external opening, usually on the perianal skin. Fistula-in-ano develops in half of the patients who undergo an incision and drainage of an anal abscess.[28] Fistulas are classified based on their relation to the anal sphincter complex and typically are divided into 5 common types: submucosal, intersphincteric, trans-sphincteric (high and low), suprasphincteric, and extrasphincteric. Submucosal fistulas typically originate at an offending crypt at the level of the dentate line, but track beneath the submucosa and do not involve the sphincter complex. These fistulas also may be opened without fear of compromising continence. Intersphincteric fistulas cross through the internal sphincter and exit into the intersphincteric plane. They do not involve the external sphincter muscle and can be opened without high risk of incontinence. Trans-sphincteric fistulas cross through the internal and external sphincter muscles to varying degrees. Low fistulas involve only the distal third of the external sphincter muscle, whereas high fistulas involve greater proportions of the external sphincter. This distinction is clinically significant because division of greater amounts of the external sphincter leads to higher rates of fecal incontinence. Suprasphincteric fistulas typically originate at the dentate line internally, cross above the external sphincter but below the puborectalis, and exit onto the perianal skin through the ischiorectal fossa. Extrasphincteric fistulas are rare and do not involve the sphincter complex. They typically arise from the pelvis or rectum above the dentate line, cross proximal to the sphincter complex into the ischiorectal fossa, and exit onto the perianal skin. These fistulas do not have an origin from the crypts and are often associated with IBD, pelvic inflammatory disease, and neoplasia.[54]

Treatment

Treatment of fistula-in-ano is surgical, and the course of the fistulous tract influences the type of surgery (Fig. 129-7). The most common treatment is a fistulotomy, or unroofing of the tunnel. Fistulotomy should not be performed if the tract traverses a substantial portion of the external sphincter, in which case its division will result in incontinence. Fistulas that are appropriate for fistulotomy can be unroofed, however, and the base curetted and allowed to heal from the bottom up. The cure rate for uncomplicated fistulas not associated with Crohn's disease approaches 100%.

A fistula that involves a substantial portion of the anal sphincter requires special treatment to avoid incontinence; therapeutic options are transanal advancement flap, skin advancement flap, fibrin glue injection, or collagen plug insertion. Transanal advancement flaps are a common surgical repair for these complex fistulas. Studies have found success rates varying from 65% to 75%. Rates of incontinence after a flap repair range from 9% to 35%. Alterations in continence tend to occur in patients older than age 50.[55]

Because traditional methods to repair complex fistulas have varied in their rates of incontinence, investigations into less invasive procedures have been performed. Fibrin glue from commercial fibrin sealant has been used to close anal fistulas. The principle of its sealant properties is based on clot formation, and knowledge of the clotting cascade allows understanding of its mode of action. Fibrin glue is a mixture of fibrinogen, thrombin, and calcium ions that, when combined, act to form a soluble clot because fibrinogen is cleaved into fibrin. This soluble clot is transformed into an insoluble, stable clot as the thrombin and calcium activate factor XIII. This reaction seals the fistula tract within 30 to 60 seconds as the glue sets. The glue also stimulates the migration and proliferation of fibroblasts and pluripotent endothelial cells to heal the fistula. Between days 7 and 14, plasmin that is present in the surrounding tissue lyses the fibrin clot as the tract is replaced by synthesized collagen. Studies have reported success rates for fistula closing of 59% to 92%, with most groups reporting a long-term success rate of less than 33%. The fistula tract is first curetted aggressively, and the fibrin product is injected via the external opening until it is seen emerging in the anal canal.[54] Few complications have been reported with this method and continence should not be affected.

Anal fistula plugs made from collagen are another option for treatment of complex fistulas (Fig. 129-8). The biological plug is made of lyophilized porcine small intestinal submucosa, which has an inherent resistance to infection, generates no foreign-body or giant cell reaction, and is repopulated by host cell tissue within 3 months. Its conical shape allows for added mechanical stability because high pressures within the anal canal maintain the plug in its proper position, avoiding dislodgement during straining. In the initial report by Armstrong, healing occurred in 83% of patients, with a median follow-up of 12 months; other groups, however, reported short-term success rates of 30% to 60%.[54]

A seton is a rubber band–like material that is threaded through a fistula, after which its 2 ends are tied loosely external to the outside skin (Fig. 129-9). Setons may be used to allow a fistulous tract to drain before surgical repair and thus

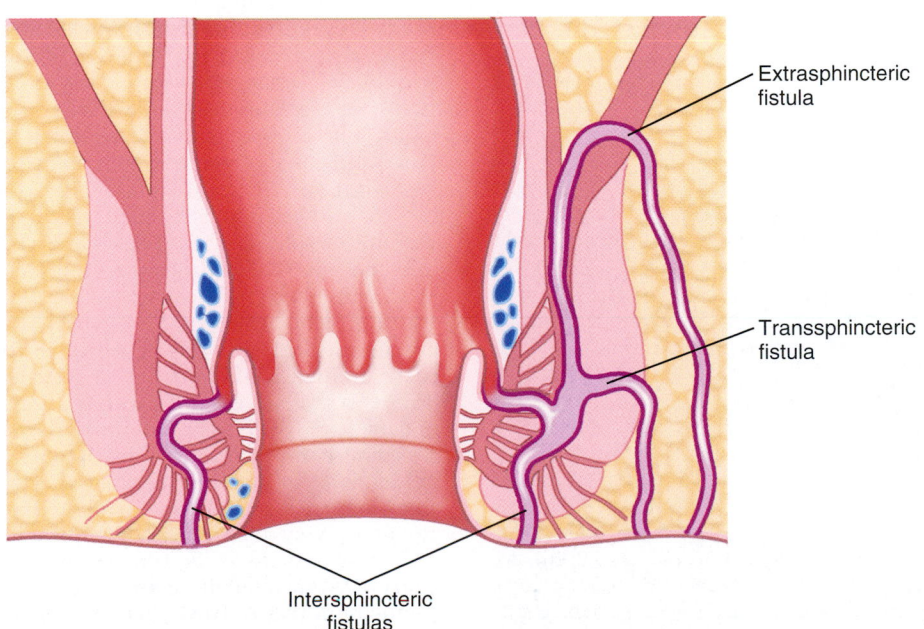

Extrasphincteric fistula

Transsphincteric fistula

Intersphincteric fistulas

FIGURE 129-7. Schematic depiction of the classification of fistula-in-ano. Fistulotomy is not appropriate for extrasphincteric fistulas, because it would leave the patient incontinent.

to prevent accumulation of pus; however, they can also be therapeutic if used as a cutting seton. In this latter approach, the seton is tightened gradually over weeks to months until it gradually cuts through muscle. This technique allows the fistulous tract to be unroofed gradually as the cut ends of the muscle scar close to their usual location, thereby lessening the chance of incontinence.[1] Setons also may be used as prolonged treatment of an anal fistula to prevent recurrent abscess formation. In this situation, the seton is tied loosely around the fistula tract, its presence preventing closure of any part of the fistula. The patient will have some minor continuous drainage but is unlikely to develop further abscess formation. This technique is considered when a patient has anal Crohn's disease, multiple fistulas, has had failed multiple procedures in the past, or is a poor candidate for surgery.

More novel approaches designed to surgically extirpate or interrupt anal fistulas include the "coring out" procedure, or fistulectomy and ligation of the intersphincteric fistula tract (LIFT) procedure. The LIFT procedure is compelling because it does not involve dividing any sphincter muscle. An incision is made in the intersphincteric groove below the fistula, and dissection is carried proximally between the sphincters up to the fistula tract. Placing a fistula probe through the fistula facilitates its identification. The tract is identified and is then suture ligated with absorbable suture material. Studies have revealed success rates ranging from 57% to 82%.[54]

Special Fistulas

Fistulas resulting from Crohn's disease may pose a difficult dilemma. Just as the cause of Crohn's disease is multifactorial, the treatment is multidisciplinary. Fistulizing Crohn's disease involves the anus in one third of patients (see Chapter 115). It may cause variable degrees of inflammatory stigmata, such as abscesses, fistulas, fissures, ulcerations, strictures, and large skin tags. Treatment of an acute Crohn's abscess follows the same rules as for any other abscess—it requires drainage. In the long term, treatment may include antibiotics and immunosuppressive medications. Once the active infection is controlled, biologic agents may be used to help resolve any remaining inflammation. Once anti-TNF therapy starts and the perineal inflammation begins to respond, setons can be removed and fistulas then followed to document closure. In the absence of active perineal disease or proctitis, any fistulas should be managed using 1 or more of the sphincter-preserving techniques. Repeat surgery may be necessary to ultimately achieve success; draining setons may be used chronically, and diversion with colostomy or ileostomy may be an option.[1]

The surgical management of fistula-in-ano is driven by the amount of sphincter complex that is involved with the tract, and the potential coexistence of Crohn's disease. Sphincter-sparing methods have lower success rates than non-sphincter-sparing techniques but come with little or no risk to fecal continence. The first line of treatment of this disease should focus on methods that do not require any sphincter division. These techniques do not prevent a more aggressive surgical approach if they fail. Submucosal fistulas can be treated by fistulotomy with little risk. Intersphincteric and trans-sphincteric fistulas may be treated with fistulotomy as first-line management if the patient has perfect continence preoperatively and no previous history of sphincter injury.[54]

Anterior fistulas in women must be approached with caution. Almost all are related to obstetric injury, and few are cryptoglandular in origin. The local tissue is scarred and too rigid for successful treatment with advancement flaps. The anovaginal septum is usually very thin. Repair of the sphincter in conjunction with repair of the fistula to give more tissue

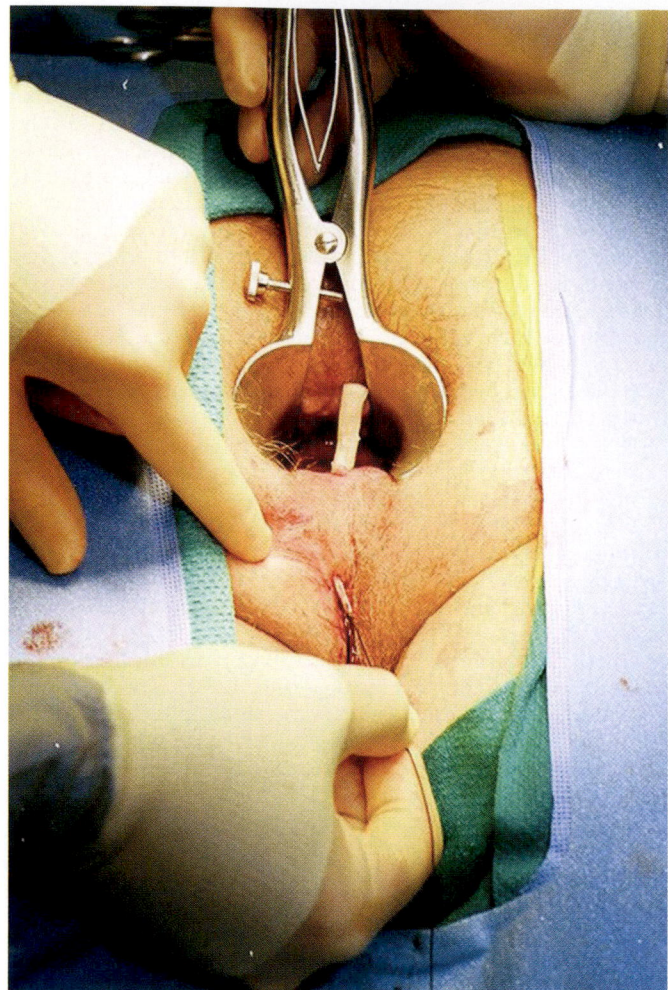

FIGURE 129-8. Anal fistula plug being placed through an anterior anal fistula tract. Once it is pulled snugly through the tract, the plug is secured internally and the internal opening closed. Excess plug projecting externally is also trimmed.

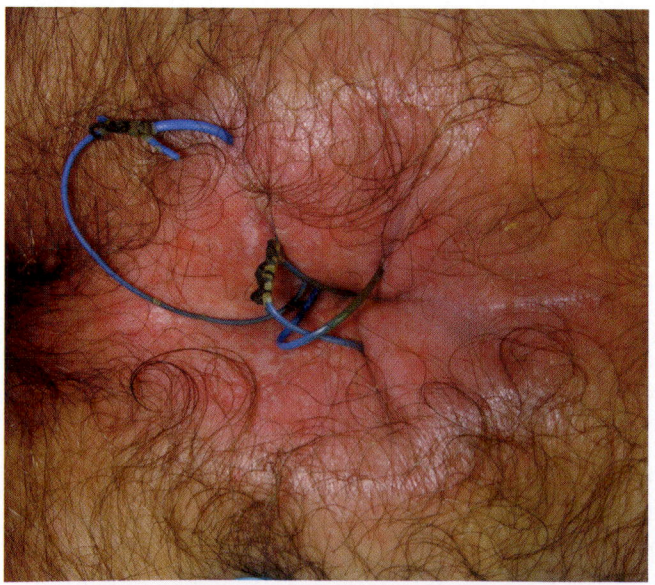

FIGURE 129-9. Blue setons placed through fistulous tracts in a patient with anal Crohn's disease.

bulk to the anovaginal septum is the procedure of choice in this challenging situation.

ANAL MALIGNANCIES

Anal cancers are rare and account for 1.5% of GI cancers in the United States, with about 6200 new cases each year.[56] The incidence has increased 2% to 3% every year since the early 1980s, largely because of the increased incidence of anal cancer in HIV-infected patients, in whom the incidence has risen from 19.0/100,000 per year (1992-1995) to 78.2/100,00 per year (2000-2003).[56] This rising incidence has not been slowed by HAART. Almost 80% of anal cancers are squamous cell cancers, 16% are adenocarcinomas, and 4% are other types.[57] Adenocarcinoma of the anal canal behaves like adenocarcinoma of the rectum and is treated similarly. Patients undergo abdominoperineal resection with chemoradiation therapy when the tumor is large, invades other organs, or has nodal involvement.

Most anal cancers are squamous cell carcinomas. Those arising in the distal anal canal usually are keratinizing, whereas those arising in the transitional mucosa are often nonkeratinizing. In the past, the 2 nonkeratinizing types were referred to as *transitional cell carcinoma* and *cloacogenic carcinoma*. Today these are all considered to be variants of squamous cell carcinoma with differing degrees of glandular and adnexal differentiation. They may be heterogeneous microscopically, but all exhibit similar clinical behavior. Anal bleeding is the most common symptom (45%), followed by the sensation of a mass (30%); 20% of patients have no symptoms.[58] The development of anal cancer is associated with HPV and HIV infections, history of receptive anal intercourse, sexually transmitted diseases, cervical cancer, and use of immunosuppressive medication after solid organ transplantation.[59] HPV is found in 86% to 100% of anal cancers[60] but is not found in rectal adenocarcinoma. HPV can be found in normal-appearing anal skin but is rarely found in normal-appearing rectal mucosa.

Anal Margin Cancers

Cancers that arise distal to the anal verge (anal margin) are considered skin cancers and are treated as such. Small lesions (<4 cm^2) with no fixation to deeper tissues are excised widely. Treated patients are then followed closely for 5 years. If the disease recurs, chemoradiation therapy is started. Squamous cell cancer of the anal margin that is deeply invading is treated by chemoradiation.

Anal Canal Cancers

Abdominoperineal resection was the standard treatment for anal cancers until 1974, when Norman Nigro and colleagues presented their results with combined radiation and chemotherapy and showed that cure was possible without the need for permanent colostomy.[61] This led to a regimen of external beam radiation, with fluorouracil and mitomycin C, as the treatment of choice; surgery is reserved for residual or recurrent cancer. Cisplatin has been substituted for mitomycin to reduce toxicity, with similar local success rates, though the rate of colostomy is higher (10% vs. 19%),[62] with an overall survival at 5 years of 75%. Patents with persistent or recurrent squamous cell carcinoma of the anal canal are treated with an abdominoperineal resection, which leads to cure in about 50% of patients. Recurrence has also been treated with additional chemoradiation, depending upon initial radiation dosage.[58]

Melanoma

The anus is the third most common location for melanoma after the skin and eye, and it is as deadly in the anal region as elsewhere. Surgical excision offers the best chance for cure, and even this treatment has poor results. Median survival is about 20 months, with no difference between those undergoing abdominoperineal resection and those undergoing wide local excision.[63] There is a survival advantage to complete resection. When an R0 resection is performed, the 5-year survival is 19%, compared with 6% when surgical margins are involved.[64] Given these findings, local excision should probably be performed when negative margins can be obtained, with radical excision when this is not possible. US examination may be useful in determining depth of invasion and assessing feasibility of local resection.

Squamous Intraepithelial Lesions

These HPV-associated lesions have been known by a variety of terms: *anal intraepithelial neoplasia* (AIN), *Bowen's disease*, *squamous cell carcinoma in situ*, or *anal squamous intraepithelial lesion*. The terms all pertain to the spectrum of changes due to HPV infection seen in the anal mucosa as it takes on an increasingly dysplastic appearance on the path to invasive anal cancer. The most recent attempt to standardize the nomenclature for these conditions was published in 2012 and represents a consensus opinion of the College of American Pathologists and the American Society of Colposcopy and Cervical Pathology.[65] They recommend the terms *low-grade squamous intraepithelial lesion* (LSIL) and *high-grade squamous intraepithelial lesion* (HSIL). In this system, a lesion formerly known as AIN 1 is now LSIL, whereas a lesion formerly known as AIN 3 is now HSIL. LSIL includes condyloma acuminata, and progression of LSIL to invasive cancer is rare. HSIL is clearly a premalignant condition and is treated by excision or local destruction. AIN 2 lesions are intermediate, and their malignant potential uncertain. Immunohistochemistry assessment for p16 may be useful because the presence of this marker can define the lesion as HSIL. Regardless of the terminology used, it is important to understand that HPV infection can lead to malignant transformation, and that such infection may identify a patient as being at increased risk for developing anal cancer.

Disagreement continues regarding the treatment of HSIL,[66] which consists of 2 approaches. One approach is active intervention, in which progression of HSIL to invasive cancer is prevented by tissue destruction (e.g., cautery or infrared coagulation) of the HSIL. Adherents to this approach argue that this histopathologic sequence is analogous to that of cervical cancer and should be approached similarly.[67] High-risk patients can be screened by anal pap smears and evaluated with high-resolution anoscopy. This technique utilizes a colposcope to assess the anal canal; 3% acetic acid and Lugol's solution is used to aid in the identification of abnormal mucosa, which is then biopsied and destroyed. Recurrence is common, and long-term follow-up is needed. Proponents of this approach argue that progression from HSIL to invasive cancer is reduced or eliminated. Detractors argue that such benefit has not been convincingly demonstrated. In addition to the controversy, it is a labor-intensive endeavor and requires a dedicated set of providers and a compliant patient to properly implement. An alternative approach to the patient with HSIL is close observation with physical examination every 6 months, and ansocopy with biopsy of suspicious areas to exclude invasive malignancy.[68,69]

TABLE 129-3 Treatment Options for Anal Warts

Treatment	Success Rate	Comments
Podophyllin	20%-50%	May need repeat applications Skin irritation can occur Not used in the anal canal Poorly absorbed by keratinized lesions (most chronic warts are keratinized)
Trichloroacetic or dichloroacetic acid	75%	Can be used in the anal canal Care is required to control the size of the slough
Cryotherapy	75%	Can be used in the anal canal Care is required to limit the size of the wound Fumes from the therapy can contain active HPV*
Topical 5-fluorouracil	50%-75%	Probably better used after surgical excision to decrease the frequency of recurrence
Imiquimod	75% in women 33% in men	Cannot be used in the anal canal; works better in women then in men
Surgical excision (usually combined with cautery)	60%-90%	Fumes from the cautery may contain HPV* May need to be done in more than one session to avoid excising or burning excessive anoderm if a thick carpeting of lesions is present
Intralesional interferon-α	>70%	Injected into the base of up to 5 warts 3 times a week for 3-8 weeks Approved by the FDA for refractory condyloma
HspE7	Experimental	Promising treatment involving subcutaneous injections Fusion protein that combines immune-stimulating properties and a target antigen from HPV
External-beam radiation therapy	Variable	Reserved for giant cavitating condyloma (Buschke-Löwenstein lesions) Used as a last resort, usually when bleeding or tissue invasion cannot be controlled

*The risk of HPV transmission from such fumes is unknown.

Paget's Disease

Paget's disease is a rare intraepithelial mucinous adenocarcinoma that appears as an erythematous, eczematoid plaque that probably arises from the dermal apocrine sweat glands. The disease is more common in women than men and manifests with intractable itching. Diagnosis is by biopsy, and wide local excision is the treatment if invasion is not found. For invasive cancer, abdominoperineal resection is the treatment of choice. It is associated with underlying malignancy and mandates colonoscopy.

ANAL WARTS

Anal warts (condyloma acuminata) are caused by HPV. Over 5.5 million patients in the United States develop anal warts each year.[70] Transmission is usually sexual, although nonsexual transmission is possible.[71] There are over 80 subtypes of HPV, about 35 of which commonly occur in the anogenital area. Many patients are infected with more than 1 subtype. HPV subtypes 6 and 11 are most commonly associated with anal warts. They occur more commonly in men who have sex with men (MSM) and in immunocompromised patients. Incidence is correlated with the number of sexual partners.[66] Most HPV infections are subclinical, and the virus remains even after eradication or spontaneous involution of visible lesions. Treatment is indicated to remove visible lesions, improve

quality of life,[72] and (possibly) reduce the incidence of anal cancer.[73] Numerous treatment modalities exist (Table 129-3).

Podophyllin is a topical agent that is antimitotic. It requires repeated applications in the office,[74] and results in a cure rate of 50%.[75] It must be washed off 4 to 6 hours after application. It can cause skin irritation. Podophyllin is teratogenic in animals, and thus cannot be used in pregnancy. It can cause histologic tissue changes that can mimic cancer. Podophyllin cannot be used in the anal canal owing to extensive local irritation and to systemic absorption, which may lead to fatal toxicity.

Less toxic than podophyllin, trichloroacetic and dichloroacetic acid cause sloughing of tissue. They must be used with care to control the depth and size of the wound. Unlike podophyllin, their effect is immediate, and thus can be used in the anal canal. Their histologic effect is coagulation necrosis. Cure rates of 75% have been reported.[74,76] Retreatment is common.

Cryotherapy is useful in anal canal lesions and has success rates similar to those associated with trichloroacetic acid.[74,77] The depth and width of the wound must be monitored carefully. It can be used in conjunction with podophyllin for increased effectiveness.[78] The addition of photodynamic therapy may reduce recurrence.[79]

Topical 5-fluorouracil (5-FU) penetrates the skin and is used as a 5% cream. Success rates range from 50% to 70%.[80] It can be used as a biweekly application after surgical removal to decrease recurrence.[80]

Imiquimod cream is an immune response modifier that stimulates monocytes and macrophages to produce cytokines that affect cell growth and have an antiviral effect.[81] It can be applied as a 5% cream 3 times per week for up to 16 weeks, or as a 3.75% cream daily for up to 8 weeks. The lower concentration preserves efficacy and lowers the risk of side effects of skin irritation and pruritus.[82] Efficacy of imiquimod and cryotherapy are similar.[83]

Catechins are green tea extracts that are effective against HPV. Their mechanism of action is unclear, and antiviral and immunostimulatory properties have both been invoked. A commercial preparation is available (Veregen), which is applied 3 times a day for up to 16 weeks. A clearance rate of 58% is reported.[84]

Surgical excision and cautery yield the highest success rate, with cure rates of 63% to 91%; laser seems to offer no advantage. Disadvantages of cautery include the need for anesthesia and the presence of bioactive HPV that is vaporized into the air in a cautery-induced plume.[85] Immune status seems to influence recurrence rates of condyloma. One study found significantly more recurrences in a shorter period for patients with immune systems compromised by HIV, leukemia, idiopathic lymphopenic syndrome, organ transplant, or chemotherapy.[86]

Interferon-α is approved by the FDA for injection therapy of refractory condyloma acuminata. Up to 5 lesions can be treated at a time with injection of 10^6 units 3 times per week for 3 to 8 weeks. Recurrence rates are 20% to 40%.[87] It can also be used as an adjuvant to surgery. Topical interferon is ineffective.[88]

Patients with compromised immune systems (e.g., organ transplant, HIV infection) are particularly susceptible to HPV, and such lesions are more likely to recur after treatment and more likely to progress to dysplasia than in immunocompetent patients. HPV-related dysplasia can occur in the absence of visible warts.[89] These patients also have a very high incidence of anal cancer. Patients with severe dysplasia (HSIL) should undergo, at minimum, regular examinations including anoscopy. Anal cytology has been recommended for this group of patients, though the role of this test is still evolving.

Great progress in the prevention of warts has recently been made with vaccination against HPV. Quadrivalent HPV vaccine became available in the United States in June 2006. The vaccine is directed against HPV type 6 and 11, which cause about 90% of warts, and types 16 and 18, which are present in most anal cancers. Vaccination has been associated with a reduction in warts in young women by 34% in California,[90] over 25% in Sweden,[91] and nearly 90% in Australia.[92] Concomitant reductions have been seen in men, though they are less often vaccinated.[93] This vaccine may used in patients at high risk for anal cancer and may be protective against HSIL. Vaccination is not effective once warts are established.[94]

Buschke-Löwenstein tumors are a rare variant of anal warts. These lesions appear as giant condylomata that can grow rapidly, invade locally, and cause extensive destruction of surrounding tissue. Treatment is surgical excision, if possible. They have also been treated with chemoradiation and with laser ablation.[95]

PRURITUS ANI

Pruritus ani results from irritation of the skin of the perianal region and anus. The intensity of anal itching increases from moisture, pressure, and rubbing caused by clothing and sitting. At worst, anal itching causes intolerable discomfort that often is accompanied by burning and soreness. It is estimated that up to 5% of the population of the United States experiences this type of discomfort daily.[1]

The primary type of this condition is the classic syndrome of idiopathic pruritus ani, whereas the secondary type implies an identifiable cause or a specific diagnosis. Because pruritus ani can be caused by premalignant or malignant lesions, all patients with pruritus must undergo thorough history and physical examination.

Symptoms

Symptoms, which usually start insidiously, are characterized by the occasional awareness of an uncomfortable perianal sensation. The anal skin is richly endowed with sensory nerves, but the perceptions of individual patients vary. Some patients feel an itch, whereas others sense burning. Often the patient is more aware of the problem at night or in hot, humid weather. The itching also may be exaggerated by friction from clothing, especially wool, and perspiration; conversely, applying cool compresses counters irritation, and heat avoidance, mental distraction, and lubrication of the skin surface ease the itching. With time, the condition may progress to an unrelenting, intolerably tormenting burning soreness compounded by the urge to scratch, claw, and otherwise irritate the area in a futile effort to obtain relief.

Diagnosis

Because the diagnosis is one of exclusion, inquiries about diabetes, psoriasis, family history of eczema, use of topical medications (e.g., glucocorticoids), seborrhea, antibiotic use, vaginal discharge or infection, acholic stools, dark urine, or anal intercourse may suggest etiology. Stress and anxiety may exaggerate pruritus ani. When taking a history, the physician should be sensitive, show concern, and encourage the patient to openly express or consider factors that may be contributing to the discomfort.[96]

In the early stages of pruritus ani, examination may reveal only minimal erythema and excoriations. As symptoms progress, the perianal skin becomes thin, friable, tender, blistered, ulcerated, and weeping. In the later stages, the skin is raw, red, lichenified, and oozing or pale, with exaggeration of the radiating folds of anal skin. Often, secondary bacterial or fungal infection is present. Careful local anorectal examination may distinguish an inciting factor, but a detailed skin examination of the entire body may provide the diagnosis. Adjunctive laboratory and radiologic testing may be required to diagnose a primary cause. If there is any suspicion of premalignant or malignant lesions, biopsy is warranted. It is also important to note that mucosal prolapse associated with hemorrhoids or other benign anorectal pathology (e.g., fistula-in-ano, fissures) can be the cause of pruritus. Leakage of stool due to fecal incontinence and leakage of mucus are common sources of pruritus. Treatment should be directed at the offending pathology.

Treatment

Therapy for idiopathic pruritus ani is nonspecific and often changes over the course of time. Treatment is mainly symptomatic and directed toward decreasing moisture in the perianal area to regain clean, dry, and intact perianal skin. Reassurance that there is no underlying pathology, particularly carcinoma, is often as effective in producing a "cure" as any of the physical or medicinal modalities used.[96] Providing detailed patient education is also very important. Patients are instructed to cleanse the anus and perineum several times daily, especially after bowel movements. Although cleanliness is stressed, use of medicated soaps in the perianal region is discouraged. Coffee, tea, colas, chocolate, beer, citrus fruits, alcohol, dairy products, and tomatoes may contribute to the symptoms of pruritus, and serial elimination of each item for 2 weeks may help identify the offending substance.

Other nonspecific therapy includes shaving hirsute patients. Estrogens may be useful in postmenopausal women. Wearing loose-fitting clothes and undergarments made of cotton may be helpful as well. Topical agents such as zinc oxide or glucocorticoid creams have been used with good results in some patients. It is important to note that long-term use of glucocorticoid creams is discouraged because of the thinning of the skin it can cause, which may result in even more future problems. Most patients will respond to these regimens, but relapse is common and requires re-education of the patient.

Anal tattooing with methylene blue solution has been described in cases of refractory pruritus ani. Eusebio and associates reported on this modality in 23 patients, 13 of whom had complete relief; 8 had incomplete relief but were much improved, and 2 had no improvement.[97] Three cases of skin necrosis resulted in modification of the technique, and treatment of an additional 11 patients was without complication and with good results. The treatment is known to cause relative cutaneous hypoesthesia; certain individuals have found this sensation very disagreeable. Skin changes of severe pruritus in all cases rapidly and dramatically regressed and resolved.[12] Anal tattooing is a good option for practitioners to keep in their armamentarium of treatment for pruritus ani.[97]

ANAL STENOSIS

Anal stenosis, narrowing of the anal canal, is an uncommon disabling condition that most commonly results from anorectal surgery, in particular, radical hemorrhoidectomy; it is seen in 5% to 10% of cases after radical hemorrhoidectomy and is due to scarring of the anoderm.[98] Treatment, both medical and surgical, is based on severity of the stenosis. Mild stenosis can be managed conservatively with stool softeners or fiber supplements. Daily digital or mechanical anal dilatations may be used with commercial medical dilators or even candles. Sphincterotomy may be quite adequate for a patient with mild narrowing, but for more severe anal stenosis, a formal anoplasty should be performed.

Etiology

Ninety percent of anal stenosis is caused by overzealous hemorrhoidectomy. Removal of large areas of anoderm and hemorrhoidal rectal mucosa, without sparing of adequate mucocutaneous bridges, leads to scarring and progressive chronic stricture. Surgeons have modified their surgical techniques in an attempt to reduce the incidence of anal stenosis. Other causes of anal stenosis are trauma, IBD, radiation therapy, sexually transmitted diseases, and TB.

Diagnosis

Diagnosis is usually straightforward. The patient typically reports difficult or painful bowel movements and may also have bleeding or narrow stools. Suspicion of anal canal stenosis is heightened by a history of hemorrhoidectomy, Crohn's disease, or excessive laxative use. Physical examination confirms the diagnosis. Visual examination of the anal canal and perianal skin, along with an attempt at digital rectal examination, is usually sufficient to establish the presence of anal

stenosis. It is important to identify the cause of the stricture in order to determine proper therapy; malignant disease must be treated by excision or resection, and anal Crohn's disease should be treated accordingly (see Chapter 115).

Treatment

The best treatment of postsurgical anal stenosis is prevention. Nonoperative treatment is recommended for mild stenosis and for initial care of moderate stenosis. With severe stenosis, conservative treatment can lead to good results, but surgery is almost always necessary. The use of stool softeners and fiber supplements, with adequate intake of fluids, is the basis of nonoperative treatment. Anal dilatation is also important and can be performed daily both digitally and with graduated mechanical dilators. Patients are instructed to sit down on the commode, bear down gently, and gradually insert the smallest dilator with ample lubrication. If the patient can persist with self-dilation on a regular basis, the result is usually excellent. Moderate stenosis is generally treated initially in the same fashion as mild stenosis. Lateral internal sphincterotomy may be quite adequate for a patient with a mild degree of narrowing. This allows the associated scarred anoderm to be resected. For more severe anal stenosis, a formal anoplasty should be performed to treat the loss of anal canal tissue. Various types of flaps have been described for anal stenosis, which allows delivery of the more pliable anoderm into the anal canal to replace the scarred lining at that level.[98]

UNEXPLAINED ANAL PAIN

Unexplained anal pain refers to pain in the anorectal region in the absence of an underlying anatomic abnormality. Diagnosis is based largely on symptoms and physical findings.

Coccygodynia

Coccygodynia is pain or aching in the coccyx. It usually results from trauma or arthritis. Movement of the coccyx on digital rectal exam can reproduce the pain. Treatment includes sitz baths, NSAIDs, and stool softeners.[99] Symptoms may last for weeks or months. A supporting pillow or cushion may be helpful. If symptoms persist, injection of local anesthetics or glucocorticoids may be used.[100] Refractory cases may benefit from coccygectomy.[101]

Levator Ani Syndrome and Proctalgia Fugax

Anal pain syndromes can be subdivided into proctalgia fugax, which is by definition fleeting, and chronic proctalgia, defined as pain that is chronic or recurring for at least 12 weeks in the preceding year, with episodes lasting at least 20 minutes and the exclusion of underlying pathology. Chronic proctalgia is termed *levator ani syndrome* (LAS) if there is tenderness on digital rectal exam when pressure is applied to the puborectalis, and unspecified functional anorectal pain if there is no tenderness.[102]

LAS typically affects women younger than 45 years of age. The pain is described as a vague tenderness or poorly localized aching sensation high in the rectum. It does not usually awaken the patient from sleep, and may be worse with defecation or sitting; walking or lying down may help.[103] Symptoms may be associated with obstetrical injury to the levator ani muscle.[104] Proctalgia fugax more often occurs in young men. It is usually seen in early adulthood and subsides by middle age. The pain last seconds or minutes and then disappears. Pain is described as a sharp cramp or stabbing pain and can awaken the patient from sleep.[99,105] The pathogenesis is thought to involve anal smooth muscle dysfunction, perhaps triggered by stressful events.[103] The frequency of symptoms may be increased in patients with other functional GI disorders. Physical examination is normal.[106] LAS and proctalgia fugax are probably not the same entity. In the literature, however, the terms are sometimes used interchangeably.

Treatment

No specific therapy is usually all that is needed for proctalgia fugax. The patient can be reassured of the benignity of his or her symptoms, which usually resolve spontaneously in seconds to minutes. Salbutamol inhaler use has been successfully reported for proctalgia fugax, though symptoms usually resolve before therapy can be initiated.[107] Topical nitroglycerin 0.2% applied at the onset of proctalgia fugax has been used successfully.[108]

Chronic proctalgia is initially treated successfully with reassurance, sitz baths, perineal strengthening exercises, regulation of bowel habits, and NSAIDs.[99] If such treatment is unsuccessful, sublingual nifedipine (10 mg) or clonidine (150 μg) may be used.[109] Botulinum toxin injection has been tried but has not improved pain.[110] Biofeedback, levator massage, and electrogalvanic stimulation have all been used with success.[111] Linearly polarized near-infrared irradiation therapy also has been used in patients with LAS to good effect.[112] Benzodiazepines have been recommended in the past, but their popularity has declined because of their abuse potential and the availability of better and safer treatment options. Clonidine, an α_2-adrenergic agonist, relaxes smooth muscle and has been used successfully.[113] The dose is 150 mg twice daily for 3 days, then 75 mg twice daily for 2 days, then 75 mg daily for 2 days. Diltiazem, a calcium channel blocker, relaxes smooth muscle and has also has been effective at a dose of 80 mg twice daily.[114] Amitriptyline 25 mg nightly can be used, increasing the dose to 50 mg after 2 weeks, if needed.

HIDRADENITIS SUPPURATIVA

Hidradenitis is an acute or chronic infection of the apocrine glands of the skin (Fig. 129-10). It can occur wherever apocrine sweat glands are found (e.g., axillary, mammary, inguinal, genital, perianal, and periumbilical areas). A follicular disease, hidradenitis traditionally has been considered the result of keratotic debris plugging the apocrine gland. Plugging is followed by bacterial proliferation, suppurative infection, gland rupture, and spread of inflammation to the surrounding subcutaneous tissues. Numerous tracts and pits develop, and the tissues become fibrotic and thickened from the persistent inflammatory response. The axilla is the most common site, followed by the anogenital region. Clinical features include recurrent abscesses, chronic draining sinuses, and indurated, scarred skin and subcutaneous tissues. The spectrum of severity ranges from mild disease with spontaneous regression to severe involvement at multiple sites. A number of factors have been implicated in the development and perpetuation of hidradenitis, including the use of depilatories, close shaving, poor personal hygiene, tight-fitting and synthetic clothing, and antiperspirant use.

Diagnosis of hidradenitis suppurativa is based on clinical presentation. Clinically, patients may complain of burning, itching, and hyperhidrosis. The affected areas have a purplish appearance with drainage of watery pus. In advanced cases, numerous fistulous tracts are readily identified. Over time, multiple abscesses and sinus tracts develop in the subcutaneous region to form a honeycomb-like pattern.

Treatment

For early limited disease, emphasis should be placed on incision and drainage of infections and prevention of recurrences. Oral antibiotics should be targeted against *Staphylococcus* and *Streptococcus*. Although not proved, frequent cleansing and warm water soaking, avoidance of tight-fitting and synthetic clothing, and avoidance of chemical irritants may reduce the severity of active disease. When tracts are well established and superficial, they can be unroofed. For more extensive and deeper disease, wide excision may be required. Wound closure can be tailored to the specific conditions of the patient. In cases of large wounds, flaps or skin grafts can be used. Healing by secondary intention requires less delicate wound care but usually takes longer for complete healing to be accomplished. Close follow-up is needed in all of these patients.

PILONIDAL DISEASE

Pilonidal disease is a common condition that affects many patients, leading to discomfort and inconvenience. It is believed to be an acquired infectious process, with high significant morbidity; for example, patients frequently are prevented from working or attending school for extended periods of time. Sacrococcygeal pilonidal disease occurs predominantly in young men at a ratio of 3:1 over women.[1] Factors associated with the development of pilonidal disease are obesity, increased sweating activity, and local trauma. The prevailing theory of pathogenesis is that hair in the gluteal cleft, along with desquamated epithelium, is propelled into the base of the cleft, where the barbs of the hair shafts prevent them from being expelled (Fig. 129-11). This sets up a granulomatous reaction that creates a sinus. Pilonidal disease is essentially a foreign-body reaction. Histopathology demonstrates foreign-body giant cells associated with hair shafts within a background of chronic granulation tissue lining the abscess cavities and sinus tracts. Midline pits normally are lined with squamous epithelium; in pilonoidal disease most are lined with only granulation tissue. Hair in the form of broken hair shafts is found in the cavities in at least 50% of cases.[1]

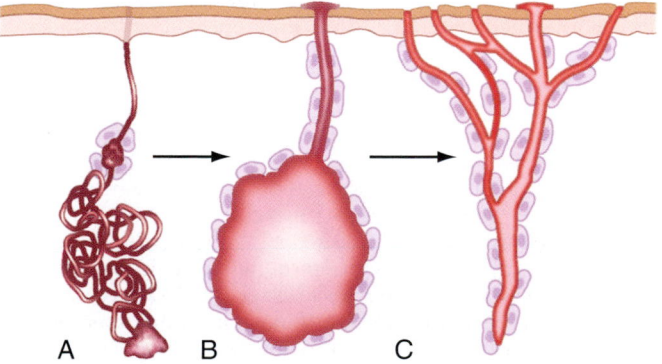

FIGURE 129-10. Pathogenesis of hidradenitis suppurativa, an inflammatory disease of the apocrine sweat glands and adjacent connective tissue. *A,* The initiating event is occlusion of the apocrine duct by a keratinous plug. *B,* Bacteria are trapped beneath the keratinous plug and multiply to form an abscess, which can rupture into adjacent tissue. *C,* The end result is recurrent abscesses, chronic draining sinuses, and indurated scarred skin and subcutaneous tissues. Often, multiple tracts are interconnected and lead to the skin.

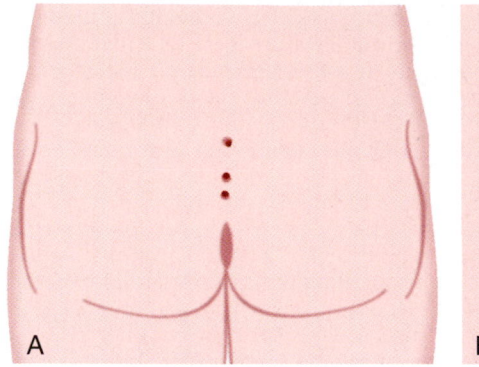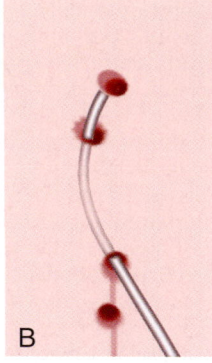

FIGURE 129-11. Pilonidal disease. On examination, there may be multiple pits or external openings in the intergluteal cleft proximal to the anus (A). The openings often communicate with each other (B). A probe can be passed between the communicating network of tracts. Trapped loose hair is usually found in these tracts. One successful treatment option is to unroof all the tracts.

Pilonidal disease is a common condition that can present as an acute abscess, sinus tract, or complex disease with chronic recurring abscesses and extensive branching sinus tracts. Patients may present to the surgeon with asymptomatic small midline pits in the gluteal cleft or as an obvious painful abscess. An acute abscess is the presenting finding in approximately 50% of patients with pilonidal disease. The diagnosis is made by identifying the abscess, which characteristically is several centimeters cephalad to the anus, or seeing tiny openings in the intergluteal cleft over the sacrum.

Surgical management of pilonidal disease depends on the clinical presentation. In mild cases, successful treatment has been achieved simply by shaving the hair on a regular basis to prevent the hair from embedding in the intergluteal cleft. Abscesses require prompt drainage. Complex cases may require wide excision with extensive reconstructive procedures. When extensive surgical débridement is needed, vacuum-assisted closure devices have been shown to decrease length of time until the wound is healed. In caring for the patient, the surgeon should strive for complete wound healing with minimal patient disability, low recurrence rate, and early return to activities of daily living. Postoperative wound care requires diligent attention to gluteal hygiene to reduce the incidence of secondary hair invading the healing wound.

Malignant degeneration of chronic pilonidal wounds is a rare complication. Most such tumors are squamous cell carcinomas that are locally invasive and aggressive. Inguinal lymph node metastasis may be present in 14% of patients. The presence of carcinoma in a pilonidal wound is an indication for wide en bloc excision of the mass, including the sacral fascia. Flap techniques are usually required to close the defect. Local recurrence rates seem lower when radiation therapy is added to surgical resection.

RECTAL FOREIGN BODY

Most foreign bodies in the rectum have been placed via the anus for sexual stimulation. Patients then present when they or their partner cannot retrieve the object. Foreign bodies can also be inserted during sexual assault, in which case the exam should include appropriate sample collection.[115] An accurate history is often difficult to obtain because patients are usually embarrassed.[116] It is important to know what the object is, how long it has been in place, and whether the patient has abdominal symptoms suggesting perforation. Plain abdominal films should be obtained both to see the object and to check for free intra-abdominal air. If free air is seen, a laparotomy is almost unavoidable.

Ease of removal depends upon the object. Cylindrical objects such as dildos and vibrators can usually be removed at the bedside. Using 1 hand to place pressure on the lower abdomen while an examining finger directs the object may be successful. If not, the appropriate tool varies with the type of object to be retrieved, and it is best to practice retrieval of the same or a similar object outside of the patient to facilitate safe removal. Plastic objects can usually be grasped with a tenaculum, which can usually be found in the emergency department. Glass objects can sometimes be removed with obstetrical forceps or vacuum extractors.[117] Bottles may allow insertion of an achalasia balloon to allow traction to be applied.[118] Some objects are amenable to endoscopic retrieval with a snare or grasping (alligator or rat-tooth) forceps. Removal is sometimes helped with IV sedation and local anesthetic infiltrated into the perianal tissue. Sometimes air instillation above the object with a Foley catheter facilitates removal. If this is not successful, the patient should be taken to the operating room. Often the relaxation obtained with anesthesia allows removal the foreign body to be removed transanally.

Laparotomy is used for those objects that cannot otherwise be removed and in patients suspected having sustained a perforation. At surgery the object should be guided to the rectum for transanal removal. If this is not possible, a colotomy is performed. A temporary colostomy may be required depending upon the degree of peritoneal contamination and the extent of colon injury.

The rectum must be examined after removal of the foreign body. This may be done via sigmoidoscopy, CT scan with rectal contrast, or with a water-soluble contrast enema.[119] Reliable patients may be sent home with instructions to return or to call if abdominal pain, fever, or tenderness occurs. Overnight observation may be appropriate for some patients following foreign-body removal.

SEXUALLY TRANSMITTED DISEASES

Sexually transmitted diseases (STDs), often called *venereal diseases,* are exceeded only by the common cold and influenza in the spectrum of infectious diseases. As sexual freedom has become commonplace and homosexual intercourse has increased, the occurrence of STDs has increased correspondingly. Intestinal disease and anorectal disease among homosexuals and bisexuals have emerged as public health problems. National health organizations have devised diagnostic and treatment regimens to assist physicians in providing the appropriate care for these patients.[96]

Site and route of infection determine the symptoms caused by STDs. Infections of the distal anal canal, anoderm, and perianal skin are similar to infections in the other parts of the genitalia and perineum caused by the same organisms. These infections typically result from anoreceptive intercourse, but in some instances represent contiguous spread from genital infections. Proctitis from sexually transmitted organisms is almost always acquired from anal intercourse. Direct or indirect fecal-oral contact produces infection with organisms that cause proctocolitis or enteritis, but which are generally thought of as food or waterborne diseases instead of STDs. While it appears that male homosexual activity and the use of the anorectum for sexual gratification are increasing, data regarding the frequency of these behaviors are limited.[5]

Promiscuity is another definite risk factor for the spread of STDs. Monogamous homosexuals have no higher risk than do monogamous heterosexuals, but exposure to STDs may become vast as the number of sexual partners increases among promiscuous individuals. STDs most frequently found in the homosexual population are gonorrhea, syphilis, chlamydia, herpes simplex, and condyloma acuminata (genital warts). It is thought that the anoderm is quite susceptible to these infections.[96]

Gonorrhea

Gonorrhea is the most common reportable infectious disease in the United States. Many patients are asymptomatic, and asymptomatic rectal infection constitutes the main reservoir of gonococcal disease in homosexual men. Peak incidence for all forms of gonorrhea is in the late teens for females and early 20s for males. Anorectal transmission in homosexual men and in some women is by anoreceptive intercourse with an infected partner. From 35% to 50% of women with gonococcal cervicitis have concomitant rectal infection, which is believed a result of contiguous spread from the genital infection. Oral-anal sex has been suggested as another mode of anorectal gonococcal infection.[96]

In men, the urethra is the most common site of infection, manifesting after an incubation period of 3 to 5 days. Dysuria is the chief complaint, and a creamy yellow discharge can be expressed from the urethra. Women do not have this type of urethral discharge, although the cervix may be red and have some discharge. Gonococcal proctitis results from anogenital sexual exposure. Presenting symptoms include anal itching and irritation, painful defecation, a sensation of rectal fullness, constipation, and anal discharge, which may be copious. External inspection of the anus is generally unremarkable; however, nonspecific erythema and ulceration may occur. Women who engage in anal sex also may have these symptoms.[96]

The anorectal or genital discharge can be cultured on a modified Thayer-Martin plate, which has a sensitivity of approximately 70%. A positive Gram stain of a cervical discharge raises suspicion, but culture is the confirmatory test. Culture of the rectum may be obtained via anoscopy. Complications of gonorrhea include Bartholin's gland abscess, epididymitis, pelvic inflammatory disease, pharyngitis, cutaneous abscess, and disseminated infection with chills, fever, joint pain, and macular rash.[96]

Treatment of anorectal gonococcal infection consists of ceftriaxone (125 mg intramuscularly) or ciprofloxacin (500 mg orally), ofloxacin (400 mg orally), or levofloxacin (250 mg orally).[120] Quinolone resistance has increased over the past decade. Because of the high rate of concomitant infection with chlamydia, patients treated for gonococcal infections should be given appropriate treatment for chlamydia at the same visit, or measures to exclude chlamydial infection should be taken. Sexual partners from the past 60 days should be treated, and patients should abstain from intercourse until treatment is completed and symptoms have resolved.[5]

Chlamydia

Chlamydia is the most commonly reported STD in the United States, with an annual incidence of approximately 3 million cases per year. Aggressive screening programs have been credited with the recent decline of the chlamydia infection rate.[5]

Anorectal transmission of chlamydia is through anoreceptive intercourse, although secondary involvement can occur as a later manifestation of genital infection. There are many immunotypes of *Chlamydia trachomatis*, and the more serious venereal lymphogranulomatosis can be linked to types L1, L2, and L3. The incubation period is 5 days to 2 weeks. Chlamydia is found most often in the urethra, pharynx, and anorectum of male homosexuals. In women, chlamydial infections present as cervicitis, urethral syndrome, endometritis, and salpingitis. Chlamydia can produce an aggressive infection with perianal, anal, and rectal ulceration. Chlamydial proctitis may present with rectal pain and discharge. Anoscopy and sigmoidoscopy demonstrate friable rectal mucosa and ulcers, findings that may be difficult to distinguish from Crohn's disease. Perianal abscesses, fistulas, and strictures also may occur. Lymphadenopathy develops in draining nodal basins, including the iliac, perirectal, inguinal, and femoral regions, several weeks after initial infection.[5]

The best method to diagnose *Chlamydia* infection is to isolate the organism in cell culture. Proper specimen collection increases diagnostic yield and consists of swabbing the affected tissues. In patients whose clinical presentation is consistent with a chlamydial proctitis, a rectal Gram stain that shows polymorphonuclear leukocytes without visible gonococci is presumptive for the diagnosis.[5]

For uncomplicated infection, the best treatment is doxycycline 100 mg orally twice daily for 7 days, or azithromycin 1 g in a single oral dose.[121] In patients with HIV and chlamydia, prolonged treatment may be necessary. Management of sexual contacts is the same as for gonorrhea. Abstinence from sexual intercourse for 7 days after treatment is recommended.[5]

Syphilis

Syphilis is an STD caused by the spirochete *Treponema pallidum*. It can present in 1 of several progressive stages: primary (chancre or proctitis), secondary (condyloma latum), or tertiary.[5]

The infection is transmitted by sexual contact and introduction of the spirochetes through the intact mucous membrane or a break in the skin. The mouth, genitals, and anus are common sites of infection and harbor the primary lesion—the chancre—which appears within 2 to 10 weeks. The chancre may be painful or painless. Anal ulcers are frequently painful, in contrast to genital ulcers. Anal ulcers are without exudate. Inguinal lymphadenopathy is significantly notable. The primary lesion heals spontaneously; however, 2 to 10 weeks later, secondary lesions start to appear as a red maculopapular rash anywhere on the body. Flat, pale lesions, condylomata lata, may be found around the genitals or the anus. Both primary and secondary lesions are infectious. The exudate of lesions in the early stages may be tested by dark-field examination for the presence of spirochetes. Latent or late syphilis, occurring over 1 year after the infection, is detected by serologic testing, because the recognizable primary and secondary lesions are absent. Late disease may lead to cardiovascular, central nervous system, or nephritic disease, and hepatic syphilis.[96,122]

Diagnosis

Diagnosis in the primary or secondary stage of disease is made by visualization of spirochetes on dark-field microscopic exam of lesional scrapings. Alternatively, spirochetes may be demonstrated on Warthin-Starry silver stain of biopsy specimens.[96]

T. pallidum is sensitive to penicillin. Benzathine penicillin G, 2.4 million units given intramuscularly, will maintain treponemicidal levels for 2 weeks. It is also common to give a second injection 1 week later. Patients who are allergic to penicillin may be treated with doxycycline.

HSV

HSV is a DNA virus of the family Herpesviridae that includes varicella-zoster virus, EBV, and cytomegalovirus (CMV). HSV may include several clinical syndromes. HSV type 1 causes dermatitis, eczema, keratoconjunctivitis, encephalitis, and labial inflammation. HSV type 2 causes genital and anal infections and neonatal infections. Manifestations of HSV at primary infection include fever, malaise, and lymphadenopathy. Primary infections are usually worse than subsequent recurrent infections. Transmission is via close contact with an individual who is shedding the virus, and infection results from penetration of mucosal surfaces or breaks in the skin. Clinical infection presents first with systemic symptoms such as fever, headache, and myalgias, followed by local symptoms including pain and pruritus. Vesicles appear over the anogenital area, increase in size and number, and eventually ulcerate and coalesce.

Anorectal involvement by HSV-2 is acquired by anorectal intercourse and is second only to gonorrhea as a cause of proctitis in homosexual men. Herpetic infection of the anorectum results in severe anal pain, tenesmus, hematochezia, dysuria, and rectal discharge. The definitive diagnostic laboratory test is viral isolation and tissue culture, which is accomplished from cultures taken from ulcerations or rectal swabs. The presence of multinucleated giant cells with intranuclear inclusion bodies (ground glass appearance) on Pap smear or Tzank prep are less sensitive than is viral culture. Direct immunofluorescence has also been used for diagnosing HSV.

Acyclovir was the first oral antiherpes agent. Oral acyclovir 200 mg 5 times daily for 5 days shortens the duration of virus shedding and thus aids in clearing of the lesions. Herpes proctitis responds to a larger dose of acyclovir (400 mg) given orally 5 times a day. Valacyclovir and famciclovir are other antiviral agents that can be used against HSV.[96]

HIV

HIV belongs to the lentivirus genus of the retroviridae family, one of the genuses (see Chapter 34). The clinical characteristics of HIV infection are long incubation time, systemic involvement, and association with immune suppression. The HIV infection affects T-helper lymphocytes and macrophages in such a way that there is an absolute reduction in numbers. CD4 counts have been used to indirectly define the state of the immune deficiency. Progressively lower CD4 counts lead to clinicopathologic changes and worsening of health status.[96]

Transmission of HIV occurs through sexual contact, exposure to blood products, and mother-to-child perinatal exposure. Anorectal disease is the most common indication for surgery in HIV-infected patients, and in 5% of patients, their anorectal complaint is the presenting symptom of their HIV infection.[5,123]

Anal fissures that occur in HIV-positive patients must be distinguished from idiopathic AIDS-related anal ulcers and ulcerating STDs such as HSV or syphilis. Anal fissures in this patient population may present differently from the HIV-negative population. They may be lateral to the midline and may be caused by opportunistic infections or underlying malignancy. In fact, on examination of the HIV-positive patient, these atypical fissures may serve as a clue to warrant more extensive workup than those seen in the HIV-negative population. Treatment of fissures in HIV-positive patients includes controlling diarrhea when possible and encouraging abstinence from anoreceptive intercourse. Perianal suppurative diseases are common conditions in AIDS patients. Abscesses should be drained using small incisions, and placement of a mushroom catheter lessens recurrent sepsis. Hemorrhoid treatment is essentially the same for HIV-positive as for HIV-negative patients. One thing to bear in mind is poor wound healing in HIV-positive patients. Morandi and coworkers found that at 32 weeks after hemorrhoidectomy, 50% of AIDS patients had incompletely healed wounds.[123] The overall complication rate was significantly higher in the AIDS group than in the HIV-positive group without AIDS. Also, studies have shown that CD4 counts below 50 cells/mm^3 are associated with significant risk of impaired wound healing.[123] Because of this, and the increased risk of sepsis, we do not perform RBL in patients with CD4 counts below 200 cells/mm^3. (See previous section on Treatment of Internal Hemorrhoids)

ACKNOWLEDGMENT

Special thanks to Peter Marcello, who wrote this chapter in the previous edition of this text.

KEY REFERENCES

Full references for this chapter can be found on www.expertconsult.com.

1. Bailey HR, Billingham RP, Stamos MJ, et al. Colorectal surgery. Philadelphia: Saunders; 2013.
3. Nelson H, Cima R. Anus. In: Townsend CM, Beauchamp RD, Evers BM, Mattox KL, editors. Sabiston textbook of surgery: The biological basis of modern surgical practice. Philadelphia: Saunders; 2008. pp 1444-9.
5. Beck DE, Roberts PL, Saclarides TJ, Senagore AJ, editors. The ASCRS textbook of colon and rectal surgery. 2nd ed. New York: Springer; 2011.
10. Orkin BA. When are " hemorrhoids" really hemorrhoids? A prospective study. Dis Colon Rectum 2000; 43:A35.
14. Keighley MRB, Williams NS. Surgery of the anus, rectum & colon. 3rd ed. Philadelphia: Saunders; 2008.
17. Rivadeneira DE, Steele SR, Ternent C, et al. Practice parameters for the management of hemorrhoids (revised 2010). Dis Colon Rectum 2011; 54:1059-64.
61. Nigro ND, Vaitkevicius VK, Considine B Jr. Combined therapy for cancer of the anal canal: A preliminary report. Dis Colon Rectum 1974; 17:354-6.
73. Palefsky JM, Rubin M. The epidemiology of anal human papillomavirus and related neoplasia. Obstet Gynecol Clin North Am 2009; 36:187-200.
90. Bauer HM, Wright G, Chow J. Evidence of human papillomavirus vaccine effectiveness in reducing genital warts: An analysis of California public family planning administrative claims data, 2007-2010. Am J Public Health 2012; 102:833-5.

SECTION

XI

Additional Treatments for Patients with Gastrointestinal and Liver Disease

CHRISTINA M. SURAWICZ AND LAWRENCE J. BRANDT

PROBIOTICS

In the United States, probiotics and prebiotics are over-the-counter products that are widely used but not subject to FDA oversight. The most commonly used probiotics are bacteria that belong to the *Lactobacillus* (*L. acidophilus*, *L. bulgaricus*, *L. reuteri*, *L. casei*, and *L. rhamnosus* GG), *Bifidobacterium*, and *Streptococcus thermophilus* groups, and *Saccharomyces boulardii*, which is a yeast. Probiotics are available as single strain or multi-strain products. The definition of a probiotic, according to the Food and Agriculture Organization of the United Nations is "live organisms which, when administered in adequate amounts, confer a health benefit on the host." Characteristics of a probiotic should include resistance to gastric acid and bile, so that viable organisms can survive passage through the GI tract and be recoverable in stool. Each strain of probiotic is unique with specific enzymes, metabolic products, and other properties,[1] and ideally each would be identified by its genus and strain, the numbers of viable organisms in the products, and a statement about its expected shelf-life. Rigorous randomized controlled trials (RCTs) should be performed to prove efficacy and safety; however, at this time there is no regulation by the FDA to ensure that this is done with any consistency. The ability to do rigorous RCTs on these products is hampered by the great variability in whether organisms are present singly or as part of a group of related or unrelated organisms, in their stated but perhaps inaccurate concentrations, and in their shelf life.

Prebiotics are poorly digestible dietary substances such as polysaccharides and oligosaccharides which, after selective fermentation, allow specific changes in the composition and/or function of the microbiota that are believed to confer health benefits upon the host. The selective fermentation products of these substances can favor the growth of beneficial organisms such as *Bifidobacteria* in the intestine and the products of metabolism such as short chain fatty acids (SCFAs) can lower the luminal pH (which may inhibit growth of pathogens)[2] and modulate properties of the immune system, including gut-associated lymphoid immune cells.[3] Prebiotics also increase fecal weight, increase calcium absorption, and shorten transit time through the GI tract.[1]

The combination of a probiotic and a prebiotic is called a *synbiotic*.

Mechanisms of Action

There are many mechanisms of action of probiotics, most of which have been observed in animals, with few studies in humans. Probiotics can result in alterations of the microbiota. The production of metabolites via carbohydrate digestion by a probiotic can inhibit pathogens by lowering intraluminal pH, by inhibiting the adherence and translocation of bacteria, and by the production of bacteriocins (antimicrobial peptides).[4] Effects on the microbiota are complex and help correct intestinal dysbiosis and commensal depletion. In part, benefits of probiotic administration result from binding of the probiotic to the intestinal mucosa, with resultant competitive inhibition of binding sites and prevention of pathogen binding. In addition, intestinal barrier function is enhanced by increased mucin production and binding of probiotics with Toll-like receptors on the epithelial cells to activate protein kinase C, which results in tightening of tight junctions.[5] As an example, *Lactobacillus* GG was shown to alter muc-2 mucin gene expression in human enterocytes.[6] Moreover, probiotics can enhance immune function by a variety of mechanisms, including increasing production of immunoglobulin (Ig)A antibodies and cytoprotective molecules, and modulating expression of cytokines.[4,7] Many effects on the immune system have been documented in animals. For example, 1 of several animal studies showed that *Lactobacillus* strains could induce interleukin (IL)-6, IL-2, and TNF production from murine dendritic cells.[8] Another found that *Bifidobacteria* could affect the production of immunoglobulins in lactating mice.[9] Studies of probiotics in humans are limited, and while some studies have been done with human epithelial cells in vitro, much work remains to be done in vivo to define their modes of action.

Efficacy in GI Diseases

An ambitious meta-analysis of 11 species of probiotics evaluated their efficacy in the prevention and/or treatment of 8 major GI diseases and concluded that there was efficacy in treatment of infectious diarrhea, antibiotic-associated diarrhea (AAD), *Clostridium difficile* infection (CDI), Hp, IBS, and pouchitis; there was a lack of efficacy for traveler's diarrhea (TD) and necrotizing enterocolitis.[10] Some of these results conflict with meta-analyses of individual diseases, and results of all studies should be interpreted with caution. Rigorous blinded RCTs of specific probiotics are needed to provide robust data on efficacy, adverse events, and cost benefit before widespread use can be recommended for many products on an evidence-based approach (Tables 130-1 and 130-2); despite lack of data, these products are widely used.

Infectious Diarrhea

Many probiotics have been studied for the prevention and treatment of infectious diarrhea, including *L. reuteri* SD2112 and *B. lactis* Bb-12, *Lactobacillus* GG, *Saccharomyces boulardii*, and mixtures of *Lactobacillus* spp. with *B. bifidum*.

TABLE 130-1 Indications, Efficacy, and Quality of Evidence for Probiotics in GI Diseases

Indication	Efficacy and Quality of Evidence
Infectious diarrhea	
Prevention	Moderate
Treatment	High
Traveler's diarrhea prevention	Moderate
Antibiotic-associated diarrhea prevention	High
Clostridium difficile infection (CDI)	
Prevention	Moderate
Treatment	None
Recurrent CDI treatment	Low to moderate
IBD	
UC treatment	Moderate
Pouchitis treatment and prevention	High
Crohn's disease treatment	Low
IBS treatment	Moderate

TABLE 130-2 Indications for Commonly Used Probiotics in the USA

Probiotic	Indication
Lactobacillus rhamnosus GG	Prevention of AAD
Lactobacillus reuteri	Treatment of infectious diarrhea in children
Saccharomyces boulardii	Prevention of AAD Treatment of RCDI
E. coli Nissle strain 1917 VSL #3	Treatment of UC Treatment and prevention of pouchitis
Bifidobacter infantis 35624	Treatment of IBS Treatment of UC

AAD, antibiotic-associated diarrhea; RCDI, recurrent *Clostridium difficile* infection.

Prevention

Probiotics may have a role in prevention of infectious diarrhea in children.[11,12] One meta-analysis pooled data from 34 RCTs of several different probiotics and concluded that probiotics gave a 35% decrease in infectious diarrhea.[13] At this time, however, the American Academy of Pediatrics (AAP) does not recommend the routine use of probiotics to prevent infectious diarrhea in children.

Treatment

There are many RCTs of various probiotics for the treatment of acute infectious diarrhea. A Cochrane review of probiotic therapy for acute infectious diarrhea evaluated 63 studies, of which 56 were in infants and children[14]; it concluded that probiotics decrease the mean duration of diarrhea by 25 hours, and decrease stool frequency on day 2. Despite the fact that specific products were not recommended, the AAP supports their use in the course of acute infectious diarrhea because studies suggest a 1-day shortening of the duration of diarrhea.[13]

Traveler's Diarrhea (TD)

TD is a good model to evaluate prevention of acute infectious diarrhea in adults. A meta-analysis of 12 studies of probiotics concluded that there was efficacy in TD for *S. boulardii* as well as for a mixture of *L. acidophilus* and *B. bifidum*.[15] Another meta-analysis found that probiotics reduced the risk of TD by 8%[16] with little variability among different strains: *L. rhamnosus* GG, *L. acidophilus*, *L. bulgaricus*, and *S. boulardii*. However, a third meta-analysis of probiotics for a variety of GI diseases concluded there was no efficacy for TD.[10] The variability in results can reflect many factors including type and dose of probiotic, the risk of TD in the environment, the subject's risk of TD (genetic, behaviors), and the wide variety of organisms that can cause TD.

Antibiotic-Associated Diarrhea and Clostridium difficile Infection

Antibiotic-Associated Diarrhea

Diarrhea is a common side effect of antibiotics and occurs in 10% to 20% of patients treated with these agents. There is good evidence in the form of meta-analyses for efficacy of 2 probiotics (*L. rhamnosus* GG and *S. boulardii*) in the prevention of AAD in both children and adults. A 2006 meta-analysis suggested that probiotics reduce the risk of AAD[17] and was supported by a Cochrane analysis of single and multistrain probiotics that found an overall decrease in the incidence of AAD from 19% in the control group to 9% in the probiotic group with a number needed to treat (NNT) of 7.[18] A meta-analysis of 34 studies comprising 4138 patients concluded that there was a significant effect of probiotics in the prevention of AAD, with an NNT of 8. The effect remained significant when grouped by probiotic species, patient age, and duration of antibiotics and probiotic therapy.[19] A larger meta-analysis pooled data from 63 RCTs with 11,811 participants and found a statistically significant benefit in reducing AAD, with a relative risk of 0.58 and a NNT of 13.[20] In summary, the evidence favors a benefit for probiotics in the prevention of AAD.

Clostridium difficile Infection

Prevention of *Clostridium difficile* Infection. Several probiotics including *C. butyricum*, *L. plantarum* 299v, and mixtures containing a variety of bacteria have been studied in the prevention of CDI. An RCT of a yogurt drink that contained *L. casei*, *L. bulgaricus*, and *S. thermophilus* given to hospitalized patients receiving antibiotics found a significant reduction in CDI cases, with none in the treatment group and 17% in the placebo group who developed the infection.[21] In an RCT of a proprietary probiotic formula that contained *L. acidophilus* CL1285 and *L. casei* LBC80R given to patients receiving antibiotics, it was shown that patients who received 2 capsules had the lowest rate of AAD (15.5%), compared with those who received 1 capsule (28.2%) or placebo (44.1%). There also was less CDI in the 2-capsule group (1.2%) compared with the 1-capsule (9.4%) and placebo (23.8%) groups.[22] While most prior meta-analyses did not find any efficacy in prevention of CDI,[13] a more recent one pooled data from 3818 patients in 20 trials, and found that probiotics reduced the incidence of CDI by 66%, with minimal adverse effects.[23] The probiotics were *Bifidobacterium* spp., *Lactobacillus* spp., *Streptococcus* spp., and *S. boulardii*. Trials that used multiple species of the probiotics had a larger effect.

Treatment of *Clostridium difficile* Infection. There are no data to support treatment of initial episodes or severe episodes of CDI with probiotics.

Treatment of Recurrent *Clostridium difficile* Infection (RCDI). *S. boulardii* was shown to decrease recurrences of CDI in patients with multiple recurrences when given as an adjunct to antibiotics.[24,25] In 1 study, *S. boulardii* or placebo was given as adjunctive therapy with antibiotics to patients with CDI. In patients with a first episode of CDI there was no difference in recurrence rates with *S. boulardii* or placebo. In patients who already had had a recurrence, however, *S. boulardii* was associated with a lower recurrence rate compared with placebo (34.6% vs. 64.7%).[24] A later trial evaluated just patients with RCDI and showed that *S. boulardii* decreased recurrence rates only in those patients treated with high-dose vancomycin (2 g/day) in whom recurrence was seen in 16.7% compared with 50% in placebo-treated patients. In patients treated with a lower dose of vancomycin or metronidazole, however, recurrence rates were in the range of 44.7% to 51% for both *S. boulardii*- and placebo-treated patients.[25] Small controlled trials of *L. plantarum* 299v and of *Lactobacilllus* GG have not shown significant efficacy in treating RCDI.

IBD

UC and Crohn's disease (CD) constitute a group of chronic inflammatory conditions of unknown etiology called IBD. Genetic and environmental factors are implicated in the pathogenesis of IBD, as is the intestinal microbiota, which has led to interest in probiotics to treat IBD. Multiple probiotics have been used to treat or prevent flares of UC, pouchitis, and CD.

UC

There are numerous small, controlled and uncontrolled trials of probiotics to treat acute UC and to maintain remission. Some trials are of probiotics as single products; others are as an adjunct to standard therapy. The probiotics studied include VSL#3, *E. coli Nissle* 1917, *Bifidobacteria*, and fermented milk. Treatment with *E. coli Nissle* 1917 was shown to be equivalent to mesalamine for maintenance and remission of UC in 2 controlled trials.[26,27] Small uncontrolled studies suggest a benefit of other probiotics including *Lactobacillus* GG, VSL #3, and *B. longum* combined with a prebiotic. One systematic review concluded that adding a probiotic to standard therapy did not improve induction of remission in patients with mild to moderate UC.[28] Another meta-analysis evaluated 4 RCTs (2

of *E. coli Nissle* 1917, 1 of *Lactobacillus* GG, and 1 of a mixture of *L. acidophilus* LA-5 and *B. animalis* subsp. *lactis* BB-12) and found that probiotics might improve maintenance of remission when given with standard therapy but that better trials were needed.[29]

The use of parasites to treat IBD evolved from the observation that IBD is uncommon in underdeveloped areas of the world. It has been proposed that exposure to intestinal parasites stimulates the immune response and that loss of this exposure could promote the development of autoimmune diseases including IBD.[30] Helminths produce immune regulatory products and can strengthen immune regulatory circuitry in their hosts. In animal models of colitis, helminths were able to inhibit disease development.[31] Several RCTs to test helminth therapy in humans with IBD are underway. One helminth carefully chosen for safety is *Trichiuris suis* (pig whipworm) given as its ova (TSO).[32] One RCT of 54 patients with severe UC given TSO showed improvement in 43% compared with 17% of placebo-treated patients.[33]

Pouchitis

Pouchitis is inflammation of the ileal pouch in patients with UC who have had a colectomy. It occurs in 15% to 50% of patients and may be chronic. Antibiotics and probiotics are used as part of standard therapy for pouchitis. Probiotics have been used to prevent initial episodes in postoperative patients as well as to treat and maintain remission. A small study of *Lactobacillus* GG failed to show any benefit in pouchitis. In a study of prevention of a first episode of pouchitis, patients treated with VSL#3 had a lower rate of pouchitis (19%) than those given placebo (40%) in the first year after surgery,[34] and in another study, meta-analysis concluded that VSL #3 is effective to prevent the first episodes of pouchitis.[35] A meta-analysis of 5 RCTs found greater efficacy of VSL#3 compared with placebo.[36] Several studies also show efficacy of VSL#3 in treating and maintaining remission of pouchitis. A clinical guideline for management of pouchitis recommends antibiotics or VSL #3 to prevent recurrence.[37]

Crohn's Disease

Several small trials have tested probiotics in CD, including *S. boulardii*, *Lactobacillus* mixtures, and *E. coli Nissle* 1917. A meta-analysis of probiotics to maintain remission and prevent clinical and endoscopic relapse in CD evaluated 8 RCTs, and found no efficacy.[38] An open study of TSO to treat active CD resulted in remission in 70% of subjects.[39]

IBS

IBS is a heterogeneous group of symptoms, with many different treatment approaches. The rationale for using probiotics is based, in part, on small studies often with conflicting results that show an altered microbiota in IBS patients, and that the microbiota in patients with IBS differs from that of controls[40,41]; this has led to interest in the use of probiotics to treat IBS. Probiotics are thought to modulate the colonic microbiota, their metabolic products and their cytokine responses, ultimately with control of symptoms. In patients with IBS, *B. infantis* 35624 restored IL-10/IL-12 ratios to normal. This change was not seen with placebo nor with *L. salivarus*.[42] In a large trial of patients with IBS, *B. infantis* was associated with improvement in abdominal pain, bloating, and difficulty in having bowel movements.[43] VSL#3 was found to decrease flatulence, but had no effect on abdominal pain or urgency.[44] Other probiotics that have been studied include *L. acidophilus* SDC, *Lactobacillus* GG, and mixtures of bacteria.

Several meta-analyses have evaluated the uses of probiotics in IBS. One of 2 meta-analyses published in 2008 of 122 trials and 1404 subjects found that probiotic use was associated with improvement in global IBS symptoms.[45] The other evaluated 8 RCTs, and also concluded that probiotics could improve IBS symptoms.[46] Yet another meta-analysis of probiotics in IBS that evaluated 19 RCTs and pooled 1650 patients found probiotics to be significantly better than placebo in improving symptoms, with a NNT of 4. They studied a variety of products including *Lactobacillus*, *Bifidobacterium*, *Streptococcus*, and combinations of bacteria. Overall, there was a statistically significant benefit for improvement of IBS symptoms, especially pain and flatulence.[47] At this time, *Bifidobacteria* and *Lactobacilli* at concentrations above 1×10^8 CFU are most promising to have efficacy. Finally, a systematic review and meta-analysis of 14 RCTs concluded that probiotics may have a role in the treatment of symptomatic IBS, but that current evidence was weak and that better trials are needed to define who will benefit, and what type and dose of specific species and strains should be used.[48]

Safety

While probiotics are used widely and adverse effects are uncommon, there is no systematic reporting system for probiotics. Most studies did not report a statistically significant increase in adverse events compared with controls, but it has been questioned if probiotics are safe in immunosuppressed individuals. There are isolated case reports of bacteremia with *Lactobacillus* and fungemia with *S. boulardii*. A case-review study found sepsis, liver abscess, and endocarditis from *Lactobacillus* GG, to occur mostly in patients with severe illness.[49] The same paper reviewed *S. boulardii* fungemia and found numerous cases, some related to ingestion of *S. boulardii*, but others resulting from suspected contamination of central lines when the product capsules were opened, and the lyophilized yeast was allowed to become airborne. Again, most, but not all, cases were in immunosuppressed individuals.[35] Two systematic reviews and an Agency for Healthcare Research and Quality study have evaluated the safety of probiotics and concluded that adverse effects are uncommon, but serious infections with *Lactobacilli* or *S. boulardii* can occur.[50-52] Given this conclusion, it is prudent to avoid probiotics in individuals who are immunosuppressed or severely ill.

FECAL MICROBIOTA TRANSPLANTATION

Fecal transplantation was first performed by mouth in China during the 4th century to treat food poisoning and severe diarrhea,[53] and for almost 300 years veterinarians have instilled stool into the stomach or rectum to treat horses with diarrhea or via the stomach (rumen) to treat a variety of diseases in ruminants. Its clinical use as reported in the English language dates back to a 1958 case series of 4 patients with staphylococcal pseudomembranous enterocolitis who were given fecal retention enemas as an adjunct to conventional treatment.[54] The rationale for fecal microbiota transplantation (FMT) lies in the belief that certain diseases such as recurrent CDI result from a perturbed ecologic imbalance in the microbiota of the intestinal tract dysbiosis and that reintroduction of normal flora via donor feces corrects the imbalance and restores phylogenetic richness, thereby enabling recovery of normal bowel function and health; this theory is supported by clinical and laboratory data.[54-57]

Recurrent *Clostridium difficile* Infection

The first use of FMT for confirmed recurrent CDI, which is its most common indication today, was in 1983,[58] and now over 1000 such cases have been reported in the world's literature.

Details of how to perform FMT are beyond the scope of this chapter but may easily be found in the literature.[59,60] Suffice it to say that the first step is to determine if a patient would benefit from FMT and, if so, to choose an appropriate donor. In the near future, donor selection may become moot, as results with frozen specimens from standard (universal) donors already have shown results just as good as those of using donors selected by the recipients.[60]

Regardless of the route of administration, worldwide, mean cure rates to date are consistently around 91%,[60] and FMT is effective even in patients with the *C. difficile* NAP1/BI/027 strain.[61] In 2011, of 325 cases of FMT performed worldwide for recurrent *C. difficile* infection (CDI), approximately 75% had been administered by colonoscopy or retention enema, and 25% by nasogastric or nasoduodenal tube, or by EGD.[60,62,63] In case series reported throughout the world, FMT done via upper tract endoscopy, NG or nasoduodenal tube, had CDI resolution rates in the range of 76% to 79%.[60,63] In the only RCT to date involving FMT, however, the cure rate was 81% (13 of 16) after 1 FMT infusion of 500 mL given by nasoduodenal tube and 94% after a second infusion.[64] In fact, the study was terminated early because the rate of cure was so superior to that of vancomycin (31%) or vancomycin with a bowel lavage (23%) that it was considered unethical to continue; there were no serious adverse effects; only transient diarrhea, cramping, and belching. In 2014, a systematic review reported on FMT for CDI in 20 case series, 15 case reports, and the randomized trial cited above with resolution rates of diarrhea determined by site of administration: stomach (81%), duodenum/jejunum (86%), cecum/ascending colon (93%) and 84% (distal colon).[65] Thus, regardless of route, FMT appears to be safe, with no serious adverse effects or complications directly attributed to the procedure yet published.[66]

In the only long-term follow-up of FMT to date, data collected from 77 patients who had had FMT at 5 different medical centers and who were followed for more than 3 months had a 91% primary cure rate and a 98% secondary cure rate, the latter defined as cure enabled by use of antibiotics to which the patient had not responded to before the FMT or by a second FMT.[66] Most of these patients (97%) stated they would have another FMT were they to develop CDI again, and 58% said they would choose to have FMT rather than antibiotics. Of the 77 subjects, 4 developed an autoimmune disease (RA, Sjögren syndrome, idiopathic thrombocytopenic purpura, and peripheral neuropathy) at some time after the FMT, although a clear relationship between the new disease and FMT was not evident. Safety of FMT in immunosuppressed patients needs to be established, although experience suggests immunocompromise is not of concern.[67] Nonetheless, safety remains the prime consideration, and more well-designed controlled trials are necessary to confirm the efficacy of FMT, and to determine the optimal route of administration among other variables.

Use of stool for such transplants is but the initial step in our attempt to "correct" a perturbed intestinal microbiota. In 1 study, a standardized filtered, previously frozen preparation of stool from a "universal donor" has been used with great success,[60] and in another study, a synthetic stool composed of 33 bacterial strains cultured from the feces of a healthy donor cured 2 patients with refractory CDI.[68]

FMT also has been used in a limited numbers of patients to treat severe and complicated CDI manifest by toxic megacolon or ileus with rapid success and no adverse FMT-related sequelae.[69,70]

Other Diseases

FMT also has been used to treat non-CDI GI disorders including UC, CD, IBS, and constipation, and there is a growing literature on an altered intestinal microbiome in these disorders.[71-73] Use of FMT for non-GI disease has been successful in a wide range of disorders, albeit only in a scattering of isolated case reports and small clinical series including Parkinson's disease,[74] fibromyalgia, chronic fatigue syndrome,[75] multiple sclerosis,[76] myoclonus dystonia,[77] obesity,[78] insulin resistance and the metabolic syndrome,[79] and childhood regressive autism[80] among others. Rigorous studies of FMT in these areas are needed to determine whether FMT is efficacious therapy and, if so, who is the optimal candidate, what route should be used, and how often FMT should be delivered, among other considerations.

FMT is a highly effective means of curing recurrent CDI, and its role in treating other GI and non-GI diseases is just beginning to be studied. Well-designed clinical trials with carefully performed studies of the intestinal microbiota are needed to ensure patient safety and to identify patients and diseases that are most likely to respond to FMT. Although there do not appear to be any significant short-term adverse effects, the possibility of long-term effects remains of concern. We do not yet have an inkling of the long-term effects of changing one's population of commensal microbiota if even for, as shown by limited studies, a relatively short time period of months.

KEY REFERENCES

Full references for this chapter can be found on www.expertconsult.com.

1. Guarner F, Khan AG, Garisch J, et al. World Gastroenterology Organisation Global Guidelines: Probiotics and prebiotics October 2011. J Clin Gastroenterol 2012; 46:46881. www.worldgastroenterology.org/.../Probiotics_FINAL_20111128.pd.
10. Ritchie ML, Romanuk TN. A meta-analysis of probiotic efficacy for gastrointestinal diseases. PLosONE 2012; 7:e34938.
19. Videlock EJ, Cremonini F. Meta-analysis: Probiotics in antibiotic-associated diarrhea. Aliment Pharmacol Ther 2012; 35:1355-69.
20. Hempel S, Newberry SJ, Maher AR, et al. Probiotics for the prevention and treatment of antibiotic-associated diarrhea. A systematic review and meta-analysis. JAMA 2012; 307:1959-69.
23. Johnston BC, Ma SSY, Goldenberg JZ, et al. Probiotics for the prevention of *Clostridium difficile*–associated diarrhea. A systematic review and meta-analysis. Ann Intern Med 2012; 157:878-88.
29. Gordon NK, Fagbemi AO, Thomas AG, Akobeng AK. Probiotics for maintenance of remission in ulcerative colitis. Cochrane Summaries 2011; CD007443.
32. Summers RW, Elliott DA, Qadir K, et al. *Trichuris suis* seems to be safe and possibly effective in the treatment of inflammatory bowel disease. Am J Gastroenterol 2003; 98:2034-41.
47. Moayyedi P, Ford AC, Talley NJ, et al. The efficacy of probiotics in the treatment of irritable bowel syndrome: A systematic review. Gut 2010; 59:325-32.
49. Segarra-Newnham M. Probiotics for *Clostridium difficile*–associated diarrhea: Focus on *Lactobacillus rhamnosus* GG and *Saccharomyces boulardii*. Ann Pharmacother 2007; 41:1212-21.
56. Lawley TD, Clare S, Walker AW, et al. Targeted restoration of the intestinal microbiota with a simple, defined bacteriotherapy resolves relapsing *Clostridium difficile* disease in mice. PLoS Pathog 2012; 8:e1002995.
59. Bakken JS, Borody T, Brandt LJ, et al. Fecal Microbiota Transplantation (FMT) Workgroup. Treating *Clostridium difficile* infection with fecal microbiota transplantation. Clin Gastroenterol Hepatol 2011; 9:1044-9.
60. Gough E, Shaikh H, Manges AR. Systematic review of intestinal microbiota transplantation (fecal bacteriotherapy) for recurrent *Clostridium difficile* infection. Clin Infect Dis 2011; 53:994-1002.
62. Brandt LJ, Reddy S. Fecal microbiota transplantation for recurrent *Clostridium difficile* infection. J Clin Gastroenterol 2011; 45:S159-67.
64. Van Nood E, Vrieze A, Nieuwdorp M, et al. Duodenal infusion of donor feces for recurrent *Clostridium difficile*. N Engl J Med 2013; 368:407-15.
65. Cammarota G, Ianiro G, Gasbarrini A. Fecal microbiota transplantation for the treatment of Clostridium difficile infection: a meta-analysis. J Clin Gastroenterol 2014 epub ahead of print 2014.
66. Brandt LJ, Aroniadis OC, Mellow M, et al. Long-term follow-up of colonoscopic fecal microbiota transplant for recurrent *Clostridium difficile* infection. Am J Gastroenterol 2012; 107:1079-87.

131
Complementary and Alternative Medicine

DAVID J. HASS

DEFINITION AND EPIDEMIOLOGY

Complementary and alternative medicine (CAM) is defined broadly as practices neither taught widely in medical schools nor generally available in U.S. hospitals.[1] However, this is rapidly changing with the advent of integrative health care centers within many academic centers. The prevalence of CAM therapies has increased at an exponential rate both in national and international medical communities. A study by Eisenberg and associates[1] demonstrated that among the U.S. population, CAM use increased from 33.8% in 1990 to 42.1% in 1997. In the 2007 National Health Interview Survey (NHIS) from a sample of 23,393 subjects, nearly 40% of individuals detailed that they had used a CAM therapy within the past year.[2] Estimated annual expenditures for CAM therapies are in excess of $27 billion, a sum equivalent to patients' out-of-pocket expenditures for all U.S. physician-based services.[1]

In a study by Ganguli and colleagues, at least 50% of gastroenterology outpatients in a community setting were shown to have implemented CAM therapies to help ameliorate their symptoms.[3] Given the widespread use of these modalities and the continuing trend of their increased utilization, an understanding of CAM therapies, including their potential risks and benefits, is necessary for the practicing gastroenterologist. A thorough knowledge of these practices will allow physicians to provide more comprehensive medical care and can help further therapeutic rapport between physicians and their patients.

TYPES OF THERAPIES

There are a wide variety of CAM therapies, and those most commonly employed for GI and hepatic disease are defined in Box 131-1. Regardless of which therapy is employed, the overall philosophy of CAM takes the uniform holistic approach that all disease results from disturbances at a combination of physical, psychological, social, and spiritual levels. Thus, a CAM modality is used to restore balance and to facilitate the body's own healing responses, thereby ameliorating troublesome symptoms.[4]

The National Center for Complementary and Alternative Medicine (NCCAM) divides CAM therapies into 4 major domains. The first domain is mind-body medicine, which includes hypnosis, meditation, biofeedback, and cognitive behavioral therapy. Biologically based practices constitute the second domain and include substances within our natural environment that are used to strengthen and heal the human body, such as prebiotics, probiotics, and dietary supplements. Manipulative and body-based practices encompass the third domain and involve manipulation and movement of 1 or more parts of the body as a means of achieving healing; examples include massage, chiropractic manipulation, and reflexology. The final domain within CAM therapy comprises "energy medicine," namely acupuncture, magnetic therapy, and Reiki.

Two additional disciplines of note include traditional Chinese medicine (TCM) and Ayurvedic medicine. TCM has a heritage some 2000 years old and concerns itself with bringing a patient into balance through practices that affect the opposing forces of yin and yang. Ayurvedic medicine is a traditional Indian practice, also based on the premise of balance; it is a comprehensive medical discipline aimed at integrating mind, body, and spirit to achieve contentment, prevention of disease, and good health. Practitioners use naturally occurring substances such as oils and herbs, as well as various treatments including fasting, yoga, and meditation, to achieve harmony in an individual patient.

DEMOGRAPHY OF COMPLEMENTARY AND ALTERNATIVE MEDICINE (CAM) USERS

Certain patients are more likely to use CAM therapies than are others. Women and Caucasians tend to use CAM more

BOX 131-1 Common CAM Therapies for GI and Hepatic Diseases

Acupuncture
Based on the principles of Chinese medicine, *qi* is energy, which circulates among organs along channels called *meridians*. Through placement of needles at specifically defined locations (points), the flow of *qi* is restored to appropriate levels and the health of specific organs is improved.

Ayurveda
Holistic system of medicine from India that provides diet and lifestyle recommendations to improve overall health

Colonic Irrigation Therapy
Cleansing of the colon through various oral and enema preparations to improve "digestive health"

Herbal Medicine
Ingestion of various herbal therapies or supplements to improve physiologic function

Homeopathy
Based on the principle "like should be cured with like." Administration of a diluted solution that, when given to a healthy person in an undiluted form, causes symptoms identical to those experienced by the ill person.

Hypnosis
Induction of a deeply relaxed state during which therapeutic suggestions are made to alter behavior and enhance relief of symptoms

Meditation, Relaxation
A process of reflection and contemplation that allows one to focus thoughts to help alleviate symptoms

Reflexology
Areas on the feet correspond to organs of the body. Massage and pressure applied to these regions can improve symptoms throughout the body.

---

often than do men and African Americans, respectively. Patients with higher levels of education, higher annual incomes, and comorbid medical conditions also are more likely to resort to CAM therapies.[1,3] Although knowledge of these demographics assists the gastroenterologist in determining which patients are likely to be using CAM therapies, it is also important to understand each patient's rationale and motivation for choosing a particular therapeutic modality.

RATIONALE FOR USE

Digestive disorders rank among the most common disease states for which people seek the advice of complementary practitioners. The attraction of CAM therapies is multifaceted. First, they provide patients who might not have a medical background with a sense of control over their own bodies and health. Second, they provide patients with therapeutic alternatives when conventional medical therapies have failed to alleviate their symptoms or cure diseases such as terminal cancer. Last, CAM therapies are attractive to patients who feel dissatisfied with the ways their physicians demonstrate understanding of their illnesses or handle their complaints.

GI DISORDERS AMENABLE TO COMPLEMENTARY AND ALTERNATIVE THERAPIES

The majority of research on CAM therapies and GI illness encompasses trials that involve IBS, functional dyspepsia, and liver disease, although studies to investigate the role of CAM therapies for IBD are increasing continually. Supplement and herbal therapies are the most common modalities implemented for digestive disorders.

This chapter focuses on the 7 areas in gastroenterology and hepatology that are addressed most often by CAM therapies: nausea and vomiting, functional dyspepsia, IBS, IBD, diarrhea and constipation, liver disease, and GI malignancies. For each area, data that support the most commonly used CAM modalities are reviewed, along with their potential benefits and adverse effects (AEs).

Nausea and Vomiting

Nausea and vomiting have a wide array of causes ranging from viral gastroenteritis to pregnancy. These symptoms can be quite distressing, and patients often resort to CAM therapies to seek symptomatic improvement. In 1 study of pregnant women with nausea and vomiting, 61% reported using CAM therapies for relief.[5] Several complementary modalities have been used to help ameliorate nausea and vomiting, and range from herbal medicines to relaxation techniques (Table 131-1).

Ginger

Ginger (*Zingiber officinale*) is the herbal supplement most commonly used to relieve nausea and vomiting and derives its name from the Sanskrit word for "horn," which describes the twisted, gnarled shape of its roots. Several mechanisms have been postulated to explain the antiemetic effect of ginger. Animal studies have demonstrated that 1 component of the herb, 6-gingerol, improves GI motility,[6] and another component, galanolactone, is a 5-hydroxytryptamine $(HT)_3$ antagonist,[7] similar to ondansetron, an antiemetic agent used to treat chemotherapy-induced nausea and vomiting.

The antiemetic effect of ginger has been studied in various clinical conditions, including morning sickness, seasickness, chemotherapy-induced nausea, and postoperative nausea. Although no more effective than placebo for preventing experimentally induced motion sickness, ginger has been documented to reduce vertigo induced by caloric stimulation of the inner ear's vestibular apparatus.[8-10] In a systematic review of randomized controlled trials (RCTs) that evaluated the efficacy of ginger for nausea and vomiting, Ernst and Pittler demonstrated that ginger was superior to placebo and equal in efficacy to metoclopramide for postoperative nausea and emesis. Furthermore, ginger relieved symptoms better than did placebo agents for the treatment of seasickness, morning sickness of pregnancy, and chemotherapy-induced nausea and vomiting.[11] The dose of ginger prescribed in most of these studies ranged from 0.5 to 1 g/day, which is roughly equal to one quarter teaspoon of ground ginger.

Although ginger is a natural supplement with therapeutic effect, its potential AEs must be taken into consideration before advocating it for relief of symptoms. First, ginger has been shown to inhibit platelet aggregation by inhibiting

TABLE 131-1 CAM Therapies for Nausea and Vomiting

Therapy	Proposed Mechanism of Action	Evidence	Adverse Effects
Ginger (Zingiber officinale)	Enhances GI motility; 5-HT$_3$ receptor antagonist[6,7]	Efficacy over placebo in RCTs for postoperative and chemotherapy-induced nausea, morning sickness, sea sickness[11]	Inhibits thromboxane synthase, thereby causing an increased risk of bleeding with concurrent antithrombotic or antiplatelet agents[12] Questionable safety in pregnancy
Pyridoxine (vitamin B$_6$)	Unclear	RCTs reveal mixed results in the treatment of morning sickness[16]	Decreases serum levels of levodopa, phenobarbital, and phenytoin[17] Allergic reactions Taken in excess (>250 mg/day), can cause peripheral neuropathy, dermatoses, photosensitivity, and dizziness[18]
Acupuncture	Placement of needles at specifically defined locations (points) to restore the flow of qi and improve the health of specific organs	RCTs demonstrate efficacy for relief of symptoms following chemotherapy, surgery, and morning sickness[21-23]	Infectious complications, perforations of internal organs, and spinal cord injury[24-32]
Relaxation therapy	Process of reflection and contemplation allows one to focus thoughts to help alleviate symptoms	Effective as an adjunctive therapy to standard antiemetic agents for chemotherapy-induced symptoms[33]	None reported

5-HT, 5-hydroxytryptamine; RCT, randomized controlled trial.

thromboxane synthase. Therefore, if patients are taking warfarin, aspirin, NSAIDs, or clopidogrel concurrently, the risk of bleeding is increased.[12] Second, although not proved in animal studies, ginger has been documented to be potentially mutagenic in laboratory assays, thereby raising questions about its safety in pregnancy.[13,14]

Pyridoxine (Vitamin B$_6$)

The water-soluble vitamin pyridoxine is another CAM therapy used to relieve the nausea and vomiting associated with pregnancy,[15] and it was 1 of the most commonly employed CAM agents in a survey of pregnant Canadian women with these complaints, 29% of whom reported using it.[5] In a RCT, Vutyavanich and colleagues reported that pyridoxine (30 mg daily) resulted in a significant reduction in nausea, but no statistically significant reduction in vomiting.[16]

Although the mechanism of action of pyridoxine is not established, certain drug interactions and AEs have been noted. Pyridoxine has been documented to decrease serum levels of levodopa, phenobarbital, and phenytoin when administered with these agents.[17] Allergic reactions to pyridoxine also have been documented, and when taken in excess (>250 mg/day), pyridoxine has been reported to cause peripheral neuropathy, dermatoses, photosensitivity, and dizziness.[18,19]

Acupuncture and Acupressure

Acupuncture is another CAM modality commonly used to treat nausea and vomiting. In Chinese subjects, the P6 acupuncture point stimulated for relief of these symptoms is named neiguan, meaning "medial pass." This acupuncture point is anatomically located 3 fingerbreadths above the proximal palmar crease on the volar aspect of the wrist in the midline. To date, more than 30 published trials have evaluated the role of stimulating the P6 acupuncture point to relieve nausea and vomiting.[20] In a systematic review, acupuncture was demonstrated to be superior to placebo in ameliorating nausea and vomiting; the results were consistent despite numerous investigators, diverse patient populations, and various forms of acupuncture point stimulation.[19] Trials have demonstrated that acupuncture effectively relieved nausea and vomiting associated with chemotherapy,[21] surgery,[22] and pregnancy.[23]

The data supporting use of acupuncture and acupressure are impressive; however, gastroenterologists must recognize the difficulties of applying traditional placebo-RCT methodology to test the efficacy of acupuncture. The nature of this complementary modality is such that each patient's regimen is individualized for relief of his or her specific symptoms, thereby precluding standardization of the treatment and calling into question the validity of the studies.

Several AEs have been noted with acupuncture, mainly from infection secondary to improper handling of needles or their reuse without sterilization.[24] Such infections have included HBV, HCV, and HIV[25-27]; bacterial endocarditis secondary to Propionibacterium acnes[28]; and bacteremia from Staphylococcus aureus and Pseudomonas aeruginosa with a consequent psoas abscess.[29] Two fatalities have been documented in which acupuncture was thought to have led to staphylococcal sepsis.[30] Although improperly sterilized needles seem to be the only risk factor for the aforementioned infections, it is difficult to prove such infections were a direct result of acupuncture, because patients might not have divulged other personal potential risk factors such as sexual preference or IV drug use.[31] Other risks reported to be associated with acupuncture therapy include perforation of an organ during placement of the needles, with resultant pneumothorax, hemopericardium with tamponade, and spinal cord injury.[24,31,32]

Relaxation Therapy

Relaxation therapies have been used for chemotherapy-induced nausea and vomiting. It has been reported that side effects related to chemotherapy are somewhat conditioned and are developed as a form of associative learning[33]; the anxiety experienced during chemotherapy sessions can serve as a conditioning cue that leads to physiologic reactions. Through progressive muscle relaxation therapy, a patient's anxiety can be alleviated and physical symptoms averted. Relaxation therapies often are used as an adjunct to standard antiemetic medications.[31]

Functional Dyspepsia

Functional dyspepsia is defined as pain or discomfort in the epigastric area in the absence of demonstrable structural or physiologic abnormalities. Because symptoms tend to be short in duration and relatively mild, dyspepsia often is self-managed[34]; therefore, CAM therapies clearly are appealing. Herbal therapy has been a mainstay of CAM treatments for functional dyspepsia. The most common supplement therapies for functional dyspepsia, including their active ingredients, proposed mechanisms of action, and AEs, are listed in Table 131-2.

Banana (*Musa sapientum*) has been evaluated for the treatment of functional dyspepsia in prospective open trials. This supplement is thought to promote gastric mucus secretion and has been documented to have anti-ulcerogenic properties in animals.[35] In a study by Arora and Sharma,[36] treatment with banana powder reduced symptoms in 75% of patients in the treatment group compared with 25% of those in the placebo group (P < 0.05). Causes of organic dyspepsia were excluded through various endoscopic and laboratory methods before subjects were included in the study. The only AE reported was pruritus in the treatment group.[36]

Capsaicin, derived from the dried fruit of *Capsicum annuum* (red pepper), is an herbal supplement. Its mechanism of action is selective impairment of pain (C-type) fibers, which carry pain sensation from the abdominal viscera to the central nervous system.[37] In 1 study, 2.5 mg of red pepper powder given daily improved epigastric pain, nausea, and bloating, whereas placebo did not.[37] Although abdominal pain and diarrhea occurred initially in patients treated with capsaicin, these AEs were self-limited and of no serious clinical consequence.

Greater celandine (*Chelidonium majus*) was investigated in functional dyspepsia by Ritter and colleagues in a double-blind RCT.[38] Celandine accounted for a 34% greater reduction in symptoms compared with placebo (P = 0.003).[38] This agent is thought to contain a variety of alkaloids that also have a spasmolytic effect on smooth muscle.[39] Despite its apparent efficacy, celandine has many AEs, including xerostomia, insomnia, diarrhea, and fatigue. Idiosyncratic hepatotoxicity

TABLE 131-2 Herbal Supplements for Functional Dyspepsia

Herbal Supplement	Proposed Mechanism of Action	Evidence	Adverse Effects
Banana (*Musa sapientum*)	Anti-ulcerogenic; promotes gastric mucus secretion[35,36]	Open-label trial demonstrates efficacy[36]	Pruritus
Capsaicin (*Capsicum annuum*)	Selectively impairs activity of CNS nociceptive C-type pain fibers[37]	RCT demonstrates efficacy over placebo[37]	Abdominal pain, diarrhea
Celandine (*Chelidonium majus*)	Contains alkaloids, which have a spasmolytic effect on smooth muscle[39]	RCT demonstrates efficacy over placebo[38]	Xerostomia, insomnia, diarrhea, fatigue, hepatotoxicity[40]
Liu-jun-zi-tang	Increases gastric emptying, plasma somatostatin, and gastrin levels; promotes gastric relaxation[34,41]	RCT demonstrates efficacy over placebo[41]	Interstitial pneumonitis[42]
Peppermint and caraway	Inhibits gastric smooth muscle contraction[43,44]	RCTs demonstrate efficacy over placebo[34,45]	Diarrhea, nausea, vomiting, allergic contact dermatitis, contact urticaria, asthma exacerbations, and atrial fibrillation[46-48]
Shenxiahewining	Unknown	RCT demonstrates efficacy over control medication[34]	None reported
STW 5 (Iberogast)	Alters GI motility; smooth muscle relaxant[43]	RCTs demonstrate efficacy over placebo[50-53]	Potential for hepatotoxicity, increased bleeding risk, potentiation of sedatives and anxiolytics; altered metabolism of drugs metabolized by CYP3A4 and uridine diphosphate-glucuronyl transferase[40,67,68]
Turmeric (*Curcuma longa*)	Increases biliary secretion, promotes contraction of gallbladder; antispasmodic agent[49]	RCT documents efficacy over placebo[34]	Nausea, vomiting, fatigue, headache

CNS, Central nervous system; CYP3A4, cytochrome P450 3A4; RCT, randomized controlled trial.
Data adapted from Coon JT, Ernst E. Systematic review: Herbal medicinal products for non-ulcer dyspepsia. Aliment Pharmacol Ther 2002; 16:1689-99.

also has been described with celandine, but it resolved without complication in most cases when the supplement was discontinued.[40]

Liu-jun-zi-tang, also known as TJ-43, is a Chinese herbal medicine that has been used to relieve functional dyspepsia and is a combination of several extracts including *Actractylodis laneae rhizoma*, *Ginseng radix*, *Pinelliae* tuber, Hoelen, *Zizyphi fructus*, *Aurantii nobilis pericarpium*, *Glycyrrhizae radix*, and *Zingiberis rhizoma*.[34] Multiple mechanisms of action have been proposed, including increased gastric emptying, elevated serum levels of gastrin and somatostatin,[41] and relaxation of gastric smooth muscle.[42] One RCT compared TJ-43, 2.5 g 3 times daily, with placebo for 7 days in patients with functional dyspepsia. The treatment group displayed greater reductions in epigastric fullness, reflux, and nausea compared with the group treated with placebo (P < 0.05).[41] The only AE noted with TJ-43 was 1 case of drug-induced interstitial pneumonitis, which resolved after therapy was discontinued.[34]

Peppermint *(Mentha piperita)* and caraway *(Carum carvi)* are the supplements that have been investigated most thoroughly for treating functional dyspepsia. Their proposed mechanism of action is thought to be inhibition of smooth muscle contractions by direct blockade of smooth muscle calcium channels.[43,44] Several placebo-controlled trials have compared variable, fixed doses of these agents ranging from 180 to 270 mg for peppermint and 100 to 150 mg daily for caraway, and showed statistically significant improvement in symptoms such as bloating and epigastric pain when treatment and placebo groups were compared.[34,45] AEs seen with these supplements include diarrhea, nausea, vomiting, allergic contact dermatitis, contact urticaria,[46] asthma exacerbations, and atrial fibrillation.[47,48]

Shenxiahewining is a mixture of Chinese herbs, specifically *Ginseng radix*, *Pinelliae* tuber, *Coptidis rhizoma*, *Zingiberis rhizoma exsiccatum*, and *Glycyrrhizae radix*, in a 3:9:3:3:3 ratio.[34] In an RCT performed in China, 92% of patients treated with shenxiahewining reported improvement in symptoms compared with 20% of a control group. No important AEs were noted.[34]

Turmeric *(Curcuma longa)* is an agent that also has been documented to have therapeutic efficacy in alleviating functional dyspepsia. This agent is thought to increase biliary secretion, promote contraction of the gallbladder, and act as an antispasmodic.[49] In a placebo-controlled trial performed in Thailand, turmeric (2 g/day) was found to significantly improve dyspeptic symptoms (P = 0.003).[34]

Another agent that has been studied for the treatment of functional dyspepsia is STW 5, also known as Iberogast. This agent is an herbal preparation composed of bitter candytuft *(Iberis umbellata)*, chamomile *(Matricaria chamomilla)*, peppermint, caraway fruit, licorice root *(Glycyrrhiza glabra)*, lemon balm leaves *(Melissa officinalis)*, celandine *(Chelidonium majus)*, angelica root *(Angelica archangelica)*, and milk thistle *(Silybum marianum)*. In a meta-analysis performed by Melzer and colleagues,[50] evaluating 3 double-blind RCTs, STW 5 in a dosage of 1 mL 3 times daily for 4 weeks was more effective than placebo to improve the study patients' most bothersome dyspeptic symptoms. Twenty-six percent of patients in the placebo group compared with 7% in the STW 5 group reported that their symptom remained "severe" or "very severe" after treatment. Specifically, STW 5 appeared more effective in providing symptomatic relief to patients with predominant epigastric pain and gastroesophageal reflux symptoms.[50]

von Armin and colleagues[51] also have demonstrated in the largest double-blind RCT evaluating STW 5 that a significantly higher percentage of patients with functional dyspepsia who are prescribed STW 5 are free from their symptoms compared with a placebo group.[51] Pilichiewicz and coworkers showed

that STW 5 affects gastric motility in a region-dependent manner, inducing gastric fundic relaxation and antral contraction.[52] Although no AEs have been reported for STW 5, individual components of the preparation are known to have potential toxicities, details of which are addressed in the next section.

Data on the supplement therapies above suggest that some of those studied could be useful for patients with functional dyspepsia. Peppermint, caraway, and STW 5 are the most extensively evaluated to date and, given their encouraging safety profiles, warrant further study.[34]

IBS

IBS is defined as abdominal discomfort and altered bowel function in the absence of structural and biochemical abnormalities (see Chapter 122).[53] Symptoms include pain, bloating, cramping, constipation, and diarrhea. In a systematic review citing only studies that used Rome criteria for diagnosis, IBS prevalence was found to vary between 5% and 10% of various populations, with a pooled prevalence of 7%.[53] Patients with IBS often are frustrated that laboratory, radiologic, and endoscopic examinations fail to reveal an "organic" source of their discomfort, and they therefore often employ CAM therapies to help ameliorate their symptoms.

Many CAM therapies have been investigated for the treatment of IBS (Table 131-3), of which herbal supplement therapy and probiotics have been evaluated most extensively. Psyllium *(Plantago isphagula)* is the most commonly prescribed dietary supplement for patients with IBS. This fiber product acts as an osmotic bulking agent and decreases bowel transit time. There have been 3 placebo-controlled trials of psyllium use in IBS,[54-56] but only 1 fulfilled the 5 Rome criteria for appropriate study methodology (randomization, concealed allocation, placebo control, double blinding, and appropriate follow-up of study patients). Two additional trials compared psyllium with "active" agents, but neither trial was of high quality.[57,58] In general, the evidence that stool frequency, consistency, and ease of passage were better with psyllium than with placebo was modest. There were no statistically significant differences in AEs among psyllium, lactulose, and placebo.

Although psyllium appears to be fairly harmless, allergic hypersensitivity reactions to psyllium have been documented, and impaired absorption of certain medications taken concomitantly, such as lithium and carbamazepine, also has been reported.[59-61] Cases of acute esophageal obstruction that have occurred with psyllium-based agents suggest that dysphagia might preclude its use and that history of difficulty swallowing should be sought before beginning therapy with this agent.[62]

Other supplemental therapies have been used for IBS. Peppermint oil, as previously discussed, is prescribed for its smooth muscle relaxant capabilities. In a meta-analysis by Pittler and Ernst,[63] peppermint oil significantly improved symptoms of IBS compared with placebo treatment. Although statistical significance was demonstrated in this study, flaws in trial methodology preclude evidence-based acceptance of the efficacy of peppermint oil in IBS treatment. A subsequent systematic review of 4 trials by Ford and associates demonstrated significant and consistent improvement in IBS symptoms compared with placebo,[64] lending support to the use of peppermint oil in the treatment for IBS.

STW 5 also has been used to treat patients with IBS. Placebo-controlled trials have demonstrated that STW 5 improves symptoms of IBS and reduces the severity of abdominal pain.[65] Multiple mechanisms of action of STW 5 are postulated; certain components are thought to alter GI motility,

TABLE 131-3 CAM Therapies for IBS

Therapy	Proposed Mechanism of Action	Evidence	Adverse Effects
Acupuncture	Placement of needles at specifically defined locations (points) to restore the flow of *qi* and to improve the health of specific organs	RCT demonstrates superiority of acupuncture to sham[81] RCT demonstrates equivalency to sham but superiority over medical therapy[82]	Infectious complications, perforations of internal organs, spinal cord injury[23-31]
Ayurvedic medicine	Holistic system of Indian medicine providing dietary and lifestyle recommendations improve overall health	RCT demonstrates efficacy over placebo but with significant dropout rates in the trials[83]	None reported
Chinese herbal medicine	Unknown	RCT demonstrates efficacy over placebo[77,78]	None reported
Hypnotherapy	Gut-related imagery; patient's thoughts are focused toward inhibition of gastric acid secretion[77,78]	RCT demonstrates efficacy over placebo[77,78]	None reported
Peppermint oil	Inhibits smooth muscle contraction[43,44]	RCTs reveal possible efficacy over placebo, but flaws noted in studies[65]	Diarrhea, nausea, vomiting, allergic contact dermatitis, contact urticaria, asthma exacerbations, and atrial fibrillation[46-48]
Probiotic therapy	Alters intestinal microbiota	RCT demonstrates efficacy over placebo[71,72]	None reported
Psyllium	Osmotic bulking agent; decreases bowel transit time	RCT demonstrates efficacy for relief of constipation[53]	Allergic reactions, impaired absorption of medications (lithium, carbamazepine), acute esophageal obstruction[56-63]
STW 5 (Iberogast)	Alters GI motility; smooth muscle relaxant[44]	RCT demonstrates efficacy over placebo[65]	Potential for hepatotoxicity, increased bleeding risk, potentiation of sedatives and anxiolytics, altered metabolism of drugs metabolized by CYP3A4 and uridine diphosphate-glucuronyl transferase[40,66-68]

CYP3A4, cytochrome P450 3A4; RCT, randomized controlled trial.

and others are thought to act as smooth muscle relaxants.[60] Although no AEs have been reported for STW 5, individual components of the preparation are known to have potential toxicities: celandine is known to be hepatotoxic at certain doses (>10 mg/day)[40]; chamomile is known to contain a coumarin derivative, which increases the risk of bleeding if prescribed concurrently with warfarin, aspirin, or NSAIDs, and chamomile can potentiate the central nervous system depressant effects of benzodiazepines and barbiturates,[66,67] which often are prescribed to patients with IBS; milk thistle is known to inhibit cytochrome P450 3A4 (CYP3A4) and uridine diphosphoglucuronosyl transferase and thus could alter the metabolism of many pharmacologic agents.[68]

Chinese herbal medicine has been used for IBS symptoms, and RCTs have demonstrated a statistically significant benefit of its use over placebo. Patients treated with Chinese herbal medicine reported improvement in their symptoms and an overall improvement in their quality of life.[69]

Probiotics are microorganisms that promote health benefits through alterations of intestinal microbiota (see Chapter 130).[70] Patients with infectious and inflammatory disease states such as pseudomembranous colitis and IBD, as well as patients with IBS, also have had benefit from these agents. Evidence from RCTs has demonstrated that ingestion of *Lactobacillus plantarum* resulted in significant reductions in abdominal pain and flatulence in patients with IBS.[71,72]

A report of fermented milk that contains *Bifidobacterium animalis* showed this probiotic improves abdominal distention and associated symptoms in patients with constipation-predominant IBS.[73] In addition, a systematic review of probiotics demonstrated that *Bifidobacterium infantis* 35624 (Align) significantly improves abdominal pain, bloating, distention, and the sensation of incomplete evacuation.[74]

Nonpharmacologic, central-acting therapies such as cognitive behavioral therapy, hypnotherapy, and mindfulness training are evidenced-based complementary modalities that also have been shown to improve global symptoms of IBS. The effectiveness of these therapies is based on their aim to reduce over-reactivity to stressors and maladaptive coping behaviors.

Hypnotherapy has been documented to have a significant therapeutic effect on symptoms of IBS. Through the use of gut-directed metaphorical imagery, patients imagine the normalization of GI function and develop improvement in their symptoms. Studies report an overall symptom improvement rate between 50% and 80%.[75] Gut-directed hypnotherapy allows individuals to focus on their specific somatic symptoms and bring forward a deeper sense of being able to mitigate the effect of noxious visceral stimuli. Clinical remission of IBS symptoms for up to 3 months has been documented in patients treated with hypnotherapy. A recent review of 11 studies showed hypnotherapy to significantly improve IBS symptoms, including quality-of-life scores and overall function.[76] Although the efficacy of gut-directed hypnotherapy has become more apparent in recent literature, studies have suggested that its effectiveness may be lower when therapy is provided outside of highly specialized research centers.[77] Women and those younger than 50 years of age seem to respond best to this modality. Hypnotherapy has proved effective in the pediatric IBS population as well, 1 study having documented that successful treatment of functional abdominal pain or IBS was accomplished in 85% of children treated with hypnotherapy compared with 25% of patients treated with placebo.[78]

Mindfulness training (MT), defined as a nonjudgmental acceptance and interested awareness of the moment-to-moment experience of sensations, perceptions, emotions, and other forms of mental activity, also has recently been shown effective in the treatment of IBS.[79] In a prospective RCT, Gaylord and coworkers demonstrated that participation in a group program of MT compared with enrollment in a functional bowel disease support group resulted in greater reductions in IBS symptom severity immediately after treatment, and that the therapeutic effect was sustained at a follow up 3 months later. This trial effectively demonstrated that MT has a substantial therapeutic effect on bowel symptom severity, health-related quality of life, and stress reduction.[79] From a physiologic standpoint, MT is thought to help modulate visceral perception by decreasing activation of the central arousal and corticolimbic networks. MT is a promising and safe therapeutic approach for the treatment of IBS; however, additional prospective studies are needed to assess the durability of the effect seen in recent studies.

In earlier trials, acupuncture had been shown to be superior to sham therapy and fiber supplementation in patients with IBS,[80,81] but a more recent meta-analysis of sham-controlled RCTs by Manheimer and colleagues, found that acupuncture is, in fact, no more effective for IBS symptom severity or quality-of-life indices compared with sham acupuncture.[82] Acupuncture was, however, deemed superior to pharmacologic antispasmodic therapies, although this effect was limited to trials that did not include a control arm, and the effects were modest at best.[82] The medications used in these trials were not those accepted as mainstays of treatment for this condition, and therefore, these data also do not support the efficacy of acupuncture in the treatment of IBS.

Lastly, Ayurvedic medicine (see Box 131-1) also has demonstrated efficacy in relief of IBS symptoms. The largest trial of Ayurvedic medicine, however, had a significant dropout rate and should be interpreted with caution.[83]

IBD

Crohn's disease is currently believed to be driven by an overactive intestinal mucosal immune system interacting with the intestinal microbiota,[84] in combination with an ineffective mucosal barrier to potential dietary and environmental toxins (see Chapter 115). Given the chronic and persistent nature of Crohn's disease, many patients turn to CAM therapies when conventional treatment does not offer complete symptomatic relief. Current data suggest that up to one third of all patients with IBD resort to CAM therapies to help ameliorate their symptoms. The most commonly used CAM therapies among IBD patients are supplements, followed by homeopathy and massage. Current federally supported research includes investigation of the relationship between stress and IBD flares, the role of diet in the natural history of IBD, and the effect of green tea extract on the clinical course of UC.

Probiotics are often employed by certain subgroups of patients with IBD (see Chapter 130). Typically, those having had total proctocolectomy with ileal pouch-anal anastomosis (IPAA) claim the greatest benefit from these agents. Probiotics are thought to act via various mechanisms. Some of these organisms have been shown to produce butyrate, a short-chain fatty acid important for colonocyte health–particularly the epithelial cells in the rectum and descending colon–as well as to have important immunomodulatory activity, activating T cells to down-regulate proinflammatory cytokines.[85] Although the cause of pouchitis remains unknown, alteration in the intestinal microbiota appears to play an important role.[86]

VSL #3 is a probiotic agent that consists of 4 strains of *Lactobacillus*, 3 strains of *Bifidobacterium*, and 1 strain of *Streptococcus*. VSL #3 is thought to act by increasing tissue levels of interleukin (IL)-10 and decreasing levels of proinflammatory cytokines, such as IL-1 and TNF.[87] In RCTs, administration of VSL #3 reduced the frequency of pouchitis in IBD patients after IPAA, and it decreased the number of flares of pouchitis in patients known to have chronic pouchitis.[82,88] In 1 RCT, VSL #3 appeared effective to prevent endoscopic recurrence of IBD compared with placebo.[89]

VSL #3 has also recently been shown to induce remission in patients with mild to moderately active UC. Sood and colleagues demonstrated in a multicenter double-blind RCT that 6 weeks into treatment with VSL #3, patients treated with this probiotic experienced a statistically significant improvement in the UC disease activity index (UCDAI) compared with the placebo group. In addition, 42.9% of patients treated with VSL #3 compared with 15.7% of patients receiving placebo achieved remission ($P < 0.001$).[90] No AEs have been noted with VSL #3 in any of the studies evaluated.

Saccharomyces boulardii is a nonpathogenic yeast originally isolated from the litchi fruit, and it is another probiotic shown to decrease the relapse rate of Crohn's disease.[91] S. boulardii exerts its beneficial effect by acting as a trophic agent on intestinal mucosa and by triggering the release of immunoglobulin (Ig)A.[84] In 1 study, clinical relapses over a 6-month period were observed in 37% of patients who received mesalamine alone and in 6% of patients treated with mesalamine plus S. boulardii.[84]

Another supplemental therapy used to treat IBD is fish oil. Fish oil contains high amounts of omega-3 fatty acids, which, compared with other fatty acids commonly found in many foods, serve as precursors of less proinflammatory cytokines. In patients with UC who have frequent disease exacerbations, disease activity scores were improved to a greater extent in patients who received fish oil than in those who consumed other forms of fat[92]; however, RCTs have failed to demonstrate that fish oil is effective in maintaining remission.[93] No trial has yet documented fish oil to be effective in maintaining remission of Crohn's disease or in lowering an individual patient's Crohn's disease activity index (CDAI).[92]

Turmeric is a spice that originates from the root *Curcuma longa*, a member of the ginger family, traditionally used in Indian and Chinese herbal medicine. This is another complementary agent reported to be effective in the treatment of

IBD. A pure curcumin preparation was administered in an open-label study to patients with ulcerative proctitis or Crohn's disease. All proctitis patients improved, with reductions in concomitant medications in 4 patients. Four of 5 patients with Crohn's disease had lowered CDAI scores and erythrocyte sedimentation rates. This encouraging study warrants further evaluation of this agent with double-blind, placebo-controlled follow-up studies.[94]

Hanai and coworkers performed an RCT in which 43 patients who had UC in remission received curcumin (2 g daily for 6 months) and compared results with a similar group of patients who received placebo[95]; 4.65% of those receiving curcumin suffered relapse versus 20.5% of individuals who received placebo, a statistically significant difference.[95] Both of the aforementioned studies revealed a potential therapeutic benefit for turmeric; however, larger prospective trials are warranted before making definitive recommendations regarding its therapeutic efficacy.

The mechanism of action of turmeric is multifactorial: it protects lipids from peroxidation and thereby prevents the formation of free radical species; it inhibits lipopolysaccharide-induced nitric oxide synthase (iNOS) gene expression, thus decreasing TNF-α and IL-1β production; it inhibits nuclear factor (NF)-κB activation and cytokines thought to be integral to the pathophysiology of IBD; and it inhibits the synthesis of proinflammatory prostaglandins and leukotrienes through inhibiting arachidonic acid uptake by macrophages.[96] Curcumin has been found in most studies to be safe even in high doses, and in animal studies there has been no evidence of mutagenicity or chromosomal damage.[97] Turmeric does exhibit an inhibitory effect on platelet aggregation, and therefore, patients who are maintained on NSAIDs or antiplatelet agents should be closely monitored.[97]

Vitamin D also has been shown in recent literature to potentially have an anti-inflammatory effect in Crohn's disease. Data presented by Boothe and colleagues revealed that patients given high-dose vitamin D supplementation (10,000 IU/day) experienced statistically significant greater reduction in the Harvey-Bradshaw Index compared with individuals who received standard vitamin D supplementation ($P < 0.04$).[98] Patients' concurrent treatment regimens were held relatively constant during the study period, thereby suggesting that vitamin D had a significant clinical impact in Crohn's disease, with no coexistent toxicity. Vitamin D is known to reduce levels of TNF-α, and this likely is 1 of the means by which its therapeutic efficacy is postulated.[98]

Andrographis paniculata, a member of the plant family Ancanthaceae, is a complementary therapy used in China, India, and across the Asian continent. In vitro, *A. paniculata* extract has demonstrated inhibitory activity against TNF-α, IL-1β, and NF-κB.[99] A previous pilot study also demonstrated equivalent efficacy of *A. paniculata* extract to mesalamine for UC.[100] In a recent double-blind RCT,[101] participants who received *A. paniculata* extract at a dose of of 1800 mg daily were noted to have increased mucosal healing, with trends for greater induction of remission, compared with those who received placebo. The extract was well tolerated and appears to be a novel oral therapy that could serve as an alternative treatment to glucocorticoids, immunomodulators, and biologic therapies for UC.[101]

Hypnosis has also been demonstrated to have a potential benefit in the treatment of UC. In a study performed by Mawdsley and associates, the effect of hypnotherapy on systemic and rectal mucosal inflammatory responses was shown to reduce the median serum IL-6 level and rectal mucosal release of substance P and IL-13 levels. Reduction of these proinflammatory mediators provides a rationale for RCTs of hypnotherapy in the treatment of IBD.[102]

Diarrhea and Constipation

Altered bowel habits often lead to the use of CAM therapies. Within the discipline of CAM, practitioners often group the symptoms of diarrhea and constipation together under the term *colonic health*. Although several CAM modalities have been reported to promote and improve colonic health, herbal supplements are considered the mainstay of treatment. These supplements range from anthraquinone-based stimulant laxatives (e.g., aloe [*Aloe barbadensis*]) to osmotic laxatives (e.g., magnesium citrate) to extracts of papaya (*Carica papaya*) and raspberry (*Rubus udaeus*). The most commonly used, including their proposed mechanisms of action, possible medication interactions, and reported AEs, are listed in Table 131-4. As discussed later, because the supplement industry is not regulated, the content and potency of many of these agents are not standardized, which should give practitioners pause before prescribing them. Probiotics also are employed often to prevent diarrhea (see Chapter 130). A meta-analysis performed by D'Souza and colleagues described the clinical efficacy of various strains of *Lactobacillus* (*Lactobacillus bulgaricus*, *Lactobacillus acidophilus*, *Lactobacillus casei*, and *Lactobacillus* GG) and *S. boulardii* in the prevention of antibiotic-associated diarrhea (see Chapters 112 and 130).[103] Castagliuolo and colleagues described the protective effects of *S. boulardii* on *Clostridium difficile*-induced diarrhea in humans; the mechanism of this action is the proteolytic digestion of toxin A and B molecules by a protease secreted by *S. boulardii*.[104] Another study reported that *S. boulardii* stimulates intestinal IgA in response to infection with *C. difficile*.[105] *S. boulardii* also has been shown to prevent relapses of pseudomembranous colitis (see Chapters 112 and 130) and to maintain intestinal mucosal barrier function against enteropathogenic *Escherichia coli*.[106,107] VSL #3 has been demonstrated in an RCT to be effective in preventing radiation-induced diarrhea.[108]

Ernst and colleagues have reviewed the various CAM therapies that have been used to treat constipation. Biofeedback, a treatment technique in which people are trained to use signals from their own bodies to help recognize a relaxed state, has demonstrated clear efficacy for the treatment of constipation.[109] Pelvic floor dyssynergia, an often-neglected cause of chronic constipation, is a result of inappropriate contraction or failed relaxation of the puborectalis and external anal sphincter muscles during defecation (see Chapter 19). Pelvic floor dyssynergia is considered a form of maladaptive learning,[110] and biofeedback is thought to help retrain the body to alleviate this condition.

Sensory training involves simulated defecation through the use of a water-filled balloon that is inserted into the rectum and then slowly withdrawn as the patient is asked to concentrate on relaxing the muscles that are behaving inappropriately.[110] Anal manometry and electromyography, which record muscle activity either from intraluminal probes or perianal surface electrodes, are alternative means by which sensory feedback can be provided to the patient with pelvic floor dyssynergia. More than 70% of adult patients with this disorder improve following biofeedback training.[110] Further studies are needed, however, to assess the long-term efficacy of biofeedback.

Abdominal massage therapy has shown mixed results in the treatment of constipation. Ernst[111] reviewed the data from an RCT for abdominal massage as a treatment for constipation and found that although some data suggested a significant increase in the number of days with bowel movements, and decrease in the number of episodes of fecal incontinence and number of enemas given, the trials were of poor quality and were methodologically flawed. The trials were not blinded and were subject to observer bias; only 1 study was

TABLE 131-4 Herbal Supplements Claimed to Promote "Colonic Health"

Supplement	Proposed Mechanism of Action	Possible Interactions	Adverse Events
Aloe (*Aloe barbadensis*)	Anthraquinone stimulant laxative; increases bowel motility	Potentiation of cardiac glycosides; reduced action of glucocorticoids	GI spasm, bloating, hypokalemia, arrhythmias, pseudomelanosis coli
Apple pectin	Dietary fiber; binds bile acids (unknown mechanism)	None reported	None reported
Cascara sagrada (*Rhamnus purshianus*)	Anthraquinone stimulant laxative; increases bowel motility	Potentiation of cardiac glycosides; reduced action of glucocorticoids	GI spasm, bloating, hypokalemia, arrhythmias, pseudomelanosis coli
Chamomile (*Matricaria chamomilla*)	Unknown mechanism	Increased risk of bleeding with concurrent warfarin, aspirin, and other NSAIDs; potentiation of CNS depressant medications	Increased risk of bleeding; lethargy with potentiation of CNS depressants
Clove (*Syzygium aromaticum*)	Spasmolytic and local anesthetic	None reported	None reported
Echinacea	Promotes immune function through increased cytokine activity, increasing T-helper cell population	Acetaminophen (secondary to glutathione depletion)	Allergic reactions have been reported; potential hepatotoxicity if administered with acetaminophen
Fennel (*Foeniculum vulgare*)	Stimulates GI motility	None reported	Allergic reactions have been reported
Fenugreek (*Trigonella foenum-graecum*)	Unknown mechanism	Increased risk of bleeding with concurrent warfarin, aspirin, and other NSAIDs	Increased risk of bleeding; galactorrhea (secondary to interaction at dopamine receptors)
Ginger (*Zingiber officinale*)	Enhances GI motility; 5-HT$_3$ receptor antagonist; inhibits platelet aggregation by inhibiting thromboxane synthase	Increased risk of bleeding with concurrent warfarin, aspirin and other NSAIDs, clopidogrel	Increased risk of bleeding
Hibiscus (*Hibiscus sabdariffa*)	Laxative (unknown mechanism)	None reported	None reported
Magnesium citrate	Osmotic laxative	None reported	Hypermagnesemia: prolonged QT interval on ECG, hypotension, hyporeflexia
Marshmallow (*Althaea officinalis*)	Immune stimulant, anti-inflammatory	Can delay absorption of other medications	None reported
Oat bran (*Avena sativa*)	Decreases cholesterol and prostaglandin synthesis	None reported	None reported
Oregon grape (*Berberis vulgaris*)	Source of vitamin C; stimulates immune system; stimulates intestinal peristalsis	None reported	None reported
Papaya (*Carica papaya*)	Promotes healing of GI ulceration and improves pancreatic function	Increased risk of bleeding with concurrent warfarin, aspirin, and other NSAIDs	Increased risk of bleeding, decreased testicular weight, interrupted estrous cycle in mice
Psyllium (*Plantago isphagula*)	Osmotic bulking agent; decreases bowel transit time; generates short-chain fatty acids	Impaired absorption of medications	Allergic reactions have been reported; impaired vitamin B$_{12}$, lithium, carbamazepine absorption; esophageal obstruction

CNS, central nervous system.

TABLE 131-4 Herbal Supplements Claimed to Promote "Colonic Health"—cont'd

Supplement	Proposed Mechanism of Action	Possible Interactions	Adverse Events
Raspberry (Rubus idaeus)	Unknown	None reported	None reported
Rhubarb (Rheum palmatum)	Anthraquinone stimulant laxative; increases bowel motility	Potentiation of cardiac glycosides; reduced action of glucocorticoids	GI spasm, bloating, hypokalemia, arrhythmias, pseudomelanosis coli
Senna (Cassia senna)	Anthraquinone stimulant laxative; increases bowel motility	Potentiation of cardiac glycosides; reduced action of glucocorticoids	GI spasm, bloating, hypokalemia, arrhythmias, pseudomelanosis coli
Spirulina	Green algae; contains Mg	None reported	None reported
Valerian (Valeriana officinalis)	Spasmolytic agent	Interacts at GABA receptor: potentiation of CNS depressant medications	Lethargy; withdrawal from valerian is similar to withdrawal from benzodiazepines
Yellow dock (Rumex crispis)	Laxative (unknown mechanism)	None reported	None reported

ECG, electrocardiogram; GABA, γ-aminobutyric acid; 5-HT₃, 5-hydroxytryptamine-3.
Derived from Hass DJ, Lewis JD. Quality of manufacturer provided information on safety and efficacy claims for dietary supplements. Pharmacoepidemiol Drug Saf 2006; 15:1-9.

randomized. Therefore, further RCTs are needed to determine whether massage is effective in patients with chronic constipation.

Homeopathy has been suggested to have clinical efficacy in the treatment of postoperative ileus (see Chapter 124). A meta-analysis of studies of patients with ileus after abdominal and gynecologic surgery revealed that homeopathic treatment with agents such as opium poppy (Papaver somniferum L.) and chaparral (Raphanus sativus) significantly reduced the time to normal intestinal peristalsis compared with placebo treatment.[112] The underlying principle of homeopathy is "like cures like," and these supplements, in diluted doses, are thought to ameliorate slowed intestinal transit because they themselves are known to cause constipation. This meta-analysis, however, did not enable definitive conclusions, because several of the trials included were reported in publications that are not peer reviewed, thereby raising suspicion as to the quality of the data.

Lastly, colonic irrigation therapy has gained popularity among patients interested in complementary therapies. "Colonics," as they are colloquially termed, differ from enemas because they are not self-administered but rather are given by a practitioner who has a certain degree of training, via a device that controls water flow, temperature, and pressure.[113] The rationale for this practice derives from "autointoxication," a concept popularized by Sir Arbuthnot Lane in the late 1800s and early 1900s that toxins originating in the intestine can enter the circulation and poison the body. There are no large RCTs thoroughly evaluating the efficacy of colonic irrigation therapy. AEs of colonic irrigations have been reported, including amebiasis and rectal perforation.[114,115]

Liver Disease

CAM therapies are commonly used to treat conditions such as nonalcoholic fatty liver disease (NAFLD), nonalcoholic steatohepatitis (NASH), hepatitis B, hepatitis C, and alcoholic liver disease. One study of U.S. outpatients with chronic liver disease reported that 41% had used some form of CAM therapy in the preceding 4 weeks.[116] As with the other GI conditions already discussed, most therapies used for chronic liver disease have been herbal supplements. Table 131-5 details the commonly employed supplements, their mechanisms of action, levels of evidence to support their use, and AEs.

Silymarin

Milk thistle (Silybum marianum), the CAM compound most commonly used for liver disease, has been employed for many disorders, including alcoholic liver disease, chronic viral hepatitis, and drug-induced hepatitis. Silymarin, the active ingredient, is derived from the milk thistle plant. Its mechanism of action is not defined fully but appears to be multifaceted: it is thought to act as an antioxidant to prevent glutathione depletion[117]; it has anti-inflammatory activity and decreases formation of leukotrienes, prostaglandins, and TNF-α[118] in animal studies; and it has been shown to block proliferation of hepatic stellate cells and production of procollagen III, suggesting a role to slow fibrosis in chronic liver disease.[119]

Silymarin has been evaluated in several trials of alcoholic liver disease. Ferenci and colleagues,[120] in an RCT of cirrhotic patients treated with 420 mg of silymarin or placebo, demonstrated an improved 4-year survival in the treatment group compared with the placebo-treated group. Patients with alcoholic liver disease and early cirrhosis (Child-Turcotte-Pugh class A) were more likely to benefit than were those with Child-Turcotte-Pugh class B or C. This trial, however, did not confirm a clear benefit of silymarin, because patients were not randomized properly: the placebo group contained patients with more advanced cirrhosis (Child-Turcotte-Pugh class C) than did the treatment group. In addition, the degree of abstinence from alcohol among the study participants was not followed, and the dropout rate was high. A larger, more rigorously defined study by Pares and colleagues[121] failed to demonstrate a survival benefit in alcoholic cirrhotic patients treated with 450 mg of daily silymarin compared with a group treated with placebo.

The Hepatitis C Antiviral Long-term Treatment against Cirrhosis (HALT-C) Trial was designed to determine whether

TABLE 131-5 CAM Therapies for Chronic Liver Disease

Therapy	Proposed Mechanism of Action	Evidence	Adverse Effects
Chinese herbal medicine (CHM)	Antioxidant; inhibition of stellate cell activation in animal studies; increased interferon production[131,132]; inhibition of HBV DNA polymerase[133]	Trials suggest that combination therapy of interferon and CHM might help increase clearance of HBsAg, HBeAg, HBV DNA; methodologic flaws preclude recommendation for use without further investigation	Hepatotoxicity, autoimmune hepatitis, interstitial pneumonitis, immune thrombocytopenic purpura
Licorice (Glycyrrhiza glabra)	Activates CYP450 phase I detoxification reactions, enhances endogenous interferon production, inhibits TNF-α[124,141]	RCTs demonstrate a biochemical effect; no demonstrable morbidity or mortality benefit[142]	Pseudoaldosteronism effects: hypokalemia, sodium retention, hypertension; potential digitalis toxicity if taken concurrently[144]
Milk thistle (Silybum marianum)	Antioxidant, anti-inflammatory, possibly antifibrotic effects[117-119]	Trials suggest benefit over placebo for improving serum aminotransferase levels. No data to support morbidity or mortality benefit[120,121,123-126]	Nausea, diarrhea, dyspepsia, headache, arthralgias, skin reactions, impotence, anaphylaxis; inhibits CYP3A4 and uridine diphosphate-glucuronyl transferase[123,124]
Picrorrhiza kurroa	Antioxidant, anti-inflammatory, antiviral effects[124]	Only one trial details efficacy in acute HBV infection; paucity of data precludes recommendations[148]	None reported
S-adenosyl-L-methionine (SAMe)	Involved in glutathione synthesis; acts as an antioxidant[128]	Methodologic flaws in trials assessing efficacy. No definitive data to support its use in alcoholic hepatitis	Dry mouth, nausea, akathisia; reported to block platelet aggregation in vitro
Thymic extracts	Unknown	Trials suggest that combination therapy with interferon yields higher virologic response rate than interferon alone or placebo[139]	Nausea, vomiting, rare thrombocytopenia[140]

CYP450, cytochrome P450; HBeAg, hepatitis B e antigen; HBsAg, hepatitis B surface antigen; RCT, randomized, controlled trial.

maintenance interferon therapy could slow disease progression in patients in whom prior interferon treatment had failed to eradicate HCV. Seeff and colleagues[122] examined the use and potential effects of silymarin in the HALT-C patient population. Among all participants, 67% had never used silymarin, 16% used it in the past, and 17% used it at baseline. Silymarin use varied widely with gender and ethnicity; men were more frequent users than women; non-Hispanic whites were more frequent users than African Americans and Hispanics. Silymarin use correlated strongly with higher education. No beneficial effect of silymarin was found on serum ALT or HCV RNA levels. Univariate analysis showed significantly fewer liver-related symptoms and better quality-of-life parameters in users than nonusers.

A systematic review of RCTs of silymarin in various hepatic diseases (hepatitis B, hepatitis C, alcoholic liver disease) also drew no firm conclusions about its therapeutic efficacy. Approximately one half of the trials demonstrated a significant biochemical response to silymarin, specifically a decrease in serum aminotransferase levels; however, this response did not translate into a statistically significant mortality or morbidity benefit. Favorable trends toward a decrease in the frequency of hepatic encephalopathy and GI bleeding were suggested by these trials, but a statistically significant difference was not reached between those treated with silymarin and those treated with placebo.[123,124]

Reddy and colleagues evaluated the use of silymarin in 1 of the original studies from the SyNCH (Silymarin in NASH and C Hepatitis) study group, a randomized multicenter, double-blind, placebo-controlled trial funded by the NCCAM. This was a phase I/II trial, the objectives of which were to examine the impact of silymarin on noncirrhotic patients who were nonresponders to traditional antiviral medications for HCV, and to evaluate its impact on patients with NASH who failed to respond to conventional treatment. The hope of this study was to define the role of silymarin in the treatment of these difficult-to-treat clinical conditions for which conventional medicine had failed to yield therapeutic results;[125] there did not appear to be a significant morbidity or mortality benefit of silymarin in the treatment of HCV. Extensive data on the effect of silymarin in the treatment of NASH are to date unpublished.[125]

In the most rigorous trial to date, Fried and colleagues of the SyNCH study group performed a multicenter double-blind, placebo-controlled trial that investigated patients with chronic HCV in whom interferon-based therapies had previously failed. Patients received 420 mg of silymarin, 700 mg of silymarin, or placebo 3 times daily for 24 weeks. No statistically significant differences were seen among treatment and placebo groups, definitively demonstrating that silymarin, even at 3 to 5 times the usual dose is ineffective in treating patients with chronic HCV.[126]

The reported AEs of silymarin include nausea, diarrhea, dyspepsia, headache, arthralgias, skin reactions, impotence, and anaphylaxis. Most important, milk thistle has been shown to inhibit CYP3A4 and uridine diphosphoglucuronosyl transferase, thereby potentially leading to interactions with traditional prescription medications such as quinine, lidocaine, certain calcium channel blocking agents, and cyclosporine, all of which are metabolized in part by CYP3A4.[123,124]

S-Adenosyl-L-Methionine

S-Adenosyl-L-methionine (SAMe) acts as a methyl donor for many biochemical reactions and participates in the synthesis of glutathione, the predominant biochemical antioxidant.[127] This compound has been studied most in the treatment of alcoholic liver disease. A systematic review of 8 placebo-controlled trials of patients treated for alcoholic liver disease revealed that SAMe had no statistically significant effect on mortality, liver-related mortality, or rate of liver transplantation,[124] and the methodological quality of these trials was poor. Further evaluation of SAMe in more properly designed trials is needed.[124]

SAMe also has been evaluated in the treatment of cholestasis of pregnancy. In several controlled trials, SAMe reduced pruritus and serum bilirubin levels during pregnancy, thereby suggesting possible efficacy.[128] The safety of this agent in pregnancy has been demonstrated in RCTs.[129]

Chinese Herbal Medicine

Chinese herbal medicine (CHM) is the most common CAM therapy used for treating HBV, and it is the therapy that has been evaluated most rigorously. HBV is a significant global health problem (see Chapter 79).[130] Given the large number of people affected and high rate of endemic HBV infection in some parts of the world such as Asia, it is not surprising that CAM therapies are often used to treat illness associated with HBV.

Many different herbal combinations have been used to treat HBV infection. For example, TJ-9, known as xiao-chai-hu-tang in China, is a combination of 7 herbs: *Bupleurum* root, *Pinellia* tuber, *Scutellaria* root, jujube fruit, ginger rhizome, ginseng root, and *Glycyrrhiza* root. This agent is thought to act as an antioxidant as well as an inhibitor of stellate cell fibrosis.[131,132] Another example of CHM is *Phyllanthus amarus*, the mechanism of action for which appears to be inhibition of HBV DNA polymerase.[133]

A systematic review of 9 RCTs that evaluated CHM revealed that compared with placebo treatment, the CHM compound fuzheng jiedu tang significantly increased the rate of clearance of hepatitis B surface antigen (HBsAg), hepatitis B e antigen (HBeAg), and HBV DNA. *P. amarus* and kurorinone were comparable to interferon treatment in clearing these serologic markers.[134] The quality of the aforementioned trials was poor, however, and thus no definitive conclusion can be reached at present regarding the efficacy of these agents for chronic HBV infection.

A review of the effects of CHM on asymptomatic HBsAg-positive carriers with normal aminotransferase levels evaluated 3 RCTs, all of which were of poor methodological quality. The compound Jianpi Wenshen recipe was found to have beneficial effects on clearance of HBsAg and HBeAg and on seroconversion of HBeAg to antibody to HBeAg.[135] Given the flaws in the methodology of the trials evaluated, however, a

recommendation for use of this agent cannot be endorsed without further investigation.

A meta-analysis of 27 RCTs compared CHM alone, CHM combined with interferon, and interferon alone for chronic HBV infection.[136] The absence of a strict placebo group in these trials is of concern. In China, where most CHM is used for HBV infection, CHM often is used as an adjunct or alternative to interferon therapy. Therefore, these trials were designed to assess the efficacy of CHM in conditions that replicate common clinical practice.[132] Patients who received CHM alone were more likely to clear HBsAg than were those treated with interferon alone. CHM was equivalent in efficacy to interferon in achieving clearance of HBeAg and HBV DNA. Patients who received combined therapy were more likely than those treated with interferon alone to achieve seroconversion for HBsAg and HBeAg and to clear HBV DNA.[132]

Although these trials appear to favor the use of CHM as a potential adjunct therapy to interferon, most of the trials were of poor methodological quality. In addition, most of the studies had a follow-up of only 3 months for assessing treatment outcomes. The studies that were reviewed were published in Chinese journals, and many details regarding blinding and randomization of the subjects in the trials were omitted, raising additional concerns regarding methodological quality.[132]

CHM also has been studied for the treatment of HCV infection. A systematic review of 10 randomized trials evaluated the efficacy of CHM in patients with chronic HCV infection. The results of the trials were disappointing in that none of the herbal agents employed was found to increase the rate of HCV RNA clearance. In addition, 9 of the 10 trials showed no improvement in serum aminotransferase levels.[137]

AEs of CHM include hepatotoxicity; however, given the lack of manufacturing uniformity in content and potency of these agents, definitive causality has not been established.[138] Cases of interstitial pneumonitis, autoimmune hepatitis, and acute thrombocytopenic purpura also have been reported.[124]

Thymic Extract

The efficacy and safety of thymic extract in treating HCV infection has been evaluated in 5 RCTs. Patients who received thymosin-1, a synthetic polypeptide, in combination with interferon therapy were more likely to have complete virologic response than were those patients treated with interferon alone or with placebo.[139] Reported AEs included nausea and vomiting, and 1 case of thrombocytopenia.[140]

Licorice (Glycyrrhiza glabra)

Licorice (*G. glabra*) therapy has been evaluated for treatment of chronic HCV infection. The active component of licorice, glycyrrhizin, is thought to activate cytochrome P450 phase I detoxification reactions, stimulate endogenous interferon, and inhibit TNF-α.[124,141] In an RCT, Suzuki and colleagues[142] demonstrated that daily injections of Stronger Neo-Minophagen C, a compound of glycyrrhizin, glycine, and cysteine, decreased serum aminotransferase levels compared with placebo. A morbidity or mortality benefit was not demonstrated. Furthermore, the follow-up period in this trial was only 1 month, making it extremely difficult to assess any long-term AEs of *G. glabra*. Given that this study was published in 1983, the presence of HCV was not determined in the study population; inclusion criteria merely necessitated histologic evidence of chronic hepatitis. It is not clear, in fact, that the study population had HCV infection.

Another RCT evaluated the effects of *G. glabra* in patients with chronic HCV infection[143] and compared the efficacy of combined ursodeoxycholic acid and glycyrrhizin with glycyrrhizin alone. There was a statistically significant biochemical improvement in the treatment group, but the trial lacked a placebo arm, thereby making definitive conclusion of therapeutic and clinically relevant efficacy beyond placebo effect uncertain.

AEs with *G. glabra* are thought to be secondary to the active metabolite of licorice root, glycyrrhizin, which inhibits 11-β-hydroxysteroid dehydrogenase. This inhibition leads to a pseudoaldosterone effect, resulting in hypokalemia, sodium retention, and hypertension[144]; hypokalemia can increase the risk of toxicity from some drugs, such as digitalis.

Ayurvedic Medicine

Picrorrhiza kurroa is an Indian herb commonly used in traditional Ayurvedic medicine. It has been used for many GI conditions and also is often used for hepatic disease. The active ingredients, picroside and kutkoside,[145] are thought to act as antioxidants, anti-inflammatory agents, and inhibitors of proinflammatory cytokines.[124] Various studies have described possible cancer chemopreventive and antiviral qualities of these agents.[146,147] One trial demonstrated a beneficial biochemical effect of *P. kurroa* in reducing serum aminotransferase levels in patients with acute HBV infection.[148] Clearly, more data are needed before any recommendation can be made regarding this agent.

Liv 52 is an Indian Ayurvedic medication that has been marketed specifically for the treatment of liver disease. It is composed of *Capparis spinosa* (capers), *Cichorium intybus* (wild chicory), *Terminalia arjuna* (arjuna), *Solanum nigrum* (black nightshade), *Achillea millefolium* (yarrow), and *Tamarix gallica* (tatarisk).[149] This agent has demonstrated efficacy in protecting rats from carbon tetrachloride and alcohol-induced liver injury, as well as improving liver function in patients with acute viral hepatitis. This agent was withdrawn from the U.S. market, however, after an RCT demonstrated decreased survival in patients with alcoholic hepatitis compared with placebo-treated patients.[150]

Acupuncture

Acupuncture has been demonstrated in a study by Li and colleagues to have gained popularity in patients with chronic hepatitis; approximately 9% of patients report implementing this therapy. There are no convincing data detailing the effectiveness of acupuncture in treatment of either chronic hepatitis B or C. Li and colleagues have demonstrated that acupuncture is useful as an adjunctive therapy to ameliorate postoperative pain in patients with pain from hepatocellular carcinoma and secondary to hepatic capsule inflammation.[151]

GI Malignancies

Estimates are that up to 64% of adult oncology patients have used CAM therapies at some point during their treatment.[152] The motivation for these therapies in oncology patients is similar to the rationale cited by other patient populations: CAM therapies are appealing as a result of a failure of conventional medicine to control or cure disease, and they provide patients with a mechanism for feeling in more control of their therapeutic plan. Textbooks have been dedicated to this subject, and the discussion that follows just highlights the most commonly employed CAM therapies.

A systematic review of the beneficial effect of green tea consumption to reduce the incidence of GI malignancy[153] demonstrated that green tea did help prevent colonic adenomatous polyp formation and chronic atrophic gastritis. No definitive supporting evidence, however, was found to conclude that green tea had a similar beneficial effect on the incidence of GI malignancy.

Garlic is thought to inhibit the development of gastric cancer through several proposed mechanisms. An antibacterial effect against Hp has been demonstrated and is attributable to the thiosulfinate component of this agent.[154] Kaempferol, a flavonol present in high concentration in garlic, also contributes to the detoxification of carcinogenic compounds.[155] Published studies suggest that garlic might protect against the development of gastric and colonic carcinomas. Most of the literature, however, consists of observational studies that cannot be used to confirm a therapeutic effect of garlic. Additional therapeutic intervention trials are needed to substantiate the claim that garlic is chemopreventive.[156]

Vitamins C and E are antioxidants that might reduce the incidence of colorectal cancer. In an epidemiologic study of colorectal cancer patients, long-term use of vitamins C and E did not provide a mortality benefit. In a subgroup analysis, however, use of vitamin C for more than 10 years was associated with a decreased risk of death from colorectal cancer before 65 years of age and a decreased risk of rectal cancer mortality at any age.[157]

Other dietary factors also could play a role in preventing malignancy. In Mediterranean countries there is a lower incidence of breast, endometrial, colorectal, and prostate cancer compared with Western countries. These cancers have been postulated to have a relationship to diet, in that a low consumption of fruits and vegetables and a high consumption of red meat correlate with cancer incidence. A traditional Mediterranean diet contains low amounts of red meat and high amounts of fruits, vegetables, and olive oil. By statistical modeling, some epidemiologists estimate that up to 25% of colorectal cancer could be prevented in Western countries if diets were changed to reflect Mediterranean practices.[158]

Several CAM therapies have been implemented to help ameliorate pain in patients with metastatic disease. Acupuncture has shown promise for the treatment of the pain associated with gastric cancer.[159] *Lycopodium clavatum*, a type of fern moss, has been reported to be an effective homeopathic treatment for rectal cancer pain.[160] Meditation and relaxation therapies are practiced commonly by many cancer patients, not only to ameliorate physical pain, but also to help cope with the depression that commonly accompanies malignant disease.

SAFETY AND REGULATION OF CAM THERAPIES

With the increasing popularity of CAM therapies, it is important that physicians understand their mechanisms of action as well as the data supporting their efficacy. Although some medical schools and residency programs are increasingly offering education programs in CAM therapies, curricula should be mandated to include information on these modalities so as to familiarize medical professionals with these practices early in their careers. A study by Mikail and colleagues[161] reported that only 16% of medical residents surveyed routinely asked their patients about their use of herbal therapy. It is equally important that health care professionals also understand the lack of regulatory mechanisms for these modalities, so that effective safety measures can be employed to protect the welfare of patients.

A study was performed recently to presented in 2012 evaluated and compared the general knowledge base of CAM therapies between gastroenterology fellows-in-training and attending physicians.[162] Any demonstrated differences would help in determining where to target a formalized curriculum on the subject matter so as to maximize educational efforts. Attending physicians demonstrated a more comprehensive knowledge base; however, over 90% of participants rated their knowledge of CAM therapies as "no knowledge" or "minimal." A majority of respondents indicated an interest in having formal instruction in CAM therapies, with supplement therapies being the topic they most wished to learn more about. By incorporating complementary therapies into the curriculum of gastroenterology postgraduate education, individuals will acquire a more thorough knowledge base of CAM therapies, which will allow them to care for their patients in a more comprehensive fashion.

In the United States, total yearly sales of herbal supplements are approximately $13.9 billion and steadily increasing. An estimated 15 million adults take prescription medications concurrently with herbal supplements.[1] Therefore, the safety of concurrent administration of herbal supplements and traditional allopathic medications is a concern to many physicians. In 1994, the U.S. Congress implemented the Dietary Supplement Health and Education Act (DSHEA), legislation written to prevent the FDA from regulating dietary supplements "excessively" and to ensure that safe and appropriately labeled supplements remain available to those persons who wish to use them.

DSHEA officially defines a "dietary supplement" as:

A product (other than tobacco) that is intended to supplement the diet that bears or contains one or more of the following dietary ingredients: a vitamin, a mineral, an herb or other botanical, an amino acid, a dietary substance for use by man to supplement the diet by increasing total daily intake, or a concentrate, metabolite, constituent, extract or combination of these ingredients.[163]

Additional FDA guidelines specify that supplement manufacturers themselves are responsible for determining the safety of their products and for providing the evidence, if asked, to substantiate the claims made by their individual products. Approval from the FDA is not required before marketing of most of these agents unless the supplement is deemed "new." A new supplement is defined as an agent not marketed before October 15, 1994; however, no definitive list exists of products marketed before this date. Therefore, the responsibility rests with the manufacturer to determine if its product is in fact a new supplement. This rule creates an obvious conflict of interest in that new supplements require clinical research and capital expenditures to substantiate their efficacy, and manufacturers would prefer that supplement therapies be considered previously marketed.

Additionally, supplement manufacturers are not required to report AEs that occur with use of their products. It is the responsibility of the FDA to prove that products are unsafe before their use can be restricted.[162] The FDA relies on physicians and other health care professionals to report suspected AEs before an inquiry can be established for a particular agent. Therefore, it is of utmost importance that all health care professionals be aware of their patients' use of supplements, both to provide safe care and to know when to suspect AEs or medication interactions. Suspected AEs events or medication interactions can be reported online at http://www.fda.gov/medwatch.

Resources for health care professionals regarding CAM therapies have become much more accessible. Information regarding definitions of CAM therapies, as well as efficacy of the various modalities, can be found at the following websites:

www.nccam.nih.gov
www.fda.gov
www.cochrane.org
www.NaturalDatabase.com

All health care professionals should be aware of these resources so as to effectively and safely prescribe medications and care for patients from a comprehensive standpoint. It is hoped that through continued educational efforts at all levels of medical training, the data regarding the efficacy of CAM therapies, as well as their potential benefits and dangers, will be increasingly understood. Health care professionals and their patients will then be able to maintain a healthy therapeutic rapport while at the same time incorporating these therapeutic modalities, if they are clinically appropriate, in a safe and efficacious manner.

KEY REFERENCES

Full references for this chapter can be found on www.expertconsult.com.

1. Eisenberg DM, Davis RB, Ettner SL, et al. Trends in alternative medicine use in the United States, 1990-1997. JAMA 1998; 280:1569-75.
8. Koretz RL, Rotblatt M. Complementary and alternative medicine in gastroenterology: The good, the bad, and the ugly. Clin Gastroenterol Hepatol 2004; 2:957-67.
11. Ernst E, Pittler MH. Efficacy of ginger for nausea and vomiting: A systematic review of randomized clinical trials. Br J Anaesth 2000; 84:367-71.
34. Coon JT, Ernst E. Systematic review: Herbal medicinal products for non-ulcer dyspepsia. Aliment Pharmacol Ther 2002; 16:1689-99.
50. Melzer J, Rosch W, Reichling J, et al. Meta-analysis: Phytotherapy of functional dyspepsia with the herbal drug preparation STW 5 (Iberogast). Aliment Pharmacol Ther 2004; 20:1279-87.
53. Brandt LJ, Bjorkman D, Fennerty MB, et al. Systematic review on the management of irritable bowel syndrome in North America. Am J Gastroenterol 2002; 97(Suppl 11):S7.
65. Madisch A, Holtmann G, Plein K, Hotz J. Treatment of irritable bowel syndrome with herbal preparations: Results of a double-blind, randomized, placebo-controlled, multi-center trial. Aliment Pharmacol Ther 2004; 19:271-9.
74. Brenner DM, Moeller M, Chey WD. Schoenfeld P. The utility of probiotics in the treatment of irritable bowel syndrome: A systematic review. Am J Gastroenterol 2007; 104:1033-49.
75. Whorwell PJ, Prior A, Colgan SM. Hypnotherapy in severe irritable bowel syndrome: Further experience. Gut 1987; 28:423-25.
77. Lindfors P, Unge P, Arvidsson P, et al. Effects of gut directed hypnotherapy on IBS in different clinical settings—Results from two randomized controlled trials. Am J Gastroenterol 2012; 107:276-85.
95. Hanai H, Iida T, Takeuchi K, et al. Curcumin maintenance therapy for ulcerative colitis: Randomized, multicenter, double-blind, placebo-controlled trial. Clin Gastroenterol Hepatol 2006; 4:1502-6.
101. Sandborn WJ, Targan SR, Byers VS, et al. *Andrographis paniculata* extract (HMPL-004) for active ulcerative colitis. Am J Gastroenterol 2012; 108:90-8.

124. Levy C, Seeff LD, Lindor KD. Use of herbal supplements for chronic liver disease. Clin Gastroenterol Hepatol 2004; 2:947-56.

126. Fried MW, Navarro VJ, Afdhal N, et al. Effect of silymarin (milk thistle) on liver disease in patients with chronic hepatitis C unsuccessfully treated with interferon therapy: A randomized controlled trial. JAMA 2012; 308:274-82.

149. Verma S, Thuluvath PJ. Complementary and alternative medicine in hepatology: Review of the evidence of efficacy. Clin Gastroenterol Hepatol 2007; 5:408-16.

CHAPTER OUTLINE

The purpose of this chapter is to gain an understanding of the complex physical and psychosocial care needs of seriously ill patients. Common GI symptoms, important aspects of setting appropriate life goals of care, and communication skills are reviewed.

WHAT IS PALLIATIVE MEDICINE?

Palliative care is an approach that improves the quality of life of seriously ill patients and their families through the prevention and relief of suffering. Integral to this care is the early identification, impeccable assessment, and treatment of pain and other problems, including their physical, psychosocial, and spiritual needs.[1] Currently, palliative care is offered to patients only in the very late stages of serious illness.[2] It should, however, be offered concurrently with curative therapies from the time of diagnosis, because many patients suffer in silence not only from their illness but from treatment-related symptoms and consequences. In fact, data show that concurrent curative and palliative treatments may prolong lifespan.[3]

Most patients want to die gently at home with comfort and dignity[4,5] and are able to articulate some or all of the following goals[6]:

Freedom from pain and other distressing symptoms
Having a sense of personal control over end-of-life decisions
Avoiding inappropriate prolongation of the dying process
Finding meaning and purpose in life
Saying goodbye to friends and families
Quality palliative care for seriously ill persons who endure complex physical and psychosocial problems are best provided by a team of multidisciplinary clinicians, including physicians, nurses, social workers, chaplains, and bereavement counselors. The interdisciplinary palliative care team works in concert with, and does not replace, the primary medical team. Thus, the ultimate goal of palliative care is to prevent and relieve suffering and to optimize quality of life for patients and their families, regardless of whether their anticipated prognosis is on the order of days, months, years, or decades.

HOSPICE VERSUS PALLIATIVE CARE

Palliative medicine is the medical subspecialty that provides a complete set of options for pain and symptom management in all seriously ill patients; it can easily incorporate concurrent curative therapies like bone-marrow transplant and liver transplant into the treatment plan as needed. Hospice care shares the philosophy of palliative care to give utmost importance to patient-centered care and shared decision making to provide care that is congruent with the patient's goals and values. However, hospice care in the United States is also a financial reimbursement system for patients with an anticipated lifespan of 6 months or less and is largely defined by the Medicare Hospice Benefit (MHB). As such, hospice care has defined regulations and admission criteria. Under the MHB, patients are eligible for a specific set of services if the physician certifies that the patient has 6 months or less to live, if the disease follows its usual course, and if the goal of treatment is oriented toward comfort rather than cure.[7] It is important to note that MHB does *not* require patients to relinquish heroic life-prolonging measures, future hospitalizations, or participation in research. Prognosis is based on the attending

BOX 132-1 What Is Palliative Care?

Provides relief from pain and other distressing symptoms

Affirms life and regards dying as a normal process

Intends neither to hasten nor postpone death

Integrates psychological and spiritual aspects of patient care

Offers a support system to help patients live as actively as possible until death

Offers a support system to help the family cope during the patient's illness and in their own bereavement

Uses a team approach to address the needs of patients and their families, including bereavement counseling, if indicated

Enhances quality of life and may also positively influence the course of illness

Is applicable early in the course of illness, in conjunction with other therapies that are intended to prolong life, such as chemotherapy or radiation therapy, and includes those investigations needed to better understand and manage distressing clinical complications

Adapted from WHO, 2008.

physician's clinical judgment regarding the normal course of the person's illness; if the patient lives beyond the expected 6 months, the hospice benefit through Medicare may be continued by recertifying the patient under MHB. Although hospice care can be provided in special residential facilities or in long-term care facilities, currently most hospice care in the U.S. is provided in the patient's home.

In contrast to hospice care, and because palliative care is a medical subspecialty, billing for reimbursement is similar to any other medical subspecialty (e.g., gastroenterology or cardiology). Simply put, all hospice care is palliative, but not all palliative care is hospice care (Box 132-1). To truly provide seamless care of patients who are seriously ill, communities need both palliative care and hospice services.

EXPLORING THE GOALS OF CARE

Exploring patient-defined goals of care is the first step in determining the most appropriate therapeutic interventions in any serious illness. It is also important to engage the family in provision of care that is consonant with the patient's stated wishes, because many patients lose their decision-making capacity in advanced illness.[9] An organized approach to goal setting can help the clinician and patient achieve clearly articulated goals. Goal setting is best accomplished through meeting with the patient and family or surrogate decision-maker (Box 132-2). Before a goal-setting meeting, the clinician should review the disease course, the patient's response to prior treatments, and the potential for further disease-modifying treatments, and then develop a realistic short- and long-term vision for the future clinical course, including a general sense of prognosis. With this in mind, the clinician can begin to review treatment options and help the patient decide which treatments are most likely to help meet his or her specific goals. All therapeutic options should be examined in light of the question, "Does the intervention match or assist with the patient's treatment goals?"[10] As the burden of decision making increases near the end of life, it is important for physicians to understand their central role in helping patients make decisions. A model of shared decision making[9] in which the physician provides guidance and recommendations generally is preferred to a paternalistic approach or, at the opposite extreme, to one in which numerous treatment options are

presented with no guidance[11] about how each option may relate to the patient's goals of care.

PROGNOSTICATION

Physicians' estimates of patient survival are important to physicians as well as to patients and families in all phases of a patient's life, because they influence both medical and nonmedical decisions. This is especially true at the end of life when patients and families have to make numerous personal, fiscal, and social arrangements in anticipation of impending death.

Despite the great need for accurate prognosis, prognostication remains an elusive clinical art. Numerous empirical studies have revealed a consistent optimistic bias,[12] with most physicians overestimating anticipated lifespan by a factor of 3. Physicians' prognostic "radars" are further skewed when they are more connected with the patient. Consequently, patients who are in great need of quality palliative care are referred too late to palliative care services and thus are deprived of access to good symptom management.

There are 2 key tasks in prognosticating: (1) formulating the prognosis by reviewing patient-specific medical factors and disease-specific actuarial estimation of survival; and (2) communicating the prognosis to patients and families while providing ongoing support.

Given that prognostication is challenging, many physicians are uncomfortable with this task and often avoid providing realistic prognostic information, or may continue to offer ineffective treatment options that can convey false hope and unrealistic expectations to patients and families. When pressed by patients, physicians then typically overestimate survival. If the imminence of death is not discussed honestly, patients might be more likely to accept costly, burdensome, and futile treatments.[13]

Prognostication guidelines are well established for cancer.[14,15] The single best prognostic variable in cancer is performance status.[14,15] For example, patients with a Karnofsky Performance Status (KPS) of 40 (disabled; requires special care and assistance) live on average less than 50 days, and patients with a KPS of 20 live an average of only 10 to 20 days (Table 132-1).[14] Put another way, patients who are either bed-fast or spending more than 50% of the day resting or in bed because of the effects of the serious illness generally have a prognosis of 3 months or less. Specific symptoms provide further information: symptoms with an independent predictive value for a poor prognosis are shortness of breath, anorexia, difficulty swallowing, and weight loss.[14]

Prognostic criteria for non-cancer diagnoses have been published and are especially useful to help physicians know when to refer patients for hospice services.[16] Specific to gastroenterology, for example, general criteria have been established for chronic liver disease (Box 132-3). Beyond guidelines, data show that the question[17-20] "Would I be surprised if this patient died in the next year?" is helpful in identifying patient with poor prognosis.

No matter what type of cancer or non-cancer fatal illness a person has, a "common final clinical pathway" occurs in most patients.[14] Signs and symptoms that predict a prognosis of hours to days are decreased or fluctuating levels of consciousness, a precipitous clinical decline, decreased oral intake, and inability to turn over in bed.[15] Patients close to death typically exhibit periods of apnea, retained oropharyngeal secretions (the death rattle), fever, and cool or mottled extremities.[15]

Discussing prognosis with patients and families is a key skill in palliative care. The first step is to form a clear mental

---

BOX 132-2 Process Steps for a Goal-Setting Family Meeting

1. Determine the reasons for convening a family conference.
   Clarify the goals of care and review the patient's medical condition.
   Decide on future levels of care and treatments, and resolve family conflicts.
2. Determine who should and who will be present for the conference.
   Include appropriate health care providers (e.g., nurse, chaplain, social worker, physician consultants, primary care physician).
   Ask the patient, or health care power of attorney, who he or she would like to participate (e.g., the designated health care power of attorney, appropriate family members, clergy, lawyer, friend).
   Family and other participants should be given significant time (often 48 hours) to prepare for the meeting.
3. Determine whether the patient has decision-making capacity:
   Able to understand information about diagnosis and treatment?
   Able to evaluate alternatives and compare risks and benefits?
   Able to communicate a choice—verbally, in writing, or with a nod or gesture?
4. Choose the proper physical setting.
5. Introduce yourself, explain your relationship to the patient, and invite all participants to do the same.
6. Identify the legal decision maker, if available.*
7. Review the goals and purpose of the meeting.
8. Establish ground rules:
   Everyone will have the opportunity to talk.
   No interruptions are permitted.
9. Review the patient's current medical condition.
   "What is your understanding of ____'s present condition?" or "What have you been told about ____'s condition?"
   Review with the patient and family the current medical condition (e.g., expected prognosis and potential treatment plans). Avoid medical jargon.
   Invite questions.
   Defer treatment decision-making until all questions about the patient's medical status have been asked to the extent possible.

10. Family discussion guidelines include the following:
    When the patient can speak for himself or herself:
    Ask the patient what he or she is considering.
    Ask the patient what type of support he or she would like from family members and from the health care team.
    Invite discussion from other family members.
    When the patient cannot speak for himself or herself:
    Describe the goal of substituted decision-making (i.e., to speak on behalf of the patient by making those choices we believe the patient would make if he or she could speak).
    Ask each family member what he or she believes the patient would choose if he or she were able to speak on his or her own behalf.
    Ask each family member what his or her own wishes are for the patient.
    Allow patient and family and other important people to the patient (e.g., clergy, friends, lawyer) time alone if they wish to talk before making a decision.
    If there is a clear consensus of opinion, the meeting can be concluded. If there is no consensus, see No. 11.
11. Follow these guidelines when there is no consensus.
    Ask the family to discuss the issue on their own and schedule a follow-up meeting (use time as an ally).
    Ask each family member on what values his or her decision is based and how the decision will affect the patient and the other family members.
    Review again the goals you are trying to reach: What would the patient say if he or she were able to speak?
    Discuss other resources to support decision-making.
12. Bring the conference to conclusion.
    Summarize the meeting for the family, including areas of agreement and disagreement.
    Decide if the decisions made lead to related issues that should be addressed while the family is present (e.g., "do not resuscitate" order, continuation or withdrawal of treatments, discharge planning).
    Provide a plan for follow-up, and offer to schedule further meetings with the family.
    Document a summary of the meeting in the medical record.
    Discuss relevant issues with all health team members.

*Laws governing surrogate decision making vary from state to state.
Adapted from Weissman DE, Ambuel B. Establishing treatment goals, withdrawing treatments. In: Weissman DE, Ambuel B, Hallenback J, editors. Improving end-of-life care. 3rd ed. Milwaukee: Medical College of Wisconsin; 2000. p 101.

---

picture of the overall status of health and prognosis of the patient by carefully reviewing all the medical records and correlating physical examination and other data with the current patient history (with special importance to gauging symptom burden, mood, and functional status). Next, physicians are advised to start by asking patients if they previously have been given prognostic information, if they have a sense of how much time is left, and whether they would like to discuss prognosis. If a patient indicates that he or she wishes to discuss prognostic information, and given that the prognostic ability of doctors is not very accurate, it is important to provide an estimate as a range, such as a few days to a few weeks or a few weeks to a few months, rather than "Mr. Jones, you have only 6 months to live."[7] Once the time frame is presented, important future goals can be determined by asking, "What do you want or need to do in the time that is left?" (e.g., important events, saying goodbye to loved ones). This allows the clinician to aim the information at the level of the patient and family.[15]

KEY PROGNOSTIC VARIABLES AND TOOLS

MELD Scores

The MELD score (see Chapter 97) is a numeric scale used to prioritize patients for liver transplantation.[22-26] It is calculated by a formula using the serum bilirubin, INR, and serum creatinine. The MELD score has been validated for short-term and intermediate-term mortality in a heterogeneous group of patients with liver disease.[21] Modifications of the MELD score using serum sodium values are thought to enhance its prognostic ability for patients with cirrhosis. A recent study demonstrated that the MELD score and its sodium-based variants (MELD-Na, MELDNa, and MESO) are effective tools to predict mortality of patients with decompensated cirrhosis for short and intermediate periods.[27] Of these, MELDNa and MESO scores are superior for predicting 3- and 6-month survival.

TABLE 132-1 Karnofsky Performance Scale

%	Level of Functional Capacity
100	Normal, no complaints, no evidence of disease
90	Able to carry on normal activity; minor symptoms or signs of disease
80	Normal activity with effort; some symptoms or signs of disease
70	Cares for self; unable to carry on normal activity or to do active work
60	Requires occasional assistance but is able to care for most needs
50	Requires considerable assistance and frequent medical care
40	Disabled, requires special care and assistance
30	Severely disabled; hospitalization is indicated although death is not imminent
20	Hospitalization is necessary; patient is very sick; active supportive treatment is necessary
10	Moribund, fatal processes are progressing rapidly
0	Dead

From Karnofsky, DA, Burchenal, JH. The clinical evaluation of chemotherapeutic agents in cancer. In: MacLeod CM, editor. Evaluation of chemotherapeutic agents. New York: Columbia University Press; 1949. p 196.

BOX 132-3 Hospice Eligibility Criteria for End-Stage Liver Disease

The patient is *not* a transplant candidate and opts for comfort care *and*
The patient has:
    Prothrombin time >5 sec over control or INR >1.5 *and*
    Serum albumin <2.5 g/dL *and* one or more of the following conditions:
        Ascites refractory to treatment, or the patient is not compliant with treatment
        SBP
        Hepatorenal syndrome, elevated serum creatinine and BUN, oliguria (<400 mL/day), urine sodium concentration <10 mEq/L, cirrhosis, and ascites
        Hepatic encephalopathy refractory to treatment, or the patient is not compliant with treatment
        Recurrent variceal bleeding despite intensive therapy
Supporting documentation (as applicable):
    Progressive malnutrition
    Muscle wasting with reduced strength and endurance
    Continued active alcoholism (>80 g ethanol/day)
    Hepatocellular carcinoma
    HBsAg positivity

BUN, blood urea nitrogen; HBsAg, hepatitis B surface antigen.
Adapted from Standards and Accreditation Committee. Medical guidelines for determining prognosis in selected noncancer diseases. 2nd ed. Arlington, Va.: National Hospice Organization; 1996.

Hepatorenal Syndrome

Hepatorenal syndrome (see Chapter 94) refers to functional renal failure in end-stage liver disease and is classified into 2 types, each with a different prognosis. Type 1 hepatorenal syndrome exhibits a rapidly progressive reduction of renal function, and manifests clinically as acute renal failure. Patients with type 1 hepatorenal syndrome have a median survival of 2 weeks. Type 2 hepatorenal syndrome exhibits moderate renal failure with steady or slowly progressive renal failure. These patients present with refractory ascites and have a median survival of 4 to 6 months.

Malignant Ascites

Only 10% of patients who have ascites have malignancy as the primary cause; epithelial malignancies (ovary, breast, endometrial, colon, gastric, and pancreatic) cause 80% of cases. Ascites is an indicator of poor prognosis, and patients with malignant ascites have a median survival of 4 months. If the malignant ascites and the underlying malignancy are chemoresponsive, survival may be prolonged. Ascites is very distressing to patients and should be managed aggressively to optimize patients' quality of life (see Chapter 93).

Hepatic Encephalopathy

Survival in patients with hepatic encephalopathy (see Chapter 94) is very short: approximately 20% to 40% at 1 year and 15% at 3 years of follow-up.

COMMON THEMES IN PALLIATING GI AND HEPATIC DISEASES

A complete review of symptoms commonly experienced by patients being cared for by palliative medicine physicians is beyond the scope of this chapter. Some of the more common symptoms of patients with advanced GI and hepatic disease, and common GI symptoms experienced by all patients at end of life, are discussed briefly in the following sections. As with all interventions, the benefit and burden of each treatment need to be evaluated in light of each patient's goals of care. If an intervention does not help advance a patient's individual goals of care, it should be withheld or withdrawn.[22]

Abdominal Pain

Freedom from pain is a central goal of palliative medicine. Abdominal pain can occur as 1 of 3 types: somatic, visceral, or neuropathic.

Diagnosis

Somatic pain typically is described as dull and achy; abdominal wall stretching from ascites is a common example. Patients describe visceral abdominal pain as poorly localized; it can be diffuse (e.g., with peritonitis), referred (e.g., pain that is felt in the shoulder from hepatic disease), or colicky (e.g., with bowel or bile duct obstruction).[28] Visceral pain associated with ailments such as gallstones, acute pancreatitis, acute appendicitis, and diverticulitis are the most common reasons for visits to outpatient and inpatient GI clinics.[29] Data suggest that GI nociception is mediated predominantly by spinal visceral afferents.

Spinal mesenteric and serosal nerve endings (combination of chemo- and mechanonociceptors) mediate acute pain

Simple Descriptive Pain Intensity Scale*

No pain — Mild pain — Moderate pain — Severe pain — Very severe pain — Worst possible pain

0–10 Numeric Pain Intensity Scale*

0 — 1 — 2 — 3 — 4 — 5 — 6 — 7 — 8 — 9 — 10
No pain — Moderate pain — Worst possible pain

Visual Analog Scale (VAS)†

No pain — Pain as bad as it could possibly be

FIGURE 132-1. Pain intensity scales. *If used as a graphic rating scale, a line 10 cm long is recommended. †A line 10 cm long is recommended for VAS scales. *(From Agency for Health Care Policy and Research. Management of cancer pain: Adults. Rockville, Md.: U.S. Department of Health and Human Services, Public Health Services; 1994.)*

By mouth	When giving pain medications, the oral route is always preferred over other routes, such as transdermal, intravenous, or subcutaneous routes
By the clock	Chronic basal pain usually is best treated with scheduled long-acting pain medications, plus short-acting pain medications on an as-needed basis for incidental or breakthrough pain
By the ladder	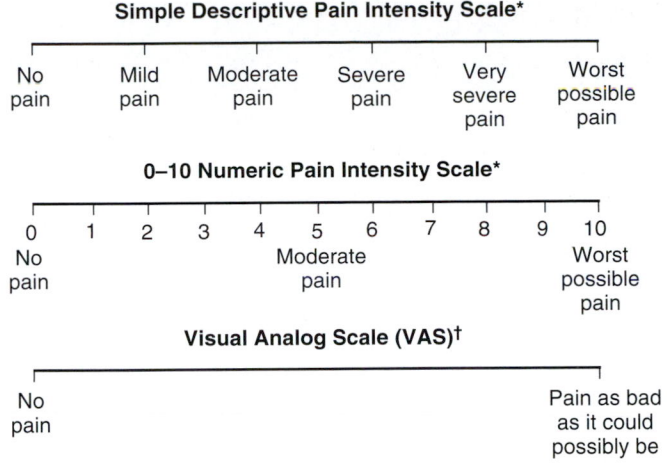

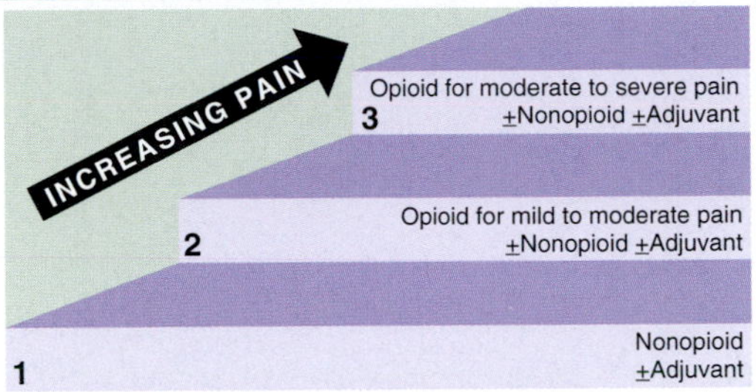

Pain Ladder from the WHO

FIGURE 132-2. Recommended approach to opioid therapy for patients with chronic severe pain. *(From Periyakoil VS. Opioid conversion. Stanford palliative care online curriculum 2008. [cited 2009 June 23] Available at: http://endoflife.stanford.edu.)*

caused by bowel distension or ischemia. Mucosal endings probably have a greater role after sensitization that results from inflammatory states. Neuropathic abdominal pain arises from direct damage to peripheral or autonomic nerves near the spinal cord, the celiac or lumbar plexus, or more peripheral nerves. Neuropathic pain usually is described as tingling, burning, throbbing, sharp, or lancinating; abdominal pain from pancreatic cancer invading the celiac plexus is a common example.[28]

It is important to distinguish between pain types, because treatments for each type of pain may differ. A thorough pain assessment is the first step. Questions to be asked include location, duration, temporal pattern, and pain modifiers.[30] Patients should be asked to rate the pain on a numeric or visual analog scale or from mild to severe (Fig. 132-1). Other important questions are drug and nondrug treatments that have been used, including their efficacy and toxicity. Finally, clinicians should assess the impact of the pain on the patient's activities of daily living, the patient's understanding of the cause of pain, and the patient's specific goals for pain relief (e.g., improved sleep).[31]

Treatment

Nonpharmacologic therapies (e.g., relaxation exercises, imagery, and judicious use of heat and cold) and over-the-counter medications (e.g., NSAIDs and acetaminophen) often are adequate for mild pain. Opioids are the drugs of choice for moderate to severe pain[28] seen in patients with serious illness. Short-acting opioids taken orally (morphine sulfate immediate release, oxycodone, hydrocodone, and hydromorphone) reach their peak effect in 60 to 90 minutes and provide analgesic benefit for 2 to 4 hours (Fig. 132-2, Table 132-2).[28] There is no ceiling dose of opioids, and the dose is limited mainly by their side effects. Combination products containing an opioid with acetaminophen, aspirin, or NSAIDs have a ceiling based on the toxicity profile of the nonopioid.[28]

Long-acting oral opioid preparations (morphine or oxycodone sustained action) provide 8 to 12 hours of analgesia.[28] Transdermal fentanyl offers 72 hours of pain relief and is a good option for patients with stable opioid requirements who cannot take oral medications.[31] Transdermal fentanyl takes 12 to 24 hours to reach full effect, and analgesia and toxicities last for up to 24 hours after removal of a patch.[31] A small percentage of patients need to replace the patch before 72 hours; cases of withdrawal occurring between 48 and 72 hours have been reported.[26,32]

Seriously ill patients who are receiving a long-acting opioid preparation typically need a short-acting opioid for breakthrough pain. One method for calculating the size of the dose for breakthrough pain is to take 10% to 20% of the 24-hour daily opioid dose and give it every 1 to 4 hours as needed.[28] For example, if a patient is using 120 mg/day of long-acting morphine, an appropriate breakthrough dose would be morphine sulfate immediate release, 15 mg orally every 1 to 4 hours as needed.

The oral route is preferred for opioid administration based on availability, cost, and ease of use.[28] For those with dysphagia, many of the short-acting oral opioids come in concentrated solutions.[28] Fentanyl also comes in a buccal tablet and in a candy matrix on an applicator stick that can be twirled against the buccal mucosa for absorption; it has a quick onset and is an option for breakthrough pain.[28,33] Morphine and hydromorphone can be administered rectally in the same dosages as used orally, with analgesic benefit similar to that in the oral route.[28]

Most long-acting oral morphine and oxycodone preparations are too large to put into NG or gastrostomy tubes, and crushing them destroys their long-acting properties. Long-acting opioid analgesia for patients with gastrostomy tubes can be provided using methadone (liquid formulation or by crushing the solid pill), using a special formulation of morphine in which the tiny pellets in the capsule are coated with a polymer that gives them extended release, or by using a fentanyl transdermal patch. The sustained-action formulation of morphine or other opioids should *not* be crushed and delivered through the gastrostomy tube; the time-release formulation is on the outer coating of the pill, and when crushed, the

TABLE 132-2 Common Opioids			
Drug	**Oral Dose***	**Parenteral Dose***	**Conversion Ratio to Oral Morphine**
Morphine sulfate	30 mg	10 mg	Parenteral morphine is about 3 times as potent as oral morphine
Oxycodone	20 mg	N/A	Oral oxycodone is about 1.5 times as potent as oral morphine
Hydrocodone	20 mg	N/A	Oral hydrocodone is about 1.5 times as potent as than oral morphine
Hydromorphone	7 mg	1.5 mg	Oral hydromorphone is about 4-7 times as potent as oral morphine Parenteral hydromorphone is about 20 times as potent as oral morphine
Fentanyl	N/A Fentanyl has poor oral bioavailability Transmucosal forms are available	15 µg/hr	Transdermal fentanyl is about 80 times as potent as oral morphine[†]
Meperidine[‡]	300 mg	75 mg	Oral meperidine is about one tenth as potent as oral morphine Parenteral meperidine is about one half as potent as oral morphine (mg for mg)

*Doses of opioids shown here are common usual doses; however, the actual effective dose varies from patient to patient and depends on many individual factors.
[†]Based on studies converting the dose of morphine the equivalent dose of to fentanyl; there are no observational studies converting the dose of fentanyl to the equivalent dose of morphine.
[‡]Meperidine is not a recommended drug in a palliative care setting and should be avoided. If a patient with chronic pain is on meperidine, convert the meperidine to an equivalent analgesic dose of another opioid listed in this table.
N/A, not applicable.
From Periyakoil VS. Opioid conversion. Stanford palliative care online curriculum 2008. [cited 2009 June 23] Available at: http://endoflife.stanford.edu.

coating is destroyed. The effect is like giving a bolus dose of the immediate-release formulation, which may be risky and should be avoided.

Patients who are unable to take medications by oral, sublingual, transdermal, or rectal routes or patients in need of rapid pain control benefit from an IV or subcutaneous infusion.[28] Dosage by the subcutaneous route is equivalent to that by the IV route.[28] Morphine or hydromorphone can be given subcutaneously, either as periodic injections or by a continuous infusion.[28] Intramuscular injections are never indicated; they are unnecessarily painful, and their absorption can be erratic.[28]

Opioid toxicities are predictable and often resolve without treatment. Opioids can cause nausea when the drug is initiated or the dose is increased, but this almost always resolves within a few days. Nausea that occurs when patients have been on a stable dosage of opioid for a prolonged period (>1 week) rarely is related to the opioid but can occur in patients on very high doses.[34] There is no proven best treatment for opioid-induced nausea, but starting with a low-cost dopamine antagonist (e.g., prochlorperazine) is a reasonable first step.

Pain is the antidote to the sedative effects of opioids, and respiratory depression represents the most serious end result of opioid-induced sedation. Tolerance develops rapidly to opioid-induced sedation, and patients with severe pain can easily tolerate many grams per day of morphine or other opioids, with no sedation or respiratory depression. Risk factors for respiratory depression include rapid IV bolus dosing, high doses in opioid-naïve patients, simultaneous use of other sedating medications, and poor hepatic or renal function. Patients with hepatic or renal insufficiency might need lower opioid doses given at longer intervals; short-acting opioids are preferred over long-acting agents in these patients. A physician's fear of causing respiratory depression in patients

who are dying is not sufficient justification for withholding opioids; pain or palliative care experts should be consulted to assist in patient care.

Tolerance does not develop to opioid-induced pruritus and constipation. Prophylaxis for opioid-induced constipation should begin at the onset of opioid therapy; preferred first treatment is a senna preparation. Pruritus is largely an idiosyncratic reaction, best treated by rotating opioids in hope of finding a less itch-producing product. True allergic reactions are rare and are heralded by bronchospasm.

Tolerance to the analgesic effects of opioids is uncommon; in most patients, increasing pain indicates increasing pathology.[35] Physical dependence is universal: all patients on chronic opioids for more than several weeks can be expected to develop some signs of opioid withdrawal if the opioid is discontinued or an antagonist is administered.[36] A difficult diagnostic dilemma can arise in patients with underlying abdominal pain, because cramping abdominal pain is a symptom of opioid withdrawal. Psychological dependence (i.e., addiction) is rare in patients who have chronic pain and no history of addiction; the hallmark of addiction is the use of drugs despite their harmful effects and the patient's loss of control over drug use.[36] A physician's fear of causing addiction in a dying patient is not a rational reason to withhold opioids.[36]

Many patients benefit from adjuvant analgesics, defined as non-opioid drugs used to enhance the effectiveness of opioids or drugs specifically used for neuropathic pain.[28] Examples include NSAIDs or glucocorticoids for somatic pain[33,37] and tricyclic antidepressants and antiseizure drugs for neuropathic pain.[38] When oral and IV medications fail to provide adequate analgesia, anesthetic procedures should be explored, including autonomic blockade (e.g., celiac plexus block[39]) or epidural or intrathecal anesthesia.[40] All patients can benefit

TABLE 132-3 Adjuvant Therapies for Neuropathic Pain

Medication Class	Starting Dose	Titration	Maximum Dosage	Duration of Adequate Trial
Tricyclic Antidepressants				
Nortriptyline (best tolerated in older adults)	25 mg at bedtime	Increase by 25 mg daily every 3-7 days as tolerated	150 mg daily (therapeutic range is 50-150 ng/mL serum)	6-8 wk, with at least 2 wk at maximum tolerated dosage
Desipramine	75 mg daily in divided doses (25 mg daily in older adults)	Increase to 100 mg daily in single or divided doses	300 mg daily in adults and 100-150 mg/day in older adults (therapeutic range is 50-300 ng/mL serum, but older adults can manifest toxicity at higher end of the therapeutic range)	6-8 wk, with at least 2 wk at maximum tolerated dosage
Serotonin/Norepinephrine Reuptake Inhibitors				
Duloxetine	30 mg daily	Increase to 60 m daily after 1 wk	60 mg twice daily	4 wk
Venlafaxine	37.5 mg once or twice daily	Increase by 75 mg each wk	225 mg daily	4-6 wk
Calcium Channel $\alpha2\delta$ Ligand				
Gabapentin	100-300 mg at bedtime, or 100-300 mg 3 times a day	Increase by 100-300 mg 3 times a day every 1-7 days as tolerated	3600 mg (1200 mg 3 times a day); reduce if impaired renal function	3-8 wk for titration + 2 wk at maximum dosage
Pregabalin	50 mg 3 times a day or 75 mg twice daily	Increase to 300 mg daily after 3-7 days, then by 150 mg daily every 3-7 days as tolerated	600 mg daily (200 mg 3 times a day or 300 mg twice daily); reduce if impaired renal function	4 wk
Opioid and Opioid Agonists				
Morphine	Low-risk patient: 0.3 × wt (kg) High-risk patient: 0.1 × wt (kg)	After 1-2 wk, convert total daily dose to long-acting opioid analgesic and continue short-acting med as needed	No maximum dose with careful titration; use longer intervals for renal or hepatic insufficiency	4-6 wk
Oxycodone, methadone, others	Use equianalgesic dosages for other opioids	As for morphine	As for morphine	4-6 wk
Tramadol	50 mg once or twice daily	Increase by 50-100 mg daily in divided doses every 3-7 days as tolerated	400 mg daily (100 mg 4 times a day); in patients >75 yr, 300 mg daily	4 wk
Topical Agent				
Lidocaine patch (5%)	Max 3 patches daily for a maximum of 12 hr	None needed	Maximum of 3 patches daily for a maximum of 12-18 hr	3 wk

Adapted from Periyakoil VS, Pan XP, Lee S, Scheufler J. The American Geriatrics Society Annual Scientific Meeting. Preconference session: Latest updates in hospice & palliative medicine: A skill-based hands-on workshop for interdisciplinary clinicians booklet, April 29-May 2, 2009, Chicago, Ill.

from nonpharmacologic treatments, including relaxation exercises, imagery, and judicious use of heat or cold.[41] An abbreviated list of adjuvant analgesics for neuropathic pain is provided in Table 132-3.

Acute and chronic abdominal pain are covered in Chapters 11 and 12, respectively.

Nausea and Vomiting

Nausea is a highly prevalent and challenging symptom to manage in seriously ill patients.[34,42] Causes of nausea and vomiting in this population are often multifactorial and result from GI causes (gastroparesis, gastric compression, dysmotility, constipation, bowel obstruction), central nervous system causes (brain metastases, anxiety, vestibular dysfunction), hepatic or renal dysfunction, and medications (opioids). Cancer chemotherapy and radiation therapy also often precipitate nausea. Many palliative care experts favor a mechanistic approach[43] to management based on the likely etiology, and target therapy based on the specific neurotransmitter involved (Table 132-4); others recommend an empirical approach. Evidence supporting the existing consensus-based

TABLE 132-4 Targeted Treatment of Nausea

Mediator/Receptor	Triggering Event(s)	Site Involved	Antiemetic Medication(s)
Neurokinin 1 (NK1) (substance P)	Chemotherapy	CTZ	Aprepitant
Dopamine (D_2)	Opioid	CTZ	Prochlorperazine, haloperidol, chlorpromazine, domperidone
5-HT_3	Radiotherapy	CTZ	Ondansetron, granisetron, dolasetron, palonosetron High-dose metoclopramide Mirtazapine
5-HT_4	Bowel obstruction, radiation enteritis, chemotherapy	Various sites in intestine	Metoclopramide
Cannabinoid (CB) receptors: CB_1 in CNS, CB_2 in PNS	Anxiety	Cortex	Dronabinol, nabilone
Histamine	Dysequilibrium	Vestibular apparatus	Cyclizine, promethazine, dimenhydrinate
Acetylcholine (muscarinic)	Stasis	Intestine	Metoclopramide, domperidone
IL-1, IL-2, TNF-α	Tumor, infection, inflammation	Immune system	Megestrol, glucocorticoids, thalidomide, lenalinomide

5-HT, 5-hydroxytryptamine (serotonin); CNS, central nervous system; CTZ, chemoreceptor trigger zone; IL, interleukin; PNS, peripheral nervous system.
From Periyakoil VS. Opioid conversion. Stanford palliative care online curriculum 2008. [cited 2009 June 23] Available at: http://endoflife.stanford.edu.

guidelines for managing nausea and vomiting in patients with advanced cancer is sparse. Well-designed studies of the impact of standard management and novel agents on nausea and vomiting in seriously ill populations are needed.[44]

Nausea and vomiting are covered in Chapter 15.

Anorexia and Cachexia

Anorexia is defined as loss of appetite, especially from disease; cachexia is defined as weight loss and wasting, particularly of muscle mass, and is accompanied by the general debility that can occur with chronic illness.[45] These entities often are combined into the *anorexia-cachexia syndrome*, a term that usually refers to cancer-related anorexia and cachexia,[46] although this symptom complex can occur in patients with serious illness from any cause. Anorexia-cachexia syndrome is reported in up to 80% of cancer patients and represents a poorly understood neuroendocrine and metabolic disorder.[46,47]

Involuntary weight loss is associated with decreased functional status, decreased response to chemotherapy, and decreased survival. Although the anorexia-cachexia syndrome itself is not painful, patients and families experience emotional suffering, given the cultural significance of food intake; the loss of weight and inability to eat are a daily reminder of the illness experience and impending death.[47,48] The syndrome contributes to fatigue, increased complications of antineoplastic treatments, and decreased survival. Weight loss itself is an independent risk factor for mortality.[47]

Aggressive nutritional supplementation in patients with advanced malignancy provides no survival benefit, no improvement in tumor shrinkage, and only minimal decrease in toxicity from antineoplastic treatments.[47] Patients and families often want to continue enteral or parenteral nutrition and hydration to provide the sense of "offering comfort" and to prevent their loved one from "starving to death."[49] Attempts to provide such hydration and nutrition, however, can make

the goal of comfort harder to achieve in the dying patient. A Cochrane review in 2008[50] of medically assisted nutrition for palliative care patients concluded that there were not enough studies done to make any conclusive clinical recommendations. NG and gastrostomy tubes are uncomfortable at the end of life, and IV delivery of nutrition necessitates IV access. Physical or chemical restraints are commonly needed to maintain access as patients get more confused and try to pull out uncomfortable tubes. Nutrition and hydration increase the patient's fluid volume, which in patients close to death can worsen ascites, pleural effusions, and peripheral edema.[51]

Appetite stimulants have a limited role in patients with advanced cancer. Indications for starting an appetite stimulant include a prognosis of longer than 4 weeks combined with the patient's interest in regaining appetite. No drug has shown efficacy in prolonging survival or improving quality of life in population-based research, although individual patients might gain weight and have a greater sense of well-being.[48] The progestational agent megestrol acetate has been well studied.[52] At doses of 160 to 800 mg/day, megestrol results in a greater than 5% weight gain in 20% to 30% of patients with advanced cancer, the weight gain being adipose tissue, not muscle[52]; if improvement is not seen in 2 to 4 weeks, discontinuation of the drug is appropriate.[52] A Cochrane systematic review of anorexia-cachexia done in 2013 reviewed 35 trials and concluded that megestrol improves appetite and is associated with slight weight gain in patients with cancer, AIDS, and with other underlying pathology. Megestrol is, however, also associated with side effects including edema and thromboembolic events, and deaths were more common in patients who received megestrol.[53] Glucocorticoids can lead to weight gain, but the well-known toxicities of these agents often preclude anything but their short-term use.[48] Other agents currently under investigation include human recombinant growth hormone, eicosapentaenoic acid, dronabinol and other cannabinoids, testosterone, thalidomide, ATP, and NSAIDs.[52,54]

Most importantly, patients and families should be educated about the benefits and burdens of the treatment, and if expected side effects will erode the quality of life, it is important to stop such orexigenics in patients with limited prognosis.

Constipation

Constipation[55-59] is a very common and highly distressing symptom in palliative care patients. It was reported in more than 50% of patients[55,56] on a palliative care or hospice unit, a percentage that probably underestimates its true prevalence.[57] In seriously ill and dying patients, the most common precipitants of constipation are poor fluid intake, immobility, autonomic failure, and use of opioid and anticholinergic medications.

More than 90% of patients on opioid medications experience constipation.[59] Opioids bind to mu receptors on intestinal smooth muscle, suppressing peristalsis and raising anal sphincter tone. In 1 study, patients using transdermal fentanyl used laxatives less than patients using oral morphine, indicating that transdermal fentanyl may be less constipating than other opioids.[60] Although a stool softener can help lubricate hard stool, a bowel stimulant such as senna usually is necessary both as a prophylactic drug for opioid-induced constipation and for initial therapy of established constipation. A commonly recommended regimen in the hospice literature is to start with senna, escalating as necessary; if no bowel movement is obtained in 3 days, bisacodyl or an enema (phosphosoda) is recommended.[58] More refractory constipation can be relieved with magnesium citrate, a sorbitol-based product, or small doses of polyethylene glycol. Fiber supplements can lead to obstipation or obstruction and are not recommended for palliative care unless patients also are able to ingest large quantities of water.

Orally administered opioid antagonists may be effective in reversing opioid-related constipation in patients for whom other therapies are not effective.[57] Parenteral opioid antagonists that do not cross the blood-brain barrier are most effective in reversing the opioid effects on the intestine. Methylnaltrexone[61,62] has been approved by the FDA for chronic opioid-induced constipation. The methylation of naltrexone prevents it from crossing the blood-brain barrier and thereby reversing the central analgesic effects of opioids.

When patients are actively dying—that is, death is expected within 1 to 2 weeks—and they have no abdominal symptoms, aggressive drug therapy to cause laxation on a regular basis is not indicated. In fact, laxatives that cause cramping or any suppositories or enemas usually increase patient discomfort and, therefore, should be withheld (Table 132-5).

Constipation is covered in Chapter 19.

Diarrhea

Diarrhea is less common than constipation and is reported in up to 10% of hospice patients.[55] Although the differential diagnosis for diarrhea is broad, 2 common causes in the palliative care patient are overuse of laxative therapy and diarrhea secondary to leakage of stool around a fecal impaction.[56,57]

Treatment is directed at the cause of diarrhea. Octreotide[63] is useful for refractory diarrhea (particularly with endocrine tumors such as VIPomas and gastrinomas), although it is quite costly. Replacement of pancreatic enzymes is helpful in cases of malabsorption following pancreatic cancer surgery. Cholestyramine (to bind bile salts) and aspirin (to reduce prostaglandin synthesis, thus decreasing water and electrolyte secretion) may be beneficial in secretory diarrhea induced by radiation colitis.[64] Opioids or opioid-like medications (e.g., loperamide) might offer the best symptomatic relief for diarrhea. Diarrhea erodes patients' quality of life and dignity (if the patient becomes too weak to do toileting and needs help or has fecal incontinence) and needs to be aggressively managed.

Diarrhea is covered in Chapter 16.

TABLE 132-5 Laxatives in Palliative Care

Class	Laxative(s)	Side Effects	Relevance to Palliative Care
Bulk-forming agents	Bran, psyllium, calcium polycarbophil, methyl cellulose	Impaction above strictures, bloating	Patients with serious illnesses are often unable to consume a large amount of fiber. Because these patients often eat and drink little, fiber supplements can worsen constipation
Emollient, softener	Docusate sodium	Rash	Constipation in a palliative care setting is multifactorial, and emollients per se are often ineffective in reversing the underlying malfunction
Osmolar agents	Sorbitol, lactulose	Abdominal bloating, flatulence	Many patients dislike the sickly sweet taste, which can exacerbate their nausea
	Polyethylene glycol	Nausea, bloating, cramping	Patients might be unable to drink large volumes of the constituted solution
	Magnesium citrate, magnesium sulfate	Magnesium toxicity (with renal insufficiency)	Unpleasant taste can exacerbate nausea
Stimulant agents	Bisacodyl, senna	Colicky pain	First-line laxatives in all patients taking opioids
Chloride channel activator	Lubiprostone	Nausea	Easy to swallow, small capsule, well tolerated

From Periyakoil VS. Opioid conversion. Stanford palliative care online curriculum 2008. [cited 2009 June 23] Available at: http://endoflife.stanford.edu.

Intestinal Obstruction

Malignant bowel obstruction is seen most commonly as a complication of cancers of the colon, ovary, pancreas, and stomach.[65] Obstruction results from either intraluminal or extraluminal tumor. Benign causes such as adhesions, radiation bowel damage, IBD, opioid-induced impaction, or hernia also can cause obstruction.[65-67] Intestinal obstruction can occur in the small or large bowel or in both sites, and multifocal obstructions are common.[66,67]

Symptoms of intestinal obstruction are nausea, vomiting, abdominal distention, constipation, and colicky abdominal pain.[68] NG suction is used to provide temporary relief; in many cases, just a few days of NG suction may convert a complete obstruction to a partial one or might even resolve an obstruction.[69] Surgery with resection and a primary anastomosis or just a diverting stoma (e.g., colostomy, ileostomy) or endoluminal stenting are the preferred options for managing obstruction; the morbidity from major abdominal surgery in cancer patients with bowel obstruction is high.[70]

NG tubes are uncomfortable and therefore not desirable for long-term use. Although a venting gastrostomy tube may be a less desirable option than directly bypassing the obstruction, it can provide great symptomatic relief and avoid the need for prolonged NG intubation, especially in patients who have only weeks to live and are eating for pleasure. Although partly digested food passes out of the tube, patients can still enjoy tastes and experience the psychological and communal benefit of eating.

Despite the advances in surgery and the growing use of endoluminal stents, such procedures are not possible for many patients.[65] Medical management using drugs is effective at reducing the symptom burden of inoperable obstructions. The goals of pharmacologic therapy are to reduce distressing symptoms, avoid the need for parenteral hydration, and remove NG suction. Pharmacologic treatments consist of a cocktail of drugs including opioids for abdominal pain, dopamine antagonist antiemetics such as phenothiazines or butyrophenones for nausea, and antisecretory drugs (octreotide) to reduce colicky pain and reduce intestinal secretions.[71-75] A recent review[76] that looked at 15 RCTs or observational reports on the use of octreotide concluded that octreotide is the first-choice antisecretory agent for malignant bowel obstruction. A prokinetic agent such as metoclopramide can provide relief for an incomplete or functional obstruction but should be avoided in complete obstruction.[69]

Intestinal obstruction is covered in Chapter 123.

Jaundice

Although jaundice[77] is usually an ominous sign in patients with cancer, it might have a correctable cause. The goal of pursuing an evaluation of jaundice is to determine if there are conditions amenable to treatment in which the burden-to-benefit ratio is favorable, given the underlying extent of cancer. Interventional procedures[78] for biliary obstruction, such as surgical bypass of the biliary tract or endoscopic placement of biliary stents, may be useful early in the disease course when patients have a good performance status, but their utility becomes less as performance status declines and the burden of stent placement with its potential for various complications increases.

Pruritus commonly is associated with jaundice. Cool temperatures, lower humidity, and topical agents like astringents, moisturizers, and steroid creams can provide relief. Both H_1 and H_2 antihistamines, phenothiazines, and bile acid resins have been used with some effectiveness. Opioid antagonists also have been used to treat pruritus, but their systemic use

reverses analgesia in many patients receiving opioids.[79-83] Other drugs shown to be effective in pruritus include butorphanol and nalfurafine (κ-opioid receptor agonists), mirtazapine (α_2-receptors and 5-HT$_2$ and 5-HT$_3$ serotonin antagonist), methylnaltrexone (peripherally acting opioid receptor antagonist), gabapentin and pregabalin (GABA analog), and aprepitant (neurokinin-1 antagonist). Gabapentin and butorphanol are effective in palliating uremic pruritus, which usually does not respond to antihistamines. Rifampin has been used to palliate pruritus, but its use may be limited by its risk for causing hepatitis.

Jaundice is covered in Chapter 21.

Ascites

Between 15% and 50% of patients with cancer develop ascites, most commonly from ovarian, endometrial, breast, colon, stomach, and pancreatic cancers.[84,85] Malignant ascites portends a poor prognosis, with a 1-year survival of 40% and 3-year survival of less than 10%.[77] The well-known list of nonmalignant causes of ascites, including portal vein thrombosis, congestive heart failure, nephrotic syndrome, and pancreatitis, should be considered before assuming malignancy is the reason for the patient's ascites. Symptoms of ascites include an increase in abdominal girth, bloating, abdominal wall pain, nausea, anorexia, and dyspnea.

Paracentesis should be performed to evaluate new-onset ascites if the intervention will lead to a change in therapy or if the paracentesis will provide symptomatic benefit. Repeated therapeutic paracentesis, with or without an indwelling peritoneal catheter, is the most commonly used invasive treatment for malignant ascites.[77] Peritoneovenous shunts[86] have a better success rate in patients with nonmalignant ascites than in patients with malignant ascites but are infrequently used today. Octreotide has been reported to provide symptomatic benefit in malignant ascites, but its cost may be prohibitive.[87,88]

Ascites is covered in Chapter 93.

Hepatic Encephalopathy

Hepatic encephalopathy is associated with poor prognosis. Two studies[88,89] have shown that the cumulative survival in these patients was very short: approximately 20% to 40% at 1 year and 15% at 3 years of follow-up. Hepatic encephalopathy due to hepatic metastases is uncommon unless there is an overwhelming liver tumor burden, and is usually a terminal event. Aggressive attempts at reversal usually are futile except for a very short-term benefit, which for some patients may be needed to help bring family closure. When death is near, clinicians should use opioid analgesics and other sedating medication liberally for control of distressing symptoms, even if such treatments worsen the encephalopathy. Family and staff counseling at this time are important to ensure that all parties share the same goals of care.

Hepatic encephalopathy is covered in Chapter 94.

GI Bleeding

Few events are as traumatic for families caring for their loved one as observing a massive GI hemorrhage.[89] If GI bleeding is considered a likely future event, the key is to discuss care options and to develop a plan to provide patients and families with a sense of control for what can seem to be an out-of-control situation. If the patient has advanced disease and is dying, the focus should be toward comfort rather than toward diagnostic and therapeutic interventions. Having dark-colored towels and sheets available to camouflage the bleeding is helpful, along with a rapidly acting sedating medication for emergency use. Some experts recommend chlorpromazine 25 mg given as a slow IV push or a 50-mg suppository rectally. Education and support of the family is of great importance, especially when the patient is dying at home.

GI bleeding is covered in Chapter 20.

KEY REFERENCES

Full references for this chapter can be found on www.expertconsult.com.

1. World Health Organization. WHO definition of palliative care. Available at: http://www.who.int/cancer/palliative/definition/en/. Accessed April 28, 2013.

11. Christakis NA, Lamont EB. Extent and determinants of error in physicians' prognoses in terminally ill patients: Prospective cohort study. West J Med 2000; 172:310-3.

14. Lamont EB, Christakis NA. Prognostic disclosure to patients with cancer near the end of life. Ann Intern Med 2001; 134:1096-105.

20. Said A, Williams J, Holden J, et al. Model for end stage liver disease score predicts mortality across a broad spectrum of liver disease. J Hepatol 2004; 40:897-903.

21. Srikureja W, Kyulo NL, Runyon BA, et al. MELD score is a better prognostic model than Child-Turcotte-Pugh score or Discriminant Function score in patients with alcoholic hepatitis. J Hepatol 2005; 42:700-6.

22. Huo TI, Wu JC, Lin HC, et al. Evaluation of the increase in model for end-stage liver disease (DeltaMELD) score over time as a prognostic predictor in patients with advanced cirrhosis: Risk factor analysis and comparison with initial MELD and Child-Turcotte-Pugh score. J Hepatol 2005; 42:826-32.

23. Huo TI, Lin HC, Huo SC, et al. Comparison of four model for end-stage liver disease–based prognostic systems for cirrhosis. Liver Transpl 2008; 14:837-44.

32. Bruera E, Sweeney C. Chronic nausea and vomiting. In: Berger AM, Portenoy RK, Weissman DE, editors. Principles and practice of palliative care and supportive oncology. 2nd ed. Philadelphia: Lippincott Williams & Wilkins; 2002. p 222.

36. Farrar JT, Portenoy RK. Neuropathic cancer pain: The role of adjuvant analgesics. Oncology (Williston Park) 2001; 15:1435-42, 45.

39. Abrahm JL. Nonpharmacologic strategies for pain and symptom management. In: Abrahm JL, editor. A physician's guide to pain and symptom management in cancer patients. Baltimore: Johns Hopkins University Press; 2000. p 247.

59. Chappell D, Rehm M, Conzen P. Methylnaltrexone for opioid-induced constipation in advanced illness. N Engl J Med 2008; 359:1071.

74. Kichian K, Bain VG. Jaundice, ascites and hepatic encephalopathy. In: Doyle D, Hank SG, Cherny N, Calman K, editors. Oxford textbook of palliative medicine. 4th ed. Oxford: Oxford University Press; 2004. p 507.

75. Baron TH. Palliation of malignant obstructive jaundice. Gastroenterol Clin North Am 2006; 35:101-12.

86. Ripamonti CI, Easson AM, Gerdes H. Management of malignant bowel obstruction. Eur J Cancer 2008; 44:1105-15.

INDEX

Page numbers followed by "f" indicate figures, "t" indicate tables, and "b" indicate boxes.

Food poisoning *(Continued)*
   Campylobacter spp. in, 1930
   Clostridium botulinum in, 1935
   Clostridium perfringens in, 1933-1934
   from fish, 1936-1937
   Listeria species in, 1934
   patient approach in, 1930-1931, 1932t, 1933b
   rates of, 1931t
   Salmonella spp. in, 1930
   Staphylococcus aureus in, 1931-1933
Food protein-induced enterocolitis syndrome, 154
Food supplements, malabsorption caused by, 1811
Foramen of Winslow hernia, 422
Foregut, formation of, 1658f
Foreign bodies
   endoscopy for, therapeutic, 681
   impaction of, 427f
   rectal, 2334
Formulas, nutritional, infant, for glycogen storage disease type I, 1284
Forrest classification, for bleeding peptic ulcers, 307
Foveolar hyperplasia, in reactive gastropathy, 880, 880f
Fractalkine, 26
Fracture, proton pump inhibitors and, 889
Frey procedure, for chronic pancreatitis, in pain control, 1018-1019
Fructose
   absorption of, 1753
   hepatic metabolism of, 1236
   incomplete absorption of, 1809-1810
   intolerance of, 1809-1810
   malabsorption of, in irritable bowel syndrome, 2146
Fruits, gastric cancer and, 906
Fucosylated alpha fetoprotein, in hepatocellular carcinoma, 1607
Full liquid diets, 100
Fumagillin, for *Enterocytozoon bieneusi* infection, 1966
Fumarylacetoacetate hydrolase (FAH), in tyrosinemia, 1290-1291, 1291f
Functional abdominal pain syndrome, 177-183
   biopsychosocial issues, 350
   biopsychosocial model of, 178, 178f
   central nervous system in, 177
   clinical features of, 180-181
   clinical implications of, 180
   diagnosis of, 181, 181f
   differential diagnosis of, 181
   epidemiology of, 177
   history in, 180
   pathophysiology of, 178-180
   patient behavior in, 180-181
   physical examination in, 181
   Rome III diagnostic criteria for, 177, 177b
   treatment of, 181-183
     mental health referral and psychological, 183
     patient-physician relationship in, 181-182
     pharmacotherapy, 182-183
     plan for, 182
   visceral pain transmission in
     ascending, 178-179
     descending modulation of pain, 179
   visceral sensitization in, 179

Functional constipation, 271b, 275t
Functional dyspepsia, 196-200
   classification/diagnostic criteria for, 196b
   epidemiology of, 198
   frequency of symptoms in, 197f
   genetic predisposition of, 199
   infection in, 199
   new drug development for, 203-204
   pathogenetic factors in, 199-200
   pathophysiology of, 198-199
   proton pump inhibitor therapy for, 203t
   psychological interventions for, 204-205
   psychosocial factors in, 199-200
   Rome III criteria for, 197f
   treatment for, 202-205
     pharmacologic, 202-204
Functional fecal retention, 268, 276
Fundic gland, polyps of, proton pump inhibitors and, 751
Fundoplication
   in Barrett's esophagus, 758
   failure of, 753
   gastric motility disorders after, 831
   for gastroesophageal reflux disease, 752, 752f
   pseudoachalasia after, 721
Fungal diseases, causes of hepatic granulomas, 612t
Fungal infection
   in acute liver failure, 1596
   after solid organ transplantation, 557
   gastritis in, 875
   hematopoietic cell transplantation after, 569
   intestinal, after transplantation, 559
   liver, in hematopoietic cell transplantation, 563
   peritonitis in, 642
Fungal liver abscess, after hematopoietic cell transplantation, 563
Fungi, hepatic, 1388
Furazolidone, for giardiasis, 1962
Furosemide, for ascites, 1572-1573
Fusidic acid, for *Clostridium difficile*-associated diarrhea and colitis, 1950-1951

G
G phase, cell cycle, 3
G protein-coupled receptors (GPCRs), 40
G proteins, 40
   signaling pathways of, 40t
Gabapentin
   for irritable bowel syndrome, 2150t, 2151
   for neuropathic pain, 2365t
Gabexate, for acute pancreatitis, 978
Gag reflex, 712
Galactose
   hepatic metabolism of, 1236
   malabsorption of, congenital, 1677
Galactose elimination capacity test, 1251
Galanin, 1732
Gallbladder
   adenomas of, 1161f, 1163-1164
   adenomyomas of, 1159, 1162-1163, 1199
   adenomyomatosis of, 1159-1162, 1160f-1162f
   agenesis of, 1060
   anatomy of, 1058f, 1059-1060
   arterial supply of, 1059
   carcinoma of, 1192-1196
   cholesterolosis of, 1157-1159, 1158f
   development of, 1056f

Gallbladder *(Continued)*
   developmental anomalies of, 1060
   in diabetes mellitus, 599
   disorders of, in cystic fibrosis, 959-960
   double, 1060
   dyskinesia, 1076, 1078-1079
   "folded," 1060
   "ghost" triad, 1061-1062
   Hartmann's pouch of, 1058f, 1059
   in hematopoietic cell transplantation, 563
   heterotopia of, 1199
   hydrops of, 1076, 1127
   innervation of, 1059
   kinked, 1060
   lymph vessels of, 1059
   malpositions of, 1060
   mesenchymal tumors of, 1199
   multiple, 1060
   papillomas of, 1162
   pediatric disorders of, 1073-1076
   polyps of, 1162-1165, 1163t
     clinical features of, 1164, 1164f
     definition of, 1162
     diagnosis of, 1164, 1164f
     epidemiology of, 1162
     inflammatory, 1163
     miscellaneous, 1164
     natural history of, 1164-1165
     pathology of, 1162-1164
     in primary sclerosing cholangitis, 1165
     treatment of, 1165
   polyps of, adenomatous, gallbladder carcinoma and, 1193
   porcelain, in gallstone disease, 1133
   in pregnancy, 650
   pseudotumors of, 594
   small, in cystic fibrosis, 960
   strawberry, 1158
   in systemic lupus erythematosus, 585
   tumors of, 1184-1200
   varices of, 1534
   venous drainage of, 1059
   wall of, thickened, in acute acalculous cholecystitis, 1155, 1156f
Gallbladder adenocarcinoma
   adenomyomatosis and, 1160-1161, 1161f
   progression to, 1164
Gallbladder carcinoma, 1192-1196
   clinical features and diagnosis of, 1194, 1195f
   diagnosed during laparoscopic cholecystectomy, 1196, 1196f
   epidemiology of, 1192
   etiology of, 1192-1193, 1193b
   gallstone disease and, 1150-1151
   gallstones and, 1192-1193
   pathogenesis of, 1194
   pathology of, 1193-1194
   progression to, 1194
   risk factors for, 1192-1193, 1193b
   staging of, 1194, 1195t
   treatment of, 1194-1196, 1196f
Gallbladder disease
   in obesity, 107
   in somatostatinoma, 520
Gallbladder sludge
   in acute acalculous cholecystitis, 1155
   dissolution of, 1157
Gallstone disease, 1100-1133, 1122t-1123t
   after bariatric surgery, 1121
   age and, 1101-1102

Hepatoblast, 1217
Hepatoblastoma, 1615-1616
  clinical features of, 1615-1616
  diagnosis of, 1616
  epidemiology of, 1615
  etiology and pathogenesis of, 1615
  liver transplantation for, 1637
  pathology of, 1616
  treatment and prognosis of, 1616
Hepatoblasts, proliferation of, 1055-1056
Hepatocavopathy, obliterative, 1393
Hepatocellular adenoma, 1618-1620
  clinical features of, 1619
  diagnosis of, 1619
  epidemiology of, 1618
  etiology and pathogenesis of, 1618-1619,
    1619f
  in glycogen storage disease type I, 1284
  pathology of, 1619-1620, 1620f
  treatment and prognosis of, 1620
Hepatocellular carcinoma, 1603-1614
  aflatoxin B$_1$ and, 1605
  age and, 1603-1604
  in alcoholic liver disease, 1420, 1421f
  alpha fetoprotein in, 1607
  ascites in, 1553, 1562, 1606
  in autoimmune hepatitis, 1508, 1510
  in cirrhosis, 1605
  clinical features of, 1606-1607, 1606t
  computed tomography in, 1608, 1608f
  des-γ-carboxy prothrombin in, 1607
  diagnosis of, 1607-1609
  epidemiology of, 1603-1604, 1604f
  etiology of, 1604-1606
  fibrolamellar, 1610, 1637
  fibrolamellar, in pregnancy, 663
  fucosylated alpha fetoprotein in, 1607
  geographic distribution of, 1603
  gross appearance of, 1609-1610
  in hemochromatosis, 1268, 1605
  hepatic angiography in, 1609
  in hepatitis B, 1309, 1316, 1316b,
    1604-1605
  in hepatitis C, 1344, 1605
  in HIV infection, 1606
  hypercalcemia in, 1607
  hypoglycemia in, 1606-1607
  imaging of, 1608-1609
  laparoscopy in, 1609
  magnetic resonance imaging in, 1608,
    1609f
  MELD score in, 1637
  metastasis of, 1610
  microscopic appearance of, 1610
  moderately differentiated appearance of,
    1610
  molecular pathways in, 1606, 1606b
  natural history of, 1610
  oral contraceptive and, 1606
  paraneoplastic manifestations of,
    1606-1607, 1606b
  pathogenesis of, 1604-1606
  pathology of, 1609-1610
  pityriasis rotunda in, 1607
  polycythemia in, 1607
  positron emission tomography in, 1609
  in pregnancy, 663
  prevention of, 1613-1614
  progenitor cell, 1610
  prognosis of, 1610
  rash in, 1607
  risk factors for, 1604b
  serum tumor markers of, 1607-1608

Hepatocellular carcinoma (Continued)
  smoking and, 1606
  staging of, 1610
  surveillance of, 1613, 1613t
  treatment of, 1610-1613, 1612t
    chemoembolization for, 1612-1613
    chemotherapy for, 1613
    liver transplantation for, 1612
    local ablation for, 1612
    surgical resection for, 1611-1612
  treatment of, liver transplantation for,
    1637
  ultrasonography for, 1608
  undifferentiated appearance of, 1610
  well-differentiated appearance of, 1610
  in Wilson disease, 1605
Hepatocellular nodules, classification of,
    614b
Hepatocytes, 1223-1226
  cell junctions of, 1224, 1224f
  copper transport by, 1271f
  cytoskeleton, 1224
  differentiation of, 1217
  endocytosis in, 1225-1226
  endoplasmic reticulum of, 1225
  exocytosis in, 1225-1226
  glucose regulation by, 1234-1236
  Golgi complex of, 1225
  ground-glass, in hepatitis B, 1318, 1318f
  lysosomes of, 1225
  mitochondria of, 1225
  nucleus of, 1224-1225
  peroxisomes of, 1225
  plasma membranes of, 1223-1224
  regenerative response of, 1228
  transplantation of, for glycogen storage
    disease type I, 1285
  transport between nucleus and
    cytoplasm, 1224-1225
Hepatoerythropoietic porphyria (HEP),
    388t, 1288t, 1289
Hepatogenous diabetes, 600
Hepatolithiasis, 1180
Hepatomegaly
  in alcoholic liver disease, 1416, 1417t
  in glycogen storage disease type I, 1284
  in HIV/AIDS, 551b
  in nonalcoholic fatty liver disease, 1432
Hepatopathy, congestive, 1404-1405
Hepatoportal sclerosis, 1534-1535
Hepatopulmonary syndrome, 1583-1587
  clinical features and diagnosis of,
    1584-1586
  liver transplantation for, 1586, 1631-1632
  pathophysiology of, 1584, 1584f
  screening for, 1585, 1585f
  treatment of, 1586
Hepatorenal syndrome, 1580-1583
  in alcoholic liver disease, 1425
  cardiac dysfunction in, 1581
  classification of, 1582
  clinical features and diagnosis of,
    1581-1582, 1581b, 1582t
  pathophysiology of, 1580-1581, 1581f
  prevention and treatment of, 1582-1583,
    1583b
  prognosis in, 2362
  renal arterial vasoconstriction in,
    1580-1581
  splanchnic arterial vasodilatation in,
    1580
  type 1, 1582
  type 2, 1582

Hepatotoxicity, 1446, 1468t, 1482t-1483t
  Liver disease, 85-86
  of adulterated cooking oils, 1485-1486
  of anesthetic agents, 1478-1481, 1480t
  of antidiabetic drugs, 1466
  of antiretroviral agents, 1460-1461
  of aspirin, 1461
  of azathioprine, 1476-1477
  of black cohosh, 1491
  of carbon tetrachloride, 1481-1483
  of chemical agents, 1481-1485, 1482b
  of Chinese herbal medications, 1490-1491
  of cocaine, 1486
  of contaminated food, 1485-1486
  of copper, 1485
  of desflurane, 1480
  of drugs of abuse, 1484
  of foodstuffs, 1485, 1487
  of germander, 1490
  of haloalkane compounds, 1480, 1481t
  of halogenated aromatic compounds,
    1484
  of halothane, 1479-1480
  of herbal medicines, 1490-1491
  of iron, 1485
  of isoflurane, 1480
  of isoniazid, 1465
  of kava kava, 1488t-1489t, 1491
  of metals, 1485
  of methotrexate, 1474-1476
  of methoxyflurane, 1480
  of minocycline, 1463
  of monoamine oxidase inhibitors, 1467
  of mushrooms, 1481, 1486-1487, 1486t
  of niacin, 1459
  of nitroaliphatic compounds, 1484
  of nitroaromatic compounds, 1483-1484
  of non-nucleoside reverse transcriptase
    inhibitors, 1461
  of nonhalogenated organic compounds,
    1483
  of nucleoside (nucleotide) reverse
    transcriptase, 1460-1461
  of nutritional supplements, 1488-1492
  of pennyroyal, 1490
  of pesticides, 1484-1485
  of phosphorus, 1485
  of polychlorinated biphenyls, 1484
  of protease inhibitors, 1461
  of pyrrolizidine, 1490
  of selective serotonin reuptake inhibitors
    (SSRIs), 1467
  of sevoflurane, 1480
  of thiazolidinediones, 1466
  of thorium dioxide, 1485
  of tricyclic antidepressants, 1467
  of trinitrotoluene, 1483-1484
  of valproic acid, 1460
  of vinyl chloride, 1483
  of vitamin A, 1487-1488
Hepcidin, in hereditary hemochromatosis,
    1262-1263, 1263f
Hephaestin, in hereditary
    hemochromatosis, 1262
Herbal medicines, 2345b
  Chinese
    hepatotoxicity of, 1490-1491
    for irritable bowel syndrome, 2152-
      2153, 2349, 2349t
    for liver disease, 2354t, 2355
  for colonic health, 2352t-2353t
  for functional dyspepsia, 2347t
  hepatotoxicity of, 1488t-1489t, 1490-1491

Histamine H$_2$ receptor antagonists, for Zollinger-Ellison syndrome, 514-515

Histiocytosis, Langerhans cell, in children, 1072

Histoplasmosis
gastritis in, 875
hepatic, 1388

HITChip (Human intestinal tract chip), 30

HIV/AIDS, 2336
abdominal pain in, 173, 549, 549t
anorectal disease in, 549-550, 550b
bacillary angiomatosis and, 1376
bacillary peliosis hepatis in, 553
biliary tract in, 553
cholangiopathy in, 1167-1168
cholecystitis in, acalculous, 553
Clostridium difficile infection in, 1945
cytomegalovirus, 552
esophagitis in, 543, 543f
diarrhea in, 545-548
differential diagnosis of, 545b
drug-induced, 548
evaluation and management of, 545-548, 546f-547f, 546t, 548b
drug induced liver disease and, 1447t
dysphagia in, 543-545
esophageal ulceration in
bacterial, 544
nonspecific, 543, 544f
gastrointestinal bleeding in, 550
gastrointestinal consequences of infection with, 542-554
gastrointestinal symptoms in, evaluation of, 542-543
GBV-C virus infection with, 1367-1368, 1368f
hemorrhoids in, 2322
hepatitis A in, 552, 1308
hepatitis B in, 551, 1328
hepatitis C in, 552, 1346, 1351
hepatobiliary disease in, 550-553
hepatocellular carcinoma in, 1606
herpes simplex virus in, 543-544, 544f
jaundice in, 553
liver test abnormalities in, 550-551
mucocutaneous disorders of, 379-380
Mycobacterium avium complex in, diarrhea and, 548f
odynophagia in, 543-545
opportunistic disorders on, CD4 lymphocyte count and, 543f
pancreatic, in children, 951
papillary stenosis in, 553, 553f
peritonitis associated with, 642
tropical malabsorption and, 1882-1883
tuberculosis in, intestinal, 1927

HIV-associated lipodystrophy, 380

HIV-associated non-Hodgkin's lymphoma, 485

H$^+$,K$^+$-ATPase pumps, in intestinal ion transport, 1723

HLA (human leukocyte antigen)
amebiasis and, 1956
in autoimmune hepatitis, 1497t
in microscopic colitis, 2299
in primary biliary cirrhosis, 1514
in primary sclerosing cholangitis, 1169

HLA-DQ2, in celiac disease, 1853

HLA-DQ8, in celiac disease, 1853

HLA-DR3, in autoimmune hepatitis, 1499t

HLA-DR4, in autoimmune hepatitis, 1499t

Homeopathy, 2345b
for postoperative ileus, 2353

Homeostasis, tissue, 6-8

Homocysteine, in alcoholic liver disease, 1413

Hooking maneuver, in slipping rib syndrome, 177

Hookworm infection, 1973-1976

Hordeins, 1852

Hormonal therapy
for colon ischemia, 2090
for colonic angioectasia, 622-623
for intestinal endometriosis, 2312

Hormone replacement therapy, colorectal cancer and, 2255

Hormones
defining, 36-37
gastrointestinal, 1684
of gastrointestinal tract, 38b
importance of, 50-53
and neurotransmitters, 36-38

Hospice care, 2359-2360
eligibility criteria for end-stage liver disease, 2362b

Hospitalized patients
aggressive nutritional support in, 81-82
with decompensated alcoholic liver disease, 82
energy recommended for, 58-61
undergoing radiation therapy, 82

Host defense factors, against enteric infection, 1896-1897

Host-microbe
age-sensitive relationships, 31
dialogue, language of, 32-33
spatial relationships, 30

Hourglass stomach, in syphilis, 874, 874f

Houston, valves of, 1651

Howel-Evans syndrome, in gastrointestinal malignancies, 390

Howship-Romberg sign, in obturator hernia, 420

HspE7, for anal warts, 2330t

Human chorionic gonadotropin
hyperemesis gravidarum and, 652
in pancreatic endocrine tumors, 503-504

Human fecal microbiota, 29f

Human gastrointestinal microbiota, characteristics of, 30-33

Human homeobox gene 9, in pancreatic development, 930

Human intestinal microbiome, characteristics of, 31t

Human Microbiome Project, 13

Human papillomavirus infection, esophagitis in, 771

Human secretin, 44

Human sodium-dependent multivitamin transporter (hSMVT), 1767f

Huntington's chorea, gastrointestinal manifestations of, 604t

Hyaluronan, in hepatic fibrosis, 1250-1251

Hycanthone, hepatotoxicity of, 1461

Hydatid cyst, hepatic, 1387f

Hydralazine, granulomatous hepatitis from, 1469t

Hydration status, in nutritional assessment techniques, 77

Hydrazine, hepatotoxicity of, 1484

Hydrochloric acid secretion, by parietal cells, 842, 846f

Hydrochlorofluorocarbons, hepatotoxicity of, 1483

Hydrocodone, in palliative care, 2363, 2364t

Hydrocortisone, for Crohn's disease, 2012

Hydrogen breath test
in irritable bowel syndrome, 2148
small intestinal bacterial overgrowth, 1829

Hydrogen peroxide
chemical colitis from, 2305, 2305f

Hydrogen sulfide, odoriferous gas from, 245

Hydrolases, brush border membrane, 1755, 1757f

Hydromorphone, in palliative care, 2363, 2364t

Hydrops, of gallbladder, 1076

Hydrothorax, hepatic, liver transplantation and, 1632

3β-Hydroxy-Δ^5-C$_{27}$-steroid dehydrogenase/isomerase (3β- HSD) deficiency, 1296-1297

Hydroxycut, hepatotoxicity of, 1491

5-hydroxyindoleacetic acid (5-HIAA), as carcinoid tumor marker, 2206

Hydroxymethylglutaryl-coenzyme A (HMG-CoA) reductase inhibitors, 1464

15-Hydroxyprostaglandin dehydrogenase (15-PGDH), 2253

5-hydroxytryptamine (5-HT), and irritable bowel syndrome, 2145

5-hydroxytryptamine receptor-4 (5-HT-4), for ileus, 2178

5-Hydroxytryptamine$_4$ agonists, for constipation, 292-293

Hygiene theory of appendicitis, 2114

Hymenolepis nana/diminuta infection, 1981-1982
clinical features and pathophysiology of, 1981-1982
diagnosis and treatment of, 1982
epidemiology of, 1981
life cycle of, 1981

Hyoid bone, 702, 702f

Hyperammonemia
coma from, in urea cycle defects, 1295
differential diagnosis of, 1578, 1579b
glutamine synthesis and, 1578
in hepatic encephalopathy, 1577-1578
idiopathic, and coma, 569
in urea cycle defects, 1293

Hyperbaric oxygen therapy, for radiation enteritis, 672

Hyperbilirubinemia
in autoimmune hepatitis, 1496, 1505
conjugated or mixed, jaundice in, 340
differential diagnosis of, 338t
evaluation of, 1244-1245, 1244f, 1245t
management of, 343f
postoperative, 1480-1481, 1481t
therapy for, 347
unconjugated, jaundice in, 338-340

Hypercalcemia
acute pancreatitis in, 977
constipation in, 278
in esophageal cancer, 776
familial hyperparathyroidism with, pancreatitis in, 967
gastric acid secretion in, 850-851
in hepatocellular carcinoma, 1607
in VIPoma, 518

Hypercholesterolemia, in glycogen storage disease type I, 1284

Hypercoagulability, in ulcerative colitis, 2060-2061

Jejunum
adenoma of, in familial adenomatous polyposis, 2238-2239
anatomy of, 1649
in digestion and absorption, short bowel syndrome and, 84
diverticulosis of, 2190
nutrient absorption in, 87t
Jin bu huan, hepatotoxicity of, 1490-1491
Johanson-Blizzard syndrome, pancreatic insufficiency in, 966
Joints, disease of, in obesity, 108-109
Jump sign, in myofascial pain syndrome, 176-177
Juvenile hereditary hemochromatosis, 1261-1262
Juvenile polyposis syndrome, 2239t, 2245
colorectal cancer in, 2233, 2233f
gastric cancer in, 907
SI tumors and, 2199
Juvenile rheumatoid arthritis, gastrointestinal manifestations of, 580t, 582
Juxtacardiac gastric diverticulum, 403f
Juxtapapillary diverticula (JPD), 403, 404f

K

K-ras gene, 8-9
in colorectal adenoma, 2218
diversity of signaling through, 11f
mutations in, 2197
colorectal cancers, testing for, 14
Kaposi's sarcoma, in HIV/AIDS, 380, 380f, 552
Karnofsky Performance Status (KPS), 2360, 2362t
Karyopherins, 1225
Kasai's portoenterostomy, in biliary atresia, 1066f
Katayama syndrome, 1385
Kato-Katz thick smear, in schistosomiasis, 1987
Kava kava, hepatotoxicity of, 1488t-1489t, 1491
Kawasaki's disease, 2100
pancreatitis in, 951
Kayser-Fleischer rings, in Wilson disease, 1273
Kegel exercises, in rectocele, 276
Keratosis palmaris et plantaris, in gastrointestinal malignancies, 390
Ketoconazole
drug interactions of, with proton pump inhibitors, 889
hepatotoxicity of, 1465
Ketogenesis, during starvation, 72
Ketotifen, for irritable bowel syndrome, 2152, 2152t
Kidney, transplant, 557-558
Kidney disease, 107
polycystic, portal hypertension in, 1535
Kidney stones
calcium oxalate, in short bowel syndrome, 1843, 1843f
Kidneys, in protein-energy malnutrition, 76
Killian's triangle, 701-702
in Zenker's diverticula, 397
Kinase inhibitors, for ulcerative colitis, 2049
KIT gene
in gastrointestinal stromal tumors, 488
immunostaining, 488f
KIT proto-oncogene, 2208

Klatskin tumors, 1184, 1185f, 1188f, 1211, 1614
Klebsiella oxytoca infection, antibiotic-associated diarrhea in, 1939
Klippel-Trenaunay syndrome, 631-632
Knudson's 2-hit hypothesis, of tumor suppressor genes, 9f
Kock pouch, 2063f, 2065
Köhlmeier-Degos disease, 386
Korsakoff's psychosis, 1775
KRAS2 oncogene, pancreatic cancer and, 1029
Kupffer cells
in alcoholic liver disease, 1411-1412
in liver, 595, 595f
in nonalcoholic fatty liver disease, 1429
sinusoidal, 1220-1221, 1227
Kwashiorkor, in children, 74

L

L-Ornithine-L-aspartate, for hepatic encephalopathy, 1580
L-type calcium channels, 1698
Laboratory testing, nutritional therapy, 89-90
Lactase, 222-223
deficiency of
acquired primary, rates of, 1809b
congenital, 1677
in cystic fibrosis, 955
secondary, 148
Lactase-phlorizin hydrolase (LPH gene), polymorphisms of, 1808
Lactate, in ascites, 1562
Lactate dehydrogenase, in ascitic fluid, 1561-1562
Lacteals, 1657
Lactic acidosis, in short bowel syndrome, 1843
Lactic acidosis syndrome, 551
Lactitol, 222-223
Lactobacillus acidophilus, 1726
CL1285, for *Clostridium difficile* infection prevention, 2340-2341
for traveler's diarrhea, 2340
Lactobacillus bulgaricus
for *Clostridium difficile* infection prevention, 2340-2341
for traveler's diarrhea, 2340
Lactobacillus casei
for *Clostridium difficile* infection prevention, 2340-2341
LBC80R, for *Clostridium difficile* infection prevention, 2340-2341
Lactobacillus GG
for antibiotic-associated diarrhea, 1939-1940
for *Clostridium difficile*-associated diarrhea and colitis, 1952-1953
for ulcerative colitis, 2341
Lactobacillus rhamnosus GG
for antibiotic-associated diarrhea prevention, 2340
for traveler's diarrhea, 2340
Lactose, 83
deficiency of
acquired primary, 1808
transient, in premature infants, 1808
intolerance of, 1730, 1808-1809
hydrogen breath test for, 1809
malabsorption of, 1808-1809, 1809f
hydrogen breath test for, 1809

Lactulose, 222-223, 234
for constipation, 289
for hepatic encephalopathy, 1579-1580
for urea cycle defects, 1294
Lactulose hydrogen breath test (LHBT), 1690
for small intestinal bacterial overgrowth, 1829
Ladd's bands, 1666, 2165
Laimer's triangle, 704
Lambert-Eaton myasthenic syndrome, chronic intestinal pseudo-obstruction in, 2188
Lamina propria, 24, 1652
of esophagus, 691, 692f
of stomach, 800
Lamina propria mononuclear cells (LPMCs), 24
Lamivudine
for hepatitis B, 1324
in liver transplantation, 1634
pegylated interferon with, 1326
in pregnancy, 1327
resistance to, 1324
Lamivudine therapy, for hepatitis D, 1358-1359
Langerhans cell histiocytosis, 592-593
in children, 1072
Lansoprazole
drug interactions with, 889
mechanism of action, 889
for NSAID ulcer prophylaxis, 892
for peptic ulcer disease, 889
Laparoscopic adhesiolysis, for chronic abdominal pain, 183
Laparoscopic pyloromyotomy, for infantile hypertrophic pyloric stenosis, 806
Laparoscopic treatment, of small bowel obstruction, 2161
Laparoscopy
in acute mesenteric ischemia, 2081
in appendicitis, 2118
in ascites of unknown origin, 647, 647f
in evaluation of peritoneal diseases, 647-648
in hepatocellular carcinoma, 1609
in ileal pouch-anal anastomosis, 2073-2074
in ileostomy, 2073-2074
ileus after, 2176-2177
with lysis of adhesions, 183
in pancreatic cancer, 1034
for perforated peptic ulcers, 898
with peritoneal lavage, for gastric cancer, 917
for peritonitis, 640
staging, 647-648
Laparotomy
hernias after, 417-418
for peritonitis, 640
Laplace's law, 1530, 2166
Large-volume diarrhea, 226
Larva migrans, visceral, 1382
Laryngitis, reflux, 741-742, 742f
Larynx, in swallowing, 702
Late dumping syndrome, 86
Lateral sclerosis, in amyotrophic, esophageal motility disorders, 713
Latex agglutination assay, for *C. difficile*, 1947